W9-CJP-982

Koneman's Color Atlas and Textbook of Diagnostic Microbiology

Koneman's Color Atlas and Textbook of Diagnostic Microbiology

Sixth Edition

Washington C. Winn, Jr., MD, MBA
Director, Clinical Microbiology Laboratory
Fletcher Allen Health Care
Professor of Pathology
University of Vermont College of Medicine
Burlington, Vermont

Stephen D. Allen, MD
Professor of Pathology and Laboratory Medicine,
    Indiana University School of Medicine
Director, Division of Clinical Microbiology,
    Clarian Health—Methodist, Indiana University,
    and Riley Hospitals
Chief, Clinical Microbiology Laboratory,
    Roudebush Veterans Affairs Hospital
Pathologist, Wishard Memorial Hospital
Indianapolis, Indiana

William M. Janda, PhD, D(ABMM)
Associate Professor of Pathology
Director, Clinical Microbiology Laboratory
University of Illinois Medical Center
Chicago, Illinois

Elmer W. Koneman, MD
Professor Emeritus
University of Colorado School of Medicine
Denver, Colorado

Gary W. Procop, MD, MS
Section Head, Clinical Microbiology
The Cleveland Clinic Foundation
Cleveland, Ohio

Paul C. Schreckenberger, PhD, D(ABMM)
Professor of Pathology
Director, Clinical Microbiology
Loyola University Medical Center
Maywood, Illinois

Gail L. Woods, MD
Professor and Medical Director of Clinical
    Laboratories
Department of Pathology
University of Arkansas for Medical Scienc
Little Rock, Arkansas

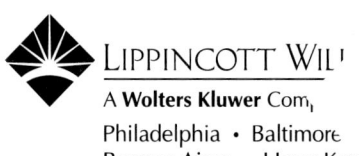
LIPPINCOTT WIL'
A **Wolters Kluwer** Com
Philadelphia · Baltimore
Buenos Aires · Hong Kon

Acquisitions Editor: Peter Darcy
Managing Editor: Nancy Peterson
Project Management: Anne Seitz, Hearthside Publishing Services
Marketing Manager: Mary Martin
Production Editor: Julie Montalbano
Designer: Risa Clow
Compositor: Maryland Composition
Printer: Quebecor—Taunton

Library of Congress Cataloging-in-Publication Data

Koneman's color atlas and textbook of diagnostic microbiology / Washington C. Winn Jr. ...
[et al.].-- 6th ed.
    p. ; cm.
  Rev. ed. of: Color atlas and textbook of diagnostic microbiology / Elmer W. Koneman ...
[et al.]. 5th ed. c1997.
  Includes bibliographical references and index.
  ISBN 0-7817-3014-7
  1. Diagnostic microbiology--Atlases.   I. Winn, Washington C. II. Koneman, Elmer W.,
1932- III. Title: Color atlas and textbook of diagnostic microbiology.
  [DNLM: 1. Microbiology--Laboratory Manuals. 2. Laboratory Techniques and Procedures.
QW 25 K816 2006]
QR67.C64 2006
616.9′041--dc22
                                                                        2005008049

Dedication

In Remembrance of Our Former Colleagues and Co-Authors

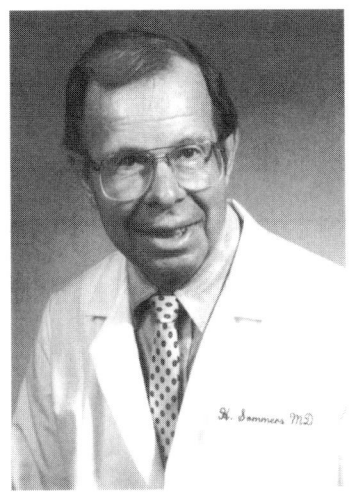

Herbert M. Sommers, MD
Professor of Pathology
Northwestern University Medical School
Director of Microbiology Laboratory
Northwestern Memorial Hospital
Chicago, Illinois

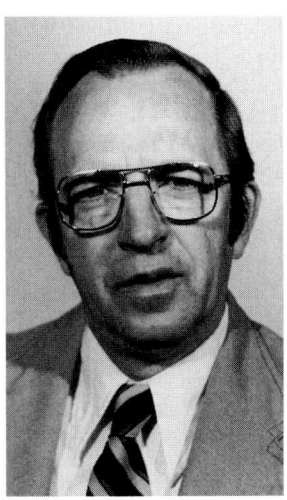

V.R. Dowell, Jr., PhD
Chief, Anaerobic Bacteriology Branch
Hospital Infections Program
Centers for Disease Control
Atlanta, Georgia

Foreword

It has been said that clinical microbiology is both an art and a science. Scientific information regarding the metabolic, physiologic, and genetic characteristics of microorganisms has provided the basis for clinical laboratory tests to identify isolates. The recognition of characteristic microscopic and macroscopic morphologies of microorganisms is considered to be the art of clinical microbiology that is essential to the initial selection of the tests most appropriate for identifying clinical isolates. The process of identifying the cause of an infection is, however, far more complex. It is initiated by the patient's physician, whose assessment of the patient's history, signs and symptoms, and physical findings suggests a tentative diagnosis of infection that, in turn, prompts the collection of specimens that are thought to be most likely to confirm the diagnosis. It is essential that the clinical microbiologist work with physicians to establish specimen-collection guidelines according to the suspected cause and site of the infection. It is also the clinical microbiologist's responsibility to ensure that specimens are not only properly collected and contained but also are transported to the laboratory as expeditiously as possible.

Given the fact that specimens are collected by a wide variety of healthcare providers, it is also essential that the clinical microbiologist establish criteria for specimen rejection, either because the specimen has been improperly collected or the test requested is not appropriate for the specimen submitted. Communication between the microbiologist and the physician is important in such instances, not only to ensure that another specimen is submitted but also to educate the physician as to what the most appropriate specimen is.

Once an appropriate specimen has been received in the laboratory, the microbiologist must have established processing guidelines to ensure that the relevant tests are carried out. Laboratory workers need to be able to distinguish between indigenous flora and potential pathogens because of the obvious tendency of physicians to ascribe clinical significance to anything the laboratory reports. Similarly, discretion needs to be exercised in the selection of microorganisms to undergo antimicrobial susceptibility testing, as well as in the selection of antimicrobial agents to be tested.

As if the aforementioned problems were not enough, additional challenges facing the microbiology laboratory are those imposed by increasing cost constraints and the centralization of laboratories. The former requires that the utmost care be exercised in the selection of tests and procedures used in the laboratory, while the latter poses problems in specimen transport and communication.

The objective of *Koneman's Color Atlas and Textbook of Diagnostic Microbiology* is to provide the scientific information required to understand the structural, physiological, pathogenetic, and clinical manifestations of organisms causing infectious disease and to present guidelines and procedures for the laboratory diagnosis of these diseases. The text provides detailed approaches to specimen collection and transport, procedures for specimen processing, tests used for organism identification, and charts and tables listing test reactions required for organism identification. Charts, tables, and figures are interspersed to highlight key points made in the text. Color photomicrographs of organisms and photographs of colonies on solid media are provided to enhance the laboratory worker's ability to recognize characteristic organism morphologies. As such, this book is the most comprehensive guide on diagnostic microbiology available today and should be required reading for physicians specializing in infectious diseases, pathologists, clinical microbiologists, and medical technologists.

John A. Washington, M.D.

Preface

The sixth edition of this text represents a continued evolution in our attempt to communicate the increasingly complex and challenging field of diagnostic microbiology to our audience. Elmer Koneman, one of the founding authors and the driving force behind the first five editions, has elected not to continue as the coordinating author. In recognition of his enormous contributions, his fellow authors unanimously insisted that the text be renamed *Koneman's Color Atlas and Textbook of Diagnostic Microbiology*. Fortunately, Dr. Koneman agreed to continue as a contributing author, so his expertise remains an important part of the book. We welcome two new authors to this edition: Gary Procop, MD, and Gail Woods, MD. Their diverse experience brings ''new blood'' and additional perspectives to the work—always important for the continued growth of any textbook.

The general organization of the text remains similar to that of previous editions, but some significant changes have been made to reflect the dynamic nature of our field. Chapters 1 and 2, the introduction to clinical microbiology, have been extensively revised, with greater emphasis on the whole field and less concentration on bacteriology. A new color plate has been added to illustrate artifacts in Gram-stained smears, emphasizing the importance of knowing what is *not* real. Expanded discussion of management and regulatory issues in the diagnostic microbiology laboratory reflects the reality of modern medical practice. In addition, we have addressed the most difficult but critically important ''soft'' issues that all clinical microbiologists face daily: What do we work up, when do we work it up, and how extensively do we work it up? With increasingly scarce financial and personnel resources, these challenges have become as important as the more traditional scientific issues.

The traditional techniques that are still important for clinical laboratories receive appropriate attention in this edition, but the increasing importance of immunologic methods (Chapter 3) and particularly molecular techniques (Chapter 4) justifies explicit discussion of principles, as well as expanded coverage in individual chapters as appropriate. Where immunologic and/or molecular approaches have become the norm in diagnostic laboratories, the text has been updated to reflect these changes. Discussion of methods that are obsolete or rapidly becoming archaic have been eliminated or significantly condensed.

The introduction to bacteriology, still the lynchpin of clinical laboratories, follows as Chapter 5 and sets the stage for the subsequent chapters on this vast field. The chapter on *Haemophilus* spp. has been integrated into the discussion of other fastidious Gram-negative bacilli. Conversely, consideration of the aerobic actinomycetes, an increasingly complicated group of bacteria, has been separated from discussion of other Gram-positive bacilli.

The increasing frequency with which ectoparasites are submitted to diagnostic laboratories for identification has been acknowledged with an expanded discussion of tick identification in an appendix, including several new color plates.

The philosophy behind the book remains the same: Our goal is to provide an extensive but practical discussion of the science and art of diagnostic microbiology. We strongly believe that it is essential to integrate the clinical problems and challenges with the tools that we in the laboratory use to provide the information that our clinical colleagues need to serve their patients. Serving the patient is the core of medical practice both in the clinic and in the laboratory. We also believe that rigorous documentation of the primary sources behind the concise discussions is crucial.

The intended audience is twofold. The first group is students of microbiology and medicine, particularly those interested in infectious diseases. The book provides a comprehensive review for graduate students, residents in pathology, and fellows in infectious disease. For undergraduate students the mass of material may appear overwhelming, but that is real life. The dedicated teacher is essential for guiding the beginning student, who will then have a resource to carry on into the graduate environment or the workplace, rather than a superficial and outmoded introduction for the bookshelf.

The second, equally important audience is laboratory professionals for whom the text can represent the initial resource for updating competence or troubleshooting problems in clinical practice.

To facilitate understanding of the subject matter, we continue to employ tables, detailed charts, summary text boxes, and extensive illustrations, many in full color. Each chapter begins with a detailed outline—the chapter at a glance.

We are all greatly indebted to a variety of mentors, colleagues, and students who have challenged and inspired us. We are particularly indebted to John A. Washington who generously agreed to contribute a Foreword for this edition. Two of our former co-authors, the late V.R. Dowell, Jr., and Herbert Sommers, are very much in our memory. We could not have done this without their fundamental work on previous editions. To recognize their contributions, we dedicate this edition to their memory.

Acknowledgments

We are, first of all, indebted to our colleagues in the microbiology laboratories at our respective institutions for their important roles in our professional life. They have challenged us, inspired us, and educated us. We hope this book serves to repay their contributions in some small part. Additionally, we are grateful to the members of our families for their forbearance while we struggled to meet deadlines when we could have been spending time with them. Their support and encouragement at home are integral to our activities at work.

We would like to acknowledge the editorial and scientific guidance of J. Stephen Dumler, MD; James Versalovic, MD, PhD; P. Rocco Lasala, MD; Deborah Reardon, MT(ASCP); Ann Croft, BS, MT(ASCP); Linda Marler, MT(ASCP), MS; and Janet Reynolds, MT(ASCP), MS. In particular we thank Fred W. Westenfeld, MT(ASCP)SM; Frederick C. Patterson; and Jean A. Siders, MT(ASCP), MS, for their substantial contributions to this and previous editions. It would be considerably diminished without their input.

Brief Contents

CHAPTER 1

Introduction to Microbiology: Part I: The Role of the Microbiology Laboratory in the Diagnosis of Infectious Diseases: Guidelines to Practice and Management   1

CHAPTER 2

Introduction to Microbiology: Part II: Guidelines for the Collection, Transport, Processing, Analysis, and Reporting of Cultures From Specific Specimen Sources   67

CHAPTER 3

Laboratory Diagnosis by Immunologic Methods   111

CHAPTER 4

Molecular Microbiology   132

CHAPTER 5

Medical Bacteriology: Taxonomy, Morphology, Physiology, and Virulence   166

CHAPTER 6

The *Enterobacteriaceae*   211

CHAPTER 7

The Nonfermentative Gram-Negative Bacilli   303

CHAPTER 8

Curved Gram-Negative Bacilli and Oxidase-Positive Fermenters: Campylobacteraceae and Vibrionaceae   392

CHAPTER 9

Miscellaneous Fastidious Gram-Negative Bacilli   429

CHAPTER 10

Legionella   549

CHAPTER 11

Neisseria Species and *Moraxella catarrhalis*   566

CHAPTER 12

Gram-Positive Cocci: Part I: Staphylococci and Related Gram-Positive Cocci   623

CHAPTER 13

Gram-Positive Cocci: Part II: Streptococci, Enterococci, and the "Streptococcus-Like" Bacteria   672

CHAPTER 14

Aerobic and Facultative Gram-Positive Bacilli   765

CHAPTER 15

Aerobic Actinomycetes   858

CHAPTER 16

The Anaerobic Bacteria   877

CHAPTER 17

Antimicrobial Susceptibility Testing   945

ix

Chapter 18

Mycoplasmas and Ureaplasmas   1022

Chapter 19

Mycobacteria   1064

Chapter 20

Spirochetal Infections   1125

Chapter 21

Mycology   1151

Chapter 22

Parasitology   1244

Chapter 23

Diagnosis of Infections Caused by Viruses, *Chlamydia*, *Rickettsia*, and Related Organisms   1327

Appendix I

Ectoparasites and Other Invertebrates in the Clinical Laboratory: A Brief Guide[*]   1420

Appendix II

Free-Living Amebae   1437

Charts   1442

Color Plates

Index   I-1

---

[*] With contributions by Fred Westenfeld and Fred Patterson

Expanded Contents

CHAPTER 1
Introduction to Microbiology

Part I: The Role of the Microbiology Laboratory in the Diagnosis of Infectious Diseases: Guidelines to Practice and Management

INTRODUCTION	2
Outline of the Book	2
The World of Infectious Disease	2
THE TRIAD OF INFECTIOUS DISEASE	2
The Infectious Agent	3
Classes of Infectious Agents	3
Interactions Between Hosts and Infectious Agents	4
Purpose of Infectious Agents in Nature	4
Virulence	4
The Environment	5
The Infected Host	5
Innate Humoral (Noncellular) Defenses	6
Innate Cellular Defenses	7
Types of Inflammation	7
Adaptive Immunologic Cellular Defenses	7
Adaptive Immunologic Noncellular (Humoral) Defenses	8
Clinical Signs and Symptoms of Infection	8
Indirect Effects of Infectious Agents on Humans	9
PHASES OF THE DIAGNOSTIC CYCLE	9
Preanalytic Phase	10
Specimen Collection	10
Specimen Transport	14
Specimen Receipt and Preliminary Observations	14
Criteria for Rejection of Specimens	14
Cost-Effective Approaches in the Preanalytic Phase	15
Analytic Phase	15
Microscopic Examination	15
Processing Specimens	27
Interpretation of Cultures	33
Procedures for Preliminary Identification of Bacterial Isolates	38
Identification of Organisms Other Than Bacteria	39
Testing of Susceptibility to Antimicrobial Agents	39
Cost-Effective Approaches in the Analytic Phase	39
Postanalytic Phase	43
Reporting Results	43
Interactions With Epidemiologists	44
Analysis of Results	44
Maintenance of Samples and Records	44

ADMINISTRATIVE ASPECTS OF THE MICROBIOLOGY LABORATORY	45
Government Regulations	45
Risk Management	47
Laboratory Safety	47
General Safety Rules and Regulations	47
Routine Safety Precautions	48
Biologic Agents	50
Universal Precautions	51
Shipping of Specimens and Etiologic Agents	55
Nonbiologic Hazards	56
Bioterrorism	58
Quality Assurance	58
Quality Control	59
Components of a Quality Control Program	60
Monitoring Laboratory Equipment	60
Monitoring Culture Media, Reagents, and Supplies	61

CHAPTER 2
Introduction to Microbiology

Part II: Guidelines for the Collection, Transport, Processing, Analysis, and Reporting of Cultures from Specific Specimen Sources

INFECTIONS OF THE RESPIRATORY TRACT	68
Infections of the Upper Respiratory Tract	71
Indigenous Flora	71
Pharyngitis	72
Infections of the Oral Cavity Other Than Pharyngitis	73
Infections of the Nasopharynx and Nasopharyngeal Cultures	74
Otitis Media and Sinusitis	74
Epiglottitis	74
Laryngitis	74
Other Infections of the Upper Respiratory Tract	74
Infections of the Lower Respiratory Tract	75
Tracheobronchitis	75
Bronchiolitis	75
Pneumonia	75
Chronic Pneumonia	76
Empyema	76
Pneumonia in Special Populations	76
Collection of Specimens for the Diagnosis of Lower Respiratory Infection	76
Laboratory Diagnosis of Pneumonia	78

INFECTIONS OF THE GASTROINTESTINAL TRACT 79
Lower Intestinal Infections 79
Clinical Symptoms 79
Collection of Fecal Specimens 81
Epidemiologic Considerations in the Evaluation of Patients With Gastroenteritis 81
Upper Intestinal Infections 81
Clinical Symptoms 81
Obtaining Specimens From the Upper Gastrointestinal Tract 82

URINARY TRACT INFECTIONS 82
Clinical Signs and Symptoms 82
Host Factors 83
Collection of Urine Samples for Culture 83
Midstream Urine Specimens 83
Other Voided Urine Specimens 84
Catheter Collections 85
Suprapubic Aspiration 85
Culture of Urine Specimens 85
Screening Tests for Urinary Tract Infection 86
Screening Tests for Bacteriuria 86
Screening Tests for Pyuria 86

INFECTIONS OF THE GENITAL TRACT 87
Sexually Transmitted Infections 87
Urethritis and Cervicitis 87
Genital Ulcer Disease 88
Genital Infections Transmitted by Nonsexual Means 88
Vaginitis and Vaginosis 88
Infections of the Upper Female Genital Tract 89
Systemic Complications of Genital Infections 89
Diagnosis of Genital Tract Infections 89
Diagnosis of Urethritis, Cervicitis, and Vaginitis 89
Diagnosis of Genital Ulcer Disease and Venereal Warts 90
Collection of Genital Specimens 90

INFECTIONS OF THE BONES AND JOINTS 91
Clinical Presentation 91
Diagnosis of Infections of the Bones and Joints 91

INFECTIONS OF THE CENTRAL NERVOUS SYSTEM 92
Meningitis 92
Encephalitis and Brain Abscess 93
Diagnosis of Central Nervous System Infections 93
Collection of Specimens 93
Assessing the Inflammatory Response and Microscopic Techniques 93
Direct Detection of Antigen and Nucleic Acid 94
Serologic Diagnosis 95
Diagnosis by Culture 95

WOUNDS, ABSCESSES, AND CELLULITIS 95
Clinical Presentation 95
Diagnosis of Wound Infections, Abscesses, and Cellulitis 95
Collection of Specimens 95
Microscopic Examination of Specimens 96
Culture 96

EYE INFECTIONS 96
Clinical Presentation 96
Conjunctivitis 96
Keratitis 97
Uveitis and Endophthalmitis 97

Diagnosis of Eye Infections 97
Collection of Specimens 97
Microscopic Examination 97
Culture 97

INFECTIONS OF THE BLOOD 97
Clinical Presentation and Pathogenesis 97
Bacteremia and Septicemia 97
Types of Bacteremia 97
Intravascular Infection 98
Catheter-Associated Bacteremia and Sepsis 100
Collection of Blood Cultures 100
Contamination With Skin Flora 100
Number and Timing of Cultures 101
Culture Media 101
Systems for Processing Blood Cultures 102
Manual Blood Culture Systems 102
Lysis-Centrifugation Blood Culture System 103
Automated and Computerized Blood Culture Systems 103
Comparative Studies 104
Special Considerations 105
Fastidious Organisms and Endocarditis 105
Catheter-Associated Bacteremia and Sepsis 105
Tissues and Biopsies 105

CHAPTER 3
Laboratory Diagnosis by Immunologic Methods

ANTIGENS AND ANTIBODIES: BASIC DEFINITIONS 112
MONOCLONAL ANTIBODIES 113
TYPES OF ANTIGEN-ANTIBODY REACTIONS USED IN DIAGNOSTIC SEROLOGY 114
Precipitin Reactions 114
Complement Fixation and Hemagglutination Inhibition 116
Agglutination Reactions 116
SOLID-PHASE IMMUNOASSAY METHODS 119
Enzyme Immunoassays for Antibody Detection 119
Enzyme Immunoassay Antibody Capture Methods for IgM Detection 122
Enzyme Immunoassays for Antigen Detection 122
IMMUNOFLUORESCENCE TECHNIQUES 125
Immunofluorescence Techniques for Antigen Detection 125
Immunofluorescence Techniques for Antibody Detection 125

CHAPTER 4
Molecular Microbiology

NUCLEIC ACIDS—THE BASICS OF DNA AND RNA 133
Structure of DNA 133
Structure of RNA 134
Function of DNA—Information Storage 135
Function of RNA—Information Transfer 135
Reading (Transcription) and Interpretation (Translation) of the Genetic Code 135

SIGNAL-AMPLIFICATION METHODS   137
Nucleic-Acid Probes   137
Clinical Applications   137
Hybrid Capture   137
Clinical Applications   138
Branched DNA   139
Clinical Applications   139
In Situ **Hybridization**   139
Clinical Applications   140

NUCLEIC-ACID AMPLIFICATION   141
Basics of the Polymerase Chain Reaction   141
Clinical Applications   143
Other Methods of Nucleic-Acid Amplification 143
Clinical Applications   144
Modifications of PCR   144
RT-PCR   144
Clinical Applications   145
Broad-Range PCR   145
Clinical Applications   145
Multiplex PCR   146
Clinical Applications   146
Nested PCR   146
Clinical Applications   146

POSTAMPLIFICATION ANALYSIS   147
Traditional Methods of Detection   147
Gel Electrophoresis/Southern Blot Analysis   147
Enzymatic Detection of Amplified Products   147
Clinical Applications   148
Reverse Hybridization   148
Clinical Applications   148
DNA Sequencing   148
Traditional DNA Sequencing   149
Clinical Applications   149
Sequencing by Synthesis (Pyrosequencing)   149
Clinical Applications   150
Microarray Analysis   150
Clinical Applications   151

REAL-TIME NUCLEIC-ACID AMPLIFICATION   151
Methods of Detecting the Products of Real-Time Amplification 151
SYBR Green   151
Hybridization Probes   151
Clinical Applications   154

STRAIN TYPING   156
Non-Amplification-Based Typing   156
Pulsed-Field Gel Electrophoresis   156
Amplification-Based Typing   157
PCR-RFLP   157
Rep-PCR   158
Clinical Applications of Microbial Typing   158

CONCLUSION   158

CHAPTER 5
Medical Bacteriology: Taxonomy, Morphology, Physiology, and Virulence

TAXONOMY: CLASSIFICATION, NOMENCLATURE, AND IDENTIFICATION OF BACTERIA   167

The Naming of Bacteria   167
Phenotypic Identification of Bacteria   168
Phylogenetic Criteria for Classification of Bacteria 168

BASIC BACTERIAL ANATOMY AND PHYSIOLOGY   177
Bacterial Size and Shape   177
Nuclear Structure, DNA Replication, Transcription, and Translation   178
Cytoplasm   181
Cytoplasmic Membrane   182
Bacterial Cell Wall Structure   182
Gram-Positive Bacterial Cell Walls   184
Gram-Negative Bacterial Cell Walls   185
"Acid-Fast" Bacterial Cell Walls   188
Bacterial Endospores   189
Bacterial Surface Structures   190
Capsules   190
Flagella   190
Fimbriae (Pili)   191
Genetic Exchange and Recombination in Bacteria 192
Requirements for Bacterial Growth and Metabolism 195
Carbon   195
Carbon Dioxide   195
Oxygen   195
Nitrogen   195
Growth Factors   196
Kinetics of Bacterial Cell Growth   196
General Bacterial Metabolism and Energy Generation 196
Fermentation   196
Utilization of Pyruvate   198

BACTERIAL VIRULENCE FACTORS AND PATHOGENICITY   200
Definitions and Concepts   200
Requirements for Pathogenicity   203
Virulence Factors of Microorganisms   204
Adhesins   204
Aggressins   204
Exotoxins and Endotoxins   205
Bacterial Superantigens   207

CHAPTER 6
The *Enterobacteriaceae*

CHARACTERISTICS FOR PRESUMPTIVE IDENTIFICATION   213
Screening Characteristics   213
Carbohydrate Utilization   213
Cytochrome Oxidase Activity   215
Nitrate Reduction   216

CULTURE MEDIA USED FOR DETECTION OF CARBOHYDRATE FERMENTATION   216
Use of Kligler Iron Agar and Triple Sugar Iron Agar   216
Biochemical Principles   217

SELECTION OF PRIMARY ISOLATION MEDIA   218
Chemicals and Compounds Used in Selective Media   219
Selective Isolation Media   221

Highly Selective Isolation Media Used Primarily for
Gastrointestinal Specimens   222
Enrichment Media   222
Guidelines for Choosing Selective Isolation Media   222

DIFFERENTIAL IDENTIFICATION CHARACTERISTICS   223

Indole Production   224
Methyl Red Test   224
Voges-Proskauer Test   225
Citrate Utilization   225
Urease Production   225
Decarboxylation of Lysine, Ornithine, and Arginine   225
Phenylalanine Deaminase Production   226
Hydrogen Sulfide Production   226
Motility   227

TAXONOMY OF THE ENTEROBACTERIACEAE   228

Classification of *Enterobacteriaceae* by Tribes   228
Key Identification Characteristics for the Most Common Species   228
  Tribe *Escherichieae*   235
  Tribe *Edwardsielleae*   250
  Tribe *Salmonelleae*   251
  Tribe *Citrobactereae*   258
  Tribe *Klebsielleae*   259
  Tribe *Proteeae*   267
  Tribe *Yersinieae*   269
  Tribe *Erwinieae*   274
Miscellaneous New Genera of *Enterobacteriaceae*   274
  Identification Characteristics of Newer *Enterobacteriaceae*   277
  Clinical Significance of Newer *Enterobacteriaceae*   277

QUICK SCREENING METHODS FOR RAPID IDENTIFICATION   282

Commercial Screening Kits   282
Chromogenic Agar Media   283

CLASSIC IDENTIFICATION SYSTEMS   284

Checkerboard Matrix   284
Branching Flow Diagrams   284
Computer-Aided Schemes   285

NUMERIC CODING SYSTEMS   285

Reading Octal Codes in Numeric Code Registers   286
Estimated Frequency of Occurrence   287
Calculation of Likelihood   287
Resolving Discrepancies   287

PACKAGED KIT IDENTIFICATION SYSTEMS   287

Overview of Packaged Systems   287
Specific Identification Systems   289
  API 20E   289
  BBL Crystal Enteric/Nonfermenter ID System   289
  RapID onE System   289
  Enterotube II   290
  Micro-ID   291
  Biolog GN2 Microplate   291
  MicroScan System   291
  Sensititre System   291

SEMIAUTOMATED AND AUTOMATED IDENTIFICATION SYSTEMS   292

MicroScan Walkaway   292
Vitek System   292
Sensititre Gram-Negative AutoIdentification System   293
The Phoenix System   293
The OmniLog ID System   293

CHAPTER 7
The Nonfermentative Gram-Negative Bacilli

Part I: Metabolism of the Nonfermenters

FERMENTATIVE AND OXIDATIVE METABOLISM   309

The Embden-Meyerhof-Parnas Pathway   309
The Entner-Doudoroff Pathway   311
The Warburg-Dickens Hexose Monophosphate Pathway   312

INITIAL CLUES THAT AN UNKNOWN ISOLATE IS A NONFERMENTER   312

Lack of Evidence for Glucose Fermentation   312
Positive Cytochrome Oxidase Reaction   312
Failure to Grow on MacConkey Agar   313

TESTS USED IN THE IDENTIFICATION OF NONFERMENTERS   313

Utilization of Glucose   313
Motility   313
Pigment Production   314
Hydrolysis of Urea   314
Nitrate Reduction   315
Denitrification of Nitrates and Nitrites   315
Indole Production   315
Decarboxylation   315
Esculin Hydrolysis   315
Flagella Stains   315
  Leifson Method   315
  Ryu Method   316
  Wet-Mount Technique   316
  Flagellar Morphology   316

Part II: Taxonomy, Biochemical Characteristics, and Clinical Significance of Medically Important Genera of Nonfermenters

ORGANISMS THAT ARE MOTILE WITH POLAR FLAGELLA   316

Pseudomonads   316
Family *Pseudomonadaceae*   317
  Genus *Pseudomonas*—rRNA Group I   317
Family *Burkholderiaceae*   323
  rRNA Group II   323
  Genus *Burkholderia*—*Pseudomallei* Group   323
  Genus *Ralstonia* and Genus *Cupriavidus*   328
  Genus *Pandoraea*   329
  Genus *Inquilinus*   331
  Genua *Lautropia*   331

Family *Comamonadaceae* — 331
rRNA Group III — 331
Acidovorans Group — 331
Facilis-Delafieldii Group — 332
Family *Caulobacteraceae* — 332
rRNA Group IV — 332
Brevundimonas-Diminuta Group — 332
Family *Xanthomonadaceae* — 332
rRNA Group V — 332
Genus *Stenotrophomonas* — 332
Family *Sphingomonadaceae* — 334
Genus *Sphingomonas* — 334
Family *Oceanospirillaceae* — 334
Genus *Balneatrix* — 334
Family *Oxalobacteraceae* — 334
Genus *Massilia* — 334
Genus *Herbaspirillum* — 334
Family *Alteromonadaceae* — 336
Genus *Shewanella*—Hydrogen Sulfide-Producing Group — 336
Genus *Alishewanella*—Halophilic Group — 337
Family *Halomonadaceae* — 337
Genus *Halomonas* — 337
Family *Methylobacteriaceae* — 337
Genus *Methylobacterium* — 337
Genus *Roseomonas* — 338
Unnamed Species — 339
Laribacter hongkongensis — 339

ORGANISMS THAT ARE MOTILE WITH PERITRICHOUS FLAGELLA — 340
Family *Alcaligenaceae* — 340
Genus *Alcaligenes* — 340
Genus *Achromobacter* — 340
Genus *Bordetella* — 343
Genus *Kerstersia* — 344
Genus *Oligella* — 344
Family *Rhizobiaceae* — 344
Genus *Rhizobium* (Formerly *Agrobacterium*) — 344
Family *Brucellaceae* — 345
Genus *Ochrobactrum* — 345

ORGANISMS THAT ARE NONMOTILE AND OXIDASE-POSITIVE — 345
Family *Flavobacteriaceae* — 345
Chryseobacterium, Empedobacter, and Unnamed CDC Groups — 346
Weeksella and *Bergeyella* — 348
Genus *Myroides* — 348
Family *Sphingobacteriaceae* — 348
Sphingobacterium and *Pedobacter* — 348
Family *Moraxellaceae* — 349
Genus *Moraxella* — 349
Genus *Psychrobacter* and CDC EO Groups — 350
Family *Neisseriaceae* — 353
Genus *Neisseria* — 353
Gilardi Rod Group 1 — 353

ORGANISMS THAT ARE NONMOTILE AND OXIDASE-NEGATIVE — 353
Genus *Acinetobacter* — 353
CDC Group NO-1 — 355
Bordetella holmesii (CDC Group NO-2) — 355
CDC Group EO-5 — 355

Part III: Approach to Recovery and Identification of Nonfermenters
LEVELS OF SERVICE IN IDENTIFICATION OF NONFERMENTERS — 355
GUIDELINES FOR RECOVERY OF NONFERMENTERS — 356
IDENTIFICATION OF MOST COMMON SPECIES — 356
Pseudomonas aeruginosa — 356
Acinetobacter baumannii — 357
Stenotrophomonas maltophilia — 357
METHODS FOR IDENTIFICATION USING CONVENTIONAL TESTS — 357
Weyant (CDC), Gilardi, and Pickett Identification Schemes — 358
Practical Approach to Identification of Nonfermenters — 358
Computer-Aided Schemes — 359
COMMERCIAL KIT SYSTEMS — 359
The Oxi/Ferm Tube — 359
The API 20E System — 362
The API 20NE System — 362
The Remel N/F System — 362
The Crystal Enteric/Nonfermenter System — 367
The RapID NF Plus System — 367
The Biolog System — 373
AUTOMATED IDENTIFICATION SYSTEMS — 373
The Vitek Legacy System — 373
The Vitek 2 System — 374
The Microscan Walkaway-96, Walkaway-40, and Autoscan-4 Systems — 375
The Sensititre AP80 System — 375
The Phoenix System — 375
SELECTION OF A SYSTEM — 375

CHAPTER 8
Curved Gram-Negative Bacilli and Oxidase-Positive Fermenters: *Campylobacteraceae* and *Vibrionaceae*

Part I: Curved Rods: *Campylobacter, Wolinella, Arcobacter Helicobacter,* and Related Bacteria

HISTORICAL BACKGROUND — 393
CLASSIFICATION OF CAMPYLOBACTER AND RELATED TAXA — 393
Campylobacter Species — 395
Campylobacter jejuni Subsp. *jejuni* — 395
Other *Campylobacter* Species — 398
Former *Wolinella* and *Bacteroides* Species Included in the Family *Campylobacteraceae* — 402
Genus *Arcobacter* — 403
Genus *Helicobacter* — 403
H. pylori — 404
Other Medically Important *Helicobacter* Species — 404
Nonhuman *Helicobacter* Species — 405
Other Microaerophilic Gram-Negative Bacilli — 405

DEFINITIVE IDENTIFICATION OF CAMPYLOBACTERS *AND RELATED* BACTERIA — 406

Rapid Identification of Campylobacters From Colonies and From Stool Specimens — 406
Nonculture Tests — 406
Direct Detection Methods — 407
Culture and Isolation of *Helicobacter pylori* — 407
Specimens for Recovery of *H. pylori* — 407
Isolation Procedure — 407
Identification of *H. pylori* — 407
Biopsy Urease Test (CLO Test) — 408
Noninvasive Tests To Diagnose *H. pylori* Infection — 408
Accuracy of Invasive and Noninvasive Tests To Diagnose *H. pylori* Infection — 408
Enterohepatic Helicobacters — 408

Part II: The Families *Vibrionaceae* and *Aeromonadaceae*

PHYLOGENY OF THE VIBRIONACEAE — 408
Genus *Vibrio* — 408
Taxonomy — 409
Description and Associated Clinical Syndromes of *Vibrio* Species of Human Importance — 409
Methods for Laboratory Isolation of *Vibrios* — 414
Biochemical Characterization and Laboratory Identification of *Vibrio* Species — 416

GENERA LISTONELLA, PHOTOBACTERIUM *AND* SHEWANELLA — 417

AEROMONAS *AND* PLESIOMONAS — 417
Genus *Aeromonas* — 417
Taxonomy — 419
Clinical Significance — 419
Aeromonas Species in Medicinal Leeches — 420
Laboratory Recovery of *Aeromonas* Species From Clinical Specimens — 420
Laboratory Identification of *Aeromonas* Species — 420
Genus *Plesiomonas* — 422
Laboratory Isolation and Identification — 422

GENUS CHROMOBACTERIUM — 422

CHAPTER 9
Miscellaneous Fastidious Gram-Negative Bacilli

HAEMOPHILUS *SPECIES* — 431
Taxonomy of *Haemophilus* and Related Organisms — 431
Haemophilus influenzae — 433
Haemophilus influenzae Type B Vaccines — 433
Infections Caused by *Haemophilus* Species — 435
Meningitis — 435
Epiglottitis — 439
Otitis Media — 439
Sinusitis — 440
Bronchitis and Chronic Obstructive Pulmonary Disease — 440
Pneumonia — 440
Bacteremia and Infectious Complications of Bacteremia — 441
Endocarditis — 441
Urogenital, Maternal, and Perinatal Infections — 441
Ocular Infections — 442
Brazilian Purpuric Fever — 442
Miscellaneous *Haemophilus influenzae* Infections — 443

Haemophilus parainfluenzae — 443
Haemophilus aphrophilus and *Haemophilus paraphrophilus* — 444
Other *Haemophilus* Species — 444
Haemophilus ducreyi — 444
Laboratory Diagnosis of *Haemophilus* Infections — 444
Direct Examination of Clinical Specimens — 444
Culture of *Haemophilus* Species — 445
Identification of *Haemophilus* Species — 446
Laboratory Diagnosis of *Haemophilus ducreyi* Infection — 449
Antimicrobial Susceptibility of *Haemophilus* Species — 451

ACTINOBACILLUS *SPECIES* — 452
Actinobacillus actinomycetemcomitans — 452
Clinical Significance — 452
Cultural Characteristics and Identification — 453
Antimicrobial Susceptibility — 455
Actinobacillus ureae — 455
Actinobacillus hominis — 458
Animal Species in the Genus *Actinobacillus* — 458

PASTEURELLA *AND* MANNHEIMIA SPECIES — 458
Taxonomy and Characteristics of the Genus *Pasteurella* — 458
Pasteurella multocida — 459
Clinical Significance and Virulence — 459
Cultural Characteristics and Identification — 462
Antimicrobial Susceptibility — 464
Other *Pasteurella* Species Isolated From Human Infections — 465
Pasteurella pneumotropica ("*Actinobacillus pneumotropica*") — 465
Pasteurella aerogenes ("*Actinobacillus aerogenes*") — 465
Pasteurella dagmatis — 465
Pasteurella canis and *Pasteurella stomatis* — 466
Pasteurella bettyae — 466
Pasteurella caballi — 466
Pasteurella gallinarum — 466
Mannheimia Species (Formerly the "*Pasteurella haemolytica*/*Pasteurella granulomatis*" Complex) — 467

CARDIOBACTERIUM HOMINIS — 467
Taxonomy — 467
Clinical Significance — 468
Cultural Characteristics and Identification — 468
Antimicrobial Susceptibility — 468

EIKENELLA CORRODENS — 470
Taxonomy and Virulence — 470
Clinical Significance — 470
Cultural Characteristics and Identification — 471
Antimicrobial Susceptibility — 471

KINGELLA *AND* SUTTONELLA *SPECIES* — 472
Taxonomy — 472
Clinical Significance — 472
Cultural Characteristics and Identification — 473
Antimicrobial Susceptibility — 474

HUMAN CAPNOCYTOPHAGA *SPECIES* — 474
Taxonomy — 474
Clinical Significance — 474
Cultural Characteristics and Identification — 475
Antimicrobial Susceptibility — 475

CANINE CAPNOCYTOPHAGA *SPECIES* — 477
Taxonomy — 477
Clinical Significance — 477
Cultural Characteristics and Identification — 477
Antimicrobial Susceptibility — 478

DYSGONOMONAS *SPECIES* 479
CDC GROUPS EF-4A AND EF-4B 479
SIMONSIELLA *SPECIES* 481
STREPTOBACILLUS MONILIFORMIS 481
  Taxonomy 481
  Clinical Significance 481
  Cultural Characteristics and Identification 481
  Antimicrobial Susceptibility 482
BRUCELLA *SPECIES* 482
  Epidemiology of Brucellosis 482
  Taxonomy of *Brucella* Species 484
  Virulence of *Brucella* Species 484
  Clinical Spectrum of Brucellosis 486
  Serologic Diagnosis of Brucellosis 486
  Isolation and Cultural Characteristics 488
  Identification of *Brucella* Species 488
  Treatment of Brucellosis 490
FRANCISELLA TULARENSIS 491
  Epidemiology of Tularemia 491
  History and Taxonomy 491
  Virulence of *F. tularensis* 492
  Clinical Spectrum of Tularemia 493
  Isolation and Cultural Characteristics 494
  Serologic Diagnosis of Tularemia 495
  Treatment of Tularemia 495
BARTONELLA *SPECIES* 497
  Taxonomy and Epidemiology of *Bartonella* Species 497
  Clinical Significance of *Bartonella* Species 499
    Oroya Fever and Verruga Peruana 500
    "Classical" and "Urban" Trench Fever 500
    Bacillary Angiomatosis 501
    Peliosis 501
    Fever and Bacteremia 502
    Endocarditis 502
    Cat-Scratch Disease (CSD) 503
    Miscellaneous Infections 504
  Detection, Isolation, and Identification of *Bartonella* Species 505
    Specimen Types 505
    Culture 505
    Gram Stain and Colony Morphology 505
    Identification Methods 505
  Serologic Diagnosis of *Bartonella* Infections 507
  In Vitro Antimicrobial Susceptibility 509
AFIPIA *SPECIES* 510
  Taxonomy and Clinical Significance 510
  Isolation and Identification 510
  Antimicrobial Susceptibility 510
BORDETELLA *SPECIES* 510
  Background and Taxonomy of *Bordetella* Species 510
  Epidemiology of Pertussis 512
  Clinical Significance of *Bordetella pertussis* 512
  Pertussis Vaccines 513
  Clinical Significance of Other *Bordetella* Species 516
    Bordetella parapertussis 516
    Bordetella bronchiseptica 516
    Bordetella hinzii 517
    Bordetella holmesii 517
    Bordetella trematum 517

  Isolation and Identification of *Bordetella* Species 517
    Specimens and Culture Media 517
    Direct Fluorescent Antibody Test 518
    Cultural Characteristics and Identification 519
  New Technologies for Detection and Identification of *Bordetella pertussis* 519
  Serologic Tests for Diagnosis of Pertussis 521
  Treatment of Pertussis 522
  Antimicrobial Susceptibility Testing of *Bordetella* Species 522

CHAPTER 10
Legionella

TAXONOMY AND CHARACTERISTICS OF THE GENUS LEGIONELLA 550
CLINICAL AND PATHOLOGIC SPECTRUM OF LEGIONELLOSIS 551
  Predisposing Factors 552
  Pathology and Pathogenesis 552
EPIDEMIOLOGIC AND ECOLOGIC ASPECTS OF LEGIONELLOSIS 553
  Incidence 553
  Legionellaceae in the Environment 553
    Natural Habitats 553
    Man-Made (Artificial) Aquatic Habitats 554
  Legionellosis in Travelers 554
  Nosocomial Outbreaks of Legionellosis 555
LABORATORY DIAGNOSIS 555
  Selection, Collection, and Transport of Clinical Specimens 555
  Direct Examination of Clinical Specimens 556
    Gross Examination and Microscopic Examination of Stained Materials 556
    Microscopic Examination of Stained Materials 556
    Direct Fluorescent Antibody (DFA) Procedure 556
    Antigen Detection in Urine and Body Fluids 557
DETECTION OF LEGIONELLA IN CLINICAL SPECIMENS 557
  Isolation of *Legionella* Species From Clinical Specimens 557
    Biopsy, Surgical Removal, and Autopsy Tissue 557
    Pleural Fluid and Transtracheal Aspirates 557
    Acid-Wash Decontamination Procedure for Sputum and Other Contaminated Specimens 557
    Blood Cultures 557
  Identification of *Legionella* Species 558
  Antimicrobial Susceptibility and Treatment 558
  Serum Indirect Immunofluorescent Antibody Test 560
  Molecular Diagnosis 560
ENVIRONMENTAL MICROBIOLOGY STUDIES 561
  Isolation of *Legionella* From Environmental Samples 561
  Typing of *Legionella* Isolates 561

CHAPTER 11
Neisseria Species and *Moraxella catarrhalis*

TAXONOMY OF THE FAMILY NEISSERIACEAE AND THE FAMILY MORAXELLACEAE 568
GENERAL CHARACTERISTICS OF THE GENUS NEISSERIA 569

CLINICAL SIGNIFICANCE OF NEISSERIA SPECIES — 570
Neisseria gonorrhoeae — 570
Epidemiology — 570
Infections Caused by N. gonorrhoeae — 573
Neisseria meningitidis — 578
Epidemiology — 578
Infections Caused by N. meningitidis — 580
Meningococcal Prophylaxis and Meningococcal Vaccines — 582
Other Neisseria Species — 584

CLINICAL SIGNIFICANCE OF MORAXELLA CATARRHALIS — 585

ISOLATION OF NEISSERIA SPECIES — 588
Neisseria gonorrhoeae — 588
Direct Gram-Stained Smears — 588
Specimen Collection — 588
Specimen Transport — 589
Selective Culture Media: Inoculation and Incubation — 590
Neisseria meningitidis — 591
Laboratory Safety — 591
Direct Gram-Stained Smears and Direct Capsular Antigen Tests — 591
Specimen Collection and Transport — 591
Isolation and Incubation — 591

IDENTIFICATION OF NEISSERIA SPECIES — 592
Colony Morphology — 592
Gram Stain and Oxidase Test — 593
Superoxol Test — 593
Differentiation of Other Organisms on Selective Media — 593
Presumptive Criteria for Identification of N. gonorrhoeae — 593
Identification Tests for Neisseria Species — 593
Carbohydrate-Utilization Tests — 594
Conventional CTA Carbohydrates — 594
Rapid Carbohydrate-Utilization Test — 594
RIM-Neisseria Test (Rapid Identification Method-Neisseria) — 594
Other Carbohydrate-Utilization Methods. — 594
Chromogenic Enzyme Substrate Tests — 594
Gonochek II — 595
BactiCard Neisseria — 595
Immunologic Methods for Culture Confirmation of N. gonorrhoeae — 596
Direct Fluorescent Monoclonal Antibody Test — 596
Coagglutination Tests — 596
GonoGen II Test — 596
Multitest Identification Systems — 597
DNA Probe Test for Culture Confirmation of N. gonorrhoeae — 597
Nucleic Acid Hybridization and Amplification Tests for N. gonorrhoeae — 597
Molecular Methods for Detection of N. meningitidis — 599

CULTURAL CHARACTERISTICS OF NEISSERIA SPECIES — 600
Neisseria gonorrhoeae — 600
Neisseria meningitidis — 602
Other Neisseria Species — 603
Neisseria lactamica — 603
Neisseria cinerea — 603
Neisseria flavescens — 603
Neisseria subflava Biovars, Neisseria mucosa, and Neisseria sicca — 603
Neisseria polysaccharea — 604
Neisseria elongata Subspecies — 604
Neisseria gonorrhoeae Subspecies kochii ("Neisseria kochii") — 604
Atypical and Non-Human Neisseria Species — 604

CULTURAL CHARACTERISTICS AND IDENTIFICATION OF MORAXELLA CATARRHALIS — 604

ANTIMICROBIAL SUSCEPTIBILITY OF NEISSERIA SPECIES — 605
Neisseria gonorrhoeae — 605
Neisseria meningitidis — 607

ANTIMICROBIAL SUSCEPTIBILITY OF MORAXELLA CATARRHALIS — 608

CHAPTER 12
Gram-Positive Cocci

Part I: Staphylococci and Related Gram-Positive Cocci

TAXONOMY OF STAPHYLOCOCCI AND RELATED GRAM-POSITIVE COCCI — 624

CLINICAL SIGNIFICANCE OF STAPHYLOCOCCI AND RELATED GRAM-POSITIVE COCCI — 625
Staphylococcus aureus Subsp. aureus — 625
Coagulase-Negative Staphylococci — 638
Staphylococcus epidermidis — 638
Staphylococcus saprophyticus Subsp. saprophyticus — 641
Other Coagulase-Negative Staphylococci — 642
Micrococcus Species and Related Genera — 642
Rothia mucilaginosa — 642

ISOLATION AND PRELIMINARY DIFFERENTIATION OF STAPHYLOCOCCI AND RELATED GRAM-POSITIVE COCCI — 643
Direct Gram-Stained Smears — 643
Isolation From Clinical Specimens — 643
Colony Morphology — 643
The Catalase Test — 644
Methods for Differentiating Micrococci and Staphylococci — 644
Fermentation of Glucose — 644
Susceptibility to Lysostaphin — 645
Production of Acid From Glycerol in the Presence of Erythromycin — 645
Susceptibility to Furazolidone — 645
Modified Oxidase Test — 645
Susceptibility to Bacitracin — 645

IDENTIFICATION OF STAPHYLOCOCCUS AUREUS — 645
Slide Coagulase Test — 645
Tube Coagulase Test — 646
Alternative Coagulase Test Procedures — 646
Latex Agglutination — 646
Passive Hemagglutination — 646
Additional Confirmatory Tests — 647
Deoxyribonuclease (DNase) Test — 647
Thermostable Endonuclease Test — 648
Mannitol Fermentation — 648
Other Methods for Identification of Staphylococcus aureus — 648
Rapid Tests for Detection of Methicillin Resistance — 648
Differentiation of Coagulase-Positive Staphylococci of Veterinary Origin — 648

IDENTIFICATION OF COAGULASE-NEGATIVE STAPHYLOCOCCI 649
Conventional Identification Methods 649
Production of Phosphatase for Identification of *Staphylococcus epidermidis* 650
Pyrrolidonyl Arylamidase Activity 650
Susceptibility to Polymyxin B 652
Ornithine Decarboxylase Test (ODC) 652
Urease Production 655
Acetoin Production 655
Susceptibility to Deferoxamine 655
Susceptibility to Novobiocin for Identification of *Staphylococcus saprophyticus* 655
Commercial Identification Systems 655
RapiDEC Staph 656
API Staph-IDENT 656
API Staph 656
API ID32 Staph 656
Vitek Gram-Positive Identification (GPI) Card 657
MicroScan Rapid Pos Combo Panel 657
MicroScan Pos ID Panel 657
BBL Crystal Gram-Positive (GP) Identification System 657
Staf-Sistem 18-R 658
Staph-Zym 658
Microbact Staphylococcal 12S 658
Microbial Identification System 658
Biolog Microplate Identification System 658
Molecular Identification and Typing Methods for Staphylococci 658
Identification of *Micrococcus* and Related Species 661
Identification of *Rothia mucilaginosa* 661

LABORATORY APPROACH TO THE IDENTIFICATION OF STAPHYLOCOCCI 661

Chapter 13
Gram-Positive Cocci

Part II: Streptococci, Enterococci, and the "Streptococcus-Like" Bacteria
GENERAL CHARACTERISTICS OF THE STREPTOCOCCI 674
GROUP A β-HEMOLYTIC STREPTOCOCCI (STREPTOCOCCUS PYOGENES) 676
Virulence Factors 676
Clinical Significance 679
GROUP B β-HEMOLYTIC STREPTOCOCCI (STREPTOCOCCUS AGALACTIAE) 683
Virulence Factors 683
Clinical Significance 684
GROUP C AND GROUP G β-HEMOLYTIC STREPTOCOCCI 688
GROUP F β-HEMOLYTIC STREPTOCOCCI 689
OTHER STREPTOCOCCI IN THE "PYOGENIC COCCI" GROUP 689
STREPTOCOCCUS PNEUMONIAE 689
Virulence Factors 689
Pneumococcal Vaccines 690
Clinical Significance 691

VIRIDANS STREPTOCOCCI 693
THE ANGINOSUS GROUP: STREPTOCOCCUS ANGINOSUS, STREPTOCOCCUS CONSTELLATUS, AND STREPTOCOCCUS INTERMEDIUS 695
GROUP D STREPTOCOCCI: THE "STREPTOCOCCUS BOVIS/STREPTOCOCCUS EQUINUS COMPLEX" AND RELATED SPECIES 697
STREPTOCOCCUS SUIS 698
OTHER VIRIDANS STREPTOCOCCI ISOLATED FROM ANIMALS 700
MISCELLANEOUS STREPTOCOCCI 700
ENTEROCOCCUS SPECIES 700
Taxonomy 700
Virulence Factors 701
Clinical Significance 701
Genus *Melissococcus* 704
THE "STREPTOCOCCUS-LIKE" BACTERIA 704
Abiotrophia and *Granulicatella* Species 704
Aerococcus and *Helcococcus* Species 705
Leuconostoc Species 706
Pediococcus and *Tetragenococcus* Species 706
Gemella Species 707
Vagococcus Species 707
Alloiococcus Species 708
Globicatella Species 708
Facklamia Species 708
Dolosigranulum, *Ignavigranum*, and *Dolosicoccus* Species 709
Eremococcus Species 709
Genus *Lactococcus* 709
ISOLATION AND IDENTIFICATION OF STREPTOCOCCI AND "STREPTOCOCCUS-LIKE" BACTERIA 709
Direct Gram-Stained Smears 709
Culture Media 710
Hemolysis on Blood Agar 710
Nonculture, Direct Detection Techniques for Group A β-Hemolytic Streptococci in Pharyngeal Specimens 711
Nonculture, Direct Detection Techniques for Group B β-Hemolytic Streptococci and *Streptococcus pneumoniae* 712
Colony Morphology and Catalase Testing 713
Recognition and Preliminary Characterization of Streptococci and the "Streptococcus-Like" Bacteria 713
Presumptive Identification of Streptococci 715
Susceptibility to Bacitracin 715
Susceptibility to Sulfamethoxazole-Trimethoprim (SXT) 715
CAMP Test and Pigment Production 717
Hydrolysis of Sodium Hippurate 717
Bile-Esculin Test 717
Salt-Tolerance Test (6.5% NaCl Broth) 717
Leucine Aminopeptidase (LAP) Test 718
Pyrrolidonyl Arylamidase (PYR) Test 718
Susceptibility to Optochin 718
Bile-Solubility Test 718
Commercial Presumptive Identification Tests 718

Serologic Identification of β-Hemolytic Streptococci 718
Capillary Precipitin Test 718
Coagglutination 718
Latex Agglutination 719
Serologic Identification of *Streptococcus pneumoniae* 719
Biochemical Characteristics for Identification of
Groupable Streptococci 719
Identification of the Viridans Streptococci 719
Sanguis Group 722
Mitis Group 722
Mutans Group 722
Salivarius Group 722
Anginosus Group 725
Bovis Group 726
Identification of *Streptococcus suis* and Other Streptococci
Isolated From Animals 726
Identification of *Enterococcus* Species 726
Identification of *Abiotrophia* and *Granulicatella* Species 731
Identification of *Aerococcus* and *Helcococcus* Species 731
Identification of *Leuconostoc*, *Pediococcus*, and
Tetragenococcus Species 734
Identification of *Gemella* Species 736
Identification of *Vagococcus* Species 736
Identification of *Alloiococcus*, *Globicatella*, *Facklamia*,
Dolosigranulum, *Ignavigranum*, and *Dolosicoccus* Species 738
Identification of *Lactococcus* Species 742
Commercially Available Systems for Identification of Streptococci,
Enterococci, and Selected "Streptococcus-Like" Bacteria 742
API Rapid Strep 743
BBL Crystal Gram-Positive Identification System 743
Rapid ID 32 Strep 744
RapID STR 744
Vitek Gram-Positive Identification (GPI) Card 744
Microscan Gram-Positive Breakpoint Combo Panel 745

Chapter 14

Aerobic and Facultative Gram-Positive Bacilli

LISTERIA *SPECIES AND* LISTERIA MONOCYTOGENES 766
Taxonomy of the Genus *Listeria* 766
Virulence Factors of *L. monocytogenes* 768
Epidemiology of *L. monocytogenes* 768
Clinical Significance of *L. monocytogenes* 768
Isolation of *L. monocytogenes* From Clinical Specimens 770
Identification of *Listeria* Species 770
Antimicrobial Susceptibility and Treatment of *Listeria* Infections 773
Pathogenicity of Other *Listeria* Species 773

ERYSIPELOTHRIX *SPECIES:* ERYSIPELOTHRIX RHUSIOPATHIAE *AND* ERYSIPELOTHRIX TONSILLARUM 773
Taxonomy of the Genus *Erysipelothrix* 773
Virulence Factors of *E. rhusiopathiae* 774
Clinical Significance of *E. rhusiopathiae* 774
Isolation and Identification of *E. rhusiopathiae* 775
Antimicrobial Susceptibility of *E. rhusiopathiae* 775

BACILLUS *SPECIES AND RELATED GENERA* 775
Taxonomy and the Taxonomic Dissection of the Genus *Bacillus* 775
Bacillus anthracis 776

Epidemiology of Anthrax 776
Virulence Factors of *B. anthracis* 777
Clinical Presentations of Anthrax 777
Treatment of Anthrax 778
Prevention of Anthrax 778
Bacillus cereus 778
Virulence Factors of *B. cereus* 778
B. cereus Gastroenteritis 779
Opportunistic *Bacillus* Species Infections 779
Bacteremia and Endocarditis 779
Infections in Compromised Hosts 780
Ocular Infections 780
Musculoskeletal Infections 780
Nosocomial Infections 780
Laboratory Safety, Specimen Collection, and Processing 781
Isolation and Identification of *Bacillus* Species: The
"*Bacillus cereus* Group": *B. anthracis*, *B. cereus*,
B. thuringiensis, and *B. mycoides* 781
Antimicrobial Susceptibility of *Bacillus* Species 783

CORYNEBACTERIUM *SPECIES* 783
Introduction and Taxonomy 783
Identification of *Corynebacterium* Species and the
Coryneform Bacteria 785
Antimicrobial Susceptibility Testing of *Corynebacterium*
Species and the Coryneform Bacteria 797
Members of the Genus *Corynebacterium* Isolated From Humans 797
Corynebacterium amycolatum 798
Corynebacterium diphtheriae 803
Corynebacterium jeikeium 807
Corynebacterium pseudodiphtheriticum 808
Corynebacterium striatum 808
Corynebacterium urealyticum 808
Corynebacterium Species Associated With Animals 809
Corynebacterium Species Isolated From Foods and
the Environment 810

OTHER CORYNEFORM BACTERIA 810
Actinobaculum Species 810
Actinomyces Species Isolated From Humans 811
Actinomyces Species Isolated From Animals 817
Arcanobacterium Species 817
Arthrobacter Species 823
Brevibacterium Species 823
Cellulomonas, *Cellulosimicrobium*, and *Oerskovia* Species 826
Dermabacter Species 828
Exiguobacterium Species 828
Leifsonia Species 830
Microbacterium (*Aureobacterium*) Species 830
Rothia and "*Rothia*-Like" Species (CDC Group 4) 832
Turicella Species 834

GARDNERELLA VAGINALIS 834
Taxonomy and Cellular Morphology 834
Virulence Factors of *G. vaginalis* 835
Clinical Significance of *G. vaginalis* 835
Isolation and Identification 836
Antimicrobial Susceptibility 838

LACTOBACILLUS *SPECIES* 838
Taxonomy and Epidemiology 838
Clinical Significance 839
Isolation and Identification 840
Antimicrobial Susceptibility 840

Chapter 15
Aerobic Actinomycetes

INTRODUCTION, CLASSIFICATION, AND
TAXONOMY 858
THE NOCARDIOFORM GROUP 860
Nocardia 860
Epidemiology, Pathology, and Pathogenesis 861
Clinical Disease 862
Rhodococcus 863
Epidemiology, Pathology, and Pathogenesis 863
Clinical Disease 863
Other Nocardioform Bacteria 863
THE MADUROMYCETES AND
THERMOMONOSPORAS 864
Actinomadura 864
Epidemiology 864
Clinical Disease and Pathology 864
Nocardiopsis 864
THE STREPTOMYCETES 865
Streptomyces 865
THERMOPHILIC ACTINOMYCETES 865
MISCELLANEOUS ACTINOMYCETES 865
Oerskovia 865
Dermatophilus 865
Tropheryma whipplei 865
History and Taxonomy 865
Ecology 866
Clinical Disease and Pathology 866
LABORATORY DIAGNOSIS OF INFECTIONS
CAUSED BY AEROBIC ACTINOMYCETES 866
Primary Isolation 866
Differentiation of Nocardia From Other Genera of
Aerobic Actinomycetes 867
Identification of Thermophilic Actinomycetes 871
Identification of Tropheryma whipplei 871
In Vitro Susceptibility of Nocardia and Related Bacteria to
Antimicrobial Agents and Therapy of Infections 871

Chapter 16
The Anaerobic Bacteria

RELATIONSHIPS OF BACTERIA TO OXYGEN 878
Oxygen Tolerance 879
Oxidation-Reduction Potential 879
HABITATS 880
TAXONOMIC CLASSIFICATION AND
NOMENCLATURE 880
HUMAN INFECTIONS 887
ISOLATION OF ANAEROBIC BACTERIA 890
Selection of Specimens for Culture 890
Collection and Transport of Specimens 891
Anaerobic Blood Culture (Summary of Guidelines for
Traditional Broth and Instrumented Systems) 891
Direct Examination of Clinical Materials 892
Selection and Use of Media 893

ANAEROBIC SYSTEMS FOR THE
CULTIVATION OF ANAEROBIC BACTERIA 895
Anaerobic Jar Techniques 895
Use of the Anaerobic Glove Box 897
The Roll-Streak System 897
Anaerobic Disposable Plastic Bags 898
Use of the Anaerobic Holding Jar 898
INCUBATION OF CULTURES 898
INSPECTION AND SUBCULTURE OF
COLONIES 900
AEROTOLERANCE TESTS 900
PRELIMINARY REPORTING OF RESULTS 901
DETERMINATION OF CULTURAL AND
BIOCHEMICAL CHARACTERISTICS FOR
DIFFERENTIATION OF ANAEROBIC
ISOLATES 901
Presumptive Identification 901
Use of Differential Agar Media 901
Presumpto Plates 902
Antimicrobial Susceptibility Plates 904
Characterization of Anaerobes Using Conventional Biochemical
Tests in Large Tubes 904
Alternative Procedures 905
The Nagler Test and the CAMP Test for C. perfringens 905
Packaged Microsystems 905
Commercial Packaged Kits for Identification of Anaerobes
After 4 Hours of Incubation 905
DETERMINATION OF METABOLIC PRODUCTS
BY GAS-LIQUID CHROMATOGRAPHY 906
Identification of Volatile Fatty Acids 906
Analysis of Nonvolatile Acids 908
Gas-Liquid Chromatography Controls 909
IDENTIFICATION OF ANAEROBIC BACTERIA 909
Anaerobic Gram-Negative Non–Spore-Forming Bacilli 912
Classification and Nomenclature 912
Presumptive or Preliminary Group Identification of Bacteroides,
Prevotella, Porphyromonas, and Fusobacterium 913
Identification of the Anaerobic Cocci 924
Identification of the Anaerobic Non–Spore-Forming
Gram-Positive Bacilli 927
Propionibacterium Species 927
Bifidobacterium Species 927
Lactobacillus Species 930
Actinomyces Species 930
Eubacterium Species 930
Mobiluncus and Bacterial Vaginosis 931
Additional Genera and Species of Anaerobic Non–Spore-Forming
Gram-Positive Bacilli 931
Identification of Clostridium Species 931
Histotoxic Clostridia Involved in Clostridial Myonecrosis or
Gas Gangrene 932
Miscellaneous Clostridia in Other Clinical Settings 935
Clostridium difficile–Associated Intestinal Disease 936
Botulism 937
Tetanus 938

ANTIMICROBIAL SUSCEPTIBILITY TESTING OF ANAEROBIC BACTERIA   939
Methods for Antimicrobial Susceptibility Testing of Anaerobes   939

CHAPTER 17
Antimicrobial Susceptibility Testing

HISTORICAL INTRODUCTION   946
BACTERIAL RESISTANCE TO ANTIMICROBIAL AGENTS   947
Mechanistic Variables   947
Mechanisms of Resistance   949
  Transport of Antimicrobial Agents Across the Cell Wall and Cell Membranes   949
  Antibiotics That Interfere With Formation of Bacterial Cell Walls: The β-Lactam and Glycopeptide Antibiotics   955
  Antimicrobial Agents That Do Not Exert Their Effect on Cell Walls   961
  Interactions Among Resistance Mechanisms   963

LABORATORY GUIDANCE OF ANTIMICROBIAL THERAPY   963
TESTS FOR DETERMINING INHIBITORY ACTIVITY OF ANTIMICROBIAL AGENTS   968
Indications   968
Choice of Test   968
Selection of Antimicrobial Agents   970
Standardization   970
  Growth Medium   970
  pH   970
  Serum   970
  Cation Concentration   975
  Atmosphere   975
  Temperature   975
  Inoculum   975
  Antimicrobial Agents   975
  Quality Control   976
Quality Assurance   977
Interpretation of Results   977
Selection of Antimicrobial Agents to Be Reported   981
Macrodilution Broth Susceptibility Test   982
Agar Dilution Susceptibility Test   982
Disk Diffusion Susceptibility Test   983
  Development of a Standardized Disk Diffusion Procedure   986
  Interpretation of Results   987
  Quality Control   989
  Limitations   989
Microbroth Dilution Susceptibility Test   989
Commercial Systems   993
  Vitek (BioMérieuxVitek, Hazelwood, MO) and MicroScan (Dade International, West Sacramento, CA)   993
  Epsilometer Test (Etest; AB Biodisk, Sweden)   996

SPECIAL ISSUES IN SUSCEPTIBILITY TESTING   996
β-Lactamases   996
  Staphylococcus Species   1001
  Haemophilus Species   1002
  Neisseria gonorrhoeae   1002
  Moraxella (Branhamella) catarrhalis   1002
  Enterococcus Species   1002
  Extended-Spectrum β-Lactamases   1003
Staphylococcus Species   1004

β-Lactam Antibiotics (Oxacillin-Resistant Staphylococcus Species)   1004
  Vancomycin   1007
  Macrolides, Lincosamides, and Streptogramins   1008
  Fluoroquinolones   1008
Haemophilus Species   1008
  Penicillin Antibiotics   1009
  Chloramphenicol   1009
  Cephalosporins   1009
  Trimethoprim-Sulfamethoxazole   1009
Streptococcus pneumoniae   1009
  Penicillin and Other β-Lactam Antibiotics   1009
  Multiple Resistance   1010
  Macrolides and Lincosamides   1010
Neisseria gonorrhoeae   1011
Neisseria meningitidis   1011
Enterococcus Species   1011
  Aminoglycoside Antibiotics   1012
  β-Lactam Antibiotics   1012
  Vancomycin   1012
Listeria monocytogenes   1013
Streptococcus pyogenes (Group A β-Hemolytic Streptococcus)   1013
  Penicillin   1013
  Erythromycin   1013
  Fluoroquinolones   1013
Streptococcus agalactiae (Group B β-Hemolytic Streptococcus)   1014
Viridans Streptococci   1014
Other Gram-Positive Bacteria   1014
Pseudomonas aeruginosa, Burkholderia cepacia, and Stenotrophomonas maltophilia in Patients With Cystic Fibrosis   1014
Direct Susceptibility Testing   1014

CHAPTER 18
Mycoplasmas and Ureaplasmas

TAXONOMY OF MYCOPLASMAS AND UREAPLASMAS   1023
VIRULENCE FACTORS OF HUMAN MYCOPLASMAS   1026
CLINICAL SIGNIFICANCE OF THE HUMAN MYCOPLASMAS   1027
Mycoplasma pneumoniae   1027
Mycoplasma hominis and Ureaplasma urealyticum   1028
Mycoplasma genitalium   1033
Mycoplasma fermentans   1034
Mycoplasma penetrans   1037
Mycoplasma pirum   1038
Mycoplasma primatum   1039
Mycoplasma spermatophilum   1039
Human Infections Due to Mycoplasma Species of Animal Origin   1039
Hemotrophic Mycoplasma Species   1039

CULTURE OF HUMAN MYCOPLASMAS FROM CLINICAL SPECIMENS   1040
General Considerations   1040
Specimen Collection   1041
Transport Media   1041
Media for Culture of Mycoplasmas   1041
Isolation and Identification of Mycoplasma pneumoniae   1042
Noncultural Detection of Mycoplasma pneumoniae   1043
Isolation and Identification of the Genital Mycoplasmas   1044

Noncultural Detection of the Genital Mycoplasmas 1045
Commercial Mycoplasma Culture Systems 1047
Isolation of Mycoplasmas on Routine Culture Media 1048

SEROLOGIC TESTS FOR DIAGNOSIS OF MYCOPLASMA PNEUMONIAE INFECTIONS 1048

SEROLOGIC TESTS FOR GENITAL MYCOPLASMAS 1050

ANTIMICROBIAL SUSCEPTIBILITY AND TREATMENT OF MYCOPLASMA INFECTIONS 1051

DIAGNOSIS AND TREATMENT OF HEMOTROPHIC MYCOPLASMA INFECTIONS IN ANIMALS 1054

CHAPTER 19
Mycobacteria

TRENDS IN CLINICAL TUBERCULOSIS 1065
Worldwide Increase in the Incidence of Tuberculosis 1065
Impact of Coinfection With HIV and Mycobacterium tuberculosis 1066
Persons at Risk for Tuberculosis 1066
Rapidly Progressive Disease 1066
Implementation of More Aggressive Infection Control and Epidemiologic Measures 1067

TRENDS IN THE LABORATORY DIAGNOSIS OF TUBERCULOSIS 1067
Use of Molecular Techniques 1067
Use of Automated Instruments 1067
Use of Broth Culture Media 1067
Inoculation of Clinical Specimens to Agar-Based Culture Media 1067
Use of p-nitro-acetylamino-hydroxypropiophenone (NAP) 1068
Applications of Gas-Liquid Chromatography, High-Performance Liquid Chromatography, and Mass Spectrometry 1068
Use of the Lysis-Centrifugation System Blood Culture Tube 1068

THE CLINICAL LABORATORY 1068
Optimizing the Detection and Identification of Mycobacteria 1068
Laboratory Safety 1068

SPECIMEN COLLECTION 1069
Respiratory Specimens 1069
Blood Cultures 1069
Stool Specimens 1070
Miscellaneous "Sterile" Specimens 1070

LABORATORY APPROACH TO THE RECOVERY AND IDENTIFICATION OF MYCOBACTERIA 1071
Specimen Preparation 1072
Digestion and Decontamination 1072
Centrifugation 1074
Bone Marrow and Biopsy Specimens 1074
Miscellaneous Liquid Specimens 1075
Staining of Acid-Fast Bacilli 1075

CULTURE OF SPECIMENS FOR RECOVERY OF MYCOBACTERIA 1077
Culture Media 1077
Nonselective Culture Media for Recovery of Mycobacteria 1077
Media of Cohen and Middlebrook 1078
Selective Media 1078
Incubation 1079

RAPID METHODS FOR ESTABLISHING A DIAGNOSIS 1079
Sensitivity of Acid-Fast Smears 1079
Gas-Liquid and High-Performance Liquid Chromatography 1080
Use of Broth Culture Medium 1080

AUTOMATED DETECTION SYSTEMS 1080
BACTEC AFB System 1081
Mycobacteria Growth Indicator Tube (MGIT) and MGIT 960 1081
MB/BacT Mycobacteria Detection System 1082
The ESP Culture System II 1082
The BACTEC MYCO/F Lytic 1083

MANUAL DETECTION SYSTEMS 1083
Septi-Chek AFB System 1083

IDENTIFICATION OF MYCOBACTERIA USING CONVENTIONAL METHODS 1085
Optimal Temperature for Isolation and Rates of Growth 1085
Pigment Production 1086
Niacin Accumulation 1086
Reduction of Nitrates to Nitrites 1086
Tween 80 Hydrolysis 1087
Catalase Activity 1087
Arylsulfatase Activity 1087
Urease Activity 1087
Pyrazinamidase 1087
Iron Uptake 1087
Growth Inhibition by Thiophene-2-carboxylic Acid Hydrazide 1087
Growth in 5% Sodium Chloride 1087
Growth on MacConkey Agar 1090

CLASSIFICATION OF MYCOBACTERIA 1090
Laboratory Identification of Mycobacteria and Related Clinical Syndromes 1091
Review of Mycobacterium Species: Laboratory Aspects and Clinical Correlations 1091
Mycobacterium tuberculosis Complex 1091
Photochromogens 1093
Scotochromogens 1095
Nonphotochromogens 1099
Rapid Growers 1104
Other Mycobacteria 1104

THE DETECTION AND IDENTIFICATION OF MYCOBACTERIA BY MOLECUAR METHODS 1106
Signal-Amplification Methods 1107
Nucleic-Acid Probes 1107
In Situ Hybridization 1107
Nucleic-Acid Amplification Methods 1108
Commercially Available Applications 1108
Home-Brew PCR Assays, Including Real-Time PCR 1109
Postamplification Analysis 1110
Reverse Hybridization 1110
DNA Sequencing 1111
Microarray Analysis 1111
Strain Typing and DNA Fingerprinting 1111

SUSCEPTIBILITY TESTING 1113

SHORT-COURSE THERAPY 1115
American Thoracic Society Recommendations 1117

SUMMARY 1117

CHAPTER 20
Spirochetal Infections

TAXONOMY	1126
TREPONEMA	1126
Treponema pallidum Subspecies *pallidum*	1126
Incubation Period	1127
Primary Syphilis	1127
Secondary Syphilis	1127
Latent Syphilis	1127
Late Syphilis	1127
Epidemiology	1128
Immunity	1129
Treponema pallidum Subspecies *pertenue*	1129
Treponema pallidum Subspecies *endemicum*	1130
Treponema carateum	1130
Laboratory Diagnosis of Treponemal Infections	1130
Serologic Tests	1131
Innovations: Provisional and Investigative Tests	1133
BORRELIA	1134
Relapsing Fever	1134
Epidemiology	1134
Clinical Disease	1135
Laboratory Diagnosis	1135
Lyme Disease	1135
Epidemiology	1137
Clinical Disease	1139
Laboratory Diagnosis	1140
LEPTOSPIRA	1143
Leptospirosis	1144
Epidemiology	1144
Clinical Disease	1144
Laboratory Diagnosis	1144
SPIRILLUM MINOR *(RAT-BITE FEVER)*	1146

CHAPTER 21
Mycology

PATIENTS AT RISK FOR FUNGAL INFECTIONS	1153
General Signs and Symptoms Suggesting Fungal Infection	1153
CLINICAL CATEGORIZATION OF FUNGAL INFECTIONS	1153
Common Mycologic Terms	1155
LABORATORY APPROACH TO THE DIAGNOSIS OF FUNGAL INFECTIONS	1156
Specimen Collection and Transport	1158
Specimen Processing	1160
Direct Examination	1160
Preparation of Mounts for Study	1162
Selection and Inoculation of Culture Media	1162
Incubation of Fungal Cultures	1165
LABORATORY APPROACH TO THE PRESUMPTIVE IDENTIFICATION OF FUNGAL ISOLATES	1166
Extent of Laboratory Genus/Species Identification	1166
Genus and Species Identification of the Major Groups of Fungi	1168
Zygomyces Species and Zygomycosis	1168
Histopathology of Infections Caused by the Zygomycetes	1171

HYALINE MOLDS AND HYALOHYPHOMYCOSIS	1172
***Aspergillus* Species and Aspergillosis**	1174
Laboratory Presentation	1174
Colony Morphology	1174
Microscopic Features	1174
Aspergillus fumigatus	1175
Aspergillus flavus	1175
Aspergillus niger	1175
Aspergillus terreus	1176
Aspergillus nidulans	1177
Histopathology	1177
Diagnosis Using Nonculture Techniques	1179
Additional Rapidly Growing Hyaline Molds	1181
Colony Characteristics	1181
Genera of Hyaline Filamentous Molds Producing Conidia in Chains	1181
Penicillium Species	1181
Paeciliomyces Species	1182
Scopulariopsis Species	1182
Identification of Hyaline Molds Producing Conidia in Clusters	1182
Acremonium Species	1182
Fusarium species	1183
Gliocladium Species	1183
Trichoderma Species	1184
Identification of the Genera of Hyalohyphomycetes Producing Conidia Singly	1184
Scedosporium Species	1185
Chrysosporium Species	1186
Sepedonium Species	1186
Beauveria Species	1187
IDENTIFICATION OF THE DERMATOPHYTES	1187
Identification of *Microsporum* Species	1189
Microsporum canis	1189
Microsporum gypseum	1190
Microsporum nanum	1190
Identification of *Trichophyton* Species	1190
Trichophyton mentagrophytes	1190
Trichophyton rubrum	1190
Trichophyton tonsurans	1191
Trichophyton verrucosum	1191
Epidermophyton floccosum	1192
Diagnosis by Nonculture Techniques	1192
THE DIMORPHIC FUNGI	1192
***Blastomyces dermatitidis* and Blastomycosis**	1194
Laboratory Presentation	1196
Diagnosis Using Nonculture Techniques	1197
***Coccidioides immitis* and Coccidioidomycosis**	1199
Laboratory Presentation	1199
***Histoplasma capsulatum* and Histoplasmosis**	1199
Laboratory Presentation	1200
Diagnosis Using Nonculture Techniques	1202
***Sporothrix schenckii* and Sporotrichosis**	1203
Laboratory Presentation	1203
Diagnosis Using Nonculture Techniques	1203
***Paracoccidioides immitis* and Paracoccidioidomycosis**	1203
Laboratory Presentation	1206
Diagnosis Using Nonculture Techniques	1206
DEMATIACEOUS FUNGI	1208
Agents of Phaeohyphomycosis	1208
Laboratory Presentation	1208

Macroconidia With Transverse and Longitudinal
  Septa (Muriform)   1208
  Alternaria Species   1209
  Ulocladium Species   1209
  Stemphylium Species   1210
  Epicoccum Species   1210
Macroconidia With Transverse Septa   1210
  Bipolaris Species   1210
  Drechslera Species   1210
  Curvularia Species   1210
  Exserohilum Species   1210
Macroconidia Borne Singly or Via Special Conidiation   1210
  Nigrospora Species   1211
  Phoma Species   1211
  Chaetomium Species   1211

AGENTS OF CHROMOMYCOSIS
AND MYCETOMA   1211
  Cladophialophora (Cladosporium) carrionii   1214
  Phialophora verrucosum   1215
  Phialophora richardsiae   1215
  Fonsecaea pedrosoi   1215
  Exophiala jeanselmei   1216

THE LABORATORY IDENTIFICATION
OF YEASTS   1216
  Germ Tube   1216
  Cornmeal Agar Preparations   1218
  Growth Patterns of Yeasts on Cornmeal Agar   1219
  CHROMagar   1219
  Candida albicans   1219
  Candida tropicalis   1220
  Candida parapsilosis   1220
  Candida kefyr (pseudotropicalis)   1220
  Other Emerging Pathogenic *Candida* Species   1220
  Candida Species and Candidiasis   1221
  Species That Produce True Hyphae   1221
  Species That Fail to Produce True Hyphae   1224
  Cryptococcosis and *Cryptococcus neoformans*   1224
  Diagnosis by Nonculture Methods   1226
  Miscellaneous Non-Hyphae-Forming Yeasts of
    Medical Importance   1226
  Candida (Torulopsis) glabrata   1226
  Rhodotorula Species   1226
  Saccharomyces Species   1226
  Hansenula anomala   1228
  Malassezia furfur   1228
  Laboratory Identification of ''Black Yeasts''   1229
  Aureobasidium pullulans   1229
  Phaeoannellomyces werneckii   1229
  Packaged Yeast-Identification Systems   1230
  Antifungal Susceptibility Testing   1230

SEROLOGIC DIAGNOSIS OF FUNGAL
DISEASES   1232

CHAPTER 22
Parasitology

RISK AND PREVENTION OF PARASITIC
INFECTIONS   1247

CLINICAL MANIFESTATIONS OF PARASITIC
DISEASE   1247
COLLECTION, TRANSPORT, AND
PROCESSING OF SPECIMENS   1248
  Fecal Specimens   1248
  Preservation of Clinical Specimens   1249
  Visual Examination   1249
  Processing Fresh Stool Specimens for Ova and Parasite Examination 1249
  Examination of Intestinal Specimens Other Than Stool   1253
  Examination of Extraintestinal Specimens   1254
  Sputum   1254
  Urine and Body Fluids   1254
  Tissue Biopsies and Aspirates   1254
  Corneal Scrapings or Biopsy   1254
  Muscle Biopsy   1254
  Blood   1254

IDENTIFICATION AND DIFFERENTIATION OF
PARASITES   1255
  Life Cycles of Human Parasites   1256

INTESTINAL PROTOZOA   1256
  The Intestinal Amoebae   1258
  Amebiasis and *Entamoeba histolytica*   1258
  Entamoeba histolytica versus *Entamoeba coli*   1260
  Serologic Diagnosis of Amebiasis   1260
  Nonpathogenic *Entamoeba histolytica*: *Entamoeba dispar*   1261
  Other Intestinal Amoebae   1262
  Protozoa of Uncertain Classification   1262
  Intestinal Flagellates   1263
  Giardia lamblia   1263
  Other Intestinal Flagellates   1266
  Ciliates: *Balantidium coli*   1267
  Coccidia   1267
  Cryptosporidium parvum   1267
  Cyclospora cayetanensis   1270
  Isospora belli   1271
  Sarcocystis Species   1271
  Phylum *Microsporum*: *Microsporidium* Species   1272

NEMATODES   1273
  Ascariasis and *Ascaris lumbricoides*   1274
  Trichuriasis and *Trichuris trichiura* (Whipworm)   1274
  Enterobius vermicularis   1275
  Hookworms   1276
  Strongyloidiasis and *Strongyloides stercoralis*   1279
  Trichostrongylus Species   1279
  Capillaria philippinensis   1280

CESTODES   1281
  Taenia solium and *Taenia saginata*   1282
  Diphyllobothrium latum: The Giant Fish Tapeworm   1284
  Hymenolepis Species   1285
  Dipylidium caninum   1286

TREMATODES   1286
  Schistosomes   1287
  Fasciola hepatica and *Fasciolopsis buski*   1288
  Clonorchis sinensis   1290
  Paragonimus westermani   1292

BLOOD AND TISSUE PARASITES   1292
  Malaria   1294
  Babesia   1298
  Hemoflagellates: *Leishmania* Species and *Trypanosoma* Species   1298
  Leishmaniasis and *Leishmania* Species   1299
  Trypanosomiasis   1299

Filarial Nematodes and Filariasis ... 1303
Onchocerciasis and *Onchocerca volvulus* ... 1305
Dracunculiasis ... 1306
Dirofilariasis ... 1306
Tissue Protozoan Infections ... 1306
Toxoplasma gondii ... 1306
Pneumocystis carinii ... 1311
Miscellaneous Larval Tissue Parasite Infections ... 1311
Trichinosis ... 1312
Visceral Larval Migrans ... 1312
Cutaneous Larva Migrans—Toxocara ... 1314
Anisakiasis ... 1314
Gnathostomiasis ... 1315
Angiostrongyliasis ... 1315
Echinococcosis (Hydatid Disease) ... 1315
Multiceps Species—Coenurosis ... 1316
Sparganosis: *Spirometra mansonoides* ... 1316

*SEROLOGIC DIAGNOSIS OF PARASITIC
    INFECTIONS* ... 1318
*DRUGS COMMONLY USED IN THE
    TREATMENT OF PARASITIC DISEASES* ... 1321

CHAPTER 23

Diagnosis of Infections Caused by Viruses,
Chlamydia, *Rickettsia*, and Related Organisms

INTRODUCTION ... 1329
Historical Review ... 1329
Evolution of Cell-Culture Techniques ... 1329
Evolution of Diagnostic Virology Services ... 1329
Levels of Service ... 1330

TAXONOMY AND NOMENCLATURE ... 1330
*CLINICAL MANIFESTATIONS OF VIRAL
    INFECTIONS* ... 1333
Orthomyxoviruses ... 1335
Paramyxoviruses ... 1342
Parainfluenza Viruses ... 1342
Mumps Virus ... 1344
Measles Virus ... 1344
Respiratory Syncytial Virus ... 1344
Other Paramyxoviruses ... 1344
Picornaviruses ... 1344
Rhabdoviruses ... 1345
Arenaviruses ... 1346
Filoviruses ... 1346
Togaviruses ... 1347
Bunyaviruses ... 1348
California Encephalitis Viruses ... 1348
Hantaviruses ... 1348
Human Gastroenteritis Viruses ... 1349
Rotaviruses ... 1350
Caliciviruses ... 1350
Astroviruses ... 1350
Enteric Adenoviruses ... 1350
Coronaviruses ... 1350
Coltiviruses ... 1351
Retroviruses ... 1351
Herpesviruses ... 1356
Herpes Simplex Virus ... 1356

Cytomegalovirus ... 1358
Epstein-Barr Virus ... 1359
Varicella-Zoster Virus ... 1359
Human Herpesviruses-6 and -7 ... 1359
Human Herpesvirus-8 ... 1360
B Virus ... 1360
Adenoviruses ... 1360
Poxviruses ... 1361
Papovaviruses ... 1361
Papillomaviruses ... 1362
Polyomaviruses ... 1364
Parvoviruses ... 1364
Hepatitis Viruses ... 1364
Hepatitis A Virus ... 1365
Hepatitis B Virus ... 1365
Hepatitis C Virus ... 1365
Hepatitis D Virus ... 1366
Hepatitis E Virus ... 1366
Prion Diseases (Transmissible Spongiform Encephalopathies) ... 1366

*CLINICAL CLASSIFICATION OF VIRAL
    INFECTIONS* ... 1367
DIAGNOSIS OF VIRAL INFECTIONS ... 1367
Collection of Specimens for Diagnosis ... 1369
Transportation and Storage of Specimens ... 1373
Isolation of Viruses in Culture ... 1373
Preparation and Maintenance of Cell Cultures ... 1373
Contamination of Cell Cultures ... 1375
Technical Aspects of Cell Culture ... 1377
Selection of Cell Cultures for Isolation of Viruses ... 1380
Inoculation and Incubation of Cell Cultures ... 1380
Detection of Virus and Provisional Identification ... 1381
Cytopathic Effect ... 1381
Hemagglutination and Hemadsorption ... 1383
Light Microscopy ... 1387
Electron Microscopy ... 1387
Biochemical Differentiation ... 1387
Cell Association ... 1389
Detection of Viral Antigens ... 1389
Artifacts and Non-Virus-Induced Changes ... 1389
Definitive Identification of Isolates ... 1390
Storage of Viral Isolates ... 1391
Summary of Detection and Identification of Viruses in Culture ... 1391

*DIRECT DETECTION OF VIRUSES IN CLINICAL
    SPECIMENS* ... 1392
Light Microscopic Detection of Inclusions ... 1392
Electron Microscopic Detection of Viral Particles ... 1393
Immunologic Detection of Viral Antigen ... 1393
Respiratory Viruses ... 1393
Herpes Group Viruses ... 1393
Other Viruses ... 1394
Molecular Techniques ... 1394
Human Immunodeficiency Virus ... 1394
Hepatitis C Virus ... 1395
Hepatitis B Virus ... 1396
Human Papillomaviruses ... 1396
Parvovirus B19 ... 1396
West Nile Virus ... 1396
Herpes Simplex Virus ... 1396
Cytomegalovirus ... 1397
Enteroviruses ... 1397

SARS Coronavirus 1397
Other Viral Infections 1397
Selection of Tests for Rapid Diagnosis 1397

SEROLOGIC DIAGNOSIS OF VIRAL INFECTIONS 1397

Human Immunodeficiency Virus 1398
Hepatitis B Virus and Epstein-Barr Virus 1399
Hepatitis A Virus 1401
Hepatitis C Virus 1401
Parvovirus 1402
Herpes Simplex Virus 1402
Varicella-Zoster Virus 1402
Cytomegalovirus 1402
West Nile Virus 1402
Rubella 1402
SARS Coronavirus 1402
Anti-IgM Antibodies 1402
Miscellaneous Serologic Procedures 1403
Diagnosis of Other Viral Infections 1403
Antiviral Susceptibility Testing 1403

INFECTIONS WITH CHLAMYDIA SPECIES 1403

Chlamydia trachomatis 1403
Clinical Features and Epidemiology 1403
Collection of Specimens 1403
Isolation of Chlamydia trachomatis in Cell Culture 1405
Direct Detection of Chlamydia trachomatis in Clinical Specimens 1405
Serologic Diagnosis 1406
Other Methods for Diagnosis 1406
Diagnosis of Sexual Abuse 1406
Chlamydia psittaci 1406
Chlamydia pneumoniae 1406

INFECTIONS WITH RICKETTSIA, COXIELLA, EHRLICHIA, AND ANAPLASMA 1407

Rickettsia and Coxiella 1407
Clinical Features and Epidemiology 1407
Collection of Specimens 1408
Isolation of Rickettsia and Coxiella in Culture 1408
Direct Detection of Antigen and Nucleic Acid in Clinical Specimens 1409
Serologic Diagnosis 1409
Ehrlichia and Anaplasma Species 1409

Appendix I   1420

Appendix II   1437

Charts

Chart 1-1   Catalase   1443
Chart 1-2   Bile-Solubility Test   1443
Chart 1-3   The Slide Coagulase Test   1444
Chart 1-4   Indole Test   1445
Chart 1-5   Cytochrome Oxidase Test   1447
Chart 1-6   PYR Test   1448
Chart 3-1   Complement Fixation (CF) Test   1448
Chart 3-2   Hemagglutination Inhibition (HAI) Test   1450
Chart 6-1   o-Nitrophenyl-β-D-Galactopyranoside   1451
Chart 6-2   Nitrate Reduction: General Applications   1452
Chart 6-3   Methyl Red   1453
Chart 6-4   Voges-Proskauer Test   1454
Chart 6-5   Citrate Utilization   1456
Chart 6-6   Urease: Conventional   1457

Chart 6-7   Decarboxylases   1459
Chart 6-8   Phenylalanine Deaminase   1461
Chart 7-1   Oxidative-Fermentative Test (Hugh and Leifson)   1462
Chart 7-2   Flagellar Stain   1463
Chart 7-3   Fluorescence-Denitrification   1465
Chart 7-4   Esculin Hydrolysis Test   1466
Chart 8-1   The CAMP Test   1468
Chart 9-1   Test for X and V Factor Requirements   1469
Chart 11-1   Rapid Carbohydrate Utilization Test for Identification of Neisseria Species   1470
Chart 12-1   Furazolidone Disk Test   1471
Chart 12-2   Novobiocin Disk Test   1471
Chart 13-1   Bacitracin and SXT Susceptibility Tests   1472
Chart 13-2   Bile-Esculin Test   1473
Chart 13-3   Optochin Susceptibility Test   1474
Chart 13-4   Salt-Tolerance Test   1474
Chart 14-1   Loefflers' Methylene Blue Stain   1475
Chart 14-2   Loefflers' Serum Medium   1476
Chart 14-3   Tinsdales' Agar (as Modified by Moore and Parsons)   1477
Chart 14-4   Cystine-Tellurite Blood Agar   1478
Chart 15-1   Hydrolysis of Xanthine, Hypoxanthine, Tyrosine, and Casein   1478
Chart 17-1   Disk Diffusion (Bauer-Kirby) Susceptibility Test for Nonfastidious Bacteria   1480
Chart 17-2   Performance of Microbroth Dilution Susceptibility Tests with Nonfastidious Bacteria   1481
Chart 17-3   Gradient Diffusion Test (Etest) for Bacterial Susceptibility   1482
Chart 18-1   Diene's Stain Procedure for Identification of Mycoplasmas   1483
Chart 18-2   Hemadsorption Test for Identification of Mycoplasma pneumoniae   1484
Chart 18-3   Manganous Chloride-Urea Test for Identification of Ureaplasma urealyticum   1484
Chart 18-4   Medium for Isolation of Mycoplasma pneumoniae   1485
Chart 18-5   Medium for Isolation of the Genital Mycoplasmas   1487
Chart 18-6   Tetrazolium Reduction Test for the Presumptive Identification of Mycoplasma pneumoniae   1488
Chart 19-1   Digestion and Decontamination: N-Acetyl-L-cysteine–Sodium Hydroxide (NALC)   1489
Chart 19-2   Carbol Fuchsin Stains   1491
Chart 19-3   Fluorescent Stain: Auramine O; Auramine-Rhodamine   1492
Chart 19-4   NAP Test (p-Nitro-α-Acetylamino-β-Hydroxypropiophenone); (BACTEC)   1494
Chart 19-5   Arylsulfatase   1496
Chart 19-6   Assessment of Photoreactivity of Mycobacteria   1497
Chart 19-7   Catalase 68°C   1499
Chart 19-8   Growth on MacConkey Agar   1500
Chart 19-9   Inhibition by Thiophene-2-carboxylic Acid Hydrazide (T$_2$H, 1μg/mL)   1501
Chart 19-10   Iron Uptake   1502
Chart 19-11   Niacin Accumulation   1502
Chart 19-12   Nitrate Reduction: Mycobacteria   1504
Chart 19-13   Pyrazinamidase   1505
Chart 19-14   Sodium Chloride Tolerance: Mycobacteria   1506
Chart 19-15   Tween-80 Hydrolysis   1507
Chart 19-16   Urease: Mycobacteria   1508
Chart 19-17   DNA Probes for the Identification of Mycobacteria   1509
Chart 19-18   Detection, Identification, and Drug Susceptibility Testing of M. tuberculosis by Radiometric Instrumentation   1511

Chart 20-1   Darkfield Microscopy of Genital Lesions   1513

Chart 20-2   Venereal Disease Research Laboratory (VDRL) Slide Test on Serum   1514

Chart 20-3   Rapid Plasma Reagin (RPR) Card Test   1517

Chart 20-4   Fluorescent Treponemal Antibody Absorption Test (FTA-ABS)   1521

Chart 22-1   Fecal Concentration Techniques for the Recovery of Intestinal Parasites   1525

Chart 22-2   Trichrome-Staining Technique for Fecal Smears   1528

Chart 22-3   Preparation of Thin and Thick Blood Smears   1529

Chart 22-4   Calibration of the Ocular Micrometer   1531

Chart 22-5   Cellulose Tape Preparation for Pinworm Examination   1533

Chart 23-1   Hemadsorption (HAD) Test   1534

Chart A-1   Formulations of Commonly Used Stool Preservatives   1535

Color Plates

Index

List of Color Plates

Color Plate 1-1

Gram Stain Evaluation of Sputum Smears

Color Plate 1-2

Miscellaneous Stains Used in Microbiology

Color Plate 1-3

Presumptive Bacterial Identification Based on Observing Microscopic Cellular Morphology in Stained Smear Preparations

Color Plate 1-4

Pitfalls and Artifacts in Gram's Stain

Color Plate 1-5

Presumptive Bacterial Identification Based on Observing Colonial Morphology

Color Plate 6-1

Presumptive Identification of the *Enterobacteriaceae*

Color Plate 6-2

Appearance of the *Enterobacteriaceae* Colonies on MacConkey and EMB Agars

Color Plate 6-3

Appearance of the *Enterobacteriaceae* on XLD and HE Agar Plates

Color Plate 6-4

Differential Characteristics of the *Enterobacteriaceae*

Color Plate 6-5

Human Plague/Chromogenic Agar

Color Plate 6-6

Commercial Identification Systems

Color Plate 7-1

Important Characteristics for Distinguishing Nonfermentative Gram-Negative Bacilli

Color Plate 7-2

Tests Used in the Identification of Nonfermentative Gram-Negative Bacilli

Color Plate 7-3

Colonial and Microscopic Morphology of Certain Nonfermentative Bacilli

Color Plate 7-4

Colonial and Microscopic Morphology of Certain Nonfermentative Bacilli (*continued*)

Color Plate 7-5

Colonial and Microscopic Morphology of Certain Nonfermentative Bacilli (*continued*)

Color Plate 8-1

Laboratory Identification of *Campylobacter* Species

Color Plate 8-2

Laboratory Identification of *Vibrio cholerae* and Other *Vibrio* Species

Color Plate 9-1

Identification of *Haemophilus* Species

Color Plate 9-2

Identification of *Haemophilus* Species (*continued*)

Color Plate 9-3

Actinobacillus, *Cardiobacterium*, and *Eikenella* Species

Color Plate 9-4

Kingella, *Capnocytophaga*, and *Dysgonomonas* Species

Color Plate 9-5

Pasteurella, *Brucella*, and *Bordetella* Species

Color Plate 10-1

Laboratory Diagnosis of Legionellosis

Color Plate 11-1

Identification of *Neisseria* Species

Color Plate 11-2

Identification of *Neisseria* Species and *Moraxella catarrhalis*

Color Plate 12-1

Identification of Staphylococci and Related Species

Color Plate 12-2

Identification of Staphylococci

Color Plate 12-3

Identification of Staphylococci (*continued*)

Color Plate 13-1

Identification of Streptococci

Color Plate 13-2

Identification of Streptococci and Enterococci

Color Plate 13-3

Identification of Streptococci and Enterococci and Streptococcus-Like Bacteria

Color Plate 13-4

Identification of Enterococci and Viridans Group Streptococci

Color Plate 14-1

Listeria and *Erysipelothrix* Species

Color Plate 14-2

Erysipelothrix and *Bacillus* Species

Color Plate 14-3

Corynebacterium Species

Color Plate 14-4

Corynebacterium Species (*continued*)

Color Plate 14-5

Corynebacterium Species (*continued*)

Color Plate 14-6

Corynebacterium, *Arcanobacterium*, and *Brevibacterium* Species

Color Plate 14-7

Rothia, *Cellulosimicrobium*, *Cellulomonas/ Microbacterium*, and *Lactobacillus* Species

Color Plate 14-8

Lactobacillus and *Gardnerella* Species

Color Plate 15-1

Identification of Aerobic and Facultatively Anaerobic Gram-Positive Bacilli

Color Plate 16-1

Identification of Anaerobic Bacteria: Gram-Negative Bacilli

Color Plate 16-2

Identification of Anaerobic Bacteria: Gram-Positive, Non–Spore-Forming Organisms

Color Plate 16-3

Identification of Anaerobic Bacteria: Clostridia

Color Plate 16-4

Identification of Anaerobic Bacteria: Clostridia (*continued*)

Color Plate 16-5

Identification of Anaerobic Bacteria: Use of Presumpto Quadrant Plates and Disks on Anaerobic Blood Agar

Color Plate 18-1

Mycoplasmas and Ureaplasmas

Color Plate 19-1

The Laboratory Identification of *Mycobacterium tuberculosis*

Color Plate 19-2

Laboratory Identification of *Mycobacterium* Species Other Than *M. tuberculosis*

Color Plate 19-3

Clinical Manifestations of Select Mycobacterial Diseases

Color Plate 20-1

Laboratory Diagnosis of Spirochetal Diseases

Color Plate 21-1

Colony Morphology of *Zygomycetes* Species and Select *Aspergillus* Species

Color Plate 21-2

Colony Morphology of Commonly Encountered Hyaline Molds

Color Plate 21-3

Colony Morphology of Commonly Encountered Dematiaceous Molds

Color Plate 21-4

Colony Morphology of Dermatophytes

Color Plate 21-5

Colony Morphology of Dimorphic Fungi

Color Plate 21-6

Morphology of Commonly Recovered Yeasts

Color Plate 22-1

Artifacts: "Nobody Knows the Rubble I've Seen"

Color Plate 22-2

Intestinal Amoeba/Flagellates

Color Plate 22-3

Flagellates

Color Plate 22-4

Coccidia

Color Plate 22-5

Nematodes

Color Plate 22-6

Cestodes

Color Plate 22-7

Trematodes

Color Plate 22-8

Plasmodium

Color Plate 22-9

Babesiosis/Leishmaniasis/Trypanosomiasis

Color Plate 22-10

Filaria

Color Plate 22-11

Tissue Parasites

Color Plate 23-1

Viral Inclusion

Color Plate 23-2

Diagnosis of Infections Caused by Viruses, *Chlamydia,* and *Ehrlichia*

Color Plate A-1

Identification of Ticks

Color Plate A-2

Identification of Ticks and Other Arthropods

Color Plate A-3

Identification of Miscellaneous Arthropods

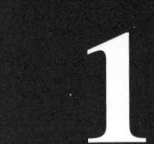
Introduction to Microbiology

Part I: The Role of the Microbiology Laboratory in the Diagnosis of Infectious Diseases: Guidelines to Practice and Management

Introduction

Outline of the Book
The World of Infectious
Disease

The Triad of Infectious Disease

The Infectious Agent

Classes of Infectious Agents
Interactions between Hosts and
Infectious Agents
Purpose of Infectious Agents in
Nature
Virulence

The Environment
The Infected Host

Innate Humoral (Noncellular)
Defenses
Innate Cellular Defenses
Types of Inflammation
Adaptive Immunologic Cellular
Defenses
Adaptive Immunologic Noncellular
(Humoral) Defenses
Clinical Signs and Symptoms of
Infection
Indirect Effects of Infectious
Agents on Humans

Phases of the Diagnostic Cycle

Preanalytic Phase

Specimen Collection
Specimen Transport
Specimen Receipt and
Preliminary Observations
Criteria for Rejection of
Specimens
Cost-Effective Approaches in the
Preanalytic Phase

Analytic Phase

Microscopic Examination
Processing Specimens
Interpretation of Cultures
Procedures for Preliminary
Identification of Bacterial Isolates
Identification of Organisms Other
Than Bacteria
Testing of Susceptibility to
Antimicrobial Agents
Cost-Effective Approaches in the
Analytic Phase

Postanalytic Phase

Reporting Results
Interactions With Epidemiologists
Analysis of Results
Maintenance of Samples and
Records

Administrative Aspects of the Microbiology Laboratory

Government Regulations
Risk Management
Laboratory Safety

General Safety Rules and Regulations
Routine Safety Precautions
Biologic Agents

Universal Precautions
Shipping of Specimens and Etiologic Agents
Nonbiologic Hazards

Bioterrorism
Quality Assurance
Quality Control

Components of a Quality Control Program
Monitoring Laboratory Equipment
Monitoring Culture Media, Reagents, and Supplies

Introduction
Outline of the Book

There are almost as many ways to look at the world of infectious disease as there are infectious agents. In this book we will concentrate on the detection and identification of infectious agents in the clinical laboratory, followed by determination of susceptibility to antimicrobial agents if appropriate. Conceptually, the book is divided into three sections. The first two chapters cover general principles of infectious diseases and laboratory diagnosis. In the second section, immunologic and molecular techniques that have virtually universal applicability are presented. Finally, the third and largest section consists of extensive discussion of groups of infectious agents and the diseases that they produce. General principles of bacteriology are illuminated in a separate chapter because of the diversity of organisms in this large group of human pathogens.

The World of Infectious Disease

For most of human existence infectious diseases have been the predominant cause of illness and death, not only limiting improvements in personal comfort but also thwarting the advancement of general societal well-being. Not until the twentieth century did improvements in living conditions, sanitation, and medical intervention pull developed societies out of the quagmire of infectious disease. Unfortunately the beneficiaries of these advances have been concentrated in wealthy countries, leaving out the majority of the world. The challenge is for the world community to extend these achievements around the globe.

By the 1950s the successes of modern medicine and public health seemed so impressive that many prominent scientists were prompted to predict the conquest of infectious disease and the eradication of pestilence as a cause of misery from the face of the earth. William H. Stewart, Surgeon General of the United States, famously stated in 1969, "It is time to close the book on infectious diseases." It is the misfortune of us all that those wise men greatly underestimated the adaptability of the multitudinous life forms that share Earth with us—both infectious agents and predators, such as arthropods. Likewise, they

could not foresee the unanticipated negative consequences of major medical advances that prolonged human life, sometimes with unfortunate effects on host defense mechanisms. Nor did they appreciate the effects of human incursion farther into the environment or the consequences of free movement of plants and animals, including humans, around the globe. As a result, the list of new or newly rejuvenated infectious diseases that have plagued us since those erroneous predictions is long and still growing. A partial accounting is given in Table 1-1.

The Triad of Infectious Disease

In order to understand infectious diseases the student must appreciate the interactions among three entities:

1. **The affected host**. From our anthropomorphic point of view this host will usually be a human. The veterinarian will be concerned with animal hosts, while a botanist will focus on plants. The affected host may even itself be an infectious agent.
2. **An infectious agent**. This designation is the broadest description for a variety of life forms that interact intimately with others.
3. **The environment**. The natural environment, both animate and inanimate, is essential for maintenance of most infectious agents and for transmission of infectious agents from one host to another.

An amusing and readable but highly educational view of these relationships has been presented as a fantastical assembly of bacteria that have come together to voice their complaints about the "spin" humans have placed on their relationships.[54] *The Other End of the Microscope: The Bacteria Tell Their Story* by E.W. Koneman turns our traditional view of the world on its head.

A more traditional, but also eminently readable elucidation of the complex interconnections between humans and infectious agents was prepared by Cedric Mims, the distinguished British microbiologist. It has been updated by colleagues and is an outstanding way to explore the fascinating subject of pathogenesis further.[69]

Table 1-1 Newly Recognized Infectious Diseases and Newly Identified Pathogens Since the "Conquest of Infectious Diseases"*

YEAR	AGENT	DISEASE(S)
1977	Ebola virus	Ebola hemorrhagic fever
	Legionella spp.	Legionnaires' disease
	Hantaan virus	Hemorrhagic fever with renal symptoms
	Campylobacter jejuni	Gastroenteritis
1982	*Escherichia coli* 0157 (verotoxin-producing)	Hemorrhagic colitis; hemolytic uremic syndrome
	Borrelia burgdorferi	Lyme disease
1983	*Helicobacter pylori*	Gastric/duodenal ulcer
	Human immunodeficiency virus	Acquired immunodeficiency syndrome
1989	Hepatitis C virus	Non-A, non-B hepatitis
1991	*Ehrlichia chaffeensis*	Human monocytic ehrlichiosis
	Guanarito virus	Venezuelan hemorrhagic fever
1993	Sin nombre virus	Hantavirus pulmonary syndrome
	Bartonella henselae	Cat scratch disease; Bacillary angiomatosis
1994	Human herpesvirus 8	Kaposi's sarcoma
	Anaplasma (Ehrlichia) phagocytophilum	Human granulocytic anaplasmosis (ehrlichiosis)
1995	Hendra virus	Respiratory disease; meningoencephalitis
1996	Australian lyssavirus	Human rabies
1997	Influenza virus H5N1	Avian influenza in humans
1999	Nipah virus	Respiratory illness; meningoencephalitis
	Influenza virus H9N2	New variant of avian influenza in humans
2001	Human metapneumovirus	Respiratory illness
2003	SARS coronavirus	Severe acute respiratory syndrome

* with contributions by Joseph McDade, PhD

The Infectious Agent
CLASSES OF INFECTIOUS AGENTS

Infectious agents can be divided into a finite number of types. Most are free-living and contain all the machinery for the maintenance of their kind; they are referred to as **microbes**. Bacteria, fungi, parasites, and viruses are the traditional infectious agents.

1. **Bacteria** contain the largest number of species that are pathogenic for humans. They are single-celled and contain both DNA and RNA, but they are not differentiated into nucleus and cytoplasm; they reproduce by binary fission. There are a few families of bacteria, most notably the *Rickettsiaceae*, *Anaplasmataceae*, and *Chlamydiaceae* that lack all the machinery necessary for replication and must interact with a host cell to reproduce.
2. **Fungi** are single and multicelled agents that are further differentiated into a defined nucleus and cytoplasm. **Yeast** are single-celled fungi that reproduce by binary fission. **Molds** or **moulds** are more complex multicelled organisms that reproduce by both sexual and asexual means. Some fungi have both yeast and mold phases; they are referred to as dimorphic fungi.

3. **Parasites** are a large and very complex group of microbes. They include single-celled animals, such as the protozoa, and very complex, multicelled organisms that have well-defined organs and tissues, such as gastrointestinal tracts and genital systems. Some of these parasites are, in effect, small animals. Others, typically members of the protozoa, lack the machinery for independent reproduction and must obtain needed substances from a host.
4. **Viruses** comprise a large number of infectious agents that are, strictly speaking, not microbes because they do not have complete genetic machinery for their own propagation. With rare exceptions viruses contain either DNA or RNA, but not both. They must, therefore, infect another life form, including humans, animals, plants, bacteria, and even other viruses. They represent the simplest form of infectious agent. Microbes reproduce by multiplying—after division of their genetic material, they divide into two new identical forms. In contrast, viruses reproduce by replication—they make copies of their nucleic acid, after which the new genomes are packaged individually, all within the confines of an infected cell.

In addition to the traditional infectious agents, more evolved members of the animal kingdom, such as insects, may be considered a kind of parasitic agent if their existence is intimately related to a host. At the other extreme, the entirely unconventional **prions** contain no nucleic acid and, therefore, cannot replicate according to the established laws of nature. Yet their abnormal protein structure results in a process that looks for all the world like an infection with a replicating cycle.

INTERACTIONS BETWEEN HOSTS AND INFECTIOUS AGENTS

If an infectious agent and its host exist together and each is neither rewarded nor damaged, the process is called **commensalism** and the agent is referred to as a **commensal**.

If the infectious agent derives benefit from the host, but causes no harm to the host, the infectious agent is designated a **saprobe** (or **saprobic**). If both host and infectious agent benefit from the encounter, the process is called **symbiosis** or **mutualism**.

On the other hand, if the host is damaged by the infectious agent with or without benefit to the infectious agent the process is caused **parasitism** and the infectious agent is designated a **parasite** (a more general use of the word than the class of infectious agents known as parasites.). Infectious agents of all types may be parasites.

When microbes exist on body surfaces, either external (skin or hair) or internal (upper respiratory and gastrointestinal tracts), they are described as **colonizing flora**. The relationship of the colonizing flora to the host may be commensal, saprobic, or parasitic. It may even change from one time to another if there is an alteration in the virulence of the microbe or a diminution in the ability of the host to resist infection.

An organism that has demonstrated the ability to cause infections regularly is referred to as a **pathogen**. If the microbe produces disease on occasion, it is often termed a **potential pathogen**. A potential pathogen is described as an **opportunistic agent** if it produces infection only in individuals who have compromised defense mechanisms.

Infectious agents also have several types of relationships to their hosts at the cellular level. Free-living microbes (some bacteria, fungi, and parasites) exist extracellularly and can grow in vitro in the absence of cells. Facultatively intracellu-lar microbes can grow in the absence of cells in vitro; in vivo they grow either intracellularly or extracellularly, but often have a special relationship to macrophages. Obligately intracellular infectious agents lack all of the machinery necessary for an extracellular existence; they must have a host cell to supply the needed substance(s). These relationships are summarized in Table 1-2.

PURPOSE OF INFECTIOUS AGENTS IN NATURE

Although it may not seem that way to the victim of an infectious agent, the tormentors were not put on earth to make life miserable for humans. Bacteria are carnivores. They are an essential component in the disintegration of dead tissue. In addition, they play a major role in many chemical reactions in nature and have been utilized for such unpleasant duties as decontaminating toxic spills.

In contrast, fungi are vegetarians. They play a major role in removing decaying vegetation. Nobody who loves bread, beer, wine, or cheese needs to be reminded about the importance of yeast in our society. And, of course, higher fungi serve as a food source—from mushrooms to truffles.

VIRULENCE

Virulence is the sum of characteristics that give infectious agents a leg up in the battle with their chosen hosts (or victims). It is not an all or none phenomenon; there are widely varying degrees of virulence. Most discussions of virulence focus on microbial factors, but it is actually the balance of all three members of the triad that is most important.[11]

The most virulent organism will not cause disease if it does not have access to a susceptible host, for one of two reasons:

1. The organism exists in a different environmental compartment from potential hosts. After the yellow fever virus cycle in urban mosquitoes was interrupted, transmission of disease stopped until humans entered a previously unrecognized cycle of yellow fever in species of mosquitoes that lived in the jungle.
2. All of the available hosts have developed protective immunity. For instance many viral infections that elicit protective immunity, such as measles virus,

Table 1-2 Relationships of Infectious Agents and Their Hosts at the Cellular Level		
RELATIONSHIP	INFECTIOUS AGENTS	EXAMPLES
Free-living	Most bacteria, fungi, and parasites	*Staphylococcus, Enterobacteriaceae, Candida, Aspergillus,* Protozoa, Helminths
Facultatively intracellular	Certain bacteria, mycobacteria, certain fungi	*Legionella, Brucella, Mycobacterium tuberculosis,* Dimorphic fungi
Obligately intracellular	Certain bacteria, fungi, and protozoa; viruses	*Rickettsia, Ehrlichia, Anaplasma; Toxoplasma gondii;* influenza virus

"burn out" after all the susceptible persons have been infected. Only after a new generation of uninfected—and therefore susceptible—individuals grows up can there be a new epidemic.

Conversely, an organism that produces mild or no disease in immunocompetent individuals (intrinsically low virulence) may produce devastating disease in an individual whose immune system has been compromised.

One could argue that the most successful infectious agents are those that have the best survival strategies, which may include minimal or absent virulence. Particularly for obligate intracellular pathogens, an agent that destroys its hosts rapidly will soon put itself out of business. As an example, it has been hypothesized that Epstein-Barr virus is designed to insinuate itself into long-lived memory lymphocytes and has developed strategies for minimizing negative effects on its host.[113]

An organism may, however, be virulent for its human host, but survive because it has a permissive relationship with other hosts. For instance, humans may be lethally infected, while other vertebrate hosts suffer little or no ill effect.

Virulence may result from factors that are operative at virtually any stage of the infectious process. If one thinks in the broadest terms, virulence must include characteristics beyond those that foster the promotion of disease in an infected host. Some examples are summarized in Table 1-3.

A number of excellent references are available for readers who desire more detailed information.[36,41,53,55,62,100,101]

The Environment

The host range of some infectious agents is limited to humans. Maintenance of such organisms requires access to a new susceptible host and the ability to survive during the transfer. Environmental factors are, therefore, of relatively little importance.

Most infectious agents, however, have a phase in which they live free in the environment, infect nonhuman hosts, and/or pass through a vector, usually an arthropod, between various vertebrate hosts. Some of the interactions may become extremely complex, with multiple transfers through different phases of the environment; for instance, the several developmental stages of parasites in a series of animal hosts.

The link between the infectious agent and the ultimate host is the environment. The transfer to a new host requires a portal of entry. The most common routes of transmission and portals of entry are summarized in Table 1-4. Some of the terms used to describe infectious diseases in populations are defined in Box 1-1.

The Infected Host

Once an individual has been infected, a variety of host responses are usually elicited. The response may be localized

Table 1-3 Selected Virulence Factors

CATEGORY	VIRULENCE FACTOR	EXAMPLE
Survival in environment	Intracellular replication in free-living-amoebae	*Legionella* spp.
	Resistance to desiccation	Variola virus
Effective transfer/transmission	Motile forms that can seek out a susceptible host	Cercaria of schistosomes
	Adaptation to a vector that can transmit infection	*Rickettsia rickettsii* in ticks
Evasion of host defenses	Lysis of polymorphonuclear inflammatory cells	*Streptococcus pyogenes* leukocidins
	Destruction of tissue	Proteases of *Pseudomonas aeruginosa*
	Destruction of tissue	Invasion of blood vessels by *Aspergillus fumigatus*
	Destruction of immune lymphocytes	Human immunodeficiency virus
	Antigenic modulation to subvert humoral immunity (antibodies)	Antigenic shift and drift of influenza virus; antigenic variation of *Borrelia recurrentis* or *Trypanosoma brucei*
Sequestration in an inaccessible site	Intracellular location in macrophages	*Mycobacterium tuberculosis*
	Intracellular location in neurons of spinal ganglia	Varicella-zoster virus or herpes simplex virus
Resistance to antimicrobial agents	Resistance to disinfectants	*Pseudomonas aeruginosa* and antiseptics
	Resistance to fixatives	Prions and formaldehyde
	Resistance to antiinfective agents	*Staphylococcus aureus* and methicillin
	Resistance to antiviral agents	Human immunodeficiency virus; cytomegalovirus

Table 1-4 Common Routes of Transmission and Portals of Entry for Infectious Agents

SOURCE OF AGENT	MECHANISM FOR ENTRY	PORTAL OF ENTRY	EXAMPLE
Infected human	Aerosol	Respiratory	Influenza virus
Infected human	Direct contact	Cutaneous	Herpes simplex in wrestlers
Infected human	Sexual intercourse	Genital	Syphilis; gonorrhea
Infected human or patient	Oral or nasopharyngeal secretions to eye	Ocular	Bacterial or viral conjunctivitis
Infected human	Transfusion of blood products	Intravascular	Hepatitis viruses
Contaminated environment	Food or water	Gastrointestinal	Enteric bacterial and viral pathogens
Contaminated environment	Cooling tower drift	Respiratory	Legionnaires' disease
Infected animal	Animal bite	Cutaneous	Rabies
Infected tick	Tick bite	Cutaneous	Lyme disease
Patient	Aspiration of endogenous flora	Respiratory	Bacterial pneumonia
Patient	Spillage of intestinal flora through a damaged bowel wall	Gastrointestinal	Bacterial peritonitis
Patient	Migration of bacteria from oropharynx to middle ear through eustachian tube	Ear	Bacterial otitis media

at the site of infection or may be generalized (systemic). The local reaction to infection takes the form of inflammation. **Inflammation** is a general term that refers to the abnormal alteration of tissues or organs caused by injury or destruction of tissue. Inflammation has both immunologic and nonimmunologic components. In each case the defense may be cellular or noncellular (humoral). The suffix ''-itis'' is used to indicate inflammation; when attached to the anatomic site, it describes a disease process. For instance appendicitis is an inflammatory process that affects the appendix, whereas hepatitis is inflammation of the liver (hepar), and endocarditis is inflammation of the endocardium (lining of the chambers of the heart).

Box 1-1 Categories of Infectious Diseases

Communicable disease: An illness that can be transmitted from an external source, animate or inanimate, to a patient

Contagious disease: An illness that can be transmitted from patient to patient

Iatrogenic infection: An infection that is produced by medical interventions

Infectious disease: An illness caused by a replicating or multiplying external agent

Nosocomial infection: An infection that is acquired in a health-care facility

Opportunistic infection: An infection in a patient with compromised defenses by an agent of low virulence that would not produce infection in a normal patient

Subclinical infection: An infection that produces an immunologic response, but no clinical symptoms (also called asymptomatic infection)

Innate and adaptive immunity are the two major arms of the immune response.[104,27,28,63] The innate response is the more primitive of the two. It provides an immediate response against invading microbes, regardless of their immunologic makeup. The receptors that make contact between the invader and the cellular defender are compounds called lectins that are widely distributed in nature. The innate response is limited by the lack of an amplification method for specific defenses. Rather, the innate defenses send signals that activate the second arm, which is called adaptive immunity. To use a military analogy, the innate immune response is a lightly armed border patrol that signals succeeding ranks of the regular army when it senses that an invader has crossed the national boundary.

The adaptive immune response is immunologically specific. It responds to material that is sensed as nonself or ''foreign'' by multiplying the number of defenders with weapons specifically directed against that particular foe. That is, it adapts to a very defined threat, rather than reacting universally to all threats. Once activated, the adaptive immune response serves as mission control for the rest of the campaign until victory, defeat, or occasionally stalemate results.

INNATE HUMORAL (NONCELLULAR) DEFENSES

The most basic defenses in this category are the mucus that lines all mucosal surfaces (for example, gastric mucus and the surfactant lining of the pulmonary membrane) and the fluids that sweep potential pathogens out (for example, the flow of biliary fluid, tears, and urine). In addition, certain antibacterial compounds, such as lysozyme, may help to diminish bacterial numbers. Finally, some ''primitive'' or ''preimmunologic'' humoral defenses play an important role in host defense. As a group these compounds are referred to as acute-phase reactants.[36] The first to be identified, in 1930, was C-reactive protein, which was found to react with pneumococcal C-polysaccharide. Components of the clotting system fall into this category. Importantly, the alternate pathway of the complement system is an early defense against some bacterial infections before specific antibodies develop. Finally, the innate cellular defenses produce a variety of inflammatory modulators that include chemoattractants for other inflammatory cells. These compounds are the means by which cells talk to each other; they are called **cytokines** (sometimes referred to as chemokines or lymphokines).[25] The first recognized cytokine (Interleukin 1 or IL-1), which is the main mediator responsible for the febrile response, is produced by monocytes and macrophages.[30] Cytokines also play a prominent role in the adaptive immune response, as described below.

INNATE CELLULAR DEFENSES

The primary nonimmunologic cells are fixed tissue macrophages (histiocytes), their circulating counterparts (monocytes), and polymorphonuclear neutrophils. The tissue macrophages are the primary defenses against some infectious invaders. For instance, the alveolar macrophages are very effective in disposing of invading bacteria; those organisms that can survive in macrophages (e.g., mycobacteria or *Legionella* spp.) have a competitive advantage. Tissue macrophages in the liver, spleen, and lymph nodes make up the reticuloendothelial system; they are critical for removing circulating particles, including infectious agents, from the blood. Patients whose spleens have been removed or whose livers have been damaged are at increased risk of many serious bacterial infections.

A second cellular defense is an effector cellular system called natural killer (NK) cells. It is primarily active against microbes.

Last, but not least, the physical barriers of the skin, the respiratory tract, the gastrointestinal tract, and the genitourinary tract play an important role in resisting infection. The disastrous infectious consequences of burn wounds are testimony to the effectiveness of the skin. In the respiratory tract the physical barrier of the respiratory epithelium is complemented by the action of the cilia on the surface, which propel foreign material out of the respiratory tract. In conjunction with the noncellular lining this defense is referred to as "the mucociliary escalator."

TYPES OF INFLAMMATION[121]
Acute Suppurative (or Purulent) Inflammation. An acute suppurative infection elicits a response in which pus is formed. Pus is a liquid material that contains large numbers of inflammatory cells and has a specific gravity exceeding 1.013. The initial and dominant cellular combatant is the polymorphonuclear neutrophil.[61] Later, macrophages enter the area to help clean up the debris and fibroblasts may be activated in the process of healing (fibrosis or scar tissue).

Cellulitis is often used to describe involvement of loose subcutaneous connective tissue in which the purulent exudate spreads between layers of the involved tissues. **Necrosis** refers to cell death or dissolution of tissue, which may be caused by destructive enzymes or by restriction of nutrients from the site, usually by blockage of blood flow. **Abscess** is the term used when segmented neutrophils become localized in a walled-off area of suppurative inflammation, with resultant destruction of tissue.

Purulent inflammation is a hallmark of infections caused by bacteria and some fungi, although certain viruses and parasites may also produce an acute or suppurative inflammatory response. Abscesses, however, are almost exclusively caused by bacteria and some yeast. The humoral immune response is often prominent in suppurative infections.

Granulomatous Inflammation. Granulomatous infection is a subtype of chronic infection in which granulomas are formed. A **granuloma** can be most simply defined as focal collections of large activated macrophages or histiocytes that have an increased capacity for phagocytosis and digestion of foreign particles. These cells are also called "epithelioid" cells because they occasionally line up in a manner that recalls squamous epithelium. Macrophages often aggregate to form multinucleated giant cells. Other cellular components of granulomas are lymphocytes and fibroblasts. Activation of the macrophages is produced by products of immunologically specific lymphocytes.

Certain granulomas contain a particular type of necrosis, called caseous necrosis, in which the tissue has a cheeselike consistency. (It is remarkable how often pathologists have used food analogies to describe disease processes.) The presence of multinucleated giant cells and caseous necrosis are characteristic of tuberculosis, but they may also be seen in certain other infections, particularly dimorphic fungal infections. If the granuloma is solid and the cells are intact, it is described as nonnecrotizing or noncaseous.

Granulomas are found in mycobacterial and fungal infections, some bacterial infections, and some parasitic infections. The immunologic correlate of granulomas is cell-mediated immunity.

Lymphohistiocytic Inflammation. Some infections, particularly those caused by viruses, elicit an inflammatory response composed of lymphocytes and macrophages. Both humoral and cellular immune responses are involved.

Atopic Inflammation. Allergic reactions are mediated by a different group of cells—eosinophils, basophils, and mast cells (fixed tissue basophils). The inciting allergen may be chemical, such as the familiar grasses and pollens that make life seasonally miserable for individuals who react to them.[52] Certain pathogens, particularly parasites, also elicit an eosinophilic inflammatory response.

ADAPTIVE IMMUNOLOGIC CELLULAR DEFENSES

The Grand Central Station of immunologic defenses is the lymphocyte, of which there are two primary classes. The B lymphocyte and plasma cell are responsible for producing immunologically specific antibodies, which comprise the humoral immune system.

The capo di capi of the immune system, however, is the T lymphocyte, which is responsible for cellular immunity. T lymphocytes are divided into (1) helper lymphocytes (CD 4 phenotype), which are responsible for immunologic memory and secretion of cytokines to modulate the immune response, and (2) suppressor lymphocytes (CD 8 phenotype), which are cytotoxic and responsible for eliminating foreign cellular material (including cells infected with viruses). The suppressor lymphocytes are sometimes referred to dramatically as "killer T cells." CD4 lymphocytes are further subdivided into type 1 (Th1) cells and type 2 (Th1) cells based on the types of cytokines they secrete.

ADAPTIVE IMMUNOLOGIC NONCELLULAR (HUMORAL) DEFENSES

These humoral defenses are driven and produced by the immunologically specific cells. The sophisticated communication system that coordinates activity of all host defenses consists of chemicals produced by lymphocytes that are called **cytokines**.[25] Cytokines also function as effector molecules for the cytotoxic lymphocytes.

Another important humoral defense is the complement system, which consists of a cascade of enzymes that eventually result in a group of compounds (C7-8-9) that are known collectively as the attack complex.[117,116] They are effector molecules that are critical in defense against certain pathogens, such as meningococci. The complement system functions in a manner similar to the clotting system. Intermediate components of the system, particularly C3a and C5a, are extremely important as chemoattractants, i.e., they recruit the various inflammatory cells to the site of an infection.

The complement system has two arms, which converge at C3; beyond that point the pathway is the same. The classical arm is immunologically specific; it is triggered by complexes of antigen and corresponding antibodies. The alternate arm (formerly called the properdin system) and the more recently recognized lectin-binding system are not immunologically specific and form part of the innate immune response.

On occasion the immune response can go awry. In normal development it recognizes the constituents of the host as "self" the phenomenon is known as tolerance.[51] The dark side is exposed when normal tissue components are mistaken as "foreign" or "nonself" and are attacked. Rheumatic fever is the classic example of unintentional damage, caused when the immune response mistakes myosin of the cardiac muscle fibers for the very similar M protein of *Streptococcus pyogenes*.[93] In addition, there is often "collateral damage" (to use the military euphemism) when normal tissue is damaged or even destroyed in the process of eliminating an invading infectious agent or tumor. This aberrant response is referred to as autoimmunity.[26] In addition, defects in the innate immune system may cause serious disease and aberrant inflammatory responses.[57]

Control of infectious agents and surveillance of cells for neoplastic change produced the immune system. We cannot survive without it and are at great risk when it is diminished either by natural defects or by chemicals. The chemicals may be encountered in the environment or may be administered therapeutically because they are required for medical care. The classic example is the recipient of an organ transplant. In order to prevent the body from rejecting the foreign transplant, the immune system must be suppressed, at least temporarily. In the process, defenses against invading microbes and tumor cells are compromised, sometimes with disastrous consequences.[88]

The complexity of the immune system is a beautiful thing. Its intricacies are staggering and are still not completely understood. The interested reader is referred to several excellent reviews of the subject.[104,27,28,63]

CLINICAL SIGNS AND SYMPTOMS OF INFECTION

Signs and symptoms of infection may be generalized or systemic on the one hand; on the other hand, they may be focal or localized to a given organ or organ system. Early Greek and Roman physicians recognized four cardinal signs of inflammation:

1. Dolor (pain)
2. Calor (heat)
3. Rubor (redness)
4. Tumor (swelling)

The underlying mechanisms predisposing to these signs are incompletely known. The initiating pathophysiologic mechanism is the dilation of blood vessels caused by a complex cascade of vasoactive amines and other chemical mediators.[23] The local release of chemical mediators results in (1) increased blood flow with venous and capillary congestion (calor and rubor) and (2) increased permeability of vessels with fluid, blood, and proteins escaping into the extracellular spaces (dolor and tumor). Segmented neutrophils are attracted to the area of irritation by chemotactic substances and escape through the permeable vasculature into the extracellular spaces (pus formation).

General or Systemic Signs and Symptoms of Infection. In the acute phase of infection, the patient may experience fever (often high-grade and spiking), chills, flushing (vasodilation), and an increase in pulse rate. Patients with subacute or chronic infections may present with minimal or vague symptoms—intermittent low-grade fever, weight loss or fatigability, and lassitude. Toxic reactions to bacterial products may produce eczematous or hemorrhagic skin reactions or a variety of neuromuscular, cardiorespiratory, or gastrointestinal signs and symptoms—initial indicators of an underlying infectious disease.

Radiographic manifestations of infectious disease include pulmonary infiltrates, fibrous thickening of cavity linings, gas and swelling in soft tissues, radiopaque masses, or accumulation of fluid within body cavities and organs.

Laboratory values suggesting an infectious disease in patients with minimal or early symptoms include an elevation in the erythrocyte sedimentation rate, peripheral blood leukocytosis or monocytosis, and alterations in plasma proteins. Elevations in gamma globulins, the presence of certain reactants such as C-reactive protein, or the production of type-specific antibodies may also indicate infection.

Local Signs of Infection. The cardinal signs of inflammation are the unmistakable manifestations of local infection. Localized redness and heat and the production of a swelling or tumorous mass can usually be observed, either visually if present on the external surfaces, or from radiographs or other noninvasive techniques (ultrasonography, computed tomography scans, nucleomagnetic resonance, etc.). If nerve endings are irritated or stretched by the expanding mass or by chemical irritants, pain may be experienced either in the immediate area or in other sites through complementary efferent pathways (known as "referred" pain). The presence of a draining sinus and the secretion of a purulent exudate are also indications of a local inflammatory or infectious process. Any of these signs and symptoms should direct the physician to collect material for direct microscopic examination and culture.

The specific signs and symptoms of infection manifest in the several organ systems (respiratory, gastrointestinal, urinary tract, genital, or other) will be presented in detail in Chapter 2 where these individual sites of infection are discussed.

INDIRECT EFFECTS OF INFECTIOUS AGENTS ON HUMANS

As humans have battled against infectious agents, many changes in our genetic makeup have resulted. The development of the immune system is the most dramatic and important, but other examples can be found. Malaria is one of the most prevalent and devastating infections in the world, although not common in the United States. The appearance of hemoglobin S, which results in less severe infections by *Plasmodium falciparum*,[58] probably was an adaptive change.

Unfortunately, when the infectious challenge no longer exists, the negative consequences of this hemoglobin, manifested as sickle cell disease, are preeminent. Similarly, the Duffy blood group antigen is required for entry of *P. vivax* merozoites into red blood cells. Although it is a highly prevalent antigen, the recognition of this biologic phenomenon has provided clues for construction of vaccines to block entry of malarial parasites into their target cells.[65]

Phases of the Diagnostic Cycle

It is useful to think of laboratory testing as a series of events (Figure 1-1). Traditionally, microbiologists have concentrated, as have other laboratory workers, on the scientific measurement—the analytic phase. It is now very clear that what happens before the measurement (preanalytic phase) and after the scientific determination is complete (postana-

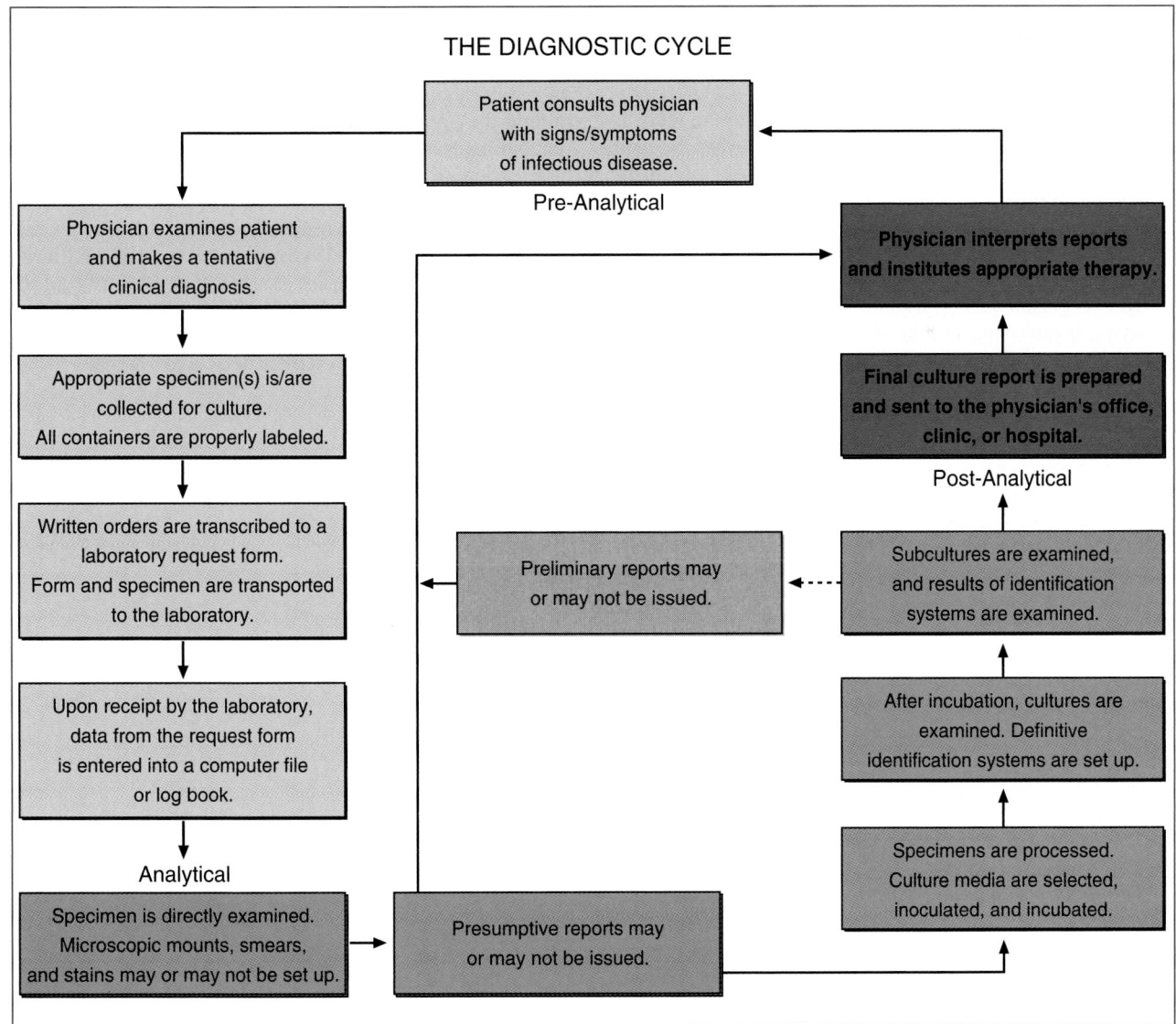

Figure 1-1 The clinical and laboratory diagnosis of infectious diseases: A schematic overview of the diagnostic cycle.

lytic phase) are just as important as the accuracy of the measurement. Monitoring of performance throughout the whole cycle is part of quality assurance for the laboratory,[84] as discussed later in this chapter.

Preanalytic Phase
SPECIMEN COLLECTION

Once an infectious disease is suspected, appropriate tests must be ordered. Culture, serologic detection of antigens or antibodies, and/or molecular detection of nucleic acids are all possible diagnostic approaches. As discussed in Chapters 3 and 4, direct detection of antigen and nucleic acid in clinical specimens and use of these approaches for identification of isolated organisms are utilized with increasing frequency. Pathologists, microbiologists, and medical technologists are available in most institutions and communities to assist physicians in selecting the proper specimens for culture and in ordering the appropriate tests to achieve the maximum recovery or detection of microorganisms.

The proper collection and transport to the laboratory of a specimen for examination is a critically important step in the ultimate confirmation that a microorganism is responsible for the infectious disease process.[68] A poorly collected specimen not only may result in failure to recover important agents, but may also lead to incorrect or even harmful therapy if treatment is directed toward a commensal or contaminant organism. For example, assume that *Klebsiella pneumoniae*, a recognized cause of human pneumonia, as the species name would indicate, was recovered from the sputum of a patient with clinical pneumonia. *Klebsiella pneumoniae* is also known to colonize the nasopharynx. If the sputum in this theoretical case was improperly collected and consisted primarily of saliva, the recovery of *K. pneumoniae* might not reflect the true cause of the pneumonia, but merely nasopharyngeal colonization. Treatment for *K. pneumoniae* could be improper and might, by chance, be effective only if the bacterial species causing the pneumonia had an antibiotic susceptibility pattern similar to that of *K. pneumoniae*. If *Pseudomonas aeruginosa* had actually been the causal agent, the therapy selected may have been in error. This theoretical scenario actually happened in Pennsylvania in 1976. Attendees at the annual convention of the Pennsylvania American Legion were infected at the convention hotel in Philadelphia, but became ill after they returned to their homes. They were treated with ineffective antibiotics directed against enteric bacilli that were colonizing the upper respiratory tract. The actual pathogen, *Legionella pneumophila*, was not known at the time and unfortunately the wrong therapeutic approach was employed based on the misleading laboratory results.[33]

The following are fundamentals to be considered when collecting specimens:

1. The material must be from the actual site of infection, collected with a minimum of contamination from adjacent tissues, organs, or secretions. For example, throat swabs for streptococcal screening should be taken from the peritonsillar fossae and posterior pharyngeal wall, avoiding contact of the swab with other areas in the mouth. Contamination of sputum or lower respiratory specimens with oropharyngeal secretions must also be minimized. Other situations where an improperly collected specimen may produce misleading results include:

a. Failure to culture the depths of a wound or draining sinus without touching the adjacent skin
b. Inadequate cleansing of the periurethral tissue and perineum before collecting a clean-catch urine sample from a woman
c. Contamination of an endometrial sample with vaginal secretions
d. Failure to reach deep abscesses with aspirating needles or cannulas.

Swabs are, by and large, inferior in the collection of most specimens; the use of aspiration needles and catheters should be encouraged. Protected discard containers for collection of ''sharps'' should be readily accessible and appropriate devices to minimizing injury when removing needles must be provided.

2. Optimal times for collection of specimens must be established to provide the best chance of recovering causative microorganisms. Knowledge of the natural history and pathophysiology of the infectious process is important for determining the optimal time to collect the specimen. Although typhoid fever is now a rare disease in the United States, the progression of the infectious process in this disease is a prime example of the importance of proper timing of specimens (Figure 1-2). The causative bacterium can be recovered optimally from the blood during the first week of illness. Culture of the feces or urine is usually positive during the second and third weeks of illness. Serum agglutinins begin to rise during the second week of illness, reaching a peak during the fifth week; they remain detectable for many weeks

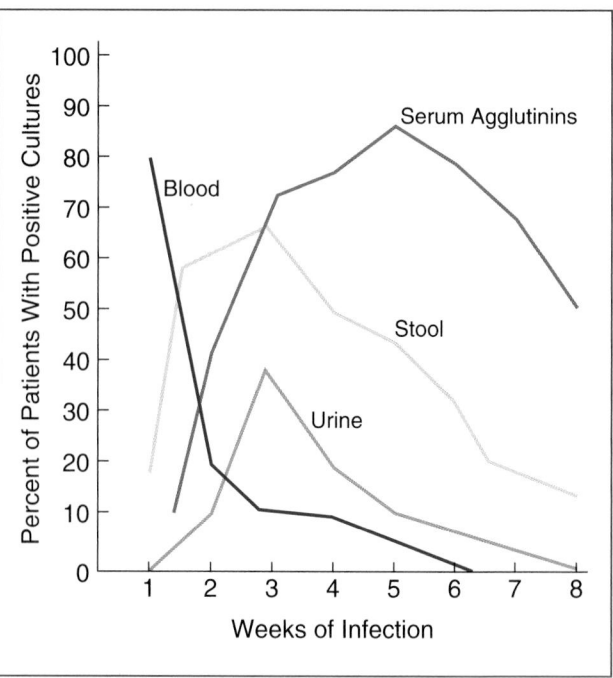

Figure 1-2 Diagnosis of typhoid fever by culture and serology.

after clinical remission of the disease, but are infrequently used diagnostically in modern laboratories.

Twenty-four hour collections of clinical materials for culture, particularly of sputum and urine, should not be done, because the risk of contamination or overgrowth of rapidly growing commensal bacteria is greater than if "spot" specimens are submitted to the laboratory.

3. A sufficient quantity of specimen must be obtained to perform the tests requested. Guidelines should be established to define a sufficient volume of material for testing. In most active bacterial infections, sufficient quantities of pus or purulent secretions are produced that volume should not be a problem. All too often, however, an unknowing clinician may submit a tiny sample, while discarding the remainder of a voluminous specimen.

In chronic or mild forms of infection, it may be difficult to procure sufficient material. Submission of a dry swab or scant secretions to the laboratory with the hope that something will grow is frequently an exercise in futility and, possibly, of considerable cost to the patient. Worse still, the lesion may be incorrectly considered to be uninfected on the basis of a falsely negative culture.

All too frequently, 0.5 mL or less of material labeled "sputum" or "bronchial washings" is delivered to the laboratory with a request for routine, AFB, and fungal cultures. Such specimens may not represent pulmonary secretions from the site of infection, and the low volume may be insufficient to enable performance of all the procedures requested. Tubes containing holding broth such as physiologic saline (nonnutrient) or phosphate yeast glucose (PYG) (nutrient) can be provided. The physician can directly inoculate whatever amount of material can be collected. In this way, the specimen can be divided in the laboratory for inoculation to a variety of primary isolation media. In some institutions, several tubes are provided, each containing culture media optimal for the recovery of mycobacteria, fungi, and viruses. If the secretions obtained are minimal, the physician must choose which tube to inoculate based on clinical considerations.

When the sample size is too small to fulfill all of the requests adequately, it is worth a telephone call to the clinician so that priorities for culture may be established. The report should indicate that the material submitted for examination was scanty.

4. Appropriate collection devices, specimen containers, and culture media must be used to ensure optimal recovery of microorganisms. Sterile containers should be used for collection of most specimens. It is also important that containers be constructed for ease of collection, particularly if the patients are required to obtain their own specimens. Narrow-mouthed bottles are poorly designed for collection of sputum or urine samples. The containers should also be provided with tightly fitted caps or lids to prevent leakage or contamination during transport.

Swabs are commonly used for obtaining many types of cultures; however, they are generally inferior to other methods for collecting specimens, and their use should be discouraged as much as possible. If swabs are used, certain precautions should be taken. Cotton swabs may contain residual fatty acids, and calcium alginate may emit toxic products that may inhibit certain fastidious bacteria. Swabs tipped with Dacron or Rayon polyester are often better choices. Specimens should

not be allowed to remain in contact with the swab any longer than necessary. In addition to toxicity, the ability of swabs to absorb and then release specimens varies with the material used to construct the swabs.

Swabs should be placed in a transport medium or moist container to prevent drying and death of bacteria. Good recovery of most bacterial species from these tubes has been demonstrated for up to 48 hours or longer. The use of culture tubes containing semisolid Stuart's or Amies' transport medium, with or without charcoal, also serves as an adequate means for holding swab cultures during transport. There are a few exceptions to this guideline. Skin scrapings and nail clippings for recovery of dermatophytic fungi should be submitted dry in a clean container to prevent the overgrowth of bacteria. Throat swabs for recovery of *Streptococcus pyogenes* may be submitted in transport media, but recovery of this "drought-resistant" bacterium is actually improved if the swab is submitted dry because other bacteria that colonize the oropharynx die off.

The ability to collect a specimen of virtually anything with a swab is an even larger problem than toxicity and retention of material. Whereas an aspirate or biopsy guarantees a specimen that will yield interpretable results, positive or negative, a swab may have been used to sample either an inflammatory process or colonizing flora. At times the true pathogen may be hiding in a mix recovered by swab, but it is often impossible to be sure. An organism that is a documented pathogen and never colonizes humans can be interpreted, but those criteria are very rarely met. In Figure 1-3 the results of culturing an aspirate and a swab from the same site are compared.

It is possible to perform a smear and a culture from a single swab if the glass slide is flamed to sterilize it before the smear is prepared. Many laboratories, however, require

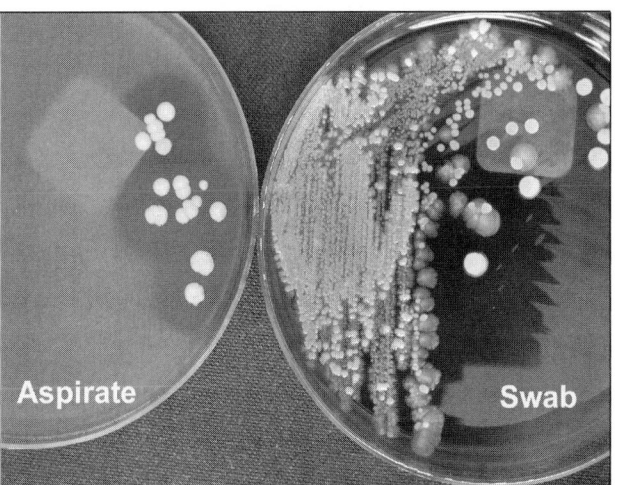

Figure 1-3 Comparison of aspirated pus and swab specimens. An infected joint site was sampled with a swab and with aspirated material. The aspirate yielded a pure culture of coagulase-positive *Staphylococcus*. The staphylococcus was also recovered in the specimen collected by swabbing, but it was mixed in with other contaminating flora. Interpretation of the aspirate was straightforward; determining the significance of the swab culture is problematic, even with the presence of a potential pathogen.

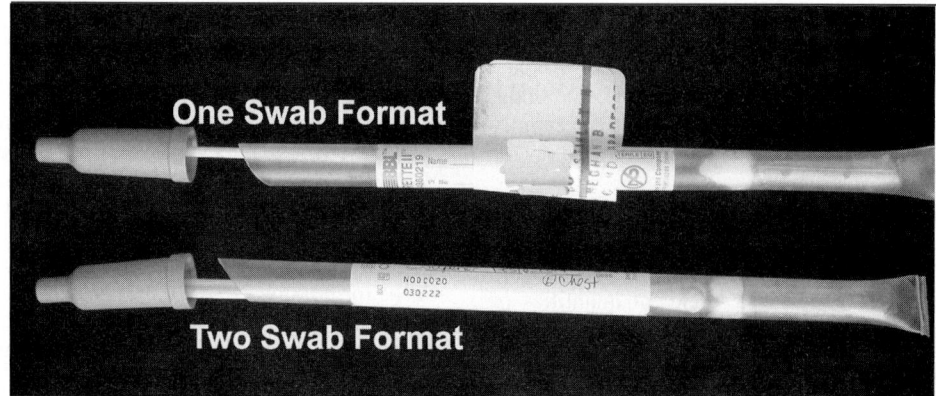

Figure 1-4 Swab transport systems. The simplest system contains a single swab in a transport tube that contains a nonnutrient medium to maintain moisture (top). A similar system is available with two swabs in a single transport tube (bottom); in this case one swab can be used for culture and the second swab for a direct smear.

that two swabs be submitted for smear and culture, so that there will be adequate material for both. In that case it is wise to provide two-swab transport systems to caregivers in order to minimize the instances where a single swab accompanies a request for smear and culture (Figure 1-4).

In particular, the use of swabs for collection of specimens for recovery of anaerobic bacteria is discouraged; rather, aspiration with a needle and syringe is recommended. In either event, the collected specimens must be protected from exposure to ambient oxygen and kept from drying until they can

be processed in the laboratory. Selected transport systems suitable for anaerobic specimens are listed in Table 1-5.

Constant education is required to discourage inappropriate use of swabs, a propensity that seems to have been imprinted on our brains at birth. The education can be as instructions for collection of specimens in a laboratory services directory, as newsletters, and as comments on reports for specimens that were submitted on swabs.

The operating room is one place where there is virtually no excuse for collection of a specimen with a swab. A campaign

Table 1-5 Transport Containers for Anaerobic Specimens	
CONTAINER	RATIONALE OR DESCRIPTION
Syringe and needle for aspiration	Fresh exudate or liquid specimens can be transported to the laboratory after bubbles are carefully expelled from the syringe and the tip of the needle is inserted into a sterile stopper. This procedure is valid only if the specimen can be transported to the laboratory without delay. This practice is under question because of the chance of HIV transmission from needlestick injury.
Tube or vial	Tube or vial contains semisolid holding medium, an atmosphere of 5% CO_2, a reducing agent, and resazurin indicator to give visual indication of anaerobiosis. The tube is used primarily for insertion of swab specimens; the vials are used for inoculation of liquid specimens.
Swab/plastic jacket system	Plastic tube or jacket is fitted with a swab and contains either Cary–Blair, Amies transport, or prereduced (PRAS) medium. The culturette system also includes a vial or chamber separated by a membrane that contains chemicals resulting in generation of CO_2 catalysts, and desiccants to "scavenger" any residual O_2 that may get into the system.
Bio-bag or plastic pouch	Transparent plastic bag containing a CO_2-generating system, palladium catalyst cups, and an anaerobic indicator. The bag is sufficiently large to enclose an inoculated Petri dish containing prereduced media, or a biochemical identification microtube tray such as for performing Minitek tests. Bag or pouch is sealed after inoculated plates have been inserted and the CO_2-generating system is activated. The advantage of these systems is that the plates can be directly observed through the thin, clear plastic of the bag for visualization of early growth of colonies.

should be undertaken to remove swabs from the operating room and prevent their reimportation. Communication with the operating room nurses is a useful means for accomplishing that goal. At the University of Vermont we were forced to devise our own approach to specimen collection in the operating room, because adequate resources were not available commercially. Sterile vials that have a screw-on top with a rubber diaphragm are prepared in the laboratory. A thin layer of nonnutrient agar with a redox indicator is placed in the bottom of the vial to maintain moisture. The vial is then placed in a package that can be autoclaved, so that a sterile vial can be emptied from the package onto the instrument tray in the operating room by a circulating nurse. The surgeon can then inject material through the diaphragm or place tissue into the vial after unscrewing the top. Tissue is sufficiently anaerobic that the system is perfectly suitable for anaerobes as well as facultative organisms. Without the outer envelope the vial works well as a general transport system (Figure 1-5).

Regardless of the transport system used, the major task is to reduce to a minimum the time delay between collection of specimens and inoculation of media. For example, if rectal swabs are used for the recovery of *Shigella* species from patients with bacillary dysentery, the material collected should optimally be inoculated directly onto the surface of MacConkey medium or into gram-negative (GN) enrichment broth. Even the use of a holding or transport medium may jeopardize the recovery of certain strains. Urethral or cervical secretions obtained for the recovery of *Neisseria gonorrhoeae* also should be inoculated directly onto the surface of chocolate agar and one of several selective culture media. Alternatively, a commercially available transport system that includes a tablet for generation of CO_2 can be employed (BD BBL™ Jem-

bec™ system; BD, Franklin Lakes, NJ) for the recovery of *N. gonorrhoeae*. Similarly, upper respiratory specimens intended for isolation of *Bordetella pertussis* should be inoculated onto fresh Bordet-Gengou, Regan-Lowe charcoal agar[94], or an equivalent at the bedside or in the clinic, unless an appropriate transport system (such as Regan-Lowe medium) is used.

5. Whenever possible, obtain cultures before the administration of antibiotics. Obtaining cultures before the use of antibiotics is particularly recommended for recovery of organisms that are usually highly susceptible to antibiotics, such as β-hemolytic streptococci from throat specimens, *N. gonorrhoeae* from genitourinary samples, or *Haemophilus influenzae* or *N. meningitidis* from cerebrospinal fluid. Administration of antibiotics does not necessarily preclude recovery of microorganisms from clinical specimens, however; even a compromised specimen is better than none at all, as long as clinicians understand that the results must be viewed with circumspection.

6. Smears should be performed in addition to cultures in most instances. Smears provide extremely useful information that supplements the culture. There are occasions when the smear is arguably more useful than the culture, as in examination of expectorated sputum. Smears allow assessment of the inflammatory nature of the specimen and provide an indication as to whether the results of culture are meaningful clinically. For instance, a wound specimen that does not contain polymorphonuclear neutrophils and yields mixed bacterial flora on culture cannot be considered valid. The clinician who trusts the results of this culture is likely practicing self-delusion.

In addition, Gram's smear provides an indication of the microbial flora. A smear that contains many gram-negative bacilli that fail to grow in a conventional aerobic culture indicates that the culture conditions were not optimal or the organisms were nonviable. Suboptimal culture conditions include the wrong atmosphere of incubation (anaerobes) or the wrong media (fastidious organisms, such as *Legionella* or *Bordetella*). Microbes could be nonviable because of appropriate antimicrobial therapy or because of an effective inflammatory response.

The federal fraud and abuse regulations require that a laboratory perform only the tests that have been requested. Mechanisms for enhancing appropriate use of the laboratory in the preanalytical phase are discussed below.

7. The culture container must be properly labeled. Each culture container must have a legible label, with the following minimum information:

Patient name
Patient identification number
Source of specimen
Clinician
Date/hour collected

Use the patient's full name and avoid initials. The identification number may be the hospital number, clinic or office number, home address, or social security number, depending on the circumstances. The clinician's name or office contact is necessary should consultation or early reporting be required. The specimen source should be noted so that special

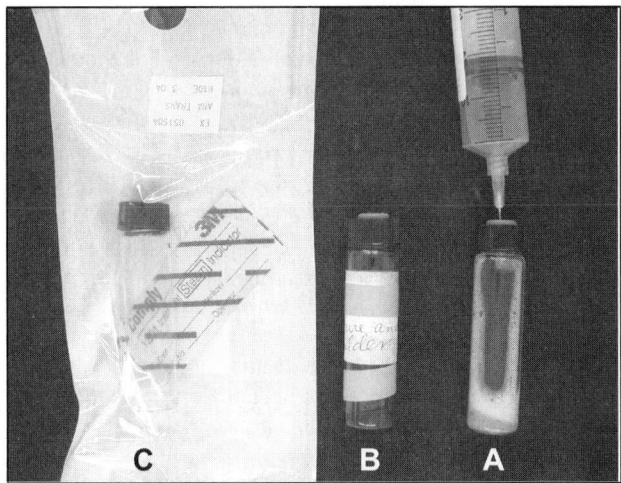

Figure 1-5 Transport system for aerobic and/or anaerobic culture. A vial is closed with a screw cap that contains a rubber diaphragm. A layer of agar in the bottom of the vial maintains moisture; a redox indicator in the agar visually displays the oxygenation of the atmosphere. Vial A contains aspirated fluid that has been inoculated through the rubber diaphragm. Vial B contains a resected graft segment that has been placed into the uncapped vial at surgery. Vial C has been sterilized in an envelope made for surgical instruments; it is ready for use in a sterile field.

culture media can be selected if required. The date and time of collection should appear on the label to assess the timeliness of processing. Other potentially useful information includes the clinical diagnosis and the antibiotic treatment history of the patient.

SPECIMEN TRANSPORT

The primary objective in the transport of diagnostic specimens, whether within the hospital, from the clinic, or externally by mail to a distant reference laboratory, is to maintain the sample in as near its original state as possible. Quality control guidelines for manufacturers of devices used for collection and transport of specimens have been developed by the Clinical and Laboratory Standards Institute (CLSI).[85] Potential hazards to specimen handlers are minimized by using tightly fitting collection devices that are confined within proper protective containers. To maintain the integrity of the specimen, adverse environmental conditions, such as exposure to extremes of heat and cold, rapid changes in pressure (during air transport), or excessive drying should be avoided. If prolonged delay is expected before the specimen can be processed (e.g., more than 4 days), it is generally preferable to freeze the specimen at $-70°C$. A freezer at $-20°C$ may be used for many specimens if the periods of storage are brief, but it must not be a frost-free type. Many virologists believe that specimens for viral culture (and isolated viruses) should never be stored at $-20°C$.

Sputum samples that have been collected primarily for recovery of mycobacteria and fungi may be shipped without further treatment if collected in sterile propylene or polyethylene containers. To avoid breakage during transport, do not use glass containers.

Most fluid specimens should be transported to the laboratory as quickly as possible. In a hospital setting, a maximum 2-hour time limit between collection and delivery of specimens to the laboratory is recommended.[5,49] This time limit poses a problem for specimens collected in physicians' offices. Urine transport containers containing a small amount of boric acid may be used if rapid transport is not possible. Alternatively, urine specimens may be refrigerated for up to 24 hours before they are cultured. A holding or transport medium can be used for most other specimens, following the manufacturer's instructions. Stuart, Amies, and Carey-Blair transport media are most frequently used (Box 1-2).

These media are essentially solutions of buffers with carbohydrates, peptones and other nutrients and growth factors excluded, designed to preserve the viability of bacteria during transport without allowing their multiplication. Sodium thioglycolate is added as a reducing agent to improve recovery of anaerobic bacteria, and the small amount of agar provides a semisolid consistency to prevent oxygenation and spillage during transport. Sodium borate solution can be recommended as a preservative for shipping specimens suspected of containing mycobacteria to distant laboratories.[98] Sucrose-phosphate-glutamate is a good transport buffer medium for recovery of certain viruses, such as herpesvirus. Culturette swabs have also been used successfully for viral specimens in some facilities.[107]

SPECIMEN RECEIPT AND PRELIMINARY OBSERVATIONS

In most clinical laboratories an area is designated for the receipt of specimens. Initial observations and handling should be performed in a biological safety cabinet (see below) because of the increasing possibility that laboratory personnel may incur a laboratory-acquired infection from specimens that contain pathogens. Personnel should wear protective clothing as appropriate—laboratory coats, rubber gloves and, in some instances, custom-fitted masks. Previously, these precautions were taken only for specimens carrying hazard labels. It is not possible, however, to determine if a patient may be harboring a transmissible agent or if a given sample contains a highly contagious pathogen. It is prudent, therefore, to practice special care when handling all specimens (universal precautions).

The processing of specimens includes the following: (1) the entry of essential data into a log book or computer database; (2) visual examination and determination of whether all criteria for acceptance are met (see section on criteria for specimen rejection immediately below); and (3) for certain specimens, the microscopic examination of direct mounts or stained smears to establish a presumptive diagnosis.

CRITERIA FOR REJECTION OF SPECIMENS

Criteria for rejection of unsuitable specimens for culture must be established in all laboratories.[112] Although general guidelines exist and accrediting agencies have established standards, each laboratory director must decide which parameters to utilize, depending on local conditions. Request slips and specimen labels must be checked to see that all essential information is included and is internally consistent. Should there be a problem, collection of a fresh sample is the best course of action. If the specimen cannot be re-collected, a responsible person should be contacted to make corrections. A comment should be entered on the final report that the specimen was received with a (specified) problem, and the name of the person who corrected the problem should be appended. If the type of specimen can be ascertained, it may be acceptable in certain cases to issue a report: ''specimen appears to be ----------.'' If not, the specimen should be rejected. Whenever discrepancies occur, a written record of how the situation was handled and names of the individual contacted should be entered on the back of the requisition, in a log, or in the computer database.

A list of specimen types or culture requests that should

Box 1-2 Stuart's Transport Medium	
Sodium chloride	3 g
Potassium chloride	0.2 g
Disodium phosphate	1.25 g
Monopotassium phosphate	0.2 g
Sodium thioglycollate	1.0 g
Calcium chloride, 1% aqueous	10.0 g
Magnesium chloride, 1% aqueous	10.0 g
Agar	4.0 g
Distilled water to equal	1.0 L
pH = 7.3	

appear on the reject list and should not be processed further appears in Box 1-3.

When a specimen is to be rejected, the person who submitted the specimen should be contacted and made aware of the problem. Every effort should be made not to reject specimens that are difficult to re-collect, such as cerebrospinal fluid or bronchial washings. If a problem cannot be resolved expeditiously, cultures should be set up to avoid losing the integrity of the specimen. The decision can be made afterward whether to report the results. If appropriate, the condition of the specimen should be indicated on the report. The clinician will then have the responsibility for interpreting the report in light of the qualifying information.

Rejection criteria should be clearly listed in the laboratory service directory. Instruction of hospital personnel on the importance of submitting relevant specimens for culture should be conducted when possible. Recurring problems and their solutions should be published in laboratory newsletters or other publications that may reach hospital personnel and staff physicians.

COST-EFFECTIVE APPROACHES IN THE PREANALYTIC PHASE

Cost-effectiveness in clinical microbiology was a dirty word for many years. It was considered antiacademic, impure, or even dangerous by traditional microbiologists. Another way to view the issue, however, is the application of clinical relevance to diagnostic microbiology. The point is not to identify every organism that might be recovered or to perform susceptibility tests on every organism that will grow in the laboratory. The point is to provide clinicians with information that will allow them to provide the best care for their patients. In the process, the work can usually be done more economically than if everything possible is done. Thus, clinical relevance usually equals cost-effectiveness. Cost-effectiveness does not mean cheap; it means the best value for money.

The father of the drive for clinical relevance in diagnostic microbiology laboratories is Raymond Bartlett, a distinguished pathologist and the director of the microbiology laboratory at Hartford Hospital in Connecticut for many years. His seminal book on the subject is still worthwhile reading for clinical microbiologists.[5,6] All of those who have followed Dr. Bartlett owe him a debt of gratitude.

Clinical relevance and cost-effectiveness should inform laboratory practice at every stage in the process. Some suggestions for the preanalytical phase are detailed in Table 1-6. Substantial savings in materials and time can be achieved.[70] Conditions vary in every institution, so each laboratory director must decide which possibilities are appropriate.

Analytic Phase
MICROSCOPIC EXAMINATION

The reasons for performing microscopic examination of clinical materials have been emphasized.[5,7]

1. The number and percentage of segmented neutrophils that are present indicate the magnitude and type of inflammatory response. The quality of the specimens can be validated.
2. The observation of bacteria, mycelial elements, yeast forms, parasitic structures, or viral inclusions may provide sufficient information to render an immediate presumptive diagnosis.
3. Direct microscopic examination may also give immediate presumptive evidence that species of anaerobic bacteria are present. With these clues in hand the clinician can make more rational decisions about initial antimicrobial therapy.

The examination of wet mounts of unstained materials by phase contrast or darkfield microscopy is useful for demonstrating motility, spirochetes and endospores. Giemsa's, Wright's, or acridine orange stains may be helpful in observing bacterial forms that stain poorly or that have little contrast with background material.

Direct Gram's stains of clinical material may also be used to determine whether a specimen is representative

---

Box 1-3 Specimen Types or Culture Requests That Should Be Rejected

1. Any specimen received in formalin. The only exception might be large specimens in which the time of exposure to formalin is short (less than 1 hour). In these instances, the tissue should be bisected with a sterile knife or scissors and an innermost portion sampled for culture.
2. Twenty-four-hour sputum collections. It is difficult to prevent contamination, and individual collections containing a high concentration of microorganisms will be diluted out by subsequent, less-concentrated samples.
3. Smears of secretions from uterine cervix, vaginal canal, or anus for Gram's stain detection of *Neisseria gonorrhoeae*.
4. A single swab submitted for multiple requests; for example, "aerobes, anaerobes, fungus, and tuberculosis."
5. Submission in an improper, nonsterile, or obviously contaminated container in which portions of the specimen have leaked out. Any leaking container having a biohazard label should be handled with extreme care.
6. Culture plates that are overgrown or dried out. One exception might be a culture plate obtained for the recovery of one of the pathogenic fungi (see Chapter 19). At times, one of the slower-growing pathogenic fungi will still grow on top of bacteria or another mold. Consultation with the physician may be in order.
7. Specimens that are obviously contaminated, as evidenced by the presence of foreign materials, such as barium, colored dyes, or oily chemicals.
8. The following specimens are not acceptable for anaerobic culture: gastric washings, midstream urine, prostatic secretions collected transurethrally, feces (except for the recovery of *Clostridium* species associated with gastrointestinal disease—*C. difficile, C. perfringens, C. septicum*), ileostomy or colostomy swabs, throat, nose, or other oropharyngeal specimens (except specimens obtained from deep tissue during oral surgery), superficial skin, and environmental cultures.

Table 1-6 Cost-Effective Approaches in the Preanalytical Phase of Testing

ACTION	RATIONALE	COMMENTS
Selective culturing of CSF for fungi[70]	Low yield in immunocompetent patients who have normal CSF chemistry and cell count values	*Cryptococcus neoformans* may produce chronic infection without pleocytosis in the CSF.
Selective culturing of CSF for mycobacteria[70]	Low yield in immunocompetent patients who have normal CSF chemistry and cell count values	In populations with a low risk of tuberculosis the yield will be even less.
Selective culturing of feces for bacterial pathogens or examination for O&P[70,105]	Low yield in patients who have been hospitalized more than 3 days	
Selective culturing of endo-tracheal suction aspirates or expectorated sputum[70]	Recovery of contaminating oropharyngeal flora increased if more tan 10 squamous epithelial cells per low power field observed	Several different criteria have been applied by investigators.
Selective use of broth back-up for bacterial cultures	Questionable usefullness except for tissue biopsies and certain fluids, such as patients with CSF shunts or receiving chronic peritoneal dialysis	Broth cultures may be used in other situations if they are examined only when an organism seen in smears is not recovered on plates. They should never be performed on specimens from mucosal surfaces.
Non-use of bacterial antigen tests on CSF[70,111]	Poor sensitivity and specificity limit usefulness	
Selective culturing of perito-neal fluid	Pattern of organisms recovered and susceptibility profiles predictable in patients with secondary peritonitis (community-acquired)	Cultures indicated in primary peritonitis (spontaneous bacterial peritonitis) and in peritonitis acquired in the hospital
Selective culturing of throat specimens	*Streptococcus pyogenes* is the major cause of pharyngitis: "routine culture" with multiple media will likely provide misleading information.	Culture for *Corynebacterium diphtheriae, Neisseria gonorrhoeae,* or herpes simplex virus should be requested specifically if appropriate. *Arcanobacterium hemolyticum* causes pharyngitis in older children and adolescents, but is isolated on media for recovery of *Streptococcus pyogenes*
Selective culturing for anae-robic bacteria	Anaerobic cultures should be performed routinely only on tissues or aspirated fluid/pus	Never perform anaerobic cultures on specimens from sites that may be contaminated with mucosal flora or feces.
Limits on frequency of culture	Throat, urine, wound limited to one per 24 hours; Blood limited to two to three cultures (10 to 20 ml per culture) per 24 hours	Culture no more often than 48 to 72 hours (time required to evaluate the first specimen) should be suggested
Limits on frequency of O&P exams	Yield from exams for *Giardia* minimal after three specimens, which should be collected every other day	Less than three exams probably adequate for other intestinal parasites
Limits on frequency of testing for *C. difficile*[96]	Yield after two negative exams minimal	
Limits on testing of CSF for herpes simplex DNA[106,110]	Yield minimal if CSF cell counts normal and no evidence of focal lesions by MRI examination	Exceptions have been described, especially in children.
Limits on duplicate specimens submitted from the same site on the same day	Either pool the specimens or select the best specimen (based on Gram's stain and/or transport time)	If there is any uncertainty as to the equivalence of the specimens, consult the clinician before processing; when in doubt, process separately immediately and consult at leisure; Preserve specimens for at least 24 hours
Limits on repeat specimens from a *nonsterile* site within a defined time period	Refer subsequent specimens to the previous evaluation; if the subsequent specimen has been inoculated to media and substantial differences from the original specimen are present, consult clinician about further action	Preserve specimen for at least 24 hours; preserve inoculated plates that are incompletely evaluated for a defined period (e.g., 7 days)
Elimination of culture of in-dwelling urinary catheter tips[114]	Reject the specimen for culture	Inform the clinician that urine should be submitted.

CSF = cerebrospinal fluid; O&P = ova and parasites; MRI = magnetic resonance imaging.
For more information the reader should consult references[48,67].

Box 1-4 Bartlett's Grading System for Assessing the Quality of Sputum Samples

No. of Neutrophils Per 10 × Low-Power Field	Grade
<10	0
10–25	+1
>25	+2
Presence of mucus	+1
No. of Epithelial Cells Per 10 × Low-Power Field	
10–25	−1
>25	−2
Total*	

Average the number of epithelial cells and neutrophils in about 20 or 30 separate 10× microscopic fields and then calculate the total. A final score of 0 or less indicates lack of active inflammation or contamination with saliva. Repeat sputum specimens should be requested.

of the site of infection. This technique has been applied to the evaluation of sputum samples. From the relative numbers of squamous epithelial cells and segmented neutrophils in direct Gram's stains of sputum samples, Bartlett[5] has devised a grading system for evaluating sputum samples (Box 1-4). Using this system, negative numbers are assigned to a smear when squamous epithelial cells are observed, indicating contamination with oropharyngeal secretions (saliva). Positive numbers are assigned for the presence of segmented neutrophils, indicating the presence of active inflammation. The magnitude of these negative and positive determinations depends on the relative numbers of epithelial cells and segmented neutrophils as shown in the outline of Bartlett's grading system. A final score of 0 or less indicates either lack of inflammatory response or presence of significant salivary contamination, thus invalidating the specimen. Representative photomicrographs of gram-stained sputum preparations illustrating this grading system are shown in Color Plate 1-1.

A similar grading system has been proposed by Murray and Washington[72] (Box 1-5). The large number of epithelial cells in groups 1 to 4 of this system indicates contamination with oropharyngeal secretions and invalidates the samples.

Box 1-5 Murray and Washington's Grading System for Assessing the Quality of Sputum Samples

	Epithelial Cells Per Low-Power Field	Leukocytes Per Low-Power Field
Group 1	25	10
Group 2	25	10–25
Group 3	25	25
Group 4	10–25	25
Group 5	<10	25

Only group 5 specimens are considered clinically relevant. In a clinical study, Van Scoy[115] recommended that sputum samples containing more than 25 neutrophils be accepted for culture even if more than 10 epithelial cells are present (group 4). These suggested criteria for evaluation of sputum have been evaluated by applying them to matched pairs of respiratory secretion obtained by expectoration and by transtracheal aspiration, a technique that bypasses the oropharyngeal flora.[39]

The sputum grading system cannot be employed if pulmonary infections caused by mycobacteria, most fungi, *Legionella* spp., and viruses are suspected. Additionally, the significance of polymorphonuclear neutrophils is altered in a few situations: (1) when the patient is neutropenic from disease or therapy, (2) when the patient does not mount an effective inflammatory response, and (3) where a foreign body causes irritation to a mucosal surface. Neutropenia can result from an inherited deficiency or because the inflammatory cells or their precursors are destroyed, either by a disease process or by chemotherapy for a disease. In some conditions the ability of neutrophils to migrate to the site of an infection is impaired. From the information ordinarily supplied by clinicians, it is rarely possible for the clinical microbiologist to determine whether a patient is neutropenic. One of the exceptions is the incompletely understood deficiency in mobilization of neutrophils that is found in infancy.[24] The exact age at which a full neutrophilic response can be mounted is not clearly defined, but in the very youngest children (less than 2 months of age) decisions to reject specimens or evaluate isolates incompletely should not be based on the absence of neutrophils in the specimen.

The two situations in which foreign bodies modify the interpretation of neutrophils are the lower respiratory tract with an endotracheal catheter in place and the lower urinary tract with an indwelling catheter, such as a Foley catheter. In each of these situations the presence of neutrophils in a specimen may reflect irritation from the catheter rather than from an infectious agent (although both factors may be present). In the respiratory tract the inflammation may come from local infection (tracheitis) rather than pneumonia, even if there is an infectious element. In the lower urinary tract the presence of leukocytes cannot be used as an indication of a clinically important infection if a catheter is in place[108] or even if repeated intermittent catheterization is performed[40]. The critical determinant for therapy of urinary tract infections in the chronically catheterized patient is whether the infection is symptomatic (see Chapter 2). In the respiratory tract neutrophils cannot be used as an indication of pneumonia; the diagnosis of pneumonia is made clinically and radiographically, as discussed in Chapter 2.

Microscopic Techniques. A number of techniques may be used in the direct microscopic examination of clinical specimens, either to demonstrate the presence of microorganisms or to observe certain biochemical, physiologic, or serologic characteristics. The techniques commonly used in clinical microbiology laboratories are outlined in Table 1-7. Because the refractive index of bacteria and other microorganisms is similar to that of the mounting medium, they are not visible when examined by brightfield illumination. Therefore, certain manipulations of the light source may be necessary.

Table 1-7 Techniques for Direct Examination of Unstained Specimens

METHODS AND MATERIALS	PURPOSE	TECHNIQUES
Saline Mount Sodium chloride, 0.85% (aqueous) Glass microscope slides, 3 × 1-inch Coverslips Paraffin–petrolatum mixture (Vaspar)	To determine biologic activity of microorganisms, including motility or reactions to certain chemicals, or serologic reactivity in specific antisera. The latter includes the quellung (capsular swelling) reaction used to identify different capsular types of *Streptococcus pneumoniae* and *Haemophilus influenzae*.	Disperse a small quantity of the specimen to be examined into a drop of saline on a microscope slide. Overlay a coverslip and examine directly with a 40 × or 100 × (oil immersion) objective of the microscope, closing the iris diaphragm to reduce the amount of transmitted light. To prevent drying, ring the coverslip with a small amount of paraffin–petrolatum before overlaying the specimen drop on the slide.
Hanging-drop Procedure Hanging-drop glass side (This is a thick glass slide with a central concave well.) Coverslip Physiologic saline or water Paraffin-petrolatum mixture	The hanging-drop mount serves the same purpose as the saline mount, except there is less distortion from the weight of the coverslip and a deeper field of focus into the drop can be achieved. This technique is generally used for studying the motility of bacteria.	A small amount of paraffin-petrolatum mixture is placed around the lip of the well on the undersurface of the hanging-drop slide. Cells from a bacterial colony to be examined are placed in the center of the coverslip, into a small drop of saline or water. The slide is inverted and pressed over the coverslip, guiding the drop of bacterial suspension into the center of the well. The slide is carefully brought to an upright position for direct examination under the microscope.
Iodine Mount Lugol's iodine solution: Iodine crystals, 5 g Potassium iodide, 10 g Distilled water, 100 mL Dissolve KI in water and add iodine crystals slowly until dissolved. Filter and store in tightly stoppered bottle. Dilute 1 : 5 with water before use. Microscope slides, 3 × 1-inch Coverslips	Iodine mounts are usually used in parallel with saline mounts when examining feces or other materials for intestinal protozoa or helminth ova. The iodine stains the nuclei and intracytoplasmic organelles so that they are more easily seen. Iodine mounts cannot be used to the exclusion of saline mounts because iodine paralyzes the motility of bacteria and protozoan trophozoites.	A small amount of fecal matter or other material is mixes in a drop of the iodine solution on a microscope slide. This is mixed to form an even suspension, and a coverslip is placed over the drop. The mount is then examined directly under a microscope. If this is to be delayed or if a semipermanent preparation for future study is desired, the edges of the coverslip can be sealed with the paraffin–petrolatum mixture.
Potassium Hydroxide (KOH) Mount Potassium hydroxide, 10% (aqueous) Microscrope slides, 3 × 1-inch Coverslips	The KOH mount is used to aid in detecting fungus elements in thick mucoid material or in specimens containing keratinous material, such as skin scales, nails, or hair. The KOH dissolves the background keratin, unmasking the fungus elements to make them more apparent.	Suspend fragments of skin scales, nails, or hair in a drop of 10% KOH. Add coverslip over the drop and let sit at room temperature for about a half hour. The mount may be gently heated in the flame of a Bunsen burner to accelerate the clearing process. Do not boil. Examine under a microscope for fungal hyphae or spores.
India Ink Preparation India Ink (Pelikan brand) or Nigrosin (granular)* Microscope slides, 3 × 1-inch Coverslips	India ink or nigrosin preparations are used for the direct microscopic examination of the capsules of many microorganisms. The fine granules of the India ink or nigrosin give a semiopaque background against which the clear capsules can easily be seen. This technique is particularly useful in visualizing the large capsules of *Cryptococcus neoformans* in cerebrospinal fluid, sputum, and other secretions.	Centrifuge the cerebrospinal fluid or other fluid specimens lightly to concentrate any microorganisms in the sediment. Emulsify a small quantity of the sediment into a drop of India ink or nigrosin on a microscope slide and overlay with a coverslip. Do not make the contrast emulsion too thick, or the transmitted light may be completely blocked. Examine the mount directly under a microscope, using the 10 × objective for screening and the 40 × objective for confirmation of suspicious encapsulated microorganisms.
Darkfield Examination Compound microscope equipped with a darkfield condenser Microscope slides, 3 × 1-inch Coverslips Physiologic saline Applicator sticks or curet Paraffin-petrolatum mixture	Darkfield examinations are used to visualize certain delicate microorganisms that are invisible by brightfield optics and stain only with great difficulty. This method is particularly useful in demonstrating spirochetes from suspicious syphilitic chancres for *Treponema pallidum*.	The secretion to be examined is obtained from the patient. In the case of a chancre, the top crust is scraped away with a scalpel blade and a small quantity of serous material is placed on a microscope slide. Ring a coverslip with paraffin–petrolatum mixture and place over the drop of material.

Table 1-7 *Continued*

METHODS AND MATERIALS	PURPOSE	TECHNIQUES
		Examine the mount directly under a microscope fitted with a darkfield condenser with a 40 × or 100 × objective. Spirochetes will appear as motile, bright "corkscrews" against a black background.
Neufeld's Quellung Reaction Homologous anticapsular serum Physiologic saline Microscope slides, 3 × 1-inch Coverslips	When species of encapsulated bacteria are brought into contact with serum containing homologous anticapsular antibody, their capsules undergo a change in refractive index to produce "swelling" that is visible by microscopic examination. This serologic procedure is useful in identifying the various types of *Streptococcus pneumoniae* and *Haemophilus influenzae* in biologic fluids or in cultures.	A loopful of material, such as emulsified sputum, body fluid, or broth culture, is spread over a 1-cm area in two places on opposite ends of a microscope slide. A loopful of specific anticapsular typing serum is spread over the area of one of the dried preparations; the opposite area is overlaid with a loopful of saline to serve as a control. Each area is overlaid with a coverslip and examined under the 100 × (oil immersion) objective of the microscope. Organisms showing a positive reaction appear surrounded with a ground-glass, refractile halo owing to capsular swelling. Compare the test preparation with the saline control where no capsular swelling occurs.

* Available from Harleco Co., Philadelphia, PA.

Often it is helpful to reduce the amount of light entering the field by closing the iris diaphragm, thereby increasing the contrast between the object being observed and the background. The common practice of lowering the condenser to achieve this effect should be discouraged.

Direct Stains. Biologic stains are generally required to visualize bacteria adequately and demonstrate the fine detail of internal structures. The introduction of stains in the mid-19th century was, in large part, responsible for the major advances that have occurred in clinical microbiology and in other fields of diagnostic microscopy during the past 100 years. Today we are so dependent on biologic stains that it is difficult to realize how the study of bacteria could have progressed before their introduction. The chemical formulas, components and purposes of the stains commonly used in the microbiology laboratory are shown in Table 1-8.

Stains consist of aqueous or organic preparations of dyes or groups of dyes that impart a variety of colors to microorganisms, plant and animal tissues, or other substances of biologic importance. Dyes may be used as direct stains of biologic materials, as indicators of pH shifts in culture media, as oxidation-reduction indicators to demonstrate the presence or lack of anaerobic conditions, or to demonstrate physiologic functions of microorganisms using so-called supravital techniques.

Almost all biologically useful dyes are derivatives of coal tar. The fundamental chemical structure of most dyes is the benzene ring. Dyes are generally composed of two or more benzene rings connected by well-defined chemical bonds (chromophores) that are associated with color production. Although the underlying mechanism of the color development is not totally understood, it is theorized that certain chemical radicals have the property of absorbing light of different wavelengths, acting as chemical prisms. Some of the more common chromophore groupings found in dyes are: C=C, C=O, C=S, C=N, N=N, N=O, and NO_2. (Note the presence of these groups in the chemical formulas of the stains shown in Table 1-8.) The depth of color of a dye is proportional to the number of chromophore radicals in the compound.

Dyes differ from one another in the number and arrangement of these rings and in the substitution of hydrogen atoms with other molecules. For example, there are three key single substitutions for one hydrogen atom of benzene that constitute the basic structure of most dyes: (1) substitution of a methyl group to form toluene (methylbenzene), (2) substitution of a hydroxyl group to form phenol (carbolic acid), and (3) the substitution of an amine group to form aniline (phenylamine). Most stains used in microbiology are derived from aniline and are called aniline dyes.

All biologic dyes have a high affinity for hydrogen. When all the molecular sites that can bind hydrogen are filled, the

Table 1-8 Common Biologic Stains Used in Bacteriology

STAIN	CHEMICAL FORMULA	INGREDIENTS		PURPOSE
Loeffler's methylene blue	Tetramethyl thionin	Methylene blue Ethyl alcohol, 95% Distilled water	0.3g 30 mL 100 mL	This is a simple direct stain used to a variety of microorganisms, specifically used to detect bacteria in cerebrospinal fluid smears in suspected cases of bacterial meningitis.

Gram's stain	Crystal Violet (Hexamethylpararosanilin)
	
	Dimethyl Phenosafranin
		Crystal violet
		  Crystal violet
		  Ethyl alcohol, 95%
		  NH₄ oxalate
		  Distilled water
		Gram's iodine
		  Potassium iodide
		  Iodine crystals
		  Distilled water
		Decolorizer
		  Acetone
		  Ethyl alcohol, 95%
		Counterstain
		  Safranin 0
		  Ethyl alcohol, 95%
		  Add 100 mL to distilled water
			
			2 g
			20 mL
			0.8 g
			100 mL
			
			2 g
			1 g
			100 mL
			
			50 mL
			50 mL
			
			2.5 g
			100 mL
			
			100 mL
				This is a different stain used to demonstrate the staining properties of bacteria of all types.
				Gram-positive bacteria retain the crystal violet dye after decolorization and appear deep blue.
				Gram-negative bacteria are not capable of retaining the crystal violet dye after decolorization and are counterstained red by the safranin dye.
				Gram-staining characteristics may be atypical in very young, old, dead, or degenerating cultures.
				Staining of cyst forms of *Pneumocystis carinii* (Gram-Weigert modification).

Ziehl-Neelsen acid-fast stain	Carbolfuchsin (Triaminotriphenylmethane)	Carbolfuchsin
		  Phenol crystals
		  Alcohol, 95%
		  Basic fuchsin
		  Distilled water
		Acid alcohol, 3%
		  HCl, concentrated
		  Alcohol, 70%
		Methylene blue
		  Methylene blue
		  Glacial acetic
		  Distilled water
			
			2.5 mL
			5 mL
			0.5 g
			100 mL
			
			3 mL
			100 mL
			
			0.5 g
			0.5 mL
			100 mL
				Acid-fast bacilli are so called because they are surrounded by a waxy envelope that is resistant to staining. Either heat or a detergent (Tergitol) is required to allow the stain penetrate the capsule. Once stained, acid-fast bacteria resist decolorization, whereas other bacteria are destined with the acid alcohol.

Fluorochrome	Auramine O
	
	Rhodamine B
	
	Acridine orange (AO)
		Auramine O
		Rhodamine B
		Glycerol
		Phenol
		Distilled water
		
		AO powder
		Sodium acetate
		  buffer (pH 3.5)
		  (Add about 90 mL
		  1 M HCl to 100 mL
		  1 M Na acetate)
			1.5 g
			0.75 g
			75 mL
			10 mL
			50 mL
			
			20 mg
			
			190 mL
				This fluorochrome dye stains mycobacteria selectively by binding to the mycolic acid in the cell wall. This stain demonstrates mycobacteria better than conventional acid-fast stains and permits screening of smears at lower magnification because organisms are more easily seen.
				
				Acridine orange is a stain particularly well adapted for the demonstration of bacteria in blood culture broth, cerebrospinal fluid, urethral smears, or other exudates where they may be present in relatively small numbers, as low as 10^4 CFU mL, or when they are obscured by a heavy background of polymorphonuclear leukocytes or other debris. At pH below 4.0, bacteria and yeast cells stain brilliant orange against a black, light green, or yellow background.

Table 1-8 *Continued*

STAIN	CHEMICAL FORMULA	INGREDIENTS		PURPOSE
Wright's–Giemsa	Polychrome methylene blue Methylene blue Methylene azure Eosin Methylene azure B	Powdered Wright's stain Powdered Giemsa stain Glycerin Absolute methyl alcohol Mix in brown bottle and let stand 1 month before using.	9 g 1 g 90 mL 2910 mL	Wright's–Giemsa is commonly used for staining the cellular elements of the peripheral blood smear. It is useful in microbiology for the demonstration of intracellular organisms such as *Histoplasma capsulatum* and *Leishmania* species (see Color Plate 1-2*G*) The stain is also useful in demonstrating intracellular inclusions in direct smears of skin or mucous membranes, such as corneal scrapings for trachoma.
Lactophenol aniline blue	Aniline blue	Phenol crystals Lactic acid Glycerol Distilled water Dissolve ingredients, then add: Aniline blue	20 g 20 g 40 mL 20 mL 0.05 g	Because of the sulfonic groups, the dye is strongly acidic and has been used as a counterstain for unfixed tissues, bacteria, and protozoa, in combination with other dyes. Currently used for the direct staining of fungal mycelium and fruiting structures which take on a delicate light blue color.

dye is in its reduced state and is generally colorless. In the colorless state, the dye is called a leuko compound. Looking at this concept from the opposite view, a dye retains its color only as long as its affinities for hydrogen are not completely satisfied. Because oxygen generally has a higher affinity for hydrogen than many dyes, color is retained in the presence of air. This allows certain dyes, such as methylene blue, to be used as an oxidation-reduction indicator in an anaerobic environment, because the indicator becomes colorless in the absence of oxygen.

In broad terms, dyes are referred to as acidic or basic, designations not necessarily indicating their pH reactions in solution, but rather, whether a significant part of the molecule is anionic or cationic. From a practical standpoint, basic dyes stain structures that are acidic, such as the nuclear chromatin in cells; acidic dyes react with basic substances, such as cytoplasmic structures. If both nuclear and cytoplasmic structures are to be stained in a given preparation, combinations of acidic and basic dyes may be used. A common example is the hematoxylin (basic) and eosin (acidic), or H & E, stain used in the examination of tissue sections.

The Use of Stains in Microbiology. Microbiologists are encouraged to perform direct microscopic examination on specimens submitted for culture. Not only may it be possible to provide the physician with a rapid presumptive diagnosis, but also the detection of specific microorganisms may serve as a guide for selecting appropriate culture media and provide a valuable quality control comparison with isolates recovered.

The positive findings for various staining procedures and diseases in selected specimens that are submitted to microbiology laboratories are listed in Table 1-9. The following is a brief description of the stains most commonly used.

Gram's Stain. Gram's stain, discovered a little over 100 years ago by Hans Christian Gram, is most commonly used for direct microscopic examination of specimens and subcultures (the formula can be found in Table 1-8). The staining procedure is explained in Box 1-6.

Crystal violet (gentian violet) serves as the primary stain, binding to the bacterial cell wall after treatment with a weak solution of iodine, which serves as the mordant to bind the dye. Some bacterial species, because of the chemical nature of their cell walls, have the ability to retain the crystal violet even after treatment with an organic decolorizer, such as a mixture of equal parts of acetone and 95% ethyl alcohol. Dye-retaining bacteria appear blue-black when observed under the microscope and are called gram-positive. Certain bacteria lose the crystal violet primary stain when treated with the decolorizer, presumably because of the high lipid content of their cell wall. These decolorized bacteria then pick up the safranin counterstain and appear red when observed under the microscope; they are called gram-negative (Color Plate 1-2A). The visualization of certain fastidious gram-negative bacilli can be improved by adding 0.05% carbolfuchsin to the safranin counterstain. These gram reactions, when observed in conjunction with the morphologic

Table 1-9 Diagnosis of Infectious Disease by Direct Examination of Culture Specimens

SPECIMEN	SUSPECTED DISEASE	LABORATORY PROCEDURE	POSITIVE FINDINGS
Throat culture	Diphtheria	Gram's stain	Delicate pleomorphic gram-positive bacilli in Chinese letter arrangement
		Methylene blue stain	Light-blue-staining bacilli; with prominent metachromatic granules
	Acute streptococcal pharyngitis	Direct fluorescent antibody technique (after 4–6 hours incubation in Todd-Hewitt broth)	Fluorescent cocci in chains; use positive and negative controls with each stain
Oropharyngeal ulcers	Vincent's disease	Gram's stain	Presence of gram-negative bacilli and thin, spiral-shaped bacilli
Sputum Transtracheal aspirates Bronchial washings	Bacterial pneumonia	Gram's stain	Variety of bacterial types; *Streptococcus pneumoniae* with capsules particularly diagnostic
	Tuberculosis Pulmonary mycosis	Acid-fast stain Gram's stain, Wright-Giemsa's stain or Calcofluor white Gram-Weigert stain	Acid-fast bacilli Budding yeasts, pseudohyphae, true hyphae, or fruiting bodies
Cutaneous wounds or purulent drainage from subcutaneous sinuses	Bacterial cellulitis	Gram's stain	Variety of bacterial types; suspect anaerobic species
	Gas gangrene (myonecrosis)	Gram's stain	Gram-positive bacilli suggesting *Clostridium perfringens;* spores usually not seen
	Actinomycotic mycetoma	Direct saline mount Gram's stain or modified acid-fast stain	"Sulfur granules" Delicate, branching gram-positive filaments; *Nocardia* species may be weakly acid-fast
	Eumycotic mycetoma	Direct saline mount Gram's stain or lactophenol cotton blue mount	White, grayish, or black grains True hyphae with focal swellings or chlamydospores
Cerebrospinal fluid	Bacterial meningitis	Gram's stain	Small gram-negative pleomorphic bacilli (*Haemophilus* species) Gram-negative diplococci *(Neisseria meningitidis)* Gram-positive diplococci *(Streptococcus pneumoniae)*
		Methylene blue stain	Bacterial forms that stain blue-black
		Acridine orange stain	Bacterial forms that glow brilliant orange under ultraviolet illumination
	Pneumococcal meningitis	Quellung reaction (type specific antisera)	Swelling and ground-glass apperance of bacterial capsules
	Cryptococcal meningitis	India ink or nigrosin mount	Encapsulated yeast cells with buds attached by thin thread
	Listeriosis	Gram's stain Hanging-drop mount	Delicate gram-positive bacilli Bacteria with tumbling motility

Table 1-9 *Continued*

SPECIMEN	SUSPECTED DISEASE	LABORATORY PROCEDURE	POSITIVE FINDINGS
Urine	Yeast infection	Gram's stain or Wright-Giemsa stain	Pseudohyphae or budding yeasts
	Bacterial infection	Gram's stain	Variety of bacterial types
	Leptospirosis	Darkfield examination	Loosely coiled motile spirochetes
Purulent urethral discharge	Gonorrhea	Gram's stain	Intracellular gram-negative diplococci
	Chlamydial infection	Direct fluorescent antibody stain of smear	Elementary bodies
Purulent vaginal discharge	Yeast infection	Direct mount or Gram's stain	Pseudohyphae or budding yeasts
	Trichomonas infection	Direct mount	Flagellates with darting motility
	Gardnerella vaginalis	Pap stain or Gram's stain Measure pH of vaginal secretions	"Clue cells" or pH of vaginal secretions > 5.5
Penile or vulvar ulcer (chancre)	Primary syphilis	Darkfield mount of chancre secretion	Tightly coiled motile spirochetes
	Chancroid	Gram's stain of ulcer secretion or aspirate of inguinal bubo	Intracellular and extracellular small gram-negative bacilli
Eye	Purulent conjunctivitis	Gram's stain	Variety of bacterial species
	Trachoma	Giemsa stain of corneal scrapings	Intracellular perinuclear inclusion clusters
Feces	Purulent enterocolitis	Gram's stain	Neutrophils and aggregates of staphylococci
	Cholera	Direct mount of alkaline peptone water enrichment	Bacilli with characteristic darting motility; no neutrophils
	Parasitic disease	Direct saline or iodine mounts Examine purged specimens	Adult parasites or parasite fragments; protozoa or ova
Skin scrapings, nail fragments, or plucked hairs	Dermatophytosis	10% KOH mount	Delicate hyphae or clusters of spores
	Tinea versicolor	10% KOH mount or lactophenol cotton blue mount	Hyphae and spores resembling spaghetti and meatballs
Blood	Relapsing fever *(Borrelia)*	Wright's or Giemsa stain Darkfield examination	Spirochetes with typical morphology
	Blood parasites: malaria, trypanosomiasis, filariasis	Wright's or Giemsa stain Direct examination of anticoagulated blood for the presence of microfilaria	Intracellular parasites (malaria, babesia) Extracellular forms: trypanosomes or microfilaria

form (cocci and bacilli) and arrangement of bacterial cells, can be used to make presumptive identifications.

Common applications of Gram's stain have been reviewed by Friedly.[34] Gram-positive cocci in clusters suggest staphylococci; in chains, they suggest streptococci. Gram-positive, lancet-shaped diplococci, when seen in smears made from sputum samples, are characteristic of *Streptococcus pneumoniae*; these characteristics cannot be used diagnostically in other specimens, because enterococci are similar in appearance. Gram-negative, kidney-shaped diplococci are characteristic of *Neisseria* species. Large, gram-positive bacilli suggest *Bacillus* or *Clostridium* species; small gram-

Box 1-6 Gram's Stain Technique

1. Make a thin smear of the material for study and allow to air dry.
2. Fix the material to the slide by passing the slide three or four times through the flame of a Bunsen burner so that the material does not wash off during the staining procedure. Some workers now recommend the use of alcohol for the fixation of material to be gram-stained (flood the smear with methanol or ethanol for a few minutes).
3. Place the smear on a staining rack and overlay the surface with crystal violet solution.
4. After 1 minute (less time may be used with some solutions) of exposure to the crystal violet stain, wash thoroughly with distilled water or buffer.
5. Overlay the smear with Gram's iodine solution for 1 minute. Wash again with water.
6. Hold the smear between the thumb and forefinger and flood the surface with a few drops of the acetone–alcohol decolorizer, until no violet color washes off. This usually takes 10 seconds or less.
7. Wash with running water and again place the smear on the staining rack. Overlay the surface with safranin counterstain for 1 minute. Wash with running water.
8. Place the smear in an upright position in a staining rack, allowing the excess water to drain off and the smear to dry.
9. Examine the stained smear under the 100× (oil) immersion objective of the microscope. Gram-positive bacteria stain dark blue; gram-negative bacteria appear pink-red.

positive bacilli suggest *Listeria* species or one of the coryneforms (diphtheroids) if "Chinese-letter" arrangements are observed. Curved, gram-negative rods in diarrheal stool specimens suggest *Vibrio* species or, if corkscrew forms are also seen, *Campylobacter* species. Gram-negative bacilli are the bacteria most commonly encountered in clinical laboratories and include the *Enterobacteriaceae*, the nonfermentative bacilli, *Haemophilus* species, and a variety of fastidious species. Selected gram-stained images are included in Color Plate 1-3, which is discussed in more detail in a later section of this chapter.

Gram's stain is a deceptively simple procedure. Staining can be performed quickly and easily. Preparation and interpretation of the smears is another matter, however. Considerable experience and careful training are essential for good performance. A casual observer of Gram's stain will not do as well as someone who views them regularly and has the opportunity to check the morphologic findings against the resulting culture. An excellent example of this fact of life is an interesting study that evaluated the performance of medical housestaff and experienced microbiologists in the diagnosis of community-acquired pneumonia.[31] The housestaff were better at obtaining purulent sputum than were nursing personnel, but their preparation and interpretation of the smears was inferior to that of the microbiologists.

There are some microbiologic and technical reasons for the importance of experience. Most of the time bacterial morphology matches the classic descriptions. Unfortunately, on occasion the bacteria haven't read the rule book. With good training, practice, and a willingness to learn from mistakes the microbiologist will learn the pitfalls. Some of the classic "traps" that Gram's stain can present are summarized in Table 1-10. A cardinal rule is that the final interpretation must be made on the basis of staining

Table 1-10 Pitfalls in the Interpretation of Gram's Stains

ORGANISM	CLASSIC PRESENTATION	VARIANT PRESENTATION	COMMENTS
Streptococcus pneumoniae	Gram-positive, lancet-shaped, diplococci	Elongated cocci, resembling short bacilli	May be misinterpreted as mixed o ganisms
Acinetobacter spp.	Gram-negative coccobacilli	Gram-negative cocci	May be mistaken for *Neisseria* spp. and reported as gram-negative cocci; search the smear to find some organisms that demonstrate elongated forms, which are not seen in *Neisseria*
		Gram-positive cocci	May be mistaken for *Streptococcus pneumoniae* and reported as gram positive cocci; in addition to a cocal form cells retain crystal violet tenaciously during decolorization
Clostridium perfringens	Boxcar shaped gram-positive bacilli	Gram-variable or gram-negative bacilli	May be mistaken for gram-negative bacilli; the boxcar shape is a clue that the organism is gram-positive; other clostridia and *Bacillus* spp. may also appear similar
Yeast, especially *Cryptococcus neoformans*	Gram-positive round or oval cells with budding	Gram-variable cells	May be mistaken for artifacts; size and shape distinguish them from bacteria

color, bacterial morphology, and known variants. To complicate matters still further a variety of artifacts can resemble infectious agents and be reported mistakenly as a microbe. Some of these potential sources of error are illustrated in Color Plate 1-4. If the possibility of an artifact is considered, a useful maneuver is to stain another smear with acridine orange (see below); with this stain it can be established whether the structure contains DNA and is, therefore, biologic. Although the staining procedure is simple, the decolorization step can cause problems if not performed properly. If acetone is used as the decolorizer, particular care must be taken because it acts very quickly. Under-decolorization can be monitored by observing the nuclei of inflammatory cells; if they are not completely gram-negative, the smear has not been adequately decolorized. The only recipe for detecting over-decolorization is cross-checking the gram reaction and the morphology of the bacteria. If the quality assurance program (see below) includes a review of smears that do not correlate with cultures, improper decolorization and nonbacterial artifacts that have been reported erroneously can be detected and the reader of the smear can learn from the mistake.

Gram's stain can also be used to identify nonbacterial forms such as trichomonads, strongyloides larvae, *Pneumocystis jiroveci* (*carinii*) cysts, and *Toxoplasma gondii* trophozoites, although it is not as sensitive as other special stains used for visualizing these organisms. These various applications demonstrate the versatility of Gram's stain.

Acid-Fast Stains. Mycobacteria are coated with a thick, waxy material that resists staining; once stained, however, the bacterial cells resist decolorization by strong organic solvents such as acid-alcohol. Consequently, these bacteria are known as acid-fast, a phenomenon first discovered in 1881 by Ziehl and Neelsen.

Special treatment is required for the primary stain, carbolfuchsin, to penetrate the waxy material of the acid-fast bacilli. Heat is used in the conventional Ziehl-Neelsen technique. After the carbolfuchsin is overlaid on the surface of the smear to be stained, the flame of a Bunsen burner is passed back and forth beneath the slide. The smear is heated to steaming, stopping short of boiling. The Kinyoun modification of the acid-fast stain is called the "cold method" because a surface-active detergent, such as Tergitol, is used rather than heat treatment.

With either of these stains, the acid-fast bacilli appear red against either a green or blue background depending on the counter-stain used (Color Plate 1-2B). Although this method is satisfactory for most mycobacteria, certain weakly acid-fast strains of rapidly growing species (*Mycobacterium fortuitum/chelonae* complex) may stain better with the Ziehl-Neelsen method (further discussion can be found in Chapter 19). In addition, certain bacteria, such as *Nocardia* spp., characteristically exhibit partial or weak acid-fastness.

Fluorescent Stains. Fluorescein isothiocyanate (FITC) and tetramethylrhodamine isethionate (TMRI) are two commonly used fluorochromes that, on excitation with ultraviolet or short-wavelength visible light, emit light waves in the visible range, with absorption maxima of 490 nm and 555 nm, respectively. These fluorochromes bind chemically with a variety of proteins, including antigens and antibodies, providing a label or tag by which immunologic reactions can be visualized in direct smears of biological fluids or secretions and in tissue sections. Fluorochrome/protein ratios vary with different reagents for optimal staining of the desired objects with a minimum of nonspecific background distraction. The current development of monoclonal antibodies, which are monospecific for their respective antigens, has led to the preparation of fluorescent reagents for direct and indirect detection of several pathogens: *Chlamydia trachomatis*, *Legionella* species, *Treponema pallidum*, *Toxoplasma gondii*, and several viruses, including varicella-zoster, herpes simplex, influenza, cytomegalovirus, and respiratory syncytial viruses, among others.

Fluorescence microscopy is an exacting technique that requires a microscope of high quality, the proper combination of microscope objectives, bright and darkfield condensers, a mercury arc or halogen ultraviolet light source, and appropriate combinations of exciter and barrier or suppression filters.[21] Achromatic objectives are satisfactory for most applications, except in research applications where expensive apochromatic lenses may be needed to achieve maximum illumination and resolution. The selection of microscope slides and coverslips of proper thickness and the use of low-fluorescing immersion oils and mounting fluids are critical for optimal performance.

The choice of filters in fluorescence microscopy is also critical to successful work. Four filters are required in sequence: (1) one to absorb heat (to prevent damage to the exciter filter), (2) an exciter filter with a wave bandwidth appropriate for the wavelength of light produced by the excited fluorochrome, (3) a red-absorbing filter to block any red light emitted by the blue excitation filters, and (4) a barrier filter to absorb any of the residual short-wavelength incident excitation light (which would damage the eyes of the microscopist), allowing only the longer-wavelength visible light to pass. Suboptimal performance of a fluorescence microscope system is often due to poor selection of filter combinations. Manufacturers of fluorescence equipment provide information and consultation so that users can achieve optimal performance. Fluorescence systems that employ (1) epi-illumination, (2) blue light halogen lamps that do not require expensive transformers, and (3) interference filters with maximum absorption peaks at the longer visible wavelengths are now available within a price range acceptable to most clinical laboratory directors.

Fluorochrome Stains for Mycobacteria. The fluorochrome dyes auramine and rhodamine can be used to demonstrate acid-fast bacilli. Viewed by fluorescence microscopy, the bacterial cells appear yellow, red, or orange (depending on the filter combination and dyes used); the background is dark when potassium permanganate is the counterstain (Color Plate 1-2C). Use of the fluorescence procedure facilitates the screening of smears, particularly when a $25 \times$ objective is utilized. This objective provides magnification low enough to scan wide microscopic fields, yet sufficiently high to see the yellow light points emanating from the fluorescing bacterial cells (Color Plate 1-2C). Higher magnification can be used to confirm suspicious objects observed with the $25 \times$ lens.

The acid-fast stains can also be used to identify nonbacterial microorganisms. The oocysts of *Cryptosporidium* species and *Isospora belli*, two coccidian organisms that have been incriminated as important etiologic agents of gastroenteritis, are acid-fast and can be readily detected in appropriately stained preparations of stool (Color Plate 1-2J).

Acridine Orange. The acridine orange (AO) stain is used with increasing frequency in microbiology laboratories to detect bacteria in smears prepared from fluids and exudates in which bacteria are expected to be in low concentration (10^3 to 10^4 colony-forming units [CFU]/mL) or are trapped within a heavy aggregate of background debris, making them difficult to visualize by conventional staining procedures. The AO stain was originally used by microbiologists to demonstrate bacteria in soil samples. As in the application of fluorochrome dyes for studying acid-fast bacilli, smears stained with AO and examined under ultraviolet light can be more rapidly and efficiently screened at low-power magnifications ($100\times$), utilizing study at magnifications of $450\times$ or higher when suspicious forms are visualized. The stain detects both living and dead bacteria, but does not indicate whether they are gram-negative or gram-positive. Once bacteria have been detected using the AO stain, a Gram's stain must be used to determine their differential-staining characteristics (Color Plate 1-2D).

Lauer and associates have found the AO stain to be more sensitive than Gram's stain in detecting bacteria in CSF sediments, particularly when gram-negative bacteria are present.[56] The AO stain has also been useful to screen urine specimens for significant bacteriuria.[45] In Box 1-7 preparation of an AO stain is outlined.

Toluidine Blue and Methylene Blue. Toluidine blue, a dye closely related to azure A and methylene blue, is used for staining lung biopsy imprints and respiratory secretions to detect *Pneumocystis jiroveci* (*carinii*) rapidly. Methylene blue stains may be performed on spinal fluid sediments along with Gram's stains. The gram-negative bacterial cells of *H. influenzae* and *N. meningitidis* often do not stand out against the red-staining background in Gram's stains. With methylene blue, polymorphonuclear leukocytes stain blue; the bacterial cells are also deep blue and easier to detect against the light gray-staining background (Color Plate 1-2E). Methylene blue stains should be considered as an adjunct to Gram's stains in laboratories where the inaccessibility to a

fluorescence microscope precludes the use of the AO procedure.

Calcofluor White. Calcofluor white, a colorless dye used in industry to whiten textiles and paper, has two properties that make it useful in microbiology: (1) binding to β1-3, β1-4-polysaccharides (specifically cellulose and chitin); and (2) fluorescence when exposed to long-wavelength ultraviolet and short-wavelength visible light. Calcofluor white is a valuable fluorochrome stain for the rapid detection of fungi in wet mounts, smears, and tissue sections, because the cell walls of fungi and plants are rich in chitin. The stain has been most useful in detecting yeast cells, hyphae, and pseudohyphae in skin and mucous membrane scrapings. When mixed with 10% potassium hydroxide, mounts of skin scrapings can be screened for dermatophytes rapidly. Viewed microscopically under ultraviolet light, fungal structures display a brilliant apple-green or a ghostly blue-white (Color Plate 1-2F), depending on the wavelength of the exciter light and the filter combinations used. The fungi are readily differentiated from background debris, cells, and tissue fragments. Calcofluor white has the added advantage that tissue sections can be stained subsequently with periodic acid-Schiff stain (PAS), Gomori methenamine silver (GMS), or other special stains without interference, should confirmation of findings or the availability of permanent slides be desired. The calcofluor white-staining technique is rapid and provides good definition of fungal fine structures and better contrast from the background than the widely used lactophenol aniline blue stain.[42]

Silver Impregnation Stains. Certain bacteria, e.g., spirochetes (including the etiologic agent of Lyme disease, *Borrelia burgdorferi*) and the small bacillary organisms associated with cat scratch disease (*Bartonella henselae* and *Bartonella quintana*), are not readily stained by conventional methods. These organisms are either too slender to be visualized by brightfield microscopy, they are not present in sufficient concentrations to be detected, or their chemical composition does not interact with the stains. Darkfield microscopy has been used to identify *Treponema pallidum*, the etiologic agent of syphilis, and other nontreponemal spirochetes, such as *Leptospira interrogans*, the cause of leptospirosis. One limitation of the darkfield procedure is the necessity to examine wet, moist specimens containing living organisms very quickly, because visualization of the moving bacteria is essential to detection. The silver stain has been used to observe these organisms in tissue sections and immunofluorescent reagents are available for some pathogens, such as *T. pallidum*.

The Warthin-Starry, Dieterle, and Steiner silver impregnation stains have been used for years to demonstrate spirochetes in formalin-fixed tissue sections. They perform equivalently.

Wright's-Giemsa's Stain. The Wright's-Giemsa's stain is commonly used for staining the cellular elements of the peripheral blood smear. This stain has little use for staining bacteria, but is used primarily to detect the intracellular yeast forms of *Histoplasma capsulatum* or the intracellular amastigotes of *Leishmania* species or *Trypanosoma cruzi* (Color Plate 1-2G). The stain is also helpful for demonstrating certain intracellular viral inclusions (see Table 1-8).

Periodic Acid-Schiff. The periodic acid-Schiff stain is based on the oxidation of hexoses and hexosamines by periodic acid, which breaks their pyranose rings, producing dialde-

---

Box 1-7 Preparation of an AO Stain

Ingredients: AO powder 20 mg, sodium acetate buffer 290 mL, HCl 1M

Reagent preparation: Add 20 mg AO powder (JT Baker Chemical Co., Phillipsburg NJ) to 290 mL of sodium acetate buffer (stock solution of 100 mL of 2 molar [M]CH$_2$COONa.3H$_2$O and 90 mL of 1 M HCl); 1 M HCl should be added as necessary to maintain the differential staining of the bacteria against the background debris.[56] The staining solution should be stored in a brown bottle at room temperature.

Procedure: The stain is performed by flooding air-dried and methanol-fixed smears of the material to be examined with the AO stain for 2 minutes, followed by a washing with tap water. The stained slides are dried and examined with a microscope equipped with an ultraviolet light source.

hydes that react with Schiff reagent. Schiff reagent is a triphenylmethane dye prepared from basic fuchsin or p-rosaniline by reduction with sulfuric acid. Most substances that contain hexoses or hexosamines are PAS-positive, staining red against a green or blue background, depending on the counterstain used. The stain is most frequently used for staining tissue sections to demonstrate fungi (Color Plate 1-2H).

PROCESSING SPECIMENS

After a specimen for culture has been received in the microbiology laboratory, the following decisions must be made:

1. Select primary culture media appropriate for the particular specimen.
2. Determine the temperature and atmosphere of incubation to recover all organisms of potential significance.
3. Determine which of the isolates recovered on primary media require further characterization.
4. Determine whether antimicrobial susceptibility tests are required.

No single approach can be expected to serve the needs of all laboratories and clinical settings. The protocol in a 50-bed rural community hospital will differ from that used in a large, multidepartment medical center. Everyone recognizes, however, the difficulties in maintaining quality services in the face of more and more stringent demands for containment of costs. Laboratory directors and supervisors must weed out much of the clinically irrelevant work that was performed in the past. One hopes that the day of the ''panculture'' (the indiscriminate ordering of cultures from all accessible body sites in the hope of recovering a pathogen) is over. For the past several decades many microbiologists have been attempting to practice what Bartlett calls ''processing control'':[5] ''restricting the processing and reporting of culture specimens to the production of predictably useful information.''

Selection of Primary Culture Media. Only a few media are required for daily use in the diagnostic laboratory. Agar plates are commonly used. Inoculation of broth media for primary recovery of organisms should be limited to those few specimens for which supplemental broth media have proven useful (see Table 1-6). The past practice of inoculating thioglycolate broth routinely to recover anaerobes or as an enrichment procedure to recover fecal pathogens has been abandoned in most laboratories. In almost all instances recovery of an organism in broth culture after 4 or 5 days of incubation will have little clinical relevance. Incubation of broths for prolonged periods also leads to the frequent recovery of contaminants.[71] Bacterial isolates in very low concentrations are rarely significant, and the prolonged time for recovery will usually render the information irrelevant for effective management. In some laboratories broth media are inoculated for certain types of specimens, but they are examined only if growth is not detected on agar plates or if bacterial morphotypes observed in a direct smear of patient material are not recovered on agar.

There are situations in which broth cultures are useful or even essential. The most obvious one is in the culture of blood, where a single pathogen is expected in most situations and commensal flora are not expected. A few other clinical situations meet these guidelines and broth cultures may be useful: spontaneous bacterial (primary) peritonitis (as opposed to peritonitis after disruption of an abdominal viscus),[9] peritoneal infections in patients who are receiving peritoneal dialysis,[2] and septic arthritis.[46]

Media may be selective or nonselective. Nonselective media are free of inhibitors and support the growth of most microorganisms encountered in clinical laboratories. Five percent sheep blood agar is the most commonly used nonselective medium and is included in the battery of primary isolation media for virtually every clinical specimen. Horse blood agar, sheep blood agar supplemented with additives such as IsoVitaleX (or a similar supplement that includes nicotinamide adenine dinucleotide [NAD] and a heme product), or chocolate agar (agar to which partially hemolyzed blood or hemoglobin powder has been added) is necessary for the recovery of *Haemophilus influenzae* because it has no inhibitory effects on bacterial growth and is a rich source of factor X. Chocolate agar is also important for recovery of *Neisseria gonorrhoeae*.

Blood agar can be made selective by adding antibiotics or inhibitory chemicals. It is a general rule that inhibitory agars should not be used alone, because they usually inhibit the organisms of interest—just less so than other flora. Often the inhibition is only partial, so growth on a selective agar should not be taken as proof that the targeted organism has been isolated. For instance, enterococci and yeast often break through and produce small colonies on MacConkey agar, especially if the formulation does not include crystal violet.

Media can also be made differential by addition of certain dyes or other chemicals, thus providing some clues to the identity of the isolated microbes. Some of the commonly used inhibitory and differential agars are summarized in Table 1-11.

Techniques for Transfer and Culturing of Clinical Specimens. Once a specimen has ''passed'' the various criteria for rejection and has been accepted for culture, appropriate portions must be transferred to the culture media described previously. This activity is usually carried out in a designated part of the laboratory. The transfer of all specimens to culture media should be carried out in a biologic safety cabinet (see below). The best policy is to handle all specimens as if they were highly infectious. Personnel should be required to wear rubber gloves when handling most specimens; the wearing of a surgical mask is optional, but is unnecessary for most operations in the diagnostic microbiology laboratory (except for mycobacteriology).

The inoculation area should be equipped with all of the necessary implements and stocked with appropriate culture media. Most media must be refrigerated for prolonged storage, but must be allowed to warm to room temperature before inoculation.

Although full-time personnel working in the setup area may have memorized the culture media required for each specimen type, it is essential to have appropriate charts and instructions posted on a bulletin board or included in a bench manual for use by those who perform the tasks infrequently. Every attempt should be made to use well-trained personnel, under close supervision, for the processing of specimens.

Table 1-11 Commonly Used Differential and Inhibitory Agars

INHIBITORY (I) OR DIFFERENTIAL (D) AGAR	ADDED COMPOUNDS (I OR D)	ORGANISMS INHIBITED	ORGANISMS ENRICHED	COMMENTS/CHAPTER REFERENCE
Bacteroides bile esculin (BBE) (I, D)	Bile salts (I); esculin (D)	Most bacteria	*Bacteroides fragilis* group	Bile stimulatory for *B. fragilis*
Campy-BAP (I)	Bacitracin, novobiocin, colistin, cephalothin, polymyxin B (I)	Most bacteria	*Campylobacter jejuni*	Incubation at 42°C also selects for *C. jejuni*
CCFA (I, D)	Cycloserine, Cefoxitin (I); Fructose (D)	Most bacteria	*Clostridium difficile*	Yellow colonies; very inhibitory
CHROMagar (D)	Various (D)	NA	Various	Identification of colonies suggested by color
CIN (I)	Cefsulodin, Irgasan, novobiocin (I)	Most bacteria	*Yersinia* spp., *Aeromonas* spp.	Several formulations available
CNA (I)	Colistin, nalidixic acid (I)	Gram-negative bacteria	Gram-positive bacteria	Most strains of *Staphylococcus saprophyticus*[34] and some strains of *S. aureus* are inhibited
EMB (I, D)	Eosin (I); eosin, methylene blue, lactose, sucrose (D)	Gram-positive bacteria	Gram-negative bacteria	Slightly selective (inhibitory); lactose or sucrose fermenting organisms produce blue-black colonies (sucrose fermenters, such as *Yersinia enterocolitica*, appear identical to lactose fermenters); strong lactose fermenters (such as *Escherichia coli* or *Candida kefyr*) produce a characteristic green sheen
Hektoen enteric (HE) (I, D)	Bile salts (I); lactose, sucrose, salicin, bromthymol blue, acid fuchsin (D); sodium thiosulfate, ferric ammonium citrate for hydrogen sulfide production (D)	Gram-positive bacteria	Enteric pathogens*	Moderately inhibitory; lactose (sucrose, salicin) fermenters produce green colonies; hydrogen sulfide producers form black colonies
LKV (I)	Kanamycin, vancomycin (I)	Aerobic bacteria; anaerobic gram-positive bacteria	Anaerobic gram-negative bacilli, particularly *Bacteroides*	Laked blood added as a source of nutrients; vancomycin-resistant enterococci may be selected on this medium
MacConkey (I, D)	Bile salts, crystal violet (I); lactose, neutral red (D)	Gram-positive bacteria	Enteric pathogens*	Moderately inhibitory (selective); lactose fermenters produce red colonies; formulations without crystal violet available
Mannitol-salt (I, D)	NaCl (I); Mannitol, phenol red (D)	Gram-negative bacteria; gram-positive bacteria other than *Staphylococcus*	*Staphylococcus aureus*	Coagulase negative staphylococci grow on salt agar, but do not ferment mannitol
Mycobiotic/Mycosel (I)	Chloramphenicol, cycloheximide (I)	Bacteria; saprophytic fungi (and a few fungal pathogens)	Dermatophytes, dimorphic fungi	

Table 1-11 *Continued*

INHIBITORY (I) OR DIFFERENTIAL (D) AGAR	ADDED COMPOUNDS (I OR D)	ORGANISMS INHIBITED	ORGANISMS ENRICHED	COMMENTS/CHAPTER REFERENCE
PC (*Pseudomonas [Burkholderia] cepacia*) (I, D)	Crystal violet, bile salts for gram-positive bacteria (I); polymyxin B, ticarcillin for gram-negative bacteria (I); pyruvate (D)	Gram-positive bacteria; most gram-negative bacteria	*Burkholderia cepacia*	Highly selective; pink colonies not completely specific for *B. cepacia*
PEA (I)	Phenylethyl alcohol (I)	Gram-negative bacteria	Gram-positive bacteria	
Salmonella-Shigella (SS) (I, D)	Bile salts, brilliant green (I); lactose, neutral red (D); sodium thiosulfate, ferric ammonium citrate for hydrogen sulfide (D)	Gram-positive bacteria	Enteric pathogens*	More inhibitory (selective) than MacConkey and EMB agars; *Shigella* spp. may be inhibited
Sorbitol-MacConkey (I, D)	Bile salts, crystal violet (I); sorbitol, neutral red (D)	Gram-positive bacteria	*Escherichia coli* O157 (sorbitol negative)	Screening agar for verotoxin-producing *E. coli*
TCBS (I, D)	Sodium thiosulfate, sodium citrate, NaCl for gram-negative bacteria (I); bile salts, NaCl for gram-positive bacteria (I); sucrose, thymol-blue-bromthymol blue (D)	Gram-positive bacteria; most gram-negative bacteria	*Vibrio spp.*	Sucrose fermenting species appear yellow; species that utilize citrate appear blue
GC selective media (Modified Thayer-Martin, Martin-Lewis, etc.) (I)	Vancomycin for gram-positive bacteria (I); colistin for gram-negative bacteria (I); trimethoprim for swarming *Proteus* (I); nystatin, amphotericin B, or anisomycin for yeast (I); supplements for growth	Gram-positive bacteria; gram-negative bacilli	*Neisseria gonorrhoeae, N. meningitidis*	Multiple formulations available. Some strains of *N. gonorrhoeae* are inhibited by vancomycin. Optimally, chocolate agar should also be inoculated
XLD (I, D)	Bile salts, NaCl (I); lactose, sucrose, xylose, phenol red (D); sodium thiosulfate, ferric ammonium citrate for hydrogen sulfide production (D)	Gram-positive bacteria	Enteric pathogens*	Performs similarly to Hektoen enteric agar

* Enteric pathogens = Salmonella, spp., Shigella spp., and Yersinia spp.

Errors or misjudgments made during this phase of the diagnostic cycle can negate all the expertise one may apply in the reading and interpretation of cultures. Expert microbiologists and technologists are often caught short in making a definitive diagnosis because inadequate or incorrect media were selected for a specimen.

Techniques for Culturing Specimens. The equipment required for the primary inoculation of specimens is relatively simple. A Nichrome or platinum inoculating wire or loop is recommended (Figure 1-6), with one end inserted into a cylindrical handle for easy use. The surface of agar media in Petri plates may be inoculated with the specimen by several methods, one of which is shown in Figure 1-7. The primary inoculation can be made with a loop, swab, or other suitable device. Once the primary inoculum is made, a loop or straight wire can be used to spread the material into the four quadrants of the plate, as illustrated in Figure 1-8. The inoculum is successively streaked with a back-and-forth motion into each quadrant by turning the plate at 90-degree angles. The loop or wire should be sterilized between each successive quadrant streak. The purpose of this process is to dilute the inoculum sufficiently on the surface of the agar medium so that well-isolated colonies of bacteria, known as colony-forming units (CFU) can be obtained. The isolated

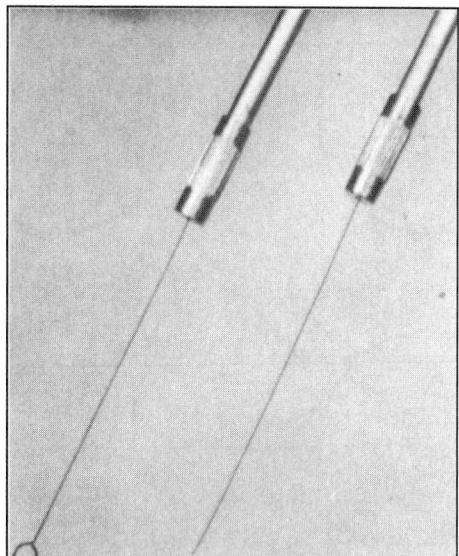

Figure 1-6 Loop and straight wires commonly used for the transfer and inoculation of specimens and cultures.

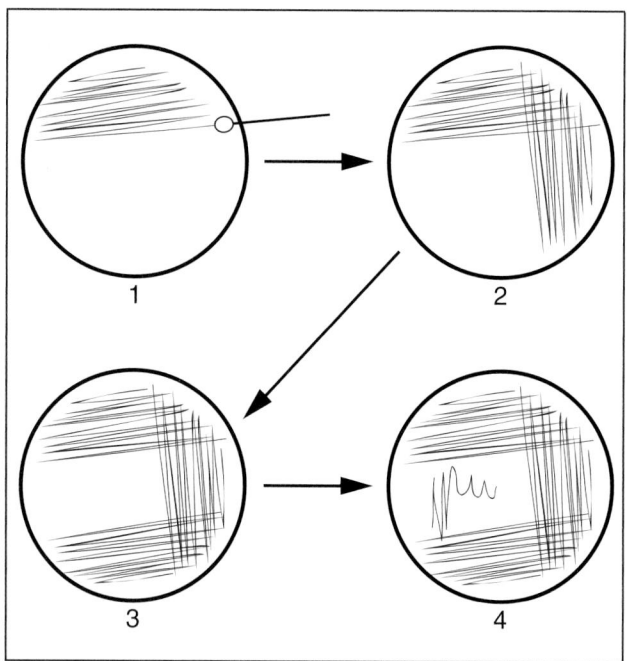

Figure 1-8 Streaking pattern for the inoculation of specimens onto culture plates to obtain isolated bacterial colonies.

colonies can then be subcultured individually to other media to obtain pure populations for further study. When streaking blood agar plates with throat swabs submitted for streptococcal screens, multiple stabs should be made in the areas of inoculation to unmask the oxygen-labile hemolysins, enhancing the detection of β-hemolytic streptococci. Also, bits of tissue that have been submitted for the recovery of fungi should be submerged beneath the surface of the agar. The initial growth of many species of fungi is enhanced in the microaerophilic atmosphere just beneath the agar surface.

The streaking technique used to inoculate agar media for semiquantitative colony counts is illustrated in Figure 1-9. Nonferrous (Nichrome or platinum) or disposable plastic inoculating loops, calibrated to contain either 0.01 or 0.001

mL of fluid, are immersed into an uncentrifuged urine sample. The loop is then carefully removed and the entire volume delivered to the surface of an agar plate by making a single streak across the center. The inoculum is spread evenly at right angles to the primary streak; then the plate is turned 90 degrees and the inoculum is spread to cover the entire surface. In some laboratories, two plates are inoculated, one with the 0.01- and the other with the 0.001-mL loop, serving as a quality control check. Although the inoculating loops are calibrated to deliver the volume of urine prescribed, accuracy has an error rate of as much as ±50%, particularly when using the 0.001-mL loop.[1] Vertical sampling from a small container may deliver only 50% of the prescribed volume; horizontal sampling at a 45-degree angle from a large

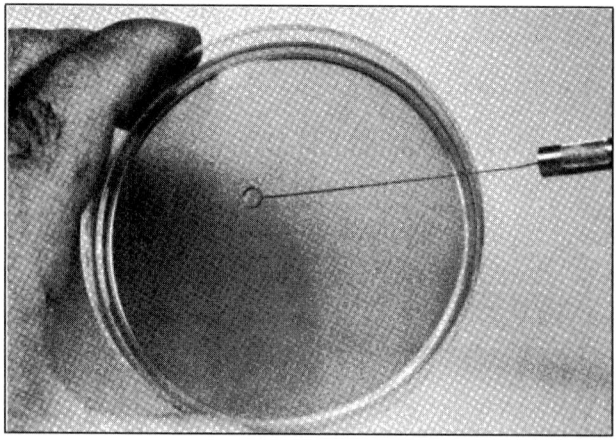

Figure 1-7 The surface of an agar plate being inoculated with a specimen contained within an inoculating loop. Inoculation is accomplished by first touching the surface of the agar in one small area, then streaking the surface with a back and forth motion in a pattern shown in Figure 1-8.

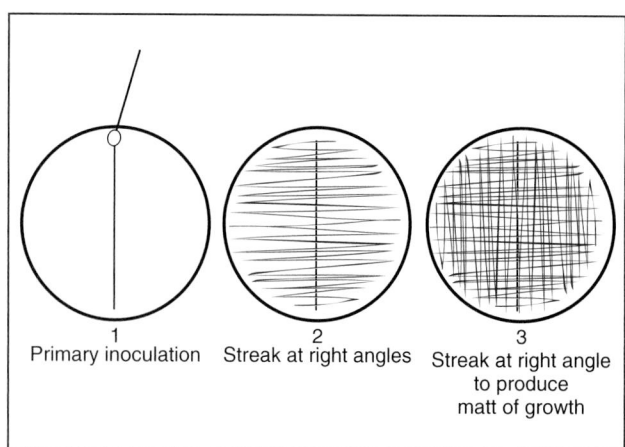

| 1 | 2 | 3 |
| Primary inoculation | Streak at right angles | Streak at right angle to produce matt of growth |

Figure 1-9 Culture plates demonstrating streaking patterns of specimens for which a semiquantitative bacterial count is to be performed.

container may deliver 150% of volume. Microbiologists should be aware of these potential errors and derive a standard angle for sampling in their laboratory, based on the volume of containers being used.

Accuracy and precision studies on the volume of inoculum can be done (1) photometrically, by adding a loop of gentian violet sampled from a 60-mL reservoir of dye to 2 mL of water in a cuvette and reading it in a spectrophotometer set at 590 nm, or (2) manometrically, by noting the change in weight when a loop of water is delivered to a filter paper disk placed in the pan of a highly sensitive analytical balance. Devices are available to deliver a standard inoculum from fluid samples.[59]

After 18 to 24 hours of incubation, the number of bacteria in urine samples is estimated by counting the number of colonies on the surface of the agar. As illustrated in Figure 1-10, approximately 50 colonies are present. If a 0.001-mL loop had been used to inoculate the medium, the number of colonies would be multiplied by 1,000. Therefore, the count in this illustration is 50,000 CFU/mL.

Semiquantitative techniques are used most commonly with urine, but have been employed in other situations also. Quantitating the bacteria recovered from the lower respiratory tract by bronchoscopic techniques may help in interpretation of these cultures.[20] When bacteria were present at a concentration greater than 10^3-10^4 CFU, the probability that they were causing pneumonia was greater than when lesser quantities were present. Considerable work can be avoided by not evaluating small quantities of contaminating throat flora.

Semiquantitative cultures are commonly employed to evaluate the likelihood that intravascular catheters are the

source of a bacteremia. Although a variety of techniques has been employed, the most prevalent approach is to roll the resected segment of catheter on the surface of agar.[60] There is a statistical association of isolated bacteria with catheter-related bacteremia if more than 15 colonies of the bacterium are present. In this approach the catheter is removed in order to perform the test. Quantitation of bacteria in blood drawn through an intravascular catheter, which is left in place, has also been used to assess the role of the catheter in an infectious process.[32]

Quantitation may also be useful in virology for determining the significance of a virus, such as cytomegalovirus, that can produce persistent infection.[10] In addition, the effectiveness of antiviral chemotherapy can be monitored by following the quantity of virus present.[47] Many of the quantitative tests for viral disease (viral loads) employ molecular detection of nucleic acid rather than culture.

Media in tubes may be liquid, semisolid (0.3% to 0.5% agar) or solid (1% to 2% agar). Semisolid agar is suitable for motility testing. Broth medium in a tube can be inoculated by the method shown in Figure 1-11. The tube should be tipped at an angle of approximately 30 degrees and an inoculating loop touched to the inner surface of the glass, just above the point where the surface of the broth makes an acute angle. When the culture tube is returned to its upright position, the area of inoculation is submerged beneath the surface. Laboratory directors and microbiology supervisors must determine which specimens should be transferred to broth cultures routinely (see Table 1-6).

Slants of agar medium are inoculated by first stabbing the depth of the agar, followed by streaking the slant from bottom to top with an S-motion as the inoculating wire is removed (Figures 1-12 and 1-13). When inoculating semisolid tubed agar for motility testing, it is important that the inoculating wire be removed along the exact track used to stab the medium. A fanning motion can result in a growth

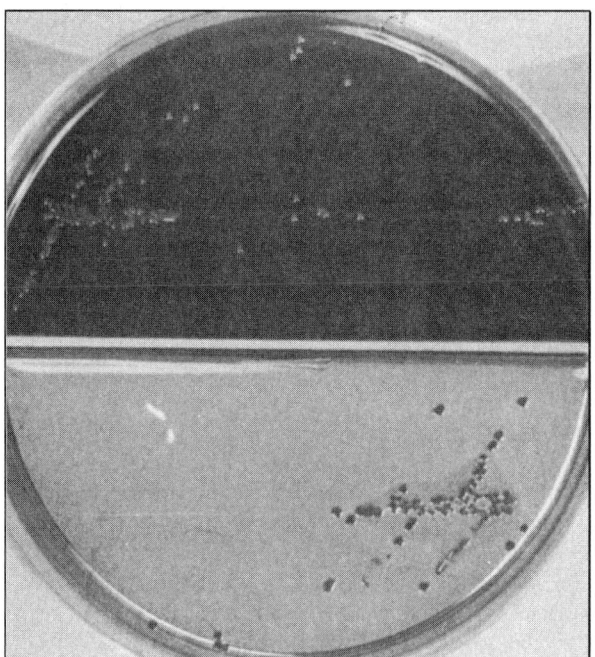

Figure 1-10 Blood agar-MacConkey agar biplate previously streaked for a semiquantitative colony count as illustrated in Figure 1-9. Approximately 50 colonies appear on each side of the plate. If a 0.001 mL calibrated semiquantitative urine inoculating loop had been used for streaking each medium, the colony count would be 50,000 colony forming units (CFU) per mL.

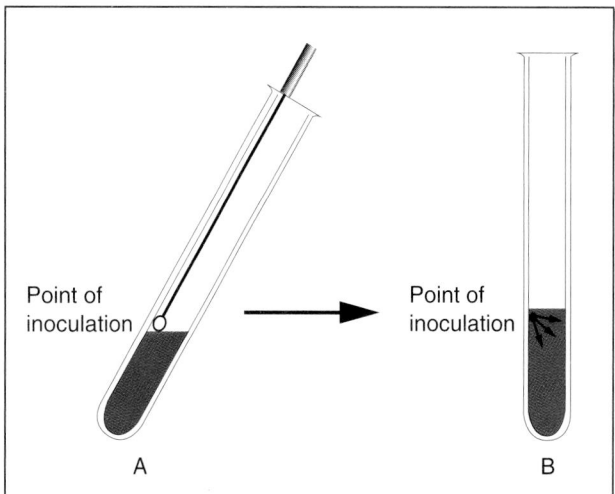

Figure 1-11 Technique for inoculating a tube of broth medium. (**A**) Slant the tube and inoculate the tube by touching the moist inner surface of the glass tube at the acute angle of the meniscus. (**B**) Return the tube to an upright position, which has the effect of submerging the point of inoculation under the surface.

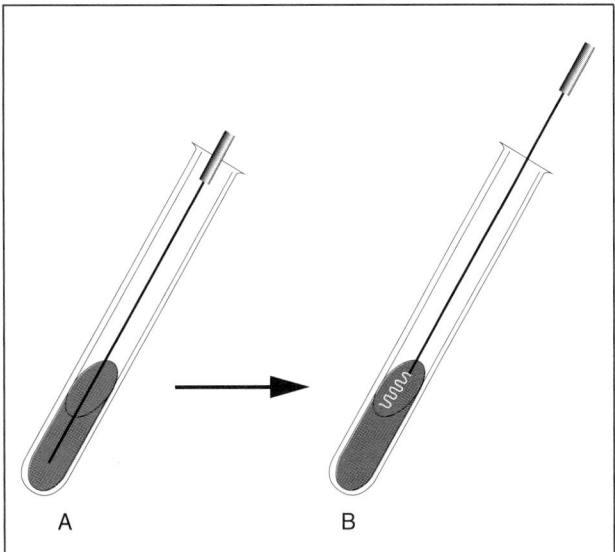

Figure 1-12 The technique for inoculating an agar slant with a straight inoculating wire: (**A**) Stab the deep of the agar slant to within 2–3 mm of the bottom of the glass. If the bottom of the glass is touched, atmospheric air may enter, negating the anaerobic conditions. (**B**) Slowly remove the wire and streak the agar surface with a back and forth "S" motion.

pattern along the stab line that may be falsely interpreted as bacterial motility.

Certain specimens may require centrifugation or filtering to concentrate any microbes present. Tenacious, mucoid sputum samples can be liquefied with N-acetylcysteine (Mucomyst, WellSpring Pharmaceutical Corp., Neptune, NJ) to facilitate even streaking of the agar surface. Sputum samples to be processed for the recovery of *Mycobacterium* spp. must also be treated with sodium hydroxide to minimize the overgrowth of bacterial contaminants. Other specimens, such as

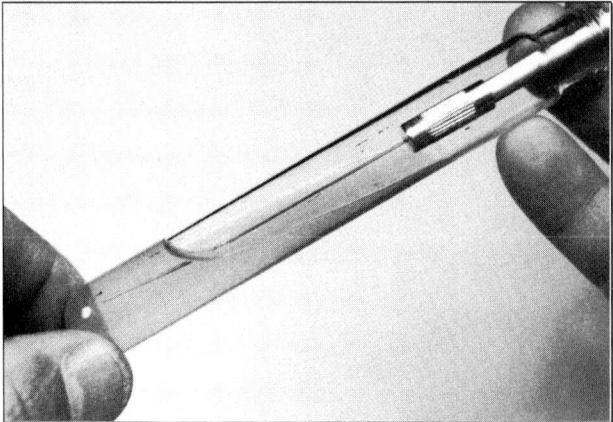

Figure 1-13 The technique for inoculating an agar deep with a straight wire, as illustrated in Figure 1-12A. The deep of the medium is stabbed with the wire to within 2–3 mm of the bottom of the tube; then, after slowly removing the needle, the agar surface is streaked with a back and forth "S" motion, as illustrated in Figure 1-12B.

urine and stool suspensions submitted for the recovery of mycobacteria, can also be briefly treated with NaOH to eliminate colonizing bacteria. Similarly, antibiotics can be added to control bacterial overgrowth in culture media and cell monolayers used for the recovery of viruses.

Body fluids, such as those obtained by thoracentesis and paracentesis, should first be allowed to settle, after which aliquots of the sediment are centrifuged to concentrate further any bacteria that are present. Requests may be made to provide blood culture bottles for the direct inoculation of certain specimens, as previously discussed. This practice is appropriate in those few situations where small numbers of a single pathogen are expected. It should be discouraged in other situations for several reasons:

1. If mixed bacterial species are present, bacteria that grow more rapidly will overgrow their slower cousins in the broth.
2. The semiquantitative relationships of isolated bacterial types that may be seen on agar plates are lost in a broth culture.
3. The direct smear that is so important to assessment of the inflammatory nature of the specimen and the types of bacteria present are lost if the entire specimen is inoculated into a broth.

Cerebrospinal fluid specimens, particularly for the recovery of *Cryptococcus neoformans*, should be centrifuged and portions of the sediment transferred to appropriate culture media; or preferably, the fluid should be passed through a 0.45-μm microbiological filter to trap any of the larger yeast cells that may be present.

Microorganisms differ in their optimal temperatures of incubation. In small laboratories, where resources may be limited, it may not be possible to provide all of the incubation temperatures optimal for growth of all clinical isolates. Most microorganisms grow at 35°C; thus, if only one incubator is provided, it should be set at 35°C. Even organisms such as *Campylobacter jejuni*, which grows optimally at 42°C, will grow at 35°C if an additional 24 or 48 hours of incubation are allowed. In this case, however, the differential effect of incubation at higher temperatures where other bacteria do not grow is lost. The growth of most organisms is enhanced by an atmosphere of 5% to 10% CO_2. If only an ambient air, non-CO_2 incubator is available, the culture tubes and plates can be placed in a candle extinction jar and the entire assembly placed in the incubator. Conversely, an ambient air environment can be maintained in a CO_2 incubator by placing the cultures into a holding jar with a tightly fitted lid (an anaerobic jar or chamber is suitable). It should be realized, however, that organisms such as *C. jejuni*, which requires a reduced oxygen tension of 5% or below, will have difficulty growing in a candle jar, in which the oxygen concentration is in the range of 10%.

Many microorganisms grow optimally within a narrow temperature range; others have a relatively wide spectrum within which they can be recovered. The optimum temperature for growth of *C. jejuni* at 42°C was just mentioned. Most fungi grow best at 30°C; however, most can be recovered at room temperature or 35°C on appropriate media. *Yersinia enterocolitica* grows optimally at slightly above room temperature. Most strains will also grow, however, at 35°C, even though colonies may appear small or require an additional

24-hour incubation period. Thus, only infrequently will access to a single incubator compromise the ability of a microbiologist to recover most clinically important bacteria. In large laboratories where several incubation temperatures can be provided, recovery of organisms will often be more rapid, and the appearance of colonies more true to form. Occasionally, incubation at room temperature for an extended time may be necessary to demonstrate certain biochemical or physical characteristics, such as pigment production and motility. These various adjustments will be learned through experience and by trial and error.

Probably more important than the specific temperature of incubation is prevention of wide fluctuations in temperature. Incubators should be carefully controlled for temperature, with no more than ± 1–2° fluctuations from day to day. Incubators should be located or protected so that control dials cannot be easily disturbed by cleaning personnel during off hours.

Humidity control within the incubator is also important. Most organisms grow maximally when the humidity is 70% or higher, and culture media tend to deteriorate more rapidly when undue drying occurs. The recovery of *H. pylori*, in particular, and to a lesser extent, *N. gonorrhoeae* requires an atmosphere with high humidity. Most incubators purchased during recent years have built-in water reservoirs by which humidity in the chamber can be regulated. If not, open pans of water can be placed on shelves to provide moisture through evaporation. Incubators must also be checked periodically for inadvertent spills that can cause contamination or a buildup of chemicals from reagents that may be inhibitory to bacterial growth.

INTERPRETATION OF CULTURES

Interpretation of primary cultures after 24 to 48 hours of incubation requires considerable skill. From initial observations the microbiologist must assess the nature of isolated colonies and decide whether additional procedures are required. The relevant parameters include the characteristics and relative number of each type of colony recovered on agar media; the purity, gram reaction, and morphology of the bacteria in each type of colony; and changes in the media, which reflect metabolic activities of the bacteria in adjacent colonies.

In the process of collecting specimens from patients or in handling those specimens in the laboratory extraneous organisms may be introduced from the environment or from the indigenous flora of the individuals who handle the culture. In blood cultures, for instance, resident skin flora is frequently encountered and must be interpreted carefully. In addition, "contaminants" may be introduced in the process of manufacturing or handling microbiologic products, such as agar plates. It may be apparent that a colony is extraneous if it is present on the second or third streak area of a plate—with no growth on the initial inoculation zone. These colonies can usually be ignored, although special attention must be given to important pathogens that are unusual "contaminants." A more difficult challenge arises when a single colony of a typical skin organism, such as coagulase-negative *Staphylococcus*, is found in the primary inoculation zone. There is, of course, a 1/3 or 1/4 probability of a plate contaminant ending up in the first zone. If the specimen is a critical one, such as cerebrospinal fluid and has been retained in the laboratory, it can be reinoculated on to the surface of agar. Although it is

not appropriate to ignore the isolate in this situation, it is appropriate to append a comment that a single colony was recovered and was not reisolated from the specimen. The clinician can then put the laboratory and clinical facts together before making a final interpretation of the significance.

Unusual situations present themselves on occasion. For instance, mixed organisms that resemble indigenous upper respiratory tract flora may be recovered from a normally sterile site. It is hard to avoid the suspicion that someone "sneezed" on the plate, but further evaluation must depend on evaluation of all factors, perhaps in consultation with the clinician. A most unusual laboratory phenomenon is illustrated in Figure 1-14.

Characteristics of Macroscopic Colonies. Assessment of gross colony characteristics is usually performed by inspecting growth on the surface of agar plates. This examination is carried out by holding the plate in one hand and observing the surface of the agar for the presence of bacterial growth (Figure 1-15). Standard culture plates are 100 mm in diameter and are convenient to hold in one hand. Each plate must be studied carefully, because the bacteria initially recovered from specimens are often in mixed culture and a variety of colonial types may be present. Pinpoint colonies of slow-growing bacteria may be overlooked among larger colonies, particularly if there is any tendency for growth to spread over the surface of the plate.

During examination, plates should be tilted in various directions, under bright, direct illumination, so that light is reflected from various angles. We highly recommend use of a hand lens or a dissecting microscope to assist in the detection of tiny or immature colonies and to observe their characteristics better (Figure 1-16). Blood agar plates should also be examined with transilluminating bright light from behind the plate to detect hemolytic reactions in the agar (Figure 1-17).

Figure 1-18 provides terms and illustrations helpful when

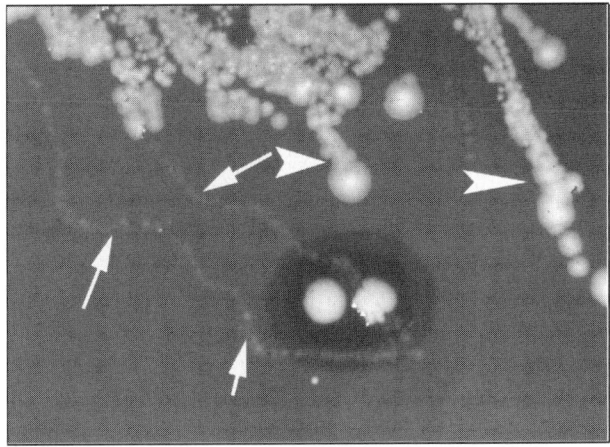

Figure 1-14 An agar plate, which had been inoculated with a skin specimen, contains mixed bacterial flora. An irregular, meandering track of bacteria can be seen among the isolated colonies (arrow). In addition, unusual linear patterns of mature colonies may represent the same process (arrowheads). The most likely explanation is that an insect that was present in the specimen carried bacterial cells around the plate. Free-living amoebae have also been described to produce this phenomenon.

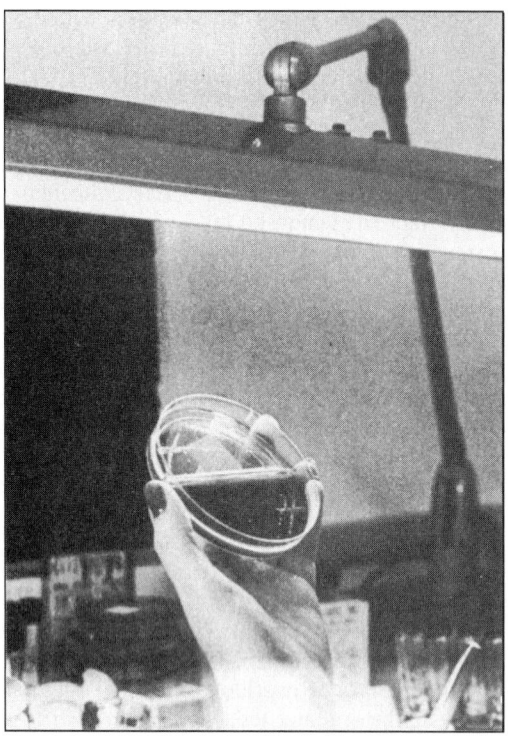

Figure 1-15 The technique for examining the surface of an agar plate by direct, oblique-reflected light.

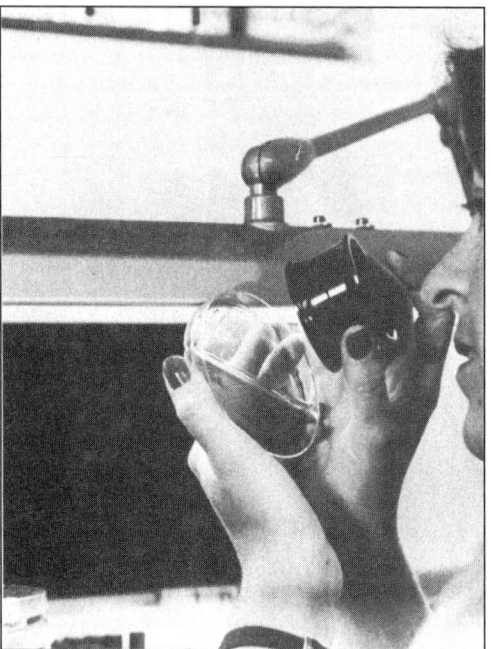

Figure 1-16 The technique, using a hand lens, for examining colonies growing on the surface of an agar plate.

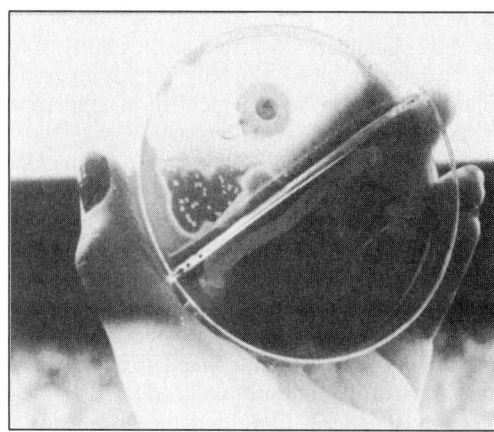

Figure 1-17 The technique for examining colonies growing on the surface of an agar plate, using transmitted light. This technique is helpful in assessing the hemolytic properties of colonies growing on blood agar.

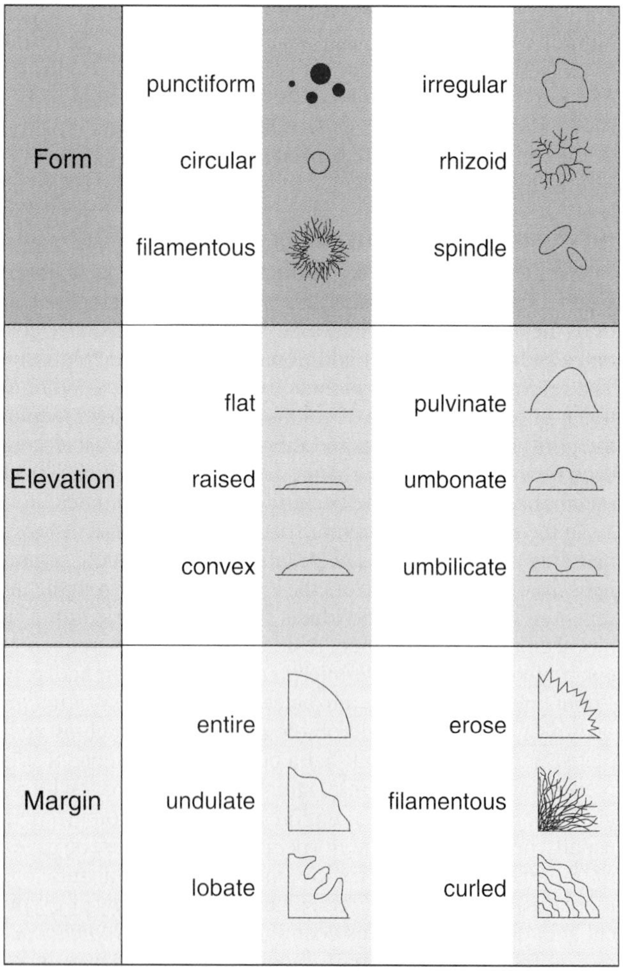

Form	punctiform		irregular	
	circular		rhizoid	
	filamentous		spindle	
Elevation	flat		pulvinate	
	raised		umbonate	
	convex		umbilicate	
Margin	entire		erose	
	undulate		filamentous	
	lobate		curled	

Figure 1-18 Illustrations of a variety of morphologic colony forms, with labels of terms for each.

Box 1-8 Characteristics of Colonies Used in the Identification of Bacteria

Size: diameter in millimeters

Form: punctiform, circular, filamentous, irregular, rhizoid, spindle-like

Elevation: flat, raised, convex, pulvinate, umbonate, umbilicate

Margin (edge of colony): entire, undulant, lobate, erose, filamentous, curled

Color: white, yellow, black, buff, orange, other

Surface: glistening, dull, other

Density: opaque, translucent, transparent, other

Consistency: butyrous, viscid, membranous, brittle, other

See also Fig. 1-18 and Color Plate 1-5.

Box 1-9 Reactions in Agar Media Used in the Identification of Bacteria

Hemolysis on blood agar

Alpha: partial clearing of blood around colonies with green discoloration of the medium; outline of red blood cells intact

Beta: zone of complete clearing of blood around colonies owing to lysis of the red blood cells

Gamma: no change in the medium around the colony; no lysis or discoloration of the red blood cells

Alpha prime: halo of incomplete lysis immediately surrounding colonies, with a second zone of complete hemolysis at the periphery

Pigment production in agar medium

Water-soluble pigments discoloring the medium

Pyocyanin

Fluorescent pigments

Nondiffusable pigments confined to the colonies

Reaction in egg yolk agar

Lecithinase: zone of precipitate in medium surrounding colonies

Lipase: "pearly layer," an iridescent film in and immediately surrounding colonies, visible by reflected light

Proteolysis: clear zone surrounding colonies

Box 1-10 Changes in Differential Media

Various dyes, pH indicators, and other ingredients are included in differential plating media to serve as indicators of enzymatic activities and aid in identifying bacterial isolates.

describing bacterial colonies. Additional guidelines are outlined in Boxes 1-8 through 1-10.

Although difficult to describe specifically, odors produced by the action of certain bacteria in plating media and in liquid media can be very helpful in the tentative identification of the microorganisms involved (Table 1-12). Sniffing should always be performed with caution, by raising the lid of the Petri dish slightly to detect the odor. Laboratory workers are cautioned that a few species have demonstrated the ability to infect laboratory workers and should not be sniffed at all. If there is a suspicion that *Bacillus anthracis, Francisella tularensis, Burkholderia pseudomallei, Brucella* spp., or *Neisseria meningitidis* might be present, the culture should be removed to a biological safety cabinet, where all subsequent work can be done without danger of transmission to the worker. Of course, plates and tubes should never be opened in the mycobacteriology laboratory or when molds are present in the mycology laboratory. Some odors, such as those of *Nocardia* and *Streptomyces*, are so strong that they can be smelled even without removing the lid of the Petri dish.

By assessing the described colonial characteristics and action on media, the microbiologist can make a preliminary identification of the bacteria isolated by primary culture. These characteristics are helpful in selecting other appropriate differential media and tests to complete the identification of the isolates. In Table 1-13 some of the commonly encountered colonial types are listed, along with the groups of bacteria associated with each, additional tests required for definitive identification, and reference to the relevant frame in Color Plate 1-5.

Table 1-12 Characteristic Odors of Selected Microbes*

MICROBE	ODOR
Alkaligenes faecalis (*odorans*)	Freshly cut apples
CDC EF-4	Popcorn-like
Candida spp.	Yeast
Citrobacter spp.	Dirty sneakers
Clostridium difficile	Putrid, fecal
Corynebacterium spp., DF-3	Fruity
Eikenella corrodens	Bleach
Haemophilus spp.	Wet fur
Nocardia spp.	Musty basement
Pasteurella multocida	Pungent (indole)
Peptostreptococcus anaerobius	Fecal
Pigmented *Bacteroides* group	Acrid
Proteus spp.	Burnt chocolate
Pseudomonas aeruginosa	Grape juice
Staphylococcus spp.	Dirty sneakers
Streptococcus spp.	Butter
Streptomyces spp.	Musty basement

* Certain organisms (not listed here) pose a hazard if smelled. See text for discussion.

Table 1-13 Preliminary Bacterial Identification by Colonial Types

COLONIAL TYPE	BACTERIAL GROUP	ADDITIONAL TESTS	FRAME OF PLATES ILLUSTRATING TYPE
Convex, entire edge, 2–3 mm, creamy, yellowish, zone of β-hemolysis	*Staphylococcus*	Catalase Coagulase DNase Mannitol utilization Tellurite reduction Novobiocin resistance Furazolidone resistance	1–5A
Convex or pulvinate, translucent, pinpoint in size, butyrous, wide zone of β-hemolysis	*Streptococcus*	Catalase A disk 6.5% NaCl tolerance Bile-esculin CAMP test Hippurate hydrolysis L-Pyrrolidonyl-β-naph-thylamide (PyR)	1–5B, C
Umbilicate or flat, translucent, butyrous or mucoid, broad zone of α-hemolysis	*Pneumococcus*	P disk Bile solubility	1–5G
Pulvinate, semiopaque, gray, moist to somewhat dry, β-hemolysis may or may not be present	*Escherichia coli* and other Enterobacteriaceae	Multiple tests Indole Methyl red Voges-Proskauer reaction Citrate Decarboxylases Urease Phenylalanine Carbohydrate fermenta-tions	1–5D
Flat, gray; spreading as thin film over agar surface; burned chocolate odor	*Proteus*	Phenylalanine deaminase Urease Lysine deaminase	
Flat, opaque, gray to green-ish, margins erose or spreading, green-blue pig-ment, grapelike odor	*Pseudomonas*	Cytochrome oxidase Fluorescence of carbo-hydrate assimilations Denitrification DNase Hydrolysis of acetamide Growth at 42°C	

The initial inspection of colonies for preliminary identification of bacteria is one of the cornerstones of diagnostic microbiology and is discussed in detail in later chapters devoted to specific groups of pathogenic bacteria and other microorganisms.

Separation of Bacterial Morphotypes in Mixed Cultures.

When agar plates are struck for isolation, it will be a simple matter to select isolated colonies for subculture. On occasion, however, growth may be so crowded that it is difficult to pick individual isolated colonies. Several manipulations are available to the microbiologist in this eventuality (Table 1-14).

Gram's Stain Examination of Cultures:.

Preliminary impressions, based on observation of colony characteristics, can be further confirmed by studying gram-stained smears, a technique that is relatively simple to perform. The top and center of the colony to be studied is first touched with the end of a straight inoculating wire, taking care not to touch the adjacent agar (Figure 1-19). The portion of the colony to be sampled is emulsified in a small drop of water or physi-

Table 1-14 Techniques for Preparation of Pure Isolates from Mixed Cultures

TECHNIQUE	DESCRIPTION
Straight subculture	Carefully touch the surface of the desired colony with the tip of an inoculating needle (not a loop); streak a new plate for isolation
Use of selective media	Subculture the colony of interest onto an agar that will inhibit growth of the unwanted colonies; e.g., subculture of a gram-negative bacillus onto MacConkey agar to separate it from gram-positive cocci
Use of inhibitory chemicals incorporated into agar (analogous to selective media)	Subculture the colony of interest onto an agar that contains antibiotics or chemicals that will inhibit growth of the unwanted colonies
Use of antibiotic disks (analogous to an agar plate containing antibiotics but more flexible)	Subculture the colony of interest onto the surface of an agar plate and position an antibiotic-impregnated disk that is designed to inhibit the unwanted bacteria

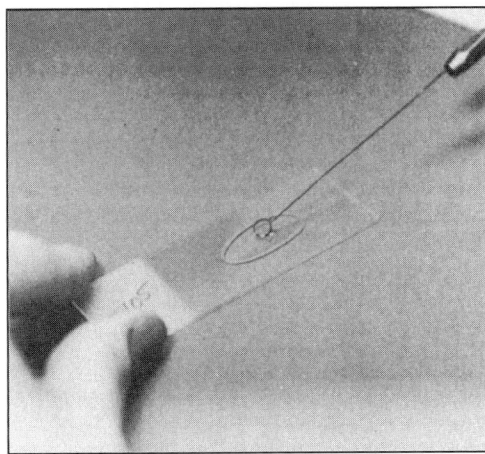

Figure 1-20 The technique for preparing a smear for Gram's stain. The top portion of an isolated bacterial colony, as illustrated in Figure 1-19, is touched with an inoculating wire or loop, then the tip of the loop is submerged in a drop or water or physiologic saline on a glass slide. The inoculum is then emulsified and the preparation is left to air-dry before heat fixation and staining.

ologic saline on a microscope slide to disperse the individual bacterial cells (Figure 1-20). After the slide has air dried, the bacterial film is fixed to the glass surface either by using heat, quickly passing the slide four or five times through the flame of a Bunsen burner, or by flooding with methanol or ethanol for a few minutes. The fixed smear is then placed on a staining rack and Gram's stain is performed as described in Box 1-6.

The stained smear should be examined microscopically

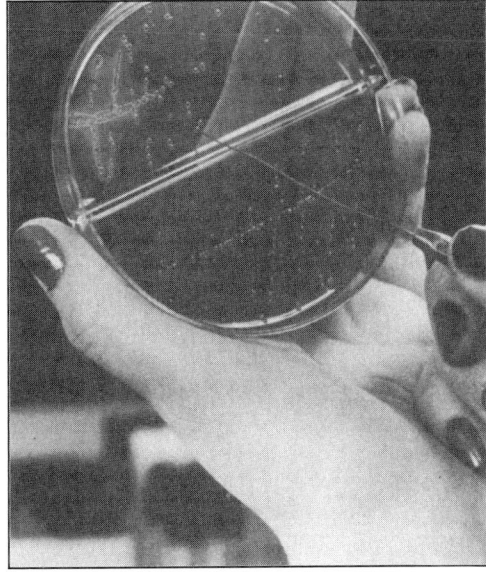

Figure 1-19 The technique for picking an isolated bacterial colony with a straight wire for subculture to another medium.

using an oil immersion objective. In addition to the Gram's stain reaction of the bacterial cells (gram-positive bacteria appear blue; gram-negative bacteria appear red or pink), three other characteristics are helpful in making a preliminary identification of isolates: (1) size and shape of the bacterial cells, (2) arrangement of the bacterial cells, and (3) presence or lack of specific structures or organelles (spores, metachromatic granules, swollen bodies, or other features).

In making a preliminary identification of bacterial isolates, the microbiologist should evaluate each of these characteristics. A series of photomicrographs of several stains illustrating a number of the morphologic cells types and spatial arrangements of bacteria commonly encountered in clinical laboratories is shown in Color Plate 1-X3.

With the information derived from the examination of bacterial colonies and gram-stained smears of cells, the microbiologist now can be guided to the particular tests most likely to provide the correct identification. For example, a raised, creamy, yellow hemolytic colony on blood agar that consists of gram-positive cocci in clusters is most likely *Staphylococcus* (see Color Plate 1-3C). A pinpoint translucent β-hemolytic colony on blood agar that consists of gram-positive cocci in chains is most probably a streptococcus (see Color Plate 1-3D).

The microbiologist soon learns, however, not to rely solely on the examination of gram-stained smears because the staining reactions may be variable, particularly with very young or older colonies. Gram's stain morphology of bacteria is most characteristic when smears are prepared from a young broth subculture (4–6 hours), a time when the bacterial cells are in log phase of growth. Often the Gram's stain morphology is less characteristic when smears are prepared from colonies growing on agar surfaces.

Microbiologists should provide as much preliminary information to the physician as possible. In selected cases, such as when observing bacteria in a blood culture broth or directly in infected CSF, this type of preliminary information can be quite useful in directing specific antibiotic therapy before the final identification or antimicrobial susceptibility test results are available.

PROCEDURES FOR PRELIMINARY IDENTIFICATION OF BACTERIAL ISOLATES

Most tests used to assess the biochemical or metabolic activity of bacteria for the purpose of identifying an isolate are performed by inoculating the primary isolate onto a series of differential test media or into solutions. The initial observation and interpretation of culture media should be used to determine whether the microorganism(s) recovered merit further identification and whether antibiotic susceptibility tests should be performed.

Direct Biochemical Procedures for Making Preliminary Bacterial Identifications. Certain preliminary observations or a direct rapid test can be performed on select colonies. Frequently, an isolate can be identified to a level that is clinically useful based on these assessments alone. For example, the lactose-utilizing properties of gram-negative bacilli can be directly evaluated from MacConkey agar by observing the red pigmentation of the colonies; H_2S production may be detected on Hektoen and XLD agars by observing colonies with black centers. The decarboxylation of lysine can also be suspected when observing colonies growing on XLD agar. A red halo around the colony, indicating an alkaline pH shift, indicates the decarboxylation of lysine.

The following are direct tests that can be performed on isolated colonies recovered on primary culture plates:

The Catalase Test A few drops of 3% hydrogen peroxide are placed directly on a colony. Rapid effervescence indicates production of molecular oxygen and a positive test (see Chart 1-1). Accurate results may be difficult to obtain if the test is performed on colonies growing on blood agar because of the presence of peroxidase in erythrocytes. The peroxidase reaction produced by erythrocytes is delayed and weak, however, and can usually be readily differentiated from the immediate and highly active reactions produced by catalase-positive bacteria. The catalase test is most often used to differentiate staphylococci (positive) from streptococci (negative) or *Bacillus* spp. (positive) from *Clostridium tertium* (negative).

The Bile Solubility Test Two methods for determining bile solubility are commonly used. As an initial screen, a few drops of a 10% solution of sodium deoxycholate solution are placed on colonies suspected of being *Streptococcus pneumoniae*. Pneumococcal colonies lyse completely and disappear after about 30 minutes (see Chart 1-2). This test is sometimes difficult to interpret; the tube test is more straightforward. An inoculum from the unknown bacterial colony can be suspended in a 10% solution of deoxycholate (bile salts) until turbidity is achieved. The clearing of the turbidity within 30 to 60 minutes after incubation at 35°C indicates bile solubility (see Chart 1-2). A control viridans streptococcus, which does not dissolve in bile, should be tested concurrently. Alternatively, a rapid latex agglutination test for pneumococci may be used.

The Slide Coagulase Test A colony suspected of being *Staphylococcus* species is emulsified in a drop of rabbit plasma on a glass slide. Bacterial clumping within 2 minutes indicates the presence of bound coagulase and constitutes a positive test result (see Chart 1-3). A negative slide coagulase test should be followed with a conventional tube coagulase test. Agglutination tests for detection of staphylococcal protein A can also be used as a marker for *Staphylococcus aureus*. Many laboratories base their identification of staphylococci on the presence or absence of coagulase. In that case the report should indicate the presence of coagulase-positive or coagulase-negative staphylococci, rather than an imputed species name (e.g., *S. aureus*).

The Direct Spot Indole Test A small portion of the colony to be tested is transferred from a nonselective medium, such as blood or chocolate agar, to a strip of filter paper that has been saturated with Kovac's reagent or p-dimethylamino cinnamaldehyde (PACA) solution. The immediate development of a red color with Kovac's reagent indicates the presence of indole and a positive test (see Chart 1-4). PACA is more sensitive than Kovac's reagent, and a positive test reaction is indicated by the rapid development of a blue color. In many laboratories, dry-appearing, lactose-positive, spot indole-positive colonies appearing after 24 hours of incubation on MacConkey agar, particularly on isolates from the urinary tract, are presumptively identified as *E. coli*, and further tests are usually not performed. In these cases the spot indole must be performed on colonies growing on parallel blood agar plates, because the pigmentation of the lactose-positive colonies on MacConkey agar will make interpretation of the color reaction difficult.

Cytochrome Oxidase Test A portion of the colony to be tested is smeared on the reagent-impregnated area of an oxidase test strip. The immediate development of a blue color indicates cytochrome oxidase activity and a positive test result (see Chart 1-5). Cytochrome oxidase tests are useful for the initial categorization of many bacterial species that have distinctive colonial morphology. Oxidase-positive colonies can be discounted as belonging to the *Enterobacteriaceae*, which are uniformly negative. Bacterial species that produce cytochrome oxidase include *Aeromonas* spp., *Plesiomonas* spp., *Pseudomonas* spp. and *Pasteurella* spp.

MUG Test Other direct tests can be used to screen for certain organisms from primary isolation plates, offering potential savings on time-consuming and costly differentiation procedures. One is the MUG (4-methylumbelliferyl-β-D-glucuronidase) test, based on detecting the capability of the unknown organism to produce β-glucuronidase. This test can be used as a screen for *E. coli* instead of the spot indole test. A heavy suspension of the unknown organism is inoculated into the MUG reagent, which has been suspended in tubes or impregnated in dehydrated disks. The reagent will fluoresce from release of 4-methylumbelliferone if glucuronidase is present. Indole can also be detected by adding Kovac's indole reagent to the MUG tube, making this combination test a valuable method for screening lactose-fermenting enteric bacilli.

PYR Test L-pyrrolidonyl-β-naphthylamide (PyR) substrate provides a simple method for the rapid identification of enterococci. After 4 hours of incubation following heavy inoculation of the substrate with a liquid suspension of the unknown organism prepared from a primary isolation plate, the production of a red color after adding N,N-methylamino cinnamaldehyde reagent is indicative of enterococci (group A streptococci are also PyR-positive, but can usually be differentiated by morphologic criteria; see Chart 1-6).

Identification of Bacteria to the Level of Species and Selection of Differential Characteristics. The final characterization of an unknown bacterial isolate is usually accomplished by testing for enzyme systems that are characteristic of each species. These enzyme systems are detected by inoculating a small portion of a well-isolated bacterial colony into a series of culture media that contain specific substrates and chemical indicators. By this means the microbiologist can detect changes in pH produced by utilization of chemical substrates or color changes produced by specific by-products. The clinical microbiologist must select appropriate sets of differential characteristics that will permit the identification of each group of bacteria. One of the major advances in diagnostic microbiology has been the miniaturization of biochemical systems, so that multiple characteristics can be examined expeditiously and relatively inexpensively. Probabilistic models for the identification can be developed based on multiple characteristics. Before these advances a small number of tests was performed in macroscopic tubes or plates, followed by subsequent testing based on the initial results. This process was slow, expensive, and more prone to error than modern approaches.[87]

IDENTIFICATION OF ORGANISMS OTHER THAN BACTERIA

Fungi. Yeast share many characteristics with bacteria and similar approaches are used. Urease testing (including a rapid version) can be used to examine respiratory isolates, because the most frequent pathogen (*Cryptococcus neoformans*) produces urease, whereas the most frequent commensal yeast isolate (*Candida* spp.) does not contain this enzyme with rare exceptions. Yeast are identified by morphologic characteristics in addition to assimilation and/or fermentation of carbohydrates. Variations on the approaches used for bacteria are commonly employed for yeast.

The mainstay of identification of mold isolates, however, is morphologic study of asexual reproductive characters. Biochemical testing plays a subsidiary role.

Mycobacteria. As specialized bacteria, the approaches to identification are similar for these organisms. The biochemical testing, however, is considerably more difficult with mycobacteria than with conventional bacteria. Most laboratory directors choose to refer specimens to specialized laboratories and/or use molecular probes for commonly isolated species.

Parasites. With occasional exceptions characterization of parasites is by morphologic study. Culture of parasites is uncommonly performed.

Viruses. As obligate intracellular pathogens, viruses require a very different diagnostic approach. Characterization of antigens and nucleic acids are the predominant techniques used for viral diagnosis.

TESTING OF SUSCEPTIBILITY TO ANTIMICROBIAL AGENTS

In many respects determining the susceptibility of pathogens to appropriate antimicrobial agents is the most important task performed in diagnostic microbiology laboratories.

Box 1-11 Factors Involved in Susceptibility Testing

Factor	Criteria
Isolate	Potential pathogen from a valid specimen (not likely to represent colonizing flora)
Susceptibility	Not predictable for infectious agent and antimicrobial
Clinical situation	Antimicrobial therapy indicated
Interpretive standards	Validated criteria available for determining the clinical significance of the result

Some of the factors that must be evaluated when susceptibility testing is considered are summarized in Box 1-11.

Antimicrobial susceptibility testing is most often used for guidance in therapy of bacterial and mycobacterial infections (see Chapters 17 and 19). It is the job of clinical microbiologists to ensure to the greatest extent possible that testing is done on appropriate isolates by valid methods. The easiest course of action is to give in to an insistent clinician who demands testing of an isolate for which there are no interpretive standards, but the microbiologist must resist that temptation, recruiting knowledgeable colleagues for support if necessary.

Testing of anaerobic bacteria, fungi, and viruses may be required in certain situations, but is not necessary routinely. If these agents are tested, it is important that a sophisticated clinician, who will be able to interpret the results properly, be involved in care of the patient.

Use of Antimicrobial Susceptibility Results for Quality Control of Identification Results. Some bacteria have predictable susceptibility to certain agents and need not be tested. Many more have characteristic susceptibility patterns that are not sufficiently absolute to obviate testing. These patterns can be used, however, as a check on the taxonomic characterization. For instance, *Klebsiella pneumoniae* is typically resistant to ampicillin, but susceptible to first generation cephalosporins. In contrast, *Enterobacter* spp. are usually resistant to both groups of antibiotics. If an isolate is identified as *Enterobacter*, but is susceptible to these agents, the results should be questioned. Tests both for identification and for susceptibility should be repeated, as either, both, or neither result might be erroneous. Optimally a different method should be used for the repeat test from that used initially.

COST-EFFECTIVE APPROACHES IN THE ANALYTIC PHASE

In the analytical phase resources can be utilized efficiently by concentrating on several areas. It is possible to use abbreviated protocols for identifying certain organisms (Table 1-15). NCCLS has provided consensus recommendations for certain approaches.[80] Other means for optimizing resources are summarized in Table 1-16. The philosophical underpinning of these approaches is the focus on results that can be interpreted

Table 1-15 Abbreviated Identification of Bacteria and Yeast

SITUATION	ABBREVIATED TEST PROTOCOL	IDENTIFICATION
Gram-negative, nonswarming, oxidase-negative, β-hemolytic on sheep blood agar*	No additional tests	*Escherichia coli*
Gram-negative, nonswarming, oxidase-negative, nonhemolytic on sheep blood agar, lactose-fermenter*	PYR negative	*Escherichia coli*
Gram-negative, nonswarming, oxidase-negative, non-hemolytic on sheep blood agar, lactose-nonfermenter*	MUG positive	*Escherichia coli*
Small gram-negative bacilli or cocco-bacilli from respiratory or cerebrospinal fluid specimens; growth in 5% CO_2 on chocolate agar, but not sheep blood agar*	Rapid test for porphyrin synthesis negative	*Haemophilus influenzae* (cannot differentiate from *Haemophilus hemolyticus*, an uncommon human pathogen)
Gram-negative diplococci, oxidase-positive, growth on both chocolate and sheep blood agars*	Rapid butyrate esterase or DNAse positive	*Moraxella catarrhalis*
Gram-negative bacilli, oxidase-negative, lactose-nonfermenter, swarming growth on chocolate or sheep blood agar*	Indole positive	*Proteus vulgaris*
Gram-negative bacilli, oxidase-negative, lactose-nonfermenter, swarming growth on chocolate or sheep blood agar*	Indole negative; ampicillin susceptible	*Proteus mirabilis*
Gram-negative bacilli, oxidase-negative, lactose-nonfermenter, swarming growth on chocolate or sheep blood agar*	Indole negative; ampicillin resistant; maltose negative; ornithine positive	*Proteus mirabilis*
Gram-negative bacilli, oxidase-negative, lactose-nonfermenter, swarming growth on chocolate or sheep blood agar*	Indole negative; ampicillin resistant; maltose positive; ornithine negative	*Proteus penneri*
Gram-negative bacilli, oxidase-positive, typical smell of Concord grapes, typical colonial morphology (metallic sheen, green/reddish/black, mucoid)*	No additional tests	*Pseudomonas aeruginosa* (rare isolates of *Aeromonas* may be similar but are spot indole positive)
Gram-positive cocci in clusters; catalase positive; creamy, opaque, yellowish colonies on sheep blood agar (color accentuated on chocolate agar)*	Slide coagulase and/or 4-hour tube coagulase positive	*Staphylococcus aureus* (Coagulase positive *Staphylococcus*); rarely other staphylococci may be positive in one or other coagulase tests
Gram-positive cocci in pairs and short chains, catalase negative or occasionally weakly positive; non-β-hemolytic on sheep blood agar*	PYR positive	*Enterococcus* spp.; failure to grow well for susceptibility tests suggests the isolate may be another genus
Gram-positive cocci in pairs and chains; catalase negative; usually narrow zone of beta hemolysis*	Rapid hippurate hydrolysis positive; spot CAMP test positive; or latex agglutination positive with specific antiserum	*Streptococcus agalactiae* (Group B); β-hemolytic enterococci may be hippurate positive, but are also PYR positive
Gram-positive cocci in pairs and short chains; catalase negative; α-hemolytic on sheep blood agar; colonies typically either mucoid or "checker" shaped	Spot bile or tube bile solubility positive; Pneumoslide positive; Quellung positive; or latex agglutination positive with specific antiserum	*Streptococcus pneumoniae*
Gram-positive cocci in pairs and chains; catalase negative; β-hemolytic on sheep blood agar with a wide zone of hemolysis; colonies usually dry and small relative to hemolysis*	PYR positive or latex agglutination positive with specific antiserum	*Streptococcus pyogenes* (Group A); occasional strains of β-hemolytic enterococci have different colony morphology and are agglutination negative
Small gram-negative bacilli; oxidase-positive; pitting agar, "Mexican hat" or "dewdrop" colony appearance on sheep blood agar; odor of bleach	No additional tests	*Eikenella corrodens*

Table 1-15 *Continued*

SITUATION	ABBREVIATED TEST PROTOCOL	IDENTIFICATION
Gram-negative regular bacilli or coccobacilli with large (>1mm) colonies on anaerobic blood agar and similar size on LKV and BBE agars; no growth on chocolate agar in 5% CO_2*	No additional tests essential; disk pattern may be used (penicillin resistant; kanamycin resistant; rifampin susceptible) as additional evidence	*Bacterioides fragilis* group
Gram-negative, thin, pointed, fusiform bacilli; breadcrumb or opalescent colonies on anaerobic blood agar; no growth on BBE agar; no growth on chocolate agar in 5% CO_2*	Spot indole positive	*Fusobacterium nucleatum*
Gram-negative bacilli; small (<1mm) colonies on anaerobic blood agar and BBE agar after at least 48 hours incubation; no growth on chocolate agar in 5% CO_2; black dot in colony center from H_2S production*	Catalase strongly positive	*Bilophila wadsworthia*
Small coccobacillary gram-negative bacilli; black colonies (or brick red fluorescence under long wavelength UV light) on LKV agar; small translucent or opaque colonies on anaerobic BAP agar; no growth on chocolate agar in 5% CO_2*	No additional tests needed	*Prevotella* spp.; *Prevotella intermedia* if spot indole positive
Small coccobacillary gram-negative bacilli; small translucent or opaque colonies on anaerobic BAP agar with brick red fluorescence under long wavelength UV light; no growth on chocolate agar in 5% CO_2*	Spot indole positive	*Porphyromonas* spp.
Thin gram-negative bacilli; flat, transparent colonies that pit the agar on anaerobic BAP agar; no growth on LKV agar; no growth on chocolate agar incubated in 5% CO_2; catalase negative; urease positive*	No additional tests needed	*Bacteroides ureolyticus*
Tiny gram-negative diplococci; small (<1mm) transparent to opaque colonies on anaerobic BAP agar with red fluorescence under long wavelength UV light; no growth on BBE agar; no growth on chocolate agar in 5% CO_2*	No additional tests needed	*Veillonella* spp.
Large, boxcar-shaped, blunt ended gram-positive or gram-variable bacteria; large (>2mm) irregular colonies with a double zone of β-hemolysis on anaerobic BAP; no growth on LKV or BBE agars; no growth on chocolate agar in 5% CO_2; catalase negative*	No additional tests needed	*Clostridium perfringens*
Thin gram-positive bacilli with swollen, subterminal spores; smoothly swarming growth on anaerobic BAP agar; no growth on LKV or BBE agars; no growth on chocolate agar in 5% CO_2; catalase negative; spot indole negative*	No additional tests needed	*Clostridium septicum*
Thin gram-positive bacilli with subterminal spores; equivalent growth on anaerobic BAP agar and on chocolate agar in 5% CO_2; catalase negative	No additional tests needed	*Clostridium tertium*
Pleomorphic, coryneform gram-positive bacilli; small (1 to 2 mm) enamel-white opaque colonies on anaerobic BAP agar; catalase positive; spot indole positive*	No additional tests needed	*Propionibacterium acnes*
Budding yeast cells*	Germ tube test positive in < 3 hours; or mycelial projections from colonies on blood-containing media at <48 hours incubation	*Candida albicans*
Spherical budding yeast cells; often mucoid colonies*	Rapid phenol oxidase test positive	*Cryptococcus neoformans* (Cryptococcus can be excluded on rapid urease negative colonies)

* *From consensus recommendations in reference[80].*

Table 1-16 Some Suggested Approaches to Optimizing Laboratory Identifications

CATEGORY	PROPOSED POLICY*
Repeat specimens from a *nonsterile* site within a defined time period	Refer subsequent specimens to the previous evaluation; if the subsequent specimen has been inoculated to media and substantial differences from the original specimen are present, consult clinician about further action
Mixed flora from a *nonsterile* site, especially if submitted on a swab; inflammation minimal or no Gram's smear available	Report as mixed gram-positive/gram-negative flora
Mixed flora from a *nonsterile* site, especially if submitted on a swab; moderate to heavy inflammation present	Report as mixed gram-positive/gram-negative flora; append a comment to consult the laboratory within X days for further processing
Mixed flora from a *nonsterile* site, especially if submitted on a swab; moderate to heavy inflammation present; single predominant potential pathogen present	Report identification of predominant pathogen and presence of mixed flora; either perform antimicrobial susceptibility tests on predominant pathogen or append a comment to consult the laboratory for susceptibility testing
Yeast isolated in mixed culture with bacteria from a *nonsterile* or *potentially contaminated* site, such as a wound or peritoneal fluid	Report presence of yeast; consider appending a comment to consult the laboratory for further processing
Mixed flora from urine specimens obtained by clean catch or in dwelling catheter	Report as mixed gram-positive/gram-negative flora; append comment suggesting 1) repeat collection with an in-and-out catheter if clinically indicated and the patient does not have an indwelling catheter or 2) notifying the laboratory if the patient has an indwelling catheter and requires antimicrobial therapy
Mixed flora with a single predominant pathogen from urine specimens obtained by clean catch or indwelling catheter	Evaluate predominant pathogen; append a comment indicating presence of mixed flora
Mixed vaginal flora present	Report only presence or absence of documented vaginal pathogens that are best documented by culture; i.e., *Listeria monocytogenes*, *Streptococcus agalactiae* (in women of childbearing age), *Streptococcus pyogenes*, *Staphylococcus aureus* (if toxic-shock syndrome suspected), and yeast. Susceptibility testing rarely indicated.
Mixed flora from intravascular catheter	Report mixed gram-positive/gram-negative flora and consider appending a comment to consult the laboratory for further processing
Recovery of bacteria that resemble *Haemophilus influenzae* or *Moraxella catarrhalis* from expectorated sputum	Proceed with identification and report the result only if the organism is found in a concomitant Gram's stain associated with polymorphonuclear neutrophils

* It is good policy to preserve specimens that are not evaluated completely for at least 24 hours. Preserve agar plates that have not been evaluated completely for a period of time. Seven days is a convenient period to preserve the plates, because all plates from a day can be stored together and discarded one week later.

correctly and that will lead to the best treatment for the patient. One conceptual principle is to think about specimens in two broad categories: (1) those from which isolated agents are highly likely to be pathogens and (2) those from which isolated agents cannot be interpreted with confidence. If a microbiologist gives equal attention to these two categories, it is entirely possible that so many resources will have been squandered on specimens of questionable significance that the most important specimens will be shortchanged.

It is the job of each microbiologist to make decisions for the local laboratory, depending on the local environment. A prime consideration is to avoid providing results that may be misinterpreted. A report of "Mixed flora; interpretation difficult" is likely to stimulate collection of an additional (and hopefully better) specimen or treatment of the patient

based on the pathogens that are likely causes of the particular infection. Putting a name on an isolated organism that is, in fact, colonizing or contaminating flora gives that organism more apparent credibility than it deserves. Adding antimicrobial susceptibility results compounds the difficulty. A baseball analogy may be used to illustrate common deficiencies:

1. Specimen submitted on a swab: Strike One
2. No polymorphonuclear neutrophils present or no Gram's smear requested: Strike Two
3. Mixed bacterial flora present: Strike Three
4. You're Out!

The question becomes "What is mixed bacterial flora?" Common sense and a solid grounding in the principles of diagnostic microbiology are essential to the decision, which must be made individually on each specimen. For instance, *Streptococcus pyogenes* is an important pathogen, no matter how many other species are present; any β-hemolytic colonies should be evaluated for the presence of the Group A streptococcal antigen. As a guideline Schreckenberger and Miller have suggested the "Rule of Three."[67,103] They suggest that one or two potential pathogens should be evaluated even in the presence of commensal flora, but three or more potential pathogens should not be evaluated.

The "Rule of Three" guideline is a useful aid, but sound judgment should be used. For instance, the rule should not be applied automatically to biopsied tissue or aspirated fluids and pus. In the urinary tract, a mixture of three or more organisms of any variety suggests contamination with vaginal or perineal flora; even if a potential pathogen is a part of the mixture and does not predominate, it is difficult to be confident that the analysis will provide valid information. Sometimes the quantitative relationship of the organisms in the mixture can provide a clue. If one or possibly two organisms clearly predominate, it is often reasonable to evaluate those organisms and report the presence of mixed flora in addition.

It should be noted that when a microbiologist examines an agar plate and determines that mixed bacterial types are present, it is actually mixed bacterial colonial types (morphotypes) that are being observed. These visually distinctive colonies often represent different species (or even genera), but they may also represent phenotypic variants of a single genotypic organism. The only way to be sure that multiple bacterial species have been isolated is to identify all of them, by which time, of course, all the work will have been done. In practice, we must use judgment as to whether the colonies are sufficiently different to justify characterizing the growth as mixed and recognize that we may be wrong on occasion.

One sensible approach to these situations is to offer the clinician a chance to request that the isolates be evaluated or to initiate a dialogue preemptively, either through a verbal phone report or a written communication on the laboratory record. It is a simple matter to store plates for which consultation has been requested or which contained mixed flora. If the plates are taped together each day and stored for seven days, the outdated specimens can be discarded easily. Should a dispute arise as to further evaluation of a specimen, it is a much more tenable position for the microbiologist if the specimen has been retained than if it has been discarded.

The techniques and interpretations of the foregoing procedures are discussed in greater detail in subsequent chapters. In an era of stringent cost containment, it is imperative that microbiologists apply their skills of observation and use a few select characteristics to identify bacterial species presumptively whenever possible. Developing this microbiologic "sixth sense" can also be helpful in verifying the results obtained from packaged kit systems or from automated instruments. On occasion, the biotype numbers issued by these systems may be in conflict with colonial characteristics, gram stain morphology, and/or biochemical "spot tests." Continued study may be in order to prevent issuing an erroneous report.

Postanalytic Phase
REPORTING RESULTS

Reports of microbiology culture results should be issued as soon as useful information becomes available. Each laboratory director must establish those results that will be considered "urgent" or "panic values." In addition, some results may be considered "important," but not necessarily "urgent." Some typical "urgent" and "important" results are listed in Table 1-17. The construction of such a list will vary greatly, depending on such factors as the capability of the institutional information systems and the practice patterns of clinicians who use the laboratory. In addition to the

---

Table 1-17 Suggested List of "Urgent" and "Important" Reports*

"URGENT" REPORTS	"IMPORTANT" REPORTS
Positive blood cultures	Positive tissues and fluids other than blood and cerebrospinal fluid
Positive cerebrospinal fluid cultures	Stool pathogens
Positive acid-fast smears	Positive parasites other than *Plasmodium* spp.
Mycobacterium tuberculosis	Positive sexually transmitted pathogens
Plasmodium spp., especially *P. falciparum*	*Streptococcus agalactiae* if recovered via predelivery culture protocol
Streptococcus pyogenes from a normally sterile site or genital site	*Streptococcus pyogenes* from throat cultures
Streptococcus agalactiae from a genital site of a woman at term	Positive viral pathogens
Herpes simplex virus from a genital site of a woman at term	Positive dimorphic fungi
	Positive antigen or nucleic acid tests performed drectly on clinical specimens

This list is a suggested model and should be modified as appropriate for local conditions.

defined categories, the clinician should have the opportunity to request a telephoned result on any culture at the time the examination is requested.

''Urgent'' results must always be telephoned to the caregiver. ''Important'' results may be reported by telephone, fax, computer, or paper. The most important consideration is that all parties understand the rules. If all laboratory results are available immediately and conveniently to users of the laboratory services, clinicians may find it much more convenient to get all but urgent results electronically. Confidentiality of patient data must be assured anytime a report might be viewed by unauthorized personnel; e.g., faxing reports only to office machines that are secure. It is good practice to have a protocol for telephone reports that specifies backup recipients if the primary caregiver is not available; this protocol should be acceptable to both clinicians and laboratory workers.

Timely preliminary and interim reports should be issued as a matter of policy. For example, preliminary reports on negative bacterial cultures should be issued within 48 hours. The timing of initial reports on other types of agents will vary with the speed of growth; e.g., weekly for mycobacteria, twice the first week followed by weekly for fungi. An interim report of ''negative culture'' may be helpful, because the physician may wish to reevaluate the case pending the final report. Final reports should be issued as soon as possible; for most bacterial cultures 48 hours is a reasonable goal.

INTERACTIONS WITH EPIDEMIOLOGISTS

Microbiologists play an important role in safeguarding the health of patients and the public at large.[38,89] Certain infectious agents must be reported to public health authorities by law; the list of agents varies by state and should be available in the laboratory. The reports may be written or, increasingly, electronic. Within the institution similar relationships must be cultivated with hospital (or health-care system) epidemiologists. The epidemiologists will review certain laboratory results on a regular basis. In addition, microbiologists should remain alert for unusual patterns of isolates that deserve mention to the epidemiologists for consideration of further investigation. On occasion, molecular characterization of isolates may increase the quality of epidemiologic investigations. The additional testing may be performed locally or in a referral laboratory, depending on available expertise.

ANALYSIS OF RESULTS

It is incumbent on the laboratory director to provide feedback to clinicians on some important parameters of laboratory performance (Box 1-12). If local information systems have the capability, feedback should be made optimally to individual clinicians or groups of clinicians (such as practice groups). The ultimate quality control tool for caregivers is to receive a report card on their use of the laboratory and results on their patients (such as frequency and rate of positive examinations) compared to other clinicians. Such reports are daunting to design because of the difficulty in being sure that the practitioners being compared serve patient groups that are truly equivalent. Studies of turnaround time (TAT) are more problematic in microbiology than in other areas of the laboratory

---

Box 1-12 Parameters of Laboratory Performance and Clinical Results

Activity	Parameters
Blood cultures	Frequency and rate of recovery of ''skin organisms''/''contaminants''
	Frequency and rate of submission of single cultures
	Frequency and rate of recovery of potential pathogens
Direct examination of clinical specimens	Analysis of turnaround time
Antimicrobial susceptibility testing	Summaries of % susceptibility of important bacterial pathogens

---

because of the delays inherent in generating microbiologic results. Certain examinations, such as direct examinations of clinical specimens, do lend themselves to TAT analysis. Summaries of antimicrobial susceptibility results should be provided on a yearly basis.

MAINTENANCE OF SAMPLES AND RECORDS

Local and national guidelines for storage of requisitions and reports must be followed. They differ by specimen type and clinical situation.

Sterile body fluids and tissue should be maintained at room or refrigerator temperatures until the culture has been completely evaluated; cerebrospinal fluid should be stored at room temperature because of the lability of *Neisseria meningitidis* at 4°C. Ideally, tissue should be frozen at $-70°C$ for potential future use, although this action will be difficult for many laboratories. It will not be necessary to return to the freezer often. On occasion, however, subsequent analysis (e.g., after histologic examination of tissue) suggests the need to culture for mycobacteria, viruses, or fungi after an initial request for bacterial culture only. In that situation, the frozen tissue represents an invaluable resource with which a specific etiologic diagnosis may be obtained and appropriate susceptibility testing performed.

Blood culture isolates should be maintained for at least 30 days. Ideally, all positive cultures should be retained for a period (e.g., 7 days) to allow further evaluation, such as molecular typing or additional susceptibility tests, if clinically indicated. Once again, freezing of important or unusual isolates at $-70°C$ is a luxury, but a potentially useful one. If isolates are maintained, careful and rigorous ''weeding'' of the cultures must be done to maintain space for storage of future isolates. A variety of methods has been described for storage of microbial isolates.[95] We have found the simple expedient of placing into a sterile vial an excised block of agar with intact colonies on the surface a simple and effective method of preserving even the most fastidious of bacterial and yeast isolates. Fungi can be maintained as ''water cultures'' at room temperature. Viruses must be frozen at $-70°C$.

Administrative Aspects of the Microbiology Laboratory

The focus of this book is on the science of microbiology as applied to diagnosis and treatment of infectious diseases. In the trenches, however, it is impossible to separate the business of microbiology from the science. One of the strengths of clinical microbiology laboratories is the sophistication of support systems for the scientific process. Research laboratories have much to learn from the planned maintenance and rigorous quality control of their diagnostic counterparts. The reader is referred to an extensive exploration of laboratory management in theory and action.[37]

Government Regulations

In the United States the government is involved in virtually every aspect of laboratory testing. Although some issues are directly related to specific sets of regulations, all aspects of laboratory management derive from governmental imperatives in one way or the other. In many cases leaders in the private and academic laboratory industry developed the framework and defined the standards, which were then adopted by the government and made applicable to all laboratories. The federal agencies and quasigovernmental agencies involved in laboratory and medical regulation are summarized in Box 1-13.

The authority for regulatory involvement in laboratory medicine derives from the Clinical Laboratory Improvement Act of 1967 (CLIA '67). This legislation authorized the regulation of hospital and commercial clinical laboratories. For 20 years laboratories in other settings were exempt. The Clinical Laboratory Improvement Amendments of 1988 (CLIA '88) extended the mandate to include governmental laboratories, public health laboratories and physicians' office laboratories that perform laboratory testing for human disease. Testing for research purposes (results not used in the care of patients) and veterinary medicine do not fall under governmental purview.

Several categories of testing were established in the CLIA '88 regulations (Table 1-18), and many other regulations depend on the category in which a test is placed. The CDC is charged with the task of assigning each test to a complexity category. An advisory group that is composed of individuals from government, industry, medical groups, clinical and public health laboratories, and consumers advises the government on these decisions (Clinical Laboratory Improvement Advisory Committee—CLIAC).

Detailed specifications for personnel qualifications, proficiency testing, and quality control are delineated in the regulations for all laboratories that perform nonwaived testing.

Box 1-13 Agencies Involved in Laboratory and Medical Practice

Agency	Area of Responsibility
Center for Medicare and Medicaid Services (CMS)	Establishes the rules for accreditation, licensure, and inspection of laboratories; Sets reimbursement rates for services to Medicare
Centers for Disease Control and Prevention (CDC)	Participates in categorization of test complexity; Provides recommendations on a variety of issues, including laboratory techniques and bioterrorism preparedness
National Institute of Occupational Health and Safety (NIOSH); a division of CDC	Responsible for regulations on protection from chemical and biological hazards
Occupational Health and Safety Administration (OSHA)	Responsible for regulations on workplace safety
Food and Drug Administration (FDA)	Responsible for approving medicines and medical devices; FDA "clears" medical devices, but does not "approve" them
Veterans Affairs Department	Responsible for the health and welfare of eligible veterans, including a national network of hospitals and clinics
International Air Transport Association (IATA)	An international organization of air carriers; involved in promulgation of rules on safe shipment of infectious agents by air
Clinical and Laboratory Standards Institute (CLSI) (formerly National Committee for Clinical Laboratory Standards [NCCLS])	A voluntary organization of academia, industry, and government; its goal is to improve laboratory performance; although advisory, the recommendations often become standards of laboratory practice
American Medical Association (AMA)	Largest organization of physicians in the United States; responsible for developing coding of laboratory tests and medical procedures, which serve as the basis for reimbursement
Joint Commission for the Accreditation of Healthcare Organizations (JCAHO)	Inspects and accredits hospitals and hospital laboratories, home health-care agencies, long-term health-care facilities, and others

Table 1-18 Complexity Categories of Laboratory Testing Under CLIA '88

CATEGORY	DESCRIPTION	PERSONNEL REQUIREMENTS	PROFICIENCY TESTING	QUALITY CONTROL	COMMENTS
High Complexity	Tests requiring the greatest analytical skill and judgment	Most stringent; requires equivalent of Associates Degree	Required	Required	High and moderate complexity testing are jointly considered nonwaived testing
Moderate Complexity	Tests requiring analytical skill and judgment but at a somewhat lower level	Less stringent; requires training which may be on the job	Required	Required	There is a complex formula for categorizing tests as to level of complexity
Provider Performed Microscopy	Microscopic examinations by certain groups of clinicians	Defined provider groups; cannot be delegated to other personnel	Required if applicable	Required if applicable	This is a subcategory of moderate complexity testing
Waived Testing	Simple tests that are not likely to have adverse consequences if performed incorrectly	None	Not required	Must follow manufacturers instructions	Most laboratory workers have a hard time understanding how a test could be worth doing if a wrong answer causes no harm

For more detailed information see the CMS Web site: http://www.cms.hhs.gov/clia/appendc.asp

Several consequences of the CLIA '88 regulations have devolved.

1. Most physicians have stopped performing all but the most basic testing because the regulatory requirements are considered too burdensome.
2. There is constant pressure from physician groups (other than pathologists) to loosen the regulations and allow performance of more complex tests without stringent controls.
3. Manufacturers strive to have their instruments and products placed into the waived category, so they can market them to physicians as simple tests without rigorous requirements for control and documentation.

Accreditation and Laboratory Inspection. The CLIA '88 regulations provide for licensure of laboratories after inspection by state inspectors or by another organization that has been "deemed" by CMS to provide equivalent—or stricter—standards. The two organizations that are most commonly used by clinical laboratories for accreditation and inspection are JCAHO and CAP. In every case the laboratory must be evaluated biennially. Laboratories that utilize JCAHO are usually located in hospitals, and the inspection of the laboratory is performed at the same time as the hospital inspection. In this case, the inspectors are "professional inspectors," usually with a medical or nursing background rather than training in laboratory medicine specifically. The CAP was the first organization to evaluate laboratories; before the entry of the government into the process. Initially, accreditation was voluntary and viewed as an educational means to self-improvement. The CAP philosophy is based on peer evaluation. Each laboratory that is inspected must provide a team to inspect another similar laboratory in turn.

The inspectors are, therefore, "volunteers" who are practicing laboratory professionals.

Each organization that inspects laboratories has a set of standards for evaluation; these standards must be submitted to CMS for approval. In some states accreditation by a state agency must also be performed if a laboratory does business in that state.

Proficiency Testing. An integral part of continuing accreditation is participation in proficiency testing. Specimens are sent to participating laboratories as unknowns on a periodic basis. The laboratory evaluates the specimens and returns the answers to the accrediting agency, after which the results are evaluated and a grade provided. Once again, CAP initiated this protocol many years before CLIA '67. The rules are now set by the government, although there is some freedom to work within them. The best programs provide an educational experience as part of the exercises. NCCLS has provided guidance for improving laboratory performance through proficiency testing.[78] If an external source for proficiency testing samples is not available for an analyte, another method for assessing performance must be developed in the laboratory. A variety of methods exists, including exchanging samples between laboratories and constructing a panel of challenges within the laboratory.[81]

In CLIA '88 some seemingly obvious rules were codified: the protocol for proficiency tests must be as close to that used for clinical specimens as feasible (including the use of the same testing personnel) and laboratory personnel cannot compare results before submitting the answers—in other words, no cheating!

Personnel Qualifications. Detailed specifications for personnel at all levels are provided in the CLIA '88 regulations for laboratories that perform nonwaived testing.

Procedure Manuals. Although there is not a rigid prescription for preparation of written policies and procedures, some general principles must be followed.[82] Policies must be clearly stated—and followed. Procedures should include the principle of the test and references as well as instructions for performance. Manuals must be available to all workers who will need to refer to them.

Space Requirements. The regulations do not specify detailed space requirements. Rather they indicate that the space must be adequate to perform the work satisfactorily. Informal guidelines for general laboratories[75] and for microbiology laboratories[120] have been described, however; they can serve as a useful guide when constructing a new facility or evaluating the adequacy of an existing laboratory.

Reference or Referral Laboratories. It is a rare laboratory that will be able to fulfill all the requests made by clinicians. Some specimens must be sent to a specialized laboratory for further testing.[76] Selection of the referral laboratory or laboratories should not be done casually. The available choices should be evaluated carefully in conjunction with the medical staff as appropriate. Price is not the only determinant, or even the most important factor. The selection should be reviewed on a regular basis.

Patient Confidentiality. The Health Insurance Portability and Accountability Act of 1996 (HIPAA) provides safeguards for the confidentiality of information and allows patients to have access to their medical records. For the laboratory, however, CLIA '88 regulations supersede the HIPAA requirements. Laboratory results may be released to authorized individuals—the person who requested the test or who is responsible for using the results. In some jurisdictions laboratories may accept requests for testing directly from patients.

Risk Management

Most health-care facilities are currently involved in risk management. In fact, many hospitals and clinics have established formal risk management offices, fully funded and staffed, to help reduce to a minimum the chances for accidents and high-risk practices that might cause harm to employees and patients alike. Although the major impetus for this practice may be directed toward reducing costly workers'' compensation claims and malpractice suits, in a larger sense risk management efforts are to help ensure a safe working environment and an atmosphere in which patients can receive the latest that medical technology has to offer, without fear of being harmed.[97]

Working in conjunction with the quality assurance committee, a risk manager is assigned to investigate cases in which quality management falls below the established thresholds or situations in which employees or patients may be at undue risk. After reviewing the details of the situation with the appropriate representatives of the department involved and after gathering the necessary data, the risk manager submits a condensed report to the quality assurance committee along with recommendations for corrective actions. A dialogue continues between the risk manager and the committee chairman until an appropriate plan of action is agreed upon. The department's compliance with the corrective action plans is then monitored.

Although the major focus of risk management is directed toward patient care, the clinical laboratory participates in seeing that all laboratory operations are in compliance with the overall practices and policies of the institution. If equipment or instruments are damaged because of fire or electrical accidents, if personnel are injured, or if workers contract serious laboratory-acquired infections, work flow may be disrupted laboratory reports may be delayed. Thus, for the most part, laboratory risk management is related to implementing and monitoring laboratory safety practices, directed more to employees than to patients. Liability for injury clearly rests with the employer, even though the negligence leading to the injury is that of a fellow worker.[50] For this reason risk managers are insistent on conducting safety-oriented education courses and seeing that all rules and regulations pertaining to laboratory safety are both implemented and followed.

The other major area that is of increasing concern to risk managers is financial. There are strict regulations covering conflicts of interest, fraudulent billing, and unlawful enticements for business (such as kickbacks). Billing of government programs (Medicare and Medicaid) must utilize a set of test codes, called Current Procedural Terminology (CPT) codes. Most other insurers also utilize these codes. They are revised and published yearly by the AMA, which has been charged by the government with this task. Input into the construction of the codes can be provided by any person or organization, but the operative committee of the AMA is drawn from its constituent societies. In the field of laboratory medicine these are CAP and American Society for Clinical Pathology (ASCP).

Laboratory Safety

Although it is the legal responsibility of hospital and laboratory managers to provide for a safe working environment, employees must also bear the responsibility for adhering to safety standards outlined in the Laboratory Safety Manual, to bring to the attention of the supervisor any hazards or potential hazards that may be encountered during work activities, and to seek immediate medical attention for any potentially job-related injury.[50]

One person in the laboratory should be designated the safety officer, whose duties are to see that safety standards and guidelines are written and published, that employees are informed of these standards through regularly scheduled laboratory safety courses and in-service briefings, and that a system is in place to monitor compliance. The safety officer will work closely with the hospital risk manager to reconcile and correct any breaches of conduct or any irregularities discovered.

GENERAL SAFETY RULES AND REGULATIONS

Laboratory workers are advised not to take unnecessary risks. Carelessness, negligence, and unsafe practices may result in serious injuries, not only to the individual, but to coworkers and patients as well. The following are general considerations that will make working in microbiology laboratories less of a risk.[73] Each laboratory director is responsible for ensuring that laboratory policies and procedures follow current legal requirements (federal, state, and local) and standards of good laboratory practice.

1. Each employee should be instructed on the location and operation of all safety equipment and facilities, such as fire blankets, fire extinguishers, showers,

and eye wash fountains. Each of these must be readily accessible in the laboratory.

2. Personal protective equipment (surgical gloves, lab coats, etc.) should be worn when indicated. Laboratory coats should be worn (with buttons closed) at all times while in the laboratory, and removed when leaving the laboratory. Masks that are individually fitted for each individual must be used for some manipulations that might result in the generation of infectious aerosols with important pathogens, such as *Mycobacterium tuberculosis.*

3. Personal habits and grooming must be put in perspective. Long hair must be tied such that it will not interfere with equipment or reagents. Application of cosmetics in the work area is prohibited. Sandals and open style shoes do not afford proper foot protection and are not acceptable. Smoking is prohibited in the laboratory. Fingers, pencils, and other implements do not belong in the mouth. Horseplay and practical jokes should not be tolerated.

4. Contact lenses, especially the soft type, absorb certain solvents and may be a hazard after splashes and spills. Employees are strongly advised not to wear contact lenses in the laboratory, or to wear safety glasses when working with caustic or infective materials.

5. Eating or storing food and beverages in the laboratory or in refrigerators used for specimens or laboratory materials is not permitted. A refrigerator should be designated specifically to store food and drink.

6. Pipetting by mouth of any material is absolutely prohibited. A variety of suitable pipetting aids are available.

7. Laboratory personnel with current skin infections, acute respiratory infections, or other contagious diseases should avoid patient contact.

8. It is important that laboratory workers know the characteristics of all materials in use, so appropriate precautions can be taken during use and during disposal. The manufacturer is required to provide this information in material safety data sheets (MSDS). These sheets should be easily available to everyone in the laboratory.

9. Appropriate labels and signs must be placed on all specimens or instruments and in all areas of the laboratory where they are necessary for maintenance of a safe work environment.

10. Types and levels of decontamination are summarized in Table 1-19. It is important to match the type of disinfection or sterilization to the biohazard.[18,19,119]

ROUTINE SAFETY PRECAUTIONS
Centrifugation

1. Before centrifuging any item, check tubes, vials, or bottles for cracks. Periodically replace the rubber cushions in the bottoms of the trunnions and remove any broken glass that may have accumulated.

2. Make sure that the centrifuge is properly balanced before use. Check the trunnion rings and tube carriers to be sure the weights match.

3. Wait for the centrifuge to come to a complete stop before opening the lid to remove samples. Use only the braking device to bring the rotation to a more rapid and complete stop.

4. Should breakage of a tube occur in the centrifuge, first turn off the instrument, wait at least 20 minutes before opening the lid, and, after donning mask and gloves, thoroughly clean and disinfect the inside of the centrifuge.

5. As part of the routine maintenance program, each centrifuge should be thoroughly cleaned with a suitable disinfectant on each day of use. Preventive maintenance of all working parts should be on a regular schedule as appropriate.

6. If potentially infectious material is centrifuged, the specimen must be placed in a closed carrier (sealed dome centrifuge tubes).

Needles and Glassware

1. Discard all chipped or cracked glassware in appropriate containers.

2. Pick up broken glass with a brush and pan; do not use hands.

3. Glass articles should not be discarded in the sink or loosely in a wastebasket where paper articles are being discarded. They can cut the fingers and hands of individuals removing the refuge. They should be placed in a container designed for sharp objects.

4. Used needles and lancets (sharps) must be placed into appropriate used-needle containers for safe disposal. These sharps containers should be replaced periodically; they should be monitored to prevent overfilling.

5. Avoid removing needles or exchanging needles on syringes as much as possible. The practice of changing needles before discharging venepuncture blood into blood culture bottles has been abandoned in most hospitals.

Electrical Safety

1. All personnel must know the location of master switches and circuit breaker boards. Do not attempt to repair any instrument while it is still plugged in.

2. Plugs or cords that are broken, frayed, or worn should not be used.

3. Outlets must not be overloaded. Never use gang-type plugs.

4. All cord and plug-type electrical equipment should have grounded power cords and plugs. All shocks, including small tingles, must be immediately investigated.

5. Extension cords should be used only in compliance with the overall hospital policies and procedures.

Table 1-19 Types of Decontamination, Disinfection, and Sterilization*

LEVEL*	EPA/FDA CATEGORY	CDC CATEGORY	EXAMPLE	TYPE OF ORGANISMS	EXAMPLES
1	Hospital disinfectant	Low-level disinfectant	Quaternary ammonium compounds	Vegetative bacteria	*Staphylococcus* spp. *Pseudomonas* spp.
				Enveloped or midsized viruses	Human immunodeficiency virus Herpes simplex virus Hepatitis viruses B & C Coronavirus
2	Hospital disinfectant with tuberculocidal claim	Intermediate-level disinfectant	Quaternary ammonium compounds with alcohol; phenolics; iodophors; chlorine containing products	Fungi	*Aspergillus* spp. *Candida* spp.
				Nonlipid or small viruses	Enteroviruses Rhinoviruses
				Mycobacteria	*Mycobacterium tuberculosis*
3	Sterilant/high-level disinfectant	High-level disinfectant	Glutaraldehyde; hydrogen peroxide	Bacterial spores	*Bacillus* spp.
4	Sterilization	Sterilization	Ethylene oxide; autoclave	All agents	

* Agents at each level are also effective against organisms killed by agents in lower levels. Prions require separate consideration; consult reference[99]. Adapted from references[18,19].

Corridor Cautions

1. Open doors into corridors with caution. Watch out for swinging doors. If there is a window in the door, look out to be certain the way is clear before opening the doors.
2. Keep to the right when approaching corridor intersections and when using stairways. Walk, never run, in halls, rooms, and stairwells. Appropriately placed mirrors provide images of potential traffic on crossing corridors.
3. Watch for hall hazards such as beds, carts, or tables. Watch out for articles on the floor, such as paper clips, electrical cords, loose tiles, and spilled liquids. Only one side of the corridor should be used for the temporary storage of movable equipment.

Lifting

1. Back injuries are among the most frequent causes of debilitating illness among personnel. Avoid lifting heavy objects when possible. Always get help.
2. If you must lift objects alone, exercise the following precautions:

a. Have a good footing. Keep feet about 10 inches apart.
b. Bend at the knees to grasp the object.
c. Keep the object close to you and get a firm hold.
d. Keep the arms and back as straight as possible and lift gradually upward by straightening the legs.

Handling Specimens and Spills

1. Specimens should be collected in sturdy containers with adequate closure to prevent spillage or leakage. All specimens must be considered a potential hazard.
2. Cuts on hands should be adequately covered with adhesive bandages. Wear disposable gloves if the work activity involves contact with blood, serum, plasma, other fluids, or tissues.
3. If a sample shows evidence of breakage, leakage, or soiling inside a specimen container, put on gloves and transfer as much of the specimen as possible to a second sterile container. Also rewrite any pertinent information from the old onto the new container.

4. Blood-contaminated specimen requisitions should be rejected. Handle such a requisition only with gloves if processing is necessary in an emergency. Notify the requestor that such contaminated materials present a health hazard.

5. Wash hands thoroughly with soap and water several times a day and, particularly, after handling specimens before leaving for a coffee or lunch break.

6. Spills must be handled according to the nature of the material involved.

Handling of Wastes and Hazardous Material

1. Set aside certain sinks in the laboratory to dispose of blood or urine specimens. Hand washing should not be allowed in these sinks.

2. Biohazard bags (so labeled) must be used to dispose of all potentially contaminated samples—blood tubes, specimen containers, pipettes, pipette tips, reaction vessels, stoppers, and such. Leave sufficient room at the top so that the bag can be easily closed and secured with an elastic band. It is good practice to double bag hazardous waste.

3. Dispose of glassware and sharps in appropriate hard-walled containers. When filled, such containers should be sealed with tape and placed in appropriate labeled waste boxes for proper disposal.

4. Remove filled biohazard bags to designated waste areas as frequently during the day as necessary to avoid buildup.

5. Immerse contaminated reusable glassware into disinfectant solution. Thoroughly rinse with water and autoclave before reusing.

6. At the end of each day or after a spill all work surfaces must be disinfected with an agent that is effective against the agents expected at that site. All equipment that is removed from the laboratory should be decontaminated first. In addition, laminar flow safety cabinets must be decontaminated (preferably by a technician certified in care of this equipment) before any maintenance is done or filters changed.

BIOLOGIC AGENTS

Classification of Biologic Agents. The CDC and National Institutes of Health have categorized infectious organisms into risk groups,[99] which are summarized in Table 1-20 The document can be ordered from the government printing office or downloaded from the internet: (http://www.cdc.gov/od/ohs/biosfty/bmbl4/bmbl4toc.htm).

Physical Containment of Biohazards. The physical barriers to infection in the laboratory are either personal or institutional. The personal barriers include good hygiene (e.g., separate facilities for food or for hand washing) and protective equipment (e.g., splash shields, goggles, gloves, gowns, and masks). Institutional barriers are structural (e.g., isolated facilities, doors, and locks) and technological (e.g., air handling and filtration). Biological safety cabinets (BSC) are a critical component of protection for workers. It is important to recognize that BSC and chemical hoods serve very different purposes. It is possible to construct a BSC that can be used as a chemical hood, but only certain types of BSC should be used for chemicals and chemical hoods should not be used for infectious agents.

The classification of BSCs is summarized in Table 1-21 and depicted in Figures 1-21 through 1-25. Most clinical laboratories use Type II A BSCs for processing of specimens and for work with isolates, especially those that present an aerosol hazard. Type I hoods are rarely used today; type III hoods are not commonly employed in diagnostic laboratories. In the Class II and III cabinets air is directed across the work surface from the top of the cabinet in a laminar fashion, minimizing contamination of the samples from aerosolized agents. These devices are sometimes referred to as laminar flow safety cabinets. The downward laminar flow also protects the work from unfiltered air that is drawn in through the front portal in the Class II cabinets; the front intake air is directed by the laminar flow into the sump below the work surface where it is filtered before eventually joining the downward laminar flow.

The velocity of the airflow in Class I and II BSCs must be validated by a certified technician at least yearly or whenever repair work is done. The cabinet must be decontaminated by a certified technician before any manipulations that require compromise of the contaminated area are undertaken (e.g., changing filters, replacing or repairing motors, or moving the cabinet).

Common infectious hazards in diagnostic laboratories: Although most agents encountered in a clinical laboratory have the potential for causing diseases in laboratory workers, a relatively small number fulfill that potential. Miller and associates[66] describe a 25-year experience of laboratory-acquired human infections at the National Animal Disease Center (NADC) in Ames, Iowa, an institution where research on domestic diseases of livestock and poultry is conducted. The level of risk among workers is probably somewhat greater than in the average clinical laboratory. From 1960 to 1985, 128 laboratory exposures to zoonotic organisms were reported at NADC. Thirty-four laboratory-associated infections resulted. Brucellosis accounted for 47% of the cases, leptospirosis for 27%, and mycobacteriosis for 9%. Salmonella spp. and Chlamydia spp., Newcastle disease virus (not a human pathogen), and *Trichophyton* spp. accounted for the other laboratory-acquired infections at NADC.

The 10 most frequent laboratory-acquired infections from accumulated studies are 1) brucellosis, 2) Q-fever, 3) typhoid fever, 4) tularemia, 5) tuberculosis, 6) typhus, 7) infectious hepatitis, 8) Venezuelan equine encephalitis, 9) coccidioidomycosis, and 10) psittacosis.[90,91,92,118] Some of these infections are difficult to prevent, although zero infections should always be the goal. In some circumstances, however, a means to prevent the infection is not hard to see, at least in retrospect. For instance, a 22-year-old medical technology student contracted typhoid fever with complications after working with *Salmonella typhi* as an unknown organism.[44] Even worse, 22% of the technologists in a laboratory developed gastroenteritis from *Shigella sonnei*. Typing of the isolate revealed that all the strains were identical to one that

Table 1-20 Classification of Biologic Agents by Risk*

BIOSAFETY LEVEL (BSL)	CLASS OF AGENTS	EXAMPLES OF AGENTS	PRACTICES	SAFETY EQUIPMENT (PRIMARY BARRIERS)	FACILITIES (SECONDARY BARRIERS)
1	Not known to cause disease consistently in healthy adults		Standard microbiological practices	None required	Open bench top sink required
2	Associated with human disease Hazard = percutaneous injury, ingestion, or mucous membrane exposure	*Enterobacteriaceae* *Candida* spp. *Mycobacterium avium* complex Herpes simplex virus	BSL-1 plus: • Limited access • Biohazard warning signs • "Sharps" precautions • Biosafety manual defining any waste decontamination or medical surveillance practices	Class I or II BSCs or other physical containment devices used for all manipulations of agents that cause splashes or aerosols of infectious materials PPEs: laboratory coats, gloves, face protection as needed	BSL-1 plus: • Autoclave available
3	Indigenous or exotic agents with potential for aerosol transmission Disease may have serious or lethal consequences	*Mycobacterium tuberculosis* *Franciscella tularensis* West Nile virus	BSL-2 practices plus: • Controlled access • Decontamination of all waste • Decontamination of lab clothing before laundering • Baseline serum	Class I or II BSCs or other physical containment devices used for all manipulations of agents that cause splashes or aerosols of infectious materials PPEs: laboratory coats, gloves, face protection as needed	BSL-2 plus: • Physical separation from access corridors • Self-closing, double-door access • Exhausted air not recirculated • Negative airflow into laboratory
4	Dangerous or exotic agents which pose high risk of life-threatening diseases, aerosol-transmitted laboratory infections Or related agents with unknown risk of transmission	Arenaviruses that produce hemorrhagic fever (e.g., Lassa, Junin, Machupo) Filoviruses that produce hemorrhagic fever (e.g., Marburg, Ebola)	BSL-3 practices plus: • Clothing change on entering • Shower on exit • All material decontaminated on exit from facility	All procedures conducted in Class III BSCs or Class I or II BSCs in combination with full-body, air-supplied, positive pressure personnel suit	BSL-3 plus: • Separate building or isolated zone • Dedicated supply and exhaust, vacuum, and decon systems • Other requirements listed in Reference[99]

BSL = Biosafety level; BSC = Biological safety cabinet; PPE = Personal protective equipment.
* The safety level of many agents is increased when manipulations that might reasonably be expected to generate aerosols are performed or when large volumes of materials are employed. For some Level 2 agents a higher level is indicated when cultures known to contain the agent are manipulated. A separate classification is used for agents in naturally or experimentally infected animals.
Adapted from reference[99].

had been given to a student as an unknown.[64] Some agents that would not be encountered in a clinical laboratory may cause infection in research workers,[22,43,4] sometimes when manipulations that produce aerosols are performed without adequate containment.

UNIVERSAL PRECAUTIONS

Ironically, laboratory workers are at considerably less risk of acquiring infections than are their clinical colleagues. There are several reasons for this phenomenon. Patients sneeze and cough; culture plates do not. Unless procedures

Table 1-21 Comparison of Biological Safety Cabinets

TYPE	FACE VELOCITY (LFPM)	AIRFLOW PATTERN	RADIONUCLIDES/ TOXIC CHEMICALS	BIOSAFETY LEVELS	PRODUCT (SPECIMEN) PROTECTION
Class 1 Open front	75	In at front; rear and top through HEPA filter (Figure 1-21)	No	2, 3	No
Class II Type A	75	70% recirculated through HEPA filter; exhaust through HEPA filter (Figure 1-22)	No	2, 3	Yes
Class II Type B1	100	30% recirculated through HEPA filter; exhaust via HEPA filter and hard ducted (Figure 1-23)	Yes (low levels/volatility)	2, 3	Yes
Class II Type B2	100	No recirculation; total exhaust via HEPA filter and hard ducted (Figure 1-24)	Yes	2, 3	Yes
Class II Type B3	100	Same as IIA, but plena under negative pressure to room and exhaust air is ducted	Yes	2, 3	Yes
Class III	NA	Supply air inlets and exhaust through 2 HEPA filters (Figure 1-25)	Yes	3, 4	Yes

Lfpm = linear feet per minute; HEPA = high energy particulate.
From reference[99].

that produce large aerosols are performed in the laboratory, the risk for workers is relatively low. Physicians and nurses are much more likely to use sharp objects, such as instruments and needles than are laboratory personnel. In modern medicine the greatest infectious risks are blood-borne pathogens. Once again, it is ironic that microbiology workers are at lower risk than colleagues in other areas of the laboratory, such as chemistry and hematology, where large numbers of blood specimens are handled daily. The most important laboratory infections are human immunodeficiency virus (HIV), hepatitis B virus, and hepatitis C virus. Of these agents hepatitis C virus is the most prevalent in most hospitals, because an effective vaccine is available for hepatitis B virus and the incidence of HIV in the general population is low. It is fortunate that an effective vaccine for hepatitis B virus exists, because the risk of an unimmunized worker contracting this infection is far greater than infection with hepatitis C virus or HIV.

Recommendations for minimizing blood-borne infections have been promulgated by CDC[14–17], by the NCCLS,[79] and by laboratory workers.[8]

The risks of contracting the major blood-borne pathogens are summarized in Table 1-22.[17]

It is usually not possible to predict in advance those individuals who are likely sources of risk, so the concept of **universal precautions** has arisen. That is, every specimen is considered a risk. Specifying some specimens as risky increases the possibility that a false sense of security will be engendered.

The CDC and OSHA have established the following universal precautions:[12]

1. Blood and body fluids from all patients must be handled as infectious material. All patients should be assumed to be infectious for HIV and other blood-borne pathogens.
2. All specimens of blood and body fluids should be put in a well-constructed container, with a secure lid, to prevent leaking during transport.
3. All persons who process blood and body fluid specimens (e.g., removing tops from vacuum tubes) should wear gloves—plus a face shield (or a mask with glasses or goggles)—if blood or body fluids are expected to splatter.
4. Workers must change gloves and wash hands when finished processing specimens.
5. Workers should never pipette by mouth; they must use mechanical devices.
6. Use of needles and syringes should be limited to situations in which there is no alternative.
7. Laboratory work surfaces should be decontaminated with an appropriate chemical germicide after a spill of blood or other body fluids and when work activities are completed.
8. Contaminated materials used in laboratory tests should be decontaminated before reprocessing or be placed in bags and disposed of in accordance with institutional policies.
9. All persons should wash their hands after completing laboratory activities and should remove protective clothing before leaving the laboratory.

The recommendations for dealing with exposures vary by agent; recommendations are reviewed regularly by CDC

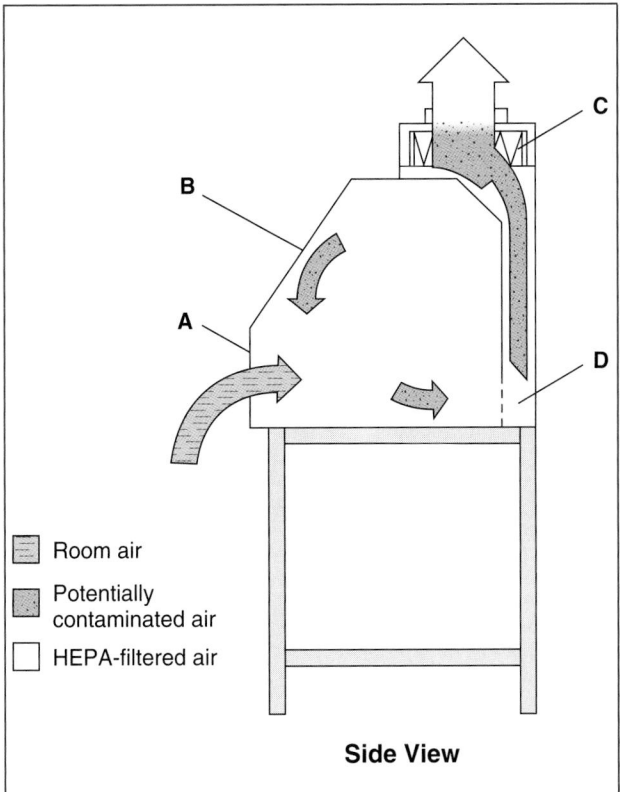

Figure 1-21 Design of class I biological safety cabinet. These negative pressure cabinets draw air from the room into the cabinet at a velocity of 75 lfpm and exhaust it through a HEPA filter to the room or to the outside through a duct. It does not protect the specimen or sample from contamination with material present in room air. It may be used for toxic or radiologic chemicals only if it is vented to the outside. Adapted from reference [99].

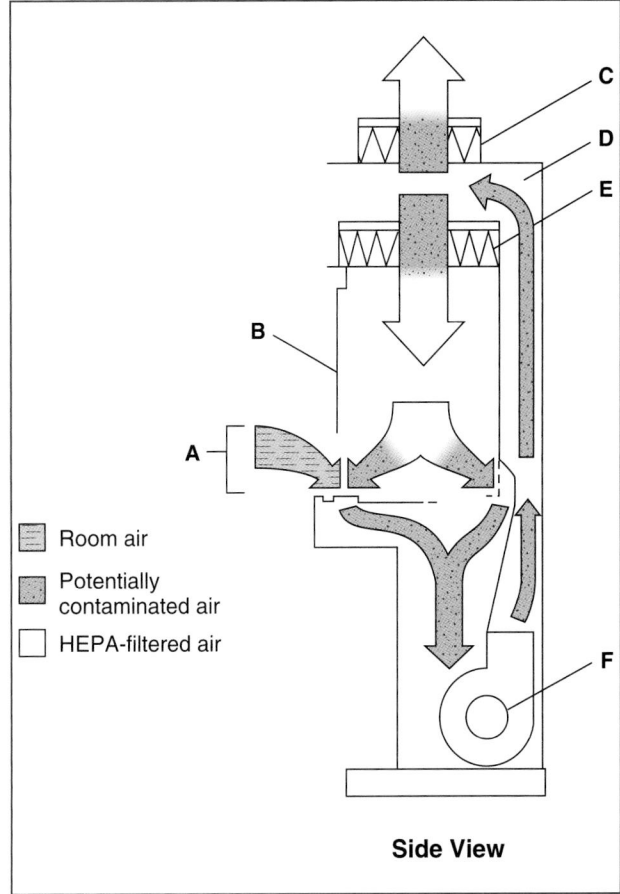

Figure 1-22 Design of class II A biological safety cabinet. Air is drawn from the room into the cabinet through the front opening (A), typically at a velocity of 75 lfpm. It is then recirculated through a plenum (D) and a HEPA filter; a portion of the air, typically 70%, is recirculated into the workspace; the remainder is exhausted through the HEPA filter (C) to the room. If the remainder is exhausted through a negative pressure plenum to the outside of the building, the cabinet is classified as class III B3. The work can be viewed through a glass sash (B). Adapted from reference [99].

and altered as necessary. In general, the source patient should be tested to determine if a risk exists and the injured worker should be followed to determine if infection has resulted. Postexposure immunization and/or prophylactic antiviral chemotherapy are appropriate in certain situations. It must be emphasized strongly that primary attention should be given to prevention, so that the problem of an accident never presents itself. Prevention can take the form of immunizing at-risk personnel and minimizing the exposure to ''sharps'' (needles, scalpel blades, broken glass, etc.), which are the most common sources of injury.

Cleaning Spills of Infectious Materials. The recommended protocol for cleaning up skills of infectious material is:[79]

1. Wear gloves (preferably heavy-weight, puncture-resistant utility gloves), gowns, and masks.
2. If there are fragments of glass or other objects, they should be removed without touching them directly before proceeding.
3. Wear shoe covers that are impermeable to water if the spill is large.
4. Cover the spill with absorbent material and add con-

centrated disinfectant. After waiting ten minutes, proceed with cleanup.

5. If aerosols may have been generated, as in a broken centrifuge tube, turn the centrifuge off but leave it closed for at least 30 minutes to allow any aerosols to settle.
6. Absorb the bulk of the spill with disposable materials before proceeding with disinfection.
7. Clean the spill site of all visible contaminating material with an aqueous detergent solution or a 10% solution of household bleach.
8. Decontaminate the site with an appropriate disinfectant (see Table 1-19).
9. Absorb the disinfectant material and rinse the site with water. Dry the site a final time to prevent slipping.
10. Dispose of all materials in a biohazard container.

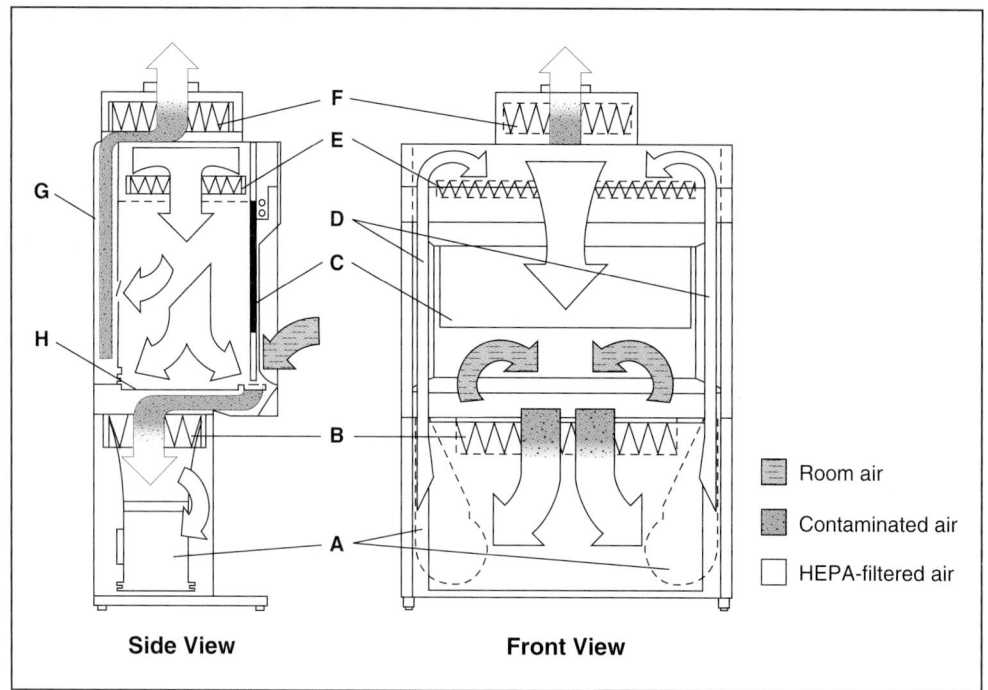

Figure 1-23 Design of Class II B1 biological safety cabinet. Air enters the cabinet from the room through the front opening at a velocity of 100 lfpm. It is then recirculated (typically 30%) through a sump (A) and recirculating plenum (D), passing through HEPA filters (B and E) before being exhausted (G) through a HEPA filter (F) into negative pressure ducts to the outside. Because of minimal recirculation limited quantities of low-level chemicals can be used in addition to biologic agents. The work can be viewed through a glass sash (C). Adapted from reference [99].

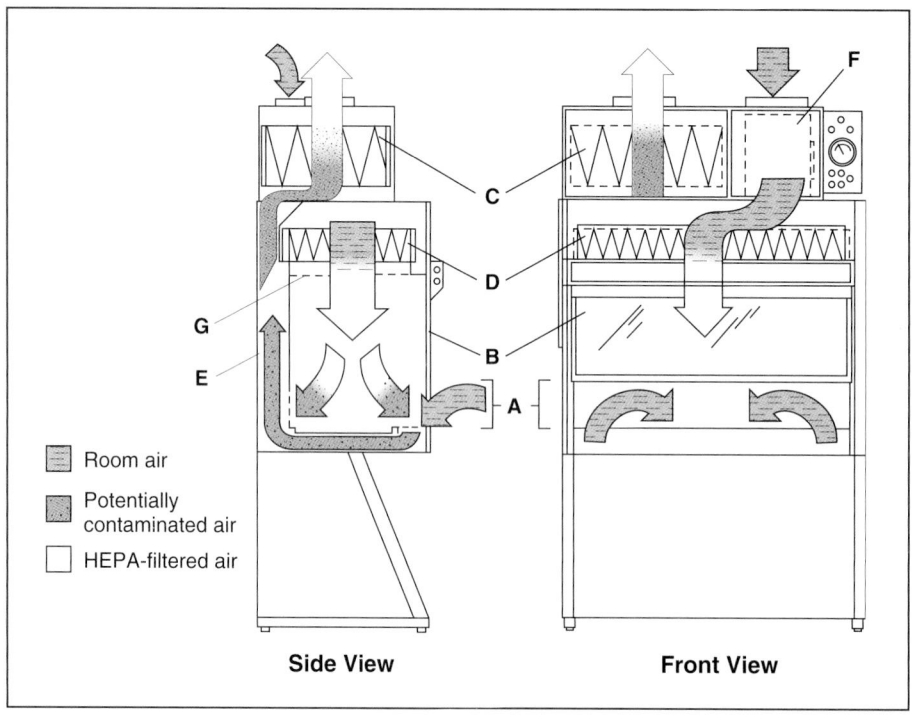

Figure 1-24 Design of Class II B2 biological safety cabinet. Air enters the cabinet from the room through the front opening (A) and is drawn into a cabinet plenum (E) before being exhausted to the outside through a HEPA filter (C) and a negative pressure duct system. Simultaneously room air enters the cabinet through a second portal (F) and a HEPA filter (D), after which it passes down across the work area and then joins the outflow stream in the cabinet plenum (E). The work can be viewed through a glass sash (B). Toxic chemicals can be used in this cabinet that recirculates no air. Adapted from reference [99].

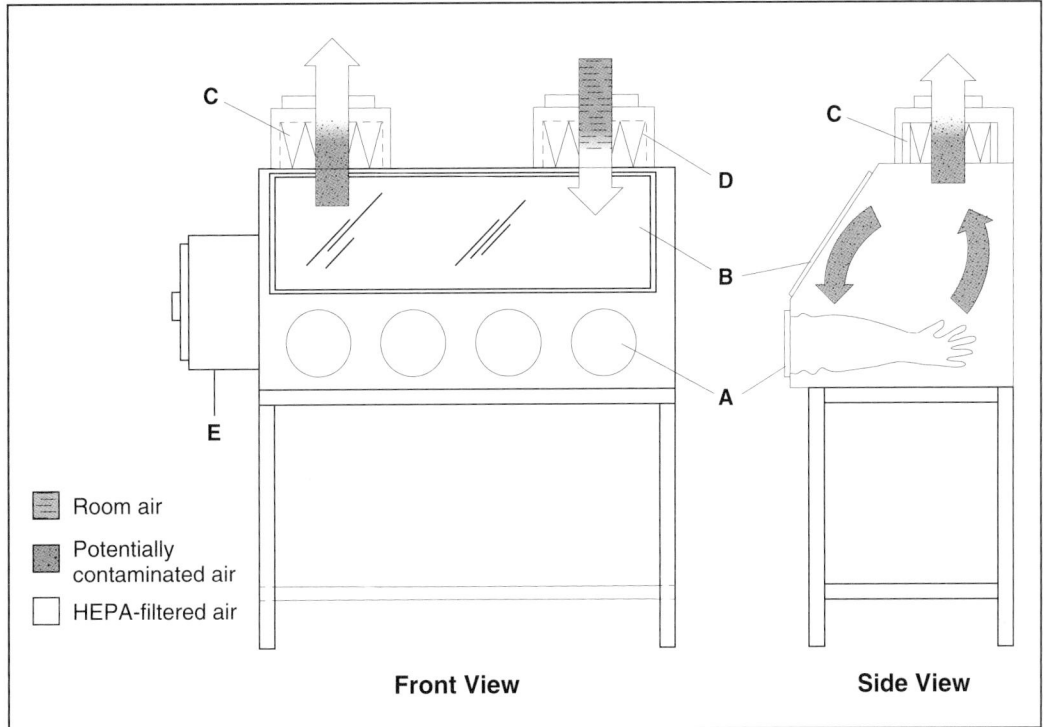

Figure 1-25 Design of Class III biological safety cabinet. This cabinet functions as a totally enclosed glove box with recirculating air. The hazardous agents are totally contained within the box, so the worker is not exposed. The same effect can be achieved if a Class II cabinet is used in conjunction with a biological suit connected to an air supply for the worker, essentially putting the worker into the box. Air enters through a portal and HEPA filter (D) before exhausting out through a HEPA filter (C) into a negative pressure duct system and the outside environment. The worker manipulates the samples through sealed gloves (A) and views the work through a glass shield (B). Samples are passed into the box through an interlock (E). The disadvantages of this approach include the difficulty of performing fine manipulations through thick rubber gloves, but expensive ''space suit'' systems for protection of the worker are less essential. Adapted from reference [99].

If a BSL-3 agent is spilled outside of a biological safety cabinet, evacuate the area for at least sixty minutes, and notify the appropriate authorities.

SHIPPING OF SPECIMENS AND ETIOLOGIC AGENTS

All microbiology specimens to be transported through the United States mail must be packaged under strict regulations specified by the Department of Transportation (DOT) and the International Air Transport Association (IATA). Isolated organisms (etiologic agents) other than biosafety level 1 (see Table 1-20) and diagnostic specimens reasonably expected to contain those etiologic agents must be appropriately packaged and labeled.

Specimens must be prepared to withstand shocks or pressure changes that may occur during handling and cause the

Table 1-22 Risks of Contracting Certain Blood-Borne Viral Infections After Needle Stick Exposure to Blood*

VIRUS	STATUS OF SOURCE PATIENT	OUTCOME	RISK
Hepatitis B	Positive for HBsAg and HBeAg	Clinical hepatitis	22–31%
	Positive for HBsAg and negative for HBeAg	Clinical hepatitis	1–6%
		Seroconversion	23–37%
Hepatitis C	Seropositive	Seroconversion	0–7%
HIV	Seropositive	Seroconversion	0.3%

The risk after contact of blood with mucous membranes is less well defined, but less than after needle sticks.
Data from reference[17].

contents to leak. A leaking container not only predisposes the specimen to potential contamination, but may also expose handlers or personnel at the receiving site to pathogenic agents. Figure 1-26 illustrates the proper packaging and labeling of etiologic agents. The primary container (test tube, vial) must be fitted with a watertight cap and surrounded by sufficient packing material to absorb the fluid contents should a leak occur. In turn, this container is placed in a water-tight secondary container, preferably constructed of metal, fitted with a screw-cap lid. The primary and secondary containers are then enclosed in an outer shipping carton constructed of corrugated fiberboard, cardboard, or Styrofoam.

Dry ice is considered a hazardous material. A shipping carton containing dry ice as a refrigerant for a specimen must be marked **"DRY ICE FROZEN MEDICAL SPECIMEN."** The packaging should be such that carbon dioxide gas can escape, preventing a buildup of pressure that could rupture the container. The dry ice should be placed outside the secondary container along with shock-absorbent material in such a manner that the secondary container does not become loose inside the outer container as the dry ice sublimates.

In addition to the address label, the outer container must also have the etiologic agents/biomedical material label (with its red logo against a white background) affixed as well as a notice to the carrier, as illustrated in Figure 1-27.

NONBIOLOGIC HAZARDS
Chemicals

1. A chemical hygiene plan should be constructed for the laboratory.[73] Guidelines for managing laboratory waste are available.[83]
2. Flash point: volatile combustible substances give off vapors along the surface of the liquid. The flash point is the lowest possible temperature at which a sufficient concentration of vapors is produced for a flame to occur. Volatile substances are collectively referred to as ignitables. The classification based on flash points and boiling points is:
   a. Flammables
      1) Class IA: Flash point, <73°F (22°C); boiling point, <100°F (38°C)
      2) Class IB: Flash point, <73°F (22°C); boiling point, >100°F (38°C)
      3) Class IC: Flash point, >72°F (21°C) and <100°F (38°C)

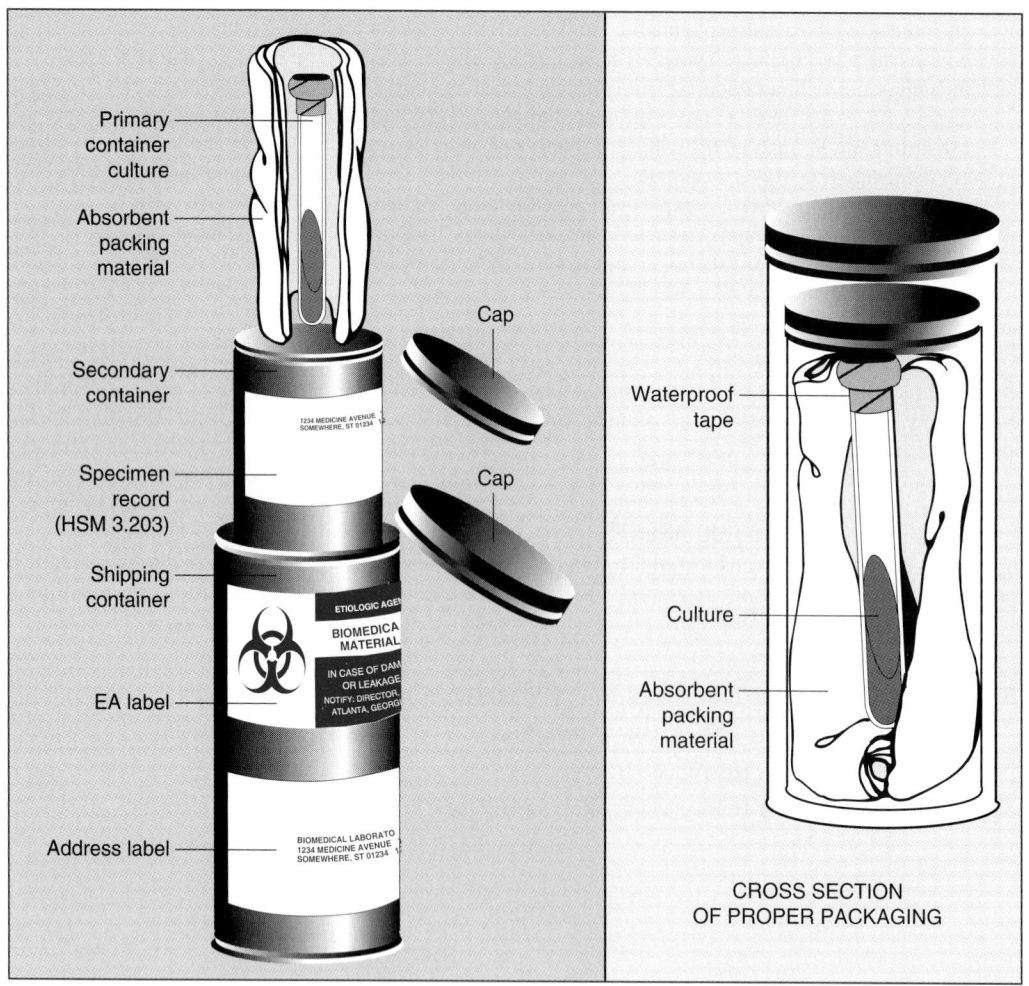

Figure 1-26 Proper technique for packaging of biologically hazardous materials.

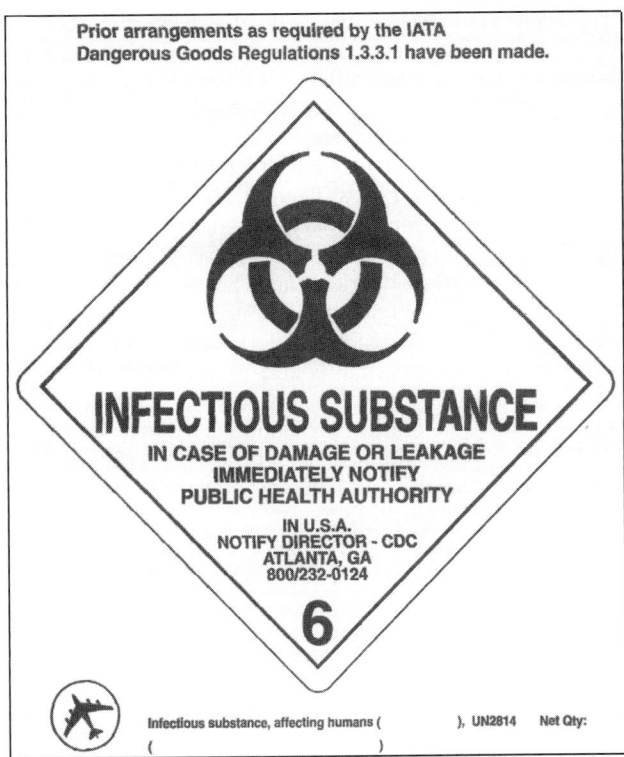

Prior arrangements as required by the IATA Dangerous Goods Regulations 1.3.3.1 have been made.

INFECTIOUS SUBSTANCE

IN CASE OF DAMAGE OR LEAKAGE IMMEDIATELY NOTIFY PUBLIC HEALTH AUTHORITY

IN U.S.A.
NOTIFY DIRECTOR - CDC
ATLANTA, GA
800/232-0124

6

Infectious substance, affecting humans (   ), UN2814   Net Qty:
(   )

Figure 1-27 Etiologic agents logo and "notice to carrier" that must be affixed to the outside of any package containing potentially hazardous or infectious materials.

b. Combustibles:
   1) Class IIIA: Flash point, >140°F (60°C) and <200°F (94°C)
   2) Class IIIB: Flash point, >200°F (94°C)

A number of combustible materials may be found in the microbiology laboratory, although not in the quantities that are used in some other areas. A particular hazard is diethyl ether, which can form explosive peroxides after exposure to air. Ether has been used in some parasitology concentration procedures. Other alternatives that eliminate this hazard are now available. If it is necessary to use ether, the smallest quantity possible should be stored appropriately.

3. Corrosive chemicals are defined as agents that have a pH <2.1 or >12.5 or that can corrode steel (SAE 1020) more than 0.25 inches per year at a temperature of 130°F. In the laboratory the most common corrosives are strong acids, such as hydrochloric acid. Acid bottle carriers must be used for concentrated acids in quantities greater than 500 ml.
4. Incompatible chemicals (identified from MSDS) must not be used or stored together.
5. Storage safety cans and cabinets must be located away from sources of heat, flame, sparks, and exits. Storage areas should be adequately ventilated and of limited access to personnel.
6. All containers should be clearly labeled with
   a. Content
   b. Hazard warnings

c. Special precautions
d. Date received/prepared
e. Date opened/put in use
f. Expiration date
g. Manufacturer

7. In case of a liquid chemical spill[83,73]:
   a. Determine the nature of the hazard, consulting the MSDS if necessary. If the spill is an emergency, evacuate the area. If the material is a fire hazard, eliminate all sources of ignition.
   b. Notify the appropriate personnel and obtain additional help if necessary. Identify any need for personal protective devices.
   c. Confine the spill to as small an area as possible.
   d. Neutralize acids with disodium carbonate. Neutralize alkalis with 1% boric acid. For larger amounts of acids or bases, flush with large amounts of water after neutralization.
   e. Clean any areas that have been splashed by the spill.
   f. For flammable and toxic liquid spills, use an absorbent to reduce the vapor pressure and prevent possible ignition of the liquid.

8. Disposal of chemicals:
   a. Wear rubber gloves, a rubber apron, and goggles.
   b. Remove all items from the sink designated for disposal. Start a nonsplashing stream of cold water into the sink.
   c. Slowly pour the liquid as close to the drain as possible without splashing. Only quantities less than 500 mL can be disposed of in the sink drain.
   d. Continue to run cold water for several minutes after completion.
   e. Dispose of water-soluble organic solvents (methanol, acetone) as described in the foregoing. For water-insoluble organic liquids, only quantities less than 100 mL can be disposed of as just described. For quantities over 100 mL, consult with the hospital safety officer or the local Environmental Health and Safety Office.

9. Radiologic hazards: Formerly, clinical laboratories used radiochemicals, primarily for immunoassays. These procedures have been almost completely replaced by enzyme immunoassays. If any radioactive materials are used in the laboratory, appropriate regulations must be strictly followed. There is usually an institutional safety officer for radioactive materials, often in the Department of Radiology.

10. Carcinogens: Careful attention to safety issues is necessary for those chemicals that have been shown to have some neoplastic potential, sometimes only in laboratory animals. In the microbiology laboratory the most likely compound to fall in this category is formaldehyde. Formalin is a commercial stabilized solution of formaldehyde, usually used as a 10% buffered solution (4% formaldehyde). Formaldehyde is combustible as well as a potential carcinogen. Local regulations for storage, use, and disposal differ. The work area should be well ventilated; preferably a chemical exhaust hood should

be used. The College of American Pathologists requires monitoring of formaldehyde vapors in the workspace; if acceptable levels are found, the test need not be repeated unless conditions change.

11. Mercury: Elemental mercury is a significant health hazard. In the microbiology laboratory it will be most often encountered in thermometers and in some fixatives for parasitology smears. Although only small quantities are involved, many institutions have elected, either voluntarily or because of local laws, to eliminate mercury entirely.

Fire

1. Every hospital employee is responsible for preventing fires and assisting in minimizing losses should fire occur.
2. Keep work areas free of trash accumulation and excess flammable materials. Corridors, passageways, aisles, and stairs must be kept free of obstructions that may inhibit exit or add fuel to a fire.
3. Be aware of ignition sources, open flames, heating elements, and sparks gaps (motors, light switches, friction, and static). More than 22% of hospital fires are caused by faulty wiring.
4. Personnel should be instructed in the differences in, and use of, fire extinguishers for the four classes of fire:
    a. Class A: Fires involving ordinary combustible materials such as wood, paper, cloth, and plastics; use a pressurized water extinguisher (type A).
    b. Class B: Fires involving flammable liquids, such as alcohol, gasoline, kerosene, and grease; use a carbon dioxide extinguisher (type B).
    c. Class C: Fires involving energized electrical equipment in which a resulting shock hazard owing to electrical conductivity may exist. Never use a water extinguisher; use a dry chemical type extinguisher (type C).
    d. Class D: Fires involving combustible metals, such as magnesium and potassium. Special techniques are required. Immediately call the local fire station.
5. Fire blankets are used to smother clothing by wrapping the victim in the blanket. If clothing should catch fire, drop to the ground and roll to smother the flame against the floor. **Do not run for the blanket**—airflow will only fan the flames and result in more serious injury. Similarly, a fire blanket should be used on the floor; wrapping the blanket around a standing person only creates a chimney for the flames.
6. Comply with all local fire regulations. Participate in periodic fire drills as conducted by the hospital. Each employee should know the fire drill procedure and the evacuation route for their area of the laboratory.

Bioterrorism

The possibility of terrorists using chemical, biological, or radiological agents has been real for many years, but the possibility took on new significance after 1) the tragedy at the World Trade Center and 2) the discovery of letters that contained anthrax spores and had been sent through the postal service soon thereafter. All laboratories are now required to limit certain agents to absolutely essential use and to provide the government with an inventory of those agents. In addition, each laboratory must prepare a plan for dealing with bioterrorism. Very few diagnostic laboratories will have one of the select agents on hand (see Table 1-23). The primary responsibility for dealing with most of these organisms falls to reference laboratories, public health laboratories, and other government laboratories. The primary job of the diagnostic laboratory is to recognize the possibility of one of the listed agents in the normal course of doing business, after which the agent is referred to a designated support facility and the proper authorities are notified. If terrorism is suspected, the investigation will quickly take on a criminal component. The categories of potential bioterrorism agents are summarized in Table 1-23.[13]

The national preparedness plan for terrorism envisions a multilevel categorization of laboratories with a graded responsibility for evaluating potential threats. The classification of laboratories is detailed in Table 1-24. The original four categories have been compressed to three.[13]

Quality Assurance

Constant attention to the quality of work is a hallmark of good clinical laboratories. Quality Assurance is the broad umbrella that covers several activities. The names for the programs sometimes seem to change as frequently as those of the bacteria. Quality improvement or total quality improvement have given way to quality assurance, but the basic message is that microbiologists must constantly look at what they are doing and improve the processes. Quality control is a traditional element that will be discussed separately.

Quality assurance can be accomplished entirely internally or may be done as part of an external program. National consensus guidelines are available.[84,77] It should encompass all phases of the diagnostic cycle.[84]

Many of the features of a quality assurance program were discussed in the section on laboratory accreditation, which includes quality programs as a critical feature. Internal activities include documentation of the clinical performance of tests (which must be done for each new test introduced into the laboratory) or documentation of the utilization of the laboratory by clinicians. The performance of technical personnel in each task for which they are responsible must be documented. The comparability of morphologic observations among technologists performing the same tasks must be evaluated. Formal evaluation of the competencies of all personnel who perform laboratory tests (including nurses and physicians) is required for all nonwaived tests. The testing can take a number of forms: e.g., direct observation, written tests, or ''wet'' tests, using laboratory samples. National consensus guidelines for setting up the program have been published.[86]

Evaluating laboratory performance can be improved by comparing your performance to that of your peers, using an external program. The College of American Pathologists offers two such programs.[122,102] A parameter that is chosen for evaluation is referred to as an indicator.

The first program, called Q-Probes, consists of one-time

Table 1-23 Classification of Biologic and Chemical Agents With Potential for Terrorism

CATEGORY OF AGENT	DESCRIPTION OF CATEGORY	EXAMPLES
Category A	• Easily disseminated or transmitted person-to-person • Cause high mortality with potential for major public health impact • Might cause public panic and social disruption AND • Require special action for public health preparedness	• Variola major (smallpox virus) • *Bacillus anthracis* (anthrax) • *Yersinia pestis* (plague) • *Clostridium botulinum* toxin (botulism) • *Francisella tularensis* (tularemia) • Filoviruses (Marburg and Ebola viruses) • Arenaviruses causing hemorrhagic fever
Category B	• Moderately easy to disseminate • Moderate morbidity and low mortality • Require enhanced disease surveillance	• *Coxiella burnetii* (Q fever) • *Brucella* spp. (brucellosis) • *Burkholderia mallei* (glanders) • Alphaviruses (e.g., eastern and western encephalomyelitis viruses) • Ricin toxin from *Ricinus communis* (castor beans) • ε-toxin of *Clostridium perfringens* • Staphylococcal enterotoxin B • *Salmonella* spp. • *Shigella dysenteriae* • *Escherichia coli* (O157:H7) • *Vibrio cholerae* • *Cryptosporidium parvum*
Category C	Emerging agents with: • Availability • Ease of production and dissemination • Potential for high morbidity, mortality, and public health impact	• Nipah virus • Hantaviruses • Tick-borne hemorrhagic fever viruses • Tick-borne encephalitis viruses • Yellow fever virus • Multidrug resistant *Mycobacterium tuberculosis*

Adapted from reference[13].

studies on a single issue, such as the frequency of skin organisms in blood cultures. Each participating laboratory submits the results of a study that has been performed according to a defined protocol. The results of all participants are analyzed carefully and a critique is provided to all who have submitted results.

In contrast, the Q-tracks program is a repetitive monitor of a limited number of indicators that have been judged to be particularly useful for assessment of laboratory performance. For instance, laboratory turnaround time for a particular analyte might be studied over time. It is then possible to plot performance over time in relation to peers.

A laboratory can also judge its performance against peers by participating in proficiency testing, as discussed previously.[78,109] Proficiency testing was initially provided by the College of American Pathologists as an educational tool for improving laboratory performance. After the introduction of the two CLIA laws, proficiency testing became a mandated part of doing business.

Quality Control

Quality control in the narrow sense has consisted of an on-going, systematic assessment of work to ensure that the final product conforms to previously established tolerance limits of precision and accuracy.[3] Laboratory directors and supervisors must now realize that quality control is only one facet in the larger arena of quality assurance. Interested readers can access the current requirements of the College of American Pathologists for quality control (as well as safety and other important management issues) by downloading the Laboratory General Checklist from the College Web site (http://www.cap.org).

In a broad sense, quality control in microbiology is more

Table 1-24 Classification of Laboratories Involved in Investigation of Biological or Chemical Terrorism

LEVEL	DESCRIPTION	EXAMPLES
A	• Early detection of intentional dissemination of biological or chemical agents • Initial processing of clinical specimens	• Hospital or public health laboratories • Low level biosafety facilities
B (formerly B and C)	• Core capacity for isolation and characterization of select bioterrorism agents • Serve to minimize higher level laboratories from being overwhelmed with specimens • Advanced capacity for rapid identification of select agents, using culture and molecular techniques • Participate in test development and evaluation	• Local and state public health laboratories • High level federal laboratories • Academic medical centers
C (formerly D)	• Highest level of containment and sophistication • Ability to detect engineered agents	• Select group of federal laboratories • Academic laboratories operating at highest containment level under federal contract

Adapted from reference[13].

an art than a science. It involves intangible items such as common sense, good judgment, and constant attention to detail. Programs should be organized, with well-defined objectives in mind.

COMPONENTS OF A QUALITY CONTROL PROGRAM

A basic microbiology quality control program lists several specific items that must be considered when implementing the various phases of the program. Bartlett[5] developed a quality control program and discusses different levels of activity ranging from basic to most advanced. Using his outline, a supervisor can select the level of activity that is appropriate for the personnel and volume of work in any given laboratory.

The Commission on Laboratory Inspection and Accreditation of the College of American Pathologists (CAP) has established standards for accreditation of medical laboratories, including an inspection checklist for microbiology laboratories. This checklist provides microbiology supervisors with valuable guidelines for making a point-by-point assessment of the quality control needs in their laboratories. Many of the requirements are embedded in the federal regulations of CLIA '88.

Regulations are constantly under review and may be revised. In January, 2004, for instance, CMS issued revised regulations on ''equivalent quality control.'' This revision allows reduced frequency of certain quality control tasks after validation in the laboratory that defined criteria have been satisfied. Some of the changes are more stringent than those of some deemed accreditation agencies, such as CAP; others are less stringent. By law the deemed agencies must have standards that are at least as stringent as CMS, but their standards may be more stringent.

At the onset, a quality control coordinator must be selected. The duties of the coordinator must be clearly established and appropriate authority conferred to the extent that problems can be efficiently handled when they arise. It is the coordinator's responsibility to establish the minimal

standards for quality control that are to be met by the laboratory and to outline the several steps to be taken for daily monitoring and surveillance of all facets of the program.

The coordinator should see that all activities are clearly described in a quality control manual, in which should also be outlined clearly:

1. Details of all quality control practices, such as the procedures and schedules for monitoring equipment function
2. Monitoring of all media and reagents for reactivity, expiration dates, reaction patterns of appropriate challenge organisms
3. All proficiency testing results.

Appropriate forms must be designed to collect data in the form of columns of numbers, graphs, or diagrams so that any item that is out of control can be detected quickly. The coordinator also must review all control records and verify that all measurements that are out of control—and the resulting corrective actions—are clearly noted. A brief review of the several components of a quality control program follows.

MONITORING LABORATORY EQUIPMENT

A preventive maintenance program to ensure proper functioning of all electrical and mechanical equipment should be established in all microbiology laboratories. Equipment should be checked at prescribed time intervals; certain working parts should be replaced after a specified period of use, even though they may not appear worn. A brief list of some of the equipment, the monitoring procedures to be carried out, and the frequency and tolerance limits is shown in Table 1-25. Assignments should be made among laboratory personnel to ensure that all inspections are carried out and all data are recorded accurately onto charts or in maintenance manuals. It is important to detect upward or downward

Table 1-25 Quality Control Surveillance Procedures of Commonly Used Microbiology Equipment

EQUIPMENT	PROCEDURE	SCHEDULE	TOLERANCE LIMITS
Refrigerators	Recording of temperature*	Daily or continuous	2°C–8°C
Freezers	Recording of temperature*	Daily or continuous	–8°C to –20°C
			–60°C to –75°C
Incubators	Recording of temperature*	Daily or continuous	35.5°C ± 1°C
Incubators (CO_2)	Measuring of CO_2 content	Daily or twice daily	5%–10%
	Use blood gas analyzer or Fyrite[†] device		
Water baths	Recording of temperature*	Daily	36°C–38°C
			55°C–57°C
Heating blocks	Recording of temperature*	Daily	±1°C of setting
Autoclaves	Test with spore strip (*Bacillus stearothermophilus*)	At least weekly	No growth of spores in subculture indicates sterile run
pH meter	Test with pH-calibrating solutions	With each use	±0.1 pH units of standard being used
Anaerobic jars	Methylene blue indicator strip	With each use	Conversion of strip from blue to white indicates low O_2 tension
Anaerobic glove box	*Clostridium novyi* type B culture	Run periodically	Growth indicates very low O_2 tension. It is used only where extremely low O_2 tension is required.
	Methylene blue indicator solution	Continuously or daily	Solution remains colorless if O_2 tension is low.
Serology rotator	Count revolutions per minute	With each use	180 RPM ± 10 RPM
Centrifuges	Check revolutions with tachometer	Monthly	Within 5% of dial indicator setting
Safety hoods	Measure air velocity[‡] across face opening	Semiannually or quarterly	50 ft of airflow per minute ± 5 ft/min

* *Each monitoring thermometer must be calibrated against a standard thermometer.*
[†] *Bacharach Instrument Co., Pittsburgh, PA.*
[‡] *Velometer Jr., Alnor Instrument Co., Chicago, IL.*

trends immediately, so appropriate corrective action can be taken before serious errors result. The temperature of incubators, refrigerators, freezers, water baths, and heating blocks must be determined and recorded daily with a thermometer calibrated by the Bureau of Standards or with one that has been checked against a calibrated thermometer. The concentration of CO_2 in all CO_2 incubators must also be determined daily. For any reading that falls outside of the established quality control range, the cause must be determined and the defect quickly corrected.

MONITORING CULTURE MEDIA, REAGENTS, AND SUPPLIES

All media and reagents must be checked against appropriate controls for the proper reactivity. It has been recognized that many modern commercial media perform with a high degree or reliability. Consensus recommendations have been developed for the necessity of local quality control.[74] The

few media with occasional quality control problems (e.g., chocolate agar, media for *Campylobacter jejuni*, and Thayer-Martin agar) should be subjected to control tests in each laboratory. Many others need not be tested if the manufacturer of the media provides documentation that the appropriate reactivity has been observed.

A list of suggested organisms and acceptable results for the culture media most commonly used in clinical laboratories is found in Table 1-26. Quality control stock organisms may be maintained in the laboratory by subculturing bacterial isolates recovered as part of the routine work. Alternatively, and more conveniently, dried stock organisms may be purchased from culture collections, such as ATCC (American Type Culture Collection, 12301 Parklawn Dr., Rockville MD) or from commercial vendors. Each batch of media should be checked for reactivity and for appropriate support of microbial growth, either by the manufacturer or in the local laboratory.

Table 1-26 Quality Control of Commonly Used Media: Suggested Control Organisms and Expected Reactions

MEDIUM	CONTROL ORGANISMS	EXPECTED REACTIONS
Blood agar	Group A *Streptococcus*	Good growth, β-hemolysis
	S. pneumoniae	Good growth, α-hemolysis
Bile–esculin agar	*Enterococcus* species	Good growth, black
	α-Hemolytic	No growth; no discoloration of media
	Streptococcus, not group D	
Chocolate agar	*Haemophilus influenzae*	Good growth
	Neisseria gonorrhoeae	Good growth
Christensen urea agar	*Proteus mirabilis*	Pink throughout (positive)
	Klebsiella pneumoniae	Pink slant (partial positive)
	Escherichia coli	Yellow (negative)
Simmons citrate agar	*K. pneumoniae*	Growth or blue color (positive)
	E. coli	No growth, remains green (negative)
Cystine trypticase (CTA) agar	*N. gonorrhoeae*	Yellow (positive)
Dextrose	*Branhamella catarrhalis*	No color change (negative)
Sucrose	*Escherichia coli*	Yellow (positive)
	N. gonorrhoeae	No color change (negative)
Maltose	*Salmonella* species, or *N. meningitidis*	Yellow (positive)
	N. gonorrhoeae	No color change (negative)
Lactose	*N. lactamicus*	Yellow (positive)
	N. gonorrhoeae	No color change (negative)
Decarboxylases		
Lysine	*K. pneumoniae*	Bluish (positive)
	Enterobacter sakazakii	Yellow (negative)
Arginine (dihydrolase)	*E. cloacae*	Bluish (positive)
	Proteus mirabilis	Yellow (negative)
Ornithine	*P. mirabilis*	Bluish (positive)
	K. pneumoniae	Yellow (negative)
Deoxyribonuclease	*Serratia marcescens*	Zone of clearing (add 1 N HCl)
(DNase)	*E. cloacae*	No zone of clearing
Eosin–methylene blue agar	*E. coli*	Good growth, green metallic sheen
	K. pneumoniae	Good growth, purple colonies, no sheen
	Shigella flexneri	Good growth, transparent colonies (lactose negative)
Hektoen enteric agar	*Salmonella typhimurium*	Green colonies with black centers
	S. flexneri	Green transparent colonies
	E. coli	Growth slightly inhibited, orange colonies
Indole (Kovac's)	*E. coli*	Red (positive)
	K. pneumoniae	No red color (negative)
Kligler iron agar	*E. coli*	Acid slant/acid deep
	Shigella flexneri	Alkaline slant/acid deep
	Pseudomonas aeruginosa	Alkaline slant/alkaline deep
	Salmonella typhimurium	Alkaline slant/black deep
Lysine iron agar	*S. typhimurium*	Purple deep and slant, + H_2S

Table 1-26 *Continued*

MEDIUM	CONTROL ORGANISMS	EXPECTED REACTIONS
	Shigella flexneri	Purple slant, yellow deep
	P. mirabilis	Red slant, yellow deep
MacConkey agar	*E. coli*	Pink colonies (lactose positive)
	P. mirabilis	Colorless colonies, no spreading
	Enterococcus species	No growth
Malonate	*E. coli*	No growth
	K. pneumoniae	Good growth, blue (positive)
Motility (semisolid agar)	*P. mirabilis*	Media cloudy (positive)
	K. pneumoniae	No feather edge on streak line (negative)
Nitrate broth or agar	*E. coli*	Red on adding reagents
	Acinetobacter lwoffi	No red (negative)
Phenylethyl alcohol blood agar	*Streptococcus* species	Good growth
	E. coli	No growth
o-Nitrophenol-β-D-galactopyra-noside (ONPG)	*Serratia marcescens*	Yellow (positive)
	Salmonella typhimurium	Colorless (negative)
Phenylalanine deaminase	*P. mirabilis*	Green (add 10% FeCl$_3$)
	E. coli	No green (negative)
Salmonella–Shigella (SS) agar	*S. typhimurium*	Colorless colonies, black centers
	E. coli	No growth
Voges–Proskauer	*K. pneumoniae*	Red (add reagents)
	E. coli	No development (negative)
Xylose–lysine–dextrose (XLD) agar	*Salmonella* species	Red colonies (positive lysine)
	E. coli	Yellow colonies (positive sugars)
	Shigella species	Transparent colonies (negative)

* From Microbiology Checklist, College of American Pathologists, Revised October 14, 2003.

Table 1-27 Quality Control of Selected Reagents and Media*

MEDIA OR REAGENTS	FREQUENCY	CONTROLS
Gram's stain	Each new batch of stains and at least weekly	Gram-positive and gram-negative organism
Other nonimmunologic, nonfluorescent stains	Each day of use and each new batch, lot number, and shipment	Appropriate reactivity
Fluorescent stains	Each time of use	Appropriate reactivity
Catalase, coagulase, oxidase, bacitracin, optochin, ONPG, X or V or XV disks, identification systems	Each new batch, lot number, or shipment	Positive and negative controls
Antisera (Salmonella & Shigella)	Each new batch, lot number, and shipment when prepared or opened and once every 6 months thereafter	Positive and negative controls
β-lactamase (other than Nitrocefin)	Each day of use	Positive and negative controls
β-lactamase (Nitrocefin)	Each new batch, lot number, or shipment	Positive and negative controls
Nucleic acid probes	Each day of use	Positive and negative controls
AFB stains	Each day of use	Positive and negative controls
Antimicrobial susceptibility tests	Daily or weekly if criteria met (see Chapter 17)	Appropriate organisms

From Microbiology Checklist, College of American Pathologists, Revised October 14, 2003.

Culture tubes, plates of media, and reagents must bear a label that clearly indicates the content and the dates of preparation and expiration. ''Coded'' culture tubes, plated media, and reagents should be referenced in such a way that even nonlaboratory personnel would be able to interpret the code. Clearly defined quality control rules apply to antimicrobial susceptibility testing.

Each batch of tubed or plated media must also undergo sterility testing, particularly media in which components are added after sterilization. Sterility checks must be done both visually and by subculture. Certain selective media, for example, may sufficiently suppress the visible growth of bacteria; however, viable organisms may appear on subculture. Prepared media should also be observed for other signs of deterioration, such as discoloration, turbidity, color changes, evidence of freeze/thawing, and status of hydration.

The frequency with which quality control testing of media and reagents (including serologic reagents) is performed is clearly defined by various accrediting agencies. Some of the rules for quality control of media and reagents are displayed in Table 1-27. Recommendations for quality control are not static. It is important to follow current recommendations, at least in part because changes are as likely to result in less work as in more work.

REFERENCES

1. Albaers AC, Fletcher RD. Accuracy of calibrated-loop transfer. J Clin Microbiol 1983;18:40–42.
2. Alfa MJ, et al. Improved detection of bacterial growth in continuous ambulatory peritoneal dialysis effluent by use of BacT/Alert FAN bottles. J Clin Microbiol 1997;35:862–866.
3. August MJ, et al. Quality control and quality assurance practices in clinical microbiology. Cumitech 1990;3A.
4. Barry M, et al. Brief report: treatment of a laboratory-acquired Sabia virus infection. N Engl J Med 1995;333:294–296.
5. Bartlett RC. A plea for clinical relevance in microbiology. Am J Clin Pathol 1974;61:867–872.
6. Bartlett RC, ed. Medical Microbiology: Quality Cost and Clinical Relevance. New York, John Wiley, 1974.
7. Bartlett RC. Leadership for quality: laboratory scientists have an unprecedented opportunity to contribute to the leadership required to introduce effective quality management. ASM News 1991;57:15–21.
8. Beltrami EM, et al. Risk and management of blood-borne infections in health care workers. Clin Microbiol Rev 2000;13:385–407.
9. Bobadilla M, et al. Improved method for bacteriological diagnosis of spontaneous bacterial peritonitis. J Clin Microbiol 1989;27:2145–2147.
10. Caliendo AM, et al: Comparison of quantitative cytomegalovirus (CMV) PCR in plasma and CMV antigenemia assay: clinical utility of the prototype AMPLICOR CMV MONITOR test in transplant recipients. J Clin Microbiol 2000;38:2122–2127.
11. Casadevall A, Pirofski L. Host-pathogen interactions: the attributes of virulence. J Infect Dis 2001;184:337–344.
12. Centers for Disease Control. Guidelines for prevention of transmission of human immunodeficiency virus and hepatitis B virus to health-care and public-safety workers. MMWR Morb Mortal Wkly Rep 1989;38:1–37.
13. Centers for Disease Control. Biological and chemical terrorism: strategic plan for preparedness and response. Recommendations of the CDC strategic planning workgroup. MMWR Morb Mortal Wkly Rep 2000;49(RR-4):1–14.
14. Centers for Disease Control. Appendix A. Practice recommendations for health-care facilities implementing the U.S. public health service guidelines for management of occupational exposures to bloodborne pathogens. MMWR Recomm Rep 2001;50(RR-11):43–44.
15. Centers for Disease Control. Appendix B. Management of occupational blood exposures. MMWR Recomm Rep 2001;50(RR-11):45–46.
16. Centers for Disease Control. Appendix C. Basic and expanded HIV postexposure prophylaxis regimens. MMWR Recomm Rep 2001;50(RR-11):47–52.
17. Centers for Disease Control. Updated U.S. public health service guidelines for the management of occupational exposures to HBV, HCV, and HIV and recommendations for postexposure prophylaxis. MMWR Recomm Rep 2001;50(RR-11):1–42.
18. Centers for Disease Control. Appendix A. Regulatory framework for disinfection and sterilants. MMWR Morbid Mortal Wkly Rep 2003;52(RR-17):62–64.
19. Centers for Disease Control. Appendix C. Methods for sterilizing and disinfecting patient-care items and environmental surfaces. MMWR Morbid Mortal Wkly Rep 2003;52(RR-17):66.
20. Chastre J, et al. Prospective evaluation of the protected specimen brush for the diagnosis of pulmonary infections in ventilated patients. Am Rev Respir Dis 1984;130:924–929.
21. Cherry WB, Moody MD. Fluorescent-antibody techniques in diagnostic bacteriology. Bacteriol Rev 1965;29:222–250.
22. Conomy JP, et al. Airborne rabies encephalitis: demonstration of rabies virus in the human central nervous system. Neurology 1977;27:67–69.
23. Cotran RS, Kumar V, Collins T, Robbins SL. Robbins Pathologic Basis of Disease. 6th Ed. Philadelphia: WB Saunders, 1999
24. Crain EF, Gershel JC. Urinary tract infections in febrile infants younger than 8 weeks of age. Pediatrics 1990;86:363–367.
25. Curfs JH, et al. A primer on cytokines: sources, receptors, effects, and inducers. Clin Microbiol Rev 1997;10:742–780.
26. Davidson A, Diamond B. Autoimmune diseases. N Engl J Med 2001;345:340–350.
27. Delvies PJ, Roitt IM. The immune system: first of two parts. N Engl J Med 2000;343:37–49.
28. Delvies PJ, Roitt IM. The immune system: first of two parts. N Engl J Med 2000;343:37–49.
29. Delvies PJ, Roitt IM. The immune system: second of two parts. N Engl J Med 2000;343:108–117.
30. Dinarello CA, Cannon JF, Wolff SM. New concepts on the pathogenesis of fever. Rev Infect Dis 1988;10:168–189, 1988.
31. Fine MJ, et al. Evaluation of housestaff physicians' preparation and interpretation of sputum Gram stains for community-acquired pneumonia. J Gen Intern Med 1991;6:189–198.
32. Flynn PM, et al. Differential quantitation with a commercial blood culture tube for diagnosis of catheter-related infection. J Clin Microbiol 1988;26:1045–1046.
33. Fraser DW, et al. Legionnaires' disease: description of an epidemic of pneumonia. N Engl J Med 1977;297:1189–1197.
34. Friedly G. Importance of bacterial stains in the diagnosis of infectious disease. J Med Technol 1985;1:823–833.
35. Fung JC, et al. Growth of coagulase-negative staphylococci on colistin-nalidixic acid agar and susceptibility to polymyxins. J Clin Microbiol 1984;19:714–716.
36. Gabay C, Kushner I. Acute-phase proteins and other systemic responses to inflammation. N Engl J Med 1999;340:448–454.
37. Garcia LS (Ed.) Clinical Laboratory Management. American Society for Microbiology, Washington DC, 2004.
38. Gavin PJ, et al. The role of molecular typing in the epidemiologic investigation and control of nosocomial infections. Pathol Case Rev 2003;8:163–171.
39. Geckler RW, et al: Microscopic and bacteriological comparison of paired sputa and transtracheal aspirates. J Clin Microbiol 1977;6:396–399.
40. Gribble MJ, et al. Pyuria: its relationship to bacteriuria in spinal cord injured patients on intermittent catheterization. Arch Phys Med Rehabil 1989;70:376–379.
41. Guerrant RL, Walker DH, Weller PF: Tropical Infectious Diseases. Philadelphia: Churchill Livingstone, 1999.
42. Hageage GJ Jr, Harrington BJ. Use of calcofluor white in clinical mycology. Lab Med 1984;15:109–115.
43. Hall CJ, et al. Laboratory outbreak of Q fever acquired from sheep. Lancet 1982;1:1004–1006.
44. Hoerl D, et al. Typhoid fever acquired in a medical technology teaching laboratory. Lab Med 1988;19:166–168.
45. Hoff RG, et al. Bacteriuria screening by use of acridine orange-stained smears. J Clin Microbiol 1984;21:513–516.
46. Hughes JG, et al. Culture with BACTEC Peds Plus/F Bottle compared with conventional methods for detection of bacteria in synovial fluid. J Clin Microbiol 2001;39:4468–4471.
47. Hughes MD, et al. Monitoring plasma HIV-1 RNA levels in addition to CD4 + lymphocyte count improves assessment of antiretroviral therapeutic response. ACTG 241 Protocol Virology Substudy Team. Ann Intern Med 1997;126:929–938.
48. Isenberg HD. Clinical Microbiology Procedures Handbook. 2nd Ed. Washington, DC: ASM Press, 2004.

49. Isenberg HD, Washington JA, Doern G, Amsterdam D. Collection, handling and processing of specimens. In Balows A, ed. Manual of Clinical Microbiology. 5th ed. Washington, DC: American Society for Microbiology, 1991: 15–28.

50. James AN. Legal realities and practical applications in laboratory safety management. Lab Med 1988;19:84–87.

51. Kamradt T, Mitchison NA. Tolerance and autoimmunity. N Engl J Med 2001; 44:655–664.

52. Kay AB. Allergy and allergic diseases: first of two parts. N Engl J Med 2001; 44:30–37.

53. Knipe DM, Howley PM. Fields Virology. 4th Ed. Philadelphia: Lippincott Williams & Wilkins, 2001.

54. Koneman EW. The Other End of the Microscope: The Bacteria Tell Their Story. Washington, DC: ASM Press, 2002.

55. Kwon-Chung KJ, Bennett JE. Medical Mycology. Philadelphia: Lea & Febiger, 1992.

56. Lauer BA, et al. Comparisons of acridine orange and Gram stains for detection of microorganisms in cerebrospinal fluid and other clinical specimens. J Clin Rev 1981;14:201–205.

57. Lekstrom-Himes JA, Gallin JI. Immunodeficiency diseases caused by defects in phagocytes. N Engl J Med 2000;343:1703–1714.

58. Lell B, et al. The role of red blood cell polymorphisms in resistance and susceptibility to malaria. Clin Infect Dis 1999;28:794–799.

59. Lund ME, Hawkinson RW. Evaluation of the prompt inoculation system for preparation of standardized bacteria inocula. J Clin Microbiol 1985;18:84–91.

60. Maki DG, et al. A semiquantitative culture method for identifying intravenous-catheter-related infection. N Engl J Med 1977;296:1305–1309.

61. Malech HL, Gallin JI. Current concepts in immunology. Neutrophils in human diseases. N Engl J Med 1987;317:687–694.

62. Mandell GL, Bennett JE, Dolin R. Principles and Practice of Infectious Diseases. 5th Ed. Philadelphia: Churchill Livingstone, 2000.

63. Medzhitov R, Janeway C. Advances in immunology: innate immunity. N Engl J Med 2000;343:338–344.

64. Mermel LA, et al. Outbreak of *Shigella sonnei* in a clinical microbiology laboratory. J Clin Microbiol 1997;35:3163–3165.

65. Michon P, et al. Naturally acquired and vaccine-elicited antibodies block erythrocyte cytoadherence of the *Plasmodium vivax* Duffy binding protein. Infect Immun 2000;68:3164–3171.

66. Miller CD, et al. A twenty-five year review of laboratory-acquired human infections at the National Animal Disease Center. Am Ind Hyg Assoc J 1987;48: 271–275.

67. Miller JM. A Guide to Specimen Management in Clinical Microbiology, 2nd Ed. Washington, DC: ASM Press, 1998.

68. Miller JM, Holmes HT, Krisher K. General principles of specimen collection and handling. In Murray PR, Baron EJ, Jorgensen JH, Pfaller MA, Yolken RH, eds. Manual of Clinical Microbiology. 8th Ed. Washington, DC: ASM Press, 2003: 55–66.

69. Mims CA, Nash A. Stephen J. Mims' Pathogenesis of Infectious Disease. 5th Ed. Burlington, MA: Elsevier, 2000.

70. Morris AJ, et al. Cost and time savings following introduction of rejection criteria for clinical specimens. J Clin Microbiol 1996;34:355–357.

71. Morris AJ, et al. Clinical impact of bacteria and fungi recovered only from broth cultures. J Clin Microbiol 1995;33:161–165.

72. Murray PR, Washington JA II. Microscopic and bacteriologic analysis of expectorated sputum. Mayo Clin Proc 1975;50:339–344.

73. National Committee for Clinical Laboratory Standards. Clinical laboratory safety; approved guideline (GP17-A). 1996.

74. National Committee for Clinical Laboratory Standards. Quality assurance for commercially prepared microbiological culture media: approved standard. 2nd Ed. (M22-A2). 1996.

75. National Committee for Clinical Laboratory Standards. Clinical laboratory design: approved guideline (GP18-A). 1998.

76. National Committee for Clinical Laboratory Standards. Selecting and evaluating a referral laboratory: approved guideline (GP09-A). 1998.

77. National Committee for Clinical Laboratory Standards. Continuous quality improvement: essential management approaches: approved guideline (GP22-A). 1999.

78. National Committee for Clinical Laboratory Standards. Using proficiency testing (PT) to improve the clinical laboratory: approved guideline (GP27-A). 1999.

79. National Committee for Clinical Laboratory Standards. Protection of laboratory workers from occupationally acquired infections: approved guideline. 2nd Ed. (M29-A2). 2001.

80. National Committee for Clinical Laboratory Standards. Abbreviated identification of bacteria and yeast: approved guideline (M35-A). 2002.

81. National Committee for Clinical Laboratory Standards. Assessment of laboratory tests when proficiency testing is not available: approved guideline (GP29-A). 2002.

82. National Committee for Clinical Laboratory Standards. Clinical laboratory technical procedures manuals: approved guideline. 4th ed. (GP02-A4). 2002.

83. National Committee for Clinical Laboratory Standards. Clinical laboratory waste management: approved guideline. 2nd Ed. (GP05-A2). 2002.

84. National Committee for Clinical Laboratory Standards. Application of a quality system model for laboratory services: approved guideline. 2nd Ed. (GP26-A2). 2003.

85. National Committee for Clinical Laboratory Standards. Quality control of microbiological transport systems: approved standard (M40-A). 2003.

86. National Committee for Clinical Laboratory Standards. Training and competence assessment: approved guideline. 2nd ed. (GP21-A2). 2004.

87. O'Hara CM, Weinstein MP, Miller JM. Manual and automated systems for detection and identification of microorganisms. In Murray PR., Baron EJ, Jorgensen JH, Pfaller MA, Yolken RH, eds. Manual of Clinical Microbiology. 8th Ed. Washington, DC: ASM Press, 2003: 185–207.

88. Patel R, Paya CV. Infections in solid-organ transplant recipients. Clin Microbiol Rev 1997;10:86–124.

89. Peterson LR, Brossette SE. Hunting health care-associated infections from the clinical microbiology laboratory: passive, active, and virtual surveillance. J Clin Microbiol 2002;40:1–4.

90. Pike RM. Laboratory-associated infections: summary and analysis of 3921 cases. Health Lab Sci 1976;13:105–114.

91. Pike RM. Past and present hazards of working with infectious agents. Arch Pathol Lab Med 1978;102:333–336.

92. Pike RM. Laboratory-associated infections: incidence, fatalities, causes and prevention. Annu Rev Microbiol 1979;33:41–66.

93. Quinn A, et al. Induction of autoimmune valvular heart disease by recombinant streptococcal m protein. Infect Immun 2001;69:4072–4078.

94. Regan J, Lowe F. Enrichment medium for the isolation of *Bordetella*. J Clin Microbiol 1977;6:303–309.

95. Reimer LG, Carroll KC. Procedures for the storage of microorganisms. In Murray PR., Baron EJ, Jorgensen JH, Pfaller MA, Yolken RH, eds. Manual of Clinical Microbiology. 8th Ed. Washington, DC: ASM Press, 2003: 67–73.

96. Renshaw AA, et al. The lack of value of repeated *Clostridium difficile* cytotoxicity assays. Arch Pathol Lab Med 1996;120:49–52.

97. Richards P, Rathbun K. Medical Risk Management: Preventive Strategies for Health Care Providers. Rockville, MD: Aspen Press, 1983.

98. Richards WD, Wright HS. Preservation of tissue specimens during transport to mycobacteriology laboratories. J Clin Microbiol 1983;17:393–395.

99. Richmond JY, McKinney RW. Biosafety in Microbiological and Biomedical Laboratories. 4th Ed. Washington, DC: U.S. Government Printing Office, 1999.

100. Ryan KJ, Ray CG. Sherris Medical Microbiology: An Introduction to Infectious Diseases. 4th Ed. Columbus, OH: McGraw Hill/Appleton & Lange, 2003.

101. Salyers AA, Whitt DD. Bacterial Pathogenesis: A Molecular Approach. 2nd Ed. Washington, DC: ASM Press, 2001.

102. Schifman RB. Q-probes (short-term studies of the laboratory's role in quality care): nosocomial infections data analysis and critique. Coll Am Pathol 1990;1–14.

103. Schreckenberger PC. Questioning dogmas: proposed new rules and guidelines for the clinical laboratory. ASM News 2001;67:388–389.

104. Schwartz RS. Shattuck lecture: diversity of the immune repertoire and immunoregulation. N Engl J Med 2003;348:1017–1026.

105. Siegel DL, et al. Inappropriate testing for diarrheal diseases in the hospital. JAMA 1990;263:979–982.

106. Simko JP, et al. Differences in laboratory findings for cerebrospinal fluid specimens obtained from patients with meningitis or encephalitis due to herpes simplex virus (HSV) documented by detection of HSV DNA. Clin Infect Dis 2002; 35:414–419.

107. Smith TF, et al. Isolation of viruses from single throat swabs processed for diagnosis of Group A beta-hemolytic streptococci by fluorescent antibody technic. Am J Clin Pathol 1973;60:707–710.

108. Steward DK, et al. Failure of the urinalysis and quantitative urine culture in diagnosing symptomatic urinary tract infections in patients with long-term urinary catheters. Am J Infect Control 1985;13:154–160.

109. Strand CL. Proficiency testing: one important component of continuous quality improvement. Am J Clin Pathol 1994;102:393–394.

110. Tang YW, et al. Effective use of polymerase chain reaction for diagnosis of central nervous system infections. Clin Infect Dis 1999;29:803–806.

111. Tarafdar K, et al. Lack of sensitivity of the latex agglutination test to detect bacterial antigen in the cerebrospinal fluid of patients with culture-negative meningitis. Clin Infect Dis 2001;33:406–408.

112. Thomson RJ Jr, Miller JM. Specimen collection, transport and processing: bacteriology. In Murray PR., Baron EJ, Jorgensen JH, Pfaller MA, Yolken RH, eds. Manual of Clinical Microbiology. 8th Ed. Washington, DC: ASM Press, 2003: 286–330.

113. Thorley-Lawson DA, Gross A. Mechanisms of disease: persistence of the Epstein-Barr virus and the origins of associated lymphomas. N Engl J Med 2004; 350:1328–1337.

114. Uehling DT, Hasham AI. Significance of catheter tip cultures. Invest Urol 1977; 15:57–58.

115. Van Scoy RE. Bacterial sputum cultures: a clinician's viewpoint. Mayo Clin Proc 1977;52:39–41.

116. Walport MJ. Complement: second of two parts. N Engl J Med 2001;344: 1140–1144.

117. Walport MJ. Complement: first of two parts. N Engl J Med 2001;344: 1058–1066.

118. Wedam AG, et al. Handling of infectious agents. J Am Vet Med Assoc 1972; 161:1557–1565.

119. Widmer AF, Frei R. Decontamination, disinfection, and sterilization. In Murray PR., Baron EJ, Jorgensen JH, Pfaller MA, Yolken RH, eds. Manual of Clinical Microbiology. 8th Ed. Washington, DC: ASM Press, 2003: 77–108.

120. Wilson ML, Reller LB. Laboratory design. In Murray PR., Baron EJ, Jorgensen JH, Pfaller MA, Yolken RH, eds. Manual of Clinical Microbiology. 8th ed. Washington, DC: ASM Press, 2003: 22–30.

121. Winn WC Jr, Kissane JM. Bacterial infections. In Damjanov I, Linder J, eds. *Anderson's Textbook of Pathology*. 10th Ed. St. Louis: Mosby, 1995: 747–865.

122. Zarbo RJ, et al. Q-tracks: a College of American Pathologists program of continuous laboratory monitoring and longitudinal tracking. Arch Pathol Lab Med 2002;126:1036–1044.

Introduction to Microbiology
Part II: Guidelines for the Collection, Transport, Processing, Analysis, and Reporting of Cultures from Specific Specimen Sources

Infections of the Respiratory Tract

Infections of the Upper Respiratory Tract

Indigenous Flora
Pharyngitis
Infections of the Oral Cavity Other Than Pharyngitis
Infections of the Nasopharynx and Nasopharyngeal Cultures
Otitis Media and Sinusitis
Epiglottitis
Laryngitis
Other Infections of the Upper Respiratory Tract

Infections of the Lower Respiratory Tract

Tracheobronchitis
Bronchiolitis
Pneumonia
Chronic Pneumonia
Empyema
Pneumonia in Special Populations

Collection of Specimens for the Diagnosis of Lower Respiratory Infection
Laboratory Diagnosis of Pneumonia

Infections of the Gastrointestinal Tract

Lower Intestinal Infections

Clinical Symptoms
Collection of Fecal Specimens
Epidemiologic Considerations in the Evaluation of Patients with Gastroenteritis

Upper Intestinal Infections

Clinical Symptoms
Obtaining Specimens from the Upper Gastrointestinal Tract

Urinary Tract Infections

Clinical Signs and Symptoms
Host Factors
Collection of Urine Samples for Culture

Midstream Urine Specimens
Other Voided Urine Specimens
Catheter Collections
Suprapubic Aspiration

Culture of Urine Specimens
Screening Tests for Urinary Tract Infection

Screening Tests for Bacteriuria
Screening Tests for Pyuria

Infections of the Genital Tract

Sexually Transmitted Infections

Urethritis and Cervicitis
Genital Ulcer Disease

Genital Infections Transmitted by Nonsexual Means

Vaginitis and Vaginosis
Infections of the Upper Female Genital Tract

Systemic Complications of Genital Infections
Diagnosis of Genital Tract Infections

Diagnosis of Urethritis, Cervicitis, and Vaginitis
Diagnosis of Genital Ulcer Disease and Venereal Warts
Collection of Genital Specimens

Infections of the Bones and Joints

Clinical Presentation
Diagnosis of Infections of the Bones and Joints

Infections of the Central Nervous System

Meningitis
Encephalitis and Brain Abscess
Diagnosis of Central Nervous System Infections

Collection of Specimens
Assessing the Inflammatory Response and
    Microscopic Techniques
Direct Detection of Antigen and Nucleic Acid
Serologic Diagnosis
Diagnosis by Culture

Wounds, Abscesses, and Cellulitis

Clinical Presentation
Diagnosis of Wound Infections, Abscesses, and
    Cellulitis

Collection of Specimens
Microscopic Examination of Specimens
Culture

Eye Infections

Clinical Presentation

Conjunctivitis
Keratitis
Uveitis and Endophthalmitis

Diagnosis of Eye Infections

Collection of Specimens
Microscopic Examination
Culture

Infections of the Blood

Clinical Presentation and Pathogenesis

Bacteremia and Septicemia
Types of Bacteremia
Intravascular Infection
Catheter-Associated Bacteremia and Sepsis

Collection of Blood Cultures

Contamination With Skin Flora
Number and Timing of Cultures
Culture Media

Systems for Processing Blood Cultures

Manual Blood Culture Systems
Lysis-Centrifugation Blood Culture System
Automated and Computerized Blood Culture Systems

Comparative Studies
Special Considerations

Fastidious Organisms and Endocarditis
Catheter-associated Bacteremia and Sepsis
Tissues and Biopsies

I n this chapter we focus on the steps necessary for the diagnosis of infections. In each of the sections that follow, signs and symptoms of infections that involve the major organ systems will be presented. Procedures for collection, transport, and processing of specimens are described. This information is summarized in Table 2-1. In other words, this chapter will consider the preanalytical phase of the diagnostic cycle. Later phases will be consid-

ered only briefly, because they are the subject of most of the succeeding chapters.

Infections of the Respiratory Tract

The respiratory tract is divided into the upper tract (the nose, throat, oropharynx, and nasopharynx) and the lower tract (the larynx, trachea, bronchi, bronchioles, and alveolar

Table 2-1 The Diagnosis of Bacterial Infections at Different Body Sites

SITE OF INFECTION	PRESENTING SIGNS AND SYMPTOMS	SPECIMENS TO CULTURE	BACTERIAL SPECIES POTENTIALLY ASSOCIATED WITH INFECTIONS
Respiratory tract	Upper tract—nose sinuses: Headache Pain and redness over malar area Rhinitis Radiograph: Sinus consolidation, fluid levels, or membrane thickening	Acute: Nasopharyngeal swab Sinus washings Chronic: Sinus washings Surgical biopsy specimen	*Streptococcus pneumoniae* *Streptococcus*, β-hemolytic group A *Staphylococcus aureus* *Haemophilus influenzae* *Klebsiella* spp. and other *Enterobacteriaceae* *Bacteroides* spp. and other anaerobes (sinus)
	Upper tract—throat and pharynx: Redness and edema of mucosa Exudation of tonsils Pseudomembrane formation Edema of uvula Gray coating of tongue/"strawberry tongue" Enlargement of cervical nodes	Swab of posterior pharynx Swab of tonsils (abscess) Nasopharyngeal swab	*Streptococcus*, β-hemolytic group A *Corynebacterium diphtheriae* *Neisseria gonorrhoeae* *Bordetella pertussis*
	Lower tract—lungs and bronchi: Cough: bloody or profuse Chest pain Dyspnea Consolidation of lungs: Rales and rhonchi Diminished breath sounds Dullness to percussion Radiographic infiltrates Cavity lesions Empyema	Sputum (poor return) Blood Bronchoscopy secretions Transtracheal aspirate Lung aspirate or biopsy	*Streptococcus pneumoniae* *Haemophilus influenzae* *Staphylococcus aureus* *Klebsiella pneumoniae* and other *Enterobacteriaceae* *Moraxella catarrhalis* *Legionella* spp. *Mycobacterium* spp. *Fusobacterium nucleatum, Prevotella melaninogenicus* and other anaerobes *Bordetella* species
Middle ear	Serous or purulent drainage Deep pain in ear and jaw Throbbing headache Red bulging tympanic membrane	Acute: No culture Nasopharyngeal swab Tympanic membrane aspirate Chronic: Drainage of external meatus	Acute: *Streptococcus pneumoniae* and other streptococci *Haemophilus influenzae* Chronic: *Pseudomonas aeruginosa* *Proteus* spp. Anaerobic bacteria
Gastrointestinal tract	Upper—stomach and duodenum: Gastritis and peptic ulcer disease	Gastric or duodenal biopsy	*Helicobacter pylori*
	Lower—small and large intestine: Diarrhea Dysentery Purulent Mucous Bloody Cramping abdominal pain	Stool specimen Rectal swab or rectal mucus Blood culture (typhoid fever)	*Campylobacter jejuni* and other *Campylobacter* spp. *Salmonella* spp. *Shigella* spp. *Escherichia coli* (toxigenic strains) *Vibrio cholerae* and other *Vibrio* spp.

(Continued)

Table 2-1 *Continued*

SITE OF INFECTION	PRESENTING SIGNS AND SYMPTOMS	SPECIMENS TO CULTURE	BACTERIAL SPECIES POTENTIALLY ASSOCIATED WITH INFECTIONS
			Yersinia species
			Clostridium difficile (demonstration of toxin)
Urinary tract	Urinary bladder infection:	Clean-catch midstream urine	*Enterobacteriaceae*
	Pyuria	Catheterized urine	*Escherichia coli*
	Dysuria	Suprapubic aspiration of urine	*Klebsiella* spp.
	Hematuria		*Proteus* spp.
	Pain and tenderness; suprapubic or lower abdomen		*Enterococcus* spp.
	Kidney infection:		*Pseudomonas aeruginosa*
	Back pain		*Staphylococcus aureus, S. epidermidis,* and *S. saprophyticus*
	Tenderness: costovertebral angle (CVA)		
Genital tract	Males:	Urethral discharge	*Neisseria gonorrhoeae* (*N. meningitidis*)
	Urethral discharge: serous or purulent	Prostatic secretions	
	Burning on urination		*Haemophilus ducreyi*
	Terminal hematuria		*Treponema pallidum* (syphilis)
			Mobiluncus spp. and other anaerobes
			Gardnerella vaginalis
	Females:	Uterine cervix	Nonbacterial:
	Purulent vaginal discharge	Rectum (anal sphincter swab)	*Trichomonas vaginalis*
	Burning on urination	Urethral swab	*Candida albicans*
	Lower abdominal pain, spasm, and tenderness	Darkfield examination	*Mycoplasma* spp.
			Chlamydia trachomatis
	Mucous membrane chancre or chancroid		Herpes simplex virus
Central nervous system	Headache	Spinal fluid	*Neisseria meningitidis*
	Pain in neck and back	Subdural aspirate	*Haemophilus influenzae*
	Stiff neck	Blood culture	*Streptococcus pneumoniae*
	Straight-leg raising: positive	Throat or sputum culture	*Streptococcus*, β-hemolytic groups A and B (group B in infants)
	Kernig sign		*Enterobacteriaceae*: debilitated patients, infants, and postcraniotomy
	Nausea and vomiting		
	Stupor to coma		*Listeria monocytogenes*
	Petechial rash		
Eye	Conjunctival discharge: serous or purulent	Purulent discharge	*Haemophilus* spp.
		Lower cul-de-sac	*Moraxella* supp.
	Conjunctival redness (hyperemia): pink eye	Inner canthus	*Neisseria gonorrhoeae*
			Staphylococcus aureus
	Ocular pain and tenderness		*Streptococcus pneumoniae*
			Streptococcus pyogenes
			Pseudomonas aeruginosa (report immediately)
Blood	Spiking fever	Blood: two to three cultures; repeat as needed	*Streptococcus* spp.
	Chills		Group A—all ages

Table 2-1 *Continued*

SITE OF INFECTION	PRESENTING SIGNS AND SYMPTOMS	SPECIMENS TO CULTURE	BACTERIAL SPECIES POTENTIALLY ASSOCIATED WITH INFECTIONS
	Cardiac murmur (endocarditis)	Any suspected primary site of infection:	*S. viridans* (endocarditis)
			Groups A, B, D—neonates
	Petechiae: skin and mucuous membranes	Cerebrospinal fluid	*S. pneumoniae*
		Respiratory tract	*Staphylococcus aureus*
	"Splinter hemorrhages" of nails	Skin—umbilicus	*Listeria monocytogenes*
	Malaise	Skin—ear	*Corynebacterium jeikeium*
		Wounds	*Haemophilus influenzae*
		Urinary tract	HACEK (*Haemophilus* species, *Actinobacillus actinomycetem comitans, Cardiobacterium hominis, Eikenella corrodens,* and *Kingella* species) Group (see Chapter 8)
			Escherichia coli and other "coliforms"
			Salmonella typhi
			Pseudomonas aeruginosa
			Bacteroides fragilis and other anaerobic bacteria
Wounds	Discharge: serous or purulent	Aspirate of drainage	*Staphylococcus aureus*
	Abscess: subcutaneous or submucosal	Deep swab of purulent drainage	*Streptococcus pyogenes*
	Redness and edema	Tissue biopsy	*Clostridium* spp., *Bacteroides* spp., and other anaerobic bacteria
	Crepitation (gas formation)		*Enterobacteriaceae*
	Pain		*Pseudomonas aeruginosa*
	Ulceration or sinus formation		*Enterococcus* species
Bones and joints	Joint swelling	Joint aspirate	*Staphylococcus aureus*
	Redness and heat	Synovial biopsy	*Haemophilus influenzae*
	Pain on motion	Bone spicules or bone marrow aspirate	*Streptococcus pyogenes*
	Tenderness on palpation		*Neisseria gonorrhoeae*
	Radiograph: synovitis or osteomyelitis		*Streptococcus pneumoniae*
			Enterobacteriaceae
			Mycobacterium species

air sacs of the lungs). For purposes of this discussion, the middle ear (connected to the posterior pharynx through the eustachian tube), the salivary glands (connected to the oral cavity by draining ducts), and the paranasal sinuses (connected to the nasal cavity by draining ducts) are considered part of the upper respiratory tract.

Infections of the Upper Respiratory Tract
INDIGENOUS FLORA

Diagnosis of upper respiratory infections is complicated by the presence of most pathogens in the normal individual in the absence of symptoms. Even *S. pyogenes* may be found, usually in small numbers, in the throats of asymptomatic individuals. The major exception to this rule is *Neisseria gonorrhoeae*, which is found only as a sexually transmitted infection. The oropharyngeal flora of normal individuals is comprised mainly of viridans streptococci. β-hemolytic streptococci, *Staphylococcus aureus, Haemophilus influenzae, Streptococcus pneumoniae, Moraxella catarrhalis,* many anaerobic bacteria including *Fusobacterium* spp. and *Actinomyces israelii,* yeast including *Candida albicans,* adenoviruses, and herpes simplex virus all inhabit the upper respiratory tract without causing disease. In patients who are sick and have been admitted to the hospital the indigenous flora switches from gram-positive (predominantly streptococci) to gram-negative (*Enterobacteriaceae* and *Pseudomonas* spp.).[129] The reason for this alteration appears to be the loss of fibronectin, which enhances binding of gram-positive bacteria, from the surfaces of oropharyngeal epithelial cells.[276,327]

PHARYNGITIS

Acute pharyngitis is the most common infection of the upper respiratory tract. By far the most important pathogen is *Streptococcus* pyogenes (group A β-hemolytic *Streptococcus*). Viral infection is the other common cause of pharyngitis.[25]

Streptococcal Pharyngitis. *Streptococcus pyogenes* pharyngitis may be suggested clinically by observing an inflamed and edematous pharyngeal mucosa in a patient who reports throat pain, difficulty swallowing, and secondary symptoms such as fever, headache, tender anterior cervical lymph nodes, and occasionally a scarlatiniform rash. Purulent exudates over the posterior pharynx and tonsillar area may also be observed. The clinical presentations of streptococcal and nonstreptococcal pharyngitis overlap broadly.[26] Although diagnosis by clinical criteria alone has been advocated, the prevailing opinion is that it is impossible to determine the cause from clinical observations and that diagnostic support from the laboratory is required.[27]

The presence of a tough, fibrinous, gray membrane (''pseudomembrane''), pus exuding from abscesses or from draining sinuses, and mucosal ulcerations suggest an infectious disease other than acute streptococcal pharyngitis; a diagnostic approach different from that required for streptococcal disease is necessary.

β-Hemolytic streptococci other than group A (groups C and G) produce symptoms similar to, but milder than those of group A strains.[25] They are not associated with rheumatic fever as a noninfectious sequela. Although group A strains may be found in the oropharynx occasionally in small numbers, group C and G strains are regular colonizers. It is, therefore, more difficult to interpret isolation of these organisms. If they are recovered in pure culture or as the predominant flora, it is reasonable to report their presence with a note about their clinical significance and interpretation.

The gold standard for diagnosis of streptococcal pharyngitis is bacterial culture on sheep blood agar. Rapid methods for detection of group A streptococcal antigen are widely used in laboratories and at the point of care in offices and clinics. Most of the assays have high specificity, but the sensitivity is not good enough to depend on a negative result.[25] Thus, a negative rapid test should be followed by a bacterial culture. The primary advantages of antigen tests is that they allow expedited treatment of patients who are detected, thus reducing the period of discomfort and allowing the patient to return to school or work sooner. The frequency of noninfectious sequelae (rheumatic fever and glomerulonephritis) is not increased by using conventional culture for diagnosis. The rapid antigen tests add expense and many of them are classified as moderately complex (see Chapter 1)—with attendant investment of time and effort by clinical staff. There is little justification for performing

''rapid'' tests in a central laboratory, because the patient will already have gone home by the time the result is available. Each clinician must make a determination as to the utility of performing the antigen tests.

Diphtheria. Diphtheria is now extremely rare in the United States.[25] It is primarily an infection of children, in whom it occurs in sporadic outbreaks, but adults may become infected, particularly those in lower socioeconomic groups.[111] The thick blue-white or gray membrane that covers the posterior pharynx, with marked edema of the underlying and surrounding tissues, can usually be differentiated from the fire-red throat of acute streptococcal pharyngitis. The diagnosis is made by culture of the membrane on Loeffler's medium or tellurite selective medium. Specimens for culture of *Corynebacterium diphtheriae* are best referred to a reference or public health laboratory (see Chapter 14).

Arcanobacterium haemolyticum Pharyngitis. This bacterium causes acute pharyngitis that closely mimics streptococcal pharyngitis, including a scarlatiniform rash in many patients. It usually affects adolescents and young adults, in contrast to β-hemolytic streptococci, which typically cause disease in young children.[25] *Arcanobacterium* (formerly *Corynebacterium*) *haemolyticum* is better isolated on human blood agar than on sheep blood agar, but can be recovered in the clinical laboratory. It may be dismissed as a non–group A streptococcus if Gram's stain and/or a catalase test are not performed (see Chapter 14).

Gonococcal Pharyngitis. Oropharyngeal infection by *Neisseria gonorrhoeae* is usually asymptomatic, but clinical symptoms may be present and may be associated with disseminated disease.[25] It should be suspected in women and homosexual men who practice fellatio. Clinicians must indicate this possibility so that media for recovery of gonococcus can be inoculated.

Viral Pharyngitis. The most common viral cause of pharyngitis is Epstein-Barr virus. After a nonspecific, febrile prodromal phase an acute pharyngitis with tonsillar enlargement, a white exudates, and cervical lymphadenopathy ensues. Palatal petechiae may be present.[25] Subsequently, systemic signs and symptoms of infectious mononucleosis, including hematologic abnormalities, hepatosplenomegaly, and generalized lymphadenopathy make the diagnosis more obvious. In the early stages the pharyngitis may suggest streptococcal disease, but adolescents and young adults are most commonly symptomatically infected. The diagnosis is serologic. A similar illness may occur as part of the acute retroviral syndrome, caused by human immunodeficiency virus, but the onset is more acute and exudates are not seen. A disseminated maculopapular rash is common in the acute retroviral syndrome, but it is rarely seen in infectious mononucleosis unless ampicillin has been administered.

Adenoviruses produce an acute pharyngitis that resembles streptococcal pharyngitis closely. Conjunctivitis often is present in addition, a clue to the etiology (pharyngoconjunctival fever). Some serotypes of Coxsackie A virus produce acute pharyngitis with vesicles in the posterior pharynx as part of hand, foot, and mouth disease. The infection typically occurs in children and is readily diagnosed clinically by the occurrence of cutaneous and mucosal vesicles. Herpes simplex virus pharyngitis has been described in young adults, but this virus is found in asymptomatic individuals, as is adenovirus. More details about the viral infections are found in Chapter 23.

Other Infectious Causes of Pharyngitis. *Mycoplasma pneumoniae* and *Chlamydia pneumoniae* have been described as causes of pharyngitis, but more commonly cause disease in the lower respiratory tract. *Candida* spp., especially *C. albicans*, produces a tenacious, creamy exudate when it infects the oropharynx, but does not produce prominent pharyngitis. Cytomegalovirus may cause the infectious mononucleosis syndrome, and a number of respiratory viruses may cause pharyngeal discomfort as part of an acute respiratory illness.

Although there is some disagreement in the medical literature, most microbiologists consider *Haemophilus influenzae* and *Staphylococcus aureus* to be colonizing flora rather than etiologic agents of pharyngitis. They may be recovered in culture when the true cause is an agent, such as a virus, that has not been sought. For this reason the request of ''Full Throat Culture'' should be discouraged. The default test should be a ''Streptococcal Culture'' or ''Streptococcal Screen.''

INFECTIONS OF THE ORAL CAVITY OTHER THAN PHARYNGITIS

Gingivitis and dental caries are caused by bacteria, but are primarily a concern for dentists, rather than physicians. In actuality, bacteria cause very few infections of the nasal and oral cavities, other than pharyngitis. Given the impossibility of collecting a surface culture of these spaces without including the abundant indigenous flora, cultures of lesions for bacteria will not produce interpretable results.

Necrotizing, ulcerative gingivostomatitis (Vincent's infection, Vincent's angina, or ''trench mouth'') is a synergistic infection caused by multiple oral anaerobic bacteria. It is rarely encountered today. Culture is not indicated. The condition may be accompanied by sepsis and metastatic infection, however, so blood cultures should be obtained in suspected cases. Observing gram-negative fusiform bacilli and spirochetes in gram-stained smears prepared from an ulcerative buccal or gingival ulcer is helpful for presumptive diagnosis of Vincent's angina. Cultures of the mouth and oral cavity are rarely helpful because of the presence of many species of commensal anaerobes.

Capnocytophaga spp., fusiform bacteria that are normally present in the oropharynx, have also been associated with ulcerations of the oral mucosa and positive blood cultures, particularly in patients with severe neutropenia.[308] These organisms may be recovered on selective media for pathogenic *Neisseria* because of their resistance to vancomycin, colistin, and trimethoprim. By using a selective medium similar in formulation to selective *Neisseria* medium, Rummens and associates[236] recovered *Capnocytophaga* spp. from 96% of oropharyngeal cultures compared with only a 6% recovery on chocolate agar plates inoculated in parallel.

If the clinical history reveals a long-standing, nonhealing mucosal ulcer in the oral cavity, the possibility of the cutaneous extension of a systemic fungal disease must be considered. A biopsy of tissue for histologic study and direct examination of exudative material may be required. White patches on the oral mucosa or the more extensive involvement of the

oral cavity with production of a thick, curdlike exudate may be caused by *Candida* spp., especially *C. albicans*, a diagnosis that can be made by observing pseudohyphae and budding blastoconidia in a gram-stained smear of the exudate.

Herpes simplex virus, almost exclusively serotype 1, may produce an acute gingivostomatitis as a part of primary infection. Most individuals are exposed as children and young adults. The vesicular lesions occur on the skin of the face and the mucosa of the lips, but they may extend into the anterior portions of the mouth. The diagnosis may be made by demonstrating infected cells in a stained smear (Tzanck preparation) or by culture.

Collection of Throat Cultures. The proper method for obtaining a throat swab specimen is shown in Figure 2-1. A bright light from over the shoulder of the specimen collector should be focused into the oral cavity so that the swab can be guided to the posterior pharynx. The patient is instructed to tilt the head back and breathe deeply. The tongue is gently de-

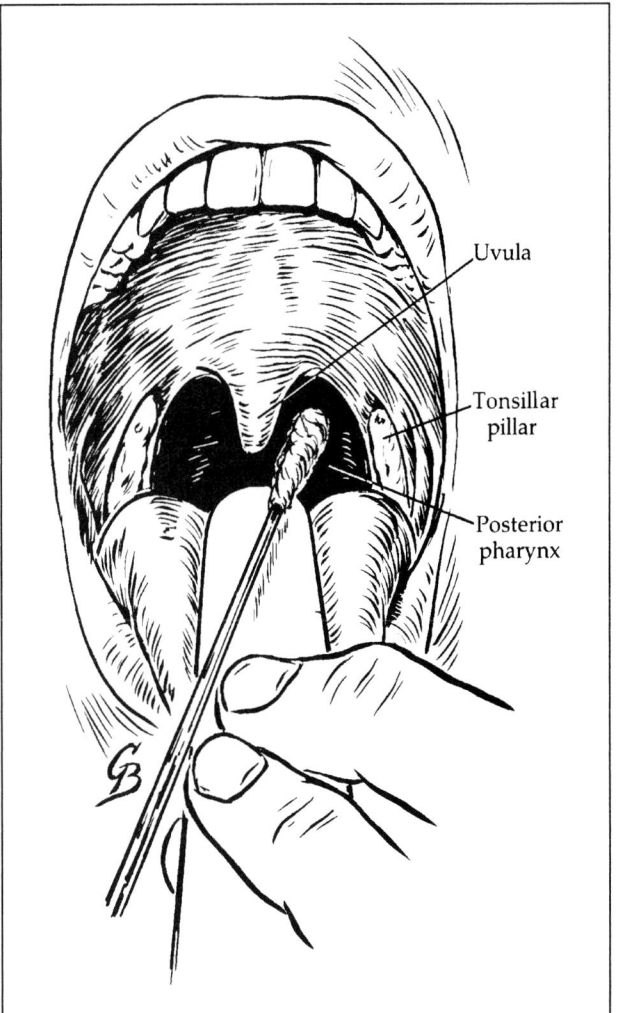

Uvula

Tonsillar pillar

Posterior pharynx

Figure 2-1 Throat culture technique. The patient is asked to open the mouth widely and phonate an ''ah.'' The tongue is gently depressed with a tongue blade and a swab is guided over the tongue into the posterior pharynx. The mucosa behind the uvula and between the tonsillar pillars is swabbed with a gentle sweeping motion.

pressed with a tongue blade to visualize the tonsillar fossae and posterior pharynx. The swab is extended between the tonsillar pillars and behind the uvula. Care should be taken not to touch the lateral walls of the buccal cavity or the tongue to minimize contamination with commensal bacteria. Having the patient phonate a long ''ah'' serves to lift the uvula and helps prevent gagging. The tonsillar areas and the posterior pharynx should be firmly rubbed with the swab. Any purulent exudate should also be sampled.

After collection, the swab should be placed immediately into a sterile tube or other suitable container for transport to the laboratory. If the recovery of only group A β-hemolytic streptococci is desired (i.e., a ''strep screen''), swabs may be allowed to dry during transport without compromising the recovery of viable organisms. Some reference laboratories recommend that swab tips be placed in a desiccant, such as silica gel, to suppress survival of commensal organisms and improve the recovery of *Streptococcus pyogenes*. Swabs for the recovery of viral agents should be placed in a special transport medium (see Chapter 23), although some microbiologists have found swabs in transport medium designed for bacteria to be acceptable for viral culture.[264]

INFECTIONS OF THE NASOPHARYNX AND NASOPHARYNGEAL CULTURES

The most frequent infection of the nasopharynx is the ''common cold,'' usually caused by one of more than 100 serotypes of rhinovirus. This infection is rarely life-threatening, although we now recognize that the lower respiratory tract and even other organ systems may be affected.[75] The common cold is, however, a major cause of morbidity and the large numbers of lost workdays makes it a potent economic force. The ubiquity of this infection is illustrated by the fact that, although very few of us will have had tuberculosis or hemorrhagic fever, we will all have experienced the discomfort of the common cold. The predominant symptom is coryza (runny nose). Fever is not a part of the infection. Laboratory studies are not necessary, because the illness is self-limited and specific therapy is not yet available.

Obtaining nasopharyngeal specimens is of little practical value, except in a few defined situations. Nasopharyngeal swabs are of limited value for establishing the diagnosis of acute otitis media[248] or bacterial sinusitis,[81] but they are the specimen of choice for the isolation of *Bordetella pertussis*, the etiologic agent of whooping cough.[120] Nasopharyngeal swabs and aspirates are equally effective for the diagnosis of viral respiratory infections,[91] although some virologists prefer aspirates for recovery of respiratory syncytial virus.

Nasopharyngeal specimens are obtained under direct vision using over-the-shoulder illumination. With the thumb of one hand, gently elevate the tip of the nose. Moisten the tip of a small flexible nasopharyngeal wire swab with sterile water or saline and gently insert it into one of the nares. Guide the swab backward and upward along the nasal septum until a distinct feel of resistance indicates that the posterior pharynx has been reached. Gently remove the swab. If while guiding the swab undue resistance is met, attempt the procedure through the opposite nares. Leave the swab in contact with the posterior nasopharynx for 15–30 seconds if the patient can tolerate the discomfort.

OTITIS MEDIA AND SINUSITIS

The middle ear and the paranasal sinuses are connected to the upper airway by ducts. Infections, primarily caused by viruses and bacteria, result when pathogens that populate the nose and throat make their way into the normally sterile worlds of ear and sinus.[85,105,304] Acute infections are caused by respiratory viruses and by certain bacteria—*Streptococcus pneumoniae*, *Moraxella catarrhalis*, and *Haemophilus influenzae*.[114] When the infection becomes chronic, facultatively aerobic gram-negative bacilli, anaerobic bacteria, and fungi assume a prominent role in a polymicrobial infection.[66,85] It is virtually impossible to obtain an interpretable specimen by sampling the airway.

Sampling these structures for culture is difficult. Fortunately, the pathogens in acute disease are predictable, so antimicrobial therapy can be initiated without the necessity of invasive procedures. In chronic diseases, invasive procedures and surgical approaches may be required.

EPIGLOTTITIS

Acute bacterial epiglottitis, which was most commonly caused by *Haemophilus influenzae* type B,[180] is a life-threatening infection, but has fortunately been virtually eliminated by immunization. Swelling of the epiglottis can block the airway unless relieved by tracheostomy. Most historians believe that George Washington died from acute epiglottitis, which was treated by repeated bleeding.[192] The youngest of his three consulting physicians wanted to try the newly developed technique of tracheostomy, but he was overruled by his ''wiser'' superiors. The diagnosis of epiglottitis must be made clinically, because touching the epiglottis to obtain a sample can aggravate the obstruction. In *Haemophilus* epiglottitis blood cultures were frequently positive.

LARYNGITIS

Acute laryngitis and (more commonly) laryngotracheobronchitis (croup) are most commonly caused by respiratory viruses. *Mycoplasma pneumoniae* is another common cause.[65]

OTHER INFECTIONS OF THE UPPER RESPIRATORY TRACT

Infection of the soft tissues of the head and neck usually originate in the oral cavity and are caused by organisms that reside there normally. Retropharyngeal abscesses and infection of the retropharyngeal space (quinsy) are infectious complications of streptococcal tonsillitis and pharyngitis. Compression of the airway can result; it represents a medical emergency.[102] Sampling of peritonsillar abscesses must be done by percutaneous aspiration to avoid contamination with oropharyngeal flora.

Similarly, dental infections can extend into the adjacent soft tissues, resulting in abscesses, or into bone, causing osteomyelitis. Chronic draining infections of the neck may be caused by *Actinomyces israelii* (actinomycosis),[35,311] a component of the oropharyngeal flora in a minority of individuals. Material from the draining sinus must be collected by aspiration or curetting; a swab is not adequate to recover the concretions (sulfur granules) in which the bacteria are concentrated. Alternatively, gauze may be placed over the draining sinus to collect the granules that become enmeshed in the interstices of the cloth. Draining material can be placed in a Petri dish, diluted with water, and examined for the concretions. If the granules are crushed, demonstration of branching gram-positive bacilli establishes the diagnosis. The crushed granule can then be cultured anaerobically to determine the specific cause.

Historically, mycobacterial infection also caused cervical lymphadenopathy, and the lymph nodes often drained to the surface of the skin (scrofula). It was commonly caused by *Mycobacterium bovis*, which entered the body through the oropharynx after being ingested in contaminated milk. Pasteurization eradicated the infection. Tuberculous lymphadenopathy usually follows primary pulmonary disease. Today the most common mycobacterial infection of cervical lymph nodes is caused by *Mycobacterium avium* complex (MAC) and primarily affects young children.[21] In contrast to other mycobacterial infections, which require antimicrobial therapy, MAC infection in children can be treated effectively by surgical excision of the affected nodes.

The most common infection of the salivary glands in past years was mumps, but effective immunization has essentially eliminated the infection. Bacterial infection is uncommon.

Infections of the Lower Respiratory Tract

The lower respiratory tract consists of all structures below the larynx: trachea (tracheitis), bronchi and bronchioles (bronchitis and bronchiolitis), and the distal air spaces (pneumonia).

TRACHEOBRONCHITIS

Acute infections can be caused by bacteria or viruses. In children, viral and mycoplasmal agents predominate.[65] Symptoms include cough, fever, and varying degrees of sputum production. A distinctive illness, characterized by an inspiratory whoop, is caused by *Bordetella pertussis* or *B. parapertussis*, which usually produces a milder illness.[31] The characteristic whoop of whooping cough is not present in the initial phases of illness, however. Apneic spells (absence of breathing) are common, but not lethal. Adenoviruses may produce a similar syndrome, although their etiologic role is controversial. *Chlamydia pneumoniae*, a more recently recognized pathogen, can cause acute bronchitis as well as pneumonia.

Chronic tracheobronchitis is symptomatically similar to acute disease, but more prolonged and less intense. Bacteria predominate, particularly *Streptococcus pneumoniae*, nonencapsulated *Haemophilus influenzae*, and *Moraxella catarrhalis*.

Prolonged acute disease may overlap with chronic bronchitis. *Mycoplasma pneumoniae* has classically been associated with a lingering cough, but it is now recognized that *Bordetella pertussis* can produce chronic illness in older children, adolescents, and adults[252] and *Chlamydia pneumoniae* may result in a lingering illness.[108]

Viral infections are usually not diagnosed with laboratory support unless the illness is sufficiently severe to require hospitalization. Whooping cough and *Chlamydia* infection are diagnosed by culture or, increasingly, by molecular methods. Chronic bronchitis is usually evaluated by sputum culture if the illness is sufficiently severe. Special requests must be made if *Bordetella*, *Mycoplasma*, or *Chlamydia* is considered.

BRONCHIOLITIS

Infection of the smallest airways before the air spaces is dominated by viruses and *Mycoplasma pneumoniae*.[113,325] Bronchiolitis affects infants and young children primarily and it occurs most commonly during the winter months. After a prodromal period of upper respiratory infections, primarily coryza, the predominant symptoms are cough, wheezing, and stridor (difficulty breathing). The differential diagnosis may include asthma and physical obstructions, such as foreign bodies. The illness is self-limited and laboratory diagnosis is required only if the patient is sufficiently ill to require hospitalization.

PNEUMONIA

The most serious infection of the respiratory tract is pneumonia, which is centered on the distal air spaces from the alveolar ducts to the alveolar sacs. The symptoms of pneumonia include fever, cough, varying degrees of sputum production, dyspnea (shortness of breath; difficulty breathing), and chest pain. Chest pain may be diffuse, vague and constant, or localized and intermittent, accentuated by deep respiration if pleuritis is present. Shortness of breath and dyspnea usually indicate involvement of the terminal bronchioles and alveoli in a more diffuse pneumonic process. Physical signs pointing to the lower respiratory tract include rales and rhonchi, diminished breath sounds, and localized dullness to percussion in cases of lobar pneumonia.[69]

Pneumonia has been broadly divided into several types: atypical pneumonia, acute pneumonia, and chronic pneumonia. In addition, aspiration pneumonia, lung abscess, and empyema require special consideration. Finally, from a management perspective pneumonia may be classified epidemiologically: outpatient pneumonia (''walking pneumonia'') and pneumonia requiring hospitalization; community-acquired pneumonia versus hospital-acquired pneumonia; pneumonia in immunosuppressed patients; pneumonia in cystic fibrosis; and pneumonia at the extremes of life. The distinction between lobar pneumonia, classically caused by *Streptococcus pneumoniae* (pneumococcus) and *Klebsiella pneumoniae* serotype 1 (Friedlander's pneumonia), and multifocal pneumonia, caused by other bacteria, is less useful clinically, because there is extensive overlap between the two patterns.

The type of pneumonia produced is a combination of microbial factors and the status of host defense mechanisms. Most pneumonia results from inhalation of respiratory pathogens or aspiration (usually microscopic and subclinical) of contents of the upper respiratory tract. As the colonizing flora of the oropharynx change, so will the nature of organisms that infect the lung.

Atypical Pneumonia. Atypical pneumonia was defined in the 1930s as lower respiratory infection that did not resemble the classic lesions that had been described. The major difference is that sputum production is minimal in atypical pneumonia. Infection is often milder than in classic pneumonia, but not necessarily so. The primary pathogens responsible for atypical pneumonia are *Mycoplasma pneumoniae, Chlamydia pneumoniae,* and *Legionella* spp.

Acute Pneumonia. Acute pneumonia in the outpatient setting (community-acquired pneumonia) is a combination of atypical pneumonia and classic pneumonia caused by oropharyngeal bacteria. The most important ''classic'' pathogen remains pneumococcus; other contributors are *Haemophilus influenzae* (now predominantly nontypeable strains), and *Moraxella catarrhalis.*[11,171,185]

Viral pneumonia is rare in immunocompetent adults. Viral pneumonia will develop in a small percentage of previously healthy adults with influenza. In this situation, secondary bacterial infection (superinfection) is the major threat. Acute viral pneumonia is a more important consideration in young children, in whom it overlaps with bronchiolitis, caused by respiratory syncytial virus and parainfluenzavirus type 3. The most common cause of viral pneumonia in the immunosuppressed population is cytomegalovirus.

Acute pneumonia in the hospital is caused most commonly by *Enterobacteriaceae, Pseudomonas* spp., and *Staphylococcus aureus.*[38] The shift in etiologic agents reflects changes in the nature of colonizing flora in the upper airways (See Chapter 1).

Aspiration Pneumonia. Although most pneumonia is caused by aspiration of oropharyngeal contents, massive aspiration causes a distinctive picture of focal pneumonia, affecting the dependent portions of the lung when standing or lying down (lower lobes and superior segment of the upper lobe). The infecting organisms in the outpatient are a mixture of aerobic (primarily gram-positive) and anaerobic bacteria.[8] In the hospitalized patient, aspiration pneumonia reflects the gram-negative character of the upper airways.

CHRONIC PNEUMONIA

As the name implies, the course of chronic pneumonia is prolonged. Symptoms are usually less dramatic than in acute pneumonia. As a result, diagnosis may be delayed for weeks or months, because nonspecific signs and symptoms such as low-grade fever, malaise (feeling ''poorly''), and weight loss may be the only manifestations of infection. The etiologic agents in chronic pneumonia are mycobacterial and fungal, but smoldering bacterial infection is also a major player. *Candida* spp. are notably absent from the list of pulmonary pathogens, except as a part of disseminated candidiasis in immunosuppressed patients.

Lung Abscess. Closely related to aspiration pneumonia is lung abscess, sometimes called putrid lung abscess, because of the fecal odor of the infecting anaerobic bacteria.[8,9] The formation of abscesses is also a function of microbial virulence factors. *Staphylococcus aureus, Enterobacteriaceae,* and *Pseudomonas* spp. often cause destructive lesions. Certain fungi, primarily *Aspergillus* spp. and Zygomycetes, characteristically invade blood vessels. Thrombosis ensues and tissue death results when oxygenation is blocked, a process called infarction. *Pseudomonas aeruginosa* also has the capacity to produce vasculitis. When an infectious agent and thrombosis are present together, the process is called a septic infarct and is particularly destructive. The thrombosis can occur in situ or can result from a blood clot that travels through the bloodstream to the lung (an embolus).

Granulomas are another type of destructive lesion (see Chapter 1). They are typically produced by mycobacteria, especially *Mycobacterium tuberculosis* and by dimorphic fungi, particularly *Histoplasma capsulatum, Blastomyces dermatitidis,* and *Coccidioides immitis.*

EMPYEMA

Inflammation of the pleura (the mesothelial membrane that lines the lung and the chest wall) is common in pneumonia (pleurisy) and may produce an exudation of fluid (pleural effusion).[2] If the pleural effusion itself becomes infected, a thick pus results in empyema. The causes are those of bacterial pneumonia. Healing may result in obliteration of the pleural cavity.

PNEUMONIA IN SPECIAL POPULATIONS

Pneumonia in the elderly is more of a threat than in younger adults, but the list of pathogens is similar. *S. pneumoniae* is the most frequent agent.[162,200] It is now recognized that some agents such as respiratory syncytial virus, thought to be etiologic agents in children, also infect adults and the elderly.

Immunosuppressed patients are at risk for many pathogens that do not cause disease regularly in immunocompetent individuals. Among these opportunistic pathogens are parasites, including *Toxoplasma gondii;* viruses, including cytomegalovirus; fungi, including *Aspergillus* spp., Zygomycetes, *Cryptococcus neoformans,* and *Pneumocystis jiroveci* (*carinii*); and mycobacteria, such as *Mycobacterium avium* complex.[253]

A special category of compromised individuals is those with cystic fibrosis.[95] A progression of pathogens follows these patients throughout the course of their illness: *Staphylococcus aureus, Haemophilus influenzae,* and *Pseudomonas aeruginosa.* Strains of *P. aeruginosa* in cystic fibrosis have a characteristic mucoid character that is seen much less frequently in other patients. More recently, *Burkholderia cepacia, Stenotrophomonas maltophilia* (both previously species of *Pseudomonas*), and *Alcaligenes* spp. have become major concerns in cystic fibrosis because the infections are difficult to treat and the pathogens are easily spread from one individual to another.

Allergic bronchopulmonary disease is most often caused by *Aspergillus fumigatus.*[98] This versatile, although opportunistic pathogen can produce invasive disease in immunosuppressed patients, mycetoma (fungus ball) in preexisting cavities, as well as an immunologic reaction in individuals with an atopic (allergic) predisposition.[90,93] Hyphae are found in the air spaces, where they produce an inflammatory reaction but do not invade tissue in allergic aspergillosis.

COLLECTION OF SPECIMENS FOR THE DIAGNOSIS OF LOWER RESPIRATORY INFECTION

Expectorated Sputum. The simplest and least expensive specimen for the diagnosis of lower respiratory infections is expectorated sputum. The utility of this approach is the subject of considerable argument, because of the difficulty some patients have mobilizing lower respiratory secretions and the frequency with which the specimen is contaminated by oropharyngeal flora as it passes through the mouth.[225]

When the specimen is collected carefully, however, it can provide useful information for initial therapy of community-acquired pneumonia.[235]

The patient should be instructed carefully on the proper collection of sputum, rather than saliva. Having patients brush their teeth and gargle with water immediately before obtaining the specimen reduces the number of contaminating oropharyngeal bacteria. Spada and colleagues[268] showed a 1-log decrease in the mean concentration of contaminating bacteria from $3.6 \pm 7.5 \times 10^8$ to $3.7 \pm 7.2 \times 10^7$ in sputum samples obtained from patients immediately following a simple mouth wash. Avoid using proprietary mouthwashes or gargles that may contain antibacterial substances. Once the specimen is collected it should be submitted to the laboratory promptly rather than sitting at the bedside.

Early-morning sputum samples should be obtained because they contain pooled overnight secretions in which pathogenic bacteria are more likely to be concentrated. Twenty-four-hour collections should be discouraged because there is not only a greater likelihood of contamination, but bacterial pathogens that may be in high concentration in one sample potentially become diluted with the addition of subsequent, more watery specimens. When sputum production is scant, induction with nebulized saline may be effective in producing a sample more representative of the lower respiratory tract. Avoid the use of "saline for injection," many preparations of which contain antibacterial substances.[227]

Special sputum collection devices are commercially available through laboratory supply companies, or a sterile wide-mouth jar with a tightly fitted screw-cap lid can be used. To prevent contamination of the outside of the container, the patient should be instructed to press the rim of the container under the lower lip to catch all of the expectorated cough sample.[3]

Endotracheal Aspirate. The lower respiratory tract may be sampled by introducing a catheter through the larynx into the trachea. If an endotracheal tube is in place or there is a tracheotomy, aspirating tracheal secretions is simple. It is often assumed that endotracheal aspirates avoid some of the contamination problems of expectorated sputum. In fact, intubation introduces the possibility of contamination because oral secretions can dribble down the pathway of the endotracheal tube. These specimens must, therefore, be interpreted with the same care as that taken with expectorated sputum. It has been suggested that quantitative cultures of tracheal aspirates may provide better data (see the discussion of bronchoalveolar lavage below).[22] The quantitative technique involved performing a dilution of sputum that had been liquefied enzymatically before plating onto agar. A simpler semiquantitative approach, in which the sputum was washed twice with saline and struck onto agar as usual (see Chapter 1), correlated closely with the quantitative technique. This technique has not been widely adopted, but most laboratories use the semiquantitative technique (although few go through the washing steps).

Translaryngeal (Transtracheal) Aspiration. Translaryngeal aspiration is an invasive technique that was introduced to avoid contamination problems. Technical difficulties with proper performance and too frequent complications have reduced the frequency with which this approach is used.

Rigid Bronchoscopy. The rigid bronchoscope was capable of sampling only the central airways. Although it is adequate for mycobacterial cultures, it is not appropriate for organisms that colonize the oropharynx and infect the distal tract. It is seldom used today.

Flexible Bronchoscopy. Fiberoptic bronchoscopy is a technique frequently used for obtaining transbronchial biopsies, washings, and brushings, particularly in patients with lung abscesses or other suspected deep pulmonary infections. The bronchial brush technique uses a telescoping double catheter plugged with polyethylene glycol at the distal end to protect a small bronchial brush. This technique is recommended for the optimal recovery of aerobic and anaerobic bacteria, both facultative and obligate anaerobes, from deep-seated pulmonary lesions.[10] Discrete sampling of focal lesions may be accomplished after fluoroscopic localization of the tip of the bronchoscope. Specimens that cannot be cultured immediately should be placed into a holding-transport medium for delivery to the laboratory. The success of this procedure depends on the following: 1) obtaining ample brush material from the distal bronchioles and alveoli to make several slides, 2) preparing a full set of special stains and multiple cultures, and 3) searching for more than one type of microorganism.

Bronchoalveolar Lavage. Bronchoalveolar lavage involves the injection of 30 to 50 mL of physiologic saline through a fiberoptic bronchoscope that has been threaded into the peripheral bronchiolar ramifications. The saline is then aspirated and submitted for smear preparation and culture. Semiquantitative or quantitative cultures of respiratory secretions obtained by protected bronchial brush and alveolar lavage techniques have been recommended for diagnosis of pneumonia in intubated patients undergoing ventilation.[50] Organisms that are present in concentrations greater than 10^3 to 10^4 colony-forming units (CFU)/mL and specimens that demonstrate intracellular bacteria in more than 25% of the inflammatory cells present are indicators of pneumonia that requires specific treatment. Unfortunately, the experience with quantitative microbiology of respiratory secretions has been highly variable.[290] One group of investigators found high specificity if a cutoff of 10^5 CFU/mL was used for fluid obtained by bronchoalveolar lavage, but the sensitivity was only 33%, largely because of prior antimicrobial therapy.[269] They concluded that at this bacterial concentration, pneumonia could be diagnosed reliably, but a negative result did not exclude the diagnosis.

Lung Puncture and Biopsy. Percutaneous aspiration or needle biopsy may be performed blindly or under fluoroscopic guidance, particularly if a localized lesion is present.[291] Open lung biopsy is the most invasive approach and is reserved for situations in which other measures have failed.

Additional procedures may be helpful in determining the etiology of respiratory infections when cultures are negative or nonrevealing. Blood cultures should always be obtained during the acute phases of pneumonia. *Streptococcus pneumoniae* may be recovered from the blood in 25–30% of patients with pneumococcal pneumonia, often when sputum cultures are negative.[194]

If sputum is not produced it is possible to detect bacterial antigen of *Legionella pneumophila* serogroup 1 and *Streptococcus pneumoniae* in urine specimens.[20,195] The antigen may be excreted for days, weeks, or even months, so a positive test does not absolutely document a recent infection. Careful correlation with clinical information is required.

LABORATORY DIAGNOSIS OF PNEUMONIA

The etiologic diagnosis of pneumonia is a cooperative enterprise that requires microbiologists, radiologists, and clinicians. The diagnosis of pneumonia is a clinical one, using history, the stethoscope, and chest radiographs. With a few important exceptions, such as recovery of *Mycobacterium tuberculosis*, pneumonia is *not* diagnosed in the microbiology laboratory. Clinicians who send a sputum specimen to the laboratory without having a clinical diagnosis of pneumonia in hand are asking for confusing, or even misleading, information. Once a diagnosis of pneumonia has been made, the laboratory can help a clinician define the etiology and select appropriate therapy.[42]

Sputum samples should be processed as soon after collection as possible. A significant decrease in recoverable organisms from sputum samples after 20 hours of refrigeration has been found,[210] although there was no compromise in the number or quality of epithelial cells and segmented neutrophils. A decline in the number of viable tubercle bacilli that could be recovered from sputum after storage at room temperature for several days has also been found,[208] although the concentration of acid-fast bacilli seen in acid-fast stains was not reduced after 20 days.

The quality of sputum samples should also be assessed using one of the grading systems described in Chapter 1. There is controversy about the value of providing presumptive bacterial identifications based on morphologic criteria. Bartlett and coworkers[13] first suggested that categories of bacteria could be defined accurately by morphology in Gram-stained smears of sputum. For example, the morphologic identification of staphylococci, "bacteroides-haemophilus," and bacteria of mixed morphology were made with 75% accuracy if the sputum specimens were of high quality. It has been demonstrated[295] that semiquantitative enumeration of the bacteria in Gram-stained sputum cannot be reproduced from one technologist to another (or even with the same technologist examining smears on repeated occasions) and that such estimations should not be reported. One possible explanation for this observation is the variability of smears from one area to the next. On the other hand, a more optimistic report[97] suggests that Gram's stains of high-quality sputum specimens, performed in a select population of adults with community-acquired pneumonia, may provide clinicians with enough information to initiate empiric antibiotic therapy. In either event, considerable experience on the part of the observers and regular correlation of laboratory results with clinical indicators is necessary before Gram's stain interpretations of sputum samples will be of value.

A useful quality assurance tool is the comparison of Gram's stains and cultures. If organisms seen in the smears do not grow in culture or if organisms that grow in moderate to heavy quantities are not seen in the smear, the smear should be reviewed. Gram's stain is relatively insensitive (approximately 10^5 CFU/mL must be present to be visualized), so small numbers of bacteria in the culture may well not be seen in the smear. If the smear has been misinter-

preted, it should be reviewed with the reader as an educational tool. If the smear was correctly interpreted, this may be a clue that additional approaches to culture should be considered.

The grading systems for sputum samples do not apply in lower respiratory tract infections caused by *Legionella* spp., mycobacteria, fungi, and viruses. Purulent inflammatory cell responses are not necessarily elicited in these infections.

The semiquantitation of stainable tubercle bacilli in sequential examinations of sputum by acid-fast smears is of value for determining the efficacy of antituberculous drug therapy. A decrease from 4+ to 1+ to rare or even to an absence of bacilli over a 4- to 6-week course of therapy indicates good drug response and may be used to determine when it may be safe to discharge a patient to home care.

The importance of the microorganisms recovered from respiratory samples must always be evaluated in light of clinical information. Interpretation of sputum cultures is particularly difficult because they are neither specific nor sensitive in the evaluation of lower respiratory infections. Lentino and Lucks[156] have succinctly stated the problem based on their experience in a study of 249 patients with suspected pneumonia (Box 2-1).

Establishing the bacterial etiology of acute and chronic bronchitis can also be difficult, because so many species of bacteria can be found as normal flora or commensals in the respiratory tract (Table 2-2). The recovery of *Streptococcus pneumoniae*, *Klebsiella pneumoniae*, *Haemophilus influenzae*, and *Moraxella* (*Branhamella*) *catarrhalis* as the predominant microorganism from respiratory secretions, particularly when Gram-stained smears support their presence and/or the organisms are also recovered from concomitant blood cultures, supports their role in the development of acute pneumonia.[69,332] Induced sputum samples, collected after inhalation of nebulized saline, may be required to increase the yield of detection of certain organisms, particularly *Pneumocystis jiroveci* (*carinii*).

If pulmonary infections caused by mycobacteria, fungi, human parasites, or viruses are suspected, special techniques must be used to recover the etiologic agents, as outlined in

---

Box 2-1 Interpretation of Sputum Cultures: Observations of Lentino and Lucks[156]

1. Using the sputum quality-grading system of Bartlett and of Murray and Washington as outlined in Chapter 1, 48% of the sputum cultures submitted to their laboratory did not pass the quality grade and were more reflective of oral secretions.
2. 26.5% of purulent sputum samples were from patients showing no radiologic or clinical evidence for pneumonia.
3. 40% of sputum samples obtained from patients with evidence of pneumonia were not deeply expectorated, again more reflective of oral secretions.
4. Only 10.8% of patients producing nonpurulent sputa had pneumonia.
5. Only 56.8% of patients with pneumonia produced purulent sputum.

Table 2-2 Selected Commensal Flora and Potential Pathogens in the Respiratory Tract

COMMENSAL FLORA	POTENTIAL PATHOGENS
α/γ-Hemolytic streptococci	Adenovirus
β-Hemolytic streptococci, other than group A	Anaerobes (as part of mixed infection)
Candida spp.	*Bordetella pertussis*
Coagulase-negative staphylococci	*Chlamydia pneumoniae*
Corynebacterium spp. (diphtheroids)	*Chlamydia psittaci*
Haemophilus parainfluenzae	*Corynebacterium diphtheriae*
Neisseria spp.	*Cryptococcus neoformans*
	Cytomegalovirus
	Enterobacteriaceae
	Haemophilus influenzae
	Herpes simplex virus
	Legionella spp.
	Moraxella catarrhalis
	Mycobacterium spp.
	Mycoplasma pneumoniae
	Myxoviruses and paramyxoviruses
	Neisseria gonorrhoeae
	Neisseria meningitidis
	Pneumocystis jiroveci (*carinii*)
	Pseudomonas aeruginosa
	Staphylococcus aureus
	Streptococcus pneumoniae
	Streptococcus pyogenes (group A)

the chapters devoted to each of these groups of microbes. Although the recovery of certain fungi, such as the dimorphic pathogens, usually indicates disease, other fungi, such as *Aspergillus* species, must be recovered repeatedly from successive samples before the diagnosis can be confirmed. The presence of fungal hyphae is less likely to represent environmental contamination. Diagnosis of viral pneumonia will be attempted most frequently in immunosuppressed patients and in children who are sufficiently ill to require admission to the hospital.

The use of blood culture, urinary antigen detection, and quantitative culture techniques has been discussed above. Modern molecular techniques are now available for expedited diagnosis of viral and mycobacterial infections; the number of situations in which these approaches will be applicable is unlikely to expand in the future. Measurement of a soluble triggering receptor that is found on myeloid cells has been proposed as a useful approach,[94] but the promising results require confirmation.

Infections of the Gastrointestinal Tract
Lower Intestinal Infections

CLINICAL SYMPTOMS

The most common presenting symptom of lower intestinal tract infections is diarrhea.[287] Although diarrhea is diffi-

cult to define quantitatively, patients usually know when they have bowel movements in excess of normal and when the stool takes on a form that is softer or more liquid than usual. The diarrhea may be accompanied by cramping abdominal pain of varying severity. "Gastroenteritis" is a term used to describe the several types of lower gastrointestinal infection.

"Dysentery" is a term used to describe the condition in which diarrhea is accompanied by cramping abdominal pain and tenesmus (painful straining when passing a stool). Dysentery results from "enteroinvasive" microorganisms that penetrate the mucosa and cause inflammation of the intestinal wall. The stools often contain inflammatory cells and red blood cells; there may be grossly visible blood.

At the opposite end of the spectrum are the nonpainful, profusely watery diarrheal syndromes caused by viruses and by some parasites and bacteria. Most acute, watery diarrheal syndromes resolve spontaneously within a week. If symptoms persist without explanation, parasites, such as *Giardia lamblia*, and noninfectious etiologies should be considered. The stools produced by *Giardia* are often foul-smelling, greasy, and float in the toilet bowl.

A special, and fortunately uncommon category is enteric fever. This syndrome is classically caused by *Salmonella typhi*, although other species and serovars of *Salmonella* may produce a similar disease. Enteric fever is characterized by fever, first remitting and later constant headache, abdominal pain, splenomegaly, relative bradycardia (low pulse rate), and leukopenia. Diarrhea is not prominent; in fact, constipation may be more common at the outset. In addition, some invasive pathogens may be associated with systemic disease and metastatic infection in other organs, particularly in patients with underlying illnesses, such as chronic liver disease.

Certain infectious agents are associated with discrete risk factors or clinical features. Some agents, such as microsporidia, occur almost exclusively in severely immunosuppressed patients. *Clostridium difficile* produces disease almost exclusively in patients who have been treated with antimicrobial agents that alter the normal gastrointestinal flora. Many of the agents are transmitted through contaminated food and water.[48] The major syndromes of lower gastrointestinal disease are summarized in Table 2-3.

In most communities the most commonly identified agents of gastroenteritis are *Campylobacter jejuni*, *Salmonella* spp., *Giardia lamblia*, rotaviruses, and noroviruses (Norwalk-like viruses, for which laboratory testing is not readily available).[62] When all is said and done, however, the diagnostic yield from stool cultures in most clinical laboratories is a disappointing 1.5 to 5.6 percent.[287]

Some agents of gastroenteritis require prompt treatment, e.g., *Shigella* spp.; for others specific therapy is not available, e.g., viruses; for still others therapy is indicated only if complicated disease or enteric fever is present, e.g., *Salmo-*

nella spp. Physicians are most likely to order stool cultures if one of the following conditions is present[115]:

1. The patient has acquired immunodeficiency syndrome
2. The patient has traveled recently to a developing country
3. Presence of bloody stools
4. Diarrhea has been present for more than 3 days
5. Diarrhea has required intravenous rehydration
6. Fever is present

Laboratories differ greatly in the sophistication of their evaluation of fecal specimens. In a survey of 388 clinical laboratories during 1999 most microbiologists examined feces for the presence of *Salmonella* spp., *Shigella* spp., and *Campylobacter* spp. In contrast, approximately 50% of sites included *Escherichia coli* O157:H7, *Vibrio* spp., and *Yersinia* spp. in their diagnostic protocol.[298] Examination of stools for parasites was performed in only 59% of 455 laboratories surveyed; specimens were sent to a reference laboratory for testing.[132] Examination of feces for *Cryptosporidium* spp., *Cyclospora cayetanensis*, and microsporidia was performed only on specific request in 89% of these laboratories. It is very important for each laboratory to indicate the pathogens sought when the results are reported to the clinician. A report of "No enteric pathogens isolated" is no

Table 2-3 The Major Gastroenteritis Syndromes and Most Common Etiologic Agents				
SYNDROME	BACTERIA	VIRUSES	PARASITES	COMMENTS
Inflammatory diarrhea, including dysentery	*Shigella* spp., enteroinvasive *E. coli*, enterohemorrhagic *E. coli*, *Salmonella enteritidis*, *Campylobacter jejuni*, *Vibrio parahaemolyticus*, *Clostridium difficile*	None	*Entamoeba histolytica*	Involves colon; fecal leukocytes often present
Noninflammatory diarrhea	Enterotoxigenic *E. coli*, Enteroaggregative *E. coli*, *Vibrio cholerae*, *Clostridium perfringens*, *Bacillus cereus*, *Staphylococcus aureus*	Norovirus, rotavirus, enteric adenovirus, astrovirus, etc.	*Giardia lamblia*, *Cryptosporidium parvum*, *Isospora belli*, *Cyclospora cayetensis*, microsporidia	Involves proximal small bowel; fecal leukocytes usually absent
Diarrhea with systemic disease, including enteric fever	*Salmonella typhi*, other *Salmonella* spp., *Yersinia enterocolitica*, *Campylobacter* spp.	None	None	Involves distal small bowel; fecal mononuclear leukocytes may be present

Adapted from reference[104].

longer acceptable. In a survey of almost 3,000 physicians in five states 28% of physicians did not know whether the laboratory tested for *Escherichia coli* O157:H7 and 40% did not know whether *Yersinia* spp. or *Vibrio* spp. had been tested.[115]

COLLECTION OF FECAL SPECIMENS

The collection of diarrheal stools is not difficult. Specimens for detection of all pathogens should be collected in clean (not necessarily sterile), wide-mouthed containers that can be covered with a tight-fitting lid. The containers should be free of preservatives, detergents, and metal ions. Contamination with urine should also be avoided. If an intestinal parasite such as *Entamoeba histolytica*, *Giardia lamblia*, or *Cryptosporidium* spp. is suspected, a small portion of stool sample should be placed in preservatives, such as polyvinyl alcohol (or a mercury-free alternative) and 10% formalin. Stool specimens for detection of viruses should not be added to viral transport medium because the viral particles may be diluted out beyond the sensitivity of detection of the system being used.

In some instances, the collection of a rectal swab rather than feces may be necessary, particularly in newborns or in severely debilitated adults. Rectal swabs may be more effective than feces for recovery of certain strains of *Shigella*, because these organisms are susceptible to cooling and drying. Swabs have also been reported to be more effective than stool specimens[183] for recovery of *Clostridium difficile* in hospitalized patients. The rectal swab should be inserted just beyond the anal sphincter, avoiding direct contact with fecal material in the rectum. The swabs should be inoculated immediately onto culture media or placed in a suitable transport system to prevent drying. Rectal swabs are also necessary for diagnosis of rectal gonococcal infection.

EPIDEMIOLOGIC CONSIDERATIONS IN THE EVALUATION OF PATIENTS WITH GASTROENTERITIS

A detailed medical history should be taken, including recent travel, exposure to potentially contaminated food or water, and the presence of similar disease in friends or family. In particular, travel to countries outside the United States, where certain diarrheal diseases may be endemic, should be solicited. The most common cause of "traveler's diarrhea" (also called "Montezuma's revenge," "Delhi belly," and other colorful names) is enterotoxigenic *E. coli*,[1] but other important pathogens, such as *Entamoeba histolytica*, are also more common outside the United States. Poor-quality water and food supplies, marginal cold-storage facilities, and contamination from people preparing foods in countries outside the United States put travelers at risk. In these days of global commerce, however, staying at home is not free of risk either. Epidemics of gastroenteritis have been reported as a result of contaminated food,[48] usually vegetables or fruit that are not cooked before eating, that has been imported from other countries. For instance, a multistate outbreak of *Cyclospora* infection was traced to raspberries imported from Central America only after reports accumulated at national reference centers.[116] It is important to remember that bacteria commonly found on poultry (which will be killed during cooking) may cause disease if uncooked food,

Table 2-4 Association of Gastrointestinal Infections With Specific Factors

FACTOR	INFECTIOUS AGENT(S)
Backpacking and drinking from mountain streams	*Giardia lamblia*
Dairy products	*Salmonella* spp., *Campylobacter* spp., *Yersinia* spp., *Listeria monocytogenes*
East Coast and Gulf Coast	Halophilic vibrios; e.g., *Vibrio parahaemolyticus*, *Vibrio vulnificus*
Egg and potato salads, pastries	*Staphylococcus aureus*
Eggs	*Salmonella* spp.
Fresh fruit	*Cryptosporidium* spp; *Cyclospora* spp.
Fried rice	*Bacillus cereus*
Hamburger	*Escherichia coli* O157:H7
Immunosuppressed patients	*Cryptosporidium* spp., *Isospora belli*, *Mycobacterium avium* complex, *Strongyloides stercoralis* hyperinfection, cytomegalovirus, *Candida* spp.
Shellfish	*Vibrio* spp., noroviruses, hepatitis A virus

such as vegetables, come in contact with the chopping boards or counters that were used for preparation of the poultry.

Certain locales, foods, and clinical settings are particularly associated with specific pathogens (Table 2-4). Any combination, including ones not previously reported, are possible, however, emphasizing the importance of the careful clinical history and reporting of cases to public health authorities.

Upper Intestinal Infections

The upper gastrointestinal tract consists of the esophagus, stomach, and proximal duodenum (from the oropharynx to the intestine).

CLINICAL SYMPTOMS

Esophagitis is associated with difficulty swallowing and pain on swallowing (dysphagia) and by pain that radiates to the back. The gastroesophageal mucosa is at particular risk of ulceration. The most common infectious agents in this site are *Candida albicans* and herpes simplex virus, both of which produce erosive disease.

When the stomach and gastroesophageal junction are involved, symptoms include anorexia, a feeling of nausea (occasionally with overt vomiting), and upper abdominal pain. Because of the very low pH of the gastric acid, 99.9% of ingested bacteria are killed within 30 minutes of exposure;

therefore, gastritis from direct invasion of the stomach wall is rare. Upper gastrointestinal infection, therefore, is most commonly caused by viruses and bacterial toxins. Gastric acid also has an important role to play in protecting the lower gastrointestinal tract from bacterial infection. Antacid therapy, which neutralizes the low gastric pH and gastrectomy, in which most of the acid-forming mucosa is removed, predispose individuals to enteric infections from a variety of bacterial species. Guerrant[103] reports that the dose of *V. cholerae* required to cause infection in normal people (10^8 organisms per milliliter) was reduced to only 10^4/mL in volunteers who were given bicarbonate to neutralize gastric acidity.

Helicobacter pylori (formerly *Campylobacter pylori*) has been associated with gastritis and peptic ulcer disease.[152,174,284] The organism has the unique biochemical property of rapidly and avidly hydrolyzing urea and releasing ammonium ions. The bacterial cells can presumably surround themselves with an alkaline cloud, thereby making it possible to survive the highly acid environment of the gastric mucosa. The infectious etiology of peptic ulcer eluded detection for so long because it does not have the classic signs and symptoms of an infectious disease. The knowledge of this infectious ''noninfectious'' disease has opened new vistas on the spectrum of illness that microbes can produce.

A major factor in upper gastrointestinal infection is ingestion of microbes and/or preformed microbial toxins in food and drink, commonly known as food poisoning. The acute and often fulminant gastritis, accompanied by generalized weakness and vomiting, that may be experienced after ingesting food heavily contaminated with organisms such as *Staphylococcus aureus*, *Salmonella* spp., *Clostridium perfringens*, and *Bacillus cereus*, does not result from direct bacterial invasion of the stomach wall; rather, it results from the direct emetic action of preformed neurotoxins on the central autonomic nervous system.

OBTAINING SPECIMENS FROM THE UPPER GASTROINTESTINAL TRACT

Gastric specimens for culture are only rarely obtained and are limited to those few situations for which a diagnosis may not be possible by other means. The bacterial agents of acute toxic food poisoning may be recovered from vomitus material.

Gastric biopsies are performed to detect *Helicobacter pylori*.[280,297] Biopsy specimens may be cultured for the recovery of *H. pylori*, a procedure rarely performed in clinical laboratories; tested for the presence of urease activity, a presumptive clue to the presence of *H. pylori;* or examined histologically for the presence of gastritis and spiral bacteria. Alternatively, serologic examination may be undertaken.

Aspirations of duodenal contents may be helpful in making the diagnosis of giardiasis and strongyloidiasis if repeated stool examinations have failed to detect a pathogen. The use of the commercial ''string test'' (Enterotest, HDC, Milpitas, CA) is an alternative to passing a gastric tube. The Enterotest is a capsule containing a tightly wound string. The string is unraveled for a short distance and the end taped to the patient's cheek; then the capsule is swallowed. In about 30 to 60 minutes, when the capsule has reached the upper duodenum, the string is carefully removed and any mucus adhering to the strand is milked onto the surface of a glass slide for direct microscopic examination.

Urinary Tract Infections

The urinary tract is divided into an upper portion, composed of the kidneys, renal pelves, and ureters, and a lower portion, made up of the urinary bladder and the urethra. Upper urinary tract infections are most commonly ascending; that is, they originate in the urinary bladder and ascend through the ureters to the kidneys. Normally, the vesicourethral valve prevents reflux of urine from the urinary bladder into the ureters. Individuals with urogenital anomalies or with overdistention of the urinary bladder from outflow obstruction, neurogenic malfunctions, or pressure from an enlarged uterus during pregnancy are particularly susceptible to ascending urinary tract infections. Infections of the renal pelvis (pyelitis) and kidney (pyelonephritis) are the most common complications. The infections can be acute or can be recurrent with chronic inflammatory damage.

Upper urinary tract infections less commonly result from hematogenous spread of bacteria into the renal cortex in patients with septicemia. Multifocal abscesses or acute suppurative pyelonephritis are common manifestations.

Urinary tract infections are sometimes divided into uncomplicated and complicated categories.[273,307] Uncomplicated infection is acute cystitis or pyelonephritis in a young woman without underlying urinary tract or systemic disease. If the diagnosis is cystitis, empiric antimicrobial therapy can be instituted without resorting to a culture, because *Escherichia coli* is responsible for almost all of these infections. A urinalysis or test for leukocyte esterase should be performed to demonstrate that the process is inflammatory; if polymorphonuclear neutrophils are absent, a culture should be performed before initiating therapy. A follow-up culture (''test of cure'') is not necessary unless symptoms persist.

Cystitis or pyelonephritis in males, children, chronically catheterized patients, and women with recurrent infection, urologic abnormalities, or underlying disease is considered a complicated infection. Both urinalysis and urine culture are required for complicated cystitis and all cases of pyelonephritis.[273,307]

Clinical Signs and Symptoms

The cardinal clinical manifestations of upper urinary tract infections are fever (often with chills) and flank pain. Frequency, urgency, and dysuria are more suggestive of infections of the urinary bladder and urethra. In some patients with pyelonephritis or other upper urinary tract infections, however, symptoms consistent with lower tract infections develop first. The differentiation is important because the approach to antimicrobial chemotherapy differs for the two conditions.[273,307]

Lower urinary tract infections typically involve the urinary bladder and/or the urethra. The symptoms are similar for infections in the two sites, so the process is sometimes called the acute urethral syndrome.[275] Frequent and painful urination of small amounts of turbid urine (frequency and dysuria) and suprapubic heaviness or pain are the usual clinical manifestations. Vaginitis in women and prostatitis in men can produce similar symptoms, but can usually be differentiated clinically. Diagnosis is particularly difficult in elderly persons, in whom fever or leukocytosis may not develop during an infection.

There has been much discussion about the significance of asymptomatic bacteriuria. Although this phenomenon has been documented in many types of patients and clinical scenarios, serious medical problems that necessitate treatment of the bacteriuria occur in only a few situations: pregnant women, women who are undergoing invasive genitourinary procedures, and recipients of renal transplants during the early posttransplantation period.[203]

Host Factors

The prevalence of urinary tract infections varies with the gender and age of the patient. In neonates and infants, urinary tract infections are more common in boys, with an overall prevalence of about 1%. Most of these infections are associated with congenital anomalies. By the time children attend school, there is a higher prevalence in girls compared with boys.[279] This ratio remains consistent into adulthood. High rates of incidence occur in certain conditions, such as diabetes or pregnancy. In the elderly, higher rates of occurrence can be expected for both women (20%) and men (10%) in whom predisposing conditions exist, such as obstructive uropathy from the prostate in men, poor emptying of the bladder from uterine prolapse in women, and procedures that require instrumentation in both men and women.

By far the most common population at risk for both symptomatic urinary tract infection and asymptomatic bacteriuria, however, is sexually active women.[278] Although asymptomatic infection in this group does not clearly produce serious medical problems, it may be a predictor of future symptomatic infection.[203] Women are more susceptible to infection than men because of the shorter length of the female urethra. Perineal bacterial flora that originate in the gastrointestinal tract are the usual pathogens, especially if the bacteria possess factors that facilitate their binding to the uroepithelium.[238] Sexual intercourse facilitates entry of the bacteria into the female urethra.

A second population that is at increased risk of infection is the chronically catheterized patient.[271] A foreign body, such as an indwelling urinary catheter, guarantees colonization of the catheter within 5 days of placement. The resulting asymptomatic bacteriuria is not harmful per se, but it does put the patient at risk for developing symptomatic infection, including pyelonephritis and urosepsis. When the patient is also afflicted with dementia, as many elderly individuals are, it may be difficult to ascertain whether the infection is symptomatic. Without fever and leukocytosis the only indicators may be subtle changes in personality or mentation. The best person to assess these characteristics may be the primary caregivers, rather than the physician who sees the patient intermittently.

Collection of Urine Samples for Culture

Except for the urethral mucosa, which supports the growth of a microflora, the normal urinary tract is usually devoid of bacteria.[135] Urine can easily become contaminated

Table 2-5 Some Commensal Flora and Potential Pathogens in the Urinary Tract

COMMENSAL FLORA	POTENTIAL PATHOGENS
α/β-Hemolytic streptococci	*Corynebacterium urealyticum* (D2)[a]
Bacillus spp.	*Enterococcus* spp.
Coagulase-negative staphylococci	*Enterobacteriaceae*[a]
Diphtheroids	*Pseudomonas* spp.
Lactobacillus spp.	*Staphylococcus aureus*
	Staphylococcus epidermidis (elderly men)
	Staphylococcus saprophyticus (young women)

[a] *Proteae and Corynebacterium urealyticum are urea splitters, alkalinizing the urine and predisposing to stone formation.*

with bacteria from the vaginal canal, the perineum, or indigenous bacterial flora in the urethra. Table 2-5 lists selected microorganisms that are considered contaminants and potential pathogens in the urinary tract.

MIDSTREAM URINE SPECIMENS

Urine samples are most commonly collected by sampling the midstream flow by the clean-catch technique. Urine collection from women by this technique requires personal supervision for best results.[29] The periurethral area and perineum are first cleansed with two or three gauze pads saturated with soapy water, using a forward-to-back motion, followed by a rinse with sterile saline or water. Bradbury offers evidence that failure to clean the periurethral area and perineum in females may not adversely affect the quality of midstream urine samples for culture. Despite this counsel, we still recommend that the following cleaning procedure be carried out when collecting urine specimens for culture from females.

The labia should be held apart during voiding, and the first few milliliters of urine passed into a bedpan or toilet bowl to flush out bacteria from the urethra (Fig. 2-2). The midstream portion of urine is then collected in a sterile, wide-mouthed container that can be covered with a tightly fitted lid. The soapy water preparation is usually not required for men; rather, simple cleansing of the urethral meatus immediately before voiding and then collection of the midstream sample is usually sufficient.

Patients seen in a clinician's office or in a clinic are frequently asked to obtain their own urine sample. This practice is acceptable if the patient is given precise instructions for properly collecting the specimen. It is recommended that these instructions be printed on a card that the patient can retain after receiving the verbal description. When the patient does not seem to comprehend or when language is a barrier, the nurse or office assistant should read through the instructions point by point or provide direct assistance in collecting the sample. An example of an instruction card is given in Box 2-2.

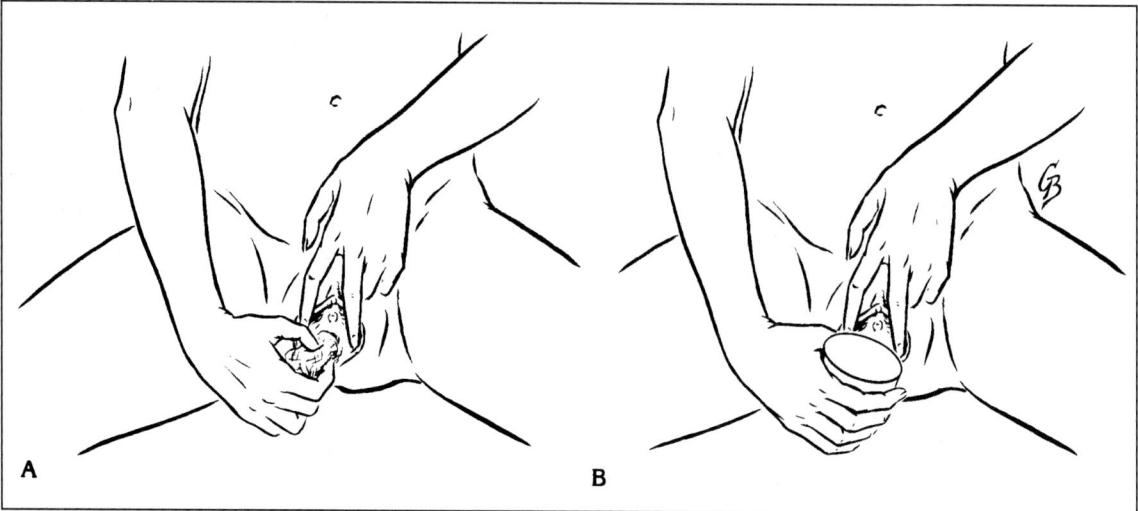

Figure 2-2 Midstream clean-catch urine collection. **(A)** The labia are separated with the fingers and cleansed with a 4 × 4-inch gauze pad saturated with green soap. **(B)** The midstream portion of the urine is collected in a sterile container.

The accuracy of the urine collection procedure can be monitored over time by noting the frequency with which urine colony counts range between 10,000 and 100,000 CFU/mL. Most patients will have colony counts that fall outside this range. Those free of infection will have no bacteria or fewer than 10^2 CFU/mL. Infected patients will have 100,000 CFU/mL or more. The frequency of intermediate counts should not exceed 5–10% if the urine collection procedures have been performed properly. Specimens should be processed within 2 hours after collection to achieve accurate colony counts.

The B-D Urine Collection Kit (Becton-Dickinson, Cockeysville, MD), designed to maintain the bacterial population in urine at room temperature for 24 hours, has been equally as effective as overnight refrigeration of specimens.[122] Although some decrease in colony count may be noted after prolonged storage, the system is recommended for transport of urine samples for which processing will be delayed up to 24 hours. Transport systems using boric acid (which is in included in the B-D Urine Collection Kit additives) may offer an alternative method for home or remote collection of urine samples. Jewkes and associates[128] conclude from a study of 84 children that urine collection in boric acid minimizes contamination, although growth of potential bacterial pathogens may also be inhibited in a small number of cases.

Collection of valid clean-catch urine specimens for culture from incontinent elderly men residing in nursing homes also poses a problem. Nicolle and colleagues[204] reported success in diagnosing urinary tract infections in this population of patients by using an external collection device consisting of a sterile condom and leg bag. Before applying the condom, the glans penis was cleaned with soap and water and rinsed with sterile saline. The leg bag was examined every 10 to 15 minutes until a specimen was obtained. Because contamination with low counts of bacteria occurred in almost 50% of the patients, rapid transport of the specimens to the laboratory and immediate transfer to culture media were required. Bacterial counts greater than 10^5 CFU/mL, particularly if obtained on two successive collections, had a high correlation with other indicators of urinary tract infection.

OTHER VOIDED URINE SPECIMENS

The purpose of the midstream technique is to collect urine that has been sitting in the bladder, discarding the initial portion that has been in contact with the urethra—and presumably contaminated with urethral flora. If one is investigating urethritis, however, it is actually the initial portion of voided urine that is of interest. Alternatively (although more

---

Box 2-2 Instructions for Obtaining Clean-Catch Urine Specimens (Females)

1. Remove underclothing completely and sit comfortably on the seat, swinging one knee to the side as far as you can.
2. Spread yourself with one hand, and continue to hold yourself spread while you clean yourself and collect the specimen.
3. Wash. Be sure to wash well and rinse well before you collect the urine sample. Using each of four separate 4 × 4-inch sterile sponges soaked in 10% green soap, wipe from the front of your body toward the back. Wash between the folds of the skin as carefully as you can.
4. Rinse. After you have washed with each soap pad, rinse with a moistened pad with the same front-to-back motion. Do not use any pad more than once.
5. Hold yourself apart and allow the first few drops of urine to pass into the toilet bowl. Hold the cup on the outside and pass the remaining urine into the cup.
6. Place the lid on the container or ask the nurse to do so for you.

painfully), a swab may be inserted into the distal urethra to collect the specimen. The primary application of initial voided urine specimens is the diagnosis of urethritis caused by *Neisseria gonorrhoeae* and *Chlamydia trachomatis.*[130]

If one is considering the diagnosis of acute prostatitis, however, prostatic secretions are the material of interest. The most common technique is differential culturing of urine before and after prostatic massage. A 10-fold increase in bacterial numbers after massage of the prostate suggests the diagnosis.[68]

CATHETER COLLECTIONS

Catheterization for the express purpose of obtaining a urine specimen should be avoided if possible because of the risk of introducing bacterial pathogens. In a study of 105 women with suspected urinary tract infection,[305] the culture results obtained from midstream, clean-catch urine samples did not differ in sensitivity, specificity, or positive or negative predictive values from parallel in-out (I&O) catheter specimens collected immediately after the midstream samples. Catheterization should be restricted to patients who are unable to produce an adequate midstream sample, and it should be performed with meticulous attention to aseptic technique. The first several milliliters of urine from the catheter should be discarded to wash out any organisms that may have lodged in the catheter tip during transit through the urethra.

Urine samples can be obtained from an indwelling catheter using a no. 28 needle and a syringe. Be sure to disinfect the area where the needle puncture is to be made. Urine can be aspirated through the soft rubber connector between the catheter and the collecting tubing. Urine samples should not be obtained from catheter bags. Although it is tempting to use wet diapers or bags as a source of urine in infants, obtaining an interpretable specimen by these means is a major challenge. Foley catheter tips are unsuitable for culture because they are invariably contaminated with urethral or colonizing organisms.[294]

SUPRAPUBIC ASPIRATION

Suprapubic aspirations are reserved almost exclusively for neonates and small children. This technique is illustrated in Figure 2-3. The procedure is best performed when the bladder is full. The suprapubic skin overlying the urinary bladder is disinfected and sterile drapes are put in place. In the immediate site where the tap is to be made, an anesthetic solution, such as 1% lidocaine HCl, is injected subcutaneously. With the point of a sharply tapered surgical blade, a small incision is made through the epidermidis. Through this wound, an 18-gauge, short-bevel spinal needle is gently extended into the urinary bladder and 10 mL of urine is aspirated into the syringe.

Culture of Urine Specimens

Both selective and nonselective media are required. A combination of 5% sheep blood agar and MacConkey agar is usually sufficient for the recovery of the organisms listed in Table 2-5. Microbiologists whose laboratories serve primarily ambulatory patients, in whom *Escherichia coli*

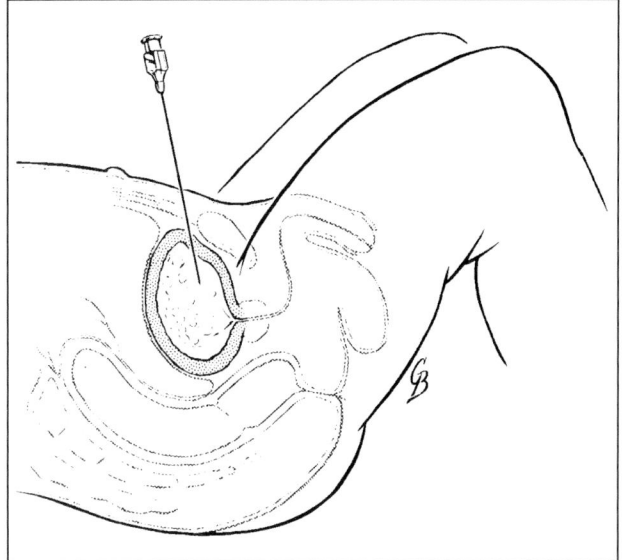

Figure 2-3 Suprapubic urinary bladder aspiration. A needle is directed percutaneously into the urinary bladder just above the symphysis pubis. Urine can be removed with a syringe.

is the most common pathogen expected, prefer to use eosin-methylene blue (EMB) agar because of the distinctive morphology of *E. coli* on that media. Although some microbiologists incorporate a medium selective for gram-positive bacteria as well (e.g., colistin-nalidixic acid [CNA] blood agar or phenylethyl alcohol [PEA] agar), the yield from this addition is probably not worth the expense.[43] In many laboratories, inoculation of duplicate plates with both 0.01-mL- and 0.001-mL-calibrated loops is performed for comparison of counts as a quality control check and to facilitate counting colonies.

After delivering the inoculum from the calibrated loop, the surface of each agar plate should be completely streaked over all quadrants as demonstrated in Chapter 1 so that semi-quantitative colony counts can be performed after incubation. A colony count of 10^5 CFU/mL or greater is the criterion most commonly used to determine whether identification and susceptibility testing of an isolate should be performed. When the colony count is between 10^4 and 10^5 CFU/mL, or when multiple species are recovered, the decision to make identifications and perform susceptibility tests must be made by each laboratory director, often on a case-by-case basis. Some microbiologists use 10^4 CFU/mL as the decision point, because the calibrated loops tend to underestimate the colony count. Similarly, a pure culture is required in some laboratories, while two pathogens will be evaluated in others. (See Chapter 1 for further discussion of evaluating mixed cultures.)

Cultures of catheterized or suprapubic urine specimens are usually analyzed in detail, even with low colony counts or with the recovery of multiple organism types. Colony counts as low as 10^2 CFU/mL of enteric gram-negative bacilli may be significant in female patients with the acute urethral syndrome[274,275]; however, the physician must alert the laboratory in suspected cases, because semiquantitative urine culture techniques are not designed to detect such low colony counts. The significance of these ''low-colony-count'' infections has been documented only in women infected with enteric bacilli. Contamination is even more of an issue when evaluating small numbers of organisms. In one study contaminated specimens were increased by 19% when a 0.01-mL loop was used.[43] Discussion with the clinician about the course of action is appropriate.

Screening Tests for Urinary Tract Infection

The literature on screening tests for urinary tract infection is voluminous, contradictory, and confusing. It is useful to consider that screening for bacteriuria is a very different task from screening for inflammation.[323] The two will be considered separately.

With the exception of the few situations in which asymptomatic bacteriuria is clinically important, the end point of interest is symptomatic urinary tract infection. Many studies use the presence of 10^5 bacteria as a surrogate end point, but this approach is flawed. It is perhaps useful to think of the problem in the terms used to describe the approach to pneumonia. The diagnosis of urinary tract infection is made by evaluating clinical symptoms and/or testing for the presence of an inflammatory response. Once an infection has been documented, microbiologic culture is useful to determine the etiology of that infection.

SCREENING TESTS FOR BACTERIURIA

The presence of bacteriuria at concentrations that suggest urinary tract infection can be assessed by microscopic examination of the urine, by tests for bacterial products, and by cultures. None of the tests detect low colony counts in urine with adequate sensitivity.

Microscopic Examination. Gram's stain is an inexpensive method to estimate bacteriuria. In one study the presence of at least one organism per oil-immersion field in uncentrifuged urine had a sensitivity of 94% and a specificity of 90% for detecting colony counts of at least 10^5 CFU/mL.[309] This approach has the advantage that the gram reactivity of the organisms can be characterized. Gram stain of urine is not used in most clinical laboratories as a screening test, however, because methodically reviewing the smears is too labor-intensive. Examining unstained centrifuged urine as part of the urinalysis has been reported to have a sensitivity similar to Gram's stain on uncentrifuged urine,[43] but this experience has not been universal, and most clinicians do not depend on urinalysis for detection of bacteriuria. Differentiating bacteria from other particles in unstained preparations at moderate magnifications can be a challenge. A useful quality assurance tool is comparison of the results of culture and urinalysis.

Tests for Bacterial Products. One common approach is the use of a reagent-impregnated dipstick, designed to detect the presence of urine nitrite (Griess test) and indirectly to estimate the number of segmented neutrophils by detecting leukocyte esterase activity (Ames, Elkhart, IN; Chemstrips, Biodynamics/Boehringer-Mannheim, Indianapolis, IN).[214] The rationale for the nitrite test is that most urinary tract infections are caused by nitrate-reducing members of the family *Enterobacteriaceae* (particularly *Escherichia coli*). This test lacks accuracy when used alone.[131,191] False-posi-

tive results may occur if the specimen has been delayed in transit and overgrown with nitrate-reducing bacteria or from drug interference; false-negative results are encountered if the organism causing the infection does not reduce nitrates (e.g., *Enterococcus* spp.) or if the patient is on a vegetable-free diet (loss of an important source of nitrate).

The sensitivity of the combination nitrite-leukocyte esterase strip with bacteriuria at a level of 10^5 CFU/mL is in the range of 79–93%, with a specificity of approximately 82–98%.[131,214] In a multicenter study of 298 urine specimens with colony counts of fewer than 10^5 CFU/mL,[212] the LN strip detected 81% of cases. In a subset of 204 specimens with pyuria in addition to colony counts fewer than 10^5 CFU/mL (i.e., both inflammation and bacteria), however, the detection rate was increased to 95%.

An alternative approach is detection of catalase, which is produced by most uropathogens, marketed as Uriscreen (Diatech Diagnostics, Allston, MA). It appears to function similarly to nitrite and suffers from the same defects. If the pathogens in a particular population of patients produce catalase, a negative catalase test effectively excludes high-colony-count bacteriuria; it offers no advantage over a test for leukocyte esterase.[212,301]

Detection of Bacteriuria by Culture. Conventional culture is a simple and economic approach to screening. Although it does require 24-hour incubation, the decision to treat is rarely urgent. Some clinicians prefer to inoculate a urine dip slide in the office, rather than send the urine to a laboratory for culture. The dip slide (SOLAR-CULT; Solar Biologicals, Ogdensburg, NY; Uricult, Orion Diagnostica, Espoo, Finland) is a paddle coated on each side with an agar intended to recover gram-positive and gram-negative bacteria. The paddle is dipped into the urine, drained, replaced in its container, and incubated. The quantity of growth is assessed by comparison to a chart. The dipslides are not waived tests; a clinician who uses them must meet the requirements for nonwaived tests, even if the bacteria are not identified and tested for susceptibility. The advantage of this approach is simplicity and economy for negative specimens. The disadvantage is the difficulty obtaining subcultures for subsequent evaluation of colonies. In the post-CLIA 1988 era (see Chapter 1) many clinicians prefer the most straightforward approach of sending the original specimen to a diagnostic laboratory.

SCREENING TESTS FOR PYURIA

Leukocyte esterase (LE) is produced by polymorphonuclear neutrophils. A reagent strip, impregnated with buffered indoxyl carboxylic acid ester and a diazonium salt, can be used to detect leukocyte esterase activity in the urine. One advantage of this test is that leukocytes need not be viable for LE activity to be detected. When performed alone, this test correlated with 10 or more white blood cells per high-power field (WBC/HPF) in the urine, with a sensitivity in the range of 88% and a specificity of 94%.[149] False-positive LE test findings may result from high urinary levels of ascorbic acid or albumin (>300 mg/dL) or from the effects of preservatives and detergents. Most false-negative results occur when urine WBC counts are in the marginal range of 5 to 10/HPF. Kierkegaard and associates[139] report that 35%

of urine samples in their study turned from positive (30 WBC/HPF) to negative (10 WBC/HPF or fewer) when the urine was delayed in transit for ≥3 hours. Thus, the LE test may better reflect pyuria than does microscopic enumeration of neutrophils when the interval between collection and processing cannot be controlled.

A useful option to offer clinicians is that of performing a urine culture only if the leukocyte esterase test is positive (i.e., if an inflammatory process is present). This approach is obviously not appropriate in the few situations in which asymptomatic bacteriuria is of concern or if the patient has neutropenia. The option to order a urine culture regardless of documented pyuria should be offered if the patient has the symptoms of an acute urinary tract infection.

Infections of the Genital Tract

The genital tract consists of external and internal genitalia in both sexes. In males, the internal genitalia include the testes, epididymis, seminal vesicles, and urethra (the prostate was discussed above). In the female, the internal genitalia are ovaries, fallopian tubes, uterus (primarily endometrium), uterine cervix, and the vagina with its accessory glands. The external genitalia consist of the penis and the labia.

Infections can be divided conceptually into sexually transmitted infections, peripartum infections, and vaginitis. The commensal flora and common pathogens of the genital tract are summarized in Table 2-6.

Sexually Transmitted Infections[46]
URETHRITIS AND CERVICITIS

The most common sexually transmitted infection is caused by *Chlamydia trachomatis*, which causes urethritis and cervicitis. In men the symptoms primarily relate to urethritis: pain on urination and urethral discharge. Asymptomatic infections occur, but are less common than in women. In women a distinctive mucopurulent cervicitis is a common manifestation of infection, in addition to acute urethritis.[36]

Table 2-6 Commensal Flora and Selected Etiologic Agents in the Genital Tract

ANATOMIC SITE	COMMENSAL FLORA	SEXUALLY TRANSMITTED DISEASE (STD) ETIOLOGIES	NON-STD ETIOLOGIES
Urethra	*Enterobacteriaceae*, α/γ-streptococci, *Enterococcus* spp., diphtheroids, coagulase-negative staphylococcus, anaerobes (distal 1–2 cm)	*Chlamydia trachomatis* *Neisseria gonorrhoeae*	
External genitalia and perineal skin	Diphtheroids, coagulase-negative staphylococci, *Micrococcus* spp., yeast, *Acinetobacter* spp., *Enterobacteriaceae*	Herpes simplex virus, type 1; human papillomavirus; *Treponema pallidum; Haemophilus ducreyi;* granuloma inguinale; lymphogranuloma venereum (*Chlamy diatrachomatis*, serotypes L1–L3)	Herpes simplex virus, type 1; *Candida* spp.; *Streptococcus pyogenes*
Vagina	*Lactobacillus* spp., anaerobes, *Enterobacteriaceae*, α/γ-streptococci, *Enterococcus* spp., diphtheroids, coagulase negative staphylococcus (varies with age)	Human papillomavirus	*Candida* spp., bacterial vaginosis, *Trichomonas vaginalis; Staphylococcus aureus* (toxic-shock syndrome)
Endocervix	Normally sterile or minimally contaminated with vaginal flora	Human papillomavirus; herpes simplex virus, type 2; *Neisseria gonorrhoeae, Chlamydia trachomatis*	Herpes simplex virus, type 1; cytomegalovirus
Endometrium, fallopian tube, ovaries	Normally sterile	*Neisseria gonorrhoeae, Chlamydia trachomatis*	Mixed aerobic-anaerobic infection (ascending); *Streptococcus pyogenes, Listeria monocytogenes, Streptococcus agalactiae; Actinomyces israelii* (in patients with intrauterine contraceptive devices)
Systemic infections with genital portal of entry		Human immunodeficiency virus (HIV), hepatitis B virus, hepatitis C virus	

The most serious complications of these infections is pelvic inflammatory disease, which can produce inflammatory scarring of the fallopian tubes that leads to infertility and ectopic pregnancies. Especially in the case of *C. trachomatis*, infection may be asymptomatic, so that screening of sexually active women is necessary to prevent these serious complications.[45]

GENITAL ULCER DISEASE

Herpes Simplex Virus. Several infectious agents, most sexually transmitted, produce ulcerated lesions in the external and/or internal genitalia.[188] By far the most common is herpes simplex virus. The initial infection is frequently asymptomatic,[87] and asymptomatic shedding of virus occurs in a small percentage of both women and men.[302] In fact, the rate of viral shedding is very similar, whether a clinically evident or an asymptomatic infection has occurred.[303] Clinical disease is most frequently accompanied by vesicular lesions with an erythematous base on the glans penis, vulva, perineum, buttocks, or cervix. The vesicles are painful, may ulcerate, and may be accompanied by systemic symptoms—fever, malaise, anorexia, and tender bilateral inguinal adenopathy.

Herpes simplex virus has two serotypes, which produce infections that differ both epidemiologically and clinically. Type 1 virus produces initial infections in infants, children, and adolescents. The infections are primarily in the upper half of the body, but approximately one third of genital infections are caused by this serotype. It may infect the genital tract by autoinoculation from oral secretions, so sexual transmission is not necessary. In contrast, acquisition of type 2 virus is associated with sexual activity, and its presence implies sexual contact with an infected person. The relative prevalence of the two serotypes varies geographically.[263] Infection with type 2 virus is unfortunately increasing in the United States.[142] The presence or absence of symptoms after infection with type 2 virus is modified by preexisting antibody to type 1 virus[329] and may be influenced by characteristics of the infecting strain.

Herpesvirus establishes latency in the spinal ganglia after a primary infection. Reactivation of genital herpes infection is more common and illness is more severe if the infecting strain is type 2 than if it is type 1. In both cases recurrences decrease in frequency over time.[19]

Other Genital Ulcers. In addition to herpes simplex type 2, other genital ulcer syndromes include syphilis, chancroid (caused by *Haemophilus ducreyi*)[232]; lymphogranuloma venereum (caused by L1, L2, and L3 serotypes of *Chlamydia trachomatis*)[249]; granuloma inguinale (caused by *Calymmatobacterium granulomatis*) and trauma.[232] The chancres of syphilis differ from those of herpes in that they are painless and have indurated margins with a clean base.[259] Chancroid ulcers, in contrast to syphilitic chancres, are painful and, in contrast to herpetic ulcers, do not have indurated margins. The primary pustule of lymphogranuloma venereum may resemble herpes simplex; however, this condition is usually recognizable by the massive bilateral necrotizing inguinal adenopathy. The primary lesion of granuloma inguinale is a subcutaneous nodule that erodes the surface, from which a beefy red, painless, elevated granulomatous lesion develops.

Although these other agents of genital ulcers are relatively uncommon in most areas of the United States, they are unfortunately making a comeback. In particular, syphilis[47] and chancroid[188,189] must be considered in the differential diagnosis in certain geographic areas and in certain patient populations. Chancroid, in particular, may be underreported.[246]

Interactions between Genital Ulcers and Human Immunodeficiency Virus (HIV) Infection. Patients with genital ulcers of several etiologies are at increased risk for acquiring HIV. Conversely, men who are infected with HIV shed type 2 herpes simplex virus more frequently than non-HIV-infected men (even if they have sex with men)[243] and are also quite likely more efficient at shedding HIV in the genital tract if they have ulcerative herpetic lesions.[242]

Venereal Warts. Human papillomaviruses (HPVs) produce exophytic excrescences in squamous epithelium of the skin (common warts and plantar warts) and mucosal surfaces of the respiratory and genital tracts.[110] Symptomatic anogenital warts are usually caused by genotypes 6 and 11. Condyloma acuminatum are cauliflowerlike excrescences that occur on moist mucosal surfaces, most commonly the vulva, vagina, and anus. Keratotic and smooth pustular lesions occur on dry skin, while asymptomatic ''flat warts'' may be found in either smooth or dry areas. Untreated infections usually regress spontaneously, but latent or subclinical infection is probably common. The more serious manifestation of HPV infection is the cellular dysplasia and neoplasia that is produced by certain genotypes, particularly types 16 and 18.[23]

Genital Infections Transmitted by Nonsexual Means
VAGINITIS AND VAGINOSIS

Vaginitis is caused by a limited number of infectious agents, but noninfectious irritants can also cause inflammation, especially if the vaginal mucosa is atrophic.[266] The disease often involves the vulva (vulvovaginitis); mixed infections are not uncommon. Classic presentations are described below. Unfortunately, the symptoms overlap sufficiently that it is not possible to make a definitive diagnosis clinically.[241] It is necessary to document the etiologic agent microbiologically. As many as half of vaginal infections do not have a demonstrable etiology.[241]

Trichomonas vaginalis classically produces a copious, frothy yellow or yellow-green discharge that collects in the posterior vaginal fornix. The discharge in candidiasis is typically more thick and curdlike, and the vaginal mucosa tends to be erythematous. The most common agent is *Candida albicans*, but other species of *Candida* and even other genera can infect the vagina on occasion.

Bacterial Vaginosis. *Gardnerella vaginalis*, initially thought to be associated with bacterial vaginosis, actually works synergistically with anaerobic bacteria of the genera *Bacteroides*, *Peptococcus*, and *Mobiluncus* to produce the characteristic malodorous discharge.[270] The recovery of *G. vaginalis* in the absence of mixed anaerobic flora and symptoms of bacterial vaginosis probably constitutes normal vaginal flora. It has been reported[74] that bacterial vaginosis (defined by clinical criteria) was not present in 55% of women from whom *G. vaginalis* was isolated. The importance of recognizing bacterial vaginosis clinically and establishing a laboratory diagnosis is emphasized.[118] In a study of 49 women with preterm labor, out of a subset of 12 who had concomitant bacterial vaginosis, 8 (67%) had a 2.1-fold increased risk for preterm birth before 37 weeks of gestation. Bacterial vaginosis was also associated with low birth weight.

INFECTIONS OF THE UPPER FEMALE GENITAL TRACT

These infections result from entry of vaginal flora into the upper tract.[44,117] The etiologic agents are, therefore, a mixture of aerobic and anaerobic bacteria. An association between *Actinomyces israelii* and endometritis in women using plastic intrauterine contraceptive devices has been clearly documented.[71] The etiology is thought to involve the formation of a calcium carbonate nidus on the plastic, in which the *Actinomyces* species grow. Women using copper devices are rarely infected, presumably because the metal is mildly bacteriostatic. If *A. israelii* is present, the infections are more chronic and recalcitrant than if it is absent. The role of *Mycoplasma* spp. and *Ureaplasma* spp. in genital infections is controversial.

In the postpartum period, infection is a common cause of fever and even sepsis (puerperal infections).[80] The most devastating of these infections are caused by *Clostridium perfringens*, typically after an illegal abortion with nonsterile instruments, and *Streptococcus pyogenes*, the classic cause of puerperal fever. One of the milestones of epidemiology and infection control was the study of puerperal fever by Semmelweis, who proved that the infection was carried to pregnant patients from the autopsy room by physicians who did not wash their hands.[127] The medical staff responded by ostracizing him; over a hundred years later medical personnel still have not absorbed the simple lesson of adequate handwashing.

Systemic Complications of Genital Infections

Infections in many organ systems may spill over into the bloodstream, resulting in disseminated infection and distant metastatic disease. In women genital infectious agents may also be spread through the peritoneal cavity and toxins may produce extragenital effects after being absorbed through the mucosa. Dissemination of pathogens through the bloodstream occurs with *Neisseria gonorrhoeae*, *Treponema pallidum*, and any of the agents of upper tract infection. *Chlamydia trachomatis* and *Neisseria gonorrhoeae* produce a perihepatitis, known as Fitz-Hugh-Curtis syndrome.[140,326] *Haemophilus ducreyi*[231] and the lymphogranuloma venereum serotypes of *C. trachomatis*[133] spread to regional lymph nodes, where they produce swollen, painful, suppurative lesions called buboes (as in bubonic plague). In addition, the granulomas of lymphogranuloma venereum may also be found in the rectal mucosa in individuals who practice receptive anal intercourse.[219] Granuloma inguinale, also known as donovanosis, does not produce regional lymphadenopathy,[14] but some variants of the infection may produce scarring that can result in lymphatic blockage, lymphedema, and even elephantiasis of the external genitals.[251] Rarely,

extragenital donovanosis can occur in any part of the body.[221] Finally, herpes simplex virus migrates through the peripheral nerves to the sacral ganglia, as mentioned previously. Reactivation of the virus can result in aseptic meningitis as well as recurrent genital disease.

Genital infections can also affect the fetus and the newborn infant. Some infections, primarily viral, will cross the placenta and infect the developing fetus.[217] These congenital infections include the rubella virus, cytomegalovirus, parvovirus, varicella-zoster virus, and HIV virus, as well as *Toxoplasma gondii* and *Treponema pallidum*. Other agents infect the neonate as it traverses the vagina (or in utero if an ascending infection causes chorioamnionitis). These infectious agents, mainly bacterial, include *Neisseria gonorrhoeae* (conjunctivitis); *Chlamydia trachomatis* (conjunctivitis and neonatal pneumonia); and agents of neonatal sepsis, prominently herpes simplex virus,[141] *Streptococcus agalactiae*, *Escherichia coli*, and *Listeria monocytogenes*.[119]

Diagnosis of Genital Tract Infections
DIAGNOSIS OF URETHRITIS, CERVICITIS, AND VAGINITIS
Urethritis and Cervicitis. The traditional approach to diagnosis of gonococcal urethritis is to examine a Gram-stained preparation of the smear for the presence of intracellular gram-negative, biscuit-shaped diplococci. Although the presenting symptom in females may be a urethral discharge, clinical manifestations are usually more complex, and varying degrees of exudative cervicitis, vaginitis, salpingitis, and pelvic inflammatory disease may be present. Examination of a Gram-stained smear of cervical or urethral exudate alone is not sufficient to establish the diagnosis in the female because the cell morphology and staining characteristics of other bacterial species mimic the gonococci. Gram's stain is, therefore, recommended only for males with urethral discharge.[130]

Definitive diagnosis requires recovery of the etiologic agent in culture or demonstration of bacterial antigen/nucleic acid. If sexual abuse is under consideration or if medicolegal questions are likely to arise, culture (with chain-of-custody documentation of the specimen) is recommended because of the absolute specificity of this approach. Detection of antigen has been superseded by molecular approaches. Molecular diagnosis is more sensitive than culture for *C. trachomatis* and equivalent for *N. gonorrhoeae*.[130]

Vaginitis. The quickest and least expensive method for diagnosis of vaginal infections is a wet preparation of vaginal secretions. It is possible to detect yeast of *Candida* spp., motile *Trichomonas vaginalis* (only if the specimen is examined promptly), and the clue cells of bacterial vaginosis by examining a drop of unstained secretions microscopically.

Bacterial vaginosis may be diagnosed by several means. Elevated levels of vaginal fluid sialidase activity, probably derived from enzymatic activity of *Bacteroides* species and *Prevotella* species,[30] and an elevation of vaginal fluid pH above 4.5 in conjunction with high levels of *G. vaginalis* (as determined by a specific DNA probe)[54,255] were other markers useful in confirming the diagnosis of bacterial vaginosis. Cook and associates[54] found that a persistent elevated pH and high polyamine and fatty acid levels in vaginal secretions along with clue cells in small numbers were valuable residual abnormalities predicting recurrence of bacterial vaginosis. Clue cells are vaginal epithelial cells that are covered with bacteria, causing a change in the refractile index of the cells; they are a result of the altered bacterial flora in bacterial vaginosis. False-positive rates as high as 18.5% have been reported because other bacteria can also attach to epithelial cells. A 10% false-negative rate has been reported owing to inhibition of bacterial attachment by IgA. However, when the clue cell test is combined with the amine production or "whiff" test, the predictive negative value of 99% provides a good screen for the absence of bacterial vaginosis. Amine production is detected by mixing equal volumes of genital fluid and 10% KOH; perception of a fishy odor is a positive result.[173]

Microscopic examination for clue cells can be performed with a wet mount or a stained preparation, using the Papanicolaou (Pap) or Gram stains. With Gram's stain the characteristic shift from predominantly gram-positive bacilli (*Lactobacillus* spp.) to mixed flora is also useful for making the diagnosis.[181] As discussed previously, culture is not useful for diagnosis of vaginosis. By extension, enzymatic or molecular methods for demonstration of selected microbes, such as *G. vaginalis*, are not useful either.

If it is not possible to examine a specimen quickly, there is a convenient and sensitive method for diagnosis of *T. vaginalis* infections. The InPouch TV Test (Biomed Diagnostics, White City, OR) consists of nutrient medium in a plastic pouch. After introduction of vaginal secretions, the pouch is resealed. It can then be examined immediately as a wet preparation and/or incubated for subsequent periodic observation of motile trophozoites. Although less sensitive than culture or a wet preparation (in which the motility of the parasites facilitates detection), trichomonads can be visualized with Gram's stain or the Pap stain.

Culture for bacterial pathogens has a limited role in diagnosis of vaginitis. In patients with recalcitrant or recurrent infections fungal culture may be used to demonstrate small numbers of yeast that were not seen in a direct smear.

DIAGNOSIS OF GENITAL ULCER DISEASE AND VENEREAL WARTS

Diagnosis of genital ulcer disease may be by direct microscopy, immunofluorescence microscopy, molecular methods, or culture, depending on the organism and the clinical situation. Herpetic ulcers may be sampled for viral culture or for demonstration of characteristic viral cytopathology. Herpes simplex virus produces multinucleated giant cells with intranuclear inclusions. They can be visualized after staining with Wright's stain (or Wright-Giemsa stain), hematoxylin-eosin stain, or the Pap stain (the Tzanck test). Alternatively, immunofluorescence or immunoperoxidase reagents can be used to stain viral antigen in epithelial cells or demonstrate the antigen in an enzyme immunoassay.[267]

The Donovan bodies of granuloma inguinale can be visualized (with difficulty) by staining the intracellular bacteria in mononuclear cells, using Wright's stain (or an equivalent), hematoxylin-eosin (used for primary histologic study of biopsies), or the Pap stain.[61,233] The classic technique for the diagnosis of chancroid used rabbit blood agar, which is not available in most microbiology laboratories.[109] Fortu-

nately, *Haemophilus ducreyi* can be cultivated on a variant of the enriched chocolate agar used for *Neisseria gonorrhoeae*.[59,109] If the modified media are not available, enriched chocolate agar may be substituted. *Haemophilus ducreyi* is labile and does not survive well in transport. If standard transport media, such as Amies media, are used and the specimen is refrigerated, however, the bacteria can be recovered with acceptable accuracy.[60] Lymphogranuloma venereum is usually diagnosed serologically, but the agent can be cultivated if material from a suppurative regional lymph node is cultured for *Chlamydia trachomatis*.[249]

The diagnosis of primary syphilis was classically made by darkfield microscopy of scrapings from the ulcer base.[151] The scrapings must be examined immediately, because visualization depends on having live, motile treponemes. Immunofluorescence reagents that react with *Treponema pallidum* have been available from the Centers for Disease Control and Prevention, but their continued availability is unsure. With these reagents a dried smear can be stained after transport to the laboratory.[125] Serologic diagnosis should also be attempted, but even the fluorescent treponemal antibody absorption (FTA-ABS) procedure may be negative very early in the infection. If syphilis is a consideration and initial tests are negative, follow-up serologic examination with the standard serologic tests for syphilis should be done.

Diagnosis of venereal warts must be made by molecular means because human papillomaviruses do not grow in cell culture and serologic responses are not dependable. If venereal warts are the problem, the laboratory must be informed so that "low-risk" (for cervical neoplasia) genotypes, particularly types 6 and 11, are assayed.[110] More commonly, moderate- to high-risk genotypes are sought as a means of evaluating precursors of cervical cancer.

COLLECTION OF GENITAL SPECIMENS

Collection of Urethral Specimens from Males. When urethral discharge is scant and intracellular diplococci are not seen in a random sample, collecting an early-morning specimen before urination may be helpful. Exudate may be expressed from the urethral orifice by gently "milking" the penis; if material is not readily obtained, the tip of a narrow-diameter cotton, rayon, or Dacron swab on a plastic or aluminum shaft may be inserted 3 to 4 cm into the anterior urethra. The swab should be left in place for a few seconds to allow the fibers to become saturated with the exudate. If a culture for *Chlamydia trachomatis* is being obtained, the swab should be rotated 360 degrees to dislodge some of the epithelial cells.

Collection kits designed for each commercial assay are supplied by the manufacturer. If nucleic-acid amplification methods are used, urine is a satisfactory specimen that is simpler to obtain and more acceptable to the patient than is a urethral swab. The first portion of the urine, which contains urethral cells and bacteria that have been washed out, is collected, in contrast to the midstream urine that is obtained for the diagnosis of cystitis. The manufacturers of kits vary in the specifics of their recommendations for culture.

Collection of Genital Specimens from Females. In females with signs and symptoms of acute genital infection, samples are most commonly obtained from the uterine cervix and the urethra. Cervical specimens are collected with the aid of a speculum after clearing off the cervical mucus with a large swab. A smaller swab with a plastic shaft and a Dacron or polyester tip is recommended for obtaining the specimen.[168] The tip of the swab is inserted a few millimeters past the cervical os, rotated firmly to obtain both exudate and cervical cells, and removed, taking care not to touch the lateral walls of the vaginal canal. Urethral samples may be obtained by milking the urethra and collecting the discharge or, if no discharge is observed, by inserting a small urogenital swab into the urethra and leaving it in place for a few seconds to saturate the fibers with exudate.

As it is for males, urine is a satisfactory specimen for diagnosis of infection in women. Although slightly less sensitive than cervical specimens, it is less invasive and may obviate the need for a speculum exam. Specific recommendations vary by manufacturer.

Vaginal secretions can be aspirated or collected with a swab. Specimens from the upper tract are difficult to obtain from below without contaminating the specimen with vaginal flora. Endometrial specimens are best obtained by inserting the swab through a narrow-bore catheter that has been introduced into the cervical canal, as illustrated in Figure 2-4. By using this technique, there is less chance of contaminating the specimen from secretions of the cervical os or the vaginal

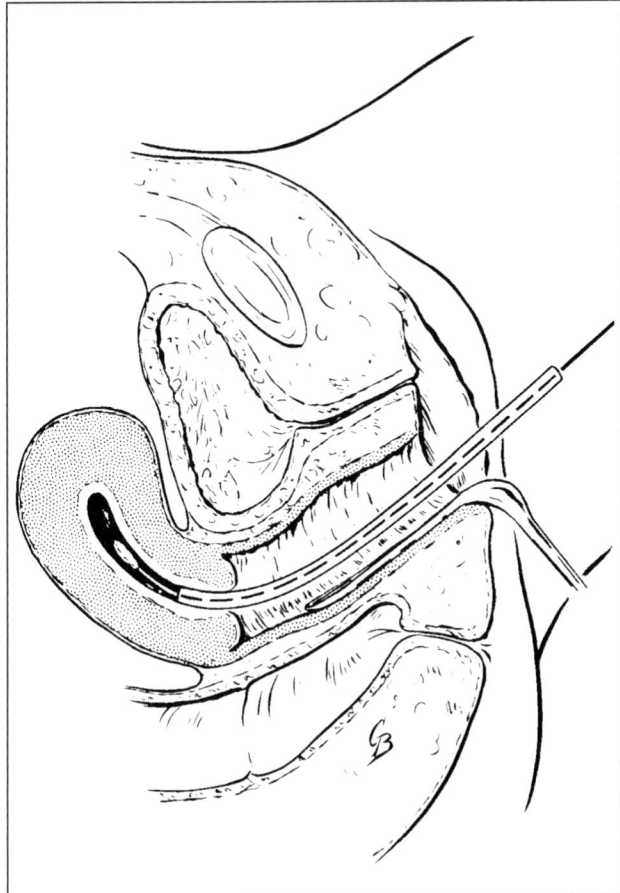

Figure 2-4 Endometrial culture technique. Through a speculum, a catheter is introduced into the cervical os and a swab extended through the catheter into the endometrial cavity. This helps prevent contamination of the swab by contact with the vaginal wall or the cervical os.

canal.[175] For specimens from the fallopian tubes and ovaries, laparoscopy or surgical approaches are necessary.

Collection of Specimens from Genital Ulcers. Ulcers should be cleaned to remove surface debris and contaminating bacteria. For darkfield examination or preparation of smears, a scalpel blade should be used to abrade the base of the ulcer and transfer the material onto a glass slide. For culture, either a washing of the base or a cotton swab may be used.[109] If intact vesicles are present, a swab may be used to collect fluid for Tzanck preparations or herpes culture. Swabs for bacterial culture may be placed in Amies' or Stuart's transport media

---

Infections of the Bones and Joints
Clinical Presentation

Infections of the bones and joints may develop after bacteremic spread of the pathogen from a distant site, by direct extension from an adjacent infection, or by introduction from the environment through trauma. The most common pathogenic organism in bacteremic spread is *Staphylococcus aureus*, but other microbes may also reach the skeletal system by this route, including *Borrelia burgdorferi* (Lyme disease) and agents of systemic mycosis, such as *Blastomyces dermatitidis* and *Coccidioides immitis*. Infections that originate in adjacent tissue are often polymicrobial and include anaerobic bacteria. Traumatic lesions reflect the environmental flora that were introduced at the time of injury.

The symptoms of septic arthritis are fever, pain, and swelling of the affected joint(s).[257] Osteomyelitis may be associated with local pain and tenderness and with restriction of movement.[157] Systemic symptoms may be present in both sites. If the affected bone is in the extremity, the problem is usually evident. In acute vertebral osteomyelitis there is often point tenderness over the affected vertebra. If, however, the infection is subacute, there may be nonlocalized back pain or no local symptoms at all, especially in the elderly.[57] Osteomyelitis may become chronic; septic arthritis is less likely to enter a chronic phase.

Diagnosis of Infections of the Bones and Joints

Diagnosis of osteomyelitis must be accomplished by surgical biopsy of the affected bone. The fluid in a septic joint may be aspirated for microscopic examination and culture. Joint fluid clots readily, so special approaches are necessary. The fluid may be inoculated directly into blood culture bottles[123,147] or into the Isolator system,[331] an effective method for recovering single pathogens. Alternatively, the fluid may be inoculated into a sterile tube that contains sodium polyanethol sulfonate (SPS), the anticoagulant commonly added to blood culture bottles; after transport to the laboratory, the unclotted fluid can be processed as usual. If clotted joint fluid is received in the laboratory, cell counts cannot be performed, but the clot can be homogenized for Gram's stain and culture. It is essential to include chocolate agar when joint fluid is cultured, because fastidious bacteria are prominent pathogens. For infections that are thought to have originated with a bacteremia, blood cultures may yield the pathogen.[57] On occasion, recovery of *Staphylococcus aureus* from blood in the absence of a clear source may be the first clue to vertebral osteomyelitis.

Infections of the Central Nervous System

The most common infections of the central nervous system (CNS) are encephalitis (brain), myelitis (spinal cord), encephalomyelitis, and meningitis (membranous covering of the brain and spinal cord). Often both meningitis and encephalitis (meningoencephalitis) are part of the same infectious process. Less commonly, adjacent infections of soft tissue (e.g., epidural abscess) and bone (osteomyelitis) may impinge on the nervous system. Infections of the peripheral nervous system, which include neuroborreliosis (a variant of Lyme disease), leprosy, and tuberculosis, are infrequent.

Meningitis

Patients with early acute meningitis may experience an influenzalike syndrome—sore and stiff neck, headache, low-grade fever, and lethargy. In elderly, debilitated, or immunosuppressed patients an unexpected alteration in mental status may be the only clue. Various degrees of confusion, agitation, disorientation, or coma may be observed. A positive Brudzinski's sign (resistance to passive neck flexion) and Kernig's sign (inability to extend the leg when the thigh is flexed at a 90-degree angle with the trunk) are signs of meningeal irritation. Subacute or chronic meningitis caused by tuberculosis or fungal infections may present with signs of increased intracranial pressure (papilledema, nausea, vomiting) and mental changes, such as disorientation, confusion, personality change and stupor.[184]

The cerebrospinal fluid (CSF) is normally water-clear, has no more than five lymphocytes per milliliter, has a glucose concentration between 45 and 100 mg/dL depending on the level of blood sugar, a protein concentration between 14 and 45 mg/dL, and is sterile. The classic alterations attributable to meningitis are summarized in Table 2-7. Bacterial infections, which typically are accompanied by large numbers of polymorphonuclear neutrophils, are often called septic or purulent meningitis, whereas infections without a pronounced neutrophil response (mycobacterial, viral, and most fungal infections) are called aseptic meningitis.[53] The common lay term ''spinal meningitis'' is not inaccurate, but it is not informative because it is rare for only one segment of the meninges to be infected; the term is often used for meningococcal meningitis, but obviously any agent can affect the spinal membranes.

Infectious agents can get to the CNS through the blood-stream or by direct extension from adjacent structures. Herpesviruses and rabies virus reach the CNS by retrograde extension up peripheral nerves from spinal ganglia, but this route is unusual for other agents.

Meningitis is most prevalent in certain age groups or in patients with various underlying diseases. Meningitis in the neonate most commonly results from infection that is acquired from the mother in utero or during vaginal delivery.[7,333] *Streptococcus agalactiae* and *Escherichia coli* are the organisms most often recovered; *Listeria monocytogenes*, various members of the *Enterobacteriaceae*, *Pseudomonas* spp., *Flavobacterium meningosepticum*, *Staphylococcus aureus*, and miscellaneous anaerobic bacteria are recovered less frequently. For reasons that are unknown *Citrobacter koseri* (*diversus*) can cause a devastating meningoencephalitis in the neonate.[100] Herpes simplex virus type 2 produces sepsis and meningitis in neonates after acquisition during vaginal delivery.[286]

Neisseria meningitidis causes infections in all age groups. *Haemophilus influenzae* type B was the most common cause of acute bacterial meningitis in the 6-month to 5-year age group, but this infection has been virtually eradicated by an effective vaccine. *Streptococcus pneumoniae* meningitis results from bacteremia or extension of infection from adjacent sinuses or the middle ear.

In adults, *S. pneumoniae* is the most common cause of bacterial meningitis. In young adults, *N. meningitidis* is also common. In the elderly, meningitis follows Shakespeare's ages of man, with the pathogens of the neonatal period making a reappearance. *E. coli* and other gram-negative bacilli are high in prevalence[184] and *S. agalactiae* is also a factor.[72]

Viral meningitis in all age groups is caused primarily by enteroviruses.[223] A large number of viruses that are transmitted by ticks and mosquitoes (arthropodborne viruses or arboviruses) cause CNS disease uncommonly,[41] although the recent appearance of West Nile virus in the United States has stimulated interest.[201]

Cryptococcus neoformans, *Listeria monocytogenes*, and *Mycobacterium tuberculosis* cause indolent or chronic forms of meningitis in both intact hosts and in those with altered defenses. Recurrent aseptic meningitis (Mollaret's meningitis) is typically caused by herpes simplex virus,[285] but the diagnosis must be made by molecular means. *E. coli*, *K. pneumoniae*, and staphylococci are most commonly recovered from patients with posttraumatic or postsurgical meningitis. Approximately 50% of acute meningitis associated with ventricular shunts is caused by coagulase-negative staphylococci.[184]

Table 2-7 Cerebrospinal Fluid Abnormalities in Meningitis

PARAMETER	BACTERIA	MYCOBACTERIA	FUNGI	VIRUSES	EXCEPTIONS
Polymorphonuclear neutrophils	High to very high	High	High	Absent to elevated early; usually absent late	May be absent in *Cryptococcus neoformans*
Monocytes	Variable	Variable	Variable	Usually present	
Glucose	Low	Low	Low	Normal	May be low in herpes simplex infections
Protein	High	High	High	Elevated	

Naegleria fowleri, a free-living amoeba, produces a necrotizing meningoencephalitis, particularly in patients who swim in warm, brackish water.[166]

Encephalitis and Brain Abscess

Brain abscess and encephalitis are the most serious infections of the CNS.[176,224,321] Encephalitis is most commonly caused by viruses, although it can also be produced by other agents, such as *Mycoplasma pneumoniae*. The etiologic agent of most encephalitis syndromes is unknown.[96] Herpes simplex virus type 1 is the most frequently documented cause of sporadic encephalitis. The reactivated virus travels up the olfactory nerve to the temporal lobe of the brain, where it produces a necrotizing encephalitis that is distinctive because of the anatomic location. The diagnosis is unlikely in the absence of evidence of temporal lobe disease or a pleocytosis (inflammatory response) in the CSF, although exceptions have been described, particularly in children.[145]

Varicella-zoster virus produces a localized encephalitis uncommonly, usually in the setting of a patient with ophthalmic zoster (a recrudescent infection, usually years after chickenpox). The virus travels up the fifth cranial nerve and produces a necrotizing infection, often with vasculitis and presumably small vascular infarcts.[143] The clinical presentation can even mimic that of noninfectious stroke. Other types of sporadic or epidemic encephalitis affect the brain diffusely; clinical and radiographic data are not diagnostic of a particular etiology, which must be made with microbiologic or molecular techniques. Rabies, fortunately extremely rare, is uniformly fatal; if associated with an animal bite, the diagnosis is obvious, but contact with an animal is not always obvious and the diagnosis may not be made until autopsy.[205]

Anaerobic bacteria are frequently recovered from brain abscesses; anaerobic streptococci, *Porphyromonas melaninogenica*, *Bacteroides* spp., *Fusobacterium nucleatum*, *Eubacterium* spp., and *Propionibacterium acnes* are the most commonly encountered species. The aerobic bacteria most commonly recovered include α/γ-hemolytic streptococci, *Staphylococcus aureus*, *Streptococcus pneumoniae*, and gram-negative bacilli, both *Enterobacteriaceae* and nonfermentative organisms. *Nocardia* spp. and the dematiaceous fungus *Cladosporium bantianum* (*Xylohypha bantiana*) (formerly *Cladosporium trichoides*) may also produce brain abscesses.[250] A necrotizing encephalitis can result from extension of a zygomycetes fungus from a sinus into the eye and brain, particularly in patients with neoplastic or immunosuppressive disease and in diabetic patients who are experiencing ketoacidosis.[172]

Brain abscess may result from bacteremic spread, particularly in patients with bacterial endocarditis (usually a single organism),[199] or there may be direct extension from an infection in an adjacent sinus or in the middle ear (often polymicrobial).[234] Most viridans streptococci are recovered as part of a polymicrobial infection, but one particular streptococcus, known variously as ''*Streptococcus milleri*'' or as *Streptococcus anginosus/constellatus* group, causes abscesses in several organs, including the brain, as a sole pathogen.[51]

Several parasitic infections can cause necrotizing infection or a mass lesion in the brain. These include *Acanthamoeba* spp. and related free-living amoebae,[166] *Taenia solium* and related cysticerci,[254] and *Toxoplasma gondii*.[83] Cerebral malaria, caused by *Plasmodium falciparum*, is an often fatal complication in which the cerebral capillaries are blocked.[112,265]

Diagnosis of Central Nervous System Infections
COLLECTION OF SPECIMENS

CNS specimens for culture include CSF (obtained either by subdural tap, ventricular aspiration, or lumbar puncture), brain abscess (obtained by aspirate), and brain tissue (obtained by surgical biopsy). The spinal tap technique is illustrated in Figure 2-5.

CSF obtained from lumbar spinal puncture is the most common CNS specimen received in the laboratory. Usually, three separate tubes of CSF fluid are submitted:

Tube 1 for cell counts and differential stains
Tube 2 for Gram's stain and culture
Tube 3 for protein and glucose or for special studies, such as VDRL (Venereal Disease Research Laboratory; a serologic test for syphilis), cryptococcal antigen, or cytology, depending on the clinical situation.

ASSESSING THE INFLAMMATORY RESPONSE AND MICROSCOPIC TECHNIQUES

An orderly approach to the processing and culture of CSF specimens should be implemented. Examining stained smears of CSF sediment and performing direct antigen detection tests may be helpful both in establishing a presumptive diagnosis and in providing guidelines for the selection of culture media. Microorganisms can often be detected in Gram-stained or methylene-blue–stained CSF smears if they are present in concentrations of at least 10^4–10^5/mL. Methylene blue appears to be more sensitive than Gram's stain, but the assessment of the Gram reaction is important. It is recommended, therefore, that both a Gram-stained and a methylene blue–stained smear be prepared in parallel. Gram-negative organisms are often better observed in the methylene blue–stained smear because the deep blue–staining cells are easier to differentiate from the background debris.[58] Safranin stains the background red in Gram's stain, tending to obscure any pink-staining bacteria. Addition of 0.05% basic fuchsin to the safranin counterstain improves the staining of gram-negative organisms. Smalley and Bradley[261] suggest that the leukocyte esterase (LE) test may substitute for the performance of cell counts on body fluids suspected of harboring bacteria. In a study of 63 culture-positive peritoneal fluids, 85.7% also had positive LE reactions. Six of the nine culture-positive and LE-negative fluids grew only a few colonies of coagulase-negative staphylococci, isolates of questionable clinical significance. DeLozier and Auerbach[64] reported an overall sensitivity of 84.4% and a specificity of 98.1% using the dipstick LE test on spinal fluids collected from 800 patients with suspected meningitis. The sensitivity of LE in culture-proved cases of bacterial meningitis was only 73%. They concluded that the LE is an adjunct to, but not a substitute for,

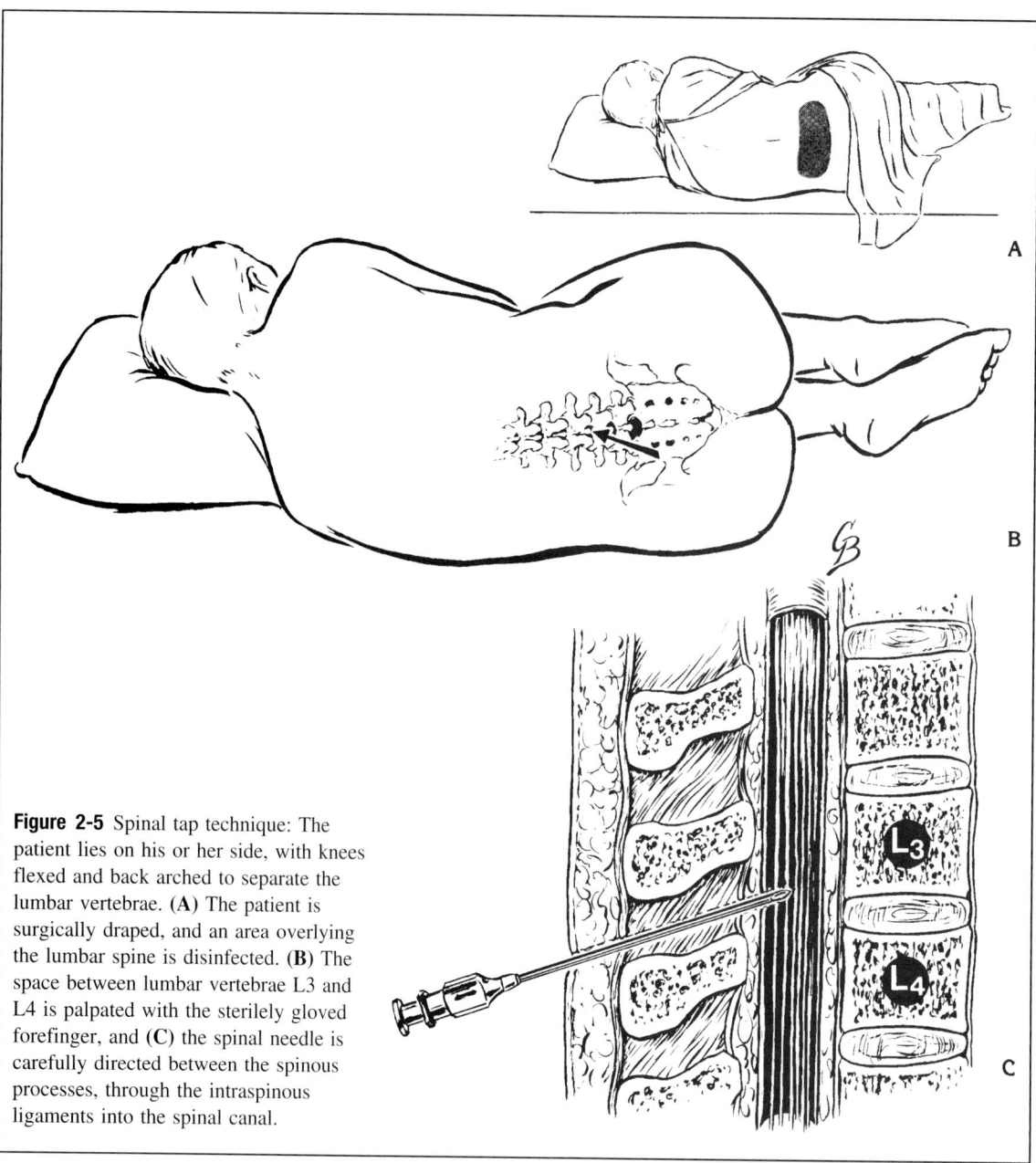

Figure 2-5 Spinal tap technique: The patient lies on his or her side, with knees flexed and back arched to separate the lumbar vertebrae. (**A**) The patient is surgically draped, and an area overlying the lumbar spine is disinfected. (**B**) The space between lumbar vertebrae L3 and L4 is palpated with the sterilely gloved forefinger, and (**C**) the spinal needle is carefully directed between the spinous processes, through the intraspinous ligaments into the spinal canal.

CSF cell count and chemistry determination in the initial laboratory assessment of bacterial meningitis.

DIRECT DETECTION OF ANTIGEN AND NUCLEIC ACID

The initial enthusiasm for the rapid diagnosis of bacterial meningitis by antigen detection has been tempered by more recent experiences.[229] When latex particle agglutination tests for *H. influenzae* type b, *Streptococcus agalactiae*, *Neisseria meningitidis*, and *S. pneumoniae* were performed on 1,540 CSF specimens obtained from patients with suspected acute bacterial meningitis, antigen was detected in only 27 samples.[222] The positive antigen results were helpful only in the treatment of neonates with group B streptococcal infections.

These authors considered the latex test not to be cost-effective. In addition, occasional false-positive agglutination results in an unacceptably poor predictive value of a positive result. Use of these tests has declined dramatically and cannot be recommended.

In contrast, direct detection of cryptococcal antigen in the spinal fluid is almost as sensitive as culture and has replaced the insensitive India ink test in most laboratories. Latex agglutination and enzyme immunoassay kits have been developed. In a study of 218 CSF specimens, which included 16 retrospective and 6 prospective cases of known cryptococcosis, two latex antigen kits performed with 100% sensitivity compared to culture.[328] False-positive tests occur occasionally, caused at least in part by the presence of rheumatoidlike factors in specimens. Treatment of the sample with pronase decreases spurious reactions, but does not completely eliminate them.[237] The sensitivity of latex tests on serum, but not on CSF, is increased by treating with pronase.[107]

Molecular techniques have been developed for diagnosis of selected infections, primarily those caused by herpes simplex virus and enteroviruses.[240,296] Although not yet routine in diagnostic laboratories, these tests are becoming the diagnostic standard because of increased sensitivity and speed of detection.

SEROLOGIC DIAGNOSIS

Serology is a useful diagnostic tool for West Nile virus. Detection of IgM in CSF is currently the method of choice in selected laboratories where the performance of the test is carefully controlled and monitored.[170,216] It has a secondary role for other agents of viral encephalitis, such as other arthropodborne viruses, which are difficult to culture. Unfortunately, it has no role in the most common infections, those caused by herpes simplex viruses, enteroviruses, fungi, and bacteria.

DIAGNOSIS BY CULTURE

Culture is the diagnostic standard for bacteria and fungi. Culture of viruses is limited by restricted availability, slow growth of common enteroviral pathogens, and inability to recover herpes simplex virus from CSF in cases of encephalitis. Molecular methods are preferred for viral agents. The most important question in meningitis is whether a bacterial agent that could be treated with antibiotics is present, so bacterial culture is essential.

In preparing CSF specimens for culture, the fluid should be centrifuged to concentrate any bacteria that may be present. Centrifugation is also recommended for the recovery of *Mycobacterium tuberculosis* in cases of suspected tubercular meningitis. A total volume of at least 6 mL (which need not be collected all at once) must be processed to have any chance to recover mycobacteria.[288] As an alternative to centrifugation for the recovery of cryptococci, the CSF can be passed through a 0.45-μm bacterial filter (Millipore, Bedford MA) to concentrate the yeast cells. The filters should be placed face down on the surface of the agar and moved to a new location every 3 or 4 days to permit the detection of colonial growth.

An excellent review of the approach to the laboratory diagnosis of meningitis has been published by Gray and Fedorko.[101]

Wounds, Abscesses, and Cellulitis
Clinical Presentation

The accumulation of pus, either within an abscess or exuding from a sinus tract or from a mucocutaneous surface, is one of the cardinal indicators of local sepsis. Varying degrees of redness, pain, and swelling may also be present. Exogenous wound infections include those associated with traumatic injury or decubitus pressure ulcers (bedsores),[160] animal or human bites,[86,283] burns,[63,179] or foreign bodies in the skin or mucous membranes.

Endogenous wounds and abscesses may be associated with appendicitis, cholecystitis, cellulitis, dental infections, osteomyelitis, empyema, septic arthritis, sinusitis, or other internal infections. Many of these processes are nosocomial (acquired in healthcare institutions), contracted after invasive procedures, surgical manipulations, or placement of prostheses. Others derive from hematogenous spread from primary sites of infection. Finally, there may be direct extension of bacteria from adjacent sites of infection or from ruptured viscera, particularly the large intestine. Anaerobic bacteria are commonly a problem when the infectious site is adjacent to the intestine or when the wound is contaminated with fecal flora.[202]

Certain bacteria are associated with particular clinical situations. *Pasteurella multocida* is commonly found in wounds that result from animal bites.[86,283] *Pseudomonas aeruginosa* is a common pathogen when a penetrating injury of the foot occurs in patients who are wearing sneakers.[126] *Pseudomonas aeruginosa*, *Candida* spp., and a variety of filamentous fungi are particular problems in burn wounds,[164] but herpes simplex virus can also cause serious infections in these patients.[89] Aerobic gram-positive bacteria (including *Staphylococcus aureus* and *Streptococcus pyogenes*), strict anaerobic bacteria, and aerobic gram-negative bacilli frequently cause infections in patients with diabetes.[134]

Many wounds and abscesses are polymicrobial, particularly those that result from fecal spillage, bedsores, and infections in diabetic patients. There is considerable dispute about the value of identifying and testing the antimicrobial susceptibility of multiple isolates, even if the specimen is a biopsy of tissue. Problems of sampling make it difficult to ensure that all pathogenic species have been recovered. A particularly instructive example of this phenomenon is a study of abscesses, in which multiple cultures of each specimen were performed over a 24-hour period; 11 of 37 total anaerobic strains were not recovered in the initial plating.[12] A case can be made, therefore, for empiric therapy based on the likely pathogens expected in a particular clinical situation.[28]

Cellulitis is a soft-issue infection that spreads through the planes of the connective tissue rather than producing a mass lesion as an abscess does. It is often possible to see the redness and feel the heat and swelling of the process by palpation of the overlying skin.[281] Cellulitis is most commonly caused by staphylococci and streptococci, but in certain situations, gram-negative bacilli and anaerobic bacteria are implicated.

Diagnosis of Wound Infections, Abscesses, and Cellulitis
COLLECTION OF SPECIMENS

Surface wounds are often colonized with environmental bacteria, and swab samples often do not reflect the true cause of the infectious process. Biopsy of tissue, curettage of a draining wound, or aspiration of loculated fluid/pus from the depths of wounds and abscesses are the most desirable methods for collecting material to examine. The site from which the culture is to be obtained should first be decontaminated with surgical soap and 70% ethyl or isopropyl alcohol, after which the wound is washed well with sterile saline and dried. In the past the aspirating syringe was often used as the transport container, provided the needle was capped. This procedure is discouraged now because of the risk that a bloodborne virus will be transmitted by a needlestick. The needle can be removed safely and replaced with a nonsharp syringe cap, using implements designed for this purpose. In any event, if a delay of more than 30 minutes is anticipated before processing, the specimen should be transferred to a transport container (see Chapter 1). If such a small amount of fluid is obtained that the entire specimen is within the needle, recap the needle carefully, secure the cap, and transport the syringe and needle in a puncture-proof container, along with notification that a needle is contained within. In the laboratory the needle can be rinsed with broth to obtain material for culture.

If material cannot be obtained with a needle and syringe, a surface culture may be taken.[28] Swabs are used most commonly, but velvet pads and filter paper disks have also been used. Careful cleaning of the site should be done, as described above (although not all studies have demonstrated a major difference in the results between washed and unwashed wounds). It may be necessary either to separate the wound margins with the thumb and forefinger of one hand (wearing a sterile glove) or to make a small opening in a closed abscess with a scalpel blade before extending the tip of the swab deeply into the depths of the lesion with the other hand. Care should be taken not to touch the adjacent skin margins. The swab should then be placed immediately into an appropriate transport container. It is possible, but unlikely, that a surface culture will not recover a bacterial pathogen that is present deeper in the wound; it is far more likely that a surface culture will recover colonizing microbes in addition to the true pathogens. Fungi and viruses (particularly in burn wounds), however, may be recovered only from biopsied tissue.

Aspiration of material from an area of cellulitis with or without first injecting sterile normal saline may be attempted, but the results are usually unsatisfactory. Punch biopsies may provide more satisfactory results, but experience with this method is limited.[281] Blood cultures are usually not useful in this clinical situation.[211] Commonly, the therapeutic approach is defined by empiric knowledge of the pathogens expected in a given clinical situation.

MICROSCOPIC EXAMINATION OF SPECIMENS

Gram's stain should be performed on all specimens (see Chapter 1). Morphologic clues to the etiology may suggest additional diagnostic procedures beyond those requested by the clinician; (e.g., anaerobic or fungal cultures). If a biopsy of tissue is received, histologic examination should include stains for bacteria and fungi and an examination of hematoxylin-eosin stains for viral inclusions.

CULTURE

Both selective and enriched nonselective media should be used to recover both eugonic and fastidious bacterial species. Anaerobic culture is appropriate if tissue or aspirated material has been obtained.

Quantitative microbial cultures have been advocated for culture of wounds to determine the significance of isolates, predict the likelihood of burn wound sepsis, and determine the probability that wound healing will proceed smoothly. Quantitative culture of biopsied tissue is complex, expensive, and time-consuming; tissue must be weighed on an analytic balance, homogenized in a measured amount of broth, diluted serially, and inoculated onto multiple agar plates. These maneuvers are difficult for most laboratories to accomplish. It is clear that infections by *Streptococcus pyogenes* are clinically important, no matter what the quantity of bacteria present.[230] Investigators have not been unanimous in their endorsement of this approach. The problem is complicated still further by the evidence that a single biopsy of a wound will not give an accurate picture of the microbial flora of chronic wounds.[245]

There are data that support the use of surface cultures rather than biopsies.[28] Similarly, semiquantitative cultures (as performed routinely by serial streaking of quadrants on agar plates) have provided information that is equivalent to the more difficult quantitative approaches.[40] Obviously, if no microbes are recovered, a qualitative culture provides the same information as a quantitative one.

Eye Infections
Clinical Presentation

Infectious agents may attack any part of the eye, either from the outside or the inside. External infections usually involve the superficial structures—the conjunctiva and the cornea—unless there has been a penetrating injury that introduces microbes into the globe.

CONJUNCTIVITIS

The conjunctiva is a thin membrane that covers the eyelid (palpebral conjunctiva) and reflects onto the outer surface of the eyeball, the sclera (bulbar conjunctiva). The central cornea is not covered. The conjunctiva is the target of many microbes, most of which inhabit the upper respiratory tract. Inflammation (conjunctivitis) produces redness (pink eye), itching, and a discharge, which may be mucous or purulent.[155,282] The exudates in bacterial infection are particularly sticky and encrusted, so the eyelids may stick together. Acute noninfectious inflammation may also develop in patients with seasonal allergies. Conjunctivitis is highly contagious; the infection can be transferred easily to the other eye or to other individuals by contact (e.g., rubbing the infected eye and then the normal eye).

The most common bacterial pathogens are *Staphylococcus aureus*, *Haemophilus influenzae*, *Streptococcus pneumoniae*, and *Pseudomonas aeruginosa*. Acute conjunctivitis can result from two sexually transmitted pathogens, *Chlamydia trachomatis* and *Neisseria gonorrhoeae*, which can affect sexually active adults or neonates who acquire the infection during vaginal delivery. The most common viral etiology is adenovirus, which can cause epidemic disease, with or without pharyngitis (epidemic pharyngoconjunctival fever).

KERATITIS

Keratitis, inflammation of the cornea, is a much more serious infection than conjunctivitis. Rather than the temporary discomfort of conjunctivitis, keratitis can result in scarring and blindness. It is caused by infectious agents in every class. The most common bacterial agent is *Staphylococcus aureus*.[158] Filamentous molds, especially *Fusarium* spp. and *Aspergillus* spp., and yeast, most commonly *Candida* spp. produce a lesion that may resemble bacterial infection, delaying diagnosis and appropriate treatment.[144] Herpes simplex virus can cause an ulcerative lesion called dendritic keratitis because of the branching pattern of the lesions.[167] Reactivated varicella-zoster virus (shingles) can produce a similar keratitis if it affects the ocular branch of the trigeminal (fifth cranial) nerve.[277] In people who wear contact lenses *Acanthamoeba* spp. (a free-living amoeba) can produce ulcerative lesions that are frequently very painful.[166]

Interstitial keratitis, produced when blood vessels grow into the cornea from the conjunctiva, is the most common cause of blindness in the world. Trachoma is a form of chronic keratoconjunctivitis that is produced by *C. trachomatis*.[133] The scarring that can result from recurrent disease has 6 six million people worldwide. The World Trachoma Initiative aims to eliminate this treatable infection by 2020. In parts of Africa a filarial parasite, *Onchocerca volvulus*, which is transmitted by black flies (*Simulium* spp.), produces an intense inflammatory response when migrating worms die, resulting in river blindness.[106] Other causes of interstitial keratitis include *Treponema pallidum* (syphilis),[153] *Mycobacterium leprae* (leprosy), and *M. tuberculosis* (tuberculosis).

Keratitis (and blindness) can also be produced by noninfectious injury, such as trauma, ultraviolet radiation (the reason for not looking directly at the sun, particularly during an eclipse), and conditions that diminish the tears that lubricate the cornea.

UVEITIS AND ENDOPHTHALMITIS

The most serious infections are those that affect the interior of the eye. Endogenous infections reach the eye through the bloodstream. A variety of bacteria, fungi, and viruses may be responsible. Exogenous infections are usually associated with penetrating trauma to the eye. A special category is post-surgical infection.

Diagnosis of Eye Infections
COLLECTION OF SPECIMENS

Conjunctivitis is usually diagnosed with a swab of the affected conjunctiva, which can be placed in an appropriate transport medium. All other infections are appropriately collected by an ophthalmologist. Keratitis is addressed by scrapings of the affected lesion; if a bacterial or fungal etiology is suspected, material is often inoculated directly onto appropriate media by the clinician. Specimens for the diagnosis of endophthalmitis must be collected surgically.

MICROSCOPIC EXAMINATION

Depending on the pathogen suspected, Gram's stain, Calcofluor White, or Wright's stain (or equivalent) should be performed. If tissue is obtained surgically, appropriate stains for infectious agents should be done.

CULTURE

The appropriate media to inoculate depends on the clinical assessment of the most likely etiologies. For certain pathogens, such as the agents of syphilis, leprosy, and onchocerciasis, the diagnosis must be made microscopically or serologically.

Infections of the Blood
Clinical Presentation and Pathogenesis

BACTEREMIA AND SEPTICEMIA

The suffix ''-emia'' refers to the circulatory system. Bacteremia, fungemia, and viremia are states in which bacteria, fungi, and viruses, respectively, circulate through the vascular system. Signs and symptoms may be present, but are not invariable. If the patient is not aware of the circulating microbes, the condition is termed ''silent'' or ''subclinical.'' In contrast, septicemia (sepsis) is a clinical syndrome characterized by fever, chills, malaise, tachycardia, hyperventilation, and toxicity or prostration. Septicemia results when circulating bacteria multiply at a rate that exceeds their removal by phagocytes. The symptoms are produced by microbial toxins and/or cytokines produced by inflammatory cells.[209] It now appears that the immunostimulation of cytokines is followed by a series of important immunosuppressive events.[121] Failure of multiple organs is an important component of fatal sepsis, but the pathogenetic mechanisms that lead to death remain unclear.

Sepsis is traditionally associated with gram-negative bacteria, which contain endotoxin.[178] It is now well appreciated, however, that gram-positive bacteria can also cause the sepsis syndrome.[6,78]

TYPES OF BACTEREMIA

Bacteremia may be transient, intermittent, or continuous, reflecting several mechanisms by which bacteria enter the bloodstream. Transient bacteremia occurs when organisms, often members of the normal flora, are introduced into the blood by minimal trauma to membranes (e.g., brushing of teeth, straining during bowel movements, or medical procedures[154]). Intermittent bacteremia occurs when bacteria from an infected site are periodically released into the blood from extravascular abscesses, spreading cellulitis, or infections of body cavities, such as empyema, peritonitis, or septic arthritis. Continuous bacteremia usually occurs when the infection is intravascular, such as infected endothelium (bacterial endocarditis or aneurysms) or infected hardware (arteriovenous fistulas, intraarterial catheters, or indwelling cannulas). The source of organisms may not be determined, however, in up to one third of bacteremias.

Bacteremia may result from an infection in an organ or tissue (secondary bacteremia). Often, however, the primary site is not evident (primary bacteremia). In this situation it is possible that a transient bacteremia was not efficiently cleared by host defense mechanisms. At least in the case of *Staphylococcus aureus* it appears that colonizing bacteria in the nose may be the source of the systemic infection.[299]

The factors that trigger dissemination from the anterior nares remain unclear, but spread to the skin and subsequent infection of wounds or intravascular devices is one possibility.

When an infection in an organ spills over into the blood (e.g., bacteremic pneumococcal pneumonia), the severity of the infection is often increased and the prognosis for the patient worsened.[198] Conversely, bacteremia can result in disseminated infection in distant organisms, a phenomenon that is termed ''metastatic infection.''

Bacteremia can also be classified as community-acquired or nosocomial. It can occur in immunocompetent or immunosuppressed hosts. The types of organisms and the prognosis of the resulting infection vary greatly depending on these factors, as well as on the age of the patient.[84,162,185,258]

A variety of bacteria is recovered from the bloodstream, both gram-positive[213] and gram-negative.[67] Over the past several decades there has been a clear shift in the nature of the infecting flora. The number of anaerobic isolates has decreased over that time, whereas the number of isolates of yeast and clinically significant coagulase-negative staphylococci has increased.[319] For reasons that are unclear bacteremias with nonfermenting gram-negative bacilli are more often polyclonal (more than one molecular type) than are bacteremias with other gram-negative bacilli.[320]

Some specific microbes have distinct clinical significance. *Clostridium septicum* is frequently associated with neoplastic disease, particularly carcinoma of the colon,[146] and may result in distant metastatic abscesses. Similarly, bacteremic *Streptococcus bovis* is commonly associated with endocarditis and with colonic disease, including carcinoma of the colon.[17] Rarely, episodes of *Clostridium perfringens* bacteremia result in sudden, dramatic hemolysis, which can be rapidly fatal[292]; the hemolysis is caused by clostridial toxins, but it is unclear why the fatal hemolysis occurs only in a small proportion of clostridial bacteremias.

Risk Factors and Prognosis. Several mechanisms play a role in the removal of microorganisms from the bloodstream. In healthy and immunocompetent hosts, a sudden influx of bacteria is usually cleared from the blood within 30 to 45 minutes. The liver and spleen play the primary role in clearing bacteria; intravascular neutrophils play only a minor role. Encapsulated bacteria are more difficult to eliminate, but specific antibodies (opsonins) enhance clearance.[34] Patients who are debilitated, immunodeficient, or immunocompromised are at increased risk because circulating bacteria may not be cleared from the blood for hours.

Other risk factors have been investigated by Weinstein and associates.[316] In their study of 500 episodes of bacteremia and fungemia, the overall mortality rate was 42%, with approximately half of these deaths attributed directly to septicemia. Risk factors and the relative mortality rates for each are shown in Table 2-8. Bryan[37] also emphasizes how positive blood cultures identify a population of patients at high risk of death; patients with positive blood cultures were 12 times more likely to die during hospitalization than those with negative blood cultures. From these experiences, it is imperative that the laboratory perform blood cultures correctly and report accurate results as soon as possible.

The timely detection of bacteremia and fungemia, followed by expeditious identification of pathogens and determination of susceptibility to antimicrobial agents can have great diagnostic and prognostic importance. The mortality rate from septicemia may be 40% or higher in certain populations of hospitalized patients,[316] Although underlying diseases are important determinants of fatal outcomes, approximately half of the deaths can be attributed directly to the infection.[37] Prompt initiation of appropriate antimicrobial therapy is demonstrably important for preventing morbidity and mortality.[161] Initial therapy must be empirically based on likely pathogens and typical patterns of antimicrobial susceptibility. The microbiology laboratory plays its most important role when the actual pathogen and/or the antimicrobial susceptibility deviate from that predicted by the clinician. The fatality rate for patients who are treated appropriately is significantly less than that for patients who receive ineffective antibiotics.[319] Prompt correction of the empirically chosen course of action is dependent on speedy provision of data by the laboratory. In addition to all important quality issues a financial case can also be made for expeditious provision of results.[18] Any activity that reduces complications and shortens hospital stay will result in major financial savings for the institution as well as improved care for the patient.

INTRAVASCULAR INFECTION

The most common intravascular infection is endocarditis, infection of the endothelial lining of the heart.[16,239,310] The earlier division of illness into acute and subacute forms is no longer considered useful. Although almost any organism can produce endocarditis on occasion, the majority of infecting organisms are gram-positive. Most important among these are the viridans streptococci of the oral cavity and *Staphylococcus aureus*. Patients are most at risk if they have endocardial abnormalities and dental procedures.[73] Endocardial damage was formerly most commonly the result of rheumatic fever. With the virtual disappearance of that disease, congenital or developmental abnormalities, such as bicuspid aortic valves and prolapsed mitral valves, have assumed greater importance. Fibrin-platelet thrombi on the surface of abraded endocardium serve as a landing site for the bacteria that transiently circulate in all of us (e.g., after brushing our teeth). Certain microbes, particularly streptococci and enterococci, have an enhanced ability to adhere to these thrombi.[56] The thrombi and associated bacteria form excrescences (vegetations), which can be visualized by radiographic or echographic techniques. Uninfected and infected thrombi cause marantic and infective endocarditis, respectively.

Although gram-positive bacteria are the most common etiologic agents of endocarditis, some fastidious gram-negative bacilli[33,77] and some fungi[5,186] can produce the infection. The gram-negative bacteria of the HACEK group (*Haemophilus aphrophilus*, *Actinobacillus actinomycetemcomitans*, *Eikenella corrodens*, and *Kingella kingae*) are particularly likely to infect heart valves. Fungi and some of these gram-negative bacilli are notable for their propensity to form large vegetations that can break off and travel through the bloodstream to distant sites (septic emboli). Most cases of endocarditis involve the left side of the heart, which is the high-pressure side of the system. If, however, bacteria are directly injected into the venous system, as oc-

Table 2-8 Mortality Rates and Risk Factors Associated With Bacteremia[316]

CONDITION	MORTALITY (%)	RELATIVE RISK OF DEATH
Age of Patient		
20	13.8	1.00
21–40	32.8	2.33
41–50	42.9	3.06
>50	49.8	3.55
Type of Organism		
Nonfermenters	27.7	6.84
(*Pseudomonas aeruginosa*)		
Enterobacteriaceae		
Escherichia coli	35.5	3.36
Klebsiella pneumoniae	48.0	4.52
Gram-positive cocci		
Staphylococcus aureus	32.7	3.08
Streptococcus pneumoniae	22.0	2.08
Enterococci	45.5	4.28
Unimicrobial bacteremia	37.7	
Polymicrobial bacteremia	63.0	5.96
Fungi	67.7	
Source of Infection		
Intravenous catheter	1.1	1.00
Genitourinary	14.9	1.35
Foley catheter	37.8	3.38
Surgical wound (and burns)	42.9	3.88
Abscess	51.2	4.65
Respiratory infection	52.3	4.73
Predisposing Conditions		
Surgery	16.3	0.78
Trauma	27.3	1.30
Diabetes mellitus	30.0	1.43
Corticosteroids	33.3	1.59
Renal failure	37.5	1.79
Neoplasm	42.1	2.01
Cirrhosis	71.5	3.40

curs with illicit intravenous injection of drugs, left-sided endocarditis, often caused by *Pseudomonas aeruginosa*, may result.[322]

In a minority of patients with signs and symptoms of endocarditis it is difficult or impossible to isolate an etiologic agent (culture-negative endocarditis). Diseases that cause marantic endocarditis may be responsible, but certain microbes are not readily recovered by conventional blood culture techniques. Prominent among these agents are *Chlamydia pneumoniae*, *Coxiella burnetii* (Q fever) and *Bartonella* spp.,[32,92,177,293] but other agents, such as *Legionella* spp. may be responsible less commonly.

Patients who have recently implanted intravascular hardware are usually infected with bacteria that are indigenous to the skin, most commonly coagulase-negative staphylococci and diphtheroids, or, less commonly, ones that cause wound infection, such as gram-negative bacilli, *Staphylococcus aureus*, or fungi.[215] Prosthetic-valve endocarditis occurs in 3–6% of patients who receive either mechanical or bioprosthetic (valves made from animal tissues) grafts[300]; the infections can be divided conceptually into early (<60 days after surgery) and late stages. In the early stage the skin and wound microbes predominate. In late stages the organisms that infect native valves are found.

The most serious complications of endocarditis are rupture of a cardiac valve with resultant heart failure and metastatic disease caused by embolization of pieces of the infected vegetation. Sudden cardiac decompensation is a particular problem in endocarditis caused by *Staphylococcus aureus*, which may represent a surgical emergency. Renal failure and strokes can result from septic emboli to the kidney and brain, respectively.

CATHETER-ASSOCIATED BACTEREMIA AND SEPSIS

A special kind of intravascular infection has been the result of technologic advances that allow the life-saving use of indwelling vascular catheters. Catheters may simply be the portal of entry for bacteria that colonize the skin adjacent to the entry point or they may serve as a foreign body that harbors microbial microcolonies. Sepsis and serious metastatic disease may result from catheter-related infections.[220] In patients with neoplastic disease, intravascular catheters may be in place for prolonged periods; this group of patients, who may have profound neutropenia, are at great risk for serious and life-threatening infection.[76] In addition to the effects on quality of care and quality of life, catheter-related infections put a major financial burden on institutions.[4] Although central venous catheters are most commonly used and are most commonly the route of infection, intraarterial catheters may also present a risk.[272]

The most common organism found in catheter-related infections is coagulase-negative *Staphylococcus*, which is a common indigenous bacterium on the skin and possesses characteristics, such as the presence of slime, that facilitate colonization of catheters.[124] The most serious infections, however, are caused by *Staphylococcus aureus* and gram-negative bacilli.

Collection of Blood Cultures

The critical factors that must be decided by laboratory directors include the type of collection, number and timing of blood cultures, the volume of blood to be cultured, the amount and composition of the culture medium, when and how frequently to subculture, and the interpretation of results.[226,228,319]

CONTAMINATION WITH SKIN FLORA

Every precaution should be taken to minimize the percentage of contaminated blood cultures.[313] Isolates of *Corynebacterium* spp., *Propionibacterium acnes*, and *Bacillus* spp. other than *B. anthracis* are almost always contaminants. Most isolates of gram-negative bacilli, yeast, β-hemolytic streptococci, *Streptococcus pneumoniae*, *Enterococcus* spp., and *Staphylococcus aureus* are clinically significant. The most problematic isolates are coagulase-negative staphylococci, because these species are increasingly causes of true bacteremia but are also indigenous flora of the skin.

A quality assurance monitor tracing the incidence of contaminated samples should be performed regularly in all microbiology laboratories. Less than 3% of blood cultures should be contaminated. Bates and associates[15] estimate that a contaminant blood culture can lead to an increase of as much

as 20–39% in a patient's hospital bill from an extended stay for intravenous antibiotic therapy and additional tests. They also emphasize the need for paired blood culture sets to indicate likely contamination if only one turns positive. If collection technique is good and contamination minimized, the cost of contaminants becomes acceptable.[306] Inappropriate antibiotic use can be discouraged by a laboratory policy that single isolates of coagulase-negative staphylococci not be tested for antimicrobial susceptibility routinely. Several approaches to this determination are provided by Weinstein.[313]

A variety of techniques have been proposed for determining whether an isolate of coagulase-negative *Staphylococcus* represents contamination. Unfortunately, none works well. Neither the number of positive bottles,[190] identification of the isolate to the level of species,[315] time to initial positivity,[137] or the number of other negative sets[137] distinguished clinically significant from insignificant isolates. Species of coagulase staphylococci other than *S. epidermidis*, *S. capitis*, and *S. haemolyticus* were almost always clinically insignificant, but these three species accounted for 98% of the significant isolates and 89% of the insignificant isolates.[315] The only way to determine with certainty whether two or more isolates represent the same strain is to perform molecular typing, a technique that is not available in most laboratories. Use of clinical data in combination with the antibiogram of the strains[137] or a combination of antibiogram and biochemical pattern (as opposed to identification)[313] have been proposed as means for determining whether multiple isolates represent multiple contaminants or a single infecting strain.

To reduce the chance of introducing contaminating organisms from the skin, the venipuncture site should ideally be prepared as follows: 1) wash with soap, 2) rinse with sterile water, 3) apply 1–2% tincture of iodine or povidone-iodine and allow to dry for 1–2 minutes (povidone-iodine) or 30 seconds (tincture of iodine), and 4) remove the tincture of iodine with a 70% alcohol wash. In practice, the soap wash is usually omitted; however, the combined use of iodine compound and alcohol to disinfect the venipuncture site is essential. If the site must again be palpated after the iodine-alcohol preparation, the finger must be disinfected or a sterile glove worn. If povidone-iodine is used, step 4 must be omitted. Be sure, however, that the povidone-alcohol solution is dry before making the venipuncture. A packaged skin preparation kit performed similarly to individual iodophor and alcohol pledgets.[324] Healthcare personnel are almost always in a hurry, so there is a strong temptation not to allow the prolonged contact required for povidone-iodine solutions. Tincture of iodine, which is effective after contact with the skin for 30 seconds, has obvious advantages and has been reported to be more effective than povidone-iodine,[159] but is less acceptable to personnel. Other disinfectants have been suggested for preparation of venipuncture sites,[313] but have not been widely accepted.

Blood cultures may be obtained either by using a needle and syringe (Figure 2-6) or by a closed system, consisting of a vacuum bottle and double-needle collection tube. Obtaining blood for culture from indwelling intravenous or intraarterial catheters should be discouraged. Although some authors have found a good correspondence between cultures drawn through a catheter or by venipuncture, most investigators have found a significantly increased risk of recovering

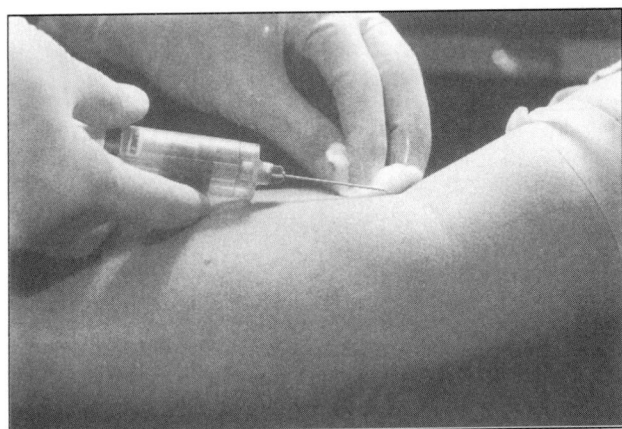

Figure 2-6 Venipuncture technique for blood culture using a sterile needle and syringe. A tourniquet is applied to the upper arm above the venipuncture site to distend the antecubital veins. The site has previously been prepared with tincture of iodine and alcohol. The blood is removed with the syringe and needle and injected into an appropriate blood culture bottle. Rubber gloves must be worn during this procedure.

skin organisms if an intravascular catheter is used.[39,82] The hope is that a patient will be saved the discomfort of a venipuncture, but recovery of a coagulase-negative staphylococcus may actually result in more discomfort from additional venipunctures undertaken to address the questionable isolate.[313] If an intravascular catheter is used, a second culture should be drawn by venipuncture for comparison.

The practice of changing needles after the venipuncture and before injecting the blood into culture bottles has been replaced by direct injection with the original phlebotomy needle, because hepatitis or HIV infections can be acquired from accidental needlesticks. The majority of investigators who have studied this issue have concluded that there is no significant difference in blood culture contamination rates between patients for whom needles were switched between phlebotomy and injection of the bottles and those for whom needles were not switched. [49,148,262] A meta-analysis of the issue did reveal more frequent contamination when needles were not changed, but the risk of acquiring a bloodborne viral infection greatly outweighs the benefits gained from changing needles.

One important factor in the quality of blood culture collection that is often overlooked is the training of the collectors. Multiple investigators have demonstrated that a trained phlebotomy team can obtain blood cultures with fewer instances of contamination than random individuals, no matter what their educational level.[312,313]

NUMBER AND TIMING OF CULTURES

The number of specimens collected is less important than the total volume of blood cultured. Multiple studies have documented the importance of volume; most are consonant with the finding that the yield increases to approximately 30 mL of blood in adults.[318] If a set of two bottles, each containing 10 mL of blood is submitted, two sets will satisfy the volume criterion. If the bottles only hold 5 mL each, or if

a full complement of blood is not inoculated by the clinician, a correspondingly greater number of sets must be collected to satisfy the volume requirement. One exception may be community-acquired pneumonia in otherwise healthy children, in which a single aerobic culture may be sufficient.[207]

In a study of hospital blood culture practices, Schifman and associates[244] discovered that the incidence of solitary blood cultures ranged from 1% to 99%, with a median of 26%. They estimated that as many as 18,000 episodes of bacteremia might be missed annually because an inadequate volume of blood was collected. Between 20% and 30% of the solitary blood cultures they reviewed were not clinically indicated; most of the others were ordered by physicians who were unaware that one culture was not sufficient. Focused intervention and global education reduced solitary blood cultures from 40% to 24% in one hospital, and unnecessary collections were reduced from 38% to 12.5% in another institution. Unfortunately, the improvement of performance after education has a short half-life; constant monitoring (e.g., as part of an ongoing quality assurance program), is required. Solitary blood cultures present the additional problem that single isolates of coagulase-negative staphylococcus are difficult to interpret, as described above.

Blood cultures should be drawn before the use of systemic antimicrobials if possible. If therapy has been started, cultures should still be obtained, but negative results must be interpreted with circumspection.

Traditional guidelines were that multiple cultures should be taken at different times if intravascular infection and continuous bacteremia was suspected. Most authorities now believe that there is little to be gained by spacing cultures over time. Fever is often a somewhat delayed response to the entry of bacteria into the blood system, so collection of the specimens as soon as possible after a fever spike makes sense. At least two venipunctures should be performed, but all necessary specimens (usually two to three sets, each containing two bottles) can be collected at one time.[150]

After collecting an adequate volume of blood and initiating antimicrobial therapy, there is nothing to be gained by collecting additional specimens until the results of the initial sets are known.[99] The practice of a standing order for daily cultures should not be condoned. Most bacterial isolates are recovered by continuous monitoring systems within 72 hours, so it is reasonable to wait at least 3 days before collecting specimens again. A good rule is that it is preferable to consider the possibility of another cause rather than blindly repeating a nonproductive diagnostic approach. If clinical conditions change, however, additional specimens are indicated. "Breakthrough bacteremia" (positive cultures and new or persistent symptoms in the face of antimicrobial therapy) suggest the possibility of antimicrobial resistance and are a poor prognostic sign.[317] It should be remembered, however, that newer blood culture media that contain resins for removal of antimicrobial agents may result in the apparent persistence of pathogens; the symptomatic status of the patient is of critical importance.

CULTURE MEDIA

The media used in blood culture bottles are multipurpose and nutritionally enriched: tryptic or trypticase soy, supplemented peptone, brain-heart infusion, Columbia CNA agar, and brucella broths are commonly used. All are commercially available; however, variations in the composition of the same type of medium by different manufacturers makes comparisons and conclusions about the comparative yields of bacteria from each difficult to assess.

Most commercially available blood culture media contain the anticoagulant sodium polyanetholsulfonate (SPS) in concentrations varying from 0.025% to 0.05%. In addition to its anticoagulant properties (anticoagulation is a desired effect because certain bacteria do not survive well within the clot, where phagocytosis by neutrophils and macrophages remains active), SPS also inactivates neutrophils and certain antibiotics, including streptomycin, kanamycin, gentamicin, and polymyxin, and precipitates fibrinogen, β-lipoproteins, β1-C globulin, and other components of serum complement. SPS may also inhibit the growth of certain bacteria—*Peptostreptococcus anaerobius*, *Neisseria gonorrhoeae*, and *N. meningitidis*. The inhibitory effect of SPS can be neutralized by adding gelatin to the medium, to a final concentration of 1%.

Many current blood culture bottles incorporate synthetic antibiotic-removing resins Recovery of pathogens (but also skin contaminants) is clearly improved by these additions.[313] In a study of 6,839 paired blood cultures,[136] the use of resin media significantly improved the recovery of members of the family *Enterobacteriaceae*, *Enterococcus* spp., *Streptococcus pneumoniae*, and viridans streptococci.

Traditionally, blood culture sets consisted of a bottle designed to recover aerobic bacteria and one engineered for anaerobic bacteria. In truth, all types of bacteria were always recovered in both bottles; once again, the microbes forgot to read the textbook. The change in the pattern of bacteremias over time described above has led some investigators to suggest that an "anaerobic" bottle be limited to situations in which anaerobes might be expected (e.g., in patients with abdominal disease processes).[193] Recovery rates from three different paired bottle systems were compared: 1) one aerobic and one anaerobic bottle (5 mL of blood each); 2) two aerobic bottles (5 mL each); and 3) two aerobic bottles plus an extra anaerobic bottle when anaerobic infection was clinically suspected. The third approach had the largest yield of isolates. From their data, these investigators concluded that the use of two aerobic bottles with selective culturing for anaerobes will potentially increase the number of clinically important isolates by at least 6%.[193] The policy of substituting a second "aerobic" bottle for the "anaerobic" bottle has not caught on, probably in part because of the difficulty of deciding which patients would benefit from the practice and the impossibility of leaving the decision to the clinical staff. It has been pointed out that many facultatively anaerobic bacteria (the majority of human pathogens) grow well in the "anaerobic" bottle.[52] It should be noted that the policy at one institution, where a decreasing incidence of anaerobic bacteremias had also been documented,[70] included two aerobic components in addition to the nonvented "anaerobic" bottle.

Blood cultures for mycobacteria and fungi should be considered in appropriate clinical situations, such as when patients who are infected with HIV are frequently cultured. Dimorphic fungi and filamentous molds require special attention.[165] In recent studies, however, most *Candida* spp.

Box 2-3 Guidelines for Obtaining Blood Cultures[a]

Ideally a trained phlebotomy team should collect all blood cultures according to established protocols. The frequency of likely contaminants in cultures collected by each member of the team should be monitored so that team members can improve their performance.

Blood cultures are indicated when a serious febrile illness that will require antimicrobial therapy is present or when an infection in an organ system might be elucidated by isolating a pathogen from the blood (e.g., meningitis or pneumonia).

Compare the name on the requisition with the stated identity of the patient. Establish the site(s) for venipuncture and clean the site with an iodine compound followed by alcohol (preceded by surgical soap and water if possible).

Collect a sufficient number of cultures so that at least 30 mL has been inoculated into the chosen bottles. There should be at least two venipuncture sites, but all venipunctures may be collected at one session.

Use all available safety devices, such as needles with safety features, a safety transfer device for inoculating blood into bottles, and a tube holder adapter when a winged collection device is used. Dispose of all sharps in a protected container.

Do not force blood into the bottles.

Transmit the inoculated bottles to the laboratory as quickly as possible.

[a] *Adapted from reference*[79].

---

were recovered effectively in systems designed for bacteria.[182]

A summary of recommendations for collecting blood cultures is presented in Box 2-3.

Systems for Processing Blood Cultures[206]
MANUAL BLOOD CULTURE SYSTEMS

Two of the manual commercial systems are variations on the classic agar-broth combination bottles, known as Castañeda bottles. For laboratories that do not have the resources for a more automated system that monitors bacterial growth continuously, they represent a reasonable choice.

The Oxoid Signal System. The Oxoid (Ogdensburg, NY) Signal System is a single-bottle blood culture system that uses the production of CO_2 to detect early bacterial growth. The main blood culture bottle is similar to those used in other broth systems; however, the system uses a second plastic chamber, known as the signal chamber, which is fitted at the bottom with a long needle. After the blood sample to be cultured has been inoculated into the main bottle, the signal chamber is connected by inserting the needle through the rubber stopper and positioning it below the surface of the culture medium. Growing and metabolizing bacteria produce CO_2. The resulting increase in pressure forces liquid into the signal chamber, which can be directly visualized and used to prepare Gram's stain and subculture. This system has been evaluated favorably.[197,247] A higher than normal number of false-positive results and a lower than normal yield of anaerobes remain problems. Weinstein and coworkers[314] found an improved yield of organisms with newly designed bottles that have an increased head-gas space and are subjected to agitation.

BBL Septi-Chek Blood Culture System. The Septi-Chek biphasic agar-slide system (BD Diagnostic Systems, Sparks, MD) is also widely used. The system uses a standard blood culture bottle that contains either brain-heart infusion broth or trypticase soy broth. The bottle is designed for connection to a second plastic chamber that contains a paddle with agar surfaces. After the primary bottle is inoculated with the blood sample to be cultured, the plastic-contained ''slide'' is screwed on. This slide contains a trisurface paddle faced with chocolate, MacConkey, and malt agar strips. The first ''subculture'' is made after 4 to 6 hours of incubation at 35°C by inverting the bottle and allowing broth to enter the slide's chamber, thereby flooding the agar surfaces. The bottle is then again placed upright for continued incubation. The bottle can be inverted again at regular intervals to reinoculate the agar media on the paddle.

LYSIS-CENTRIFUGATION BLOOD CULTURE SYSTEM

Wampole Isostat/Isolator Microbial System. The Isolator system is widely accepted as an alternative blood culture method that is particularly useful for recovery of fastidious or slow-growing organisms. It is the method of choice for filamentous molds, dimorphic fungi, *Malassezia furfur*, and *Legionella* spp.[24] There was a reduction of mean recovery time for yeasts from 4.9 days using a conventional biphasic broth-agar system to 2.12 days with the Isolator. The mean recovery time of 8.0 days for *Histoplasma capsulatum* compared with 24.14 days for the conventional biphasic system. An overall 36.6% increase in the recovery rate of fungi from blood cultures was documented when the Isolator system was used. This method should be considered when other fastidious organisms, such as *Bartonella henselae*,[163,260] are suspected, especially if conventional systems have had negative results. The Isolator Microbial System (Wampole Laboratories, Princeton, NJ) is a special tube that contains saponin, a chemical that lyses both the red and the white blood cells. Approximately 7.5 to 10 mL of blood are added to the tube, which is then thoroughly mixed by inverting the tube several times, so that the lysis reaction can go to completion. The tube is then placed into an angle centrifuge and spun at 3,00 rpm for 15 minutes to concentrate any microorganisms that may be present. After centrifugation, the sediment is aspirated and subcultured to appropriate media. A small version that does not require centrifugation is available for use in infants and young children; the use of the pediatric version for adults should be discouraged or prohibited because an insufficient volume of blood is cultured.

The Isolator system is also the method of choice when quantitative cultures of blood are desired. The CFU/mL can be calculated from the volume of blood processed and the number of colonies present on the agar surfaces.[330]

A twofold to eightfold increase in contamination rates over conventional systems is the major problem with the use of the Isolator. It has been suggested that contamination can be reduced by using dry agar plates, disinfecting the work area, and processing samples in a vertical laminar air hood.[138]

Examination of Manual Systems. Blood culture bottles should be incubated at 35°C and examined visually for evidence of growth (hemolysis, gas production, or turbidity) during the first 6 to 18 hours after collection. For those using conventional broth media, bottles should be examined against bright fluorescent bulbs or with incandescent transmitted light. The surface of the sedimented blood layer should be examined because discrete colonies may be detected. Blind subcultures to chocolate agar plates should be made from all blood culture bottles (agar-broth and continuous monitoring systems excluded) within 12 to 24 hours after collection, after which the plates are incubated aerobically in 5–10% CO_2 at 35°C. Blind anaerobic subcultures are usually not done in most laboratories. It is generally agreed, however, that both aerobic and anaerobic subcultures of all visually positive blood culture bottles should be set up. In a study of 20,155 blood culture bottles (trypticase soy broth and thiol broth),[196] only 32 trypticase soy bottles and 10 thiol bottles turned positive after 7 days of incubation. Fifteen of the 32 trypticase isolates and all of the thiol isolates were either recovered in other cultures or were not considered clinically significant, indicating that holding manual blood cultures beyond 7 days is unnecessary.

The routine microscopic examination of macroscopically negative blood culture bottles after 24 hours of incubation is probably not indicated because the number of organisms that can be detected by Gram's stain (about 10^5 CFU) is not appreciably less than the 10^6 to 10^7 CFUs required to produce visible turbidity of the broth.[228] Acridine orange stains are more sensitive, detecting 10^3 to 10^4 CFU/mL. Tierney and associates report a 16.8% increase in the early detection of septicemia by examining macroscopically negative blood culture broths with the acridine orange stain.[289]

AUTOMATED AND COMPUTERIZED BLOOD CULTURE SYSTEMS

The introduction of continuous-reading, automated, and computerized blood culture systems represents an important advance in clinical microbiology practice. Three such systems, the BacT/Alert (Organon Teknika, Durham NC), the BACTEC 9240/9120 (BD Diagnostic Systems), and the TREK ESP Culture System II (TREK Diagnostic Systems, Cleveland, OH) are commonly used in the United States. Each of these systems alerts the microbiologist that a culture is positive, after which the relevant bottles can be removed for Gram's stain and subculture. The media selected for subculture can be chosen based on the gram reaction and morphology of the microbes. If organisms are not visualized, a blind subculture should be performed and the bottle returned to the instrument for continued incubation. Multiple studies have demonstrated that bottles need be incubated only for 5 days when the continuous monitoring systems are used. In the future it may be possible to reduce the incubation time even further.[55]

The BacT/Alert Blood Culture System. As the first continuous-monitoring blood culture system developed and marketed in the United States, the BacT/Alert system has been implemented in many clinical laboratories. Each blood culture bottle has the capacity to receive 10 mL of blood. As microorganisms grow in the blood-broth mixture, CO_2 is liberated. A CO_2-sensitive chemical sensor that is separated from the blood-broth mixture by a unidirectional CO_2-permeable membrane is bonded to the bottom of each bottle. In the presence of CO_2, the color of the sensor turns from green to yellow, although the light-sensitive detector built into the instrument reacts before a color change is apparent.

Each bottle is placed bottom down into a receiving well in the data unit, directed by a bar code on the bottle label, which is integrated in the computer to match the patient identification data for each. Each data unit is a cabinet about the size of a small refrigerator which serves as a self-contained incubator, shaker, and detection device, with a capacity to hold either 240 or 120 bottles, depending on the model. Up to five modules can be linked through the same computer controls, yielding a total of 1,440 bottles that can be monitored. The wells are arranged in two rows within a horizontal rack that gently rocks back and forth when the door to the data unit is closed. As each rack holds 20 bottles, 12 racks are contained in the 240-bottle data unit. At 10-minute intervals, a light beam from emitting diodes (one for each well) is projected through an excitation filter to reflect off the CO_2-sensitive sensor in the bottom of each bottle. The reflecting light is directed through an emission filter to a photosensitive detector that, in turn, is connected to a computer compiler. As soon as the accumulation of CO_2 is sufficient in the bottle to alter the sensor, an audible or visible ''alert'' is generated, and the position of the positive bottle is immediately flagged by the computer. Positive bottles can be immediately removed and further processed. A graph can be brought on the computer screen at any time to monitor the progress of CO_2 production.

The BACTEC 9240/9120 Blood Culture System. The BACTEC system consists of a self-contained incubator, agitator, and detection device, similar in appearance to the BacT/Alert system. There are two sizes: model 9240 holds 240 bottles and model 9120 holds 120 bottles; up to five modules can be linked to the same computer control unit. Similar to the BacT/Alert, each bottle has a sensor disk bonded to the inner surface of the bottom. The one operational difference between the BacT/Alert and the BACTEC systems is that the latter uses fluorescent, rather than spectral light to detect changes in the concentration of CO_2 in the broth-blood mixture. As CO_2 is produced in each bottle, its sensor emits a fluorescent light that passes an emission filter on the way to a light-sensitive diode. Bottles are placed bottom down into receiving wells that are monitored once every 10 minutes. The voltage of the current reading of the diode is compared with the previous reading. If the voltage change exceeds a preset delta value, the microcomputer flags the bottle as positive. The position of the positive bottle is indicated on the computer screen so that bottle can be pulled for further processing. A graph illustrating the progress of CO_2 production can be brought up on the computer screen at any time.

The TREK ESP Culture System II. The ESP blood culture system (TREK Diagnostic Systems, Cleveland, OH) differs from the BacT/Alert and the BACTEC 9240/9120 system in the following ways: 1) the production of CO_2 is monitored manometrically, 2) both gas consumption and production

are monitored, and 3) changes in the concentrations of H_2 and O_2 in addition to CO_2 are detected.

The data unit is also a cabinet that serves as a self-contained incubator, agitator, and detector. Units with a capacity of 128 or 384 bottles are currently available, although more than one module can be linked to a central computer system. After inoculation of up to 10 mL of venous blood, each bottle is fitted with a disposable connector, which includes a recessed needle that penetrates the septum of the blood culture bottle. Each bottle is then placed in a defined position on a carrying rack that is aligned such that the connector attaches directly to a sensing probe located at the top of each position. Once the bottle is properly aligned, the pressure of the head gas is continuously monitored. A reading is taken every 12 minutes. When the change in reading exceeds a delta value, lights are illuminated that indicate the position of any positive bottle.

A reading may occur during a phase of consumption of H_2 and O_2. Oxygen consumption is accelerated at the time replicating organisms enter the log phase of growth. A reading may be possible, therefore, early in the incubation period before a detectable amount of CO_2 is produced. Testing multiple gases is a theoretical advantage for the ESP system, especially for the detection of asaccharolytic microorganisms that may not produce sufficient CO_2 to trip the indicator. The performance of the media that are available with each system is, however, at least as important as the detection mechanism.

Comparative Studies

The comparative performance of these blood culture systems has been extensively studied. Depending on the design of the study, the spectrum of microorganisms being recovered from clinical specimens, the volume of blood being cultured, and the exact types of bottles and media formulations being compared, one system may emerge as superior or inferior to another. Improvements in formulations of media, sensitivity of detectors, and design of instruments continue to be made; the results of a study performed some months ago may not necessarily reflect the current technology. Therefore, each laboratory director and supervisor must weigh published and verbal comments from individuals who have used the system and the needs of the local laboratory when determining whether a new system should be implemented.

The advantages of continuous-monitoring blood culture systems include a decrease in laboratory workload, a decrease in the number of false-positive results and pseudobacteremia (because of decreased handling and sampling of the bottles), and a significant increase in the speed of detection and in the rate of microbial recovery. Disadvantages include a limited database for some systems, a limited selection of media, the large size of the instruments (for laboratories in which space is an issue), and last, but not least, expense. The decrease in laboratory workload is primarily because a technologist's time can be dedicated to processing only the positive cultures instead of loading and unloading instruments or subculturing and observing mostly negative specimens. An adjustment in staffing during off hours must be made because cultures may become positive at any time of day. Each laboratory director must decide the hours during which the instrument will be attended.

Special Considerations
FASTIDIOUS ORGANISMS AND ENDOCARDITIS

Although most pathogens are detected in a few days, some fastidious microbes grow slowly. Some of these organisms produce endocarditis. It is, therefore, appropriate to prolong incubation beyond the routine cutoff period when requested by the clinician. An additional problem is that some pathogens do not generate sufficient CO_2 to trigger the detector. A useful maneuver in either of these situations is blind staining of bottles with acridine orange after incubation for 7 days and/or the total period of incubation. Acridine orange is preferred to Gram's stain because it is more sensitive and the smear can be examined more quickly.

CATHETER-ASSOCIATED BACTEREMIA AND SEPSIS

Two basic approaches have been taken to the diagnosis of catheter-associated bacteremia. One requires removal of the catheter; the other does not.[187]

The initial suggestion for diagnosis—and probably the most common approach even today—was a semiquantitative procedure.[169] The tip of the catheter is rolled across the surface of an agar plate and the resulting colonies are counted after overnight incubation. A statistical association of >15 CFU with catheter-associated sepsis was established and subsequently confirmed by other investigators, Variations on this procedure have included culturing multiple segments, sonication of the catheter tip, and washing the interior of the catheter,[256] but the simplicity of the original procedure has appealed to most microbiologists.

The second approach is performance of quantitative blood cultures, simultaneously collected through the catheter and by venipuncture.[88,218] The theory is that if the catheter is secondarily infected by a bacteremia from another source, fewer CFUs will be detected in the blood drawn through the catheter than in that collected by venipuncture. If the catheter was the source of the bacteremia, the reverse will obtain. The simplest method for performing the quantitative cultures is to use the Isolator blood collection system.[88]

The advantage of the quantitative culture technique is that the catheter can be left in place if it is not implicated in the bacteremia. It should be noted, however, that it is possible to change a catheter over a wire, so that it is not necessary to perform a new procedure to maintain vascular access; in that case a decision about removing the new catheter can be made after the results of culturing the first catheter are known.[187] In either case an intravascular catheter is left in place if the catheter is exonerated as the cause of the sepsis.

TISSUES AND BIOPSIES

Tissue samples for culture should be delivered promptly to the laboratory in a suitably capped, sterile container. If the sample is very small, it may be placed on a piece of sterile, moistened filter paper. Gauze is sometimes used, but it may be very difficult to recover the specimen from the interstices of the gauze. Specimens that have been placed in formalin are not suitable for culture, although it may be possible to rescue the situation if the exposure time has been short and the culture can be obtained from a central portion of the tissue not exposed to formalin.

Bone marrow cultures may be helpful in establishing the diagnosis of granulomatous diseases such as brucellosis, histoplasmosis, and tuberculosis. Using the Isolator system to process the bone marrow samples may be improve the recovery of bacteria, particularly if the infections are caused by intracellular organisms.

REFERENCES

1. Travelers' diarrhea. NIH Consensus Development Conference. JAMA 1985; 253:2700–2704.
2. Alfageme I, et al. Empyema of the thorax in adults. Etiology, microbiologic findings, and management. Chest 1993;103:839–843.
3. Allen BW, Darrell JH. Contamination of specimen container surfaces during sputum collection. J Clin Microbiol 1983;36:479–481.
4. Arnow PM, et al. Consequences of intravascular catheter sepsis. Clin Infect Dis 1993;16:778–784.
5. Atkinson JB, et al. Cardiac fungal infections: review of autopsy findings in 60 patients. Hum Pathol 1984;15:935–942.
6. Aube H, et al. Risk factors for septic shock in the early management of bacteremia. Am J Med 1992;93:283–288.
7. Bale JF Jr, Murph JR. Infections of the central nervous system in the newborn. Clin Perinatol 1997;24:787–806.
8. Bartlett JG. Anaerobic bacterial infections of the lung and pleural space. Clin Infect Dis 1993;16:Suppl 4:S248–S255.
9. Bartlett JG. Bacteriologic diagnosis in anaerobic pleuropulmonary infections. Clin Infect Dis 1993;16:Suppl 4:S443–S445.
10. Bartlett JG. Should fiberoptic bronchoscopy aspirates be cultured? Am Rev Respir Dis 1976;114:73–78.
11. Bartlett JG, et al. Community-acquired pneumonia in adults: guidelines for management: The Infectious Diseases Society of America. Clin Infect Dis 1998;26: 811–838.
12. Bartlett JG, et al. Anaerobes survive in clinical specimens despite delayed processing. J Clin Microbiol 1976;3:133–136.
13. Bartlett RC, et al. Quality assurance of gram-stained direct smears. Am J Clin Pathol 1979;72:984–990.
14. Bassa AG, et al. Granuloma inguinale (donovanosis) in women. An analysis of 61 cases from Durban, South Africa. Sex Transm Dis 1993;20:164–167.
15. Bates DW, et al. Contaminant blood cultures and resource utilization (The true consequences of false-positive results). JAMA 1991;265:365–369.
16. Bayer AS. Infective endocarditis. Clin Infect Dis 1993;17:313–320.
17. Beeching NJ, et al. *Streptococcus bovis* bacteraemia requires rigorous exclusion of colonic neoplasia and endocarditis. Q J Med 1985;56:439–450.
18. Beekmann SE, et al. Effects of rapid detection of bloodstream infections on length of hospitalization and hospital charges. J Clin Microbiol 2003;41: 3119–3125.
19. Benedetti JK, et al. Clinical reactivation of genital herpes simplex virus infection decreases in frequency over time. Ann Intern Med 1999;131:14–20.
20. Benin AL, et al. Trends in legionnaires disease, 1980–1998: declining mortality and new patterns of diagnosis. Clin Infect Dis 2002;35:1039–1046.
21. Benjamin DR. Granulomatous lymphadenitis in children. Arch Pathol Lab Med 1987;111:750–753.
22. Bergmans DC, et al. Reproducibility of quantitative cultures of endotracheal aspirates from mechanically ventilated patients. J Clin Microbiol 1997;35: 796–798.
23. Beutner KR, Tyring S. Human papillomavirus and human disease. Am J Med 1997;102:9–15.
24. Bille J, et al. Clinical evaluation of the lysis-centrifugation blood culture system for the detection of fungemia and comparison with a conventional biphasic broth blood culture system. J Clin Microbiol 1984;19:126–128.
25. Bisno AL. Acute pharyngitis. N Engl J Med 2001;344:205–211.
26. Bisno AL, et al. Practice guidelines for the diagnosis and management of group A streptococcal pharyngitis. Infectious Diseases Society of America. Clin Infect Dis 2002;35:113–125.

27. Bisno AL, et al. Diagnosis of strep throat in adults: are clinical criteria really good enough? Clin Infect Dis 2002;35:126–129.

28. Bowler PG, et al. Wound microbiology and associated approaches to wound management. Clin Microbiol Rev 2001;14:244–269.

29. Bradbury SM. Collection of urine specimens in general practice: to clean or not to clean? J R Coll Gen Pract 1988;38:363–365.

30. Briselden AM, et al. Sialidases (neuraminidases) in bacterial vaginosis and bacterial vaginosis-associated microflora. J Clin Microbiol 1992;30:663–666.

31. Brooksaler F, Nelson, JD. Pertussis: a reappraisal and report of 190 confirmed cases. Am J Dis Child 1967;114:389–396.

32. Brouqui P, et al. Chronic *Bartonella quintana* bacteremia in homeless patients. N Engl J Med 1999;340:184–189.

33. Brouqui P, Raoult D. Endocarditis due to rare and fastidious bacteria. Clin Microbiol Rev 2001;14:177–207.

34. Brown EJ, et al. The role of antibody and complement in the reticuloendothelial clearance of pneumococci from the bloodstream. Rev Infect Dis 1983;5(Suppl 4):S797–S805.

35. Brown JR. Human actinomycosis: a study of 181 subjects. Hum Pathol 1973;4:319–330.

36. Brunham RC, et al. Mucopurulent cervicitis: the ignored counterpart in women of urethritis in men. N Engl J Med 1984;311:1–6.

37. Bryan CS. Clinical implications of positive blood cultures. Clin Microbiol Rev 1989;2:329–353.

38. Bryan CS, Reynolds KL. Bacteremic nosocomial pneumonia: analysis of 172 episodes from a single metropolitan area. Am Rev Respir Dis 1984;129:668–671.

39. Bryant JK, Strand CL. Reliability of blood cultures collected from intravascular catheter versus venipuncture. Am J Clin Pathol 1987;88:113–116.

40. Buchanan K, et al. Comparison of quantitative and semiquantitative culture techniques for burn biopsy. J Clin Microbiol 1986;23:258–261.

41. Calisher CH. Medically important arboviruses of the United States and Canada. Clin Microbiol Rev 1994;7:89–116.

42. Carroll KC. Laboratory diagnosis of lower respiratory tract infections: controversy and conundrums. J Clin Microbiol 2002;40:3115–3120.

43. Carroll KC, et al. Laboratory evaluation of urinary tract infections in an ambulatory clinic. Am J Clin Pathol 1994;101:100–103.

44. Casey BM, Cox SM. Chorioamnionitis and endometritis. Infect Dis Clin North Am 1997;11:203–222.

45. Centers for Disease Control and Prevention. Recommendation for the prevention and management of *Chlamydia trachomatis* infections, 1993. MMWR Morb Mortal Wkly Rep 1993;42:1–39.

46. Centers for Disease Control and Prevention. 1998 guidelines for treatment of sexually transmitted diseases. MMWR Morb Mortal Wkly Rep 1998;47:1–111.

47. Centers for Disease Control and Prevention. Primary and secondary syphilis-United States, 2000–2001. MMWR Morb Mortal Wkly Rep 2002;51:971–973.

48. Centers for Disease Control and Prevention. Diagnosis and management of foodborne illnesses: a primer for physicians and other health care professionals. MMWR Morb Mortal Wkly Rep 2004;53(RR-4):1–29.

49. Chapnick EK, et al. Technique for drawing blood for cultures: is changing needles truly necessary? South Med J 1991;84:1197–1198.

50. Chastre J, et al. Diagnosis of nosocomial bacterial pneumonia in intubated patients undergoing ventilation: comparison of the usefulness of bronchoalveolar lavage and the protected specimen brush. Am J Med 1988;85:499–506.

51. Clarridge JE III, et al. Streptococcus intermedius, Streptococcus constellatus, and Streptococcus anginosus (''Streptococcus milleri group'') are of different clinical importance and are not equally associated with abscess. Clin Infect Dis 2001;32:1511–1515.

52. Cockerill FR III, et al. Analysis of 281,797 consecutive blood cultures performed over an eight-year period: trends in microorganisms isolated and the value of anaerobic culture of blood. Clin Infect Dis 1997;24:403–418.

53. Connolly KJ, Hammer SM. The acute aseptic meningitis syndrome. Infect Dis Clin North Am 1990;4:599–622.

54. Cook RL, et al. Clinical, microbiological and biochemical factors in recurrent bacterial vaginosis. J Clin Microbiol 1992;30:870–877.

55. Cornish N, et al. Reassessment of the incubation time in a controlled clinical comparison of the BacT/Alert aerobic FAN bottle and standard anaerobic bottle used aerobically for the detection of bloodstream infections. Diagn Microbiol Infect Dis 1998;32:1–7.

56. Crawford I, Russell C. Comparative adhesion of seven species of streptococci isolated from the blood of patients with sub-acute bacterial endocarditis to fibrin-platelet clots in vitro. J Appl Bacteriol 1986;60:127–133.

57. Cunha BA. Osteomyelitis in elderly patients. Clin Infect Dis 2002;35:287–293.

58. Daly JA, et al. Evaluation of the Wayson variation of a methylene blue staining procedure for the detection of microorganisms in cerebrospinal fluid. J Clin Microbiol 1985;21:919–921.

59. Dangor Y, et al. A simple medium for the primary isolation of *Haemophilus ducreyi*. Eur J Clin Microbiol Infect Dis 1992;11:930–934.

60. Dangor Y, et al. Transport media for *Haemophilus ducreyi*. Sex Transm Dis 1993;20:5–9.

61. de Boer AL, et al. Cytologic identification of Donovan bodies in granuloma inguinale. Acta Cytol 1984;28:126–128.

62. de Wit MA, et al. Etiology of gastroenteritis in sentinel general practices in The Netherlands. Clin Infect Dis 2001;33:280–288.

63. Deitch EA, Desforges JF. The management of burns. N Engl J Med 1990;323:1249–1253.

64. DeLozier JS, Auerbach PS. The leukocyte esterase test for detection of cerebrospinal fluid leukocytosis and bacterial meningitis. Ann Emerg Med 1989;18:1191–1198.

65. Denny FW, et al. Croup: an 11-year study in a pediatric practice. Pediatrics 1983;71:871–876.

66. DeShazo RD, et al. Fungal sinusitis. N Engl J Med 1997;337:254–259.

67. Diekema DJ, et al. Survey of bloodstream infections due to gram-negative bacilli: frequency of occurrence and antimicrobial susceptibility of isolates collected in the United States, Canada, and Latin America for the SENTRY Antimicrobial Surveillance Program, 1997. Clin Infect Dis 1999;29:595–607.

68. Domingue GJ Sr, Hellstrom WJ. Prostatitis. Clin Microbiol Rev 1998;11:604–613.

69. Donowitz GR, Mandell GL. Acute pneumonia. In: Mandell GL, Douglas RG Jr, Bennett JE, Eds. Principles and Practice of Infectious Diseases. 3rd Ed. New York: Churchill Livingstone,1990:540–555.

70. Dorsher CW, et al. Anaerobic bacteremia: decreasing rate over a 15 year period. Rev Infect Dis 1991;13:633–636.

71. Duguid H, et al. *Actinomyces* and intrauterine devices. JAMA 1982;248:1579–1580.

72. Dunne DW, Quagliarello V. Group B streptococcal meningitis in adults. Medicine (Baltimore) 1993;72:1–10.

73. Durack DT, et al. Apparent failures of endocarditis prophylaxis. Analysis of 52 cases submitted to a national registry. JAMA 1983;250:2318–2322.

74. Echenbach DA, et al. Diagnosis and clinical manifestations of bacterial vaginosis. Am J Obstet Gynecol 1988;158:819–828.

75. El Sahly HM, et al. Spectrum of clinical illness in hospitalized patients with ''Common Cold'' virus infections. Clin Infect Dis 2000;31:96–100.

76. Elishoov H, et al. Nosocomial colonization, septicemia, and Hickman/Broviac catheter-related infections in bone marrow transplant recipients: a 5-year prospective study. Medicine (Baltimore) 1998;77:83–101.

77. Ellner JJ, et al. Infective endocarditis caused by slow-growing fastidious gram-negative bacteria. Medicine (Baltimore) 1979;56:145–158.

78. Elting LS, et al. Septicemia and shock syndrome due to viridans streptococci: a case-control study of predisposing factors. Clin Infect Dis 1992;14:1201–1207.

79. Ernst DJ. Controlling blood culture contamination rates. Med Lab Observ 2004;36:14–18.

80. Eschenbach DA, Wager GP. Puerperal infections. Clin Obstet Gynecol 1980;23:1003–1037.

81. Evans FO, et al. Sinusitis of the maxillary antrum. N Engl J Med 1975;293:735–739.

82. Everts RJ, et al. Contamination of catheter-drawn blood cultures. J Clin Microbiol 2001;39:3393–3394.

83. Falangola MF, et al. Histopathology of cerebral toxoplasmosis in human immunodeficiency virus infection: a comparison between patients with early-onset and late-onset acquired immunodeficiency syndrome. Hum Pathol 1994;25:1091–1097.

84. Fein AM. Pneumonia in the elderly: overview of diagnostic and therapeutic approaches. Clin Infect Dis 1999;28:726–729.

85. Finegold SM, et al. Bacteriologic findings associated with chronic bacterial maxillary sinusitis in adults. Clin Infect Dis 2002;35:428–433.

86. Fleisher GR. The management of bite wounds. N Engl J Med 1999;340:138–140.

87. Fleming DT, et al. Herpes simplex virus type 2 in the United States, 1976 to 1994. N Engl J Med 1997;337:1105–1111.

88. Flynn PM, et al. Differential quantitation with a commercial blood culture tube for diagnosis of catheter-related infection. J Clin Microbiol 1988;26:1045–1046.

89. Foley FD, et al. Herpesvirus infection in burned patients. N Engl J Med 1970;282:652–656.

90. Fraser RS. Pulmonary aspergillosis: pathologic and pathogenetic features. Pathol Annu 1993;28:231–277.

91. Frayha H, et al. Nasopharyngeal swabs and nasopharyngeal aspirates equally effective for the diagnosis of viral respiratory disease in hospitalized children. J Clin Microbiol 1989;27:1387–1389.

92. Gdoura R, et al. Culture-negative endocarditis due to *Chlamydia pneumoniae*. J Clin Microbiol 2002;40:718–720.

93. Gefter WB. The spectrum of pulmonary aspergillosis. J Thorac Imaging 1992;7:56–74.

94. Gibot S, et al. Soluble triggering receptor expressed on myeloid cells and the diagnosis of pneumonia. N Engl J Med 2004;350:451–458.

95. Gilligan PH. Microbiology of airway disease in patients with cystic fibrosis. Clin Microbiol Rev 1991;4:35–51.

96. Glaser CA, et al. In search of encephalitis etiologies: diagnostic challenges in the California Encephalitis Project, 1998–2000. Clin Infect Dis 2003;36:731–742.

97. Gleckman R, et al. Sputum gram stain assessment in community-acquired bacteremic pneumonia. J Clin Microbiol 1988;26:846–849.

98. Golbert TM, Patterson, R. Pulmonary allergic aspergillosis. Ann Intern Med 1970;72:395–403.

99. Grace CJ, et al. Usefulness of blood culture for hospitalized patients who are receiving antibiotic therapy. Clin Infect Dis 2001;32:1651–1655.

100. Graham DR, Band JD. *Citrobacter diversus* brain abscess and meningitis in neonates. JAMA 1981;245:1923–1925.

101. Gray LD, Fedorko DP. Laboratory diagnosis of bacterial meningitis. Clin Microbiol Rev 1992;5:130–145.

102. Grodinsky M. Retropharyngeal and lateral pharyngeal abscesses: an anatomic and clinical study. Ann Surg 1939;110:177–199.

103. Guerrant RL. Gastrointestinal infections and food poisoning: principles and definition of syndromes. In: Mandell GL, Douglas RG Jr, Bennett JE, Eds. Principles and Practice of Infectious Diseases. 3rd Ed. New York: Churchill Livingstone,1990:839.

104. Guerrant RL, Steiner TS. Principles and syndromes of enteric infection. In: Mandell GL, Bennett JE, Dolin R, eds. Principles and Practice of Infectious Diseases. 5th Ed. Philadelphia: Churchill Livingstone, 2000:1076–1093.

105. Gwaltney JM Jr, et al. The microbial etiology and antimicrobial therapy of adults with acute community-acquired sinusitis: a fifteen-year experience at the University of Virginia and review of other selected studies. J Allergy Clin Immunol 1992;90(Pt 2):457–461.

106. Hall LR, Pearlman E. Pathogenesis of onchocercal keratitis (river blindness). Clin Microbiol Rev 1999;12:445–453.

107. Hamilton JR, et al. Performance of cryptococcus antigen latex agglutination kits on serum and cerebrospinal fluid specimens of AIDS patients before and after pronase treatment. J Clin Microbiol 1991;29:333–339.

108. Hammerschlag MR, et al. Persistent infection with *Chlamydia pneumoniae* following acute respiratory illness. Clin Infect Dis 1992;14:178–182.

109. Hammond GW, et al. Comparison of specimen collection and laboratory techniques for isolation of *Haemophilus ducreyi*. J Clin Microbiol 1978;7:39–43.

110. Handsfield HH. Clinical presentation and natural course of anogenital warts. Am J Med 1997;102:16–20.

111. Harnisch JP, et al. Diphtheria among alcoholic urban adults: a decade of experience in Seattle. Ann Intern Med 1989;111:71–82.

112. Hearn J, et al. Immunopathology of cerebral malaria: morphological evidence of parasite sequestration in murine brain microvasculature. Infect Immun 2000;68:5364–5376.

113. Henderson FW, et al. The etiologic and epidemiologic spectrum of bronchiolitis in pediatric practice. J Pediatr 1979;95:183–190.

114. Hendley JO. Otitis media. N Engl J Med 2002;347:1169–1174.

115. Hennessy TW, et al. Survey of physician diagnostic practices for patients with acute diarrhea: clinical and public health implications. Clin Infect Dis 2004;38(Suppl 3):S203–S211.

116. Herwaldt BL, Ackers ML. An outbreak in 1996 of cyclosporiasis associated with imported raspberries. N Engl J Med 1997;336:1548–1556.

117. Holmes KK, et al. Salpingitis: overview of etiology and epidemiology. Am J Obstet Gynecol 1980;138:893–900.

118. Holst E, et al. Bacterial vaginosis and vaginal microorganisms in idiopathic premature labor and association with pregnancy outcomes. J Clin Microbiol 1994;32:176–186.

119. Hoogkamp-Korstanje JA, et al. Analysis of bacterial infections in a neonatal intensive care unit. J Hosp Infect 1982;3:275–284.

120. Hoppe JE. Methods for isolation of *Bordetella pertussis* from patients with whooping cough. Eur J Clin Microbiol Infect Dis 1988;7:616–620.

121. Hotchkiss RS, Karl IE. The pathophysiology and treatment of sepsis. N Engl J Med 2003;348:138–150.

122. Hubbard WA, et al. Comparison of the B-D urine culture kit with a standard culture method and with MS-2. J Clin Microbiol 1983;17:327–331.

123. Hughes JG, et al. Culture with BACTEC Peds Plus/F bottle compared with conventional methods for detection of bacteria in synovial fluid. J Clin Microbiol 2001;39:4468–4471.

124. Ishak MA, et al. Association of slime with pathogenicity of coagulase-negative staphylococci causing nosocomial septicemia. J Clin Microbiol 1985;22:1025–1029.

125. Ito F, et al. Specific immunofluorescence staining of *Treponema pallidum* in smears and tissues. J Clin Microbiol 1991;29:444–448.

126. Jacobs RF, et al. *Pseudomonas* osteochondritis complicating puncture wounds of the foot in children: a 10-year evaluation. J Infect Dis 1989;160:657–661.

127. Jay V. Ignaz Semmelweis and the conquest of puerperal sepsis. Arch Pathol Lab Med 1999;123:561–562.

128. Jewkes FE, et al. Home collection of urine specimens-boric acid bottles or Dipslides? Arch Dis Child 1990;65:286–289.

129. Johanson WG Jr, et al. Changing pharyngeal bacterial flora of hospitalized patients. Emergence of gram-negative bacilli. N Engl J Med 1969;281:1137–1140.

130. Johnson RE, et al. Screening tests to detect *Chlamydia trachomatis* and *Neisseria gonorrhoeae* infections-2002. MMWR Recomm Rep 2002;51(RR-15):1–38.

131. Jones C, et al. Inability of the Chemstrip LN compared with quantitative urine culture to predict significant bacteriuria. J Clin Microbiol 1986;23:160–162.

132. Jones JL, et al. Survey of clinical laboratory practices for parasitic diseases. Clin Infect Dis 2004;38 Suppl 3:S198–S202.

133. Jones RB, Batteiger BE. *Chlamydia trachomatis* (Trachoma, perinatal infections, lymphogranuloma venereum, and other genital infections). In: Mandell GL, Bennett JE, Dolin R, Eds. Mandell, Douglas, and Bennett's Principles and Practice of Infectious Diseases. 5th Ed. Philadelphia: Churchill Livingstone, 2000: 1989–2004.

134. Joshi N, et al. Infections in patients with diabetes mellitus. N Engl J Med 1999; 341:1906–1912.

135. Kaye E. Antibacterial activity of human urine. J Clin Invest 1968;42:2374–2390.

136. Kelly MT, et al. Clinical comparison of Isolator and BACTEC 660 resin media for blood culture. J Clin Microbiol 1990;28:1925–1927.

137. Khatib R, et al. Coagulase-negative staphylococci in multiple blood cultures: strain relatedness and determinants of same-strain bacteremia. J Clin Microbiol 1995;33:816–820.

138. Kiehn TE, Camarata R. Comparative recoveries of *Mycobacterium avium/Mycobacterium intracellulare* from isolator lysis-centrifugation and BACTEC 13A blood culture systems. J Clin Microbiol 1988;26:760–761.

139. Kierkegaard H, et al. Falsely negative urinary leucocyte counts due to delayed examination. Scand J Clin Lab Invest 1980;40:259–261.

140. Kimball MW, Knee S. Gonococcal perihepatitis in a male. The Fitz-Hugh-Curtis syndrome. N Engl J Med 1970;282:1082–1084.

141. Kimberlin DW. Neonatal herpes simplex infection. Clin Microbiol Rev 2004; 17:1–13.

142. Kimberlin DW, Rouse DJ. Genital herpes. N Engl J Med 2004;350:1970–1977.

143. Kleinschmidt-DeMasters BK, Gilden DH. Varicella-zoster virus infections of the nervous system: clinical and pathologic correlates. Arch Pathol Lab Med 2001;125:770–780.

144. Klotz SA, et al. Fungal and parasitic infections of the eye. Clin Microbiol Rev 2000;13:662–685.

145. Kohl S. Herpes simplex virus encephalitis in children. Pediatr Clin North Am 1988;35:465–483.

146. Koransky JR, et al. *Clostridium septicum* bacteremia: its clinical significance. Am J Med 1979;66:63–66.

147. Kortekangas P, et al. Synovial fluid culture and blood culture in acute arthritis: a multi-case report of 90 patients. Scand J Rheumatol 1995;24:44–47.

148. Krumholz HM, et al. Blood culture phlebotomy: switching needles does not prevent contamination. Ann Intern Med 1990;113:290–292.

149. Kusumi RK, et al. Rapid detection of pyuria by leukocyte esterase activity. JAMA 1981;245:1653–1655.

150. Lamy B, et al. What is the relevance of obtaining multiple blood samples for culture? A comprehensive model to optimize the strategy for diagnosing bacteremia. Clin Infect Dis 2002;35:842–850.

151. Larsen SA, et al. Laboratory diagnosis and interpretation of tests for syphilis. Clin Microbiol Rev 1995;8:1–21.

152. Lee A, Hazell SL. *Campylobacter pylori* in health and disease: an ecological prospective. Microbial Ecol Health Dis 1988;1:1–16.

153. Lee ME, Lindquist TD. Syphilitic interstitial keratitis. JAMA 262:2921–2921, 1989.

154. Lefrock JL, et al. Transient bacteremia associated with sigmoidoscopy. N Engl J Med 1973;289:467–469.

155. Leibowitz HM. The red eye. N Engl J Med 2000;343:345–351.

156. Lentino JR, Lucks DA. Nonvalue of sputum culture in the management of lower respiratory tract infections. J Clin Microbiol 1988;25:758–762.

157. Lew DP, Waldvogel FA. Osteomyelitis. N Engl J Med 1997;336:999–1007.

158. Liesegang TJ. Bacterial keratitis. Infect Dis Clin North Am 1992;6:815–829.

159. Little JR, et al. A randomized trial of povidone-iodine compared with iodine tincture for venipuncture site disinfection: effects on rates of blood culture contamination. Am J Med 1999;107:119–125.

160. Livesley NJ, Chow AW. Infected pressure ulcers in elderly individuals. Clin Infect Dis 2002;35:1390–1396.

161. Lodise TP, et al. Outcomes analysis of delayed antibiotic treatment for hospital-acquired *Staphylococcus aureus* bacteremia. Clin Infect Dis 2003;36:1418–1423.

162. Loeb M. Pneumonia in older persons. Clin Infect Dis 2003;37:1335–1339.

163. Lucey D, et al. Relapsing illness due to *Rochalimaea henselae* in immunocompetent hosts: implication for therapy and new epidemiological associations. Clin Infect Dis 1992;14:683–688.

164. Luterman A, et al. Infections in burn patients. Am J Med 1986;81:45–52.

165. Lyon R, Woods G. Comparison of the BacT/Alert and Isolator blood culture systems for recovery of fungi. Am J Clin Pathol 1995;103:660–662.

166. Ma P, et al. *Naegleria* and *Acanthamoeba* infections: a review. Rev Infect Dis 1990;12:490–513.

167. Mader TH, Stulting RD. Viral keratitis. Infect Dis Clin North Am 1992;6: 831–849.

168. Mahony JB, Phernesky MA. Effect of swab type and storage temperature in the isolation of *Chlamydia trachomatis* from clinical specimens. J Clin Microbiol 1985;22:865–867.

169. Maki DG, et al. A semiquantitative culture method for identifying intravenous-catheter-related infection. N Engl J Med 1977;296:1305–1309.

170. Malan AK, et al. Evaluations of commercial West Nile virus immunoglobulin G (IgG) and IgM enzyme immunoassays show the value of continuous validation. J Clin Microbiol 2004;42:727–733.

171. Mandell LA, et al. Canadian guidelines for the initial management of community-acquired pneumonia: an evidence-based update by the Canadian Infectious Diseases Society and the Canadian Thoracic Society. Clin Infect Dis 2000;31: 383–421.

172. Marchevsky AM, et al. The changing spectrum of disease, etiology, and diagnosis of mucormycosis. Hum Pathol 1980;11:457–464.

173. Marquez-Davila G, Martinez-Barreda CE. Predictive value of the ''clue cells'' investigation and the amine volatilization test in vaginal infections caused by *Gardnerella vaginalis*. J Clin Microbiol 1985;22:686–687.

174. Marshall BJ, Warren JR. Unidentified curved bacilli in the stomach of patients with gastritis and peptic ulceration. Lancet 1984;1:1311–1315.

175. Martens MG, et al. Comparison of two endometrial sampling devices. Cotton-tipped swab and double-lumen catheter with a brush. J Reprod Med 1989;34: 875–879.

176. Mathisen GE, Johnson JP. Brain abscess. Clin Infect Dis 1997;25:763–779.

177. Maurin M, Raoult D. Q fever. Clin Microbiol Rev 1999;12:518–553.

178. Maury E, et al. Circulating endotoxin during initial antibiotic treatment of severe gram-negative bacteremic infections. J Infect Dis 1998;178:270–273.

179. Mayhall CG. The epidemiology of burn wound infections: then and now. Clin Infect Dis 2003;37:543–550.

180. MayoSmith MF, et al. Acute epiglottitis in adults: an eight-year experience in the state of Rhode Island. N Engl J Med 1986;314:1133–1139.

181. Mazzulli T, et al. Reproducibility of interpretation of Gram-stained vaginal smears for the diagnosis of bacterial vaginosis. J Clin Microbiol 1990;28: 1506–1508.

182. McDonald LC, et al. Controlled comparison of BacT/ALERT FAN aerobic medium and BACTEC fungal blood culture medium for detection of fungemia. J Clin Microbiol 2001;39:622–624.

183. McFarland LV, et al. Rectal swab cultures for *Clostridium difficile* surveillance studies. J Clin Microbiol 198725:2241–2242.

184. McGee ZA, Baringer JR. Acute meningitis. In: Mandell GL, Douglas RG Jr, Bennett JE, eds. Principles and Practice of Infectious Diseases. 3rd Ed. New York, Churchill Livingstone, 1990:741–755.

185. McIntosh K. Community-acquired pneumonia in children. N Engl J Med 2002; 346:429–437.

186. Melgar GR, et al. Fungal prosthetic valve endocarditis in 16 patients: an 11-year experience in a tertiary care hospital. Medicine (Baltimore) 1997;76:94–103.

187. Mermel LA, et al. Guidelines for the management of intravascular catheter-related infections. Clin Infect Dis 2001;32:1249–1272.

188. Mertz KJ, et al. Etiology of genital ulcers and prevalence of human immunodeficiency virus coinfection in 10 US cities. J Infect Dis 1998;178:1795–1798.

189. Mertz KJ, et al. An investigation of genital ulcers in Jackson, Mississippi, with use of a multiplex polymerase chain reaction assay: high prevalence of chancroid and human immunodeficiency virus infection. J Infect Dis 1998;178:1060–1066.

190. Mirrett S, et al. Relevance of the number of positive bottles in determining clinical significance of coagulase-negative staphylococci in blood cultures. J Clin Microbiol 2001;39:3279–3281.

191. Monte-Verde D, Nosanchuk JS. The sensitivity and specificity of nitrite testing for bacteriuria. Lab Med 1981;12:755–757.

192. Morens DM. Death of a president. N Engl J Med 1999;341:1845–1849.

193. Morris AJ, et al. Rationale for selective use of anaerobic blood cultures. J Clin Microbiol 1993;31:2110–2113.

194. Mufson MA. *Streptococcus pneumoniae*. In: Mandell GL, Douglas RG Jr, Bennett JE, eds. Principles and Practice of Infect Disease. 4th Ed. New York: Churchill Livingstone, 1990:Chapter 178.

195. Murdoch DR, et al. Evaluation of a rapid immunochromatographic test for detection of *Streptococcus pneumoniae* antigen in urine samples from adults with community-acquired pneumonia. J Clin Microbiol 2001;39:3495–3498.

196. Murray PR. Determination of the optimum incubation period of blood culture broths for the detection of clinically significant septicemia. J Clin Microbiol 1985;85:481–485.

197. Murray PR, et al. Comparative evaluation of the Oxoid signal and Roche septi-chek blood culture systems. J Clin Microbiol 1988;26:2526–2530.

198. Musher DM, et al. Bacteremic and nonbacteremic pneumococcal pneumonia: a prospective study. Medicine (Baltimore) 2000;79:210–221.

199. Mylonakis E, Calderwood SB. Infective endocarditis in adults. N Engl J Med 2001;345:1318–1330.

200. Mylotte JM. Nursing home-acquired pneumonia. Clin Infect Dis 2002;35: 1205–1211.

201. Nash D, et al. The outbreak of West Nile virus infection in the New York City area in 1999. N Engl J Med 2001;344:1807–1814.

202. Nichols RL, Smith JW. Wound and intraabdominal infections: microbiological considerations and approaches to treatment. Clin Infect Dis 1993;16:Suppl 4: S266–S272.

203. Nicolle LE. Asymptomatic bacteriuria: important or not? N Engl J Med 2000; 343:1037–1039.

204. Nicolle LE, et al. Urine specimen collection with external devices for diagnosis of bacteriuria in elderly incontinent men. J Clin Microbiol 1988;26:1115–1119.

205. Noah DL, et al. Epidemiology of human rabies in the United States, 1980 to 1996. Ann Intern Med 1998;128:922–930.

206. O'Hara CM, Weinstein MP, Miller JM. Manual and automated systems for detection and identification of microorganisms. In: Murray PR, Baron EJ, Jorgensen JH, et al., eds. Manual of Clinical Microbiology. 8th Ed. Washington, DC: ASM Press, 2003:185–207.

207. Paisley JW, Lauer BA. Pediatric blood cultures. Clin Lab Med 1994;14:17–30.

208. Paramasivan CN, et al. Effect of storage of sputum specimens at room temperature on smear and culture results. Tubercle 1983;64:119–121.

209. Parrillo JE. Pathogenetic mechanisms of septic shock. N Engl J Med 1993;328: 1471–1477.

210. Penn RL, Silberman R. Effects of overnight refrigeration on the microscopic evaluation of sputum. J Clin Microbiol 1984;19:161–163.

211. Perl B, et al. Cost-effectiveness of blood cultures for adult patients with cellulitis. Clin Infect Dis 1999;29:1483–1488.

212. Pezzlo MT, et al. Detection of bacteriuria and pyuria by URISCREEN a rapid enzymatic screening test. J Clin Microbiol 1992;30:680–684.

213. Pfaller MA, et al. Survey of blood stream infections attributable to gram-positive cocci: frequency of occurrence and antimicrobial susceptibility of isolates collected in 1997 in the United States, Canada, and Latin America from the SENTRY Antimicrobial Surveillance Program. SENTRY Participants Group. Diagn Microbiol Infect Dis 1999;33:283–297.

214. Pfaller MA, Koontz FP. Laboratory evaluation of leukocyte esterase and nitrite tests for the detection of bacteriuria. J Clin Microbiol 1985;21:840–842.

215. Piper C, et al. Prosthetic valve endocarditis. Heart 2001;85:590–593.

216. Prince HE, et al. Utility of the Focus Technologies West Nile virus immunoglobulin M capture enzyme-linked immunosorbent assay for testing cerebrospinal fluid. J Clin Microbiol 2004;42:12–15.

217. Prober CG, Arvin AM. Perinatal viral infections. Eur J Clin Microbiol 1987;6: 245–261.

218. Quilici N, et al. Differential quantitative blood cultures in the diagnosis of catheter-related sepsis in intensive care units. Clin Infect Dis 1997;25:1066–1070.

219. Quinn TC, et al. *Chlamydia trachomatis* proctitis. N Engl J Med 1981;305: 195–200.

220. Raad II, Bodey GP. Infectious complications of indwelling vascular catheters. Clin Infect Dis 1992;15:197–208.

221. Rajam RV, et al. Systemic donovanosis. Br J Vener Dis 1954;30:73–80.

222. Rathore MH, et al. Latex particle agglutination tests on the cerebrospinal fluid: a reappraisal. J Fla Med Assoc 1995;82:21–23.

223. Ratzan KR. Viral meningitis. Med Clin North Am 1985;69:399–413.

224. Rautonen J, et al. Prognostic factors in childhood acute encephalitis. Pediatr Infect Dis J 1991;10:441–446.

225. Reimer LG, Carroll KC. Role of the microbiology laboratory in the diagnosis of lower respiratory tract infections. Clin Infect Dis 1998;26:742–748.

226. Reimer LG, et al. Update on detection of bacteremia and fungemia. Clin Microbiol Rev 1997;10:444–465.

227. Rein MF, Mandell GL. Bacterial killing by bacteriostatic saline solutions: potential for diagnostic error. N Engl J Med 1973;289:794–795.

228. Reller LB, et al. Cumitech 1A. Blood Cultures II. American Society for Microbiology, Washington, DC, 1982.

229. Ringelmann R, et al. Role of immunological tests in diagnosis of bacterial meningitis. Antibiot Chemother 1992;45:68–78.

230. Robson MC, et al. Wound healing alterations caused by infection. Clin Plast Surg 1990;17:485–492.

231. Ronald AR, Plummer FA. Chancroid and *Haemophilus ducreyi*. Ann Intern Med 1985;102:805–807.

232. Ronald AR, Plummer FA. Chancroid and granuloma inguinale. Clin Lab Med 1989;9:535–543.

233. Rosen T, et al. Granuloma inguinale. J Am Acad Dermatol 1984;11:433–437.

234. Rosenfeld EA, Rowley AH. Infectious intracranial complications of sinusitis, other than meningitis, in children: 12-year review. Clin Infect Dis 1994;18: 750–754.

235. Roson B, et al. Prospective study of the usefulness of sputum gram stain in the initial approach to community-acquired pneumonia requiring hospitalization. Clin Infect Dis 2000;31:869–874.

236. Rummens JL, et al. Isolation of *Capnocytophaga* species with a new selective medium. J Clin Microbiol 1985;22:375–378.

237. Sachs MK, et al. Failure of dithiothreitol and pronase to reveal a false-positive

cryptococcal antigen determination in cerebrospinal fluid. Am J Clin Pathol 1991;96:381–384.

238. Sandberg T, et al. Virulence of *Escherichia coli* in relation to host factors in women with symptomatic urinary tract infection. J Clin Microbiol 1988;26: 1471–1476.

239. Sandre RM, Shafran SD. Infective endocarditis: review of 135 cases over 9 years. Clin Infect Dis 1996;22:276–286.

240. Sauerbrei A, Wutzler P. Laboratory diagnosis of central nervous system infections caused by herpesviruses. J Clin Virol 2002;25:Suppl 51.

241. Schaaf VM, et al. The limited value of symptoms and signs in the diagnosis of vaginal infections. Arch Intern Med 1990;150:1929–1933.

242. Schacker T, et al. Frequent recovery of HIV-1 from genital herpes simplex virus lesions in HIV-1-infected men. JAMA 1998;280:61–66.

243. Schacker T, et al. Frequency of symptomatic and asymptomatic herpes simplex virus type 2 reactivations among human immunodeficiency virus-infected men. J Infect Dis 1998;178:1616–1622.

244. Schifman RB, et al. Solitary blood cultures as a quality assurance indicator. Qual Assur Util Rev 1991;6:132–137.

245. Schneider M, et al. Quantitative assessment of bacterial invasion of chronic ulcers. Statistical analysis. Am J Surg 1983;145:260–262.

246. Schulte JM, et al. Chancroid in the United States, 1981–1990: evidence for underreporting of cases. MMWR CDC Surveill Summ 1992;41:57–61.

247. Schwabe LD, et al. A comparison of Oxoid Signal with nonradiometric BACTEC NR-660 for detection of bacteremia. Diagn Microbiol Infect Dis 1990;13:3–8.

248. Schwartz R, et al. The nasopharyngeal culture in acute otitis media: a reappraisal of its usefulness. JAMA 1979;241:2170–2173.

249. Scieux C, et al. Lymphogranuloma venereum: 27 cases in Paris. J Infect Dis 1989;160:662–668.

250. Seaworth JB, et al. Brain abscess caused by a variety of *Cladosporium trichoides*. Am J Clin Pathol 1983;79:747–752.

251. Sehgal VN, Sharma HK. Pseudoelephantiasis of the penis following donovanosis. J Dermatol 1990;17:130–131.

252. Senzilet LD, et al. Pertussis is a frequent cause of prolonged cough illness in adults and adolescents. Clin Infect Dis 2001;32:1691–1697.

253. Sepkowitz KA. Opportunistic infections in patients with and patients without acquired immunodeficiency syndrome. Clin Infect Dis 2002;34:1098–1107.

254. Shandera WX, et al. Neurocysticercosis in Houston, Texas: a report of 112 cases. Medicine (Baltimore) 1994;73:37–52.

255. Sheiness D, et al. High levels of *Gardnerella vaginalis* detected with an oligonucleotide probe combined with elevated pH as a diagnostic indicator of bacterial vaginosis. J Clin Microbiol 1992;30:642–648.

256. Sherertz RJ, et al. Diagnosis of triple-lumen catheter infection: comparison of roll plate, sonication, and flushing methodologies. J Clin Microbiol 1997;35: 641–646.

257. Shirtliff ME, Mader JT. Acute septic arthritis. Clin Microbiol Rev 2002;15: 527–544.

258. Siegman-Igra Y, et al. Reappraisal of community-acquired bacteremia: a proposal of a new classification for the spectrum of acquisition of bacteremia. Clin Infect Dis 2002;34:1431–1439.

259. Singh AE, Romanowski B. Syphilis: review with emphasis on clinical, epidemiologic, and some biologic features. Clin Microbiol Rev 1999;12:187–209.

260. Slater LN, et al. A newly recognized fastidious gram-negative pathogen as a cause of fever and bacteremia. N Engl J Med 1990;323:1587–1593.

261. Smalley DL, Bradley ME. Correlation of leukocyte esterase activity and bacterial isolation from body fluids. J Clin Microbiol 1984;20:1186–1186.

262. Smart D, et al. Effect of needle changing and intravenous cannula collection on blood culture contamination rates. Ann Emerg Med 1993;22:1164–1168.

263. Smith JS, Robinson NJ. Age-specific prevalence of infection with herpes simplex virus types 2 and 1: a global review. J Infect Dis 2002;186:Suppl 28.

264. Smith TF, et al. Isolation of viruses from single throat swabs processed for diagnosis of group A beta-hemolytic streptococci by fluorescent antibody technic. Am J Clin Pathol 1973;60:707–710.

265. Snow RW, et al. Relation between severe malaria morbidity in children and level of *Plasmodium falciparum* transmission in Africa. Lancet 1997;349:1650–1654.

266. Sobel JD. Vaginitis. N Engl J Med 1997;337:1896–1903.

267. Solomon AR. New diagnostic tests for herpes simplex and varicella zoster infections. J Am Acad Dermatol 1988;18:218–221.

268. Spada EL, et al. Proposal of an easy method to improve routine sputum bacteriology. Respiration 1989;56:137–146.

269. Speich R, et al. Low specificity of the bacterial index for the diagnosis of bacterial pneumonia by bronchoalveolar lavage. Eur J Clin Microbiol Infect Dis 1998; 17:78–84.

270. Spiegel CA. Bacterial vaginosis. Clin Microbiol Rev 1991;4:485–502.

271. Stamm WE. Catheter-associated urinary tract infections: epidemiology, pathogenesis, and prevention. Am J Med 1991;91:65S–71S.

272. Stamm WE, et al. Indwelling arterial catheters as a source of nosocomial bacteremia: an outbreak caused by *Flavobacterium* species. N Engl J Med 1975;292: 1099–1102.

273. Stamm WE, Hooton TM. Management of urinary tract infections in adults. N Engl J Med 1993;329:1328–1334.

274. Stamm WE, et al. Treatment of the acute urethral syndrome. N Engl J Med 1981;304:956–958.

275. Stamm WE, et al. Causes of the acute urethral syndrome in women. N Engl J Med 1980;303:409–415.

276. Stanislawski L, et al. Role of fibronectin in attachment of *Streptococcus pyogenes* and *Escherichia coli* to human cell lines and isolated oral epithelial cells. Infect Immun 1985;48:257–259.

277. Starr CE, Pavan-Langston D. Varicella-zoster virus: mechanisms of pathogenicity and corneal disease. Ophthalmol Clin North Am 200215:7–15.

278. Strom BL, et al. Sexual activity, contraceptive use, and other risk factors for symptomatic and asymptomatic bacteriuria. A case-control study. Ann Intern Med 1987;107:816–823.

279. Stull TL, LiPuma JJ. Epidemiology and natural history of urinary tract infections in children. Med Clin North Am 1991;75:287–297.

280. Suerbaum S, Michetti P. *Helicobacter pylori* infection. N Engl J Med 2002;347: 1175–1186.

281. Swartz MN. Cellulitis. N Engl J Med 2004;350:904–912.

282. Syed NA, Hyndiuk RA. Infectious conjunctivitis. Infect Dis Clin North Am 1992;6:789–805.

283. Talan DA, et al. Bacteriologic analysis of infected dog and cat bites. N Engl J Med 1999;340:85–92.

284. Taylor DE, et al. Isolation and characterization of *Campylobacter pyloridis* from gastric biopsies. Am J Clin Pathol 1987;87:49–54.

285. Tedder DG, et al. Herpes simplex virus infection as a cause of benign recurrent lymphocytic meningitis. Ann Intern Med 1994;121:334–338.

286. Terni M, et al. Aseptic meningitis in association with herpes progenitalis. N Engl J Med 1971;285:503–504.

287. Thielman NM, Guerrant RL. Acute infectious diarrhea. N Engl J Med 2004; 350:38–47.

288. Thwaites GE, et al. Improving the bacteriological diagnosis of tuberculous meningitis. J Clin Microbiol 2004;42:378–379.

289. Tierney BM, et al. Early detection of positive blood cultures by the acridine orange staining technique. J Clin Microbiol 1983;18:830–833.

290. Torres A, Ewig S. Diagnosing ventilator-associated pneumonia. N Engl J Med 2004;350:433–435.

291. Torres A, et al. Diagnostic value of nonfluoroscopic percutaneous lung needle aspiration in patients with pneumonia. Chest 1990;98:840–844.

292. Tsai IK, et al. *Clostridium perfringens* septicemia with massive hemolysis. Scand J Infect Dis 1989;21:467–471.

293. Tunkel AR. Evaluation of culture-negative endocarditis. Hosp Pract 1993;28: 59–66.

294. Uehling DT, Hasham AI. Significance of catheter tip cultures. Invest Urol 1977; 15:57–58.

295. Valenstein PN. Semiquantitation of bacteria in sputum gram stains. J Clin Microbiol 1988;26:1791–1794.

296. van Vliet KE, et al. Multicenter evaluation of the Amplicor Enterovirus PCR test with cerebrospinal fluid from patients with aseptic meningitis. J Clin Microbiol 1998;36:2652–2657.

297. Versalovic J. *Helicobacter pylori*. Pathology and diagnostic strategies. Am J Clin Pathol 2003;119:403–412.

298. Voetsch AC, et al. Laboratory practices for stool-specimen culture for bacterial pathogens, including *Escherichia coli* O157:H7, in the FoodNet sites, 1995–2000. Clin Infect Dis 2004;38(Suppl 3):S190–S197.

299. von Eiff C, et al. Nasal carriage as a source of *Staphylococcus aureus* bacteremia. N Engl J Med 2001;344:11–16.

300. Vongpatanasin W, et al. Prosthetic heart valves. N Engl J Med 1996;335: 407–416.

301. Waisman Y, et al. The validity of the uriscreen test for early detection of urinary tract infection in children. Pediatrics 1999;104:e41.

302. Wald A, et al. Genital shedding of herpes simplex virus among men. J Infect Dis 2002;186:Suppl 9.

303. Wald A, et al. Reactivation of genital herpes simplex virus type 2 infection in asymptomatic seropositive persons. N Engl J Med 2000;342:844–850.

304. Wald ER. Sinusitis. N Engl J Med 1992;326:319–323.

305. Walter FG, Knopp RK. Urine sampling in ambulatory women: midstream cleancatch versus catheterization. Ann Emerg Med 1989;18:166–172.

306. Waltzman ML, Harper M. Financial and clinical impact of false-positive blood culture results. Clin Infect Dis 2001;33:296–299.

307. Warren JW, et al. Guidelines for antimicrobial treatment of uncomplicated acute bacterial cystitis and acute pyelonephritis in women. Infectious Diseases Society of America (IDSA). Clin Infect Dis 1999;29:745–758.

308. Warren SS, Allen SD. Clinical, pathogenic and laboratory features of *Capnocytophaga* infections. Am J Clin Pathol 1986;86:513–518.

309. Washington JA II, et al. Detection of significant bacteriuria by microscopic examination of urine. Lab Med 1981;12:294–296.

310. Watanakunakorn C, Burkert T. Infective endocarditis at a large community

teaching hospital, 1980–1990: a review of 210 episodes. Medicine (Baltimore) 1993;72:90–102.

311. Weese WC, Smith IM. A study of 57 cases of actinomycosis over a 36-year period: a diagnostic ''failure'' with good prognosis after treatment. Arch Intern Med 1975;135:1562–1568.

312. Weinbaum FI, et al. Doing it right the first time: quality improvement and the contaminant blood culture. J Clin Microbiol 1997;35:563–565.

313. Weinstein MP. Blood culture contamination: persisting problems and partial progress. J Clin Microbiol 2003;41:2275–2278.

314. Weinstein MP, et al. The effect of altered headspace atmosphere on yield and speed of detection of the Oxoid Signal blood culture system versus BACTEC radiometric system. J Clin Microbiol 1990;28:795–797.

315. Weinstein MP, et al. Clinical importance of identifying coagulase-negative staphylococci isolated from blood cultures: evaluation of MicroScan Rapid and Dried Overnight Gram-Positive panels versus a conventional reference method. J Clin Microbiol 1998;36:2089–2092.

316. Weinstein MP, et al. The clinical significance of positive blood cultures: a comprehensive analysis of 500 episodes of bacteremia and fungemia in adults. II. Clinical observations, with special reference to factors influencing prognosis. Rev Infect Dis 1983;5:54–70.

317. Weinstein MP, Reller LB. Clinical importance of ''breakthrough'' bacteremia. Am J Med 1984;76:175–180.

318. Weinstein MP, et al. The clinical significance of positive blood cultures: a comprehensive analysis of 500 episodes of bacteremia and fungemia in adults. I. Laboratory and epidemiologic observations. Rev Infect Dis 1983;5:35–53.

319. Weinstein MP, et al. The clinical significance of positive blood cultures in the 1990s: a prospective comprehensive evaluation of the microbiology, epidemiology, and outcome of bacteremia and fungemia in adults. Clin Infect Dis 1997; 24:584–602.

320. Wendt C, Grunwald WJ. Polyclonal bacteremia due to gram-negative rods. Clin Infect Dis 2001;33:460–465.

321. Whitley RJ, Kimberlin DW. Viral encephalitis. Pediatr Rev 1999;20:192–198.

322. Wieland M, et al. Left-sided endocarditis due to *Pseudomonas aeruginosa*: a report of 10 cases and review of the literature. Medicine (Baltimore) 1986;65: 180–189.

323. Wilson ML, Gaido L. Laboratory diagnosis of urinary tract infections in adult patients. Clin Infect Dis 2004;38:1150–1158.

324. Wilson ML, et al. Comparison of iodophor and alcohol pledgets with the mediflex blood culture prep kit II for preventing contamination of blood cultures. J Clin Microbiol 2000;38:4665–4667.

325. Wohl ME, Chernick V. State of the art: bronchiolitis. Am Rev Respir Dis 1978; 118:759–781.

326. Wolner-Hanssen P, et al. Isolation of *Chlamydia trachomatis* from the liver capsule in Fitz-Hugh-Curtis syndrome. N Engl J Med 1982;306:113–113.

327. Woods DE, et al. Role of fibronectin in the prevention of adherence of *Pseudomonas aeruginosa* to mammalian buccal epithelial cells. J Infect Dis 1981;143: 784–790.

328. Wu TC, Koo SY. Comparison of three commercial cryptococcal latex kits for detection of cryptococcal antigen. J Clin Microbiol 1983;18:1120–1127.

329. Xu F, et al. Seroprevalence and coinfection with herpes simplex virus type 1 and type 2 in the United States, 1988–1994. J Infect Dis 2002;185:1019–1024.

330. Yagupsky P, Nolte FS. Quantitative aspects of septicemia. Clin Microbiol Rev 1990;3:269–279.

331. Yagupsky P, Press J. Use of the isolator 1.5 microbial tube for culture of synovial fluid from patients with septic arthritis. J Clin Microbiol 1997;35:2410–2412.

332. Yuen KY, Seto WH, Ong SG, et al. The significance of *Branhamella catarrhalis* in bronchopulmonary infection—a case-control study. J Infect 1989;19: 2511–2516.

333. Ziai M, Haggerty RJ. Neonatal meningitis. N Engl J Med 1958;259:314–320.

Laboratory Diagnosis by Immunologic Methods

Antigens and Antibodies: Basic Definitions

Monoclonal Antibodies

Types of Antigen-Antibody Reactions Used in Diagnostic Serology

Precipitin Reactions
Complement Fixation and
    Hemagglutination Inhibition
Agglutination Reactions

Solid-Phase Immunoassay Methods

Enzyme Immunoassays for
    Antibody Detection

Enzyme Immunoassay Antibody
    Capture Methods for IgM
    Detection
Enzyme Immunoassays for
    Antigen Detection

Immunofluorescence Techniques

Immunofluorescence Techniques
    for Antigen Detection
Immunofluorescence Techniques
    for Antibody Detection

In clinical microbiology laboratories, culture of microorganisms from patient specimens remains the principal method for the diagnosis of infectious diseases. During the 1940s and 1950s, serologic techniques, such as Oudin and Ouchterlony immunodiffusion, that were developed in research settings were introduced into clinical laboratories. Subsequently, other methods that exploited basic immunologic concepts, such as complement fixation, were introduced as methods for retrospectively documenting the host immune response to infection. The development of radioimmunoassay, enzyme immunoassay, and hybridoma technology has completely altered the role of serology in the diagnosis of infectious diseases. Through the efforts of many scientists and laboratory workers, methods that were originally developed for antibody detection were reconfigured for direct detection of microbial antigens in patient specimens. These newer immunoserologic techniques have expanded the role of the laboratory in patient care and have gained widespread acceptance as helpful diagnostic tools for both laboratorians and physicians. All of these techniques, however, have their foundations in certain basic immunologic concepts. After a brief review of these concepts, the newer applications of immunoserology to patient care will be discussed.

Antigens and Antibodies: Basic Definitions

An **antigen** is a substance that evokes the formation of antibodies in an animal that is immunized with that particular antigen. An antigen is generally immunogenic, i.e., it has the capability to stimulate antibody formation and it is also able to specifically combine with the antibodies that are formed against it. Not all molecular structures composing the antigen are equally immunogenic; molecular structures that are immunogenic and that are recognized by antibodies are called **immunodominant antigenic determinants** or **epitopes**. The unique characteristics of each antigen depend on the types and sequences of amino acids in proteins; the chemical and structural composition of polysaccharides, glycoproteins, and nucleic acids; and their secondary, tertiary, and quaternary structures. Different molecules may share antigenic determinants and will be recognized by antibodies directed against these determinants. For example, the C1 portions of the light chains of the various immunoglobulin classes (discussed below) contain common antigenic determinants that allow them to be recognized by the same antibodies. These antigen-antibody combinations are termed ''cross-reactive.'' Cross-reactions of antibodies with common or closely related antigens may be clinically important in some disease states. For example, it is believed that the cardiac damage that occurs during the development of rheumatic heart disease may be related to the cross-reactivity of the cell-surface antigens of group A β-hemolytic streptococci and several antigenic moieties in myocardial, endocardial, and valvular heart tissues, myocardial sarcolemma, and skeletal muscle (see Chapter 12).[136,150] In this model, antibodies developed during acute streptococcal pharyngitis may subsequently bind to these cross-reactive epitopes in heart tissue. This binding activates the complement cascade, resulting in immunologically mediated damage to cardiac muscle and adjacent tissues. A similar mechanism is believed to operate in the pathogenesis of poststreptococcal glomerulonephritis. Antibodies elicited by ''nephritogenic'' group A streptococci may react with renal tissue to produce glomerular injury, and, indeed, several similarities between antigenic constituents of group A streptococci and human kidney tissue have been reported.[8,79] In addition, monoclonal antibodies produced against human glomerular tissues also cross-react with some group A streptococcal M proteins, suggesting that the pathogenic mechanisms of these poststreptococcal sequelae are similar.[51]

Antibodies belong to a group of structurally related glycoprotein molecules found in the blood and extracellular fluids and are known collectively as **immunoglobulins (Igs)**. These molecules are produced by B lymphocytes that express surface-bound Igs of a single specificity. When the antigen receptors on these cells encounter the appropriate binding ligand, the B cells proliferate and start to secrete soluble antibodies against the target antigen. Individual plasma cells produce large amounts of single antibody molecules that have the same antigen-binding specificities. In addition, some B cells function as antigen-processing cells that subsequently present the antigen to T lymphocytes, stimulating additional antibody production and the induction of cellular immune responses.[36] The genesis of the cellular and humoral immune responses and the cellular interactions that result in the production of specific antibodies are beyond the scope of this book and may be found in other resources devoted to immunology and immunogenetics.[36]

Immunoglobulins (Igs) can be divided into five classes based on their structure: **IgG, IgM, IgA, IgD, and IgE** (Fig. 3-1). IgG molecules have a molecular weight of about 150 kilodaltons (kDa), are composed of two light chains and two heavy chains, and have two sites for binding to specific antigen (Fab sites). The non-antigen-binding site, composed of portions of the two heavy chains, is called the Fc region. Molecules of the IgG class are actively transported across the placenta and provide passive immunity to the newborn infant at a time when the infant's immune mechanisms are in development. IgGs are divided into four subclasses—IgG$_1$, IgG$_2$, IgG$_3$ and IgG$_4$.[36] IgG$_1$ is the major immunoglobulin in serum and is able to fix and, therefore, activate complement. IgG$_2$ and IgG$_4$ are the major immunoglobulins produced in response to polysaccharide antigens and, therefore, to encapsulated bacteria such as *Streptococcus pneumoniae* and *Haemophilus influenzae* type b. IgG$_3$ is produced in greater quantities during the secondary immune response and is particularly important in viral neutralization. IgM molecules have a molecular weight of about 950 kDa and are composed of five monomers, each of which resembles a single IgG molecule. The five monomeric structures are joined to each other by disulfide bonds on the Fc region of each monomer and by a 15-kDa molecule called the J-chain, which is necessary for aggregation of the pentameric structure.[115] IgM is the first immunoglobulin class produced by the fetus and is the first immunoglobulin to appear in the circulation following immunization or infection.[15] This antibody species is also able to fix complement. The appearance of IgM in the serum is transient, and its presence usually indicates recent infection. However, IgM responses may be noted during reactivation of latent viral infections and during reinfection with the same or closely related agents.[35] In addition, IgM antibodies may persist for weeks to months, depending on the agent's and host's immune competence. Unlike serum IgG, IgM does not cross the placenta, so demonstration of IgM against an infectious agent (e.g., rubella) in fetal or cord blood indicates a congenital or perinatally acquired infection. Serum IgG appears 4 to 6 weeks after infection and usually persists for life. IgA antibodies occur either as monomers (160 kDa) or dimers (400 kDa) and account for about 15% of the total serum immunoglobulin. IgA is the principal antibody class found on mucosal surfaces and in extracellular secretions (e.g., colostrum, saliva, tears, mucin, intestinal, respiratory, and genital tract secretions). IgD is similar in structure to IgG, has a molecular weight of 175 kDa, and comprises only about 0.2% of the total serum immunoglobulin. This antibody class is found primarily on the surfaces of immature B lymphocytes and acts as a cellular antigen receptor. IgE is a 190-kDa immunoglobulin present in only trace amounts in serum. This immunoglobulin is noncovalently bound by its Fc region to mast cells and basophils. Binding of antigen to IgE activates the degranulation of these cells, leading to the synthesis of peptide mediators of hypersensitivity. Therefore, IgE antibodies play major roles in allergic reactions (e.g., anaphylaxis). These antibodies also may be transiently or persistently elevated in serum during certain intestinal helminth infections.[65]

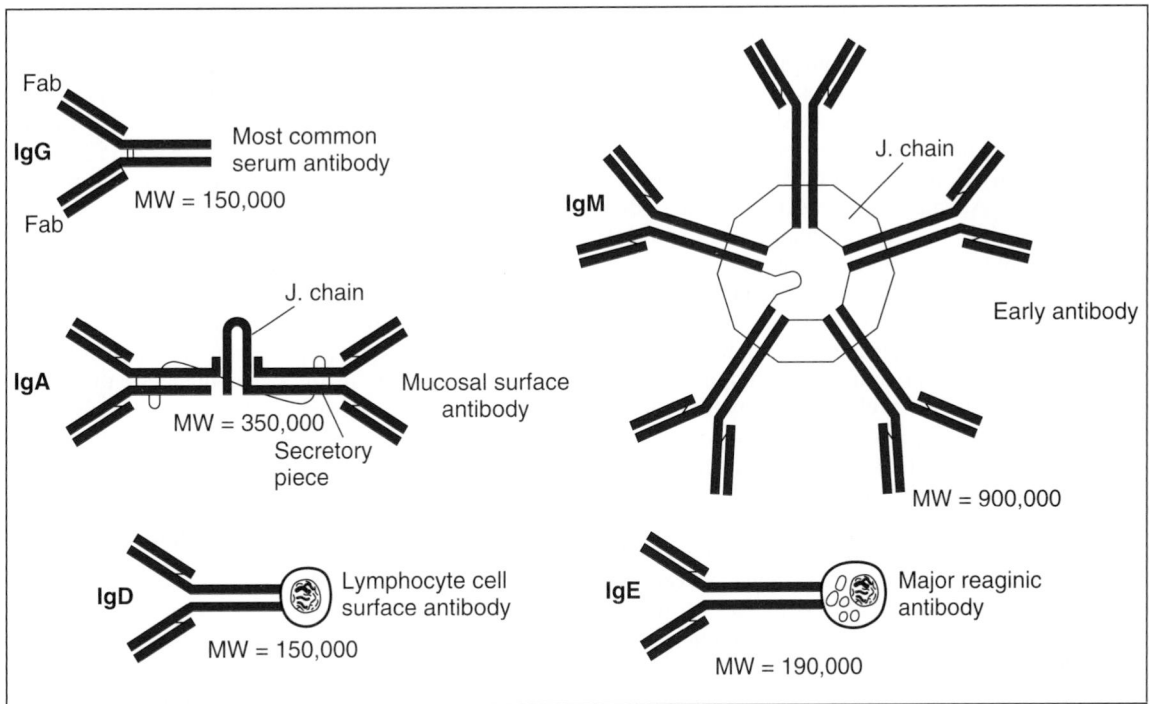

Figure 3-1 Classes of human immunoglobulins. Antibodies belong to five structural and functional classes, designated IgG, IgM, IgA, IgD, and IgE. The basic structural unit of members in each class consists of two pairs of polypeptides (two heavy chains and two light chains) joined by disulfide bonds, and each unit has two antigen-combining sites. Some Ig types have other structural components (J chain in IgM, secretory piece in IgA).

Serologic diagnosis of infections with bacterial, viral, fungal, or parasitic agents in the clinical laboratory is accomplished by detection of specific antibodies in patient serum specimens. As mentioned, IgM is the first antibody to appear after infection, so a serologic diagnosis of recent infection may be obtained by performing an IgM-specific test on a single serum specimen collected early in the clinical course. Diagnosis of recent infection can also be made by the detection of IgG antibodies in paired specimens. The first specimen is collected within 5 to 7 days after the onset of symptoms, while the second is collected during convalescence 2 to 4 weeks later. A fourfold or greater rise in the antibody titer between the acute and the convalescent specimen suggests a recent or intercurrent infection. The antibody titer is defined as the reciprocal of the dilution of serum that still gives a positive test for the presence of antibodies. For example, if an acute-phase specimen is reactive at the highest dilution of 1 to 8 (titer of 8), and the convalescent specimen is reactive up to a dilution of 1 to 64 (titer of 64), the second specimen's titer is greater than fourfold the titer of the first specimen ($8 \times 4 = 32$, and $64 > 32$). This fourfold rise in titer suggests infection with the agent within the recent past. Use of a fourfold rise in titer to delineate recent infection is based on normal test variation and is predicated on testing of both acute and convalescent specimens in the same procedure at the same time. Single serum specimens may be tested to determine the immune status of individuals to certain agents (e.g., rubella, varicella-zoster, etc.); in these cases, test performance may include not only positive and negative

controls, but additional sera of known reactivity to serve as calibrators for the interpretation of test results.

Serologic diagnosis of infectious diseases is characteristically retrospective, as some time must elapse between infection with an agent and the presence of a detectable immune response. However, serologic procedures have broadened in scope to include not only the detection of antibodies in serum, but also the detection of antigens in a variety of specimen types. For the rest of this chapter, methods for serologic detection of both antibodies and antigens will be addressed in general terms, with specific applications of these methods being addressed in subsequent chapters.

Monoclonal Antibodies

Antigens, by their nature as macromolecules having primary, secondary, tertiary and quaternary structures, constitute a "mosaic" of antigenic determinants. An outgrowth of basic serologic principles and techniques has been the attempt to "purify" antigens to reduce the heterogeneity of antibodies developed against them. Antigen molecules with only a single epitope are rarely encountered; rather, hundreds or even thousands of potential antigenic determinants may exist on a cell surface or within the mix of other substances. When these mixed antigens are injected into an animal, an equal number of lymphocyte clones are stimulated. Even though each clone produces a specific antibody, the final result is a highly heterogeneous mixture of antibody molecules, the specificity and affinity of which are often unknown and difficult to control from batch to batch. When these **polyclonal antisera** are used in immunologic test systems involving infectious agents, cross-reactivity may be noted either because antigenic determinants are shared by different species or because mutations may have led to the evolution of epitopes sufficiently close in specificity to produce detectable cross-reactions. Attempts to produce pure antibodies through absorption with cross-reacting antigens or to prepare "clonal" from "polyclonal" antisera via techniques such as affinity column chromatography have been only partially successful.

As the science of serologic testing evolved, the view was held that the availability of an antibody with a high degree of molecular homogeneity and with a specificity for a single, antigenic epitope without cross-reactivity would solve many of the problems encountered in the use of polyclonal antibodies. Highly specific **monoclonal antibodies**, the product of a single clone of lymphoid cells, gradually emerged as a by-product of the investigations in cell fusion and hybridoma technology conducted by Kohler and Milstein.[76] Because of their discovery, it is now possible to isolate cloned lines of individual lymphocytes that produce unique, monospecific antibody molecules. Thus, monoclonal antibodies refer to a uniform, homogeneous, molecular species of immunoglobulin, rather than to a heterogeneous array of immunoglobulins, as is produced during the immune response. The principal feature of this technology was not that a single line of monoclonal antibody-producing cells could be isolated, but rather that these mouse lymphocytes could be "fused" with mouse myeloma cells to produce hybrid cells with two inherent properties: 1) the capability of producing monospecific antibodies (acquired from the parent lymphocytes) and, 2) the ability to grow permanently in culture (the characteristic "immortality" acquired from the myeloma cells). Thus, individual monoclonal antibodies can now be produced in a continuous and almost endless supply. The production of monoclonal antibodies involves the seven steps listed below. Additional information and details regarding these steps are found in Box 3-1:

1. Selection of antigen (need not be purified);
2. Immunization of the animal;
3. Fusion of animal splenic lymphocytes with myeloma cells;
4. Formation of antibody-producing hybrids;
5. Cloning of desired isolated hybridomas;
6. Screening for antibodies by use of selective techniques;
7. Mass production of desired monoclonal antibodies.

Monoclonal antibodies have been produced against many clinically relevant antigens, and the current applications of these antibodies are far too numerous to cite in detail here.[101] Microbiologists must keep up with current publications to determine which developments in this area may be of use in their laboratories. Monoclonal antibodies have been developed for a wide variety of viruses, bacteria, parasites, and fungi, and reagents and conjugates prepared with them are now used in many commercially available enzyme immunoassay and immunofluorescence test kits. In addition to the direct detection of microbial structural antigens (e.g., capsular polysaccharides, outer-membrane-protein antigens),

monoclonal antibodies have also been developed for the detection of virulence factors produced by microorganisms, such as toxins produced by *Shigella* species, adherence-mediating fimbriae of uropathogenic *Escherichia coli*, enterotoxins produced by some serotypes of *E. coli*, and toxins A and B produced by *Clostridium difficile*, among others.[31,34,39,88,121] This approach introduces a totally new way of looking at the relationship of microorganisms and infectious diseases. Instead of the conventional focus on detection and identification of the organisms themselves, these reagents allow the specific detection of microbial virulence factors that may be shared by several bacterial species associated with a given symptom complex. For example, it may be more important to know that an enteric toxin is the cause of hyperosmotic diarrhea, rather than receiving the information that the patient is infected with *Shigella* species or an enterotoxigenic *E. coli* strain.

Types of Antigen-Antibody Reactions Used in Diagnostic Serology
Precipitin Reactions

The basic type of antigen-antibody reaction is the precipitin reaction. This reaction is found in test systems that allow the free diffusion of antigen and antibody fronts toward one another. At a critical point of interface, where the concentrations are optimal, a visible precipitate composed of combined antigens and antibodies forms. In a **single-diffusion** system, antibody is incorporated into an agar gel into which antigen is allowed to diffuse. In the tube (Oudin) immunodiffusion method, antigen is overlaid onto agar containing antisera, and one or more precipitin lines form at zones of equivalence.[103] In **radial immunodiffusion,** antibody is incorporated into agar that is coated onto a glass slide. Material containing antigen is then placed into a circular well cut into the agar. During incubation, the antigen diffuses into the agar and a ring of precipitate forms. The square of the radius of the ring is directly proportional to the amount of antigen present in the material. Using a constant dilution of antiserum, semiquantitative antigen concentrations may be determined by comparing the diameters of the precipitin reaction produced by solutions of known antigen concentrations with that of the ring produced by an unknown solution.[92,107] The most commonly used conventional immunodiffusion procedure is **double diffusion.** In this technique, antigen and antibody are place in wells adjacent to one another, and the materials diffuse out and toward one another. A line of precipitate then forms between the wells when concentrations of equivalence are reached. Double diffusion may require incubation for up to 48 hours before an interpretable result is obtained. **Countercurrent immunoelectrophoresis (CIE)** uses double diffusion technology, but uses an electric current running through the agarose support matrix to speed up the migration of the antigen and antibody toward one another. These methods may be used for the detection of either antibody or antigen in body fluids.

One precaution in performing precipitin procedures is to recognize the possibility of false-negative reactions due to prozone or postzone phenomena. If antibody is in excess (i.e., in concentrations far in excess of available antigen), a false-negative (prozone) reaction occurs because molecular lattices, which make up the visible precipitate, do not form.

Box 3-1 Procedure for Production of Monoclonal Antibodies

1. **Selection of Antigen**

   Monoclonal antibodies can be produced against any substance recognized as an antigen by the immune system of the animal being injected. Using a pure antigen is ideal. In fact, certain antigens, such as chemically purified drugs used for assays (e.g., digoxin), may be homogeneous. Even so, one can never guarantee that an antigenic determinant will consist of only one epitope. The fact that impure antigens can be used in monoclonal antibody production is a chief advantage over conventional methods used to produce polyclonal antibodies.

2. **Animal Immunization**

   The chief objectives in the immunization procedure are to prime the immune system of the animal to avidly recognize all antigens injected, to maximally stimulate B-lymphocyte clones, and to have the spleen cells divide at a high rate. In the production of monoclonal antibodies, the BALB/cj mouse strain is most commonly used. The antigen is injected subcutaneously or intraperitoneally, with the simultaneous injection of Freund's adjuvant. Injections are repeated at weekly intervals and a final "booster" injection is given intravenously approximately 3 days prior to harvesting the spleen cells. At the end of the injection schedule, the animal is killed and the spleen is aseptically removed.

3. **Fusion of Splenic Lymphocytes and Myeloma Cells**

   The animal spleen is placed in sterile culture medium containing antibiotics. The splenic tissue is teased to release cells and to form a slurry. This material is passed through a mesh to obtain single cells. Ficoll is added and the slurry is centrifuged to remove red blood cells. Polyethylene glycol (PEG) is added to the slurry to reduce cell-to-cell surface tension; this brings the cells into close proximity to one another, allowing their membranes to fuse. Dimethylsulfoxide (DMSO) is added to the fusion mixture to maximize cell contact even more. Finally, the cells are packed into a pellet by gently centrifuging the mixture for 5 minutes. Thus, at the end of these steps, the preparation consists of unfused myeloma cells, unfused lymphocytes and a few fused hybrid lymphocyte-myeloma cells (it should be recognized that splenic lymphocytes and myeloma cells fuse with a frequency of only about 1 per 10^5 or 10^6 cells).

4. **Selection of Hybrid Lymphocyte-Myeloma Cells**

   Unfused myeloma cells rapidly outgrow the hybrids and must be removed in some manner. The myeloma cells used for fusion are grown in the presence of 8-azoguanine, a drug that causes the cells to permanently switch off the production of hypoxanthine phosphoribosyl transferase (HRPT), an enzyme that is needed to continue growth. If these HRPT-negative cells are suspended in a medium containing hypoxanthine, aminopterin, and thymidine (HAT medium), only the hybridoma cells will grow successfully. The hybridoma cells inherit HRPT from the splenic lymphocytes with which they have fused and will survive. The unfused myeloma cells, unable to synthesize DNA because of inability to produce HRPT, will be killed by the aminopterin in the selective HAT medium. It should also be remembered that unfused splenic lymphocytes do not survive beyond a few days in culture medium; therefore, the fused hybrid lymphocyte-myeloma cells alone survive in the HAT medium.

5. **Cloning the Hybridoma Cells**

   The single hybrid cells producing the desired antibody must be isolated and grown as a clone. Two techniques can be used: 1) limiting dilution and 2) growth in an agar gel medium. In the limiting or doubling dilution technique, the suspension of hybrids (after maximum growth) is diluted and distributed into a series of sterile wells in a microtiter plate. The dilutions are so calculated that each well contains an average of only one cell that can then be replaced as a single antibody-producing clone. In the alternative method, using agarose gel supplemented with serum, amino acids, and antibiotics, the dividing hybrid cells form tiny, spherelike clusters. These spheres can be selected with a Pasteur pipette and transferred to microtube wells for further culture and ultimately for assay to determine whether the desired antibody is being produced.

6. **Screening for Desired Antibodies**

   In the fusion step of the procedure of producing monoclonal antibodies, many lymphocytes other than those producing the desired monoclonal antibodies may have fused. In fact, less than 5% of the hybrid cells out of those selected actually produce the desired specific antibodies. Thus, assays of the selected cell lines are required to determine if the desired antibody is being produced. Radioimmunoassays, enzyme-linked immunosorbent assay (ELISA), precipitin techniques, and blotting techniques can be used for this phase of the procedure.

7. **Mass Production of Monoclonal Antibodies**

   Once the desired clone of hybrid cells has been selected, the next step is the production of large quantities of monoclonal antibodies. The peritoneal cavity of mice, preferably the same strain that was used for the initial immunization step, can be used to grow the selected hybrid cell clone. First, the peritoneal cavity is injected with an organic irritant, such as pristeane, to produce a chemical peritonitis. Next, the selected hybrid cell line is injected into the peritoneal cavity. Within days, a tumor known as a hybridoma develops. This tumor produces large quantities of monoclonal antibodies that can be harvested by aspirating the ascitic fluid from the mouse's peritoneal cavity. A tumor-bearing mouse will survive for 4 to 6 weeks, during which time large quantities of antibody can be harvested. Hybridomas can also be grown in tissue cultures in which highly purified antibodies are produced without the potential for contamination from serum, nonspecific interference from ascites proteins, or cross-reactivity of histoincompatibility antibodies derived from the mouse tissues.

In contrast, postzone reactions occur when antigen is in excess and binding sites on the antibody become saturated with antigen such that the lattice formation characteristic of precipitin reactions does not occur. In cases in which high concentrations of antigen or antibody are anticipated, false-negative prozone or postzone phenomena, respectively, can be avoided by performing repeated tests on serial dilutions of the specimen. The zone of equivalence is defined as the range of reactant ratios that results in maximum precipitation of both antigens and antibodies.

All of the methods described above have been used for the detection of bacterial antigens in body fluids such as cerebrospinal fluid (CSF); however, CIE was the only method that gained acceptance in clinical practice because of the relative rapidity of the test (30–60 minutes). However, even this method has been replaced by rapid latex agglutination and coagglutination procedures (see below). Double diffusion methods are still used as an aid in the diagnosis of systemic fungal infections such as aspergillosis, blastomycosis, histoplasmosis, and coccidioidomycosis (i.e., fungal immunodiffusion testing).[57,68] In fungal immunodiffusion, purified antigens from these systemic fungal pathogens are reacted with patient and control sera containing antibodies in double diffusion tests. The development of precipitin lines of identity with the positive control sera and with the patient's serum indicates the presence of antifungal antibodies. The presence or absence of certain precipitin bands (e.g., the H and M bands seen in *Histoplasma capsulatum* infection, anti-A antigen bands in *Blastomyces dermatitidis* infection) may have diagnostic and prognostic significance for patient treatment.[57,68,69] Although highly specific, these tests suffer from inadequate sensitivity and their use has been eclipsed by newer serologic (e.g., antigen detection, radioimmunoassays, latex agglutination, enzyme immunoassays) and molecular diagnostic methods (e.g., gene amplification).[23,45,78,93,141,142]

Immunodiffusion is also the basis for the exoantigen test for identification of systemic fungal pathogens. In this method, an agar slant growing a mycelial culture of the organism to be identified is extracted with a mixture of water and merthiolate overnight. This aqueous extract is concentrated and reacted in a double diffusion test with antisera against *H. capsulatum*, *B. dermatitidis*, *C. immitis*, and *Aspergillus* species along with appropriate antigen controls. After 24 hours of incubation, the immunodiffusion plate is examined for lines of identity between the mycelial extract, the fungal antisera, and control antigens for each organism.[70] Although this method is still used for identification of systemic fungal pathogens, the availability of nucleic-acid probes for these agents offers certain advantages, including the use of younger, less mature colonies, clear-cut results, rapid turnaround time, and specific identification.[104,105,130]

Complement Fixation and Hemagglutination Inhibition

Over the past three decades, serologic methods for the diagnosis of infectious diseases have changed significantly. Older methods include **complement fixation** (**CF**) and **hemagglutination inhibition** (**HAI**).[129,135] CF and HAI can be used to identify either viral antigens (i.e., usually for identification of viruses in tissue cultures) or to detect antibodies in patient serum and certain other specimen types (e.g., CSF).

The principal of the CF test is quite straightforward (Fig. 3-2). In order to detect antibodies in patient serum, the serum specimen is first heated at 56°C for 30 minutes to inactivate endogenous complement, and an aliquot is placed in the well of a microtiter plate. A titered amount of complement and antigen (specific for the antibody to be detected) are added to the microwell, mixed, and incubated overnight. If antibody in the patient serum ''recognizes'' the antigen, the two molecules combine, and complement becomes ''fixed' to this antigen-antibody complex. If antibody against that antigen is not present, no immune complexes form and complement remains free or ''unfixed.'' In the next step, red blood cells (RBCs; generally from sheep) that are ''sensitized'' with anti-RBC antibodies are added to the microtiter well. If the complement was bound to immune complexes during the first step, it is not available to bind to the antibody-coated erythrocytes, so the sensitized RBCs are not lysed and settle to the bottom of the well as a ''button.'' On the other hand, if immune complexes were not formed during the first step, complement is free to bind to the antibody-coated RBCs, resulting in lysis of the erythrocytes. Lysis of the cells produces a diffuse reddish discoloration of the reactants within the microtiter well. Although CF is still of value in the diagnosis of certain infections (influenza and parainfluenza virus infections, *C. immitis* meningitis), the procedure has been largely supplanted by enzyme immunoassays and indirect fluorescent antibody procedures for antibody detection.[69,143,151] CF may also be used to identify viruses grown in culture; however, direct and indirect fluorescent antibody immunoassays are more rapid and have essentially replaced the CF test for this purpose. The CF procedure is presented in Chart 3-1.

Erythrocytes have also been used as antigen carriers for detection of antiviral antibodies. Certain viruses (e.g., rubella, influenza, and parainfluenza viruses, respiratory syncytial virus, measles, mumps) have surface antigens that are hemagglutinins; that is, they bind to RBCs and form cross-linkages that result in macroscopic agglutination. Antibodies directed against the specific virus can inhibit macroscopic agglutination of erythrocytes ''sensitized'' with viral antigens. This reaction is the basis of the HAI assay (Fig. 3-3).[129] Patients with infections caused by hemagglutinating viruses can be diagnosed retrospectively by detecting a four-fold or greater rise in the titer of antibodies that inhibit the ability of the virus to agglutinate erythrocytes. Although antibody detection for rubella and other viral agents is now done by latex agglutination, enzyme immunoassay, or indirect immunofluorescence in most hospital settings, HAI is still performed in some public health and reference laboratories for surveillance and diagnosis (e.g., serology for *Flaviviridae*, *Bunyaviridae*, alphaviruses).[124] The HAI procedure is presented in Chart 3-2.

Agglutination Reactions

Agglutination reactions can be defined as the specific immunochemical aggregation of particles (erythrocytes, latex particles, staphylococcal cells) coated with antigen or antibody that can be used to detect either soluble antibodies

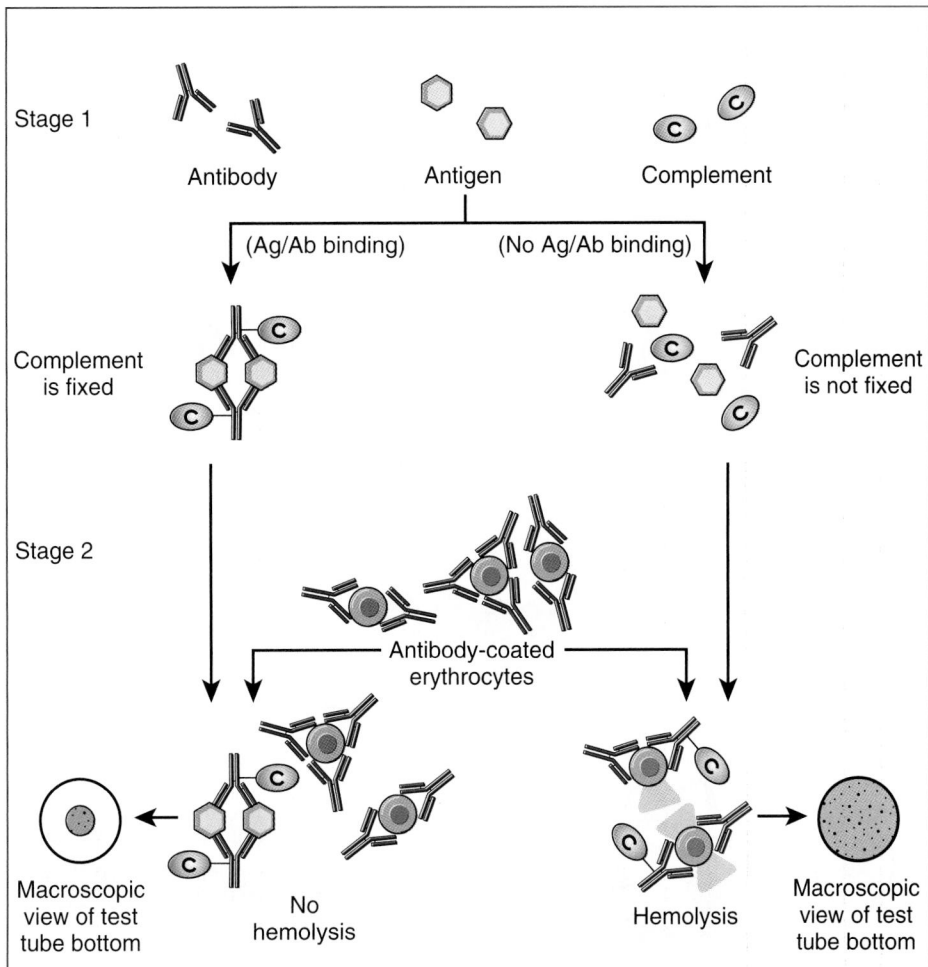

Figure 3-2 Complement fixation testing. Antigen, antibody, and complement are mixed in stage one. If the antigen and antibody bind, complement is fixed and will be unable to act on antibody-coated erythrocytes added in stage two. The final reaction appears as an absence of hemolysis. If the antigen and antibody do not bind in stage one, complement is not fixed and remains free to act on the antibody-coated erythrocytes added in stage two. The final result appears as hemolysis of the erythrocytes. Unhemolyzed cells settle into a button in the center of the bottom of the test tube, whereas hemolyzed cells produce a reddish discoloration of fluid with very few if any cells settled in the center of the bottom of the tube. Ag/Ab, antigen-antibody. Redrawn from Leland DS. Clinical Virology. Philadelphia: Saunders, 1996.

or antigens, respectively. Antigens or antibodies are attached to these particles either by intramolecular electrical forces or by covalent bonds. Clumping of the carrier particles occurs as an indicator of antigen-antibody interactions occurring on the surface of the carriers. Initially, erythrocytes were used as carriers. These erythrocytes had to be treated with tannic acid or other agents to stabilize the cell membrane and then formalinized to increase the nonspecific absorption of peptides, proteins, and polysaccharides. For example, in the passive hemagglutination (PHA) test for detection of rubella antibodies, the erythrocytes are treated with formaldehyde-pyruvate aldehyde so that rubella virus antigen can be adsorbed onto the membrane surfaces. For some proteins, chemical coupling agents were used to covalently link the proteins to the red cells; these agents worked for some pro-

teins but not for others. In 1955, uniformly sized (i.e., 0.81 nm diameter) polystyrene latex beads were "discovered" to be the ideal carrier for antibody molecules, since the hydrophobic surfaces of the beads specifically and irreversibly bind to the Fc region of IgG molecules. Antigens such as complex polysaccharides and proteins could also be linked to latex beads via sulfate groups that are present on the surface of the beads as a result of the manufacturing process. At present, latex beads are the most commonly used carriers in agglutination assays. Latex agglutination tests are usually performed on slides or plastic-coated cardboard cards. Latex beads coated with specific antibodies are the basis for cryptococcal antigen latex agglutination tests (CALAS, Meridian Diagnostics, Cincinnati, OH; Crypto LA International Biological Labs, Cranbury, NJ; Pastorex Cryptococcus, Sanofi-

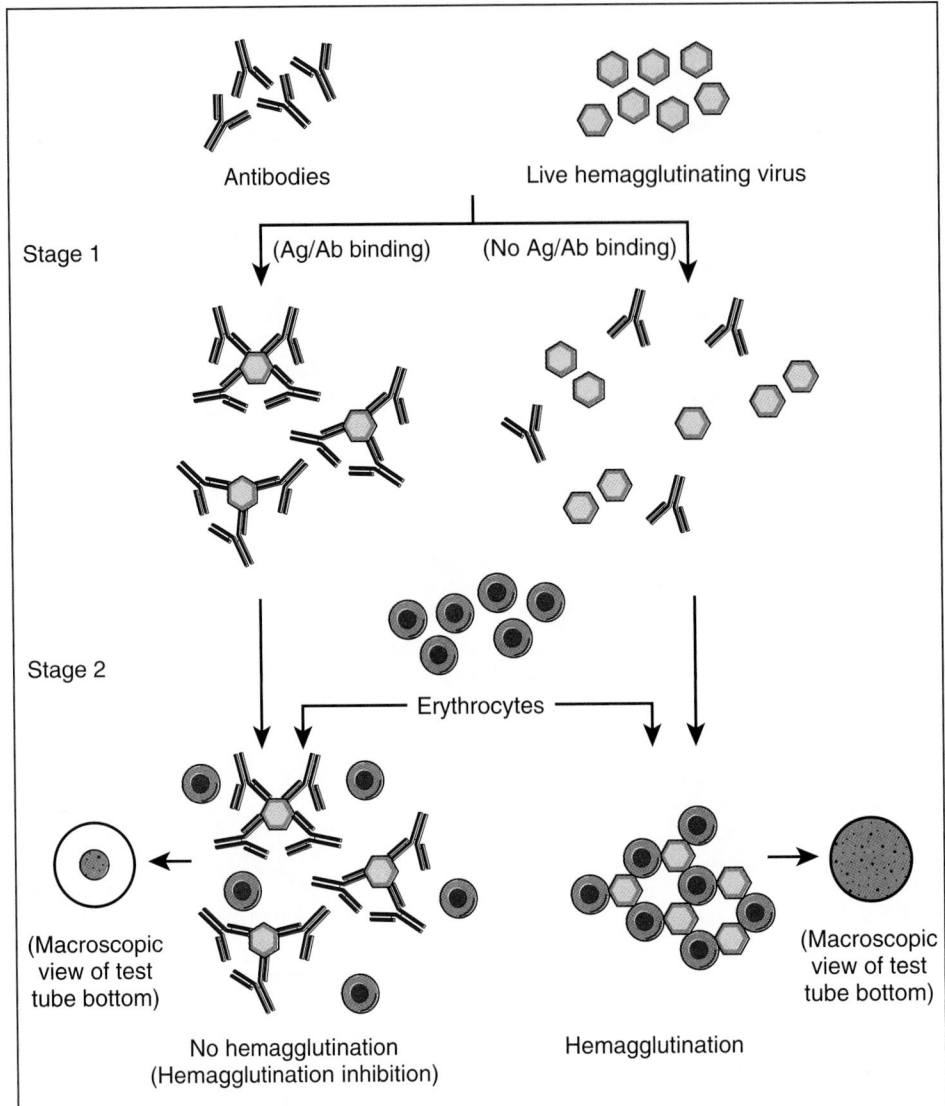

Figure 3-3 Hemagglutination inhibition testing is performed in two stages. In stage one, hemagglutinating viruses and antibodies are mixed In stage two, erythrocytes are added. If the antibodies bind to the virus in stage one, the virus is inhibited and fails to hemagglutinate the erythrocytes. If the antibodies do not bind to the virus in stage one, the virus remains active and hemagglutinates the erythrocytes in stage two. Hemagglutination appears as a layer or "shield" of tiny aggregates in the bottom of the tube. Unagglutinated cells settle into a button in the center of the bottom of the tube. Ag/Ab, antigen-antibody. Redrawn from Leland DS. Clinical Virology. Philadelphia: Saunders, 1996.

Diagnostics Pasteur, Marnes-la-Coquette, France), particle agglutination assays for direct detection of group A streptococci in throat swab specimens, commercial products for serologic grouping of β-hemolytic streptococci (e.g., Streptex, Abbott-Murex, Abbott Park, IL), and kits used for detecting bacterial capsular antigens in CSF and serum.[22,25,26,44,62,111,123] Latex particles also can be conjugated to antigens, thereby allowing latex agglutination to be used for the qualitative detection of antibodies. Latex agglutination kits are commercially available for the detection of antibodies to a variety of agents, including rubella virus, cytomegalovirus, and varicella-zoster virus.[6,41,50,61,94,96,110,127,128] These tests

are convenient, rapid, easy to perform, detect both IgG and IgM antibodies, and are fairly comparable in sensitivity and specificity to other methods of antibody detection. Latex agglutination tests are used mostly for determining immune status, although they may perform less well with sera having titers near those that are generally regarded as separating "immune" from "nonimmune."[124,127]

Staphylococci may also be used as carrier agents. Strains of *Staphylococcus aureus* (for example, ATCC 12498) have a high content of protein A in their cell wall. This protein is able to specifically bind the Fc region of IgG, leaving the Fab regions available for binding of antigen.[43] Because of the nature of protein A and its specific interaction with IgG molecules as a functional carrier, staphylococcal coagglutination is used primarily for antigen detection and is the method used in some commercial kits for serologic grouping of β-hemolytic streptococci.[55] Following extraction of antigen from the organisms by chemical or physical means, the antibody-coated staphylococci are mixed with the extract. Visible agglutination of the staphylococcal cells is a positive test.[55] Commercial coagglutination tests are also available for culture confirmation of *Neisseria gonorrhoeae* (Phadebact GC Monoclonal Antibody test, Karo Bio Diagnostics AB, Huddinge, Sweden; Gonogen I, New Horizons Diagnostics, Columbia, MD).[64]

Agglutination reactions are more sensitive than precipitin reactions because of the direct nature of the antigen-carrier-antibody interaction. The sensitivity and the ability of these reactions to occur at high dilutions allows semiquantitative measurements of antigens or antibodies to be made. In the case of antibodies, semiquantitative results can be derived by determining the highest dilution of serum that produces a visible agglutination reaction. Changes in agglutination titers in acute and convalescent specimens may provide retrospective serologic diagnoses in a manner similar to CF or HAI methods.[94,96] For semiquantitative antigen concentration assays, an end-point titer in a patient specimen (e.g., CSF) may be compared with end-point agglutination titers obtained with a serially diluted preparation of a known concentration of antigen. Titers in sequential specimens can directly influence patient care and clinical management. For example, decreasing CSF titers of capsular polysaccharide antigen is directly related to therapeutic responses in *Cryptococcus neoformans* meningitis.[32] Conversely, rising or persistently elevated antigen titers are poor prognostic signs that indicate persistent, recurring, or relapsing infection.

Another type of agglutination reaction is the basis of a technique called **immune electron microscopy (IEM)**. This technique is used for visual detection of viral agents that are noncultivable, such as hepatitis A and some of the newer agents of hepatitis in stool filtrates.[40,60] Specific antiviral antibodies are used to cause aggregation of the viral particles; these aggregates are detected by the electron microscope more easily than individual, dispersed virions. The immunospecific aggregation of the viral particles increases electron microscopic detection of viral agents by 100- to 1,000-fold, thereby allowing detection of as few as 10^5 to 10^6 particles/mL of stool filtrate.

Solid-Phase Immunoassay Methods
Enzyme Immunoassays for Antibody Detection

''Solid-phase immunoassay'' refers to the binding of either antigen or antibody to a variety of solid materials, such as polystyrene microtube wells or plastic beads. For example, solid-phase immunoassays designed for the detection of antibody in an unknown sample have antigen bound to the solid phase (Fig. 3-4). The initial reaction occurs when the specimen to be tested is incubated for a prescribed time in contact with the solid phase. Specific antibody binds to the immobilized antigen. After the reaction mixture is washed to remove any extraneous materials, an antiglobulin conjugated

with a ''tag'' is added and incubated in the reaction vessel. In **radioimmunoassay (RIA)** procedures, the tag is a radioactive isotope (e.g., ^{32}P or ^{125}I); in **enzyme immunoassay (EIA)** methods, the tag is an enzyme. In commercially available EIA systems for detecting human antibodies, the conjugate is frequently alkaline phosphatase—or horseradish peroxidase—labeled antihuman immunoglobulin raised in goats. If the initial antigen-antibody reaction has occurred, the antiglobulin (with its radioactive or enzyme tag) binds to the antibody. The final step in these assays is the detection of radioactive or enzymatic activity. This is done with a scintillation counter, which detects either β or γ emissions, or by the addition of an enzyme substrate that generally yields a colored end product that is detected visually or with a spectrophotometer. A positive reaction indicates that antibody was present in the original sample, and the intensity of the reaction is proportional to the concentration of antibody in the specimen. A diagrammatic representation of an EIA for detection of rubella antibodies is shown in Fig. 3-4.

The chemistry of antibody conjugates used in EIA techniques is not limited to antigen-antibody interactions, as exemplified by the use of avidin, streptavidin, and biotin. Avidin and streptavidin are glycoproteins purified from egg white and *Streptomyces avidinii*, respectively. Biotin is a component of the B_2 vitamin complex. Avidin molecules are able to stoichiometrically bind biotin residues in much the same way as an antibody-antigen interaction. In EIA formats, goat antihuman globulin attached to biotin molecules can be used as the conjugate to detect human antibodies that have bound to an antigen fixed to the solid phase. After a wash step, enzyme-labeled avidin (or streptavidin) is added. After incubation and washing, addition of the enzyme substrate yields a colored end product. Alternatively, biotinylated antiglobulin may be detected by added unlabeled avidin; after a wash step, biotinylated enzyme is added. The biotinylated enzyme binds to the avidin; after washing, addition of the enzyme substrate yields a colored end product.

Most RIAs use a competitive-type assay system. In the quantitative test for antibodies, the solid-phase system is first standardized using an unlabeled bound antigen and a standard concentration of antibody that is labeled with a radioactive tag. The unknown sample, containing the (unlabeled) antibody to be detected, is added to the assay system. The amount of labeled antibody displaced from the antigen is proportional to the amount of unlabeled antibody present in the test sample. Antibody concentrations in the unknown samples are determined by comparison on a standard curve derived by determining the degree of inhibition of binding of labeled antibody mixed with dilutions of quantified, unlabeled antibodies. The approach is similar when antigens are being detected by this method, except that a labeled antigen is used to quantitate free antigen in the specimen. RIA has achieved wide use in clinical chemistry, clinical endocrinology, and toxicology, but has not found significant routine applications in clinical microbiology. Although RIA has exceptional sensitivity and specificity, radioactive waste disposal and the inherent instability of certain radionuclides has limited the expansion of RIA techniques in modern clinical pathology service laboratories. Commercially available EIA test kits for the detection of antibodies in serum have become

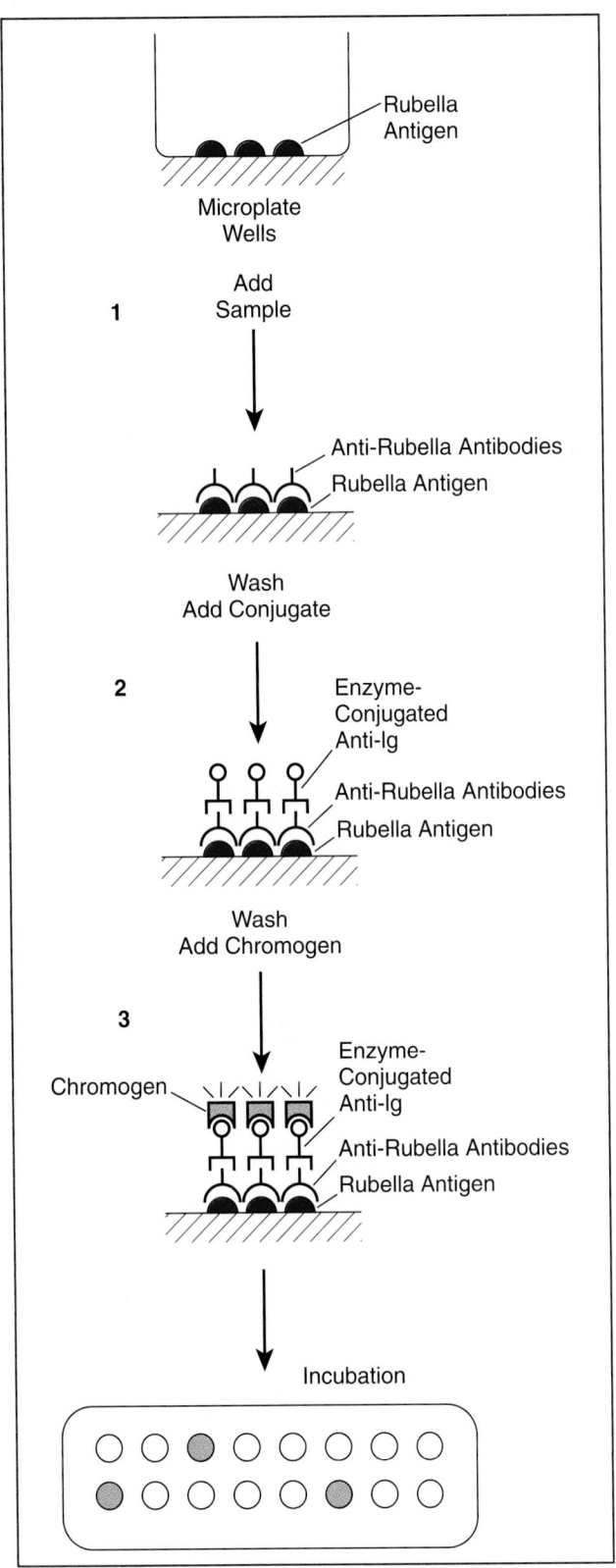

Microplate
Wells

Rubella
Antigen

1 Add
Sample

Anti-Rubella Antibodies
Rubella Antigen

Wash
Add Conjugate

2 Enzyme-
Conjugated
Anti-Ig

Anti-Rubella Antibodies
Rubella Antigen

Wash
Add Chromogen

3 Enzyme-
Conjugated
Anti-Ig

Chromogen

Anti-Rubella Antibodies
Rubella Antigen

Incubation

Figure 3-4 Principles of enzyme immunoassay (EIA). This figure shows the EIA procedure for the detection of antibodies against rubella virus. Purified rubella antigens are absorbed onto microplate wells. In step 1, serum is added and incubated. Antirubella antibodies, if present, bind to the antigen. Following a wash step, antihuman immunoglobulin that is conjugated with

more widely available over the past 10 years, and they have supplanted, in many cases, the more time-consuming and laborious procedures like CF and HIA for viral serology.[5,12, 30,41,81,84,94,96,110] EIA methods are the recommended formats for the newer serologic tests, such as the screening tests for detection of antibodies to HIV-1 and HIV-2.[49]

Serologic procedures for detection of antibody that have EIA technology as their basis have also been modified to increase their utility as specific diagnostic or confirmatory test methods. The Western immunoblot procedure for HIV-1 antibodies is an example of such a modification (Fig. 3-5).[49,117] In the original HIV-1 Western immunoblot procedure, HIV-1 grown in tissue culture is partially purified away from the cell culture and solubilized by detergent treatment. Using polyacrylamide gel electrophoresis, the HIV-1 proteins are fractionated on the basis of molecular weight, with the low-molecular-weight proteins migrating farther than the high-molecular-weight proteins and glycoproteins. A sheet of nitrocellulose paper is placed on the gel and the HIV-1 proteins are electrophoretically "transblotted" or transferred onto the nitrocellulose sheet. This sheet is then cut into strips for use as the "solid phase" in the assay. Serum that is repeatedly reactive in the HIV-1 EIA screening test is diluted and incubated with the nitrocellulose strip. If present, HIV-1 antibodies will bind to specific viral antigens on the strip. After washing, the strips are incubated with goat anti-human antibodies that are conjugated with horseradish peroxidase or alkaline phosphatase. After another wash step, enzyme substrate is added to the strip. At this time, colored bands will appear on the strip in areas where an initial antibody-antigen reaction has occurred. The position of these bands and comparison of the patterns with positive control samples enables reactivity of a given sample with specific viral antigens to be assessed and an interpretation to be made.[49]

Immunoblot techniques can also be used to assess the specificities of antibodies against other infectious agents. For example, EIAs that are used to detect antibodies against herpes simplex viruses (HSVs) are not able to differentiate HSV-1- or HSV-2-specific antibodies (e.g., Vidas, BioMérieux-Vitek, Hazelwood, MO; Bio Whittaker, Walkersville, MD).[3] Immunoblot methods can be used to differentiate prior infection with HSV type 1 or 2 by analyzing the reactions of patient serum with antigen immunoblots prepared from HSV-1 or HSV-2 and looking for positive reactions with those antigens that are virus-specific.[4] Immunoblot methods have also been used to detect rubella virus–specific antibodies in cases of suspected congenital rubella.[152] Immunoblot technology has also been evaluated as a test format for the diagnosis of syphilis.[16] Using this assay, antibodies directed against immunodeterminant *Treponema pallidum* antigens with molecular weights of 15.5, 17, 44.5, and 47 kDa are diagnostic of acquired syphilis when an anti-IgG conjugate is used.[100] When developed with an anti-IgM con-

an enzyme is added (step 2). After a second wash step, a chromogenic enzyme substrate is added. Absorbances for individual wells are read spectrophotometrically, and test results are interpreted by comparison, with positive and negative controls performed in the same test.

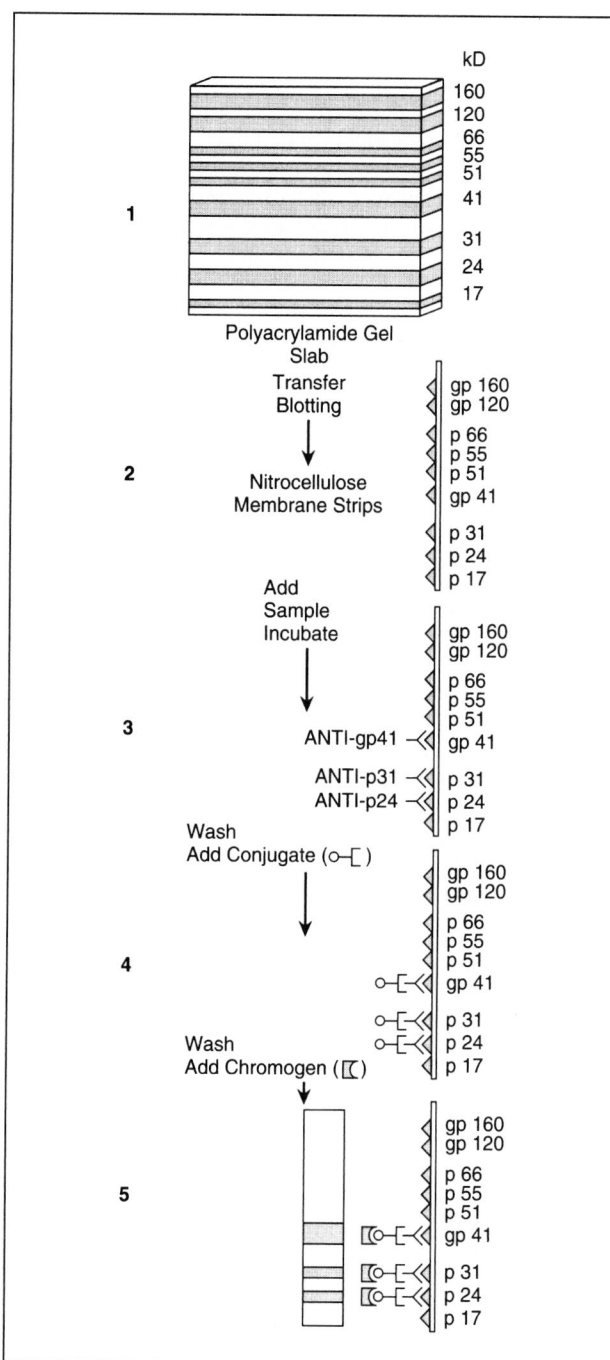

jugate, the immunoblot procedure has been shown to be a sensitive and specific assay for the diagnosis of congenital syphilis.[86] Owing to the relative insensitivity of EIA and immunofluorescence techniques, Western immunoblot procedures have also emerged as the most sensitive and specific method for serodiagnosis of Lyme disease caused by *Borrelia burgdorferi*, and diagnostic criteria based on immunoblot banding patterns have been established.[38,66,91]

Because of the gravity of HIV-1 disease and the need to make a specific diagnosis, both EIA and immunoblot test systems for the detection of HIV-1 antibodies have undergone several modifications since their introduction in 1984.[117] Initially, test kit manufacturers used lysates prepared from HIV-1-infected cultured T-lymphocyte cell lines as the source for antigens in both the first-generation EIA and immunoblot procedures. Biologic false-positive reactions were seen, caused by the reactivity of antibodies directed against HLA (human leukocyte antigen) proteins that are expressed by the lymphoid cell lines used to grow the virus.[10,77] Subsequently, recombinant antigens were obtained by cloning viral genes into bacteria or yeast expression systems using plasmid vectors. Use of these antigens resulted in the development of tests (second-generation EIAs) with even greater specificity than the first-generation assays. In these assays, cross-reactions with contaminating bacterial or yeast antigens, however, may be a cause of false-positive reactions. Purification and amino acid sequencing of retroviral antigens then led to the use of synthetic peptides as antigens in the EIA procedure (third-generation assays). These antigens can be produced in large quantities and show little lot-to-lot variability. Because of their purity, indeterminate or atypical reactions due to contaminating components in lysate- and recombinant-based tests are minimized. However, it was shown that tests using synthetic envelope antigens may not detect anti-HIV-1 antibodies in patients infected with the highly divergent viral strains, such as HIV-1 group O.[28,87,118] While the first- and second-generation assays detected primarily IgG, the third-generation assays detect all classes of antibody (i.e., IgG, IgM, and IgA) to HIV-1 present in serum or saliva. Third-generation HIV-1 EIAs also differ slightly from earlier assays in their methodology; synthetic viral antigens fixed to the solid phase initially "capture" anti-HIV-1 antibodies, and the bound antibodies are detected by adding enzyme-labeled HIV-1 antigen instead of an enzyme-labeled antiglobulin.[49] Because of their high specificity, synthetic antigen-based assays are able to differentiate anti-HIV-1 and anti-HIV-2 antibodies easily.

The availability of recombinant and synthetic antigens that produce sensitive and specific reactions has also led to the development of new screening and supplemental tests for HIV-1/HIV-2 antibodies. Rapid (10–15 minutes) "dot blot" EIAs have been developed using synthetic and recombinant antigens. In these assays, viral antigens are bound to

Figure 3-5 Western blot technique for detection of anti-HIV-1 antibodies. In step 1, virus that is grown in tissue culture is solubilized, partially purified, and subjected to electrophoresis in a polyacrylamide slab gel. This separates the viral proteins and glycoproteins by their molecular weights. In step 2, the antigens in the gel are electrophoretically "transblotted" onto a nitrocellulose sheet, which is then cut into strips. The strips are then incubated (step 3) with the test sample (serum). After washing away unbound material, an enzyme-labeled conjugate is added (step 4). This material binds to antibodies from the serum sample that have bound to the strip. After another wash step, the enzyme's chromogen substrate is added, and colored bands appear on the strip at the sites of initial antibody reactivity. In this diagram, reactivity is shown with gp41, p24, and p31,

confirming that the serum sample contains anti-HIV-1 antibodies. Reprinted, with permission, from Sandler SG. Xxxxx. In: DeVita VI Jr, Hellman S, Rosenberg SA, eds. AIDS Etiology, Diagnosis, Treatment, and Prevention. 2nd Ed. Philadelphia: Lippincott, 1988:128.

a membrane in a reaction cartridge. If antibodies are present in the test serum, they bind to the antigens on the membrane. Following a wash step, an antihuman IgG/IgM enzyme conjugate is added to the cartridge. If antibodies were bound in the previous step, the conjugate binds to the antigen-antibody complex. Unbound conjugate is removed by a wash step, and addition of enzyme substrate results in a color reaction directly on the membrane. Most of these assays have positive and negative control spots on the membrane to indicate whether the test was performed correctly and to establish the validity of the test. One of these assays, the SUDS test (Abbott-Murex), has been licensed by the FDA as a diagnostic test for HIV-1 antibodies. Other dot blot immunoassays have been developed that also detect antibodies to both HIV-1 and HIV-2.[27] Application of purified synthetic antigens to nitrocellulose in banded patterns on plastic support strips has also led to the development of second- and third-generation supplemental "Western immunoblot–like" assays that can be used in place of the viral lysate–based immunoblot procedure. These tests have been labeled line immunoassays (LIAs).[74,108] EIA methods using recombinant or synthetic antigens are also revolutionizing the traditional laboratory approach to the diagnosis of other infections, such as Epstein-Barr virus infection and syphilis.[59,149]

Enzyme Immunoassay Antibody Capture Methods for IgM Detection

EIA methods for antibodies detect primarily IgG. However, specific IgM detection methods can be used to differentiate recent from past infections because only IgM is present early in the course of most infections. Methods specific for IgM detection obviate the need for testing of acute and convalescent specimens for specific IgG. In congenital infections, detection of specific IgM in fetal/neonatal blood indicates active infection rather than transplacental antibodies. Initially, EIA formats for IgM detection used an enzyme-labeled anti-IgM antibody as the conjugate. However, if IgG and IgM are present in the same specimen, the smaller, more numerous IgG molecules effectively compete for binding sites on the antigen fixed to the solid phase, resulting in no binding of the anti-IgM conjugate and a false-negative IgM test result. In addition, rheumatoid factor in the specimen may interfere with the assay as well. Rheumatoid factors are antibodies primarily of the IgM class that are directed against IgGs of any specificity. If serum contains both IgG and rheumatoid factor, the smaller, specific IgG molecules bind to the antigen on the solid phase, and the rheumatoid factors, in turn, bind to the IgG. Addition of a labeled anti-IgM conjugate results in its binding to the rheumatoid factor, with the subsequent generation of a false-positive result on addition of the enzyme substrate.

In order to detect IgM in patient sera, several methods have been developed to separate IgM from IgG. Ion exchange column chromatography and gel filtration separate immunoglobulin classes based on molecular size and charge. Using buffers of varying ionic strength, IgM can be eluted from these columns and separated from IgG. Sucrose gradient density centrifugation also separates the molecules based on size, with IgM molecules traversing further in the sucrose gradient than the lighter, smaller IgG molecules.

Serum specimens may also be treated with anti-IgG antibodies, resulting in binding of IgG into immune complexes and effectively preventing these antibodies from reacting in IgM assays. Staphylococcal protein A, either mixed directly with the serum specimen or incorporated into a gel filtration column, may also be used to "bind up" IgG molecules in patient specimens. However, these separation methods pose other technical problems. None of the methods are totally effective in separating IgM from IgG, so IgG interference with IgM detection may still be a problem even after specimen pretreatment. In addition, all of these techniques result in dilution of the serum specimen. Since IgM may be present in very low levels, specimen dilution may result in false-negative IgM test results even when agent-specific IgM is actually present. Accurate and reliable laboratory testing for IgM is of considerable importance for the diagnosis of congenital rubella syndrome since the risk of serious damage to the fetus is substantial. Termination of pregnancy is the recommended approach if congenital rubella syndrome is diagnosed antepartum.

The IgM detection method of choice is an "antibody capture" method (see Fig. 3-6). In this modification, IgG directed against IgM is bound to the solid phase. Incubation of the specimen results in binding of all IgM in the specimen aliquot to the immobilized IgG. After a wash step, the specific antigen is added to the microtiter well and becomes bound to IgM antibody molecules having that particular antigenic specificity. Subsequent addition of an enzyme-labeled IgG antibody conjugate directed against another epitope of the antigen results in indirect, enzymatic labeling of the antigen-specific IgM, yielding a colored end product after the addition of enzyme substrate. Captured rheumatoid factor or IgM antibodies of other antigenic specificities do not bind the conjugate to produce a colored end product.

Enzyme Immunoassays for Antigen Detection

EIA formats may also be modified for the detection of antigens rather than antibodies. In this case, a "capture" antibody is fixed to the solid phase (Fig. 3-7). Incubation with a specimen containing the antigen results in binding of the antigen to the antibody. After a wash step, incubation with an enzyme-labeled (or biotinylated) antibodies against a second epitope of the antigen results in binding of that antibody. After washing, enzyme substrate (or enzyme conjugated to avidin) is added. Addition of the enzyme substrate yields a colored end product. Antigen-detection EIA methods have been used to detect bacterial antigens of several agents in diverse specimen types, including capsular antigens of *S. pneumoniae*, *H. influenzae* type b, and *N. meningitidis* in CSF, *Legionella* and *S. pneumoniae* antigens in urine, Shiga-like-toxins produced by enterohemorrhagic *E. coli*, and *Clostridium difficile* toxins in stool specimens, and chlamydial antigens in endocervical specimens.[7,33,89,90,97,119,122,123,148] In virology, EIA methods have been developed for the direct detection of rotavirus in stool filtrates, respiratory syncytial virus in lower respiratory tract specimens, and detection of the p24 antigen in serum during acute primary HIV infection.[39,42,54,58,72,80,120,134,137,138] The availability of EIAs for the detection of *Entamoeba histolytica/dispar*, *Giardia lamblia*, and *Cryptosporidium parvum* antigens di-

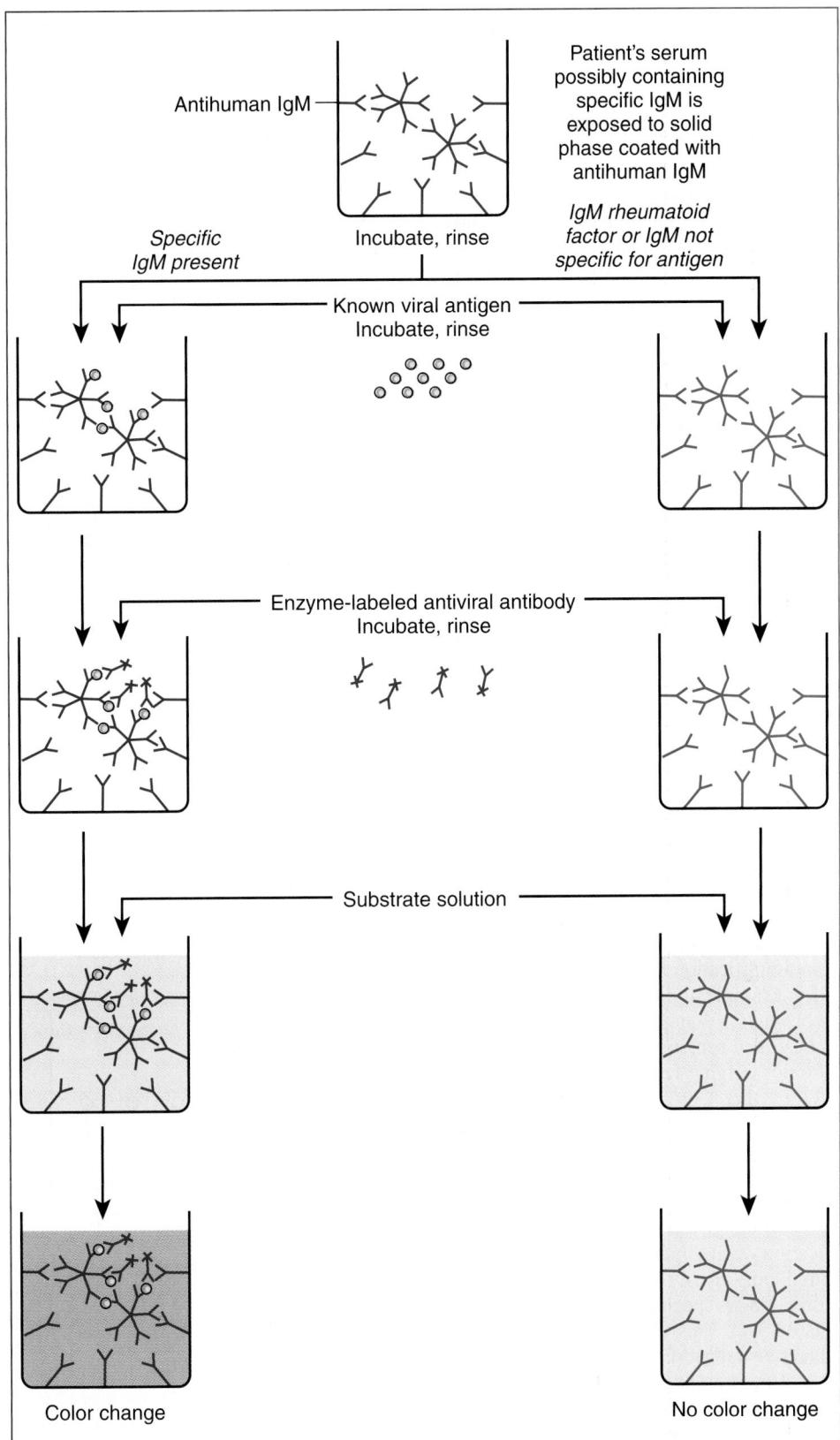

Figure 3-6 IgM capture enzyme immunoassay. Patient's serum possibly containing IgM is exposed to antihuman IgM attached to a solid phase. Any IgM in the serum is "captured" or bound by the antihuman IgM. Subsequent steps in the assay (addition of known viral antigen, enzyme-labeled antiviral antibodies, and substrate) are performed to determine the specificity of the captured IgM. Captured IgM of the proper specificity will produce a final result of color change. Captured IgM of other specificity, including rheumatoid factor, will not produce an end result of color change. Redrawn from Leland DS. Clinical Virology. Philadelphia: Saunders, 1996.

rectly in stool specimens has brought EIA technology into a diagnostic area that has seen relatively little innovation since the introduction of specimen preservation and staining techniques.[1,11,47,71,102,153] In mycology, the *Histoplasma* antigen test and cryptococcal antigen tests are currently the only antigen-detection tests that are routinely available.[44,141,142] The Premier cryptococcal antigen EIA (Meridian Diagnostics, Cincinnati, OH) uses a polyclonal capture immunoglobulin and a monoclonal detection antibody and can be performed on both CSF and serum specimens with no pretreatment steps.[44] A diagram of a typical antigen capture assay for detection of *Chlamydia trachomatis* antigen is presented in Fig. 3-7.

Another significant modification of antigen detection using EIA methods is the development of membrane EIAs for antigen detection. These assays use a nitrocellulose membrane to absorb the antigen from the clinical specimen. Sequential addition of conjugate and substrate results in the subsequent appearance of a colored reaction product directly on the membrane. One advantage of these assays is the presence of internal positive controls on the membrane along with the test reaction. These controls determine if the test was performed correctly, and expected control results must be observed on the membrane for the test to be considered valid. At present, membrane EIA tests are available for direct detection of group A streptococci in throat swab specimens, respiratory syncytial virus (RSV) and influenza in lower respiratory tract secretions, rotavirus in stool specimens, and *C. trachomatis* in endocervical specimens. Although these tests provide a rapid result, several studies have indicated that they are 15–20% less sensitive and have reduced specificities compared with antigen-detection microtiter EIAs, immunofluorescence assays, molecular detection methods (e.g., direct probe or amplification methods) or culture.[20,37,82,114,116,133,134,139] For example, the Clearview rapid EIA for detection of *C. trachomatis* (Wampole Laboratories, Cranbury, NJ) has demonstrated sensitivities ranging from 62% to 95% and specificities ranging from 86.9% to 99% compared with cell culture, direct probe assay, or polymerase chain reaction.[2,9,75,83,125,131] The lower sensitivities of this assay indicate that from 5% to 38% of chlamydial infections will not be detected, while the low specificities suggest that this test may not be useful for routine diagnosis of chlamydial infections, particularly in low-prevalence populations.[122]

Another modification of EIA methods for antigen detection is the optical immunoassay (OIA) for detection of group A streptococci in throat swab specimens. (Biostar, Boulder, CO) (see Color Plate 13-1). This assay is performed on a slide that allows direct visualization of a physical change in the thickness of thin films resulting from binding reactions between the capture antibody on the slide and the antigen from the specimen. After extraction of the antigen from the swab, an enzyme-labeled rabbit anti–group A streptococcal antibody is added to the extract. This mixture is placed on the slide to allow the antigen-antibody complex to bind to anti–group A streptococcal antibodies on the slide. After a 2-minute incubation, enzyme substrate is added. After washing, the reaction is read by examining the hue of light reflected from the slide surface. Presence of streptococcal antigen in the specimen is determined by the presence of a purple spot, while absence of antigen is indicated by the retention

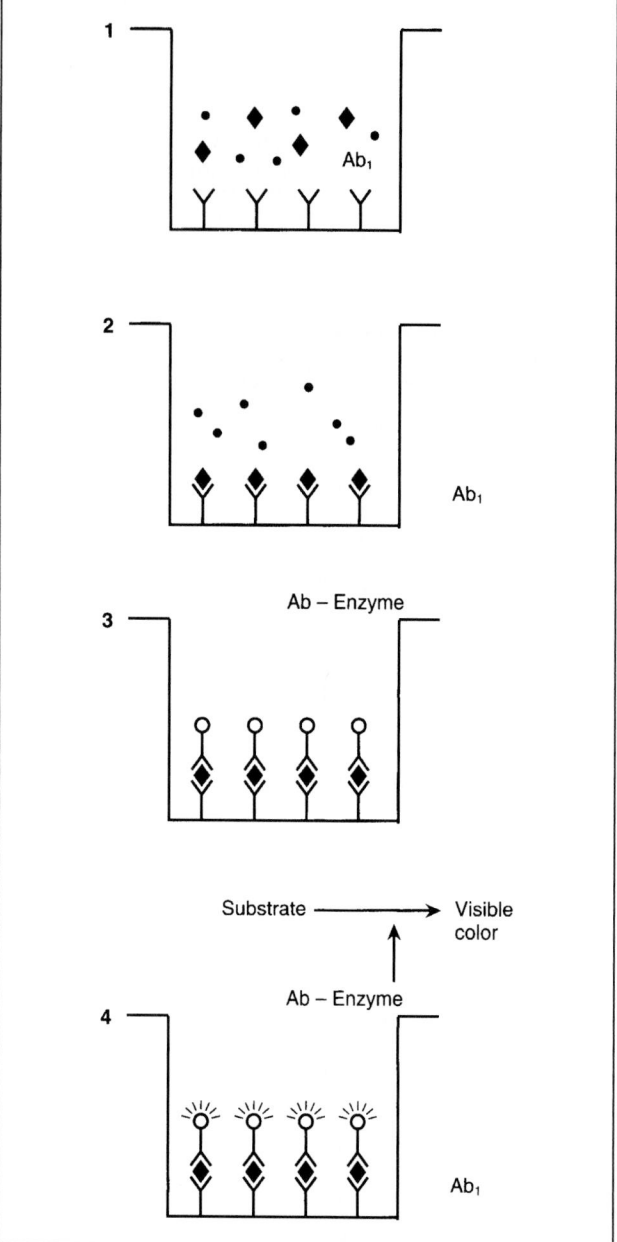

Figure 3-7 Enzyme immunoassay antigen capture technique for *Chlamydia trachomatis*. In this technique, antibody directed against the antigen to be detected is bound to the solid phase. Endocervical swab specimen washings are added to the well (step 1). Chlamydiae present in the urogenital sample are "captured" by the solid-phase antibody. After a wash step, antichlamydia antibody that is conjugated to an enzyme is added (step 2) and reacts with the solid-phase antibody-bound antigen. After another wash step, enzyme substrate is added (step 3), and a visible color is detected.

of a gold color on the reaction slide. The sensitivities and specificities of the Strep A OIA test have ranged from 81.0% to 98.9% and 95.0% to 98.6%, respectively.[24,29,56,114] Since the OIA for group A streptococci was released, OIAs for detection of group B streptococci and *C. trachomatis* have also been marketed. An evaluation of the OIA for *C. tra-chomatis* conducted by Pate et al. reported a sensitivity and specificity of 73.8% and 100%, respectively, when compared with PCR.[106] For detection of group B streptococci in vaginal specimens, none of the rapid tests (i.e., OIA, other EIAs, or latex agglutination) have demonstrated sufficient sensitivity for detecting low levels of colonization when compared with the broth method recommended by the CDC.[17,18,52,53,147] Consequently, none of these methods is recommended for screening of pregnant women for group B streptococcal colonization.

Immunofluorescence Techniques

Immunofluorescence provides an alternative to EIA as a means for detecting and localizing antigens in making the diagnosis of bacterial, fungal, parasitic, and viral diseases. This technique may also be used to detect antibodies for retrospective diagnosis of infectious diseases. Fluorescence is defined as the radiation of energy when light of a shorter wavelength (the ''excitation'' wavelength) incites the electrons of a molecule to a higher-energy state for a very short time. As the electrons return to the preexcitation or ground state, the energy is released as light of a longer wavelength. In fluorescence immunoassays, specific antibody is conjugated to a compound capable of photoexcitation and subsequent fluorescence (usually fluorescein isothiocyanate [FITC] or rhodamine derivatives), resulting in a sensitive tracer with unaltered immunologic reactivity. The conjugated antiserum is added to cells or tissues on a slide and becomes fixed to antigens, forming a stable immune complex. Nonreacting materials are removed by washing, and the preparation is then dried and observed with a fluorescence microscope equipped with an appropriate light source and barrier filters. Antigens bound specifically to fluorescent antibody can be detected as bright apple-green or orange-yellow objects against a dark background, depending on the fluorochrome being used. Immunofluorescence techniques may be direct or indirect. Direct immunofluorescence tests are usually used for antigen detection, while the indirect method can be used for both antigen and antibody detection (i.e., serology).

Immunofluorescence Techniques for Antigen Detection

Direct immunofluorescence techniques (also called **direct fluorescent antibody [DFA]**) techniques) (Fig. 3-8) involve application of the labeled conjugate to the material being examined, followed by a 15- to 30-minute period of incubation in a humid environment at 35 to 37°C to allow the antigen-antibody reaction to occur. After a wash step to remove unbound conjugate, the preparation is air-dried and mounted for observation under a microscope fitted with an appropriate fluorescent light source and barrier filters. In the **indirect fluorescent antibody (IFA)** procedure (Fig. 3-9), the material to be examined is first overlaid with an excess of unlabeled immune serum directed at the antigen and allowed to react for 30 to 45 minutes at 35 to 37°C. The specimen is washed with phosphate-buffered saline solution and then reacted with tagged antiserum against the species of immunoglobulin used in the initial reaction (e.g., fluores-

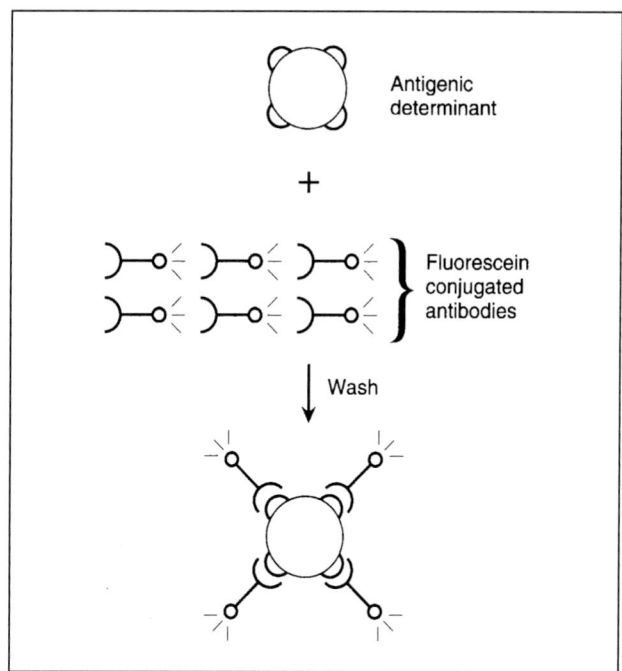

Figure 3-8 Schematic diagram of a direct immunofluorescence assay (DFA). In the DFA method, the antigen (e.g., respiratory specimens for respiratory syncytial virus, urogenital specimen for chlamydia) is placed in the well of an fluorescent antibody slide and reacted directly with a fluorescein-conjugated monoclonal antibody directed against the antigen. After incubation and washing, the slide is examined for characteristic fluorescence.

cein-conjugated antihuman antibody raised in goats). After washing the background free of extraneous material, the presence of microscopic fluorescence indicates the presence of antigen. DFA tests are simple and rapid to perform with fewer nonspecific reactions; however, they may be less sensitive than indirect procedures. IFA methods are more sensitive and produce brighter fluorescence; however, they may be less specific and are subject to increased cross-reactivity.[13] Reagents for either DFA or IFA detection of antigens are commercially available for a variety of agents, including *T. pallidum, C. trachomatis,* herpes simplex viruses, varicella-zoster virus, respiratory viruses (i.e., influenza, respiratory syncytial virus, parainfluenza viruses), *Pneumocystis carinii, G. lamblia,* and *C. parvum.*[14,19,21,48,63,95,98,99,126,132,139,140,145,146,153] Some reagents can be used for both direct detection of organisms in clinical specimens (e.g., endocervical smears, cells scraped from the base of vesicular lesions, sputum, bronchoalveolar lavages, diarrheal stools) and for identification of isolates recovered in culture (e.g., respiratory viruses, herpes simplex viruses, and varicella-zoster).

Immunofluorescence Techniques for Antibody Detection

IFA assays can be used for detection of antibodies in much the same way as the CF or HAI tests (Fig. 3-10). IFA tests are most often used for retrospective diagnosis of viral

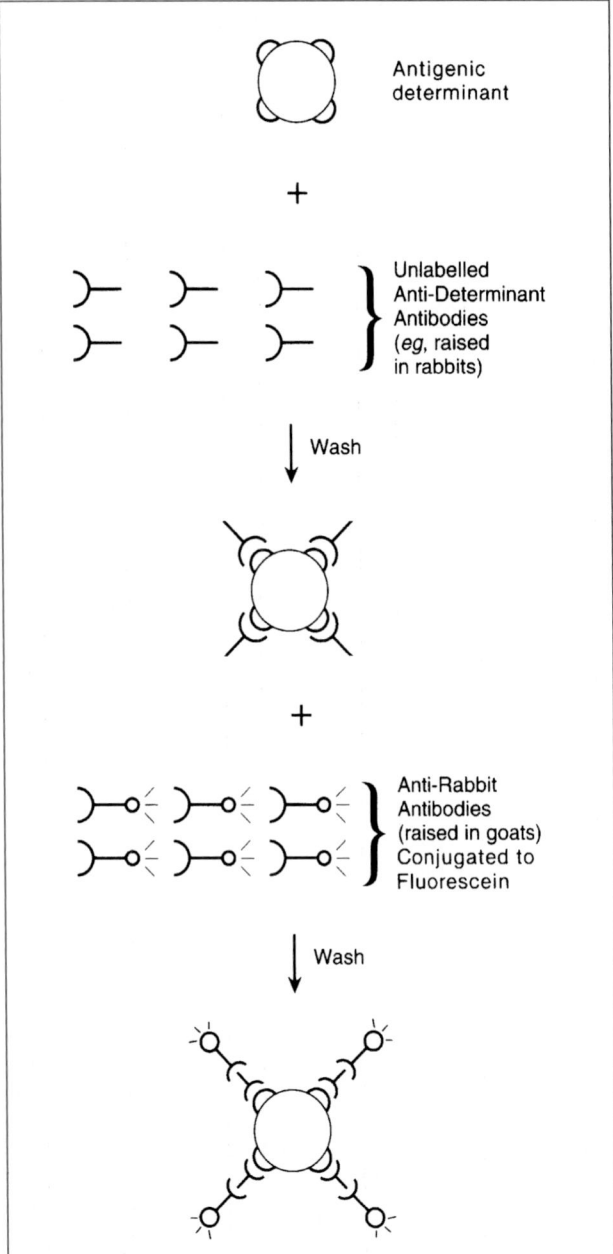

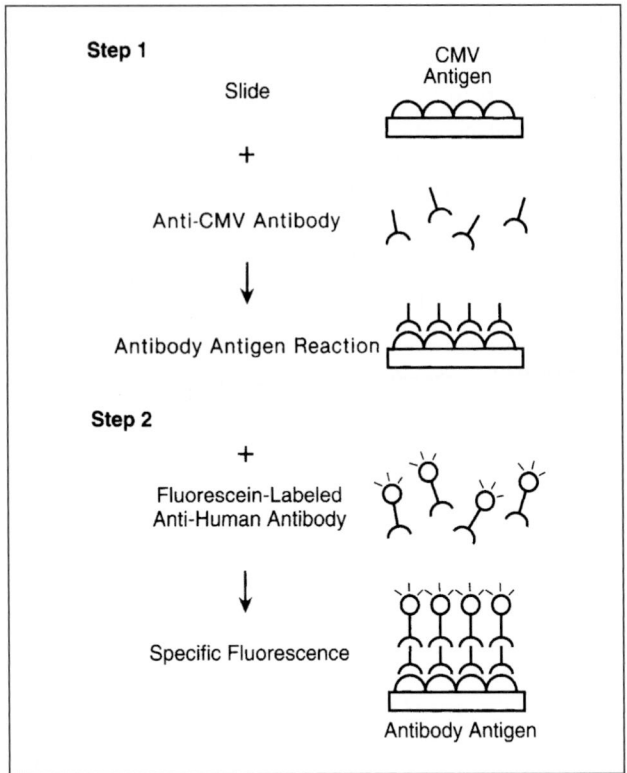

Figure 3-10 Indirect fluorescent antibody (IFA) method for antibody detection. In this method, antigen (e.g., cytomegalovirus [CMV]-infected tissue culture cells) is fixed onto a fluorescent antibody slide and reacted with patient serum. If anti-CMV antibodies are present, they bind to the antigens on the slide. After a washing step, a fluorescein-conjugated goat antihuman antibody is overlaid on the slide. This results in labeling of the CMV-infected cells on the slide and indicates the presence of anti-CMV antibodies in the initial serum specimen. Titers can be determined by performing the assay with twofold dilutions of serum and reading for the highest serum dilution resulting in a proscribed degree of fluorescence.

Figure 3-9 Schematic diagram of an indirect immuno-fluorescence assay (IFA) for antigen detection. In this method, the specimen (e.g., sputum for *Legionella*) is reacted with an excess of unlabeled antibodies directed against the antigen. After a wash step, fluorescein-conjugated antibodies directed against the species of antibody used in the initial reaction (e.g., fluorescein-labeled antirabbit IgG raised in goats) are overlaid on the fluorescent antibody slide. After washing, the slide is examined for specific fluorescence. With *Legionella*, for example, unlabeled rabbit antibodies against a large number of serotypes can be used for the first step in the procedure, while only a single fluorescein-conjugated goat antirabbit Ig is required for the second step. If *Legionella* organisms were to be detected by a DFA method, separate fluorescein-labeled conjugates for each serotype would be required.

infections by looking either for seroconversion or for a four-fold increase in antibody titer between acute and convalescent specimens. In the IFA procedure, slides with virus-infected tissue culture cells fixed in discrete FA (fluorescent antibody) test slide wells are overlaid with serial dilutions of patient serum. After incubation and washing, a fluorescein-labeled goat or rabbit antibody directed against human immunoglobulin (conjugate) is added to each of the slide areas containing the viral antigens. After washing, the slides are inspected with a fluorescence microscope, and an end point (i.e., the highest dilution of serum producing positive immunofluorescence) is determined. Changes in titer may be determined by inspection of slides reacted with serial dilutions of acute- and convalescent-phase sera that are performed together in the same test. Indirect assays can also be performed using enzyme-labeled conjugates (e.g., horseradish peroxidase) instead of fluorochrome-tagged reagents. Enzyme conjugate tests produce a colored precipitate that is read with a light microscope instead of a fluorescence microscope. Most laboratories that use IFA for serology will screen sera at a dilution of 1:8 or 1:10. If a positive reaction is obtained at this dilution, further twofold dilutions are prepared and each dilution is tested by IFA until an end-point dilution is reached. The reciprocal of the highest serum dilution showing fluorescence is the titer of that specimen for the antibody in question. Fig. 3-10 shows an IFA procedure for detection of antibodies to CMV.

The diagnoses of certain viral infections such as Epstein-Barr virus infection rely totally on serologic detection of antigens or antibodies because these agents do not grow in cell culture lines used in routine clinical microbiology laboratories. Epstein-Barr virus (EBV) is a member of the Family *Herpesviridae* and causes infectious mononucleosis. The specific immune response to EBV infection is characterized by the sequential appearance of certain antibodies, such as anti-VCA (viral capsid antigen) IgM and IgG, and antibodies against Epstein-Barr nuclear antigen (EBNA) and early antigen (EA) (see Chapter 22). Although anti-VCA IgM and then IgG appear during acute infection, anti-EBNA antibodies are absent during acute infection, appear during convalescence, and are maintained for life. Therefore, the presence of anti-EBNA in serum is indicative of past rather than current infection. Because EBNA is present in low levels in EBV-infected cells, the sensitive **anticomplement immunofluorescence (ACIF) test** is often used for its detection (Fig. 3-11).[113] In ACIF, an EBV-infected lymphoblastic cell line is used as the source of antigen. Raji cells are usually used for this purpose because these cells express only EBNA antigens; VCA is not expressed and EA is rarely detectable in this cell line.[85] These cells are fixed to a slide and reacted with patient serum. Specific anti-EBNA antibodies, if present, bind to the nuclear antigen. After a wash step, complement is overlaid on the cells. If specific anti-EBNA antibodies have reacted in the first step, complement binds to the immune complexes. After another wash step, fluorescein-conjugated anticomplement antibodies are overlaid on the

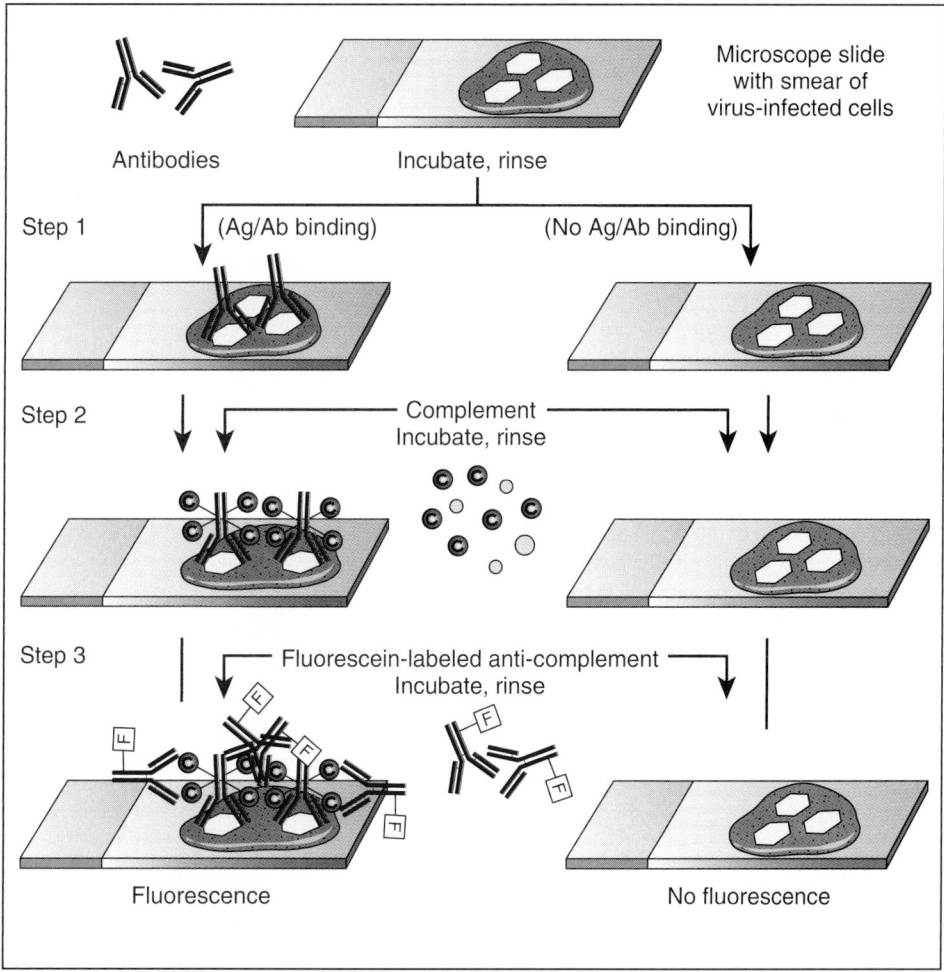

Figure 3-11 Anticomplement immunofluorescence. In step 1, antibodies are exposed to virus-infected cells fixed on a microscope slide. In step 2, complement is added and binds to antigen-antibody (Ag/Ab) complexes formed in step 1. In step 3, fluorescein-labeled anticomplement is added and binds to complement that bound in step 2, and fluorescence is seen. If antibodies do not bind in step 1, complement cannot bind in step 2, fluorescein-labeled anticomplement cannot bind in step 3, and no fluorescence is seen. Redrawn from Leland DS. Clinical Virology. Philadelphia: Saunders, 1996.

cells. The presence of nuclear fluorescence indicates the presence of EBNA and indicates past infection with EBV. ACIF is also used for determining immune status, detection of antibodies to CMV, and for demonstrating seroconversion following immunization with viral vaccines (e.g., varicella-zoster virus).[5,30,46,73,109,112]

Another immunofluorescence assay called the **fluorescent antibody to membrane antigen (FAMA) test** is the test of choice for determining immune status for certain viruses such as varicella-zoster virus (VZV), largely because of its exquisite sensitivity.[46,144] In this assay, patient serum is serially diluted in microtiter wells, and cultured cells infected with VZV are added to the diluted serum. After incubation, the microtiter tray is centrifuged to force the cells to the bottom of the wells and washed twice, with intervening centrifugation steps. A working dilution of fluorescein-conjugated antihuman IgG is the added to the wells and incubated. After a few wash/centrifugation steps, the cells are harvested, fixed to the wells of an FA slide, and examined with a fluorescence microscope. The FAMA test is more sensitive than CF or EIA, but it requires live, virus-infected cells for its performance.[5,30,50,128]

Immunofluorescence and enzyme immunoassay approaches each have their own advantages and disadvantages. EIA methods for antigen detection are advantageous in high-volume laboratories where many samples are examined daily for a single determinant (e.g., *C. trachomatis* or respiratory syncytial virus).[67,132] Although DFA techniques are more labor-intensive, the ability to directly observe the background cellular elements in certain direct antigen procedures to determine the adequacy of the specimen is a distinct advantage. For example, since *C. trachomatis* preferentially infects cervical columnar epithelial cells, the presence of squamous epithelial cells and/or segmented neutrophils, erythrocytes, and mucus indicates that the specimen is inadequate for diagnostic purposes. Adequate specimens show a preponderance of intact cuboidal and columnar epithelial cells. This assessment can be made with the direct fluorescent antibody test and incorporated into the laboratory report, allowing the physician to weigh clinical evidence of chlamydial infection along with the possibility that a negative report may actually reflect an inadequately collected endocervical specimen. These determinations cannot be made with nonvisual tests such as antigen-capture EIAs for *Chlamydia trachomatis* and most molecular assays.

REFERENCES

1. Addis DG, Mathews HM, Stewart JM, et al. Evaluation of a commercially available enzyme-linked immunosorbent assay for *Giardia lamblia* antigen in stool. J Clin Microbiol 1991;29:1137–1142.
2. Arumainayagam JT, Matthews RS, Uthayakumar S, Clay JC. Evaluation of a novel solid-phase immunoassay, Clearview Chlamydia, for the rapid detection of *Chlamydia trachomatis*. J Clin Microbiol 1990;28:2813–2814.
3. Ashley R, Cent A, Maggs V, et al. Inability of enzyme immunoassays to discriminate between infections with herpes simplex virus types 1 and 2. Ann Intern Med 1991;115:520–526.
4. Ashley RL, Militoni J, Lee F, et al. Comparison of Western blot (immunoblot) and glycoprotein G-specific immunodot enzyme assay for detecting antibodies to herpes simplex virus types 1 and 2 in human sera. J Clin Microbiol 1988; 26:662–667.
5. Balfour HH, Edelman CK, Dirksen CL, et al. Laboratory studies of acute varicella and varicella immune status. Diagn Microbiol Infect Dis 1988;10:149–158.
6. Beckwith DG, Halstead DC, Alpaugh K, et al. Comparison of a latex agglutination test with five other methods for determining the presence of antibody against cytomegalovirus. J Clin Microbiol 1985;21:328–331.
7. Bibb WF, Arnow PM, Thacker L, McKinney RM. Detection of soluble *Legionella pneumophila* antigens in serum and urine by enzyme-linked immunosorbent assay with monoclonal and polyclonal antibodies. J Clin Microbiol 1984; 20:478–482.
8. Bisno AL, Wood JW, Lawson J, et al. Antigens in urine of patients with glomerulonephritis and in normal human serum which cross-react with group A streptococci: identification and partial characterization. J Lab Clin Med 1978;91: 500–513.
9. Blanding J, Hirsch L, Stranton N, et al. Comparison of Clearview Chlamydia, the PACE 2 assay, and culture for detection of *Chlamydia trachomatis* from cervical specimens in a low-prevalence population. J Clin Microbiol 1993;31: 1622–1625.
10. Blanton M, Balakrishnan K, Dumaswala U, et al. HLA antibodies in blood donors with reactive screening tests for antibody to the immunodeficiency virus. Transfusion 1987;27:118–119.
11. Boone JH, Wilkins TD, Nash TE, et al. TechLab and Alexon Giardia enzyme-linked immunosorbent assay kits detect cyst wall protein 1. J Clin Microbiol 1999;37:611–614.
12. Booth JC, Hannington G, Bakir TMF, et al. Comparison of enzyme-linked immunosorbent assay, radioimmunoassay, complement fixation, anticomplement immunofluorescence, and passive haemagglutination techniques for detecting cytomegalovirus IgG antibody. J Clin Pathol 35:1345–1348, 1982.
13. Brown SL, Bibb WF, McKinney RM. Retrospective examination of lung tissue specimens for the presence of *Legionella* organisms: comparison of an indirect fluorescent antibody system with direct fluorescent antibody testing. J Clin Microbiol 19:468–472, 1984.
14. Brumback BG, Farthing PG, Castellino SN. Simultaneous detection of and differentiation between herpes simplex and varicella-zoster viruses with two fluorescent probes in the same test system. J Clin Microbiol 31:3260–3263, 1993.
15. Buckley RH, Dees SC, O'Fallon WM. Serum immunoglobulins: I. Levels in normal children and in uncomplicated childhood allergy. Pediatrics 1968;41: 600–611.
16. Byrne RE, Laske S, Bell M, et al. Evaluation of a *Treponema pallidum* Western immunoblot assay as a confirmatory test for syphilis. J Clin Microbiol 1992; 30:115–122.
17. Carroll KC, Ballou D, Varner M, et al. Rapid detection of group B streptococcal colonization of the genital tract by a commercial optical immunoassay. Eur J Clin Microbiol Infect Dis 1996;15:206–210.
18. Centers for Disease Control. Prevention of perinatal group B streptococcal disease: a public health perspective. MMWR Morb Mortal Wkly Rep 45(RR-7): 1–24.
19. Cheeseman SH, Pierik LT, Leombruno D, et al. Evaluation of a commercially available direct immunofluorescence staining reagent for detection of respiratory syncytial virus in respiratory secretions. J Clin Microbiol 1986;24:155–156.
20. Chernesky M, Castriciano S, Mahony J, et al. Ability of Testpack Rotavirus enzyme immunoassay to diagnose rotavirus gastroenteritis. J Clin Microbiol 1988;26:2459–2461.
21. Chernesky MA, Mahony JB, Castriciano S, et al. Detection of *Chlamydia trachomatis* antigens by enzyme immunoassay and immunofluorescence in genital specimens from symptomatic and asymptomatic men and women. J Infect Dis 1986;154:141–148.
22. Chuck SL, Sande MA. Infections with *Cryptococcus neoformans* in the acquired immunodeficiency syndrome. N Engl J Med 1989;321:794–799.
23. Collins MH, Jiang B, Croffie JM, et al. Hepatic granulomas in children: a clinicopathologic analysis of 23 cases including polymerase chain reaction for *Histoplasma*. Am J Surg Pathol 1996;20:332–338.
24. Dale JC, Vetter EA, Contezac JM, et al. Evaluation of two rapid antigen assays, Biostar Strep OIA and Pacific Biotech CARD O.S. and culture for detection of group A streptococci in throat swabs. J Clin Microbiol 1994;32:2698–2701.
25. Daley JA, Seskin KC. Evaluation of rapid, commercial latex agglutination techniques for serogrouping β-hemolytic streptococci. J Clin Microbiol 1988;26: 2429–2431.
26. Daum RS, Siber GR, Kamon JS, Russell RR. Evaluation of a commercial latex particle agglutination test for rapid diagnosis of *Haemophilus influenzae* type b infection. Pediatrics 1982;69:466–471.
27. DeCock KM, Maran M, Kouadio JC, et al. Rapid tests for distinguishing HIV-1 and HIV-2. Lancet 1990;336:757–759.
28. DeLeys R, Vanderborght RB, Vanden Haesevelde M, et al. Isolation and partial characterization of an unusual human immunodeficiency retrovirus from two persons of west central African origin. J Virol 1990;64:1207–1216.

29. Della-Latta P, Whittier S, Hosmer M, et al. Rapid detection of group A streptococcal pharyngitis in a pediatric population with optical immunoassay. Pediatr Infect Dis J 1994;13:742–743.

30. Demmler G, Steinberg S, Blum G, et al. Rapid enzyme linked immunosorbent assay for detecting antibody to varicella-zoster virus. J Infect Dis 1988;157:211–212.

31. DeRee JM, Schwillens P, van den Borch JF. Monoclonal antibodies for serotyping of the P fimbriae of uropathogenic *Escherichia coli*. J Clin Microbiol 1986;24:121–125.

32. Diamond RD, Bennett JE. Prognostic factors in cryptococcal meningitis: a study of 111 cases. Ann Intern Med 1981;80:175–177.

33. Dominguez JA, Gali N, Pedroso P, et al. Comparison of the Binax *Legionella* urinary antigen enzyme immunoassay (EIA) with the Biotest *Legionella* urine antigen EIA for detection of *Legionella* antigen in both concentrated and nonconcentrated urine samples. J Clin Microbiol 1998;36:2718–2722.

34. Donohue-Rolfe A, Kelley MA, Bennish M, et al. Enzyme-linked immunosorbent assay for shigella toxin. J Clin Microbiol 1986;24:65–58.

35. Drew WL. Controversies in viral diagnosis. Rev Infect Dis 1986;8:814–824.

36. Dwyer JM. The specific immune response. In: Root RK, Waldvogel F, Corey L, Stamm WE, eds. Clinical Infectious Diseases: A Practical Approach. New York: Oxford University Press, 1999:91–108.

37. Englund JA, Piedra PA, Jewell A, et al. Rapid diagnosis of respiratory syncytial virus infection in immunocompromised adults. J Clin Microbiol 1996;34:1649–1653.

38. Engstrom SM, Shoop E, Johnson RC. Immunoblot interpretation criteria for serodiagnosis of early Lyme disease. J Clin Microbiol 1995;33:419–427.

39. Fedorko DP, Engler HD, O'Shaughnessy EM, et al. Evaluation of two rapid assays for detection of *Clostridium difficile* toxin A in stool specimens. J Clin Microbiol 1999;37:3044–3047.

40. Feinstone SM, Kapikian AZ, Purcell RH. Hepatitis A: detection by immune electron microscopy of a virus-like antigen associated with acute illness. Science 1973;182:1026–1028.

41. Ferraro MJ, Kallas, WM, Welch KP, et al. Comparison of a new, rapid enzyme immunoassay with a latex agglutination test for qualitative detection of rubella antibodies. J Clin Microbiol 1987;25:1722–1724.

42. Flander RT, Lindsay PD, Chairez R, et al. The evaluation of clinical specimens for the presence of respiratory syncytial virus antigen using an enzyme immunoassay. J Med Virol 1986;19:1–9.

43. Forsgren A, Sjoguist J. "Protein A" from *Staphylococcus aureus* I. Pseudo immune reaction with human globulin. J Immunol 1966;97:822.

44. Gade W, Hinnefeld SW, Babcock LS, et al. Comparison of the Premier Cryptococcal antigen enzyme immunoassay and the latex agglutination assay for detection of cryptococcal antigens. J Clin Microbiol 1991;29:1616–1619.

45. Gade W, Ledman DW, Wethington R. Serological responses to various *Coccidioides* antigen preparations in a new enzyme immunoassay. J Clin Microbiol 1992;30:1907–1912.

46. Gallo D, Schmidt NJ. Comparison of anti-complement immunofluorescence and fluorescent antibody to membrane antigen test for determination of immunity status to varicella-zoster virus and for serodifferentiation of varicella-zoster and herpes simplex virus infections. J Clin Microbiol 1981;14:539–543.

47. Garcia LS, Shimizu RY. Evaluation of nine immunoassay kits (enzyme immunoassay and direct fluorescence) for detection *of Giardia lamblia* and *Cryptosporidium parvum* in human fecal specimens. J Clin Microbiol 1997;35:1526–1529.

48. Garcia LS, Shum AC, Bruckner DA. Evaluation of a new monoclonal antibody combination reagent for direct fluorescence detection of *Giardia* cysts and *Cryptosporidium* oocysts in human fecal specimens. J Clin Microbiol 1992;30:3255–3257.

49. George JR, Schochetman G. Detection of HIV infection using serologic techniques. In: Schochetman G, George JR, eds. AIDS Testing: A Comprehensive Guide to Technical Medical, Social, Legal, and Management Issues. New York: Springer-Verlag, 1994:62–102.

50. Gershon A, Steinberg S, LaRussa P. Detection of antibodies to varicella-zoster virus by latex agglutination. Clin Diagn Virol 1994;2:271–277.

51. Goroncy-Bermes P, Dale JB, Beachey EH, Opferkuch W. Monoclonal antibody to human renal glomeruli cross-reacts with streptococcal M protein. Infect Immun 1987;55:2416–2419.

52. Granato PA, Petosa MT. Evaluation of a rapid screening test for detecting group B streptococci in pregnant women. J Clin Microbiol 1991;29:1536–1538.

53. Green M, Dashefsky B, Wald ER, et al. Comparison of two antigen assays for rapid intrapartum detection of vaginal group B streptococcal colonization. J Clin Microbiol 1993;31:78–82.

54. Halstead DC, Todd S, Fritch G. Evaluation of five methods for respiratory syncytial virus detection. J Clin Microbiol 1990;28:1021–1025.

55. Hamilton JR. Comparison of Meritec Strep with Streptex for direct colony grouping of β-hemolytic streptococci from primary isolation and subculture plates. J Clin Microbiol 1988;26:692–695.

56. Harbeck RJ, Teague J, Crossen GR, et al. Novel, rapid optical immunoassay technique for detection of group A streptococci from pharyngeal specimens: comparison with standard culture methods. J Clin Microbiol 1993;31:839–844.

57. Heiner DC. Diagnosis of histoplasmosis using precipitin reactions in agar gel. Pediatrics 1958;22:616–627.

58. Henrard DR, Wu S, Phillips J, et al. Detection of p24 antigen with and without immune complex dissociation for longitudinal monitoring of human immunodeficiency virus type 1 infection. J Clin Microbiol 1995;33:72–75.

59. Hinderer W, Lang D, Rothe M, et al. Serodiagnosis of Epstein-Barr virus infection by using recombinant viral capsid antigen fragments and autologous gene fusion. J Clin Microbiol 1999;37:3239–3244.

60. Humphrey CD, Cook EH Jr, Bradley DW. Identification of enterically transmitted hepatitis virus particles by solid phase immune electron microscopy. J Virol Methods 1990;29:177–188.

61. Hursh DA, Abbot AD, Sun R, et al. Evaluation of a latex particle agglutination assay for the detection of cytomegalovirus antibody in patient serum. J Clin Microbiol 1989;27:2878–2879.

62. Ingram DL, Pearson AW, Occhiuti AR. Detection of bacterial antigens in body fluids with the Wellcogen *Haemophilus influenzae* b, *Streptococcus pneumoniae*, and *Neisseria meningitidis* (ACYW135) latex agglutination tests. J Clin Microbiol 1983;18:1119–1121.

63. Ito F, George RW, Hunter EF, et al. Specific immunofluorescent staining of pathogenic treponemas with a monoclonal antibody. J Clin Microbiol 1992;30:831–838.

64. Janda WM, Wilcoski LM, Mandel KL, et al. Comparison of monoclonal antibody-based methods and a ribosomal ribonucleic acid probe test for *Neisseria gonorrhoeae* culture confirmation. Eur J Clin Microbiol Infect Dis 1993;12:177–184.

65. Jarrett EE, Miller H. Production and activities of IgE in helminth infections. Prog Allergy 1982;31:178–184.

66. Johnson BJB, Robbins KE, Bailey RE, et al. Serodiagnosis of Lyme disease: accuracy of a two-step approach using a flagella-based ELISA and immunoblotting. J Infect Dis 1996;174:346–353.

67. Kao C-L, McIntosh K, Fernie B, et al. Monoclonal antibodies for the rapid diagnosis of respiratory syncytial virus infection by immunofluorescence. Diagn Microbiol Infect Dis 1984;2:199–206.

68. Kaufman L. Laboratory methods for the diagnosis and confirmation of systemic mycoses. Clin Infect Dis 1992;14(Suppl 1):S23–S29.

69. Kaufman L, Sekhon AS, Moledina N, et al. Comparative evaluation of commercial Premier EIA and microimmunodiffusion and complement fixation for *Coccidioides immitis* antibodies. J Clin Microbiol 1995;33:618–619.

70. Kaufman L, Standard PG. Specific and rapid identification of medically important fungi by exoantigen detection. Annu Rev Microbiol 1987;41:209–225.

71. Kehl KSC, Cicirello H, Havens PL. Comparison of four different methods for detection of *Cryptosporidium* species. J Clin Microbiol 1995;33:416–418.

72. Kellog JA. Culture vs. direct antigen assays for detection of microbial pathogens from lower respiratory tract specimens suspected of containing the respiratory syncytial virus. Arch Pathol Lab Med 1991;115:451–458.

73. Kettering JD, Schmidt NJ, Gallo D, Lennette EH. Anti-complement immunofluorescence test for antibodies to human cytomegalovirus. J Clin Microbiol 1977;6:627–632.

74. Kline RL, McNairn D, Holodniy M, et al. Evaluation of Chiron HIV-1/HIV-2 recombinant immunoblot assay. J Clin Microbiol 1996;43:2650–2653.

75. Kluytmans JAJW, Goessens WHF, Mouton JW, et al. Evaluation of Clearview and Magic Lite tests, polymerase chain reaction, and cell culture for detection of *Chlamydia trachomatis* in urogenital specimens. J Clin Microbiol 1993;31:3204–3210.

76. Kohler G, Milstein C. Continuous culture of fused cells secreting antibodies of predefined specificity. Nature 1975;256:495–497.

77. Kuhnl P, Seidl S, Holzberger G. HLA DR4 antibodies cause false-positive HTLV-III antibody ELISA results. Lancet 1985;1:1222–1223.

78. Lambert RS, George RB. Evaluation of enzyme immunoassay as a rapid screening test for histoplasmosis and blastomycosis. Am Rev Respir Dis 1987;136:316–319.

79. Lange CF. Chemistry of cross-reactive fragments of streptococcal cell membrane and human glomerular basement membrane. Transplant Proc 1969;1:959–963.

80. Lange J, Goudsmit J. Decline of antibody reactivity to HIV core proteins secondary to increased production of HIV antigen. Lancet 1987;1:448.

81. LaRussa P, Steinberg S, Waithe E, et al. Comparison of five assays for antibody to varicella-zoster virus and the fluorescent-antibody-to-membrane-antigen test. J Clin Microbiol 1987;25:2059–2062.

82. Laubscher B, van Melle G, Dreyfuss N, et al. Evaluation of a new immunologic test for rapid detection of group A streptococci, the Abbott Testpack Strep A Plus. J Clin Microbiol 1995;33:260–261.

83. Lauderdate T-L, Landers L, Thorneycroft I, Chapin K. Comparison of the PACE II assay, two amplification assays, and Clearview EIA for detection of *Chlamydia trachomatis* in female endocervical and urine specimens. J Clin Microbiol 1999;37:2223–2229.

84. Leland DS, Barth KA, Cunningham EB, et al. Evaluation of four methods for

cytomegalovirus antibody detection tests for use by a bone marrow transplant service. J Clin Microbiol 1989;27:176–178.

85. Lennette ET. Epstein-Barr Virus. In: Murray PR, Baron EJ, Pfaller MA, et al., eds. Manual of Clinical Microbiology. 7th Ed. Washington, DC: ASM Press, 1999:912–918.

86. Lewis LL, Taber LH, Baughn RE. Evaluation of immunoglobulin M Western blot analysis in the diagnosis of congenital syphilis. J Clin Microbiol 1990;28:296–302.

87. Loussert-Ajaka I, Ly TD, Chaix ML. HIV-1/HIV-2 seronegativity in HIV subtype O infected patients. Lancet 1994;323:1393–1395.

88. Lyerly DM, Neville HD, Evans DT, et al. Multicenter evaluation of the *Clostridium difficile* TOX A/B TEST. J Clin Microbiol 1998;36:184–190.

89. Mackenzie AMR, Lebel P, Orrbine E, et al. Sensitivities and specificities of Premier *E. coli* O157 and Premier EHEC enzyme immunoassays for diagnosis of infection with verotoxin (shiga-like toxin)-producing *Escherichia coli*. J Clin Microbiol 1998;36:1608–1611.

90. Macone AB, Arakere G, Letourneau JM, et al. Comparison of a new rapid enzyme-linked immunosorbent assay with latex particle agglutination for the detection of *Haemophilus influenzae* type b infections. J Clin Microbiol 1985;21:711–714.

91. Magnarelli LA, Miller JN, Anderson JF, Riviere GR. Cross-reactivity of nonspecific treponemal antibody in serologic tests for Lyme disease. J Clin Microbiol 1990;28:1276–1279.

92. Mancini G, Carbonara AO, Heremans JF. Immunochemical quantitation of antigens by single radial immunodiffusion. Immunochemistry 1965;2:235–237.

93. Martins TB, Jaskowski TD, Mouritsen CL, Hill HR. Comparison of commercially available enzyme immunoassay with traditional serological tests for detection of antibodies to *Coccidioides immitis*. J Clin Microbiol 1995;33:940–943.

94. Mayo DR, Brennan T, Sirpenski SP, et al. Cytomegalovirus antibody detection by three commercially available assays and complement fixation. Diagn Microbiol Infect Dis 1985;3:455–459.

95. McDonald JC, Quennec P. Utility of a respiratory virus panel containing a monoclonal antibody pool for screening of respiratory specimens in nonpeak respiratory syncytial virus season. J Clin Microbiol 1993;31:2809–2911.

96. McHugh TM, Casavant CH, Wilber JC, et al. Comparison of six methods for the detection of antibody to cytomegalovirus. J Clin Microbiol 1985;22:1014–1019.

97. Moncada J., Schachter J, Bolan G, et al. Evaluation of Syva's enzyme immunoassay for the detection of *Chlamydia trachomatis* in urogenital specimens. Diagn Microbiol Infect Dis 1992;15:663–668.

98. Ng VL, Virani NA, Chaisson RE, et al. Rapid detection of *Pneumocystis carinii* using a direct fluorescence monoclonal antibody stain. J Clin Microbiol 1990;28:2228–2233.

99. Ng VL, Yajko DM, McPhaul LW, et al. Evaluation of an indirect fluorescent-antibody stain for detection of *Pneumocystis carinii* in respiratory specimens. J Clin Microbiol 1990;28:975–979.

100. Norris SJ, Treponema pallidum Polypeptide Research Group. Polypeptides of *Treponema pallidum*: progress toward understanding their structural, functional, and immunologic roles. Microbiol Rev 1993;57:750–779.

101. Nowinski RC, Tam MR, Goldstein LC, et al. Monoclonal antibodies for diagnosis of infectious diseases in humans. Science 1983;219:637–644.

102. Ong SJ, Cheng MY, Liu KH, Horng CH. Use of the ProSpecT microplate enzyme immunoassay for the detection of pathogenic and nonpathogenic *Entamoeba histolytica* in faecal specimens. Trans R Soc Trop Med Hyg 1996;90:248–249.

103. Oudin J. Methode d'analyse immunochimique par precipitation specifique en milieu gelifie. CR Acad Sci 1946;222:115–116.

104. Padhye AA, Smith G, McLaughlin D et al. Comparative evaluation of a chemiluminescent DNA probe and an exoantigen test for rapid identification of *Histoplasma capsulatum*. J Clin Microbiol 1992;30:3108–3111.

105. Padhye AA, Smith G, Standard PG, et al. Comparative evaluation of chemiluminescent DNA probe assays and exoantigen tests for rapid identification of *Blastomyces dermatitidis* and *Coccidioides immitis*. J Clin Microbiol 1994;32:867–870.

106. Pate MS, Dixon PB, Hardy K, et al. Evaluation of the Biostar Chlamydia OIA assay with specimens from women attending a sexually transmitted disease clinic. J Clin Microbiol 1998;36:2183–2186.

107. Petrie GF. A specific precipitin reaction associated with the growth on agar plates of meningococcus, pneumococcus, and B. dysenteria (Shiga). Br J Exp Pathol 1932;13:380–394.

108. Pollet DE, Saman EL, Peeters DC, et al. Confirmation and differentiation of antibodies to human immunodeficiency virus 1 and 2 with a strip-based assay including recombinant antigens and synthetic peptides. Clin Chem 1991;37:1700–1707.

109. Preissner C, Steinberg S, Gershon A, Smith TF. Evaluation of the anticomplement immunofluorescence test for detection of antibody to varicella-zoster virus. J Clin Microbiol 1982;16:373–376.

110. Pruneda RC, Dover JC. A comparison of two passive agglutination procedures with enzyme-linked immunosorbent assay for rubella antibody status. Am J Clin Pathol 1986;86:768–770.

111. Radestsky M, Wheeler RC, Roe MH, et al. Comparative evaluation of kits for rapid diagnosis of group A streptococcal disease. Pediatr Infect Dis 1985;4:274–281.

112. Rao N, Waruszewski DT, Armstrong JA, et al. Evaluation of anti-complementary immunofluorescence test in cytomegalovirus infection. J Clin Microbiol 1977;6:633–638.

113. Redman BM, Klein G. Cellular localization of an Epstein-Barr virus (EBV)-associated complement-fixing antigen in producer and non-producer lymphoblastoid cell lines. Int J Cancer 1973;11:499–520.

114. Roe M, Kishyama C, Davidson K, et al. Comparison of Biostar Strep A OIA optical immune assay, Abbott Test-Pack Plus Strep A, and culture with selective media for diagnosis of group A streptococcal pharyngitis. J Clin Microbiol 1995;33:1551–1553.

115. Roth RA, Koshland ME. Identification of a lymphocyte enzyme that catalyzes pentamer immunoglobulin M assembly. J Biol Chem 1981;256:4633–4639.

116. Rothbarth PH, Hermes M-C, Schrijnemakers P. Reliability of two new test kits for rapid diagnosis of respiratory syncytial virus infection. J Clin Microbiol 1991;29:824–826.

117. Sarngadharan MG, Popovic M, Bruch L, et al. Antibodies reactive with human T-lymphotropic retroviruses (HTLV-III) in the serum of patients with AIDS. Science 1984;224:506–508.

118. Schable C, Zekeng L, Pau CP, et al. Sensitivity of United States HIV antibody tests for detection of HIV-1 group O infections. Lancet 1994;344:1333–1334.

119. Schachter J, Jones RB, Butler RC, et al. Evaluation of the Vidas Chlamydia test to detect and verify *Chlamydia trachomatis* in urogenital specimens. J Clin Microbiol 1997;35:2102–2106.

120. Schupbach J, Boni J. Quantitative and sensitive detection of immune-complexed and free HIV antigen after boiling of serum. J Virol Methods 1993;43:247–256.

121. Scotland SM, Willshaw GA, Said B, et al. Identification of *Escherichia coli* that produces heat-stable enterotoxin ST^A by a commercially available enzyme-linked immunoassay and a comparison of the assay with infant mouse and DNA probe tests. J Clin Microbiol 1989;27:1697–1699.

122. Sellors J, Mahoney J, Jang D, et al. Rapid, on-site diagnosis of chlamydial urethritis in men by detection of antigens in urethral swabs and urine. J Clin Microbiol 1991;29:407–409.

123. Sippel JE, Hider PA, Controni G. Use of Directigen latex agglutination test for detection of *Haemophilus influenzae*, *Streptococcus pneumoniae*, and *Neisseria meningitidis* antigens in cerebrospinal fluid from meningitis patients. J Clin Microbiol 1984;20:884–886.

124. Skendzel LP, Wilcox KR, Edson DC. Evaluation of assays for the detection of antibodies to rubella: A report based on data from the College of American Pathologists Surveys of 1982. Am J Clin Pathol 1983;80:594–598.

125. Skulnick M, Small GW, Simor AE, et al. Comparison of the Clearview Chlamydia test, Chlamydiazyme, and cell culture for detection of *Chlamydia trachomatis* in women with a low prevalence of infection. J Clin Microbiol 1991;29:2086–2088.

126. Spada B, Biehler K, Chegas P, et al. Comparison of rapid immunofluorescence assay to cell culture isolation for the detection of influenza A and B viruses in nasopharyngeal secretions from infants and children. J Virol Methods 1991;33:305–310.

127. Steece RS, Talley MS, Skeels MR, et al. Comparison of enzyme-linked immunosorbent assay, hemagglutination inhibition, and passive latex agglutination for determination of rubella immune status. J Clin Microbiol 1985;21:140–142.

128. Steinberg SP, Gershon AA. Measurement of antibodies to varicella-zoster virus by using a latex agglutination test. J Clin Microbiol 1991;29:1527–1529.

129. Stewart GL. Parkman PD, Hopps HE, et al. Rubella virus hemagglutination-inhibition test. N Engl J Med 1967;276:554–557.

130. Stockman L, Clark KA, Hunt JM, Roberts GD. Evaluation of commercially available acridinium ester-labeled chemiluminescent DNA probes for culture identification of *Blastomyces dermatitidis*, *Coccidioides immitis*, *Cryptococcus neoformans*, and *Histoplasma capsulatum*. J Clin Microbiol 1993;31:845–850.

131. Stratton NJ, Hirsch L, Harris F, et al. Evaluation of the rapid Clearview Chlamydia test for direct detection of chlamydiae from cervical specimens. J Clin Microbiol 1991;29:1551–1553.

132. Tam MR, Stamm WE, Handsfield HH. Culture independent diagnosis of *Chlamydia trachomatis* using monoclonal antibodies. N Engl J Med 1984;310:1146–1150.

133. Thomas EE, Book LE. Comparison of two rapid methods for detection of respiratory syncytial virus (Test Pack RSV and Ortho Elisa) with direct immunofluorescence and virus isolation for the diagnosis of pediatric RSV infection. J Clin Microbiol 1991;29:632–635.

134. Thomas EE, Puterman ML, Kawano E, Curran M. Evaluation of seven immunoassays for detection of rotavirus in pediatric stool specimens. J Clin Microbiol 1988;26:1189–1193.

135. U.S. Public Health Service. Standardized diagnostic complement fixation method and adaptation to micro test. In: U.S. Public Health Service Public Health Monograph 74, Washington DC: Government Printing Office, 1965.

136. Van de Rijn I, Zabriskie JB, McCarty M. Group A streptococcal antigens cross-

reactive with myocardium. Purification of heart-reactive antibody and isolation and characterization of the streptococcal antigen. J Exp Med 1977;146:579–599.

137. Von Sydow M, Gaines H, Sonnerborg A, et al. Antigen detection in primary HIV infection. Br Med J 1988;295:238–240.

138. Wall R, Denning D, Amos A. HIV antigenaemia in acute HIV infection. Lancet 1987;1:566.

139. Waner JL, Todd SJ, Shalaby J, et al. Comparison of Directigen FLU-A with viral isolation and direct immunofluorescence for the rapid detection and identification of influenza A virus. J Clin Microbiol 1991;29:470–482.

140. Waner JL, Whitehurst NJ, Downs T, Graves DG. Production of monoclonal antibodies against parainfluenza 3 virus and their use in diagnosis by immunofluorescence. J Clin Microbiol 1985;22:535–538.

141. Wheat LJ, Connolly-Springfield P, Kohler RB, et al. *Histoplasma capsulatum* polysaccharide antigen detection in diagnosis and management of disseminated histoplasmosis in patients with acquired immunodeficiency syndrome. Am J Med 1989;87:396–400.

142. Wheat LJ, Kohler RB, Tewari RP. Diagnosis of disseminated histoplasmosis by detection of *Histoplasma capsulatum* antigen in serum and urine specimens. N Engl J Med 1986;314:83–88.

143. Wieden MA, Lundergan LL, Blum J, et al. Detection of coccidioidal antibodies by 33-kDa spherule antigen, *Coccidioides* EIA, and standard serologic tests in sera from patients being evaluated for coccidioidomycosis. J Infect Dis 1996; 173:1272–1277.

144. Williams V, Gershon A, Brunell P. Serologic response to varicella-zoster membrane antigens measured by indirect immunofluorescence. J Infect Dis 1974; 130:669–672.

145. Wolfson JS, Waldron MA, Sierra LS. Blinded comparison of a direct immunofluorescent monoclonal antibody staining method for identification of *Pneumocystis carinii* in induced sputum and bronchoalveolar lavage specimens of patients infected with human immunodeficiency virus. J Clin Microbiol 1990;28: 2136–2138.

146. Wong DT, Welliver RC, Riddlesberger KR, et al. Rapid diagnosis of parainfluenza virus infection in children. J Clin Microbiol 1982;16:164–167.

147. Wust J, Hebisch G, Peters K. Evaluation of two enzyme immunoassays for rapid detection of group B streptococci in pregnant women. Eur J Clin Microbiol Infect Dis 1993;12:124–127.

148. Yolken RH, Davis D, Winkelstein J, et al. Enzyme immunoassay for detection of pneumococcal antigen in cerebrospinal fluid. J Clin Microbiol 1984;20:802–805.

149. Young H, Moyes A, Seagar L, McMillan A. Novel recombinant-antigen enzyme immunoassay for serological diagnosis of syphilis. J Clin Microbiol 1998;36: 913–917.

150. Zabriskie JB, Freimer EH. An immunological relationship between group A streptococcus and mammalian muscle. J Exp Med 1966;124:661–678.

151. Zartarian M, Peterson EM, De la Maza LM. Detection of antibodies to *Coccidioides immitis* by enzyme immunoassay. Am J Clin Pathol 1997;107:148–153.

152. Zhang T, Mauracher CA, Mitchell LA, Tingle A. Detection of rubella virus-specific immunoglobulin G (IgG), IgM, and IgA antibodies by immunoblot assays. J Clin Microbiol 1992;30:824–830.

153. Zimmerman SK, Needham CA. Comparison of conventional stool concentration and preserved-smear methods with Merifluor *Cryptosporidium*/*Giardia* direct immunofluorescence assay and ProSpecT *Giardia* EZ microplate assay for detection of *Giardia lamblia*. J Clin Microbiol 1995;33:1942–1943.

Molecular Microbiology

Nucleic Acids—The Basics of DNA and RNA

Structure of DNA
Structure of RNA
Function of DNA—Information Storage
Function of RNA—Information Transfer

Reading (Transcription) and Interpretation (Translation) of the Genetic Code

Signal-Amplification Methods

Nucleic-Acid Probes

Clinical Applications

Hybrid Capture

Clinical Applications

Branched DNA

Clinical Applications

In Situ Hybridization

Clinical Applications

Nucleic-Acid Amplification

Basics of the Polymerase Chain Reaction

Clinical Applications

Other Methods of Nucleic-Acid Amplification

Clinical Applications

Modifications of PCR

RT-PCR

Clinical Applications
Broad-Range PCR
Clinical Applications
Multiplex PCR
Clinical Applications
Nested PCR
Clinical Applications

Postamplification Analysis

Traditional Methods of Detection

Gel Electrophoresis/Southern Blot Analysis
Enzymatic Detection of Amplified Products
Clinical Applications

Reverse Hybridization

Clinical Applications

DNA Sequencing

Traditional DNA Sequencing
Clinical Applications
Sequencing by Synthesis (Pyrosequencing)
Clinical Applications
Microarray Analysis
Clinical Applications

Real-Time Nucleic-Acid Amplification

Methods of Detecting the Products of Real-Time Amplification

SYBR Green
Hybridization Probes
Clinical Applications

Strain Typing

Non-Amplification-Based Typing

Pulsed-Field Gel Electrophoresis

Amplification-Based Typing

PCR-RLFP
Rep-PCR
Clinical Applications of Microbial Typing

Conclusion

Microbiologists have always searched and continue to search for more rapid and efficient ways to detect and characterize microorganisms. The molecular techniques, introduced into the clinical microbiology laboratory long ago, have provided some of the most powerful tools to date. The migration of modern molecular diagnostic methods from the basic science research laboratories into clinical laboratories has been underway for more than a decade. These assays have revolutionized the microbiology laboratory and have changed the way we detect, characterize, and quantify microorganisms directly in clinical specimens and from cultures. Over the past 15 years, these techniques have progressed from once cumbersome, highly technical, labor-intensive assays to user-friendly tests that are so rapid that it is, in some instances, possible to achieve test results within an hour from the start of the assay, directly from the clinical specimen.

The molecular assays used by the early molecular microbiologist were often used for the detection of only fastidious or uncultivable microorganisms or to determine the cause of significant outbreaks. However, as these assays became easier to use and less expensive, they have been exploited for the detection and characterization of more common microorganisms.

Molecular microbiology may be separated into three categories. The first is the detection of microorganisms without the use of nucleic acid amplification. These applications rely on the amplification of a signal generated, usually light or a color, which is the result of the successful hybridization of a nucleic acid probe with the target nucleic acid molecule. The second is the detection, characterization, and in some instances, quantification of microorganisms using one of a variety of nucleic acid amplification methods that are currently available. Finally, molecular methods have been used extensively to determine the relatedness among microorganisms (i.e., strain typing), which have become a critical tool for the hospital and public health epidemiologist. These technologies, in one way or another, all use nucleic acid chemistry. Therefore, we will begin this chapter with a review of the basics of nucleic acids.

It would be impractical and beyond the scope of this book to review all the molecular assays that have been used in the assessment of microorganisms. Therefore, tests that have proven most useful in the clinical laboratory, tests that are commercially available, and some newer assays that hold particular promise are covered in greater detail. There are now many different types of nucleic acid amplification. The polymerase chain reaction (PCR), which is the forerunner of the other types of nucleic acid amplification assays, and

may on occasion be used in a generic sense in this textbook, is a surrogate term for nucleic acid amplification. This is done for practicality and the flow of the text, but the reader should know that the use of other types of nucleic acid amplification chemistries is also feasible.

Nucleic Acids—The Basics of DNA and RNA
Structure of DNA

Deoxyribonucleic acid (DNA) is a long molecule composed of two strands. Each strand of DNA is a polymer, which means that each strand is composed of repeating similar subunits. The repeating subunits, or the building blocks, of DNA are nucleotide monophosphates. The two strands that compose the DNA molecule have direction determined by their organic chemistry, and they are oriented in directions opposite to one another. The two strands of an intact DNA molecule interact through hydrogen bonds and are termed complementary. The basic configuration of DNA is depicted in Figure 4-1.

There are four kinds of nucleotide monophosphates that make up DNA; they are named according to the type of base they contain. Each nucleotide monophosphate is, in turn, made up of three molecules: the sugar deoxyribose, a phosphate, and a nucleotide base (Fig. 4-2). The backbone of each of the two strands of the DNA molecule consists of alternating deoxyribose sugar and phosphate molecules that are covalently bonded to one another. The nucleotide bases extend from the sugar molecule into the central aspect of the double-stranded DNA molecule. The positions and the orientation of nucleic acids are determined by convention according to the numbering of the carbon molecules of the sugar. The nucleotide base is attached to the sugar at the 1' carbon position. The bridging phosphate molecules are attached at the 3' and 5' carbons, which gives the strand its particular orientation, the importance of which will become clear later in the text. The four nucleotide bases present in DNA are adenine (A) and guanine (G), both of which are purine molecules, and thymine (T) and cytosine (C), both of which are pyrimidine molecules. The purine adenine present on one strand of DNA forms two hydrogen bonds with the pyrimidine thymine on the opposite strand of DNA. These nucleotides are said to be complementary. Similarly the guanine on one DNA strand forms three hydrogen bonds with the complementary cytosine on the opposite strand of DNA.

The structure of DNA is often depicted as a ladder, for simplicity, wherein the rungs of the ladder are made up of complementary bases of the two strands of DNA and the sides of the ladder are understood to represent the alternating

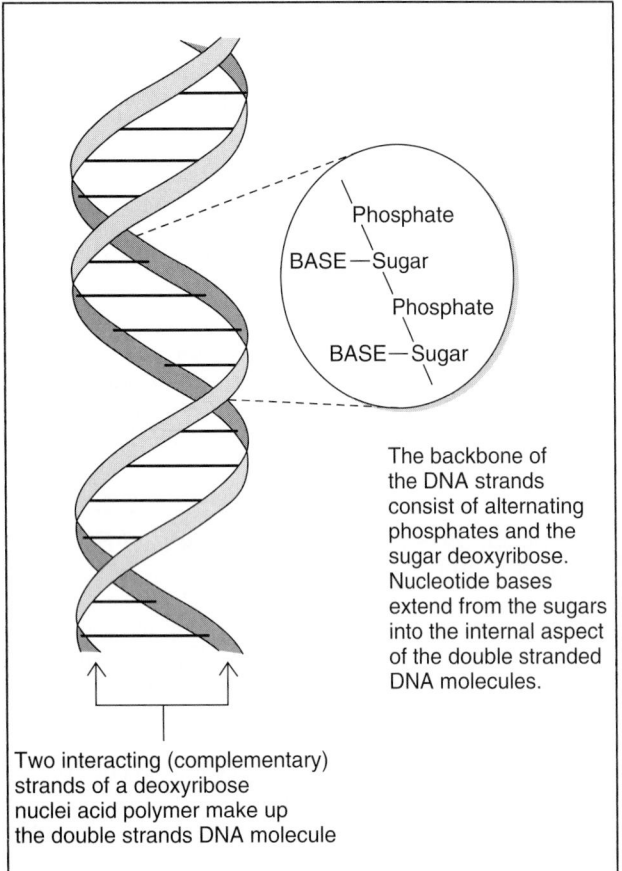

Figure 4-1 Structure of DNA. The structure of DNA has been described as a double helix. DNA is a double-stranded polymer that consists of nucleotides as the basic repetitive unit; nucleotides, in turn, consist of a sugar (deoxyribose), a phosphate, and one of four bases.

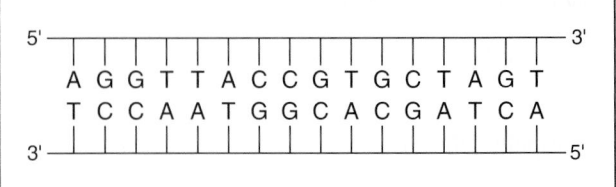

Figure 4-3 Simplified drawing of DNA. The complex structure of DNA is often simplified to that of a ladderlike structure, wherein the rungs of the latter are depicted as the complementary nucleotide bases. This often is simplified even further, wherein only the top strand of DNA is depicted in a 5′ to 3′ direction and the presence of the complementary strand is understood.

length can be packed into very small spaces. The actual structure of DNA is the classic double helix described by James Watson and Francis Crick in 1953 (http://nobelprize.org/medicine/laureates/1962/). The two strands of DNA held together by hydrogen bonds as previously described, exists as a left-handed, helical molecule with major and minor grooves. A knowledge of the basic structure of DNA and the replication of this molecule was pivotal in the development of what are now commonly used nucleic acid amplification-based tests.

Structure of RNA

There are many types of RNA molecules in the cell, but we will confine this discussion to the most commonly described forms, which are messenger RNA (mRNA), transfer RNA (tRNA), and ribosomal RNA (rRNA). The building blocks of RNA are similar to those of DNA. RNA is also a polymer, but it is single-stranded. The backbone of this molecule also consists of alternative sugar and phosphate molecules, but for RNA the sugar is ribose. Like DNA, nucleotide bases are covalently bonded to the sugar molecule. In RNA, however, the nucleotide base thymine is replaced by the base uracil. Although most RNA molecules are single-stranded, they may fold back on themselves and form complementary hydrogen bonds, thereby creating a secondary structure.

sugar phosphate molecules (Fig. 4-3). In life, DNA does not exist, except perhaps temporarily, as a linear molecule. Rather, it is supercoiled; the entire length of the DNA molecule is often greater than the length of the cell that contains it. DNA, therefore, must be supercoiled so that its extensive

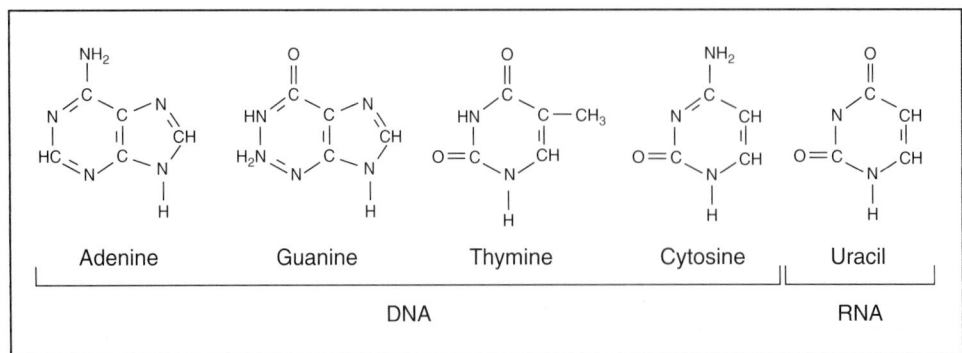

Figure 4-2 Nucleotide bases of DNA and RNA. The four nucleotide bases present in DNA are adenine (A) and guanine (G), both of which are purines, and thymine (T) and cytosine (C), both of which are pyrimidines. Uracil (U) is present in RNA in place of thymine.

Function of DNA—Information Storage

The genes that encode for the vast majority of the structural and functional proteins of the cell are contained in the cell's chromosomal DNA. If the cell requires more protein for its cytoskeleton or if it needs more of an enzyme to metabolize a sugar, it can make more by opening, reading, and using the message in the DNA (see the next section). The DNA has, therefore, been referred to as the blueprint of the cell, which is an apt analogy. When a cell divides, the new cell must also have a copy of the DNA blueprint in order to preserve its structure and perform its functions.

It is important to understand the basics of DNA replication, since many of these principles are used in the PCR and in some other methods of nucleic acid amplification. DNA replication begins with the relaxation of the supercoiled DNA molecule. Then, the more linearized portion of the double helix is at least partially separated into its two component strands. It is as if the rungs of the schematic DNA ladder were sawed down the middle and the two sides of the ladder pulled apart (Fig. 4-4). DNA helicase is an enzyme important in separating the two strands of DNA. One limitation in DNA synthesis, which is performed by DNA polymerase, is that it occurs only from the 5′ to 3′ direction. Therefore, only one strand of DNA can be made in a continuous manner in the 5′ to 3′ direction. This strand, because it is synthesized continuously and more rapidly than the opposing strand, is termed the leading strand. The lagging strand is replicated in sections, since the 5′ end becomes available for synthesis only after DNA helicase has performed its function. The discontinuous portions of DNA that are synthesized on the lagging strand are ligated or annealed one to another by DNA ligase, which makes that final lagging strand a continuous strand of DNA. The end result in the replication of DNA is the creation of two daughter strands of DNA from one parent DNA molecule (Fig. 4-5). Each of the new daughter molecules of DNA consists of one strand from the parent DNA molecule and one newly synthesized strand that is complementary to the parent strand. Each of the newly synthesized double-stranded DNA molecules are perfect matches of the parent DNA molecule, unless an error occurs in replication. DNA replication must precede cell

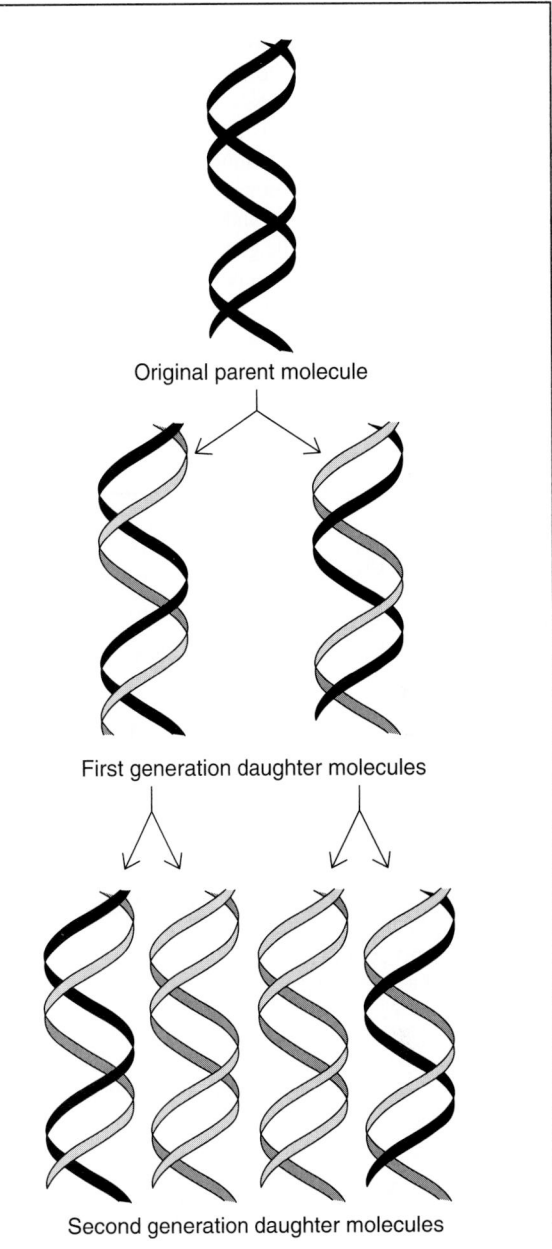

Figure 4-5 Products of DNA replication. Each of the first-generation daughter molecules of DNA contains one strand from the parent molecule and one newly synthesized strand. Two of the daughter molecules of the second generation of DNA replication contain one of the original parent strands and two consist of entirely newly synthesized DNA.

division, so that each new cell formed has a full complement of DNA.

Function of RNA—Information Transfer
READING (TRANSCRIPTION) AND INTERPRETATION (TRANSLATION) OF THE GENETIC CODE

The nucleic acids and proteins of the cell interact in the formation of new proteins, which form the structure and per-

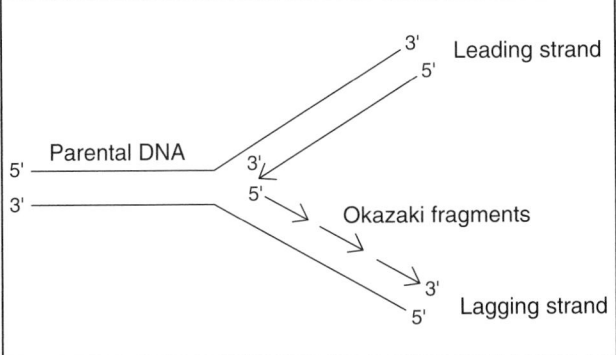

Figure 4-4 DNA replication. DNA replication occurs in a 5′ to 3′ direction. Therefore, one strand, the leading strand, is continuously synthesized, whereas the opposite strand is segmentally synthesized in Okazaki fragments.

form the functions of the cell. The first step in protein synthesis is the "rewriting," or transcription, of the genetic message so that it can be transported to the ribosome. The message, which is encoded by the DNA, is transcribed in the form of an RNA molecule, which is aptly termed messenger RNA (mRNA). This occurs in a manner similar to DNA synthesis, but uses a different set of enzymes. Briefly, the DNA strand is unwound and a single-stranded RNA molecule is created that is complementary to the gene being transcribed. This may or may not undergo additional processing (transcriptional processing), depending on the type of cell in which it is occurring. The message is then read or the genetic code is translated by the cellular machinery. This involves other types of RNA molecules, such as tRNA, rRNA, and a variety of proteins.

The translation of the message into a protein occurs on a complicated superstructure composed of proteins and rRNA termed the ribosome. The mRNA becomes associated with the ribosome and is processed three bases at a time. These three base pair segments are called codons, and they encode for particular amino acids. The codons on the mRNA are complementary to anticodons on a portion of the tRNA. Particular tRNAs transport or transfer particular amino acids to the ribosome, the site of protein synthesis. The amino acid molecules are situated so that peptide bonds may be enzymatically formed between them. Eventually, a chain of amino acids is formed (a peptide), which through continued extension, secondary structure folding, and posttranslational modifications becomes a protein (Fig. 4-6). The reader who is interested in

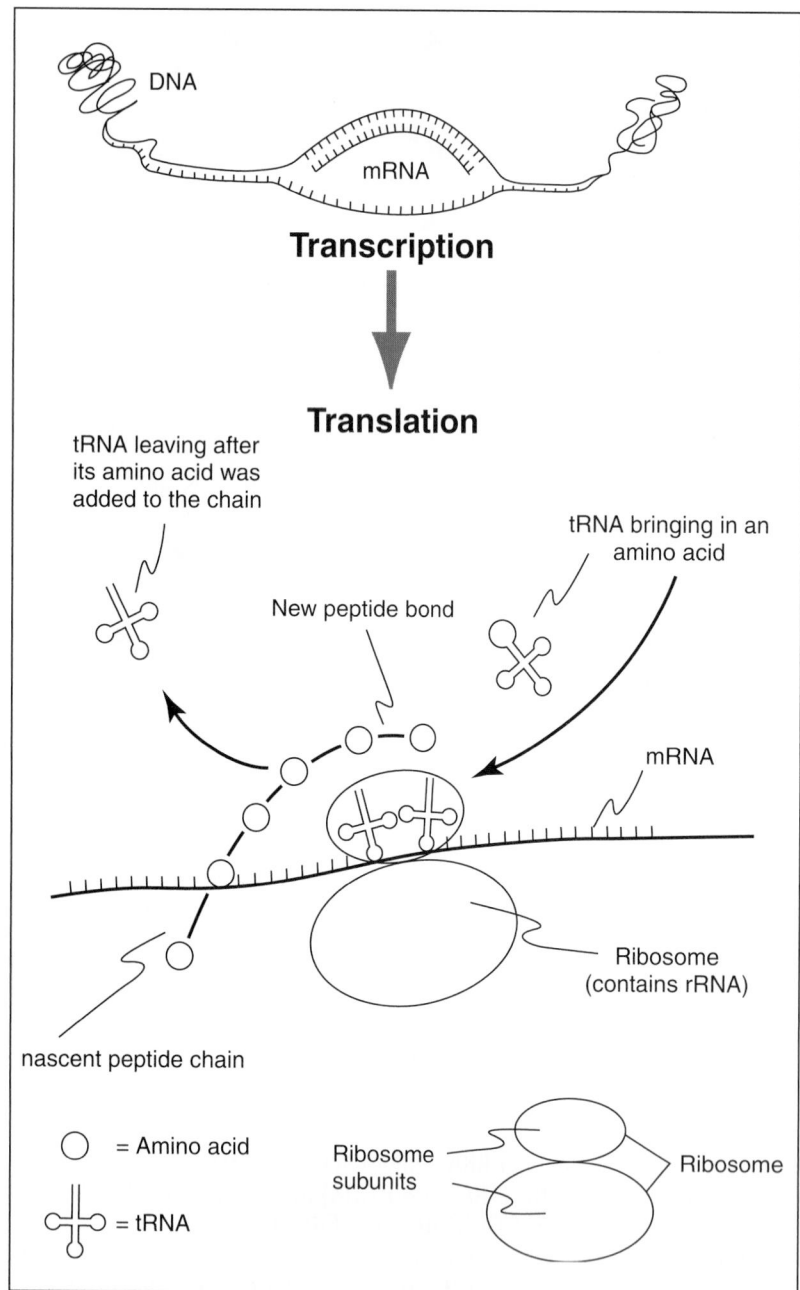

Figure 4-6 Schematic of transcription and translation. In the most basic representation, the genetic message in DNA is rewritten or transcribed (transcription) into messenger RNA (mRNA), which is used as the substrate for translation (the forming of proteins from the genetic code).

obtaining a more thorough understanding of these processes is directed to textbooks of biochemistry and molecular biology.[5,333]

Signal-Amplification Methods

The signal-amplification methods described combine some type of nucleic acid, usually a probe, with a generation of a signal. The signal is often amplified through an enzymatic reaction. The signal from fluorescence in situ hybridization (FISH), however, may be directly observed, following the hybridization of the fluorescently labeled probe to its complementary nucleic acid target. A variety of chemical and enzymatic modifications may be applied to FISH or chromogenic in situ hybridization if further amplification of the signal is necessary, but are beyond the scope of this book. We will discuss four types of signal amplification in this section: nucleic acid probes, Hybrid Capture, branched-chain DNA, and in situ hybridization.

Signal amplification is usually considered to be less sensitive than nucleic acid amplification methods. One exception may be FISH, wherein a single copy of a target molecule may be identified in a large population of other cells. This application of FISH is more useful in anatomic pathology specimens or research, wherein a minor subpopulation of cells may be of clinical importance. Signal-amplification technologies have several advantages over nucleic acid amplification methods. These procedures are far less likely to produce false-positive results secondary to contamination compared with traditional nucleic acid amplification assays. However, signal contamination or the bleed over of a strong signal from one reaction chamber into an adjacent well has been reported.

Nucleic-Acid Probes

Nucleic-acid probes were the first molecular assays to become commonplace in many laboratories. The probes, termed AccuProbes, are commercially available for the detection numerous microorganisms from Gen-Probe (San Diego, CA). These are DNA probes that contain a chemiluminescent label and target the rRNA of the microorganism of interest, which is a useful target since the rRNA is present in greater quantities than the rDNA genes that encode for it. This is an example of biologic amplification, or the amplification of a nucleic acid that occurs during the normal course of cellular events or secondary to microorganism growth. This proprietary chemistry allows for the differentiation of the hybridized from the nonhybridized probe. When the stable DNA-RNA hybrid is treated with the detection reagents provided, light is produced secondary to a chemical reaction. The presence of a certain amount of light that exceeds a predetermined threshold value is considered a positive reaction and indicates the presence of the microorganism to which the probe was designed to hybridize.

CLINICAL APPLICATIONS

AccuProbe genetic probes are available for the direct detection of bacteria in clinical specimens or as a rapid and specific method of identifying microorganisms in culture. The products available for the direct detection of bacteria in clinical specimens are the PACE products (GenProbe, Inc., San Diego, CA) for the detection of N. gonorrhoeae and C. trachomatis, and an assay for the direct detection of group A Streptococcus. The PACE products, at the time of their introduction represented a significant advance in sensitivity compared with culture for these fastidious pathogens.[45,116] However, these products are slightly less sensitive than the nucleic acid amplification assays with which they must now compete.[38,116,194] The group A Streptococcus assay is an easy-to-use test that has approximately the same sensitivity and specificity as culture. Although the product may be more expensive than the materials needed for culture, the savings in the labor required for subculturing and confirmatory testing, such as latex agglutination, makes the Group A Streptococcus Direct Test (Gen-Probe) an attractive option.[38]

Today, genetic probes remain a useful option for the rapid identification of a variety of microorganisms in culture, many of which would otherwise require complicated and time-consuming tests for identification. The most useful of these in many laboratories have been for the rapid identification of mycobacteria and the dimorphic fungi. Genetic probes are commercially available for the Mycobacterium tuberculosis complex, M. kansasii, M. gordonae, and the M. avium–intracellulare complex.[72,112,234] Genetic probes are also available for Histoplasma capsulatum, Blastomyces dermatitidis, and Coccidioides immitis.[128,151] The use of these probes for the characterization of cultures that contain mycobacteria or fungi suspected to be dimorphic fungi, respectively, significantly diminishes the time to identification for the clinical laboratory when compared with routine, traditional methods. Although more expensive, these may save money for the laboratory, when cost of both materials and labor are considered.

A variety of AccuProbes are also available for the identification of certain bacteria in culture. These include assays for Campylobacter, group A and group B Streptococcus, Haemophilus influenzae, Streptococcus pneumoniae, Staphylococcus aureus, Listeria monocytogenes, and N. gonorrhoeae.[60] These assays, when performed from cultures, have sensitivities and specificities in the high 90s to 100%. The advantage of using these assays is time savings. The disadvantage is higher cost.

Hybrid Capture

Hybrid Capture (Digene, Gaithersburg, MD) is a signal-amplification technology that consists of the retention (capture) of a DNA-RNA molecular complex (a hybrid) in a tube or microtiter plate (Fig. 4-7). Initially, the specimen is processed to prepare the DNA. The RNA probes used are complementary to the DNA molecule from the microorganism of interest. The detection of a DNA-RNA hybrid complex is useful, since this complex exists only transiently in nature, primarily during transcription. If the complex is not present, the specimen is considered negative. The DNA-RNA hybrid, if present, is introduced into a tube or the well of a microtiter plate, the walls of which have been coated with a monoclonal antibody that recognizes a DNA-RNA hybrid. This antibody captures and immobilizes the complex

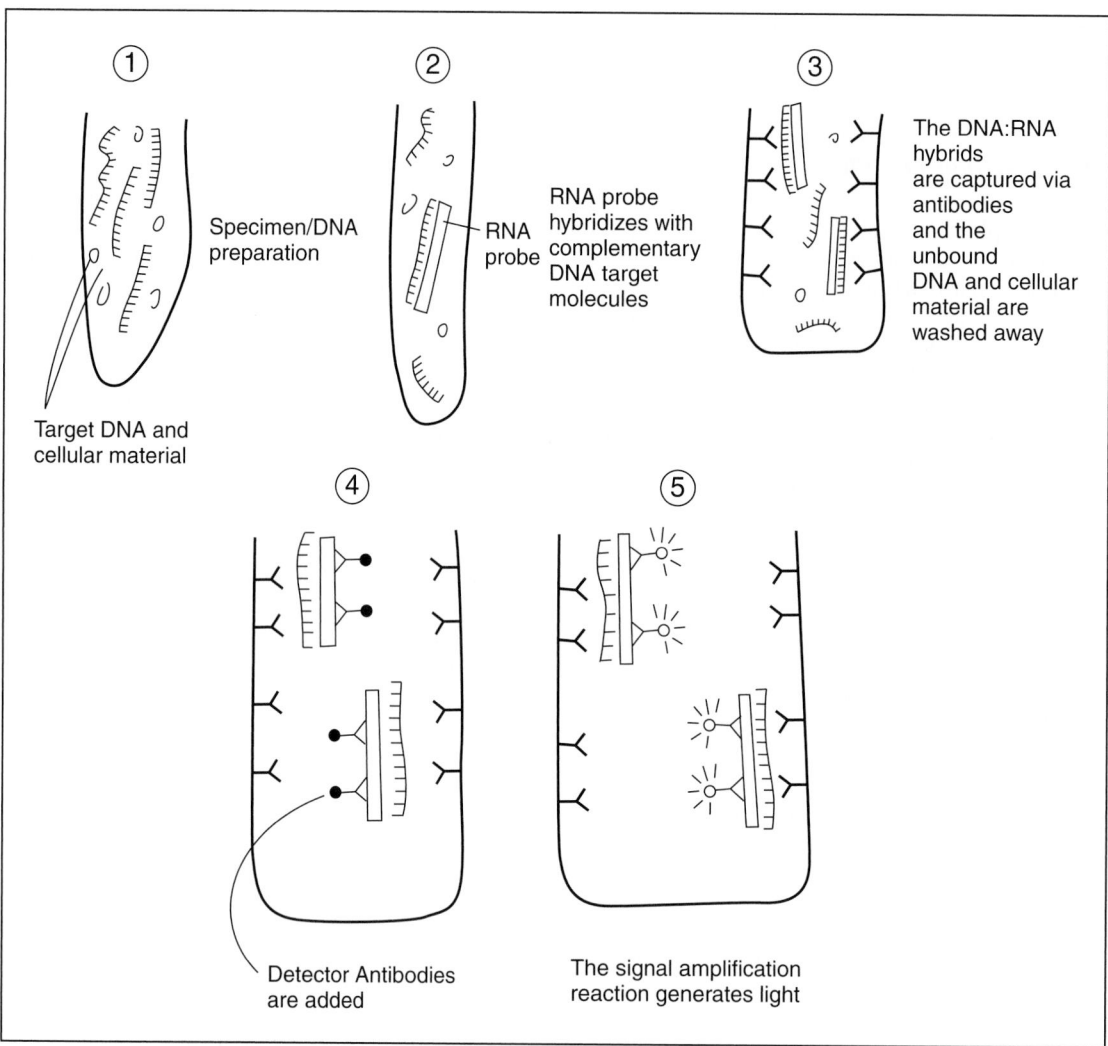

Figure 4-7 Hybrid Capture technology. Hybrid capture technology is a signal-amplification assay. It has become a popular way to detect high-risk HPV subtypes and to determine the CMV viral load in the blood.

and allows the other constituents of the processed clinical specimen to be washed away. Next, another antibody is added that also recognizes the DNA-RNA complex, but this antibody is labeled with a reporter molecule and able to generate a signal in the form of light. Light above a certain threshold is considered a positive reaction.

CLINICAL APPLICATIONS

There are Hybrid Capture (HC) assays commercially available for the detection of high-risk human papillomavirus (HPV) subtypes, *Neisseria gonorrhoeae* and *Chlamydia trachomatis*, and cytomegalovirus (CMV). The high-risk HPV assay has become an important supplemental assay for women with cytologic diagnoses of atypical squamous cells of undetermined significance (ASCUS). A meta-analysis showed that the HCII assay had a greater sensitivity and equivalent specificity compared with a repeat Pap smear for the detection of women with cervical intraepithelial neoplasia type 2 (CIN 2) lesions or higher, whose initial Pap smear

was interpreted as ASCUS.[7] In addition, it has been added to the recommendations of the American College of Obstetricians and Gynecologists as an adjunct to cytologic screening for women over 30 years old.[2] The strength of this assay is its high sensitivity and its high negative predictive value.[149] It has been found by some to even be comparable to PCR; however, others have found it slightly less sensitive.[28,46] Although this is a highly useful assay, both the sensitivity and the specificity have been questioned.[65,273] de Cremoux et al. showed that some of the false-positive reactions with this assay were due to probe cross-reactivity with low-risk HPV subtypes, whereas others were likely due to "signal contamination" or bleed over of the fluorescent signal from a strongly positive wells into an adjacent well that contained negative specimens.[65] The final role that the molecular detection and classification of HPV will play in the routine screening of women for the enhanced detection of dysplasia and carcinoma remains to be determined. It seems, however, that HPV testing in some form is here to stay.

The hybrid capture has also been used successfully for the detection of *N. gonorrhoeae* and *C. trachomatis.*[61,62,227,305,350] This assay has been reported to be more sensitive than culture, which is not surprising given the fastidious nature of these pathogens, and more sensitive than genetic probe analysis.[62] Rigorous comparisons between Hybrid Capture for the detection of *N. gonorrhoeae* and *C. trachomatis* compared with nucleic-acid amplification assays have yet to be accomplished.

Hybrid capture technology may also be used to detect the CMV and HBV in the blood. The HBV test is a qualitative assay, whereas the CMV Hybrid Capture test is quantitative.[349] The amount of signal generated in the assay is proportional to the amount of target present. When the data generated is used in conjunction with the quantitative standards provided by the manufacturer, a viral load may be calculated. The CMV viral load, by this and other methods, has been found useful for monitoring patients who have received solid organ and stem cell (bone marrow) tranplants.[247,367] When compared with PCR, the hybrid capture technology is less 1.5–2.0 log less sensitive than PCR; the specificities of PCR and hybrid capture in this comparison were 100% and 93.8%, respectively.[32]

Branched DNA

Branched-DNA technology is used for the detection and quantification of pathogens such as HIV, HBV, and HCV. This technology consists of a variety of branched DNA (bDNA) probes and signal-amplification reporter molecules. In brief, the organism-specific bDNA oligonucleotide probes hybridize to the target nucleic-acid molecule and this complex is captured onto a solid substrate. Branched-DNA oligonucleotide reporter molecules, which are conjugated to reporter enzymes, are added. These, in turn, generate a chemiluminescent signal after the addition of the appropriate substrate. The amount of signal, as with the hybrid capture assay, is proportional to the amount of target nucleic acid, which means quantitative results can be generated when this assay is performed with quantitative standards.[301,348]

CLINICAL APPLICATIONS

Although a very useful and highly reproducible technology, a large number of clinical assays that use this technology have not been developed. This technology has been used most successfully for the detection and quantification of the HIV, HBV, and HCV.[42,81,255,375] It has become the standard of care to monitor the viral loads of patients infected with HIV. The VERSANT HIV-1 RNA 3.0 (Bayer Diagnostics, Tarrytown, NY) has been found to be a highly reproducible assay with wide linear range (75–500 copies of HIV-1 RNA) that is useful for quantitative HIV-1 viral load measurements, even when compared with reverse transcriptase (RT)-PCR.[80,110] Similarly, multicenter evaluations of the VERSANT Hepatitis B DNA 3.0 assay and the VERSANT HCV RNA 3.0 assay found that these assays and this technology were reproducible, had a wide dynamic range, and demonstrated results comparable with other commonly used assays.[79,255,375] Although the sensitivity of the bDNA assays may be slightly less than that for PCR, there is overall a good correlation between viral loads generated by these different assays.[59,231]

In Situ Hybridization

In situ hybridization has been used in the molecular pathology for many years to detect chromosomal translocations (i.e., t9;22), gene amplifications (i.e., Her2/neu) and for the identification of infectious agents.[215] These once complex methods are becoming easier to use, and semiautomated platforms are available. *In situ* hybridization by be separated into fluorescent *in situ* hybridization (FISH), wherein the oligonucleotide probe is labeled with a fluorophore that is detected by direct fluorescence microscopy, and chromogenic *in situ* hybridization (CISH), wherein the oligonucleotide probe is labeled in such a way that an enzymatic reaction generates a color that can be viewed using traditional light microscopy. More recently several studies have demonstrated the feasibility and potential advantages of *in situ* assays in the clinical microbiology laboratory.[148,158,170,239,240,285]

Some of the first *in situ* hybridization assays used were for the detection of viruses through direct hybridization of an oligonucleotide probe and the viral nucleic acids. These have been used to confirm the identify the particular virus associated with a certain a cytologic effect (i.e., CMV as a cause of a Cowdry type A intranuclear inclusion), as well as to differentiate viruses that produce identical cytopathic effects (i.e., HSV and VZV).[26] This technology may also be used to differentiate the high-risk and low-risk HPV subtypes.[323]

In situ hybridization has also proven useful as a technology that allows for the demonstration of the certain viruses with neoplasia, such as HPV with dysplasia/squamous-cell carcinoma of the uterine cervix, Epstein-Barr virus (EBV) with posttransplantation lymphoproliferative disorders and Burkitt's lymphoma, and human herpesvirus 8 (HHV-8) with Kaposi's sarcoma.[323,355,36,195] The direct visualization of the virally infected cells in the focus of pathology helps support the etiologic role of the detected organism with the disease. Although the detection of viruses using *in situ* hybridization has proven useful in the molecular pathology laboratory, it is uncommon to find these technologies used in clinical virology laboratories.

In situ hybridization may also be used for the detection of bacteria, mycobacteria, fungi, and parasites. When *in situ* hybridization is used to detect these organisms the microbial rRNA may be used as the target for the hybridization probe. This may advantageous over a DNA target for two reasons. First, there are many more copies of rRNA in the cell than there are copies of the genes that encode for the ribosomes (rDNA), which increases the sensitivity of the assay. Second, the presence of rRNA helps denote the presence of a viable organism, wherein the detection of DNA, particularly by methods such as PCR, may occur even after the organism is nonviable (i.e., killed by antimicrobial therapy).

Prior to the relatively recent introduction of FISH into the clinical microbiology laboratory, these technologies have been used by environmental microbiologists to identify and enumerate *Legionella*, *E. coli*, and other bacteria in water samples and biofilms.[208,207,264] Veterinary microbiologists have also used these techniques to study a variety of diseases.[184,199] The molecular pathologist has used the *in situ* hybridization to study *Helicobacter pylori* in gastric biopsies, *Chlamydia* in a variety of disease states, and *Legionella pneumophila* in fixed respiratory specimens.[16,14,159,124,21,106]

The ability to rapidly characterize mycobacteria as tuberculosis or nontuberculous mycobacteria has been the goal of many assays. The mycobacteria are excellent candidates for identification by molecular methods, since some of these cause severe disease and are slow-growing in culture (i.e., *M. tuberculosis*), and some are fastidious (i.e., *M. genevense* and *M. haemophilum*) or cannot be cultivated on artificial media (i.e., *M. leprae*). FISH using peptide nucleic-acid probes has been used successfully for the rapid identification of *M. tuberculosis* in smears from mycobacterial cultures and directly in respiratory samples that contained acid-fast bacilli.[244,330,331] Traditional *in situ* applications have also been used in histologic sections to definitely identify *M. leprae*.[8]

Fungi and parasites have also been characterized by *in situ* hybridization. *In situ* hybridization assays have been described for the identification of *Aspergillus* species, which is important given the increasing importance of non-*Aspergillus* hyaline septate molds, such as *Fusarium* and *Pseudallescheria*, that are pathogenic to humans and have antifungal susceptibility profiles that are different from most *Aspergillus* species.[135,248,380] These methods are especially important when the excised material was not submitted for culture or if the mold fails to grow in culture. Chromogenic *in situ* hybridization, using a tyramide signal amplification method, has also been applied to the difficult histologic differential diagnosis of morphologically similar yeast and yeastlike forms in human tissues.[141] These methods were less sensitive than the methenamine silver stain for the detection of some of the fungi, but they demonstrated 100% specificity with species-specific identification.[141] Another fungus that has been studied using *in situ* hybridization is *Pneumocystis jiroveci*.[140] The use of *in situ* hybridization for the detection of this fungus may hold some advantages, since both the trophozoite and cyst forms may be detected, rather than only the cyst form, which is the case with some histochemical stains, such as Gomori's methenamine silver (GMS) stain.

CLINICAL APPLICATIONS

Most of the work to date regarding the use of *in situ* hybridization for the detection of microorganisms in clinical specimens has been done in molecular pathology laboratories in fixed, often paraffin-embedded specimens. However, this technology holds perhaps even greater promise for routine use in the clinical microbiology laboratory. Jansen et al.[158] and Kempf et al.[170] simultaneously published articles investigating the use of *in situ* hybridization for the rapid identification of organisms present in positive blood culture bottles. A variety of probes were used, all of which were directed against specific target sequences present in bacterial rRNA. Some probes were genus- and family-inclusive probes (i.e., all staphylococci or all Enterobacteriaceae, respectively), whereas others were specific for particular species (i.e., *Staphylococcus aureus* or *Escherichia coli*). The majority of these probes were highly accurate for the identification of the bacteria responsible for the positive blood cultures. One attractive feature of these assays was that the

selection of the *in situ* hybridization probes to be used could be directed based on the findings of the Gram stain. Another attractive feature was the time to detection, which may be as little a 2–3 hours. Kempf et al. compared the time to identification for *in situ* hybridization to traditional methods for 115 positive blood cultures they examined. They found an approximate time savings of 26 hours for the identification of staphylococci (62 of 62 identified by *in situ* hybridization [ISH]), 46 hours for streptococci (19 of 20 identified by ISH), and 40 hours for gram-negative bacilli (28 of 30 identified by ISH).[170] Overall, they concluded that with a limited number of *in situ* hybridization probes, the cause of 96.5% of positive blood cultures could be identified within 2.5 hours, whereas conventional culture took between 1 and 3 days.[170]

In situ hybridization has also been used for the direct detection of pathogenic bacteria directly in clinical specimens. Hogardt et al. used *in situ* hybridization to detect and identify the bacteria likely to be present in the respiratory specimens of patients with cystic fibrosis.[148] They tested for *Pseudomonas aeruginosa*, *Burkholderia cepacia*, *Stenotrophomonas maltophilia*, *Haemophilus influenzae*, and *Staphylococcus aureus* using *in situ* hybridization. The *in situ* hybridization assays performed directly on the clinical specimen demonstrated 90% sensitivity and 100% specificity compared with culture, even in the complicated milieu of respiratory specimens from patients with cystic fibrosis.[148] It is conceivable that a battery of *in situ* hybridization probes may be useful for the detection of pathogens that are commonly associated with particular diseases, such as bacterial meningitis and community-acquired pneumonia.

Another method of ISH, which uses a peptide nucleic-acid (PNA) probe rather than a DNA probe has been developed and is commercially available. Peptide nucleic-acid probes have properties that may be advantageous over DNA probes with regard to penetration, when hybridization is performed on intact organisms, and for greater differentiation, particularly of single nucleotide polymorphisms.[329] AdvanDx (Woburn, MA) is a supplier of PNA ISH kits for the rapid detection of *S. aureus*, *Candida albicans*, and *E. faecalis*. Several studies have examined this assay and found it to be useful for differentiating *S. aureus* from coagulase-negative staphylococci in blood culture bottles that signal positive and contain gram-positive cocci in clusters in the Gram stain.[39,239,240]

In situ hybridization has also been shown to be useful for the rapid identification and differentiation of clinically important yeast in positive blood cultures. Kempf et al. differentiated *C. albicans*, *C. glabrata*, *C. krusei*, and *C. parapsilosis* using four ISH probes.[170] Similarly, the *Candida albicans* PNA FISH assay (AdvanDx) has been shown to differentiate *C. albicans* from non–*C. albicans* yeast in positive blood cultures[241,285] (Fig. 4-8). The rapid and accurate differentiation of yeast is important, since some non-*Candida albicans* species, such as *C. glabrata* and *C. krusei*, are more likely to be resistant to fluconazole, a common drug used to treat *C. albicans* infections.[343]

Traditional and PNA *in situ* hybridization has also been used for the rapid differentiation of mycobacteria. The mycobacteria are obvious targets for differentiation by molecular methods, since members of this group cause severe dis-

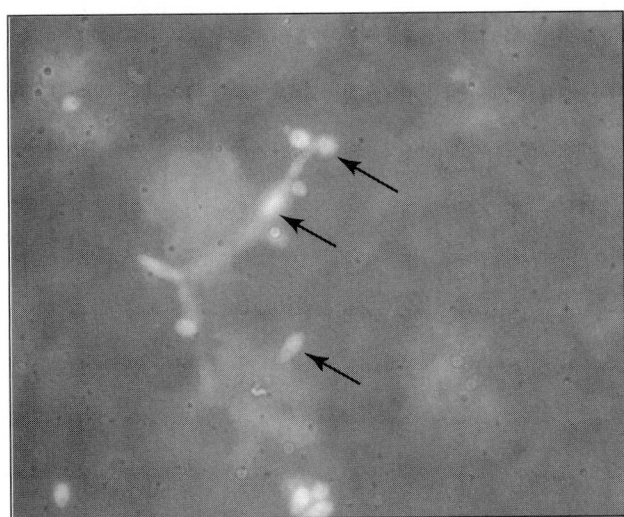

Figure 4-8 *Candida albicans* PNA FISH. The yeast and pseudohyphae (*arrows*) fluoresce apple green and are easily detected against the red background using the *Candida albicans* PNA FISH (AdvanDx).

ease (i.e., *M. tuberculosis*), many are slow-growing, and one at least, *M. leprae*, has not been cultivated on artificial media. *In situ* hybridization has been used to differentiate *M. tuberculosis* from non-tuberculous mycobacteria in cultures that become positive, as well as directly from positive acid-fast smears and in histologic sections.[331,379] The confirmation of *M. leprae* in histologic sections has also been achieved with *in situ* hybridization.[8]

There has been limited use of *in situ* hybridization when studying parasites and parasitic diseases, but some uses have been described.[156,251,346,381] There has been even less use in the clinical parasitology laboratory. *In situ* hybridization has been used to detect the most common microsporidia, *Enterocytozoon bieneusi*, which causes gastroenteritis in patients with AIDS.[356] Peptide nucleic-acid FISH has been used to detect circulating trypanosomes of patients with African sleeping sickness.[275]

In situ hybridization is a molecular diagnostic tool that is new to most clinical microbiology laboratories. Depending on the availability of commercial products, this technology could influence the way we practice clinical microbiology. The rapid time to detection, and the ability to selectively choose probes to be used based on the findings of the Gram stain or the characteristics of the patient population under consideration makes this technology attractive as a diagnostic tool.

Nucleic-Acid Amplification
Basics of the Polymerase Chain Reaction

The polymerase chain reaction, first described by Kary Mullis in 1983, exploits the basic biochemistry of DNA replication, with the end goal of amplification of a particular portion of DNA.[232,233] The portion of DNA that is amplified usually contains diagnostically useful information. The PCR reaction mixture consists of the target DNA for amplification

and the master mix. The master mix, in turn, consists of oligonucleotide DNA primers, the four nucleotide triphosphates, thermostable DNA polymerase, magnesium chloride and water or buffers. The polymerase chain reaction consists of three phases, which are repetitive, which is the basis for the "chain reaction" portion of the name. These three phases are: 1) DNA denaturation—or the separation of the two strands of DNA, 2) primer annealing, and 3) primer extension—the portion of the reaction wherein DNA synthesis occurs.

Denaturation of the template DNA molecule or separation of the two individual strands that compose the parent double-stranded DNA molecule is the first step of PCR. This is accomplished by elevating the temperature of the reaction mixture to approximately 95°C. At this temperature, the double-stranded DNA is physically separated into single strands. This occurs because the elevated thermal energy breaks the hydrogen bonds that hold the two strands of DNA together at lower temperatures. Thermal denaturation of DNA is favored over chemical denaturation, since it is readily reversible by cooling.

The next step in PCR, primer annealing, begins when the reaction mixture is cooled and the oligonucleotide primers, which flank the area to be amplified, hybridize with the single strands of the template DNA molecule. The oligonucleotide primers are short pieces of DNA, usually between 12 and 20 nucleotides in length, which are necessary to start or prime the DNA synthesis reaction. One primer is the same sense as the upper strand of DNA and is termed the forward primer, as denoted (Fig. 4-9), whereas the other is the same sense as the opposite stand of DNA and is termed the reverse primer. The primers hybridize to the target through traditional Watson and Crick base pairing, so the primer annealing temperature should be less than or equal to the T_M, or melting temperature, of the primers used; for simplicity, the T_M is the temperature at which the primers anneal.

When choosing a set of primers, number of technical factors must be considered, many of which are now included in primer design software programs. These are dealt with by industrial scientists when we purchase commercially available PCR kits. Most of the details of primer design are beyond the scope of this book, however a few points deserve mention. If a single DNA-amplification product, also known as an amplicon, is desired, then the primers should be chosen to hybridize with a single region of the DNA molecule of interest. It is important that the primers do not hybridize with other areas of the molecule from the same organism, or with the DNA of another species that may be present in the specimen preparation. For example, if the molecular microbiologist is attempting to detect *Legionella pneumophila* in clinical specimens, then they should choose a region unique to this microorganism that is not present in the human genome. This has been done successfully by targeting the macrophage infectivity potentiator (*mip*) gene, which contains regions unique enough to differentiation *L. pneumophila* from other bacteria, and is not a constituent of the human genome.[284,370] Cross-reactivity with the human genome would, at best, nonspecifically exhaust the primers and nucleotide triphosphate bases in the reaction mixture, and could, at worst, result in a false-positive PCR reaction, depending on the detection system used.

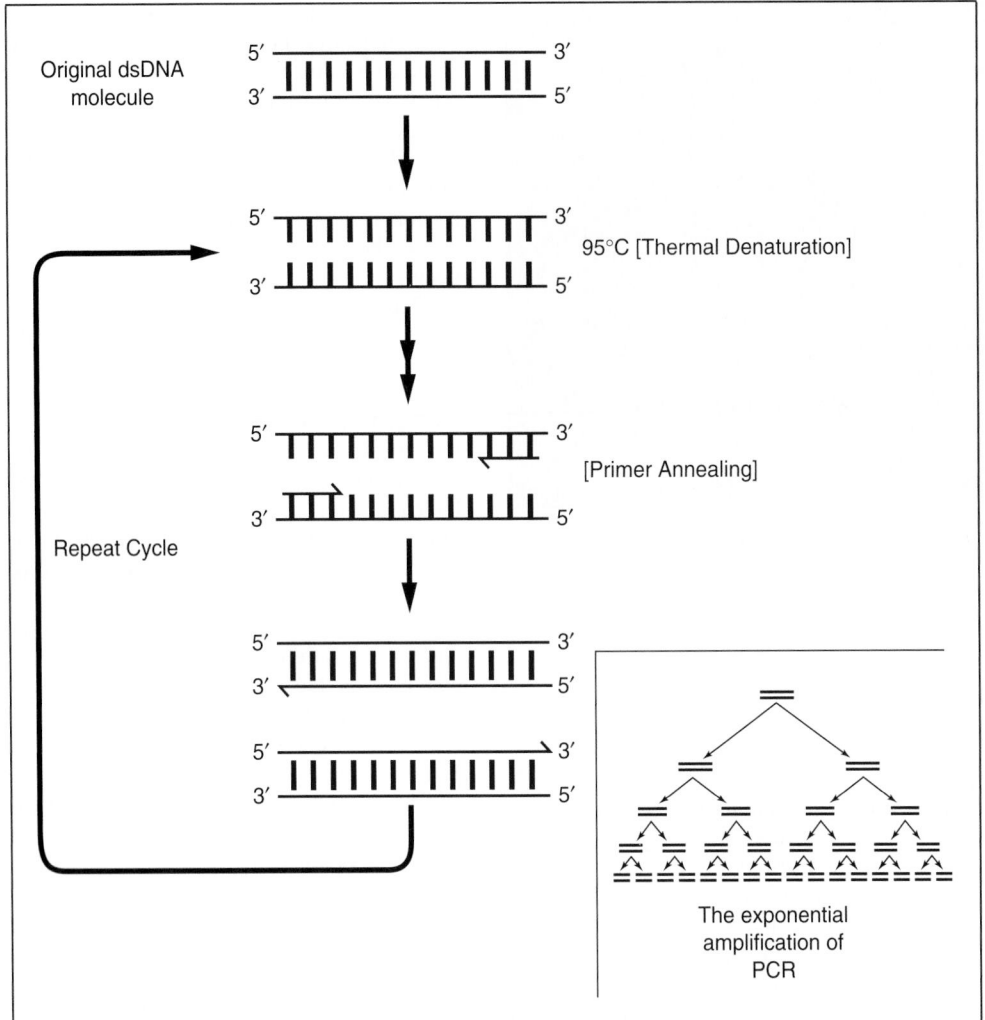

Figure 4-9 Polymerase chain reaction. The polymerase chain reaction is a repetitive cycling of thermal denaturation, primer annealing, and extension of the primers through the action of DNA polymerase (not shown here). The reaction results in the exponential production of new DNA molecules, the beginning and end of which are determined by the positions of the forward and reverse primers.

The presence of the products of PCR amplification is often first assessed by examining the products following gel electrophoresis and staining with ethidium bromide. The presence of a single band in the gel is good preliminary evidence of the specificity of the reaction. The presence of multiple bands suggests that the primers are nonspecific and/or the stringency conditions of the reaction are not optimal (Fig. 4-10). In some instances, the specificity may be improved by changing the reaction conditions, such as salt concentration or primer annealing temperature. The easiest of these to change is the primer annealing temperature. The specificity of the binding of the primers to the target DNA molecule will increase as the annealing temperature used approaches the T_M of the primers, a more stringent condition.

The synthesis of a new strand of DNA that is complementary to the parent strand of DNA is accomplished by DNA polymerase after primer annealing is complete. The discovery of a thermostable DNA polymerase enzyme afforded the

cycling of this reaction in a closed tube, without the need to add new enzyme after each thermal nucleic-acid denaturation step. DNA polymerase synthesizes the new complementary strand at a rate of approximately 25 bp/sec. This is important to determine how long the extension phase of the reaction should last, which is based on the length of the amplicon. After the appropriate amount of time has elapsed to allow for complete extension of the amplicon, the reaction mixture is again cycled to 95°C for another cycle of the PCR.

In this manner, the target portion from one molecule of DNA is amplified exponentially to form millions of amplicons. This exponential increase of the target region of DNA explains the exquisite sensitivity of the PCR reaction and the ability of diagnostic tests that use such methods to detect a very low number of pathogens. This extreme sensitivity also explains the great caution that must be taken when working with amplified DNA, since each of the amplified molecules, if released into the environment could contami-

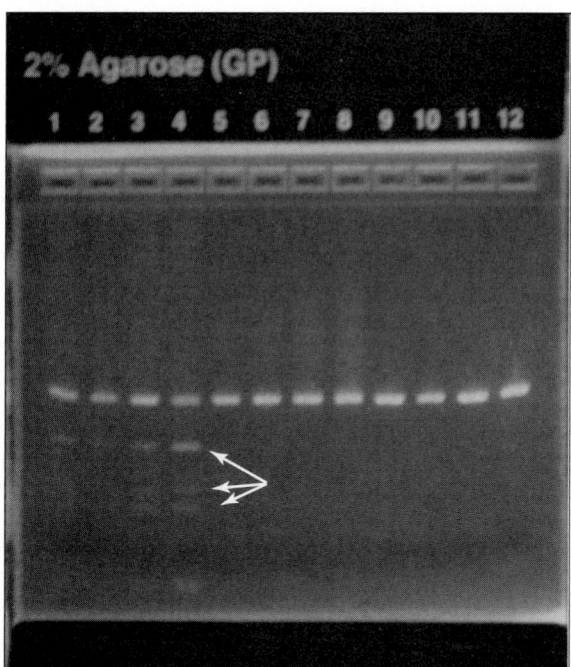

Figure 4-10 Nonspecific nucleic-acid amplification. Nonspecific nucleic-acid amplification may occur during the polymerase chain reaction or other nucleic-acid amplification assays if the primers hybridize to an alternative site or bind with one another and form primer-dimers. Nonspecific amplification and primer dimers may be minimized through careful assay design and optimization of the reaction conditions. Lanes 1–5 all demonstrate nonspecific amplification bands, but these are most prominent in lane 5 (*arrows*).

nate a clinical specimen (amplicon contamination) and result in a false-positive reaction. Although PCR sounds as if a single copy of target DNA should be detectable, in practice, there are numerous PCR inhibitors in clinical specimens that limit the sensitivity of these assays. Although nucleic-acid extraction is not covered in detail here, the preamplification processing of clinical specimens, to purge them of inhibitors and prepare them for nucleic-acid amplification, is likely as important as the amplification reaction itself.

CLINICAL APPLICATIONS

The introduction of PCR into the diagnostic laboratory represented a significant advance in medicine. PCR-based assays have allowed laboratory workers to detect organisms that could not be cultured as well as those that were fastidious and/or slow-growing. The early methods of detecting the products of PCR, however, were laborious and time-consuming (see Postamplification Analysis,'' below). Early PCR-based assays, therefore, were reserved for only the most significant of pathogens. The development of automated and semiautomated PCR platforms and easier, more timely methods of detection increased the use of these technologies, which continues today, for a wider variety of pathogens. Almost every microorganism of clinical interest has been detected and studied by PCR.

Apart from detection, PCR provided researcher with a tool to examine the presence or absence of particular genetic elements within populations, and, when coupled with DNA sequencing, allowed researchers to examine the composition and variability of genes of interest. Reverse-transcriptase PCR (see below) allowed researchers to detect RNA viruses and to measure the genetic response (i.e., the mRNA) of organisms and eukaryotic cells to a variety of stimuli.

Commercial assays, which have received FDA approval, are available to detect two of the most common sexually transmitted bacteria, *N. gonorrhoeae* and *C. trachomatis*.[176,192] Although extremely useful because of an exquisite sensitivity that far exceeds culture, these assays are not perfect.[132] The specificity of these assays, although extremely high, is not 100%, which means in a population of low prevalence the positive predictive value is suboptimal and false-positive results may occur, and confirmatory testing is recommended.[70,337,351] Furthermore, the commercially available *N. gonorrhoeae* PCR assay, as well as the assay that used strand displacement amplification (see below) have been shown to have the capacity to cross-react with certain nongonococcal *Neisseria* species, which could cause a false-positive reaction,[4,84,86] FDA-approved PCR assays are commercially available for the rapid identification of *M. tuberculosis* in acid-fast bacillus (AFB) smear–positive respiratory specimens.[98,282] FDA-approved modifications that use rapid-cycle PCR are available for the rapid detection of group B *Streptococcus* and methicillin-resistant *S. aureus* (see ''Real-Time Nucleic-Acid Amplification,'' below). FDA-approved assays that use RT-PCR (see below) are available for the detection and quantification of RNA viruses, such as HIV and HCV. There are other FDA-approved assays and a wide variety of commercially available analyte-specific reagent (ASR) and research use only (RUO) kits available for the study of a variety of human pathogens.

Other Methods of Nucleic-Acid Amplification

There are several different methods of nucleic-acid amplification that have been devised, many to avoid licensing fees associated with PCR. Commercial diagnostic kits for several microbial pathogens are available. One of the first of these to be marketed, which is no longer available, used the ligase chain reaction. This method was the first commercially available nucleic-acid amplification assay to become available and widely used for the detection of *N. gonorrhoeae* and *C. trachomatis*. The non-PCR methods that are currently commercially available are the nucleic-acid sequence-based amplification (NASBA) (bioMérieux, Durham, NC) and transcription-medicated amplification (TMA) (GenProbe, San Diego, CA), which are basically the same technology, and strand-displacement amplification (SDA) (BD Diagnostic Systems, Sparks, MD).

The ligase chain reaction in its purest form is really a signal-amplification reaction that relies on the ligation or connection of two probes that anneal contiguously on the template DNA strand. This technology, when combined with limited extension by DNA polymerase, was the basis of the Abbott products (LCx *Neisseria gonorrhoeae* or LCx *Chlamydia trachomatis* assays, Abbott Park, IL) for the detection of *N. gonorrhoeae* and *C. trachomatis*. The use of the two-probe system necessary for the ligase contributed to its excellent sensitivity. The drawback of this assay was the lack of an internal control. Given the absence of this technology from the commercial market, it will not be discussed further.

Both NASBA and TMA are commercially available assays that are examples of transcription-mediated amplification. These isothermal assays use three enzymes: reverse transcriptase (RT), RNase H, and T7 DNA-dependent RNA polymerase. In short, the RT enzyme makes a cDNA copy of the target molecule, which is usually RNA. The primer that is used to create the strand of complementary DNA to the target RNA molecule contains the T7 RNA polymerase binding sequence on the 5′ end of the molecule. The RNA portion of the DNA-RNA hybrid is then hydrolyzed by RNase H. The second primer then binds and creates the complementary strand of the DNA molecule, thereby completing the cDNA molecule. This cDNA molecule has the T7 RNA polymerase binding sequence incorporated into it and serves as the template for T7 RNA polymerase, which transcribes numerous copies of RNA, which may be detected by a variety of methods.

Strand-displacement amplification is an isothermal reaction that relies on the ability of the DNA polymerase to displace one strand of DNA at the site of a single-strand nick and proceed with DNA replication or amplification in this assay. This technology, although efficient, requires special conditions and endonucleases that will generate a nick in only one of the strands of the double-stranded DNA molecule, rather than producing a cutting through of both strands of DNA, which is the mode of action for most restriction endonucleases.

CLINICAL APPLICATIONS

There are FDA-approved commercial assays available for the detection of *N. gonorrhoeae* and *C. trachomatis* that use TMA and SDA.[4] Akduman et al. examined over 3,500 urine specimens using the BDProbeTec-SDA assay (BD Bioscience) and reported a sensitivity of 99.2%, a specificity of 99.3%, a positive predictive value of 84.9%, and a negative predictive value of 99.9%. With regard to different amplification assays, these authors, like others, recommend the need to confirm positive results, given the positive predictive value. The BDProbeTec-SDA assay has an internal amplification control, which is useful for identifying potentially false-negative reactions secondary to amplification inhibition.

The APTIMA (Gen-Probe) line of products are FDA-approved, commercially available TMA assays for the detection of *N. gonorrhoeae* and/or *C. trachomatis*. Gaydos et al. studied the APTIMA II combo (GenProbe) and compared the sensitivity and specificity of this assay from endocervical swabs versus urine specimens.[104] For *C. trachomatis*, they found a sensitivity and specificity from endocervical swabs of 94.2% and 97.6%, respectively, compared with a sensitivity and specificity from the first-catch urine of 94.7% and 98.9%, respectively. For *N. gonorrhoeae*, they found a sensitivity and specificity from endocervical swabs of 99.2% and 98.7%, respectively, and a sensitivity and specificity from first-catch urine specimens of 91.3% and 99.3%, respec-

tively. The APTIMA assays do not have an internal control for amplification, but rather use a target capture system, which they claim virtually eliminates inhibition and negates the need for an internal control.

The Nuclisens HIV-1 QT assay is an FDA-approved assay that use the NASBA technology for measuring HIV viral loads. The Nuclisens CMV pp67 assay for monitoring CMV levels has been cleared by the FDA. This has been compared with a CMV antigenemia in a study of bone marrow transplant recipients, and found to be a suitable replacement for the more labor-intensive antigenemia assay.[108] A submission trial is underway with a NASBA-based assay for the rapid detection of enteroviruses from the cerebrospinal fluid (CSF). A variety of home-brew assays have been designed using the NASBA technology and the Basic Kit (bioMérieux), which supports these assays and is commercially available. These have been particularly useful for the detection of RNA viruses, such as enteroviruses and the West Nile virus, but like TMA, NASBA has also been used to detect bacteria, by directly targeting rRNA or other specific mRNAs.[11,75,185,198] Landry et al., in a comparison with RT-PCR for the detection of enterovirus from clinical specimens, found the NASBA assay to be slightly more sensitive and that it had a shorter turnaround time.[186]

Modifications of PCR

A number of modifications have been made to the standard PCR reaction, which have expanded the use of this test, and broadened the spectrum of the microorganisms that may be detected using these molecular methods.[82,254,361] Several of these modifications are well standardized and have been introduced as routinely used techniques in the clinical laboratory. Of the modifications, the techniques that will be described here are RT-PCR, broad-range PCR, multiplex PCR, and nested PCR. The most recent modification, real-time PCR, will be covered under a separate heading.

RT-PCR

Retroviruses are RNA viruses that as a part of their life cycle make a DNA copy of their RNA genome. This feat is accomplished by the reverse transcriptase (RT) enzyme. The addition of an RT step prior to PCR makes it possible to amplify and detect RNA targets. This may be accomplished in either a two-step or single-step reaction. A separate RT enzyme is used prior to the addition of the DNA polymerase in the two-step RT-PCR reaction, whereas a single thermostable DNA polymerase that also possesses significant RT activity is used in the single-step reaction.[235] The cDNA created by reverse transcriptase may be formed using specific oligonucleotide primers or random oligonucleotide hexamers. The PCR then proceeds as previously described.

RT-PCR is particularly useful for detecting RNA viruses, but it may also be used to detect other microorganisms by targeting the ribosomal RNA.[24,166,376] The detection of mRNA is useful for studying the genetic expression of both microorganisms and human host cells. As with PCR, quantitative results may be obtained with RT-PCR, and form the basis for HIV and HCV viral load testing with this technology.[299] Other nucleic-acid amplification technologies that preferentially amplify RNA, such as NASBA and TMA, are technologies competitive with RT-PCR.

CLINICAL APPLICATIONS

The detection of RNA viruses has likely been the most important of the clinical applications for RT-PCR to date. Quantitative RT-PCR assays have become commonplace for the detection of HCV and HIV.[107,255] The quantitative nature of nucleic-acid amplification, when used in conjunction with external quantitative standards, is commonly used to determine the amount of these viruses present in the patient's blood, which is commonly known as the "viral load." Viral load data are important for monitoring the response of the individual patient to therapy. For instance, a patient infected with the HIV virus should demonstrate an increasing CD4 T-lymphocyte count and a diminishing HIV viral load, when treated with appropriate antiretroviral therapy.

RT-PCR has also been used for the detection for the viral causes of meningitis and meningoencephalitis, such as enteroviruses and the West Nile virus.[127,145,150,155,169,358] Several studies have demonstrated the advantages of the rapid detection of enteroviruses from the CSF of patients with meningitis.[276,328] These have examined the advantages of performing these assays in a rapid manner to avoid unnecessary hospitalizations, unnecessary antibiotic use, and unnecessary ancillary procedures—to improve patient care and reduce costs.

The dengue viruses, the Hanta virus, human metapneumovirus, and the severe acute respiratory syndrome (SARS) coronavirus, among others have been detected using RT-PCR.[77,168,260,302] The use of RNA-based amplification techniques for the detection of rRNA in bacteria, parasites, and fungi, may be advantageous over detection of the rDNA gene by traditional PCR, since the presence of RNA is more likely associated with the presence of a viable organisms.

BROAD-RANGE PCR

The specificity of a primer set is determined by a variety of factors. Some of these factors are technical, such as the degree to which the primers hybridize with their target (i.e., avidity), which is determined by the composition of the reaction mixture (i.e., salt concentration) and the complementarity of the primers with respect to their target sequence (i.e., 100% complementarity = a perfect match). The specificity of a PCR may also reflect the uniqueness of the complementary sequence with which the primers hybridize. In many instances, it is desirable to choose a highly unique (signature) sequence, if one is attempting to detect a single microorganism. For example, it has been shown that the gene that encodes for the *Coccidioides*-specific antigen is a useful target for the detection of *Coccidioides* and the differentiation of this organism from other fungi.[246] Failure to produce a species-specific assay may result in undesired cross-reactivity with closely related species. This is the case with two of the FDA-approved, commercially available nucleic-acid amplification assays designed to detect *N. gonorrhoeae*, which are known to be capable of cross-reacting with certain commensal *Neisseria* species.[84,86]

Alternatively, there may be interest in a detecting the presence of a larger group of microorganisms, rather than a single type. The primers of such an assay are designed to detect all the organisms in the group of interest while attempting to exclude as many organisms as possible that are not in this group. This would be considered a "broad-range"

PCR assay. For example, a primer set that detected only one of the many enteroviruses capable of causing meningitis would be of little value for diagnosing or excluding enteroviral meningitis. In this case, the regions that are conserved among all the clinically relevant enteroviruses would be potential sites for primer and probe annealing. Both specific and broad-range primers are useful, with their utility being dictated by the particular clinical question that is being addressed by the assay. There are many advantages of using broad-range primers, but there are limitations, too.

The main reason and principal advantage of using a set of broad-range PCR primers is that any of the members of a large group may be detected in a single reaction. When a positive reaction is obtained, the amplicon may be assessed by multiple methods to determine which member of the particular group is present. This may be done by the use of multiple probes in a Southern blot or enzyme immunoassay (EIA) format, by sequencing of the amplicon, or by microarray analysis.[97,131,213] Postamplification melt-curve analysis is a more recently described method of achieving limited differentiation following a broad-range real-time PCR (see "Real-Time Nucleic-Acid Amplification" below).[314] The limitation of this technology is that the larger the group the assay is designed to detect, the more likely it is that the reaction will also detect organisms that are phylogenetically related to, but not necessarily part of, the group of interest. For example, we have used a broad-range PCR of the detection of all clinically relevant mycobacteria, but it also will amplify the same segment of DNA from many other G-C (guanine-cytosine) rich bacteria that are closely related to this group. These limitations can be dealt with successfully by using highly specific probes, but some limitations of this type of application remain. When multiple microorganisms are amplified there is an early exhaustion of the PCR primers. In addition, it is often difficult to obtain useful information from DNA sequencing because a meaningless mixed sequence will result, unless one is able to identify a sequence that is conserved in the group of interest but is not present in the contaminating organisms.

CLINICAL APPLICATIONS

Any group of related microorganisms, the members of which are of clinical interest, is a candidate for broad-range PCR. As previously mentioned, broad-range primers have proven useful for detecting the enteroviruses that cause aseptic meningitis.[272,276,328] One limitation of some broad-range assays for the detection of enterovirus is cross-reactivity of rhinovirus.[186] This should not be a significant problem if only CSF is examined, but may result in false-positive reactions if respiratory specimens, for example, are examined.

Possibly the most commonly used targets for broad-range PCRs have been the genes that encode for the bacterial, fungal, and parasite ribosomal subunits (rDNA).[128,138,309] These genes are particularly useful for both broad-range PCR and taxonomic categorization of microorganisms because they possess both highly conserved and variable regions. The highly conserved regions are excellent sites for broad-range primers, whereas the variable regions that lie in between may be used as target sites for species-specific probes or may be assessed by DNA sequencing. These applications have been used to help determine the cause of bacterial meningitis, infective endocarditis, bacteremia in patients with infective endocarditis, and other bacterial infections.[103,268,279,295,309] As with culture, the presence of contaminating bacteria is an issue for the interpretation of the results from a broad-range PCR.[17,115]

Not surprisingly, this type of approach has been used by many different groups for the identification of mycobacteria.[49,129,134] The most common type of postamplification analysis has been DNA sequencing, but multiple probes and DNA microarray analysis have also been used successfully for identification.

The rDNA target sites form the basis of many of the sequence-based identification systems currently used. The MicroSeq Microbial Identification System is a commercially available microbial identification system that uses broad-range primers to target the bacterial 16S rDNA and fungal D2 rDNA region (Applied Biosystems, Foster City, CA). After PCR amplification of the unknown bacterium or fungus, the sequence is obtained and submitted and matched against a database that is maintained and updated by the provider. This database has been evaluated by a number of groups regarding its usefulness in the molecular identification of a variety of pathogens from bacteria to dermatophytes.[49,129,131,219,236,268,372]

A number of other genetic targets, which like the 16S rDNA gene contain both highly conserved and variable regions, have been used for microorganism identification. These alternative targets for identification via broad-range PCR include the RNA polymerase (*rpoB*), heat-shock protein (*hsp*), and the elongation factor—Tu (*tuf*).[73,173,213] Characterization of microorganisms, particularly mycobacteria, by the *rpoB* gene is particularly of interest, since analysis of this gene also provides information regarding the resistance of mycobacteria to rifampin.[10,66,228,313]

MULTIPLEX PCR

Multiplex PCR is an alternative method to broad-range PCR for the detection of multiple pathogens.[19,105,288] In the simplest of multiplex assays, there are multiple primer sets used in a multiplex PCR reaction, each of which usually targets a particular pathogen. More complex multiplex assays could use combinations of broad-range and species-specific primer sets, for example. The advantage of multiplex reactions is that numerous pathogens may be detected in a single reaction. In some instances, one of the primer sets included in the amplification reactions may be directed against a human gene, such as β-globin, or nucleic acid that has been added to the specimen; these are as internal amplification controls for the reaction.[229] The amplification of an internal control is important to ensure that the amplification reaction was not inhibited, and it helps to ensure the accuracy of the negative results. The quantitative competitive PCR assay is one method of obtaining a quantitative result and is a type of multiplex reaction.[258,374] The limitations of multiplex PCR reactions are largely secondary to interactions between the different oligonucleotides, which compromise the sensitivity of the reaction, particularly when compared with the individual amplification reactions. The design of

highly efficient multiplex assays that have minimal oligonucleotide interactions is complicated.

CLINICAL APPLICATIONS

Multiple multiplex assays are usually designed to detect different microorganisms that cause the same types of diseases. For example, multiplex assays have been developed to detect *S. pneumoniae*, *H. influenzae*, and *N. meningitidis*, the most common causes of bacterial meningitis.[13,320] A number of multiplex assays have been described for the detection of the viral agents of meningitis and meningoencephalitis.[209,270,281] Multiplex PCR reactions are particularly useful when the number of possible pathogens is limited. Multiplex assays have also been used to detect and differentiate the polyomaviruses that infect humans, the bacteria that cause middle ear infection, the agents of atypical and typical bacterial pneumonia, and causes of viral respiratory tract infections.[53,88,121,143,261,341]

A number of multiplex assays are commercially available through Prodesse (Waukesha, WI). Examples of these include multiplex assays that detect the common respiratory viruses (Hexaplex) and the causes of atypical bacterial pneumonia (Pneumoplex).[317] The Adenoplex detects the wide variety of adenovirus subtypes that infect humans.

NESTED PCR

Nested PCR is a modification of PCR designed to increase the sensitivity of the assay reaction. This modification consists of two primer sets directed against the same target.[82,136] The first set of primers is developed in the usual manner, whereas the second set are primers are situated internally or nested with respect to the first set of primers. The traditional approach to nested PCR was to perform a number of PCR cycles, usually less than a full run would contain, and then open the reaction vessel and add the second, nested, set of primers.[90,136,288] As one may imagine, the major problem with this approach is amplicon contamination in the laboratory and a consequential loss of specificity of the assay as a clinical test. More recently, assays described as single-step nested PCR reactions have been reported, wherein both sets of primers are added to the initial reaction vessel and an extended PCR is performed. These have been performed in a real-time or homogeneous format (see below) and have demonstrated an increased sensitivity without amplicon contamination.[377] The advantages of these types of applications over nonnested reactions in the routine laboratory have yet to be proven, but may be used in the future to detect targets that are present in very low quantities.

CLINICAL APPLICATIONS

Nested PCR has been used in many PCR assays in an attempt to improve the sensitivity of the assay. Nested PCRs have proven valuable for the detection of microorganisms that may be in low quantity in the blood and tissues, such as *Rickettsia*, *Bartonella*, and similar organisms.[214,377] Not surprisingly, these have also been designed for the detection of herpesvirus and enterovirus from the CSF and have been used in the direct examination of the blood as a means of determining the cause of bacteremia.[69,96,125,174,322] Nested

PCR primers may also be used in a multiplex reaction and have been used in this manner to detect different herpesviruses, such as herpes simplex virus (HSV) and CMV.[242] This approach has also been used to detected *M. tuberculosis*, which may pose problems for nucleic-acid amplification-based detection systems when the bacilli are present in very low quantities.[243]

Postamplification Analysis

After completion of the nucleic-acid amplification reaction, the amplified product must be analyzed. The methods of analyzing the amplified product range from simply determining the size of the amplicon and the presence of any other products of amplification through gel electrophoresis to determining each nucleotide that composes the amplicon through DNA sequencing. Some methods of postamplification analysis, such as hybridization protection assays and single-stranded conformational polymorphisms are not covered here, whereas others such as restriction-fragment-length polymorphism (RFLP) analysis is covered below in the section on microbial typing.

Traditional Methods of Detection
GEL ELECTROPHORESIS/SOUTHERN BLOT ANALYSIS

Gel electrophoresis is one of the simplest ways of gaining information about the amplicon. Different types of gels may be used for gel electrophoresis, but a simple agarose gel is often used. The agarose gel is rectangular and has wells near one end. The gel is placed into a gel box and covered with buffer; newer, single-use gel electrophoresis systems are available that do not require the addition of buffer. To perform gel electrophoresis, the products of amplification are mixed with a loading dye, which is a dense, viscous, colored liquid. This helps the user visualize the placement of the mixture into the well when pipetting. After loading, an electrical current is passed through the contents of the gel box and the negatively charged DNA migrates toward the anode. The larger pieces of DNA are retarded by the gel matrix, compared with the smaller pieces of DNA. Therefore, the separation of DNA in gel electrophoresis is largely due to size. A set of DNA molecules of different known sizes, which is a commonly referred to as a ladder, is often placed in the first lane and run in concert with the samples. Through visual comparison of the migration of the amplicon(s) in the sample lanes (the area beneath the well) and the migration of the DNA molecules of varying sizes in the ladder, the user can estimate of the size of the DNA molecule(s) amplified.

The presence of a single band of the expected size is good preliminary evidence of the specificity of the amplification reaction. But the question remains: ''How can one actually be sure that the amplified product is the desired product and not the product of nonspecific amplification that just happened to be of or near the same size?'' The answer to this question using traditional methods was achieved by using specific oligonucleotide probes and performing a Southern blot. In short, after gel electrophoresis, the amplified product was transferred to nitrocellulose paper and a radiolabeled oligonucleotide probe added. After an appropriate amount of hybridization time and subsequent wash steps to remove

unbound probe, the nitrocellulose paper was exposed to x-ray film. If the expected amplicon was present, the radiolabeled probe would hybridize to its complementary sequence on the amplicon, producing an area of exposure on the x-ray film. If the amplicon was the result of nonspecific amplification, the probe would not bind and would be washed away, and the x-ray film would not contain an area of exposure on development. This procedure often took 2 to 3 days to complete, was technically complicated, and did not fit well into the clinical laboratory.

ENZYMATIC DETECTION OF AMPLIFIED PRODUCTS

The use of enzyme immunoassay technology as a method to detect the product of amplification represented a major advance in the rapid detection of specific amplified products.[338] The enzymatic reaction for the detection of the amplified products is often performed in a 96-well plate. Different methods of labeling and detecting the hybridized oligonucleotide probe may be used. The end result, however, is that the hybridized probe that has not been removed by washing generates a signal of either light or, more commonly, color [206] (Fig. 4-11). The use of an oligonucleotide probe increases the specificity of the reaction, whereas linkage with an enzymatic reaction increases the sensitivity of the reaction.[338] The amount of signal generated is proportional

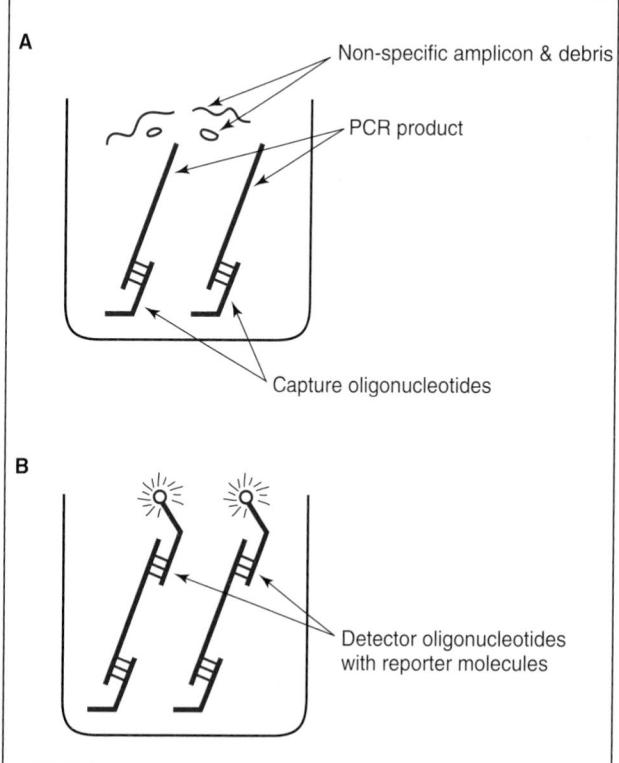

Figure 4-11 There are many methods of detecting an amplicon using enzymes. (**A**) Here, a capture probe is used to retain the specific amplicon, so that any nonspecific amplified material and cellular debris may be removed by washing. (**B**) The retained amplicon is then detected with another oligonucleotide and a signal is generated using one of many enzyme systems.

to the amount of amplicon present. When used with calibrated standards, quantitative information may be obtained.

CLINICAL APPLICATIONS

Many of the commercially available systems use a colorimetric reaction for the detection of the amplified products. There was a rapid conversion from the labor-intensive and time-consuming Southern blot to enzymatic detection following the introduction of this technology. This method of detection is used in several commercial systems and with a variety of nucleic-acid amplification chemistries. Quantitative viral load data, which is regularly generated using these systems, is obtained using this technology.

Reverse Hybridization

The Southern blot, although effective, is time-consuming and labor-intensive. In addition, multiple probes or sequencing of the amplicon would be necessary if the product of amplification was secondary to a broad-range PCR. An alternative, highly effective approach is to immobilize all the probes of interest on a nitrocellulose strip and then apply the amplicon to the strip and determine which probe hybridized with the amplicon. This is termed reverse hybridization, since the amplicon is applied to the probe that is immobilized in the nitrocellulose strip, which is opposite to how a Southern blot is performed. The assay also has the advantage of using a chromogenic reaction, rather than radioactivity to detect hybridization (Fig. 4-12).

CLINICAL APPLICATIONS

Reverse hybridization technology is commercially available as line probe assays (LiPA) (Innogenetics, Gent, Belgium, and Bayer Diagnostics, Tarrytown, NY) or reverse dot blot strips (Roche Molecular Diagnostics, Indianapolis, IN). This type of technology has been used to differentiate the various genetic subtypes of HCV (i.e., HCV genotyping), a test that provides important prognostic and therapeutic information.[51,63,252,267] The INNO-LiPA HCV II (Bayer) was found to be comparable to DNA sequencing in a direct comparison.[237] Reverse hybridization has also proven useful for screening for the most common mutations present in the HIV genome that confer resistance to antiretroviral agents.[30,67,306,334] The LiPA is technically much easier to perform than DNA sequencing, with simpler posttest analysis. However, unlike sequencing, the use of reverse hybridization allows for an assessment of only the sequences for which there are probes, and does not afford the opportunity to evaluate new mutations, which may be either silent or clinically relevant.[280] Reverse hybridization has also been used to detect HPV and identify the subtypes that are associated with a high risk of dysplasia and subsequent carcinoma.[175,193,216,253,271,353] In addition to virologic applications, reverse hybridization technology has been used to identify mycobacteria, medically important fungi, and mutations associated with mycobacterial resistance to rifampin.[1,15,35,66,147,212,217,221,224,294,304,335,342] Although highly accurate, the mycobacterial, fungal, and rifampin LiPAs are expensive and are not available in the United States.

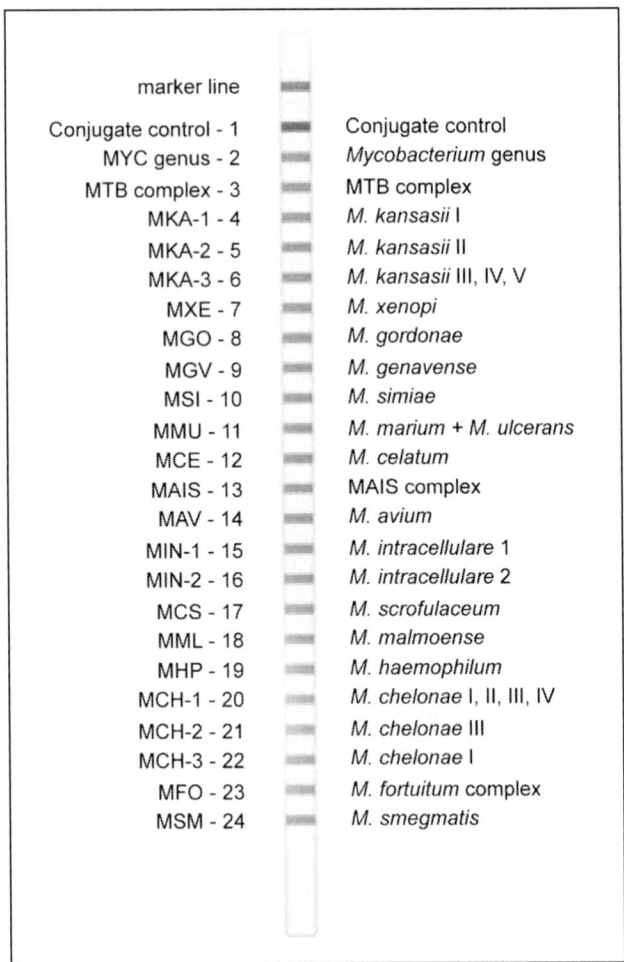

Figure 4-12 The reverse hybridization strip demonstrated shows that most clinically important mycobacteria could be identified using PCR followed by reverse hybridization of the amplicon. Similar assays are useful for determining the most frequently encountered HIV and HCV genotypes. (Photo from INNO-LiPA Mycobacteria V2 reverse-hybridization assay package insert, Innogenetics, Ghent, Belgium.)

DNA Sequencing

DNA sequencing for the analysis of an amplified product is now a common method of postamplification analysis. Although useful, this technology is more complicated than simple probe hybridization and often requires the user to have experience with sequence alignment, editing software, and genetic databases. DNA sequencing is particularly useful when analyzing a group of microorganisms to determine the areas of conservation and variability within the amplicon obtained by broad-range PCR. Analysis of these variable regions then becomes a powerful tool for the identification of microorganisms.[27,103,111,119,187,197,278,309,359,368,373] It has also proven critically useful for the analysis of genetic mutations within viral genomes, which may often be single nucleotide polymorphisms (SNPs) and may confer resistance to antiviral drugs.[50,133,179,201]

TRADITIONAL DNA SEQUENCING

Traditional DNA sequencing, once a tool used solely in research laboratories, has also become commonplace in many molecular pathology and molecular microbiology laboratories. This technology, which uses traditional Sanger sequencing or sequencing by termination, works through the incorporation of dideoxynucleotides into a growing strand of DNA. When a dideoxynucleotide is incorporated into the DNA strand, it can be extended no further. The analysis of the DNA fragments that result, which are as numerous as the nucleotides that compose the strand, provides the sequence information. In the past, this was accomplished with large gels poured between two glass plates, and the use of radioactive reporter molecules. Today, these methods have been modified to use either fluorescently labeled reporter molecules, with either a more user-friendly gel system or with capillary electrophoresis (Fig. 4-13). The sequence of long regions of DNA, up to hundreds of base pairs in length, may be readily determined by these methods.

CLINICAL APPLICATIONS

HIV genotyping is one of the principle applications of DNA sequencing in the molecular microbiology laboratory.[44,290] This is done to determine the presence of acquired mutations in the genome of HIV for a particular patient that may confer resistance to antiretroviral agents. This assay is complicated and consists of extraction of the HIV RNA, followed by four RT-PCR assays, each of which is followed by Sanger sequencing. Although nucleotide determination is largely automated in many of these systems, some manual sequence analysis of the generated sequences in still required. DNA sequencing has also been used to demonstrate resistance-associated mutations in CMV and to determine the HCV genotype.[133,139,179,201,237]

DNA sequencing has also been used successfully for the identification of bacteria, mycobacteria, *Nocardia*, and fungi. The genes that encode for the ribosomal subunits of these organisms are the most commonly used genetic targets of sequence-based identification. One of the most common uses of this approach has been for the identification of the causes of bacterial endocarditis.[103,111,120,172,222,269] Sequence-based identification, however, has also been used to determine the causative agent of infection in a variety of other infections, including sinusitis and urinary tract infections.[37,122] This technology is revolutionizing the way in which we identify slow-growing microorganisms like mycobacteria and nocardia.[48,129,171,219,250,256] It has also been used for the identification of fungal pathogens.[130,131,265] Although rDNA genes are commonly used as the genetic targets for sequence-based identification, other genes that have proven useful for characterizing microorganisms include the *rpoB*, *hsp*, and *tuf* genes, among others.[73,74,94,171,183,249,287]

SEQUENCING BY SYNTHESIS (PYROSEQUENCING)

Pyrosequencing is a relatively new method of DNA sequencing, which is sequencing by synthesis, in contrast to sequencing by dideoxynucleotide termination or Sanger sequencing.[238,291,292] This technology has been used extensively in the analysis of single nucleotide polymorphisms (SNPs) associated with genetic diseases and neoplasia; it has also been used for the identification and differentiation of microorganisms.[3,6,100,238] Unlike traditional sequencing by termination, this technology is sequencing based on nucleotide incorporation into the newly synthesized strand of DNA. In short, the PCR-amplified DNA molecule, one strand of which contains a terminal biotin that was bonded to the primer, is immobilized in the well of a microtiter plate. Processing creates a single strand. The sequencing primer and reagents are added, followed by the automated addition of each of the four nucleotides. If the nucleotide added is the next appropriate nucleotide required in the growing strand, then pyrophosphate—a natural by-product of nucleotide incorporation—is generated. The pyrophosphate is then converted into light by enzymatic reactions. The light generated is recorded by the instrument and the sequence is thereby determined (Fig. 4-14).

The primary limitations of sequencing by synthesis are its ability to generate only relatively short sequences (~30 bp), problems generating a sequence when extensive secondary structure is present, and an inability to accurately characterize regions that contain more than four of the same nucleotide in tandem (i.e., homopolymers). The advantages are ease of use (i.e., the sequencing reaction occurs in a commonly used 96-well plate) and the sequence generated is present in context, which means surrounding, known sequences may be used as a sequencing control. The key of using pyrosequencing for microorganism identification is a knowledge of focal genetic targets that provide information sufficient for the differentiation of the microorganisms of interest.

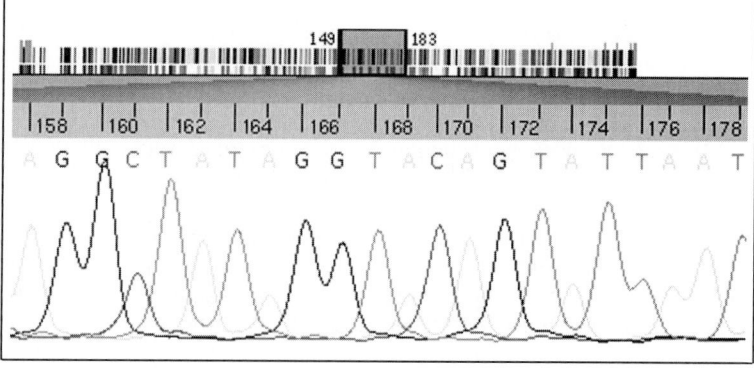

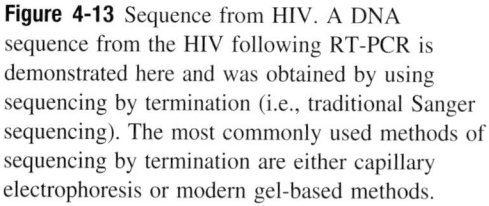

Figure 4-13 Sequence from HIV. A DNA sequence from the HIV following RT-PCR is demonstrated here and was obtained by using sequencing by termination (i.e., traditional Sanger sequencing). The most commonly used methods of sequencing by termination are either capillary electrophoresis or modern gel-based methods.

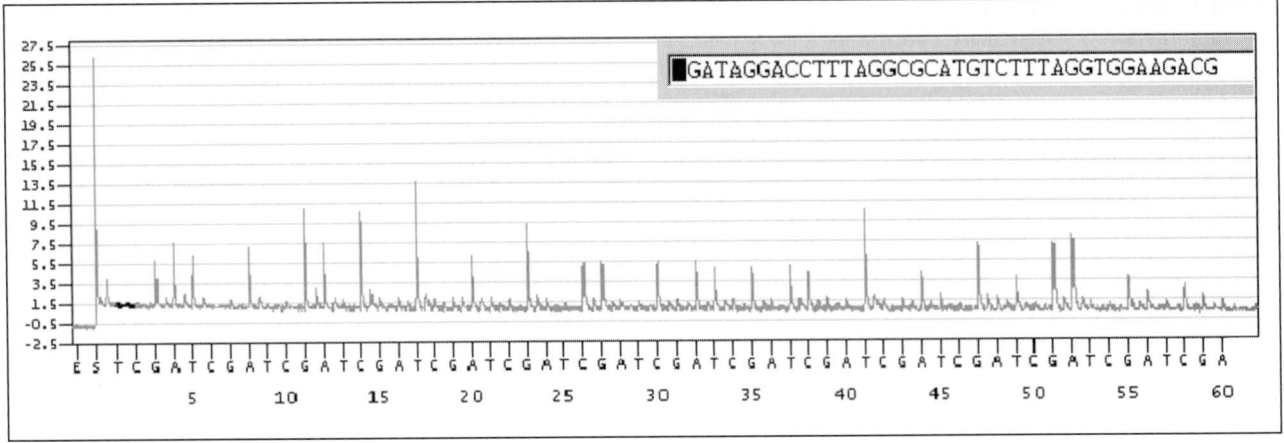

Figure 4-14 DNA sequence by pyrosequencing. This pyrogram was generated from a clinical specimen that contained acid-fast bacilli. Real-time PCR followed by pyrosequencing was performed because of the possibility of tuberculosis. The sequence generated, which is from the hypervariable region A of the 16S rDNA gene, identified the isolate as *M. intracellulare*.

CLINICAL APPLICATIONS

Applications that use sequencing by synthesis are currently being introduced into the clinical microbiology laboratory. Research applications have included the identification and typing of bacteria, such as *Helicobacter pylori* and *Listeria monocytogenes*, and have been used to differentiate bacteria into clinically relevant groups.[115,230,347] It has also been used to study linezolid resistance in the enterococci.[316] Additional uses that would likely prove useful for the clinician may include the rapid identification of bacteria that cause infections in neonates, and the rapid identification of the bacteria that cause meningitis.

Pyrosequencing has also been used to identify clinically relevant fungi, nocardiae, and mycobacteria.[109] We have used a broad-range PCR that targets the portion of the 16S rDNA that contains the hypervariable region A and have demonstrated with pyrosequencing excellent differentiation of the vast majority of the clinically relevant mycobacteria with the analysis of a region consisting of only 30 bp.[345] We chose this target because the hypervariable region A had been shown by several groups to be useful for the genetic differentiation of mycobacteria.[71,134,325] Similarly, we have targeted portions of the 16S rDNA gene that confer taxonomic information for *Nocardia* species and have achieved excellent results.[87,211]

The differentiation of viruses has also been demonstrated using this technology. An assay has been developed to determine the HCV genotype using pyrosequencing.[78] We have also used this method to differentiate the human polyomaviruses that may be recovered from human tissues and body fluids.[18]

Many of the pyrosequencing applications described for clinical microbiology laboratories use a broad-range PCR for the microorganisms of interest, followed by the investigation of a compact variable region that confers the genetic information of interest. There are many additional potential applications for sequencing by synthesis for the diagnosis of infectious disease and for the characterization of the infecting microorganisms and the host. These applications may include the identification of the causative agents of infection and the detection of resistance-associated genetic mutations. Furthermore, the characterization of SNPs or other genetic polymorphisms that may increase the risk of infection in the host could also be determined by this technology. Unfortunately, commercially available kits are not yet available, so users must rely on home-brew assays, which limits the widespread use of this technology.

MICROARRAY ANALYSIS

A wide variety of microarrays, often commonly known as "gene chips" have been used for many years in the basic sciences for many purposes, including infectious diseases.[12,24,31] These devices detect a multitude of signals simultaneously and may be used to detect genetic (DNA) differences or differences in expression (mRNA).[31] They are useful in determining which genes are expressed and which genes are silenced in response to different stimuli. These discovery tools have proven useful when studying everything from infections to cancer. Briefly, products of nucleic-acid amplification, which may be the result of broad-range PCR or RT-PCR, are applied to the microarray. The microarray consists of often thousands of hybridization sites, each of which provides information regarding the nucleotide composition of the amplicon. The signal generated from the microarray may be fluorescent or electrical. The major advantage of the microarray is its ability to examine thousands of hybridization reactions simultaneously. This feature also contributes to one of its major limitations, namely the amount of data generated from a single microarray may be overwhelming to the user and usually requires computers and advanced software packages for data analysis. The cost of microarray analysis also prohibits making it routine at this time. Although microarrays will certainly be used in the study of infectious diseases, the future of this technology in the routine clinical microbiology laboratory has yet to be determined.

CLINICAL APPLICATIONS

Microarray formats have been used extensively in discovery. They have been used to identify bacteria, mycobacteria, fungi, and viruses, to detect the genetic determinants of resistance, to study host response to infection, and to discover new drugs that may be useful to cure infections.[34,41,43,57,91,97,226,303] Regarding HIV, this technology has proven very useful for studying viral gene expression and the changes in the host-cell expression profile after infection.[157,311,336,354,363]

Microarrays, although very useful for research and discovery, have not yet been introduced into routine use in the clinical microbiology laboratory, and they are not yet commercially available for the diagnosis or assessment of patients with infections. The potential utility of microarrays in the clinical microbiology laboratory is apparent in the title of a recent article: "Chips with Everything: DNA Microarrays in Infectious Diseases."[31] How and when these technologies become available for routine use remains to be realized.

Real-Time Nucleic-Acid Amplification

Two technologic advances resulted in the development of real-time nucleic-acid amplification. The first was the development of methods of more rapid heat exchange (i.e., rapid heating and cooling) of the reaction chamber.[203] Traditional PCR, for example, occurs in a block cycler, in which the block consists of metal or some other solid material. The rate at which the solid block can be heated and cooled to the temperatures needed for PCR limits the rate at which the cycling may proceed. The rapid introduction of heated air and the removal of the heated air (cooling), which may be achieved through fans in real-time instruments, allows the cycling reaction to proceed more rapidly. The use of smaller reaction volumes also assists in the more rapid exchange of thermal energy. The second technical advance was in the development of a homogeneous reaction mixture.[203] This is a mixture in which the fluorogenic molecules that are used for the detection of the amplified products are present within the same reaction vessel in which amplification occurs. Furthermore an assessment of the fluorescence from these molecules is usually obtained by the instrument once per amplification cycle. Evidence of amplification occurs during the PCR reaction in "real-time," which is why these assays are commonly referred to as real-time PCR. This type of amplicon detection represents a significant advance in nucleic acid chemistry, since it is more rapid than traditional methods of amplicon detection. In addition, there is a significant reduction in the chance of amplicon contamination of the laboratory, since the reaction vessel does not have to be opened to analyze the amplicon. There are a variety of platforms available for real-time nucleic acid amplification.[95] In addition to real-time PCR, the NASBA reaction has been modified to a real-time format with detection using molecular beacons (see below). There is the possibility of modifying any nucleic-acid amplification technology to a real-time format.

Methods of Detecting the Products of Real-Time Amplification

There are a variety of fluorogenic molecules that may be used for the detection of amplified nucleic acids in a homogeneous or real-time reaction. These may be nonspecific and detect any amplified nucleic acid, or specific, which means they are oligonucleotides and hybridize with a specific sequence present in the amplicon. The nonspecific detection of amplicon using SYBR green, as well as the three most commonly used methods of specific amplicon detection will be covered. These are the TaqMan (Applied Biosystems, Foster City, CA) or hydrolysis probe chemistry, fluorescence resonance energy transfer (FRET) probes, and molecular beacons. Other types of detector molecules are also available, but a discussion of these is beyond the scope of this book.

SYBR GREEN

SYBR green I is a dye that binds to the minor groove of double-stranded DNA. This dye emits very little fluorescence when in the unbound state, but generates considerably more fluorescence when bound to DNA (Fig. 4-15). This property makes it useful for determining the presence of an amplified DNA product. Multiple molecules of SYBR green may bind to a single amplicon, thereby making it a sensitive method of amplicon detection. Also, this dye is much less expensive than specific oligonucleotide probes that are labeled with fluorophores. The detection of amplicons using SYBR green is useful for optimizing the PCR reaction (i.e., determining the optimal concentrations of the primers and $MgCl_2$). It is also useful to determine if amplification has occurred prior to a definitive method of postamplification analysis, such as DNA sequencing or microarray analysis. The main disadvantage of SYBR green detection is that it is nonspecific and these detector molecules will bind to any double-stranded DNA, including the products of nonspecific amplification and primer dimers. This method of detection lacks the specificity achieved with the use of an oligonucleotide probe (described below). It is for this reason that SYBR green detection should never be used as the sole method of detection in a clinical assay.

HYBRIDIZATION PROBES

There are many different types of fluorescently labeled oligonucleotide probes that may be used for amplicon detection in a real-time nucleic-acid amplification assay. The three that will be discussed are the most commonly used and cover the most important aspects of real-time detection chemistry. These are the TaqMan or hydrolysis probes, the fluorescence resonance energy transfer (FRET) probes, and molecular beacons.

TaqMan or Hydrolysis Probes. The TaqMan or hydrolysis probe detection chemistry relies on the 5′ to 3′ exonuclease activity of DNA polymerase. This function of DNA polymerase hydrolyzes any oligonucleotide that may bind to the single-stranded portion of the DNA molecule for which the complementary strand is being synthesized. In nature, this helps to ensure that only the appropriate nucleotides are incorporated into the newly synthesized strand of DNA.

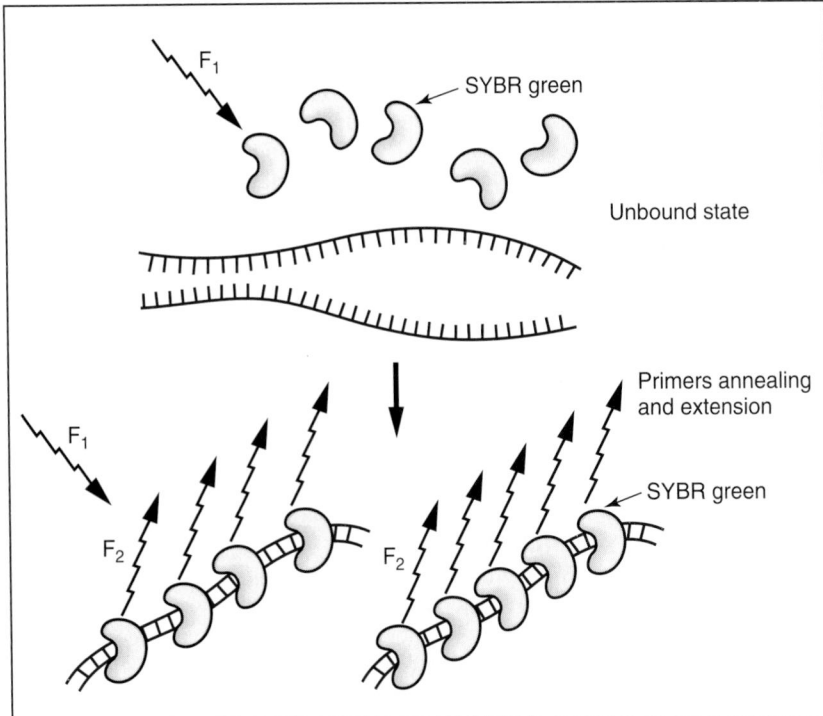

Figure 4-15 SYBR green chemistry. SYBR Green I dye binds to the minor groove of double-stranded DNA. When DNA is single-stranded there is no minor groove so SYBR green does not bind to DNA. However, after primer annealing and extension SYBR green can bind and emit light (*F2*) in response to the appropriate excitation (*F1*). SYBR green is an excellent method of measuring nonspecific amplicon generation, since the more DNA is produced by PCR results in more binding sites and therefore more fluorescence.

TaqMan or hydrolysis probe chemistries exploit this property of DNA polymerase to generate a detectable signal. The hydrolysis oligonucleotide probe is labeled with both a fluorophore and a quencher molecule. In the absence of specific target, this molecule folds up to a certain degree, which places the quencher molecule in close enough proximity to the fluorophore that the majority of any fluorescent signal emitted is immediately absorbed. When this probe binds to the complementary portion of DNA that has been generated by the previous cycles of PCR, it is hydrolyzed by DNA polymerase (Fig. 4-16). This hydrolysis affords the diffusion of the fluorophore away from the quencher molecule, and the generation of light that is not quenched and, therefore, detectable.

Fluorescence Resonance Energy Transfer (FRET) Probes.
FRET probes function through the transfer of energy. In this system, there are two detector probes used instead of one. These probes hybridize in close proximity to one another on the amplicon, with a two- to five-nucleotide gap between the two probes. The probe on the upstream side of the pair has a fluorescein molecule attached to the 3′ end of the probe, and may be termed the donor molecule. The second probe in the FRET set is situated downstream in relation to the first probe, has an acceptor molecule, usually LC640 or LC705 when used with the LightCycler system on the 5′ end of molecule, and may be termed the acceptor molecule. Other acceptor molecules may be used, but they must have the property of being excited by the wavelength of light that is emitted by the fluorescein or another donor molecule and, in turn, to emit light of another, detectable wavelength. In addition, the 5′ end of the acceptor-containing probe must be phosphorylated to prevent probe extension during PCR. Detection with the FRET probes works as follows: if the appropriate probe hybridization sequence is present in the amplicon, the FRET probes will hybridize to it. At this time,

the donor molecule (the fluorescein) is excited by light energy introduced into the system by the instrument. When the excited donor molecule returns to its base energy state, it releases light of a particular wavelength. This released light excites the nearby acceptor molecule (LC640 or

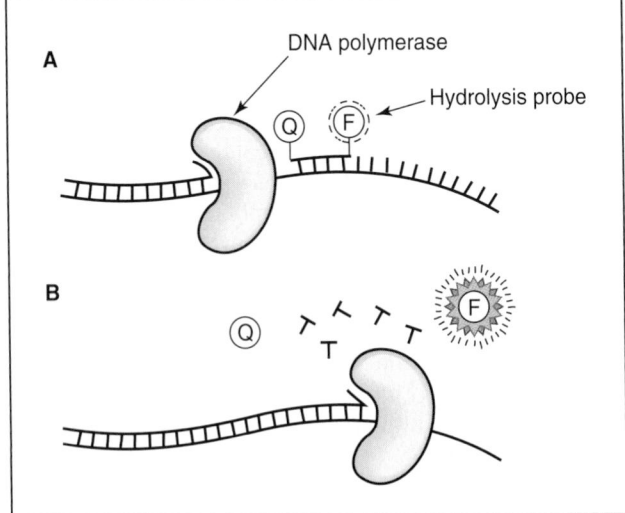

Figure 4-16 Hydrolysis probe chemistry. (**A**) The close proximity of the quencher molecule (*Q*) to the fluorescent molecule (*F*), both of which are attached to the intact hydrolysis probe, results in only minimal background fluorescence. (**B**) The hydrolysis of this probe by the exonuclease activity of DNA polymerase as extension occurs results in diffusion of the fluorophore from the quencher molecule, so that fluorescence may occur when the fluorophore is appropriately excited.

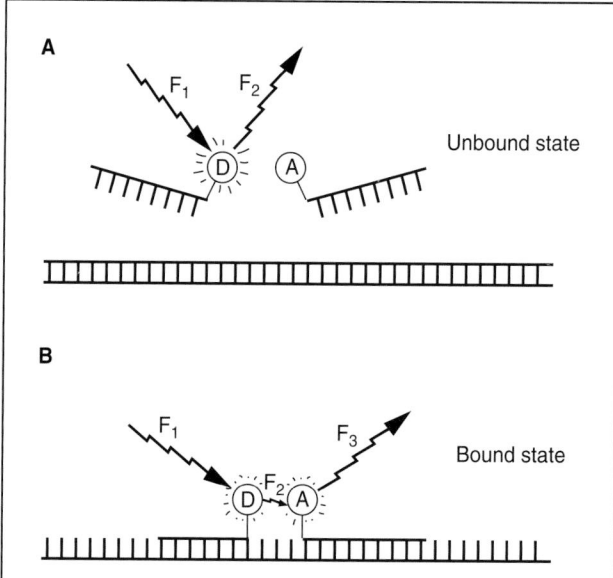

Figure 4-17 Fluorescence resonance energy transfer. Two probes, both of which are labeled with a fluorophore, are necessary to achieve fluorescence resonance energy transfer (FRET). (**A**) The excitation wavelength (*F1*) of the donor fluorophore (*D*) raises the energy state of the molecule and an emission occurs (*F2*). This does not affect the acceptor fluorophore (*A*) when the probes are not hybridized, because they are not in close proximity to one another. (**B**) When the two probes are hybridized and next to one another secondary to Watson and Crick base pairing, the donor fluorophore is near the acceptor fluorophore. The emitted light from the excited donor fluorophore (*F2*) acts as the excitation energy for the acceptor fluorophore, which in turn emits an particular wavelength of light of its own (*F3*). The presence of the emission (*F3*) from the acceptor molecule is evidence that probe hybridization has occurred.

LC705), completing resonance energy transfer. The acceptor molecule is in turn excited to a heightened energy state. When the acceptor molecule returns to its base energy state, it releases light energy that is detected by the system (Fig. 4-17). Detection using FRET-based chemistry is by its nature highly specific, since the only way to receive the final energy signal is for four independent reactions occur. These independent reactions are the hybridization of the two primers that afford amplification, and the hybridization of each of the probes that afford detection (Fig. 4-18).

The use of FRET probes also allows the user to perform a postamplification melt-curve analysis. This is possible because of the nature of FRET probe interaction and the fact that unlike taqman probes these probes are not hydrolyzed during detection. The reader will recall that the hydrogen bonds are responsible for the hybridization between the oligonucleotide probes to the complementary DNA strand. When thermal energy is added to the system that exceeds the energy of these bonds, the bonds will be broken and the probe will ''melt off'' the complementary DNA target. The point at which half the probe molecules are bound and half are unbound is the melting point or T_M of the oligonucleotide.

Melting-curve analysis is performed after the PCR reaction is complete. Initially, the reaction mixture is cooled to a point well below the T_M of the individual FRET probes so that both will hybridize if the appropriate amplified DNA is present. At this point, an excitation wavelength of light is introduced into the instrument and a signal will be generated from the FRET reaction that occurs between the juxtaposed probes. Next, the reaction mixture is then slowly heated while continuous fluorescence measurements are taken. When the reaction mixture reaches and finally exceeds the T_M of the FRET probes, there will be a precipitous loss in the fluorescence signal (Fig. 4-19). The first derivative of the slope of this curve results in a peak (Fig. 4-19). The perpendicular line that may be drawn through the center of this peak represents the experimentally derived T_M.

There are at least three important uses for melt-curve analysis. First, there should be a relatively predictable melting temperature for the expected amplicon, which may be confirmed using known standards. The demonstration of the appropriate melting temperature helps assure the user that the identification is correct, rather than a misidentification potentially obtained through the amplification and detection of a taxonomically related organism. In this vein, postamplification melt-curve analysis may be used to differentiate closely related organisms. Finally, the detection of nucleo-

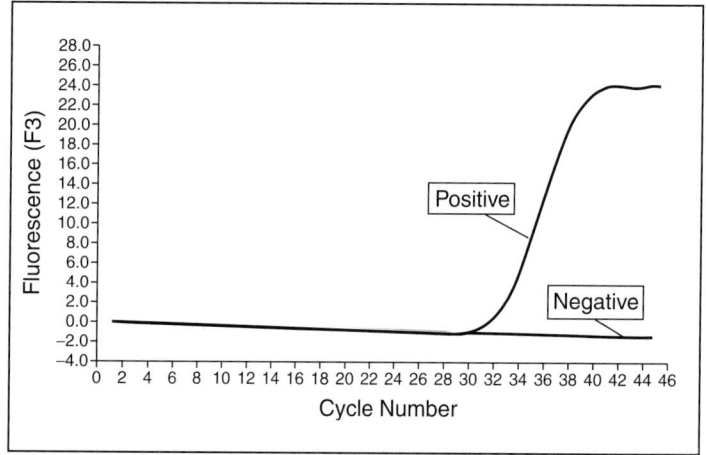

Figure 4-18 Positive and negative real-time PCR reactions. Positive real-time PCR reactions demonstrate an exponential increase in fluorescence, whereas the negative reactions retain only low, basal levels of fluorescence.

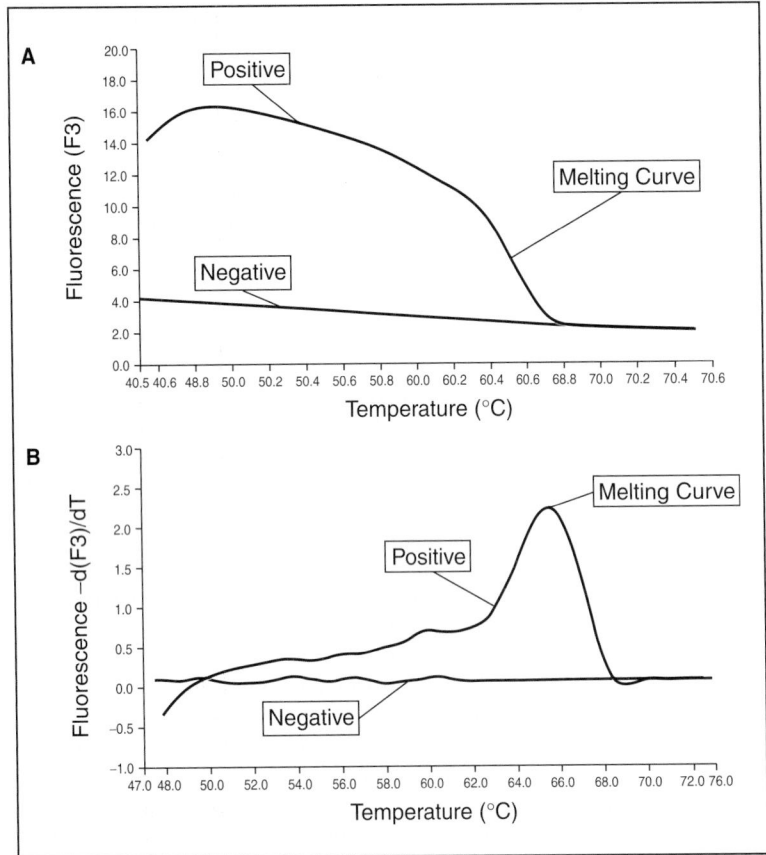

Figure 4-19 The melting curves (**A**) and the derivative of the curve (the melting peaks; **B**) are demonstrated for one positive and one negative specimen in a real-time PCR that specifically detects *Staphylococcus aureus*.

tide mismatches between the FRET probes and their corresponding probe hybridization site, just like that used for organism differentiation, may be use to detect other clinically important SNPs, such as those that may confer resistance to antimicrobials or those in the host that may denote relative susceptibility to infection.

Molecular Beacons. The next type of detector molecule to be discussed is the molecular beacon. This molecule, like the TaqMan or hydrolysis probe contains both a fluorophore and a quencher molecule. The molecular beacon, however, is larger than typical hydrolysis probes and is not hydrolyzed by the DNA polymerase in order to achieve fluorescence in the presence of the appropriate amplicon. This molecule, which is shaped like a lollipop, has a loop-and- stem configuration (Fig. 4-20). The loop portion of the molecule is the part of the molecule that is complementary to a specific part of the amplicon. The stem is a construct of complementary nucleic acids designed to keep the molecule closed (i.e., in the lollipop configuration), in the absence of a specific amplicon. The two respective ends of the molecular beacon probe molecule are the sites of attachment for the fluorophore and quencher molecules. The fluorophore is juxtaposed with the quencher molecule when the beacon is closed (i.e., when it is not in the presence of the appropriate amplicon). When the beacon is in the presence of the appropriate amplicon, the thermodynamics favor hybridization with the amplicon over the closed, semi-self-hybridized state. When the molecular beacon is hybridized, the fluorophore is spacially separated from the quencher and fluorescence can be detected by the instrument. Melting curves can be achieved with molecular beacons, but it is much more difficult to achieve the same quality of melt curve results as those achieved with FRET probes.

It may seem difficult for the molecular microbiologist to choose which type of detector molecule to use for a real-time nucleic acid amplification assay. In part this may be dictated by the type of instrumentation present in the laboratory. For example, if a SmartCycler or EasyQ is purchased, a molecular beacon would be favored, whereas for the LightCycler, FRET-probe chemistry is favored. The ABI (Applied Biosystems, Foster City, CA) and Roche (COBAS) TaqMan 48 (Roche Diagnostics, Indianapolis, IN) platforms use hydrolysis probes. Some platforms, like the RotorGene (Corbett, Corbett, Australia), are biochemically agnostic and support any type of probe chemistry. For the most part, the same ends (i.e., detection of the microorganism of interest) can be achieved by a variety of different means. The other major factor in determining the type of probe to use on a particular segment of DNA is the nucleotide composition of that segment. Factors that may influence probe selection include the G-C content of the region and the presence of secondary structure, among others.

CLINICAL APPLICATIONS

Real-time nucleic-acid amplification, most notably real-time PCR, has contributed significantly to the implementation of real-time assays for a wide variety of clinically important microorganisms. Most microorganisms that have been

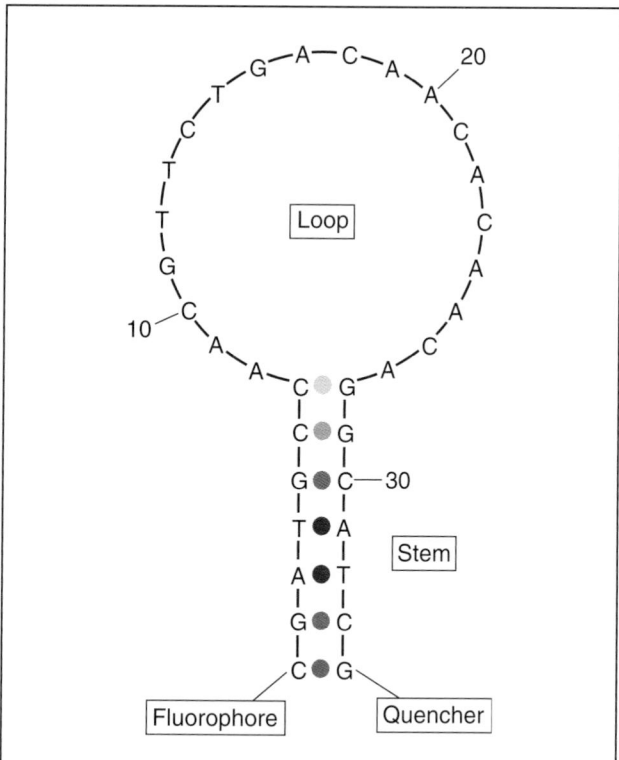

Figure 4-20 This molecular beacon was designed to detect the amplified product of a broad-range *Salmonella* PCR. It consists of 34 nucleotides and has a stem-loop configuration. This structure places the fluorophore in close proximity to the fluorescence-quenching molecule when the molecular beacon is not hybridized with its genetic target (i.e., the PCR is negative). When the appropriate amplicon is present, the thermodynamics favor hybridization over the stem-loop configuration, the molecule opens and hybridizes, and fluorescence is discernible since the fluorophore is spatially separated from the quencher.

detected in the past using traditional PCR have been detected more recently using real-time formats. These assays have been used to detect the fastidious pathogens that have traditionally been approached using PCR, as well as more common agents of infectious diseases.

Real-time assays for DNA viruses include assays for the herpesviruses, adenovirus, smallpox virus, and parvovirus B19, among others.[123,137,142,162,177,307,321,332] Postamplification melt-curve analysis has been used to differentiate HSV type 1 from HSV type 2.[369] The quantitative nature of these assays has also been used to predict disease and monitor the viral load in response to therapy.[9,113,118,162,300,362] Real-time RT-PCR and NASBA assays for RNA viruses include broad-range assays for enteroviruses that cause viral encephalitis and individual and multiplex assays for the detection of respiratory viruses.[25,52,126,169,274,319,357,358,364,366] Real-time assays have also been used to rapidly detect newly recognized and emerging viral pathogens, such as human metapneumovirus and the SARS coronavirus.[56,117,190,204,205,259,260] Some of these assays are available as analyte-specific-reagent (ASR) or research-use-only (RUO) kits.

Numerous assays have been described that detect bacteria

and the genes associated with resistance. Two real-time PCR assays have received FDA approval for use on the SmartCycler system. These are an assay for group B *Streptococcus* for prenatal screening during pregnancy and a recently released assay for the detection of methicillin-resistant *Staphylococcus aureus* (MRSA) colonization. A number of ASR kits are available for the detection of bacteria, which include kits for *Enterococcus* (specifically vancomycin-resistant enterococci {VRE}), *Staphylococcus* and MRSA, *Pseudomonas*, and *Bacillus anthracis*. In addition, the literature is replete with examples of real-time amplification assays for the detection and differentiation of a variety of microorganisms and resistance-associated genes. Many of these assays target the traditional microorganisms that do not grow on artificial media or are extremely difficult to culture, such as *T. whippelii*, *Rickettsia*, and *Bartonella* species.[89,164,377] Postamplification melt-curve analysis also has be used to differentiate the most common *Bartonella* species (Fig. 4-21). In addition to these applications, as PCR in the real-time formats has become more readily available and more user-friendly, it is being applied to commonly encountered bacteria and their mechanisms of resistance. For example, real-time PCR has been shown to be a reliable and more timely method for the differentiation of *S. aureus* from coagulase-negative staphylococci in blood-culture bottles that signal positive and contain gram-positive cocci, and is a reliable method for determining oxacillin resistance in these *S. aureus* isolates.[315]

Real-time assays for fungi include assays for organisms that cannot be cultivated in the routine clinical microbiology laboratory, such as *P. jirovecii*, and for slow-growing organisms, such as *H. capsulatum*.[152,167,189,210,218,245] Other applications have included the detection of invasive mold and yeast infection in immunocompromised patients and the detection of other systemic dimorphic fungal pathogens, such as *Coccidioides immitis* and *Penicillium marneffei*.[22,152,257,262,266,277,324]

Another important application for these assays has been for the rapid detection of mycobacteria, particularly *M. tuberculosis*. Mycobacteria are excellent candidates for detection and identification by molecular methods, since these microorganisms are slow-growing, some cause severe disease and death, and tuberculosis is a communicable disease for which transmission-control measures may be instituted. Several real-time assays have been developed for the rapid detection of *M. tuberculosis* directly from clinical specimens. Shrestha et al. describe a LightCycler assay that detects and differentiates *M. tuberculosis* from nontuberculous mycobacteria using postamplification melt-curve analysis.[314] Excellent assays for the detection of *M. tuberculosis* are also available for SmartCycler and TaqMan users.[47,68,293] Assays have also been developed for the rapid detection of resistance to commonly used drugs, such as isoniazid and rifampin.[286,297,352]

The detection and identification of parasites has also been approached using real-time nucleic-acid amplification assays. A number of assays have been described for the rapid detection of otherwise difficult to detect parasite *Toxoplasma gondii*.[54,161,196] Other applications include the detection of stool parasites, such as *Cryptosporidium* and microsporidia, the identification of tissue parasites, such as *Leishmania* and *Trypanosoma*, and the detection and differ-

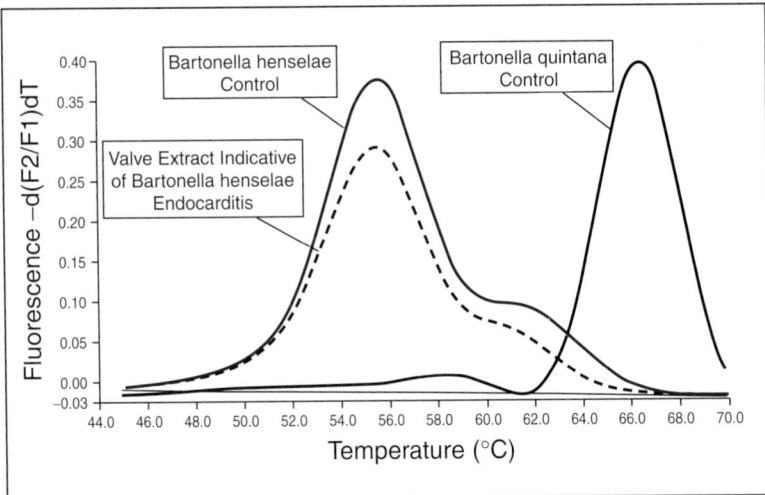

Figure 4-21 Postamplification melt-curve analysis. Postamplification melt-curve analysis may be used to differentiate closely related species. In this example, the causative agent of the culture-negative endocarditis, *Bartonella henselae*, is distinguished from *Bartonella quintana* using this technique.

entiation of the *Plasmodium* species, among many other applications.[20,29,40,58,83,93,146,220,308,365,371]

Strain Typing

Hospital microbiologists and epidemiologists may need to determine relatedness among bacteria or fungi of the same species to determine if transmission of the organism of interest has taken place in a manner that may be addressed by infection control. For example, if *Pseudomonas aeruginosa* has been isolated from four babies in a neonatal intensive-care unit, the hospital epidemiologist may wonder if these are the same bacterial strain that has been transferred from a point source or if are they different strains and the infection has occurred merely by chance. The determination that the bacteria are all of the same strain strengthens the evidence that there is a point source of transmission of the bacteria and that there is a breakdown in techniques or personal hygiene, all of which may be corrected.

Phenotypic methods of strain typing preceded genotypic methods, but many of these lack the high degree of discrimination that may be achieved by genotypic strain typing. Some others, such as bacteriophage typing, require a high degree of specialized expertise and the maintenance of considerable resources (i.e., libraries of bacteriophages). Antimicrobial susceptibility profiling, although not as definitive as some of the genotypic methods of profiling, is valuable, and uses information that is often already available because of susceptibility testing performed to guide therapy. Bacteria that have very different antimicrobial susceptibility profiles are likely not identical and therefore probably do not warrant more expensive genotypic strain typing.

The earliest molecular attempts at demonstrating relatedness among different groups of bacteria were accomplished with simple DNA-DNA hybridization studies. Groups of bacteria with high degrees of DNA homology, as determined through DNA-DNA hybridization studies, were considered to be more closely related, compared with groups that had poor DNA homology when compared with one another. For the most part, these studies confirmed what was considered to be true from phenotypic testing. For example, the DNA-

DNA hybridization studies between *Staphylococcus* and *Micrococcus*, which are in the same family, would demonstrate greater homology than would a comparison between *Staphylococcus* and *Pseudomonas*.

Plasmids are small, circular DNA molecules that are present in many bacteria and exist separately from the chromosomal DNA. Plasmids are important because they may contain genes important for virulence, including genes that impart resistance to antimicrobial agents. Plasmids may also spread from one bacterium to another via conjugation and thereby disseminate these genes. Developments in electrophoresis that allowed for the separation of plasmids from the chromosomal DNA, and the differentiation of plasmids from one another, made possible plasmid profiling as an early means of strain typing. Plasmid profiling was one of the earliest genetic methods used to determine strain relatedness.

There have been many genetic methods described for analyzing the relationship of microorganisms. Methods that are not discussed here but that have proven useful include ribotyping, random amplified polymorphic DNA (RAPD) analysis, and spoligotyping, among others. Molecular typing methods may be categorized as those that require nucleic-acid amplification for the typing process (amplification-based methods) and those that do not (non-amplification-based methods). This chapter will discuss one non-amplification-based method, pulsed-field gel electrophoresis (PFGE), which is considered by many to be the standard for microbial typing. Two amplification-based typing methods will be discussed, PCR-RFLP, which combines the strengths of PCR with the typing of restriction-fragment-length polymorphism, and Rep-PCR, a relatively new, commercially available technology that uses, for the purpose of typing, repetitive genetic elements that are occur naturally in bacteria.

Non-Amplification-Based Typing
PULSED-FIELD GEL ELECTROPHORESIS

There are many strain typing methods that vary in the degree of distinction that may be detected, cost, and ease of use. Many of the current methods of molecular strain typing rely on the use of a group of enzymes called restriction endonucleases. These enzymes are naturally occurring enzymes that cleave double-stranded DNA based on particular sequences termed restriction sites. Different enzymes cleave based on different sequences, and a variety of restriction endonucleases are commercially available. When the enzymes cleave the DNA, the two ends of the DNA produced may be either blunt or may have overhanging, so-called sticky ends. When microbial chromosomal or plasmid DNA is extracted from the organisms and exposed to one or more restriction endonucleases, it will be cleaved depending on the restriction endonucleases used and the number of restriction sites present in the DNA. The fragments of DNA that result will vary in size, and may be separated from one another by gel electrophoresis and visualized by staining with ethidium bromide. This is an RFLP analysis. Microorganisms with the same RFLP pattern are likely to be closely related, whereas those with very different RFLP patterns are less likely to be closely related. Although RFLP patterns are highly reproducible and very accurate, problems may arise in assessing the hundreds of DNA fragments that may arise following restriction enzyme digestion. PFGE was devised as a means to simplify RFLP typing.

PFGE is considered by many to be the standard form of strain typing, to which newer methods should be compared. In short, this technique begins with the extraction of the chromosomal bacterial DNA of the strains of interest, which are exposed to a variety of restriction endonucleases. The type of restriction endonucleases used is usually determined by the type of bacteria under analysis, based on previous research that has demonstrated the efficacy of these enzymes. As above, the restriction endonucleases cut the chromosomal DNA into a variety of pieces, depending on the number of restriction sites present in that particular strain. The fragments of chromosomal DNA are then separated using a specialized type of electrophoresis. The chromosomal restriction profile resulting from PFGE usually results in 5–20 fragments that range in size from 10–800 kb[338,340] (Fig. 4-22). These are visualized, photographed, and submitted for image analysis. Computer programs are then used to determine if the strains under analysis are indistinguishable or distinguishable and the degree to which these may be distinguished. The process has been termed DNA finger-

printing when the process of RFLP is combined with Southern blot transfer and probe hybridization.[338]

Amplification-Based Typing

There are a number of postamplification methods of analysis that may be used for microbial typing. These include single-stranded conformation polymorphism analysis, amplified fragment-length polymorphisms, arbitrarily primed PCR, RFLP analysis of the PCR product (PCR-RFLP), and analysis of PCR products of repetitive elements present in bacterial genomes (rep-PCR). The discussion of all these methods is beyond the scope of this book. We will briefly describe the latter two types of analysis, PCR-RFLP and rep-PCR, as examples of amplification-based methods of microbial typing

PCR-RFLP

Just as restriction endonucleases may be used to ligate the chromosomal DNA of bacteria, these enzymes may also to be used to cleave the amplicon. The selection of the endonuclease(s) used with PCR-RFLP must be chosen with care, since the amplicon is orders of magnitude smaller than the bacterial chromosome and is less likely to randomly contain restriction sites. The enzymes are often chosen based on previous knowledge of restriction sites that are variably present in the amplicons and, therefore, may be useful for the comparison of strains. The size of the amplicon and the number of potential restriction sites that it may contain imposes limitations on the differentiating capabilities of this technology.

RFLP analysis of the PCR product is commonly performed on assays directed against the rDNA. When the PCR product of an assay that targets the rDNA is analyzed by RFLP, it may be referred to as PCR ribotyping. Even when the rDNA is analyzed, it is important to target particular areas, to achieve type-specific information.[163,178] PCR-RFLP has been used to type all different kinds of microorganisms, including bacteria such as *Campylobacter* and *Borrelia* species and atypical fungi such as *Pneumocystis jiroveci*.[55,154,191] In addition to strain comparisons, PCR-RFLP patterns may be used for organism identification. The use

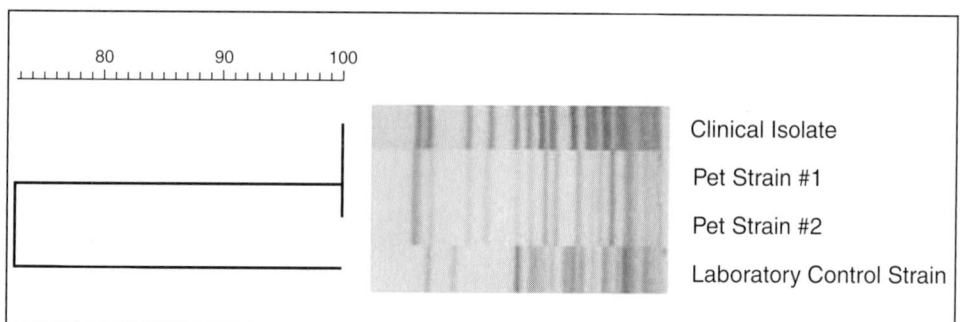

Figure 4-22 Pathogenic isolate of *Pasteurella multocida*. The analysis of a pathogenic isolate of *Pasteurella multocida* (clinical isolate) was genetically indistinguishable from two phenotypically different *P. multocida* isolates obtained from the patient's cat, but is clearly distinguishable from the laboratory control strain.

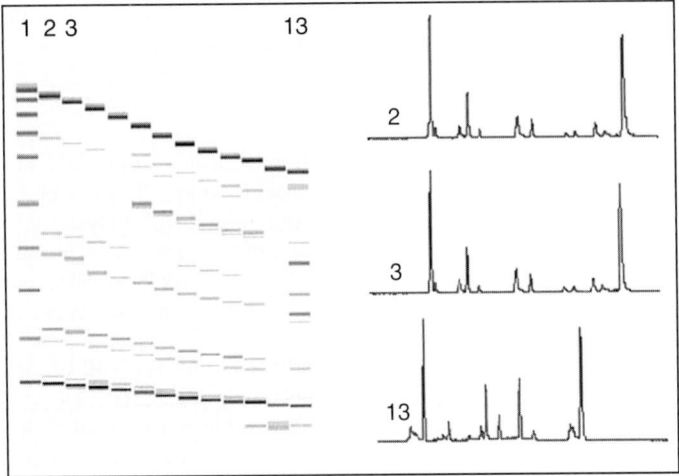

Figure 4-23 Rep-PCR of *Staphylococcus* isolates. The fragment analysis (*right*) reflects the patterns of the bands in the gel that is performed following rep-PCR. The ladder (lane 1) is used as a comparative standard. The fragments from the isolates represented in lanes 2 and 3 are indistinguishable, whereas these are clearly different from those produced by the isolate represented in lane 13.

of this technology in this manner relies on the use of highly specific PCR primers. This technique, for example, has been used to identify fastidious bacteria, such as *Bartonella* species, and difficult-to-identify parasites, such as hookworms and filarial worms.[101,102,165,283] This technology has also proven very useful for the differentiation of *Nocardia* species, which is clinically important given the differences in antimicrobial susceptibilities within this group.[200,326] The nonribosomal genes that are may be used for PCR-RFLP include either housekeeping genes, such as *rpoB*, or any gene that may contain strain-specific information for a particular group of organisms (i.e., the genes that encode for the enzymes responsible for hippurate hydrolysis for *Campylobacter jejuni*).[160,283,327]

REP-PCR

Repetitive DNA elements in prokaryotic genomes form the basis for rep-PCR. These repetitive elements are the hybridization sites for the primers used in rep-PCR. These primers, which are complementary to the interspersed repetitive sequences, generate through PCR amplification variably sized DNA fragments, which may be separated by gel electrophoresis (Fig. 4-23). The electrophoretic patterns may be used to determine the relatedness of bacterial strains that are being compared. A single primer set may be used for a variety of gram-positive and gram-negative bacteria, or more than one primer set may be used to target different repetitive elements. Rep-PCR has been used to type enterohemorrhagic *E. coli* isolates to investigate animal-to-human transmission.[92,99,310] It, like other typing techniques, has been used to track both gram-positive and gram-negative bacteria that are resistant to antimicrobial agents and of importance to the hospital epidemiologist.[23,64,312,344] The information generated through rep-PCR may also be used for microorganism identification. This technology, for example, has been used to identify organisms and examine diversity with the *Streptomyces* genus and to identify *Bartonella* species.[188,289]

CLINICAL APPLICATIONS OF MICROBIAL TYPING

Genetic comparisons of microorganisms have been used to investigate outbreaks in hospitals, in cities, and even across the nation.[33,114,182,202,223,263,378] It is common for potential nosocomial outbreaks to be investigated using genetic typing methods. A possibility of an outbreak is often suspected when the frequency of isolation of a pathogenic microorganism exceeds its usual baseline recovery rate. This may be in a particular place, such as the number of MRSA blood isolates in the hospital in general or a ward in particular, or it may be the number of *Salmonella* isolates reported to a county health department.

Given the fragility of premature babies, these techniques are commonly used to investigate outbreaks in neonatal intensive-care units.[180,225,298] Molecular typing methods are also commonly used to investigate infections caused by bacteria that are resistant to antimicrobial agents.[85,144,153,298] In some instances, genetic typing methods have been used to successfully determine the point source of an outbreak. Outbreaks and the transmission of *M. tuberculosis* are often studied using molecular typing methods.[76,181,296,318,339,360]

Public health epidemiologists from across the country are now collaborating by submitting standardized typing information obtained from strains of bacteria that cause foodborne disease into a national public database in a program called PulseNet. The PFGE fingerprint patterns are submitted from participants in all 50 states. PulseNet is designed as an early warning system for foodborne diseases. More information about this national effort to track and rapidly curtail bacterial foodborne illnesses may be obtained at www.cdc.gov/pulsenet.

Conclusion

The molecular revolution is here and is ongoing. The number of molecular applications for the detection and characterization of all types of microorganisms increases each year, with many commercial vendors seeking FDA approval for their applications. These applications include numerous signal-amplification methods, which in many instances may be not as sensitive as PCR, but are simple to use, may be less expensive, and are not burdened with the specter of potential amplicon contamination. Nucleic-acid amplification assays, and the methods to detect the products of amplification, have evolved rapidly over the past decade, culminating in the exciting applications of real-time PCR and similar technologies. Finally, the use of genetic typing of microbes to demonstrate relatedness among microorganisms continues to provide useful information regarding the transmission of infectious diseases. The standard methods, such as PFGE, continue to be useful, but amplification-based assays, such as rep-PCR, which is now commercially available, will likely find its niche given its utility, ease-of-use, and rapid turnaround time.

REFERENCES

1. Abe C, et al. [Detection of rifampin-resistant Mycobacterium tuberculosis by line probe assay (LiPA)]. Kekkaku 2000;75(10):575–581.

2. Acog Practice Bulletin. Clinical management guidelines for obstetrician-gynecologists. Number 45, August 2003. Cervical cytology screening (replaces committee opinion 152, March 1995). Obstet Gynecol 2003;102:417–427.

3. Ahmadian A, et al. Single-nucleotide polymorphism analysis by pyrosequencing. Anal Biochem 2000;280:103–110.

4. Akduman D, et al. Evaluation of a strand displacement amplification assay (BD ProbeTec-SDA) for detection of Neisseria gonorrhoeae in urine specimens. J Clin Microbiol 2002;40:281–283.

5. Alberts B, Johnson A, Lewis J, et al. Molecular Biology of the Cell. 4th Ed. New York: Garland, 2002.

6. Alderborn A, Kristofferson A, Hammerling U. Determination of single-nucleotide polymorphisms by real-time pyrophosphate DNA sequencing. Genome Res 2000;10:1249–1258.

7. Arbyn M, et al. Virologic versus cytologic triage of women with equivocal Pap smears: a meta-analysis of the accuracy to detect high-grade intraepithelial neoplasia. J Natl Cancer Inst 2004;96:280–293.

8. Arnoldi J, et al. Species-specific assessment of Mycobacterium leprae in skin biopsies by in situ hybridization and polymerase chain reaction. Lab Invest 1992; 66:618–623.

9. Asano S, et al. Monitoring herpesvirus DNA in three cases of acute retinal necrosis by real-time PCR. J Clin Virol 2004;29:206–209.

10. Asoh N, et al. Emergence of rifampin-resistant Rhodococcus equi with several types of mutations in the rpoB gene among AIDS patients in northern Thailand. J Clin Microbiol 2003;41:2337–2340.

11. Baeumner AJ, et al. RNA biosensor for the rapid detection of viable Escherichia coli in drinking water. Biosensors Bioelectronics 2003;18:405–413.

12. Baghurst PA. Chips with everything. Aust N Z J Public Health 2002;26: 106–107.

13. Balganesh M, Lalitha MK, Nathaniel R. Rapid diagnosis of acute pyogenic meningitis by a combined PCR dot-blot assay. Mol Cell Probes 2000;14:61–69.

14. Barrett DM, et al. In situ hybridization for Helicobacter pylori in gastric mucosal biopsy specimens: quantitative evaluation of test performance in comparison with the CLOtest and thiazine stain. J Clin Lab Anal 1997;11:374–379.

15. Bartfai Z, et al. Molecular characterization of rifampin-resistant isolates of Mycobacterium tuberculosis from Hungary by DNA sequencing and the line probe assay. J Clin Microbiol 2001;39:3736–3739.

16. Bashir Ms. In situ hybridization for the identification of Helicobacter pylori in paraffin was embedded tissue. J Clin Pathol 1994;47:862–864.

17. Bastien P, Chabbert E, Lachaud L. Contamination management of broad-range or specific PCR: is there any difference? J Clin Microbiol 2003;41:2272.

18. Beck RC, Kohn DJ, Tuohy MJ, et al. Detection of polyoma virus in brain tissue of patients with progressive multifocal leukoencephalopathy by real-time PCR and pyrosequencing. Diag Mol Pathol 2004;13:15–21.

19. Bej AK, Mahbubani MH, Miller R, et al. Multiples PCR amplification and immobilized capture probes for detection of bacterial pathogens and indicators in water. Mol Cell Probes 1990;4:353–365.

20. Bell A, Ranford-Cartwright L. Real-time quantitative PCR in parasitology. Trends Parasitol 2002;18:338.

21. Berlau J, et al. In situ hybridization and direct fluorescence antibodies for the detection of Chlamydia trachomatis in synovial tissue from patients with reactive arthritis. J Clin Pathol 1998;51:803–806.

22. Bialek R, et al. PCR assays for identification of Coccidioides posadasii based on the nucleotide sequence of the antigen 2/proline-rich antigen. J Clin Microbiol 2004;42:778–783.

23. Biddick R, et al. Evidence of transmission of Burkholderia cepacia, Burkholderia multivorans and Burkholderia dolosa among persons with cystic fibrosis. FEMS Microbiol Lett 2003;228:57–62.

24. Boddinghaus B, Rogall T, Flohr T, Blocker H, Bottger EC: Detection and identification of mycobacteria by amplification of rRNA. J Clin Microbiol 1990;28: 1751–1759.

25. Boivin G, et al. Multiplex real-time PCR assay for detection of influenza and human respiratory syncytial viruses. J Clin Microbiol 2004;42:45–51.

26. Botma HJ, et al. Differential in situ hybridization for herpes simplex virus typing in routine skin biopsies. J Virol Meth 1995;53:37–45.

27. Boye K, Hogdall E, Borre M.: Identification of bacteria using two degenerate 16S rDNA sequencing primers. Microbiol Res 1999;154:23–26.

28. Bozzetti M, et al. Comparison between hybrid capture II and polymerase chain reaction results among women at low risk for cervical cancer. Ann Epidemiol 2000;10:466.

29. Bretagne S. Molecular diagnostics in clinical parasitology and mycology: limits of the current polymerase chain reaction (PCR) assays and interest of the real-time PCR assays. Clin Microbiol Infect 2003;9:505–511.

30. Brites C, et al. Evaluation of viral resistance to reverse transcriptase inhibitors (RTI) in HIV-1-infected patients before and after 6 months of single or double antiretroviral therapy. Braz J Infect Dis 2001;5:177–182.

31. Bryant PA, et al. Chips with everything: DNA microarrays in infectious diseases. Lancet Infect Dis 2004;4:100–111.

32. Caliendo AM, et al. Comparison of molecular tests for detection and quantification of cell-associated cytomegalovirus DNA. J Clin Microbiol 2003;41: 3509–3513.

33. Cao V, et al. Distribution of extended-spectrum beta-lactamases in clinical isolates of Enterobacteriaceae in Vietnam. Antimicrob Agents Chemother 2002; 46:3739–3743.

34. Caveman A. ''I'll have a genome with chips, please.'' J Cell Sci 2000;113(Pt 20):3543–3544.

35. Cavusoglu C, et al. Characterization of rpoB mutations in rifampin-resistant clinical isolates of Mycobacterium tuberculosis from Turkey by DNA sequencing and line probe assay. J Clin Microbiol 2002;40:4435–4438.

36. Chan JK, et al. A study of the association of Epstein-Barr virus with Burkitt's lymphoma occurring in a Chinese population. Histopathology 1995;26:239–245.

37. Chang WN, et al. Septic cavernous sinus thrombosis due to Streptococcus constellatus infection. J Formos Med Assoc 2003;102:733–736.

38. Chapin KC, Blake P, Wilson CD. Performance characteristics and utilization of rapid antigen test, DNA probe, and culture for detection of group a streptococci in an acute care clinic. J Clin Microbiol 2002;40:4207–4210.

39. Chapin K, Musgnug M. Evaluation of three rapid methods for the direct identification of Staphylococcus aureus from positive blood cultures. J Clin Microbiol 2003;41:4324–4327.

40. Cheesman SJ, et al. Real-time quantitative PCR for analysis of genetically mixed infections of malaria parasites: technique validation and applications. Mol Biochem Parasitol 2003;131:83–91.

41. Chemlal K, Portaels F. Molecular diagnosis of nontuberculous mycobacteria. Curr Opin Infect Dis 2003;16:77–83.

42. Chernoff DN. The significance of HIV viral load assay precision: a review of the package insert specifications of two commercial kits. J Int Assoc Physicians AIDS Care (Chicago) 2002;1:134–140.

43. Chopra P, Meena LS, Singh Y. New drug targets for Mycobacterium tuberculosis. Indian J Med Res 2003;117:1–9.

44. Clarke JR. Molecular diagnosis of HIV. Expert Rev Mol Diagn 2002;2:233–9.

45. Clarke LM, Sierra MS, Daidone BJ, et al. Comparison of the Syva MicroTrak enzyme immunoassay and Gen-Probe PACE 2 with cell culture for diagnosis of cervical Chlamydia trachomatis infection in a high-prevalence female population. J Clin Microbiol 1993;31:968–971.

46. Clavel C, et al. Hybrid capture II, a new sensitive test for human papillomavirus detection. Comparison with hybrid capture I and PCR results in cervical lesions. J Clin Pathol 1998;51:737–740.

47. Cleary TJ, et al. Rapid and specific detection of Mycobacterium tuberculosis by using the Smart Cycler instrument and a specific fluorogenic probe. J Clin Microbiol 2003;41:4783–4786.

48. Cloud JL, et al. Evaluation of partial 16S ribosomal DNA sequencing for identification of nocardia species by using the MicroSeq 500 system with an expanded database. J Clin Microbiol 2004;42:578–584.

49. Cloud JL, et al. Identification of Mycobacterium spp. by using a commercial 16S ribosomal DNA sequencing kit and additional sequencing libraries. J Clin Microbiol 2002;40:400–406.

50. Coen DM: Antiviral Drug Resistance. Ann N Y Acad Sci 1990;616:224–237.

51. Comanor L, et al. Successful HCV genotyping of previously failed and low viral load specimens using an HCV RNA qualitative assay based on transcription-mediated amplification in conjunction with the line probe assay. J Clin Virol 2003;28:14–26.

52. Corless CE, et al. Development and evaluation of a ''real-time'' RT-PCR for the detection of enterovirus and parechovirus RNA in CSF and throat swab samples. J Med Virol 2002;67:555–562.

53. Corsaro D, et al. Multiplex PCR for rapid and differential diagnosis of Mycoplasma pneumoniae and Chlamydia pneumoniae in respiratory infections. Diagn Microbiol Infect Dis 1999;35:105–108.

54. Costa JM, et al. Real-time PCR for diagnosis and follow-up of Toxoplasma reactivation after allogeneic stem cell transplantation using fluorescence resonance energy transfer hybridization probes. J Clin Microbiol 2000;38: 2929–2932.

55. Costa MC, et al. Dihydropteroate synthase (DHPS) genotyping by PCR-RFLP analysis of Pneumocystis jirovecii repeated isolates from HIV-infected patients: a preliminary study. J Eukaryot Microbiol 2003;50(Suppl):607–608.

56. Cote S, Abed Y, Boivin G. Comparative evaluation of real-time PCR assays for detection of the human metapneumovirus. J Clin Microbiol 2003;41:3631–635.

57. Cummings CA, et al. Bordetella species are distinguished by patterns of substantial gene loss and host adaptation. J Bacteriol 2004;186:1484–1492.

58. Cummings KL, Tarleton Rl. Rapid quantitation of Trypanosoma cruzi in host tissue by real-time PCR. Mol Biochem Parasitol 2003;129:53–59.

59. Dai CY, et al. Clinical evaluation of the COBAS Amplicor HBV monitor test for measuring serum HBV DNA and comparison with the Quantiplex branched DNA signal amplification assay in Taiwan. J Clin Pathol 2004;57:141–145.

60. Daly JA, Clifton NL, Seskin KC, Gooch WM III. Use of rapid, nonradioactive DNA probes in culture confirmation tests to detect Streptococcus agalactiae, Haemophilus influenzae, and Enterococcus spp. from pediatric patients with significant infections. J Clin Microbiol 1991;29:80–82.

61. Darwin LH, et al. Comparison of Digene hybrid capture 2 and conventional culture for detection of Chlamydia trachomatis and Neisseria gonorrhoeae in cervical specimens. J Clin Microbiol 2002;40:641–644.

62. Darwin LH, et al. Evaluation of the Hybrid Capture 2 CT/GC DNA tests and the GenProbe PACE 2 tests from the same male urethral swab specimens. Sex Transm Dis 2002;29:576–580.

63. Davis Gl. Hepatitis C virus genotypes and quasispecies. Am J Med 1999; 107(6B):21S–26S.

64. Decre D, et al. Characterization of CMY-type beta-lactamases in clinical strains of Proteus mirabilis and Klebsiella pneumoniae isolated in four hospitals in the Paris area. J Antimicrob Chemother 2002;50:681–688.

65. De Cremoux P, et al. Efficiency of the hybrid capture 2 HPV DNA test in cervical cancer screening: a study by the French Society of Clinical Cytology. Am J Clin Pathol 2003;120:492–499.

66. De Oliveira MM, et al. Rapid detection of resistance against rifampicin in isolates of Mycobacterium tuberculosis from Brazilian patients using a reverse-phase hybridization assay. J Microbiol Methods 2003;53:335–342.

67. Derdelinckx I, et al. Performance of the VERSANT HIV-1 resistance assays (LiPA) for detecting drug resistance in therapy-naive patients infected with different HIV-1 subtypes. FEMS Immunol Med Microbiol 2003;39:119–124.

68. Desjardin LE, et al. Comparison of the ABI 7700 system (TaqMan) and competitive PCR for quantification of IS6110 DNA in sputum during treatment of tuberculosis. J Clin Microbiol 1998;36:1964–1968.

69. Dharakul T, et al. Detection of Burkholderia pseudomallei DNA in patients with septicemic melioidosis. J Clin Microbiol 1996;34:609–614.

70. Diemert DJ, Libman MD, Lebel P. Confirmation by 16S rRNA PCR of the COBAS AMPLICOR CT/NG test for diagnosis of Neisseria gonorrhoeae infection in a low-prevalence population. J Clin Microbiol 2002;40:4056–4059.

71. Dobner P, et al. Rapid identification of mycobacterial species by PCR amplification of hypervariable 16S rRNA gene promoter region. J Clin Microbiol 1996; 34:866–869.

72. Drake TA, Hindler JA, Berlin OG, Bruckner Da. Rapid identification of Mycobacterium avium complex in culture using DNA probes. J Clin Microbiol 1987; 25:1442–1445.

73. Drancourt M, et al. rpoB gene sequence-based identification of aerobic Gram-positive cocci of the genera Streptococcus, Enterococcus, Gemella, Abiotrophia, and Granulicatella. J Clin Microbiol 2004;42:497–504.

74. Drancourt M, Raoult D. rpoB gene sequence-based identification of Staphylococcus species. J Clin Microbiol 2002;40:1333–1338.

75. D'souza DH, Jaykus La. Nucleic acid sequence based amplification for the rapid and sensitive detection of Salmonella enterica from foods. J Applied Microbiol 2003;95:1343–1350.

76. Durmaz R, et al. Primary drug resistance and molecular epidemiology of Mycobacterium tuberculosis isolates from patients in a population with high tuberculosis incidence in Turkey. Microb Drug Resist 2003;9:361–366.

77. Ebihara T, et al. Human metapneumovirus infection in Japanese children. J Clin Microbiol 2004;42:126–132.

78. Elahi E, et al. Determination of hepatitis C virus genotype by Pyrosequencing. J Virol Methods 2003;109:171–176.

79. Elbeik T, et al. Multicenter evaluation of the performance characteristics of the Bayer VERSANT HCV RNA 3.0 assay (bDNA). J Clin Microbiol 2004;42: 563–569.

80. Elbeik T, et al. Comparative analysis of HIV-1 viral load assays on subtype quantification: Bayer Versant HIV-1 RNA 3.0 versus Roche Amplicor HIV-1 Monitor -version 1.5. J Acquir Immune Defic Syndr 2002;29:330–339.

81. Elbeik T, Loftus RA, Beringer S. Health care industries' perspective of viral load assays: the VERSANT HIV-1 RNA 3.0 assay. Expert Rev Mol Diagn 2002; 2:275–285.

82. Erlich HA, Gelfand D, Sninsky Jj. Recent advances in the polymerase chain reaction [Review]. Science 1991;252:1643–1651.

83. Fabre R, et al. Comparative assessment of conventional PCR with multiplex real-time PCR using SYBR Green I detection for the molecular diagnosis of imported malaria. Parasitol 2004;128(Pt 1):15–21.

84. Farrell Dj. Evaluation of AMPLICOR Neisseria gonorrhoeae PCR using cppB nested PCR and 16S rRNA PCR. J Clin Microbiol 1999;37:386–390.

85. Farrell DJ, et al. Molecular epidemiology of multiresistant Streptococcus pneumoniae with both erm(B)- and mef(A)-mediated macrolide resistance. J Clin Microbiol 2004;42(2):764–768.

86. Farrell DJ, Sheedy Tj. Urinary screening for Neisseria gonorrhoeae in asymptomatic individuals from Queensland, Australia: an evaluation using three nucleic acid amplification methods. Pathology 2001;33:204–205.

87. Farrell JJ, Tuohy JM, Brown-elliot BA, et al. Rapid Identification of Nocardia by Pyrosequencing IDSA. San Diego: Xxxxx, 2003.

88. Fedele CG, et al. Multiplex polymerase chain reaction for the simultaneous detection and typing of polyomavirus JC, BK and SV40 DNA in clinical samples. J Virol Methods 1999;82:137–144.

89. Fenollar F, et al. Quantitative detection of Tropheryma whipplei DNA by real-time PCR. J Clin Microbiol 2002;40:1119–1120.

90. Feray C, Samuel D, Thiers V, et al. Reinfection of liver graft by hepatitis C after liver transplantation. J Clin Invest 1992;89:1361–1365.

91. Fisher MA, Plikaytis BB, Shinnick Tm. Microarray analysis of the Mycobacterium tuberculosis transcriptional response to the acidic conditions found in phagosomes. J Bacteriol 2002;184:4025–4032.

92. Foley SL, et al. Evaluation of molecular typing methods for Escherichia coli O157:H7 isolates from cattle, food, and humans. J Food Prot 2004;67:651–657.

93. Fontaine M, Guillot E. Study of 18S rRNA and rDNA stability by real-time RT-PCR in heat-inactivated Cryptosporidium parvum oocysts. FEMS Microbiol Lett 2003;226:237–243.

94. Fouad AF, et al. PCR-based identification of bacteria associated with endodontic infections. J Clin Microbiol 2002;40:3223–3231.

95. Foy CA, Parkes Hc. Emerging homogeneous DNA-based technologies in the clinical laboratory. Clin Chem 2001;47:990–1000.

96. Frias C, et al. Usefulness of adding multiplex nested-polymerase chain reaction assay of cerebrospinal fluid samples to routine diagnostic testing for herpesvirus encephalitis. Eur J Clin Microbiol Infect Dis 2001;20:670–672.

97. Fukushima M, et al. Detection and identification of Mycobacterium species isolates by DNA microarray. J Clin Microbiol 2003;41:2605–2615.

98. Gamboa F, et al. Comparative evaluation of two commercial assays for direct detection of Mycobacterium tuberculosis in respiratory specimens. Eur J Clin Microbiol Infect Dis 1998;17:151–157.

99. Garcia A, Fox JG. The rabbit as a new reservoir host of enterohemorrhagic Escherichia coli. Emerg Infect Dis 2003;9:1592–1597.

100. Garcia CA, et al. Mutation detection by pyrosequencing: sequencing of exons 5–8 of the p53 tumor suppressor gene. Gene 2000;253:249–257.

101. Gasser RB, et al. Rapid delineation of closely-related filarial parasites using genetic markers in spacer rDNA. Acta Trop 1996;62:143–150.

102. Gasser RB, Stewart LE, Speare R. Genetic markers in ribosomal DNA for hookworm identification. Acta Trop 1996;62:15–21.

103. Gauduchon V, et al. Molecular diagnosis of infective endocarditis by PCR amplification and direct sequencing of DNA from valve tissue. J Clin Microbiol 2003; 41:763–766.

104. Gaydos CA, et al. Performance of the APTIMA Combo 2 assay for detection of Chlamydia trachomatis and Neisseria gonorrhoeae in female urine and endocervical swab specimens. J Clin Microbiol 2003;41:304–309.

105. Geha DJ, Uhl JR, Gustaferro CA, Persing Dh. Multiplex PCR for identification of methicillin-resistant staphylococci in the clinical laboratory. J Clin Microbiol 1994;32:1768–1772.

106. Gencay M. Chlamydia trachomatis detected in human placenta. J Clin Pathol 1997;50:852–855.

107. Germer JJ, et al. Comparison of the VERSANT HCV RNA qualitative assay (transcription-mediated amplification) and the COBAS AMPLICOR hepatitis C virus test, version 2.0, in patients undergoing interferon-ribavirin therapy. Diagn Microbiol Infect Dis 2003;47:615–618.

108. Gerna G, et al. Human cytomegalovirus immediate-early mRNAemia versus pp65 antigenemia for guiding pre-emptive therapy in children and young adults undergoing hematopoietic stem cell transplantation: a prospective, randomized, open-label trial. Blood 2003;101:5053–5060.

109. Gharizadeh B, et al. Identification of medically important fungi by the Pyrosequencing technology. Mycoses 2004;47(1–2):29–33.

110. Gleaves CA, et al. Multicenter evaluation of the Bayer VERSANT HIV-1 RNA 3.0 assay: analytical and clinical performance. J Clin Virol 2002;25(2):205–216.

111. Goldenberger D, et al. Molecular diagnosis of bacterial endocarditis by broad-range PCR amplification and direct sequencing. J Clin Microbiol 1997;35: 2733–2739.

112. Gonzalez R, Hanna BA. Evaluation of Gen-Probe DNA hybridization systems for the identification of Mycobacterium tuberculosis and Mycobacterium avium-intracellulare. Diag Microbiol Infect Dis 1987;8:69–77.

113. Gourlain K, et al. Quantitation of cytomegalovirus (CMV) DNA by real-time PCR for occurrence of CMV disease in HIV-infected patients receiving highly active antiretroviral therapy. J Med Virol 2003;69:401–407.

114. Graham Pl Iii, et al. Epidemiology of methicillin-susceptible Staphylococcus aureus in the neonatal intensive care unit. Infect Control Hosp Epidemiol 2002; 23:677–682.

115. Grahn N, et al. Identification of mixed bacterial DNA contamination in broad-range PCR amplification of 16S rDNA V1 and V3 variable regions by pyrosequencing of cloned amplicons. FEMS Microbiol Lett 2003;219:87–91.

116. Granato PA, Franz MR. Use of the Gen-Probe PACE system for the detection of Neisseria gonorrhoeae in urogenital samples. Diag Microbiol Infect Dis 1990; 3:217–221.

117. Grant PR, et al. Detection of SARS coronavirus in plasma by real-time RT-PCR. N Engl J Med 2003;349:2468–2469.

118. Greenlee DJ, et al. Quantitation of CMV by real-time PCR in transfusable RBC units. Transfusion 2002;42:403–408.

119. Greisen K, et al. PCR primers and probes for the 16S rRNA gene of most species of pathogenic bacteria, including bacteria found in cerebrospinal fluid. J Clin Microbiol 1994;32:335–351.

120. Grijalva M, et al. Molecular diagnosis of culture negative infective endocarditis: clinical validation in a group of surgically treated patients. Heart 2003;89: 263–268.

121. Grondahl B, et al. Rapid identification of nine microorganisms causing acute respiratory tract infections by single-tube multiplex reverse transcription-PCR: feasibility study. J Clin Microbiol 1999;37:1–7.

122. Grude N, et al. Identification of Aerococcus urinae in urine samples. Clin Microbiol Infect 2003;9:976–979.

123. Gu Z, et al. Multiplexed, real-time PCR for quantitative detection of human adenovirus. J Clin Microbiol 2003;41:4636–4641.

124. Gumus B, et al. Evaluation of non-invasive clinical samples in chronic chlamydial prostatitis by using in situ hybridization. Scan J Urol Nephrol 1997;431: 449–51.

125. Guney C, et al. Laboratory diagnosis of enteroviral infections of the central nervous system by using a nested RT-polymerase chain reaction (PCR) assay. Diagn Microbiol Infect Dis 2003;47:557–562.

126. Habib-Bein NF, et al. Comparison of SmartCycler real-time reverse transcription-PCR assay in a public health laboratory with direct immunofluorescence and cell culture assays in a medical center for detection of influenza A virus. J Clin Microbiol 2003;41:3597–3601.

127. Hadziyannis E, et al. Amplicor enterovirus polymerase chain reaction in patients with aseptic meningitis: a sensitive test limited by amplification inhibitors. Arch Pathol Lab Med 1999;123:882–884.

128. Hall GS, Pratt-Rippin K, Washington JA. Evaluation of a chemiluminescent probe assay for identification of Histoplasma capsulatum isolates. J Clin Microbiol 1992;30:3003–3004.

129. Hall L, et al. Evaluation of the MicroSeq system for identification of mycobacteria by 16S ribosomal DNA sequencing and its integration into a routine clinical mycobacteriology laboratory. J Clin Microbiol 2003;41:1447–1453.

130. Hall L, Wohlfiel S, Roberts GD. Experience with the MicroSeq D2 large-subunit ribosomal DNA sequencing kit for identification of filamentous fungi encountered in the clinical laboratory. J Clin Microbiol 2004;42:622–626.

131. Hall L, Wohlfiel S, Roberts GD. Experience with the MicroSeq D2 large-subunit ribosomal DNA sequencing kit for identification of commonly encountered, clinically important yeast species. J Clin Microbiol 2003;41:5099–5102.

132. Hamilton MS, et al. High frequency of competitive inhibition in the Roche Cobas AMPLICOR multiplex PCR for Chlamydia trachomatis and Neisseria gonorrhoeae. J Clin Microbiol 2002;40:4393.

133. Hamprecht K, et al. Ganciclovir-resistant cytomegalovirus disease after allogeneic stem cell transplantation: pitfalls of phenotypic diagnosis by in vitro selection of an UL97 mutant strain. J Infect Dis 2003;187:139–143.

134. Han XY, et al. Rapid and accurate identification of mycobacteria by sequencing hypervariable regions of the 16S ribosomal RNA gene. Am J Clin Pathol 2002; 118:796–801.

135. Hanazawa R, Murayama SY, Yamaguchi H. In-situ detection of Aspergillus fumigatus. J Med Microbiol 2000;49:285–290.

136. Haqqi TM, Sarkar G, David CS, Sommer SS. Specific amplification of a refractory segment of genomic DNA. Nucleic Acids Res 1988;16:11844.

137. Harder TC, et al. New LightCycler PCR for rapid and sensitive quantification of parvovirus B19 DNA guides therapeutic decision-making in relapsing infections. J Clin Microbiol 2001;39:4413–4419.

138. Harris KA, Hartley JC. Development of broad-range 16S rDNA PCR for use in the routine diagnostic clinical microbiology service. J Med Microbiol 2003; 52(Pt 8):685–691.

139. Haushofer AC, et al. Genotyping of hepatitis C virus-comparison of three assays. J Clin Virol 2003;27:276–285.

140. Hayashi Y, et al. A novel diagnostic method of Pneumocystis carinii: in situ hybridization of ribosomal ribonucleic acid with biotinylated oligonucleotide probes. Lab Invest 1990;63:576–580.

141. Hayden RT, et al. In situ hybridization for the identification of yeastlike organisms in tissue section. Diag Mol Pathol 2001;10:15–23.

142. Heim A, et al. Rapid and quantitative detection of human adenovirus DNA by real-time PCR. J Med Virol 2003;70:228–239.

143. Hendolin PH, Paulin L, Ylikoski J. Clinically applicable multiplex PCR for four middle ear pathogens. J Clin Microbiol 2000;38:125–132.

144. Henriques Normark B, et al. Clonal analysis of Streptococcus pneumoniae non-susceptible to penicillin at day-care centers with index cases, in a region with low incidence of resistance: emergence of an invasive type 35B clone among carriers. Microb Drug Resist 2003;9:337–344.

145. Hiatt B, et al. A fatal case of West Nile virus infection in a bone marrow transplant recipient. Clin Infect Dis 2003;37:129–131.

146. Higgins JA, et al. Real-time PCR for the detection of Cryptosporidium parvum. J Microbiol Methods 2001;47:323–337.

147. Hirano K, Abe C, Takahashi M. Mutations in the rpoB gene of rifampin-resistant Mycobacterium tuberculosis strains isolated mostly in Asian countries and their rapid detection by line probe assay. J Clin Microbiol 1999;37:2663–2666.

148. Hogardt M, et al. Specific and rapid detection by fluorescent in situ hybridization of bacteria in clinical samples obtained from cystic fibrosis patients. J Clin Microbiol 2000;38:818–825.

149. Hong IS, et al. Comparative analysis of a liquid-based Pap test and concurrent HPV DNA assay of residual samples: a study of 608 cases. Acta Cytol 2002; 46:828–834.

150. Huang C, et al. First Isolation of West Nile virus from a patient with encephalitis in the United States. Emerg Infect Dis 2002;8:1367–171.

151. Huffnagle KE, Gander RM. Evaluation of Gen-Probe's Histoplasma capsulatum and Cryptococcus neoformans AccuProbes. J Clin Microbiol 1993;31:419–442.

152. Imhof A, et al. Rapid detection of pathogenic fungi from clinical specimens using LightCycler real-time fluorescence PCR. Eur J Clin Microbiol Infect Dis 2003;22:558–60.

153. Ip M, et al. A longitudinal analysis of methicillin-resistant Staphylococcus aureus in a Hong Kong teaching hospital. Infect Control Hosp Epidemiol 2004;25: 126–129.

154. Iriarte P, Owen RJ. PCR-RFLP analysis of the large subunit (23S) ribosomal RNA genes of Campylobacter jejuni. Lett Appl Microbiol 1996;23:163–166.

155. Jacques J, et al. New reverse transcription-PCR assay for rapid and sensitive detection of enterovirus genomes in cerebrospinal fluid specimens of patients with aseptic meningitis. J Clin Microbiol 2003;41:5726–5728.

156. Jambou R, Hatin I, Jaureguiberry G. Evidence by in situ hybridization for stage-specific expression of the ATP/ADP translocator mRNA in Plasmodium falciparum. Exp Parasitol 1995;80:549–571.

157. Janket ML, et al. Differential regulation of host cellular genes by HIV-1 viral protein R (Vpr): cDNA microarray analysis using isogenic virus. Biochem Biophys Res Commun 2004;314:1126–1132.

158. Jansen GJ, et al. Rapid identification of bacteria in blood cultures by using fluorescently labeled oligonucleotide probes. J Clin Microbiol 2000;38: 814–817.

159. Jantos CA, et al. Low prevalence of Chlamydia pneumoniae in atherectomy specimens from patients with coronary heart disease. Clin Infect Dis 1999;28: 988–992.

160. Jauk V, et al. Phenotypic and genotypic differentiation of Campylobacter spp. isolated from Austrian broiler farms: a comparison. Avian Pathol 2003;32: 33–37.

161. Jauregui LH, et al. Development of a real-time PCR assay for detection of Toxoplasma gondii in pig and mouse tissues. J Clin Microbiol 2001;39: 2065–2071.

162. Jebbink J, et al. Development of real-time PCR assays for the quantitative detection of Epstein-Barr virus and cytomegalovirus, comparison of TaqMan probes, and molecular beacons. J Mol Diagn 2003;5:15–20.

163. Jensen MA, Webster JA, Straus N. Rapid identification of bacteria on the basis of polymerase chain reaction-amplified ribosomal DNA spacer polymorphisms. Appl Environ Microbiol 1993;59:945–952.

164. Jiang J, Temenak JJ, Richards AL. Real-time PCR duplex assay for Rickettsia prowazekii and Borrelia recurrentis. Ann NY Acad Sci 2003;990:302–310.

165. Joblet C, et al. Identification of Bartonella (Rochalimaea) species among fastidious gram-negative bacteria on the basis of the partial sequence of the citrate-synthase gene. J Clin Microbiol 1995;33:1879–1883.

166. Jou NT, Yoshimori RB, Mason GR, et al. Single-tube, nested, reverse transcriptase PCR for detection of viable Mycobacterium tuberculosis. J Clin Microbiol 1997;35:1161–1165.

167. Kaiser K, Rabodonirina M, Picot S. Real time quantitative PCR and RT-PCR for analysis of Pneumocystis carinii hominis. J Microbiol Methods 2001;45: 113–118.

168. Kantakamalakul W, et al. Prevalence of rabies virus and Hantaan virus infections in commensal rodents and shrews trapped in Bangkok. J Med Association Thailand 2003;86:1008–1014.

169. Kares S, et al. Real-time PCR for rapid diagnosis of entero- and rhinovirus infections using LightCycler. J Clin Virol 2004;29:99–104.

170. Kempf VA, Trebesius K, Autenrieth IB. Fluorescent in situ hybridization allows rapid identification of microorganisms in blood cultures. J Clin Microbiol 2000; 38:830–838.

171. Khamis A, et al. Usefulness of rpoB gene sequencing for identification of Afipia and Bosea species, including a strategy for choosing discriminative partial sequences. Appl Environ Microbiol 2003;69:6740–6749.

172. Khulordava I, et al. Identification of the bacterial etiology of culture-negative endocarditis by amplification and sequencing of a small ribosomal RNA gene. Diagn Microbiol Infect Dis 2003;46:9–11.

173. Kim BJ, et al. Differential identification of Mycobacterium tuberculosis complex and nontuberculous mycobacteria by duplex PCR assay using the RNA polymerase gene (rpoB). J Clin Microbiol 2004;42:1308–1312.

174. Kitagawa Y, et al. Rapid diagnosis of methicillin-resistant Staphylococcus aureus bacteremia by nested polymerase chain reaction. Ann Surg 1996;224: 665–671.

175. Kleter B, et al. Development and clinical evaluation of a highly sensitive PCR-reverse hybridization line probe assay for detection and identification of anogenital human papillomavirus. J Clin Microbiol 1999;37:2508–2517.

176. Knox J, et al. Evaluation of self-collected samples in contrast to practitioner-collected samples for detection of Chlamydia trachomatis, Neisseria gonorrhoeae, and Trichomonas vaginalis by polymerase chain reaction among women living in remote areas. Sex Transm Dis 2002;29:647–654.

177. Koppelman MH, et al. Quantitative real-time detection of parvovirus B19 DNA in plasma. Transfusion 2004;44:97–103.

178. Kostman JR, Edlind TD, Lipuma JJ, Stull TL. Molecular epidemiology of Pseudomonas cepacia determined by polymerase chain reaction ribotyping. J Clin Microbiol 1992;30:2084–2087.

179. Kottaridi C, et al. Elucidation of cytomegalovirus disease recurrence in an HIV-1-positive patient. J Gastroenterol 2003;38:643–646.

180. Kuboyama RH, de Oliveira HB, Moretti-Branchini ML. Molecular epidemiology of systemic infection caused by Enterobacter cloacae in a high-risk neonatal intensive care unit. Infect Control Hosp Epidemiol 2003;24:490–494.

181. Kulaga S, et al. Diversity of Mycobacterium tuberculosis isolates in an immigrant population: evidence against a founder effect. Am J Epidemiol 2004;159: 507–513.

182. Kumar R, et al. Changing pattern of biotypes, phage types and drug resistance involvement of Salmonella typhi in Ludhiana during 1980–1999. Ind J Med Res 2001;113: 175–180.

183. Kwok AY, et al. Species identification and phylogenetic relationships based on partial HSP60 gene sequences within the genus Staphylococcus. Int J Syst Bacteriol 1999;49(Pt 3):1181–92.

184. Kwon D, Chae C. Detection and localization of Mycoplasma hyopneumoniae DNA in lungs from naturally infected pigs by in situ hybridization using a digoxigenin-labeled probe. Vet Pathol 1999;36:308–313.

185. Lanciotti RS. Molecular amplification assays for the detection of flaviviruses. Adv Virus Res 2003;61:67–99.

186. Landry ML, Garner R, Ferguson D. Comparison of the NucliSens Basic kit (Nucleic Acid Sequence-Based Amplification) and the Argene Biosoft Enterovirus Consensus Reverse Transcription-PCR assays for rapid detection of enterovirus RNA in clinical specimens. J Clin Microbiol 2003;41:5006–5010.

187. Lang S, et al. Evaluation of PCR in the molecular diagnosis of endocarditis. J Infect 2004;48:269–275.

188. Lanoot B, et al. BOX-pCR fingerprinting as a powerful tool to reveal synonymous names in the genus Streptomyces: emended descriptions are proposed for the species Streptomyces cinereorectus, S. fradiae, S. tricolor, S. colombiensis, S. filamentosus, S. vinaceus and S. phaeopurpureus. Syst Appl Microbiol 2004; 27:84–92.

189. Larsen HH, et al. Development of a rapid real-time PCR assay for quantitation of Pneumocystis carinii f. sp. carinii. J Clin Microbiol 2002;40:2989–2893.

190. Lau LT, et al. A real-time PCR for SARS-coronavirus incorporating target gene pre-amplification. Biochem Biophys Res Commun 2003;312:1290–1296.

191. Lee SH, et al. Characterization of Borrelia burgdorferi strains isolated from Korea by 16S rDNA sequence analysis and PCR-RFLP analysis of rrf (5S)-rrl (23S) intergenic spacer amplicons. Int J Syst Evol Microbiol 2000;50(Pt 2): 857–863.

192. Leslie DE, et al. An assessment of the Roche Amplicor Chlamydia trachomatis/ Neisseria gonorrhoeae multiplex PCR assay in routine diagnostic use on a variety of specimen types. Commun Dis Intell 2003;27:373–379.

193. Levi JE, Kleter B, Quint WG, et al. High prevalence of human papillomavirus (HPV) infections and high frequency of multiple HPV genotypes in human immunodeficiency virus-infected women in Brazil. J Clin Microbiol 2002;40(9): 3341–3345.

194. Lewis JS, Fakile O, Foss E, et al. Direct DNA probe assay for Neisseria gonorrhoeae in pharyngeal and rectal specimens. J Clin Microbiol 1993;31:2783–2785.

195. Li JJ, et al. Localization of human herpes-like virus type 8 in vascular endothelial cells and perivascular spindle-shaped cells of Kaposi's sarcoma lesions by in situ hybridization. Am J Pathol 1996;148:1741–1748.

196. Lin MH, et al. Real-time PCR for quantitative detection of Toxoplasma gondii. J Clin Microbiol 2000;38:4121–4125.

197. Loeffler J, et al. Identification of rare Candida species and other yeasts by polymerase chain reaction and slot blot hybridization. Diagn Microbiol Infect Dis 2000;38:207–212.

198. Loens K, et al. Detection of Mycoplasma pneumoniae by real-time nucleic acid sequence-based amplification. J Clin Microbiol 2003;41:4448–4450.

199. Loy JK, et al. Molecular phylogeny and in situ detection of the etiologic agent of necrotizing hepatopancreatitis in shrimp. Appl Environ Microbiol 1996;62: 3439–3445.

200. Lungu O, et al. Differentiation of Nocardia from rapidly growing Mycobacterium species by PCR-RFLP analysis. Diagn Microbiol Infect Dis 1994;18:13–18.

201. Lurain NS, et al. Sequencing of cytomegalovirus UL97 gene for genotypic antiviral resistance testing. Antimicrob Agents Chemother 2001;45:2775–2780.

202. Macdonald DM, et al. Escherichia coli O157:H7 outbreak linked to salami, British Columbia, Canada, 1999. Epidemiol Infect 2004;132:283–289.

203. Mackay IM. Real-time PCR in the microbiology laboratory. Clin Microbiol Infect 2004;10:190–212.

204. Mackay IM, et al. Molecular assays for detection of human metapneumovirus. J Clin Microbiol 2003;41:100–105.

205. Maertzdorf J, et al. Real-time reverse transcriptase PCR assay for detection of human metapneumoviruses from all known genetic lineages. J Clin Microbiol 2004;42:981–986.

206. Mantero G, Zonaro A, Albertini A, et al. DNA enzyme immunoassay: general method for detecting products of polymerase chain reaction. Clin Chem 1991; 37:422–429.

207. Manz W, et al. In situ identification of Legionellaceae using 16S rRNA-targeted oligonucleotide probes and confocal laser scanning microscopy. Microbiology 1995;141:29–39.

208. Manz W, et al. In situ identification of bacteria in drinking water and adjoining biofilms by hybridization with 16S and 23S rRNA-directed fluorescent oligonucleotide probes. Appl Environ Microbiol 1993;59:2293–2299.

209. Markoulatos P, et al. Laboratory diagnosis of common herpesvirus infections of the central nervous system by a multiplex PCR assay. J Clin Microbiol 2001; 39:4426–4432.

210. Martagon-Villamil J, et al. Identification of Histoplasma capsulatum from culture extracts by real-time PCR. J Clin Microbiol 2003;41:1295–1298.

211. Martagon-Villamil J, Farrell JJ, Rehm SJ, et al. Nocardia abscessus: mediastinal involvement and superior vena cava syndrome. Speciation by pyrosequencing. Poster presentation. Infectious Diseases Society of America. 41st Annual Meeting. October 9–12, 2003. San Diego.

212. Martin C, et al. Development of a PCR-based line probe assay for identification of fungal pathogens. J Clin Microbiol 2000;38:3735–3742.

213. Martineau F, et al. Development of a PCR assay for identification of staphylococci at genus and species levels. J Clin Microbiol 2001;39:2541–2547.

214. Massung RF, Slater KG. Comparison of PCR assays for detection of the agent of human granulocytic ehrlichiosis, Anaplasma phagocytophilum. J Clin Microbiol 2003;41:717–722.

215. McNicol AM, Farquharson MA. In situ hybridization and its diagnostic applications in pathology. J Pathol 1997;182:250–261.

216. Melchers WJ, et al. Short fragment polymerase chain reaction reverse hybridization line probe assay to detect and genotype a broad spectrum of human papillomavirus types. Clinical evaluation and follow-up. Am J Pathol 1999;155: 1473–1478.

217. Meletiadis J, et al. Evaluation of a polymerase chain reaction reverse hybridization line probe assay for the detection and identification of medically important fungi in bronchoalveolar lavage fluids. Med Mycol 2003;41:65–74.

218. Meliani L, et al. Real time quantitative PCR assay for Pneumocystis jirovecii detection. J Eukaryot Microbiol 2003;50(Suppl):651.

219. Mellmann A, et al. Evaluation of RIDOM, MicroSeq, and Genbank services in the molecular identification of Nocardia species. Int J Med Microbiol 2003;293: 359–370.

220. Menotti J, et al. Development of a real-time PCR assay for quantitative detection of Encephalitozoon intestinalis DNA. J Clin Microbiol 2003;41:1410–1413.

221. Mijs W, et al. Evaluation of a commercial line probe assay for identification of mycobacterium species from liquid and solid culture. Eur J Clin Microbiol Infect Dis 2002;21:794–802.

222. Millar B, et al. Molecular diagnosis of infective endocarditis—a new Duke's criterion. Scand J Infect Dis 2001;33:673–680.

223. Miller AC, et al. Clonal relationships in a shelter-associated outbreak of drug-resistant tuberculosis: 1983–1997. Int J Tuberc Lung Dis 2002;6:872–878.

224. Miller N, Infante S, Cleary T. Evaluation of the LiPA MYCOBACTERIA assay

for identification of mycobacterial species from BACTEC 12B bottles. J Clin Microbiol 2000;38:1915–1919.

225. Miranda-Novales G, et al. An outbreak due to Serratia marcescens in a neonatal intensive care unit typed by 2-day pulsed field gel electrophoresis protocol. Arch Med Res 2003;34:237–241.

226. Mitterer G, et al. Microarray-based identification of bacteria in clinical samples by solid-phase PCR amplification of 23S ribosomal DNA sequences. J Clin Microbiol 2004;42:1048–1057.

227. Modarress KJ, et al. Detection of Chlamydia trachomatis and Neisseria gonorrhoeae in swab specimens by the Hybrid Capture II and PACE 2 nucleic acid probe tests. Sex Transm Dis 1999;26:303–308.

228. Mokrousov I, et al. Allele-specific rpoB PCR assays for detection of rifampin-resistant Mycobacterium tuberculosis in sputum smears. Antimicrob Agents Chemother 2003;47:2231–2235.

229. Monpoeho S, et al. Application of a real-time polymerase chain reaction with internal positive control for detection and quantification of enterovirus in cerebrospinal fluid. Eur J Clin Microbiol Infect Dis 2002;21:532–536.

230. Monstein H, Nikpour-Badr S, Jonasson J. Rapid molecular identification and subtyping of Helicobacter pylori by pyrosequencing of the 16S rDNA variable V1 and V3 regions. FEMS Microbiol Lett 2001;199:103–107.

231. Morishima C, et al. Strengths and limitations of commercial tests for hepatitis C virus RNA quantification. J Clin Microbiol 2004;42:421–425.

232. Mullis K. The unusual origin of the polymerase chain reaction. Sci Am 1990; 262:56–65.

233. Mullis KB, Faloona FA. Specific synthesis of DNA in vitro via a polymerase-catalyzed reaction. Methods Enzymol 1987;155:335–350.

234. Musial CE, Tice LS, Stockman L, Roberts GD. Identification of mycobacteria from culture by using the Gen-Probe rapid diagnostic system for Mycobacterium avium complex and Mycobacterium tuberculosis complex. J Clin Microbiol 1988;26:2120–2123.

235. Myers TW, Gelfand DH. Reverse transcription and DNA amplification by a Thermus thermophilus DNA polymerase. Biochemistry 1991;30:7661–7666.

236. Ninet B, et al. Identification of dermatophyte species by 28S ribosomal DNA sequencing with a commercial kit. J Clin Microbiol 2003;41:826–830.

237. Nolte FS, et al. Clinical evaluation of two methods for genotyping hepatitis C virus based on analysis of the 5′ noncoding region. J Clin Microbiol 2003;41: 1558–1564.

238. Nordstrom T, et al. Method enabling pyrosequencing on double-stranded DNA. Anal Biochem 2000;282:186–193.

239. Oliveira K, et al. Direct identification of Staphylococcus aureus from positive blood culture bottles. J Clin Microbiol 2003;41:889–891.

240. Oliveira K, et al. Rapid identification of Staphylococcus aureus directly from blood cultures by fluorescence in situ hybridization with peptide nucleic acid probes. J Clin Microbiol 2002;40:247–251.

241. Oliveira K, et al. Differentiation of Candida albicans and Candida dubliniensis by fluorescent in situ hybridization with peptide nucleic acid probes. J Clin Microbiol 2001;39:4138–4141.

242. O'neill HJ, et al. Real-time nested multiplex PCR for the detection of herpes simplex virus types 1 and 2 and varicella zoster virus. J Med Virol 2003;71: 557–560.

243. Ortega-Larrocea G, et al. Nested polymerase chain reaction for Mycobacterium tuberculosis DNA detection in aqueous and vitreous of patients with uveitis. Arch Med Res 2003;34:116–119.

244. Padilla E, et al. Evaluation of a fluorescence hybridization assay using peptide nucleic acid probes for identification and differentiation of tuberculous and non-tuberculous mycobacteria in liquid cultures. Eur J Clin Microbiol Infect Dis 2000;19:140–145.

245. Palladino S, et al. Use of real-time PCR and the LightCycler system for the rapid detection of Pneumocystis carinii in respiratory specimens. Diagn Microbiol Infect Dis 2001;39:233–236.

246. Pan S, Cole Gt. Molecular and biochemical characterization of a Coccidioides immitis-specific antigen. Infect Immun 1995;63:3994–4002.

247. Pancholi P, Wu F, Della-Latta P. Rapid detection of cytomegalovirus infection in transplant patients. Expert Rev Mol Diagn 2004;4:231–242.

248. Park CS, Kim J, Montone KT. Detection of Aspergillus ribosomal RNA using biotinylated oligonucleotide probes. Diagn Mol Pathol 1997;6:255–260.

249. Patel JB, et al. Sequence-based identification of Mycobacterium species using the MicroSeq 500 16S rDNA bacterial identification system. J Clin Microbiol 2000;8:246–251.

250. Pauls RJ, et al. A high proportion of novel mycobacteria species identified by 16S rDNA analysis among slowly growing AccuProbe-negative strains in a clinical setting. Am J Clin Pathol 2003;120:560–566.

251. Pereira MC, et al. Ultrastructural distribution of poly (A) + RNA during Trypanosoma cruzi cardiomyocyte interaction in vitro: a quantitative analysis of the total mRNA content by in situ hybridization. J Eukaryot Microbiol 2000;47: 264–270.

252. Perez-Cano R, et al. Factors related to the chronicity and evolution of hepatitis

253. Perrons C, et al. Detection and genotyping of human papillomavirus DNA by SPF10 and MY09/11 primers in cervical cells taken from women attending a colposcopy clinic. J Med Virol 2002;67:246–252.

254. Persing D. Polymerase chain reaction: trenches to benches. J Clin Microbiol 1991;29:1281–1285.

255. Peter JB, Sevall JS. Molecular-based methods for quantifying HIV viral load. AIDS Patient Care STDS 2004;18:75–79.

256. Petrini B. 16S rDNA sequencing in the species identification of non-tuberculous mycobacteria. Scand J Infect Dis 2003;35:519–520.

257. Pham AS, et al. Diagnosis of invasive mold infection by real-time quantitative PCR. Am J Clin Pathol 2003;119:38–44.

258. Piatak M, Luk KC, Williams B, Lifson JD. Quantitative competitive polymerase chain reaction for accurate quantitation of HIV DNA and RNA species. BioTechniques 1993;14:70–81.

259. Poon LL, et al. Detection of SARS coronavirus in patients with severe acute respiratory syndrome by conventional and real-time quantitative reverse transcription-PCR assays. Clin Chem 2004;50:67–72.

260. Poon LL, et al. Early diagnosis of SARS coronavirus infection by real time RT-PCR. J Clin Virol 2003;28:233–238.

261. Post JC, et al. Development and validation of a multiplex PCR-based assay for the upper respiratory tract bacterial pathogens Haemophilus influenzae, Streptococcus pneumoniae, and Moraxella catarrhalis. Mol Diagn 1996;1:29–39.

262. Prariyachatigul C, et al. Development and evaluation of a one-tube seminested PCR assay for the detection and identification of Penicillium marneffei. Mycoses 2003;46:447–454.

263. Preliminary Foodnet Data On The Incidence Of Foodborne Illnesses-Selected Sites, United States, 2002. MMWR Morb Mortal Wkly Rep 2003;52:340–343.

264. Prescott AM, Fricker CR. Use of PNA oligonucleotides for the in situ detection of Escherichia coli in water. Mol Cell Probes 1999;13:261–268.

265. Pryce TM, et al. Rapid identification of fungi by sequencing the ITS1 and ITS2 regions using an automated capillary electrophoresis system. Med Mycol 2041(5):369–381.

266. Pryce TM, et al. Real-time automated polymerase chain reaction (PCR) to detect Candida albicans and Aspergillus fumigatus DNA in whole blood from high-risk patients. Diagn Microbiol Infect Dis 2003;47:487–496.

267. Qian KP, et al. Hepatitis C virus mixed genotype infection in patients on haemodialysis. J Viral Hepat 2000;7:153–160.

268. Qian Q, et al. Direct identification of bacteria from positive blood cultures by amplification and sequencing of the 16S rRNA gene: evaluation of BACTEC 9240 instrument true-positive and false-positive results. J Clin Microbiol 2001; 39:3578–3582.

269. Qin X, Urdahl KB: Pcr And Sequencing Of Independent Genetic Targets For The Diagnosis Of Culture Negative Bacterial Endocarditis. Diagn Microbiol Infect Dis 2001;40:145–149.

270. Quereda C, et al. Diagnostic utility of a multiplex herpesvirus PCR assay performed with cerebrospinal fluid from human immunodeficiency virus-infected patients with neurological disorders. J Clin Microbiol 2000;38:3061–3067.

271. Quint WG, et al. Comparative analysis of human papillomavirus infections in cervical scrapes and biopsy specimens by general SPF(10) PCR and HPV genotyping. J Pathol 2001;194:51–58.

272. Quiros E, Piedrola G, Maroto Mc. Detection of enteroviral RNA by a new single-step PCR. Scand J Clin Lab Invest 1997;57:415–419.

273. Qureshi MN, et al. Role of HPV DNA testing in predicting cervical intraepithelial lesions: comparison of HC HPV and ISH HPV. Diagn Cytopathol 2003;29: 149–155.

274. Rabenau HF, et al. Rapid detection of enterovirus infection by automated RNA extraction and real-time fluorescence PCR. J Clin Virol 2002;25:155–164.

275. Radwanska M, et al. Direct detection and identification of African trypanosomes by fluorescence in situ hybridization with peptide nucleic acid probes. J Clin Microbiol 2002;40:4295–4297.

276. Ramers C, et al. Impact of a diagnostic cerebrospinal fluid enterovirus polymerase chain reaction test on patient management. JAMA 2000;283:2680–2685.

277. Rantakokko-Jalava K, et al. Semiquantitative detection by real-time PCR of Aspergillus fumigatus in bronchoalveolar lavage fluids and tissue biopsy specimens from patients with invasive aspergillosis. J Clin Microbiol 2003;41: 4304–4311.

278. Rantakokko-Jalava K, et al. Direct amplification of rRNA genes in diagnosis of bacterial infections. J Clin Microbiol 2000;38:32–39.

279. Rantakokko-Jalava K, Jalava J. Optimal DNA isolation method for detection of bacteria in clinical specimens by broad-range PCR. J Clin Microbiol 2002;40: 4211–4217.

280. Re MC, et al. Analysis of HIV-1 drug resistant mutations by line probe assay and direct sequencing in a cohort of therapy naive HIV-1 infected Italian patients. BMC Microbiol 2001;1:30.

281. Read SJ, Mitchell JL, Fink Cg. LightCycler multiplex PCR for the laboratory

diagnosis of common viral infections of the central nervous system. J Clin Microbiol 2001;39:3056–3059.

282. Reischl U, et al. Clinical evaluation of the automated COBAS AMPLICOR MTB assay for testing respiratory and nonrespiratory specimens. J Clin Microbiol 1998;36:2853–2860.

283. Renesto P, et al. Use of rpoB gene analysis for detection and identification of Bartonella species. J Clin Microbiol 2001;39:430–437.

284. Riffard S, et al. Distribution of mip-related sequences in 39 species (48 serogroups) of Legionellaceae. Epidemiol Infect 1996;117:501–506.

285. Rigby S, et al. Fluorescence in situ hybridization with peptide nucleic acid probes for rapid identification of Candida albicans directly from blood culture bottles. J Clin Microbiol 2002;40:2182–2186.

286. Rindi L, et al. A real-time PCR assay for detection of isoniazid resistance in Mycobacterium tuberculosis clinical isolates. J Microbiol Methods 2003;55:797–800.

287. Ringuet H, et al. hsp65 sequencing for identification of rapidly growing mycobacteria. J Clin Microbiol 1999;37:852–857.

288. Roberts TC, Storch GA. Multiple PCR for diagnosis of AIDS-related central nervous system lymphoma and toxoplasmosis. J Clin Microbiol 1997;35:268–269.

289. Rodriguez-Barradas MC, et al. Genomic fingerprinting of Bartonella species by repetitive element PCR for distinguishing species and isolates. J Clin Microbiol 1995;33:1089–1093.

290. Romanelli F, Pomeroy C. Human immunodeficiency virus drug resistance testing: state of the art in genotypic and phenotypic testing of antiretrovirals. Pharmacotherapy 2000;20:151–157.

291. Ronaghi M. Pyrosequencing sheds light on DNA sequencing. Genome Res 2001;11:3–11.

292. Ronaghi M. Improved performance of pyrosequencing using single-stranded DNA-binding protein. Anal Biochem 2000;286:282–288.

293. Rondini S, et al. Development and application of real-time PCR assay for quantification of Mycobacterium ulcerans DNA. J Clin Microbiol 2003;41:4231–4237.

294. Rossau R, et al. Evaluation of the INNO-LiPA Rif. TB assay, a reverse hybridization assay for the simultaneous detection of Mycobacterium tuberculosis complex and its resistance to rifampin. Antimicrob Agents Chemother 1997;41:2093–2098.

295. Rothman RE, et al. Detection of bacteremia in emergency department patients at risk for infective endocarditis using universal 16S rRNA primers in a decontaminated polymerase chain reaction assay. J Infect Dis 2002;186:1677–1681.

296. Ruddy MC, et al. Outbreak of isoniazid resistant tuberculosis in north London. Thorax 2004;59:279–285.

297. Ruiz M, et al. Direct detection of Rifampin- and Isoniazid-resistant mycobacterium tuberculosis in Auramine-Rhodamine-positive sputum specimens by real-time PCR. J Clin Microbiol 2004;42:1585–1589.

298. Saiman L, et al. An outbreak of methicillin-resistant Staphylococcus aureus in a neonatal intensive care unit. Infect Control Hosp Epidemiol 2003;24:317–321.

299. Salomon R. Introduction to quantitative reverse transcription polymerase chain reaction. Diag Mol Pathol 1995;4:82–84.

300. Sanchez JL, Storch GA. Multiplex, quantitative, real-time PCR assay for cytomegalovirus and human DNA. J Clin Microbiol 2002;40:2381–2386.

301. Sanchez-Pescador R, Stempien MS, Urdea MS. Rapid chemiluminescent nucleic acid assays for detection of TEM-1 beta-lactamase-mediated penicillin resistance in Neisseria gonorrhoeae and other bacteria. J Clin Microbiol 1988;26:1934–1938.

302. Sa-Ngasang, A, et al. Evaluation of RT-PCR as a tool for diagnosis of secondary dengue virus infection. Jpn J Infect Dis 2003;56:205–209.

303. Sassetti CM, Boyd DH, Rubin EJ. Comprehensive identification of conditionally essential genes in mycobacteria. Proc Natl Acad Sci USA 2001;98(22):12712–12717.

304. Scarparo C, et al. Direct identification of mycobacteria from MB/BacT alert 3D bottles: comparative evaluation of two commercial probe assays. J Clin Microbiol 2001;39(9):3222–3227.

305. Schachter J, et al. Ability of the digene hybrid capture II test to identify Chlamydia trachomatis and Neisseria gonorrhoeae in cervical specimens. J Clin Microbiol 1999;37(11):3668–3671.

306. Schinazi RF, Schlueter-Wirtz S, Stuyver L. Early detection of mixed mutations selected by antiretroviral agents in HIV-infected primary human lymphocytes. Antivir Chem Chemother 2001;12(Suppl 1):61–65.

307. Schmutzhard J, et al. Detection of herpes simplex virus type 1, herpes simplex virus type 2 and varicella-zoster virus in skin lesions: comparison of real-time PCR, nested PCR and virus isolation. J Clin Virol 2004;29:120–126.

308. Schulz A, et al. Detection, differentiation, and quantitation of pathogenic leishmania organisms by a fluorescence resonance energy transfer-based real-time PCR assay. J Clin Microbiol 2003;41:1529–1535.

309. Schuurman T, et al. Prospective study of use of PCR amplification and sequencing of 16S ribosomal DNA from cerebrospinal fluid for diagnosis of bacterial meningitis in a clinical setting. J Clin Microbiol 2004;42:734–740.

310. Seurinck S, Verstraete W, Siciliano SD. Use of 16S–23S rRNA intergenic spacer region PCR and repetitive extragenic palindromic PCR analyses of Escherichia coli isolates to identify nonpoint fecal sources. Appl Environ Microbiol 2003;69:4942–4950.

311. Shaheduzzaman S, et al. Effects of HIV-1 Nef on cellular gene expression profiles. J Biomed Sci 2002;9:82–96.

312. Shannon KP, French GL. Increasing resistance to antimicrobial agents of Gram-negative organisms isolated at a London teaching hospital, 1995–2000. J Antimicrob Chemother 2004;53:818–825.

313. Sharma M, et al. Rapid detection of mutations in rpoB gene of rifampicin resistant Mycobacterium tuberculosis strains by line probe assay. Ind J Med Res 2003;17:76–80.

314. Shrestha NK, et al. Detection and differentiation of Mycobacterium tuberculosis and nontuberculous mycobacterial isolates by real-time PCR. J Clin Microbiol 2003;41:5121–5126.

315. Shrestha NK, et al. Rapid identification of Staphylococcus aureus and the mecA gene from BacT/ALERT blood culture bottles by using the LightCycler system. J Clin Microbiol 2002;40:2659–2661.

316. Sinclair A, Arnold C, Woodford N. Rapid detection and estimation by pyrosequencing of 23S rRNA genes with a single nucleotide polymorphism conferring linezolid resistance in Enterococci. Antimicrob Agents Chemother 2003;47:3620–3622.

317. Singh DV. Hexaplex PCR for rapid detection of virulence factors. Exp Rev Mol Diagn 2003;3:781–784.

318. Skotnikova OI, et al. Typing of Mycobacterium tuberculosis strains resistant to rifampicin and isoniazid by molecular biological methods. Bull Exp Biol Med 2003;136:273–275.

319. Smith AB, et al. Rapid detection of influenza A and B viruses in clinical specimens by Light Cycler real time RT-PCR. J Clin Virol 2003;28:51–58.

320. Smith K, Diggle MA, Clarke SC. Automation of a fluorescence-based multiplex PCR for the laboratory confirmation of common bacterial pathogens. J Med Microbiol 2004;53(Pt 2):115–117.

321. Sofi Ibrahim M, et al. Real-time PCR assay to detect smallpox virus. J Clin Microbiol 2003;41:3835–3839.

322. Song JH, et al. Detection of Salmonella typhi in the blood of patients with typhoid fever by polymerase chain reaction. J Clin Microbiol 1993;31:1439–1443.

323. Southern SA, Graham DA, Herrington CS. Discrimination of human papillomavirus types in low and high grade cervical squamous neoplasia by in situ hybridization. Diag Mol Pathol 1998;7:114–121.

324. Spiess B, et al. Development of a LightCycler PCR assay for detection and quantification of Aspergillus fumigatus DNA in clinical samples from neutropenic patients. J Clin Microbiol 2003;41:1811–1818.

325. Springer B, et al. Two-laboratory collaborative study on identification of mycobacteria: molecular versus phenotypic methods. J Clin Microbiol 1996;34:296–303.

326. Steingrube VA, et al. Rapid identification of clinically significant species and taxa of aerobic actinomycetes, including Actinomadura, Gordona, Nocardia, Rhodococcus, Streptomyces, and Tsukamurella isolates, by DNA amplification and restriction endonuclease analysis. J Clin Microbiol 1997;35:817–822.

327. Steinhauserova I, et al. Identification of thermophilic Campylobacter spp. by phenotypic and molecular methods. J Appl Microbiol 2001;90:470–475.

328. Stellrecht KA, et al. The impact of an enteroviral RT-PCR assay on the diagnosis of aseptic meningitis and patient management. J Clin Virol 2002;25(Suppl 1):S19–S26.

329. Stender H. PNA FISH: an intelligent stain for rapid diagnosis of infectious diseases. Expert Rev Mol Diagn 2003;3:649–655.

330. Stender H, et al. Direct detection and identification of Mycobacterium tuberculosis in smear-positive sputum samples by fluorescence in situ hybridization (FISH) using peptide nucleic acid (PNA) probes. Int J Tubercul Lung Dis 1999;3:830–837.

331. Stender H, et al. Fluorescence in situ hybridization assay using peptide nucleic acid probes for differentiation between tuberculous and nontuberculous mycobacterium species in smears of mycobacterium cultures. J Clin Microbiol 1999;37:2760–2765.

332. Stocher M, et al. Automated detection of five human herpes virus DNAs by a set of LightCycler PCRs complemented with a single multiple internal control. J Clin Virol 2003;29:171–178.

333. Stryer L. Biochemistry. 5th Ed. New York: Freeman, 2003.

334. Sturmer M, et al. Evaluation of the LiPA HIV-1 RT assay version 1: comparison of sequence and hybridization based genotyping systems. J Clin Virol 2002;25(Suppl 3):S65–S72.

335. Suffys PN, et al. Rapid identification of Mycobacteria to the species level using INNO-LiPA Mycobacteria, a reverse hybridization assay. J Clin Microbiol 2001;39:4477–4482.

336. Sui Y, et al. Microarray analysis of cytokine and chemokine genes in the brains of macaques with SHIV-encephalitis. J Med Primatol 2003;32:229–239.

337. Tabrizi SN, et al. Evaluation of real time polymerase chain reaction assays for confirmation of Neisseria gonorrhoeae in clinical samples tested positive in the Roche Cobas Amplicor assay. Sex Transm Infect 2004;80:68–71.

338. Tang YW, Procop GW, Persing DH. Molecular diagnostics of infectious diseases. Clin Chem 1997;43:2021–2038.

339. Tazi L, et al. Genetic diversity and population structure of Mycobacterium tuberculosis in Casablanca, a Moroccan city with high incidence of tuberculosis. J Clin Microbiol 2004;42:461–466.

340. Tenover FC, Arbeit RD, Goering RV, et al. Interpreting chromosomal DNA restriction patterns produced by pulsed-field gel electrophoresis: criteria for bacterial strain typing. J Clin Microbiol 1995;33:2233–2239.

341. Tong CY, et al. Multiplex polymerase chain reaction for the simultaneous detection of Mycoplasma pneumoniae, Chlamydia pneumoniae, and Chlamydia psittaci in respiratory samples. J Clin Pathol 1999;52:257–263.

342. Tortoli E, Mariottini A, Mazzarelli G. Evaluation of INNO-LiPA MYCOBACTERIA v2: improved reverse hybridization multiple DNA probe assay for mycobacterial identification. J Clin Microbiol 2003;41:4418–4420.

343. Tortorano AM, et al. The European Confederation of Medical Mycology (ECMM) survey of candidaemia in Italy: antifungal susceptibility patterns of 261 non-albicans Candida isolates from blood. J Antimicrob Chemother 2003;52:679–682.

344. Trindade PA, et al. Molecular techniques for MRSA typing: current issues and perspectives. Braz J Infect Dis 2003;7:32–43.

345. Tuohy MJ, Procop GW. The rapid identification of routine clinical Mycobacteria by Pyrosequencing™, 42nd ICAAC Meeting, San Diego, CA, 2002.

346. Unnasch TR, et al. Characterization of a putative nuclear receptor from Onchocerca volvulus. Mol Biochem Parasitol 1999;104:259–269.

347. Unnerstad H, et al. Pyrosequencing as a method for grouping of Listeria monocytogenes strains on the basis of single-nucleotide polymorphisms in the inlB gene. Appl Environ Microbiol 2001;67:5339–5342.

348. Urdea MS, Horn T, Fultz TJ, A et al. Branched DNA amplification multimers for the sensitive, direct detection of human hepatitis viruses. Nucleic Acids Symp Ser 1991;24:197–200.

349. van Der Eijk AA, et al. Paired measurements of quantitative hepatitis B virus DNA in saliva and serum of chronic hepatitis B patients: implications for saliva as infectious agent. J Clin Virol 2004;29:92–94.

350. van Der Pol B, et al. Evaluation of the digene hybrid capture II assay with the Rapid Capture System for detection of Chlamydia trachomatis and Neisseria gonorrhoeae. J Clin Microbiol 2002;40:3558–3564.

351. van Der Pol B, et al. Enhancing the specificity of the COBAS AMPLICOR CT/NG test for Neisseria gonorrhoeae by retesting specimens with equivocal results. J Clin Microbiol 2001;39:3092–3098.

352. van Doorn HR, et al. Detection of a point mutation associated with high-level isoniazid resistance in Mycobacterium tuberculosis by using real-time PCR technology with 3′-minor groove binder-DNA probes. J Clin Microbiol 2003;41:4630–4635.

353. van Doorn LJ, et al. Genotyping of human papillomavirus in liquid cytology cervical specimens by the PGMY line blot assay and the SPF(10) line probe assay. J Clin Microbiol 2002;40:979–983.

354. van 'T Wout AB, et al. Cellular gene expression upon human immunodeficiency virus type 1 infection of CD4(+)-T-cell lines. J Virol 2003;77:1392–1402.

355. Vasef MA, Ferlito A, Weiss LM. Nasopharyngeal carcinoma with emphasis on its relationship to Epstein-Barr virus. Ann Oto Rhin Laryn 1997;106:348–356.

356. Velasquez JN, et al. In situ hybridization: a molecular approach for the diagnosis of the microsporidian parasite Enterocytozoon bieneusi. Hum Pathol 1999;30:54–58.

357. Verboon-Maciolek MA, et al. Diagnosis of enterovirus infection in the first 2 months of life by real-time polymerase chain reaction. Clin Infect Dis 2003;37:1–6.

358. Verstrepen WA, Bruynseels P, Mertens AH. Evaluation of a rapid real-time RT-PCR assay for detection of enterovirus RNA in cerebrospinal fluid specimens. J Clin Virol 2002;25(Suppl 1):S39–S43.

359. Voldstedlund M, et al. Different polymerase chain reaction-based analyses for culture-negative endocarditis caused by Streptococcus pneumoniae. Scand J Infect Dis 2003;35:757–759.

360. Vukovic D, et al. Molecular epidemiology of pulmonary tuberculosis in Belgrade, Central Serbia. J Clin Microbiol 2003;41:4372–4377.

361. Wagar E. Direct hybridization and amplification applications for the diagnosis of infectious diseases. J Clin Lab Anal 1996;10:312–325.

362. Wagner HJ, et al. Longitudinal analysis of Epstein-Barr viral load in plasma and peripheral blood mononuclear cells of transplanted patients by real-time polymerase chain reaction. Transplantation 2002;74:656–664.

363. Wang Z, et al. Effects of human immunodeficiency virus type 1 on astrocyte gene expression and function: potential role in neuropathogenesis. J Neurovirol 2004;10(Suppl 1):25–32.

364. Ward CL, et al. Design and performance testing of quantitative real time PCR assays for influenza A and B viral load measurement. J Clin Virol 2004;29:179–188.

365. Wasson K, Barry PA. Molecular characterization of Encephalitozoon intestinalis (Microspora) replication kinetics in a murine intestinal cell line. J Eukaryot Microbiol 2003;50:169–174.

366. Watkins-Riedel T, et al. Rapid diagnosis of enterovirus infections by real-time PCR on the LightCycler using the TaqMan format. Diagn Microbiol Infect Dis 2002;42:99–105.

367. Weinberg A, Schissel D, Giller R. Molecular methods for cytomegalovirus surveillance in bone marrow transplant recipients. J Clin Microbiol 2002;40:4203–4206.

368. Westergren V, Bassiri M, Engstrand L: Bacteria Detected By Culture And 16s Rrna Sequencing In Maxillary Sinus Samples From Intensive Care Unit Patients. Laryngoscope 2003;113:270–275.

369. Whiley DM, et al. Detection and differentiation of herpes simplex virus types 1 and 2 by a duplex LightCycler PCR that incorporates an internal control PCR reaction. J Clin Virol 2004;30:32–38.

370. Wilson DA, et al. Detection of Legionella pneumophila by real-time PCR for the mip gene. J Clin Microbiol 2003;41:3327–3330.

371. Wolk DM, et al. Real-time PCR method for detection of Encephalitozoon intestinalis from stool specimens. J Clin Microbiol 2002;40:3922–3928.

372. Woo PC, et al. Usefulness of the MicroSeq 500 16S ribosomal DNA-based bacterial identification system for identification of clinically significant bacterial isolates with ambiguous biochemical profiles. J Clin Microbiol 2003;41:1996–2001.

373. Xu J, et al. Employment of broad-range 16S rRNA PCR to detect aetiological agents of infection from clinical specimens in patients with acute meningitis: rapid separation of 16S rRNA PCR amplicons without the need for cloning. J Appl Microbiol 2003;94:197–206.

374. Yang L, Weis JH, Eichwald E, et al. Heritable susceptibility to Borrelia burgdorferi-induced arthritis is dominant and is associated with persistence of high numbers of spirochetes in tissues. Infect Immun 1994;62:492–500.

375. Yao JD, et al. Multicenter evaluation of the VERSANT hepatitis B virus DNA 3.0 assay. J Clin Microbiol 2004;42(2):800–806.

376. Young KK, Resnick RM, Meyers TW. Detection of hepatitis C virus by a combined reverse transcription-polymerase chain reaction assay. J Clin Microbiol 1993;31:882–886.

377. Zeaiter Z, et al. Diagnosis of Bartonella endocarditis by a real-time nested PCR assay using serum. J Clin Microbiol 2003;41(3):919–925.

378. Zeana C, et al. The epidemiology of multidrug-resistant Acinetobacter baumannii: does the community represent a reservoir? Infect Control Hosp Epidemiol 2003;24:275–279.

379. Zerbi P, et al. Amplified in situ hybridization with peptide nucleic acid probes for differentiation of Mycobacterium tuberculosis complex and nontuberculous Mycobacterium species on formalin-fixed, paraffin-embedded archival biopsy and autopsy samples. Am J Clin Pathol 2001;116:770–775.

380. Zimmerman RL, et al. Ultra fast identification of Aspergillus species in pulmonary cytology specimens by in situ hybridization. Int J Mol Med 2000;5:427–429.

381. Zurita M, Bieber D, Mansour TE. Identification, expression and in situ hybridization of an eggshell protein gene from Fasciola hepatica. Mol Biochem Parasitol 1989;37:11–17.

Medical Bacteriology: Taxonomy, Morphology, Physiology, and Virulence

Taxonomy: Classification, Nomenclature, and Identification of Bacteria

The Naming of Bacteria
Phenotypic Identification of Bacteria
Phylogenetic Criteria for Classification of Bacteria

Basic Bacterial Anatomy and Physiology

Bacterial Size and Shape
Nuclear Structure, DNA Replication, Transcription, and Translation
Cytoplasm
Cytoplasmic Membrane
Bacterial Cell Wall Structure

Gram-Positive Bacterial Cell Walls
Gram-Negative Bacterial Cell Walls
"Acid-Fast" Bacterial Cell Walls

Bacterial Endospores
Bacterial Surface Structures

Capsules
Flagella
Fimbriae (Pili)

Genetic Exchange and Recombination in Bacteria
Requirements for Bacterial Growth and Metabolism

Carbon
Carbon Dioxide
Oxygen
Nitrogen
Growth Factors

Kinetics of Bacterial Cell Growth
General Bacterial Metabolism and Energy Generation

Fermentation
Utilization of Pyruvate

Bacterial Virulence Factors and Pathogenecity

Definitions and Concepts
Requirements for Pathogenicity
Virulence Factors of Microorganisms

Adhesins
Aggressins
Exotoxins and Endotoxins

Bacterial Superantigens

Over the three centuries that have passed since Leeuwenhoek first observed bacteria and protozoa with his primitive microscope, a vast amount of knowledge has been accumulated about the microbial world. Microorganisms are found in all environments, including the soil, water, and air. They are able to participate in all the vital life functions that are observed in higher, more complex life forms and are found in association with the nonliving environment and with all other living things. By their activities in these environments, microorganisms are an integral part of the balance of life. Using microorganisms, biochemical and genetic processes that occur in all forms of life have been elucidated, and the innumerable roles of microorganisms in environmental cycles are only now beginning to be fully appreciated. By necessity, subsequent chapters in this textbook deal with a relatively small number of microorganisms that are capable of causing pathology and disease in humans.

By the end of the 19th century, Louis Pasteur had experimentally dispelled the myth of spontaneous generation, and Robert Koch, among others, had shown that microorganisms were able to cause infectious diseases, such as anthrax and tuberculosis. Although current techniques allow more direct assessments of microbial virulence and pathogenicity, making Koch's original postulates somewhat inapplicable, these fundamental principles still serve as the basis for the unequivocal link between microorganisms and infectious diseases. **Koch's postulates** are outlined in Box 5-1.

Taxonomy: Classification, Nomenclature, and Identification of Bacteria

The taxonomy of bacteria specifically refers to three basic concepts: classification, nomenclature, and identification. **Classification** is the process of systematically dividing organisms into groups, with the species being the smallest and most definitive level of division. Classification also refers to the grouping of described species into genera, and on through the levels of families, orders, classes, and phyla. Historically, new species have evolved from the recognition of isolates that have phenotypic characteristics that differ from similar organisms (e.g., other members of the Family *Enterobacteriaceae*). These isolates are then compared with other organisms using a large battery of phenotypic tests. Present-day applications of molecular techniques (e.g., DNA

hybridization, DNA sequencing, and PCR-based amplification) have enabled taxonomists to identify microbial "signature sequences" and other genetic elements that establish genetic relatedness between and among different microorganisms. Based on systematic comparisons of genetic, chemotaxonomic, and phenotypic traits, new taxa would be proposed and named via publication. The process of naming organisms is delineated by rules of nomenclature.

The Naming of Bacteria

Efforts to codify the taxonomy and nomenclature of bacteria started in earnest at the beginning of the 20th century with the work of Chester, Buchanan, and others.[17,18,23,101] During the early 20th century, committees of interested microbiologists were convened to organize bacterial taxonomy, to promulgate rules regarding the validation of new bacterial names, and to establish procedures for changes in nomenclature (see Box 5-2). These discussions resulted in the publication of the International Code of Nomenclature of Bacteria in 1948. Sequential revisions of this document were published by the International Committee of Systematic Bacteriology in 1958, 1973, and 1992.[127,128] Priorities and rules for the naming of bacteria were established beginning on May 1, 1953, and in January 1, 1980, the first "Approved List of Bacterial Names" was published in the *International Journal of Systematic Bacteriology* (IJSB).[124] This list was subsequently amended and republished in 1989.[125] Quarterly issues of IJSB (now called the *International Journal of Systematic and Evolutionary Microbiology*, IJSEM) routinely list the names of new species (i.e., Validation Lists). Descriptions of new species can be published either in IJSEM or in a variety of other American and foreign journals. If the description is published in a journal other than IJSEM, the name and the literature reference containing its description must subsequently appear in an IJSEM Validation List. As of the beginning of the new millennium, 4,314 validly named prokaryotic species names have appeared either in the "Approved List of Bacterial Names," in IJSEM, or in IJSEM Validation Lists.[124,125] More recently, provisions for proposed species names that are currently nonculturable but that have been characterized by molecular methods (see below) have also been established.[98,99] New or revised species designations can be proposed by any investigator, and criteria for publication include the naming of the new species (according to the rules cited in Box 5-2), provision of a detailed description of the organism's morphologic, biochemical, and genetic characteristics, and designation of a living culture of the organism as the "type strain" of the species. This type strain is deposited in reference type culture collections (e.g., the **American Type Culture Collection [ATCC]** and the **National Type Culture Collection [NTCC]**) so the new species will be available to other investigators. Challenges to the validity of new species names are made by publishing a "request for an opinion" from the Judicial Commission of the International Union of Microbiological Societies. This commission usually refers the request to smaller committees that deal with specific groups of organisms, such as the *Enterobacteriaceae* or the *Pasteurellaceae*.

Box 5-1 Koch's Postulates

1. A given organism must be present in every case of a given infectious disease;
2. The microorganism can be isolated from specimens associated with that disease state;
3. Inoculation of the isolate into susceptible animals produces a similar disease; and
4. The same organism that is associated with the disease state can be recovered from representative specimens from the experimentally infected animal.

Box 5-2 Rules of the Nomenclature of Bacteria

1. There is only one correct name for an organism. When more than one name exists for the same species, the oldest legitimate name for that organism has precedence. Occasionally, proposed and accepted names may be changed to reflect proper latinized endings (e.g. the name *Alloiococcus otitis* being changed to *Alloicoccus otitidis*)[3,152];
2. Names that cause error or confusion should be rejected;
3. All names are in Latin or are "latinized" (i.e., given endings that agree in terms of proper usage and gender [masculine, feminine, neuter]), regardless of origin.
4. The first word of the name (genus name) is always capitalized;
5. The second word (species or specific epithet) is not capitalized;
6. Both the genus and species name, together referred to as the species, are either underlined or italicized when appearing in print; and
7. The correct name of a species or higher taxonomic designations is determined by valid publication, legitimacy of the name with regards to the rules of nomenclature, and priority of publication.
8. Genus and species names appearing in the *International Journal of Systematic and Evolutionary Microbiology, IJSEM*) (formerly *International Journal of Systematic Bacteriology, IJSB*) can be changed according to the following rules:
   a. In transferring a species from one genus to another, the species epithet is retained, (e.g., *Campylobacter pylori* became *Helicobacter pylori*);
   b. If a type strain is found to actually belong to another genus, the type strain genus is considered invalid; and
   c. If an organism is included in two or more genera or has two or more species designations, the name of the genus/species containing the correct type strain is considered the valid name.

Phenotypic Identification of Bacteria

Phenotypic identification procedures remain the principal method for identification of most isolates in the clinical microbiology laboratory (see Box 5-3). The focus of identification efforts is at the genus and species level, with no attempt to describe the hierarchy to which a given organism belongs. At present, taxonomic schemes, such as those published in the four-volume 1984–1989 edition of *Bergey's Manual of Systematic Bacteriology*, the 1994 edition of *Bergey's Manual of Determinative Bacteriology*, and various laboratory manuals and journals, reflect groupings of bacteria in nonhierarchical schemes based strictly on phenotypic characteristics.[69,77,129,133,157] In the preface to the 1994 edition of *Bergey's Manual of Determinative Bacteriology*, J.G. Holt, the editor in chief, states that ''the arrangement of the book is strictly phenotypic; no attempt has been made to offer a natural classification. The arrangement chosen is utilitarian and is intended to aid in the identification of bacteria.''[69] In this context, an operational definition of a **species** is a collection of strains that share many common phenotypic characteristics. A bacterial **strain** is derived from a single culture isolate, and a species **type strain** represents the permanent example of the species that carries the reference name and is part of a culture collection (e.g., ATCC). Species are assigned to morphologically and biochemically defined **genera**, which, in turn, are assigned to **families**, each of which also have certain morphologic, physiologic, and biochemical features. Since taxonomic decisions and controversies are arbitrated by committee, individual knowledge and bias introduced at this level make phenotypic classification above the species level somewhat arbitrary.[134] Nomenclature rules that imply a hierarchical classification have been accepted for years, however, as taxonomic convention for these nonhierarchical classification schemes. Consequently, family names have the latinized ending *-aceae* (e.g. the Family *Enterobacteriaceae*, the Family *Neisseriaceae*), order names have the ending *-ales* (i.e., Order *Eubacteriales*), and tribe names end in *-eae* (e.g., the Tribe *Proteae*). The incorporation of phenotypic data into computer-assisted databases of commercially available identification systems has provided systematic organization for the vast amount of phenotypic data that has accumulated. These data will no doubt continue to serve the clinical laboratory as the principal method for bacterial identification. The development of elegant and powerful genetic techniques, however, has made hierarchical bacterial classification not just a possibility but an inevitability.

Phylogenetic Criteria for Classification of Bacteria

Because the nucleotide sequence of DNA is unique to individual species of microorganisms, analysis of nucleic acid relatedness between and among microbes was recognized as a potential tool for unraveling bacterial taxonomy and nomenclature. Initially DNA was analyzed for its **G + C% (guanosine plus cytosine percent)** content. This analysis is limited,

Box 5-3 Methods for Characterization of Microorganisms in the Clinical Microbiology Laboratory

1. **Cellular morphology**—This includes cell size, cell shape, and the arrangement of cells with respect to one another.
2. **Staining characteristics**—This usually refers to the Gram and acid-fast stains, but may include the description of other microscopic characteristics, such as the presence of spores, metachromatic granules, vacuoles, etc.
3. **Motility**—Motility may be observed microscopically with a wet preparation, or by inoculation of semisolid motility medium.
4. **Presence or absence of spores**—The presence of spores is particularly helpful for identifying *Bacillus*, *Clostridium*, and related species. Spores can generally be discerned on Gram stains or wet preparations, but specific spore stains may be helpful from time to time.
5. **Growth characteristics;**
   a. **Rapidity of growth**—Most organisms isolated in the clinical laboratory grow within 1 to 2 days. However, certain bacteria (e.g., actinomycetes, mycobacteria) and fungi may take considerably longer.
   b. **Morphology of colonies on growth media**—Bacteria vary in their appearance on solid culture media. With experience, colony morphology on various media coupled with a few rapid tests (e.g., oxidase, catalase) is often sufficient for genus-level characterization of organisms growing from clinical specimens.
   c. **Optimal atmospheric conditions for growth**—Microorganisms can be characterized by their requirements for oxygen and, depending on this requirement, can be classified as **aerobic** (require O_2), **facultative** (can grow in the presence or absence of O_2), or **anaerobic** (optimal growth in the absence of O_2). The growth of most organisms is also stimulated by carbon dioxide, and for capnophilic organisms, CO_2 is required for growth (e.g., *Neisseria* species). Other organisms, such as *Campylobacter* species, may require atmospheres with slightly decreased O_2 tension; these organisms are termed microaerophilic.
   d. **Optimal temperature for growth**—Most organisms isolated in clinical laboratories grow optimally at 35–37°C. Ability to grow at various temperatures may be helpful in characterizing some isolates (e.g., campylobacters, certain nontuberculous mycobacteria).
   e. **Colonial morphology on selective, nonselective, and differential media**—Clinical laboratories routinely inoculate specimens onto both nonselective and selective media in order to provide optimal conditions for recovery of organisms in a specimen. Selective media use antimicrobial agents (e.g., colistin and nalidixic acid in colistin-nalidixic acid [CNA] agar) or dyes and bile salts (e.g., MacConkey agar; eosin-methylene blue agar) to inhibit growth of some organisms and to allow growth of others. In addition, some selective media are also differential, which means that the colonies growing on a given medium have an appearance that provides clues about a phenotypic characteristic or characteristics. These clues suggest the possible identity of the organism (e.g., the colorless colonies of lactose-nonfermenting colonies of *Shigella* species versus the red colonies of lactose-fermenting *E. coli* on MacConkey agar).
6. **Biochemical characteristics**—Along with cellular and colonial morphology and the appearance of colonies on selective and differential media, biochemical and enzymatic tests form the basis for most identification procedures performed in clinical microbiology laboratories. In general, biochemical characteristics refer to the formation of distinct biochemical end products from defined substrates, the production of acid from various carbohydrates, and the presence of certain bacterial enzymes as determined by chromogenic substrates or other methods.
7. **Serologic tests**—Serologic tests for bacterial identification usually involve the detection of antigens by enzyme or fluorescence immunoassays (Chapter 3). Serologic identification methods may also be used to confirm identifications obtained by other methods. For example, *Salmonella* species can be identified as such by biochemical tests, but serotyping of *Salmonella* isolates for somatic and flagellar antigens is usually performed by slide agglutination with group- and type-specific antisera.
8. **Analysis of metabolic end products or structural components of organisms**—Metabolic end product analysis is performed indirectly with virtually all microbial identification systems, in which a metabolic end product produces a visually detectable change in an indicator of some kind. However, these analyses may also be performed by other methods, such as gas chromatographic analysis of spent broth culture fluids after extraction with various organic solvents. This technique is especially helpful for genus and species identification of anaerobic bacteria. Chemotaxonomic approaches (e.g., cell wall outer membrane and peptidoglycan analysis, cell wall lipid composition, detection of electron transport components such as cytochromes and menaquinones by gas-liquid or high-pressure liquid chromatography) are also helpful but are not routine in most laboratories. Cell wall analysis has enjoyed success in some hospital laboratories as a method for differentiation and identification of the mycobacteria and related organisms.
9. **Molecular genetic analysis**—Molecular methods include G+C% content, DNA-DNA hybridization, and DNA base sequencing. Although these methods are not used routinely in hospital laboratories, they enabled the development of probe tests that are now used in many laboratories for identification of mycobacteria, chlamydiae, systemic fungi, and some bacteria. Amplification techniques (e.g., polymerase chain reaction, ligase chain reaction, strand displacement amplification, and nucleic acid sequence-based amplification) are also being used in clinical laboratories for direct detection of *Chlamydia trachomatis* and *Neisseria gonorrhoeae* and for viral load determinations in patients with HIV-1 and hepatitis C infections.

however, by the fact that two organisms with divergent DNA sequences can have similar $G + C\%$ contents.[140] Subsequently, it was found that **DNA-DNA hybridization** yielded more useful information. Double-stranded DNA can be separated into its two component strands by heat or high salt concentrations. On cooling or on lowering the salt concentration, the two single strands will reanneal or hybridize into the double-stranded forms by specific base-pairing (see below). The extent to which two single strands of DNA reanneal with one another is an indirect assessment of their relatedness.[131] Using this technique, it was found that organisms with about 15% or more sequence mismatches do not reanneal under ideal conditions, so DNA from distantly related organisms will not hybridize. Consequently, DNA-DNA hybridization has been most useful for comparing organisms at or below the species level. In this context, a **bacterial species** can be defined as a group of bacteria that exhibit greater than 70–75% DNA relatedness with 5% or less divergence in related nucleotide sequences.[131,153]

In the 1970s, geneticists began to examine ribosomal RNA sequences as a method for demonstrating microbial relatedness. This work centered on the **16S rRNA molecule**, which is a part of the 30S subunit of the bacterial ribosome (see below). This molecule is 1500 to 1800 nucleotides in length, is easily isolated from bacterial organisms, and has the same structural and functional roles in all bacterial cells. Small-subunit ribosomal RNAs have remained highly conserved during evolution; mutations in these highly conserved base sequences are usually lethal, and organisms with such mutations do not survive and propagate. In addition, since these molecules are an integral part of a complex, protein-containing structure (i.e., the bacterial ribosome), horizontal transfer of rRNAs to other organisms is rare. By examining the nucleotide sequences of the 16S rRNA, phylogenetic relationships and evolution of organisms from common ancestral types can be ascertained.[132] Ribosomal RNA sequence analysis is most useful for determining the relatedness of microorganisms above the genus level, although this technique has been used to validate existing phenotypic differences between closely related genera and species. Strains of the same species usually show greater than 97% similarity in the rRNA sequences.[131]

Since its inception, sequencing studies of small-subunit RNA has had a tremendous impact on bacterial systematics. In the late 1970s, analysis of 16S rRNA from diverse bacterial groups (i.e., methanogenic [methane-producing] bacteria, halophilic bacteria, thermoacidophilic bacteria, etc.) revealed that these organisms were completely divergent from other bacteria and from eukaryotic organisms and heralded the division of the microbial world into two domains—the *Archaea* and the *Bacteria*—and reinforced the phylogenetic separation of eukaryotic organisms into a third domain, the *Eukaryota*. The development of DNA sequencing in the late 1970s and reverse transcriptase polymerase chain reaction (PCR) technology in the early to mid-1980s enabled the amplification and sequencing of small-subunit rDNA. Extensive study and cataloging of these sequences in the 1980s and 1990s forms the basis of the proposed phylogenetic classification scheme.[55]

The publication of the second edition of *Bergey's Manual of Systematic Bacteriology* over the next several years will reflect a complete departure from the first edition in its phylogenetic classification scheme. The prokaryotic world is divided into two **Domains**—the *Archaea* and the *Eubacteria*.[158] Eukaryotic organisms are placed in Domain *Eukaryota*. *Archaea* and *Bacteria* probably evolved from an ancestral organism, as evidenced by similarities in amino acid sequences of large structural and regulatory molecules and enzymes, including adenosine triphosphatases and elongation factors that function in protein synthesis.[158] The *Archaea* include two major branches—the *Euryarchaeota* and the *Crenarchaeota*. The *Euryarchaeota* include the methanogenic bacteria, the sulfate-reducing bacteria, aerobic **halophilic** (salt-requiring) and **thermoacidophilic** (optimal growth at 50–60°C at pH less than 5) bacteria, and anaerobic **hyperthermophilic** bacteria. The *Crenarchaeota* are all **thermophilic** (optimal growth at 50–60°C), organisms that are either sulfur-reducing heterotrophs or aerobic organisms capable of oxidizing sulfur or other inorganic and organic substrates. Although *Archaea* are similar to the *Eubacteria* in size, nucleoid structure, cell growth, and division, they also differ in several respects. The genome size of the *Eubacteria* ($0.6–12 \times 10^6$ base pairs) can be up to three times larger than that of the *Archaea* ($1–4 \times 10^6$ base pairs). The *Archaea* have cell walls composed primarily of protein and lack the murein peptidoglycan found in the *Eubacteria*. Although both groups have 70S ribosomes, those of the *Archaea* are insensitive to inhibition of protein synthesis by streptomycin or chloramphenicol, but, like the *Eukaryota*, they are sensitive to inhibition by diphtheria toxin. The opposite characteristics obtain in the *Eubacteria*. In short, the *Archaea* encompasses bacteria that are environmental "extremophiles"; it contains no human pathogens.

According to the "roadmap" for the upcoming second edition of *Bergey's Manual of Systematic Bacteriology*, organisms in the Domain *Eubacteria* (or Domain *Bacteria*, as addressed in Bergey's) are divided into 23 divisions or phyla.[55] Most of these phyla are composed of environmental species, such as the thermophilic and/or photosynthetic bacteria. Human pathogens are distributed among seven different phyla. Most of the clinically significant gram-negative bacteria belong to the **Phylum *Proteobacteria***, which is divided into five classes, designated **α-, β-, γ-, δ-, and ε-Proteobacteria**. All of the enteric bacteria, most of the nonfermentative species, fastidious gram-negative coccobacilli and cocci, and the campylobacters belong to the various classes within the Phylum *Proteobacteria*. Phylum *Firmicutes* includes three classes comprising the clostridia, eubacteria, peptococci mycoplasmas, ureaplasmas, the aerobic spore-forming gram-positive bacilli (e.g., *Bacillus* and related genera), and the staphylococci. **Phylum *Actinobacteria*** includes the aerobic and anaerobic actinomycetes and related organisms, the aerobic gram-positive cocci, and several other genera of facultative gram-positive bacilli. **Phylum *Chlamydiae*** and **Phylum *Spirochaetes*** contain the chlamydias and spiral-shaped bacteria (e.g. *Borrelia*, *Treponema*, and *Leptospira*). **Phylum *Bacteroidetes*** contains *Bacteroides* group organisms (*Bacteroides*, *Porphyromonas*, and *Prevotella*), flavobacteria, sphingobacteria, and related nonfermentative gram-negative bacilli. **Phylum *Fusobacteria*** is comprised of the fusobacteria and the genus *Streptobacillus*. Box 5-4 provides a complete outline of the

Box 5-4 Hierarchical Classification of Clinically Significant Bacteria in *Bergey's Manual of Systematic Bacteriology*, Second Edition

DOMAIN BACTERIA
Phylum XII.   *Proteobacteria* phy. nov.

Class I.	**"α-Proteobacteria"**			
	Order II.	*Rickettsiales*		
		Family I	*Rickettsiaceae*	
			Genus I.	*Rickettsia*
		Family II.	*Ehrlichiaceae*	
			Genus I.	*Ehrlichia*
	Order IV.	"Sphingomonadales"		
		Family I.	"Sphingomonadaceae"	
			Genus I.	*Sphingomonas*
	Order V.	*Caulobacteriales*		
		Family I.	*Caulobacteriaceae*	
			Genus III.	*Brevundimonas*
	Order VI.	"Rhizobiales"		
		Family I.	*Rhizobiaceae*	
			Genus II.	*Agrobacterium*
		Family II.	*Bartonellaceae*	
			Genus I.	*Bartonella*
		Family III.	*Brucellaceae*	
			Genus I.	*Brucella*
			Genus III.	*Ochrobactrum*
		Family VII.	"Bradyrhizobiaceae"	
			Genus II.	*Afipia*
		Family IX.	"Methylobacteriaceae"	
			Genus I.	*Methylobacterium*
			Genus III.	*Roseomonas*
Class II.	**"β-Proteobacteria"**			
	Order I.	"Burkholderiales"		
		Family I.	"Burkholderiaceae"	
			Genus I.	*Burkholderia*
		Family II.	"Ralstoniaceae"	
			Genus I.	*Ralstonia*
		Family IV.	*Alcaligenaceae*	
			Genus I.	*Alcaligenes*
			Genus II.	*Achromobacter*
			Genus III.	*Bordetella*
			Genus VI.	*Taylorella*
		Family V.	*Comamonadaceae*	
			Genus I.	*Comamonas*
	Order IV.	"Neisseriales"		
		Family I.	*Neisseriaceae*	
			Genus I.	*Neisseria*
			Genus II.	*Alysiella*
			Genus VI.	*Eikenella*
			Genus IX.	*Kingella*
	Order V.	"Nitrosomonadales"		
		Family II.	*Spirillaceae*	
			Genus I.	*Spirillum*
Class III.	**"γ-Proteobacteria"**			
	Order II.	"Xanthomonadales"		
		Family I.	"Xanthomonadaceae"	
			Genus I.	*Xanthomonas*
			Genus VII.	*Stenotrophomonas*

(Continued)

Box 5-4 *Continued*

DOMAIN BACTERIA
Phylum XII.   *Proteobacteria* phy. nov.

Order III.	"Cardiobacteriales" Family I.	*Cardiobacteriaceae* Genus I. Genus II.	*Cardiobacterium* *Suttonella*
Order IV.	"Thiotrichales" Family III.	"Francisellaceae" Genus I.	*Francisella*
Order V.	"Legionellales" Family I.	*Legionellaceae* Genus I.	*Legionella*
	Family II.	"Coxiellaceae" Genus I. Genus II	*Coxiella* *Ricketsiella*
Order VIII.	*Pseudomonadales* Family I.	*Pseudomonadaceae* Genus I. Genus V. Genus VI. Genus X.	*Pseudomonas* *Chryseomonas* *Flavimonas* *Oligella*
	Family II.	*Moraxellaceae* Genus I. Genus II. Genus III.	*Moraxella* *Acinetobacter* *Psychrobacter*
Order IX.	"Alteromonadales" Family	"Alteromonadaceae" Genus X.	*Shewanella*
Order X.	"Vibrionales" Family I.	*Vibrionaceae* Genus I. Genus V.	*Vibrio* *Photobacterium*
Order XI.	"Aeromonadales" Family I.	*Aeromonadaceae* Genus I.	*Aeromonas*
	Family II.	*Succinivibrionaceae* Genus I. Genus II. Genus III. Genus IV.	*Succinivibrio* *Anaerobiospirillum* *Ruminobacter* *Succinimonas*
Order XII.	"Enterobacteriales" Family I.	*Enterobacteriaceae* Genus I. Genus IV. Genus VI. Genus VII. Genus VIII. Genus IX. Genus X. Genus XI. Genus XII. Genus XIII. Genus XIV. Genus XV. Genus XVI. Genus XVII. Genus XVIII. Genus XIX.	*Enterobacter* *Brenneria* *Budvicia* *Buttiauxella* *Calymmatobacterium* *Cedeceae* *Citrobacter* *Edwardsiella* *Erwinia* *Escherichia* *Ewingella* *Hafnia* *Klebsiella* *Kluyvera* *Leclercia* *Leminorella*

Box 5-4 *Continued*

DOMAIN BACTERIA
Phylum XII.   *Proteobacteria* phy. nov.

		Genus XX.	*Moellerella*
		Genus XXI.	*Morganella*
		Genus XXII.	*Obesumbacterium*
		Genus XXIII.	*Pantoea*
		Genus XXVI	*Plesiomonas*
		Genus XXVIII.	*Proteus*
		Genus XXIX.	*Providencia*
		Genus XXX.	*Rahnella*
		Genus XXXII.	*Salmonella*
		Genus XXXIII.	*Serratia*
		Genus XXXIV.	*Shigella*
		Genus XXXVI.	*Tatumella*
		Genus XXXVII.	*Trabulsiella*
		Genus XL.	*Yersinia*
		Genus XLI.	*Yokenella*
	Order XIII.	"Pasteurellales"	
		Family I.	*Pasteurellaceae*
		Genus I.	*Pasteurella*
		Genus II.	*Actinobacillus*
		Genus III.	*Haemophilus*
		Genus V.	*Mannheimia*
Class IV.	**"δ-Proteobacteria"**		
	Order II.	"Desulfovibrionales"	
		Family I.	"Desulfovibrionaceae"
		Genus I.	*Desulfovibrio*
		Genus II.	*Bilophila*
Class V.	**"ε-Proteobacteria"**		
	Order I.	"Campylobacteriales	
		"Family I.	*Campylobacteriaceae*
		Genus I.	*Campylobacter*
		Genus II.	*Arcobacter*
		Family II.	"Helicobacteriaceae"
		Genus I.	*Helicobacter*
		Genus II.	*Wolinella*

Phylum XIII.   *Firmicutes* phy. nov.

Class I.	**"Clostridia"**		
	Order I.	*Clostridiales*	
		Family I.	*Clostridiaceae*
		Genus I.	*Clostridium*
		Genus VIII.	*Sarcina*
		Family II.	"Lachnospiraceae"
		Genus I.	*Lachnospira*
		Family III.	"Peptostreptococcaceae"
		Genus I.	*Peptostreptococcus*
		Genus IV.	*Helcococcus*
		Family IV.	"Eubacteriaceae"
		Genus I.	*Eubacterium*
		Family V.	*Peptococcaceae*
		Genus I.	*Peptococcus*
		Family VII.	"Acidominococcaceae"
		Genus I.	*Acidaminococcus*
		Genus XIII.	*Veillonella*
Class II.	**Mollicutes**	*Mycoplasmatales*	
	Order I.	Family I.	*Mycoplasmataceae*
		Genus I.	*Mycoplasma*

(Continued)

Box 5-4 *Continued*

Phylum XIII.	*Firmicutes* phy. nov.			
			Genus IV.	*Ureaplasma*
	Order V.	Incertae sedis		
		Family I.	"Erysipelotrichaceae"	
			Genus I.	*Erysipelothrix*
			Genus II.	*Holdemania*
Class III.	**"Bacilli"**			
	Order I.	*Bacillales*		
		Family I.	*Bacillaceae*	
			Genus I.	*Bacillus*
			Genus II.	*Amphibacillus*
			Genus III.	*Exiguobacterium*
			Genus IV.	*Gracilibacillus*
			Genus V.	*Halobacillus*
			Genus VI.	*Saccharococcus*
			Genus VII.	*Salibacillus*
			Genus VIII.	*Virgibacillus*
		Family II.	*Planococcaceae*	
			Genus I.	*Planococcus*
			Genus III.	*Kurthia*
		Family III.	*Caryophanaceae*	
			Genus I.	*Caryophanon*
		Family IV.	"Listeriaceae"	
			Genus I.	*Listeria*
			Genus II.	*Brochothrix*
		Family V.	"Staphylococcaceae"	
			Genus I.	*Staphylococcus*
			Genus II.	*Gemella*
			Genus III.	*Macrococcus*
			Genus IV.	*Salinococcus*
		Family VI.	"Sporolactobacillaceae"	
			Genus I.	*Sporolactobacillus*
			Genus II.	*Marinococcus*
		Family VII.	"Paenibacillaceae"	
			Genus I.	*Paenibacillus*
			Genus III.	*Aneurinibacillus*
			Genus IV.	*Brevibacillus*
		Family VIII.	"Alicyclobacillaceae"	
			Genus I.	*Alicyclobacillus*
	Order II.	"Lactobacillales"		
		Family I.	*Lactobacillaceae*	
			Genus I.	*Lactobacillus*
			Genus II.	*Pediococcus*
		Family II.	"Aerococcaceae"	
			Genus I.	*Aerococcus*
			Genus II.	*Abiotrophia*
			Genus III.	*Dolosicoccus*
			Genus IV.	*Eremococcus*
			Genus V.	*Facklamia*
			Genus VI.	*Globicatella*
			Genus VII.	*Ignavigranum*
		Family III.	"Carnobacteriaceae"	
			Genus I.	*Carnobacterium*
			Genus III.	*Alloiococcus*
			Genus V.	*Dolosigranulum*
		Family IV.	"Enterococcaceae"	
			Genus I.	*Enterococcus*

Box 5-4 Continued

Phylum XIII.	*Firmicutes* phy. nov.			
			Genus II.	*Melissococcus*
			Genus III.	*Tetragenococcus*
			Genus IV.	*Vagococcus*
		Family V.	"Leuconostocaceae"	
			Genus I.	*Leuconostoc*
			Genus II.	*Oenococcus*
			Genus III.	*Weissella*
		Family VI.	*Streptococcaceae*	
			Genus I	*Streptococcus*
			Genus II.	*Lactococcus*

Phylum XIV.	*Actinobacteria* phy. nov.			
Class I.	**Actinobacteria**			
	Subclass V.	*Actinobacteridae*		
	Order I.	*Actinomycetales*		
	Suborder I.	*Actinomycineae*		
		Family I.	*Actinomycetaceae*	
			Genus I.	*Actinomyces*
			Genus II.	*Actinobaculum*
			Genus III.	*Arcanobacterium*
			Genus IV.	*Mobiluncus*
	Suborder VI.	*Micrococcineae*		
		Family I.	*Micrococcaceae*	
			Genus I.	*Micrococcus*
			Genus II.	*Arthrobacter*
			Genus V.	*Kocuria*
			Genus VII.	*Nesterenkonia*
			Genus IX.	*Rothia*
			Genus X.	*Stomatococcus*
		Family II.	*Brevibacteriaceae*	
			Genus I.	*Brevibacterium*
		Family III.	*Cellulomonadaceae*	
			Genus I.	*Cellulomonas*
			Genus II.	*Oerskovia*
		Family IV.	*Dermabacteriaceae*	
			Genus I.	*Dermabacter*
			Genus II	*Brachybacterium*
		Family V.	*Dermatophilaceae*	
			Genus I.	*Dermatophilus*
			Genus II.	*Dermacoccus*
			Genus III.	*Kytococcus*
		Family VI.	*Intrasporangiaceae*	
			Genus IV.	*Sanguibacter*
		Family VII.	*Jonesiaceae*	
			Genus I.	*Jonesia*
		Family VIII.	*Microbacteriaceae*	
			Genus I.	*Microbacterium*
			Genus II.	*Agrococcus*
			Genus III.	*Agromyces*
			Genus IV.	*Aureobacterium*
			Genus VI.	*Cryobacterium*
	Suborder VII.	*Corynebacterineae*		
		Family I.	*Corynebacteriaceae*	
			Genus I.	*Corynebacterium*
		Family II.	*Dietziaceae*	
			Genus I.	*Dietzia*

(Continued)

Box 5-4 *Continued*

Phylum XIV.	*Actinobacteria* phy.			
		Family III.	*Gordoniaceae*	
			Genus I.	*Gordonia*
			Genus II.	*Skermania*
		Family IV.	*Mycobacteriaceae*	
			Genus I.	*Mycobacterium*
		Family V.	*Nocardiaceae*	
			Genus I.	*Nocardia*
			Genus II.	*Rhodococcus*
		Family VI.	*Tsukamurellaceae*	
			Genus I.	*Tsukamurella*
	Suborder VIII.	*Micromonosporineae*		
		Family I.	*Micromonosporaceae*	
			Genus I.	*Micromonospora*
	Suborder IX.	*Propionibacterineae*		
		Family I.	*Propionibacteriaceae*	
			Genus I.	*Propionibacterium*
			Genus IV.	*Propioniferax*
		Family II.	*Nocardiopsaceae*	
			Genus I.	*Nocardioides*
	Suborder XI.	*Streptomycineae*		
		Family I.	*Streptomycetaceae*	
			Genus I.	*Streptomyces*
	Suborder XII.	Streptosporangineae		
		Family II.	*Nocardiopsaceae*	
			Genus I.	*Nocardiopsis*
		Family III	*Thermomonosporaceae*	
			Genus I.	*Thermomonospora*
			Genus II.	*Actinomadura*
	Order II.	*Bifidobacteriales*		
		Family I.	*Bifidobacteriaceae*	
			Genus I.	*Bifidobacterium*
			Genus II.	*Gardnerella*
		Family II.	Unknown affiliation	
			Genus V.	*Turicella*
Phylum XVI.	*Chlamydiae* phy. nov.			
Class I.	**"Chlamydiae"**			
	Order I.	*Chlamydiales*		
		Family I.	*Chlamydiaceae*	
			Genus I	*Chlamydia*
Phylum XVII.	*Spirochaetes* phy. nov.			
Class I.	**"Spirochaetes"**			
	Order I.	*Spirochaetales*		
		Family I.	*Spirochaetaceae*	
			Genus I.	*Borrelia*
			Genus IX.	*Treponema*
		Family II.	"Serpulinaceae"	
			Genus II.	*Serpulina*
		Family III.	*Leptospiraceae*	
			Genus I.	*Leptospira*
Phylum XX.	*Bacteroidetes* phy. nov.			
Class I.	**"Bacteroides"**			
	Order I.	"Bacteroidales"		
		Family I.	*Bacteroidaceae*	
			Genus I.	*Bacteroides*

Box 5-4 Continued

Phylum XIV.	*Bacteroidetes* phy. nov.			
		Family III.	"Porphyromonadaceae"	
			Genus I.	*Porphyromonas*
		Family IV.	"Prevotellaceae"	
			Genus I.	*Prevotella*
Class II.	**"Flavobacteria"**			
		Family I.	*Flavobacteriaceae*	
			Genus I.	*Flavobacterium*
			Genus II.	*Bergeyella*
			Genus III.	*Capnocytophaga*
			Genus V.	*Chryseobacterium*
			Genus XIV	*Weeksella*
		Family II.	"Myroidaceae"	
			Genus I.	*Myroides*
Class III.	**"Sphingobacteria"**			
	Order I.	"Sphingobacteriales"		
		Family I.	*Sphingobacteriaceae*	
			Genus I.	*Sphingobacterium*
		Family III.	"Flexibacteriaceae"	
			Genus I.	*Flexibacter*
Phylum XXI.	*Fusobacteria* phy. nov.			
Class I.	**"Fusobacteria"**			
	Order I.	"Fusobacteriales"		
		Family I.	"Fusobacteriaceae"	
			Genus I.	*Fusobacterium*
			Genus VI.	*Streptobacillus*

new classification scheme for organisms associated with humans and human disease that will appear in the forthcoming edition of *Bergey's Manual of Systematic Bacteriology*.[55]

Despite the current emphasis on molecular methods for classification, phenotypic criteria continue to be the mainstay of bacterial identification in the clinical microbiology laboratory. With the methods outlined in Box 5-3, along with various identification schemes and computer-assisted databases, most bacteria isolated in the clinical laboratory can be placed in a taxonomic framework that allows a genus and species name to be determined. This approach fulfills the role of the clinical microbiology laboratory in providing physicians with accurate and timely organism identifications and determining the susceptibility of these organisms to antimicrobial agents. Physicians, in turn, use this information to guide their selection of appropriate therapeutic interventions, to monitor the clinical response of the patient, and to evaluate the patient's clinical course.

In order to provide the reader with sufficient background information for understanding subsequent chapters regarding specific bacterial pathogens and the diseases that they cause, the next section of this chapter deals with the general morphology, physiology, and virulence mechanisms of bacteria. This discussion will provide the information necessary for understanding the nuances of morphology, staining properties, growth, metabolic features, and biochemical characteristics of the organisms discussed in subsequent chapters. The basic morphology and physiology of fungi, parasites, and viruses are presented in Chapters 20, 21, and 22, respectively.

Basic Bacterial Anatomy and Physiology

Bacteria are prokaryotic, while fungi, protozoa, and other organisms are eukaryotic. Eukaryotic cells contain a nucleus with a nuclear membrane enclosing multiple chromosomes, while prokaryotic cells have a single chromosome (nucleoid) that is not enclosed in a nuclear membrane. Eukaryotic cells also possess a variety of subcellular organelles with specialized functions, such as mitochondria (sites of aerobic respiration) and chloroplasts (sites of photosynthesis in green plants). In fact, these subcellular organelles probably evolved from prokaryotic organisms that entered the eukaryotic cells and developed symbiotic relationships with them over time by losing metabolic functions associated with a free-living existence and developing features or attributes that benefitted the "host" organism. Prokaryotic and eukaryotic cells differ substantially in many other characteristics; these are briefly described in Table 5-1.

Bacterial Size and Shape

Bacterial cells have a wide variety of sizes and shapes. Most bacteria are generally 0.2–2 μm in diameter and 1–6 μm in length, although many environmental organisms may

Table 5-1 Properties of Prokaryotic and Eukaryotic Cells

CHARACTERISTIC	PROKARYOTIC (EUBACTERIAL) CELLS	EUKARYOTIC CELLS
Major groups	Bacteria, blue-green algae	Algae, fungi, protozoa, plants, animals
Cell wall	Contains peptidoglycan, lipids, proteins	Absent; when present, contains chitin or cellulose (green plants)
Nuclear structure		
Nuclear membrane	Absent	Present
Chromosomes	Single, closed, circular, double-stranded DNA	Multiple, linear chromosomes
Ploidy	Haploid	Diploid, haploid (fungi)
Transcription/translation	Continuous, with short-lived mRNA and polyribosome (polysome) formation	Discontinuous; long-lived mRNA transcribed in nucleus and translated in cytoplasm
Histones	Absent	Present
Cytoplasm		
Ribosomes	Present; 70S (50S + 30S)	Present; 80S (60S + 40S)
Mitochondria	Absent	Present
Golgi complex	Absent	Present
Endoplasmic reticulum	Absent	Present
Cytoplasmic membrane	Present; phospholipids, no sterols (except for *Mycoplasma* species)	Present; phospholipids and sterols (cholesterol, ergosterol)
Triglyceride fats	Absent	Present
Motility	Flagella (simple)	Flagella (complex); pseudopodia; other complex locomotor organs
Energy generation	Cytoplasmic membrane–associated	Mitochondria
Sexual reproduction	Absent (unnecessary)	Present (may alternate with asexual reproductive cycles)
Recombination/gene exchange	Chromosomal or plasmid gene exchange via transformation, transduction, or conjugation	Diploid zygote formed from haploid germ cells; meiosis results in genetic recombination

be as long as 100 μm. The largest bacteria ever described, *Epulopiscium fishelsonii*, lives in the gut of the surgeonfish and measures 600 μm by 80 μm.[5] Bacteria exist in four basic morphologies: spherical cells, or **cocci**; rod-shaped cells, or **bacilli**; spiral-shaped cells, or **spirilla**; and comma-shaped cells, or **vibrios**. Arrangements of coccal cells in pairs, chains, or clusters define groups of organisms called **diplococci**, **streptococci**, and **staphylococci**, respectively (Fig. 5-1). Rod-shaped organisms may be regular in morphology, may be somewhat shorter (i.e., "**coccobacillary**"), or may appear club- or dumbbell-shaped ("**coryneform**"). Comma-shaped cells generally define a basic characteristic of certain species (e.g., *Vibrio* species). The same is true for certain other spiral-shaped bacteria (e.g., *Campylobacter, Helicobacter, Borrelia,* and *Treponema* species), in which spiral formation may be loose (about 4 coils per organism) or tight (14 to 20 coils per organism). In addition to their size, shape, and cellular arrangement, bacteria can be further differentiated on the basis of their staining characteristics with the **Gram stain**. Using this staining technique, most

bacteria can be classified as gram-positive or gram-negative. The Gram stain helps to differentiate bacteria based on their cell wall structure and is discussed later in this chapter. The structure of a generalized bacterial cell (both gram-positive and gram-negative) is depicted in Fig. 5-2.

Nuclear Structure, DNA Replication, Transcription, and Translation

The inheritable characteristics of all living organisms are determined by the structure of the genetic material. The genetic material of an individual cell is composed of **deoxyribonucleic acid (DNA)** organized into single or multiple chromosomes. Collectively, the genetic material is referred to as the organism's genome. In the vast majority of prokaryotic organisms, the **genome** is composed of a single, covalently closed, circular chromosome of double-stranded DNA (dsDNA); in some organisms (e.g., *Borrelia burgdorferi,* the streptomycetes) linear DNA is present.[29] In the *Archaea* and the *Bacteria,* this circular chromosome is not bounded by a

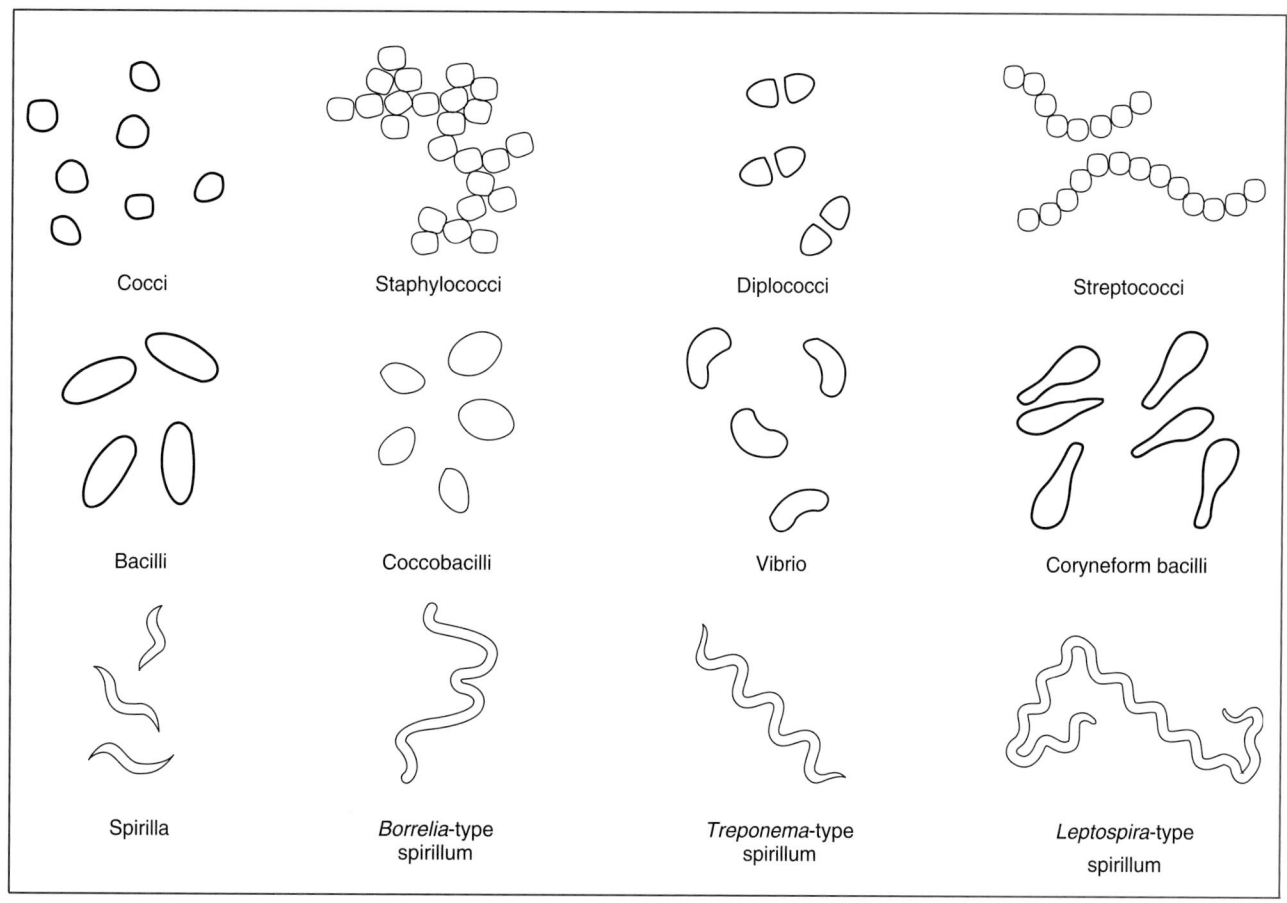

Figure 5-1 Basic morphologies of various bacteria.

membrane, but is free in the cytoplasm in a discrete central portion of the bacterial cell called the **nucleoid**.[29] Bacterial cellular DNA has a molecular weight of about 10^6 kDa, measures 300 to 1400 μm in length, and is present in the cell in a **supercoiled** state (i.e., the double-stranded molecule is twisted up on itself like a ''twisted'' rubber band). Individual genes are arranged linearly on the chromosome. The nucleoid represents about 10% of the cell volume, although DNA is only 2–3% of the cell's dry weight. In *Escherichia coli*, the chromosome contains about 5×10^6 base pairs, and its length is about 1,000 times the length of the bacterial cell in which it is contained. Unlike similar processes in eukaryotic cells, DNA replication and transcription of the DNA into messenger ribonucleic acid (mRNA) occur continually. The chromosome also appears to be attached to the inner aspect of the cell membrane at certain points. In **eukaryotic** organisms, the genetic material is organized into several **chromosomes** within the nucleus. The chromosome are, in turn, associated with several basic proteins called histones, which help to stabilize chromosomal structure. The chromosomes of eukaryotic organisms are separated from the rest of the cellular material by a **nuclear membrane**, which is composed of a lipid bilayer that is similar in composition to the cell membrane. The nuclear membrane also contains pores that allow passage of small molecules into and out of the nucleus.

Nucleic acids of all bacteria, like other organisms, are composed of **polynucleotides** (a polymer consisting of nucleotides) that are comprised of the following three components (Fig. 5-3): (1) a cyclic, five-carbon sugar (ribose in RNA; deoxyribose in DNA), (2) a purine (adenine, guanine) or pyrimidine (cytosine, thymine, uracil) base attached to the $1'$ carbon atom of the pentose by an *N*-glycosidic bond, and (3) a phosphate (PO_3) attached to the $5'$ carbon of the pentose by a phosphodiester linkage. Deoxyribose moieties are linked together via alternating phosphate groups to form a chain that has a characteristic helical coil, and the bases are directed toward the central axis of the coil. Such a structure composes a single strand of nucleic acid (ssDNA).

The double-helix structure of DNA, specifically, results from the interaction between two complementary single strands of nucleic acid. Complementarity is associated with the sequence of bases on a single strand and the hydrogen bonding that occurs between specific bases on the complementary strand (Fig. 5-4). The **purine** bases are **adenine (A)** and **guanine (G)**, and the **pyrimidine** bases are **cytosine (C)**, **thymine (T)**, and **uracil (U)** (Fig. 5-3). The purine adenine will specifically base-pair only with the pyrimidine thymine, while the purine guanosine will specifically base-pair only with the pyrimidine cytosine. Antiparallel chains of ssDNA are held together by three hydrogen bonds between C and G and two hydrogen bonds between A and T (see Fig. 5-4). Native DNA exists as a double-stranded helix, while RNA exists primarily in a single-stranded form as **messen-**

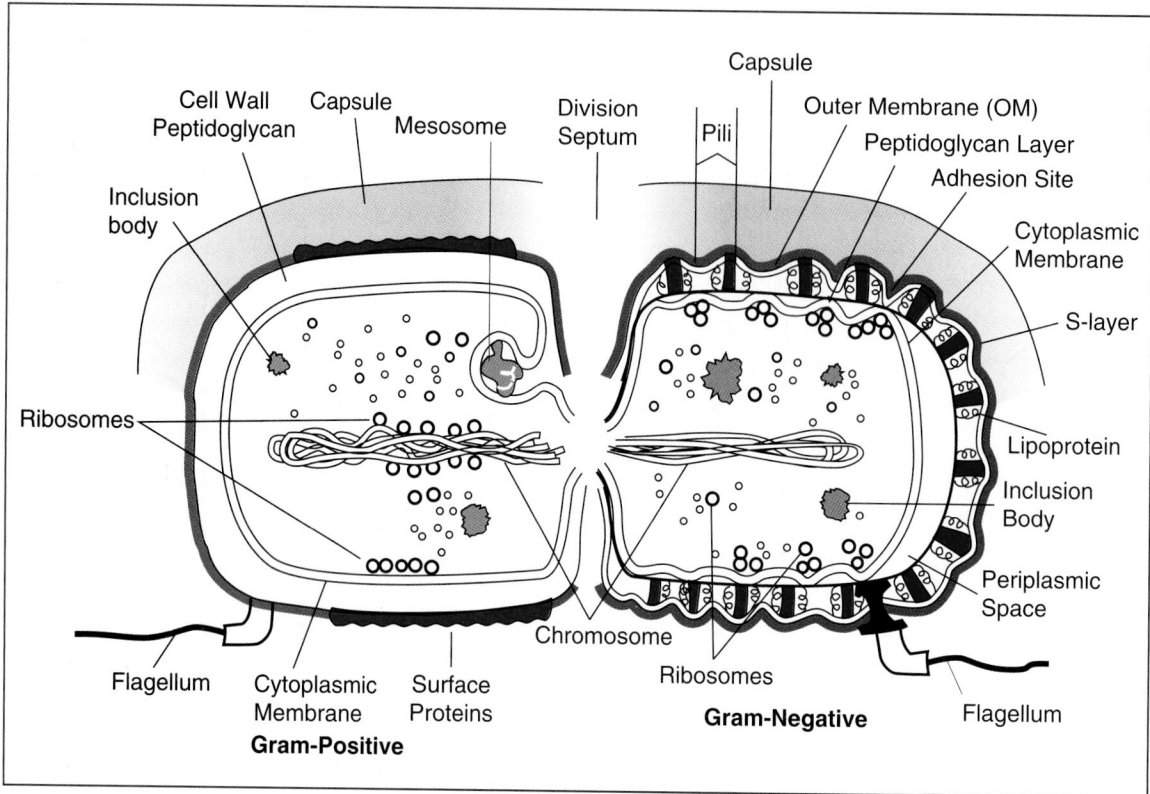

Figure 5-2 Cross-section through a generalized bacterial cell. The left half of this figure depicts the structure of a gram-positive bacterium; the right half shows the structure of a gram-negative bacterium.

ger RNA (**mRNA**) and in partially double-stranded forms in **ribosomal RNA (rRNA)** and **transfer RNA (tRNA)** molecules. In all RNA species, uracil is present in place of thymine (see Fig. 5-3). The sequence of purine and pyrimidine bases in DNA constitutes the genetic code, with specific codons (three base-pair sequences) coding for specific amino acids. Single-stranded messenger RNA (mRNA) is synthesized from double-stranded DNA during the process of **transcription** by a **DNA-dependent RNA polymerase**, in which a complementary strand of mRNA is synthesized with the "sense" strand of dsDNA as the template. The mRNA then becomes associated with **ribosomes**, which are the sites of protein synthesis.

Both prokaryotic and eukaryotic organisms harbor large numbers of ribosomes. In prokaryotic organisms, the ribosomes are 70S, while in eukaryotic organisms, the ribosomes are 80S. The "S" refers to a Svedberg unit, which is an indirect measure of the size of the ribosome as determined by its rate of sedimentation when subjected to ultracentrifugal force. The 70S bacterial ribosome has a molecular weight of about 80 kDa and exists in a dissociated state as two subunits termed the 30S and the 50S subunits. The 30S subunit contains the 16S RNA species, whereas the 50S subunit contains both 23S and 5S RNA; together, the subunits also contain about 50 ribosomal proteins. Ribosomal ribonucleic acid (rRNA) comprises 70% of the total cellular RNA. The remaining cellular RNA is found as transfer ribonucleic acid (tRNA, 16%) and messenger ribonucleic acid (mRNA, 14%).

When complexed with an mRNA transcript from the DNA, the 50S and 30S ribosomal subunits form the intact 70S ribosome found in bacterial cells. Ribosome-mRNA aggregates, termed **polyribosomes** or **polysomes,** contain all components of the protein-synthesizing system; polysomes are essentially chains of 70S ribosomes (monomers) attached to messenger RNA (mRNA). Histone or histone-like proteins that serve to stabilize the nascent polypeptides synthesized by the polysomes have only recently been found in small amounts in association with *Escherichia coli* DNA, whereas the occurrence of polyamine proteins (e.g., putrescine and spermidine) associated with bacterial DNA is well known. The mRNA is "decoded" in association with several ribosomes in a polysome-mRNA complex, where the **codon-anticodon base-pairing** occurs through molecules of tRNA during the process of **translation**. Transfer RNA molecules bear the **specific anticodons** corresponding to the codons of the mRNA and also carry the corresponding, covalently linked amino acid. The tRNA-amino acid complex interacts with the ribosome such that a peptide bond is formed between the amino acid on the tRNA and the nascent peptidyl-tRNA. Interaction of tRNA-amino acid, ribosomes, adenosine triphosphate (ATP) and several cofactors result in the formation of a specific polypeptide chain. Thus, the genetic code present in the DNA is translated into protein molecule "building blocks" or enzymes that, in turn, catalyze the synthesis and degradation of all the other cellular components. The synthesis of new DNA molecules, called **replication**, occurs by the uncoiling and "unzipping" of

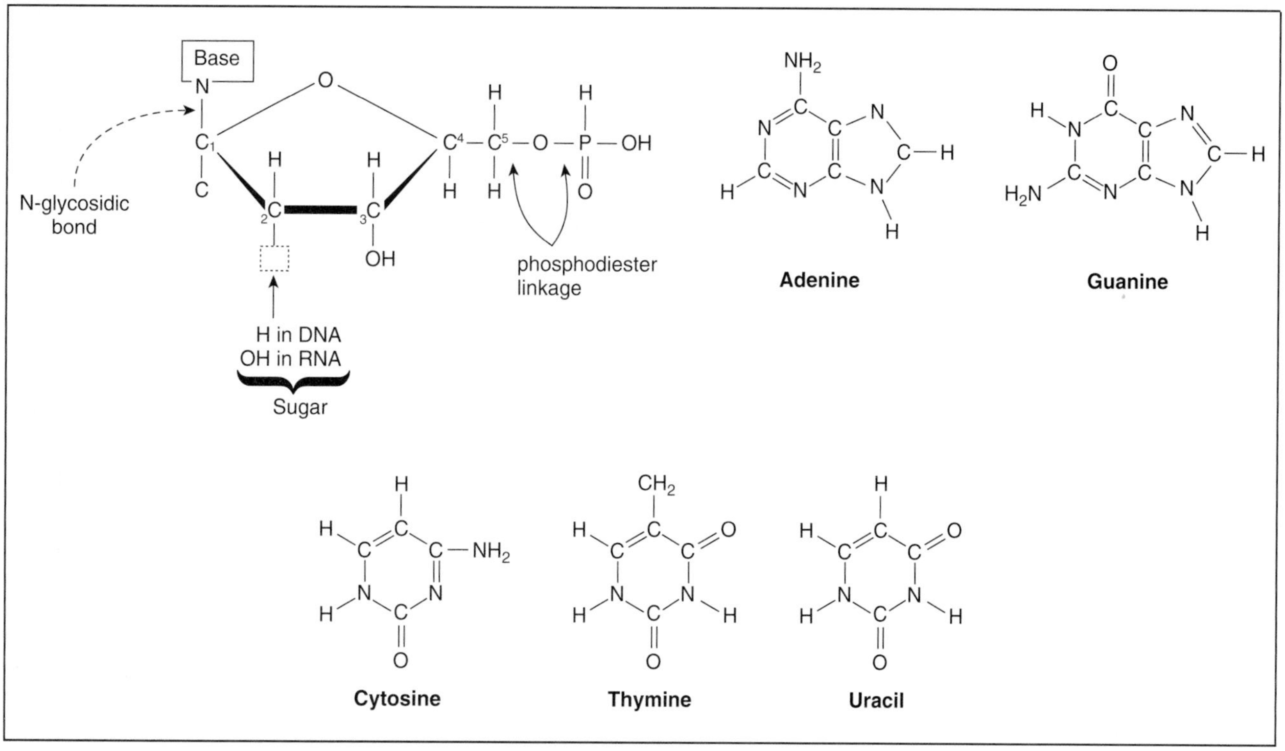

Figure 5-3 Molecular structure of polynucleotides and nucleic acid bases. Polynucleotides consist of a cyclic, 5-carbon sugar (ribose or deoxyribose), a purine or pyrimidine base attached to the 1′ carbon atom of the sugar by an *N*-glycosidic bond, and a phosphate group linked to the 5′ carbon of the sugar by a phosphodiester linkage. The structures of the two purine (adenine and guanine) and the three pyrimidine (cytosine, thymine, and uracil) bases are also shown.

the dsDNA molecule by a **DNA gyrase** enzyme, and the synthesis of complementary strands of DNA by a DNA-dependent DNA polymerase. Each new dsDNA molecule contains a single strand of the parent DNA. The relationship among DNA replication, RNA transcription, and translation of the genetic code into proteins is summarized in Fig. 5-5.

In addition to its utility for determining genetic relatedness among bacteria (see above), sequencing of rRNA molecules has revealed nucleotide sequences that are unique to individual species. Since these unique RNA sequences are also highly conserved and exist in multiple copies within the ribosomes of a bacterial cell, synthetic oligonucleotides that can hybridize with these unique sequences can be used to both detect and identify bacteria. Such an approach forms the basis for nucleic acid probe technology for direct detection of *Neisseria gonorrhoeae* and *Chlamydia trachomatis* in clinical specimens.[25,61,74,102] These probes can also be applied to organisms recovered on culture media as a method of organism identification.[60,72]

Cytoplasm

The cytoplasm is an amorphous gel containing enzymes, ions, and a variety of granules, many of which represent food and energy reserves. The cytoplasmic enzymes of prokaryotic cells function in both anabolic and catabolic processes, and many of these enzymes are associated with the inner aspect of the cell membrane (see below). Prokaryotic cells lack separate, membrane-bounded subcellular organelles, while eukaryotic cells contain a variety of subcellular structures (e.g., mitochondria, endoplasmic reticula, etc.) composed of or bounded by phospholipid bilayer membranes. Intracellular, cytoplasmic inclusions or granules represent accumulations of food reserves (polysaccharides, lipids, or polyphosphates). The numbers and types of storage granules vary with the medium and the functional state of the cells. Starch is the principle storage product among the *Neisseria* and *Clostridium* species, while glycogen is the major storage material of enteric bacteria. *Bacillus* and *Pseudomonas* species accumulate 30% or more of their dry weight as a high-molecular weight lipid called **poly-β-hydroxybutyrate**. High-molecular-weight polymers of polyphosphate known as **metachromatic granules** or **volutin** occur in *Corynebacterium* species, *Yersinia pestis*, and *Mycobacterium* species. These volutin granules appear reddish-pink when stained with methylene blue. Intracytoplasmic inclusions that are found mostly among environmental bacteria include magnetosomes and gas vesicles. **Magnetosomes** are composed of various forms of iron and impart a magnetic axis to the organism that allows it to orient itself in relation to the earth's magnetic field. **Gas vesicle**s permit the organisms to maintain buoyancy at a certain level in an aqueous environment. Both of these inclusions enable the organisms to adjust locations in response to growth conditions and nutrient concentrations.

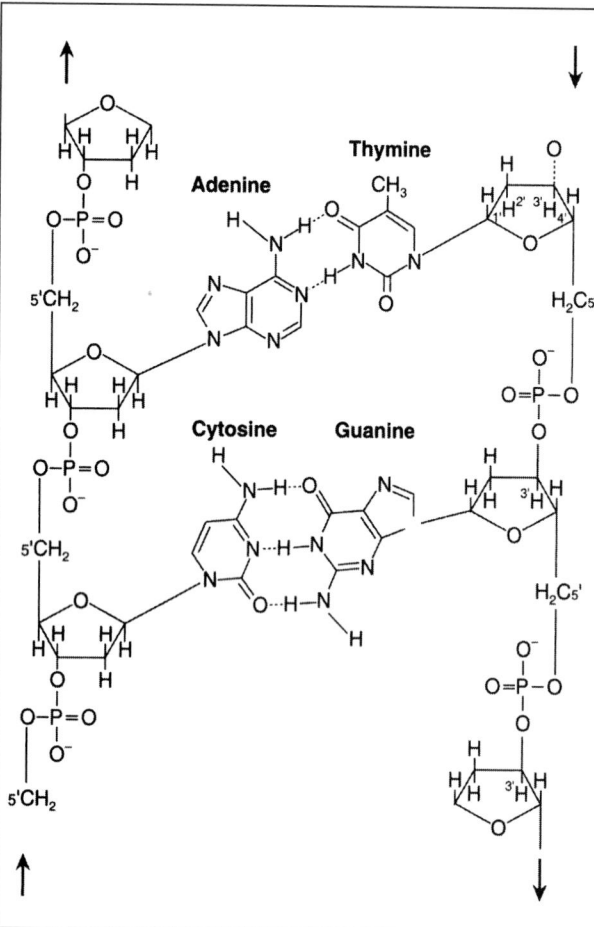

Figure 5-4 In the DNA molecule, the two polynucleotide strands of the DNA double helix are "anti-parallel," i.e., the 3′-OH terminus of one strand is adjacent to the 5′-P terminus of the complementary strand. The bases, which are directed toward the central axis of the helix, hold the two polynucleotide strands together by relatively weak hydrogen bonds. Adenine pairs with thymine via two hydrogen bonds, while cytosine pairs with guanine via three hydrogen bonds. These interactive forces between the polynucleotide strands can be overcome by thermal energy (heat) or by strong alkali in the process of denaturation.

Extrachromosomal DNA is frequently present in the cytoplasm of prokaryotic organisms in the form of **plasmids**. Plasmids exist as covalently closed circles of dsDNA that range in size from about 1 kilobase (kb) to greater than 400 kb, which is equivalent to about 10% of the size of the *E. coli* chromosome. They are generally not found in eukaryotic organisms, although some subcellular organelles in eukaryotic organisms (e.g., mitochondria) do contain DNA molecules that resemble bacterial plasmids. Plasmids are capable of autonomous replication, are inherited by progeny bacterial cells, and may contain the genetic information for a variety of structures or functions related to bacterial virulence, including genes for antimicrobial resistance, virulence-related adhesins, toxin production, and resistance to heavy metal ions. Some plasmids, termed **conjugative plasmids**, encode for enzymes that facilitate transmission of plasmids to other

bacterial cells. Some bacteria may also possess **transposons** and **insertion sequences**, which are sequences of DNA that are able to insert into different, unrelated sites on either the chromosome or a plasmid. Insertion of these elements into DNA does not require that the transposon base sequence be homologous with its insertion site (see below).

Cytoplasmic Membrane

The cytoplasm of all bacterial cells is surrounded by a cytoplasmic membrane. The bacterial cytoplasmic membrane lies immediately within the cell wall peptidoglycan layer in gram-positive bacteria, and adjacent to the periplasmic space in gram-negative bacteria (discussed below). The basic structure of the cytoplasmic membrane is a phospholipid bilayer in which various constituent proteins are embedded. The membrane is comprised of 30–60% phospholipid and 50–70% protein by weight. Most bacterial cell membranes contain phosphatidyl glycerol, phosphatidyl ethanolamine, and diphosphatidyl glycerol; they do not contain sterols (e.g., cholesterol or ergosterol). The only prokaryotic exceptions to this are the mycoplasmas and ureaplasmas, which incorporate sterols from the growth medium into their cell membranes. The fatty acids that compose the lipid portion of the phospholipid bilayer generally contain 15 to 18 carbon backbones and are usually saturated or monounsaturated.

The cell membrane of prokaryotes possesses several functions that are relegated to specialized intracytoplasmic organelles in eukaryotic organisms. The bacterial cell membrane contains enzymes that are active in cellular respiration and oxidative phosphorylation, peptidoglycan and complex lipid biosynthesis, DNA replication, and outer membrane biosynthesis in gram-negative bacteria. In phototrophic bacteria, the early events associated with light harvesting also occur at the cell membrane level. The cell membrane contains the machinery for the synthesis and secretion of enzymes and bacterial toxins and provides an insulating barrier across which energy can be built up in the form of an ion gradient or membrane potential; such energy may be used for flagellar movement, chromosomal mobilization, etc. The membrane structure allows the retention of metabolites and exclusion of many external compounds. Some membrane proteins are involved in the active transport of materials (e.g., certain monosaccharides and disaccharides) into the cytoplasm. Such specific membrane-associated carrier proteins are termed **permeases**. **Mesosomes**, which are invaginations of the cytoplasmic membrane that extend into the cytoplasm, may function to increase the available membrane surface area for catabolic and anabolic cellular enzymes. They may also function in DNA replication and DNA duplex separation in actively growing cells. However, there is also evidence suggesting that mesosomes may actually be artifacts that result from the fixation techniques used for electron microscopy.

Bacterial Cell Wall Structure

The bacterial cell wall provides structural rigidity, confers shape to the cell, and forms a physical barrier against the

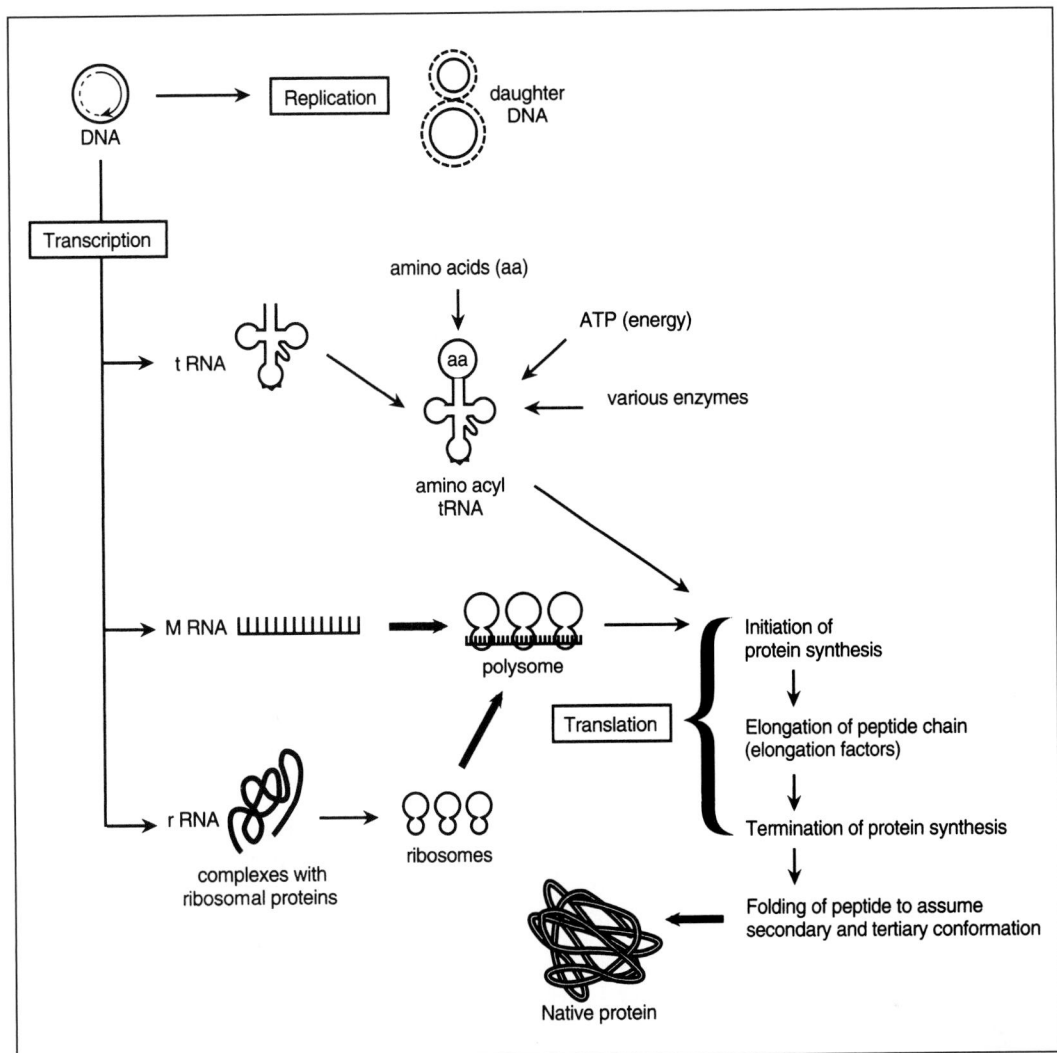

Figure 5-5 Replication, transcription, and translation of the genetic code in prokaryotic organisms. DNA is replicated by DNA-dependent DNA polymerase to produce two double-stranded DNA (dsDNA) molecules. The genetic code in the dsDNA is copied to produce a single-stranded RNA called messenger RNA (mRNA) during the process of transcription. Transfer RNA (tRNA) and ribosomal RNA (rRNA) are also transcribed. rRNA becomes complexed with specific proteins to form part of the structure of the ribosome. The mRNA becomes complexed with ribosomes to form polysomes, which are the site of protein synthesis. On the polysome, codons specific for individual amino acids are recognized by anticodons on tRNA molecules by specific base-pairing. Specific codons correspond to different amino acids attached to aminoacyl tRNA molecules. During the stages of translation, protein synthesis is initiated, polypeptide chains are elongated, and synthesis is eventually terminated with the release of a protein molecule.

outside environment. The rigid component of the cell wall of all bacteria is composed of **peptidoglycan**. Peptidoglycan is found in all bacterial species except for the cell-wall-deficient mycoplasmas and ureaplasmas. This structure is composed of a backbone of alternating carbohydrate moieties of ***N*-acetylglucosamine and *N*-acetylmuramic acid** in β-1,4 linkage (Fig. 5-6).[11] Short tetrapeptides, generally composed of identical short chains of D- and L-amino acids, are attached to the *N*-acetylmuramic acid residues via a peptide bond to the lactyl group on C3. These short chains con-

tain unusual amino acids not generally found in proteins, including D-isomers of alanine and D-glutamic acid (gram-positive bacteria), *meso*-diaminopimelic acid (*meso*-DAP) or lysine (gram-negative bacteria). Some of these tetrapeptides are, in turn, linked to one another by short peptides forming cross-bridges between adjacent peptidoglycan strands (see Fig. 5-7). The types of amino acids found and the degrees of cross-linkage are variable components of the peptidoglycan structure. For example, in *Staphylococcus aureus*, most of the *N*-acetylmuramic acid residues are cross-

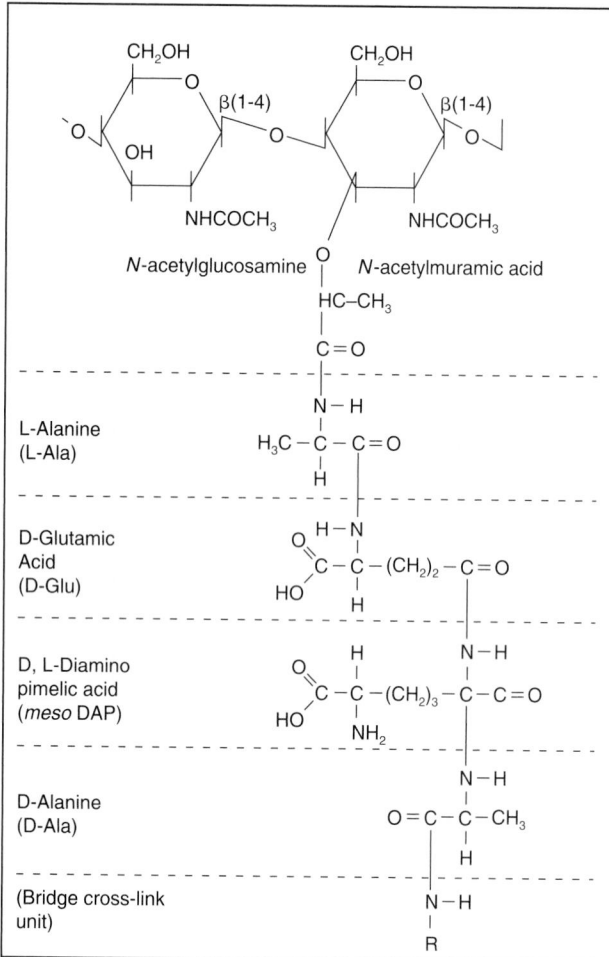

Figure 5-6 Structure of the repeating peptidoglycan unit of *Escherichia coli*.

cephalosporins inhibit bacterial cell growth by binding to the penicillin-binding proteins, thereby inhibiting polymer renewal at the inner aspect of the wall. Continuous autolytic hydrolysis of older peptidoglycan materials causes a thinning of the wall, eventually resulting in cell lysis.[75,138]

GRAM-POSITIVE BACTERIAL CELL WALLS

The gram-positive bacterial cell wall (Fig. 5-8*A*) is almost 80 nm thick and is composed mostly of several layers of peptidoglycan; in fact, anywhere from 40% to greater than 80% of the dry weight of some gram-positive cell walls may be peptidoglycan. Trapped within this peptidoglycan matrix are a variety of proteins, polysaccharides, and unique molecules called teichoic acids. Teichoic acids are polymers of either ribitol (5-carbon) or glycerol (3-carbon) units joined together by phosphodiester linkages (Fig. 5-9). Ribitol teichoic acids are associated with the cell wall, while glycerol teichoic acids are associated with the inner aspect of the bacterial cell membrane. Ribitol teichoic acids are covalently linked to the peptidoglycan via the C6 hydroxyl group of *N*-acetylmuramic acid, while the glycerol teichoic acids are linked to glycolipids of the cytoplasmic membrane. The latter molecules are termed lipoteichoic acids. They are linked to the outer lipid layer of the cell membrane and extend into the cell wall.[130] Teichoic acids of different bacteria are further modified by addition of "R" groups including ester-linked D-alanine or D-lysine residues or *O*-glycoside-linked glucose, galactose, or *N*-acetylglucosamine. Teichoic acids stabilize the cell wall, maintain the association of the wall with the cell membrane, chelate small ions necessary for cell function and cell wall integrity, and participate in cellular interaction and adherence to mucosal or other surfaces. Teichoic acids may also function in peptidoglycan synthesis and septum formation during growth and reproduction and may also play a role in the competence of some gram-positive bacteria to undergo transformation. In some organisms, the teichoic acids are antigenic and form the basis for antigenic grouping (e.g., the group D antigen in group D streptococci and members of the genus *Enterococcus*).

In the various groups of pathogenic gram-positive bacteria, other cell wall structures that are important virulence determinants may also be present. For example, M protein, a well-recognized virulence factor of group A β-hemolytic streptococci, is associated with lipoteichoic acids in the streptococcal cell wall and extends out of the wall as a fimbrial protein (see Chapter 12).[68] The group antigens of the group A, B, C, F, and G β-hemolytic streptococci are also nonteichoic acid polysaccharides that are found in the cell wall. The C polysaccharide found in the cell walls of *Streptococcus pneumoniae* is a complex lipoteichoic acid composed of ribitol and phosphate substituted at various points with *N*-acetyl-D-galactosamine, D-glucose, *N*-acetyl-2,4-diamino-2,4,6-trideoxyhexose in *O*-glycosidic linkage and choline in diester linkage.[73]

Gram-positive (and some gram-negative) bacterial cell walls also possess a cell wall component called the **S-layer**. S-layers consist of protein or glycoprotein molecules of 50–120 kDa molecular weight that self-assemble on the outer surface of the organism in oblique, square or hexagonal, packed lattice-like structures.[12,126] S-layer material may constitute up to 20% of the total cell protein. On electron microscopy, the S-layer appears as an extra "layer" on top

linked to adjacent peptidoglycan strands by five glycine residues, thereby providing a rather tight, rigid cell wall structure (Fig. 5-7*A*).[144] In gram-negative bacteria such as *E. coli*, the cross-linkage is directly between the *meso*-DAP of one peptidoglycan "chain" and the terminal D-alanyl residue on an adjacent strand (Fig. 5-7*B*). The degree of such cross-linking determines whether a cell wall structure is termed "tight" (highly cross-linked) or "loose." Among the gram-positive bacteria, there are over 100 different peptidoglycan chemotypes that differ by having various amino acid substituents attached to the lactyl group of *N*-acetylmuramic acid or that have different linkage units comprising the interpeptide bridges.[116] Slight changes in the cell wall chemotype may occur on exposure to high salt concentrations or cell-wall active antimicrobial agents such as methicillin.[35,150]

Bacterial cell wall biosynthesis is a continual process. New peptidoglycan polymers are exported from the cell and linked to preexisting cell wall polymers at the inner aspect of the cell wall by **penicillin binding proteins**.[100,105] At the same time, older peptidoglycan material overlying the newly synthesized structures are continually being removed by cell wall autolysins. Antimicrobial agents such as penicillins and

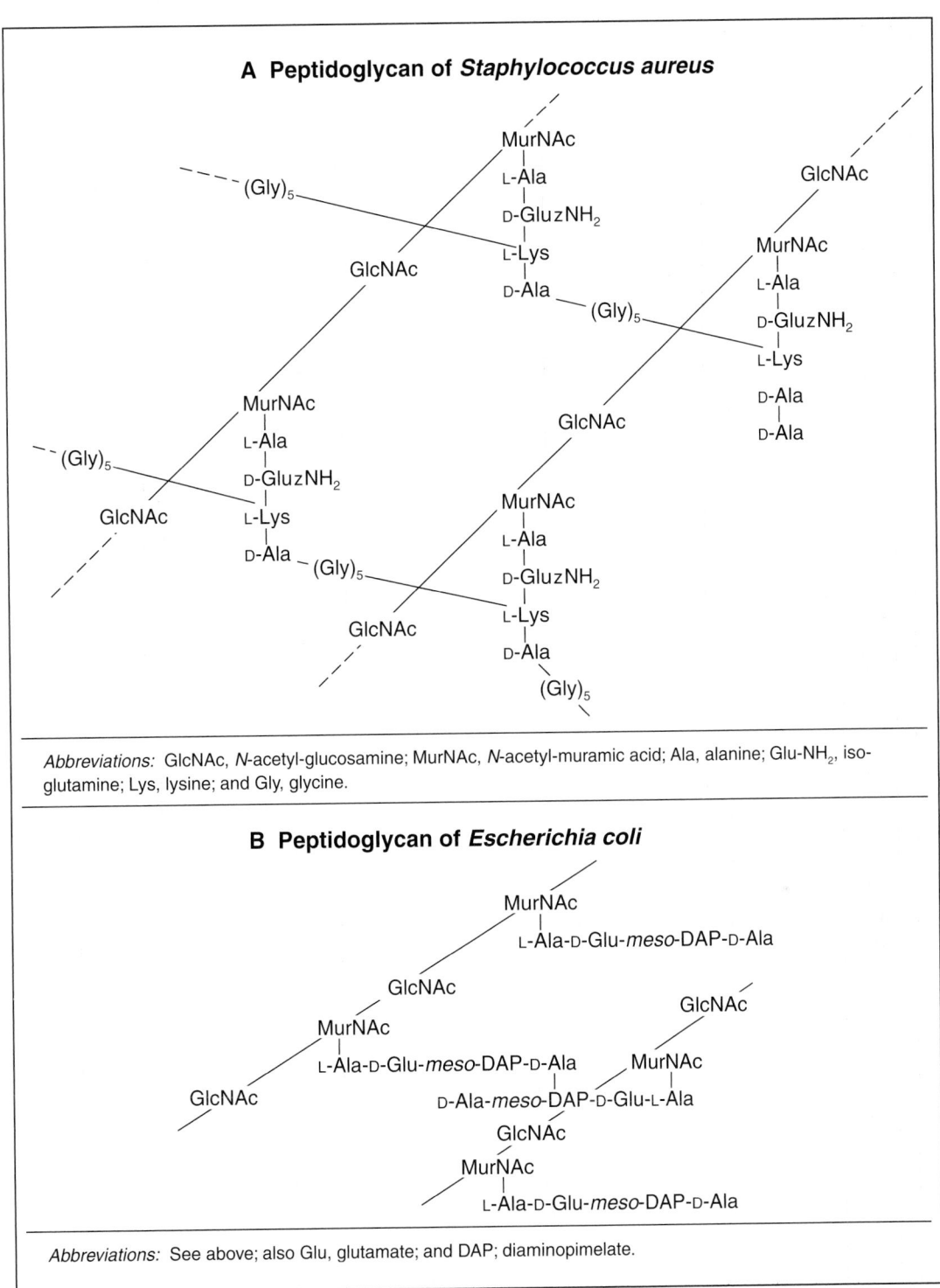

A Peptidoglycan of *Staphylococcus aureus*

Abbreviations: GlcNAc, *N*-acetyl-glucosamine; MurNAc, *N*-acetyl-muramic acid; Ala, alanine; Glu-NH₂, iso-glutamine; Lys, lysine; and Gly, glycine.

B Peptidoglycan of *Escherichia coli*

Abbreviations: See above; also Glu, glutamate; and DAP; diaminopimelate.

Figure 5-7 Structure of the peptidoglycan in *Staphylococcus aureus* (**A**) and *Escherichia coli* (**B**).

of the cell wall. Freeze-etch electron microscopic techniques have demonstrated S-layers in *Bacillus*, *Lactobacillus*, *Clostridium*, *Campylobacter*, and *Aeromonas* species. The S-layer may function to protect the organism from stressful or harsh environments. In pathogenic microorganisms, the S-layer may inhibit phagocytosis and/or prevent the binding of immunoglobulin and complement. In *Bacillus anthracis*,

it is now thought that the S-layer is this organism's major cell wall antigen and, along with the capsule and the two toxins, may contribute to virulence.[94]

GRAM-NEGATIVE BACTERIAL CELL WALLS

The cell wall of gram-negative bacteria (see Fig. 5-8*B*) is thinner than that of gram-positive bacteria but is structurally

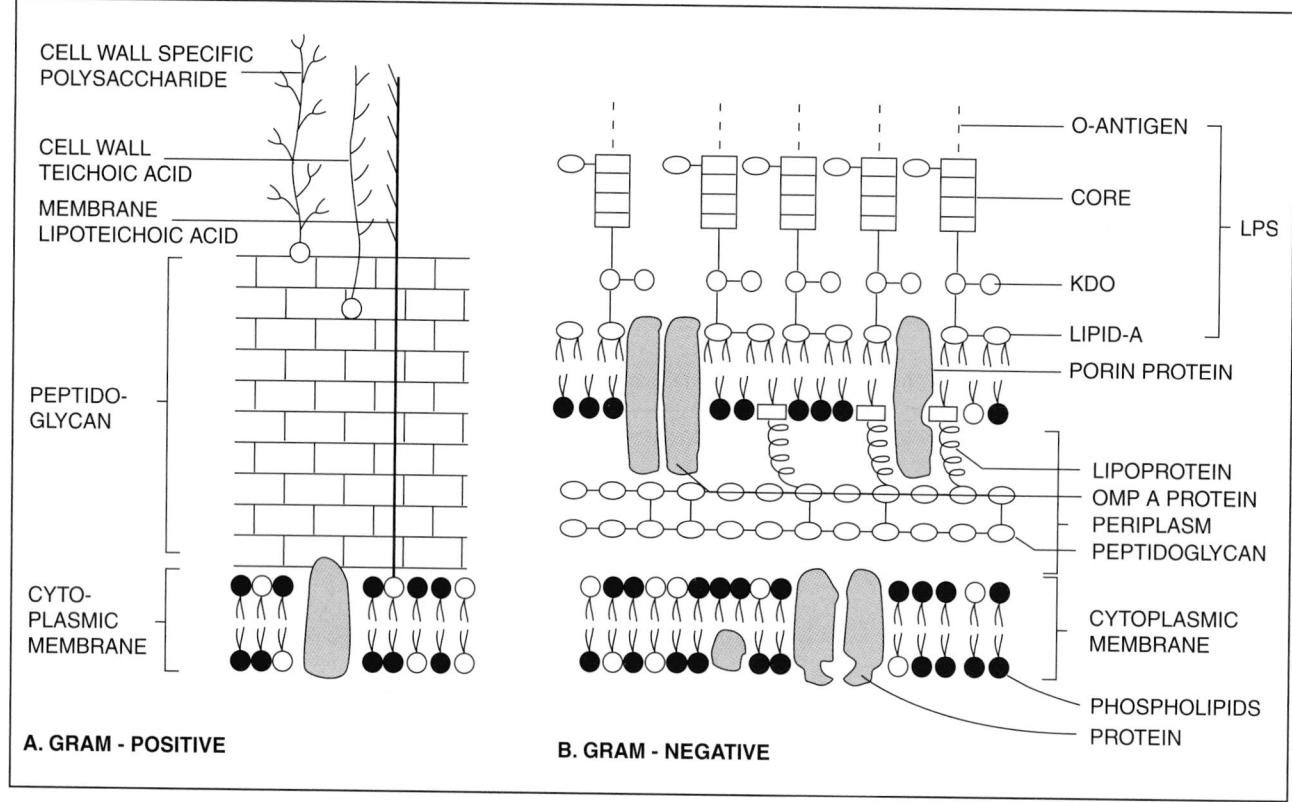

Figure 5-8 Structure of the cell wall of gram-positive (**A**) and gram-negative (**B**) bacteria. KDO, keto-deoxy-octulonate; LPS, lipopolysaccharide.

more complex. Immediately outside of the cytoplasmic membrane is the **periplasmic space**. The periplasmic space contains degradative enzymes (alkaline phosphatase, proteases, nucleosidases, β-lactamases, and aminoglycoside phosphorylases) and specific binding and transport proteins for vitamins, amino acids, and ions. A **single-unit-thick peptidoglycan layer** forms the outer border of the periplasmic space. Because the peptidoglycan layer is only one layer thick, cross-linking occurs only to adjacent peptidoglycan strands rather than to layers of peptidoglycan either deeper in or more external to the individual cell surface. Cross-links are formed from the carboxyl group of the terminal D-alanine residue on one chain to the free amino group of a *meso*-DAP residue on an adjacent chain (Fig. 5-7*B*). The peptidoglycan layer of gram-negative bacteria is fairly "loose"; i.e., only about half of the peptide chains attached to the N-acetylmuramic acid residues are actually involved in cross-linking. Moreover, cross-linking within the peptidoglycan occurs directly from the muramyl tetrapeptide on one peptidoglycan chain to the muramyl tetrapeptide of an adjacent peptidoglycan chain (i.e., no interpeptide bridges as in Fig. 5-7*A*).

Outside of the thin peptidoglycan layer is the **outer membrane**. This outer membrane has a basic structure similar to the cytoplasmic membrane; that is, a phospholipid bilayer in which various other large molecules are embedded. The outer membrane is anchored to the peptidoglycan layer by small, strongly lipophilic **murein lipoproteins** that are attached covalently to the amino group of diaminopimelic acid in the peptidoglycan and extend across the periplasmic space as an α-helical structure. The other end of this lipoprotein is noncovalently embedded in the lipid structure of the outer membrane.

A structural component that is unique to the gram-negative outer membrane is **lipopolysaccharide (LPS)** (Fig. 5-10*A*). LPS molecules are the major surface antigenic determinants (called **somatic** or **O antigens**) in gram-negative bacteria and are responsible for the endotoxin activity of

Figure 5-9 Structure of teichoic acids of gram-positive bacteria. Ribotol teichoic acid is shown on the left; glycerol teichoic acid is shown on the right. "R" group substitutions may include ester-linked D-alanine or D-lysine or *O*-glycosidic links to glucose, galactose, or N-acetylglucosamine.

Ribitol-type teichoic acid

Glycerol-type teichoic acid

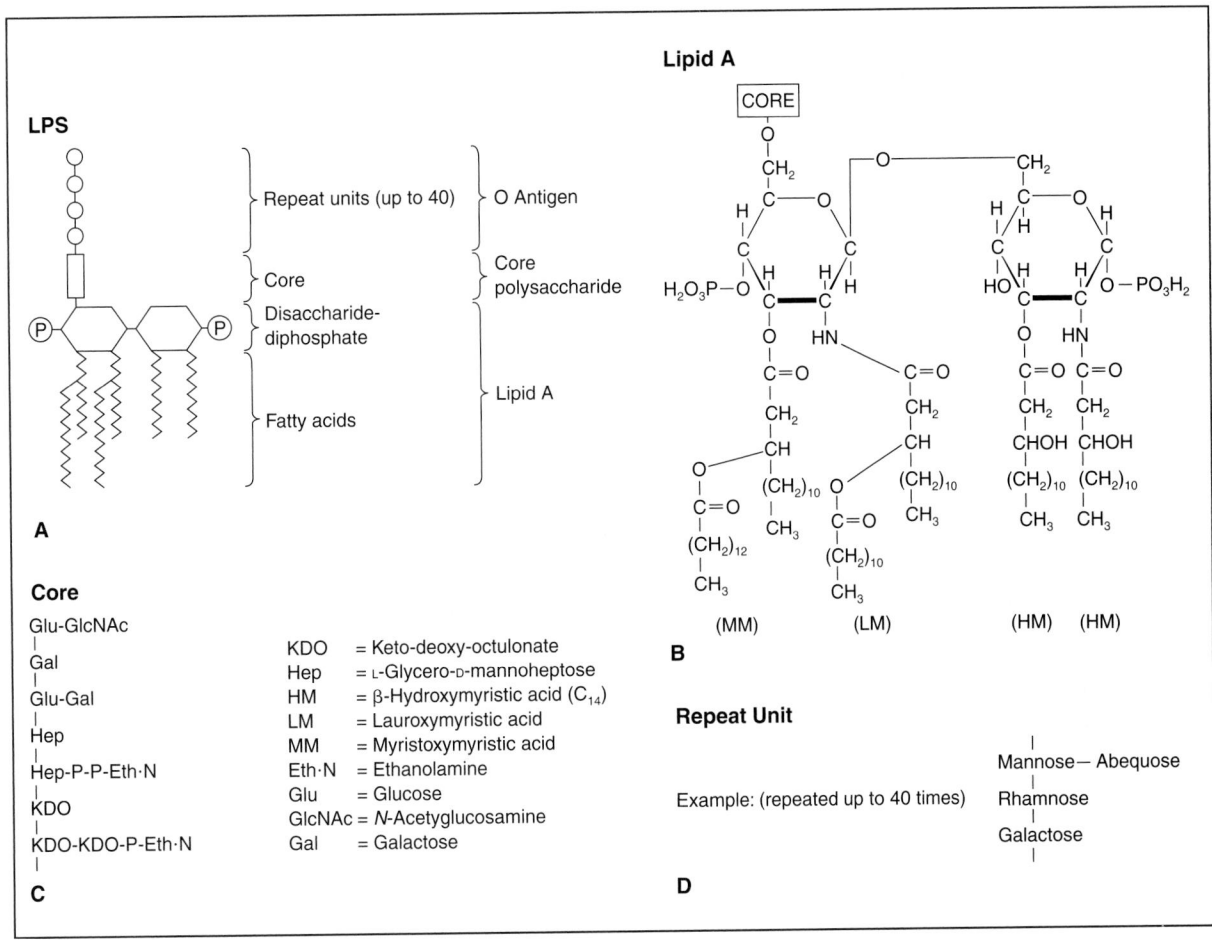

Figure 5-10 The lipopolysaccharide (LPS) of the gram-negative cell envelope. (**A**) Segment of the polymer showing the arrangements of the major constituents. (**B**) Structure of lipid A of *Salmonella typhimurium*. (**C**) Polysaccharide core. (**D**) Typical repeat unit (*Salmonella typhimurium*). (Redrawn from Brooks GF, et al. Xxxxx. Jawetz, Melnick and Adelberg's Medical Microbiology. 19th Ed. Norwalk, CT: Appleton & Lange, 1991.)

gram-negative cells. LPS molecules are high-molecular-weight, complex glycolipids consisting of three components: a complex, hydrophobic, lipid portion called **lipid A**, a **core polysaccharide region** that links lipid A to the more external structures of the molecule and that is generally similar in structure within a given bacterial genus or species, and **O-specific (somatic antigen) polysaccharide side chains**, which are regions of variable biochemical structure that impart unique serologic identity to gram-negative species. The lipid A moiety of the LPS is embedded in the outer leaflet of the outer membrane, with the core polysaccharide and the O-specific side chains projecting from the outer membrane surface like whiskers. Each *Salmonella* serotype, for example, has characteristic O-specific side chains that allow serologic confirmation of biochemical identifications and provide part of the organism's epidemiologic "fingerprint" when possible foodborne *Salmonella* outbreaks are being investigated. The structure of LPS has been studied most extensively in *Salmonella* species and *E. coli*.

Lipid A is composed of a glucosamine disaccharide in which the hydroxyl groups are esterified to uncommon β-hydroxy fatty acids like β-hydroxymyristic acid (C14), myristomyristic acid, and lauromyristic acid (Fig. 5-10*B*). Additional fatty acids may be attached via hydroxyl groups to other unsubstituted locations on the myristic acid molecule; these additional substitutions differ among the various genera of gram-negative bacteria. Attached to the lipid A portion of the LPS is the core polysaccharide. The core polysaccharide contains two unique carbohydrates: **3-deoxy-D-mannooctulosonate** (formerly called **2-keto-3-deoxyoctonoic acid [KDO]**), an eight-carbon sugar, and **heptose**, a seven-carbon sugar. Core KDO forms covalent connections between lipid A and heptose moieties in the core polysaccharide. Additional sugars (e.g., *N*-acetylglucosamine, glucose, and galactose) may also be found in the core polysaccharide. The core polysaccharide structure is fairly conserved within a given genus, but may vary from species to species. The O-specific side chains are attached to the core polysaccharide and are responsible for the antigenic specificity of individual isolates. These side chains contain a variable number (up to about 40) of repeating oligosaccharide units comprised of three to five monosaccharides each. These antigenically specific side chains often contain unusual or uncommon carbohydrate residues, including aminohexuronic acid, 6-deoxyhexoses, and 2,6-dideoxyhexoses. The lipid A moiety appears to be the principal component responsible for the manifestations of endotoxin activity in patients with gram-negative bacterial sepsis (e.g., fever, shock, vascular collapse, and hemorrhage). Endotoxin can also activate complement and can cause disseminated intravascular coagulation. The generalized structure of the LPS of *Salmonella* species is shown in Figure 5-10*A*, while the structure of lipid A, the core polysaccharides, and somatic antigens are shown in Figure 5-10*B, C,* and *D,* respectively.

Dissociation of the outer-membrane LPS can be partially accomplished by treatment of cell suspensions with ethylenediamine tetraacetic acid (EDTA), which chelates the divalent cations of the outer membrane. Subsequent treatment with lysozyme hydrolyzes the peptidoglycan layer of gram-negative bacteria, and the cells may be lysed. The dependence of the integrity of the outer membrane on calcium and magnesium ions is one of the principal reasons for the inclusion of these ions in media that is used for antimicrobial susceptibility testing.

Some gram-negative bacteria (e.g., *Haemophilus influenzae, Neisseria gonorrhoeae,* and *Bordetella pertussis*) have **lipo-oligosaccharides (LOS)** rather than LPS in their cell walls.[62,160] LOS contains lipid A and an oligosaccharide core containing KDO, but it does not have a long-chain polysaccharide O antigen as is found in the LPS of enteric bacteria.[16] These molecules, like endotoxin, possess a range of biologic activity, including general toxicity, pyrogenicity, and the unique ability to induce B-cell mitogenicity and polyclonal B-cell activation.[20] Antigenic variation seen in *N. gonorrhoeae* is partially due to high-frequency structural modulation of the LOS, which has also been shown to affect gonococcal adherence to mucosal surfaces and susceptibility to the bactericidal action of normal human serum.[119,120]

The gram-negative outer membrane also contains phospholipids and proteins. The phospholipids are similar to those found in the cytoplasmic membrane and include phosphatidyl ethanolamine and phosphatidyl glycerol. Proteins also constitute a significant portion of the outer membrane. Those that are present in greatest concentrations are called **principal or major outer membrane proteins (OMPs)**. These proteins fall into three major groups. **Porin proteins** are proteins that form trans-outer membrane channels through which lower-molecular-weight materials (e.g., amino acids, sugars, ions) are allowed into the periplasmic space. Many of these porin proteins have a "trimer" structure (i.e., three identical proteins that form a "doughnut-shaped" pore). Porins also help to limit passage of many antimicrobial agents into the cell. **Transmembrane proteins** are nonporin proteins that span the outer membrane, extend through the periplasm, and are associated with the peptidoglycan layer of the cell wall. They may function in exoenzyme production and secretion, transport of specific proteins, attachment to surfaces, or in binding of antimicrobial agents to their cell surface targets (e.g., penicillin binding proteins). **Peripheral proteins** are responsible for transmembrane transport of molecules that are also too large for porin entry. Most of these proteins are components of substrate-specific permease systems (e.g., siderophore binding

and transport of iron into the cell). Lipoproteins (see above) are the smallest of the outer membrane proteins and serve to stabilize the cell wall via covalent linkage with the peptidoglycan.

The structure of the bacterial cell wall has direct, practical importance to the microbiologist because the type of cell wall structure is largely responsible for the **Gram stain** reaction. This differential stain divides the majority of bacteria into two groups—**the gram-positive** and the **gram-negative bacteria**. In the Gram stain procedure, cells are (1) stained with **crystal violet**; (2) treated with **iodine** to form a crystal violet/iodine complex within the cell; (3) washed with an **organic solvent (acetone-alcohol)**; and (4) stained again with the red counterstain **safranin**. In gram-positive bacteria, the purple crystal violet/iodine complex is retained within the cell after washing with acid-alcohol because the thick peptidoglycan layer does not allow the crystal violet-iodine complex to be washed out of the cell. In gram-negative bacteria, the crystal violet/iodine complex is leached from the cell (i.e., the cells become colorless) because of disruption of the lipid-rich outer membrane by the acetone-alcohol organic solvent. These colorless cells must be counterstained in order to be seen under the light microscope; this counterstain is provided by safranin. Gram-positive bacteria appear blue-purple under the microscope, while gram-negative bacteria are stained red by the safranin counterstain.

Some gram-negative bacteria do not have the complex cell wall structure described above. Organisms in the *Cytophaga-Flexibacter-Flavobacterium* group have outer membranes containing ornithine-aminolipids and sulfonolipids as their principal components, along with large amounts of branched-chain fatty acids with odd-numbered carbon side chains. Organisms in *Archaea* lack a peptidoglycan structure and have instead a "pseudopeptidoglycan" composed of proteins, glycerol esters, and *N*-acetyltalosaminuronic acid (i.e., *meso*-DAP and *N*-acetylmuramic acid are absent). Some *Archaea* lack even this rudimentary peptidoglycan, having instead a thin cell wall consisting of proteins or sulfated polysaccharides.

"ACID-FAST" BACTERIAL CELL WALLS

A modification of the gram-positive cell wall is seen in organisms belonging to the genera *Mycobacterium, Nocardia,* and *Corynebacterium.* In these organisms, lipids account for as much as 60% of the dry weight of the cell wall. These organisms contain molecules called **mycolic acids** in their cell walls. Mycolic acids are large, α-substituted, β-hydroxy fatty acids that occur as esters attached to cell wall polysaccharides.[10] Mycolic acids vary in the number of carbon atoms; those with 30 carbons (C30) are found among the corynebacteria (corynemycolenic acids), those with C50 are found in *Nocardia* species (nocardic acids), and those with C90 or more constitute the mycolic acids found in the genus *Mycobacterium.* In *Mycobacterium tuberculosis,* the unique mycolic acid **6,6′-dimycolyltrehalose,** is known as **cord factor** (Fig. 5-11*A*). This molecule is associated with virulence of *M. tuberculosis* and has a wide range of biologic activities, including cell membrane cytotoxicity, inhibition of polymorphonuclear cell migration, induction

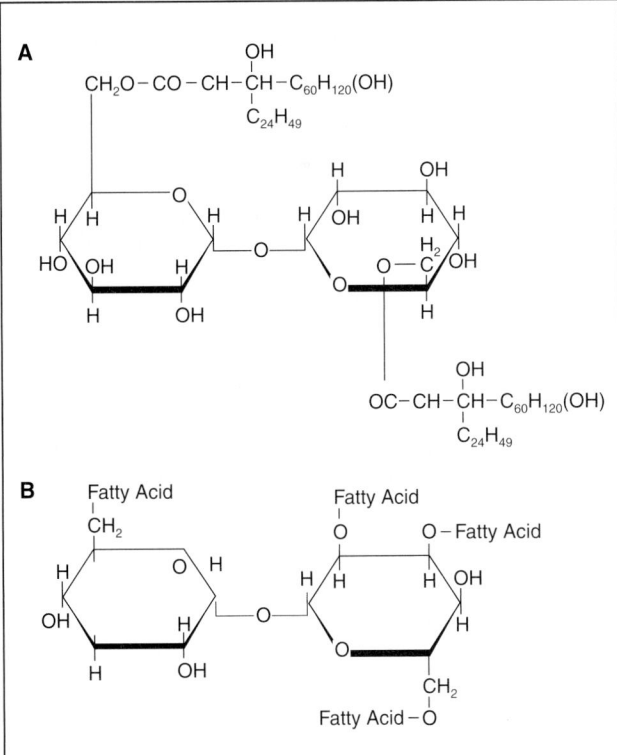

Figure 5-11 Molecular structure of specialized lipids found in the cell wall of *Mycobacterium tuberculosis*. (**A**) Molecular structure of cord factor (6,6'-dimycolyltrehalose) produced by *Mycobacterium tuberculosis*. (**B**) Molecular structure of the principal sulfolipid (2,3,6,6'-tetraacyltrehalose-2'-sulfate) of *M. tuberculosis*.

of granuloma formation, adjuvanticity, antitumor activity, and ability to activate the alternative complement pathway.

The cell membrane of mycobacteria is similar to other bacterial unit membranes except that it contains **phosphatidylinositol mannosides** and **lipoarabinomannan**. External to the membrane is the peptidoglycan layer which is composed of *N*-acetylglucosamine in β-1,4 linkage to *N*-glycolylmuramic acid.[15] The murein layer is cross-linked by tetrapeptide bridges containing L-alanine, D-glutamate, and *meso*-DAP residues. Some of the *N*-glycolylmuramic acid residues are linked by phosphodiester bonds to an overlying layer of branched-chain polysaccharide macromolecules called **arabinogalactans** (containing arabinose and galactose moieties). The distal arabinose residues of this layer are linked to the overlying mycolic acids. The hydrocarbon chains of the mycolic acids are intercalated with those of numerous other wall-associated lipids and glycolipids. These cell wall-associated lipids include those with medium (C24 to C36) and short (C12 to C20) fatty acyl groups. These wall-associated lipids include trehalose sulfolipids (Fig. 5-11*B*). The trehalose sulfolipids, typified by the principal sulfolipid of *M. tuberculosis* **2,3,6,6'-tetraacyltrehalose-2'-sulfate**, are associated with mycobacterial virulence in that these molecules may act to prevent phagosome-lysozyme fusion following phagocytosis of the mycobacterial cells, thereby allowing the organisms to survive as facultative intracellular parasites.[57,58] Protruding from the plasma membrane through the peptidoglycan, arabinogalactan, and mycolic acid layers of the wall are substituted phospholipids (phosphatidylinositol mannosides) and lipopolysaccharides (lipoarabinomannans) that are attached to the outer leaflet of the mycobacterial cell membrane. These molecules provide a noncovalent link between the cell membrane and the cell wall. Proteins that are embedded in the mycobacterial cell wall are involved in biosynthesis and construction of the cell-wall polymers and some apparently also function as porins.

Organisms that are acid-fast are stained red with the basic dye carbol fuchsin and are resistant to decolorization with acid-alcohol. Because of the hydrophobicity of the mycobacterial cell wall, penetration of the dye into the cell is enhanced by heat treatment (i.e., the Ziehl-Neelsen method) or incorporation of detergent into the dye (i.e., the Kinyoun method). Resistance to decolorization by acid alcohol (i.e., ''acid-fastness'') is associated with the mycolic acid-arabinogalactan moieties that constitute the bulk of wall materials external to the peptidoglycan layer. The soluble lipids contribute to but do not determine the acid-fast properties of mycobacterial cells, since extraction of these lipids diminishes but does not destroy acid-fastness. Mechanical disruption of the cell wall and extraction of the cell-wall lipids with ethanolic alkalis that remove both free and esterified lipids destroy the acid-fast properties of these organisms, indicating that the total lipid content of the cell wall is responsible for the acid-fast staining property.

Bacterial Endospores

Endospores are spherical or oval structures formed within certain bacterial species that represent a dormant or ''resting'' stage in the growth cycle of the organism. Among clinically significant bacteria, endospores are formed by aerobic gram-positive bacilli belonging to genus *Bacillus* and other related genera, and by the anaerobic gram-positive bacilli in the genus *Clostridium*. In these genera, endospores are formed in response to nutritional deprivation within the vegetative bacterial cell. They are highly resistant to the injurious effects of heat, drying, pressure, and many chemical disinfectants. Sterilization temperatures (i.e., 120°C for 15–20 minutes) are required to kill spores. The heat resistance of bacterial endospores is believed to be due to reduced amounts of water in the core of the spore itself. The size, shape, and location of incipient endospores in stationary phase cells of *Clostridium, Bacillus,* and related species is helpful for characterization and identification of certain species within these two genera (see Chapters 12 and 13). The endospores may be spherical, subspherical or oval in shape, they may differ in their location within the cell (i.e., central, terminal, or subterminal), and they may or may not swell the cell. Endospores generally do not stain with routine staining methods like the Gram stain, and appear as refractile, nonstaining bodies in smears.

Under the stimulus of certain environmental conditions such as the exhaustion of nutrients (i.e., glucose, nitrogen, or phosphate) or exposure to suboptimal temperatures or redox potentials, the nuclear material divides into two nucleoids, and one becomes separated from the other by a membranous septum.[67] The septum then grows together and the spore core becomes engulfed in a double membrane. Between the two membranes, a cortex layer is deposited by the membranes. This cortex consists primarily of peptidoglycan material. The cortex layer thickens and accumulates calcium ions due to the chelating activity of a unique molecule called **dipicolinic acid**. The core becomes protected by the high concentration of calcium ions tightly cross-linking the peptidoglycan material and all available water in the spore is expelled. Several layers of the spore coat (a keratin-like substance that is rich in disulfide bonds) are laid down, and the endospore is liberated on the death and lysis of the mother vegetative cell. Endospores may remain viable for prolonged periods. When the spore is placed in a favorable environment in the presence of particular stimuli (e.g., the presence of particular amino acids or carbohydrates and water), spore outgrowth occurs. Upon this stimulus, enzymes are activated which degrade the spore cortex and release the peptidoglycan material, calcium ions, and dipicolinic acid. RNA synthesis begins, followed by protein synthesis and, eventually, DNA synthesis. A new vegetative cell results.

Bacterial Surface Structures
CAPSULES

Some bacteria possess a capsule external to the outer layer of the cell wall. The capsule may be thick or thin, and may be closely or loosely associated with the external aspect of the cell wall. Loosely associated capsular material may also be referred to as a **slime layer** or **glycocalyx**. Capsular material is usually polysaccharide in nature; these polysaccharides may be polymers of single monosaccharides (glucans, dextrans, levans) or heteropolysaccharides containing both hexose and pentose sugars, plus ribitol, glycerol, or other sugar alcohols. Phosphates are also frequently present. In most cases, the capsule is synthesized at the level of the cell membrane; components are synthesized and exported out of the cell by an isoprenoid lipid ''carrier'' system, in which the components become attached to ''primer'' capsular material already present on the surface of the cell. In some cases, such as the glucan capsule of *Streptococcus mutans*, the capsule is synthesized by a class of extracellular and cell wall–associated enzymes called **glucosyltransferases** and **fructosyltransferases**.[145] The action of these enzymes on dietary sucrose creates a branched, **insoluble glucan** matrix that specifically interacts with the tooth surface and with receptors on the *S. mutans* cell. Subsequent formation of acids from dietary sucrose and from intracellular glycogen stores in *S. mutans* and other organisms leads to formation of dental caries.[28,63]

The bacterial capsule serves several functions. It protects the cell from desiccation and from toxic materials in the environment (e.g., heavy metal ions, free radicals) and promotes the concentration of nutrients at the bacterial cell surface because of its polyanionic nature. In addition, the capsule also plays a role in the adherence of bacteria to cells and mucosal surfaces. This adherence is necessary for many organisms to establish infections in appropriate hosts (discussed below). Some bacterial capsules function to protect cells from phagocytosis (in the absence of anticapsular antibodies) by polymorphonuclear leukocytes. Capsular material is usually antigenic, and the serologic detection of the capsule forms the basis of the **Quellung test** (Chapter 12), which can be used to identify and/or subtype several important human pathogenic bacteria, including *S. pneumoniae*, *H. influenzae* type b, *Klebsiella pneumoniae*, and *Neisseria meningitidis* serogroups. The capsular material of many microorganisms is synthesized in abundance and is shed into the surrounding fluid both in vivo and in vitro. This material can be detected in various body fluids. (e.g., serum, spinal fluid, and urine) during infection by encapsulated bacteria and can be specifically detected and identified by electrophoresis or agglutination tests to provide a rapid diagnosis (see Chapter 3).[122]

In recent years, the capsular structure of *Staphylococcus aureus* has been an area of interest to both basic scientists and clinical microbiologists. More than 90% of *S. aureus* strains isolated in the clinical laboratory are encapsulated, and these capsules have been divided serologically into 11 types. The types that have been characterized thus far (types 1, 2, 5, and 8) are complex *N*- and *O*-acetylated carbohydrates in β-1,4 and β-1,3 linkages.[49,96] Capsular types 5 and 8 predominate among clinical isolates, and a predominant number of oxacillin-resistant strains express the type 5 capsular polysaccharide.[6,47] Of interest to the bench microbiologist is that capsular type 5 *S. aureus* strains also may not be reliably identified by latex agglutination coagulase tests used in clinical laboratories.[46] For this reason, latex beads coated with antibodies to type 5 and 8 capsular polysaccharides are now included in some formulations of the coagulase latex agglutination test.[48]

In some bacterial species, such as *Bacillus* and related species, the capsule is polypeptide in nature. *Bacillus anthracis*, the cause of anthrax, is encapsulated in both infected tissue and when grown on media containing bicarbonate or in a >5% CO_2 environment. Both capsule formation (and toxin production) are specifically ''turned on'' by these cultural conditions, which, interestingly, reflect the same bicarbonate and CO_2 concentrations found in tissues infected with *B. anthracis*.[142] The *B. anthracis* capsule is composed of linked, α-peptide chains of D-glutamic ranging from 50 to 100 residues per chain.[142] The presence of the capsule renders *B. anthracis* resistant to phagocytosis.[90]

FLAGELLA

Bacterial flagella are long, filamentous appendages that arise at the level of the cytoplasmic membrane and extend through the cell wall into the surrounding medium. They are responsible for cellular motility. Flagella are usually found in rod-shaped, gram-negative bacteria, although motile, gram-positive rods (e.g., *Listeria* species) and cocci (some *Enterococcus* species, *Vagococcus* species) are also found. Flagella differ in their numbers and their arrangements on cells. Bacteria with a single polar flagellum are termed **monotrichous;** those with two or more flagella originating at one pole or point are **lophotrichous;** those with a single flagellum located at two different points or poles are called **amphitrichous;** and those with two or more (a tuft) flagellae at two points or poles of the cell are called **amphi-lophotrichous.** Organisms that have flagella arising over the entire cell surface are termed **peritrichous.**

In gram-negative bacteria, flagella have been demon-

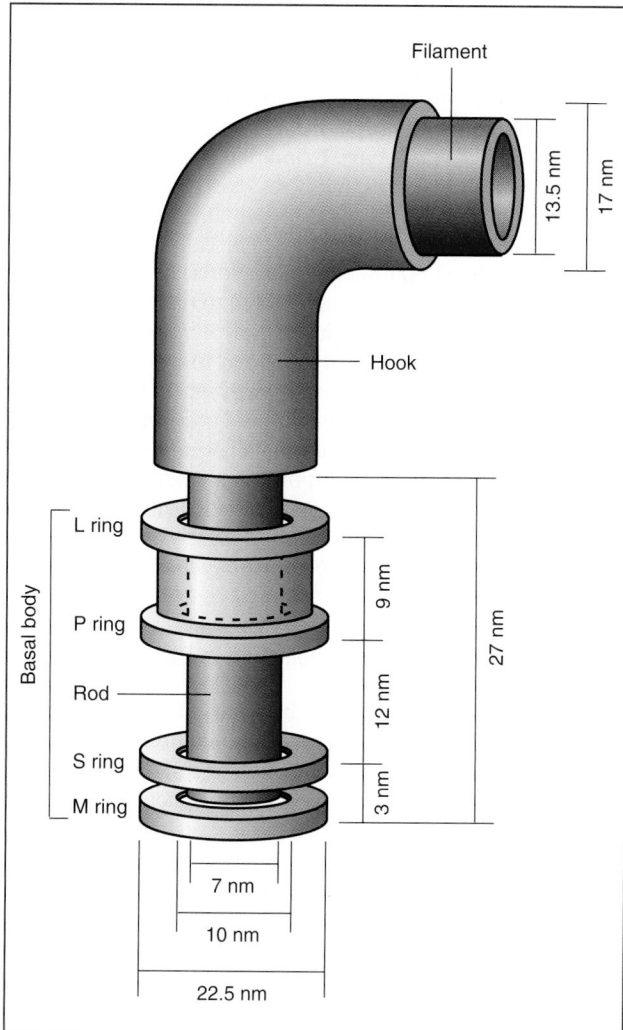

Figure 5-12 Ultrastructure of a flagellum from a gram-negative bacterium.

strated to have a complex structure consisting of three parts: the **filament**, the **hook**, and the **basal body** (Fig. 5-12). The flagellar filament is 13–17 nm in diameter and is variable in length. The filament is composed of parallel subfibrils of the 30–40-kDa subunit protein **flagellin,** which interact to form a hollow cylinder. The filament is semirigid and forms a left-handed helix as it exits the cell. Flagellin has the capacity to self-assemble. Monomers of the protein are synthesized and passed through the lumen of the cylinder. At the growing tip of the flagellum helix, the monomer undergoes a conformational change and becomes added to the distal end of the flagellum. The hook is composed of another distinct protein and acts as a "sleeve" from which the flagellar filament emerges. The hook permits the transmission of a rotary motion from the basal body to the filament. The **basal body** is composed of complex rings connected by a rod-shaped structure. The **M, S, P, and L rings** are anchored in the membrane, the periplasmic space, the peptidoglycan, and the lipopolysaccharide outer membrane, respectively. At least 10 proteins comprise the outer ring structure in gram-

negative bacteria. The ring structure attached to the cell membrane rotates as a part of an energy-dependent reaction, causing the rigid flagellar helix to turn like a propeller. The energy for this reaction is derived by the passage of protons from the outside into the cytoplasm via the basal body. The outer rings (L and P rings) evidently function as bearings, minimizing friction and leakage of materials from the cell at the points of flagellar insertion. In gram-positive bacteria, the flagellar structure is less complex and is composed of two rings. One ring structure anchors the flagellum to the plasma membrane, while the second ring structure is embedded in the thick peptidoglycan layer.

Several species of flagellated organisms are also able to alter the expressed antigenic type of flagella that they produce; this process is known as **phase variation**.[121] This refers to the ability of organisms to express two types of flagella alternately. Phase variation occurs by the differential expression of chromosomal genes that code for two variously structured flagellin proteins. This phenomenon was first recognized in enteric gram-negative bacteria such as *Salmonella* species, but also occurs in other species, such as *N. gonorrhoeae* (see below). Flagellar antigens in gram-negative bacilli are referred to as H antigens, from the German word "hauch," meaning "breath." Some organisms have slightly modified flagellar structures. Vibrio species have the typical flagellar morphology, but the flagellum is encased in a sheath derived from the outer membrane of the cell wall. In the spirochetes, the flagellum does not protrude into the environment, but lies within a sheath that is exterior to the protoplasmic cylinder of the cell body of the organism. This endoflagellum or **axial filament** arises from one pole of the cell and wraps around the cell body internal to the sheath.

Other Locomotor Organelles. Some gram-negative bacteria exhibit what is known as "gliding motility." This type of motility is most apparent when organisms are in contact with a surface. In clinical microbiology, gliding motility is seen among the *Capnocytophaga* species, which are part of the normal flora of the human oropharynx and are occasionally isolated from infectious processes (Chapter 9). Studies with *Flavobacterium johnsonii* and other organisms in the *Cytophaga-Flavobacterium-Bacteroides* group have suggested that proteins or glycoproteins located within the outer membrane adhere to the substratum and that other proteins within the cell membrane harvest proton-motive forces that cause the surface proteins to move along "tracks" within the peptidoglycan layer.[92,93] Other studies have also shown the presence of unique sulfonolipids in the outer membrane of gliding bacteria that are absent in nonmotile mutants of the same species.[1] Using spontaneous, chemically induced, and transposon-induced nonmotile mutants, several unlinked genes and operons involved with gliding motility have been identified.[71]

FIMBRIAE (PILI)

Fimbriae or pili are smaller appendages found on the surface of many gram-negative and some gram-positive bacteria. Although the terms "pili" and "fimbriae" have been used interchangeably, the latter term is now used to describe any nonflagellar hairlike appendages, while the former term is used to denote the fimbriae of gram-negative bacteria that function specifically in the transfer of DNA from one cell to another during the process of conjugation (i.e., sex pili). Fimbriae are composed of a protein called **fimbrillin** (or **pilin**), are 3 to 25 nm in diameter, and are 10 to 20 μm in length. Fimbrillin produced in gram-negative bacteria is a subunit protein of 17 to 20 kDa molecular weight. The proteins form hollow tubes that originate in the cell membrane, but that lack the basal body and hook structures of flagella. Fimbrial subunit proteins are added at the base of the structure, rather than at the tip as is seen with flagellar synthesis. Sex pili are involved in specific pair formation for exchange of genetic material during conjugation and also serve as attachment sites for bacteriophages.

Fimbriae also function as cellular organelles for attachment to cells and/or mucosal surfaces; fimbriae that serve this attachment function are often referred to as **adhesins.** Most adhesins display lectin-like binding to terminal carbohydrate residues (e.g., mannose).[70] For example, the adherence of enteric bacteria to mucosal surfaces that is mediated by type 1 (type-specific) or common pili can be inhibited by preincubation of the bacteria with mannose. Mannose attaches to the terminal portion of the adhesin and blocks adherence; therefore, type 1 pili are termed mannose-sensitive. Adhesins that are not affected by mannose are termed mannose-resistant; mannose-resistant pili are referred to as type 2. Differing lectin-like specificities are partly responsible for the tissue tropisms observed with a variety of bacterial species.

The role of fimbriae as virulence factors in gram-negative bacteria has been studied extensively in *N. gonorrhoeae* and *N. meningitidis.*[64,107] These pathogenic *Neisseria* species produce antigenically and structurally similar fimbriae that are composed of 16.5- to 21.5- kDa fimbrial subunit proteins. Virulent strains of *N. gonorrhoeae* express these surface fimbriae and are able to adhere avidly to mucosal cells in the genital tract.[151] Fimbriated organisms are also responsible for the domed type 1 and type 2 colonies produced by freshly isolated gonococci on agar media. The loss of fimbriae on repeated subculture in vitro renders these organisms unable to initiate urogenital infection because of lack of mucosal adherence. Colonies composed of nonpiliated gonococci are larger and flatter. Gonococci possess a large number of genes that code for structurally and antigenically distinct fimbrial proteins, and these proteins undergo both **phase variation** and **antigenic variation** (see Chapter 9). In phase variation between the piliated and the nonpiliated state, the *pil* genes (fimbrial structural genes) are either not expressed or the fimbrial proteins cannot be assembled into function fimbriae. In antigenic variation, new fimbrial types may emerge because of recombinational events among the 20 or so fimbrial genes present in the bacterial genome. Because of the ability of a single gonococcal strain to produce multiple, antigenically distinct fimbrial antigens, the use of fimbriae as candidate antigens for antigonococcal vaccines has been largely unsuccessful.[146]

Among the gram-positive bacteria, only a limited number of species express cell surface fimbriae, including some streptococci, corynebacteria, and *Actinomyces* species. *Actinomyces viscosus* and *Actinomyces naeslundii*, facultative gram-positive bacilli found in the oral cavity, express two type of fimbriae. Type 1 fimbriae mediate bacterial adherence to tooth surfaces via interaction with salivary acidic proline-rich proteins, while type 2 fimbriae mediate bacterial adherence to oral streptococci and various mammalian cell types, including polymorphonuclear leukocytes and erythrocytes.[24,33,56,115] These type 2 fimbriae bind to either galactose or *N*-acetylgalactosamine residues on the surface of coaggregating oral streptococci or with the oligosaccharides of mammalian cell membrane glycoproteins.[24,33,115] Unlike the fimbriae from gram-negative bacteria, fimbriae of *Actinomyces* species are covalently linked to the cell wall peptidoglycan layer.[159] The ability of oral *Actinomyces* species to adhere to buccal mucosal cells and to coaggregate with cariogenic oral streptococci facilitates biofilm formation and the initiation of dental plaque. Fimbrial coaggregates of *Actinomyces* and oral streptococci have been shown to resist phagocytosis and killing by polymorphonuclear cells, and binding of *Actinomyces* to PMNs results in the release of mediators of inflammation. Fimbria clearly play a key role in the ability of these periodontal pathogens to colonize and initiate infection.

Genetic Exchange and Recombination in Bacteria

Bacterial replication occurs by binary fission, an asexual process that does not involve recombinational events and results in the generation of two daughter cells that are identical to the parent cell. Several groups of bacteria, however, do have the ability to undergo genetic exchange and recombination with other organisms. Genetic exchange between bacteria occurs by one of three general mechanisms: transformation, transduction, and conjugation (Fig. 5-13).

Transformation involves the uptake of free DNA from the surrounding environment (Fig. 5-13A). Cells that are physiologically capable of taking up and incorporating free DNA into their genomes are termed **competent.** Competence is usually a transient state that occurs toward the late exponential phase of growth, although some organisms may be competent at all times. In competent gram-positive cells (e.g., *Bacillus subtilis*, *S. pneumoniae*), small pieces of double-stranded DNA become bound to the cell via a cell surface receptor that is expressed during the competent period. As the DNA enters the cell, one strand is hydrolyzed by a surface-bound nuclease. Recombinational events between the single-stranded DNA and homologous regions of the bacterial chromosome result in integration of the transformed DNA into the bacterial genome. If homologous regions for the transforming DNA are lacking, the DNA strand does not integrate, genes on the particular DNA strand are not expressed, and the single-stranded DNA is degraded by endogenous restriction endonucleases. *H. influenzae*, a transformation-competent gram-negative bacterium, also possess receptors for DNA on the cell surface; DNA binding occurs via the recognition of a 10- to 14-base-pair surface-expressed nucleotide sequence that allows DNA only from closely related species to bind and enter the competent cell.[123] Double-stranded DNA then enters the cell, but only one strand participates in the recombinational events that incorporate the transforming DNA into the genome of the recipient. Cells that normally do not express competence for genetic transformation can be made permeable to extracellular DNA

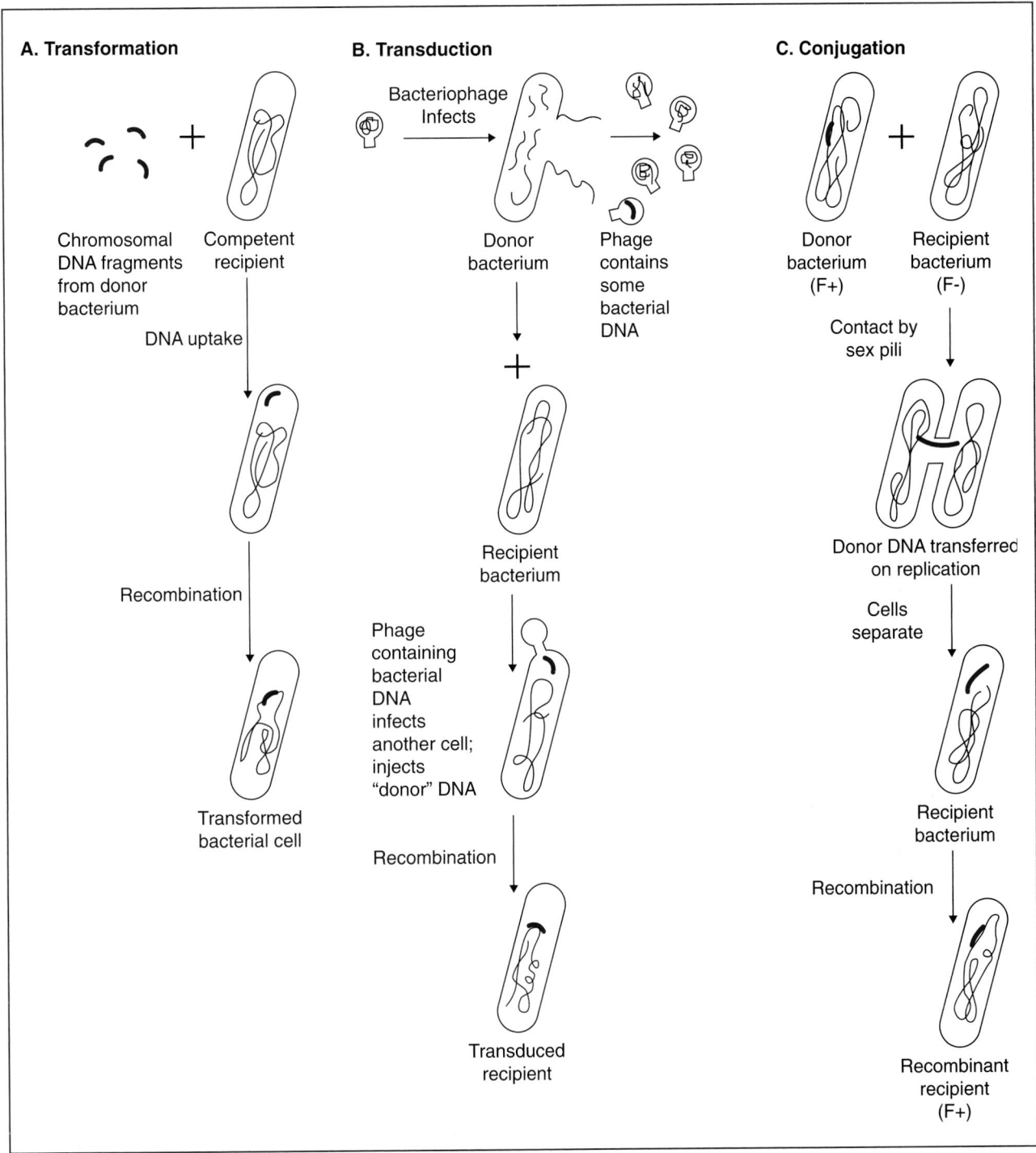

Figure 5-13 Mechanisms of gene transfer in bacteria. Microorganisms may exchange genetic material by any of three processes: transformation (**A**), transduction via bacteriophage (**B**), and conjugation (**C**).

(''artificially competent'') by treatment with $CaCl_2$ or other salt solutions at 0°C or by **electroporation,** in which cell suspensions are exposed to an electric current that induces DNA entrance into bacterial cells.

   Transduction refers to the exchange of genetic information via bacteriophages (Fig 5-13*B*). Bacteriophages (or sim-

ply ''phages'') are viruses that infect bacteria. Some bacteriophages are **lytic;** that is, after infecting the bacterial cell, the bacteriophage regulatory genes ''take over'' the cellular biosynthetic machinery, resulting in the expression of phage structural genes and the production of new phage particles that are released on lysis and death of the host bacterium.

With temperate bacteriophages, the genetic material of the bacteriophage becomes incorporated into the host cell DNA as a "prophage" and replicates along with the bacterial chromosome. Such bacteriophages are also termed **lysogenic bacteriophages,** and the bacterial cell infected with this phage is said to be **lysogenized.** On induction by exposure to certain chemicals (e.g., mitomycin C) or to ultraviolet irradiation, a lysogenic bacteriophage may be induced to begin production of new phages (i.e., the phage becomes "lytic"). Excision of the bacteriophage DNA from the bacterial cell genome results in some bacteriophages containing not only "phage-specific" genes, but also host cell genes that were located adjacent to the site of phage DNA integration in the bacterial chromosome.

The transfer of genetic information during transduction may be generalized or specialized. **Generalized transduction** refers to the accidental, random packaging of host-cell DNA into the capsid or "head" of the phage particle. Release of the mature phage particle on cell lysis and subsequent infection of another bacterial cell results in the introduction of "donor DNA" from the original host bacterium into the "recipient." Recombination of the transduced DNA with a homologous region on the chromosome of the recipient cell results in integration and subsequent expression of the transduced genes. Generalized transduction occurs with a frequency of 1 transducing phage out of 10^5 to 10^8 phage particles produced on induction from the lysogenized state, and about 1–2% of the total length of the host cell genome may be transferred by this mechanism. **Specialized transduction** refers to the packaging of specific host cell genes into the transducing prophage. This type of transduction occurs with temperate phages that have specific chromosomal integration sites, such as bacteriophage *lambda*. Only host cell genes that flank the integrated phage genome have the opportunity to become incorporated into the bacteriophage genome on induction from the lysogenic state. One specialized transducing phage is produced out of 10^5 to 10^6 new phage particles following induction.

Conjugation is the only mechanism of genetic exchange between bacteria that requires cell-to-cell contact (Fig. 5-13C). Gram-negative bacteria that are able to participate in conjugation possess a plasmid called the **F plasmid** ("fertility plasmid"). This plasmid contains an operon of genes called the *tra* region that codes for the sex pilus (or conjugative pilus) and other molecules involved in conjugation.[41] The specialized pilus functions as a vehicle for establishing contact with another bacterial cell. Once contact is established, the sex pilus apparently is retracted, thereby drawing the other cell closer. The pilus may also act as a "tube" through which DNA is passed during the conjugative process. Cells that possess F plasmids are termed F+, while cells that lack this plasmid are termed F−. Once contact of an F+ cell with an F− cell is established by the sex pilus, the circular F plasmid begins to be replicated. During this process, one of the single strands of the plasmid DNA is transferred into the recipient cell. This single strand is replicated as it enters the recipient cell, and the end result are two cells that contain complete conjugative plasmids (i.e., both become F+ cells).

In some organisms, the F plasmid becomes integrated into the host-cell genome at specific integration sites in which homologous nucleotide sequences are present. Establishment of a connection via the F pilus and subsequent conjugation results in the transfer of some F-plasmid genes plus genetic material from the host cell that is adjacent to the integration site of the F plasmid. Cells possessing an integrated F plasmid are termed **Hfr cells** (high-frequency recombinations). Matings between Hfr cells and F− cells results in transfer of part of the F genome plus some host cell genes from the donor. Recipient F− cells usually remain F− following conjugation since only part of the F plasmid from the donor Hfr cell is transferred to the recipient cell during the conjugative process. Therefore, these recipient cells will not possess the complete operon that is necessary for subsequent conjugation to occur. Recombination between the genetic material from the donor cell and homologous regions in the F− recipient enables the donor DNA to become expressed in the recipient cell. The donor cell remains Hfr, since the host-cell chromosome (containing the integrated F plasmid) is replicated during the transfer of the genomic single-stranded DNA from the Hfr to the F− cell.

Among the gram-positive bacteria, *Enterococcus faecalis* is also able to exchange plasmids via a conjugative process. However, gene transfer is not accomplished via a pilus, but by a **coaggregation** of the organisms in response to **pheromones** by the donor bacterium.[27] When exposed to plasmid-free cells (or culture filtrates from plasmid free cells), plasmid containing cells produce plasmid-encoded pheromones called **aggregation substances.** These aggregation substances are small (seven to eight amino acids) peptides. The pheromones bind to sites that are present on both recipient and donor cells, causing bacterial aggregation. Aggregation results in the establishment of the cell-to-cell connections necessary for plasmid mobilization to occur. Interestingly, enterococcal cells that contain like plasmids and similar aggregation substances respond only to pheromones from cells that have different plasmids and, therefore, produce different aggregation substances. At present, 18 different sex pheromone plasmids have been described.[66]

In addition to the mechanisms of gene transfer just described, other genetic elements also may participate in recombinational events that affect the characteristics and pathogenicity of microorganisms. **Transposable genetic elements** are pieces of DNA that can insert into different, unrelated sites on a bacterial chromosome or plasmid. Because these insertions occur randomly, mutations may be generated because of the disruption of gene sequence continuity. They have been described in *E. coli* and a wide variety of other bacteria. Unlike the mechanisms described above, regions of nucleic acid sequence homology are not required for recombination with these genetic elements to occur. Transposable genetic elements fall into two groups: insertion sequences and transposons. **Insertion sequences** are usually small pieces of DNA that carry genes coding only for their own transposition; expression of these genes is not recognized and the insertion is usually phenotypically "silent."[53] **Transposons** are larger and encode for at least one function that is recognizable as a phenotypic alteration, such as acquisition of antimicrobial resistance. Transposons described in enteric gram-negative bacteria contain genes for resistance to antimicrobial agents (e.g. aminoglycosides, tetracycline, chloramphenicol) and structural genes for the heat-stable toxin produced by some enterotoxigenic *E. coli* strains.[8]

Among clinically significant gram-positive bacteria, transposons carrying resistance genes for chloramphenicol, tetracycline, and erythromycin have been described in both *Clostridium perfringens* and *Clostridium difficile*.[2,87,88]

Requirements for Bacterial Growth and Metabolism
CARBON

Bacteria can be divided into two large groups on the basis of their carbon requirement. The **lithotrophic,** or **autotrophic,** bacteria and the **organotrophic,** or **heterotrophic,** bacteria. The lithotrophic bacteria can use carbon dioxide as the sole source of carbon and synthesize from it the carbon "skeletons" for all their organic metabolites. They require only water, inorganic salts, and CO_2 for growth, and their energy is derived either from light (photolithotrophic bacteria) or from the oxidation of one or more inorganic substances (chemolithotrophic bacteria). Organotrophic bacteria are unable to use CO_2 as their sole source of carbon but require it in an organic form, such as glucose. For these heterotrophic bacteria, a portion of the organic compound that serves as an energy source is also used for the synthesis of organic compounds required by the organism. A wide variety of other substances can also be used as exclusive or partial sources of carbon by different bacterial species. Among the most versatile bacteria are *Pseudomonas* species, some of which can use more than 100 different organic compounds as their sole source of carbon and energy. The relationships among energy sources, carbon sources, and electron donors for generation of energy are summarized in Table 5-2.

CARBON DIOXIDE

Some bacteria are able to use atmospheric carbon dioxide as a principal source of carbon for biosynthetic reactions. The energy for catalyzing this utilization may come from light energy (**photolithotrophic bacteria**) or from oxidation of inorganic molecules (**chemolithotrophic bacteria**). Organisms that require an organic source of carbon also require some CO_2 for certain macromolecular synthetic pathways, such as fatty acid biosynthesis. Carbon dioxide for these reactions is usually obtained from the breakdown of organic substrates occurring at the same time as the biosynthetic reactions.

OXYGEN

The oxygen requirement of a particular bacterium reflects the mechanism used for satisfying its energy needs. On the basis of their oxygen requirements, bacteria may be divided into five groups. **Obligate anaerobes** grow only under condition of high reducing intensity and for which oxygen is toxic. **Aerotolerant anaerobes** are anaerobic bacteria that are not killed by exposure to oxygen. **Facultative anaerobes** are capable of growth under both aerobic and anaerobic conditions. **Obligate aerobes** have an absolute requirement for oxygen in order to grow. **Microaerophilic organisms** grow the best under lower oxygen tension; higher oxygen tensions may be inhibitory. In obligate and facultative aerobes, the assimilation of glucose results in the terminal generation of the free radical superoxide (O_2^-). The superoxide is reduced by the enzyme superoxide dismutase to oxygen gas (O_2) and hydrogen peroxide (H_2O_2). Subsequently, the toxic hydrogen peroxide generated in this reaction is converted to water and oxygen gas by the enzyme catalase, which is found in aerobic and facultative bacteria, or by various peroxidases, which are found in several aerotolerant anaerobes.

NITROGEN

The nitrogen atoms of important biomolecules (i.e., amino acids, purines, pyrimidines) come from ammonium ions (NH_4^+). The generation of ammonium ions starts with the reduction of atmospheric N_2 to NH_4^+ (ammonium ion or ammonia, NH_3). NH_4^+ is then assimilated into more complex macromolecules by way of the key compounds **glutamate** and **glutamine**. Certain species of bacteria (*Rhizobium* species, *Azotobacter* species) and blue-green algae are able to "fix" atmospheric N_2 into a more readily usable organic form. Because of the strength of the triple bonds in N_2, nitrogen fixation requires cellular energy in the form of ATP and a powerful reductant. The process is catalyzed by a complex multienzyme system called the nitrogenase complex. In most nitrogen-fixing organisms, reduced ferredoxin is the source of electrons:

$$N_2 + 6e^- + 12\,ATP + 12\,H_2O \rightarrow 2\,NH_4^+ + 12\,ADP + 12\,P_i + 4H^+$$

The ability to fix nitrogen is accomplished primarily by the soil-dwelling bacteria mentioned above. However, some

---

Table 5-2 Energy and Carbon Sources of Bacteria

TYPE/EXAMPLES	ENERGY SOURCE(S)	CARBON SOURCE(S)	ELECTRON DONORS
Photolithotrophs Green sulfur bacteria Purple sulfur bacteria	Light	CO_2	Inorganic compounds (H_2S, S)
Photoorganotrophs Purple nonsulfur bacteria	Light	Organic compounds (and CO_2)	Organic compounds
Chemolithotrophs Hydrogen, sulfur, and denitrifying bacteria	Oxidation-reduction reactions	CO_2	Inorganic compounds (H_2, S, H_2S, Fe, NH_3)
Chemoorganotrophs	Oxidation-reduction reactions	Organic compounds	Organic compounds (glucose, and other carbohydrates)

bacterial species that are involved in human disease, such as *K. pneumoniae* and certain environmental clostridia (e.g., *Clostridium pasteurianicum*) are also able to fix atmospheric nitrogen.

Ammonium ions may also be generated by nitrate reduction. This is accomplished by two distinct physiologic mechanisms. **Assimilatory nitrate reduction** is a process in which nitrate is reduced to nitrite and hydroxylamine, which are then converted to ammonia for assimilation. **Dissimilatory nitrate reduction** is when nitrate serves as an alternative electron acceptor to oxygen (anaerobic respiration), with NO_2 or N_2 being the usual products. Nitrate assimilation is quite widespread in microorganisms and requires both nitrate and nitrite reductases, while dissimilatory nitrate reduction is seen only in anaerobic bacteria and facultative anaerobic bacteria growing at low oxygen tension (i.e., in a broth, for example). Ammonia generated by these mechanisms becomes incorporated into organic molecules by the action of the enzymes **glutamate dehydrogenase**, **glutamine synthetase** and **glutamic acid synthase** (Fig. 5-14). The final products of these reactions are glutamine and glutamic acid, which then become the building blocks used in other biosynthetic reactions for the synthesis of several amino acids, purines, pyrimidines, and other necessary nitrogenous compounds (Fig. 5-14).

GROWTH FACTORS

These substances promote growth of the organism and are provided by various body fluids and tissues in vivo and in the form of yeast extract and blood and/or blood products in vitro. These factors include B-complex vitamins, minerals, certain amino acids, purines, and pyrimidines. The B-complex vitamins play a catalytic role within the cell, acting either as components of coenzymes or as prosthetic groups of enzymes. Organisms that do not require an exogenous source of a given growth factor because they are capable of synthesizing their own are referred to as **prototrophic. Auxotrophic** organisms require the addition of the growth factor to culture media before growth can occur. Small amounts of a number of inorganic ions also are required by all bacteria. In addition to nitrogen, sulfur, and phosphorus, which are present as constituents of important biologic compounds, potassium, magnesium, and calcium are often functionally associated with certain anionic polymers. Magnesium divalent cations stabilize ribosomes, cell membranes, the cell wall, and nucleic acids, and are also required for the activity of many enzymes. Potassium is also necessary for the activity of a number of enzymes, and in gram-positive bacteria its concentration in the cell is influenced by the teichoic acid content of the cell wall. Most organisms also need zinc, iron, manganese, copper, and cobalt. Certain physical requirements for growth include optimal growth temperature, pH, and oxidation/reduction potential.

Kinetics of Bacterial Cell Growth

During growth in fluid culture medium, bacteria display a uniform growth curve, as expressed in logarithmic numbers of bacteria over time. A typical bacterial growth curve is shown in Figure 5-15. The lag phase is a period of physiologic adjustment and ''gearing up,'' when the cell synthes-

izes new enzymes, cofactors, and essential metabolic intermediates, and the intracellular pools of nutrients are established. During the increasing growth phase, cell growth begins as enzymatic reaction rates begin to approach their steady-state rates. During the exponential or logarithmic growth phase, cell growth and cell division are occurring at their maximal rates. This rate is influenced by temperature, the type of carbon source being used, the rate-limiting concentrations of various essential nutrients, the types of nutrients available, and the oxygen tension or redox potential. During the declining growth phase, growth eventually ceases because of exhaustion of essential nutrients from the medium or from the accumulation of substances that are inhibitory or toxic. During the stationary phase, the number of viable cells has plateaued and the numbers of new organisms produced is equal to the numbers of cells that die because of lack of nutrients. During the death phase, cells begin to lyse and die.

Clinical laboratories most often deal with bacteria growing on solid media such as blood or chocolate agars. In general, organisms are able to grow to high numbers on solid media because the acid and other inhibitory products diffuse away from the bacterial colonies during growth, and the depletion of nutrients in the vicinity of the colonies is countered by diffusion of fresh nutrients into growth areas on the agar media. However, some organisms are extremely sensitive to slight pH shifts or metabolic by-products that cause cell lysis by themselves or that activate cellular autolysins. Periodic or frequent subculture to fresh agar media is usually sufficient for short-term preservation of organism viability on solid culture media.

General Bacterial Metabolism and Energy Generation
FERMENTATION

Bacterial metabolism is a dynamic balance between biosynthesis (anabolic reactions) and degradation (catabolic reactions). Catabolic reactions, in addition to providing smaller building blocks for subsequent biosynthetic processes, provide the energy to ''drive'' the biosynthetic reactions. In these processes, energy from the hydrolysis of chemical bonds is captured in the high energy phosphate bonds of **adenosine triphosphate (ATP)**. These bonds provide for the activation and continuation of other biochemical events. Using this energy, the bacterial cell wall, proteins, nucleic acids, and other structural and regulatory macromolecules are synthesized. Utilization of carbohydrates by bacteria and the conditions under which this utilization occurs are key characteristics for broadly characterizing bacteria. In general, many tests performed in the clinical microbiology laboratory involve the detection of the end products of bacterial metabolism in spent culture fluids, either by pH indicators in the medium or by gas-liquid chromatography. The ability of a given microorganism to produce acid from a variety of carbohydrates (e.g., maltose, sucrose, mannitol, mannose, etc.) reflects the enzymatic capabilities of these organisms to initially convert such carbohydrates to glucose, which is the starting point for both aerobic and anaerobic carbohydrate catabolism.

Utilization of glucose under anaerobic conditions is termed **fermentation.** Fermentation occurs via glycolysis (also called the **hexose diphosphate** and the **Embden-**

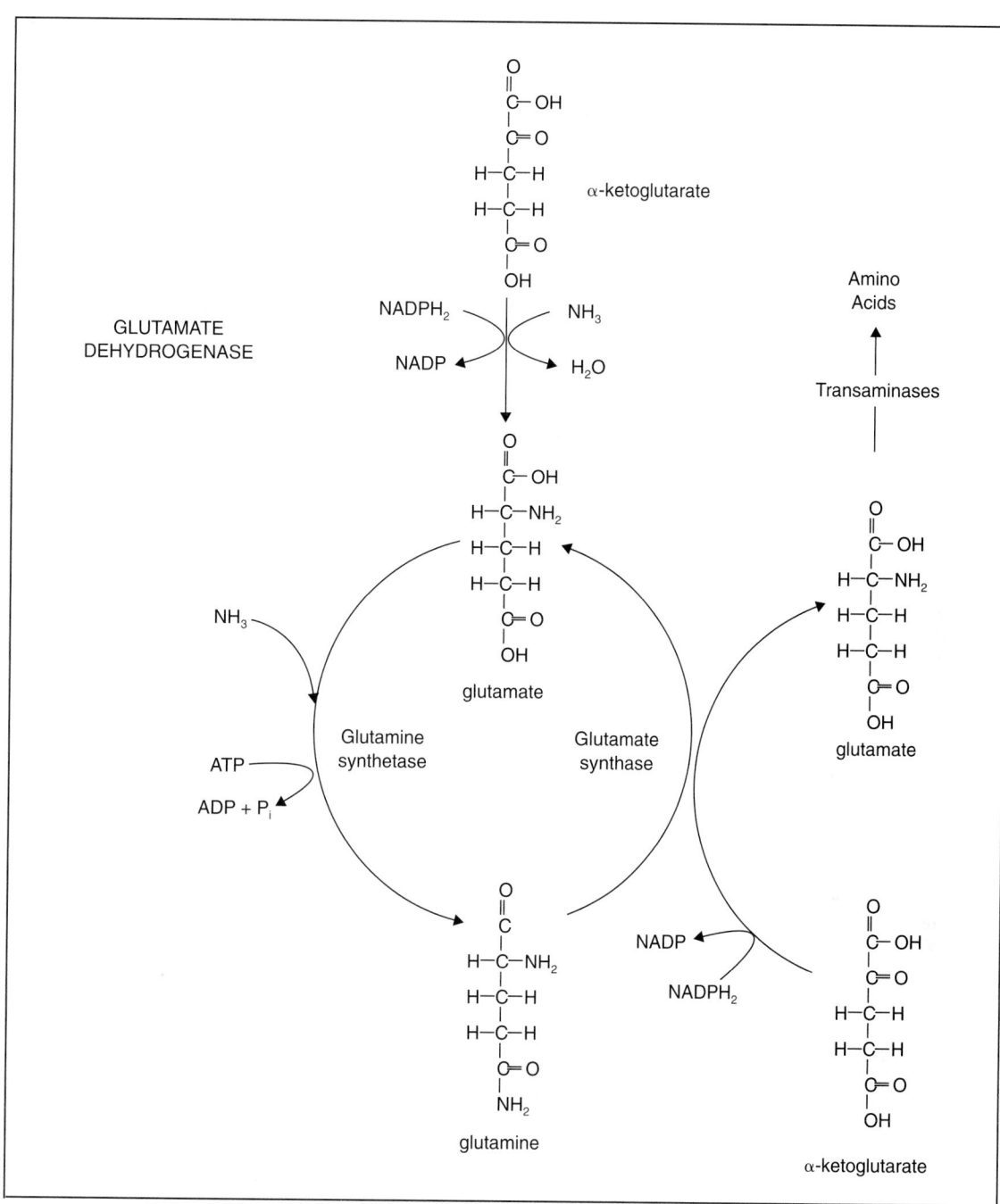

Figure 5-14 Nitrogen assimilation and metabolism via the enzymes glutamine synthetase, glutamate dehydrogenase, and glutamate synthase. This enzymatic system results in the formation of amino acids and other compounds.

Meyerhof-Parnas pathway), with the end product being pyruvic acid or pyruvate. The glycolytic pathway from glucose to pyruvate is shown in Figure 5-16. This pathway requires two ATP molecules for initial phosphorylation of glucose to glucose-6-phosphate and subsequent phosphorylation of fructose-6-phosphate to fructose-1,6-diphosphate. During glycolysis, ATP is generated at two points in the pathway. As a result of the conversion of 1,3-diphosphoglyceric acid to 3-phosphoglyceric acid, the energy derived from the oxidation of an aldehyde group is conserved as a high energy phosphate bond in ATP. The conversion of phosphoenolpyruvate to pyruvate results in the generation of another ATP molecule. Therefore, four ATP molecules are produced from every molecule of glucose during glycolysis by a process called **substrate level phosphorylation,** resulting in a net gain of two molecules of ATP. In addition to ATP, reducing power is also produced by the generation of $NADH_2$ from the cofactor NAD (nicotinamide adenine dinucleotide).

Glycolysis is not the sole pathway for carbohydrate me-

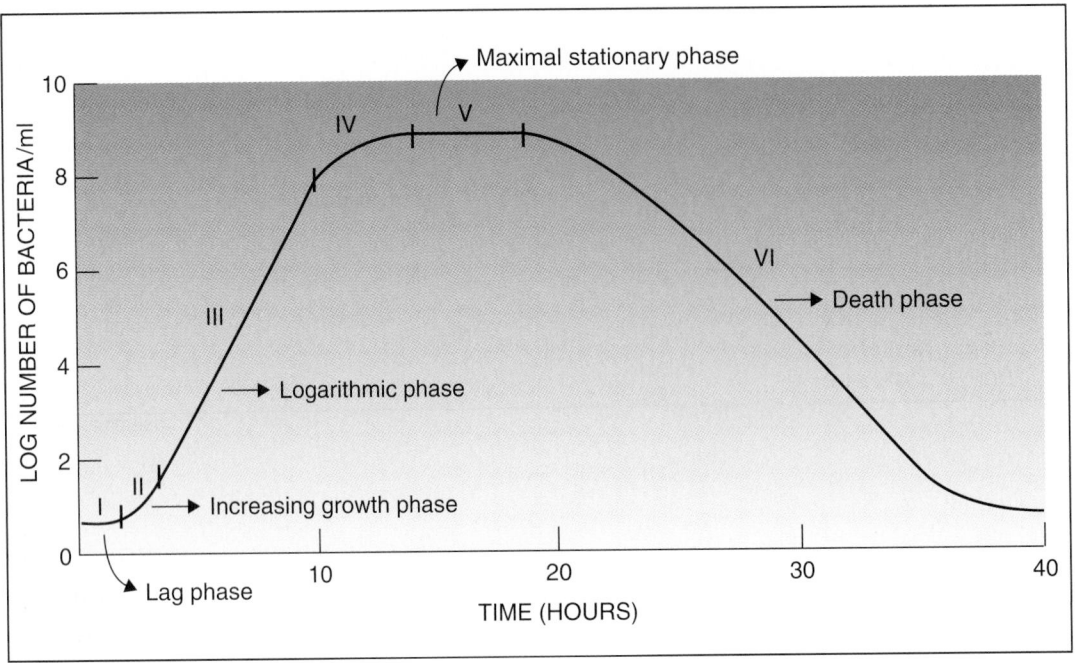

Figure 5-15 Kinetics of bacterial growth.

tabolism in most organisms. Many strictly aerobic bacteria use the Entner-Doudoroff pathway, which begins with glucose being converted to 6-phosphogluconic acid. This molecule is dehydrated to form 2-keto-3-deoxy-6-gluconate, and then hydrolyzed to pyruvate and glyceraldehyde-3-phosphate (Fig. 5-17). Pyruvate then enters the **Krebs tricarboxylic acid cycle** (see below), and the glyceraldehyde-3-phosphate is converted to pyruvate via the glycolytic cycle. Many bacteria use the pentose phosphate pathway, in which glucose-6-phosphate is oxidized to 6-phosphogluconic acid, which is then further oxidized to ribulose-5-phosphate (5-carbon), CO_2, and NADH (see Fig. 5-18). Five-carbon monosaccharides are used in the biosynthesis of nucleic acids. Some bacteria are able to metabolize 5-carbon (pentose) sugars such as xylose and arabinose. In the metabolism of 5-carbon sugars, enzymes known as transketolases and transaldolases convert these simple carbohydrates to various 3-, 4-, and 5-carbon intermediates, which, in turn, are used as building blocks for the biosynthesis of nucleic acid precursors.

UTILIZATION OF PYRUVATE

Pyruvate may enter a variety of pathways, resulting in several different end products. It is these end products that are often useful in categorizing the organisms isolated in the clinical microbiology laboratory. The metabolic pathways shown in Figures 5-19 and 5-20 include:

Pathway 1—Homolactic fermentation (homofermentative). In this pathway, the simplest of fermentations, the primary product of glucose fermentation is lactic acid. Some organisms that are considered homolactic fermenters also make small amounts of acetate, ethanol, and formate. The relative amounts of the latter products are de-

pendent on the initial pH and the buffering capacity of the medium. Generally, no gas is formed. Homolactic fermentation of glucose is characteristic of the streptococci, enterococci, pediococci, and lactobacilli.

Pathway 2—Heterolactic fermentation. Pyruvate is decarboxylated to yield acetaldehyde and CO_2, and the acetaldehyde is reduced by $NADH_2$ and alcohol dehydrogenase to form ethanol. This type of pathway is seen in *Leuconostoc* species, some lactobacilli, and yeasts.

Pathway 3—Mixed acid fermentation. In this metabolic pathway, pyruvate is metabolized to a number of different products (acetic acid, ethanol, succinic acid, formic acid). Initially, pyruvate is cleaved in the presence of coenzyme A (CoA) to form formic acid and acetyl-CoA. Some of the acetyl-CoA is reduced to acetaldehyde and then to ethanol. The acetyl group of some acetyl-CoA is transferred to phosphate, yielding acetylphosphate, which then yields its high energy bond to ADP, producing one ATP and acetic acid. Some bacteria are able to oxidize formate directly to hydrogen gas and CO_2. The nature and amounts of these acid products depend on the organism.

Pathway 4—Butanediol fermentation. Bacteria that use this pathway have an enzyme that condenses two pyruvate molecules (each with three carbons) to CO_2 and a five-carbon intermediate called α-acetolactate. The α-acetolactate is then enzymatically decarboxylated, resulting in acetoin (acetylmethylcarbinol) formation. In the presence of hydrogen ions, acetoin is further reduced to 2,3-butanediol. This reduction reaction is slowly reversible in air under alkaline conditions; the acetoin that is synthesized can be detected by the addition of α-naphthol. This is the basis of the **Voges-Proskauer (VP) test**, which uses α-naphthol in the presence of alkali to detect acetoin. This pathway is seen in the *Klebsiella-*

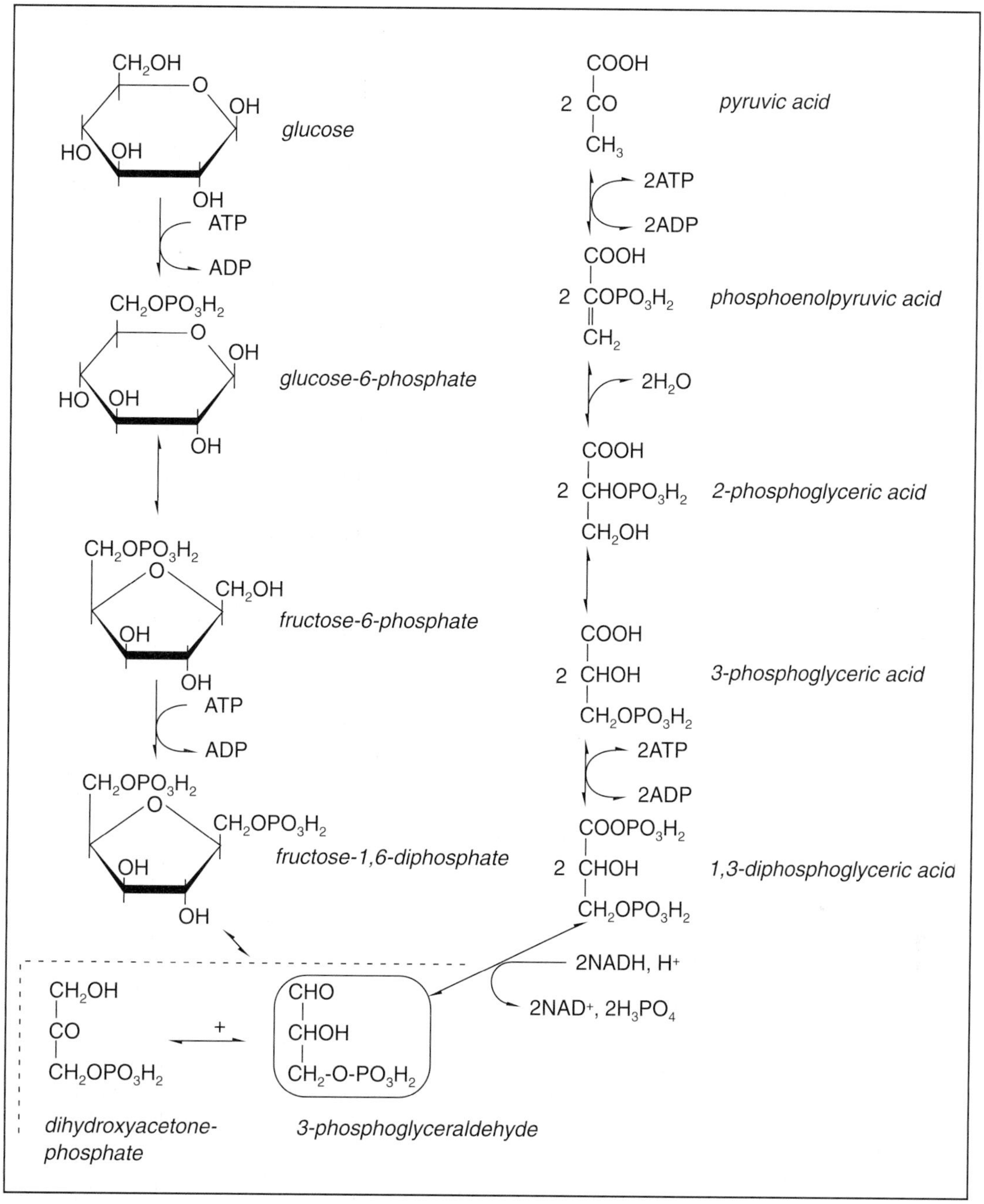

Figure 5-16 Glycolytic pathway.

Enterobacter-Serratia-Hafnia group of the Family Enterobacteriaceae. The conversion of some of the pyruvate to 2, 3-butanediol reduces the amount of acid relative to the mixed acid pathway described above and is responsible for **methyl-red (MR)** reaction used to separate *E. coli* and related organisms **(MR+/VP−)** from the *Klebsiella-Enterobacter-Serratia-Hafnia* group **(MR−/VP+)**.

Pathway 5—Butanol fermentation. This fermentation pathway is seen among members of the genus *Clostridium*. These organisms possess an enzyme that condenses two molecules of acetyl-CoA formed from pyruvate to form acetoacetyl-CoA. This molecule is reduced to in a stepwise fashion to butyryl-CoA, which can be subsequently hydrolyzed to butyric acid and ATP. Alternatively, free acetoacetate is released and decarboxylated to produce CO_2 and acetone, which may be reduced to isopropyl alcohol. In clinical microbiology laboratories performing reference work on clostridia, volatile and nonvolatile fermentation products are detected by gas-liquid chromatographic analysis of derivatives prepared from broth cultures. Detection of these metabolic end products is helpful for genus- or species-level identification of these anaerobic bacteria.

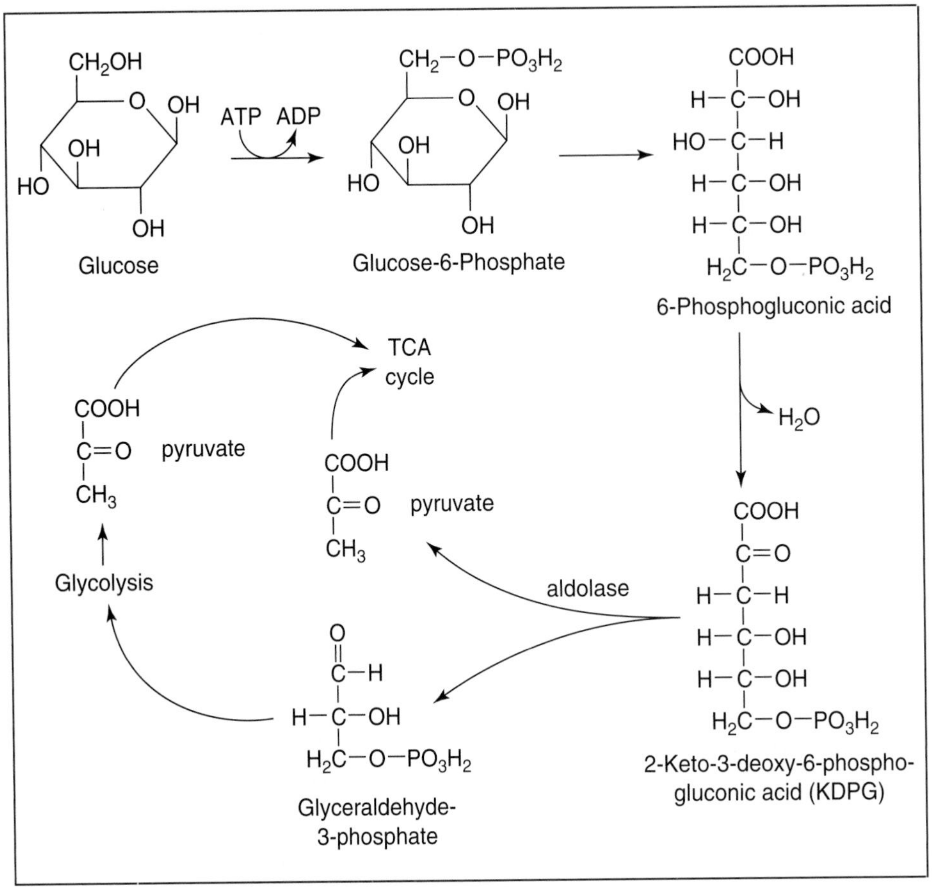

Figure 5-17 The Entner-Doudoroff pathway.

Pathway 6—Propionic acid fermentation. This is a cyclic-type of reaction in which oxaloacetate is formed from carbon dioxide, pyruvate, and ATP using a biotin-containing coenzyme. Oxaloacetate is reduced to malate, converted to fumarate and then reduced to succinic acid (succinate). Decarboxylation of succinate results in the formation of propionic acid (propionate). This pathway is seen in anaerobic gram-negative bacilli in the genus *Bacteroides* and in *Propionibacterium* species, which are gram-positive, anaerobic, non-spore-forming bacilli.

Utilization of glucose under aerobic conditions is called respiration (Fig. 5-18). Pyruvate formed during fermentation enters the Krebs cycle, during which it is broken down to CO_2 and H_2O with the generation of ATP. Oxidative decarboxylation of pyruvate yields the high-energy intermediate called acetyl-coenzyme A, which condenses with a molecule of oxaloacetate to form citrate and free coenzyme A. A series of oxidative reactions ensues with the regeneration of oxaloacetate and the generation of reducing power in the forms of reduced NAD (NADH) and reduced flavin adenine dinucleotide (FADH). These high-energy compounds subsequently enter the **electron transport chain,** which consists of alternating hydrogen and electron carriers located in sequence across the cell membrane. Transfer of protons down the electron transport chain creates a membrane potential. The energy of this potential is harnessed by a membrane-associated multienzyme system called **ATP synthase.** The subunit enzyme catalyzes the phosphorylation of ADP with inorganic phosphate. The final electron acceptor in the electron transport chain is oxygen (O_2), with the final product being H_2O. Complete oxidation of glucose via anaerobic glycolysis and the aerobic Krebs cycle results in a net gain of 38 ATP molecules per mole of glucose, as compared with the net generation of only 2 ATP molecules per mole of glucose via the glycolytic (fermentative) pathway alone. In addition to the generation of ATP during aerobic metabolism, the Krebs cycle also provides the cell with precursors or intermediate compounds used in the biosynthesis of several other cellular components, such as purines, pyrimidines, amino acids and lipids. The cycle also serves a catabolic function by providing a venue for the oxidative breakdown of these same macromolecules.

Bacterial Virulence Factors and Pathogenicity
Definitions and Concepts

Pathogenicity refers to the ability of an organism to cause disease. Organisms that are capable of causing disease under

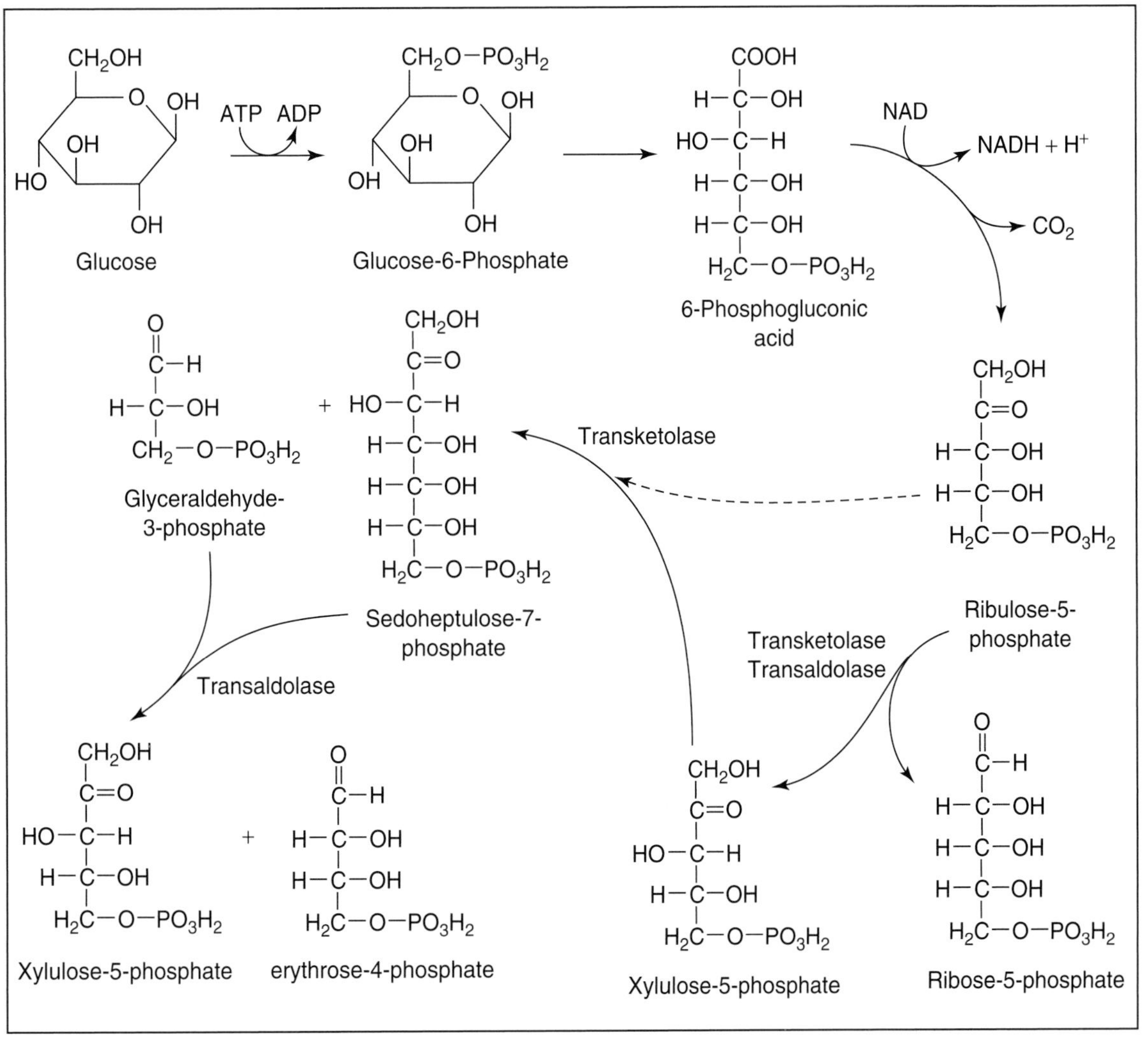

Figure 5-18 The pentose phosphate pathway.

the appropriate circumstances are called **pathogens. Virulence** usually refers to the degree of pathogenicity within a group or species of microorganisms. The virulence of a microorganism is not generally attributable to a single factor, but is dependent on several parameters that relate to the organism, the host, and the dynamic interaction between them. This balance between the host and the "potential pathogen" is an area of increasing interest among microbiologists. In general, virulence encompasses two features of a pathogenic microorganism: its **infectivity** (i.e., the ability to initiate an infection), and the **severity** of the condition produced. Highly virulent, moderately virulent, and/or avirulent strains may occur within a species or group of organisms that are generally considered to be pathogenic. Infection of the host by an organism is a necessary step in the production of disease. However, infection does not always cause disease. Colonization of a host with normal flora organisms is, in a broad sense, infection, and the colonization factors present on the surfaces of normal flora organisms (e.g., fimbriae, lipoteichoic acids, capsules, and outer-membrane proteins)

are operationally the same as those used by pathogenic microorganisms. The normal flora organisms become established in and on the host early in life and persist throughout the lifetime of the host. Infection with exogenous bacteria may be aborted by the presence of normal flora organisms that already occupy the ecologic niche of the potential pathogen. If it does occur, infection may only be apparent by the demonstration of an antibody response with elimination of the exogenous organism. In some cases an asymptomatic carrier state may result, or overt disease may develop.

Clearly, the ability of an organism to cause disease involves both microbial and host factors, and there is currently a great deal of interest in the variety of **adaptive responses** of bacteria that result in the expression of characteristics involved in disease pathogenesis. For example, *Pseudomonas aeruginosa* is a ubiquitous soil and water organism that, because of its genetic versatility, has successfully adapted to human environments, such as hospitals, to create its own particularly niche. Over the years of its coexistence with humans, *P. aeruginosa* has emerged as a nosocomial and

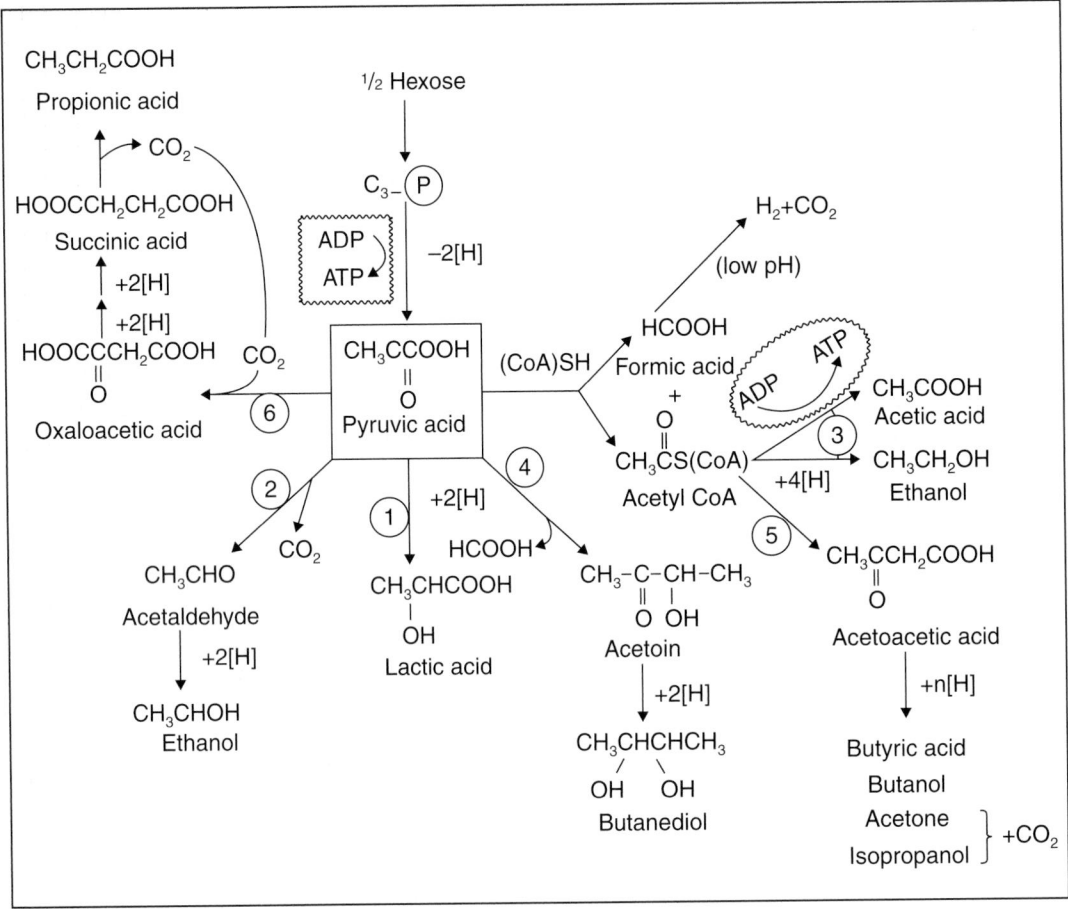

Figure 5-19 Fate of pyruvate formed during anaerobic fermentation.

opportunistic pathogen that expresses a range of genetically determined virulence factors, including several exotoxins, hemolysins, lipases, elastases, and proteases, highly mucoid alginate capsular polysaccharides, and plasmid- and transposon-mediated antimicrobial resistance.[21,85,103,136,148] These genetically determined adaptive responses have provided *P. aeruginosa* with the versatility to survive and actually thrive in potentially hostile environments. Medical progress has also enabled us to appreciate the adaptive responses of organisms that are part of the normal human flora. When host defense mechanisms are abrogated by underlying noninfectious causes or various interventions (e.g., malignancy, diabetes, immunosuppressive therapy), endogenous organisms may also cause pathology and disease due to the phenotypic expression of characteristics that reflect a new adaptive response of the organism to its host.

In recent years, **bacterial sensing mechanisms** have become a focus of research in medical microbiology. Bacteria have developed sophisticated methods for sensing their environment and regulating the expression of genes involved in virulence. **Two-component signal transduction** refers to regulatory protein pairs that function sequentially in detecting alterations in the external environment and in effecting adaptive responses in the organism. At the molecular level, this occurs by transfer of phosphate groups from sensor to

effector proteins; the phosphorylation state of the effector proteins regulates the strength and duration of the response by binding to promoters in the nucleic acid that allow the expression (i.e., transcription and subsequent translation) of bacterial genes that code for virulence factors. Two-component signal transduction sensing systems have been described in enteric gram-negative bacteria, *B. fragilis*, *B. pertussis*, *M. tuberculosis*, *Vibrio* species, and *C. perfringens*, among others.[39,135,149] Some organisms express certain virulence genes in response to threshold levels of autoinducers. These autoinducers are *N*-acylhomoserine or *N*-butyrylhomoserine lactones that are produced continually.[51,139] When the bacterial population reaches a certain threshold, enough autoinducer is present to activate transcription factors within the cells that coordinate the expression of virulence genes. This complex signaling mechanism, called **"quorum sensing,"** has been demonstrated in environmental bacteria (e.g., *Vibrio fischeri*, *Agrobacterium tumefaciens*) and in human pathogens (i.e., *P. aeruginosa*, *Yersinia enterocolitica*).[54,106,143] The transcription activators that respond to quorum sensing in these diverse microbial groups show significant amino acid sequence homology, suggesting that sensing mechanisms evolved early and were disseminated widely among microorganisms that occupy various ecologic niches.

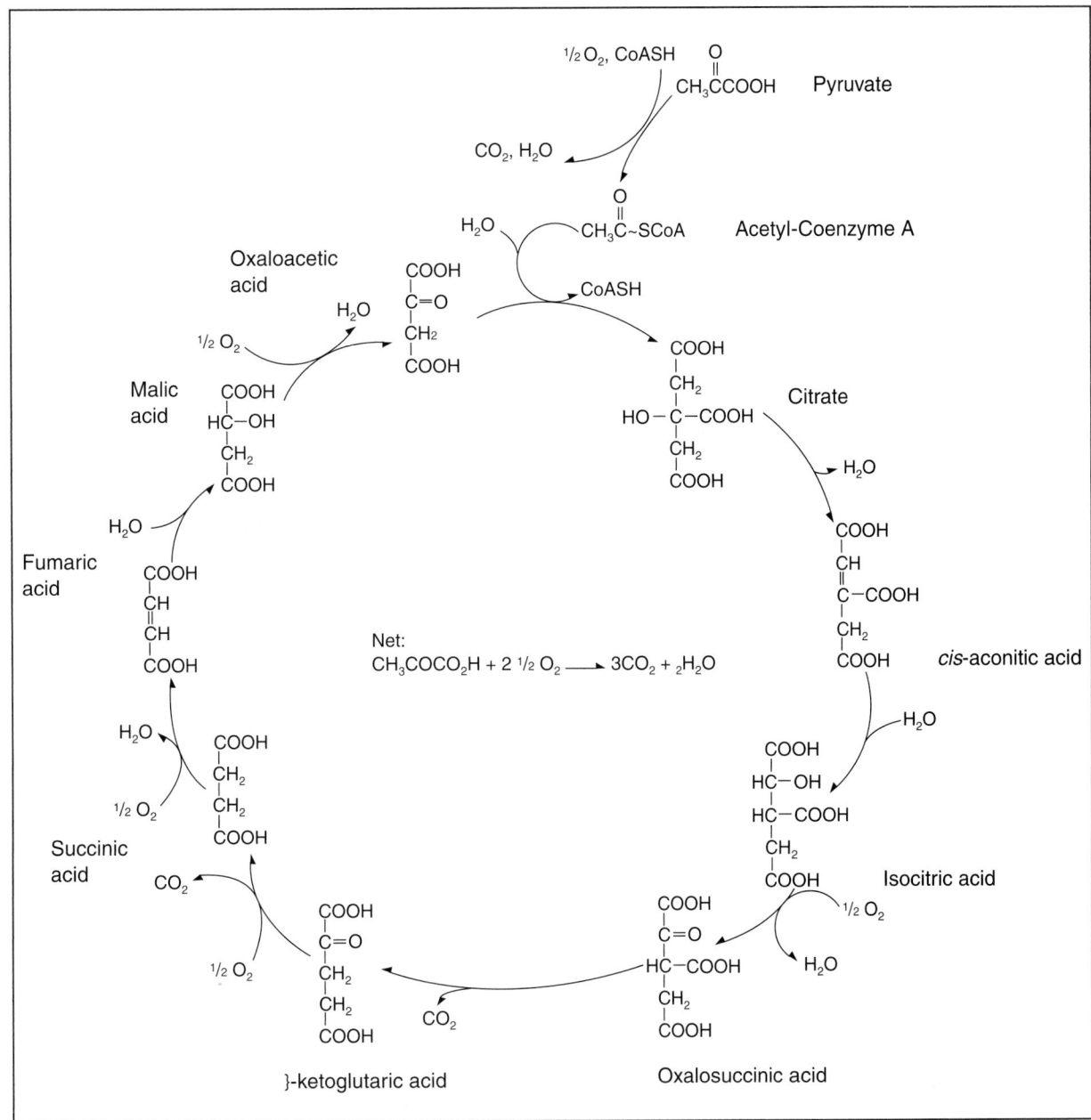

Figure 5-20 Krebs tricarboxylic acid cycle.

Requirements for Pathogenicity

The first step in the establishment of an infectious process resides in the ability of a microorganism to enter the host and to initiate infection. The initial contact depends on the ability of the organism to attach to and survive on the host's mucous membrane surfaces. Attachment occurs via interaction of various bacterial adhesins with cell surface receptors (see below). Some organisms will attach to epithelial cells without invasion of the deeper tissues. In such cases, toxins or enzymes elaborated by the organisms are usually responsible for the pathology, and the effects of toxins may be local or systemic. Certain organisms attach to the mucosal epithelial cells and subsequently penetrate this barrier. Further multiplication of the organisms in the subepithelial tissues results in tissue destruction from bacterial factors (e.g., proteases, collagenases, hyaluronidases) and from the immune response (i.e., complement-mediated cytolysis, cell-mediated immune reactions). More invasive organisms may attach, penetrate the epithelial cell surfaces, multiply, and extend into the deeper tissues; eventually gaining access to the bloodstream and causing disseminated infection. Organisms such as mycobacteria and brucellae, attach, invade, multiply, and subsequently adapt themselves to a continued existence within the host, usually by taking up residence within cells of the reticuloendothelial system.[76]

Many organisms are highly specific in the types of tissues that they may infect. For example, *N. meningitidis* can be a normal inhabitant of the throat, and the asymptomatic carrier state is well characterized. Under the appropriate circumstances, these organisms may invade the meninges and the bloodstream. *S. pneumoniae* may also inhabit the throat and nasopharynx, yet virulent strains preferentially invade the lower respiratory tract and the bloodstream, causing pneumonia and/or pneumococcal sepsis. Tissue specificities may reflect the presence of mucosal receptors for bacterial surface antigens or the presence of nutrients that serve as chemoattractants for the microorganisms (e.g., certain amino acids, ions, or carbohydrates). A classic example of this nutritional dependence is seen with *Brucella abortus*, the cause of contagious abortion in cattle. This organism has a specific growth requirement for the sugar alcohol erythritol, which is present in high concentrations in the bovine uterus and placental tissue. Hence, this organism may actually "home in" on the bovine genital tract because of this nutritional predilection.

Virulence Factors of Microorganisms

Bacterial virulence factors are structural components or products produced by bacteria that allow the organism to harm the host in some manner. Some virulence factors are cell-associated, while others may be extracellular. In addition, some of the factors involved in disease production are part of the anatomic or physiologic composition of the cell, and their roles as virulence factors are incidental to the life cycle of the organism.

ADHESINS

In order to infect a host, microorganisms must first adhere to the mucosal surface. Bacterial adherence is usually a specific process involving bacterial cell surface structures that are generally known as adhesins and complementary receptors on the surface of susceptible cells. Bacterial adhesins may include fimbriae, components of the bacterial capsule, lipoteichoic acids that project outside the peptidoglycan of the cell wall of gram-positive bacteria, outer membrane proteins or other cell-surface antigens. Specific examples of well-characterized adhesins in pathogenic microorganisms have been discussed previously and include the adherence fimbriae of *N. gonorrhoeae*, mannose-sensitive (type 1) and mannose-resistant (type 2) fimbriae of uropathogenic and enteropathogenic *E. coli*, and lipoteichoic acids of group A β-hemolytic streptococci.[64,70,107] The human cell-surface protein fibronectin is a host receptor for some bacterial pathogens.

AGGRESSINS

In order to survive and multiply within the host, many organisms produce a variety of substances that allow them to avoid or circumvent host defense mechanisms. These substances, termed aggressins, include capsules and extracellular slime substances, surface proteins and carbohydrates, en-

zymes, toxins, and other small molecules. The capsular structures of some bacteria enable the organisms to avoid phagocytosis by preventing interaction between the bacterial cell surface and phagocytic cells or by concealing bacterial cell-surface components that would otherwise interact with phagocytic cells or complement and lead to their ingestion.[34,97,154,155] Specific antibodies directed against capsular material lead to opsonization of the microorganisms. Following opsonization, encapsulated bacteria are readily and rapidly ingested and killed by phagocytic cells. Some organisms produce capsules that are structurally similar to host tissues and, therefore, are not recognized as foreign by immunosurveillance. In this manner, such organisms can evade host defenses. For example, the capsules of *E. coli* K1 and group B meningococci are composed of partially *O*-acetylated, α-2,8-linked, *N*-acetylneuraminic acid, which is structurally similar to the neuraminic acid found in tissue of the central nervous system.[91] Organisms that possess capsules that behave as aggressins include *S. aureus*, *S. pneumoniae*, *N. meningitidis*, *H. influenzae* type b, *K. pneumoniae*, group A and group B β-hemolytic streptococci, and *B. anthracis*.[34,65,90,91,97,141,142,147,154,155]

Some bacteria possess surface proteins that play roles in adherence and other virulence-associated functions. For example, the M protein of group A streptococci plays many roles in the pathogenesis of infection with this organism, including adherence, resistance to phagocytosis, intracellular invasion, impairment of complement function, and lytic effects on polymorphonuclear leucocytes.[9,36,42,43] Protein A, a cell wall protein of *S. aureus*, is able to bind immunoglobulin (IgG) molecules by their Fc region. Since antibody-mediated phagocytosis (i.e., opsonization) is Fc receptor-dependent, protein A may interfere with this process. The presence of protein A may also inhibit the activation of complement by the staphylococcal cell wall by masking the peptidoglycan moieties that are known to have complement-activating activity. Some bacteria are able to produce proteases that are able to hydrolyze and inactivate secretory immunoglobulins (IgA).[109] This immunoglobulin acts locally to prevent bacterial adherence; hydrolysis of IgA by bacterial protease therefore fosters mucosal colonization (see Chapter 3).

Some aggressins act after phagocytosis has occurred by interfering with phagosome/lysosome fusion and with the activity of the myeloperoxidase system. The mycobacteria and brucellae are able to adapt to an intracellular existence within host cells by elaborating substances that prevent intracellular destruction of organisms. In the mycobacteria, this may be due to the presence of cell-wall-associated mycosides and sulfolipids that become incorporated into the inner aspect of the phagosome and prevent lysosome/phagosome fusion.[7,26,50,57,58] *Listeria monocytogenes* expresses a surface protein called **internalin** that binds to glycoprotein receptors on epithelial cells and allows the organism to become internalized in a membrane-bound vacuole.[52,79,80] The organism then produces a hemolysin called **listeriolysin O**, which intercalates into the membrane of the vacuole and causes the formation of pores.[83,108] *L. monocytogenes* then enters the cytoplasm of the cell, where it continues to grow, thereby escaping the toxic environment with the phagolysosome. *S. aureus* secretes **catalase** and **superoxide dismutase**, which inhibit organism destruction by the myeloperoxidase system of phagocytic cells. Taking up residence within phagocytic cells by these mechanisms also contributes to virulence by protecting the organisms from destruction by specific antibodies and complement. Intracellular existence also has a significant influence on therapy. Infections with organisms such as *Brucella* species and *Francisella tularensis* must be treated with antibiotics that are able to act intracellularly (e.g., tetracyclines, aminoglycosides) in order to affect these "protected" organisms.[44]

Many bacteria produce enzymes or toxins or possess cellular constituents that have direct toxic or necrotizing effects on host inflammatory cells and other components of the immune system. Leukocidin and γ-hemolysin produced by *S. aureus* cause rounding and swelling of exposed polymorphonuclear cells and macrophages, followed by degranulation, nuclear rupture, and cell lysis.[110] The lipopolysaccharide of gram-negative bacteria may delay or blunt the acute inflammatory response, allowing the organism to establish itself within the host with relative ease. The lipid A portion of endotoxin, in particular, can activate complement and stimulate the release of various cytokines (i.e., interleukin [IL]-2, IL-6, IL-8, tumor necrosis factor α [TNF-α]) that lead to the clinical manifestations of endotoxic shock, which includes hypotension, disseminated intravascular coagulation, and death. Gram-positive bacteria possess cell wall peptidoglycan polymers and membrane teichoic acids that can cause a similar release of cytokines and can precipitate similar septic shock symptoms. Some organisms have other cell-surface properties, such as the LOS and certain surface proteins that render them resistant to the bactericidal effects of normal human serum (e.g., *N. gonorrhoeae*).[104,113] This property may facilitate dissemination of the bacteria via the bloodstream and lymphatics, leading to systemic infection or to the establishment of infected foci at sites distant from the site of the initial infection.

The invasive properties of some bacteria are attributed to the elaboration of enzymes that act extracellularly. *S. aureus*, *S. pneumoniae*, group B streptococci, and *Propionibacterium acnes* produce an enzyme called **hyaluronate lyase** (or hyaluronidase) during the exponential growth phase. This enzyme promotes the spread of the organism through the connective tissues by depolymerizing hyaluronic acid, the ground substance responsible for cell-to-cell adhesion.[40] Group A streptococci and staphylococci also elaborate enzymes that hydrolyze fibrin clots (**streptokinase** and **staphylokinase**), which also facilitate the spread of organisms in the tissues.[30,112] *C. perfringens* and other clostridia (e.g., *C. histolyticum*, *C. septicum*, *C. sordellii*, *C. novyi*, and *C. fallax*) produce cytotoxins, cytolysins, collagenases, phospholipases, hyaluronidases, and deoxyribonucleases that allow these organisms to colonize devitalized tissue, break down the collagen matrix of muscle and connective tissue, and facilitate the extension of the organisms into these tissues to cause fasciitis and gas gangrene.[86]

Iron has been shown to be an essential nutrient for many organisms, and a requirement for virulence in some bacterial pathogens. In this regard, successful pathogenic bacteria have evolved ways to obtain iron from the environment or from the iron-restricted milieu of host tissues, in which free iron is maintained at low concentrations by binding to transferrin and lactoferrin proteins. Microorganisms scavenge

this iron by the production of **siderophores**, which are small molecules that function as high-affinity iron chelators. The production of siderophores is, therefore, considered a virulence factor.[59] Other organisms have evolved lactoferrin- or transferrin-binding proteins, from which the iron is removed and transported into the cell.[111] Both *N. gonorrhoeae* and *N. meningitidis* possess outer membrane receptors for binding human transferrin, lactoferrin, and hemoglobin and periplasmic binding proteins for removal of iron from the bound carriers and transport into the cell.[4,13,81,82,84] In addition, the production of many extracellular microbial products, including **toxins**, is partially regulated at the transcriptional level by the concentrations of iron in the surrounding medium. For example, expression of the β-phage structural gene for diphtheria toxin in lysogenized *Corynebacterium diphtheriae* only occurs when iron becomes the growth-limiting substrate (see below).[117,118]

Although plasmids themselves are not virulence factors, the genes that code for many of the bacterial cell products responsible for virulence frequently reside on bacterial plasmids. **R factors** (plasmids that contain genes coding for resistance to antimicrobial agents) may be considered virulence factors because the acquisition of resistance to antimicrobial agents fosters continued growth and spread of bacterial infections in spite of therapeutic interventions. Some bacteria also contain plasmids that code for sex pili and chromosomal mobilization. These two factors enable a microorganism to transfer genetic material (either plasmid borne, chromosomal, or both) to other organisms. Plasmids may also bear the genes that code for colonization antigens, serum resistance, iron chelation and transport, toxin and hemolysin production, and undefined intracellular survival functions. Plasmids containing resistance genes have been described in many gram-negative (i.e., all genera of the *Enterobacteriaceae*, *Pseudomonas*, *Vibrio*, *Pasteurella*, *Campylobacter*, *Haemophilus*, *Neisseria*, and *Bacteroides*) and gram-positive (e.g., *Staphylococcus*, *Streptococcus*, *Enterococcus*, *Bacillus*, *Clostridium*, and *Corynebacterium*) genera.

EXOTOXINS AND ENDOTOXINS

Toxins of microbial origin fall into two groups: exotoxins and endotoxins. **Bacterial exotoxins** are the most potent biologic toxins known and are produced mostly by gram-positive bacteria, although some gram-negative bacteria elaborate them as well. Exotoxins are usually protein in nature and are heat-labile. Because they are proteins, many can be inactivated or destroyed by proteolytic enzymes. On the other hand, some exotoxins become activated only after partial hydrolysis ("nicking") by proteolytic enzymes (see below). The toxic activity of many exotoxins can be destroyed by formaldehyde treatment (**toxoid development**) and neutralized by specific antibodies. Exploitation of these properties led to the development of the diphtheria and tetanus toxoids that are used for active immunization against diphtheria and tetanus, respectively.

In general, bacterial exotoxins fall into two groups. The first group consists of **cytolytic toxins**, which act on cell membranes to cause pore formation and subsequent lysis of the cell. Examples of these toxins include the seven enterotoxins of *S. aureus*, and streptolysins O and S produced by group A streptococci. The second group consists of two-subunit, A-B, or **bipartite toxins**. These toxins contain a B (or binding) subunit that attaches to a specific host-cell receptor, and an A (or active) subunit, that passes into the cell and interacts with the target. These toxins include the cholera toxin of *V. cholerae*, the Shiga toxin of *Shigella dysenteriae*, pertussis toxin produced by *B. pertussis*, and diphtheria toxin produced by lysogenized *C. diphtheriae*. Certain diseases, such as tetanus, botulism, diphtheria, and cholera, are due almost entirely to the effects of the toxins on their target organs and tissues

Tetanus is caused by the systemic effects of tetanus neurotoxin, the toxin produced by *Clostridium tetani*. Tetanus usually occurs as a result of wound infection by *C. tetani* or, rarely, from injection of materials contaminated with *C. tetani* vegetative cells or spores.[14] Tetanus neurotoxin is released upon cell lysis after bacterial growth under anaerobic conditions (e.g., in deep puncture wounds). The toxin is translated initially as a single peptide of about 150 kDa. On release from the bacterial cell, the toxin peptide is cleaved by proteolytic enzymes to form a light (L, 50 kDa) and a heavy (H, 100 kDa) chain that are connected by a disulfide bond; under reducing conditions, the two peptides are split into separate L and H chains. The receptor-binding site of the intact toxin molecule resides in the H chain. The L chain is internalized and moves from the peripheral nerves to the central nervous system by retrograde axonal transport. When tetanus toxin reaches the neurons in the spinal cord, brain stem, and cerebellum, it becomes rapidly fixed to its receptor, a ganglioside containing stearic acid, sphingosine, glucose, galactose, *N*-acetylglucosamine, and *N*-acetyl neuraminic acid (sialic acid). The spasmogenic effect of the toxin is due to its action on presynaptic reflexes involving interneurons in the spinal cord. The toxin blocks the normal postsynaptic inhibition of spinal motor neurons following afferent impulses by preventing the release of inhibitory neurotransmitters (i.e., γ-aminobutyric acid, glycine). This presynaptic blockage of central neurons results in elevated muscle tone and hyperactive reflexes. Resulting sensitivity to excitatory impulses, unchecked by inhibitory mechanisms, produces the generalized spastic paralysis characteristic of tetanus.[14]

Botulism results from the ingestion of toxins formed by *Clostridium botulinum* growing in food, the principal vehicles being improperly canned fruits and vegetables (generally home canned), condiments, and fish products. Wound botulism is a systemic intoxication resulting from growth of *C. botulinum* and toxin production in wounds, and was reported during the 1980s and 1990s as a complication of wound infections in parenteral-drug users.[19,89] *C. botulinum* can also colonize the intestinal tract of infants and produce toxin at that site (infant botulism).[37,95] Toxin accumulates in cells of *C. botulinum* during spore germination and active vegetative cell growth, but is released only upon cell lysis. Organisms described as *C. botulinum* cluster into three groups depending on their 16S rRNA gene sequences: *C. botulinum* types B, E, and F, *C. botulinum* types C and D, and *C. botulinum* types A, F, and B. *C. botulinum* type G clusters independently from the others and is also called *C. argentinense*.[31,32] These groups correspond to seven serologic types of *C. botulinum* toxins (types A, B, C-1, D, E,

F, and G [associated with *C. argentinense*]), and each produces an immunologically type-specific toxin.[137] Toxin types A, B, E, and F are the types known to affect humans.

Native botulinum toxins are labile proteins and are complexed with nontoxin proteins to stabilize the molecules.[114] Botulinum toxin is produced as a progenitor protein with a molecular weight of about 150 kDa. These toxins are produced as inert molecules that become activated after proteolysis, but proteolytic cleavage is internal to the peptide molecules and the toxins do not change in molecular weight following activation. The active toxin, therefore, consists of a 50-kDa light (L) chain and a 100-kDa heavy (H) chain connected by a disulfide bond. After absorption from the gastrointestinal tract, the toxin reaches susceptible neurons (at neuromuscular junctions and peripheral autonomic synapses) via the bloodstream. There it becomes bound to presynaptic terminals, where it blocks the release of acetylcholine from cholinergic motor nerve endings. The hallmark of botulism includes cranial nerve involvement, bilateral and descending weakening, and paralysis of skeletal muscles and is characterized by fatigue, dizziness, nausea, blurring of vision, slurring of speech, dilatation of pupils, urinary retention, general flaccid paralysis of skeletal muscles, and respiratory paralysis.[22]

Diphtheria is another example of an illness that is due primarily to the action of a toxin. Interestingly, only strains of *C. diphtheriae* that contain a lysogenic bacteriophage (β-corynephage) are able to produce diphtheria toxin. The structural genes for the toxin (called the *tox* gene) is part of the bacteriophage's genome. The expression of the *tox* gene is regulated by an iron-activated repressor and toxin production occurs only when iron becomes the growth-limiting substrate.[117,118] In the presence of iron (Fe^{2+}), the repressor forms active dimers with Fe^{2+}, which bind to the *tox* gene promoter and inhibit *tox* gene expression. When Fe^{2+} becomes limiting, the Fe^{2+}/repressor dimer dissociates, allowing the *tox* gene to be transcribed and translated.[45,156]

The toxin molecule is formed by *C. diphtheriae* in association with the cell membrane and is secreted from the cell as a single peptide consisting of 535 amino acids with a molecular weight of about 58 kDa. On gentle proteolysis, the single peptide is cleaved into two major chains, designated as A and B, that are connected by disulfide bonds. Peptide A is a 21-kDa peptide that contains the enzymatic activity of the molecule that inhibits protein synthesis, while peptide B is a 37-kDa fragment that contains a C-terminal receptor-binding domain and an internal translocating domain. Peptide B is responsible for binding of the toxin molecule to its target receptor. On binding to the target cell via peptide B, the toxin enters the cell via receptor-mediated endocytosis. The low pH within the endosome triggers the translocation of peptide A (via interaction with the peptide B translocating domain) into the cytosol; at this time the disulfide bonds are reduced, peptide B is released, and peptide A becomes enzymatically active. Peptide A inhibits protein synthesis by the adenoribosylation of elongation factor 2, an enzyme that is required for translocation of the polypeptidyl-tRNA from the acceptor site to the donor site on the eucaryotic ribosome.[78] The adenoribosyl group is transferred from nicotinamide adenine dinucleotide (NAD) to elongation factor-2 by the peptide A toxin subunit, rendering EF-2 inactive:

$$NAD^+ + EF\text{-}2 \xrightarrow{A} \text{toxin peptide adenoribosyl phosphate:}$$

$$EF\text{-}2 \text{ complex} + \text{nicotinamide} + H^+$$

Treatment of the intact toxin with formalin renders a toxoid that cannot be split into A and B subunits. Therefore, the toxoid lacks the ability to catalyze its toxic intracellular effects, yet it retains its antigenicity. Immunity to diphtheria is generally mediated by the presence of antibodies against the toxin.

All the signs and symptoms of cholera caused by *V. cholerae* result from the rapid loss of fluid from the gut. Increased electrolyte secretion is caused by a protein enterotoxin. The 84-Da enterotoxin consists of a binding subunit (subunit B) composed of five identical 11.5-kDa monomers and a biologically active 27-kDa subunit (subunit A). The mode of action of cholera toxin is described in Chapter 8.

Endotoxins, on the other hand, are produced only by gram-negative bacteria and consist primarily of lipopolysaccharide (LPS). LPS, as described earlier, is a structural component of the gram-negative outer membrane, representing the somatic (O) antigenic determinants. Endotoxins are heat-stable, are not detoxified by formaldehyde treatment, and are only partially neutralized by specific antibodies. Compared with many of the exotoxins, endotoxin are of relatively low toxicity. Although endotoxin may escape into the surrounding fluids (as ''blebs'' on the surface of gram-negative bacteria), the whole cell generally retains the major portion of the toxic activity. The biologic and toxic activities of endotoxin are broad. Nanogram amounts of endotoxin cause fever in humans and the release of endogenous pyrogen. Larger doses cause hypotension, lowered polymorphonuclear leukocyte and platelet counts from increased margination of these cells toward the walls of small blood vessels, hemorrhage, and sometimes disseminated intravascular coagulation due to the activation of clotting mechanisms. Endotoxin is also mitogenic for B lymphocytes and stimulates the release of several cytokines from macrophages.

Bacterial Superantigens

Another group of extracellular protein toxins, such as those produced by *S. aureus* or group A β-hemolytic streptococci are able to bind to structural peptides on host T-lymphocyte receptors and macrophage class II histocompatibility antigens. This binding induces the release of cytokines. Various *S. aureus* extracellular proteins, such as toxic shock syndrome toxin 1 (TSST-1), staphylococcal enterotoxins A and B, and group A streptococcal toxins act as ''superantigens'' and induce high levels of T-cell proliferation, prompt IL-2 and TNF-α release and cause a shock syndrome.[38] Superantigens produced by various bacteria will be discussed further in subsequent chapters dealing with specific bacterial genera.

REFERENCES

1. Abbanat DR, Leadbetter ER, Godchaux W III, Escher A. Sulphonolipids are molecular determinants of gliding motility. Nature 1986;324:367–369.

2. Abraham LJ, Rood JI. Identification of Tn4451 and Tn4452, chloramphenicol resistance transposons from *Clostridium perfringens*. J Bacteriol 1987;169:1579–1584.

3. Aguirre M, Collins MD. Phylogenetic analysis of *Alloiococcus otitis* gen. nov., sp. nov., an organism from human middle ear fluid. Int J Syst Bacteriol 1992;42:79–83.

4. Anderson JE, Sparling PF, Cornelissen CN. Gonococcal transferrin-binding protein 2 facilitates but is not essential for transferrin utilization. J Bacteriol 1994;176:3162–3170.

5. Angert ER, Clements KD, Pace NR. The largest bacterium. Nature (London) 1993;362:239–241.

6. Arbeit RD, Karakawa WW, Vann WF, et al. Predominance of two newly described capsular polysaccharide types among clinical isolates of *Staphylococcus aureus*. Diagn Microbiol Infect Dis 1984;85–91.

7. Armstrong JA, D'Arcy Hart P. Phagosome-lysosome interactions in cultured macrophages infected with virulent tubercle bacilli: reversal of the usual fusion pattern and observations on bacterial survival. J Exp Med 1975;142:1–16.

8. Berg CM, Berg DE, Groisman EA. Transposable elements and the genetic engineering of bacteria. In: Berg DE, Howe MM, eds. Mobile DNA. Washington, DC: ASM Press, 1989:879–925.

9. Berkower C, Ravins M, Moses AE, Hanski E. Expression of different group A streptococcal M proteins in an isogenic background demonstrates diversity in adherence and invasion of eukaryotic cells. Mol Microbiol 1999;31:1463–1475.

10. Besra GS, Chatterjee D. Lipids and carbohydrates of *Mycobacterium tuberculosis*. In: Bloom B, ed. Tuberculosis: Pathogenesis, Protection, and Control. Washington, DC: ASM Press, 1994:285–306.

11. Beveridge TJ. Ultrastructure, chemistry, and function of the bacterial wall. Int Rev Cytol 1981;12:229–317.

12. Beveridge TJ. Bacterial S-layers. Curr Opin Struct Biol 1994;4:204–212.

13. Biswas GD, Sparling PF. Characterization of *lbpA*, the structural gene for the LF receptor in *Neisseria gonorrhoeae*. Infect Immun 1995;63:2958–2967.

14. Bleck TP. Clinical aspects of tetanus. In Simpson LL, ed.: Botulinal Toxin and Tetanus Toxin. San Diego: Academic Press, 1989:379–398.

15. Brennan PJ, Nikaido H. The envelope of mycobacteria. Ann Rev Biochem 1995;64:29–63.

16. Brodeur BR, Martin D. Antigenic analysis of the saccharide moiety of the lipooligosaccharide of *Bordetella pertussis*. Springer Semin Immunopathol 1993;15:205–215.

17. Buchanan RE. Studies in the nomenclature and classification of the bacteria. V. Subgroups and genera of the *Bacteriaceae*. J Bacteriol 1918;3:27.

18. Buchanan RE. General Systematic Bacteriology: History, Nomenclature, Groups of Bacteria. Baltimore: Williams & Wilkins, 1925.

19. Centers for Disease Control and Prevention. Wound botulism—California, 1995. MMWR Morb Mortal Wkly Rep 1995;44:890–892.

20. Chaby R, Caroff M. Lipopolysaccharides of *Bordetella pertussis* endotoxin. In: Wardlaw AC, Parton R, eds. Pathogenesis and Immunity in Pertussis. Chichester: Wiley, 1988:247–271.

21. Chen HY, Yuan M, Livermore DM. Mechanisms of resistance to β-lactam antibiotics amongst *Pseudomonas aeruginosa* isolates collected in the UK in 1993. J Med Microbiol 1995;43:300–309.

22. Cherington M. Clinical spectrum of botulism. Muscle Nerve 1998;21:701–710.

23. Chester FD. A Manual of Determinative Bacteriology. New York: Macmillan, 1901.

24. Cisar JO, Takahashi Y, Rhul RS. Specific inhibitors of a bacterial adhesion: observation from the study of gram-positive bacteria that initiate biofilm formation on the tooth surface. Adv Dent Res 1997;11:168–175.

25. Clarke LM, Sierra MF, Daidone BJ, et al. Comparison of the Syva Micro-Trak enzyme immunoassay and Gen-Probe PACE 2 with cell culture for diagnosis of cervical *Chlamydia trachomatis* infection in a high-prevalence female population. J Clin Microbiol 1993;26:1735–1737.

26. Clemens DL, Horowitz MA. Characterization of the *Mycobacterium tuberculosis* phagosome and evidence that phagosomal maturation is inhibited. J Exp Med 1995;181:257–270.

27. Clewell DB. Bacterial sex pheromone-induced plasmid transfer. Cell 1993;73:9–12.

28. Colby SM, Russell RRB. Sugar metabolism by mutans streptococci. J Appl Microbiol Symp Suppl 1997;83:80S–88S.

29. Cole ST, Saint Girons I. Bacterial genomics. FEMS Microbiol Rev 1994;14:139–160.

30. Collen D. Staphylokinase: a potent, uniquely fibrin-selective agent. Nat Med 1998;4:279–284.

31. Collins MD, East AK. Phylogeny and taxonomy of the food-borne pathogen *Clostridium botulinum* and its neurotoxins. J Appl Microbiol 1998;84:5–17.

32. Collins MD, Lawson PA, Willems A, et al. The phylogeny of the genus *Clostridium*: proposal of five new genera and eleven new species combinations. Int J Syst Bacteriol 1994;44:812–826.

33. Costello AH, Cisar JO, Kolenbrander PE, Gabriel O. Neuraminidase-dependent

hemagglutination of human erythrocytes by human strains of *Actinomyces viscosus* and *Actinomyces naeslundii*. Infect Immun 1979;26:563–572.

34. Dale JB, Washburn RG, Marques MB, Wessels MR. Hyaluronate capsule and surface M protein in resistance to opsonization of group A streptococci. Infect Immun 1996;64:1495–1501.

35. DeJonge BLM, Chang Y-S, Gage D, Tomasz A. Peptidoglycan composition of a highly methicillin-resistant *Staphylococcus aureus*. J Biol Chem 1992;267: 11248–11254.

36. Dombek PE, Sedgewick J, Lam H, et al. High frequency intracellular invasion of epithelial cells by serotype M1 group A streptococci: M1 protein-mediated invasion and cytoskeletal rearrangements. Mol Microbiol 1999;31:859–870.

37. Dodds KL. Worldwide incidence and ecology of infant botulism. In: Hauschild AHW, Dodds KL, eds: *Clostridium botulinum*: Ecology and Control in Foods. New York: Marcel Dekker, 1993:105–117.

38. Dwyer JM. The Specific Immune Response. In: Root RK, Waldvogel F, Corey L, Stamm WE, eds. Clinical Infectious Diseases: A Practical Approach. New York: Oxford University Press, 1999:91–108.

39. Dziejman M, Mekalanos JJ. Two-component signal transduction and its role in the expression of bacterial virulence factors. In: Xxxx XX, ed. Two Component Signal Transduction. Washington, DC: ASM Press, 1995:305–317.

40. Farrell AM, Taylor D, Holland KT. Cloning, nucleotide sequence determination, and expression of the *Staphylococcus aureus* hyaluronate lyase gene. FEMS Microbiol Lett 1995;130:81–85.

41. Firth N, Ippen-Ihler K, Skurray RA. Structure and function of the F factor and mechanisms of conjugation, *Escherichia coli* and *Salmonella*. In: Neidhardt FC, ed. Cellular and Molecular Biology. Washington, DC: ASM Press, 1996: 2377–2401.

42. Fischetti VA. Streptococcal M proteins: molecular design and biological behavior. Clin Microbiol Rev 1989;2:285–314.

43. Fluckiger U, Jones KF, Fischetti VA. Immunoglobulins to group A streptococcal surface molecules decrease adherence to and invasion of human pharyngeal cells. Infect Immun 1998;66:974–979.

44. Fortier AH, Leiby DA, Narayanan RB, et al. Growth of *Francisella tularensis* LVS in macrophages: the acidic intracellular compartment provides essential iron required for growth. Infect Immun 1995;63:1478–1483.

45. Fourel G, Phalipon A, Kaczorek. Evidence for direct regulation of diphtheria toxin gene transcription by an Fe^{2+}-dependent DNA-binding repressor (DtoxR) in *Corynebacterium diphtheriae*. Infect Immun 1989;57:3221–3225.

46. Fournier JM, Boutonnier A, Bouvet A. *Staphylococcus aureus* strains which are not identified by rapid agglutination procedures are of capsular serotype 5. J Clin Microbiol 1989;27:1372–1374.

47. Fournier JM, Bouvet A, Boutonnier A, et al. Predominance of capsular type 5 among oxacillin-resistant *Staphylococcus aureus*. J Clin Microbiol 1987;25: 1932–1933.

48. Fournier JM, Bouvet A, Mathieu D, et al. New latex reagent using monoclonal antibodies to capsular polysaccharide for reliable identification of both oxacillin-susceptible and oxacillin-resistant *Staphylococcus aureus*. J Clin Microbiol 1993;31:1342–1344.

49. Fournier JM, Vann WF, Karakawa WW. Purification and characterization of *Staphylococcus aureus* type 8 capsular polysaccharide. Infect Immun 1984;47: 87–93.

50. Frehel C, Rastogi N. Phagosome-lysosome fusions in macrophages infected with *Mycobacterium avium*: role of mycosides-C and other cell-surface components. Acta Leprol 1989;7(Suppl 1):173–174.

51. Fuqua WC, Winans SC, Greenberg EP, et al. Quorum sensing in bacteria: the LuxR-LuxI family of cell density-responsive transcriptional regulators. J Bacteriol 1994;176:269–275.

52. Gaillard JL, Berche LP, Frehel C, et al. Entry of *L. monocytogenes* into cells is mediated by internalin, a repeat protein reminiscent of surface antigens from gram-positive cocci. Cell 1991;65:1127–1141.

53. Galas DJ, Chandler M. Bacterial insertion sequences. In: Berg DE, Howe MM, eds. Mobile DNA. Washington, DC: ASM Press, 1989:109–162.

54. Gambello MJ, Kaye S, Iglewski BH. LasR of *Pseudomonas aeruginosa* is a transcriptional activator of the alkaline protease gene (*apr*) and an enhancer of exotoxin A expression. Infect Immun 1993;61:1180–1184.

55. Garrity GM, Holt JG. Bergey's Manual of Systematic Bacteriology: An Overview of the Road Map to the Manual. New York: Bergey's Manual Trust/Springer, 2000.

56. Gibbons RJ, Hay DI. Human salivary acidic proline-rich proteins and statherin promote the attachment of *Actinomyces viscosus* LY7 to apatitic surfaces. Infect Immun 1988;56:439–445.

57. Goren MB, Brokl O, Schaeffer WB. Lipids of putative relevance to virulence of *Mycobacterium tuberculosis*: correlation of virulence with elaboration of sulfatides and strongly acidic lipids. Infect Immun 1974;9:142–149.

58. Goren MB, D'Arcy Hart PD, Young MR, Armstrong JA. Prevention of phagosome-lysosome fusion in cultured macrophages by sulfatides of *Mycobacterium tuberculosis*. Proc Natl Acad Sci USA 1976;73:2510–2514.

59. Gorringe AR, Woods G, Robinson A. Growth and siderophore production by *Bordetella pertussis* under iron-restricted conditions. FEMS Microbiol Lett 1990;66:101–106.

60. Goto M, Oka S, Okuzumi K, et al. Evaluation of acridinium ester-labeled DNA probes for identification of *Mycobacterium tuberculosis* and *Mycobacterium avium-Mycobacterium intracellulare* complex in culture. J Clin Microbiol 1991; 29:2473–2476.

61. Granato PA, Franz MR. Use of the Gen Probe PACE system for the detection of *Neisseria gonorrhoeae* in urogenital samples. Diagn Microbiol Infect Dis 1990;13:217–221.

62. Griffiss JM, Schneider H, Mandrell RE, et al. Lipooligosaccharides: the principal glycolipids of the neisserial outer membrane. Rev Infect Dis 1988;10(Suppl 1): S87–S95.

63. Harris GS, Michalek AM, Curtiss R III. Cloning a locus involved in *Streptococcus mutans* intracellular polysaccharide accumulation and virulence testing of an intracellular polysaccharide-deficient mutant. Infect Immun 1992;60: 3175–3185.

64. Heckels JE. Structure and function of pili of pathogenic *Neisseria*. Clin Microbiol Rev 1989;2(Suppl):S66–S73.

65. Henrichsen J. Six newly recognized types of *Streptococcus pneumoniae*. J Clin Microbiol 1995;33:2759–2762.

66. Hirt H, Wirth R, Muscholl A. Comparative analysis of 18 sex pheromone plasmids from *Enterococcus faecalis*: detection of a new insertion element on pPD1 and implications for the evolution of this plasmid family. Mol Gen Genet 1996;252:640–647.

67. Hitchens AD, Slepecky RA. Bacterial spore formation as a modified cell division. Nature (London) 1969;223:804–807.

68. Hollingshead SK, Fischetti VA, Scott JR. Complete nucleotide sequence of type 6 M protein of the group A streptococcus: repetitive structure and membrane anchor. J Biol Chem 1986;261:1677–1686.

69. Holt JG, Krieg NR, Sneath PHA, Staley JT, Williams ST, eds. Bergey's Manual of Determinative Bacteriology. 9th Ed. Baltimore: Williams & Wilkins, 1994.

70. Hultgren SJ, Abraham S Caparon M, et al. Pilus and non-pilus bacterial adhesins: assembly and function in cell recognition. Cell 1993;73:897–901.

71. Hunnicutt DW, McBride MJ. Cloning and characterization of the *Flavobacterium johnsonii* (*Cytophaga johnsonii*) gliding motility genes, *gldB* and *gldC*. J Bacteriol 2000;182:911–918.

72. Janda WM, Wilcoski LM, Mandel KL, et al. Comparison of monoclonal antibody-based methods and a ribosomal ribonucleic acid probe test for *Neisseria gonorrhoeae* culture confirmation. Eur J Clin Microbiol Infect Dis 1993;12: 177–184.

73. Jennings HJ, Lugowski C, Young NM. Structure of the complex polysaccharide C-substance from *Streptococcus pneumoniae* type 1. Biochemistry 1980;19: 3712–4719.

74. Kluytmans J, Goessens W, Van Rijsoort J, et al. Improved performance of PACE 2 with modified collection system in combination with probe competition assay for detection of *Chlamydia trachomatis* in urethral specimens from males. J Clin Microbiol 1994;32:568–570.

75. Koch AL, Doyle RJ. Inside-to-outside growth and turnover of the cell wall of gram-positive rods. J Theor Biol 1985;117:137–157.

76. Kreutzer DL, Robertson DC. Surface macromolecules and virulence in intracellular parasites: comparison of cell envelope components of smooth and rough strains of *Brucella abortus*. Infect Immun 1979;23:819–828.

77. Krieg NR, Holt JG, eds. Bergey's Manual of Systematic Bacteriology. Vol. 1. Baltimore: Williams & Wilkins, 1984.

78. Krueger KM, Barbieri JT. The family of bacterial ADP-ribosylating exotoxins. Clin Microbiol Rev 1995;8:38–47.

79. Lebrun M, Mengaud H, Ohayon H, et al. Internalin must be on the bacterial surface to mediate entry of *Listeria monocytogenes* into epithelial cells. Infect Immun 1996;57:55–61.

80. Lecuit M, Ohayon H, Braun L, et al. Internalin of *Listeria monocytogenes* with an intact leucine-rich repeat region is sufficient to promote internalization. Infect Immun 1997;65:5309–5319.

81. Lee BC. Isolation of haemin-binding proteins of *Neisseria gonorrhoeae*. J Med Microbiol 1992;36:121–127.

82. Lee BC. Isolation and characterization of the haemin-binding proteins from *Neisseria meningitidis*. J Gen Microbiol 1994;140:1473–1480.

83. Lee KD, Oh YK, Portnoy DA, Swanson JA. Delivery of macromolecules into cytosol using liposomes containing hemolysin from *Listeria monocytogenes*. J Biol Chem 1996;271:7249–7252.

84. Lewis LA, Dyer DW. Identification of an iron-regulated outer membrane protein of *Neisseria meningitidis* involved in the utilization of hemoglobin complexed to haptoglobin. J Bacteriol 1995;177:1299–1306.

85. Linker A, Jones RS. A new polysaccharide resembling alginic acid isolated from pseudomonads. J Biol Chem 1966;241:3845–3851.

86. Lorber B. Gas gangrene and other *Clostridium*-associated diseases. In: Mandell GL, Bennett JE, Dolin R, eds. Mandell, Douglas, and Bennett's Principles and Practice of Infectious Diseases. Philadelphia: Churchill Livingstone, 2000: 2549–2561.

87. Lyras D, Rood JI. Transposable genetic elements and antibiotic resistance determinants from *Clostridium perfringens* and *Clostridium difficile*. In: Rood JI, McClane BA, Songer JG, Titball RW, eds.): The Clostridia: Molecular Biology and Pathogenesis. London: Academic Press, 1997:73–92.

88. Lyras D, Storie C, Huggins AS, et al. Chloramphenicol resistance in *Clostridium difficile* is encoded on Tn4453 transposons that are closely related to Tn4451 from *Clostridium perfringens*. Antimicrob Agents Chemother 1998;42:1563–1567.

89. MacDonald KL, Rutherford GW, Friedman SM, et al. Botulism and botulism-like illness in chronic drug abusers. Ann Intern Med 1985;102:616–619.

90. Makino S-I, Uchida I, Terakado N, Yoshikawa M. Molecular characterization and protein analysis of the *cap* region, which is essential for encapsulation in *Bacillus anthracis*. J Bacteriol 1989;171:722–730.

91. Masson L, Holbein BE, Ashton FE. Virulence linked to polysaccharide production in serogroup B *Neisseria meningitidis*. FEMS Microbiol Lett 1982;13:187–190.

92. McBride MJ. Bacterial gliding motility: mechanisms and mysteries. ASM News 2000;66:203–210.

93. McBride MJ, Kempf MJ. Development of techniques for the genetic manipulation of the gliding bacterium *Cytophaga johnsonii*. J Bacteriol 1996;178:583–590.

94. Mesnage S, Tosi-Couture E, Mock M, et al. Molecular characterization of the *Bacillus anthracis* main S-layer component; evidence that it is the major cell-associated antigen. Mol Microbiol 1997;23:1147–1155.

95. Midura TF, Arnon SS. Infant botulism: identification of *Clostridium botulinum* and its toxin in faeces. Lancet 1976;2:934–936.

96. Moreau MJ, Richards JC, Fournier JM, et al. Structure of the type-5 capsular polysaccharide of *Staphylococcus aureus*, Carbohydr Res 1990;201:285–297.

97. Moses AE, Wessels MR, Zalcman K, et al. Relative contributions of hyaluronic acid capsule and M protein to virulence of group A streptococcus. Infect Immun 1997;65:64–71.

98. Murray RGE, Schleifer KH. Taxonomic notes: a proposal for recording the properties of putative taxa of procaryotes. Int J Syst Bacteriol 1994;44:174–176.

99. Murray RGE, Stackebrandt E. Taxonomic note: implementation of the provisional status, *Candidatus*, for incompletely described prokaryotes. Int J Syst Bacteriol 1995;45:186.

100. Murray T, Popham DL, Setlow P. Identification and characterization of *pbpA* encoding *Bacillus subtilis* penicillin-binding protein 2A. J Bacteriol 1997;179:3021–3029.

101. Orla-Jensen S. The Lactic Acid Bacteria. Copenhagen: Host and Sons, 1919.

102. Panke ES, Yang LI, Leist PA, et al. Comparison of Gen-Probe DNA probe test and culture for the detection of *Neisseria gonorrhoeae* in endocervical specimens. J Clin Microbiol 1991;29:883–888.

103. Parmely MJ. *Pseudomonas* metalloproteases and the host-microbe relationship. In: Fick RB, ed. *Pseudomonas aeruginosa:* The Opportunist—Pathogenesis and Disease. Boca Raton, FL: CRC Press, 1993:79–84.

104. Parsons NJ, Curry A, Fox AJ, et al. The serum resistance of gonococci in the majority of urethral exudates is due to sialylated lipooligosaccharide seen as a surface coat. FEMS Microbiol Lett 1992;90:295–300.

105. Paul TR, Venter A, Blaszczak LC, et al. Localization of penicillin-binding proteins to the splitting system of *Staphylococcus aureus* septa using a mercury-penicillin V derivative. J Bacteriol 1995;177:3631–3640.

106. Pearson JP, Passador L, Iglewski BH, Greenberg EP. A second N-acylhomoserine lactone signal produced by *Pseudomonas aeruginosa*. Proc Natl Acad Sci USA 1995;92:1490–1494.

107. Pinner R, Onyango F, Perkins BA, et al. Evidence for functionally distinct pili expressed by *Neisseria meningitidis*. Infect Immun 1991;59:3169–3175.

108. Portnoy DA, Chakraborty T, Goebel W, Cossart P. Molecular determinants of *Listeria monocytogenes* pathogenesis. Infect Immun 1992;60:1263–1267.

109. Poulsen K, Reinholdt J, Jespersgaard C, et al. A comprehensive genetic study of streptococcal immunoglobulin A1 proteases: evidence for recombination within and between species. Infect Immun 1998;66:181–190.

110. Prevost G, Cribier B, Coupie P, et al. Panton-Valentine leukocidin and γ-hemolysin from *Staphylococcus aureus* ATCC 49775 are encoded by distinct genetic loci and have different biological activities. Infect Immun 1995;63:4121–4129.

111. Redhead K, Hill T, Chart H. Interaction of lactoferrin and transferrins with the outer membrane of *Bordetella pertussis*. J Gen Microbiol 1987;133:891–898.

112. Reed GL, Kussie P, Parhami-Seren B. A functional analysis of the antigenicity of streptokinase using monoclonal antibody mapping and recombinant streptokinase fragments. J Immunol 1993;150:4407–4415.

113. Rice PA. Molecular basis for serum resistance in *Neisseria gonorrhoeae*. Clin Microbiol Rev 1989;2(Suppl):S112–S117.

114. Sakaguchi G. *Clostridium botulinum* toxins. Pharmacol Ther 1983;19:165–194.

115. Sandberg AL, Ruhl S, Joralmon RA, et al. Putative glycoprotein and glycolipid polymorphonuclear leukocyte receptors for the *Actinomyces naeslundii* WVU fimbrial lectin. Infect Immun 1988;63:267–269.

116. Schleifer KH, Kandler O. Peptidoglycan types of bacterial cell walls and their taxonomic implications. Bacteriol Rev 1972;36:404–477.

117. Schmitt MP. Transcription of the *Corynebacterium diphtheriae hmuO* gene is regulated by iron and heme. Infect Immun 1997;65:4634–4641.

118. Schmitt MP, Holmes RK. Characterization of a defective diphtheria toxin repressor (*dtxR*) allele and analysis of *dtxR* transcription in wild-type and mutant strains of *Corynebacterium diphtheriae*. Infect Immun 1991;59:3903–3908.

119. Schneider H, Griffiss JM, Mandrell RE, et al. Elaboration of a 3.6 kilodalton lipooligosaccharide, antibody against which is absent from human sera, is associated with serum resistance in *Neisseria gonorrhoeae*. Infect Immun 1985;50:672–677.

120. Schneider H, Hammack CA, Apicella MA, et al. Instability of expression of lipooligosaccharides and their epitopes in *Neisseria gonorrhoeae*. Infect Immun 1988;56:942–946.

121. Silverman M, Simon M. Phase variation: genetic analysis of switching mutants. Cell 1980;19:845–854.

122. Sippel JE, Hider PA, Controni G. Use of Directigen latex agglutination test for detection of *Haemophilus influenzae*, *Streptococcus pneumoniae*, and *Neisseria meningitidis* antigens in cerebrospinal fluid from meningitis patients. J Clin Microbiol 1981;20:884–886.

123. Sisco Kl, Smith HO. Sequence-specific DNA uptake in *Haemophilus* transformation. Proc Natl Acad Sci USA 1979;76:972–976.

124. Skerman VBD, McGowan V, Sneath PHA, eds. Approved list of bacterial names. Int J Syst Bacteriol 1980;30:225–420.

125. Skerman VBD, McGowan V, Sneath PHA, eds. Approved list of bacterial names, amended edition. Washington, DC: American Society for Microbiology, 1989.

126. Sleytr UB, Beveridge TJ. Bacterial S-layers. Trends Microbiol 1999;7:253–260.

127. Sneath PHA, ed. *International Code of Nomenclature of Bacteria*, 1990 revision. Washington, DC:, American Society for Microbiology, 1990.

128. Sneath PHA, ed. *International Code of Nomenclature of Bacteria*, 1992 revision. Washington, DC: American Society for Microbiology, 1992.

129. Sneath PHA, Mair NS, Sharpe ME, Holt JG, eds. Bergey's Manual of Determinative Bacteriology. Vol 2. Baltimore: Williams & Wilkins, 1986.

130. Sorenson UB, Blom SJ, Birch-Andersen A, Henrichsen J. Ultrastructural localization of capsules, cell wall polysaccharide, cell wall proteins, and F antigen in pneumococci. Infect Immun 1988;56:1890–1896.

131. Stackebrandt E, Goebel BM. Taxonomic note: a place for DNA-DNA reassociation and 16S rRNA sequence analysis in the present species definition in bacteria. Int J Syst Bacteriol 1994;44:846–849.

132. Stackebrandt E, Liesack W. Nucleic acids and classification. In O'Donnell M, ed. Handbook of New Bacterial Systematics. London: Academic Press, 1993:152–194.

133. Staley JT, Bryant MP, Pfennig N, Holt JG, eds. Bergey's Manual of Systematic Bacteriology. Vol 3. Baltimore: Williams & Wilkins, 1989.

134. Staley JT, Krieg MR. Classification of prokaryotic organisms: an overview. In: Krieg NR, Holt JG, eds. Bergey's Manual of Systematic Bacteriology. Vol. 1. Baltimore: Williams & Wilkins, 1984:1–4.

135. Stock JB, Surette MG. Two-component signal transduction systems: structure-function relationships and mechanisms of catalysis. In: Xxxx XX, ed. Two Component Signal Transduction. Washington, DC: ASM Press, 1995:25–51.

136. Stuer JT, Jaegar KE, Winkler UK. Purification of extracellular lipase from *Pseudomonas aeruginosa*. J Bacteriol 1986;168:1070–1074.

137. Suen JC, Hatheway CL, Steigerwalt AG, Brenner DJ. *Clostridium argentinense*, sp. nov., a genetically homogenous group composed of all strains of *Clostridium botulinum* toxin type G and some non-toxigenic strains previously identified as *Clostridium subterminale* or *Clostridium hastiforme*. Int J Syst Bacteriol 1988;38:375–381.

138. Sugai M, Yamada S, Nakashima S, et al. Localized perforation of the cell wall by a major autolysin: *atl* gene products and the onset of penicillin-induced lysis of *Staphylococcus aureus*. J Bacteriol 1997;179:2958–2962.

139. Swift S, Bainton NJ, Winston MK. Gram-negative bacterial communication by N-acyl homoserine lactones: a universal language? Trends Microbiol 1994;2:193–198.

140. Tamaoka J. Determination of DNA base composition. In: Goodfellow M, O'Donnell eds. Chemical Methods in Prokaryotic Systematics. Chichester: Wiley, 1994:463–469.

141. Thakker M, Park JS, Carey V, Lee JC. *Staphylococcus aureus* serotype 5 capsular polysaccharide is antiphagocytic and enhances bacterial virulence in a murine bacteremia model. Infect Immun 1998;66:5183–59.

142. Thorne CB. *Bacillus anthracis*. In: Sonenshein AL, Hoch JA, Losick R, eds. *Bacillus subtilis* and other Gram-Positive Bacteria: Biochemistry, Physiology, and Molecular Genetics. Washington, DC: American Society for Microbiology, 1993:113–124.

143. Throup JP, Camara M, Briggs GS, et al. Characterisation of the *yenI/yenR* locus from *Yersinia enterocolitica* mediating the synthesis of two N-acylhomoserine lactone signal molecules. Mol Microbiol 1995;17:345–356.

144. Tomasz. A. The staphylococcal cell wall. In: Fischetti VA, Novick RP, Ferretti JJ, et al., eds. Gram Positive Pathogens. Washington, DC: ASM Press, 2000:351–360.

145. Tsumori H, Kuramitsu H. The role of the *Streptococcus mutans* glucosyltransfer-

ases in the sucrose-dependent attachment to smooth surfaces: essential role of the GtfC enzyme. Oral Microbiol Immunol 1997;12:274–280.

146. Tramont EC. Gonococcal vaccines. Clin Microbiol Rev 1989;2(Suppl): S74–S77.

147. Tunkel AR, Scheld WM. Pathogenesis and pathophysiology of bacterial meningitis. Clin Microbiol Rev 1993;6:118–136.

148. Vasil M, Prince RW, Shortridge VD. Exoproducts: *Pseudomonas* exotoxin A and phospholipase C. In: Fick RB, ed. *Pseudomonas aeruginosa:* The Opportunist—Pathogenesis and Disease. Boca Raton, FL: CRC Press, 1993:59–77.

149. Via LE, Curcic R, et al. Elements of signal transduction in *Mycobacterium tuberculosis*: in vitro phosphorylation and in vivo expression of the response regulator *MtrA*. J Bacteriol 178:3314–3321, 1996.

150. Vijaranakul U, Nadakavukaren MJ, DeJonge B, et al. Increased cell size and shortened interpeptide bridge of NaCl-stressed *Staphylococcus aureus* and their reversal by glycine betaine. J Bacteriol 1995;177:5116–5121.

151. Virji M, Heckels JE. The role of common and type-specific pilus antigenic domains in adhesion and virulence of gonococci for human epithelial cells. J Gen Microbiol 1984;130:1089–1095.

152. Von Graevenitz A. Revised nomenclature of *Alloiococcus otitis*. J Clin Microbiol 1993;31:472.

153. Wayne LG, Brenner DJ, Colwell RR, et al. Report of the *ad hoc* committee on reconciliation of approaches to bacterial systematics. Int J Syst Bacteriol 1987; 37:463–464.

154. Wessels MR, Moses AE, Goldberg JB, DiCesare TJ. Hyaluronic acid capsule is a virulence factor for mucoid group A streptococci. Proc Natl Acad Sci USA 1991;88:8317–8321.

155. Wessels MR, Rubens CE, Benedi VJ, Kasper DL. Definition of a bacterial virulence factor: sialylation of the group B streptococcal capsule. Proc Natl Acad Sci USA 1989;86:8983–8987.

156. White A, Ding X, Murphy JR, Ringe D. Structure of metal ion-activated diphtheria toxin repressor/*tox* operator complex. Nature 1998;394:502–506.

157. Williams ST, Sharpe ME, Holt JG, eds. Bergey's Manual of Systematic Bacteriology. Vol 4. Baltimore: Williams & Wilkins, 1989.

158. Woese CR, Kandler O, Wheelis ML. Towards a natural system of organisms: proposal for the domains *Archaea*, *Bacteria*, and *Eucarya*. Proc Natl Acad Sci USA 1990;87:4576–4579.

159. Yeung MK, Ragsdale PA. Synthesis and function of *Actinomyces naeslundii* T14V type 1 fimbriae require the expression of additional fimbria-associated genes. Infect Immun 1997;65:2629–2639.

160. Zamze SE, Moxon ER. Composition of the lipopolysaccharide from different capsular serotype strains of *Haemophilus influenzae*. J Gen Microbiol 1987;133: 1443–1451.

The *Enterobacteriaceae*

Characteristics for Presumptive Identification

Screening Characteristics

Carbohydrate Utilization
Cytochrome Oxidase Activity
Nitrate Reduction

Culture Media Used for Detection of Carbohydrate Fermentation

Use of Kligler Iron Agar and Triple Sugar Iron Agar
Biochemical Principles

Selection of Primary Isolation Media

Chemicals and Compounds Used in Selective Media
Selective Isolation Media
Highly Selective Isolation Media Used Primarily for Gastrointestinal Specimens
Enrichment Media
Guidelines for Choosing Selective Isolation Media

Differential Identification Characteristics

Indole Production
Methyl Red Test
Voges-Proskauer Test
Citrate Utilization
Urease Production
Decarboxylation of Lysine, Ornithine, and Arginine

Phenylalanine Deaminase Production
Hydrogen Sulfide Production
Motility

Taxonomy of the Enterobacteriaceae

Classification of Enterobacteriaceae by Tribes
Key Identification Characteristics for the Most Common Species

Tribe *Escherichieae*
Tribe *Edwardsielleae*
Tribe *Salmonelleae*
Tribe *Citrobactereae*
Tribe *Klebsielleae*
Tribe *Proteeae*
Tribe *Yersinieae*
Tribe *Erwinieae*

Miscellaneous New Genera of Enterobacteriaceae

Identification Characteristics of Newer *Enterobacteriaceae*
Clinical Significance of Newer *Enterobacteriaceae*

Quick Screening Methods for Rapid Identification

Commercial Screening Kits
Chromogenic Agar Media

Classic Identification Systems

Checkerboard Matrix
Branching Flow Diagrams
Computer-Aided Schemes

Numeric Coding Systems

Reading Octal Codes in Numeric Code Registers
Estimated Frequency of Occurrence
Calculation of Likelihood
Resolving Discrepancies

Packaged Kit Identification Systems

Overview of Packaged Systems
Specific Identification Systems

API 20E
BBL Crystal Enteric/Nonfermenter ID System
RapID onE System
Enterotube II

Micro-ID
Biolog GN2 Microplate
MicroScan System
Sensititre System

Semiautomated and Automated Identification Systems

MicroScan Walkaway
Vitek System
Sensititre Gram-Negative Autoldentification System
The Phoenix System
The OmniLog ID System

ram-negative bacilli belonging to the *Enterobacteriaceae* are the most frequently encountered bacterial isolates recovered from clinical specimens. Widely dispersed in nature, these organisms are found in soil and water, on plants, and, as the family name indicates, within the intestinal tracts of humans and animals. Before the advent of antibiotics, chemotherapy, and immunosuppressive measures, the infectious diseases caused by the *Enterobacteriaceae* were relatively well defined. Diarrheal and dysenteric syndromes, accompanied by fever and septicemia in classic cases of typhoid fever, were known to be caused by *Salmonella* and *Shigella* species. Classic cases of pneumonia, characterized by production of brick-red or "currant jelly" sputum, were known to be caused by Friedlander's bacillus (*Klebsiella pneumoniae*). *Escherichia coli*, *Proteus* species, and various members of the *Klebsiella–Enterobacter* group were commonly recovered from traumatic wounds contaminated with soil or vegetative matter or from abdominal wound incisions following gastrointestinal surgery.

Thus, members of the *Enterobacteriaceae* may be incriminated in virtually any type of infectious disease and recovered from any specimen received in the laboratory. Immunocompromised or debilitated patients are highly susceptible to hospital-acquired infections, either after colonization with environmental strains or following invasive procedures, such as catheterization, bronchoscopy, colposcopy, or surgical biopsies, in which mucous membranes are traumatized or transected.

Endotoxic shock is one potentially lethal manifestation of infection with gram-negative bacteria, including the *Enterobacteriaceae*. Endotoxin is a complex pharmacologically active lipopolysaccharide that is contained within the cell wall of gram-negative species. This lipopolysaccharide is structured in three layers: 1) an outer variable carbohydrate portion that determines O-antigenic specificity (e.g., various *Salmonella* serotypes), 2) a middle core polysaccharide that is structurally similar among species, and 3) a central, highly conserved lipid moiety called lipid-A. The biologic effects of endotoxin have been demonstrated experimentally: small quantities injected intravenously into animals produce fever, leukopenia, capillary hemorrhage, hypotension, and circulatory collapse—symptoms that are, to a large extent, the same as those seen in humans with gram-negative sepsis.

The limulus lysate assay, which uses a reagent prepared from the amebocytes of the horseshoe crab (*Limulus polyphemus*), has been used with varying success in the diagnosis of endotoxic shock.[154] The lysate undergoes gelation when in contact with even trace amounts of endotoxin. More promising in the diagnosis of gram-negative sepsis is the development of monoclonal antibodies that can be used in enzyme-linked immunoassay or other techniques for the detection of lipid-A. The pharmacologic effects of endotoxin can be attributed primarily to lipid-A. It is highly antigenic and has determinants common to all strains of gram-negative bacilli. Thus, the detection of circulating lipid-A in patients with gram-negative sepsis, using a monoclonal antibody, could establish a diagnosis so that presumptive therapy could be started before the causative organism is recovered and identified.

Microbiologists must be alert to the emergence of any *Enterobacteriaceae* that are resistant to multiple antibiotics. The mechanisms by which resistance may develop are discussed in more detail in Chapter 17. Antibiotic resistance may evolve in formerly susceptible clinical isolates through the transfer of plasmids known as R factors or R plasmids. The gram-negative enteric bacteria commonly possess a single, large R plasmid that encodes for resistance to several antibiotics. An increasing percentage of strains within the genera *Enterobacter, Serratia, Klebsiella*, and *Providencia*, in addition to some indole-positive strains of *Proteus* and cephalothin-resistant strains of *Escherichia coli*, possess inducible β-lactamases that impart cross-resistance to many β-lactam antibiotics.[435,436] Inactivating enzymes are often chromosomally mediated and may be responsible for "breakthrough" resistance in patients who are being treated for septicemia. Disk-diffusion susceptibility tests may not always detect resistant strains, particularly when testing the cephalosporins; thus, a broth-dilution procedure may be indicated. Detecting these resistant strains is not only important in treating the patient from whom the isolate is recovered but also has important implications for surveillance of nosocomial infections. Specific clinical syndromes of individual genera and species are discussed in later sections of this chapter.

Characteristics for Presumptive Identification

What are the initial clues that an unknown isolate recovered from a clinical specimen may belong to the *Enterobacteriaceae*? In specimens other than feces, a gram-stained preparation may reveal short, plump, gram-negative bacillary or coccobacillary cells, ranging from 0.5 to 2 fm wide to 2 to 4 fm long (see Color Plate 6-1*A*). However, species differentiation cannot be made on the basis of only Gram stain morphology.

Characteristic colonial morphology of an organism growing on a solid medium may provide a second clue. Typically, members of the *Enterobacteriaceae* produce relatively large, dull gray, dry, or mucoid colonies on sheep blood agar, the latter suggesting encapsulated strains of *Klebsiella pneumoniae* (see Color Plate 6-1*B* and *C*). Hemolysis on blood agar is variable and indistinctive. Colonies appearing as a thin film or as waves (a phenomenon known as **swarming**) suggest that the organism is motile and probably a *Proteus* species (see Color Plate 6-1*D*). Colonies that appear red on MacConkey agar or have a green sheen on eosin methylene blue (EMB) agar (see Color Plate 6-2) indicate that the organism is capable of forming acid from lactose in the medium.

Differentiation of the *Enterobacteriaceae*, however, is based primarily on the presence or absence of different enzymes coded by the genetic material of the bacterial chromosome. These enzymes direct the metabolism of bacteria along one of several pathways that can be detected by special media used in in vitro culture techniques. Substrates on which these enzymes can react are incorporated into the culture medium, together with an indicator that can detect either the utilization of the substrate or the presence of specific metabolic products. By selecting a series of media that measure different metabolic characteristics of the microorganisms to be tested, a biochemical profile can be determined for making a species identification.

Screening Characteristics

Definitive identification of the members of the *Enterobacteriaceae* may require a battery of biochemical tests. Considerable time and possible misidentification can be avoided if a few preliminary observations are made to ensure that the organism being tested belongs to this group. If the organism is a gram-negative organism of another group, it may be necessary to use a different set of characteristics than that commonly used for the identification of the *Enterobacteriaceae*. With few exceptions, all members of the *Enterobacteriaceae* demonstrate the following characteristics:

- Glucose is fermented (see Color Plate 6-1*E* and *F*)
- Cytochrome oxidase is negative (see Color Plate 6-1*G*)
- Nitrate is reduced to nitrite (see Color Plate 6-1*H*).

CARBOHYDRATE UTILIZATION

It is common for laboratory microbiologists to refer to all carbohydrates as **sugars.** This is convenient in an operational sense, although it is understood that polyhedral alcohols, such as dulcitol and mannitol, or cationic salts of acetate or tartrate are not carbohydrates and thus are not truly sugars in a chemical sense.

The term **fermentation** is also used somewhat loosely in reference to the utilization of carbohydrates by bacteria, with terms such as **lactose fermenters** and **non–lactose fermenters**. By definition, fermentation is an oxidation–reduction metabolic process that takes place in an anaerobic environment, and instead of oxygen, an organic substrate serves as the final hydrogen (electron) acceptor. In bacteriologic test systems, this process is detected by observing color changes in pH indicators as acid products are formed. Acidification of a test medium may occur through the degradation of carbohydrates by pathways other than fermentation, or there may be ingredients other than carbohydrates in some media that result in acid end products. Although most bacteria that metabolize carbohydrates are facultative anaerobes, the utilization may not always be under strictly anaerobic conditions, as is observed in the production of acid products by bacterial colonies growing on the surface of agar media. Even though all tests used to measure an organism's ability to enzymatically degrade a ''sugar'' into acid products may not be ''fermentative,'' these terms will be used in this textbook for convenience.

Basic Principles of Fermentation. Pasteur's mid 19th-century studies of the action of yeasts on wine provide the basis for our present understanding of carbohydrate fermentation. Pasteur observed that certain contaminating bacterial species produced a drop in the pH of wine (a carbohydrate substrate) from the production of a variety of acids. Full descriptions of the fermentative pathways by which a monosaccharide such as glucose is degraded evolved soon thereafter. Through a series of enzymatic glycolytic cleavages and transformations, the glucose molecule is split into a series of three carbon compounds, the most important of which is pyruvic acid. The chemical sequence by which glucose is converted to pyruvic acid is known as the **Embden–Meyerhof pathway** (EMP; Fig. 6-1). Many bacteria, including all *Enterobacteriaceae*, ferment glucose through the EMP to form pyruvic acid; the manner in which pyruvic acid is further used, however, varies among bacterial species. The alternative fates of pyruvic acid are the result of a variety of fermentation pathways, yielding quite different products (see Fig. 6-1).

Bacteria are differentiated by the carbohydrates they metabolize and the types and quantities of acids produced. These differences in enzymatic activity serve as one of the important characteristics by which the different species are recognized. It is important for students of microbiology to understand that in the glycolytic formation of pyruvic acid, adenosine triphosphate (ATP) is generated at the expense of the reduction of nicotinamide adenine dinucleotide (NAD)

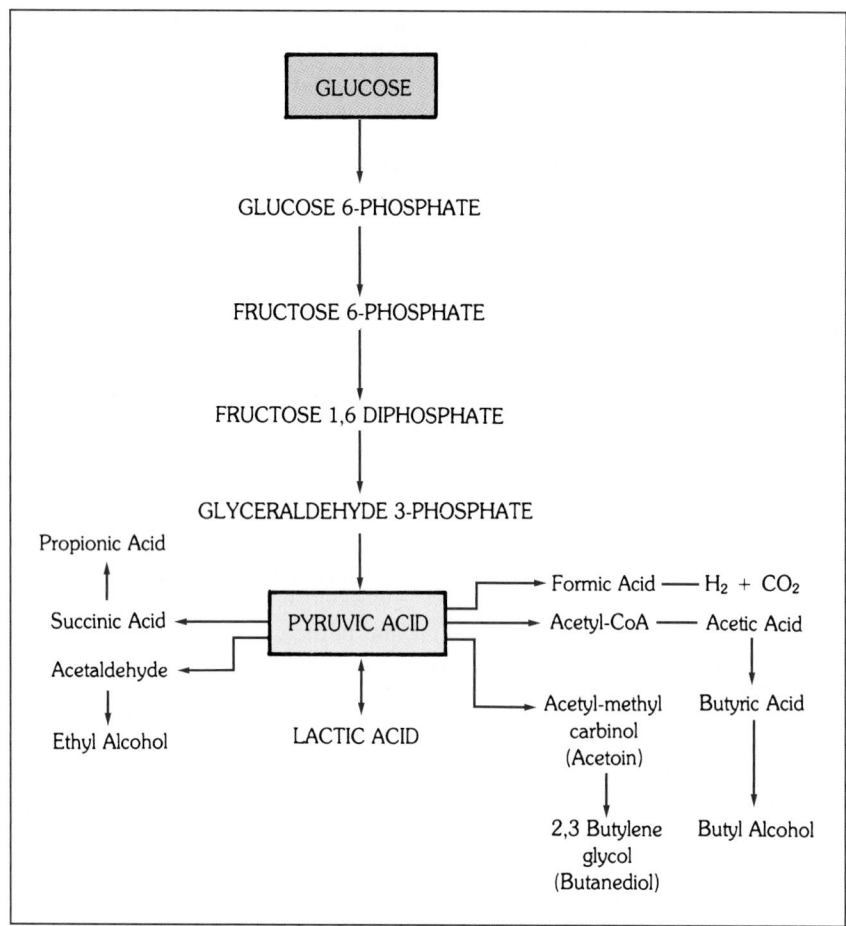

Figure 6-1 Fermentation of glucose to form pyruvate (Embden–Meyerhof pathway) and the alternative fates of pyruvic acid.

to NADH$_2$. For each glucose molecule that is fermented to form pyruvic acid, four hydrogen ions are consumed through the reduction of two NAD to two NADH$_2$. Since the total NAD in the cell is very limited, fermentation would cease very rapidly if the NADH$_2$ were not reoxidized in the further metabolism of pyruvic acid. Figure 6-2 depicts the fermentation of three molecules of glucose by means of two alternative pathways. For example, glucose fermentation by *Escherichia coli* occurs by means of the mixed acid fermentation pathway and results in the production of large quantities of acetic, lactic, and formic acids, with a marked drop in the pH of the test medium. This is detected by a positive methyl red test (see Fig. 6-2). On the other hand, the *Klebsiella–Enterobacter–Hafnia–Serratia* group metabolize pyruvic acid primarily through the butylene glycol pathway, producing acetyl methyl carbinol (acetoin) and a positive Voges-Proskauer (VP) test (see Fig. 6-2). Note that the principal end products in this latter pathway are alcohols, with only a small amount of acid produced, thus the methyl red test is usually negative for this group of organisms.

The gas resulting from fermenting bacteria is primarily a mixture of hydrogen and carbon dioxide formed through the cleavage of formic acid. It is an accepted rule of thumb that any bacterium that forms gas in carbohydrate test medium must first form acid, which is self-evident from the EMP scheme shown in Figure 6-1. Gas is best detected by using a broth carbohydrate-fermentation medium into which

small inverted Durham tubes have been placed (see Color Plate 6-1*F*). Even trace amounts of gas, which collect as bubbles under the Durham tubes, can be detected. Some species of *Enterobacteriaceae* lack the enzyme formic dehydrogenase and cannot cleave formic acid and, as a result, do not form even trace amounts of CO$_2$ (e.g., most species of *Shigella*). Conversely, organisms that use the butylene glycol pathway (i.e., are VP-positive) produce copious amounts of CO$_2$ (see Fig. 6-2). Therefore, when a large amount of gas is observed, one should consider members of the *Klebsiella–Enterobacter–Hafnia–Serratia* group as the likely identification. The formation of ethyl alcohol by microorganisms is of utmost commercial importance in the manufacture of alcoholic beverages and organic reagents; however, it is of limited usefulness in the laboratory identification of bacteria.

The bacterial fermentation of lactose is more complex than that of glucose. Lactose is a disaccharide composed of glucose and galactose, connected through an oxygen linkage known as a **galactoside bond.** On hydrolysis, this bond is severed, releasing glucose and galactose. For a bacterium to metabolize lactose, two enzymes must be present: 1) β-galactoside permease, permitting the transport of a β-galactoside, such as lactose, through the bacterial cell wall; and 2) β-galactosidase, the enzyme required to hydrolyze the β-galactoside bond once the disaccharide has entered the

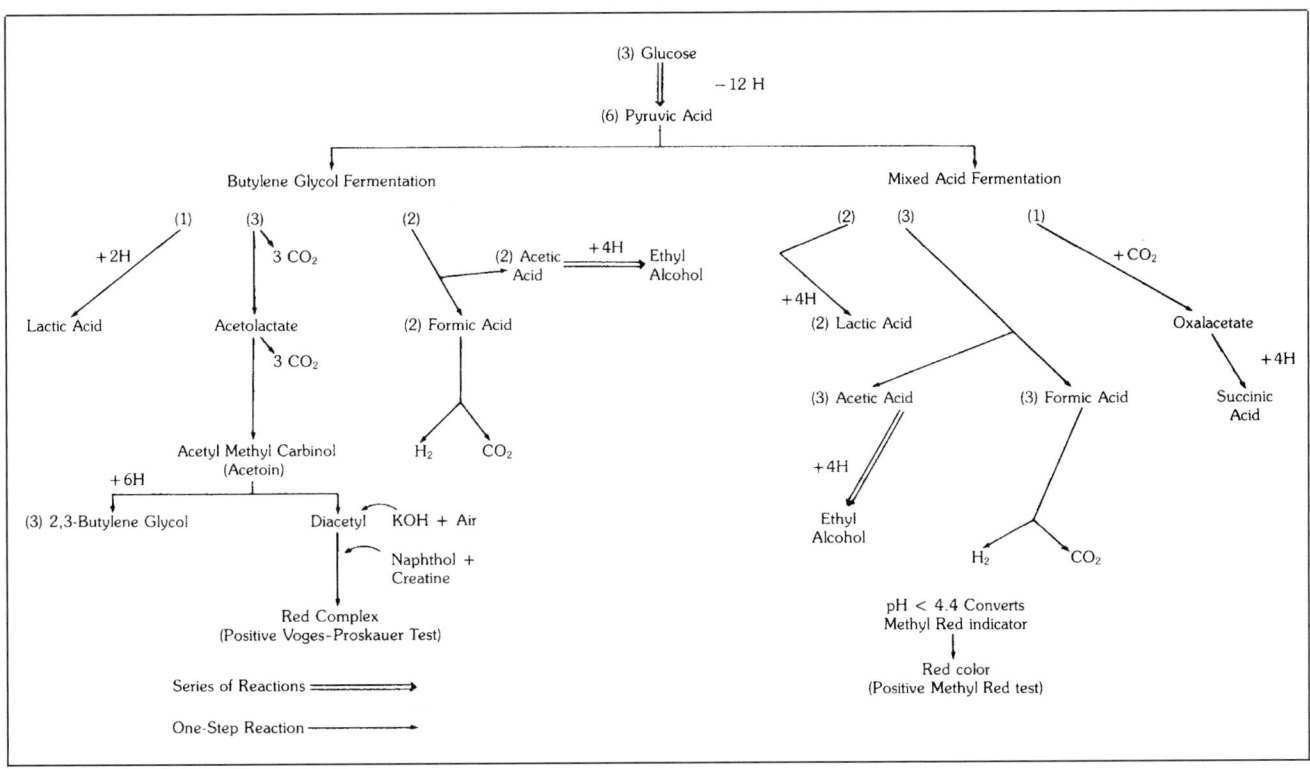

Figure 6-2 Mixed acid and butylene glycol pathways of glucose fermentation.

cell. The final acid reaction results from the degradation of glucose as shown in Figure 6-3.

Because lactose fermentation ultimately proceeds by way of glucose degradation through the EMP, it follows that any organism incapable of metabolizing glucose cannot form acid from lactose. This explains why glucose is omitted from the formulas of primary isolation media such as MacConkey agar and EMB agar: if it is not omitted, the ability to detect the lactose-fermenting capability of the test bacteria would be lost. In the test medium, the end point of lactose fermentation is the detection of acid production. A non–lactose-fermenting organism is one that lacks either one or both of the two enzymes required for lactose metabolism or lacks the ability to attack glucose. So-called late lactose-fermenters are believed to be organisms that exhibit β-galactosidase activity but show sluggish β-galactoside permease activity.

β-Galactosidase and the ONPG Test. *o*-Nitrophenyl-β-D-galactopyranoside (ONPG) is a compound structurally similar to lactose except that the glucose has been replaced by an *o*-nitrophenyl group. This rather ingenious manipulation of the molecule forms the basis for the ONPG test, which is outlined in Chart 6-1. This test detects the enzyme β-galactosidase far more quickly than does the test for lactose fermentation previously described. This is helpful in identifying late lactose fermenters that are deficient in β-galactoside permease. ONPG permeates the bacterial cell more readily than lactose and, under the action of β-galactosidase, is hydrolyzed into galactose and *o*-nitrophenol (see Chart 6-1). *o*-Nitrophenol is a chromophore that is colorless when bound to D-galactopyranoside but is yellow in its free (unbound) form (see Color Plate 6-4*A*).

ONPG test tablets that can be easily reconstituted by adding a small amount of water are available commercially and are convenient for use in the laboratory. Organisms with strong β-galactosidase activity may produce a positive test within a few minutes after inoculation of the medium. The ONPG test is most helpful for detection of β-galactosidase activity in late lactose fermenters, such as some strains of *E. coli*, in which differentiation from species of *Shigella* (except certain strains of *S. sonnei*) may otherwise be difficult. The test is also helpful in distinguishing some strains of *Citrobacter* species and *Salmonella* ser. Arizonae (ONPG-positive) from most *Salmonella* species (ONPG-negative). The ONPG test is not a substitute for the determination of lactose fermentation because only the enzyme β-galactosidase is measured.

CYTOCHROME OXIDASE ACTIVITY

Any organism that displays cytochrome oxidase activity following the procedure and test conditions outlined in Chart 1-5 is excluded from the *Enterobacteriaceae*. The developing color reaction must be interpreted within 10 to 20 seconds because many organisms, including selected members of the *Enterobacteriaceae*, may produce delayed false-positive reactions. Both oxidase-positive and oxidase-negative control organisms should be tested if there is difficulty in interpreting the cytochrome oxidase reaction. The commercial cytochrome oxidase droppers are used most often because of their convenience. The color reactions are clearly visible within 10 seconds. If metal inoculating loops or wires are used in the laboratory for transferring bacteria to the oxidase reagent, those made from stainless steel or Nichrome

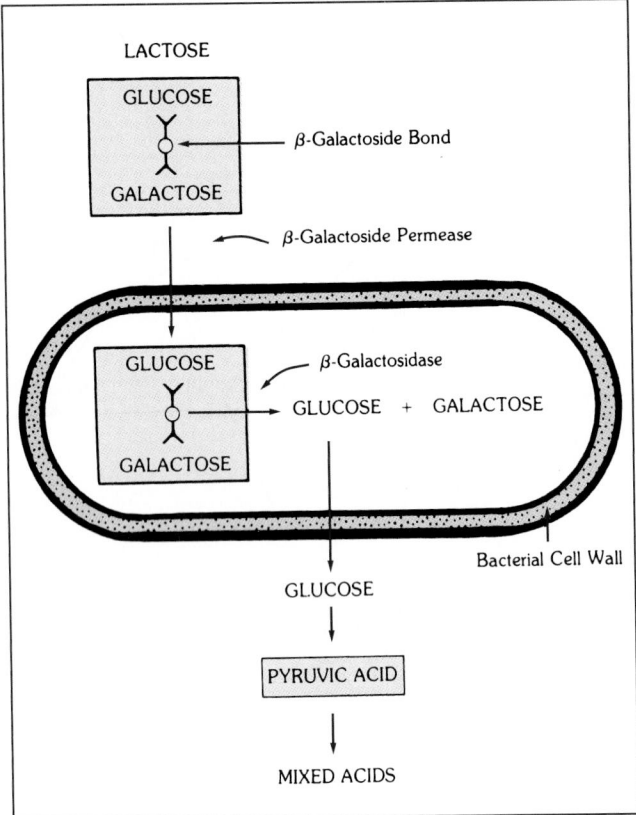

LACTOSE

GLUCOSE

— β-Galactoside Bond

GALACTOSE

← β-Galactoside Permease

GLUCOSE — β-Galactosidase

GLUCOSE + GALACTOSE

GALACTOSE

Bacterial Cell Wall

GLUCOSE

PYRUVIC ACID

MIXED ACIDS

Figure 6-3 Bacterial fermentation of lactose: Lactose, a disaccharide composed of molecules of glucose and galactose joined by a β-galactoside bond, diffuses through the bacterial cell wall under the action of β-galactoside permease. If the bacterium produces β-galactosidase, the lactose is hydrolyzed to produce glucose and galactose. The glucose is then metabolized as illustrated in Figure 6-1.

may produce false-positive reactions, owing to trace amounts of iron oxide on the flamed surface of the metal. This problem can be circumvented by using plastic or platinum inoculating loops or by using wooden applicator sticks or cotton swabs to perform the oxidase test. Tetramethyl-*p*-phenylenediamine, rather than the dimethyl derivative, is most commonly used because the reagent is more stable, more sensitive, and less toxic (see Chart 1-5 and Color Plate 6-1*G*).

NITRATE REDUCTION

All *Enterobacteriaceae*, with the exception of certain biotypes of *Pantoea agglomerans* and certain species of *Serratia* and *Yersinia*, reduce nitrate to nitrite. Because a variable period of incubation (3 to 24 hours, depending on the system used) is required to perform the nitrate reduction test, it is not commonly used to prescreen unknown bacterial isolates. Rather, the test is used in most laboratories either to confirm the correct classification of an unknown microorganism or as an aid in determining the identification of bacterial species. Details of the nitrate reduction test are presented in Chart 6-2.

Any basal medium that supports the growth of the organism and contains a 0.1% concentration of potassium nitrate (KNO_3) is suitable for performing this test. Nitrate broth and nitrate agar in a slant are the media forms most commonly used in clinical laboratories. Because the enzyme nitrate reductase is maximally active under anaerobic conditions, Zobell has recommended the use of semisolid agar.[516] Semisolid media also enhance the growth of many bacterial species and provide the anaerobic environment needed for enzyme activation. The addition of zinc dust to all negative reactions, as shown in Chart 6-2, should be a routine procedure. Most organisms capable of reducing nitrates will do so within 24 hours; some may produce detectable quantities within 2 hours. A rapid nitrate test has been described by Schreckenberger and Blazevic.[444] Both α-naphthylamine and sulfanilic acid are relatively unstable, so their reactivity should be determined at frequent intervals by testing with positive- and negative-control organisms. The diazonium compound that forms from the reaction of the reduced nitrate and reagents is also relatively unstable, and the color tends to fade; accordingly, readings should be made soon after the reagents are added (see Color Plate 6-1*H*).

Culture Media Used for Detection of Carbohydrate Fermentation

A variety of liquid or agar media can be used to measure the ability of a test organism to fermentatively utilize carbohydrates. The carbohydrate to be tested, such as glucose, is filter-sterilized and added aseptically to a basal medium to a final concentration of 0.5–1.0%. The formula of a typical basal fermentation medium contains trypticase (BBL), 10 g; sodium chloride, 5 g; phenol red, 0.018 g; and distilled water to equal 1 L. Trypticase is a hydrolysate of casein that serves as a source for carbon and nitrogen; sodium chloride is an osmotic stabilizer; and phenol red is a pH indicator that turns yellow when the pH of the medium drops below 6.8. Color Plate 6-1*F* illustrates acid fermentation reactions in purple broth medium. All of the *Enterobacteriaceae* grow well in this type of medium, and the base formula used is a matter of personal preference. In addition to producing a pH color shift in fermentation culture media, the production of mixed acids, notably butyric acid, often results in a pungent, foul odor from the culture medium. When such an odor is detected, one should immediately be suspicious of the presence of one of the *Enterobacteriaceae* (in addition, the anaerobic bacteria produce characteristic metabolic products with distinctive odors).

Use of Kligler Iron Agar and Triple Sugar Iron Agar

In practice, microorganisms that are capable of fermenting glucose are commonly detected by observing the reactions they produce when grown on Kligler iron agar (KIA) or triple sugar iron (TSI) agar (Fig. 6-4; see Color Plate 6-1*E*). If an organism cannot ferment glucose, then an alkaline-slant–alkaline-butt (no change) reaction is observed (see Fig. 6-4*A*), indicating a lack of acid production and failure of the test organism to ferment any of the sugars present. This reaction alone is sufficient to exclude an organism from the *Enterobacteriaceae*. The formula for KIA is listed in Box

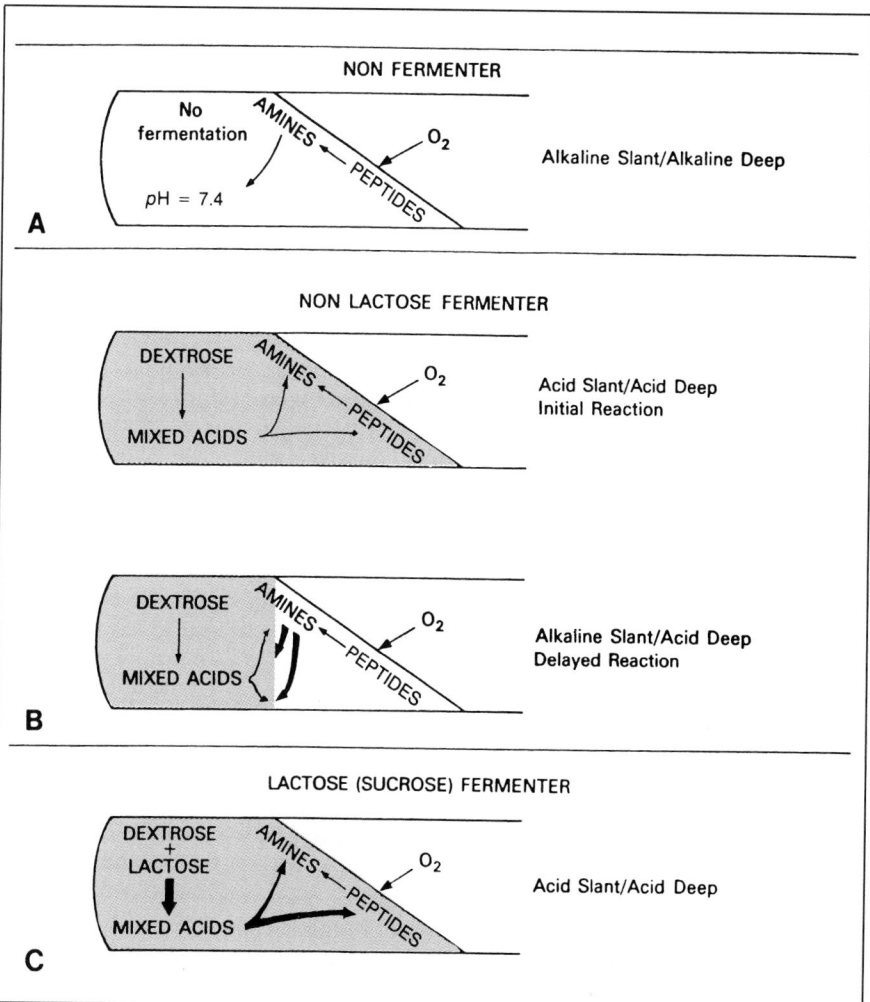

Figure 6-4 Three general types of reactions produced by bacteria growing on Kligler iron agar: (**A**) Nonfermentative bacilli that are unable to produce acids from the fermentation of glucose or lactose; there is no change in the medium (represented by *white*). (**B**) Initial acidification of both the deep and the slant of the medium (*shaded area*) by bacteria that ferment glucose, but the slant reverts back to alkaline pH as alkaline amines are formed from the oxidative decarboxylation of peptides (derived from protein in the medium) near the surface. (**C**) Complete permanent acidification of both the deep and the slant of the tube by lactose-fermenting bacteria.

6-1 (the formula for TSI is identical except that 10 g of sucrose is added).

Several observations are important in studying the formulas of KIA and TSI. The incorporation of four protein derivatives—beef extract, yeast extract, peptone, and proteose peptone—makes KIA and TSI nutritionally very rich. The lack of inhibitors permits the growth of all but the most fastidious bacterial species (excluding the obligate anaerobes). For this reason, KIA and TSI agar can be used only when testing a bacterial species selected from a single colony recovered on primary or selective agar plates. Glucose and lactose (and

sucrose in TSI medium) are evenly distributed throughout both the slant and butt (deep) portion of the tube. However, lactose is present in a concentration 10 times that of glucose (similarly, the ratio of sucrose to glucose is 10:1 in TSI medium). This 10:1 ratio is important to the understanding of the biochemical principles discussed later. Ferrous sulfate as a hydrogen sulfide detector is somewhat less sensitive than other ferric or ferrous salts; therefore, there may be discrepancies in the hydrogen sulfide readings between KIA and TSI and other test media (see Color Plate 6-4*B*). The phenol red indicator is yellow below a pH of 6.8. Because the pH of the uninoculated medium is buffered at 7.4, relatively small quantities of acid production result in a visible color change.

Biochemical Principles

The biochemical principles underlying the reactions observed in KIA or TSI agar are illustrated in Figure 6-4. Note that the molten agar is allowed to solidify in a slant. This configuration results in essentially two reaction chambers within the same tube. The **slant** portion, exposed throughout its surface to atmospheric oxygen, is aerobic; the lower portion, called the **butt** or the **deep,** is protected from the air

Box 6-1 Kligler Iron Agar	
Beef extract, 3 g	Sodium chloride, 5 g
Yeast extract, 3 g	Sodium thiosulfate, 0.3 g
Peptone, 15 g	Agar, 12 g
Proteose peptone, 5 g	Phenol red, 0.024 g
Lactose, 10 g	Distilled water to equal 1 L
Glucose, 1 g	Final pH, 7.4
Ferrous sulfate, 0.2 g	

and is relatively anaerobic. It is important when preparing the media that the slant and the deep are kept equal in length, approximately 3 cm (1.5 in.) each, so that this two-chamber effect is preserved.

KIA and TSI tubes are inoculated with a long, straight wire. The well-isolated test colony recovered from an agar plate is touched with the end of the inoculating needle, which is then stabbed into the deep of the tube, extending to within 3 to 5 mm of its bottom. When the inoculating wire is removed from the deep of the tube, the slant surface is streaked with a back-and-forth motion. Inoculated tubes are placed into an incubator at 35°C for 18 to 24 hours. The color photographs shown in Color Plates 6-1*E* and 7-1*A* reveal the reactions that are described in Box 6-2. Thus, as shown in Figure 6-4*A* and in Plate 7-1*A*, without carbohydrate fermentation, no acids are formed, and the amine production in the slant together with the alkaline buffers produce a red color throughout the medium. The bacteria that produce this type of reaction are known as **nonfermenters** (see Chapter 7).

If the KIA tube is inoculated with a glucose-fermenting organism that cannot utilize lactose, only a relatively small quantity of acid can be obtained from the 0.1% concentration of glucose in the medium. Initially, during the first 8 to 12 hours of incubation, even this amount of acid may be sufficient to convert both the deep and the slant color to yellow. Within the next few hours, however, the glucose supply is completely exhausted and the bacteria begin oxidative degradation of the amino acids within the slant portion of the tube where oxygen is present. This results in the release of amines that soon counteract the small quantities of acid present in the slant; by 18 to 24 hours, the entire slant reverts to an alkaline pH and the color returns to red. In the deep (anaerobic portion) of the tube, however, amino acid degradation is insufficient to counteract the acid formed, and the medium remains yellow. Thus, the alkaline-slant–acid-deep reaction on KIA (or TSI) is an important initial indicator that the test organism is a non–lactose-fermenter (see Fig. 6-4*B* and Color Plate 6-1*E*).

If the KIA tube is inoculated with a lactose-fermenting organism, then, even though the glucose is completely used up after the first 8 to 12 hours, fermentation continues as the organism is able to use lactose (present in 10 times the concentration of glucose). Consequently, when the tube is examined at the end of 18 to 24 hours, acid production from fermentation of lactose is still occurring and both the slant and the deep appear yellow, resulting in an acid-slant–acid-deep reaction (see Fig. 6-4*C* and Color Plate 6-1*E*).

Many microbiologists prefer TSI over KIA because the addition of sucrose to the formula helps screen for *Salmonella* and *Shigella* species, because neither of these (except rare strains) metabolizes either lactose or sucrose. Therefore, any acid–acid reaction of TSI indicates that either lactose, sucrose, or both have been fermented, excluding *Salmonella* and *Shigella*. It should also be remembered that *Yersinia enterocolitica* ferments sucrose, but not lactose; thus, on TSI the reaction will be acid–acid (similar to coliforms such as *E. coli*), but on KIA, the reaction will be alkaline–acid (similar to a non-lactose fermenter). Consequently, when screening stool specimens for *Salmonella*, *Shigella*, and *Yersinia*, some might argue that KIA is preferable to TSI.

For the detection of hydrogen sulfide, which is colorless, the medium must include an indicator. Sodium thiosulfate is the source of sulfur atoms in most media used for hydrogen sulfide production. Iron salts (ferrous sulfate and ferric ammonium citrate) incorporated in the culture media then react with hydrogen sulfide to produce an insoluble black precipitate (ferrous sulfide). An acid environment is required for an organism to produce hydrogen sulfide and, therefore, a source of hydrogen ions must be provided. Because the deep of the KIA and TSI tubes becomes acidic with glucose fermentation (hydrogen ions increase), the blackening is often first seen or confined there, particularly with non–lactose-fermenting bacteria (see Color Plate 6-1*E*). Thus, it follows that a black deep should be read as acid even if the usual yellow color is obscured by the black precipitate. KIA and TSI are less sensitive in the detection of hydrogen sulfide than other iron-containing media, such as sulfide indole motility (SIM) medium (see Color Plate 6-4*B*).

If an organism can be excluded from the *Enterobacteriaceae* before an extended battery of biochemical tests is set up, considerable time and labor will be saved. It is recommended that either a KIA or a TSI slant be set up on all isolates suspected of being one of the *Enterobacteriaceae* at the same time that differential test media of kit systems are set up. Even if an organism is a fermenter and is suspected of being one of the *Enterobacteriaceae*, a cytochrome oxidase test should be performed to exclude organisms belonging to other genera of fermenting bacteria, such as *Aeromonas, Plesiomonas, Vibrio*, and *Pasteurella* species, that are oxidase-positive.

Selection of Primary Isolation Media

Selective culture media must be used to recover the significant species of bacteria from specimens that may harbor a mixture of microorganisms. To make rational selections,

---

Box 6-2 Reactions on KIA

Alkaline Slant/Alkaline Deep (K/K)

No carbohydrate fermentation. This is characteristic of nonfermentative bacteria, such as *Pseudomonas aeruginosa*.

Alkaline Slant/Acid Deep (K/A)

Glucose fermented; lactose (or sucrose for TSI medium) not fermented. This is characteristic of non–lactose-fermenting bacteria, such as *Shigella* species.

Alkaline Slant/Acid (Black) Deep (K/A/H$_2$S)

Glucose fermented; lactose not fermented, hydrogen sulfide produced. This is characteristic of non–lactose-fermenting, hydrogen sulfide–producing bacteria, such as *Salmonella* species, *Citrobacter* species, and *Proteus* species.

Acid Slant/Acid Deep (A/A)

Glucose and lactose (or sucrose with TSI) fermented. This is characteristic of lactose-fermenting coliforms, such as *Escherichia coli* and the *Klebsiella–Enterobacter* species.

Table 6-1 Selective Differential Media for Recovery of *Enterobacteriaceae*

MEDIUM	FORMULATION		PURPOSE AND DIFFERENTIAL INGREDIENTS	REACTIONS AND INTERPRETATION
MacConkey agar (see Color Plates 6-2*A* and *B*)	Peptone Polypeptone Lactose Bile salts Sodium chloride Agar Neutral red Crystal violet Distilled water to Final pH, 7.1	17 g 3 g 10 g 1.5 g 5 g 13.5 g 0.03 g 0.001g 1 L	MacConkey agar is a differential-plating medium for the selection and recovery of the *Enterobacteriaceae* and related enteric gram-negative bacilli. The bile salts and crystal violet inhibit the growth of gram-positive bacteria and some fastidious gram-negative bacteria. Lactose is the sole carbohydrate. Lactose-fermenting bacteria produce colonies that are varying shades of red, owing to the conversion of the neutral red indicator dye (red below pH 6.8) from the production of mixed acids. Colonies of non–lactose-fermenting bacteria appear colorless or transparent.	Typical strong lactose fermenters, such as species of *Escherichia*, *Klebsiella*, and *Enterobacter*, produce red colonies surrounded by a zone of precipitated bile. Slow or weak lactose fermenters, such as *Citrobacter*, *Providencia*, *Serratia*, and *Hafnia*, may appear colorless after 24 hr or slightly pink in 24–48 hr. Species of *Proteus*, *Edwardsiella*, *Salmonella*, and *Shigella*, with rare exceptions, produce colorless or transparent colonies. Representative colonies, showing these various reactions, are shown in Color Plate 6-2.
Eosin methylene blue (EMB) agar (see Color Plate 6-2*C* through *F*)	Peptone Lactose Sucrose* Dipotassium, PO₄ Agar Eosin Y Methylene blue Distilled water to Final pH, 7.2	10 g 5 g 5 g 2 g 13.5 g 0.4 g 0.065g 1 L	EMB agar is a differential-plating medium that can be used in place of MacConkey agar in the isolation and detection of the *Enterobacteriaceae* or related coliform bacilli from specimens with mixed bacteria. The aniline dyes (eosin and methylene blue) inhibit gram-positive and fastidious gram-negative bacteria. They combine to form a precipitate at acid pH, thus also serving as indicators of acid production. Levine EMB, with only lactose, gives reactions more in parallel with MacConkey agar; the modified formula also detects sucrose fermenters.	Typical strong lactose-fermenting colonies, notably *Escherichia coli*, produce colonies that are green-black with a metallic sheen. Weak fermenters, including *Klebsiella*, *Enterobacter*, *Serratia*, and *Hafnia*, produce purple colonies within 24–48 hr. Non–lactose-fermenters, including *Proteus*, *Salmonella*, and *Shigella*, produce transparent colonies. *Yersinia enterocolitica*, a non–lactose, sucrose fermenter, produces transparent colonies on Levine EMB and purple to black colonies on the modified formula. See Color Plate 6-2.

* *Modified Holt-Harris-Teague formula. Sucrose is not contained in Levine EMB agar.*

microbiologists must know the composition of each formula and the purpose and relative concentration of each chemical or compound that is included. For example, it is not sufficient to know that bile salts are included in the formulas of a number of selective media to inhibit the growth of gram-positive and some of the more fastidious gram-negative bacteria species. For example, *Salmonella–Shigella* (SS) agar contains about five times the concentration of bile salts compared with MacConkey agar and is more inhibitory to *E. coli* and more selective for the recovery of *Salmonella* species from stool cultures.

For the recovery of the *Enterobacteriaceae* from clinical specimens that potentially harbor mixed bacteria, three general types of media are available: 1) nonselective media for primary isolation (e.g., blood agar); 2) selective or differential agars (e.g., MacConkey and Hektoen enteric agars); and 3) enrichment broths. Tables 6-1 and 6-2 compare different media commonly used in clinical practice. The formulas are complex and include ingredients that not only inhibit the growth of certain bacterial species (selective), but also detect several biochemical characteristics that are important in making a preliminary identification of the microorganisms present in the specimen (differential).

Chemicals and Compounds Used in Selective Media

Box 6-3 lists the general types of chemicals and compounds used in selective media, including brief comments on the function of each.

Table 6-2 Highly Selective Media for Recovery of *Enterobacteriaceae* from Gastrointestinal Specimens

MEDIUM	FORMULATION		PURPOSE AND DIFFERENTIAL INGREDIENTS	REACTIONS AND INTERPRETATION
Salmonella–Shigella (SS) agar	Beef extract	5 g	SS agar is a highly selective medium formulated to inhibit the growth of most coliform organisms and permit the growth of species of *Salmonella* and *Shigella* from environmental and clinical specimens. The high bile salts concentration and sodium citrate inhibit all gram-positive bacteria and many gram-negative organisms, including coliforms. Lactose is the sole carbohydrate and neutral red is the indicator for acid detection. Sodium thiosulfate is a source of sulfur. Any bacteria that produce hydrogen sulfide gas are detected by the black precipitate formed with ferric citrate (relatively insensitive). High selectivity of SS agar permits use of heavy inoculum.	Any lactose-fermenting colonies that appear are colored red by the neutral red. Rare strains of *Salmonella arizonae* are lactose fermenting, and colonies may simulate *Escherichia coli*. Growth of species of *Salmonella* is uninhibited, and colonies appear colorless with black centers, owing to hydrogen sulfide gas production. Species of *Shigella* show varying inhibition and colorless colonies with no blackening. Motile strains of *Proteus* that appear on SS agar do not swarm.
	Peptone	5 g		
	Lactose	10 g		
	Bile salts	8.5 g		
	Sodium citrate	8.5 g		
	Sodium thiosulfate	8.5 g		
	Ferric citrate	1 g		
	Agar	12.5 g		
	Neutral red	0.025 g		
	Brilliant green	0.033 g		
	Distilled water to Final pH, 7.4	1 L		
Hektoen enteric (HE) agar (see Color Plates 6-3*E* and *F*)	Peptone	12 g	HE agar is a recent formulation devised as a direct-plating medium for fecal specimens to increase the yield of species of *Salmonella* and *Shigella* from the heavy numbers of normal flora. The high bile salt concentration inhibits growth of all gram-positive bacteria and retards the growth of many strains of coliforms. Acids may be produced from the carbohydrates, and acid fuchsin reacting with thymol blue produces a yellow color when the pH is lowered. Sodium thiosulfate is a sulfur source, and hydrogen sulfide gas is detected by ferric ammonium citrate (relatively sensitive).	Rapid lactose fermenters (such as *E. coli*) are moderately inhibited and produce bright-orange to salmon-pink colonies. *Salmonella* colonies are blue-green, typically with black centers from hydrogen sulfide gas. *Shigella* appear more green than *Salmonella*, with the color fading to the periphery of the colony. *Proteus* strains are somewhat inhibited; colonies that develop are small transparent, and more glistening or watery in appearance than species of *Salmonella* or *Shigella*. See Color Plate 6-3.
	Yeast extract	3 g		
	Bile salts	9 g		
	Lactose	12 g		
	Sucrose	12 g		
	Salicin	2 g		
	Sodium chloride	5 g		
	Sodium thiosulfate	5 g		
	Ferric ammonium citrate	1.5 g		
	Acid fuchsin	0.1 g		
	Thymol blue	0.04 g		
	Agar	14 g		
	Distilled water to Final pH, 7.6	1 L		
Xylose lysine deoxycholate (XLD) agar (see Color Plate 6-3*A* through *D*)	Xylose	3.5 g	XLD agar is less inhibitory to growth of coliform bacilli than HE agar and was designed to detect shigellae in feces after enrichment in gram-negative broth. Bile salts in relatively low concentration make this medium less selective than the other two included in this table. Three carbohydrates are available for acid production, and phenol red is the pH indicator. Lysine-positive organisms, such as most *Salmonella* species, produce initial yellow colonies from xylose utilization and delayed red colonies from lysine decarboxylation. Hydrogen sulfide detection system is similar to that of HE agar.	Organisms such as *E. coli* and *Klebsiella–Enterobacter* species may use more than one carbohydrate and produce bright yellow colonies. Colonies of many species of *Proteus* are also yellow. Most species of *Salmonella* produce red colonies, most with black centers from hydrogen sulfide gas. *Shigella, Providencia,* and many *Proteus* species use none of the carbohydrates and produce translucent colonies. *Citrobacter* colonies are yellow with black centers; many *Proteus* species are yellow or translucent with black centers; salmonellae are red with black centers. See Color Plate 6-3.
	Lysine	5 g		
	Lactose	7.5 g		
	Sucrose	7.5 g		
	Sodium chloride	5 g		
	Yeast extract	3 g		
	Phenol red	0.08 g		
	Agar	13.5 g		
	Sodium deoxycholate	2.5 g		
	Sodium thiosulfate	6.8 g		
	Ferric ammonium citrate	0.8 g		
	Distilled water to Final pH, 7.4	1 L		

Box 6-3 Chemicals and Compounds Used in Selective Media

Protein hydrolysates (e.g., peptones, meat infusion, typtones, and casein): Proteins are cleaved by acids or enzymes into amino acids and peptides that can be used by bacteria to provide the carbon and nitrogen needed for bacterial metabolism.

Carbohydrates: A variety of disaccharides (e.g., lactose, sucrose, and maltose), hexoses (dextrose), and pentoses (xylose) are included in selective media for two purposes: 1) to provide a ready sources of carbon for energy and 2) to serve as substrates in biochemical reactions for identification of unknown organisms.

Buffers: Balanced monosodium and disodium or potassium phosphates are most commonly used. Buffers provide 1) a stable pH for optimal growth of microorganisms, and 2) a standard reference pH for those media in which acid or alkaline reactions are used to identify microorganisms.

Enrichments (e.g., blood, serum, vitamin supplements, and yeast extracts): Growth supplements are added to media to recover fastidious organisms. Enrichments are less commonly used for the recovery of the *Enterobacteriaceae* because most members of this group grow without them.

Inhibitors: Various different compounds may serve to inhibit the growth of certain undesired bacterial species, thus making the medium selective: 1) aniline dyes (e.g., brilliant green and eosin), 2) heavy metals (e.g., bismuth), 3) chemicals (e.g., azide, citrate, deoxycholate, selenite, and phenylethyl alcohol), and 4) antimicrobial agents (e.g., neomycin, colistin, vancomycin, and chloramphenicol). Their relative concentrations are important in determining the selectivity of the medium in which they are contained.

pH indicators: Fuchsin, methylene blue, neutral red, phenol red, and bromcresol purple are commonly used indicators in test media to measure pH shifts resulting from bacterial metabolism of given substrates.

Miscellaneous indicators: Other indicators may be included to detect specific bacterial products (e.g., ferric and ferrous ions for the detection of hydrogen sulfide).

Miscellaneous compounds and chemicals: Agar, a gelatinous extract of red seaweed, is commonly added to a medium, in varying concentrations, as a solidifying agent. Concentrations of 1–2% are used for plating media; concentrations of 0.05–0.3% are used for semisolid motility media; and trace amounts are added to anaerobic broth media to prevent convection currents and oxygen penetration. Sodium thiosulfate is commonly added to provide a source of sulfur.

Selective Isolation Media

In 1905 MacConkey[297] first described a selective differential medium (neutral red–bile salt agar) that he used to isolate gram-negative enteric bacilli from specimens containing mixtures of bacterial species. He incorporated lactose and the indicator neutral red into this medium to provide a visual means for detecting lactose utilization by the test organism. At that time, all non-spore-forming, gram-negative bacilli were still referred to as enteric organisms; however, microbiologists had recognized that certain species were more pathogenic to humans than others. The carbohydrate-utilization patterns of several species of bacteria were already known by the turn of the century, and the fermentation of lactose, in particular, was recognized as an important marker for differentiating certain enteric pathogens. Holt-Harris and Teague[227] in 1916 described a medium with eosin and methylene blue as indicators for differentiating between lactose-fermenting and non–lactose-fermenting colonies. Sucrose was included in the medium to detect members of the coliform group that ferment sucrose more readily than lactose.

MacConkey and EMB agars are only moderately inhibitory and are designed primarily to prevent growth of gram-positive bacteria from mixed cultures. Many species of fastidious gram-negative organisms are inhibited as well; however, all *Enterobacteriaceae* grow well. Table 6-1 compares the formulas, inhibitory ingredients, and key differential characteristics for MacConkey and EMB agars. Recently, a new formulation of MacConkey agar, MacConkey III, was developed by researchers at Becton-Dickinson to improve recovery of CO_2-sensitive *Enterobacteriaceae*. Although aerobic incubation is recommended for MacConkey agar, it has become common in many clinical microbiology laboratories to incubate all primary plates including MacConkey agar in a 5% CO_2 incubator in order to keep all plates together. The problem with this is that some strains of *Enterobacteriaceae* may fail to grow or show partial inhibition when incubated in CO_2 because of a decrease in pH of the medium. In one study, MacConkey III was shown to provide superior recovery and colony size in both air and CO_2 incubation to a comparator MacConkey agar.[270]

Deciding whether to use MacConkey or EMB agar is largely a matter of personal preference, because bacterial species that use lactose can be differentiated on both. MacConkey agar contains neutral red as the pH indicator and, as a result, lactose-metabolizing colonies appear pink from the production of mixed acids (see Color Plate 6-2*A* and *B*). Strong acid-producing bacteria, such as *E. coli*, form deep red colonies with a diffuse pink precipitate in the agar surrounding the colonies caused by precipitation of the bile salts in the medium that occurs at a low pH (see Color Plate 6-2*A*). Weaker acid-producing bacteria form light-pink colonies or colonies that are clear at the periphery and have pink centers, with the agar surrounding the colonies remaining clear (see Color Plate 6-1*C*). On EMB agar, strong acid-producing bacteria form colonies that have a metallic sheen (see Color Plate 6-2*C* and *D*). The appearance of the sheen, caused by precipitation of dye in the colonies, is highly suggestive of *E. coli*, although other strong acid producers, such as *Yersinia enterocolitica*, may have a similar appearance.

Highly Selective Isolation Media Used Primarily for Gastrointestinal Specimens

Media are made highly selective by the addition of a variety of inhibitors to their formulas, generally in higher concentrations than in MacConkey and EMB agars. These media are used primarily to inhibit the growth of *E. coli* and other ''coliforms,'' but they allow *Salmonella* and *Shigella* species to grow out from stool specimens.

Several selective media formulated for use in clinical laboratories are discussed here. The most commonly used are *Salmonella–Shigella* (SS) agar, xylose lysine deoxycholate (XLD) agar, and Hektoen enteric (HE) agar. These are described in Table 6-2.

Deciding which of these selective media to use for the recovery of enteric pathogens from fecal specimens depends both on personal preference and on the species to be selected. In general, these media are used in the clinical laboratory for the recovery of *Salmonella* and *Shigella* species from diarrheal stool specimens, or in public health laboratories to investigate possible fecal contamination of food and water supplies. Virtually all species of *Salmonella* grow well in the presence of bile salts, which explains why the gallbladder often serves as one reservoir for human carriers. Bile salts are added to selective media because other species of enteric bacilli, including some of the more fastidious strains of *Shigella*, grow poorly or not at all. SS and HE agars contain relatively high concentrations of bile salts and are well adapted for recovering *Salmonella* species from specimens heavily contaminated with other coliform bacilli. However, because of its inhibitory effect on the recovery of certain strains of *Shigella* species, the routine use of SS agar as a single selective medium for isolation of enteric pathogens from stool specimens is not recommended.

XLD agar contains lactose, sucrose, and xylose[471]; thus, microorganisms that ferment these carbohydrates form yellow colonies (see Color Plate 6-3A). Bacteria incapable of fermenting these carbohydrates do not produce acids and form colorless colonies (see Color Plate 6-3B). Organisms that produce hydrogen sulfide form black pigment beginning in the center of the colonies (see Color Plate 6-3C). XLD agar also contains lysine. This is important because many species of *Salmonella* will ferment xylose and, therefore, will initially produce yellow colonies on XLD, but because these same species also decarboxylate lysine, the colonies will revert to pink after the small amount of xylose in the medium is used up. Lactose and sucrose, added in excess, prevent lysine-positive coliforms from similarly reverting. Because the decarboxylation of lysine results in the formation of strongly alkaline amines, a light pink halo may appear around the colonies on XLD agar (see Color Plate 6-3C). Black colonies without a pink halo are more suggestive of a hydrogen sulfide–producing strain of *Proteus* species (see Color Plate 6-3D).

The carbohydrates in HE agar are lactose, sucrose, and salicin.[269] Microorganisms capable of fermenting these carbohydrates also form yellow colonies (see Color Plate 6-3E); asaccharolytic strains produce colonies that are translu-

cent or light green (see Color Plate 6-3F). Lactose- and sucrose-negative bacteria that acidify salicin may produce orange colonies. HE agar also contains ferric salts; thus hydrogen sulfide–producing colonies appear black. Bismuth sulfite and brilliant green agars are highly selective media that are not commonly used in clinical laboratories. They are difficult to prepare, and their shelf life is very short (48 to 72 hours). These media are specifically designed to recover *Salmonella typhi* from fecal specimens and are particularly useful when screening numerous patients in endemic areas or during an epidemic. *Salmonella* species (*S. typhi* in particular) can be suspected on these media because of the propensity to produce colonies with a black sheen.

Enrichment Media

As the name indicates, an enrichment medium is used to enhance the growth of certain bacterial species while inhibiting the development of unwanted microorganisms. Enrichment media are most commonly used in clinical laboratories for the recovery of *Salmonella* and *Shigella* species from fecal specimens. Enrichment broths are particularly helpful in the recovery of organisms from the stools of *Salmonella* carriers or from patients with light *Shigella* infections in whom the number of organisms may be as low as 200 per gram of feces. (*E. coli* and other enteric bacilli may reach massive concentrations, as high as 10^9 per gram of feces.)

Enrichment media work on the principle that *E. coli* and other gram-negative organisms, which constitute the normal fecal flora, are maintained in a prolonged **lag** phase by the inhibitory chemicals in the broth. *Salmonella* and *Shigella* species are far less inhibited, enter into a log phase of growth, and are more readily recovered from fecal samples. However, after several hours, the enrichment media no longer suppress the growth of *E. coli* and other enteric organisms, which will ultimately overgrow the culture. Thus, for maximal recovery of *Salmonella* and *Shigella* species from fecal samples, it is recommended that the enrichment broth be subcultured within 8 hours.

The two most commonly used enrichment media are selenite broth and gram-negative (GN) broth. Selenite broth is more inhibitory to the growth of *E. coli* and other enteric gram-negative bacilli than is GN broth. Thus, selenite broth is best adapted for the recovery of *Salmonella* or *Shigella* species from heavily contaminated specimens, such as feces or sewage. However, GN broth is used with greater frequency in clinical laboratories because it is less inhibitory to the growth of many of the more fastidious strains of *Shigella* species. Enrichment of fecal specimens in GN broth for 4 to 6 hours and then subculturing to HE or XLD agar is the optimal technique for the recovery of *Shigella* species in suspected cases of bacillary dysentery. The formulas and salient characteristics of these two enrichment media are summarized in Table 6-3.

Guidelines for Choosing Selective Isolation Media

The media listed in Tables 6-1 through 6-3 and the several combinations in which they can be used may be somewhat

Table 6-3 Enrichment Broths for Recovery of *Enterobacteriaceae*

BROTH	FORMULATION		PURPOSE AND DIFFERENTIAL INGREDIENTS	REACTIONS AND INTERPRETATION
Selenite broth	Peptone	5 g	Selenite F broth is recommended for the isolation of salmonellae from specimens—such as feces, urine, or sewage—that have heavy concentrations of mixed bacteria.	Within a few hours after inoculation with the specimen, the broth becomes cloudy.
	Lactose	4 g		Because coliforms or other intestinal flora may overgrow the pathogens within a few hours, subculture to *Salmonella–Shigella* (SS) agar or bismuth sulfite is recommended within 8–12 hr.
	Sodium selenite	4 g	Sodium selenite is inhibitory to *Escherichia coli* and other coliform bacilli, including many strains of *Shigella*.	
	Sodium phosphate	10 g		
	Distilled water to Final pH, 7.0	1 L	The medium functions best under anaerobic conditions, and a pour depth of at least 5 cm (2 in.) is recommended.	Overheating of the broth during preparation may produce a visible precipitate, making it unsatisfactory for use.
Gram-negative (GN) broth	Polypeptone peptone	20 g	Because of the relatively low concentration of deoxycholate, GN broth is less inhibitory to *E. coli* and other coliforms. Most strains of *Shigella* grow well. The deoxycholate and citrate are inhibitory to gram-positive bacteria.	GN broth is designed for the recovery of *Salmonella* and *Shigella* species when they are in small numbers in fecal specimens.
	Glucose	1 g		
	D-mannitol	2 g		
	Sodium citrate	5 g		The broth may become cloudy within 4–6 hr of inoculation, and subculture to HE agar or XLD agar within that time is recommended.
	Sodium deoxycholate	0.5 g	The increased concentration of mannitol over glucose limits the growth of *Proteus* species, nonetheless encouraging growth of *Salmonella* and *Shigella* species, both of which are capable of fermenting mannitol.	
	Dipotassium phosphate	4 g		
	Monopotassium phosphate	1.5 g		
	Sodium chloride	5 g		
	Distilled water to Final pH, 7.0	1 L		

confusing. The following is a guide for selecting media that may be optimal in the recovery of the *Enterobacteriaceae* from clinical specimens.

For specimens other than feces or rectal swabs, a combination of MacConkey or EMB agar and a blood agar is usually sufficient. Media with greater inhibitory properties are not routinely required because the concentration of commensal flora or contaminating organisms is relatively low in most nonenteric specimens. Subculturing to a more inhibitory medium can be done in instances in which it appears necessary.

For fecal specimens or rectal swabs, it is necessary to select only one medium from each of the groups listed in Tables 6-1 and 6-2. The approach outlined in Box 6-4 is suggested.

Differential Identification Characteristics

Although a preliminary identification of the *Enterobacteriaceae* is possible based on colony characteristics and biochemical reactions on primary isolation media, further species identification requires the determination of additional phenotypic characteristics that reflect the genetic code and unique identity of the organism being tested. It is the purpose of this discussion to review the salient features of the tests that measure these phenotypic characteristics and are commonly used in clinical laboratories. This orientation is necessary so that laboratory personnel can develop a fundamental understanding of the principles behind these procedures in order to recognize and correct any biochemical inconsisten-

---

Box 6-4 Selecting a Medium for Fecal Specimen or Rectal Swab

1. Inoculate the specimen directly to a MacConkey or EMB agar plate for primary isolation of all species of enteric gram-negative bacilli.
2. Directly inoculate either an XLD or an HE agar plate for the selective screening of *Salmonella* or *Shigella* species.
3. Enrich a small portion of the specimen by heavily inoculating either selenite or GN broth. If selenite is used, subculture to HE agar within 8 to 12 hours; if GN is used, subculture within 4 hours. *Note:* In the author's laboratory this step is not routinely performed unless screening asymptomatic patients for presence of a carrier state.
4. Incubate all plate cultures at 35°C for 24 to 48 hours. Select suspicious colonies for definitive biochemical or serologic testing.

Box 6-5 Tests Used To Measure Metabolic Characteristics of *Enterobacteriaceae*

Carbohydrate utilization
o-Nitrophenyl-β-D-galactopyranoside (ONPG) activity
Indole production
Methyl red
Voges-Proskauer test (production of acetyl methyl carbinol [acetoin])
Citrate utilization
Urease production
Decarboxylation of lysine, ornithine, and arginine
Phenylalanine deaminase production
Hydrogen sulfide production
Motility

---

cies, problems with mixed cultures, or faulty techniques. It is not possible to discuss the variety of differential tests and numerous schemes available for the final species identification of the *Enterobacteriaceae*. However, several of the tests widely used in clinical laboratories to measure the metabolic characteristics by which all but a few rare or atypical species of the *Enterobacteriaceae* can be identified are listed in Box 6-5. Carbohydrate utilization and ONPG activity have been discussed previously.

Indole Production

Indole is one of the degradation products from the metabolism of the amino acid tryptophan. Bacteria that possess the enzyme tryptophanase are capable of cleaving tryptophan, thereby producing indole, pyruvic acid, and ammonia. Indole can be detected in tryptophan test medium by observing the development of a red color after adding a solution containing *p*-dimethylaminobenzaldehyde (e.g., Ehrlich's or Kovac's reagent). The biochemistry and details of the indole test are schematically illustrated in Figure 6-5 and Chart 1-4, respectively. A color reproduction is shown in Color Plate 6-4*C*.

The choice between Ehrlich's and Kovac's reagents is one of personal preference. Ehrlich's reagent is more sensitive and is preferred when testing nonfermentative bacilli or anaerobes in which indole production is minimal. Because indole is soluble in organic compounds, xylene or chloroform should be added to the test medium before adding Ehrlich's reagent. This extraction step is less critical for Kovac's reagent because amyl alcohol is used for the diluent (ethyl alcohol is used with Ehrlich's reagent).

Methyl Red Test

A simplified schema showing only two alternative pathways (mixed acid and butylene glycol) for the metabolism of the pyruvate formed from the fermentation of glucose is shown in Figure 6-2. Bacteria that follow primarily the mixed acid fermentation route often produce sufficient acid to maintain a pH below 4.4 (the acid color breakpoint of the

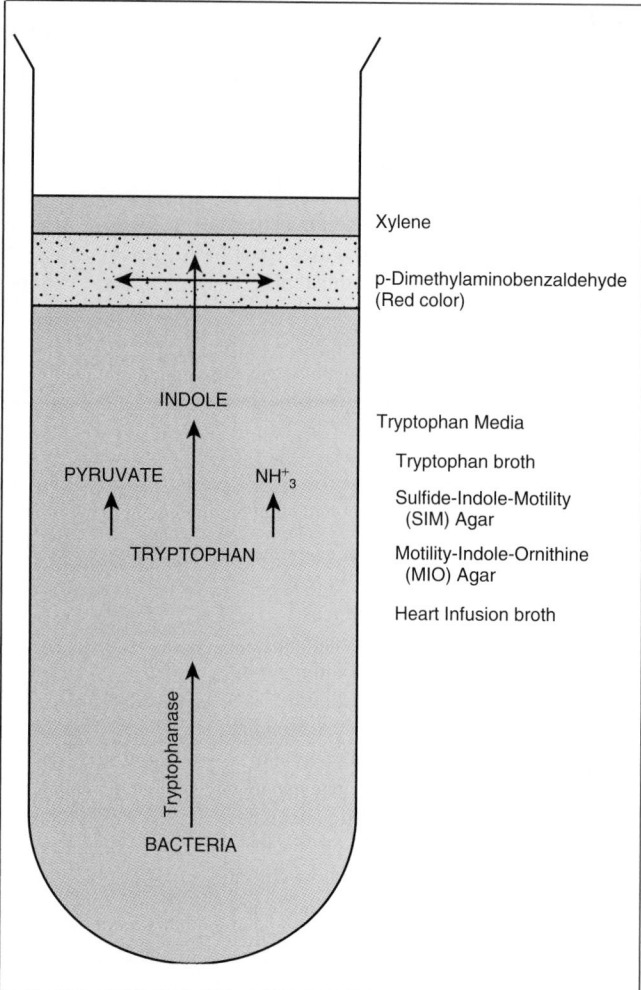

Figure 6-5 Formation of indole by tryptophanase-producing bacteria growing on a culture medium containing tryptophan. Indole is one of the immediate degradation products (in addition to pyruvic acid and ammonia) resulting from the deamination of tryptophan. Indole can be extracted from the aqueous phase of the medium by chloroform and detected by the addition of Ehrlich's reagent (dimethylaminobenzaldehyde).

methyl red indicator). The methyl red test provides a valuable characteristic for identifying bacterial species that produce strong acids from glucose.

The details of the methyl red test are shown in Chart 6-3. The test, as originally described, requires 48 to 72 hours of incubation before a valid result can be obtained, an amount of time unacceptable to most clinical microbiology laboratories. Barry and coworkers[30] have described a modification that can be read in 18 to 24 hours. A 0.5-mL aliquot of broth is used with a relatively heavy inoculum of the test organism. One or two drops of methyl red reagent are added after 18 to 24 hours of incubation at 35°C, and the development of red color indicates a positive test (see Color Plate 6-4*C*). The Barry modification is as accurate as the test originally described and saves a significant amount of time.

Voges-Proskauer Test

The details of the Voges-Proskauer test, shown in Chart 6-4, are based on the conversion of acetyl methyl carbinol (acetoin) to diacetyl through the action of potassium hydroxide and atmospheric oxygen. Diacetyl is converted into a red complex under the catalytic action of α-naphthol and creatine (see Color Plate 6-4D).

Note, in Figure 6-2, that the formation of acetoin and butylene glycol is an alternative pathway for the metabolism of pyruvic acid. Bacteria that use this pathway, such as certain strains within the *Klebsiella–Enterobacter–Serratia–Hafnia* group, produce only small quantities of mixed acids that may be insufficient to lower the pH of the methyl red medium enough to produce a color change. Consequently, most species of the *Enterobacteriaceae* that are Voges-Proskauer-positive, with rare exceptions, are methyl red–negative and vice versa (see Color Plate 6-4C and D).

Citrate Utilization

The principle of the citrate-utilization test (Chart 6-5) is to determine the ability of an organism to use sodium citrate as the sole source of carbon for metabolism and growth. The original formula, described by Koser[2] in 1923, was a broth medium containing sodium ammonium phosphate, monopotassium phosphate, magnesium sulfate, and sodium citrate. Proteins and carbohydrates were omitted as carbon and nitrogen sources. The end point of the Koser test was either the presence or lack of visible turbidity after incubation of the test organism: this end point was actually a measure of the organism's ability to use carbon from sodium citrate to produce sufficient growth to become visible. It was soon recognized, however, that nonspecific turbidity could occur in Koser's medium. Simmons[450] resolved this problem by adding agar and bromthymol blue to the Koser formula, which provided a more sensitive color end point. Simmons citrate agar medium is poured into a test tube and slanted. A light inoculum from a colony of growth of the test organism is streaked onto the surface of the agar slant. If the inoculum is too heavy, preformed organic compounds within the cell walls of dying bacteria may release sufficient carbon and nitrogen to produce a false-positive test result. When inoculating a series of tubes of differential culture media with an unknown organism, it is important that the citrate medium be streaked first to prevent carryover of proteins or carbohydrates from the other media.

The production of a blue color in the test medium after 24 hours of incubation at 35°C indicates the presence of alkaline products and a positive citrate-utilization test result (see Color Plate 6-4D). If carbon is used from sodium citrate, nitrogen is also extracted from the ammonium phosphate contained in the medium, releasing ammonia. Occasionally, visible growth is detected along the streak line before conversion of the medium to a blue color. This visible growth also indicates a positive test result. Malonate, acetate, and mucate are other anionic radicals commonly used to determine the ability of bacteria to use these simple compounds as a sole source of carbon.

The acronym IMViC (indole, methyl red, Voges-Proskauer, and citrate) was once used by sanitarians and epidemiologists to refer to the tests needed to detect fecal contamination of food and water. Public health officials have used *Escherichia coli* for many years to indicate fecal contamination. *Enterobacter aerogenes* produces colonies on primary isolation media that often cannot be distinguished from *E. coli*. However, the recovery of *E. aerogenes* from food and potable water does not necessarily signify fecal contamination because the organism is widespread in soil, grasses, and vegetative matter. Therefore, a set of biochemical characteristics was needed to differentiate the two organisms. The IMViC tests were adopted to serve this purpose. Most strains of *E. coli* are indole- and methyl red–positive, with Voges-Proskauer and citrate being negative. *E. aerogenes* typically produces exactly opposite reactions (see Color Plates 6-4C and D). Although the individual characteristics included in the IMViC battery are still used in bacterial identification systems, they are used only infrequently as a specific test set.

In view of the complexity of differentiating over 100 species of *Enterobacteriaceae* presented in the next section, it is interesting that there was a time when the major decisions in microbiology were relatively simple and could be made on the basis of only four easy-to-perform biochemical tests.

Urease Production

Microorganisms that possess the enzyme urease hydrolyze urea, releasing ammonia and producing a pink-red color change in the medium (see Color Plate 6-4E). The details of the urease test are shown in Chart 6-6.

Important differences between Stuart's urea broth and Christensen's urea agar should be noted. Stuart's broth is heavily buffered with phosphate salts at a pH of 6.8. Relatively large quantities of ammonia must be formed by the test organism before the buffer system is overcome and the medium's pH is elevated above 8.0 to produce a color change in the indicator. Stuart's broth, therefore, is virtually selective for *Proteus* species.

Christensen's urea agar[113] is less buffered than Stuart's urea broth and contains peptones and glucose. This enriched medium supports the growth of many species of bacteria that cannot grow in Stuart's broth, and the decreased buffer capacity permits the detection of smaller amounts of ammonia. Organisms that produce less urease, such as certain species of *Klebsiella, Enterobacter, Brucella,* and *Bordetella bronchiseptica,* can be tested with Christensen's urea agar. For many of these species, a positive urease reaction is first detected by a pink-to-red color change in the slant portion of the agar (see Color Plate 6-4E). The slant initially turns red because the alkaline reaction, resulting from the splitting of small quantities of urea, is augmented by the amines formed from the oxidative decarboxylation of the amino acids in the air-exposed portion of the medium.

Decarboxylation of Lysine, Ornithine, and Arginine

Many species of bacteria possess enzymes capable of decarboxylating specific amino acids in the test medium. The decarboxylase enzymes remove a molecule of CO_2 from an amino acid to form alkaline-reacting amines. The following are the amino acids most commonly tested and their amine degradation products:

Lysine → cadaverine

Ornithine → putrescine

Arginine → citrulline

A number of test systems have been described to measure this property, based on either detection of an alkaline pH shift in the test medium or direct measurement of the reaction products. For example, the amines resulting from the decarboxylation reaction can be detected with Ninhydrin reagent after extraction from the broth culture with chloroform. This is the relatively sensitive Carlquist reaction,[67] most commonly used for detecting the weak decarboxylase activity of many of the nonfermentative gram-negative bacilli and certain species of anaerobic bacteria.

The decarboxylase activity of the *Enterobacteriaceae* is most commonly measured in clinical microbiology laboratories with Møller decarboxylase broth.[328] The details of this test are shown in Chart 6-7. The end point of the reaction is the production of an alkaline pH shift in the medium and the development of a blue-purple color after incubation with the test organism (see Color Plate 6-4F). Note, in the Møller formula, included in Chart 6-7, that the medium is buffered at pH 6.0. This is more acidic than most culture media. This low pH is necessary because the decarboxylase enzymes are not optimally active until the pH of the medium drops below 5.5. The drop from 6.0 to 5.5 results from the growing bacteria that metabolize the small amount of glucose in the medium to produce mixed acids. A control tube, devoid of amino acid, must always be included when performing the decarboxylase test to ensure that this initial drop in pH has occurred. A yellow color change in the bromcresol purple indicator of the control tube shows acidification. Pyridoxal phosphate is included in the medium and acts as a coenzyme to further enhance the decarboxylase activity.

Many microbiologists prefer Falkow lysine broth[162] over the Møller medium because the Falkow test depends on only an alkaline shift in pH indicator, and neither an anaerobic nor an acid environment is required. However, this medium cannot be used to detect lysine decarboxylase activity in certain members of the *Klebsiella–Enterobacter–Serratia–Hafnia* group. They produce acetyl methyl carbinol, which interferes with the final alkaline pH shift, leading to false-negative interpretations. Modifications in this medium form the basis of the motility indole ornithine (MIO)[148] semisolid agar used in clinical microbiology laboratories. Rapid methods for detecting ornithine[171] and lysine[60] decarboxylase activity in members of the *Enterobacteriaceae* have also been described.

Edwards and Fife[150] described a solid lysine decarboxylase medium based on the Falkow formula, which includes ferric ammonium citrate and thiosulfate for the detection of hydrogen sulfide. This medium is lysine iron agar (LIA), used in many laboratories as an aid in the identification of *Salmonella* species, most of which are both hydrogen sulfide–positive and lysine decarboxylase–positive. A black deep and a purple slant with LIA are virtually indicative of *Salmonella* species. Another advantage of LIA is that *Proteus* and *Providencia* species, both of which deaminate, rather than decarboxylate, amino acids, can be detected by the development of a red color in the slant of the tube (see Color Plate 6-4G).

The lysine decarboxylase test is useful in differentiating lactose-negative *Citrobacter* species (0% positive) from *Salmonella* species (98% positive). Almost all strains of *Shigella sonnei* (more than 98%) possess ornithine decarboxylase activity, whereas only a few strains of *S. boydii* (2.5%) show such activity; *S. dysenteriae* and *S. flexneri* are ornithine-negative. The ornithine decarboxylase test is perhaps most useful in differentiating *Klebsiella* species (most species are negative) from *Enterobacter* species (most strains are positive).

Phenylalanine Deaminase Production

The phenylalanine deaminase determination is useful in the initial differentiation of *Proteus*, *Morganella*, and *Providencia* species from other gram-negative bacilli. Only members of these genera, and a few relatively rare isolates of the *Enterobacter* group, possess the enzyme responsible for the oxidative deamination of phenylalanine. The test is easily performed, as outlined in Chart 6-8. Phenylpyruvic acid may be detected in as little as 4 hours if a heavy inoculum is used; however, 18 to 24 hours of incubation are generally recommended. The phenylalanine test medium uses yeast extract as the source for carbon and nitrogen. Meat extracts or protein hydrolysates contain varying amounts of naturally occurring phenylalanine that can lead to inconsistent results. The development of a green color after addition of the ferric chloride reagent is immediate and easy to visualize (see Color Plate 6-4E).

Hydrogen Sulfide Production

The ability of certain bacterial species to liberate sulfur from sulfur-containing amino acids or other compounds in the form of H_2S is an important characteristic for their identification. The media most commonly used for the detection of H_2S and the sources for sulfur and the sulfide indicators are listed in Table 6-4. The sequence of steps leading to the production and detection of H_2S in a test system is outlined in Box 6-6.

The differences in detecting H_2S production in the different media result from alteration in one or more of these conditions. H_2S detected in one medium may not be detected in another, and it is necessary to know the test system used when interpreting identification charts. SIM medium is more sensitive than KIA for the detection of H_2S, presumably because of KIA's semisolid consistency, lack of carbohydrates to suppress H_2S formation, and use of peptonized iron as the indicator (see Color Plate 6-4B). KIA, on the other

Table 6-4 Media for the Detection of Hydrogen Sulfide (H_2S)

MEDIA	SULFUR SOURCE	H_2S INDICATOR
Bismuth sulfite	Peptones plus sulfite	Ferrous sulfate
Citrate sulfide agar	Sodium thiosulfate	Ferric ammonium citrate
Deoxycholate citrate agar	Peptones	Ferric citrate
Lysine iron agar	Sodium thiosulfate	Ferric ammonium citrate
Kligler iron agar	Sodium thiosulfate	Ferrous sulfate
Triple sugar iron agar	Sodium thiosulfate	Ferrous sulfate
Lead acetate agar	Sodium thiosulfate	Lead acetate
Salmonella–Shigella agar	Sodium thiosulfate	Ferric citrate
Sulfide–indole–motility medium	Sodium thiosulfate	Peptonized iron
Xylose–lysine–deoxycholate or Hektoen enteric	Sodium thiosulfate	Ferric ammonium citrate

hand, is more sensitive than TSI agar because sucrose is believed to suppress the enzyme mechanisms responsible for H_2S production. Lead acetate is the most sensitive indicator and should be used whenever bacteria that produce only trace amounts of H_2S are tested. Unfortunately, lead acetate, when incorporated in culture media, also inhibits the growth of many fastidious bacteria, specifically the ones that may require a sensitive detection system. These organisms can be tested for production of H_2S by draping a lead acetate–impregnated filter paper strip under the cap of a culture tube of KIA medium. In this way, the extreme sensitivity of the lead acetate indicator can be used without incorporating it directly into the medium.

With all H_2S detection systems, the end point is an insoluble, heavy metal sulfide, which produces a black precipitate in the medium or on the filter paper strip. Because hydrogen ions must be available for H_2S formation, the blackening is first seen in test media in which acid formation is maximal, that is, along the inoculation line, within the deeps of slanted agar media, or in the centers of colonies growing on agar surfaces.

Motility

Bacterial motility is another important determinant in making a final species identification. Bacteria move by means of flagella, the number and location of which vary among the different species. Flagellar stains are available for this determination (see Chapter 7).

Bacterial motility can be observed directly by placing a drop of culture broth medium on a microscope slide and viewing it under a microscope. Hanging-drop chambers are available so that the preparation can be viewed under higher magnification without danger of lowering the objectives onto the contaminated drop. This technique is used primarily for detecting the motility of bacteria species that do not grow well in semisolid agar media. However, *Enterobacteriaceae* do grow well, and tubes containing semisolid agar are most commonly used.

Motility media have agar concentrations of 0.4% or less. At higher concentrations, the gel is too firm to allow the organisms to spread freely. Combination media, such as SIM medium[298] or MIO agar[148] have found wide use in clinical microbiology laboratories because more than one characteristic can be measured in the same tube. The motility test must be interpreted first because the addition of an indole reagent may obscure the results. Because SIM medium and MIO agar have a slightly turbid background, interpretations may be somewhat difficult with bacterial species that grow slowly in these media. In these cases, a motility test medium (Box 6-7) is recommended because it supports the growth of most fastidious bacteria and has a crystal-clear appearance.

The motility test is interpreted by making a macroscopic examination of the medium for a diffuse zone of growth

---

Box 6-6 How H_2S Is Produced

1. Release of sulfide from cysteine or thiosulfate by bacterial enzymatic action
2. Coupling of sulfide (S^{2-}) with a hydrogen ion (H^1) to form H_2S
3. Detection of H_2S by iron, bismuth, or lead to produce insoluble, heavy metal sulfides that appear as a black precipitate

---

Box 6-7 Motility Test Medium (Edwards and Ewing)

Beef extract, 3 g	Agar, 4 g
Peptone, 10 g	Distilled water to equal 1 L
Sodium chloride, 5 g	Final pH, 7.3

flaring out from the line of inoculation (see Color Plate 6-4*H*). The use of tetrazolium salts in motility medium has been advocated as an aid in the visual detection of bacterial growth. Tetrazolium salts are colorless but are converted into insoluble red formazan complexes by the reducing properties of growing bacteria. In a motility test medium containing tetrazolium, the development of this red color helps trace the spread of bacteria from the inoculation line. However, these salts may inhibit certain fastidious bacteria and cannot be used in all cases. Of the *Enterobacteriaceae*, species of *Shigella* and *Klebsiella* are uniformly nonmotile. Most motile species of the *Enterobacteriaceae* can be detected at 35°C; however, *Yersinia enterocolitica*, in which flagellar proteins develop more rapidly at lower temperatures, is motile at 22°C (room temperature) but not at 35°C. *Listeria monocytogenes* is another bacterial species that requires room-temperature incubation before motility develops. *Pseudomonas aeruginosa*, an organism that grows well only in the presence of oxygen, produces a spreading film on the surface of motility agar and does not show the characteristic fanning out from the inoculation line because it does not grow in the deeper oxygen-deficient portions of the tube.

Taxonomy of the Enterobacteriaceae

The application of new technologies to study the taxonomy of microorganisms has led to a rapid increase in the number of genera and species of bacteria that fit the general criteria for *Enterobacteriaceae*. In 1972, Edwards and Ewing[149] described 11 genera and 26 species belonging to the *Enterobacteriaceae*. In 1985, Farmer and associates[165] described 22 genera comprising 69 species and 29 enteric groups. In this chapter, 31 genera and 139 species, biogroups, and unnamed enteric groups of *Enterobacteriaceae* are described.

Classification of *Enterobacteriaceae* by Tribes

The division of the *Enterobacteriaceae* into tribes is not used in the current edition of *Bergey's Manual* or in the Centers for Disease Control and Prevention (CDC) classification because the authors believe that the use of tribes is of no diagnostic significance and of questionable taxonomic significance. This argument has validity from the perspective of pure classification. Yet, for the users of this book who are new to the field of microbiology and who must orient themselves to the complex and confusing *Enterobacteriaceae*, the tribe concept proposed by Ewing[157] has certain teaching and learning advantages. We agree with Ewing that his scheme, although imperfect, represents a good compromise between practical and ideal taxonomies.

The tribe concept provides both students and practitioners with a convenient method of grouping together the major genera within the family that share similar biochemical reactions and are of similar diagnostic importance. We believe it is important that practicing microbiologists maintain a base of knowledge that is firmly grounded in the morphology, physiology, and biochemistry of medically important bacteria. Furthermore, certain phenotypic pat-

terns that allow easy subgrouping and clustering of related species must be committed to memory. This orientation is especially important if microbiologists use semiautomated and automated commercial systems with computer-assisted identification, because it serves as a quality control to validate instrument-generated information. The use of the tribe concept as an approach to learning the *Enterobacteriaceae* serves these goals well and is the approach chosen for use in this textbook for teaching the key features of the established genera of the *Enterobacteriaceae*. The current species included in the established genera, sorted by tribes, are listed in Table 6-5.

Key Identification Characteristics for the Most Common Species

Table 6-6 shows the key identification characteristics used in separating the established genera of the *Enterobacteriaceae* into seven tribes. Students should study this table and learn to categorize an unknown isolate into one of these tribes on the basis of reactions seen with these key tests. The following observations are made to assist students in identifying the most common species.

The members of the *Escherichieae* have the following key reactions: indole-positive, methyl red–positive, Voges-Proskauer–negative, citrate-negative (the classic example of mixed acid fermenters). They are negative for all the other key biochemical tests: hydrogen sulfide, phenylalanine deaminase, and urea. Note from Table 6-6 that *Shigella* species are similar to *Escherichia* species except they are negative for CO_2 gas and motility.

The *Edwardsielleae* are similar to *Escherichieae* except for the property of being hydrogen sulfide–positive. Students may wish to think of *Edwardsiella tarda* as hydrogen sulfide–positive *E. coli*. *Salmonelleae* resemble *Edwardsielleae* except that they are indole-negative and citrate-positive. *Citrobacter freundii* is similar to *Salmonella* except for being lysine-negative. *C. koseri* differs from *C. freundii* by being hydrogen sulfide–negative and indole-positive.

The *Klebsielleae* are composed of the Voges-Proskauer–positive members of the *Enterobacteriaceae*. As shown in Table 6-6 and illustrated in Figure 6-2, most members of this tribe produce copious amounts of CO_2, so much so that the deep portion of KIA and TSI slants is often pushed halfway up the tube. Notice that the *Klebsiella* species are nonmotile and that *Pantoea* is triple decarboxylase-negative (lysine-negative, arginine-negative, and ornithine-negative).

The *Proteeae* are separated from all others by virtue of being phenylalanine deaminase–positive, a feature unique to this tribe. The urea reaction for the species in the genus *Proteus* and *Morganella* as well as one of the *Providencia* species (*P. rettgeri*) is strongly positive. Both species of *Proteus* listed in Table 6-6 are hydrogen sulfide–positive and exhibit swarming motility.

The *Yersinieae* represented here by the most commonly isolated species, *Y. enterocolitica*, are very similar to members of the *Escherichieae*, except that *Y. enterocolitica* is usually urea-positive. Students may wish to think of *Y. enterocolitica* as urea-positive *E. coli*. Note that the motility for *Y. enterocolitica* is negative at 36°C but positive at 22°C.

Table 6-5 Important Recent Changes in the Established Genera of the *Enterobacteriaceae*

NEW DESIGNATION	PREVIOUS DESIGNATION	COMMENTS
Tribe I: *Escherichieae*		
Escherichia coli		Sorbitol (+) except for serotype O157:H7. All other species are sorbitol (−).
Escherichia coli inactive	Alkalescens-Dispar	Anaerogenic, lactose-negative (or delayed) and non-motile.
Escherichia albertii	New species	Associated with diarrheal disease in Bangladeshi children. Indole-negative, ferments D-mannitol but not D-xylose. Separated from *H. alvei* by negative VP test.
Escherichia blattae		Not found in human specimens.
		Isolated from cockroach feces.
Escherichia fergusonii	Enteric group 10	Found in blood, urine, and feces. Indole (+), Sorbitol (−), LAO (+,−,+), lactose (−) but ONPG (+).
Escherichia hermanii	Enteric group 11	Wounds and feces most common sources. Yellow pigmented, indole (+), sorbitol (−), LAO (−,−,+).
Escherichia vulneris	Enteric group 1 API group 2 Alma group 1	Most strains from human wounds. Over half the strains are yellow-pigmented.
Shigella		The four species of *Shigella* and *E. coli* form a single species on the basis of DNA hybridization. *S. dysenteriae* (Group A), *S. flexneri* (Group B), and *S. boydii* (Group C) are biochemically similar and must be separated by serologic methods. *S. sonnei* is ornithine (+).
Tribe II: *Edwardsielleae*		
Edwardsiella tarda	*Edwardsiella anguillimortifera* Asakusa group	Produce indole and abundant H_2S, ferment glucose and maltose but not mannitol, lactose, sucrose, or arabinose. Found in cold-blooded animals. Opportunistic human pathogen. May cause wound infections and diarrhea.
Edwardsiella tarda biogroup 1		Indole (+), H_2S (−), mannitol-, sucrose-, and arabinose-positive. Found in snakes, not a human clinical isolate.
Edwardsiella hoshinae		Indole (−), H_2S (−), isolated from birds, reptiles, and water. Several isolates from human feces.
Edwardsiella ictaluri		No human isolates, causes enteric septicemia in catfish.
Tribe III: *Salmonelleae*		
Salmonella	*S. cholerae-suis* *S. typhi* *S. enteritidis*	All subgroups (subgenera) of *Salmonella* and *Arizonae* are considered to belong to the same species. Organisms are now reported by genus and serotype, omitting reference to species.
Tribe IV: *Citrobactereae*		
Citrobacter amalonaticus	*Levinea amalonaticus*	H_2S (−), indole (+), adonitol (−), malonate (−). Found primarily in human feces, very rarely isolated from blood.
Citrobacter braakii	*Citrobacter* genomospecies 6	H_2S and indole are variable, adonitol (−), malonate (−). Isolated from human stool, urine, and wounds and from animals and food.
Citrobacter farmeri	*Citrobacter amalonaticus* biogroup 1	Found primarily in human feces. Stains of biogroup 1 ferment sucrose, raffinose, alpha-methyl-D-glucoside, and melibiose and are citrate (−). *C. amalonaticus* usually have the opposite reactions.
Citrobacter freundii		H_2S (+), indole (−), adonitol (−), malonate (−). Found in urine, throat, sputum, blood, and wounds.

(Continued)

Table 6-5 *Continued*

NEW DESIGNATION	PREVIOUS DESIGNATION	COMMENTS
Citrobacter gillenii	*Citrobacter* genomospecies 10	H_2S is variable, indole (−), adonitol (−), malonate (+). Found in human stool and food.
Citrobacter koseri	*Levinea malonatica* *Citrobacter diversus*	H_2S (−), indole (+), adonitol (+), malonate (+). Found in urine, throat, nose, sputum, and wounds. Rare cause of neonatal meningitis.
Citrobacter murliniae	*Citrobacter* genomospecies 11	H_2S is variable, indole (+), adonitol (−), malonate (−). Found in human stool and blood.
Citrobacter rodentium	*Citrobacter* genomospecies 9	H_2S (−), indole (−), adonitol (−), malonate (+). This organism has been isolated only from rodents.
Citrobacter sedlakii	*Citrobacter* genomospecies 8	H_2S (−), indole (+), adonitol (−), malonate (+). Found in human stool, blood, and wounds.
Citrobacter werkmanii	*Citrobacter* genomospecies 7	H_2S (+), indole (−), adonitol (−), malonate (+). Found in human stool and urine and in food.
Citrobacter youngae	*Citrobacter* genomospecies 5	H_2S and indole are variable, adonitol (−), malonate (−). Isolated from human stool and blood and from animals and food.

Tribe V: Klebsielleae

NEW DESIGNATION	PREVIOUS DESIGNATION	COMMENTS
Klebsiella granulomatis	*Calymmatobacterium granulomatis*	Cannot be cultured on conventional culture media. Causative agent of granuloma inguinale.
Klebsiella oxytoca	Indole (+) *K. pneumoniae*	MIO (−,+,−). Common clinical isolate.
Klebsiella pneumoniae subsp. pneumoniae		MIO (−,−,−). Common clinical isolate.
Klebsiella pneumoniae subsp. ozaenae	*Klebsiella ozaenae*	Biochemically inactive strain of *K. pneumoniae*. Causes atrophic rhinitis, a condition called ozena.
Klebsiella pneumoniae subsp. rhinoscleromatis	*Klebsiella rhinoscleromatis*	Biochemically inactive strain of *K. pneumoniae*. Causes a granulomatous disease known as rhinoscleroma.
Raoultella ornithinolytica	*Klebsiella* Group 47 *Klebsiella ornithinolytica*	MIO (−,+,+). Isolated from blood, urine, sputum, and wounds.
Raoultella planticola	*Klebsiella* species 2 *Klebsiella trevisanii* *Klebsiella planticola*	Water and plant isolates. Rare human clinical isolates.
Raoultella terrigena	*Klebsiella terrigena*	Soil and water isolates
Enterobacter aerogenes		LAO (+,−−,+). Common clinical isolate.
"*Enterobacter agglomerans* complex"	*Erwinia herbicola* *Erwinia milletiae*	Heterogeneous group of organisms representing over 13 DNA hybridization groups (HG). HG XIII has been transferred to the new genus *Pantoea* as *Pantoea agglomerans*. Organisms that are LAO-negative (referred to as "triple decarboxylase negative") and are yellow-pigmented were usually identified as *E. agglomerans* in the past.
Enterobacter amnigenus biogroup 1 *Enterobacter amnigenus* biogroup 2	Group H3	Two biogroups. Biogroup 1 ferment sucrose and raffinose, but not D-sorbitol. Biogroup 2 ferment D-sorbitol but not sucrose or raffinose. Primarily water organisms. Have been isolated from human specimens but no evidence that *E. amnigenus* can cause human infection.
Enterobacter asburiae	Enteric group 17 Atypical *Citrobacter*	Biochemically similar to *E. cloacae*. Nonmotile, VP (−), (79% + after 2 days), urea (+) (delayed). Isolated from variety of human sources: blood, urine, wounds, respiratory tract, feces.

Table 6-5 *Continued*

NEW DESIGNATION	PREVIOUS DESIGNATION	COMMENTS
Enterobacter cancerogenus	*Erwinia cancerogena* *Enterobacter taylorae* Enteric group 19	Includes organisms formerly classified as *E. taylorae*. LAO (−,+,+), adonitol, inositol, sorbitol, raffinose, and melibiose all negative. Isolated from a variety of clinical sources, including blood and spinal fluid.

Enterobacter cloacae
Enterobacter cloacae–like
  unnamed species 1
Enterobacter cloacae–like
  unnamed species 2
Enterobacter cloacae–like
  unnamed species 3		

Enterobacter cowanii	Japanese NIH Group 42	Majority of strains isolated from clinical specimens LAO (−, +, +). Common clinical isolate.
Enterobacter dissolvens	*Erwinia dissolvens*	Closely related to *E. cloacae*. Not found in human clinical specimens.
Enterobacter gergoviae	Atypical *Enterobacter aerogenes*	LAO (+,−,+). Strong urease (+). Found in environment and urine and respiratory tract of humans. Rare isolates have been recovered from blood.
Enterobacter hormaechei	Enteric group 75	LAO (−,+,+). Biochemically closest to *E. cancerogenus* except is urea (+), sucrose (+), and esculin (−). Isolates reported from blood, wounds, and sputum.
Enterobacter intermedius	Group H1 *Enterobacter intermedium*	Found in water and soil. Human isolates have been recovered from blood, stool, wound, and bile.
Enterobacter kobei	Enteric group 69 Japanese NIH Group 21	Closely related to *E. cloacae*. Majority isolated from clinical specimens.
Enterobacter nimipressuralis	*Erwinia nimipressuralis*	Closely related to *E. cloacae*. Not found in human clinical specimens.
Enterobacter pyrinus	*Erwinia pirina*	Urease (+), most closely resemble *E. gergoviae* is differentiated by its growth in potassium cyanide broth, acid production from myoinositol, and lack of acid production from raffinose. Causes brown leaf spot disease of pear trees.
Enterobacter sakazakii	Yellow-pigmented *Enterobacter cloacae*	LAO (−,+,+). Bright yellow pigment at 35°C. May cause meningitis, brain abscesses, and bacteremia in neonates.
Hafnia alvei	*Enterobacter hafniae*	Lactose (−), LAO (+,−,+). Grows at 35°C but biochemically more active at 25°C. Found in clinical specimens especially feces, occasionally from blood, sputum, urine, and wounds.
Hafnia alvei biogroup 1	"*Hafnia protea*" *Obesumbacterium proteus* biogroup 1	Not a human clinical isolate. Occurs in breweries, where it grows in beer wort.
Pantoea agglomerans	*Enterobacter agglomerans* HG XIII *Erwinia herbicola* *Erwinia milletiae*	LAO (−,−,−) some may be yellow-pigmented. Isolated from plant surfaces, seeds, and water, as well as from humans (wound, blood, urine, internal organs) and animals.
Pantoea ananatis	*Pantoea ananas* *Enterobacter agglomerans* HG VI *Erwinia ananas* *Erwinia uredovora*	Plant pathogen, causes pineapple rot
Pantoea citrea	New species	Isolated from Mandarin oranges in Japan
Pantoea dispersa	*Enterobacter agglomerans* HG III	Isolated from plant surfaces, seeds, humans, and the environment. Separated from *P. agglomerans* by negative salicin reaction.

(Continued)

Table 6-5 *Continued*

NEW DESIGNATION	PREVIOUS DESIGNATION	COMMENTS
Pantoea punctata	New species	Isolated from Mandarin oranges in Japan
Pantoea stewartii subsp. *indologenes*	*Erwinia stewartii*	Cause of leaf spot on foxtail millet and pearl millet
Pantoea stewartii subsp. *stewartii*	*Erwinia stewartii*	Causative agent of Stewart's bacterial wilt of corn
Pantoea terrea	New species	Isolated from soil in Japan
Serratia entomophila		Resembles *S. marcescens* (arabinose-negative). Insect pathogen, no human isolates reported.
Serratia ficaria		Natural habitat is figs and fig wasps. Has been reported very rarely from human clinical specimens.
"Serratia" fonticola		Not really a species of *Serratia*. A water organism, rarely isolated from human specimens, mostly from wounds.
Serratia grimesii	See *Serratia liquefaciens* group	Isolated from environment and human clinical specimens. Cannot be differentiated from other members of "*S. liquefaciens* group" by commonly used tests.
"Serratia liquefaciens group"	*Enterobacter liquefaciens* Different biogroups within the species *S. liquefaciens*	Consists of several DNA hybridization groups, including species now named *Serratia proteamaculans*, and *S. grimesii*. Cannot be separated by currently used biochemical tests. Differ from *S. marcescens* by being L-arabinose (+). Report as "*S. liquefaciens* group."
Serratia marcescens		DNase (+), gelatin (+), L-arabinose (−) (other species are positive). Common clinical isolate. Red pigment produced by some strains.
Serratia odorifera biogroup 1 *Serratia odorifera* biogroup 2		Dirty, musty odor, like potatoes. Two biogroups. Biogroup 1 is ornithine-, sucrose-, and raffinose-positive and is predominantly isolated from sputum. Biogroup 2 is negative for these three reactions and has been recovered from blood and CSF.
Serratia plymuthica	*Bacterium plymuthica*	May have red pigment. Isolated from soil, water, and sputum. Extremely rare in clinical specimens.
Serratia proteamaculans subsp. *proteamaculans*	See *Serratia liquefaciens* group	Cannot be separated from other members of "*S. liquefaciens* group" by currently used biochemical tests. Differ from *S. marcescens* by being L-arabinose (+).
Serratia quinivorans	*Serratia proteamaculans* subsp. *quinovora* see *Serratia liquefaciens* group	Isolated from plants, wild rodents, insects, and water, but not yet from human clinical specimens.
Serratia rubidaea		Red pigment produced. Rarely isolated in humans.
Tribe VI: Proteeae		
Proteus hauseri	*Proteus vulgaris* biogroup 3, DNA group 3	H$_2$S (+), indole (+); salicin and esculin are (−).
Proteus mirabilis		H$_2$S (+), indole (−), ornithine (+). Common clinical isolate.
Proteus myxofaciens		No human isolates reported. Isolated only from living and dead gypsy moths.
Proteus penneri	*Proteus vulgaris* biogroup 1	Closely related to *P. vulgaris*, except that indole (−), salicin (−), esculin (−), and chloramphenicol-resistant.
Proteus vulgaris	*Proteus vulgaris* biogroup 2	H$_2$S (+), indole (+), ornithine (−) Common clinical isolate. Indole, salicin, and esculin are positive

Table 6-5 *Continued*

NEW DESIGNATION	PREVIOUS DESIGNATION	COMMENTS
Proteus vulgaris biogroup 3		Consists of four separate genetic species and are designated DNA groups 3, 4, 5, and 6. Indole (+), but salicin and esculin (−). DNA group 3 has recently been named *Proteus hauseri*.
Morganella morganii subsp. *morganii*	*Proteus morganii*	H$_2$S (−), lysine, ornithine, and motility all variable, trehalose (−). Causes urinary tract infections and is cultured from many other body sites. Contains four biogroups designated A through D
Morganella morganii subsp. *sibonii*	*Morganella morganii* biogroup 1	H$_2$S (−), lysine, ornithine variable, trehalose and motility (+). Contains three biogroups designated E through G
Morganella morganii subsp. 3		
Providencia alcalifaciens	*Providencia alcalifaciens* biogroups 1 and 2	Urea (−), adonitol (+), inositol (−). Generally isolated from diarrheic stool, particularly in children.
Providencia heimbachae		Not a human clinical isolate. Found in penguin feces and an aborted cow fetus.
Providencia rettgeri	*Proteus rettgeri*	Urea (+), adonitol (+), inositol (+). Mostly isolated from urine of hospitalized patients and specimens from catheters.
Providencia rustigianii	*Providencia alcalifaciens* biogroup 3, *Providencia friedericiana*	Urea (−), adonitol (−), inositol (−). Rarely found in clinical specimens, mostly from human feces.
Providencia stuartii	*Providencia alcalifaciens* biogroup 4	Urea (v), adonitol (−), inositol (+). Isolated most often from urine, less often from wounds, burns, and bacteremias. May cause nosocomial outbreaks.

Tribe VII: Yersinieae

Yersinia aldovae	*Yersinia enterocolitica*–like Group X2	Biochemically similar to *Y. enterocolitica*. Isolated from surface water, drinking water, and fish.
Yersinia bercovieri	*Yersinia enterocolitica* biogroup 3B	Biochemically similar to *Y. enterocolitica*. Isolated from human feces, water, soil, and raw vegetables.
Yersinia enterocolitica		May cause diarrhea, terminal ileitis, mesenteric lymphadenitis, arthritis, and septicemia in humans.
Yersinia frederiksenii	Biogroup of *Y. enterocolitica*	Found mainly in water, sewage, and fish. Occasionally found in human feces, blood, and sputum. Rarely associated with gastrointestinal illness.
Yersinia intermedia	Biogroup of *Y. enterocolitica*	Found in fresh water, sewage, and aquatic animals. Human isolates have been from stool, blood, wounds, and urine. Probably not a cause of gastrointestinal illness.
Yersinia kristensenii	Biogroup of *Y. enterocolitica*	Found in water, soil, and animals. Human isolates have been from stool, blood, and urine. No evidence that it can cause gastrointestinal illness.
Yersinia mollaretii	*Yersinia enterocolitica* biogroup 3A	Biochemically similar to *Y. enterocolitica*. Isolated from human feces, drinking water, meat, and raw vegetables.
Yersinia pestis	*Pasteurella pestis*, *Yersinia pseudotuberculosis* subsp. *pestis*	Causative agent of plague.
Yersinia pseudotuberculosis		May cause mesenteric lymphadenitis, diarrhea, and septicemia in humans.
Yersinia rohdei		Biochemically similar to *Y. enterocolitica*. Isolated from dog feces, water, and human feces.
"*Yersinia*" *ruckeri*	"Red mouth bacterium"	Will probably be moved to a new genus. Fish pathogen. Human isolates are extremely rare.

LAO, lysine, arginine, ornithine; MIO, motility, indole, ornithine; PAD, phenylalanine deaminase; HG, hybridization group; (+) = >90% of strains positive; (−) = >90% of strains negative; (v) = variable.

Table 6-6 Key Identification Characteristics for the Most Common *Enterobacteriaceae*

	KIA	GAS	H₂S	MR	VP	IND	CIT	PAD	URE	MOT	LYS	ARG	ORN	ONPG
Tribe I: *Escherichieae*														
Genus: *Escherichia*														
E. coli	A/A	+	−	+	−	+	−	−	−	+	+	−/+	+/−	+
Genus: *Shigella*														
Groups A, B, C	Alk/A	−	−	+	−	−/+	−	−	−	−	−	−	−	−
S. sonnei	Alk/A	−	−	+	−	−	−	−	−	−	−	−	+	+
Tribe II: *Edwardsielleae*														
Genus: *Edwardsiella*														
E. tarda	Alk/A	+	+	+	−	+	−	−	−	+	+	−	+	−
Tribe III: *Salmonelleae*														
Genus: *Salmonella*	Alk/A	+	+	+	−	−	+	−	−	+	+	+/−	+	−
Tribe IV: *Citrobactereae*														
Genus: *Citrobacter*														
C. freundii	A/A; Alk/A	+	+	+	−	−	+	−	+/−	+	−	+/−	−/+	+
C. koseri	Alk/A	+	−	+	−	+	+	−	+/−	+	−	+/−	+	+
Tribe V: *Klebsielleae*														
Genus: *Klebsiella*														
K. pneumoniae	A/A	++	−	−	+	−	+	−	+	−	+	−	−	+
K. oxytoca	A/A	++	−	−	+	+	+	−	+	−	+	−	−	+
Genus: *Enterobacter*														
E. aerogenes	A/A	++	−	−	+	−	+	−	−	+	+	−	+	+
E. cloacae	A/A	++	−	−	+	−	+	−	+/−	+	−	+	+	+
Genus: *Hafnia*														
H. alvei	Alk/A	+	−	−/+	+	−	−	−	−	+	+	−	+	+
Genus: *Pantoea*														
P. agglomerans	A/A; Alk/A	−/+	−	−/+	+/−	−/+	+/−	−/+	−/+	+	−	−	−	+
Genus: *Serratia*														
S. marcescens	Alk/A	+	−	−/+	+	−	+	−	−	+	+	−	+	+
Tribe VI: *Proteeae*														
Genus: *Proteus*														
P. vulgaris	Alk/A	+/−	+	+	−	+	−/+	+	++	+*	−	−	−	−
P. mirabilis	Alk/A	+	+	+	+/−	−	+/−	+	++	+*	−	−	+	−
Genus: *Morganella*														
M. morganii	Alk/A	+	−	+	−	+	−	+	++	+	−	−	+	−
Genus: *Providencia*														
P. rettgeri	Alk/A	−	−	+	−	+	+	+	++	+	−	−	−	−
P. stuartii	Alk/A	−	−	+	−	+	+	+	−/+	+/−	−	−	−	−
P. alcalifaciens	Alk/A	+/−	−	+	−	+	+	+	−	+	−	−	−	−
Tribe VII: *Yersinieae*														
Genus: *Yersinia*														
Y. enterocolitica	Alk/A	−	−	+	−	+/−	−	−	+/−	−†	−	−	+	+

KIA, Kligler's iron agar; H₂S, hydrogen sulfide; MR, methyl red; VP, Voges-Proskauer; IND, indole; CIT, citrate; PAD, phenylalanine deaminase; URE, urease; MOT, motility; LYS, lysine; ARG, arginine; ORN, ornithine; ONPG, o-nitrophenyl-β-D-galactopyranoside; ++, strong positive reaction; +, 90% or more strains positive; −, 90% or more strains negative; +/−, 50–90% of strains positive; −/+, 50–90% of strains negative; shaded areas indicate key reactions.
* Swarming motility demonstrated on noninhibitory media.
† Nonmotile at 36°C, motile at 22°C.

Box 6-8 Key Facts To Remember for Identifying *Enterobacteriaceae*

Hydrogen sulfide–positive

Edwardsiella tarda   *Proteus vulgaris*
Salmonella species   *Proteus mirabilis*
Citrobacter freundii

Voges-Proskauer–positive

Klebsiella species   *Pantoea* species
Enterobacter species   *Serratia* species
Hafnia species

Phenylalanine deaminase–positive

Proteus species   *Providencia* species
Morganella species

Nonmotile at 36°C

Shigella species   *Klebsiella* species
Yersinia species (motile at 22°C)

Key reactions for students to remember are found in Box 6-8. When it is necessary to confirm the identification of a common *Enterobacteriaceae* with an unusual biochemical pattern or when an uncommon species is suspected, it will be necessary to consult Table 6-7, which gives the reactions of all named species of *Enterobacteriaceae* to 47 biochemical substrates.

TRIBE *ESCHERICHIEAE*

The two genera within this tribe are *Escherichia* and *Shigella*. On first reflection these two groups of bacteria would not appear to be related because of differences in growth characteristics and appearance on the enteric isolation media (*E. coli* characteristically ferments lactose, *Shigella* species do not). *E. coli* is generally biochemically active compared with *Shigella* species, which tend to be inert. However, *E. coli* and *Shigella* species are closely related genetically; in fact, all four species of *Shigella* and *E. coli* form a single species on the basis of DNA hybridization studies.[48] However, because *Shigella* species are associated with a specific disease spectrum (bacillary dysentery) and because specific typing antisera for separating *E. coli* from *Shigella* are commercially available, *Shigella* species will continue to be classified in a separate genus, at least for now. Students should note, however, that certain late lactose-fermenting, nonmotile, and biochemically inactive strains of *E. coli* can be difficult to differentiate from *Shigella* species, and rare strains of *Shigella* species (*S. flexneri*) also can produce gas from the fermentation of glucose. The pathogenic spectrum of *E. coli* is much broader than that of *Shigella* species, and toxigenic strains of *E. coli* can produce dysentery-like diarrheal syndromes indistinguishable from shigellosis. Serologic testing may be required in some instances to differentiate certain closely related strains. The key characteristics of the *Escherichieae* are given in Table 6-6.

***Genus* Escherichia.** *E. coli* is the bacterial species most commonly recovered in the clinical laboratories and has been incriminated in infectious diseases involving virtually every human tissue and organ system. *E. coli* is one of the common organisms involved in gram-negative sepsis and endotoxin-induced shock. Urinary tract and wound infections, pneumonia in immunosuppressed hospitalized patients, and meningitis in neonates are other common infections caused by *E. coli*. *E. coli* are serotyped on the basis of their O (somatic), H (flagellar), and K (capsular) surface antigens. More than 170 different O antigen serogroups are currently recognized.[339] The combination of O and H antigens defines a ''serotype'' of an isolate; for example, *E. coli* O157:H7 is a serotype of a virulent strain of *E. coli* associated with hemorrhagic colitis and hemolytic–uremic syndrome (HUS).

***E. coli* That Cause Gastroenteritis** Certain strains of *E. coli* can cause enteritis or gastroenteritis by six distinct mechanisms, resulting in six different clinical syndromes. These include enterotoxigenic *E. coli* (ETEC), enteropathogenic *E. coli* (EPEC), enteroinvasive *E. coli* (EIEC), enterohemorrhagic *E. coli* (EHEC), enteroaggregative *E. coli* (EAEC) and diffusely adherent *E. coli* (DAEC).[339] (See Table 6-8.) EPEC, EAEC, and DAEC isolates are characterized by their distinct patterns of adherence to epithelial cells in vitro. EPEC strains bind to host cells in a pattern called localized adherence, in which microcolonies form on the surfaces of the cells. EAEC isolates bind in an aggregative adherence pattern that is characterized by a stacked-brick-like arrangement on the surfaces of the cells. DAEC strains are defined by a pattern of diffuse adherence in which the bacteria uniformly cover the entire cell surface.[339] In addition to the six classes of diarrheagenic *E. coli* mentioned above, there are other potential classes, such as cytolethal distending toxin (CDT)–producing *E. coli* and cell-detaching *E. coli* (CDEC) that have yet to be fully characterized.[339]

Although assays to identify all categories of *E. coli* that cause gastroenteritis are available, in most cases it is not necessary to identify a specific *E. coli* pathogen in a particular patient. Most patients with gastroenteritis due to *E. coli* will resolve their diarrhea before seeking medical attention or their diarrhea resolves following treatment with empirical antibiotics given for other bacterial diarrheas. Therefore, with the exception of assays for the detection of EHEC (discussed below), phenotypic assays or serotyping of *E. coli* for diagnosis of diarrheagenic strains is not routinely performed in the clinical laboratory.

Pathophysiology of Enterohemorrhagic *E. coli* (EHEC) The clinical significance of EHEC was not known until 1982, when these organisms were associated with two conditions of previously unknown etiology: hemorrhagic colitis[426] and hemolytic–uremic syndrome.[257] (See Clinical Correlation Box 6-1.) *E. coli* O157:H7 was the first of several Shiga toxin–producing serotypes known to cause human illness. *E. coli* O157:H7 is so named because it expresses the 157th somatic (O) antigen identified and the 7th flagellar (H) antigen. Among the most important virulence characteristics of *E. coli* O157:H7 is its ability to produced one or more Shiga toxins (also called verocytotoxins, and formerly

Table 6-7 Biochemical Reactions of the Named Species and Unnamed Groups of the Family *Enterobacteriaceae*

"ORGANISM"[a,b]	INDOLE PRODUCTION	METHYL RED	VOGES-PROSKAUER	CITRATE (SIMMONS)	HYDROGEN SULFIDE (TSI)	UREA HYDROLYSIS	PHENYLALANINE DEAMINASE	LYSINE DECARBOXYLASE	ARGININE DIHYDROLASE	ORNITHINE DECARBOXYLASE	MOTILITY	GELATIN HYDROLYSIS (22°C)	GROWTH IN KCN	MALONATE UTILIZATION	"D-GLUCOSE, ACID"	"D-GLUCOSE, GAS"	LACTOSE FERMENTATION	SUCROSE FERMENTATION	D-MANNITOL FERMENTATION	DULCITOL FERMENTATION	SALICIN FERMENTATION
Budvicia																					
B. aquatica	0	93	0	0	80	33	0	0	0	0	27	0	0	0	100	53	87	0	60	0	0
Buttiauxella																					
B. agrestis	0	100	0	100	0	0	0	0	0	100	100	0	80	60	100	100	100	0	100	0	100
B. brennerae	0	100	0	0	0	0	0	0	0	33	100	0	100	100	100	100	0	0	100	0	100
B. ferragutiae	0	100	0	0	0	0	0	100	0	80	60	0	40	0	100	100	0	0	100	0	100
B. gaviniae	0	100	0	20	0	0	0	0	20	0	80	0	60	100	100	40	60	0	100	0	100
B. izardii	0	100	0	0	0	0	0	0	0	100	100	0	67	100	100	100	100	0	100	0	100
B. noackiae	33	100	0	33	0	0	100	0	67	0	100	0	100	100	100	100	100	0	100	0	100
B. warmboldiae	0	100	0	33	0	0	100	0	0	0	100	0	33	100	100	100	0	0	100	0	100
Cedecea																					
C. davisae	0	100	50	95	0	0	0	0	50	95	95	0	86	91	100	70	19	100	100	0	99
C. lapagei	0	40	80	99	0	0	0	0	80	0	80	0	100	99	100	100	60	0	100	0	100
C. neteri	0	100	50	100	0	0	0	0	100	0	100	0	65	100	100	100	35	100	100	0	100
Cedecea species 3	0	100	50	100	0	0	0	0	100	0	100	0	100	0	100	100	0	50	100	0	100
Cedecea species 5	0	100	50	100	0	0	0	0	50	50	100	0	100	0	100	100	0	100	100	0	100
Citrobacter																					
C. amalonaticus	100	100	0	95	5	85	0	0	85	95	95	0	99	1	100	97	35	9	100	1	30
C. braakii	33	100	0	87	60	47	0	0	67	93	87	0	100	0	100	93	80	7	100	33	0
C. farmeri	100	100	0	10	0	59	0	0	85	100	97	0	93	0	100	96	15	100	100	2	9
C. freundii	33	100	0	78	78	44	0	0	67	0	89	0	89	11	100	89	78	89	100	11	0
C. gillenii	0	100	0	33	67	0	0	0	33	0	67	0	100	100	100	100	67	33	100	0	0
C. koseri (diversus)	99	100	0	99	0	75	0	0	80	99	95	0	0	95	100	98	50	40	99	40	15
C. murliniae	100	100	0	100	67	67	0	0	67	0	100	0	100	0	100	100	67	33	100	100	33
C. rodentium	0	100	0	0	0	100	0	0	0	100	0	0	0	100	100	100	100	0	100	0	0
C. sedlakii	83	100	0	83	0	100	0	0	100	100	100	0	100	100	100	100	100	0	100	100	17
C. werkmanii	0	100	0	100	100	100	0	0	100	0	100	0	100	100	100	100	17	0	100	0	0
C. youngae	15	100	0	75	65	80	0	0	50	5	95	0	95	5	100	75	25	20	100	85	10
Edwardsiella																					
E. hoshinae	50	100	0	0	0	0	0	100	0	95	100	0	0	100	100	35	0	100	100	0	50
E. ictaluri	0	0	0	0	0	0	0	100	0	65	0	0	0	0	100	50	0	0	0	0	0
E. tarda	99	100	0	1	100	0	0	100	0	100	98	0	0	0	100	100	0	0	0	0	0
E. tarda biogroup 1	100	100	0	0	0	0	0	100	0	100	100	0	0	0	100	50	0	100	100	0	0
Enterobacter																					
E. aerogenes	0	5	98	95	0	2	0	98	0	98	97	0	98	95	100	100	95	100	100	5	100
E. amnigenus biogroup 1	0	7	100	70	0	0	0	0	9	55	92	0	100	91	100	100	70	100	100	0	91
E. amnigenus biogroup 2	0	65	100	100	0	0	0	0	35	100	100	0	100	100	100	100	35	0	100	0	100
E. asburiae	0	100	2	100	0	60	0	0	21	95	0	0	97	3	100	95	75	100	100	0	100
E. cancerogenus (*E. taylorae*)	0	5	100	100	0	1	0	0	94	99	99	0	98	100	100	100	10	0	100	0	92

ADONITOL FERMENTATION	MYO-INOSITOL FERMENTATION	D-SORBITOL FERMENTATION	L-ARABINOSE FERMENTATION	RAFFINOSE FERMENTATION	L-RHAMNOSE FERMENTATION	MALTOSE FERMENTATION	D-XYLOSE FERMENTATION	TREHALOSE FERMENTATION	CELLOBIOSE FERMENTATION	α-METHYL-D-GLUCOSIDE FERMENTATION	ERYTHRITOL FERMENTATION	ESCULIN HYDROLYSIS	MELIBIOSE FERMENTATION	D-ARABITOL FERMENTATION	GLYCEROL FERMENTATION	MUCATE FERMENTATION	"TARTRATE, JORDAN'S"	ACETATE UTILIZATION	LIPASE (CORN OIL)	DNASE (25°C)	NITRATE NITRITE	"OXIDASE, KOVACS"	ONPG TEST	YELLOW PIGMENT	D-MANNOSE FERMENTATION
0	0	0	80	0	100	0	93	0	0	0	0	0	0	27	0	20	27	0	0	0	100	0	93	0	0
0	0	0	100	100	100	100	100	100	100	0	0	100	100	0	60	100	60	0	0	0	100	0	100	0	100
67	0	0	100	100	33	100	100	100	100	0	0	100	100	67	67	67	0	0	0	0	100	0	100	0	100
0	0	100	100	0	100	100	100	100	100	40	0	100	0	0	0	60	0	0	0	0	100	0	100	0	100
100	0	0	100	0	100	60	100	100	100	0	0	100	0	80	0	80	40	0	0	0	100	0	100	0	100
0	0	0	100	33	100	100	100	100	100	0	0	100	67	0	33	100	67	0	0	0	100	0	100	0	100
0	0	0	100	0	100	100	100	100	100	33	0	100	0	0	0	100	100	0	0	0	100	0	100	0	100
0	67	0	100	0	100	100	100	100	100	0	0	100	0	0	0	0	0	0	0	0	100	0	100	0	100
0	0	0	0	10	0	100	100	100	100	5	0	45	0	100	0	0	0	0	91	0	100	0	90	0	100
0	0	0	0	0	0	100	0	100	100	0	0	100	0	100	0	0	0	60	100	0	100	0	99	0	100
0	0	100	0	0	0	100	100	100	100	0	0	100	0	100	0	0	0	0	100	0	100	0	100	0	100
0	0	0	0	100	0	100	100	100	100	50	0	100	100	100	0	0	0	50	100	0	100	0	100	0	100
0	0	100	0	100	0	100	100	100	100	0	0	100	100	100	0	0	0	50	50	0	100	0	100	0	100
0	0	99	99	5	100	99	99	100	100	2	0	5	0	0	60	96	96	86	0	0	99	0	97	0	100
0	0	100	100	7	100	100	100	100	73	33	0	0	80	0	87	100	93	53	0	0	100	0	80	0	100
0	0	98	100	100	100	100	100	100	100	75	0	0	100	0	65	100	93	80	0	0	100	0	100	0	100
0	0	100	100	44	100	100	89	100	44	11	0	0	100	0	100	100	100	44	0	0	100	0	89	0	100
0	0	100	100	0	100	100	100	100	67	0	0	0	67	0	67	67	100	0	0	0	100	0	67	0	100
99	0	99	99	0	99	100	100	100	99	40	0	1	0	98	99	95	90	75	0	0	100	0	99	0	100
0	0	100	100	33	100	100	100	100	100	0	0	0	33	0	100	100	100	33	0	0	100	0	100	0	100
0	0	100	100	0	100	100	100	100	100	0	0	0	0	0	0	100	100	0	0	0	100	0	100	0	100
0	0	100	100	0	100	100	100	100	100	0	0	17	100	0	83	100	100	83	0	0	100	0	100	0	100
0	0	100	100	0	100	100	100	100	100	0	0	0	0	0	100	100	100	100	0	0	100	0	100	0	100
0	5	100	100	10	100	95	100	100	45	0	0	5	10	5	90	100	100	65	0	0	85	0	90	0	100
0	0	0	13	0	0	100	0	100	0	0	0	0	0	0	65	0	0	0	0	0	100	0	0	0	100
0	0	0	0	0	0	100	0	0	0	0	0	0	0	0	0	0	0	0	0	0	100	0	0	0	100
0	0	0	9	0	0	100	0	0	0	0	0	0	0	0	30	0	25	0	0	0	100	0	0	0	100
0	0	0	100	0	0	100	0	0	0	0	0	0	0	0	0	0	0	0	0	0	100	0	0	0	100
98	95	100	100	96	99	99	100	100	100	95	0	98	99	100	98	90	95	50	0	0	100	0	100	0	95
0	0	9	100	100	100	100	100	100	100	55	0	91	100	0	0	35	9	0	0	0	100	0	91	0	100
0	0	100	100	0	100	100	100	100	100	100	0	100	100	0	0	100	0	0	0	0	100	0	100	0	100
0	0	100	100	70	5	100	97	100	100	95	0	95	0	0	11	21	30	87	0	0	100	0	100	0	100
0	0	1	100	0	100	99	100	100	100	1	0	90	0	0	1	75	0	35	0	0	100	0	100	0	100

(Continued)

Table 6-7 *Continued*

"ORGANISM"[a,b]	INDOLE PRODUCTION	METHYL RED	VOGES-PROSKAUER	CITRATE (SIMMONS)	HYDROGEN SULFIDE (TSI)	UREA HYDROLYSIS	PHENYLALANINE DEAMINASE	LYSINE DECARBOXYLASE	ARGININE DIHYDROLASE	ORNITHINE DECARBOXYLASE	MOTILITY	GELATIN HYDROLYSIS (22°C)	GROWTH IN KCN	MALONATE UTILIZATION	"D-GLUCOSE, ACID"	"D-GLUCOSE, GAS"	LACTOSE FERMENTATION	SUCROSE FERMENTATION	D-MANNITOL FERMENTATION	DULCITOL FERMENTATION	SALICIN FERMENTATION
Enterobacter																					
E. cloacae	0	5	100	100	0	65	0	0	97	96	95	0	98	75	100	100	93	97	100	15	75
E. cowanii	0	NA	92	100	0	0	0	0	0	0	92	0	92	0	100	100	100	100	100	100	100
E. dissolvens	0	0	100	100	0	100	0	0	100	100	0	0	100	100	100	100	0	100	100	0	100
E. gergoviae	0	5	100	99	0	93	0	90	0	100	90	0	0	96	100	98	55	98	99	0	99
E. hormaechei	0	57	100	96	0	87	4	0	78	91	52	0	100	100	100	83	9	100	100	87	44
E. intermedius	0	100	100	65	0	0	0	0	0	89	89	0	65	100	100	100	100	65	100	100	100
E. kobei (enteric group 69)	0	0	100	100	0	0	0	0	100	100	100	0	100	100	100	100	100	25	100	100	100
E. nimipressuralis	0	100	100	0	0	0	0	0	0	100	0	0	100	100	100	100	0	0	100	0	100
E. pyrinus	0	29	86	0	0	86	0	100	0	100	43	0	0	86	100	100	14	0	100	0	100
E. sakazakii	11	5	100	99	0	1	50	0	99	91	96	0	99	18	100	98	99	0	100	5	99
Escherichia																					
E. albertii	0	100	0	0	0	0	0	100	0	100	0	0	0	0	100	0	0	0	100	0	0
E. blattae	0	100	0	50	0	0	0	100	0	100	0	0	0	100	100	100	0	0	0	0	0
E. coli	98	99	0	1	1	1	0	90	17	65	95	0	3	0	100	95	95	0	98	60	40
"E. coli, inactive"	80	95	0	1	1	1	0	40	3	20	5	0	1	0	100	5	25	0	93	40	10
E. fergusonii	98	100	0	17	0	0	0	95	5	100	93	0	0	35	100	95	0	0	98	60	65
E hermannii	99	100	0	1	0	0	0	6	0	100	99	0	94	0	100	97	45	0	100	19	40
E. vulneris	0	100	0	0	0	0	0	85	30	0	100	0	15	85	100	97	15	0	100	0	30
Ewingella																					
E. americana	0	84	95	95	0	0	0	0	0	0	60	0	5	0	100	0	70	0	100	0	80
Hafnia																					
H. alvei	0	40	85	10	0	4	0	100	6	98	85	0	95	50	100	98	5	0	99	0	13
H. alvei biogroup 1	0	85	70	0	0	0	0	100	0	45	0	0	0	45	100	0	0	0	55	0	55
Klebsiella																					
K. oxytoca	99	20	95	95	0	90	1	99	0	0	0	0	97	98	100	97	100	0	99	55	100
K. pneumoniae subsp. ozaenae	0	98	0	30	0	10	0	40	6	3	0	0	88	3	100	50	30	0	100	2	97
K. pneumoniae subsp. pneumonia	0	10	98	98	0	95	0	98	0	0	0	0	98	93	100	97	98	0	99	30	99
K. pneumoniae subsp. rhinoscleromatis	0	100	0	0	0	0	0	0	0	0	0	0	80	95	100	0	0	0	100	0	98
Raoultella																					
R. (Klebsiella) ornithinolytica	100	96	70	100	0	100	0	100	0	100	0	0	100	100	100	100	100	0	100	10	100
R. (Klebsiella) planticola	20	100	98	100	0	98	0	100	0	0	0	0	100	100	100	100	100	0	100	15	100
R. (Klebsiella) terrigena	0	60	100	40	0	0	0	100	0	20	0	0	100	100	100	80	100	0	100	20	100
Kluyvera																					
K. ascorbata	92	100	0	96	0	0	0	97	0	100	98	0	92	96	100	93	98	0	100	25	100
K. cryocrescens	90	100	0	80	0	0	0	23	0	100	90	0	86	86	100	95	95	0	95	0	100
K. georgiana	100	100	0	100	0	0	0	100	0	100	100	0	83	50	100	17	83	0	100	33	100

ADONITOL FERMENTATION	MYO-INOSITOL FERMENTATION	D-SORBITOL FERMENTATION	L-ARABINOSE FERMENTATION	RAFFINOSE FERMENTATION	L-RHAMNOSE FERMENTATION	MALTOSE FERMENTATION	D-XYLOSE FERMENTATION	TREHALOSE FERMENTATION	CELLOBIOSE FERMENTATION	α-METHYL-D-GLUCOSIDE FERMENTATION	ERYTHRITOL FERMENTATION	ESCULIN HYDROLYSIS	MELIBIOSE FERMENTATION	D-ARABITOL FERMENTATION	GLYCEROL FERMENTATION	MUCATE FERMENTATION	"TARTRATE, JORDAN'S"	ACETATE UTILIZATION	LIPASE (CORN OIL)	DNASE (25°C)	NITRATE NITRITE	"OXIDASE, KOVACS"	ONPG TEST	YELLOW PIGMENT	D-MANNOSE FERMENTATION
25	15	95	100	97	92	100	99	100	99	85	0	30	90	15	40	75	30	75	0	0	99	0	99	0	100
0	0	100	0	100	100	100	100	100	100	0	0	100	100	0	100	91	100	100	0	0	100	0	100	66	100
0	0	100	100	100	100	100	100	100	100	100	0	100	100	0	0	100	0	100	0	0	100	0	100	0	100
0	0	0	99	97	99	100	99	100	99	2	0	97	97	97	100	2	97	93	0	0	99	0	97	0	100
0	0	0	100	0	100	100	96	100	100	83	0	0	0	0	4	96	13	74	0	0	100	0	95	0	100
0	0	100	100	100	100	100	100	100	100	100	0	100	100	0	100	100	100	0	0	0	100	0	100	0	100
0	0	100	100	100	100	100	100	100	100	100	0	100	100	0	0	100	0	25	0	0	100	0	100	0	100
0	0	100	100	0	100	100	100	100	100	100	0	100	100	0	0	100	0	0	0	0	100	0	100	0	100
0	100	0	100	0	100	100	0	100	100	0	0	100	0	0	0	0	0	0	0	0	100	0	100	0	100
0	75	0	100	99	100	100	100	100	100	96	0	100	100	0	15	1	1	96	0	0	99	0	100	95	100
0	0	0	100	0	0	60	0	60	0	0	0	0	0	0	0	NA	100	0	0	100	0	100	0	100	0
0	0	0	100	0	100	100	100	75	0	0	0	0	0	0	100	50	50	0	0	0	100	0	0	0	100
5	1	94	99	50	80	95	95	98	2	0	0	35	75	5	75	95	95	90	0	0	100	0	95	0	98
3	1	75	85	15	65	80	70	90	2	0	0	5	40	5	65	30	85	40	0	0	98	0	45	0	97
98	0	0	98	0	92	96	96	96	96	0	0	46	0	100	20	0	96	96	0	0	100	0	83	0	100
0	0	0	100	40	97	100	100	100	97	0	0	40	0	8	3	97	35	78	0	0	100	0	98	98	100
0	0	1	100	99	93	100	100	100	100	25	0	20	100	0	25	78	2	30	0	0	100	0	100	50	100
0	0	0	0	0	23	16	13	99	10	0	0	50	0	99	24	0	35	10	0	0	97	0	85	0	99
0	0	0	95	2	97	100	98	95	15	0	0	7	0	0	95	0	70	15	0	0	100	0	90	0	100
0	0	0	0	0	0	0	0	70	0	0	0	0	0	0	0	0	30	0	0	0	100	0	30	0	100
99	98	99	98	100	100	100	100	100	100	98	2	100	99	98	99	93	98	90	0	0	100	0	100	1	100
97	55	65	98	90	55	95	95	98	92	70	0	80	97	95	65	25	50	2	0	0	80	0	80	0	100
90	95	99	99	99	99	98	99	99	98	90	0	99	99	98	97	90	95	75	0	0	99	0	99	0	99
100	95	100	100	90	96	100	100	100	100	0	0	30	100	100	50	0	50	0	0	0	100	0	0	0	100
100	95	100	100	100	100	100	100	100	100	100	0	100	100	100	100	96	100	95	0	0	100	0	100	0	100
100	100	92	100	100	100	100	100	100	100	100	0	100	100	100	100	100	100	62	0	0	100	0	100	1	100
100	80	100	100	100	100	100	100	100	100	100	0	100	100	100	100	100	100	20	0	0	100	0	100	0	100
0	0	40	100	98	100	100	99	100	100	98	0	99	99	0	40	90	35	50	0	0	100	0	100	20	100
0	0	45	100	100	100	100	91	100	100	95	0	100	100	0	5	81	19	86	0	0	100	0	100	0	100
0	0	0	100	100	83	100	100	100	100	100	0	100	100	0	33	83	50	83	0	0	100	0	100	0	100

(Continued)

Table 6-7 *Continued*

"ORGANISM"[a,b]	INDOLE PRODUCTION	METHYL RED	VOGES-PROSKAUER	CITRATE (SIMMONS)	HYDROGEN SULFIDE (TSI)	UREA HYDROLYSIS	PHENYLALANINE DEAMINASE	LYSINE DECARBOXYLASE	ARGININE DIHYDROLASE	ORNITHINE DECARBOXYLASE	MOTILITY	GELATIN HYDROLYSIS (22°C)	GROWTH IN KCN	MALONATE UTILIZATION	"D-GLUCOSE, ACID"	"D-GLUCOSE, GAS"	LACTOSE FERMENTATION	SUCROSE FERMENTATION	D-MANNITOL FERMENTATION	DULCITOL FERMENTATION	SALICIN FERMENTATION
Leclercia																					
L. adecarboxylata	100	100	0	0	0	48	0	0	0	0	79	0	97	93	100	97	93	0	100	86	100
Leminorella																					
L. grimontii	0	100	0	100	100	0	0	0	0	0	0	0	0	0	100	33	0	0	0	83	0
L. richardii	0	0	0	0	100	0	0	0	0	0	0	0	0	0	100	0	0	0	0	0	0
Moellerella																					
M. wisconsensis	0	100	0	80	0	0	0	0	0	0	0	0	70	0	100	0	100	0	60	0	0
Morganella																					
M. morganii subsp. *morganii*	95	95	0	0	20	95	95	1	0	95	95	0	98	1	99	90	1	0	0	0	0
M. morganii subsp. *sibonii*	50	86	0	0	7	100	93	29	0	64	79	0	79	0	100	86	0	0	0	0	0
M. morganii biogroup 1	100	95	0	0	15	100	100	100	0	80	0	0	90	5	100	93	0	0	0	0	0
Obesumbacterium																					
O. proteus biogroup 2	0	15	0	0	0	0	0	100	0	100	0	0	0	0	100	0	0	0	0	0	0
Pantoea																					
P. agglomerans	20	50	70	50	0	20	20	0	0	0	85	2	35	65	100	20	40	0	100	15	65
P. dispersa	0	82	64	100	0	9	0	0	0	0	100	0	82	9	100	0	0	0	100	0	0
Photorhabdus																					
P. luminescens (23°C)	50	0	0	50	0	25	0	0	0	0	100	50	0	0	75	0	0	0	0	0	0
P. asymbiotica	0	0	0	20	0	60	0	0	0	0	100	80	20	0	100	0	0	0	0	0	0
Pragia																					
P. fontium	0	100	0	89	89	0	22	0	0	0	100	0	0	0	100	0	0	0	0	0	78
Proteus																					
P. hauseri	100	100	0	0	50	100	100	0	0	0	100	100	100	0	100	0	0	0	0	0	0
P. mirabilis	2	97	50	65	98	98	98	0	0	99	95	90	98	2	100	96	2	0	0	0	0
P. myxofaciens	0	100	100	50	0	100	100	0	0	0	100	100	100	0	100	100	0	0	0	0	0
P. penneri	0	100	0	0	30	100	99	0	0	0	85	50	99	0	100	45	1	0	0	0	0
P. vulgaris	98	95	0	15	95	95	99	0	0	0	95	91	99	0	100	85	2	0	0	0	50
Providencia																					
P. alcalifaciens	99	99	0	98	0	0	98	0	0	1	96	0	100	0	100	85	0	0	2	0	1
P. heimbachae	0	85	0	0	0	0	100	0	0	0	46	0	8	0	100	0	0	0	0	0	0
P. rettgeri	99	93	0	95	0	98	98	0	0	0	94	0	97	0	100	10	5	0	100	0	50
P. rustigianii	98	65	0	15	0	0	100	0	0	0	30	0	100	0	100	35	0	0	0	0	0
P. stuartii	98	100	0	93	0	30	95	0	0	0	85	0	100	0	100	0	2	0	10	0	2
Rahnella																					
R. aquatilis	0	88	100	94	0	0	95	0	0	0	6	0	0	100	100	98	100	0	100	88	100
Salmonella																					
S. enterica subsp *enterica* (Group I)																					
Most serotypes	1	100	0	95	95	1	0	98	70	97	95	0	0	0	100	96	1	1	100	96	0

ADONITOL FERMENTATION	MYO-INOSITOL FERMENTATION	D-SORBITOL FERMENTATION	L-ARABINOSE FERMENTATION	RAFFINOSE FERMENTATION	L-RHAMNOSE FERMENTATION	MALTOSE FERMENTATION	D-XYLOSE FERMENTATION	TREHALOSE FERMENTATION	CELLOBIOSE FERMENTATION	α-METHYL-D-GLUCOSIDE FERMENTATION	ERYTHRITOL FERMENTATION	ESCULIN HYDROLYSIS	MELIBIOSE FERMENTATION	D-ARABITOL FERMENTATION	GLYCEROL FERMENTATION	MUCATE FERMENTATION	"TARTRATE, JORDAN'S"	ACETATE UTILIZATION	LIPASE (CORN OIL)	DNASE (25°C)	NITRATE NITRITE	"OXIDASE, KOVACS"	ONPG TEST	YELLOW PIGMENT	D-MANNOSE FERMENTATION
93	0	0	100	66	100	100	100	100	100	0	0	100	100	96	3	93	83	28	0	0	100	0	100	37	100
0	0	0	100	0	0	0	83	0	0	0	0	0	0	0	17	100	100	0	0	0	100	0	0	0	0
0	0	0	100	0	0	0	100	0	0	0	0	0	0	0	0	50	100	0	0	0	100	0	0	0	0
100	0	0	0	100	0	30	0	0	0	0	0	0	100	75	10	0	30	10	0	0	90	0	90	0	100
0	0	0	0	0	0	0	0	0	0	0	0	0	0	0	5	0	95	0	0	0	90	0	10	0	98
0	0	0	0	0	0	0	0	100	0	0	0	0	0	0	7	7	100	0	0	0	100	0	0	0	100
0	0	0	0	0	0	0	0	0	0	0	0	0	0	0	100	0	100	0	0	0	90	0	20	0	100
0	0	0	0	0	15	50	15	85	0	0	0	0	0	0	0	0	15	0	0	0	100	0	0	0	85
7	15	30	95	30	85	89	93	97	55	7	0	60	50	50	30	40	25	30	0	0	85	0	90	75	98
0	0	0	100	0	91	82	100	100	55	0	0	0	0	100	27	0	9	100	0	0	91	0	91	27	100
0	0	0	0	0	0	25	0	0	0	0	0	0	0	0	0	0	50	0	0	0	0	0	0	50	100
0	0	0	0	0	0	0	0	0	0	0	0	0	0	0	0	0	60	20	0	0	0	0	0	60	100
0	0	0	0	0	0	0	0	0	0	0	0	78	0	0	0	0	0	0	0	0	100	0	0	0	0
0	0	0	0	0	0	100	100	0	0	50	0	0	0	0	0	0	0	0	0	0	100	0	0	0	0
0	0	0	0	1	1	0	98	98	1	0	0	0	0	0	70	0	87	20	92	50	95	0	0	0	0
0	0	0	0	0	0	100	0	100	0	100	0	0	0	0	100	0	100	0	100	50	100	0	0	0	0
0	0	0	0	1	0	100	100	55	0	80	0	0	0	0	55	0	85	5	45	40	90	0	1	0	0
0	0	0	0	1	5	97	95	30	0	60	1	50	0	0	60	0	80	25	80	80	98	0	1	0	0
98	1	1	1	1	0	1	1	2	0	0	0	0	0	0	15	0	90	40	0	0	100	0	1	0	100
92	46	0	0	0	100	54	8	0	0	0	0	0	0	0	92	0	69	0	0	0	100	0	0	0	100
100	90	1	0	5	70	2	10	0	3	2	75	35	5	100	60	0	95	60	0	0	100	0	5	0	100
0	0	0	0	0	0	0	0	0	0	0	0	0	0	0	5	0	50	25	0	0	100	0	0	0	100
5	95	1	1	7	0	1	7	98	5	0	0	0	0	0	50	0	90	75	0	10	100	0	10	0	100
0	0	94	100	94	94	94	94	100	100	0	0	100	100	0	13	30	6	6	0	0	100	0	100	0	100
0	35	95	99	2	95	97	97	99	5	2	0	5	95	0	5	90	90	90	0	2	100	0	2	0	100

(Continued)

Table 6-7 *Continued*

"ORGANISM"[a,b]	INDOLE PRODUCTION	METHYL RED	VOGES-PROSKAUER	CITRATE (SIMMONS)	HYDROGEN SULFIDE (TSI)	UREA HYDROLYSIS	PHENYLALANINE DEAMINASE	LYSINE DECARBOXYLASE	ARGININE DIHYDROLASE	ORNITHINE DECARBOXYLASE	MOTILITY	GELATIN HYDROLYSIS (22°C)	GROWTH IN KCN	MALONATE UTILIZATION	"D-GLUCOSE, ACID"	"D-GLUCOSE, GAS"	LACTOSE FERMENTATION	SUCROSE FERMENTATION	D-MANNITOL FERMENTATION	DULCITOL FERMENTATION	SALICIN FERMENTATION
Salmonella																					
S. serotype Choleraesuis	0	100	0	25	50	0	0	95	55	100	95	0	0	0	100	95	0	0	98	5	0
S. serotype Gallinarum	0	100	0	0	100	0	0	90	10	1	0	0	0	0	100	0	0	0	100	90	0
S. serotype Paratyphi A	0	100	0	0	10	0	0	0	15	95	95	0	0	0	100	99	0	0	100	90	0
S. serotype Pullorum	0	90	0	0	90	0	0	100	10	95	0	0	0	0	100	90	0	0	100	0	0
S. serotype Typhi	0	100	0	0	97	0	0	98	3	0	97	0	0	0	100	0	1	0	100	0	0
S. enterica subsp. salamae (Group II)	2	100	0	100	100	0	0	100	90	100	98	2	0	95	100	100	1	1	100	90	5
S. enterica subsp. arizonae (Group IIIa)	1	100	0	99	99	0	0	99	70	99	99	0	1	95	100	99	15	1	100	0	0
S. enterica subsp. diarizonae (Group IIIb)	2	100	0	98	99	0	0	99	70	99	99	0	1	95	100	99	85	5	10	1	0
S. enterica subsp. houtenae (Group IV)	0	100	0	98	100	2	0	100	70	100	98	0	95	0	100	100	0	0	98	0	60
S. enterica subsp. indica (Group VI)	0	100	0	89	100	0	0	100	67	100	100	0	0	0	100	100	22	0	100	67	0
S. bongori (Group V)	0	100	0	94	100	0	0	100	94	100	100	0	100	0	100	94	0	0	100	94	0
Serratia																					
S. entomophilia	0	20	100	100	0	0	0	0	0	0	100	100	100	0	100	0	0	100	100	0	100
S. ficaria	0	75	75	100	0	0	0	0	0	0	100	100	55	0	100	0	15	100	100	0	100
"S. fonticola"	0	100	9	91	0	13	0	100	0	97	91	0	70	88	100	79	97	21	100	91	100
S. liquefaciens group	1	93	93	90	0	3	0	95	0	95	95	90	90	2	100	75	10	98	100	0	97
S. marcescens	1	20	98	98	0	15	0	99	0	99	97	90	95	3	100	55	2	99	99	0	95
S. marcescens biogroup 1	0	100	60	30	0	0	0	55	4	65	17	30	70	0	100	0	4	100	96	0	92
S. odorifera biogroup 1	60	100	50	100	0	5	0	100	0	100	100	95	60	0	100	0	70	100	100	0	98
S. odorifera biogroup 2	50	60	100	97	0	0	0	94	0	0	100	94	19	0	100	13	97	0	97	0	45
S. plymuthica	0	94	80	75	0	0	0	0	0	0	50	60	30	0	100	40	80	100	100	0	94
S. rubidea	0	20	100	95	0	2	0	55	0	0	85	90	25	94	100	30	100	99	100	0	99
Shigella																					
S. dysenteria (Group A)	45	99	0	0	0	0	0	0	2	0	0	0	0	0	100	0	0	0	0	5	0
S. flexneri (Group B)	50	100	0	0	0	0	0	0	5	0	0	0	0	0	100	3	1	1	95	1	0
S. boydii (Group C)	25	100	0	0	0	0	0	0	18	2	0	0	0	0	100	0	1	0	97	5	0
S. sonnei (Group D)	0	100	0	0	0	0	0	0	2	98	0	0	0	0	100	0	2	1	99	0	0

ADONITOL FERMENTATION	MYO-INOSITOL FERMENTATION	D-SORBITOL FERMENTATION	L-ARABINOSE FERMENTATION	RAFFINOSE FERMENTATION	L-RHAMNOSE FERMENTATION	MALTOSE FERMENTATION	D-XYLOSE FERMENTATION	TREHALOSE FERMENTATION	CELLOBIOSE FERMENTATION	α-METHYL-D-GLUCOSIDE FERMENTATION	ERYTHRITOL FERMENTATION	ESCULIN HYDROLYSIS	MELIBIOSE FERMENTATION	D-ARABITOL FERMENTATION	GLYCEROL FERMENTATION	MUCATE FERMENTATION	"TARTRATE, JORDAN'S"	ACETATE UTILIZATION	LIPASE (CORN OIL)	DNASE (25°C)	NITRATE NITRITE	"OXIDASE, KOVACS"	ONPG TEST	YELLOW PIGMENT	D-MANNOSE FERMENTATION
0	0	90	0	1	100	95	98	0	0	0	1	0	45	1	0	0	85	1	0	0	98	0	0	0	95
0	0	1	80	10	10	90	70	50	10	0	1	0	0	0	0	50	100	0	0	10	100	0	0	0	100
0	0	95	100	0	100	95	0	100	5	0	0	0	95	0	10	0	0	0	0	0	100	0	0	0	100
0	0	10	100	1	100	5	90	90	5	0	0	0	0	0	0	0	0	0	0	0	100	0	0	0	100
0	0	99	2	0	0	97	82	100	0	0	0	0	100	0	20	0	100	0	0	0	100	0	0	0	100
0	5	100	100	0	100	100	100	100	0	8	0	15	8	0	25	96	50	95	0	0	100	0	15	0	95
0	0	99	99	1	99	98	100	99	1	1	0	1	95	1	10	90	5	90	0	2	100	0	100	0	100
0	0	99	99	1	99	98	100	99	1	1	0	1	95	1	10	30	20	75	0	2	100	0	95	0	100
5	0	100	100	0	98	100	100	100	50	0	0	0	100	5	0	0	65	70	0	0	100	0	0	0	100
0	0	0	100	0	100	100	100	100	0	0	0	0	89	0	33	89	100	89	0	0	100	0	44	0	100
0	0	100	94	0	88	100	100	100	0	0	0	0	94	0	0	88	0	100	0	0	100	0	94	0	100
0	0	0	0	0	0	100	40	100	0	0	0	100	0	60	0	0	100	80	20	100	100	0	100	0	100
0	55	100	100	70	35	100	100	100	100	8	0	100	40	100	0	0	17	40	77	100	92	8	100	0	100
100	30	100	100	100	76	97	85	100	6	91	0	100	98	100	88	0	58	15	0	0	100	0	100	0	100
5	60	95	98	85	15	98	100	100	5	5	0	97	75	0	95	0	75	40	85	85	100	0	93	0	100
40	75	99	0	2	0	96	7	99	5	0	1	95	0	0	95	0	75	50	98	98	98	0	95	0	99
30	30	92	0	0	0	70	0	100	4	0	0	96	0	0	92	0	50	4	75	82	83	0	75	0	100
50	100	100	100	100	95	100	100	100	100	0	0	95	100	0	40	5	100	60	35	100	100	0	100	0	100
55	100	100	100	7	94	100	100	100	100	0	7	40	96	0	50	0	100	65	65	100	100	0	100	0	100
0	50	65	100	94	0	94	94	100	88	70	0	81	93	0	50	0	100	55	70	100	100	0	70	0	100
99	20	1	100	99	1	99	99	100	94	1	0	94	99	85	20	0	70	80	99	99	100	0	100	0	100
0	0	30	45	0	30	15	4	90	0	0	0	0	0	0	10	0	75	0	0	0	99	0	30	0	100
0	0	29	60	40	5	30	2	65	0	0	0	0	55	1	10	0	30	8	0	0	99	0	1	0	100
0	0	43	94	0	1	20	11	85	0	0	0	0	15	0	50	0	50	0	0	0	100	0	100	0	100
0	0	2	95	3	75	90	2	100	5	0	0	0	25	0	15	10	90	0	0	0	100	0	90	0	100

(Continued)

Table 6-7 *Continued*

"ORGANISM"[a,b]	INDOLE PRODUCTION	METHYL RED	VOGES-PROSKAUER	CITRATE (SIMMONS)	HYDROGEN SULFIDE (TSI)	UREA HYDROLYSIS	PHENYLALANINE DEAMINASE	LYSINE DECARBOXYLASE	ARGININE DIHYDROLASE	ORNITHINE DECARBOXYLASE	MOTILITY	GELATIN HYDROLYSIS (22°C)	GROWTH IN KCN	MALONATE UTILIZATION	"D-GLUCOSE, ACID"	"D-GLUCOSE, GAS"	LACTOSE FERMENTATION	SUCROSE FERMENTATION	D-MANNITOL FERMENTATION	DULCITOL FERMENTATION	SALICIN FERMENTATION
Tatumella																					
T. ptyseos	0	0	5	2	0	0	90	0	0	0	0	0	0	0	100	0	0	98	0	0	55
Trabulsiella																					
T. guamensis	40	100	0	88	100	0	0	100	50	100	100	0	100	0	100	100	0	0	100	0	13
Xenorhabdus																					
X. nematophilus (25°C)	40	0	0	0	0	0	0	0	0	0	100	80	0	0	80	0	0	0	0	0	0
Yersinia																					
Y. aldovae	0	80	0	0	0	60	0	0	0	40	0	0	0	0	100	0	0	20	80	0	0
Y. bercoviera	0	100	0	0	0	60	0	0	0	80	0	0	0	0	100	0	20	100	100	0	20
Y. enterocolitica	50	97	2	0	0	75	0	0	0	95	2	0	2	0	100	5	5	95	98	0	20
Y. frederiksenii	100	100	0	15	0	70	0	0	0	95	5	0	0	0	100	40	40	100	100	0	92
Y. intermedia	100	100	5	5	0	80	0	0	0	100	5	0	10	5	100	18	35	100	100	0	100
Y. kristensenii	30	92	0	0	0	77	0	0	0	92	5	0	0	0	100	23	8	0	100	0	15
Y. mollaretii	0	100	0	0	0	20	0	0	0	80	0	0	0	0	100	0	40	100	100	0	20
Y. pestis	0	80	0	0	0	5	0	0	0	0	0	0	0	0	100	0	0	0	97	0	70
Y. pseudotuberculosis	0	100	0	0	0	95	0	0	0	0	0	0	0	0	100	0	0	0	100	0	25
Y. rohdei	0	62	0	0	0	62	0	0	0	25	0	0	0	0	100	0	0	100	100	0	0
"Y. ruckeri"	0	97	10	0	0	0	0	50	5	100	0	30	15	0	100	5	0	0	100	0	0
Yokenella																					
Y. regensburgei (Koserella trabulsii)	0	100	0	92	0	0	0	100	8	100	100	0	92	0	100	100	0	0	100	0	8
Enteric group 58	0	100	0	85	0	70	0	100	0	85	100	0	100	85	100	85	30	0	100	85	100
Enteric group 59	10	100	0	100	0	0	30	0	60	0	100	0	80	90	100	100	80	0	100	0	100
Enteric group 60	0	100	0	0	0	50	0	0	0	100	75	0	0	100	100	100	0	0	50	0	0
Enteric group 68	0	100	50	0	0	0	0	0	0	0	0	0	100	0	100	0	0	100	100	0	50
Enteric group 137	100	100	0	0	0	70	0	0	20	100	100	0	100	0	100	0	100	100	100	0	100

[a] Each number is the percentage of positive reactions after 2 days of incubation at 36°C unless otherwise indicated (gelatin liquefication and deoxyribonuclease and positive after 2 days are not considered.

[b] All Data from Centers for Disease Contol, except E. alberti[3]; E. cowanii[235]; P. hauserii[335]; and enteric group 137[492].

TSI, triple sugar iron agar; ONPG, o-nitrophenyl-β-D-galactopyrannoside; NA, not available.

ADONITOL FERMENTATION	MYO-INOSITOL FERMENTATION	D-SORBITOL FERMENTATION	L-ARABINOSE FERMENTATION	RAFFINOSE FERMENTATION	L-RHAMNOSE FERMENTATION	MALTOSE FERMENTATION	D-XYLOSE FERMENTATION	TREHALOSE FERMENTATION	CELLOBIOSE FERMENTATION	α-METHYL-D-GLUCOSIDE FERMENTATION	ERYTHRITOL FERMENTATION	ESCULIN HYDROLYSIS	MELIBIOSE FERMENTATION	D-ARABITOL FERMENTATION	GLYCEROL FERMENTATION	MUCATE FERMENTATION	"TARTRATE, JORDAN'S"	ACETATE UTILIZATION	LIPASE (CORN OIL)	DNASE (25°C)	NITRATE NITRITE	"OXIDASE, KOVACS"	ONPG TEST	YELLOW PIGMENT	D-MANNOSE FERMENTATION
0	0	0	0	11	0	0	9	93	0	0	0	0	25	0	7	0	0	0	0	0	98	0	0	0	100
0	0	100	100	0	100	100	100	100	100	0	0	40	0	0	0	100	50	88	0	0	100	0	100	0	100
0	0	0	0	0	0	0	0	0	0	0	0	0	0	0	0	0	60	0	0	20	20	0	0	60	80
0	0	60	60	0	0	0	40	80	0	0	0	0	0	0	0	0	100	0	0	0	100	0	0	0	100
0	0	100	100	0	0	100	100	100	100	0	0	20	0	0	0	0	100	0	0	0	100	0	80	0	100
0	30	99	98	5	1	75	70	98	75	0	0	25	1	40	90	0	85	15	55	5	98	0	95	0	100
0	20	100	100	30	99	100	100	100	100	0	0	85	0	100	85	5	55	15	55	0	100	0	100	0	100
0	15	100	100	45	100	100	100	100	96	77	0	100	80	45	60	6	88	18	12	0	94	0	90	0	100
0	15	100	77	0	0	100	85	100	100	0	0	0	0	45	70	0	40	8	0	0	100	0	70	0	100
0	0	100	100	0	0	60	60	100	100	0	0	0	0	0	20	0	100	0	0	0	100	0	20	0	100
0	0	50	100	0	1	80	90	100	0	0	0	50	20	0	50	0	0	0	0	0	85	0	50	0	100
0	0	0	50	15	70	95	100	100	0	0	0	95	70	0	50	0	50	0	0	0	95	0	70	0	100
0	0	100	100	62	0	0	38	100	25	0	0	0	50	0	38	0	100	0	0	0	88	0	50	0	100
0	0	50	5	5	0	95	0	95	5	0	0	0	0	0	30	0	30	0	30	0	75	0	50	0	100
0	0	0	100	25	100	100	100	100	100	0	0	67	92	0	0	0	0	25	0	0	100	0	100	0	100
0	0	100	100	0	100	100	100	100	100	55	0	0	0	0	30	0	60	45	0	0	100	0	100	0	100
0	0	0	100	0	100	100	100	100	100	10	0	100	0	10	10	60	50	50	0	0	100	0	100	25	100
0	0	0	25	0	75	0	0	100	0	0	0	0	0	0	75	0	75	0	0	0	100	0	100	0	100
0	0	0	0	0	0	50	0	100	0	0	0	0	0	0	50	0	0	0	0	100	100	0	0	0	100
0	0	100	100	100	100	100	100	100	100	80	0	100	100	0	100	100	50	100	0	0	100	0	100	0	100

all reactions of Xenorhabdus species and P. luminescens and Yersinia rucker). The vast majority of the positive reactions occur within 24 hr. Reactions that become

Table 6-8 Key Features of Diarrheagenic *E. coli*[140,339]

TERM	ABBREVIATION	PATHOGENIC PHENOTYPE	SIGNS AND SYMPTOMS
Enterotoxigenic *E. coli*	ETEC	Elaboration of secretory heat-labile (LT) and/or heat-stable (ST) entero-toxins that do not damage the mucosal epithelium. Toxin production is plasmid-mediated and most commonly involves *E. coli* serogroups 06, 08, 015, 020, 025, 027, 063, 078, 080, 085, 092, 0115, 0128ac, 0139, 0148, 0153, 0159, and 0167.[410] From 1996 to 2003, 16 outbreaks of ETEC infections occurred in the U.S. and on cruise ships. *E. coli* O169:H41 was identified in 10 outbreaks. This serotype was identified in 1 of 21 confirmed ETEC outbreaks before 1996.[32]	Associated with two major clinical syndromes: "weanling diarrhea" among children in the developing world and "traveler's diarrhea." Typically abrupt in onset with short incubation period (14–50 hr). Profuse watery diarrhea is predominant symptom (similar to *Vibrio cholerae*), usually without blood, mucus, or pus. Often accompanied by mild abdominal cramps. Dehydration and vomiting occur in some cases.
Enteropathogenic *E. coli*	EPEC	Adhere to intestinal epithelial cells in localized microcolonies producing characteristic histopathologic lesions known as "attaching and effacing lesions" (A/E lesions) serogroups 055, 086, 0111, 0119, 0126, 0127, 0128ab, and 0142 are most commonly involved.[410]	Usually occurs in infants. Characterized by low-grade fever, malaise, vomiting, and profuse, watery diarrhea, with a prominent amount of mucus, but with no gross blood. Fecal leukocytes are seen only occasionally.
Enteroinvasive *E. coli*	EIEC	Invade colonic epithelial cells. Pathogenesis virtually identical to *Shigella* species. As with *Shigella*, most strains are nonmotile, late- or non–lactose-fermenters, and anaerogenic. The most commonly involved serogroups are 028ac, 029, 0112ac, 0124, 0136, 0143, 0144, 0152, and 0164.[410]	Infection presents most commonly as watery diarrhea, indistinguishable from ETEC. Some patients present with a dysentery syndrome; hallmarks are fever and colitis. Symptoms are urgency and tenesmus; blood, mucus, and many leukocytes in stool.
Enterohemorrhagic *E. coli*	EHEC	Elaboration of Shiga toxins, an enterohemolysin, and like EPEC produce A/E lesions. Most commonly involved serogroup is O157:H7	Bloody diarrhea without white cells. Often no fever. Abdominal pain is common. May progress to HUS.
Enteroaggregative *E. coli*	EAEC	Adhere to epithelial cells in a pattern resembling a pile of stacked bricks and produce an ST-like toxin (EAST1), an LT toxin and fimbrial colonization factors called "AAFs" (aggregative adherence fimbriae).	Watery, mucoid, secretory diarrheal illness with low-grade fever and little or no vomiting. Stools usually without gross blood or fecal leukocytes. Recovered principally from children with chronic diarrhea.[340,372]
Diffusely adherent *E. coli*	DAEC	Adhere to epithelial cells in a diffuse pattern and carry a gene encoding surface fimbria designated F1845.	Majority of patients have watery diarrhea without blood or fecal leukocytes.

known as Shiga-like toxins). Shiga toxin 1 (Stx1) is indistinguishable from Shiga toxin produced by *Shigella dysenteriae* type 1. Shiga toxin 2 (Stx2) is a more divergent molecule that has multiple variants (Stx2, Stx2c, Stx2d, Stx2e, Stx2f) that are closely related to each other but more distantly related to Stx1. Some *E. coli* O157 strains produce only Stx1, some only Stx2, while others produce both. The toxins do not carry equivalent risks of causing HUS. Strains that produce only Stx2 have the highest risk; strains that produce only Stx1 have the lowest risk, while strains that make both toxins carry an intermediate risk. Both toxins are composed of five B subunits and a single A subunit. The B subunit binds to globotriaosylceramide (Gb_3), a glycolipid found in varying degrees in membranes of eukaryotic cells. The A

CLINICAL CORRELATION BOX 6-1 Hemorrhagic Colitis and Hemolytic—Uremic Syndrome

Hemolytic—uremic syndrome (HUS) is a thrombotic disease of the kidney microvasculature in which the endothelial cell is the primary site of damage. HUS is defined by a triad of features: 1) the appearance of fragmented red cells (microangiopathic hemolytic anemia), 2) reduced platelet count (thrombocytopenia), and 3) acute renal failure, evidenced by a reduced glomerular filtration rate and low urine output. HUS is the leading cause of acute renal failure in children. In its most common form, this syndrome is preceded by a diarrheal illness that presents with severe abdominal pain, vomiting, and watery diarrhea. The diarrhea subsequently becomes blood-streaked or grossly bloody, and despite evidence of colitis, the children typically have little or no fever. This constellation of signs and symptoms is called **hemorrhagic colitis.** In the most severe cases, ischemic colitis and perforation can occur. In some patients, colonic stenosis can develop following ischemic colitis. EHEC organisms colonize the large intestine via the formation of distinctive attaching and effacing lesions that provide a tight junction between the EHEC and the surface of the intestinal epithelial cells. Development of attaching and effacing lesions (A/E lesions) requires numerous genes that are located on a 35-kb chromosome pathogenicity island termed the locus on enterocyte effacement (LEE). Following colonization, EHEC produce Shiga toxins (Stxs) that translocate into the circulation, probably facilitated by the influx (transmigration) of neutrophils. Once in the circulation, Shiga toxin travels to the kidneys, where it is transferred and bound via the toxin's B subunits to neutral glycolipid globotriaosylceramide (Gb_3) receptors on target cells (i.e., glomerular endothelial and tubular epithelial cells). The toxin is then internalized and routed to the endoplasmic reticulum, where the single A subunit enzymatically inactivates the ribosomes, causing inhibition of protein synthesis and cell damage. This leads to glomerular endothelial cell swelling and detachment from the underlying basement membrane with secondary activation of both platelets and the coagulation cascade.

This sequence of events results in the classic signs of Shiga toxin—mediated HUS. The coagulation cascade results in fibrin deposition, causing narrowing of the capillaries and shearing of red cells as they attempt to push through the damaged vessels. The shearing and tearing of red cells results in the fragmented red cells typical of microangiopathic hemolytic anemia. The consumption of platelets leads to thrombocytopenia, and the anemia along with restricted blood flow to the kidneys leads to renal failure.[447] There are no treatments of proven value other than supportive care. Antibiotic treatment of children with *E. coli* O157:H7 infection increases the risk of HUS and therefore should be avoided.[508] Research is currently underway to develop specific Stx antibodies to block the binding of Stx to endothelial cells as well as synthetic Gb_3 receptor analogues that can be given orally and entrap Stx in the gut and prevent its entrance into the circulation.[256,493]

subunit is a potent cytotoxin and is responsible for cell injury. Production of Shiga toxin is not in itself sufficient to cause disease. Other virulence factors identified in *E. coli* O157 include a 60-MDa-virulence plasmid (pO157) and the locus of enterocyte effacement (LEE). The 60-MDa plasmid encodes an enterohemolysin (designated EHEC-Hly) that may allow *E. coli* O157 to use hemoglobin released by the action of EHEC-Hly as a source of iron, thereby stimulating the growth of *E. coli* O157 in the gut.[380] The LEE contains genes for an adhesion molecule (intimin) and for other factors important for the production of attaching—effacing lesions. The clinical manifestations of *E. coli* O157 infection range from asymptomatic carriage to nonbloody diarrhea, hemorrhagic colitis, hemolytic—uremic syndrome, and death. The incubation period varies from 1 to 8 days, with an average interval of 3 days between exposure and illness. Most patients with hemorrhagic colitis recover within 7 days. Illness typically begins with abdominal cramps and nonbloody diarrhea. Stool may become bloody after the first 1–2 days, with the amount of blood varying from a few small streaks to stools that are almost entirely blood. Vomiting occurs in 30–60% of cases, and fever is usually low-grade or absent.[315] Hemolytic—uremic syndrome following urinary tract infection with EHEC has been reported[323,459]; however, because of the low prevalence, routine testing of sorbitol-negative *E. coli* urinary isolates for the presence of Shiga toxin does not seem warranted.[477,505] Currently, antibiotics are not recommended for treatment of *E. coli* O157 infections because of the concern that antibiotic use will increase the production of Shiga toxins. Shiga toxin genes are bacteriophage-encoded, and antibiotics that cause bacteriophage induction (e.g., fluoroquinolones, trimethoprim-sulfamethoxazole and furazolidone) may increase Stx expression. In view of these issues, it is recommended that clinical laboratories do not report antimicrobial susceptibility results for O157 or other Shiga toxin *E. coli* isolates.[267,508]

Epidemiology of Enterohemorrhagic: *E. coli* In early 1993, the largest *E. coli* food-poisoning outbreak to date caused by *E. coli* O157:H7 occurred in the states of Washington, Idaho, California, and Nevada. Altogether, 582 culture-confirmed cases were reported, causing 171 hospitalizations, 41 cases of HUS, and 4 deaths. Hamburgers from a single fast-food restaurant chain were implicated. The source of most cases of *E. coli*–related illnesses in the United States is considered to be ground beef. Hamburgers in particular have been the cause of multiple outbreaks of disease. This is because of the high prevalence of *E. coli* O157:H7 infection in cows. For a summary of risk factors during all the steps of industrial scale beef production from farm to fork see the review by Meyer-Broseta and colleagues.[322] According to recent market-basket surveys, *E. coli* O157:H7 is present in 1.0–2.5% of meat and poultry samples. It also turns up less frequently in supermarket samples of lamb and pork, although such isolates could arise from secondary contamination in the butchering area. In the United States, cases have tended to occur in the last two thirds of the year and in states bordering Canada. Infection persists in animal reservoirs in part because the organism survives in soil for long periods. Other animals, including pigs, sheep, deer, and rabbits, can also carry EHEC, and many other foods and water can be contaminated with the feces of infected animals.[185,350] The result has been outbreaks involving municipal water supplies,[368] venison,[409] uncooked vegetables, cheese curd,[97] apple cider,[91] and alfalfa sprouts.[59,327] In addition, because incredibly low numbers of these organisms can cause illness, person-to-person spread has occurred within families and in day-care centers, among children during visits to dairy farms,[98] and petting zoos,[218] and among persons exposed to sawdust and other surfaces in county fair buildings used for showing animals.[486] Although O157:H7 is the prototypic serotype of EHEC in the United States, several other EHEC serotypes, such as O26:H11, O48:H21, O103:H2, O111:NM (nonmotile), and O145:NM, have been recognized in other countries.[153,252,293] Although non-O157 serotypes of EHEC are rare in the United States, one outbreak of hemorrhagic colitis caused by EHEC serotype O104:H21 was reported among 11 patients in Helena, Montana. in 1994.[90] Another outbreak occurred among teenage campers in Texas in June 1999, caused by EHEC serotype O111:H8, in which 55 campers became ill and HUS developed in two.[61,96] *E. coli* O111 is the second most common non-O157 STEC reported in the United States,[62] and it is among the most common reported in Europe.[65] To learn more about infections caused by EHEC, the reviews by Kaper and O'Brien,[254] Mead and Griffin,[315] Nataro and Kaper,[339] Paton and Paton,[380] and Tarr[469] may be consulted.

Detection of Enterohemorrhagic *E. coli* Isolation of *E. coli* O157:H7 is possible only during the acute phase of illness, and the organisms may not be detectable 5–7 days after onset. Since the majority of EHEC infections are caused by *E. coli* serotype O157:H7, the current laboratory approaches to detection are based on either detection of Shiga toxin–producing strains or detection of the O157:H7 serotype. The currently accepted methods for detection can be summarized as follows: 1) assays for the detection of the O157 serotype[299,376,458] or Shiga toxins[259,299,346] directly from stool; 2) direct plating on sorbitol MacConkey agar (SMAC),[306] cefixime-SMAC,[108] SMAC supplemented with cefixime and tellurite (CT-SMAC),[514] or media containing either 5-bromo-5-chloro-3-indoxyl-β-D-glucuronide,[367] or 4-methylumbelliferyl-β-D-glucuronide[476]; and 3) immunomagnetic separation (IMS) using O157-specific, antibody-coated beads, followed by bacteriologic culture.[109,255] Many laboratories in the United States and elsewhere use sorbitol–MacConkey (SMAC) agar to identify the slow sorbitol fermentation phenotype (i.e., sorbitol-negative at 24 hr) of O157:H7. SMAC agar contains 1% D-sorbitol, rather than lactose to differentiate sorbitol-negative *E. coli* strains (colonies appear colorless, similar to lactose-negative colonies on regular MacConkey agar). Suspected isolates are then confirmed with specific O157:H7 antisera. This medium, however, does not detect other, sorbitol-positive EHEC serotypes. Other detection methods such as chromogenic medium and ELISA methods for detection of Shiga toxin are more sensitive and specific but are considerably more expensive than SMAC.[346,376] Incorporation of this testing into the routine microbiology laboratory comes at a significant additional cost, and laboratories may want to limit testing to patients at highest risk. A minireview on the role of the laboratory in the diagnosis of EHEC infections has been provided by Kehl.[260]

Species Other Than *E. coli* Strains designated in the CDC classification as *E. coli* inactive are anaerogenic (non–gas-producing), lactose-negative (or delayed), and nonmotile. These strains were previously known as the Alkalescens-Dispar serotype.

E. albertii is a newly described species of indole-, D-sorbitol-, and lactose-negative enterobacterial isolates recovered from diarrheal stools of children.[233] Because these strains are not included in the databases of commercial systems at present, they are most often identified as *Hafnia*, *Salmonella*, *Escherichia coli*, or *Yersinia ruckeri*.[3] *E. albertii* most closely resemble inactive *E. coli*, although they do not resemble the Alkalescens-Dispar group because of their ability to produce gas from D-glucose. They can be separated from *H. alvei* based on acetate assimilation, negative Voges-Proskauer test, and failure to grow in potassium cyanide (KCN). In addition, *E. albertii* show weak to moderate L-prolineaminopeptidase (PYR) reactions, whereas *H. alvei* express strong PYR activity.[3] Laboratory workers should be advised that isolates recovered from stool specimens that give an unacceptable first-choice identification of *H. alvei* for an isolate that is L-rhamnose-, D-xylose- and Voges-Proskauer-negative should be further tested to rule out *E. albertii*.

E. fergusonii (formerly CDC enteric group 10) has been recovered from blood, gallbladder, urine, and feces; however, its clinical significance has not been established.[165,166,179,180,423] It is differentiated from *E. coli* by being sorbitol- and lactose-negative, but adonitol- and cellobiose-positive.

E. hermanii (formerly CDC enteric group 11) has been most commonly found in human wounds, sputum, and feces.[394] Of eight strains recovered at the University of Illinois Medical Center, five have been from wound specimens, including four leg wounds in patients with cellulitis and one finger wound, and one strain each has been recovered from urine, maxillary sinus, and blood. The isolates recovered from wounds were mixed with other pathogenic species; however, the blood, urine, and sinus isolates were present as the only isolates. Ginsberg and Daum[194] reported recovery of *E. hermanii* from blood, cerebrospinal fluid (CSF), and peritoneal fluid of a septic neonate with bowel perforation; however, other organisms were recovered from the blood, and the pathogenic role in this patient was uncertain. The only documented case of invasive disease caused by *E. hermanii* is from a neonate with bacterial infection of a cephalohematoma with meningitis documented by culture from multiple CSF specimens and fluid aspirated from an enlarging cephalohematoma.[126] *E. hermanii* strains are yellow-pigmented, indole-positive, and sorbitol-negative.[50] Because *E. hermanii* are sorbitol-negative, they appear biochemically similar to the O157 serotype of *E. coli*.

E. vulneris (formerly CDC enteric group 1) has a high propensity for causing human wound infections, particularly of the arms and legs,[54,394] which may lead to osteomyelitis.[285] In addition, there have been reports of urosepsis and intravenous catheter–related bacteremia caused by *E. vulneris*.[19,229,455] One case of *E. vulneris* bacteremia in a 40-day-old infant has been seen at the University of Illinois Medical Center. Over half of the strains are yellow-pigmented, and they are both indole- and sorbitol-negative.

Table 6-9 Differentiation of Species Within the Genus *Escherichia*

BIOCHEMICAL TEST	E. ALBERTII	E. BLATTAE	E. COLI	E. FERGUSONII	E. HERMANNII	E. VULNERIS
Indole	−	−	+	+	+	−
Methyl red	+	+	+	+	+	+
Voges-Proskauer	−	−	−	−	−	−
Citrate	−	V (50)	−	V (17)	−	−
Lysine decarboxylase	+	+	+	+	−	V (85)
Arginine dihydrolase	−	−	V (17)	−	−	V (30)
Ornithine decarboxylase	+	+	V (65)	+	+	−
ONPG	+	−	+	V (83)	+	+
Fermentation of:						
Lactose	−	−	+	−	V (45)	V (15)
Sorbitol	−	−	+[a]	−	−	−
Mannitol	+	−	+	+	+	+
Adonitol	−	−	−	+	−	−
Cellobiose	−	−	−	+	+	+
Yellow pigment	−	−	−	−	+	V (50)

[a] Strains of E. coli belonging to serotype O157:H7 are sorbitol-negative.
+, 90% or more strains positive; −, 90% or more strains are negative; V, 11–89% of strains are positive.

E. blattae, recovered from the intestinal tract of cockroaches, is indole-negative and does not ferment lactose. It has not been associated with human infections.

E. adecarboxylata has been assigned to a new genus as *Leclercia adecarboxylata*.[467] The different biochemical reactions for the recognized species of *Escherichia* are shown in Table 6-9.

Genus Shigella. *Shigella* species can be suspected in cultures because they are non–lactose-fermenters and tend to be biochemically inert. They typically do not produce gas from carbohydrates, with the exception of certain biogroups of *S. flexneri* that are aerogenic. Rare strains of *S. sonnei* can slowly ferment lactose (2%) and sucrose (1%), and most strains can decarboxylate ornithine—characteristics not shared by other *Shigella* species.

There are 4 major subgroups and 43 recognized serotypes of Shigella as shown in Box 6-9.[78] The CDC classification combines *S. dysenteriae* (group A), *S. flexneri* (group B), and *S. boydii* (group C) as ''Shigella serogroups A, B, and C'' because of their biochemical similarities. The presence of ornithine decarboxylase activity and β-galactosidase make most strains of *S. sonnei* biochemically distinct from the other *Shigella* species. The inability to ferment mannitol distinguishes *S. dysenteriae*. The differential characteristics for the four species of *Shigella* are included in Table 6-10. Isolates recovered from stool specimens from patients with diarrheal disease that are suspected of being *Shigella* species, should be biochemically categorized and the species confirmed by serologic testing. In the near future, it may be possible to detect *Shigella* species and enteroinvasive strains of *E. coli* using DNA probes selected to detect the virulence plasmids responsible for coding the gene products that initiate intracellular penetration and bowel wall invasion.[43]

Incidence and Sources of *Shigella* Infections Shigellosis is the most communicable of the bacterial diarrheas. Humans serve as the natural host, and disease is transmitted by the fecal–oral route, with as few as 200 viable organisms being able to cause disease. Between 20,000 and 30,000 cases

CLINICAL CORRELATION BOX 6-2 *Shigella* **Infection (Bacillary Dysentery)**

The term "dysentery" was used by Hippocrates to indicate a condition characterized by frequent passage of stool containing blood and mucus accompanied by straining and painful defecation.[142] Humans are the only natural host for *Shigella,* and infection occurs by ingestion. Bacillary dysentery is the most communicable of the bacterial diarrheas, with an infective dose as low as 10–100 bacteria producing disease in healthy adults.[143] Fever, watery diarrhea with cramping abdominal pain, and generalized myalgias are the most common early symptoms suggesting shigellosis.[69] Fluid and electrolyte losses may also be noted early in the illness, owing to the action of enterotoxin on the intestinal epithelial cells. After 2 or 3 days, bowel movements become less frequent and the quantity of stool decreases, but the presence of bright red blood and mucus in the feces and the onset of tenesmus (straining on stooling) indicate the dysenteric phase of illness, suggesting that bacterial penetration of the bowel has probably occurred. *Shigella* infections should be suspected in communitywide outbreaks of diarrheal illness that disproportionately affect young children. Outbreaks can occur at any time of the year, but are most common in the summer.

Table 6-10 Differentiation of Species Within the Genus *Shigella*

BIOCHEMICAL TEST	S. DYSENTERIAE	S. FLEXNERI	S. BOYDII	S. SONNEI
Serogroup	A	B	C	D
ONPG	−	−	−	+
Ornithine decarboxylase	−	−	−	+
Fermentation of:				
Lactose	−	−	−	−
Mannitol	−	+	+	+
Raffinose	−	D	−	−
Sucrose	−	−	−	−
Xylose	−	−	D	−
Indole production	D	D	D	−

+, 90% or more strains positive; −, 90% or more strains negative; D, different strains positive/negative.

of shigellosis are reported annually in the United States.[104] *S. sonnei* is the serotype most commonly associated with diarrheal disease in the U.S., accounting for 77% of the *Shigella* serogroups reported to the CDC in 2001.[78] Symptoms associated with *S. sonnei* infection tend to be mild, and some patients may be asymptomatic. *S. dysenteriae* is the least commonly recovered species in the United States, but it is the most virulent serotype and the most common serotype isolated in developing countries. The belief that *Shigella* species remain confined to the bowel and neither invade the bowel lymphatics nor extend to other organs may no longer pertain. Drow and associates[138] reported the recovery of *S. flexneri* from a splenic abscess in a patient with diabetes, indicating that extraintestinal sites of infection may be encountered. Specimens other than stool from which *Shigella* spp have been recovered include liver, mesenteric lymph nodes, CSF, synovial fluid, vaginal lesions, lungs, conjunctival sacs, corneal scrapings, blood, cutaneous lesions of the penile shaft, and urine.[141,375] Urinary tract infections (UTIs) due to *Shigella* spp. in adults are extremely rare. *Shigella* vaginitis with or without accompanying UTI has been reported in prepubertal girls.[25] Some patients experience a bloody vaginal discharge that may be confused with gonorrhea.[453] Most cases of *Shigella* vulvovaginitis are caused by *S. flexneri*.[335]

TRIBE *EDWARDSIELLEAE*

The *Edwardsielleae* were initially called the Asakusa group by Sakazaki and Murata in 1963[433] and the Bartholo-

mew group by King and Adler in 1964.[268] Ewing and associates suggested the name *Edwardsielleae* in 1965,[158] in honor of the prominent American microbiologist, P.R. Edwards. The *Edwardsielleae* consists of one genus, *Edwardsiella*, which has three species; however, only one species, *E. tarda*, is of medical importance. The chief reservoirs in nature are reptiles (especially snakes, toads, and turtles) and freshwater fish. The key characteristics that suggest *E. tarda* are given in Table 6-6.

A key feature of *E. tarda* is the production of abundant amounts of hydrogen sulfide. Except for this feature, the bacterium has biochemical properties similar to those of *Escherichia coli*. The organism also resembles some *Citrobacter* and *Salmonella* species by its production of hydrogen sulfide in TSI agar and its failure to use lactose. This failure to ferment lactose and many other carbohydrates is the basis for the species name *tarda*. A species similar to *E. tarda*, which is hydrogen sulfide–negative, but mannitol-, sucrose-, and arabinose-positive, has been designated ''*E. tarda* biogroup 1.''[169] This biotype is rarely encountered in laboratory practice and does not yet appear to have clinical significance.

E. tarda has been cited as the cause of a variety of extraintestinal infections.[117,451] The most common are wound infections resulting from trauma, often related to aquatic accidents. Also common are abscesses that may lead to bacteremia or myonecrosis.[451] Seven patients in one study had typhoidal illnesses, an important differential consideration because *E. tarda* can simulate *Salmonella typhi* in culture.[117] Most reports of enteric illness describe a mild gastroenteritis that improves without therapy in 2 to 3 days. However, Vandepitte and associates[484] reported one case of protracted diarrhea in a 2-month-old infant in whom *E. tarda* (of the same biogroup isolated from tropical aquarium fish in the home of the patient) was the only potential pathogen recovered. Marsh and Gorbach[307] reported the isolation of *E. tarda* from the stool of a patient with bloody diarrhea and sigmoidoscopic findings of multiple colonic ulcers and mucosal thickening consistent with Crohn's disease. The patient became asymptomatic after 2 days of antibiotic therapy. Iron availability has been thought to regulate the seriousness of *E. tarda* infection.[242,243] Iron overload, caused by such

Box 6-9 Subgroups, Serotypes, and Subtypes of Shigella

Subgroup	Serotypes and Subtypes
Group A: *Shigella dysenteriae*	15 serotypes (type 1 produces Shiga toxin)
Group B: *Shigella flexneri*	8 serotypes and 9 subtypes
Group C: *Shigella boydii*	19 serotypes
Group D: *Shigella sonnei*	1 serotype

Table 6-11 Differentiation of Species Within the Genus *Edwardsiella*

BIOCHEMICAL TEST	E. TARDA	E. TARDA BIOGROUP 1	E. HOSHINAE	E. ICTALURI
Indole	+	+	V (50)	−
Hydrogen sulfide	+	−	−	−
Motility	+	+	+	−
Fermentation of:				
Mannitol	−	+	+	−
Sucrose	−	+	+	−
Arabinose	−	+	V (13)	−
Trehalose	−	−	+	−

+, 90% or more strains positive; −, 90% or more strains negative; V, 11–89% of strains positive.

conditions as red cell sickling, leukemia, and cirrhosis, is associated with *E. tarda* septicemia.[242,506,511] Infection with *E. tarda* related to vascular prostheses has also been reported.[121,343] Clusters of asymptomatic *E. tarda* infections are believed to occur in humans, and at least one such cluster has been reported among seven children and a teacher in a Florida day-care center.[132]

Two other species in the genus *Edwardsiella* have been described. Grimont and associates[207] described *E. hoshinae*, initially recovered from birds, reptiles, and water. This species has also been recovered from human feces; however, it is not known to cause diarrhea. Hawke and coworkers[214] described *E. ictaluri*, an organism that has been recovered only from fish and, at present, has no clinical significance. The biochemical characterization of *Edwardsiella* species is shown in Table 6-11.

TRIBE *SALMONELLEAE*

The *Salmonelleae* contain a single genus, *Salmonella*, and are named after the American microbiologist, D.E. Salmon. Salmonellae have somatic (O) antigens that are lipopolysaccharides, and flagellar (H) antigens that are proteins. *S. typhi* also has a capsular or virulence (Vi) antigen. Biochemically, they are usually both lactose- and sucrose-negative. The key characteristics by which the genus *Salmonella* can be suspected are given in Table 6-6.

Classification of Salmonellae. From the time of the first isolation of microorganisms of the *Salmonella* group, reported in 1884 by Gaffky (*Bacterium typhosum*) and in 1886 by Salmon and Smith (*Salmonella choleraesuis*) the development of salmonella nomenclature has been very complex and a matter of dispute (Box 6-10). The salmonellae are the most complex of all the *Enterobacteriaceae*, with more than 2,400 serotypes described in the current Kauffmann-White scheme.[402] Prior to July 1, 1983, three species of *Salmonella* were used to report positive results: *S. choleraesuis*, *S. typhi*, and *S. enteritidis*, with most of the serotypes belonging to the last species, *S. enteritidis*. Presently, all former species and subgroups of *Salmonella* and *Arizona* are considered to be the same species, but can be separated into seven taxa representing six distinct subgroups. The only exception is *S. bongori*, previously know as subgenera V, which by DNA-DNA hybridization is a distinct species.[414] Thus, there are two species and six subspecies of *S. enterica* in the current system used by the CDC (Box 6-11). The differential characteristics of *Salmonella* species and subspecies are given in Table 6-12.

Salmonellae Nomenclature. Beginning in 1966, the WHO began naming serotypes only in subspecies I and dropped all existing serotype names in the other subspecies. The CDC follows this practice and uses names for serotypes in subspecies I and uses antigenic formulas for unnamed serotypes described after 1966 in subspecies II, IV, and VI and *S. bongori*. For named serotypes, to emphasize that they are not separate species, the serotype name is not italicized and the first letter is capitalized. At the first citation of a serotype the genus name is given followed by the word "serotype" or the abbreviation "ser." and then the serotype name (*Salmonella* serotype or ser. Typhimurium). Subsequently, the name may be written with the genus followed directly by the serotype name *Salmonella* Typhimurium or *S.* Typhimurium (Box 6-12).[58]

In day-to-day practice, unknown isolates from clinical specimens that are biochemically suggestive of *Salmonella* species are confirmed using polyclonal antisera containing antibodies to all the major subgroups. Subcultures of confirmed isolates are forwarded to public health laboratories, where serotype designations (e.g., *S.* serotype Typhimurium) are made based on serologic reactions to O and H determinants.

Identification of Salmonella typhi. Although most *Salmonella* serotypes cannot be distinguished by biochemical reactions, one serotype, namely *S. typhi*, does possess some unique biochemical characteristics that will allow it to be differentiated from other serotypes. First and foremost is the observation that strains of *S. typhi* produce only a trace amount of hydrogen sulfide, which is usually observed as a crescent-shaped wedge of black precipitate forming at the interface of the slant and butt in KIA or TSI media (Color Plate 6-4B). In addition, *S. typhi* strains are noted to be less active biochemically than the more common serotypes and specifically are negative in the following reactions: Simmon's citrate; ornithine decarboxylase; gas from glucose; fermentation of dulcitol, arabinose, and rhamnose; and mucate and acetate utilization. Consequently, the authors believe that it is within the capabilities of most clinical labora-

Box 6-10 Salmonella Taxonomy and Nomenclature

The antigenic formulae of *Salmonella* serotypes are defined and maintained by the World Health Organization (WHO) Collaborating Centre for Reference and Research on *Salmonella* at the Pasteur Institute in Paris, France. New serotypes are listed in annual updates of the Kauffmann-White scheme.[402,403] In this scheme, the salmonellae are grouped (A, B, C, etc.) on the basis of somatic O antigens and are subdivided into serotypes (1, 2, 3, etc.) by their flagellar H antigens, resulting in serogroups designated A, B, C_1, C_2, C_3, etc. Each unique serotype is given a name. The first salmonellae were given names that indicated the disease and/or the animal from which the organism was isolated (e.g. *Salmonella* ser. Typhi, *Salmonella* ser. Choleraesuis, etc.). New names are now given the name of the geographic location where they were first isolated (*Salmonella* ser. Canada, *Salmonella* ser. Cleveland, etc.). Initially each serotype was considered a separate species (for example, *S. canada, S. cleveland*); however, today this would result in over 2,400 species of *Salmonella*. DNA relatedness studies have demonstrated that all *Salmonella* strains and all serotypes of "*Arizona*" form a single DNA hybridization group with seven subgroups, with the exception of *S. bongori* (subgroup V) that has been shown by DNA-DNA hybridization to form a distinct species.[124,283,284,414] Since *S. choleraesuis* was already recognized as the type species of *Salmonella*, it had priority as the species designation for the six subgroups considered to comprise a single hybridization group. The name "choleraesuis," however, can lead to confusion since the name refers to both a species and a serotype. So, in 1986, the Subcommittee on *Enterobacteriaceae* of the International Committee on Systematic Bacteriology at the XIV International Congress on Microbiology unanimously recommended that the type species for *Salmonella* be changed to *S. enterica*, a name that had not been used previously as a serovar.[384] In 1987, Le Minor and Popoff[282] made a proposal as a "Request for an Opinion" to the Judicial Commission of the International Committee of Systematic Bacteriology that the genus *Salmonella* consist of only one species "*Salmonella enterica*," to include seven subspecies. *S. typhi, S. typhimurium,* and *S. enteritidis* were included in *S. enterica*. This recommendation was adopted by the CDC and many other laboratories. However, after a long delay, the Judicial Commission denied the request based on the fact that the status of *Salmonella* ser. Typhi was not adequately addressed in the Le Minor and Popoff proposal.[497,498] They were concerned that if *S. enterica* were adopted that *Salmonella* ser. Typhi would be referred to as *S. enterica* subsp. *enterica* ser. Typhi and might be missed or overlooked by physicians.[58] The Judicial Committee therefore ruled that *S. choleraesuis* be retained as the legitimate type species pending an amended request for an opinion.[497,498] Le Minor and Popoff[282] also proposed in 1987 that the seven subgenera of *Salmonella* be referred to as subspecies (subspecies I, II, IIIa, IIIb, IV, V, and VI). Most recently, Euzéby[156] proposed that the genus *Salmonella* consists of three species named *S. bongori, S. enterica,* and *S. typhi*. He further proposed the *S. enterica* be divided into six subspecies: *S. enterica* subsp. *enterica, S. enterica* subsp. *arizonae, S. enterica* subsp. *diarizonae, S. enterica* subsp. *houtenae, S. enterica* subsp. *indica,* and *S. enterica* subsp. *salamae*. As of this writing the Judicial Committee has not acted on this latest proposal.

tories to make a preliminary report of *S. typhi* or *Salmonella* species not *S. typhi* while the laboratory awaits specific serotype confirmation from their local public health laboratory. **Incidence and Sources of Salmonelloses.** Salmonellosis is a major cause of bacterial enteric illness in both humans and animals (see Clinical Correlation Box 6-3). Each year an estimated 1.4 million cases of salmonellosis occur among humans in the United States, resulting in 16,000 hospitalizations, and nearly 600 deaths.[316] Approximately 35,000 of these cases are serotyped by public health laboratories and

the results are electronically transmitted to the CDC. Human infections with salmonellae are most commonly caused by ingestion of food, water, or milk contaminated by human or animal excreta. Salmonellae are primary pathogens of lower animals (e.g., poultry, cows, pigs, pets, birds, sheep, seals, donkeys, lizards, and snakes), which are the principal source of nontyphoidal salmonellosis in humans. Interestingly, humans are the only known reservoir for *S. typhi*. Although the incidence of typhoid fever has declined in developed countries, sporadic outbreaks continue to occur. About 400 cases are reported annually in the United States.[77] About half the salmonellosis epidemics are the result of contaminated poultry and poultry products. Salmonellae in the feces of hens contaminate the surface of eggs or penetrates internally through hairline cracks. In hens with ovarian infection, the organisms may gain access to the yolk. The Egg Products Inspection Act of 1970 requires pasteurization of all bulk egg products and federally supervised inspection of shell eggs for cracks.

Historically *S.* Typhimurium has been the most frequently reported serotype, accounting for slightly more than 20% of isolates reported to the CDC annually. The three most common serotypes of *Salmonella* in 2001 were Typhimurium (22%), Enteritidis (18%), and Newport (10%), which accounted for 50% of all isolates. The largest single source outbreak of salmonellosis in U.S. history (16,000 culture

Box 6-11 Classification of *Salmonella* Species and Subspecies

There are two species of *Salmonella*: *S. enterica*, which encompasses six subspecies, and *S. bongori*

S. enterica subsp. *enterica* (I): includes most serotypes

S. enterica subsp. *salamae* (II)

S. enterica subspecies *arizonae* (IIIa)

S. enterica subsp. *diarizonae* (IIIb)

S. enterica subsp. *houtenae* (IV)

S. enterica subsp. *indica* (VI)

Salmonella bongori (formerly subspecies V)

Table 6-12 Differential Characteristics of Salmonella Species and Subspecies [modified from Ewing (1986)][157]

SPECIES	*S. ENTERICA*						*S. BONGORI*
SUBSPECIES	I *enterica*	II *salamae*	IIIA *arizonae*	IIIB *diarizonae*	IV *houtenae*	VI *indica*	
Biochemical test							
Dulcitol	+	+	−	−	−	d	+
ONPG (2 hr)	−	−	+	+	−	d	+
Malonate	−	+	+	+	−	−	−
Gelatinase	−	+	+	+	+	+	−
Sorbitol	+	+	+	+	−/+	−	+
KCN	−	−	−	−	+	−	+
D-tartrate	+	−	−	−	−	−	−
Galacturonate	−	+	−	+	+	+	+
β-glucuronidase (MUG)	D	D	−	+	−	D	−
Mucate	+	+	+	− (70%)	−	+	+
Salicin	−	−	−	−	+	−	−
Lactose	−	−	− (75%)	+ (75%)	−	D	−

+, 90% or more strains positive; −, 90% or more strains negative; D, different reactions by different serovars.

Box 6-12 *Salmonella* Nomenclature in Use at CDC

TAXONOMIC POSITION CURRENT NOMENCLATURE

Genus (italics) . . . . *Salmonella*

Species (italics) . . . . *enterica*, which includes subspecies I, II, IIIa, IIIb, IV, and VI *bongori* (formerly subspecies V)

Serotype (capitalized, not italicized)
—The first time a serotype is mentioned; the name should be preceded by the word "serotype" or "ser."

—Serotypes are named in subspecies I and designated by antigenic formulae in subspecies II, III, IV, and VI and *S. bongori* (e.g., *Salmonella* serotype (ser.) Typhimurium, *Salmonella* II 50:b:z$_6$, *Salmonella* IIIb 60:k:z)

—Members of subspecies II, IV, and VI and *S. bongori* retain their names if named before 1966 (e.g., *Salmonella* ser. Marina (IV 48:g,z$_{51}$:-)

From reference[58].

CLINICAL CORRELATION BOX 6-3 *Salmonella* Infection

Four clinical types of *Salmonella* infection may be distinguished[449]: 1) gastroenteritis, the most frequent manifestation, ranging from mild to fulminant diarrhea, accompanied by low-grade fever and varying degrees of nausea and vomiting; 2) bacteremia or septicemia without major gastrointestinal symptoms (*S. choleraesuis* is particularly invasive) characterized by high, spiking fever and positive blood cultures; 3) enteric fever, potentially caused by any strain of *Salmonella* species, usually manifested as mild fever and diarrhea, except for classic cases of typhoid fever *(S. typhi),* in which the disease progresses through a bimodal course, characterized by an early period (lasting 1 to 2 weeks) of fever and constipation, during which blood cultures are positive and stool cultures remain negative, followed by a second (diarrheic) phase during which blood cultures become negative and stool cultures positive; and 4) a carrier state in which persons with previous infection, especially with *S. typhi,* may continue to excrete the organism in their feces for up to 1 year following remission of symptoms. Of some concern are reports of lactose-positive strains of *S. virchow* causing bacteremia and meningitis.[430] Although detection of lactose-positive strains in the blood or cerebrospinal fluid would not be difficult, finding such strains in stool would pose a problem for most laboratories owing to the similarity in appearance to other lactose-positive coliforms present in stool specimens.

confirmed cases with epidemiologic data indicating that 150,000 to 200,000 persons were actually infected) occurred in 1985 in Illinois and surrounding states and was traced to a faulty valve in a major commercial milk supply firm.[82] Several *S.* Enteritidis outbreaks have occurred in the United States since 1990 that were associated with shell eggs.[83,85,87,95] An estimated 0.01% of all shell eggs contain *S.* Enteritidis. Consequently, foods containing raw or undercooked eggs (e.g., homemade eggnog or ice cream, hollandaise sauce, Caesar salad dressing, homemade mayonnaise, and runny omelettes) pose a slight risk of infection with *S.* Enteritidis.[85,87] In 1994, an outbreak of *S.* Enteritidis infection was linked to a nationally distributed ice cream brand. Illnesses were documented in 41 states, and more than 200,000 persons were estimated to have been ill.[88] The incidence of *S.* Enteritidis illness and the number of such outbreaks in the United States have decreased by almost 50% between the mid-1990s and 1999.[381] To meet the challenge of further reducing the incidence of such infections, the President's Council on Food Safety announced an Egg Safety Action Plan on December 10, 1999, with the interim goal of reducing egg-associated *S.* Enteritidis illnesses by half by 2005 and eliminating them by 2010.[406] These outbreaks serve as a constant reminder that modern technology cannot always protect against the ravages of infectious diseases that may occur in explosive and widespread epidemics.

Salmonellosis has also been associated with direct or indirect contact with reptiles (i.e., lizards, snakes, turtles). Reptiles are commonly colonized with *Salmonella* and shed the organism intermittently in their feces.[94] During the early 1970s, small pet turtles were an important source of salmonella infection in the United States. In 1975, the Food and Drug Administration prohibited the distribution and sale of small turtles, resulting in the prevention of 100,000 cases of salmonellosis annually.[119] However, since 1986, the popularity of iguanas and other reptiles that can transmit infection to humans has given rise to an increased incidence of salmonella infections caused by reptile-associated serotypes.[89,94,103] Increasing evidence now suggests that amphibians (e.g., frogs, toads, newts, and salamanders) can also pose risks for salmonellosis in humans.[319] Overall, reptile and amphibian contacts are estimated to account for 74,000 (6%) of the *Salmonella* infections that occur each year in the United States.[319] Because young children are at increased risk for reptile- and amphibian-associated salmonellosis with potentially severe complications (e.g., septicemia and meningitis), reducing exposure of infants or children younger than 5 years of age to reptiles is particularly important. For this reason reptiles and amphibians should be kept out of households that include children <5 years or immunocompromised persons, and should not be allowed in child-care centers.[103]

Emergence of Multidrug-Resistant Salmonellae.
A multidrug-resistant (MDR) strain of *S.* Typhimurium definitive type 104 (DT104) that is resistant to five antibiotics (ampicillin, chloramphenicol, streptomycin, sulfamethoxazole, and tetracycline) emerged across the United States during the 1990s.[196] In a national survey conducted by the CDC in 2000, 50% of the *S.* Typhimurium isolates were resistant to one or more drugs and 28% had a five-drug resistance pattern characteristic of the phage type DT104.[77] Similarly, since 1998, *S.* Newport has emerged as a major MDR pathogen.[208]

In 2001, 33 (26%) of 128 *S.* Newport isolates submitted to the National Antimicrobial Resistance Monitoring System (available at www.cdc.gov/narms/index.htm) were resistant to at least 9 of the 17 antimicrobial agents tested.[100]

Infections Due To Salmonella enterica Subspecies arizonae.
Salmonella enterica subsp. *arizonae* resembles salmonellae antigenically, clinically, and epidemiologically. It was first recovered in 1939 from diseased reptiles in Arizona and was initially called "*Salmonella* sp. Dar-es-salaam type, variety from Arizona."[64] It was later distinguished from *Salmonella* and placed in the new genus *Arizona*, with a single species *A. hinshawii*. However, in 1983 it was again reclassified as a serotype of the genus *Salmonella* based on DNA homology studies. Although most *Salmonella* serotypes cannot be distinguished by biochemical reactions, *Salmonella enterica* subsp. *arizonae* can be easily differentiated on the basis of having positive malonate and negative dulcitol reactions. In addition, some strains ferment lactose, and all strains are ONPG-positive. As a result of these unique biochemical reactions, a correct serotype designation can be easily made by most of the commercially available identification systems. For clinical significance see Clinical Correlation Box 6-4.

CLINICAL CORRELATION BOX 6-4 *Salmonella Arizonae*

Reptiles, particularly snakes, are the main natural reservoir of *S.* Arizonae, but humans, poultry, and other animals have also contracted disease from this organism. Human infection should trigger inquiries of a possible connection with reptiles as well as poultry and egg products. Reports of *S.* Arizonae infection in cancer patients and HIV-positive patients following consumption of snake powder capsules as a so-called folk remedy has been reported by several investigators.[20,80,161,494] A fatal case of *S.* Arizonae gastroenteritis has been reported in a child with microcephaly born to a family of snake charmers in New Delhi, India.[302]

The clinical spectrum of disease varies from benign gastroenteritis, to enteric fever and septicemia with localized infection, and is similar to that caused by other *Salmonella* serotypes. Keren et al. reported that gastroenteritis may be seen in any age group and is characterized by cramping abdominal pain, diarrhea (often watery), nausea, vomiting, and low-grade fever.[262] Diarrhea is usually self-limited and lasts from 1 to 5 days. Septicemia may follow, but has also been reported in the absence of gastroenteritis. Localized infection in diverse organ sites, such as brain, bone, liver, lung, joints, and gallbladder, is presumed, although not always documented to occur following bacteremia. Well-documented cases of osteomyelitis have also been reported.[262] The prevalence of human infections caused by *S.* Arizonae is probably underreported because the gastrointestinal symptoms are usually mild. However, this pathogen should be considered in the differential diagnoses of patients with sepsis and severe gastroenteritis who have a history of contact with reptiles, especially snakes. Ownership of reptiles should be discouraged, especially in households with children less than 5 years of age.[302]

New Methods for Recovery and Characterization of Salmonellae. In addition to the classic media discussed previously (see Tables 6-1 through 6-3), new media have been described that are intended to improve the isolation of *Salmonella* species from stool samples.

Selective and Differential Media These include novobiocin–brilliant green–glucose agar (NGB),[134] novobiocin–brilliant green–glycerol–lactose agar (NBGL),[401,429] xylose–lysine–Tergitol 4 (XLT4) medium,[326] and modified semisolid Rappaport Vassiliadis medium (MSRV).[18,133,198] The formulations and differential properties of these media are given in Table 6-13.

Chromogenic Media Chromogenic enzyme substrates are compounds that act as the substrate for specific enzymes and change color due to the action of the enzyme on the chromogenic substrate (Fig. 6-6). The first medium of this type was Rambach agar. It uses a chromogenic substrate for β-galactosidase (X-Gal, 5-bromo-4-chloro-3-indolyl-β-D-galactopyranoside) in conjunction with propylene glycol, which is fermented by *Salmonella* spp. to generate acid.[411] Rambach agar is highly specific; however, it does not detect *S.* Typhi and *S.* Paratyphi A.[144,145,395] SM-ID agar is similar to Rambach except that it incorporates two chromogenic substrates, X-Gal, for β-galactosidase, and X-GLU, for β-glucosidase. SM-ID medium detects both Typhi and Paratyphi A serotypes.[144,145,329,385,395,429] *Salmonella* chromogenic medium (SCM; Oxoid, Basingstoke, United Kingdom), contains two chromogenic substrates. The first is Magenta-cap (5-bromo-6-chloro-3-indolylcaprylate), which is hydrolyzed by *Salmonella* species to yield magenta colonies. The second substrate is X-Gal, which causes β-D-galactosidase-producing organisms to turn blue. Other colonies that do not utilize the chromogens, grow as colorless colonies.[75] ABC medium (αβ-chromogenic medium) uses two chromogenic substrates. The first substrate, 3,4-cyclohexenoesculetin-β-D-galactoside (CHE-GAL), is used to detect β-galactosidase-producing organisms that appear as black colonies in the presence of iron. The second substrate, 5-bromo-4-chloro-3-indolyl-α-D-galactopyranoside (X-α-Gal), is hydrolyzed by *Salmonella* spp. which appear as green colonies.[349,385,387] Perry and colleagues subsequently modified ABC medium with the incorporation of alafosfalin (L-alanyl-1-aminoethylphosphonic acid), a "suicide substrate," that aids in the recovery of *Salmonella* spp. by inhibiting the growth of a wide range of gram-negative bacteria.[388] COMPASS Salmonella agar (Biokar Diagnostics, Beauvais, France) utilizes two chromogenic substrates— 5-bromo-6-chloro-3-indolyl-caprylate, which detects esterase activity from *Salmonella* spp. yielding magenta colonies, and 5-bromo-4-chloro-3-indolyl-glucopyranoside, which detects β-glucosidase activity from other *Enterobacteriaceae* yielding blue colonies.[385] CHROMagar Salmonella (CHROMagar Microbiology, Paris, France; also sold by BD under the name BBL CHROMagar Salmonella, BD Diagnostics Sparks, MD) is a newer selective chromogenic medium that uses a chromogen mixture (patented substrates) that detects esterase activity of *Salmonella* spp. and β-galactosidase activity of other *Enterobacteriaceae*.[152,184,300,385] The formulas, principles and interpretations of the chromogenic agars are given in Table 6-13. Pictures of colonies

growing on CHROMagar can be found in Color Plates 6-5E through *H*)

Evaluations In a study by Ruiz and associates comparing five plating media for isolation of *Salmonella*, NBGL media had the highest sensitivity (78.4%) and positive predictive value (61%) for direct recovery of *Salmonella* from stool.[429] These authors recommend the use of SM-ID for recovery of *S.* Typhi, which is not detected on NBGL agar. Monnery and colleagues found SMID and Rambach agars to be considerably more specific than salmonella–shigella agar and Hektoen agar.[329] Dusch and Altwegg compared six media (Hektoen enteric agar [HE], Rambach agar, SM-ID medium, XLT4 agar, NBGL agar, and MSRV medium) and concluded that MSRV was the most sensitive medium tested for the isolation of nontyphoid salmonellae from stool; however, these authors noted that the semisolid nature of the medium was a disadvantage and requires careful handling in the laboratory. They noted that XLT4 had sensitivity comparable with HE and nearly 100% specificity and can be considered an alternative for the isolation of salmonellae from stools.[145] Perez and colleagues[385] compared four chromogenic media (ABC medium, COMPASS Salmonella agar, CHROMagar Salmonella agar, and SM-ID agar) with conventional Hektoen agar on 916 stool samples from inpatients at three hospitals. After 48 hr of incubation, the sensitivity before and after enrichment in selenite broth was 62.5 and 89.1% with ABC medium, 77.1 and 93.8% with COMPASS agar, 66.7 and 89.1% with CHROMagar, 68.8 and 85.9% with SM-ID agar, and 85.4 and 98.4% with Hektoen agar, respectively. Without enrichment, after 24 hr of incubation, between 45.8 and 62.5% of all the *Salmonella* isolates were detected, according to the medium used. Hektoen was significantly more sensitive than the four chromogenic media, while the sensitivities of the four chromogenic media were not significantly different from each other. With enrichment and a 48-hr incubation period, Hektoen agar again had the highest sensitivity (98.4%), while the sensitivities of COMPASS, ABC, CHROMagar and SM-ID were 93.8, 89.1, 89.1 and 85.9% respectively.

Other Rapid Detection Methods The 4-methylumbelliferyl caprylate test (MUCAP test; Biolife, Milan, Italy) is a fluorescence test for rapid identification of *Salmonella* strains directly from agar plates. The test consists of an eight-carbon-atom ester conjugated with methylumbelliferone. This substrate interacts with the salmonella C_8 esterase, leading to release of umbelliferone, which is strongly fluorescent at 365 nm. The test is performed by applying a drop of the reagent directly onto suspect colonies on the agar surface and then observing for the appearance of blue fluorescence of the colony under a Wood's lamp within 5 minutes. Several studies have shown this test to provide nearly 100% sensitivity and specificity in detecting *Salmonella* strains and offers a useful and rapid adjunct to routine biochemical characterization of *Salmonella* strains.[8,369,431,432] The Oxoid Biochemical Identification System (O.B.I.S.) Salmonella Test (Oxoid) is a rapid colorimetric spot test for the determination of pyroglutamyl aminopeptidase (PYRase) and nitrophenylalanine deaminase (NPA) activity. A sample is taken from a colony growing on an agar plate and applied to the PYR and NPA test areas on the card. A drop of buffer solution is added to both test areas, and after 5 minutes, one drop of

Table 6-13 New Media for Recovery of *Salmonella* Species From Stool

MEDIUM	FORMULATION	PRINCIPLE AND INTERPRETATION
Novobiocin-brilliant green-glucose agar (NBG)	Tryptic soy agar, 40 g Ferric ammonium citrate, 1.5 g Sodium thiosulfate pentahydrate, 5 g Phenol red (sodium salt), 80 mg Glucose, 1 g Brilliant green, 7 mg Novobiocin, 10 mg Distilled water to 1 L Final pH, 7.3	*Salmonella* colonies appear smooth and entire with medium- to large-sized, dark black, nucleated centers owing to H_2S production. In addition, reddening and a visible zone of clearing occurs in the medium around each colony. Coliforms are either inhibited or fail to produce black-centered colonies. Some *Citrobacter freundii* strains produce colonies indistinguishable from *Salmonella* species.
Novobiocin-brilliant green-glycerol-lactose agar (NBGL)	Trypticase soy agar, 40 g Ferric ammonium citrate, 1.5 g Sodium thiosulfate, 5 g Lactose, 10 g Glycerol, 10 mL Brilliant green, 7 mg Novobiocin, 10 mg Distilled water to 1 L	The detection of *Salmonella* spp. is based on the production of H_2S, resulting in black colonies. Sufficient H_2S formation is achieved only by colonies that do not produce acid from glycerol or lactose, because a low pH interferes with H_2S formation. This results in colorless colonies for most *Proteus* and *Citrobacter* species.
Rambach agar	Propylene glycol, 10 g Peptone, 5 g Yeast extract, 2 g Sodium desoxycholate, 1 g Neutral red, 0.03 g 5-Bromo-4-chloro-3-indolyl-β-D-galactopyranoside, 0.1 g Agar, 15 g Distilled water to 1 L	Detects ability of *Salmonella* spp. to metabolize propylene glycol. Suspect colonies on this medium are usually bright red. Contains moderate amount of bile salts to inhibit coliforms.
SM-ID agar	Beef extract, 3 g Bio-Polytone, 6 g Yeast extract, 2 g Bile salts, 4 g Neutral red, 0.025 g Tris buffer, 0.65 g Brilliant green, 0.3 mg Chromogen substrate 1 (galactopyranoside), 0.17 g Sodium glucuronate, 12 g Chromogen substrate 2 (glucopyranoside), 0.026 g Sorbitol, 8 g Agar 13.5 g Distilled water to 1 L Final pH, 7.6 ± 0.2	Detection of *Salmonella* spp. is based on the formation of acid from the glucuronate and on the absence of β-galactosidase. *Salmonella* serotypes produce pinkish-red colonies (sometimes with a colorless rim), whereas coliforms form other colors (green, blue, or violet) if they are positive for β-galactosidase, or they remain colorless. Contains moderate amount of bile salts to inhibit coliforms.
Modified Semisolid Rappaport-Vassiliadis Medium (MSRV)	Tryptose, 4.59 g Casein hydrolysate acid, 4.59 g Sodium chloride, 7.34 g Potassium dihydrogen phosphate, 1.47 g Magnesium chloride (anhydrous), 10.93 g Malachite green oxalate, 0.037 g Agar, 2.7 g Distilled water to 1 L Novobiocin (2% solution) added after sterilization 1 mL Final pH, 5.2 ± 2	Based on the swarming phenomenon of motile bacteria (*Salmonella* spp. and others) at reduced agar concentrations. After incubation the plates are checked for motile bacteria that appear as a halo of growth spreading out from the original inoculation point. Subcultures are taken from the edge of migration to check for purity and for further biochemical and serologic tests. Coliforms are inhibited by a combination of increased osmotic pressure, malachite green, and incubation at 41–43°C
Xylose-Lysine-Tergitol 4 (XLT4)	Bacto proteose peptone No. 3, 1.6 g Bacto yeast extract, 3.0 g L-lysine, 5.0 g Bacto xylose, 3.75 g Bacto lactose, 7.5 g Bacto saccharose, 7.5 g	This is a highly selective medium that substitutes the anionic surfactant Tergitol 4 for sodium desoxycholate found in XLD agar. The XLT4 agar completely inhibits the growth of all gram-positive bacteria and fungi, and either completely or strongly inhibits the growth of

Table 6-13 *Continued*

MEDIUM	FORMULATION	PRINCIPLE AND INTERPRETATION
	Ferric ammonium citrate, 0.8 g Sodium thiosulfate, 6.8 g Sodium chloride, 5 g Bacto agar, 18 g Bacto phenol red, 0.08 g Distilled water to 1 L Final pH, 7.4 ± 0.2	numerous gram-negative bacteria, including *Proteus, Providence,* and *Pseudomonas*. In addition, *Citrobacter* species are somewhat inhibited and very rarely produce colonies with black centers after overnight incubation. *Salmonella* colonies (H_2S-positive) appear black or black-centered with a yellow periphery after 18–24 hours of incubation. After continued incubation, the colonies become entirely black or pink to red with black centers. Rare strains of *Salmonella* that produce no H_2S display pink to pinkish-yellow colonies that can be differentiated from bright yellow nonsalmonellae colonies.

Modified ABC medium (αβ-chromogenic medium with alafosfalin)	Bacteriologic agar, 10 g
	L-Arginine, 0.1 g
	L-Aspartic acid, 0.1 g
	L-Cysteine, 0.005 g
	Glycine, 0.1 g
	L-Histidine, 0.1 g
	L-Isoleucine, 0.1 g
	L-Leucine, 0.1 g
	L-Lysine, 0.1 g
	L-Methionine, 0.005 g
	L-Phenylalanine, 0.1 g
	L-Proline, 0.1 g
	L-Serine, 0.1 g
	L-Threonine, 0.1 g
	L-Tryptophan, 0.1 g
	L-Tyrosine, 0.1 g
	L-valine, 0 .1 g
	Guanine, 0.01 g
	Uracil, 0.01 g
	Cytosine, 0.01 g
	Adenine, 0.01 g
	Sodium citrate, 6.5 g
	Magnesium sulfate, 0.1 g
	Ammonium sulfate, 1 g
	Yeast extract, 0.1 g
	Dipotassium hydrogen phosphate, 7 g
	Potassium dihydrogen phosphate, 2 g
	Chromogen Mix:
	   Ferric ammonium citrate, 0.5 g
	   X-alpha-Gal, 0.08 g
	   CHE-Gal, 0.3 g
	   IPTG, 0.03 g
	Distilled water to 1 L
	Ingredients added after sterilization:
	   Sodium deoxycholate, 0.5 g
	   Alafosfalin final concentration range in agar of 32 to 0.125 mg/L
	(Perry et al.[388])
		Salmonella yield blue colonies; other *Enterobacteriaceae* yield black colonies. Alafosfalin is taken up by bacteria at different rates via a stereospecific permease and may be cleaved intracellularly by an aminopeptidase to yield fosfalin. This released compound interferes with bacterial metabolism via interaction with the alanine racemase enzyme responsible for generating D-alanine. This interaction may result in growth inhibition.[388]

BBL™ CHROMagar™ Salmonella (sold by BD under a licensing agreement with CHROMagar, Paris, France)	Chromopeptone, 22.0 g Chromogen mix, 0.34 g Inhibitory agents, 0.02 g Agar, 15.0 g Distilled water to 1 L	*Salmonella* spp. appear as light mauve to mauve-colored colonies. *Citrobacter freundii* and other coliforms appear as light blue-green to blue-green colored colonies. Some organisms that do not hydrolyze any of the chromogenic compounds may appear as colorless colonies. (See Color Plates 6–5*E* through *H*)

Note: Rambach, XLT4, MSRV, NBG, and NBGL are not suitable for use in the isolation of typhoid Salmonella serotypes.

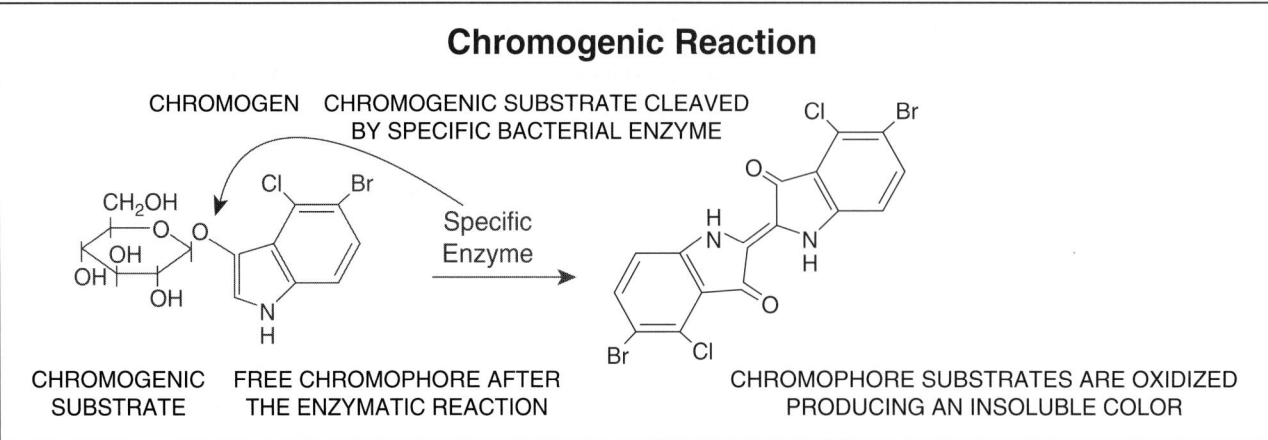

Figure 6-6 Chromogenic Reaction: artificial substrates (chromogens) release differently colored compounds upon degradation by specific bacterial enzymes.

PYR developing solution is added to the PYR test area, and one drop of NPA developing solution is added to the NPA test area. The PYRase area on the Test Card is impregnated with L-pyroglutamic acid 7-amino-4-methylcourmarin (7AMC). The enzymatic hydrolysis of the substrate produces a purple color on addition of the PYR developing solution (dimethylaminocinnamaldehyde). The NPA area on the Test Card is impregnated with nitrophenylalanine. Deamination of the reagent is shown by an orange-brown color when the NPA developing solution (0.25 M sodium hydroxide) is added. The lack of PYRase and NPA activity in *Salmonella* spp. can be used to differentiate them from *Citrobacter* spp., which possess PYRase activity[105,234,332] and *Proteus, Morganella* and *Providencia* spp. which have NPA activity.[192]

Other new techniques are being introduced that may significantly alter the future identification of *Salmonella* species, both in the clinical laboratory and in epidemiologic field studies. As an example of new applications, Olsvik and associates[370] traced the transmission of *S.* Typhimurium strains from diseased cattle in four separate herds in Norway to human farm workers, by demonstrating identical cryptic plasmid profiles for the various isolates by using restriction endonuclease digestion techniques. As these authors point out, conventional serotyping and biotyping techniques are often not sufficiently specific to determine definitively that two or more isolates from different sources are, in fact, identical. Techniques, such as restriction endonuclease analysis or genetic probes, that detect nucleotide sequences in plasmids or in chromosomal DNA and RNA will make epidemiologic and diagnostic work in microbiology much more exacting in the future. These techniques are discussed in more detail in Chapter 4.

TRIBE *CITROBACTEREAE*

Included in the *Citrobactereae* are 1 genus—*Citrobacter*—and 11 species. The genus *Citrobacter* and the species *C. freundii* were designated in 1932 by Werkman and Gillen. In 1970 Frederiksen described a new species that he named *C. koseri*. In 1971, Young and coworkers proposed

the name *Levinea malonatica* for a similar group of organisms, and in 1972 Ewing and Davis described *C. diversus*. Frederiksen examined all three strains and determined that they were phenotypically alike and proposed that the name *C. koseri* be restored as the valid name for this taxon.[176] In 1993, Brenner and colleagues, using DNA relatedness studies, showed that organisms identified as *C. freundii* consisted of a heterogeneous group representing several genetic species.[51] This work led to the establishment of 11 genomospecies within the genus *Citrobacter*, as shown in Table 6-14.

The characteristics that suggest that an isolate may belong to the genus *Citrobacter* are given in Table 6-6. The key characteristics that differentiate *C. freundii* and other H_2S-positive Citrobacters from salmonellae are growth in KCN (*Salmonella* species are negative), absence of lysine decarboxylase activity (*Salmonella* species are positive), and the hydrolysis of ONPG (*Salmonella* species are negative). The biochemical differentiation among the *Citrobacter* species is shown in Table 6-15. Human isolates of all genomospecies except *C. koseri* have been obtained predominantly from stools.[51] Farmer and coworkers,[165] who reviewed strains referred to the CDC, cited *C. freundii* as a possible cause of diarrhea (although most fecal isolates do not appear to be associated with disease) and as a cause of isolated cases of extraintestinal infections. They also cite a possible association between *C. koseri* and outbreaks of meningitis and brain abscesses in neonates and report the recovery of *C. amalonaticus* from a few blood cultures. Janda and colleagues at the Microbial Diseases Laboratory in Berkeley, California, reported that *C. freundii* was the most common species identified from all body sites except feces. In gastrointestinal specimens, *C. freundii* ranked fourth behind *C. youngae, C. braakii*, and *C. werkmanii*.[246] *C. freundii* (complex) has been reported as a cause of gastrointestinal illness associated with imported Brie cheese,[81] and isolation of a *C. freundii* strain that carries the *E. coli* O157 antigen has been reported.[35] *C. koseri* has been isolated most often from urine and respiratory tract specimens.[224,294] *C. koseri* has also been reported with increasing frequency as a cause of sporadic and epi-

Table 6-14 Former and Current Species Within the Genus *Citrobacter*

FORMER SPECIES DESIGNATION	GENOMOSPECIES	CURRENT SPECIES
C. freundii complex	1	*C. freundii*
	5	*C. youngae*
	6	*C. braakii*
	7	*C. werkmanii*
	8	*C. sedlakii*
	9	*C. rodentium*
	10	*C. gillenii*
	11	*C. murliniae*
C. diversus	2	*C. koseri*
C. amalonaticus	3	*C. amalonaticus*
C. amalonaticus biogroup 1	4	*C. farmeri*

demic meningitis in neonates and young infants.[200,273,274,378,488] Brain abscesses are found in 75% of infants with *C. koseri* meningitis, a prevalence far higher than that reported for other bacteria that cause meningitis.[201,273] One third of infants with *C. koseri* meningitis die, and at least 75% of survivors have severe neurologic impairment.[201] Other reports corroborate the tendency for *C. koseri* to cause meningitis and brain abscesses, particularly in association with the anaerobic gram-negative bacillus *Prevotella melaninogenica*.[15,125,286] *C. sedlakii* was isolated from the blood and cerebrospinal fluid of a 5-day-old premature infant seen with sepsis, meningitis, and a brain abscess at the University of Illinois Medical Center.[146] The child was treated with ampicillin, piperacillin, and cefotaxime. By day 14 the infant was clinically stable, and the therapy was changed to intravenous cefotaxime and oral cotrimoxazole. The child was discharged after 8 weeks to complete 2 more weeks of oral cotrimoxazole therapy at home. At 5½ months of age a computed tomographic scan of the brain showed resolution of all abscess cavities. Additional isolates of *C. sedlakii* at the University of Illinois have been from urine and an infected arteriovenous graft of the leg. Of 13 *C. braakii* identified at the University of Illinois Medical Center, 5 were recovered from urines, 4 from peritoneal fluids, 1 from an abdominal wound, 2 from endotracheal specimens, and 1 from a bronchial specimen. *C. farmeri* isolates at the University of Illinois have been from stool, urine, abdominal wall tissue, and aqueous fluid. Bruckner and colleagues reported a case of *C. farmeri* bacteremia in a child with short-bowel syndrome in whom a septic episode developed shortly after commencement of a total parenteral nutrition (TPN) infusion.[63] Only three *C. gillenii* isolates have been recovered at the University of Illinois from three separate sources; urine, peritoneal fluid, and a central venous catheter tip. Most *C. youngae* isolates have been recovered from urine. *C. rodentium* has been isolated only from rodents and causes a disease in laboratory mice known as transmissible murine colonic hyperplasia.[295,440]

Identification of *Citrobacter* species is hampered because the new species are not yet included in the databases of most commercial identification systems. To assist laboratories in speciating the new *Citrobacter* species, O'Hara and colleagues have published a dichotomous key using conventional biochemical tests.[358] The susceptibility pattern of isolates also offers an aid to identification. *C. koseri* has an antibiotic susceptibility pattern similar to *Klebsiella* (i.e., resistant to ampicillin and ticarcillin), whereas *C. freundii* has a pattern more typical of *Enterobacter* species (i.e., resistant to ampicillin and first-generation cephalosporins).

TRIBE *KLEBSIELLEAE*

The tribe *Klebsielleae* includes four major genera—*Klebsiella*, *Enterobacter*, *Hafnia*, and *Serratia*—each of which includes several species that are overt and opportunistic pathogens in humans. A new, fifth genus, *Pantoea*, has been added to accommodate the reclassification of the organism formerly named *Enterobacter agglomerans* biotype XIII and now called *Pantoea agglomerans*.[188] The key characteristics suggesting that an unknown isolate belongs to the *Klebsielleae* are given in Table 6-6. The biochemical differences between the major genera and species within the tribe are presented in Table 6-16.

***Genus* Klebsiella.** The genus *Klebsiella* was named after Edwin Klebs, a late-19th-century German microbiologist. The bacillus now known as *Klebsiella* was also described by Carl Friedlander, and for many years the "Friedlander bacillus" was well known as a cause of severe, often fatal, pneumonia. *K. pneumoniae* is the type species of this genus.

Taxonomic Changes in the Genus *Klebsiella* In 2001, Drancourt and colleagues[137] performed a comparative analysis of the sequences of the 16S rRNA and *rpoB* genes (encoding the bacterial RNA polymerase β-subunit) of the type stains of nine *Klebsiella* species. Their findings confirmed that *Klebsiella* is heterogeneous and composed of species that form three phyletic clusters. Cluster I comprises *K. pneumoniae* subspecies *pneumoniae*, *rhinoscleromatis*, and *ozaenae*, and *K. granulomatis*; cluster II contains *K. ornithinolytica*, *K. planticola*, *K. trevisanii*, and *K. terrigena*; and cluster III contains *K. oxytoca*.[137] On the basis of this evidence they proposed that the genus *Klebsiella* be divided into two genera, *Klebsiella* and *Raoultella* (named after the French bacteriologist Didier Raoult), and that *K. oxytoca*

Table 6-15 Differentiation of Species Within the Genus *Citrobacter*[a]

BIOCHEMICAL TEST	CITROBACTER										
	C. koseri	C. werkmanii	C. sedlakii	C. rodentium	C. gillenii	C. amalonaticus	C. farmeri	C. braakii	C. freundii	C. murliniae	C. youngae
Adonitol	+[b]	–	–	–	–	–	–	–	–	–	–
Malonate	+	+	+	+	+	–	–	–	–	–	–
Ornithine	+	–	+	+	+	+	+	+	–	–	–
Melibiose	–	–	+	–	V (67)	–	+	V (78)	+	V (33)	–
Sucrose	V (44)	–	–	–	V (33)	(V 13)	+	V (33)	+	V (33)	V (19)
Indole	+	–	+	–	–	+	+	V (33)	V (38)	+	V (14)
Dulcitol	V (38)	–	+	–	–	–	–	V (33)	V (13)	+	V (86)
H₂S	–	+	–	–	V (67)	V (13)	–	V (60)	V (75)	V (67)	V (67)

[a] Data obtained from Brenner DJ, et al.[51]
+, 90% or more strains positive; –, 90% or more strains negative; V, 11–89% of strains positive; numbers in parentheses are percentages of strains giving a positive reaction.

Table 6-16 Differentiation of the Major Genera and Species Within the Tribe *Klebsielleae*

BIOCHEMICAL TEST[a]	KLEBSIELLA		ENTEROBACTER		PANTOEA	HAFNIA	SERRATIA	
	K. pneumoniae	K. oxytoca	E. aerogenes	E. cloacae	P. agglomerans	H. alvei	S. marcescens	S. liquefaciens
Indole	–	+	–	–	V (20)	–	–	–
Motility	–	–	+	+	V (85)	V (85)	+	+
Lysine	+	+	+	–	–	+	+	+
Arginine	–	–	–	+	–	–	–	–
Ornithine	–	–	+	+	–	+	+	+
DNase (25°C)	–	–	–	–	–	–	+	V (85)
Gelatinase (22°C)	–	–	–	–	–	–	+	+
Fermentation of:								
Lactose	+	+	+	+	V (40)	–	–	–
Sucrose	+	+	+	+	V (75)	–	+	+
Sorbitol	+	+	+	+	V (30)	–	+	+
Adonitol	+	+	+	V (25)	–	–	V (40)	–
Arabinose	+	+	+	+	+	+	–	+

+, 90% or more strains positive; –, 90% or more strains negative; V, 11–89% of strains positive.

should be left as a monophyletic taxon. Species included in cluster I are retained in the genus *Klebsiella*, while species included in cluster II are transferred to the new genus *Raoultella*.[137] Granier et al. have further shown that the *K. oxytoca* taxon is divided into two clades, which correspond to two genetic groups, called oxy-1 and oxy-2.[202,203] Finally, *Calymmatobacterium granulomatis*, the presumed causative agent of donovanosis, has been reclassified as *Klebsiella granulomatis* on the basis of phylogenetic data.[73,263]

Klebsiella and *Raoultella* species are widely distributed in nature and in the gastrointestinal tracts of humans and animals. A *Klebsiella* species should be suspected when large colonies with a mucoid consistency are recovered on primary isolation plates. On MacConkey agar, the colonies typically appear large, mucoid, and red, with red pigment usually diffusing into the surrounding agar, indicating fermentation of lactose and acid production. Not all strains, however, are mucoid, and certain species of *Enterobacter* can closely simulate the *Klebsiella* species in screening tests. All *Klebsiella* and *Raoultella* species are nonmotile and most do not decarboxylate ornithine (*R. ornithinolytica* is ornithine-positive)—characteristics that are positive for most *Enterobacter* species. Many strains of *Klebsiella* and *Raoultella* hydrolyze urea slowly, producing a light-pink color in the slant of Christensen's urea agar. Production of indole from tryptophan can be used to separate the two principal species. *K. pneumoniae* is indole-negative, and *K. oxytoca* is indole-positive. Certain strains do not produce these classic reactions, which led to the naming of several additional species (Table 6-17).

K. pneumoniae is most frequently recovered from clinical specimens and can cause a classic form of primary pneumonia. It is infrequently found in the oropharynx of normal persons (1–6% carrier rate)[420]; however, a prevalence as high as 20% may occur in hospitalized patients. This colonization may prove to be the source of lung infections that generally occur in patients with debilitating conditions such as alcoholism, diabetes mellitus, and chronic obstructive pulmonary disease.[420] The pneumonia tends to be destructive, with extensive necrosis and hemorrhage, resulting in the production of sputum that may be thick, mucoid, and brick red, or thin and "currant jelly–like" in appearance. Lung abscesses, chronic cavitary disease, internal hemorrhage, and hemoptysis may be seen in severe cases. Pleuritis is commonly present, which explains why pleuritic pain is found in about 80% of patients. *K. pneumoniae* can also cause a variety of extrapulmonary infections, including enteritis and meningitis (in infants), urinary tract infections (in children and adults), and septicemia.

K. ozaenae and *K. rhinoscleromatis* are infrequent isolates that are now considered to be subspecies of *K. pneumoniae*; however, each is associated with a unique spectrum of disease. *K. ozaenae* is associated with atrophic rhinitis, a condition called ozena, and purulent infections of the nasal mucous membranes. Janda and colleagues[248] have also reported a case of corneal abscess caused by *K. ozaenae*. Reports of the isolation of *K. ozaenae* from blood, urine, and soft tissue suggests that the spectrum of disease caused by this organism is more extensive than had been thought previously.[197] *K. rhinoscleromatis* causes the granulomatous disease rhinoscleroma, an infection of the respiratory mucosa,

oropharynx, nose, and paranasal sinuses. Clinical correlations should be made when these species are recovered in cultures to determine their medical significance in individual cases. Even though these two species are no longer considered to be true species but, rather, biochemically inactive strains of *K. pneumoniae*,[48] we believe that there is medical relevance in reporting the names *K. ozaenae* and *K. rhinoscleromatis* because of the specific disease association of these two strains.

Nearly half of the isolates of *K. oxytoca* submitted to the CDC have been from feces, with the next most common source being blood.[165] The more recently named species, *R. terrigena*[236] and *R. planticola*,[24] reflect their sources in nature. *R. terrigena* closely resembles *K. pneumoniae* and has been isolated mainly from soil and water. Human isolates have been recovered from the feces of healthy humans[398] and the respiratory tract[396]; however, their capacity to cause human infection has not been shown. *R. planticola* (synonym *K. trevisanii*)[172,187] has been isolated primarily from botanical and aquatic environments. Human isolates have been recovered from the respiratory tract, urine, cerebrospinal fluid, and blood,[177,178] with the majority of isolates representing colonization, rather than infection. Studies from France and Germany suggest that up to 19% of *Klebsiella/Raoultella* species are actually *R. planticola*[330,397,399]; however, the occurrence of *R. planticola* in the United States appears to be less frequent.[504] See Table 6-17 for a listing of the characteristics by which these various species can be differentiated.

The higher incidence of infections due to *Klebsiella* species during the past decade probably reflects both an increase in nosocomial infections in debilitated or immunosuppressed patients and a trend toward greater antibiotic resistance. In the United States, *Klebsiella* accounts for 3–7% of all nosocomial bacterial infections, placing them among the eight most important infectious pathogens in hospitals.[400] *Klebsielleae* have a tendency to harbor antibiotic-resistant plasmids; thus, infections with multiply antibiotic-resistant strains can be anticipated. Virtually all clinical strains are resistant to ampicillin, carbenicillin, and ticarcillin. Of particular concern is the recent appearance of *Klebsiella* strains that possess plasmids that mediate resistance to extended-spectrum β-lactam drugs. This form of resistance is due to the production of unique β-lactamase enzymes, referred to as extended-spectrum β-lactamases, or ESBLs.[249,290] These enzymes have been seen mostly in strains of *K. pneumoniae* and *E. coli,* and cause them to be resistant to most β-lactam drugs, including the third-generation cephalosporins. A unique feature of ESBLs is their ability to escape detection with most of the commonly used susceptibility tests and the resultant concern that organisms possessing ESBLs are reported to be susceptible to antibiotics to which they are, in fact, resistant.[240,321] This subject is discussed in more detail in Chapter 17.

Klebsiella granulomatis (formerly *Calymmatobacterium granulomatis*)[73] is a fastidious gram-negative encapsulated bacillus found intracytoplasmically within macrophages. It is the etiologic agent of granuloma inguinale (also known as Donovanosis), a sexually transmitted disease involving the genitalia and surrounding sites.[424] It is found in specific geographic foci, namely New Guinea, northwest Australia,

Table 6-17 Differentiation of Species Within the Genera *Klebsiella* and *Raoultella*

BIOCHEMICAL TEST	KLEBSIELLA				RAOULTELLA		
	K. pneumoniae SUBSP. pneumoniae	*K. pneumoniae* SUBSP. ozaenae	*K. pneumoniae* SUBSP. rhinoscleromatis	*K. oxytoca*	*R. ornithinolytica*	*R. planticola*	*R. terrigena*
Indole	−	−	−	+	+	V (20)	−
Methyl red	−	+	+	V (20)	+	+	V (60)
Voges-Proskauer	+	−	−	+	V (70)	+	+
Urease	+	−	−	+	+	+	+
Lysine	+	V (40)	−	+	+	+	−
Ornithine	−	−	−	−	+	−	+
ONPG	+	V (80)	−	+	+	+	V (20)
Malonate	+	−	+	+	+	+	+
Growth at:							
5°C	−	−	−	−	+	+	+
10°C	−	−	−	+	+	+	+
41°C	+	NA	NA	+	+	+	−

+, 90% or more strains positive; −, 90% or more strains negative; V, 11–89% of strains positive; NA, results not available.
Data from Farmer JJ III, Davis BR, Hickman-Brenner FW, et al.[168]

southeast India, the Caribbean, parts of South America, parts of central Africa and the KwaZulu/Natal region of South Africa.[264] *K. granulomatis* cannot be cultured on conventional agar media, although it has been successfully grown in embryonated eggs and in a monocyte coculture system.[264] Currently, the laboratory diagnosis of granuloma inguinale relies on the observation of "Donovan bodies" in tissue smears or biopsy specimens examined by Giemsa and Wright stains. To increase the specificity of the diagnosis, Dieterle's, Warthin-Starry,[204] and rapid Giemsa (Diff Quick)[352] stains have been used. A polymerase chain reaction (PCR) for detection of donovanosis in genital specimens has been reported.[72,74] Azithromycin has emerged as the drug of choice and should be used if the diagnosis is confirmed or suspected.[351]

Genus Enterobacter. Because large amounts of gas are produced by many strains of the genus *Enterobacter*, for many years the type species was called *Aerobacter aerogenes*. The genus designation was changed to *Enterobacter* by Hormaeche and Edwards in 1960.[229a]

There are 16 species included in the genus *Enterobacter*. A recent development has been the removal of one of the biotypes of *E. agglomerans* and its placement in the genus *Pantoea*.[188] As a genus, *Enterobacter* has the general charac-

teristics of the *Klebsielleae*, but can be differentiated from most *Klebsiella* species because they are motile and ornithine-positive. The biochemical characteristics by which the medically important species can be differentiated are included in Table 6-18.

E. aerogenes and *E. cloacae* are the species most commonly encountered in clinical specimens. They are widely distributed in water, in sewage, in soil, and on vegetables. They are part of the commensal enteric flora and are not believed to cause diarrhea, although a Shiga-like toxin-producing strain of *E. cloacae* has been isolated from the feces of an infant with hemolytic–uremic syndrome.[379] They are also associated with a variety of opportunistic infections involving the urinary tract, respiratory tract, and cutaneous wounds; and, on occasion, cause septicemia and meningitis.[377]

E. sakazakii, known as yellow-pigmented *E. cloacae*,[163] has been found in several cases of neonatal meningitis and sepsis.[36,115,253,272,336,480] Fatality rates as high as 75% have been reported,[279,341] indicating that this organism can be highly virulent. Recent reports have linked *E. sakazakii* infection in neonates with contaminated powdered-milk formulas.[99,483] The bright yellow pigment (particularly intense if cultures are incubated at 25°C) and "tough" nature of the

Table 6-18 Differentiation of Clinically Important Species Within the Genus *Enterobacter*[a]

TEST	*E. AEROGENES*	*E. AMNIGENUS* BIOGROUP 1	*E. AMNIGENUS* BIOGROUP 2	*E. ASBURIAE*	*E. CANCEROGENUS*	*E. CLOACAE*	*E. COWANII*	*E. GERGOVIAE*	*E. HORMAECHEI*	*E. INTERMEDIUS*	*E. KOBEI*	*E. SAKAZAKII*
Methyl red	−	−	V (65)	+	−	−	NA	−	V (57)	+	−	−
Voges-Proskauer	+	+	+	−	+	+	+	+	+	+	+	+
Lysine	+	−	−	−	−	−	−	+	−	−	−	−
Arginine	−	−	V (35)	V (21)	+	+	−	−	V (78)	−	+	+
Ornithine	+	V (55)	+	+	+	+	−	+	V (91)	V (89)	+	+
Urease	−	−	−	V (60)	−	V (65)	−	+	V (87)	−	−	−
Motility	+	+	+	−	+	+	+	+	V (52)	V (89)	+	+
Fermentation of:												
Lactose	+	V(70)	V (35)	V (75)	−	+	+	V (55)	−	+	+	+
Sucrose	+	+	−	+	−	+	+	+	+	V (65)	V (25)	+
Adonitol	+	−	−	−	−	V (25)	−	−	−	−	−	−
Sorbitol	+	−	+	+	−	+	+	−	−	+	+	−
Raffinose	+	+	−	V (70)	−	+	+	+	−	+	+	+
Rhamnose	+	+	+	−	+	+	+	+	+	+	+	+
Melibiose	+	+	+	−	−	+	+	+	−	+	+	+
Yellow pigment	−	−	−	−	−	−	V (66)	−	−	−	−	+

+, 90% or more strains positive; −, 90% or more strains negative; V, 11–89% of strains positive; NA, not available.

[a] Table includes only Enterobacter species that have been isolated from human clinical specimens. Isolates that are triple decarboxylase negative may by Pantoea species, and isolates that are both lactose- and sucrose-negative but are lysine-positive may be Hafnia alvei (see Table 6–16).

colonies are the initial clues that this organism is present (*Pantoea agglomerans* also produces a yellow pigment, usually less intense, and often only after delayed incubation at room temperature). The decarboxylase pattern of *E. sakazakii* (lysine-negative, arginine-positive, and ornithine-positive) helps to differentiate it from *E. aerogenes* (lysine-positive, arginine-negative, and ornithine-positive) and *P. agglomerans* (lysine-, arginine-, and ornithine-negative); and *E. sakazakii* does not ferment sorbitol, in contrast to *E. cloacae*, which does.

E. gergoviae causes urinary tract infections, and additional isolates have been recovered from the respiratory tract and blood.[56] Biochemically it is closest to *E. aerogenes* (lysine-positive, arginine-negative, ornithine-positive), but is strongly urease-positive. It can be further differentiated by negative reactions in adonitol, inositol, and sorbitol, whereas *E. aerogenes* is positive for all three reactions.

E. cancerogenus (formerly called *Erwinia cancerogena*, *Enterobacter taylorae*, and CDC enteric group 19)[166,443] has been reported to cause a variety of clinical infections, including osteomyelitis after an open fracture,[502] wound infection,[415] especially after severe trauma or crush injuries,[1] urinary tract infection,[418,428] and bacteremia and pneumonia.[428] The key biochemical features are its lysine-negative, arginine-positive, and ornithine-positive reactions and its negative reactions in adonitol, inositol, sorbitol, raffinose, and melibiose. They are lactose-negative but ONPG-positive, and we have noted that colonies growing on MacConkey agar will develop purple centers after extended incubation.

E. asburiae (formerly called CDC enteric group 17, or atypical *Citrobacter*) is biochemically similar to *E. cloacae*; however, it is unique among the *Enterobacter* species by being nonmotile and Voges-Proskauer-negative. It has been reported from a variety of human sources, including blood, urine, wounds, respiratory tract, and feces.[53] One case of community-acquired pneumonia caused by *E. asburiae* has been reported.[462] We have found considerable variation in the ability of commercial identification systems to correctly identify this species.

E. amnigenus is primarily a water organism that has been isolated from human specimens.[238] A case of posttransfusion septicemia caused by *E. amnigenus* has been reported in France.[241]

E. hormaechei is a new species of *Enterobacter* named in 1989 after Estenio Hormaeche, a Uruguayan microbiologist who (with P.R. Edwards) proposed and defined the genus *Enterobacter*.[361] Formerly known as enteric group 75, it is biochemically closest to *E. taylorae* (now *E. cancerogenus*) except it is urea-positive, sucrose-positive, and esculin-negative. Isolates have been reported from blood, sputum, wounds, ear, gallbladder, and stool. In March 1993, CDC investigators identified a nosocomial outbreak of *E. hormaechei* septicemia in a neonatal intensive care unit. Five infants had positive blood cultures with *E. hormaechei*, and another infant had *E. hormaechei* tracheitis. Four additional infants were identified with *E. hormaechei* colonization. No deaths were reported. Environmental cultures showed the organism to be present on three isolettes and one doorknob.[79,499] An outbreak of *E. hormaechei* bloodstream infections were reported in three neonatal intensive care units in Rio de Janeiro. Chart review for previous procedures re-

vealed parenteral nutrition as the only common procedure.[128] A case of recurrent bacteremia caused by *E. hormaechei* has been seen at the University of Illinois Medical Center in a 2-year-old patient with a neuroblastoma involving a left supraclavicular lymph node, an adrenal gland, and a perinavel lymph node.

In 1981, CDC enteric group 69 was defined for a group of yellow-pigmented strains that resembled *E. cloacae* biochemically. In 1996, *Enterobacter kobei* was described as a new species of *Enterobacteriaceae* resembling *Enterobacter cloacae*,[276] and similar to enteric group 69, but which were negative in tests for VP, fermentation of adonitol, and yellow pigment production. DNA hybridization studies performed at the CDC and the National Institute of Health, Tokyo, have led to the conclusion that enteric group 69 species are yellow-pigmented biochemical variants of *E. kobei*.[276,359] The majority of strains of *E. kobei* were isolated from clinical specimens including blood, sputum, throat, and urine.[276,454]

Enterobacter cowanii is a new species proposed for a group of organisms referred to as NIH Group 42 (refers National Institute of Health, Tokyo).[235] *E. cowanii* strains are negative for lysine and ornithine decarboxylases and arginine dihydrolase; therefore, phenotypically they most closely resemble *Pantoea agglomerans*. Tests useful for differentiation from *P. agglomerans* are negative malonate utilization and fermentation of dulcitol and sorbitol (both negative for *P. agglomerans*). Of the nine strains studied, eight were isolated from clinical specimens: urine (four), sputum (two), blood (one), and pus (one), but their clinical significance is unknown.[235]

Four additional species (*E. intermedius*, *E. dissolvens*, *E. nimipressuralis*, and *E. pyrinus*) are found in the environment or as plant pathogens and have only rarely been found in human clinical specimens. *E. intermedius* (formerly *E. intermedium* and Group H1)[489] had not been known to occur in humans until 1987 when Prats et al. reported four strains of *E. intermedius* that had been isolated from a foot wound, blood, stool, and bile.[405] More recently O'Hara et al. reported the isolation of *E. intermedius* from the gallbladder of a patient with cholecystitis that also grew group D *Streptococcus*, and coagulase-negative *Staphylococcus*.[363]

Enterobacter species together with certain other members of the family *Enterobacteriaceae* (namely *C. freundii*, *Serratia* species, *Morganella morganii*, and *Providence* species) carry a gene for chromosomally encoded β-lactamase that can be induced by certain antibiotics, amino acids, or body fluids.[290] Unlike plasmid-mediated β-lactamases, these enzymes are not normally expressed. Only under the influence of an inducer or following mutation does the gene become activated and the enzyme expressed. It is a concern, therefore, that organisms harboring genes for inducible β-lactamases may show false susceptibility if tested in the uninduced state. Recently, methods for the detection of resistance owing to inducible β-lactamases have been described.[232] This topic is discussed further in Chapter 17.

Genus Pantoea. In the early 1970s, *P. agglomerans* (then called *Enterobacter agglomerans*) was responsible for a nationwide outbreak of septicemia caused by contaminated intravenous fluids.[303] The new genus *Pantoea* was created in 1989 with the type species being *P. agglomerans*.[188] This taxon includes the former type strains of *Enterobacter ag-*

glomerans, Erwinia herbicola, and *Erwinia milletiae*. *Pantoea* is derived from a Greek word meaning "of all sorts and sources," thus describing these bacteria that come from diverse geographic and ecologic sources. A second species, *P. dispersa*, has been isolated from plant surfaces, seeds, humans, and the environment. Both species are triple-decarboxylase-negative (lysine-negative, arginine-negative, and ornithine-negative), but can be separated by salicin, which is positive for *P. agglomerans* and negative for *P. dispersa*.[188] Five additional species found in soil and plants have been described (see Table 6-5).

Genus Hafnia. *H. alvei*, formerly *Enterobacter hafnia*, is the only species in the genus *Hafnia*. The biochemical characteristics are similar to those of *Enterobacter* species except that *H. alvei* does not produce acids from the following carbohydrates: lactose, sucrose, melibiose, raffinose, adonitol, sorbitol, dulcitol, and inositol (see Table 6-16). *H. alvei* can be distinguished from *Serratia* species because it does not produce lipase or deoxyribonuclease. We have also noted that, unlike other species of *Enterobacteriaceae*, this organism gives off a strong scent of human feces. The clinical significance of *H. alvei* is not well defined. The organism has been recovered from human feces in the absence of symptoms. Isolated cases of infection have been reported from persons in whom *H. alvei* has been recovered from wounds, abscesses, sputum, urine, blood, and other sites. In one of our laboratories (University of Illinois) *H. alvei* was isolated in pure culture from a chest wound of a patient following thoracic surgery. There is evidence to suggest that *H. alvei* may be an emerging cause of acute bacterial gastroenteritis.[10,412,413,417,425,503] However, Janda et al. have subsequently shown that the prototypal diarrheagenic stains of *Hafnia alvei* that were reported to contain the eae gene of enteropathogenic *E. coli* are in fact a category of diarrheagenic isolates belonging to the genus *Escherichia* that were misidentified as *Hafnia alvei* by the API 20E system.[233,245] These strains have been designated as the new species *Escherichia albertii* discussed previously.[233]

Genus Serratia. *Serratia* species are unique among the *Enterobacteriaceae* in producing three hydrolytic enzymes: lipase, gelatinase, and DNase. Resistance to colistin and cephalothin are additional distinguishing features. There are currently 10 species recognized, 7 of which have been recovered from human clinical specimens. The biochemical differentiation of *Serratia* species of clinical importance is shown in Table 6-19.

S. marcescens is the most important member of the genus *Serratia* and is often associated with a variety of human infections, particularly pneumonia and septicemia in patients with reticuloendothelial malignancies who are receiving chemotherapeutic agents. At one time, the organism was used as a harmless commensal to trace environmental contamination, primarily because the characteristic red pigmentation of some strains was easy to spot in culture media. However, the organism is now recognized as an important pathogen with invasive properties and a tendency to resist many commonly used antibiotics. *S. marcescens* can be a significant nosocomial opportunist, as evidenced by a recent case of childhood meningitis following the use of contaminated benzalkonium chloride disinfectant solution.[437] The species referred to as *S. liquefaciens* is now known to be not a single species but a collection of several DNA hybridization groups, including species named *S. proteamaculans* and *S. grimesii*. They are found on the surfaces of plants

Table 6-19 Differentiation of Clinically Important Species Within the Genus *Serratia*[a]

BIOCHEMICAL TEST	*S. MARCESCENS*	*S. LIQUEFACIENS*	*S. RUBIDAEA*	*S. PLYMUTHICA*	*S. FICARIA*	*S. FONTICOLA*	*S. ODORIFERA* BIOGROUP 1	2
DNase (25°C)	+	V (85)	+	+	+	−	+	+
Lipase (corn oil)	+	V (85)	+	V (70)	V (77)	−	V (35)	V (65)
Gelatinase (22°C)	+	+	+	V (60)	+	−	+	+
Lysine (Moeller's)	+	+	V (55)	−	−	+	+	+
Ornithine (Moeller's)	+	+	−	−	−	+	+	−
Odor of potatoes	−	−	V	−	+	−	+	+
Red, pink, or orange pigment	V	−	V	V	−	−	−	−
Fermentation of:								
L-Arabinose	−	+	+	+	+	+	+	+
D-Arabitol	−	−	V (85)	−	+	+	−	−
D-Sorbitol	+	+	−	V (65)	+	+	+	+
Sucrose	+	+	+	+	+	V (21)	+	−
Raffinose	−	V (85)	+	+	V (70)	+	+	−
Malonate utilization	−	−	+	−	−	+	−	−

+, 90% or more strains positive; −, 90% or more strains negative; V, 11–89% of strains positive.
[a] Data obtained from reference 193 and other sources.
Table includes only those *Serratia* species that have been isolated from human clinical specimens.

and belong to the "*Serratia liquefaciens-proteamaculans-grimesii*" complex. Strains of these species produce plant-growth–promoting chemicals, have antifungal properties, encourage the establishment of nitrogen-fixing symbionts, and act as insect pathogens.[16] Because the species that make up this hybridization group cannot be separated by currently used biochemical tests, it is suggested that members of this species be reported as "*Serratia liquefaciens* group." This group is differentiated from *S. marcescens* by virtue of its ability to ferment L-arabinose.

S. *rubidaea*, as its name would imply, produces colonies that are red-pigmented but is rarely isolated from human clinical specimens. Ursua and associates reported a case of *S. rubidaea* isolated from the bile and blood of a patient with a bile tract carcinoma who underwent invasive procedures.[482] *S. odorifera* produces a dirty, musty odor, similar to unpeeled potatoes. Two biogroups are described. Biogroup 1 is ornithine-, sucrose-, and raffinose-positive and is isolated predominantly from sputum; however, it has been reported to cause severe sepsis in elderly, compromised patients,[112,318] and catheter-associated sepsis in an adolescent patient with thalassemia major who had been splenectomized.[195] Biogroup 2 is negative for these three reactions and has been recovered from blood and cerebrospinal fluid.[165] Strains of *S. plymuthica* may be red-pigmented and have been isolated from soil, water, and human sputum specimens. Although *S. plymuthica* is generally not considered to be a cause of serious human infections, recent reports have shown that it can be a significant pathogen causing chronic osteomyelitis,[515] wound infections,[70,116] and community-acquired[416] and nosocomial bacteremia[70,136,230] and has been isolated from the peritoneal fluid of a patient with cholecystitis.[70] *S. ficaria* has a natural habitat in figs and the fig wasp.[193] Isolation of this species from human specimens is extremely rare and usually is accompanied by a history of ingestion of figs.[12,21,127] *S. entomophila* is an insect pathogen, and no human isolates have been reported. "*S.*" *fonticola* is not really a species of *Serratia* and is likely to be reclassified. It is a water organism that has been isolated rarely from human clinical specimens, mostly wounds.[44,165,391] *S. fonticola* has been recovered from the blood of a patient with a digestive neoplasm at the University of Illinois Medical Center.

TRIBE *PROTEEAE*

The *Proteeae* comprise three genera: *Proteus, Morganella,* and *Providencia.* The characteristics suggesting that an organism belongs to this tribe are given in Table 6-6. The classification, identification, and clinical significance of the Proteeae has been reviewed by O'Hara et al.[354]

Genus Proteus. DNA relatedness studies have clarified the classification of organisms within the *Proteeae.* The genus *Proteus* now includes five named species: *P. vulgaris, P. mirabilis, P. myxofaciens, P. penneri,* and *P. hauseri,* and three unnamed genomospecies that were formerly identified as members of biogroup 3 of *P. vulgaris.*[52] Strains of *P. vulgaris* have traditionally been placed into three biogroups, as follows:

Proteus biogroup 1: indole-, salicin-, esculin-negative;
    chloramphenicol-resistant

Proteus biogroup 2: indole-, salicin-, esculin-positive
Proteus biogroup 3: indole-positive, salicin- and esculin-negative

Proteus biogroup 1 is a single genetic species and is now known as *P. penneri.*[219] *Proteus* biogroup 2 is a single genetic species and will retain the name *P. vulgaris. Proteus* biogroup 3 consists of four separate genetic species that are designated DNA groups (genomovars) 3, 4, 5, and 6. DNA group 3 can be distinguished from *Proteus* DNA groups 4, 5 and 6 because it is negative for Jordan's tartrate, lipase, and DNase (Table 6-20). Since DNA group 3 can be phenotypically separated from the other *Proteus* genomospecies, it has been officially named *Proteus hauseri* to honor Gustav Hauser, the German microbiologist, who proposed the genus *Proteus* in 1885.[355] *Proteus* genomospecies 4, 5, and 6 will remain unnamed until better phenotypic differentiation can be accomplished. Biochemical separation of the *Proteus* species and DNA groups is given in Table 6-20.

The genus *Proteus* is found in soil, water, and fecally contaminated materials. *Proteus* species exhibit the characteristic feature of swarming motility, which is observed on noninhibitory agar (e.g., blood agar plate) as a wavelike spreading of the organism across the entire surface of the agar (see Color Plate 6-1*D*). Whenever swarming is observed, *Proteus* species should be suspected. *P. mirabilis* is the species most frequently recovered from humans, particularly as the causative agent of both urinary tract and wound infections. *P. vulgaris* is more commonly recovered from infected sites in immunosuppressed hosts, particularly those receiving prolonged regimens of antibiotics. As noted in Table 6-20, *P. vulgaris* is indole-positive, whereas *P. mirabilis* is indole-negative. Thus, by performing a rapid spot indole test on a characteristic swarming colony, a rapid presumptive identification of *P. mirabilis* or *P. vulgaris* can be made. The new species *P. penneri*[219] and *P. myxofaciens* are also indole-negative but are rarely encountered in clinical laboratories (the latter is a pathogen of gypsy moth larvae and has not been recovered from human specimens). Therefore, for practical purposes, the recovery of an indole-negative *Proteus* species can be presumptively identified as *P. mirabilis.* Virtually all strains of *P. mirabilis* are sensitive to ampicillin and cephalosporins, whereas *P. vulgaris* is resistant; therefore, most patients with clinical infection, from whom an indole-negative *Proteus* species is recovered, can be treated with one of the broad-spectrum penicillins or cephalosporins.

P. penneri closely resembles *P. vulgaris* but differs from *P. vulgaris* by being indole-, salicin-, and esculin-negative and by failing to produce hydrogen sulfide in TSI. When *P. penneri* is suspected, a chloramphenicol susceptibility test should be performed for identification purposes. *P. penneri* is chloramphenicol-resistant, whereas other indole-negative *Proteus* species are chloramphenicol-susceptible (see Table 6-20).[219] Documented human infections with *P. penneri* have been limited mainly to the urinary tract and wounds of the abdomen, groin, neck, and ankle.[219,278] In one report, a patient with leukemia was described, in whom a *P. penneri* bacteremia developed with a concomitant subcutaneous thigh abscess, demonstrating the invasive potential of this bacterium.[155] Microbiologists are advised to be suspicious of any *P. vulgaris* isolates that are indole-negative and hy-

Table 6-20 Differentiation of Species Within the Members of the Genus *Proteus*[a]

TEST	P. MIRABILIS	P. MYXOFACIENS	P. PENNERI	P. VULGARIS	P. HAUSERI	PROTEUS VULGARIS BIOGROUP 3 DNA Group 4	DNA Group 5	DNA Group 6
Ornithine	+	−	−	−	−	−	−	−
Indole	−	−	−	+	+	+	+	+
Esculin	−	−	−	+	−	−	−	V (9)
Salicin	−	−	−	+	−	−	−	V (9)
Lipase	+	+	V (35)	V (14)	−	+	+	V (90)
Tartrate	V (87)	+	V (89)	V (14)		+	+	+
Rhamnose	−	−	−	−		+	V (17)	−
DNase 25°C	V (50)	V (50)	V (12)	+	−	+	+	V (55)
Acetate	V (20)		V (12)	V (14)	−	−	V (12)	V (18)

[a] Data obtained from reference[355].
+, 90% or more strains positive; −, 90% or more strains negative; V, 11–89% of strains positive; numbers in parentheses are the percentages of strains giving positive reactions.

drogen sulfide-negative because these may possibly be isolates of *P. penneri*.

Genus Morganella. On the basis of genetic studies performed by Brenner and colleagues in 1978, the organism previously designated *Proteus morganii* was reassigned to the new genus *Morganella* as *M. morganii*.[48] Studies by Jensen and colleagues have shown that *M. morganii* can be further separated into three DNA relatedness groups and seven biogroups.[250] DNA relatedness group 1 contains biogroups A through D. DNA relatedness group 2 contains biogroups E and F and two thirds of biogroup G (termed biogroup G-2). DNA relatedness group 3 contains the remaining one third of biogroup G (termed biogroup G-1). Because G-1 and G-2 are phenotypically indistinguishable, Jensen and associates have proposed dividing *M. morganii* into just two subspecies based on trehalose fermentation.[250] *M. morganii* that are unable to ferment trehalose are designated *M.*

morganii subsp. *morganii*, and those that are able to utilize trehalose are designated *M. morganii* subsp. *sibonii*.

M. morganii is a cause of both urinary tract and wound infections and has been implicated as a cause of diarrhea. Serious infections reportedly caused by *M. morganii* include a case of meningitis in a patient with AIDS[308] and a case of meningitis and brain abscess in an 8-day-old infant.[487] As shown in Table 6-6, the pattern of Simmons citrate–negative, hydrogen sulfide-negative, and ornithine decarboxylase-positive is characteristic of this genus. The biochemical differentiation of the subspecies and biogroups is given in Table 6-21.

Genus Providencia. Five species of *Providencia* are now recognized: *P. alcalifaciens, P. stuartii, P. rettgeri,* and the newly described species *P. rustigianii*[220] and *P. heimbachae*.[334] All species of the genus *Providencia* deaminate phenylalanine, but only *P. rettgeri* consistently hydrolyzes urea.

Table 6-21 Differentiation of Species Within the Genus *Morganella*[a]

BIOCHEMICAL TEST	M. MORGANII SUBSP. MORGANII BIOGROUPS A	B	C	D	M. MORGANII SUBSP. SIBONII BIOGROUPS E	F	G
Lysine	−	+	−	+	+	d+	−
Ornithine	+	+	−	−	+	−	+
Trehalose	−	−	−	−	+	+	+
Tetracycline (% susceptible)	100[b]	100	14	100	0	0	21
Motility	+	−	d+	−	+	+	+

[a] Data obtained from reference[250].
[b] Strains with a zone of ≥28 mm around tetracycline were considered susceptible (minimal inhibitory concentration [MIC] correlate, ≤2 μg/mL), and those with a zone diameter ≤15 mm were considered tetracycline-resistant (MIC correlate, ≥32 μg/mL).
+, 90% or more strains positive; −, 90% or more strains negative; V, 11–89% of strains positive; d+, delayed reaction, 50–89% positive within 48 hr.

Table 6-22 Differentiation of Species Within the Genus *Providencia*

BIOCHEMICAL TEST	P. ALCALIFACIENS	P. RUSTIGIANII	P. HEINBACHAE	P. STUARTII	P. RETTGERI
Urea hydrolysis	−	−	−	V (30)	+
Citrate utilization	+	−	−	+	+
Fermentation of:					
Inositol	−	−	V (46)	+	+
Adonitol	+	−	+	−	+
Arabitol	−	−	+	−	+
Trehalose	−	−	−	+	−
Galactose	−	+	+	+	+

+, 90% or more strains are positive; −, 90% or more strains are negative.
Data obtained from[334] and other sources.

The biochemical differences of the species are shown in Table 6-22.

Except for causing urinary tract infections, for which Penner has cited several nosocomial outbreaks,[383] infections with *Providencia* species are uncommon and are limited to isolated case reports. All species may be recovered from feces; however, only *P. alcalifaciens* may be associated with diarrheal illness, usually in children.[247] Hickman-Brenner and associates[220] designated *P. rustigianii* to what was previously known as *P. alcalifaciens* biogroup 3. This organism has also been recovered from feces; however, its role in diarrheal disease is still questionable. A new species, *P. heimbachae*, has been reported from penguin feces and an aborted cow fetus.[334] There has been only one report of human *P. heimbachae* infection, from the stool of a 23-year-old woman with idiopathic diarrhea.[360]

TRIBE *YERSINIEAE*

Three species of *Pasteurella*, including the causative agent of human plague, *P. pestis*, were formally assigned to a new genus, *Yersinia*, in the eighth edition of *Bergey's Manual* and placed in the *Enterobacteriaceae*. The name for the genus *Yersinia* was derived from the French bacteriologist Alexander Yersin, who in 1894, first identified the organism now called *Y. pestis*. The key characteristics of the *Yersinieae* are given in Table 6-6.

Although *Yersinia* species qualify biochemically for inclusion in the *Enterobacteriaceae*, the cells appear small and coccobacillary in gram-stained smears and may be small and pinpoint on MacConkey agar, particularly for certain strains of *Y. pestis* and *Y. pseudotuberculosis*. Optimal growth occurs from 25 to 32°C. Colonies tend to be pinpoint in size after 24 hours of incubation on sheep blood agar. If incubation is continued at room temperature, after 48 hours, gray-white, convex colonies measuring 1 to 2 mm in diameter may be observed.

Genus *Yersinia*. *Yersinia* is the only genus in the *Yersinieae*. Three species, *Y. pestis*, *Y. pseudotuberculosis*, and *Y. enterocolitica*, were included when the genus was transferred to the *Enterobacteriaceae*. In 1980, three new species were proposed for strains that were former subgroups of *Y. enterocolitica*[34,49,57,481]: *Y. frederiksenii* is the name given to the rhamnose-positive biogroup[481]; *Y. intermedia* is the designation for those atypical strains that ferment rhamnose, raffinose, and melibiose[49]; and *Y. kristensenii* is the name for the previous sucrose-negative, trehalose-positive biogroup of *Y. enterocolitica*.[34] Presently, 11 species are included in the genus *Yersinia*; however, only three (*Y. pestis*, *Y. pseudotuberculosis*, and *Y. enterocolitica*) have been unquestionably shown to be human pathogens. One species, *Y. ruckeri*, a fish pathogen not known to cause human infection, will probably be moved to a new genus.[159] The differential characteristics for these various species are included in Table 6-23.

Plague—*Y. pestis* Plague is an infectious disease of antiquity that persists in modern times. *Y. pestis*, which undergoes an obligate flea-rodent-flea life cycle, causes bubonic plague, a rapid and highly fatal zoonotic disease that is responsible for at least three pandemics occurring in the 5–6th, 8–14th, and 19–21st centuries (Box 6-13).[389]

Epidemiology *Y. pestis* is endemic in various rodents, including rats, ground squirrels, prairie dogs, mice, and rabbits. Two epidemic forms of disease occur: urban plague, which is maintained in the urban rat population, and sylvatic plague, which is endemic in 17 Western states (Fig. 6-7) and is carried by prairie dogs, mice, rabbits, and rats. The organism is transferred from rodent to rodent or from rodent to human by fleas. Human cases have been concentrated in two principal regions in the U.S.: 1) a southwestern area that includes New Mexico, northeastern Arizona, southern Colorado, and southern Utah; and 2) a Pacific Coast region located in California, Oregon, and western Nevada (Fig. 6-7).[86] During 1988–2002, a total of 112 human cases of plague were reported from 11 western states. The majority (97) were exposed in four states (New Mexico, Colorado, Arizona, and California).[101] Approximately 80% of these exposures occurred in peridomestic environments, particularly those that provided abundant food and harbor for flea-infested, plague-susceptible rodents. Household infections occur when people, domestic animals (especially cats), and peridomestic rodents bring fleas into the house, exposing more persons. Domestic cats permitted to roam freely in areas where plague occurs in rodents are at increased risk for infection and, therefore, increase the risk for peridomestic transmission to humans. Mouth abscesses develop in infected cats, by which they pass the plague directly to people

Table 6-23 Differentiation of Species Within the Genus *Yersinia*

BIOCHEMICAL TEST	Y. PESTIS	Y. PSEUDOTUBERCULOSIS	Y. ENTEROCOLITICA	Y. FREDERIKSENII	Y. INTERMEDIA	Y. KRISTENSENII	Y. ALDOVAE	Y. BERCOVIERI	Y. MOLLARETII	Y. ROHDEI
Indole	–	–	V (50)	+	+	V (30)	–	–	–	–
Ornithine	–	–	+	+	+	+	V (40)	V (80)	V (80)	V (25)
Motility 25–28°C	–	+	+	+	+	+	+	+	+	NA
Fermentation of:										
Sucrose	–	–	+	+	+	–	V (20)	+	+	+
Rhamnose	–	V (70)	–	+	+	–	–	–	–	–
Cellobiose	–	–	V (75)	+	+	+	–	+	+	V (25)
Sorbitol	V(50)	–	+	+	+	+	V (60)	+	+	+
Melibiose	V(50)	V (70)	–	–	V (80)	–	–	–	–	V (50)

Data obtained from references 33, 496, and other sources. All tests were done at 25–28°C.
+, 90% or more strains positive; –, 90% or more strains negative; V, 11–89% of strains positive; NA, results not available.

CLINICAL CORRELATION BOX 6–5 Human Plague

When plague bacilli are introduced into a human host, the microorganisms replicate at the initial site of infection, which may be the site of the flea bite, the bloodstream, or the lung and as a result three clinical forms of human plague may occur:

1. Bubonic: Incubation period of 7 days or less after a bite from an infected flea. Bacteria spread to regional lymph nodes, usually in the groin (most common), axilla, or neck. An early sign of lymph node infection is the appearance of large, painful swellings called buboes. There is often a sudden onset of fever, chills, weakness, and headache. Within hours, patients may notice intense pain in anatomic region with buboes. Patients become prostrate and lethargic and may exhibit agitation, particularly when the bubo is disturbed. It is the mildest form of plague; however, the fatality rate in untreated cases is approximately 75%.

2. Pneumonic: This form is usually secondary to the bubonic process, although it may also result from direct exposure to respiratory droplets from another pneumonic patient or from infected cats.[151,501] Shorter incubation (2 to 3 days); patients initially have fever and malaise, then pulmonary signs develop within 1 day. In such patients, cough, chest pain, and hemoptysis are seen, with the sputum usually purulent and containing plague bacilli (Color Plate 6-5*B*, 6-5*C*). Pneumonic plague is quickly followed by sepsis and death unless antimicrobial therapy is initiated within the first day. The fatality rate exceeds 90% if untreated. Persons suspected of having pneumonic plague should be placed in respiratory isolation and reported immediately to public health authorities so that rapid diagnosis, environmental assessments, and control measures can be initiated.

3. Septicemic: Direct infection of the bloodstream by the flea bite, or spread of the plague bacillus from lymph nodes to the bloodstream can result in septicemic plague. In this form, 100% of patients become septic, with positive blood cultures. High fever, delirium, seizures in children, septic shock, and disseminated intravascular coagulation (DIC) develop. Black hemorrhagic splotches (Color Plate 6-5*A*) develop that gave plague the name "Black Death."

Diagnosis: Plague should be suspected in febrile patients who have been exposed to rodents or other mammals in known endemic areas (Fig. 6-7). The differential diagnosis of plague includes Reye's syndrome, tularemia, bacterial pneumonia, and acute surgical abdomen. A febrile course in a prostrate patient with a bubo should suggest either plague or tularemia: a bacteriologic diagnosis in such a patient can be made readily with a smear and culture of a bubo aspirate.

Treatment: Primary therapy: streptomycin; alternatively use gentamicin, tetracyclines, or chloramphenicol.[101]

Modified from Stratton.[464]

Box 6-13 History of Plague

Three major plague pandemics have occurred at intervals of 600 years, each occurring at the end of a major historical epoch: Justinian Plague at the end of Antiquity, Black Death at the end of the Middle Ages, and the Modern Pandemic at the end of the current era.

First Pandemic—The Justinian Plague (A.D. 541–544): Named after the Roman emperor of the 6th century, affected the Mediterranean Countries from 532 to 595 and resulted in more than 100 million deaths. It began in Egypt and spread through Middle East and Mediterranean Europe. After that, the 2nd–11th epidemics (A.D. 558–654) occurred in 8–12 year cycles. Eventually affecting all the "known world."

Second Pandemic—The Black Death (A.D. 1347–1351): Originated in the area of the Black Sea, spread to Sicily and eventually affected the entire area of Europe up to Great Britain, Scandinavia, and Western Russia. A total of 17–28 million Europeans died from the disease which represented 30–40% of the European population. Epidemics continued in 2–5-year cycles from 1361 to 1480, and in less frequent cycles into the 17th century. The second pandemic again encompassed all the "known world."

Third Pandemic: The Modern Pandemic: Started in 1855 in Yunnan, a Southwestern province of China. Hong Kong was affected in May 1894; Bombay in 1896; Madagascar in 1898; Egypt, Portugal, Japan, Paraguay and Eastern Africa in 1899; and Manila, Glasgow, Sydney, and San Francisco in 1900. The outbreaks in India affected more than 10 million victims between 1896 and 1918, causing the majority of the deaths that occurred during this pandemic. Local epidemics subsequently took place all over the world until the 1950s, when the pandemic ended.

Plague in the United States: After plague appeared in Hong Kong in 1894 it spread rapidly, reaching the port of San Francisco by boat in 1900. At approximately the same time it also appeared in Brazil, New Orleans, and New York. Reluctance of California health officials to admit that plague existed in Chinatown resulted in initiation of sylvatic infection. Through sylvatic infection (primarily in the ground squirrel), the infection eventually covered much of the Western U.S. (17 states), with the majority of cases occurring in Arizona, California, Colorado, New Mexico, and Oregon. Between 1947 and 1996, 390 cases of plague occurred in the U.S., resulting in 60 (15.4%) deaths. The most common form was bubonic plague (327 [84%] cases resulting in 44 [14%] deaths), followed by primary septicemic plague (49 [13%] cases and 11 [22%] deaths), and primary pneumonic plague (7 [2%] cases and 4 [57%] deaths). Seven cases and 1 death were unclassified.[93]

through licking, scratching, or biting.[404] Between 1977 and 1998, 23 human cases of cat-transmitted plague were reported in Western states, and five of those who were ill died.[183]

Travelers can acquire plague in one area and become ill in another area where plague is not endemic (i.e., peripatetic plague). Although rare, peripatetic plague is more likely to

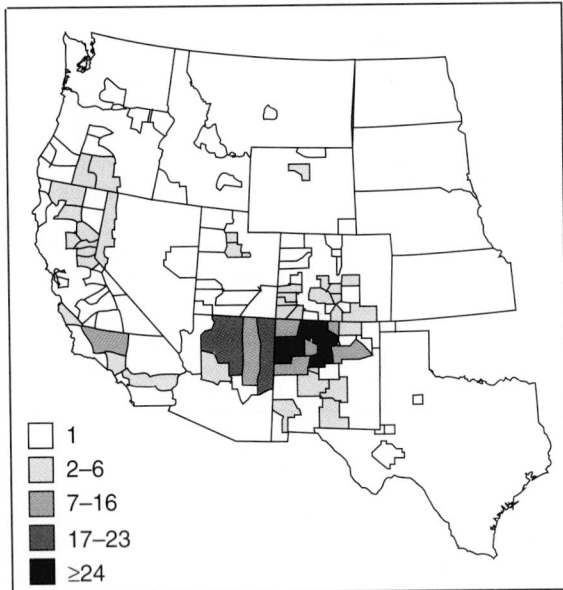

Figure 6-7 Number of plague cases, by county—western United States, 1970–2002.
Source: Centers for Disease Control and Prevention. MMWR 2003;52:725–728.

<table>
<tr><td>□</td><td>1</td></tr>
<tr><td>▨</td><td>2–6</td></tr>
<tr><td>▨</td><td>7–16</td></tr>
<tr><td>▨</td><td>17–23</td></tr>
<tr><td>■</td><td>≥24</td></tr>
</table>

Box 6-14 Epidemiology, Diagnosis, Treatment, and Prevention and Reporting of Plague (*Yersinia pestis*)

Epidemiology

- Plague is usually transmitted to humans by the bite of an infected rodent flea.
- Incubation period is 1–7 days for bubonic plague and 1–4 days for pneumonic plague.
- Case-fatality rate for untreated bubonic plague is ≥50%.
- Domestic pets (i.e., cats and dogs) can carry plague-infected fleas.
- Risks include hunting, trapping, cat ownership, and rural residence in areas where plague is endemic.
- Person-to-person transmission can occur after contact with a suppurating lesion (bubonic plague) or via respiratory droplets (pneumonic plague).
- Naturally acquired plague typically begins as bubonic plague; intentional release (i.e. terrorism) would manifest chiefly as pneumonic plague.

Clinical Findings

- Signs and symptoms include fever, chills, malaise, sore throat, and headache.
- A lymphadenitis (bubo) commonly develops; inguinal lymph nodes are affected in 90% of cases.
- Infection can progress to shock (septicemic plague) and pneumonia (pneumonic plague).

Laboratory Testing

- Bipolar staining, "safety pin" ovoid, gram-negative organisms are suggestive of plague infection.
- Direct fluorescent antibody testing or antigen capture enzyme-linked immunosorbent assay are specific tests.
- Confirmatory testing includes culture or a fourfold or greater change in antibody titer.

Recommended Treatment

- Primary therapy: streptomycin; alternatively, use gentamicin, tetracyclines, or chloramphenicol.
- Mortality from bubonic plague is reduced markedly by appropriate therapy.
- Patients with primary pneumonic plague are not likely to survive if they do not receive adequate therapy within 18 hours after onset of respiratory symptoms.

Prevention and Reporting

- Educate the public about plague symptoms, mode of transmission, and prevention methods.
- Use insect repellents.
- Rodent-proof buildings.
- Avoid handling rodents or camping near rodent burrows.
- Treat dogs and cats with insecticidesw in rural areas where plague is endemic.
- Report plague cases and sick or dead animals to health authorities.

From reference[101].

result in fatal outcomes because of delays in seeking treatment or misdiagnosis in areas where health-care providers might be less familiar with the disease.[101] In the current state of heightened awareness of possible terrorism, peripatetic cases also might be confused with those arising from an intentional release of plague bacteria. (See Box 6-14.)

Clinical Syndromes. Three clinical forms of plague are recognized: bubonic, septicemic, and pneumonic. The septicemic and pneumonic forms are usually secondary to the bubonic form, and the bubonic form is the most common in the U.S. (see Box 6-13). Bubonic plague is characterized by swelling of cervical, axillary, and inguinal lymph nodes, depending on the location of the portal of entry of the bacteria. Hematogenous dissemination of the bacteria to other organs and tissues may cause intravascular coagulation and endotoxic shock, producing dark discoloration in the extremities (Color Plate 6-5*A*; Clinical Correlation Box 6-5).

Laboratory Diagnosis. Laboratory confirmation of all forms of plague is performed either by microbiologic methods or by serologic demonstration of antigen or antibody titers. Our colleagues at the Colorado Department of Health have noted that blood cultures are positive in approximately 80% of patients with bubonic plague and 100% of patients with septicemic plague. Gram stains (Color Plate 6-5*B*) of bubo aspirates show gram-negative rods in about two thirds of cases, and Wright-Giemsa stains (Color Plate 6-5*C*) of peripheral blood smears often reveal the characteristic bipolar staining typical of yersiniae. The colonies are slow growing on ordinary media and are said to have the appearance of beaten copper when viewed under the stereoscope (Color Plate 6-5*D*). The reaction observed on TSI agar in 24 hours is similar to that seen with *Pasteurella* species (i.e., weak acid production on the slant, with little or no change in the butt). A rapid diagnostic test has been developed that uses a simple dipstick test using monoclonal antibodies to detect the F1 antigen, a protein that is specific to *Y. pestis*. The test produces reliable results within 15 minutes and could help control the disease in developing countries and perhaps speed detection and treatment of the infection during a bioterrorist attack.[107]

Infections Caused by *Y. pseudotuberculosis* *Y. pseudotuberculosis* is also endemic in a wide variety of animals, including fowl, and is responsible for mesenteric lymphadenitis, particularly in children in whom a clinical disease simulating appendicitis is manifested.[474] A septicemic form of *Y. pseudotuberculosis* infection occurs rarely and has been described mainly in patients with an underlying disorder, such as hepatic cirrhosis, hemochromatosis, or diabetes, with mortality rates as high as 75% despite antibiotic treatment.[291] Rare cases of urinary tract infection and chronic prostatitis due to *Y. pseudotuberculosis* have also been reported.[123,338] The vehicles and sources of *Y. pseudotuberculosis* infection are unknown. By virtue of its similarity to *Y. enterocolitica*, it has been presumed to be a possible foodborne pathogen, but the evidence for this is limited to a few suggestive outbreaks and two larger outbreaks, one in Canada linked to pasteurized milk[347] and one in Finland due to contaminated iceberg lettuce traced to a farm that used untreated water for spray irrigation of the fields.[348] The major biochemical tests that differentiate *Y. pseudotuberculosis* from *Y. enterocolitica* are ornithine decarboxylase, sucrose, and sorbitol. *Y. pseudotuberculosis* is negative for all three, whereas *Y. enterocolitica* is positive (Table 6-23).

Infections Caused by *Y. enterocolitica* *Y. enterocolitica* is widely distributed in aquatic and animal reservoirs, with swine serving as the major reservoir for human pathogenic strains.[46] It is the most common species of *Yersinia* recovered from clinical specimens. The portal of entry in humans is the oral digestive route, with infection occurring in the terminal ileum that anatomically is adjacent to the appendix. The organism adheres to and penetrates the ileum, causing terminal ileitis, lymphadenitis, and acute enterocolitis, with secondary manifestations of erythema nodosum, polyarthritis,[485] and less commonly, septicemia,[122,175] and endocarditis.[191] Septicemia with *Y. enterocolitica* is almost exclusively associated with patients in iron overload or those being treated with the iron-chelating agent deferoxamine.[46] Iron-loaded patients with β-thalassemia are at greatly increased risk for severe yersiniosis even when their body iron burden (as indicated by the serum ferritin level) is only moderately elevated and they are not receiving iron-chelating therapy.[6] There are six biovars (1A, 1B, 2, 3, 4, and 5) and over 50 serogroups of *Y. enterocolitica;* however, only five, designated 0:1,2a,3; 0:3; 0:5,27; 0:8; and 0:9, are generally considered pathogenic for humans.[37] Biogroup 1A lacks the virulence determinants of invasive isolates and is considered to be nonpathogenic.[46] The remaining biogroups are of human origin and can be divided into biogroup 1B, found mainly in the U.S., and biogroups 2–5, found in Europe and elsewhere. Neubauer et al. have proposed division of *Y. enterocolitica* into two subspecies: *Y. enterocolitica* subsp. *enterocolitica* for biogroup 1B and *Y. enterocolitica* subsp. *palaearctica* for European bioserovars.[344]

Association of* Y. enterocolitica *With Transfusion Reactions. *Y. enterocolitica* was recovered from a unit of donor blood submitted to the University of Illinois Hospital Microbiology Laboratory for culture following a transfusion reaction. Shaking chills and a shocklike syndrome developed in the recipient of a contaminated unit of blood after about 50 mL had been transfused. Similar cases have also been reported elsewhere, illustrating this organism's ability to grow

at cold temperatures.[38,84,92,239,461,465,478] Between November 1985 and November 1996, the CDC reported 21 cases of sepsis associated with receipt of transfused *Y. enterocolitica*-contaminated red cells.[92] Investigation of these cases has led to the conclusion that blood contamination resulted from asymptomatic *Y. enterocolitica* bacteremia in the blood donors at the time of donation. Arduino and colleagues[14] have demonstrated that *Y. enterocolitica*, when inoculated into units of packed erythrocytes and stored at 4°C, can proliferate and produce endotoxin after a lag phase of 2 to 3 weeks. It is clear from these reports that *Y. enterocolitica* should be looked for whenever transfusion-associated bacteremia or endotoxemia is suspected. To learn more, the reader is referred to the review article by Wagner and coauthors.[490]

Association of* Y. enterocolitica *With Household Preparation of Chitterlings. In countries where *Y. enterocolitica* has become an important cause of diarrhea, 0:3 is the predominant serotype, and pigs appear to be the major reservoir for infection.[470] A review of clinical isolates of *Y. enterocolitica* submitted to the Yersinia Reference Laboratory of the CDC from 1970 to 1980 and from 1986 to 1988, showed a shift in the preponderant serotype of *Y. enterocolitica* in the United States from 0:8 to 0:3. This shift coincides with an outbreak of gastroenteritis caused by *Y. enterocolitica* serotype 0:3 in Atlanta from November 1988 to January 1989. The outbreak involved 15 patients (all African American), of which 14 were infants (median age, 3 months). A febrile, diarrheal illness developed in all of them, which was strongly associated with the household preparation of chitterlings (the large intestines of pigs). Although none of the infants had direct contact with the raw chitterlings, in nearly all cases the persons caring for the infants gave a history of cleaning chitterlings.[280] *Y. enterocolitica* was cultured from unopened containers of chitterlings, from the case households as well as from containers of chitterlings purchased from local supermarkets. In 10 of the 12 exposed households, the chitterlings were prepared for a Thanksgiving, Christmas, or New Year's meal. A survey of a grocery store chain in Atlanta revealed that the sale of chitterlings is largely restricted to the period from October through January, and peaks in November. Data from other surveys support the association between chitterling preparation during the Thanksgiving to Christmas holiday period and cases of *Y. enterocolitica* infection and suggest that routine screening for *Y. enterocolitica* is warranted at certain hospitals, particularly in Black communities, and especially for children younger than 1 year of age.[4,102,281,320] Information on the safe preparation of chitterlings is available at http://www.ph.dhr.state.ga.us/epi/news/oct02/103102.shtml.[102]

Recovery of* Y. enterocolitica *From Clinical Specimens. Most strains of *Y. enterocolitica* will grow on selective enteric agars and will appear as small, lactose-negative colonies on MacConkey and SS agars in 48 hours. In some laboratories, plates of MacConkey agar inoculated with stool specimens suspected of harboring *Yersinia* species are routinely incubated at room temperature. *Y. enterocolitica*, in particular, can best be recovered from stool specimens that are incubated at 25°C. Cold enrichment of highly contaminated specimens, such as feces, by incubating cultures at 4°C for 1 to 3 weeks in phosphate-buffered saline before subculture onto enteric media, also enhances the recovery of

Y. enterocolitica.[374] Weissfeld and Sonnenwirth[500] reported that pretreatment of stool with 0.5% potassium hydroxide at a ratio of 1:2 for 2 minutes, followed by plating onto enteric agar, resulted in the recovery of the highest number of *Yersinia* isolates. The superiority of cefsulodin–irga-san–novobiocin (CIN) agar for recovery of *Y. enterocolitica* from stool suspensions containing 10^2 colony-forming units or fewer has been reported by Head and colleagues.[215] The use of cold-enrichment methods and specialized culture media, such as CIN agar, for the recovery of *Yersinia* is usually not required because, in cases of enterocolitis, the organisms are usually found in relatively high concentrations. The use of EMB agar is not recommended because *Y. enterocolitica* is sucrose-positive and will appear as a coli-form on this medium. A similar problem may also be encountered with the use of TSI, which also contains sucrose.

Identification of Y. enterocolitica. *Y. enterocolitica* is more biochemically reactive at room temperature than at 37°C. It has been our experience at the University of Illinois Hospital that isolates of *Y. enterocolitica* generally do not give an acceptable identification when set up on the Vitek system or the API 20E at an incubation temperature of 37°C. However, API 20E strips incubated at room temperature do provide an acceptable identification. This finding has been confirmed in recent published reports.[13,446] Neubauer and colleagues compared the API 20E, API Rapid 32 IDE, and PCR-based tests and found that the API 20E provided the highest sensitivity at both the genus and species level.[345] A later study by the same group found that the Vitek GNI card identified Yersinia with 96.3% accuracy to the genus level and 57.4% accuracy to the species level.[287] Although anti-sera that can actually be used to serotype strains of *Y. enterocolitica* are not readily available, Farmer and colleagues have described four simple tests that can be used to screen for pathogenic serotypes. These tests include the pyrazinami-dase test, salicin fermentation–esculin hydrolysis, D-xylose fermentation, and Congo red–magnesium oxalate (CR-MOX) agar used to determine Congo red dye uptake and calcium-dependent growth at 36°C.[164]

Antibiotic Susceptibility of Y. enterocolitica. *Y. ente-rocolitica* serogroups 0:3 and 0:9 are able to produce two chromosomally mediated β-lactamases, resulting in resistance to ampicillin, cephalothin, and carbenicillin. Serotype 0:8 strains are susceptible to ampicillin and variable for car-benicillin and cephalosporins. In vitro testing is not reliable, and the administration of broad-spectrum cephalosporins in combination with an aminoglycoside appears effective for most extraintestinal infections, including septicemia.[189] Flu-oroquinolones, alone or with aminoglycosides or extended-spectrum cephalosporins, also appear effective.[189,439] Tri-methoprim-sulfamethoxazole shows in vitro efficacy but has little effect on the clinical course (duration) of *Y. enterocoli-tica* gastroenteritis.[4,373]

Other *Yersinia* Species *Y. frederiksenii* is most commonly recovered from fresh water, foods, and nonirrigated soil and has only infrequently been recovered from human specimens. This organism can be recovered from stool specimens using MacConkey or SS agars incubated at 25°C for 48 hours, and cold-enrichment techniques are rarely required. *Y. frederiksenii* is believed to be part of the commensal flora and does not cause diarrhea. Farmer and coworkers[165] cite

a few human isolates, referred to the CDC, that were obtained from wound and respiratory samples.

Y. intermedia may also be recovered by cold enrichment from human fecal specimens, but it is probably not related to intestinal disease. Bottone[45] reviewed the medical literature to 1976, noting 21 case histories of extraintestinal infections with these atypical rhamnose-positive species. Of these cases, eight were from conjunctivitis and three were from urinary tract infections. Bottone added three more cases, representing urinary tract, conjunctival, and auxiliary abscess infections.

Farmer and coworkers[165] cite six specimens received at the CDC from which *Y. kristensenii* was recovered: four from stools, one from blood, and one from urine. Its pathogenic role has not yet been determined. Four additional new species of *Yersinia* have been described that are all biochemically similar to *Y. enterocolitica*. All are very rare human isolates. *Y. rohdei* has been isolated from dog feces, water, and human feces.[11] *Y. aldovae* (formerly *Y. enterocolitica*-like group X2) has been found in surface water, drinking water, and fish.[33] *Y. mollaretii* (formerly *Y. enterocolitica* biogroup 3A) has been isolated from human feces, drinking water, meat, and raw vegetables.[496] *Y. bercovieri* (formerly *Y. enterocolitica* biogroup 3B) has been reported from human feces, water, soil, and vegetables.[496]

TRIBE *ERWINIEAE*

The *Erwinieae* are primarily pathogens in plants and only saprophytic in humans. The species of the genus *Erwinia* may be divided into three phylogenetic groups. Cluster I represents the true erwinias and comprises *E. amylovora, E. mallotivora, E. persicinus, E. psidii. E. rhapontici,* and *E. tracheiphila.* The species of cluster II have been transferred to the genus *Pectobacterium* as *P. carotovorum* subsp. *atro-septicum, P. carotovorum* subsp. *betavasculorum, P. caroto-vorum* subsp. *carotovorum, P. carotovorum* subsp. *odori-ferum, P. carotovorum* subsp. *wasabiae, P. cacticidum, P. chrysanthemi,* and *P. cypripedii.* The members of cluster III have been classified in a new genus *Brenneria* as *B. alni, B. nigrifluens, B. paradisiaca, B. quercina, B. rubrifaciens,* and *B. salicis.*[213] *Erwinia, Pectobacterium,* and *Brenneria* species cause wilt and rotting diseases on plants, food crops, and trees or are part of the epiphytic flora. There has been one report of a urinary tract infection in an 88-year-old woman caused by *Erwinia persicinus,* which previously had been isolated only from a variety of fruits and vegetables.[362] Recently, a new phytopathogenic species isolated from diseased Erythrina trees was determined to be sufficiently different from *Erwinia, Brenneria,* and *Pectobacterium* to warrant placement in a new genus and has been designated *Samsonia erythrinae.*[466]

Miscellaneous New Genera of *Enterobacteriaceae*

Table 6-24 is a listing of the more recently described and less common species of *Enterobacteriaceae*. New genus and species designations have evolved from DNA hybridization studies and biochemical characterizations performed on atypical strains referred to the CDC and other reference laboratories for identification and classification. Many of these

Table 6-24 New Genera and Species in the Family *Enterobacteriaceae*

NEW DESIGNATION	PREVIOUS DESIGNATION	COMMENTS
Arsenophonus nasoniae	New species	Not isolated from humans. Cause of the sun-killer trait in the parasitic wasp, *Nasonia vitripennis*
Budvicia aquatica	"HG Group"	H_2S (+). Frequently found in drinking and surface water. Has been isolated from human feces, but is not associated with human disease
Buttiauxella agrestis	"Group F"	Biochemically closest to *Kluyvera*. Key reactions are IMViC (−,+,−,+), LAO (−,−,+), Sucrose (−). Isolated from water. No human isolates reported.
Buttiauxella brennerae	New species	Isolated from mollusks, water, soil, and humans
Buttiauxella ferragutiae	"Group F" Enteric group 63	Isolated from water and soil
Buttiauxella gaviniae	"Group F" Enteric group 64	Isolated from mollusks
Buttiauxella izardii	New species	Isolated from mollusks
Buttiauxella noackiae	Enteric group 59	Like *Pantoea agglomerans* except arginine-positive. Isolated from mollusks, human sputum and wounds, and food
Buttiauxella warmboldiae	New species	Isolated from snails
Cedecea davisae	"Enteric group 15–Davis subgroup"	*Cedecea* resemble *Serratia* because they are lipase (+), and resistant to colistin and cephalothin, but unlike *Serratia* are gelatin and DNase (−). *C. davisae* is most common species. Sputum is the most common source.
Cedecea lapagei		Isolated from human respiratory tract specimens.
Cedecea neteri	"*Cedecea* species 4" "*Cedecea* sp strain 002"	Isolated from blood cultures of patient with valvular heart disease.
Cedecea sp. 3	"*Cedecea* sp. strain 001"	Isolated from sputum and heart blood at autopsy.
Cedecea sp. 5	"*Cedecea* sp. strain 012"	Toe wound.
Cedecea sp. 6		
Ewingella americana	Enteric group 40	IMViC (−,+,+,+), LAO (−,−,−). Strains may formerly have been classified as *Enterobacter agglomerans* but differ by being arabinose (−). Isolated from sputum, wounds, and blood cultures.
Kluyvera ascorbata	Enteric group 8	Looks like *E. coli* except malonate, esculin, and citrate (+). Dark purple pigment on non-blood-containing media. Most common source is sputum followed by urine, stool, and blood.
Kluyvera cochleae	New species	Isolated from mollusks
Kluyvera cryocrescens	Enteric group 8	Similar to *K. ascorbata* except grows and ferments glucose at 5 °C.

(Continued)

Table 6-24 *Continued*

NEW DESIGNATION	PREVIOUS DESIGNATION	COMMENTS
Kluyvera georgiana	Enteric group 8 *Kluyvera* sp. group 3	Isolated from human sputum and throat
Leclercia adecarboxylata	Enteric group 41 *Escherichia adecarboxylata* *Enterobacter agglomerans* HG XI	IMViC (+,+,−,−), LAO (−,−,−). Yellow-pigmented. Resembles *E. coli* on MacConkey and EMB agars. Isolated from a variety of clinical specimens, food, water, and the environment.
Leminorella grimontii	Enteric group 57	H₂S (+), TDA (−), LAO (−,−,−), IMViC (−,+,−,+). Isolated from human feces and urine.
Leminorella richardii *Leminorella* species 3	Enteric group 57 Enteric group 57	Same as *L. grimontii* except for IMViC (−,−,−,−).
Moellerella wisconsensis	Enteric group 46	Looks like *E. coli* on enteric media. IMViC (−,+,−,+), LAO (−,−,−), lactose and sucrose (+). Originally isolated from stool cultures in Wisconsin.
Obesumbacterium proteus biogroup 2	*Flavobacterium proteus*	No human isolates reported. Common brewery contaminant. Grows slowly when incubated at 36°C, making it difficult to identify.
Photorhabdus luminescens subsp. *luminescens* *Photorhabdus luminescens* subsp. *akhurstii* *Photorhabdus luminescens* subsp. *laumondii* *Photorhabdus temperata* subsp. *temperata* *Photorhabdus asymbiotica*	*Xenorhabdus luminescens* New subspecies New subspecies New species and subspecies New species	Bioluminescent and biochemically inactive. Optimal growth at 25°C. All human clinical isolates belong to *P. asymbiotica*. Colonies are yellow-pigmented, produce an unusual hemolytic reaction and are negative for nitrate reduction. Isolates have been from human wounds and blood.
Pragia fontium		H₂S (+), biochemically similar to *Budvicia*. Most strains from drinking water in Czechoslovakia.
Rahnella aquatilis *Rahnella* species 2 *Rahnella* species 3	Group H2	LAO (−,−,−), nonmotile at 36°C, but motile at 25°C, PAD (weakly +), no yellow pigment. May have been identified as *E. agglomerans* in past. Isolates have been from water, foods, and various human sources.
Tatumella ptyseos	Group EF-9	Pinpoint colonies, slow-growing, relatively inert. Motile at 25°C, but nonmotile at 35°C. Flagella are polar, lateral, or subpolar rather than peritrichous. Large zones of inhibition are formed around disks containing penicillin (10 U). PAD very slow (weakly +). Isolated from human clinical specimens particularly sputum.
Trabulsiella guamensis	Enteric group 90	H₂S (+) and biochemically similar to *Salmonella*. IMViC (−,+,−,+), lysine (+) arginine (50% +), ornithine (+). Isolates have been from soil and human feces. No evidence that it causes diarrhea.

Table 6-24 *Continued*

NEW DESIGNATION	PREVIOUS DESIGNATION	COMMENTS
Xenorhabdus beddingii	*Xenorhabdus nematophilus* subsp. *beddingii*	
Xenorhabdus bovienii	*Xenorhabdus nematophilus* subsp. *bovienii*	
Xenorhabdus japonicus		
Xenorhabdus nematophilus	*Achromobacter nematophilus*	Has been isolated only from nematodes.
Xenorhabdus poinarii	*Xenorhabdus nematophilus* subsp. *poinarii*	
Yokenella regensburgei	*Koserella trabulsii*	Biochemically similar to *Hafnia alvei*. Differs by being colistin resistant and VP (−). Isolated from blood, wounds, throat, sputum, feces, and water.
	Enteric group 45	
	Japanese NIH biogroup 9 Atypical *Hafnia*	
	Hafnia species 3	
Enteric group 58		Clinical isolates have been from wounds and feces.
Enteric group 60		Biochemically inactive. Recovered from urine and sputum.
Enteric group 68		DNase (+) but otherwise biochemically different from *Serratia*. Clinical isolates have been from urines.
Enteric group 137		Closely related to *Citrobacter farmeri* and *Citrobacter amalonaticus*. Isolated from sputum, urine and wounds.[492]

IMViC, indole, methyl red, Voges-Proskauer, citrate; LAO, lysine, arginine, ornithine; MIO, motility, indole, ornithine; PAD, phenylalanine deaminase; HG, hybridization group; +, >90% of strains positive; −, >90% of strains negative; V, variable.

new genus names have been applied to bacterial strains that, at one time, were designated atypical enteric groups at the CDC. Several enteric groups remain unnamed but will probably achieve genus status in the future when a sufficient number of strains are gathered.

IDENTIFICATION CHARACTERISTICS OF NEWER *ENTEROBACTERIACEAE*

The key identifying characteristics of several of the new genera are listed in Table 6-25. Learning the new genera need not be overly difficult if one remembers that most of these bacteria represent atypical strains closely related to well-established groups. For example, the closely related genera *Buttiauxella*[173] and *Kluyvera*[167] will phenotypically present as "citrate-positive *E. coli*"; the specific characteristics by which they can be differentiated are included in Table 6-25. Bacteria belonging to *Cedecea*[170,206] resemble *Serratia* because they are lipase-positive and are resistant to cephalothin and colistin; however, unlike *Serratia*, they do not hydrolyze gelatin or DNA. *Ewingella*,[205] *Rahnella*,[237] and *Tatumella*,[225] will initially be grouped with *Pantoea agglomerans* because they are lysine-, ornithine-, and arginine decarboxylase-negative. The genera *Yokenella*[277] and *Obesumbacterium*[407] are similar to *Hafnia alvei*; *Moeller-*

ella[222] can be considered phenylalanine-negative, lactose-positive *Providencia;* and *Leminorella*[223] can be thought of as phenylalanine- and urease-negative *Proteus* species. By using this orientation, identification is made somewhat easier.

The reaction patterns of these new genera and species have been incorporated into the numerical code files of most computer-assisted identification systems. Thus, the names of these genera and species may appear in the computer-generated reports of many commercial systems. In these instances, it may be necessary to visually check the individual reactions for accuracy and assess additional characteristics using Table 6-25 or the expanded tables published by the CDC and reproduced here in Table 6-7. Careful correlation of the biochemical activity with the growth patterns and appearance of colonies on agar media is usually enough to make accurate identifications. It cannot be overemphasized that students and microbiologists must retain a fundamental orientation to the morphology, physiology, and biochemistry of bacteria if accurate identifications are to be made.

CLINICAL SIGNIFICANCE OF NEWER *ENTEROBACTERIACEAE*

The seemingly endless reclassification and changes in bacterial taxonomy and the frequent addition of new genera

Table 6-25 Differentiating Characteristics of New *Enterobacteriaceae*

GENUS	GENUS CHARACTERISTICS	SPECIES AND DIFFERENTIATING CHARACTERISTICS

Buttiauxella
Ferragut[173]
(*Group F, Gavini*
1976)

Genus characteristics		*B. AGRESTIS*	*KLUYVERA ASCORBATA*	*KLUYVERA CRYOCRESCENS*
Indole –	Indole	–	+	+
MR/VP +/–	Lysine	–	+	V (23)
Citrate +	Ascorbate	–	+	–
Lysine –	Glucose (5°C)	+	–	+
Arginine –	Sucrose	–	+	+
Ornithine +				
Sucrose –				

Cedecea
Grimont[206]
(Enteric group 15)

Genus characteristics		*C. DAVISAE*	*C. LAPAGEI*	*C. NETERI*	*SPEC 3*	*SPEC 5*
ONPG +	Ornithine	+	–	–	–	V (50)
MRVP + V (50–80)	Sucrose	+	–	+	V (50)	+
Citrate +	Sorbitol	–	–	+	–	+
Esculin +	Raffinose	–	–	–	+	+
Lipase (corn oil) +	Xylose	+	–	+	+	+
DNAse –	Melibiose	–	–	–	+	+
Gelatin –	Malonate	+	+	+	–	–
Colistin R						
Cephalothin R						

Ewingella
Grimont[205]
(Enteric group 40)

Genus characteristics		*E. AMERICANA*	*P. AGGLOMERANS*
Indole –	Arabinose	–	+
MR/VP +/+	Xylose	V (15)	+
Citrate +	Yellow pigment	–	V (75)
Lysine –			
Arginine –			
Ornithine –			

Kluyvera
Farmer[167]
(Enteric group 8)

Genus characteristics		*K. ASCORBATA*	*K. CRYOCRESCENS*
Indole +	Ascorbate	+	–
MR/VP +/–	Glucose (5°C)	–	+
Citrate +	Lysine	+	V (23)
Malonate +			
Esculin +			

Table 6-25 *Continued*

GENUS	GENUS CHARACTERISTICS	SPECIES AND DIFFERENTIATING CHARACTERISTICS

			L. ADECARBOXYLATA	*E. COLI*	*P. AGGLOMERANS*
Leclercia Tamura et al.[467] (*Escherichia* *adecarboxylata,* Enteric group 41)	Indole + MR/VP +/− Citrate − Lysine − Arginine − Ornithine −	Lysine Adonitol Malonate Yellow pigment	− + + +	+ − − −	− − V +

			L. GRIMONTII	*L. RICHARDII*	*PROTEUS SPECIES*
Leminorella Hickman-Brenner[223] (Enteric group 57)	H₂S+ Phenylalanine − Mannose − Arabinose + Xylose + L/A/O −/−/−	Methyl red Citrate Dulcitol Phenylalanine Urease Arabinose	+ + V (83) − − +	− − − − − +	+ −/V (15–65) − + + −

			M. WISCONSENSIS	*PROVIDENCIA SPECIES*
Moellerella Hickman-Brenner[222] (enteric group 46)	Indole − MR/VP +/− Citrate + Lysine − Arginine − Ornithine − Phenylalanine − Colistin R	Phenylalanine Lactose Sucrose ONPG Tyrosine	− + + + −	+ − V (15–50) − +

			O. PROTEUS 2	*HAFNIA ALVEI*	*H. ALVEI 1*
Obesumbacterium Priest[407]	Indole − MR/VP V (15)/− Citrate − Lysine + Ornithine + Motility −	Mannitol Salicin Arabinose	− − −	+ V (13) +	V (55) V (55) −

(Continued)

Table 6-25 *Continued*

GENUS	GENUS CHARACTERISTICS	SPECIES AND DIFFERENTIATING CHARACTERISTICS

Rahnella
Izard et al.[237]
("Group H2")

GENUS CHARACTERISTICS:
Indole −
MR/VP +/+
Citrate +
Urea −
Phenylalanine + wk
L/A/O −/−/−
Motility − (36°C)/+ (25°C)

	R. AQUATILIS	P. AGGLOMERANS
Motility (36°C)	−	+
Phenylalanine	+	V (20)
Yellow-pigmented	−	V (75)

Tatumella
Hollis[225]
(Biogroup EF-9)

GENUS CHARACTERISTICS:
Indole −
MR/VP −/−/(+ Coblentz)
L/A/O −/−/−
Phenylalanine + wk
Sucrose +
Gelatin −

	T. PTYSEOS	P. AGGLOMERANS
Mannitol	−	+
Phenylalanine	+	V (20)
Motility (36°C)	−	+
Penicillin	S	R

Trabulsiella
McWhorter et al.[314]
(Enteric group 90)

GENUS CHARACTERISTICS:
H$_2$S +
Indole V (40)
MR/VP +/−
Citrate +
Lysine +
Arginine V (50)
Ornithine +
KCN +

	T. GUAMENSIS	SALMONELLA SUBGROUP 4	SALMONELLA SUBGROUP 5
Dulcitol	−	−	+
Lactose	−	−	−
ONPG	+	−	+
Malonate	−	−	−
Growth KCN	+	+	+
Mucate Ferm	+	−	V (85)
D-Sorbitol	+	+	+

Yokenella
Kosako et al.[277]
(*Koserella trabulsii*)
Enteric group 45

GENUS CHARACTERISTICS:
Indole −
MR/VP +/−
Citrate +
Lysine +
Ornithine +
Cellobiose +
Melibiose +

	Y. REGENSBURGEI	H. ALVEI
VP	−	+
Citrate	+	−
Melibiose	+	−
Colistin R	+	−

and species might be discouraging for microbiology students and instructors alike. However, Farmer and associates conducted a study of scores of unclassified biogroups submitted for identification at the CDC and have brought order out of disarray in a landmark report that summarizes all of the old and new genera of *Enterobacteriaceae* known as of January 1985.[165] As these investigators point out, up to 95% of all *Enterobacteriaceae* recovered in clinical laboratories are *Escherichia coli, Klebsiella pneumoniae,* and *Proteus mirabilis;* over 99% of the isolates belong to only 23 species, leaving less than 1% as the incidence of recovery for the several newly designated species. Thus, the bacteria listed in Table 6-24 are rarely encountered in most clinical laboratories; however, as Dr. Farmer has also stated, there are at least three reasons why these new species of *Enterobacteriaceae* are important to clinical microbiologists: 1) Some species cause serious human infections; 2) others occur in clinical specimens, but their causative role in disease is uncertain; and 3) many are biochemically similar to well-established species and thus can cause problems in identification. The clinical significance of the newer species that have been recovered from human clinical specimens is summarized as follows:

The genus *Buttiauxella* now contains seven species (see Table 6-24) that occur frequently and abundantly in the intestines of snails, slugs, and other mollusks.[333] A few strains have been isolated from unpolluted soil and drinking water, surface water, sewage, soil, and fecal samples, but have not been isolated from primary sterile clinical specimens.[333] Two clinical isolates of *B. gaviniae*-like organisms have been reported from urine and leg wound specimens in Belgium. The isolates were biochemically indistinguishable from *B. gaviniae* but 16S rRNA gene sequencing was indecisive.[130]

Cedecea has been isolated from respiratory specimens,[23] blood,[170,304,386] a scrotal abscess,[22] cutaneous ulcer,[211] and lung tissue.[120] In most cases, however, an etiologic role for *Cedecea* in these infections was not proved.

Ewingella americana was described in 1983 and named in honor of the American bacteriologist, William Ewing.[205] The original strains were from human clinical specimens, including sputum, blood, throat, toe and thumb wounds, urine, and stool.[165,205] *E. americana* has been implicated in bacteremia,[135,393] catheter-related bacteremia,[301] an outbreak of nosocomial bacteremia,[392] and an outbreak of pseudobacteremia associated with nonsterile blood collection tubes.[311–313] It has also been associated with wound colonization,[31] conjunctivitis,[216] and peritonitis in a patient undergoing peritoneal dialysis.[258]

The genus *Kluyvera* presently contains four species (see Table 6-24).[333] The original isolates of *Kluyvera* species were from human clinical specimens and the environment. The most common human sources have been sputum, followed by urine, stool, throat, and blood.[167] Environmental sources noted have been sewage, soil, kitchen food, water, milk, and a hospital sink.[167] There are only a few reports of serious infections with *Kluyvera* species that involved the urinary tract,[479] the gallbladder,[475] the gastrointestinal tract,[7,160] and soft tissue of the forearm following a cut from a garbage can.[296] In addition, cases of catheter-related bacteremia[509] and mediastinitis and bacteremia following open-heart surgery[448] have been reported.

The clinical significance of *Leclercia adecarboxylata* is uncertain, but human isolates from blood, sputum, urine, stool, and wounds have been reported.[129,292,310,371,423,467,473] At the University of Illinois Hospital, *L. adecarboxylata* was found colonizing the endotrachea of a neonate and in a cystoscopic urine specimen from a patient in renal failure. In both cases, the organism was isolated along with other pathogen species; therefore, an etiologic role could not be established. In a third patient, *L. adecarboxylata* was recovered in pure culture from the blood of a patient in chronic renal failure receiving hemodialysis.

Leminorella has been isolated primarily from stool and urine.[223] Blekher and associates[39] reviewed the medical records of 14 patients from which *Leminorella* spp. were isolated and classified 43% of the cases as definite pathogens, 29% as probable pathogens, and 21% as possible pathogens. Clinical syndromes included urinary tract infections (six patients), surgical site infection (three), and primary bacteremia, peritonitis, respiratory tract infection, and soft tissue infection in one patient each. In one case of asymptomatic bacteriuria, the isolate had no clinical significance.[39] *Leminorella* spp. appear as lactose-negative colonies on primary plating media and gives an alkaline slant and a weak acid reaction with H_2S in the butt of TSI after 48 hours. Similar to *Proteus, Leminorella* species are H_2S-positive, D-mannose-negative, and tyrosine-positive, but unlike *Proteus,* they are urea- and phenylalanine-negative and L-arabinose-positive.

Moellerella wisconsensis was originally found in human stool samples, mainly from the state of Wisconsin.[222] It has also been isolated from water and animals and from clinical specimens other than stool, such as the gallbladder[353,507] and a bronchial aspirate.[491] However, the majority of isolates have been from human feces, and there is evidence that *M. wisconsensis* is associated with human diarrhea.[244] On MacConkey agar, colonies appear bright red with precipitated bile around them; thus, they are indistinguishable from *E. coli* colonies.[222] Stock and colleagues report that *M. wisconsensis* is naturally sensitive to doxycycline, minocycline, all aminoglycosides, numerous beta-lactams, all fluoroquinolones, folate-pathway inhibitors, chloramphenicol, and nitrofurantoin.[463]

Photorhabdus species are the only terrestrial bioluminescent bacteria (bacterial bioluminescence is seen primarily in marine species). The classification within the genus is complex, with three currently recognized species: *P. luminescens* (formerly, *Xenorhabdus luminescens*), *P. temperata,* and *P. asymbiotica.*[42,174] Several subspecies are recognized (Table 6-24). *Photorhabdus* spp. inhabit the gut of some insect-pathogenic nematodes, where they form a symbiotic relationship. Nematode species of this type are able to invade the larvae of susceptible insects and release *Photorhabdus* spp. The bacteria proliferate and kill the insect larvae.[190] Insect-pathogenic nematodes harboring *Photorhabdus* spp. are used as biopesticides in a number of countries, including the United States and Australia. A total of 12 human infections with *Photorhabdus* spp. have been reported from the U.S. and Australia, most often causing skin and soft-tissue infections and rarely bacteremia.[168,190,382] Colonies are formed on BAP after 24–48 hours at both 35°C and at room temperature, with a tendency to "swarm."[190] The defining characteristic is the presence of faint luminescence, which can be seen with the naked eye under conditions of total darkness. Gerrard and colleagues have observed that it is critical to allow the observer's eyes to adjust to the darkness for 10 minutes.[190] *Photorhabdus* spp. do not currently appear in the databases for either the MicroScan Rapid or overnight panels, or the Vitek GNI+ cards, which leads to misidentifications when using these systems.[190]

The genus *Rahnella* consists of three closely related species, *R. aquatilis* and two genomospecies that cannot be phenotypically differentiated from *R. aquatilis* and therefore are given the vernacular names *Rahnella* genomospecies 2 and *Rahnella* genomospecies 3.[55] The natural habitat of *Rahnella aquatilis*, as its name implies, is water, and most isolates in the original CDC collection were from water, except two isolates from humans (one from a burn wound and the other from the bronchial washing of a patient with HIV).[212] Of the few case reports of *R. aquatilis* in the literature, most describe infections in immunocompromised patients. In addition to the CDC isolates, others have reported the isolation of this organism from sputum (in a patient with chronic lymphocytic leukemia and emphysema),[114] the urinary tract (in a patient with a renal transplant),[9] from a surgical wound possibly due to a nosocomial source,[305] and from blood of immunocompromised[66,68,182,199,228] and immunocompetent[106] patients. *R. aquatilis* has also been isolated from vegetables (primarily carrots) purchased in supermarkets[209] and has been identified as the causative agent of a smoky/phenolic odor (due to the formation of guaiacol) in spoiled, refrigerated chocolate milk.[251]

Of the original strains of *Tatumella ptyseos* studied at the CDC, 30 were from sputum, 6 from throat cultures, 3 from blood, and 1 each from a tracheal aspirate, a feeding tube, a pharynx, a stool, and urine.[225] One case of *T. ptyseos* obtained from the blood culture of a neonate with presumed sepsis has been reported.[468] There are three striking differences between *T. ptyseos* and other members of the *Enterobacteriaceae*: 1) strains produce a large zone of inhibition around penicillin; 2) it has a tendency to die on some laboratory media, such as blood agar, within 7 days; and 3) usually only one flagellum (either polar, subpolar, or lateral) is observed per cell.[225]

Trabulsiella guamensis, formerly known as enteric group 90, is H_2S-positive and biochemically resembles *Salmonella* subgroups 4 and 5.[314] Strains have been isolated from vacuum cleaner dust, soil, and human feces; however, there is no evidence that it causes diarrhea. Its main interest to clinical microbiologist may be its possible misidentification as a strain of *Salmonella* (see Table 6-25).

Yokenella regensburgei was originally identified as NIH biogroup 9 by the National Institutes of Health in Japan[277] and later found to be identical to "*Koserella trabulsii*" (enteric group 45) named by workers from the CDC.[221,275] Since the name *Y. regensburgei* has priority over "*K trabulsii*" by virtue of prior publication, the use of the later name has been discontinued. In the original reports, *Y. regensburgei* had been recovered from the intestinal tracts of insects and well water, as well as human clinical specimens, including wounds of the limbs, the upper respiratory tract, urine, feces, and knee fluid.[221,277] More recently, Abbott and Janda

have reported the recovery of *Y. regensburgei* from the blood of a patient with a transient bacteremia and from a knee wound of a patient with a diagnosis of septic knee.[2] The organism most closely resembles *H. alvei*, from which it must be differentiated (see Table 6-25).

Quick Screening Methods for Rapid Identification

Escherichia coli, the bacterial isolate most frequently recovered in clinical laboratories, is often presumptively identified if an oxidase-negative, lactose-fermenting, dry colony on MacConkey agar gives a positive spot indole reaction (when tested on a colony growing on noninhibitory media, such as blood agar), particularly if the organism has been recovered in pure culture.[26] The spot indole test is also used in many laboratories for rapid speciation of swarming *Proteus* from primary isolation plates.[27] A rapid (2-minute) spot urease test has been described by Qadri and colleagues.[408] This test might be used to separate possible stool pathogens that require further biochemical testing from the nonpathogenic *Proteus–Providencia–Morganella* group. Taylor and Achanzar have reported using the catalase test (with 3% H_2O_2) as an aid in the identification of *Enterobacteriaceae*.[472] They observed vigorous catalase reactions with *Serratia, Proteus,* and *Providencia;* moderate reactions with *Salmonella, Enterobacter, Klebsiella,* and rare *Escherichia;* and weak reactions with *Shigella* and most *Escherichia.* They report using the rapid catalase test for screening suspicious colonies on enteric media that mimic stool pathogens. Colonies of *Serratia, Proteus, Providencia,* or *Pseudomonas* are quickly eliminated by vigorous catalase reactions, in contrast with salmonellae, which give weak to moderate reactions, or shigellae, which are negative and, therefore, are flagged for further workup. Chester and Moskowitz[111] have reported on the catalase activity of many of the newer members of the *Enterobacteriaceae* and further advocate the use of catalase activity as a rapid supplemental test. Mulczyk and Szewczuk[332] suggested that the test for L-pyrrolidonyl peptidase (PYR) is of great value in differentiating between *Salmonella* and *Citrobacter freundii* complex strains. Other authors have also noted the value of using the PYR test for separating *Salmonella* and *E. coli* strains (both negative from *Citrobacter* spp. (PYR+).[105,234] York and colleagues[512] have proposed an algorithm for rapid identification of *E. coli* based on spot tests for oxidase, indole, and PYR and observation of lactose fermentation on MacConkey or EMB and presence or absences of β-hemolysis on BAP (Fig. 6-8). Their algorithm permitted identification of the majority of suspected *E. coli* strains with an accuracy of greater than 99% and a 75% reduction in cost of reagents and technologist time, as well as a decrease in the time to reporting. Clearly, any of these approaches has validity in an era of cost-containment and the desire to receive test results quickly.

Commercial Screening Kits

Several commercial companies have marketed rapid detection kits for the identification of *E. coli*: E.COLI SCREEN, MUG Disk, and BactiCard *E. coli* (Remel, Lenexa, KS); Lyfo-Kwik OMI (MicroBioLogics, St. Cloud, MN); and ColiScreen (Hardy Diagnostics, Santa Maria CA).

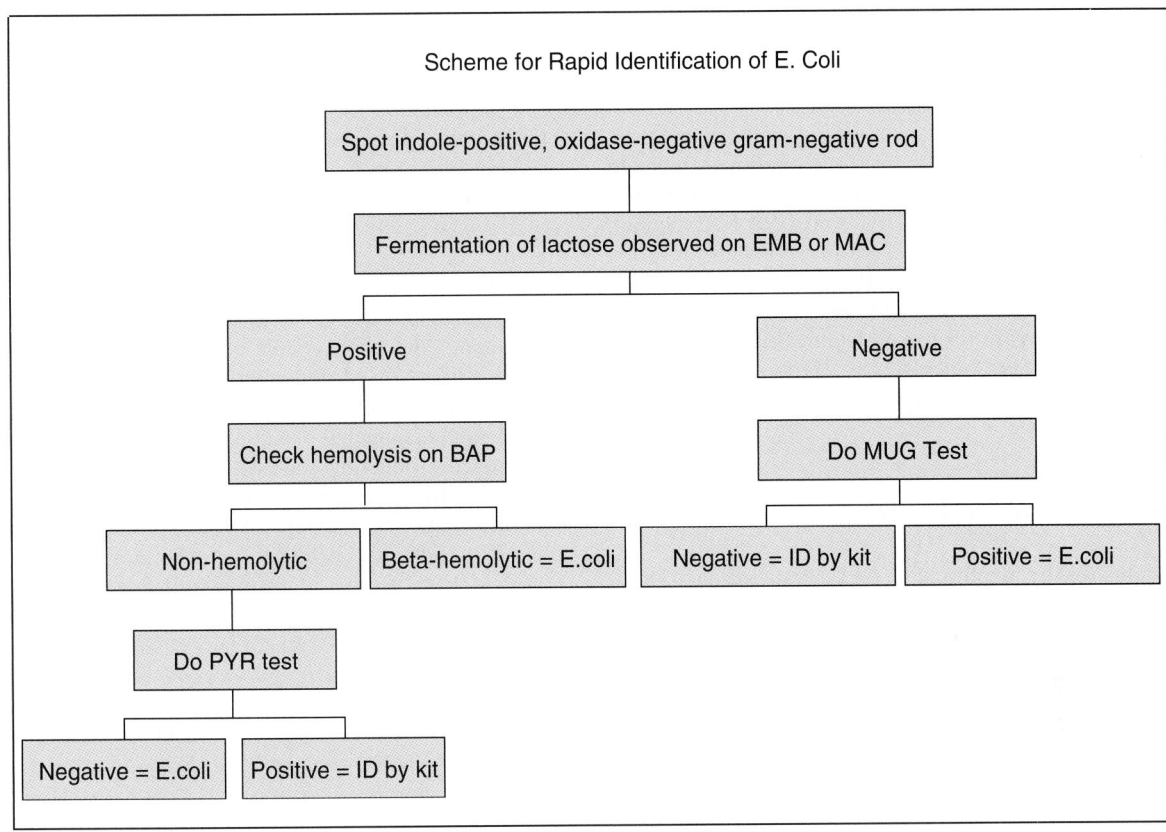

Figure 6-8 Identification scheme for the separation of *E. coli* from other indole-positive, oxidase-negative rods. BAP, blood agar plate; EMB, eosin-methylene blue; MAC, MacConkey agar; MUG, 4-methylumbelliferyl-β-D-glucuronide; PYR, L-pyrrolidonyl-β-naphthylamide; ID, identification. (Modified from York MK, et al. J Clin Microbiol 2000;38:3394–3398.)[512]

These test systems are based on the finding that the majority of strains of *E. coli* are rapidly indole-, ONPG-, and MUG (4-methylumbelliferyl-β-D-glucuronide)-positive.[147,265] The hydrolysis of MUG releases 4-methylumbelliferone, which is highly fluorescent when viewed under long-wave UV light. An interesting use of the MUG test is to screen isolates of *E. coli* for the detection of serotype O157:H7 strains, which are the Shiga-like, toxin-producing strains associated with hemorrhagic colitis. This specific serotype is both sorbitol- and MUG-negative.

Also available is the RapID SS/u System (Remel), consisting of a set of 12 single-substrate chromogenic tests selected to identify rapidly the bacteria most commonly encountered in urinary tract infections (*E. coli, Proteus* species, *Klebsiella* species, *Serratia* species, *Enterobacter* species, *Pseudomonas* species, coagulase-negative staphylococci, enterococci, and others). Answers are available in 30 minutes to 2 hours, depending on the system used and the biochemical activity of the strain being tested. Another system called OMP and NGP Wee-Tabs (KEY Scientific Products, Round Rock, TX) consists of two substrate tablets that together provide eight enzymatic tests, which, combined with urease, will identify approximately 95% of the *Enterobacteriaceae*. The tablets are rehydrated in a bacterial suspension, with results available in 2 to 4 hours. Hardy Diagnostics (Santa Maria, CA) offers the EnteroScreen4, which

is a single tube screening system for use in screening stools for *Salmonella* and *Shigella* species. This system detects lysine deaminase, lysine decarboxylase, H₂S, and urea in a single inoculation one-tube configuration.

Chromogenic Agar Media

Chromogenic agar contains artificial substrates (chromogens) that when hydrolyzed by specific microbial enzymes produce colored compounds (Fig. 6-6). The appearance of various colony types on chromogenic agar are illustrated in Color Plates 6-5*E* through *H*. Kilian and Bülow were the first to use selective chromogenic medium for the direct identification of *E. coli* in primary culture of urine.[266] Currently, several chromogenic media allowing the direct identification of *E. coli, P. mirabilis,* and *Enterococcus* spp. are marketed: CPS ID2 (bioMérieux, Hazelwood, MO),[17,71,110,217,309,347a,419,438,504a] CHROMagar Orientation (BD Diagnostics, Sparks, MD; Hardy Diagnostics, Santa Maria, CA),[17,71,139,217,231,317,366,434,438] Rainbow UTI (Biolog, Hayward, CA),[41,71,441] and Chromogenic UTI (Oxoid, Basingstoke, United Kingdom).[17,71,110] In evaluations of multiple formulations of these media, the detection rates and identification rates are very similar.[17,71,110] In one study the use of chromogenic agar allowed a >50% reduction in inoculation time and a >20% reduction in workup time.[139] To extend identification to additional species, colony characteristics on chromogenic agar can be combined with easy-to-use confirmatory spot tests that can be performed in seconds either on paper strips or directly on the agar medium.[366] One cautionary note, however, is that inocula taken from chromogenic agar plates may not be suitable for susceptibility testing with certain automated test systems. Reisner and Austin showed that susceptibility testing directly from CPS ID2 medium resulted in low error rates for all antimicrobial agents tested using the Vitek Legacy System (bioMérieux, Hazelwood, MO).[419] Laboratories using chromogenic media should check with their instrument manufacturer to determine the compatibility of using inocula from chromogenic agar for antibiotic susceptibility testing on the system in use in their laboratory.

Classic Identification Systems

Systems for the identification and naming of microorganisms are either computer-assisted or manual. Before discussing the derivation and applications of numeric coding systems, two manual bacterial identification schemes that are still in use will be reviewed: 1) the cross-hatch or checkerboard matrix, and 2) the branching or dichotomous flow charts.

Checkerboard Matrix

Table 6-7 is a comprehensive identification table formulated by Farmer and colleagues for use at the CDC to identify all named species, biogroups, and unnamed enteric groups of the *Enterobacteriaceae*. This table is a classic example of the checkerboard matrix and demonstrates its advantages and disadvantages. The matrix is large, with 48 biochemical characteristics for 30 genera, 129 species, biogroups, and unnamed enteric groups. The numbers in the intersecting squares represent the percentage of strains that are positive or reactive against the various biochemical tests (listed in the vertical columns). A reaction is generally considered positive if 90% or more of the strains are reactive, negative if 10% or fewer of the strains fail to produce a result, and variable if 11–89% of reactions are positive. The ability to determine both the positive and negative reactions for the various characteristics being measured in this type of identification system results in a high degree of diagnostic accuracy. The major disadvantage of the checkerboard matrix is the tedium involved in matching point-by-point the various reactions against those derived from the test media and constructing the patterns that best match with a specific genus, species, or biogroup.

Branching Flow Diagrams

Flow diagrams were designed to reduce the tedium of reading the checkerboard matrices and to facilitate the likely bacterial identification by tracing a series of positive and negative branch points in a dichotomous algorithm (Fig. 6-8, 6-9). With the advent of automated instruments and packaged identification systems that rely on computer-assisted

analyses of the various reactions of the characteristics being measured, flow diagrams are now used less frequently in clinical laboratories. One problem with flow diagrams has been the potential for inaccuracy if the reaction at a given branch point is either aberrant (i.e., not typical for the species), misinterpreted, or the result of the reactions of a mixed culture. Many flow diagrams are constructed to repeat some species names at several junctures to accommodate reactions that may be less than 100% or in the variable category (Fig. 6-9). However, this built-in protection does not always apply for reactions that are misinterpreted, either by an automated instrument's detection system or by the human eye.

A modification of this approach is being used in many microbiology laboratories for the preliminary screening of commonly encountered bacterial species that are associated with specific infectious disease syndromes. York and colleagues[512] have presented a simple scheme for the rapid identification of *E. coli* from EMB or MacConkey agar (Fig. 6-8). To validate this scheme, five laboratories sequentially collected 1,064 fresh, clinically significant strains with the core criteria of indole-positive, oxidase-negative, nonspreading organisms on BAP. Of the 1,064 strains tested, 1,000 were *E. coli* and 64 were non–*E. coli*. Using the scheme, three non–*E. coli* isolates were identified as *E. coli*, for an error rate of 0.3%. A total of 13 kit identifications, 657 PYR tests, and 113 MUG tests were needed to identify 1,000 *E. coli* strains with the algorithm.[512] The authors showed that the use of this rapid system saves laboratory resources, provides timely identifications, and yields rare misidentifications. The NCCLS has produced a guideline (M35-P, *Abbreviated Identification of Bacteria and Yeast: Proposed Guideline*) that describes tests that can be used to identify a number of aerobic gram-negative rods and gram-positive cocci, a number of commonly isolated anaerobes, and three species of yeast.[342] Since all methods described in the guideline yield results that are highly accurate—attaining a level of reliability equal to or better than current conventional biochemical tests, multitest systems, and automated systems—the resulting identification does not require the adjective "presumptive" qualifying the resulting identification. The genus and species (or genus only, as designated by the algorithm) can be reported without any qualifying wording.[28] Laboratory workers are referred to the NCCLS document for methodologic details about the tests chosen and for more information than is presented here.[342]

An algorithm using a KIA and LIA tube (supplemented with tryptophan for detection of indole) is used in the microbiology laboratory at the University of Illinois Hospital for the screening of enteric pathogens from stool (Fig. 6-9). Definitive biochemical and serologic procedures are performed only on isolates with reactions that are presumed to be positive, saving the cost of performing more expensive kit identifications.

In addition to saving the cost of setting up commercial test panels these dichotomous schemes coupled with a few inexpensive biochemical tests and observations offer an additional advantage over automated systems in that they require thought, reasoning, and knowledge on the part of the student or microbiologist, who are not reduced to passive observers.

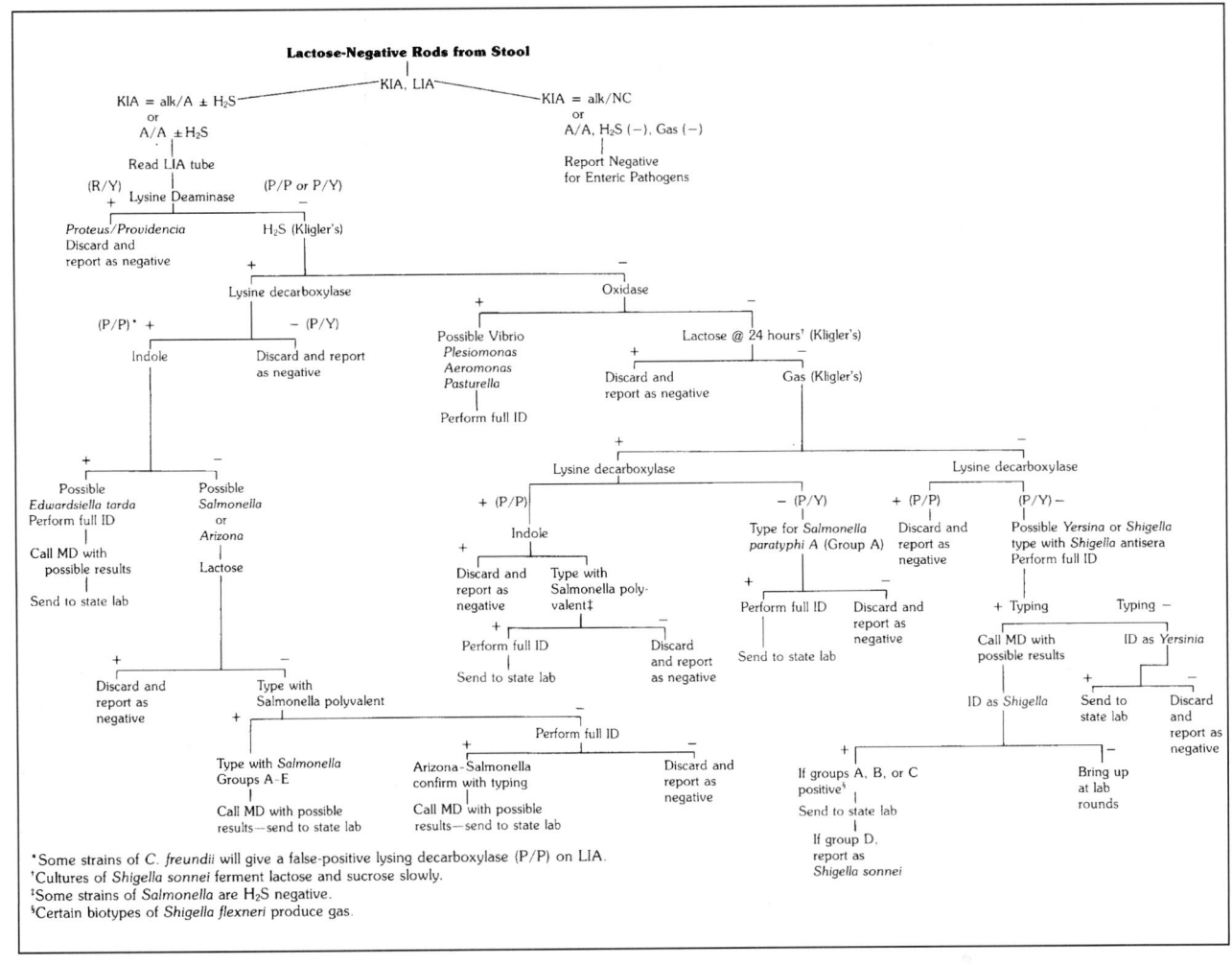

Figure 6-9 Schematic for screening of enteric pathogens from stool using KIA and modified LIA.

Computer-Aided Schemes

BioBASE (BioBASE, Boston) is a computer-enhanced numeric identification software package for use on personal computers (PCs) that allows the user to create, update, and manipulate unlimited numbers of microbial databases. Conventional biochemical reactions on an unknown isolate are entered into the appropriate database whereby the program compares the unknown profile with that of any taxon in the database. To reach an identification verdict, BioBASE calculates identification scores, modal scores, and similarity indices of each taxon and compares them with the unknown's input data. The top-scoring microorganisms are then analyzed and weighted for a decision on identification, ranging from unacceptable to excellent. Miller and Alachi evaluated this program and report it to be user-friendly, rapid and accurate, and state that it would be of value to any laboratory that uses conventional biochemicals.[324]

Numeric Coding Systems

The identification of the *Enterobacteriaceae* and many other families and groups of bacteria has been facilitated by the use of automated and packaged kit systems, by which organisms are identified with computer-assisted numeric codes. A numeric code is a system by which the several identifying characteristics of bacteria are translated into a sequence of numbers that represent one or more bacterial species. The fact that the identification of microorganisms is based on a series of positive and negative biochemical reactions makes computer programming easy because computer logic is also constructed on a sequence of positive and negative entries, using a binary numeric system. In binary logic there are only two numbers: "0" (or off) and "1" (or on). As can quickly be surmised, the identification characteristics of microorganisms can be easily translated into binary numbers by assigning a "1" to all positive reactions and a "0" to all negative reactions. This approach can be illustrated using the sequence of characteristics in the API 20E strip (bioMérieux) as a point of reference and converting the positive and negative reactions into binary numbers (Table 6-26). If the binary numbers shown in Table 6-26 are read from top to bottom and rearranged horizontally, the following 21-digit binary number is derived:

101010000111111011100

Table 6-26 Binary Conversion of Reactions of Unknown Organism on API 20-E Strip

CHARACTERISTIC	REACTION	BINARY CONVERSION
ONPG	+	1
Arginine	−	0
Lysine	+	1
Ornithine	−	0
Citrate	+	1
Hydrogen sulfide	−	0
Urease	−	0
Tryptophan deaminase	−	0
Indole	−	0
Voges-Proskauer	+	1
Gelatin	+	1
Glucose	+	1
Mannitol	+	1
Inositol	+	1
Sorbitol	+	1
Rhamnose	−	0
Sucrose	+	1
Melibiose	+	1
Amygdalin	+	1
Arabinose	−	0
Oxidase	−	0

Table 6-27 Octal Conversion of Binary Code

BINARY	CONVERSION FORMULA	OCTAL
− − −	0 + 0 + 0 =	0
+ − −	1 + 0 + 0 =	1
− + −	0 + 2 + 0 =	2
+ + −	1 + 2 + 0 =	3
− − +	0 + 0 + 4 =	4
+ − +	1 + 0 + 4 =	5
− + +	0 + 2 + 4 =	6
+ + +	1 + 2 + 4 =	7

Now convert each three-digit subset into its octal equivalent using the formula given in Table 6-27.

101 010 000 111 111 011 100

5 2 0 7 7 6 1

The number 5207761 is far easier to remember and simpler to enter into a computer than the binary number 101010000111111011100.

A simpler way of remembering how to convert each binary triplet into its corresponding octal equivalent is to assign the following values (again reading from right to left): A value of 4 to a positive reaction for the first test in each triplet, a value of 2 to a positive reaction for the second test in each triplet, a value of 1 to a positive reaction for the third test in each triplet, and a value of 0 to any negative reactions (see Table 6-27).

These octal derivatives are known as **biotype numbers,** that is, a numeric representative of a series of phenotypic characteristics expressed by and unique to a particular bacterial species. It is important that everyone using biotype numbers, particularly those who are teaching students, understand that each number in the octal system is representative of three biochemical characteristics and that the number itself represents a pattern of positive and negative reactions. There is great danger that modern microbiologists consider biotype numbers as magic figures that can be read from charts or put into computers to derive automatic organism identification, thus losing sight not only of the biochemical reactions that they represent, but also of the biochemical principles on which the discipline of microbiology is based.

Reading Octal Codes in Numeric Code Registers

All manufacturers who have packaged identification kits on the market publish numeric code registers in which hundreds of biotype numbers are matched with one or more bacterial species that are unique for that number. For example, for the biotype number 5207761, derived from the API 20E set of reactions used in the previous example, the following species are listed in the API 20E Profile Index:

Although computers are constructed to receive 1/0 bits of data from which to calculate meaningful results, the human mind cannot efficiently manipulate binary logic; therefore, binary codes must be converted into simpler mathematic systems to become usable. Conversion of the two-digit (binary) system into an eight-digit (octal) system serves this purpose. To understand the conversion of binary into octal numbers, visualize a series of three light bulbs. By turning different lights on and off, a total of eight combinations is possible, each of which can be represented by one of eight numbers ranging from 0 to 7. If all lights are off (−), the combination − − − is equivalent to octal 0. If only the left bulb is turned on (+), the combination + − − is equivalent to octal 1. Octal 2 is represented by the binary pattern − + −, and octal 3 by the pattern + + −. The octal equivalents of the eight combinations of a three-digit binary number are shown in Table 6-27.

To illustrate how binary numbers longer than three digits can be converted into their octal equivalents, use the binary number that was derived from the API 20E reactions:

101010000111111011100

Beginning from the right, because binary numbers are read from right to left, divide the binary numbers into subsets of three:

101 010 000 111 111 011 100

Serratia marcescens: acceptable identification; *S. marcescens*: 1/243; and *S. rubidaea*: 1/2,859.

The message in the API Profile Index for biotype number 5207761 for *S. marcescens* "Acceptable Identification" indicates that *S. marcescens* can be reported. This assessment is based on a computer-derived calculation of the percentage likelihood that *S. marcescens* is the correct identification compared with all the other organisms entered into the database.

Estimated Frequency of Occurrence

The frequency figures listed with each individual species name (in the previous example, 1/243 for *S. marcescens*) indicate the number of strains selected at random that would have a biotype number similar to the strain being studied. In other words, if one were to randomly test 243 *S. marcescens*, there is a chance of 1 in 243 that you will encounter this exact biochemical pattern. Whereas, if you tested 2,859 randomly selected *S. rubidaea*, you would have a 1 in 2859 chance of finding a strain of this exact biotype. This figure does not directly indicate the percentage likelihood that one of these species is the correct one, so the user cannot determine from this statistic how viable one of the choices might be.

Calculation of Likelihood

The identification of an unknown organism with a given biotype number is based on the calculation of percentage likelihood between the unknown biotype number and each taxon stored in the memory of the computer. Code registers that list percentage likelihood figures are more useful for everyday decision making in the laboratory. Any identification that has a likelihood of 90% or greater can be reported, those that are near 90% may be easily identified with one or two additional tests, and those with very low likelihood percentages can probably be discounted. The use of messages such as "excellent identification," "acceptable identification," and "very good identification" in the API system implies that there is a percentage likelihood of 90% or greater. However, when the message describes an identification as "questionable" or "doubtful" and the percentage likelihood is not given, the user is unable to make any assessments concerning the likelihood that an unknown represents a certain species. For students and microbiologists who may be trying to understand this concept for the first time, an example for calculating percentage likelihood and frequency of occurrence is given in Table 6-28.

Resolving Discrepancies

It must be pointed out that all answers derived from computer-based identification systems, whether or not they represent 90% or more confidence, must be interpreted in conjunction with other information available on the unknown organism—the colony morphology, reactions on various isolation media, cellular morphology on Gram stain, results of presumptive biochemical reactions, antibiotic susceptibility patterns, and clinical setting.

When discrepancies occur, visualization of the tubes, reaction chambers, or microcupules, in which the reactions have taken place, may be necessary. In many instances, the visual interpretation of certain reactions may differ from that detected by instruments. When recalculated, the new biotype number may indicate an alternative bacterial identification that is much more in keeping with preliminary and supplemental observations.

Also, any given species may have several biotype numbers because one or more individual reactions may be variable. Consequently, designating bacterial species by biotype numbers may have epidemiologic value in recognizing the emergence of clusters of similar isolates in a given practice setting. For example, recovery of many *E. coli* from a given environment or series of cultures may be of limited value; however, knowing that all of the organisms have the same biotype number may be invaluable. In this way, it may be possible to trace the agents causing hospital nosocomial outbreaks or communitywide epidemics to a common source. Biotype analysis may also lead to a better understanding of the relation between virulence of bacterial variants and the presence or absence of certain biochemical characteristics.

Packaged Kit Identification Systems

The concept of combining a series of differential media or substrates in a single package, selected to aid in identifying members of a group of bacteria, is a logical development. In fact, the availability of packaged identification systems evolved naturally, almost as a practical necessity. The microorganisms currently known to cause infectious diseases are not only legion, but also are often fastidious and require a large battery of biochemical tests for identification. It is beyond the capability of many laboratories to maintain the diversity of conventional media required. The compact construction (requiring little storage space), easily visible chemical reactions, long shelf life, and standardized quality control provided by the manufacturers of these kits make them very convenient for use in microbiology laboratories. They are especially useful in low-volume laboratories, where there may not be the time or the technical expertise to make many of these identifications, and where quality control is more difficult to maintain.

Overview of Packaged Systems

It has now become almost standard practice in many clinical laboratories to use one or more available packaged systems for the identification of certain groups of microorganisms. Extensive testing in diagnostic and research laboratories has demonstrated a 95% or greater agreement between most packaged identification systems and conventional methods in the identification of microorganisms. Thus, packaged systems have found wide acceptance in clinical laboratories for the following reasons:

1. Their accuracy has proved to be comparable with that of conventional identification systems. Evaluations of several systems have been made at the CDC

Table 6-28 Calculation of Frequency of Occurrence and Percentage Likelihood

The identification of an unknown profile is based on the calculation of likelihood between the unknown profile and each species of organism stored in the memory of the computer. To test your understanding of frequency of occurrence and percentage likelihood, work through the following example. For ease in explaining the calculations, this example is based on only four biochemical tests and three species.

Step 1. An unknown organism gives the following profile:

	IND	MR	VP	CIT
Unknown	+	−	+	−

Step 2. Known biochemical reactions of three species of *Enterobacteriaceae* for the four tests (shown as percentage of positive reactions).

	IND	MR	VP	CIT
Serratia marcescens	1	20	98	98
Enterobacter agglomerans	20	50	70	50
Klebsiella oxytoca	99	20	95	95

Step 3. Frequencies of occurrence of observed reactions (+ − + −) for each species.

Note: When a test result of the unknown is positive (IND and VP in this example), the probability of the positive reaction of the test listed in the database is used for the calculation. When the test result of the unknown is negative (MR and CIT), the probability of the negative reaction is 1 minus the probability of positive reactions.

	IND	MR	VP	CIT
Serratia marcescens	.01	.80	.98	.02
Enterobacter agglomerans	.20	.50	.70	.50
Klebsiella oxytoca	.99	.80	.95	.05

Step 4. Calculation of frequencies of occurrence of observed profile (+ − + −) for each species. The frequency of occurrence is calculated by multiplying together all the frequencies of occurrence of the reactions.

Serratia marcescens	= .01 × .80 × .98 × .02 =	.0001568
Enterobacter agglomerans	= .20 × v .50 × .70 × .50 =	.0350000
Klebsiella oxytoca	= .99 × .80 × .95 × .05 =	.0376200
		.0727768

Step 5. Identification percentages. Each frequency is divided by the sum of all the frequencies, then multiplied by 100 to give the %ID. The sum of the percentages of identification is equal to 100.

Serratia marcescens	%ID = (.001568/.0727768) × 100 =	0.21%
Enterobacter agglomerans	%ID = (.0350000/.0727768) × 100 =	48.1%
Klebsiella oxytoca	%ID = (.0376200/.0727768) × 100 =	51.7%

Step 6. Order of likelihood

1. *Klebsiella oxytoca*   %ID = 51.7
2. *Enterobacter agglomerans*   %ID = 48.1
3. *Serratia marcescens*   %ID = 0.21

What is the likelihood that *Klebsiella oxytoca* is the correct answer among the three species in the database?

(*Answer:* From step 5, the answer is 51.7%; however, there is a 48.1% likelihood that the unknown organism is *Enterobacter agglomerans;* therefore, additional tests would have to be set up to correctly identify this unknown organism.)

How frequently will *Klebsiella oxytoca* give this particular reaction profile?

(*Answer:* From step 4, 3.8% of the time; in other words, not very often.)

by Smith and associates.[452] In all evaluations, two criteria were used for measuring the performance of a product: 1) a comparison of each test in the product with its conventional counterpart and 2) the accuracy of identification made using the product.

2. Several of the systems have a long shelf life—6 months to 1 year—so that outdating of media, a problem particularly with conventional systems, is minimized.

3. The systems require only a minimum of space for storage and incubation.

4. Some of the systems are as easy or easier to use than conventional methods. Inoculation is simple, reactions are generally clear-cut within 24 hours, and the availability of computer-assisted file registers makes final identification easy and accurate.

Whether to use one of the packaged identification systems and which one to select is largely a matter of personal preference. The ease of inoculation, the ability to select only the characteristics to be measured, the manipulation required in adding reagents after incubation, and the availability of interpretive charts or computer databases are the main items that potential users should consider before selecting a system. If strict attention is paid to the instructions provided by the manufacturer, essentially the same degree of accuracy and reliability of performance can be attained, with only minor differences in the sensitivity of individual tests.

Specific Identification Systems
API 20E

The API 20E identification system (bioMérieux) has become the reference method against which the accuracy of other systems is compared. The 21 characteristics that can be determined by the API 20E system make it among the largest test sets of the packaged kits. The system identifies a high percentage of bacterial species within 24 hours, without the need to determine additional physiologic characteristics (Color Plate 6-6A). This system is among the most frequently used in clinical laboratories and has a large database that includes common and atypical strains. The API Profile Index, which can be used manually or with computer assistance, provides the frequency probability of several strains that must be considered for each biotype number. Thus, the accuracy of identification of the members of the *Enterobacteriaceae* is maximized. Castillo and Bruckner found that the API 20E system correctly identified 97.7% of 339 clinical and stock isolates.[76] The system is somewhat cumbersome to inoculate—a problem, however, that is overcome quickly with practice. After inoculation, the strips must be handled carefully so that the bacterial suspensions do not spill and contaminate the surrounding environment. Practice is required to interpret occasional borderline reactions, which can affect the biotype number and the final identification. Occasionally, biotype numbers may not appear in the profile register; however, the manufacturer maintains a telephone number for consultation. The design of the system,

the operating procedures, substrates included, and evaluation studies are shown in Table 6-29 (Color Plate 6-6A).

BBL CRYSTAL ENTERIC/NONFERMENTER ID SYSTEM

The BBL Crystal E/NF identification system (Becton Dickinson Microbiology Systems, Sparks, MD) is a miniaturized identification method using modified conventional and chromogenic substrates. It is intended for the identification of clinically significant aerobic gram-negative bacteria that belong to the family *Enterobacteriaceae,* as well as some of the more frequently isolated glucose-fermenting and nonfermenting gram-negative bacilli of human origin. The E/NF kit comprises 1) BBL Crystal E/NF lids, 2) BBL Crystal bases, and 3) BBL Crystal Enteric/Stool ID inoculum fluid tubes (see Color Plate 6-6B). The BBL Crystal lid contains 30 dehydrated substrates on tips of plastic prongs. The BBL Crystal base has 30 reaction wells. Test inoculum is prepared with the BBL Crystal Enteric/Stool ID inoculum fluid and is used to fill all 30 wells in the BBL Crystal base. When the lid is aligned with the base and snapped into place, the test inoculum rehydrates the dried substrates and initiates test reactions. The tests used in the Crystal system include tests for fermentation, oxidation, degradation, and hydrolysis of various substrates, including chromogen-linked substrates.

Following inoculation, panels are incubated upside-down in a non-CO_2 incubator with 40–60% humidity for 18 to 20 hours at 35 to 37°C. After incubation, panels are read upside-down using the BBL Crystal light box. The wells are examined for color changes, and a 10-digit profile number is generated. The profile number and off-line test results for indole and oxidase are entered on a PC in which the BBL Crystal ID System Electronic Codebook has been installed to obtain the identification.

In an external study involving three clinical laboratories, the reproducibility of the 30 individual E/NF substrates' ranged from 96.3% to 100%. The performance of the E/NF was evaluated with both fresh clinical isolates and challenge test strains. Of 299 fresh clinical isolates tested by the laboratories' current identification methods, the BBL Crystal ID System correctly reported 96.7%, including 16 instances in which two or three organisms were reported and required supplemental testing to resolve. Of 291 previously identified challenge strains confirmed by the laboratories' current identification methods, the BBL Crystal ID System correctly reported 96.9%, including eight instances in which two or three organisms were reported and required supplemental testing to resolve (BBL Crystal Package Insert, May 1994). In two independent evaluations of the Crystal system with fermentative organisms largely from the family *Enterobacteriaceae,* correct identification without supplemental testing was reported to be 91.6%[427] and 92.9%,[495] respectively. In a study using 626 stock challenge isolates conducted at the CDC, the Crystal system 71.1% which improved to 87.9% (88.8% for enterics; 84.3% for nonenterics) after additional tests suggested by the software program were included.[365]

RAPID ONE SYSTEM

The RapID onE system (Remel) is a qualitative micromethod using conventional and chromogenic substrates

Table 6-29 Construction, Use, and Evaluation of the API 20E Identification System

FUNCTIONAL DESIGN	OPERATING PROCEDURE	SUBSTRATES INCLUDED	EVALUATION STUDIES
The system consists of a plastic strip with 20 miniaturized cupules containing dehydrated substrates and a plastic incubation chamber with a loosely fitting lid (see Color Plate 6-6*A*). Each cupula has a small hole at the top through which the bacterial suspension can be inoculated with a pipette. Bacterial action on the substrates produces color changes that are interpreted visually.	Add 5 mL of tap water to an incubation tray to provide a humid atmosphere during incubation. Place an API 20E strip into the incubation tray. Prepare a bacterial suspension of the test organism by suspending the cells from a well-isolated colony in 5 mL of sterile 0.85% saline. The turbidity of the suspension is compared with a McFarland 0.5 standard, except for same-day identifications of the *Enterobacteriaceae*, when the suspension is matched to a 1 standard. Using a Pasteur pipette, fill each cupula with the bacterial suspension through the inoculating hole. Overlay the three decarboxylase and the urease cupules with sterile mineral oil. The unit is incubated at 35°C for 5 hr (same-day identification) or for 24–48 hr before reading results.	ONPG Arginine dihydrolase Lysine decarboxylase Ornithine decarboxylase Citrate Hydrogen sulfide Urease Tryptophan deaminase (add 10% $FeCl_3$) Indole Voges-Proskauer (add KOH and α-naphthol) Gelatin Glucose Mannitol Inositol Sorbitol Rhamnose Sucrose Melibiose Amygdalin Arabinose	Aldridge and Hodges, International Clinical Laboratories, Nashville, TN: 90.5% of stock cultures and 96.6% of clinical isolates identified. Overall accuracy 92%. (J Clin Microbiol 1981; 13:120–125.) Gooch and Hill, University of Utah, 415 cultures, same-day identification 90.2%. (J Clin Microbiol 1982;15:885–890.)

for the identification of medically important *Enterobacteriaceae* and other selected oxidase-negative, gram-negative bacteria isolated from human clinical specimens. The system comprises 1) RapID onE panels and 2) RapID onE reagent. Each RapID onE panel has 18 reaction cavities molded into the periphery of a plastic disposable tray. Reaction cavities contain dehydrated reactants, and the tray allows the simultaneous inoculation of each cavity with a predetermined amount of inoculum (see Color Plate 6-6*C*). A suspension of the test organism in RapID inoculation Fluid (2 mL) is used as the test inoculum, which rehydrates and initiates test reactions. Inoculated panels are placed into the chipboard incubation trays provided in the package and incubated at 35 to 37°C in a non-CO_2 incubator for 4 hours.

RapID onE panels contain 18 reaction cavities that provide 19 test scores. Tests labeled PRO, GGT, and PYR (cavities 15, 16, and 17) require RapID onE Reagent and are designated with a box drawn around the tests. Test 18 is bifunctional, containing two separate tests in the same cavity. This test is scored **before** the addition of reagent, providing the first test result, which is adonitol; then two drops of INOVA Spot Indole reagent is added to cavity 18 and the same cavity is scored again **after** the addition of reagent to provide the second test result, which is indole. The 19 test results plus oxidase are scored in the appropriate boxes of the report form, and a seven-digit profile code is generated.

The organism ID is obtained by finding the profile code in the RapID onE Code Compendium.

In a study conducted at the University of Illinois Medical Center, 302 of 344 (87.8%) oxidase-negative, gram-negative bacilli tested were correctly identified to the species level, with an additional 24 (7%) organisms correctly identified to the genus or group level. Six organisms gave unacceptable or no ID, eight gave questionable IDs, and four organisms (1.1%) gave incorrect IDs.[445] Kitch and colleagues reported similar findings with an overall identification rate to species or to genus level of 95.8%, with a misidentification rate of 1.3%.[271]

ENTEROTUBE II

Of all the systems, Enterotube II (Becton Dickinson Microbiology Systems, Cockeysville, MD) is the easiest to inoculate. The system takes up little space, and the risk of contamination is minimal. The color reactions are generally easy to interpret; a minor problem exists in differentiating the elevation of the wax overlay in the glucose chamber (an indicator of gas production) from artifactual shrinkage of the media during storage. A false-negative interpretation may also result if a tiny leak in the plastic allows the gas to escape as it forms. Indole and Voges-Proskauer reagents must be added with a needle and syringe through the thin plastic backing. If this is not done carefully, the added reagent can leak into other compartments, altering reactions. Thus, it is recommended that the reactions in other compartments be interpreted before adding these reagents. One additional disadvantage of the Enterotube II, compared with systems that use dry substrates, is that the incorporation of conventional agar media shortens the shelf life. The manufacturer provides a convenient computer-coding and identification system (CCIS) that lists the possible bacterial identifications for the five-digit biotype numbers that are derived from the interpretation of color changes. Details of the functional design, operating procedures, and substrates included are listed in Table 15-2, page 639, in the second edition of this book.

MICRO-ID

Micro-ID (Remel) is the ideal system for laboratories where identification of bacteria is desired within 4 to 6 hours. Inoculation of the system is relatively easy, and the units occupy little space during incubation or storage. Only one reagent (20% potassium hydroxide) needs to be added to one of the chambers before interpreting the results. Reactions are distinct and can be compared with a color guide. A profile register that lists the probable organism identification for the five-digit biotype numbers is supplied by the manufacturer, and computer comparisons can be made to search for the best fit. Accuracy is equal to or exceeds that of other packaged systems. Construction details and operating procedures for this system are listed in Table 15-2, page 642, in the second edition of this book.

BIOLOG GN2 MICROPLATE

Biolog GN2 MicroPlate (Biolog, Hayward CA) consists of a 96-well microtiter plate that tests for the ability of a microorganism to utilize (oxidize) one or more of 95 different carbon sources in the presence of a redox indicator (tetrazolium dye). One well contains no carbon and serves as a negative control or reference well. All the necessary nutrients and biochemicals are prefilled and dried into the 96 wells of the plate. Tetrazolium violet is used to colorimetrically detect the increased respiration that occurs in a cell when it is oxidizing a carbon source (see Color Plate 6-6D). Regardless of its structure, virtually any chemical substrate that is oxidized by the cell will result in formation of NADH, leading to a flow of electrons along a pathway of electron transport. Redox dyes, such as tetrazolium, tap electrons from this flow, converting the tetrazolium to a highly colored formazan. Thus, if a cell is presented with a chemical that it can oxidize, its respiration increases and the colorless dye is irreversibly reduced to a formazan, forming a purple color. If the cell is given a chemical that it cannot oxidize, no respiratory burst occurs, and no color is formed. The test yields a pattern of purple wells that constitutes a "metabolic fingerprint" of the capacities of the inoculated organism. Bochner has published a description and overview of the system.[40] Miller and Rhoden, at the CDC, have published a preliminary evaluation on the Biolog in which they report that the system performed well with many genera, but that problems were encountered with some strains of *Klebsiella*, *Enterobacter*, and *Serratia*.[325] Holmes and colleagues[226] studied 789 strains, including 55 gram-negative taxa encountered in the clinical laboratory. They reported significantly better results when plates were read manually, rather than when they were read by the automated reader. Plates read manually gave the following performances: oxidase-positive fermenters, five taxa, 64 strains, 92% correct, 3% not identified, and 5% incorrect; biochemically active nonfermenters, eight taxa, 122 strains, 88% correct, 6% not identified, and 6% incorrect; *Enterobacteriaceae*, 35 taxa, 511 strains, 77% correct, 8% not identified, and 15% incorrect; unreactive nonfermenters, seven taxa, 92 strains, 38% correct, 24% not identified, and 38% incorrect. These authors reported problems with identification of encapsulated strains of some *Enterobacter* and *Klebsiella* taxa, as well as the least biochemically active *Moraxella* and *Neisseria* strains.[226] The Biolog system is now available in a fully automated platform and is described in the next section on automated instruments.

MICROSCAN SYSTEM

The MicroScan System (Dade Behring, West Sacramento, CA) consists of plastic, standard-sized, 96-well microtiter trays in which up to 32 reagent substrates are included for the identification of the *Enterobacteriaceae* and other bacterial species (gram-positive, gram-negative, and urinary tract panels are available). Some trays, called Combo trays, also include broth microdilutions of various antibiotics in certain of the microtubes for performing susceptibility tests[131]. MicroScan panels are supplied either in a frozen state or contain dehydrated substrates that make shipping more convenient and allow for room temperature storage and a longer shelf life. Schieven and associates[442] found that both the frozen and dehydrated microdilution trays provided comparable organism identification and antimicrobial susceptibility results (only 1.3% and 4.2% discrepancy rates, respectively).

The microtubes are inoculated with a heavy suspension of the organism to be identified and incubated at 35°C for 15 to 18 hours. The panels can be interpreted visually (see Color Plate 6-6E), after which the biochemical results are converted into a seven- or eight-digit biotype number that can be translated into an identification with a code book supplied by the manufacturer. Alternatively, an automated tray reader can be used to detect bacterial growth or color changes by differences in light transmission. Differences in electronic pulses are automatically analyzed by a microcomputer that compares reaction patterns with an internal program to determine the likelihood of identifications. Rhoden and associates[422] found that the AutoScan-4, an automatic reader in the MicroScan system, correctly identified 95.4% of members of the *Enterobacteriaceae* (occasional false-negative readings for hydrogen sulfide and arginine dihydrolase reactions were the only problems resulting in misidentification). One disadvantage cited by the authors was that the instrument occasionally reports "very rare biotype," leaving the user unclear as to what rare biotype was indicated.

SENSITITRE SYSTEM

The Sensititre System (TREK Diagnostic Systems, Cleveland, OH) may be purchased as either a manual enteric identification system or in the form of an autoidentification system. The manual plate contains media for performing 23 standard biochemical tests, plus a control, which are dried in the wells of a standard-sized 96-well microtiter tray. Each tray contains four duplicate sets of biochemical wells, permitting simultaneous identification of four organisms per tray. The system contains conventional biochemical tests and is inoculated and read manually. Staneck and associates[457] reported that agreement between Sensititre and API 20E for 1415 isolates of *Enterobacteriaceae* was 94.6% at the species level.

Semiautomated and Automated Identification Systems
MicroScan Walkaway

The Walkaway (Dade MicroScan, West Sacramento CA) is a fully automated instrument that incubates any combination of up to 96 conventional or Rapid MicroScan panels simultaneously, automatically adds reagents to conventional panels when required, reads and interprets panel results, and prints results, all without operator intervention (Color Plate 6-6*F*). Rapid fluorescence panels in addition to the conventional MicroScan panels are available for use with the Walkaway instrument. The rapid panels use fluorescent labeled compounds and require only a 2-hour incubation for bacterial identification. Each fluorescent substrate consists of a fluorophore, either methylumbelliferone (MEU) or 7-amino-4-methyl-coumarin (AMC) attached to a phosphate, sugar, or amino acid compound. Two types of reactions occur: fluorogenic and fluorometric. In fluorogenic reactions, a specific enzyme, if present in the bacterial suspension, cleaves the fluorescent compound, releasing the fluorophore, which then fluoresces. For example:

$$\text{Alanine}$$

$$\underset{\text{(nonfluorescent)}}{\text{L-Alanine-AMC}} \xrightarrow{\text{Aminopeptidase}} \underset{\text{(fluorescent)}}{\text{Alanine + AMC}}$$

Fluorometric reactions detect changes in pH such as occurs with carbohydrate fermentation. The resultant acid production causes a drop in pH and a decrease in fluorescence. In addition, eight fluorogenic rate reactions are used. These reactions measure the rate of release of the fluorophore and are used in differentiating phenotypically similar species. Results of the ID reactions are converted into 15-digit biocodes for interpretation by the computer. The Walkaway colorimetric optical system has 97 photometers illuminated by a single tungsten–halogen source through 97 optical fibers. Light from the source passes through interference filters on a color wheel and is focused on the fiberoptics, 96 of which mirror the configuration of a 96-well panel. The 97th photometer provides a baseline reading to which all photometer signals are ratioed. During each read cycle, the rotating color wheel provides readings at six different wavelengths through the visible spectrum. For biochemical reactions, the computer selects the wavelength reading that best discriminates the reaction occurring in each well. A review of the Walkaway technology has been published by Clayland and colleagues.[118] Several studies have shown that the Walkaway provides accurate identification of organisms belonging to the family *Enterobacteriaceae*.[261,356,364,390,421,513]

MicroScan's fluorogenic 2-hour Rapid Negative Identification Panel has been updated to significantly increase accuracy of identification and expand the number of taxa in the database. The updated panel (Rapid Gram Negative Identification Panel 3, RNID3) consists of 36 newly formulated tests and a new database consisting of 119 taxa, covering a total of 150 species, including 12 additional new species. Achondo and associates reported that the new system has an accuracy of 98.4% (92.5% correct to species, 1.6% correct to genus, and 4.3% correct to species with additional tests) and 99.3% for clinically significant isolates (97.4% correct to species, 1.0% correct to genus, and 0.9% correct to species with additional tests).[5] The accuracy and performance of the RNID3 panel were examined in a multicenter evaluation in which a total of 405 isolates comprising 54 species were tested; 96.8% of these species were identified correctly. In the same study, 465 isolates were examined for intra- and interlaboratory identification reproducibility and gave an agreement of 99.8%.[30a]

Vitek System

The Vitek System (Legacy) (bioMérieux) was first introduced to perform automated antimicrobial susceptibility tests, with subsequent modifications to improve accuracy.[337] In 1982, the *Enterobacteriaceae*-plus Biochemical Card (EBC +) was introduced, providing for automatic identification of the *Enterobacteriaceae* within 8 hours of incubation.[29,510] An improvement to the Gram-Negative Identification Card was made in 1996. The new version card, called the GNI + Card added 20 new species to the database and provided improved performance and increased speed of identification.[47,365] Moss and coworkers reported that the GNI + identifies glucose-fermenting organisms in 2 to 8 hours and glucose-nonfermenting organisms in 4 to 12 hours, with 40.1% of the organisms tested being identified in 3 hours.[331] Hansen and colleagues evaluated the accuracy of the Vitek GNI + cards using direct inoculation from positive blood culture bottles using a suspension made by differential centrifugation of positive blood culture broth. The direct method resulted in 75% correct identifications, 9% misidentifications, and 17% nonidentifications. All misidentified isolates were *E. coli*, of which 80% were reported as *Salmonella* ser. Arizonae.[210] The Vitek Legacy system has found wide use in clinical microbiology laboratories and has generally been accepted as a reliable approach to the rapid identification of commonly encountered gram-negative bacilli.[364,390,421] The construction and operating procedures of earlier versions of the Vitek system, initially designed to perform automated antibiotic susceptibility tests, were described in some detail in the second edition of this book (Table 15-10, pages 668–670).

The VITEK 2 System (bioMérieux) is an integrated modular system that consists of a filling-sealer unit, a reader-incubator, a computer control module, a data terminal, and a multicopy printer (see Color Plate 6-6*G*). In addition, the VITEK 2 system incorporates several technical improvements that automates many procedures that are performed manually with the VITEK legacy system. The system detects bacterial growth and metabolic changes in the microwells of thin plastic cards by using a fluorescence-based technology (a colorimetric-based instrument was introduced in late 2004). The identification card for gram-negative bacilli (ID-GNB card) for the VITEK 2 is a 64-well plastic card containing 41 fluorescent biochemical tests, including 18 enzymatic tests for aminopeptidases and -osidases. Substrates used for detection of aminopeptidases are usually coupled with 7-amino-methylcoumarin (7AMC); substrates for detection of -osidases are usually coupled with 4-methylumbelliferone (4MU). In addition there are 18 fermentation tests, 2 decarboxylase tests, and 3 miscellaneous tests. There are two negative control wells, and the remaining wells are empty. Results are interpreted by the ID-GNB database after a 3-hr incubation period. In a study by Funke and colleagues, the VITEK 2 system was shown to correctly identify 84.7% of selected species representing 70 different taxa of *Enterobacteriaceae* and nonenteric bacteria within 3 hr.[181] Ling and colleagues in a much smaller study representing 31 different taxa of the most commonly recovered *Enterobacteriaceae* and non-fermenter species, obtained 95% correct identification to the species level with the VITEK 2.[289] These same researchers evaluated the VITEK 2 for rapid direct identification of gram-negative bacilli from positive blood culture bottles and reported that 97 (82.2%) of strains were correctly identified to species level and 21 (17.8%) strains were not identified. There were no misidentifications.[288] In two additional studies, O'Hara and Miller[357] reported an accuracy of 93.0% for the identification of 482 enteric stock cultures and Gavin et al.[186] reported 95.3% accuracy (*Enterobacteriaceae*, 95.9%; non-*Enterobacteriaceae*, 92.5%) with the VITEK 2.

Sensititre Gram-Negative AutoIdentification System

The Sensititre Automated Reading and Incubation System (ARIS) (TREK Diagnostic Systems) is an automated system that uses fluorescence technology to detect bacterial growth and enzyme activity. The system consists of 32 newly formulated biochemical tests, including selected classic biochemical media reformulated to yield a fluorescence signal, along with newly developed fluorescence tests. Each biochemical test medium along with an appropriate fluorescence indicator is dried into the individual wells of the Sensititre plate. Each plate is designed to test three separate organisms. Because these are dried plates, they may be stored at room temperature. All autoIdentification tests are read on the Sensititre AutoReader for the presence or absence of fluorescence. The results are transmitted to a computer for analysis and identification. Results may be read after 5 hours of incubation. If a satisfactory level of identification cannot be obtained at 5 hours, the plate may simply be reincubated and read after overnight incubation. Owing to the use of fluorescence technology, these plates cannot be read manually and can be read only on a correctly standardized Sensititre AutoReader. Company in-house data for 1,084 isolates of *Enterobacteriaceae* show overall agreement at 5 hours to be 92.4% and at 18 hours to be 93.4% when compared with standard methods (Sensititre Technical Product Information).

The Phoenix System

The Phoenix Automated Microbiology System (Becton Dickinson Microbiology Systems, Sparks, MD) is a newly developed, fully automated, identification and antimicrobial susceptibility test system. The system is comprised of disposable panels that combine both identification and antimicrobial susceptibility testing, and an instrument that performs automatic reading at 20-minute intervals during incubation (Color Plate 6-6*H*). The gram-negative identification segment uses 45 biochemical substrates, including 16 fluorogenic, 14 fermentation, 8 carbon source, 5 chromogenic, and 2 miscellaneous substrates (urea and ornithine) to identify aerobic gram-negative bacilli in 2–12 hours, with the vast majority of results provided in 4 hours or less. The instrument monitors both visible spectral changes and fluorescence intensity levels, depending on the type of substrate, interprets the results, and provides an answer when the system is confident of the identification. In a study by Stefaniuk and colleagues, the Phoenix showed a high rate of agreement with conventional identification methods, ranging from 100% for gram-positive cocci to 96% for gram-negative nonfermenters and 92.5% for Enterobacteriaceae.[460]

The OmniLog ID System

The OmniLog ID System (Biolog, Hayward, CA) is a fully automated platform for use with Biolog's proprietary carbon source utilization test method (See description of Biolog GN2 MicroPlate in previous section). The OmniLog System simultaneously incubates, reads, and interprets the Biolog MicroPlates. It continuously processes samples but allows the user complete access at any time during a sample run. A unique feature of the OmniLog System is user-defined incubation temperature, allowing organisms to be incubated at their optimal temperature to obtain maximum growth for accurate identification. The instrument begins reading the MicroPlates 4 hours after they have been placed into the Reader. The pattern is compared to the identification database, and an ID is called if enough positive reactions have developed. If no result is obtained after 6 hours, the instrument automatically continues to incubate the MicroPlate and begins reading again after 16 hours up to 24 hours. Biolog's databases contain over 1,400 different organisms including 501 gram-negative species, representing those important in both clinical and nonclinical microbiology. Many of these species cannot be identified with other identification systems.

In summary, commercial manufacturers continue to provide new systems and modifications of existing systems for the identification of microorganisms. To pass Food and Drug Administration standards, all of these systems must perform with accuracy equal to or better than reference methods. Therefore, each system can be used in clinical laboratories, but the choice depends on several variables, including volume of testing, experience of the technical staff, need for definitive identifications, and cost of operation. The *Enterobacteriaceae*, as a group, are rapidly expanding and, for the most part, are biochemically very active; therefore, they are well-suited for processing by automated and semiautomated systems. Space has allowed for only a brief overview of these systems in this book. To learn more the reader is referred to the review of automated systems written by Stager and Davis.[456] The cited references may be consulted for more detailed descriptions and evaluations of performance.

REFERENCES

1. Abbott S, Janda MJ. *Enterobacter cancerogenus* (''*Enterobacter taylorae*'') infections associated with severe trauma or crush injuries. Am J Clin Pathol 1997; 107:359–361.

2. Abbott SL, Janda JM. Isolation of *Yokenella regensburgei* (''*Koserella trabulsii*'') from a patient with transient bacteremia and from a patient with a septic knee. J Clin Microbiol 1994;32:2854–2855.

3. Abbott SL, O'Connor J, Robin T, et al. Biochemical properties of a newly described *Escherichia* species, *Escherichia albertii*. J Clin Microbiol 2003;41: 4852–4854.

4. Abdel-Haq NM, Asmar BI, Abuhammour WM, et al. *Yersinia enterocolitica* infection in children. Pediatr Infect Dis J 2000;19:954–958.

5. Achondo K, Bascomb S, Bobolis J, et al. New improved MicroScan Rapid Negative Identification Panel. Abstr Annu Meet Am Soc Microbiol 1995;C307: 53.

6. Adamkiewicz TV, Berkovitch M, Krishnan C, et al. Infection due to *Yersinia enterocolitica* in a series of patients with β-thalassemia: incidence and predisposing factors. Clin Infect Dis 1998;27:1362–1366.

7. Aevaliotis A, Belle AM, Chanione JP, Serruys E. *Kluyvera ascorbata* isolated from a baby with diarrhea. Clin Microbiol Newslett 1985;7:51.

8. Aguirre PM, Cacho JB, Folgueira L, et al. Rapid fluorescence method for screening *Salmonella* spp. from enteric differential agars. J Clin Microbiol 1990;28: 148–149.

9. Alballaa SR, Qadri SMH, Al-Furayh O, Al-Qatary K. Urinary tract infection due to *Rahnella aquatilis* in a renal transplant patient. J Clin Microbiol 1992; 30:2948–2950.

10. Albert MJ, Alam K, Islam M, et al. *Hafnia alvei*, a probable cause of diarrhea in humans. Infect Immun 1991;59:1507–1513.

11. Aleksic S, Steigerwalt AG, Bockemuhl J, et al. *Yersinia rohdei* sp. nov. isolated from human and dog feces and surface water. Int J Syst Bacteriol 1987;37: 327–332.

12. Anahory T, Darbas H, Ongaro O, et al. *Serratia ficaria*: a misidentified or unidentified rare cause of human infections in fig tree culture zones. J Clin Microbiol 1998;36:3266–3272.

13. Archer JR, Schell RF, Pennell DR, et al. Identification of *Yersinia* spp. with the API 20E system. J Clin Microbiol 1987;25:2398–2399.

14. Arduino MJ, Bland LA, Tipple MA, et al. Growth and endotoxin production of *Yersinia enterocolitica* and *Enterobacter agglomerans* in packed erythrocytes. J Clin Microbiol 1989;27:1483–1485.

15. Arthur JD, Pierce JR. *Citrobacter diversus* meningitis and brain abscess associated with *Bacteroides melaninogenicus*. Pediatr Infect Dis 1984;3:592–593.

16. Ashelford KE, Fry JC, Bailey MJ, et al. Characterization of *Serratia* isolates from soil, ecological implications and transfer of *Serratia proteamaculans* subsp. *quinovora* Grimont, et al. 1983 to *Serratia quinivorans* corrig., sp. nov. Int J Syst Evol Microbiol 2002;52:2281–2289.

17. Aspevall O, Osterman B, Dittmer R, et al. Performance of four chromogenic urine culture media after one or two days of incubation with reference media. J Clin Microbiol 2002;40:1500–1503.

18. Aspinall ST, Hindle MA, Hutchinson DN. Improved isolation of salmonellae from faeces using a semisolid Rappaport-Vassiliadis medium. Eur J Clin Microbiol Infect Dis 1992;11:936–939.s

19. Awsare SV, Lillo M. A case report of *Escherichia vulneris* urosepsis. Rev Infect Dis 1991;13:1247–1248.

20. Babu K, Sonnenberg M, Kathpalia S, et al. Isolation of salmonellae from dried rattlesnake preparations. J Clin Microbiol 1990;28: 361–362.

21. Badenoch PR, Thom AL, Coster DJ. *Serratia ficaria* endophthalmitis. J Clin Microbiol 2002;40:1563–1564.

22. Bae BHC, Sureka SB. *Cedecea davisae* isolated from scrotal abscess. J Urol 1983;130:148–149.

23. Bae BHC, Sureka SB, Ajamy JA. Enteric group 15 (Enterobacteriaceae) associated with pneumonia. J Clin Microbiol 1981;14:596–597.

24. Bagley ST, Seidler RJ, Brenner DJ. *Klebsiella planticola* sp. nov.: a new species of Enterobacteriaceae found primarily in nonclinical environments. Curr Microbiol 1981;6:105–109.

25. Baiulescu M, Hannon PR, Marcinak JF, et al. Chronic vulvovaginitis caused by antibiotic-resistant *Shigella flexneri* in a prepubertal child. Pediatr Infect Dis J 2002;21:170–172.

26. Bale MJ, McLaws SM, Fenn JP, et al. Use of and cost savings with morphologic criteria and the spot indole test as a routine means of identification of *Escherichia coli*. Diagn Microbiol Infect Dis 1984;2:187–191.

27. Bale MJ, McLaws SM, Matsen JM. The spot indole test for identification of swarming *Proteus*. Am J Clin Pathol 1985;83:87–90.

28. Baron EJ. Rapid identification of bacteria and yeast: summary of a National Committee for Clinical Laboratory Standards proposed guideline. Clin Infect Dis 2001;33:220–225.

29. Barry AL, Badal RE. Identification of Enterobacteriaceae by the AutoMicrobic system: Enterobacteriaceae biochemical cards versus Enterobacteriaceae-plus biochemical cards. J Clin Microbiol 1982;15:575–581.

30. Barry AL, Bernsohn KL, Adams AP, et al. Improved 18-hour methyl red test. Appl Microbiol 1970;20:866–870.

30a. Bascomb S, Abbott SL, Bobolis JD, et al. Multicenter evaluation of the MicroScan Rapid Gram-Negative Identification Type 3 Panel. J Clin Microbiol 1997;35:2531–2536.

31. Bear N, Klugman KP, Tobiansky L, Koornhof HJ. Wound colonization by *Ewingella americana*. J Clin Microbiol 1986;23:650–651.

32. Beatty ME, Bopp CA, Wells JG, et al. Enterotoxin-producing *Escherichia coli* O169:H41, United States. Emerg Infect Dis 2004;10:518–521.

33. Bercovier H, Steigerwalt AG, Guiyoule A, et al. *Yersinia aldovae* (formerly *Yersinia enterocolitica*-like group X2): a new species of Enterobacteriaceae isolated from aquatic ecosystems. Int J Syst Bacteriol 1984;34:166:172.

34. Bercovier H, Ursing J, Brenner DJ, et al. *Yersinia kristensenii*: a new species of Enterobacteriaceae composed of sucrose-negative strains (formerly called atypical *Yersinia enterocolitica* or *Yersinia enterocolitica*-like). Curr Microbiol 1980;4:219–224.

35. Bettelheim KA, Evangelidis H, Pearce JL, et al. Isolation of a *Citrobacter freundii* strain which carries the *Escherichia coli* O157 antigen. J Clin Microbiol 1993;31:760–761.

36. Biering G, Karlsson S, Clark NC, et al. Three cases of neonatal meningitis caused by *Enterobacter sakazakii* in powdered milk. J Clin Microbiol 1989;27: 2054–2056.

37. Bissett ML, Powers C, Abbott SL, Janda JM. Epidemiologic investigations of *Yersinia enterocolitica* and related species: sources, frequency, and serogroup distribution. J Clin Microbiol 1990;28:910–912.

38. Bjune G, Ruud TE, Eng J. Bacterial shock due to transfusion with *Yersinia enterocolitica* infected blood. Scand J Infect Dis 1984;16:411–412.

39. Blekher L, Siegman-Igra Y, Schwartz D, et al. Clinical significance and antibiotic resistance patterns of *Leminorella* spp., an emerging nosocomial pathogen. J Clin Microbiol 2000;38:3036–3038.

40. Bochner B. ''Breathprints'' at the microbial level: an automated redox-based technology quickly identifies bacteria according to their metabolic capacities. ASM News 1989;55:536–539.

41. Bochner B. Rainbow UTI System: a rapid and simple multicolor diagnostic system for common urinary tract pathogens. Abstr Annu Meet Am Soc Microbiol 1995;C374:65.

42. Boemare NE, Akhurst RJ, Mourant RG. DNA relatedness between *Xenorhabdus* spp. (*Enterobacteriaceae*), symbiotic bacteria of entomopathogenic nematodes, and a proposal to transfer *Xenorhabdus luminescens* to a new genus, *Photorhabdus* gen. nov. Int J Syst Bacteriol 1993;43:249–255.

43. Boileau CR, D'Hauteville HM, Sansonetti PJ. DNA hybridization technique to detect *Shigella* sp and enteroinvasive *Escherichia coli*. J Clin Microbiol 1984; 20:959–961.

44. Bollet C, Gainnier M, Sainty J-M, et al. *Serratia fonticola* isolated from a leg abscess. J Clin Microbiol 1991;29:834–835.

45. Bottone EJ. Atypical *Yersinia enterocolitica*: clinical and epidemiological parameters. J Clin Microbiol 1978;7:562–567.

46. Bottone EJ. *Yersinia enterocolitica*: the charisma continues. Clin Microbiol Rev 1997;10:257–276.

47. Bourbeau PP, Heiter BJ. Comparison of Vitek GNI and GNI+ cards for identification of gram-negative bacteria. J Clin Microbiol 1998;36:2775–2777.

48. Brenner DJ. Enterobacteriaceae. In: Krieg NR, Holt JG. eds. Bergey's Manual of Systematic Bacteriology. Vol 1. Baltimore: Williams & Wilkins, 1984:408–420.

49. Brenner DJ, Bercovier H, Ursing J, et al. *Yersinia intermedia*: a new species of Enterobacteriaceae composed of rhamnose-positive, melibiose-positive, raffinose-positive strains (formerly called *Yersinia enterocolitica* or *Yersinia enterocolitica*-like). Curr Microbiol 1980;4:207:212.

50. Brenner DJ, Davis BR, Steigerwalt AG, et al. Atypical biogroups of *Escherichia coli* found in clinical specimens and description of *Escherichia hermanii* sp. nov. J Clin Microbiol 1982;15:703–713.

51. Brenner DJ, Grimont PAD, Steigerwalt AG, et al. Classification of citrobacteria by DNA hybridization: designation of *Citrobacter farmeri* sp. nov., *Citrobacter youngae* sp. nov., *Citrobacter braakii* sp. nov., *Citrobacter werkmanii* sp. nov.,

Citrobacter sedlakii sp. nov., and three unnamed *Citrobacter* genomospecies. Int J Syst Bacteriol 1993;43:645–658.

52. Brenner DJ, Hickman-Brenner FW, et al. Replacement of NCTC 4175, the current type strain of *Proteus vulgaris*, with ATCC 29905: request for an opinion. Int J Syst Bacteriol 1995;45:870–871.

53. Brenner DJ, McWhorter AC, Kai A, et al. *Enterobacter asburiae* sp. nov., a new species found in clinical specimens, and reassignment of *Erwinia dissolvens* and *Erwinia nimipressuralis* to the genus *Enterobacter* as *Enterobacter dissolvens* comb. nov. and *Enterobacter nimipressuralis* comb. nov. J Clin Microbiol 1986;23:1114–1120.

54. Brenner DJ, McWhorter AC, Leete-Knutson JK, et al. *Escherichia vulneris*: a new species of Enterobacteriaceae associated with human wounds. J Clin Microbiol 1982;15:1133–1140.

55. Brenner DJ, Muller HE, Steigerwalt AG, et al. Two new *Rahnella* genomospecies that cannot be phenotypically differentiated from *Rahnella aquatilis*. Int J Syst Bacteriol 1998;48:141–149.

56. Brenner DJ, Richard C, Steigerwalt AG, et al. *Enterobacter gergoviae* sp. nov.: a new species of Enterobacteriaceae found in clinical specimens and environment. Int J Syst Bacteriol 1980;30:1:6.

57. Brenner DJ, Ursing J, Bercovier H, et al. Deoxyribonucleic acid relatedness in *Yersinia enterocolitica* and *Yersinia enterocolitica*-like organisms. Curr Microbiol 1980;4:195–200.

58. Brenner FW, Villar RG, Angulo FJ, et al. *Salmonella* nomenclature. J Clin Microbiol 2000;38:2465–2467.

59. Breuer T, Benkel DH, Shapiro RL, et al. A multistate outbreak of *Escherichia coli* O157:H7 infections linked to alfalfa sprouts grown from contaminated seeds. Emerg Infect Dis 2001;7:977–982.

60. Brooker DC, Lund ME, Blazevic DJ. Rapid test for lysine decarboxylase activity in Enterobacteriaceae. Appl Microbiol 1973;26:622–623.

61. Brooks JT, Bergmire-Sweat D, Kennedy M, et al. Outbreak of shiga toxin-producing *Escherichia coli* O111:H8 infections among attendees of a high school cheerleading camp. Clin Infect Dis 2004;38:190–198.

62. Brooks JT, Sowers EG, Wells JG, et al. Non-O157 Shiga toxin-producing *Escherichia coli* reported to CDC, 1983–2000 (abstract 856). In: Program and abstracts of the 39th Annual Meeting of the Infectious Diseases Society of America (San Francisco): Alexandria, VA: Infectious Diseases Society of America, 2001:185.

63. Bruckner DA, Colonna P, Glenn D, et al. *Citrobacter farmeri* bacteremia in a child with short-bowel syndrome. J Clin Microbiol 1997;35:3353–3354.

64. Caldwell ME, Ryerson DL. Salmonellosis in certain reptiles. J Infect Dis 1939; 65:242–245.

65. Caprioli A, Tozzi AE. Epidemiology of Shiga toxin-producing *Escherichia coli* infections in continental Europe. In: Kaper JB, O'Brien AD, eds. *Escherichia coli* O157:H7 and other Shiga toxin-producing *E. coli* strains. Washington, DC: American Society for Microbiology Press, 1998:38–48.

66. Carinder JE, Chua JD, Corales RB, et al. *Rahnella aquatilis* bacteremia in a patient with relapsed acute lymphoblastic leukemia. Scand J Infect Dis 2001; 33:471–473.

67. Carlquist PR: A biochemical test for separating paracolon groups. J Bacteriol 1956;71:339:341.

68. Caroff N, Chamoux C, Le Gallou F, et al. Two epidemiologically related cases of *Rahnella aquatilis* bacteremia. Eur J Clin Microbiol Infect Dis 1998;17: 349–352.

69. Carpenter CCJ: Shigellosis. In Wyngaarden JB, Smith LH, eds. Cecil Textbook of Medicine. 16th ed. Philadelphia: Saunders, 1982:1517–1519.

70. Carrero P, Garrote JA, Pacheco S, et al. Report of six cases of human infection by *Serratia plymuthica*. J Clin Microbiol 1995;33:275–276.s

71. Carricajo A, Boiste S, Thore J, et al. Comparative evaluation of five chromogenic media for detection, enumeration and identification of urinary tract pathogens. Eur J Clin Microbiol Infect Dis 1999;18:796–803.

72. Carter J, Bowden FJ, Sriprakash KS, et al. Diagnostic polymerase chain reaction for donovanosis. Clin Infect Dis 1999;28:1168–1169.

73. Carter JS, Bowden FJ, Bastian I, et al. Phylogenetic evidence for reclassification of *Calymmatobacterium granulomatis* as *Klebsiella granulomatis* comb. nov. Int J Syst Bacteriol 1999;49:1695–1700.

74. Carter JS, Kemp DJ. A colorimetric detection system for *Calymmatobacterium granulomatis*. Sex Transm Infect 2000;76:134–136.

75. Cassar R, Cuschieri P. Comparison of *Salmonella* chromogenic medium with DCLS agar for isolation of *Salmonella* species from stool specimens. J Clin Microbiol 2003;41:3229–3232.

76. Castillo CB, Bruckner DA. Comparative evaluation of the Eiken and API 20E systems and conventional methods for identification of members of the family Enterobacteriaceae. J Clin Microbiol 1984;20:754–757.

77. Centers for Disease Control and Prevention. *Salmonella* surveillance: annual summary, 2001. Atlanta: Department of Health and Human Services, 2002.

78. Centers for Disease Control and Prevention. *Shigella* surveillance: annual summary, 2001. Atlanta: Department of Health and Human Services, 2002.

79. Centers for Disease Control and Prevention. HIP investigates *Enterobacter hormaechei* infections. CDC/NCID Focus Fol 1993;3(5).

80. Centers for Disease Control and Prevention. *Arizona hinshawii* septicemia associated with rattlesnake powder—California. MMWR Morb Mortal Wkly Rep 1983;32:464–465.

81. Centers for Disease Control and Prevention. Gastrointestinal illness associated with imported Brie cheese—District of Columbia. MMWR Morb Mortal Wkly Rep 1983;32:533.

82. Centers for Disease Control and Prevention. Update: milkborne salmonellosis—Illinois. MMWR Morb Mortal Wkly Rep 1985;34:200.

83. Centers for Disease Control and Prevention. Update: *Salmonella enteritidis* infections and shell eggs—United States, 1990. MMWR Morb Mortal Wkly Rep 1990;39:909.

84. Centers for Disease Control and Prevention. Update: *Yersinia enterocolitica* bacteremia and endotoxin shock associated with red blood cell transfusions—United States, 1991. MMWR Morb Mortal Wkly Rep 1991;40:176–178.

85. Centers for Disease Control and Prevention. Outbreak of *Salmonella enteritidis* infection associated with consumption of raw shell eggs, 1991. MMWR Morb Mortal Wkly Rep 1992;41:369–372.

86. Centers for Disease Control and Prevention. Pneumonic plague—Arizona, 1992. MMWR Morb Mortal Wkly Rep 1992;41:737–739.

87. Centers for Disease Control and Prevention. Outbreaks of *Salmonella enteritidis* gastroenteritis—California, 1993. MMWR Morb Mortal Wkly Rep 1993;42: 793–797.

88. Centers for Disease Control and Prevention. Outbreak of *Salmonella enteritidis* associated with nationally distributed ice cream products—Minnesota, South Dakota, and Wisconsin, 1994. MMWR Morb Mortal Wkly Rep 1994;43: 740–741.

89. Centers for Disease Control and Prevention. Reptile-associated salmonellosis—selected states, 1994–1995. MMWR Morb Mortal Wkly Rep 1995;44: 347–350.

90. Centers for Disease Control and Prevention. Outbreak of acute gastroenteritis attributable to *Escherichia coli* serotype O104:H21—Helena, Montana, 1994. MMWR Morb Mortal Wkly Rep 1995;44:501–503.

91. Centers for Disease Control and Prevention. Outbreaks of *Escherichia coli* O157: H7 infection and cryptosporidiosis associated with drinking unpasteurized apple cider—Connecticut and New York, October 1996. MMWR Morb Mortal Wkly Rep 1997;46: 4–8.

92. Centers for Disease Control and Prevention. Red blood cell transfusions contaminated with *Yersinia enterocolitica*—United States, 1991–1996, and initiation of a national study to detect bacteria-associated transfusion reactions. MMWR Morb Mortal Wkly Rep 1997;46:553–555.

93. Centers for Disease Control and Prevention. Fatal human plague—Arizona and Colorado, 1996. MMWR Morb Mortal Wkly Rep 1997;46:617–620.

94. Centers for Disease Control and Prevention. Reptile-associated salmonellosis—selected states, 1996–1998. MMWR Morb Mortal Wkly Rep 1999;48: 1009–1013.

95. Centers for Disease Control and Prevention. Outbreaks of *Salmonella* serotype Enteritidis infection associated with eating raw or undercooked shell eggs—United States, 1996–1998. MMWR Morb Mortal Wkly Rep 2000;49:73–79.

96. Centers for Disease Control and Prevention. *Escherichia coli* O111:H8 outbreak among teenage campers—Texas, 1999. MMWR Morb Mortal Wkly Rep 2000; 49:321–324.

97. Centers for Disease Control and Prevention. Outbreak of *Escherichia coli* O157: H7 infection associated with eating fresh cheese curds—Wisconsin, June 1998. MMWR Morb Mortal Wkly Rep 2000;49: 911–913.

98. Centers for Disease Control and Prevention. Outbreaks of Escherichia coli O157: H7 infections among children associated with farm visits—Pennsylvania and Washington, 2000. MMWR Morb Mortal Wkly Rep 2001;50:293–297.

99. Centers for Disease Control and Prevention. *Enterobacter sakazakii* infections associated with the use of powdered infant formula—Tennessee, 2001. MMWR Morb Mortal Wkly Rep 2002;51:297–300.

100. Centers for Disease Control and Prevention. Outbreak of multidrug-resistant *Salmonella* Newport—United States, January—April 2002. MMWR Morb Mortal Wkly Rep 2002;51:545–548.

101. Centers for Disease Control and Prevention. Imported plague—New York City, 2002, MMWR Morb Mortal Wkly Rep 2003;52:725–728.

102. Centers for Disease Control and Prevention. Yersinia enterocolitica gastroenteritis among infants exposed to chitterlings—Chicago, Illinois, 2002. MMWR Morb Mortal Wkly Rep 2003;52:956–958.

103. Centers for Disease Control and Prevention. Reptile-associated salmonellosis—selected states, 1998–2002. MMWR Morb Mortal Wkly Rep 2003;52: 1206–1209.

104. Centers for Disease Control and Prevention. Summary of provisional cases of selected notifiable diseases, United States, cumulative, week ending January 3, 2004 (53rd) week. MMWR Morb Mortal Wkly Rep 2004;52:1297.

105. Chagla AH, Borczyk AA, Aldom JE, et al. Evaluation of the L-pyrrolidonyl-beta-naphthylamide hydrolysis test for the differentiation of member of the families Enterobacteriaceae and Vibrionaceae. J Clin Microbiol 1993;31:1946–1948.

106. Chang CL, Jeong J, Shin JH, et al. *Rahnella aquatilis* sepsis in an immunocompetent adult. J Clin Microbiol 1999;37:4161–4162.

107. Chanteau S, Rahalison L, Ralafiarisoa L, et al. Development and testing of a rapid diagnostic test for bubonic and pneumonic plague. Lancet 2003;361:211–216.

108. Chapman PA, Siddons CA, Zadik PM, Jewes L. An improved selective medium for the isolation of *Escherichia coli* O157. J Med Microbiol 1991;35:107–110.

109. Chapman PA, Wright DJ, Siddons CA. A comparison of immunomagnetic separation and direct culture for the isolation of verocytotoxin-producing *Escherichia coli* O157 from bovine faeces. J Med Microbiol 1994;40:424–427.

110. Chaux C, Crepy M, Xueref S, et al. Comparison of three chromogenic agar plates for isolation and identification of urinary tract pathogens. Clin Microbiol Infect 2002;8:641–645.

111. Chester B, Moskowitz LB. Rapid catalase supplemental test for identification of members of the family Enterobacteriaceae. J Clin Microbiol 1987;25:439–441.

112. Chmel H. *Serratia odorifera* biogroup 1 causing an invasive human infection. J Clin Microbiol 1988;26:1244–1245.

113. Christensen WB. Urea decomposition as a means of differentiating *Proteus* and paracolon cultures from each 72. other and from *Salmonella* and *Shigella* types. J Bacteriol 1946;52:461–466.

114. Christiaens E, Hansen W, Moinet J. Isolament des expectorations d'un patient atteint de leucemie lymphoide chronique et de broncho-emphyseme d' une Enterobacteriaceae nouvellement decrite: *Rahnella aquatilis*. Med Maladies Infect 1987;17:732–734.

115. Clark NC, Hill BC, O'Hara CM, Steingrimsson O, Cooksey RC: Epidemiologic typing of *Enterobacter sakazakii* in two neonatal nosocomial outbreaks. Diagn Microbiol Infect Dis 1990;13:467–472.

116. Clark RB, Janda JM. Isolation of *Serratia plymuthica* from a human burn site. J Clin Microbiol 1985;21:656–657.

117. Clarridge JE, Musher DM, Fainstein V, et al. Extraintestinal human infection caused by *Edwardsiella tarda*. J Clin Microbiol 1980;11:511–514.

118. Clayland BG, Clayland C, Tomfohrde KM, et al. Full spectrum automation for the clinical microbiology laboratory. Am Clin Lab 1989;May:30–34

119. Cohen ML, Potter M, Pollard R, Feldman RA. Turtle-associated salmonellosis in the United States: effect of public health action, 1970–1976. JAMA 1980;243:1247–1249.

120. Coudron PE, Markowitz SM. *Cedecea lapagei* isolated from lung tissue. Clin Microbiol Newslett 1987;9:171–172.

121. Coutlée F, Saint-Jean LA, Plante R. Infection with *Edwardsiella tarda* related to a vascular prosthesis. Clin Infect Dis 1992;14:621–622.

122. Cover TL, Aber RC. *Yersinia enterocolitica*. N Engl J Med 1989;321:16:24.

123. Crchova V, Grondin C. Urinary infection due to *Yersinia pseudotuberculosis*. Vie Med Can Fr 1973;2:3–5.

124. Crosa JH, Brenner DJ, Ewing WH, et al. Molecular relationships among the salmonellae. J Bacteriol 1973;115:307–315.

125. Curless RG. Neonatal intracranial abscess: two cases caused by *Citrobacter* and a literature review. Ann Neurol 1980;8:269–272.

126. Dahl KM, Barry J, DeBiasi RL. *Escherichia hermanii* infection of a cephalohematoma: case report, review of the literature, and description of a novel invasive pathogen. Clin Infect Dis 2002;35:e96–e98.

127. Darbas H, Jean-Pierre H, Paillisson J. Case report and review of septicemia due to *Serratia ficaria*. J Clin Microbiol 1994;32:2285–2288.

128. da Silva CL, Miranda LE, Moreira BM, et al. *Enterobacter hormaechei* bloodstream infection at three neonatal intensive care units in Brazil. Pediatr Infect Dis J 2002;21:175–177.

129. De Baere T, Wauters G, Huylenbroeck A, et al. Isolation of *Leclercia adecarboxylata* from a patient with a chronically inflamed gallbladder and from a patient with sepsis without focus. J Clin Microbiol 2001;39:1674–1675.

130. De Baere T, Wauters G, Kämpfer P, et al. Isolation of *Buttiauxella gaviniae* from a spinal cord patient with urinary bladder pathology. J Clin Microbiol 2002;40:3867–3870.

131. Degirolami PC, Eichelberger KA, Salfity LC, et al. Evaluation of the AutoScan-3 devise for reading microdilution trays. J Clin Microbiol 1983;18:1292:1295.

132. Desenclos J-C A, Junejo S, Klontz KC. A cluster of *Edwardsiella tarda* infection in a day-care center in Florida. J Infect Dis 1990;162:782–783.

133. De Smedt JM, Bolderdijk RF. Dynamics of *Salmonella* isolation with modified semi-solid Rappaport-Vassiliadis medium. J Food Prot 1987;50:658–661.

134. Devenish JA, Ciebin BW, Brodsky MH. Novobiocin–brilliant green–glucose agar: new medium for isolation of salmonellae. Appl Environ Microbiol 1986;52:539–545.

135. Devreese K, Claeys G, Verschraegen G. Septicemia with *Ewingella americana*. J Clin Microbiol 1992;30:2746–2747.

136. Domingo D, Limia A, Alarcon T, et al. Nosocomial septicemia caused by *Serratia plymuthica*. J Clin Microbiol 1994;32:575–577.

137. Drancourt M, Bollet C, Carta A, et al. Phylogenetic analyses of *Klebsiella* species delineate *Klebsiella* and *Raoultella* gen. nov., with description of *Raoultella ornithinolytica* comb. nov., *Raoultella terrigena* comb. nov. and *Raoultella planticola* comb. nov. Int J Syst Evol Microbiol 2001;51:925–932.

138. Drow DL, Mercer L, Peacock JB. Splenic abscess caused by *Shigella flexneri* and *Bacteroides fragilis*. J Clin Microbiol 1984;19:79–80.

139. D'Souza HA, Campbell M, Baron EJ. Practical bench comparison of BBL CHROMagar Orientation and standard two-plate media for urine cultures. J Clin Microbiol 2004;42:60–64.

140. Dulguer MV, Fabbricotti SH, Bando SY, et al. Atypical enteropathogenic *Escherichia coli* strains: phenotypic and genetic profiling reveals a strong association between enteroaggregative *E. coli* heat stable enterotoxin and diarrhea. J Infect Dis 2003;188:1685–1694.

141. Dupont HL. *Shigella*. Infect Dis Clin N Am 1988;2:599–605.

142. Dupont HL. *Shigella* species (bacillary dysentery). In: Mandell GL, Bennett JE, Dolin R, eds. Principles and Practice of Infectious Diseases. 5th ed. Philadelphia: Churchill Livingstone, 2000:2363–2369.

143. Dupont HL, Levine MM, Hornick RB, et al. Inoculum size in shigellosis and implications for expected mode of transmission. J Infect Dis 1989;159:1126.

144. Dusch H, Altwegg M. Comparison of Rambach agar, SM-ID medium, and Hektoen enteric agar for primary isolation of non-typhi salmonellae from stool samples. J Clin Microbiol 1993;31:410–412.

145. Dusch H, Altwegg M. Evaluation of five new plating media for isolation of *Salmonella* species. J Clin Microbiol 1995;33:802–804.

146. Dyer J, Hayani KC, Janda WM, Schreckenberger PC. *Citrobacter sedlakii* meningitis and brain abscess in a premature infant. J Clin Microbiol 1997;35:2686–2688.

147. Edberg SC, Trepeta RW. Rapid and economical identification and antimicrobial susceptibility test methodology for urinary tract pathogens. J Clin Microbiol 1983;18:1287–1291.

148. Ederer GM, Clark M. Motility–indole–ornithine medium. Appl Microbiol 1970;20:849–850.

149. Edwards PR, Ewing WH. Identification of Enterobacteriaceae. 3rd ed. Minneapolis: Burgess, 1972.

150. Edwards PR, Fife MA. Lysine–iron agar in the detection of *Arizona* cultures. Appl Microbiol 1961;9:478–480.

151. Eidson M, Tierney LA, Roollag OJ, et al. Feline plague in New Mexico: risk factors and transmission to humans. Am J Public Health 1988;78:1333–1335.

152. Eigner U, Reissbrodt R, Hammann R, et al. Evaluation of a new chromogenic medium for the isolation and presumptive identification of *Salmonella* species from stool specimens. Eur J Clin Microbiol Infect Dis 2001;20:558–565.

153. Eklund M, Scheutz F, Siitonen A. Clinical isolates of non-O157 shiga toxin—producing Escherichia coli: serotypes, virulence characteristics, and molecular profiles of strains of the same serotype. J Clin Microbiol 2001;39:2829–2834.

154. Elin RJ, Robinson RA, Levin AS, et al. Lack of clinical usefulness of the limulus test in the diagnosis of endotoxemia. N Engl J Med 1975;293:521–524.

155. Engler HD, Troy K, Bottone EJ. Bacteremia and subcutaneous abscess caused by *Proteus penneri* in a neutropenic host. J Clin Microbiol 1990;28:1645–1646.

156. Euzéby JP. Revised *Salmonella* nomenclature: designation of *Salmonella enterica* (ex Kauffmann and Edwards 1952) Le Minor and Popoff 1987 sp. nov., nom. rev. as the neotype species of the genus *Salmonella* Lignieres 1900 (Approved Lists 1980), rejection of the name *Salmonella choleraesuis* (Smith 1894) Weldin 1927 (Approved Lists 1980), and conservation of the name *Salmonella typhi* (Schroeter 1886) Warren and Scott 1930 (Approved Lists 1980). Request for an Opinion. Int J Syst Bacteriol 1999;49:927–930.

157. Ewing WH. Identification of Enterobacteriaceae. 4th ed. New York: Elsevier, 1986.

158. Ewing WH, McWhorter AC, Escobar MR, et al. *Edwardsiella*, a new genus of Enterobacteriaceae, based on a new species of *E. tarda*. Int Bull Bact Nomencl Taxon 1965;15:33–38.

159. Ewing WH, Ross AJ, Brenner DJ, Fanning GR: *Yersinia ruckeri* sp. nov., the redmouth (RM) bacterium. Int J Syst Bacteriol 1978;28:37–44.

160. Fainstein V, Hopper RL, Mills K, Bodey GP. Colonization by or diarrhea due to *Kluyvera* species. J Infect Dis 1982;145:127.

161. Fainstein V, Yancey R, Trier P, Bodey GP. Overwhelming infection in a cancer patient caused by *Arizona hinshawii*: its relation to snake pill ingestion. Am J Infect Control 1982;10:147–148.

162. Falkow S. Activity of lysine decarboxylase as an aid in the identification of *Salmonella* and *Shigella*. Am J Clin Pathol 1958;29:598–600.

163. Farmer JJ III, Asbury MA, Hickman FW, et al. *Enterobacter sakazakii:* a new species of ''Enterobacteriaceae'' isolated from clinical specimens. Int J Syst Bacteriol 1980;30:569–584.

164. Farmer JJ III, Carter GP, Miller VL, Falkow S, Wachsmuth IK. Pyrazinamidase, CR-MOX agar, salicin fermentation-esculin hydrolysis, and D-xylose fermentation for identifying pathogenic serotypes of *Yersinia enterocolitica*. J Clin Microbiol 1992;30:2589–2594.s

165. Farmer JJ III, Davis BR, Hickman-Brenner FW, et al. Biochemical identification of new species and biogroups of Enterobacteriaceae isolated from clinical specimens. J Clin Microbiol 1985;21:46–76.

166. Farmer JJ III, Fanning GR, Davis BR, et al. *Escherichia fergusonii* and *Entero-*

bacter taylorae, two new species of Enterobacteriaceae isolated from clinical specimens. J Clin Microbiol 1985;21:77–81.

167. Farmer JJ III, Fanning GR, Huntley-Carter GP, et al. *Kluyvera,* a new (redefined) genus in the family Enterobacteriaceae: identification of *Kluyvera ascorbata* sp. nov. and *Kluyvera cryocrescens* sp. nov. in clinical specimens. J Clin Microbiol 1981;13:919–933.

168. Farmer JJ III, Jorgensen JH, Grimont PAD, et al. *Xenorhabdus luminescens* (DNA hybridization group 5) from human clinical specimens. J Clin Microbiol 1989;27:1594–1600.

169. Farmer JJ III, McWhorter AC. Genus X. *Edwardsiella* Ewing and McWhorter 1965, 37[AL]. In: Krieg NR, Holt JG, eds. Bergey's Manual of Systematic Bacteriology. vol 1. Baltimore: Williams & Wilkins, 1984:486–491.

170. Farmer JJ III, Sheth NK, Hudzinski JA, et al. Bacteremia due to *Cedecea neteri* sp. nov. J Clin Microbiol 1982;16:775–778.

171. Fay GD, Barry AL. Rapid ornithine decarboxylase test for the identification of Enterobacteriaceae. Appl Microbiol 1972;23:710–713.

172. Ferragut C, Izard D, Gavini F, et al. *Klebsiella trevisanii:* a new species from water and soil. Int J Syst Bacteriol 1983;33:133–142.

173. Ferragut C, Izard D, Gavini F, et al. *Buttiauxella,* a new genus of the family Enterobacteriaceae. Zentralbl Bakteriol Parasitenkd Infektionskr Hyg Abt 1 Orig Reihe C 1981;2:33–44.

174. Fischer-Le Saux M, Viallard V, Brunel B, et al. Polyphasic classification of the genus *Photorhabdus* and proposal of new taxa: *P. luminescens* subsp. *luminescens* subsp. nov., *P. luminescens* subsp. *akhurstii* subsp. nov., *P. luminescens* subsp. *laumondii* subsp. nov., *P. temperata* sp. nov., *P. temperata* subsp. *temperata* subsp. nov. and *P. asymbiotica* sp. nov. Int J System Bacteriol 1999;49: 1645–1656.

175. Foberg U, Fryden A, Kihlstrom E, et al. *Yersinia enterocolitica* septicemia: clinical and microbiological aspects. Scand J Infect Dis 1986;18:269–279.

176. Frederiksen W. Correct names of the species *Citrobacter koseri, Levinea malonatica,* and *Citrobacter diversus:* request for an opinion. Int J Syst Bacteriol 1990;40:107–108.

177. Freney J, Fleurette J, Gruer LD, et al. *Klebsiella trevisanii* colonization and septicaemia. Lancet 1984;1:909.

178. Freney J, Gavini F, Alexandre H, et al. Nosocomial infection and colonization by *Klebsiella trevisanii.* J Clin Microbiol 1986;23:948–950.

179. Freney J, Gavini F, Ploton C, et al. Isolation of *Escherichia fergusonii* from a patient with septicemia in France. Eur J Clin Microbiol Infect Dis 1987;6:78.

180. Funke G, Hany A, Altwegg M. Isolation of *Escherichia fergusonii* from four different sites in a patient with pancreatic carcinoma and cholangiosepsis. J Clin Microbiol 1993;31:2201–2203.

181. Funke G, Monnet D, deBernardis C, et al. Evaluation of the VITEK 2 system for rapid identification of medically relevant gram-negative rods. J Clin Microbiol 1998;36:1948–1952.

182. Funke G, Rosner H. *Rahnella aquatilis* bacteremia in an HIV-infected intravenous drug abuser. Diag Microbiol Infect Dis 1995;22:293–296.

183. Gage KL, Dennis DT, Orloski KA, et al. Cases of cat-associated human plague in the western US, 1977–1998. Clin Infect Dis 2000;30:893–900.

184. Gailllot O, Di Camillo P, Berche P, et al. Comparison of CHROMagar Salmonella medium and Hektoen enteric agar for isolation of salmonellae from stool samples. J Clin Microbiol 1999;37:762–765.

185. Garcia A, Fox JG. The rabbit as a new reservoir host of enterohemorrhagic Escherichia coli. Emerg Infect Dis 2003;9:1592–1597.

186. Gavin PJ, Warren JR, Obias AA, et al. Evaluation of the Vitek 2 system for rapid identification of clinical isolates of gram-negative bacilli and members of the family Streptococcaceae. Eur J Clin Microbiol Infect Dis 2002;21:869–874.

187. Gavini F, Izard D, Grimont PAD, et al. Priority of *Klebsiella planticola* Bagley, Seidler, and Brenner 1982 over *Klebsiella trevisanii* Ferragut, Izard, Gavini, Kersters, DeLey, and Leclerc 1983. Int J Syst Bacteriol 1986;36:486–488.

188. Gavini F, Mergaert J, Beji A, et al. Transfer of *Enterobacter agglomerans* (Beijerinck 1888) Ewing and Fife 1972 to *Pantoea* gen. nov. as *Pantoea agglomerans* comb. nov. and description of *Pantoea dispersa* sp. nov. Int J Syst Bacteriol 1989;39:337–345.

189. Gayraud M, Scavizzi MR, Mollaret HH, et al. Antibiotic treatment of *Yersinia enterocolitica* septicemia: a retrospective review of 43 cases. Clin Infect Dis 1993;17:405–410.

190. Gerrard JG, McNevin S, Alfredson D, et al. *Photorhabdus* species: bioluminescent bacteria as emerging human pathogens? Emerg Infect Dis 2003;9:251–254.

191. Giamarellou H, Antoniadou A, Kanavos K, et al. *Yersinia enterocolitica* endocarditis: case report and literature review. Eur J Clin Microbiol Infect Dis 1995; 14:126–130.

192. Giammanco G, Pignato S, Agodi A. A simple chromogenic test for rapid screening of *Proteus* and *Providencia* bacteria. Microbiologica 1985;8:395–397.

193. Gill VJ, Farmer JJ III, Grimont PAD, et al. *Serratia ficaria* isolated from a human clinical specimen. J Clin Microbiol 1981;14:234–236.

194. Ginsberg HG, Daum RS. *Escherichia hermanii* sepsis with duodenal perforation in a neonate. Pediatr Infect Dis J 1987;6:300–302.

195. Glustein JZ, Rudensky B, Abrahamov A. Catheter-associated sepsis caused by *Serratia odorifera* biovar 1 in an adolescent patient. Eur J Clin Microbiol Infect Dis 1994;13:183–184.

196. Glynn MK, Bopp C, Dewitt W, et al. Emergence of multidrug-resistant *Salmonella enterica* serotype Typhimurium DT104 infections in the United States. N Engl J Med 1998;338:1333–1338.

197. Goldstein EJC, Lewis RP, Martin WJ, et al. Infections caused by *Klebsiella ozaenae:* a changing disease spectrum. J Clin Microbiol 1978;8:413–418.

198. Goossens H, Wauters G, De Boeck M, et al. Semisolid selective-motility enrichment medium for isolation of salmonellae from fecal specimens. J Clin Microbiol 1984;19:940–941.

199. Goubau P, Van Aelst F, Verhaegen J, Boogaerts M. Septicaemia caused by *Rahnella aquatilis* in an immunocompromised patient. Eur J Clin Microbiol Infect Dis 1988;7:697–699.

200. Graham DR, Anderson RL, Ariel FE, et al. Epidemic nosocomial meningitis due to *Citrobacter diversus* in neonates. J Infect Dis 1981;144:203–209.

201. Graham DR, Band JD. *Citrobacter diversus* brain abscess and meningitis in neonates. JAMA 1981;245:1923–1925.

202. Granier SA, Leflon-Guibout V, Goldstein FW, et al. Enterobacterial repetitive intergenic consensus 1R PCR assay for detection of *Raoultella* sp. isolates among strains identified as *Klebsiella oxytoca* in the clinical laboratory. J Clin Microbiol 2003;41:1740–1742.

203. Granier SA, Plaisance L, Leflon-Guibout V, et al. Recognition of two genetic groups in *Klebsiella oxytoca* taxon on the basis of the chromosomal beta-lactamase and housekeeping gene sequences as well as ERIC PCR typing. Int J Syst Evol Microbiol 2003;53:661–668.

204. Greenblatt RB, Barfield WE. Newer methods in the diagnosis and treatment of granuloma inguinale. Br J Ven Dis 1952;28:123–128.

205. Grimont PAD, Farmer JJ III, Grimont F, et al. *Ewingella americana* gen. nov. sp. nov. A new Enterobacteriaceae isolated from clinical specimens. Ann Microbiol (Paris) 1983;134A:39–52.

206. Grimont PAD, Grimont F, Farmer JJ III, Asbury MA. *Cedecea davisae* gen. nov., sp. nov. and *Cedecea lapagei* sp. nov., new Enterobacteriaceae from clinical specimens. Int J Syst Bacteriol 1981;31:317–326.

207. Grimont PAD, Grimont F, Richard C, et al. *Edwardsiella hoshinae,* a new species of Enterobacteriaceae. Curr Microbiol 1980;4:347–351.

208. Gupta A, Fontana J, Crowe C, et al. Emergence of multidrug-resistant *Salmonella enterica* serotype Newport infections resistant to expanded-spectrum cephalosporins in the United States. J Infect Dis 2003;188:1707–1716.

209. Hamilton-Miller JMT, Shah S. Identity and antibiotic susceptibility of enterobacterial flora of salad vegetables. Int J Antimicrob Agents 2001;18:81–83.

210. Hansen DS, Jensen AG, Nørskov-Lauritsen N, et al. Direct identification and susceptibility testing of enteric bacilli from positive blood cultures using VITEK (GNI+/GNS-GA). Clin Microbiol Infect 2002;8:38–44.

211. Hansen MW, Glupczynski GY. Isolation of an unusual *Cedecea* species from a cutaneous ulcer. Eur J Clin Microbiol 1984;3:152–153.

212. Harrell LJ, Cameron ML, O'Hara CM. *Rahnella aquatilis,* an unusual gram-negative rod isolated from the bronchial washing of a patient with acquired immunodeficiency syndrome. J Clin Microbiol 1989;27:1671–1672.

213. Hauben L, Moore ERB, Vauterin L, et al. Phylogenetic position of phytopathogens within the *Enterobacteriaceae.* System Appl Microbiol 1998;21:384–397.

214. Hawke JP, McWhorter AC, Steigerwalt AG, et al. *Edwardsiella ictaluri* sp. nov., the causative agent of enteric septicemia of catfish. Int J Syst Bacteriol 1981; 31:396–400.

215. Head CB, Whitty DA, Ratnam S. Comparative study of selective media for recovery of *Yersinia enterocolitica.* J Clin Microbiol 1982;16:615–621.

216. Heizmann WR, Michel R. Isolation of *Ewingella americana* from a patient with conjunctivitis. Eur J Clin Microbiol Infect Dis 1991;10:957–959.

217. Hengstler KA, Hammann R, Fahr A-M. Evaluation of BBL CHROMagar Orientation medium for detection and presumptive identification of urinary tract pathogens. J Clin Microbiol 1997;35:2773–2777.

218. Heuvelink AE, van Heerwaarden C, Zwartkruis-Nahuis JT, et al. *Escherichia coli* O157 infection associated with a petting zoo. Epidemiol Infect 2002;129: 295–302.

219. Hickman FW, Steigerwalt AG, Farmer JJ III, Brenner DJ. Identification of *Proteus penneri* sp. nov., formerly known as *Proteus vulgaris* indole negative or as *Proteus vulgaris* biogroup 1. J Clin Microbiol 1982;15:1097–1102.

220. Hickman-Brenner FW, Farmer JJ III, Steigerwalt AG, et al. *Providencia rustigianii:* a new species in the family Enterobacteriaceae formerly known as *Providencia alcalifaciens* biogroup 3. J Clin Microbiol 1983;17:1057–1060.

221. Hickman-Brenner FW, Huntley-Carter GP, Fanning GR, et al. *Koserella trabulsii,* a new genus and species of Enterobacteriaceae formerly known as enteric group 45. J Clin Microbiol 1985;21:39–42.

222. Hickman-Brenner FW, Huntley-Carter GP, Saitoh Y, et al. *Moellerella wisconsensis,* a new genus and species of Enterobacteriaceae found in human stool specimens. J Clin Microbiol 1984;19:460–463.

223. Hickman-Brenner FW, Vohra MP, Huntley-Carter GP, et al. *Leminorella,* a new genus of Enterobacteriaceae: identification of *Leminorella grimontii* sp. nov.

and *Leminorella richardii* sp. nov. found in clinical specimens. J Clin Microbiol 1985;21:234–239.

224. Hodges GR, Degener CE, Barnes WG. Clinical significance of *Citrobacter* isolates. Am J Clin Pathol 1978;70:37–40.

225. Hollis DG, Hickman FW, Fanning GR, et al. *Tatumella ptyseos* gen. nov., sp. nov., a member of the family Enterobacteriaceae found in clinical specimens. J Clin Microbiol 1981;14:79–88.

226. Holmes B, Costas M, Ganner M, et al. Evaluation of Biolog system for identification of some gram-negative bacteria of clinical importance. J Clin Microbiol 1994;32:1970–1975.

227. Holt-Harris JE, Teague O. A new culture medium for the isolation of *Bacillus typhosus* from stools. J Infect Dis 1916;18:596–600.

228. Hoppe JE, Herter M, Aleksic S, et al. Catheter-related *Rahnella aquatilis* bacteremia in a pediatric bone marrow transplant recipient. J Clin Microbiol 1993;31: 1911–1912.

229. Horii T, Suzuki Y, Kimura T, et al. Intravenous catheter–related septic shock caused by *Staphylococcus sciuri* and *Escherichia vulneris*. Scand J Infect Dis 2001;33:930–932.

229a.Hormaeche E, Edwards PR. Proposal for the rejection of the generic name *Cloaca* Castellani and Chalmers, and proposal of *Enterobacter* as a generic name with designation of type species and of its type culture, with request for an opinion. Int Bull Bacteriol. Nomencl Taxon 1960;10:75–76.

230. Horowitz HW, Nadelman RB, Van Horn KG, et al. *Serratia plymuthica* sepsis associated with infection of central venous catheter. J Clin Microbiol 1987;25: 1562–1563.

231. Houang ETS, Tam PC, Lui SL, et al. The use of CHROMagar Orientation as a primary isolation medium with presumptive identification for the routine screening of urine specimens. Acta Pathol Microbiol Immunol Scand 1999;107: 859–862.

232. Huber TW, Thomas JS. Detection of resistance due to inducible β-lactamase in *Enterobacter aerogenes* and *Enterobacter cloacae*. J Clin Microbiol 1994;32: 2481–2486.

233. Huys G, Cnockaert M, Janda JM, Swings J. *Escherichia albertii* sp. nov., a diarrhoeagenic species isolated from stool specimens of Bangladeshi children. Int J Syst Evol Microbiol 2003;53:807–810.

234. Inoue K, Miki K, Tamura K, et al. Evaluation of L-pyrrolidonyl peptidase paper strip test for differentiation of members of the family Enterobacteriaceae, particularly *Salmonella* spp. J Clin Microbiol 1996;34:1811–1812.

235. Inoue K, Sugiyama K, Kosako Y, et al. *Enterobacter cowanii* sp. nov., a new species of the family Enterobacteriaceae. Curr Microbiol 2000;41:417–420.

236. Izard D, Ferragut C, Gavini F, et al. *Klebsiella terrigena*, a new species from soil and water. Int J Syst Bacteriol 1981;31:116–127.

237. Izard D, Gavini F, Trinel PA, Leclerc H. *Rahnella aquatilis*, nouveau membre de la famille des Enterobacteriaceae. Ann Microbiol 1979;130A:163–177.

238. Izard D, Gavini F, Trinel PA, Leclerc H. Deoxyribonucleic acid relatedness between *Enterobacter cloacae* and *Enterobacter amnigenus* sp. nov. Int J Syst Bacteriol 1981;31:35–42.

239. Jacobs J, Jamaer D, Vandeven J, et al. *Yersinia enterocolitica* in donor blood: a case report and review. J Clin Microbiol 1989;27:1119–1121.

240. Jacoby GA, Han P. Detection of extended-spectrum β-lactamases in clinical isolates of *Klebsiella pneumoniae* and *Escherichia coli*. J Clin Microbiol 1996; 34:908–911.

241. Jan D, Berlie C, Babin G. Fatal posttransfusion *Enterobacter amnigenus* septicemia. Presse Med 1999;28:965.

242. Janda JM, Abbott SL. Infections associated with the genus *Edwardsiella*: the role of *Edwardsiella tarda* in human disease. Clin Infect Dis 1993;17:742–748.

243. Janda JM, Abbott SL. Expression of an iron-regulated hemolysin by *Edwardsiella tarda*. FEMS Microbial Lett 1993;111:275–280.

244. Janda JM, Abbott SL. The *Enterobacteriaceae*. Philadelphia: Lippincott-Raven, 1998.

245. Janda JM, Abbott SL, Albert MJ. Prototypal diarrheagenic strains of *Hafnia alvei* are actually members of the genus *Escherichia*. J Clin Microbiol 1999;37: 2399–2401.

246. Janda JM, Abbott SL, Cheung WKW, et al. Biochemical identification of citrobacteria in the clinical laboratory. J Clin Microbiol 1994;32:1850–1854.

247. Janda JM, Abbott SL, Woodward D, et al. Invasion of Hep-2 and other eukaryotic cell lines by providenciae: further evidence supporting the role of *Providencia alcalifaciens* in bacterial gastroenteritis. Curr Microbiol 1998;37:159–165.

248. Janda WM, Hellerman DV, Zeiger B, et al. Isolation of *Klebsiella ozaenae* from a corneal abscess. Am J Clin Pathol 1985;83:655–657.

249. Jarlier V, Nicolas M-H, Fournier G, Philippon A: Extended broad-spectrum β-lactamases conferring transferable resistance to newer β-lactam agents in Enterobacteriaceae: hospital prevalence and susceptibility patterns. Rev Infect Dis 1988;10:867–878.

250. Jensen KT, Frederiksen W, Hickman-Brenner FW, et al. Recognition of *Morganella* subspecies, with proposal of *Morganella morganii* subsp. *morganii* subsp. nov. and *Morganella morganii* subsp. *sibonii* subsp. nov. Int J Syst Bacteriol 1992;42:613–620.

251. Jensen N, Varelis P, Whitfield FB. Formation of guaiacol in chocolate milk by the psychrotrophic bacterium *Rahnella aquatilis*. Lett Appl Microbiol 2001;33: 339–343.

252. Johnson RP, Clarke RC, Wilson JB, et al. Growing concerns and recent outbreaks involving non-O157:H7 serotypes on verotoxigenic *Escherichia coli*. J Food Prot 1996;59:1112–1122.

253. Joker RN, Norholm T, Siboni KE. A case of neonatal meningitis caused by a yellow *Enterobacter*. Dan Med Bull 1965;12:128–130.

254. Kaper JB, O'Brien AD, eds. *Escherichia coli* O157:H7 and other Shiga toxin-producing *E. coli* strains. Washington DC: ASM Press, 1998.

255. Karch H, Janetzki-Mittmann C, Aleksic S, Datz M. Isolation of enterohemorrhagic *Escherichia coli* O157 strains from patients with hemolytic–uremic syndrome by using immunomagnetic separation, DNA-based methods, and direct culture. J Clin Microbiol 1996;34:516–519.

256. Karmali MA. Prospects for preventing serious systemic toxemic complications of shiga toxin-producing *Escherichia coli* infections using shiga toxin receptor analogues. J Infect Dis 2004;189:355–359.

257. Karmali MA, Steele BT, Petric M, et al. Sporadic cases of hemolytic uremic syndrome associated with fecal cytotoxin and cytotoxin-producing *Escherichia coli*. Lancet 1983;1:619–620.

258. Kati C, Bibashi E, Kokolina E, et al. Case of peritonitis caused by *Ewingella americana* in a patient undergoing continuous ambulatory peritoneal dialysis. J Clin Microbiol 1999;37:3733–3734.

259. Kehl KS, Havens P, Behnke CE, Acheson DWK. Evaluation of the premier EHEC assay for detection of Shiga toxin-producing Escherichia coli. J Clin Microbiol 1997;35:2051–2054.

260. Kehl SC. Role of the laboratory in the diagnosis of enterohemorrhagic *Escherichia coli* infections. J Clin Microbiol 2002;40:2711–2715.

261. Kelly MT, Leicester C. Evaluation of the Autoscan Walkaway system for rapid identification and susceptibility testing of gram-negative bacilli. J Clin Microbiol 1992;30:1568–1571.

262. Keren DF, Rawlings W, Murray HW, Leonard WR. *Arizona hinshawii* osteomyelitis with antecedent enteric fever and sepsis. Am J Med 1976;60:577–582.

263. Kharsany ABM, Hoosen AA, Kiepiela P, et al. Phylogenetic analysis of *Calymmatobacterium granulomatis* based on 16S rRNA gene sequences. J Med Microbiol 1999;48:841–847.

264. Kharsany ABM, Hoosen AA, Kiepiela P, et al. Growth and cultural characteristics of *Calymmatobacterium granulomatis*: the aetiological agent of granuloma inguinale (Donovanosis). J Med Microbiol 1997;46:579–585.

265. Kilian M, Bülow P. Rapid diagnosis of *Enterobacteriaceae*. I. Detection of bacterial glycosidases. Acta Pathol Microbiol Scand [B] 1976;84:245–251.

266. Kilian M, Bülow P. Rapid identification of *Enterobacteriaceae*: II. Use of a beta-glucuronidase detecting agar medium (PGUA agar) for the identification of *E. coli* in primary cultures of urine samples. Acta Pathol Microbiol Scand [B] 1979;87:271–276.

267. Kimmitt PT, Harwood CR, Barer MR. Toxin gene expression by Shiga toxin-producing *Escherichia coli*: the role of antibiotics and the bacterial SOS response. Emerg Infect Dis 2000;6:458–465.

268. King BM, Adler DL. A previously unclassified group of Enterobacteriaceae. Am J Clin Pathol 1964;41:230–232.

269. King S, Metzger WI. A new plating medium for the isolation of enteric pathogens: I. Hektoen enteric agar. Appl Microbiol 1968;16:577–578.

270. Kircher SM, Cote RJ, Dick NK, Seip WF. CO_2 incubation of MacConkey agar (MacConkey III). Abstr Annu Meet Am Soc Microbiol 2000;C274:194.

271. Kitch TT, Jacobs MR, Appelbaum PC. Evaluation of RapID onE system for identification of 379 strains in the family Enterobacteriaceae and oxidase-negative, gram-negative nonfermenters. J Clin Microbiol 1994;32:931–934.

272. Kleiman MB, Allen SD, Neal P, Reynolds J. Meningoencephalitis and compartmentalization of the cerebral ventricles caused by *Enterobacter sakazakii*. J Clin Microbiol 1981;14:352–354.

273. Kline MW. *Citrobacter* meningitis and brain abscess in infancy: epidemiology, pathogenesis, and treatment. J Pediatr 1988;113:430–434.

274. Kline MW, Mason EO, Kaplan SL. Characterization of *Citrobacter diversus* strains causing neonatal meningitis. J Infect Dis 1988;157:101–105.

275. Kosako Y, Sakazaki R. Priority of *Yokenella regensburgei* Kosako, Sakazaki, and Yoshizaki 1985 over *Koserella trabulsii* Hickman-Brenner, Huntley-Carter, Brenner, and Farmer 1985. Int J Syst Bacteriol 1991;41:171.

276. Kosako Y, Tamura K, Sakazaki R, et al. *Enterobacter kobei* sp. nov., a new species of the family Enterobacteriaceae resembling *Enterobacter cloacae*. Curr Microbiol 1996;33:261–265.

277. Kosako Y, Sakazaki R, Yoshizaki E. *Yokenella regensburgei* gen. nov., sp. nov.: a new genus and species in the family Enterobacteriaceae. Jpn J Med Sci Biol 1984;37:117–124.

277a.Koser SA. Utilization of the salts of organic acids by the colon-aerogenes group. J Bacteriol 1923;8:493-520.

278. Krajden S, Fuksa M, Petrea C, et al. Expanded clinical spectrum of infections caused by *Proteus penneri*. J Clin Microbiol 1987;25:578–579.

279. Lai KK. *Enterobacter sakazakii* infection among neonates, infants, children, and

adults: case reports and a review of the literature. Medicine (Baltimore) 2001;80:113–122.

280. Lee LA, Gerber AR, Lonsway DR, et al. *Yersinia enterocolitica* 0:3 infections in infants and children, associated with the household preparation of chitterlings. N Engl J Med 1990;322:984–987.

281. Lee LA, Taylor J, Carter GP, et al. *Yersinia enterocolitica* 0:3: an emerging cause of pediatric gastroenteritis in the United States. J Infect Dis 1991;163:660–663.

282. Le Minor L, Popoff MY. Request for an opinion: designation of *Salmonella enterica* sp. nov., nom. rev., as the type and only species of the genus *Salmonella*. Int J Syst Bacteriol 1987;37:465–468.

283. Le Minor L, Popoff MY, Laurent B, et al. Individualisation d'une septième sous-espèce de *Salmonella*: *S. choleraesuis* subsp. *indica* subsp. nov. Ann Inst Pasteur/Microbiol 1986;137B:211–217.

284. Le Minor L, Véron M, Popoff M. Taxonomie des *Salmonella*. Ann Microbiol (Inst Pasteur) 1982;133B:223–243.

285. Levine WN, Goldberg MJ. *Escherichia vulneris* osteomyelitis of the tibia caused by a wooden foreign body. Orthop Rev 1994;23:262–265.

286. Levy RL, Saunders RL. *Citrobacter* meningitis and cerebral abscess in early infancy: cure by moxalactam. Neurology 1981;31:1575–1577.

287. Linde H-J, Neubauer H, Meyer H, et al. Identification of *Yersinia* species by the Vitek GNI card. J Clin Microbiol 1999;37:211–214.

288. Ling TKW, Liu ZK, Cheng AFB. Evaluation of the VITEK 2 system for rapid direct identification and susceptibility testing of gram-negative bacilli from positive blood cultures. J Clin Microbiol 2003;41:4705–4707.

289. Ling TKW, Tam PC, Liu ZK, et al. Evaluation of VITEK 2 rapid identification and susceptibility testing system against gram-negative clinical isolates. J Clin Microbiol 2001;39:2964–2966.

290. Livermore DM. β-Lactamases in laboratory and clinical resistance. Clin Microbiol Rev 1995;8:557–584.

291. Ljungberg P, Valtonen M, Harjola VP, et al. Report of four cases of *Yersinia pseudotuberculosis* septicemia and a literature review. Eur J Clin Microbiol Infect Dis 1995;14:804–810.

292. Longhurst CA, West DC. Isolation of *Leclercia adecarboxylata* from an infant with acute lymphoblastic leukemia. Clin Infect Dis 2001;32:1659.

293. Ludwig K, Bitzan M, Zimmermann S, et al. Immune response to non-O157 vero toxin–producing *Escherichia coli* in patients with hemolytic uremic syndrome. J Infect Dis 1996;174:1028–1039.

294. Lund ME, Matsen JM, Blazevic DJ. Biochemical and antibiotic susceptibility studies of H₂S-negative *Citrobacter*. Appl Microbiol 1974;28:22–25.

295. Luperchio SA, Newman JV, Dangler CA, et al. *Citrobacter rodentium*, the causative agent of transmissible murine colonic hyperplasia, exhibits clonality: synonymy of *C. rodentium* and mouse-pathogenic *Escherichia coli*. J Clin Microbiol 2000;38:4343–4350.

296. Luttrell RE, Rannick GA, Soto-Hernandez JL, Verghese A. *Kluyvera* species soft tissue infection: case report and review. J Clin Microbiol 1988;26:2650–2651.

297. MacConkey A. Lactose-fermenting bacteria in feces. J Hyg 1905;5:333–378.

298. MacFaddin JF. Biochemical Tests for Identification of Medical Bacteria. 3rd Ed. Philadelphia: Lippincott Williams & Wilkins, 2000.

299. Mackenzie AMR, Lebel P, Orrbine E, et al. Sensitivities and specificities of Premier *E. coli* O157 and Premier EHEC enzyme immunoassays for diagnosis of infection with verotoxin (Shiga-like toxin)-producing *Escherichia coli*. J Clin Microbiol 1998;36:1608–1611.

300. Maddocks S, Olma T, Chen S. Comparison of CHROMagar Salmonella medium and xylose-lysine-desoxycholate and Salmonella-Shigella agars for isolation of *Salmonella* strains from stool samples. J Clin Microbiol 2002;40:2999–3003.

301. Maertens J, Delforge M, Vandenberghe P, et al. Catheter-related bacteremia due to *Ewingella Americana*. Clin Microbiol Infect 2001;7:103–104.

302. Mahajan RK, Khan SA, Chandel DS, et al. Fatal case of *Salmonella enterica* subsp. *arizonae* gastroenteritis in an infant with microcephaly. J Clin Microbiol 2003;41:5830–5832.

303. Maki DG, Rhame FS, Mackel DC, et al. Nationwide epidemic of septicemia caused by contaminated intravenous products: epidemiologic and clinical features. Am J Med 1976;60:471–485.

304. Mangum ME, Radisch D. *Cedecea* species: unusual clinical isolate. Clin Microbiol Newslett 1982;4:117–119.

305. Maraki S, Samonis G, Marnelakis E, Tselentis Y. Surgical wound infection caused by *Rahnella aquatilis*. J Clin Microbiol 1994;32:2706–2708.

306. March SB, Ratnam S. Sorbitol-MacConkey medium for detection of *Escherichia coli* O157:H7 associated with hemorrhagic colitis. J Clin Microbiol 1986;23:869–872.

307. Marsh PK, Gorbach SL. Invasive enterocolitis caused by *Edwardsiella tarda*. Gastroenterology 1982;82:336–338.

308. Mastroianni A, Coronado O, Chiodo F. *Morganella morganii* meningitis in a patient with AIDS. J Infect 1994;29:356–357.

309. Mazoyer MA, Orenga S, Doleans F, et al. Evaluation of CPS ID2 medium for detection of urinary tract bacterial isolates in specimens from a rehabilitation center. J Clin Microbiol 1995;33:1025–1027.

310. Mazzariol A, Zuliani J, Fontana R, et al. Isolation from blood culture of a *Leclercia adecarboxylata* strain producing an SHV-12 extended-spectrum beta-lactamase. J Clin Microbiol 2003;41:1738–1739.

311. McNeil MM, Davis BJ, Anderson RL, et al. Plasmids of *Ewingella Americana*: supplementary epidemiologic markers in an outbreak of pseudobacteremia. J Clin Microbiol 1987;25:501–503.

312. McNeil MM, Davis BJ, Anderson RL, et al. Mechanism of cross-contamination of blood culture bottles in outbreaks of pseudobacteremia associated with non-sterile blood collection tubes. J Clin Microbiol 1985;22:23–25.,

313. McNeil MM, Davis BJ, Solomon SL, et al. *Ewingella americana*: recurrent pseudobacteremia from a persistent environmental reservoir. J Clin Microbiol 1987;25:498–500.

314. McWhorter AC, Haddock RL, Nocon FA, et al. *Trabulsiella guamensis*, a new genus and species of the Family Enterobacteriaceae that resembles *Salmonella* subgroups 4 and 5. J Clin Microbiol 1991;29:1480–1485.

315. Mead PS, Griffin PM. *Escherichia coli* O157:H7. Lancet 1998;352:1207–1212.

316. Mead PS, Slutsker L, Dietz V, et al. Food-related illness and death in the United States. Emerg Infect Dis 1999;5:607–625.

317. Merlino J, Siarakas S, Robertson GJ, et al. Evaluation of CHROMagar Orientation for differentiation and presumptive identification of gram-negative bacilli and *Enterococcus* species. J Clin Microbiol 1996;34:1788–1793.

318. Mermel LA, Spiegel CA. Nosocomial sepsis due to *Serratia odorifera* biovar 1. Clin Infect Dis 1992;14:208–210.

319. Mermin J, Hutwagner L, Vugia D, et al. Reptiles, amphibians, and human *Salmonella* infection: a population-based, case-control study. Clin Infect Dis 2004;38(Suppl):S253–S261.

320. Metchock B, Lonsway DR, Carter GP, et al. *Yersinia enterocolitica*: a frequent seasonal stool isolate from children at an urban hospital in the southeast United States. J Clin Microbiol 1991;29:2868–2869.

321. Meyer KS, Urban C, Eagan JA, et al. Nosocomial outbreak of *Klebsiella* infection resistant to late-generation cephalosporins. Ann Intern Med 1993;119:353–358.

322. Meyer-Broseta S, Bastian SN, Arne PD, et al. Review of epidemiological surveys on the prevalence of contamination of healthy cattle with *Escherichia coli* serogroup O157:H7. Int J Hyg Environ Health 2001;203:347–361.

323. Miedouge M, Hacini J, Grimont F, Watine J. Shiga toxin–producing *Escherichia coli* urinary tract infection associated with hemolytic–uremic syndrome in an adult and possible adverse effect of ofloxacin therapy. Clin Infect Dis 2000;30:395–396.

324. Miller JM, Alachi P. Evaluation of new computer-enhanced identification program for microorganisms: adaption of BioBASE for identification of members of the family Enterobacteriaceae. J Clin Microbiol 1996;34:179–181.

325. Miller JM, Rhoden DL. Preliminary evaluation of Biolog, a carbon source utilization method for bacterial identification. J Clin Microbiol 1991;29:1143–1147.

326. Miller RG, Tate CR, Mallinson ET. Xylose–lysine–tergitol 4: an improved selective agar medium for the isolation of *Salmonella*. Poultry Sci 1991;70:2429–2432. (Erratum, Poultry Sci 1992;71:398.)

327. Mohle-Boetani JC, Farrar JA, Werner SB, et al. *Escherichia coli* O157 and *Salmonella* infections associated with sprouts in California, 1996–1998. Ann Intern Med 2001;135:239–247.

328. Møller V. Simplified tests for some amino acid decarboxylases and for the arginine dihydrolase system. Acta Pathol Microbiol Scand 1955;36:158–172.

329. Monnery I, Freydiere AM, Baron C, et al. Evaluation of two new chromogenic media for detection of *Salmonella* in stools. Eur J Clin Microbiol Infect Dis 1994;13:257–261.

330. Mori M, Ohta M, Agata N, et al. Identification of species and capsular types of *Klebsiella* clinical isolates, with special reference to *Klebsiella planticola*. Microbiol Immunol 1989;33:887–895.

331. Moss NS, Wilder D, Combs D, et al. Evaluation of the Vitek GNI+ Card. Abstr Annu Meet Am Soc Microbiol 1996;C389.

332. Mulczyk M, Szewczuk A. Pyrrolidonyl peptidase in bacteria: a new colorimetric test for differentiation of Enterobacteriaceae. J Gen Microbiol 1970;61:9–13.

333. Muller HE, Brenner DJ, Fanning GR, et al. Emended description of *Buttiauxella agrestis* with recognition of six new species of *Buttiauxella* and two new species of *Kluyvera*: *Buttiauxella ferragutiae* sp. nov., *Buttiauxella gaviniae* sp. nov., *Buttiauxella brennerae* sp. nov., *Buttiauxella izardii* sp. nov., *Buttiauxella noackiae* sp. nov., *Buttiauxella warmboldiae* sp. nov., *Kluyvera cochleae* sp. nov., and *Kluyvera georgiana* sp. nov. Int J Syst Bacteriol 1996;46:50–63.

334. Muller HE, O'Hara CM, Fanning GR, et al. *Providencia heimbachae*, a new species of Enterobacteriaceae isolated from animals. Int J Syst Bacteriol 1986;36:252–256.

335. Murphy TV, Nelson JD. *Shigella* vaginitis: report of 38 patients and review of the literature. Pediatrics 1979;63:511–516.

336. Muytjens HL, Zanen HC, Sonderkamp HJ, et al. Analysis of eight cases of neonatal meningitis and sepsis due to *Enterobacter sakazakii*. J Clin Microbiol 1983;18:115–120.

337. Nadler HL, Dolan C, Mele L, et al. Accuracy and reproducibility of the AutoMi-

crobic system gram-negative general susceptibility-plus card for testing selected challenge organisms. J Clin Microbiol 1985;22:355–360.

338. Naiel B, Raul R. Chronic prostatitis due to *Yersinia pseudotuberculosis*. J Clin Microbiol 1998;36:856.

339. Nataro JP, Kaper JB. Diarrheagenic *Escherichia coli*. Clin Microbiol Rev 1998; 11:142–201.

340. Nataro JP, Steiner T, Guerrant RL. Enteroaggregative *Escherichia coli*. Emerg Infect Dis 1998;4:251–261.

341. Nazarowec-White M, Farber JM. *Enterobacter sakazakii*: a review. Int J Food Microbiol 1997;34:103–113.

342. NCCLS. Abbreviated Identification of Bacteria and Yeast; Approved Guideline. NCCLS document M35-A. Wayne, PA: NCCLS, 2002.

343. Nettles RE, Sexton DJ. Successful treatment of *Edwardsiella tarda* prosthetic valve endocarditis in a patient with AIDS. Clin Infect Dis 1997;25:918–919.

344. Neubauer H, Aleksic S, Hensel A, et al. *Yersinia enterocolitica* 16S rRNA gene types belong to the same genospecies but form three homology groups. Int J Med Microbiol 2000;290:61–64.

345. Neubauer H, Sauer T, Becker H, et al. Comparison of systems for identification and differentiation of species within the genus *Yersinia*. J Clin Microbiol 1998; 36:3366–3368.

346. Novicki TJ, Daly JA, Mottice SL, Carroll KC. Comparison of sorbitol MacConkey agar and a two-step method which utilizes enzyme-linked immunosorbent assay toxin testing and a chromogenic agar to detect and isolate enterohemorrhagic *Escherichia coli*. J Clin Microbiol 2000;38:547–551.

347. Nowgesic E, Fyfe M, Hockin J, et al. Outbreak of *Yersinia pseudotuberculosis* in British Columbia—November 1998. Can Commun Dis Rep 1999;25:97–100.

347a. Nunez ML, Diaz J, Lorente I, et al. Evaluation of CPS ID2 medium for diagnosis of urinary infections. Eur J Clin Microbiol Infect Dis 1995;14:1111–1113.

348. Nuorti JP, Niskanen T, Hallanvuo S, et al. A widespread outbreak of *Yersinia pseudotuberculosis* O:3 infection from iceberg lettuce. J Infect Dis 2004;189: 766–774.

349. Nye KJ, Fallon D, Frodsham D, et al. An evaluation of the performance of XLD, DCA, MLCB, and ABC agars as direct plating media for the isolation of *Salmonella* enterica from faeces. J Clin Pathol 2002;55:286–288.

350. Ochoa TJ, Cleary TG. Epidemiology and spectrum of disease of *Escherichia coli* O157. Cur Opin Infect Dis 2003;16:259–263.

351. O'Farrell N. Donovanosis. Sex Transm Infect 2002;78:452–457.

352. O'Farrell N, Hoosen AA, Coetzee K, et al. A rapid stain for the diagnosis of granuloma inguinale. Genitourin Med 1990;66:200–201.

353. Ohanessian JH, Fourcade N, Priolet B, et al. A propos d'une infection vesiculaire par *Moellerella wisconsensis*. Med Maladies Infect 1987;6:414–416.

354. O'Hara CM, Brenner FW, Miller JM. Classification, identification, and clinical significance of *Proteus*, *Providencia*, and *Morganella*. Clin Microbiol Rev 2000; 13:534–546.

355. O'Hara CM, Brenner FW, Steigerwalt AG, et al. Classification of *Proteus vulgaris* biogroup 3 with recognition of *Proteus hauseri* sp. nov., nom. rev. and unnamed *Proteus* genomospecies 4, 5, and 6. Int J Syst Evol Microbiol 2000; 50:1869–1875.

356. O'Hara CM, Miller JM. Evaluation of the autoSCAN-W/A system for rapid (2-hour) identification of members of the family Enterobacteriaceae. J Clin Microbiol 1992;30:1541–1543.

357. O'Hara CM, Miller JM. Evaluation of the Vitek 2 ID-GNB assay for identification of members of the family *Enterobacteriaceae* and other nonenteric gram-negative bacilli and comparison with the Vitek GNI+ card. J Clin Microbiol 2003;41:2096–2101.

358. O'Hara CM, Roman SB, Miller JM. Ability of commercial identification systems to identify newly recognized species of *Citrobacter*. J Clin Microbiol 1995;33: 242–245.

359. O'Hara CM, Steigerwalt AG, Farmer JJ, et al. Proposed reclassification of CDC enteric group 69 as *Enterobacter kobei*. Abstr Annu Meet Am Soc Microbiol 2001;C435:252,

360. O'Hara CM, Steigerwalt AG, Green D, et al. Isolation of *Providencia heimbachae* from human feces. J Clin Microbiol 1999;37:3048–3050.

361. O'Hara CM, Steigerwalt AG, Hill BC, et al. *Enterobacter hormaechei*, a new species of the family Enterobacteriaceae formerly known as enteric group 75. J Clin Microbiol 1989;27: 2046–2049.

362. O'Hara CM, Steigerwalt AG, Hill BC, Miller JM, et al. First report of a human isolate of *Erwinia persicinus*. J Clin Microbiol 1998;36:248–250.

363. O'Hara CM, Steward CD, Wright JL, et al. Isolation of *Enterobacter intermedium* from the gallbladder of a patient with cholecystitis. J Clin Microbiol 1998; 36:3055–3056.

364. O'Hara CM, Tenover FC, Miller JM. Parallel comparison of accuracy of API 20E, Vitek GNI, MicroScan Walk/Away Rapid ID, and Becton Dickinson Cobas Micro ID-E/NF for identification of members of the family Enterobacteriaceae and common gram-negative, non–glucose-fermenting bacilli. J Clin Microbiol 1993;31:3165–3169.

365. O'Hara CM Westbrook GL, Miller JM. Evaluation of Vitek GNI+ and Becton Dickinson Microbiology Systems Crystal E/NF identification systems for identi-

fication of members of the family *Enterobacteriaceae* and other gram-negative, glucose-fermenting and non-glucose-fermenting bacilli. J Clin Microbiol 1997; 35:3269–3273.

366. Ohkusu K. Cost-effective and rapid presumptive identification of gram-negative bacilli in routine urine, pus, and stool cultures: evaluation of the use of CHROMagar Orientation medium in conjunction with simple biochemical tests. J Clin Microbiol 2000;38:4586–4592.

367. Okrend AJG, Rose BE, Lattuada CP. Use of 5-bromo-4-chloro-3-indoxyl-β-D-glucuronide in MacConkey sorbitol agar to aid in the isolation of *Escherichia coli* O157:H7 from ground beef. J Food Prot 1990;53:941–943.

368. Olsen SJ, Miller G, Kennedy M, et al. A waterborne outbreak of *Escherichia coli* O157:H7 infections and hemolytic uremic syndrome: implications for rural water systems. Emerg Infect Dis 2002;8:370–375.

369. Olsson M, Syk A, Wollin R. Identification of salmonellae with the 4-methylumbelliferyl caprilate fluorescence test. J Clin Microbiol 1991;29:2631–2632.

370. Olsvik O, Sorum H, Birkness K, et al. Plasmid characterization of *Salmonella typhimurium* transmitted from animals to humans. J Clin Microbiol 1985;22: 336–338.

371. Otani E, Bruckner DA. *Leclercia adecarboxylata* isolated from a blood culture. Clin Microbiol Newslett 1991;13:157–158.

372. Pabst WL, Altwegg M, Kind C, et al. Prevalence of enteroaggregative *Escherichia coli* among children with and without diarrhea in Switzerland. J Clin Microbiol 2003;41:2289–2293.

373. Pai CH, Gillis F, Tuomanen E, et al. Placebo-controlled double-blind evaluation of trimethoprim-sulfamethoxazole treatment of *Yersinia enterocolitica* gastroenteritis. J Pediatr 1984;104:308–311.

374. Pai CH, Sorger S, Lafleur L, et al. Efficacy of cold enrichment techniques for recovery of *Yersinia enterocolitica* from human stools. J Clin Microbiol 1979; 9:712–715.

375. Papasian CJ, Enna-Kifer S, Garrison B. Symptomatic *Shigella sonnei* urinary tract infection. J Clin Microbiol 1995;33:2222–2223.

376. Park CH, Vandel NM, Hixon DL. Rapid immunoassay for detection of *Escherichia coli* O157 directly from stool specimens. J Clin Microbiol 1996;34: 988–990.

377. Parodi S, Lechner A, Osih R, et al. Nosocomial *Enterobacter* meningitis: risk factors, management, and treatment outcomes. Clin Infect Dis 2003;37:159–166.

378. Parry MF, Hutchinson JH, Brown NA, et al. Gram-negative sepsis in neonates: a nursery outbreak due to hand carriage of *Citrobacter diversus*. Pediatrics 1980; 65:1105–1109.

379. Paton AW, Paton JC. *Enterobacter cloacae* producing a Shiga-like toxin II-related cytotoxin associated with a case of hemolytic–uremic syndrome. J Clin Microbiol 1996;34:463–465.

380. Paton JC, Paton AW. Pathogenesis and diagnosis of Shiga toxin-producing *Escherichia coli* infections. Clin Microbiol Rev 1998;11:450–479.

381. Patrick ME, Adcock PM, Gomez TM, et al. *Salmonella* Enteritidis infections, United States, 1985–1999. Emerg Infect Dis 2004;10:1–7.

382. Peel MM, Alfredson DA, Gerrard JG, et al. Isolation, identification, and molecular characterization of strains of *Photorhabdus luminescens* from infected humans in Australia. J Clin Microbiol 1999;37:3647–3653.

383. Penner JL. Genus XII. *Providencia* Ewing 1962, 96AL. In: Krieg NR, Holt JG, eds. Bergey's Manual of Systematic Bacteriology. Vol 1. Baltimore: Williams & Wilkins, 1984:494–496.

384. Penner JL. International Committee on Systematic Bacteriology Taxonomic Subcommittee on *Enterobacteriaceae*. Int J Syst Bacteriol 1988;38:223–224.

385. Perez JM, Cavalli P, Roure C, et al. Comparison of four chromogenic media and Hektoen agar for detection and presumptive identification of *Salmonella* strains in human stools. J Clin Microbiol 2003;41:1130–1134.

386. Perkins SR, Beckett TA, Bump CM. *Cedecea davisae* bacteremia. J Clin Microbiol 1986;24:675–676.

387. Perry JD, Ford M, Taylor J, et al. ABC medium, a new chromogenic agar for selective isolation of *Salmonella* spp. J Clin Microbiol 1999;37:766–768.

388. Perry JD, Riley G, Gould FK, et al. Alafosfalin as a selective agent for the isolation of *Salmonella* from clinical specimens. J Clin Microbiol 2002;40: 3913–3916

389. Perry RD, Fetherston JD. *Yersinia pestis*: etiologic agent of plague. Clin Microbiol Rev 1997;10:35–66.,

390. Pfaller MA, Sahm D, O'Hara C, et al. Comparison of the AutoSCAN-W/A rapid bacterial identification system and the Vitek AutoMicrobic System for identification of gram-negative bacilli. J Clin Microbiol 1991;29:1422–1428.

391. Pfyffer GE. *Serratia fonticola* as an infectious agent. Eur J Clin Microbiol Infect Dis 1992;11:199–200.

392. Pien FD, Bruce AE. *Ewingella americana*: bacteremia in an intensive care unit. Arch Intern Med 1986;146:111–112.

393. Pien FD, Farmer JJ III, Weaver RE. Polymicrobial bacteremia caused by *Ewingella americana* (family Enterobacteriaceae) and an unusual *Pseudomonas* species. J Clin Microbiol 1983;18:727–729.

394. Pien FD, Shrum S, Swenson JM, et al. Colonization of human wounds by *Escherichia vulneris* and *Escherichia hermanii*. J Clin Microbiol 1985;22:283–285.

395. Pignato S, Giammanco G, Giammanco G. Rambach agar and SM-ID medium sensitivity for presumptive identification of *Salmonella* subspecies I-VI. J Med Microbiol 1995;43:68–71.

396. Podschun R. Isolation of *Klebsiella terrigena* from human feces: biochemical reactions, capsule types, and antibiotic sensitivity. Zentralbl Bakteriol 1991;275:73–78.

397. Podschun R, Acktun H, Okpara J, et al. Isolation of *Klebsiella planticola* from newborns in a neonatal ward. J Clin Microbiol 1998;36:2331–2332.

398. Podschun R, Ullmann U. Isolation of *Klebsiella terrigena* from clinical specimens. Eur J Clin Microbiol Infect Dis 1992;11:349–352.

399. Podschun R, Ullmann U. Incidence of *Klebsiella planticola* among clinical *Klebsiella* isolates. Med Microbiol Lett 1994;3:90–95.

400. Podschun R, Ullmann U. *Klebsiella* spp. as nosocomial pathogens: epidemiology, taxonomy, typing methods, and pathogenicity factors. Clin Microbiol Rev 1998;11:589–603.

401. Poisson DM. Novobiocin, brilliant green, glycerol, lactose agar: a new medium for the isolation of *Salmonella* strains. Res Microbiol 1992;143:211–216.

402. Popoff MY, Bockemühl J, Brenner FW. Supplement 1998 (no. 42) to the Kauffmann-White scheme. Res Microbiol 2000;151:63–65.

403. Popoff MY, Le Minor L. Antigenic formulas of the *Salmonella* serovars. 7th Rev. Paris: World Health Organization Collaborating Centre for Reference and Research on *Salmonella*, Pasteur Institute, 1997.

404. Potera C. Prairie dogs plagued by *Yersinia pestis*. ASM Newslett 2000;66:718–719.

405. Prats G, Richard C, Mirelis B, Lopez P. Human isolates of *Enterobacter intermedium*. Zentralbl Bakteriol Mikrobiol Hyg [A] 1987;266:422–424.

406. President's Council on Food Safety. Egg safety from production to consumption: an action plan to eliminate *Salmonella* Enteritidis illnesses due to eggs. Washington, DC: President's Council on Food Safety, 1999.

407. Priest FG, Somerville HJ, Cole JA, et al. The taxonomic position of *Obesumbacterium proteus*, a common brewery contaminant. J Gen Microbiol 1973;75:295–307.

408. Qadri SMH, Zubairi S, Hawley HP, et al. Simple spot test for rapid detection of urease activity. J Clin Microbiol 1984;20:1198–1199.

409. Rabatsky-Ehr T, Dingman D, Marcus R, et al. Deer meat as the source for a sporadic case of Escherichia coli O157:H7 infection, Connecticut. Emerg Infect Dis 2002;8:525–527.

410. Raj P. Pathogenesis and laboratory diagnosis of *Escherichia coli*-associated enteritis. Clin Microbiol Newslett 1993;15:89–93.

411. Rambach A. New plate medium for facilitated differentiation of *Salmonella* spp. from *Proteus* spp. and other enteric bacteria. Appl Environ Microbiol 1990;56:301–303.

412. Ratnam S. Etiologic role of *Hafnia alvei* in human diarrheal illness. Infect Immun 1991;59:4744–4745.

413. Ratnam S, Butler RW, March S, et al. *Enterobacter hafniae*-associated gastroenteritis—Newfoundland. Can Dis Wkly Rep 1979;5:231–232

414. Reeves MW, Evins GM, Heiba AA, et al. Clonal nature of *Salmonella typhi* and its genetic relatedness to other salmonellae as shown by multilocus enzyme electrophoresis and proposal of *Salmonella bongori* comb. nov. J Clin Microbiol 1989;27:313–320.

415. Reina J, Alomar P. *Enterobacter taylorae* wound infection. Clin Microbiol Newslett 1989;11:134–135.

416. Reina J, Borrell N, Llompart I. Community-acquired bacteremia caused by *Serratia plymuthica*: case report and review of the literature. Diagn Microbiol Infect Dis 1992;15:449–452.

417. Reina J, Hervas J, Borrell N. Acute gastroenteritis caused by *Hafnia alvei* in children. Clin Infect Dis 1993;16:443.

418. Reina J, Salva F, Gil J, Alomar P. Urinary tract infection caused by *Enterobacter taylorae*. J Clin Microbiol 1989;27:2877.

419. Reisner BS, Austin EF. Evaluation of CPS ID 2 chromogenic agar as a single medium for urine culture. Diagn Microbiol Infect Dis 1997;28:113–117.

420. Reynolds HY, Pneumonia due to *Klebsiella* (Friedlanders pneumonia). In: Wyngaarden JB, Smith LH, eds. Cecil Textbook of Medicine. 16th ed. Philadelphia: Saunders, 1982:1430–1432.

421. Rhoads S, Marinelli L, Imperatrice CA, Nachamkin I. Comparison of MicroScan WalkAway system and Vitek system for identification of gram-negative bacteria. J Clin Microbiol 1995;33:3044–3046.

422. Rhoden DL, Smith PB, Baker CN, et al. AutoSCAN-4 system for identification of gram-negative bacilli. J Clin Microbiol 1985;22:915–918.

423. Richard C. Nouvelles Enterobacteriaceae rencontrees en bacteriologie medicale: *Moellerella wisconsensis, Koserella trabulsii, Leclercia adecarboxylata, Escherichia fergusonii, Enterobacter asburiae, Rahnella aquatilis*. Ann Biol Clin 1989;47:231–236.

424. Richens J. The diagnosis and treatment of donovanosis (granuloma inguinale). Genitourin Med 1991;67:441–452.

425. Ridell J, Siitonen A, Paulin L, et al. *Hafnia alvei* in stool specimens from patients with diarrhea and healthy controls. J Clin Microbiol 1994;32:2335–2337.

426. Riley LW, Remis RS, Helgerson SD, et al. Hemorrhagic colitis associated with a rare *Escherichia coli* serotype. N Engl J Med 1983;308:681–685.

427. Robinson A, McCarter YS, Tetreault J. Comparison of Crystal enteric/nonfermenter system, API 20E system, and Vitek automicrobic system for identification of gram-negative bacilli. J Clin Microbiol 1995;33:364–370.

428. Rubinstien EM, Klevjer-Anderson P, Smith CA, et al. *Enterobacter taylorae*, a new opportunistic pathogen: report of four cases. J Clin Microbiol 1993;31:249–254.

429. Ruiz J, Nunez M-L, Diaz J, et al. Comparison of five plating media for isolation of *Salmonella* species from human stools. J Clin Microbiol 1996;34:686–688.

430. Ruiz J, Nunez M-L, Sempere MA, Diaz J, Gomez J. Systemic infections in three infants due to a lactose-fermenting strain of *Salmonella virchow*. Eur J Clin Microbiol Infect Dis 1995;14:454–456.

431. Ruiz J, Sempere MA, Varela MC, Gomez J. Modification of the methodology of stool culture for *Salmonella* detection. J Clin Microbiol 1992;30:525–526.

432. Ruiz J, Varela MC, Sempere MA, et al. Presumptive identification of *Salmonella enterica* using two rapid tests. Eur J Clin Microbiol Infect Dis 1991;10:649–651.

433. Sakazaki R, Murata Y. The new group of *Enterobacteriaceae*: the Asakusa group. Jpn J Bacteriol 1963;17:616–617.

434. Samra Z, Heifetz M, Talmor J, et al. Evaluation of use of a new chromogenic agar in detection of urinary tract pathogens. J Clin Microbiol 1998;36:990–994.

435. Sanders CC, Moellering RC Jr, Martin RR, et al. Resistance to cefamandole: a collaborative study of emerging clinical problems. J Infect Dis 1982;145:118–125.

436. Sanders CC, Sanders WE Jr. Emergence of resistance during drug therapy with newer beta lactam antibiotics: role of inducible beta lactamases and implications for the future. Rev Infect Dis 1983;5:639–648.

437. Sautter RL, Mattman LH, Legaspi RC. *Serratia marcescens* meningitis associated with a contaminated benzalkonium chloride solution. Infect Control 1984;5:223–225.

438. Scarparo C, Piccoli P, Ricordi P, et al. Comparative evaluation of two commercial chromogenic media for detection and presumptive identification of urinary tract pathogens. Eur J Clin Microbiol Infect Dis 2002;21:283–289.

439. Scavizzi MR, Gayraud M, Hornstein MJ, et al. In-vitro and in-vivo activities of antibiotics on *Yersinia enterocolitica*. J Antimicrob Chemother 1996;38:1108–1109.

440. Schauer DB, Zabel BA, Pedraza IF, et al. Genetic and biochemical characterization of *Citrobacter rodentium* sp. nov. J Clin Microbiol 1995;33:2064–2068.

441. Schieven BC. Evaluation of Rainbow UTI system for rapid isolation and identification of urinary pathogens. Abstr Annu Meet Am Soc Microbiol 1995;C375:65.

442. Schieven BC, Hussain Z, Lannigan R. Comparison of American MicroScan dry frozen microdilution trays. J Clin Microbiol 1985;22:495–496.

443. Schønheyder HC, Jensen KT, Frederiksen W. Taxonomic notes: synonymy of *Enterobacter cancerogenus* (Urosevic 1966) Dickey and Zumoff 1988 and *Enterobacter taylorae* Farmer et al. 1985 and resolution of an ambiguity in the biochemical profile. Int J Syst Bacteriol 1994;44:586–587.

444. Schreckenberger PC, Blazevic DJ. Rapid methods for biochemical testing of anaerobic bacteria. Appl Microbiol 1974;28:759–762.

445. Schreckenberger P, Montero M, Heldt N. Evaluation of the RapID E Plus Panel for Identification of *Enterobacteriaceae*. Abstr Ann Mtg Am Soc Microbiol 1993;C309:500.

446. Sharma NK, Doyle PW, Gerbasi SA, Jessop JH. Identification of *Yersinia* species by the API 20E. J Clin Microbiol 1990;28:1443–1444.

447. Siegler RL. Postdiarrheal Shiga toxin–mediated hemolytic uremic syndrome. JAMA 2003;290:1379–1381.

448. Sierra-Madero J, Pratt K, Hall GS, et al. *Kluyvera* mediastinitis following open-heart surgery: a case report. J Clin Microbiol 1990;28:2848–2849

449. Silverblatt FJ, Weinstein R. Enterobacteriaceae. In: Mandell GL, Douglas RG Jr, Bennett JE, eds. Principles and Practice of Infectious Disease 2nd Ed. New York: Wiley, 1985:226–1236.

450. Simmons JS. A culture medium for differentiating organisms of typhoid-colon aerogenes groups and for isolation of certain fungi. J Infect Dis 1926;39:209–214.

451. Slaven EM, Lopez FA, Hart SM, Sandersw CV. Myonecrosis caused by *Edwardsiella tarda*: a case report and case series of extraintestinal *E. tarda* infections. Clin Infect Dis 2001;32:1430–1433.

452. Smith PB. Performance of Six Bacterial Identification Systems. Atlanta: Centers for Disease Control, Bacteriology Division, 1975.

453. Smith RD, McNamara JJ, Ladd M. *Shigella* and child abuse. Pediatrics 1986;78:953–954.

454. Søgaard P, Kjaeldgaard P. Two isolations of enteric group 69 from human clinical specimens. Acta Pathol Microbiol Immunol Scand [B] 1986;94:365–367.

455. Spaulding AC, Rothman AL. *Escherichia vulneris* as a cause of intravenous catheter–related bacteremia. Clin Infect Dis 1996;22:728–729.

456. Stager CE, Davis JR: Automated systems for identification of microorganisms. Clin Microbiol Rev 1992;5:302–327.

457. Staneck JL, Vincelette J, Lamothe F, et al. Evaluation of the sensitite system for identification of Enterobacteriaceae. J Clin Microbiol 1983;17:647–654.

458. Stapp JR, Jelacic S, Yea Y-L, et al. Comparison of *Escherichia coli* O157:H7 antigen detection in stool and broth cultures to that in sorbitol-MacConkey agar stool cultures. J Clin Microbiol 2000;38:3404–3406.

459. Starr M, Bennett-Wood V, Bigham AK, et al. Hemolytic–uremic syndrome following urinary tract infection with enterohemorrhagic *Escherichia coli*: case report and review. Clin Infect Dis 1998;27:310–315.

460. Stefaniuk E, Baraniak A, Gniadkowski M, et al. Evaluation of the BD Phoenix automated identification and susceptibility testing system in clinical microbiology laboratory practice. Eur J Clin Microbiol Infect Dis 2003;22:479–485.

461. Stenhouse MAE, Milner LV. *Yersinia enterocolitica*: a hazard in blood transfusion. Transfusion 1982;22:396–398.

462. Stewart JM, Quirk JR. Community-acquired pneumoniae caused by *Enterobacter asburiae*. Am J Med 2001;111:82–83.

463. Stock I, Falsen E, Wiedemann B. *Moellerella wisconsensis*: identification, natural antibiotic susceptibility and its dependency on the medium applied. Diagn Microbiol Infect Dis 2003;45:1–11.

464. Stratton CW. An overview of plague: pathogenesis and clinical manifestations. Antimicrob Infect Dis Newslett 1997;16:49–51.

465. Strobel E, Heesemann J, Mayer G. Bacteriological and serological findings in a further case of transfusion-mediated *Yersinia enterocolitica* sepsis. J Clin Microbiol 2000;38:2788–2790.

466. Sutra L, Christen R, Bollet C, et al. *Samsonia erythrinae* gen. nov., sp. nov., isolated from bark necrotic lesions of *Erythrina* sp., and discrimination of plant-pathogenic *Enterobacteriaceae* by phenotypic features. Int J Syst Evol Microbiol 2001;51:1291–1304.

467. Tamura K, Sakazaki R, Kosako Y, Yoshizaki E. *Leclercia adecarboxylata* gen. nov., comb. nov., formerly known as *Escherichia adecarboxylata*. Curr Microbiol 1986;13:179–184.

468. Tan SC, Wong YH, Jegathesan M, et al. The first isolate of *Tatumella ptyseos* in Malaysia. Malays J Pathol 1989;11:25–27.

469. Tarr PI. *Escherichia coli* O157:H7: clinical, diagnostic, and epidemiological aspects of human infection. Clin Infect Dis 1995;20:1–10.

470. Tauxe RV, Vandepitte J, Wauters G, et al. *Yersinia enterocolitica* infections and pork: the missing link. Lancet 1987;1:1129–1132.

471. Taylor WI. Isolation of *Shigellae*: I. Xylose lysine agars: new media for isolation of enteric pathogens. Am J Clin Pathol 1965;44:471–475.

472. Taylor WI, Achanzar D. Catalase test as an aid to the identification of Enterobacteriaceae. Appl Microbiol 1972;24:58–61.

473. Temesgen Z, Toal DR, Cockerill FR III. *Leclercia adecarboxylata* infections: case report and review. Clin Infect Dis 1997;25:79–81.

474. Tertti R, Vuento R, Mikkola P, et al. Clinical manifestations of *Yersinia pseudotuberculosis* infection in children. Eur J Microbiol Infect Dis 1989;8:587–591.

475. Thaller R, Berlutti F, Thaller MC. A *Kluyvera cryocrescens* strain from a gallbladder infection. Eur J Epidemiol 1988;4:124–126.

476. Thompson JS, Hodge DS, Borczyk AA. Rapid biochemical test to identify verocytotoxin-positive strains of *Escherichia coli* serotype O157. J Clin Microbiol 1990;28:2165–2168.

477. Thorpe CM, Acheson DWK. Testing of urinary *Escherichia coli* isolates for Shiga toxin production. Clin Infect Dis 2001;32:1517–1518.

478. Tipple MA, Bland LA, Murphy JJ, et al. Sepsis associated with transfusion of red cells contaminated with *Yersinia enterocolitica*. Transfusion 1990;30: 207–213.

479. Tristram DA, Forbes BA. *Kluyvera*: a case report of urinary tract infection and sepsis. Pediatr Infect Dis J 1988;7:297–298.

480. Urmenyi AMC, White-Franklin A. Neonatal death from pigmented coliform infection. Lancet 1961;1:313–315.

481. Ursing J, Brenner DJ, Bercovier H, et al. *Yersinia frederiksenii*: a new species of Enterobacteriaceae composed of rhamnose-positive strains (formerly called atypical *Yersinia enterocolitica* or *Yersinia enterocolitica*-like). Curr Microbiol 1980;4:213–217.

482. Ursua PR, Unzaga MJ, Melero P, et al. *Serratia rubidaea* as an invasive pathogen. J Clin Microbiol 1996;34:216–217.

483. Van Acker J, De Smet F, Muyldermans G, et al. Outbreak of necrotizing enterocolitis associated with *Enterobacter sakazakii* in powdered milk formula. J Clin Microbiol 2001;39:293–297.

484. Vandepitte J, Lemmens P, De Swert L. Human edwardsiellosis traced to ornamental fish. J Clin Microbiol 1983;17:165–167.

485. van der Heijden IM, Res PCM, Wilbrink B, et al. *Yersinia enterocolitica*: a cause of chronic polyarthritis. Clin Infect Dis 1997;25:831–837.

486. Varma JK, Greene KD, Reller ME. An outbreak of *Escherichia coli* O157 infection following exposure to a contaminated building. JAMA 2003;290: 2709–2712.

487. Verboon-Maciolek M, Vandertop WP, Peters ACB, et al. Neonatal brain abscess caused by *Morganella morganii*. Clin Infect Dis 1995;20:471.

488. Vogel LC, Ferguson L, Gotoff SP. *Citrobacter* infections of the central nervous system in early infancy. J Pediatr 1978;93:86–88.

489. von Graevenitz A. Revised nomenclature of *Campylobacter laridis*, *Enterobacter intermedium*, and ''*Flavobacterium branchiophila*.'' Int J Syst Bacteriol 1990;40:211.

490. Wagner SJ, Friedman LI, Dodd RY. Transfusion-associated bacterial sepsis. Clin Microbiol Rev 1994;7:290–302.

491. Wallet F, Fruchart A, Bouvet PJM, Courcol RJ. Isolation of *Moellerella wisconsensis* from bronchial aspirate. Eur J Clin Microbiol Infect Dis 1994;13: 182–183.

492. Warren JR, Farmer JJ III, Dewhirst FE, et al. Outbreak of nosocomial infections due to extended-spectrum β-lactamase-producing strains of enteric group 137, a new member of the family *Enterobacteriaceae* closely related to *Citrobacter farmeri* and *Citrobacter amalonaticus*. J Clin Microbiol 2000;38:3946–3952.

493. Watanabe M, Matsuoka K, Kita E, et al. Oral therapeutic agents with highly clustered globotriose for treatment of shiga toxigenic *Escherichia coli* infections. J Infect Dis 2004;189:360–368.

494. Waterman SH, Juarez G, Carr SJ, Kilman L. *Salmonella arizona* infections in Latinos associated with rattlesnake folk medicine. Am J Public Health 1990;80: 286–289.

495. Wauters G, Boel A, Voorn GP, et al. Evaluation of a new identification system, Crystal enteric/non-fermenter, for gram-negative bacilli. J Clin Microbiol 1995; 33:845–849.

496. Wauters G, Janssens M, Steigerwalt AG, Brenner DJ. *Yersinia mollaretii* sp. nov. and *Yersinia bercovieri* sp. nov., formerly called *Yersinia enterocolitica* biogroups 3A and 3B. Int J Syst Bacteriol 1988;38:424–429.

497. Wayne LG. Judicial Commission of the International Committee on Systematic Bacteriology. Int J Syst Bacteriol 1991;41:185–187.

498. Wayne LG. Actions of the Judicial Commission of the International Committee on Systematic Bacteriology on Requests for Opinions published between January 1985 and July 1993. Int J Syst Bacteriol 1994;44:177–178.

499. Wenger PN, Tokars JI, Brennan P, et al. An outbreak of *Enterobacter hormaechei* infection and colonization in an intensive care nursery. Clin Infect Dis 1997;24:1243–1244.

500. Weissfeld AS, Sonnenwirth AC. Rapid isolation of *Yersinia* spp. from feces. J Clin Microbiol 1982;15:508–510

501. Werner SB, Weidmer CE, Nelson BC, et al. Primary plague pneumonia contracted from a domestic cat at South Lake Tahoe, Calif. JAMA 1984;251: 929–931.

502. Westblom TU, Coggins ME. Osteomyelitis caused by *Enterobacter taylorae*, formerly enteric group 19. J Clin Microbiol 1987;25:2432–2433.

503. Westblom TU, Milligan TW. Acute bacterial gastroenteritis caused by *Hafnia alvi*. Clin Infect Dis 1992;14:1271–1272.

504. Westbrook GL, O'Hara CM, Roman SB, et al. Incidence and identification of *Klebsiella planticola* in clinical isolates with emphasis on newborns. J Clin Microbiol 2000;38:1495–1497.

504a. Willinger B, Manafi M. Evaluation of a new chromogenic agar medium for the identification of urinary tract pathogens. Lett Appl Microbiol 1995;20:300–302.

505. Wilson D, Tuohy M, Procop GW: The low prevalence of Shiga-toxin production among sorbitol non-fermenting *Escherichia coli* urinary tract isolates does not warrant routine screening. Clin Infect Dis 2000;31:1313.

506. Wilson JP, Waterer RR, Wofford JD Jr, Chapman SW. Serious infections with *Edwardsiella tarda*, a case report and review of the literature. Arch Intern Med 1989;149:208–210.

507. Wittke J-W, Aleksic S, Wuthe H-H. Isolation of *Moellerella wisconsensis* from an infected human gallbladder. Eur J Clin Microbiol 1985;4:351–352.

508. Wong CS, Jelacic S, Habeeb RL, Watkins SL, Tarr PI. The risk of the hemolytic–uremic syndrome after antibiotic treatment of *Escherichia coli* O157:H7 infections. N Engl J Med 2000;342:1930–1936.

509. Wong VK. Broviac catheter infection with *Kluyvera cryocrescens*: a case report. J Clin Microbiol 1987;25:1115–1116.

510. Woolfrey BF, Lally RT, Ederer MN, et al. Evaluation of the AutoMicrobic system for identification and susceptibility testing of gram-negative bacilli. J Clin Microbiol 1984;20:1053–1059.

511. Wu M-S, Shyu R-S, Lai M-Y, et al. A predisposition toward *Edwardsiella tarda* bacteremia in individuals with preexisting liver disease. Clin Infect Dis 1995; 21:705–706.

512. York MK, Baron EJ, Clarridge JE, et al. Multilaboratory validation of rapid spot tests for identification of *Escherichia coli*. J Clin Microbiol 2000;38:3394–3398.

513. York MK, Brooks GF, Fiss EH. Evaluation of the autoSCAN-W/A rapid system for identification and susceptibility testing of gram-negative fermentative bacilli. J Clin Microbiol 1992;30:2903–2910.

514. Zadik PM, Chapman PA, Siddons CA. Use of tellurite for the selection of verocytotoxigenic *Escherichia coli* O157. J Med Microbiol 1993;39:155–158.

515. Zbinden R, Blass R. *Serratia plymuthica* osteomyelitis following a motorcycle accident. J Clin Microbiol 1988;26:1409–1410.

516. Zobell CE. Factors influencing the reduction of nitrates and nitrites by bacteria in semisolid media. J Bacteriol 1932;24:273–281.

The Nonfermentative Gram-Negative Bacilli

Part I: Metabolism of the Nonfermenters

Fermentative and Oxidative Metabolism

The Embden-Meyerhof-Parnas Pathway
The Entner-Doudoroff Pathway
The Warburg-Dickens Hexose Monophosphate Pathway

Initial Clues That an Unknown Isolate Is a Nonfermenter

Lack of Evidence For Glucose Fermentation
Positive Cytochrome Oxidase Reaction
Failure to Grow on MacConkey Agar

Tests Used in the Identification of Nonfermenters

Utilization of Glucose
Motility
Pigment Production
Hydrolysis of Urea
Nitrate Reduction

Denitrification of Nitrates and Nitrites
Indole Production

Decarboxylation
Esculin Hydrolysis
Flagella Stains

Leifson Method
Ryu Method
Wet-Mount Technique
Flagellar Morphology

Part II: Taxonomy, Biochemical Characteristics, and Clinical Significance of Medically Important Genera Nonfermenters

Organisms That Are Motile With Polar Flagella

Pseudomonads
Family *Pseudomonadaceae*

Genus *Pseudomonas*—rRNA Group I

Family *Burkholderiaceae*

rRNA Group II
Genus *Burkholderia*—*Pseudomallei* Group
Genus *Ralstonia* and *Cupriavidus*
Genus *Pandoraea*
Genus *Inquilinus*
Genua *Lautropia*

Family *Comamonadaceae*

rRNA Group III
Acidovorans Group
Facilis-Delafieldii Group

Family *Caulobacteraceae*

rRNA Group IV
Brevundimonas-Diminuta Group

Family *Xanthomonadaceae*

rRNA Group V
Genus *Stenotrophomonas*

Family *Sphingomonadaceae*

Genus *Sphingomonas*

Family *Oceanospirillaceae*

Genus *Balneatrix*

Family *Oxalobacteraceae*

Genus *Massilia*
Genus *Herbaspirillum*

Family *Alteromonadaceae*

Genus *Shewanella*—Hydrogen Sulfide–Producing
Group
Genus *Alishewanella*—Halophilic Group

Family *Halomonadaceae*

Genus *Halomonas*

Family *Methylobacteriaceae*

Genus *Methylobacterium*
Genus *Roseomonas*

Unnamed Species
Laribacter hongkongensis

Organisms That Are Motile With Peritrichous Flagella

Family *Alcaligenaceae*

Genus *Alcaligenes*

Genus *Achromobacter*
Genus *Bordetella*
Genus *Kerstersia*
Genus *Oligella*

Family *Rhizobiaceae*

Genus *Rhizobium* (Formerly *Agrobacterium*)

Family *Brucellaceae*

Genus *Ochrobactrum*

Organisms That Are Nonmotile and Oxidase-Positive

Family *Flavobacteriaceae*

Chryseobacterium, Empedobacter, and Unnamed
CDC Groups
Weeksella and *Bergeyella*
Genus *Myroides*

Family *Sphingobacteriaceae*

Sphingobacterium and *Pedobacter*

Family *Moraxellaceae*

Genus *Moraxella*
Genus *Psychrobacter* and CDC EO Groups

Family *Neisseriaceae*

Genus *Neisseria*
Gilardi Rod Group 1

Organisms That Are Nonmotile and Oxidase-Negative

Genus *Acinetobacter*
CDC Group NO-1
Bordetella holmesii (CDC Group NO-2)
CDC Group EO-5

Part III: Approach to Recovery and Identification of Nonfermenters

Levels of Service in Identification of Nonfermenters

Guidelines for Recovery of Nonfermenters

Identification of Most Common Species

Pseudomonas aeruginosa
Acinetobacter baumannii
Stenotrophomonas maltophilia

Methods for Identification Using Conventional Tests

Weyant (CDC), Gilardi, and Pickett Identification Schemes
Practical Approach to Identification of Nonfermenters
Computer-Aided Schemes

Commercial Kit Systems

The Oxi/Ferm Tube

The API 20E System
The API 20NE System
The Remel N/F System
The Crystal Enteric/Nonfermenter System
The RapID NF Plus System
The Biolog System

Automated Identification Systems

The Vitek Legacy System
The Vitek 2 System
The Microscan Walkaway-96, Walkaway-40, and Autoscan-4 Systems
The Sensititre AP80 System
The Phoenix System

Selection of a System

The nonfermentative gram-negative bacilli are a group of aerobic, non–spore-forming bacilli that either do not use carbohydrates as a source of energy or degrade them through metabolic pathways other than fermentation. Within this group are several genera and species of bacteria with special growth requirements that are not discussed in this chapter. The dividing line between what is a "nonfermenter" and what may otherwise be designated a "fastidious," "unusual," or "miscellaneous" non–glucose-fermenting, gram-negative bacillus (discussed in Chapter 9) is based more on convention than on well-defined genetic or phenotypic characteristics. The term **nonfermentative gram-negative bacilli** is used in this chapter to mean all aerobic gram-negative rods that show abundant growth within 24 hours on the surface of Kligler iron agar (KIA) or triple sugar iron (TSI) medium, but neither grow in nor acidify the butt of these media.

The genera of nonfermenters to be discussed in this chapter include *Achromobacter, Acidovorax, Acinetobacter, Agrobacterium, Alcaligenes, Alishewanella, Balneatrix, Bergeyella, Bordetella, Brevundimonas, Burkholderia, Chryseobacterium, Comamonas, Cupriavidus, Delftia, Empedobacter, Flavobacterium, Laribacter, Methylobacterium, Moraxella, Myroides, Ochrobactrum, Oligella, Pandoraea, Parococcus, Pedobacter, Pseudomonas, Psychrobacter, Ralstonia, Rhizobium, Roseomonas, Shewanella, Sphingobacterium, Sphingomonas, Stenotrophomonas, Weeksella,* and a few organisms that currently carry only Centers for Disease Control and Prevention (CDC) alphanumeric designations. Also included in this chapter are a few species of *Neisseria* that appear as gram-negative rods and must be differentiated from similar-appearing nonfermenting bacilli. The genera *Eikenella, Brucella,* and *Francisella,* although they possess the general characteristics of nonfermenters, are grouped in this book with the fastidious, gram-negative bacilli and are discussed in Chapter 9. The currently accepted organism nomenclature and a listing of previous designations are presented in Table 7-1. The synonyms for several bacterial species either previously or currently having CDC alphanumeric designations are presented in Table 7-2.

As more information accumulates, reclassification of bacteria between genera and species and the creation of new designations must be accepted as part of scientific progress. DNA homology studies often play a larger role in the ultimate classification of bacteria than a scheme based on phenotypic characteristics alone. For example, within the genus *Pseudomonas* several biovars and pathovars are now recognized, arranged according to recombinant RNA (rRNA) and DNA homologies.[560] Despite refinements, clinical microbiologists must still recognize and classify clinical laboratory isolates based on morphologic and biochemical characteristics. Microbiologists must also keep abreast of changes in bacterial nomenclature so that current names can be used in everyday practice and research data gathered from various investigations using previous designations will not be misinterpreted.

PART I: METABOLISM OF THE NONFERMENTERS

Bacteria that derive their energy from organic compounds are known as **chemoorganotrophs.** Most of the bacteria encountered in clinical medicine derive energy from the utilization of carbohydrates by one of several metabolic pathways. Detection and measurement of various metabolic products are necessary to identify bacterial species that may be the cause of infectious disease. Some bacteria, such as members of the genus *Moraxella*, do not metabolize carbohydrates but rather derive energy from the degradation of other organic compounds, such as amino acids, alcohols, and organic acids. Some free-living bacteria, such as the nitrogen-fixing groups or those capable of oxidizing sulfur

Table 7-1 Nomenclature for Gram-Negative Nonfermentative Bacilli

CURRENT USAGE	PREVIOUS DESIGNATIONS	COMMENTS
Achromobacter Groups B, E, and F		Unnamed *Achromobacter* species
Achromobacter denitrificans	*Alcaligenes xylosoxidans* subsp. *denitrificans* *Alcaligenes denitrificans* subsp. *denitrificans* CDC Vc	Subspecies designation no longer used
Achromobacter piechaudii	*Alcaligenes piechaudii*	New species isolated primarily from human clinical specimens, but some strains from the environment. Clinical significance not known. One report of otitis media caused by this organism
Achromobacter xylosoxidans	*Alcaligenes xylosoxidans* subsp. *xylosoxidans* *Achromobacter xylosoxidans* *Alcaligenes denitrificans* subsp. *xylosoxidans* CDC IIIa and IIIb	Subspecies designation no longer used
Acinetobacter baumannii	*Acinetobacter calcoaceticus* var. *anitratus* *Achromobacter anitratus* *Bacterium anitratum* *Herellea vaginicola* Morax-Axenfeld bacillus *Moraxella glucidolytica* var. *nonliquefaciens* *Pseudomonas calcoacetica*	Species name given to *Acinetobacter* genospecies 2. Produces acid from glucose. Can be separated from *Acinetobacter calcoaceticus* (genospecies1) by growth at 41°C and 44°C, production of β-xylosidase, and utilization of malate (*A. baumannii*–positive and *A. calcoaceticus*–negative) Laboratories that do not perform these tests may choose to report these organisms as *A. calcoaceticus-A. baumannii* complex. Most *Acinetobacter* strains isolated from human clinical specimens belong to this species
Acinetobacter lwoffii	*Acinetobacter calcoaceticus* var. *lwoffi* *Achromobacter lwoffi* *Mima polymorpha* *Moraxella lwoffi*	Species name given to *Acinetobacter* genospecies 8. Non–glucose-oxidizing strain found in human clinical specimens
Alcaligenes faecalis	CDC VI *Alcaligenes odorans*	*Alcaligenes odorans* was proposed at a later date for an organism that is a strain of the earlier-named *Alcaligenes faecalis*.
Bergeyella zoohelcum	*Weeksella zoohelcum* CDC IIj	Rapid urea–positive. Associated with dog and cat bites
Bordetella bronchiseptica	*Alcaligenes bronchicanis* *Alcaligenes bronchiseptica* *Bordetella bronchicanis* *Brucella bronchiseptica* *Haemophilus bronchiseptica*	Rapid urea–positive
Bordetella hinzii	*Bordetella avium*–like *Alcaligenes faecalis* type II TC (turkey coryza) bacterium type II *Alcaligenes* sp. strain C_2T_2	New species isolated from respiratory tracts of chickens and turkeys. Human isolates reported from respiratory tract, ear discharge, and feces
Bordetella holmesii	CDC nonoxidizer group 2 (NO-2)	New species isolated from blood cultures. Oxidase-negative, nonmotile; brown soluble pigment produced on heart infusion tyrosine agar

Table 7-1 *Continued*

CURRENT USAGE	PREVIOUS DESIGNATIONS	COMMENTS
Bordetella trematum		New species isolated from wounds and ear discharge Oxidase-negative, motile
Brevundimonas diminuta	*Pseudomonas diminuta* CDC Ia	
Brevundimonas vesicularis	*Pseudomonas vesicularis* *Corynebacterium vesiculare*	
Burkholderia cepacia complex	*Pseudomonas cepacia* *Pseudomonas multivorans* *Pseudomonas kingae* CDC EO-1	Yellow pigment. Recovered from numerous water sources and wet surfaces. Respiratory pathogens in patients with cystic fibrosis
		Consists of at least nine genetic species that are difficult to separate phenotypically
Burkholderia gladioli	*Pseudomonas gladioli* *Pseudomonas marginata*	Primarily plant pathogen. Has been reported from sputum of patients with cystic fibrosis
Burkholderia pseudomallei	*Pseudomonas pseudomallei*	Cause of melioidosis in humans
Chryseobacterium indologenes	*Flavobacterium indologenes* CDC IIb	
Chryseobacterium meningosepticum	*Flavobacterium meningosepticum* CDC IIa	Highly pathogenic for premature infants
Comamonas terrigena	Various species of *Vibrio* E. Falsen group 10 *Aquaspirillum aquaticum*	
Comamonas testosteroni	*Pseudomonas testosteroni* *Pseudomonas desmolytica* *Pseudomonas dacunhae* *Pseudomonas cruciviae*	
Cupriavidus pauculus	*Wautersia paucula* *Ralstonia paucula* CDC Group IVc-2	Rapid urease positive
Delftia acidovorans	*Comamonas acidovorans* *Pseudomonas acidovorans* *Pseudomonas desmolytica* *Pseudomonas indoloxidans* *Achromobacter cystinovorum*	Orange indole reaction. Due to production of anthranilic acid from tryptone
Empedobacter brevis	*Flavobacterium breve*	
Flavobacterium species		Several species previously included in the genus *Flavobacterium* have been reclassified as members of new or other genera; remaining species widely distributed in soil and freshwater habitats and are not found in human clinical specimens
Methylobacterium mesophilicum	*Pseudomonas mesophilica* *Pseudomonas methanica* *Vibrio extorquens* *Mycoplana rubra* *Protaminobacter* spp. *Chromobacterium* spp. *Beijerinckia* spp.	Slow-growing pink-pigmented rods. Do not stain well, appear amorphous, with many nonstaining vacuoles
Moraxella atlantae	CDC M-3	

(Continued)

Table 7-1 *Continued*

CURRENT USAGE	PREVIOUS DESIGNATIONS	COMMENTS
Moraxella lacunata	*Moraxella liquefaciens*	
Moraxella nonliquefaciens	*Bacillus duplex nonliquefaciens*	
Moraxella osloensis	*Mima polymorpha* var. *oxidans*	Large colonies with a tendency to spread; indole-negative
Myroides odoratus	*Flavobacterium odoratum*	
Myroides odoratimimus	CDC M-4F	
Neisseria weaveri	*Moraxella* sp. M-5 CDC M-5	Clinical isolates associated with dog bites
Neisseria elongata subsp. *nitroreducens*	*Moraxella* sp. M-6 CDC M-6	Catalase-negative. Clinical isolates associated with endocarditis
Ochrobactrum anthropi	CDC Vd-1, Vd-2 *Achromobacter* spp. biotypes 1 and 2. *Achromobacter* groups A, C, and D.	Only isolates have been from human clinical specimens.
Oligella ureolytica	CDC IV e	Rapid urea-positive and phenylalanine deaminase–positive
Oligella urethralis	CDC M-4	Clinical isolates have been from ear and urinary tract infections.
Pandoraea	New genus comprising five species	Isolated from human clinical samples (mostly patients with cystic fibrosis) and the environment
Pseudomonas aeruginosa	*Pseudomonas pyocyanea* *Bacterium aeruginosa*	Belongs to fluorescent group, grows at 42°C. Most common clinical isolate
Pseudomonas fluorescens		Belongs to fluorescent group, gelatin-positive
Pseudomonas luteola	CDC Ve-1 *Chryseomonas luteola* *Chryseomonas polytricha*	Yellow-pigmented, oxidase-negative, esculin-positive
Pseudomonas mendocina	CDC Vb-2	
Pseudomonas oryzihabitans	CDC Ve-2 *Flavimonas oryzihabitans* *Pseudomonas lacunogenes*	Clinical isolates associated with septicemia and prosthetic-valve endocarditis. Yellow-pigmented, oxidase-negative, esculin-negative
Pseudomonas putida		Belongs to fluorescent group, gelatin-negative
Pseudomonas stutzeri	CDC Vb-1	Wrinkled colonies. Ubiquitous in soil and water. Rarely associated with infection
Psychrobacter phenylpyruvicus	*Psychrobacter phenylpyruvica* *Moraxella phenylpyruvica* CDC group M-2	Phenylalanine deaminase positive, grows at 4°C, tolerates NaCl concentrations up to 9%
Ralstonia pickettii	*Burkholderia pickettii* *Pseudomonas pickettii* CDC Va-1, Va-2	Slow-growing, pinpoint colonies after 24 hours on blood agar (BAP). Rarely associated with infection
Ralstonia mannitolilytica	*Pseudomonas thomasii* (Va-3)	Mannitol-positive
Rhizobium radiobacter	CDC Vd-3 *Agrobacterium radiobacter* *Agrobacterium tumefaciens* *Agrobacterium biovar 1*	
Roseomonas sp.	CDC "pink coccoid group"	Includes three named (*R. gilardii, R. cervicalis, R. fauriae*) and three unnamed genomospecies. Pink, often mucoid colonies, weakly staining gram-negative, plump, coccoid rods

Table 7-1 *Continued*

CURRENT USAGE	PREVIOUS DESIGNATIONS	COMMENTS
Shewanella putrefaciens *Shewanella algae*	*Pseudomonas putrefaciens* *Alteromonas putrefaciens* *Achromobacter putrefaciens* CDC Ib-1, Ib-2	H_2S-positive. *S. algae* is the predominant human clinical isolate and requires NaCl for growth.
Sphingobacterium multivorum	CDC IIk-2 *Flavobacterium multivorum*	Yellow-pigmented, oxidase-positive, esculin-positive, mannitol-negative, rarely associated with serious infection
Sphingobacterium spiritivorum	*CDC IIk-3* *Flavobacterium spiritivorum* *Flavobacterium yabuuchiae* *Sphingobacterium versatilis*	Yellow-pigmented, oxidase-positive, esculin-positive, mannitol-positive. Most common sources for isolation have been blood and urine
Sphingomonas paucimobilis	*Pseudomonas paucimobilis* CDC IIk-1	Yellow-pigmented, oxidase-positive, esculin-positive, slow-growing. Found in a variety of clinical specimens
Stenotrophomonas maltophilia	*Xanthomonas maltophilia* *Pseudomonas maltophilia* CDC group I	Oxidase-negative, lysine- and DNAse-positive, can be recovered from almost any clinical site. May cause opportunistic infections
Weeksella virosa	CDC IIf *Flavobacterium genitale*	Mucoid and sticky. Difficult to remove from agar. Clinical isolates have been associated with urinary and vaginal infections.

or iron, can derive energy from simple inorganic chemicals. These so-called **chemolithotrophs** are seldom implicated as causes of disease in humans.

Space in this textbook permits only a brief summary of the metabolic pathways used by the nonfermenters, enough to gain a working understanding of terms such as **aerobic, anaerobic, fermentation,** and **oxidation.** These metabolic processes not only define the taxonomic niche of bacteria but also determine the tests and procedures used in the laboratory identification of microorganisms. Textbooks by Doelle[192] and Thimann[737] should be consulted for a more detailed discussion of bacterial metabolism and physiology, and the text by MacFaddin[465] provides a review of the biochemistry of the various tests and reactions used in making identifications.

Fermentative and Oxidative Metabolism

The bacterial degradation of carbohydrates proceeds by several metabolic pathways in which hydrogen ions (electrons) are successively transferred to compounds of higher redox potential, with the ultimate release of energy in the form of adenosine triphosphate (ATP). All six-, five-, and four-carbon carbohydrates are initially degraded to pyruvic acid, an initial intermediate. Glucose is the main carbohydrate source of carbon for bacteria, and degradation proceeds by three major pathways: the Embden-Meyerhof-Parnas, the Entner-Doudoroff, and the Warburg-Dickins (hexose mono-

phosphate) pathways. As shown in Figure 7-1, glucose is converted to pyruvic acid in each of these three pathways by a different set of degradation steps. Bacteria use one or more of these pathways for glucose metabolism depending on their enzymatic composition and the presence or lack of oxygen.

The Embden-Meyerhof-Parnas Pathway

Because glucose is degraded without oxygen, the Embden-Meyerhof-Parnas (EMP) pathway has also been called the **glycolytic** or **anaerobic** pathway, used primarily by anaerobic bacteria and, to some degree, by facultatively anaerobic bacteria as well. The intermediate steps in the EMP pathway include the initial phosphorylation of glucose, conversion to fructose phosphate, and cleavage to form two molecules of glyceraldehyde phosphate, which, through a series of intermediate steps (not shown in Fig. 7-1), forms pyruvic acid. The EMP pathway is discussed more thoroughly in Chapter 6.

Historically, the EMP pathway has also been termed the **fermentative pathway.** Fermentation and anaerobic metabolism have been considered synonymous ever since Pasteur demonstrated that acids and alcohols are the major end products of carbohydrate degradation when oxygen is excluded from the system. According to a current concept, fermentative metabolism is said to exist in a glycolytic system when organic compounds serve as the final hydrogen (electron)

Table 7-2 CDC Lettered and Numbered Bacterial Groups: Synonyms

CDC DESIGNATIONS	CURRENT USAGE	CDC DESIGNATIONS	CURRENT USAGE
I	*Stenotrophomonas maltophilia*	HB-3,4	*Actinobacillus actinomycetemcomitans*
Ia	*Brevundimonas diminuta*	HB-5	*Pasteurella bettyae*
Ib-1	*Shewanella putrefaciens*	M-1	*Kingella kingae*
Ib-2	*Shewanella algae*	M-2	*Psychrobacter phenylpyruvicus*
IIa	*Chryseobacterium meningosepticum*	M-3	*Moraxella atlantae*
IIb	*Chryseobacterium indologenes*	M-4	*Oligella urethralis*
IIc	CDC group IIc	M-4f	*Myroides odoratus/odoratimimus*
IId	*Cardiobacterium hominis*	M-5	*Neisseria weaveri*
IIe	CDC group IIe	M-6	*Neisseria elongata* subsp. *nitroreducens*
IIf	*Weeksella virosa*	TM-1	*Kingella denitrificans*
IIg	CDC group IIg	DF	*Dysgonic fermenter*
IIh	CDC group IIh	DF-1	*Capnocytophaga ochracea*
IIi	CDC group IIi		*Capnocytophaga gingivalis*
IIj	*Bergeyella zoohelcum*		*Capnocytophaga sputigena*
IIk-1	*Sphingomonas paucimobilis*	DF-2	*Capnocytophaga canimorsus*
IIk-2	*Sphingobacterium multivorum*	DF-2-like	*Capnocytophaga cynodegmi*
IIk-3	*Sphingobacterium spiritivorum*	DF-3	Unnamed
IIIa, IIIb	*Achromobacter xylosoxidans*	EO	*Eugonic oxidizer*
IVa	*Bordetella bronchiseptica*	EO-1	*Burkholderia cepacia*
IVb	*Bordetella parapertussis*	EO-2	*Paracoccus yeei*
IVc	Unnamed	EO-3	Unnamed
IVc-2	*Cupriavidus pauculus*	EO-5	Unnamed
IVd	Pseudomonas-like group 2	EF	*Eugonic fermenter*
IVe	*Oligella ureolytica*	EF-1	Pseudomonas-like group 2
Va-1	*Ralstonia pickettii*	EF-3	*Vibrio vulnificus*
Va-2	*Ralstonia pickettii*	EF-4	*Pasteurella*-like
Va-3	*Ralstonia mannitolilytica*	EF-5	*Photobacterium damsela*
Vb-1	*Pseudomonas stutzeri*	EF-6	*Vibrio fluvialis*
Vb-2	*Pseudomonas mendocina*	EF-9	*Tatumella ptyseos*
Vb-3	*Pseudomonas stutzeri*–like	EF-13	*Vibrio hollisae*
Vc	*Achromobacter denitrificans*	EF-19	*Comamonas terrigena*
Vd-1	*Ochrobactrum anthropi*	EF-26	*Bordetella*-like species
Vd-2	*Ochrobactrum anthropi*	NO	Nonoxidizer
Vd-3	*Rhizobium radiobacter*	NO-1	CDC group NO-1
Ve-1	*Pseudomonas luteola*	NO-2	*Bordetella holmesii*
Ve-2	*Pseudomonas oryzihabitans*	WO	Weak oxidizer
VI	*Alcaligenes faecalis*	WO-1	Unnamed
HB-1	*Eikenella corrodens*	WO-2	*Pandoraea* sp.
HB-2	*Haemophilus aphrophilus*		

acceptor. Thus, as shown in the EMP pathway outlined in the left column of Figure 7-1, pyruvic acid acts as an intermediate hydrogen acceptor but is then oxidized by giving up its hydrogen ions to sodium lactate to form lactic acid or to other organic salts to form one of several so-called mixed acids. These acids are the end products of glucose metabo-

lism by the EMP pathway, accounting for the drop in pH in fermentation tests used for identifying bacteria. Bacteria that possess the appropriate enzyme systems can further degrade these mixed acids into alcohols, CO_2, or other organic compounds.

Although these biochemical principles seem somewhat

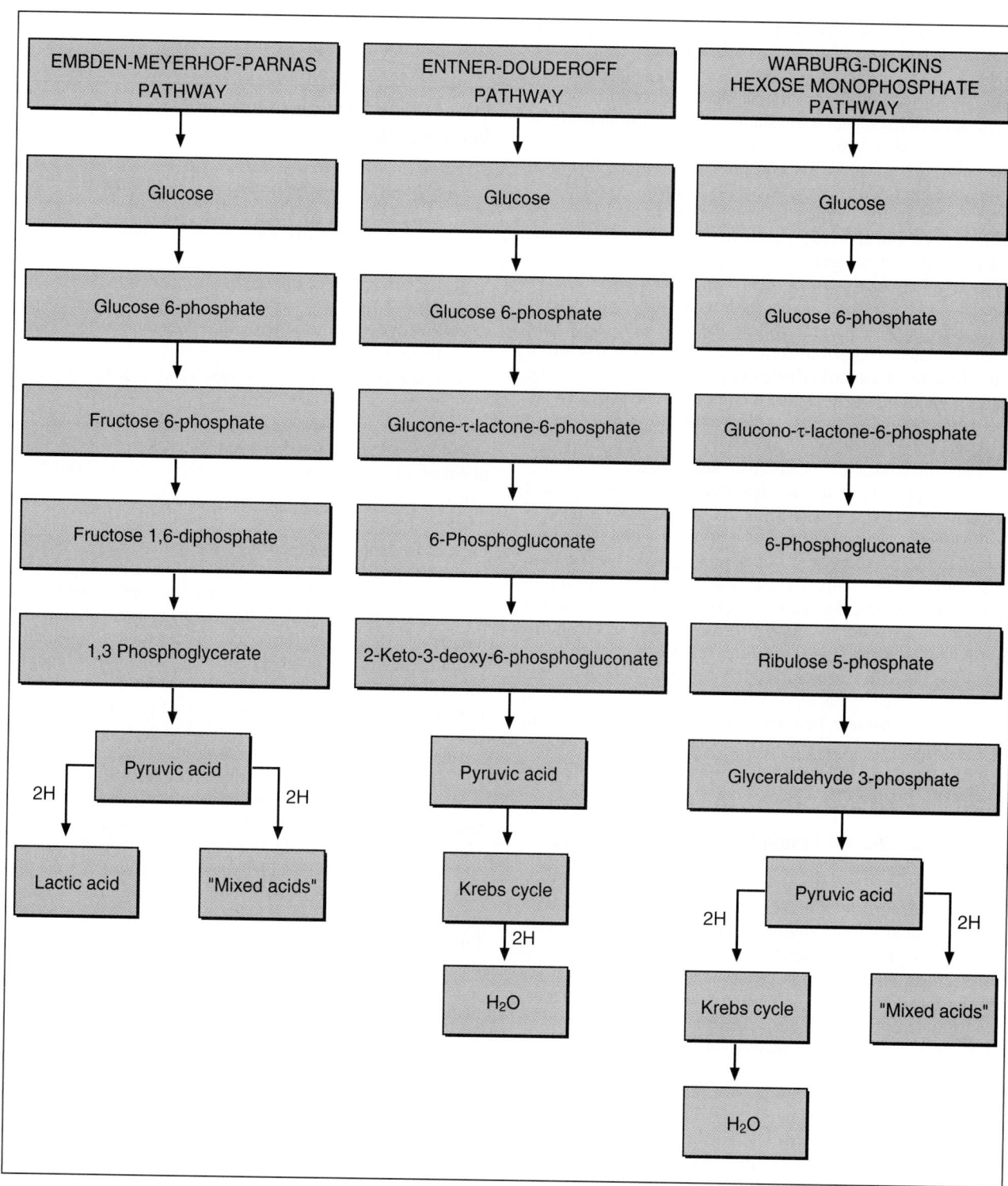

Figure 7-1 Metabolic pathways for the bacterial degradation of glucose.

removed from the daily work in the laboratory, microbiologists must have a basic understanding of bacterial metabolism when designing or interpreting test procedures that compare fermentation with oxidation. Fermentation must be determined in test systems that exclude oxygen. The glycolytic products formed by fermentation have relatively strong acidity, which is easily detected by pH indicators, and large

amounts of gas may be produced. This is not true for the Entner-Doudoroff pathway.

The Entner-Doudoroff Pathway

The Entner-Doudoroff (ED) pathway is also termed the **aerobic pathway** because oxygen is required for glycolysis to occur. Note in the center column of Figure 7-1 that glucose is not converted into two triose carbon molecules as in the EMP pathway; rather, it is oxidized to 6-phosphogluconate and 2-keto-3-deoxy-6-phosphogluconate before forming pyruvic acid. Some bacteria use shunt pathways through which glucose is oxidized directly into glucuronic and ketoglucuronic acid without an initial phosphorylation step. In either event, the intermediate pyruvic acid is formed. "Oxidation" refers more to the manner in which pyruvic acid transfers its hydrogen ions than to the pathway by which it is formed. Lacking the dehydrogenase enzymes necessary to oxidize pyruvic acid to lactic acid or other "mixed acids," oxidative bacteria transfer the available hydrogen ions from pyruvic acid into the Krebs cycle, where the ions ultimately link with elemental oxygen to form water. Thus, the **oxidative metabolism of carbohydrates** is presently defined as the energy-yielding reactions that require molecular oxygen (or other nonorganic elements) as the terminal hydrogen (electron) acceptor.

This difference in metabolism necessitates alternative, practical approaches to the identification of oxidative and fermentative bacteria. The acids that are formed in the ED pathway (glucuronic acid and its derivatives) and those produced in the Krebs cycle (citric acid and its derivatives) are extremely weak compared with the mixed acids resulting from fermentation. Because the end product of oxidative metabolism is water, gas is not formed from carbohydrates by oxidative organisms. Therefore, test systems with more sensitive detectors of acid production must be used when studying oxidative bacteria, which are discussed in detail later in this chapter. Test systems designed to detect acid production from fermentative bacteria often cannot be applied to oxidative organisms that produce insufficient acids to convert the pH indicator.

The Warburg-Dickens Hexose Monophosphate Pathway

Facultatively anaerobic bacteria have the capacity to grow on the surface of an agar plate in the presence of oxygen or in an anaerobic environment. Just because a microorganism can grow in an aerobic environment does not necessarily mean that oxygen is metabolically used. That is, not all aerobes are oxidative. The term **aerotolerant** is more appropriate for nonoxidative bacteria that are capable of growing in the presence of oxygen but grow better in an anaerobic environment.

Many of the facultative anaerobes can use either the EMP or the ED pathway, depending on the environmental conditions in which they are growing. The hexose monophosphate pathway (HMP), as shown in the right-hand column of Figure 7-1, is actually a hybrid of the EMP and ED pathways. Note that the initial steps in the degradation of glucose in the HMP pathway parallel those of the ED pathway; however, later in the HMP scheme, glyceraldehyde 3-phosphate is formed as the precursor of pyruvic acid, similar to the EMP pathway. These organisms appear fermentative in test systems, even though the EMP pathway is not strictly used.

Note in Figure 7-1 that ribulose 5-phosphate is the precursor to formation of glyceraldehyde 3-phosphate in the HMP pathway. Ribulose is a pentose and, for this reason, the HMP pathway has also been referred to as the pentose cycle. It provides the major avenue by which pentoses are metabolized by a number of bacterial species.

Initial Clues That an Unknown Isolate Is a Nonfermenter

The microbiologist may suspect that an unknown gram-negative bacillus is a member of the nonfermenter group by observing one or more of the following characteristics:

1. Lack of evidence for glucose fermentation (see Color Plate 7-1A)
2. Positive cytochrome oxidase reaction (see Color Plate 7-1B)
3. Failure to grow on MacConkey agar (see Color Plate 7-1C)

Additional characteristics used to make preliminary identification of the nonfermenters are presented in Color Plate 7-1.

Lack of Evidence for Glucose Fermentation

Acids produced by nonfermenters are considerably weaker than the mixed acids derived from fermentative bacteria; thus, the pH in fermentation test media in which a nonfermenter is growing may not drop sufficiently to convert the pH indicator. The initial clue that an unknown organism is a nonfermenter is usually the lack of acid production in either KIA or TSI media, manifested in each instance as an alkaline (red) slant and an alkaline deep (see Color Plate 7-1A). Initially, it is important that an unknown organism be classified by its mode of glucose utilization to select the correct set of biochemical characteristics to make a definitive identification. Microbiologists who use packaged commercial identification kits and bypass inoculation of the unknown organism to KIA or TSI tubes may not know whether to select a fermentative or oxidative system. Therefore, before setting up differential systems, it is recommended that the oxidative-fermentative (OF) characteristic of all unknown isolates of gram-negative bacilli be assessed by inoculating a KIA or TSI slant.

Positive Cytochrome Oxidase Reaction

Any colony of a gram-negative bacillus growing on blood agar or other primary isolation media that is cytochrome oxidase–positive can be suspected of belonging to the nonfermentative group (see Color Plate 7-1B). However, not all oxidase-positive, gram-negative bacilli are nonfermenters. Therefore, the mode of glucose utilization must still be measured (again demonstrating the importance of setting up a KIA or TSI tube). Cultures of oxidase-positive fermenters, such as *Pasteurella* species, *Aeromonas* species, *Plesiomonas* species, *Vibrio* species, and others, may be mistaken for nonfermenters, making identification more difficult. The procedure for performing the cytochrome oxidase test is given in Chart 1-5. To test the oxidase activity of nonfermenters, the CDC recommends using a 0.5% aqueous solution of tetramethyl-*p*-phenylene-diamine hydrochloride. This solution is good for 1 week if stored in a dark bottle in the refrigerator at 4 to 10°C. A few drops of reagent can be used to flood the surface of agar medium on which bacterial colonies are growing. The development of a blue color within a few seconds indicates a positive test. Negative reactions can be confirmed using the more sensitive Kovac's method, in which a loopful of organisms is mixed with a few drops of reagent on a piece of filter paper (see Color Plate 7-1*B*). The development of a dark blue color within 10 seconds indicates a positive test result.

Failure to Grow on MacConkey Agar

While all members of the *Enterobacteriaceae* grow on MacConkey agar, some nonfermenters do not grow on Mac-Conkey agar. Therefore, a gram-negative bacillus that grows on blood agar but grows poorly or not at all on MacConkey agar should be suspected of belonging to the nonfermentative group. This guideline, however, is far from absolute, because many of the fastidious gram-negative bacilli also do not grow on MacConkey agar. The ability of bacteria to grow on MacConkey agar is determined by inspecting with reflected light the surface of plates that have been inoculated and then incubated for 24 to 48 hours. Organisms that grow well produce colonies that are 3 mm or more in diameter and easy to see. Poorly growing strains produce either widely scattered, tiny pinpoint colonies or absolutely no growth (see Color Plate 7-1*C*).

Tests Used in the Identification of Nonfermenters
Utilization of Glucose

Most conventional culture media designed to detect acid production from fermentative bacteria, such as the *Enterobacteriaceae*, are not suitable for the study of nonfermentative bacilli. They do not support the growth of many strains, and the acids produced are often too weak to convert the pH indicator. Hugh and Leifson[350] were the first to design an OF medium that accommodated the metabolic properties of the nonfermentative bacilli, as outlined in Chart 7-1.

Note that the Hugh-Leifson OF medium contains 0.2% peptone and 1.0% carbohydrate, so that the ratio of peptone to carbohydrate is 1:5, in contrast with the 2:1 ratio found in media used for carbohydrate fermentation. The decrease in peptone minimizes the formation of oxidative products from amino acids, which tend to raise the pH of the medium and may neutralize the weak acids produced by the nonfermentative bacilli. On the other hand, the increase in carbohydrate concentration enhances acid production by the microorganism. The semisolid consistency of the agar, the use of bromthymol blue as the pH indicator, and the inclusion of a small quantity of diphosphate buffer are all designed to enhance the detection of acid.

Two tubes of each carbohydrate medium are required for the test. The medium in one tube is exposed to air; the other is overlaid with sterile mineral oil or melted paraffin (Fig. 7-2). Oxidative microorganisms produce acid

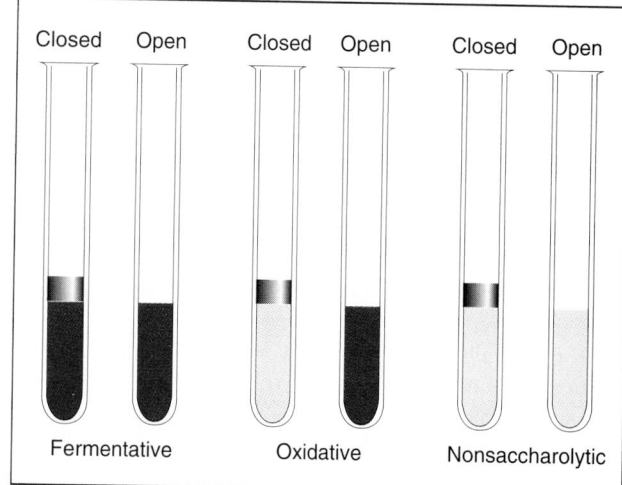

Figure 7-2 The oxidative-fermentative (OF) test. Fermentative organisms produce acid in both the closed and open tubes (*dark blue*); oxidative organisms produce acid only in the open tube. Asaccharolytic organisms that do not use carbohydrates produce no change in either tube.

only in the open tube exposed to atmospheric oxygen; fermenting organisms produce acid in both tubes; and nonsaccharolytic bacteria are inert in this medium, which remains at an alkaline pH after incubation. Color Plate 7-1*D* shows the OF reaction of an oxidative nonfermenter, with only the open tube showing the yellow color of acid production.

The OF test has limitations. Slow-growing nonfermentative bacilli may not produce color changes for several days, and species that produce amides from amino acids may cause weak acid reactions to reverse with time, thereby confusing the final interpretation. It is important that the Hugh-Leifson formula be strictly followed when performing the OF test (see Chart 7-1).

Motility

A semisolid agar medium for detecting motility of fermentative organisms may not be suitable for nonfermenting species that grow only on the surface of the agar. If a semisolid agar medium is used for nonfermentative bacilli, stab-inoculate only the upper 4 mm of the medium and make an initial reading within 4 to 6 hours. Many motile strains of nonfermentative bacilli show only an early, faint haziness near the surface of the agar, which tends to disappear with prolonged incubation. Readings should again be made at 24 and 48 hours to detect the motility of slowly growing strains. Incubation at 25°C enhances the motility of some strains. We have found that Motility B Medium with tetrazolium (Remel, Lenexa, KS) works particularly well for demonstrating motility with the nonfermenting bacilli (see Color Plate 7-1*E*).

The hanging-drop preparation may be more accurate in detecting motility of many species of nonfermentative bacilli. In this technique, a loopful of a 6- to 24-hour, actively growing broth culture that has been incubated at 25°C is placed in the center of a No. 1 coverslip that is inverted and suspended over the concavity of a depression slide. A more practical approach (preferred by the author) is to remove a small amount of growth from the surface of an 18- to 24-hour BAP and apply to the surface of a dry glass slide. A drop of saline is added to the inoculum on the slide and a coverslip is place over the drop. In either method the organisms are view under a 40× objective with reduced light for the presence of motility. True motility must be differentiated from brownian movement or the flow of fluid beneath the coverslip. Motile bacteria show directional movement and change in position relative to each other; when brownian movement is the cause of the motion, they maintain the same relative positions. The use of flagellar stains (see Chart 7-2), discussed later in this chapter, is also helpful in differentiating certain motile species (Fig. 7-3).[130,429]

Pigment Production

A number of pigments are produced by nonfermenters, some of which are helpful in making a species identification (see Color Plate 7-1F). Water-insoluble pigments include carotenoids (yellow-orange), violacein (violet or purple), and phenazines (red, maroon, yellow) that impart distinctive colors to the colonies. Water-soluble and diffusible pigments include fluorescein (pyoverdin), pyocyanin, pyorubin, melanin, and miscellaneous other pigmented byproducts that discolor the culture medium. "Tech" and "Flo" media[398] were developed to enhance formation of the water-soluble pigments pyocyanin and pyoverdin (see Color Plate 7-1G). These media have special peptones

and an increased concentration of magnesium and sulfate ions to enhance pigment production. King and coworkers[398] found that the kind of peptone used in the basal medium markedly affected pigment production. Bacto peptone (Difco Laboratories, Detroit, MI) proved to be superior for the production of pyocyanin but had an inhibitory effect on the elaboration of fluorescein, whereas proteose peptone 3 (Difco) enhanced the production of fluorescein and inhibited the formation of pyocyanin. An increase in phosphate concentration causes enhanced production of fluorescein but decreases pyocyanin production. Pigment production can also be enhanced by growing organisms in gelatin-, potato-, or milk-containing media and by incubating them at 25 to 30°C. Pyoverdin may be demonstrated on Flo agar by observing fluorescence under ultraviolet light (using a Wood's lamp) or by the appearance of a yellow pigment in the media in visible light (see Color Plate 7-1G and H).

Hydrolysis of Urea

Urea hydrolysis is presented in detail in Chart 6-6. Because many of the urea-splitting nonfermenters require enriched media for growth, Christensen's urea agar slants are used. Positive results may be achieved more rapidly by using a heavy inoculum. Bacterial species, such as *Bordetella bronchiseptica*, that avidly split urea may produce a red color change within 4 hours; weak reactors may require up to 48 hours before a positive reaction can be visualized. The appearance of a faint, delayed, pink tinge in the upper slant portion of the medium probably indicates nonspecific amino

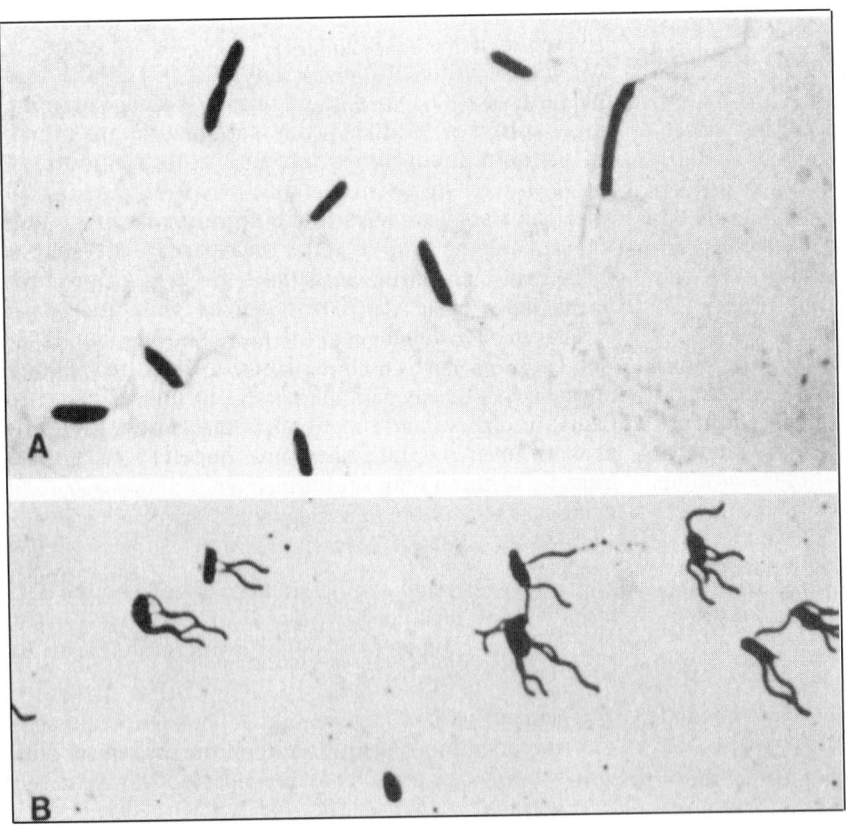

Figure 7-3 Bacteria stained with flagellar stains. (**A**) Positive flagellar stain of bacilli with polar flagella (original magnification, ×900). (**B**) Positive flagellar stain of bacilli with peritrichous flagella (original magnification, ×900).

acid degradation and should be read as a negative test result (see Color Plate 7-2*A*).

Nitrate Reduction

The basic principles and procedures for performing the nitrate reduction test are presented in Chart 6-2. The reduction of nitrate to nitrite is only the first step in a biochemical process used by some microorganisms to release oxygen—a final hydrogen acceptor at the end point of oxidative metabolism. The nitrate reduction test for nonfermenters is performed in a similar manner to that for other organisms, the end point being the appearance of a red color on addition of sulfanilic acid and α-naphthylamine to an overnight culture in nitrate-containing media. If a red color does not develop, either nitrate has not been reduced or reduction has proceeded beyond the nitrite stage to the formation of other compounds or to nitrogen gas (denitrification). The appearance of a red color on the addition of a small quantity of zinc dust indicates the residual presence of nitrates, denoting a negative test result; the absence of color indicates that the nitrate has been reduced to compounds other than nitrites (usually nitrogen gas), indicating that the original test was positive.

Denitrification of Nitrates and Nitrites

Certain nonfermenters have the capability of reducing either nitrate or nitrite (or both) to gaseous nitrogen (see Chart 7-3). Nitrate-nitrite broth, with an inverted Durham tube or an agar slant, may be used. Because the media contain no carbohydrates, any gas that forms is derived from the nitrate or the nitrite, indicating a positive denitrification test. The broth test is easier to interpret because the collection of gas within the inverted Durham tube is readily visualized. In agar slants, the collection of gas bubbles, usually in the depths of the butt, indicates a positive test result. Most denitrifying media contain both nitrates and nitrites. In rare instances (e.g., in the identification of *Alcaligenes faecalis*, which denitrifies nitrites but not nitrates), separate denitrification tests may be in order. Combination fluorescence-denitrification or fluorescence-lactose-denitrification media are available; however, the reactions may vary from those produced in the media recommended by the CDC (see Color Plate 7-2*B*).

Indole Production

The basic principles and procedure for determination of indole production are presented in Chart 1-4. Minor modifications may be required when detecting indole production by certain weak-reacting nonfermenters. An enriched tryptophan-containing medium, usually heart infusion broth, may be required. Because only small quantities of indole are formed by some nonfermenters, extraction of the culture media by layering a small quantity of xylene or chloroform on the surface may be helpful. Care should be taken to add only a small quantity of extractant because even minimal dilution may lower the concentration of indole below the sensitivity of detection by either Ehrlich's or Kovac's re-

agent. The appearance of a fuchsia color at the interface of the surface of the medium (or the extractant) with the reagent indicates indole formation and constitutes a positive test result. One organism, *Delftia (Comamonas) acidovorans*, produces a distinctive "pumpkin orange" indole reaction owing to the formation of anthranilic acid, rather than indole, from tryptophan (see Color Plate 7-2*C*).[486]

Decarboxylation

The Møller method for detecting decarboxylation of an amino acid (described in Chapter 6) is based on a change in pH. The development of an alkaline purple color in the test medium, following inoculation with the test organism and incubation at 35°C for 24 to 48 hours, constitutes a positive test result (see Chart 6-7). Many nonfermenters display only weak decarboxylase activity and may produce insufficient amines to convert the pH indicator system. This potential shortcoming in the Møller method can be overcome by using only small quantities of substrates (1 to 2 mL) and a heavy inoculum of pregrown organisms in which a high concentration of enzymes has already accumulated. The sensitivity of detection is also increased by overlaying the culture medium with 4 mm of petrolatum. It is essential that uninoculated, amino acid–free substrate controls be used to compare the color reactions. The initial conversion of the medium to a yellow color as acids accumulate from the small amount of glucose in the medium is not seen with nonfermenters; rather, the end-point reactions are read comparing the strong alkaline purple color reactions with the lighter blue-green hue of the controls (see Color Plate 7-2*D*). Tubes should be incubated at 35°C for up to 5 days before interpreting the reaction as negative. Other systems that use Ninhydrin reagent as an indicator may be more sensitive in detecting decarboxylase activity because the compound reacts directly with the amines to form a purple color.

Esculin Hydrolysis

Esculin hydrolysis is used primarily as a differential characteristic to distinguish between the two *Brevundimonas* species and some of the yellow-pigmented pseudomonads. An esculin medium without bile is recommended for testing of the nonfermenters, because some nonfermenter species are inhibited by bile. Esculin agar slants are inoculated with the unknown isolate and incubated at 35°C for 24 to 48 hours. Esculin in the medium fluoresces when observed with a Wood's lamp. When esculin is hydrolyzed, the medium turns reddish black and fluorescence is lost, indicating a positive test result (see Color Plate 7-2*E* and Chart 7-4).

Flagella Stains

Although usually not required, flagellar stains are occasionally useful in identifying certain motile nonfermentative bacilli, particularly when biochemical reactions are weak or equivocal.

LEIFSON METHOD

Reliable results may be obtained using Leifson's staining technique, described in Chart 7-2, if the considerations described in Box 7-1 are given strict attention.[130,429]

Box 7-1 Considerations When Preparing a Leifson Stain

1. The slides must be scrupulously clean. Slides should be soaked in acid dichromate or acid alcohol (3% concentrated hydrochloric acid in 95% ethyl alcohol) for 3 to 4 days. Final cleaning can be done immediately before use by heating the slides in the blue flame of a Bunsen burner.
2. Bacteria must be grown in a carbohydrate-free medium. A low pH may inhibit formation of flagella, and any acid formation in the medium may be detrimental. The pH of the staining solution should be maintained at 5.0 or higher.
3. Bacteria should be stained during the active log phase of growth, usually within 24 or 48 hours. Room-temperature incubation for 24 to 48 hours may be required to promote full development of flagella in some species.
4. Care should be taken not to transfer agar to the slide because it may interfere with the staining reaction. Washing the bacteria to be stained two or three times in water (lightly centrifuging between washes) before adding to the slides may help remove surface-staining inhibitors.

RYU METHOD

The use of the Ryu flagella stain, which is easy to perform and gives good results, is also recommended.[410,654] The procedure for this method is given in Chart 7-2.

WET-MOUNT TECHNIQUE

Heimbrook and colleagues[299] have described use of the wet-mount technique of Mayfield and Innis[493] and the stain of Ryu[654] as a rapid, simple way of staining flagella. In this approach, the test bacteria are grown on a noninhibitory medium for 16 to 24 hours. A faintly turbid suspension is made by first touching an applicator stick or wire to a colony on the plate and then touching a drop of water on a slide. A coverslip is placed over the drop, and the slide is examined for motile cells. After 5 to 10 minutes, or when about half of the cells are attached to the glass slide or coverslip, two drops of the Ryu stain (described in Chart 7-2) are applied to the edge of the coverslip and allowed to flow under the coverslip by capillary action. The cells are examined for the presence of flagella after 5 to 15 minutes at room temperature.

FLAGELLAR MORPHOLOGY

The number and arrangement of flagella on the bacterial cell can be an aid in identification of the species. The following types of flagellar arrangements can be observed:

- Polar
- Monotrichous—single flagellum at one or both poles
- Multitrichous—two or more flagella at one or both poles
- Subpolar—flagella near pole with base of flagella at right angle to long axis
- Lateral—flagella projecting from middle of bacterial cell

- Peritrichous—flagella haphazardly arranged all around bacterial cell

Representative bacteria stained with flagellar stains are shown in Figure 7-3.

PART II: TAXONOMY, BIOCHEMICAL CHARACTERISTICS, AND CLINICAL SIGNIFICANCE OF MEDICALLY IMPORTANT GENERA OF NONFERMENTERS

In the space available here, it is possible to provide only a brief summary of the medically important nonfermenters. Several references can be consulted for an in-depth discussion of the identifying features and clinical syndromes caused by this group of organisms.[244,247,257,327,403,545,570,671,802]

Unlike the *Enterobacteriaceae* the nonfermenting gram-negative bacilli do not fit conveniently into a single family of well-characterized genera, and the correct taxonomic placement of many nonfermentative, gram-negative bacilli (NFBs) remains unresolved. Consequently, the study of nonfermenters is often confusing for the beginning microbiologist. The major genera of nonfermenting, gram-negative bacilli have been classified into at least 15 families. including *Alcaligenaceae (Alcaligenes, Achromobacter, Bordetella, Oligella), Alteromonadaceae (Alishewanella, Shewanella), Brucellaceae (Ochrobactrum), Burkholderiaceae (Burkholderia, Cupriavidus, Pandoraea, Ralstonia,), Caulobacteraceae (Brevundimonas), Comamonadaceae (Comamonas, Acidovorax, Delftia), Flavobacteriaceae (Flavobacterium, Bergeyella, Chryseobacterium, Empedobacter, Myroides, Weeksella), Methylobacteriaceae (Methylobacterium, Roseomonas), Moraxellaceae (Moraxella, Acinetobacter, Psychrobacter), Oceanospirillaceae (Balneatrix), Pseudomonadaceae (Pseudomonas), Rhizobiaceae (Rhizobium, Agrobacterium), Sphingobacteriaceae (Sphingobacterium Pedobacter), Sphingomonadaceae (Sphingomonas),* and *Xanthomonadaceae (Stenotrophomonas).*[237] In addition, there are a number of clinically important nonfermenters that are not yet assigned to a family and whose taxonomic position is still uncertain.

One approach to studying the nonfermenters is to group them on the basis of the presence or absence of motility and on the type of flagella present in strains that are motile. With this approach, the medically important nonfermenters can be grouped as in Box 7-2.

Organisms That Are Motile With Polar Flagella
Pseudomonads

The genus *Pseudomonas* and some closely related genera, many of which were formerly placed in the genus *Pseudomonas*, make up a group often referred to as the pseudomonads. Members of this group share the characteristics of being straight or slightly curved, gram-negative bacilli that are strict aerobes; most strains are motile by means of one of more polar flagella; they utilize glucose and other carbo-

Box 7-2 Medically Important Nonfermenters

Motile With Polar Flagella

Family *Pseudomonadaceae*
(rRNA group I)
  Genus *Pseudomonas*
Family *Burkholderiaceae*
(rRNA group II)
  Genus *Burkholderia*
  Genus *Cupriavidus*
  Genus *Lautropia*
  Genus *Pandoraea*
  Genus *Ralstonia*
Family *Comamonadaceae*
(rRNA group III)
  Genus *Comamonas*
  Genus *Acidovorax*
  Genus *Delftia*
Family *Caulobacteraceae*
(rRNA Group IV)
  Genus *Brevundimonas*
Family *Xanthomonadaceae*
(rRNA Group V)
  Genus *Stenotrophomonas*
Family *Sphingomonadaceae*
  Genus *Sphingomonas*
Family *Oceanospirillaceae*
  Genus *Balneatrix*
Family *Alteromonadaceae*
  Genus *Alishewanella*
  Genus *Shewanella*
Family *Oxalobacteraceae*
  Genus *Herbaspirillum*
  Genus *Massilia*
Family *Methylobacteriaceae*
  Genus *Methylobacterium*
  Genus *Roseomonas*
Organisms Whose Taxonomic Position Is Uncertain
  CDC Groups Ic, O-1, O-2, O-3, Vb-3

Motile With Peritrichous Flagella

Family *Alcaligenaceae*
  Genus *Achromobacter*
  Genus *Alcaligenes*
  Genus *Bordetella* (*B. avium, B. bronchiseptica, B. hinzii,*
    B. trematum)

  Genus *Kerstersia*
  Genus *Oligella* (*O. ureolytica*)
Family *Rhizobiaceae*
  Genus *Rhizobium*
Family *Brucellaceae*
  Genus *Ochrobactrum*
Family *Halomonadaceae*
  Genus *Halomonas*

Nonmotile, Oxidase-Positive

Family *Flavobacteriaceae*
  Genus *Flavobacterium*
  Genus *Bergeyella*
  Genus *Chryseobacterium*
  Genus *Empedobacter*
  Genus *Myroides*
  Genus *Weeksella*
Family *Sphingobacteriaceae*
  Genus *Sphingobacterium*
  Genus *Pedobacter*
Family *Moraxellaceae*
  Genus *Moraxella*
  Genus *Psychrobacter*
Family *Neisseriaceae*
  Genus *Neisseria*
Family *Alcaligenaceae*
  Genus *Oligella* (*O. urethralis*)
Family *Rhodobacteraceae*
  Genus *Paracoccus* (EO-2)
Organisms Whose Taxonomic Position Is Uncertain
  CDC groups EO-3, EO-4, EF-4b
  CDC groups IIc, IIe, IIg, IIh, IIi,
  Gilardi rod group 1

Nonmotile, Oxidase-Negative

Family *Moraxellaceae*
  Genus *Acinetobacter*
Family *Alcaligenaceae*
  Genus *Bordetella* (*B. pertussis, B. parapertussis,*
    B. trematum)
Organisms Whose Taxonomic Position Is Uncertain
  CDC group NO-1
  CDC group EO-5

---

hydrates oxidatively; and are usually cytochrome oxidase-positive. The key differentiating features of the pseudomonad group are given in Table 7-3.

Palleroni[560] separated the pseudomonads into five ribosomal RNA homology groups based on rRNA-DNA homology studies. Gilardi, on the other hand separated the pseudomonads into seven major groups based on phenotypic characteristics: fluorescent, stutzeri, alcaligenes, pseudomallei, acidovorans, facilis–delafieldii, and diminuta.[250] An updated scheme that combines some of the features of both

the genotypic and phenotypic classification is outlined in Box 7-3.

Family *Pseudomonadaceae*
GENUS *PSEUDOMONAS*—rRNA GROUP I

Although most of the pseudomonads were originally classified in the genus *Pseudomonas*, it is now known that each of the five rRNA groups represents taxonomically distinct genetic groups, and as a result different genus names have been assigned to each of the rRNA groups. Only the mem-

Table 7-3 Key Characteristics of Pseudomonads

	OXIDASE	MOTILITY	PYOVERDIN	YELLOW	GLUCOSE	MALTOSE	LACTOSE	MANNITOL	ARGININE	LYSINE	NO₃→NO₂	NO₃→N₂	UREA	ONPG	DNASE	ACETAMIDE	ESCULIN	H₂S IN KIA	POLYMYXIN
Genus *Pseudomonas*																			
Fluorescent group																			
P. aeruginosa	+	+	+	−	+	V	−	V	+	−	+	V	V	−	−	+	−	−	S
P. fluorescens	+	+	+	−	+	V	−	+	+	−	V	−	V	−	−	−	−	−	S
P. putida	+	+	+	−	+	V	−	V	+	−	−	−	V	−	−	−	−	−	S
Stutzeri group																			
P. stutzeri	+	+	−	−	+	+	−	V	+	−	+	+	V	−	−	−	−	−	S
P. mendocina	+	+	−	−	+	−	−	V	+	−	+	+	V	−	−	−	−	−	S
CDC group Vb-3	+	+	−	−	+	+	−	+	+	−	+	+	V	−	−	−	−	−	S
Alcaligenes group																			
P. alcaligenes	+	+	−	−	−	−	−	−	−	−	V	−	V	−	−	−	NA	−	S
P. pseudoalcaligenes	+	+	−	−	−	−	−	−	V	V	+	+	−	−	−	V	−	−	S
Pseudomonas sp. group 1	+	+	−	−	−	−	−	−	V	−	+	+	−	−	−	−	NA	−	S
Yellow-pigmented group																			
P. luteola	−	+	−	+	+	+	+	+	+	−	V	−	V	+	−	−	+	−	S
P. oryzihabitans	−	+	−	+	+	+	+	+	−	−	−	+	V	−	−	−	−	−	S
Genus *Burkholderia*																			
B. pseudomallei	+	+	−	−	+	+	+	+	+	−	+	+	V	−	−	−	V	−	R
B. cepacia complex	w	+	−	V	+	+	+	+	−	V	V	−	V	V	V	V	V	−	R
B. gladioli	−	+	−	+	+	−	−	+	−	−	V	−	+	+	−	−	−	−	R
Genus *Ralstonia*																			
R. pickettii Va-1	+	+	−	−	+	+	+	−	−	−	V	V	+	−	−	−	−	−	R
R. pickettii Va-2	+	+	−	−	+	−	−	−	−	−	V	+	+	−	−	−	−	−	R
R. mannitolilytica	+	+	−	−	+	+	+	+	−	−	V	V	+	−	−	−	−	−	R
Genus *Delftia*																			
D. acidovorans	+	+	−	−	−	−	−	+	−	−	+	−	−	−	−	+	−	−	S
Genus *Brevundimonas*																			
B. diminuta	+	+	−	−	w	−	−	−	−	−	−	−	−	−	V	−	V	−	V
B. vesicularis	+	+	−	+	w	V	V	+	−	−	+	−	−	V	−	−	+	−	S
Genus *Stenotrophomonas*																			
S. maltophilia	−	+	−	−	+	+	+	−	−	+	V	−	−	+	+	+	+	−	S
Genus *Shewanella*																			
S. algae	+	+	−	−	+	−	−	−	−	−	+	−	−	−	+	−	−	+	S
S. putrefaciens	+	+	−	−	+	+	V	+	−	−	+	−	−	−	+	−	V	+	S
Genus *Sphingomonas*																			
S. paucimobilis	+	+	−	+	+	+	+	−	−	−	−	−	−	+	−	−	+	−	S

+, 90% or more strains positive; −, 90% or more strains negative; V, 11–89% of strains positive; w, weak positive; S, susceptible; R, resistant; ONPG, orthonitrophenyl-β-D-galactopyranoside. Key reactions are shaded. Data from reference[249].

Box 7-3 Phenotypic Classification of the Pseudomonads (Polar-Flagellated NFBs)

RNA Group I

Fluorescent Group
  Pseudomonas aeruginosa
  Pseudomonas fluorescens
  Pseudomonas putida
Stutzeri Group
  Pseudomonas stutzeri
  Pseudomonas mendocina
  CDC Group Vb-3
Alkaligenes Group
  Pseudomonas alcaligenes
  Pseudomonas pseudoalcaligenes
  Pseudomonas species group 1

rRNA Group II

Pseudomallei Group (Colistin-Resistant Group)
  Burkholderia mallei
  Burkholderia pseudomallei
  Burkholderia cepacia complex
  Burkholderia gladioli
  Pandoraea species
  Ralstonia species
  Cupriavidus species

rRNA Group III

Weak Oxidizer Group
  Comamonas acidovorans
  Comamonas terrigena
  Comamonas testosteroni
  Acidovorax delafieldii
  Acidovorax facilis
  Acidovorax temperans
  Lautropia mirabilis
  CDC WO-1

rRNA Group IV

Diminuta Group
  Brevundimonas diminuta
  Brevundimonas vesicularis

rRNA Group V

Stenotrophomonas maltophilia

Yellow-Pigmented Group

Pseudomonas luteola
Pseudomonas oryzihabitans
Sphingomonas paucimobilis

H$_2$S-Positive Group

Shewanella putrefaciens
Shewanella algae

Halophilic Group

Alishewanella fetalis
Halomonas venusta
CDC halophilic nonfermenter group 1

---

bers of rRNA group I retain the genus designation of *Pseudomonas*.

Fluorescent Group. The species within this group are all characterized by the production of a water-soluble pyoverdin pigment that fluoresces white to blue-green under long-wavelength (400-nm) ultraviolet light. Production of fluorescent pigments is particularly enhanced in media with a high phosphate concentration.[398] Although all three members of this group produce pyoverdin, only one species, *P. aeruginosa*, produces the distinctive blue, water-soluble pigment pyocyanin (see Color Plate 7-1*G*). The key biochemical features that separate the members of the fluorescent group are given in Table 7-4.

Pseudomonas aeruginosa produces a characteristic appearance when grown on BAP. It appears as large gray colonies with a spreading periphery and exhibits β-hemolysis. Colonies often have an alligator skin appearance and exhibit a metallic sheen (Color Plate 7-2*F*). Rapid identification of *P. aeruginosa* in culture can be made whenever the following characteristics are observed: typical colony morphology (Color Plate 7-2*F*), production of diffusible pigments (Color Plate 7-2*G*), the presence of a fruity odor, and oxidase positivity (Box 7-4).[529] We have occasionally observed strains that produce a pungent, ''rotten-potato'' odor. There has been at least one report of a nosocomial outbreak caused by strains of malodorous *P. aeruginosa*.[417]

Pseudomonas aeruginosa is the pseudomonad most frequently recovered from clinical specimens. *P. aeruginosa* infection is especially prevalent among patients with burn wounds, cystic fibrosis, acute leukemia, organ transplants, and intravenous drug addiction.[69] Infections commonly occur at any site where moisture tends to accumulate—tracheostomies, indwelling catheters, burns, the external ear (''swimmer's ear''), and weeping cutaneous wounds. The exudation of bluish pus, with a grape-like odor from the production of pyocyanin, is characteristic. *P. aeruginosa* also causes urinary tract and lower respiratory tract infections; the latter can be severe and even life-threatening in immunocompromised hosts. The organism can also cause devastating infections of the eye. Pseudomonas keratitis, infection of corneal ulcers, and endophthalmitis must be approached as a medical emergency that can be fulminant and threaten permanent loss of vision. Individual cases of endocarditis, meningitis, brain abscess, and infections of bones and joints from hematogenous spread appear with regular frequency in the literature.[69] Most cases of endocarditis require valve replacement because the infection is difficult to eradicate.[622] *P. aeruginosa* dermatitis and otitis externa outbreaks associated with swimming-pool and hot-tub use are well described. The CDC reported at least 75 cases during six outbreaks occurring between 1997 and 1998.[47] Sporadic *P. aeruginosa* infections following ear piercing have also been reported.[381]

P. aeruginosa produces several substances that are thought to enhance the colonization and infection of host tissue.[69] These substances, together with a variety of virulence factors, including lipopolysaccharide (LPS), exotoxin A, leukocidin, extracellular slime, proteases, phospholipase, and several other enzymes (Box 7-5), make *P. aeruginosa* the most clinically significant bacteria among the NFBs. An unusual mucoid morphotype of *P. aeruginosa* is frequently

Table 7-4 Key Characteristics of the Fluorescent Group

TEST	P. AERUGINOSA	P. FLUORESCENS	P. PUTIDA
Pyoverdin	+	+	+
Pyocyanin	+	−	−
Acetamide	V	−	−
Growth at 42°C	+	−	−
NO$_3$ reduction	V (74)	V (19)	−
Gelatin hydrolysis	V (46)	+	−

+, 90% or more strains positive; −, 90% or more strains negative; V, 11–89% of strains positive; ++, strong positive reaction; numbers in parentheses are percentages of strains giving positive reaction. Data from reference[249].

recovered from respiratory secretions of patients with cystic fibrosis who are chronically infected with *P. aeruginosa* (see Color Plate 7-2*H*). The mucoid morphotype is due to the production of large amounts of a polysaccharide (called alginate) that surrounds the cell. The production of alginate is ultimately responsible for the poor prognosis and high mortality rates among patients with cystic fibrosis. Comprehensive reviews of this subject are available.[255,492,518]

Treatment of *P. aeruginosa* infections can be difficult. A relatively narrow spectrum of antimicrobials is effective against *P. aeruginosa*, including the carboxypenicillins (carbenicillin, ticarcillin), the ureidopenicillins (mezlocillin, piperacillin), the antipseudomonal cephalosporins (ceftazidime), monobactams (aztreonam), carbapenems (imipenem, meropenem), quinolones (ciprofloxacin, levofloxacin), and aminoglycosides (gentamicin, tobramycin, amikacin). Almost all strains are resistant to other penicillins and cephalosporins, including ampicillin, cefuroxime, and cefotax-

Box 7-4 Minimum Requirements for Definitive Identification of *P. aeruginosa*

Identification based on all of the following:
1. Gram-negative rod
2. Oxidase-positive
3. Typical smell (fruity grape-like odor or corn tortilla)
4. Recognizable colony morphology
   a. On blood or chocolate agar appear as large colonies with metallic sheen, mucoid, rough, or pigmented (pyocyanin) and often β-hemolytic (Color Plate 7-2*F*)
   b. On MacConkey, appear as lactose-negative with green pigmentation, or metallic sheen (Color Plate 7-2*G*)

Limitations:
1. Rare *Aeromonas* isolates may resemble *P. aeruginosa* (lacking the typical smell) but will be spot indole-positive (*P. aeruginosa* are indole-negative).
2. Some *Burkholderia cepacia* isolates from patients with cystic fibrosis may exhibit morphotypes that resemble *P. aeruginosa*.

From reference[529].

Box 7-5 Virulence Factors of *Pseudomonas aeruginosa*

Virulence Factor	Biologic Activity
Alginate	Capsular polysaccharide that allows infecting bacteria to adhere to lung epithelial cell surfaces and form biofilms which, in turn, protect the bacteria from antibiotics and the body's immune system
Pili	Surface appendages that allow adherence of organism to GM-1 ganglioside receptors on host epithelial cell surfaces
Neuraminidase	Removes sialic acid residues from GM-1 ganglioside receptors, facilitating binding of pili
Lipopolysaccharide	Produces endotoxin, causes sepsis syndrome: fever, shock, oliguria, leukopenia or leukocytosis, disseminated intravascular coagulation, metabolic abnormalities
Exotoxin A	Tissue destruction, inhibition of protein synthesis; interrupts cell activity and macrophage response
Enterotoxin	Interrupts normal gastrointestinal activity, leading to diarrhea
Exoenzyme S	Inhibits protein synthesis
Phospholipase C	Destroys cytoplasmic membrane; destroys pulmonary surfactant; inactivates opsonins
Elastase	Cleaves immunoglobulins and complement components, disrupts neutrophil activity
Leukocidin	Inhibits neutrophil and lymphocyte function
Pyocyanins	Suppress other bacteria and disrupt respiratory ciliary activity; cause oxidative damage to tissues, particularly oxygenated tissues such as lung

ime.[233,451] *P. aeruginosa* has the capacity to carry multiresistance plasmids, and this feature has led to the appearance of some *P. aeruginosa* strains that are resistant to all reliable antibiotics.[451]

P. fluorescens and *P. putida* occur in water and soil and may exist in water sources in the hospital environment. Both may exist as normal pharyngeal flora and are rare opportunistic pathogens in humans. *P. putida* has been reported to cause catheter-related sepsis in patients with cancer[10,490] and septic arthritis.[466,469] Both species have been associated with bacteremia from transfused blood.[389,521,605,672,726,733] Of increasing importance are reports of *P. fluorescens* pseudobacteremias, the presence of positive blood cultures in the absence of true bacteremia and any related symptoms, most often attributed to contaminated catheters and catheter-related devices.[527,699]

Stutzeri Group. The organisms in the stutzeri group are all soil denitrifiers and can grow anaerobically in nitrate-containing media, with production of nitrogen gas. Strains are motile by way of polar monotrichous flagella. They can grow with NH_4 as the sole source of nitrogen and acetate as the sole source of carbon for energy. Characteristics that differentiate members of the stutzeri group are given in Table 7-5.

P. stutzeri (formerly CDC group Vb-1) is ubiquitous in soil and water and has been recovered from humus, manure, straw, sewage, stagnant water, baby formula, hospital equipment, eye cosmetics, and various clinical specimens.[243,250,570] It has only rarely been associated with infections, such as otitis media,[243] conjunctivitis,[570] pneumonia,[97,100,553] septic arthritis,[468] endocarditis,[639] meningitis in an HIV-positive patient,[634] infections of synthetic vascular grafts,[238] infections of traumatic wounds,[243,253] and vertebral osteomyelitis.[619] It is susceptible to most antibiotics. Freshly isolated colonies are adherent and have a characteristic wrinkled appearance (see Color Plate 7-3A), which may be lost after repeated laboratory subculture. *P. stutzeri* comprises a heterogeneous set of strains that includes at least 10 genomic groups without taxonomic status called genomovars.[129,235,646,649,677] However, the *P. stutzeri* genomovars are characterized by a high level of heterogeneity of phenotypic properties, which does not allow the taxa to be split into different species.[646,647,648] Only one of the described *P. stutzeri* genomovars has been reclassified and validly published, as the new species *Pseudomonas balearica*.[58] No human clinical isolates of *P. balearica* have yet been reported.

P. mendocina (formerly CDC group Vb-2) and the unnamed species CDC group Vb-3 are rarely isolated from clinical specimens. *P. mendocina* colonies are smooth and have the appearance and consistency of butter. One case each of mitral-valve endocarditis in a patient following aortic-valve replacement,[21] and tricuspid-valve endocarditis in a patient with a congenital heart defect[367] have been reported. CDC group Vb-3 isolates resemble *P. stutzeri* except they are arginine-positive. Potvliege and colleagues[602] have reported a case of Vb-3 septicemia in a patient with multiple myeloma.

Alcaligenes Group. Organisms in the alcaligenes group are characterized by being asaccharolytic or only weakly saccharolytic in OF glucose medium. Members of this group include *P. alcaligenes*, *P. pseudoalcaligenes*, and *Pseudomonas* species CDC group 1. The latter unnamed species is similar to *P. alcaligenes*, except that *Pseudomonas* species group 1 strains reduce both nitrate and nitrite to gas.[250] Characteristics that differentiate this group from other similar alkaline pseudomonads are given in Table 7-6. Although members of this group are recovered from clinical specimens, their ability to act as human pathogens has only rarely been documented. There have been reports of *P. alcaligenes*

Table 7-5 Key Characteristics of the Stutzeri Group

TEST	*P. STUTZERI* VB-1	*P. MENDOCINA* VB-2	CDC GROUP VB-3
Oxidase	+	+	+
OF glucose	A	A	A
OF maltose	A	−	A
OF lactose	−	−	−
OF mannitol	V (70)	−	A
NO_3 reduction	+	+	+
NO_3 to gas	+	+	+
Arginine	−	+	+
Lysine	−	−	−
Starch hydrolysis	+	−	V (75)
Polymyxin B	S	S	S
Wrinkled colonies	+	−	−

+, 90% or more strains positive; −, 90% or more strains negative; V, 11–89% of strains positive; ++, strong positive reaction; A, acid reaction; S, susceptible. Numbers in parentheses are percentages of strains giving positive reactions.
Data are from reference[249].

Table 7-6 Key Characteristics of Alkaline Pseudomonads[a]

TEST	COMAMONAS				DELFTIA	PSEUDOMONAS		BREVUNDIMONAS	
	C. terrigena	C. aquatica	C. kerstersii	C. testosteroni	D. acidovorans	P. alcaligenes	P. pseudoAlcaligenes	B. diminuta	B. vesicularis
Oxidase	+	+	+	+	+	+	+	+	+
Growth on MacConkey agar	+ (91)	NA	NA	+	+	+	+	+	V (26)
OF glucose	Alk	Alk	Alk	Alk	Alk	Alk	Wk (19)	Wk (29)	Wk (57)
OF fructose	Alk	Alk	Alk	Alk	A	Alk	A	Alk	Alk
OF mannitol	Alk	Alk	Alk	Alk	A	Alk	Alk	Alk	Alk
NO$_3$ reduction	+	+	+	+	+	V (61)	+	−	−
NO$_3$ to gas	·	−	−	−	−	−	−	−	V (38)
Gelatin hydrolysis	−	−	−	−	−	−	−	−	+
Esculin hydrolysis	−	−	−	−	−	−	−	−	+
Starch hydrolysis	−	−	+	+	−	V (16)	NA	V (58)	NA
Tyrosine hydrolysis	+	−	NA	−	NA	NA	−	NA	+
DNAse	−	NA	NA	−	−	−	−	V (12)	−
Acetamide	−	NA	−	−	+	−	−	−	−
Indole	−	−	−	−	Orange[b]	−	−	−	−
PYR[c]	+	−	−	+	+ (96)	V	−	V (12)	S
Susceptibility to 250 μg deferoxamine[d]	S	S	S	R	R	V	V	S(92)	−
Alkaline phosphatase	−	−	−	−	−	−	−	+	+
Assimilation on API ID 32 GN of:									
3-Hydroxybenoate	−	−	−	+	NA	NA	NA	NA	NA
4-Hydroxybenoate	+	V	+	+	NA	NA	NA	NA	NA
L-Alanine	+	−	−	+	NA	NA	NA	NA	NA
Growth at 42°C	−	−	+	−	V (8)	V (48)	V (75)	V (19)	−
Flagellar arrangement	Polar or bipolar tufts, long wavelength (3.0 μm)					Single polar, normal wavelength (1.5 μm)		Single polar, short wavelength (0.5 μm)	

[a] Data are from references[249,793].

[b] Pumpkin orange color develops on addition of Kovacs reagent due to formation of anthranilic acid from tryptophan

[c] PYR data from Laffineur K et al.[419a]

[d] Procedure described by Lindsay JA and Riley TV[444a]

+, 90% or more strains positive; −, 90% or more strains negative; V, 11–89% of strains positive; A, acid reaction; Alk, alkaline reaction; Wk, weak acid; S, susceptible; R, resistant. Numbers in parentheses are percentages of strains giving positive reactions.

causing eye infections, empyema, and one case of fatal endocarditis.[750]

Yellow-Pigmented Group.

Pseudomonas Luteola This species has been previously known as *Chromobacterium typhiflavum*, CDC group Ve-1, *Pseudomonas luteola*, *Pseudomonas polytricha*, and *Chryseomonas luteola*.[332] The taxonomic placement was resolved in 1997 when the species was placed back into the genus *Pseudomonas*.[14] *P. luteola* is motile by means of multitrichous polar flagella, is oxidase-negative, and grows on both MacConkey and blood agar media, producing yellow-pigmented colonies that are often wrinkled and become adherent to the agar (Color Plate 7-3*B*). The biochemical features that differentiate *P. luteola* from other yellow-pigmented pseudomonads are given in Table 7-11. It is a rare clinical isolate and has been recovered from a variety of clinical specimens, including wound, cervix, urine, and throat specimens.[250] Isolates recovered from clinical specimens at the University of Illinois Hospital have been from the cornea, sputum, leg, endometrial cavity, and blood. It is often isolated with other organisms and judged not to be clinically significant. In one study, only 14 strains of *P. luteola* were found among 565 clinical isolates of nonfermenters over a 2-year period.[570] Reports of serious infections caused by *P. luteola* include bacteremia,[59,123,154,210,225,608,612] endocarditis,[549] meningitis,[123,415] leg ulceration,[746] osteomyelitis,[608] and peritonitis.[148,608]

Pseudomonas Oryzihabitans This organism has been described formerly as *Chromobacterium typhiflavum*, *Pseudomonas oryzihabitans*, CDC group Ve-2, and *Flavimonas oryzihabitans*.[332] The taxonomic placement was resolved in 1997 when the species was placed back into the genus *Pseudomonas*.[14] *P. oryzihabitans* has characteristics similar to *Chryseomonas luteola* in that these organisms are also motile and oxidase-negative and form yellow-pigmented colonies on blood agar medium. Like *P. luteola*, colonies of *P. oryzihabitans* form rough or wrinkled colonies. This organism can be differentiated from *P. luteola* by negative reactions for esculin hydrolysis and orthonitrophenyl-β-D-galactopyranoside (ONPG) and the feature of having a single polar flagellum. Additional differential characteristics are given in Table 7-11. *P. oryzihabitans* has also been recovered from a variety of clinical sites, including wounds, sputum, ear, eye, urine, peritoneal fluid, inhalation-therapy equipment, and blood.[225,252,400,430,441,593,608] More recently, infections with this organism have been related to the presence of an intravascular catheter in immunocompromised patients.[462,481,636,772] At the University of Illinois Hospital, this organism has been recovered from sputum, urine, prostatic secretion, skin, and blood. *P. oryzihabitans* also appears to be an emerging pathogen in peritonitis related to continuous ambulatory peritoneal dialysis, with several cases now reported in the literature.[9,57,211,212,692] Other predisposing factors for *P. oryzihabitans* infections include indwelling intravascular catheters, artificial grafts, intravenous drug abuse, severe head trauma requiring surgery, and bone marrow transplantation.[116]

Family *Burkholderiaceae*
rRNA GROUP II

rRNA Group II consists of organisms that have been placed in the genera *Burkholderia*,[258,824] *Ralstonia*,[825] *Pand-*

oraea,[133] and *Cupriavidus*[752a]and have been referred to in the past as the *Pseudomallei* group. All species in this group are easily separated from other groups of pseudomonads by the property of exhibiting resistance to the polymyxin group of antibiotics (polymyxin B and colistin). The biochemical characteristics used to distinguish the members of this group are given in Tables 7-7, 7-8, and 7-9. This group comprises many species, including several plant-associated species. Only those that have been associated with human disease are included in this textbook. Two of the pathogenic species, *B. pseudomallei* and *B. mallei* are listed as category B biothreat agents by the CDC's Strategic Planning Workgroup because of their availability and potential to cause illnesses with high morbidity and mortality.[651]

GENUS *BURKHOLDERIA—PSEUDOMALLEI* GROUP

B. mallei is an obligate parasite of animals (primarily horses, mules, and donkeys) causing a respiratory tract infection known as glanders. The acute form of the disease can kill a horse in a couple of weeks. In rare instances, it can be transmitted to humans, usually through an abrasion of the skin.[780] A case of laboratory-acquired glanders occurred in 2000.[110] Glanders shares with anthrax and plague the distinction of use in war. There is documentation that *B. mallei* was used as a biowarfare agent in World War I.[803] *B. mallei* is a small gram-negative coccobacillus. On sheep blood agar it appears as smooth, gray, translucent colonies in 2 days, without pigment or distinctive odor. It is the only nonmotile species in the genus. Other differentiating features are given in Table 7-7.

B. pseudomallei causes melioidosis, a glanders-like disease in animals and humans (Box 7-6). From the rRNA and DNA-DNA results of Yabuuchi et al. it is evident the *B. mallei* and *B. pseudomallei* belong to a single genomospecies, but it has been proposed that these two species be kept separate for epidemiologic and zoonotic reasons.[824] *B. pseudomallei* grows well on standard laboratory media and often produces wrinkled colonies and thus morphologically may resemble *P. stutzeri*. The organism, has a specific ecologic niche, existing in soil and stagnant water in an area of latitudes 20° north and south of the equator, primarily in Thailand, Vietnam, and parts of northern Australia.[153,160] Recent reports confirm that it is endemic in China, Taiwan, and Laos, but the true incidence in most countries is unknown.[158,344] Very few cases of melioidosis have been reported from the Indian subcontinent despite similarities in environmental conditions with Southeast Asian countries, although, a case of melioidosis brain and lung abscess after travel to Sri Lanka was reported in 1999.[572] Most infections are asymptomatic or present as a self-limited, short-term, flu-like illness and can be diagnosed only by serology.[31] It is estimated that thousands of U.S. military personnel became infected with *B. pseudomallei* while serving in Southeast Asia in the 1960s and 1970s. Serologic surveys have revealed positive titers for this organism in 1–9% of U.S. soldiers returning from Vietnam.[131,402,710] Thus, with an estimated 3 million military personnel serving in Vietnam from 1965 to 1973, as many as 250,000 may have become infected with *B. pseudomallei*.[513] An important feature of this disease is its ability to produce latent infection that can reactivate many years after primary exposure. For this reason, melioidosis has been dubbed the "Vietnamese time bomb" be-

Table 7-7 Key Characteristics of *Burkholderia mallei, B. pseudomallei,* and *P. stutzeri*

TEST	P. STUTZERI	B. PSEUDOMALLEI	B. MALLEI
Oxidase	+	+	V
Motility	+	+	–
Growth on MacConkey agar	+	+	V
OF glucose	A	A	A
OF maltose	A	A	V
OF lactose	–	A	V
OF mannitol	V	A	V
NO₃ reduction	+	+	+
NO₃ to gas	+	+	–
Arginine	–	+	+
Lysine	–	–	–
Starch hydrolysis	+ (92)	–	NA
Polymyxin B	S	R	R
Wrinkled colonies	+	+	–
Pigment	Gray or slightly yellow	Cream or tan	Gray

+, 90% or more strains positive; –, 90% or more strains negative; V, 11–89% of strains positive; ++, strong positive reaction; A, acid reaction; S, susceptible; R, resistant; NA, not available. Numbers in parentheses are percentage of strains giving positive reaction
Data from reference[249,802].

cause the disease may still be incubating in American veterans of the Vietnam conflict.[267,513]

Infections are acquired by contact with the organism either by inhalation of dust or direct contact through breaks in the skin. Three forms of melioidosis have been described: 1) acute disease, presenting as septicemia with metastatic lesions; 2) subacute disease, presenting as a tuberculosis-like pneumonia with cellulitis and lymphangitis; and 3) chronic disease, presenting as a localized chronic cellulitis (Box 7-6). There has been one report of *B. pseudomallei* lymphadenitis and mediastinitis in a patient with chronic granulomatous disease.[198] Diabetes mellitus has been shown to be a risk factor for the development of bacteremic melioidosis.[723] It is important to treat suspected cases with antibiotics before any treatment of patients, such as draining lesions, in order to avoid sepsis. The mortality rate is 95% in patients with acute disease who are not treated. *B. pseudomallei* is intrinsically resistant to many antibiotics, including the penicillins, first- and second-generation cephalosporins, macrolides, rifamycins, colistin, and the aminoglycosides.[161,364] It is generally susceptible to chloramphenicol, the tetracyclines, trimethoprim-sulfamethoxazole, ureidopenicillins, third-generation cephalosporins, carbapenems, and (unusual for a pseudomonad) amoxicillin-clavulanate.[805,829] The fluoroquinolones have only weak activity, and have proved very disappointing in clinical trials.[30,115] This unusual antibiotic profile (i.e., gentamicin- and colistin-resistant and amoxicillin-clavulanate–susceptible) in an oxidase-positive gram-negative rod is useful for confirming the identification of *B. pseudomallei* in the microbiology laboratory.[162] Ceftazidime has been the treatment of choice for treating severe melioidosis, but response to high-dose parenteral treatment is slow.[805] Carbapenem antibiotics have been shown to be highly active against *B. pseudomallei* in vitro,[161,703] and in one study imipenem alone was shown to be an effective treatment for acute severe melioidosis, resulting in fewer treatment failures than ceftazidime alone.[696] In another study, the use of combination therapy with cefoperazone-sulbactam plus trimethoprim-sulfamethoxazole or ceftazidime plus trimethoprim-sulfamethoxazole appeared to be equally efficacious for treatment of severe melioidosis.[120]

Definitive diagnosis of melioidosis, which has been called "the great mimicker," depends on the isolation and identification of *B. pseudomallei* from clinical specimens. The organism grows readily on most routine laboratory media and can be recovered from blood using standard blood culture techniques.[820] Selective agars, either Ashdown's selective agar (ASA)[28] or *Burkholderia pseudomallei* selective agar (BPSA),[339] or selective broths[788] are recommended for isolation of *B. pseudomallei* from nonsterile body sites, particularly sputum in clinically suspected cases of melioidosis, and for follow-up during treatment of the disease.[821] The biochemical properties useful in identifying this organism are given in Table 7-7. Two biotypes of *B. pseudomallei* are categorized by their ability to assimilate L-arabinose.[700] The arabinose non-assimilators (Ara–) are virulent and can be isolated from both clinical specimens and the environment, whereas the arabinose assimilators (Ara+) are usually avirulent and with rare exceptions are found only in the environment.[433,700] Identification of *B. pseudomallei* is usually not difficult in laboratories in areas where the organism is endemic. However, with the increase in international travel and the threat of bioterrorism, it has become more likely that laboratories in areas where *B. pseudomallei* is not en-

Box 7-6 Epidemiology, Diagnosis, Treatment, and Prevention and Reporting of Melioidosis (*Burkholderia pseudomallei*)

Epidemiology

- Melioidosis is an infectious disease caused by the bacterium *Burkholderia pseudomallei*.
- It is clinically and pathologically similar to glanders disease caused by *Burkholderia mallei*.
- Melioidosis is predominantly a disease of tropical climates, especially in Southeast Asia, where it is endemic, with the greatest concentration of cases reported in Vietnam, Cambodia, Laos, Thailand, Malaysia, Myanmar (Burma), and northern Australia.
- The bacteria causing melioidosis are found in contaminated water and soil. Infection is acquired by inhalation of dust, ingestion of contaminated water, and contact with contaminated soil especially through skin abrasions, and for military troops, by contamination of war wounds. Person-to-person transmission can occur.
- Glanders is contracted by humans from infected domestic animals.
- *Burkholderia pseudomallei* and *Burkholderia mallei* are considered potential agents for biological warfare and biological terrorism.

Clinical Findings

- Four clinical presentations of melioidosis are described:
  - *Acute, localized infection:* This form of infection is generally localized as a nodule and results from inoculation through a break in the skin. The acute form of melioidosis can produce fever and general muscle aches, and may progress rapidly to infect the bloodstream.
  - *Pulmonary infection:* This form of the disease can produce a clinical picture of mild bronchitis to severe pneumonia. The onset of pulmonary melioidosis is typically accompanied by a high fever, headache, anorexia, and general muscle soreness. Chest pain is common, but a nonproductive or productive cough with normal sputum is the hallmark of this form of melioidosis.
  - *Acute bloodstream infection:* Patients with underlying illness such as HIV, renal failure, and diabetes are affected by this type of the disease, which usually results in septic shock. The symptoms generally include respiratory distress, severe headache, fever, diarrhea, development of pus-filled lesions on the skin, muscle tenderness, and disorientation. This is typically an infection of short duration, and abscesses will be found throughout the body.
  - *Chronic suppurative infection:* Chronic melioidosis is an infection that involves the organs of the body. These typically include the joints, viscera, lymph nodes, skin, brain, liver, lung, bones, and spleen.
- The incubation period (time between exposure and appearance of clinical symptoms) is not clearly defined, but may range from 2 days to many years.

Laboratory Testing

- Organisms appearing as small gram-negative rods may be observed in direct Gram stain from respiratory specimens or abscess materials.
- *Burkholderia pseudomallei* can be recovered from the blood, urine, sputum, or skin lesions using standard laboratory media incubated at 35 to 37°C in ambient atmosphere.
- Detecting and measuring antibodies to the bacteria in the blood is another means of diagnosis.

Recommended Treatment

- For acute or chronic infections, parenteral administration of imipenem or ceftazidime for 2–4 weeks followed by oral therapy with amoxicillin-clavulanate or a combination of doxycycline and trimethoprim-sulfamethoxazole for 3–6 months is recommended.[344]
- Treatment should be initiated early in the course of the disease. Although bloodstream infection with melioidosis can be fatal, the other types of the disease are nonfatal.

Prevention and Reporting

- There is no vaccine for melioidosis.
- Prevention of the infection in endemic-disease areas can be difficult, since contact with contaminated soil is so common. Persons with diabetes and skin lesions should avoid contact with soil and standing water in these areas. Wearing boots during agricultural work can prevent infection through the feet and lower legs.
- Laboratory-acquired infections have been documented. In healthcare settings, using common precautions while handling blood and body fluids can prevent transmission.
- All patient specimens and culture isolates should be handled while wearing gloves and gowns in a biosafety cabinet. Plates should be taped shut when incubating. "Sniffing" of plates containing *B. pseudomallei* is dangerous and should not be done.
- Report possible cases of melioidosis to health authorities

From the CDC (http://www.cdc.gov/ncidod/dbmd/diseaseinfo/melioidosis_g.htm) and the American Society for Microbiology (http://www.asm.org/policy/index.asp?bid=6342).

demic could encounter this organism. Since many laboratories rely on commercial identification systems, Lowe and colleagues compared the accuracy of four systems, the manual APE 20NE and 20E, and the automated Vitek 1 and 2 systems (bioMérieux Inc. Hazelwood, MO) for their ability to correctly identify 103 strains of *B. pseudomallei*. The API 20NE, API 20E, and Vitek 1 systems gave the correct identification in 98%, 99%, and 99% of the cases, respectively. The Vitek 2 failed to identify a large number of the *B. pseudomallei* strains largely due to differences in the biochemical reactions achieved compared to expected values in the data-base.[460] Koh and colleagues, using 47 strains of *B. pseudomallei*, tested a relatively new automated identification system, the BD Phoenix System. Although *B. pseudomallei* is not in the Phoenix database only 4 strains were read as no identification. The remaining strains were all incorrectly identified with high confidence as *B. cepacia* (34), *Burkholderia/Ralstonia* spp. (6), or another nonfermenter species (3).[412]

Rapid latex agglutination tests for detection of *B. pseudomallei* antigen in urine[186,701,702] have been developed that offer a simple, rapid, and highly specific method for diagnosing melioidosis and are particularly useful in areas with limited laboratory facilities.

Laboratory workers are advised to use biologic safety hoods when working with this organism because laboratory-acquired infection with *B. pseudomallei* has been reported.[29,279,594,667] Additional information on the clinical and laboratory features of melioidosis can be found in other published reviews.[158–160,428,805]

Burkholderia cepacia is a phytopathogen that causes onion bulb rot in plants and foot rot (jungle rot) in humans.[732] Since the early 1980s *B. cepacia* has emerged as a cause of opportunistic human infections, particularly in patients with chronic granulomatous disease[73,419,551] and cystic fibrosis.[262,356,694,738] Recent taxonomic advances have demonstrated that *B. cepacia* is actually a cluster of at least nine closely related genomic species (or genomovars) now called the *B. cepacia* complex and includes *B. cepacia* (genomovar I), *B. multivorans* (genomovar II), *B. cenocepacia* (genomovar III), *B. stabilis* (genomovar IV), *B. vietnamiensis* (genomovar V), *B. dolosa* (genomovar VI), *B. ambifaria* (genomovar VII), *B. anthina* (genomovar VIII), and *B. pyrrocinia* (genomovar IX), which can be differentiated on the basis of molecular and biochemical tests.[137,139,142,258,302,754,756,757,759,773] Although all genomovars of *B. cepacia* complex have been cultured from the sputa of patients with cystic fibrosis (CF), *B. cenocepacia* (genomovar III) and *B. multivorans* (genomovar II) account for the majority of the isolates recovered from patients in North America[448,568,709] and Europe.[3,188,479] Patients with cystic fibrosis who are colonized with these genomotypes have a higher mortality in the year following colonization and have a more precipitous decline in overall pulmonary function following colonization.[437] These bacteria are also those most frequently associated with epidemic spread and with ''cepacia syndrome,'' which is manifested by severe progressive respiratory failure and bacteremia.[26,142,187,269,472,445,817] In addition, several epidemiologic studies have indicated that certain *B. cepacia* complex strains are transmissible between patients and that cross-infection probably occurs by direct person-to-person spread.[108,268,446,447,698] Virulence markers such as the cable (cbl) pilus encoded by the cable pilin subunit gene (*cblA*) that mediates adherence to mucus glycoproteins and enhances adherence to epithelial cells,[263,658,659,721] and the *B. cepacia* epidemic strain marker (BCESM)[471] designated such because of its association with *B. cepacia* strain types infecting multiple patients with CF, occur almost exclusively in *B. cenocepacia*.

B. cepacia complex has been isolated from numerous water sources and wet surfaces, including detergent solutions and intravenous fluids. Hospital outbreaks of *B. cepacia* infection are usually due to a single contaminated source such as anesthetics,[72] disinfectants,[565,705] intravenous solutions,[193,766] nebulizer solutions,[287,351] mouthwash,[109] and medical devices, including respiratory therapy equipment.[459,794] Disinfectants in which *B. cepacia* will grow include povidone-iodine, quaternary ammonium compounds, and chlorhexidine.[61,151,705] Pseudobacteremias (false-positive blood cultures) have been reported following the use of *B. cepacia*–contaminated disinfectant solutions.[61,151,559,565] *B. cepacia* can also grow in distilled water with a nitrogen source owing to the ability of this organism to fix CO_2 from air. Clinical infections include pneumonia and pneumonitis

in patients receiving contaminated anesthetics, urinary tract infection in patients receiving contaminated irrigation fluids following catheterization or cystoscopy, septicemia following heart surgery, endocarditis caused by contaminated heart valves, conjunctivitis, and septic arthritis.[559] Peritonitis following peritoneal dialysis has been associated with povidone-iodine solution contaminated with *B. cepacia*.[565] Infections involving the central nervous system include one case of bacteremia secondary to a contaminated Holter ventriculoatrial shunt in a child with congenital hydrocephalus[49] and a case of brain abscesses secondary to chronic suppurative otitis media in an adult.[307]

Selective media with bacteriostatic dyes, antibiotics, or low pH have been described for the selective isolation of *B. cepacia*. These include *Pseudomonas cepacia* medium (PCM), containing crystal violet, polymyxin B and ticarcillin[256]; OFPBL medium, containing polymyxin B and bacitracin and lactose[796]; and *Burkholderia cepacia* selective agar (BCSA), containing lactose, sucrose, polymyxin B, gentamicin, and vancomycin.[300] Comparative evaluations of these media have shown that the recovery of *B. cepacia* from patients with cystic fibrosis is enhanced with their use.[301,767,774,819] Overall, BCSA (predominantly used in the United States) and Mast *B. cepacia* medium (predominantly used in Europe) have been found to be the most suitable for growth of all *B. cepacia* complex isolates.[774,819]

Identification of *B. cepacia* in the clinical laboratory is problematic because *B. cepacia* is not a single phenotype but a complex of at least nine separate genetic species.[496] Commercial identification systems have performed poorly in identifying these organisms. Kiska et al. compared four commercial systems, including the RapID NF Plus (Remel), API Rapid NFT (renamed API 20NE (bioMérieux), Vitek GNI (bioMérieux), and Uni-N/F Tek (Remel). Correct identification for *B. cepacia* was 86% for Uni-N/F Tek, 81% for RapID NF Plus, 50% for Vitek GNI, and 43% for API 20NE.[404] van Pelt and colleagues reported that 90% of *B. cepacia* strains were identified correctly with the API 20NE and Vitek GNI, with 68% identified correctly with the MicroScan WalkAway overnight urine combo type 1 panels.[767] Shelly et al. evaluated the performance of nine different commercial systems used in 108 clinical microbiology laboratories from 91 U.S. cities that referred isolates to a CF reference laboratory for confirmatory testing using a polyphasic approach that included genus- and species-specific rRNA-based PCR assays.[682] Positive predictive values ranged from 71% to 98%; negative predictive values ranged from 50% to 82%, and all systems gave misidentifications for *B. cepacia* complex. The species most frequently misidentified as *B. cepacia* was *Burkholderia gladioli*. Brisse et al.[85] compared the BD Phoenix and Vitek 2 automated instruments for identification of isolates of the *B. cepacia* complex. Rates of correct identification were 50% for BD Phoenix and 53% for Vitek 2 when all *B. cepacia* complex isolates were considered, but differed markedly for *B. cenocepacia* (genomovar III) (71% for Phoenix and 38% for Vitek 2) and *B. multivorans* (genomovar II) (58% for Phoenix and 89% for Vitek 2). The results of these studies support the recommendation that when using commercial systems for identification of *B. cepacia* complex isolates, results should be confirmed by performing supplemental biochemical tests (Table 7-8) or by molecular methods.

Table 7-8 Key Characteristics of *Burkholderia cepacia* Complex and Related Species

TEST	B. CEPACIA[a] I	B. MULTIVORANS[a] II	B. CENOCEPACIA[a] III	B. STABILIS[a] IV	B. VIETNAMIENSIS[a] V	B. DOLOSA[a,b] VI	B. AMBIFARIA[a,c] VII	B. ANTHINA[d] VIII	B. PYRROCINIA[e] IX	B. GLADIOLII[a]	PANDORAEA[a,h] SPECIES	INQUILINUS LIMOSUS[f]	RALSTONIA PICKETTII
Oxidase	100[c]	100	100	100	100	100	100	100	+	0	67	+	100
Catalase	+	+	+	+	+	+	+	+	+	+	+	+	D[g]
Lipase	+	+	+	+	+	+	+	+	+	+	–	+	+
OF glucose	100	100	95	100	100	100	100	100	+	100	11	0	100
OF maltose	39	98	78	93	97	100	100	100	V	0	0	NA	92
OF lactose	61	100	79	93	97	100	100	100	+	0	0	43	92
OF xylose	87	98	88	44	75	100	100	100	NA	96	0	NA	83
OF sucrose	87	0	88	0	94	0	95	V	+	0	0	0	0
OF adonitol	70	91	79	78	0	100	100	V	NA	93	0	NA	0
10% Lactose	100	100	36	100	100	NA	NA	NA	NA	8		75	0
ONPG	100	98	99	100	100	100	100	V	–	100	0	0	0
Lysine	100	53	99	100	100	0	100	V	+	0	0	0	0
Ornithine	30	0	71	100	0	0	0	0	NA	0	0	0	17
Nitrate-reduced	4	94	31	4	47	100	67	V	+	33	11	38	33
Gelatin	74	2	55	93	0	0	94	0	V	70	0	NA	0
Esculin	56	2	33	0	0	0	56	V	V	11	63	25	100
Urease	91	100	8	60	100	0	0	NA	–	75	R	R	R
Colistin, 10 µg	R	R	R	R	R	R	R	R	R	R	R	R	50
Growth on MacConkey	83	96	84	93	83	100	100	100	+	96	100	NA	83
Growth at 42°C	43	100	84	0	100	100	26	V	–	4	89	100	NA
Malonate utilization	100	90	42	100	100	NA	NA	NA	NA	0	NA	NA	NA
Yellow pigmented	78	2	3	0	0	0	0	0	–	44	0	0	0

[a] Data from references 302,757.
[b] Data from reference 137.
[c] Data from reference 199.
[d] Data from reference 754.
[e] Data from reference 715a.
[f] Data from references 136,595.
[g] The catalase reaction for R. pickettii is often weak or delayed (Schreckenberger P: personal observation)
[h] Data from reference 153.

+, 90% or more strains positive; –, 90% or more strains negative; V, 11–89% of strains positive; S, susceptible; R, resistant; NA, not available; D, different results reported. Oxidation test results were recorded after 3 days of incubation. Roman numerals represent genomovars of B. cepacia complex.

Unlike other common pseudomonads, *B. cepacia* is resistant to aminoglycoside antibiotics but is usually susceptible to trimethoprim-sulfamethoxazole, which has become the drug of choice in treating *B. cepacia* infections. Daniel et al. performed in vitro susceptibility studies on 36 *B. cepacia* blood isolates and found that most strains were susceptible to minocycline (94.4%), ceftazidime (86.1%), ciprofloxacin (83.3%), and trimethoprim-sulfamethoxazole (83.3%).[168] In two- and three-drug synergy studies performed by Bonacorsi and colleagues, the addition of ciprofloxacin significantly enhanced the killing activities of piperacillin, imipenem, and meropenem, while the three-drug combination of β-lactam–ciprofloxacin–tobramycin gave the most consistently synergistic effect.[71] Aaron and colleagues also performed in vitro testing using multiple antibiotic combinations for *B. cepacia* isolates.[1] They reported that using double-antibiotic combinations improved bactericidal activity for the following drug combinations: meropenem-minocycline, meropenem-amikacin, and meropenem-ceftazidime. Triple-antibiotic combinations that contained tobramycin, meropenem, and an additional antibiotic were most effective and were bactericidal against 81% and 93% of isolates. In another study Nzula and colleagues showed that antibiotic minimal inhibitory concentrations (MICs) vary widely for the different strains of the *B. cepacia* complex.[541] While all strains were resistant to polymyxin B, MICs for chloramphenicol ranged from 4 to 128 mg/L and those for trimethoprim from 0.25 to 64 mg/L, with the majority of strains exhibiting resistance. Similarly, the MIC ranges for tobramycin, ciprofloxacin, and ceftazidime varied widely, suggesting the need for laboratories to perform susceptibility testing on individual isolates. Vermis et al. noted that the MICs of clinical isolates originating from patients with CF were higher than those isolated from patients who did not have CF and that in general, *B. cepacia* complex isolates were most sensitive to rifampicin, trimethoprim-sulfamethoxazole, and imipenem and most resistant to polymyxin B.[774]

For further information on the biology, taxonomy, mechanisms of virulence, and epidemiology of *B. cepacia*, several excellent reviews can be consulted.[142,255,269,369,445,470,774]

B. gladioli (formerly named *P. marginata*) is primarily a plant pathogen causing "flower rot" in gladiolus and other plants. It is one of the few pseudomonads that is negative for cytochrome oxidase, and it produces nonfluorescent yellow colonies after 48 to 72 hours of incubation. It has been reported to cause human pulmonary disease and sometimes bacteremia and soft-tissue infections in patients with CF,[43,127,274,370,374,390,514] chronic granulomatous disease,[306,643] diabetes,[686] and other immunologic deficiencies.[274] There has been one report of *B. gladioli* keratitis and endophthalmitis in an elderly patient with diabetes mellitus.[629]

B. gladioli usually grows as yellow colonies because of production of a diffusible, nonfluorescent yellow pigment. Biochemical tests that enable differentiation from *B. cepacia* complex include negative reactions for lysine, maltose, and lactose. Most strains are oxidase-negative or weakly oxidase-positive and catalase-positive. Further differentiating characteristics are given in Table 7-8. Laboratory workers should be aware that phenotypic methods for differentiation of *B. gladioli* from the organisms of the *B. cepacia* complex are unreliable and may lead to misidentification.[132] Commercial identification systems often fail to discriminate *B. gladioli* from related species.[682,767] Therefore, molecular-based methods should be used when confirmation of an isolate as *B. gladioli* is deemed necessary.[51,132,804] The antibiotic susceptibility pattern may also serve as a clue that an organism might be *B. gladioli*, since it tends to be susceptible to aminoglycosides, imipenem, ciprofloxacin, and trimethoprim-sulfamethoxazole and resistant to aztreonam and cephalosporins.[643]

GENUS *RALSTONIA* AND GENUS *CUPRIAVIDUS*

Palleroni[560] and later Li et al.[439] demonstrated two DNA homology groups within the *Pseudomonas* RNA homology group II. In 1992 Yabuuchi proposed the generic name *Burkholderia* for seven species but noted that *B. pickettii* and *B. solanacearum* were similar to each other and different from the other five *Burkholderia* species named at the time.[824] In 1995 Yabuuchi et al. proposed the transfer of *B. pickettii*, *B. solanacearum*, and *Alcaligenes eutrophus* to the new genus *Ralstonia* with *R. pickettii* serving as the type species.[825] Subsequently, several new species or new combinations were added to the genus *Ralstonia*. Comparative 16S rDNA sequence analysis now indicates that two distinct sublineages exist within the genus *Ralstonia*. The first, which is called the *Ralstonia eutropha* lineage, is comprised of *R. basilensis*, *R. campinensis*, *R. eutropha*, *R. gilardii*, *R. metallidurans*, *R. oxalatica*, *R. paucula*, *R. repiraculi*, and *R. taiwanensis*. The second is the *Ralstonia pickettii* lineage, which is comprised of *R. insidiosa*, *R. mannitolytica*, *R. pickettii*, *R. solanacearum*, and *R. syzygii*. This separation is supported by phenotypic differences. Members of the *R. eutropha* lineage have peritrichous flagella, do not produce acids from glucose and are colistin-susceptible, in contrast to members of the *R. pickettii* lineage, that have one or more polar flagella, produce acid from several carbohydrates and are colistin-resistant (see Box 7-7).[175,763] Vaneechoutte and colleagues proposed that the species of the *R. eutropa* lineage be reclassified into the new genus *Wautersia*.[763] Subsequently, DNA-DNA hybridization experiments and an evaluation of phenotypic characteristics, DNA base ratios and 16S rRNA gene sequences demonstrated that *Wautersia eutropha* the type species of the genus *Wautersia*, is a later synonym of *Cupriavidus necator*, the type species of the genus *Cupriavidus*. Therefore, all members of the genus *Wautersia* are reclassified into the genus *Cupriavidus*.[752a]

Box 7-7 Characteristics for Differentiation of *Ralstonia* and *Cupriavidus*		
Characteristic	**Ralstonia**	**Cupriavidus**
Flagellation	Polar, 1–4	Peritrichous
Colistin (10-μg disks)	Resistant	Susceptible
Acid from carbohydrates	Positive	Negative

Ralstonia pickettii was created for a group of clinical isolates[609] and also turned out to include strains of CDC groups Va-1 and Va-2, which were regarded as two different biovars of *R. pickettii*.[586] Shortly before this, King et al.[395] reported that *R.* (*"Pseudomonas"*) *pickettii* contained several biovars, including the strains originally isolated from St. Thomas Hospital, London,[579,580] which had been designated "*Pseudomonas thomasii*," although the name was never validly published. In 1994, Pickett[583] noted that *R. pickettii* should be recognized as having three biovars designated biovar Va-1, biovar Va-2, and biovar 3/*thomasii*. De Baere et al.[175] subsequently confirmed by DNA-DNA hybridization that *R. pickettii* biovar 3/*thomasii* was a separate species and proposed the name *Ralstonia mannitolytica*, later corrected to *Ralstonia mannitolilytica*.[449]

B. pickettii is rarely associated with human infections, but it has been reported to cause nosocomial infections, including bacteremia and urinary tract infections. In 1983, five infants in the special-care nursery of a hospital in Chicago became colonized with *B. pickettii* following endotracheal suctioning with saline from commercially prepared saline in 5-mL unit-dose vials. Subsequently, four additional hospitals reported respiratory colonization of infants and adults with *B. pickettii* following the use of the same brand of saline vials.[107] This outbreak demonstrates the ability of *B. pickettii* to survive and grow in commercially prepared "sterile" saline despite pertinent Food and Drug Administration (FDA) regulations and company programs for identifying such contamination. More recent nosocomial outbreaks have occurred with contaminated respiratory care solutions,[418] heparin solutions,[487] "sterile" saline for injection,[121] distilled water,[382,485] and a contaminated water irrigation system.[833] Pseudo-outbreaks have also been reported due to contaminated blood-culture bottle caps,[75] and water splashed from a sink.[298] There have been only a few reports of primary infection cause by *R. pickettii*, including one case of vertebral osteomyelitis and diskitis in a patient receiving long-term hemodialysis,[799] bacteremia in a cord-blood-transplant recipient,[814] and meningitis in a presumably healthy rancher,[297] in which an obvious contaminating source for the infection could not be found.

R. pickettii is slow-growing and produces only pinpoint colonies on blood agar plates after 24 hours. All strains are urease-positive and some strains may be catalase-negative. Motility is weak or delayed and may not be detectable. Biovar Va-1 can be separated from Va-2 by the oxidation of lactose and maltose. For additional biochemical characteristics see Table 7-9.

R. mannitolilytica is the name give to organisms formerly classified as *R. pickettii* biovar 3/*thomasii* (see discussion above).[175] It has been recovered from the sputum of patients with CF[143,220] and one case each of recurrent meningitis and hemoperitoneum.[762] It can be distinguished from all described *Ralstonia* species by its acidification of D-arabitol and mannitol and its lack of nitrate reduction and of alkalinization of tartrate.

R. insidiosa strains have been isolated from the environment as well as human clinical samples, including respiratory secretions of patients with cystic fibrosis.[135,763] Strains of *R. solanacearum* and *R. syzygii* have not been isolated

from human clinical specimens. Characteristics for identification of *Ralstonia* species of human origin are given in Table 7-9.

The genus *Cupriavidus* is composed of former *Ralstonia* species that are asaccharolytic, colistin-susceptible, and motile, with peritrichous flagella (Box 7-7) and includes: *C. basilensis, C. campinensis, C. gilardii, C. metallidurans, C. necator* (type species formerly *Ralstonia eutropha*), *C. oxalaticus, C. pauculus, C. respiraculi,* and *C. taiwanensis*.[752a]

C. gilardii (formerly *Ralstonia gilardii*) was named in honor of G.L. Gilardi, an American microbiologist who contributed much to our knowledge of NFBs. It is phenotypically similar to *Alcaligenes faecalis,* and was referred to as *A. faecalis*–like by Gilardi. It is a gram-negative, nonfermenting, asaccharolytic bacillus that is motile by means of peritrichous flagella,[792] although in the original description by Coenye et al. they were described as being motile by means of a single polar flagellum[134] Catalase and oxidase are positive. Nitrate and nitrite are not reduced. It can be differentiated from *A. faecalis* by the absence of nitrite reduction and failure to grow on acetamide and in 6.5% NaCl. Human isolates have been from the respiratory tract, a furuncle, cerebrospinal fluid (CSF), bone marrow, and blood.[134,792]

C. pauculus (formerly *Ralstonia paucula* and CDC group IV c-2) is an oxidase-positive, nonsaccharolytic gram-negative rod that is motile by means of peritrichous flagella and is strongly urease-positive. It therefore phenotypically resembles *Alcaligenes, Bordetella,* and *Oligella ureolytica,* from which it must be differentiated (see Table 7-9). Most reports of human infection have been cases of bacteremia in immunocompromised patients.[13,22,24,152,156,491,504,538,611,660,736,837] There have also been two cases of peritonitis following continuous ambulatory peritoneal dialysis, one with accompanying septicemia[837] and one with a mixed infection with IVc-2 and *Alcaligenes faecalis*[291]; and one case of tenosynovitis of the hand following a cat bite.[522] In the latter case it is not clear whether the source of the infectious agent was the cat bite or the tap water used to rinse the lesion.

C. respiraculi (formerly *Ralstonia respiraculi*) has been recovered from the respiratory tract of patients with CF, although the isolates did not grow on BCSA.[144] Characteristics that differentiate *C. respiraculi* from other *Cupriavidus*-species are given in Table 7-9.

C. taiwanensis (formerly *Ralstonia taiwanensis*) has also been isolated from the sputum of a patient with CF.[118] It is an nonsaccharolytic gram-negative rod that is oxidase-, catalase-, nitrate-, and esculin-positive. Additional biochemical characteristics are given in Table 7-9.

GENUS *PANDORAEA*

In 2000, Coenye et al. described a new genus, *Pandoraea* (referring to Pandora's box in Greek mythology) of gram-negative nonfermenters isolated primarily from sputa of patients with cystic fibrosis and from soil.[133] Originally, this genus contained five named species (*P. apista, P. norimbergensis, P. pnomenusa, P. pulmonicola,* and *P. sputorum*) and one unnamed genomic species.[133] More recently, three new (yet unnamed) *Pandoraea* genomospecies, previously classified as CDC weak oxidizer group 2 (WO-2), were

Table 7-9 Key Characteristics of *Ralstonia* and *Cupriavidus* and Phenotypically Similar Nonfermenters[a]

TEST	RALSTONIA				CUPRIAVIDUS				ALCALIGENES	BORDETELLA
	R. pickettii Biovar VA-1	R. pickettii Biovar VA-2	R. mannitolilytica Biovar 3/thomasii	R. insidiosa	C. gilardii	C. pauculus	C. respiraculi	C. taiwanensis	A. faecalis	B. bronchiseptica
Oxidase	D[b]	D[b]	D[d]	+	+	+	+	+	+	+
Catalase	D[c]	D[b]	V (87)[d]	+	+	+	+	+	+	+
Lipase	+	+	+	+	−	+	−	+	−	−
OF glucose	+	+	+	+	−	−	−	−	−	+
OF maltose	+	−	+	−	−	−	−	−	−	−
OF lactose	+	−	+	−	−	−	−	−	−	−
OF xylose	+	+	+	+	−	−	−	−	−	+
OF sucrose	−	−	−	−	−	−	−	−	−	−
OF adonitol	NA	NA	NA	NA	−	−	−	−	−	−
OF mannitol	−	−	+	−	−	−	−	−	−	−
10% lactose	V (81)[e]	−	+	NA	−	−	−	−	−	−
ONPG	−	−	−	−	−	−	−	−	−	−
Lysine	−	−	−	−	−	−	−	−	−	−
Ornithine	−	−	−	−	−	−	−	−	−	−
Nitrate-reduced	+ (87)[e]	+ (100)[e]	− (20)[e]	+	V[f]	−	V	+	−	+ (100)[e]
Nitrite-reduced	NA	NA	NA	NA	−	−	NA	NA	+	−
Gelatin	V (77)[e]	V (40)[e]	− (80)[e]	−	−	−	−	NA	− (4)[e]	−
Esculin	−	−	−	NA	−	−[d]	NA	+	−[d]	−[d]
Urease	+	+	+	V	−	++	−	−	−[d]	++
Colistin 10 µg	R	R	R	R	S	S	S (97)[e]	S	S (100)[e]	S (96)[e]
Deferoxamine[g]	S	S	R	NA	R	R	NA	NA	S	R
PYR[h]	+	+	+	+	−/+w	+	+	NA	−	−
Growth on MacConkey	+ (77)[e]	+	+	NA	NA	(90)[e]	+ (90)[e]	NA	+	+
Growth at 42°C	V (26)[e]	V (60)[e]	+ (60)[e]	NA	+	V (68)[e]	V (68)[e]	−	V (67)[e]	V (46)[e]
Growth in 6.5% NaCl	−	−	−	NA	−	−	−	NA	+	−
Growth on acetamide	−	−	−	NA	NA	−	−	NA	+	−
Malonate utilization	+	+	−	NA	V	NA	NA	NA	+	+
Yellow-pigmented	V (36)[d]	NA	V (33)[d]	NA	−	−	−	NA	−	−

[a] Except where noted data from references[18,134,135,144,792].
[b] De Baere et al.[175] report these reactions positive, Vandamme et al.[755a] report these reactions negative.
[c] The catalase reaction for R. pickettii is often weak or delayed (Schreckenberger P: personal observation).
[d] Data from reference[802].
[e] Data from reference[249].
[f] Data from reference[763].
[g] Procedure described in reference[444a].
[h] PYR data from reference[419a].

+, 90% or more strains positive; −, 90% or more strains negative; V, 11–89% of strains positive; numbers are percentage of strains giving positive reaction; S, susceptible; R, resistant; NA, not available; +w, weak reaction; ++, strong positive reaction; D, different results reported; PYR, added.[166] *Pandoraea* spp. have been isolated mainly from the respiratory secretions of patients with CF but have also been found in other clinical samples, including blood and lung tissue.[371,507,718] Epidemic spread of *P. apista* from an index patient to five other patients with cystic fibrosis participating in winter camps and/or who had been hospitalized has been reported.[371] At present, the prevalence, patient-to-patient transmissibility, and clinical impact of *Pandoraea* organisms in patients with CF are unknown because the usual manual and automated phenotypic identification methods used in most clinical laboratories are not satisfactory in identifying *Pandoraea* spp.[138,507] *Pandoraea* species will usually grow well on *B. cepacia*–selective medium and therefore, can be misidentified as members of the *B. cepacia* complex. *Pandoraea* species grow well on BAP after overnight incubation at 35°C. Isolated colonies appear circular, convex, semiopaque, entire, and smooth and are 0.5 to 1 mm in diameter. Hemolysis is variable. All species are motile, with polar flagella, and are positive for growth on Mac-Conkey agar, production of catalase, and alkalinization of citrate. All species are negative for reduction of nitrite; denitrification; indole production; gelatin, esculin, and Tween hydrolysis; lysine and ornithine decarboxylase; and arginine dihydrolase, β-galactosidase, and DNase activity. No acid is produced from OF base mannitol, lactose, sucrose, maltose, or fructose. Strains produce weak acid or are negative in OF glucose.[133,166] For features that differentiate *Pandoraea* from phenotypically similar organisms see Table 7-8.

GENUS *INQUILINUS*

Inquilinus limosus is a nonmotile, rod-shaped gram-negative bacterium that measures 1.5 to 2 μm in width by 3.5 μm in length. It grows at 35 and 42°C but poorly at 25°C. It forms very slimy, nonpigmented colonies on nonselective media. Growth on MacConkey agar is very slight after 3 days. It is polymyxin B–resistant and lipase-positive, making it appear phenotypically similar to the *B. cepacia* complex (Table 7-8).[136,595] All strains are positive for oxidase, catalase, β-glucosidase, phosphatase, proline aminopeptidase, pyrrolidonyl aminopeptidase, and acetoin production and negative for lysine, arginine, ornithine, denitrification, indole, citrate and glucose utilization.[136] All strains have been recovered from respiratory secretions of patients with CF. The pathogenicity is unknown.

GENUS *LAUTROPIA*

Lautropia mirabilis is a motile facultatively anaerobic gram-negative coccus that ferments glucose, fructose, sucrose, and mannitol; reduces nitrate and nitrite; and produces positive reactions for oxidase, urease, and, sometimes weakly, catalase.[240] Phylogenetic characterization based on 16S rRNA gene sequence analysis places this species in the β-subgroup of the *Proteobacteria*, separate from all other described genera, but most closely related to *Burkholderia*.[240] Interestingly, the cellular fatty acid (CFA) composition of *L. mirabilis* is most similar to the CFA of *Acidovorax delafieldii*, *Comamonas terrigena*, and CDC weak oxidizer group 1 (WO-1).[163] Coccoid morphology and the ability to ferment glucose separates *L. mirabilis* from *C. terrigena*, *A. delafieldii*, and WO-1 and members of the *Burkholderia*

group. *L. mirabilis* displays extremely polymorphic cell morphology. At least three colony morphologies are seen: 1) flat, dry, circular colonies in young cultures, 2) larger, wrinkled, crisp, and crater forms on prolonged incubation, and 3) smooth, glistening, raised, round, mucoid colonies. The colony diameter varies between pinpoint and more than 5 mm, and colonies are usually adherent to the agar.[240] *L. mirabilis* has been recovered from oral and upper respiratory sites,[240] the sputum of a patient with cystic fibrosis,[56] and the oral cavities of children infected with HIV.[650] Its pathogenic potential is unknown.

Family *Comamonadaceae*
ᴿRNA GROUP III

Willems and colleagues have proposed that the organisms belonging to rRNA group III be recognized as a new bacterial family, the *Comamonadaceae*.[806]

ACIDOVORANS GROUP

This group consists of the organisms formerly named *Pseudomonas acidovorans*, *Pseudomonas testosteroni*, and *Comamonas terrigena*. In 1987 Tamaoka[730] proposed that the organisms known as *Pseudomonas acidovorans* and *P. testosteroni* be placed in the genus *Comamonas*, along with the species *C. terrigena*. Subsequently, *C. acidovorans* was placed into a new genus *Delftia* as the type species *D. acidovorans*.[797] All are motile by way of a polar tuft of up to six flagella, with the distinctive feature of having a long wavelength (3.0 μm between the top of adjacent waves). Acid is not produced in OF glucose medium, and thus these organisms are grouped among the alkaline pseudomonads (see Table 7-6). As a group, the comamonads have a wide geographical distribution and are common soil and water saprophytes. They have been isolated from animal sources, foodstuffs, hospital equipment, and human clinical specimens, but they are rarely clinically significant. *D. acidovorans* is the most common of this group to be isolated from clinical specimens. It can be easily distinguished from other alkaline pseudomonads because of the production of a weak acid or neutral reaction in OF fructose and OF mannitol. It is acetamide-positive and reduces nitrate without gas formation. It is indole-negative, but most strains produce an orange color in the medium on the addition of Kovacs' reagent (so-called orange indole) because of the production of anthranilic acid from tryptone (see Color Plate 7-2C).[486] The orange indole reaction can also be demonstrated by adding a drop of Kovacs' reagent to colonies growing on the surface of blood agar plates. When the indole test is performed with xylene extraction and the addition of Ehrlich's reagent, these same strains produce a vivid yellow reaction in the test medium. *D. acidovorans* has been isolated from a variety of clinical specimens and is usually considered to be nonpathogenic. Isolates recovered from patients at the University of Illinois hospital have been from sputum, urine, the right and left ureters of a transplanted kidney, renal preservation fluid, corneal scrapings from a patient who had undergone multiple previous eye surgeries, and the blood of a patient with tuberculosis. There are reports in the literature of *D. acidovorans* associated with catheter-related bacteremia,[103,104,209] suppurative otitis,[618] urinary tract infection,[183] ocular infections,[431,715] and peritonitis in a patient who had undergone continuous ambulatory peritoneal dialysis.[455] A case of *D. acidovorans* endocarditis has also been described in a 42-year-old intravenous drug abuser.[338]

C. testosteroni is an uncommon isolate in the clinical laboratory, despite its wide environmental distribution. Eighteen cases of *C. testosteroni* infections have been reviewed by Barbaro and colleagues.[41] They report that the organism was most often found in association with anatomic abnormalities of the gastrointestinal tract, with perforation of the appendix being the most common. Other previously published reports describe *C. testosteroni* as a cause of sepsis,[35] central venous catheter-related infection,[432] and meningitis in a patient with recurrent cholesteatoma.[23] Coenye recovered *C. testosteroni* from the respiratory secretions of two patients with cystic fibrosis.[136]

C. terrigena actually comprises three genotypically separate groups. *C. terrigena* DNA group 1 retains the name *C. terrigena*, while *C. terrigena* DNA group 2 (containing *Aquaspirillum aquaticum* and some E. Falsen [EF] group 10 strains) is renamed *C. aquatica* and *C. terrigena* DNA group 3 (containing some former EF group 10 strains) is renamed *C. kerstersii*.[793] *C. terrigena* is not considered a human pathogen, although Sonnenwirth reported the isolation of *C. terrigena* from two blood cultures of a patient with endocarditis; however, the role of the organism as a pathogen in this patient was uncertain.[706]

FACILIS–DELAFIELDII GROUP

Willems and colleagues have proposed a new genus, *Acidovorax*, which contains the following three species: *Acidovorax facilis* (formerly *Pseudomonas facilis*), *Acidovorax delafieldii* (formerly *Pseudomonas delafieldii*), and *Acidovorax temperans* (for several former *Pseudomonas* and *Alcaligenes* strains).[807] These three species form a separate group within the rRNA group III complex. Two of the species, *A. delafieldii* and *A. temperans*, have been isolated from clinical specimens; however, no information regarding the clinical significance of these organisms is available.[250,807] *A. delafieldii* is probably the same as CDC group WO-1 and *A. temperans* is probably the same as CDC group WO-1A.[802] *Acidovorax* species are oxidase-positive, motile, and utilize carbohydrates oxidatively. For additional differentiating features, consult the published report by Willems and colleagues.[807]

Family *Caulobacteraceae*
rRNA GROUP IV

All species in rRNA group IV have been transferred to the new genus *Brevundimonas* (meaning bacterium with short-wavelength flagella).[673]

BREVUNDIMONAS-DIMINUTA GROUP

The genus *Brevundimonas* includes nine species of which only two, *B. diminuta* and *B. vesicularis,* are found in human clinical specimens. They are grouped with the alkaline pseudomonads because they are nonreactive or only weakly reac-tive in most carbohydrates (see Table 7-6). This group is characterized by the presence of a single, tightly coiled (wavelength of 0.6 to 1.0 μm), polar flagellum. *B. vesicularis* is slow-growing and usually requires 48 hours of incubation for colonies to be observed on sheep blood agar, producing dark-yellow- to orange-pigmented colonies (Color Plate 7-3*C*). Most strains fail to grow on MacConkey agar. *B. vesicularis* can be separated from all other species of alkaline pseudomonads by virtue of a strong esculin hydrolysis reaction. At the University of Illinois, we have isolated *B. vesicularis* from peritoneal dialysate fluid, a renal dialysis machine, an oral abscess, and a scalp wound. Others have reported isolating this species from cervical specimens,[555] blood,[122,242,542,596,764] and a case of botryomycosis, a rare, chronic suppurative, granulomatous condition affecting the skin.[95] *B. vesicularis* has also been recovered from hospital environmental samples including a shower hose[413] and a hydrotherapy pool.[33] There is one published report of a patient with *B. diminuta* bacteremia in a patient with cirrhosis.[122] *B. diminuta* has been isolated in pure culture from the blood of three patients at the University of Illinois Hospital. One patient had diabetes, another had right middle lobe pneumonia, and a history was not obtained on the third. All isolates were nonpigmented, grew well on MacConkey agar, and were DNase-positive with the UNI-N/F system (Remel, Lenexa KS). Moss and Kaltenbach have reported that glutaric acid is produced by *B. diminuta* but not by *B. vesicularis* when the organisms are grown on trypticase soy agar.[516]

Family *Xanthomonadaceae*
rRNA GROUP V
GENUS *STENOTROPHOMONAS*

The genus *Stenotrophomonas* was created in 1993 to accommodate *Xanthomonas maltophilia* (formerly *Pseudomonas maltophilia*).[561] Several recent studies have shown that there is considerable genetic diversity within *S. maltophilia* and that this species consists of at least nine genomic groups.[146,295] In addition, four new *Stenotrophomonas* species have been described: *Stenotrophomonas africana*,[199a] *Stenotrophomonas nitritireducens*,[221] *Stenotrophomonas acidaminiphila*,[34] and *Stenotrophomonas rhizophila*.[810] *S. africana* was proposed for a single isolate recovered from CSF. Phenotypically, it was determined to be almost identical to *S. maltophilia,* except for the property of being *cis*-aconitate assimilation–negative.[199a] However, based on extensive molecular analyses Coenye and colleagues have determined that *S. africana* is a strain of the species *S. maltophilia;* therefore, the species name *S. africana* is disallowed.[145] Of the remaining species, only *S. maltophilia* is associated with human infection.

S. maltophilia is a motile rod, possesses polar multitrichous flagella, and can be easily distinguished from other pseudomonads by virtue of being lysine- and DNAse-positive and oxidase-negative (see Table 7-10). *S. maltophilia* are susceptible to colistin and polymyxin B. This property can be used to distinguish *S. maltophilia* from *B. cepacia,* which is also lysine-positive but is resistant to colistin and polymyxin B and DNase-negative. *S. maltophilia* vigorously attacks OF maltose but is usually negative or only weakly

Table 7-10 Key Characteristics of *S. maltophilia* and *B. cepacia* Complex

TEST	*S. MALTOPHILIA*	*B. CEPACIA* COMPLEX
Oxidase	−	+ (93)
Motility	+	+
Growth on MacConkey agar	+	+
OF glucose	A or Wk	A
OF maltose	A	A
OF lactose	V (86)	A
OF mannitol	−	A
NO3 reduction	V (42)	V (37)
NO3 to gas	−	−
Arginine	−	−
Lysine	+	V
Esculin hydrolysis	+	V (67)
ONPG	+ (93)	V (79)
DNase	+	−
Polymyxin B	S	R
Pigment	Gray, slight yellow, lavender	Gray, chartreuse, yellow

Data from reference[249,802].

+, 90% or more strains positive; −, 90% or more strains negative; V, 11–89% of strains positive; ++, strong positive reaction; A, acid reaction; Wk, weak acid; S, susceptible; R, resistant; NA, not available. Numbers in parentheses are percentage of strains giving positive reaction.

positive in OF glucose in 24 hours. Colonies may appear pale yellow or lavender gray on blood agar medium (see Color Plate 7-3*D*). We have noted rare strains of *S. maltophilia* that will be slowly oxidase-positive but have all the other biochemical features characteristic of *S. maltophilia*. Students of microbiology should be aware that rare strains possessing aberrant characteristics may be recovered from clinical specimens.

S. maltophilia is ubiquitous and can be recovered from almost any clinical site. It occasionally causes opportunistic infections and is emerging as an important hospital-acquired pathogen.[391,488,520] The most common site for recovery of *S. maltophilia* is the respiratory tract, although in most patients these isolates do not appear to be clinically significant. An increasing incidence of *S. maltophilia* has been reported in some CF centers in recent years,[40,91,260,377,749] and an association between *S. maltophilia* colonization and lung damage has been observed.[40,377] The use of selective media has been shown to increase the isolation rates of *S. maltophilia* from the sputa of patients with CF.[184,384] In patients who do not have CF, *S. maltophilia* has been reported to cause a wide spectrum of disease, including pneumonia,[597] bacteremia,[16,227,407,416,501,519,597,676] endocarditis,[283] catheter-related infections,[208] cholangitis,[566] urinary tract infection,[769] meningitis,[567,597] and serious wound infections, particularly in patients with cancer.[770] Morrison and colleagues[511] have studied the spectrum of clinical disease in patients with hospital-acquired *S. maltophilia* infections and report both an increasing rate of nosocomial isolation and a crude mortality rate of 43% in all patients from whom the organism was cultured. Risk factors associated with death

for patients with an *S. maltophilia* isolate included the following: patient in intensive care unit, age older than 40 years, and a pulmonary source for the *S. maltophilia* isolate.[511] A comprehensive review of infections associated with *S. maltophilia* has been written by Denton and Kerr.[185]

Another important feature in the rising incidence of *S. maltophilia* infections may be the unique antibiotic susceptibility profile of the organism. *S. maltophilia* is inherently resistant to most of the commonly used antipseudomonal drugs, including aminoglycosides and many β-lactam agents, including those effective against *P. aeruginosa*.[533,564,768] Thus, colonization may be favored by the use of broad-spectrum antipseudomonal therapy. Interestingly, *S. maltophilia* is inherently susceptible to trimethoprim-sulfamethoxazole, a drug that has no activity against *P. aeruginosa* or most other *Pseudomonas* species.[125,219] In addition to the problem of inherent resistance, there are problems related to susceptibility testing of *S. maltophilia*. Some automated methods (i.e., Vitek Legacy; bioMérieux, Hazelwood, MO) have programmed software that will prevent the reporting of susceptibility results if the test organism is known to be *S. maltophilia*. Trailing end points can be observed in agar-dilution and microdilution tests, and false susceptible readings with disk diffusion assays have occurred with aminoglycosides (should be uniformly resistant) and ciprofloxacin.[310,564] Studies on the use of the E test (discussed in Chapter 17) for antimicrobial susceptibility testing of *S. maltophilia* have noted the presence of tiny microcolonies or a haze of translucent growth within the area of inhibition that if missed could lead to false susceptibility results.[564,830] To learn more, the reader is referred to the review written by Robin and Janda.[630]

Family *Sphingomonadaceae*[414]
GENUS *SPHINGOMONAS*

The genus *Sphingomonas* was described by Yabuuchi et al. in 1990[827] and was emended by Takeuchi et al. in 1993.[728] Organisms in this genus are gram-negative, non–spore-forming rods that have a single polar flagellum when they are motile. They are yellow, are obligately aerobic, and produce catalase. Bacteria belonging to the genus *Sphingomonas* are ubiquitous in soil, water, and sediments, and strains isolated from these environments are known to be decomposers of aromatic compounds and, therefore, are expected to be used for bioremediation of the environment.[39] It is now known that members of the genus *Sphingomonas* can be divided into four phylogenetic groups, each representing a different genus. Consequently, three new genera, *Sphingobium*, *Novosphingobium*, and *Sphingopyxis*, in addition to the genus *Sphingomonas* have been created to accommodate the four phylogenetic groups.[727] The emended genus *Sphingomonas* contains at least 23 species, of which only *S. paucimobilis*, designated the type species, and *S. parapaucimobilis* are thought to be important clinically.

S. paucimobilis, formerly known as *Pseudomonas paucimobilis* and as CDC group IIk-1, is the most common species found in human clinical specimens. It is a gram-negative, motile rod with a polar flagellum. However, few cells are actively motile in broth culture, thus making motility a difficult characteristic to demonstrate. Motility occurs at 18 to 22°C but not at 37°C.[560] The oxidase reaction is positive, although Gilardi has reported that only 90% of the strains are oxidase-positive.[248] Colonies grown on blood agar medium are yellow-pigmented; however, this species is slow-growing, and only small colonies may be observed after 24 hours of incubation. Growth occurs at 37°C but not at 42°C, with optimal growth occurring at 30°C.[560] Isolates are strongly esculin hydrolysis–positive and produce a zone of inhibited growth around a vancomycin disk (30 µg) placed on BAP (Schreckenberger P: personal observation). Additional biochemical features are given in Table 7-11. *S. paucimobilis* has been isolated from a variety of clinical specimens, including blood, CSF, urine, wounds, vagina, and cervix, and from the hospital environment.[323,614] Community-acquired bacteremia and peritonitis have also been reported in patients receiving long-term ambulatory peritoneal dialysis.[512] There have been a few reports of nosocomially acquired *S. paucimobilis* infections from contamination of hemodialysis fluids,[96] contamination of a hospital water system,[575] contamination during in vitro processing of bone marrow for transplantation,[426] and catheter-related sepsis.[177,345,661,662] There has also been a report of *S. paucimobilis* bacteremia that was accompanied by septic shock in a burn patient.[101] Most strains are susceptible to tetracycline, chloramphenicol, trimethoprim-sulfamethoxazole, and aminoglycosides; their susceptibility to other antimicrobial agents, including fluoroquinolones, varies.[217,345,614]

The cellular and colonial characteristics of *S. parapaucimobilis* are similar to those of *S. paucimobilis*. It is differentiated from *S. paucimobilis* by blackening of lead acetate paper suspended over Kligler iron agar, ability to grow and alkalinize Simmons' citrate medium, and a negative extracellular deoxyribonuclease reaction.[827] Clinical isolates have been obtained from the sputum, urine, and vagina.[827]

Family *Oceanospirillaceae*
GENUS *BALNEATRIX*

Balneatrix is a new genus consisting of a single species, *B. alpica*.[170] This bacterium was first isolated in 1987 during an outbreak of pneumonia and meningitis among persons who attended a hot (37°C) spring spa in Southern France.[102,170,348] Thirty-five cases of pneumonia and two cases of meningitis occurred. Isolates from eight patients were recovered from blood, CSF, and sputum, and one from water. The bacterium is described as gram-negative, straight or curved rods, motile by a single polar flagellum, strictly aerobic, and growing at a wide range of temperatures (20 to 46°C). Colonies are 2 to 3 mm in diameter, convex, and smooth. The center of the colonies is pale yellow after 2 to 3 days and pale brown after 4 days. The organism grows on chocolate and tryptic soy agars but not on MacConkey agar. It is oxidase-positive and nonfermentative but oxidatively utilizes glucose, mannose, fructose, maltose, sorbitol, mannitol, glycerol, and inositol. Indole is produced, and nitrate is reduced to nitrite. Gelatin is weakly hydrolyzed, and lecithinase is positive. The following substrates are not utilized: arginine, lysine, ornithine, urease, esculin, acetamide, starch, and ONPG (Table 7-11).[102,170] *B. alpica* is reported to be susceptible to penicillin G and to all other β-lactam antibiotics and to all aminoglycosides, chloramphenicol, tetracycline, erythromycin, sulfonamides, trimethoprim, ofloxacin, and nalidixic acid. It is resistant to clindamycin and vancomycin.[102]

Family *Oxalobacteraceae*
GENUS *MASSILIA*

The genus *Massilia* consists of a single species, *M. timonae* that is an actively motile (with lateral as well as single polar flagella), strictly aerobic gram-negative rod. The original description by La Scola and colleagues[423] described the type strain as being oxidase-negative and arginine dihydrolase–positive, however, Lindquist et al. reported that the type strain as well as four additional human isolates tested oxidase-positive and arginine-negative.[443] Colonies appear pale yellow and are distinctly tenacious on agar media and have a tendency to form pellicles on the surface of liquid medium.[423] Acid is produced oxidatively from some carbohydrates. Lindquist and colleagues reported that when grown in OF medium without added carbohydrate, the strains produced a distinctly alkaline reaction. Consequently, a neutral reaction in a tube with carbohydrate was interpreted as weakly positive for acid production.[443] Additional biochemical reactions are given in Table 7-11. Isolates have been recovered from a surgical wound, CSF, the femur of a 29-year-old with osteomyelitis, and from the blood of three other patients.[423,443,697] *M. timonae* is susceptible to most antibiotics, with resistance reported to ampicillin, cephalothin, and aztreonam.[423,697]

GENUS *HERBASPIRILLUM*

This genus consists of small spiral-shaped bacteria from herbaceous seed-bearing plants. *Herbaspirillum* species are

Table 7-11 Key Characteristics of Yellow-Pigmented Pseudomonads

	PSEUDOMONAS		SPHINGOMONAS		"AGROBACTERIUM"	BALNEATRIX	MASSILIA	CDC GROUPS	
TEST	P. luteola[a]	P. oryzihabitans[a]	S. paucimobilis[a]	S. parapaucimobilis[b]	Yellow Group[c]	B. alpica[d]	M. timonae[e]	O-1[c]	O-2[c]
Oxidase	−	−	+ (94)	+	+	+	+	V (77)	+
Motility	+	+	+ (92)	+	+	+	+	+	+ (20)
Growth on MacConkey agar	+	+	− (10)	−		−	+	+	
OF glucose	A	A	A	A	V (50)	A	+	V (40)	− (10)
OF xylose	A	A	A	A	A	NA	Wk	Wk	V (84)
OF maltose	A	A	A	A	A	A	A	−	−
OF mannitol	A	A	−	−	A	A	A	−	A
Indole	−	−	−	−	−	+	−	−	−
Esculin	+	−	+	+	+	−	−	+	
ONPG	+	−	+	+	V (30)	−	+	NA	V (64)
DNase	−	−	+	−	−	−	NA	NA	NA
Citrate	+	+	−	+	−	NA	+	−	NA
H₂S lead acetate	V (12)	+	−	+	−	−	+	+	−
3-ketolactose	NA	NA	NA	NA	+	NA	NA	NA	+
Lipase	NA	NA	+	+	−	NA	NA	NA	NA
Polymyxin B	S	S	S (89)	V	NA	S	S	NA	NA
Pigment	Dull yellow	Dull yellow	Deep yellow	Deep yellow	Yellow	Yellow	Straw	Yellow	Yellow
Flagella	Multitrichous	Single polar	Single polar	Single polar	Single polar	Single polar	Single polar	1–2 polar	1–2 polar

[a] Data from reference[249].
[b] Data from references[414,827].
[c] Data from references[724,802].
[d] Data from reference[170].
[e] Data from reference[443].

+, 90% or more strains positive; −, 90% or more strains negative; V, 11–89% of strains positive; S, susceptible; A, acid reaction; NA, results not available. Numbers in parentheses are percentages of strains giving positive reaction.

335

gram-negative, generally curved, and sometimes helical bacilli. Individual cells are 0.6 to 0.7 μm wide and 1.5 to 5.0 μm in length and have one to three or more flagella on one or both poles.[38] A group of clinical isolates previously described as EF-1, has been shown by molecular hybridization to belong to the genus *Herbaspirillum* and is designated as a new unnamed species, *Herbaspirillum* species 3.[38] The organism is oxidase- and urease-positive; catalase is weak or variable. Other reactions are given in Table 7-12. Isolates have been recovered from the respiratory tract, feces, urine, ear, eye, and wound sites.[38] Antibiotic susceptibility data are not available.

Family *Alteromonadaceae*
GENUS *SHEWANELLA*—HYDROGEN SULFIDE–PRODUCING GROUP

In 1985 MacDonell and Colwell proposed the new genus *Shewanella*, composed of three species: *S. putrefaciens* (formerly *Pseudomonas putrefaciens*, *Alteromonas putrefaciens*, and CDC group Ib), *S. hanedai*, and *S. benthica*.[464] Currently, there are at least 22 species included in the genus *Shewanella* most of which are associated with aquatic and marine habitats; however, the type species, *S. putrefaciens*, has been recovered from human clinical specimens. The CDC recognizes two biotypes of *S. putrefaciens* based on the requirement of NaCl for growth, oxidation of sucrose and maltose, and the ability to grow on *Salmonella-Shigella* (SS) agar.[802] Owen et al.[557] have shown that organisms identified as *S. putrefaciens* comprise at least four clearly sepa-

rated genomic groups (I–IV). Based on the taxonomic proposals of Nozue and colleagues[539] and Simidu et al.,[693] strains belonging to Owen's genomic group IV (synonymous with CDC biotype 2) should be identified as *S. alga* (corrected to *S. algae*).[745] Khashe and Janda[392] have reported that *S. algae* is the predominant human clinical isolate (77%), while *S. putrefaciens* (CDC biotype 1) represents the majority of nonhuman isolates (89%). *S. algae* requires NaCl for growth, while *S. putrefaciens* does not (Table 7-13). Strains of *S. putrefaciens* and *S. algae* are oxidase-positive and motile by means of polar flagella. They are easily distinguished because they are the only nonfermenters that produce hydrogen sulfide in KIA and TSI media. All strains are positive for ornithine decarboxylase, nitrate reductase, and DNase. Colonies produce an orange-tan pigment on blood agar medium. Although they are infrequent clinical isolates, *S. putrefaciens* and *S. algae* have been associated with skin ulcers,[17,119,176,180,195,558,832] ear infections,[243,334,784] eye infections,[92] arthritis and osteomyelitis,[436,600] bacteremia,[84,195,357,394,484,558,668,760] infective endocarditis,[189] and peritonitis in patients undergoing continuous ambulatory peritoneal dialysis.[157] Several isolates recovered at the University of Illinois Microbiology laboratory have been from stool, sacral decubitus ulcer, ulcer of leg tissue, bile, vitreous fluid, and blood. Many of the infections reported to be caused by *S. putrefaciens* were probably caused by *S. algae*.[195,777] Shewanellae are generally susceptible to most antimicrobial agents effective against gram-negative rods, except penicillin and cephalothin.[217,780] Re-

---

Table 7-12 Curved Pseudomonads

TEST	*LARIBACTER HONGKONGENSIS*[a]	CDC GROUP O-3[b]	*HERBASPIRILLUM SPECIES* 3[c]
Oxidase	+	+	+
Catalase	+	+ or weak	NA
Motility	+	+	+
Growth on MacConkey agar	+	V (38)	NA
OF glucose	−	A	A
OF xylose	−	A	A
OF mannitol	−	−	A
Arginine	+	−	NA
Urea	+	−	NA
NO₃ to NO₂	+	V (8)	NA
Indole	−	−	NA
Esculin	−	+	−
Citrate	−	−	+
Pigment	−	−	−
Flagella	Bipolar	Single polar	1–3 polar

[a] Data from reference[812].
[b] Data from reference[164].
[c] Data from reference[38].
+, 90% or more strains positive; −, 90% or more strains negative; V, 11–89% of strains positive; S, susceptible; A, acid reaction; NA, results not available. Numbers in parentheses are percentages of strains giving positive reaction.

Table 7-13 Halophilic and/or Hydrogen Sulfide–Positive Pseudomonads

| TEST | SHEWANELLA[a] | | ALISHEWA-NELLA[b] | HALOMO-NAS[c] | CDC[d] |
	S. putrefaciens	S. algae	A. fetalis	H. venusta	Halophilic Nonfermenter Group 1
Oxidase	+	+	+	+	+
Motility	+ p. 1–2	+ p. 1–2	−	+ pe	+ pe
Growth on MacConkey agar	+	+	+	+	+
Growth in 6.5% NaCl	−	+	+	+	+
H$_2$S (TSI butt)	+ (93)	+ (100)	−	NA	−
Growth at 42°C	−	+	+	NA	V (17)
OF glucose	Wk	−	−	+	V (83)
OF maltose	−	−	−	+	V (67)
OF lactose	−	−	−	−	−
OF mannitol	−	−	−	V (80)	V (67)
NO$_3$ reduction	V (80)	+	+	+	V (33)
NO$_3$ to gas	−	−	NA	NA	−
Ornithine	+	+	NA	−	−
Esculin hydrolysis	−	−	+	+	−
Gelatin hydrolysis	+	+	+	−	−
DNase	+	+	NA	NA	NA

[a] Data from references[249,392,802].
[b] Data from reference[778].
[c] Data from reference[781].
[d] Unpublished data from the CDC.
+, 90% or more strains positive; −, 90% or more strains negative; V, 11–89% of strains positive; ++, strong positive reaction; A, acid reaction; Wk, weak acid. Numbers in parentheses are percentages of strains giving positive reactions; S, susceptible; R, resistant; NA, not available; p, polar flagella; pe, peritrichous flagella.

cent investigations have noted that the mean MICs of *S. algae* to penicillin, ampicillin and tetracycline were higher than the corresponding MICs of *S. putrefaciens*.[392,777]

GENUS *ALISHEWANELLA*—HALOPHILIC GROUP

Alishewanella fetalis is a halophilic gram-negative rod that grows at temperatures between 25 and 42°C, with optimal growth at 37°C. NaCl is required for growth. It can withstand NaCl concentrations up to 8%, but it does not grow at 10% NaCl, which helps differentiate this species from *S. algae,* which can grow in 10% NaCl.[778] Also, unlike *S. algae*, it is esculin hydrolysis–positive. It is oxidase- and catalase-positive and asaccharolytic. It does not produce H$_2$S in the butt of TSI and KIA. Other reactions are given in Table 7-13. It has been isolated from a human fetus at autopsy; however, its association with clinical infection is unknown.[778]

Family *Halomonadaceae*
GENUS *HALOMONAS*

Halomonas venusta was originally described as *Alcaligenes venustus*,[52] but later transferred to the new genus *Deleya*, as *Deleya venusta*, by Baumann and colleagues.[53] In 1996 Dobson and Franzmann proposed combining the genus

Deleya into a more broadly defined genus, *Halomonas*.[191] von Graevenitz and colleagues were the first to report a human infection caused by *H. venusta* in a wound that originated from a fish bite.[781] They reported that the organism grew on BAP and MacConkey agars and appeared as mucoid, colorless colonies. Positive reactions occurred with nitrate, urea, and esculin. Additional biochemical reactions are given in Table 7-13. *H. venusta* are reported to be susceptible to most antibiotics.[781]

CDC Halophilic Nonfermenter Group 1 consists of six phenotypically similar isolates received by the CDC between 1971 and 1998 that are similar to *H. venusta* except for esculin hydrolysis and CFA composition. Five of these are from human blood cultures, the sixth is from a hip wound culture (CDC: unpublished data).

Family *Methylobacteriaceae*
GENUS *METHYLOBACTERIUM*

Methylobacterium species are gram-negative, pink-pigmented bacteria that have the ability to facultatively utilize methane.[277] Fourteen species of *Methylobacterium* (*M. aminovorans, M. chloromethanicum, M. dichloromethanicum, M. extorquens, M. fujisawaense, M. lusitanum, M. mesophilicum, M. organophilum, M. radiotolerans, M. rhode-*

sianum, M. rhodinum, M. suomiense, M. thiocyanatum, and *M. zatmanii*) and additional unassigned biovars are recognized on the basis of carbon assimilation type, electrophoretic type, and DNA-DNA homology grouping.[237,277,278,747] *M. mesophilicum*, formerly classified as *Pseudomonas mesophilica* and *Vibrio extorquens*, is the species most often isolated from human clinical specimens. Isolates are reported to be oxidase-positive and motile; however, the oxidase reaction may be weak, and motility may be difficult to demonstrate. In our experience, all isolates seen have appeared nonmotile. Other key reactions include positive tests for catalase, urease, and amylase (Table 7-14). Additional differentiating characteristics can be found in the article by Urakami and colleagues.[747] Isolates are slow-growing on ordinary media, with the best growth occurring on Sabouraud's agar, buffered charcoal–yeast extract agar, or Middlebrook 7H11 agar.[250] Optimal growth occurs from 25 to 30°C. Colonies are dry and appear pink or coral in incandescent light (Color Plate 7-3*E*). Under UV light, colonies appear dark, owing to the absorption of UV light. Although classified as a gram-negative rod, this species often does not stain well, or it may show variable results on Gram staining. Individual cells contain large, nonstaining vacuoles that give this organism a unique microscopic appearance[704] (see Color Plate 7-3*F*). *M. mesophilicum* has been reported to cause chronic skin ulcers,[421] central catheter infection,[663] bacteremia in immunocompromised patients,[87,251,254,380,704] synovitis,[450] and peritonitis in a patient undergoing continuous ambulatory peritoneal dialysis.[653] Isolates have also been reported from bronchial washings[222] and from the cornea of a patient receiving corticosteroids.[206] Isolates recovered from patients at the University of Illinois Hospital have been from blood, leg tissue, and an appendectomy wound. In an immunocompromised patient, one case of bacteremia and fever due to *M. zatmanii* has been reported.[337] Tap water has been implicated as a possible mode of transmission for methylobacteria in the hospital environment because they have been reported

to exhibit resistance to chlorination.[304,624] To learn more see the review by Truant and colleagues.[744]

GENUS *ROSEOMONAS*

Roseomonas is a newly proposed genus of pink-pigmented bacteria that phenotypically and genotypically resemble *Methylobacterium* species but are separable from the latter by their inability to oxidize methanol, to assimilate acetamide, and by lack of absorption of long-wave UV light.[626] Members of the genus are nonfermentative, weakly staining, gram-negative, plump coccoid rods, appearing in pairs or short chains, to mainly cocci with only an occasional rod (see Color Plate 7-3*G*). They grow on 5% sheep blood agar, chocolate agar, buffered charcoal yeast extract (BCYE) agar, Sabouraud's agar, and almost always (91%) on Mac-Conkey agar. Growth occurs at 25, 35, and usually 42°C. Growth appears as pinpoint, pale-pink, shiny, raised, entire, and often mucoid colonies after 2 to 3 days of incubation at 35°C (Color Plate 7-3*H*). All strains are weakly oxidase-positive (often after 30 seconds) or oxidase-negative, catalase-positive, and urease-positive (see Table 7-14). The genus *Roseomonas* was first described in 1993 to include three named species, *R. gilardii, R. cervicalis,* and *R. fauriae,* and three unnamed genomospecies (genomospecies 4, 5, and 6).[626] More recently, Han et al. proposed a new species, *Roseomonas mucosa,* and a new subspecies, *R. gilardii* subspecies *rosea* (in differentiation from *R. gilardii* subspecies *gilardii*).[289] *Roseomonas* species have been reported in several single-case reports from blood or catheter-related infections.[5,173,482,625,688,719] One case of vertebral osteomyelitis caused by *Roseomonas* species,[525] and two cases of peritonitis, one due to *R. gilardii*[664] and one due to *R. fauriae*[64] in patients undergoing continuous ambulatory peritoneal dialysis have also been reported. In multiple-case reports about 60% of the isolates recovered have been from blood with about 20% from wounds, exudates, and abscesses, and about 10% from genitourinary sites.[173,438,717] At the University of

---

Table 7-14 Key Characteristics of Pink-Pigmented Pseudomonads[a]

TEST	*METHYLOBACTERIUM* SPP.	*ROSEOMONAS* SPP.
Oxidase	+	+
Motility	+	V
Growth on MacConkey agar	−	+
OF glucose	V	V
OF methanol	+	−
NO$_3$ reduction	V	V
Starch hydrolysis	+	+
Urea	+	+
Colonies appear dark when exposed to long-wave UV light	+	−
Colonial morphology	Dry, coral	Mucoid, pink
Gram stain morphology	Vacuolated rods	Coccoid rods

[a] *Data from references*[249,802].

+, 90% or more strains positive; −, 90% or more strains negative; V, 11–89% of strains positive.

Illinois Hospital, we have recovered 21 clinical isolates of pink-pigmented bacteria, mostly from blood; 16 of these fit the description of *Roseomonas* and 5 have been identified as *Methylobacterium*. We have noted that the *Roseomonas* grow very well on Sabouraud's agar, producing light pink mucoid (sometimes runny) colonies. The organisms do not appear black when viewed under UV light.

Unnamed Species

Some organisms possessing characteristics of the Pseudomonads have not been officially named. These are included below.

- **_Pseudomonas_-like Group 2.** This is an unclassified group of *Pseudomonas*-like organisms that previously had been included in CDC group IVd. Strains are oxidase-positive and motile. Colonies on blood agar are reported to have a sticky consistency and are difficult to remove.[250] Other identifying characteristics include growth on MacConkey agar; oxidation of glucose, xylose, mannitol, and lactose; hydrolysis of urea; and negative reactions for indole, nitrate, esculin hydrolysis, and oxidation of sucrose and maltose.[179] Isolates are similar to *B. gladioli* but do not oxidize dulcitol or inositol.[802] The majority of strains (66%) are colistin-resistant.[249] Human clinical isolates have been recovered from the respiratory tract, blood, spinal fluid, feces, urine, and dialysate.[250,270,395,408]

- **CDC Group WO-1.** This is the designation given to a group of weakly oxidative (WO) gram-negative rods isolated primarily from clinical specimens. They oxidize mannitol and glucose, often weakly and sometimes delayed (3 to 7 days), and reduce nitrate. Most strains are motile, with one or two polar flagella; however, motility is usually delayed in motility medium or is detected only by wet preparation. Strains are usually oxidase- and catalase-positive. Some strains produce soluble pigment (yellow, tan, amber, olive green, or brown). Other differentiating characteristics can be found in the article by Hollis and colleagues.[314] CDC WO-1 strains that oxidize xylose and are citrate-positive are probably *Acidovorax delafieldii*, whereas, strains WO-1A that are xylose-negative and citrate-negative are probably *Acidovorax temperans*.[802] Isolates characterized at the CDC have been from blood (33%), CSF (10%), urine, lung, wound, and some environmental sources.[314]

- **CDC Group 1c.** Members of CDC group 1c are gram-negative slender short to long, motile rods with one to two polar flagella. The organisms grow well on MacConkey, SS, and usually cetrimide agars; oxidize glucose and maltose; reduce nitrate to nitrite without gas; produce H_2S on lead acetate paper (usually strong); are arginine dihydrolase–positive; are urease- and citrate-variable; are esculin and gelatin hydrolysis-negative; and grow well at 25, 35, and usually 42°C. Most isolates have come from human sources, including urine, sputum, blood, and other sites.[802] Antibiotic susceptibility data are not available.

- **CDC Groups O-1, O-2 and O-3.** CDC groups O-1, O-2, and O-3 are phenotypically similar, motile, and usually oxidase-positive, gram-negative rods. Groups O-1 and O-2 are yellow-pigmented and most closely resemble

Agrobacterium yellow group and *Sphingomonas* species (Table 7-11). These organisms grow poorly or not at all on MacConkey agar, usually hydrolyze esculin, but are otherwise inactive. All are motile, although motility may be difficult to demonstrate. O-1 appear as uniformly short gram-negative rods, O-2 appear as slightly pleomorphic rods, with some cells appearing thin in the central portion with thickened ends, and O-3 cells appear as thin, medium to slightly long curved rods with tapered ends (sickle-like).[164,802] O-3 is the only group in which yellow growth pigment is not produced and the only group of predominantly curved rods (Table 7-12). Gram stain of colonies after 18–24 hours on heart infusion agar show thin, medium to slightly long curved rods with tapered ends (sickle-like) that sometimes form rosettes.[164] Most isolates of O-3 grow well on CAMPY CVA (*Campylobacter* agar with cefoperazone, vancomycin, and amphotericin B) plates under microaerophilic conditions, thus, creating the potential for misidentification of O-3 organisms as *Campylobacter*.[164] Isolates of all three O groups have been from a variety of clinical sources. One case of group O1-associated pneumonia complicated by bronchopulmonary fistula and bacteremia has been reported.[607] Antibiotic susceptibility data have been reported only for group O-3. All isolates tested were susceptible to the aminoglycosides, trimethoprim-sulfamethoxazole, and imipenem. Resistance was noted to most β-lactams and variable susceptibility was noted for chloramphenicol, tetracycline, ciprofloxacin, and amoxicillin-clavulanate.[164]

- **Agrobacterium Yellow Group.** Organisms in this group are represented by slender, medium to long gram-negative rods that produce a yellow insoluble growth pigment and most closely resemble *Sphingomonas paucimobilis* and CDC group O-1 and O-2 organisms. Growth on MacConkey agar is variable, motility occurs via a single polar flagellum, and oxidase and catalase are positive; glucose, xylose, lactose, sucrose, and maltose are oxidized, but not mannitol. Carbohydrate reactions may be weak and /or late.[802] A positive 3-ketolactonate reaction and negative lipase and DNase reactions differentiate this organism from *S. paucimobilis* (Table 7-11). Isolates have been from blood and peritoneal fluid.[112,724,802]

- **OFBA-1.** OFBA-1 is an unclassified medium to long gram-negative, motile rod with 1 to 2 polar flagella that has the unusual property of producing acid in OF base medium without carbohydrate, thus the acronym "OFBA," meaning "OF Base Acid." The organism most closely resembles *P. aeruginosa* biochemically because of β-hemolysis, growth at 42°C, presence of arginine dihydrolase, nitrate reduction to gas, and utilization of most carbohydrates.[783,802] Unlike *P. aeruginosa* it is negative for pyocyanin and pyoverdin production and acetamide hydrolysis. Isolates have been recovered from blood, leg ulcer, abdominal wound, bronchial wash, and a catheter tunnel infection in a patient on continuous ambulatory peritoneal dialysis.[783,802]

Laribacter hongkongensis

Based on phylogenetic affiliation, this bacterium belongs to the *Neisseriaceae* family and is a facultatively anaerobic, nonsporulating bacillus. On Gram stain the organisms appear as gram-negative seagull-shaped or spiral rods. It grows on sheep blood agar as nonhemolytic, gray colonies 1 mm in diameter after 24 hours of incubation at 37°C in ambient air. Growth also occurs on MacConkey agar and at 25 and 42°C. No enhancement of growth is observed with 5% CO_2. Most strains are motile with bipolar flagella. All strains are oxidase-, catalase-, urease-, and arginine dihydrolase–positive and reduce nitrate, but do not ferment, oxidize, or assimilate any carbohydrates (Table 7-12).[812,836] *L. hongkongensis* has been isolated from the blood and pleural fluid of a 54-year-old patient with cirrhosis[836] and from the stools of patients with community-acquired diarrhea.[424,812,813] Woo and colleagues have reported an association between *L. hongkongensis* and community-acquired diarrhea, eating fish, and travel[813]; however, a causative role has not been shown.[215] *L. hongkongensis* has been reported from countries in Asia (China and Japan), Europe (Switzerland), Africa (Tunisia), and Central America (Cuba), suggesting that the bacterium is found worldwide.[813] However, as of this writing, no isolates have been reported from North America.

Organisms That Are Motile With Peritrichous Flagella
Family *Alcaligenaceae*

This family includes the clinically relevant genera *Alcaligenes*, *Achromobacter*, *Bordetella*, *Kerstersia*, and *Oligella*.[182,237] Members of the family *Alcaligenaceae* are gram-negative rods that are usually oxidase-positive, grow on MacConkey agar, and are motile by means of peritrichous flagella. The biochemical features that differentiate the members of this family, as well as certain other nonfermenters with similar biochemical characteristics, are given in Tables 7-15 and 7-16.

GENUS *ALCALIGENES*

The taxonomy of the genus *Alcaligenes* is closely intertwined with the taxonomy of the genus *Achromobacter*, and several *Alcaligenes* species have now been reclassified as *Achromobacter* species.[823] *A. faecalis* is the most frequently isolated member of the *Alcaligenaceae* in the clinical laboratory. Members of this species produce strong alkaline reactions in all carbohydrate media. Most strains form characteristic colonies with a thin, spreading irregular edge (see Color Plate 7-4*A*). Some strains (previously named ''*A. odorans*'') produce a characteristic fruity odor (sometimes described as the odor of green apples) and cause a greenish discoloration of blood agar medium. A key biochemical feature of this species is its ability to reduce nitrite but not nitrate. *A. faecalis* exists in the soil and water and has been isolated from many types of clinical specimens. It is a rare cause of acute otitis, urinary tract infection, and bacteremia.[4,66] Most infections are opportunistic and are acquired from moist items, such as nebulizers, respirators, and lavage fluids. It is often found in mixed cultures, particularly in samples of diabetic ulcers of the feet and lower extremities, and its clinical significance is difficult to determine.

GENUS *ACHROMOBACTER*

The genus *Achromobacter* was described in 1981 by Yabuuchi and Yano[826] and originally contained a single species, *Achromobacter xylosoxidans*. Based on taxonomic studies, Yabuuchi et al. transferred the species *Alcaligenes ruhlandii* and *Alcaligenes piechaudii* to the genus *Achromobacter* and proposed the transfer of *Alcaligenes denitrificans* to the genus *Achromobacter* as *Achromobacter xylosoxidans* subsp. *denitrificans*,[823] thus automatically creating a second subspecies, *Achromobacter xylosoxidans* subsp. *xylosoxidans*. However, the reclassification of *Alcaligenes denitrificans* as a subspecies of *Achromobacter xylosoxidans* contradicted previous work that showed that the two taxa are distinct species.[755] Accordingly, Coenye and colleagues have proposed that *Alcaligenes denitrificans* be reclassified as *Achromobacter denitrificans*.[140] In this textbook, we treat these organisms as separate species, referring to them as *Achromobacter xylosoxidans* and *Achromobacter denitrificans*, respectively. For identification purposes, the *Achromobacter* species can be divided into the asaccharolytic and saccharolytic species based on their ability to oxidize OF glucose (Tables 7-15 and 7-16).

Asaccharolytic *Achromobacter* Species. *A. piechaudii* was first described in 1986.[399] It can be distinguished from other species of *Alcaligenes* by its abilities to reduce nitrate but not nitrite and to grow in 6.5% sodium chloride (see Table 7-15). Although this species is reported to have been isolated mainly from human clinical material, there are only rare reports of a possible pathogenic role for this species. One case of chronic ear discharge in a man with diabetes[571] and one case of recurrent bacteremia in association with an intravenous catheter in an immunocompromised elderly man[379] have been reported.

A. denitrificans strains are found in the soil but can occasionally be found in human clinical specimens. Isolates have been reported from blood collection tubes, blood, ear, CSF, and urine.[780] An organism that is biochemically similar to *A. xylosoxidans* subsp. *denitrificans*, known as *Alcaligenes*-like group 1, has been recovered from blood, brain abscess, urine, bronchial wash, knee joint, and water, suggesting that it may have greater potential to cause human infection. It can be differentiated from *A. denitrificans* by cellular fatty acid composition, failure to grow on SS agar, failure to alkalinize tartrate and acetamide, and a positive urease reaction (Table 7-15).[802]

Two novel asaccharolytic *Achromobacter* species, *A. insolitus* and *A. spanius* have been recently described by Coenye et al.[141] These two species are found rarely in human clinical specimens. They are both oxidase- and catalase-positive and reduce nitrate without the formation of gas. They are both asaccharolytic and are biochemically difficult to separate from each other and from other *Achromobacter* species and from *Alcaligenes faecalis*.[141] *A. ruhlandii* is a soil commensal and is not known to be pathogenic to humans.[386]

Saccharolytic *Achromobacter* Species. *A. xylosoxidans* is easily distinguished from the genus *Alcaligenes* and the asaccharolytic *Achromobacter* species by acidification of OF glucose and xylose (thus, the species name). It has been isolated from many types of specimens, most frequently blood,[4,200,265,795] but also from CSF, bronchial washings,

Table 7-15 Key Characteristics of Alcaligenes, Asaccharolytic Achromobacters, Kerstersia, Bordetella, and Related Species[a]

	ALCALIGENES	ACHROMOBACTER		CDC	KERSTERSIA		BORDETELLA			OLIGELLA	CUPRIAVIDUS	
TEST	A. faecalis	A. denitrificans	A. piechaudii	Alcaligenes-like Group 1[b,c]	K. gyiorum[d]	B. trematum[e]	B. hinzii	B. avium	B. bronchiseptica	O. ureolytica	C. pauculus	C. gilardii[f]
Oxidase	+	+	+	+	−	−	+	+	+	+	+	+
Motility	+	+	+	+	V	+	+	+	+	V (84)	+	+
Growth on MacConkey agar	+	+	+	+	NA	+	+	+	+	V (79)	+	NA
OF glucose	−	−	−	−	−	−	−	−	−	−	−	−
OF xylose	−	−	−	−	−	−	−	−	−	−	−	−
NO₃ to NO₂	−	+	+	+	−	V (66)	−	−	+ (92)[b]	+	V (11)[b]	−
NO₃ to N₂	−	+	−	+	−	V (11)	−	−	−	V (58)	−	−
NO₂ to N₂	+	+	−	+	−	NA	−	−	−	V (63)	−	−
Urea	−	V (31)	−	V (75)	−	−	−	−	++	++	++	−
PAD	−	−	−	NA	NA	NA	V (15)	−	V (25)	+	V (7)	NA
Acetamide	+	V (45)	V (42)	−	−	V (89)	+	+	−	V (11)	−	−
6.5% NaCl	+	−	+	V (13)	V	NA	−	−	−	−	−	−
Malonate	+	+[g]	V (29)[g]	NA	−	+	+	−	+	NA	NA	NA
Flagella	pe	pe	pe	pe	NA	pe	pe	pe	pe	pe	pe	1–2 p

[a] Unless otherwise stated, data are from reference[249].
[b] Percentage positive derived from reference[802].
[c] Similar to A. denitrificans, can be differentiated by inability to grow on SS agar.
[d] Data from reference[140].
[e] Data from reference[755].
[f] Data from reference[134].
[g] Data from reference[399].

+, 90% or more strains positive; −, 90% or more strains negative; V, 11–89% of strains positive; pe, peritrichous flagella; p, polar flagella; NA, results not available. Numbers in parentheses are percentages of strains giving positive reactions.

Table 7-16 Key Characteristics of *Ochrobactrum*, *Rhizobium*, and Saccharolytic *Achromobacter* Species[a]

TEST	OCHROBACTRUM O. anthropi O. intermedium[b]	RHIZOBIUM R. radiobacter	AGROBACTERIUM "Agrobacterium Yellow Group"[c]	ACHROMOBACTER Group B	Group E	Group F	A. xylosoxidans	OFBA-1[d]
Oxidase	+	+	+	+	+	+	+	+
Motility	+; pe	+; pe	+; p, 1–2[e]	+; p, L	+; p, L	+	+; pe	+; p, 1–2
Growth on MacConkey agar	+	+	+	+	+	−	+	+
OF glucose	+	+	+	+	+	+	+	+
OF xylose	+	+	+	+	+	+	+	+
OF lactose	−	+	+	−	−	−	−	+
OF mannitol	V (50)	+	−	+	−	+	−	+
OF adonitol	+	+	−	−	−	+	−	NA
OF dulcitol	+	+	−	−	−	+	−	NA
ONPG	−	+	V (40)[f]	+	+	−	−	−
NO₃ to NO₂	+ (98)	V (84)	V (40)[f]	+ (100)[g]	+ (100)[g]	+[f]	+ (99)	+ (100)[g]
NO₃ to N₂	+ (91)	− (8)	NA	+ (100)[g]	+ (100)[g]	NA	V (69)	+ (100)[g]
NO₂ to N₂	+ (99)[f]	V (38)[g]	−[f]	+ (100)[g,h]	+ (100)[g,h,i]	−[f]	V (51)[f]	NA
Urea	+	+	−	+	+	+	−	V (50)
PAD	+	+	−	NA	NA	NA	−	+
Acetamide	−	−	NA	NA	NA	NA	V (66)	−
Esculin	V (40)	+	+	+	+	+	−	−
Pigment	−	−	Yellow	−	−	−	−	−

[a] Unless otherwise stated, data are from reference[249].
[b] Colistin resistance has been suggested to differentiate *O. intermedium* (colistin-resistant) from *O. anthropi* (colistin-sensitive)[771].
[c] Data from reference[724].
[d] Data from reference[783].
[e] Motile at room temperature, nonmotile at 37°C.[724]
[f] Data from reference[327].
[g] Data from reference[802].
[h] When tested at 48 hours of incubation, nitrite reduction may only be observed in media containing ≤0.01% nitrite.
[i] Holmes reports nitrite reduction negative for *Achromobacter* group E[327].
+, 90% or more strains positive; −, 90% or more strains negative; V, 11–89% of strains positive; p, polar flagella; L, lateral flagella; pe, peritrichous flagella; NA, results not available. Numbers in parentheses are percentages of strains giving positive reactions.

urine, pus, and wounds.[353,779,780] It may be an opportunistic pathogen that has been reported to cause nosocomial infections, including pneumonia, bacteremia, and meningitis, in patients with underlying disease.[510,620,708] It has been reported that *A. xylosoxidans* colonizes the respiratory tract of intubated children and patients with cystic fibrosis and that colonization of patients with CF is associated with an exacerbation of pulmonary symptoms.[201,657]

Holmes and colleagues separated achromobacters into six groups (A–F) based on genetic patterns.[319] *Achromobacter* groups A, C, and D constitute a single species and were found to be identical to *Ochrobactrum anthropi*.[328] *Achromobacter* groups B and E constitute biotypes of a single new genus and species that has yet to be named.[317,318,322] *Achromobacter* group F is genetically distinct from groups B and E.[317,318] The biochemical tests useful for separation of *Achromobacter* groups A–F from phenotypically similar bacteria have been reported by Holmes and coworkers.[327] *Achromobacter* groups B and E can be separated from *O. anthropi* by the properties of being *O*-nitrophenol-galactoside (ONPG)- and esculin-positive and failing to produce acid from adonitol and dulcitol.[322] *Achromobacter* Group F are similar to *O. anthropi* except they do not produce gas from nitrate and fail to grow on MacConkey agar (see Table 7-16). *Achromobacter* group B has been isolated from the blood of patients with septicemia[317,321,363] and one patient with replacement-valve endocarditis.[495] Isolates of *Achromobacter* groups E and F have also been recovered from blood.[317,318]

GENUS *BORDETELLA*

Currently the genus *Bordetella* comprises eight species, four are motile with peritrichous flagella (*B. avium*, *B. bronchiseptica*, *B. hinzii*, *B. trematum* [Table 7-15]) and four are nonmotile (*B. holmesii*, *B. pertussis*, *B. parapertussis*, *B. petri* [Table 7-21]). The three most common human species, *B. pertussis*, *B. parapertussis*, and *B. bronchiseptica*, cannot be differentiated genotypically through DNA homology studies and are likely subspecies or strains of a single species with different host adaptations.[569] Phenotypically they behave quite differently, however; *B. bronchiseptica* is motile by means of peritrichous flagella and grows readily on ordinary media, whereas *B. pertussis* and *B. parapertussis* are both nonmotile. *B. pertussis* requires special media for growth, whereas, *B. parapertussis* will grow on blood, chocolate, and MacConkey agars. *B. pertussis* and *B. parapertussis* are the etiologic agents of whooping cough and are discussed in detail in Chapter 9 with the fastidious gram-negative rods.

Colonies of *B. bronchiseptica* grow well on blood and MacConkey agar and in 24 hours appear as smooth, translucent, colorless colonies about 1.5 mm in diameter. On Gram stain, the organisms appear small and coccobacillary. They have the distinguishing biochemical feature of rapidly converting Christensen's urea agar (see Color Plate 7-2*A*). Other distinguishing features are given in Table 7-15. *B. bronchiseptica* is found in the respiratory tract of domestic and wild mammalian animals including dogs, cats, rabbits, rodents, horses, and pigs ("bronchiseptica" is derived from the Greek word *bronchus*, meaning "trachea"). It is an infre-

quent isolate in the clinical laboratory, and only a few cases of human infections have been reported in the literature.[241] Pedersen and coworkers[570] reported the recovery of only 12 strains of *B. bronchiseptica* from a total of 565 nonfermenters, all of which were from respiratory specimens obtained from patients who were free of infections. Most symptomatic cases have been in animal caretakers who presented with mild pertussis-like symptoms. Ghosh[241] reported a case of fatal *B. bronchiseptica*–induced septicemia and bronchopneumonia in a malnourished patient with alcoholism, which indicates that the organism can be virulent under the right circumstances. Woolfrey and Moody reviewed 25 cases of human *B. bronchiseptica* infection associated with sinusitis, tracheobronchitis, acute pneumonia, pneumonia with septicemia, septicemia, and whooping cough.[818] For the whooping cough cases, it is likely that *B. bronchiseptica* acted as a colonizer and not as the cause. *B. bronchiseptica* has been reported to cause pneumonia in patients with AIDS,[8,178,181,203,234,456,498,534,816] acute leukemia,[264] cystic fibrosis,[787] and thoracic trauma[613] and following bone marrow[54,126] and heart transplantation.[117] There have been two reports of bronchitis caused by *B. bronchiseptica*, one in an elderly woman[576] and one in an immunosuppressed patient.[497] Most strains of *B. bronchiseptica* are sensitive to most antibiotics, with the exception of ampicillin, cefamandole, and cefoxitin.[266]

B. avium is a pathogen for birds causing coryza or rhinotracheitis in poultry, especially in turkeys.[387] Similar to the species in the *B. bronchiseptica* complex, *B. avium* exhibits a strong tropism for the ciliated epithelium of the upper respiratory tract.

Bordetella hinzii was formerly referred to as *Alcaligenes faecalis* type II, or *B. avium*–like, and has been isolated from the respiratory tracts of chickens and turkeys in various parts of the world. Human isolates have been recovered from blood,[149,378] and sputum,[232,758] including repeated isolations from the sputum of a patient with cystic fibrosis.[231] *B. hinzii* has also been isolated from multiple biliary specimens collected over 6 months from a liver-transplant recipient with cholangitis.[27] *B. hinzii* are motile and oxidase-positive and must be distinguished from phenotypically similar organisms, as shown in Table 7-15.

B. holmesii strains have been recovered mostly from human blood.[280,444,494,508,535,683,731,801] Shepard and colleagues at the CDC analyzed the clinical histories of 30 patients with *B. holmesii* bacteremia whose isolates were submitted to CDC for identification. Of the 26 patients for whom data were available, 22 (85%) were anatomically or functionally asplenic. *B. holmesii* was the only organism isolated from the blood samples in 25 (96%) of the 26 patients.[683] Despite initial reports that *B. holmesii* does not cause respiratory disease, patients may be either infected or colonized with *B. holmesii* in their nasopharynx. Scientist from the Massachusetts State Laboratory Institute reported the isolation of *B. holmesii*, but not *B. pertussis*, from 32 nasopharyngeal specimens collected over a 3-year period from patients with pertussis-like symptoms.[494,831] Loeffelholz et al. demonstrated that *B. holmesii* gave strong positive results with their *B. pertussis* IS*481* PCR assay, thus confounding the diagnostic reliability of such assays.[454] Russell and colleagues reported a case of interstitial and lobar pneumonia with progression to pulmonary fibrosis caused by *B.*

holmesii.[652] *B. holmesii* is reported to be susceptible to amikacin, ampicillin, cefazolin, cefotaxime, ceftazidime, chloramphenicol, gentamicin, mezlocillin, trimethoprim-sulfamethoxazole, imipenem, ciprofloxacin, and piperacillin-tazobactam.[731] *B. holmesii* was formerly classified as CDC group NO-2 and is nonmotile and oxidase-negative, making it phenotypically similar to *Acinetobacter* species and CDC group NO-1 (Table 7-21). Additional morphologic and phenotypic characteristics are given under the heading ''Organisms That Are Nonmotile and Oxidase-Negative.''

B. petrii is nonmotile and oxidase-positive. It has been isolated only from the environment and is the only member of the genus capable of anaerobic growth.[786]

B. trematum is oxidase- negative and motile with peritrichous flagella. Growth occurs on MacConkey agar and malonate is utilized. Other biochemical reactions are given in Table 7-15. Strains have been isolated from ear infections and wounds of humans, but not from respiratory specimens.[755] Dorittke et al. had described the isolation of a ''*B. avium*–like organism'' from a patient with chronic otitis media, whereby the respective isolate (strain LMG 13506) was later reclassified as *B. trematum*.[197,755] Daxboeck et al. reported the isolation of *B. trematum* from a diabetic foot ulcer; however, there was no evidence for a causative role of the organism in the foot infection.[172]

GENUS *KERSTERSIA*

Coenye and colleagues have described a novel genus, *Kerstersia* gen. nov. that consists of a single species *K. gyiorum* (Greek *gyion,* meaning ''limb'': referring to the fact that the majority of strains were isolated from human leg wounds).[140] They appear as gram-negative, small (1–2 μm long), coccoid cells that occur singly, in pairs or in short chains. On nutrient agar, colonies are flat or slightly convex, with smooth margins and color ranging from white to light brown. Growth occurs at 28 and 42°C, motility is strain-dependent, and all strains are asaccharolytic. All strains are catalase-positive but are negative for oxidase, arginine, lysine and ornithine decarboxylase, β-galactosidase, gelatinase, amylase, urease, DNase, reduction of nitrate and nitrite, and hydrolysis of esculin (Table 7-15). Strains have been isolated from various human specimens, including feces, sputum, and leg and ankle wounds. Pathogenicity is unknown.[140]

GENUS *OLIGELLA*

The genus *Oligella* consists of two species: *O. urethralis* (formerly *Moraxella urethralis* and CDC group M-4) and *O. ureolytica* (formerly CDC group IVe).[644]

Colonies of *O. ureolytica* are first seen as slow-growing on blood agar medium, producing pinpoint colonies after 24 hours but large colonies after 3 days of incubation. Colonies are white, opaque, entire, and nonhemolytic. *O. ureolytica* strains phenotypically resemble asaccharolytic *Achromobacter* species, *Bordetella bronchiseptica,* and *Cupriavidus pauculus,* in that they are nonsaccharolytic, oxidase-positive, and motile by means of peritrichous flagella. They differ from *Achromobacter* species by their ability to rapidly hydrolyze urea in Christensen's urea agar. Additional differen-

tiating features are shown in Table 7-15. Most isolates have been obtained from human urine, often in patients with long-term indwelling catheters. One case of bacteremia has been reported in a patient with obstructive uropathy.[632] *O. ureolytica* bacteremia has also been reported in a patient with AIDS[477] and in an 18-month-old child with pneumonia.[427] *O. ureolytica* was recovered from a patient at the University of Illinois Hospital who presented with a facial wound with facial impetigo and cellulitis. *O. ureolytica* tends to be susceptible to most antibiotics, although there is one report of a highly resistant strain that demonstrated in vitro resistance to the penicillins, cephalosporins, imipenem, meropenem, ciprofloxacin, and trimethoprim-sulfamethoxazole, but was susceptible to the aminoglycosides, tetracycline, and levofloxacin.[427]

O. urethralis is similar to *Moraxella* species in that isolates are coccobacillary, oxidase-positive, nonmotile, gram-negative bacteria. Colonies are smaller than those of *M. osloensis* and are opaque to whitish. *O. urethralis* and *M. osloensis* share additional biochemical similarities, e.g., accumulation of poly-β-hydroxybutyric acid and failure to hydrolyze urea, but can be differentiated on the basis of nitrite reduction, growth at 42°C and alkalinization of formate, itaconate, proline, and threonine (all positive in *O. urethralis*, negative in *M. osloensis*).[591] Cellular fatty acid analysis can also be used to differentiate these two species.[802] Biochemical features that help differentiate *O. urethralis* from *Moraxella* species are shown in Table 7-19. As the name indicates, *O. urethralis* is most frequently recovered from urethral specimens and is considered a commensal of the genitourinary tract, however, in rare cases it may lead to urosepsis.[606] There has been one report of *O. urethralis* infectious arthritis in a case clinically mimicking gonococcal arthritis.[499]

Family *Rhizobiaceae*

The only medically important member of the family *Rhizobiaceae* is the genus *Rhizobium*. However, members of the genus *Rhizobium* are phenotypically similar to saccharolytic *Achromobacter* species and *Ochrobactrum anthropi*, from which they must be differentiated. Characteristics that are useful in separating these organisms are given in Table 7-16.

GENUS *RHIZOBIUM* (FORMERLY *AGROBACTERIUM*)

The former genus *Agrobacterium* contained several species of plant pathogens occurring worldwide in soils.[385] As a result of a large number of comparative studies, four distinct species of *Agrobacterium* were recognized: *Agrobacterium radiobacter* (formerly *A. tumefaciens* and CDC group Vd-3), *Agrobacterium rhizogenes* (subsequently transferred to the genus *Sphingomonas* as *S. rosa*),[728a] *Agrobacterium vitis*,[552] and *Agrobacterium rubi*.[666] The separation of the phenotypically indistinguishable species *A. tumefaciens* and *A. radiobacter* was based on the presence of a plant tumor-inducing plasmid, present in *A. tumefaciens* and absent in *A. radiobacter*. Genetic studies showed that the two species were the same, and a proposal was made to reject the name *A. tumefaciens* and to designate *A. radiobacter* as the type species for the genus *Agrobacterium*.[666] Young and colleagues[834,835] proposed an emended description of the genus *Rhizobium* to include all species of *Agrobacterium*. Following this proposal the new combinations are *Rhizobium radiobacter, R. rhizogenes, R. rubi,* and *R. vitis*.[834] Farrand and colleagues have presented evidence from classical and molecular comparisons that support the conclusion that agrobacteria biovars 1 and 3 are sufficiently different from members of the genus *Rhizobium* to warrant retention of the genus *Agrobacterium*.[216] No doubt the final chapter on the classification of *Agrobacterium radiobacter* has not been written and the controversy is likely to continue for some years; however, for the purposes of this textbook we have decided to accept the arguments set forth by Young and colleague[835] and will refer to this bacterium as *Rhizobium radiobacter*.

The key biochemical tests used in differentiating *R. radiobacter* from the closely related species *Ochrobactrum anthropi* are given in Table 7-16. Key features for this group of organisms are a rapid urease reaction and a positive test for phenylalanine deaminase. Colonies of *R. radiobacter* grow optimally at 25 to 28°C but will grow at 35°C as well. They appear circular, convex, smooth, and nonpigmented to light beige on blood agar. Colonies may be wet-looking and become extremely mucoid and pink on MacConkey agar with prolonged incubation (Color Plate 7-4*B*). *R. radiobacter* is occasionally isolated from clinical specimens but only rarely linked with human infection. In cases of reported human infection, *Rhizobium* has been most frequently isolated from blood,[68,94,202,205,207,224,288,475,598,603,635,808] followed by peritoneal dialysate,[294,633,635] urine,[7,635] and ascitic fluid.[610] The majority of cases have occurred in patients with transcutaneous catheters or implanted biomedical prostheses, and effective treatment often requires removal of the device.[68,202,205,207,224,288,598,603,635,808] Lai and colleagues examined the medical records of 13 patients with *R. radiobacter* infections during the period 1996–2002. Ten (76%) had underlying hematologic malignancy or solid-organ cancer. Six (46%) had febrile neutropenia during the course of their infection. Fifty-four percent of the infections were catheter-related bacteremia, and 92% were hospital-acquired.[420] Two cases of *R. radiobacter* endophthalmitis subsequent to cataract extraction have also been reported.[503,526] Antimicrobial susceptibility is variable, and requires testing of individual isolates. Lai et al. reported that all isolates tested in their series were susceptible to cefepime, piperacillin-tazobactam, carbapenems, and ciprofloxacin.[420]

Family *Brucellaceae*
GENUS *OCHROBACTRUM*

Ochrobactrum anthropi is the name given to the urease-positive "*Achromobacter*" species formerly designated CDC group Vd-1 and Vd-2 and *Achromobacter* groups A, C, and D of Holmes et al.[327,328] Subsequent studies have shown, however, that biogroup C and some strains belonging to biogroup A constitute a homogeneous DNA-DNA hybridization group separate from *O. anthropi* that has been given the new species designation of *Ochrobactrum intermedium*.[771] Both *Ochrobactrum* species are closely related to *Brucella* spp., with *Ochrobactrum intermedium* occupying a phylogenetic position that is intermediate between *O. an-*

thropi and *Brucella*.[771] The two species share identical phenotypic properties. They are oxidase-positive, saccharolytic, and motile by means of peritrichous flagella. Good growth is observed on routine media in 24 hours. Colonies are about 1 mm in diameter and appear circular, low convex, smooth, shining, and entire. Isolates we have observed grow readily on MacConkey agar and appear mucoid. Key tests useful in distinguishing *O. anthropi* from related organisms include their ability to hydrolyze urea, inability to hydrolyze esculin, and a negative ONPG test. Additional biochemical tests useful in differentiating *O. anthropi* from *Rhizobium* species and saccharolytic *Achromobacter* species are shown in Table 7-16. There are no biochemical tests currently available that separate *O. intermedium* from *O. anthropi;* however, it has been suggested that colistin (polymyxin E) and polymyxin B resistance can be used to separate *O. intermedium* (resistant) from *O. anthropi* (susceptible).[771] One case of pyogenic liver infection due to *O. intermedium* has been reported[505]; however, because of the close phenotypic similarity between *O. anthropi* and *O. intermedium*, it is possible that certain infections thought to be caused by *O. anthropi* were actually caused by *O. intermedium*.

All strains of *O. anthropi* have thus far been recovered from human clinical specimens (*anthropi* is derived from Greek and means "of a human being"). Strains have been isolated predominantly from blood, wounds, urogenital tracts or urine, respiratory tracts, ears, feces, an eye, and CSF.[18,46,86,113,328,362,474,765] Of particular concern are recent reports of central venous catheter (CVC)-related sepsis caused by *O. anthropi*.[6,128,272,286,383,401,655,714] Isolation of this organism from blood should raise suspicion of CVC-related infection. There has been one report of septic shock following peripheral venous infusion of a solution contaminated with *O. anthropi*,[388] and a report of nosocomial bacteremia in five organ-transplant recipients following infusion of contaminated antithymocyte globulin.[214] Two cases of infective endocarditis due to *O. anthropi* have been reported.[473,637] *O. anthropi* is reported to be susceptible to aminoglycosides, carbenicillin, fluoroquinolones, imipenem, tetracycline, and trimethoprim-sulfamethoxazole but resistant to other antimicrobial agents.[65,249,383,780]

Organisms That Are Nonmotile and Oxidase-Positive
Family *Flavobacteriaceae*

Vandamme and colleagues have reported that none of the established species of flavobacteria were closely related to the type species *F. aquatile;* therefore, they proposed that the generically misclassified organisms *F. balustinum, F. gleum, F. indologenes, F. indoltheticum, F. meningosepticum,* and *F. scophthalmum* be included in a new genus, *Chryseobacterium,* with *C. gleum* as the type species.[752] These same authors reported that *Flavobacterium breve* represented a distinct genetic taxon and proposed the name *Empedobacter brevis* for this species.[752] Furthermore, *Flavobacterium odoratum* was found to comprise two distinct species, which have been renamed *Myroides odoratus* and *Myroides odoratimimus*.[751] French researchers working together with Vandamme's group in Belgium published an emended description of the family *Flavobacteriaceae* and an emended classification and description of the genus *Flavobacterium*.[62] An outline of the current classification and nomenclature for the medically important members of the family *Flavobactericeae* is given in Box 7-8.[237]

Interestingly, none of the remaining *Flavobacterium* species are found in human clinical specimens, and none are indole-positive—a feature that has been synonymous with the genus *Flavobacterium* in the past. The key differentiating features of the clinically significant members of the family *Flavobacteriaceae* and related bacteria are given in Table 7-17. Most species produce yellow-pigmented colonies on blood agar medium, and all are oxidase-positive. All species are nonmotile and negative for nitrate reduction, and most species fail to grow on MacConkey agar. Most species (except *Weeksella virosa*) are polymyxin-resistant, a property they share with the pseudomallei group discussed elsewhere in this chapter. Only the clinically significant members of the *Flavobacteriaceae*

Box 7-8 Description of Medically Important Members of the Family *Flavobacteriaceae*

Genus I. *Flavobacterium*
  Type genus consisting of 29 species isolated from aquatic environments. Not associated with human clinical specimens
Genus IV. *Bergeyella*
  B. zoohelcum
Genus V. *Capnocytophaga*
  C. ochracea
  C. canimorsus
  C. cynodegmi
  C. gingivalis
  C. granulosa
  C. haemolytica
  C. sputigena
Genus VII. *Chryseobacterium*
  C. gleum
  C. balustinum
  C. defluvii
  C. indologenes
  C. indoltheticum
  C. joostei
  C. meningosepticum[a]
  C. miricola
  C. scophthalmum
Genus X. *Empedobacter*
  E. brevis
Genus XV. *Myroides*
  M. odoratus
  M. odoratimimus
Genus XXIII. *Weeksella*
  W. virosa

---

[a] Author's note at press time: Chryseobacterium meningosepticum *has recently been transferred to a new genus with the name* Elizabethkingia meningoseptica.

will be discussed further in this chapter. The taxonomic dilemma of *Flavobacterium* and *Sphingobacterium* has been reviewed in detail elsewhere.[62,685,752,822]

CHRYSEOBACTERIUM, EMPEDOBACTER, AND UNNAMED CDC GROUPS

These former *Flavobacterium* species occur naturally in soil, water, plants, and foodstuffs. In the hospital environment they exist in water systems and on wet surfaces. They are readily distinguished from other nonfermenters by their ability to produce indole in tryptophan broth (see Color Plate 7-2C). Often the indole reaction is weak and difficult to demonstrate; therefore, the more sensitive Ehrlich method (discussed earlier in this chapter) should be used. *C. indologenes* is easily recognized by the production of dark yellow colonies (Color Plate 7-4C). *C. meningosepticum*, in contrast, produces colonies with a very pale yellow pigment that may not be evident on initial examination of colonies at 24 hours. Colonies of *Empedobacter brevis* are pale yellow. Pigment production may be augmented by incubating the culture for an additional 24 hours at room temperature. The *Chryseobacterium* species generally grow poorly, or not at all, on MacConkey agar and are considered to be glucose oxidizers, although most strains will slowly ferment glucose after prolonged incubation. Microscopically, cells of *C. meningosepticum*, *C. indologenes*, and groups IIe, IIh, and IIi are thinner in their central than in their peripheral portions and include filamentous forms; IIh cells are significantly smaller than those of other species. It should be emphasized that test results (e.g. DNase, indole, urea, starch hydrolysis) in this group are dependent on the choice of medium, reagent, and length of incubation.[582] *Chryseobacterium indologenes*, *C. gleum*, and CDC Group IIb are tabulated individually in Table 7-17. Group IIb is genetically heterogeneous and includes strains of *C. indologenes*, *C. gleum*, and probably additional genomospecies. Additional DNA-DNA hybridization studies will be required to resolve this issue. Phenotypic separation between *C. indologenes* and *C. gleum* has been difficult; however, acid production from xylose and growth at 41°C are consistently positive in DNA groups clustering around the type strain of *C. gleum*.[748] Additional characteristics separating the members of this group of organisms can be found in Table 7-17.

C. meningosepticum (formerly *Flavobacterium meningosepticum* and CDC group IIa)[a] is the species most often associated with significant disease in humans. In adults it has been reported to cause pneumonia, endocarditis, wound infections, postoperative bacteremia, and meningitis, usually in patients with severe underlying illness.[32,67,124,150,228,293,305,440,476,550,628,684,735,798] It is highly pathogenic for premature infants and has been associated with neonatal meningitis.[124,150,239,296,325,396,467,599,628,739] Although neonatal meningitis is only rarely encountered it is important to diagnose the disease accurately because epidemics may occur in nurseries, and a mortality rate as high as 55% has been reported.[780]

C. indologenes (formerly *F. indologenes* and CDC group IIb) is the most frequent human isolate, although it rarely has clinical significance.[780] It has been documented to cause bacteremia in hospitalized patients with severe underlying disease, although the mortality is relatively low even among

Table 7-17 Key Characteristics of the Indole-Positive Nonfermenters[a]

TEST	CHRYSEOBACTERIUM				CDC GROUPS					WEEKSELLA	BERGEYELLA	EMPEDOBACTER
	C. meningosepticum[b]	C. gleum[b]	C. indologenes[b]	IIb[c]	IIc[d]	IIe[c]	IIg[c]	IIh[b]	IIi[b]	W. virosa[b]	B. zoohelcum[b]	E. brevis[b]
Oxidase	+	+	+	+	+	+	+	+	+	+	+	+
Motility	-	-	-	-	-	-	-	-	-	-	-	-
Growth on MacConkey agar	V (26)	V (50)	-	V (54)	-	-	+	-	-	V (79)	+	V (80)
OF glucose	+	+	+	+	+	D[e]	-	+	+	-	-	-
OF mannitol	+	-	V (10)	V (10)	-	-	-	-	-	-	-	-
Indole	+	+	+	+	+	+	+	+	+	+	+	+
NO₃ to NO₂	-	V (67)	V (14)	V (22)	+ (90)	-	-	-	-	-	-	-
NO₂ to N₂	NA	+	-	V (20)	+ (90)	-	+	-	-	-	-	-
Gelatin	+	+	+	V (78)	V (20)	-	-	D[f]	-	-	-	+
Starch	V (8)	+	+	+	NA	+	NA	+	V (14)	-	-	V (40)
Esculin	+	+	+	V (70)	+	-	-	+	+	NA	NA	-
ONPG	+	+	V (41)	V (57)	NA	NA	NA	-	+	NA	NA	-
DNase	+	V (17)	V (7)	NA	NA	-	NA	V (78)	-	V (13)	-	+
Urea	-	+	V (10)	V (14)	NA	-	-	NA	-	-	+	-
Penicillin	R	R	12% S	NA	NA	S	NA	67% S	57% S	S	S	R
Polymyxin	R	R	3% S	NA	NA	S	NA	22% S	R	S	R	R
Pigment	Pale yellow	Yellow-orange	Yellow-orange	Yellow-orange	Tan to buff	-	-	-	-, or yellow	Butterscotch	-	Pale yellow

[a] Data from references[249,802].
[b] Percentage positive derived from reference[249].
[c] Percentage positive derived from reference[802].
[d] Data from reference[313].
[e] Gilardi[249] reports glucose-negative; Weyant[802] reports glucose-positive or delayed positive.
[f] Gilardi[249] reports gelatin-positive; Weyant[802] reports gelatin-negative.
+, 90% or more strains positive; −, 90% or more strains negative; V, 11–89% of strains positive; pe, peritrichous flagella; p, polar flagella; S, susceptible; R, resistant; NA, results not available; D, different results reported. Numbers in parentheses are percentages of strains giving positive reactions.

patients who were administered antibiotics without activity against *C. indologenes*.[341] Nosocomial infections due to *C. indologenes* have been linked to the use of indwelling devices during a hospital stay.[343,346,540] Rare cases of pneumonia, meningitis, pyomyositis, keratitis, and bacteremia have been reported.[276,341,343,461] *C. indologenes* recovered in the microbiology laboratory at the University of Illinois Hospital have been mostly from wounds and tracheal cultures; one isolate was recovered from the blood of a neonate delivered by cesarean section. The infant did not have sepsis and was later discharged from the hospital.

Empedobacter brevis (formerly *Flavobacterium breve*) and the unnamed CDC groups IIe, IIg, IIh, and IIi are rarely recovered from clinical material, and little is known about their involvement in clinical disease. Janknecht et al. reported an outbreak of *E. brevis* endophthalmitis in a series of patients who had cataract extractions performed on the same day by the same surgeon, suggesting that the source of infection may be anything from the lens to the sterilization process.[358] One case of meningitis caused by CDC group IIe has been reported,[790] and the phenotypic characteristics of several clinical isolates of CDC groups IIc and IIg have also been reported.[311,313]

The appropriate choice of effective antimicrobial agents for treatment of chryseobacterial infections is difficult. *Chryseobacterium* spp. are inherently resistant to many antimicrobial agents commonly used to treated infections caused by gram-negative bacteria (aminoglycosides, β-lactam antibiotics, tetracyclines, chloramphenicol) but are often susceptible to agents generally used for treating infections caused by gram-positive bacteria (rifampin, clindamycin, erythromycin, sparfloxacin, trimethoprim-sulfamethoxazole, and vancomycin).[217,707,780] While early investigators recommended vancomycin for treating serious infection with *C. meningosepticum*,[296,599] recent studies have shown greater in vitro activity of minocycline, rifampin, trimethoprim-sulfamethoxazole, and quinolones.[67,223,707] Further complicating the choice of appropriate antimicrobial therapy is the fact that MIC breakpoints for resistance and susceptibility of chryseobacteria have not been established by the Clinical Laboratory Standards Institute (formerly, the National Committee for Clinical Laboratory Standards) and the results of disk diffusion testing have been shown to be unreliable in predicting antimicrobial susceptibility to *Chryseobacterium* species.[2,114,223,782] The Etest has been shown to be a possible alternative to the standard agar dilution method for testing cefotaxime, ceftazidime, amikacin, minocycline, ofloxacin, and ciprofloxacin but not piperacillin.[340] Definitive therapy for clinically significant isolates should be guided by individual susceptibility patterns determined by an overnight MIC method.

WEEKSELLA AND BERGEYELLA

The genus *Weeksella* as originally proposed contained two species, *W. virosa* (formerly CDC group IIf) and *W. zoohelcum* (formerly CDC group IIj).[330,331] Vandamme and colleagues have shown that these two species represent separate genetic taxa and thus proposed the reclassification of one of these species, *W. zoohelcum*, as *Bergeyella zoohelcum*.[752] Both species are oxidase-positive, fail to grow on MacConkey agar, and are nonpigmented, nonsaccharolytic, and indole-positive. Both species have the unusual feature

of being susceptible to penicillin, which allows them to be easily differentiated from the related genera (see Table 7-17). *W. virosa* (derived from the Latin word for "slimy") forms mucoid, sticky colonies that are difficult to remove from agar. Colonies are at first observed to be nonpigmented but further incubation may result in a butterscotch pigmentation. *W. virosa* is urease-negative and polymyxin B–susceptible. It has been recovered primarily from the urogenital tract of women, but there is as yet no evidence that it can play a pathogenic role.[330,480,616,617] There has been one report from Spain of spontaneous peritonitis caused by *Weeksella virosa*.[70]

A key differentiating feature of *B. zoohelcum* is the production of an intense urease reaction in Christensen's urea agar. *B. zoohelcum* forms sticky colonies that are at first nonpigmented but may form tan to yellow-colored colonies with prolonged incubation. It is penicillin-susceptible but polymyxin B–resistant. *B. zoohelcum* is part of the normal oral and nasal flora of dogs and cats.[665] It is not surprising, therefore, that the majority of human isolates have been the result of dog or cat bites.[331,506,615,689,802] It has been a cause of septicemia in elderly patients with severe skin infections who allowed a cat to sleep on top of their legs,[406,536] and a cause of pneumonia in a patient exposed to a dog that was a carrier of the organism.[282] There is one report of meningitis due to *B. zoohelcum* following multiple dog bites.[83]

GENUS MYROIDES

Vancanneyt et al.[751] determined that the organism formerly classified as *Flavobacterium odoratum* consisted of a heterogeneous group that comprised two distinct species for which they proposed the names *Myroides odoratus* and *Myroides odoratimimus*. Cells of both species are gram-negative rods 0.5 μm in diameter and 1 to 2 μm long. Various colony types may occur, but most colonies are yellow-pigmented and form effuse, spreading colonies that may be confused with the colony morphology of a *Bacillus* specie (Color Plate 7-4*D*)s. A characteristic fruity odor (similar to that of *A. faecalis*) is produced by most strains. *Myroides* grow on most media, including MacConkey agar. Growth occurs at 18 to 37°C but not at 42°C. They are asaccharolytic but are oxidase-, catalase-, urease-, and gelatinase- positive. Indole is not produced, and nitrite (but not nitrate) is reduced (Table 7-18). There are no routine phenotypic tests for differentiating the two *Myroides* species, their differences being confined to assimilation tests and cellular fatty acids.[751] Organisms identified as *M. odoratus* have been reported mostly from urine but have also been found in wound, sputum, blood, and ear specimens.[329,828] Clinical infection with *Myroides* spp. is exceedingly rare; however, cases of rapidly progressive necrotizing fasciitis and bacteremia[347] and recurrent cellulitis with bacteremia[36,275] have been reported. Most strains are resistant to penicillins, cephalosporins, aminoglycosides, aztreonam, and carbapenems.[329]

Family Sphingobacteriaceae
SPHINGOBACTERIUM AND PEDOBACTER

The sphingobacteria are yellow-pigmented, oxidase-positive, and nonmotile. They are differentiated from chryseobacteria and weeksellae by their failure to produce indole from tryptophan, and are separated from *Myroides* species

Table 7-18 Key Characteristics of *Myroides*, *Sphingobacterium*, and *Flavobacterium mizutaii*[a]

TEST	MYROIDES M. odoratus, M. odoratimimus	SPHINGOBACTERIUM S. multivorum	SPHINGOBACTERIUM S. spiritivorum	SPHINGOBACTERIUM S. thalpophilum	FLAVOBACTERIUM F. mizutaii
Oxidase	+	+	+	+	+
Motility	–	–	–	–	–
Growth on MacConkey[b]	V (91)	+	V (46)	+	–
OF glucose	–	+	+	+	+
OF mannitol	–	–	+	+	–
Indole	–	–	–	–	–[c]
NO₃ to NO₂	–	–	–	+	–
NO₂ to N₂	V (46)	NA	NA	NA	+
Gelatin	+	–	–	V (86)	–
Starch	–	V (79)	–	+	–
Esculin	–	+	+	+	+
ONPG	NA	+	+	+	+
DNase	+	–	+	+	–
Urea	+	+	+	+	–
Penicillin	19% S	R	R	R	R
Polymyxin	R	R	R	R	R
Pigment	Pale yellow	Pale yellow	Pale yellow	Pale yellow	Yellow

+, 90% or more strains positive; –, 90% or more strains negative; V, 11–89% of strains positive; S, susceptible; R, resistant; NA, results not available. Numbers in parentheses are percentages of strains giving positive reactions.
[a] Data from references[249,802].
[b] Growth on MacConkey from reference[802].
[c] Very weak pink color may be observed in the xylene layer[802].

by their ability to produce acid in OF glucose. The currently described species of *Sphingobacterium* are: *S. multivorum* (formerly *Flavobacterium multivorum*, CDC group IIk-2), *S. spiritivorum* (includes species formerly designated *Flavobacterium spiritivorum*, *F. yabuuchiae*, and CDC group IIk-3), *S. antarcticum*, *S. faecium*, *S. thalpophilum*, and unnamed species *Sphingobacterium* genomospecies 1 and 2.[237,333,687,729,822] The former *Sphingobacterium* species *S. heparinum* and *S. piscium* have been placed in a new genus *Pedobacter* as *P. heparinus* and *P. piscium*.[713] The genus *Pedobacter* contains several species of heparinase-producing bacteria found in soil, activated sludge, or fish, but not from human sources. *S. multivorum* and *S. spiritivorum* are the two species most frequently recovered from human clinical specimens. They can be distinguished from the similar organism *Sphingomonas paucimobilis* (formerly IIk-1) by lack of motility and resistance to polymyxin B. Additional differentiating features of these bacteria are given in Table 7-18. *S. multivorum* has been isolated from various clinical specimens but has only rarely been associated with serious infections, including peritonitis and septicemia.[25,190,226,326,601] Blood and urine have been the most common sources for the isolation of *S. spiritivorum*.[324,483,743] *S. thalpophilum* has been recovered from wounds, blood, eye, abscess, and abdominal incision.[802] A positive nitrate test and growth at

42°C differentiates *S. thalpophilum* from other *Sphingobacterium* species. The organism formerly known as *Sphingobacterium mizutaii* has been transferred to the genus *Flavobacterium*,[237,333] but is included with the sphingobacteria in Table 7-18 because it is indole-negative and phenotypically resembles the *Sphingobacterium* species. *F. mizutaii* has been isolated from blood, CSF, and wound specimens and can be differentiated from *Sphingobacterium* species by its failure to grow on MacConkey agar and its usual lack of urease activity.[802] *Sphingobacterium* species are generally resistant to aminoglycosides and polymyxin B, while they are susceptible in vitro to the quinolones and trimethoprim-sulfamethoxazole. Susceptibility to β-lactam antibiotics is variable, requiring testing of individual isolates.[707]

Family *Moraxellaceae*

The family *Moraxellaceae*, as currently constructed, contains three genera: *Moraxella*, *Acinetobacter*, and *Psychrobacter*.[237,577]

GENUS *MORAXELLA*

Several key features make one suspect that an unknown nonfermenter may belong to the genus *Moraxella*. After 24 hours on blood agar, the colonies tend to be small and pinpoint (usually less than 0.5 mm in diameter), with poor or no growth on MacConkey agar. The bacterial cells appear as tiny, gram-negative diplococci or diplobacilli in gram-stained preparations, and have a tendency to resist decolorization.[169] Both the cytochrome oxidase and catalase reactions are positive (the former rules out *Acinetobacter* species; the latter rules out *Kingella* species). The inability of *Moraxella* species to form acid from carbohydrates also eliminates most *Neisseria* species from consideration. Most *Moraxella* species are extremely sensitive to low concentrations of penicillin. Examination of Gram-stained smears prepared from the outer zone of inhibition around the penicillin susceptibility disk can be used to distinguish *Neisseria* species (which retain their coccal morphology) from *Moraxella* species (which produce elongated, pleomorphic forms; see Color Plate 7-4*E* and *F*).[106] All *Moraxella* species are nonmotile.

The *Moraxella* species of medical importance are *M. lacunata, M. nonliquefaciens, M. osloensis, M. atlantae* (CDC group M-3), and *M. catarrhalis*. *M. catarrhalis* is covered along with the pathogenic *Neisseria* species in Chapter 11. CDC groups M-2 and M-4 have been named *Psychrobacter phenylpyruvicus* and *Oligella urethralis*, respectively, and are covered later in this section. CDC groups M-5 and M-6 have both been placed in the genus *Neisseria*, even though their microscopic appearance is that of gram-negative rods. Group M-5 has been designated *Neisseria weaveri*,[316] and group M-6 has been named *Neisseria elongata* subsp. *nitroreducens*.[273] These species, along with other recently described *Moraxella* species such as *M. canis*[359] and *M. lincolnii*,[753] are difficult to distinguish from the established species of *Moraxella*. Animal species include *M. bovis*, isolated from healthy cattle and other animals, including horses, *M. boevrei* and *M. caprae* (goats), *M. caviae* (guinea pigs), *M. cuniculi* (rabbits), and *M. ovis* (sheep).

Table 7-19 provides some useful differential tests for identification of the medically important *Moraxella* species. *M. atlantae, M. lacunata*, and *M. nonliquefaciens* are similar in many of their features. Growth of *M. atlantae* is stimulated by bile salts and sodium desoxycholate, while *M. lacunata* and *M. nonliquefaciens* are not. Only *M. lacunata* liquefies gelatin while both *M. lacunata* and *M. nonliquefaciens* reduce nitrate to nitrite.[81,585] Separation of *M. lacunata* and nonspreading *M. nonliquefaciens* may prove difficult, because gelatin hydrolysis (with any method) and liquefaction of Loeffler slants may take more than 1 week. In some instances, fatty acid analysis may help determine the species.[802] Because many strains of *Moraxella* are somewhat fastidious and biochemical reactions are often negative or equivocal, many laboratories choose to simply report members of this group as ''*Moraxella* species.''

Moraxella species are normal flora on mucosal surfaces and are considered to have low pathogenic potential. They occur most frequently in the respiratory tract and less commonly in the genital tract and occasionally may cause systemic infection. *M. lacunata*, which has been known since the turn of the century to cause conjunctivitis, is fastidious and requires either enriched nonpeptone media or the addition of oleic acid or rabbit serum to counteract a toxic proteo-

lytic effect. In addition to conjunctivitis, this species has been reported to cause keratitis, chronic sinusitis, and endocarditis.[524,627,741] *M. nonliquefaciens* also may require serum supplements for optimal growth. It is part of the normal flora in the human upper respiratory tract and is frequently isolated from the nasal cavity. It has been isolated from the blood, eye, CSF, lower respiratory tract, and other local sites[80,271,741] and has been associated with endophthalmitis[204,425,453] and septic arthritis.[368] Atypical mucoid strains of *M. nonliquefaciens* have been recovered from sputum samples of three patients with chronic lung disease.[171] *M. osloensis* is commonly recovered from clinical specimens and does not require growth supplements. It is usually not pathogenic when isolated from humans; however, isolated cases of sinusitis, conjunctivitis, bronchitis, septic arthritis, osteomyelitis, peritonitis, meningitis, endocarditis, CVC infection, and septicemia have been reported.[89,218,290,640,678,720] *M. atlantae* grows slowly in culture medium, producing colonies with a tendency to form a spreading zone after 48 hours of incubation.[81] They are a rare cause of bacteremia in immunocompromised patients.[88,174]

M. canis is a new species that resides in the upper respiratory tracts of dogs and cats. Human isolates have been from blood,[359] lymph node,[761] and a dog bite wound.[359] *M. canis, M. catarrhalis, M. cuniculi, M. caviae*, and *M. ovis* belong to the coccoid moraxellae, which in contrast to the bacillary moraxellae, all exhibit DNase activity. Isolates of *M. canis* resemble *M. catarrhalis* on Gram stain; however, their colony morphology on sheep blood agar more closely resembles that of members of the *Enterobacteriaceae* (large, smooth colonies).[359] Some isolates may also produce very slimy colonies resembling colonies of *Klebsiella pneumoniae*.[359] The production of a brown pigment on starch-containing Mueller-Hinton agar is also typical of most *M. canis* strains.[359] *M. lincolnii* has been isolated mainly from the respiratory tract of humans.[753]

Most *Moraxella* strains are susceptible to penicillin and its derivatives, cephalosporins, tetracyclines, quinolones, and aminoglycosides.[217,641,707] Production of β-lactamase has been reported only rarely in *Moraxella* species other than *M. catarrhalis*.[368,524,641] Because of the fastidious nature of many *Moraxella* species and the predictability of the antibiotic profile, antibiotic susceptibility testing, except for β-lactamase testing, is usually not performed on clinical isolates.

GENUS *PSYCHROBACTER* AND CDC EUGONIC OXIDIZER (EO) GROUPS

The *Psychrobacter* species that are important clinically are *P. immobilis* and *P. phenylpyruvicus* (formerly *Moraxella phenylpyruvica*).[82]

Psychrobacter phenylpyruvicus. *P. phenylpyruvicus* is both urea- and phenylalanine deaminase–positive, features that help to distinguish it from *Moraxella* species and *Oligella urethralis* (Table 7-19). Laboratorians should be aware that *P. phenylpyruvicus* can phenotypically resemble *Brucella* species, and there have been several reports of *Brucella* species misidentified as *P. phenylpyruvicus* in commercial identification systems.[42,50,573] The differentiation of *P. phenylpyruvicus* and *Brucella* spp. requires microscopy (*Brucella* are

Table 7-19 Key Characteristics of *Moraxella*, *Oligella urethralis*, and *Moraxella*-Like Species

| TEST | MORAXELLA | | | | | | | PSYCHROBACTER | OLIGELLA | NEISSERIA | | GILARDI ROD GROUP 1[a,h] |
	M. atlantae[a]	M. canis[a,b,c]	M. catarrhalis[a]	M. lacunata[a]	M. lincolnii[a,d]	M. nonliquefaciens[a]	M. osloensis[a]	P. phenylpyruvicus[a]	O. urethralis[a]	N. weaveri[a,e]	elongata subsp. nitroreducens[a,f,g]	
Oxidase	+	+	+	+	+	+	+	+	+	+	+	+
Catalase	+	+	+	+	+	+	+	+	+	+	−	+
Growth on MacConkey agar	+	+	−	−	−	V(10)	V(70)	V(86)	+	V(45)	V(54)	+
Motility	−	−	−	−	−	−	−	−	−	−	−	−
OF Glucose	−	−	−	−	−	−	−	−	−	−	V(23)	−
Urea	−	−	−	−	−	−	−	+	−	−	−	−
PAD	−	−	V(68)	V(17)	NA	−	V(14)	+	+	V(71)	−	+
Gelatin	−	−	−	V(42)	−	−	−	−	−	−	−	−
NO₃ reduced	−	+	+(92)	+	−	+	V(24)	V(68)	−	−	+	−
NO₂ reduced	−	V	V(86)	−	V	−	−	−	+	+	+	−
DNase	−	+	+	−	−	−	−	−	−	−	−	−
Penicillin	S	S	R	S	S	S	92% S	73% S	S	S	S	S
Cell shape	CB	C	C	CB	CB	CB	CB	CB	CB	R	R	R

[a] Data from reference 802.
[b] Data from reference 359.
[c] *M. canis* produces a brown pigment when grown on starch-containing Mueller-Hinton agar.[359]
[d] Data from reference 753.
[e] Data from reference 11.
[f] Data from reference 273.

[g] *N. elongata* subsp. *elongata* is catalase-, glucose-, and nitrate-negative and nitrite-positive. *N. elongata* subsp. *glycolytica* is catalase-positive, weakly glucose-positive or glucose-negative, nitrate-negative and nitrite-positive. *N. elongata* subsp. *nitroreducens* is catalase-negative and weakly glucose-positive or glucose-negative and reduces nitrate and nitrite.[11,316]

[h] Data from reference 515.

+, 90% or more strains positive; −, 90% or more strains negative; V, 11–89% of strains positive; NA, not available; C, coccus; CB, coccobacillus; R, rod. Numbers in parentheses are percentages of strains giving positive reactions.

tiny coccobacilli) and tests for acidification of xylose and glucose.[584,588] *P. phenylpyruvicus* is asaccharolytic, whereas *Brucella* spp. utilize xylose and usually glucose when a sufficiently sensitive method for detecting acidification of glucose is used.[584] *P. phenylpyruvicus* is a rare cause of infections in humans but has been reported to cause endocarditis,[284,742] peritonitis,[111] and a fungating lesion of the foot.[393]

Psychrobacter immobilis, Paracoccus yeei (EO-2) and CDC Groups EO-3 and EO-4. The classification of this group of EOs and saccharolytic *Psychrobacter immobilis* strains is incomplete. Members of this group are aerobic, gram-negative (sometimes appearing gram-variable), coccoid to short, thick or slightly thick rods that grow, sometimes poorly, on MacConkey agar. All are strongly oxidase-positive, nonmotile, and indole-negative and utilize glucose, xylose, and lactose[517] (see Table 7-20). Daneshvar et al.[167] proposed the name *Paracoccus yeeii* (later changed to *yeei* in accordance with the international code for bacterial nomenclature)[213] for the former CDC group EO-2. CDC groups EO-3 and EO-4 remain unnamed. *P. yeei* grows on both BAP and MacConkey agars and appears as mucoid to very mucoid, non-pigmented colonies after 48 hours incubation (Color Plate 7-4*G*). *P. yeei* also has a distinctive O-shaped cellular morphology on Gram stain examination owing to the presence of vacuolated or peripherally stained cells (Color Plate 7-4*H*).[517] This O-shaped morphology is not observed with *P. immobilis* or EO-3 or EO-4 strains. EO-3 and EO-4 strains have a definite yellow, nondiffusible pigment that is not observed with either *P. immobilis* or *P. yeei*.[517]

Most strains of *P. immobilis* grow lightly or not at all at 35°C and grow best at 20°C.[349] *P. immobilis* is divided into saccharolytic and asaccharolytic strains. Saccharolytic *P. immobilis* strains share all of the characteristics of the asaccharolytic strains (Table 7-20), except that glucose, xylose, and lactose, but not sucrose and maltose, are oxidized. Asaccharolytic strains are phenotypically similar to *P. phenylpyruvicus*. The diagnosis of *P. immobilis* can be confirmed by transformation studies, cellular fatty acid profile, and optimal growth temperatures <35°C.[517,802] Many strains of *P. immobilis* have an odor resembling that of phenylethyl alcohol (PEA) agar (roses)[349] and are resistant to penicillin but susceptible to most other antibiotics.[259,452]

All four groups have been recovered from clinical specimens. *P. yeei* has been isolated from various human wound infections and blood.[167,229] EO-3 has been reported to cause peritonitis in a patient on continuous peritoneal dialysis.[155] EO-4 has been recovered from blood, urine and a nasal sinus, but the clinical significance of these isolates is unknown.[800] One case of ocular infection and one case of infant meningitis have been reported to be caused by *P. immobilis*.[259,452]

CDC Group EF-4b. EF-4b along with EF-4a were originally designated eugonic fermenter group 4 (EF-4); however, EF-4b does not ferment glucose, does not hydrolyze arginine, and does not produce gas from nitrate, which separates it from the glucose-fermenting strains now designated CDC Group EF-4a (see Chapter 9). EF-4b strains are coccoid to short rods that are nonmotile and oxidase- and catalase-positive. Colonies on culture plates are nonpigmented and reported to smell like popcorn. Most isolates have been re-

Table 7-20 Key Characteristics of *Psychrobacter immobilis*, *Paracoccus yeei*, EO-3, EO-4, and EF-4b[a]

| | *PSYCHROBACTER* | *PARACOCCUS* | CDC GROUPS | | |
	P. immobilis	*P. yeei* (EO-2)	EO-3	EO4	EF-4B
Oxidase	+	+	+	+	+
Motility	−	−	−	−	−
Growth on MacConkey agar	V(40)	V(64)	+	V(67)	V(65)
OF glucose	−[b]	+	+	+	+
OF xylose	−[b]	+	+	+	−
NO$_3$ to NO$_2$	V(40)	+	−	−	+
Growth at					
25°C	+	V(73)	+	+	V(88)
35°C	V(40)	+	+	+	+
42°C	V(20)	V(36)	V(14)	−	V(69)
O-shaped cells	−	+	−	−	−
Yellow pigment	−	−	+	V(83)	−
Odor	Rose-like	−	−	−	Popcorn

[a] Data from reference[802].
[b] Saccharolytic *P. immobilis* strains share all of the characteristics of the asaccharolytic strains listed here except that glucose, xylose, and lactose, but not sucrose and maltose are oxidized[802].
+, 90% or more strains positive; −, 90% or more strains negative; V, 11–89% of strains positive; NA, results not available. Numbers in parentheses are percentages of strains giving positive reactions.

covered from human infections following dog and cat bites.[802] Antibiotic susceptibility resembles that of EF-4a.

Family *Neisseriaceae*
GENUS *NEISSERIA*

Some *Neisseria* species appear rod-shaped on Gram stain and as such may not be recognized initially as *Neisseria* species. Two such species are *N. weaveri* and *N. elongata*, both of which must be differentiated from other phenotypically similar NFBs (see Table 7-19). The coccoid members of the genus *Neisseria* are covered in Chapter 11.

Neisseria weaveri is found as normal oral flora in dogs and is associated with human wound infections resulting from dog bites.[11,44,271,316] It has also been isolated from blood,[11,99] sputum, and bronchial washings[11,562] and from eye, peritoneal, and chest fluids.[11] There is one report of a wound infection in a child after being bitten by a white Siberian tiger.[98] *N. weaveri* appear as aerobic, gram-negative, broad, plump, medium-to-large, straight rods of varying length, with a tendency to grow in chains or longer rods in broth cultures.[11] Growth occurs at 25 and 35°C, and most strains grow at 42°C. Colonies are gray-white, with an entire border, flat, somewhat glistening, and smooth. *N. weaveri* is nonmotile, strongly positive for oxidase and catalase, and negative for carbohydrate utilization. Nitrite is reduced, but not nitrate, and it is weakly positive for phenylalanine deaminase (Table 7-19).[11] It is susceptible to penicillin, colistin, and vancomycin.

N. elongata subsp. *elongata* and *N. elongata* subsp. *glycolytica* are considered to be transient colonizers of the human upper respiratory tract and urogenital tract; however, *N. elongata* subsp. *elongata* has been reported to cause human endocarditis,[15,528] and *N. elongata* subsp. *glycolytica* has been isolated from human wounds and blood cultures.[12,336] Most human infections are due to *N. elongata* subsp. *nitroreducens,* which has been associated with a variety of human infections but is most often associated with bacteremia and endocarditis,[194,273,285,309,354,375,409,500,574,592,638,695,716,811] and rarely with osteomyelitis.[236,811] It was first known as CDC group M-6, but was recognized as a unique subspecies of *N. elongata* named ''*nitroreducens*'' because it reduces nitrates and nitrites to amines without the formation of gas.[273] Other characteristics of the organism include negative catalase, urease, and indole reactions; a positive oxidase reaction; and lack of acid production from carbohydrates (Table 7-19). *N. elongata* subsp. *nitroreducens* is typically susceptible to aminopenicillins, carbenicillin, cephalosporins, aminoglycosides, trimethoprim-sulfamethoxazole, and polymyxin, and it is variably susceptible to penicillin.[194]

GILARDI ROD GROUP 1

This group consists of nonfastidious, nonoxidative, gram-negative, oval to medium-length and sometimes pleomorphic rods. The cultural and biochemical characteristics of these organisms are most similar to CDC group M-5, now called *Neisseria weaveri*. All Gilardi rod group 1 strains are strongly positive in the phenylalanine deaminase reaction, producing a deep green color in the agar slant, whereas M-5 isolates, when positive, give a weak to moderate reaction. All M-5 isolates reduce 0.01% nitrite, whereas all Gi-

lardi rod group 1 isolates are negative.[249,515] Other differentiating characteristics are given in Table 7-19. Isolates of Gilardi rod group 1 have been recovered from a variety of human sources, including leg, arm, and foot wounds; an oral lesion; urine; and blood; however, their pathogenic potential has yet to be determined.[515]

Organisms That Are Nonmotile and Oxidase-Negative
GENUS *ACINETOBACTER*

The genus *Acinetobacter* is currently classified in the family *Moraxellaceae* and consists of bacteria that are nonmotile, oxidase-negative, gram-negative coccobacilli.[237,645] In 1986, Bouvet and Grimont provided a new classification that distinguished 12 different groups (genomospecies) within the genus *Acinetobacter* based on DNA-DNA hybridization and nutritional characteristics.[76] In 1989, Tjernberg and Ursing[740] described three additional DNA groups coded 13 through 15; concurrently, Bouvet and Jeanjean[78] described five DNA groups of proteolytic *Acinetobacter* species that they number 13 through 17. However, two of the DNA groups described by Tjernberg and Ursing differ phenotypically from the DNA groups described by Bouvet and Jeanjean. Thus, different DNA groups have the same number, which adds to the confusion surrounding the present subdivision of the genus. Currently there are at least 25 genomospecies described within the genus *Acinetobacter*.[352,530,531]

Genomospecies 1 is the type species and is named *A. calcoaceticus.* It is isolated principally from soil. Genomospecies 2 is named *A. baumannii;* it includes isolates previously referred to as *A. calcoaceticus* var. *anitratus*. The designation *anitratus* is considered invalid and should no longer be used. Genomospecies 4 is named *A. haemolyticus;* genomospecies 5 is named *A. junii;* genomospecies 7 is named *A. johnsonii;* genomospecies 8 is named *A. lwoffii;* and genomospecies 12 is named *A. radioresistens*. Most of the remaining genomospecies are unnamed. A scheme of phenotypic tests has been described for *Acinetobacter* genomospecies 1 through 12.[76] Because of problems in separating the saccharolytic strains belonging to DNA groups 1, 2, 3, and 13 using phenotypic tests, some laboratories have chosen to report members of this group as ''*Acinetobacter calcoaceticus*–*A. baumannii* complex,'' or ''saccharolytic *Acinetobacter*.'' Similarly, laboratories may wish to report the nonsaccharolytic members of this genus as ''nonsaccharolytic *Acinetobacter*'' (see Table 7-21).

One initial clue that a nonfermenter isolate may belong to the genus *Acinetobacter* is the Gram-stain morphology: gram-negative coccobacillary cells often appearing as diplococci (see Color Plate 7-5A). This similarity in appearance to *Neisseria gonorrhoeae* led to the archaic taxonomic genus designation ''*Mima*'' (to mimic). Students and laboratory workers should also be aware of the fact that *Acinetobacter* species may initially appear as gram-positive cocci in direct smears of clinical specimens and in smears prepared from positive blood-culture bottles.[169,292] After 24 hours of growth on blood agar, the colonies are between 0.5 and 2 mm in diameter, translucent to opaque (never pigmented),

Table 7-21 Key Characteristics of *Acinetobacter, Bordetella holmesii, Bordetella parapertussis,* and CDC Groups NO-1 and EO-5[a]

TEST	*ACINETOBACTER BAUMANNII*	*ACINETOBACTER LWOFFII*	CDC GROUP NO-1	*BORDETELLA HOLMESII* (NO-2)	*BORDETELLA PARAPERTUSSIS*[b]	CDC GROUP EO-5[c]
Oxidase	−	−	−	−	−	−
Motility	−	−	−	−	−	−
Growth on MacConkey agar	+	+	V(20)	+	+	−
Growth at 42°C	+	−	V(15)	−	V(18)	−
OF glucose	+	−	−	−	−	+
NO₃ reduced	−	−	+	−	−	−
Gelatin	V	V	−	−	−	−
Urea	V	V	−	−	+	+
Pigmentation	−	−	−	Brown, soluble	Brown, soluble	Yellow pigment produced by some strains

[a] *Except where noted, data are from reference[802].*
[b] *Grows slowly on blood agar producing minuscule colonies, β-hemolysis, and a brown, water-soluble pigment[802].*
[c] *Data from reference[165].*
+, 90% or more strains positive; −, 90% or more strains negative; V, 11–89% of strains positive. Numbers in parentheses are percentages of strains giving positive reactions.

convex, and entire. Most strains grow well on MacConkey agar and produce a faint pink tint (see Color Plate 7-5*B*). Certain glucose-oxidizing acinetobacters may also cause a unique brown discoloration of heart infusion agar with tyrosine or blood agar into which glucose is incorporated.[690,802] We have also observed this phenomenon on MacConkey and Mueller-Hinton agars with a clinical isolate of *A. baumannii* (Color Plate 7-5*C*). Differential and selective media have been described for isolation of *Acinetobacter* spp. from contaminated specimens.[335,360] Presumptive identification of *Acinetobacter* species can be made on the basis of the lack of cytochrome oxidase activity, lack of motility, and resistance to penicillin.

A. baumannii is saccharolytic and acidifies most OF carbohydrates; in particular, definitive identification is made by demonstrating the rapid production of acid from lactose (1% and 10% concentrations). In contrast, *A. lwoffii* is asaccharolytic. Genomospecies 7, *A. johnsonii*, is also asaccharolytic but can be separated from all other *Acinetobacter* species by its failure to grow at 37°C. Additional differentiating features of the 12 genomospecies can be found in the article by Bouvet and Grimont.[76]

A. baumannii is the most commonly found species in human clinical specimens, followed by *A. lwoffii, A. haemolyticus, A. johnsonii,* genomospecies 3, and genomospecies 6.[79,373,675,740] *A. johnsonii, A. lwoffii,* and *A. radioresistens* are nonsaccharolytic *Acinetobacter* species that occur as natural inhabitants of human skin.[79,675] A variety of human infections caused by *Acinetobacter* species has been reviewed by Lyons,[463] including pneumonia (most often related to endotracheal tubes or tracheostomies),[93] endocarditis, meningitis, skin and wound infections, peritonitis (in patients receiving peritoneal dialysis), and urinary tract infections. Sporadic cases of conjunctivitis, osteomyelitis, and synovitis have also been reported.[261] It is now recognized

that *Acinetobacter* spp. play a significant role in the colonization and infection of hospitalized patients. They have been implicated in a variety of nosocomial infections, including bacteremia, urinary tract infection, and secondary meningitis, but their predominant role is as agents of nosocomial pneumonia, particularly ventilator-associated pneumonia in patients confined to hospital intensive-care units.[60,775]

A. baumannii is the species most often responsible for hospital-acquired infections.[55,457,775] A biotyping system for differentiating 17 biotypes of *A. baumannii* based on the utilization of six substrates has been established and may be useful for epidemiologic studies.[77] Other species, such as *A. johnsonii, A. lwoffii,* and *A. radioresistens,* seem to be natural inhabitants of the human skin and may also be commensals in the oropharynx and vagina.[79] *A. lwoffii* has been more commonly associated with meningitis than other *Acinetobacter* species.[691] *A. ursingii* has been shown to cause bloodstream infections in hospitalized patients.[458,530,532] *A. junii* is a rare cause of ocular infection[604] and bacteremia, particularly in pediatric patients.[63,376,442] A case of community-acquired *Acinetobacter radioresistens* bacteremia in an HIV-positive patient has also been reported.[776] *A. schindleri* have been recovered from a variety of human specimens (vaginal, cervical, throat, nasal, ear, conjunctiva, and urine) but are mostly regarded as clinically nonsignificant.[530,532]

Acinetobacter species tend to be resistant to a variety of antibiotics, although one species, *A. lwoffii,* tends to be more sensitive than the others. There is almost universal resistance to penicillin, ampicillin, and cephalothin, and most strains are resistant to chloramphenicol.[463,674] Variable susceptibility to second- and third-generation cephalosporins and to trimethoprim-sulfamethoxazole has been reported. We have noticed an increased trend toward aminoglycoside resistance among the *Acinetobacter* species in recent years and multiply resistant strains, including carbapenem-resistant *Acinet-*

obacter species have been reported in nosocomial outbreaks.[74,342,478,815]

Antimicrobial susceptibility testing for *Acinetobacter* species is problem-prone. Swenson and colleagues at the CDC have shown that results obtained using standardized microbroth dilution do not agree with results obtained with the standardized disk diffusion method for certain antibiotics. Very major errors were frequent with the β-lactam and β-lactam inhibitor combination antibiotics with the microbroth dilution method typically showing greater resistance.[725] At present, there are no data to indicate which method provides more clinically relevant information.

Combined treatment with an aminoglycoside and ticarcillin or piperacillin is synergistic and may be effective in serious infections. For multiply resistant *Acinetobacter* infections, several studies have demonstrated clinical efficacy of sulbactam in combination with ampicillin or cefoperazone.[303,361,365,434,563] The only other antibacterial agent that has been shown to be active against multiply resistant *Acinetobacter* is colistin.[105,366,435] For a review of the clinical features, molecular epidemiology and antimicrobial susceptibility of nosocomial *Acinetobacter* infections consult the reviews by Bergogne-Berezin and Towner[60] and Wisplinghoff et al.[809]

CDC GROUP NO-1

An unnamed species of a fastidious, nonoxidative, gram-negative rod, designated CDC group NO-1 (nonoxidizer-1), has been isolated from human wounds resulting primarily from dog or cat bites.[37,312,372] This organism is nonmotile, oxidase-negative, and asaccharolytic. They appear as coccoid to medium-sized gram-negative rods that form small colonies on sheep blood agar. They resemble *Acinetobacter* spp. phenotypically but can be readily separated from *Acinetobacter* by a positive nitrate reduction test. Cellular fatty acids and ubiquinone analysis are also useful in differentiating NO-1 from *Acinetobacter* species.[312] Other phenotypic characteristic are given in Table 7-21. They are susceptible to a variety of antimicrobial agents, including the aminoglycosides, β-lactam antibiotics, tetracyclines, quinolones, and sulfonamides. Fifty percent of isolates are reported to be resistant to trimethoprim.[312]

BORDETELLA HOLMESII (CDC GROUP NO-2)

B. holmesii was formerly classified as CDC group NO-2, and is described as a gram-negative, small coccoid and short rod, with medium-width longer rods occasionally observed. They are asaccharolytic, oxidase-negative, nonmotile, and fastidious, and they produce a brown soluble pigment (see Table 7-21).[801] The lack of oxidase activity and the production of a brown soluble pigment differentiate *B. holmesii* from *B. pertussis*, *B. bronchiseptica*, and *B. avium*; the lack of urease activity differentiates this species from *B. parapertussis*. A negative nitrate reaction differentiates it from NO-1 strains, and the production of a brown soluble pigment differentiates it from *Acinetobacter* species. Information on the clinical significance of *B. holmesii* and its association with disease in humans was presented elsewhere in this chapter under the heading "Genus *Bordetella*."

CDC GROUP EO-5

CDC EO-5 are glucose oxidizing gram-negative rods that have a biochemical profile similar to *A. baumannii*.[165] They are nonmotile and oxidase-negative, but unlike *Acinetobacter* species, they fail to grow on MacConkey agar. Some strains produce a yellow soluble pigment. Cellular fatty acid analysis is also useful in differentiating EO-5 strains from *Acinetobacter*. Other characteristics are given in Table 7-21. Isolates have been recovered from blood, peritoneal fluid, transtracheal aspirate, gallbladder, and an arm wound.[165] Antibiotic susceptibility data are not available.

PART III: APPROACH TO RECOVERY AND IDENTIFICATION OF NONFERMENTERS

Levels of Service in Identification of Nonfermenters

The level to which species identification of nonfermenters is performed depends on the size and purpose of the individual laboratory. Reference laboratories, or universities and clinics where students and residents are being trained, may be required to identify all clinically relevant nonfermenters to the species level. Laboratories that provide services primarily for the medical community may be prepared to identify only the more frequently encountered species, sending the rare isolates to a reference laboratory. In the analysis of bacteriology specimens circulated by the CDC for their microbiology performance evaluation programs, Griffin and associates[281] found that laboratories for which the volume of specimen testing is small (fewer than 80 samples per week) average about double the error rate of laboratories handling more than 1,200 specimens per week. They conclude that this difference in performance is constant and that a laboratory cannot necessarily correct its performance, for many of the reasons listed in Box 7-9. They recommend that laboratories limit testing to procedures that can be done well and make arrangements with a reference laboratory to provide services for testing specimens that are received infrequently. Factors that contribute to the difficulties in identifying nonfermenters are listed in Box 7-9.

Box 7-9 Factors Contributing to the Difficulties in Identifying Nonfermenters

1. Most species are only infrequently encountered.
2. Because of this infrequency, laboratory personnel may not be familiar with many of the nonfermenters.
3. Many of the conventional culture media are not suitable for identifying nonfermenters.
4. Many species grow slowly, and biochemical reactivity is weak, requiring considerable experience to interpret equivocal reactions.
5. Quality control of culture media may be difficult, and, because of infrequent use, outdating becomes a problem.
6. Packaged commercial kit systems often have low accuracy in the identification of the more fastidious strains of nonfermenters, requiring the use of additional media.

Several commercial packaged systems for the identification of nonfermenters (discussed later in this chapter) are currently available[315,405,546,548,556,631,711,791]; however, because these systems depend on bacterial growth and on the formation of biochemical products in conventional media or in marginally nutritious substrates, only the more biochemically active species can be identified with an acceptable degree of accuracy. The accuracy of performance is also improved with the use of one of several automated or semiautomated bacterial identification systems, primarily because they rely on automatic instrument readings and recording of results, eliminating the subjective bias inherent in the visual interpretation of equivocal end points. These instruments have the advantage of making identifications several hours faster than conventional methods.

Guidelines for Recovery of Nonfermenters

With the previous discussion in mind, each laboratory director must develop a logical approach to the identification of nonfermenters in his or her laboratory. The following guidelines are helpful in the laboratory approach to the recovery and identification of nonfermentative gram-negative bacilli:

1. Except for *P. aeruginosa* (and the rarely encountered *B. mallei* and *B. pseudomallei*), the nonfermenters have a low degree of virulence and most often cause nosocomial infections in patients who are debilitated or immunocompromised. This narrow niche of infectivity indicates that infections will be uncommon (except for the relatively high incidence of *P. aeruginosa* and *Acinetobacter baumannii*, as discussed earlier). However, because an increasingly higher proportion of hospitalized patients have serious underlying illness, nonfermenters are being recovered with increasing frequency from clinical specimens and must be considered as important agents for many infectious diseases. Specific conditions or diseases predisposing patients to infection with nonfermenters include the following:
   a. Malignancies (particularly of the reticuloendothelial system) and instrumentation and surgery—catheterizations (particularly urinary tract and indwelling intravascular), tracheostomy, lumbar puncture, dialyses, lavages, and placement of shunts and prostheses
   b. Prolonged corticosteroid, antibiotic, antimetabolic, and anticancer therapy
   c. Underlying metabolic or chronic infectious diseases (e.g., an apparent link exists between cystic fibrosis and infections caused by *B. cepacia* or mucoid *P. aeruginosa*)
   d. Burns, open wounds, and various exudative lesions
2. Most nonfermenters have their natural habitat in several environments that serve as potential reservoirs for human infections:
   a. Various water reservoirs that are prevalent in hospitals—humidifiers, mist tents and nebulizers, water baths, disinfectant and irrigation solutions, distilled water lines, hand creams, body lotions, and so on. These solutions often come in direct contact with mucous membranes and other body surfaces in the course of patient treatment.
   b. Implements, such as anesthetic equipment, forceps, and thermometers, that may be stored in disinfectant solutions; and mops, sponges, and towels.
   c. Moist intertriginous parts of the skin, such as the toe webs, groin, axilla, and antecubital fossa. Infections from these sources tend to be more prevalent in the summer.
   d. Various domestic animals predisposing caretakers to infection.
3. Certain nonfermenters have a propensity for causing specific infections, discussed elsewhere in this chapter. Septicemia may be found with virtually any species; pneumonitis or bronchitis, septic arthritis, urinary tract infections, postoperative and posttraumatic wound infections, and conjunctivitis may also be caused by most species of nonfermenters. Some species, particularly of *Pseudomonas*, may produce cytotoxic and lytic toxins that make some of these infections locally severe and potentially life-threatening.
4. Clinical isolates that are gram-negative bacilli on Gram stain can be suspected of being nonfermenters if they produce small colonies on blood agar, grow poorly or not at all on MacConkey agar, do not convert either the slant or the deep of KIA or TSI media, and are cytochrome oxidase-positive.
5. Many species of nonfermenters also tend to have certain patterns of multiresistance to antibiotics. These patterns are learned through experience and may provide an initial clue that one is dealing with one of the nonfermenters, or may point to a specific genus.

Identification of Most Common Species

The identification of the three most commonly recovered clinical species, *Pseudomonas aeruginosa*, *Acinetobacter baumannii*, and *Stenotrophomonas maltophilia* is addressed first. Most strains can be identified easily on the basis of only a few observations and chemical tests. Not only does the rapid identification of these common isolates provide the physician with immediate information, but it also relieves the laboratory of performing a battery of time-consuming and expensive secondary tests.

Pseudomonas aeruginosa

More than 95% of *P. aeruginosa* strains recovered from clinical specimens can be identified by observing the presence of the following primary characteristics:

- Large colonies, grapelike odor
- Pyocyanin is produced
- Colonies are oxidase-positive (within 10 seconds)

Most strains produce pyocyanin, a water-soluble green phenazine pigment that imparts a greenish color to the culture medium. In fact, observing the presence of pyocyanin may be the only characteristic required to identify *P. aeruginosa*, because no other nonfermenter synthesizes this pigment. Reyes and coworkers[621] have shown that 98% of the *P. aeruginosa* strains isolated in their laboratory produced pyocyanin on Tech agar[398] within 48 hours and suggest that the use of Tech agar is a satisfactory alternative to the use of extensive identification schemes when *P. aeruginosa* is suspected (see Color Plate 7-1*G*). They note that some mucoid strains of *P. aeruginosa* from patients with CF may not produce pigment and, therefore, may be misidentified if pigment production is the only criterion used for identification of these aberrant strains. Detecting the grapelike odor is also a helpful clue when examining the growth on agar plates. The colonies are large, may be mucoid or dry, and often spread (see Color Plate 7-2*F,G,H*). A few strains of *P. aeruginosa* may produce pigments with other colors— pyorubin (red), pyomelanin (brown to black), and pyoverdin (yellow).

Fluorescein pigment can be visualized by observing the growth on certain media using a long-wavelength ultraviolet light source (e.g., Wood's lamp; see Color Plate 7-1*H*). Media containing proteose peptone 3 (Difco Laboratories, Detroit MI) and cations, such as magnesium or manganese, enhance fluorescein synthesis. King's medium B, Sellers' medium, and Mueller-Hinton agar are also suitable for demonstrating fluorescence. The constricted gram-negative fermenter (GNF) tube (Remel, Lenexa, KS) permits visual observation of the yellow pigment, and the ultraviolet light may not be needed. In our experience, combination fluorescence-lactose-denitrification (FN or FLN) media is less sensitive for ultraviolet detection of fluorescein pigment. Fluorescence may be enhanced if cultures are incubated at 20 to 30°C rather than at 35 to 37°C.[246] The following additional characteristics are helpful in identifying non–pigment-producing strains of *P. aeruginosa*:

- Growth at 42°C
- Alkalinization of acetamide
- Denitrification of nitrates and nitrites
- Motile with polar, monotrichous flagellum

Variants producing mucoid or dwarf colonies with atypical biochemical reactions may also be encountered, occasionally making identification difficult. Although a flagellar stain is not needed to identify most strains, assessment of flagellar morphology may be helpful in these cases.

In summary, most strains of *P. aeruginosa* can be identified easily by observing the typical large colonies, with a blue-green discoloration on primary isolation media, and further confirmed by detecting a typical grapelike odor. Demonstration of fluorescein pigment and cytochrome oxidase activity helps to confirm the final identification, and additional tests are usually not required. The typical characteristics by which *P. aeruginosa* is identified are shown in Table 7-4.

Acinetobacter baumannii

A. baumannii is the second most frequent nonfermenter encountered in clinical laboratories, but with only about one tenth the frequency of *P. aeruginosa*. The following are the characteristics by which a presumptive identification can be made:

- Appear as cocci or coccobacilli on Gram stain
- Grow well on MacConkey agar (colonies may have a slightly pinkish tint, a helpful characteristic when present)
- Do not produce cytochrome oxidase
- Exhibit rapid utilization of glucose, with production of acid
- Exhibit rapid utilization of 10% lactose, with production of acid
- Are nonmotile
- Are penicillin-resistant

The initial clue is the observation of tiny (1.0 × 0.7 μm) diplococci on Gram stains prepared directly from clinical materials. When Gram stains are prepared from agar or broth cultures, the cells may appear larger and more like coccobacilli (see Color Plate 7-5*A*). *Acinetobacter* species are not pigmented when grown on blood agar, a helpful characteristic in differentiating them from certain other nonfermenters, such as occasional oxidase-negative, nonmotile strains of *Burkholderia cepacia*. However, colonies growing on MacConkey agar may produce a faint pink tint or a deeper cornflower blue when observed on eosin methylene blue agar (see Color Plate 7-5*B*). Resistance to penicillin helps distinguish *A. baumannii* from the highly penicillin-sensitive *Moraxella* species, which also usually appear as coccobacilli on Gram stain. Most strains of *Moraxella* species are also cytochrome oxidase-positive. *A. lwoffii* is nonsaccharolytic and can be differentiated from *A. baumannii* because it produces no acid when grown in media that contain carbohydrates.

Stenotrophomonas maltophilia

S. maltophilia is the third most frequently encountered nonfermenter in clinical laboratories. The following are the characteristics by which a presumptive identification can be made:

- Good growth on blood and MacConkey agars
- Do not produce cytochrome oxidase
- Produce acid in OF maltose but may be negative in OF glucose
- Lysine decarboxylase-positive
- DNase-positive
- Some strains have yellow pigment

The antibiotic susceptibility pattern can also be a clue to the identification of *S. maltophilia*, which is typically resistant to most antibiotics, including the aminoglycosides, but is susceptible to trimethoprim-sulfamethoxazole and colistin.

Methods for Identification Using Conventional Tests

If an unknown nonfermentative gram-negative bacillus is not *Pseudomonas aeruginosa, Acinetobacter baumannii,*

Box 7-10 Approach to Selecting a Conventional Test

1. Positive- and negative-reaction results delineated in the identification table must be based on the procedures and formulas listed in the laboratory procedure manual. That is, the media and procedures must be the same as those used to generate the results in a table of reactions used for identification.
2. All of the reactions listed in the identification table must be at a confidence level of 90% or higher and derived from a database of a sufficiently large number of organisms to be statistically significant.
3. All tests must be performed under standard quality-control surveillance to ensure that the reagents, reactions, and end points are as close as possible to those on which the table was originally based.

---

or *Stenotrophomonas maltophilia*, additional characteristics must be determined to make a species identification. Several schemes are currently being used in clinical laboratories. In many laboratories, hybrids of the test procedures used in published schemes are used. Which approach to select is largely one of personal preference, past experience, and the local availability of the culture media required to perform the various tests, providing the criteria listed in Box 7-10 are met.

Weyant (CDC), Gilardi, and Pickett Identification Schemes

Except for the packaged commercial systems, the schemes designed by Pickett,[581,587,589,590] Gilardi,[244–248] and Weyant and associates[802] (based on the identification charts originally derived by Elizabeth King at the CDC[397]) have the largest databases. The authors of each of the three identification schemes (Weyant, Gilardi, and Pickett) have separately published several scores of individual identification tables, procedures, and other information relating to the nonfermenters. The information has become too voluminous to include in this textbook, and simplification of the material is necessary to address the needs of students and new microbiologists. Therefore, the identification tables used in these schemes will not be included here; rather, only the unique approaches these researchers have devised are discussed. Interested readers are referred to the second and third editions of this book or to the references cited earlier for a complete listing of the identification tables and charts used in those systems.

CDC Scheme—Weyant and Associates. In answer to the problem of how to identify nonfermenters in the clinical laboratory without doing all the tests that are done in a reference laboratory, Weyant and colleagues[802] have published a three-part guide that includes: 1) an identification key for gram-negative aerobes, 2) a set of 12 identification tables, and 3) a numerical code book by which derived biotype numbers can be linked to species names. They also include procedures and media formulas for all of the biochemical

tests cited in the identification manual. To correctly interpret results from a given identification table, one must use the same procedures on which the reactions are based. The manual is entitled: "Identification of Unusual Pathogenic Gram-Negative Aerobic and Facultatively Anaerobic Bacteria," and is available from Lippincott Williams & Wilkins.[802]

The Gilardi Scheme. Gilardi's approach to the identification of nonfermentative gram-negative bacilli evolved over 20 years into an extensive system that is outlined in several detailed charts and tables included in a series of publications.[244–248] Yet, the system is no more complex than the nonfermenters themselves, and the latest approach, directed to small and medium-sized laboratories, reflects the progressive trend toward greater simplicity and practicality.[247]

The Gilardi approach is based on two fundamental principles that have made it practical for use in clinical laboratories: 1) the media and tests are readily available in most clinical laboratories and are frequently the same as those used for the identification of other groups of bacteria, including the *Enterobacteriaceae*, and 2) identification of most clinical isolates can be made in two stages—the first, through the use of a primary battery of media and reactions that are sufficient in the majority of cases, and a secondary battery, available when the first is inadequate.[245] The reader is referred to the publications cited in the foregoing references for a full list of the differential media and scope of reactions in the primary and secondary battery of tests leading to the identification of most clinically significant nonfermenters.

The Pickett Scheme. More than three decades ago, Pickett was among the first to bring some order to the identification of nonfermenters.[581,587,589,590] His system was designed to identify rapidly the two most frequently recovered nonfermenters: *Pseudomonas aeruginosa* and *Acinetobacter baumannii*. Pickett advocated the use of a heavy inoculum prepared in an aqueous suspension from overnight growth of bacteria (log phase growth) that was inoculated into buffered single substrates for testing the acidification of carbohydrates and the alkalinization of amides and organic salts. The rationale behind adding the heavy inoculum to the differential test substrates was to introduce a high concentration of preformed enzymes or other metabolic products that could be detected more quickly by the end-point indicator, allowing most reactions to be read within 24 hours.

Pickett designed identification tables for several groups of nonfermenters that are similar to the Weyant–CDC scheme. These tables were published in their entirety in the second edition of this book and are not reprinted here. Also included in the second edition are the formulas for reagents and substrates and a description of all procedures necessary to perform the differential tests required for each identification table. The substrates required to perform these tests are available in dehydrated tablet form from Key Scientific Products (Round Rock, TX) and in reconstituted form from Hardy Diagnostics (Santa Maria, CA).

Practical Approach to Identification of Nonfermenters

The approach used in this book was devised by one of us (P.C. Schreckenberger)[669] and requires that the various clinically important nonfermentative bacilli be divided into four functional groups based on an immediate assessment of their motility and ability to produce cytochrome oxidase (Table 7-22). Once having accomplished this subgrouping, definitive identifications can be made by referring to the identification Tables 7-23 through 7-35 and following the instructions given with the tables. The biochemical tests used in this identification guide are all conventional biochemical formulations and are available commercially from most media manufacturers. Note that in working with these tables, a given species of a nonfermenting bacillus may appear in more than one table because a particular organism may not be 100% positive or negative for a given characteristic; therefore, some redundancy is built into the scheme so that an unknown bacillus will be identified regardless of the test result obtained with the variable screening test. By following these tables, the microbiologist should be able to definitively identify over 95% of nonfermentative bacilli that will be recovered from clinical specimens.

Computer-Aided Schemes

BioBASE (BioBASE, Boston, MA) is a DOS-based computer program for computer-aided identification of microorganisms.[502] The system enables the user to create and access hundreds of microbial databases and switch between them, depending on the primary characteristics of the microbial isolates being studied. Included with the software is the database, published by Holmes and colleagues,[327] that includes 66 taxa of nonfermenters identified using 83 phenotypic tests. Identification of bacterial isolates can be based on all or some selected tests.

Pibwin (Probabilistic Identification of Bacteria for Windows). This program provides probabilistic identification of unknown bacterial isolates against identification matrices of known strains. The program has three major functions: 1) the identification of an unknown isolate, 2) the selection of additional tests to distinguish between possible strains if identification is not achieved, and 3) the storage and retrieval of results. To do this the program makes use of Excel files to store identification matrices that have either been published in the literature or created by the user. It also has some utility functions for assessing the usefulness of identification matrices and for converting matrices into different formats. PIBWIN was developed by Trevor Bryant, University of Southampton UK and can be accessed at http://www.som.soton.ac.uk/staff/tnb/pib.htm. A non-fermenting gram-negative rod identification matrix utilizing the PIBWIN program has been developed by P.C. Schreckenberger and A.P. Schreckenberger. The identification matrix can be accessed at www.pschreck.com.

Commercial Kit Systems

Packaged kit systems have been designed for, or adapted to, the identification of the nonfermentative bacilli. These kits share many of the attributes of packaged systems in general; that is, they are convenient to use, have a long shelf life, and preclude the need for fresh supplies of media and reagents. The packaged systems also provide standardized

techniques that are accurate and give reproducible results equal to or better than conventional procedures, with the exceptions discussed later in this chapter.

Inherent problems in the use of many of the currently available packaged kits for identifying nonfermenters include the 1) tendency for organisms that exhibit weak or delayed biochemical activity to produce false-negative reactions, 2) less than optimal design of many systems for cultivation of certain nonfermenters, and 3) inclusion of some differential tests that may not be applicable to the identification of nonfermenters. Whereas members of the *Enterobacteriaceae* usually grow rapidly and exhibit active enzymatic activity on a variety of substrates that can readily be detected with kit systems, most nonfermenter species are slow-growing and relatively inactive enzymatically. The microbiologist needs considerable experience to interpret some incomplete or weak reactions that may be encountered in the use of these systems.

It is with these perspectives in mind that the following seven kit systems are discussed. They were selected because accumulated experience has delineated their applications and limitations. These seven systems are the following:

- Oxi/Ferm Tube (Becton Dickinson Microbiology Systems, Cockeysville MD)
- API 20E (BioMérieux, Hazelwood MO)
- API 20NE (BioMérieux)
- Remel Uni-N/F System (Remel, Lenexa. KS)
- Crystal Enteric/Nonfermenter System (Becton Dickinson Microbiology Systems)
- RapID NF Plus (Remel)
- Biolog System (Biolog, Hayward CA)

The Oxi/Ferm Tube

Details of the functional design, operating procedures, and substrates included in Oxi/Ferm tube are presented in the third edition of this book. Studies designed to evaluate the performance of the Oxi/Ferm tube in identifying clinically significant nonfermentative bacilli have shown that the more commonly encountered species—*P. aeruginosa*, *S. maltophilia*, and *Acinetobacter* species—were identified with a relatively high degree of accuracy when compared with conventional methods. The overall accuracy drops significantly, however, when all nonfermenters are considered. The overall identification accuracy of the Oxi/Ferm in these studies ranged from 50% to 95% depending on the species tested, whether readings were taken after 24 or 48 hours of incubation, and whether supplemental tests were used to obtain the correct identifications.[20,90,199,308,320,355,411,523,537,543,544,547,554,642,679] In these studies, the highest percentage of discrepancies occurred with the fastidious or rarely encountered strains and resulted most often from false-negative Oxi/Ferm reactions for citrate, hydrogen sulfide, arginine dihydrolase, nitrate reduction, OF glucose, and urease.[308,355,523,537,547] Problems in the detection of N_2 gas under the wax overlay in the denitrification chamber were also noted.[20,355,679]

The design of the Oxi/Ferm tube appears to limit its performance with slow-growing or weakly reactive organisms.

Table 7-22 Practical Approach to the Identification of Nonfermenters

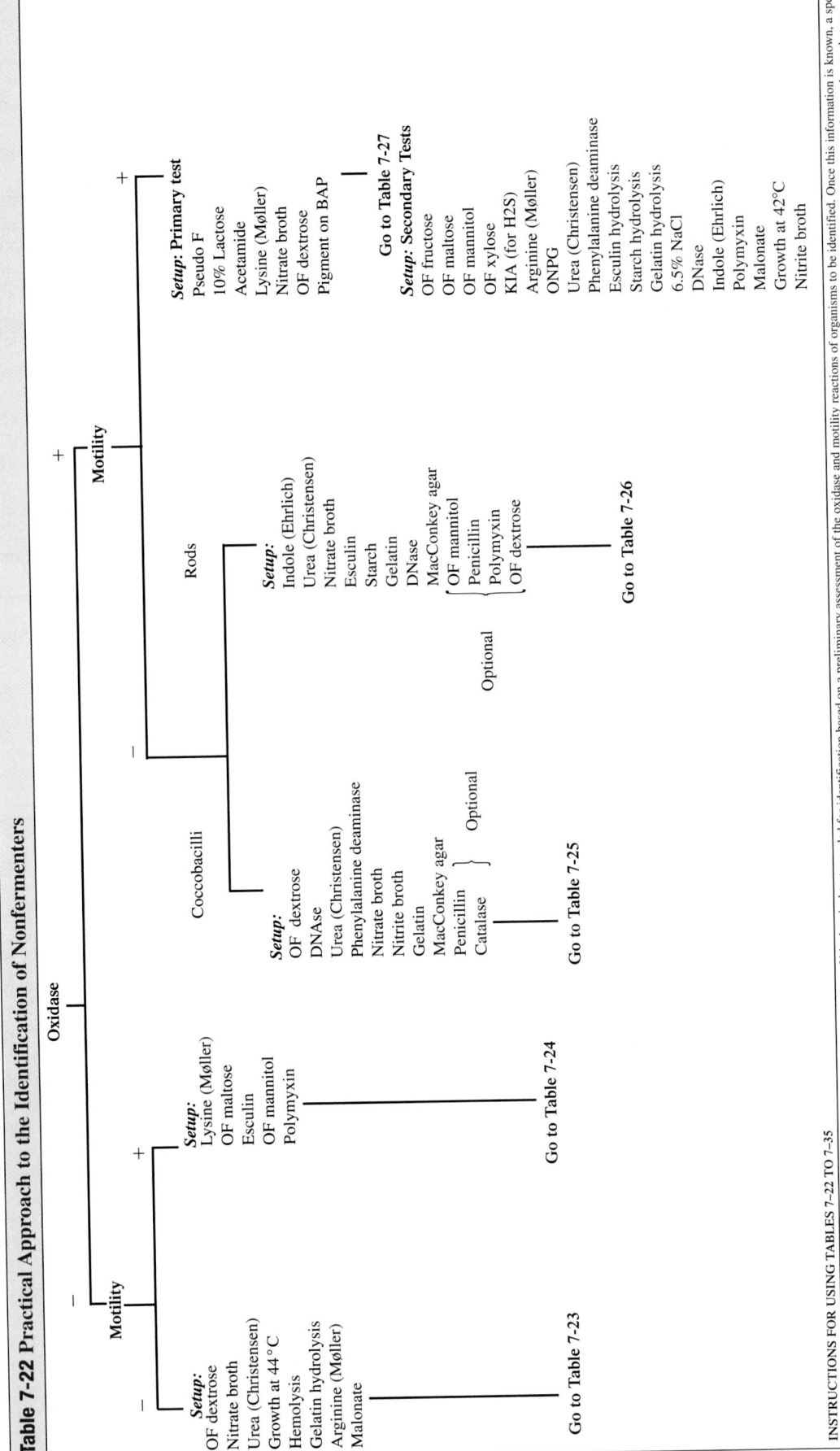

INSTRUCTIONS FOR USING TABLES 7–22 TO 7–35

This approach to the identification of nonfermenters is designed to minimize the number of biochemical tests needed for identification based on a preliminary assessment of the oxidase and motility reactions of organisms to be identified. Once this information is known, a specific battery of tests is performed to complete the identification of the organism. For organisms that are both oxidase-positive and motile, a two-step approach is used, based on the reactions obtained in a primary test battery followed by additional supplemental tests that are specified in the designated tables. Depending on the needs and resources available, the user of this guide may wish to set up all of the tests included in the primary and secondary batteries whenever a motile, oxidase-positive nonfermenter is encountered in order to obtain a definitive identification in the shortest time possible. As a general rule when working with NFBs, a heavy inoculum should be used and reactions should be held 48 hours before the final reading is taken.

STEPS TO FOLLOW

1. Determine the motility and oxidase reactions and follow the flow diagram in Table 7–22.

2. Set up the specified biochemical tests and go to the table indicated to complete the identification.

3. To use Tables 7–23 to 7–35, begin with the first biochemical test listed on the left hand side of the table and locate the shaded box or boxes in the upper left-hand corner.

4. If a single box is shaded, and if the reaction given matches the reaction obtained with your specimen, you are done. The organism identification is listed in the same row to the left of the box.

5. If multiple boxes are shaded and the reaction matches that of your specimen, use the reactions to the right of the shaded boxes to determine the correct identification.

6. If the reaction obtained with your specimen does *not* match that in the shaded box or boxes, proceed to the next column on the right and find the shaded box or boxes in this column. Repeat steps 4 and 5 until you reach a definitive identification.

7. Special consideration must be given to shaded boxes that contain a variable (V) reaction sign. In these rare cases, you must treat the variable reaction in the shaded box as both a match and a nonmatch.

Table 7-23 Oxidase-Negative, Nonmotile Nonfermenters[a]

ORGANISM[b]	GENOMO-SPECIES	YELLOW PIGMENT	UREASE	NITRATE REDUCED	BROWN SOLUBLE PIGMENT	GROWTH AT 37°C	GROWTH AT 44°C	HEMOLYSIS SHEEP BLOOD	GELATIN HYDROLYSIS	OF DEXTROSE	ARGININE	MALONATE
CDC EO-5		+	+	–	–	+	–	NA	–	+	–	NA
Bordetella parapertussis		–	+	–	–	+	NA	NA	NA	–	–	NA
CDC NO-1		–	–	+	–	+	NA	+	NA	–	NA	NA
Bordetella holmesii (NO-2)		–	–	–	+[c]	+	–	–	–	–	–	NA
Acinetobacter johnsonii	7	–	–	–	–	–	–	–	–	–	–	NA
Acinetobacter baumannii	2	–	–	–	–	+	+[d]	–	–	–	V(35)	V(13)
Acinetobacter haemolyticus	4	–	–	–	–	+	–	+	+	+	+	+
Acinetobacter spp.	6	–	–	–	–	+	–	+	+	V(52)	+	–
Acinetobacter spp.	10	–	–	–	–	+	–	+	+	V(66)	+	–
Acinetobacter calcoaceticus	1	–	–	–	–	+	–	–	–	+	–	–
Acinetobacter spp.	3	–	–	–	–	+	–	–	–	+	+	+
Acinetobacter spp.	12	–	–	–	–	+	–	–	–	+	+	V(87)
Acinetobacter junii	5	–	–	–	–	+	–	–	–	V(33)	+	+
Acinetobacter lwoffii	8/9	–	–	–	–	+	–	–	–	–	+	–
Acinetobacter spp.	11	–	–	–	–	+	–	–	–	–	–	–

[a] Data from reference[76,312,801]

[b] All organisms included in this table appear as gram-negative coccobacilli on Gram stain.

[c] Brown soluble pigment produced when grown at 35°C on heart infusion tyrosine agar.

[d] Must also be OF dextrose positive

+, 90% or more strains positive; –, 90% or more strains negative; V, 11–89% of strains positive; NA, results not available; Numbers in parentheses are percentages of strains giving positive reactions.

Table 7-24 Oxidase-Negative, Motile Nonfermenters

ORGANISM	LYSINE DECARBOXYLASE	OF MALTOSE	OF MANNITOL	ESCULIN	POLYMYXIN	PIGMENT
Stenotrophomonas maltophilia	+	+	–	+	S	Yellow Lavender
Burkholderia cepacia complex	+	+	+	V(67)	R	Yellow
Burkholderia gladioli	–	–	+	–	R	Yellow
Bordetella trematum	–	–	–	–	NA	Gray-white
Sphingomonas paucimobilis	–	+	–	+	V(89)	Deep yellow
Pseudomonas luteola	–	+	+	+	S	Dull yellow
Pseudomonas oryzihabitans	–	+	+	–	S	Dull Yellow

Data from reference[249].
+, 90% or more strains positive; –, 90% or more strains negative; V, 11–89% of strains positive; ++, strong positive reaction; NA, results not available; R, resistant; S, susceptible. Numbers in parentheses are percentages of strains giving positive reactions.

The inoculating needle can hold only a relatively small amount of inoculum, and it has been demonstrated that a heavy inoculum is essential to elicit detectable biochemical products from many of the nonfermenters. Many of the nonfermenters are strict aerobes, and the environment within the confined chambers in the Oxi/Ferm tube may not support optimal growth. The test organisms are delivered into the central depths of the medium in each chamber, where they are minimally exposed to atmospheric oxygen. With surface growth lacking, it is difficult to determine if a negative reaction reflects biochemical inactivity or the inability of the organism to grow in the medium. Some of the media in the Oxi/Ferm tube are incapable of supporting the growth of the more fastidious strains of nonfermenters (e.g., citrate agar is not found in most identification systems for nonfermenters). To some extent, these shortcomings have hampered the acceptance of the Oxi/Ferm tube in many clinical laboratories.

The API 20E System

The API 20E system, originally designed for identification of the *Enterobacteriaceae,* has been extended to include the identification of common nonfermentative bacilli as well. To maximize the use of the API 20E for nonfermenters, six additional tests are added to generate a nine-digit profile number (Box 7-11). Studies performed with nonfermenters have shown that although the API 20E system identifies *P. aeruginosa, S. maltophilia,* and *Acinetobacter* species with up to 99% accuracy, particularly after 48 hours of incubation, the performance with other less common nonfermenters was often less than acceptable.[20,90,199,308,509,537,543,544,554,680,789] Incorrect identifications occurred most often because of false-negative reactions for citrate, gelatin liquefaction, motility, arginine dihydrolase, ONPG, nitrate reduction, and urease tests.[20,199,308,537] In the specific study by Hofherr and associates,[308] 12.2% of 836 individual biochemical reactions differed between the API system and conventional methods (53% involved citrate utilization and gelatin liquefaction tests). In other cases, identifications were not possible because the biotype number derived from the 20E strip was not listed in the API Profile Index.[680]

The API 20NE System

The API 20NE is a modification of the API 20E strip. The construction of the plastic strip is the same as in the 20E system; however, the substrates have been changed to include 8 conventional tests and 12 assimilation tests that are based on the observation of microbial growth in the presence of a single source of carbon (see Color Plate 7-5D). A description of the operating procedure and substrates included is given in Box 7-11. Positive and negative reactions are converted to a 7-digit biotype number, and organism identifications are made either from a computerized database or from a profile list provided by the manufacturer. Users of this system should note that the database is constructed on the basis of reactions obtained at an incubation temperature of 30°C (instead of the conventional 35 to 37°C) with final readings taken after 48 hours of incubation. Kiska et al.[404] tested 150 nonfermenters isolated from patients with cystic fibrosis and reported an overall correct identification rate of 57%, including 43% of the *B. cepacia* isolates. The overall performance of the API 20NE has shown it to be one of the better-performing commercial systems for the identification of nonfermenters.[19,422,489,785,791]

The Remel N/F System

The Remel N/F (formerly Uni-N/F) system, as described in Box 7-12 and shown in Color Plate 7-5E, includes three components:

1. A constricted GNF tube that detects glucose fermentation and N_2 (below the constriction) and fluorescein production on the slant (above the constriction).
2. A nonconstricted 42P tube that is used to test for growth at 42°C and pyocyanin pigment production.
3. A circular UNI-N/F Tek plate that consists of 11 independently sealed peripheral wells, containing conventional agar, with which the following characteristics can be determined: utilization of glucose, xylose, mannitol, lactose, and maltose; acetamide assimilation; hydrolysis of esculin and urea; DNase and ONPG activity. One of the peripheral wells is a carbohydrate growth control. A center well contains

Table 7-25 Indentification of Oxidase-Positive, Nonmotile Coccobacilli[a]

ORGANISM	CHARACTERISTIC ODOR OR APPEARANCE	OF DEXTROSE	DNASE	UREASE	PHENYLALANINE DEAMINASE	GELATIN HYDROLYSIS	NITRATE REDUCED	GROWTH ON MAC-CONKEY AGAR	NITRITE REDUCED	CATALASE	GROWTH AT 35°C
Psychrobacter immobilis	Odor of PEA agar (roses)	+	−	+	+	−	V(86)	V	NA	+	−
CDC EO-2	O-shaped cells[b]	+	−	+	NA	−	+	V(82)	NA	+	−
CDC EO-3	Yellow colonies (100)	+	−	+	NA	−	−	+	NA	+	+
CDC EO-4	Yellow colonies (83)	+	NA	+	NA		−	+	NA	+	+
M. canis		−	+	−	−	−	+	+	NA	+	+
M. catarrhalis		−	+	−	V	−	+	+	V	+	+
Psychrobacter phenylpyruvicus[c]		−	−	+	+	−	V(89)	−	+	weak	+
O. urethralis	Small coccoid cells	−	−	−	+	−	−	+	−		+
M. lacunata		−	−	−	−	−	−	V(83)	+	+	+
M. nonliquefaciens		−	−	−	−	+	+	−	−	weak	+
M. osloensis		−	−	−	−	−	V(26)	V(17)	−	+	+
M. atlantae	Spreading or pitting colonies	−	−	−	−	−	−	V(49)	V(20)	weak	+
M. lincolnii	Coccus-like to plump rods	−	−	−	NA	−	−	+	V	weak or −	+

[a] Data from references[249,349,515,517,753]

[b] Gram stain smears show coccoid-to-short thick rods that are frequently vacuolated. Cells have unstained centers but are peripherally stained and appear as O's.

[c] Brucella species may be misidentified as Psychrobacter phenylpyruvicus in some commercial identification systems.

+, 90% or more strains positive; −, 90% or more strains negative; V, 11–89% of strains positive; NA, results not available. Numbers in parentheses are percentages of strains giving positive reactions.

Table 7-26 Identification of Oxidase-Positive, Nonmotile Rod-Shaped Bacilli[a]

ORGANISM	ODOR OR CHARACTERISTIC, ODOR, OR APPEARANCE	INDOLE	UREASE	NITRATE REDUCTION	ESCULIN HYDROLYSIS	GELATIN HYDROLYSIS	STARCH HYDROLYSIS	DNASE HYDROLYSIS	GROWTH ON MACCONKEY AGAR	OF MANNITOL	OF DEXTROSE	PENICILLIN	POLYMYXIN
Sphingobacterium multivorum	Pale yellow	−	+	−	+	−	V(79)	−	V(17)	−	+	R	R
Sphingobacterium spiritivorum	Pale yellow	−	+	−	+	−	V(51)	+	−	+	+	S(33)	S(89)
Sphingomonas paucimobilis	Bright yellow	−	−	−	+	−	−	−	V(10)	+	+	S(19)	R
Myroides odoratus	Yellow-green fruity odor	−	+	−	−	+	−	+	V(78)	−	−	S	S
Neisseria weaveri	Gray-white colonies, strongly catalase +	−	−	−	−	−	NA	−	V(42)	−	−	S	S
Neisseria elongata subsp. nitroreducens	Catalase-	−	−	+	−	−	NA	−	V(20)	−	−	S	S
Gilardi rod group 1	Strong PAD +	+	++	−	−	+	NA	−	+	+	+	NA	NA
Bergeyella zoohelcum	No pigment	+	−	+	+	V	NA	NA	−	−	−	S	R
CDC group IIc	No pigment	+	−	−	−	−	−	V(13)	−	−	−	S	S
Weeksella virosa	Colonies stick to agar	+	−	−	−	+	V(40)	+	+[b]	−	Delayed	R	R
Empedobacter brevis	Pale Yellow	+	−	−	−	+	+	−	−	−	Delayed	S	S
CDC group IIe	No pigment	+	−	−	−	−	NA	−	+	−	−	NA	S
CDC group IIg	No pigment	+	−[b]	−	+	−[b]	+	V(78)	−[b]	−	Delayed	S(67)	S(22)
CDC group IIh	No pigment	+	−	−	+	−	V(14)	−	−	−	Delayed	S(57)	R
CDC group IIi	NA	+	−	−	+	+	−	+	V(26)	Delayed	Delayed	R	R
Chryseobacterium meningosepticum	Pale yellow	+	−	−	+	+	−	−	−	−	Delayed	R	R
Chryseobacterium indologenes	Deep yellow	+	−	−	+	+	+	−	−	−	Delayed	R	R

[a] Data from references[179a,240,311].

[b] Different results reported, reaction used here is that reported by CDC.[179a]

+, 90% or more strains positive; −, 90% or more strains negative; V, 11–89% of strains positive; NA, results not available; R, resistant; S, susceptible; PAD, phenylalanine deaminase. Numbers in parentheses are percentages of strains giving positive reactions.

Note: Balneatrix alpica is pale yellow and indole-positive but is excluded from this table because it is motile (see Tables 7-32 and 7-34).

Table 7-27 Screening Tests for Species Identification of Oxidase-Positive, Motile Nonfermenters

						−	+	Fluorescence (Pseudo F agar under UV light)
					−	+		10% Lactose
				−	+			Acetamide
			−	+				Lysine (Møller)
		−	+					Pigment on blood agar
	−	+						Gas from nitrate or nitrate
−	+							OF dextrose
See Table 7–35	See Table 7–34	See Table 7–33	See Table 7–32	See Table 7–31	See Table 7–30	See Table 7–29	See Table 7–28	

Table 7-28 Identification of Fluorescent Nonfermenters

ORGANISM	ACETAMIDE	GROWTH 42°C	GELATIN
Pseudomonas aeruginosa	+	+	+
P. fluorescens	−	−	+
P. putida	−	−	−

+, 90% or more of strains positive; −, 90% or more of strains negative.

Table 7-29 Identification of Strongly Lactose-Positive Nonfermenters (Oxidase +, Motility +, Fluorescein −)

ORGANISM	LYSINE	OF MANNITOL	UREASE	ONPG	POLYMYXIN B
Burkholderia cepacia complex	+	+	V(45)	V(79)	R
Burkholderia pseudomallei	−	+	V(43)	−	R
Rhizobium radiobacter	−	+	+	+	S
Ralstonia mannitolilytica (Va-3)	−	+	+	−	R
Ralstonia pickettii (Va-1)	−	−	+	−	R
Sphingomonas paucimobilis	−	−	−	+	S(89)

Data from reference[249].

+, 90% or more strains positive; −, 90% or more strains negative; V, 11–89% of strains positive; R, resistant; S, susceptible. Numbers in parentheses are percentages of strains giving positive reactions.

Note: Acinetobacter baumannii and Sphingobacterium species are strongly lactose-positive, but are excluded from this table because they are nonmotile (see Tables 7-23 and 7-26).

Table 7-30 Identification of Acetamide Positive Nonfermenters (Oxidase +, Motility +, Fluorescein −, 10% Lactose −)

ORGANISM	ARGININE	OF DEXTROSE	OF FRUCTOSE	OF MANNITOL	NITRATE-REDUCED	NITRITE TO GAS	MALONATE	NITRATE TO GAS	ORANGE INDOLE
Pseudomonas aeruginosa	+	+	V(89)	V(68)	V(74)	NA	NA	V(60)	−
Burkholderia cepacia complex	−	+	+	+	V(37)	NA	NA	−	−
Achromobacter xylosoxidans	−	+	V(9)	−	+	NA	NA	V(69)	−
Delftia acidovorans	−	−	+	+(92)	+	NA	NA	−	+
Achromobacter denitrificans	−	−	−	−	+	+	+	+	−
Achromobacter piechaudii	−	−	−	−	+	−	+	−	−
Oligella ureolytica	−	−	−	−	+	V(63)	−	V(58)	−
Alcaligenes faecalis	−	−	−	−	−	+	+	−	−
Bordetella hinzii	−	−	−	−	−	−	+	−	−
Bordetella avium	−	−	−	−	−	−	−	−	−

Data from references[249,758]; data for alkalinization of malonate also from reference[40a].
+, 90% or more strains positive; −, 90% or more strains negative; V, 11–89% of strains positive; ++, strong positive reaction; NA, results not available; R, resistant; S, susceptible. Numbers in parentheses are percentages of strains giving positive reactions.

Table 7-31 Identification of Lysine-Positive Nonfermenters

ORGANISM	POLYMYXIN B	DNASE	OF MANNITOL
Burkholderia cepacia complex	R	−	+
Stenotrophomonas maltophilia	S	+	−

+, 90% or more of strains are positive; −, 90% or more of strains are negative; R, resistant; S, susceptible.
Note: Occasional strains of S. maltophilia may be oxidase-positive.

a medium for detecting indole and hydrogen sulfide production.

The UNI-N/F Tek plate is well constructed to test for most nonfermenters. The plate includes media that closely resemble conventional formulations and will support the growth of many of the more fastidious strains. The organism suspension is inoculated to the surface of the agar wedges, where not only are the organisms exposed to atmospheric oxygen, but the colonial growth can also be directly viewed. Thus, negative test reactions owing to no growth can be distinguished from those owing to biochemical inactivity, and the user can determine directly whether other organisms may be contaminating the inoculum.

The ability of the Remel N/F system to detect *P. aeruginosa* by the use of the supplemental constricted GNF tube and the nonconstricted 42P tube saves time. If the test organism is other than *P. aeruginosa*, 1 drop of a heavy suspension prepared from the slant of the GNF tube is delivered into each of the peripheral chambers in the UNI-N/F Tek plate, and the center well is stab-inoculated. The plate is incubated at 35°C for 24 hours, and the various reactions are interpreted visually.

About 90% of *P. aeruginosa* were identified by researchers with the two screening tubes after 24 hours of incubation, increasing to approximately 98% after 48 hours incubation.[20,45,90,411,681,789] The capability to screen out *P. aeruginosa* without using a full set of biochemical tests is considered a distinct advantage by most users. Some of the problems cited with the UNI-N/F system were as follows: The screening tubes identified only about one third of the strains of *P. fluorescens* and *P. putida*, and further testing was necessary.[20,45,90,422,681] Problems were also encountered in the interpretation of the N_2 gas reaction in the GNF tube and the indole test.[20,789] Only a low percentage of identification was possible with organisms such as *B. cepacia* and CDC group IV, and with many of the nonoxidative and non-saccharolytic strains.[789] Supplemental tests, such as Gram stain morphology, hanging-drop motility, and flagellar stains were needed to identify these strains. The researchers, nonetheless, report that the UNI-N/F system is convenient to use, gives a high overall percentage of nonfermentative bacilli identifications in 24 hours, and performed better in identifying nonfermenters than either the Oxi/Ferm or API 20E systems.[20,45,90,411,422,681,789] Kiska and associates reported that the Uni-N/F system correctly identified 72% of the NFBs encountered in patients with cystic fibrosis, including 86% of the *B. cepacia* isolates. The identification percentage for *B. cepacia* isolates was the highest among the four test kits studied.[404] We have found that the Uni-N/F system performs

comparably with the Crystal Enteric/Nonfermenter and the IDS RapID NF Plus systems. (Schreckenberger PC, Anderson RR, Pierson C, Debusscher J, Brown W: unpublished data).

The Crystal Enteric/Nonfermenter System

The Crystal Enteric/NonFermenter ID kit was described in Chapter 6. The nonfermenter database includes 24 taxa of nonfermenters representing 10 different genera. Twenty additional taxa are included in a group called "Miscellaneous Gram-Negative Bacilli," that consists of a group of oxidase-positive species that are relatively inactive and indistinguishable from each other in the Crystal E/NF System. Included in this group are some medically relevant species of *Alcaligenes, Burkholderia, Comamonas, Moraxella, Ochrobactrum, Oligella*, and *Pseudomonas*. In a study by Wauters and coworkers[791] the overall correct identification of 201 nonfermenters (including 31 different species) was 75.9% with the Crystal E/NF compared with 75.3% for the API 20NE. Of note is that only 36 of 45 *P. aeruginosa* strains were correctly identified by the Crystal E/NF compared with 41 of 45 by the API 20NE. The overall percentage of incorrect identifications for nonfermenters was substantially higher for the API (13.8%) than for the Crystal (6.3%). The authors noted that an advantage of Crystal over the API system is that both fermenters and nonfermenters can be tested in the same panel. In addition the API 20NE may require 48 hours of incubation, whereas the Crystal E/NF requires only 18 hours of incubation. Robinson and colleagues[631] studied 131 nonenteric bacilli on the Crystal E/NF including 11 species of nonfermenters; however, three species (*P. aeruginosa, A. baumannii, S. maltophilia*) accounted for 90% of the nonfermenters tested. The Crystal system correctly identified all of the *P. aeruginosa, A. baumannii*, and *S. maltophilia* species tested, but correctly identified only 8 of the 13 (61.5%) remaining nonfermenter species tested. Our own evaluation showed an overall identification rate to the species level of 62.5%. (Schreckenberger PC, Anderson RR, Pierson C, Debusscher J, Brown W: unpublished data.)

The RapID NF Plus System

The RapID NF Plus System (Remel) is a micromethod using conventional and chromogenic substrates for the identification of medically important glucose-nonfermenting gram-negative bacteria and other selected glucose-fermenting gram-negative bacteria not belonging to the family En-

Table 7-32 Identification of Pigmented Nonfermenters[a] (Oxidase +, Motility +, Fluorescein −, 10% Lactose −, Acetamide −, Lysine −)

ORGANISM	COLOR	KIA/H₂S	OF FRUCTOSE	GAS FROM NITRATE	INDOLE	OF MANNITOL	ESCULIN HYDROLYSIS	GROWTH IN 6.5% NACL
Roseomonas spp.[b]	Pink	−	+	−	−	V	−	−
Methylobacterium spp.[b]	Pink	−	V(50)	−	−	−	−	−
Shewanella alga	Tan	+	−	NA	−	−	−	+
Shewanella putrefaciens	Tan	+	V	−	−	−	−	−
Massilia timonae	Pale Yellow	−	−	−	−	−	+	−
Brevundimonas vesicularis	Tan/orange	−	−	−	−	−	+	−
Pseudomonas stutzeri	Yellow	−	+	+	−	V(70)	−	+
Balneatrix alpica	Pale Yellow	−	+	−	+	+	−	NA
Burkholderia cepacia	Yellow	−	+	−	−	+	V(67)	−
Sphingomonas paucimobilis	Yellow	−	+	−	−	−	+	−

[a] Data from references[170,249,392,443,626].

[b] Methylobacterium species appear as dark colonies under long-wave UV light due to absorption of UV light. Roseomonas species do not absorb UV light and do not appear dark.

Note: All of these pigments develop only as the culture ages. Most strains of Chryseobacterium spp. and Sphingobacterium spp. are also pigmented (yellow); however, these organisms are excluded from this table because they are nonmotile (see Table 7-26).

+, 90% or more strains positive; −, 90% or more strains negative; V, 11–89% of strains positive; NA, results not available. Numbers in parentheses are percentages of strains giving positive reactions.

Table 7-33 Identification of Denitrifying Nonfermenters (Oxidase +, Motility +, Fluorescein −, 10% Lactose −, Acetamide −, Lysine −, Pigment −)

ORGANISM	OXIDATION OF DEXTROSE	POLYMYXIN B	ONPG	6.5% NACL	PHENYLALANINE DEAMINASE	ARGININE	STARCH HYDROLYSIS	OXIDATION OF MALTOSE	UREASE
Oligella ureolytica	−	S	−	−	+	−	−	−	++
Pseudomonas sp. CDC group 1	−	S	−	−	−	V(50)	−	−	−
A. denitrificans	−	S(83)	−	−	−	−	−	−	V(31)
R. pickettii (Va-1)	+	R	−	−	−	−	V(48)	+	+
R. pickettii (Va-2)	+	R	−	−	V(40)	−	V(12)	−	+
Rhizobium radiobacter	+	S	+	−	+	−	V(16)	+	+
P. stutzeri (Vb-1)	+	S	−	+	V(55)	−	+	+	V(17)
P. mendocina (Vb-2)	+	S	−	+	V(50)	+	−	V(50)	V(50)
CDC Vb-3	+	S	−	+	V(56)	+	V(75)	V(88)	V(31)
Ochrobactrum anthropi	+	S	−	−	+	V(36)	−	V(50)	+
P. aeruginosa	+	S	−	−	−	+	−	V(12)	V(66)
A. xylosoxidans	+	S	−	−	−	−	−	−	−

Data from reference[249].

+, 90% or more strains positive; −, 90% or more strains negative; V, 11–89% of strains positive; R, resistant; S, susceptible. Numbers in parentheses are percentages of strains giving positive reactions. Note: A. denitrificans can be separated from Pseudomonas spp. CDC group 1 on the basis of flagellar morphology. Achromobacter has peritrichous flagella, Pseudomonas group 1 has a single polar flagellum.

Table 7-34 Identification of Dextrose Positive Nonfermenters (Oxidase +, Motility +, Fluorescein −, 10% Lactose −, Acetamide −, Lysine −, Pigment −, Denitrification −)

ORGANISM	PIGMENT OF COLONIES	KIA H₂S	INDOLE	OF FRUCTOSE	ONPG	OF XYLOSE	DNASE	GROWTH IN 6.5% NACL	PHENYLALANINE DEAMINASE	ARGININE	GROWTH AT 42°C	GELATIN HYDROLYSIS	ESCULIN HYDROLYSIS
Methylobacterium	Pink	−	−	V	−	V	−	−	−	−	−	−	−
Shewanella putrefaciens	−	+	−	V	−	−	+	−	−	−	V	V	−
Balneatrix alpica	Pale yellow	−	+	+	−	NA	−	−	NA	+	+	weak +	−
A. xylosoxidans	−	−	−	−	−	+	−	−	−	−	V(86)	−	−
Brevundimonas diminuta	−	−	−	−	−	−	V(12)	−	V(16)	−	V(19)	V(58)	−
Rhizobium radiobacter	−	−	−	+	+	+	−	−	+	−	V(13)	−	+
Pseudomonas-like group 2	−	−	−	+	+	+	−	−	+	−	−	−	−
P. pseudoalcaligenes	−	−	−	+	−	−	−	−	V(21)	V(36)	V(75)	−	−
Acidovorax delafieldii	−	−	−	+	−	+	+	+	−	+	−	+	−
CDC Vb-3	−	−	−	+	−	+	−	−	V(56)	+	V(75)	−	−
O. anthropi	−	−	−	+	−	+	−	−	+	V(36)	V(10)	−	V(40)
R. pickettii (VA-1)	−	−	−	+	−	+	−	−	−	−	V(26)	V(77)	−
P. aeruginosa	−	−	−	+	−	V(85)	−	−	−	+	+	V(46)	−
P. fluorescens	−	−	−	+	−	+	−	−	−	+	−	+	−
P. putida	−	−	−	+	−	+	−	−	−	+	−	−	−

Data from references[170,249].
+, 90% or more strains positive; −, 90% or more strains negative; V, 11–89% of strains positive. Numbers in parentheses are percentages of strains giving positive reactions.
flagellum.

Table 7-35 Identification of Dextrose Negative Nonfermenters[a] (Oxidase +, Motility +, Fluorescein −, 10% Lactose −, Acetamide −, Lysine −, Pigment −, Denitrification −, Dextrose −)

ORGANISM	PINK PIGMENTED COLONIES	KIA H$_2$S	OF FRUCTOSE	UREASE	NO$_3$ TO NO$_2$	NO$_2$ TO GAS	STARCH HYDROLYSIS	PHENYLALANINE DEAMINASE	DNASE	ARGININE	FLAGELLAR ARRANGEMENT
Methylobacterium[b]	+	−	V	+	V	NA	+	−	−	−	Polar monotrichous
Roseomonas[b]	+	−	+	+	−	NA	+	V(17)	−	−	Variable
Shewanella putrefaciens/alga[c]	−	+	V	−	V	NA	−	−	+	−	Polar, 1–2
P. pseudoalcaligenes	−	−	+	−	+	NA	−	V(21)	−	V(36)	Polar, 1–2
O. ureolytica	−	−	−	++	+	V(63)	−	+	−	−	Peritrichous
B. bronchiseptica	−	−	−	++	+	−	−	V(25)	−	−	Peritrichous
Cupriavidus pauculus	−	−	−	++	−	−	V(16)	−	−	−	Peritrichous
Brevundimonas diminuta	−	−	−	−	−	NA	−	V(16)	V(12)	−	Polar monotrichous
B. hinzii	−	−	−	−	+	−	−	V(15)	−	−	Peritrichous
P. alcaligenes	−	−	−	V(21)	V(61)	V(10)	V(16)	V(20)	−	V(7)	Polar monotrichous
C. testosteroni	−	−	−	−	+	V(11)	−	V(30)	−	−	Polar multitrichous
A. piechaudii	−	−	−	−	+	−	−	−	−	−	Peritrichous

[a] Data from refrence[249].
[b] Methylobacterium species appear as dark colonies under long-wave UV light due to absorption of UV light. Roseomonas species do not absorb UV light and do not appear dark.
[c] Shewanella alga grow in 6.5% NaCl, Shewanella putrefaciens do not grow in 6.5% NaCl.
+, 90% or more strains positive; −, 90% or more strains negative; V, 11–89% of strains positive; ++, strong positive reaction; NA, results not available. Numbers in parentheses are percentages of strains giving positive reactions.

Box 7-11 API 20E and API 20NE Systems for Identifying Nonfermenters

Functional Design	Operating Procedure	Substrates Included
Each system consists of a plastic strip with 20 miniaturized cupules containing dehydrated substrates and a plastic incubation chamber with a loosely fitting lid (see Color Plates 6-6*A* and 7-5*D*). Each cupule has a small hole at the top through which the bacterial suspension can be inoculated with a pipette. Bacterial action on the substrates produces turbidity or color changes that are interpreted visually.	*For both systems:* Add 5 mL of tap water to an incubation tray to provide a humid atmosphere during incubation. Place the strip into the incubation tray. Prepare a bacterial suspension of the test organism by suspending the cells from a well-isolated colony in 5 mL of sterile 0.85% saline. The turbidity must be equivalent to a 0.5 McFarland standard.	API 20E: ONPG Arginine dihydrolase Lysine decarboxylase Ornithine decarboxylase Citrate Hydrogen sulfide Urease Tryptophan deaminase (add 10% $FeCl_3$) Indole Voges-Proskauer (add KOH and α-naphthol) Gelatin Glucose Mannitol

API 20E: With a Pasteur pipette, fill each cupule with the bacterial suspension through the inoculating hole. Overlay the three decarboxylase and the urease cupules with sterile mineral oil. The unit is incubated at 35°C for 24 or 48 hours before reading results according to the following rules: after 24 hours, if the glucose is positive, add reagents, perform an oxidase test, and generate a 7-digit profile number to look up in the white section of the Profile Index; if glucose is negative, but three or more other reactions are positive before adding reagents, proceed as above; if glucose is negative and fewer than three other tests are positive, do not add reagents, reincubate strip for additional 24 hours and inoculate OF glucose, motility medium, and MacConkey agar. After 48 hours, add reagents, perform oxidase test, and generate a 9-digit profile number to look up in the blue section of the Profile Index.

API 20NE: With a Pasteur pipette, fill the tube portion of the first eight cupules (NO_3 through PNPG) with the bacterial suspension. Inoculate an ampule of AUX medium with four drops of the same saline suspension. Mix well. With a new sterile pipette inoculate the assimilation tests GLU through PAC (cupules with colored lines) by filling the tube and cupule until a flat liquid surface without a meniscus is obtained. Add mineral oil to the GLU, ADH, and URE cupules. Incubate strip for 24 hours at 29–31°C. After 24 hours, add nitrate reagents to NO_3 cupule and TRP reagent to TRP cupule. Read and record reactions. Assimilation tests are recorded as positive if there is visible growth in the cupule portion of the tube. A 7-digit profile number is generated. If a good identification is not obtained or profile number is not found in codebook, the test strip may be incubated for an additional 24 hours. To do so, immediately cover the NO_3 and TRP cupules with mineral oil. Record the NO_3, TRP, and GLU test results after 24 hours; do not read these tests after 48 hours.

Inositol
Sorbitol
Rhamnose
Sucrose
Melibiose
Amygdalin
Arabinose
Supplemental Tests:
Oxidase
NO_2
N_2 gas
Motility
MacConkey agar
OF glucose-oxidative
OF glucose-fermentative
API 20NE:
Biochemical Tests:
NO_3 Nitrate reduction
TRP Tryptophanase
GLU Glucose fermentation
ADH Arginine dihydrolase
URE Urease
ESC Esculin hydrolysis
GEL Gelatinase
PNPG β-Galactosidase
Assimilation Tests:
GLU D-Glucose
ARA L-Arabinose
MNE D-Mannose
MAN D-Mannitol
NAG N-Acetyl-D glucosamine
MAL Maltose
GNT D-Gluconate
CAP Caprate
ADI Adipate
MLT L-Malate
CIT Citrate
PAC Phenylacetate

Box 7–12 The Remel N/F System for Identifying Nonfermenters

Functional Design	Operating Procedure	Substrates Included

This system consists of two tubes of media poured on a slant and a wheel, including 13 compartments, 12 peripheral and 1 central, containing a variety of media substrates (Color Plate 7-5*E*).
 	
The two tubes are used to screen for *P. aeruginosa*. The nonconstricted tube is incubated at 42°C to observe for growth and pyocyanin pigment production; the constricted GNF tube is used to screen for fluorescence, glucose fermentation, and N$_2$.
 	
The wheel is used to determine several biochemical characteristics. Each of the peripheral media compartments has a small pore through which a bacterial suspension can be inoculated. The medium in the central compartment is open to the air and is inoculated directly. A plastic lid covers the unit to prevent evaporation during incubation.
	Initially stab-inoculate the two tubes, using a straight inoculating wire that has been touched to the surface of a well-isolated colony of the test bacterium growing on an agar plate. Incubate the tubes for 18–24 hours at 35°C.
	
	If the reactions in the tubes are not consistent with *P. aeruginosa*, prepare a heavy bacterial suspension by emulsifying the entire growth from the slant of the GNF tube into 2 mL of sterile distilled water. Add 1 drop to each of the 12 peripheral wells through the inoculating pore and deeply stab-inoculate the agar medium in the center of the wheel. Replace the plastic lid on the wheel and incubate the unit at 35°C for 18–24 hour. Color reactions are interpreted visually and identifications made using a logic scheme or computer program supplied by the manufacturer.
		Nonconstricted tube agar slant:
		  42°C growth and pyocyanin pigment production
		Constricted tube
		  GNF medium
		    Glucose fermentation
		    N$_2$
		    Fluorescence
		Wheel
		  Peripheral compartments
		    Growth control
		    Glucose
		    Xylose
		    Mannitol
		    Lactose
		    Maltose
		    Acetamide
		    Esculin
		    Urea
		    DNAse
		    ONPG
		  Central compartment
		    Agar media:
		      Hydrogen sulfide
		      Indole

terobacteriaceae. The tests used in the RapID NF Plus System are based on the microbial degradation of specific substrates detected by various indicator systems. The reactions used are a combination of conventional tests and single-substrate chromogenic tests. The system is described in Box 7-13 and shown in Color Plate 7-5*F*. In the study by Kitch and colleagues,[405] 90.1% of all strains were identified correctly to species without additional tests. Kiska and associates[404] showed that the NF Plus correctly identified 80% of the NFBs recovered from patients with cystic fibrosis, including 81% of the *B. cepacia* isolates. This was the highest overall identification rate of the four commercial systems included in the study.[404] In the study by Schreckenberger and coworkers, the overall correct identification to species was 61.8%. (Schreckenberger PC, Anderson RR, Pierson C, Debusscher J, Brown W: unpublished data.) The RapID NF Plus system is currently the only nonautomated 4-hour test system available for the identification of nonfermenters.

The Biolog System

The Biolog System (Biolog, Hayward CA) was described in Chapter 6. The gram-negative database version 4.01 contains approximately 275 species and biogroups of nonfermenting gram-negative rods. Holmes and associates[315] have evaluated the Biolog System, using 214 strains of nonfermenters representing 15 species. They report that after 4 hours of incubation, 20% of the nonfermenters were correctly identified to the species level using the automated reader; however, after 24 hours of incubation 54% and 66% of the nonfermenters were correctly identified to the species level by automated and manual reading, respectively, using version 3.01A software. The authors note that no other commercial bacterial identification system has as many taxa in a single database as that supplied by Biolog, but because there are so many, even the large number of tests available may not be adequate, in practice, for discriminating all pairs of taxa.[315]

Automated Identification Systems
The Vitek Legacy System

The Vitek Legacy System (bioMérieux), described in Chapter 6, has also been used with success in the identification of the nonfermenters most frequently encountered in the clinical laboratory. Pfaller and coworkers[578] tested 91 NFBs, with 90.1% identified correctly. Fifteen percent were identified at 4 hours, an additional 45% were identified 5 to 8 hours, and an additional 40% were identified at 9 to 18 hours. Colonna and associates[147] tested 142 NFBs and found 79.6% agreement with the API NFT. Kiska and colleagues[404] evaluated four identification systems, including the Vitek GNI card, for identification of NFBs from patients with cystic fibrosis. A total of 150 isolates were tested in-

Box 7-13 RapID NF Plus System for Identifying Nonfermenters

Functional Design	Operating Procedure	Substrates Included

The system consists of 10 reaction cavities molded into the periphery of a plastic disposable tray (see Color Plate 7-5*F*). Reaction cavities contain dehydrated reactants, and the tray allows the simultaneous inoculation of each cavity with a predetermined amount of inoculum. When the test inoculum is added to the reaction cavity, the test substrate is rehydrated and the test reaction is initiated. After incubation for 4 hours, each test cavity is examined for reactivity by noting the development of a color. In some cases, reagents must be added to the test cavities to provide a color change. The resulting pattern of positive and negative test reactions is used as the basis for identification of the test isolate by comparison of test results to reactivity of known organisms stored in a computer generated database.	*Preparation of Inocula:* Test organisms must be grown in pure culture and should be examined by Gram stain and oxidase before use in the RapID NF System. Test organisms may be removed from a variety of selective and nonselective agar growth media. Plates used for inocula preparation should preferably be 18–24 hours old. Using a cotton swab or inoculating loop, remove organisms from agar plate and suspend in RapID Inoculation Fluid to achieve a visual turbidity of at least a 1 but not in excess of a 3 McFarland turbidity standard. Suspensions should be mixed thoroughly and used within 15 minutes of preparation.
	
	Inoculation of Panels: Peel back the panel lid over the inoculation port. With a Pasteur pipette, gently transfer the entire contents of the inoculation fluid into the upper right-hand corner of the panel. Reseal the inoculation port by pressing the peel tab back in place. After adding the test suspension, tilt the panel back away from the test cavities at approximately a 45-degree angle. While tilted back, gently rock the panel from side to side to evenly distribute the inoculum along the rear baffles. While maintaining a level horizontal position, slowly tilt the panel forward toward the reaction cavities until the inoculum flows along the baffles into the reaction cavities. Incubate panels at 35–37°C in a non-CO_2 incubator for 4 hours.
	
	Reading Panels: Place panel on the benchtop and peel back the label lid over the reaction cavities. Without the addition of any reagents, read and score cavities 1 through 10, reading from left to right and record on report form. Record color of cavity 10 (GLU) in space provided on report pad. Then add 2 drops of NF Plus Reagent to cavities 4–8, 2 drops of Innova Spot Indole Reagent to cavity 9, and 2 drops of Innova Nitrate A reagent to cavity 10. Allow at least 30 seconds but no more than 3 minutes for color development. Record results in appropriate boxes on report form. Look up in Code Compendium or computer database.
		Arginine dihydrolase
		Aliphatic thiol utilization
		Triglyceride hydrolysis
		Enzymatic hydrolysis of glycoside or phosphoester linked nitrophenyl substrates releases yellow *o*- or *p*-nitrophenol:
		    p-Nitrophenyl-phosphoester
		    p-Nitrophenyl-*N*-acetyl-β, D-glucosaminide
		    p-Nitrophenyl-α, D-glucoside
		    p-Nitrophenyl-β, D-glucoside
		    o-Nitrophenyl-β, D-galactoside
		Urea hydrolysis
		Glucose utilization
		Enzymatic hydrolysis of substrate linked β-naphthylamide substrates releases free β-naphthylamine which is detected with the RapID NF Plus Reagent
		    Proline β-naphthylamide
		    Pyrrolidine β-naphthylamide
		    γ-Glutamyl β-naphthylamide
		    Tryptophan β-naphthylamide
		    N-Benzyl-arginine-β-naphthylamide
		Tryptophan utilization with formation of indole
		Sodium nitrate reduction
		The above tests together with oxidase provide 18 test parameters.

cluding 58 *B. cepacia*, 30 *S. maltophilia*, 24 *A. xylosoxidans*, 14 *P. aeruginosa*, and 24 other NFBs. The Vitek correctly identified only 50% of the *B. cepacia* isolates and 60% of the isolates overall. O'Hara and coworkers[548] tested 23 nonfermenters (8 *Acinetobacter*, 10 *P. aeruginosa*, 5 *S. maltophilia*) and reported 100% correct identification with the Vitek GNI card and version R07.1 software. Rhoads and associates[623] tested 80 *A. baumannii* and 39 *P. aeruginosa* and reported correct identification of 100% and 84.6%, respectively, with the Vitek GNI card and version AMS-R08.2 software. Sung and colleagues evaluated the GNI + for identification of 301 isolates of NFBs representing 25 different species. Correct identification to the species level at initial testing was 71.8%, improving to 92.3% after additional testing was performed as recommended by the manufacturer's protocol.[722]

The Vitek 2 System

The Vitek 2 System is described in detail in Chapter 6. The original Vitek 2 card for gram-negative bacteria identification has been redesigned to improve the identification of fermenting and nonfermenting bacilli. The new card contains 47 tests (26 that had been included in the previous card and

21 new tests), compared with 41 in the established Vitek 2 ID-GNB card. The database for the new card has been expanded to 159 taxa compared with only 101 for the original Vitek 2 card. In a study performed by Funke et al., 133 of 144 (92.4%) NFBs were correctly identified with the new Vitek 2 cards.[230]

The Microscan Walkaway-96, Walkaway-40, and Autoscan-4 Systems

These three systems (manufactured by Dade Behring, West Sacramento, CA), described in Chapter 6, all have an extensive database that includes many species of NFBs. Pfaller and colleagues,[578] using WalkAway-96 Rapid Gram Negative Panel, reported that 92.3% of the nonenteric bacilli were identified correctly with a likelihood of more than 85%. Tenover and colleagues[734] evaluated the Walkaway-96 (formerly called the autoSCAN-W/A) for its ability to identify 310 well-characterized non-glucose-fermenting gram-negative bacilli. In their study, two types of identification panels were tested: the dried colorimetric Neg ID type 2 panel (DCP) and the rapid fluorometric Neg ID panel (RFP). Results with the DCP showed that 41.3% of 286 organisms were identified correctly, with a confidence of more than 85%, whereas 22.4% were misidentified with the same degree of confidence (major errors). Fifteen percent of the organisms were reported as unidentified. Problems in identifying relatively common nonfermentative bacilli, such as *P. fluorescens*, *P. putida*, and *S. maltophilia* were reported with the DCP panel. The researchers reported better results with the RFP panels, in which 77.1% of 239 isolates were correctly identified, whereas 25% were misidentified. The researchers further noted that the results with the RFP panels were available in 2 hours; thus, if an organism cannot be identified, additional biochemical tests can be inoculated on the same day, and little time is lost in identifying the organisms. Colonna and colleagues at UCLA tested 142 NFBs using the 2-hour rapid Neg ID panel and reported 74.6% agreement with the API NFT.[147] O'Hara and colleagues[548] at the CDC tested 23 strains of NFBs, including 8 *Acinetobacter*, 10 *P. aeruginosa*, and 5 *S. maltophilia*, and reported 100% accuracy with the Walkaway Neg combo 3 panel and version 17.02 software. Rhoads and coworkers[623] reported 97.5% and 82.1% correct identification of *A. baumannii* and *P. aeruginosa* isolates, respectively, using the Walkaway-96 system with urine combo 6 and negative combo 16 and version 20.20 software. Sung and colleagues compared the MicroScan Walkaway (W/A) using conventional (overnight) Neg Combo type 12 panels, with the Vitek GNI + for identification of 301 isolates of NFBs representing 25 different species. The W/A correctly identified 71.4% of the isolates to the species level at initial testing improving to 96.0% after additional testing that was recommended by the manufacturer's protocol.[722] Saiman et al. evaluated the ability of the MicroScan Autoscan to identify *P. aeruginosa* isolates recovered from patients with cystic fibrosis.[656] Using Negative Combo type 15 panels read after 20 to 24 hours and again at 48 hours of incubation they were able to correctly identify 57% (108 or 189) of nonmucoid strains and 40% (24 of 60) mucoid strains. The most common misidentification was *Pseudomonas fluorescens/putida*.[656]

In 1997, MicroScan updated the Rapid Gram-Negative Identification panels from the Type 2 panel to the Type 3 panel in order to improve identification accuracy and to remove the need for mineral oil overlay for the decarboxylase tests, and to increase the shelf-life from 1 year to 2 years. The identification database for the revised panel was updated to include 119 taxa. In a multicenter evaluation of the new type 3 panel 91.3% (63 of 69) NFBs were correctly identified to the species level.[48] In a study performed at the University of Illinois at Chicago, 92.2% (71 of 77) NFBs representing 10 species were correctly identified to the species level with the Rapid Gram Negative type 3 panels.[670]

The Sensiture AP80 System

The Sensitire AP80 Identification panels (TREK Diagnostic Systems, Cleveland, OH) can be inoculated and incubated offline and then read in the Sensitire Autoreader, or can be inoculated and placed in the ARIS (Automated Reading and Incubation System) Instrument described in Chapter 6. The AP80 panel permits the identification of gram-negative bacilli in as little as 5 hours, with the option of additional overnight incubation if needed or desired. Colonna and coworkers tested 142 NFBs using the Sensitire AP80 panels and reported 71.1% agreement with the API NFT.[147] Staneck and colleagues[711] tested 144 nonenteric isolates including 135 nonfermenters representing eight species. Ninety-three percent of the isolates tested consisted of just three species (68 *P. aeruginosa*, 33 *Acinetobacter*, 25 *S. maltophilia*). Correct identification was obtained for 99.2% of these three species and for 95.1% of all nonenterics tested. The small number of nonfermenter species tested in this study makes it difficult to evaluate the performance of this system for routine clinical laboratory testing of the nonfermenters.

The Phoenix System

The Phoenix Automated Microbiology System (Becton Dickinson Microbiology Systems) is a newly developed, fully automated, identification and antimicrobial susceptibility test system. Details of the system are presented in Chapter 6. To date, only a few studies have been published that evaluate the system for identification of NFBs. Stefaniuk et al. tested 54 NFBs (22 *P. aeruginosa*, 17 *Acinetobacter*, 15 *S. maltophilia*) and reported 96.3% (52 of 54) agreement with standard methods.[712] Donay and colleagues tested 56 NFBs representing 7 species and reported 89.3% correct identification with the Phoenix compared to a reference ID.[196]

Selection of a System

Clinical microbiologists must evaluate parameters such as accuracy, cost-effectiveness, and effects on work flow when deciding whether to use a commercially manufactured system for identifying nonfermenters. The commercial systems perform with levels of accuracy equal to or better than conventional methods in identifying *P. aeruginosa*, *Acinetobacter* species, and *S. maltophilia*; however, these metabolically active organisms can also be identified easily by using a few simple biochemical tests described earlier in this chapter. Many laboratories have adopted one of the commercial systems as a matter of convenience. However, because of the reported low sensitivity and specificity in the identification of many of the more fastidious and biochemically inactive nonfermenters, supplemental conventional differential media must still be kept on hand. Therefore, the definitive identification of most nonfermenters still requires considerable technical experience and access to a variety of fresh culture media kept under strict quality control. Because relatively few nonfermenters, particularly strains of species other than the three mentioned in the foregoing, are encountered in most medium-sized or small laboratories, the services of a reference laboratory should be seriously considered. Identifying nonfermenters is not difficult if the microbiologist is willing to devote the time and dedication necessary to achieve an acceptable level of accuracy. Packaged systems can be recommended, provided one understands their shortcomings and is willing to set up supplemental tests to identify weakly reactive or fastidious strains.

REFERENCES

1. Aaron SD, Ferris W, Henry DA, et al. Multiple combination bactericidal antibiotic testing for patients with cystic fibrosis infected with *Burkholderia cepacia*. Am J Respir Crit Care Med 2000;161:1206–1212.
2. Aber RC, Wennersten C, Moellering RC Jr. Antimicrobial susceptibility of flavobacteria. Antimicrob Agents Chemother 1978;14:483–487.
3. Agodi A, Mahenthiralingam E, Barchitta M, et al. *Burkholderia cepacia* complex infection in Italian patients with cystic fibrosis: prevalence, epidemiology, and genomovar status. J Clin Microbiol 2001;39:2891–2896.
4. Aisenberg G, Rolston KV, Safdar A. Bacteremia caused by *Achromobacter* and *Alcaligenes* species in 46 patients with cancer (1989–2003). Cancer 2004;101: 2134–2140.
5. Alcala L, Vasallo FJ, Cercenado E, et al. Catheter-related bacteremia due to *Roseomonas gilardii* sp. nov. J Clin Microbiol 1997;35:2712.
6. Alnor D, Frimodt-Moller, Espersen F, et al. Infections with the unusual human pathogens *Agrobacterium* species and *Ochrobactrum anthropi*. Clin Infect Dis 1994;18:914–920.
7. Alos JI, de Rafael L, Gonzalez-Palacios R, et al. Urinary tract infection probably caused by *Agrobacterium radiobacter*. Eur J Clin Microbiol 1985;4:596–597.
8. Amador C, Chiner E, Calpe JL, et al. Pneumonia due to *Bordetella bronchiseptica* in a patient with AIDS. Rev Infect Dis 1991;13:771–772.
9. Amber IJ, Reimer LG: *Pseudomonas* sp. group Ve-2 bacterial peritonitis in a patient on continuous ambulatory peritoneal dialysis. J Clin Microbiol 1987;25: 744–745.
10. Anaissie E, Fainstein V, Miller P, et al. *Pseudomonas putida*: newly recognized pathogen in patients with cancer. Am J Med 1987;82:1191–1194.
11. Andersen BM, Steigerwalt AG, O'Connor SP, et al. *Neisseria weaveri* sp. nov., formerly CDC group M-5, a gram-negative bacterium associated with dog bite wounds. J Clin Microbiol 1993;31:2456–2466.
12. Andersen BM, Weyant RS, Steigerwalt AG, et al. Characterization of *Neisseria elongata* subsp. *glycolytica* isolates obtained from human wound specimens and blood cultures. J Clin Microbiol 1995;33:76–78.
13. Anderson RR, Warnick P, Schreckenberger PC. Recurrent CDC Group IVc-2 bacteremia in a human with AIDS. J Clin Microbiol 1997;35:780–782.
14. Anzai Y, Kudo Y, Oyaizu H. The phylogeny of the genera *Chryseomonas*, *Flavimonas*, and *Pseudomonas* supports synonymy of these three genera. Int J Syst Bacteriol 1997;47:249–251.
15. Apisarnthanarak A, Dunagan WC, Dunne WM.: *Neisseria elongata* subsp. *elongata*, as a cause of human endocarditis. Diagn Microbiol Infect Dis 2001;39: 265–266.
16. Apisarnthanarak A, Mayfield JL, Garison T, et al. Risk factors for *Stenotrophomonas maltophilia* bacteremia in oncology patients: a case-control study. Infect Control Hosp Epidemiol 2003;24:269–274.
17. Appelbaum PC, Bowen AJ. Opportunistic infection of chronic skin ulcers with *Pseudomonas putrefaciens*. Br J Dermatol 1978;98:229–231.
18. Appelbaum PC, Campbell DB. Pancreatic abscess associated with *Achromobacter* group Vd biovar 1. J Clin Microbiol 1980;12:282–283.
19. Appelbaum PC, Leathers DJ. Evaluation of the rapid NFT system for identification of gram-negative, nonfermenting rods. J Clin Microbiol 1984;20:730–734.
20. Appelbaum PC, Stavitz J, Bentz MS, et al. Four methods for identification of gram-negative nonfermenting rods: organisms more commonly encountered in clinical specimens. J Clin Microbiol 1980;12:271–278.
21. Aragone MDR, Maurizi DM, Clara LO, et al. *Pseudomonas mendocina*, an environmental bacterium isolated from a patient with human infective endocarditis. J Clin Microbiol 1992;30:1583–1584.
22. Arance A, Montes A, Cisnal M, et al. CDC group IV c-2 infection in a stem cell transplant recipient. Bone Marrow Transplant 1997;20:1005–1006.
23. Arda B, Aydemir S, Yamazhan T, et al. *Comamonas testosteroni* meningitis in a patient with recurrent cholesteatoma. APMIS 2003;111:474–476.
24. Arduino S, Villar H, Veron MT, et al. CDC group IV c-2 as a cause of catheter-related sepsis in an immunocompromised patient. Clin Infect Dis 1993;17: 512–513.
25. Areekul S, Vongsthongsri U, Mookto T, et al. *Sphingobacterium multivorum* septicemia: a case report. J Med Assoc Thai 1996;79:395–398.
26. Aris RM, Routh JC, LiPuma JJ, et al. Lung transplantation for patients with cystic fibrosis with *Burkholderia cepacia* complex. Am J Respir Crit Care Med 2001;164: 2102–2106.
27. Arvand M, Feldhues R, Mieth M, et al. Chronic cholangitis caused by *Bordetella hinzii* in a liver transplant recipient. J Clin Microbiol 2004;42:2335–2337.
28. Ashdown LR. An improved screening technique for isolation of *Pseudomonas pseudomallei* from clinical specimens. Pathology 1979;11:293–297.
29. Ashdown LR. Melioidosis and safety in the clinical laboratory. J Hosp Infect 1992;21:301–306.
30. Ashdown LR, Currie BJ. Melioidosis: when in doubt leave the quinolone alone! Med J Aust 1992;157:427–428.
31. Ashdown LR, Johnson RW, Koehler JM, et al. Enzyme-linked immunosorbent assay for the diagnosis of clinical and subclinical melioidosis. J Infect Dis 1989; 160:253–260.
32. Ashdown LR, Previtera S. Community acquired *Flavobacterium meningosepticum* and septicaemia. Med J Aust 1992;156:69–70.
33. Aspinall ST, Graham R. Two sources of contamination of a hydrotherapy pool by environmental organisms. J Hosp Infect 1989;14:285–292.
34. Assih EA, Ouattara AS, Thierry S, et al. *Stenotrophomonas acidaminiphila* sp. nov., a strictly aerobic bacterium isolated from an upflow anaerobic sludge blanket (UASB) reactor. Int J Syst Evol Microbiol 2002;52:559–568.
35. Atkinson BE, Smith DL, Lockwood WR. *Pseudomonas testosteroni* septicemia. Ann Intern Med 1975;83:369–370.
36. Bachman KH, Sewell DL, Strausbaugh LJ. Recurrent cellulitis and bacteremia caused by *Flavobacterium odoratum*. Clin Infect Dis 1996;22:1112–1113.
37. Bailie WE, Stowe EC, Schmitt AM. Aerobic bacterial flora of oral and nasal fluids of canines with reference to bacteria associated with bites. J Clin Microbiol 1978;7:223–231.
38. Baldani JI, Pot B, Kirchhof G, et al. Emended description of *Herbaspirillum*; inclusion of [*Pseudomonas*] *rubrisubalbicans*, a milk plant pathogen, as *Herbaspirillum rubrisubalbicans* comb. nov.; and classification of a group of clinical isolates (EF group 1) as *Herbaspirillum* species 3. Int J Syst Bacteriol 1996;46: 802–810.
39. Balkwill DL, Drake GR, Reeves RH, et al. Taxonomic study of aromatic-degrading bacteria from deep-terrestrial-subsurface sediments and description of *Sphingomonas aromaticivorans* sp. nov., *Sphingomonas subterranea* sp. nov., and *Sphingomonas stygia* sp. nov. Int J Syst Bacteriol 1997;47:191–201.
40. Ballestero S. Virseda I, Escobar H, et al. *Stenotrophomonas maltophilia* in patients with cystic fibrosis. Eur J Clin Microbiol Infect Dis 1995;14:728–729.
40a. Balows A, Hausler Jr. WJ, Herrmann KL, Isenberg HD, Shadomy HJ. eds. Manual of Clinical Microbiology. Ed. 5. Washington DC: American Society for Microbiology, 1991.
41. Barbaro DJ, Mackowiak PA, Barth SS, et al. *Pseudomonas testosteroni* infections: eighteen recent cases and a review of the literature. Rev Infect Dis 1987; 9:124–129.
42. Barham WB, Church P, Brown JE, et al. Misidentification of *Brucella* species with use of rapid bacterial identification systems. Clin Infect Dis 1993;17: 1068–1069.
43. Barker PM, Wood RE, Gilligan PH. Lung infection with *Burkholderia gladioli* in a child with cystic fibrosis: acute clinical and spirometric deterioration. Pediatr Pulmonol 1997;23:123–125.
44. Barnham M, Holmes B. Isolation of CDC group M-5 and *Staphylococcus intermedius* from infected dog bites. J Infect 1992;25:332–334.
45. Barnishan J, Ayers LW. Rapid identification of nonfermentative gram-negative rods by the Corning N/F system. J Clin Microbiol 1979;9:239–243.

46. Barson WJ, Cromer BA, Marcon MJ. Puncture wound osteochondritis of the foot caused by CDC group Vd. J Clin Microbiol 1987;25:2014–2016.

47. Barwick RS, Levy DA, Craun GF, et al. Surveillance for waterborne-disease outbreaks—United States, 1997–1998. MMWR CDC Surveill Summ 2000;49:1–21.

48. Bascomb S, Abbott SL, Bobolis JD, et al. Multicenter evaluation of the MicroScan rapid gram-negative identification type 3 panel. J Clin Microbiol 1997;35:2531–2536.

49. Basset DCJ, Dickson JAS, Hunt GH. Infection of Holter valve by Pseudomonas-contaminated chlorhexidine. Lancet 1973;1:1263–1264.

50. Batchelor BI, Brindle RJ, Gilks GF. Biochemical mis-identification of Brucella melitensis and subsequent laboratory-acquired infections. J Hosp Infect 1992;22:159–162.

51. Bauernfeind A, Schneider I, Jungwirth R, et al. Discrimination of Burkholderia gladioli from other Burkholderia species detectable in patients with cystic fibrosis by PCR. J Clin Microbiol 1998;36:2748–2751.

52. Baumann L, Baumann P, Mandel M, et al. Taxonomy of aerobic marine eubacteria. J Bacteriol 1972;110:402–429.

53. Baumann L, Bowditch RD, Baumann P. Description of Deleya gen. nov. created to accommodate the marine species Alcaligenes aestus, A. pacificus, A. cupidus, A. venustus, and Pseudomonas marina. Int J Syst Bacteriol 1983;33:793–802.

54. Bauwens JE, Spach DH, Schacker TW, et al. Bordetella bronchiseptica pneumonia and bacteremia following bone marrow transplantation. J Clin Microbiol 1992;30:2474–2475.

55. Beck-Sague CM, Jarvis WR, Brook JH, et al. Epidemic bacteremia due to Acinetobacter baumannii in five intensive care units. Am J Epidemiol 1990;132:723–733.

56. Ben Dekhil SM, Peel MM, Lennox VA, et al. Isolation of Lautropia mirabilis from sputa of a cystic fibrosis patient. J Clin Microbiol 1997;35:1024–1026.

57. Bendig JWA, Mayes PJ, Eyers DE, et al. Flavimonas oryzihabitans (Pseudomonas oryzihabitans; CDC Group Ve-2): an emerging pathogen in peritonitis related to continuous ambulatory peritoneal dialysis? J Clin Microbiol 1989;27:217–218.

58. Bennasar A, Rosselló-Mora R, Lalucat J, et al. 16S rRNA gene sequence analysis relative to genomovars of Pseudomonas stutzeri and proposal of Pseudomonas balearica sp. nov. Int J Syst Bacteriol 1996;46:200–205.

59. Berger SA, Siegman–Igra Y, Stadler J, et al. Group VE-1 septicemia. J Clin Microbiol 1983;17:926–927.

60. Bergogne-Berezin E, Towner KJ. Acinetobacter spp. as nosocomial pathogens: microbiological, clinical, and epidemiological features. Clin Microbiol Rev 1996;9:148-165.

61. Berkelman RL, Lewin S, Allen JR, et al. Pseudobacteremia attributed to contamination of povidone-iodine with Pseudomonas cepacia. Ann Intern Med 1981;95:32–36.

62. Bernardet J-F, Segers P, Vancanneyt M, et al. Cutting a Gordian knot: emended classification and description of the genus Flavobacterium, emended description of the family Flavobacteriaceae, and proposal of Flavobacterium hydatis, nom. nov. (basonym, Cytophaga aquatilis Strohl and Tait 1978). Int J Syst Bacteriol 1996;46:128–148.

63. Bernards AT, de Beaufort AJ, Dijkshoorn L, et al. Outbreak of septicaemia in neonates caused by Acinetobacter junii investigated by amplified ribosomal DNA restriction analysis (ARDRA) and four typing methods. J Hosp Infect 1997;35:129–140.

64. Bibashi E, Sofianou D, Kontopoulou K, et al. Peritonitis due to Roseomonas fauriae in a patient undergoing continuous ambulatory peritoneal dialysis. J Clin Microbiol 2000;38:456–457.

65. Bizet C, Bizet J. [Comparative susceptibility of Ochrobactrum anthropi, Agrobacterium tumefaciens, Alcaligenes faecalis, Alcaligenes denitrificans subsp. denitrificans, Alcaligenes denitrificans subsp. xylosidans and Bordetella bronchiseptica against 35 antibiotics including 17 beta-lactams.] Pathol Biol (Paris) 1995;43:258–263.

66. Bizet J, Bizet C. Strains of Alcaligenes faecalis from clinical material. J Infect 1997;35:167–169.

67. Block KC, Nadarajah R, Jacobs R. Chryseobacterium meningosepticum: an emerging pathogen among immunocompromised adults. Medicine (Baltimore) 1997;76:30–41.

68. Blumberg DA, Cherry JD. Agrobacterium radiobacter and CDC group Ve-2 bacteremia. Diagn Microbiol Infect Dis 1989;12:351–355.

69. Bodey GP, Bolivar R, Fainstein V, et al. Infections caused by Pseudomonas aeruginosa. Rev Infect Dis 1983;5:279–313.

70. Boixeda D, de Luis DA, Meseguer MA, et al. A case of spontaneous peritonitis caused by Weeksella virosa. Eur J Gastroenterol Hepatol 1998;10:897–898.

71. Bonacorsi S, Fitoussi F, Lhopital S, et al. Comparative in vitro activities of meropenem, imipenem, temocillin, piperacillin, and ceftazidime in combination with tobramycin, rifampin, or ciprofloxacin against Burkholderia cepacia isolates from patients with cystic fibrosis. Antimicrob Agents Chemother 1999;43:213–217.

72. Borghans JGA, Hosli MTC, Olsen H, et al. Pseudomonas cepacia bacteraemia

73. due to intrinsic contamination of an anaesthetic. Acta Path Microbiol Scand Sect B 1979;87:15–20.

73. Bottone EJ, Douglas SD, Rausen AR, et al. Association of Pseudomonas cepacia with chronic granulomatous disease. J Clin Microbiol 1975;1:425–428.

74. Bou G, Cervero G, Dominguez MA, et al. PCR-based DNA fingerprinting (REP-PCR, AP-PCR) and pulsed-field gel electrophoresis characterization of a nosocomial outbreak caused by imipenem- and meropenem-resistant Acinetobacter baumannii. Clin Microbiol Infect 2000;6:635–643.

75. Boutros N, Gonullu N, Casetta A, et al. Ralstonia pickettii traced in blood culture bottles. J Clin Microbiol 2002;40:2666–2667.

76. Bouvet PJM, Grimont PAD. Taxonomy of the genus Acinetobacter with the recognition of Acinetobacter baumannii sp. nov., Acinetobacter haemolyticus sp. nov., Acinetobacter johnsonii sp. nov., and Acinetobacter junii sp. nov. and emended descriptions of Acinetobacter calcoaceticus and Acinetobacter lwoffi. Int J Syst Bacteriol 1986;36:228–240.

77. Bouvet PJM, Grimont PAD. Identification and biotyping of clinical isolates of Acinetobacter. Ann Inst Pasteur Microbiol 1987;138:569–578.

78. Bouvet PJM, Jeanjean S. Delineation of new proteolytic genomic species of the genus Acinetobacter. Res Microbiol 1989;140:291–299.

79. Bouvet PJM, Jeanjean S, Vieu J–F, et al. Species, biotype, and bacteriophage type determinations compared with cell envelope protein profiles for typing Acinetobacter strains. J Clin Microbiol 1990;28:170–176.

80. Bovre K. Genus II. Moraxella Lwoff 1939, 173 emend. Henriksen and Bovre 1968, 391^{AL}. In: Krieg NR, Holt JG, eds. Bergey's Manual of Systematic Bacteriology. Vol. 1. Baltimore: Williams & Wilkins, 1984:296–303.

81. Bovre K, Fuglesang JE, Hagen N, et al. Moraxella atlantae sp. nov. and its distinction from Moraxella phenylpyrouvica. Int J Syst Bacteriol 1976;26:511–521.

82. Bowman JP, Cavanagh J, Austin JJ, et al. Novel Psychrobacter species from Antarctic ornithogenic soils. Int J Syst Bacteriol 1996;46:841–848.

83. Bracis R, Seibers K, Julien RM. Meningitis caused by Group IIj following a dog bite. West J Med 1979;131:438–440.

84. Brink AJ, Van Straten A, Van Rensburg AJ. Shewanella (Pseudomonas) putrefaciens bacteremia. Clin Infect Dis 1995;20:1327–1332.

85. Brisse S, Stefani S, Verhoef J, et al. Comparative evaluation of the BD Phoenix and VITEK 2 automated instruments for identification of isolates of the Burkholderia cepacia complex. J Clin Microbiol 2002;40:1743–1748.

86. Brivet F, Guibert M, Kiredjian M, et al. Necrotizing fasciitis, bacteremia, and multiorgan failure caused by Ochrobactrum anthropi. Clin Infect Dis 1993;17:516–518.

87. Brown MA, Greene JN, Sandin RL, et al. Methylobacterium bacteremia after infusion of contaminated autologous bone marrow. Clin Infect Dis 1996;23:1191–1192.

88. Buchman AL, Pickett MJ. Moraxella atlantae bacteraemia in a patient with systemic lupus erythematosus. J Infect 1991;23:197–199.

89. Buchman AL, Pickett MJ, Mann L, et al. Central venous catheter infection caused by Moraxella osloensis in a receiving patient home parenteral nutrition. Diagn Microbiol Infect Dis 1993;17:163–166.

90. Burdash NM, Bannister ER, Manos JP, et al. A comparison of four commercial systems for the identification of nonfermenting gram-negative bacilli. Am J Clin Pathol 1980;73:564–569.

91. Burns JL, Emerson J, Stapp JR, et al. Microbiology of sputum from patients at cystic fibrosis centers in the United States. Clin Infect Dis 1998;27:158–163.

92. Butt AA, Figueroa J, Martin DA. Ocular infection caused by three unusual marine organisms. Clin Infect Dis 1997;24:740.

93. Buxton AE, Anderson RL, Werdegar D, et al. Nosocomial respiratory tract infection and colonization with Acinetobacter calcoaceticus. Am J Med 1978;65:507–513.

94. Cain JR. A case of septicaemia caused by Agrobacterium radiobacter. J Infect 1988;16:205–206.

95. Calegari L, Gezuele E, Torres E, et al. Botryomycosis caused by Pseudomonas vesicularis. Int J Dermatol 1996;35:817–818.

96. Calubiran OV, Schoch PE, Cunha BA. Pseudomonas paucimobilis bacteraemia associated with haemodialysis. J Hosp Infect 1990;15:383–388.

97. Campos-Herrero MI, Bordes A, Rodriguez H, et al. Pseudomonas stutzeri community-acquired pneumonia associated with empyema: case report and review. Clin Infect Dis 1997;25:325–326.

98. Capitini CM, Herrero IA, Patel R, et al. Wound infection with Neisseria weaveri and a novel subspecies of Pasteurella multocida in a child who sustained a tiger bite. Clin Infect Dis 2002;34:E74–E76.

99. Carlson P, Kontiainen S, Anttila P, et al. Septicemia caused by Neisseria weaveri. Clin Infect Dis 1997;24:739.

100. Carratala J, Salazar A, Mascaro J, et al. Community-acquired pneumonia due to Pseudomonas stutzeri. Clin Infect Dis 1992;14:792.

101. Casadevall A, Freundlich LF, Pirofski L. Septic shock caused by Pseudomonas paucimobilis. Clin Infect Dis 1992;14:784.

102. Casalta JP, Peloux Y, Raoult D, et al. Pneumonia and meningitis caused by a

new nonfermentative unknown gram-negative bacterium. J Clin Microbiol 1989; 27:1446–1448.

103. Castagnola E, Conte M. Venzano P, et al. Broviac catheter-related bacteraemias due to unusual pathogens in children with cancer: case reports with literature review. J Infect 1997;34:215–218.

104. Castagnola E, Tasso L, Conte M, et al. Central venous catheter-related infection due to *Comamonas acidovorans* in a child with non-Hodgkin's lymphoma. Clin Infect Dis 1994;19:559–560.

105. Catchpole CR, Andrews JM, Brenwald N, et al. A reassessment of the in-vitro activity of colistin sulphomethate sodium. J Antimicrob Chemother 1997;39: 255–260.

106. Catlin BW. Cellular elongation under the influence of antibacterial agents: way to differentiate coccobacilli from cocci. J Clin Microbiol 1975;1:102–105.

107. Centers for Disease Control and Prevention. *Pseudomonas pickettii* colonization associated with a contaminated respiratory therapy solution—Illinois. Morb Mortal Wkly Rep 1983;38:495.

108. Centers for Disease Control and Prevention. *Pseudomonas cepacia* at summer camps for persons with cystic fibrosis. Morb Mortal Wkly Rep 1993;42: 456–459.

109. Centers for Disease Control and Prevention. Nosocomial *Burkholderia cepacia* infection and colonization associated with intrinsically contaminated mouthwash—Arizona, 1998. Morb Mortal Wkly Rep 1999;47:926–928.

110. Centers for Disease Control and Prevention. Laboratory-acquired human glanders—Maryland, May 2000. Morb Mortal Wkly Rep 2000;49:532–535.

111. Chagla AH, Haque KN. Peritonitis due to *Moraxella phenylpyruvica*. Clin Microbiol Newslett 1988;10:103.

112. Chalandon Y, Roscoe DL, Nantel SH. *Agrobacterium* yellow group: bacteremia and possible septic arthritis following peripheral blood stem cell transplantation. Bone Marrow Transplant 2000;26:101–104.

113. Chang HJ, Christenson JC, Pavia AT, et al. *Ochrobactrum anthropi* meningitis in pediatric pericardial allograft transplant recipients. Clin Infect Dis 1996;173: 656–660.

114. Chang J-C, Hsueh P-R, Wu J-J, et al. Antimicrobial susceptibility of flavobacteria as determined by agar dilution and disk diffusion methods. Antimicrob. Agents Chemother 1997;41:1301–1306.

115. Chaowagul W, Suputtamongkul Y, Smith MD, et al. Oral fluoroquinolones for maintenance treatment of melioidosis. Trans R Soc Trop Med Hyg 1997;91: 599–601.

116. Chaudhry HJ, Schoch PE, Cunha BA. *Flavimonas oryzihabitans* (CDC Group Ve-2). Infect Control Hosp Epidemiol 1992;13:485–488.

117. Chauncey JB, Schaberg DR. Interstitial pneumonia caused by *Bordetella bronchiseptica* in a heart transplant patient. Transplantation 1990;49:817–819.

118. Chen W-M, Laevens S, Lee T-M, et al. *Ralstonia taiwanensis* sp. nov., isolated from root nodules of *Mimosa* species and sputum of a cystic fibrosis patient. Int J Syst Evol Microbiol 2001;51:1729–1735.

119. Chen Y-S, Liu Y-C, Yen M-Y, et al. Skin and soft-tissue manifestations of *Shewanella putrefaciens* infection. Clin Infect Dis 1997;25:225–229.

120. Chetchotisakd P, Porramatikul S, Mootsikapun P, et al. Randomized, double-blind, controlled study of cefoperazone-sulbactam plus cotrimoxazole versus ceftazidime plus cotrimoxazole for the treatment of severe melioidosis. Clin Infect Dis 2001;33:29–34.

121. Chetoui H, Melin P, Struelens MJ, et al. Comparison of biotyping, ribotyping, and pulsed-field gel electrophoresis for investigation of common-source outbreak of *Burkholderia pickettii* bacteremia. J Clin Microbiol 1997;35: 1398–1403.

122. Chi C-Y, Fung C-P, Wong W-W, et al. *Brevundimonas bacteremia*: two case reports and literature review. Scand J Infect Dis 2004;36:59–77.

123. Chihab W, Alaoui AS, Amar M. *Chryseomonas luteola* identified as the source of serious infections in a Moroccan University Hospital. J Clin Microbiol 2004; 42:1837–1839.

124. Chiu C-H, Waddingdon M, Hsieh W-S, et al. Atypical *Chryseobacterium meningosepticum* and meningitis and sepsis in newborns and the immunocompromised, Taiwan. Emerg Infect Dis 2000;6:481–486.

125. Chow AW, Wong J, Bartlett KH. Synergistic interactions of ciprofloxacin and extended-spectrum beta-lactams or aminoglycosides against multiply drug-resistant *Pseudomonas maltophilia*. Antimicrob Agents Chemother 1988;32:782–784.

126. Chow KW, Wulffraat NM, Wolfs TFW, et al. *Bordetella bronchiseptica* respiratory infection in a child after bone marrow transplantation. Pediatr Infect Dis 1999;J 18:481–482.

127. Christenson JC, Welch DF, Mukwaya G, et al. Recovery of *Pseudomonas gladioli* from respiratory tract specimens of patients with cystic fibrosis. J Clin Microbiol 1989;27:270–273.

128. Cieslak TJ, Robb ML, Drabick CJ, et al. Catheter-associated sepsis caused by *Ochrobactrum anthropi*: report of a case and review of related nonfermentative bacteria. Clin Infect Dis 1992;14:902–907.

129. Cladera AM, Bennasar A, Barcelo M, et al. Comparative genetic diversity of

Pseudomonas stutzeri genomovars, clonal structure, and phylogeny of the species. J Bacteriol 2004;186:5239–5248.

130. Clark WA. A simplified Leifson flagella stain. J Clin Microbiol 1976;3:632–634.

131. Clayton AJ, Lisella RS, Martin DG. Melioidosis: a serologic survey in military personnel. Milit Med 1973;138:24–26.

132. Clode FE, Metherell LA, Pitt TL. Nosocomial acquisition of *Burkholderia gladioli* in patients with cystic fibrosis. Am J Respir Crit Care Med 1999;160: 374–375.

133. Coenye T, Falsen E, Hoste B, et al. Description of *Pandoraea* gen. nov. with *Pandoraea apista* sp. nov., *Pandoraea pulmonicola* sp. nov., *Pandoraea pnomenusa* sp. nov., *Pandoraea sputorum* sp. nov. and *Pandoraea norimbergensis* comb. nov. Int J Syst Evol Microbiol 2000;50:887–899.

134. Coenye T, Falsen E, Vancanneyt M, et al. Classification of *Alcaligenes faecalis*-like isolates from the environment and human clinical samples as *Ralstonia gilardii* sp. nov. Int J Syst Bacteriol 1999;49:405–413.

135. Coenye T, Goris J, De Vos P, et al. Classification of *Ralstonia pickettii*-like isolates from the environment and clinical samples as *Ralstonia insidiosa* sp. nov. Int J Syst Evol Microbiol 2003;53:1075–1080.

136. Coenye T, Goris J, Spilker T, et al. Characterization of unusual bacteria isolated from respiratory secretions of patients with cystic fibrosis and description of *Inquilinus limosus* gen. nov., sp. nov. J Clin Microbiol 2002;40:2062–2069.

137. Coenye T, LiPuma JJ, Henry D, et al. *Burkholderia cepacia* genomovar VI, a new member of the Burkholderia cepacia complex isolated from patients with cystic fibrosis. Int J Syst Evol Microbiol 2001;51:271–279.

138. Coenye T, Liu L, Vandamme P, et al. Identification of *Pandoraea* species by 16S ribosomal DNA-based PCR assays. J Clin Microbiol 2001;39:4452–4455.

139. Coenye T, Mahenthiralingam E, Henry D, et al. *Burkholderia ambifaria* sp. nov., a novel member of the *Burkholderia cepacia* complex including biocontrol and cystic fibrosis-related isolates. Int J Syst Evol Microbiol 2001;51: 1481–1490.

140. Coenye T, Vancanneyt M, Cnockaert MC, et al. *Kerstersia gyiorum* gen. nov., sp. nov., a novel *Alcaligenes faecalis*-like organism isolated from human clinical samples, and reclassification of *Alcaligenes denitrificans* Rüger and Tan 1983 as *Achromobacter denitrificans* comb. nov. Int J Syst Evol Microbiol 2003;53: 1825–1831.

141. Coenye T, Vancanneyt M, Falsen E, et al. *Achromobacter insolitus* sp. nov. and *Achromobacter spanius* sp. nov., from human clinical samples. Int J Syst Evol Microbiol 2003;53:1819–1824.

142. Coenye T, Vandamme P, Govan JRW, et al. Taxonomy and identification of the *Burkholderia cepacia* complex. J Clin Microbiol 2001;39:3427–3436.

143. Coenye T, Vandamme P, LiPuma JJ. Infection by *Ralstonia* species in patients with cystic fibrosis: identification of *R. pickettii*, and *R. mannitolilytica* by polymerase chain reaction. Emerg Infect Dis 2002;8:692–696.

144. Coenye T, Vandamme P, LiPuma JJ. *Raltonia respiraculi* sp. nov., isolated from the respiratory tract of patients with cystic fibrosis. Int J Syst Evol Microbiol 2003;53:1339–1342.

145. Coenye T, Vanlaere E, Falsen E, et al. *Stenotrophomonas africana* (Drancourt et al. 1997) is a later synonym of *Stenotrophomonas maltophilia* (Hugh 1981) Palleroni and Bradbury 1993. Int J Syst Evol Microbiol 2004;54:1235–1237.

146. Coenye T, Vanlaere E, LiPuma JJ, et al. Identification of genomic groups in the genus *Stenotrophomonas* using gyrB RFLP analysis. FEMS Immunol Med Microbiol 40:181–185, 2004.

147. Colonna P, Nikolai D, Bruckner D: Comparison of MicroScan autoSCAN-W/A, Radiometer Sensititre and Vitek systems for rapid identification of gram-negative bacilli. Abstracts of the 90th Annual Meeting of the American Society for Microbiology. Washington DC: American Society for Microbiology, 1990: 370.

148. Connor BJ, Kopecky RT, Frymoyer PA, et al. Recurrent *Pseudomonas luteola* (CDC Group Ve-1) peritonitis in a patient undergoing continuous ambulatory peritoneal dialysis. J Clin Microbiol 1987;25:1113–1114.

149. Cookson BT, Vandamme P, Carlson LC, et al. Bacteremia caused by a novel *Bordetella* species, "*B. hinzii*." J Clin Microbiol 1994;32:2569–2571.

150. Coyle-Gilchrist MM, Crewe P, Roberts G. *Flavobacterium meningosepticum* in the hospital environment. J Clin Pathol 1976;29:824–826.

151. Craven DE, Moody B, Connolly MG, et al. Pseudobacteremia caused by povidone-iodine solution contaminated with *Pseudomonas cepacia*. N Engl J Med 1981;305:621–623.

152. Crowe HM, Brecher SM. Nosocomial septicemia with CDC group IVc-2, an unusual gram-negative bacillus. J Clin Microbiol 1987;25:2225–2226.

153. Currie BJ, Fisher DA, Howard DM, et al. Endemic melioidosis in tropical northern Australia: a 10-year prospective study and review of the literature. Clin Infect Dis 2000;31:981–986.

154. Dalamaga M, Karmaniolas K, Chavelas C, et al. *Pseudomonas luteola* cutaneous abscess and bacteraemia in a previously healthy man. Scand J Infect Dis 2004; 36:495–497.

155. Daley D, Neville S, Kociuba K. Peritonitis associated with a CDC group EO-3 organism. J Clin Microbiol 1997;35:3338–3339.

156. Dan M, Berger SA, Aderka D, et al. Septicemia caused by the gram-negative

bacterium CDC IVc-2 in an immunocompromised human. J Clin Microbiol 1986;23:803.

157. Dan M, Gutman R, Biro A. Peritonitis caused by *Pseudomonas putrefaciens* in patients undergoing continuous ambulatory peritoneal dialysis. Clin Infect Dis 1992;14:359–360.

158. Dance DA. Melioidosis. Curr Opin Infect Dis 2002;15:127–132.

159. Dance DAB. Melioidosis. Rev Med Microbiol 1990;1:143–150.

160. Dance DAB. Melioidosis: The tip of the iceberg. Clin Microbiol Rev 1991;4: 52–60.

161. Dance DA, Wuthiekanun V, Chaowagul W, et al. The antimicrobial susceptibility of *Pseudomonas pseudomallei*: emergence of resistance in vitro and during treatment. J Antimicrob Chemother 1989;24:295–309.

162. Dance DA, Wuthiekanun V, Naigowit P, et al. Identification of *Pseudomonas pseudomallei* in clinical practice: use of simple screening tests and API 20NE. J Clin Pathol 1989;42:645–648.

163. Daneshvar MI, Douglas MP, Weyant RS. Cellular fatty acid composition of *Lautropia mirabilis*. J Clin Microbiol 2001;39:4160–4162.

164. Daneshvar MI, Hill B, Hollis DG, et al. CDC group O-3: phenotypic characteristics, fatty acid composition, isoprenoid quinone content, and in vitro antimicrobic susceptibilities of an unusual gram-negative bacterium isolated from clinical specimens. J Clin Microbiol 1998;36:1674–1678.

165. Daneshvar MI, Hollis DG, Moss CW, et al. Eugonic oxidizer group 5: an unusual gram-negative nonfermenter isolated from clinical specimens. Abstracts of the 98th General Meeting of the American Society for Microbiology. Washington DC: American Society for Microbiology, 1998:165.

166. Daneshvar MI, Hollis DG, Steigerwalt AG, et al. Assignment of CDC weak oxidizer group 2 (WO-2) to the genus *Pandoraea* and characterization of three new *Pandoraea* genomospecies. J Clin Microbiol 2001;39:1819–1826.

167. Daneshvar MI, Hollis DG, Weyant RS, et al. *Paracoccus yeeii* sp. nov. (formerly CDC group EO-2), a novel bacterial species associated with human infection. J Clin Microbiol 2003;41:1289–1294.

168. Daniel C-T, Chang S-C, Chen Y-C, et al. In vitro activities of antimicrobial agents, alone and in combinations, against *Burkholderia cepacia* isolated from blood. Diagn Microbiol Infect Dis 1997;28:187–191.

169. Das K, Shah S, Levi MH. Misleading Gram stain from a patient with *Moraxella (Branhamella) catarrhalis* bacteremia. Clin Microbiol Newslett 1997;19:85–88.

170. Dauga C, Gillis M, Vandamme P, et al. *Balneatrix alpica* gen. nov., sp. nov., a bacterium associated with pneumonia and meningitis in a spa therapy centre. Res Microbiol 1993;144:35–46.

171. Davis JM, Whipp MJ, Ashhurst-Smith C, et al. Mucoid nitrate-negative *Moraxella nonliquefaciens* from three patients with chronic lung disease. J Clin Microbiol 2004;42:3888–3890.

172. Daxboeck F, Goerzer E, Apfalter P, et al. Isolation of *Bordetella trematum* from a diabetic leg ulcer. Diabet Med 2004;21:1247–1248.

173. De I, Rolston KVI, Han XY: Clinical significance of *Roseomonas* species isolated from catheter and blood samples: analysis of 36 cases in patients with cancer. Clin Infect Dis 2004;38:1579–1584.

174. De Baere T, Muylaert A, Everaert E, et al. Bacteremia due to *Moraxella atlantae* in a cancer patient. J Clin Microbiol 2002;40:2693–2695.

175. De Baere T, Steyaert S, Wauters G, et al. Classification of *Ralstonia pickettii* biovar 3/''thomasii'' strains (Pickett 1994) and of new isolates related to nosocomial recurrent meningitis as *Ralstonia mannitolytica* sp. nov. Int J Syst Evol Microbiol 2001;51:547–558.

176. Debois J, Degreef H, Vandepitte J, et al. *Pseudomonas putrefaciens* as a cause of infection in humans. J Clin Pathol 1975;28:993–996.

177. Decker CF, Hawkins RE, Simon GL. Infections with *Pseudomonas paucimobilis*. Clin Infect Dis 1992;14:783–784.

178. Decker GR, Lavelle JP, Kumar PN, et al. Pneumonia due to *Bordetella bronchiseptica* in a patient with AIDS. Rev Infect Dis 1991;13:1250–1251.

179. Dees SB, Hollis DG, Weaver RE, et al. Cellular fatty acid composition of *Pseudomonas marginata* and closely associated bacteria. J Clin Microbiol 1983;18: 1073–1078.

179a. Dees SB, Moss CW, Hollis DG, Weaver RE. Chemical characterization of *Flavobacterium odoratum*, *Flavobacterium breve*, and Flavobacterium-like groups IIe, IIh, and IIf. J Clin Microbiol 1986;23:267–273.

180. Degreef H, Debois J, Vandepitte J. *Pseudomonas putrefaciens* as a cause of infection of venous ulcers. Dermatologica 1975;151:296–301.

181. de la Fuente J, Albo C, Rodriguez A, et al. *Bordetella bronchiseptica* pneumonia in a patient with AIDS. Thorax 1994;49:719–20.

182. De Ley J, Segers P, Kersters K, et al. Intra- and intergeneric similarities of the *Bordetella* ribosomal ribonucleic acid cistrons: proposal for a new family, *Alcaligenaceae*. Int J Syst Bacteriol 1986;36:405–414.

183. Del Mar Ojeda-Vargas M, Suarez-Alonso A, de Los Angeles Perez-Cervantes M, et al. Urinary tract infection associated with *Comamonas acidovorans*. Clin Microbiol Infect 1999;5:443–444.

184. Denton M, Hall MJ, Todd NJ, et al. Improved isolation of *Stenotrophomonas maltophilia* from the sputa of patients with cystic fibrosis using a selective medium. Clin Microbiol Infect 2000;6:397–398.

185. Denton M, Kerr KG. Microbiological and clinical aspects of infection associated with *Stenotrophomonas maltophilia*. Clin Microbiol Rev 1998;11:57–80.

186. Desakorn V, Smith MD, Wuthiekanun V, et al. Detection of *Pseudomonas pseudomallei* antigen in urine for the diagnosis of melioidosis. Am J Trop Med Hyg 1994;51:627–633.

187. De Soyza A, McDowell A, Archer L, et al. *Burkholderia cepacia* complex genomovars and pulmonary transplantation outcomes in patients with cystic fibrosis. Lancet 2001;358:1780–1781.

188. De Soyza A, Morris K, McDowell A, et al. Prevalence and clonality of *Burkholderia cepacia* complex genomovars in UK patients with cystic fibrosis referred for lung transplantation. Thorax 2004;59:526–528.

189. Dhawan B, Chaudhry R, Mishra BM, et al. Isolation of *Shewanella putrefaciens* from a rheumatic heart disease patient with infective endocarditis. J Clin Microbiol 1998;36:2394.

190. Dhawan VK, Rajashekaraiah KR, Metzger WI, et al. Spontaneous bacterial peritonitis due to a group IIk-2 strain. J Clin Microbiol 1980;11:492–495.

191. Dobson SJ, Franzmann PD. Unification of the genera *Deleya* (Baumann et al. 1983), *Halomonas* (Vreeland et al. 1980), and Halovibrio (Fendrich 1988) and the species *Paracoccus halodenitrificans* (Robinson and Gibbons 1952) into a single genus, *Halomonas*, and placement of the genus *Zymobacter* in the family *Halomonadaceae*. Int J Syst Bacteriol 1996;46:550–558.

192. Doelle H. Bacterial Metabolism. Ed. 2. New York: Academic Press, 1975.

193. Doit C, Loukil C, Simon A-M, et al. Outbreak of *Burkholderia cepacia* bacteremia in a pediatric hospital due to contamination of lipid emulsion stoppers. J Clin Microbiol 2004;42:2227–2230.

194. Dominguez EA, Smith TL. Endocarditis due to *Neisseria elongata* subspecies *nitroreducens*: case report and review. Clin Infect Dis 1998;26:1471–1473.

195. Dominguez H, Vogel BF, Gram L, et al. *Shewanella alga* bacteremia in two patients with lower leg ulcers. Clin Infect Dis 1996;22:1036–1039.

196. Donay J-L, Mathieu D, Fernandes P, et al. Evaluation of the automated Phoenix system for potential routine use in the clinical microbiology laboratory. J Clin Microbiol 2004;42:1542–1546.

197. Dorittke C, Vandamme P, Hinz KH, et al. Isolation of a *Bordetella avium*-like organism from a human specimen. Eur J Clin Microbiol Infect Dis 1995;14: 451–454.

198. Dorman SE, Gill VJ, Gallin JI, et al. *Burkholderia pseudomallei* infection in a Puerto Rican patient with chronic granulomatous disease: case report and review of occurrences in the Americas. Clin Infect Dis 1998;26:889–894.

199. Dowda H. Evaluation of two rapid methods for identification of commonly encountered nonfermenting or oxidase-positive, gram-negative rods. J Clin Microbiol 1977;6:605–609.

199a. Drancourt M, Bollet C, Raoult D. *Stenotrophomonas africana* sp. nov., an opportunistic human pathogen in Africa. Int J Syst Bacteriol 1997;47:160–163.

200. Duggan JM, Goldstein SJ, Chenoweth CE, et al. *Achromobacter xylosoxidans* bacteremia: report of four cases and review of the literature. Clin Infect Dis 1996;23:569–576.

201. Dunne WM Jr, Maisch S. Epidemiological investigation of infections due to *Alcaligenes* species in children and patients with cystic fibrosis: use of repetitive-element-sequence polymerase chain reaction. Clin Infect Dis 1995;20:836–841.

202. Dunne WM Jr, Tillman J, Murray JC. Recovery of a strain of *Agrobacterium radiobacter* with a mucoid phenotype from an immunocompromised child with bacteremia. J Clin Microbiol 1993;31:2541–2543.

203. Dworkin MS, Sullivan PS, Buskin SE, et al. *Bordetella bronchiseptica* infection in human immunodeficiency virus-infected patients. Clin Infect Dis 1999;28: 1095–1099.

204. Ebrigh T JR, Lentino JR, Juni E. Endophthalmitis caused by *Moraxella nonliquefaciens*. Am J Clin Pathol 1982;77:362–363.

205. Edmond MB, Riddler SA, Baxter CM, et al. *Agrobacterium radiobacter*: a recently recognized opportunistic pathogen. Clin Infect Dis 1993;16:388–391.

206. Egbert JE, Feder JM, Rapoza PA, et al. Keratitis associated with *Pseudomonas mesophilica* in a patient taking topical corticosteroids. Am J Ophthalmol 1990; 116:445–446.

207. Ekelund B, Johnsen CR, Nielsen PB. Septicemia with *Agrobacterium* species from a permanent vena cephalica catheter: a case report. Acta Pathol Microbiol Immunol Scand Sect B 1987;95:323–324.

208. Elting LS, Bodey GP. Septicemia due to *Xanthomonas* species and non-*aeruginosa Pseudomonas* species: increasing incidence of catheter-related infections. Medicine (Baltimore) 1990;69:296–306.

209. Ender PT, Dooley DP, Moore RH. Vascular catheter-related *Comamonas acidovorans* bacteremia managed with preservation of the catheter. Pediatr Infect Dis J 1996;15:918–920.

210. Engel JM, Alexander FS, Pachucki CT. Bacteremia caused by CDC Group Ve-1 in previously healthy patient with granulomatous hepatitis. J Clin Microbiol 1987;25:2023–2024.

211. Esteban J, Martin J, Ortiz A, et al. *Pseudomonas oryzihabitans* peritonitis in a patient on continuous ambulatory peritoneal dialysis. Clin Microbiol Infect 2002; 8:607–608.

212. Esteban J, Valero-Moratalla ML, Alcazar R, et al. Infections due to *Flavimonas*

oryzihabitans: case report and literature review. Eur J Clin Microbiol Infect Dis 1993;12:797–800.

213. Euzeby J. Validation of publication of new names and new combinations previously effectively published outside the IJSEM. Int J Syst Evol Microbiol 2003; 53:935–937.

214. Ezzedine H, Mourad M, Van Ossel C, et al. An outbreak of *Ochrobactrum anthropi* bacteraemia in five organ transplant patients. J Hosp Infect 1994;27: 35–42.

215. Farmer JJ III, Gangarosa RE, Gangarosa EJ. Does *Laribacter hongkongensis* cause diarrhoea, or does diarrhoea ''cause'' *L hongkongensis*? Lancet 2004;363: 1923–1924.

216. Farrand SK, van Berkum PB, Oger P. *Agrobacterium* is a definable genus of the family *Rhizobiaceae*. Int J Syst Evol Microbiol 2003;53:1681–1687.

217. Fass RJ, Barnishan J. In vitro susceptibility of nonfermentative gram-negative bacilli other than *Pseudomonas aeruginosa* to 32 antimicrobial agents. Rev Infect Dis 1980;2:841–853.

218. Feigin RD, San Joaquin V, Middelkamp JN. Septic arthritis due to *Moraxella osloensis*. J Pediatr 1969;75:116–117.

219. Felegie TP, Yu VL, Rumans LW, et al. Susceptibility of *Pseudomonas maltophilia* to antimicrobial agents, singly and in combination. Antimicrob Agents Chemother 1979;16:833–837.

220. Ferroni A, Sermet-Gaudelus I, Abachin E, et al. Use of 16S rRNA gene sequencing for identification of nonfermenting gram-negative bacilli recovered from patients attending a single cystic fibrosis center. J Clin Microbiol 2002;40: 3793–3797.

221. Finkmann W, Altendorf K, Stackebrandt E, et al. Characterization of N_2O-producing *Xanthomonas*-like isolates from biofilters as *Stenotrophomonas nitritireducens* sp. nov., *Luteimonas mephitis* gen. nov., sp. nov. and *Pseudoxanthomonas broegbernensis* gen. nov., sp. nov. Int J Syst Evol Microbiol 2000;50: 273–282.

222. Flournoy DJ, Petrone RL, Voth DW. A pseudo-outbreak of *Methylobacterium mesophilica* isolated from patients undergoing bronchoscopy. Eur J Clin Microbiol Infect Dis 1992;11:240–243.

223. Fraser SL, Jorgensen JH: Reappraisal of the antimicrobial susceptibilities of *Chryseobacterium* and *Flavobacterium* species and methods for reliable susceptibility testing. Antimicrob. Agents Chemother. 1997;41:2738–2741.

224. Freney J, Gruer LD, Bornstein N, et al. Septicemia caused by *Agrobacterium* sp. J Clin Microbiol 1985;22:683–685.

225. Freney J, Hansen W, Etienne J, et al. Postoperative infant septicemia caused by *Pseudomonas luteola* (CDC group Ve-1) and *Pseudomonas oryzihabitans* (CDC group Ve-2). J Clin Microbiol 1988;26:1241–1243.

226. Freney J, Hansen W, Ploton C, et al. Septicemia caused by *Sphingobacterium multivorum*. J Clin Microbiol 1987;25:1126–1128.

227. Friedman ND, Korman TM, Fairley CK, et al. Bacteraemia due to *Stenotrophomonas maltophilia*: an analysis of 45 episodes. J Infect 2002;45:47–53.

228. Fujita Y, Hata Y, Irino S. Respiratory infection caused by *Flavobacterium meningosepticum*. Lancet 1990;335:544.

229. Funke G, Frodl R, Sommer H. First comprehensively documented case of *Paracoccus yeei* infection in a human. J Clin Microbiol 2004;42:3366–3368.

230. Funke G, Funke-Kissling P. Evaluation of the new Vitek 2 card for identification of clinically relevant gram-negative rods. J Clin Microbiol 2004;42:4067–4071.

231. Funke G, Hess T, von Graevenitz A, et al. Characteristics of *Bordetella hinzii* strains isolated from a cystic fibrosis patient over a 3-year period. J Clin Microbiol 1996;34:966–969.

232. Gadea I, Cuenca-Estrella M, Benito N, et al. *Bordetella hinzii*, a ''new'' opportunistic pathogen to think about. J Infect 2000;40:298–299.

233. Gales AC, Jones RN, Turnidge J, et al. Characterization of *Pseudomonas aeruginosa* isolates: occurrence rates, antimicrobial susceptibility patterns, and molecular typing in the global SENTRY antimicrobial surveillance program, 1997–1999. Clin Infect Dis 32(Suppl 2): 2001;S146–S155.

234. Garcia San Miguel L, Quereda C, Martinez M, et al. *Bordetella bronchiseptica* cavitary pneumonia in a patient with AIDS. Eur J Clin Microbiol Infect Dis 1998;17:675–6.

235. Garcia-Valdes E, Castillo MM, Bennasar A, et al. Polyphasic characterization of *Pseudomonas stutzeri* CLN100 which simultaneously degrades chloro- and methylaromatics: a new genomovar within the species. Syst Appl Microbiol 2003;26:390–403.

236. Garner J, Briant RH. Osteomyelitis caused by a bacterium known as M-6. J Infect 1986;13:298–300.

237. Garrity GM, Bell JA, Lilburn TG. Taxonomic outline of the Procaryotes. Bergey's Manual of Systematic Bacteriology. Ed. 2. Release 5.0., May 2004, New York: Springer-Verlag, 2004.

238. George LJ, Cunha BA. *Pseudomonas stutzeri* synthetic vascular graft infection. Heart Lung 1990;19:203–205.

239. George RM, Cochran CP, Wheeler WE. Epidemic meningitis of the newborn caused by flavobacteria. Am J Dis Child 1961;101:296–304.

240. Gerner-Smidt P, Keiser-Nielsen H, Dorsch M, et al. *Lautropia mirabilis* gen.

nov., sp. nov., a gram-negative motile coccus with unusual morphology isolated from the human mouth. Microbiology 1994;140:1787–1797.

241. Ghosh JK, Tranter J. *Bordetella bronchiseptica* infections in man: review and case report. J Clin Pathol 1979;32:546–548.

242. Gilad J, Borer A, Peled N, et al. Hospital-acquired *Brevundimonas vesicularis* septicaemia following open-heart surgery: case report and literature review. Scand J Infect Dis 2000;32:90–91.

243. Gilardi GL. Infrequently encountered *Pseudomonas* species causing infection in humans. Ann Intern Med 1972;77:211–215.

244. Gilardi GL, ed. Glucose Nonfermenting Gram-Negative Bacteria in Clinical Microbiology. West Palm Beach, FL: CRC Press, 1978.

245. Gilardi GL. Identification of *Pseudomonas* and related bacteria. In: Gilardi GL, ed. Glucose Nonfermenting Gram-Negative Bacteria in Clinical Microbiology. West Palm Beach, FL: CRC Press, 1978:15–44.

246. Gilardi GL. Identification of miscellaneous glucose nonfermenting gram-negative bacteria. In: Gilardi GL, ed. Glucose Nonfermenting Gram-Negative Bacteria in Clinical Microbiology. West Palm Beach, FL: CRC Press, 1978: 45–55.

247. Gilardi GL. Nonfermentative Gram-Negative Rods: Laboratory Identification and Clinical Aspects. New York: Marcel Dekker, 1985.

248. Gilardi GL. Cultural and biochemical aspects for identification of glucose-nonfermenting gram-negative rods. In: Gilardi GL, ed. Glucose Nonfermenting Gram-Negative Bacteria in Clinical Microbiology. West Palm Beach, FL: CRC Press, 1978:17–84.

249. Gilardi GL. Identification of Glucose-Nonfermenting Gram-Negative Rods. New York: North General Hospital, 1990.

250. Gilardi GL. *Pseudomonas* and related genera. In: Balows A, ed. Manual of Clinical Microbiology. Ed. 5. Washington DC: American Society for Microbiology, 1991:429-441.

251. Gilardi GL, Faur YC. *Pseudomonas mesophilica* and an unnamed taxon, clinical isolates of pink-pigmented oxidative bacteria. J Clin Microbiol 1984;20: 626–629.

252. Gilardi GL, Hirschl S, Mandel M. Characteristics of yellow-pigmented nonfermentative bacilli (groups Ve-1 and Ve-2) encountered in clinical bacteriology. J Clin Microbiol 1975;1:384–389.

253. Gilardi GL, Mankin HJ. Infection due to *Pseudomonas stutzeri*. NY State J Med 1973;73:2789–2791.

254. Gilchrist MJR, Kraft JA, Hammond JG, et al. Detection of *Pseudomonas mesophilica* as a source of nosocomial infections in a bone marrow transplant unit. J Clin Microbiol 1986;23:1052–1055.

255. Gilligan PH. Microbiology of airway disease in patients with cystic fibrosis. Clin Microbiol Rev 1991;4:35–51.

256. Gilligan PH, Gage PA, Bradshaw LM, et al. Isolation medium for the recovery of *Pseudomonas cepacia* from respiratory secretions of patients with cystic fibrosis. J Clin Microbiol 1985;22:5–8.

257. Gilligan PH, Lum G, Vandamme PAR, Whittier S. *Burkholderia, Stenotrophomonas, Ralstonia, Brevundimonas, Comamonas, Delftia, Pandoraea,* and *Acidovorax*. In: Murray PR, Baron EJ, Jorgensen JH, et al., eds. Manual of Clinical Microbiology. Ed. 8. Washington DC: ASM Press, 2003:729–748.

258. Gillis M, Van TV, Bardin R, et al. Polyphasic taxonomy in the genus *Burkholderia* leading to an emended description of the genus and proposition of *Burkholderia vietnamiensis* sp. nov. for N_2-fixing isolates from rice in Vietnam. Int J Syst Bacteriol 1995;45:274–289.

259. Gini GA. Ocular infection caused by *Psychrobacter immobilis* acquired in the hospital. J Clin Microbiol 1990;28:400–401.

260. Gladman G, Connor PJ, Williams RF, et al. Controlled study of *Pseudomonas maltophilia* in cystic fibrosis. Arch Dis Child 1993;67:192–195.

261. Glew RH, Moellering RC, Kunz LJ. Infections with *Acinetobacter calcoaceticus (Herellea vaginicola)*: Clinical and laboratory studies. Medicine 1977;56:79–97.

262. Goldmann DA, Klinger JD. *Pseudomonas cepacia*: biology, mechanisms of virulence, epidemiology. J Pediatr 1986;108:806–812.

263. Goldstein R, Sun L, Jiang RZ, et al. Structurally variant classes of pilus appendage fibers coexpressed from *Burkholderia (Pseudomonas) cepacia*. J Bacteriol 1995;177:1039–1052.

264. Gomez L, Grazziutti M, Sumoza D, et al. Bacterial pneumonia due to *Bordetella bronchiseptica* in a patient with acute leukemia. Clin Infect Dis 1998;26: 1002–1003.

265. Gomez-Cerezo J, Suarez I, Rios JJ, et al. *Achromobacter xylosoxidans* bacteremia: a 10-year analysis of 54 cases. Eur J Clin Microbiol Infect Dis 2003;22: 360–363.

266. Goodnow RA. Biology of *B. bronchiseptica*. Microbiol Rev 1980;44:722–738.

267. Goshorn RK. Recrudescent pulmonary melioidosis: a case report involving the so-called ''Vietnamese time bomb.'' Indiana Med 1987;80:247–249.

268. Govan JRW, Brown PH, Maddison J, et al. Evidence for transmission of *Pseudomonas cepacia* by social contact in cystic fibrosis. Lancet 1993;342:15–19.

269. Govan JRW, Hughes JE, Vandamme P. *Burkholderia cepacia*: medical, taxonomic and ecological issues. J Med Microbiol 1996;45:395–407.

270. Graber CD, Jervey LP, Ostrander WE, et al. Endocarditis due to a lanthanic,

unclassified gram-negative bacterium (group IVd). Am J Clin Pathol 1968;49:220–223.

271. Graham DR, Band JD, Thornsberry C, et al. Infections caused by *Moraxella, Moraxella urethralis, Moraxella*-like groups M-5 and M-6, and *Kingella kingae* in the United States, 1953–1980. Rev Infect Dis 1990;12:423–431.

272. Gransden WR, Eykyn SJ. Seven cases of bacteraemia due to *Ochrobactrum anthropi*. Clin Infect Dis 1992;15:1068–1069.

273. Grant PE, Brenner DJ, Steigerwalt AG, et al. *Neisseria elongata* subsp. *nitroreducens* subsp. nov., formerly CDC group M-6, a gram-negative bacterium associated with endocarditis. J Clin Microbiol 1990;28:2591–2596.

274. Graves M, Robin T, Chipman AM, et al. Four additional cases of *Burkholderia gladioli* infection with microbiological correlates and review. Clin Infect Dis 1997;25:838–842.

275. Green BT, Green K, Nolan PE. *Myroides odoratus* cellulitis and bacteremia: case report and review. Scand J Infect Dis 2001;33:932–934.

276. Green BT, Nolan PE. Cellulitis and bacteraemia due to *Chryseobacterium indologenes*. J Infect 2001;42:219–220.

277. Green PN, Bousfield IJ. Emendation of *Methylobacterium* Patt, Cole, and Hanson 1976; *Methylobacterium rhodinum* (Heumann 1962) comb. nov. corrig.; *Methylobacterium radiotolerans* (Ito and Iizuka 1971) comb. nov. corrig.; and *Methylobacterium mesophilicum* (Austin and Goodfellow 1979) comb. nov. Int J Syst Bacteriol 1983;33:875–877.

278. Green PN, Bousfield IJ, Hood D. Three new *Methylobacterium* species: *M. rhodesianum* sp. nov., *M. zatmanii* sp. nov., and *M. fujisawaense* sp. nov. Int J Syst Bacteriol 1988;38:124–127.

279. Green RN, Tuffnell PG. Laboratory acquired melioidosis. Am J Med 1968;44:599–605.

280. Grieg JR, Gunda SS, Kwan JTC. *Bordetella holmesii* bacteraemia in an individual on haemodialysis. Scand J Infect Dis 2001;33:716–717.

281. Griffin CW III, Mehaffey MA, Cook EC, et al. Relationship between performance in three of the Centers for Disease Control microbiology proficiency testing programs and the number of actual patient specimens tested by participating laboratories. J Clin Microbiol 1986;23:246–250.

282. Grimault E, Glerant JC, Aubry P, et al. [Uncommon site of *Bergeyella zoohelcum*: apropos of a case]. Rev Pneumol Clin 1996;52:387–389.

283. Gutierrez Rodero F, Masia MM, Cortes J, et al. Endocarditis caused by *Stenotrophomonas maltophilia*: case report and review. Clin Infect Dis 1996;23:1261–1265.

284. Guttigoli A, Zaman MM. Bacteremia and possible endocarditis caused by *Moraxella phenylpyruvica*. South Med J 2000;9:708–709.

285. Haddow LJ, Mulgrew C, Ansari A, et al. Neisseria elongata endocarditis: case report and literature review. Clin Microbiol Infect 2003;9:426–430.

286. Haditsch M, Binder L, Tschurtschenthaler G, et al. Bacteraemia caused by *Ochrobactrum anthropi* in an immunocompromised child. Infection 1994;22:291–292.

287. Hamill RJ, Houston ED, Georghiou PR, et al. An outbreak of *Burkholderia* (formerly *Pseudomonas*) *cepacia* respiratory tract colonization and infection associated with nebulized albuterol therapy. Ann Intern Med 1995;122:762–766.

288. Hammerberg O, Bialkowska-Hobrzanska H, Gopaul D. Isolation of *Agrobacterium radiobacter* from a central venous catheter. Eur J Clin Microbiol Infect Dis 1991;10:450–452.

289. Han XY, Pham AS, Tarrand JJ, et al. Bacteriologic characterization of 36 strains of *Roseomonas* species and proposal of *Roseomonas mucosa* sp. nov. and *Roseomonas gilardii* subsp *rosea* subsp nov. Am J Clin Pathol 2003;120:256–264.

290. Han XY, Tarrand JJ. *Moraxella osloensis* blood and catheter infections during anticancer chemotherapy: clinical and microbiologic studies of 10 cases. Am J Clin Pathol 2004;121:581–587.

291. Hansen W, Glupczynski Y. Group IV c-2 associated peritonitis. Clin Microbiol Newslett 1985;7:43.

292. Harrington BJ. Letter to the Editors. Clin Microbiol Newlsett 1997;19:191.

293. Harrington SP, Perlino CA. *Flavobacterium meningosepticum* sepsis: disease due to bacteria with unusual antibiotic susceptibility. Southern Med J 1981;74:764–766.

294. Harrison GAJ, Morris R, Holmes B, et al. Human infections with strains of *Agrobacterium*. J Hosp Infect 1990;16:383–388.

295. Hauben L, Vauterin L, Moore ERB, et al. Genomic diversity of the genus *Stenotrophomonas*. Int J Syst Bacteriol 1999;49:1749–1760.

296. Hawley HB, Gump DW. Vancomycin therapy of bacterial meningitis. Am J Dis Child 1973;126:261–264.

297. Heagney MA. An unusual case of bacterial meningitis caused by *Burkholderia pickettii*. Clin Microbiol Newslett 1998;20:102–103.

298. Heard S, Lawrence S, Holmes B, et al. A pseudo-outbreak of *Pseudomonas* on a special care baby unit. J Hosp Infect 1990;16:59–65.

299. Heimbrook ME, Wang WLL, Campbell G. Staining bacterial flagella easily. J Clin Microbiol 1989;27:2612–2615.

300. Henry DA, Campbell ME, LiPuma JJ, et al. Identification of *Burkholderia cepacia* isolates from patients with cystic fibrosis and use of a simple new selective medium. J Clin Microbiol 1997;35:614–619.

301. Henry D, Campbell M, McGimpsey C, et al. Comparison of isolation media for recovery of *Burkholderia cepacia* complex from respiratory secretions of patients with cystic fibrosis. J Clin Microbiol 1999;37:1004–1007.

302. Henry DA, Mahenthiralingam E, Vandamme P, et al. Phenotypic methods for determining genomovar status of *Burkholderia cepacia* complex. J Clin Microbiol 2001;39:1073–1078.

303. Higgins PG, Wisplinghoff H, Stefanik D, et al. In vitro activities of the β-lactamase inhibitors clavulanic acid, sulbactam, and tazobactam alone or in combination with β-lactams against epidemiologically characterized multidrug-resistant *Acinetobacter baumannii* strains. Antimicrob Agents and Chemother 2004;48:1586–1592.

304. Hiraishi A, Furuhata K, Matsumoto A, et al. Phenotypic and genetic diversity of chlorine-resistant *Methylobacterium* strains isolated from various environments. Appl Environ Microbiol 1995;61:2099–107.

305. Hirsh BE, Wong B, Kiehn TE, et al. *Flavobacterium meningosepticum* bacteremia in an adult with acute leukemia: use of rifampin to clear persistent infection. Diagn Microbiol Infect Dis 1986;4:65–69.

306. Hoare S, Cant AJ. Chronic granulomatous disease presenting as severe sepsis due to *Burkholderia gladioli*. Clin Infect Dis 1996;23:411.

307. Hobson R, Gould I, Govan J. *Burkholderia (Pseudomonas) cepacia* as a cause of brain abscesses secondary to chronic suppurative otitis media. Eur J Clin Microbiol Infect Dis 1995;14:908–911.

308. Hofherr L, Votava H, Blazevic DJ. Comparison of three methods for identifying nonfermenting gram-negative rods. Can J Microbiol 1978;24:1140–1144.

309. Hofstad T, Hope O, Falsen E. Septicaemia with *Neisseria elongata* spp. *nitroreducens* in a patient with hypertrophic obstructive cardiomyopathia. Scand J Infect Dis 1998;30:200–201.

310. Hohl P, Frei R, Aubry P. In vitro susceptibility of 33 clinical case isolates of *Xanthomonas maltophilia*. Inconsistent correlation of agar dilution and of disk diffusion test results. Diagn Microbiol Infect Dis 1991;14:447–450.

311. Hollis DG, Daneshvar MI, Moss CW, et al. Phenotypic characteristics, fatty acid composition, and isoprenoid quinone content of CDC group IIg bacteria. J Clin Microbiol 1995;33:762–764.

312. Hollis DG, Moss CW, Daneshvar MI, Meadows L, et al. Characterization of Centers for Disease Control group NO-1, a fastidious, nonoxidative, gram-negative organism associated with dog and cat bites. J Clin Microbiol 1993;31:746–748.

313. Hollis DG, Moss CW, Daneshvar MI, Wallace-Shewmaker PL. CDC group IIc: phenotypic characteristics, fatty acid composition, and isoprenoid quinone content. J Clin Microbiol 1996;34:2322–2324.

314. Hollis DG, Weaver RE, Moss CW, et al. Chemical and cultural characterization of CDC group WO-1, a weakly oxidative gram-negative group of organisms isolated from clinical sources. J Clin Microbiol 1992;30:291–295.

315. Holmes B, Costas M, Ganner M, et al. Evaluation of Biolog System for identification of some gram-negative bacteria of clinical importance. J Clin Microbiol 1994;32:1970–1975.

316. Holmes B, Costas M, On SLW, et al. *Neisseria weaveri* sp. nov. (formerly CDC group M-5), from dog bite wounds of humans. Int J Syst Bacteriol 1993;43:687–693.

317. Holmes B, Costas M, Wood AC, Kersters K. Numerical analysis of electrophoretic protein patterns of ''*Achromobacter*'' group B, E and F strains from human blood. J Appl Bacteriol 1990;68:495–504.

318. Holmes B, Costas M, Wood AC, Owen RJ, et al. Differentiation of *Achromobacter*-like strains from human blood by DNA restriction endonuclease digest and ribosomal RNA gene probe patterns. Epidemiol Infect 1990;105:541–551.

319. Holmes B, Dawson CA. Numerical taxonomic studies on *Achromobacter* isolates from clinical material. In: Leclerc H, ed. Gram Negative Bacteria of Medical and Public Health Importance: Taxonomy–Identification–Applications. Paris, Les Editions INSERM, 1983:331–341.

320. Holmes B, Dowling J, Lapage SP. Identification of gram-negative nonfermenters and oxidase-positive fermenters by the Oxi/Ferm tube. J Clin Pathol 1979;32:78–85.

321. Holmes B, Lewis R, Trevett A. Septicaemia due to *Achromobacter* group B: a report of two cases. Med Microbiol Lett 1992;1:177–184.

322. Holmes B, Moss CW, Daneshvar MI. Cellular fatty acid compositions of ''*Achromobacter* groups B and E.'' J Clin Microbiol 1993;31:1007–1008.

323. Holmes B, Owen RJ, Evans A, et al. *Pseudomonas paucimobilis*, a new species isolated from human clinical specimens, the hospital environment, and other sources. Int J Syst Bacteriol 1977;27:133–146.

324. Holmes B, Owen RJ, Hollis DG. *Flavobacterium spiritivorum*, a new species isolated from human clinical specimens. Int J Syst Bacteriol 1982;32:157–165.

325. Holmes B, Owen RJ, McMeekin TA. Genus *Flavobacterium*. In: Krieg NR, Holt JG, eds. Bergey's Manual of Systematic Bacteriology. Vol. 1. Baltimore: Williams & Wilkins, 1984:353–361.

326. Holmes B, Owen RJ, Weaver RE. *Flavobacterium multivorum*, a new species isolated from human clinical specimens and previously known as group IIk, biotype 2. Int J Syst Bacteriol 1981;31:21–34.

327. Holmes B, Pinning CA, Dawson CA. A probability matrix for the identification

of gram-negative, aerobic, non-fermentative bacteria that grow on nutrient agar. J Gen Microbiol 1986;132:1827–1842.

328. Holmes B, Popoff M, Kiredjian M, et al. *Ochrobactrum anthropi* gen. nov., sp. nov. from human clinical specimens and previously known as group Vd. Int J Syst Bacteriol 1988;38:406–416.

329. Holmes B, Snell JJS, Lapage SP. *Flavobacterium odoratum*: a species resistant to a wide range of antimicrobial agents. J Clin Pathol 1979;32:73–77.

330. Holmes B, Steigerwalt AG, Weaver RE, Brenner DJ. *Weeksella virosa* gen. nov., sp. nov. (formerly group IIf), found in human clinical specimens. Syst Appl Microbiol 1986;8:185–190.

331. Holmes B, Steigerwalt AG, Weaver RE, Brenner DJ. *Weeksella zoohelcum* sp. nov. (formerly group IIj), from human clinical specimens. Syst Appl Microbiol 1986;8:191–196.

332. Holmes B, Steigerwalt AG, Weaver RE, Brenner DJ. *Chryseomonas luteola* comb. nov. and *Flavimonas oryzihabitans* gen. nov., comb. nov., *Pseudomonas*-like species from human clinical specimens and formerly known, respectively, as groups Ve-1 and Ve-2. Int J Syst Bacteriol 1987;37:245–250.

333. Holmes B, Weaver RE, Steigerwalt AG, et al. A taxonomic study of *Flavobacterium spiritivorum* and *Sphingobacterium mizutae*: proposal of *Flavobacterium yabuuchiae* sp. nov. and *Flavobacterium mizutaii* comb. nov. Int J Syst Bacteriol 1988;38:348–353.

334. Holt HM, Sogaard P, Gahrn-Hansen B. Ear infections with *Shewanella alga*: a bacteriologic, clinical and epidemiologic study of 67 cases. Clin Microbiol Infect 1997;3:329–334.

335. Holton J. A note on the preparation and use of a selective and differential medium for the isolation of the *Acinetobacter* spp. from clinical sources. J Appl Bacteriol 1983;66:24–26.

336. Hombrouck-Alet C, Poilane I, Janoir-Jouveshomme C, et al. Utilization of 16S ribosomal DNA sequencing for diagnosis of septicemia due to *Neisseria elongata* subsp. *glycolytica* in a neutropenic patient. J Clin Microbiol 2003;41:3436–3437.

337. Hornei B, Luneberg E, Schmidt-Rotte H, et al. Systemic infection of an immunocompromised patient with *Methylobacterium zatmanii*. J Clin Microbiol 1999;37:248–250.

338. Horowitz H, Gilroy S, Feinstein S, et al. Endocarditis associated with *Comamonas acidovorans*. J Clin Microbiol 1990;28:143–145.

339. Howard K, Inglis TJJ: Novel selective medium for isolation of *Burkholderia pseudomallei*. J Clin Microbiol 2003;41:3312–3316.

340. Hsueh P-R, Chang J-C, Teng L-J, et al. Comparison of Etest and agar dilution method for antimicrobial susceptibility testing of *Flavobacterium* isolates. J Clin Microbiol 1997;35:1021–1023.

341. Hsueh P-R, Hsiue T-R, Wu J-J, et al. *Flavobacterium indologenes* bacteremia: clinical and microbiological characteristics. Clin Infect Dis 1996;23:550–555.

342. Hsueh P-R, Teng L-J, Chen C-Y, et al. Pandrug-resistant *Acinetobacter baumannii* causing nosocomial infections in a university hospital, Taiwan. Emerg Infect Dis 2002;8:827–832.

343. Hsueh P-R, Teng L-J, Ho S-W, et al. Clinical and microbiological characteristics of *Flavobacterium indologenes* infections associated with indwelling devices. J Clin Microbiol 1996;34:1908–1913.

344. Hsueh P-R, Teng L-J, Lee L-N, et al. Melioidosis: an emerging infection in Taiwan? Emerg Infect Dis 2001;7:428–433.

345. Hsueh P-R, Teng L-J, Yang P-C, et al. Nosocomial infections caused by *Sphingomonas paucimobilis*: clinical features and microbiological characteristics. Clin Infect Dis 1998;26:676–681.

346. Hsueh P-R, Teng L-J, Yang P-C, et al. Increasing incidence of nosocomial *Chryseobacterium indologenes* infections in Taiwan. Eur J Clin Microbiol Infect Dis 1997;16:568–574.

347. Hsueh P-R, Wu J-J, Hsiue T-R, et al. Bacteremic necrotizing fasciitis due to *Flavobacterium odoratum*. Clin Infect Dis 1995;21:1337–1338.

348. Hubert B, De Mahenge A, Grimont F, et al. An outbreak of pneumonia and meningitis caused by a previously undescribed gram-negative bacterium in a hot spring spa. Epidemiol Infect 1991;107:373–381.

349. Hudson MJ, Hollis DG, Weaver RE, et al. Relationship of CDC group EO-2 and *Psychrobacter immobilis*. J Clin Microbiol 1987;25:1907–1910.

350. Hugh R, Leifson E. The taxonomic significance of fermentative versus oxidative metabolism of carbohydrates by various gram-negative bacteria. J Bacteriol 1953;66:24–26.

351. Hutchinson GR, Parker S, Pryor JA, et al. Home-use nebulizers: a potential primary source of *Burkholderia cepacia* and other colistin-resistant, gram-negative bacteria in patients with cystic fibrosis. J Clin Microbiol 1996;34:584–587.

352. Ibrahim A, Gerner-Smidt P, Liesack W. Phylogenetic relationship of the twenty-one DNA groups of the genus *Acinetobacter* as revealed by 16S ribosomal DNA sequence analysis. Int J Syst Bacteriol 1997;47:837–841.

353. Igra-Siegman Y, Chmel H, Cobbs C. Clinical and laboratory characteristics of *Achromobacter xylosoxidans* infection. J Clin Microbiol 1980;11:141–145.

354. Imperial HL, Joho KL, Alcid DV. Endocarditis due to *Neisseria elongata* subspecies *nitroreducens*. Clin Infect Dis 1995;20:1431–1432.

355. Isenberg HD, Sampson–Scherer J. Clinical laboratory evaluation of a system approach to the recognition of nonfermentative or oxidase-producing gram-negative, rod-shaped bacteria. J Clin Microbiol 1977;5:336–340.

356. Isles A, Macluskey I, Corey M, et al. *Pseudomonas cepacia* infection in cystic fibrosis: an emerging problem. J Pediatr 1984;104:206–210.

357. Iwata M, Tateda K, Matsumoto T, et al. Primary *Shewanella alga* septicemia in a patient on hemodialysis. J Clin Microbiol 1999;37:2104–2105.

358. Janknecht P, Schneider CM, Ness T. Outbreak of *Empedobacter brevis* endophthalmitis after cataract extraction. Graefes Arch Clin Exp Ophthalmol 2002;240:291–295.

359. Jannes G, Vaneechoutte M, Lannoo M, et al. Polyphasic taxonomy leading to the proposal of *Moraxella canis* sp. nov. for *Moraxella catarrhalis*-like strains. Int J Syst Bacteriol 1993;43:438–449.

360. Jawad A, Hawkey PM, Heritage J, et al. Description of Leeds *Acinetobacter* Medium, a new selective and differential medium for isolation of clinically important *Acinetobacter* spp., and comparison with Herellea agar and Holton's agar. J Clin Microbiol 1994;32:2353–2358.

361. Jellison TK, McKinnon PS, Rybak MJ. Epidemiology, resistance, and outcomes of *Acinetobacter baumannii* bacteremia treated with imipenem-cilastatin or ampicillin-sulbactam. Pharmacotherapy 2001;21:142–148.

362. Jelveh N, Cunha BA. *Ochrobactrum anthropi* bacteremia. Heart Lung 1999;28:145–146.

363. Jenks PJ, Shaw EJ. Recurrent septicaemia due to ''*Achromobacter* Group B.'' J Infect 1997;34:143–145.

364. Jenney AW, Lum G, Fisher DA, et al. Antibiotic susceptibility of *Burkholderia pseudomallei* from tropical northern Australia and implications for therapy of melioidosis. Int J Antimicrob Agents 2001;17:109–113.

365. Jiménez-Mejías ME, Pachón J, Becerril B, et al. Treatment of multidrug-resistant *Acinetobacter baumannii* meningitis with ampicillin/sulbactam. Clin Infect Dis 1997;24:932–935.

366. Jiménez-Mejías ME, Pichardo-Guerrero C, Márquez-Rivas FJ, et al. Cerebrospinal fluid penetration and pharmacokinetic/pharmacodynamic parameters of intravenously administered colistin in a case of multidrug-resistant *Acinetobacter baumannii* meningitis. Eur J Clin Microbiol Infect Dis 2002;21:212–214.

367. Johansen HK, Kjeldsen K, Høiby N. *Pseudomonas mendocina* as a cause of chronic infective endocarditis in a patient with situs inversus. Clin Microbiol Infect 2001;7:650–652.

368. Johnson DW, Lum G, Nimmo G, et al. *Moraxella nonliquefaciens* septic arthritis in a patient undergoing hemodialysis. Clin Infect Dis 1995;21:1039–1040.

369. Jones AM, Dodd ME, Webb AK. *Burkholderia cepacia*: current clinical issues, environmental controversies and ethical dilemmas. Eur Respir J 2001;17:295–301.

370. Jones AM, Stanbridge TN, Islaska BJ, et al. *Burkholderia gladioli*: recurrent abscesses in a patient with cystic fibrosis. J Infect 2001;42:69–71.

371. Jorgensen IM, Johansen HK, Frederiksen B, et al. Epidemic spread of *Pandoraea apista*, a new pathogen causing severe lung disease in patients with cystic fibrosis. Pediatr Pulmonol 2003;36:439–446.

372. Kaiser RM, Garman RL, Bruce MG, et al. Clinical significance and epidemiology of NO-1, an unusual bacterium associated with dog and cat bites. Emerg Infect Dis 2002;8:171–174.

373. Kämpfer P. Grouping of *Acinetobacter* genomic species by cellular fatty acid composition. Med Microbiol Lett 1993;2:394–400.

374. Kanj SS, Tapson V, Davis RD, et al. Infections in patients with cystic fibrosis following lung transplantation. Chest 1997;112:924–930.

375. Kaplan LJ, Flaherty J. Centers for Disease Control Group M-6: a cause of destructive endocarditis. J Infect Dis 1991;164:822–823.

376. Kappstein I, Grundmann H, Hauer T, et al. Aerators as a reservoir of *Acinetobacter junii*: an outbreak of bacteraemia in paediatric oncology patients. J Hosp Infect 2000;44:27–30.

377. Karpati F, Malmborg AS, Alfredsson H, et al. Bacterial colonization with *Xanthomonas maltophilia*: a retrospective study in a cystic fibrosis patient population. Infection 1994;22:258–263.

378. Kattar MM, Chavez JF, Limaye AP, et al. Application of 16S rRNA gene sequencing to identify *Bordetella hinzii* as the causative agent of fatal septicemia. J Clin Microbiol 2000;38:789–794.

379. Kay SE, Clark RA, White KL, et al. Recurrent *Achromobacter piechaudii* bacteremia in a patient with hematological malignancy. J Clin Microbiol 2001;39:808–810.

380. Kaye KM, Macone A, Kazanjian PH. Catheter infection caused by *Methylobacterium* in immunocompromised hosts: report of three cases and review of the literature. CID 1992;14:1010–1014.

381. Keene WE, Markum AC, Samadpour M. Outbreak of *Pseudomonas aeruginosa* infections caused by commercial piercing of upper ear cartilage. JAMA 22004;91:981–985.

382. Kendirli T, Ciftci E, Ince E, et al. *Ralstonia pickettii* outbreak associated with contaminated distilled water used for respiratory care in a paediatric intensive care unit. J Hosp Infect 2004;56:77–78.

383. Kern WV, Oethinger M, Kaufhold A, et al. *Ochrobactrum anthropi* bacteremia: report of four cases and short review. Infection 1993;21:306–310.

384. Kerr KG, Denton M, Todd NJ, et al. A novel selective culture medium for the isolation of *Stenotrophomonas maltophilia*. Eur J Clin Microbiol Infect Dis 1996;15:607–608.

385. Kersters K, De Ley J. Genus III. *Agrobacterium* Conn 1942, 359^AL. In: Krieg NR, Holt JG, eds. Bergey's Manual of Systematic Bacteriology. Vol. 1. Baltimore: Williams & Wilkins, 1984:244–254.

386. Kersters K, De Ley J. Genus *Alcaligenes* Castellani and Chalmers 1919, 936^AL. In: Krieg NR, Holt JG, eds. Bergey's Manual of Systematic Bacteriology. Vol. 1. Baltimore: Williams & Wilkins, 1984:pp 361–373.

387. Kersters K, Hinz K-H, Hertle A, et al. *Bordetella avium* sp. nov., isolated from the respiratory tracts of turkeys and other birds. Int J Syst Bacteriol 1984;34:56–70.

388. Kettaneh A, Weill F-X, Poilane I, et al. Septic shock caused by *Ochrobactrum anthropi* in an otherwise healthy host. J Clin Microbiol 2003;41:1339–1341.

389. Khabbaz RF, Arnow PM, Highsmith AK, et al. *Pseudomonas fluorescens* bacteremia from blood transfusion. Am J Med 1984;76:62–68.

390. Khan SU, Gordon SM, Stillwell PC, et al. Empyema and bloodstream infection caused by *Burkholderia gladioli* in a patient with cystic fibrosis after lung transplantation. Pediatr Infect Dis J 1996;15:637–639.

391. Khardori N, Elting L, Wong E, et al. Nosocomial infections due to *Xanthomonas maltophilia* (*Pseudomonas maltophilia*) in patients with cancer. Rev Infect Dis 1990;12:997–1003.

392. Khashe S, Janda JM. Biochemical and pathogenic properties of *Shewanella alga* and *Shewanella putrefaciens*. J Clin Microbiol 1998;36:783–787.

393. Kikuchi I, Arao T, Oiwa T. Surgical treatment of fungating lesion of foot due to *Moraxella phenylpyruvica*. Case report. Plast Reconstr Surg 1978;61:911–916.

394. Kim JH, Cooper RA, Welty-Wolf KE, et al. *Pseudomonas putrefaciens* bacteremia. Rev Infect Dis 1989;11:97–104.

394a. Kim KK, Kim MK, Lim JH, et al. Transfer of *Chryseobacterium meningosepticum* and *Chryseobacterium miricola* to *Elizabethkingia* gen. nov. as *Elizabethkingia meningoseptica* comb. nov. and *Elizabethkingia miricola* comb. nov. Int J Syst Evol Microbiol 2005;55:1287–1293.

395. King A, Holmes B, Phillips I, et al. A taxonomic study of clinical isolates of *Pseudomonas pickettii*, 'P. thomasii' and 'group IVd' bacteria. J Gen Microbiol 1979;114:137–147.

396. King EO: Studies of a group of previously unclassified bacteria associated with meningitis in infants. Am J Clin Pathol 1959;31:241–247.

397. King EO. The Identification of Unusual Pathogenic Gram-Negative Bacteria. Atlanta: Centers for Disease Control, 1964.

398. King EO, Ward MK, Raney DE. Two simple media for the demonstration of pyocyanin and fluorescein. J Lab Clin Med 1954;44:301–307.

399. Kiredjian M, Holmes B, Kersters K, et al. *Alcaligenes piechaudii*, a new species from human clinical specimens and the environment. Int J Syst Bacteriol 1986;36:282–287.

400. Kiris S, Over U, Babacan F, et al. Disseminated *Flavimonas oryzihabitans* infection in a diabetic patient who presented with suspected multiple splenic abscesses. Clin Infect Dis 1997;25:324–325.

401. Kish MA, Buggy BP, Forbes BA. Bacteremia caused by *Achromobacter* species in an immunocompromised host. J Clin Microbiol 1984;19:947–948.

402. Kishimoto RA, Brown GL, Blair EB, et al. Melioidosis: serologic studies on U.S. army personnel returning from Southeast Asia. Milit Med 1971;136:694–698.

403. Kiska DL, Gilligan PH. *Pseudomonas*. In: Murray PR, Baron EJ, Jorgensen JH, et al., eds. Manual of Clinical Microbiology. Ed. 8. Washington DC: ASM Press, 2003:719–728.

404. Kiska DL, Kerr A, Jones MC, et al. Accuracy of four commercial systems for identification of *Burkholderia cepacia* and other gram-negative nonfermenting bacilli recovered from patients with cystic fibrosis. J Clin Microbiol 1996;34:886–891.

405. Kitch T, Jacobs MR, Appelbaum PC. Evaluation of the 4-hour RapID NF Plus method for identification of 345 gram-negative non-fermentative rods. J Clin Microbiol 1992;30:1267–1270.

406. Kivinen PK, Lahtinen M-R, Ruotsalainen E, et al. *Bergeyella zoohelcum* septicaemia of a patient suffering from severe skin infection. Acta Derm Venereol 2003;83:74–75.

407. Klausner JD, Zukerman, C, Limaye AP, et al. Outbreak of *Stenotrophomonas maltophilia* bacteremia among patients undergoing bone marrow transplantation: association with faulty replacement handwashing soap. Infect Control Hosp Epidemiol 1999;20:756–758.

408. Knuth BD, Owen MR, Latorraca R. Occurrence of an unclassified organism group IVd. Am J Med Technol 1969;35:227–232.

409. Kociuba K, Munro R, Daley D. M-6 endocarditis: report of an Australian case. Pathology 1993;25:310–312.

410. Kodaka H, Armfield AY, Lombard GL, Dowell VR. Practical procedure for demonstrating bacterial flagella. J Clin Microbiol 1982;16:948–952.

411. Koestenblatt EK, Larone DH, Pavletich KJ. Comparison of the Oxi/Ferm and N/F systems for identification of infrequently encountered nonfermentative and oxidase-positive fermentative bacilli. J Clin Microbiol 1982;15:384–390.

412. Koh TH, Ng LSY, Ho JLF, et al. Automated identification systems and *Burkholderia pseudomallei*. J Clin Microbiol 2003;41:1809.

413. Koide M, Miyata T, Nukina M, et al. A strain of *Pseudomonas vesicularis* isolated from shower hose which supports the multiplication of Legionella. Kansenshogaku Zasshi 1989;63:1160–1164.

414. Kosako Y, Yabuuchi E, Naka T, et al. Proposal of *Sphingomonadaceae* fam. nov., consisting of *Sphingomonas* Yabuuchi et al. 1990, *Erythrobacter* Shiba and Shimidu 1982, *Erythromicrobium* Yurkov et al. 1994, *Porphyrobacter* Fuerst et al. 1993, *Zymomonas* Kluyver and van Niel 1936, and *Sandaracinobacter* Yurkov et al. 1997, with the type genus *Sphingomonas* Yabuuchi et al. 1990. Microbiol Immunol 2000;44:563–575.

415. Kostman JR, Soloman F, Fekete T. Infections with *Chryseomonas luteola* (CDC Group Ve-1) and *Flavimonas oryzihabitans* (CDC Group Ve-2) in neurosurgical patients Rev. Infect Dis 1991;13:233–236.

416. Labarca JA, Leber AL, Kern VL, et al. Outbreak of *Stenotrophomonas maltophilia* bacteremia in allogenic bone marrow transplant patients: role of severe neutropenia and mucositis. Clin Infect Dis 2000;30:195–197.

417. Labarca JA, Pegues DA, Wagar EA, et al. Something's rotten: a nosocomial outbreak of malodorous *Pseudomonas aeruginosa*. Clin Infect Dis 1998;26:1440–1446.

418. Labarca JA, Trick WE, Peterson CL, et al. A multistate nosocomial outbreak of *Ralstonia pickettii* colonization associated with an intrinsically contaminated respiratory care solution. Clin Infect Dis 1999;29:1281–1286.

419. Lacy DE, Spencer DA, Goldstein A, et al. Chronic granulomatous disease presenting in childhood with *Pseudomonas cepacia* septicaemia. J Infect 1993;27:301–304.

419a. Laffineur K, Janssens M, Charlier J, et al. Biochemical and susceptibility tests useful for identification of nonfermenting gram-negative rods. J Clin Microbiol 2002;40:1085–1087.

420. Lai C-C, Teng L-J, Hsueh P-R, et al. Clinical and microbiological characteristics of *Rhizobium radiobacter* infections. Clin Infect Dis 2004;38:149–153.

421. Lambert WC, Pathan AK, Imaeda T, et al. Culture of *Vibrio extorquens* from severe, chronic skin ulcers in a Puerto Rican woman. J Am Acad Dermatol 1983;9:262–268.

422. Lampe AS, van der Reijden TJK. Evaluation of commercial test systems for the identification of nonfermenters. Eur J Clin Microbiol 1984;3:301–305.

423. La Scola B, Birtles RJ, Mallet M-N, et al. *Massilia timonae* gen. nov., sp. nov., isolated from blood of an immunocompromised patient with cerebellar lesions. J Clin Microbiol 1998;36:2847–2852.

424. Lau SKP, Woo PCY, Hui W-T, et al. Use of cefoperazone MacConkey agar for selective isolation of *Laribacter hongkongensis*. J Clin Microbiol 2003;41:4839–4841.

425. Laukeland H, Bergh K, Bevanger L. Posttrabeculectomy endophthalmitis caused by *Moraxella nonliquefaciens*. J Clin Microbiol 2002;40:2668–2670.

426. Lazarus HM, Magalhaes-Silverman M, Fox RM, et al. Contamination during in vitro processing of bone marrow for transplantation: clinical significance. Bone Marrow Transplant 1991;7:241–246.

427. Lechner A, Bruckner DA. *Oligella ureolytica* in blood culture: contaminant or infection? Eur J Clin Microbiol Infect Dis 2001;20:142–143.

428. Leelarasamee A, Bovornkitti S. Melioidosis: review and update. Rev Infect Dis 1989;11:413–425.

429. Leifson E. Atlas of Bacterial Flagellation. New York:, Academic Press, 1960.

430. Lejbkowicz F, Belavsky L, Kudinsky R, et al. Bacteraemia and sinusitis due to *Flavimonas oryzihabitans* infection. Scand J Infect Dis 2003;35:411–414.

431. Lema I, Gomez-Torreiro M, Rodriguez-Ares MT. *Comamonas acidovorans* keratitis in a hydrogel contact lens wearer. CLAO J 2001;27:55–56.

432. Le Moal G, Paccalin M, Breux JP, et al. Central venous catheter-related infection due to *Comamonas testosteroni* in a woman with breast cancer. Scand J Infect Dis 2001;33:627–628.

433. Lertpatanasuwan N, Sermsri K, Petkaseam A, et al. Arabinose-positive *Burkholderia pseudomallei* infection in humans: case report. Clin Infect Dis 1999;28:927–928.

434. Levin AS: Multiresistant *Acinetobacter* infections: a role for sulbactam combinations in overcoming an emerging worldwide problem. Clin Microbiol Infect 2002;8:144–153.

435. Levin AS, Barone A, Penco J, et al. Intravenous colistin as therapy for nosocomial infections caused by multidrug-resistant *Pseudomonas aeruginosa* and *Acinetobacter baumannii*. Clin Infect Dis 1999;28:1008–1011.

436. Levy P-Y, Tessier JL. Arthritis due to *Shewanella putrefaciens*. Clin Infect Dis 1998;26:536.

437. Lewin LO, Byard PJ, Davis PB. Effect of *Pseudomonas cepacia* colonization on survival and pulmonary function of patients with cystic fibrosis. J Clin Epidemiol 1990;43:125–131.

438. Lewis L, Stock F, Williams D, et al. Infections with *Roseomonas gilardii* and review of characteristics used for biochemical identification and molecular typing. Am J Clin Pathol 1997;108:210–216.

439. Li X, Dorsch M, Del Dot T, et al. Phylogenetic studies of the rRNA group II pseudomonads based on 16S rRNA gene sequences. J Appl Bacteriol 1993;74:324–329.

440. Lin P-Y, Chu C, Su L-H, et al. Clinical and microbiological analysis of blood-

stream infections caused by *Chryseobacterium meningosepticum* in nonneonatal patients. J Clin Microbiol 2004;42:3353–3355.

441. Lin R-D, Hsueh P-R, Chang J-C, et al. *Flavimonas oryzihabitans* bacteremia: clinical features and microbiological characteristics of isolates. Clin Infect Dis 1997;24:867–873.

442. Linde H-J, Hahn J, Holler E, et al. Septicemia due to *Acinetobacter junii*. J Clin Microbiol 2002;40:2696–2697.

443. Lindquist D, Murrill D, Burran WP, et al. Characteristics of *Massilia timonae* and *Massilia timonae*-like isolates from human patients, with an emended description of the species. J Clin Microbiol 2003;41:192–196.

444. Lindquist SW, Weber DJ, Mangum ME, et al. *Bordetella holmesii* sepsis in an asplenic adolescent. Pediatr Infect Dis J 1995;14:813–815.

444a. Lindsay JA, Riley TV. Susceptibility of desferrioxamine: a new test for the identification of *Staphylococcus epidermidis* J Med Microbiol 1991;35:45–48.

445. LiPuma JJ. *Burkholderia cepacia*. Management issues and new insights. Clin Chest Med 1998;19:473–486.

446. LiPuma JJ, Dasen SE Nielson DW, et al. Person-to-person transmission of *Pseudomonas cepacia* between patients with cystic fibrosis. Lancet 1990;336: 1094–1096.

447. LiPuma JJ, Marks-Austin KA, Holsclaw DS Jr, et al. Inapparent transmission of *Pseudomonas (Burkholderia) cepacia* among patients with cystic fibrosis. Pediatr Infect Dis J 1994;13:716–719.

448. LiPuma JJ, Spilker T, Gill LH, et al. Disproportionate distribution of *Burkholderia cepacia* complex species and transmissibility markers in cystic fibrosis. Am J Respir Crit Care Med 2001;164:92–96.

449. List Editor, IJSEM. Notification that new names and new combinations have appeared in volume 51, part 2, of the IJSEM. Int J Syst Evol Microbiol 2001; 51:795–796.

450. Liu J-W, Wu J-J, Chen H-M, et al. *Methylobacterium mesophilicum* synovitis in an alcoholic. Clin Infect Dis 1997;24:1008–1009.

451. Livermore, DM: Multiple mechanisms of antimicrobial resistance in *Pseudomonas aeruginosa*: our worst nightmare? Clin Infect Dis 2002;34:634–640.

452. Lloyd-Puryear M, Wallace D, Baldwin T, et al. Meningitis caused by *Psychrobacter immobilis* in an infant. J Clin Microbiol 1991;29:2041–2042.

453. Lobue TD, Deutsch TA, Stein RM: *Moraxella nonliquefaciens* endophthalmitis after trabeculectomy. Am J Ophthalmol 1985;99:343–345.

454. Loeffelholz MJ, Thompson CJ, Long KS, et al. Detection of *Bordetella holmesii* using *Bordetella pertussis* IS*481* PCR assay. J Clin Microbiol 2000;38:467.

455. Lopez-Menchero R, Siguenza F, Caridad A, et al. Peritonitis due to *Comamonas acidovorans* in a CAPD patient. Perit Dial Int 1998;18:445–446.

456. Lorenzo-Pajuelo B, Villanueva JL, Rodriguez-Cuesta J, et al. Cavitary pneumonia in an AIDS patient caused by an unusual *Bordetella bronchiseptica* variant producing reduced amounts of pertactin and other major antigens. J Clin Microbiol 2002;40:3146–54.

457. Lortholary O, Fagon J-Y, Hoi AB, et al. Nosocomial acquisition of multiresistant *Acinetobacter baumannii*: risk factors and prognosis. Clin Infect Dis 1995;20: 790–796.

458. Loubinoux J, Mihaila-Amrouche L, Le Fleche A, et al. Bacteremia caused by *Acinetobacter ursingii*. J Clin Microbiol 2003;41:1337–1338.

459. Loukil C, Saizou C, Doit C, et al. Epidemiologic investigation of *Burkholderia cepacia* acquisition in two pediatric intensive care units. Infect Control Hosp Epidemiol 2003;24:707–710.

460. Lowe P, Engler C, Norton R. Comparison of automated and nonautomated systems for identification of *Burkholderia pseudomallei*. J Clin Microbiol 2002; 40:4625–4627.

461. Lu PC, Chan JC. *Flavobacterium indologenes* keratitis. Ophthalmologica 1997; 211:98–100.

462. Lucas KG, Kiehn TE, Sobeck KA, et al. Sepsis caused by *Flavimonas oryzihabitans*. Medicine (Baltimore) 1994;73:209–214.

463. Lyons RW. Ecology, clinical significance and antimicrobial susceptibility of *Acinetobacter* and *Moraxella*. In: Gilardi GL. ed. Nonfermentative Gram-Negative Rods: Laboratory Identification and Clinical Aspects.: New York: Marcel Dekker, 1985159–179.

464. Macdonell MT, Colwell RR. Phylogeny of the *Vibrionaceae*, and recommendation for two new genera, *Listonella* and *Shewanella*. Syst Appl Microbiol 1985; 6:171–182.

465. MacFaddin JF. Biochemical Tests for Identification of Medical Bacteria. Ed. 3. Philadelphia: Lippincott Williams & Wilkins, 2000.

466. MacFarlane L, Oppenheim BA, Lorrigan P. Septicaemia and septic arthritis due to *Pseudomonas putida* in a neutropenic patient. J Infect 1991;23:346–347.

467. Maderazo EG, Bassaris HP, Quintiliani R. *Flavobacterium meningosepticum* meningitis in a newborn infant. Treatment with intraventricular erythromycin. J Pediatr 1974;85:675–676.

468. Madhavan T. Septic arthritis with *Pseudomonas stutzeri*. Ann Intern Med 1974; 80:670–671.

469. Madhavan T, Fisher EJ, Cox F, et al. *Pseudomonas putida* and septic arthritis. Ann Intern Med 1973;78:971–972.

470. Mahenthiralingam E, Baldwin A, Vandamme P. *Burkholderia cepacia* complex infection in patients with cystic fibrosis. J Med Microbiol 2002;51:533–538.

471. Mahenthiralingam E, Simpson DA, Speert DP. Identification and characterization of a novel DNA marker associated with epidemic *Burkholderia cepacia* strains recovered from patients with cystic fibrosis. J Clin Microbiol 1997;35: 808–816.

472. Mahenthiralingam E, Vandamme P, Campbell ME, et al. Infection with *Burkholderia cepacia* complex genomovars in patients with cystic fibrosis: virulent transmissible strains of genomovar III can replace *Burkholderia multivorans*. Clin Infect Dis 2001;33:1469–1475.

473. Mahmood MS, Sarwari AR, Khan MA, et al. Infective endocarditis and septic embolization with *Ochrobactrum anthropi*: case report and review of literature. J Infect 2000;40:287–290.

474. Manfredi R, Nanetti A, Ferri M, Calza L, et al. *Ochrobactrum anthropi* as an agent of nosocomial septicemia in the setting of AIDS. Clin Infect Dis 1999; 28:692–694.

475. Manfredi R, Nanetti A, Ferri M, Mastroianni A, et al. Emerging gram-negative pathogens in the immunocompromised host: *Agrobacterium radiobacter* septicemia during HIV disease. Microbiologica 1999;22:375–382.

476. Mani RM, Kuruvila KC, Batliwala PM, et al. *Flavobacterium meningosepticum* as an opportunist. J Clin Pathol 1978;31:220–222.

477. Manian FA. Bloodstream infection with *Oligella ureolytica*, Candida krusei, Bacteroides species in a patient with AIDS. Clin Infect Dis 1993;17:290–291.

478. Manikal VM, Landman D, Saurina G, et al. Endemic carbapenem-resistant *Acinetobacter* species in Brooklyn, New York: citywide prevalence, interinstitutional spread, and relation to antibiotic usage. Clin Infect Dis 2000;31:101–106.

479. Manno G, Dalmastri C, Tabacchioni S, et al. Epidemiology and clinical course of *Burkholderia cepacia* complex infections, particularly those caused by different *Burkholderia cenocepacia* strains, among patients attending an Italian cystic fibrosis center. J Clin Microbiol 2004;42:1491–1497.

480. Mardy C, Holmes B. Incidence of vaginal *Weeksella virosa* (formerly group IIf). J Clin Pathol 1988;41:211–214.

481. Marin M, Garcia de Viedma D, Martin-Rabadan P, et al. Infection of Hickman catheter by *Pseudomonas* (formerly *Flavimonas*) *oryzihabitans* traced to a synthetic bath sponge. J Clin Microbiol 2000;38:4577–4579.

482. Marin M, Marco Del Pont J, Dibar E, et al. Catheter-related bacteremia caused by *Roseomonas gilardii* in an immunocompromised patient. Int J Infect Dis 2001;5:170–171.

483. Marinella MA. Cellulitis and sepsis due to *Sphingobacterium*. JAMA 2002;288: 23.

484. Marne C, Pallares R, Sitges-Serra A. Isolation of *Pseudomonas putrefaciens* in intra-abdominal sepsis. J Clin Microbiol 1983;17:1173–1174.

485. Maroye P, Doermann HP, Rogues AM, et al. Investigation of an outbreak of *Ralstonia pickettii* in a paediatric hospital by RAPD. J Hosp Infect 2000;44: 267–272.

486. Marraro RV, Mitchell JL, Payet CR. A chromogenic characteristic of an aerobic pseudomonad species in 2% tryptone (indole) broth. J Am Med Technol 1977; 39:13–19.

487. Marroni M, Pasticci MB, Pantosti A, et al. Outbreak of infusion-related septicemia by *Ralstonia pickettii* in the oncology department. Tumori 2003;89: 575–576.

488. Marshall WF, Keating MR, Anhalt JP, et al. *Xanthomonas maltophilia*: an emerging nosocomial pathogen. Mayo Clin Proc 1989;64:1097–1104.

489. Martin R, Siavoshi F, McDougal DL: Comparison of rapid NFT system and conventional methods for identification of nonsaccharolytic gram-negative bacteria. J Clin Microbiol 1986;24:1089–1092.

490. Martino R, Martinez C, Pericas R, et al. Bacteremia due to glucose non-fermenting gram-negative bacilli in patients with hematological neoplasias and solid tumors. Eur J Clin Microbiol Infect Dis 1996;15:610–615.

491. Martino R, Pericas R, Romero P, et al. CDC group IV c-2 bacteremia in stem cell transplant recipients. Bone Marrow Transplant 1998;22:401–402.

492. May TB, Shinabarger D, Maharaj R, et al. Alginate synthesis by *Pseudomonas aeruginosa*: a key pathogenic factor in chronic pulmonary infections of patients with cystic fibrosis. Clin Microbiol Rev 1991;4:191–206.

493. Mayfield CI, Innis WE. A rapid, simple method for staining bacterial flagella. Can J Microbiol 1977;23:1311–1313.

494. Mazengia E, Silva EA, Peppe JA, et al. Recovery of *Bordetella holmesii* from patients with pertussis-like symptoms: use of pulsed-field gel electrophoresis to characterize circulating strains. J Clin Microbiol 2000;38:2330–2333.

495. McKinley KP, Laundy TJ, Masterton RG. *Achromobacter* group B replacement valve endocarditis. J Infect 1990;20:262–263.

496. McMenamin JD, Zaccone TM, Coenye T, et al. Misidentification of *Burkholderia cepacia* in US cystic fibrosis treatment centers: an analysis of 1,051 recent sputum isolates. Chest 2000;117:1661–1665.

497. Meis JFGM, van Griethuijsen AJA, Muytjens HL. *Bordetella bronchiseptica* bronchitis in an immunosuppressed patient. Eur J Clin Microbiol Infect Dis 1990;9:366–367.

498. Mesnard R, Guiso N, Michelet C, et al. Isolation of *Bordetella bronchiseptica* from a patient with AIDS. Eur J Clin Microbiol Infect Dis 1993;12:304–306.

499. Mesnard R, Sire JM, Donnio PY, et al. Septic arthritis due to *Oligella urethralis.* Eur J Clin Microbiol Infect Dis 1992;11:195–196.

500. Meuleman P, Erard K, Herregods MC, et al. Bioprosthetic valve endocarditis caused by *Neisseria elongata* subspecies *nitroreducens.* Infection 1996;24:258–260.

501. Micozzi A, Venditti M, Monaco M, et al. Bacteremia due to *Stenotrophomonas maltophilia* in patients with hematologic malignancies. Clin Infect Dis 2000;31:705–711.

502. Miller JM, Alachi P. Evaluation of new computer-enhanced identification program for microorganisms: adaption of BioBASE for identification of members of the family Enterobacteriaceae. J Clin Microbiol 1996;34:179–181.

503. Miller JM, Novy C, Hiott M. Case of bacterial endophthalmitis caused by an *Agrobacterium radiobacter*-like organism. J Clin Microbiol 1996;34:3212–3213.

504. Moissenet D, Tabone M-D, Girardet J-P, et al. Nosocomial CDC group IV c-2 bacteremia: epidemiological investigation by randomly amplified polymorphic DNA analysis. J Clin Microbiol 1996;34:1264–1266.

505. Möller LVM Arends JP, Harmsen HJM, et al. *Ochrobactrum intermedium* infection after liver transplantation. J Clin Microbiol 1999;37:241–244.

506. Montejo M, Aguirrebengoa K, Ugalde J, et al. *Bergeyella zoohelcum* bacteremia after a dog bite. Clin Infect Dis 2001;33:1608–1609.

507. Moore JE, Reid A, Millar BC, et al. *Pandoraea apista* isolated from a patient with cystic fibrosis: problems associated with laboratory identification. Br J Biomed Sci 2002;59:164–166.

508. Morris JT, Myers M. Bacteremia due to *Bordetella holmesii.* Clin Infect Dis 1998;27:912–913.

509. Morris MJ, Young VM, Moody MR. Evaluation of a multitest system for identification of saccharolytic pseudomonads. Am J Clin Pathol 1978;69:41–47.

510. Morrison AJ, Boyce K. Peritonitis caused by *Alcaligenes denitrificans* subsp. *xylosoxidans:* case report and review of the literature. J Clin Microbiol 1986;24:879–881.

511. Morrison AJ, Hoffmann KK, Wenzel RP. Associated mortality and clinical characteristics of nosocomial *Pseudomonas maltophilia* in a university hospital. J Clin Microbiol 1986;24:52–55.

512. Morrison AJ, Shulman JA. Community-acquired bloodstream infection caused by *Pseudomonas paucimobilis*: case report and review of literature. J Clin Microbiol 1986;24:853–855.

513. Morrison RE, Lamb AS, Craig DB, et al. Melioidosis: a reminder. Am J Med 1988;84:965–967.

514. Mortensen JE, Schidlow DV, Stahl EM. *Pseudomonas gladioli* (*marginata*) isolated from a patient with cystic fibrosis. Clin Microbiol Newslett 1988;10:29–30.

515. Moss CW, Daneshvar MI, Hollis DG. Biochemical characteristics and fatty acid composition of Gilardi Rod Group 1 bacteria. J Clin Microbiol 1993;31:689–691.

516. Moss CW, Kaltenbach CM. Production of glutaric acid: a useful criterion for differentiating *Pseudomonas diminuta* from *Pseudomonas vesiculare.* Appl Microbiol 1974;27:437–439.

517. Moss CW, Wallace PL, Hollis DG, et al. Cultural and chemical characterization of CDC groups EO-2, M-5, and M-6, *Moraxella* (*Moraxella*) species, *Oligella urethralis, Acinetobacter* species, and *Psychrobacter immobilis.* J Clin Microbiol 1988;26:484–492.

518. Moss RB. Cystic fibrosis: pathogenesis, pulmonary infection, and treatment. Clin Infect Dis 1995;21:839–851.

519. Muder RR, Harris AP, Muller S, et al. Bacteremia due to *Stenotrophomonas* (*Xanthomonas*) *maltophilia*: a prospective, multicenter study of 91 episodes. Clin Infect Dis 1996;22:508–512.

520. Muder RR, Yu VL, Dummer JS, Vinson C, Lumish RM. Infections caused by *Pseudomonas maltophilia.* Arch Intern Med 1987;147:1672–1674.

521. Murray AE, Bartzokas CA, Shepherd AJ, et al. Blood transfusion-associated *Pseudomonas fluorescens* septicaemia: is this an increasing problem? J Hosp Infect 1987;9:243–248.

522. Musso D, Drancourt M, Bardot J, et al. Human infection due to the CDC group IVc-2 bacterium: case report and review. Clin Infect Dis 1994;18:482–484.

523. Nadler H, George H, Barr J. Accuracy and reproducibility of the Oxi-Ferm system in identifying a select group of unusual gram-negative bacilli. J Clin Microbiol 1978;9:180–185.

524. Nagano N, Sato J, Cordevant C, et al. Presumed endocarditis caused by BRO β-lactamase-producing *Moraxella lacunata* in an infant with Fallot's tetrad. J Clin Microbiol 2003;41:5310–5312.

525. Nahass RG, Wisneski R, Herman DJ, et al. Vertebral osteomyelitis due to *Roseomonas* species: case report and review of the evaluation of vertebral osteomyelitis. Clin Infect Dis 1995;21:1474–1476.

526. Namdari H, Hamzavi S, Peairs RR. *Rhizobium (Agrobacterium) radiobacter* identified as a cause of chronic endophthalmitis subsequent to cataract extraction. J Clin Microbiol 2003;41:3998–4000.

527. Namnyak S, Hussain S, Davalle J, et al. Contaminated lithium heparin bottles as a source of pseudobacteraemia due to *Pseudomonas fluorescens,* J Hosp Infect 1999;41:23–28.

528. Nawaz T, Hardy DJ, Bonnez W. *Neisseria elongata* subsp. *elongata,* a cause of human endocarditis complicated by pseudoaneurysm. J Clin Microbiol 1996;34:756–758.

529. National Committee for Clinical Laboratory Standards. Abbreviated Identification of Bacteria and Yeast; Approved Guideline. NCCLS document M35-A. Wayne, PA: NCCLS, 2002.

530. Nemec A, De Baere T, Tjernberg I, et al. *Acinetobacter ursingii* sp. nov. and *Acinetobacter schindleri* sp. nov., isolated from human clinical specimens. Int J Syst Evol Microbiol 2001;51:1891–1899.

531. Nemec A, Dijkshoorn L, Cleenwerck I, et al. *Acinetobacter parvus* sp. nov., a small-colony-forming species isolated from human clinical specimens. Int J Syst Evol Microbiol 2003;53:1563–1567.

532. Nemec A, Dijkshoorn L, Jezek P. Recognition of two novel phenons of the genus *Acinetobacter* among non-glucose-acidifying isolates from human specimens. J Clin Microbiol 2000;38:3937–3941.

533. Neu HC, Saha G, Chin N-X. Resistance of *Xanthomonas maltophilia* to antibiotics and the effect of beta-lactamase inhibitors. Diagn Microbiol Infect Dis 1989;12:283–285.

534. Ng VL, Boggs JM, York MK, et al. Recovery of *Bordetella bronchiseptica* from patients with AIDS. Clin Infect Dis 1992;15:376–377.

535. Njamkepo E, Delisle F, Hagege I, et al. *Bordetella holmesii* isolated from a patient with sickle cell anemia: analysis and comparison with other *Bordetella holmesii* isolates. Clin Microbiol Infect 2000;6:131–136.

536. Noell F, Gorce MF, Garde C, et al. Isolation of *Weeksella zoohelcum* in septicaemia. Lancet 1989;2:332.

537. Nord C-E, Wretlind B, Dahlback A. Evaluation of two test kits—API and Oxi/Ferm tube—for identification of oxidative-fermentative gram-negative rods. Med Microbiol Immunol 1977;163:93–97.

538. Noyola DE, Edwards MS. Bacteremia with CDC group IV c-2 in an immunocompetent infant. Clin Infect Dis 1999;29:1572.

539. Nozue H, Hayashi T, Hashimoto Y, et al. Isolation and characterization of *Shewanella alga* from human clinical specimens and emendation of the description of *S. alga* Simidu et al., 1990, 335. Int J Syst Bacteriol 1992;42:628–634.

540. Nulens E, Bussels B, Bols A, et al. Recurrent bacteremia by *Chryseobacterium indologenes* in an oncology patient with a totally implanted intravascular device. Clin Microbiol Infect 2001;7:391–393.

541. Nzula S, Vandamme P, Govan JRW. Influence of taxonomic status on the in vitro antimicrobial susceptibility of the *Burkholderia cepacia* complex. J Antimicrob Chemother 2002;50:265–269.

542. Oberhelman RA, Humbert JR, Santorelli FW. *Pseudomonas vesicularis* causing bacteremia in a child with sickle cell anemia. South Med J 1994;87:821–822.

543. Oberhofer TR. Comparison of the API 20E and Oxi/Ferm systems in identification of nonfermentative and oxidase-positive fermentative bacteria. J Clin Microbiol 1979;9:220–226.

544. Oberhofer TR. Use of the API 20E, Oxi/Ferm and Minitek systems to identify nonfermentative and oxidase-positive fermentative bacteria: seven years of experience. Diagn Microbiol Infect Dis 1983;1:241–256.

545. Oberhofer TR. Manual of Nonfermenting Gram-Negative Bacteria. New York: Wiley, 1985.

546. Oberhofer TR. Rapid identification of glucose-nonfermenting gram-negative rods with commercial miniaturized kits. In: Gilardi GL, ed. Nonfermentative Gram-Negative Rods: Laboratory Identification and Clinical Aspects. New York: Marcel Dekker, 1985:85–116.

547. Oberhofer TR, Rowen JW, Cunningham GF, et al. Evaluation of the Oxi/Ferm tube system with selected gram-negative bacteria. J Clin Microbiol 1977;6:559–566.

548. O'Hara CM, Tenover FC, Miller JM. Parallel comparison of accuracy of API 20E, Vitek GNI, MicroScan Walk/Away Rapid ID, and Becton Dickinson Cobas Micro ID-E/NF for identification of members of the family Enterobacteriaceae and common gram-negative, non-glucose-fermenting bacilli. J Clin Microbiol 1993;31:3165–3169.

549. O'Leary T, Fong IW. Prosthetic valve endocarditis caused by group Ve-1 bacteria. J Clin Microbiol 1984;20:995.

550. Olsen H, Frederiksen WC, Siboni KE. *Flavobacterium meningosepticum* in 8 non-fatal cases of postoperative bacteraemia. Lancet 1965;1:1294–1296.

551. O'Neil KM, Herman JH, Modlin JF, et al. *Pseudomonas cepacia*: an emerging pathogen in chronic granulomatous disease. J Pediatr 1986;108:940–942.

552. Ophel K, Kerr A. *Agrobacterium vitis* sp. nov. for strains of *Agrobacterium* biovar 3 from grapevines. Int J Syst Bacteriol 1990;40:236–241.

553. Ostergaard L, Andersen PL. Etiology of community-acquired pneumonia: evaluation by transtracheal aspiration, blood culture, or serology. Chest 1993;104:1400–1407.

554. Otto LA, Blachman U. Nonfermentative bacilli: evaluation of three systems for identification. J Clin Microbiol 1979;10:147–154.

555. Otto LA, Deboo BS, Capers EL, et al. *Pseudomonas vesicularis* from cervical specimens. J Clin Microbiol 1978;7:341–345.

556. Otto LA, Pickett MJ: Rapid method for identification of gram-negative, nonfermentative bacilli. J Clin Microbiol 1976;3:566–575.

557. Owen RJ, Legros RM, Lapage SP. Base composition, size and sequence similarities of genome deoxyribonucleic acids from clinical isolates of *Pseudomonas putrefaciens*. J Gen Microbiol 1978;104:127–138.

558. Pagani L, Lang A, Vedovelli C, et al. Soft tissue infection and bacteremia caused by *Shewanella putrefaciens*. J Clin Microbiol 2003;41:2240–2241.

559. Pallent LJ, Hugo WB, Grant DJW, et al. *Pseudomonas cepacia* as contaminant and infective agent. J Hosp Infect 1983;4:9–13.

560. Palleroni NJ. Family I. *Pseudomonadaceae*. In: Krieg NR, Holt JG, eds. Bergey's Manual of Systematic Bacteriology. Vol. 1. Baltimore: Williams & Wilkins, 1984:141–219.

561. Palleroni NJ, Bradbury JF. *Stenotrophomonas*, a new bacterial genus for *Xanthomonas maltophilia* (Hugh 1980) Swings et al. 1983. Int J Syst Bacteriol 1993; 43:606–609.

562. Panagea S, Bijoux R, Corkill JE, et al. A case of lower respiratory tract infection caused by *Neisseria weaveri* and review of the literature. J Infect 2002;44:96–98.

563. Pandey A, Kapil A, Sood S, et al. In vitro activities of ampicillin-sulbactam and amoxicillin-clavulanic acid against *Acinetobacter baumannii*. J Clin Microbiol 1998;36:3415–3416.

564. Pankuch GA, Jacobs MR, Rittenhouse SF, et al. Susceptibilities of 123 strains of *Xanthomonas maltophilia* to eight β-lactams (including β-lactam-β-lactamase inhibitor combinations) and ciprofloxacin tested by five methods. Antimicrob Agents Chemother 1994;38:2317–2322.

565. Panlilio AL, Beck-Sague CM, Siegel JD, et al. Infections and pseudoinfections due to povidone-iodine solution contaminated with *Pseudomonas cepacia*. Clin Infect Dis 1992;14:1078–1083.

566. Papadakis KA, Vartivarian SE, Vassilaki ME, et al. *Stenotrophomonas maltophilia*: an unusual cause of biliary sepsis. Clin Infect Dis 1995;21:1032–1034.

567. Papadakis KA, Vartivarian SE, Vassilaki ME, et al. *Stenotrophomonas maltophilia* meningitis. Report of two cases and review of the literature. J Neurosurg 1997;87:106–108.

568. Parke JL, Gurian-Sherman D. Diversity of the *Burkholderia cepacia* complex and implications for risk assessment of biological control strains. Annu Rev Phytopathol 2001;39:225–258.

569. Parkhill J, Sebaihia M, Preston A, et al. Comparative analysis of the genome sequences of *Bordetella pertussis*, *Bordetella parapertussis* and *Bordetella bronchiseptica*. Nat Genet 2003;35:32–40.

570. Pedersen MM, Marso E, Pickett MJ. Nonfermentative bacilli associated with man: III. Pathogenicity and antibiotic susceptibility. Am J Clin Pathol 1970;54: 178–192.

571. Peel MM, Hibberd AJ, King BM, et al. *Alcaligenes piechaudii* from chronic ear discharge. J Clin Microbiol 1988;26:1580–1581.

572. Peetermans WE, van Wijngaerden E, van Eldere J, et al. Melioidosis brain and lung abscess after travel to Sri Lanka. Clin Infect Dis 1999;28:921–922.

573. Peiris V, Fraser S, Fairhurst M, et al. Laboratory diagnosis of *Brucella* infection: some pitfalls. Lancet 1992;339:1415–1416.

574. Perez RE. Endocarditis with *Moraxella*-like M-6 after cardiac catheterization. J Clin Microbiol 1986;24:501–502.

575. Perola O, Nousiainen T, Suomalainen S, et al. Recurrent *Sphingomonas paucimobilis*-bacteraemia associated with a multi-bacterial water-borne epidemic among neutropenic patients. J Hosp Infect 2002;50:196–201.

576. Petrocheilou-Paschou V, Georgilis K, Kostis E, et al. Bronchitis caused by *Bordetella bronchiseptica* in an elderly woman. Clin Microbiol Infect 2000;6: 147–148.

577. Pettersson B, Kodjo A, Ronaghi M, et al. Phylogeny of the family *Moraxellaceae* by 16S rDNA sequence analysis, with special emphasis on differentiation of *Moraxella* species. Int J Syst Bacteriol 1998;48:75–89.

578. Pfaller MA, Sahm D, O'Hara C, et al. Comparison of the AutoSCAN-W/A rapid bacterial identification system and the Vitek AutoMicrobic system for identification of gram-negative bacilli. J Clin Microbiol 21991;9:1422–1428.

579. Phillips I, Eykyn S. Contaminated drip fluids. BMJ 1972;1:746.

580. Phillips I, Eykyn S, Laker M. Outbreak of hospital infection caused by contaminated autoclave fluids. Lancet 1972;1:1258–1260.

581. Pickett MJ. Nonfermentative Gram-Negative Bacilli: A Syllabus for Detection and Identification. Los Angeles: Scientific Development Press, 1980.

582. Pickett MJ. Methods for identification of flavobacteria. J Clin Microbiol 1989; 27:2309–2315.

583. Pickett MJ. Typing of strains from a single-source outbreak of *Pseudomonas pickettii*. J Clin Microbiol 1994;32:1132–1133.

584. Pickett MJ. Identification of *Brucella* species with a procedure for detecting acidification of glucose. Clin Infect Dis 1994;19:976.

585. Pickett MJ. Moraxellae: differential features for identification of *Moraxella atlantae*, *M. lacunata*, and *M. nonliquefaciens*. Med Microbiol Lett 1994;3: 397–400.

586. Pickett MJ, Greenwood JR. A study of the Va-1 group of pseudomonads and its relationship to *Pseudomonas pickettii*. J Gen Microbiol 1980;120:439–446.

587. Pickett MJ, Hollis DG, Bottone EJ. Miscellaneous gram-negative bacteria. In: Balows A, ed. Manual of Clinical Microbiology. Ed. 5. Washington, DC: American Society for Microbiology, 1991:410–428.

588. Pickett MJ, Nelson EL. 1955. Speciation within the genus *Brucella* IV. Fermentation of carbohydrates. J Bacteriol 1995;69:333–336.

589. Pickett MJ, Pedersen MM. Characterization of saccharolytic nonfermentative bacteria associated with man. Can J Microbiol 1970;16:351–362.

590. Pickett MJ, Pedersen MM. Nonfermentative bacilli associated with man: II. Detection and identification. Am J Clin Pathol 1970;54:164–177.

591. Pickett MJ, von Graevenitz A, Pfyffer GE, et al. Phenotypic features distinguishing *Oligella urethralis* from *Moraxella osloensis*. Med Microbiol Lett 1996;5: 265–270.

592. Picu C, Mille C, Popescu GA, et al. Aortic prosthetic endocarditis with *Neisseria elongata* subspecies *nitroreducens*. Scand J Infect Dis 2003;35:280–282.

593. Pien FD, Chung EYS. Group Ve infection: case report of group Ve-2 septicemia and literature review. Diagn Microbiol Infect Dis 1986;5:177–180.

594. Pike RM. Laboratory-associated infections: summary and analysis of 3921 cases. Health Lab Sci 1976;13:105–114.

595. Pitulle C, Citron DM, Bochner B, et al. Novel bacterium isolated from a lung transplant patient with cystic fibrosis. J Clin Microbiol 1999;37:3851–3855.

596. Planes AM, Ramirez A, Fernandez F, et al. *Pseudomonas vesicularis* bacteraemia. Infection 1992;0:367–368.

597. Platsouka E, Routsi C, Chalkis A, et al. *Stenotrophomonas maltophilia* meningitis, bacteremia and respiratory infection. Scand J Infect Dis 2002;4:391–392.

598. Plotkin GR. *Agrobacterium radiobacter* prosthetic valve endocarditis. Ann Intern Med 1980;3:839–840.

599. Plotkin SA, McKitrick JC. Nosocomial meningitis of the newborn caused by a *Flavobacterium*. JAMA 1966;98:194–196.

600. Pope TL Jr, Teague WG Jr, Kossack R, et al. *Pseudomonas* sacroiliac osteomyelitis: diagnosis by gallium citrate Ga 67 scan. Am J Dis Child 1982;36:649–650.

601. Potvliege C, Dejaegher-Bauduin C, Hansen W, et al. *Flavobacterium multivorum* septicemia in a hemodialyzed patient. J Clin Microbiol 1984;9:568–569.

602. Potvliege C, Jonckheer J, Lenclud C, et al. *Pseudomonas stutzeri* pneumonia and septicemia in a patient with multiple myeloma. J Clin Microbiol 1987;5: 458–459.

603. Potvliege C, Vanhuynegem L, Hansen W. Catheter infection caused by an unusual pathogen *Agrobacterium radiobacter*. J Clin Microbiol 1989;7:2120–2122.

604. Prashanth K, Ranga MPM, Rao VA, et al. Corneal perforation due to *Acinetobacter junii*: a case report. Diagn Microbiol Infect Dis 2000;7:215–217.

605. Puckett A, Davison G, Entwistle CC, et al. Post-transfusion septicaemia 1980–1989: importance of donor arm cleansing. J Clin Pathol 1992;5:155–157.

606. Pugliese A, Pacris B, Schoch PE, et al. *Oligella urethralis* urosepsis. Clin Infect Dis 1993;7:1069–1070.

607. Purcell BK, Dooley DP. Centers for Disease Control and Prevention group O1 bacterium-associated pneumonia complicated by bronchopulmonary fistula and bacteremia. Clin Infect Dis 1999;9:945–946.

608. Rahav G, Simhon A, Mattan Y, et al. Infections with *Chryseomonas luteola* (CDC group Ve-1) and *Flavimonas oryzihabitans* (CDC group Ve-2). Medicine (Baltimore) 1995;4:83–88.

609. Ralston E, Palleroni NJ, Doudoroff M. *Pseudomonas pickettii*, a new species of clinical origin related to *Pseudomonas solanacearum*. Int J Syst Bacteriol 1973;23:15–19.

610. Ramirez FC, Saeed ZA, Darouiche RO, et al. *Agrobacterium tumefaciens* peritonitis mimicking tuberculosis. Clin Infect Dis 1992;15:938–940.

611. Ramos JM, Soriano F, Bernacer M, et al. Infection caused by the nonfermentative gram-negative bacillus CDC group IV c-2: case report and literature review. Eur J Clin Microbiol Infect Dis 1993;12:456–458.

612. Rastogi S, Sperber SJ. Facial cellulitis and *Pseudomonas luteola* bacteremia in an otherwise healthy patient. Diagn Microbiol Infect Dis 1998;32:303–305.

613. Reina J, Bassa A, Llompart I, Borrell N, et al. Pneumonia caused by *Bordetella bronchiseptica* in a patient with a thoracic trauma. Infection 1991;19:46–48.

614. Reina J, Bassa A, Llompart I, Portela D, et al. Infections with *Pseudomonas paucimobilis*: report of four cases and review. Rev Infect Dis 1991;13: 1072–1076.

615. Reina J, Borrell N. Leg abscess caused by *Weeksella zoohelcum* following a dog bite. Clin Infect Dis 1992;14:1162–1163.

616. Reina J, Gil J, Alomar P. Isolation of *Weeksella virosa* (formerly CDC group IIf) from a vaginal sample. Eur J Clin Microbiol Infect Dis 1989;8:569–570.

617. Reina J, Gil J, Salva F, et al. Microbiological characteristics of *Weeksella virosa* (formerly CDC Group IIf) isolated from the human genitourinary tract. J Clin Microbiol 1990;28:2357–2359.

618. Reina J, Llompart I, Alomar P. Acute suppurative otitis caused by *Comamonas acidovorans*. Clin Microbiol Newslett 1991;13:38–39.

619. Reisler RB, Blumberg H. Community-acquired *Pseudomonas stutzeri* vertebral osteomyelitis in a previously healthy patient: case report and review. Clin Infect Dis 1999;29:667–669.

620. Reverdy ME, Freney J, Fleurette J. Nosocomial colonization and infection by *Achromobacter xylosoxidans*. J Clin Microbiol 1984;19:140–143.
621. Reyes EAP, Bale MJ, Cannon WH, et al. Identification of *Pseudomonas aeruginosa* by pyocyanin production in Tech agar. J Clin Microbiol 1981;13:456–458.
622. Reyes MP, Lerner AM. Current problems in the treatment of infective endocarditis due to *Pseudomonas aeruginosa*. Rev Infect Dis 1983;5:314.
623. Rhoads S, Marinelli L, Imperatrice CA, et al. Comparison of MicroScan WalkAway System with Vitek System for identification of gram-negative bacteria. J Clin Microbiol 1995;33:3044–3046.
624. Rice EW, Reasoner DJ, Johnson CH, et al. Monitoring for methylobacteria in water systems. J Clin Microbiol 2000;38:4296–4297.
625. Richardson JD. Failure to clear a *Roseomonas* line infection with antibiotic therapy. Clin Infect Dis 1997;25:155.
626. Rihs JD, Brenner DJ, Weaver RE, et al. *Roseomonas*, a new genus associated with bacteremia and other human infections. J Clin Microbiol 1993;31:3275–3283.
627. Ringvold A, Vik E, Bevanger LS. *Moraxella lacunata* isolated from epidemic conjunctivitis among teen-aged females. Acta Ophthalmol 1985;63:427–431.
628. Rios I, Klimek JJ, Maderazo E, et al. *Flavobacterium meningosepticum* meningitis: report of selected aspects. Antimicrob Agents Chemother 1978;14:444–447.
629. Ritterband D, Shah M, Cohen K, et al. *Burkholderia gladioli* keratitis associated with consecutive recurrent endophthalmitis. Cornea 2002;21:602–603.
630. Robin T, Janda MJ. *Pseudo-*, *Xantho-*, *Stenotrophomonas maltophilia*: an emerging pathogen in search of a genus. Clin Microbiol Newslett 1996;18:9–13.
631. Robinson A, McCarter YS, Tetreault J. Comparison of Crystal Enteric/Nonfermenter System, API 20E System, and Vitek Autimicrobic System for identification of gram-negative bacilli. J Clin Microbiol 1995;33:364–370.
632. Rockhill RC, Lutwick LI. Group IVe-like gram-negative bacillemia in a patient with obstructive uropathy. J Clin Microbiol 1978;8:108–109.
633. Rodby RA, Glick E. *Agrobacterium radiobacter* peritonitis in two patients maintained on chronic peritoneal dialysis. Am J Kidney Dis 1991;18:402–405.
634. Roig P, Orti A, Navarro V. Meningitis due to *Pseudomonas stutzeri* in a patient infected with human immunodeficiency virus. Clin Infect Dis 1996;22:587–588.
635. Roilides E, Mueller BU, Letterio JJ, et al. *Agrobacterium radiobacter* bacteremia in a child with human immunodeficiency virus infection. Pediatr Infect Dis J 1991;10:337–338.
636. Romanyk J, Gonzalez-Palacios R, Nieto A. A new case of bacteraemia due to *Flavimonas oryzihabitans*. J Hosp Infect 1995;29:236–237.
637. Romero Gomez MP, Peinado Esteban AM, Sobrino Daza JA, et al. Prosthetic mitral valve endocarditis due to *Ochrobactrum anthropi*: case report. J Clin Microbiol 2004;42:3371–3373.
638. Rose RC, Grossman AM, Giles JW. Infective endocarditis due to the CDC group M6 bacillus. J Tenn Med Assoc 1990;83:603–604.
639. Rosenberg I, Leibovici L, Mor F, et al. *Pseudomonas stutzeri* causing late prosthetic valve endocarditis. J R Soc Med 1987;80:457–459.
640. Rosenthal SL: Clinical role of *Acinetobacter* and *Moraxella*. In: Gilardi GL, ed. Glucose Nonfermenting Gram-Negative Bacteria in Clinical Microbiology. West Palm Beach, FL: CRC Press, 1978:105–117.
641. Rosenthal SL, Freundlich LF, Gilardi GL, et al. In vitro antibiotic sensitivity of *Moraxella* species. Chemotherapy 1978;24:360–363.
642. Rosenthal SL, Freudlich LF, Washington W. Laboratory evaluation of a multitest system for identification of gram-negative organisms. Am J Clin Pathol 1978;70:914–917.
643. Ross JP, Holland SM, Gill VJ, et al. Severe *Burkholderia (Pseudomonas) gladioli* infection in chronic granulomatous disease: report of two successfully treated cases. Clin Infect Dis 1995;21:1291–1293.
644. Rossau R, Kersters K, Falsen E, et al. *Oligella*, a new genus including *Oligella urethralis* comb. nov. (formerly *Moraxella urethralis*) and *Oligella ureolytica* sp. nov. (formerly CDC group IVe): relationship to *Taylorella equigenitalis* and related taxa. Int J Syst Bacteriol 1987;37:198–210.
645. Rossau R, van Landschoot A, Gillis M, et al. Taxonomy of *Moraxellaceae* fam. nov., a new bacterial family to accommodate the genera *Moraxella*, *Acinetobacter*, and *Psychrobacter* and related organisms. Int J Syst Bacteriol 1991;41:310–319.
646. Rosselló R, Garcia-Valdés E, Lalucat J, et al. Genotypic and phenotypic diversity of *Pseudomonas stutzeri*. Syst Appl Microbiol 1991;14:150–157.
647. Rosselló R, Garcia-Valdés E, Macario AJL, et al. Antigenic diversity of *Pseudomonas stutzeri*. Syst Appl Microbiol 1992;15:617–623.
648. Rosselló-Mora RA, Lalucat J, Dott W, et al. Biochemical and chemotaxonomic characterization of *Pseudomonas stutzeri* genomovars. J Appl Bacteriol 1994;76:226–233.
649. Rosselló-Mora RA, Lalucat J, Moore ERB: Strain JM300 represents a new genomovar within *Pseudomonas stutzeri*. Syst Appl Microbiol 1996;19:596–599.
650. Rossmann SN, Wilson PH, Hicks J, et al. Isolation of *Lautropia mirabilis* from oral cavities of human immunodeficiency virus-infected children. J Clin Microbiol 1998;36:1756–1760.
651. Rotz LD, Khan AS, Lillibridge SR, et al. Public health assessment of potential biological terrorism agents. Emerg Infect Dis 2002;8:225–230.
652. Russell FM, Davis JM, Whipp MJ, et al. Severe *Bordetella holmesii* infection in a previously healthy adolescent confirmed by gene sequence analysis. Clin Infect Dis 2001;33:129–130.
653. Rutherford PC, Narkowicz JE, Wood CJ, et al. Peritonitis caused by *Pseudomonas mesophilica* in a patient undergoing continuous ambulatory peritoneal dialysis. J Clin Microbiol 1988;26:2441–2443.
654. Ryu E. A simple method of staining bacterial flagella. Kitasato Arch Exp Med 1937;14:218–219.
655. Saavedra J, Garrido C, Folgueira D, et al. *Ochrobactrum anthropi* bacteremia associated with a catheter in an immunocompromised child and review of the pediatric literature. Pediatr Infect Dis J 1999;18:658–660.
656. Saiman L, Burns JL, Larone D, et al. Evaluation of MicroScan Autoscan for identification of *Pseudomonas aeruginosa* isolates from patients with cystic fibrosis. J Clin Microbiol 2003;41:492–494.
657. Saiman L, Chen Y, Tabibi S, et al. Identification and antimicrobial susceptibility of *Alcaligenes xylosoxidans* isolated from patients with cystic fibrosis. J Clin Microbiol 2001;39:3942–3945.
658. Sajjan US, Sun L, Goldstein R, et al. Cable (cbl) type II pili of cystic fibrosis-associated *Burkholderia (Pseudomonas) cepacia*: nucleotide sequence of the cblA major subunit pilin gene and novel morphology of the assembled appendage fibers. J Bacteriol 1995;177:1030–1038.
659. Sajjan US, Xie H, Lefebre MD, et al. Identification and molecular analysis of cable pilus biosynthesis genes in *Burkholderia cepacia*. Microbiology 2003;149:961–971.
660. Salar A, Carratala J, Zurita A, et al. Bacteremia caused by CDC group IV c-2 in a patient with acute leukemia. Haematologica 1998;83:670–672.
661. Salazar R, Martino R, Sureda A, et al. Catheter-related bacteremia due to *Pseudomonas paucimobilis* in neutropenic cancer patients: report of two cases. Clin Infect Dis 1995;20:1573–1574.
662. Saltissi D, MacFarlane DJ. Successful treatment of *Pseudomonas paucimobilis* haemodialysis catheter-related sepsis without catheter removal. Postgrad Med J 1994;70:47-48.
663. Sanders JW, Martin JW, Hooke M, et al. *Methylobacterium mesophilicum* infection: case report and literature review of an unusual opportunistic pathogen. Clin Infect Dis 2000;30:936–938.
664. Sandoe JAT, Malnicki H, Loudon KW. A case of peritonitis caused by *Roseomonas gilardii* in a patient undergoing continuous ambulatory peritoneal dialysis. J Clin Microbiol 1997;35:2150–2152.
665. Saphir DA, Carter GR. Gingival flora of the dog with special reference to bacteria associated with bites. J Clin Microbiol 1976;3:344–349.
666. Sawada H, Ieki J, Oyaizu H, et al. Proposal for rejection of *Agrobacterium tumefaciens* and revised descriptions for the genus *Agrobacterium* and for *Agrobacterium radiobacter* and *Agrobacterium rhizogenes*. Int J Syst Bacteriol 1993;43:694–702.
667. Schlech WF, Turchik JB, Westlake RE, et al. Laboratory-acquired infection with *Pseudomonas pseudomallei* (melioidosis). N Engl J Med 1981;305:1133–1135.
668. Schmidt U, Kapila R, Kaminski Z, et al. *Pseudomonas putrefaciens* as a cause of septicemia in humans. J Clin Microbiol 1979;10:385–387.
669. Schreckenberger PC. Practical Approach to the Identification of Glucose-Nonfermenting Gram-Negative Bacilli: A Guide to Identification. Ed. 3. Maywood, IL: Loyola University, 2005.
670. Schreckenberger PC, Connell S, Skinner J, et al. Comparison of MicroScan Rapid Gram-Negative Identification Type 3 (RNID3) Panel with Vitek GNI and API 20E for Identification of Gram-Negative Bacilli. Abstracts of the General Meeting of the American Society for Microbiology. Washington, DC: American Society for Microbiology, 1998:156.
671. Schreckenberger PC, Daneshvar MI, Weyant RS, Hollis DG. *Acinetobacter, Achromobacter, Chryseobacterium, Moraxella*, and other nonfermentative gram-negative rods. In: Murray PR, Baron EJ, Jorgensen JH, et al., eds. Manual of Clinical Microbiology. Ed. 8. Washington DC: ASM Press, 2003:749–779.
672. Scott J, Boulton FE, Govan JRW, et al. A fatal transfusion reaction associated with blood contaminated with *Pseudomonas fluorescens*. Vox Sang 1988;54:201–204.
673. Segers P, Vancanneyt M, Pot B, et al. Classification of *Pseudomonas diminuta* Leifson and Hugh 1954 and *Pseudomonas vesicularis* Busing, Doll, and Freytag 1953 in *Brevundimonas* gen. nov. as *Brevundimonas diminuta* comb. nov. and *Brevundimonas vesicularis* comb. nov., respectively. Int J Syst Bacteriol 1994;44:499–510.
674. Seifert H, Baginski R, Schulze A, et al. Antimicrobial susceptibility of *Acinetobacter* species. Antimicrob Agents Chemother 1993;37:750–753.
675. Seifert H, Dijkshoorn L, Gerner-Smidt P, et al. Distribution of *Acinetobacter* species on human skin: comparison of phenotypic and genotypic identification methods. J Clin Microbiol 1997;35:2819–2825.
676. Senol E, Des-Jardin J, Stark PC, et al. Attributable mortality of *Stenotrophomonas maltophilia* bacteremia. Clin Infect Dis 2002;34:1653–1656.
677. Sepulveda-Torres LC, Zhou J, Guasp C, et al. Pseudomonas sp. strain KC represents a new genomovar within *Pseudomonas stutzeri*. Int J Syst Evol Microbiol 2001;51:2013–2019.

678. Shah SS, Ruth A, Coffin SE. Infection due to *Moraxella osloensis*: case report and review of the literature. Clin Infect Dis 2000;30:179–181.

679. Shayegani M, Lee AM, McGlynn DM. Evaluation of the Oxi/Ferm tube system for identification of nonfermentative gram-negative bacilli. J Clin Microbiol 1978;7:533–538.

680. Shayegani M, Maupin PS, McGlynn DM. Evaluation of the API 20E system for identification of nonfermentative gram-negative bacteria. J Clin Microbiol 1978;7:539–545.

681. Shayegani M, Maupin PS, Parsons LM, et al. Evaluation of the N/F system for identification of nonfermentative gram-negative bacilli using a reference laboratory population. Lab Med 1981;12:177–182.

682. Shelly DB, Spilker T, Gracely EJ, et al. Utility of commercial systems for identification of *Burkholderia cepacia* complex from cystic fibrosis sputum culture. J Clin Microbiol 2000;38:3112–3115.

683. Shepard CW, Daneshvar MI, Kaiser RM, et al. *Bordetella holmesii* bacteremia: a newly recognized clinical entity among asplenic patients. Clin Infect Dis 2004;38:799–804.

684. Sheridan RL, Ryan CM, Pasternack MS, et al. Flavobacterial sepsis in massively burned pediatric patients. Clin Infect Dis 1993;17:185–187.

685. Shewan JM: Taxonomy and ecology of *Flavobacterium* and related genera. Annu Rev Microbiol 1983;37:233–252.

686. Shin JH, Kim SH, Shin MG, et al. Bacteremia due to *Burkholderia gladioli*: case report. Clin Infect Dis 1997;25:1264–1265.

687. Shivaji S, Ray MK, Rao NS, et al. *Sphingobacterium antarcticus* sp. nov., a psychrotrophic bacterium from the soils of Schirmacher Oasis, Antarctica. Int J Syst Bacteriol 1992;42:102–106.

688. Shokar NK, Shokar GS, Islam J, et al. *Roseomonas gilardii* infection: case report and review. J Clin Microbiol 2002;40:4789–4791.

689. Shukla SK, Paustian DL, Stockwell PJ, et al. Isolation of a fastidious *Bergeyella* species associated with cellulitis after a cat bite and a phylogenetic comparison with *Bergeyella zoohelcum* strains. J Clin Microbiol 2004;42:290–293.

690. Siau H, Yuen K-Y, Ho P-L. Identification of acinetobacters on blood agar in presence of D-glucose by unique browning effect. J Clin Microbiol 1998;36:1404–1407.

691. Siegman-Igra Y, Bar-Yosef S, Gorea A, et al. Nosocomial *Acinetobacter* meningitis secondary to invasive procedures: report of 25 cases and review. Clin Infect Dis 1993;17:843–849.

692. Silver MR, Felegie TP, Sorkin MI. Unusual bacterium, group Ve-2, causing peritonitis in a patient on continuous ambulatory peritoneal dialysis. J Clin Microbiol 1985;21:838–839.

693. Simidu U, Kita-Tsukamoto K, Yasumoto T, et al. Taxonomy of four marine bacterial strains that produce tetrodotoxin. Int J Syst Bacteriol 1990;40:331–336.

694. Simmonds EJ, Conway SP, Ghoneim ATM, et al. *Pseudomonas cepacia*: a new pathogen in patients with cystic fibrosis referred to a large centre in the United Kingdom. Arch Dis Child 1990;65:874–877.

695. Simor AE, Salit IE. Endocarditis caused by M6. J Clin Microbiol 1983;17:931–933.

696. Simpson AJH, Suputtamongkol Y, Smith MD. Comparison of imipenem and ceftazidime as therapy for severe melioidosis. Clin Infect Dis: 1999;29:381–387.

697. Sintchenko V, Jelfs P, Sharma A, et al. *Massilia timonae*: an unusual bacterium causing would infection following surgery. Clin Microbiol Newslett 2000;22:149–151.

698. Smith DL, Gumery LB, Smith EG, et al. Epidemic of *Pseudomonas cepacia* in an adult cystic fibrosis unit: evidence of person-to-person transmission. J Clin Microbiol 1993;31:3017–3022.

699. Smith J, Ashhurst-Smith C, Norton R. *Pseudomonas fluorescens* pseudobacteraemia: a cautionary lesson. J Paediatr Child Health 2002;38:63–65.

700. Smith MD, Angus BJ, Wuthiekanun V, et al. Arabinose assimilation defines a nonvirulent biotype of *Burkholderia pseudomallei*. Infect Immun 1997;65:4319–4321.

701. Smith MD, Wuthiekanun V, Walsh AL, Pitt TL. Latex agglutination test for identification of *Pseudomonas pseudomallei*. J Clin Pathol 1993;46:374–375.

702. Smith MD, Wuthiekanun V, Walsh AL, Teerawattanasook N, et al. Latex agglutination for rapid detection of *Pseudomonas pseudomallei* antigen in urine of patients with melioidosis. J Clin Pathol 1995;48:174–176.

703. Smith MD, Wuthiekanun V, Walsh AL, White NJ. In-vitro activity of carbapenem antibiotics against beta-lactam susceptible and resistant strains of *Burkholderia pseudomallei*. J Antimicrob Chemother 1996;37:611–615.

704. Smith SM, Eng RHK, Forrester C. *Pseudomonas mesophilica* infections in humans. J Clin Microbiol 1985;21:314–317.

705. Sobel JD, Hashman N, Reinherz G, et al. Nosocomial *Pseudomonas cepacia* infection associated with chlorhexidine contamination. Am J Med 1982;73:183–186.

706. Sonnenwirth AC. Bacteremia with and without meningitis due to *Yersinia enterocolitica*, *Edwardsiella tarda*, *Comamonas terrigena*, and *Pseudomonas maltophilia*. Ann NY Acad Sci 1970;174:488–502.

707. Spangler SK, Visalli MA, Jacobs MR, et al. Susceptibilities of non-*Pseudomonas aeruginosa* gram-negative nonfermentative rods to ciprofloxacin, ofloxacin, levofloxacin, D-ofloxacin, sparfloxacin, ceftazidime, piperacillin, piperacillin-tazobactam, trimethoprim-sulfamethoxazole, and imipenem. Antimicrob Agents Chemother 1996;40:772–775.

708. Spear JB, Fuhrer J, Kirby BD. *Achromobacter xylosoxidans* (*Alcaligenes xylosoxidans* subsp. *xylosoxidans*) bacteremia associated with a well-water source: case report and review of the literature. J Clin Microbiol 1988;26:598–599.

709. Speert DP, Henry D, Vandamme P, et al. Epidemiology of *Burkholderia cepacia* complex in patients with cystic fibrosis, Canada. Emerg Infect Dis 2002;8:181–187.

710. Spotnitz M, Rudnitzky J, Rambaud JJ. Melioidosis pneumonitis. JAMA 1967;202:950-954.

711. Staneck JL, Weckbach LS, Tilton RC, et al. Collaborative evaluation of the Radiometer Sensititre AP80 for identification of gram-negative bacilli. J Clin Microbiol 1993;31:1179–1184.

712. Stefaniuk E, Baraniak A, Gniadkowski, et al. Evaluation of the BD Phoenix automated identification and susceptibility testing system in clinical microbiology laboratory practice. Eur J Clin Microbiol Infect Dis 2003;22:479–485.

713. Steyn PL, Segers P, Vancanneyt M, et al. Classification of heparinolytic bacteria into a new genus, *Pedobacter*, comprising four species: *Pedobacter heparinus* comb. nov., *Pedobacter piscium* comb. nov., *Pedobacter africanus* sp. nov. and *Pedobacter saltans* sp. nov. proposal of the family *Sphingobacteriaceae* fam. nov. Int J Syst Bacteriol 1998;48:165–177.

714. Stiakaki E, Galanakis E, Samonis G, et al. *Ochrobactrum anthropi* bacteremia in pediatric oncology patients. Pediatr Infect Dis J 2002;21:72–74.

715. Stonecipher KG, Jensen HG, Kasti PR, et al. Ocular infections associated with *Comamonas acidovorans*. Am J Ophthalmol 1991;112:46–49.

715a. Storms V, Van Den Vreken N, Coenye T, et al. Polyphasic characterisation of *Burkholderia cepacia*-like isolate leading to the emended description of *Burkholderia pyrrocinia*. Syst Appl Microbiol 2004;27:517–526.

716. Struillou L, Raffi F, Barrier JH. Endocarditis caused by *Neisseria elongata* subspecies *nitroreducens*: case report and literature review. Eur J Clin Microbiol Infect Dis 1993;12:625–627.

717. Struthers M, Wong J, Janda JM. An initial appraisal of the clinical significance of *Roseomonas* species associated with human infections. Clin Infect Dis 1996;23:729–733.

718. Stryjewski ME, LiPuma JJ, Messier RH, et al. Sepsis, multiple organ failure, and death due to *Pandoraea pnomenusa* infection after lung transplantation. J Clin Microbiol 2003;41:2255–2257.

719. Subudhi CP, Adedeji A, Kaufmann ME, et al. Fatal *Roseomonas gilardii* bacteremia in a patient with refractory blast crisis of chronic myeloid leukemia. Clin Microbiol Infect 2001;7:573–575.

720. Sugarman B, Clarridge J. Osteomyelitis caused by *Moraxella osloensis*. J Clin Microbiol 1982;15:1148–1149.

721. Sun L, Jiang RZ, Steinbach S, et al. The emergence of a highly transmissible lineage of cbl+ *Pseudomonas* (*Burkholderia*) *cepacia* causing CF centre epidemics in North America and Britain. Nat Med 1995;1:661–666.

722. Sung LL, Yang DI, Hung CC, et al. Evaluation of autoSCAN-W/A and the Vitek GNI+ AutoMicrobic System for identification of non-glucose-fermenting gram-negative bacilli. J Clin Microbiol 2000;38:1127–1130.

723. Suputtamongkol Y, Chaowagul W, Chetchotisakd P, et al. Risk factors for melioidosis and bacteremic melioidosis. Clin Infect Dis 1999;29:408–413.

724. Swann RA, Foulkes SJ, Holmes B, et al. "*Agrobacterium* yellow group" and *Pseudomonas paucimobilis* causing peritonitis in patients receiving continuous ambulatory peritoneal dialysis. J Clin Pathol 1985;38:1293–1299.

725. Swenson JM, Killgore GE, Tenover FC. Antimicrobial susceptibility testing of *Acinetobacter* spp. by NCCLS broth microdilution and disk diffusion methods. J Clin Microbiol 2004;42:5102–5108.

726. Tabor E, Gerety RJ. Five cases of pseudomonas sepsis transmitted by blood transfusions. Lancet 1984;1:1403.

727. Takeuchi M, Hamana K, Hiraishi A. Proposal of the genus *Sphingomonas sensu stricto* and three new genera, *Sphingobium*, *Novosphingobium* and *Sphingopyxis*, on the basis of phylogenetic and chemotaxonomic analyses. Int J Syst Evol Microbiol 2001;51:1405–1417.

728. Takeuchi M, Kawai F, Shimada Y, et al. Taxonomic study of polyethylene glycol-utilizing bacteria: emended description of the genus *Sphingomonas* and new descriptions of *Sphingomonas macrogoltabidus* sp. nov., *Sphingomonas sanguis* sp. nov. and *Sphingomonas terrae* sp. nov. Syst Appl Microbiol 1993;16:227–238.

728a. Takeuchi M, Sakane T, Yanagi M, et al. Taxonomic study of bacteria isolated from plants: proposal of *Sphingomonas rosa* sp. nov., *Sphingomonas pruni* sp. nov., *Sphingomonas asaccharolytica* sp. nov., and *Sphingomonas mali* sp. nov. Int J Syst Bacteriol 1995;45:334–341.

729. Takeuchi M, Yokota A. Proposals of *Sphingobacterium faecium* sp. nov., *Sphingobacterium piscium* sp. nov., *Sphingobacterium heparinum* comb. nov., *Sphingobacterium thalpophilum* comb. nov. and two genospecies of the genus *Sphingobacterium*, and synonymy of *Flavobacterium yabuuchiae* and *Sphingobacterium spiritivorum*. J Gen Appl Microbiol 1992;38:465–482.

730. Tamaoka J, Ha D-M, Komagata K. Reclassification of *Pseudomonas acidovor-*

ans den Dooren de Jong 1926 and *Pseudomonas testosteroni* Marcus and Talalay 1956 as *Comamonas acidovorans* comb. nov. and *Comamonas testosteroni* comb. nov., with an emended description of the genus *Comamonas.* Int J Syst Bacteriol 1987;37:52–59.

731. Tang, Y-W, Hopkins MK, Kolbert CP, et al. *Bordetella holmesii*-like organisms associated with septicemia, endocarditis, and respiratory failure. Clin Infect Dis 1998;26:389–392.

732. Taplan D, Bassett DCJ, Mertz PM. Foot lesions associated with *Pseudomonas cepacia.* Lancet 1971;2:568–571.

733. Taylor M, Keane CT, Falkiner FR. *Pseudomonas putida* in transfused blood. Lancet 1984;2:107.

734. Tenover FC, Mizuki TS, Carlson LG. Evaluation of autoSCAN-W/A automated microbiology system for the identification of non-glucose-fermenting gram-negative bacilli. J Clin Microbiol 1990;28:1628–1634.

735. Teres D. ICU-acquired pneumonia due to *Flavobacterium meningosepticum.* JAMA 1974;228:732.

736. Thayu M, Baltimore RS, Sleight BJ, et al. CDC group IV c-2 bacteremia in a child with recurrent acute monoblastic leukemia. Pediatr Infect Dis J 1999;18: 397–398.

737. Thimann KV. The Life of Bacteria: Their Growth, Metabolism and Relationships. Ed. 2. New York: Macmillan, 1963.

738. Thomassen MJ, Demko CA, Klinger JD, et al. *Pseudomonas cepacia* colonization among patients with cystic fibrosis: a new opportunist. Am Rev Respir Dis 1985;131:791–796.

739. Thong ML, Puthucheary SD, Lee EL. *Flavobacterium meningosepticum* infection: an epidemiological study in a newborn nursery. J Clin Pathol 1981;34: 429–433.

740. Tjernberg I, Ursing J. Clinical strains of *Acinetobacter* classified by DNA–DNA hybridization. APMIS 1989;97:595–605.

741. Tonjum T, Caugant DA, Bovre K. Differentiation of *Moraxella nonliquefaciens, M. lacunata,* and *M. bovis* by using multilocus enzyme electrophoresis and hybridization with pilin-specific DNA probes. J Clin Microbiol 1992;30:3099–3107.

742. Tripodi MF, Adinolfi LE, Rosario P, et al. First definite case of aortic valve endocarditis due to *Moraxella phenylpyruvica.* Eur J Clin Microbiol Infect Dis 2002;21:480–482.

743. Tronel H, Plesiat P, Ageron E, et al. Bacteremia caused by a novel species of *Sphingobacterium.* Clin Microbiol Infect 2003;9:1242–1244.

744. Truant AL, Gulati R, Giger O, et al. *Methylobacterium* species: an increasingly important opportunistic pathogen. Lab Med 1998;29:704–710.

745. Truper HG, De Clari L. Taxonomic note: necessary correction of specific epithets formed as substantives (Nouns) ''in apposition.'' Int J Syst Bacteriol 1997;47: 908–909.

746. Tsakris A, Hassapopoulou H, Skoura L, et al. Leg ulcer due to *Pseudomonas luteola* in a patient with sickle cell disease. Diagn Microbiol Infect Dis 2002; 42:141–143.

747. Urakami T, Araki H, Suzuki K-I, et al. Further studies of the genus *Methylobacterium* and description of *Methylobacterium aminovorans* sp. nov. Int J Syst Bacteriol 1993;43:504–513.

748. Ursing J, Bruun B. Genotypic heterogeneity of *Flavobacterium* group IIb and *Flavobacterium breve,* demonstrated by DNA-DNA hybridization. APMIS 1991;99:780–786.

749. Valdezate S, Vindel A, Maiz L, et al. Persistence and variability of *Stenotrophomonas maltophilia* in patients with cystic fibrosis, Madrid, 1991–1998. Emerg Infect Dis 2001;7:113–122.

750. Valenstein P, Bardy GH, Cox CC, et al. *Pseudomonas alcaligenes* endocarditis. Am J Clin Pathol 1983;79:245–247.

751. Vancanneyt M, Segers P, Torck U, et al. Reclassification of *Flavobacterium odoratum* (Stutzer 1929) strains to a new genus, *Myroides,* as *Myroides odoratus* comb. nov. and *Myroides odoratimimus* sp. nov. Int J Syst Bacteriol 1996;46: 926–932.

752. Vandamme P, Bernardet J-F, Segers P, et al. New perspectives in the classification of the flavobacteria: description of *Chryseobacterium* gen. nov., *Bergeyella* gen. nov., and *Empedobacter* nom. rev. Int J Syst Bacteriol 1994;44:827–831.

752a. Vandamme P, Coenye T: Taxonomy of the genus *Cupriavidus*: a tale of lost and found. Int J Syst Evol Microbiol 2004;54:2285–2289.

753. Vandamme P, Gillis M, Vancanneyt M, et al. *Moraxella lincolnii* sp. nov., isolated from the human respiratory tract, and reevaluation of the taxonomic position of *Moraxella osloensis.* Int J Syst Bacteriol 1993;43:474–481.

753a. Vandamme P, Goris J, Coenye T, et al. Assignment of Centers for Disease Control group IVc-2 to the genus *Ralstonia* as *Ralstonia paucula* sp. nov. Int J Syst Bacteriol 1999;49:663–669.

754. Vandamme P, Henry D, Coenye T, et al. *Burkholderia anthina* sp. nov. and *Burkholderia pyrrocinia,* two additional *Burkholderia cepacia* complex bacteria, may confound results of new molecular diagnostic tools. FEMS Immunol Med Microbiol 2002;33:143–149.

755. Vandamme P, Heyndrickx M, Vancanneyt M, et al. *Bordetella trematum* sp. nov., isolated from wounds and ear infections in humans, and reassessment of

Alcaligenes denitrificans Rüger and Tan 1983. Int J Syst Bacteriol 1996;46: 849–858.

756. Vandamme P, Holmes B, Coenye T, et al. *Burkholderia cenocepacia* sp. nov.—a new twist to an old story. Res Microbiol 2003;154:91–96.

757. Vandamme P, Holmes B, Vancanneyt M, et al. Occurrence of multiple genomovars of *Burkholderia cepacia* in patients with cystic fibrosis and proposal of *Burkholderia multivorans* sp. nov. Int J Syst Bacteriol 1997;47:1188–1200.

758. Vandamme P, Hommez J, Vancanneyt M, et al. *Bordetella hinzii* sp. nov., isolated from poultry and humans. Int J Syst Bacteriol 1995;45:37–45.

759. Vandamme P, Mahenthiralingam E, Holmes B, et al. Identification and population structure of *Burkholderia stabilis* sp. nov. (formerly *Burkholderia cepacia* genomovar IV). J Clin Microbiol 2000;38:1042–1047.

760. Vandepitte J, Debois J. *Pseudomonas putrefaciens* as a cause of bacteremia in humans. J Clin Microbiol 1978;7:70–72.

761. Vaneechoutte M, Claeys G, Steyaert S, et al. Isolation of *Moraxella canis* from an ulcerated metastatic lymph node. J Clin Microbiol 2000;38:3870–3871.

762. Vaneechoutte M, De Baere T, Wauters G, et al. One case each of recurrent meningitis and hemoperitoneum infection with *Ralstonia mannitolilytica.* J Clin Microbiol 2001;39:4588–4590.

763. Vaneechoutte M, Kämpfer P, De Baere T, et al. *Wautersia* gen. nov., a novel genus accommodating the phylogenetic lineage including *Ralstonia eutropha* and related species, and proposal of *Ralstonia [Pseudomonas] syzygii* (Roberts et al. 1990) comb. nov. Int J Syst Evol Microbiol 2004;54:317–327.

764. Vanholder R, Vanhaecke E, Ringoir S. *Pseudomonas* septicemia due to deficient disinfectant mixing during reuse. Int J Artif Organs 1992;15:19–24.

765. van Horn KG, Gedris CA, Ahmed T, et al. Bacteremia and urinary tract infection associated with CDC group Vd biovar 2. J Clin Microbiol 1989;27:201–202.

766. van Laer F, Raes D, Vandamme P, et al. An outbreak of *Burkholderia cepacia* with septicemia on a cardiology ward. Infect Control Hosp Epidemiol 1998;19: 112–113.

767. van Pelt C, Verduin CM, Goessens WHF, et al. Identification of *Burkholderia* spp. in the clinical microbiology laboratory: comparison of conventional and molecular methods. J Clin Microbiol 1999;37:2158–2164.

768. Vartivarian S, Anaissie E, Bodey G, et al. A changing pattern of susceptibility of *Xanthomonas maltophilia* to antimicrobial agents: implications for therapy. Antimicrob Agents Chemother 1994;38:624–627.

769. Vartivarian SE, Papadakis KA, Anaissie EJ. *Stenotrophomonas (Xanthomonas) maltophilia* urinary tract infection: a disease that is usually severe and complicated. Arch Intern Med 1996;156:433–435.

770. Vartivarian SE, Papadakis KA, Palacios JA, et al. Mucocutaneous and soft tissue infections caused by *Xanthomonas maltophilia*: a new spectrum. Ann Intern Med 1994;121:969–973.

771. Velasco J, Romero C, Lopez-Goni I, et al. Evaluation of the relatedness of *Brucella* spp. and *Ochrobactrum anthropi* and description of *Ochrobactrum intermedium* sp. nov., a new species with a closer relationship to *Brucella* spp. Int J Syst Bacteriol 1998;48:759–768.

772. Verhasselt B, Claeys G, Elaichouni A, et al. Case of recurrent *Flavimonas oryzihabitans* bacteremia associated with an implanted central venous catheter (Port-A-Cath): assessment of clonality by arbitrarily primed PCR. J Clin Microbiol 1995;33:3047–3048.

773. Vermis K, Coenye T, LiPuma JJ, et al. Proposal to accommodate *Burkholderia cepacia* genomovar VI as *Burkholderia dolosa* sp. nov. Int J Syst Evol Microbiol 2004;54:689–691.

774. Vermis K, Vandamme PAR, Nelis HJ. *Burkholderia cepacia* complex genomovars: utilization of carbon sources, susceptibility to antimicrobial agents and growth on selective media. J Appl Microbiol 2003;95:1191–1199.

775. Villegas MV, Hartstein AI. *Acinetobacter* outbreaks, 1977–2000. Infect Control Hosp Epidemiol 2003;24:284–295.

776. Visca P, Petrucca A, De Mori P, et al. Community-acquired *Acinetobacter radioresistens* bacteremia in an HIV-positive patient. Emerg Infect Dis 2001;7: 1032–1035.

777. Vogel BF, Jorgensen K, Christensen H, et al. Differentiation of *Shewanella putrefaciens* and *Shewanella alga* on the basis of whole-cell protein profiles, ribotyping, phenotypic characterization, and 16S rRNA gene sequence analysis. Appl Environ Microbiol 1997;63:2189–2199.

778. Vogel BF, Venkateswaran K, Christensen H, et al. Polyphasic taxonomic approach in the description of *Alishewanella fetalis* gen. nov., sp. nov., isolated from a human foetus. Int J Syst Evol Microbiol 2000;50:1133–1142.

779. von Graevenitz A. Clinical role of infrequently encountered nonfermenters. In: Gilardi GL, ed. Glucose Nonfermenting Gram-Negative Bacteria in Clinical Microbiology. West Palm Beach, F:, CRC Press, 1978:119–153.

780. von Graevenitz A. Ecology, clinical significance, and antimicrobial susceptibility of infrequently encountered glucose-nonfermenting gram-negative rods. In: Gilardi GL, ed. Glucose Nonfermenting Gram-Negative Bacteria in Clinical Microbiology. West Palm Beach, F:, CRC Press, 1978:181–232

781. von Graevenitz A, Boewman J, Del Notaro C, et al. Human infection with *Halomonas venusta* following fish bite. J Clin Microbiol 2000;38:3123–3124.

782. von Graevenitz A, Grehn M. Susceptibility studies on *Flavobacterium* II-b. FEMS Microbiol Lett 1977;2:289–292.

783. von Graevenitz A, Pfyffer GE, Pickett MJ, et al. Isolation of an unclassified non-fermentative gram-negative rod from a patient on continuous ambulatory peritoneal dialysis. Eur J Clin Microbiol Infect Dis 1993;12:568–570.

784. von Graevenitz A, Simon G. Potentially pathogenic, nonfermentative, H₂S-producing gram-negative rod (1b). Appl Microbiol 1970;19:176.

785. von Graevenitz A, Zollinger–Iten J. Evaluation of pertinent parameters of a new identification system for non-enteric gram-negative rods. Eur J Clin Microbiol 1985;4:108–112.

786. von Wintzingerode F, Schattke A, Siddiqui RA, et al. *Bordetella petrii* sp. nov., isolated from an anaerobic bioreactor, and emended description of the genus *Bordetella*. Int J Syst Evol Microbiol 2001;51:1257–65.

787. Wallet F, Perez T, Armand S, et al. Pneumonia due to *Bordetella bronchiseptica* in a cystic fibrosis patient: 16S rRNA sequencing for diagnosis confirmation. J Clin Microbiol 2002;40:2300–2301.

788. Walsh AL, Wuthiekanun V, Smith MD, et al. Selective broths for the isolation of *Pseudomonas pseudomallei* from clinical samples. Trans R Soc Trop Med Hyg 1995;89:124.

789. Warwood NM, Blazevic DJ, Hofherr L. Comparison of the API 20E and Corning N/F systems for identification of nonfermentative gram-negative rods. J Clin Microbiol 1979;10:175–179.

790. Watson KC, Muscat I. Meningitis caused by a *Flavobacterium*-like organism (CDC IIe strain). J Infect 1983;7:278–279.

791. Wauters G, Boel A, Voorn GP, et al. Evaluation of a new identification system, Crystal Enteric/Non-Fermenter, for gram-negative bacilli. J Clin Microbiol 1995; 33:845–849.

792. Wauters G, Claeys G, Verschraegen G, et al. Case of catheter sepsis with *Ralstonia gilardii* in a child with acute lymphoblastic leukemia. J Clin Microbiol 2001;39:4583–4584.

793. Wauters G, de Baere T, Willems A, et al. Description of *Comamonas aquatica* comb. nov. and *Comamonas kerstersii* sp. nov. for two subgroups of *Comamonas terrigena* and emended description of *Comamonas terrigena*. Int J Syst Evol Microbiol 2003;53:859–862.

794. Weems JJ Jr. Nosocomial outbreak of *Pseudomonas cepacia* associated with contamination of reusable electronic ventilator temperature probes. Infect Control Hosp Epidemiol 1993;14:583–586.

795. Weitkamp J-H, Tang Y-W, Haas DW, et al. Recurrent *Achromobacter xylosoxidans* bacteremia associated with persistent lymph node infection in a patient with hyper-immunoglobulin M syndrome. Clin Infect Dis 2000;31:1183–1187.

796. Welch DF, Muszynski MJ, Pai CH, et al. Selective and differential medium for recovery of *Pseudomonas cepacia* from the respiratory tracts of patients with cystic fibrosis. J Clin Microbiol 1987;25:1730–1734.

797. Wen A, Fegan M, Hayward C, et al. Phylogenetic relationships among members of the *Comamonadaceae*, and description of *Delftia acidovorans* (den Dooren de Jong 1926 and Tamaoka et al. 1987) gen. nov., comb nov. Int J Syst Bacteriol 1999;49:567–576.

798. Werthamer S, Weiner M. Subacute bacterial endocarditis due to *Flavobacterium meningosepticum*. Am J Clin Pathol 1972;57:410–412.

799. Wertheim WA, Markovitz DM. Osteomyelitis and intervertebral discitis caused by *Pseudomonas pickettii*. J Clin Microbiol 1992;30:2506–2508.

800. Weyant RS, Daneshvar MI, Jordan JG, et al. Eugonic oxidizer group 4: an unusual gram-negative bacterium isolated from clinical specimens. Abstracts of the 99th General Meeting of the American Society for Microbiology. Washington, DC: American Society for Microbiology, 1999:144.

801. Weyant RS, Hollis DG, Weaver RE, et al. *Bordetella holmesii* sp. nov., a new gram-negative species associated with septicemia. J Clin Microbiol 1995;33:1–7.

802. Weyant RS, Moss CW, Weaver RE, et al. Identification of Unusual Pathogenic Gram-Negative Aerobic and Facultatively Anaerobic Bacteria. Ed. 2. Baltimore: Williams & Wilkins, 1996.

803. Wheelis M. First shots fired in biological warfare. Nature 1998;395:213.

804. Whitby PW, Pope LC, Carter KB, et al. Species-specific PCR as a tool for the identification of *Burkholderia gladioli*. J Clin Microbiol 2000;38:282–285.

805. White NJ. Melioidosis. Lancet 2003;361:1715–1722.

806. Willems A, De Ley J, Gillis M, et al. *Comamonadaceae*, a new family encompassing the acidovorans rRNA complex, including *Variovorax paradoxus* gen. nov., comb. nov., for *Alcaligenes paradoxus* (Davis 1969). Int J Syst Bacteriol 1991;41:445–450.

807. Willems A, Falsen E, Pot B, et al. *Acidovorax*, a new genus for *Pseudomonas facilis*, *Pseudomonas delafieldii*, E. Falsen (EF) Group 13, EF Group 16, and several clinical isolates, with the species *Acidovorax facilis* comb. nov., *Acidovorax delafieldii* comb. nov., and *Acidovorax temperans* sp. nov. Int J Syst Bacteriol 1990;40:384–398.

808. Wilson APR, Ridgway GL, Ryan KE, et al. Unusual pathogens in neutropenic patients. J Hosp Infect 1988;11:398–400.

809. Wisplinghoff H, Edmond MB, Pfaller MA, et al. Nosocomial bloodstream infections caused by *Acinetobacter* species in United States hospitals: clinical features, molecular epidemiology, and antimicrobial susceptibility. Clin Infect Dis 2000;31:690–697.

810. Wolf A, Fritze A, Hagemann M, et al. *Stenotrophomonas rhizophila* sp. nov., a novel plant-associated bacterium with antifungal properties. Int J Syst Evol Microbiol 2002;52:1937–1944.

811. Wong JD, Janda JM. Association of an important *Neisseria* species, *Neisseria elongata* subsp. *nitroreducens*, with bacteremia, endocarditis, and osteomyelitis. J Clin Microbiol 1992;30:719–720.

812. Woo PC, Kuhnert P, Burnens AP, et al. *Laribacter hongkongensis*: a potential cause of infectious diarrhea. Diagn Microbiol Infect Dis 2003;47:551–556.

813. Woo PC, Lau SKP, Teng JLL, et al. Association of *Laribacter hongkongensis* in community-acquired gastroenteritis with travel and eating fish: a multicentre case-control study. Lancet 2004;363:1941–1947.

814. Woo PC, Wong SS, Yuen KY: *Ralstonia pickettii* bacteraemia in a cord blood transplant recipient. New Microbiol 2002;25:97–102.

815. Wood CA, Reboli AC. Infections caused by imipenem-resistant *Acinetobacter calcoaceticus* biotype *anitratus*. J Infect Dis 168:1602–1603, 1993.

816. Woodard DR, Cone LA, Fostvedt K. *Bordetella bronchiseptica* infection in patients with AIDS. Clin Infect Dis 1995;20:193–194.

817. Woods CW, Bressler AM, LiPuma JJ, et al. Virulence associated with outbreak-related strains of *Burkholderia cepacia* complex among a cohort of patients with bacteremia. Clin Infect Dis 2004;38:1243–1250.

818. Woolfrey BF, Moody JA. Human infection associated with *Bordetella bronchiseptica*. Clin Microbiol Rev 1991;4:243–255.

819. Wright RM, Moore JE, Shaw A, et al. Improved cultural detection of *Burkholderia cepacia* from sputum in patients with cystic fibrosis. J Clin Pathol 2001; 54:803–805.

820. Wuthiekanun V, Dance D, Chaowagul W, et al. Blood culture techniques for the diagnosis of melioidosis. Eur J Clin Microbiol 1990;9:654–658.

821. Wuthiekanun V, Dance DA, Wattanagoon Y, et al. The use of selective media for the isolation of *Pseudomonas pseudomallei* in clinical practice. J Med Microbiol 1990;33:121–126.

822. Yabuuchi E, Kaneko T, Yano I, et al. *Sphingobacterium* gen. nov., *Sphingobacterium spiritivorum* comb. nov., *Sphingobacterium multivorum* comb. nov., *Sphingobacterium mizutae* sp. nov., and *Flavobacterium indologenes* sp. nov.: glucose-nonfermenting gram-negative rods in CDC groups IIk-2 and IIb. Int J Syst Bacteriol 1983;33:580–598.

823. Yabuuchi E, Kawamura Y, Kosako Y, et al. Emendation of genus *Achromobacter* and *Achromobacter xylosoxidans* (Yabuuchi and Yano) and proposal of *Achromobacter ruhlandii* (Packer and Vishniac) comb. nov., *Achromobacter piechaudii* (Kiredjian et al.) comb. nov., and *Achromobacter xylosoxidans* subsp. *denitrificans* (Rüger and Tan) comb. nov. Microbiol Immunol 1998;42:429–438.

824. Yabuuchi E, Kosako Y, Oyaizu H, et al. Proposal of *Burkholderia* gen. nov. and transfer of seven species of the genus *Pseudomonas* homology group II to the new genus, with the type species *Burkholderia cepacia* (Palleroni and Holmes 1981) comb. nov. Microbiol Immunol 1992;36:1251–1275.

825. Yabuuchi E, Kosako Y, Yano I, et al. Transfer of two *Burkholderia* and an *Alcaligenes* species to *Ralstonia* gen. nov.: proposal of *Ralstonia pickettii* (Ralston, Palleroni and Doudoroff 1973) comb. nov., *Ralstonia solanacearum* (Smith 1896) comb. nov. and *Ralstonia eutropha* (Davis 1969) comb. nov. Microbiol Immunol 1995;39:897–904.

826. Yabuuchi E, Yano I. *Achromobacter* gen. nov. and *Achromobacter xylosoxidans* (ex Yabuuchi and Ohyama 1971) nom. rev. Int J Syst Bacteriol 1981;31:477–478.

827. Yabuuchi E, Yano I, Oyaizu H, et al. Proposals of *Sphingomonas paucimobilis* gen. nov. and comb. nov., *Sphingomonas parapaucimobilis* sp. nov., *Sphingomonas yanoikuyae* sp. nov., *Sphingomonas adhaesiva* sp. nov., *Sphingomonas capsulata* comb. nov., and two genospecies of the genus *Sphingomonas*. Microbiol Immunol 1990;34:99–119.

828. Yagci A, Cerikcioglu N, Kaufmann ME, et al. Molecular typing of *Myroides odoratimimus* (*Flavobacterium odoratum*) urinary tract infections in a Turkish hospital. Eur J Clin Microbiol Infect Dis 2000;19:731–732.

829. Yamamoto T, Naigowit P, Dejsirilert S, et al. In vitro susceptibilities of *Pseudomonas pseudomallei* to 27 antimicrobial agents. Antimicrob Agents Chemother 1990;34:2027–2029.

830. Yao JDC, Louie M, Louie L, et al. Comparison of E test and agar dilution for antimicrobial susceptibility testing of *Stenotrophomonas* (*Xanthomonas*) *maltophilia*. J Clin Microbiol 1995;33:1428–1430.

831. Yih WK, Silva EA, Ida J, et al. *Bordetella holmesii*-like organisms isolated from Massachusetts patients with pertussis-like symptoms. Emerg Inf Dis 1999;5:441–443.

832. Yohe S, Fishbain JT, Andrews M: *Shewanella putrefaciens* abscess of the lower extremity. J Clin Microbiol 1997;35:3363.

833. Yoneyama A, Yano H, Hitomi S, et al. *Ralstonia pickettii* colonization of patients in an obstetric ward caused by a contaminated irrigation system. J Hosp Infect 2000;46:79–80.

834. Young JM Kuykendall LD, Martinez-Romero E, et al. A revision of *Rhizobium* Frank 1889, with an emended description of the genus, and the inclusion of all

species of *Agrobacterium* Conn 1942 and *Allorhizobium undicola* de Lajudie et al. 1998 as new combinations: *Rhizobium radiobacter, R. rhizogenes, R. rubi, R. undicola* and *R. vitis*. Int J Syst Evol Microbiol 2001;51:89–103.

835. Young JM, Kuykendall LD, Martinez-Romero E, et al. Classification and nomenclature of *Agrobacterium* and *Rhizobium*—a reply to Farrand et al. (2003). Int J Syst Evol Microbiol 2003;53:1689–1695.

836. Yuen, K-Y, Woo PCY, Teng JLL, et al. *Laribacter hongkongensis* gen. nov., sp. nov., a novel gram-negative bacterium isolated from a cirrhotic patient with bacteremia and empyema. J Clin Microbiol 2001;39:4227–4232.

837. Zapardiel J, Blum G, Caramelo C, et al. Peritonitis with CDC group IV c-2 bacteria in a patient on continuous ambulatory peritoneal dialysis. Eur J Clin Microbiol Infect Dis 1991;10:509–511.

Curved Gram-Negative Bacilli and Oxidase-Positive Fermenters: *Campylobacteraceae* and *Vibrionaceae*

Part I: Curved Rods: *Campylobacter, Wolinella, Arcobacter, Helicobacter,* and Related Bacteria

Historical Background

Classification of *Campylobacter* and Related Taxa

Campylobacter Species

Campylobacter jejuni Subsp. jejuni
Other Campylobacter Species
Former Wolinella and Bacteroides Species Included in the Family Campylobacteraceae

Genus *Arcobacter*
Genus *Helicobacter*

H. pylori

Other Medically Important
Helicobacter Species
Nonhuman Helicobacter Species
Other Microaerophilic Gram-Negative Bacilli

Definitive Identification of Campylobacters and Related Bacteria

Rapid Identification of Campylobacters From Colonies and From Stool Specimens

Nonculture Tests
Direct Detection Methods

Culture and Isolation of *Helicobacter pylori*

Specimens for Recovery of H. pylori
Isolation Procedure
Identification of H. pylori
Biopsy Urease Test (CLO Test)
Noninvasive Tests To Diagnose H. pylori Infection

Accuracy of Invasive and Noninvasive Tests To
    Diagnose *H. pylori* Infection
Enterohepatic Helicobacters

Part II: The Families *Vibrionaceae* and "*Aeromonadaceae*"

Phylogeny of the *Vibrionaceae*

Genus *Vibrio*

Taxonomy
Description and Associated Clinical Syndromes of
    Vibrio Species of Human Importance
Methods for Laboratory Isolation of *Vibrios*

Biochemical Characterization and Laboratory
    Identification of *Vibrio* Species

Genera *Listonella*, *Photobacterium*, and *Shewanella*

Aeromonas and *Plesiomonas*

Genus *Aeromonas*

Taxonomy
Clinical Significance
Aeromonas species in Medicinal Leeches
Laboratory Recovery of *Aeromonas* Species From
    Clinical Specimens
Laboratory Identification of *Aeromonas* Species

Genus *Plesiomonas*

Laboratory Isolation and Identification

Genus *Chromobacterium*

PART I: CURVED RODS: CAMPYLOBACTER, WOLINELLA, ARCOBACTER, HELICOBACTER, *AND RELATED BACTERIA*

Historical Background

The microorganism presently classified as *Campylobacter jejuni* was discovered in 1931 by Jones and coworkers[157] as the causative agent of winter dysentery in cattle. Twenty-six years lapsed before King described a group of microaerophilic, motile curved rods isolated from the blood of children with acute dysentery, which she designated "related vibrios" because they were similar in many respects to *Vibrio fetus*.[174] King astutely mentioned that the vibrios isolated from the blood of children might be closely related to the organism described as *V. jejuni* by Jones in 1931 and that the organism might be more important as a cause of childhood diarrheal syndromes of unknown etiology than previously realized.

This was a prophetic statement; nevertheless, another 15 years passed before this association was substantiated in the laboratory. In 1972, Dekeyser and colleagues[71] isolated the "related vibrios" from the feces of patients with acute enteritis using a filtration technique that allowed the small, curved rods to pass through the membrane but retained larger fecal microorganisms. Several other reports followed, linking related vibrios (*V. fetus*, subsp. *jejuni*; *C. jejuni*) with gastroenteritis in humans, with a distribution throughout the world.[26,27,164] This relative incidence has since been the experience in most clinical laboratories, although during the past several years, the rates of recovery have declined to some degree.

The history of the discovery of *Helicobacter pylori* (formerly named *Campylobacter pyloridis* and then *C. pylori*) is even more circuitous. Warren and Marshall are credited with the "discovery" of the organism in Perth, Australia, in 1982[328]; however, many previous descriptions of spiral organisms in biopsy specimens of human gastric mucosa have appeared in the literature dating back to the beginning of this century.[105,180] Only after successful cultivation of this bacterium using the unique "*Campylobacter* atmosphere" has serious attention been paid to this organism, which may be the most common cause of human gastrointestinal infection as well as the most frequent cause of gastritis.[257]

Classification of Campylobacter *and Related Taxa*

Classification of the microaerophilic gram-negative bacilli has changed considerably over the past few decades. Vandamme and associates,[317,320] using a variety of molecular techniques including DNA-rRNA hybridization, 16S ribosomal RNA (rRNA) sequence analysis, and immunotyping analysis, determined that the *Campylobacter* species and related taxa belong to the same phylogenetic group, which they named rRNA superfamily VI. Five genera, including *Campylobacter*, *Arcobacter*, *Helicobacter*, *Wolinella*, and "*Flexispira*" (which subsequently has been placed in the genus *Helicobacter*) were included in rRNA superfamily VI. Characteristics that differentiate between these related genera are listed in Table 8-1. Solnick and colleagues have also described two uncultivable human gastric spiral organ-

Table 8-1 Characteristics for Differentiating *Arcobacter, Campylobacter, Wolinella, Helicobacter,* **and** *"Flexispira"*

GENUS	NITRATE REDUCTION	GROWTH ON 0.5% GLYCINE	HYDROLYSIS OF UREA	GROWTH AT 15° C	GROWTH AT 30° C	GROWTH AT 42° C	CELL MORPHOLOGY	FLAGELLAR SHEATHS
Arcobacter	+	NA	V	+	+	−	Curved and spiral rods	Absent
Campylobacter	+	V	−	−	+	V	Curved and spiral rods	Absent
Wolinella	+	−	−	−	−	W	Spiral	Absent
Helicobacter	V	+	V	−	V	V	Curved and spiral rods	Present
"Flexispira"	−	+	+	−	−	+	Straight fusiform rods	Present

+, 90% or more of strains are positive; −, 90% or more of strains are negative; V, 11%–89% of strains are positive; W, weak reaction.
Modified from Vandamme P, Falsen E, Rossau R, et al: Revision of Campylobacter, Helicobacter, *and* Wolinella *taxonomy: Emendation of generic descriptions and proposal of* Arcobacter *gen. nov. Int J Syst Bacteriol 41 : 88–103, 1991.*

isms, "*Gastrospirillum hominis*" 1 and 2, that they have identified as helicobacters by 16S rRNA analysis and provisionally named "*Helicobacter heilmannii*".[287]

Studies of Thompson and coworkers[311] showed that bacterial species included in rRNA superfamily VI could be separated into three distinct rRNA clusters. They reported that only those organisms comprising rRNA group I (*C. fetus, C. coli, C. jejuni, C. lari, C. hyointestinalis, C. concisus, C. mucosalis, C. sputorum,* and *C. upsaliensis*) were the true campylobacters. Paster and Dewhirst[252] found a close relationship between *Wolinella curva, Wolinella recta, Bacteroides gracilis, Bacteroides ureolyticus,* and the true campylobacters that made up the rRNA homology group I and suggested that all members of the campylobacter cluster should be placed in the genus *Campylobacter.* Vandamme and colleagues[320] confirmed the findings of Thompson and coworkers[311] and Paster and Dewhirst[252] and proposed an amended description of the genus *Campylobacter* to include all organisms placed in homology group I and the transfer of *W. curva* and *W. recta* to the genus *Campylobacter* as *C. curvus* and *C. rectus,* respectively. Most recently, Vandamme and coworkers[316] proposed the reclassification of *B. gracilis* as *Campylobacter gracilis.* However, while [*B. ureolyticus*] is considered a member of the family *Campylobacteraceae,* it has not as yet been renamed and remains a species *incertae sedis* pending the isolation and characterization of additional *B. ureolyticus*-like bacteria.

The rRNA cluster II contained a homogeneous group of organisms for which Vandamme and associates[320] proposed the genus designation of *Arcobacter.* The genus *Arcobacter* currently includes *Arcobacter nitrofigilis* (formerly *Campylobacter nitrofigilis*), *Arcobacter cryaerophilus* (formerly *Campylobacter cryaerophila*), *Arcobacter (Campylobacter) butzleri,* and *Arcobacter skirrowii.*[172,322]

rRNA cluster III contained members of three different genera: *Helicobacter, Wolinella,* "*Flexispira,*" and an unnamed species, CLO-3. Vandamme and associates emended the description of the genus *Helicobacter* and proposed the transfer of *Campylobacter cinaedi* and *C. fennelliae* to the genus *Helicobacter* as *H. cinaedi* and *H. fennelliae,* respectively.[320] "*Flexispira*" is now included in the genus *Helicobacter. Wolinella succinogenes* remains as the only species of the genus *Wolinella.*

Campylobacter Species

Campylobacter species are microaerophilic (require decreased O_2) and capnophilic (require increased CO_2), curved spiral bacteria, motile by means of a single unsheathed polar flagellum. These organisms are nonfermentative and nonoxidative in their metabolism, deriving energy from the use of amino acids and four- and six-carbon Krebs' cycle intermediates. These organisms used to be classified with *Vibrio* species, until DNA homology studies showed that they were unrelated to the vibrios. Even among the currently recognized *Campylobacter* species, much genotypic and phenotypic diversity exists. The organisms inhabit a wide variety of ecologic niches and environments. Most species are found in animals (cattle, swine) and cause infertility and abortion.

CAMPYLOBACTER JEJUNI SUBSP. *JEJUNI*

Clinical Significance. *C. jejuni* subsp. *jejuni* is the most important human pathogen among the campylobacters. It has worldwide distribution, and in industrialized countries is recovered from diarrheal stool samples from two to seven more times frequently than *Salmonella* or *Shigella.*[10] It is also ubiquitous in domestic animals—house pets may carry the organism, and the vast majority of chickens, turkeys, and waterfowl are colonized.[119] Ingestion of raw milk,[56,324] partially cooked poultry,[119] or contaminated water[48,163] are the common sources for human infections.[107] Enteritis with this organism is characterized by crampy abdominal pain, bloody diarrhea, chills, and fever. For most persons, the infection is self-limited and resolves in 3 to 7 days. The organism may continue to be excreted by convalescing patients for 2 weeks to 1 month. In cases of severe disease, the patient may be treated with oral erythromycin.

Although enteritis and diarrheal syndromes remain the most common manifestations of *Campylobacter* infections, other diseases have emerged during the past few years. Cases of septic arthritis, meningitis, and proctocolitis secondary to *C. jejuni* have been reported.[263] There have now been several reports that associate *C. jejuni* infection with Guillain-Barré syndrome (GBS), an acute demyelinating disease of the peripheral nerves.[122,182,270,290] Data from both serologic and culture studies show that between 20–40% of patients with GBS are infected with *C. jejuni* 1 to 3 weeks prior to the onset of neurological symptoms.[11] The risk of developing GBS after *C. jejuni* infection, however, is quite small (<1 case of GBS/1,000 *C. jejuni* infections).[10] There is no relation between the severity of gastrointestinal symptoms and the likelihood of developing GBS after infection with *C. jejuni*; and in fact, even asymptomatic infections may trigger GBS.[11] In the United States and Japan, 30–80% of *C. jejuni* isolates from patients with GBS belong to Penner serotype 0:19.[11,108] Recently, infection with *C. jejuni* has been associated with immunoproliferative small intestinal disease (also called alpha chain disease).[191] A review of the epidemiology, pathogenesis, and clinical features of *C. jejuni* infection has been written by Allos.[10]

Presumptive Identification From Stool. It may be possible to make a presumptive diagnosis of *Campylobacter* enteritis by observing characteristic gram-negative, curved, S-shaped, gull-winged, or long spiral forms in Gram-stained preparations of diarrheal stools (see Color Plate 8-1*A*). One could consider examining wet mounts or stained smears of all diarrheal stool specimens for polymorphonuclear leukocytes and the presence of bacterial forms suggestive of *Campylobacter* species. Stool specimens for *Campylobacter* species are not further processed in some laboratories unless polymorphonuclear leukocytes are present. The rationale for this practice is that it is unlikely that *Campylobacter* species will be recovered in clinically significant numbers in stool specimens devoid of leukocytes. The expenditure of time and use of special culture media for specimens in which there is little chance to recover significant microbes is not considered cost effective.

Methods for Laboratory Isolation. Successful isolation of *C. jejuni* from stool depends on the use of selective media (e.g., Campy-Thio, Campy-BAP), incubation at an elevated temperature (42°C), and the proper incubation atmosphere (5%

oxygen, 10% CO_2, 85% nitrogen). A membrane filtration technique that is used with nonselective blood agar plates has been reported to be as effective as the use of selective media for the isolation of *C. jejuni*.[295] This method has the advantage of allowing the isolation of antibiotic-sensitive campylobacters. For the past several decades, the selective culture media and special incubation conditions necessary to recover *Campylobacter* species have been used in most clinical microbiology laboratories.

Various procedures can be used to provide a suitable gaseous atmosphere for cultivating microaerophilic campylobacters. These include evacuation-replacement procedures, disposable gas generators, and the use of the Fortner principle. Two of these procedures, which have been used successfully by various investigators, are outlined in Table 8-2. The use of a CO_2 incubator is not recommended for cultivating campylobacters because only strains that are very aerotolerant grow in the atmosphere provided. Likewise, a candle extinction jar is not recommended because the oxygen level (12% to 17%) is too high for optimal growth of campylobacters.[201,327]

Several selective media have been developed to allow for the isolation of *C. jejuni* from fecal samples. Merino and colleagues[217] evaluated the efficacy of seven selective *Campylobacter* isolation media. The names of these media, their composition, and a summary of the evaluation of each are included in Table 8-3. Butzler selective medium, Blaser medium (Campy-BAP), and Skirrow blood agar have been used in most clinical laboratories. However, Merino and colleagues[217] found that Preston *Campylobacter* blood-free medium with cefoperazone yielded the greatest number of *C. jejuni* isolations. Karmali and colleagues[165] found that a blood-free, charcoal-based selective medium (CSM), consisting of Columbia agar base, activated charcoal, hematin, sodium pyruvate, cefoperazone, vancomycin, and cycloheximide, is more selective than Skirrow's medium and has a higher isolation rate of *C. jejuni* from mixed cultures. Charcoal, hematin, ferrous sulfate, and sodium pyruvate serve as substitutes for blood in growth media for campylobacters. Casein is added to help grow certain strains of nalidixic acid-resistant thermophilic campylobacters that are environmental organisms.

Endtz and colleagues[82] compared a semisolid blood-free selective motility medium[117] with two blood-free CSM, two blood-based media (Skirrow medium and Blaser's Campy-BAP), and the membrane filter technique. They found that CSM was the single best medium; however, the highest isolation rates were observed when CSM was used in combination with any other media or the filter technique. Endtz and colleagues also reported that extending the incubation time from 48 to 72 hours led to an increase in the isolation rate regardless of the medium used.[82]

Rectal swabs or swab samples of the stool specimen can be inoculated directly to a small area on the surface of one of the recommended selective agar media. Formed stool specimens may also be processed by emulsifying a small portion (peanut sized) in phosphate-buffered saline or broth before inoculating 1 or 2 drops to the surface of the agar with a Pasteur pipette; similarly, 1 or 2 drops of liquid stool specimens can be inoculated directly.

An outline of a procedure that will allow isolation of enteric campylobacters from fecal samples is shown in Box 8-1. This technique is consistent with current information from the literature about requirements for cultivation of these bacteria and should be suitable for use in most clinical laboratories.

An alternative membrane filter technique, as described by Steele and McDermott,[295] may be used in combination with a Campy-selective medium with equivalent results (see Color Plate 8-1*B* and Box 8-2).

Routine use of enrichment selective "Campy broth" is generally not recommended. Enrichment broths may be beneficial if stool specimens are delayed in transit or left at room temperature too long. Each laboratory director must decide whether an enrichment broth will be beneficial based on local disease patterns and how well the collection and transport of quality specimens can be monitored. Since campylobacters are microaerophilic, they tend to grow best near the top of the tube. If a *Campylobacter* broth is used, the following procedure for subculture should be followed:

Use a Falcon brand polyethylene plastic pipette that can be inverted. Place the tip of the pipette 1 inch below the surface of the medium and continuously withdraw sample as you remove the pipette. Invert the pipette to facilitate mixing of the sample, place 3 drops on a Campy-BAP plate

---

Table 8-2 **Procedures Used by Various Investigators to Create a Microaerophilic Environment Suitable for Cultivating *Campylobacter* Species**

INVESTIGATORS	PROCEDURE
Luechtefeld et al.[201] Evacuation-replacement	Evacuated 75% of air from an anaerobic jar and refilled to atmospheric pressure with a mixture of 10% CO_2 and 90% N_2. Six plates of media were incubated in one jar.
Herbert et al.* Ecacuation-replacement	Evacuated 75% of air from a modified pressure cooker by twice evacuating the container to -15 in. (-38 cm) Hg and refilling with a mixture of 10% CO_2 and 90% N_2 to atmospheric pressure. Plates occupied no more than one-half the volume of the container.

* Herbert GA, Hollis DG, Weaver RE, et al: 30 years of campylobacters: Biochemical characteristics and a biotyping proposal for Campylobacter jejuni. J Clin Microbiol 15: 1065–1073, 1982.

Table 8-3 Formulas for Selective Media for Isolation of *Campylobacter jejuni*

MEDIUM	BASE	ADDITIVES
Butzler's selective medium	Fluid thioglycollate medium (Difco Laboratories, Detroit MI)	Agar (3%) Sheep blood (10%) Bacitracin (25,000 IU/L) Novobiocin (5 mg/L) Colistin (10,000 IU/L) Cephalothin (15 mg/L) Actidione (50 mg/L)
Skirrow's blood agar	Blood agar base No. 2 (Oxoid)	Lysed horse blood (7%) Vancomycin (10 mg/L) Polymyxin B (2,500 IU/L) Trimethoprim (5 mg/L)
Blaser's medium (Campy-BAP)	Brucella agar base (Becton Dickinson, Microbiology Systems, Cockeysville, MD)	Sheep blood (10%) Vancomycin (10 mg/L) Trimethoprim (5 mg/L) Polymyxin B (2500 IU/L) Cephalothin (15 mg/L) Amphotericin B (2 mg/L)
Preston Campylobacter selective medium	Nutrient broth No. 2 (Oxoid CM67) 1.2% New Zealand agar	5% Saponin-lysed horse blood Trimethoprim (10 μg/mL) Polymyxin B (5 IU/mL) Rifampin (10 μg/mL) Cycloheximide (100 μg/mL)
Preston Campylobacter blood-free medium	Nutrient broth No. 2 (Oxiod CM67) 1.2% New Zealand agar	Bacteriologic charcoal Sodium deoxycholate Ferrous sulfate Sodium pyruvate Casein hydrolysate Cefoperazone (32 mg/L)
Butzler virion medium	Columbia agar base (Oxoid CM331)	Defibrinate sheep blood Cefoperazone (15 mg/L) Rifampin (10 mg/L) Colistin (10,000 U/L) Amphotericin B (2 mg/L)
Modified Preston	Nutrient broth No. 2 (Oxoid)	7% defibrinated horse blood Cefoperazone (32 mg/L) Amphotericin B (2 mg/L) Campylobacter growth supplement (Oxoid)
Charcoal-based blood-free selective	Columbia agar base (GIBCO)	Activated charcoal (Oxoid) Hematin (0.032 g/L) Sodium pyruvate (0.1 g/L) Vancomycin (20 mg/L) Cefoperazone (32 mg/L) Cycloheximide (100 mg/L)

Data from Karmali MA, Simer AE, Roscoe M, et al: Evaluation of a blood-free, charcoal-based, selective medium for the isolation of Campylobacter organisms from feces. J Clin Microbiol 23: 456–459, 1986; and Merino FJ, Agulla A, Villasante PA, et al: Comparative efficacy of seven selective media for isolating Campylobacter jejuni. J Clin Microbiol 24: 451–452, 1986.

Box 8-1 Procedure for Isolating *C. jejuni* and Other Enteric *Campylobacter* Species From Fecal Specimens

1. Using a fecal sample or a swab sample in Cary-Blair medium, prepare a turbid suspension of the feces in 10 mL of brain-heart infusion broth. Immediately inoculate one or two plates (two plates are preferable) of a *Campylobacter*-selective medium (best results are obtained with CSM as noted in text); streak to obtain isolated colonies; and hold in a nitrogen-holding jar (see Chapter 14) until the remaining media are inoculated.

2. Lightly centrifuge the specimen (at approximately 1000*g*) for 5 minutes.

3. Remove about 5 mL of the supernatant with a syringe and filter through a sterile 0.65-μL Millipore filter, as described by Butzler.[41] Discard the first 3 mL of fluid and use 1 or 2 drops of the remainder to inoculate two plates of chocolate agar without selective agents or a blood agar medium such as the Centers for Disease Control (CDC) anaerobe blood agar that will support the growth of *Campylobacter*. Streak for isolation.

4. Incubate one set of Campy-selective agar and chocolate agar plates at 42°C in an atmosphere of 5% O_2, 10% CO_2, and 85% N_2 and the remaining plates at 35°C to 37°C in the same gaseous atmosphere.

5. Inspect the plates after 24, 48, and 72 hours of incubation for colonies characteristic of *Campylobacter* species and identify the isolates with the techniques described in the text. Plates not showing growth after 24 or 48 hours of incubation should be returned for an additional 24 to 48 hours in the same incubator and gaseous atmospheric conditions, as described above.

Box 8-2 Steele and McDermott Membrane Filter Technique

1. Mix 1 g stool in 10 mL of sterile saline containing glass beads. Vortex for 30 seconds.

2. Place a 47-mm, 0.45 Gelman cellulose triacetate membrane filter (Gelman No. 63069) centrally onto the surface of a nonselective *Brucella* agar plate containing 5% sheep blood.

3. Place 8 to 10 drops of fecal suspension on the surface of the filter with a Pasteur pipette. Take care to ensure that the drops do not extend to the edge of the filter.

4. Remove filter and discard 30 minutes after the suspension is applied.

5. Incubate plate in Campy environment as described previously.

---

and streak for isolation. Incubate as you would a primary culture plate.

Identification From Culture. The appearance of colonies on one of the selective *Campylobacter* agars that has been incubated at 42°C in the gaseous environment described previously is already presumptive evidence that the organism is one of the thermophilic *Campylobacter* species (most commonly *C. jejuni*). The morphology of *Campylobacter* species on selective agar varies from flat, gray, irregular-shaped colonies that may be either dry or moist to colonies that are round and convex and glistening with entire edges (Color Plate 8-1*C, D*). There is a tendency for colonies to form confluent growth along the streak lines on the agar surface. Hemolytic reactions are not observed on blood agar. The identification can be further confirmed by performing rapid catalase and cytochrome oxidase tests (*C. jejuni, C. coli,* and *C. lari* are positive for both). On occasion, thermophilic bacterial species other than *Campylobacter* species, notably *Pseudomonas aeruginosa,* may break through and grow on the selective media. It is unlikely, however, that *P. aeruginosa* would be confused with *C. jejuni*. The colony morphology of the two organisms is different; and if there were any question, a Gram stain would quickly differentiate *Campylobacter* species from *P. aeruginosa*.

Gram-stained preparations from colonies of *C. jejuni* after 24 to 48 hours incubation on blood agar show characteristic gram-negative, curved, "S"-shaped, gull-winged, or long spiral forms (see Color Plate 8-1*A*). Coccoid forms are more commonly seen in older cultures of *C. jejuni,* particularly after colonies have been exposed to ambient air. Strict adherence to usual Gram stain timing is important because *Campylobacter* species are typically faintly staining. For this reason, one could consider extending the staining time of the safranin counterstain to at least 10 minutes to allow for greater staining intensity.

Once isolated, both subspecies of *C. jejuni* can be easily identified since they are the only campylobacters that hydrolyze hippurate (see Color Plate 8-1*E* and Table 8-4). In addition, this species is resistant to cephalothin and usually is susceptible to nalidixic acid, although resistant isolates are occasionally encountered (see Color Plate 8-1*F*).

OTHER *CAMPYLOBACTER* SPECIES

C. coli. *C. coli* is closely related to *C. jejuni* and also is an important foodborne pathogen in humans.[303] It shares several cultural characteristics with *C. jejuni,* including susceptibility to nalidixic acid and resistance to cephalothin. *C. coli* can be differentiated from *C. jejuni* by the hippurate hydrolysis test (*C. jejuni* hydrolyzes hippurate; *C. coli* does not). The report when this organism is recovered in laboratories in which the hippurate test is not performed should read, "*C. jejuni/coli.*" It is estimated that *C. coli* accounts for 5–10% of cases of *Campylobacter* enteritis in humans.[228] A case of urinary tract infection caused by quinolone-resistant *C. coli* has also been reported.[251]

C. concisus. *C. concisus* is capable of anaerobic growth and requires hydrogen or formate for growth. The organism is isolated most commonly from human gingival crevices. However, it also may cause gastrointestinal disease, especially in immunocompromised patients.[1,190,318] Recovery of

Table 8-4 Differential Characteristics of Campylobacters and Related Taxa of Medical Importance

ORGANISM	CATALASE	NITRATE	HYDROGEN SULFIDE TRIPLE SUGAR IRON	UREASE	INDOXYL ACETATE	HIPPURATE	GROWTH 25°C	37°C	42°C	Mac-Conkey	0.1% TMAO	1.5% NaCl	1% Glycine	SUSCEPTIBILITY* Nalidixic Acid	Cephalothin
RNA Group I															
Campylobacter coli	+	+	–	–	+	–	–	+	+	+	–	–	+	V	R
C. concisus	–	+	+	–	–	–	–	+	C	+	–	–	C	R	R
C. curvus	–	+	+	–	V	V	–	+	V	V	NA	NA	+	C	S
C. fetus subsp. fetus	+	+	–	–	–	–	+	+	–	+	–	V	+	V	S
C. fetus subsp. venerealis	V	+	–	–	–	–	+	+	–	+	–	V	–	V	S
C. gracilis	–	+	–	–	V	–	–	+	V	V	NA	NA	+	V	S
C. helveticus	–	+	–	–	+	–	–	+	+	–	–	NA	V	S	S
C. hyointestinalis subsp. hyointestinalis	+	+	+	–	–	–	V	+	+	+	+	–	+	R	S
C. hyointestinalis subsp. lawsonii	+	+	+	–	–	–	–	+	+	V	NA	NA	V	R	S
C. jejuni subsp. jejuni	+	+	–	–	+	+	–	+	+	–	–	–	+	V	R
C. jejuni subsp. doylei	V	–	–	–	+	+	–	+	W	–	–	–	+	S	S
C. lari	+	+	–	–	–	–	–	+	+	+	+	+	+	R	R
C. mucosalis	–	+	+	–	–	–	C	+	+	+	C	C	C	C	S
C. rectus	–	+	+	–	+	–	–	+	W	–	NA	NA	+	V	S
C. showae	+	+	+	–	V	–	–	+	V	+	NA	NA	V	S	S
C. sputorum biovar bubulus	–	+	+	–	–	–	–	+	C	–	+	+	+	R	S
C. sputorum biovar fecalis	+	+	+	–	–	–	–	+	+	+	+	+	+	R	S
C. sputorum biovar sputorum	–	+	+	–	–	–	–	+	+	–	C	+	+	V	S
C. upsaliensis	–(w)	+	–	–	+	–	–	+	+	–	–	–	C	S	S

(Continued)

399

Table 8-4 *Continued*

ORGANISM	CATALASE	NITRATE	HYDROGEN SULFIDE TRIPLE SUGAR IRON	UREASE	INDOXYL ACETATE	HIPPURATE	GROWTH							SUSCEPTIBILITY*	
							25°C	37°C	42°C	Mac-Conkey	0.1% TMAO	1.5% NaCl	1% Glycine	Nali-dixic Acid	Cephal-othin
RNA Group II															
Arcobacter butzleri	−(w)	+	−	−	+	−	+	+	V	+	NA	V	+	V	R
A. cryaerophilus	+	+	−	−	+	−	+	+	−	−	−	+	−	V	R
A. nitrofigilis	+	+	+	V	−	−	+	+	−	−	NA	+	−	S	S
A. skirrowii	+	+	−	−	+	−	+	+	V	−	NA	−	V	S	V
RNA Group III															
Helicobacter cinaedi (CLO-1)	+	+	−	−	C	−	−	+	−	−	−	−	+	S	S
H. fennelliae (CLO-2)	+	−	−	−	+	−	−	+	+	−	−	−	+	S	S
CLO-3	+	−	−	−	+	−	−	+	+	NA	NA	NA	+	S	R
H. pullorum	+	+	−	−	−	−	−	+	+	NA	−	NA	NA	S	R
H. pylori	+	−	−	++	−	−	−	+	C	−	−	NA	V	R	S
Helicobacter sp. strain flexispira	C	−	−	++	−	−	−	+	+	NA	NA	NA	−(w)	R	R

*Susceptibility to antibiotics determined with 30-µg disks.

+, 90% or more of strains are positive; −, 90% or more of strains are negative; V, 11%–89% of strains are positive; ++, strong positive reaction; NA, results not available; C, contradictory reports in literature; R, resistant; S, susceptible; TMAO, trimethylamine oxide.

Data from references 8, 14, 17, 36, 84, 91, 115, 135, 172, 245, 256, 261, 275, 292, 293, 296, 313, 317, 320, 322.

400

C. concisus from stool specimens requires use of the filter method (discussed elsewhere in this chapter).

C. fetus Subsp. fetus. *C. fetus* subsp. *fetus* is primarily associated with infective abortion in cattle and sheep and is an infrequent cause of human infections. Infections usually result in systemic illness and usually affect debilitated persons with chronic hepatic, renal, or neoplastic disease, or with compromised immune function.[49,256] *C. fetus* subsp. *fetus* has been reported to cause proctitis and proctocolitis in homosexual men[74]; premature labor and neonatal sepsis in humans[50]; septic abortion[298]; neonatal meningitis[185]; prosthetic hip joint infection[19,333]; and both native and prosthetic valve endocarditis.[88] The organism was not previously believed to cause gastroenteritis, but, because of its susceptibility to cephalothin and its failure to grow at 42°C, it may not be recovered in clinical laboratories where selective media and increased incubation temperatures are used as a screen for *C. jejuni;* therefore, its etiologic role in this infection is not known.[127]

C. fetus Subsp. venerealis. *C. fetus* subsp. *venerealis* comprises part of the normal genital tract flora of bulls but has not been associated with human infection.[283]

C. helveticus. *C. helveticus* is a thermophilic catalase-negative *Campylobacter* that has been isolated from the feces of domestic cats and dogs.[292] Of note is the fact that almost half of the *Campylobacter* isolates found in cats belong to *C. helveticus*.[39] Colonies of *C. helveticus* are adherent on blood agar and can be separated from other thermophilic species (*C. jejuni, C. coli,* and *C. lari*) by virtue of a negative catalase reaction. It is indoxyl acetate positive and susceptible to both nalidixic acid and cephalothin.

C. hyoilei. *C. hyoilei* is the name for a group of similar bacteria isolated from intestinal lesions of pigs with proliferative enteritis.[8] No human isolates have been reported.

C. hyointestinalis. *C. hyointestinalis,* closely related to *C. fetus* subsp. *fetus,* was initially found only in animals, principally as a cause of ileitis in swine,[110] but more recently has been reported from human clinical specimens. In one report, *C. hyointestinalis* was isolated from stool specimens of four persons, all of whom were experiencing nonbloody, watery diarrhea. The youngest (8 months) and the oldest (79 years) persons were female, and the other two were homosexual men.[80] A case of a 52-year-old woman with chronic myeloid leukemia and nonbloody, watery diarrhea associated with this organism has been reported from France,[220] and an isolate from the rectal culture of a homosexual man with proctitis has been reported in the United States.[90] *C. hyointestinalis* will not be recovered on many *Campylobacter* media formulations because it is susceptible to cephalosporins such as cephalothin and cefoperazone. Although it will grow at 42°C, growth is more luxuriant at 35°C.[90] The organism is also resistant to nalidixic acid, is hippurate negative, and produces hydrogen sulfide in triple sugar iron agar. The production of hydrogen sulfide in triple sugar iron agar is dependent on the test being incubated in a microaerophilic environment containing hydrogen.[110]

A group of ''*C. hyointestinalis*-like'' organisms obtained from porcine stomachs have been described. These isolates are sufficiently different from *C. hyointestinalis* to warrant creation of a separate subspecies classification, *C. hyointestinalis* subsp. *lawsonii*.[245] The creation of this new subspecies

necessitates that the description of *C. hyointestinalis* be emended to *C. hyointestinalis* subsp. *hyointestinalis*. *C. hyointestinalis* subsp. *lawsonii* can be separated from subsp. *hyointestinalis* by its failure to grow in 1.5% bile. *C. hyointestinalis* subsp. *lawsonii* has been isolated from the intestines and stomachs of pigs; hamster intestines; and the feces of cattle, deer, and humans; but its pathogenicity is not known.[245]

C. jejuni Subsp. doylei. A new subspecies of *C. jejuni* has been isolated from human clinical specimens including gastric epithelium biopsies[166] and feces from children with diarrhea.[296] The pathogenicity of the organism remains unknown. *C. jejuni* subsp. *doylei* can be distinguished readily from other campylobacters because it does not reduce nitrates and hydrolyzes hippurate.[296] It is susceptible to cephalothin and therefore will not be recovered on media containing cephalosporin-type antibiotics.

C. lari. Formerly named *C. laridis,* the organism now known as *C. lari* is thermophilic, halotolerant, and nalidixic acid resistant; otherwise, it shares several features with *C. jejuni* and *C. coli*.[282] Anaerobic growth in the presence of 0.1% trimethylamine oxide (TMAO) and failure to hydrolyze indoxyl acetate help to identify this species (reagents available from Sigma Chemical Co., St. Louis, MO). Many laboratories rely on resistance to nalidixic acid to separate *C. lari* from *C. jejuni* and *C. coli;* however, *C. jejuni* resistant to nalidixic acid are being seen with increased frequency. *C. lari* is endemic in sea gulls but is an infrequent human pathogen. However, occasionally it causes enteritis simulating *C. jejuni* infections and rarely, bacteremia, especially in immunocompromised persons.[21,58,209,230,306]

C. mucosalis. *C. mucosalis,* formerly classified as *C. sputorum* subsp. *mucosalis,* produces a yellow pigment and is catalase negative. Phenotypically, this species is very similar to *C. sputorum* biovars *sputorum* and *bubulus* but is able to grow at 25°C. Unlike the majority of campylobacters, this species requires hydrogen and formate as an electron donor for growth, an essential requirement of *C. concisus, C. mucosalis, C. curvus,* and *C. rectus*.[317] Figura and colleagues[92] reported what was thought to be the first isolation of *C. mucosalis* from children with enteritis. However, this finding has been disputed and the isolates have been shown by molecular probe studies to be *C. concisus*.[186,188,242] These two species are difficult to separate on the basis of biochemical tests alone and it has been suggested that molecular methods must be used for the precise identification of these two species.[188] On[242] has suggested the use of several media containing various inhibitory agents for separating *C. concisus* and *C. mucosalis*. There are as yet no confirmed reports associating *C. mucosalis* with human infection.

C. showae. *C. showae* is a recently described species isolated from human gingival crevices.[84] The organism appears as a straight rod with round ends and contains two to five unsheathed unipolar flagella—a feature that is unique among campylobacters. The organism grows in a microaerophilic atmosphere in the presence of fumarate with formate or H_2, but prefers to grow under anaerobic conditions. Because of the limited number of reliable biochemical traits that can be used to differentiate closely related *Campylobacter* species, serologic or molecular tests or protein profiles may be required to positively identify isolates of this species.[84] An association with human disease has not been shown.

C. sputorum. *C. sputorum* is capable of anaerobic growth and can be recovered from the oral cavity and gingival crevices of humans. This organism is not recognized as an agent of human disease, although a few clinical isolates have been reported. Three biovars are described: *C. sputorum* bv. *bubulus, C. sputorum* bv. *sputorum,* and *C. sputorum* bv. *fecalis.*[269]

C. upsaliensis. *C. upsaliensis* is catalase negative or only weakly positive and thus has been referred to as the CNW strain of *Campylobacter.* However, because weak catalase reactions may also occur for *C. jejuni* subsp. *doylei,* the CNW designation no longer holds. Except for the lack of or weak production of catalase, this organism shares several characteristics with pathogenic campylobacters. It is thermophilic (grows at 42°C) and is highly susceptible to drugs that are present in selective isolation media, making them unsuitable for the isolation of *C. upsaliensis.*[297] Goossens and coworkers[116] reported the isolation of 99 strains of *C. upsaliensis* by the filter method, with only 4 strains recovered simultaneously from selective media.

Domestic pets may serve as the reservoir of this species, which was first isolated from healthy dogs, dogs with diarrhea, and, later, from asymptomatic cats.[102,276] Data from some reports suggest that this organism may be an opportunistic agent of infections in children. Lastovica and associates[187] reported the recovery of *C. upsaliensis* from blood cultures of 16 patients, 10 of whom were 10 months old or younger. Walmsley and Karmali[326] reported the isolation of this organism from the stools of six children. Other reports have associated the isolation of *Campylobacter upsaliensis* from the blood of patients with serious underlying disease.[43,60] There has been one report of *C. upsaliensis* isolated from the blood and fetoplacental material of an 18-week pregnant woman who suffered a spontaneous abortion.[120] The patient had no underlying disease, and her only previous

pregnancy was uneventful. Numerical analysis of protein profiles revealed that strains isolated from the patient and a healthy household cat were almost identical, implying that the cat might have been the source of the infection.[120] The only report of *C. upsaliensis* from a site other than blood or stool was from a case of a breast abscess in which *C. upsaliensis* was recovered along with a *Peptostreptococcus* species from purulent exudate obtained through fine-needle aspiration of the infected site.[109] Sandstedt and Ursing[275] have described *C. upsaliensis,* including its phenotypic characteristics and clinical significance.

FORMER *WOLINELLA* AND *BACTEROIDES* SPECIES INCLUDED IN THE FAMILY *CAMPYLOBACTERACEAE*

Tanner and colleagues, in their studies of the taxonomy of the anaerobic, agar-pitting, gram-negative bacilli, placed the nonmotile strains into the genus *Bacteroides* and the motile strains into the group of "anaerobic vibrios" (including *Wolinella recta, W. curva,* and *Campylobacter concisus*).[304,305] The nonmotile strains are separated on the basis of urease production into *B. ureolyticus* (urease positive) and *B. gracilis* (urease negative; see Table 8-5). These species are all now included in the family *Campylobacteraceae* and are considered true campylobacters.[317,320]

C. gracilis. The name *Bacteroides gracilis* was proposed by Tanner et al.[304] for a group of agar-corroding bacteria that were originally considered to be anaerobic. In 1995, Vandamme and colleagues proposed the transfer of this organism to the genus *Campylobacter* as *C. gracilis.*[316] These bacteria are found in the gingival crevices of humans and have been isolated primarily from sites of deep tissue infection. Johnson and colleagues have reported that 83% of the specimens in which *C. gracilis* was isolated were obtained from patients with serious visceral or head and neck infections.[155] *C. gracilis* is microaerophilic and asaccharolytic and resembles campylobacters in almost all phenotypic characteristics. In-

Table 8-5 Characteristics Useful for Differentiating *Campylobacter curvus, C. rectus, C. gracilis,* [*Bacteroides ureolyticus*], and *Wolinella succinogenes*

CHARACTERISTIC	*C. CURVUS*	*C. RECTUS*	*C. GRACILIS*	[*B. UREOLYTICUS*]	*W. SUCCINOGENES*
Source	Human clinical	Human clinical	Human clinical	Human clinical	Bovine rumen
Morphology					
Helical or curved cells dominate	+	−	−	−	+
Straight cells dominate	−	+	+	+	−
Cells with tapered ends	+	−	−	−	+
Motility	+	+	−	−	+
Urease	−	−	−	+	−
Growth in 1% glycine	+	+	NA	NA	−
Indoxyl acetate hydrolysis	+	+	V	NA	−

+, 90% or more of strains are positive; −, 90% or more of strains are negative; V, 11% to 89% of strains are positive; NA, results not available.
Modified from Tanner ACR, Listgarten MA, Ebersole JL: Wolinella curva sp. nov.: "Vibrio succinogenes" of human origin. Int J Syst Bacteriol 34:275–282, 1984.

dividual cells stain gram-negative and are small and un-branched, often having both tapered and rounded ends. Growth is stimulated in broth cultures by formate and fumarate. They may be differentiated from other campylobacters by the absence of flagella and the absence of oxidase activity.[304] *C. gracilis* isolates appear less susceptible to antimicrobial agents than the closely related species [*B. ureolyticus*], with only 67% of the isolates reported to be susceptible to penicillin.[155] A selective medium for isolation of *C. gracilis* has been described that contains tryptic soy agar base, formate, fumarate, nitrate, and two selective agents, nalidixic acid and teicoplanin.[194]

Bacteroides ureolyticus. Ribosomal RNA sequence analysis clearly places [*B. ureolyticus*] as a member of the family *Campylobacteraceae,* however, it is not clear whether it branches outside the *Campylobacter* cluster (and should be placed in a new genus) or inside the *Campylobacter* cluster (and should be included in the genus *Campylobacter*).[316] [*B. ureolyticus*] differs from campylobacters in its fatty acid composition, its proteolytic metabolism, and its ability to hydrolyze urea.[316] [*B. ureolyticus*] strains have been isolated from patients with superficial ulcers, soft-tissue infections, nongonococcal nonchlamydial urethritis, and periodontal disease.[76,77,95,96] In a study by Johnson and colleagues, [*B. ureolyticus*] strains were found to be uniformly susceptible to penicillins, cephalosporins, erythromycin, clindamycin, chloramphenicol, metronidazole, and aminoglycosides.[155]

C. curvus. *C. curvus* was originally named *Wolinella curva.*[305,320] Cells stain gram negative and are short and slightly curved. Helical or straight cells may also occur. Strains exhibit rapid, darting motility and are asaccharolytic. The organism grows anaerobically and in 5% O_2 atmospheres containing H_2. No growth occurs in air enriched with 10% CO_2. All cultures require formate and fumarate for broth growth. Some strains exhibit a corroding morphology on agar media. Isolates have been recovered exclusively from human sources and include dental root canal, alveolar abscess, and blood.[305] Characteristics useful in distinguishing *C. curvus* from similar species are given in Table 8-5.

C. rectus. *C. rectus* was originally named *Wolinella recta.*[304,320] Microscopically, the cells appear small and straight with rounded ends and stain gram negative. Strains exhibit rapid, darting motility and are asaccharolytic. Growth is anaerobic; however, some strains can grow in a 5% O_2 atmosphere but not in air enriched with 10% CO_2. Growth in broth is stimulated by formate and fumarate. Nitrates and nitrites are reduced, and both oxidase and catalase are negative. Additional identifying characteristics are given in Table 8-5. *C. rectus* is found in the gingival crevices of humans.[304] Spiegel and Telford[291] reported isolating this organism along with *Actinomyces viscosus* from an actinomycotic chest wall mass. Two isolates of *C. rectus* have been recovered from patients at the University of Illinois Hospital, one from a lung nodule of a patient with an 18-year history of alcohol abuse and an 8-month history of right-sided chest pain and another from the blood culture of a patient with a lung mass.

Genus *Arcobacter*

Arcobacter species are aerotolerant; they grow in the presence of atmospheric levels of oxygen.[244] Other characteristics useful in distinguishing aerotolerant "*Campylobacter*" species from other campylobacters include hydrolysis of indoxyl acetate; growth at 15°C, 25°C, and 36°C but not 42°C; and the inability to hydrolyze hippurate (see Table 8-4). Vandamme and colleagues have shown that the arcobacters can be separated into five major groups, which were identified by DNA-DNA hybridization data as *A. cryaerophilus* (two distinct subgroups), *A. butzleri, A. nitrofigilis,* and *A. skirrowii.*[322]

A. cryaerophilus. *A. cryaerophilus* (formerly *C. cryaerophila*) grows well under aerobic conditions, although it may require microaerophilic conditions for initial isolation. Optimal growth occurs at 30°C, and the organism will not grow at 42°C. Biochemically, this species resembles *C. fetus* subsp. *fetus;* however, *A. cryaerophilus* is indoxyl acetate positive, whereas *C. fetus* subsp. *fetus* is not (see Table 8-4). Most strains are sensitive to nalidixic acid and resistant to cephalothin. In a report by Borczyk and colleagues[30] comparing growth of *A. cryaerophilus* on CMS, Skirrow's blood agar, and cefsulodin irgasan novobiocin (CIN) agar, it was noted that the most luxuriant growth was obtained on CIN agar incubated for 24 to 48 hours at 25°C and 36°C. Isolates resembling *A. cryaerophilus* have been recovered from humans. One case of *A. cryaerophilus* isolated from the stool of a man infected with human immunodeficiency virus (HIV) with intermittent diarrhea was reported, however, this strain was subsequently found to be *A. butzleri.*[307,308]

A. nitrofigilis. *A. nitrofigilis* (formerly *Campylobacter nitrofigilis*) is a cryophilic species that grows optimally at 25°C. It is urea positive and nonpathogenic for humans.

A. butzleri. Kiehlbauch and colleagues at the CDC[172] have reported that the strains of aerotolerant campylobacters do not make up a homogeneous group. The majority of human isolates, both from within and outside the United States, make up a distinct DNA homology group that they named *Campylobacter butzleri* (changed to *Arcobacter butzleri* following the acceptance of the new genus designation for this group of organisms).[322] Strains of *A. butzleri* can be separated from *A. cryaerophilus* by demonstrating aerotolerance at both 30°C and 36°C (*A. cryaerophilus* is aerotolerant at 30°C but not at 36°C). In addition, *A. butzleri* grows on MacConkey agar and in glycine- and nitrate-containing media (reducing nitrate to nitrite) and in 1.5% and 3.5% NaCl. *A. cryaerophilus* gives the opposite reactions.[172] The majority of isolates of *A. butzleri* from humans have been from stools of patients with diarrheal illness;[172,195,321] however, the organism rarely has been isolated from abdominal contents, peritoneal fluid, and blood.[172,332]

A. skirrowii. *A. skirrowii* is the newest species of *Arcobacter* to be described. Strains have been isolated mainly from the preputial fluids of bulls; other strains have been isolated from aborted fetuses and diarrheic feces from cows, pigs, and sheep. The clinical significance of this new species has not been established.

Genus *Helicobacter*

(Proposed names that are not yet validated by the International Committee on Systematic Bacteriology are enclosed in quotation marks.)

The genus *Helicobacter* comprises 23 formally validated

species. *Helicobacter* species are strict microaerophiles with a spiral or helical morphology. Many species exhibit strong urease activity. *Helicobacter* species strain ''flexispira'' (formerly ''*Flexispira rappini*'') is the name proposed for an organism that is closely related to *Helicobacter* but is cigar-shaped rather than curved and fusiform shaped. Species included in the genera *Helicobacter* possess sheathed flagella. No *Campylobacter* or *Wolinella* species possess sheathed flagella (see Table 8-1).

H. PYLORI

This species was initially called *Campylobacter pyloridis* and then *Campylobacter pylori*. Molecular analysis provided evidence showing that this organism does not belong to the genus *Campylobacter*.[115] Features that distinguish this organism from campylobacters are its multiple sheathed flagella, its strong hydrolysis of urea, and its unique fatty acid profile (a high percentage of 14:0 acid, a low percentage of 16:0 acid, and the presence of 3-OH-18:0 acid). 16S rRNA sequencing has shown that this organism is closely related to *Wolinella succinogenes*. However, there are many differences in biochemical features and growth characteristics between *H. pylori* and *W. succinogenes* that indicate that these species should not be in the same genus. *W. succinogenes* is catalase negative, is urease negative, does not possess γ-glutamyltranspeptidase or alkaline phosphatase activity, and does not grow at 30°C or on 0.5% glycine; *H. pylori* has the opposite characteristics.

H. pylori is found only on the mucus-secreting epithelial cells of the stomach. Evidence suggests that *H. pylori* is the causative agent of active chronic antral gastritis[207] and is a major factor in the pathogenesis of peptic ulcer disease.[257] Additionally, there is strong evidence that *H. pylori* is linked to gastric adenocarcinoma and to the development of gastric non-Hodgkin's lymphoma.[250,288] *H. pylori* gastritis is widespread in many countries in the world and may be one of the most common chronic human infections. The case for *H. pylori* as a causative agent of duodenal ulcer remains controversial. For excellent reviews see the work of Blaser,[25] Buck,[36] and Dunn and colleagues.[78]

H. pylori strains are microaerophilic (10% CO_2, 5% O_2, 85% N_2) and will also grow in air with increased (10%) CO_2 content. The optimum temperature for isolation is 35°C to 37°C, although some strains will grow at 42°C. High humidity has also been found to favor growth. Most strains take 3 to 5 days to grow, with occasional isolates requiring 7 days of incubation before growth is evident. They can be cultured on nonselective blood-containing media, producing small, translucent, gray colonies. The characteristic Gram stain (small, curved, slightly plump bacilli) and positive reactions for catalase, oxidase, and urease provide an identification.

OTHER MEDICALLY IMPORTANT HELICOBACTER SPECIES

Several species of *Helicobacter* other than *H. pylori* have been isolated from humans and are associated with human disease.[145,286,288] These include *H. cinaedi, H. fennelliae, H. canadensis, H. canis, H. winghamensis, H. pullorum, Helicobacter* species strain flexispira (''*Flexispira rappini*''), *H.*

heilmanni (''*Gastrospirillum hominis*''), and the unnamed *Helicobacter* species CLO-3 (see Table 8-6).[97,215,288,293]

H. cinaedi. *H. cinaedi*, originally designated as CLO-1, and formerly known as ''*Campylobacter cinaedi*,'' has been isolated from rectal swabs taken from symptomatic as well as asymptomatic homosexual men.[91,313] This organism has also been described as a cause of bacteremia in two homosexual men with concurrent tuberculosis,[254] in patients with acquired immunodeficiency syndrome (AIDS),[61,70,273] and in another who was HIV seropositive but did not have AIDS.[236] Reports, however, suggest that *C. cinaedi* infections are not restricted to homosexual or bisexual men. For example, Vandamme and associates[319] have reported the isolation of *H. cinaedi* from the blood of two women without any record of sexual contact with homosexuals and from the stools of three children, two of whom were girls.

Orlicek and colleagues have reported a case of septicemia and meningitis caused by *H. cineadi* in a neonate.[246] Since *H. cinaedi* has been identified as a normal intestinal inhabitant of hamsters[111,299] and the mother of the newborn cared for pet hamsters during the first two trimesters of her pregnancy, it is likely that the hamsters served as a reservoir for the transmission of the organism to the mother and that the newborn most likely became colonized with *H. cinaedi* during the birth process.[246] Kielbauch and colleagues reported that the clinical spectrum of illness associated with *H. cinaedi* infection includes fever, bacteremia, and recurrent cellulitis, with most patients having signs of systemic infection including leukocytosis, and often thrombocytopenia.[173] These same authors report that treatment with a penicillin, tetracycline, or aminoglycoside may be more effective than treatment with cephalosporins, erythromycin or ciprofloxacin.[173] Burman and coworkers have also reported the association of skin infections and arthritis due to *H. cinaedi* bacteremia.[38] Most blood isolates are recovered in automated blood culture instruments after 5 or more days of incubation. In general, organisms are not seen on initial Gram staining of the blood culture material but can be visualized by darkfield or acridine orange staining. *H. cinaedi* grows only at 37°C, shows intermediate resistance to cephalothin (30-μg disk) and reduces nitrate to nitrite. Additional genotypic and phenotypic characteristics can be found in the report by Kiehlbauch and colleagues.[171] The only known natural reservoir of *H. cinaedi* found so far is the intestinal tract of hamsters, which may serve as a reservoir of human infections.[111,299]

H. fennelliae. Originally designated CLO-2, and formerly known as ''*Campylobacter fennelliae*,''[313] this organism has the distinctive odor of hypochlorite cleaning powders.[91] It is susceptible to cephalothin and does not reduce nitrates to nitrite. As with *H. cinaedi, H. fennelliae* has been isolated from rectal swabs taken from symptomatic and asymptomatic homosexual men.[91] There is one report of this organism being isolated from the blood of a 31-year-old bisexual man with a history of intravenous drug abuse and a positive HIV serology.[236]

CLO-3. An unnamed species originally described by Fennell and coworkers,[91] CLO-3 can be separated from the other CLOs by its ability to grow at 42°C, its resistance to cephalothin, and its inability to reduce nitrate (see Table 8-4). One

Table 8-6 *Helicobacter* **Species and Related Organisms**

SPECIES	HOSTS	SITE OF ISOLATION
H. acinonychis	Cheetahs	Gastric mucosa
H. bilis	Mice	Bile, liver, intestine
H. bizzozeronii	Dogs	Gastric mucosa
H. canis	Dogs, humans	Feces
H. cinaedi	Humans, hamsters	Blood, rectal swabs (humans), intestines (hamsters)
H. felis	Cats, dogs	Gastric mucosa
H. fennelliae	Humans	Blood, rectal swabs
H. hepaticus	Mice	Liver, intestine
H. muridarum	Rats, mice	Intestine
H. mustelae	Ferrets	Gastric mucosa
H. nemestrinae	Pigtailed macaque monkeys	Gastric mucosa
H. pametensis	Wild birds (tern, gull), pigs	Feces
H. pullorum	Chickens, humans	Intestines, liver (chickens), feces (humans)
H. pylori	Humans, monkeys, cats	Gastric mucosa
Helicobacter sp. strain flexispira	Sheep, dogs, humans	Liver (sheep), stomach (dogs), feces (humans)
"*H. heilmannii*"	Cheetahs, humans	Gastric mucosa
CLO-3	Humans	Rectal swabs

isolate has been reported from a rectal swab obtained from a symptomatic homosexual man.[91]

Helicobacter *Sp.* Strain *flexispira* ("Flexispira rappini").
Helicobacter species strain "flexispira" (formerly "*Flexispira rappini*") is the proposed name[35] of an organism that is urease positive and possibly genomically closely related to *H. pylori*.[320] However, it is a straight organism rather than a spiral one and is fusiform with a corrugated surface owing to the presence of periplasmic fibers. It has multiple, bipolar flagella. It does not possess alkaline phosphatase or grow at 30°C but does grow at 42°C and is resistant to metronidazole (5 µg), whereas *H. pylori* has the opposite characteristics.[115] It is separated from the campylobacters by negative reactions for catalase and nitrate and an inability to grow in 1% glycine.[14] *Helicobacter* species strain "flexispira" has been isolated from stool specimens of humans with symptoms of gastroenteritis and from blood cultures, from stool of dogs,[14,268] and from aborted ovine fetuses.[175,176,268,289,309]

"Helicobacter heilmannii" ("Gastrospirillum hominis").
"*Helicobacter heilmannii*" is an uncultivated spiral bacterium found in human gastric mucosa that is larger and more tightly coiled than *H. pylori*. The organism is helical, 3.5–7.5 fm long and 0.9 µm in diameter with truncated ends flattened at the tips, six to eight tight spirals, and up to 12 sheathed flagella 28 nm in diameter at each pole.[212] McNulty and colleagues proposed the name "*G. hominis*." However, Solnick and coworkers[287] have shown that "*Gastrospirillum*"

is a member of the *Helicobacter* genus and have proposed the name "*H. heilmannii*" after Konrad Heilmann, a German histopathologist who described the first large series of patients infected with the organism.[128] Heilmann and Borchard reported the prevalence of "*Gastrospirillum*" infection in patients presenting for endoscopy to be less than 1%.[128] "*H. heilmannii*" appears to be ubiquitous in domestic animals, suggesting that human infection may be acquired as a zoonosis.[75,100,129] Human infection with this bacterium may be accompanied by chronic gastritis similar to that seen with infection by *H. pylori*.[72,94,128,192,212,222,286]

NONHUMAN *HELICOBACTER* SPECIES

A number of *Helicobacter* species have been isolated from animals. Among these are *H. acinonychis*,[79] *H. bilis*,[104] *H. bizzozeronii*,[123] *H. canis*,[294] *H. felis*,[253] *H. hepaticus*,[99] *H. muridarum*,[193] *H. mustelae*,[98,103,115] *H. nemestrinae*,[34] and *H. pullorum*.[40,293] These bacteria are generally found in the stomach or the lower gastrointestinal tract.[101] When present in the stomach, these helicobacters are usually associated with gastritis in the host animal. Some of these strains have also been isolated from humans (see Table 8-6).

OTHER MICROAEROPHILIC GRAM-NEGATIVE BACILLI

Wolinella succinogenes. This is the type species of the genus *Wolinella*, presently defined as being anaerobic, catalase negative, and hydrogen sulfide positive.[304] However, it has been shown that *W. succinogenes* is oxidase positive and is capable of using O_2 as a terminal electron acceptor under microaerophilic conditions (2% O_2) but not under atmospheric levels of O_2. These findings, along with additional evidence on the electron transport system, indicate that *W. succinogenes* is not an anaerobe but is an H_2-requiring microaerophile.[311] *W. succinogenes* has not been associated with human infections.

Sutterella wadsworthensis. Wexler and colleagues have proposed the name *S. wadsworthensis* for a group of bacteria that were originally identified as *C. gracilis* but differed in genetic and biochemical characteristics from typical *C. gracilis* strains.[331] These organisms are gram-negative straight rods that grow in a microaerophilic atmosphere or under anaerobic conditions. They are differentiated from *C. gracilis* and *Campylobacter* species by being oxidase-, urease-, and indoxyl acetate-negative; resistant to 20% bile disks; and by not reducing tetrazolium tetrachloride under aerobic conditions. They have been isolated mainly from human infections of the gastrointestinal tract.[331]

Definitive Identification of Campylobacters and Related Bacteria

The colonial morphology and Gram-stain characteristics of *C. jejuni* as described earlier also pertain to most other *Campylobacter* species. However, definitive species identification depends on the determination of the phenotypic characteristics presented in Table 8-4 or, when these tests do not provide a species identification, molecular techniques.

The differential susceptibility to nalidixic acid and cephalothin may be useful in differentiating the more commonly encountered *Campylobacter* species according to the scheme in Box 8-3 if the isolate is susceptible to nalidixic acid. Because isolates of *C. jejuni* and *C. coli* resistant to nalidixic acid are encountered with increasing frequency, these tests have become less helpful.

Luechtefeld and Wang[202] also found that resistance of *C. jejuni* to triphenyltetrazolium chloride (TTC) is helpful in distinguishing *C. fetus*. The test for hippurate hydrolysis is useful in separating *C. jejuni* from the closely related species *C. coli*. Most strains of *C. jejuni* hydrolyze hippurate to benzoic acid and glycine.[126] The rapid procedure of Hwang and Ederer for hippurate hydrolysis, described in Chapter 12, is suitable for testing clinical isolates of *Campylobacter* spe-

cies. Morris and associates[223] describe a more sensitive method for detecting benzoic acid using gas liquid chromatography (GLC). This application is an extension of the procedure previously reported by Kodaka and colleagues,[179] who used hippurate formate fumarate medium to detect not only hippurate hydrolysis by GLC but the utilization of formate and fumarate as well.

Mills and Gherna[219] described the use of a rapid test for detecting hydrolysis of indoxyl acetate by *Campylobacter* species. Studies have shown that all strains of *C. jejuni, C. coli, C. curvus, C. helveticus, C. rectus, C. showae, C. upsaliensis, Arcobacter butzleri, A. cryaerophilus,* and *Helicobacter fennelliae* hydrolyze indoxyl acetate, whereas most other campylobacters are negative.[135,219,243,261] Several additional biochemical and physical characteristics may be helpful in separating the various *Campylobacter* and *Campylobacter*-like species (see Table 8-4). An extensive review of identification methods for campylobacters, helicobacters, and related organisms has been published by On.[243]

Rapid Identification of Campylobacters From Colonies and From Stool Specimens

In most instances the appearance of small, tan to gray, watery colonies that tend to flatten on *Campylobacter*-selective agar, and that exhibit characteristic "S"-shape and gull-wing morphology on Gram stain and are oxidase and catalase positive, will be sufficient to establish the diagnosis of campylobacteriosis in patients with diarrheal syndromes.

Hodge and coworkers[136] advocate the use of direct immunofluorescence techniques in the rapid screening of stool specimens from patients with an acute diarrheal syndrome. This approach has the potential for removing the guesswork involved in interpreting gram-stained smears. However, these reagents are not commercially available.

NONCULTURE TESTS

Latex agglutination tests have been used for the identification of *Campylobacter* species. These tests use isolated colonies to identify *C. jejuni* and *C. coli* but not distinguish between the two.[138,229] The ability of these tests to correctly identify *C. lari* is variable.

Nucleic acid probes can also be used for culture confirmation of *Campylobacter* species.[262] AccuProbe *Campylobacter* Culture Identification Test (Gen-Probe, Inc., San Diego, CA) is a DNA probe-based test that provides rapid

---

Box 8-3 Definitive Identification of Most Commonly Encountered Campylobacters

	NALIDIXIC ACID	CEPHALOTHIN	TTC*	HIPPURATE HYDROLYSIS	INDOXYL ACETATE HYDROLYSIS
C. jejuni subsp. *jejuni*	V	R	R	+	+
C. coli	S	R	R	−	+
C. fetus subsp. *fetus*	R	S	S	−	−
C. lari	R	R	S	−	−

* TTC, triphenyltetrazolium chloride.

identification of *C. jejuni, C. coli,* and *C. lari* directly from bacterial colonies.[310] The probe is nonradiometric and is labeled with a chemiluminescent acridinium ester. Reactions are read in a luminometer.

DIRECT DETECTION METHODS

Enzyme immunoassays for assessing virulence properties of *C. jejuni* and for direct detection of *Campylobacter* antigen in stool specimens (ProSpecT Campylobacter, Alexon-Trend, Inc., Ramsey, MN) have been developed.[134,177] The commercially available ProSpecT Campylobacter test is less sensitive than culture (sensitivity, 80% to 96% in published studies) but is highly specific for *C. jejuni/C. coli.*[81,134,312] The assay does cross-react with *C. upsaliensis*; however, this species is uncommonly encountered in the clinical laboratory. Several investigators have developed PCR tests for direct detection of *Campylobacter* species in stool specimens.[181,199,204] However, before these tests can be transferred to the clinical laboratory, a technically simple and practical procedure for DNA extraction from stool specimens that eliminates PCR inhibitors is needed.

Culture and Isolation of *Helicobacter pylori*
SPECIMENS FOR RECOVERY OF *H. PYLORI*

For the diagnosis of *H. pylori*-associated gastritis, histologic staining and culturing of biopsy specimens has been considered the "gold standard."[18] Suitable specimens include gastric and duodenal biopsies. Specimens should be fresh and not delayed in transport for more than 3 hours. Specimens may be kept for up to 5 hours if stored at 4°C.

Tissue should be kept moist by the addition of 2 mL or less of sterile isotonic saline.

ISOLATION PROCEDURE

Grinding of specimens in a ground-glass grinder yields heavier growth than mincing or rubbing the specimen onto an agar surface. Material should be inoculated onto a nonselective blood agar medium, such as Brucella, brain-heart infusion (BHI), or tryptic soy agar plates with 5% sheep or horse blood added. Poor growth is observed on commercially prepared chocolate agar plates; therefore, this medium is not recommended. Because these bacteria are susceptible to cephalothin, *H. pylori* will not grow on any selective medium containing cephalosporins. Many laboratories have had good results using modified Thayer-Martin agar as a selective medium for isolation of *H. pylori* in mixed cultures. Plates are incubated at 37°C in a humid, microaerophilic environment. Growth is usually observed in 3 to 5 days. Unpublished data from experiments conducted at the University of Illinois Hospital Microbiology Laboratory are shown in Table 8-7. Because of the potential hazard of using an anaerobic jar without a catalyst, we recommend the use of the Campy GasPak jar (column 2 in Table 8-7). Growth occurred in the Campy GasPak jar but not in the Poly Bag with Campy gas mixture (column 4 in Table 8-7), presumably because the water added in the former system provides the necessary humidity for growth.

IDENTIFICATION OF *H. PYLORI*

Colonies of *H. pylori* are small, gray, translucent, and weakly β-hemolytic. Gram stain reveals pale-staining,

---

Table 8-7 Comparison of Culture Media and Atmospheric Conditions for Growth of *Helicobacter pylori*

	CONDITIONS OF INCUBATION*				
AGAR MEDIA	Anaerobe Jar (No Catalyst)	Campy GasPak Jar	Anaerobe Jar (Catalyst)	Poly Bag (Campy Gas Mixture)†	Atmos-Pheric air With 5% CO_2
Brucella with 5% sheep blood	Best growth β-hemolytic	Very good growth β-hemolytic	No growth	No growth	No growth
Tryptic soy with 5% sheep blood	Very good growth	Good growth	No growth	No growth	No growth
Brain–heart infusion with 5% horse blood	Very good growth	Good growth	No growth	No growth	No growth
Chocolate (Becton Dickinson Microbiology Systems, Cockeysville, MD)	No growth	No growth	No growth	No growth	No growth
Chocolate (GIBCO)	Small colonies	Small colonies	No growth	No growth	No growth
Chocolate (freshly prepared)	Very small colonies	Very small colonies	No growth	No growth	No growth
Campy-BAP (Blaser's)	No growth	No growth	No growth	No growth	No growth

All cultures were incubated at 37°C and read after 5 days.
† 5% O_2, 10% CO_2, 85% N_2
Data from K. Ristow, University of Illinois Hospital, Chicago IL.

curved, gram-negative bacteria with characteristic gull-wing and "U" shapes. Presumptive identification can be made with positive reactions for oxidase and catalase and an extremely rapid (within minutes) urease reaction. Additional identifying characteristics are listed in Table 8-4.

BIOPSY UREASE TEST (CLO TEST)

A more rapid but somewhat less sensitive and specific technique than the previously mentioned tests is the biopsy urease test (CLO test). In this test, a medium containing urea and a pH-sensitive dye is inoculated with the mucosal biopsy specimen. If urease is present in the specimen, urea is split and ammonia causes a rise in pH and subsequent change in the color of the indicator. This test may produce false-negative results if only a small number of organisms are present or false-positive results if other urea-splitting organisms are present in the specimen.[213]

NONINVASIVE TESTS TO DIAGNOSE *H. PYLORI* INFECTION

H. pylori infection may be diagnosed by invasive assays that require endoscopy (culture, stain, PCR, CLO test), or by noninvasive assays in which endoscopy is not necessary. Included in the latter category are the urease method, antigen detection, and serology.

Urease Method. Two urease methods have been described. The first method, called the urea breath test, requires that the patient ingest ^{14}C-labeled urea dissolved in water, followed by collection of breath samples that are analyzed for the presence of ^{14}CO$_2$ at 60 minutes. A second method utilizes radiolabeled urea containing ^{15}N.[154] After oral ingestion, radiolabeled urea is broken down into ammonia and carbon dioxide by *H. pylori* urease in the stomach. The ammonia is absorbed into the blood and excreted in the urine. The amount of [^{15}N]urea, reflecting the magnitude of *H. pylori* infection, is evaluated by measuring the abundance and excretion rate of ^{15}N in ammonia in the urine. The sensitivity of the ^{15}NH$_4$ excretion test is reported to be 96% with 100% specificity when compared to patients who were *H. pylori* positive by culture and Gram stain.[154]

Antigen Detection. An enzyme immunoassay for direct detection of *H. pylori* antigen in stool specimens is commercially available to be used for diagnosis and follow-up (Premier Platinum HpSA, Meridian Bioscience, Cincinnati, OH). Studies have shown that the test sensitivity is approximately 89% and the specificity, 94 to 95%.[205,221]

Serologic Methods. Serologic tests for detecting antibody to *H. pylori* have been used mainly for epidemiologic studies but can also be used to monitor the efficacy of treatment. The principle format is the ELISA test for the detection of IgG, although latex agglutination tests are available. IgA and IgM can also be detected but are less useful diagnostically. One inherent problem is attempting to establish a baseline for positivity since the prevalence of persons with elevated antibody titers is relatively high in certain populations. In an extensive study of Army recruits, Smoak et al.[285] found an overall positivity rate of 26.3%. This rate increased from 24.0% in age group 17 to 18 years to 43% in age group 24 to 26 years. Seropositivity for blacks was 44%, for hispanics 38%, and for whites 14%.

ACCURACY OF INVASIVE AND NONINVASIVE TESTS TO DIAGNOSE *H. PYLORI* INFECTION

Cutler and colleagues[68] evaluated the accuracy of several tests for determining *H. pylori* infection including the urea breath test (UBT), measurement of serum IgG and IgA antibody levels, and antral biopsy specimens for CLO test, histology, and Warthin-Starry stain. They found that the Warthin-Starry stain had the best sensitivity and specificity, although the CLO test, UBT, and IgG levels were not statistically different in determining the correct diagnosis. They concluded that the noninvasive UBT and IgG serology tests are as accurate in predicting *H. pylori* status in untreated patients as the invasive tests of CLO and Warthin-Starry. The absence of chronic antral inflammation accurately excludes *H. pylori* infection.[68]

ENTEROHEPATIC HELICOBACTERS

Most intestinal helicobacters recovered from humans (e.g., *H. canadensis*, *H. cinaedi*, *H. fennelliae*) are urease negative. Differentiating these catalase-positive, urease-negative helicobacters from enteric campylobacters like *C. jejuni* can be problematic. Temperature studies may be helpful, as *H. cinaedi* and *H. fennelliae* will not grow at 42°C (*C. jejuni* and *C. coli* do). *C. jejuni* and *C. coli* also hydrolyze indoxyl acetate, whereas *H. cinaedi* does not. *H. pullorum* usually can be distinguished from *C. lari* based on its resistance to nalidixic acid.

PART II: THE FAMILIES VIBRIONACEAE AND "AEROMONADACEAE"

Phylogeny of the Vibrionaceae

The name *Vibrionaceae* was originally proposed by Veron in 1965 with the intent of grouping a number of non-enteric, fermentative, gram-negative rods that were oxidase positive and motile by means of polar flagella. This grouping was intended as a convenience for the purpose of differentiating these organisms from the *Enterobacteriaceae* and did not necessarily imply a taxonomic relationship among the included species. The *Vibrionaceae* once included four genera: *Vibrio*, *Aeromonas*, *Photobacterium*, and *Plesiomonas*. However, in the past few decades a variety of methods for nucleic acid analysis have revolutionized microbial taxonomy and have resulted in the restructuring of this family along phylogenetic lines and the establishment of two new genera, *Listonella* and *Shewanella*, and a new family, *Aeromonadaceae*.[66,203,271] The correct phylogenic placement of the genus *Plesiomonas* remains unresolved at this time.

Genus *Vibrio*

Vibrio species have both historical and contemporary interest. *V. cholerae* is the etiologic agent of Asiatic cholera in humans, a potentially severe diarrheal disease that has been the scourge of humanity for centuries. The organism was first described and named by Pacini in 1854; 32 years later Koch isolated the organism, which he called "Kommabacillus'' because of the characteristic curved or comma-shaped appearance of the individual bacterial cells.

Seven cholera pandemics have occurred since 1816–1817. The most recent pandemic, caused by *V. cholerae* O1, biotype El Tor, began in 1961 in Indonesia, rapidly spread to Asia, Europe, Africa, and the South Pacific, and reached South and then Central America in 1991. In addition, a number of minor epidemics of diarrheal syndromes and extraintestinal infections caused by non-01 serogroups of *V. cholerae* and by several newly described halophilic species have been reported in the United States in several Gulf Coast states since the early 1970s.[143,162] Most infections have occurred following ingestion of contaminated and poorly cooked seafood. Wound infections have also been reported following trauma while swimming or working in infected waters or on exposure to marine animals.[143]

The point of this discussion is that clinical microbiologists cannot discount *Vibrio* species as a possible isolate from diarrheal stool specimens and must remain informed on how to recover and identify the various species. Those working in inland laboratories will have fewer potential encounters than those working in the Gulf Coast hospitals; nevertheless, with open world travel and shipping of seafoods to inland markets, everyone must remain alert.

TAXONOMY

The strains of *Vibrio cholerae* that have been recovered from classic cases of pandemic cholera agglutinate in what has been designated 01 antiserum. Strains not agglutinating in this antiserum are called either non-01 *V. cholerae* (if this species is determined biochemically) or a variety of other vibrio species names, such as *V. parahemolyticus, V. mimicus,* and so on. Since the non-01 species usually do not cause diarrheal syndromes as severe or potentially life threatening as 01 species, or more commonly may be associated with extraintestinal infections, early differentiation between the two groups can be of considerable clinical importance. Although 35 or more distinct *Vibrio* species have been identified, all but 11 are environmental organisms, called ''marine vibrio species,'' and have not been associated with human infections.[152]

DESCRIPTION AND ASSOCIATED CLINICAL SYNDROMES OF *VIBRIO* SPECIES OF HUMAN IMPORTANCE

The species that are recovered from humans and potentially cause disease can be divided into two groups, namely, *Vibrio cholerae* and the non-cholera vibrios.

Vibrio cholerae. *Vibrio cholerae* is the etiologic agent of epidemic and pandemic cholera in humans. Within the species of *V. cholerae*, there is much dissimilarity among the strains in both their pathogenic and epidemic potential (Table 8-8). The strains can be divided according to differences in their cell wall composition (somatic O antigen), which forms the basis of the serotyping scheme that classifies the organisms into 139 different serogroups. All share a common flagellar (H) antigen. It was determined in the mid-1930s that all of the pandemic strains were agglutinated with a single antiserum that has been designated 01. The 01 type *V. cholerae* strains can be further separated into one of three serogroups: Inaba, Ogawa, and Hikojima. These serogroups are important for epidemiologic studies. For example, the current pandemic of cholera that began 1961 is caused by the Ogawa serogroup, whereas a focus of cholera that is endemic in the Gulf Coast region of the United States is associated with a *V. cholerae* 01 Inaba serotype.[168] In January 1991, epidemic cholera appeared simultaneously in several coastal cites of Peru and has since been reported in Ecuador, Chile, Colombia, Brazil, and the United States. This outbreak is apparently also due to a strain other than the pandemic strain and has been identified as 01 serotype Inaba, biotype El Tor.[51]

Epidemic strains of serovar 01 may be further divided into the classic and El Tor biovars. El Tor is an actively hemolytic biotype of *V. cholerae* that was isolated at the El Tor Quarantine Station in Egypt. The El Tor strain has been found to be hardier and better capable of surviving in the environment; furthermore, chronic carriers of the El Tor strain have been reported in the literature.[167] The El Tor vibrio is now recognized as a biotype of *V. cholerae* and is responsible for most current epidemic outbreaks of classic cholera. The present pandemic of cholera that began in 1961 is caused by the El Tor biovar, as are the Gulf Coast and South American outbreaks. The classic biovar has almost

Table 8-8 Characteristics of *Vibrio cholerae*

CLASSIFICATION METHOD	EPIDEMIC-ASSOCIATED	NOT EPIDEMIC-ASSOCIATED
Serogroups	1	Non 01 (serogroups 02–0138)*
Biotypes	Classical, El Tor	Biotypes not applicable to non-01 strains
Serotypes	Inaba, Ogawa, Hikojima	These three serotypes not applicable to non-01 strains
Toxin	Produce cholera toxin	Usually do not produce cholera toxin; sometimes produce other toxins*

* A serogroup designated 0139 Bengal emerged in Calcutta, Bangladesh and parts of India in 1992 that produces cholera toxin in quantities similar to that produced by V. cholerae 01 and has spread in epidemic proportions across the Indian subcontinent.

disappeared except for rare isolations in India. Studies from Bangladesh indicate that the classic biotype has ree-merged.[152]

Cholera: World History There have been seven pandemics of cholera in recorded history; the last three pandemics are known to be due to the *Vibrio cholerae* serogroup 01. The seventh pandemic of cholera, caused by the El Tor vibrio, originated in Clebes, Indonesia, in 1961 and subsequently spread worldwide, reaching the South American continent in 1991. The emergence and rapid spread of cholera caused by a new serotype designated 0139 Bengal in October 1992 in nine countries (India, Bangladesh, Pakistan, Thailand, Nepal, Malaysia, Burma, Saudi Arabia, and China) suggests the possibility for the beginning of the eighth pandemic.[7a,89,206,300] For a synopsis of the cholera pandemics of the 19th and 20th centuries, the reader is referred to the review published by Lacey.[183]

Toxigenic *Vibrio cholerae* 0139 Bengal In October 1992, an epidemic of cholera-like illness began in Madras, India and spread to Calcutta and Bangladesh and many other places in India and in southeast Asia.[224] The strain could not be identified as any of the 138 known types of *V. cholerae* and thus represented a new serogroup, 0139 (synonym Bengal to indicate its first isolation from the coastal areas of the Bay of Bengal).[7a] The strain caused large epidemics of cholera in Bangladesh, India, and neighboring countries and, for a time, largely replaced *V. cholerae* 01 strains in affected areas. From 1996 to 2002, most cases of cholera in Bangladesh were caused by *V. cholerae* O1 biotype El Tor, but in March 2002, V. cholerae O139 re-emerged as the predominant pathogen.[89] There are three important points to consider with regard to this new serotype: 1) the symptoms associated with *V. cholerae* 0139 infection suggest it is indistinguishable from cholera caused by *V. cholerae* 01 and should be treated with the same rapid fluid replacement, 2) the rapid spread of *V. cholerae* 0139 suggests that preexisting immunity to *V. cholerae* 01 offers little or no protective benefit, and travelers to affected areas should not assume that cholera vaccination is protective against the *V. cholerae* 0139 strain, and 3) laboratory identification methods for *V. cholerae* 01 depend on detection of the 01 antigen on the surface of the bacterium, and therefore do not identify this new strain.[53] The phenotypic, serologic, and toxigenic traits of *V. cholerae* 0139 Bengal have been reported by Nair and coworkers.[231]

Cholera: Western Hemisphere In January 1991, epidemic cholera, which had not been reported in South America in the 20th century, appeared simultaneously in several coastal cities of Peru and rapidly spread throughout South and Central America.[121,249]

In the United States, a small environmental focus of potentially epidemic *V. cholerae* exists along the Gulf Coast.[169] Cholera caused by this strain have in most cases been linked to undercooked crab or raw oysters harvested from the Gulf Coast. In 1973, the first case of cholera in the United States since 1911 was reported from Texas.[330] This was followed in 1978 by the report of 11 cases in Louisiana and in 1981 with two additional outbreaks in Texas involving 18 cases.[23] Crabs harvested from nearby estuaries were found to be the vehicle of infection in the Louisiana cases, while the largest of the two Texas outbreaks was traced to contamination of

cooked rice following accidental rinsing with water from the environment containing the outbreak strain.[167] It is now known that 44 toxigenic *V. cholerae* 01 infections were acquired in the United States between 1973 and 1987.[152] All resulted from exposures in Louisiana and Texas near the Gulf Coast. In 1991, 26 cases of cholera were reported in the U.S.; 18 were linked to the South American outbreak.[52] In 1992, 103 cholera cases were reported in the U.S.; 75 were associated with an outbreak on board an Aerolineas Argentinas flight between Argentina and Los Angeles in February 1992. In 1993 and 1994, 22 and 47 cholera cases were reported in the U.S., respectively. Of these, 65 (94%) were associated with foreign travel. Three of these were culture-confirmed cases of *V. cholerae* 0139 in travelers to Asia.[54] From 1995 to 2000, 14 cases of cholera were reported; 6 were associated with the endemic environmental focus and 8 with imported seafood.[225]

V. cholerae non-01 serotypes have been associated with isolated cases of diarrheal disease, although the majority of non-01 strains do not produce cholera toxin but appear to produce an enterotoxin different from cholera toxin. Strains have also been isolated from wounds and systemic infections. Safrin and coworkers,[274] in a review of cases of non-01 *V. cholerae* bacteremia, reported that the case-fatality rate for 13 cases in which the outcome was known was 61.5%. The majority of known cases have occurred in immunocompromised patients, particularly those with hematologic malignancy or cirrhosis. Pitrak and Gindorf[260] reported a case of bacteremic cellulitis caused by non-01 *V. cholerae* that was acquired in a freshwater inland lake in northern Illinois.

Pathophysiology of Vibrio Cholerae-Induced Gastroenteritis. *V. cholerae* is the prototype of diarrheal syndromes in which disease is caused not by tissue invasion of microorganisms but through the production of toxins that interrupt normal intraintestinal exchanges of water and electrolytes. Toxigenic strains produce a toxin that binds to a receptor on the epithelial cell membrane and activates adenylate cyclase, causing increased levels of cyclic adenosine monophosphate (cAMP) and hypersecretion of salt and water, resulting in the characteristic "rice water" diarrhea of cholera. Box 8-4 provides a brief account of the step-by-step sequence for *V. cholerae*-induced gastroenteritis. Figure 8-1 is a schematic illustration of the mode of action of the cholera toxin. For a comprehensive review of cholera including pathogenesis and virulence factors, the reader is referred to publications by Kaper and colleagues and Sack and colleagues.[161,272]

Treatment and Prevention of Vibrio Cholerae Infections. Most *V. cholerae* are rapidly killed by tetracycline; however, fluid secretion may persist for several hours after treatment from the effect of toxin already bound to the mucosal cells. Correction of fluid and electrolyte losses is essential with as much as 1 liter or more of fluid per hour required. Antibiotic therapy (e.g., trimethoprim-sulfamethoxazole or tetracycline) will help shorten the duration of the diarrhea and reduce the period of carriage, however, antibiotics should be considered ancillary to vigorous rehydration. Additionally, antimicrobial-resistant strains of *V. cholerae* have emerged during the past few decades.[225,,272] The risk for cholera and traveler's diarrhea can be reduced by following the general rule "boil it, cook it, peel it, or forget it." In particular, travelers should not consume 1) unboiled or untreated water

---

Box 8-4 Events Leading to *V. cholerae*-Induced Gastroenteritis

1. Organisms ingested in contaminated water must first pass the highly acidic secretions in the stomach. An estimated 10^{10} organisms per milliliter are required to survive gastric passage in healthy persons; only about 100 organisms per milliliter are required in hypochlorhydric persons, either because of previous gastrectomy or from ingestion of antacids in treatment of gastric ulcer disease.

2. To cause disease, *V. cholerae* bacterial cells must adhere to the gastric and intestinal mucosal epithelial cells. These bacteria are motile and secrete mucin, two properties that aid in the penetration of the protective mucin layer that coats the surface of the gastroenteric mucosa. Bacterial attachment is a complex mechanism requiring the recognition by the bacterial cells of a surface marker on the epithelial cells to which they can bind.

3. *V. cholerae* produces an enterotoxin molecule composed of two subunits; an A (active) subunit and a B (binding) subunit. The A subunit is composed of two peptides: A_1 with toxin activity and A_2, which facilitates penetration of the A subunit into the cell. The B subunit binds the toxin molecule to cholera toxin specific G_{M1} ganglioside receptors on the intestinal epithelial cell membrane. There are five B subunits per toxin molecule, arranged in a ring around a central core that contains the enzyme A_1. Initial binding occurs rapidly, followed by a slow conformational change in the toxin molecule, leading to internalization of the A_1 enzyme into the host cell; thus, there is a short lag phase (15 to 60 minutes) between the time cholera-infected water is ingested and the onset of symptoms. Through a series of steps, A_1 catalyzes the ADP-ribosylation of the G_s (stimulatory) regulatory protein, locking it in the active state. The G_s protein acts to return adenylate cyclase from its inactive to active form, which in turn causes an intracellular rise in cyclic-AMP (cAMP; see Fig. 8–1).[218]

4. Cyclic AMP prevents the reabsorption of sodium ions across the brush-border membrane of the intestinal epithelial cell and the excretion of sodium bicarbonate and potassium into the bowel lumen. The intestinal chyle has high concentrations of sodium and chloride (isotonic), bicarbonate (twice that of plasma), and potassium (three to five times that of plasma). Water, therefore, is passively passed from the epithelial cells into the intestinal lumen in response to high osmotic pressure gradients, following the old adage, "where goes the sodium, there goes the water."

5. Thus, there is diffuse fluid secretion from the gut epithelial cells and the accumulation of large quantities of water in the intestinal lumen. The rate of fluid production increases between 3 and 10 hours after exposure. Fluid loss persists for up to 5 days in patients who receive no antibiotics, after which the bacterial cells are washed from the bowel by an unknown host mechanism. The result is varying degrees of dehydration and electrolyte imbalance that can lead to metabolic acidosis, hypokalemia, shock, and death in extreme cases.

---

and ice made from such water; 2) food and beverages from street vendors; 3) raw or partially cooked fish and shellfish, including ceviche; and 4) uncooked vegetables. Cold seafood salads may be particularly risky. Considerable work has been done regarding development of oral cholera vaccines.[272] Two oral vaccines are licensed in several countries outside the United States. One consists of killed *V. cholerae* plus the cholera B subunit, the other is an avirulent mutant of *V. cholerae*. Currently no cholera vaccine is commercially available in the United States.

Non-Cholera Vibrios. Most cases of Vibrio infections in the United States have been caused by nonepidemic species other than *V. cholerae*. The natural habitat and geographic distribution, the culture media required for optimal recovery, the key biochemical reactions, and the clinical syndromes associated with the non-cholera species of human importance are listed in Table 8-9. The term *non-cholera* is probably a misnomer because many strains can cause severe diarrheal disease in addition to extraintestinal infections that can result in fatal septicemia. In most infections, symptoms are less severe and shorter in duration than is experienced in classic epidemic cholera.

Certain species of non-cholera vibrios can produce enterotoxins similar to those described for *V. cholerae*. In addition, some species cause invasive disease and more closely simulate *Shigella* dysentery; other species, *V. vulnificus* in particular, may invade the intestinal lymphatics and result in septicemia. Extraintestinal *Vibrio* infections are most commonly cutaneous wounds or otitis externa, where breaks in the skin have become contaminated while swimming or boating in infected marine waters or after handling contaminated raw seafood.[214,281] The following is a brief account of the microbiology and clinical syndromes associated with each of the non-cholera *Vibrio* species.

V. alginolyticus *V. alginolyticus* was originally classified as biotype 2 of *V. parahaemolyticus*. Most clinical isolates are recovered from superficial wounds[83,210,258,279] or the external ear.[124,152] Conjunctivitis,[197] acute gastroenteritis,[265] bacteremia[29,83,149] and necrotizing fasciitis[114] caused by *V. alginolyticus* have also been reported.

V. carchariae *V. carchariae* is a pathogen of sharks, but has been reported in one case of human wound infection in an 11-year-old girl who was attacked by a shark while wading in knee-deep water off the South Carolina coast.[255] *V. carchariae* can be differentiated from biochemically similar species (*V. alginolyticus, V. parahaemolyticus, V. vulnificus*) by negative gelatin hydrolysis at 22°C, negative motility at 36°C, and negative ornithine decarboxylase reaction. The other species have the opposite reactions.

V. cincinnatiensis Human infection caused by this *Vibrio* species is rare. It has been recovered from blood and cerebrospinal fluid of a 70-year-old patient with bacteremia and meningitis.[31] The patient was treated with ampicillin (day 1) and moxalactam for 9 days, followed by an uneventful recovery.

V. damsela (Photobacterium damsela) *V. damsela* was formerly called CDC Group EF-5. It has been reported as the cause of human wound infections, primarily after exposure to saltwater.[64,139,226] Most strains are resistant to penicillin and sensitive to gentamicin, chloramphenicol, and tetracycline. MacDonell and Colwell[203] proposed transfer of

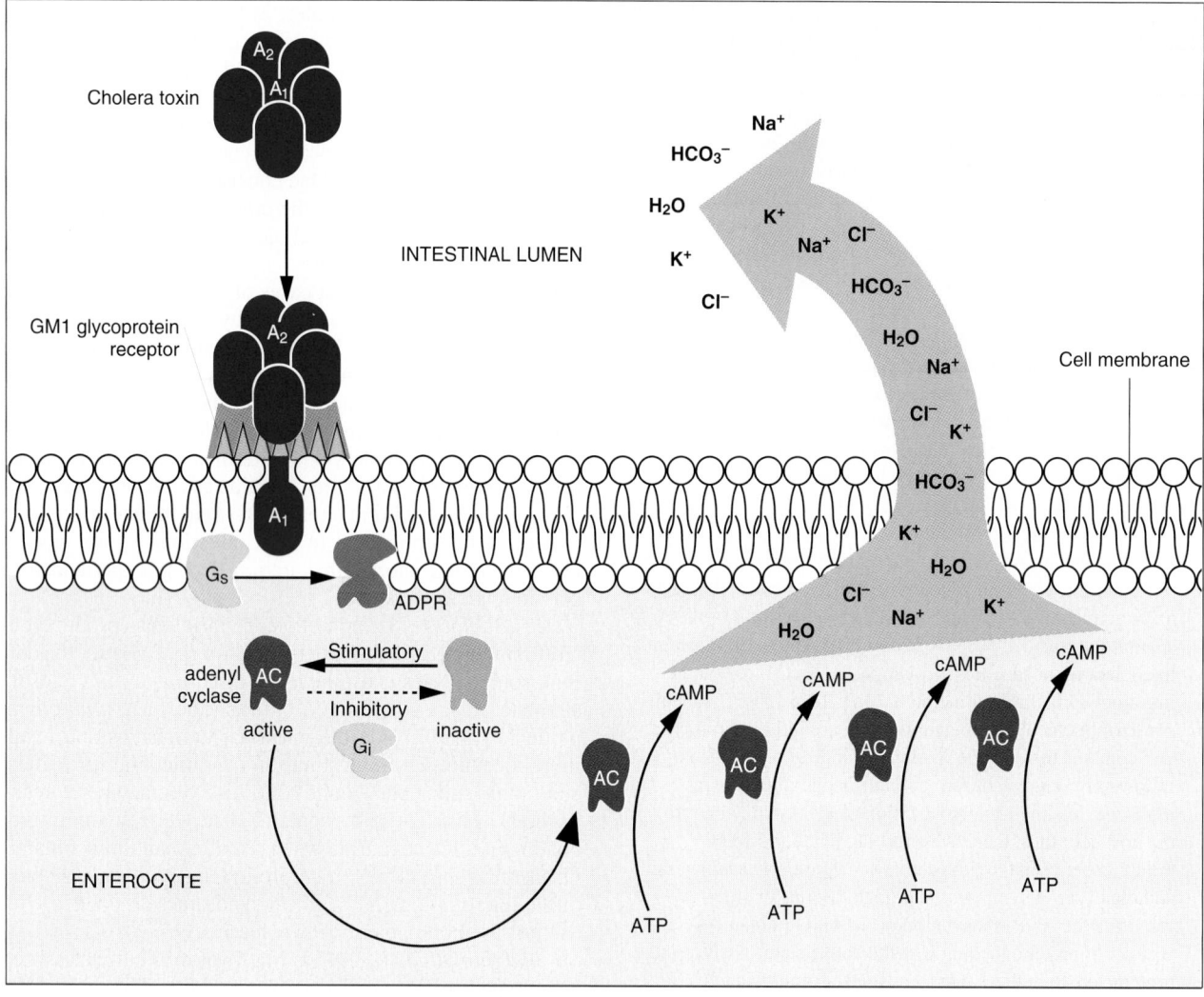

Figure 8-1 The action of cholera toxin (see Box 8-4 for details).

V. damsela to the genus *Listonella*. Subsequently, Smith and colleagues proposed that *L. damsela* should be reassigned to the genus *Photobacterium*.[284]

V. fluvialis Formerly designated as CDC Group EF-6, *V. fluvialis* has been isolated from humans with diarrhea. This species was isolated from fecal cultures of more than 500 patients with diarrhea at the Cholera Research Laboratory in Bangladesh during a 9-month period from 1976–1977.[144] In the United States, the organism has been isolated from a wound of a patient in Hawaii, from water and sediment in the New York Bay, from shellfish in Louisiana, from water and shellfish in Pacific Northwest estuaries, from an 81-year-old man from Laredo, Texas, with diarrheal illness,[302] from the stool of a 1-month old infant,[131] and from the stool of a 43-year-old man with a history of AIDS.[137]

V. furnissii Formerly designated *V. fluvialis* biogroup 2, *V. furnissii* has been isolated from patients with acute gastroenteritis in at least two outbreaks of food poisoning[33] and from the stool of a 1-month old infant.[133]

V. hollisae Formerly designated CDC Group EF-13, *V. hollisae* has most commonly been isolated from stool specimens of persons with diarrhea and abdominal pain and a history of eating raw seafood.[4,130,226] Rare cases of systemic infection caused by *V. hollisae* have been described and most often involve bacterial sepsis in persons with underlying immune deficiencies.[200,264] Evidence suggests that *V. hollisae* may share with *V. vulnificus* a predilection for bloodstream invasion in persons with liver abnormalities.[264]

V. metschnikovii *V. metschnikovii*, formerly CDC Enteric Group 16, is often isolated from the environment but rarely isolated from human clinical specimens. The first documented case of human infection was from the blood of a patient with cholecystitis at Cook County Hospital in Chicago.[153] More recently, Hansen and colleagues reported two cases of *V. metschnikovii* septicemia: one fatal case involving a patient with liver cirrhosis, renal insufficiency, and diabetes; and another in an 82-year-old woman with respiratory problems and an infected leg lesion, who was treated successfully.[125] Human isolates referred to the CDC for identification include two isolates from urine and four isolates from unknown sources.[86]

Table 8-9 Characteristics of Clinically Important *Vibrio* Species Other Than *V. cholerae*

SPECIES	NATURAL HABITAT, GEOGRAPHIC DISTRIBUTION; MODES OF HUMAN INFECTION	MEDIA FOR OPTIMAL GROWTH IN LABORATORY CULTURES	KEY BIOCHEMICAL REACTIONS		CLINICAL SYNDROMES
V. alginolyticus	Habitat: Marine environment Infection: Exposure of traumatized skin to seawater or infected animals	NaCl supplement needed for growth on nonselective media. Grows on blood agar and enteric media. Yellow colonies on thiosulfate citrate bile sucrose (TCBS) agar.	Lysine Arginine Voges-Proskauer 8%, NaCl 10% NaCl	+ − + + V	Associated with soft tissue infections; seems to also have an etiologic role in wound and ear infections.

V. damsela CDC Group EF-5 (transferred to genus *Photobacterium*)	Habitat: Marine environment
	
	Infection: Exposure of broken skin or traumatic wounds to infected marine animals or contaminated seawater.
		Requires 1% NaCl in nonselective culture media. Good growth on blood agar. Green colonies on TCBS agar. Optimum growth 25°C.	Arginine
			Voges-Proskauer
			Ferment:
			  Glucose
			  Mannitol
			  Galactose
			  Trehalose
				+
				+
				
				+
				−
				+
				+
					Associated with human wound infections.

V. fluvialis	Habitat: Worldwide—endemic in Bangladesh. In United States—Gulf Coast, New York, and Pacific Northwest estuaries. Infection: Ingestion or contact with contaminated water.	Na⁺ supplement of culture media less critical than other halophilic *Vibrio* species. Yellow colonies on TCBS agar.	Arginine 6% NaCl Glucose (gas) Hydrolysis of esculin Aminovalerate Glutarate	+ + − − − 	Cholera-like gastroenteritis and diarrheal syndrome—watery diarrhea, vomiting, dehydration; probably enterotoxin induced.
V. furnissii	Habitat: Endemic in the marine waters and estuaries in Asia. Infection: Ingestion or contact with contaminated water.	Na⁺ supplement for optimal growth in nonselective culture media. Yellow colonies on TCBS agar.	Glucose (gas) Hydrolysis of esculin Aminovalerate Glutarate	+ − − +	Isolated from patients with diarrhea and gastroenteritis, particularly tourists returning from Asia.
V. hollisae	Habitat: Marine environment in Gulf Coast and Chesapeake Bay states. Infection: Consumption of raw seafood.	1%–2% NaCl supplement needed for growth. Poor growth on TCBS or MacConkey agars. Screen for oxidase-positive colonies on blood agar.	Indole Lysine Arginine Ornithine Motility (after 7 days) Urea	+ − − − − −	Isolated from patients with diarrhea and gastroenteritis. Invasion of bloodstream reported in persons with liver abnormalities.
V. metschnikovii	Habitat: Worldwide in fresh and brackish marine waters, rivers, sewage; also in shrimp, crabs, and lobsters. Infection: Cause of fowl cholera; exposure or ingestion of contaminated water or animals.	Grows well on most laboratory isolation media. Sodium supplement not as critical as other halophilic vibrios. Yellow colonies on TCBS agar.	Oxidase Nitrate Voges-Proskauer	− − +	Associated with rare and isolated cases of human infections: septicemia, urinary tract infections, wounds, peritonitis.
V. mimicus	Habitat: Coastal waters, and oysters and shrimp. Infection: Ingestion of undercooked seafood (particularly oysters).	Grows on enteric isolation media. Green colonies on TCBS.	Sucrose Mannitol Ornithine Lipase	− + + V	Diarrheal syndrome related to production of heat-labile and heat-stable toxins; also swimmer's ear infections.

(Continued)

Table 8-9 *Continued*

SPECIES	NATURAL HABITAT, GEOGRAPHIC DISTRIBUTION; MODES OF HUMAN INFECTION	MEDIA FOR OPTIMAL GROWTH IN LABORATORY CULTURES	KEY BIOCHEMICAL REACTIONS		CLINICAL SYNDROMES
V. mimicus, cont.			Voges-Proskauer	−	
			Polymyxin	S	
V. parahaemolyti-cus	Habitat: Worldwide distribution in fresh and sea waters. Endemic in Japan. Infection: Ingestion of contaminated seafood—raw fish and shellfish.	Growth slow on nonselective media. Screen for oxidase-positive colonies on blood agar. Green colonies on TCBS agar.	Lysine	+	Acute gastroenteritis—nausea, vomiting, abdominal cramps, fever, chills. Positive Kanagawa test. Extraintestinal: wounds and septicemia.
			Arginine	−	
			Voges-Proskauer	−	
			Lactose	−	
			Salicin	−	
			Urease	V	
			Indole	+	
V. vulnificus (Lactose-positive *Vibrio*)	Habitat: Coastal water and estuaries. Infection: Ingestion of raw oysters; exposure of traumatic wounds to infected marine animals or contaminated water.	1% NaCl needed for growth. Growth good on blood agar. Green (85%) or yellow (15%) colonies on TCBS agar.	Lactose	+	Life-threatening septicemia; 50% fatality rate. High association with preexistent liver disease. Wounds are painful, with skin and muscle necrosis.
			Lysine	+	
			Arginine	−	
			Salicin	+	

S, susceptible, 90% or greater; V, variable, 11%–89%; +, positive, 90% or greater; −, negative, 90% or greater negative.

V. mimicus Formerly classified as sucrose-negative *V. cholerae*, *V. mimicus* has been isolated from shellfish and water as well as from human diarrheal stools and ear infections.[69,281]

V. parahaemolyticus *V. parahaemolyticus* causes gastroenteritis in humans following ingestion of contaminated seafood,[225] the mechanism of which has not been elucidated. Since 1996, pandemic spread of *V. parahaemolyticus* infections due to a single clone has been reported in several Asian countries.[315] Symptoms include watery and sometimes bloody diarrhea, abdominal cramps, nausea, vomiting, headache, low-grade fever, and chills. The illness is usually mild to moderate and self-limiting, with a duration of 2 to 3 days. Extraintestinal infections by *V. parahaemolyticus* have also been described, mostly from wounds in contact with seawater, although primary septicemia rarely has been reported.[225] A urea-positive biotype has appeared and has been the cause of several recent outbreaks, often associated with ingestion of contaminated raw oysters.[5,184,237,239] Janda and associates[152] reveal that 70% of the *V. parahaemolyticus* cultures submitted for identification to the Microbial Diseases Laboratory in the Berkeley, California, Department of Health Laboratory were urease positive. Similar findings have been reported in the Pacific Northwest.[170]

More than 95% of *V. parahaemolyticus* strains that have been isolated from patients with diarrhea are Kanagawa positive; that is, they hemolyze human erythrocytes on Wagatsuma agar.[160] The hemolysin is both cytotoxic and cardiotoxic. Only about 1% of strains isolated from marine environments are Kanagawa positive.[152] The implication is that Kanagawa hemolysin activity is associated with the pathogenesis of *V. parahaemolyticus* gastroenteritis. However, the association of Kanagawa hemolysin with pathogenesis has never been proven, and in fact Honda and coworkers[142] report that 11 of 12 *V. parahaemolyticus* isolates recovered from patients in a 1985 gastroenteritis outbreak in the Maldives were Kanagawa negative.

Rehydration is usually the only treatment required.

V. vulnificus Formerly CDC Group EF-3, *V. vulnificus* was first termed *lactose-positive Vibrio* by Hollis and coworkers in 1976.[139] *V. vulnificus* is a particularly virulent species associated with wound infections after exposure to contaminated seawater and primary septicemias and death following consumption of contaminated seafood (usually raw oysters).[55,57,225] A high fatality rate (40–60%) is associated with septic infections.[152] The organisms reach the bloodstream by invading the intestinal mucosa. Patients with hepatic disease are particularly susceptible to septicemia.[24,85,301]

Medical conditions that predispose to *V. vulnificus* bacteremia include liver dysfunction and syndromes leading to increased iron deposition: chronic cirrhosis, hepatitis, thalassemia major, hemochromatosis, and a history of heavy alcohol consumption.[152] The chief symptoms associated with sepsis are fever, chills, and vomiting, which begin about 38 hours after ingesting raw oysters. Diarrhea often is not a component of the syndrome.

METHODS FOR LABORATORY ISOLATION OF *VIBRIOS*

There are four possible approaches to the laboratory approach to the isolation of *Vibrio* species from clinical specimens:

1. Use normal procedures and make no specific effort to search for *Vibrio* species.

2. Use normal procedures and plating media, and look for oxidase-positive colonies.

3. Incorporate thiosulfate citrate bile sucrose (TCBS) agar as an extra plate for stool cultures and also for other likely specimens such as those from wounds, blood, eye, and ear.

4. Use other special procedures to enhance the isolation of *V. cholerae, V. parahaemolyticus,* and other *Vibrio* species.

For laboratories in the American Midwest, where positive cultures for *Vibrio* species may be few, the first or second approaches may be most appropriate. In laboratories near oceans, particularly those located in endemic areas, the third or fourth approach may be indicated. However, disadvantages to the routine use of TCBS agar, include the increased cost for a relatively low return, and some *Vibrio* species or strains may not grow well on TCBS agar. It is helpful for laboratory personnel to be informed when clinical cases of cholera or extraintestinal *Vibrio* infections are suspected. In these cases, the use of a selective medium or alkaline broth enrichment, to be discussed in a later section, may still be in order.

Specimen Collection, Processing, and Media Selection.
Laboratory personnel should be notified if the physician suspects a cholera syndrome or extraintestinal infections with *Vibrio* species. Specimens should be collected as early in the disease as possible. In the acute diarrheal stages of disease, specimens may be collected from the rectum with a soft rubber catheter or a rectal swab or from a small portion of the passed liquid stool. Culturing of vomitus also may be productive of organisms, particularly in the early stages of disease.

Specimens should be transported in closed containers to preserve moisture and transferred to culture media as soon as possible. *Vibrio* species are generally quite sensitive to drying, exposure to sunlight, and the development of an acid pH. They also are easily inhibited by the normal intestinal flora or contaminating organisms. If cultures cannot be set up immediately, *Vibrio* species will remain viable in Cary-Blair semisolid transport medium for an extended time. The use of buffered glycerol saline transport medium should be avoided. If a transport medium is not available, a 2 × 1/2-inch strip of thick blotting paper can be soaked in the fecal specimen, placed in a sealed plastic bag, and then mailed to the nearest reference laboratory.[168] Specimens suspicious for harboring *Vibrio* species should be inoculated to 5% sheep blood and MacConkey agar. Whether to also inoculate a plate of TCBS agar and/or a tube of alkaline peptone water enrichment must be determined by each laboratory supervisor depending on the prevalence of *Vibrio*-related diseases in any given locale. If TCBS agar is not used, hemolytic colonies that appear on sheep blood agar after overnight incubation should be tested for cytochrome oxidase activity. Either representative colony can be individually touched and spot tested for the oxidase reaction using Kovac's reagent or one or two drops of Kovac's reagent can be dropped in an area on the surface of the plate where suspicious colonies are present. The rapid development of a blue color is indicative of a positive test. Oxidase-positive colonies can be transferred to TCBS agar for further species identification using biochemical and other characteristics.

Alkaline peptone water (APW) enrichment broths should be subcultured to TCBS agar for further evaluation of colonies that grow after an additional 24 to 48 hours of incubation. APW, which contains 1% peptone and 1% NaCl at pH 8.6, is a simple-to-use enrichment broth that can be recommended in situations where low concentrations of organisms in the specimen are anticipated (e.g., in convalescent stages of disease). The high pH of the medium serves to suppress the growth of many commensal intestinal bacteria while allowing uninhibited multiplication of *V. cholerae.* Subcultures to TCBS or gelatin agar should be made within 12 to 18 hours since other organisms can begin to overgrow the broth after prolonged incubation. APW is also an excellent transport medium if specimens cannot be immediately delivered to the laboratory for processing. It is recommended that about 1 mL of liquid or 1 gram of formed stool be placed into 10 mL of APW in a screw-capped tube; alternatively, rectal swabs can be placed into a tube containing 1 to 2 ml of APW.[168]

Presumptive Identification of Vibrio Species Based on Colonial and Microscopic Morphology.
Vibrios grow readily on most isolation media; growth of all species is enhanced by adding 1% NaCl to the medium. Colonies are typically smooth, convex, creamy in consistency, gray-white, and have entire margins. Rough colonies are occasionally encountered that adhere to the agar. Certain marine vibrios are able to swarm on the surface of agar media, associated with the formation of long cells with lateral flagella. This phenomenon is not seen with most human isolates.

Microscopically, straight or curved gram-negative bacilli are observed (see Color Plate 8-2*D*). The curved character of the cells may be best seen in early stationary phase in broth cultures; in log phase, straight and rounded coccoid forms are intermixed. Although a presumptive diagnosis of cholera can be made by observing large numbers of curved bacilli in direct gram-stained stool specimens, recovery of the organism in culture is needed to make a definitive identification.

The differential reactions on TCBS agar are helpful in making a presumptive identification of *V. cholerae, V. alginolyticus, V. parahaemolyticus,* and *V. vulnificus.* After 18 to 24 hours of incubation on TCBS agar, *V. cholerae* grow as smooth, yellow colonies, 2 to 4 mm in diameter with an opaque center and transparent periphery (see Color Plate 8-2*A*). The colonies of *V. alginolyticus,* which also ferment sucrose, will also produce yellow colonies on TCBS agar; *V. parahaemolyticus* and *V. vulnificus,* which do not utilize sucrose, produce blue-green colonies (see Color Plate 8-2*B*). On gelatin agar, *V. cholerae* grow as transparent colonies surrounded by an opaque halo indicating liquefaction of gelatin (see Color Plate 8-2*C*). O'Brien and Colwell have described a modified taurocholate-tellurite gelatin agar for the differentiation of *V. cholerae* (β-galactose positive) versus *V. parahaemolyticus* (β-galactose negative) based on the hydrolysis of 4-methylumbelliferyl-β-D-galactose, in addition to determination of gelatin hydrolysis and tellurite reduction.[240]

BIOCHEMICAL CHARACTERIZATION AND LABORATORY IDENTIFICATION OF *VIBRIO* SPECIES

Members of the genus *Vibrio* are facultative anaerobes capable of both respiratory and fermentative metabolism. However, because they grow and react in carbohydrate test media designed for fermentative metabolism, they are classified with the fermenters. The natural habitat for *Vibrio* species is aquatic, in both fresh and salt water. The growth and biochemical reactivity of most species are enhanced in differential test media supplemented with 1% to 2% sodium chloride.

Most *Vibrio* species produce cytochrome oxidase, a characteristic that separates them from the Enterobacteriaceae. Therefore, *Vibrio* species are included in the group of oxidase-positive fermenters—*Aeromonas* species, *Plesiomonas* species, and *Chromobacterium* species—from which they must be differentiated (Table 8-10). Since *V. cholerae* ferments glucose, an acid-deep/alkaline-slant reaction is seen on Kligler iron agar. Since sucrose is also fermented, an acid-deep/acid slant reaction is seen on triple sugar iron agar. *V. cholerae* produces both lysine and ornithine decarboxylases.

Those laboratory workers who use lysine iron agar to screen stool isolates will note that *V. cholerae*, *A. hydrophila*, and *P. shigelloides* all produce a purple slant/purple deep reaction because of the decarboxylation of lysine. Arginine can be used to separate *V. cholerae* (negative) from both *Aeromonas* and *Plesiomonas* (positive). Most strains of *A.*

hydrophila hydrolyze esculin, differentiating it from the other organisms included in Table 8-10. Differences in the utilization of lactose, sucrose, mannitol, and inositol also serve to differentiate these genera.

V. cholerae, including the El Tor biotype, can be distinguished from other *Vibrio* species by the ability to produce a positive string test (see Color Plate 8-2*E*). To perform this test, bacterial colonies are mixed with a few drops of 0.5% sodium deoxycholate on a glass slide. An inoculating loop is immersed into the mixture and pulled away from the drop. *V. cholerae* produces a long string that becomes more tenacious after 60 seconds or more (other vibrios may give an initial string reaction that diminishes or disappears 45 to 60 seconds later). A positive slide agglutination with polyvalent O antiserum is also helpful in differentiating *V. cholerae* from other closely related strains (see Color Plate 8-2*F*). The El Tor biotype can be distinguished from classic strains of *V. cholerae* by several characteristics (Table 8-11). El Tor strains are actively β-hemolytic on blood agar (see Color Plate 8-2*G*) and are capable of agglutinating chicken erythrocytes (see Color Plate 8-2*H*). The chicken erythrocytes test is performed by mixing a loopful of washed chicken erythrocytes (2.5% suspension in saline) with bacterial cells from a pure culture to be tested. Visible clumping of the erythrocytes indicates the El Tor biotype, in contrast to classic 01 strains of *V. cholerae* that do not have this property. Classic strains of *V. cholerae* are susceptible to 50 IU of polymyxin B in the disk diffusion test; El Tor strains are

Table 8-10 Oxidase-Positive, Fermentative, Gram-Negative Bacilli: Differential Characteristics of *Aeromonas hydrophila, Plesiomonas shigelloides, Chromobacterium violaceum*, and *Vibrio cholerae*

CHARACTERISTIC	A. HYDROPHILA	P. SHIGELLOIDES	C. VIOLACEUM	V. CHOLERAE
Kligler iron agar (slant/deep/hydrogen sulfide)	K/A/–	K – A/A/–	K/A/–	K/A/–
Catalase	+	+	+	+
Esculin	+	–	–	–
Motility	+	+	+	+
ONPG	+	+	–	+
Indole	+	+	–	+
Voges-Proskauer	(+)	–	–	(–)
Lysine decarboxylase	+	+	–	+
Ornithine decarboxylase	–	+	–	+
Carbohydrates:				
Lactose	(–)	(+)	–	–
Sucrose	+	–	(–)	+
Mannitol	+	–	–	+
Inositol	–	+	–	–
Growth in peptone, 1% with:				
0% NaCl	+	+	+	+
7% NaCl	–	–	–	–
11% NaCl	–	–	–	–

+, 90% or more of strains are positive; (+), 51%–89% of strains are positive; (–), 10%–50% of strains are positive; –, less than 10% of strains are positive; V, variable; K/A, alkaline/acid; K – A/A, alkaline to acid/acid; ONPG, o-nitrophenyl-β-D-galactopyranoside.

Table 8-11 Differentiation Between *Vibrio cholerae* Biotypes

TEST	CLASSIC	EL TOR
String test	+	+
β-Hemolytic on sheep blood agar	−	+
CAMP test	−	+
Voges-Proskauer test	−	+
Chicken red blood cell agglutination	−	+
Susceptibility to 50 U polymyxin B	S	R
Phage IV susceptibility	S	R

+, positive test; −, negative test; S, susceptible; R, resistant.

resistant. El Tor strains also are Voges-Proskauer positive, whereas classic strains of *V. cholerae* are Voges-Proskauer negative. Lesmana and coworkers described using a modified CAMP test to differentiate the classical biotype (CAMP negative) from the EL Tor biotype (CAMP strong positive).[196] *V. cholerae* 0139 strains also demonstrate a strong positive CAMP reaction, whereas non-01 and non-0139 isolates give a weak positive CAMP reaction. The test is performed by inoculating a beta-lysin-producing *S. aureus* strain (ATCC 25178) onto a 5% sheep blood agar plate by making a single straight line streak and then inoculating the *Vibrio* species to be tested in a line perpendicular to and a few millimeters from the *S. aureus* streak. Plates are incubated in a candle jar at 37°C for 18 to 20 hours and observed for zones of synergistic hemolysis (see Chart 8-1). For laboratories capable of performing phage IV susceptibility tests, El Tor strains are resistant to this phage.

As an initial first step in the identification of *Vibrio* species, Kelly and colleagues[168] have devised a dichotomous scheme for separating the *Vibrio* species into six groups based on their reactions with seven tests: requirement for 1% NaCl for growth in nutrient broth, oxidase production, reduction of nitrate to nitrite, *myo*-inositol fermentation, and production of arginine dihydrolase, lysine decarboxylase, and ornithine decarboxylase. Their scheme is reproduced in Table 8-12. Grouping the species this way will provide simple presumptive identification of most clinical isolates. Additional key reactions and clinical correlation can be obtained by consulting Table 8-9. Overman and associates[248] recommended the use of the API 20E strip for performing the biochemical tests necessary to make identifications of the more commonly encountered members of the *Vibrionaceae*. However, a more recent evaluation of commercially available identification systems showed that the six methods evaluated correctly identified only 63 to 81% of the *Vibrio* tested to the species level.[241] For *V. cholera* in particular accuracy ranged from 50 to 97%. Thus the authors concluded that extreme care should be taken in interpreting results of commercial systems for identification of *Vibrio* species.

Nonculture Methods. An immunochromatographic dipstick test for rapid detection of *V. cholerae* O1 and O139 from stool specimens has been developed. In an evaluation of the test in Madagascar and Bangladesh, where cholera is endemic, sensitivity ranged from 94 to 100% and specificity, from 84 to 100%.[235] Bhuiyan and colleagues modified the procedure by performing a 4-hour enrichment in alkaline peptone water prior to the dipstick assay.[22] With this added step, the sensitivity and specificity, respectively, were 96% and 92% for *V. cholerae* O1 and 93% and 98% for *V. cholerae* O139.

Genera Listonella, Photobacterium, *and* Shewanella

MacDonell and Colwell[203] proposed restructuring of the *Vibrionaceae* to include the establishment of two new genera, *Listonella* and *Shewanella*, within the family. Through rather complex 5S rRNA ribonucleotide sequencing studies and cluster analysis, these authors concluded that several *Vibrio* species, notably *V. anguillarum*, *V. pelagius*, and *V. damsela* should be transferred to a proposed new genus *Listonella* as *L. anguillara*, *L. damsela*, and *L. pelagia*. They also conclude from these studies that *Alteromonas* (*Pseudomonas*) *putrefaciens* and *Alteromonas hanedai* should comprise the new genus *Shewanella* along with a proposed new species, *Shewanella benthica*. Subsequent to the work of MacDonnell and Colwell, Smith and colleagues proposed that *L. damsela* be reassigned to the genus *Photobacterium* as *P. damsela* based on phenotypic data.[284] Members of the genera *Listonella*, *Photobacterium*, and *Shewanella* are associated with marine environment and are pathogenic for fish.

Members of the genus *Shewanella* (notably *S. putrefaciens*) are straight or curved, gram-negative bacilli, motile by means of a single polar flagellum. Characteristic colonies are dome-shaped, circular, slightly viscous or mucoid, and usually red-brown or salmon-pink. They possess cytochrome oxidase activity and produce abundant hydrogen sulfide in Kligler iron agar. Nitrates are reduced to nitrites and gelatinase, ornithine decarboxylase, and DNase tests are positive. *S. putrefaciens* has been recovered from human clinical specimens and is discussed in detail in Chapter 5 of this text.

Aeromonas and Plesiomonas

Several years ago, *Aeromonas* species were included along with *Vibrio* species and *Plesiomonas shigelloides* in the *Vibrionaceae*.[20] However, based on molecular genetic evidence, *Aeromonas* species have been placed in a separate family, *Aeromonadaceae*.[66,203] It has also been proposed that *Plesiomonas* be placed in the genus *Proteus*. Phenotypic differences between *Vibrio*, *Aeromonas*, and *Plesiomonas* species are listed in Table 8-10.[112]

Genus *Aeromonas*

As the species name hydrophila (''water loving'') indicates, the natural habitat of *Aeromonas* species is fresh water or seawater, where they commonly cause infectious diseases in cold-blooded aquatic animals. These bacteria also reside

Table 8-12 Eight Key Differential Tests to Divide the 12 Clinically Significant *Vibrio* Species Into 6 Groups

REACTIONS OF THE SPECIES IN:

TEST	GROUP 1 *V. cholerae*	GROUP 1 *V. mimicus*	GROUP 2 *V. metschnikovii*	GROUP 3 *V. cincinnatiensis*	GROUP 4 *V. hollisae*	GROUP 4 *V. damsela*	GROUP 5 *V. fluvialis*	GROUP 5 *V. furnissii*	GROUP 6 *V. alginolyticus*	GROUP 6 *V. parahaemolyticus*	GROUP 6 *V. vulnificus*	GROUP 6 *V. carchariae*
Growth in nutrient broth:												
With no NaCl added	+	+	−	−	−	−	−	−	−	−	−	−
With 1% NaCl added	+	+	+	+	+	+	+	+	+	+	+	+
Oxidase	+	+	−	+	+	+	+	+	+	+	+	+
Nitrate nitrite	+	+	−	+	+	+	+	+	+	+	+	+
myo-Inositol fermentation	−	−	V	+	−	−	−	−	−	−	−	−
Arginine dihydrolase	−	−	V	−	−	+	+	+	−	−	−	−
Lysine decarboxylase	+	+	V	V	−	V	−	−	+	+	+	+
Ornithine decarboxylase	+	+	−	−	−	−	−	−	V	+	V	−

All data are for reactions within 2 days at 35°C to 37°C: +, most strains (generally 90%–100%) are positive; −, most strains are negative (generally 0–10% positive); V, between 10%–89% are positive.
Key test results are boxed.
From Kelly MT, Hickman-Brenner FW, Farmer JJ III: Vibrio. In Balows A (ed): Manual of Clinical Microbiology, 5th ed, pp 384–395. @TFN:Washington DC, American Society for Microbiology, 1991.

in sink traps and drainpipes and can be recovered from tap water faucets and distilled water supplies, which are potential sources of organisms involved in nosocomial infections.

TAXONOMY

The genus *Aeromonas* has undergone considerable taxonomic and nomenclature revisions during the past several years. Only five species were recognized in 1988.[151] By 2000, the number of valid published genomospecies had risen to 14.[158] The currently named species are listed in Table 8-13. In the mid-1970s, the genus *Aeromonas* was divided into two groups: psychrophilic and mesophilic. *A. salmonicida*, a fish pathogen, is the only species in the psychrophilic group. It is nonmotile and does not grow at 37°C. The mesophilic group of motile species are potential human pathogens.

CLINICAL SIGNIFICANCE

Four categories of human infections have been described: gastroenteritis, cellulitis and wound infections, septicemia, and miscellaneous. However, as our knowledge of *Aeromonas* has grown, the miscellaneous category of diseases they cause has expanded.[147]

Janda and others[146-148] have reviewed the infectious disease spectrum of *Aeromonas* species and concluded that there is strong evidence supporting *Aeromonas* species as a causative agent of diarrhea, although the data are not absolute. On one hand, they cite several reports indicating that there is little significant difference between symptomatic and asymptomatic persons who harbor *Aeromonas* species in their stools.[93,140,314] In contrast, other reports link *Aeromonas* species with gastroenteritis.[37,118] Watson and associates[329] proposed that the virulence factors of *Aeromonas* species that cause intestinal infections are similar to those of other enteric pathogens, that is, adherence of bacterial cells to intestinal mucosa, toxin production and mucosal invasion. About 20% of their patients with intestinal infections from *Aeromonas* species had symptoms of dysentery similar to those caused by *Shigella* species and by invasive strains of *Campylobacter jejuni*. Most of the invasive strains included in their study, as determined by invasiveness in cell culture, were *A. sobria*; a minority were *A. hydrophila*. The majority of *A. sobria* and *A. hydrophila* produce a cholera-like extractable toxin (Asao toxin) that causes watery diarrhea.[59,238] The previous notion that *A. caviae* does not produce an enterotoxin, is not invasive, and is not considered to be a human pathogen[113] may be questioned in light of a few reports in which this species was found to be a cause of gastroenteritis.[12,106,233,234]

Wounds, ranging in severity from mild, primarily cutaneous infections (e.g., cellulitis) to severe infections involving muscle, joints, and/or bone, are the second most common infection caused by *Aeromonas* species, after gastroenteritis. Clinical settings associated with *Aeromonas* wound infections include lacerations/abrasions associated with water sports, puncture wounds or other penetrating injury, crush injuries (e.g., motor vehicle accident), and invasive medical procedures (e.g., intraabdominal surgery, catheterization).[147] In a fraction of cases, no preceding trauma or precipitating event is recognized.

Table 8-13 Species in the Genus *Aeromonas*

AEROMONAS SPECIES	ISOLATED FROM: Humans/Pathogen	ASSOCIATED DISEASE Gastrointestinal	Other*
A. hydrophila	Yes/yes	✓	✓
A. caviae	Yes/yes	✓	✓
A. media	Yes/yes	✓	
A. eucrenophila	Yes/no		
A. veronii			
biovar *sobria*	Yes/yes	✓	✓
biovar *veronii*	Yes/yes	✓	✓
A. jandaei	Yes/yes	?	✓
A. trota	Yes/no		
A. schubertii	Yes/yes		
A. encheleia	Yes/no		
A. allosaccharophila	Yes/no		
A. sobria	No/no		
A. popoffii	No/no		
A. bestiarum	Yes/no		
A. salmonicida	Yes/no		

* *Predominantly septicemia and wounds, including wounds associated with the use of medicinal leeches. Infrequently, Aeromonas species have been cultured from eye, respiratory, bone, and urinary tract infections; meningitis; cholecystitis; endocarditis; and peritonitis.*

Four categories of persons who develop *Aeromonas* septicemia have been proposed, based on portal of entry, underlying disease state, immune status, and exposure to fresh water. The two most common of these groups are immunocompromised adults and infants less than 2 years of age who have complicating underlying medical conditions (e.g., malignancy, hepatobiliary disease, diabetes) and *Aeromonas* in their gastrointestinal tract. *Aeromonas* septicemia in these groups of patients can be rapidly fatal, especially in those with hepatic cirrhosis or underlying malignancy.[189] A third group are persons who develop secondary *Aeromonas* sepsis from trauma-related myonecrosis. The fourth, and smallest, group includes adults with no underlying defects and are exposed to freshwater sources. *Aeromonas* bacteremia in burn patients also has been described.[16] Most cases of *Aeromonas* septicemia in humans are caused by one of four species: *A. hydrophila, A. veronii, A. caviae,* and *A. jandaei.*[147,178] *A. schubertii* also has been responsible for a few cases of bacteremia.

Miscellaneous *Aeromonas* infections uncommonly occur. These include urinary tract infections, hepatobiliary disease, meningitis, ear infections, endocarditis, hemolytic uremic syndrome, peritonitis, respiratory tract disease, and ocular infections.[15,28,42,63,227]

Recently described *Aeromonas* species of clinical significance include *A. schubertii*[132] (formerly CDC Enteric Group 501, mannitol, sucrose and indole negative), which has been incriminated as the cause of wound infections;[47] *A. veronii*[133] (formerly CDC Enteric Group 77, ornithine decarboxylase positive), which has been reported to cause bacteremia, wound infections and diarrhea;[6,133,159] and *A. jandaei* (formerly genospecies DNA Group 9 *A. sobria,* sucrose, esculin and cellobiose negative).[46] *A. trota* has a unique biochemical profile, including negative reactions for esculin hydrolysis, arabinose fermentation, and the Voges-Proskauer test; positive reactions for cellobiose fermentation, lysine decarboxylation, and citrate utilization; and susceptibility to ampicillin.[45,65] This finding may invalidate the use of ampicillin-containing selective media (discussed in the next section) for screening stool specimens for *Aeromonas* species. *A. trota* has been isolated almost exclusively from fecal specimens. *A. allosaccharophila* is another new mesophilic *Aeromonas* species that has been isolated from diseased elvers (young eels) and from the stool of a patient with diarrhea.[208] *A. allosaccharophila* most closely resembles *A. sobria,* but may be distinguished from the latter in utilizing L-arabinose and L-histidine as sole carbon sources. In addition, this species is unique in its ability to produce acid from or utilize D-melibiose and D-raffinose, or L-rhamnose.[208]

AEROMONAS SPECIES IN MEDICINAL LEECHES

The medicinal leech *Hirudo medicinalis* has enjoyed a revival as a treatment for venous congestion following microvascular or plastic surgery. Unfortunately, *Aeromonas* species are present in the leech gut, where they aid in the breakdown of ingested red blood cells. As a result, an increasing number of *Aeromonas* infections have been associated with leech application.[156,247,278] Although some of the reported patients had relatively trivial episodes of wound drainage, other patients had significant episodes of cellulitis,

abscess, tissue loss, and sepsis.[7,198,216] It has been recommended that leech applications be restricted to tissue with arterial perfusion to minimize contamination of necrotic tissue with *Aeromonas*. Furthermore, the prophylactic administration of antibiotics has been proposed when leeches are applied.[198]

LABORATORY RECOVERY OF *AEROMONAS* SPECIES FROM CLINICAL SPECIMENS

Differential or selective agars should be utilized when *Aeromonas* is suspected as the etiologic agent of gastroenteritis or when fecal specimens are submitted for workup on patients whose peak of diarrheal symptoms has subsided (Box 8-5). Most strains grow on selective enteric media as lactose fermenters and, therefore, may be overlooked as unimportant or commensal enteric organisms.

LABORATORY IDENTIFICATION OF *AEROMONAS* SPECIES

Aeromonas species are cytochrome oxidase positive and can be quickly excluded from the *Enterobacteriaceae* by performing an oxidase test. A drop or two of tetramethyl-*p*-phenylenediamine-dihydrochloride (oxidase reagent) can be placed on surface colonies and observed for the evolution of a black discoloration characteristic of the colonies of *Aeromonas* species. Mesophilic *Aeromonas* species are motile with polar rather than peritrichous flagella similar to *Pseudomonas* species; however, *Aeromonas* species can be differentiated from the latter because they utilize glucose fermentatively rather than oxidatively and most *Aeromonas* species are indole positive (*Pseudomonas* species are negative). The phenotypic characteristics of *Aeromonas* species,[44] reviewed by Altwegg and colleagues[13] and more recently by Abbott and colleagues,[2] are summarized in Table 8-14. Janda and Duffey[151] point out that one pitfall in the identification of *Aeromonas* species is that some of the min-

---

> ### Box 8-5 Selective Agars Used To Culture *Aeromonas*
>
> 1. Blood agar (with or without ampicillin): blood agar can be made selective by incorporation of 10 μg/mL ampicillin. Janda and associates[150] recommend the use of a selective sheep blood agar containing ampicillin (SB-A agar) to improve the recovery of *Aeromonas* species from stool specimens.
> 2. Alkaline peptone water (APW, pH 8.6): initially developed for isolation of *Vibrio* species, APW can be used to recover aeromonads present in low numbers (10 CFU/mL) in stools. After overnight enrichment, APW is subcultured to the agar medium of choice.
> 3. CIN agar: originally developed for the isolation of *Yersinia enterocolitica,* CIN agar is also suitable for recovery of *Aeromonas* from feces.
> 4. Enteric agars: deoxycholate, MacConkey, and xylose lysine deoxycholate gave the highest overall plating efficiencies of eight routine enteric agars tested for recovery of *Aeromonas* species from feces.[73]

Table 8-14 Differentiation of *Plesiomonas shigelloides* and Clinically Important *Aeromonas* Species

ORGANISM	HEMOLYSIS SHEEP BLOOD	OXIDASE	MOTILITY	DNASE	INDOLE	VOGES-PROSKAUER	DECARBOXYLASE Lysine	DECARBOXYLASE Ornithine	DECARBOXYLASE Arginine	ESCULIN	GAS FROM GLUCOSE	L-arabinose	FERMENTATION Sucrose	FERMENTATION Mannitol	FERMENTATION Inositol
A. hydrophila complex															
A. hydrophila	+	+	+	+	+	+	+	−	+	+	+	+	+	+	−
A. caviae complex															
A. caviae	−	+	+	+	+	−	−	−	+	+	−	+	+	+	−
A. media	NA	+	−	+	v	−	−	−	+	+	−	+	−	NA	NA
A. eucrenophila	NA	+	+	+	NA	−	−	−	+	+	+	v	v	+	−
A. sobria	+	+	+	+	+	+	+	−	+	+	+	v	+	+	−
A. veronii biotype sobria	+	+	+	+	+	+	+	−	+	−	v	−	+	+	−
A. veronii biotype veronii	+	+	+	+	+	+	+	+	−	+	+	−	+	+	−
A. jamdaei	+	+	+	NA	+	+	+	−	+	−	+	−	−	+	−
A. schubertii	v	+	+	+	−	v	+	−	+	−	−	−	−	−	−
A. trota	+	+	+	NA	+	−	+	−	+	−	+	−	−	−	−
P. shigelloides	−	+	+	−	+	−	+	+	+	−	−	−	−	−	+

+, 90% or more of strains are positive; −, 90% or more of strains are negative; V, 11%–89% of strains are positive; NA, results not available. Shaded areas indicate key reactions.
Data from references[3, 9, 13, 32, 45, 132, 133, 151, 280].

iaturized, semiautomated test kit systems cannot efficiently distinguish between *Aeromonas* species and *Vibrio fluvialis*. The latter is only rarely encountered in clinical laboratories, however, and can be differentiated from *Aeromonas* species by demonstrating the ability of *V. fluvialis* to grow in 6.5% salt solutions, to produce yellow colonies on TCBS agar (sucrose positive), and to be sensitive to the vibriostatic agent 0/129.[151]

Namdari and Bottone[232] also describe the suicide phenomenon for the rapid differentiation of *Aeromonas* species. This phenomenon is expressed when unknown strains are grown in broth media containing 0.5% glucose. The supplied glucose suppresses the tricarboxylic acid cycle, resulting in accumulation of acetic acid and cell death. *A. hydrophila* is nonsuicidal, aerogenic and esculin positive; *A. sobria* is suicide variable, aerogenic and esculin negative; and *A. caviae* is suicidal, anaerogenic and esculin positive. Further studies on the biochemical characteristics and serologic properties of the genus *Aeromonas* have been published by Janda and colleagues and Abbott and colleagues.[2,148]

Genus *Plesiomonas*

The term *plesiomonas* is derived from the Greek word meaning "neighbor," indicating a close association with *Aeromonas*. However, as mentioned before, *Aeromonas* species have been reclassified within their own family and *Plesiomonas* is believed to be more closely related to *Proteus* than *Aeromonas*,[203,271] and is now included in the family *Enterobacteriaceae*. *P. shigelloides* is the only species in the genus.

P. shigelloides is ubiquitous in surface waters and in soil and commonly infects various cold-blooded animals (frogs, snakes, turtles, lizards). Humans become infected primarily by ingesting contaminated or unwashed food. Although less frequently recovered from human feces than *Aeromonas* species, *Plesiomonas*-induced gastroenteritis has been reported in children[211] and in adults.[140] In the latter study, 28 of 31 patients with gastroenteritis had no other organisms to account for the acute symptoms. In Thailand a carrier rate as high as 5.5% has been reported.[259]

Plesiomonas-related gastroenteritis in humans usually manifests as a mild watery diarrhea in which the stools are free of blood and mucin. Severe colitis or a cholera-like illness may be seen in patients who are immunosuppressed or who have gastrointestinal malignancies.[267] The infection is more prevalent in the subtropical and tropical regions of the world and during the warm summer months. Pathogenicity is probably related to the production of an enteropathogenic enterotoxin; Sanyal and colleagues demonstrated that 13 clinical strains they studied produced significant fluid accumulation in the ileal loop test.[277] *P. shigelloides*-associated diarrhea has occurred in epidemics but also in isolated cases. It has been described after uncooked shellfish consumption and as a cause of travelers' diarrhea.[141] A few isolated cases of extraintestinal infections including septicemia, neonatal meningitis, cellulitis, septic arthritis, and acute cholecystitis have also been reported.[32,62,266] There are also reports of an overwhelming postsplenectomy infection with *P. shigelloides* in a patient cured of Hodgkin's disease[67] and a *P. shigelloides*-associated persistent dysentery and pseudo-

membranous colitis in a 42-year-old Bangladeshi woman.[323] The clinical disease spectrum and pathogenic factors associated with *Plesiomonas* infections have been reviewed by Brenden and colleagues.[32]

LABORATORY ISOLATION AND IDENTIFICATION

P. shigelloides is a straight, rounded, short, motile gram-negative bacillus with polar, generally lophotrichous flagella (*Vibrio* species and *Aeromonas* species are monotrichous). The organism grows well on sheep blood agar and on most enteric media. Isolates are nonhemolytic on sheep blood agar; and in 24 hours at 30°C to 35°C (growth is optimum at 30°C); colonies average 1.5 mm in diameter and are gray, shiny, smooth, and opaque and may be slightly raised in the center. *P. shigelloides* is readily isolated on enteric agars such as MacConkey, deoxycholate, Hektoen, and xylose lysine deoxycholate. However, ampicillin-containing selective media that are frequently used for the isolation of *Aeromonas* species are not suitable for the isolation of *P. shigelloides*.[325]

Glucose is fermented; therefore, the deep of Kligler iron agar or triple sugar iron agar tubes will appear yellow. *P. shigelloides* will appear as a non-lactose fermenter on MacConkey agar and may be confused with *Shigella* species. The cytochrome oxidase reaction is positive, and indole is produced. *P. shigelloides* decarboxylates arginine, lysine, and ornithine. It does not produce DNAse or extracellular proteases, and it ferments inositol but not mannitol. These are key characteristics by which it is separated from *Aeromonas* species. Additional key identifying characteristics are listed in Table 8-14.

P. shigelloides can be resistant to penicillin, ampicillin, carbenicillin, and other β-lactamase sensitive penicillins. Most strains are susceptible to the aminoglycosides, chloramphenicol, tetracycline, trimethoprim-sulfamethoxazole, and the quinolones, ciprofloxacin and norfloxacin.[32,266]

Genus Chromobacterium

Brief mention of the genus *Chromobacterium* is made here because some strains are oxidase-positive fermenters and can be confused with *Aeromonas* species and *Vibrio* species. *Chromobacterium violaceum* is the species most commonly encountered in clinical laboratories, although it is seldom associated with human disease. *C. violaceum* grows well on blood agar, and most strains produce abundant violet pigment that makes recognition easy. Select biochemical characteristics are shown in Table 8-10. In addition, the ability of the organism to utilize citrate, reduce nitrates, and strongly hydrolyze casein is also helpful in making a final definitive identification.

REFERENCES

1. Aabenhus R, Permin H, On SL, Andersen LP. Prevalence of *Campylobacter concisus* in diarrhea of immunocompromised patients. Scand J Infect Dis 2002; 34:248–252.

2. Abbott SL, Cheung WKW, Janda JM. The genus *Aeromonas*: biochemical characteristics, atypical reaction, and phenotypic identification schemes. J Clin Microbiol 2003;41:2348–2357.

3. Abbott SL, Cheung WKW, Kroske-Bystrom S, Malekzadeh T, Janda JM. Identification of *Aeromonas* strains to the genospecies level in the clinical laboratory. J Clin Microbiol 1992;30:1262–1266.

4. Abbott SL, Janda JM. Severe gastroenteritis associated with *Vibrio hollisae* infection: report of two cases and review. Clin Infect Dis 1994;18:310–312.

5. Abbott SL, Powers C, Kaysner CA, Takeda, Ishibashi M, Joseph SW, Janda JM. Emergence of a restricted bioserovar of *Vibrio parahaemolyticus* as the predominant cause of *Vibrio*-associated gastroenteritis on the west coast of the United States and Mexico. J. Clin Microbiol 1989;27:2891–2893.

6. Abbott SL, Serve H, Janda JM. Case of *Aeromonas veronii* (DNA Group 10) bacteremia. J Clin Microbiol 1994;32:3091–3092.

7. Abrutyn E. Hospital-associated infection from leeches. Ann Intern Med 1988; 109:356–358.

7a. Albert MJ: Minireview. *Vibrio cholerae* 0139 Bengal. J Clin Microbiol 1994; 32:2345–2349.

8. Alderton MR, Korolik V, Coloe PJ, Dewhirst FE, Paster BJ. *Campylobacter hyoilei* sp. nov., associated with porcine proliferative enteritis. Int J Syst Bacteriol 1995;45:61–66.

9. Allen DA, Austin B, Colwell RR. *Aeromonas media,* a new species isolated from river water. Int J Syst Bacteriol 1983;33:599–604.

10. Allos BM. *Campylobacter jejuni* infections: update on emerging issues and trends. Clin Infect Dis 2001;32:1201–1206.

11. Allos BM, Blaser MJ. *Campylobacter jejuni* and the expanding spectrum of related infections. Clin Infect Dis 1995;20:1092–1101.

12. Altwegg M. *Aeromonas caviae:* An enteric pathogen? Infection 1985;13: 228–230.

13. Altwegg M, Steigerwalt AG, Altwegg-Bissig R et al. Biochemical identification of *Aeromonas* genospecies isolated from humans. J. Clin Microbiol 1990;28: 258–264.

14. Archer JR, Romero S, Ritchie AE et al. Characterization of an unclassified microaerophilic bacterium associated with gastroenteritis. J Clin Microbiol 1988; 26:101–105.

15. Baddour LM, Baselski VS. Pneumonia due to *Aeromonas hydrophila* complex: epidemiologic, clinical, and microbiologic features. South Med J 1988;81: 461–463.

16. Barillo DJ, McManus AT, Cioffi WG, McManus WF, Kim SH, Pruitt BA Jr. *Aeromonas* bacteraemia in burn patients. Burns 1996;22:48–52.

17. Barrett TJ, Patton CM, Morris GK. Differentiation of *Campylobacter* species using phenotypic characterization. Lab Med 1988;19:96–102.

18. Barthel JS, Everett ED. Diagnosis of *Campylobacter pylori* infections: The "gold standard" and the alternatives. Rev Infect Dis 1990;12:S107–S114.

19. Bates CJ, Clarke TC, Spencer. Prosthetic hip joint infection due to *Campylobacter fetus* [letter]. J Clin Microbiol 1994;32:2037.

20. Baumann P, Schubert RHW. Family II. *Vibrionaceae* Vernon 1965, 5245^AL. In Krieg NR, Holt JG (eds): Bergey's Manual of Systematic Bacteriology, vol 1, pp 516–550. Baltimore, Williams & Wilkins, 1984.

21. Benjamin J, Leaper S, Owen RJ et al. Description of *Campylobacter laridis,* a new species comprising the nalidixic acid resistant thermophilic *Campylobacter* (NARTC) group. Curr Microbiol 1983;8:231–238.

22. Bhuiyan NA, Qadri F, Farugue ASG, Malek MA, Salam MA, Nato F, Fournier JM, Chanteau S, Sack DA, Nair GB. Use of dipsticks for rapid diagnosis of cholera caused by *Vibrio cholerae* O1 and O139 from rectal swabs. J Clin Microbiol 2003;41:3939–3941.

23. Blake PA, Allegra DT, Synder JD et al. Cholera—a possible endemic focus in the United States. N Engl J Med 1980;302:305–309.

24. Blake PA, Merson MH, Weaver RE, Hollis DG, Heublein PC. Disease caused by a marine vibrio: clinical characteristics and epidemiology. N Engl J Med 1979;300:1–4.

25. Blaser MJ. *Heliobacter pylori*: its role in disease. Clin Infect Dis 1992;15: 386–393.

26. Blaser MJ, Berkowitz ID, Laforce FM et al. *Campylobacter* enteritis: Clinical and epidemiological features. Ann Intern Med 1979;91:179–185.

27. Blaser MJ, Wells JG, Feldman RA et al. *Campylobacter* enteritis in the United States. Ann Intern Med 1983;98:360–365.

28. Bogdanovic R, Cobeljic M, Markovic V et al. Haemolytic-uraemic syndrome associated with *Aeromonas hydrophila* enterocolitis. Pediatr Nephrol 1991;5: 293–295.

29. Bonner JR, Coker AS, Berryman CR, Pollock HM. Spectrum of Vibrio infections in a Gulf coast community. Ann Intern Med 1983;99:464–469..

30. Borczyk A, Rosa SD, Lior H. Enhanced recognition of *Campylobacter cryaerophila* in clinical and environmental specimens. Presented before the annual meeting of the American Society for Microbiology, 1991, abstract C-267, p 386.

31. Brayton PR, Bode RB, Colwell RR et al. *Vibrio cincinnatiensis* sp. nov., a new human pathogen. J Clin Microbiol 1986;23:104–108.

32. Brenden RA, Miller MA, Janda JM. Clinical disease spectrum and pathogenic factors associated with *Plesiomonas shigelloides* infections in humans. Rev Infect Dis 1988;10:303–316.

33. Brenner DJ, Hickman-Brenner FW, Lee JV et al. *Vibrio furnissii* (formerly aerogenic biogroup of *Vibrio fluvialis*), a new species isolated from human feces and the environment. J Clin Microbiol 1983;18:816–824.

34. Bronsdon MA, Goodwin CS, Sly LI et al. *Helicobacter nemestrinae* sp. nov., a spiral bacterium found in the stomach of a pigtailed macaque (*Macaca nemestrina*). Int J Syst Bacteriol 1991;41:148–153.

35. Bryner JH, Littleton J, Gates C et al. Paper presented before the XIV International Congress of Microbiology, Manchester, England, 1986.

36. Buck GE. *Campylobacter pylori* and gastroduodenal disease. Clin Microbiol Rev 1990;3:1–12.

37. Burke V, Gracey M, Robinson J et al. The microbiology of childhood gastroenteritis: *Aeromonas* species and other infective agents. J Infect Dis 1983;148: 68–74.

38. Burman WJ, Cohn DL, Reves RR, Wilson ML. Multifocal cellulitis and monoarticular arthritis as manifestations of *Heliobacter cinaedi* bacteremia. Clin Infect Dis 1995;20:564–570.

39. Burnens AP, Angeloz-Wick B, Nicolet J. Comparison of *Campylobacter* carriage rates in diarrhoeic and healthy pet animals. Zentralblatt fur Veterinarmedizin 1992;39:175–180.

40. Burnens AP, Stanley J, Morgentsern R, Nicolet J. Gastroenteritis associated with *Helicobacter pullorum* [letter]. Lancet 1994;344:1569–1570.

41. Butzler JP. Infections with *Campylobacter.* In Williams JD, Heremann W (eds): Modern Topics in Infectious Diseases, pp. 214–239. London, Medical Books Ltd, 1978.

42. Carta F, PinnaA, Zanetti S, Carta A, Sotgiu M, Fadda G. Corneal ulcer caused by Aeromonas species. Am J Ophthalmol 1994;118:530–531.

43. Carnahan AM, Beadling J, Watsky D, Ford N. Detection of *Campylobacter upsaliensis* from a blood culture by using the BacT/Alert system. J Clin Microbiol 1994;32:2598–2599.

44. Carnahan AM, Behram S, Joseph SW. Aerokey II: a flexible key for identifying clinical *Aeromonas* species. J Clin Microbiol 1991;29:2843–2849.

45. Carnahan AM, Chakraborty T, Fanning GR et al. *Aeromonas trota* sp. nov., an ampicillin-susceptible species isolated from clinical specimens. J Clin Microbiol 1991;29:1206–1210.

46. Carnahan AM, Fanning GR, Joseph SW. *Aeromonas jandaei* (formerly genospecies DNA group 9 *A. sobria*), a new sucrose-negative species isolated from clinical specimens. J Clin Microbiol 1991;29:560–564.

47. Carnahan AM, Marii MA, Fanning GR et al. Characterization of *Aeromonas shubertii* strains recently isolated from traumatic wound infections. J Clin Microbiol 1989;27:1826–1830.

48. Centers for Disease Control. Waterborne *Campylobacter* gastroenteritis, Vermont. MMWR 1978;27:207.

49. Centers for Disease Control. *Campylobacter* sepsis associated with "nutritional therapy"—California. MMWR 1981;30:294–295.

50. Centers for Disease Control. Premature labor and neonatal sepsis caused by *Campylobacter fetus* subspecies *fetus*—Ontario. MMWR 1984;33:483–489.

51. Centers for Disease Control. Cholera—Peru, 1991. MMWR 1991;40:108–110.

52. Centers for Disease Control. Cholera—New Jersey and Florida. MMWR 1991; 40:287–289.

53. Centers for Disease Control. Imported cholera associated with a newly described toxigenic *Vibrio cholerae* 0139 strain—California, 1993. MMWR 1993;42: 501–503.

54. Centers for Disease Control. Update: *Vibrio cholerae* 01—western hemisphere, 1991–1994, and *V. cholerae* 0139—Asia, 1994. MMWR 1995;44:215–219.

55. Centers for Disease Control. *Vibrio vulnificus* infections associated with eating raw oysters—Los Angeles, 1996. MMWR 1996;45:621–624.

56. Centers for Disease Control. Outbreak of *Campylobacter jejuni* infections associated with drinking unpasteurized milk procured through a cow-leasing program—Wisconsin, 2001. MMWR 2002;51:548–549.

57. Chiang SR, Chuang YC. Vibrio vulnificus infection: clinical manifestations, pathogenesis and antimicrobial therapy. J Microbiol Immunol Infect 2003;36: 81–88.

58. Chiu C-H, Kuo C-Y, Ou JT. Chronic diarrhea and bacteremia caused by *Campylobacter lari* in a neonate [letter]. Clin Infect Dis 1995;21:700–701.

59. Chopra AK, Houston CW, Genaux CT et al. Evidence for production of an enterotoxin and cholera toxin cross-reactive factor by *Aeromonas hydrophila.* J Clin Microbiol 1986;24:661–664.

60. Chusid MJ, Wortmann DW, Dunne WM. "*Campylobacter upsaliensis*" sepsis in a boy with acquired hypogammaglobulinemia. Diagn Microbiol Infect Dis 1990;13:367–369.

61. Cimolai N, Gill MJ, Jones A et al. "*Campylobacter cinaedi*" bacteremia: Case report and laboratory findings. J Clin Microbiol 1987;25:942–943.

62. Claesson Beb, Holmlund Dew, Lindhagen CA et al. *Plesiomonas shigelloides* in acute cholecystitis: A case report. J Clin Microbiol 1984;20:985–987.

63. Clark NM, Chenoweth CE. *Aeromonas* infection of the hepatobiliary system: report of 15 cases and review of the literature. Clin Infect Dis 2003;37:506–513.

64. Clarridge JE, Zighelboim-Daum S. Isolation and characterization of two hemolytic phenotypes of *Vibrio damsela* associated with a fatal wound infection. J Clin Microbiol 1985;21:302–306.

65. Collins MD, Martinez-Murcia AJ, Cai J. *Aeromonas enteropelogenes* and *Aeromonas ichthiosmia* are identical to *Aeromonas trota* and *Aeromonas veronii*, respectively, as revealed by small-subunit rRNA sequence analysis. Int J Syst Bacteriol 1993;43:855–856.

66. Colwell RR, MacDonell MT, De Ley J. Proposal to recognize the family *Aeromonadaceae* fam. nov. Int J Syst Bacteriol 1986;36:473–477.

67. Curti AJ, Lin JH, Szabo K. Overwhelming postsplenectomy infection with *Plesiomonas shigelloides* in a patient cured of Hodgkin's disease: A case report. Am J Clin Pathol 1985;83:522–524.

68. Cutler AF, Havstad S, Ma CK, Blaser MJ, Perez-Perez GI, Schubert TT. Accuracy of invasive and noninvasive tests to diagnose *Helicobacter pylori* infection. Gastroenterol 1995;109:136–141.

69. Davis BR, Fanning GR, Madden JM et al. Characterization of biochemically atypical *Vibrio cholerae* strains and designation of a new pathogenic species, *Vibrio mimicus*. J Clin Microbiol 1981;14:631–639.

70. Decker CF, Martin GI, Barham WB, Paparello SF. Bacteremia due to *Campylobacter cinaedi* in a patient infected with the human immunodeficiency virus [letter]. Clin Infect Dis 1992;15:178–179.

71. Dekeyser P, Gossuin-Detrain M, Butzler JP et al. Acute enteritis due to related vibrio: First positive stool cultures. J Infect Dis 1972;125:390–392.

72. Dent JC, McNulty CAM, Uff JC, Wilkinson SP, Gear MWL. Spiral organisms in the gastric antrum. Lancet 1997;ii:96.

73. Desmond E, Janda JM. Growth of *Aeromonas* species on enteric agars. J Clin Microbiol 1986;23:1065–1067.

74. Devlin HR, McIntyre L. *Campylobacter fetus* subsp. *fetus* in homosexual males. J Clin Microbiol 1983;18:999–1000.

75. Dubois A, Tarnawski A, Newell DG, Fiala N, Wojciech D, Stachura J, Krivan H, Heman-Ackah LM. Gastric injury and invasion of parietal cells by spiral bacteria in rhesus monkeys. Gastroenterol 1991;100:884–889.

76. Duerden BI, Eley A, Goodwin L, Magee JT, Hindmarch JM, Bennett KW. A comparison of *Bacteroides ureolyticus* isolates from different clinical sources. J Med Microbiol 1989;29: 63–73.

77. Duerden BI, Goodwin L, O'Neil TCA. Identification of *Bacteroides* species from adult periodontal disease. J Med Microbiol 1987;24:133–137.

78. Dunn BE, Cohen H, Blaser MJ. *Helicobacter pylori*. Clin Microbiol Rev 1997;10:720–741.

79. Eaton KA, Dewhirst FE, Radin MJ, Fox JG, Paster BJ, Krakowka S, Morgan DR. *Helicobacter acinonyx* sp. nov., isolated from cheetahs with gastritis. Int J Syst Bacteriol 1993;43:99–106.

80. Edmonds P, Patton CM, Griffin PM et al. *Campylobacter hyointestinalis* associated with human gastrointestinal disease in the United States. J Clin Microbiol 1987;25:685–691.

81. Endtz HP, Ang CW, Van Den Braak N, Luijendijk A, Jacobs BC, de Man P, van Duin JM, van Belkum A, Verbrugh HA. Evaluation of a new commercial immunoassay for rapid detection of *Campylobacter jejuni* in stool samples. Eur J Clin Microbiol Infect Dis 2000;19:794–797.

82. Endtz HP, Ruijs GJHM, Zwinderman AH et al. Comparison of six media, including a semisolid agar, for the isolation of various *Campylobacter* species from stool specimens. J Clin Microbiol 1991;29:1007–1010.

83. English, VL, Lindberg RB. Isolation of *Vibrio alginolyticus* from wounds and blood of a burn patient. Am J Med Technol 1977;43:989–993.

84. Etoh Y, Dewhirst FE, Paster BJ, Yamamoto A, Goto N. *Campylobacter showae* sp. nov., isolated from the human oral cavity. Int J Syst Bacteriol 1993;43: 631–639.

85. Farmer JJ III. *Vibrio* (''*Beneckea*'') *vulnificus,* the bacterium associated with sepsis, septicemia, and the sea. Lancet 1979;2:903.

86. Farmer JJ III, Hickman-Brenner FW, Fanning GR et al. Characterization of *Vibrio metschnikovii* and *Vibrio gazogenes* by DNA-DNA hybridization and phenotype. J Clin Microbiol 1988;26:1993–2000.

87. Farmer JJ III, Hickman-Brenner FW, Kelly MT. *Vibrio*. In Lennette EH (ed): Manual of Clinical Microbiology, 4th ed, pp. 282–301. Washington, DC, American Society for Microbiology, 1985.

88. Farrugia DC, Eykyn SJ, Smyth EG. *Campylobacter fetus* endocarditis: two case reports and review. Clin Infect Dis 1994;18:443–446.

89. Farugque SM, Chowdhury N, Kamruzzaman M, Ahmad QS, Faruque ASG, Salam MA, Ramamurthy T, Nair GB, Weintraub A, Sack DA. Reemergence of epidemic *Vibrio cholerae* O139, Bangladesh. Emerg Infect Dis 2003;9:1116–1122.

90. Fennell CL, Rompalo AM, Totten PA et al. Isolation of ''*Campylobacter hyointestinalis*'' from a human. J Clin Microbiol 1986;24:146–148.

91. Fennell CL, Totten PA, Quinn TC et al. Characterization of *Campylobacter*-like organisms isolated from homosexual men. J Infect Dis 1984;149:58–66.

92. Figura N, Guglielmetti P, Zanchi A, Partini N, Armellini D, Bayeli PF, Bugnoli M, Verdiani S. Two cases of *Campylobacter mucosalis* enteritis in children. J Clin Microbiol 1993;31:727–728.

93. Figura N, Marri L, Verdiani S et al. Prevalence, species differentiation, and toxigenicity of *Aeromonas* strains in cases of childhood gastroenteritis and in controls. J Clin Microbiol 1986;23:595–599.

94. Fisher R, Samisch W. ''*Gastrospirillum hominis*'': another four cases. Lancet 1990;i:59.

95. Fontaine EAR, Borriello SP, Taylor-Robinson D, Davies HA. Characteristics of a gram-negative anaerobe isolated from men with nongonococcal urethritis. J Med Microbiol 1984;17:129–140.

96. Fontaine EAR, Bryant TN, Taylor-Robinson D, Borriello SP, Davies HA. A numerical taxonomic study of anaerobic gram-negative bacilli classified as *Bacteroides ureolyticus* isolated from patients with nongonococcal urethritis. J Gen Microbiol 1986;132:3137–3146.

97. Fox JG, Chien CC, Dewhirst FE, Paster BJ, Shen Z, Melito PL, Woodward DL, Rodgers FG. *Helicobacter canadensis* sp. nov. isolated from humans with diarrhea as an example of an emerging pathogen. J Clin Microbiol 2000;38: 2546–2549.

98. Fox JG, Chilvers T, Goodwin CS et al. *Campylobacter mustelae*, a new species resulting from the elevation of *Campylobacter pylori* subsp. *mustelae* to species status. Int J Syst Bacteriol 1989;39:301–303.

99. Fox JG, Dewhirst FE, Tully JG, Paster BJ, Yan L, Taylor NS, Collins Jr MJ, Gorelick PL, Ward JM. *Helicobacter hepaticus* sp. nov., a microaerophilic bacterium isolated from livers and intestinal mucosal scrapings from mice. J Clin Microbiol 1994;32:1238–1245.

100. Fox JG, Lee A. Gastric *Campylobacter*-like organisms: their role in gastric disease of laboratory animals. Lab Animal Sci 1989;39:543–553.

101. Fox JG, Lee A. The role of *Helicobacter* species in newly recognized gastrointestinal tract diseases of animals. Lab Anim Sci 1997;47:222–255.

102. Fox JG, Maxwell KO, Taylor NS, Runsick CD, Edmonds P, Brenner DJ. ''*Campylobacter upsaliensis*'' isolated from cats as identified by DNA relatedness and biochemical features. J Clin Microbiol 1989;27:2376–2378.

103. Fox JG, Taylor NS, Edmonds P et al. *Campylobacter pylori* subsp. *mustelae* subsp. nov. isolated from the gastric mucosa of ferrets (*Mustela putorius furo*), and an emended description of *Campylobacter pylori*. Int J Syst Bacteriol 1988; 38:367–370.

104. Fox JG, Yan LL, Dewhirst FE, Paster BJ, Shames B, Murphy JC, Hayward A, Belcher JC, Mendes EN. *Helicobacter bilis* sp. nov., a novel *Helicobacter* species isolated from bile, livers, and intestines of aged, inbred mice. J Clin Microbiol 1995;33:445–454.

105. Freedberg AS, Barron LE. The presence of spirochetes in human gastric mucosa. Am J Dig Dis 1940;7:443–445.

106. Fritsche D, Dahn, R, Hoffmann G. *Aeromonas punctata* subsp. *caviae* as the causative agent of acute gastroenteritis. Zentralbl Bakteriol Mikrobiol Hyg [A] 1975;233:232–235.

107. Frost JA. Current epidemiological issues in human campylobacteriosis. Symp Ser Soc Appl Microbiol 2001;90:85S–95S.

108. Fujimoto S, Yuki N, Itoh T, Amako K. Specific serotype of *Campylobacter jejuni* associated with Guillain-Barre Syndrome [letter]. J Infect Dis 1992;165: 183.

109. Gaudreau C, Lamothe F. *Campylobacter upsaliensis* isolated from a breast abscess. J Clin Microbiol 1992;30:1354–1356.

110. Gebhart CJ, Edmonds P, Ward GE et al. ''*Campylobacter hyointestinalis*'' sp. nov.: A new species of *Campylobacter* found in the intestines of pigs and other animals. J Clin Microbiol 1985;21:715–720.

111. Gebhart CJ, Fennell CL, Murtaugh MP, Stamm WE. *Campylobacter cinaedi* is normal intestinal flora in hamsters. J Clin Microbiol 1989;27:1692–1694.

112. George WL, Jones MJ, Nakata MM. Phenotypic characteristics of *Aeromonas* species isolated from adult humans. J Clin Microbiol 1986;23:1026–1029.

113. George WL, Nakata MM, Thompson J et al. *Aeromonas*-related diarrhea in adults. Arch Intern Med 1985;145:2207–2211.

114. Gomez JM, Fajardo R, Patino JF, Arias CA. Necrotizing fasciitis due to *Vibrio alginolyticus* in an immunocompetent patient. J Clin Microbiol 2003;41: 3427–3429.

115. Goodwin CS, Armstrong JA, Chilvers T et al. Transfer of *Campylobacter pylori* and *Campylobacter mustelae* to *Helicobacter* gen. nov. as *Helicobacter pylori* comb. nov. and *Helicobacter mustelae* comb. nov., respectively. Int J Syst Bacteriol 1989;39:397–405.

116. Goossens H, Pot B, Vlaes L et al. Characterization and description of ''*Campylobacter upsaliensis*'' isolated from human feces. J Clin Microbiol 1990;28: 1039–1046.

117. Goossens H, Vlaes L, Galand I et al. Semisolid blood-free selective-motility medium for the isolation of campylobacters from stool specimens. J Clin Microbiol 1989;27:1077–1080.

118. Gracey M, Burke V, Robinson J. *Aeromonas*-associated gastroenteritis. Lancet 1982;2:1304–1306.

119. Grant IH, Richardson NJ, Bokkenheuser VD. Broiler chickens as potential source of *Campylobacter* infections in humans. J Clin Microbiol 1980;11:508–510.

120. Gurgan R, Diker KS. Abortion associated with *Campylobacter upsaliensis*. J Clin Microbiol 1994;32:3093–3094.

121. Guthmann JP. Epidemic cholera in Latin America: spread and routes of transmission. J Trop Med Hyg 1995;98:419–427.

122. Hadden RDM, Gregson NA. Guillain-Barre syndrome and *Campylobacter jejuni* infection. Symp Ser Appl Microbiol 2001;90:145S–154S.

123. Hanninen M-L, Happonen I, Saari S, Jalava K. Culture and characteristics of *Helicobacter bizzozeronii*, a new gastric *Helicobacter* sp. Int J Syst Bacteriol 1996;46:160–166.

124. Hansen W, Crokaert F, Yourassowsky E. Two strains of *Vibrio* species with unusual biochemical features isolated from ear tracts. J Clin Microbiol 1979;9:152–153.

125. Hansen W, Freney J, Benyagoub H, Letouzey M-N, Gigi J, Wauters G. Severe human infections caused by *Vibrio metschnikovii*. J Clin Microbiol 1993;31:2529–2530.

126. Harvey SM. Hippurate hydrolysis by *Campylobacter fetus*. J Clin Microbiol 1980;11:435–437.

127. Harvey SM, Greenwood JR. Probable *Campylobacter fetus* subsp. *fetus* gastroenteritis. J Clin Microbiol 1983;18:1278–1279.

128. Heilmann KL, Borchard F. Gastritis due to spiral shaped bacteria other than *Helicobacter pylori*: clinical, histological, and ultrastructural findings. Gut 1991;32:137–140.

129. Henry GA, Long PH, Burns JL, Charbonneau DL. Gastric spirillosis in beagles. Am J Vet Res 1987;48:831–836.

130. Hickman FW, Farmer JJ III, Hollis DG et al. Identification of *Vibrio hollisae* sp. nov. from patients with diarrhea. J Clin Microbiol 1982;15:395–401.

131. Hickman-Brenner FW, Brenner DJ, Steigerwalt AG, et al. *Vibrio fluvialis* and *Vibrio furnissii* isolated from a stool sample of one patient. J Clin Microbiol 1984;20:125–127.

132. Hickman-Brenner FW, Fanning GR, Arduino MJ et al. *Aeromonas schubertii*, a new mannitol-negative species found in human clinical specimens. J Clin Microbiol 1988;26:1561–1564.

133. Hickman-Brenner FW, MacDonald KL, Steigerwalt AG et al. *Aeromonas veronii*, a new ornithine decarboxylase-positive species that may cause diarrhea. J Clin Microbiol 1987;25:900–906.

134. Hindiyeh M, Jense S, Hohmann S, Benett H, Edwards C, Aldeen W, Croft A, Daly J, Mottice S, Carroll KC. Rapid detection of *Campylobacter jejuni* in stool specimens by an enzyme immunoassay and surveillance for *Campylobacter upsaliensis* in the greater Salt Lake City area. J Clin Microbiol 2000';38:3076–3079.

135. Hodge DS, Borczyk A, Wat L-L. Evaluation of the indoxyl acetate hydrolysis test for the differentiation of campylobacters. J Clin Microbiol 1990;28:1482–1483.

136. Hodge DS, Prescott JF, Shewen PE. Direct immunofluorescence microscopy for rapid screening of *Campylobacter* enteritis. J Clin Microbiol 1986;24:863–865.

137. Hodge Jr TW, Levy CS, Smith MA. Diarrhea associated with *Vibrio fluvialis* infection in a patient with AIDS. Clin Infect Dis 1995;21:237–238.

138. Hodinka RL, Gilligan PH. Evaluation of the Campyslide agglutination test for confirmatory identification of selected *Campylobacter* species. J Clin Microbiol 1988;26:47–49.

139. Hollis DG, Weaver RE, Baker CN et al. Halophilic *Vibrio* species isolated from blood cultures. J Clin Microbiol 1976;3:425–431.

140. Holmberg SD, Farmer JJ III. *Aeromonas hydrophila* and *Plesiomonas shigelloides* as causes of intestinal infections. Rev Infect Dis 1984;6:633–639.

141. Holmberg SD, Wachsmuth IK, Hickman-Brenner FW et al. *Plesiomonas* enteric infections in the United States. Ann Intern Med 1986;105:690–694.

142. Honda S-I, Goto I, Minematsu I et al. Gastroenteritis due to Kanagawa-negative *Vibrio parahaemolyticus*. Lancet 1987;1:331–332.

143. Hughes JM, Hollis DG, Gangarosa EJ et al. Noncholera *Vibrio* infections in the United States: Clinical, epidemiological, and laboratory features. Ann Intern Med 1978;88:602–606.

144. Huq MI, Alam AKMJ, Brenner DF et al. Isolation of *Vibrio*-like group EF-6 from patients with diarrhea. J Clin Microbiol 1980;11:621–624.

145. Husmann M, Gries C, Jehnichen P, Woelfel T, Gerken G, Ludwig W, Bhakdi S. *Helicobacter* sp. strain *Mainz* isolated from an AIDS patient with septic arthritis: case report and nonradioactive analysis of 16S rRNA sequence. J Clin Microbiol 1994;32: 3037–3039.

146. Janda JM. Recent advances in the study of the taxonomy, pathogenicity and infectious syndromes associated with the genus *Aeromonas*. Clin Microbiol Rev 1991;4:397–410.

147. Janda JM, Abbott SL. Evolving concepts regarding the genus *Aeromonas*: an expanding panorama of species, disease presentations, and unanswered questions. Clin Infect Dis 1998;27:332–344.

148. Janda JM, Abbott SL, Khashe S, Kellogg GH, Shimada T. Further studies on biochemical characteristics and serologic properties of the genus *Aeromonas*. J Clin Microbiol 1996;34:1930–1933.

149. Janda JM, Brenden R, DeBenedetti JA et al. *Vibrio alginolyticus* bacteremia in an immunocompromised patient. Diagn Microbiol Infect Dis 1986;5:337–340.

150. Janda JM, Dixon A, Raucher B et al. Value of blood agar for primary plating and clinical implications of simultaneous isolation of *Aeromonas hydrophila* and *Aeromonas caviae* from a patient with gastroenteritis. J Clin Microbiol 1984; 20:1221–1222.

151. Janda JM, Duffey PS. Mesophilic aeromonads in human disease: Current taxonomy, laboratory identification, and infectious disease spectrum. Rev Infect Dis 1988;5:980–997.

152. Janda JM, Powers C, Bryant RG et al. Current perspectives on the epidemiology and pathogenesis of clinically significant *Vibrio* spp. Clin Microbiol Rev 1988; 1:245–267.

153. Jean-Jacques W, Rajashekaraiah KR, Farmer JJ III et al. *Vibrio metschnikovii* bacteremia in a patient with cholecystitis. J Clin Microbiol 1981;14:711–712.

154. Jicong W, Guolong L, Zhenhua Z, Yanglong M, Qiang C, Jingchuan W, Sulong Y. $^{15}NH_4$1 excretion test: a new method for detection of *Helicobacter pylori* infection. J Clin Microbiol 1992;30:181–184.

155. Johnson CC, Reinhardt JF, Edelstein MAC, Mulligan ME, George WL, Finegold SM. *Bacteroides gracilis*, an important anaerobic bacterial pathogen. J Clin Microbiol 1985;22:799–802.

156. Jones BL, Wilcox MH. *Aeromonas* infections and their treatment. J Antimicrob Chemother 1995;35:453–461.

157. Jones FS, Orcutt M, Little RB. Vibrios (*Vibrio jejuni* n. sp.) associated with intestinal disorders of cows and calves. J Exp Med 1931;53:853–864.

158. Joseph SW, Carnahan AM. Update on the genus *Aeromonas*. ASM News 2000; 66:218–223.

159. Joseph SW, Carnahan AM, Brayton PR et al. *Aeromonas jandaei* and *Aeromonas veronii* dual infection of a human wound following aquatic exposure. J Clin Microbiol 1991;29:565–569.

160. Joseph SW, Colwell RR, Kaper JB. *Vibrio parahaemolyticus* and related halophilic vibrios. Crit Rev Microbiol 1982;10:77–124.

161. Kaper JB, Morris Jr JG, Levine MM. Cholera. Clin Microbiol Rev 1995;8: 48–86.

162. Kaper JB, Nataro JP, Roberts NC et al. Molecular epidemiology of non-01 *Vibrio cholerae* and *Vibrio mimicus* in the U.S. gulf coast region. J Clin Microbiol 1986; 23:652–654.

163. Kapperud G, Espeland G, Wahl E, Walde A, Herikstad H, Gustavsen S, Tveit I, Natas O, Bevanger L, Digranes A. Factors associated with increased and decreased risk of *Campylobacter* infection: A prospective case-control study in Norway. Am J Epidemiol 2003;158:234–242.

164. Karmali MA, Fleming PC. *Campylobacter* enteritis. Can Med Assoc J 1979; 120:1525–1532.

165. Karmali MA, Simor AE, Roscoe M et al. Evaluation of a blood-free, charcoal-based, selective medium for the isolation of *Campylobacter* organisms from feces. J Clin Microbiol 1986;23:456–459.

166. Kasper G, Dickgiesser N. Isolation from gastric epithelium of *Campylobacter*-like bacteria that are distinct from ''*Campylobacter pyloridis*.'' Lancet 1985;1:111–112.

167. Kelly MT. Cholera: A worldwide perspective. Pediatr Infect Dis 1986;5:S101–S105.

168. Kelly MT, Hickman-Brenner FW, Farmer JJ III. *Vibrio*. In Balows A (ed): Manual of Clinical Microbiology, 5th ed, chap 37, pp 384–395. Washington, DC, American Society for Microbiology, 1991.

169. Kelly MT, Peterson JW, Sarles HE Jr et al. Cholera on the Texas gulf coast. JAMA 1982;247:1598–1599.

170. Kelly MT, Stroh EMD. Urease-positive, Kanagawa-negative *Vibrio parahaemolyticus* from patients and the environment in the Pacific northwest. J Clin Microbiol 1989;27:2820–2822.

171. Kiehlbauch JA, Brenner DJ, Cameron DN, Steigerwalt AG, Makowski JM, Baker CN, Patton CM, Wachsmuth IK. Genotypic and phenotypic characterization of *Helicobacter cinaedi* and *Helicobacter fennelliae* strains isolated from humans and animals. J Clin Microbiol 1995;33:2940–2947.

172. Kiehlbauch JA, Brenner DJ, Nicholson MA et al. *Campylobacter butzleri* sp. nov. isolated from humans and animals with diarrheal illness. J Clin Microbiol 1991;29:376–385.

173. Kiehlbauch JA, Tauxe RV, Baker CN, Wachsmuth IK. *Helicobacter cinaedi*-associated bacteremia and cellulitis in immunocompromised patients. Ann Inter Med 1994;121:90–93.

174. King EO. Human infections with *Vibrio fetus* and a closely related vibrio. J Infect Dis 1957;101:119–128.

175. Kirkbride CA, Gates CE, Collins JE. Abortion in sheep caused by a non-classified, anaerobic, flagellated bacterium. Am J Vet Res 1986;47:259–262.

176. Kirkbride CA, Gates CE, Collins JE et al. Ovine abortion associated with an anaerobic bacterium. J Am Vet Med Assoc 1985;186:789–791.

177. Klipstein FA, Engert RF, Short HB. Enzyme-linked immunosorbent assays for virulence properties of *Campylobacter jejuni* clinical isolates. J Clin Microbiol 1986;23:1039–1043.

178. Ko W-C, Chuang Y-C. *Aeromonas* bacteremia: review of 59 episodes. Clin Infect Dis 1995;20:1298–1304.

179. Kodaka H, Lombard GL, Dowell VR Jr. Gas-liquid chromatography technique for detection of hippurate hydrolysis and conversion of fumarate to succinate by microorganisms. J Clin Microbiol 1982;16:962–964.

180. Krienitz W. Ueber das Auftreten von Spirochaeten verschiedener Form im Mageninhalt bei Carcinoma Ventriculi. Dtsch Med Wochenschr 1906;22:872.

181. Kulkarni SP, Lever S, Logan JMJ, Lawson AJ, Stanley J, Shafi MS. Detection of campylobacter species: a comparison of culture and polymerase chain reaction based methods. J Microbiol Immunol Infect 2000;33:241–247.

182. Kuroki S, Haruta T, Yoshioka M, Kobayashi Y, Nukina M, Nakanishi H. Guillain-Barre syndrome associated with *Campylobacter* infection. Pediatr Infect Dis J 1991;10:149–151.

183. Lacey SW. Cholera: calamitous past, ominous future. Clin Infect Dis 1995;20:1409–1419.

184. Lam S, Yeo M. Urease-positive *Vibrio parahaemolyticus* strain. J Clin Microbiol 1980;12:57–59.

185. La Scolea LJ. *Campylobacter fetus* subsp. *fetus* meningitis in a neonate. Clin Microbiol Newsl 1985;7:125–126.

186. Lastovica A, Le Roux A, Warren R, Klump H. Clinical isolates of *Campylobacter mucosalis* [letter]. J Clin Microbiol 1993;31:2835–2836.

187. Lastovica AJ, Le Roux E, Penner JL. ''*Campylobacter upsaliensis*'' isolated from blood cultures of pediatric patients. J Clin Microbiol 1989;27:657–659.

188. Lastovica AJ, Le Roux E, Warren R, Klump H. Additional data on clinical isolates on *Campylobacter mucosalis* [letter]. J Clin Microbiol 1994;32:2338–2339.

189. Lau SM, Peng MY, Chang FY. Outcomes of *Aeromonas* bacteremia in patients with different types of underlying disease. J Microbiol Infect 2000;33:241–247.

190. Lauwers S, Van Etterijck R, Breynaert J et al. Isolation of *C. upsaliensis* and *C. concisus* from human faeces. Presented before the annual meeting of the American Society for Microbiology, 1991, abstract C-266, p 386.

191. Lecuit M, Abachin E, Martin A, Poyart C, Pochart P, Suarez F, Bengoufa D, Feuillard J, Lavergne A, Gordon JI, Berche P, Guillevin L, Lortholary O. Immunoproliferative small intestinal disease associated with *Campylobacter jejuni*. N Engl J Med 2004;350:239–248.

192. Lee A. Human gastric spirilla other than *C. pylori*. In: Blaser MJ, ed. *Campylobacter pylori* in gastritis and peptic ulcer disease. New York, Igaku-Shoin Medical Publishers, 1989; pp. 225–240.

193. Lee A, Phillips MW, O'Rourke JL, Paster BJ, Dewhirst FE, Fraser GJ, Fox JG, Sly LI, Romaniuk PJ, Trust TJ, Kouprach S. *Helicobacter muridarum* sp, nov., a microaerophilic helical bacterium with a novel ultrastructure isolated from the intestinal mucosa of rodents. Int J Syst Bacteriol 1992;42:27–36.

194. Lee K, Baron EJ, Summanen P, Finegold SM. Selective medium for isolation of *Bacteroides gracilis*. J Clin Microbiol 1990;28:1747–1750.

195. Lerner J, Brumberger V, Preac-Mursic V. Severe diarrhea associated with *Arcobacter butzleri*. Eur J Clin Microbiol Infect Dis 1994;13:660–662.

196. Lesmana M, Albert MJ, Subekti D, Richie E, Tjaniadi P, Walz SE, Lebron CI. Simple differentiation of *Vibrio cholerae* 0139 from *V. cholerae* 01 and non-01, non-0139 by modified CAMP test. J Clin Microbiol 1996;34:1038–1040.

197. Lessner AM, Webb RM, Rabin B. *Vibrio alginolyticus* conjunctivitis. Arch Ophthalmol 1985;103:229–230.

198. Lineaweaver WC, Hill MK, Buncke GM, Follansbee S, Buncke HJ, Wong RKM, Manders EK, Grotting JC, Anthony J, Mathes SJ. *Aeromonas hydrophila* infections following use of medical leeches in replantation and flap surgery. Ann Plast Surg 1992;29:238–244.

199. Linton D, Lawson AJ, Owen RJ, Stanley J. PCR detection, identification to species level, and fingerprinting of *Campylobacter jejuni* and *Campylobacter coli* direct from diarrheic samples. J Clin Microbiol 1997;35:2568–2572.

200. Lowry PW, McFarland LM, Threefoot HK. *Vibrio hollisae* septicemia after consumption of catfish [letter]. J Infect Dis 1986;154:730–731.

201. Luechtefeld NW, Reller LB, Blaser MJ et al. Comparison of atmospheres of incubation for primary isolation of *Campylobacter fetus* subsp. *jejuni* from animal specimens: 5% oxygen versus candle jar. J Clin Microbiol 1982;15:53–57.

202. Luechtefeld NW, Wang W-LL. Hippurate hydrolysis by and triphenyltetrazolium tolerance of *Campylobacter fetus*. J Clin Microbiol 1982;15:137–140.

203. MacDonell MT, Colwell RR. Phylogeny of the *Vibrionaceae*, and recommendation for two new genera, *Listonella* and *Shewanella*. Syst Appl Microbiol 1985;6:171–182.

204. Maher M, Finnegan C, Collins E, Ward B, Carroll C, Cormican M. Evaluation of culture methods and a DNA probe-based PCR assay for detection of *Campylobacter* species in clinical specimens. J Clin Microbiol 2003;41:2980–2986.

205. Makristathis A, Pasching E, Schutze K, Wimmer M, Rotter ML, Hirschl AM. Detection of *Helicobacter pylori* in stool specimens by PCR and antigen enzyme immunoassay. J Clin Microbiol 1998;36:2772–2774.

206. Mandal BK. Epidemic cholera due to a novel strain of *V. cholerae* non 01—the beginning of a new pandemic? J Infect 1993;27:115–117.

207. Marshall BJ. *Campylobacter pyloridis* and gastritis. J Infect Dis 1986;153:650–657.

208. Martinez-Murcia AJ, Esteve C, Garay E, Collins MD. *Aeromonas allosaccharophila* sp, a new mesophilic member of the genus *Aeromonas*. FEMS Microbiol lett 1992;91:199–206.

209. Martinot M, Jaulhac B, Moog R, De Martino S, Kehrli P, Monteil H, Piemont Y. *Campylobacter lari* bacteremia. Clin Microbiol Infect 2001;4:96–97.

210. Matsiota-Bernard P, Nauciel C. *Vibrio alginolyticus* wound infection after exposure to sea water in an air crash. Eur J Clin Microbiol Infect Dis 1993;12:474–475.

211. McNeeley D, Ivy P, Craft JC et al. *Plesiomonas*: Biology of the organism and diseases in children. Pediatr Infect Dis 1984;3:176–181.

212. McNulty CAM, Dent JC, Curry A, Uff, JS, Ford GA, Gear MWL, Wilkinson SP. New spiral bacterium in gastric mucosa. J Clin Pathol 1989;42:585–591.

213. McNulty CAM, Dent JC, Uff JS et al. Detection of *Campylobacter pylori* by the biopsy urease test: An assessment in 1445 patients. Gut 1989;30:1058–1062.

214. McTighe AH. Pathogenic *Vibrio* species: Isolation and identification. Lab Management August 1982, pp. 43–46.

215. Melito PL, Munro C, Chipman PR, Woodward DL, Booth TF, Rodgers FG. *Helicobacter winghamensis* sp. nov., a novel *Helicobacter* sp. isolated from patients with gastroenteritis. J Clin Microbiol 2001;39:2412–2417.

216. Mercer NSG, Beere DM, Bornemisza AJ, Thomas P. Medical leeches as sources of wound infection. Br Med J 1987;294:937.

217. Merino FJ, Agulla A, Villasante PA et al. Comparative efficacy of seven selective media for isolating *Campylobacter jejuni*. J Clin Microbiol 1986;24:451–452.

218. Middlebrook JL, Dorland RB. Bacterial toxins: Cellular mechanisms of action. Microbiol Rev 1984;48:199–221.

219. Mills CK, Gherna RL. Hydrolysis of indoxyl acetate by *Campylobacter* species. J Clin Microbiol 1987;25:1560–1561.

220. Minet J, Grosbois B, Megraud F. *Campylobacter hyointestinalis*: An opportunistic enteropathogen? J Clin Microbiol 1988;26:2659–2660.

221. Monteiro L, de Mascarel A, Sarrasqueta AM, Bergey B, Barberis C, Talby P, Roux D, Shouler L, Goldfain D, Lamouliatte H, Megraud F. Diagnosis of *Helicobacter pylori* infection: noninvasive methods compared to invasive methods and evaluation of two new tests. Am J Gastroenterol 2001;96:353–358.

222. Morris A, Ali MR, Thomsen L, Hollis B. Tightly spiral shaped bacteria in the human stomach: another cause of active chronic gastritis? Gut 1990;31:139–143.

223. Morris GK, El Sherbeeny MR, Patton CM et al. Comparison of four hippurate hydrolysis methods for identification of thermophilic *Campylobacter* sp. J Clin Microbiol 1985;22:714–718.

224. Morris Jr JG. Vibrio cholerae 0139 Bengal: emergence of a new epidemic strain of cholera. Infect Agents Dis 1995;4:41–46.

225. Morris Jr JG. Cholera and other types of vibriosis: a story of human pandemics and oysters on the half shell. Clin Infect Dis 2003;37:272–280.

226. Morris JG Jr, Wilson R, Hollis DG et al. Illness caused by *Vibrio damsela* and *Vibrio hollisae*. Lancet 1982;i:1294–1296.

227. Munoz P, Fernandez-Baca V, Pelaez T, Sanchez R, Rodriguez-Creixems M, Bouza E. *Aeromonas* peritonitits. Clin Infect Dis 1994;18:32–37.

228. Nachamkin I. Campylobacter infections. Current Opinion in Infectious Diseases 1993;6:72–76.

229. Nachamkin I, Barbagallo S. Culture confirmation of *Campylobacter* spp. by latex agglutination. J Clin Microbiol 1990;28:817–818.

230. Nachamkin I, Stowell C, Skalina D et al. *Campylobacter laridis* causing bacteremia in an immunocompromised host. Ann Intern Med 1984;101:55–57.

231. Nair GB, Shimada T, Kurazono H et al. Characterization of phenotypic, serological, and toxigenic traits of *Vibrio cholerae* 0139 Bengal. J Clin Microbiol 1994;32:2775–2779.

232. Namdari H, Bottone EJ. Suicide phenomenon in mesophilic aeromonads as a basis for species identification. J Clin Microbiol 1989;27:788–789.

233. Namdari H, Bottone EJ. Microbiological and clinical evidence supporting the role of *Aeromonas caviae* as a pediatric enteric pathogen. J Clin Microbiol 1990;28:837–840.

234. Namdari H, Bottone EJ. Cytotoxin and enterotoxin production as factors delineating enteropathogenicity of *Aeromonas caviae*. J Clin Microbiol 1990;28:1796–1798.

235. Nato F, Boutonnier A, Rajerison M, Grosjean P, Dartevelle S, Guenole A, Bhuiyan NA, Sack DA, Nair GB, Fournier JM, Chanteau S. One-step immunochromatographic dipstick tests for rapid detection of *Vibrio cholerae* O1 and O139 in stool samples. Clin Diagn Lab Immunol 2003;10:476–478.

236. Ng VL, Hadley WK, Fennell CL et al. Successive bacteremias with ''*Campylobacter cinaedi*'' and ''*Campylobacter fennelliae*'' in a bisexual male. J Clin Microbiol 1987;25:2008–2009.

237. Nolan CM, Ballard J, Kaysner CA et al. *Vibrio parahaemolyticus* gastroenteritis: An outbreak associated with raw oysters in the Pacific northwest. Diagn Microbiol Infect Dis 1984;2:119–128.

238. Notermans S, Havelaar A, Jansen W et al. Production of ''Asao toxin'' by *Aeromonas* strains isolated from feces and drinking water. J Clin Microbiol 1986;23:1140–1142.

239. Oberhofer TR, Podgore JK. Urea-hydrolyzing *Vibrio parahaemolyticus* associated with acute gastroenteritis. J Clin Microbiol 1982;16:581–583.

240. O'Brien M, Colwell RR. Modified taurocholate-tellurite-gelatin agar for improved differentiation of *Vibrio* species. J Clin Microbiol 1985;22:1011–1013.

241. O'Hara CM, Sowers EG, Bopp CA, Duda SB, Strockbine NA. Accuracy of six

commercially available systems for identification of members of the family *Vibrionaceae*. J Clin Microbiol 2003;41:5654–5659.

242. On SLW. Confirmation of human *Campylobacter concisus* isolates misidentified as *Campylobacter mucosalis* and suggestions for improved differentiation between the two species. J Clin Microbiol 1994;32:2305–2306.

243. On SLW. Identification methods for campylobacters, helicobacters, and related organisms. Clin Microbiol Rev 1996;9: 405–422.

244. On SLW. Taxonomy of *Campylobacter, Arcobacter, Helicobacter* and related bacteria: current status, future prospects and immediate concerns. Symp Ser Soc Appl Microbiol 2001;90:1S–15S.

245. On SLW, Bloch B, Holmes B, Hoste B, Vandamme P. *Campylobacter hyointestinalis* subsp. *lawsonii* subsp. nov., isolated from the porcine stomach, and an emended description of *Campylobacter hyointestinalis*. Int J Syst Bacteriol 1995; 45:767–774.

246. Orlicek SL, Welch DF, Kuhls T. Septicemia and meningitis caused by *Helicobacter cinaedi* in a neonate. J Clin Microbiol 1993;31:569–571.

247. Ouderkirk JP, Bekhor D, Turett GS, Murali R. *Aeromonas* meningitis complicating medicinal leech therapy.

248. Overman TL, Kessler JF, Seabolt JP. Comparison of API 20E, API Rapid E, and API Rapid NFT for identification of members of the family *Vibrionaceae*. J Clin Microbiol 1985;22:778–781.

249. Pan-American Health Organization. Cholera in the Americas. Epidemiol Bull 1995;16:11–13.

250. Parsonnet J, Isaacson PG. Bacterial infection and MALT lymphoma. N Engl J Med 2004;350:213–215.

251. Pascual A, Martinez-Martinez L, Garcia-Gestoso ML, Romero J. Urinary tract infection caused by quinolone-resistant *Campylobacter coli*. Eur J Clin Microbiol Infect Dis 1994;13:690–691.

252. Paster BJ, Dewhirst FE. Phylogeny of campylobacters, wolinellas, *Bacteroides gracilis*, and *Bacteroides ureolyticus* by 16S ribosomal ribonucleic acid sequencing. Int J Syst Bacteriol 1988;38:56–62.

253. Paster BJ, Lee A, Fox JG et al. Phylogeny of *Helicobacter felis* sp. nov., *Helicobacter mustelae*, and related bacteria. Int J Syst Bacteriol 1991;41:31–38.

254. Pasternak J, Bolivar R, Hopfer RL et al. Bacteremia caused by *Campylobacter*-like organism in two male homosexuals. Ann Intern Med 1984;101:339–341.

255. Pavia AT, Bryan JA, Maher KL et al. *Vibrio carchariae* infection after a shark bite. Ann Intern Med 1989;111:85–86.

256. Penner JL. The genus *Campylobacter:* A decade of progress. Clin Microbiol Rev 1988;1:157–172.

257. Peterson WL. *Helicobacter pylori* and peptic ulcer disease. N Engl J Med 1991; 324:1043–1048.

258. Pezzlo M, Valter PJ, Burns MJ. Wound infection associated with *Vibrio alginolyticus*. Am J Clin Pathol 1979;71:476–478.

259. Pitarangsi E, Echeverria P, Whitmire R et al. Enteropathogenicity of *Aeromonas hydrophila* and *Plesiomonas shigelloides:* Prevalence among individuals with and without diarrhea in Thailand. Infect Immun 1982;35:666–673.

260. Pitrak DL, Gindorf JD. Bacteremic cellulitis caused by non-serogroup 01 *Vibrio cholerae* acquired in a freshwater inland lake. J Clin Microbiol 1989;27: 2874–2876.

261. Popovic-Uroic T, Patton CM, Nicholson MA et al. Evaluation of the indoxyl acetate hydrolysis test for rapid differentiation of *Campylobacter, Helicobacter,* and *Wolinella* species. J Clin Microbiol 1990;28:2335–2339.

262. Popovic-Uroic T, Patton CM, Wachsmuth IK, Roeder P. Evaluation of an oligonucleotide probe for identification of Campylobacter species. Lab Med 1991; 22:533–539.

263. Quinn TC, Goodell SE, Fennell C et al. Infections with *Campylobacter jejuni* and *Campylobacter*-like organisms in homosexual men. Ann Intern Med 1984; 101:187–192.

264. Rank EL, Smith IB, Langer M. Bacteremia caused by *Vibrio hollisae*. J Clin Microbiol 1988;26:375–376.

265. Reina J, Fernandez-Baca V, Lopez A. Acute gastroenteritis caused by *Vibrio alginolyticus* in an immunocompetent patient. Clin Infect Dis 1995;21: 1044–1045.

266. Reinhardt JF, George WL. *Plesiomonas shigelloides*-associated diarrhea. JAMA 1985;253:3294–3295.

267. Rolston KVI, Hopfer RL. Diarrhea due to *Plesiomonas shigelloides* in cancer patients. J Clin Microbiol 1984;20:597–598.

268. Romero S, Archer JR, Hamacher ME et al. Case report of an unclassified microaerophilic bacterium associated with gastroenteritis. J Clin Microbiol 1988;26: 142–143.

269. Roop RM II, Smibert RM, Johnson JL et al. DNA homology studies of the catalase-negative campylobacters and ''*Campylobacter fecalis*,'' an emended description of *Campylobacter sputorum,* and proposal of the neotype strain of *Campylobacter sputorum.* Can J Microbiol 1985;31:823–831.

270. Ropper AH. *Campylobacter* diarrhea and Guillain-Barre syndrome. Arch Neurol 1988;45:655–656.

271. Ruimy R, Breittmayer V, Elbaze P, Lafay B, Boussemart O, Gauthier M, Christen R. Phylogenetic analysis and assessment of the genera *Vibrio, Photobacter-*

ium, Aeromonas, and *Plesiomonas* deduced from small-subunit rRNA sequences. J Syst Bacteriol 1994;44:416–426.

272. Sack DA, Sack RB, Nair GB, Siddique AK. Cholera. Lancet 2004;363:223–233.

273. Sacks SL, Labriola AM, Gill VJ, Gordin FM. Use of ciprofloxacin for successful eradication of bacteremia due to *Campylobacter cinaedi* in a human immunodeficiency virus-infected person. Rev Infect Dis 1991;13:1066–1068.

274. Safrin S, Morris JG, Adams M et al. Non-01 *Vibrio cholerae* bacteremia: Case report and review. Rev Infect Dis 1988;10:1012–1017.

275. Sandstedt K, Ursing J. Description of *Campylobacter upsaliensis* sp. nov. previously known as the CNW group. Syst Appl Microbiol 1991;14:39–45.

276. Sandstedt K, Ursing J, Walder M. Thermotolerant *Campylobacter* with no or weak catalase activity isolated from dogs. Curr Microbiol 1983;8:209–213.

277. Sanyal SC, Saraswathi B, Sharma P. Enteropathogenicity of *Plesiomonas shigelloides*. J Med Microbiol 1980;13:401–409.

278. Sartor C, Limouzin-Perotti F, Legre R, Casanova D, Bongrand M, Sambuc R, and Drancourt M. Nosocomial infections with *Aeromonas hydrophila* from leeches. Clin Infect Dis 2002;35:e1–e5.

279. Schmidt U, Chmel H, Cobbs C. *Vibrio alginolyticus* infections in humans. J Clin Microbiol 1979;10:666–668.

280. Schubert RHW, Hegazi M. *Aeromonas eucrenophila* species nova *Aeromonas caviae,* a later and illegitimate synonym of *Aeromonas punctata*. Zentralbl Bakteriol Mikrobiol Hyg [A] 1988;268:34–39.

281. Shandera WX, Johnston JM, Davis BR et al. Disease from infection with *Vibrio mimicus,* a newly recognized *Vibrio* species. Clinical characteristics and epidemiology. Ann Intern Med 1983;99:169–171.

282. Skirrow MB, Benjamin J: ''1001'' Campylobacters. Cultural characteristics of intestinal campylobacters from man and animals. J Hyg (Cambridge) 1980;85: 427–442.

283. Smibert RM. Genus *Campylobacter* Sebald and Veron 1963, 907[AL]. In Krieg NR, Holt HG (eds): Bergey's Manual of Systematic Bacteriology, vol 1, pp 111–118, Baltimore, Williams & Wilkins, 1984.

284. Smith SK, Sutton DC, Fuerst JA, Reichelt JL. Evaluation of the genus *Listonella* and reassignment of *Listonella damsela* (Love et al.) MacDonell and Colwell to the genus *Photobacterium* as *Photobacterium damsela*. Int J Syst Bacteriol 1994;41:529–534.

285. Smoak BL, Kelley PW, Taylor DN. Seroprevalence of *Helicobacter pylori* infections in a cohort of US Army recruits. Am J Epidemiol 1994;139:513–519.

286. Solnick JV. Clinical significance of *Helicobacter* species other than *Helicobacter pylori*. Clin Infect Dis 2003;36:349–354.

287. Solnick JV, O'Rourke J, Lee A, Paster BJ, Dewhirst FE, Tompkins LS. An uncultured gastric spiral organism is a newly identified *Helicobacter* in humans. J Infect Dis 1993;168:379–385.

288. Solnick JV, Schauer DB. Emergence of diverse *Helicobacter* species in the pathogenesis of gastric and enterohepatic diseases. Clin Microbiol Rev 2001; 14:59–97.

289. Sorlin P, Vandamme P, Nortier J, Hoste B, Rossi C, Pavlof S, Struelens MJ. Recurrent ''Flexispira rappini'' bacteremia in an adult patient undergoing hemodialysis: case report. J Clin Microbiol 1999;37:1319–1323.

290. Sovilla J-Y, Regli F, Francioli PB. Guillain-Barre syndrome following *Campylobacter jejuni* enteritis: report of three cases and review of the literature. Arch Intern Med 1988;148:739–741.

291. Spiegel CA, Telford G. Isolation of *Wolinella recta* and *Actinomyces viscosus* from an actinomycotic chest wall mass. J Clin Microbiol 1984;20:1187–1189.

292. Stanley J, Burnens AP, Linton D, On SLW, Costas M, Owen RJ. *Campylobacter helveticus* sp. nov., a new thermophilic species from domestic animals: characterization and cloning of a species-specific DNA probe. J Gen Microbiol 1992; 138:2293–2303.

293. Stanley J, Linton D, Burnens AP, Dewhirst FE, On SLW, Porter A, Owen RJ, Costas M. *Helicobacter pullorum* sp. nov.—genotype and phenotype of a new species isolated from poultry and from human patients with gastroenteritis. Microbiol 1994;140:3441–3449.

294. Stanley J, Linton D, Burnens AP, Dewhirst FE, Owen RJ, Porter A, On SLW, Costas M. *Helicobacter canis* sp. nov., a new species from dogs: an integrated study of phenotype and genotype. J Gen Microbiol 1993;139:2495–2504.

295. Steele TW, McDermott SN. Technical note: The use of membrane filters applied directly to the surface of agar plates for the isolation of *Campylobacter jejuni* from feces. Pathology 1984;16:263–265.

296. Steele TW, Owen RJ. *Campylobacter jejuni* subsp. *doylei* subsp. nov., a subspecies of nitrate-negative campylobacters isolated from human clinical specimens. Int J Syst Bacteriol 1988;38:316–318.

297. Steele TW, Sangster N, Lanser JA. DNA relatedness and biochemical features of *Campylobacter* spp. isolated in central and south Australia. J Clin Microbiol 1985;22:71–74.

298. Steinkraus GE, Wright BD. Septic abortion with intact fetal membranes caused by *Campylobacter fetus* subsp. *fetus*. J Clin Microbiol 1994;32:1608–1609.

299. Stills Jr HF, Hook RR, Kinden DA. Isolation of *Campylobacter*-like organism from healthy Syrian hamsters (Mesocricetus auratus). J Clin Microbiol 1989; 27:2497–2501.

300. Swerdlow DL, Ries AA. *Vibrio cholerae* non-01—the eighth pandemic? Lancet 1993;342:382–383.
301. Tacket CO, Brenner F, Blake PA. Clinical features and an epidemiological study of *Vibrio vulnificus* infections. J Infect Dis 1984;149:558–561.
302. Tacket CO, Hickman F, Pierce GV et al. Diarrhea associated with *Vibrio fluvialis* in the United States. J. Clin Microbiol 1982;16:991–992.
303. Tam CC, O'Brien SJ, Adak GK, Meakins SM, Frost JA. *Campylobacter coli*—an important foodborne pathogen. J Infect 2003;47:28–32.
304. Tanner ACR, Badger S, Lai C-H et al. *Wolinella* gen. nov., *Wolinella succinogenes* (*Vibrio succinogenes* Wolin et al.) comb. nov., and description of *Bacteroides gracilis* sp. nov., *Wolinella recta* sp. nov., *Campylobacter concisus* sp. nov., and *Eikenella corrodens* from humans with periodontal disease. Int J Syst Bacteriol 1981;31:432–445.
305. Tanner ACR, Listgarten MA, Ebersole JL. *Wolinella curva* sp. nov.: "*Vibrio succinogenes*" of human origin. Int J Syst Bacteriol 1984;34:275–282.
306. Tauxe RV, Patton CM, Edmonds P et al. Illness associated with *Campylobacter laridis*, a newly recognized *Campylobacter* species. J Clin Microbiol 1985;21:222–225.
307. Taylor DN, Kiehlbauch JA, Tee W, Pitarangsi C, Echeverria P. Isolation of group 2 aerotolerant *Campylobacter* species from Thai children with diarrhea. J Infect Dis 1991;163:1062–1067.
308. Tee W, Baird R, Dyall-Smith M et al. *Campylobacter cryaerophila* isolated from a human. J Clin Microbiol 1988;26:2469–2473.
309. Tee W, Leder K, Karroum E, Dyall-Smith M. "*Flexispira rappini*" bacteremia in a child with pneumonia. J Clin Microbiol 1998;36:1679–1682.
310. Tenover FC, Carlson L, Barbagallo S, Nachamkin I. DNA probe culture confirmation assay for identification of thermophilic Campylobacter species. J Clin Microbiol 1990;28:1284–1287.
311. Thompson LM III, Smibert RM, Johnson JL et al. Phylogenetic study of the genus *Campylobacter*. Int J Syst Bacteriol 1988;38:190–200.
312. Tolcin R, LaSalvia MM, Kirkley BA, Vetter EA, Cockerill F, Procop GW. Evaluation of the Alexon-Trend ProSpecT Campylobacter Microplate Assay. J Clin Microbiol 2000;38:3853–3855.
313. Totten PA, Fennell CL, Tenover FC et al. *Campylobacter cinaedi* (sp. nov.) and *Campylobacter fennelliae* (sp. nov): Two new *Campylobacter* species associated with enteric disease in homosexual men. J Infect Dis 1985;151:131–139.
314. Travis LB, Washington JA II. The clinical significance of stool isolates of *Aeromonas*. Am J Clin Pathol 1986;85:330–336.
315. Tuyet DT, Thiem VD, von Seidlein L, Chowdhury A, Park E, Canh DG, Chien BT, Tung TV, Naficy A, Rao MR, Ali M, Lee H, Sy TH, Nichibuchi M, Clemens J, Trach DD. Clinical, epidemiological, and socioeconomic analysis of an outbreak of *Vibrio parahaemolyticus* in Khanh Hoa Province, Vietnam. J Infect Dis 2002;186:1615–1620.
316. Vandamme P, Daneshvar MI, Dewhirst FE, Paster BJ, Kersters K, Groossens H, Moss CW. Chemotaxonomic analyses of *Bacteroides gracilis* and *Bacteroides ureolyticus* and reclassification of *B. gracilis* as *Campylobacter gracilis* comb. nov. Int J Syst Bacteriol 1995;45:145–152.

317. Vandamme P, De Ley J. Proposal for a new family, *Campylobacteraceae*. Int J Syst Bacteriol 1991;41:451–455.
318. Vandamme P, Falsen E, Pot B et al. Identification of EF group 22 campylobacters from gastroenteritis cases as *Campylobacter concisus*. J Clin Microbiol 1989;27:1775–1781.
319. Vandamme P, Falsen E, Pot B et al. Identification of *Campylobacter cinaedi* isolated from blood and feces of children and adult females. J Clin Microbiol 1990;28:1016–1020.
320. Vandamme P, Falsen E, Rossau R et al. Revision of *Campylobacter, Helicobacter,* and *Wolinella* taxonomy: Emendation of generic descriptions and proposal of *Arcobacter* gen. nov. Int J Syst Bacteriol 1991;41:88–103.
321. Vandamme P, Pugina P, Benzi G, Van Etterijck R, Vlaes L, Kersters K, Butzler J-P, Lior H, Lauwers S. Outbreak of recurrent abdominal cramps associated with *Arcobacter butzleri* in an Italian school. J Clin Microbiol 1992;30:2335–2337.
322. Vandamme P, Vancanneyt M, Pot B, Mels L, Butzler J-P, Goossens H. Polyphasic taxonomic study of the emended genus *Arcobacter* with *Arcobacter butzleri* comb. nov. and *Arcobacter skirrowii* sp. nov., an aerotolerant bacterium isolated from veterinary specimens. Int J Syst Bacteriol 1992;42:344–356.
323. Vanloon FPL, Rahim Z, Chowdhury KA et al. Case report of *Plesiomonas shigelloides*-associated persistent dysentery and pseudomembranous colitis. J Clin Microbiol 1989;27:1913–1915.
324. Vogt RL, Little AA, Patton CM, et al. Serotyping and serology studies of campylobacteriosis associated with consumption of raw milk. J Clin Microbiol 1984;20:998–1000.
325. Von Graevenitz A, Bucher C. Evaluation of differential and selective media for isolation of *Aeromonas* and *Plesiomonas* spp. from human feces. J Clin Microbiol 1983;17:16–21.
326. Walmsley SL, Karmali MA. Direct isolation of atypical thermophilic *Campylobacter* species from human feces on selective agar medium. J Clin Microbiol 1989;27:668–670.
327. Wang W-LL, Luechtefeld NW. Effect of incubation atmosphere and temperature on isolation of *Campylobacter jejuni* from human stools. Can J Microbiol 1983;29:468–470.
328. Warren JR, Marshall BJ. Unidentified curved bacilli on gastric epithelium in active gastritis. Lancet 1983;1:1273–1275.
329. Watson IM, Robinson JO, Burke V, et al. Invasiveness of *Aeromonas* spp. in relation to biotype, virulence factors, and clinical features. J Clin Microbiol 1985;22:48–51.
330. Weissman JB, DeWitt WE, Thompson J, et al. A case of cholera in Texas, 1973. Am J Epidemiol 1974;100:487–498..
331. Wexler HM, Reeves D, Summanen PH, Molitoris E, McTeague M, Duncan J, Wilson KH, Finegold SM. *Sutterella wadsworthensis* gen. nov., sp. nov., bile-resistant microaerophilic *Campylobacter gracilis*-like clinical isolates. Int J Syst Bacteriol 1996;46:252–258.
332. Yan JJ, Ko WC, Huang AH, Chen HM, Jin YT, Wu JJ. *Arcobacter butzleri* bacteremia in a patient with liver cirrhosis. J Formos Med Assoc 2000;99:166–169.
333. Yao JDC, Ng HMC, Campbell I. Prosthetic hip joint infection due to *Campylobacter fetus*. J Clin Microbiol 1993;31:3323–3324.

Miscellaneous Fastidious Gram-Negative Bacilli

Haemophilus Species

Taxonomy of *Haemophilus* and Related Organisms
Haemophilus influenzae
Haemophilus influenzae Type B Vaccines
Infections Caused by *Haemophilus* Species

Meningitis
Epiglottitis
Otitis Media
Sinusitis
Bronchitis and Chronic Obstructive Pulmonary Disease
Pneumonia
Bacteremia and Infectious Complications of Bacteremia
Endocarditis
Urogenital, Maternal, and Perinatal Infections
Ocular Infections
Brazilian Purpuric Fever
Miscellaneous *Haemophilus influenzae* Infections

Haemophilus parainfluenzae
Haemophilus aphrophilus and *Haemophilus paraphrophilus*
Other *Haemophilus* Species
Haemophilus ducreyi
Laboratory Diagnosis of *Haemophilus* Infections

Direct Examination of Clinical Specimens
Culture of *Haemophilus* Species

Identification of *Haemophilus* Species
Laboratory Diagnosis of *Haemophilus ducreyi* Infection
Antimicrobial Susceptibility of *Haemophilus* Species

Actinobacillus Species

Actinobacillus actinomycetemcomitans

Clinical Significance
Cultural Characteristics and Identification
Antimicrobial Susceptibility

Actinobacillus ureae
Actinobacillus hominis
Animal Species in the Genus *Actinobacillus*

Pasteurella and Mannheimia Species

Taxonomy and Characteristics of the Genus *Pasteurella*
Pasteurella multocida

Clinical Significance and Virulence
Cultural Characteristics and Identification
Antimicrobial Susceptibility

Other *Pasteurella* Species Isolated From Human Infections

Pasteurella pneumotropica ("*Actinobacillus pneumotropica*")
Pasteurella aerogenes ("*Actinobacillus aerogenes*")

Pasteurella dagmatis
Pasteurella canis and *Pasteurella stomatis*
Pasteurella bettyae
Pasteurella caballi
Pasteurella gallinarum

Mannheimia Species (Formerly the "*Pasteurella haemolytica/Pasteurella granulomatis*" Complex)

Cardiobacterium Hominis

Taxonomy
Clinical Significance
Cultural Characteristics and Identification
Antimicrobial Susceptibility

Eikenella corrodens

Taxonomy and Virulence
Clinical Significance
Cultural Characteristics and Identification
Antimicrobial Susceptibility

Kingella and Suttonella Species

Taxonomy
Clinical Significance
Cultural Characteristics and Identification
Antimicrobial Susceptibility

Human Capnocytophaga Species

Taxonomy
Clinical Significance
Cultural Characteristics and Identification
Antimicrobial Susceptibility

Canine Capnocytophaga Species

Taxonomy
Clinical Significance
Cultural Characteristics and Identification
Antimicrobial Susceptibility

Dysgonomonas Species

CDC Groups EF-4A and EF-4B

Simonsiella Species

Streptobacillus moniliforms

Taxonomy
Clinical Significance
Cultural Characteristics and Identification
Antimicrobial Susceptibility

Brucella Species

Epidemiology of Brucellosis
Taxonomy of *Brucella* Species
Virulence of *Brucella* Species
Clinical Spectrum of Brucellosis
Serologic Diagnosis of Brucellosis
Isolation and Cultural Characteristics
Identification of *Brucella* Species
Treatment of Brucellosis

Francisella tularensis

Epidemiology of Tularemia
History and Taxonomy
Virulence of *F. tularensis*
Clinical Spectrum of Tularemia
Isolation and Cultural Characteristics
Serologic Diagnosis of Tularemia
Treatment of Tularemia

Bartonella Species

Taxonomy and Epidemiology of *Bartonella* Species
Clinical Significance of *Bartonella* Species

Oroya Fever and Verruga Peruana
"Classical" and "Urban" Trench Fever
Bacillary Angiomatosis
Peliosis
Fever and Bacteremia
Endocarditis
Cat-Scratch Disease (CSD)
Miscellaneous Infections

Detection, Isolation, and Identification of *Bartonella* Species

Specimen Types
Culture
Gram Stain and Colony Morphology
Identification Methods

Serologic Diagnosis of *Bartonella* Infections
In Vitro Antimicrobial Susceptibility

Afipia Species

Taxonomy and Clinical Significance
Isolation and Identification
Antimicrobial Susceptibility

Bordetella Species

Background and Taxonomy of *Bordetella* Species
Epidemiology of Pertussis

Clinical Significance of *Bordetella pertussis*

Pertussis Vaccines

Clinical Significance of Other *Bordetella* Species

  Bordetella parapertussis
  Bordetella bronchiseptica
  Bordetella hinzii
  Bordetella holmesii
  Bordetella trematum

Isolation and Identification of *Bordetella* Species

Specimens and Culture Media
Direct Fluorescent Antibody Test
Cultural Characteristics and Identification

New Technologies for Detection and Identification of *Bordetella pertussis*

Serologic Tests for Diagnosis of Pertussis

Treatment of Pertussis

Antimicrobial Susceptibility Testing of *Bordetella* Species

Haemophilus *Species*

Members of the genus *Haemophilus* are small, nonmotile, gram-negative bacilli that require factors present in blood for growth; the genus name is derived from the Greek words meaning "blood-loving." Some *Haemophilus* species require X factor, which is not a single substance, but a group of heat-stable tetrapyrrole compounds that are provided by several iron-containing pigments (e.g., hemin, hematin, protoporphyrin IX). These compounds are used in the synthesis of catalases, peroxidases, and cytochromes of the electron transport system. Most *Haemophilus* species also require V factor, which is nicotinamide adenine dinucleotide (NAD, coenzyme I) or nicotinamide adenine dinucleotide phosphate (NADP, coenzyme II). Both X and V factors are found within red blood cells, including the sheep erythrocytes found in blood agar formulations routinely used in clinical laboratories. Sheep blood also contains enzymes that slowly hydrolyze V factor.[59] Consequently, V-factor-dependent hemophili do not grow on sheep blood agar in which the erythrocytes are intact. Gentle heating during addition of blood to the molten agar base in the preparation of chocolate agar results in the lysis of erythrocytes, liberation of X and V factors, and inactivation of enzymes that hydrolyze V factor. Even though most *Haemophilus* species are unable to grow on sheep blood agar, tiny colonies of these organisms may be observed growing around colonies of other hemolytic organisms in mixed cultures (e.g., *Staphylococcus aureus*); lysis of the erythrocytes releases X factor, whereas V factor is synthesized and provided to the hemophili by the staphylococci themselves. Although most laboratories rely on chocolate agar for the recovery of *Haemophilus* species from clinical specimens, these organisms also grow on agar containing 5% horse or rabbit blood. The hemolysis observed on these media is helpful for species identification.

Taxonomy of *Haemophilus* and Related Organisms

The genus *Haemophilus* is classified in the Family *Pasteurellaceae*, which also includes the genera *Actino-bacillus*, *Pasteurella*, *Mannheimia*, *Phocoenobacter*, and *Lonepinella*.[38,425,455,686,975] Sequencing studies of 16S ribosomal RNA (rRNA) from these organisms have demonstrated the phylogenetic diversity of the species currently included in the *Pasteurellaceae*. At present, these genera are classified in the proposed order "Pasteurellales" in the γ-division of the *Proteobacteria*.[455] With the exception of *Actinobacillus actinomycetemcomitans*, *Actinobacillus ureae*, and *Actinobacillus hominis*, members of the genus *Actinobacillus* are primarily animal isolates. *Pasteurella* and *Mannheimia* species also are animal isolates that are occasionally recovered from humans. *Mannheimia* is a new genus that was created in 1999 to accommodate the trehalose-negative "*Pasteurella haemolytica*" complex and *Pasteurella granulomatis*.[38] *Phocoenobacter* and *Lonepinella* are new genera that include isolates from porpoises and the environment, respectively.[425,975] Characteristics for differentiation of the various genera within the family *Pasteurellaceae* are presented in Table 9-1. Members of the genera *Actinobacillus*, *Pasteurella*, and *Mannheimia* will be discussed later in this chapter.

The genus *Haemophilus* includes nine species found in humans and five from animals (Box 9-1). Species from humans are associated with the upper respiratory tract, except for *Haemophilus ducreyi*, which is the cause of the sexually transmitted disease chancroid. *H. aphrophilus* and *H. paraphrophilus* are found primarily in the gingival sulci and in dental plaque. *H. aphrophilus* is the only species that does not require X or V factors; the biochemically similar *H. paraphrophilus* requires V factor for growth. Although chemotaxonomic data and multilocus enzyme electrophoresis analysis suggest that these two organisms are separate species, DNA homology, hybridization, genetic transformation, and ribotyping studies indicate that these organisms represent phenotypically similar strains of the same species.[969,1154,1280] Recently, sequencing of the *infB* (elongation factor 2) gene from *Haemophilus* species indicated that all species that required X and V factors were closely related, that *H. parainfluenzae* constituted a heterogeneous group within the genus, and that *H. aphrophilus*, *H. paraphrophilus*, and *Actinobacillus actinomycetemcomitans* were only remotely related to the type species, *H. influenzae*.[550] *H. ducreyi* differs in several respects from other members of

Table 9-1 Characteristics for Differentiation of Members of the Family *Pasteurellaceae*

CHARACTERISTIC	HAEMOPHILUS	ACTINOBACILLUS	PASTEURELLA	MANNHEIMIA	LONIPINELLA	PHOCOENOBACTER
Hemolysis	V	V	-	V	-	-
Catalase	V	V	+	+	-	-
Oxidase	V	V	V	+	-	+
Requirement for X factor	V	-	-	-	-	-
Requirement for V factor	+[a]	V	V	-	-	-
Indole	V	-	+[b]	-	-	-
Urease	V	+	V	-	-	-
Acetoin production	-	-	-	-	+	+
ODC	V	-	V	V	-	-
Acid produced from:						
Glucose	+	+	+	+	+	+
L-Arabinose	-	V	-	V	V	NA
Meso-inositol	-	-	-	V	-	-
D-Mannitol	-	V	V	+	-	-
D-Mannose	V	V	+	-	NA	-
D-Melibiose	-	V	-	-	V	-
D-Sorbitol	-	-	V	V	NA	-
Trehalose	-	V	V	-	NA	-

[a] *H. aphrophilus* and *H. ducreyi are negative.*
[b] *P. avium is indole-negative.*
+, *positive reaction;* −, *negative reaction; V, variable reaction; NA, data not available.*

Box 9-1 Members of the Genus *Haemophilus*

Human Species	Animal Species
H. influenzae*	*H. parasuis* (swine)
H. parainfluenzae	*H. paragallinarum* (poultry)
H. haemolyticus	*H. paracuniculus* (rabbits)
H. parahaemolyticus	*H. haemoglobinophilus* (dogs)
H. aphrophilus	*H. felis* (cats)
H. paraphrophilus	
H. paraphrophaemolyticus	
H. segnis	
H. ducreyi	

* *Includes the former species H. aegyptius as H. influenzae biogroup aegyptius.*

the genus and was originally assigned to genus *Haemophilus* because of its X factor requirement. DNA hybridization studies have shown that *H. ducreyi* is only distantly related to *H. influenzae* and the other hemophili; however 16S rRNA sequencing has confirmed its membership in the Family *Pasteurellaceae*.[313,1099]

Haemophilus influenzae

Haemophilus species are part of the normal bacterial flora of the oropharynx and nasopharynx in more than 85% of adults.[901] Most oropharyngeal isolates are nonencapsulated *H. influenzae* and *H. parainfluenzae*, although encapsulated *H. influenzae* (capsular serotypes a, b, c, d, e, and f) may be found as part of the normal upper respiratory tract flora of both children and adults. Prior to the availability of *H. influenzae* type b conjugate vaccines, 2–6% of children carried capsular serotype b strains and as many as 60% of children in day-care centers were colonized in the oropharynx.[901] The recovery of *H. influenzae* from sputum specimens may reflect the presence of these organisms as normal flora. However, in chronic respiratory ailments (e.g., bronchitis, chronic obstructive pulmonary disease), both encapsulated (typeable) and nonencapsulated (nontypeable) *H. influenzae* may cause severe infections.[325,725,910,1134] Infections caused by hemophili, their clinical manifestations, and appropriate specimens for culture are summarized in Box 9-2.

Among the hemophili, *H. influenzae* serotype b is considered the most pathogenic of the six capsular serotypes (i.e., types a, b, c, d, e, and f) The type b polysaccharide is the only capsular type that contains two pentose monosaccharides rather than hexose sugars as subunit carbohydrates. The native type b capsule is composed of a linear teichoic acid containing ribose, ribitol (a five-carbon sugar alcohol), and phosphate linked by phosphodiester bonds, and is called PRP (polyribosyl-ribitol-phosphate) (Figure 9-1). Although virulence of *H. influenzae* type b is multifactorial, the PRP capsule is of singular importance. Animal studies with isogenic strains transformed with DNA coding for capsule production confirmed that type b strains were more virulent

than the other capsular types.[1436] The PRP capsule allows the organism to resist phagocytosis and intracellular killing by neutrophils. Anti–type b antibodies promote complement-dependent phagocytosis and killing (opsonization) of these organisms in vitro and in vivo.[1294] In addition to the type b capsule, *H. influenzae* possesses several virulence factors, most of which are related to adherence, colonization, and invasion. Some of these factors are found in both typeable and nontypeable strains, while others are found only in nontypeable *H. influenzae* isolates. The virulence factors found in type b and nontypeable *H. influenzae* are presented in Box 9-3.

Haemophilus influenzae Type B Vaccines

Prior to the introduction of effective vaccines against *H. influenzae* type b, this organism caused approximately 16,000 cases of invasive disease each year in children 5 years of age and younger.[666,901] The majority of systemic type b infections occurred in children aged 2 years and younger. Inadequate levels of protective, anti-PRP bactericidal antibodies at this age play a major role in the development of disease. During the immediate newborn period, immunity to *H. influenzae* type b is acquired by transplacental antibodies that are lost within the first few months of life. These antibodies reappear following exposure to type b organisms or to other microbial antigens that engender cross-reactive antibodies. Most individuals in whom systemic *H. influenzae* type b disease develops have low or undetectable levels of anti-PRP capsular antibodies. The antigenic capabilities of native, purified PRP were exploited in the first *H. influenzae* type b vaccine preparations. Purified PRP elicited antibodies in older children, but failed to elicit a response in children less than 2 years of age, the group most at risk for serious illness.[547] Furthermore, PRP did not predictably elicit a ''booster'' response on subsequent antigenic challenge. This failure was due to the T-cell-independent nature of the primary immune response to polysaccharide antigens.[782] Clinical trials were subsequently undertaken with four PRP/protein conjugate vaccines.[305,306,547,999] The conjugates consisted of native PRP conjugated covalently to tetanus toxoid (PRP-T), diphtheria toxoid (PTP-D), an outer-membrane-protein (OMP) complex from *Neisseria meningitidis* (PRP-OMP), and to CRM197, a ''nontoxic'' diphtheria toxin isolated from a mutant strain of *Corynebacterium diphtheriae* (PRP-HbOC). Using this approach, presumably the immunogenicity of the PRP material would be enhanced, since conjugation of carbohydrate moieties to proteins as haptens elicits a T-cell-dependent immune response with the generation of memory cells.[782] After the development of these unique conjugates, large-scale clinical efficacy trials were instituted. Clinical trials conducted with the various conjugate vaccines in the U.S., the United Kingdom, Finland, and other countries over the past decade have reported efficacies of 95–100%, depending on the dosage and study immunization schedules.[138,547,999]

At present, four basic conjugate vaccines are licensed: PRP-HbOC, PRP-OMP, and PRP-T, and PRP-D. HbOC, PRP-OMP, and PRP-T are licensed for use in children younger than 12 months of age, and all four are licensed

Box 9-2 Infectious Diseases Associated With *Haemophilus* Species

Disease	Species	Specimens for Culture	Clinical Manifestations
Meningitis	*H. influenzae type b* (rarely other capsular types)	CSF; blood	Meningeal signs (headache, stiff neck), generally insidious onset; fever, seizures; usually seen in children 1 month to 2 years of age
Epiglottis	*H. influenzae* type b (rarely other capsular types)	Blood; laryngeal secretions	Rapid onset and progression of sore throat; dysphagia and upper airway obstruction; red and swollen epiglottis; may require tracheostomy to establish airway
Otitis media	*H. influenzae* (usually nontypeable strains)	Swab of drainage in the ear canal; needle aspiration or myringotomy; suspected systemic disease may require collection of CSF or blood cultures	Pain and fullness in the ears; usually bilateral; bulging, opaque tympanic membranes; fever, irritability, and vomiting may be noted; concomitant systemic disease should be suspected
Acute sinusitis	*H. influenzae* (usually nontypeable strains); rarely, *H. parainfluenzae*	Sinus aspirates; surgical specimens	Frontal headaches; facial pain; swelling and redness of suborbital and periorbital tissues; sinus empyema
Acute pharyngitis or laryngotracheobron-chitis	*H. influenzae* type b	Posterior pharyngeal swab; laryngeal secretions	Inflamed mucous membranes with swelling and yellow exudates; sore throat with stridor and cough; similar to croup if the laryngeal mucosa is involved
Bronchitis	*H. influenzae* (often nontypeable strains)	Sputum; transtracheal aspirates; bronchial washings	Persistent, nonproductive cough; wheezing and dyspnea; disease is usually chronic with periodic purulent exacerbations
Pneumonia	*H. influenzae* type b; nontypeable strains recovered from elderly patients	Sputum; tracheal aspirates; bronchial washings	Cough, sputum production, and pleuritic pain; distribution tends to be lobar or segmental, simulating pneumococcal pneumonia; bacteremic pneumonia caused by nontypeable strains seen in elderly patients
Endocarditis	*H. aphrophilus; H. paraphrophilus; H. parainfluenzae*; rarely, *H. influenzae*	Blood	Chills, spiking fevers, leukocytosis, and secondary complications, such as anemia, weight loss, malaise, and anorexia; mitral and aortic valves most commonly involved; high incidence of arterial embolization
Genital tract infection and postpartum bacteremia; neonatal sepsis with meningitis	*H. influenzae* (nontypeable); *H. parainfluenzae; H. influenzae* cryptic genospecies	Urethral and endocervical specimens; blood; fetal tissues; CSF	Urethritis characterized by thin, mucoid discharge; organisms may be recovered from cervical and blood cultures of women with postpartum fever; may also be cultured from multiple genital sites (e.g., Bartholin's glands, endometrium); placenta, amniotic fluid, and neonatal body fluids
Conjunctivitis	*H. influenzae* biogroup aegyptius	Conjunctival swab specimen	Characterized by mucopurulent conjunctival discharge; hyperemic conjunctivae, and diffusely injected sclera; spread to others by infectious secretions on towels and hands
Brazilian purpuric fever	*H. influenzae* biogroup aegyptius (BPF clone)	Blood; conjunctival swabs; skin lesions; oropharynx	Fever, abdominal pain with vomiting; petechial and hemorrhagic skin lesions; symptoms mimic meningococcal meningitis, but meningitis is not present; previous or concurrent conjunctival infection with BPF clone or *H. influenzae* biogroup aegyptius usually found
Chancroid	*H. ducreyi*	Swabs obtained from genital ulcers; aspirates from buboes; endocervical swab specimens	Sexually transmitted disease, characterized by painful, ulcerative genital lesions and enlarged, suppurative inguinal lymph nodes; may progress to abscess and fistula formation if left untreated

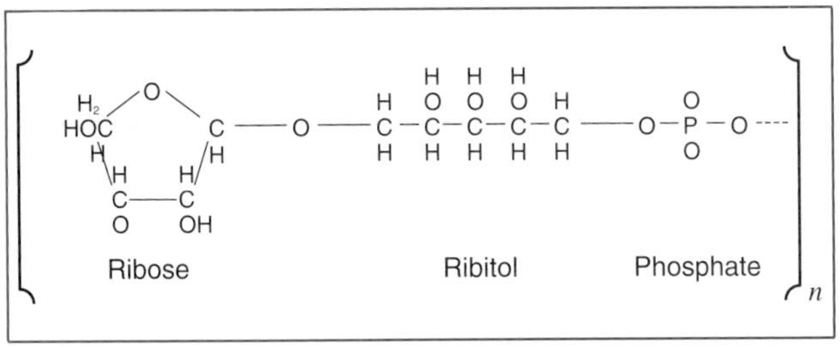

Figure 9-1 Structure of the repeating unit of the *Haemophilus influenzae* type b capsular polysaccharide polyribose-ribitol-phosphate (PRP). This molecule consists of the five-carbon monosaccharide ribose, linked by an ester bond to ribitol, a five-carbon sugar alcohol which, in turn, is linked to a phosphate group.

for children older than 12 months of age (Box 9-4). Three combination vaccines—DTP-HbOC, DTP-PRP-T, and DTaP-PRP-T—are also available. The first two contain diphtheria and tetanus toxoids and whole-cell pertussis vaccine, while the latter contains diphtheria and tetanus toxoids and an acellular pertussis vaccine. These combination vaccines can be used for the primary diphtheria, tetanus, pertussis, and *H. influenzae* type b vaccination series, except for DTaP-PRP-T, which is licensed only for use as the fourth dose of the primary series because of decreased immunogenicity in younger children.[207,210,212] The Committee on Infectious Diseases of the American Academy of Pediatrics and the Immunization Practices Advisory Committee of the Centers for Disease Control and Prevention (CDC) have issued recommendations regarding *H. influenzae* type b vaccine administration.[209,212] At present, the inclusion of *H. influenzae* type b vaccines admixed with other vaccines (e.g., acellular pertussis vaccine, polio vaccine, hepatitis B vaccine), the use of alternative administration schedules, and the persistence of antibody following administration of different vaccines are under evaluation.[195,202,306,699] General guidelines for vaccine administration are presented in Box 9-5.

During the vaccine efficacy trials, surveillance data collected during 1992, when approximately 67% of enrolled children aged 12 to 24 months had received at least one dose of conjugate vaccine, already suggested inordinate decreases in the incidence of serious *H. influenzae* type b disease. Indeed, large decreases in incidence among children less than 18 months of age were noted long before the conjugate vaccines were in widespread use in young infants.[913] These findings suggested that the conjugate vaccines not only prevented disease by inducing active immunity but also decreased oropharyngeal carriage of *H. influenzae* type b. Indeed, this has been demonstrated in studies in Europe and the U.S.[913,914,1246] The vaccines may provide additional protection for unvaccinated infants by reducing their risk of exposure to *H. influenzae* type b from older vaccinated contacts. Ongoing surveillance in populations of both children and adults will be needed to assess whether immunity engendered by the conjugate vaccines is long-term, or whether there will be an increase in the proportion of both older children and adults who are susceptible to *H. influenzae* type b infections as time passes.

Although long-term experience with these vaccines in

children born prematurely or with underlying diseases is not yet available, a few studies suggest that they may not be as effective in such individuals. In a study of 22 premature infants with a median gestational age of 28 weeks, administration of PRP-OMP at 2 and 4 months of chronologic age resulted in only 27% and 55% of the infants demonstrating anti-PRP levels greater than 1 μg/mL after the first and second vaccine dose, respectively.[1351] This antibody response was significantly lower than that seen in term infants. A follow-up study of extremely preterm infants conducted 7 years after receipt of vaccine found that the preterm children had lower antibody titers to several vaccine antigens than full-term vaccine recipients.[693] In a study of 19 HIV-1-infected children who were immunized with a single dose of PRP-T or HbOC at a mean age of 28 months, only 7 had levels of anti-PRP antibodies that indicated immunity.[1006] Another study conducted among HIV-infected African children also found that the response to vaccine was significantly reduced.[806] It is postulated that the poor vaccine response in HIV-infected individuals is due to the T-cell-depleted state of the patients and the T-cell-dependent nature of the immune response to the conjugate vaccines. *H. influenzae* type b conjugate vaccines are immunogenic in HIV-seropositive adults, but the ability to develop protective levels of antibody is related to baseline CD4 T-cell counts and IgG levels.[338,1220]

Infections Caused by *Haemophilus* Species
MENINGITIS

In the prevaccine era, *H. influenzae* was the most common cause of bacterial meningitis in children between 1 month and 2 years of age, with the peak incidence between 6 and 12 months of age.[666] Between the ages of 2 and 6 years, *H. influenzae* and *Neisseria meningitidis* occurred with equal frequency; *H. influenzae* meningitis was uncommon in children older than 6 years of age. More than 90% of isolates obtained from these cases belonged to capsular serotype b.[901] Clinically, *H. influenzae* type b meningitis closely resembles meningococcal meningitis. Prior nasopharyngeal colonization in a susceptible host leads to invasion of the bloodstream and subsequent seeding of the meninges. Symptoms of an upper respiratory tract infection of viral etiology and otitis media often precede the development of meningitis.[1247] Onset of signs and symptoms may be abrupt or insidious, with the latter being the most common pattern. Children present with fever, malaise, and occasionally vomiting; nuchal rigidity is often absent. In some children peripheral and/or cranial nerve palsies and seizures may develop. A high index of suspicion, aggressive diagnostic approaches (i.e., lumbar puncture for collection of cerebrospinal fluid [CSF], collection of blood cultures, and early administration of appropriate antimicrobial therapy), and close communication with the laboratory are essential for proper diagnosis. Although relatively unusual, complications of *H. influenzae* type b meningitis include brain abscess, subdural effusion, pericarditis, septic arthritis, and localized infections at other body sites due to hematogenous dissemination.[218,401] At present, most cases of *H. influenzae* type b meningitis occur in patients who have not been immunized.[933]

H. influenzae meningitis in adults is uncommon and usually complicates underlying conditions, such as CSF leakage

Box 9-3 Virulence Factors of *Haemophilus influenzae*

Capsule

The genetic basis of PRP capsule production is complex and involves both capsular and noncapsular genetic determinants. The *capB* genes exist in the chromosome as a duplication of two identical 17–18 kb segments that are joined by a short 1–1.3 kb region.[583,732] This short region contains *bexA*, which codes for a protein required for export of the capsular material to the cell surface.[734] This duplicate-gene arrangement is found in more than 98% of *H. influenzae* type b strains. In contrast, *cap* genes in *H. influenzae* types a, c, d, e, and f exist as single-copy genes, although recent evidence suggests that invasive non-type b *H. influenzae* strains may also display *cap* gene amplification.[959] Capsule-deficient type b strains lack the *capB* locus duplication and possess only a single copy of this gene.[732] The theoretical evolutionary advantage imparted by the duplicated *capB* genotype is the availability of a ready template for rapid amplification of type b capsular gene sequences under environmental conditions in which it may be advantageous to produce more capsular material. An examination of 36 invasive clinical isolates of *H. influenzae* type b from Finland and 14 strains from Washington, D.C., showed that, indeed, amplification of *capB* genes occurs commonly in vivo.[582] Fifteen of the 36 Finnish strains and 5 of the 14 U.S. strains contained three to five copies of the *capB* gene. Strains with multiple gene copies produced more type b capsular polysaccharide; the single strain that possessed five copies made four to five times the amount of type b capsular material as the wild-type strain. Interestingly, encapsulation of type b organisms is associated with decreased adherence to and invasion of human cells.[1228] Type b capsule-deficient mutants resulting from loss of a copy of the duplication at the *capB* locus showed a 50-fold increase in adherence to human epithelial cells and a nearly 300-fold increase in invasive capabilities. Restoration of encapsulation by transformation resulted in a large decrease in both adherence and invasion.

Fimbrial Adhesin

Fimbriae are found on encapsulated type b strains and on about 30–40% of nontypeable strains.[465,466] Some fimbriae mediate both hemagglutination and adherence to human mucosal cells, but actually inhibit mucosal cell invasion.[397] *H. influenzae* fimbriae are composed of a 24-kDa major protein (HifA) and two minor proteins of 20.6 (HifD) and 45.5kDa (HifE) molecular weight.[466,845,1232] The HifE protein is located at the tips of the fimbriae; mutations in the *hifE* gene result in the production of fimbriae that have reduced ability to hemagglutinate and to adhere to epithelial cells.[466,845,1224] Together, intact fimbriae mediate adherence by binding to glycoproteins and glycolipids on the eukaryotic cell surface and to respiratory mucin proteins.[393,735] The genes for these proteins (*hifA*, *hifD*, and *hifE*) exist as a single-copy cluster along with two genes (*hifC* and *hifB*) that code for proteins involved in fimbrial assembly (HifC) and protection of the nascent fimbrial proteins from degradation during export from the cell (HifB).[1232] Fimbriae composed of another fimbrial protein, called P5-fimbrin, have also been identified on nontypeable *H. influenzae* strains and in strains of the cryptic genospecies found in the genital tract.[491] This 36.4-kDa protein shows sequence homology with the P5 outer membrane protein (see below) and also adheres to human oropharyngeal cells, mucin, and eustachian tube mucus in the chinchilla otitis media model.[947] Although this protein shows considerable interstrain heterogeneity among nontypeable isolates, conserved epitopes of P5-fimbrin have been identified as possible vaccine candidate antigens.[947] Recently, the entire fimbrial gene cluster of the cryptic genital tract genospecies of *H. influenzae* was described and found to consist of five genes (*ghfA* through *ghfE*) that are homologous to the *hif* gene cluster of other *H. influenzae* strains.[183]

HMW1 and HMW2 Adhesins

HMW1 (160 kDa) and HMW2 (155 kDa) are high-molecular-weight protein adhesins that are found on 70–80% of nontypeable *H influenzae* and mediate adherence to epithelial cells.[1230] These proteins are related structurally and functionally to the filamentous hemagglutinin of *Bordetella pertussis*.[87] The genes for these proteins are also arranged as clusters on the chromosome along with genes coding for proteins that export, localize, and activate these large outer membrane proteins (OMPs).[88] In a study of nontypeable, matched middle-ear and nasopharyngeal isolates from children with otitis media, strains possessing HMW1 and HMW2 predominated; strains not expressing these adhesins expressed either hia adhesin (see below) or hemagglutinating fimbriae.[727] Although these proteins are fairly heterogeneous from strain to strain, animal immunization studies with purified HMW1/HMW2 showed some protection from otitis media on challenge with the homologous strain.[86] Isolates from different anatomic sites/or associated with different clinical conditions (e.g., otitis media-associated vs. COPD-associated strains) may differ in the level of expression of HMW adhesin genes.[1313] These proteins possess surface-exposed epitopes that may be useful for developing recombinant synthetic peptide-based vaccines for nontypeable *H. influenzae*.[89]

Hap Adhesin

Hap is a 155-kDa nonfimbrial adhesin that is found in all *H. influenzae* strains and mediates adherence and invasion of epithelial cells.[1227] The hap protein has both adhesive and protease activities and is related to but distinct from the IgA protease of *H. influenzae*. This molecule is synthesized, secreted, and undergoes autoproteolytic cleavage with the release of the adhesive domain from the cell surface.[408] Interaction of the hap adhesive domain with fibronectin, laminen, or collagen inhibits proteolytic cleavage of hap and promotes bacterial adherence to these proteins. Because of its proteolytic activity, this molecule may also act after cellular invasion. Intranasal immunization of mice with hap adhesin inhibits nasopharyngeal colonization.[296]

Box 9-3 *Continued*

Hia and Hsf Adhesins

Some nontypeable strains that lack HMW1/HMW2 adhesins possess another nonfimbrial protein called Hia.[90] Hia is a 115-kDa protein adhesin that is structurally similar to the Hsf protein, a minor adhesin found in type b strains.[1225,1226] The hia protein is synthesized and secreted intact and remains fully cell-associated with the bacterial outer membrane.[1225] Hsf proteins exist on the cells as short, thin fibrillar surface appendages that are distinct from fimbriae. The hsf gene locus of type b strains shows sequence homology with the hia locus of nontypeable strains.

Opacity-associated Protein A (OapA)

OapA is a 47-kDa adhesin protein found in all *H. influenzae* strains. This protein has been shown to mediate adherence to epithelial cells in culture and is required for pharyngeal colonization in animal models.[1026,1355] On transparent growth medium, OapA is responsible for an opaque colonial morphology.

Haemocin

More than 90% of *H. influenzae* type b strains also produce a bacteriocin called a "haemocin."[788,789] Bacteriocins are proteins that are produced by a variety of bacterial species and that are able to inhibit the growth of strains of the same or related species. Haemocin is not produced by encapsulated non-type b or nontypeable *H. influenzae* strains, although most of these organisms are susceptible to its lethal effects.[788] Haemocin production may contribute to the ability of *H. influenzae* type b strains to effectively compete with nontypeable strains in nasopharyngeal colonization.

IgA Protease

H. influenzae produces an IgA1 protease that inactivates human immunoglobulin A1, which accounts for over 90% of the IgA present in the oropharynx.[687] This molecule is distinct from the Hap adhesin, which has some sequence homology with IgA protease. Although 97% or more of nontypeable *H. influenzae* strains possess the IgA protease gene *(iga)*, protease activity is greater in clinical isolates from sputum, blood, and CSF than in strains isolated from throat swabs of asymptomatic carriers.[1333]

Lipooligosaccharide

H. influenzae strains possess an outer membrane-associated lipopolysaccharide (LPS) that consists of lipid A joined via 2-keto-3-deoxyoctulosonic acid (KDO) to a core polysaccharide polymer consisting of neutral monosaccharides. However, it differs from the LPS of enterics and other organisms in that it lacks the repeating terminal side chains (the "O" or somatic antigens).[85] Therefore, the LPS of *H. influenzae* is more accurately termed a lipooligosaccharide (LOS). LOS Lipid A possesses all of the endotoxic activities of LPS lipid A, including mitogenicity, pyrogenicity in rabbits, platelet aggregation, and lethality in the mouse endotoxemia model. In the LOS, neutral core oligosaccharides—glucose, galactose, glucosamine, and heptose—vary in their amounts and their structural relationships both between strains and within a given strain. LOS phase variation at the genetic level occurs by changes in the numbers of short genomic four-nucleotide sequences (i.e., 5'-CAAT-3') that result in shifts in the codon/anticodon reading frame.[569] In addition, the LOS of many *H influenzae* strains is sialylated and, therefore, structurally and antigenically similar to the sialylated oligosaccharides of human glycolated sphingolipids. This LOS modification helps the organism evade opsonization and phagocytosis by mimicry of molecular structures normally found in the host. *H. influenzae* LOS is also being investigated as a potential antigen for nontypeable *H. influenzae* vaccine development. Detoxified LOS conjugated to either *H. influenzae* outer membrane proteins or to tetanus toxoid is immunogenic, and active immunization with these conjugates reduced the incidence of otitis media due to nontypeable *H. influenzae* in the chinchilla model.[506,1398] Analysis of the genetic loci responsible for LOS biosynthesis and structure have revealed that expression of certain loci (e.g., the *lic2B* gene) may be associated with enhanced virulence.[1008]

Outer Membrane Proteins

H. influenzae strains have six to eight OMPs in the cell wall outer membrane. Research on *H. influenzae* OMPs has focused on those that might be useful as components of a vaccine against nontypeable *H. influenzae*. OMPs designated P2 and P6 have generated the most interest as potential vaccine antigens. P2, the major OMP of *H. influenzae*, comprises more than 50% of the OMP content. This protein has a molecular weight of between 38- to 40-kDa, exists in the outer membrane as a trimer, and functions as a porin; therefore, it is partially exposed on the surface of nontypeable strains.[911,1176] Antibodies directed against the P2 protein are bactericidal and protective against challenge infection in animal models. Epitopes of P2 are also immunogenic in humans and are targets for bactericidal antibodies that appear during nontypeable *H influenzae* infections.[911] Amino acid sequence analysis of purified P2 protein indicate that the portions of the molecule that are buried within the outer membrane are conserved in their amino acid sequences, whereas surface-exposed epitopes are highly variable in sequence from strain to strain.[106,1176] In addition, exposed P2 epitopes on individual respiratory isolates change over time as a result of single, sequential base changes in P2 structural genes.[358] Using animal models and monoclonal antibody technology, it has been shown that the principal anti-P2 response is directed against a single, surface-exposed "loop" of the P2 molecule.[1417] Changes in the amino acid sequence within this region result in immunologic elimination of organisms having the "recognized" P2 phenotype. This recognized phenotype is supplanted over time with organisms expressing the slightly altered P2 phenotype. Such a mechanism may partially explain the chronic nature of some infections associated with nontypeable *H. influenzae* (e.g., sinusitis, COPD). In considering P2 proteins as candidate vaccine antigens, analysis of P2 OMPs from a variety of *H. influenzae* strains will be necessary to identify epitopes that are conserved structurally and immunologically.[911]

(Continued)

Box 9-3 Continued

P6 is a protein that comprises 1–5% of the OMP content and is present on the surface of both typeable and nontypeable strains.[930] It has a molecular weight of 16.6 kDa and is actually a peptidoglycan-associated lipoprotein.[912] Antibodies directed against P6 are bactericidal and are protective against challenge in the infant rat model and in the chinchilla model of otitis media.[317,912] In the mouse model of otitis media, intranasal immunization with purified P6 resulted in the induction of both P6-specific mucosal IgA and cell-mediated immune responses.[702] Amino acid sequence analysis of the P6 protein and nucleotide sequencing of the P6 gene from type b and nontypeable strains showed greater than 97% homology, indicating that the P6 gene is highly conserved at the genetic level.[930] Bactericidal antibodies directed against P6 are present in normal human serum. Because of its conserved nature and its demonstrated immunogenicity in animals and humans, P6 OMP warrants further investigation as a potential candidate for inclusion in a vaccine against nontypeable *H. influenzae*. Additional studies have shown that the genetic loci encoding P2 do not undergo high rates of genetic variation in the coding sequences, but may show variation in areas where repetitive sequences are located.[574]

Box 9-4 Currently Licensed *Haemophilus influenzae* Type B Conjugate Vaccines

Vaccine	Manufacturer	Carbohydrate	Carrier Proteins
PRP-D	Pasteur Merieux	Medium-sized PRP	Diphtheria toxoid
PRP-HbOC	Wyeth Lederle	Small PRP oligosaccharide	Nontoxic mutant diphtheria toxin (CRM_{197})
PRP-T	Pasteur Merieux	Large-sized PRP	Tetanus toxoid
PRP-OMP	Merck & Co.	Medium-sized PRP	OMP complex of *Neisseria meningitidis* serogroup B

Box 9-5 Guidelines for Administration of *Haemophilus influenzae* Type B Conjugate Vaccines[207,209,210,212]

1. All children should receive one of the conjugate vaccines licensed for use in infants (HbOC, PRP-OMP, or PRP-T), beginning at 2 months of age. If PRP-OMP is used for the first vaccination, another dose is administered at 4 months, with a third dose at 12–15 months of age. For the HbOC and PRP-T vaccines, three doses are given at 2-month intervals (i.e., 2, 4, and 6 months) with a fourth dose at 12–15 months of age. For the 12–15-month dose, any of the conjugate vaccines may be used. These vaccines can be administered during visits when other vaccines (e.g., measles, mumps, rubella) are being given, and infants scheduled to receive both HbOC and DTP can be given the combination vaccine, HbOC-DTP. In general, conjugate vaccines should be administered in a separate syringe and at a separate site from DTP or other vaccinations.

2. For children for whom immunization is not started until 7–11 months of age, HbOC, PRP-OMP, or PRP-T should be given at that time, with a second dose of the same vaccine administered 2 months later. A third booster dose of any of the conjugate vaccines is given at 12–18 months of age.

3. For children in whom vaccination is started at 12–14 months of age, PRP-D, HbOC, PRP-OMP, or PRP-T may be given. Two doses should be administered with the second dose being given at least 2 months after the first.

4. For unvaccinated children aged 15 month to 5 years, a single dose of any of the licensed conjugate vaccines is recommended.

5. The immunization series for premature infants is based on chronologic age and should be commenced at 2 months of age.

6. For infants who have had their primary series of immunizations for diphtheria, tetanus, and/or pertussis deferred to 1 year of age (e.g., children with certain neurologic disorders), PRP-OMP vaccine may present an advantage since this vaccine is immunogenic in the absence of diphtheria or tetanus toxoids. The combo vaccine DTP-HbOC should not be used for immunization of infants in whom pertussis vaccination is contraindicated. This would include infants with a history of immediate reactions to DTP or the development of encephalopathy (alterations of consciousness, seizures) within 7 days of receipt of DTP vaccine.

7. For children 12 months to 5 years of age with underlying immunologic impairment (e.g., those with bone marrow transplants, sickle cell diseases, splenectomy, neoplastic diseases requiring chemotherapy) who have received a primary series of injections and a booster dose at 12 months of age or older, additional doses of vaccine are not required, although some have advocated the administration of an additional dose prior to undergoing a cycle of chemotherapy or splenectomy. For children 12–59 months of age with these underlying conditions who are unvaccinated, two doses of any conjugate vaccine administered 2 months apart are recommended.

8. Unvaccinated children with sickle cell disease or asplenia who are older than 5 years of age may be given one dose of any conjugate vaccine. Two doses of any vaccine given 1–2 months apart are suggested for children with HIV infection, malignancies, bone marrow transplants, and IgG2 deficiency. Vaccine efficacy data on children less than 12 months of age with immunoglobulin subclass deficiency or HIV infection currently is limited.

9. In children who have had invasive *H. influenzae* type b disease before the age of 2 years, prior immunization should be disregarded and conjugate vaccine should be readministered during convalescence according to the age-appropriate schedules outlined above. Children in whom *H. influenzae* disease develops after the age of 2 years do not require reimmunization, since the infection itself induces a protective immune response in immunologically normal children of this age.

following head trauma or neurosurgical procedures. Meningitis may also result from direct extension from a contiguous focus of infection in the sinuses or the middle ear.[1134,1210] Debilitating underlying diseases, such as diabetes, chronic alcoholism, pneumonia, HIV infection, and other immunodeficiency states also predispose adults to *H. influenzae* meningitis.[325,725] Approximately half of the cases of meningitis in adults are due to nontypeable *H. influenzae* strains, while the other half are caused by type b and other encapsulated strains.[910,1210]

H. influenzae is spread via respiratory secretions, and an increased risk of secondary, invasive disease exists for unvaccinated or incompletely vaccinated household contacts 4 years of age and younger. In this latter group, this risk may be greater than 500-fold.[998] Rifampin, the drug of choice for chemoprophylaxis, eradicates oropharyngeal carriage and, therefore, transmission of the organism. According to the American Academy of Pediatrics, prophylaxis should be administered to all household members (including adults) when the household contains a contact or contacts younger than 48 months whose immunization status is incomplete.[1005] The AAP defines a contact as a child who is a member of the immediate household or who has spent 4 or more hours each day with the index case for at least 5 of the 7 days preceding the onset of disease. The dosage of rifampin for children is 20 mg/kg once daily for 4 days and for adults 600 mg twice daily for 2 days.[998] Rifampin must be given to close contacts within 7 days after disease onset in the index case in order to be effective. All members of a household with an immunized child less than 12 months of age (i.e., children who have not yet received the 12–15-month ''booster'') should receive rifampin. Chemoprophylaxis is not necessary when all household contacts younger than 48 months of age have completed their immunization series. Children attending day-care facilities who are contacts of index cases should receive rifampin prophylaxis if they are unvaccinated or incompletely vaccinated and are exposed to the index case for 25 or more hours in the week prior to disease onset in the index case.

H. influenzae meningitis as a complication of CSF shunt infections has also been reported in recent years.[779,1390] These infections have occurred mostly in infants and children and have involved ventriculoperitoneal, ventriculoatrial, and lumboperitoneal shunt types. Although shunt infections caused by *Staphylococcus epidermidis* or *Staphylococcus aureus* usually develop from intraoperative or perioperative contamination of the shunt and ventricular CSF, *H. influenzae* shunt infections apparently result from seeding of the shunt and the CSF during bacteremia. Patients presenting with signs and symptoms of meningitis often have other infections associated with *H. influenzae*, such as otitis media. Shunt fluid isolates have either been capsular type b strains or have been nontypeable. While shunt infections caused by gram-positive bacteria require removal/replacement of the foreign body to effect cure, systemic antimicrobial therapy without shunt removal is often successful in eliminating type b strains, although medical therapy alone has been less successful in treatment of shunt infections caused by nontypeable strains.[779,1390]

EPIGLOTTITIS

H. influenzae type b has historically been associated with epiglottitis, which is a cellulitis of the supraglottic tissues that results in obstructive laryngeal edema.[901] Epiglottitis seldom occurs in infants, and is typically seen in children between 2 and 7 years of age and in adult males 20–30 years of age. The presentation is usually acute, with severe sore throat, dysphagia, fever, and swelling of the epiglottis above the larynx at the base of the tongue.[1259] In children, this abrupt onset helps to clinically differentiate epiglottitis from croup caused by various viral agents (e.g., respiratory syncytial virus, parainfluenzaviruses) and from whooping cough caused by *Bordetella pertussis*. As the disease progresses, swallowing becomes increasingly difficult and is associated with drooling, inspiratory stridor, and incipient respiratory distress. Nasotracheal intubation and vigorous administration of antimicrobial and supportive therapy may be life-saving in cases of airway obstruction. Although posterior pharyngeal cultures are not helpful because of the presence of other nasopharyngeal flora, *H. influenzae* type b will usually be recovered from blood cultures. Epiglottitis may also occur in adults; in these individuals, fever, sore throat, dysphagia, and respiratory distress are the presenting signs and symptoms.[1389] The introduction of effective vaccine strategies has also affected the incidence of epiglottitis.[904,1248] In a Swedish study, a comparison of the mean annual incidence of epiglottitis in the prevaccination period (1987–1991) to the incidence in 1996 showed decreases of 95% in children 0 to 4 years of age, 83% in children 5 to 9 years of age, and 30% in children 15 years of age and older.[454] Despite effective vaccines, however, epiglottitis due to *H. influenzae* type b has been reported in children who have received the entire series of vaccinations.[1341]

OTITIS MEDIA

Otitis media refers to inflammation of the middle ear and is operationally divided into two syndromes: acute otitis media (fluid in the middle ear accompanied by signs and symptoms of acute infection) and otitis media with effusion (fluid in the middle ear without signs and symptoms).[1097] Acute otitis media can be further classified as uncomplicated, persistent, recurrent, or chronic.[1011] Otitis media occurs most frequently in children aged 6 months to 5 years, with the highest incidence among children less than 3 years of age. The high incidence of this infection in young children reflects the underdeveloped protective mechanisms of the eustachian tube. Acute otitis media usually occurs as a complication of viral infection (e.g., respiratory syncytial virus [RSV], parainfluenzaviruses). Symptoms of otitis media include ear pain, hearing loss, and sometime discharge from the external otic canal. Signs include fever, irritability, headache, and occasionally nausea and vomiting. In patients with acute otitis media, pneumatic otoscopy reveals a red, opacified bulging tympanic membrane that is relatively immobile. In otitis media with effusion, bulging or decreased membrane mobility are noted, but the membrane appears only slightly inflamed. Definitive etiologic diagnosis requires needle aspiration of middle ear fluid (tympanocentesis), which is not performed routinely. If drainage is present, however, it should be collected for culture. Simultaneous culture of CSF and blood may be necessary if systemic signs and symptoms are present.

The most common bacterial causes of acute otitis media are *Streptococcus pneumoniae*, *H. influenzae*, and *Moraxella catarrhalis*, with one quarter to one third being caused by *H. influenzae*.[143,689] Over 90% of *H. influenzae* strains recovered from appropriately collected specimens are nontypeable, with the remaining 10% being type b.[395] Up to one fourth of children with otitis media caused by type b organisms will also have concomitant bacteremia and/or meningitis.[145] Complications include recurrent acute otitis media, persistence of middle ear effusions necessitating insertion of drainage tubes, hearing impairment, mastoiditis, meningitis, chronic otitis media, brain abscess, and sepsis.[775] Interestingly, only 20–30% of middle ear fluid specimens collected from children with otitis media with effusion will have positive bacterial cultures, although the role of fastidious, slow-growing organisms (e.g., *Alloiococcus otitidis*) as causes of this infection are only now being appreciated.[561] Amoxicillin/clavulanate combined with amoxicillin (PO), cefuroxime axetil (PO), or ceftriaxone (IM) have been recommended as the antimicrobial agents of choice for treatment of recurrent and persistent otitis media.[576,1011]

SINUSITIS

Acute sinusitis is characterized by persistent cold symptoms, purulent nasal and postnasal discharge, cough, fever, headache, and often facial pain.[1200] This acute presentation blends into a condition called chronic sinusitis, which is characterized by the persistence of the above signs and symptoms beyond 3 months' duration, with cough and purulent nasal drainage being the principal symptoms.[1145] A sensation of facial fullness or the presence of edema or discoloration around the eyes may indicate extension of the infectious process from the sinuses into the soft tissues of the orbit. Diagnosis of sinusitis is made most often by an assessment of signs and symptoms, with imaging techniques (i.e., radiography, computed tomography, magnetic resonance imaging) being used occasionally for visualizing the ethmoid and sphenoid sinuses and for determining orbital involvement. In studies in which specimens were obtained either surgically or by needle aspiration of the maxillary sinus spaces, *H. influenzae* and *S. pneumoniae* are the organisms most frequently isolated. Careful bacteriologic studies of patients with acute sinusitis have clearly demonstrated *H. influenzae* as the leading etiologic agent in 20–25% of adults and in 36–40% of children, respectively.[179,1200] These agents often represent secondary invaders following viral sinus infection (e.g., rhinovirus). Most *H. influenzae* isolates from patients with acute sinus infections are nontypeable.[395,910] *H. influenzae* plays a minor role in the pathogenesis of chronic sinusitis. A recent study of frontal sinus aspirates collected from 30 consecutive patients found that *H. influenzae* was present in only 9% of 35 cultures.[1145]

BRONCHITIS AND CHRONIC OBSTRUCTIVE PULMONARY DISEASE

Chronic bronchitis is an ill-defined clinical entity involving inflammation of the bronchi without significant lung involvement, and is characterized by a persistent, generally nonproductive cough, wheezing, and shortness of breath.[1256,1381] This condition is exceedingly common, particularly among males over age 40 years who smoke. Environmental factors (e.g., air pollution) and concomitant viral infections further irritate and inflame the respiratory mucosa, rendering them more susceptible to bacterial colonization and leading to the production of purulent sputum.[1381] In patients with stable chronic bronchitis, the lower airways are often colonized with multiple strains of nontypeable *H. influenzae;* during acute exacerbations the numbers of these organisms increase.[80,887] The occurrence of chronic cough and sputum production for at least three consecutive months for more than 2 years in succession is termed chronic obstructive pulmonary disease, or COPD.[1159,1256] Patients with severe exacerbations of chronic bronchitis and COPD present with dyspnea, hypoxia, and usually a low-grade fever. During exacerbations, sputum production is increased and the consistency changes from mucoid to mucopurulent to purulent.[1159,1381] Gram staining of properly collected sputum specimens generally shows many PMNs associated with a particular bacterial morphotype (e.g., the pale-staining coccobacilli of *H. influenzae*). The most common agents recovered from purulent sputum are nontypeable strains of *H. influenzae*, followed by *S. pneumoniae* and *M. catarrhalis*.[876,887,988] In patients with *H. influenzae*–associated disease, nontypeable strains can be isolated from the lower airways even between exacerbations of symptoms.[80,767] During exacerbations, empiric therapy with oral antimicrobial agents that cover *H. influenzae* and the other organisms are usually prescribed, along with bronchodilators and other supportive measures. In patients with severe airway obstruction who are producing increased amounts of purulent sputum, antimicrobial therapy significantly shortens the duration of symptoms.[326] Drugs that have demonstrated efficacy in this setting have included extended-spectrum cephalosporins, tetracyclines, quinolones (e.g., ciprofloxacin, prulifloxacin), and newer macrolides.[326] Chronic bronchitis, acute exacerbations of purulent bronchitis, COPD, and pneumonia may represent stages in a continuum of pathologic pulmonary processes in which nontypeable *H. influenzae* strains are a primary player. No doubt, various host factors (e.g., immune status, other pulmonary compromises, prior or concurrent viral infections) also contribute to the pathogenesis of this ill-defined condition.[1159]

PNEUMONIA

H. influenzae pneumonia can be another manifestation of systemic *H. influenzae* infection, or it may develop as a complication of COPD. *H. influenzae* pneumonia in patients with systemic disease (i.e., meningitis, epiglottitis, bacteremia, otitis media) is lobar, segmental, and purulent—characteristics similar to pneumococcal pneumonia. In these cases, encapsulated type b organisms are the usual etiologic agents. Nontypeable *H. influenzae* are important causes of pneumonia with and without bacteremia, particularly in elderly patients with underlying respiratory conditions such as chronic bronchitis, COPD, and bronchiectasis, or with systemic diseases, including immunodeficiency, diabetes, alcoholism, and neoplastic disease.[325,725,1134] In addition, bacteremic pneumonia due to *H. influenzae* capsular types other than type b have also been reported in patients with underlying conditions that impair local or systemic host defense mechanisms.[590] Definitive diagnosis of *H. influenzae* pneumonia is clouded by the presence of the organism in the upper respiratory tract of healthy individuals. Coughed, expectorated sputum specimens may provide inadequate or misleading results; bronchial washings, bronchoscopy, or bronchoalveolar lavage specimens may be necessary for definitive cultural diagnosis.

BACTEREMIA AND INFECTIOUS COMPLICATIONS OF BACTEREMIA

Bacteremia is a frequent and early manifestation of acute *H. influenzae* type b meningitis, but some infants may present with bacteremia without evidence of meningitis. The acute presentation is seen mostly in children with underlying disease (e.g., sickle cell disease) and includes fever, lethargy, and an increased peripheral neutrophil count. Bacteremia may seed the soft tissues, joints, and bone, resulting in cellulitis, septic arthritis, and osteomyelitis, respectively.[901] Cellulitis often appears in children as violaceous or reddish-blue swellings on the cheeks and periorbital areas of the face. Facial and periorbital cellulitis associated with *H. influenzae* type b has virtually disappeared since the introduction of the type b conjugate vaccines.[25,414] Cellulitis has also been described in adults in association with type b and nontypeable *H. influenzae* bacteremias.[772] Septic arthritis is characterized by pain, swelling, and decreased mobility of the infected joint.[770] Hematogenous osteomyelitis presents with constitutional symptoms, swelling, and bone pain. Although *H. influenzae* type b is still touted as the leading cause of septic arthritis in children beyond the neonatal period but less than 2 years of age, a retrospective study on 38 children with culture-documented septic arthritis between 1991 and 1997 revealed only one case due to type b *H. influenzae*.[803] This β-lactamase-negative strain was isolated in 1992 from an unimmunized 14-month-old child. Howard et al. reviewed 851 cases of septic arthritis and osteomyelitis from 1977 through 1997 in Ontario, and found that hematogenous *H. influenzae* type b septic arthritis and osteomyelitis accounted for 30% and 3% of these respective infections prior to 1992, but only one case of type b septic arthritis and no cases of osteomyelitis were seen from 1992 to 1997.[607] These results indicate that widespread vaccination has resulted in the virtual disappearance of type b organisms as etiologic agents of these complications of bacteremia.

H. influenzae bacteremia may also occur in neonates and the elderly. Acute neonatal sepsis due to *H. influenzae* has been reported as a distinct clinical entity.[440] In these cases, meningitis may or may not be present. Most cases of neonatal infection result from maternal-fetal or maternal-perinatal transmission (see below). Only 20% of isolates from bacteremias occurring during the neonatal period are type b strains, with the remainder being nontypeable.[440] Although *H. influenzae* type b sepsis has been reported in elderly adults, the majority of isolates from these individuals are nontypeable strains, with the respiratory tract as the usual source.[549,725,1134] Nontypeable *H. influenzae* bacteremia occurs mostly in older patients with underlying diseases (e.g., alcoholism, systemic lupus erythematosus [SLE], rheuma-

toid arthritis, diabetes, malignancies) and is associated with a variety of complications, including cellulitis, septic arthritis, osteomyelitis, empyema, intraabdominal infections, pyelonephritis, and endocarditis.[126,154,319,325,725,1134,1136]

ENDOCARDITIS

H. parainfluenzae, *H. aphrophilus*, and *H. paraphrophilus* are the *Haemophilus* species most frequently isolated from patients with endocarditis and intravascular infections, with typeable and nontypeable *H. influenzae* being relatively uncommon.[20,130,272,301,335,459,500,532] The incidence of endocarditis is highest in young to middle-aged adults. Although the mortality associated with properly treated *Haemophilus* endocarditis is usually about 10–15%, higher rates (25–50%) reported in the earlier literature probably reflected difficulties in recovering these fastidious organisms from blood cultures, resulting in inappropriate or inadequate antimicrobial therapy. Patients usually have a subacute clinical course with low-grade fever, malaise, chills, and respiratory tract symptoms. Preexisting or underlying valvular disease is found in only about half the cases, with the presence of a heart murmur being the only suggestive finding in these patients. Peripheral stigmata of endocarditis, such as Roth's spots, Janeway lesions, and splinter hemorrhages are usually absent. Disseminated intravascular coagulation and pulmonary hemorrhage have been reported, and both hematuria and anemia may be seen with this infection.[1177] Echocardiography studies have demonstrated that *H. aphrophilus* endocarditis is associated with a high incidence of valvular vegetations and septic complications resulting from embolization to the large arteries. Risk factors for endocarditis with *Haemophilus* species include the presence of dental or oral lesions (i.e., periodontitis, trauma, penetrating oral wounds), antecedent dental manipulations or oral surgery, diseased or damaged cardiac valves (e.g., rheumatic heart disease, congenital defects, previous cardiac surgery), and the presence of prosthetic valves.[130,272] *H. parainfluenzae* has also been implicated in cases of polymicrobial endocarditis in intravenous drug users.[1051] These patients typically present with right-sided endocarditis, tricuspid valve vegetations on echocardiography, and clinical and radiographic evidence of septic pulmonary embolization. *H. parainfluenzae* has also been associated with sustained bacteremia resulting from infection of vascular implants, such as pacemaker wires.[1096]

UROGENITAL, MATERNAL, AND PERINATAL INFECTIONS

Haemophilus species, particularly nontypeable *H. influenzae* and *H. parainfluenzae*, have been recognized as uncommon causes of urethritis, female genital tract infections, prepubertal vulvovaginitis, obstetrical and gynecologic infections, postpartum bacteremia, and neonatal sepsis with and without meningitis.[287,288,726,979,1038,1234] Sturm reported that either *H. influenzae* or *H. parainfluenzae* was the only organisms (including chlamydiae and ureaplasmas) recovered from 10% of 242 episodes of nongonococcal urethritis in 234 men; *Haemophilus* species were not recovered from asymptomatic men.[1234] In a study conducted in Houston between 1976 and 1981, *H. influenzae* was recovered from blood cultures of 16 women with postpartum bacteremia and 36 neonates with bacteremia or meningitis.[1346] Another 50 *H. influenzae* isolates not associated with bacteremia or meningitis were cultured from genital sites (vagina, endometrium, cervix, Bartholin's glands, fallopian tubes, male urethra, and prostatic fluid) and fetal tissues (amniotic fluid, placental tissues). Of these isolates, 94% were serologically nontypeable. Quentin and colleagues recovered *Haemophilus* species from genital cultures of 83 women over a 90-month period.[1038] Of the 83 women, 42 had significant bacterial genital tract infections, including endometritis, salpingitis, and Bartholin's gland abscesses. Genital tract infection was linked to the presence of intrauterine devices in 62% of the patients with endometritis and in four of six patients with salpingitis, suggesting that the genital hemophili may behave as opportunistic agents in genital sites. Prenatal and perinatal acquisition of *Haemophilus* species from the maternal genital tract was also associated with prematurity, premature rupture of membranes, amnionitis, and neonatal sepsis in this and other studies.[287,979]

Biotyping of genital isolates (see below) has shown that nontypeable biotype IV *H. influenzae* and biotype I and II *H. parainfluenzae* strains are frequent inhabitants of the genital tract and are the ones that cause localized genital tract infections and postpartum maternal and neonatal systemic infections.[1038] Additional studies of serologically nontypeable *H. influenzae* strains recovered from these infections have suggested the existence of a novel, cryptic genospecies of *H. influenzae*.[1036–1038] This genospecies types biochemically as biotype IV (i.e., indole-negative, urease-positive, and ornithine decarboxylase–positive) but is distinct by other phenotypic and genetic criteria. These strains possess peritrichous fimbriae, have a distinctive OMP profile on polyacrylamide gel electrophoresis, express a variant P6 OMP (see Box 9-3), and display a unique enzyme pattern on multilocus enzyme electrophoresis.[913,1037] DNA-DNA hybridization and ribosomal DNA restriction-fragment-length polymorphism studies indicate that these isolates are clonal and genetically homogeneous, share less than 70% overall genomic similarity with *H. influenzae sensu stricto*, and are most closely related to strains of *H. haemolyticus*.[1037] Currently, this cryptic genospecies cannot be phenotypically differentiated from other *H. influenzae* biotype IV strains. This pathogen is being further characterized to determine the properties that contribute to its virulence in genital tract and neonatal infections.[1094]

OCULAR INFECTIONS

H. influenzae causes ocular infections that vary widely in severity, including conjunctivitis, scleritis, and endophthalmitis. *H. influenzae* causes a contagious, acute conjunctivitis colloquially called "pinkeye." Localized outbreaks of acute conjunctivitis occur among persons who share towels, handkerchiefs, or other objects that come in direct contact with the skin of the face or eyes. The diffuse pink color of the sclera and the presence of a serous or purulent discharge is virtually diagnostic of Haemophilus conjunctivitis. Hemorrhagic conjunctivitis may also occur as part of the clinical presentation of invasive *H. influenzae* type b disease.[994] *H. influenzae* endophthalmitis is uncommon but may occur as an iatrogenic complication of ocular surgery (e.g., following glaucoma-filtering procedures).[21,1146] Sykes and colleagues reported on three cases of *H. influenzae* scleritis.[1240] These

elderly patients presented with severely decreased visual acuity, pain, and nodular scleral abscesses from which *H. influenzae* was recovered in culture. *H. influenzae* may also be isolated from superinfected herpetic corneal ulcers and from corneal specimens of patients with atopic keratoconjunctivitis.[1181]

Historically, isolates from conjunctival infections were designated as a separate species called "*H. aegyptius*." Phenotypically, these isolates are similar to *H. influenzae* biotype III. The distinctive clinical presentation, biochemical characteristics, and serologic studies have been used to support the status of "*H. aegyptius*" as a separate species within the genus. However, genomic nucleotide studies have demonstrated significant sequence homology between "*H. aegyptius*" and *H. influenzae*, so this organism is now called *H. influenzae* biogroup *aegyptius*. A unique, highly virulent clone of *H. influenzae* biogroup *aegyptius* emerged in the early 1980s as a causative agent of a clinical syndrome called Brazilian purpuric fever.

BRAZILIAN PURPURIC FEVER

During the 1980s, a subgroup of strains that were phenotypically indistinguishable from *H. influenzae* biotype III ("*H. aegyptius*") were recognized in association with outbreaks of a severe illness called Brazilian purpuric fever (BPF).[157,158,541] BPF was first reported in 1984 in the rural town of Promissao, São Paulo State, Brazil, when 10 children (ages from 3 months to 8 years) died from an acute illness characterized by a high fever, abdominal pain with vomiting, a petechial/purpuric rash, hypotensive shock, and vascular collapse. A subsequent outbreak among 10 children in the nearby town of Serrana resulted in four additional deaths.[159] Blood cultures from these children grew *H. aegyptius*. Although BPF resembled meningococcal disease, meningitis was not part of the clinical presentation. During epidemiologic investigations, cases were found to have had recent or concurrent purulent conjunctivitis.[157] Since the initial outbreaks, sporadic cases have been reported in other areas of Brazil and in central and western Australia.[159,847,1375]

Outbreak-associated *H. aegyptius* strains recovered from blood and/or conjunctival cultures have been studied extensively and possess several characteristics not found in *H. aegyptius* isolated from cases of purulent conjunctivitis without BPF.[167,201,384,1022,1367] These characteristics include serologic nontypeability, the presence of a unique 24-kDa plasmid, a distinctive 25-kDa OMP, a unique immunoglobulin A1 protease, and resistance to the bactericidal effects of normal human serum. The 25-kDa OMP is a fimbrial protein with 71% sequence homology with the major *H. influenzae* type b fimbrial protein; cloning and sequencing of fimbrial genes from these strains have demonstrated 82% sequence homology with fimbrial genes of reference *H. influenzae* type b strains.[1229,1367,1374] Erythrocyte agglutination and agglutination-inhibition studies have also shown that this fimbrial protein binds to the same red cell surface receptor as the *H. influenzae* type b fimbrial protein.[1231] BPF strains possess a stable, highly conserved cell surface epitope of the 48-kDa P1 OMP that is not present in non-BFP-associated strains.[771] These studies concluded that the outbreaks of BPF were caused by a unique clone of *H. aegyptius* that has been designated "*H. influenzae* biogroup *aegyptius.*" Isolates that have been recovered from subsequent outbreaks or sporadic cases of BPF in Brazil apparently lack the 24-kDa plasmid, and Australian BPF strains also do not have some of the unusual markers.[733] The Australian strains apparently represent a second BFP clone.[839] BPF cases or outbreaks have not been reported elsewhere, although this diagnosis was suspected in a 17-month-old male from Connecticut who presented with purulent conjunctivitis, fever, lethargy, and a positive blood culture with nontypeable *H. influenzae* biotype III.[1331] Postmortem examinations of liver, spleen, and lymph nodes established that overwhelming Epstein-Barr infection was the cause of the child's illness.

Studies on BPF isolates have also suggested that the organisms possess a capsule, even though they are nontypeable. Carlone and coworkers reported that DNA from BPF isolates hybridized with a probe containing DNA sequences involved in *H. influenzae* capsular polysaccharide synthesis (i.e. *cap* gene sequences).[201] However, Dobson and colleagues found that the probe used in the earlier studies contained sequences that were homologous not only to the *cap* genes of typeable *H. influenzae* strains, but the probe also contained sequences of an insertion element (IS*1016*) that is present in BFP-related *H. influenzae* biogroup *aegyptius* strains but not in non-BPF *H. influenzae* strains.[337] Transposition of the IS*1016* sequences from a plasmid into the genome of the BPF clone may have contributed to virulence by altering transcription and expression of genes adjacent to the insertion site.[337] In vivo studies using an infant rat model and in vitro studies with a human microvascular endothelial cell line also have shown that BPF-associated strains of *H. influenzae* biogroup *aegyptius* are more virulent and cytotoxic than non-BPF-associated *H. influenzae* strains.[1105,1370] Based on multilocus enzyme electrophoresis methods, biogroup *aegyptius* isolates form three distinct lineages within the species *H. influenzae*. The BPF isolates are not closely related genetically to non-BPF biogroup *aegyptius* strain but do show a close genetic relationship with encapsulated *H. influenzae* capsular serotype c.[620,916]

MISCELLANEOUS *HAEMOPHILUS INFLUENZAE* INFECTIONS

H. influenzae type b may cause other uncommon infections; in some cases, recovery of *Haemophilus* species was unexpected. Periorbital and facial cellulitis, a frequent finding in children with type b bacteremia, has been reported in adults with bacteremia and respiratory tract infections.[356] *H. influenzae* has been isolated from abdominal infections (i.e., peritonitis, pancreatic abscesses, appendicitis), and hepatobiliary tract infections (i.e., cholecystitis, pyogenic liver abscess).[67,953,1034] Bacteremic epididymitis and orchitis due to *H. influenzae* was also diagnosed in a patient with HIV-1 disease.[290]

Although sporadic infections due to encapsulated non-type b *H. influenzae* occurred prior to the availability of the type b vaccine, serious infections caused by both non-type b capsular serotypes and nontypeable strains of *H. influenzae* are being increasingly recognized in the vaccine era.[2,548] In 2001, five cases of invasive disease caused by *H. influenzae* serotype a were seen over a 10-month period in Utah.[2] These children (median age, 12 years) presented with meningitis, bacteremia, and, in one case, purpura fulminans. Examination of available isolates with molecular techniques revealed that three of the four available isolates contained a deletion in the IS*1016-bex* A gene, a characteristic also found in virulent serotype b strains. Examination of 48 invasive non-type b *H. influenzae* by restriction endonuclease typing showed that type a strains segregated into two major clonal groups, while type e and type f strains, respectively, represented single clones. The researchers proposed that the increased incidence of non-type b encapsulated *H. influenzae* reflected either the emergence of hypervirulent clones or the limited genetic diversity among non-type b strains.[970] In a study conducted in Brazil before and during the introduction of active immunization, the incidence of *H. influenzae* type a meningitis increased eightfold during the time in which the incidence of type b meningitis had decreased by 69%.[1070] As mentioned previously, bacteremic *H. influenzae* infections occurring in the vaccine era are largely due to nontypeable strains.[325,395,910] These infections generally occur in individuals with significant underlying disease (e.g., Hodgkin's disease, acute lymphocytic leukemia) and in those with underlying defects in immunoglobulin production.

Haemophilus parainfluenzae

H. parainfluenzae is an uncommon agent of human infections. Besides endocarditis (see section on "Endocarditis," above), *H. parainfluenzae* has been isolated from cases of bacteremic epiglottitis, bronchitis, sinusitis, otitis media, COPD, pneumonia, empyema, peritonitis, cellulitis, abscesses, neonatal sepsis; native and prosthetic joint infections, genital and biliary tract infections, and brain abscess.[24,68,123,232,435,573,633,962,987,1013,1031,1349] Olk et al., reported a case of *H. parainfluenzae* vertebral osteomyelitis that became clinically apparent 3 months after the patient underwent nasal septoplasty; presumably this surgical procedure caused a bacteremia that seeded the lumbosacral vertebrae.[967] This organism has also been isolated on rare occasions as a cause of urinary tract infection in adults.[895] McClain and coworkers reported a case of *H. parainfluenzae* purulent urethritis in a 24-year-old male that was accompanied by bacteremia with the same organism, and *H. parainfluenzae* prostatitis has also been reported in a 29-year-old man with HIV-1 infection.[258,843] Rare *H. parainfluenzae* hepatobiliary tract infections, including liver abscess, have been reported in both children and adults.[24,438,616] In these latter infections, it was postulated that *H. parainfluenzae* gained access to the hepatobiliary tree from the intestinal tract rather than via a hematogenous route. This is supported by the lack of documented *H. parainfluenzae* bacteremia in the patients, and the fact that *H. parainfluenzae* has been recovered from the gastrointestinal tract much more frequently than other haemophili.[850]

Haemophilus aphrophilus and *Haemophilus paraphrophilus*

H. aphrophilus and *H. paraphrophilus* are indigenous to the oral cavity, where they are minor components of the healthy periodontal flora.[1268] Among the hemophili, *H.*

aphrophilus and *H. paraphrophilus*, along with *H. parainfluenzae*, are the species most commonly associated with endocarditis (see section on "Endocarditis," above). In addition, these bacteria also cause head and neck infections (i.e., sinusitis, otitis media, epiglottitis, brain abscess), infections resulting from hematogenous dissemination (i.e., pneumonia, empyema, septic arthritis, vertebral osteomyelitis, cellulitis, endophthalmitis, meningitis, necrotizing fasciitis), abdominal infections (i.e., hepatobiliary tract infections, cholecystitis, abdominal abscesses), and wound infections.[275,332,377,650,663,880,1371] Neutropenia, malignancy, and cancer chemotherapy are predisposing factors for infections with these organisms.[377] *H. aphrophilus* and *H. paraphrophilus* resemble other fastidious gram-negative bacteria culturally and are part of the "HACEK" group, which includes hemophili (H), *Actinobacillus* (A), *Cardiobacterium* (C), *Eikenella* (E), and *Kingella* (K) species. These organisms will be discussed later in this chapter.

Other *Haemophilus* Species

H. haemolyticus, *H. parahaemolyticus*, and *H. paraphrohaemolyticus* are part of the normal respiratory tract flora and are rarely associated with infections. *H. segnis* has been isolated from dental plaque and the upper respiratory tract. In 1981, Bullock and Devitt reported on the isolation of *H. segnis* from blood and pus of a pancreatic abscess in a 29-year-old alcoholic male.[188] Subsequently, Welch et al. described the isolation of *H. segnis*, in both pure and mixed cultures, from five cases of acute appendicitis.[1362] This organism was also recovered, along with anaerobic organisms, from a cutaneous umbilical abscess of a 70-year-old women.[252] Further investigation of these fastidious organisms is needed for a more complete appreciation of their pathogenic potential.

Haemophilus ducreyi

H. ducreyi is the causative agent of chancroid, a highly contagious sexually transmitted infection characterized by painful genital and perianal ulcers and tender inguinal lymphadenopathy.[1088] Chancroid is a major cause of genital ulcer disease in Latin America, Africa, East and Southeast Asia, and India. Outbreaks of chancroid have been reported in a number of coastal cities in the United States and Canada. In these outbreaks, prostitutes have been the usual reservoir, with the exchange of sex for money or drugs (e.g., crack cocaine) being a major behavioral risk factor. In these outbreaks, male-to-female case ratios of 3:1 to 25:1 have been observed.[241]

Although several potential virulence factors have been identified in *H. ducreyi*, at present their roles in pathogenesis are poorly understood. All strains appear to have fine, tangled, surface fimbriae, 40-kDA and 18-kDa OMPs, lipooligosaccharide, and a cytotoxin/hemolysin.[12,13,169,1211,1284,1394] The role of these molecules in disease pathogenesis is currently not clear. *H. ducreyi* also has a specific growth requirement for iron, and, although it lacks siderophores, the organism has a receptor on its surface that binds hemoglobin and is essential for iron uptake.[370] In vitro, *H. ducreyi* is able to attach, invade, and cause cytopathic effects in cultured human foreskin cells, and several animal models for chancroid have been developed to study virulence and pathogenicity, including rabbit, piglet, primate and human volunteer models.[14,23,1235]

Genital lesions caused by this organism are also called "soft chancres" because, unlike the primary lesion (chancre) of syphilis, the borders of the lesion are ragged and pliable rather than sharply demarcated and indurated (see Color Plate 9-2B).[1088] After an incubation period of 4 to 7 days, the lesions begin as tender erythematous papules that become pustular, eroded, and ulcerated within the next 48 to 72 hours. In males, chancroid lesions are usually tender, painful, and are covered with a yellow-gray exudate overlying a beefy, bleeding base. In males, one to three lesions are usually present on the external genitalia; in uncircumcised men, these lesions are often found beneath the foreskin. In females, multiple lesions may be present on the labia, within the vagina, and in the perianal area. Lesions may coalesce to form large ulcerative areas that may become superinfected. Extragenital chancroid is uncommon, but lesions have been described on the glabrous skin, in the mouth, and on the conjunctivae. In about half of the infected patients, painful unilateral inguinal lymphadenopathy develops. These enlarged lymph nodes may actually suppurate through the overlying skin to form large inguinal abscesses, draining fistulas, and sinus tracts.

In undeveloped countries, infection with *H. ducreyi* is associated with transmission of human immunodeficiency virus type 1 (HIV-1) and type 2 (HIV-2). Studies in Africa have provided evidence that chancroid is a risk factor for heterosexual transmission of HIV-1, the etiologic agent of AIDS.[729,1178] Genital ulcers due to chancroid and other agents (e.g., syphilis) apparently render women more susceptible to infection with HIV-1 following heterosexual contact with infected men, and the presence of genital ulcers in HIV-1 infected women also increases the probability that their male sexual partners will become infected. Genital ulcers due to chancroid and other diseases, such as lymphogranuloma venereum, apparently facilitate the passage of the virus into vaginal secretions. In Kenya, for example, it appears that perhaps one third of HIV-1 infections in prostitutes and at least half of the HIV-1 infections in their male clients are significantly related to concomitant infection with *H. ducreyi*.[729]

Laboratory Diagnosis of *Haemophilus* Infections
DIRECT EXAMINATION OF CLINICAL SPECIMENS
Gram Stain. A rapid presumptive diagnosis of *H. influenzae* meningitis can be made by direct examination of CSF using the Gram's stain. If sufficient (i.e., more than 1–2 mL) CSF is received, the specimen is centrifuged to obtain a pellet of material for examination and culture. Cytocentrifugation of CSF specimens enhances detection of small numbers of organisms and considerably increases the sensitivity of the Gram stain in comparison with conventionally centrifuged or uncentrifuged specimens.[227] On Gram stain preparations, *Haemophilus* organisms appear as small, pale-staining, gram-negative coccobacilli (see Color Plate 9-1A). Occasionally, slender filamentous cells may be observed. Although *H. influenzae* may be the likely pathogen on the basis

of the gram-stain appearance and the patient's clinical presentation, the organisms cannot be identified on the basis of the gram-stained smear alone. Furthermore, a negative Gram's stain does not rule out the possibility of *Haemophilus* infection because very few organisms may be present in the specimen. Gram stain smears of other specimen types may also be useful for presumptive diagnosis. In a 2000 study, the sensitivity and specificity of the sputum gram stain for diagnosis of community-acquired *H. influenzae* pneumonia were 82% and 99%, respectively, if the specimen was judged as adequate by sputum screening criteria.[1098]

Detection of Type B Capsular Antigen. For rapid diagnosis of *H. influenzae* type b infections, immunologic techniques are available for the detection of the type b PRP capsular antigen in CSF, serum, and urine (Chapter 3). Commercially available methods include latex particle agglutination (LA) and staphylococcal protein A coagglutination (COA) techniques. Commercial LA kits include the Directigen Meningitis Combo Test Kit (BD Biosciences, Sparks, MD) and the Wellcogen Bacterial Antigen Kit (Murex Diagnostics, Dartford, England). The commercial COA test is the Phadebact CSF test (Boule Diagnostics, Huddinge, Sweden). All of these kits contain reagents for detecting *H. influenzae* group b PRP antigen along with reagents for *S. pneumoniae*, *N. meningitidis*, and group B streptococcal antigen detection in body fluids. Several studies have compared LA and COA for their relative sensitivities and specificities in detecting *H. influenzae* type b PRP antigen in various body fluids from patients with meningeal and nonmeningeal infections.[271,820,1359] Most studies indicate that LA and COA are generally more sensitive and detect smaller amounts of antigen than countercurrent immunoelectrophoresis (CIE), the older method for detection of bacterial antigens in body fluids.

Despite the performance of these tests in clinical trials that led to their approval for use, many laboratories have discontinued offering these tests routinely. Aside from the high cost of the latex/COA reagents themselves, their diagnostic and prognostic utility has not been borne out after years of experience. Perkins et al. reviewed all latex tests performed over a 10-month period at two hospitals and found 57 positive results.[1001] Review of these cases revealed that 31 results were false-positives, 22 were true-positives, and 4 were indeterminate. False-positive tests were noted most often with urine specimens. Patients with false-positive test results received unnecessary treatment that resulted in prolonged hospitalization and additional complications. Furthermore, among the 22 cases with true-positive LA results, there was no instance in which the antimicrobial therapy or clinical treatment of the patient was altered on the basis of the LA result. These tests may be most useful in cases of suspected meningitis for which the initial gram stain is negative and/or the CSF cultures are negative after 48 hours.[410] The recommended method for optimal direct detection of *H. influenzae* in CSF depends on careful inspection of a gram-stained smear prepared from a cytocentrifuged specimen. Latex methods are also much less sensitive for direct detection than molecular approaches. Singhi and colleagues examined the CSF from 107 children with suspected meningitis; 79% of these children had also received antibiotics.[1179] *H. influenzae* type b was isolated in 14 cases, the latex agglu-

tination test was positive in 23 cases, and PCR for *H. influenzae* type b was positive in 37 cases, including all those that were culture- or latex agglutination-positive.

CULTURE OF *HAEMOPHILUS* SPECIES

Optimal recovery of *Haemophilus* species from clinical specimens depends on proper collection and transport of specimens, and the use of appropriate culture media and incubation environments. Because these organisms are fastidious, specimens containing them should not be exposed to drying or to temperature extremes. Crucial specimens such as CSF should be hand-carried to the clinical laboratory as soon after collection as possible. Conventional sheep blood agar is not suitable for recovery of *Haemophilus* species that require V factor for growth because of the presence of V factor–inactivating enzymes in native sheep blood.[59] Rabbit or horse blood does not contain these enzymes, and agar media containing either of these blood products will support the growth of most *Haemophilus* species. Regardless of the media used, isolation of *Haemophilus* requires incubation at 35 to 37°C in a moist environment with increased CO_2 (3–5%). This atmosphere is provided by modern CO_2 incubators or by candle extinction jars. Primary isolation of *Haemophilus* species from clinical specimens is accomplished by using chocolate agar, *Haemophilus* isolation agar, or the staphylococcus streak technique.

Chocolate Agar. Chocolate agar is prepared by adding sheep blood to an enriched agar base when the temperature of the medium is high enough to lyse the red cells without inactivating the NAD in the blood lysate (i.e., about 80°C). Most clinical laboratories purchase chocolate agar and other bacteriologic media from commercial vendors. Commercially prepared ''chocolate agar'' usually contains a synthetic mixture of hemin and a ''cocktail'' of chemically defined growth factors that are added to GC (gonococcal) agar base medium. GC agar base contains proteose peptone, cornstarch. monobasic and dibasic phosphate buffers, sodium chloride, and agar. The chemically defined supplement contains NAD, vitamins (B_{12}, thiamine hydrochloride), minerals (iron, magnesium), amino acids that are required for growth of fastidious bacteria (cysteine, glutamine), and glucose. These supplements are available commercially under the trade names IsoVitalex (BD Biosciences) and GCHI Enrichment (Remel Laboratories, Lenexa, KS).

The disadvantage of using chocolate agar for primary isolation of *Haemophilus* species is that the medium does not allow the determination of hemolytic properties, which help to differentiate *H. haemolyticus* and *H. parahaemolyticus* from *H. influenzae* and *H. parainfluenzae*, respectively. However, it is an excellent medium for the recovery of other fastidious organisms, such as *N. meningitidis* and *N. gonorrhoeae*, from specimens that are not commonly contaminated with other organisms, such as CSF or joint fluid. Because *Haemophilus* species are common inhabitants of the upper respiratory tract (including both hemolytic and nonhemolytic species), many laboratories have adopted *Hemophilus* isolation agar for recovery of these organisms from respiratory specimens. Selective chocolate agar based–media containing various antibiotics (e.g., vancomycin, bacitracin, and clindamycin) have been described but are not widely used.[950]

Haemophilus *Isolation Agar.* Commercial vendors market antibiotic-containing media for the selective isolation of *Haemophilus* species from respiratory tract specimens. These media contain beef heart infusion, peptones, yeast extract, and defibrinated horse blood (5%) containing both X and V factors. Bacitracin (300 μg/mL) is added to inhibit the other normal respiratory tract flora, including staphylococci, micrococci, neisseriae, and streptococci. Besides the selective recovery of *Haemophilus* species from heavily mixed cultures, hemolytic properties of the hemophili can be determined directly on primary isolation.

Staphylococcus *Streak Technique.* Many bacteria and yeasts synthesize and secrete NAD during growth on bacteriologic media. In mixed cultures, *Haemophilus* species that require V factor may grow as pinpoint colonies around the colonies of these other microorganisms. This phenomenon is called satellitism. Satellitism provides a technique for detecting these organisms in mixed cultures as well as a presumptive test for genus-level identification. A colony of a possible *Haemophilus* species is subcultured to a sheep blood agar plate and streaked as a lawn. Using an inoculating wire, a single streak of an NAD-producing organism, such as *S. aureus*, is made through the inoculum of the possible *Haemophilus*. After overnight growth in a CO_2-enriched environment at 35 to 37°C, tiny moist gray colonies of the hemophili may be observed within the hemolytic area adjacent to the staphylococcal growth. X factor–dependent hemophili will also grow as satellite colonies because hemin and hematin are released from the lysed red blood cells by the action of staphylococcal hemolysins (see Color Plate 9-1*C*). This method may be used for presumptive identification of *Haemophilus* species when species-level identification is not required or essential (e.g., upper respiratory tract specimens).

IDENTIFICATION OF *HAEMOPHILUS* SPECIES

Colony Morphology and Cultural Characteristics. On chocolate agar, colonies of *H. influenzae* are smooth and blue-gray in color; heavily encapsulated strains may appear mucoid (see Color Plate 9-1*B*). Most strains produce convex, smooth, entire colonies of 1–2 mm after overnight growth. Some strains will have an ''*E. coli*'' odor because of the production of indole. *H. parainfluenzae* colonies are usually smaller, light gray, and have a matte appearance on growth media. Oxidase and catalase reactions for these organisms are usually positive, although the oxidase reaction may be delayed. Colonies of *H. aphrophilus* and *H. paraphrophilus* are small after 24 hours of incubation; 48 to 72 hours of incubation is often required before colony morphology can be ascertained and sufficient growth is available for preliminary identification tests. On chocolate agar, colonies are 0.5 to 1 mm in diameter, convex, granular, and have a yellowish pigment (see Color Plates 9-1*D*, 9-1*E*, and 9-1*F*). A distinct ''grade-school paste'' odor may be detected. *H aphrophilus* does not require V factor and will grow on sheep blood agar and on BHI or trypticase-soy agar without supplementation. *H. paraphrophilus* is biochemically similar to *H. aphrophilus*, except that V factor is required for growth. These organisms are oxidase-negative, although weak or delayed positive reactions may be observed with some isolates. Both *H. aphrophilus* and *H. paraphrophilus* are also catalase-

negative, a characteristic that helps differentiate them from *Actinobacillus actinomycetemcomitans*, which resembles these other fastidious organisms (see Color Plates 9-1*C* and 9-1*D*).

Identification Procedures. Commonly encountered *Haemophilus* species are identified by their hemolytic reactions on horse blood agar and their growth requirements for X and V factors (Table 9-2). Filter paper disks or strips impregnated with X factor, V factor, or both, are routinely used to determine these factor requirements. The organism to be identified is streaked as a lawn on media deficient in growth factors, such as trypticase-soy agar. It is important when selecting colonies from primary culture plates for this test that none of the chocolate agar or other blood-containing media is transferred to the factor determination plate. Suspending the organism in factor-deficient broth before plate inoculation is one way to reduce carryover of growth factors and consequent false-positive results. The X and V factor disks or strips are placed on the agar surface about 1 to 2 cm apart. If a disk/strip containing both factors is also used, the disks may be more widely spaced on the agar surface. The plates are incubated in 5–7% CO_2 at 35°C for 18 to 24 hours, and the patterns of growth around the disks/strips are observed. Differentiation of *Haemophilus* species is then made on the basis of the growth patterns shown in Chart 9-1 and in Color Plates 9-1*D* and 9-1*E*.

Doern and Chapin evaluated the performance of trypticase-soy agar, brain-heart infusion agar, nutrient agar, and Mueller-Hinton agar in the factor disk identification of 187 *H. influenzae* isolates.[341] They found that 95.7%, 92.5%, 56.1%, and 71.1% of isolates were correctly identified on the four media, respectively. False-positive readings of growth around V factor disks (resulting in misidentifications of *H. influenzae* as *H. parainfluenzae*) on brain-heart infusion agar and failure of strains to grow on Mueller-Hinton and nutrient agars were the principal findings of the study. Trypticase-soy agar was recommended as the medium of choice for performance of the growth factor determination procedure.

Although interpretation of factor requirement tests are generally clear-cut, misidentifications caused by confusing *H. influenzae* with *H. parainfluenzae* and vice versa have been reported owing to inconsistent results in X factor determinations. The following reasons were cited for these inaccuracies: 1) the presence of varying trace amounts of hemin in the basal medium used for the factor determination test; 2) the carryover of X factor in inocula taken from colonies growing on blood-containing medium; and 3) the fastidious nature of some *H. parainfluenzae* strains and the consequent difficulty in reading factor tests for these strains. The δ-aminolevulinic acid (ALA)-porphyrin test circumvents many of the problems described above for the determination of X factor requirements.[684,909] This test is a direct assessment of the ability of *Haemophilus* strains to synthesize protoporphyrin intermediates in the biosynthetic pathway to hemin from the precursor compound δ-aminolevulinic acid. Strains that require exogenous X factor for growth (i.e., *H. influenzae* and *H. haemolyticus*) are incapable of synthesizing protoporphyrins from ALA and, consequently are negative with this test. Strains that do not require exogenous X factor for growth (i.e., *H. parainfluenzae* and *H. parahaemolyticus*) possess the enzymes that synthesize protoporphyrin compounds from the ALA substrate and are, consequently,

Table 9-2 Characteristics for Identification of Human *Haemophilus* Species

SPECIES BIOTYPE	HEMO-LYSIS	REQUIREMENT FOR: X	REQUIREMENT FOR: V	ALA TEST	INDOLE TEST	UREASE TEST	ORNITHINE DE-CARBOXYLASE	ACID PRODUCTION FROM: Glucose	Sucrose	Lactose	Fructose	Ribose	Xylose	Mannose
H. influenzae														
Biotype I	−	+	+	−	+	+	+	+	−	−	−	+	+	−
Biotype II	−	+	+	−	+	+	−	+	−	−	−	+	+	−
Biotype III*	−	+	+	−	−	+	−	+	−	−	−	+	+	−
Biotype IV	−	+	+	−	−	+	+	+	−	−	−	+	+	−
Biotype V	−	+	+	−	+	−	+	+	−	−	−	+	+	−
Biotype VI	−	+	+	−	−	−	+	+	−	−	−	+	+	−
Biotype VII	−	+	+	−	+	+	−	+	−	−	−	+	+	−
Biotype VIII	−	+	+	−	−	−	−	+	−	−	−	+	+	−
Biogroup *aegyptius*	−	+	+	−	−	+	−	+	−	−	−	+w	−	−
H. parainfluenzae†														
Biotype I	−	−	+	+	−	−	+	+	+	−	+	−	−	+
Biotype II	−	−	+	+	−	+	+	+	+	−	+	−	−	+
Biotype III	−	−	+	+	−	+	−	+	+	−	+	−	−	+
Biotype IV	−	−	+	+	+	+	+	+	+	−	+	NA	NA	+
Biotype VI	−	−	+	+	+	−	+	+	+	−	+	NA	NA	V
Biotype VII	−	−	+	+	+	+	−	+	+	−	NA	−	−	NA
Biotype VIII	−	−	+	+	+	−	−	+	+	−	NA	−	−	NA
H. haemolyticus	+	+	+	−	V	+	−	+	−	−	+w	+	V	−
H. parahaemolyticus	+	−	+	+	−	+	V	+	+	−	+	−	−	−
H. segnis	−	−	+	+	−	−	−	+	+w	−	+w	−	−	−
H. aprophilus	−	−	−	+	−	−	−	+	+	+	+	+	−	+
H. paraprophilus	−	−	+	+	−	−	−	+	+	+	+	+	−	+
H. paraphrophaemo-lyticus	+	−	+	+	−	+	−	+	+	−	+	−	−	−
H. ducreyi	+w	+	−	−	−	−	−	−	−	−	−	−	−	−

+, positive; −, negative; +w, weak positive; v, variable; NA, not available.
* Biotyping reactions are identical with those of *H. influenzae* biogroup *aegyptius*, but the biogroup *aegyptius* strains are *xylose-negative.*
† Biotype V strains of *H. parainfluenza* are identical to *H. segnis.*

ALA-porphyrin test–positive. In addition, both *H. aphrophilus* and *H. paraphrophilus* are ALA-porphyrin test–positive. ALA-impregnated filter paper disks (BD Biosciences; Remel Laboratories) or growth media containing the ALA reagent (Remel Laboratories) may also be used to perform the ALA-porphyrin test (see Color Plates 9-1*F* and 9-1*G*). With the disk method, the impregnated disk is moistened with water and inoculated with organisms from growth media. After 4 hours of incubation, the disk is observed under an ultraviolet lamp (Wood's light). Brick-red fluorescence in the area of organism deposition indicates a positive test result; bluish fluorescence constitutes a negative test result. With the ALA agar medium, the organism is inoculated onto the medium and incubated overnight. The next day the growth is examined under a Wood's light for brick-red fluorescence.

Tests for hemolysis on horse blood agar, factor requirements, and the ALA porphyrin test have been incorporated into commercially available sectored-plate systems for identification of *Haemophilus* species. These include the Haemophilus ID II Triplate and the *Haemophilus* ID Quad plate (Remel). The triplate is a three-sectored plate containing horse blood agar, agar containing V factor, and agar containing ALA-agar. Following inoculation and overnight incubation, the plate is read by inspecting the blood agar sector for hemolysis, looking for growth in the V-factor sector, and looking for brick-red fluorescent growth in the ALA -sector under Wood's light illumination. The quad-plate contains four sectors contain factor-supplemented Mueller-Hinton medium with horse blood, X factor–enriched medium, V factor–enriched medium, and medium containing both X and V factors, respectively. Based on the hemolytic reaction and the pattern of growth in the remaining quadrants, the isolate can be identified.

Serotyping of Haemophilus influenzae.
The easiest technique for serotyping isolates is slide agglutination. A dense suspension of the organism is prepared in saline. Single drops of the suspension are placed in each of a series of circles on a glass slide corresponding to the number of sera to be tested, plus a saline control. Type-specific antisera are added to each of the test circles, and the slide is rotated. Rapid (i.e., less than 1 minute) agglutination of organisms by a specific antiserum and the absence of agglutination in the saline control identifies the isolate as a specific serotype. Polyvalent and type-specific antisera for all six *H. influenzae* serotypes are commercially available from BD Biosciences. Serotyping of clinical isolates by slide agglutination must be carefully performed with reliable reagents that are quality-controlled with organisms of known serotype. In a recent study, the CDC found significant discrepancies between results of serologic typing performed at state health departments and detection of capsular genes by PCR (see below). In an examination of 141 *H. influenzae* isolates from state health departments, 56 (40%) of isolates identified as a particular serotype were nontypeable by PCR, and two isolates reported as types b and f were found to be types f and e, respectively, by PCR.[743] Furthermore, of 40 isolates identified as *H. influenzae* type b by slide agglutination, 27 (68%) did not contain capsular type b genes. Institution of strict quality-control guidelines in three health department "test" laboratories resulted in significant improvement, with an

overall agreement of 94% between the slide agglutination results and capsular gene PCR.

A coagglutination culture confirmation test (Phadebact *Haemophilus* Test, Boule Diagnostics) is available for simultaneous identification and serotyping of *H. influenzae* type b from primary culture media. This kit contains a vial of staphylococcal cells sensitized with type b antisera (test reagent) and a second vial of staphylococci sensitized with antisera to types a, c, d, e, and f (control reagent). Colonies from growth media are mixed with each of the two reagents on a cardboard slide. After mixing, the slide is rocked for 30 to 60 seconds. Visible agglutination of the mixture with the type b test reagent but not the control reagent identifies the isolate as *H. influenzae* type b. A positive reaction in the control reagent indicates that the organism belongs to capsular type a, c, d, e, or f. This test has been shown to be highly sensitive and specific for identifying type b *H. influenzae*.[495]

Serotyping may also be performed by incorporation of type-specific antisera in optically clear agar medium that is supplemented with X and V factors.[84] In this format, the capsular type is detected by the formation of an antigen-antibody precipitation reaction (i.e., a "halo") surrounding the colony. This approach may be used to simultaneously serotype a large number of strains by spot-inoculating the strains on the agar surface using a Steers replicator. The antiserum agar method may also be used for detecting *H. influenzae* type b oropharyngeal carriage. When used for this purpose, bacitracin is added to inhibit other oropharyngeal organisms.[84]

Molecular methods can be used for capsular typing of *H. influenzae*. Falla and colleagues developed a PCR-based method using primers and probes derived from capsule-type specific DNA sequences cloned from the capsular gene clusters (i.e., the *cap* loci) of all six *H. influenzae* serotypes.[394,487] When these tools were used in conjunction with those for the capsule export gene *bexA*, capsulate, noncapsulate, and capsule-deficient type b mutants could be differentiated from one another. Primer and probes developed from randomly amplified DNA have also been identified to characterize nontypeable *H. influenzae* by PCR techniques.[651] This technique has been applied to investigations of outbreaks of respiratory tract disease associated with nontypeable *H. influenzae* and was validated as an acceptable epidemiologic method when compared to both OMP profile and rRNA gene restriction analyses.[651]

Biotyping of Haemophilus influenzae and Haemophilus parainfluenzae.
In his taxonomic study of the genus, Kilian introduced biochemical tests for identifying and characterizing haemophili.[685] Biotypes are determined with three tests—indole production, urease, and ornithine decarboxylase. *H. influenzae* strains could be divided into seven biotypes that were independent of serotype (i.e., type b, non–type b, or nontypeable).[496,952,1204] Seven *H. parainfluenzae* biotypes have also been described using these methods. Biotyping reactions for *Haemophilus* species are included in Table 9-2. Box 9-6 describes the media and procedures used for conventional biotyping (see Color Plate 9-1*H*).

Biotyping of *Haemophilus* species has demonstrated that specific biotypes are associated with different infections, sources, antigenic properties, and antimicrobial resistance

Box 9-6 Media and Procedures for Biotyping *H. influenzae* and *H. parainfluenzae*

Indole test

A heavy suspension of the organism is prepared in 0.05 M phosphate buffer (pH 8.0) containing 0.1% tryptophan. After 4 hours of incubation at 35°C, a few drops of Kovac's reagent are added and the suspension is shaken. A red color in the upper alcohol layer is a positive test result; a yellow color is a negative test result. Heavily inoculated indole-tryptone broth used for enterics may also be used, with the addition of Kovac's reagent after overnight incubation.

Urease test

A balanced salts solution (0.1% KH_2PO4, 0.1% K_2HPO_4, 0.5% NaCl, and 0.5 mL of a 2% solution of phenol red) is prepared (100 mL), adjusted to pH 7.0, and autoclaved. Filter-sterilized, aqueous urea (10 mL) is added, and the solution is dispensed onto sterile tubes in small amounts. To perform the test, a heavy suspension of the organism is prepared in the medium. The development of a red color in the medium after 4 hours of incubation is a positive test result. Heavily inoculated Christensen's urea agar slants may also be used for this test.

Ornithine decarboxylase test

Standard Moeller's ornithine decarboxylase broth is used along with a tube of Moeller's decarboxylase broth base as a negative control. A heavy inoculum is used and each tube is overlaid with sterile mineral oil. Results are best read after overnight incubation, although most positive tests are apparent after 4 to 6 hours and are generally available after 4 hours of incubation; negative tests should be reincubated overnight.

patterns. Oberhofer and Back examined 464 *H. influenzae* and 83 *H. parainfluenzae* and found that *H. influenzae* biotype I was recovered mostly from CSF, blood, and respiratory tract secretions, and that most were from infants less than 1 year old.[952] *H. influenzae* biotypes II and III were also recovered from conjunctival and sputum cultures from children aged 1 to 5 years and from adults older than 20 years of age. Although most serotype b strains belonged to biotype I, nontypeable strains were mostly biotype II and III. In their 1979 study, Oberhofer and Back noted an association between *H. influenzae* biotypes II and III and ocular infections; this observation was corroborated in a 2002 study in San Francisco.[21,952] As discussed above, biotype IV *H. influenzae* are emergent pathogens in obstetric, gynecologic, perinatal, and neonatal infections. The cryptic genospecies associated with maternal-neonatal infections also biotypes as *H. influenzae* biotype IV and underscores the shortcomings of phenotypic methods for strain typing. The cryptic genospecies can be distinguished from biotype IV strains only by molecular genetic approaches that are not readily available in clinical microbiology laboratories. These isolates may also be less reliably biotyped by commercial identification systems. Quentin et al. evaluated four systems for their ability to identify/biotype 188 genital and neonatal isolates.[1035] Of these, 167 (88%) were correctly identified and biotyped, 8 were misidentified, and 13 were biotyped incorrectly by at least one system. DNA-DNA hybridization analyses of the 21 discrepant isolates revealed that 15 of them were the genital tract cryptic genospecies.

Biochemical and Kit Methods for Haemophilus *Identification.*
Carbohydrate fermentation tests can also be used for identification of *Haemophilus* species (see Table 9-2). These methods bypass the technical problems associated with factor requirement determinations that were discussed earlier. Acid production from several carbohydrates (i.e., sucrose, fructose, ribose, xylose, and mannose) can be used to separate *H. influenzae* from *H. parainfluenzae*. In addition to

growth factor requirements, a limited battery of tests is also necessary for differentiating and identifying *H. aphrophilus*, *H. paraphrophilus*, and *H. segnis*. Lactose fermentation or o-nitrophenyl-β-D-galactopyranoside (ONPG) hydrolysis are useful for identifying *H. aphrophilus* and *H. paraphrophilus*; both these organisms are positive with these tests, while other *Haemophilus* species (and *Actinobacillus actinomycetemcomitans*) are negative (see Color Plates 9-2*G* and 9-2*H*). *H. segnis* produced weak or delayed acidification of sucrose and fructose, and is negative in all three biotyping reactions.

Carbohydrate utilization is determined in heavily inoculated semisolid cysteine-tryptic digest agar containing 1% filter sterilized carbohydrates. Acid production is usually apparent in 4 to 18 hours. Reagent-impregnated urease and ornithine decarboxylase disks (Remel Laboratories) and the spot indole test can be used for rapid (1 hour) biotyping of individual isolates, if necessary.

Kit identification systems that use modified conventional tests and chromogenic enzyme substrates also can be used to identify and simultaneously biotype *Haemophilus* species. The RapID NH panel (Remel Laboratories), the Vitek *Neisseria-Haemophilus* Identification (NHI) card (bioMerieux-Vitek, Hazelwood, MO), the *Haemophilus-Neisseria* Identification (HNID) panel (Dade/MicroScan, West Sacramento, CA) and the API NH strip (bioMerieux, La Balme-les-Grottes, France) identify these organism within 4 hours of inoculation (see Color Plates 9-2*A* and 9-2*C*).[341,628,629,909] ONPG and/or lactose are included for differentiation of *H. aphrophilus/paraphrophilus*; testing for a V factor requirement separates these two species.

Laboratory Diagnosis of *Haemophilus ducreyi* Infection

Cotton, Rayon, Dacron, or calcium alginate swabs may be used to collect specimens from chancroid ulcers. Ideally, specimens should be collected from the base and undermined margins of the ulcer; the organism is usually not recoverable from bubo pus. Transport media have not been evaluated for their ability to maintain clinical isolates of *H. ducreyi*, and specimens may harbor only small numbers of organisms. Therefore, media should be inoculated directly. Gram-stained smears of the suppurative exudate from the genital lesions of chancroid may be noncontributory because of the low sensitivity and specificity of the Gram stain. When seen on the direct smears, *H. ducreyi* appear as pale-staining gram-negative coccobacilli, often arranged in clustered groups (''school-of-fish'') or loosely coiled parallel chains (''railroad tracks'') (Figure 9-2). They may be found inside and outside of polymorphonuclear cells. Because genital lesions and suppurative nodes or abscesses may become superinfected with other bacteria (particularly fusobacteria, staphylococci, and streptococci), diagnosis by gram-stained smear is difficult, and culture should be attempted. Diagnosis of chancroid is frequently made on clinical and epidemiologic grounds; however, syphilis, genital herpes simplex virus infection, and lymphogranuloma venereum must be included in the differential diagnosis. A monoclonal antibody directed against *H. ducreyi* has been described and used in an indirect immunofluorescence test to detect organisms directly in smears prepared from genital ulcers.[1141] DNA probes for *H. ducreyi* have also been produced and used in research settings for identification of the organism and for direct detection in specimens from experimentally infected animals.[986]

H. ducreyi may be difficult to recover in culture, and several media have been evaluated for this purpose.[773] These media include GC agar base supplemented with 2% hemoglobin, 5% fetal-calf serum, and 1% IsoVitalex or GCH1 enrichment (Remel), and Mueller-Hinton agar supplemented with 5% chocolatized horse blood plus 1% IsoVitalex enrichment.[773,948] Totten and Stamm described a new clear plate and broth media for *H. ducreyi* that contains GC agar base, 1% XV factor enrichment (PML Microbiologicals, Tualatin, OR), 10% fetal-calf serum, and catalase (Sigma Chemical, St. Louis, MO).[1285] The catalase is added as a source of hemin. The broth has a similar composition, but

GC broth instead of agar is used as the basal medium. Commercial chocolate agar media will generally support the growth of *H. ducreyi;* vancomycin disks may be placed in various quadrants of a chocolate plate to help detect the organisms in mixed cultures.[536,773,1236] Most strains of *H. ducreyi* have vancomycin minimal inhibitory concentrations (MICs) of 32 to 128 μg/mL, but some strains have MICs as low as 4 μg/mL. Therefore, it may be advantageous to inoculate media with and without vancomycin and to collect multiple appropriate specimens. Media are incubated at 33 to 35°C in 5–7% CO_2 or in a candle jar with high humidity. Better growth may be obtained using a microaerophilic environment, where cultures are placed in a Gas-Pak jar with two carbon dioxide/hydrogen-gas-generating envelopes and no catalyst.[1236] Cultures are inspected daily for 10 days. Most isolates from clinical specimens produce visible growth in 2 to 4 days.

Colonies of *H. ducreyi* are small, nonmucoid, and gray, yellow, or tan in color. The colonies can characteristically be ''nudged'' along the agar surface with a bacteriologic loop, are difficult to pick up, and produce a nonhomogeneous, ''clumpy'' suspension in saline. On Gram stain, the organisms appear as gram-negative coccobacilli, usually in close association with one another. *H. ducreyi* is catalase-negative and oxidase-positive; the oxidase reaction is usually delayed and develops only after 15 to 20 seconds with the tetramethyl-*p*-phenylenediamine dihydrochloride reagent. Because of the fastidious nature of *H. ducreyi*, growth factor requirements cannot be demonstrated with factor-impregnated disk or strip techniques. The ALA-porphyrin test is negative, indicating that exogenous hemin is required for growth. The organism is biochemically inert, except for positive nitrate reduction and alkaline phosphatase tests. Hannah and Greenwood tested 64 *H. ducreyi* strains with the RapID NH system; all isolates were correctly identified by this system, with the phosphatase and nitrate reduction tests being the only positive reactions for all isolates tested (see Color Plate 9-2C).[536] In an evaluation with 25 *H. ducreyi* isolates, Shawar et al found that all strains produced unique and consistent enzymatic reactions on the RapID ANA system (bioMerieux-Vitek), which is a 4-hour system used for the identification of clinically significant anaerobic bacteria (see Chapter 14).[1169] These investigators also reported that *H. ducreyi* strains are susceptible to sodium polyanetholsulfonate (SPS) as determined by a disk susceptibility method. They suggested that simple growth characteristics, SPS susceptibility, and aminopeptidase profiles obtained with the enzymatic RapID ANA system could be used for clinical laboratory identification of *H. ducreyi*. Other investigators have shown that *H. ducreyi* strains have consistent aminopeptidase profiles that may be useful for laboratory identification.[1310]

Molecular methods and non-growth-dependent techniques have also been developed for identification or direct detection of *H. ducreyi*.[773] Roggen and coworkers developed an enzyme immunoassay (EIA) that uses polyclonal antibodies against a 29-kDa species-specific membrane antigen and a 30- to 34-kDa immunotype-specific membrane antigen as the capture antibodies.[1084] This EIA reacted with all *H. ducreyi* isolates tested and was also able to detect the organisms directly in clinical specimens. PCR has also been used to detect *H. ducreyi*. Chui et al reported on the development

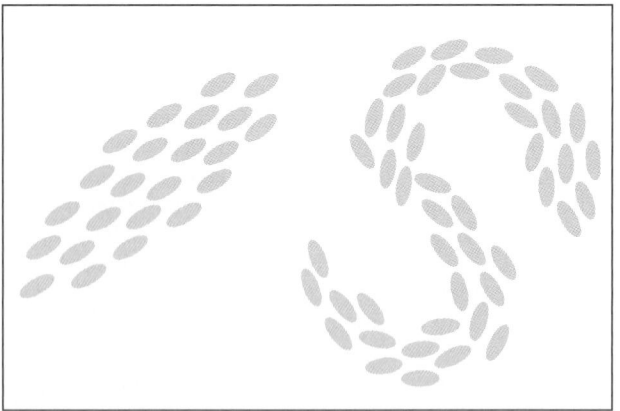

Figure 9-2 Gram-stained morphology of *Haemophilus ducreyi*. On gram-stained smears prepared from lesions of chancroid or from colonial growth, the organisms may appear in loose clusters (i.e., ''school of fish'' [left]) or as loosely coiled clusters of gram-negative bacilli lined up in parallel (i.e., ''railroad tracks'' [right]).

of a primer set and two DNA probes specific for *H. ducreyi* based on the published nucleotide sequences of the 16S rRNA of the organism.[255] The primer set and probes were 100% sensitive in detecting 51 strains of *H. ducreyi* that were isolated on six continents over a 15-year period. The PCR-based direct detection procedure was tested on 100 clinical specimens and showed a sensitivity of 83% to 98% and a specificity of 51% to 67%, depending on the number of amplification cycles.[255] Another group of investigators also developed a PCR-based assay for direct detection of *H. ducreyi*, but the sensitivity and specificity of the test were disappointing.[648] These workers found that failure of PCR to detect *H. ducreyi* probably resulted from nonspecific inhibition of the *Taq* DNA polymerase by material in the specimen. Gu et al. engineered a PCR test for *H. ducreyi* that used 16S and 23S rRNA intergenic spacer regions as the target sequences for detection.[505] Lastly, Orle and colleagues developed a multiplex PCR assay for the direct detection of *H. ducreyi*, *Treponema pallidum*, and herpes simplex virus types 1 and 2 directly in genital ulcers.[973]

Antimicrobial Susceptibility of *Haemophilus* Species

Until about 1973, antimicrobial susceptibility testing of *H. influenzae* was unnecessary because virtually all clinically significant isolates were susceptible to ampicillin, the drug of choice for meningitis and bacteremia caused by this organism. By 1974, some strains of *H. influenzae* had become resistant to ampicillin because of the production of plasmid-mediated β-lactamase enzymes that inactivate ampicillin. Plasmid-mediated β-lactamases have been found in type b, encapsulated non–type b, and nontypeable *H. influenzae* and in *H. parainfluenzae* strains. These organisms harbor a 3.0 MDA transposon that carries the gene for a TEM-1 type β-lactamase enzyme. Rare *H. influenzae* strains produce a second type of β-lactamase, called ROB-1.[303] Over the past 25 years, the prevalence of β-lactamase-positive strains has been slowly increasing throughout the world.[403] A survey of respiratory tract isolates of *H. influenzae* collected during 1997 throughout the U.S. and Canada reported that 34.2% of 837 isolates from 27 U.S. medical centers and 31.3% of 240 isolates from 7 Canadian centers were β-lactamase-positive.[342] A second recent collaborative susceptibility survey of U.S. isolates conducted as part of the SENTRY Surveillance Program found that 35% of 1,032 *H. influenzae* isolates were β-lactamase-positive.[1273] In the 2002 LIBRA surveillance project, β-lactamase-positive *H. influenzae* accounted for 32.2% of 2,791 isolates.[649] In all these studies, more than 99% of the strains were susceptible to amoxicillin-clavulanate, regardless of β-lactamase production. Clavulanate inactivates the β-lactamase, rendering the organisms susceptible to the amoxicillin included in this combination antibiotic.

Rare *H. influenzae* strains have been isolated that are resistant to ampicillin, but do not produce β-lactamases.[822,859] In these strains, resistance is due to alterations in cell-wall penicillin-binding proteins or in permeability of the cell membrane to the agent.[859] These strains display diminished susceptibility to third-generation cephalosporins and to β-lactam/β-lactamase inhibitor combinations.[857,859] Although initial studies with these strains suggested that disk diffusion methods might not accurately detect ampicillin resistance in these strains, changes in the test medium (i.e., *Haemophilus* Test Medium [HTM]) and modifications of the interpretive criteria have addressed these problems.[652,653,858] Fortunately, these ampicillin-resistant, β-lactamase-negative strains are very uncommon. A 2000–2001 *H. influenzae* surveillance study detected only 9 (0.6%) β-lactamase-negative, ampicillin-resistant strains among 1,434 isolates.[668] The ampicillin MIC for these nine isolates was 4 μg/mL; all isolates were susceptible to amoxicillin-clavulanate, cefuroxime, cefprozil, the macrolides, and the fluoroquinolones.

Chloramphenicol, the agent formerly used as an alternative to ampicillin in the treatment of meningitis, remains highly active against *H. influenzae*, with 99.0% of the isolates tested in a U.S./Canadian collaborative study being susceptible.[342] Concerns about its potential toxicity and issues regarding drug interactions have limited the use of this agent both in the U.S. and in developing countries.[1119] Resistance to chloramphenicol has also appeared in these microorganisms.[190,831] Most chloramphenicol-resistant *H. influenzae* produce chloramphenicol acetyltransferase (CAT), which catalyzes the transfer of two acetyl groups from acetyl coenzyme A to active sites on the chloramphenicol molecule, thus preventing the antimicrobial from performing its normal function of inhibiting bacterial protein synthesis.[831] Although CAT-producing strains of *H. influenzae* apparently produce the enzyme constitutively (i.e., under all growth conditions), CAT production by other *Haemophilus* species is inducible, requiring exposure to the drug for enzyme production.[831] Other chloramphenicol-resistant strains demonstrate a relative impermeability to chloramphenicol because of the loss of a major OMP that allows entry of the drug into the cell.[190]

At present, the third-generation cephalosporins are the recommended therapy for treatment of serious *Haemophilus* infections because of the excellent activity of these agents both in vitro and in vivo.[1119] In the U.S./Canada studies, Surveillance Network Database and Alexander Project reports, and SENTRY surveillance studies, all *H. influenzae* isolates were susceptible to the cephalosporins cefpodoxime, cefotaxime, ceftriaxone and cefixime.[342,403,669,1273] Besides amoxicillin, cefaclor was the only agent that was adversely affected by β-lactamase production. Although 92.5–97.2% of β-lactamase-negative *H. influenzae* were susceptible to cefaclor, only 54.0–76.9% of β-lactamase-positive strains were susceptible.[342,1273]

Infections associated with nontypeable *H. influenzae* such as exacerbations of chronic bronchitis, COPD, and otitis media are often treated with ampicillin or amoxicillin if susceptibility to these agents has been documented. Otherwise, oral macrolides, sulfonamides, or fluoroquinolones are often prescribed for these infections. Among the macrolide agents, azithromycin is the most active against *H. influenzae*, with 99.8% of strains being susceptible to azithromycin, as compared with 61.4–91.7% being susceptible to clarithromycin.[342,1273] Trimethoprim-sulfamethoxazole is also frequently given for these infections, but only 77.3–87.5% of strains are susceptible to this agent. The fluoroquinolones, however, have excellent activity against *H. influenzae*. Large collaborative studies have reported that strains of *H. influenzae* are susceptible to ciprofloxacin, ofloxacin, levofloxacin, sparfloxacin, gatifloxacin, grepafloxacin, gemifloxacin, moxifloxacin, and trovafloxacin.[107,323,451,694,1273] Although most *H. influenzae* strains have ciprofloxacin MICs of ≤0.06 μg/mL, isolates with elevated ciprofloxacin MICs (MIC, ≥0.12 μg/mL) have been reported recently.[128,129]

H. parainfluenzae, *H. aphrophilus*, and *H. paraphrophilus* are usually susceptible to third-generation cephalosporins, the quinolones, chloramphenicol, tetracyclines, and the aminoglycosides. Agents such as ceftriaxone, cefotaxime, and ciprofloxacin have been effective in patients with serious central nervous system (CNS) infections, brain abscesses, and endocarditis.[1332] Although most strains are susceptible to penicillin and ampicillin, resistant strains, including β-lactamase-producing strains, have been reported.[650]

When isolates from various parts of the world are examined, *H. ducreyi* strains display a wide range of plasmid-mediated resistance to antimicrobial agents, including ampicillin, tetracycline, sulfonamides, chloramphenicol, and the older aminoglycosides. Third-generation cephalosporins (i.e., cefotaxime, ceftriaxone, cefixime), the fluoroquinolones (i.e., ciprofloxacin), and the macrolides (i.e., erythromycin, azithromycin) show excellent activity against *H. ducreyi* in vitro, while many strains are resistant to tetracyclines and trimethoprim-sulfamethoxazole.[698,824,1309] Many of these agents have been used with success for the treatment of chancroid.[79,815,824,1295] However, because of treatment failures in HIV-infected patients, there is some concern about the clinical efficacy of single-dose or short-course therapies (e.g., with IM ceftriaxone, PO azithromycin) in individuals with chancroid who are also immunodeficient.[148,1296]

Antimicrobial susceptibility of *Haemophilus* species can be determined by disk diffusion and either broth or agar dilution procedures. Susceptibility testing methods are described in Chapter 15.

Actinobacillus Species

Actinobacillus species are small, gram-negative, nonmotile, non-spore-forming, bacilli that are found predominantly in animals. Three species—*A. actinomycetemcomitans*, *A. ureae*, and *A. hominis*—are found in humans. Besides the association with animals, these organisms are similar to members of the genus *Pasteurella* in many of their cultural and phenotypic characteristics. In 1986, the former *Pasteurella* species, *P. ureae*, was formally transferred to the genus *Actinobacillus* as *Actinobacillus ureae;* other species (e.g., *A. capsulatus*, *A. muris*, and *A. seminis*) clearly belong to other genera based on DNA-rRNA hybridization and 16S rRNA sequencing.[331,921,1009]

A. actinomycetemcomitans, the principal human isolate, shares many cultural and biochemical characteristics with the hemophili. Transformation, DNA hybridization, and immunodiffusion studies have demonstrated that *A. actinomycetemcomitans* is more closely related to *H. aphrophilus*, *H. paraphrophilus*, and *H. segnis* than to the other *Actinobacillus* species.[1258] In 1985, a proposal was made to transfer *A. actinomycetemcomitans* to the genus *Haemophilus* as "*Haemophilus actinomycetemcomitans.*"[1024] However, this proposal was rejected because of a lack of similarity to the type species of genus *Haemophilus* (i.e., *H. influenzae*). Others have argued that *A. actinomycetemcomitans* and *H. aphrophilus* should not be included in the genus *Haemophilus* because they do not require X or V factors. However, recently described species from swine—*A. minor*, *A. porcinus*, and *A. indolicus*—are V factor–dependent, as is *A. pleuropneumoniae*. At present, *Actinobacillus* species, including *A. actinomycetemcomitans*, remain in the family *Pasteurellaceae*, which is now included among the γ-Proteobacteria.[455]

Actinobacillus actinomycetemcomitans

A. actinomycetemcomitans is a part of the normal flora of the oral cavity, particularly in the gingival and supragingival crevices. Based on reactions of specific monoclonal antibodies with exposed, cell-surface carbohydrate moieties of the cell-wall lipopolysaccharide (LPS), this species can be divided into six serotypes, designated a through f.[471] Serotypes a, b, and c are the most prevalent, comprising more than 80% of oral strains with equal frequencies.[1117] Although it has been suggested that certain serotypes (e.g., serotype b) may be associated with specific forms of periodontal disease, biotyping and rRNA gene probe studies have demonstrated significant phenotypic and genomic heterogeneity among strains belonging to the same serotype.[65,344,1116] Different strains within the same serotype may also be detected with arbitrarily primed PCR and PCR–restriction-fragment-length polymorphism analyses.[344] Additional studies using sequence analysis of 16S rRNA genes, and PCR assays for leukotoxin, cytolethal distending toxin, major fimbrial subunit antigen, and serotype-specific O-polysaccharide genes have shown that *A. actinomycetemcomitans* strains can be divided into three lineages consisting of all serotype b strains, all serotype c strains, and strains belonging to serotypes a, d, e, and f.[665] All of these serotypes and lineages have been isolated from patients with periodontal disease, suggesting that all have pathogenic potential.

CLINICAL SIGNIFICANCE

A. actinomycetemcomitans is associated with actinomycotic infections, endocarditis, bacteremia, wound infections, and dental infections. The organism's name is derived from its recognized "concomitant" isolation with *Actinomyces* species from abscesses and other infections.[28,738,897,1434] Along with the other HACEK bacteria, *A. actinomycetemcomitans* is a cause of subacute bacterial endocarditis.[234,270,664,1221] Native-valve endocarditis usually occurs in individuals with prior valve damage caused by congenital heart diseases, including congenital aortic stenosis, bicuspid aortic valve disease, atrioventricular septal defect, and mitral valve insufficiency due to rheumatic heart disease. Prosthetic mitral and aortic valve endocarditis have also been reported in individuals with porcine and mechanical valves and pacemakers; localized complications have included pericarditis and paravalvular abscess.[1315,1379] Predisposing factors in the development of *A. actinomycetemcomitans* endocarditis include poor dentition and recent dental manipulations.[40,234] *A. actinomycetemcomitans* endocarditis usually follows an indolent course. Fever, weight loss, chills, cough, and night sweats are common, along with a heart murmur. Hepatosplenomegaly and conjunctival or splinter hemorrhages are variably present. Systemic complications include septic emboli, coronary arteritis, vasculitis, congestive heart failure, valvular damage requiring prosthetic valve placement or replacement, infectious complications of hematogenous dissemination (e.g., endophthalmitis, glomerulonephritis, septic arthritis), and death.[664,757,1163,1171,1221,1327]

A. actinomycetemcomitans is a recognized pathogen in the development of periodontitis. This organism is causally related to a type of early-onset periodontitis called **localized juvenile periodontitis** or **LJP**.[516] LJP is a disease of older children and young adults (ages 12–26 years) that is characterized by rapid degeneration and destruction of the alveolar bone supporting the first permanent molars and incisors. Subgingival bone loss in these areas results in the development of deep gingival pockets that bleed readily with probing. During the development of this condition, there is ordinarily minimal plaque and calculus accumulation and little apparent gingival inflammation.[516] Progression of bone loss to involve adjacent teeth leads to generalized juvenile periodontitis or rapidly progressive periodontitis.

Epidemiologic and immunologic studies suggest that LJP and other severe periodontal diseases have racial and/or genetic components that predispose individuals to these severe endogenous infections. A survey of over 11,000 subjects aged 14 to 17 years found that blacks had a much higher prevalence of LJP than whites (2.64% vs. 0.17%).[792] Black males were almost three times more likely to have LJP than black females, while white females were three time more likely to have LJP than white males. Patients with LJP also produce abnormally high levels of prostaglandin E_2, and the inflammatory cytokine tumor necrosis factor α (TNF-α) in the crevicular fluids surrounding the teeth.[516] These factors are produced by local monocytes and macrophages in response to bacterial products. Cultured monocytes and macrophages from patients with LJP produce three to six times the amount of these cytokines than similar cells from patients who do not have LJP on exposure to lipopolysaccharide.[1167] These inflammatory cytokines induce bone resorption by osteoclasts, leading to alveolar bone loss, and down-regulation of neutrophil chemotaxis. Clones of *A. actinomycetemcomitans* that produce large amounts of leukotoxin may be associated with early-onset forms of periodontitis and may be distinct among different racial and geographical populations.[540,544] Clearly, LJP and severe generalized periodontitis are multifactorial diseases that result from the interplay of genetic, environmental, and microbial factors.

Periodontal disease associated with *A. actinomycetemcomitans* evokes both systemic and localized immune responses. Patients with LJP produce high titers of serum IgG to *A. actinomycetemcomitans* serotype antigens, which are O-side chain oligosaccharides in the cell-wall lipopolysaccharide.[504] The LPS of the organism also induces localized gingival inflammation and allows the organism to establish itself in subgingival plaque. In addition to a potent leukotoxin and an LPS, *A. actinomycetemcomitans* produces several other properties that contribute to its virulence as a periodontal pathogen (Box 9-7) Some of these factors also stimulate the production of antibodies in serum and crevicular fluid.[504] The immune response to microbial antigens may help to limit the periodontal process, and failure to stimulate humoral or cell-mediated responses against the organism

and/or its products may be partially responsible for progression to more severe, generalized periodontal disease.[1120] In addition to LJP and other generalized forms of periodontitis disease, *A. actinomycetemcomitans* is also implicated in the pathogenesis of Papillon-Lefevre syndrome, which is an inherited disease characterized by hyperkeratosis of the palms and soles and extensive periodontal destruction resulting in the loss of both primary and permanent teeth.[1321]

Other infections caused by *A. actinomycetemcomitans* result from contiguous spread of the organism from its habitat in the oral cavity or from hematogenous dissemination during bacteremia. These infections include brain abscess, cervical lymphadenitis, cellulitis, septic arthritis, osteomyelitis, vertebral diskitis, subcutaneous, mediastinal, chest wall and intraabdominal abscesses, urinary tract infections, and vertebral osteomyelitis.[226,404,533,664,881,924,1434] Morris and Sewell reported a case of necrotizing pneumonia due to *A. actinomycetemcomitans* and *Actinomyces israelii* in a 46-year-old male 3 months after the extraction of several teeth due to advanced periodontal disease.[897] Kuijper and colleagues reported a case of disseminated actinomycosis in which both *A. actinomycetemcomitans* and *Actinomyces meyeri* were recovered from subcutaneous skin lesions and from cerebral abscesses.[738] The patient had had slowly progressive pulmonary lesions during the preceding 6 years that were suspected but not proven to be the source of both organisms. Pulmonary infections with *A. actinomycetemcomitans* in the absence of *Actinomyces* species are rare, with only four cases reported before 1990 in the English literature. In a case reported by Yuan and coworkers, the infection involved the lung, the soft tissue of the chest wall, and the overlying ribs and sternum.[1425] Septic embolization of the organism from a primary pulmonary focus may also occur.[1322] The portals of entry for these various types of infections have included oral lesions, prior pulmonary infections, skin abrasions, thoracotomy sites, and urinary tract instrumentation.

CULTURAL CHARACTERISTICS AND IDENTIFICATION

A. actinomycetemcomitans grows slowly on chocolate and blood agars, with visible colonies appearing after 48 to 72 hours (see Color Plate 9-3*B*). Colonies are small, smooth, translucent, nonhemolytic, and have slightly irregular edges. Fresh clinical isolates are adherent to the agar and are difficult to emulsify. With prolonged incubation (i.e., 5 to 7 days), colonies may develop a central density that appears as a four- or six-pointed star. This characteristic is lost on repeated subculture, and the colonies become less adherent. As with *H. aphrophilus*, growth in broth is scant and adherent to the sides of the tube. On Gram stain the organisms appear as pale-staining, gram-negative coccobacilli. Longer cells may be noted with repeated subcultures.

Characteristics for identification of *A. actinomycetemcomitans* include lack of growth on MacConkey and other enteric agars, and positive reactions for catalase production and nitrate reduction. The organism is oxidase-negative (occasional strains may be weakly positive) and urease-negative, does not produce indole, and does not require X or V factors. Lysine and ornithine decarboxylase and arginine dihydrolase reactions are negative. Most strains strongly ferment glucose, fructose and mannose (see Color Plate 9-3*C*);

Box 9-7 Virulence Factors of *Actinobacillus actinomycetemcomitans*

Fimbriae

Fresh isolates of *A. actinomycetemcomitans* possess many long fimbriae that are maximally produced under anaerobic conditions and lost on serial subculture.[618,1140] These fimbriae are composed of a 52- to 54-kDa subunit protein. Fimbriated cells aggregate spontaneously, demonstrate increased adherence to hydroxyapatite beads, and promote adherence to and colonization of oral mucosal surfaces and tissues, respectively.[873]

Leukotoxin

The leukotoxin is a 116-kDa protein that binds to cell membranes of neutrophils, monocytes, and T-lymphocytes.[1245] The toxin induces pore formation in cell membranes, causes degranulation of lysosomal contents to the polymorphonuclear cell surface, induces cleavage and fragmentation of chromosomal DNA, possibly by activation of endogenous nucleases, and protects the organism from phagocytosis.[644,816,1245] Production of leukotoxin in the supragingival area may result in localized degranulation of polymorphonuclear cells (PMNs) and release of lysosomal contents that may enhance inflammation and cause the localized immunosuppression central to the development of periodontal lesions of LJP. This toxin is encoded by a gene operon consisting of four genes (*ltxC, ltxA, ltxB,* and *ltxD*), of which *ltxA* is the structural gene.[711] The ltxC protein is required for activation of the leukotoxin protein, while the *ltxB* and *ltxD* gene products are involved in secretion of the toxin polypeptide.[546] Essentially all *A. actinomycetemcomitans* strains contain the leukotoxin operon, but the level of leukotoxin produced by different strains varies.[610,710] Some highly leukotoxic strains of *A. actinomycetemcomitans* produce 10 to 20 times more leukotoxin than minimally leukotoxic strains because of the presence of a 530-bp deletion within the toxin promoter region or because of the presence of an insertion sequence element adjacent to the leukotoxin promoter region.[178,546] These highly toxic clones are found in the same age groups as is LJP and are associated with severe periodontitis.[1426]

Cytolethal Distending Toxin

A gene locus in *A. actinomycetemcomitans* was recently identified that had greater than 90% sequence identity with the cytotoxin distending gene (*cdt*) locus of some pathogenic *E. coli* strains and *H. ducreyi*.[840] Strains possessing the genes produced toxin in vitro, while naturally occurring toxin-negative strains had large deletions within the *cdt* gene locus itself. In vitro, cytolethal distending toxin causes distention and death of Chinese hamster ovary and other cell lines and is able to cause cell cycle arrest of lymphocytes.[1254] The role of this toxin in disease production is under investigation.

Cellular Invasion

A. actinomycetemcomitans is able to actively invade human cells and cell lines.[863] This ability protects the organism from humoral and cellular immune factors and from the effects of some antimicrobial agents. Cellular invasion by *A. actinomycetemcomitans* involves both actin-dependent and actin-independent pathways.[176] Invasiveness is not associated with any particular strain type as defined by restriction-fragment-length polymorphism analysis, and leukotoxin production is seen more frequently in noninvasive strains of *A. actinomycetemcomitans*.[768]

Bone-resorption-inducing Antigen

A surface polysaccharide antigen of *A. actinomycetemcomitans* has been shown to stimulate bone resorption in a mouse bone culture system and to induce osteoclast-like cells in mouse marrow cultures.[1297] Alveolar bone loss during the pathogenesis of LJP may partially reflect the activity of this antigen in vivo.

Immunosuppressive Fraction

Ochiai and colleagues isolated and purified an immunosuppressive fraction (ISF) from *A. actinomycetemcomitans*, immunized animals with ISF, and performed adoptive transfer experiments to provide sensitized T-cells to unimmunized mice.[955] These ISF-induced T-cells exerted an immunosuppressive effect on B-cell function and on the production of antibodies against *A. actinomycetemcomitans*. ISF may act as a virulence factor to suppress localized antibody production, thereby preventing opsonization and microbial clearance.

Lipopolysaccharide Endotoxin

The endotoxin of *A. actinomycetemcomitans* possesses all the properties of endotoxins from other bacteria. In the gingival crevices, lipopolysaccharide also stimulates osteoclasts to initiate bone-resorption, activates complement, and induces lysosomal release from PMNs.

Immunoglobulin-degrading Enzymes and Fc-binding Components

Enzymes that are able to degrade immunoglobulins G, M, and A are also produced by *A. actinomycetemcomitans*, thus preventing opsonization by antibody.[501] In addition, cell-associated and extracellular components are produced that are able to bind the Fc region of immunoglobulin molecules.[1279] Release of these molecules from the organisms may contribute to periodontitis by interfering with opsonization of bacteria, with the phagocytic activity of polymorphonuclear cells, and with fixation of complement. This binding component is apparently a 25- to 32-kDa OMP related to the OmpA of *E. coli*.[874]

Collagenases and Proteases

A. actinomycetemcomitans and other oral microbes produce collagenases and proteases that may act on connective tissue and basement membrane collagens.[457] These enzymes may function to facilitate spread of the organism in the soft tissue and to generate small peptides that may have biologic activity as mediators of inflammation.

acid production from maltose, mannitol, and xylose varies. *A. actinomycetemcomitans* can be differentiated from *H. aphrophilus* in that the former is catalase-positive and ONPG-negative, and acid is not produced from lactose, sucrose, or trehalose (see Table 9-3).

Molecular methods for detection and identification of *A. actinomycetemcomitans* have also been described.[343,1071] Genetic studies have shown that the gene for the 23S rRNA is split into two smaller forms in *A. actinomycetemcomitans*, while the transcript is continuous in *H. aphrophilus, H. paraphrophilus, H. segnis,* and *H. influenzae.*[1028] Recognition of this atypical RNA pattern on polyacrylamide gel electrophoresis can provide accurate identification/strain differentiation. Direct probe- and amplified probe-based methods have also been developed for detection of *A. actinomycetemcomitans* and other periodontal pathogens directly in subgingival plaque samples.[712,1287] Amplification of the *lktA* gene, the structural gene for the *A. actinomycetemcomitans* leukotoxin, has also been used for identification and direct detection of the organism in gingival fluid and subgingival plaque.[415,486] While typing and characterization of *A. actinomycetemcomitans* strains may be accomplished by serology, other traditional and molecular-based methods that have been used include antibiogram typing, biotyping based on fermentation of mannose, mannitol, and xylose, sodium dodecyl sulfate–polyacrylamide gel electrophoresis (SDS-PAGE) of OMPs, restriction endonuclease analysis of whole chromosomal DNA, restriction-fragment-length polymorphisms, and ribotyping.[65,534,1239,1314] Molecular-based assays may be of particular value for differentiating atypical strains of *A. actinomycetemcomitans* (e.g., catalase-negative strains) from hemophili and for epidemiologic studies.[1071]

ANTIMICROBIAL SUSCEPTIBILITY

Strains of *A. actinomycetemcomitans* are susceptible to third-generation cephalosporins (e.g., ceftriaxone, cefuroxime, cefixime, cefotaxime, ceftazidime, cefepime), fluoroquinolones (e.g., ciprofloxacin, ofloxacin, levofloxacin, clinafloxacin), tetracycline, doxycycline, azithromycin, trimethoprim-sulfamethoxazole, rifampin, and the aminoglycosides.[736,807,981,982,983] Although amoxicillin shows good activity against *A. actinomycetemcomitans*, between 30% and 40% of strains are resistant to benzylpenicillin.[70,736,807,980] Penicillin-resistant strains do not produce β-lactamase enzymes, so resistance is presumably due to altered penicillin-binding proteins.[980] Amoxicillin-clavulanate does not demonstrate any greater activity than amoxicillin alone, which further supports the lack of β-lactamase activity.[807] In vitro susceptibility to amoxicillin does not necessarily predict a favorable clinical outcome, and because of this, the third-generation cephalosporins (i.e., ceftriaxone) are considered the drugs of choice for empiric therapy of serious infections such as endocarditis.[1382] In vitro studies indicate that combinations of antimicrobial agents for the treatment of *A. actinomycetemcomitans* endocarditis may be synergistic, additive, or antagonistic.[993] Hence, the efficacy of combination therapy cannot be predicted and must be determined for individual strains by either an agar dilution technique or Etest.[982]

Treatment of *A. actinomycetemcomitans*–associated periodontal disease involves subgingival debridement, scaling, root planing, and antimicrobial therapy directed against periodontitis-associated bacteria. Successful treatment depends partially on the eradication and suppression of *A. actinomycetemcomitans* and other bacteria from deep periodontal pockets. The currently recommended regimen includes either tetracycline, doxycycline, or combination therapy with amoxicillin and metronidazole.[517] Although most strains have remained susceptible to tetracyclines—the agents of choice for many years—plasmid-associated, *tetb*-mediated tetracycline resistance in *A. actinomycetemcomitans* has been reported.[1081] The amoxicillin-metronidazole combination is associated with fewer treatment failures and effectively eradicates and suppresses subgingival growth of *A. actinomycetemcomitans*.[1316] Because most strains of *A. actinomycetemcomitans* are resistant to metronidazole in vitro, the success of combination therapy may be partly due to the activity of amoxicillin on *A. actinomycetemcomitans* and the broad activity of metronidazole against coinfecting anaerobic periodontal organisms (i.e., *Prevotella* and *Porphyromonas* species). Fluoroquinolones (e.g., ciprofloxacin, moxifloxacin) may also be effective agents for the treatment of *A. actinomycetemcomitans*–associated periodontal infections.[697,907]

Actinobacillus ureae

Genetic and phenotypic studies have shown that several *Pasteurella* species (i.e., "*P. ureae,*" "*P. pneumotropica,*" and "*P. aerogenes*") are closely related to animal species in the genus *Actinobacillus*.[331,386,920] Phenotypic similarities include similar oxidase and catalase reactions, reduction of nitrate to nitrite, growth on MacConkey agar, production of urease, and fermentation of several carbohydrates. At present *P. ureae* is the only species that has formally been transferred to the genus *Actinobacillus* as *Actinobacillus ureae*.[921]

A. ureae is an uncommon commensal of the human respiratory tract and a rare isolate from several types of human infections, including bacteremia, endocarditis, meningitis, bone marrow infection, atrophic rhinitis, bronchitis, pneumonia, conjunctivitis, otitis media, and peritonitis.[71,131,149,156,691,943] In most cases an underlying or predisposing condition is present, such as postsurgical infection, diabetes, periodontal disease, emphysema and alcohol-associated cirrhosis of the liver. Cases of meningitis have been associated with previous skull trauma (assault, cranial surgery) and with underlying disease, including HIV infection.[661,691]

A. ureae is a pleomorphic gram-negative bacillus; on staining, some strains form distinct filaments. After 24 hours of growth on blood agar in a CO_2-enriched atmosphere, colonies are smooth, 1 mm in diameter, and nonhemolytic. Some isolates may appear mucoid. The organism is oxidase-positive and catalase-positive, reduces nitrate to nitrite, does not grow on MacConkey agar, and hydrolyzes urea rapidly. No indole is produced, and the decarboxylase and dihydrolase reactions are negative. Acid is produced from glucose, maltose, sucrose, and mannitol; no acid is produced from lactose and xylose. The other biochemically similar *Actinobacillus* species may be differentiated from *A. ureae* by acid production from additional carbohydrates (e.g., lactose and xylose) and by the abilities of the former species to grow on MacConkey agar (Tables 9-3 and 9-4). Molecular methods have

Table 9-3 Biochemical Characteristics for Identification of *Haemophilus aphrophilus*, *Haemophilus paraphrophilus*, and *Actinobacillus* Species Isolated From Humans

CHARACTERISTIC	H. APHROPHILUS	H. PARAPHROPHILUS	A. ACTINOMYCETEMCOMITANS	A. UREAE	A. HOMINIS
Hemolysis, SBA	–	–	–	–	–
Oxidase	–[a]	–[a]	–[a]	+	+
Catalase	–	–	+	+	–
NO₃ reduced to NO₂	+	+	+	+	+
Requires X factor	–	–	–	–	–
Requires V factor	–	+	–	–	–
Indole	–	–	–	–	–
Urease	–	–	–	+	+
ODC	–	–	–	–	–
ONPG hydrolysis	+	+	–	–	+
Acid produced from:					
Glucose	+	+	+	+	+
Maltose	+	+	+[b]	+[a]	+
Fructose	+	+	+	NA	NA
Sucrose	+	+	–	+	+
Lactose	+	+	–	–	+
Xylose	–	–	V	–	+
Mannitol	–	–	V[c]	+	+
Mannose	+	+	+	V	–
Galactose	+	–	V	–	+
Melibiose	–	+	–	–	+
Trehalose	+	+	–	–	+
Melezitose	–	+	NA	NA	NA
Raffinose	+	–	–	–	+

[a] *A few strains may produce weak or delayed positive reactions.*
[a] *Rare strains may be maltose-negative.*
[a] *Most strains are mannitol-positive.*
+ *positive reactive;* – *, negative reaction; V, variable reaction; NA, data not available; ODC, orotidine-5'-phosphate decarboxylase.*

Table 9-4 Biochemical Characteristics for Identification of *Actinobacillus* Species of Animal Origin

SPECIES	HEMOLYSIS, SBA	OXIDASE	CATALASE	GROWTH, MACCONEY AGAR	NITRATE REDUCTION	INDOLE	UREASE	ODC	PHOSPHATASE	ONPG	REQUIREMENT FOR V FACTOR
A. lignieresii	−	V+	V	V	+	−	+	−	+	V	−
A. equuli subsp. equuli	−	+/+w	+/+w	V	+	−	+	−	NA	+	NA
A. equuli subsp. haemolyticus	+	+	+	V	+	−	+	−	NA	+	NA
A. arthritidis	−	+	+	V	+	−	+	−	+	+	−
A. suis	+	V+	V	V	+	−	+	−	+	V+	−
A. capsulatus	−	+	+	+	+	−	+	−	+	+	+
A. maris	−	+	+	−	+	−	+	−	+	+	−
A. pleuropneumoniae	+	V	V	−	+	−	+	−	+	−	+
A. rossii	V	V	+	V+	+	−	+	−	+	V+	−
A. seminis	−	+	+	−	+	−	−	−	+	−	−
A. delphinicola	−	+	+	−	+	−	−	V	+	−	−
A. scotiae	−	+	+	−	+	−	+	V	+	+	−
A. succinogenes	−	+	+	NA	+	−	+	V	NA	NA	−
A. minor	−	NA	−	NA	+	−	−	NA	+	+	+
A. porcinus	−	NA	−	NA	+	−	−	−	NA	+	+
A. indolicus	−	NA	−	NA	+	+	−	−	NA	+	+

SPECIES	GLU	MAL	SUC	LAC	XYL	MNTL	TRE	MANN	ARAB	SORB	GAL	INOS	RAFF	MEL	SAL
A. lignieresii	+	+	+	V	+	+	+	+	V−	V−	+	−	V	−	−
A. equuli subsp. equuli	+	+	+	+	+	+	+	+	V−	V	V	−	V	+	−
A. equuli subsp. haemolyticus	+	+	+	+	+	+	+	+	V−	V	V	−	+	+	−
A. arthritidis	+	+	NA	NA	+	NA	+	NA	V	+	NA	+	+	NA	NA
A. suis	+	+	+	+	+	−	+	+	V+	+	V+	Vw+	+	+	+
A. capsulatus	+	+	+	+	+	+	+	+	−	+	+	−	+	+	+
A. maris	+	+	+	+	−	+	+	+	−	−	Vw+	Vw+	+	+w	+
A. pleuropneumoniae	+	V−	+	V	+	+	−	+	+	−	+w	+	+	−	−
A. rossii	+	V	−	V	+	−	−	−	V	V	V	V	V−	−	−
A. seminis	+	V	−	+	−	V	−	V	+	+	+	+	V−	−	−
A. delphinicola	+	−	−	+	−	−	−	+	V	V	V	V	−	−	−
A. scotiae	+	−	+	+	−	−	−	+	−	V	V	−	−	−	−
A. succinogenes	+	+	+	+	+	+	−	+	+	+	+	−	+	+	+
A. minor	+	+	+	+	NA	+	NA	+	V	+	+	V	+	+	+
A. porcinus	+	V	V	V	NA	V	NA	V	V	V	NA	−	V	NA	NA
A. indolicus	+	+	+	V	NA	NA	NA	+	−	V	+	−	+	NA	NA

+, positive reaction; −, negative reaction; V, variable reaction; V+, variable but most strains positive; V−, variable but most strains negative.

+w, weak positive reaction; Vw+, variable but most strains weakly positive; Glu, glucose; Mal, maltose; Suc, sucrose; Lac, lactose; Xyl, xylose; Mntl, mannitol; Tre, trehalose; Mann, mannose; Arab, arabinose; Sorb, sorbitol; Gal, galactose; Inos, inositol; Raff, raffinose; Mel, melibiose; Sal, salicin.

been used for the diagnosis of *A. ureae* meningitis.[1373] *A. ureae* strains are susceptible to most antimicrobial agents, including penicillin, ampicillin, cephalothin, cefoxitin, tetracycline, trimethoprim-sulfamethoxazole and the aminoglycosides.

Actinobacillus hominis

A. hominis is a rare human isolate that has been recovered from sputum specimens of individuals with chronic lung disease and from empyema fluid.[441] Wust and colleagues reported on two patients with hepatic failure, one due to chronic hepatitis B infection and the other to alcoholic cirrhosis, in which *A. hominis* septicemia occurred as the terminal event in their illness.[1400] In a study conducted in Copenhagen on 36 patients with *A. hominis* lower respiratory tract infection and/or bacteremia, chronic alcoholism, cardiovascular disease, drug addiction, chronic psychiatric disorders, and chronic obstructive pulmonary disease were frequent predisposing factors.[442] Characteristics for identification are included in Table 9-2.

Animal Species in the Genus Actinobacillus

Members of the genus *Actinobacillus* and their animal associations include *A. lignieresii* (horses), *A. equuli* (subspecies *equuli* and *haemolyticus*) (primarily horses), *A. suis* (swine), *A. capsulatus* (rabbits), *A. maris* (mice), *A. seminis* (sheep, rams), *A. delphinicola* (sea mammals), *A. scotiae* (porpoises), *A. succinogenes* (bovine rumen), and *A. arthritidis* (horses).[38,250,251,424,426,508,1194] *A. pleuropneumoniae*, *A. suis*, *A. rossii*, *A. minor*, *A. porcinus*, and *A. indolicus* are found in the respiratory tract of swine.[884,1194] Also included in this group are other uncommonly isolated unnamed taxa (i.e., Bisgaard taxa 5, and 8, and *Actinobacillus* genomospecies 2 [formerly certain strains of Bisgaard taxon 9]). *A. lignieresii* causes granulomatous infections in the oral cavity and gastrointestinal tracts of cattle and pneumonic and cutaneous infections in sheep and other ungulates. *A. equuli* causes bacteremia, peritonitis, nephritis, osteomyelitis, and arthritis in horses and swine and both localized and systemic infections in monkeys, calves, dogs and rabbits. *A. suis* causes septicemia, pneumonia, and arthritis in swine and horses.[997] *A. capsulatus* causes arthritis in rabbits, and *A. pleuropneumoniae* is an important agent causing a highly contagious pneumonia in pigs. *A. muris* is found in the genital tract of mice, *A. rossii* is found in the vaginas of postparturient sows and aborted piglets, and *A. seminis* is a cause of epididymitis and sterility in sheep.[1194] Human infections with animal species of *Actinobacillus* usually occur as a result of animal-related trauma. *A. lignieresii*, *A. equuli*, and *A. suis* have been recovered from human clinical specimens, including horse and sheep bite wounds, joint fluid, blood, and sputum.[64,109,385,997] Ashhurst-Smith and colleagues reported a case of *A. equuli* bacteremia and sepsis in a butcher after sustaining a knife cut at work.[64] Although this patient had a prosthetic mitral valve in place, endocarditis was not a complication. The remaining *Actinobacillus* species have not been isolated from human clinical specimens. Characteristics for

identifying *Actinobacillus* species of animal origin are presented in Table 9-4.

Pasteurella and Mannheimia Species
Taxonomy and Characteristics of the Genus Pasteurella

Pasteurella species are members of the family *Pasteurellaceae* (see Table 9-1).[205,331,425,975] At present, the taxonomic structure of the family *Pasteurellaceae* is complicated and unclear, and taxonomists are attempting to unravel the relationships among the members of the described genera and the proper assignment of various species to these genera.[38,254,313,331] The delineation of these genera was previously based on DNA hybridization studies, with species showing greater than 50% homology being included in the same genus with little regard for phylogenetic origin and phenotypic characterization.[918,919,920,1197] Since 1985, new species within the family *Pasteurellaceae* have been assigned to genus *Actinobacillus* or genus *Pasteurella* in a more or less arbitrary fashion. Examination of 16S rRNA sequences has shown that the ''older'' species of *Pasteurella*—*P. pneumotropica*, *P. aerogenes*, *P. ureae*, and the ''*P. haemolytica* group''—are not closely related to the type species of *Pasteurella* (*P. multocida sensu stricto*) or to each other and probably belong in either the genus *Actinobacillus* or in new genera.[331,918,1194] Formal restructuring of the family began in 1986, when *P. ureae* was reassigned to the genus *Actinobacillus* as *A. ureae*.[921] In 1999, members of the ''*P. haemolytica* group'' (including *P. haemolytica sensu stricto* and *P. granulomatis*) were placed in the new genus *Mannheimia* or reclassified as the previously described species *P. trehalosi*.[38] These studies have also resulted in the transfer of *Haemophilus pleuropneumoniae* to the genus *Actinobacillus* as *A. pleuropneumoniae* and the transfer of ''*Haemophilus avium*'' and other unclassified V factor–dependent isolates to the genus *Pasteurella* (i.e., *P. avium*, *P. volantium*).[919,1019] Like *P. aerogenes* and *P. pneumotropica*, ''species'' such as *P. caballi* and *P. bettyae* are also of undetermined taxonomic status.

Members of the genus *Pasteurella* have certain phenotypic characteristics in common.[205,918–920] *Pasteurella* species are nonmotile, gram-negative, facultatively anaerobic coccobacilli or rods. Most species are oxidase-positive, catalase-positive, and alkaline phosphatase-positive and reduce nitrate to nitrite. *Pasteurella* species also produce acid from glucose, fructose, mannose, and sucrose, and none of them hydrolyzes starch or salicin. All species have similar cell wall fatty acids, which are primarily $C_{16:1w7c}$, $C_{16:0}$ and $C_{14:0}$. All species are usually susceptible to penicillins, cephalosporins, and tetracyclines. Members of the genus *Pasteurella* and animal-associated *Actinobacillus* species are difficult to distinguish phenotypically.[920] Like the Pasteurelleae, animal *Actinobacillus* species are characteristically oxidase- and catalase-positive gram-negative coccobacilli that reduce nitrate to nitrite. Several members of both genera also produce urease. The habitats and clinical significance of *Pasteurella* and *Mannheimia* species are described in Box 9-8, and the biochemical characteristics that are useful for their identification are

Box 9-8 Currently Recognized *Pasteurella* and *Mannheimia* Species

Species/Subspecies	Habitat and Clinical Significance in Humans
***Pasteurella* Species**	
P. multocida subsp. *multocida*	Respiratory tract of nonhuman mammals; clinical isolate from infections in humans
P. multocida subsp. *septica*	Same as above
P. multocida subsp. *gallicida*	Same as above; also associated with fowl cholera
P. pneumotropica	Respiratory tracts of guinea pigs, rats, hamsters, cats, and dogs; rarely isolated from humans
P. aerogenes	Normal flora in the intestinal tract of swine; human infection following a pig bite
P. bettyae	Human Bartholin's gland and finger abscesses; may be associated with genital ulcer disease; postpartum bacteremia; pneumonia and pleural effusion in patients with AIDS
P. dagmatis	Respiratory tracts of dogs and cats; animal bite wounds and systemic infections in humans
P. canis	Respiratory tracts of dogs and calves; dog-bite wounds in humans
P. stomatis	Respiratory tract of dogs; dog-bite wound infections
P. caballi	Equine isolate causing pneumonia, wound infection; single human wound infection reported
P. gallinarum	Respiratory tracts of chickens and hens; two reported cases of bacteremia in humans
P. anatis	Intestinal tract flora of ducks
P. langaaensis	Respiratory tract flora of chickens and other fowl
P. avium	Respiratory tract flora of healthy fowl
P. lymphangitidis	Bovine lymphangitis
P. mairi	Spontaneous abortion in sows; sepsis in piglets
P. testudinis	Pathogen in some species of desert tortoises
P. trehalosi	Septicemia in adolescent lambs
Pasteurella sp. new species 1	Upper respiratory tract flora of dogs and cats; associated with dog- and cat-bite wounds; human endocarditis also reported
***Mannheimia* Species**	
M. haemolytica	Pneumonic infections in cattle; mastitis in ewes; septicemia in goats and sheep; upper respiratory tract flora of ruminants; rare human infections reported
M. glucosida	Upper respiratory tract flora in cattle and sheep
M. granulomatis	Progressive granulomatous disease (panniculitis) in cattle; bronchopneumonia and conjunctivitis in leprine species and deer
M. ruminalis	Normal flora in the rumen of sheep and cattle
M. varigena	Pneumonia, mastitis, and septicemia in cattle; also found as part of the upper respiratory, rumen, and intestinal flora of cattle; respiratory tract flora of swine; sepsis, enteritis, and pneumonia in swine

presented in Table 9-5 and Table 9-6, respectively. The present discussion will be restricted to organisms that have been associated with human disease.

Pasteurella multocida
CLINICAL SIGNIFICANCE AND VIRULENCE

P. multocida is the most frequently recovered *Pasteurella* species from human specimens; it is also recovered from a wide variety of animals. The organism can be cultured from the oral cavities of healthy domesticated cats (70–90%) and dogs (40–66%), and is also found in a wide variety of other animals, including cattle, horses, swine, sheep, fowl, rodents, rabbits, monkeys, lions, panthers, lynx, birds, reindeer, and buffalo.[1250] In some animals, this organism causes serious infections, including shipping fever and hemorrhagic septicemia in cattle, cholera in fowl, atrophic rhinitis in swine, and pleuritis, pneumonia, abscess formation, chronic rhinitis, otitis media, and septicemia in laboratory rabbits. The majority of human infections are wound infections and cellulitis associated with cat bites and scratches. Occasionally, *P. multocida* may be found in the nasopharynx of healthy

individuals who have frequent exposure to animals. Immunocompromised patients, particularly those with liver diseases (e.g., cirrhosis), solid tumors, or hematologic malignancies, may have bacteremia with this organism from localized infections (e.g., bite wounds), and bacteremia may seed other sites, leading to pneumonia, meningitis, or other complications. Additional information on the clinical spectrum of *P. multocida* is presented in Box 9-9.

Virulence factors have been investigated primarily with *P. multocida* strains that are associated with economically important diseases in animals, such as atrophic rhinitis in swine. Some *P. multocida* strains are encapsulated, and five capsular groups, designated as groups A, B, D, E, and F, have been described. These capsular groups can be divided into somatic serotypes 1 to 16.[1286] Most human isolates of *P. multocida* belong to capsular group A and, to a lesser extent, group D. Strains of *P. multocida* that cause atrophic rhinitis produce a 145-kDa dermonecrotic toxin that is an essential virulence factor for the development of this progressive respiratory tract infection.[777] Toxin production is associated primarily with capsular types A and D, and the

Table 9-5 Biochemical Characteristics for Identification of *Pasteurella* Species

SPECIES	HEMOLYSIS, SBA	OXI-DASE	CATA-LASE	GROWTH, MACCONKEY AGAR	NITRATE REDUCTION	INDOLE	UREASE	ODC	PHOS-PHATASE	ONPG	REQUIREMENT FOR V FACTOR
P. multocida subsp. *multocida*	–	+	+	–	+	+	–	+	NA	–	–
P. multocida subsp. *septica*	–	+	+	–	+	+	–	+	NA	–	–
P. multocida subsp. *gallicida*	–	+	+	–	+	+	–	+	NA	–	–
P.(A.) pneumotropica	–	+	+	V	+	+	+	+	NA	–	–
P.(A.) aerogenes	–	+	+	+	+	–	+	V	NA	–	–
P. bettyae	–	V	–	V	+	+	–	–	+	–	–
P. dagmatis	–	+	+	–	+	+	+	–	+	–	–
P. canis	–	+	+	–	+	V	–	+	+	–	–
P. stomatis	–	+	+	–	+	+^{w}	–	–	+	–	–
P. caballi	–	+	–	–	+	–	–	V	+	+	–
P. gallinarum	–	+	+	–	+	–	–	–	+	–	–
P. anatis	–	+^{w}	+	+	+	–	–	–	+	+	–
P. langaaensis	–	+^{w}	–	–	+	–	–	–	+	+	–
P. avium	–	+	+^{w}	–	+	–	–	–	+	–	+
P. lymphangitidis	–	–	+	V	–	–	+	–	+	–	–
P. mairi	V	+	V$^+$	V	+	–	+	V$^+$	+	V	–
P. testudinis	+	+	+	V	–	+	–	–	–	V+	–
Pasteurella new sp. 1	–	+	+	–	+	+	+	–	NA	NA	–
Pasteurella species A	–	+	+	–	NA	–	–	–	NA	NA	+
Pasteurella species B	–	+	+	–	NA	+	–	+	NA	NA	–

SPECIES	GLU	MAL	SUC	LAC	XYL	MNTL	TRE	MANN	ARAB	SORB	GAL	INOS	RAFF	DULC
P. multocida subsp. *multocida*	+	-	NA	-[a]	V	+	V	NA	-	+	+	NA	NA	-
P. multocida subsp. *septica*	+	-	NA	-[a]	+	+	+	NA	-	-	+	NA	NA	-
P. multocida subsp. *gallicida*	+	-	NA	-[a]	+	+	-	NA	V	+	+	NA	NA	+
P.(A.) pneumotropica	+	+	NA	V[b]	+[c]	-	+	NA	-	-	+	NA	NA	
P.(A.) aerogenes	+[d]	+	NA	V[b]	+[-]	-	-	NA	-	-	NA	NA	NA	-
P. bettyae	+	V	-	-	-	-	-	V	-	-	-	-	-	NA
P. dagmatis	+	+	+	-	-	-	+	+	-	-	+	-	+[w]	NA
P. canis	+	-	+	-	V-	-	V	+	-	-	+	-	-	NA
P. stomatis	+	-	+	-	-	-	+	+	-	-	+	-	-	NA
P. caballi	+	+	+	+	+	+	-	+	-	-	+	-	+	NA
P. gallinarum	+	-	+	-	V	-	+	+	-	-	+	-	V[+]	NA
P. anatis	+	-	+	+	+	+	+	+	-	-	+	-	+[w]	NA
P. langaaensis	+	-	+	+	-	+	+	+	-	-	+	-	-	NA
P. avium	+	-	-	V	V	-	-	+	-	-	+	-	-	NA
P. lymphangitidis	+	V	V	-	+	V[+]	V-	+	+	V	+	V	-	NA
P. mairi	+	V	+	V-	V	V	V	+	+	V[+]	+	+	-	NA
P. testudinis	+	V[+]	+	V-	+	V	V	-	V	V	V[+]	NA	V	NA
Pasteurella new species 1	+[e]	+	-	-	-	-	NA	NA	NA	NA	NA	NA	NA	NA
Pasteurella species A	+	V	NA	V[+]	V	V	+	NA	+	-	NA	NA	-	NA
Pasteurella species B	+	+	NA	-	+	-	+	NA	-	-	NA	NA	-	NA

[a] *Rare strains may be lactose-positive.*
[b] *Most reactions are negative for the indicated organisms.*
[c] *Rare strains may be xylose-negative.*
[d] *Gas produced from glucose by most strains.*
[e] *Some strains form small amounts of gas from carbohydrates.*

+, *positive reaction;* −, *negative reaction;* V, *variable reaction;* V[+], *variable reaction, most strains positive;* V[−], *variable reaction, most strains negative;* +[w], *weak positive reaction;* SBA, *sheep blood agar;* ODC, *ornithine decarboxylase;* Glu, *glucose;* Mal, *maltose;* Suc, *sucrose;* Lac, *lactose;* Xyl, *xylose;* Mnl, *mannitol;* Tre, *trehalose;* Mann, *mannose;* Arab, *arabinose;* Sorb, *sorbitol;* Gal, *galactose;* Inos, *Inositol;* Raff, *raffinose;* Dulc, *dulcitol.*

Table 9-6 Biochemical Characteristics for Identification of *Mannheimia* Species

CHARACTERISTIC	*M. HAEMOLYTICA*	*M. GLUCOSIDA[a]*	*M. GRANULOMATIS*	*M. RUMINALIS[b]*	*M. VARIGENA[c]*
Hemolysis, bovine blood	β	β	−	−	β
Oxidase	+$^-$	+	+$^-$	+	+
Nitrate reduction	+	+	+	+	+
Alkaline phosphatase	+	+	+	+	+
Citrate	−	−	−	−	−
Motility	−	−	−	−	−
Urease	−	−	−	−	−
Indole	−	−	−	−	V
Arginine dihydrolase	−	−	−	−	−
Ornithine decarboxylase	−	V^d	−	−	+$^-$
Gas from glucose	V	V	V	V	V
Acid from:					
Adonitol	−	−	−	−	−
Amygdalin	−	+	V	−	−
Arabinose	−	V^e	−	−	+
Arbutin	−	+	V	−	−
Cellobiose	−	+	V	−	−
Dextrin	+	+	V	V	V
Esculin	−	+	V	−	−
Gentabiose	−	V^f	V	−	−
Meso-inositol	V	+	V	−	V
Maltose	+	+	V	V	V
Mannitol	+	+	+	+	+
Mannose	−	−	−	−	−
Melibiose	−	−	−	−	V
Salicin	−	+	V	−	−
Sorbitol	+	+	+	V	−
Trehalose	−	−	−	−	−
Xylose	+	+	V	V	+
β-Glucosidase	−	+	+	−	V
β-Galactosidase	V	+	V	+	V
β-Xylosidase	V	V	−$^+$	−	V
β-Fucosidase	+	V	−	−	V
Source	Cattle, sheep	Sheep	Cattle, deer	Cattle, sheep^a	Cattle, swine

^{a} *Divided into 9 biovars, A–I.*
^{b} *Divided into 2 biovars, 1, 2.*
^{c} *Divided into 2 biovars, 1, 2.*
^{d} *Biovars A–E, and I are positive; biovars F, G, and H are negative.*
^{e} *Biovars A, C, D, G, and I are positive, biovars B, E, F, and H are negative.*
^{f} *Biovars A, B, D-H are positive, biovars C and I are negative.*
+, *positive reaction;* −, *negative reaction;* V, *variable reaction;* +$^-$, *most strains positive, rare strains negative;* −$^+$, *most strains negative, rare strains positive.*

toxin gene, *toxA*, is located in a conserved region of the *P. multocida* chromosome. Phenotypic and genotypic analysis of toxigenic strains have shown that these strains are not clonal, and no significant differences could be found between toxigenic strains of porcine or human origin when investigated by biochemical, serologic, or genomic typing methods.[347] Molecular methods have been developed for the direct detection of the *toxA* gene in veterinary *P. multocida* isolates.[777] The role of the dermonecrotic toxin in human disease is not known. Clinical isolates of *P. multocida* also produce lipases, which also may be potential virulence factors for this organism.[1027]

CULTURAL CHARACTERISTICS AND IDENTIFICATION

P. multocida is not difficult to isolate and identify, although knowledge of the specimen type and a history of exposure to animals increase the index of suspicion that this organism may be present. *P. multocida* grows well on chocolate and sheep blood agar, forming smooth, gray colonies that are 0.5 to 2.0 mm after 24 hours of incubation in CO_2 (see Color Plates 9-5*A* and 9-5*B*). The organism is nonhemolytic and does not grow on MacConkey agar, eosin-methylene blue (EMB) agar, or other types of selective or differential enteric media. Isolates from respiratory tract specimens may be mucoid. A characteristic odor (like *E. coli*, but more pungent) is

Box 9-9 Clinical Spectrum of Human *Pasteurella multocida* Infections

Wound Infections and Cellulitis

Local wound infections in humans are associated with cat bites, cat scratches, or dog bites. These infections are characterized by the rapid development of pain, erythema, swelling, cellulitis with or without abscess formation, and purulent or serosanguineous drainage at the site of the wound.[1366] Regional lymphadenopathy occurs in 30–40% of cases, and systemic signs of infection may or may not be present. Serious localized complications (e.g., septic arthritis, osteomyelitis) most frequently follow cat bites, where the wound may be deep, forceful, and traumatic to underlying tissues. Since most bite wounds are on the hands, bone and joint complications are usually seen at these sites. Serious wound infections requiring wide excisional debridement (e.g., necrotizing fasciitis) may also develop in patients with underlying diseases such as diabetes.[531,1424] Occasionally, this organism may be found in wounds that are not associated with animal bites or obvious animal exposure. Wound infections with *P. multocida* have also occurred as a result of a dog or cat licking open or partially healed wounds.[278] The bacterium has been isolated from decubitus ulcers, periocular abscesses, and from postsurgical abdominal and orthopedic wound infections.[615]

Bone and Joint Infections

Bone and joint infections result from implantation of *P. multocida* into the bone and joint spaces by a traumatic (usually cat) bite, by hematogenous seeding of the joint spaces, or by contiguous spread from an adjacent cellulitis. *P. multocida* septic arthritis is often associated with preexisting joint disease, rheumatoid arthritis, and use of corticosteroids; infections are usually more severe in patients with underlying diseases (e.g., cancer, gout,).[191,402] Hematogenous spread of *P. multocida* may result in infected joint prostheses as well.[817,1249] Osteomyelitis can occur from direct extension of soft-tissue infection or by traumatic inoculation of the organisms into the bone periosteum at the time of the bite.

Respiratory Tract Infections

P. multocida can also be recovered from the upper and lower respiratory tract, where it may exist as a commensal or as a cause of epiglottitis, pneumonia, empyema, lung abscess, adult respiratory distress syndrome, bronchitis, sinusitis, tonsillitis, and otitis media.[160,470,786,864,974,1383] Individuals with *P. multocida* colonization of the respiratory tract often have a history of occupational or recreational exposure to animals. Most symptomatic patients usually have some preexisting compromise of the upper airways or lungs (e.g., chronic obstructive pulmonary disease, chronic bronchitis or sinusitis, bronchiectasis, lung carcinoma, AIDS). Symptoms of *P. multocida* pneumonia include an insidious or abrupt onset with fever, malaise, shortness of breath, and pleuritic chest pain. On chest x-ray, lobar consolidation, with mostly lower lobe involvement, is the most common presentation. Complications include the development of pleural effusions and empyema. Upper respiratory tract infection with *P. multocida* may have unusual clinical presentations. A case of *P. multocida* tonsillitis was reported in a patient following accidental ingestion of a broth culture of the organism, and another case of tonsillitis was reported in a woman whose cat habitually licked her toothbrush.[1045,1433]

Endocarditis

P. multocida can be a rare cause of both native- and prosthetic valve endocarditis.[458,932,1318] Patients usually do not have a history of underlying or preexisting heart disease, although a history of cat or dog exposure and underlying disease (i.e., hepatitis, cirrhosis) is commonly found. With this infection, the aortic valve is involved more frequently than the mitral valve. Endocarditis due to *P. multocida* is usually subacute in its clinical presentation, as indicated by a 1-week to 4-month lag from the onset of symptoms to etiologic diagnosis. The single case of prosthetic-valve endocarditis occurred in a 72-year-old woman with a Carpentier-Edwards valve implant for aortic stenosis 3 years prior to the onset of disease.[932] The patient responded to penicillin and ampicillin-sulbactam, and valve replacement was not required.

Central Nervous System Infections

Central nervous system infections caused by *P. multocida* have included meningitis, subdural empyema, and brain abscess.[147,499,760,1338] The clinical presentation of *P. multocida* meningitis is similar to that caused by other agents; the CSF is usually purulent, and gram-negative coccobacilli are observed on Gram stains. CNS infections have been reported in elderly individuals with underlying disease and in infants. Cases of meningitis in infants have usually been associated with nontraumatic exposure to animals. In one case, a 7-month-old infant with meningitis had no direct exposure to the pet cat (e.g., bites, scratches, or licks), but his 2-year-old brother, whose hands had been licked by the pet dog, often comforted the baby by allowing him to suck on his fingers.[1338]

Eye Infections

P. multocida has been isolated from rare cases of conjunctivitis, periocular abscess with cellulitis, keratitis, and endophthalmitis. Purulent conjunctivitis was diagnosed in a poodle owner who did not recall receiving any bites or scratches from the animal.[1271] *P. multocida* keratitis and corneal ulcers usually occur following corneal lacerations from cat or dog scratches.[1241] *P. multocida* endophthalmitis has occurred following penetrating injuries from cat scratches or as an immediate or delayed postoperative complication of cataract or lens implantation surgery.[95,580] This infection may result in the loss of visual acuity or the need for enucleation of the eye.

Box 9-9 *Continued*

Sepsis and Bacteremia

P. multocida sepsis and bacteremia may occur by spread of the organism from a localized bite wound or it may originate from an infected site elsewhere.[1043] In some cases, the initial wound may be so innocuous (e.g., a minor scratch from a dog's paw) that it is ignored until signs and symptoms of sepsis supervene. Bacteremia occurs predominantly in the settings of preexisting liver disease (e.g., cirrhosis) or other underlying conditions, such as solid neoplasms, hematologic malignancies, systemic lupus erythematosus, and HIV infection.[77,177,194,406,1043] However, profound sepsis due to *P. multocida* has been seen following animal bites in individuals with no underlying disease.[1108] In patients with bacteremia, hematogenous dissemination may result in intraabdominal infection, meningitis, pneumonia, septic arthritis, bursitis, and vertebral osteomyelitis.[1043] Fatal biliary *P. multocida* sepsis in a patient with cirrhosis complicated by the development of Waterhouse-Friderichsen syndrome has also been described.[619]

Intraabdominal Infections

P. multocida is an infrequent cause of intraabdominal infections, including postsurgical wound infections, spontaneous bacterial peritonitis, appendicitis, intraabdominal abscesses, and splenic/hepatic abscesses.[485,594,1043,1251] Patients in whom these infections develop invariably have underlying diseases such as cirrhosis, solid organ tumors, and/or hematologic malignancies. Clinically, peritonitis caused by *P. multocida* is similar to that caused by enteric bacteria, with abdominal pain, fever, gastrointestinal bleeding, and hypotension. *P. multocida* is recovered from paracentesis fluid on culture, although direct Gram stains of the fluid are frequently negative. Because most patients with peritonitis usually have concurrent bacteremia, seeding of the peritoneal cavity is believed to be via the hematogenous route in most cases, although peritoneal infection associated with upper endoscopy has been reported.[701] Although most cases of peritonitis are associated with animal contact, some patients do not recall or have no significant exposure to cats or dogs.[103] Continuous ambulatory peritoneal dialysis-associated peritonitis caused by *P. multocida* is unusual but has been reported.[795,915] In some cases, the organism was introduced into the peritoneal cavity by cat bites or scratches on the peritoneal dialysis tubing.[662,991]

Obstetric, Gynecologic, and Urinary Tract Infections

P. multocida may occasionally colonize the female lower genital tract and can cause serious gynecologic or perinatal infections, including meningitis, in the newborn. Female genital tract and neonatal infections have included diffuse genital tract infection, tubo-ovarian abscess, Bartholin's gland abscess, intrauterine device-related endometritis, intrauterine infection followed by septic abortion, chorioamnionitis with neonatal sepsis, pneumonia and/or meningitis.[215,796,1073,1343] Most patients have some sort of underlying disease or immune compromise, including previous cranial trauma, neurosurgery, hepatic cirrhosis, postoperative wound infection, cervical carcinoma, and congenital genitourinary tract malformations. Puerperal sepsis, with isolation of the organism from the blood and endocervical discharge has also been described in a previously healthy women with nontraumatic exposure to the family cat.[1336] In this case, PCR "fingerprinting" proved the genotypic identity of the isolates from the patient and from the oral cavity of her cat. Rare urinary tract infections may be caused by *P. multocida*. These cases are most often cat-associated, and patients usually have abnormal urologic anatomy as a result of surgery.[790]

frequently noted, perhaps because of the formation of large amounts of indole by the organism. *P. multocida* is oxidase-positive, catalase positive, ornithine decarboxylase-positive, indole-positive, and urease-negative. The spot indole test using the *p*-aminocinnamaldehyde reagent is usually strongly positive (see Color Plate 9-5*C*). *P. multocida* produces acid, but no gas, from glucose, sucrose and mannitol, but not from maltose or lactose. For typical isolates recovered from likely sources, such as a cat bite or scratch, the demonstration of oxidase-positive, gram-negative bacilli that are strongly spot indole-positive and fail to grow on MacConkey agar is usually sufficient to identify the organism as *P. multocida*. *P. multocida* strains may be further broken down into three subspecies (subspecies *multocida*, *septica*, and *gallicida*) based on acid production from sorbitol and dulcitol (see Table 9-5). Strains of *P. multocida* subsp. *multocida* are also α-glucosidase-negative, while strains of *P. multocida* subsp. *septica* are α-glucosidase-positive.[613] Feline isolates of subspecies *septica* may actually constitute a separate species.[737] Identification to the subspecies level is of interest in the study of veterinary isolates but not particularly relevant or important for human clinical isolates. As with many other organisms, molecular techniques for species and subspecies identification have been described.[737,865]

ANTIMICROBIAL SUSCEPTIBILITY

Antimicrobial susceptibility testing indicates that *P. multocida* isolates are broadly susceptible to a variety of antimicrobial agents in vitro. The organism is susceptible to penicillin, ampicillin, amoxicillin-clavulanate, broad-spectrum penicillins (i.e., ticarcillin, piperacillin, mezlocillin), expanded-spectrum cephalosporins (i.e., cefotaxime, cefoperazone, cefuroxime, ceftazidime, ceftizoxime), tetracyclines, and chloramphenical.[476,899,944] Less activity has been noted with the first-generation cephalosporins, such as cephalothin and cefazolin, and with the semisynthetic penicillins.[476,944] Aminoglycosides have moderate to poor activity against *P. multocida* strains in vitro, and the organism is resistant to vancomycin and clindamycin.[477] Among the macrolide antibiotics, azithromycin, clarithromycin, roxithromycin, and dirithromycin have greater activity against *P. multocida* than does erythromycin.[477–480] *P. multocida* strains are also very susceptible to the fluoroquinolones and oxazolidinones, but clinical data supporting their efficacy as chemotherapeutic agents is limited.[479,480] Animal isolates of *P. multocida* are often resistant to tetracycline because of the presence of a transposon-associated *tet(H)* tetracycline-resistance determinant.[538]

Although disk diffusion susceptibility results for *P. multocida* strains usually correlate with those obtained by agar and broth dilution techniques, discrepancies have been noted with aminoglycosides and erythromycin. With these agents, disk diffusion tests often indicate greater resistance to these drugs than quantitative procedures. Despite in vitro susceptibility of *P. multocida* to many agents, clinical experience with many of them is limited and, therefore, precludes their being recommended for empiric therapy. At present, penicillin and the expanded-spectrum parenteral cephalosporins remain the agents of choice for treatment of infections caused by *P. multocida*. Resistance to penicillin via plasmid-mediated β-lactamase production is fairly uncommon in *P. multocida*, and was reported first among animal isolates.[791] In 1991, the first β-lactamase-producing *P. multocida* isolate from a human was recovered from a respiratory tract specimen.[1093] This isolate was resistant to penicillin, ticarcillin, cephalothin, sulfonamides, and tetracyclines; clavulanate and sulbactam reduced the MICs of the isolate to β-lactam drugs by 64-fold. This β-lactamase was characterized as a ROB-1-type β-lactamase according to substrate and inhibition specificities and isoelectric point determinations. In 2001, a *P. multocida* strain of human origin was isolated that was resistant to penicillin because of production of a TEM-1 β-lactamase encoded by a 4.3-Kb plasmid.[922]

Other *Pasteurella* Species Isolated From Human Infections
PASTEURELLA PNEUMOTROPICA ("*ACTINOBACILLUS PNEUMOTROPICA*")

P. pneumotropica is part of the respiratory tract flora of dogs, cats, rats, and mice. In laboratory rodents, the organism causes lower respiratory tract infections. Humans acquire the organism via traumatic exposure to animals, such as through dog and cat bites. Human infections attributed to *P. pneumotropica* include meningitis, bacteremia with shock, bone and joint infections, wound infection, cellulitis, and upper respiratory tract infection.[63,436,444,872,1083] Bilateral interstitial pneumonia due to *P. pneumotropica* was also documented in a 27-year-old patient with AIDS who lived at home with several dogs.[292] *P. pneumotropica* peritonitis resulting from contamination of dialysis tubing by a pet hamster was recently reported in a patient receiving continuous ambulatory dialysis.[196] Specimens yielding positive cultures have included wound drainage, bone fragments, joint fluid, throat swabs, urine, pleural fluid, and blood.

After 24 hours of incubation, colonies of *P. pneumotropica* on blood agar are variable in size (0.5–1 mm in diameter), smooth, convex, and nonhemolytic. They are urease-positive, indole-positive, and ornithine decarboxylase-positive (see Table 9-5). The latter two identification tests help to differentiate *P. pneumotropica* from *A. ureae*, which is negative for these two reactions (see Table 9-3). Some strains of *P. pneumotropica* will grow on MacConkey agar. The positive urease test and differential reactions for maltose

and mannitol help to differentiate this organism from *P. multocida*.

A "species" that is closely related to *P. pneumotropica* was given the provisional names *Pasteurella* sp. new species 1, *Pasteurella* "gas," or the SP group.[205] This species has also been isolated from animal bites, miscellaneous specimens from humans, and oropharyngeal specimens from dogs and cats. This organism resembles *P. pneumotropica* in cultural characteristics and biochemical reactions. Colonies tend to be slightly larger than those of *P. pneumotropica* after 24 hours of incubation. Like *P. pneumotropica*, it is indole-, urease-, and maltose-positive, but it can be differentiated by lack of ornithine decarboxylase activity and failure to produce acid from xylose. Urease, ornithine decarboxylase, and acid production from maltose are helpful for differentiating this species from *P. multocida*. Urease-negative "*P. pneumotropica*–like" isolates have also been referred to as *Pasteurella* species taxon 16.[140] Some isolates of *Pasteurella* "gas" produce small amounts of gas from glucose and other carbohydrates. Some members of this taxon, plus some other "*P. pneumotropica*–like" organisms have been reclassified as *P. dagmatis* (see Table 9-5). *P. pneumotropica* isolates are usually susceptible to penicillin; ampicillin; first-, second-, and third-generation cephalosporins; piperacillin; tetracycline; erythromycin; chloramphenicol; and ciprofloxacin. Most strains are susceptible to the aminoglycosides and trimethoprim-sulfamethoxazole.[292]

PASTEURELLA AEROGENES ("*ACTINOBACILLUS AEROGENES*")

P. aerogenes is a part of the oropharyngeal and intestinal flora of swine.[842] Rare human infections have resulted from bites, tusk wounds, or other occupational exposures to pigs and boars.[369] This organism is also associated with abortion and stillbirth in animals, including pigs, dogs, and rabbits. *P. aerogenes* was isolated from the ears and throat of a stillborn child delivered by a women in the 31st week of pregnancy.[1274] The same organism was isolated from vaginal cultures following the delivery. On investigation, the authors learned that the woman worked as an assistant on a pig farm in Denmark. It was not known whether the organism infected the fetus hematogenously or by an ascending genital tract infection. *P. aerogenes* vertebral osteomyelitis was also diagnosed in a 67-year-old male with immunocompetence who had no history of animal exposure.[1039]

P. aerogenes produces smooth, convex, circular, nonhemolytic colonies on blood agar and also grows on MacConkey agar. It is indole-negative and urease-positive; most isolates also produce ornithine decarboxylase (see Table 9-5) As the name implies, this species is "aerogenic," meaning that gas is produced from glucose during fermentation. *P. aerogenes* isolates recovered from human wounds have been susceptible to ampicillin, cephalothin, cefotaxime, cefuroxime, aminoglycosides, ciprofloxacin, and tetracycline.[369] Strains recovered from animals may be resistant to ampicillin and cephalothin because of β-lactamase production and are also frequently resistant to tetracyclines.

PASTEURELLA DAGMATIS

P. dagmatis is part of the oral flora of dogs and cats and is associated with bites and scratches from these animals.

In a series of 32 bacterial isolates from dog-bite wounds submitted to an Australian reference laboratory, three were identified as *P. dagmatis*.[996] Of 159 *Pasteurella* strains submitted to a veterinary laboratory in Denmark, five isolates were identified as *P. dagmatis*. These strains were isolated from a case of cellulitis (1), a groin abscess (1), a throat abscess (1), and dog-bite wounds (2).[592] *P. dagmatis* has also been isolated from cat-bite wounds.[1430] The organism is a rare cause of endocarditis, with three cases reported in the literature.[510,1095,1202] In one of these reports, endocarditis was complicated by vertebral osteomyelitis.[1202] This patient was a 55-year-old female who worked in an animal welfare agency and had sustained multiple cat bites and scratches from strays. *P. dagmatis* pneumonia was also documented in a 54-year-old female patient with squamous-cell carcinoma of the pharynx, where the organism was isolated in pure culture from a sputum specimen.[1047] This patient also kept close company with a dog as a part of the support system offered by her social worker. *P. dagmatis* bacteremia was also found in a 50-year-old male with a long-standing history of diabetes,[392] in whom *P. multocida* cellulitis of the toe and bacteremia had developed 1 year earlier. At that time, his infection was traced to his dachshund, who had licked an open blister on the patient's foot. On his second hospital admission, *P. dagmatis* was recovered from blood cultures; again the infection was likely due to loving licks from his Yorkshire terrier! This organism may also cause peritonitis in patients on continuous ambulatory peritoneal dialysis.[1347] *P. dagmatis* isolates from these human infections have been susceptible to penicillin, ampicillin, ticarcillin, cephalosporins and cephamycins, aminoglycosides, tetracycline, ciprofloxacin, and trimethoprim-sulfamethoxazole.[392,1047,1202]

PASTEURELLA CANIS AND PASTEURELLA STOMATIS

Both *P. stomatis* and *P. canis* have also been isolated from wound infections resulting from dog bites.[592,1025,1250] *P. canis* strains are divided into two biotypes; biotype 1 is found in the oral cavity of dogs, whereas biotype 2 has been recovered from calves.[918] In the study conducted by Holst and colleagues, 28 of 159 strains examined were identified as *P. canis;* all of these were from dog-bite wounds and belonged to biotype 1.[592] Ten of the 159 strains were identified as *P. stomatis;* eight were from dog-bite wounds and two were from abscesses. In the eight *P. stomatis* wound infections, *P. multocida* or *P. canis* were coisolated with *P. stomatis*. Abscess formation and osteomyelitis due to *P. canis* may also be complications of bite-wound infection.[539] *P. canis* and *P. stomatis* are susceptible to ampicillin, amoxicillin-clavulanate, cephalothin, cefotaxime, linezolid, the aminoglycosides, tetracycline, piperacillin, and the fluoroquinolones.[478,479,480,592,1025] Recent taxonomic evidence suggests that *P. canis* is misnamed and should be reclassified with *P. multocida*.[660]

PASTEURELLA BETTYAE

P. bettyae (formerly known as CDC group HB-5 and then as *P. bettii*) has been isolated primarily from the genitourinary tract and related specimens (i.e., vagina, cervix, urethra, and amniotic fluid).[75,1194] In 1989, a cluster of five patients with urethritis, pelvic inflammatory disease, or Bartholin's gland abscesses was identified in Tennessee in which *P. bettyae* was isolated as the etiologic agent. This outbreak suggested that the organism may be a sexually transmitted pathogen.[75] *P. bettyae* may also be associated with genital ulcer disease. In a study performed in Rwanda, the organism was isolated from 25 (3.6%) of 675 patients (204 women and 471 men) with genital ulcer disease, but from only 1 of 983 patients without genital ulcer disease.[150] Of 145 men with a urethral discharge but without genital ulcers, *P. bettyae* was isolated from only 1 patient. In 1996, *P. bettyae* was isolated from blood cultures of a 25-year-old woman with peripartum bacteremia and as a cause of fatal pneumonia and pleural effusion in a 40-year-old man with HIV infection.[896,1168]

P. bettyae is a gram-negative coccobacillus that grows on both blood agar and chocolate agar; ability to grow on MacConkey agar is variable. After 24 hours of incubation in a CO_2 environment, colonies are pinpoint, nonhemolytic, smooth, and white. The organism is oxidase-variable or delayed, although positive results are usually obtained with the tetramethylphenylene diamine reagent. The catalase reaction is negative. Nitrate is reduced to nitrite, but not to gas, and urease is not produced. Acid is formed from glucose (along with gas) and occasionally maltose and mannose, but not from maltose, sucrose, lactose, mannitol, and xylose (see Table 9-5). The organism produces indole after overnight incubation in tryptone broth; the amount of indole formed may be small, so xylene extraction of the broth and use of Ehrlich's indole reagent are often required for its detection.

P. bettyae isolates are usually susceptible to ampicillin, cephalosporins, aztreonam, imipenem, fluoroquinolones, aminoglycosides, trimethoprim, and trimethoprim-sulfamethoxazole and are resistant to erythromycin, clindamycin, vancomycin, and tetracycline. All five isolates recovered in the Tennessee cluster were susceptible to ampicillin, whereas 7 of the 24 isolates tested from the Rwanda study were ampicillin-resistant and produced a β-lactamase.[75,150]

PASTEURELLA CABALLI

P. caballi is an inhabitant of the upper respiratory tract of horses. It has also been isolated in pure and/or mixed culture from equine infections including endocarditis, pneumonia, peritonitis, wounds, abscesses, and the genital tract infections.[256,1144] Documented cases of human *P. caballi* infection include a boil-like fluctuant finger lesion that occurred with no previous traumatic injury in a 28-year-old veterinarian who worked with horses and ponies, and a cutaneous infection of a horse-bite wound in a 56-year-old man.[139,387] *P. caballi* strains are broadly susceptible to antimicrobial agents; some strains, however, are resistant to lincomycin, streptomycin, and sulfonamides and are intermediate in susceptibility to penicillin G.[1144] The isolate obtained from the veterinarian was susceptible to all antimicrobials tested except penicillin and the sulfonamides.[139]

PASTEURELLA GALLINARUM

P. gallinarum is a gram-negative coccobacillus that inhabits the respiratory tract of domestic fowl. The first report of a human infection with *P. gallinarum* appeared in 1995, when the organism was recovered from blood cultures of a

12-year-old Saudi male in whom endocarditis had developed 10 years after surgical repair of a ventricular septal defect.[15] The isolate was susceptible to penicillin, ampicillin, and cefotaxime, and the patient responded to 6 weeks of therapy with the latter two agents. The patient did not report any bites, scratches, or contact with animals. The second report appeared in 1999 from Japan, when *P. gallinarum* was isolated from blood cultures of a 34-year-old man with acute gastroenteritis.[47] This isolate was susceptible to ampicillin, cefazolin, cefotaxime, azithromycin, imipenem, norfloxacin, and the aminoglycosides, and the patient responded to cefazolin therapy. Gastroenteritis developed 2 days after the patient ate a chicken at a barbecue, and the authors suggested that this meal may have been the source of *P. gallinarum* in the patient. However, this isolate may have been misidentified.[437] In 2002, *P. gallinarum* was isolated from the blood, urine, and CSF of a 4-day-old neonate as a result of a septic home delivery.[3] The isolate was susceptible to penicillin, cefotaxime, and the aminoglycosides.

The biochemical characteristics of *P. bettyae*, *P. dagmatis*, *P. canis*, *P. stomatis*, *P. caballi*, and *P. gallinarum* are presented in Table 9-4 along with those of other animal Pasteurelleae.

Mannheimia Species (Formerly the "*Pasteurella haemolytica/Pasteurella granulomatis*" Complex)

P. haemolytica strains are recognized as prominent pathogens in domesticated animals, causing severe diseases and major economic losses in the cattle, sheep, swine, and poultry industries. Historically, *P. haemolytica* strains were divided into two biotypes designated A (cattle-associated) and T (sheep-associated).[205] Biotype A strains produced acid from arabinose but not trehalose, while biotype T strains produced acid from trehalose but not arabinose. These biotypes were each divided into 17 serotypes, with serotypes 1, 2, 5–9, 11–14, 16, and 17 belonging to biotype A, and serotypes 3, 4, 10, and 15 belonging to biotype T. In 1985, *P. haemolytica sensu stricto* was excluded from the genus *Pasteurella* on the basis of DNA-DNA hybridization studies, and DNA-rRNA hybridization confirmed its exclusion from the *Pasteurella*, *Haemophilus*, and *Actinobacillus* genera.[918] Genotypic investigations of trehalose-positive "*P. haemolytica*" (biotype T) strains has resulted in their reclassification as *Pasteurella trehalosi*, even though they show marginal genetic affinity with the genus *Pasteurella*.[1194] Examinations of many diverse, trehalose-negative (biotype A) "*P. haemolytica*" strains by phenotypic criteria, multilocus enzyme electrophoresis, ribotyping, and 16S rRNA sequencing has resulted in the proposal of a new genus, *Mannheimia*, to accommodate the trehalose-negative isolates of the "*P. haemolytica*" complex and "*P. granulomatis*".[304,1069] Based on 16S rRNA sequencing, four distinct related clusters corresponding to five new species have been delineated in the new genus *Mannheimia*: *M. haemolytica* and *M. glucosida* (cluster I), *M. ruminalis* (cluster II), *M. granulomatis* (cluster III) and *M. varigena* (cluster IV).[38] These new species are most closely related to genus *Actinobacillus* (particularly *A. lignieresii*) and "*P. trehalosi*." *Mannheimia* species can be separated from genus *Pasteurella* by failure of the former species to produce acid from mannose and from most animal-associated *Actinobacillus*

species by being urease-negative. *Mannheimia* species are mannitol-positive, which separates them from members of the genus *Haemophilus*, which are mannitol-negative. The biochemical characteristics of genus *Mannheimia* and *Mannheimia* species are presented in Table 9-1 and Table 9-6, respectively.

M. haemolytica strains are well recognized as the etiologic agent of bovine pneumonic pasteurellosis or "shipping fever" and a variety of other infections in cattle, sheep, pigs, and hares.[37] In cattle, this infection is triggered by overcrowding, stress, immunosuppression, and concomitant viral respiratory tract infection. *M. haemolytica* strains isolated from cattle with pneumonic pasteurellosis produce a leukotoxin that is species-specific and has cytolytic activity against ruminant lymphoid cells.[570,571] The leukotoxin is a 105- to 108-kDa protein that belongs to the RTX toxin family, which also includes the *E. coli* hemolysin, the *B. pertussis* adenylate cyclase/hemolysin, and the *A. pleuropneumoniae* Apx toxin.[1114] RTX (repeats in toxin) refers to the presence of characteristic, glycine-rich repeat units at the C-terminus of the peptide molecule. At low concentrations, *M. haemolytica* leukotoxin activates neutrophils, induces formation of inflammatory cytokines, and causes cytoskeletal changes that lead to apoptosis.[1222] At higher concentrations, the toxin causes pore formation in the cell membranes that result in cell swelling and lysis. In vitro, the leukotoxin causes cytopathic changes in the bovine alveoli, where it is associated with the membranes of degenerating macrophages and neutrophils. Leukotoxin-negative mutants of *M. haemolytica* show a significant reduction in virulence in animal models in comparison with leukotoxin-producing strains.[1264]

Members of the former "*P. haemolytica*" complex are rarely isolated from humans, and infections have usually resulted from occupational or recreational exposure to animals. Rivera and colleague reported a case of aortic graft infection due to both "*P. haemolytica*" biotype A (*M. haemolytica*) and group C β-hemolytic streptococci in a 50-year-old man.[1076] Yaneza and colleagues reported a case of endocarditis caused by this organism.[1415] The patient had no contact with cattle or other farm animals. *M. haemolytica* isolates are susceptible to penicillin, ampicillin, amoxicillin-clavulanate, macrolides (i.e., azithromycin, clarithromycin, erythromycin), chloramphenicol, the aminoglycosides, and the fluoroquinolones and are resistant to linezolid.[478–480]

Cardiobacterium hominis
Taxonomy

C. hominis is the only species in the genus *Cardiobacterium*. This organism, originally called CDC group IID, was christened *Cardiobacterium hominis* by Slotnick and Doughtery in 1964.[1190] These workers demonstrated its unique biochemical features and antigenic unrelatedness to other fastidious gram-negative and gram-positive bacteria. The organism possesses a typical gram-negative cell wall with an unusually dense outer layer and terminal and tufted polar caps that are adherent to the cell membrane.[1067] These properties may explain the atypical appearance of the organism on Gram stains (see below). In 1990, Dewhirst and coworkers examined *Cardiobacterium* strains by 16S rRNA sequence analysis and found that this organism and *Kingella indologenes* were closely related to one another and differed significantly from reference strains of other fastidious organisms.[330] They proposed the family *Cardiobacteriaceae* to include *C. hominis*, *Kingella indologenes*, and the related soil organism *Dichelobacter nodosus*. Phenotypic similarities also supported the genetic relatedness of *C. hominis* and *K. indologenes*.[186] *K. indologenes* was removed from the family *Neisseriaceae*, renamed *Suttonella indologenes*, and placed in the family *Cardiobacteriaceae* along with *Cardiobacterium* and *Dichelobacter* species.[330] The *Cardiobacteriaceae* belong to the proposed order "Cardiobacteriales" in the γ subdivision of the Proteobacteria.[455][see below]

Clinical Significance

C. hominis is an organism of very low virulence and has the unique characteristic of causing endocarditis almost exclusively; about 50 cases of endocarditis have been reported in the literature.[295,1397] The organism is a part of the normal respiratory tract flora, but it is rarely noted in respiratory tract specimens because of its slow rate of growth. As with the other HACEK organisms, *C. hominis* enters the bloodstream and usually infects previously diseased or damaged heart valves (e.g., rheumatic heart disease, ventricular septal defects). However, *C. hominis* endocarditis may also develop in individuals with no evidence of previous heart disease. About 20% of reported *C. hominis* infections have involved various types of prosthetic cardiac valves; these have included aortic homograft tissue valves, porcine xenograft aortic and mitral valves, mechanical aortic and mitral valves (Starr-Edwards, Björk-Shiley, and Carpentier-Edwards valves), and pacemaker leads.[45,949,1030,1265] Patients are usually middle-aged to elderly and have either poor dentition or a history of recent dental procedures. In one case report, prosthetic valve endocarditis developed following upper gastrointestinal endoscopy.[1030] The infection follows a very subacute course, with an insidious onset, low-grade fevers, and vague symptoms that may linger for 7 to 9 months before a diagnosis is made. In those with prolonged, low-grade illness, splenomegaly, conjunctival and splinter hemorrhages, hematuria, and anemia may be present. *C. hominis* tends to form large, friable vegetations on the heart valves, so the most serious complications include septic embolization, mycotic aneurysms, and congestive heart failure.[249,295,781,903] *C. hominis* bacteremia and sepsis without endocarditis may also occur in immunocompromised patients.[1089] Isolation of *C. hominis* from specimens other than blood cultures is rare. In 1983, Francioli and colleagues diagnosed cardiobacterial meningitis in a patient as a complication of endocarditis, and in 1991, Rechtman and Nadler reported the recovery of *C. hominis* along with *Clostridium bifermentans* from an abdominal abscess and from the blood of a 65-year-old male with diabetes and an aggressive adenocarcinoma of the kidney and caecum.[432,1052] In 1998, Nurnberger and colleagues reported a case of *C. hominis* infection of a pacemaker atrial lead without valvular involvement that was complicated by presumed hematogenous vertebral osteomyelitis; the organism was isolated from blood cultures but was not recovered from a biopsy of the involved vertebrae.[949]

Cultural Characteristics and Identification

C. hominis may be recovered in essentially all commercially available blood culture media. The organism grows slowly, producing no visible change in the blood culture medium (e.g., hemolysis, pellicle formation, turbidity). Blind subcultures of macroscopically negative blood culture bottles to chocolate and blood agars should be performed. In a recent case report, the organism was recovered only after blind subculture on the 10th day of incubation.[801] Gram stains of positive blood bottles may not reveal the organism; low-speed centrifugation of an aliquot of the medium to remove red blood cells with subsequent high-speed centrifugation to pellet small numbers of organisms may aid in their visualization. On Gram stains, the organisms may appear gram-variable, with a tendency for the cells to retain the crystal violet dye at the poles. Individual cells may appear swollen at one or both ends, resulting in teardrop-, dumbbell-, and lollipop-shaped organisms. Frequently, the cells will assume rosette-like clusters or line up in "picket fence" arrangements in their orientation with one another (see Color Plate 9-3D). The morphology of the individual cells is dependent on the type of culture medium used; in media containing yeast extract, cells appear as uniform, gram-negative bacilli with rounded ends.

On blood and chocolate agars *C. hominis* grows as very small, glistening, opaque colonies, generally after 48 to 72 hours at 35°C in 5–7% CO_2 (see Color Plate 9-3E). Some strains may also pit the agar on further incubation. No growth is observed on MacConkey agar or other enteric selective and/or differential agars. *C. hominis* is oxidase-positive and catalase-, nitrate-, and urease-negative. The positive oxidase and negative catalase reduction reactions help to differentiate this organism from *H. aphrophilus/paraphrophilus* and *A. actinomycetemcomitans*, but are similar to reactions seen for *Eikenella*, *Kingella*, and *Suttonella*. The most helpful feature for identifying this organism is the production of indole. Tryptone broth should be heavily inoculated (with a swab) and incubated for 48 hours. Extraction with xylene or chloroform and use of Ehrlich's reagent rather than Kovac's reagent allows detection of the small amounts of indole produced by this organism. The spot-indole reagent (*p*-amino cinnamaldehyde) may not reliably detect indole production by *C. hominis*. Hydrogen sulfide production can be detected using lead acetate strips. *C. hominis* produces acid from glucose, fructose, sucrose, mannose, and sorbitol; acid production from maltose and mannitol is variable, with most strains producing positive reactions. Lactose, xylose, galactose, trehalose, and raffinose are not fermented. Phenotypically, *C. hominis* is very similar to *S. indologenes* (Table 9-7).[186] *C. hominis* can also be differentiated from *S. indologenes*, *E. corrodens*, and *Kingella* species by cellular fatty acid analysis.[1344] As with other agents of bacterial endocarditis, molecular methods have been used successfully for the detection of *C. hominis* directly in clinical specimens.[903,939]

Antimicrobial Susceptibility

As with the other members of the HACEK group, antimicrobial susceptibility testing is difficult because of the organism's fastidious requirements and slow growth rate. Breakpoints and optimal media and incubation requirements have

<table>
<thead>
<tr><th colspan="7">**Table 9-7 Biochemical Characteristics for Identification of *Cardiobacterium hominis*, *Eikenella corrodens*, *Kingella* Species, and *Suttonella indologenes***</th></tr>
<tr><th>CHARACTERISTIC</th><th>C. HOMINIS</th><th>E. CORRODENS</th><th>K. KINGAE</th><th>K. DENITRIFICANS</th><th>K. ORALIS</th><th>S. INDOLOGENES</th></tr>
</thead>
<tbody>
<tr><td>Hemolysis, SBA</td><td>−</td><td>−</td><td>+[a]</td><td>−</td><td>−</td><td>−</td></tr>
<tr><td>Oxidase</td><td>+</td><td>+</td><td>+</td><td>+</td><td>+</td><td>+</td></tr>
<tr><td>Catalase</td><td>−</td><td>−[b]</td><td>−</td><td>−</td><td>−</td><td>−</td></tr>
<tr><td>NO$_3$ to NO$_2$</td><td>−</td><td>+</td><td>−</td><td>+</td><td>−</td><td>−</td></tr>
<tr><td>NO$_2$ to N$_2$ gas</td><td>+</td><td>−</td><td>+</td><td>+</td><td>−</td><td>+</td></tr>
<tr><td>Indole</td><td>+</td><td>−</td><td>−</td><td>−</td><td>−</td><td>+</td></tr>
<tr><td>Urease</td><td>−</td><td>−</td><td>−</td><td>−</td><td>−</td><td>−</td></tr>
<tr><td>Ornithine decarboxylase</td><td>−</td><td>+</td><td>−</td><td>−</td><td>−</td><td>−</td></tr>
<tr><td>Hydrolysis of esculin</td><td>−</td><td>−</td><td>−</td><td>−</td><td>−</td><td>−</td></tr>
<tr><td>Hydrolysis of ONPG</td><td>−</td><td>−</td><td>−</td><td>−</td><td>−</td><td>−</td></tr>
<tr><td>Gas from glucose</td><td>−</td><td>−</td><td>−</td><td>−</td><td>−</td><td>−</td></tr>
<tr><td>Acid produced from:</td><td></td><td></td><td></td><td></td><td></td><td></td></tr>
<tr><td>Glucose</td><td>+</td><td>−</td><td>+</td><td>+</td><td>+</td><td>+</td></tr>
<tr><td>Maltose</td><td>+[c]</td><td>−</td><td>+</td><td>−</td><td>−</td><td>+</td></tr>
<tr><td>Fructose</td><td>+</td><td>−</td><td>−</td><td>−</td><td>−</td><td>+</td></tr>
<tr><td>Sucrose</td><td>+</td><td>−</td><td>−</td><td>−</td><td>−</td><td>+</td></tr>
<tr><td>Lactose</td><td>−</td><td>−</td><td>−</td><td>−</td><td>−</td><td>−</td></tr>
<tr><td>Xylose</td><td>−</td><td>−</td><td>−</td><td>−</td><td>−</td><td>−</td></tr>
<tr><td>Mannitol</td><td>+[c]</td><td>−</td><td>−</td><td>−</td><td>−</td><td>−</td></tr>
<tr><td>Mannose</td><td>+</td><td>−</td><td>−</td><td>−</td><td>−</td><td>+</td></tr>
<tr><td>Galactose</td><td>−</td><td>−</td><td>−</td><td>−</td><td>−</td><td>−</td></tr>
<tr><td>Trehalose</td><td>−</td><td>−</td><td>−</td><td>−</td><td>−</td><td>−</td></tr>
<tr><td>Raffinose</td><td>−</td><td>−</td><td>−</td><td>−</td><td>−</td><td>−</td></tr>
<tr><td>Sorbitol</td><td>+</td><td>−</td><td>−</td><td>−</td><td>−</td><td>−</td></tr>
</tbody>
</table>

[a] Most strains produce a "soft" β-hemolysis on sheep blood agar.
[b] Rare strains may be weakly catalase-positive.
[c] Rare strains may be maltose-negative, mannitol-negative, or both.

not been established for *C. hominis* or other fastidious organisms. Strains of *C. hominis* are generally susceptible to most antimicrobial agents, including penicillin, ampicillin, cephalothin, third-generation cephalosporins (i.e., cefixime, cefuroxime, cefotaxime, ceftriaxone, ceftazidime, and cefepime), imipenem, meropenem, the fluoroquinolones (e.g., ciprofloxacin, clinafloxacin, levofloxacin, ofloxacin and trovafloxacin), aminoglycosides, chloramphenicol, rifampin, and tetracycline.[736] Patients with *C. hominis* endocarditis have usually been treated with penicillin alone or penicillin combined with an aminoglycoside. Cures have also been achieved with cefazolin and ciprofloxacin monotherapy.[249,1335] At present, the recommended treatment includes the third-generation cephalosporins.[1382] β-Lactamase-producing, penicillin-resistant strains of *C. hominis* are rare and have been reported twice. In 1994, a β-lactamase-producing strain of *C. hominis* was isolated from a case of endocarditis in a 76-year-old man.[769] This strain was susceptible to tetracycline, rifampin, vancomycin, and imipenem and was resistant to erythromycin, trimethoprim-sulfamethoxazole, gentamicin, amoxicillin, ticarcillin, cefotaxime, and piperacillin. The patient responded to vancomycin/rifampin, followed by amoxicillin-clavulanate. The second β-lactamase-producing isolate was recovered from a 66-year-old woman.[801] This isolate was resistant to penicillin and ampicillin, and was susceptible to amoxicillin-clavulanate, cefotaxime, ceftriaxone, gentamicin, ciprofloxacin, and trimethoprim-sulfamethoxazole. Many strains are also resistant to vancomycin and erythromycin; this fact is of some importance, since these agents are occasionally used for dental prophylaxis for patients who are allergic to penicillin.[1029] Most patients with native-valve endocarditis due to *C. hominis* are successfully treated with antibiotics alone, although some may require partial valve resection or valve replacement because of hemodynamic compromise, embolic phenomena, progressive cardiac failure, or mycotic aneurysms.[249,1265]

Eikenella corrodens
Taxonomy and Virulence

Originally, the genus *Eikenella* (formerly CDC group HB-1) defined isolates that were considered to be facultative strains of the anaerobic species *Bacteroides corrodens*. Subsequently, it was demonstrated that these organisms were phenotypically and genetically distinct. The obligately anaerobic species was renamed *Bacteroides ureolyticus* and the facultative anaerobes were placed in the new monospecific genus *Eikenella* as *E. corrodens*. A key characteristic that separates the anaerobic species from the facultative species is urease activity, with the anaerobic *B. ureolyticus* being urease-positive and *E. corrodens* being urease-negative. *B. ureolyticus* is also susceptible to clindamycin and metronidazole, while *E. corrodens* is resistant to these agents. Based on 16S ribosomal RNA sequencing and rRNA-DNA hybridization, it was shown that *E. corrodens* is related to *Neisseria* species; *E. corrodens* is now included in the emended family *Neisseriaceae* in the proposed order "Neisseriales" in the β-subgroup of the Proteobacteria.[329,1100]

Efforts have been made to define virulence factors of *E. corrodens*. In 1988, Yamazaki and his colleagues described

a lectin-like protein on the surface of *E. corrodens* strains that functioned in adherence of the bacteria to human crevicular epithelial cells and interacted with a galactose-bearing receptor on the epithelial cell surface.[1414] This molecule also agglutinated red blood cells. Recent work has demonstrated that *E. corrodens* expresses type 4 pili and exhibits phase variation involving the irreversible transition from piliated to nonpiliated variants.[1328,1329] On agar media, piliated variants form small, pitting colonies, while nonpiliated variants produce larger, nonpitting colonies. Pilus formation is controlled by the *pilA* locus, which includes four genes: *pilA1*, *pilA2*, *pilB*, and *hagA*. The *pilA1* and *pilA2* loci code for the structural proteins of the type IV pili, *pilB* codes for a pilus assembly protein, and *hagA* codes for a hemagglutinin.[1328,1329] Piliated cells synthesize and export the pilus proteins to the cell surface, while nonpiliated variants synthesize pili but do not export them to the cell surface. In addition, piliated cells display "twitching motility" and are competent to undergo natural transformation, while nonpiliated cells lack these features. *E. corrodens* also possesses a principal OMP with an apparent molecular weight of 33 to 42 kDa.[812] This protein can trigger the release of lysosomal enzymes by macrophages and also can stimulate or depress macrophage activity in a dose-dependent manner. Like other gram-negative bacteria, *E. corrodens* has an outer membrane lipopolysaccharide (LPS) that has similar biologic activities to the LPS found in enteric bacteria.[1032] Surface antigens of *E. corrodens* broadly cross-react with other organisms, including *K. kingae*, *K. denitrificans*, and *Moraxella bovis*.[230]

Clinical Significance

E. corrodens is a part of the normal flora of the mouth and upper respiratory tract. In the oral cavity, *E. corrodens* may play a role in certain types of periodontal disease. Suda and colleagues found that the highest prevalence of *E. corrodens* in subgingival plaque samples occurred in young patients with periodontal disease, while the prevalence was lowest in individuals with no periodontal disease.[1237] In healthy persons, the prevalence of the organism in deep gingival specimens decreased with the age of the individual. Among those with periodontal, disease, the highest prevalence was found in those under 20 years of age with juvenile periodontitis, followed by those with postjuvenile periodontitis, prepubertal periodontitis, rapidly progressive periodontitis, and adult periodontitis.[1237] In addition to periodontal disease, *E. corrodens* may play a role in other oral infections, including gingivitis, periapical abscesses, and root canal infections.

E. corrodens has been isolated from a variety of human infections.[990,1170] These include ocular infections (e.g., canaliculitis, periorbital cellulitis, corneal ulcerations, endophthalmitis, lacrimal abscesses), head and neck infections (e.g., sinusitis, otitis, media, mastoiditis, brain abscess, subdural/extradural empyema, cranial osteomyelitis, submandibular abscess), pleuropulmonary infections (e.g., aspiration pneumonia, mixed bacterial lung abscesses, empyema), intraabdominal infections (e.g., hepatic abscess), and skeletal infections (e.g., vertebral osteomyelitis).[46,62,66,560,566,609,654,655,]

[695,1130] Pulmonary infection with *E. corrodens* is seen in the settings of immunosuppression, propensity for pulmonary aspiration, and the presence of underlying lung disease resulting in compromised local defense mechanisms.[609,655,688] *E. corrodens* has also been implicated along with obligately anaerobic species (i.e., *Actinomyces* or *Arachnia* species) in the pathogenesis of a condition called chronic diffuse sclerosing osteomyelitis, which is a mixed infection of the mandible that has distinctive radiologic and tomographic scan patterns and occurs primarily in young women.[827] By extension from periodontal, middle ear, or sinus infections, the organism may enter the CNS, leading to meningitis, brain or paraspinal abscesses, and subdural empyema.[174]

E. corrodens is an uncommon isolate from several other serious infections. *E. corrodens* bacteremia and endocarditis have been seen in immunocompromised hosts, intravenous drug abusers, and individuals with previous valvular damage who had recently had extensive dental work.[554,968] However, endocarditis has also been seen in healthy individuals with no recognized risk factors.[1353] Prosthetic valve endocarditis and infections of indwelling vascular prostheses associated with *E. corrodens* have also been reported.[307,554] *E. corrodens* bacteremia with or without endocarditis may also occur in individuals with underlying diseases such as rheumatoid arthritis and hematologic malignancies.[391,886] *E. corrodens* may also be recognized in subcutaneous abscesses and soft-tissue cellulitis in intravenous drug users. These infections result from the use of saliva for cleansing of the skin prior to drug injection.[39,488,968] *E. corrodens* may also cause cellulitis and osteomyelitis of the hand resulting from "clenched fist injuries" (i.e., fist fights), chronic nail-biting, and human bites.[152,934] Traumatic implantation of the organism into the subcutaneous tissue can result in extension of the infection into the bones and joints with the development of osteomyelitis and septic arthritis. In these settings the organism is often recovered in mixed culture with other facultative organisms (α- and β-hemolytic streptococci, *Staphylococcus aureus*, coagulase-negative staphylococci, enteric gram-negative bacilli and obligate anaerobes [*Peptostreptococcus* species, oral *Bacteroides*, *Prevotella*, and *Porphyromonas* species]). *E. corrodens* vertebral diskitis may also occur as a complication of spinal surgery.[36] In 2000, an unusual case of *E. corrodens* vertebral osteomyelitis was reported in a 65-year-old male in whom the paravertebral space was inoculated by a fish bone that had transgressed the patient's pharynx.[764] Bacteremic *E. corrodens* infections resulting in hematogenous cellulitis, septic arthritis, vertebral osteomyelitis, intervertebral diskitis, paraspinal abscess, and chorioamnionitis have also been reported.[35,36,376,416,764,1040] *E. corrodens* also survives in the gastrointestinal tract and may be recovered from abdominal, splenic, hepatic, and pancreatic abscesses and peritoneal infections along with facultative and anaerobic gut flora.[56,654,1046,1218] *E. corrodens* has been isolated from gynecologic infections, including chorioamnionitis, endometritis and cervicitis resulting from colonization of intrauterine devices.[35,638]

Cultural Characteristics and Identification

E. corrodens will grow on both blood and chocolate agar and does not grow on MacConkey agar. Colonies are small (0.5–1.0 mm) after 48 hours. About 50% of isolates may "pit" the agar as they grow, and both pitting and nonpitting variants may be observed in the same culture (see Color Plates 9-3*E* and 9-3*G*). A pale yellow pigment (observed best on a white swab swept through growth on a chocolate agar plate) is usually produced, and most strains have an odor suggestive of sodium hypochlorite (i.e., laundry bleach). On Gram stain the organisms appear as regular, slender gram-negative bacilli or coccobacilli with rounded ends (see Color Plate 9-3*F*).

Biochemical characteristics of both pitting and nonpitting *E. corrodens* strains are fairly uniform. The organisms are oxidase-positive and catalase-negative, although rare strains may be weakly catalase-positive. The organism reduces nitrate to nitrite and does not require X or V factors, although hemin is necessary for aerobic growth. Nonpitting isolates may be mistaken for *Haemophilus* species and, when tested with X and V factor disks, display growth around the X but not the V disk. Indole and urease are not produced, but most strains are lysine decarboxylase- and ornithine decarboxylase-positive (see Color Plate 9-3*H*). Unlike the other organisms in the HACEK group, *E. corrodens* is asaccharolytic. The phenotypic characteristics of *E. corrodens* are presented in Table 9-7, along with the other oxidase-positive, catalase-negative fastidious HACEK bacteria.

As with many of the organisms involved in periodontal infection, molecular approaches for detection, identification, and typing of *E. corrodens* have been explored. *E. corrodens*–specific DNA probes, as well as probes for other periodontal pathogens, have been designed by analysis of 16S rRNA, identification of unique nucleotide sequences, and chemical synthesis of probe molecules that are complementary to these species-specific sequences.[787] These probes have been used for direct detection of the organism in subgingival plaque samples of patients with gingivitis and periodontitis. Epidemiologic methods, including SDS-PAGE, pulsed-field gel electrophoresis, restriction endonuclease analysis, and arbitrarily primed PCR techniques have also been applied to *E. corrodens* to determine relatedness to other bacteria and strain differences among clinical *E. corrodens* isolates.[229,230,231,1217]

Antimicrobial Susceptibility

Routine antimicrobial susceptibility testing *of E. corrodens* is difficult because of the organism's fastidious nature. Testing is usually done by agar dilution, which is impractical for routine clinical laboratories. In 1998, Alcala and colleagues reported a broth microdilution procedure for *E. corrodens* using *Haemophilus* test medium.[8] Depending on the antimicrobial agent, between 75 and 97% agreement (± 1 log$_2$ dilution) was noted between the microbroth and agar dilution procedures. Most *E. corrodens* strains are susceptible to ampicillin, amoxicillin, and tetracyclines and are resistant to the penicillinase-resistant penicillins, clindamycin, vancomycin, erythromycin, metronidazole, and the aminoglycosides.[481,804] Penicillin susceptibility may vary from strain to strain. Most isolates are variably susceptible to the first-generation cephalosporins, with cefazolin being the most active.[481] *E. corrodens* is also susceptible to cefoxitin, ceftriaxone, cefepime, ciprofloxacin, and the carbapenems (imipenem, meropenem).[8,481,736,1170] Rare, β-lactamase-positive strains have been reported.[481,744] The *E. corrodens* β-lactamase enzyme is highly cell-associated, shows little activity against cephalosporins, and is strongly inhibited by clavulanate and sulbactam.[744]

Kingella and *Suttonella* Species
Taxonomy

The type species of the genus *Kingella*, *K. kingae*, was originally described in the 1960s and at that time was called CDC group M-1. Early descriptions of this organism suggested a relationship with the moraxellae, except that these strains were catalase-negative.[1195] CDC group M-1 was renamed *Moraxella kingii* and subsequently this name was taxonomically amended to *Moraxella kingae*.[155] Because of significant genetic, chemotaxonomic, and phenotypic differences, Henriksen and Bovre recommended that *M. kingae* be removed from the genus *Moraxella* and renamed as the new genus and species *Kingella kingae* in the family *Neisseriaceae* in 1976.[562] In that same year, Snell and LaPage proposed the transfer of two other moraxella-like, oxidase-positive, catalase-negative, saccharolytic species to the genus *Kingella*.[1196] These new species included the organism previously called ''TM-1'' described by Hollis, Wiggins, and Weaver (*Kingella denitrificans*), and indole-positive strains that had originally been isolated from cases of conjunctivitis (*Kingella indologenes*).[586,1196] Based on 16S rRNA sequence comparisons, Dewhirst and colleagues showed that *K. indologenes* was more closely related to *C. hominis* than to the other *Kingella* species or to the other members of the family *Neisseriaceae*.[330] Also, despite the similar phenotypic characteristics of *C. hominis* and *K. indologenes*, the G + C content of their DNA differed enough to warrant separate genus and species status. Consequently, *K. indologenes* was removed from the family *Neisseriaceae* and placed as the only species in the new genus *Suttonella* as *Suttonella indologenes* (after the Australian microbiologist R.G.A. Sutton) in the family *Cardiobacteriaceae* in the γ-subgroup of the Proteobacteria.[330,455] *K. kingae* and *K denitrificans* remain in the emended family *Neisseriaceae*, which is also in the γ-subgroup of the Proteobacteria.[1100] In 1993, Dewhirst and colleagues described a new *Kingella* species that was recovered from human dental plaque of a patient with adult periodontitis.[328] This new species was named *Kingella orale* and subsequently was emended to *Kingella oralis*. This organism constitutes 0.4% of the total microbiota in dental plaque from periodontally healthy individuals and about 4.6% of the microbiota in dental plaque from adult and juvenile patients with periodontitis.[228]

Clinical Significance

Although they are part of the normal upper respiratory and genitourinary tract flora of humans, *Kingella* species, and *K. kingae* in particular, are increasingly being recognized as important human pathogens. Since its initial description, *K. kingae* was considered to be a rare cause of infection in patients with endocarditis. However, during the past decade, *K. kingae* has emerged as a significant pathogen in pediatric patients, causing primarily bacteremia and os-

teoarticular infections.[351] This organism can be isolated from the upper respiratory tract of infants and children; almost 75% of children over 6 months of age have been found to carry the organism in their oropharynx at some time.[1406,1407] The prevalence of the organism in the respiratory tract is highest among children aged 6 months to 4 years, which parallels the ages having the highest attack rates for invasive disease.[1407] Carriage rates are lower among children less than 6 months and greater than 4 years of age. Studies in day-care-center populations have demonstrated that *K. kingae* can be transmitted from child-to-child by the respiratory route in this setting.[1189] The portal of entry for the organism into the bloodstream is probably via breaches in the oropharyngeal mucosa.

Bone and joint infections are the most common clinical manifestations of *K. kingae* infection in children; these infections present as bacteremia, septic arthritis, osteomyelitis, diskitis, tenosynovitis, and dactylitis.[133,339,902,1403,1404] In fact, with the availability of effective vaccines against *H. influenzae* type b, *K. kingae* has essentially replaced *H. influenzae* as the most common gram-negative bacterium causing osteoarticular infections in children less than 3 years of age.[339] Most infants with systemic *K. kingae* infections present with low-grade fevers; viral upper respiratory tract infections and stomatitis are also frequently present.[27,133,339] In most cases, *K. kingae* septic arthritis is an acute infection, with patients usually presenting within 3 days of the appearance of signs and symptoms. These children are usually febrile, and the involved joints are swollen, tender, and display decreased ranges of motion. Blood cultures from these patients are frequently negative.[339] *K. kingae* septic arthritis is usually a monoarthritis, with the most frequently involved joints being the knee, hip, and ankle. Osteomyelitis due to *K. kingae* is usually an indolent infection that follows a subacute course, with patients usually presenting 7 to 10 days after the appearance of symptoms. *K. kingae* osteomyelitis usually affects the femur and other long bones and the tibia, ulna, radius, and calcaneus bones. Patients with osteomyelitis of the long bones usually are unable to bear weight on the affected limb, and there is local tenderness over the involved bone.[902] Hematogenous seeding of the intervertebral disk leads to spondylitis and intervertebral diskitis.[339,751,1403] Disk space infections can involve the lumbar, thoracic, lumbosacral, or thoracolumbar space.[751,1404] Children with invasive *K. kingae* infections often have significant underlying conditions such as acute lymphocytic leukemia or congenital heart disease. Although rare, bone and joint infections due to *K. kingae*, including intervertebral diskitis and septic arthritis, have been diagnosed in adults.[389,852]

As with the other HACEK bacteria, *K. kingae* and the other *Kingella* species are rare causes of bacteremia and endocarditis. *K. kingae* endocarditis occurs primarily in persons with underlying heart disease or cardiac prostheses, as do the other fastidious bacteria discussed thus far, although cases in people with no previous heart disease have been reported.[214,405,1363,1387] Unlike bone and joint infections, *K kingae* endocarditis is seen more in adults and school-age children, although cases in young children do occur.[1363,1404] Complications, including pericarditis, pericardial abscess, mycotic aneurysm, cerebral infarction, and congestive heart failure, may occur during the clinical course of *K. kingae* disease. Immunocompromised patients are noted to have poor oral hygiene, pharyngitis, or mucosal ulcerations due to treatment for other conditions (e.g., radiation therapy). *K. kingae* bacteremia without endocarditis has also been reported in immunocompetent adults following dental manipulations.[1086] Additional complications of *K. kingae* bacteremia and bone infections include meningitis, hematogenous endophthalmitis, soft-tissue infection, and corneal abscess.[200,883,1087,1312] *K. kingae* endocarditis with meningitis has been reported in a woman with systemic lupus erythematosus, and *K. kingae* bacteremia has been reported as the immediate cause of death in a patient with AIDS.[1300,1387] *K. kingae* has been isolated from blood and sputum specimens of patients with pneumonia, epiglottitis, and tracheobronchitis.[678] Septicemia with *K. kingae* may also mimic systemic neisserial infections (i.e., meningococcemia or disseminated gonococcal infection) in its clinical presentation. Redfield et al. reported a case of *K. kingae* bacteremia in a 4-year-old boy with acute lymphocytic leukemia who presented with skin lesions and joint involvement suggestive of disseminated gonococcal infection.[1053] Acute *K. kingae* meningitis in a patient with sickle cell anemia, *K. kingae* bacteremia presenting as meningococcemia in a male with cirrhosis, and a "DGI-like" arthritis-dermatitis syndrome due to *K. kingae* septicemia in a previously healthy 21-year-old woman also have been reported.[1164,1283]

K. denitrificans and *S. indologenes* have rarely been isolated from clinically significant infections. *K. denitrificans* constitutes a part of the normal respiratory and genitourinary tract flora and has been documented as a rare cause of septicemia and native- and prosthetic-valve endocarditis.[543] The ages of the patients with endocarditis ranged from 22 to 66 years, and all but one had either preexisting valvular disease or prosthetic valves in place. Patients often had undergone dental procedures without prophylaxis or had concomitant respiratory tract infections. *K. denitrificans* has been recovered from the empyema fluid of a patient with bronchogenic carcinoma, from the bone marrow of an AIDS patient, and from the amniotic fluid of a 23-year-old woman with chorioamnionitis.[805,870,882] *S. indologenes* has been isolated from human eye infections and was first reported in association with a case of prosthetic valve endocarditis in 1987.[634,1196] *K. oralis* has not been associated with any infectious process.

Cultural Characteristics and Identification

Kingella species are plump, short (2–3 by 0.3 μm), gram-negative bacilli or coccobacilli that sometimes occur in pairs or short chains. They are oxidase-positive and, unlike *Neisseria* and *Moraxella* species, they are catalase-negative. All species grow on chocolate and blood agars and do not grow on MacConkey agar or other enteric media. A selective medium for recovery of *K. kingae* from respiratory tract specimens has been described; it is composed of trypticase soy agar containing 5–7% sheep blood and vancomycin (2 μg/mL).[1406] The vancomycin inhibits the gram-positive oropharyngeal bacterial flora and facilitates detection of the β-hemolysis produced by the organism. All *Kingella* and *Suttonella* species are oxidase-positive and catalase-negative, and none of them produce lysine or ornithine decarboxylases, arginine dihydrolase, or urease.

K. kingae is β-hemolytic on sheep blood agar; the hemolytic reaction is "soft," resembling that of group B streptococci, and may only be noted in areas of confluent growth or after the removal of the colony from the agar surface (see Color Plate 9-4*A*). On prolonged incubation, some strains of *K. kingae* (and *K. denitrificans*) may "pit" the agar like *E. corrodens*. *K. kingae* produces acid from glucose and maltose only. *K. denitrificans* was originally called "TM-1" and was first recognized by its ability to grow on Thayer-Martin medium (see Color Plate 9-4*B*).[586] *K. denitrificans* produces acid only from glucose in supplemented media, rapid carbohydrate degradation tests, and various kit systems, and it is also prolyl-aminopeptidase-positive (see Color Plate 9-4*C*). Because of these characteristics, *K. denitrificans* may be misidentified as *N. gonorrhoeae*, particularly in specimens from the oropharyngeal and genitourinary tract. This organism, unlike the other species in the genus, reduces nitrate to nitrite, and most strains will also reduce nitrite to nitrogen gas on prolonged incubation. *S. indologenes* produces acid from glucose, maltose, and sucrose, but not from lactose, and is distinguished by its ability to produce indole. Like *C. hominis*, this characteristic should be determined in tryptone broth with xylene extraction and addition of Ehrlich's indole reagent. *S. indologenes* may be differentiated from *C. hominis*, which it closely resembles, by its appearance on Gram stain, positive alkaline phosphatase activity, and failure to produce acid from mannitol and sorbitol.[186,330] *K. oralis* produces acid from glucose only, but may be differentiated from *K. denitrificans* by its failure to reduce nitrate and nitrite and the absence of prolyl-aminopeptidase activity.[328] *E. corrodens* may be differentiated from both *C. hominis* and *Kingella* species by its Gram stain morphology, failure to ferment carbohydrates, and positive ornithine and lysine decarboxylase reactions. Biochemical reactions for identification of *Kingella* species and *S. indologenes* are presented in Table 9-6.

Although identification of these organisms is straightforward once they are isolated, some workers have reported difficulty in the recovery of *K. kingae* from clinical specimens, particularly joint fluid specimens, from patients with arthritis and osteomyelitis. Yagupsky and coworkers found that direct plating of aspirates was much less sensitive for recovering *K. kingae* than inoculation of BACTEC blood culture media.[1405] Among 100 specimens cultured by both methods, 34 grew significant organisms; 10 of the 11 *K. kingae* isolates that were obtained grew only in the BACTEC medium and were not recovered on direct plating. The discrepancy in the isolation rate of *K. kingae* was not observed for other organisms causing bone and joint infections. *K. kingae* has also been detected in blood and synovial fluids using the BacT/Alert system (Organon Tenia) and the pediatric Isolator 1.5 microbial tube (Wampole Laboratories, Cranbury, NJ).[765,1412] Using pooled synovial fluids seeded with small inocula of 24 different *K. kingae* isolates, Host and coworkers detected 100% of the 24 isolates using the BacT/Alert Aerobic and BacT/Alert Pedi-BacT aerobic bottles, 88% using the BacT/Alert FAN aerobic bottle, and 63% using the BACTEC Plus Aerobic F bottle.[604] Improved recovery of *K. kingae* from joint fluid specimens inoculated into blood culture media may be due to the dilution of inhibitory factors in synovial fluid by the culture medium (e.g., broth-based blood culture systems) or by removal of the organisms from the synovial fluid milieu (e.g., Isolator cultures). In any case, inoculation of osteoarticular fluids into blood culture bottles should be the standard for the processing of these specimens in the clinical laboratory.[902,1404] Molecular methods (e.g., PCR) have also been used for the direct detection of *K kingae* in joint fluid.[1213]

Antimicrobial Susceptibility

K. kingae strains are susceptible to penicillin, ampicillin, oxacillin, cephalosporins of all generations, chloramphenicol, the aminoglycosides, trimethoprim-sulfamethoxazole, and ciprofloxacin. Some strains may be relatively resistant to erythromycin, and most are resistant to clindamycin, lincomycin, and vancomycin.[133,636,736] Isolates of *K. denitrificans* have antimicrobial susceptibilities similar to those of *K. kingae*; growth of *K. denitrificans* on Thayer-Martin agar indicates that they are resistant to vancomycin and colistin.[586] The *K. indologenes* endocarditis isolate reported by Jenny et al. was susceptible to ampicillin, cefazolin, and tobramycin.[634] In 1993, Sordillo and colleagues recovered a *K. kingae* strain from the blood of a 29-year-old AIDS patient that produced β-lactamase and was highly resistant to ampicillin, cefazolin, and ticarcillin, but was susceptible to β-lactamase-resistant agents and combination drugs containing β-lactamase inhibitors (clavulanate and sulbactam).[1203] Among five cases of *K. kingae* infection reported from Iceland in 1997, three of the five isolates produced β-lactamase enzymes and were resistant to penicillin and ampicillin.[133]

Human Capnocytophaga *Species*
Taxonomy

Capnocytophaga species were originally described by Prévost in 1956 at the Pasteur Institute. At first, these organisms were believed to be indole-negative, fermentative variants of *Fusobacterium nucleatum;* they were named "*F. nucleatus* var. *ochraceus.*" Analysis of the G + C content of similar strains revealed that these organisms were more closely related to bacteria called "*Ristella* species" than to the fusobacteria, and proposed that *F. nucleatus* var. *ochraceus* strains be reclassified as *Ristella ochracea.*[593] At the same time, Loesche was examining isolates of "*Bacteroides oralis*" from the human oral cavity; some of these strains had "fusiform" morphologies suggestive of fusobacteria.[761] He suggested the name "*Bacteroides oralis* var. *elongatus*" for these strains. Although the original isolates of Prevot have been lost, further examination of "*Ristella ochracea*" and "*Bacteroides oralis* var. *elongatus*" confirmed that these names described the same organism, and the name was changed to "*Bacteroides ochraceus.*"[1199] During the early 1960s, Elizabeth O. King at the CDC was also studying several thin, fusiform gram-negative isolates recovered from human clinical specimens. These strains were designated CDC group DF-1, with "DF" meaning "dysgonic fermenter." This refers to the poor fermentative capabilities of these organisms in medium not supplemented with serum. These strains were not anaerobic in their metabolism, but showed a distinct requirement for CO_2 for growth on agar media.

During the late 1970s, workers at the University of Massachusetts and at the Forsyth Dental Center in Boston published studies on a group of fusiform, gram-negative bacilli that required CO_2 for both aerobic and anaerobic growth and demonstrated gliding motility.[593,761,1199,1377] These organisms appeared to have a role in the pathogenesis of human periodontal diseases and were named *Capnocytophaga* species, reflecting the organism's "consumption" or requirement for CO_2 for growth. Laboratory groups at UCLA and the Wadsworth VA Hospital compared strains and concluded that the *Capnocytophaga* species of the Boston investigators, CDC group DF-1, and "*Bacteroides ochraceus*" were different names for the same organisms.[935,1378] The type species of this group was named *Capnocytophaga ochracea.* Related isolates studied at the same time were named *Capnocytophaga sputigena* and *Capnocytophaga gingivalis.* Subsequent research studies using other methods (e.g., cellular fatty acid analysis; aminopeptidase profiles) supported the species status of *Capnocytophaga,* the synonymity of the various "species" described by United States and European scientists, and the inclusion of three separate species within the genus.[308] In 1994, two new human *Capnocytophaga* species—*C. granulosa* and *C. haemolytica*—were identified in human dental plaque specimens.[257,1413] Based on 16S rRNA analysis, the five *Capnocytophaga* species found in humans are classified in the family *Flavobacteriaceae* along with *Flavobacterium*, *Chryseobacterium*, and *Weeksella* species, in the proposed order "Flavobacteriales" in the phylum *Bacteroidetes.*[455,1305]

Clinical Significance

Capnocytophaga species are gliding, gram-negative bacteria that are a part of the normal oropharyngeal flora. These organisms may play a role (along with *A. actinomycetemcomitans*) in the pathogenesis of localized juvenile periodontitis and other periodontal diseases. *Capnocytophaga* species may also be agents of sepsis in patients with malignancies, granulocytopenia and other severe underlying illnesses (e.g., myeloblastic leukemia, acute lymphocytic leukemia, adenocarcinoma, multiple myeloma, Hodgkin's disease, endometrial carcinoma).[132,484,731] Bacteremic episodes often coincide with periods of profound granulocytopenia due to the hematologic malignancies (especially acute myelogenous leukemia or acute lymphocytic leukemia) and to administration of cytotoxic chemotherapy. Mucositis and oral ulcerations are characteristically found in profoundly immunosuppressed patients, thereby establishing an efficient entry route for the organism into the bloodstream.[83,731] *Capnocytophaga* species are mostly isolated from respiratory sources (i.e., gingival crevices, periodontal pockets) and are occasionally isolated from blood and CSF.[690] Rarely, isolates may be recovered from the lower respiratory tract, lung abscesses, wound infections, pleural/peritoneal fluids, joint fluid, bone, conjunctival, and corneal and vitreal specimens.[374,551,985,1106,1269,1352,1384] *Capnocytophaga* species have been isolated from female genital tract infections as causes of serious intrauterine, intraamniotic, and perinatal infections (e.g., endometritis, amnionitis, chorioamnionitis), preterm abortion, congenital bacteremia, and neonatal sepsis.[7,352,400,838,860] Endocarditis, cervical lymphadenitis, empyema, lung abscess, sinusitis, vertebral osteomyelitis, subphrenic abscess, pyonephrosis, liver abscess, osteomyelitis, and clenched-fist injuries involving *Capnocytophaga* species have been reported in both immunocompromised and nonimmunocompromised patients.[192,360,374,985,1156,1266,1354] In 1995, the first case of *Capnocytophaga* species (*C. sputigena*) as a cause of continuous ambulatory peritoneal dialysis–related peritonitis was documented in a 73-year-old man with end-stage renal disease.[388] In 2000, the newly described species—*C. granulosa*—was isolated from an abscess in an immunocompetent patient.[363]

Studies of virulence factors produced by *Capnocytophaga* have focused on their recognized role in periodontal disease. Isolates from oral lesions produce various aminopeptidases, proteases, elastases, and chymotrypsin-like enzymes.[457,1212] These enzymes may function as virulence factors directly by causing degradation of periodontal tissue and indirectly by their action on proteins in dental plaque that generate small molecules having known inflammatory potential in periodontal disease (e.g., bradykinin). These molecules cause increases in vascular permeability, polymorphonuclear cell accumulation, and pain. *C. ochracea* and *C. sputigena* produce neuraminidase, an enzyme produced by many other microorganisms and considered to contribute to virulence.[885] With regard to both periodontal disease and sepsis, *Capnocytophaga* species produce a dialyzable substance that alters the microscopic appearance of neutrophils and markedly inhibits chemotaxis in vitro.[1174,1311] This substance may act locally in the oropharyngeal tissue to abrogate neutrophil cell function in patients who are already immunocompromised. Extracts prepared from sonicated cells of *Capnocytophaga* species contain a 14-kDa protein substance that causes dose-dependent inhibition of lymphocyte proliferation in response to mitogens.[954] *Capnocytophaga* species also secrete IgA proteases, allowing the disabling of the mucosal immune response.[433] Extracellular polysaccharide production may also contribute to virulence by inhibiting the T-lymphocyte response to mitogens and antigens.[151] Finally, the LPS of *Capnocytophaga* species may render some strains resistant to the bactericidal effects of normal human serum.[1380]

Cultural Characteristics and Identification

Capnocytophaga species are slow-growing, with colonies becoming visible generally after 48 hours of incubation and developing a characteristic morphology after this time. All species require a CO_2-enriched environment for growth; this may be provided in a CO_2 incubator or a candle jar. The colonies of the organism are yellow, tan, or slightly pinkish and have marginal fingerlike projections (gliding motility) appearing as a film surrounding the central area of the colony (see Color Plate 9-4*D*). The central parts of the colonies also have a moist, mottled appearance. *Capnocytophaga* species grow on blood and chocolate agar, but not on MacConkey agar. Good growth may also be observed on modified Thayer-Martin agar because of the organisms' resistance to vancomycin, colistin, and trimethoprim. The organisms are gram-negative, long (2.5–7.5 by 0.5 μm), fusiform in shape, and appear straight or slightly curved (see Color Plate 9-4*E*). Pleomorphism, with swollen or large coccal cells, is characteristic in older cultures. All species are catalase-

negative and oxidase-negative, and produce acid from glucose, maltose, sucrose, and mannose, but not from ribose, xylose, mannitol, or sorbitol.[1199] Indole and urease are not produced, and both lysine and ornithine decarboxylase and arginine dihydrolase reactions are negative. *Capnocytophaga* species produce characteristic, uniform profiles on cellular fatty acid analysis that allow genus-level but not species-level identification.[308] Species are identified by an expanded battery of tests (e.g., nitrate and nitrite reduction, starch and dextran hydrolysis, etc.). The newly described species *C. haemolytica* is β-hemolytic on sheep blood and is the only human hemolytic species.[1413] *C. granulosa* strains form intracellular granular inclusions that stain with carbol fuchsin when the organisms are grown anaerobically in peptone-yeast glucose broth under anaerobic conditions.[1413] These two newly described species can also be differentiated from the three previously described human *Capnocytophaga* species by determination of various aminopeptidase activities. *C. ochracea* strains have been shown to cross-react with certain latex agglutination reagents (i.e., Serobact *Legionella*, Disposable Products, Adelaide, Australia) used for identification of *Legionella* species.[233] Biochemical characteristics of the five species of *Capnocytophaga* associated with humans are shown in Table 9-8.

Antimicrobial Susceptibility

Capnocytophaga species are generally susceptible to erythromycin, clindamycin, tetracycline, and the fluoroquinolones and are variably susceptible to penicillin, aztreonam, colistin, and metronidazole.[55,1091,1109] *Capnocytophaga* strains that are resistant to penicillin produce novel β-lactamase enzymes that confer resistance to expanded-spectrum cephalosporins and penicillins.[430,1092] These β-lactamase-producing strains are highly resistant to penicillin, amoxicillin, and cefazolin; addition of clavulanate results in a 64-fold decrease in the amoxicillin MIC for over 90% of the β-lactamase producing strains.[1091] These strains are also less susceptible to cefuroxime, cefotaxime, and ceftazidime than β-lactamase-negative strains.[1091] Imipenem appears to be active against both β-lactamase-positive and β-lactamase-negative *Capnocytophaga* isolates. *Capnocytophaga* species are usually resistant to aminoglycosides (i.e., gentamicin, tobramycin, amikacin, netilmicin), trimethoprim, colistin, and vancomycin, although some strains may be susceptible.[1091,1109] Gomez-Garces et al. reported a case of fatal bacteremia caused by a ciprofloxacin-resistant β-lactamase producing strain of *C. sputigena* that was resistant to all β-lactams (except cefoxitin) and aminoglycosides, but was susceptible to tetracycline, erythromycin, clindamycin, aztreonam, and imipenem.[484] Generally, immunocompromised patients and those with granulocytopenia are treated empirically with a combination of a β-lactam antibiotic and an aminoglycoside, and cidal levels of antimicrobials are usually required for an optimal therapeutic response. Therefore, rapid recognition by the microbiologist of the salient features of this organism is important. The intrinsic resistance of *Capnocytophaga* species to aminoglycosides and the production of β-lactamase enzymes by some clinical isolates (detected by the nitrocefin test) should be reported to the physician as soon as possible.

Table 9-8 Biochemical Characteristics of *Capnocytophaga ochracea, C. gingivalis, C. sputigena, C. haemolytica,* and *C. granulosa*

CHARACTERISTIC	C. ochracea	C. GINGIVALIS	C. SPUTIGENA	C. HAEMOLYTICA	C. GRANULOSA
Hemolysis, SBA	−	−	−	β (lost on subculture)	−
Oxidase	−	−	−	−	−
Catalase	−	−	−	−	−
Gliding motility	+	+	+	+	+
Growth on MacConkey agar	−	−	−	−	−
NO$_3$ to NO$_2$	−	v	−	+	−
NO$_2$ to N$_2$ gas	−	−	−	−	−
Indole	−	−	−	−	−
Urease	−	−	−	−	−
Arginine dihydrolase	−	−	−	−	−
Lysine decarboxylase	−	−	−	−	−
Ornithine decarboxylase	−	−	−	−	−
Hydrolysis of esculin	v	−	−	+	−
Hydrolysis of glycogen	v	−	−	+	−
Hydrolysis of starch	+	−	−	+	+
Hydrolysis of dextran	+	v	−	v	−
Gas from glucose	−	−	−		
Acid produced from:					
Glucose	+	+	+	+	+
Maltose	+	+	+	+	+
Fructose	v[a]	v	v[b]	NA	NA
Sucrose	+	+	+	+	+
Lactose	+	v	−	+	+
Xylose	−	−	−	−	−
Mannitol	−	−	−	−	−
Trehalose	−	−	−	NA	NA
Mannose	+	+	+	+	+
Raffinose	v	v	v	NA	NA
Galactose	v[a]	−	−	NA	NA
Ribose	−	−	−	−	−
Arabinose	−	−	−	NA	NA
Salicin	−	−	−	NA	NA
Sorbitol	−	−	−	−	−
L-Alanyl-aminopeptidase	2+	2+	3+	−	1+
L-Arginine-aminopeptidase	2+	2+	3+	−	2+
L-γ-Glutamylaminopeptidase	1+	1+	1+	−	1+
L-Leucyl-aminopeptidase	2+	2+	3+	−	2+
L-Lysyl-aminopeptidase	2+	2+	3+	−	2+
N-α-benzoyl-DL − arginylaminopeptidase	−	1+	−	−	−

[a] *Most strains positive.*
[b] *Most strains negative.*
+, *positive reaction;* −, *negative reaction; v, variable reaction; NA, not available; 1+ to 4+, intensity of aminopeptidase reactions.*

Canine Capnocytophaga *Species*
Taxonomy

CDC group DF-2 was originally isolated in 1976 from blood and spinal fluid cultures of a patient who had become symptomatic after suffering a dog bite.[146] Subsequently, several reports describing similar organisms were published and, through 1987, over 150 isolates of the organism, designated CDC group DF-2 (for dysgonic fermenter) were sent to the Special Bacteriology Branch of the CDC.[567] In 1989, DF-2 and a group of "DF-2-like" organisms were classified as *Capnocytophaga* species based on phenotypic characteristics and DNA relatedness studies.[165] CDC group DF-2 is now called *Capnocytophaga canimorsus* (Latin for "dog bite") and the "DF-2-like" strains are called *Capnocytophaga cynodegmi* (Greek for "dog bite"). Of these two species *C. canimorsus* is isolated far more frequently and appears be more virulent. Studies in cultured mouse macrophages have shown that *C. canimorsus* is phagocytized, multiplies intracellularly, and causes cell death within 48 hours, whereas *C. cynodegmi* demonstrates no cytotoxic effects.[413] Although these organisms are genotypically and phenotypically different from the *Capnocytophaga* species isolated from humans, they are similar to them with respect to Gram stain morphology, cellular fatty acids, gliding-type motility, and cultural conditions for growth. *C. canimorsus* and *C. cynodegmi* are classified with the human *Capnocytophaga* species in the family *Flavobacteriaceae* in the phylum *Bacteroidetes*.[455]

Clinical Significance

C. canimorsus infections are generally associated with dog bites or close contact with dogs.[606,785,1003,1113] Kullberg et al. reviewed over 60 cases of *C. canimorsus* infection and found that 47% of patients had a history of a dog bite and 27% reported contact with dogs without bites or scratches.[739] The most serious clinical manifestations occur in individuals with underlying diseases or conditions that predispose them to severe infection with the organism. These conditions include hepatic disease secondary to alcoholism (e.g., cirrhosis), previous splenectomy related to other medical circumstances, Hodgkin's disease, hairy-cell leukemia, pulmonary fibrosis, malabsorption syndrome, renal disease, chronic obstructive pulmonary disease, peptic ulcer disease, Waldenström's macroglobulinemia, and the use of systemic or topical corticosteroids.[542,567,739,825,1078,1107] The frequently noted association of systemic *C. canimorsus* infection with asplenia strongly suggests that the reticuloendothelial system plays an important role in containing the spread of the organism. Major clinical features of *C. canimorsus* infection include wound infection with cellulitis, meningitis, bacteremia with septic shock, renal failure, hemorrhagic skin lesions reminiscent of meningococcal disease, pneumonia with empyema, and both native and prosthetic valve endocarditis.[31,142,217,714,766,938] Fulminant *C. canimorsus* sepsis may clinically resemble overwhelming meningococcal disease, with the development of disseminated intravascular coagulation, purpura fulminans, rapidly evolving hemorrhagic skin lesions, symmetrical peripheral gangrene, and the

Waterhouse-Friderichsen syndrome.[542,739,877] Unusual presentations and complications of *C. canimorsus* sepsis have included precipitous hypotension complicated by adult respiratory distress syndrome, pleuritis, myocardial infarction, musculocutaneous mononeuropathy, and thrombotic thrombocytopenic purpura without disseminated intravascular coagulation.[82,217,367,411,608,709] Gastrointestinal and renal complications include acute abdominal presentations, unrelenting secretory diarrhea, the hemolytic-uremic syndrome, and dialysis-related peritonitis.[213,322,905,995,1139,1278] *C. canimorsus* has been isolated from the oropharynx and saliva of dogs and, in at least one case of sepsis, the strain recovered from the patient's blood was also recovered from gingival swab specimens from the patient's dog.[825] Eye infections, including angular blepharitis, chronic corneal ulcers, corneal ulcer with perforation, and endophthalmitis caused by *C. canimorsus* have also been reported.[242,324,468,1010,1435] In one case the patient had sustained a scratch on the cornea from his dog that was treated with, among other things, topical prednisone. Interestingly, a few cases of *C. canimorsus* infection, including keratitis and systemic infection, have occurred in individuals who sustained bites and/or scratches from domestic cats.[204,242,810,989,1302]

Cultural Characteristics and Identification

C. canimorsus is usually recovered from blood cultures, although other specimens (wound cultures, aspirates from cellulitis, CSF) may also yield the organism. *C. cynodegmi* has been recovered from dogs' mouths or from localized dog-bite wounds.[165] In cases of high-grade bacteremia, the bacteria may actually be observed on smears of peripheral blood.[877] The organism has been recovered in several types of blood culture media, and growth is generally slow. The lysis-centrifugation method (Isolator) has also been used successfully for recovery of *C. canimorsus*.[1277] In most reports, cultures become positive 3 to 7 days after collection. The organism grows on both blood and chocolate agar that is incubated at 35°C and in a CO_2 incubator or a candle jar with increased humidity.[559] Poor growth on routine sheep blood agar has been attributed to the use of a trypticase-soy base; better growth is seen when a heart infusion base is used. Heltberg and coworkers found that media supplemented with cysteine supported the best growth.[559] Commercial supplemented chocolate agars containing IsoVitalex (which contains cysteine) or other similar enrichments are satisfactory. Pinpoint colonies appear after 3 or 4 days of incubation. After a few more days the colonies appear circular, smooth, and convex (see Color Plate 9-4F). On Gram stain, the bacteria appear as thin, fusiform bacilli that are 2 to 4 μm in length (see Color Plate 9-4G). Some cells may appear slightly curved. Like the other fastidious bacteria discussed thus far, no growth is observed on MacConkey agar. *C. canimorsus* and *C. cynodegmi* are catalase- and oxidase-positive. These two reactions differentiate them from the other *Capnocytophaga* species, which are both oxidase- and catalase-negative. Both canine species are also arginine dihydrolase–positive and ONPG-positive. Lysine and ornithine decarboxylase tests are negative. *C. canimorsus* and *C. cynodegmi* are differentiated by carbohydrate utilization tests, with the latter organism producing acid from a wider

Table 9-9 Biochemical Characteristics of *Capnocytophaga canimorsus* (DF−2), *C. cynodegmi* (DF-2-like), and Other *Capnocytophaga* Species

CHARACTERISTIC	C. CANIMORSUS	C. CYNODEGMI	CAPNOCYTOPHAGA SPP*
Hemolysis, SBA	−	−	−
Oxidase	+	+	−
Catalase	+	+	−
Gliding motility	+	+	+
Growth on MacConkey agar	−	−	−
NO₃ to NO₂	−	v	v
NO₂ to N₂ gas	v	v	−
Indole	−	−	−
Urease	−	−	−
Arginine dihydrolase	+	+	−
Lysine decarboxylase	−	−	−
Ornithine decarboxylase	−	−	−
Hydrolysis of esculin	v	+	v
Hydrolysis of ONPG	+	+	v
Acid produced from:			
Glucose	+	+	+
Maltose	+	+	+
Fructose	v	+	v
Sucrose	−	+	+
Lactose	+	+	v
Xylose	−	−	−
Mannitol	−	−	−
Mannose	v	+	+
Raffinose	−	+	v
Inulin	−	+	NA
Galactose	+	v	v
Melibiose	−	+	−
Hydrolysis of glycogen	+	v	v
Hydrolysis of starch	+	+	v

* *C. ochracea, C. gingivalis, and C. sputigena.*
+, *positive reaction;* −, *negative reaction; v, variable reaction; NA, not available.*

variety of sugars. Table 9-9 shows the biochemical reactions of *C. canimorsus* and *C. cynodegmi* along with the general biochemical characteristics of the other *Capnocytophaga* species discussed previously. The term "dysgonic" means that biochemical test media for identification, including the basal medium for carbohydrate fermentation, should be supplemented with serum (three to five drops per 5 ml broth) to obtain reliable and consistent reactions.

Antimicrobial Susceptibility

Slow growth of *C. canimorsus* on agar medium and failure of some strains to grow in certain types of broth media have generally precluded adequate studies of the antimicrobial susceptibility of this organism. Nonstandardized studies using disk diffusion procedures designed for more rapidly growing bacteria had previously reported that *C. canimorsus* strains were susceptible to most antimicrobials, but were resistant to aminoglycosides. In 1988, Verghese and associates reported on a broth dilution technique using Schaedler broth as the growth medium.[1326] All eight *C. canimorsus* strains tested were susceptible to all antibiotics except aztreonam. These antimicrobial agents included penicillin, erythromycin, ticarcillin, piperacillin, cefazolin, cefoperazone, cefotaxime, ceftazidime, chloramphenicol, trimethoprim-sulfamethoxazole, and fluoroquinolones. Susceptibility of *C. canimorsus* to sulfonamides and aminoglycosides is unclear at present, since in vitro results with these agents appear to be method-dependent. Antibiotics that are generally more active against gram-positive organisms, such as vancomycin, clindamycin, erythromycin, and rifampin were also active against *C. canimorsus*. These data support the clinical efficacy observed with penicillin (mean penicillin MIC, 0.04 ± 0.01 μg/mL for all strains tested).

Dysgonomonas Species

CDC group DF-3 is an uncommon clinical isolate that has recently been classified in the new genus *Dysgonomonas* as *D. capnocytophagoides*.[581] Biochemically, this organism resembles certain *Capnocytophaga* species (its species epithet means "Capnocytophaga-like"), but 16S rRNA sequencing studies indicate genetic relatedness to *Bacteroides distasonis*, *Bacteroides uniformis*, *Bacteroides forsythus*, and *Prevotella melaninogenica*, which are anaerobic gram-negative bacilli.[581,1305] The first two reports of this organism in association with human disease were published in 1988. In one case, *D. capnocytophagoides* was isolated in pure culture from multiple stool specimens of an elderly woman with common variable hypogammaglobulinemia of long standing.[1342] In the second case, *D. capnocytophagoides* was recovered in blood cultures from a 24-year-old man with relapsed acute lymphocytic leukemia who had profound granulocytopenia resulting from intensive chemotherapy and radiation.[57] In 1991, Gill and coworkers at the National Cancer Institute screened stool specimens from 690 patients and found 11 with moderate to heavy growth of *D. capnocytophagoides*.[464] Of these 11 patients, 4 had a history of prolonged diarrhea and were treated; diarrhea had been documented in the other 7 patients, but the organisms cleared spontaneously. Blum and colleagues recovered *D. capnocytophagoides* from the stool of eight patients during a year-long period.[144] All patients were immunocompromised or had severe underlying disease, including three patients with HIV infection and two with inflammatory bowel disease. Among these patients, the clinical spectrum of *D. capnocytophagoides* ranged from chronic diarrhea with a clinical response to antimicrobial therapy to an asymptomatic carrier state.[144] Other investigators have also noted the association of enteric *D. capnocytophagoides* infection with both HIV infection and common variable hypogammaglobulinemia.[552] This organism has also been isolated from soft-tissue abscesses, decubitus ulcers, and the urinary tract of compromised patients.[81,853,1149]

D. capnocytophagoides is most easily recovered from stool specimens using cefoperazone-vancomycin-amphotericin blood agar incubated at 35°C in 5–7% CO_2. Nonselective blood agar should also be inoculated, since some strains fail to grow on this selective *Campylobacter* medium.[464] The organism has also been recovered on blood agar containing kanamycin and vancomycin following anaerobic incubation.[853] *D. capnocytophagoides* grows relatively slowly, with pinpoint colonies being visible after 24 hours of incubation. After 48 to 72 hours the colonies are gray-white, smooth, and nonhemolytic, and some strains produce a sweet odor during growth on agar media (see Color Plate 9-4H).[57,121,144,464,1342] On Gram stains the organisms appear as small gram-negative coccobacilli. Both oxidase and catalase reactions are negative, nitrate is not reduced, and urea is not

hydrolyzed. Indole is produced in tryptone broth, and esculin is hydrolyzed. Lysine and ornithine decarboxylases and arginine dihydrolase are not produced. This bacterium produces acid fermentatively from glucose, xylose, and maltose; most strains also produce acid from sucrose and lactose but do not produce acid from mannitol (Table 9-10). Some "DF-3-like" strains have also been described that are consistently sucrose-negative and slightly hemolytic.[300] Gas-liquid chromatography is also useful for identification, since all strains consistently demonstrate 12- and 13-methyltetradecanoate, with minor amounts of tetradecanoate and hexadecanoate in their cell wall.[121,144,300,1345] In addition to *D. capnocytophagoides*, two other *Dysgonomonas* species have been described. A single isolate of an organism designated *Dysgonomonas gadei*, was isolated from a human gallbladder, and *Dysgonomonas mossii* was recovered from human clinical specimens.[581,759]

Antimicrobial susceptibility of *D. capnocytophagoides* isolates has been determined by disk diffusion, broth dilution, and Etest methods.[57,144,552,853,1342] *D. capnocytophagoides* strains are resistant to several agents, including penicillin, ampicillin, ampicillin-sulbactam, aztreonam, aminoglycosides, cephalosporins (including cephalothin, cefoxitin, ceftriaxone, cefoperazone, and ceftazidime), erythromycin, ciprofloxacin, and vancomycin. Most isolates are susceptible to trimethoprim-sulfamethoxazole, rifampin, and chloramphenicol, and variably susceptible to piperacillin, clindamycin, tetracycline, and imipenem. Patients usually respond to therapy with trimethoprim-sulfamethoxazole, clindamycin, or tetracycline.[144,464]

CDC Group EF-4A and EF-4B

Formerly a group of uncertain taxonomic affiliation, these bacteria are now classified as unnamed members of the family *Neisseriaceae*.[1100] CDC group EF-4 (eugonic fermenter 4) is part of the normal oral flora of cats and dogs, and may also cause purulent cutaneous and pulmonary infections in these animals.[285,1368] EF-4 has been isolated from human wounds resulting from scratches and bites from cats and dogs and from the blood of a 65-year-old woman with metastatic small-cell carcinoid of the liver.[359,1250] The patient owned a dog, but she did not recollect a dog bite. EF-4 was coisolated with *Pasteurella multocida* from an eye laceration and vitreous fluid of an 8-year-old girl after being scratched on the face by her cat, and was recovered from purulent ear drainage of a 36-year-old man who was repeatedly licked on his ears by his pet Dalmatians.[1082,1317]

CDC group EF-4 is a gram-negative coccobacillus that grows on both blood and chocolate agars; some strains may also grow on MacConkey agar. After 24 hours of incubation, the colonies are about 1 mm in diameter, opaque, smooth, yellowish, have an entire edge, and are weakly α-hemolytic or nonhemolytic. Some strains have a distinct "popcorn"-like odor. In the single bacteremic case, EF-4 was detected radiometrically by the BACTEC system after 2 days of incubation. The organism is nonmotile, oxidase-positive and catalase-positive, and reduces nitrate to nitrite. Some strains may also reduce nitrite to nitrogen gas.[186] The organism does

Table 9-10 Biochemical Characteristics for Identification of *Dysgonomonas* Species and CDC Groups EF-4A and EF-4B

CHARACTERISTIC	*D. CAPNOCYTOPHAGOIDES*	*D. GADEI*	*D. ROSSII*	GROUP EF-4A	GROUP EF-4B
Hemolysis, SBA	−	−/α	−	−/α^w	−/α^w
Oxidase	−	−	−	+	+
Catalase	−	+	v	+	+
Motility	−	−	−	−	−
Growth on MacConkey agar	−	−	−	v	v
NO$_3$ to NO$_2$	−	−	−	+	+
NO$_2$ to N$_2$ gas	NA	NA	NA	v	v
Indole	v	v	+	−	−
Acetoin	−	−	−	NA	NA
Urease	−	−	−	−	−
Gelatin hydrolysis	NA	−	−	v	−
Alkaline phosphatase	+	+	+	NA	NA
Arginine dihydrolase	−	−	−	+	−
Ornithine decarboxylase	NA	NA	NA	NA	NA
Esculin hydrolysis	+	+	+	−	−
Gas from glucose	−	−	−	−	−
Acid produced from:					
Glucose	+	+	+	+^{a}	+^{b}
Adonitol	−	−	NA	NA	NA
L-Arabinose	+	+	NA	NA	NA
Cellobiose	NA	+	NA	NA	NA
Dulcitol	−	−	NA	NA	NA
Erythritol	NA	−	NA	NA	NA
Fructose	NA	+	+	NA	NA
Glycogen	NA	−	NA	NA	NA
Inositol	−	−	+^{w}	NA	NA
Lactose	+	+	+	−	−
Maltose	+	NA	+	−	−
Mannitol	−	−	+^{w}	−	−
Mannose	+	+	+	NA	NA
Melezitose	NA	+	NA	NA	NA
Melibiose	+	+	NA	NA	NA
Raffinose	+	+	v	NA	NA
Rhamnose	NA	+	+^{w}	NA	NA
Ribose	NA	+^{w}	NA	NA	NA
Salicin	NA	+	+	NA	NA
Sorbitol	−	−	NA	NA	NA
Starch	NA	+	NA	NA	NA
Sucrose	+	+	+	−	−
Trehalose	−	+	+	NA	NA
Xylose	+	+	+	−	−
β-glucuronidase	−	+	−	NA	NA
N-acetyl-β-glucosaminidase	−	+	+	NA	NA
α-fucosidase	−	+	+	NA	NA

+, *positive reaction;* −, *negative reaction;* +^{w}, *weak positive reaction;* v, *variable reaction;* NA, *data not available.*
^{a} *glucose fermented*
^{b} *glucose oxidized*

not produce urease or indole. EF-4 strains are divided into subgroups EF-4a and EF-4b based on carbohydrate utiliza-tion (see Table 9-10). EF-4a strains ferment glucose, do not produce acids from other carbohydrates, and are arginine dihydrolase-positive.[537,1368] EF-4b strains similarly produce acid oxidatively rather than fermentatively from glucose only. EF-4b strains also do not reduce nitrate all the way to gas and are arginine dihydrolase–negative.[537] Most EF-4 isolates are susceptible to penicillin, ampicillin, cefazo-lin, chloramphenicol, tetracycline, erythromycin, clarithromycin, trimethoprim-sulfamethoxazole, the quinolones, and the aminoglycosides.

Simonsiella Species

Simonsiella species are fastidious, aerobic gram-negative bacilli that have the unusual morphologic characteristic of existing in multicellular arrangements measuring 20–50 by 4–8 μm. These arrangements consist of six to eight cells, with the long axis of the individual bacilli at right angles to the axis of the cell group. The cell group exhibits gliding motility and forms pale yellow colonies on blood agar after 18 to 24 hours at 37°C. The genus *Simonsiella* contains three species: *S. muelleri* is found in the human oral cavity, while *S. crassa* and *S. steedae* are found in the oral cavities of sheep and dogs/cats, respectively. *S. muelleri* was isolated from a gastric aspirate from a neonate, but has not been implicated as a human pathogen.[1372] The genus is classified in the Family *Neisseriaceae*.[1100]

Streptobacillus moniliformis
Taxonomy

S. moniliformis is the only member of the genus *Streptobacillus,* and its present taxonomic positive is uncertain. Based on 16S rRNA sequencing studies, *S. moniliformis* is currently classified in the proposed family ''Fusobacteriaceae'' in the proposed class ''Fusobacteria'' of the phylum *Fusobacteria*.[455]

Clinical Significance

Streptobacillus moniliformis is a fastidious gram-negative bacillus that is normally found in the oropharynx of rodents and can be transmitted to humans by bites from these animals. Rodents are the natural reservoir of *S. moniliformis* and play a key role in organism transmission. The organism is found in the upper respiratory tracts of wild rats, laboratory rats and mice, and domesticated rodents (e.g., guinea pigs, gerbils) and may cause disease in these animals.[692,713] The organism may also be carried by animals that catch or feed on rodents, such as dogs or cats.

In humans, *S. moniliformis* causes a disease called ''rat-bite fever,'' or Haverhill fever when it is acquired by ingestion of the organism. The latter name comes from Haverhill, Massachusetts, where this organism was recovered from blood cultures of several patients during a local outbreak of the disease.[745,1165] At present, most cases involve bites from rats or exposure to rodents, and many of these infections occur in children.[497,963] After an incubation period of 7 to 10 days following the bite of a rat or the ingestion of food or water contaminated with rat excrement, there is an abrupt onset of high fever, chills, headache, muscle aches, vomiting, and other constitutional symptoms.[963] A few days after disease onset, a rash appears on the extremities (including the palms and soles), and severe joint pain, migratory, non-symmetric polyarthritis, or frank septic arthritis may develop in about 50% of patients.[294,523,577,591,1112] Typically the rash is pink-red and maculopapular, although it may also be petechial, purpuric, or pustular.[113] Cutaneous and subcutaneous abscesses with pitting edema have also been described in association with this infection.[523,1282,1319] The disease may resolve spontaneously with no residual symptoms or may develop into a chronic, periodically febrile condition. Complications related to systemic dissemination via the bloodstream include endocarditis, pneumonia with pleural effusion, septicemia, brain abscess, amnionitis, prostatitis, pancreatitis, cutaneous and genital tract abscesses, and death.[199,333,399,1014,1090,1110,1158] Arthritic symptoms may persist for years after resolution and/or treatment of the infection. Without a clue as to the origin of infection, rat-bite fever or Haverhill fever may resemble viral infection, syphilis, leptospirosis, disseminated gonococcal infection, meningococcemia, typhoid, or Rocky Mountain spotted fever.[1021,1399] Diagnosis may also be problematic because cases have been reported in patients with no history of rodent bites or direct exposure to rodents.[417] On the other hand, review of 45 cases occurring in California over the past 30 years revealed that rat-bite fever was suspected in 75% of the cases in which a tentative diagnosis was given.[497] Because of the fastidious nature of the organism and the difficulties involved with culture, retrospective diagnoses of *S. moniliformis* infection have been made on occasion by serologic techniques, including detection of serum agglutinins and complement-fixing antibodies against the bacillary form of the organism. However, serologic tests for this infection are not readily available, and most serologic approaches have been used to assess presence of the organism in laboratory rodent colonies.

Cultural Characteristics and Identification

S. moniliformis is a fastidious, pleomorphic gram-negative bacillus that tends to form long, thin, filamentous single cells. These thin (about 1 μm) cells may be over 100 μm in length and may fold into loops and coils. Occasionally, these organisms may stain gram-variable. On prolonged incubation, bulbous or sausage-shaped swelling may appear along the filament, causing the organism to resemble a string of beads. On enriched, serum-containing media, the organisms appear as regular, thin, gram-variable fusiform bacteria with rounded or pointed ends. The organism may also lose its cell wall and exist as an ''L-form ('cell wall deficient').'' In fact, there is genetic, phenotypic, serologic, and structural evidence suggesting that this organism is taxonomically related to the mycoplasmas and ureaplasmas, which also lack a typical bacterial cell wall.[1399] *S. moniliformis* is microaerophilic, and growth in liquid medium usually requires supplementation with serum (10–20%), blood, or ascites fluid.

Diagnosis of rat-bite or Haverhill fever is made by recovery of *S. moniliformis* from blood cultures; synovial fluid, skin lesions, and abscess material.[366,1165,1166] Because the organism is inhibited by the anticoagulant SPS, blood (10 mL) must be anticoagulated with citrate (10 mL of sodium citrate, 2.5%) prior to processing.[745,1166] The organism has also been successfully recovered in SPS-containing blood culture media with resins (e.g., BACTEC Peds-Plus, BD Biosciences).[591] The citrated blood cells are sedimented by centrifugation and the packed cells are inoculated onto agar medium (heart infusion agar) containing 10–20% sterile decomplemented horse serum and 0.5% yeast extract. The inoculum is gently spread over the agar surface. A broth medium of similar ingredients (heart infusion broth with 10–20% serum and yeast extract) is also inoculated with the packed cells. Isolation of *S. moniliformis* has also been accomplished using a biphasic medium of trypticase-soy broth containing a trypticase-soy agar slant. Media is incubated at 35°C in a candle jar or a CO_2 incubator. Other specimens, (citrated joint fluid, aspirates, abscess material, etc.) may be cultured in the same manner.

In broth medium the organism grows as small "puff balls" near the bottom of the tube or bottle and overlying the red cells and stroma. Accumulation of acid in broth media may kill the organism, so frequent subculture is necessary to maintain viability. On serum-enriched agar medium, growth may appear within 2 to 3 days, or may require a week or more. Colonies are small (1–2 mm in diameter), convex, gray-white, smooth, and buttery in consistency. Microscopic L-phase variants form spontaneously under or around the existing colonies; the typical "fried-egg" morphology with a dense center similar to the morphology of *Mycoplasma* species can be observed with a dissecting microscope. Identification of *S. moniliformis* is accomplished by observing the typical gram-negative, filamentous morphology on Gram staining and by performing biochemical identification tests in serum supplemented medium.[366,1399] Carbohydrate utilization tests may be performed in nutrient broth containing 1% filter-sterilized carbohydrates and 0.5% sterile horse serum. These tests should be incubated for 3 weeks before reading, although reliable and reproducible results have been obtained when cultures were incubated for only 1 week before test interpretation. Rapid identification of the organism may also be accomplished by fatty acid profile analyses using gas-liquid chromatography (GLC), by detection of enzymatic activities for various aminopeptidases and glycosidases using the API-ZYM strip (BioMerieux, Inc.), and by protein patterns obtained by PAGE.[286,366,1104] Fatty-acid methyl esters detected by GLC include hexadecanoic acid ($C_{16:0}$), linoleic acid ($C_{18:2}$), and octadecanoic acids ($C_{18:1}$, $C_{18:0}$).[366,591,1104] PAGE techniques may also be useful for strain typing of clinical isolates.[286] The reactions of *S. moniliformis* in various biochemical identification tests are shown in Table 9-11. Broad-range PCR-based amplification of a part of the 16S rRNA gene followed by amplicon sequencing has been developed for detection of *S. moniliformis* in rodent colonies, turkey flocks, and humans.[113,153] This method was used to diagnose rat-bite fever in a symptomatic 11-year-old boy in whom fever, vomiting, rash, and arthritis developed after being bitten by his pet rat. Cultures from blood, CSF, and urine were negative, but fluid from a cutaneous blister was positive by the amplification/sequencing assay.[113]

Antimicrobial Susceptibility

In vitro antimicrobial susceptibility data indicate that *S. moniliformis* is susceptible to penicillin, ampicillin, extended-spectrum and penicillinase-resistant penicillins (azlocillin, mezlocillin, piperacillin, oxacillin), cephalosporins (cefazolin, cefixime, cefotaxime, cefoxitin, cefpirome, ceftazidime), erythromycin, clindamycin, tetracycline, rifampin, imipenem, and vancomycin.[366,1399] The organism is intermediate in susceptibility to the aminoglycosides, chloramphenicol, and ciprofloxacin, and it is generally resistant to nalidixate, norfloxacin, colistin, and trimethoprim-

Table 9-11 Biochemical Characteristics of *Streptobacillus moniliformis*

CHARACTERISTIC	REACTION
Oxidase	−
Catalase	−
Nitrate reduction	−
Indole	−
Urease	−
Esculin hydrolysis	+
Production of H_2S (lead acetate)	+
Alkaline phosphatase	+
Gas production from glucose	−
Acid produced from:	
Glucose	+
Maltose	+
Fructose	+
Sucrose	v
Lactose	v
Xylose	−
Mannitol	−
Mannose	+

+, positive reaction; −, negative reaction; v, variable reaction.

sulfamethoxazole. The drug of choice for treatment is procaine penicillin G, although cephalothin, tetracycline, and other cephalosporins have also demonstrated clinical efficacy.

Brucella Species
Epidemiology of Brucellosis

Brucellosis (infection with *Brucella* species) is worldwide in distribution and has been known historically as undulant fever, Bang's disease, Gibraltar fever, Mediterranean fever, and Malta fever. The organism was first isolated in 1887 by Sir David Bruce, who recovered a suspect organism from splenic cultures of British soldiers dying of Malta fever.[1042] Later, it was found that milk, cheese, and other foods made with goats' milk were the sources of infection in these soldiers. Similar organisms were recovered from cattle, pigs, and humans exposed to these animals and their products. Brucellosis became recognized as a zoonosis of great economic importance and concern to the livestock industry in many parts of the world. In developed countries, some human infections are associated with meat-packing and dairy-related occupations.[1421] In the U.S., the majority of reported cases in recent years have come from California, Iowa, Virginia, and Texas, reflecting the animal husbandry, cattle, and dairy industries central to the economy of those states.

Brucellosis is transmitted among animals via the gastrointestinal tract, skin, and mucous membranes. Following infection, organisms reach the lymph nodes and bacteremia occurs. In some animals (e.g., *B. abortus* infection in cattle), the organisms proliferate in the uterus and in the mammary glands. Growth of the organism in the chorionic membranes of the pregnant animal leads to abortion. Many animals recover from the infection spontaneously, but continue to shed the bacteria for varying times in urine, vaginal secretions, and milk.

Brucella species are named for their primary host species and are further subdivided into biovars based on serologic agglutination with "smooth lipopolysaccharide (S-LPS)"-associated antigens M and A (see below). *B. melitensis* is found primarily in goats and sheep, but may also be found in cattle because of indirect contact with infected sheep and goat flocks that have contaminated pastures from which fodder was harvested for lactating cows.[1172] *B. melitensis* is divided into three biovars (1–3). *B. abortus* is pathogenic for cattle, but can also infect sheep, goats, canines, horses, and humans. The species is comprised of seven biovars (1–6, and 9 [biovars 7 and 8 are no longer valid]). *B. suis* contains five biovars; biovars 1, 2, and 3 are found in swine, while biovar 4 is found in reindeer and caribou in the Arctic regions of North America and Russia, and biovar 5 causes infections in rodents. *B. suis* biovar 1 has also become established in cattle herds in Brazil and Columbia.[1172] *B. canis* strains comprise a single biovar and occur in dogs (especially beagles) in the U.S., Mexico, Argentina, Spain, China, Japan, and Tunisia. *B. ovis* and *B. neotomae* each contain a single biovar and are found in rams and wood rats, respectively. Antigenic variation among existing biovars has been demonstrated for every *Brucella* species, establishing that biovar classifications require further study and expansion. *B. melitensis*, *B. abortus*, and *B. suis* are associated with human disease, with *B. melitensis* considered the most virulent species, followed by *B. suis* and B. abortus. *B. canis* rarely causes infections in humans, and reported infections have often been laboratory-associated. The protean complications associated with *Brucella* infections are not generally seen in human *B. canis* infections.

In 1994, a previously unrecognized *Brucella* species was isolated from marine mammals and a dolphin in Scotland and California, respectively.[170,261,422] Subsequently, additional isolates were obtained from seals, porpoises, and otters.[626] These isolates comprised at least two biovars corresponding to phocene or cetacean origins, respectively, and were tentatively named "*Brucella maris*."[626] Isolates obtained from aborted bottlenose dolphin fetuses were also characterized, and the name "*Brucella delphini*" was proposed for these isolates.[868] Serologic surveys of seal, porpoise, dolphin, and whale species have shown that antibodies against *Brucella* species are widely distributed among marine mammals.[639,1291] Molecular analysis has shown that isolates from whales, seals, porpoises, and dolphins are *Brucella* species but differ from each other and from other extant *Brucella* species in many respects, including LPS structure and OMPs.[100,170,635] The insertion element IS*711*, which is found in all *Brucella* species, is also found in marine isolates, but the element is in a different chromosomal location.[262] Whereas recognized *Brucella* species contain two *omp2* genes comprised of one copy each of *omp2a* and *omp2b*, or two *omp2a* genes, marine brucellae carry two *omp2b* gene copies Sequencing of these genes also revealed significant heterogeneity among the marine isolates, indicat-

ing that these organisms encompass more than a single species ("*B. maris*"), as had been proposed.[261,263] Based on host preferences and polymorphism at the *omp2* locus, Cloeckaert and coworkers have proposed two new species, "*B. pinnipediae*" and "*B. cetaceae*," to include the characterized seal and dolphin isolates, respectively.[263] Some evidence also suggests that these new species may have extended pathogenic potential. Rhyan and colleagues inoculated six cattle with a *Brucella* isolate from a harbor seal, and found that all animals seroconverted in tests used for detection of *B. abortus* antibodies. Two of the cattle aborted, and the brucellae were isolated from the stillborn fetuses, indicating that these strains are pathogenic for terrestrial mammals as well.[1068] Additional work is needed to delineate the phylogenetic relationships among these new species and to ascertain their relationships with currently recognized species in the genus.[423]

In the U.S., the incidence of human brucellosis has declined steadily as a result of control measures implemented in the livestock industry. These measures include vaccination of young animals, and slaughter of sick animals or older animals with serologic evidence of infection.[1421] At the time that the Federal-State Cooperative Brucellosis Eradication Program and routine dairy pasteurization began in 1945, over 5,000 human cases were reported to the CDC annually. In 1981, the reported annual domestic incidence of human brucellosis had dropped to 185 cases, and since that time, less than 200 cases per year have been reported. However, human brucellosis is probably underdiagnosed and underreported, with estimates that at least 25 cases go unrecognized for every case that is diagnosed.[1042] Over the past two decades, many domestically acquired brucella infections have been diagnosed among individuals living in Texas and California who have ingested Mexican cheese prepared from unpasteurized goat's milk.[245,1267] With increasing availability and popularity of international travel, many brucellosis cases diagnosed in U.S. residents occur in people who have visited countries where the organism is endemic in ovine/bovine herds and unpasteurized dairy products (e.g., whey, butter, yogurts, sauces). Infection partly reflects participation in aspects of a foreign culture that are so appealing to travelers (i.e., "living like the natives do").[1042] Humans may also become infected by contact with infected animals, products of conception (especially veterinarians, zoo workers), or body fluids of animals. Human-to-human transmission is rare. *Brucella* infections have been transmitted via blood transfusions and bone marrow transplantations from infected donors.[17,383] Neonatal infection can be acquired by the transplacental route, during delivery, or via the ingestion of contaminated breast milk.[984]

Brucellosis is found scattered throughout areas of both the eastern and western hemispheres. Indigenous animal and human infections occur in the Mediterranean region, the Arabian gulf, the Indian subcontinent, Latin America, Asia, and parts of Mexico. *B. abortus* is found worldwide, and *B. suis* is endemic in the southern U.S., Southeast Asia, and Latin America. *B. canis* infections have been diagnosed in Latin America, Central Europe, and Japan. Bovine and swine brucellosis caused by *B. melitensis* and *B. suis*, respectively, have been identified in all countries of Central America, with caprine and ovine *B. melitensis* infection being restricted to Guatemala.[892] Northern Europe, Denmark, and Norway have no animal infections because of successful control/eradication programs, but southern European countries still have *B. melitensis* in ovine and caprine populations and, consequently, report high numbers of human infections.[382,472] These countries have also seen resurgence of *B. suis* biovar 2 infection in swine because of spillover from the wild boar population.[472] Brucellosis in animals and humans remains a problem in the Balkan region of Central and Southeast Europe. *B. melitensis* infection occurs widely among sheep, goats, and humans and *B. abortus* is found in cattle herds in Greece and Macedonia.[1252] *B. melitensis* infection in sheep and goat herds and *B. suis* biovar 2 infection in swine are found in Yugoslavia and Croatia, respectively.[1252] Romania has successfully eradicated *B. abortus* infection in cattle, and the incidence of infections in sheep and swine remains low.[336]

The countries with the highest incidence of both animal and human brucellosis are Saudi Arabia, Iran, Syria, the Palestinian Authority, Jordan, and Oman. In the Near East region, the disease occurs in all domestic animals, including cattle, sheep, goats, camels, horses, swine, and buffaloes. *B. melitensis* biovar 3 (Egypt, Israel, Tunisia, Turkey, Jordan), *B. melitensis* biovar 2 (Saudi Arabia, Turkey), and *B. melitensis* biovar 1 (Libya, Oman, Israel) account for most disease, but infections with *B. abortus* biovars 1, 2, 3, and 6 have been reported in Egypt, Iran, Turkey, and the Sudan, respectively.[1055] *B. abortus* biovars have emerged as the predominant species in Yemen. Human infections acquired in these regions are usually due to *B. melitensis*, particularly biovar 3.[1055]

Brucella species also pose an occupational hazard to laboratory workers because of laboratory accidents, spills, or inappropriate manipulations of specimens or cultures containing *Brucella* organisms.[502] In 2000, Yagupsky and others described seven laboratory-acquired cases of *B. melitensis* infection at a medical center in southern Israel.[1411] This outbreak was caused by three different *B. melitensis* biovars, indicating multiple exposures, and the infections occurred over a 3-month period when 10% of 530 positive blood cultures grew *Brucella* species. On investigation, no sources or breaches in laboratory safety were found. Brucellosis also was diagnosed in seven hospital employees (six bacteriology technologists and a pathologist) over a 9-year period at a hospital in Riyadh, Saudi Arabia.[855] Infections were diagnosed by serologic tests, along with compatible clinical signs and symptoms. Resulting morbidity included relapse in two patients and complications (septic phlebitis, infected prostheses, epididymo-orchitis, and lumbar spondylitis) in four others. Infections in the technologists were traced to the handling of *Brucella* cultures. In a report from Italy, 12 laboratory workers became infected after accidental breakage of a centrifuge tube.[412] These individuals were treated and monitored by serologic testing. Even though the laboratories involved in these accidents used class II biologic safety cabinets for manipulations of specimens and cultures, the risk for laboratory-acquired infections is significant, particularly in laboratories located in endemic regions. Strict adherence to safety protocols and procedures in all laboratories and vigilance and care when handling specimens/cultures is an absolute requirement for prevention of laboratory-acquired infections of any kind. Following the outbreak at

the Riyadh hospital, the laboratory response included the installation of a Biosafety Level 3 facility.[855]

Taxonomy of *Brucella* Species

For many years, the taxonomic position of *Brucella* species was uncertain. In 1985, Verger and colleagues used DNA-DNA hybridization techniques to investigate 51 *Brucella* strains representing all species and found that all of the isolates had greater than $96 \pm 4\%$ homology with each other.[1325] These scientists proposed that all brucellae belonged to a single species (*Brucella melitensis*) and that the recognized species should be regarded as biovars of *B. melitensis* (i.e., *B. melitensis* biovars Melitensis, Abortus, Suis, and Canis). Multilocus enzyme electrophoretic analysis of *Brucella* strains also supported this monospecific genus proposal.[448] This proposal has not been generally accepted because of biochemical and serologic differences among the species, the divergent host ranges displayed by these species, recognized differences in virulence, and the presence of species-specific OMPs and genes that substantiate the status of extant species.[893] Molecular genetic studies (i.e., restriction endonuclease mapping) subsequently revealed gene polymorphisms that were able to differentiate *B. abortus*, *B. melitensis*, *B. suis*, and *B. canis* along conventional species lines, although these methods could not delineate biovars within species.[18] One of the polymorphic genes that help to differentiate species within the brucellae is the *omp2* porin gene, which codes for a 36-kDa OMP that is responsible for determining susceptibility to the dyes used for conventional species identification.[407]

Studies on the genetic relationships of brucellae have revealed other unique features of the genus. Unlike other bacteria, *Brucella* species have two chromosomes except for *B. suis* biovar 3, which has a single chromosome.[656] The genome of *B. melitensis* strain 16M was recently sequenced and is composed of 3,294,935 base pairs (bp) distributed over two circular chromosomes of 2,117,144 bp and 1,177,787 bp, respectively.[315,316] Each chromosome encodes functions that are essential for replication and survival of the organism, hence their classification as chromosomes and not plasmids. Endogenous plasmids, transformation, and conjugation have not been described in *Brucella* species. DNA-RNA hybridization and 16S rRNA sequencing studies have determined that *Brucella* species are related to *Agrobacterium*, endosymbiotic *Rhizobium* and *Mesorhizobium* species, and *Bartonella* species, and are phylogenetically closest to *Ochrobactrum* and *Phyllobacterium* species, which are free-living chemoautotrophic pathogens of tropical plants.[589,992] *Brucella* species are most closely related to *O. anthropi* hybridization group 2, for which the new species name *O. intermedium* has been proposed.[1320] The genetic relatedness of these organisms is so close that *O. anthropi* is reactive in a PCR-based assay that is "specific" for *Brucella* species.[297] *Brucella* species are now classified in the α_2 subgroup of the *Proteobacteria* in the family *Brucellaceae* in the proposed order "Rhizobiales."[455,894]

Virulence of *Brucella* Species

Brucella species undergo antigenic variation or "dissociation" on subculture. The colonies switch from a "smooth" to a "rough" morphology that results in a loss of virulence and diminished reactivity with *Brucella*-specific antibodies. On the molecular level, antigenic variation is the result of decreased expression of genes encoding the additional glycosylation of the polysaccharide moieties of the cell-wall lipopolysaccharide (LPS).[730] Organisms that are in the smooth phase possess a smooth-type LPS (S-LPS) and are resistant to intracellular killing by polymorphonuclear cells (PMNs), presumably by inhibiting lysosomal degranulation and the respiratory burst associated with PMN activation.[19,1072] Other than the antigenic variation of LPS and its relation to virulence, *Brucella* species do not produce exotoxins and very little else is known regarding additional virulence mechanisms in *Brucella* species.

The LPS of *B. melitensis*, *B. abortus*, and *B. suis* contains two major antigenic determinants called A (for "Abortus") and M (for "Melitensis").[189] In addition to providing markers for biovar determinations, these molecules also have a role in organism virulence, as monoclonal antibodies directed against the S-LPS are protective in animal challenge models, and smooth isolates that have lost S-LPS by transposon mutagenesis have attenuated pathogenicity for mice.[888] The S-LPS O (somatic antigen) chains from smooth *B. melitensis* and smooth *B. abortus* strains are both composed of polymers of 4,6-dideoxy-4-formamido-D-mannose (i.e., N-formyl-D-perosamine). In *B. abortus* S-LPS, the O chain contains about 100 residues, nearly all of which are $\alpha_{1,2}$-linked, with a small percentage being $\alpha_{1,3}$-linked (A determinants). In *B. melitensis* O chains, $\alpha_{1,2}$ and $\alpha_{1,3}$ linkages occur in a 4:1 ratio (M determinants). The serodominant A antigen tends to be rod-shaped, the shape being determined by the five consecutive $\alpha_{1,2}$-linked residues, whereas the serodominant M antigen is "kinked" in shape because the fourth residue is linked to the fifth by an $\alpha_{1,3}$ linkage. The common expression of nonterminal $\alpha_{1,2}$-linked N-formyl-D-perosamine is responsible for the cross-reactivity seen between S-LPS of smooth *B. abortus* and smooth *B. melitensis* strains and the cross-reactivity that is seen with other species (e.g., *Vibrio cholerae* O:1, *Yersinia enterocolitica* O:9, *Escherichia coli* O:157, *Salmonella* O:30 and *Stenotrophomonas maltophilia*).[189] Slide agglutination or EIA with either polyclonal or monoclonal antibodies specific for A or M epitopes are used to determine the A or M antigen predominance and the serovar designations of *Brucella* strains.[189,453] Strains of *B. abortus*, *B. melitensis*, and *B. suis* can be A antigen-positive, M antigen-positive or both A and M antigen-positive. A and M antigenic determinants are not found in *B. canis* or *B. ovis;* these species are characteristically rough, do not display phase variation, and have a restricted host range.

Brucella species are facultative intracellular organisms, and their disease spectrum is partially explained by the ability of the organism to evade host defense mechanisms by virtue of intracellular existence. Brucellae are transmitted to humans by three principal routes: direct contact with infected animal tissues, ingestion of contaminated meats or dairy products, and inhalation of aerosolized organisms.[283,1042] Once inside the host, the organisms are phagocytized but are able to survive within these cells, presumably by adenine and guanine monophosphate–mediated suppression or inactivation of the intracellular myeloperoxidase-peroxide defense mechanisms and by the production of superoxide

dismutase, which blocks formation of toxic oxygen radicals.[173,198] The organisms are carried into the lymph nodes and the bloodstream and become sequestered in various parts of the reticuloendothelial system—liver sinusoids, spleen, and bone marrow.[856] In these sites, the PMNs eventually degenerate and release the intracellular organisms. The bacteria, in turn, are endocytosed by macrophages and monocytes. Multiplication continues within these cells, and eventually the cells are killed, releasing the organisms. The "undulant" waxing-and-waning fever pattern seen in brucellosis is associated with the periodic release of bacteria and their components from phagocytic cells. Release of bacteria into the peripheral circulation results in hematogenous seeding of other organs and tissues, thereby leading to the protean clinical manifestations of human brucellosis. Relapses and recurrences of illness are kept in check to some degree by a balance between the virulence of the organism and the presence of an intact, functional cellular immune response. As with other intracellular pathogens, humoral antibodies are produced, but cellular immune defense mechanisms are required to contain the intracellular bacteria. Cytokines produced by activated macrophages, including tumor necrosis factor α (TNF-α), TNF-γ, and interleukin-1 (IL-1) and IL-2, are known to influence macrophage-mediated antibrucella activity during induction of cell-mediated immune responses.[284] Caron and colleagues have shown that brucellae synthesize and release a high-molecular-weight protein factor that specifically inhibits TNF-α expression in activated human macrophages. This inhibition likely contributes to the ability of *Brucella* species to evade human host defenses and maintain an intracellular existence.[203] Interestingly, intracellular ribosomal protein antigens designated L7/L12 have been found to stimulate protective cell-mediated immune responses along with delayed-type hypersensitivity.[966] Consequently, these proteins are being investigated for their potential as candidate vaccine antigens. The clinical spectrum of brucellosis depends on many factors, including the immune status of the host, the presence of other underlying diseases or conditions, and the species of infecting organisms. The greater virulence of *B. melitensis* and *B. suis* has been supported by in vivo studies with experimentally infected animals and by in vitro work examining phagocytosis, intracellular survival, and lymphocyte responses to the different species. Disease caused by *B. abortus* and *B. canis* are insidious in their onset, but tend to cause milder constitutional symptoms and less severe complications.

Because these organisms are infectious via the aerosol route, as evidenced by laboratory-acquired infections, *Brucella* species are one of several bacteria that are viewed as potential agents of biological warfare and bioterrorist activity. Brucellae could be delivered effectively by aerosol dispersal and are able to survive in both soil and water for several weeks, thereby providing both immediate and delayed periods of infectivity. The U.S. investigated *B. suis* as a potential weapon during the 1940s and 1950s, and it is likely that other nations have made similar efforts.[253] Reports of unusual clinical presentations, along with spurious serologic tests for brucella antibodies, have prompted investigations involving the CDC and FBI regarding possible bioterrorist activity with *Brucella* species.[211] Vaccination against brucellae is not available, as the existing *B. abortus* vaccine is licensed for veterinary use only. Postevent pro-phylactic therapy with doxycycline and rifampin has been effective in preventing disease in exposed individuals.[434]

Clinical Spectrum of Brucellosis

Brucella infections may be difficult to diagnose because of the wide spectrum of clinical manifestations associated with them.[1042,1421] Following an incubation period of about 2 to 3 weeks (range, 1 week to 2–3 months), the onset of symptoms may be abrupt or may develop over a period of several days to more than a week. Fever, night sweats, chills, and malaise, often accompanied by severe headache, myal-gias, and arthralgias, are the nonspecific symptoms seen in most cases of brucellosis. Most individuals with bacteremic present with a febrile illness alone or with both fever and arthritis.[856] Lymphadenopathy, splenomegaly, and hepato-megaly may also be present.[10,923] Cutaneous manifestations and vascular complications (e.g., erythema nodosum–like lesions, maculopapular or papulonodular rashes; deep-vein thrombosis) may be noted in some patients, with ulcerative mucocutaneous lesions and subcutaneous abscesses being more uncommon.[54,267,854,867,958] ''Undulant fever'' is syn-onymous with brucellosis (especially that caused by *B. meli-tensis*) because of the periodic fevers that may occur over weeks, months, or even years.[1421] Fevers tend to occur in the evening and night, with normal temperatures maintained during the day, over a period of 2 to 3 weeks. After this, several days may ensue when the patient is afebrile and feels relatively well, only to experience another cycle of waxing/waning fevers. These symptoms may come and go over pro-longed periods because of the containment of the organisms in granulomas in tissue and the subsequent release of organ-isms (or organism components like LPS) back into the circu-lation. Therefore, the disease presents nonspecifically and assumes the characteristics of a debilitating, chronic illness. Chronicity is usually due to persisting foci of infection, such as suppurative lesions in the joints, bones, liver, or spleen. These patients are frequently pan-cultured to determine an etiology for a ''fever of unknown origin.'' Acute and chronic brucellosis may lead to complications that affect several organ systems, including the skeletal system, the central ner-vous system, the respiratory tract, the hepatobiliary and gas-trointestinal tracts, the cardiovascular system, and the genitourinary tract.[274] In immunocompromised hosts on chemotherapy, prolonged febrile neutropenia that fails to re-spond to broad-spectrum antimicrobial coverage is sugges-tive of brucella infection, particularly in regions where brucella infection is endemic.[1135] Additional details on the clinical presentations and complication of brucellosis are presented in Box 9-10.

Various types of hematologic dyscrasias also may be present owing to the residency of the organism in the reticu-loendothelial system, including the lymph nodes, bone mar-row, and spleen. These may include granuloma and abscess formation directly in these tissues or peripheral hematologic manifestations.[73,923] Small, poorly defined noncaseating granulomas may be found in the bone marrow in about 70% of cases, along with nonspecifically reactive histiocytes.[9] Leukopenia, pancytopenia, microangiopathic hemolytic ane-mia, and severe thrombocytopenia have all been observed

in patients with brucellosis.[9,334,1162,1422] On occasion, hema-tologic abnormalities may predominate in early infection, thereby masking the infectious etiology of the disease and mimicking primary hematologic diseases.[334] These hemato-logic abnormalities are transient, and normalize following successful antimicrobial therapy for the bacterial infection.

Serologic Diagnosis of Brucellosis

Serologic testing is also helpful for diagnosis of brucel-losis, with the serum agglutination test (SAT) being the most widely used. The SAT uses a standardized commercial *B. abortus* antigen (BD Biosciences), is performed as a tube dilution test, and detects agglutinogens of the IgG and IgM classes.[1420] Incorporation of dithiothreitol or 2-mercaptoeth-anol into the tube test inactivates IgM, thereby providing an IgG-specific agglutinin titer. Studies have shown that, upon infection, IgM antibodies are produced during the first 7 to 10 days, followed by a decline in IgM and a switch to IgG production after the second week. Most patients with active brucellosis will have SAT titers of ≥160; these titers subse-quently fall with adequate therapy.[672]

As with many other serologic tests, less labor-intensive and subjective methods like EIAs have been exploited for serologic diagnosis of *Brucella* infections. EIAs for detect-ing IgM, IgG, and IgA antibodies against *Brucella* have been described that use whole *B. abortus* cells, *B. abortus* smooth LPS, *B. abortus* protein extracts, and smooth LPS from *B. melitensis* as the solid-phase antigen.[52,977,1420] Ariza and co-workers compared SAT with EIA methods for detection of *Brucella*-specific IgG, IgM, and IgA in 761 sera obtained from 75 patients with brucellosis.[52] The EIA method in this study incorporated *B. abortus* S-LPS as the antigen. These workers found that the EIA methods were just as sensitive and more specific than standard serologic tests for brucel-losis. Initial IgM titers were higher in patients who presented to their physician earlier in the clinical course, while patients who had been ill for some time prior to seeking medical attention tended to have high IgG titers and lower IgM titers. On receipt of adequate antimicrobial therapy, the serum IgG titers decreased fourfold to eightfold over the subsequent 3 to 6 months. Subsequent increases in EIA IgG and IgA were seen in patients with relapsing disease. Persistence of high levels of IgG or a slower decrease in titers following treat-ment in patients without relapse was associated with the presence of focal infection.[52] Antibrucellar IgM and IgG may also be present during bacteremic periods.[977] In brucel-losis control and eradication programs, the SAT and other serologic methods, such as complement fixation, and MAT (a microplate adaptation of the SAT), are also used.[101] In 1993, Goldbaum and coworkers in Argentina characterized an 18-kDa cytoplasmic protein that was present in all smooth and rough *Brucella* species examined.[473] Sera from patients with active brucella infections reacted with this antigen in an EIA-based assay, while patients who did not have brucel-losis or who had inactive disease were negative with this test. This EIA could also differentiate healthy vaccinated cattle from vaccinated cattle who had been infected with a wild-type, disease-producing strain. This antigen has been purified by affinity chromatography, and the gene for the antigen has been cloned in *E. coli*, with retention of the

Box 9-10 Clinical Spectrum of Brucellosis

Osteoarticular Infections

Bone and joint involvement, including arthritis, bursitis, sacroiliitis, spondylitis, and osteomyelitis, is the most commonly described complication of brucellosis and is seen most often following bacteremia with *B. melitensis*.[11,1062,1201] Arthritis and sacroiliitis are associated with acute disease in pediatric patients, while spondylitis, vertebral osteomyelitis, osteitis, and paravertebral abscess are seen more frequently in chronic infections in older individuals and in those with underlying disease (e.g., human immunodeficiency virus [HIV] infection).[11,94,446,1201] Patients with spondylitis usually present with fever, malaise, lower back pain, and difficulty walking. Bone scans, computed tomography, and magnetic resonance imaging are often helpful for detecting bone invasion and complications such as paraspinal abscess.[811,1201] Brucellar osteomyelitis may also involve both joint and nonjoint prosthetic implants.[813,927]

Central Nervous System Infections

Neurobrucellosis occurs in less than 5% of cases and initially presents as encephalitis, meningitis, meningoencephalitis, meningomyelitis, or cerebellar ataxia.[4,519] Patients will usually have CSF pleocytosis, elevated protein, and low-to-normal glucose in the CSF. Patients with acute meningitis present with headache, vomiting, fever, and nuchal rigidity, and papilledema, visual symptoms, and cranial nerve palsies may develop in some patients. Thrombosis of blood vessels may lead to cerebral infarction and hemorrhage, encephalitis, myelitis, and peripheral neuropathy.[4] Epidural spinal abscesses, subdural empyema, paraspinal abscesses, intermedullary dermoid cysts, and brain abscesses are rare but do occur occasionally.[268,1000,1132,1173] Infection of the CNS resulting in colonization of a ventriculoperitoneal shunt and the subsequent development of *B. melitensis* peritonitis has also been documented.[30] Culture of brucellae from the CSF is negative more than 75% of the time, although blood cultures may be positive.[519] Brucellar CNS disease can also be diagnosed by serologic testing of the CSF. Treatment usually involves triple antibiotic therapy, including an aminoglycoside, and must be continued for 8 to 12 weeks.[4,519]

Respiratory Tract Infections

Pulmonary *Brucella* infections may result from hematogenous dissemination and seeding of the lungs or by direct inhalation of the organisms in aerosols.[1131] Clinical manifestations of pulmonary brucellosis may include bronchitis, bronchopneumonia, lung abscess, pulmonary nodules, hilar lymphadenopathy, interstitial pneumonitis, empyema, and pleural effusions.[1,679] Patients usually present with headache, malaise, myalgia, and a nonproductive cough.[1131] Only 40% of patients with a cough have abnormal chest x-rays.

Gastrointestinal/Hepatobiliary Tract Infections

Gastrointestinal, hepatobiliary, and/or hepatosplenic brucellosis occurs as a manifestation of acute systemic infection in over 70% of patients with brucellosis. Symptoms include abdominal pain, nausea, vomiting, anorexia, diarrhea, or constipation. Infections of long standing may result in more extensive gastrointestinal pathology, including colitis, enterocolitis, spontaneous bacterial peritonitis, pancreatitis, cholecystitis, hepatosplenic abscesses, and splenic infarcts.[273,274,320,742,875,957,1115,1121] Liver involvement may be reflected only by elevations in liver enzymes, but is usually more extensive, particularly in *B. melitensis* and *B. suis* infections. Infections with these two species are associated with the formation of caseating hepatic granulomas and microabscesses, while *B. abortus* tends to produce noncaseating granulomas in the liver. The management of suppurative complications of chronic hepatosplenic brucellosis requires combined surgical and medical approaches for optimal clinical response.[53,1416] In 2002, *B. melitensis* peritonitis associated with chronic ambulatory peritoneal dialysis was described in a male patient in Turkey.[1263] The patient likely became infected by ingestion of unpasteurized cheese a month earlier. The patient relapsed following therapy with doxycycline and rifampin; cure was obtained with continued antimicrobial therapy and removal of the Tenckhoff catheter.

Genitourinary Tract Infections

Brucellae may infect the genitourinary tract, usually as a consequence of systemic infection, in which they may cause epididymitis, prostatitis, orchitis, and renal granulomas.[72,659,928] Although renal involvement is fairly uncommon, glomerulonephritis and pyelonephritis have been reported. Brucellae cause abortion in infected animals by localization in the chorioamniotic membranes of the placenta, but there is little evidence supporting a role for these organisms in spontaneous abortion in humans.[976] However, the organisms may rarely be isolated from amniotic fluid and placental tissues of humans with brucellosis.[1421] Malone and colleagues described maternal brucellosis infection that resulted in preterm labor, chorioamnionitis, placental abruption, and delivery of the infant at 25 weeks' gestational age.[814] *B. abortus* was isolated from maternal blood and amniotic fluid. A 1998 case report details the first account of sexual transmission of *B. abortus*.[1270]

Cardiovascular Infections

Cardiovascular brucellosis is a rare complication, occurring in less than 2% of infected patients.[219,1115] Interestingly, brucella endocarditis is the main cause of death related to this disease.[521] Endocarditis may occur with both native and prosthetic valves; aortic valve involvement occurs the most frequently.[5,58,1044] Complications of *Brucella* endocarditis include septic embolization, mycotic aneurysms, myocarditis, pericarditis, and the necessity for surgical intervention for prosthetic valve placement or replacement.[5,58,219,521] *B. melitensis* infection of a pacemaker and associated leads has also been reported in a 45-year-old sheep shearer who had just undergone 45 days of therapy for treatment of brucellosis.[310] In 1999, Ying and colleagues described a case of serologically confirmed *B. canis* endocarditis that occurred in a 49-year-old man upon return from Kuwait.[1419]

Ocular Infections

Ocular infections are unusual, late complications of brucella infection and include optic neuritis, uveitis, keratitis, endophthalmitis, and infection of the lacrimal glands.[16,105,373] Optic neuritis is associated with loss of vision, fever, temporal headache and retrobulbar pain. Endophthalmitis results from hematogenous dissemination, and positive cultures have been obtained from both aqueous and vitreous humors.

recombinant molecule's reactivity with animal and human sera containing anti-brucella antibodies.[474] This molecule has been characterized as a lumazine synthase, an enzyme involved in riboflavin biosynthesis.

Al-Shamahy and Wright recently reported on an antigen detection EIA for brucellosis.[22] The test used monoclonal antibodies against the brucella LPS and was performed on serum specimens. As few as 100 brucella organisms or 10^5 fg/mL LPS could be detected. This assay was challenged with 1,607 sera from random blood donors, 146 patients with brucellosis, 20 patients at risk for *Brucella* infection, and 264 sera from patients with infections other than brucellosis. The sensitivity of the assay was 100% compared with positive blood cultures; specificity of the assay was 99.5% among random blood donors and 99.2% for patients. These data indicated that antigen detection using this assay was an acceptable alternative to blood culture for the diagnosis of *Brucella* infection

Isolation and Cultural Characteristics

Because *Brucella* species infect the reticuloendothelial system, the specimens of choice in suspected cases of brucellosis primarily include blood and bone marrow specimens. In one study of 50 patients eventually diagnosed with brucellosis, culture of blood and bone marrow were positive in 70% and 92% of the patients, respectively.[490] The high rate of positive bone marrow cultures is consistent with the sequestration of these bacteria in the reticuloendothelial system. Other specimens (e.g., tissue, biopsies, CSF, etc.) may occasionally be submitted for culture from patients in whom complicated disease is suspected.

Because of the documented risk of laboratory-acquired infections due to *Brucella* species, all work with specimens suspected of harboring *Brucella* and all manipulations of *Brucella* cultures should be performed in a biologic safety cabinet with recommended precautions for Biosafety Level 3 organisms (e.g., mycobacteria, *Francisella tularensis*).[265,412,502,1299,1300] Procedures that are known to generate aerosols (aspiration of liquid with syringes, mixing on a "vortex" mixer, vigorous bulb pipetting, etc.) should be kept to a minimum. Obviously, to comply with these guidelines, close communication among the laboratory director, the technologists, and the physicians caring for patients with possible brucellosis is necessary. The clinician should alert the clinical laboratory personnel when a diagnosis of brucellosis is being considered so that the laboratory staff can take the necessary safety precautions.

For isolation of *Brucella* species, blood and bone marrow specimens are inoculated into aerobic and anaerobic bottles. Because of the slow growth of the organisms, conventional blood cultures should be incubated at 35°C for 4 to 6 weeks with blind subcultures to chocolate and blood agar (see Color Plate 9-5D). Laboratories using either radiometric or continuously monitored, nonradiometric blood culture instruments usually recover *Brucella* species from blood cultures after 5 to 7 days of incubation.[361,978,1402] Yagupsky evaluated the ability of the nonradiometric BACTEC 9240 instrument to detect growth of *Brucella* species and found that 21 (78.8%) of 27 positive cultures were detected by the 9240 instrument within 7 days; the remainder were detected by blind subcul-

ture after 2 to 3 weeks incubation.[1409] The BACTEC 9240 also detected 14 of 15 positive *Brucella* cultures from synovial fluids inoculated into Peds Plus culture bottles; all 14 positive cultures were detected within 3 to 7 days.[1408] The organism has also been successfully recovered after 12 days of incubation using the Septi-Chek system, in which the aerobic blood culture bottle is fitted with a "paddle" containing chocolate and blood agar media and "subcultures" are performed by inverting the bottle so the medium washes over the agar paddle.[492] The BacT/Alert standard aerobic, BacT/Alert FAN, and BacT/Alert enhanced aerobic bottles also support rapid growth of brucellae as evidenced by simulated blood culture studies.[1238] Rapid recovery of *Brucella* species from blood cultures has also been accomplished with the Isolator lysis-centrifugation method.[1410]

Identification of *Brucella* Species

A presumptive identification of a possible *Brucella* species can be made when a slow-growing, faintly staining, minute coccobacillus is recovered from blood or bone marrow cultures of a "compatible" patient; that is, one with a history of possible occupational exposure, "exotic" travel, or ingestion of uncooked meats or unpasteurized dairy products. *Brucella* species grow slowly on blood and chocolate agars, but not on MacConkey, EMB, or other "enteric" media. Good growth will also be obtained on buffered charcoal-yeast extract agar used for isolation of *Legionella* species.[1041]

All *Brucella* species are aerobic and require oxygen for recovery from clinical specimens. Although production of acid from carbohydrates may be demonstrated under certain conditions, their metabolism is largely oxidative. Strains of *Brucella* are both oxidase- and catalase-positive; most brucellae reduce nitrate to nitrite, and some may also reduce nitrite to gas. All species are indole-negative and VP-negative. Conventional identification methods for *Brucella* species include the requirement of CO_2 for growth, production of urease and H_2S (using lead acetate strips), and sensitivity to the dyes basic fuchsin, thionine, and thionine blue (Table 9-12). Dye sensitivity is used not only to aid in identifying the species, but, in the case of *B. abortus* and *B. suis*, is also helpful for determining the biovar of the organism. *B. abortus* and *B. suis* are subdivided into biovars on the basis of biochemical and serologic differences, while the biovars (actually serovars) of *B. melitensis* are defined solely on the basis of serologic differences, since they are classically resistant to basic fuchsin, thionine, and thionine blue. The recognition of serologically confirmed strains of *B. melitensis* that are thionine-sensitive suggests that the conventional identification scheme needs to be modified and that new, less cumbersome identification methods are needed.[282] *B. melitensis*, *B. suis*, and *B. abortus* produce urease; with a heavy inoculum, *B. suis* strains usually will be urease-positive on Christensen's urea medium within 5 minutes. Identification of *Brucella* species has also been accomplished by coagglutination and colony dot-blot using a genus-specific monoclonal antibody that detects the A or M antigens of *B. melitensis*, *B. abortus*, and *B. suis*.[1334]

At present, *Brucella* species are not included in the data-

Table 9-12 Biochemical Characteristics for the Identification of *Brucella* Species

SPECIES	BIOTYPE	CO₂ REQUIREMENT	H₂S	UREASE	BASIC FUCHSIN 20 µg	THIONINE 20 µg	THIONINE 40 µg	THIONINE BLUE 2 µg/mL	SEROLOGIC AGGLUTINATION* A	M	R	COMMON HOST
B. melitensis	1	–	–	Variable	+	+	+	+	–	+	–	Sheep
	2	–	–	Variable	+	+	+	+	+	–	–	Sheep
	3	–	–	Variable	+	+	+	+	+	+	–	Sheep
B. abortus	1	+/v	+	1–2 h	+	–	–	+	+	–	–	Cattle
	2	+/v	+	1–2 h	–	–	–	–	+	–	–	Cattle
	3	+/v	+	1–2 h	+	+	+	+	+	–	–	Cattle
	4	+/v	+	1–2 h	+/v	–	–	+	–	+	–	Cattle
	5	–	–	1–2 h	+	–	+	+	–	+	–	Cattle
	6	–	+/v	1–2 h	+	–	+	+	+	–	–	Cattle
	7	–	+	1–2 h	+	–	+	+	–	+	–	Cattle
B. suis	1	–	+	0–30 min	–/v	+	+	–/v	+	–	–	Pigs
	2	–	–	0–30 min	–	–	+	–	+	–	–	Pigs, horses
	3	–	–	0–30 min	+	+	+	+	+	–	–	Pigs
	4	–	–	0–30 min	–/v	+	+	–	+	+	–	Reindeer
	5	–	–	0–30 min	–	+	+	NA	–	+	–	Rodents
B. canis		+	–	0–30 min	–	+	+	–/v	–	–	+	Dogs
B. ovis		–	–	–	–/v	+	–	–	–	–	+	Sheep
B. neotomae		–	+	0–30 min	–	–	–	+	+	–	–	Wood rat

+, positive; −, negative; +/v, variable, but most strains positive; −/v, variable, but most strains negative; NA, not available.
* A, monospecific *B. abortus* antiserum; M, monospecific *B. melitensis* antiserum; R, Anti−rough *Brucella* serum.

bases of any of the commercially available kit systems for identifying gram-negative organisms, and the inadvertent use of these kits may delay diagnosis and treatment. *Brucella* organisms have been misidentified as *Moraxella phenylpyruvica* by the API 20NE nonenteric identification system, as *Moraxella* species by the MicroScan Negative COMBO type 5 system (Dade-MicroScan, West Sacramento, CA), and as *Haemophilus influenzae* biotype IV by the *Haemophilus-Neisseria* identification (HNID) panel (Dade-MicroScan).[91,99] In one case, brucellosis subsequently developed in the technologist who inoculated an API 20NE strip with a *B. melitensis* isolate.[99] Preliminary studies on the identification of *Brucella* species with the Biolog carbon substrate utilization identification system indicated that all *Brucella* species oxidized 3 of the 95 substrates on the panel, and that *B. melitensis*, *B. abortus*, and *B. suis* could be differentiated from one another by differential oxidation of seven additional substrates.[1391] Using the results of seven tests on the Biotype 100 (bioMerieux, Marcy-l'Etoile, France), a manually inoculated carbon substrate assimilation gallery, Lopez-Merino et al. were able to identify 85.6% of 92 *Brucella* strains; specificity varied from 97.4% to 100%, depending on the species.[799] These workers emphasized that the Biotype 100 must be inoculated in a biologic safety cabinet.

In 1994, Bricker and Halling at the U.S. Department of Agriculture developed a PCR test that was able to identify and differentiate several *Brucella* species and biovars, including *B. abortus* biovars 1, 2, and 4, all three biovars of *B. melitensis*, *B. suis* biovar 1, and all *B. ovis* biovars.[171] This assay exploited the existence of an insertion sequence IS711 (also called IS6501) that is unique to *Brucella* species and is found at species-specific and biovar-specific regions of the chromosome. The species and biovars identified by this assay constitute most of those seen in the U.S. in both animal and human infections. These workers subsequently augmented their PCR assay with additional primers to allow rapid discrimination between pathogenic strains and the *B. abortus* vaccine strains (S19 and RB51) in previously vaccinated livestock.[172,390] This assay is called the AMOS PCR because it detects *Brucella* "**A**bortus, **M**elitensis, **O**vis, and **S**uis, respectively. Cytoplasmic protein-specific gene probes have also been developed for the differentiation of certain *B. melitensis*, *B. suis*, and *B. ovis* biovars. These molecular approaches are useful for species and biovar identification in diagnostic laboratories and for epidemiologic, veterinary, and taxonomic purposes.[26,1324]

In addition to the AMOS PCR, other PCR-based assays using the same or other amplification targets have been developed for identification and direct detection of *Brucella* species in clinical specimens. Herman and DeRidder described a dot-blot hybridization test for identification of *Brucella* species using synthetic primers and probes for a conserved, genus-specific DNA sequence.[563] Fox and colleagues analyzed amplicon polymorphisms following PCR amplification of the 16S–23S ribosomal DNA spacer region and found that, while the products were unique to the genus *Brucella*, the interspace profiles of the four major species were identical.[431] A PCR assay using primers specific for a 223-bp region of the DNA sequence that encodes a 31-kD immunogenic *B. abortus* protein was developed by Casanas and others in Spain.[206] This assay was tested with sera from 31 patients with brucellosis and 45 healthy controls; brucella DNA was detected in 30 of 31 patients and was 100% specific.[1432] PCR assays have also been developed using the 16S rRNA of *B. abortus* and the gene for a *B. abortus* outer membrane protein (*omp-2*) as amplification targets.[926] Real-time PCR assays have also been described using primers derived from the genus-specific IS711 insertion site and from species- and biovar-specific signature sequences.[1054] These 30-minute assays using the LightCycler method were tested with known strains and field isolates and identified all biovars of *B. abortus*, *B. melitensis*, and *B. suis* biovar 1.

Treatment of Brucellosis

The treatment of human brucellosis is a controversial area because of the spectrum of disease, the possibility/likelihood of chronic infection, and the development of complications.[1042] Despite in vitro susceptibility to many antimicrobial agents, in vitro results do not translate to clinical efficacies and outcomes in patients. Successful treatment requires prolonged antimicrobial therapy, usually with a combination of agents, and, in some cases, surgical intervention is also indicated. The administration of agents that penetrate and have activity within phagocytic cells are prerequisites for therapy, since brucellae are facultative intracellular pathogens. Traditionally, oral tetracycline for 6 weeks combined with intramuscular streptomycin or gentamicin daily for 2–3 weeks was the recommended therapy for brucellosis.[1421] Doxycycline (a tetracycline derivative with greater lipid solubility and a longer serum half-life) and rifampin administered orally for at least 6 weeks is also recommended for treatment. Treatment of brucellosis with newer cephalosporin monotherapy, such as ceftriaxone, has resulted in failures and cannot be recommended.[746] The fluoroquinolones generally show good activity against *Brucella* species in vitro.[700] A randomized, prospective study evaluated the efficacy of ciprofloxacin versus rifampin plus doxycycline in the treatment of acute brucellosis. After treatment for 45 days, five of the six patients treated with ciprofloxacin relapsed, despite in vitro susceptibility and low MICs of the *B. melitensis* isolates.[747] In a Turkish study, the clinical efficacy of a combination of ofloxacin and rifampin for 6 weeks was comparable to that achieved with the doxycyclinerifampin combination.[6] Fluoroquinolone agents and the newer cephalosporins may show better clinical efficacy when used in combination with other agents.[1290]

Treatment of neurobrucellosis and endocarditis require combination therapy and frequently surgical interventions. In neurobrucellosis, streptomycin regimens are contraindicated because this drug does not reach therapeutic levels in the CNS. Combination therapies with two or three drugs (e.g., doxycycline, rifampin, and trimethoprim-sulfamethoxazole) that penetrate the CNS and are active against the infecting isolate are recommended. Adequate therapy of brucella endocarditis, like that caused by other bacterial agents, requires that bactericidal levels of antimicrobial agents be administered. The combination of doxycycline with rifampin and trimethoprim-sulfamethoxazole has been used successfully in the treatment of brucella endocarditis. Although cases of brucella endocarditis have been cured with antimicrobial chemotherapy alone, surgical intervention (i.e., valve replacement) combined with antibiotic therapy is the best approach.[521,1421]

Francisella tularensis
Epidemiology of Tularemia

Tularemia, the infectious disease caused by the fastidious gram-negative coccobacillus *Francisella tularensis*, is a disease of animals that humans acquire by contact with them.[372] Reservoirs of the bacterium in nature include rabbits, rodents, squirrels, muskrats, beavers, voles, deer, lemmings, and raccoons and domestic animals such as cattle, sheep, swine, and horses. Swine, horses and cattle are fairly resistant to infection, while sheep are relatively susceptible. The organism is transmitted among animals by ticks and biting flies such as deer flies. Transovarial transmission of *F. tularensis* also occurs in the tick, thereby providing a renewing source of the organism in the environment. Infections in humans are most commonly acquired by bites from infected ticks, deer flies, and mosquitoes, or by direct contact with blood or internal organs of infected animals.[1157] Among ticks, at least 13 different species are known to be naturally infected with *F. tularensis*, with the dog tick (*Dermacentor variabilis*) and the wood tick (*Dermacentor andersoni*) being the most common in North America. Among hunters, infections have occurred following skinning, dressing, and eating infected animals, including rabbits, hares, beavers, muskrats, and squirrels. Contaminated water is also an important source of the organism in the environment, and infections in humans have occurred following ingestion of water from wells in which infected animal carcasses have been found.[111] A large 1999–2000 outbreak of tularemia in Kosovo was traced to contaminated food and water, with rodents being identified as the source of the organism.[1061] Infections acquired by the airborne route have occurred following inhalation of dust and hay containing rodent feces and carcasses. Human infections have also been acquired from exposure to or bites from domestic cats. In these cases, contamination of the mouth or claws of the cat following killing and feeding on prey is the likely mode of acquisition of the organism, although cats may also acquire systemic infections.[78] One case has been described in which a veterinary surgeon contracted ulceroglandular tularemia after he cut his finger while performing a hysterectomy on a cat.[1143] *F. tularensis* is highly contagious—as few as 10 to 50 organisms administered intradermally or via the aerosol route are enough to cause infection, and the organism can easily penetrate minute, inapparent breaks in the skin.[372] Tularemia has also been acquired from laboratory accidents that have occurred during processing of infected specimens, isolation and identification of the organism, and manipulation of large numbers of organisms in research settings.

Prior to World War II, tularemia was relatively common, but the incidence steadily declined during the 1950s. Although the disease has been reported throughout the U.S., the vast majority of cases now occur in the south and south-central states (i.e., Missouri, Arkansas, Oklahoma, and Texas). Most cases occur during the summer months or midwinter, and correspond to peaks of vector-associated disease and hunting-associated disease, respectively.[624] Males are more commonly infected than females, which is related to the infection's association with certain occupations (e.g., farmers, large-animal veterinarians, hunters, and sheep shearers and herders).[1157]

Recently, issues have been raised concerning the potential use of *F. tularensis* as an agent of biological warfare and bioterrorism.[182,321,1077] In the U.S., *F. tularensis* was investigated as a potential means of biological warfare agent in the 1950s and 1960s, prior to the termination of the U.S. offensive bioterrorist program, and it is likely that other countries have investigated this agent as well.[253] At Fort Detrick, animals and both civilian and military human volunteers were exposed to aerosols containing *F. tularensis* to determine the infectivity of the agent delivered in this fashion and to assess the efficacy of vaccines, prophylactic therapies, and treatment methods.[253] Because of these investigations, a live attenuated *F. tularensis* vaccine became available from the U.S. Public Health Service and the World Health Organization as an investigational new drug. *F. tularensis* LVS (live vaccine strain) affords good protection against the pneumonic form of tularemia and modifies signs and symptoms of the ulceroglandular form.[1183] Kaufmann and colleagues at the CDC recently published a best- and worst-case scenario if *F. tularensis* organisms were released as an aerosol cloud as a part of a bioterrorist event.[674] If the infective aerosol dose of *F. tularensis* is 50 to 100 organisms, and assuming an 82.5% attack rate, exposure of 100,000 people would result in 82,500 cases of pneumonic tularemia. With a 6.2% death rate, 6,188 deaths would be expected, with an economic impact of between $465 million and $562 million!

History and Taxonomy

Tularemia was first described in 1911 by McCoy as a cause of a plague-like disease in rodents during his investigations of possible bubonic plague in the rodent population in the San Francisco area following the devastating earthquake of 1906. McCoy and Chapin subsequently isolated the causative agent and named it *Bacterium tularense* after Tulare County, California, the site of their laboratory.[372] From 1912 through 1925, Edward Francis was studying the human disease called "deer fly fever" and made the connection between this illness and the "plague-like disease" described by McCoy in rodents. He investigated the modes of transmission, studied the causative agent, and coined the name "tularemia." This name reflects that of Tulare County, where McCoy and Chapin isolated the organism, and the "bacteremia" that occurs as a manifestation of infection. For his pioneering work on the cultivation of the organism and methods for serologic diagnosis, the associated clinical syndromes, and the recognition of the principal reservoirs and vectors, Francis received the 1959 Nobel Prize in science, and the name of the organism was changed from *Bacterium tularense* to *Francisella tularensis* in his honor.

Like several other organisms described in this chapter, the taxonomic position of *Francisella* is uncertain.[368] Over the years, it has been provisionally classified as genus "*Bacterium*" and included with the brucellae and pasteurellae. However, genetic, phenotypic, and cell-wall analyses have demonstrated no relationship to *Brucella* or *Pasteurella* species, or to the tickborne members of the genus *Yersinia* (i.e., *Y. pestis*). Consequently, *Francisella* was accepted as a new genus in the mid-1960s. Examination of 16S rRNA sequences has established that *F. tularensis* belongs in the γ-subdivision of the Proteobacteria and in the upcoming edition of *Bergey's Manual* it is included as the only genus in the proposed family "*Francisellaceae*" in the proposed order "Thiotrichales."[455]

F. tularensis can be divided into four subspecies that can all can cause tularemia, although they differ in their virulence for humans and rabbits.[450,646] *F. tularensis* subsp. *tularensis* (also called *F. tularensis* subsp. *nearctica* or biovar type A) predominates in North America but is not commonly found in Europe (although this subspecies was recently recognized in Slovakia), is associated with ticks and rabbits, and is virulent in both rabbits and humans.[512,646] This biogroup is characterized phenotypically by acid production from glycerol and possession of citrulline ureidase.[819,1128] *F. tularensis* subsp. *holarctica* (formerly called *F. tularensis* subsp. *palaearctica* or biovar type b) has been isolated in Europe, Asia, Japan, and North America, is associated with water-borne infection in rodents and tick and mosquito vectors, and is intermediate in virulence in humans and minimally virulent in rabbits.[29,624] Disease due to subspecies *holarctica* may be more common in the U.S. than previously thought.[1298] Subspecies *holarctica* strains are glycerol-negative and do not usually produce citrulline ureidase. *F. tularensis* subsp. *mediaasiatica* was suggested for strains isolated in the central Asian focus of the Soviet Union, and *F. tularensis* biogroup *palaearctica japonica* was suggested for isolates from Japan.[1128] Initially, all four were proposed as separate species by Soviet scientists, but this proposal has not been generally accepted. Central Asian and Japanese strains have been shown to have low virulence for rabbits (like biogroup *holarctica/palaearctica*), but are clearly more closely related to *F. tularensis* subspecies *tularensis* based on 16S rRNA analysis.[1128] Recent data using two insertion sequence elements to type strains by restriction-fragment-length polymorphisms revealed that Japanese strains of *F. tularensis* subsp. *holarctica* (*palaearctica*) may actually represent another subspecies.[1272]

A second *Francisella* species, isolated from water in Utah in 1951 was previously classified as a *Pasteurella* species, and was renamed as *Francisella novicida* in 1959.[368,749] Genetic studies subsequently determined that *F. novicida* was not a separate species, but constituted another subspecies of *F. tularensis* (subspecies *novicida*), since the degree of 16S rRNA similarity was 99.6%.[418,585] *F. tularensis* subspecies *novicida* has been isolated from water containing dead muskrats and from humans on two occasions.

A "third" (but actually second) *Francisella* species called *F. philomiragia* includes bacterial strains formerly called "philomiragia bacteria" that were mistakenly included with the yersiniae as "*Y. philomiragia*."[585] These organisms show genetic and antigenic relatedness to *F. tularensis* subspecies and have similar cell-wall fatty acid and ubiquinone constituents. Analysis of the 16S rRNA of these organisms has corroborated the present differentiation of the genus into two species—*F. tularensis* and *F. philomiragia*.[418,419] *F. philomiragia* is considerably less virulent than *F. tularensis* and has been isolated mostly from animals (e.g., muskrats) and water. Over a 12-year period, 14 human isolates of *F. philomiragia* were submitted to the Special Bacteriology Branch of the CDC. Of these 14 isolates, five

were from patients with chronic granulomatous disease, five were from individuals who nearly drowned in saltwater, two were from unknown human sources, and single isolates were from a patient with Hodgkin's disease and a patient with myeloid metaplasia.[585,1155,1364] In 1997, Sicherer and colleagues reported on a 15th patient with *F. philomiragia* bacteremia who also had chronic granulomatous disease.[1175] These cases have defined the clinical spectrum of *F. philomiragia* as a rare agent of necrotizing pneumonia, bacteremia, and meningitis.[585,1155,1364]

In 1997, another possible *Francisella* species was recognized as an endosymbiont in ovarian tissue of female *Dermacentor andersoni* ticks, but has not been detected in male ticks.[929] The relation of this organism, designated the "*D. andersoni* symbiont" (DAS), and *Francisella* species is based on the presence of a specific membrane antigen and 16S rRNA sequences that are similar to those of *F. tularensis*. Investigation of obligately endosymbiotic bacteria found in *Paramecium tetraurelia* found that one of these endosymbionts, *Caedibacter taeniospiralis*, forms a novel evolutionary lineage with the γ-Proteobacteria and shares 87% similarity in its 16S rRNA sequences with the family *Francisellaceae*.[104] These endosymbionts are being further characterized.

Virulence of *F. tularensis*

The factors responsible for the virulence of *F. tularensis* are not known. The organism produces no identifiable exotoxins but does possess an inapparent capsule containing carbohydrate, protein, and lipid. The capsule functions in protecting the organism from complement-mediated lysis and may also be antiphagocytic. Removal of the capsule by mutation or biochemical methods abolishes virulence of the organism and renders it susceptible to the bactericidal activity of normal human serum.[1127] The LPS of the organism has a unique structure, induces less cellular toxicity, and is less active in the *Limulus* amebocyte lysate assay for endotoxin than other gram-negative bacteria.[1129,1330] In experimental infections established in mice, the organisms can only be recovered from tissue of the reticuloendothelial system and from the cellular components of the peripheral blood.[421] This may explain the infrequent recovery of this organism from blood cultures collected by venipuncture. Natural infection or immunization with *F. tularensis* LVS (live vaccine strain) engenders long-lasting cell-mediated and humoral resistance to reinfection, with the cell-mediated immune response being the most important protective mechanism.[1262] Persistence of cell-mediated, protective immunity with a concomitant decline in humoral immunity has been demonstrated in individuals who were naturally infected 25 years earlier.[381]

Studies performed with mutants of the LVS strain suggest that the principal virulence factor of *F. tularensis* is the ability to invade and multiply within macrophages, hepatocytes, and other cells of the reticuloendothelial system (RES).[127,421,498,1262] The organism is phagocytized by these cells and lives within iron-enriched, acidified vacuoles. Other RES-associated cells (e.g., natural killer cells) are stimulated to produce interferon-γ before the appearance of *F. tularensis*–specific T-lymphocytes; interferon-γ stimulates the production of nitric oxide within the macrophages, which, in turn, inhibits intracellular growth of *F. tularensis* and limits its spread within the RES.[41] The ability to induce nitric oxide production by macrophages in the mouse model is modulated by the expression of LPS phase variation. This variation includes structural modifications of both the LPS somatic (O) antigens and the core lipid A antigens.

Upon cutaneous infection of a susceptible host, the organism multiplies locally for 3 to 7 days, producing a local ulcer. The bacteria spread to the regional lymph nodes and disseminate via the lymphohematogenous route to involve multiple organs. An initial acute inflammatory response ensues, with the accumulation of neutrophils, fibrin, and macrophages. Mononuclear cells are able to engulf the organisms without opsonizing antibodies, while polymorphonuclear cells cannot. Lymphocytes and macrophages migrate into the infected tissues, engulf the organisms, and form granulomas in multiple sites (i.e., lymph nodes, bone marrow, spleen, liver, and lungs). Organisms remain viable within these macrophages by inhibition of phagosome-lysosome fusion, and utilization of iron from host cells.[420] Cell-mediated immunity appears 7 to 10 days after infection, with IgM, IgG, and IgA agglutinating antibodies appearing during the subsequent 2 weeks.[723,1262] Lysis of cells harboring organisms by immune effector cells in the liver and other organs releases organisms from intracellular compartments, thereby enabling them to infect other cells. If left untreated, suppuration of involved lymph nodes in various tissues results in additional manifestations of systemic disease.

Clinical Spectrum of Tularemia

The clinical spectrum of tularemia is dependent on the mode of acquisition of the organism, the innate virulence of the infecting strain, and immunocompetence of the host. After infection, there is an incubation period of 2 days to 3 weeks, followed by the acute onset of fever, chills, malaise, headache, sore throat, and sometimes diarrhea. Fevers may wax and wane but usually remain elevated for 4 to 5 weeks in the absence of treatment. During this time weight loss, lymphadenopathy, and chronic illness develop. Patients who are infected with less virulent strains may have a mild illness that resolves spontaneously, while in others chronic, debilitating, multisystem infections develop.

Tularemia can be divided into six major syndromes that are delineated by the mode of organism acquisition and, therefore, the degree of systemic involvement.[1085] **Ulceroglandular tularemia** is the most common form (21–85% of cases). The patient presents with an ulcerated skin lesion, usually at the site of a tick bite, along with painful regional lymphadenopathy. In adults with tick bite–associated infection, inguinal and cervical lymphadenopathy are most common, while cervical and occipital lymphadenopathy are seen predominantly in children. Animal-associated lymphadenopathy is usually cervical, since the initial lesion(s) is frequently on the upper extremities. Other symptoms (e.g., headache, fever, chills, sweating, coughing) also are present. **Glandular tularemia** (3–20% of cases) is characterized by lymphadenopathy and fever, but a skin lesion is not readily apparent. In these cases, the lesion may have healed or may be so innocuous that it goes unnoticed. In both ulceroglandu-

lar and glandular tularemia, the enlarged lymph nodes may suppurate and require surgical drainage. **Oculoglandular tularemia** (2–5% of cases) results from inoculation of the organism into the conjunctivae via direct inoculation with contaminated hands or by splashes or aerosols. This clinical form is characterized by severe granulomatous conjunctivitis; loss of visual acuity; preauricular, submandibular, and cervical lymphadenopathy; and systemic manifestations of fever and malaise.[1219] **Oropharyngeal tularemia** (2–12% of cases) describes cases in which the primary lesion is in the oropharynx. This disease form results from ingestion of contaminated food or water. The patient presents with severe headache, bilateral tonsillitis, and exudative pharyngitis suggestive of severe streptococcal pharyngitis, diphtheria, or Vincent's disease. Deep cervical lymphadenitis, usually in the form of an isolated, persistent swollen lymph node, appears a week or two after organism acquisition.[579,945] **Typhoidal tularemia** (5–30 % of cases) presents with an abrupt onset of fever, chills, headache, sore throat, vomiting, and abdominal pain and tenderness. No initial skin lesion or lymphadenopathy is apparent, and the infection is probably acquired by ingestion of contaminated water or food.[579] Typhoidal tularemia is the only form in which diarrhea is a prominent part of the clinical presentation. The diarrhea is usually loose and watery with no blood, although focal bowel necrosis with bloody stools may be seen, particularly in children. Secondary pleuropulmonary disease, with pulmonary infiltrates and pleural effusions, develops in almost half of the patients with typhoidal tularemia. In this form, blood and sputum may be culture-positive and the mortality rate is usually high. **Pneumonic tularemia** (8–20% of cases) may occur as a complication of all of the other disease forms because of seeding of the respiratory tract during bacteremia, or as a clinical entity resulting from inhalation of the organisms in an aerosol.[108] Radiographic examinations may show involvement of one or more lobes, with pleural effusions, pneumonic infiltrates, abscess formation, pulmonary nodules, and hilar lymphadenopathy.[463,925] Symptoms include fever, cough with minimal sputum production, and pleuritic chest pain. Clinically, pneumonic tularemia resembles tuberculosis; atypical pneumonias due to *Legionella*, *Chlamydia pneumoniae*, *Chlamydia psittaci*, *Coxiella burnetii*; and fungal pneumonia.[463] Pneumonic tularemia tends to be more severe in patients with underlying conditions, such as malnourishment, alcoholism, renal disease, chronic granulomatous disease, and HIV infection.[818] Complications such as hepatosplenomegaly, renal failure, and rhabdomyolysis occur more frequently in these individuals. Pneumonic tularemia is usually seen in adults and is associated with certain occupations (e.g., sheep shearers, animal husbandry workers, laboratory workers), farming activities (e.g., threshing), lawn mowing, and brush cutting.[1243] This association is likely due to the presence of rodent feces or infected animal remains in hay.[579] Suppuration of enlarged lymph nodes may be a late complication in up to 50% of patients with lymphadenopathy.[624]

Manifestations of multiple clinical types of tularemia may occur in individual patients, and additional disease complications have been described. Plourde et al. reported a case of glandular tularemia with some features of typhoidal disease in a child who had sustained an insect bite on the left shoulder blade.[1018] Inguinal lymphadenopathy, rather than lymphadenopathy near the site of the insect bite was found, and abdominal distention and severe, watery diarrhea developed, both of which are features of typhoidal disease. Cooper and colleagues reported an unusual case of chronic *F. tularensis* infection of a knee prosthesis in a 68-year-old man with degenerative joint disease 6 months after a tick bite.[281] Meningitis is a rare complication of *F. tularensis* infection, with only five pediatric and seven adult cases reported in the literature between 1931 and 1998.[1079] These patients may or may not have significant nonmeningeal disease (glandular or typhoidal tularemia). CSF findings are consistent with a bacterial meningitis (i.e., low glucose with high protein), and show a predominance of lymphocytes on Gram stain of the CSF. In 1996 Pittman and coworkers described the first case of *F. tularensis* ventriculoperitoneal shunt infection in a 5-year-old boy with myelomeningocoele.[1016] Signs and symptoms were limited to the CNS, and there was no other systemic involvement. Two weeks prior to presentation, the child had been with friends who were skinning a rabbit. The patient responded successfully to intrathecal gentamicin with shunt replacement. LeDoux reported a case of presumptive *F. tularensis* CNS disease in a 61-year-old man whose clinical presentation was predominantly gait ataxia.[763] In 2000, Tancik and Dillaha reported the first published case of *F. tularensis* native valve endocarditis in a 42-year-old male from Arkansas.[1255] The patient responded to a 4-week course of gentamicin. Severe disease is also associated with compromised host status, as evidenced by a rapidly fatal infection in a patient with neutropenia who had undergone bone marrow transplantation.[1137]

Isolation and Cultural Characteristics

Because this organism can penetrate through small breaks in the skin, it is considered potentially dangerous to handle specimens or cultures of *F. tularensis* in the laboratory. As with brucellosis, tularemia may not be suspected at the time a patient presents to the clinician, so considerable time may be spent handling specimens and cultures before this diagnosis is considered. For laboratories working with clinical materials of human and animal origin, Biosafety Level 2 practices, containment equipment, and facilities are recommended, while Biosafety Level 3 and Animal Biosafety Level 3 practices are required for working with live cultures or performing experimental studies in animal.[1299,1300] In the routine clinical microbiology laboratory, all specimens and cultures should be processed in a class II biologic safety cabinet, gloves should be worn during all procedures, and any procedures that may generate aerosols should be avoided. With the looming threat of bioterrorism, screening tests for *F. tularensis* and other bioterrorism agents must be incorporated into laboratory bench procedures in order to permit rapid presumptive identification of an isolate so that it can be referred to level B laboratories for definitive identification.[1077] Persons with confirmed laboratory exposure should be treated prophylactically.

F. tularensis may be isolated from primary ulcers, lymph node aspirates and biopsies, sputum, bone marrow, and tissue biopsies (e.g., liver, spleen). Specimens should be kept at 4–8°C until processing. Specimens may also be placed in Amies transport medium with charcoal or in Stuart medium at room temperature prior to processing. The organisms have also been isolated from peripheral blood specimens, usually in the setting of preexisting, underlying disease. Positive blood cultures have been found in patients with typhoidal, pneumonic and oropharyngeal tularemia, and in the single report of *F. tularensis* endocarditis.[579,945,1033,1298,1348] In case reports describing *F. tularensis* bacteremia, growth of the organism was found after 3 to 7 days of incubation using the BACTEC radiometric system. However, in the single case of endocarditis, *F. tularensis* was recovered after 9 days with the BACTEC system.[1255] *F. tularensis* was isolated after 12 days of incubation from a BACTEC nonradiometric aerobic blood culture bottle (BACTEC NR6A) that was inoculated with a 10–20-μL volume of a percutaneous fine-needle aspirate of an inguinal lymph node.[175] If tularemia is suspected clinically, broth blood cultures should be incubated beyond the standard 5- to 7-day incubation period used in many laboratories.

F. tularensis is a small, pale-staining, gram-negative coccobacillus (see Color Plate 9-4*E*). Classically, the organism has a growth requirement for cysteine, cystine, or other sulfhydryl-containing compounds, and the preferred medium for isolation was glucose-cysteine blood agar. However, *F. tularensis* will grow on commercially available chocolate agar and modified Thayer-Martin agar, since these hemin-containing media are supplemented with a growth enrichment (e.g., IsoVitaleX; BD Biosciences) that contains cysteine, cystine, and other nutrients required by fastidious bacteria.[1348] Like the brucellae, this organism is also able to grow on buffered charcoal-yeast extract (BCYE) agar, the medium used for isolation of *Legionella* species.[1365] *F. tularensis* has also been isolated from a biopsy of a cutaneous lesion by the centrifugation shell-vial technique using human embryonic lung fibroblasts.[428] Although the organism failed to grow on subculture on bacteriologic media, the identity of the organism was determined by PCR analysis of the organism growing in the shell vial.

In 1994, Bernard and coworkers at the National Laboratory for Bacteriology in Ontario, Canada, reported on seven isolates that were submitted to the Canadian reference lab as *Haemophilus* species or as unidentified fastidious gram-negative bacteria that were identified as *F. tularensis*.[122] These strains lacked the cysteine requirement of classical *F. tularensis* strains. These atypical isolates were oxidase- and catalase-negative, agglutinated strongly in *Francisella* agglutinating serum, and were unreactive in all other phenotypic tests, including those used for biogroup determinations. Cellular fatty acid analysis of these strains revealed the presence of long-chain (i.e., C_{18}–C_{26}) saturated and unsaturated fatty acids, and large amounts of 3-hydroxy-octadecanoate (3OH-$C_{18:0}$), a fatty acid that is unique to *F. tularensis*.[368,631] These unusual hydroxy fatty acids comprise part of the lipid A structure in the organism's LPS. Consequently, these organisms may be identified readily by cellular fatty acid analysis using the Microbial Identification (MIDI) System and Library Generation System (LGS) software (MIDI, Newark, NJ). Clarridge and colleagues have also isolated two nonfastidious *F. tularensis* strains from blood culture of patients with pneumonia.[260] These isolates grew on both chocolate and blood agar and were identified as *F. tularensis* by phenotypic characteristics, 16S rRNA gene sequencing, and rDNA probe hybridization. These strains also failed to agglutinate in commercial *F. tularensis* antisera. Strains of *F. tularensis* biogroup *novicida*, and *F. philomiragia* do not demonstrate a requirement for cysteine.

F. tularensis is obligately aerobic; growth is stimulated by increased CO_2 and may require 2 to 5 days of incubation at 35 to 37°C before colonies are visible on agar medium. Colonies on chocolate agar are gray, smooth, buttery, and about 2 mm in diameter after 3 days of incubation. *F. tularensis* subsp. *tularensis* grows more slowly than the other subspecies. Colonies of *F. philomiragia* are larger, whiter, and mucoid. Characteristics for presumptive identification of *Francisella* species are shown in Table 9-13. *F. tularensis* biogroups are oxidase-negative, weakly catalase-positive, grow poorly (if at all) on MacConkey agar, and are inert biochemically. *F. philomiragia* isolates are oxidase-positive. Species identification is usually confirmed by agglutination tests using specific rabbit polyclonal antisera. Cultures should be examined over a 10- to 14-day period.

Studies using spiked blood cultures and experimentally infected mice initially suggested the utility of PCR as a method for detection and identification of *F. tularensis* in clinical specimens from humans.[346,657,798] These assays were able to detect both *tularensis* and *holarctica* subspecies at sensitivities equal to 1 cfu/μL of blood. Subsequently, a multiplex PCR assay targeting both the 16S rRNA gene and a 17-kDa lipoprotein gene was successfully developed for direct detection of *F. tularensis* in swabs from ulceroglandular tularemia lesions.[642,1182] The lipoprotein gene is conserved among *F. tularensis* strains and does not show sequence similarities with other known prokaryotic sequences published in current gene banks.[642] PCR performed on wound specimens was able to provide a rapid diagnosis in patients with suspected ulceroglandular tularemia who were negative on culture and had not yet seroconverted.[642,667] In response to the need for epidemiologic tools for investigating outbreaks of tularemia, PCR approaches have also been developed to detect infection directly in experimental animals and in insect vectors and to provide methods for typing and discrimination of strains.[311,398,450,568,645,1272]

Several other novel techniques for rapid detection/identification of *F. tularensis* have been developed as a direct result of concerns over the use of *F. tularensis* in bioterrorism and biological warfare. Grunow and colleagues developed a standard EIA and a handheld immunochromatographic assay that used monoclonal antibodies against LPS antigen as the capture antibody for detecting *F. tularensis* subsp. *tularensis* and *F. tularensis* subsp. *holarctica* directly in veterinary specimens.[503] Antigen-capture EIAs using time-resolved fluorometry have also been developed for detection of several bioterrorism-associated agents in both clinical and environmental samples.[1004] Emanuel and coworkers developed a fluorogenic PCR-based method for detection of *F. tularensis* in infected mice. This assay could be performed using a handheld thermocycler designed for field use; results were available within 4 hours.[375]

Because strains belonging to the different *F. tularensis* biogroups are antigenically homogeneous, the subspecies are differentiated from one another on the basis of phenotypic criteria or subspecies-specific probes for 16S rRNA.[418] Strains of *F. tularensis* subsp. *tularensis* produce acid in media containing glucose, maltose, or glycerol as a carbon source, and hybridize with an oligonucleotide probe for subspecies *tularensis*-specific 16S rRNA sequences. Subspecies *holarctica* strains produce acid from glucose and maltose, but not from glycerol, and hybridize with a probe that is specific for subspecies *holarctica* 16S rRNA sequences. Both subspecies *mediaasiatica* and subspecies *palaearctica japonica* strains hybridize with the biogroup *tularensis*-specific probe; however, subspecies *mediaasiatica* strains produce acid from glycerol (and sucrose), while subspecies *palaearctica japonica* strains acidify media containing either glucose or glycerol (see Table 9-13). Serologic methods can distinguish between subspecies *tularensis* and *novicida* strains, but not between subspecies *tularensis* and *holarctica* strains. Citrulline ureidase, an enzyme that correlates with virulence of *F. tularensis*, is found in virulent strains of subspecies *tularensis*, some *holarctica* strains, and *mediaasiatica* strains.[819,1128] The enzyme is not found in attenuated *tularensis* strains and in most subspecies *holarctica* strains with low virulence. Phenotypic testing of these organisms is problematic, since reactions are often delayed or variable. Specific primers, probes, and PCR methods have been developed that are able to distinguish *F. tularensis* subsp. *holarctica* from strains of other *F. tularensis* subspecies, including *F. tularensis* subsp. *tularensis*.[450,646]

Serologic Diagnosis of Tularemia

Because tularemia may not be considered as a diagnosis until late in the clinical course, and since culture for the organism is often not successful, serologic testing is the most common method for diagnosis of this infection.[124] The antibody response to *F. tularensis* infection is influenced to some degree by the clinical form of the disease, and may have an impact on serologic results depending on the method used.[1242] The conventional serologic test is the tube agglutination (TA) test. This test uses formalin-killed whole cells as the antigen (BD Biosciences). Antibodies of the IgM, IgG, and IgA classes do not usually appear until 2 weeks after infection. Antibodies of all classes appear simultaneously. A single tube agglutination titer of ≥160 with compatible disease or a fourfold rise in titer between acute and convalescent serum specimens (collected 14 days apart) constitutes a presumptive etiologic diagnosis. A positive TA test is not helpful if there is a history of previous infection or vaccination, since antibodies of the IgM class persist for years. The TA procedure has been adapted to a microagglutination (MA) procedure using safranin-stained, formalinized *F. tularensis* organisms as the antigen. Sato and coworkers demonstrated that the MA test was more sensitive than the standard TA test, detecting anti–*F. tularensis* antibodies of the IgM class 9 days earlier than the TA test.[1138] Enzyme-linked immunosorbent assays (ELISAs) for detection of tularemia-specific antibodies have been developed using purified OMP antigens of the organism that seem to evoke early and strong immune responses that are minimally influenced by the clinical presentation.[124,125]

Treatment of Tularemia

The drug of choice for treatment of tularemia is the aminoglycoside streptomycin, with gentamicin being an alterna-

Table 9-13 Biochemical Characteristics for Identification of *Francisella tularensis* Subspecies and *Francisella philomiragia*

CHARACTERISTIC	*F. TULARENSIS* SUBSP *TULARENSIS*	*F. TULARENSIS* SUBSP. *HOLARCTICA*	*F. TULARENSIS* SUBSP. *NOVICIDA*	*F. TULARENSIS* SUBSP. *MEDIAASIATICA*	*F. TULARENSIS* SUBSP. *PALEARCTICA-JAPONICA*	*F. PHILOMIRAGIA*
Oxidase	−	−	−	−	−	+
Catalase	+w	+w	+w	+w	+w	+w
Motility	−	−	−	−	v	−
Growth on MacConkey agar	v	−	v	NA	NA	v
Growth, 6.5% NaCl	−	−	v	NA	NA	+w
H₂S in TSI agar	−	−	−	−	−	−
Urease	−	−	−	−	−	−
Nitrate reduction	−	−	−	−	−	−
Acid from:						
Glucose	+	+	+	−	NA	+w
Maltose	+	+	v	−	NA	+w
Sucrose	−	−	+	+	NA	+w
Glycerol	+	+	+	+	+	NA
Cysteine/cystine requirement	+	+	−	−	−	−
Citrulline ureidase	+−	−+	+	+	−	NA

+, positive reaction; −, negative reaction; v, variable reaction; +ᵂ, weak positive reaction; +⁻, most strains positive, rare strains negative;
−⁺, most strains negative, rare strains positive; NA, data not available.

tive agent.[379,624] However, clinical relapse after treatment with gentamicin has been reported.[379,1074] Other regimens, such as tetracycline and chloramphenicol, have been used but are associated with higher relapse rates, especially if administered early in the clinical course. The initial clinical response to treatment with tetracyclines is dramatic (i.e., patients defervesce rapidly), but relapse rates after therapy are over 12%, twice as much as the relapse rate seen with gentamicin therapy.[379,1142] Intravenous therapy with erythromycin has also been used successfully, but in vitro data suggests that *F. tularensis* strains are not predictably susceptible.[1365] Scheel et al. found that 14 of 22 Scandinavian strains were resistant to erythromycin, roxithromycin, and clarithromycin in vitro.[1142] Etest methods have also been used to demonstrate macrolide resistance in *F. tularensis*.[642] Many strains are susceptible to rifampin in vitro, but stable spontaneous mutants with rifampin MICs of >32 μg/mL have been recovered within zones of rifampin inhibition of susceptible strains.

While some in vitro studies using broth dilution methods have reported low MICs for β-lactams when tested against *F. tularensis*, other studies using agar dilution have concluded that *F. tularensis* is resistant to β-lactam antimicrobial agents.[76,1142] In a study of 22 animal and human *F. tularensis* isolates using the agar dilution method with blood-cysteine-glucose agar, all strains were resistant not only to penicillin and cephalothin, but also to cefuroxime, ceftazidime, aztreonam, imipenem, and meropenem, with a MIC of >32 μg/mL for all drugs.[1142] Ikaheimo and colleagues used Etest strips on cysteine-heart agar plates for testing 20 human isolates and 18 isolates from dead animals.[617] All strains were susceptible to the agents that have been used for treatment (i.e., streptomycin, tetracycline), but were resistant to β-lactams and penems, including ceftriaxone, ceftazidime, cefpirome, imipenem, meropenem, and piperacillin-tazobactam. Clinical experience with the use of some third-generation cephalosporins for tularemia indicates that they are not effective. Cross and Jacobs reported on eight cases of documented failures with outpatient use of ceftriaxone in the treatment of tularemia.[291] Even though MICs of ceftazidime are lower for *F. tularensis* than those of ceftriaxone, there is currently no evidence to suggest that this drug would be useful either.[379]

F. tularensis strains are susceptible to fluoroquinolones in vitro and there considerable clinical data supporting the utility of these agents for treatment.[379,647,1143,1244] Susceptibility to several fluoroquinolones has been demonstrated in vitro using agar dilution and Etest methods on enriched blood- and cysteine-supplemented media.[617,1142] Syrjala and colleagues reported on three patients with pneumonic tularemia and one with ulceroglandular tularemia who were successfully treated with ciprofloxacin; one other patient with ulceroglandular tularemia responded to norfloxacin therapy.[1244] Scheel et al. successfully treated relapsed ulceroglandular tularemia with ciprofloxacin after the patient had completed a 10-day course of amoxicillin and a 3-week course of doxycycline.[1143] Limaye and Hooper recently reviewed 10 cases of tularemia, including ulceroglandular, pneumonic, and typhoidal forms, that were treated with ciprofloxacin or levofloxacin and found favorable outcomes with no relapses in all cases.[780] A 14-day course of oral ciprofloxacin was found to be effective for treatment of 12

pediatric patients with ulceroglandular infection; culture of the lesions was successful in seven patients and all isolates had ciprofloxacin MICs of 0.03 μg/mL.[643]

Isolates of *F. philomiragia* are usually susceptible to the aminoglycosides, the fluoroquinolones, and tetracycline and variably susceptible to amoxicillin-clavulanate, rifampin, and erythromycin. Most strains produce β-lactamase enzymes and are resistant to ampicillin, and some strains may be resistant to cefazolin, cefotaxime, and trimethoprim-sulfamethoxazole.[585,1155,1175]

Bartonella Species
Taxonomy and Epidemiology of *Bartonella* Species

In the 1984 edition of *Bergey's Manual of Systematic Bacteriology*, the order *Rickettsiales* included three families: *Rickettsiaceae*, *Bartonellaceae*, and *Anaplasmataceae*.[1075] The *Rickettsiaceae* included three genera: *Rickettsia*, *Coxiella*, and *Rochalimaea*.[1357] Although the rickettsias and coxiellas could not be cultivated outside of specific host cells, members of the genus *Rochalimaea* were rod-shaped organisms that could be grown in cell-free media. The family *Bartonellaceae* included two genera—*Bartonella* and *Grahamella*.[1357] Members of the genus *Bartonella* were capable of infecting humans and characteristically grew in close association with the surfaces of vertebrate erythrocytes, while members of the genus *Grahamella* grew within the erythrocytes of nonhuman vertebrates. Only a single *Bartonella* species (*B. bacilliformis*), two *Grahamella* species (*G. talpae* and *G. peromysci*), and two *Rochalimaea* species (*R. quintana* and *R. vinsonii*) had been described up to 1984. Historically, *R. quintana* causes trench fever in humans, and *R. vinsonii* has only been isolated from voles living on Grosse Isle, Quebec, Canada.[1356]

In the early 1990s, several unusual clinical entities—particularly bacillary angiomatosis and peliosis hepatis—were described in patients with HIV infection. Organisms that stained with the Warthin-Starry silver stain could be seen on sectioned biopsies from these unusual cutaneous and visceral lesions, but they were extremely difficult to grow in culture. These organisms were eventually isolated on freshly prepared agar media or in cell cultures after prolonged incubation and were characterized by molecular and genetic techniques. These fastidious bacteria were found to be members of the genus *Rochalimaea* and included *R. quintana*, the classical etiologic agent of trench fever, and a new species that was given the name *R. henselae*.[1187,1188] In 1993, elegant taxonomic studies by Brenner and colleagues confirmed that *Rochalimaea* species were more closely related to *Bartonella bacilliformis* and supported the unification of *Rochalimaea* and *Bartonella*.[168] Consequently, all of the members of the genus *Rochalimaea* were transferred to the genus *Bartonella* as *Bartonella quintana*, *Bartonella vinsonii*, *Bartonella henselae*, and *Bartonella elizabethae*.

In 1995, three new *Grahamella* species were described along with 16S rRNA analyses and comparisons with the extant *Grahamella* and *Bartonella* species. Based on genetic and phenotypic criteria, Birtles and his colleagues at the Central Public Health Laboratory in London proposed that genus *Grahamella* also be unified with genus *Bartonella*, the latter name taking nomenclatural precedence.[136] This unification resulted in five additional *Bartonella* species found in rodents: *B. talpae*, *B. peromysci*, *B. grahamii*, *B. taylorii*, and *B. doshiae*.[136] Genetic analyses by 16S rRNA sequencing and DNA hybridization techniques confirmed that *Bartonella* is the only genus in the family *Bartonellaceae*. This family resides in the proposed order ''Rhizobiales,'' which is in the α_2 subgroup of the class *Proteobacteria*.[455,956] Close relatives include *Afipia*, *Brucella*, and *Agrobacterium tumefaciens*.

The discovery of *B. henselae* and *B. quintana* as opportunistic human pathogens, the evidence for *B. henselae* as the causative agent of cat-scratch disease, and the likelihood of vectorborne transmission of these bacteria among both animals and humans has prompted extensive studies on the epidemiology of these organisms and their roles as emerging human and veterinary pathogens. Using conventional cultural and serologic approaches and novel molecular and genetic techniques, several new *Bartonella* species have been discovered and described during the past several years. In 1993, a unique isolate dubbed *B. elizabethae* was recovered from a patient with endocarditis.[299] In 1996, Drancourt et al. identified a second genotype among *B. henselae* isolates involved in cat-scratch disease (CSD) and endocarditis, and a proposal was made to divide *B. henselae* into two geno/serogroups—*B. henselae* Houston, 16S type I and *B. henselae* Marseilles, 16S type II—based on 16S rDNA sequences and chemotaxonomic examinations of cellular proteins by SDS-PAGE.[118,353] In 1995, Clarridge and colleagues in Houston published a description of their laboratory approach for diagnosis of CSD and included case presentations of two patients with this disease.[259] Although *B. henselae* was recovered from both patients, a different *Bartonella* species was isolated from a kitten that belonged to one of the patients. In 1996, this isolate was given the name *B. clarridgeiae* in honor of Dr. Jill Clarridge, and in 1997 Kordick and associates described the first case of CSD caused by *B. clarridgeiae*.[717,758] During a survey to determine the prevalence of *B. henselae* in cats in the San Francisco Bay area, another new *Bartonella* species was isolated from two cats.[357] These two isolates were 97–100% related to one another by DNA sequencing, but only 68–92% related to the type strain (Houston-1) and to other clinical isolates of *B. henselae*. This new species was named *B. koehlerae*. In 2000, a fourth cat-associated species, (''*B. weissii*'') was isolated from felines in Utah and Illinois; this organism was identical to another species—''*B. bovis*''—found in beef cattle in North Carolina.[119,164]

Studies conducted over the past 10 to 15 years have established that *Bartonella* species constitute a unique group of bacteria found in a wide variety of wild and domesticated animals. These animals may be asymptomatic or may develop significant disease, including chronic bacteremia. Infected animals serve as reservoirs and potential sources of additional animal or human infections.[162] In 1995, a novel *Bartonella* species was described by workers at the College of Veterinary Medicine at North Carolina State University as a cause of canine endocarditis. Phenotypic and genotypic characterization of this agent confirmed its relatedness to the ''vole agent,'' *B. vinsonii*, and this organism was christened *B. vinsonii* subsp. *berkoffii*.[163,719] This subspecies apparently represents a previously unrecognized cause of cardiac arrhythmias, endocarditis, myocarditis, syncope, and sudden death in dogs.[161] In 2000, *B. vinsonii* subsp. *berkhoffii* was detected by PCR analysis of valvular tissue as the cause of human endocarditis in a 35-year-old male, who also had contact with several animals, including a dog.[1102] In 1999, another *B. vinsonii* subspecies, designated *B. vinsonii* subsp. *arupensis*, was isolated from blood cultures of a cattle rancher in Wyoming with an acute febrile illness having a marked neurologic component.[1358] This organism is closely related to *B. vinsonii* subsp *berkhoffii* and to *B. vinsonii* subsp. *vinsonii* and to isolates from naturally infected mice.[605]

Serosurveys and blood culture studies among small mammals, ruminants, and other wildlife have resulted in the descriptions of several new *Bartonella* species. During a survey to determine potential reservoirs of *Bartonella* species in wild mammals, another new species, designated *B. alsatica*, was isolated from blood cultures of wild rabbits (*Oryctolagus cuniculus*) trapped in the Alsace region of France near the Rhine River.[557] The new species *B. schoenbuchii*, *B. bovis*, *B. capreoli*, and *B. birtlesii* have been isolated from blood cultures of roe deer, dairy cattle, reindeer, and small mammals, respectively.[119,120,309] Isolation of bartonellae from rodents and other wild mammals has prompted searches for these bacteria in tick populations. Among DNA extracts from 109 *Ixodes ricinus* ticks collected from Roe deer in the Netherlands, 70% contained 16S rRNA gene sequences for *Bartonella* or species closely related to *Bartonella*.[1150] *Bartonella* gene sequences also have been detected in extracts prepared from *Ixodes* and *Dermacentor* ticks that were collected from six California counties.[221,222]

Bartonella infection is widespread and highly prevalent in rodent populations in different localities. The recently described species *B. tribocorum* was isolated from the blood of two wild rats (*Rattus norvegicus*) that were also trapped in the Alsace region of France.[558] A field study of seven rodent species from 12 geographical areas in the southeastern U.S. found *Bartonella* species in blood cultures of 42.2% of 279 rodents tested.[724] These isolates represented 14 phenotypic variants that clustered into seven phylogenetic groups, four of which contained previously described *Bartonella* species. *Bartonella* species were also isolated from the blood of 19.3% of 325 *Rattus norvegicus* and from 11.8% of 92 *Rattus rattus* from 13 areas of the U.S. and Portugal.[371] Genetic analyses of isolates from Peruvian rats and from rats (*R. norvegicus*) captured in Louisiana and Maryland revealed gene sequences identical to those of *B. elizabethae*, which has been recovered only from a case of human endocarditis.[299] Ellis and coworkers suggested that *Rattus* species, and perhaps other rodents, are the reservoir for *B. elizabethae*, and that the presence of antibodies against *B. elizabethae* among inner-city intravenous drug users reflected infection with this or a related *Bartonella* species.[277,371] In a study of 200 sera from ''street people'' using a free clinic in downtown Los Angeles, the seroprevalence of antibodies to *B. elizabethae*, *B. quintana*, and *B. henselae* were 13.6%, 12.5%, and 9.5%, respectively.[1191]

Bartonellae have also been isolated from free-ranging wild and domestic ruminants and wild and domesticated canine species in North America. Chang and colleagues isolated *Bartonella* species from 49% of 128 cattle in California and Oklahoma, 90% of 42 mule deer in California, and 15%

of 100 elk from California and Oregon.[220] Seroepidemiologic studies of *B. vinsonii* subsp. *berkhoffii* infection in 869 coyotes inhabiting both coastal and inland regions throughout California during 1994 through 1998 found antibody prevalences ranging from 51% in central regions of the state to 34% in southern and 7% in northern regions.[224] The clustered distribution of seropositivity also suggested that *B. vinsonii* subsp. *berkhoffii* infection was vectorborne among these animals. A recent epidemiologic study was conducted among coyotes in Santa Clara County, California, following the development of *Bartonella*-associated infection in a child after suffering a coyote bite. Among 109 coyotes from central coastal California, 28% of the animals were bacteremic with *B. vinsonii* subsp. *berkhoffii* and 76% had species-specific antibodies.[223] Molecular analysis of citrate synthase gene sequences, 16S rRNA, and the 16S–23S intergenic spacer regions established that 6 of the 31 isolates were identical to the *B. vinsonii* subsp. *berkhoffii* type strain isolated from a dog with endocarditis, while the remaining 25 were similar to strains isolated from healthy dogs. Based on these studies, it is likely that coyotes are the principal wildlife reservoir of *B. vinsonii* subsp. *berkhoffii*. Seven of the 31 bacteremic coyotes were also seronegative for *Bartonella* antibodies.[223]

The involvement of *B. henselae* and *B. clarridgeiae* in CSD has prompted investigations into the prevalence and pathogenicity of these organisms in domestic cats, the reservoir for both organisms. Studies have dealt with isolation and detection of these organisms in the feline bloodstream and with seroepidemiology. In a study conducted in San Francisco, Koehler et al. found that 41% of blood specimens from 61 impounded or pet cats were culture-positive for *B. henselae*; kittens were more likely to be bacteremic.[705] Chomel and colleagues also studied 205 cats living in Northern California and found that 39.5% of them had sustained *B. henselae* bacteremia; 52% of these bacteremic cats had more than 1,000 cfu of bacteria per milliliter of blood cultured.[243] Among these animals, 81% tested positive for *B. henselae* antibodies, with bacteremic cats having higher antibody titers than nonbacteremic cats. Heller and associates in France performed blood cultures on 94 stray cats from 10 cat colonies and found that 53% of the animals were bacteremic with a *Bartonella* species.[556] Of the 50 isolates obtained, 35 were *B. henselae* or a *B. henselae* variant, and 15 were *B. clarridgeiae*. Gurfield and associates performed an epidemiologic study on 436 domestic cats in France and found that 5 (1.1%) were coinfected with *B. henselae* and *B. clarridgeiae*, while 2 (0.5%) were coinfected with two strains of *B. henselae* showing variations in the sequence of the 16S rRNA gene.[511] In a study of 100 cats from 89 households in Freiburg, Germany, 13% were bacteremic with *B. henselae* or a *B. henselae* variant.[1123] In a study of one healthy dog and eight healthy cats (all without fleas) in a single household, *B. clarridgeiae* was isolated from one cat twice and *B. henselae* was isolated from a second cat four times over a 3-year period.[715] Over a 16-month period, *B. vinsonii* subsp. *berkhoffii* was isolated from the dog on 8 of 10 attempts at culture. The owner of these animals was seronegative despite her frequent contact with the animals.

Seroprevalence studies have also documented a high rate of *Bartonella* infection among cats in various parts of the world. An examination of banked sera from 592 cats in the Baltimore area yielded a *B. henselae* seroprevalence of 14.7%, and a Swiss seroprevalence study of 728 cats found that 8.3% had antibodies against *B. henselae*, with no significant differences in seroprevalence among sick versus healthy animals.[240,469] A study conducted in Denmark found that 45.5% of 92 shelter or stray cats had antibodies against *B. henselae*.[244] Interestingly, a similar seroepidemiologic study on prevalence of *Bartonella* antibodies in domestic cats conducted in Sweden found that 25% of 292 cats had antibodies to *B. elizabethae*, with the highest prevalence (46%) being found in cats living in Stockholm. The authors pointed out that *B. elizabethae* was the most common agent found in human patients in the same geographical region.[575]

Bartonella species, particularly *B. henselae*, have also been sought in cat fleas (*Ctenocephalides felis*), the presumed vector responsible for transmission of bartonellae among cats and possibly to humans. In a survey of 113 cats from shelters in the Netherlands, 50% were seropositive for *Bartonella* species; 22% of the cats also had positive blood cultures.[115] Seven of 27 DNA extracts from cat fleas removed from these cats contained *Bartonella* DNA. Chomel and coworkers detected *B. henselae* DNA in 34% of 132 fleas removed from 47 cattery cats, 89% of whom were bacteremic with *B. henselae*.[246] These workers also demonstrated that cat fleas removed from bacteremic cats were able to transmit *B. henselae* to specific pathogen-free cats. However, pathogen-free kittens housed together with bacteremic cats without fleas did not become infected with *B. henselae*. *B. henselae* can multiply to high numbers in the cat flea, and the organism can remain viable in flea feces for at least 3 days.[409]

In cats, bacteremia with *B. henselae* or *B. clarridgeiae* is usually asymptomatic, and the presence of overt disease appears to be strain-dependent. Kordick and colleagues inoculated 18 specific pathogen-free cats with *B. henselae* or *B. clarridgeiae* and found that, despite persistent bacteremia, clinical signs and symptoms were minimal.[716] *Bartonella* DNA could be detected by PCR in the blood, brain, lymph nodes, myocardium, liver, and kidneys of infected animals. O'Reilly and coworkers inoculated nine cats with a virulent *B. henselae* strain and found that all nine became bacteremic within 14 days after infection; one animal remained bacteremic up to 18 weeks after infection.[971] Anti–*B. henselae* antibodies developed in all of the animals. In another study of 19 cats belonging to 14 patients with CSD, 17 had positive blood cultures and 13 remained culture-positive for *Bartonella* during the ensuing 12 months.[720] A study of three naturally infected cats over a 2-year period found relapsing bacteremias in all three with intervals of 3 to 19 months between relapses.[658] Following bacteremic episodes, increases in *B. henselae*–specific antibody titers also were noted. Serial blood isolates of *B. henselae* from individual bacteremic cats were shown to have different restriction-fragment-length polymorphisms over time. The emergence of genetically distinct organisms during peaks of recurrent bacteremia in these animals may contribute to the establishment of persistent infections in these animals.

Clinical Significance of *Bartonella* Species

Bartonella species are associated with infections in the compromised host, particularly patients with HIV-1 infection. *Bartonella* infections now include several well-described conditions, including classical and urban trench fever, bacillary angiomatosis with cutaneous and/or systemic involvement, peliosis hepatis, relapsing fever with bacteremia, endocarditis, and cat-scratch disease. The type species of the genus *Bartonella*, *B. bacilliformis* causes Oroya fever, a geographically restricted febrile illness. The unfolding epidemiology of these organisms and the expanding literature on the variety of species and their associations with animal, insect vectors, and human disease is largely due to the elegant laboratory approaches based on both ''traditional'' culture methods and ''cutting-edge'' molecular-based technologies.[755]

OROYA FEVER AND VERRUGA PERUANA

These two clinical entities are manifestations of infection with *Bartonella bacilliformis*.[808,809] These infections are geographically restricted because of the limited habitats of the principal sandfly vector *Lutzomyia verrucarum*. The reservoir of the organism is unknown, although humans with asymptomatic bacteremia may serve as the reservoir. Infections are seen in river valleys of the west Andes Mountains at altitudes between 2000 and 8000 feet in Peru, Ecuador, and Columbia. This infection is also known as Carrion's disease after Daniel Carrion, a Peruvian medical student in whom the disease developed after inoculating himself with material from an infectious lesion. Following the bite of an infected female vector, symptoms of Oroya fever develop in from 3 weeks to 3 months, although asymptomatic infection may also occur. Disease onset may be abrupt or insidious. The patient may have anorexia, headache, malaise, and a slight fever lasting 2–7 days or more. When the onset is abrupt, the patient may present with fever, severe headache, chills, and mental status changes. Severe anemia ensues caused by destruction of red cells by the organisms. Jaundice, hepatosplenomegaly, and generalized lymphadenopathy appear, along with severe muscle and joint pain.[722] Opportunistic infections (e.g., bacteremic salmonellosis, gram-negative sepsis) or reactivated latent infections (e.g., toxoplasmosis, histoplasmosis) develop in about 30% of patients caused by cellular immune compromise. Dyspnea, angina, and pneumocystosis may develop, as well as delirium and coma. During this phase, the organisms may be isolated from the blood and can actually be seen on blood smears within red blood cells. Acute infection during pregnancy often results in abortion or both maternal and fetal death. Untreated, the fatality rate of Oroya fever may be as high as 90% but with treatment fatalities are reduced to less than 10%. This ''critical'' stage lasts from 2 to 4 weeks, at which time the organisms disappear from the circulation, the fever normalizes, and the anemia corrects itself.

After resolution of Oroya fever, pain in the bones, joints, and muscles may persist to the stage of verruga development. This stage is characterized by the appearance of nodular lesions on exposed parts of the body, on mucous membranes, or in internal organs.[48] These nodules develop over a period of 1–2 months and may persist for months to years. The lesions are red to purple in color, are nontender if not secondarily infected, and may appear in crops. The ''verrugas'' may be sessile, plaque-like, miliary, nodular, pedunculated,

or confluent.[48] Joint pain and fever usually subside after the appearance of the skin lesions, and anemia is usually not present during this stage of the disease. In tissue specimens from verruga lesions, *B. bacilliformis* can be seen with the Warthin-Starry or Giemsa stain and can be cultured from the cutaneous lesions and, occasionally from the blood and bone marrow. Oroya fever has been treated with a variety of agents, including penicillin, tetracycline, and streptomycin, with chloramphenicol considered the drug of choice.[809] Good responses have also been obtained with ciprofloxacin. Streptomycin was the drug of choice for treatment of the cutaneous disease, but rifampin and ciprofloxacin produce good clinical responses and can be given orally instead of by intramuscular injection.

''CLASSICAL'' AND ''URBAN'' TRENCH FEVER

B. quintana is the agent of trench fever, a louseborne, debilitating febrile illness that affected almost 1 million people, including German and allied military personnel during World War I. After the war, trench fever continued to occur in Spain, France, Italy, parts of eastern Europe, North Africa, and China. *B. quintana* has also been detected in lice obtained from regions of Peru and South America, where trench fever had not been documented previously.[1048] Serologic tests indicate the presence of the organism in Bolivia and Mexico as well.[96] The organism is transmitted by the human body louse, *Pediculus humanis*, which has increased in prevalence worldwide during the past 10 to 15 years, particularly in developing countries and in areas of great social, political, and economic turmoil, such as the former Soviet Union and regions of Eastern Europe. The bacterium infects the louse, which then sheds organism-laden feces that contaminate the bite wound. In humans, fever, malaise, shaking chills, drenching sweats, and severe neck, back, and leg pain develop after an incubation period of 5 to 20 days. Conjunctivitis, retroorbital pain, and shin-bone pain are characteristic; splenomegaly and a macular rash have been observed in some patients. The fever may subside rapidly or may last 4 to 5 days. Fevers lasting up to 5 days may wax and wane repeatedly, or the fever may persist unabated for several weeks. The disease is usually not severe and is self-limited. Patients have a rapid response to treatment with tetracyclines and/or chloramphenicol.

''Urban'' trench fever is a clinical entity that has been documented among homeless persons in urban areas. This infection is associated with fever, night sweats, prolonged or intermittent bacteremia, louse infestation, and high antibody titers against *B. quintana*. The appearance of *B. quintana* infection among homeless individuals in urban areas has prompted investigations of emergent trench fever and other louseborne illnesses among indigent people in several cities.[180,181,427,1103,1207] The role of body lice in the transmission of urban trench fever has been confirmed by several epidemiologic and laboratory investigations. In one study, lice were collected from 268 persons at the Moscow Municipal Disinfection Center and subjected to PCR analysis for detection of the *B. quintana gltA* (citrate synthase) gene sequence.[1111] *B. quintana* DNA was detected in 12.3% of the lice samples studied. This and other studies have confirmed the pivotal role of *P. humanus* in the epidemiology of re-emergent, 21st-century trench fever.[961]

BACILLARY ANGIOMATOSIS

Bacillary angiomatosis (BA) is a bacterial infection caused by *B. henselae* and *B. quintana* that results in unusual widespread vascular proliferation; it is seen most commonly in patients with advanced HIV disease.[61,276,456,879,1017,1133] This infection has also been reported in patients with immunosuppression who have undergone transplantation, individuals receiving cancer chemotherapy, and patients undergoing long-term corticosteroid treatment.[1151,1281] BA has also been diagnosed in immunocompetent adults and children.[1192,1260] Patients with AIDS who have BA usually have CD4 counts of less than 200 cells/µL when lesions appear. The disease is distinct from Kaposi's sarcoma (KS) and other vascular neoplasms in that the lesions begin as small papules that gradually enlarge to form rounded, red to violaceous purple nodules having a small collar of epithelium.[264] KS lesions are usually light pink to brown or black and are plaque-like rather than nodular, although on some body surfaces, BA lesions may initially develop as flat, hyperpigmented, indurated plaques.[264] BA and KS can coexist in the same patient.[1214] BA lesions develop as discrete lesions that enlarge and coalesce to form larger nodules. The lesions are initially smooth and then may ulcerate and crust over. Some lesions are located more deeply in the subcutaneous tissues (e.g., liver, spleen) and may involve the bone and bone marrow, forming large osteolytic lesions.[707] Bone involvement with BA is painful, usually affects the radius, fibula, and tibia, and is associated primarily with *B. quintana* infection.[708] An erythematous, cellulitic plaque-like lesion may be observed in the skin over and surrounding bone lesions. Visceral involvement may occur as disseminated vascular lesions or as bacillary peliosis hepatis when the liver is involved. Lesions of extracutaneous BA have been documented in mucosal surfaces of the upper and lower respiratory and gastrointestinal tracts, the conjunctivae and orbit, the heart, the diaphragm, the biliary tract, muscles, liver, spleen, lymph nodes, the genital tract, and the central nervous system.[611,614,704,908,1185,1209,1292] Internal BA lesions may become large enough to cause compression or obstruction of internal organs, with constitutional signs and symptoms that include fever, anorexia, vomiting, and weight loss. Histopathological diagnosis of BA requires the collection of punch or excisional biopsies for cutaneous and subcutaneous lesions, while excision is usually used for deep-seated lesions. Besides histopathology, biopsies may also be submitted for culture and analysis by electron microscopy and molecular methods.

Histologically, BA lesions are composed of large, cuboidal, endothelial cells lining blood vessels. These cells extend into the vascular lumen and are associated with aggregates of purplish granular material representing clusters of bacteria.[1208] There is also a dense inflammatory infiltrate of neutrophils. BA lesions can be histologically differentiated from KS lesions in that there are no bizarre, jagged blood vessels as seen in KS, and the inflammatory infiltrate consists of lymphocytes, histiocytes, and neutrophils as opposed to plasma cells.[1393] When biopsied tissue sections are stained with the Warthin-Starry silver stain, clumps and tangled masses of interstitial bacteria are seen. *B. henselae* and, in some cases, *B. quintana* have been isolated from the blood, skin lesions, bone, visceral organs, and brains of patients with BA.[707,762,1065,1066,1188,1361] In a 1997 case-control study of 49 patients with BA in San Francisco, 53% were infected with *B. henselae* and 47% with *B. quintana*.[708] Infection with *B. henselae* was epidemiologically linked with exposure to cats and cat fleas, while infection with *B. quintana* was associated with low income, homelessness, and exposure to lice. Some investigators and clinicians believe that BA may be a manifestation of CSD peculiar to the compromised host.[676,706,866] In vitro studies of *Bartonella* have established that these organisms are able to stimulate angiogenesis, the physiologic process that results in the formation of new blood vessels, and to affect the migration and proliferation of endothelial cells.[449,703]

Cutaneous BA usually responds to treatment with erythromycin, using a dose of 500 mg four times a day.[1393] Antimicrobial therapy should be continued for at least 6 weeks; longer courses may be necessary since lesions often recur after the cessation of therapy. Parenteral therapy may be required to treat relapses of cutaneous infection and disseminated infections. If the BA lesions are confined to the skin, they may be excised surgically. Good clinical responses to other antibiotics, including rifampin, tetracyclines (i.e., doxycycline, minocycline, tetracycline), other macrolides (i.e., azithromycin, clarithromycin), chloramphenicol, trimethoprim-sulfamethoxazole, vancomycin, norfloxacin, and ciprofloxacin with gentamicin have also been reported, but relapse is common following cessation of therapy. Drugs that inhibit cell-wall biosynthesis (e.g., penicillins and cephalosporins) are not useful in the treatment of BA.

PELIOSIS

Before the appearance of the AIDS epidemic, peliosis of the internal visceral organs was rare and had only been described in patients with carcinoma or tuberculosis or in persons being treated with anabolic steroids. Peliosis hepatis is characterized by the presence of cystic, blood-filled lesions that are scattered throughout the parenchyma of the liver.[1393] Increasing numbers of cases of peliosis involving the liver and spleen (splenic peliosis) have been reported in association with HIV infection.[708,1002] Most patients with hepatic or splenic peliosis also have BA, and bacteria similar to those seen on Warthin-Starry–stained biopsies of BA are also seen within the blood-filled cysts that are present in the liver and spleen. Most patients with bacillary peliosis hepatis present with weight loss, abdominal pain, intractable nausea, anemia, diarrhea, fever, hepatosplenomegaly, and lymphadenopathy. Severe intraperitoneal bleeding with hypovolemic shock has also been reported as an unusual manifestation of bacillary parenchymal peliosis.[800] Liver enzymes are usually elevated, with alkaline phosphatase levels being as high as 5 to 10 times as the normal value.[1002] Parenchymal bacillary peliosis of other internal organs (i.e., heart, larynx, lungs, adrenals, cervix, ovaries, pineal gland, and choroid plexus) has been reported as well. Peliosis hepatis appears to be associated exclusively with *B. henselae* infection and is believed by some to be another manifestation of BA.[826]

FEVER AND BACTEREMIA

B. henselae bacteremia has been described in patients with HIV, patients with AIDS, pharmacologically immunosuppressed recipients of allogeneic transplants, and immunocompetent hosts with no known risk factors for immunosuppressive diseases.[1057,1187,1361] In AIDS patients, *B. henselae* bacteremia has been detected in those with and those without focal BA or peliosis. Immunocompromised patients present with relapsing fevers, weight loss, malaise, and fatigue; relapse following therapy often occurs in these individuals. In HIV-infected patients, *B. henselae* may also cause a generalized, inflammatory disease of the reticuloendothelial system; organisms may be detected histopathologically or by molecular techniques in necrotic, inflammatory lesions in the spleen, liver, heart, bone marrow and lymph nodes.[1186] In immunocompetent, HIV-negative individuals, *B. henselae* bacteremia presents with an abrupt onset of fever with accompanying joint and muscle pain; some patients may manifest signs and symptoms of CNS involvement (i.e., headache, photophobia, and meningismus). *B. henselae* has been documented serologically as the cause of "fevers of unknown origin" in both children and adults.[625,1293] These patients present with fever, anorexia, headache, and other constitutional symptoms.

Persistent *B. quintana* bacteremia was a recognized symptom of classical trench fever and is a frequent manifestation of reemergent "trench fever" among the homeless and alcoholic residents of urban environments. Fever and bacteremia caused by *B. quintana* was first documented in 10 homeless, inner-city patients in Seattle who were HIV antibody–negative but had chronic alcoholism as an underlying disease.[1207] All of these individuals presented with fever, two had splenomegaly, two reported a recent cat scratch, and endocarditis developed in one (see below).[1206] Brouqui and colleagues documented *B. quintana* bacteremia in 10 (14%) of 71 homeless patients in France.[181] Five of these patients had chronic bacteremia, as evidenced by multiple positive blood cultures over several weeks, and 8 patients with bacteremia were afebrile. In addition, 30% of the patients had high titers of anti–*B. quintana* antibodies, and recent infections (bacteremia or seroconversion) were detected in 17 patients (24%). In this study, homeless patients with *B. quintana* bacteremia were more likely to have had exposure to lice, and to have headaches, leg pain, and lower platelet counts than those who did not have bacteremia or were seronegative for *B. quintana* antibodies.[180,181] Interestingly, *B. quintana* DNA was detected by PCR in lice from 3 of 15 patients from whom they were collected. Of these three patients, two were bacteremic and one was seropositive but not bacteremic. Serologic studies have also demonstrated a high prevalence of *Bartonella* infections among inner-city intravenous drug users. Comer and colleagues reported that 37.5% of serum specimens collected from 630 intravenous drug users in Baltimore reacted with at least one *Bartonella* antigen (i.e., *B. henselae*, *B. quintana*, or *B. elizabethae*) by immunofluorescence assay (IFA).[277]

Immunocompetent patients usually have a rapid response to a short (10 days or less) course of therapy, and generally do not relapse; in some cases infections may resolve without antimicrobial therapy.[625] However, Lucey and colleagues reported on two immunocompetent patients who had relapsing illness with positive blood cultures for *B. henselae*.[802] Interestingly, both of these patients had experienced tick bites prior to becoming ill. These two cases were the first in which transmission of *B. henselae* by insects was epidemiologically suggested. Drancourt, Raoult, and others reported two patients with bacteremia and chronic granulomatous mediastinal adenopathy from whom *B. quintana* was recovered from blood and bone marrow cultures.[355,1049] These patients were middle-aged women who were seronegative for HIV antibodies, had underlying diseases (i.e., corticosteroid treatment, chronic renal failure requiring hemodialysis), had exposure to cats, kittens, and cat fleas, and were successfully treated with parenteral aminoglycosides.[355,1049] Interestingly, neither patient mounted a detectable serologic response against *B. quintana*.

ENDOCARDITIS

Bartonella species, and *B. quintana* in particular, have been isolated from several cases of "culture negative" endocarditis.[429,518,627,1206] Endocarditis due to *B. quintana* was first reported in 1993 in a 50-year-old, HIV-1 infected homosexual male who presented with night sweats, weight loss, and fatigue.[1205] On physical examination, mild renal insufficiency, splenomegaly, anemia, and a holosystolic heart murmur were noted, and echocardiography revealed mitral and aortic valve vegetations. Subsequently, *B. quintana* was documented as a cause of bacteremia in 10 febrile, homeless, alcoholic patients in Seattle; in one of these patients aortic valve endocarditis developed.[1206] Even after 21 days of therapy, *B. quintana* was still detectable in the tissues by PCR. *B. quintana* was also recovered as the cause of endocarditis in three homeless, alcoholic men in France.[354] All of these patients required aortic and/or mitral valve replacement. *B. quintana* endocarditis has also been reported in an immunocompetent adult.[184] In 1993, Hadfield and coworkers described the first case of endocarditis caused by *B. henselae* in a 59-year-old HIV-negative man with a history of alcohol abuse, and another case of *B. henselae* endocarditis was reported in 1995 in a previously healthy 41-year-old man.[520,588] Both of these patients required valve replacement surgery. Since then, *B. henselae* has been identified as the cause of both native and prosthetic valve endocarditis in several immunocompetent patients.[312,378,696] *B. elizabethae* was first reported as a cause of endocarditis in an immunocompetent 31-year-old man.[299] This infection resolved with valve replacement and treatment with vancomycin and imipenem. In 1996, Raoult and colleagues reported on 22 new cases of *Bartonella* endocarditis in French patients who were diagnosed by serologic, culture, and molecular techniques.[1050] Of the 22 patients, 11 were alcoholics, 9 were homeless, 13 had preexisting valvular injuries, and 4 had histories of cat exposure. Most patients had aortic valve vegetations, and embolic complications developed in many, with all but two patients requiring valvular surgery. Implicated organisms included *B. quintana* (5 patients), *B. henselae* (4), and an undetermined *Bartonella* species (13). The latter 13 patients were diagnosed by serologic tests that could not distinguish between *B. quintana* and *B. henselae*. In this study, *B. quintana* endocarditis was associated with homeless patients with chronic alcoholism with no previously existing valvular damage, while *B. henselae* endocarditis occurred mostly in patients with preexisting valvular pathology and a history of contact with cats. *Bartonella* endocarditis has been successfully treated with combinations of parenteral amoxicillin and gentamicin, parenteral vancomycin with ofloxacin and netilmicin followed by oral ofloxacin, rifampin, and pristinomycin, and with parenteral ceftriaxone followed by a prolonged course of oral erythromycin.[354,1050,1207]

Bartonella species also cause endocarditis and other cardiac diseases in dogs. Breitschwerdt and colleagues in North Carolina described a case of endocarditis involving the aortic and mitral valves in a 3-year-old spayed Labrador retriever.[163] A fastidious gram-negative bacillus was isolated from the dog's blood using the lysis-centrifugation method, and DNA extracted from the involved heart valves were amplified by PCR technology and compared with other *Bartonella* species. DNA hybridization, 16S rRNA sequencing, cellular fatty acid analysis, and phenotypic testing of the isolate characterized the organism as a new *Bartonella* species that most closely resembled *B. vinsonii*. The name *B. vinsonii* subsp. *berkhoffii* was proposed for this new organism.[719] This agent represents a new veterinary pathogen causing cardiac arrhythmia, myocarditis, and endocarditis in dogs, and has recently been reported as the agent of asymptomatic endocarditis in a human.[161,1102] *B. henselae*, *B. elizabethae*, and *B. clarridgeiae* have now been detected by molecular techniques in blood specimens from dogs, and *B. clarridgeiae* was recently recovered as the cause of endocarditis in a male neutered boxer with a systolic heart murmur and severe valvular aortic stenosis.[247,862] Wild and domesticated canines may be reservoirs for all of these agents.[862]

CAT-SCRATCH DISEASE (CSD)

CSD is a common cause of lymphadenopathy, particularly in children and adolescents. It occurs throughout the world, with most cases occurring between September and March; in warm climates, peak occurrences may occur in July and August. About 90% of patients have a history of exposure to cats, and a cat scratch or a cat bite will have occurred in about 75–80% of these persons.[97] Kittens seem to be implicated more frequently than adult cats, and transmission appears to be by direct contact, since the disease generally follows a bite, scratch, or lick from a young cat. About 3 to 10 days after the scratch or bite occurs, a primary erythematous papule or pustule forms. These lesions persist for about 2 to 3 weeks. During this time, low-grade fever may be present in one third of patients, with malaise and fever being noted in about one fourth of cases.[97] About 10% will have headache and muscle aches with a sore throat, and a faint rash lasting 1 to 2 weeks may also be seen. Regional lymphadenopathy develops in over 90% of patients, the location of which is dependent on the site of the cat bite or scratch. Since most lesions are on the upper extremities, the adenopathy usually develops in axillary, cervical, or submandibular areas. Single-node involvement occurs in about half of the patients. Noncontiguous or generalized lymphadenopathy and hepatosplenomegaly are uncommon, but may be confused with malignancy (i.e., lymphoma) when they are present.[461,677] Affected lymph nodes usually exhibit

granulomas, stellate microabscesses, and follicular hyperplasia. Clusters of bacillary organisms are often seen in sections of lymph node biopsies that are stained with the Warthin-Starry silver impregnation stain. The enlarged lymph nodes usually regress spontaneously over several months, although up to 20% of patients may show lymphadenopathy for 12 to 24 months.

Although uncommon, CSD may have atypical presentations and complications. These manifestations include the oculoglandular syndrome of Parinaud, which presents as an ocular granuloma or conjunctivitis with preauricular lymphadenopathy, osteomyelitis, epitrochlear mass mimicking rhabdomyosarcoma, and hepatic and splenic microabscesses and granulomas.[51,494,612,1323] The oculoglandular syndrome usually results from a cat scratch, lick or bite on the eyelid or conjunctivae, although autoinoculation from the primary lesion into the eye may also occur. CSD encephalopathy and aseptic meningitis are rare complications that may occur 1 to 6 weeks after regional lymphadenopathy becomes apparent and are characterized by encephalitis, seizures, myelitis, and neuropathy.[460,941,1392] The patient may exhibit headache, mental status changes, seizures, convulsions, combative behavior, and/or coma.[522] Retinitis associated with CSD has also been reported, including a case of *B. henselae* bacteremia that resulted in acute loss of vision.[797,1392] Systemic CSD may also cause multifocal osteomyelitis at sites that are remote from the initial scratch or bite.[728,878] Pulmonary manifestations of CSD are extremely rare.[821]

CSD is usually a self-limited illness that does not generally respond to targeted antimicrobial therapy. Despite the in vitro susceptibility of *B. henselae* to many antimicrobial agents, their use for treatment of CSD has not resulted in clear-cut benefits for the patient. Only the aminoglycosides, and gentamicin in particular, have demonstrated effectiveness in the treatment of suppurative complications of CSD.[97,917] Chia et al. reported on four patients with CSD who were successfully treated with a 5- to 10-day course of azithromycin., including one patient in whom treatment with doxycycline and cefazolin had failed.[239] Successful treatment of CSD with azithromycin may be related not only to the in vitro susceptibility of *Bartonella* species to this agent, but also to the penetration and intracellular accumulation of azithromycin within neutrophils and macrophages, resulting in ratios of 40:1 for intracellular:extracellular drug concentrations.[239,846] Ciprofloxacin has also been used successfully for the treatment of CSD, again presumably because of its intracellular accumulation.[584]

Microbiologic and serologic studies conducted over the past several years have established that *B. henselae* is the bacterial agent responsible for CSD. In 1988, English and associates at the Armed Forces institute of Pathology (AFIP) isolated a gram-negative organism from the lymph nodes of 10 patients with CSD.[380] One of these isolates plus three others recovered at the CDC from the lymph nodes of children with CSD were further characterized and proposed as a new genus *Afipia* (named after the AFIP), with the species name *felis* reflecting its association with CSD. Based on these studies, *A. felis* was postulated to be the causative agent of CSD. At the same time, several investigators were examining the etiology of BA, peliosis, and bacteremia in HIV-infected patients with new and powerful molecular methods.

Using highly conserved oligonucleotide primers from the bacterial 16 rRNA genes, Relman and colleagues were able to demonstrate and amplify bacterial DNA sequences in BA tissues from AIDS patients and showed that these sequences were genotypically related to *Rochalimaea* species, specifically *R. (B.) quintana*.[1065] Slater and his colleagues also recovered a *Rochalimaea*-like organism from blood cultures of febrile immunocompromised adults that had 16S rRNA gene sequences that were similar to those described by Relman's group.[1187] This and other work established that the newly described *Rochalimaea* species, *R. (B.) henselae*, and the old agent of trench fever, *R. (B.) quintana*, were the causes of BA, peliosis hepatis, and bacteremia in AIDS patients.[1057,1188]

In 1992, Regnery and colleagues isolated *R. (B.) henselae* from the blood of an asymptomatic cat on two occasions, and using IFA antibody techniques, the same research group demonstrated that 88% of patients with CSD had high antibody titers to *R. (B.) henselae* antigens and not *A. felis* antigens.[1058,1059] PCR and similar techniques were used subsequently by several research groups to demonstrate the presence of *B. henselae* DNA and the absence of *B. quintana* and *A. felis* DNA in purulent material from the suppurative lymph nodes of patients with CSD.[32,34,489] Using IFA techniques, Zangwill and his collaborators found that 84% of 45 patients with CSD had anti-*R. (B.) henselae* antibodies, compared with 3% of 112 control patients. Furthermore, 81% of cats belonging to CSD patients also were seropositive, compared with 38% of 29 control animals.[1427] This study also reported that the risk of CSD was greater for individuals with kittens than for those with adult cats, that individuals with bites and scratches from kittens were at higher risk for CSD than those with wounds from adult cats, and that the risk of CSD was also greater if the kitten had fleas.[1427] Also in 1993, Dolan and coworkers grew *B. henselae* from the lymph nodes of two immunocompetent patients with CSD.[345] Bacilli observed in biopsies from suppurative lymph nodes have also been identified as *B. henselae* by immunocytochemical staining with antibodies against *B. henselae*.[869] Several additional studies have confirmed the studies cited above and, although the role of *A. felis* in CSD has not been completely characterized, *B. henselae* is very likely the predominant cause of CSD.[116,462] In 1999, *A. felis* was isolated from the water supply of a French hospital in association with species of free-living amoebae, leading the authors to suggest that previous recoveries of *A. felis* from CSD lymph node specimens on two occasions could have been due to water contamination and ineffective sterilization procedures.[756] The etiologic role of *B. henselae* in CSD has been further strengthened by the large number of epidemiologic studies on *B. henselae* infection in domestic cats (see section on "Epidemiology," above).

In 1997, a second *Bartonella* species, *B. clarridgeiae*, was also described in association with a case of CSD.[717] In this case, CSD developed in a veterinarian after a bite wound from a 6-week-old cat. Blood cultures collected from the patient and serologic tests (IFA) for *B. henselae*, *B. quintana*, and *B. elizabethae* antibodies were negative. However, the patient's serum reacted in an IFA test with a *Bartonella* isolate recovered from blood cultures obtained from the cat.

Serologic evidence for *B. clarridgeiae* infection was also obtained from a patient with CSD who had constitutional symptoms, a history of exposure to cats and cat scratches, and a large chest wall abscess.[821] Although cultures from the patient remained negative, *B. clarridgeiae* was isolated from the blood of one of the patient's cats.

MISCELLANEOUS INFECTIONS

Since the discovery of the association of *Bartonella* species with CSD, BA, and peliosis hepatis, several other manifestations of *B. henselae* infection have been reported in both immunocompromised and immunocompetent hosts. In most of these infections, an association with young cats has been documented, lending further credence to the possibility that uncommon clinical manifestations of *B. henselae* infection represent part of a continuum in the clinical presentation of CSD. These manifestations have included neuroretinitis without the oculoglandular syndrome of Parinaud, isolated unilateral and diffuse lymphadenitis, severe myocarditis, and neurologic disease associated with rapidly progressive dementia.[844,1153,1392] Meininger and colleagues described a healthy man in whom chronic active myocarditis due to *B. henselae* developed; it resulted in heart failure and the need for heart transplantation.[851] The association of *Bartonella* with AIDS-related dementia was elucidated by a serologic study conducted in Los Angeles by Schwartzman and colleagues in which both cat ownership and neuropsychological decline and dementia were associated significantly with the presence of IgM antibodies to *B. henselae*.[1152] Caniza and coworkers described a case of opportunistic pulmonary infection due to *B. henselae* in a 19-year-old female recipient of a kidney transplant.[197] Tissue from pulmonary nodules of this patient were negative on culture but contained 16S rRNA specific for *R. henselae* by PCR. All eight of the domestic cats that lived with the patient had positive blood cultures for *B. henselae*; PCR analysis of these isolates established that the feline isolates were identical to those found in the lung tissue of the patient. *B. henselae* infection has also been responsible for intraocular and retinal inflammation and optic disk edema resulting in substantial loss of visual acuity.[1337] Golnick et al. reported four patients who presented with vision loss resulting from intraocular inflammation, swelling of the optic nerve, and retinal detachment.[482] Patients had elevated titers against *B. henselae* and responded to treatment with resulting improvements in vision. Neuroretinitis has also been diagnosed in a patient with serologic evidence of infection with *B. elizabethae*.[960] In an unusual case, bilateral neuroretinitis accompanied by severe headache and behavioral changes was diagnosed in a 55-year-old woman with insulin-dependent diabetes mellitus and hypothyroidism. PCR analysis of DNA extracted from intraocular fluids revealed the presence of a 16S rRNA gene sequence that showed 100% homology with *B. grahamii*, a species normally found in rodents in Europe and North America.[680] The patient owned a dog but had no history of exposure to cats, rodents, or other animals. The patient also had serologic evidence of *B. henselae* infection by EIA, which was likely due to cross-reactivity with *B. grahamii*. She responded to therapy with daily oral doxycycline and rifampin for 4 weeks. Intraorbital and retinal infections with

B. henselae have also been diagnosed by detection of DNA in intraocular specimens.[482,1350]

Detection, Isolation, and Identification of *Bartonella* Species
SPECIMEN TYPES

Specimens that may be submitted for recovery of *Bartonella* species include blood, biopsy specimens of suspected cutaneous or systemic BA lesions, lymph node biopsies, and aspirates. Specimens collected early in the clinical course are preferable, particularly lymph node biopsy specimens from patients with suspected CSD. Late-stage, suppurative lymph nodes may not yield organisms because of the intense local cellular immune response.[60] Tissue specimens should be homogenized and plated on culture media. Lysis-centrifugation methods have been reported to enhance recovery of these fastidious bacteria from blood specimens. Blood may also be submitted in sterile lithium heparin tubes. With heparinized blood specimens, freezing the blood and then thawing it at room temperature prior to direct plating may also enhance recovery. Since the organisms produce little or no CO_2 during growth, detection of *Bartonella* species in automated blood culture systems (e.g., BACTEC; Bacti/Alert, etc.) may be problematic. Isolates have been recovered from BACTEC high-volume aerobic resin PLUS 26 bottles, although the organisms did not register growth indices above the positive threshold.[802] Therefore, staining smears prepared from inoculated bottles with the acridine orange fluorescent stain after 8 days incubation has been recommended.[349,748]

CULTURE

Bartonella species may be isolated by plating onto appropriate agar media or by cocultivation in cell culture. Cell culture methods are performed with shell vials containing a human endothelial-cell monolayer (e.g., ECV 304 cell line) or other cell types (e.g., Vero cells, HeLa cells, L292 cells).[354,707,1049,1428] Specimens processed by this technique have included biopsy specimens from cutaneous and osseus BA lesions and heparinized blood. Koehler and colleagues used a bovine endothelial cell line (i.e., CPA cells, ATTC cell line #207) to isolate both *B. henselae* and *B. quintana* from minced tissue biopsies of BA lesions.[707] After 9 to 36 days of incubation, the turbid culture supernatants were subcultured to agar media for subsequent growth and identification. Drancourt and colleagues used ECV 304 cells (a continuous human endothelial cell line) to recover *B. quintana* from blood specimens of homeless patients with endocarditis.[354] With this technique, organisms can be detected in the shell vial by immunofluorescence and identified by PCR or other molecular techniques. Broth-enrichment recovery of *Bartonella* species has also been performed with a defined medium containing RPMI 1640 (a tissue culture-type liquid medium) supplemented with hemin, amino acids, and pyruvate.[1388] This medium was used to successfully recover *B. henselae* from human and cat blood and from lymph node biopsies of patients with CSD.

Agar-based culture methods include culture on heart infusion agar containing 5% horse or rabbit blood. Blood-supplemented BHI, tryptic soy, and Columbia agars and enriched chocolate agar may also support growth. Freshly prepared media are essential for optimal recovery. Selective media are not available, and media containing antimicrobial agents should not be used. Inoculated plates are incubated in a humid atmosphere at 35 to 37°C for at least 21 days, although some *Bartonella* strains may require up to 45 days of incubation before growth is apparent.[755] Subcultures from slow-growing primary cultures may require 15 to 20 days before good growth is obtained. Most bartonellae do not grow under anaerobic conditions, at temperatures of 25 or 42°C, or in the absence of hemin and CO_2. *B. bacilliformis* is exceptional, in that this species favors a lower growth temperature (i.e., 25–28°C) and does not require supplemental CO_2 for growth.

GRAM STAIN AND COLONY MORPHOLOGY

On primary isolation, *Bartonella* species appear initially as white, small adherent colonies that vary in size and shape. Some strains of *B. henselae*, *B. quintana*, and *B. elizabethae* may pit the agar surface during growth. Characteristically, *B. henselae* colonies are white, dry, adherent, "cauliflower-like," embedded in the agar, and morphologically heterogeneous. With multiple passages, the colonies become less dry, less adherent, larger, and tend to grow faster. Colonies of *B. elizabethae* resemble *B. henselae* except that weak or partial hemolysis may be noted around colonies growing on heart infusion agar with 5% rabbit blood.[299] Colonies of *B. bacilliformis* differ from the others species in that they are initially small, smooth, and translucent and remain so on serial subculture. On Gram stain, *Bartonella* organisms appear as small, slightly curved, pleomorphic, gram-negative bacilli that measure about 1–2.5 by 0.5–0.6 μm and display "twitching" motility when mounted in saline.

IDENTIFICATION METHODS

In general, *Bartonella* species are biochemically inert and are nonreactive in routine biochemical identification tests, including oxidase, catalase, indole, urease, decarboxylase, and nitrate reduction tests. Several presumptive and definitive methods for identifying *Bartonella* species are available, including phenotypic methods, chemotaxonomic methods using fatty acid analysis, and molecular techniques (e.g., PCR, nucleic acid sequencing, etc.). Species-specific monoclonal antibodies have been evaluated for rapid identification of *B. quintana*.[776]

Presumptive identification of *Bartonella* species, including *B. henselae*, *B. quintana*, and *B. vinsonii*, may be determined with commercial identification systems that use chromogenic enzyme substrates to detect preformed bacterial enzymes (e.g., Microscan Rapid Anaerobe Panel, Vitek *Neisseria-Haemophilus* Identification card, IDS RapID ANA II panel, API AnIDENT panel, Microscan HNID Panel).[1360] These systems produced biochemical reaction patterns that were unique within their own databases, but only the reactions on the Microscan Rapid Anaerobe Panel were able to separate *B. henselae* and *B. quintana* at the species level. This panel distinguished all species tested, generating unique biotype codes for each species (Table 9-14).

Bartonella species may be identified by gas-liquid chro-

Table 9-14 Biochemical Characteristics for Identification of *Bartonella* Species

CHARACTERISTIC	*B. BACILLIFORMIS*	*B. QUINTANA*	*B. HENSELAE*	*B. ELIZABETHAE*	*B. CLARRIDGEIAE*	*B. GRAHAMII*	*B. VINSONII* SUBSP. *VINSONII*	*B. VINSONII* SUBSP. *BERKHOFFII*	*B. VINSONII* SUBSP. *ARUPENSIS*
Optimal growth temperature	25–30°C	35–37°C	35–37°C	35–37°C	35–37°C	35–37°C	35–37°C	35–37°C	35–37°C
Hemolysis	−	−	−	+w	−	−	−	−	−
Oxidase	−	v	−	−	−	−	v	−	−
Catalase	+	v	−	−	−	−	v	v	−
Nitrate reduction	−	−	−	−	−	−	−	−	−
Urease	−	−	−	−	−	−	−	−	−
Indole	−	−	−	−	−	−	−	−	−
Acetoin	−	−	−	−	−	+	−	NA	NA
O/F Glucose[a]	−/−	−/−	−/−	−/−	−/−	−/−	−/−	−/−	−/−
Flagella	+	−	−	−	+	−	−	−	−
Twitching motility	−	+	+	−	+	−	−	−	−
Major cell fatty acids	$C_{18:1\omega7C}$, $C_{16:0}$, $C_{16:1\omega7C}$, $C_{12:0}$	$C_{18:1\omega7C}$, $C_{16:0}$, $C_{18:0}$	$C_{18:1\omega7C}$, $C_{18:0}$, $C_{16:0}$	$C_{18:1\omega7C}$, $C_{17:0}$, $C_{16:0}$	$C_{18:1\omega7C}$, $C_{16:0}$, $C_{18:0}$	NA	$C_{18:\omega7C}$, $C_{18:0}$, $C_{17:0}$, $C_{16:0}$, $C_{15:0}$	$C_{18:1\omega7C}$, $C_{18:0}$, $C_{16:0}$, $C_{15:0}$	$C_{18:1\omega7C}$, $C_{16:0}$, $C_{17:0}$, $C_{18:0}$
Bis-p-Nitrophenyl-phosphate	+	v	+	+	NA	NA	+	+	+
L-Arginine-β-naphthylamidase	+	+	+	+	+	NA	+	+	+
Glycine-β-naphthylamidase	+	+	+	+	+	NA	+	+	+
Glycylglycine-β-naphthylamidase	+	+	+	+	NA	NA	+	+	+
L-Leucine-β-naphthylamidase	+	+	+	+	NA	+	+	+	+
L-Lysine-β-naphthylamidase (acidic)	+	−	+	+w	NA	NA	−	+	−
L-Lysine-β-naphthylamidase (basic)	+	+	+	+	NA	NA	+	+	+
DL-Methionine-β-naphthylamidase	+	+	+	+	NA	NA	+	+	+w
L-Proline-β-naphthylamidase	−	+	+	−	+	v	v	+	−
L-Pyrrolidonyl-β-naphthylamidase	−	−	−	−	NA	−	−	−	−
L-Tryptophan-β-naphthylamidasethylamidase	+	+	+	+	NA	NA	+	+	+

[a] Oxidation/fermentation of glucose.

+, positive reaction; −, negative reaction; v, variable reaction; +w, weak positive reaction; NA, data not available matographic analysis of cellular fatty acids (see Table 9-14).[1361] All *Bartonella* species contain greater than 50% $C_{18:1}$ isoacids, 16–25% $C_{18:0}$, and 16–22% $C_{16:0}$, with minor amounts of $C_{13:1}$ and $C_{17:0}$ fatty acids. *B. henselae* isolates lack cellular fatty acids $C_{15:0}$ and $C_{12:0}$, which are present in isolates of *B. vinsonii* and *B. bacilliformis*, respectively. *B. quintana* could be differentiated from most *B. henselae* isolates by the presence of less than 20% $C_{18:0}$ in *B. quintana* and greater than 20% $C_{18:0}$ in *B. henselae*. The cellular fatty acid composition of *B. elizabethae* is most similar to that of *B. vinsonii* and includes $C_{15:0}$ (not found in *B. henselae* or *B. quintana*) and larger amounts (21%) of $C_{17:0}$ than *B. henselae* (3%), *B. quintana* (1%), and *B. vinsonii* (9%). *B. elizabethae* also contains smaller amounts of cellular fatty acid $C_{16:0}$ (13%) than the other species, which contain from 17% to 20% $C_{16:0}$ cellular fatty acids.[299]

Definitive identification of *Bartonella* species is best accomplished by amplification-based molecular methods. PCR amplification of various genes (e.g., citrate synthase, heat-shock proteins, riboflavin synthesis genes, cell division genes) or 16S–23S rRNA intergenic spacer regions and restriction endonuclease analysis of the amplicons have been used successfully for this purpose.[69,641,823,1431] Matar and colleagues used PCR along with primers in the 16S rRNA and 23S rRNA genes to amplify the spacer region between the 16S rRNA gene and a part of the 23S rRNA gene, followed by *Alu*I and *Hae*III restriction-enzyme cleavage.[830] This approach resulted in characteristic restriction profiles for *B. bacilliformis*, *B. vinsonii*, and *B. quintana*, and two profiles for *B. henselae*, suggesting that this method may be useful both for identifying *Bartonella* species and for subtyping isolates of *B. henselae*. Amplification of part of the citrate synthase gene (*gltA*) followed by restriction-enzyme digestion and analysis has been used to identify both *Bartonella* and *Rickettsia* species belonging to the typhus and spotted fever groups.[641,946,1057] Using this method, Joblet and colleagues found that *gltA* gene amplification followed by digestion with *Taq*I and *Aci*I restriction enzymes allowed differentiation of the various *Bartonella* species.[641] Birtles and Raoult determined the sequence of a 940-bp fragment of the citrate synthase-encoding gene (*gtlA*) and found that these sequences were also helpful for constructing phylogenetic trees for determining relationships between validly described *Bartonella* species and uncharacterized *Bartonella* strains.[137] Similar phylogenetic analyses have been delineated by sequence analysis of the 60-kDa heat-shock protein gene, *groEL*.[823] Primer oligonucleotides were also designed based on localized sequence differences within the *ribC* DNA region (riboflavin synthesis genes). These sequences were then used to develop species-specific PCR assays for identification of *B. henselae*, *B. quintana*, *B. bacilliformis*, and *B. clarridgeiae*.[112] Jensen and associates developed an identification method that used PCR to amplify the 16S–23S rRNA intergenic spacer region.[637] This procedure resulted in products of unique size for each *Bartonella* species, thereby allowing species differentiation without the need for restriction-fragment-length polymorphism (RFLP) analysis or sequencing of amplicons. Rodriguez-Barradas and coworkers developed a similar "repetitive element" PCR identification method using primers derived from either repetitive extragenic or intergenic consensus sequences.[1080] Because

these sequences already exist in multiple, discontinuous copies that resulted in multiple discontinuous amplicons following amplification, subsequent treatment with restriction endonucleases prior to PAGE was not necessary. Using DNA extracted from cultured organisms, this method could identify different *Bartonella* species and could also be used for subtyping *B. henselae* strains.[1080] Handley and Regnery at the CDC reported a PCR-dependent identification method based on amplification of restriction-endonuclease-cleaved segments.[535] The enzymes used in this procedure resulted in large fragments that could be annealed with primers corresponding to base sequences adjacent to endonuclease restriction sites for subsequent PCR and resolution by PAGE. Several PCR-based identification methods have also been described that exploit species-specific base sequence variations in the 16S rDNA operon.[135,302,837,956,1065,1124]

In addition to culture confirmation, molecular approaches have been developed for direct detection of *Bartonella* species in clinical specimens. Matar and colleagues reported a PCR-RFLP method for simultaneous detection and identification of bartonellae directly in clinical specimens, including lymph node biopsies and aspirates, skin, subcutaneous nodules and other tissues.[829] This method involved the use of PCR primers from conserved regions of the 16S rDNA gene, followed by *Dde*I and *Mse*I restriction-endonuclease digestion and analysis of the amplicons. Sander and Penno used PCR to generate biotinylated amplicons of the 16S rRNA gene region and immobilized the amplicons in streptavidin-coated microtiter wells. Hybridization of these amplicons with species-specific digoxigenin-labeled 16S rDNA oligonucleotide probes and subsequent addition of antidigoxigenin peroxidase in a modified EIA format provided rapid identification of both *B. henselae* and *B. quintana*.[1124] This method could both detect and quantify both species directly in clinical specimens in concentrations as low as 10^3 cfu/mL. Avidor and colleagues evaluated PCR-mediated 16S rRNA gene amplification followed by *B. henselae* probe hybridization with PCR-based amplification of either *gltA* (citrate synthase) or *htrA* (heat-shock protein genes) followed by RFLP analysis of amplicons for direct detection of *B. henselae* in clinical specimens.[69] *B. henselae* DNA was detected in 100% of 32 pus and lymph node specimens by the 16S rRNA PCR/probe identification method, and in 94% and 69% by the *gltA*/RFLP and *htrA*/RFLP methods, respectively. These investigators suggested that direct testing by *gltA*/RFLP was preferable and easier since species-specific hybridization (via probe) was not necessary with this method.[69]

Serologic Diagnosis of *Bartonella* Infections

Because *Bartonella* species are difficult to grow in culture, serologic methods have been used to document infection with these organisms. Regnery and colleagues at the CDC developed an indirect immunofluorescence assay for *B. henselae* and found that 88% of patients with CSD had anti–*B. henselae* titers of 64 or greater.[1059] In 1995, Dalton and colleagues, also at the CDC, cocultured *B. henselae*, *B. quintana*, and *B. elizabethae* in Vero cell monolayers and used these organism to prepare slides for IFA testing.[298] Of 91 patients whose illness met a strict clinical definition of

CSD, 95% had IFA titers of 64 or greater to either *B. henselae* or *B. quintana*. Because *B. quintana* had not been associated with CSD, it was believed that positive titers against *B. quintana* represented serologic cross-reactions between the two species. Cross-reactions between *B. elizabethae* and the other two *Bartonella* species were observed only with specimens having extremely high titers against *B. henselae* or *B. quintana*. Vero cell–cocultivated *B. bacilliformis* organisms were also used to develop an IFA procedure for diagnosis of bartonellosis in endemic regions of South America. The IFA was found to be 82% sensitive in detecting antibodies in acute-phase sera of 106 patients with slide-positive (i.e., organisms observed in erythrocytes on a Giemsa-stained thin smear), PCR-positive, or culture-confirmed bartonellosis.[216] Based on the high point prevalence of 45% observed before and during the study period, the IFA test had a positive predictive value of 89%.

Bergmans and others in the Netherlands evaluated the detection of anti–*B. henselae* IgM and IgG using both IFA and EIA as tools for diagnosis of CSD and found significant variability depending on the source of the bacterial antigens for preparation of the IFA slides.[117] In this study, sera from 21 patients with ''possible CSD'' (patients fulfilling only one of four clinical criteria for CSD) and 22 with ''probable'' CSD (patients fulfilling two of four clinical criteria) were examined. When *B. henselae* cells cocultivated in Vero cells were used as the IFA antigen, the sensitivity of IgG detection was only 31.8% for sera from patients with ''probable CSD'' and 33.3% for patients with ''possible CSD.'' When *B. henselae* grown on agar media was used as the IFA antigen, the corresponding sensitivities of the assay for the two patient groups were 40.9% and 14.3%, respectively. Sensitivities of less than 50% were also seen for IgM determinations made by IFA in both groups of patients, regardless of whether agar-grown or cocultivated *B. henselae* organisms were used as the antigen. Specificities of both the IgG and IgM assays were assessed using sera from healthy blood donors and ranged from 95% to 100%. These investigators concluded that more work was needed before IFA could be reliably used as a method for serodiagnosis of CSD. In their report of *B. quintana* endocarditis in three homeless men, Drancourt and associates found that all three had high IgG titers against *B. quintana* by a microimmunofluorescence technique.[354] Titers were higher when the *B. quintana* cells used for the procedure were cocultivated in the ECV endothelial cell line (titers of 6,400–12,800) than when the cells were from cultures grown on 5% sheep blood agar (titers of 400–800).

IFA slides prepared with either blood agar–derived or cell-associated *B. henselae* as the antigen are available commercially and have been evaluated. Zbinden and associates studied two commercial IFA kits that use blood agar-derived organisms (MRL-BA, MRL Diagnostics, Cypress, CA; Virion Institut, Virion, Switzerland) and cell-associated organisms (MRL Vero/*Bartonella* IgG Substrate slides, MRL Diagnostics; Bion *B. henselae* slides, Bios, Germany).[1429] These commercial slides were compared with their in-house IFA that used Vero cell–cocultivated *B. henselae* as the antigen. In general, kits that used agar-grown *B. henselae* antigen showed higher titers (less specificity) than kits using cell-associated organisms. The MRL-Vero *B. henselae* kit

alone was then compared with the in-house system. Using a cut-off titer of 256 and sera from 26 patients with CSD and 240 controls, the MRL-Vero IFA kit showed a sensitivity of 84.5% and a specificity of 93.4%.[1429] Similar results were found in a second evaluation of the MRL IFA test.[836]

EIA has also been evaluated as a serologic method for diagnosis of CSD. Barka and colleagues at Specialty Laboratories (Santa Monica, CA) developed an EIA for detection of specific IgG, IgM, and IgA using *B. henselae* cells grown on agar as the solid-phase antigen.[92] Of serum specimens from 40 confirmed cases of CSD (by clinical history, culture, and/or histopathology), 38 (95%) had elevated levels of antibodies against *B. henselae*. Although none of the 40 patients with CSD in this study had *B. henselae*–specific IgM or IgA in the absence of IgG, the authors stated that they had observed *B. henselae*–specific IgM as the only marker in some patients and had also seen IgG seroconversion in the presence of IgM occur over a 2- to 3-week period.[92] Positive EIA results were not observed in any of 92 specimens from patients with documented high antibody titers for other agents, including *Afipia felis*, *Rickettsia typhi*, *Rickettsia rickettsii*, *Borrelia burgdorferi*, *Yersinia pestis*, *Chlamydia trachomatis*, rubella virus, and cytomegalovirus.

Several factors have an impact on the ability of serologic testing to provide a diagnosis of *Bartonella* infections, not all of which are clear at present. In HIV-infected patients with manifestations of *Bartonella* infection, a significant antibody response may not be observed because of HIV-related immunosuppression. Failure to mount an antibody response has also been observed in immunocompetent patients, as evidenced by the absence of an antibody response in a host with chronic lymphadenopathy and positive blood cultures for *B. quintana*.[1049] Failure to detect antibodies may also be due to antigenic heterogeneity of the organisms themselves. Antigenically different strains of *B. henselae* have been recovered from patients with endocarditis and from cats; these strains were not only serologically different, but were also noted to be different by protein profiles and 16S rDNA sequences.[118,353] Recently, Sander and colleagues investigated the antigenicity of the flagellin (FlaA) of *B. clarridgeiae*, the only *Bartonella* species that possesses flagella.[1126] Antibodies to FlaA were detected in 3.9% of 724 serum samples from patients with CSD and/or lymphadenopathy and in none of 100 serum samples from healthy controls. With the recognition of *B. clarridgeiae* as a possible agent of CSD, detection of antibodies against FlaA may prove useful for the diagnosis of CSD caused by this species. Using recombinant DNA technology, a 17-kDa protein has been isolated from *B. henselae* that is specifically reactive with sera from patients with CSD and may have value as a diagnostic serologic reagent.[33] A *B. henselae*–specific proliferative cellular immune response can also be demonstrated on stimulation of lymphocytes from patients with CSD who have *B. henselae* antigens.[60] This assay may be useful for diagnosis of cases in which serologic results are equivocal.

Serologic cross-reactions have also been noted between *Bartonella* species and other organisms, including *Coxiella burnetii* (the causative agent of Q fever) and *Chlamydia* species.[354,754,832] In patients with *B. quintana* endocarditis, titers of greater than 256 were observed against *C. pneumoniae* and titers of 64 were observed against both *C. psittaci* and *C.*

trachomatis.[354] Although absorption of the serum specimens with *C. pneumoniae* did not reduce the titers against *B. quintana,* absorption with *B. quintana* successfully quenched reactivity with *C. pneumoniae.* In another study, more than 50% of patients with chronic Q fever had significant antibody titers to *B. henselae.* Cross-absorption and immunoblot studies established that reactivity with *B. henselae* resulted from cross-reactions with *C. burnetii* antibodies; absorption of serum with *C. burnetii* removed reactivity with *B. henselae* antigen, while adsorption with *B. henselae* only removed the reactivity against *B. henselae.*[754] Absorption of sera with *C. pneumoniae* or *B. quintana* removed anti-*C. pneumoniae* antibodies, while adsorption with *C. pneumoniae* did not change titers against *B. quintana.*[832] In the case of *Bartonella* endocarditis, specific titers may be high, with the titers against these other agents being significantly lower, suggesting that misdiagnoses should not occur provided that antibodies against all of these agents are sought simultaneously. As mentioned above, serum with high anti–*B. henselae* titers may also cross-react with other *Bartonella* species as well.

Seroprevalence studies for *Bartonella* species have been performed in several human populations. In a study conducted in Sweden, Holmberg et al. examined 126 human serum samples that had been submitted for *Bartonella* serology and 100 serum specimens from healthy blood donors (controls) using an IFA method (positive titer of ≥64).[587] Among these specimens, 4% of the 100 controls and 8.3% of the 126 patient specimens were positive. Among the donor specimens, three were positive for *B. elizabethae* antibodies, and one was positive for both *B. henselae* and *B. elizabethae.* In the patient group, 14 specimens from 9 patients were reactive; three patients showed fourfold increases in titer on sequential specimens. These three patients had evidence of *Bartonella*-associated disease (e.g., relapsing, suppurative lymphadenopathy; visceral lesions showing chronic granulomatous inflammation) and had histories of exposure to cats and rodents. All sera also demonstrated weak positive IFA reactions for *Chlamydia pneumoniae;* this probably reflects the cross-reactivity described above. Noah et al. performed IFA tests for *Bartonella* species on sera collected from 351 veterinarians attending a veterinary conference in Ohio.[942] Among these 351, 7.1% had a positive titer for *B. henselae* or *B. quintana.*

Commercially available kits for serodiagnosis of *Bartonella* infection are available from several vendors (see above). Some serologic tests may also be able to distinguish antibodies directed against different *Bartonella* species (i.e., *B. henselae* and *B. quintana*).[1125,1184] IFA serology for *Bartonella* species is available from commercial laboratories, including Associated Regional University Pathologists (ARUP, Salt Lake City UT), Specialty Laboratories (Santa Monica, CA), and Microbiology Reference Laboratory (MRL Diagnostics)

In Vitro Antimicrobial Susceptibility

Using an agar dilution method, Maurin and Raoult tested the in vitro susceptibility of *B. henselae,* *B. quintana,* and *B. vinsonii* to a variety of antimicrobial agents.[835] These organisms were susceptible to ampicillin, third-genera-tion cephalosporins (i.e., cefotaxime, ceftriaxone), tetracyclines (i.e., doxycycline, minocycline), macrolides, rifampin, trimethoprim-sulfamethoxazole, and aminoglycosides (i.e., gentamicin, amikacin). MICs for oxacillin, cephalothin, clindamycin, chloramphenicol, and the fluoroquinolones (i.e., ciprofloxacin, perfloxacin, ofloxacin) were near the maximum concentrations of drug available in the serum. A subsequent study by the same research group used an agar dilution procedure with blood-supplemented Columbia agar to determine the in vitro susceptibilities of nine *B. quintana,* three *B. henselae,* and single isolates of *B. elizabethae* and *B. bacilliformis.*[833] Plates were incubated for 5 days at 37°C in a 5% CO_2 atmosphere before interpretation. All of the strains tested were susceptible to β-lactams (i.e., penicillin G, amoxicillin, ticarcillin, cefotetan, cefotaxime, ceftazidime, ceftriaxone, imipenem), macrolides (i.e., erythromycin, azithromycin, clarithromycin, roxithromycin), doxycycline, aminoglycosides (i.e., gentamicin, tobramycin, amikacin), and rifampin. Strains appeared less susceptible to the semisynthetic penicillins (i.e., oxacillin), first-generation cephalosporins (i.e., cephalothin), and clindamycin. Susceptibilities of these 14 isolates to the fluoroquinolones (i.e., perfloxacin, ciprofloxacin, and sparfloxacin) were variable. Sobraques and colleagues tested four strains of *B. bacilliformis* using an agar dilution procedures and found that all strains were broadly susceptible to antimicrobial agents, including β-lactams, aminoglycosides, chloramphenicol, rifampin, macrolides, tetracyclines, and fluoroquinolones.[1198]

Other in vitro susceptibility studies on *Bartonella* species have focused on the ability of antimicrobial agents to inhibit growth of the organisms in a cell culture environment. Ives et al. studied the susceptibility of *Bartonella* species to several macrolide antimicrobial agents using a Vero cell monolayer cocultivation method.[621,622] Organism inhibition by different concentrations of antimicrobial agents was assessed by visual enumeration of organisms as determined by specific immunofluorescence in comparison with cultures without antibiotics after 5 days of incubation. Using this method, individual isolates of *B. henselae,* *B. quintana* and *B. elizabethae* were susceptible to erythromycin, clarithromycin, azithromycin, dirithromycin and roxithromycin.[621,622] These workers also pointed out that both erythromycin and doxycycline are concentrated in phagocytic cells, reaching levels that exceed the achievable serum concentrations. Although the growth of organisms phagocytized by neutrophils and macrophages would likely be inhibited because of the high drug levels attained in these cells, different species or strains of *Bartonella* may behave differently within endothelial cells or other types of cells. Kordick et al. found that all strains of *B. henselae* and *B. clarridgeiae* recovered from naturally and experimentally infected bacteremic cats were susceptible to doxycycline, enrofloxacin, and ciprofloxacin.[718] However, successful treatment (defined by failure to detect bacteremia by culture or by PCR) occurred in only 9 of 14 cats who received enrofloxacin and in 2 of 8 cats who were treated with doxycycline. These workers concluded that standard agar dilution susceptibility tests on *Bartonella* species do not provide any clear-cut information on the therapeutic efficacy of the agents, since there is very little information on the cellular tropisms of *B. henselae* and *B. clarridgeiae* in cats. Kordick et al. postulated that feline cells infected with *Bartonella* may be functionally impaired to the extent that antimicrobials are not taken up or are compartmentalized away from the organisms themselves.[718]

The bactericidal activities of these agents against *B. henselae* have also been examined with Schaedler medium supplemented with blood, hemin, and vitamin K and with cocultivation techniques using either a human endothelial cell line or a murine macrophage cell line.[917] Amoxicillin, cefotaxime, ceftriaxone, doxycycline, erythromycin, rifampin and ciprofloxacin were shown to be bacteriostatic for *Bartonella* species, but only the aminoglycosides (gentamicin, tobramycin, and amikacin) were bactericidal.[917]

Afipia Species
Taxonomy and Clinical Significance

Organisms subsequently assigned to the genus *Afipia* were first isolated from lymph node aspirates of patients with CSD using a cell culture method.[380] Subsequently, Brenner and colleagues proposed that these organisms were the likely causative agent of CSD and named the type strain *Afipia felis*, after the Armed Forces Institute of Pathology, where the organism was originally isolated.[166] A second, similar organism was recovered from a tibial biopsy of a 69-year-old male at the Cleveland Clinic, and a third isolate was subsequently recovered from sputum, bone marrow, and a wrist abscess. The latter two isolates were assigned to the genus *Afipia* as *A. clevelandensis*, and *A. broomeae*, respectively.[166] Three unnamed *Afipia* genospecies—Afipia genospecies 1, 2, and 3—were also described at that time. These were isolated from a human pleural fluid specimen, a human bronchial wash specimen, and water, respectively.[166] With the discovery of *B. henselae* as the primary agent of CSD and the isolation of *A. felis* from the water supply of a French hospital in 1999, *Afipia* species are now believed to be fastidious, water-associated bacteria that are capable of intracellular existence in free-living amoebae.[750,756] In 2002, three additional isolates christened *A. birgiae*, *A. massiliensis*, and *Afipia felis* genospecies A were isolated from the water supply of Timone Hospital Centre in Marseilles, France.[752] In this milieu, these organisms may play a role in nosocomial infections, as indicated by the isolation of these organisms from water samples collected in intensive care units and by the presence of specific antibodies to these organisms in 11 of 85 patients in intensive care units who had nosocomial pneumonia.[753] *Afipia* species are classified in the α_2 subgroup of the Proteobacteria within the family *Bradyrhizobiaceae*.[455,752,1376]

Isolation and Identification

Afipia species are gram-negative, oxidase-positive, weakly catalase-positive bacilli that are motile because they possess a single polar, subpolar, or lateral flagellum. The organisms grow on buffered charcoal-yeast extract (BCYE) agar, on chocolate and blood agar, and in nutrient broth, but do not grow in the presence of 6.5% NaCl in broth and rarely grow on MacConkey agar. Good growth is obtained after incubation at 25 to 30°C for 3–4 days. Scant growth is obtained after incubation at 35°C and no growth is observed

at 42°C. After 72 hours of growth on blood agar, colonies of *Afipia* species are gray-white, glistening, nonhemolytic, convex, and opaque with an entire edge. All species and genospecies are oxidase- and urease-positive and are negative in reactions for hemolysis, gas production from nitrate, indole production, H_2S production (triple sugar ion agar [TSI] method), gelatin hydrolysis, and esculin hydrolysis. Acid is not produced oxidatively or fermentatively from glucose, lactose, sucrose, or maltose. Characteristics for identification of *Afipia* species are shown in Table 9-15.

Afipia species can also be identified by cell-wall fatty acid analysis. Members of the genus contain *cis*-octadec-11-enoic ($C_{18:1\omega7C}$), 11-methyloctadec-12-enoic ($C_{Br19:1}$), and usually 9,10-methylenehexadecanoate and 11,12-methyleneoctadecanoate. The presence of $C_{Br19:1}$ as a major cell-wall fatty acid is a key characteristic of *Afipia* species, because this fatty acid is found in only trace quantities in some *Pseudomonas* and *Brucella* species.[166,752]

Antimicrobial Susceptibility

A. felis is resistant to ampicillin, cefazolin, cefamandole, cefoperazone, cephalothin, clindamycin, erythromycin, penicillin, tetracycline, and ciprofloxacin.[166,834] Intermediate susceptibility to piperacillin, sulfamethoxazole-trimethoprim, ticarcillin, and vancomycin has been reported.[166,834] *A. felis* is susceptible to cefoxitin, cefotaxime, mezlocillin, the aminoglycosides, imipenem, and rifampin. Although *Afipia* genospecies 3 has the lowest MICs among the species, all others species showed higher MICs to most agents, including the cephalosporins (all generations), ampicillin, extended-spectrum penicillins, β-lactam/β-lactamase inhibitor combinations, tetracyclines, and the aminoglycosides. Imipenem showed the lowest MICs for all tested species.[166,834]

Bordetella Species
Background and Taxonomy of *Bordetella* Species

The genus *Bordetella* contains seven species: *B. pertussis*, *B. parapertussis*, *B. bronchiseptica*, *B. avium*, *B. hinzii*, *B. holmesii*, and *B. trematum*.[681,1015,1303,1304,1369] Genetic studies have shown that these organisms are very closely related to each other. In fact, DNA hybridization techniques indicate that these organisms may not be sufficiently different from one another to justify the assignment of individual species, although definite genetic, phenotypic, and immunologic differences exist among them.[682] In the past, the bordetellae have been classified with other bacterial species, including *Haemophilus*, *Brucella*, and *Alcaligenes*. In the 1984 edition of *Bergey's Manual of Determinative Bacteriology*, both *Bordetella* and *Brucella* species were included among the genera of uncertain affiliation.[1015] After extensive DNA-rRNA hybridization and phenotypic analyses, De Ley and coworkers proposed the family *Alcaligenaceae* to include *Alcaligenes* and *Bordetella* species.[314] The genetic relatedness of *Bordetella* species to the genus *Alcaligenes* is also supported by the finding that *B. pertussis* and *B. bronchiseptica* both produce a siderophore called **alcaligin** that is almost identical to that produced by *Alcaligenes denitrificans*.[891] Members of the genus *Bordetella* are small, gram-

Table 9-15 Biochemical Characteristics for Identification of *Afipia* Species

CHARACTERISTIC	A. FELIS	A. FELIS GENOSPECIES A	A. CLEVELANDENSIS	A. BROOMEAE	A. BIRGIAE	A. MASSILIENSIS	AFIPIA GENOSPECIES 1	AFIPIA GENOSPECIES 2	AFIPIA GENOSPECIES 3	AFIPIA GENOSPECIES 3-RELATED
Hemolysis, SBA	−	−	−	−	−	−	−	−	−	−
Oxidase	+	+	+	+	+	+	+	+	+	+
Catalase	$+^w$	$+^w$	$+^w$	$+^w$	$+^w$	$+^w$	$+^w$	$+^w$	$+^w$	$+^w$
Motility	+	+	+	−	−	+	+	+	+	+
Growth on BCYE agar, 30°C	+	+	+	+	+	+	+	+	+	+
Growth on BCYE agar, 35°C	+	+	$+^w$	+	−	−	+	+	+	−
Growth on BCYE agar, 37°C	+	+	−	+	+	−	+	+	+	−
Growth on BCYE agar, 42°C	−	−	−	−	−	−	−	−	−	−
Nitrate reduction	+	+	−	−	+	+	−	−	−	+
Citrate	−	−	−	−	−	−	+	−	−	+
Urease	+	+	+	+	−	+	+	+	+	+
Esculin hydrolysis	−	−	−	−	−	−	−	−	−	−
Arginine dihydrolase	−	−	−	−	−	−	−	−	−	−
ONPG hydrolysis	−	−	−	−	−	−	−	−	−	−
H₂S production	−	−	−	−	−	−	−	−	−	−
Acid production from:										
Glucose	−	−	−	−	−	−	+	+	−	−
Maltose	−	−	−	−	−	−	−	−	−	−
Fructose	−	−	−	−	−	−	−	−	−	−
Sucrose	−	−	−	−	−	−	−	−	−	−
Mannitol	−	−	−	−	−	−	+	+	−	−
Mannose	−	−	−	−	−	−	+	+	−	−
Arabinose	−	−	−	−	−	−	+	+	−	−
N-Acetyl-glucosamine	−	−	−	−	−	−	+	+	−	−

+, positive reaction; −, negative reaction; $+^w$, weak positive reaction.

negative coccobacilli on primary isolation. On subculture, they tend to become more pleomorphic. They are obligately aerobic, grow optimally at 35 to 37°C, do not use carbohydrates, and are inactive in most biochemical tests. *B. pertussis*, *B. parapertussis*, and *B. holmesii* are nonmotile, whereas *B. bronchiseptica*, *B. avium*, and *B. hinzii* are motile via peritrichous flagella. These organisms do not require hemin or NAD. However, primary isolation of *B. pertussis*, in particular, requires the addition of charcoal, ion exchange resins, or 15–20% blood to neutralize the growth-inhibiting effects of substances such as unsaturated fatty acids, sulfides, peroxides, and heavy metals.[602] *B. parapertussis* is somewhat less exacting in its growth requirements, but isolation still requires the use of the same special media used for *B. pertussis*. The remaining species are less fastidious and will grow on routinely used agar media, including blood, chocolate, and MacConkey agars. Sequence analyses of 16S rRNA of the described *Bordetella* species has confirmed the common phylogeny with the genus *Alcaligenes*, and the genus *Bordetella* now resides in the β_2 subdivision of the Proteobacteria in the family *Alcaligenaceae* along with the genera *Achromobacter*, *Pelistega*, *Sutterella*, and *Taylorella*.[455]

The genus *Bordetella* includes species isolated from both humans and other animals. Humans are the only recognized host of *B. pertussis*, and *B. parapertussis* was also thought to be found only in humans. In 1994, however, a *B. parapertussis*–like isolate was recovered from the respiratory tracts of both healthy and pneumonic lambs in Scotland and New Zealand.[1020] *B. parapertussis* is capable of causing a pertussis-like illness in humans. *B. bronchiseptica* is found in a variety of animals (e.g., nonhuman primates, dogs, cats, rabbits, horses, turkeys, swine, foxes, opossums) and is occasionally found in humans, primarily as an opportunistic agent. As the name suggests, *B. avium* is found in birds and causes rhinotracheitis in turkeys.[681] *B. hinzii* was formerly called ''*B. avium*–like bacterium,'' turkey coryza bacterium type II, *Alcaligenes faecalis* type II, and *Alcaligenes* species strain C2T2; this organism was formally assigned to the genus *Bordetella* in 1995.[1304] *B. holmesii* was formerly called CDC nonoxidizer group 2 (NO-2). Characterization of these isolates by DNA-DNA hybridization, 16S rRNA sequencing, and cellular fatty acid/ubiquinone analysis established their relationship to genus *Bordetella*.[1369] Since 1995, *Bordetella trematum* has been described as a new species that is found in human wounds and ear infection, and novel ''*Bordetella-holmesii*–like'' strains have been isolated from patients with bacteremia, endocarditis, and respiratory tract infections.[1257,1303,1418]

Epidemiology of Pertussis

Pertussis continues to be an endemic disease of worldwide importance, with over 350,000 deaths attributed to the disease each year. Humans are the only known host of *B. pertussis*, and transmission occurs via direct contact with aerosolized droplets from infected, coughing individuals. The attack rate is very high, with greater than 90% of susceptible individuals becoming infected after significant exposures.[141] For unknown reasons, disease among children occurs more often in females than in males and tends to occur in epidemic cycles of 3 to 5 years Prior to the availability

of the whole-cell killed vaccine, most cases of pertussis occurred among children from 1 to 5 years of age. After 1947, when the diphtheria-pertussis-tetanus (DPT) vaccine was licensed and recommended by the American Academy of Pediatrics, the highest incidence of disease shifted to children less than 1 year old. In the U.S. during the early 1990s, between 40% and 50% of reported pertussis cases occurred in children who were less than 1 year old.[207,208] Similar incidence rates have been reported in other countries that have maintained vaccination protocols. For example, during the 15-month period from July 1993 through October 1994, 65% of index cases of pertussis in a French medical center occurred in children less than 1 year of age.[93] Currently, those at highest risk for pertussis include infants 6 months of age and less who have not received the full three-dose child vaccination series and undervaccinated preschool-aged children. The greatest amount of pertussis-related mortality also occurs primarily among infants; surveillance data collected from 1992 through 1993 showed that infants less than 1 year of age accounted for 42% of the reported cases and 87% of the reported deaths.[141,208] In countries where vaccination is not commonly practiced, the 1-to-5 year age group remains at highest risk.

In 1993, over 6,300 pertussis cases were reported to the CDC, representing an 82% increase over cases reported the previous year and the highest incidence of disease since 1967.[98] The principal factor contributing to the resurgence in pertussis is the growth of a large population of susceptible adults; this resurgence is reflected in the increasing numbers of pertussis cases occurring in patients who are greater than 10 years old.[98] Because of the atypical presentation of pertussis in older individuals, the disease is often unrecognized and treatment is either not given or is delayed or incomplete. These infected individuals, however, are an important source for transmission of *B. pertussis* to others, especially to infants and young children who are not adequately immunized.

Clinical Significance of *Bordetella pertussis*

B. pertussis causes the syndrome called pertussis or ''whooping cough.'' The organism is acquired via droplet infection and is highly contagious, with an attack rate of greater than 90% in nonimmunized individuals. Partial immunization of children against pertussis may alter the classical clinical presentation. Furthermore, the presentation and diagnosis of pertussis in young children (i.e., less than 1 year old) may be complicated by concomitant viral respiratory tract infections, including influenza and respiratory syncytial viruses in particular.[900] Classically, clinical pertussis in unvaccinated children can be divided into three stages. The **prodromal** or **catarrhal stage** begins 5 to 10 days after acquisition of the organism and is characterized by nonspecific ''cold'' or ''flu'' symptoms. The disease is highly communicable at this stage since large numbers of organisms are present in the upper respiratory tract. Cultures collected at this time have the greatest likelihood of being positive. A cough appears late in this stage and increases in persistence, severity, and frequency. This evolves into the **paroxysmal** or **spasmodic stage** after 7 to 14 days.[236] This stage is characterized by the ''staccato cough'' with the prolonged inspiratory ''whoop'' heard at the end of the coughing spell.

During this stage, there is no fever or other systemic signs and symptoms. Inspiratory efforts are futile during the coughing paroxysm, and the "whoop" is caused by the inspiration of air through the swollen and narrowed glottis. The coughing spell is frequently accompanied by cyanosis and vomiting. This stage may be so severe that intermittent ventilatory assistance may be required. Complications that may occur during the course of the disease include secondary bacterial infections, otitis media, CNS symptoms such as convulsions and high fever, particularly with the presence of intervening secondary infections, encephalopathy, cerebellar ataxia, inguinal hernia, and rectal prolapse associated with the severe coughing.[447,1160] The cause of encephalopathy associated with complicated pertussis is not known because of the unavailability of a suitable animal model, but suggested mechanisms include anoxia secondary to the coughing paroxysms, hypoglycemia secondary to the toxic effects of pertussis toxin (PT), and intracerebral hemorrhage. The **convalescent stage** generally begins within 4 weeks of onset and, during this time, there is a decrease in the frequency and severity of the coughing spells. (See Box 9-11.)

Atypical pertussis seen in adults is attributed to the fact that most adults were immunized as children and that waning immunologic recall results in a modified, less severe illness.[1401] As mentioned previously, adults with symptomatic but unrecognized pertussis are often the source of the organism for pediatric cases.[134,236,972] Studies of pertussis in adults have focused on individuals with persistent cough and have used culture/molecular and serologic methods to demonstrate the presence of the organisms or significant titer increases against unique antigens of *B. pertussis*, respectively. In a study of 130 university students reporting to the student health service with a cough of 6 days' duration or greater, 26% were found to have serologic evidence of recent *B. pertussis* infection.[871] A subsequent study with this student population found that 15% of 319 students with cough of ≥5 days' duration had serologic evidence of *B. pertussis* infection; 17 of these individuals also had serologic evidence of coexisting viral, *Chlamydia pneumoniae*, or *Mycoplasma pneumoniae* infections.[623] A study conducted among U.S. Marine Corps trainees who reported 7 or more days of cough found that 17% had acute *B. pertussis* infection.[632] In another study, 51 health care workers were evaluated annually over a 5-year period (1984–1989) for rises in antibody titers to four pertussis-specific antigens (PT, FHA, pertactin, and fimbriae).[327] Of these individuals, 90% had a significant increase in antibody titer to one or more of the antigens between two consecutive years during the 5-year period of the study. In a study performed with 246 German adults with a coughing illness of greater than 14 days' duration, evidence of *B. pertussis* infection was found in 64 (26%); 5 had positive nasopharyngeal cultures and 59 were diagnosed on the basis of serologic testing and/or PCR.[1148] A Danish study conducted with 201 patients with coughs persisting for a mean of 6.5 weeks found that 4 patients (2%) were culture-positive for *B. pertussis* and 11 (5.5%) were positive by PCR (including the 4 culture-positive patients).[134] Serologic evidence of pertussis infection was also demonstrated in 100 adults aged ≥65 years who were studied over a 3-year period. Between 3.3% and 8% of this population had pertussis infec-

tions each year, and between 37.5% and 50% were symptomatic as a result of the infection.[578]

The clinical spectrum of pertussis in adults has been described in several studies. In a study performed at UCLA, the two principal clinical diagnoses entertained for individuals found to have pertussis were nonspecific upper respiratory tract infection (39%) and bronchitis (48%).[871] In a study conducted in Germany on 64 adults with documented *B. pertussis* infection, only 39% were thought to have pertussis and 14% were thought not to have pertussis clinically; other diagnoses included upper respiratory tract infections, nasopharyngitis, pharyngitis, adenoiditis, and sinusitis. However, of the 64 patients, 70% had a paroxysmal cough, 38% had an inspiratory whoop, and 17% experienced posttussive vomiting.[1148] Another German study of 84 adults with pertussis found persistent (>21 days) cough in 81%, spasmodic coughing in 65%, and choking in 56%.[1023] Eighteen patients had complications, including otitis media, pneumonia, urinary incontinence, cervical lymphadenopathy, acute hearing loss, rib fractures, and inguinal hernia. Pertussis-associated encephalopathy has also been documented in adult pertussis.[530] Although uncommon, acute *B. pertussis* infections in adults has been described; in one case, acute pertussis was diagnosed in a 53-year-old male who acquired the organism from his son, who had been immunized and had a mild case of whooping cough.[1193]

B. pertussis has also been isolated from adults with underlying disease such as HIV infection. Ng and coworkers isolated *B. pertussis* from bronchoalveolar lavage and transbronchial biopsy specimens of three patients with AIDS.[936,937] These organisms were recovered on media for isolation of *Legionella*. Doebbeling et al. reported the isolation of *B. pertussis* from the upper respiratory tract of a 25-year-old HIV-positive patient with a 4-month history of paroxysmal cough; a similar case was also reported in a 60-year-old patient with AIDS in Belgium.[269,340] Despite these case reports, pertussis is believed to be relatively rare in HIV-infected individuals, with an estimated prevalence of nasopharyngeal carriage of less than 6.5 cases per 10,000 patients.[266] In a very unusual case, *B. pertussis* was isolated from a blood culture of a 31-year-old man with Wegener's granulomatosis, a condition associated with chronic pneumonia and the development of pulmonary nodules and cavitary lung lesions.[630] Pertussis has also been recovered from the respiratory tracts of infants with other underlying problems, such as necrotizing enterocolitis, chronic lung disease and adenoviral pneumonia.[493,1161]

Pertussis Vaccines

The original whole-cell pertussis vaccine was administered along with diphtheria and tetanus toxoids and aluminum-coated adjuvants (DwPT). After licensure, widespread use of whole-cell vaccine resulted in declines in pertussis in countries with mandatory immunization, and additional evidence of efficacy accrued as a result of diminished immunization programs in some countries. For example, an upswing in reported pertussis in Denmark occurred a few years after vaccine preparations that used smaller amounts of antigen were introduced. Diminished public acceptance of immunization in Great Britain beginning in the mid-1970s re-

Box 9-11 Virulence Factors of *Bordetella pertussis*

Pertussis Toxin

Pertussis toxin (PT) is a major virulence factor of *B. pertussis*. PT is a single protein of 105–117 kDa molecular weight that has a wide spectrum of biologic activity and is produced only by *B. pertussis*. PT is synthesized with an N-terminal signal sequence that mediates secretion of toxin into the periplasmic space. In the periplasm, the signal peptide is removed and the subunits fold and assemble into the complete toxin.[289] PT is a hexamer consisting of an enzymatic, toxic moiety (A protomer) and a nontoxic heteropentameric moiety (B oligomer). The B oligomer is responsible for binding of the toxin to susceptible cells and transporting the A protomer across the eucaryotic cell membrane.[289] The B subunit is composed of two dimers—polypeptides S2 and S4 and polypeptides S3 and S4—joined by another polypeptide called S5. PT also functions as an adhesin in its ability to bind to ciliated cells and macrophages. The A subunit contains a single polypeptide, designated S1, that has adenosine diphosphate ribosyltransferase activity.[670] This enzyme transfers ADP-ribose groups from NAD to the Gi (inhibitory) regulatory proteins that normally function in cell signal transduction. The activity of PT is believed to be responsible for many of the clinical signs and symptoms of pertussis, although this has not been unequivocally demonstrated, and there are no data regarding the target or targets affected by PT in tissue. Biologic effects of PT include the sensitization of mice to histamine, the production of lymphocytosis, activation of pancreatic islet cells, and stimulation of immune responses.[564,565] Antibody directed against PT is protective for mice when challenged by either intracerebral or respiratory tract inoculation. The genes for the PT peptides are arranged as an operon; this operon is present in *B. pertussis*, *B. parapertussis*, and *B. bronchiseptica*, but the genes are neither transcribed nor translated in the latter two species.[50,1216] Antibody directed against PT is also protective in animal models of pertussis. PT is the only molecule that is represented in every acellular pertussis vaccine formulated thus far.

Filamentous Hemagglutinin

Filamentous hemagglutinin (FHA) is a cell-surface adhesin of 220-kDa molecular weight that has hemagglutinating activity and, along with PT, mediates adhesion of *B. pertussis* to eukaryotic cells in vitro and to ciliated cells of the upper respiratory tract.[1064,1306] FHA has multiple binding activities that enable *B. pertussis* to adhere to and, in some cases, invade different cell types, including macrophages, at different stages of infection and in concert with other adhesins.[889] Binding of FHA to macrophages leads to phagocytosis of the organisms without the oxidative burst associated with phagocytosis of other microorganisms. This unusual circumstance may be critical for intracellular survival of *B. pertussis*. Antibody against FHA provides some immunity against respiratory but not intracerebral challenge in animals, presumably by inhibiting attachment of the organisms.

Pertactin

Pertactin describes several surface-associated cell-membrane proteins found in three *Bordetella* species. Pertactin P.69 of *B. pertussis* has a molecular weight of 69 kDa, and homologous proteins of slightly different molecular weights are found in *B. parapertussis* (pertactin P.70) and *B. bronchiseptica* (pertactin P.68). Pertactins are encoded and produced as slightly larger proteins that are proteolytically cleaved to yield the mature molecules. *B. pertussis* pertactin was originally called P69 or 69K protein; the true molecular weight has been determined to be about 60.5 kDa after it was found that pertactin was derived from posttranslational processing of a larger precursor protein. The pertactin of *B. pertussis* functions along with FHA to mediate attachment of the bacterium to tissue culture cells by helping the FHA molecule achieve a conformation that maximizes bacterium-cell binding.[49] Antibodies against pertactin P.69 protect mice against infection with *B. pertussis* administered by the aerosol route, but protection against intracerebral challenge requires antibodies against both P.69 and FHA.

Adenylate Cyclase-Hemolysin

B. pertussis produces an adenylate cyclase-hemolysin (AC-H), a bifunctional 177-kDa protein of that is secreted into the medium and possesses both adenylate cyclase and hemolytic activities.[683] The protein is able to bind to susceptible cells and is translocated into the cell intact. Inside the target cell, the molecule is proteolytically cleaved. Activation of the adenylate cyclase activity by the eukaryotic protein calmodulin results in intracellular accumulation of cAMP. This accumulation may suppress expression of the local immune response by inhibiting neutrophil chemotaxis and phagocytosis.[565]

Tracheal Cytotoxin

Tracheal cytotoxin (TCT) is a small molecule of about 921 Da that is composed of a disaccharide tetrapeptide derived from the cell-wall peptidoglycan. The molecule contains glucosamine, muramic acid, alanine, glutamic acid, and diaminopimelic acid in a 1 : 1 : 2 : 1 : 1 ratio and is released into the culture supernatant during the logarithmic growth phase.[279] TCT specifically damages and kills the ciliated epithelial cells lining the airways where the organism attaches and may contribute to the characteristic cough of clinical pertussis. TCT has also been shown to adversely affect polymorphonuclear cell function at low concentrations, and is toxic to these cells at higher concentrations.[293] TCT also elicits interleukin-1 production and induces nitric oxide synthase, which is believed to mediate damage to the respiratory tract epithelium.[555] TCT and other similar muramyl peptides have several other biologic activities, including pyrogenicity and adjuvanticity.

Box 9-11 *Continued*

Heat-Labile Toxin (Dermonecrotizing Toxin)

B. pertussis also produces a heat-labile toxin (HLT, or dermonecrotizing toxin) that is a single polypeptide of about 140 kDa. HLTs produced by *B. pertussis*, *B. parapertussis*, and *B. bronchiseptica* are similar in their biologic properties and are physicochemically and serologically indistinguishable, whereas HLT produced by *B. avium* is slightly different in these respects. HLT induces contraction of blood vessels due to specific constrictive effects on vascular smooth muscle tissue and causes hemorrhagic necrosis in mice and guinea pigs. Although its role in the pathogenesis of pertussis, if any, is not known, constrictive effects of HLT on the highly vascularized tissues of the respiratory tract could lead to local inflammation and may explain some of the respiratory tract pathology associated with pertussis.

Lipooligosaccharide

Like other gram-negative bacteria, *B. pertussis* possesses lipopolysaccharide (LPS, or endotoxin) in its cell-wall outer membrane. Like some other bacterial pathogens, the endotoxin of *B. pertussis* is actually a lipooligosaccharide (LOS). This LOS contains lipid A and an oligosaccharide core with 2-keto-3-deoxyoctulosonic acid, but lacks the long-chain polysaccharide "O" antigens found in LPS molecules. The role of LOS in the pathogenesis of pertussis is not known, although it has the usual properties associated with LOS of many organisms, including pyrogenicity, adjuvanticity, induction of interferon production, and mitogenicity and polyclonal activation of B-cells. *B. pertussis* LOS may be at least partially responsible for the reactogenicity associated with the whole-cell pertussis vaccine.

Heat Labile "O" Agglutinogens

Bordetella species also possess specific antigens termed "O" agglutinogens on the bacterial cell surface. Fourteen heat-labile agglutinogens (AGGs) have been described for *Bordetella* species. These agglutinogens are associated with fimbriae and apparently are also involved in the mediation of attachment to target cells. AGGs 1 through 6 are found in *B. pertussis*; AGG 1 is common to all *B. pertussis* strains, with AGGs 2 through 6 being present in various combinations in different strains.

---

sulted in pertussis reaching epidemic proportions among children less than 5 years of age in the late 1970s. Although experience has suggested clinical efficacies of 80% or greater, wide variations in the performance of different whole-cell vaccine preparations became apparent only during prospective clinical efficacy studies conducted with potential acellular pertussis vaccines. In addition, publicity surrounding reports of encephalopathy and permanent neurologic sequelae that were temporally related to receipt of DwPT vaccine accelerated efforts to develop acellular or "subunit" vaccines. Characterization of subcellular components of *B. pertussis* enabled the manufacture of several acellular vaccines consisting of one or more antigens, and, beginning in the early 1990s, at least seven different acellular vaccine efficacy trials were underway. Acellular pertussis vaccines evaluated in these trials included detoxified PT along with one or more of the other immunogenic components, such as FHA, fimbriae, or pertactin P.69. Efficacies ranging from 71% to 97% were obtained with both the acellular and whole-cell vaccines. In general, one- and two-component acellular vaccine performed less well than vaccines with three to five antigens, and the whole-cell vaccines performed as well as or better than the acellular products, although the acellular vaccines were associated with significantly lower rates of reactogenicity.[365,515,778,965,1012,1147,1261,1288] In 1999 four acellular *B. pertussis* vaccines were licensed for use in the U.S. These include:

1. ACEL-IMMUNE (Wyeth-Lederle Vaccines and Pediatrics): a tetravalent vaccine containing PT, FHA, fimbriae, and pertactin

2. TriPedia (Connaught Laboratories, Inc.): contains PT and FHA

3. Infanrix (SmithKline Beecham Biologicals): contained PT, FHA, and pertactin

4. Certiva (North American Vaccines): contains only PT

At present, both whole-cell and acellular vaccines are administered along with diphtheria and tetanus toxoids as DwPT (with the whole-cell vaccine) or as DaPT (with acellular pertussis vaccines). The immunization schedule consists of three doses of DwPT or DaPT by intramuscular injection at 4- to 8-week intervals, typically at 2 months, 4 months, and 6 months of age, with a fourth dose 6 to 12 months later.[209] A fifth dose is recommended at 4 to 6 years of age. The host immune response following receipt of acellular pertussis vaccines is directed against the defined antigens contained in the individual vaccine, while the response following receipt of the whole-cell vaccine is directed against predominantly outer membrane and fimbrial antigens. In general, studies have demonstrated that multicomponent vaccines containing pertactin and fimbrial antigens in addition to PT and FHA elicit a brisker immune response than vaccines containing only PT and FHA.[209,965] These vaccines also appear to be highly immunogenic when administered along with other childhood immunizations. Halperin and colleagues investigated the immune responses of 180 infants who were immunized with a three-component acellular pertussis vaccine, diphtheria and tetanus toxoids, inactivated poliovirus vaccine, and the *H. influenzae* type b-tetanus toxoid conjugate vaccine. The *H. influenzae* type b vaccine was administered in the same or in a separate syringe from the other vaccines. This study found that all the vaccines, including the *B. pertussis* vaccine, were safe, well-tolerated, and immunogenic regardless of the number of vaccines included in the injection.[529]

Other issues related to the use of pertussis subunit vaccines include efficacy of the vaccines in adults and young infants at risk for pertussis. Although *B. pertussis* is not a significant cause of respiratory illness in most adults, epidemiologic studies have repeatedly implicated infected adults as the source and transmitter of the organism to the child.[235,236,237] In addition, outbreaks of pertussis have occurred among adult caregivers exposed to children with pertussis in day-care situations. Because whole-vaccine reactogenicity may be more severe in adults than in children, acellular component vaccines are also undergoing investigations of their immunogenicity in previously vaccinated or unvaccinated adults. Several studies in adult populations have shown that acellular pertussis vaccines, when given alone or when combined with diphtheria and tetanus toxoid, produce minimal adverse effects and engender brisk antibody responses to PT, FHA, pertactin and fimbrial antigens present in the vaccine with no interference with the immune responses to either tetanus or diphtheria toxoids.[364,675, 972,1101] Guidelines for immunization of adults at risk for pertussis are currently being developed. Pertussis may also be seen in young infants because of suboptimal levels of transplacental antibodies from pertussis-susceptible mothers. A study of an acellular pertussis vaccine in young infants showed that the vaccine did not prevent infection in these children, but did substantially ameliorate the development of severe symptoms.[42]

Because of the relatively recent licensure of the acellular pertussis vaccines, there are few data on the duration of protection afforded by the acellular vaccines. However, the data that have been published indicate that antibody levels following immunization with acellular vaccines remain high for several years. Okada and coworkers examined anti pertussis antibody levels in three groups of children 5 to 7 years after the last inoculation.[964] Children in these four groups included those who had received four doses of DwPT (75 children), three doses of DwPT and a booster with DaPT (90), or four doses of DaPT (131). This study found that antibody titers after vaccination with DaPT were equivalent to or better than those who received DwPT.[964] A 10-year follow-up study of 207 Japanese children who had received either a two-component acellular pertussis vaccine (FHA and PT) or the whole-cell pertussis vaccine found that 77% of the vaccinees still had measurable antibodies, regardless of the type of vaccine they received.[1276]

Before moving on to a discussion of isolation techniques and identification methods for *B. pertussis* and other *Bordetella* species, the pathogenetic capabilities of *B. parapertussis*, *B. bronchiseptica*, *B. hinzii*, *B. holmesii*, and *B. trematum* will be addressed.

Clinical Significance of Other *Bordetella* Species
BORDETELLA PARAPERTUSSIS

B. parapertussis is associated with a pertussis-like illness in humans as well, but it is generally less severe in clinical presentation.[114,595,828] Children with *B. parapertussis* infection had shorter durations of coughing, bronchospasm,

whooping, vomiting, apnea, and cyanosis.[595,828] However, outbreaks of *B. parapertussis* have been reported in which the illness has been quite severe and resulted in death, particularly in very young children. Wirsing von Konig and Finger compared the severity of disease in 33 children with *P. parapertussis* infection to 331 patients with *B. pertussis* infection and found that the frequency of paroxysmal coughing, whooping, and vomiting were almost identical in the two groups.[1385] Heininger and colleagues also compared *B. pertussis* infection in 76 patients with *B. parapertussis* infection in 38 patients matched by age and sex.[553] They also found that the illness caused by *B. parapertussis* was typical of pertussis but much less severe, and that, unlike pertussis, lymphocytosis was not a characteristic of the infection, presumably because of the absence of the lymphocytosis-promoting activity of PT. Decreased pathogenicity in *B. parapertussis* may indeed be due to lack of expression of PT and other virulence factors. Interestingly, when genes coding for certain pertussis virulence factors (e.g., PT and FHA) are transferred into *B. parapertussis* by genetic techniques, the organism becomes capable of producing pertussis-like characteristics in vitro (e.g., anaphylaxis, histamine sensitivity, and leukocytosis), suggesting that the presence of virulence genes and their regulation may be the primary difference between these genetically ''identical'' species.

BORDETELLA BRONCHISEPTICA

B. bronchiseptica causes respiratory tract infections in various animal species (e.g., infectious tracheobronchitis or ''kennel cough'' in dogs, pneumonia in cats, atrophic rhinitis and bronchopneumonia in pigs and piglets, pneumonia, otitis media in rabbits and guinea pigs) and may be isolated as a commensal from the human upper respiratory tract. Humans often acquire the organism from domesticated animals, and nosocomial transmission from patient-to-patient may also occur.[507,1223] *B. bronchiseptica* is an unusual cause of infections primarily in immunocompromised hosts.[1395] Sepsis, meningitis following head trauma, peritonitis, bronchitis, and pneumonia caused by *B. bronchiseptica* have been reported in patients with underlying liver disease, alcoholism, asplenia, hematologic malignancy, chronic renal failure, chronic asthma, systemic lupus erythematosus, and severe hypertension.[193,225,483,1007,1395] Bauwens et al. described a case of bacteremia and pneumonia in 20-year-old female following bone marrow transplantation for acute myelogenous leukemia.[102] Choy and colleagues also described a case of *B. bronchiseptica* pneumonia in a 7-year-old boy 28 days after bone marrow transplantation for an X-linked hyper-IgM syndrome.[248] Reina and colleagues reported a case of pneumonia due to *B. bronchiseptica* in a 37-year-old patient who had sustained serious chest injury in an automobile accident and required intubation.[1060] Infiltrates developed on chest x-ray within 72 hours, and culture of the endotracheal aspirate grew the organism in pure culture. *B. bronchiseptica* may occasionally cause severe infections, such as pneumonia with shock, in immunocompetent patients.[1253] Since 1991, several cases of *B. bronchiseptica* pneumonia have been reported in patients with AIDS.[362,452,861] Rare reports of endocarditis caused by *B. bronchiseptica* have also appeared in the literature. In one such case, the patient presented with fever and a dermatitis around a recent surgical incision. It turned out that the patient's dog frequently nipped and licked the area of dermatitis surrounding the incision, suggesting a canine origin for the organism.[1180] In fact, this organism used to be called *B. bronchicanis* because of its residence in the upper respiratory tract of dogs!

BORDETELLA HINZII

B. hinzii was proposed as a new species in 1995, although the organism had been described informally when it was isolated from sputum and multiple blood cultures collected from a 42-year-old patient with AIDS who had no respiratory tract symptoms.[280,1304] This *B. avium*–like organism has been isolated from the respiratory tract of chickens and turkeys in addition to respiratory tract specimens from humans.[1304] *B. hinzii* strains were isolated on eight occasions over a 3-year period from an adult patient with cystic fibrosis in association with acute exacerbations of his chronic pulmonary disease; the organism could not be eradicated from the patient's respiratory tract despite appropriate chemotherapy.[443] In 2000, fatal *B. hinzii* bacteremia was reported in a 69-year-old man with cholestasis, and *B. hinzii* was isolated along with *Nocardia asteroides* complex organisms from bronchoalveolar lavage fluid of an AIDS patient.[445,671] Although avian exposure of the respiratory tract could be ruled out in the AIDS patient, possible acquisition from avian exposure or gastrointestinal colonization followed by ascending cholangitis were suggested as possible modes of pathogenesis in the bacteremic patient. Another as-yet unnamed ''*B. avium*–like'' isolate was recovered in mixed culture from a patient with chronic otitis media. This isolate was distinct in its antimicrobial resistance pattern, protein and fatty acid composition, and both DNA-DNA and DNA-rRNA hybridizations.[348] *B. avium* has not been isolated from human specimens or infections.

BORDETELLA HOLMESII

B. holmesii, described originally as CDC non-oxidizer group 2 (NO-2), has been isolated from blood cultures of patients with acute febrile illnesses, endocarditis, sickle cell anemia complicated by arthritis, diabetes, prior splenectomies, Hodgkin's disease, and respiratory insufficiency.[1369] Of the 15 cases described in this report, underlying disease was present in seven cases, three occurred in asplenic patients, and one patient had been bitten by a dog. The strains described in this 1995 report had been isolated in Switzerland, Saudi Arabia, and the U.S. In 1996, Lindquist and colleagues isolated *B. holmesii* from multiple blood cultures of a 12-year-old male who presented with fever, headache, and a history significant for splenectomy 4 years earlier.[784] Although the normal habitat of *B. holmesii* is unknown, the patient had frequent and prolonged contact with hunting dogs and had recently suffered a fish-hook injury to his thumb. Tang and others at the Mayo Clinic reported the isolation of *B. holmesii*–like organism from three patients with septicemia, endocarditis, and respiratory failure.[1257] Risk factors in these three patients included underlying asplenia, Hodgkin's disease, and severe cardiomyopathy, respectively. *B. holmesii* was also isolated from a 10-month-old infant who presented to the emergency room with fever

and irritability.[898] Originally diagnosed as having a viral syndrome, *B. holmesii* was recovered from a single aerobic blood culture within 36 hours. Follow-up found the infant to be afebrile and asymptomatic. *B. holmesii* has also been isolated from multiple blood cultures of a 24-year-old male who presented with dry cough and fever and a history remarkable for neonatal-onset sickle cell anemia, hepatitis C, tibial osteomyelitis at 6 years of age, and frequent abdominal crises requiring multiple transfusions until the age of 8 years.[940] Recently, *B. holmesii* strains have been isolated from respiratory tract specimens of patients suspected of having pertussis.[841,1418] Of 10,996 specimens submitted from January 1995 through December 1998 to the Massachusetts State Laboratory Institute in Boston for culture of *Bordetella* species, 32 specimens grew *B. holmesii*, while 740 and 96 specimens were positive for *B. pertussis* and *B. parapertussis*, respectively.[841]

BORDETELLA TREMATUM

B. trematum, another recently described species, has been recovered from human wound specimens and from cases of chronic otitis media.[1303] This species was found to be genetically and chemotaxonomically more closely related to type strain of genus *Bordetella* (*B. pertussis*) than to the type strain of the genus *Alcaligenes* (*A. faecalis*).

Isolation and Identification of *Bordetella* Species
SPECIMENS AND CULTURE MEDIA

Because *B. pertussis* preferentially attaches to the ciliated epithelium in the upper respiratory tract, the specimen of choice is a nasopharyngeal aspirate. Nasopharyngeal aspirates are collected with an infant-size feeding tube connected to a mucus trap. The tip of the feeding tube is threaded into one nostril along the floor of the nasopharynx until it reaches the posterior pharynx. Once the tube is in place, gentle suction is applied. Following aspiration, saline (1 mL) is flushed through the tubing into the trap.[525] For swab specimens, a small-tipped, nasopharyngeal swab is passed posteriorly through each nostril until the swab tip reaches the posterior nasopharynx. Each swab is left in place and gently rotated for 30 seconds to 1 minute so that organisms adsorb onto the swab. Swabs for culture or molecular diagnosis must be composed of Dacron with plastic shafts. Cotton-tipped swabs should not be used because some cotton fibers are inhibitory for cultures. Calcium alginate and aluminum leached from metal swab shafts are also inhibitory for PCR-based assays for *B. pertussis* detection.[1339] Nasopharyngeal swabs collected along with an aspirate may provide the highest yield of positive cultures. Regular throat cultures are not appropriate for isolation of *B. pertussis*. Specimens for bordetellae also require special transport media for optimal organism recovery. Regan-Lowe transport medium may be used for aspirates and swab specimens and has the advantage of serving as both a transport and an enrichment medium (see below).

Special media are required for the isolation of *B. pertussis*. The classic medium used for this organism is Bordet-Gengou (BG) agar. This medium is prepared from potatoes to impart a high starch content. The starch neutralizes toxic materials that may be present in the agar or in the specimen itself. Peptones are omitted from the medium, since these proteins are also inhibitory. BG agar also contains glycerol as a stabilizing agent. Although ''homemade'' BG agar base is superior, dehydrated basal medium is commercially available (Remel Laboratories; BD Biosciences) The base is prepared ahead and stored under refrigeration. If pertussis is suspected, the laboratory must be notified in advance of receiving the specimen, since the final medium must be freshly made. To prepare the medium for use, the potato/glycerol agar base is melted, and 30 mL of defibrinated sheep blood per 100 mL of agar base medium (~23% blood w/v) is added. In older formulations, cephalexin (final concentration, 40 μg/mL) was added to media to inhibit contaminant gram-positive organisms. Methicillin (2.5 μg/mL) or oxacillin (0.625 μg/mL) may be substituted. Both nonselective and selective medium should be inoculated, since some *B. pertussis* strains may be slightly inhibited by cephalexin.

In 1977, Regan and Lowe described a medium containing charcoal and horse blood that has demonstrated superiority to BG agar in several studies.[1056] Although originally described as a transport/enrichment medium, Regan-Lowe agar formulations are available both as a semisolid transport/enrichment medium and as a solid medium for organism isolation. The formula for Regan-Lowe (RL) medium is shown in Box 9-12.

The semisolid transport/enrichment medium is identical in formula to the isolation medium shown above, except that the charcoal agar is present in half-strength (i.e., 25.5 g/L) and is dispensed into sterile screw-capped tubes rather than into 100-mm Petri dishes. It is also recommended that some of the medium be prepared without cephalexin so that both selective and nonselective medium is available for recovery of the organisms.

Optimally, media should be directly inoculated at the time of specimen collection onto both selective (with cephalexin, methicillin, or oxacillin, see above) and nonselective media (see Color Plate 9-5*G*). If a transport system is used, the Regan-Lowe (RL) semisolid medium is optimal, since Stuart and Amies transport medium formulations are not suitable for maintaining the viability of *B. pertussis*. Specimens transported in semisolid RL medium can be subcultured on receipt to RL isolation medium or BG medium with and without cephalexin (or oxacillin/methicillin). The transport medium is then incubated along with the primary plates and subcultured to RL agar after 48 hours of enrichment at 35°C in ambient humidified air.[601] Contrary to widely held beliefs and practices, ambient air is superior to a CO_2-enriched incubation environment. Plates should be incubated for at least 7–10 days. In a study conducted in Canada, however, 7

(16%) of 44 *B. pertussis* isolates and 2 (50%) of 4 *B. parapertussis* isolates were obtained after only 12 days of incubation.[673]

Various other media formulations for isolating *B. pertussis* have been reported in the literature.[44,601,602,741] Many of these have been modifications of the Regan-Lowe formula—that is, a charcoal agar base supplemented with defibrinated blood plus antibiotics such as lincomycin. Hoppe and Schlagenhauf found that horse blood encouraged abundant, more rapid growth of *B. pertussis* than sheep blood, and that both were clearly superior to human blood.[601] The organism will also grow on buffered charcoal yeast extract (BCYE) agar, the medium used for the isolation of *Legionella* species. Ng et al. unexpectedly isolated *B. pertussis* from bronchoalveolar lavage and transbronchial biopsy specimens of three AIDS patients on BCYE agar in their search for *Legionella* organisms in these patients.[937] A blood-free medium called cyclodextrin solid medium (CSM) has also been described.[44] This medium contains a compound called heptakis (2,6-*O*-dimethyl)-β-cyclodextrin in a synthetic broth base containing glutamate, proline, balanced salts, TRIS buffer, Casamino acids, and ʟ-cysteine. Heptakis-cyclodextrin was found to stimulate the growth of *B. pertussis* and to suppress the growth of the normal oropharyngeal flora. This medium can also be made selective by the inclusion of cephalexin (final concentration, 5 μg/mL). In a study of 40 specimens from 29 patients with clinical pertussis, *B. pertussis* was recovered from 100% of the specimens cultured on selective CSM medium, but from only 65% of the specimens cultured on selective BG agar.[44] CSM medium was also demonstrated to have a longer refrigerated shelf life than BG agar.

DIRECT FLUORESCENT ANTIBODY TEST

In addition to culture, direct fluorescent antibody (DFA) tests are also used to detect *B. pertussis* directly on smears prepared from nasopharyngeal specimens. Although DFA tests do provide rapid results, it is well accepted that culture on appropriate media is more sensitive than DFA.[528,1233,1423] Depending on when in the clinical course the specimens are collected, the DFA test may not detect small numbers of organisms that will be picked up on culture. Some workers have found the DFA test to be unacceptably insensitive and nonspecific, particularly when commercially available polyclonal antisera are used. Halperin and associates found that only 6 of 20 cases positive by culture were DFA-positive, and that only 4 of the 12 DFA-positive, culture-negative cases were confirmed by serologic testing of acute and convalescent serum speciemens.[528] Added to this are the inherent difficulties with interpretation and subjectivity of fluorescence techniques. Furthermore, it has been demonstrated that polyclonal *Legionella* antisera for direct fluorescent antibody detection of these organisms will also react with some *B. pertussis* and *B. bronchiseptica* strains, resulting in false-positive immunofluorescence results for *Legionella* species.[110,640,936] The DFA test for detection of *B. pertussis* should be used in conjunction with, not in place of, culture.

DFA testing may be done using polyclonal or monoclonal antibodies. The monoclonal antibody (Accu-Mab, Alta-Chem Pharma, Edmonton, Alberta, Canada) is directed

Box 9-12 Regan-Lowe Medium for Isolation of *Bordetella pertussis* (Per 1 L of Distilled Water)	
Charcoal agar (Oxoid CM 119)	51 g
Horse blood, defibrinated	100 mL
Cephalexin (omit for nonselective agar)	0.04 g
Amphotericin B (optional)	0.05 g

against a lipooligosaccharide epitope and is a dual-fluorochrome reagent for detection of both *B. pertussis* and *B. parapertussis* in the same specimen. To perform the DFA test, nasopharyngeal swab specimens or material from a nasopharyngeal aspirate are placed in a sterile tube containing a small amount (0.5 mL) of Casamino acids. After vigorous mixing, four to eight smears are prepared. Layering of drops of the material and allowing drying between drops should yield a smear with a visible film of material on it. After drying and heat-fixing, the slides may be stained. Properly titered *B. pertussis* and *B. parapertussis* conjugates should be used; because of the high specificity of the conjugates, one can be used as the nonspecific staining/negative control for the other in the staining procedure. The polyclonal conjugates are available from BD Biosciences. Positive and negative control smears are prepared from PBS/saline suspensions (equal to a McFarland #1) of stock cultures grown on antibiotic-free BG or RL medium. These suspensions yield smears with 10 to 100 organisms per oil-immersion field. On DFA, the organisms appear as small, coccobacilli with bright, apple-green peripheral fluorescence (see Color Plate 9-5*E*). They may appear singly, in pairs or in clusters. In smears prepared from highly tenacious specimens, the organisms may appear adherent to the mucous strands. Smears of specimens are examined at 400×; suspicious areas are examined under oil for confirmation. Gram stains of simultaneously prepared smears may also help to confirm the morphology of organisms that fluoresce with the antibodies.

CULTURAL CHARACTERISTICS AND IDENTIFICATION

On culture, colonies of *B. pertussis* may be observed after 2 to 4 days. Growth is usually apparent sooner on antibiotic-free medium, but this is not always the case. Plates are examined under a dissecting microscope (10×) with oblique incident light to determine colony characteristics. Fresh clinical isolates of *B. pertussis* on BG agar appear as smooth, shiny colonies with a high, domed profile. Classically, they are described as resembling small droplets of mercury (see Color Plate 9-4*G*). Colonies on BG may be slightly β-hemolytic, particularly in the more confluent areas of growth or after prolonged incubation. On RL agar medium, colonies are small, domed, and shiny, with a white mother-of-pearl opalescence (see Color Plates 9-5*G* and 9-5*H*). *B. parapertussis* colonies grow more rapidly, are more β-hemolytic on BG agar, and are gray or slightly brown in color. *B. bronchiseptica* colonies are apparent within 24 hours, are large, flatter, and have a dull rather than a shiny appearance. The latter species resembles a nonfermentative gram-negative rod (like an *Alcaligenes* species) in the appearance of its colonies and the production of a distinct "non-fermenter" odor. Gram stain morphology of these organisms also differ. *B. pertussis* appears as small, pale-staining, coccobacilli, while *B. parapertussis* and *B. bronchiseptica* are more definitely rod-shaped. Because of the pale staining of the organisms, the safranin counterstain should be left on the slide for at least 2 minutes (see Color Plate 9-5*F*).

Once isolated, *B. pertussis* is generally identified by the fluorescent antibody test, since the organism is quite inert

in biochemical identification tests (Table 9-16).[524] Serologic methods may be used to identify *B. parapertussis* as well, but biochemical methods may provide a presumptive identification. *B. pertussis*, *B. bronchiseptica*, *B. hinzii*, and *B. avium* are oxidase-positive with Kovac's oxidase reagent, while *B. parapertussis*, *B. holmesii*, and *B. trematum* are oxidase-negative. *B. parapertussis*, *B. bronchiseptica*, *B. hinzii*, and *B. holmesii* are catalase-positive, while *B. pertussis* is variable for catalase production. Both *B. parapertussis* and *B. bronchiseptica* are urease-positive, with the latter species producing a positive test in 4 hours or less. *B. hinzii* is variable for urease production, while *B. pertussis*, *B. holmesii*, *B. avium*, and *B. trematum* are urease-negative. Both *B. parapertussis* and *B. holmesii* produce a soluble brown pigment on agar media, while *B. pertussis*, *B. bronchiseptica*, *B. hinzii*, *B. trematum*, and *B. avium* do not. Other characteristics for the identification of *Bordetella* species are shown in Table 9-16.

New Technologies for Detection and Identification of *Bordetella pertussis*

Several newer technologies have also been applied to the identification and the direct detection of *B. pertussis* in clinical specimens.[906] Monoclonal antibodies developed against *B. pertussis* LPS and FHA have been used in "dot-blot" and enzyme-linked immunosorbent assay formats for identification of *B. pertussis* from isolated colonies.[513,514,1122] Various rapid methods for direct detection of *B. pertussis* antigens and virulence factors in nasopharyngeal specimens have also been described. Monoclonal antibodies prepared against *B. pertussis* PT, FHA, and LPS have been developed and tested in enzyme-immunoassay formats as "antigen-capture" tests for direct detection of these pertussis-specific virulence factors in clinical specimens.[439,513,514] In vitro tissue culture assays, such as the Chinese hamster ovary cell cytotoxicity test performed directly on upper respiratory tract specimens, have also been described as rapid, sensitive, and specific assays for diagnosis of pertussis.[527] Purified PT, FHA, and other proteins have also been exploited as antigens for use in antibody detection assays as diagnostic tools and for immune status surveys (see section on "Serologic Tests for Diagnosis of Pertussis," below).

With the genetic characterization of *B. pertussis* and its virulence factors and the cloning of the genes for these proteins, genes and/or species-specific PCR primers and probes have been developed for both direct detection of organisms in nasopharyngeal specimens and for identification of organisms recovered in culture. PCR-based assays have, in fact, become the tests of choice for diagnosis of pertussis due to their exquisite sensitivity and specificity. Nucleic acid target sequences specific for *B. pertussis* have been identified and primers and probes have been developed for detection of these targets by PCR. PCR target sequences include the *B. pertussis*–specific repeated insertion sequence IS*481*, the pertussis toxin gene promoter region, the adenylate cyclase gene, and structural genes for unique *B. pertussis* porin proteins.[187,350,467,783,849,931,1063,1275,1307,1340] The use of a combination of primers and restriction enzymes may allow for simultaneous detection of and discrimination between *B. pertussis* and *B. parapertussis*. Some target sequences used

Table 9-16 Biochemical Characteristics for Identification of *Bordetella* Species

CHARACTERISTIC	*B. PERTUSSIS*	*B. PARAPERTUSSIS*	*B. BRONCHISEPTICA*	*B. AVIUM*	*B. HINZII*	*B. HOLMESII*	*B. TREMATUM*
Oxidase	+	−	+	+	+	−	−
Catalase	+	+	+	+	+	+[a]	+
Motility	−	−	+	+	+	−	+
Nitrate reduction	−	−	+	−	−	−	v
Urease	−	+ (24 hours)	+ (4 hours)	−	v	−	−
Citrate	−	+	+	+	+	NA	NA
Brown pigment in heart infusion agar with L-tyrosine (1 g/L)	−	+	−	−	−	+	NA
Growth on:							
Bordet-Gengou agar	2–6 days	1–3 days	1–2 days	2 days	2 days	2 days	2 days
Regan-Lowe agar	3–6 days	2–3 days	1–2 days	1–2 days	2 days	2 days	2 days
Blood agar	No growth	1–3 days	1–2 days	2 days	2 days	2 days	2 days
Chocolate agar	No growth	1–3 days	+	2 days	2 days	2 days	2 days
MacConkey agar	No growth	v	+	+	+	3–7 days	2 days

+, *positive reaction;* −, *negative reaction;* v, *variable reaction.*
[a] *Weak/delayed reaction.*

for PCR, such as the IS*481* insertion sequence of *B. pertussis*, have also been detected in other *Bordetella* species such as *B. holmesii*.[794] The nested PCR technique uses a 239-bp sequence of the PT promoter region as a target.[1063] This sequence is found in *B. pertussis*, *B. parapertussis*, and *B. bronchiseptica* and is amplified during thermal cycling. Species identification is completed by amplicon cleavage with restriction endonucleases and analysis on agarose gel electrophoresis with ethidium bromide staining.[951] Each species produces a characteristic restriction- fragment pattern. Amplicon detection following PCR amplification has also been modified with the use of probe-specific product capture techniques.[187,931] In one format, amplicons are denatured and placed in microwells containing a single-stranded capture probe. After washing, a solution-phase alkaline phosphatase-conjugated detector probe is added that reacts with a portion of the captured, denatured amplicon.[931] PCR-based identification methods may also be used to identify isolates in cases in which biochemical and/or serologic tests give inconclusive results.[1215] Recommendations for a standardized approach to epidemiologic typing of *B. pertussis* isolates have included a combination of serologic and molecular techniques, including LPS and fimbrial serotyping, DNA fingerprinting by pulsed-field gel electrophoresis, and sequencing of the genes for pertactin (PRN) and the S1 subunit of PT.[890] Restriction-enzyme analysis and ribotyping have also been used for differentiation of *B. hinzii* and *B. avium*.[1118]

PCR-based methods have been compared with DFA and conventional culture in several studies. In a recent Canadian study, Tilley and colleagues found that PCR had a sensitivity of 95% compared with culture (36%), and DFA testing using both polyclonal (11.4%) and monoclonal (8.3%) reagents.[1275] In a PCR validation study conducted during a pertussis vaccine trial in Sweden, PCR analysis of 2,421 nasopharyngeal aspirates using the PT promoter region as a target had a sensitivity of 94.3% and a diagnostic specificity of 99%.[1063] Nelson et al. reported that PCR and culture had sensitivities of only 86% and 58%, respectively; the interval between disease onset and specimen collection and the immune status of the patient being tested were the factors that most affected the sensitivity of both assays.[931] Loeffelholz and colleagues compared culture, DFA, and PCR for the IS*481* sequence on 319 consecutive specimens, which resulted in 59 specimens being positive for one or more tests. Based on chart reviews and patient evaluations according to a CDC pertussis case definition, the sensitivities of culture, DFA, and PCR were 15.2%, 52.2%, and 93.5%, with corresponding specificities of 100%, 98.2%, and 97.1%, respectively.[793] This study pointed out that several positive PCR results were obtained on specimens from individuals who did not meet the case definition, but had symptoms consistent with typical and atypical pertussis.

Molecular methods have also identified insertion sequences, and, therefore, molecular identification methods, for *B. parapertussis* and *B. bronchiseptica*.[1308] IS*1002* is an insertion sequence found along with IS*481* in *B. pertussis* and has 61.5% sequence identity with IS*481*. IS*1002* is also found in human *B. parapertussis* isolates, but is absent in ovine *B. parapertussis* isolates. Another insertion sequence, IS*1001*, is found all human and ovine *B. parapertussis* and in *B. bronchiseptica* isolates that are recovered from animals

but is not found in *B. pertussis*. Direct detection of IS*1001*, an insertion sequence found in *B. parapertussis*, has been used to develop a PCR-based detection/identification technique for this organism.[783] Phylogenetic analysis of these insertion sequences suggests that human and ovine *B. parapertussis* strains probably evolved independently from *B. bronchiseptica* strains, and that *B. parapertussis* probably acquired IS*1002* from *B. pertussis*.

Serologic Tests for Diagnosis of Pertussis

With the availability of discrete pertussis antigens, like PT and FHA, serologic methods to determine the immune responses to specific antigens following clinical infection or immunization have been investigated and developed. Several components of *B. pertussis* are immunogenic and engender brisk antibody responses. Guiso and colleagues used Western blot analysis to examine the host response to several *B. pertussis* antigens, including PT, FHA, adenylate cyclase-hemolysin, and pertactin, in 27 children with suspected pertussis.[509] Of these children, 19 were diagnosed as having pertussis by serologic testing and 10 were culture-positive. Convalescent sera from all 19 patients were positive for anti-PT, anti-FHA, and anti-H-AC antibodies by Western immunoblot, while only 1 convalescent serum specimen demonstrated antipertactin antibodies. He and coworkers examined pooled and purified antigens of *B. pertussis* in an enzyme-linked immunoassay format to determine the antigen or antigens that would provide the most sensitive test having a specificity of at least 99%.[545] They found that the sensitivities of the EIA using PT alone, FHA alone, or pertactin alone were 92%, 85%, and 62%, respectively; the sensitivity of the EIA with a pool of these antigens was 85%. The adenylate cyclase of *B. pertussis* has also been purified and used as the antigen in a EIA-based serologic test, which showed that high titers of anti–adenylate cyclase antibodies are produced after infection and after immunization with whole-cell vaccines.[396] Functional assays for antibody-mediated inhibition of biologic effects of organism virulence factors have also been developed. For example, Kaslow et al. described direct and indirect methods for measuring the inhibition of PT-mediated ADP-ribosyltransferase activity following both immunization and infection with *B. pertussis*.[670]

Serologic tests for pertussis have attracted a great deal of scientific interest in recent years because of the development and testing of acellular pertussis vaccines that use purified antigens rather than whole cells.[238,524,526] Prior to the initiation of large vaccine efficacy trials, antibody detection tests for pertussis were performed with inactivated whole cells, whole-cell sonicates, or crude acellular extracts of *B. pertussis* as antigens; interpretation of serologic tests using these antigens was often difficult. As a part of several vaccine trials conducted under the auspices of the World Health Organization (WHO), pertussis serology was further developed as a semistandardized enzyme immunoassay procedure and was included in the case definition of pertussis adopted by the WHO.[1396] Currently, most antibody assays for diagnosis of pertussis use purified antigens, such as PT, FHA, pertactin, and fimbrial antigens, in an EIA format. Antibody directed against PT is specific for *B. pertussis*, while anti-FHA antibodies are also produced following infection with *B. par-*

apertussis. In addition, other organisms may also engender antibodies that cross-react with *B. pertussis* FHA. (e.g., non-typeable *H. influenzae*). Following natural infection, antibodies usually appear 10 days to 2 weeks after the onset of symptoms, with anti-PT and anti-FHA IgG antibodies being detected in over 90% and IgA antibodies being detected in 20–40% of infected individuals. Immune responses to other antigens (e.g., pertactin, fimbrial antigens) tend to be more variable and may be found in 20–60% of infected persons.

Immune responses to pertussis are influenced by the vaccination status and the age of the host.[906] In the case definition of pertussis developed by the WHO, serologic confirmation requires paired sera (showing seroconversion from negative to positive, or a fourfold titer increase), along with clinical criteria (i.e., a spasmodic cough for more than 21 days).[1396] Trollfors et al. performed pertussis serologic testing on a group of nonvaccinated Swedish children with clinical (i.e., cough ≥21 days and cough <21 days) and nonserologic evidence of *B. pertussis* infection (i.e., positive culture, PCR). Among those with cough for ≥21 days, levels of anti-PT and anti-FHA increased 400-fold and 68-fold, respectively. More than 90% of the children had significant titer increases to both antigens if the acute specimen was obtained within 14 days of disease onset.[1289] However, serologic testing may not be useful in the treatment of an acutely ill patient because production of specific antibodies may be delayed, particularly in infants. In a recent study of a group of unvaccinated pediatric patients fitting the WHO case definition of pertussis, only 7–14% of all children had high concentrations of anti-PT IgG in the acute specimen.[1386] Specimens collected 5 to 10 weeks after the onset of coughing had a diagnostic sensitivity of 81–89% when age-specific reference values regarding prevalence of pertussis in infants (<1 year old), toddlers (1–4 years), and schoolchildren (5–10 years) were applied.[1386] In vaccinated children, the secondary immune response results in rapid increases in antibody titer, so that significant titer changes between sequential specimens may not be seen. Serologic testing on vaccinated populations may be diagnostically useful, however, since a high titer from the secondary immune response in a single serum specimen may indicate infection in "real time." This approach may be useful for diagnosing pertussis in adolescents and adults, since pertussis often is not included in the initial differential diagnosis of nonpediatric respiratory infections; consequently, attempts at culture or PCR are made late in the clinical course. After analysis of data from a large population-based study conducted in the Netherlands, De Melker and colleagues found that anti-PT IgG levels of at least 100 U/mL in an EIA assay are diagnostic of recent or active *B. pertussis* infection; in most cases, this antibody level was achieved within 4 weeks of disease onset.[318] Units of PT per milliliter of serum are determined by calibration of EIA assays with FDA-prepared antigen (Food and Drug Administration Laboratory for Pertussis, Rockville, MD)

In addition to EIA, particle agglutination tests for antibody detection have also been described. Aoyama and colleagues developed a particle agglutination assay with PT-sensitized poly(γ-methyl-L-glutamate) as the solid particle for detection of anti-PT antibodies.[43] Anti-PT antibodies were detected in all of 21 vaccine recipients after receipt of each vaccination. In addition, a significant increase (more than fourfold) in anti-PT antibodies was detected in 76% of 51 patients with confirmed pertussis within 4 weeks of disease onset, compared with 67% of the 51 who were detected with EIA.[43]

Treatment of Pertussis

Pertussis is generally treated with erythromycin (estolate form, 40 mg/kg/day; ethylsuccinate form, 50–60 mg/kg/day) for a period of at least 2 weeks to prevent relapse. Shorter courses (e.g., 7–10 days) may not eliminate the organism from the upper respiratory tract. Administration of this antibiotic even during the paroxysmal stage shortens the severity and the duration of illness. Strains of *B. pertussis* are susceptible to erythromycin in vitro, having MICs ranging from 0.02 to 0.12 µg/mL. Erythromycin-resistance in *B. pertussis* was not seen until 1995, when the first case of pertussis caused by an erythromycin-resistant *B. pertussis* strain was reported in a 2-month-old child in Yuma, Arizona.[774] When there was no clinical improvement after a 12-day course of erythromycin, disk testing of the isolate showed no zones of inhibition around the erythromycin, clarithromycin, and clindamycin disks. Agar dilution testing revealed an erythromycin MIC of >64 µg/mL. However, erythromycin-resistant strains remain relatively uncommon. In a survey of 47 isolates from children collected in the intermountain west region of the U.S. from January 1985 through June 1997, only one strain was erythromycin-resistant (MIC, 32 µg/mL) on agar dilution testing.[721] Other drugs such as azithromycin have been used in open noncomparative studies and successfully eliminate the organism from the respiratory tract, but the balance of clinical experience indicates that erythromycin is superior.[74] Trimethoprim-sulfamethoxazole (TMP-SMX) also is able to eradicate *B. pertussis* from the nasopharynx and was used successfully to treat the child with the erythromycin-resistant isolate. Although TMP-SMX may be a useful alternative to erythromycin, the dosage and duration of therapy have not been ascertained.[598,774] The fluoroquinolones also have generally good activity against *B. pertussis*, but clinical trials have not been performed since fluoroquinolone use is contraindicated in children; these agents may be useful for treatment of adults with pertussis infection.[603]

In addition to antimicrobial chemotherapy, other therapeutic methods have been investigated for pertussis. Recently, a phase I trial was conducted on the safety, pharmacology, and response to treatment of pertussis with intravenous pertussis immune globulin (P-IGIV). This pooled plasma product contains a sevenfold higher concentration of anti-PT immunoglobulin than conventional immune serum globulin. Among 26 children with confirmed pertussis, treatment with P-IGIV resulted in declines in lymphocytosis and paroxysmal coughing by the third day after P-IGIV transfusion for all treated subjects with no adverse effects.[185]

Antimicrobial Susceptibility Testing of *Bordetella* Species

Although standardized procedures are not available, several methods have been developed and evaluated for in vitro antimicrobial susceptibility testing of *Bordetella* species. Agar dilution susceptibility testing has been performed with a number of media, including Mueller-Hinton agar with 5% horse blood, Bordet-Gengou agar with 5% or 20% horse blood, and Regan-Lowe agar.[572,599] Hoppe and Paulus evaluated Bordet-Genou agar with 5% horse blood, oxoid charcoal agar with 5% horse blood, and Mueller-Hinton agar with 5% horse blood for in vitro agar dilution testing and found that Mueller-Hinton with horse blood provided the most consistent results.[599] MICs determined on charcoal-containing media were onefold to fivefold higher for clinical isolates, control strains, and *S. aureus* ATCC 29213, due to inactivation of some antimicrobial agents by charcoal. Using the agar dilution method, *B. pertussis* is susceptible to a wide variety of antimicrobial agents in vitro, including β-lactams (i.e., ampicillin/amoxicillin), macrolides (i.e., azithromycin, clarithromycin, erythromycin, roxithromycin), sulfonamides (i.e., trimethoprim/sulfamethoxazole), rifampin, and fluoroquinolones (i.e., ciprofloxacin, ofloxacin, temafloxacin, trovafloxacin).[596,597,600,603,721,740] Among the fluoroquinolones, levofloxacin is more active against *B. pertussis* (MIC, 1 μg/mL) than against *B. parapertussis* strains (MIC, >2 μg/mL).[600] Most *B. pertussis* strains are resistant to tetracycline.

Etest strips (AB Biodisk, Piscataway, NJ) and modified disk diffusion methods have also been evaluated for antimicrobial susceptibility testing of *B. pertussis*. Korgenski and Daly found essential agreement between agar dilution MICs and Etest MICs for 89.1% of 46 isolates (i.e., the Etest MIC was within ± 1 doubling dilution of the agar dilution MIC, while the remaining 10.9% had Etest MICs that were >1 doubling dilution different than the agar dilution MIC.[721] Hill and colleagues also evaluated the Etest using both Bordet-Gengou with 20% horse blood and Regan-Lowe agar and found that the Etest method produced results similar to those of their reference agar dilution procedure (using Bordet-Genou agar with 20% horse blood) for erythromycin, rifampin, and chloramphenicol; trimethoprim-sulfamethoxazole MICs using Etest were lower than those obtained with agar dilution.[572] These same workers also tested a disk diffusion procedure using Regan-Lowe with a standardized inoculum (0.5 McFarland standard) and found that this method accurately detected erythromycin resistance.[572] Resistant strains (MIC, >256 μg/mL) produced no zones around the standard erythromycin disk, while susceptible strains (MIC, ≤0.06 μg/mL) produced zones of at least 42 mm. Standardization of susceptibility testing for these organisms is needed for investigation of new antimicrobial agents against the bordetellae, and it may gain additional clinical relevance if erythromycin resistance becomes more widespread.

B. parapertussis strains are more resistant to antimicrobial agents than *B. pertussis*. As a part of the Multicenter Pertussis Surveillance Project, agar dilution antimicrobial susceptibility data was collected on 46 *B. parapertussis* and 11 *B. bronchiseptica* isolates.[740] Although the *B. parapertussis* strains were susceptible to erythromycin, trimethoprim-sulfamethoxazole, and ciprofloxacin, most were resistant to amoxicillin and all were resistant to rifampin and tetracycline. Levofloxacin, ciprofloxacin, and cefpirome, a broad-spectrum cephalosporin, are more active against *B. pertussis* than against *B. parapertussis*.[600] Among the macrolides, both erythromycin and azithromycin are active against *B. parapertussis*, with 90% of strains having MICs

for erythromycin and azithromycin of 0.5 μg/mL and ≤0.06 μg/mL, respectively.[596,828]

The other *Bordetella* species tend to be more resistant to antimicrobial agents than either *B. pertussis* or *B. parapertussis*. In the multicenter study, 82% of the *B. bronchiseptica* isolates were susceptible to trimethoprim-sulfamethoxazole and 27% were susceptible to ciprofloxacin; all *B. bronchiseptica* strains were resistant to amoxicillin, erythromycin, rifampin, and tetracycline.[740] *B. hinzii* isolates are resistant to ampicillin, ampicillin-sulbactam, cefazolin, ceftriaxone, cefotaxime, cefuroxime, cefotetan, aztreonam, ciprofloxacin, and tobramycin, and are susceptible to cephalothin, ceftazidime, cefepime, imipenem, tetracycline, trimethoprim-sulfamethoxazole, levofloxacin, gentamicin, and amikacin.[443,671] Isolates of *B. holmesii* are susceptible to amoxicillin, amoxicillin-clavulanate, cefazolin, cefotaxime, ceftazidime, gentamicin, tobramycin, amikacin, imipenem, tetracycline, erythromycin, rifampin, ciprofloxacin, and trimethoprim-sulfamethoxazole, and are resistant to penicillin.[784,940,1257]

REFERENCES

1. Abu-Ekteish F, Kakish K. Pneumonia as the sole presentation of brucellosis. Respir Med 2001;95:766–767.
2. Adderson EE, Byington CL, Spencer L, et al. Invasive serotype a *Haemophilus influenzae* infections with a virulence genotype resembling *Haemophilus influenzae* type b: emerging pathogen in the vaccine era. Pediatrics 2001;108: E18.
3. Ahmed K, Sein PP, Shahnawaz M, Hoosen AA. *Pasteurella gallinarum* neonatal meningitis. Clin Microbiol Infect 2002;8:55–57.
4. Akdeniz H, Irmak H, Anlar O, Demiroz AP. Central nervous system brucellosis: presentation, diagnosis, and treatment. J Infect 1998;36:297–301.
5. Akinci E, Gol MK, Balbay Y. A case of prosthetic mitral valve endocarditis caused by *Brucella abortus*. Scand J Infect Dis 2001;33:71–72.
6. Akova M, Uzun O, Akalin HE, et al. Quinolones in treatment of human brucellosis: comparative trial of ofloxacin-rifampin versus doxycycline-rifampin. Antimicrob Agents Chemother 1993;7:1831–1834.
7. Alanen A, Laurikanien E. Second-trimester abortion caused by *Capnocytophaga sputigena*: case report. Am J Perinatol 1999;16:181–183.
8. Alcala L, Garcia-Garrote F, Cercenado E, et al. Comparison of broth microdilution method using *Haemophilus* test medium and agar dilution method for susceptibility testing of *Eikenella corrodens*. J Clin Microbiol 1998;36: 2386–2388.
9. Al-Eissa YA, Assuhaimi SA, Al-Fawaz IM, et al. Pancytopenia in children with brucellosis: clinical manifestations and bone marrow findings. Acta Haematol 1993;89:132–136.
10. Al-Eissa YA, Kambal AM, Al-Nasser MN, et al. Childhood brucellosis: a study of 102 cases. Pediatr Infect Dis 1990;J 9:74–79.
11. Al-Eissa YA, Kambal AM, Alrabeeah AA, et al. Osteoarticular brucellosis in children. Ann Rheum Dis 1990;49:896–900.
12. Alfa MJ, DeGagne P. Attachment of *Haemophilus ducreyi* to human foreskin fibroblasts involves LOS and fibronectin. Microb Pathog 1997;22:39–46.
13. Alfa MJ, DeGagne P, Totten PA. *Haemophilus ducreyi* hemolysin acts as a contact cytotoxin and damages human foreskin fibroblasts in cell culture. Infect Immun 1996;64:2349–2352.
14. Alfa MJ, Stevens MK, DeGagne P, et al. Use of tissue culture and animal models to identify virulence-associated traits of *Haemophilus ducreyi*. Infect Immun 1995;63:1754–1761.
15. Al Fadel Saleh M, Al-Madan MS, Erwa HH, et al. First case of human infection caused by *Pasteurella gallinarum* causing infective endocarditis in an adolescent 10 years after surgical correction for truncus arteriosus. Pediatrics 1995; 95:944–948.
16. Al-Faran MF. *Brucella melitensis* endogenous endophthalmitis. Ophthalmologica 1990;201:19–22.

17. Al-Kharfy TM. Neonatal brucellosis and blood transfusion: case report and review of the literature. Ann Trop Paediatr 2001;21:349–352.

18. Allardet-Servent A, Bourg G, Ramuz M, et al. DNA polymorphism in strains of the genus *Brucella*. J Bacteriol 1988;170:4603–4607.

19. Allen CA, Adams G, Ficht TA. Transposon-derived *Brucella abortus* rough mutants are attenuated and exhibit reduced intracellular survival. Infect Immun 1998;66:1008–1016.

20. Almeda FQ, Tenorio AR, Barkatullah S, et al. Infective endocarditis due to *Haemophilus aphrophilus* treated with levofloxacin. Am J Med 2002;113:702–704.

21. Alrawli AM, Chern KC, Cevallos V, et al. Biotypes and serotypes of *Haemophilus influenzae* ocular isolates. Br J Ophthalmol 2002;86:276–277.

22. Al-Shamahy HA, Wright SG. Enzyme-linked immunosorbent assay for brucella antigen detection in human sera. J Med Microbiol 1998;47:169–172.

23. Al-Tawfiq JA, Harezlak J, Katz BP, Spinola SM. Cumulative experience with *Haemophilus ducreyi* 35000 in the human model of experimental infection. Sex Transm Dis 2000;27:111–114.

24. Alvarez M, Patel C, Rey L, et al. Biliary tract infections caused by *Haemophilus parainfluenzae*. Scand J Infect Dis 1999;31:212–213.

25. Ambati BK, Ambati J, Azar N, et al. Periorbital and orbital cellulitis before and after the advent of *Haemophilus influenzae* type b vaccination. Ophthalmology 2000;107:1450–1453.

26. Amin AS, Hamdy ME, Ibrahim AK. Detection of *Brucella melitensis* in semen using the polymerase chain reaction assay. Vet Microbiol 2001;83:37–44.

27. Amir J, Yagupsky P. Invasive *Kingella kingae* infection associated with stomatitis in children. Pediatr Infect Dis J 1998;17:757–758.

28. Amrikachi M, Krishnan B, Finch CJ, Shahab I. *Actinomyces* and *Actinobacillus actinomycetemcomitans*-*Actinomyces*-associated lymphadenopathy mimicking lymphoma. Arch Pathol Lab Med 2000;124:1502–1505.

29. Anda P, Segura del Pozo J, Diaz Garcia JM, et al. Waterborne outbreak of tularemia associated with crayfish fishing. Emerg Infect Dis 2001;7(3Suppl):575–582.

30. Andersen HK, Mortensen A. Unrecognized neurobrucellosis giving rise to *Brucella melitensis* peritonitis via a ventriculoperitoneal shunt. Eur J Clin Microbiol Infect Dis 1992;11:953–954.

31. Andersen JK, Pedersen M. Infective endocarditis with involvement of the tricuspid valve due to *Capnocytophaga canimorsus*. Eur J Clin Microbiol Infect Dis 1992;11:831–832.

32. Anderson B, Kelly C, Threlkel R, et al. Detection of *Rochalimaea henselae* in cat-scratch disease skin test antigens. J Infect Dis 1993;168:1034–1036.

33. Anderson B, Lu E, Jones D, et al. Characterization of a 17-kilodalton antigen of *Bartonella henselae* reactive with sera from patients with cat scratch disease. J Clin Microbiol 1995;33:2358–2365.

34. Anderson B, Sims K, Regnery R, et al. Detection of *Rochalimaea henselae* DNA in specimens from cat scratch disease patients by PCR. J Clin Microbiol 1994;32:942–948.

35. Andres MT, Martin MC, Fierro JF, Mendez FJ. Chorioamnionitis and neonatal septicaemia caused by *Eikenella corrodens*. J Infect 2002;44:133–134.

36. Ang MS, Ngan CC. *Eikenella corrodens* discitis after spinal surgery: case report and literature review. J Infect 45:272–274, 2002.

37. Angen O, Ahrens P, Bisgaard M. Phenotypic and genotypic characterization of *Mannheimia* (*Pasteurella*) *haemolytica*-like strains isolated from diseased animals in Denmark. Vet Microbiol 2002;84:103–114.

38. Angen O, Mutters R, Caugant DA, et al. Taxonomic relationships of the [*Pasteurella*] *haemolytica* complex as evaluated by DNA-DNA hybridizations and 16S rRNA sequencing with proposal of *Mannheimia haemolytica* gen. nov., comb. nov., *Mannheimia granulomatis* comb. nov., *Mannheimia glucosida* sp. nov., *Mannheimia ruminalis* sp. nov., and *Mannheimia varigena* sp. nov. Int J Syst Bacteriol 1999;49:67–86.

39. Angus BJ, Green ST, McKinley JJ, et al. *Eikenella corrodens* septicaemia among drug injectors: a possible association with ''licking wounds.'' J Infect 1994;28:102–103.

40. Anolik R, Berkowitz RJ, Campos JM, et al. *Actinobacillus* endocarditis associated with periodontal disease. Clin Pediatr 1981;20:653–655.

41. Anthony LSD, Morrisey PJ, Nano FE. Growth inhibition of *Francisella tularensis* live vaccine strain by IFN-γ-activated macrophages is mediated by reactive nitrogen intermediates derived from L-arginine metabolism. J Immunol 1992;148:1829–1834.

42. Aoyama T, Iwata T, Iwai Y, et al. Efficacy of acellular pertussis vaccine in young infants. J Infect Dis 1993;167:483–386.

43. Aoyama T, Kato T, Takeuchi Y, et al. Simple, speedy, sensitive, and specific serodiagnosis of pertussis by using a particle agglutination assay. J Clin Microbiol 1997;35:1859–1861.

44. Aoyama T, Murase Y, Iwata T, et al. Comparison of blood-free (cyclodextrin solid medium) with Bordet-Gengou medium for clinical isolation of *Bordetella pertussis*. J Clin Microbiol 1986;23:1046–1048.

45. Apisarnthanarak A, Johnson RM, Braverman AC, et al. *Cardiobacterium hominis* bioprosthetic valve endocarditis presenting as septic arthritis. Diagn Microbiol Infect Dis 2002;42:79–81.

46. Arana E, Vallcanera A, Santamaria JA, et al. *Eikenella corrodens* skull infection: a case report with review of the literature. Surg Neurol 1998;47:389–391.

47. Arashima Y, Kato K, Kakuta R, et al. First case of *Pasteurella gallinarum* isolation from blood of a patient with symptoms of acute gastroenteritis in Japan. Clin Infect Dis 1999;29:698–699.

48. Arias-Stella J, Lieberman PH, Erlandson RA, et al. Histology, immunochemistry, and ultrastructure of the verruga in Carrion's disease. 1986;Am J Surg Pathol 10:595–610.

49. Arico B, Nuti S, Scarlato V, et al. Adhesion of *Bordetella pertussis* to eucaryotic cells requires a time-dependent export and maturation of filamentous hemagglutinin. Proc Natl Acad Sci USA 1993;90:9204–9208.

50. Arico B, Rappuoli R. *Bordetella parapertussis* and *Bordetella bronchiseptica* contain transcriptionally silent pertussis toxin genes. J Bacteriol 1987;169:2847–2853.

51. Arisoy E S, Correa AG, Wagner ML, Kaplan S. Hepatosplenic cat-scratch disease in children: selected clinical features and treatment. Clin Infect Dis 1999;28:778–784.

52. Ariza J, Pellicer T, Pallares R, et al. Specific antibody profile in human brucellosis. Clin Infect Dis 1992;14:131–140.

53. Ariza J, Pigrau C, Canas C, et al. Current understanding and management of chronic hepatosplenic suppurative brucellosis. Clin Infect Dis 2001;32:1024–1033.

54. Ariza J, Servitje O, Pallares R, et al. Characteristic cutaneous lesions in patients with brucellosis. Arch Dermatol 1989;125:380–383.

55. Arlet G, Sanson-Le Pors M-J, Casin IM, et al. In vitro susceptibility of 96 *Capnocytophaga* strains, including a β-lactamase producer, to new β-lactam antibiotics and six quinolones. Antimicrob. Agents Chemother 1987;31:1283–1284.

56. Arnon R, Ruzal-Shapiro C, Salen E, et al. *Eikenella corrodens*: a rare pathogen in a polymicrobial hepatic abscess in an adolescent. Clin Pediatr (Phila) 1999;38:429–432.

57. Aronson NE, Zbick CJ. Dysgonic fermenter 3 bacteremia in a neutropenic patient with acute lymphocytic leukemia. J Clin Microbiol 1988;26:2213–2215.

58. Arslan H, Korkmaz ME, Kart H, Gul C. Management of *Brucella* endocarditis of a prosthetic valve. J Infect 1998 ;37:70–71.

59. Artman M, Frankl G. Nicotinamide adenine dinucleotide and nicotinamide adenine dinucleotide phosphate splitting enzyme(s) of sheep and rabbit erythrocytes: their effect on the growth of *Haemophilus*. Can J Microbiol 1982;28:696–702.

60. Arvand M, Mielke MEA, Sterry K, Hahn H. Detection of specific cellular immune response to *Bartonella henselae* in a patient with cat scratch disease. Clin Infect Dis 1998;27:1633–1634.

61. Arvand M, Wendt C, Regnath T, et al. Characterization of *Bartonella henselae* isolated from bacillary angiomatosis lesions in a human immunodeficiency virus-infected patient in Germany. Clin Infect Dis 1998;26:1296–1299.

62. Asensi V, Alvarez M, Carton JA, et al. *Eikenella corrodens* brain abscess after repeated periodontal manipulations cured with imipenem and neurosurgery. J Infect 2002;30:240–242.

63. Ashdown LR. Mottarelly IW. Acute painful cellulitis caused by a *Pasteurella pneumotropica*-like bacterium in Northern Queensland. Med J Aust 1990;152:333–334.

64. Ashhurst-Smith C, Norton R, Thoreau, Peel MM. *Actinobacillus equuli* septicemia: an unusual zoonotic infection. J Clin Microbiol 1998;36:2789–279.

65. Asikainen S, Chen C, Slots J. *Actinobacillus actinomycetemcomitans* genotypes in relation to serotypes and periodontal status. Oral Microbiol Immunol 1995;10:65–68.

66. Assefa D, Dalitz E, Handrick W, et al. Septic cavernous sinus thrombosis following infection of ethmoidal and maxillary sinuses: a case report. Int J Pediatr Otorhinolaryngol 1994;29:249–255.

67. Astagneau P, Goldstein FW, Francoual S, et al. Appendicitis due to both *Streptococcus pneumoniae* and *Haemophilus influenzae*. Eur J Syst Bacteriol 1992;11:559–560.

68. Auten GM, Levy CS, Smith MA. *Haemophilus parainfluenzae* as a rare cause of epidural abscess: case report and review. Rev Infect Dis 1993;13:609–612.

69. Avidor B, Kletter Y, Abulafia S, et al. Molecular diagnosis of cat scratch disease: a two-step approach. J Clin Microbiol 35:1924–1930, 1997.

70. Avila-Campos MJ, Cavalho MAR, Zelante F. Distribution of biotypes and antimicrobial susceptibility of *Actinobacillus actinomycetemcomitans*. Oral Microbiol Immunol 10:382–384, 1995.

71. Avlami A, Papalambrou C, Tzivra M, et al. Bone marrow infection caused by *Actinobacillus ureae* in a rheumatoid arthritis patient. J Infect 35:298–299, 1997.

72. Aygen B, Sumerkan B, Dogany M, Schmen E. Prostatitis and hepatitis due to *Brucella melitensis:* a case report. J Infect 1998;36:111–112.

73. Aysha MH, Shayib MA. Pancytopenia and other haematological findings in brucellosis. Scand J Haematol 1986;36:335–338.

74. Bace A, Zrnic T, Begovac J, et al. Short-term treatment of pertussis with azithromycin in infants and young children. Eur J Clin Microbiol Infect Dis 1999;18:296–298.

75. Baddour LM, Gelfand MS, Weaver RE, et al. CDC group HB-5 as a cause of genitourinary tract infection in adults. J Clin Microbiol 1989;27:801–805.

76. Baker CN, Hollis DG, Thornsberry C. Antimicrobial susceptibility testing of *Francisella tularensis* with a modified Mueller-Hinton broth. J Clin Microbiol 1985;22:212–215.

77. Baker D, Stahlman GC. *Pasteurella multocida* infection in a patient with AIDS. J Tenn Med Assoc 84:325–326, 1991.

78. Baldwin CJ, Panciera RJ, Morton RJ, et al. Acute tularemia in three domestic cats. J Am Vet Med Assoc 1991;199:1602–1605.

79. Ballard RC, Ye H, Matta A, et al. Treatment of chancroid with azithromycin. Int J STD AIDS 1996;7(Suppl 1):9–12.

80. Bandi V, Apicella MA, Mason E, et al. Nontypeable *Haemophilus influenzae* in the lower respiratory tract of patients with chronic bronchitis. Am J Respir Crit Care Med 2001;164:2114–2119.

81. Bangsborg JM, Frederiksen W, Bruun B. Dysgonic fermenter 3-associated abscess in a diabetic patient. J Infect 1990;20:237–240.

82. Bannerjee TK, Grubb W, Otero C, et al. Musculocutaneous mononeuropathy complicating *Capnocytophaga canimorsus* infection. Neurology 1993;43:2411–2412.

83. Baquero F, Fernendez J, Dronda F, et al. Capnophilic and anaerobic bacteremia in neutropenic patients: an oral source. Rev Infect Dis 1990;12(Suppl 2):S157–S160.

84. Barbour ML, Crook DW, Mayon-White RT. An improved antiserum agar method for detecting carriage of *Haemophilus influenzae* type b. Eur J Clin Microbiol Infect Dis 1993;12:215–217.

85. Barenkamp SJ. Outer membrane proteins and lipopolysaccharides of nontypeable *Haemophilus influenzae*. J Infect Dis 1992;165(Suppl 1):S181–S184.

86. Barenkamp SJ. Immunization with high-molecular-weight adhesion proteins of nontypeable *Haemophilus influenzae* modifies experimental otitis media in chinchillas. Infect Immun 1996;64:1246–1251.

87. Barenkamp SJ, Leininger E. Cloning, expression, and DNA sequence analysis of genes encoding nontypeable *Haemophilus influenzae* high-molecular-weight surface-exposed proteins related to filamentous hemagglutinin of *Bordetella pertussis*. Infect Immun 1992;60:1302–1313.

88. Barenkamp JS, St Geme JW III. Genes encoding high-molecular-weight adhesion proteins of nontypeable *Haemophilus influenzae* are part of gene clusters. Infect Immun 1994;62:3320–3328.

89. Barenkamp SJ, St Geme JW III. Identification of surface-exposed B-cell epitopes on high-molecular-weight adhesion proteins of nontypeable *Haemophilus influenzae*. Infect Immun 1996;64:3032–3037.

90. Barenkamp SJ, St Geme JW III. Identification of a second family of high-molecular-weight adhesion proteins expressed by nontypeable *Haemophilus influenzae*. Mol Microbiol 1996;19:1215–1223.

91. Barham WB, Church P, Brown JE, et al. Misidentification of *Brucella* species with use of rapid bacterial identification systems. Clin Infect Dis 1993;17:1068–1069.

92. Barka NE, Hadfield T, Patnaik M, et al. EIA for detection of *Rochalimaea henselae*-reactive IgG, IgM, and IgA antibodies in patients with suspected cat scratch disease. J Infect Dis 1993;167:1503–1504.

93. Baron S, Njamkepo E, Grimprel E, et al. Epidemiology of pertussis in French hospitals in 1993 and 1994: thirty years after a routine use of vaccination. Pediatr Infect Dis J 1998;17:412–418.

94. Basaranoglu M, Mert A, Tabak F, et al. A case of cervical *Brucella* spondylitis with paravertebral abscess and neurological deficits. Scand J Infect Dis 1999;31:214–215.

95. Baskar B, Desai SP, Parsons MA. Postoperative endophthalmitis due to *Pasteurella multocida*. Br J Ophthalmol 1997;81:172–173.

96. Bass JW, Vincent JM, Person D. The expanding spectrum of *Bartonella* infections: I. Bartonellosis and trench fever. Pediatr Infect Dis 1997;16:2–10.

97. Bass JW, Vincent JM, Person D. The expanding spectrum of *Bartonella* infections: II. Cat-scratch disease. Pediatr Infect Dis J 1997;16:163–179.

98. Bass JW, Wittler RR. Return of epidemic pertussis in the United States. Pediatr Infect Dis J 1994;13:343–345.

99. Batchelor BI, Brindle RJ, Gilks GF, et al. Biochemical misidentification of *Brucella melitensis* and subsequent laboratory-acquired infections. J Hosp Infect 1992;22:159–162.

100. Baucheron S, Grayon M, Zygmunt MS, Cloeckaert A. Lipopolysaccharide heterogeneity in *Brucella* strains isolated from marine mammals. Res Microbiol 2002;153:277–280.

101. Baum M, Zamir O, Bergman-Rios R, et al. Comparative evaluation of microagglutination test and serum agglutination test as supplementary diagnostic methods for brucellosis. J Clin Microbiol 1995;33:2166–2170.

102. Bauwens JE, Spach DH, Schacker W, et al. *Bordetella bronchiseptica* pneumonia and bacteremia following bone marrow transplantation. J Clin Microbiol 1992;30:2474–2475.

103. Beales IL. Spontaneous bacterial peritonitis due to *Pasteurella multocida* without animal exposure. Am J Gastroenterol 1999;94:1110–1111.

104. Beier CL, Horn M, Michel R, et al. The genus *Caedibacter* comprises endosymbionts of *Paramecium* spp. related to the Rickettsiales (α-proteobacteria) and to *Francisella tularensis* (γ-proteobacteria). Appl Environ Microbiol 2002;68:6043–6050.

105. Bekir NA, Gungor K, Namiduru M. *Brucella melitensis* dacryoadenitis: a case report. Eur J Ophthalmol 2000;10:259–261.

106. Bell J, Grass S, Jeanteur D, Munson RS Jr. Diversity of the P2 protein among nontypeable *Haemophilus influenzae*. Infect Immun 1994;62:2639–2643.

107. Bell JM, Turnidge JD, Pfaller MA, Jones RN. In vitro assessment of gatifloxacin spectrum and potency tested against *Haemophilus influenzae*, *Moraxella catarrhalis*, and *Streptococcus pneumoniae* isolates from Asia-Western Pacific component of the SENTRY antimicrobial surveillance program (1998–1999). Diagn Microbiol Infect Dis 2002;43:315–318.

108. Bellido-Casado J, Perez-Castrillon JL, Bachuller-Luque P, et al. Report on five cases of tularaemic pneumonia in a tularaemia outbreak in Spain. Eur J Clin Microbiol Infect Dis 2000;19:218–220.

109. Benaoudia F, Escande F, Simonet M. Infection due to *Actinobacillus lignieresii* after a horse bite. Eur J Clin Microbiol Infect Dis 13:439–440, 1994.

110. Benson RF, Lanier-Thacker W, Plikaytis BB, et al. Cross-reactions in *Legionella* antisera with *Bordetella pertussis* strains. J Clin Microbiol 1987;25:594–596.

111. Berdal BP, Mehl R, Haaheim H, et al. Field detection of *Francisella tularensis*. Scand J Infect Dis 2000;32:287–291.

112. Bereswill S, Hinkelmann S, Kist M, Sander A. Molecular analysis of riboflavin synthesis genes in *Bartonella henselae* and use of the *ribC* gene for differentiation of *Bartonella* species by PCR. J Clin Microbiol 1999;37:3159–3166.

113. Berger C, Altwegg M, Meyer A, Nadal D. Broad range polymerase chain reaction for diagnosis of rate-bite fever caused by *Streptobacillus moniliformis*. Pediatr Infect Dis J 2001;20:1181–1182.

114. Bergfors E, Trollfors B, Taranger J, et al. Parapertussis and pertussis: differences and similarities in incidence, clinical course, and antibody responses. Int J Infect Dis 1999;3:140–146.

115. Bergmans AMC, DeJong CMA, Van Amerongen G, et al. Prevalence of *Bartonella* species in domestic cats in the Netherlands. J Clin Microbiol 1997;35:2256–2261.

116. Bergmans AMC, Groothedde JW, Schellekens JFP, et al. Etiology of cat scratch disease: comparison of polymerase chain reaction detection of *Bartonella* (formerly *Rochalimaea*) and *Afipia felis* DNA with serology and skin tests. J Infect Dis 1995;171:916–923.

117. Bergmans AMC, Peeters MF, Schellekens JFP, et al. Pitfalls and fallacies of cat scratch disease serology: evaluation of *Bartonella henselae*-based indirect immunofluorescence assay and enzyme-linked immunoassay. J Clin Microbiol 1997;35:1931–1937.

118. Bergmans AMC, Schellekens JFP, Van Embden JDA, Schouls LM. Predominance of two *Bartonella henselae* variants among cat-scratch disease patients in the Netherlands. J Clin Microbiol 1996;34:254–260.

119. Bermond D, Boulouis HJ, Heller R, et al. *Bartonella bovis* Bermond, et al. sp. nov. and *Bartonella capreoli* sp. nov., isolated from European ruminants. Int J Syst Evol Microbiol 2002;52:383–390.

120. Bermond D, Heller R, Barrat F, et al. *Bartonella birtlesii* sp. nov., isolated from small mammals (*Apodemus* spp.). Int J Syst Evol Microbiol 2000;50:1973–1979.

121. Bernard K, Cooper C, Tessier S, Ewan EP. Use of chemotaxonomy as an aid to differentiate among *Capnocytophaga* species, CDC group DF-3, and aerotolerant strains of *Leptotrichia buccalis*. J Clin Microbiol 1991;29:2263–2265.

122. Bernard K, Tessier S, Winstanley J, et al. Early recognition of atypical *Francisella tularensis* strains lacking a cysteine requirement. J Clin Microbiol 1994;32:551–553.

123. Betriu C, Coronel F, Martin P, Picazo JJ. Peritonitis caused by *Haemophilus parainfluenzae* in a patient undergoing continuous ambulatory peritoneal dialysis. J Clin Microbiol 1999;37:3074–3075.

124. Bevenger L, Maeland JA, Naess AI. Agglutinins and antibodies to *Francisella tularensis* outer membrane antigens in the early diagnosis of disease during an outbreak of tularemia. J Clin Microbiol 1988;26:433–437.

125. Bevanger L, Maeland JA, Naess AI. Competitive enzyme immunoassay for antibodies to a 43,000-molecular-weight *Francisella tularensis* outer membrane protein for the diagnosis of tularemia. J Clin Microbiol 1989;27:922–926.

126. Bezwada HP, Nazarian DG, Booth RE Jr. *Haemophilus influenzae* infection complicating a total knee arthroplasty. Clin Orthop 2002;402:202–205.

127. Bhatnagar N, Getachew E, Straley S, et al. Reduced virulence of rifampicin-resistant mutants of *Francisella tularensis*. J Infect Dis 1994;170:841–847.

128. Biedenbach DJ, Jones RN. Evaluation of in vitro susceptibility testing criteria for gemifloxacin when tested against *Haemophilus influenzae* with reduced susceptibility to ciprofloxacin and ofloxacin. Diagn Microbiol Infect Dis 2002;43:232–236.

129. Biedenbach DJ, Jones RN, Pfaller MA. Activity of BM284756 against 2,681 recent clinical isolates of *Haemophilus influenzae* and *Moraxella catarrhalis*: report from the SENTRY antimicrobial surveillance program (2000) in Europe, Canada, and the United States. Diagn Microbiol Infect Dis 2001;39:245–250.

130. Bieger RC, Brewer NS, Washington JA. *Haemophilus aphrophilus*: a microbiologic and clinical review and report of 42 cases. Medicine (Baltimore) 1978; 57:345–355.

131. Bigel ML, Berardi-Grassias LD, Furioll J. Isolation of *Actinobacillus ureae* (*Pasteurella ureae*) from a patient with otitis media. Eur J Clin Microbiol Infect Dis 1988;7:206–207.

132. Bilgrami S, Bergstrom SK, Peterson DE, et al. *Capnocytophaga* bacteremia in a patient with Hodgkin's disease following bone marrow transplantation: case report and review. Clin Infect Dis 1992;14:1045–1049.

133. Birgisson H, Steingrimsson O, Gudnason T. *Kingella kingae* infections in paediatric patients: 5 cases of septic arthritis, osteomyelitis, and bacteraemia. Scand J Infect Dis 1997;29:495–498.

134. Birkebaek NH, Kristiansen M, Seefeldt T, et al. *Bordetella pertussis* and chronic cough in adults. Clin Infect Dis 1999;29:1239–1242.

135. Birtles RJ. Differentiation of *Bartonella* species using restriction endonuclease analysis of PCR-amplified 16S rRNA genes. FEMS Microbiol Lett 1995;129: 261–266.

136. Birtles RJ, Harrison TG, Saunders NA, et al. Proposals to unify the genera *Grahamella* and *Bartonella*, with descriptions of *Bartonella talpae* comb. nov., *Bartonella peromysci* comb. nov., and three new species, *Bartonella grahamii* sp. nov., *Bartonella taylori* sp. nov., and *Bartonella doshiae* sp. nov. Int J Syst Bacteriol 1995;45:1–8.

137. Birtles RJ, Raoult D. Comparison of partial citrate synthase gene (*gltA*) sequences for phylogenetic analysis of *Bartonella* species. Int J Syst Bacteriol 1996;46:891–897.

138. Bisgaard KM, Kao A, Leake J, et al. *Haemophilus influenzae* invasive disease in the United States, 1994–1995: near disappearance of a vaccine-preventable childhood disease. Emerg Infect Dis 1998;4:229–237.

139. Bisgaard M, Heltberg O, Frederiksen W. Isolation of *Pasteurella caballi* from an infected wound on a veterinary surgeon. APMIS 1991;99:291–294.

140. Bisgaard M, Mutters R. Characterization of some previously unclassified ''*Pasteurella*'' spp. obtained from the oral cavity of dogs and cats and description of a new species tentatively classified with the family *Pasteurellaceae* Pohl 1981 and provisionally called taxon 16. Acta Pathol Microbiol Immunol Scand Sect B 1986;94:177–184.

141. Black S. Epidemiology of pertussis. Pediatr Infect Dis J 1997;16(4 Suppl): S85–S89.

142. Blanche P, Sicard D, Meyniard O, et al. *Capnocytophaga canimorsus* lymphocytic meningitis in an immunocompetent man who was bitten by a dog. Clin Infect Dis 1994;18:654–655.

143. Block SL. Causative pathogens, antibiotic resistance and therapeutic considerations in acute otitis media. Pediatr Infect Dis J 1997;16:449–456.

144. Blum RN, Berry CD, Phillips MG. Clinical illnesses associated with isolation of dysgonic fermenter 3 from stool samples. J Clin Microbiol 1992;30:396–400.

145. Blumer J. Clinical perspectives on sinusitis and otitis media. Pediatr Infect Dis J 1998;17:S68–S72.

146. Bobo RA, Newton EJ. A previously undescribed gram-negative bacillus causing septicemia and meningitis. Am J Clin Pathol 1976;65:564–569.

147. Boerlin P, Siegrist HH, Burnens AP, et al. Molecular identification and epidemiological tracing of *Pasteurella multocida* meningitis in a baby. J Clin Microbiol 2000;38:1235–1237.

148. Bogaerts J, Kestens L, Martinez Tello W, et al. Failure of treatment for chancroid in Rwanda is not related to human immunodeficiency virus infection: in vitro resistance of *Haemophilus ducreyi* to trimethoprim-sulfamethoxazole. Clin Infect Dis 1995;20:924–930.

149. Bogaerts J, LePage P, Kestelyn P, et al. Neonatal conjunctivitis caused by *Pasteurella ureae*. Eur J Clin Microbiol 1985;4:427–428.

150. Bogaerts J, Verhaegen J, Tello WM, et al. Characterization, in vitro susceptibility, and clinical significance of CDC group HB-5 from Rwanda. J Clin Microbiol 1990;28:2196–2199.

151. Bolton RW, Kluever EA, Dyer JK. In vitro immunosuppression mediated by an extracellular polysaccharide from *Capnocytophaga ochracea*: influence on macrophages. J Periodontal Res 1985;20:251–259.

152. Bonnet M, Bonnet E, Alric L, et al. Severe knee arthritis due to *Eikenella corrodens* following a human bite. Clin Infect Dis 1997;24:80–81.

153. Boot E, Oosterhuis A. Thuis HC. PCR for the detection of *Streptobacillus moniliformis*. Lab Anim 2002;36:200–208.

154. Borenstein DG, Simon GL. *Haemophilus influenzae* septic arthritis in adults. Medicine (Baltimore) 1986;65:191–201.

155. Bovre K, Henriksen SD, Jonsson V. Correction of the specific epithet *kingii* in the combinations *Moraxella kingii* Henriksen and Bovre 1968 and *Pseudomonas kingii* Jonsson 1970 to *kingae*. Int J Syst Bacteriol 1974;24:307.

156. Brass EP, Wray LM, McDuff T. *Pasteurella ureae* meningitis associated with endocarditis: report of a case and review of the literature. Eur Neurol 1983; 22:138–141.

157. Brazilian Purpuric Fever Study Group. Brazilian purpuric fever: epidemic purpura fulminans associated with antecedent purulent conjunctivitis. Lancet 1987; 2:757–761.

158. Brazilian Purpuric Fever Study Group. *Haemophilus aegyptius* bacteremia in Brazilian purpuric fever. Lancet 1987;2:761–763.

159. Brazilian Purpuric Fever Study Group. Brazilian purpuric fever identified in a new region of Brazil. J Infect Dis 1992;165(Suppl 1):S16–S19.

160. Breen D, Schonell A, Au T, Reiss-Levy E. *Pasteurella multocida*: a case report of bacteremic pneumonia and a 10-year laboratory review. Pathology 2000; 32:152–153.

161. Breitschwerdt EB, Atkins CE, Brown TT, et al. *Bartonella vinsonii* subsp. *berkhoffii* and related members of the α-subdivision of the *Proteobacteria* in dogs with cardiac arrhythmias, endocarditis, or myocarditis. J Clin Microbiol 1999;37:3618–3626.

162. Breitschwerdt EB, Kordick DL. *Bartonella* infection in animals: carriership, reservoir potential, pathogenicity, and zoonotic potential for human infection. Clin Microbiol Rev 2000;13:428–438.

163. Breitschwerdt EB, Kordick DL, Malarkey DE, et al. Endocarditis in a dog due to infection with a novel *Bartonella* subspecies. J Clin Microbiol 1995;33: 154–160.

164. Breitschwerdt EB, Sontakke S, Cannedy A, et al. Infection with *Bartonella weissii* and detection of *Nanobacterium* antigens in a North Carolina beef herd. J Clin Microbiol 2001;39:879–882.

165. Brenner DJ, Hollis DG, Fanning R, et al. *Capnocytophaga canimorsus* sp. nov. (formerly CDC group DF-2), a cause of septicemia following dog bite, and *C. cynodegmi* sp. nov., a cause of localized wound infection following dog bite. J Clin Microbiol 1989;27:231–235.

166. Brenner DJ, Hollis DG, Moss CW, et al. Proposal of *Afipia* gen. nov., with *Afipia felis* sp. nov., (formerly the cat-scratch disease bacillus), *Afipia clevelandensis* sp. nov. (formerly the Cleveland Clinic Foundation strain), *Afipia broomeae* sp. nov., and three unnamed genospecies. J Clin Microbiol 1991; 29:2450–2460.

167. Brenner DJ, Mayer LW, Carlone GM, et al. Biochemical, genetic, and epidemiologic characterization of *Haemophilus influenzae* biogroup *aegyptius* (*Haemophilus aegyptius*) strains associated with Brazilian purpuric fever. J Clin Microbiol 1988;26:1524–1534.

168. Brenner DJ, O'Connor SP, Winkler HH, et al. Proposals to unify the genera *Bartonella* and *Rochalimaea*, with descriptions of *Bartonella quintana* comb. nov., *Bartonella vinsonii* comb. nov., *Bartonella henselae* comb. nov., and *Bartonella elizabethae* comb. nov., and to remove the Family *Bartonellaceae* from the Order Rickettsiales. Int J Syst Bacteriol 1993;43:777–786.

169. Brentjiens RJ, Ketterer M, Apicella MA, Spinola SM. Fine tangled pili expressed by *Haemophilus ducreyi* are a novel class of pili. J Bacteriol 1996; 178:808–816.

170. Bricker BJ, Ewalt DR, MacMillan AP, et al. Molecular characterization of *Brucella* strains isolated from marine mammals. J Clin Microbiol 2000;38: 1258–1262.

171. Bricker BJ, Halling SM. Differentiation of *Brucella abortus* bv. 1, 2, and 4, *Brucella melitensis*, *Brucella ovis*, and *Brucella suis* bv. 1 by PCR. J Clin Microbiol. 1994;32:2660–2666.

172. Bricker BJ, Halling SM. Enhancement of the *Brucella* AMOS PCR assay for differentiation of *Brucella abortus* vaccine strains S19 and RB51. J Clin Microbiol 199533:1640–1642.

173. Bricker BJ, Tabatabai LB, Judge BA, et al. Cloning expression, and occurrence of the *Brucella* Cu-Mn dismutase. Infect Immun 1990;58:2933–2939.

174. Brill CB, Pearlstein LS, Kaplan JM, Mancall EL. CNS infection caused by *Eikenella corrodens*. Arch Neurol 39:431–432, 1982.

175. Brion JP, Recule C, Croize J, et al. Isolation of *Francisella tularensis* from lymph node aspirate inoculated into a non-radiometric blood culture system. Eur J Clin Microbiol Infect Dis 1996;15:180–181.

176. Brissette CA, Fives-Taylor PM. *Actinobacillus actinomycetemcomitans* may utilize either actin-dependent or actin-independent mechanisms of invasion. Oral Microbiol Immunol 1999;14:137–142.

177. Brivet F, Guibert M, Barthelemy P, et al. *Pasteurella multocida* sepsis after hemorrhagic shock in a cirrhotic patient: possible role of endoscopic procedures and gastrointestinal translocation. Clin Infect Dis 1994;18:842–843.

178. Brogan JM, Lally ET, Poulsen K, et al. Regulation of *Actinobacillus actinomycetemcomitans* leukotoxin expression: analysis of the promoter regions of leukotoxic and minimally leukotoxic strains. Infect Immun 1994;62:501–508.

179. Brook I. Bacteriology of acute and chronic frontal sinusitis. Arch Otolaryngol Head Neck Surg 2002;128:583–585.

180. Brouqui P, Houpikian P, DuPont HT, et al. Survey of the seroprevalence of *Bartonella quintana* in homeless people. Clin Infect Dis 1996;23:756–759.

181. Brouqui P, LaScola B, Roux V, Raoult D. Chronic *Bartonella quintana* bacteremia in homeless patients. N Engl J Med 1999;340:184–189.

182. Broussard LA. Biological agents: weapons of warfare and bioterrorism. Mol Diagn 2001;6:323–333.

183. Bruant G, Gousset N, Quentin R, Rosenau A. Fimbrial *ghf* gene cluster of genital strains of *Haemophilus* spp. Infect Immun 2002;70:5438–5445.

184. Bruneel F, D'estanque J, Fournier PE, et al. Isolated right-sided *Bartonella quintana* endocarditis in an immunocompetent adult. Scand J infect Dis 1998; 30:424–425.

185. Bruss JB, Malley R, Halperin S, et al. Treatment of severe pertussis: a study of the safety and pharmacology of intravenous pertussis immunoglobulin. Pediatr Infect Dis J 1999;18:505–511.

186. Bruun B, Ying Y, Kirkegaard E, Frederiksen W. Phenotypic differentiation of *Cardiobacterium hominis*, *Kingella indologenes*, and CDC group EF-4. Eur J Clin Microbiol 1984;3:230–235.

187. Buck GE. Detection of *Bordetella pertussis* by rapid-cycle PCR and colorimetric microwell hybridization. J Clin Microbiol 1996;34:1355–1358.

188. Bullock DW, Devitt PG. Pancreatic abscess and septicaemia caused by *Haemophilus segnis*. J Infect 1981;3:82–85.

189. Bundle DR, Cherwonogrodzky JW, Gidney JW, et al. Definition of *Brucella* A and M epitopes by monoclonal typing reagents and synthetic oligosaccharides. Infect Immun 1992;57:2829–2836.

190. Burns JL, Mendelman PM, Levy J, et al. A permeability barrier as a mechanism of chloramphenicol resistance in *Haemophilus influenzae*. Antimicrob Agents Chemother 1985;27:46–54.

191. Butt TS, Khan A, Ahmad A, et al. *Pasteurella multocida* infectious arthritis with acute gout after a cat bite. J Rheumatol 1997;24:1649–1652.

192. Buu-hoi AY, Joundy S, Acar JF. Endocarditis caused by *Capnocytophaga ochracea*. J Clin Microbiol 1988;26:1061–1062.

193. Byrd LH, Anama L, Gutkin M, et al. *Bordetella bronchiseptica* peritonitis associated with continuous ambulatory peritoneal dialysis. J Clin Microbiol 1981;14:232–233.

194. Caldeira L, Dutschmann L, Carmo G, et al. Fatal *Pasteurella multocida* infection in a systemic lupus erythematosus patient. Infection 1993;21:254–255.

195. Campbell JD, Lagos R, Levine MM, Losonsky GA. Standard and alternative regimens of *Haemophilus influenzae* type b conjugate vaccine (polyribosylribitol phosphate-tetanus toxoid conjugate vaccine) elicit comparable antibody avidities in infants. Pediatr Infect Dis J 2002 ;21:822–826.

196. Campos A, Taylor JH, Campbell M. Hamster bite peritonitis: *Pasteurella pneumotropica* peritonitis in a dialysis patient. Pediatr Nephrol 2000;15:31–32.

197. Caniza MA, Granger DL, Wilson KH, et al. *Bartonella henselae*: etiology of pulmonary nodules in a patient with depressed cell-mediated immunity. Clin Infect Dis 1995;20:1505–1511.

198. Canning PC, Roth JA, Deyoe BL. Release of 5′-guanosine monophosphate and adenine by *Brucella abortus* and the intracellular survival of the bacteria. J Infect Dis 1986;154:464–470.

199. Carbeck RB, Murphy JF, Britt EM. Streptobacillary rat-bite fever with massive pericardial effusion. JAMA 1967;201:133–134.

200. Carden SM, Colville DJ, Gonis G, Gilbert GL. *Kingella kingae* endophthalmitis in an infant. Austral NZ J Ophthalmol 1991;19:217–220.

201. Carlone GM, Gorelkin L, Gheesling LL, et al. Potential virulence-associated factors in Brazilian purpuric fever. J Clin Microbiol 1989;27:609–614.

202. Carlsson RM, Claesson BA, Fagerlund E, et al. Antibody persistence in five-year-old children who received a pentavalent combination vaccine in infancy. Pediatr Infect Dis J 2002;21:535–541.

203. Caron E, Gross A, Liautard J-P, Dornand J. *Brucella* species release a specific, protease-sensitive, inhibitor of TNF-α expression, active on human macrophage-like cells. J Immunol 1996;156:2885–2893.

204. Carpenter PD, Heppner BT, Gnann JW. DF-2 bacteremia following cat bites: report of two cases. Am J Med 1987;82:621–623.

205. Carter GR. Genus I. *Pasteurella* Trevisan 1887. 94AL. Nom. cons. Opin. 13, Jud. Comm. 1954, 153. In: Krieg NR, Holt JG, eds. Bergey's Manual of Systematic Bacteriology. Vol. 1. Baltimore: Williams & Wilkins, 1984:552–557.

206. Casanas MC, Queipo-Ortuno MI, Rodriguez-Torres A, et al. Specificity of a polymerase chain reaction assay of a target sequence on the 31-kilodalton *Brucella* antigen DNA used to diagnose human brucellosis. Eur J Clin Microbiol Infect Dis 2001;20:127–131.

207. Centers for Disease Control and Prevention. Recommendations of the Immunization Practices Advisory Committee (ACIP): Recommendations for use of *Haemophilus* b conjugate vaccines and a combined diphtheria-tetanus-pertussis and *Haemophilus* b vaccine. MMWR Morb Mortal Wkly Rep 1993;42:RR-13.

208. Centers for Disease Control and Prevention. Summary of notifiable diseases, United States, 1993. MMWR Morb Mortal Wkly Rep 1993;42:952–960.

209. Centers for Disease Control and Prevention. Pertussis vaccination: use of acellular pertussis vaccines among infants and young children. Recommendations of the Advisory Committee on Immunization Practices. MMWR Morb Mortal Wkly Rep 1997;46(RR-7):1–25.

210. Centers for Disease Control and Prevention. Unlicensed use of combination of *Haemophilus influenzae* type b conjugate vaccine and diphtheria and tetanus toxoid and acellular pertussis vaccine for infants. MMWR Morb Mortal Wkly Rep 1998;47:787.

211. Centers for Disease Control and Prevention. Suspected brucellosis case prompts investigation of possible bioterrorism-related activity—New Hampshire and Massachusetts, 1999. MMWR Morb Mortal Wkly Rep 2000;49:509–512.

212. Centers for Disease Control and Prevention. Recommended childhood immunization schedule: United States, January-December, 2000. American Academy of Pediatrics Committee in Infectious Diseases. Pediatrics 2000;105:148–151.

213. Chadha V, Warady BA. *Capnocytophaga canimorsus* peritonitis in a pediatric peritoneal dialysis patient. Pediatr Nephrol 1999;13:646–648.

214. Chakraborty RN, Meigh RE, Kaye GC. *Kingella kingae* prosthetic valve endocarditis. Indian Heart J 1999;51:438–439.

215. Challapalli M, Covert RF. Infectious diseases casebook: *Pasteurella multocida* early onset septicemia in newborns. J Perinatol 1997;17:248–249.

216. Chamberlin J, Laughlin L, Gordon S, et al. Serodiagnosis of *Bartonella bacilliformis* infection by indirect immunofluorescence antibody assay: test development and application in an area of bartonellosis endemicity. J Clin Microbiol 2000;38:4269–4271.

217. Chambers GW, Westblom TU. Pleural infection caused by *Capnocytophaga canimorsus*, formerly CDC group DF-2. Clin Infect Dis 1992;15:325–326.

218. Chan PC, Lu CY, Lee PI, et al. *Haemophilus influenzae* type b meningitis with subdural effusion: a case report. J Microbiol Immunol Infect 2002;35:61–64.

219. Chan R, Hardiman RP. Endocarditis caused by *Brucella melitensis*. Med J Aust 1993;158:631–632.

220. Chang C-c, Chomel BB, Kasten RW, et al. *Bartonella* spp. isolated from wild and domestic ruminants in North America. Emerg Infect Dis 2000;6:306–311.

221. Chang C-c, Chomel BB, Kasten RW, et al. Molecular evidence of *Bartonella* spp. in questing adult *Ixodes pacificus* ticks in California. J Clin Microbiol 2001;39:1221–1226.

222. Chang C-c, Hayashidani H, Pusterla N, et al. Investigation of *Bartonella* infection in ixodid ticks from California. Comp Immunol Microbiol Infect Dis 2002 ; 25:229–236.

223. Chang C-c, Kasten RW, Chomel BB, et al. Coyotes (*Canis latrans*) as the reservoir for a human pathogenic *Bartonella* sp.: molecular epidemiology of *Bartonella vinsonii* subsp. *berkhoffii* infection in coyotes from central coastal California. J Clin Microbiol 2000;38:4193–4200.

224. Chang C-c, Yamamoto K, Chomel BB, et al. Seroepidemiology of *Bartonella vinsonii* subsp. *berkhoffii* infection in California coyotes, 1994–1998. Emerg Infect Dis 1999;5:711–715.

225. Chang KC, Zakheim RM, Cho CT, et al. Post-traumatic purulent meningitis due to *Bordetella bronchiseptica*. J Pediatr 1975;86:639–640.

226. Chao C-L, Chang S-C, Sheu J-C, et al. Transdiaphragmatic *Actinobacillus actinomycetemcomitans* infection: case report. Clin Infect Dis 1994;19: 958–960.

227. Chapin-Robertson K, Dahlberg SE, Edberg SC. Clinical and laboratory analyses of cytospin-prepared gram stains for recovery and diagnosis of bacteria from sterile body fluids. J Clin Microbiol 1992;30:377–380.

228. Chen C. Distribution of a newly described species, *Kingella oralis*, in the human oral cavity. Oral Microbiol Immunol 1996;11:425–427.

229. Chen C, Ashimoto A. Clonal diversity of oral *Eikenella corrodens* within individual subjects by arbitrarily primed PCR. J Clin Microbiol 1996;34: 1837–1839.

230. Chen C-KC, Potts TV, Wilson ME. A homologies shared among *Eikenella corrodens* isolates and other corroding bacilli from the oral cavity. J Periodontal Res 1990;25:106–112.

231. Chen C-CK, Sunday GJ, Zambon JJ, Wilson ME. Restriction endonuclease analysis of *Eikenella corrodens*. J Clin Microbiol 1990;28:1265–1270.

232. Chen RV, Bradley JS. *Haemophilus parainfluenzae* sepsis in a very low birth weight premature infant: a case report and review of the literature. J Perinatol 1999;19:315–317.

233. Chen S, Hicks L, Yuen M, et al. Serological cross-reaction between *Legionella* spp. and *Capnocytophaga ochracea* by using latex agglutination test. J Clin Microbiol 1994;32:3054–3055.

234. Chen Y-C, Chang S-C, Luh K-T, et al. *Actinobacillus actinomycetemcomitans* endocarditis: a report of four cases and review of the literature. Q J Med 1991; 81:871–878.

235. Cherry JD. Comparative efficacy of acellular pertussis vaccines: an analysis of recent trials. Pediatr Infect Dis J 1997;16:S90–S96.

236. Cherry JD. Pertussis in the preantibiotic and prevaccine era, with emphasis on adult pertussis. Clin Infect Dis 1999;28(Suppl 2):S107–S111.

237. Cherry JD. Epidemiological, clinical, and laboratory aspects of pertussis in adults. Clin Infect Dis 1999;28(Suppl 2):S112–S117.

238. Cherry JD, Beer T, Chartrand SA, et al. Comparison of values of antibody to *Bordetella pertussis* antigens in young German and American men. Clin Infect Dis 1995;20:1271–1274.

239. Chia JKS, Nakata MN, Lami JLM, et al. Azithromycin for the treatment of cat-scratch disease. Clin Infect Dis 1998;26:193–194.

240. Childs JE, Rooney JA, Cooper JL, et al. Epidemiologic observations on infec-

tion with *Rochalimaea* species among cats living in Baltimore, Md. J Am Vet Med Assoc 1994;204:1775–1778.

241. Chirgwin K, DeHovitz JA, Dillon S, McCormack WM. HIV infection, genital ulcer disease, and crack cocaine use among patients attending a clinic for sexually transmitted diseases. Amer J Public Health 1991;81:1576–1579.

242. Chodosh J. Cat's tooth keratitis: human corneal infection with *Capnocytophaga canimorsus*. Cornea 2001;0:661–663.

243. Chomel BB, Abbott RC, Kasten RW, et al. *Bartonella henselae* in domestic cats in California: risk factors and association between bacteremia and antibody titers. J Clin Microbiol 1995;3:2445–2450.

244. Chomel BB, Boulouis HJ, Petersen H, et al. Prevalence of *Bartonella* infection in domestic cats in Denmark. Vet Res 2002;3:205–213.

245. Chomel BB, DeBess EE, Mangiamele DM, et al. Changing trends in the epidemiology of human brucellosis in California from 1973–1992: a shift toward foodborne transmission. J Infect Dis 1994;70:1216–1223.

246. Chomel BB, Kasten RW, Floyd-Hawkins K, et al. Experimental transmission of *Bartonella henselae* by the cat flea. J Clin Microbiol 1996;4:1952–1956.

247. Chomel BB, MacDonald KA, Kasten RW, et al. Aortic valve endocarditis in a dog due to *Bartonella clarridgeiae*. J Clin Microbiol 2001;39:3548–3554.

248. Choy KW, Wulffraat NM, Wolfs TF, et al. *Bordetella bronchiseptica* respiratory infection in a child after bone marrow transplantation. Pediatr Infect Dis J 1999;18:481–483.

249. Christen RD. *Cardiobacterium hominis* endocarditis in a patient with a hypersensitivity reaction to penicillin. Successful treatment with partial resection of the posterior mitral valve leaflet and antibiotic therapy with cefazolin. Infection 1990;18:291–293.

250. Christensen H, Bisgaard M, Angen O, Olsen JE. Final classification of Bisgaard taxon 9 as *Actinobacillus arthritidis* sp. nov. and recognition of a novel genomospecies for equine strains of *Actinobacillus lignieresii*. Int J Syst Evol Microbiol 2002;52:1239–1246.

251. Christensen H, Bisgaard M, Olsen JE. Reclassification of equine isolates previously reported as *Actinobacillus equuli*, variants of *A. equuli*, *Actinobacillus suis* or Bisgaard taxon 11 and proposal of *A. equuli* subsp. *equuli* subsp. nov. and *A. equuli* subsp. *haemolyticus* subsp. nov. Int J Syst Evol Microbiol 2002; 52:1569–1576.

252. Christensen JJ, Kirkegaard E, Korner B. *Haemophilus* isolated from unusual anatomical sites. Scand J Infect Dis 1990;22:437–444.

253. Christopher GW, Cieslak TJ, Pavlin JA, Eitzen MM Jr. Biological warfare: a historical perspective. JAMA 1997;278:412–417.

254. Chuba PJ, Bock R, Graf G, et al. Comparison of 16S RNA sequences from the Family *Pasteurellaceae*: phylogenetic relatedness by cluster analysis. J Gen Microbiol 1988;134:1923–1930.

255. Chui L, Albritton W, Paster B, et al. Development of the polymerase chain reaction for diagnosis of chancroid. J Clin Microbiol 1993;31:659–664.

256. Church S, Harrigan KE, Irving AE, Peel MM. Endocarditis caused by *Pasteurella caballi* in a horse. Aust Vet J 1998;76:528–530.

257. Ciantar M, Spratt DA, Newman HN, Wilson M. *Capnocytophaga granulosa* and *Capnocytophaga haemolytica*: novel species in subgingival plaque. J Clin Periodontol 2001;28:701–705.

258. Clairmont GJ, Zon LI, Groopman JE. *Haemophilus parainfluenzae* prostatitis in a homosexual man with chronic lymphadenopathy and HTLV-III infection. Am J Med 1987;82:175–178.

259. Clarridge JE III, Raich TJ, Pirwani D, et al. Strategy to detect and identify *Bartonella* species in routine clinical laboratory yields *Bartonella henselae* from human immunodeficiency virus-positive patient and unique *Bartonella* strain from his cat. J Clin Microbiol 1995 ;33:2107–2113.

260. Clarridge JE III, Raich TJ, Sjostedt A, et al. Characterization of two unusual clinically significant *Francisella* strains. J Clin Microbiol 1996;34:1995–2000.

261. Clavareau C, Wellemans V, Walravens K, et al. Phenotypic and molecular characterization of a *Brucella* strain isolated from a mink whale (*Balaenoptera acutorostrata*). Microbiology 1999;144:3267–3273.

262. Cloeckaert A, Grayon M, Grepinet O. An IS711 element downstream of the bp26 gene is a specific marker of *Brucella* spp. isolated from marine mammals. Clin Diagn Lab Immunol 2000;7:835–839.

263. Cloeckaert A, Verger JM, Grayon M, et al. Classification of *Brucella* spp. isolated from marine animals by DNA polymorphism at the *omp2* locus. Microbes Infect 2001;3:729–738.

264. Cockerell CJ, LeBoit PE. Bacillary angiomatosis: a newly characterized, pseudoneoplastic, infectious, cutaneous vascular disorder. J Am Acad Dermatol 1990;22:501–512.

265. Coggin JH Jr. Bacterial pathogens. In: Fleming DO, Hunt DL, eds. Biological Safety: Principles and Practices. 3rd Ed. Washington, DC: ASM Press, 2000: 65–88.

266. Cohn SE, Knorr KL, Gilligan PH, et al. Pertussis is rare in human immunodeficiency virus disease. Am Rev Respir Dis 1993;147:411–413.

267. Cokca F, Azap A, Meco O. Bilateral mammary abscess due to *Brucella melitensis*. Scand J Infect Dis 1999;31:318–319.

268. Cokca F, Meco O, Arasil E, et al. An intramedullary dermoid cyst abscess

due to *Brucella abortus* biotype 3 at T11-L2 spinal levels. Infection 1994;22: 359–360.

269. Colebunders R, Vael C, Blot K, et al. *Bordetella pertussis* as a cause of chronic respiratory infection in an AIDS patient. Eur J Clin Microbiol Infect Dis 1994; 13:313–315.

270. Collazos J, Diaz F, Ayarza R, et al. *Actinobacillus actinomycetemcomitans*: a cause of pulmonary-valve endocarditis of 18 month's duration with unusual manifestations. Clin Infect Dis 1994;18:115–116.

271. Collins JK, Kelly MT. Comparison of Phadebact coagglutination, Bactigen latex agglutination, and counterimmunoelectrophoresis for detection of *Haemophilus influenzae* type b antigens in spinal fluid. J Clin Microbiol 1983;17: 1005–1008.

272. Coll-Vinent B, Suris X, Lopez-Soto A, et al. *Haemophilus aphrophilus* endocarditis: case report and review. Clin Infect Dis 1995;20:1381–1383.

273. Colmenero JD, Queipo-Ortuno MI, Maria Reguera J, et al. Chronic hepatosplenic abscesses in brucellosis: clinicotherapeutic features and molecular diagnostic approach. Diagn Microbiol Infect Dis 2002;42:159–167.

274. Colmenero JD, Reguera JM, Martos F, et al. Complications associated with *Brucella melitensis* infection: a study of 530 cases. Medicine (Baltimore) 1996; 75:195–211.

275. Colson P, LaScola B, Champsaur P. Vertebral infections caused by *Haemophilus aphrophilus*: case report and review. Clin Microbiol Infect 2001;7:107–113.

276. Colson P, LeBrun L, Drancourt M, et al. Multiple recurrent bacillary angiomatosis due to *Bartonella quintana* in an HIV-infected patient. Eur J Clin Microbiol Infect Dis 1996;15:178–179.

277. Comer JA, Flynn C, Regnery RL, et al. Antibodies to *Bartonella* species in inner-city intravenous drug users in Baltimore Md. Arch Intern Med 1996;156: 2491–2495.

278. Cook PP. Persistent postoperative wound infection with *Pasteurella multocida*: case report and literature review. Infection 1995;23:252.

279. Cookson BT, Cho HL, Herwaldt LA, et al. Biological activities and chemical composition of purified tracheal cytotoxin of *Bordetella pertussis*. Infect Immun 1989;57:2223–2229.

280. Cookson BT, Vandamme P, Carlson C, et al. Bacteremia caused by a novel *Bordetella* species, ''B. hinzii.'' J Clin Microbiol 1994;32:2569–2571.

281. Cooper CL, Van Caeseele P, Canvin J, Nicolle LE. Chronic prosthetic device infection with *Francisella tularensis*. Clin Infect Dis 1999;29:1589–1591.

282. Corbel MJ. Identification of dye-sensitive strains of *Brucella melitensis*. J Clin Microbiol 1991;29:1066–1068.

283. Corbel MJ. Brucellosis: an overview. Emerg Infect Dis 1997;3:213–221.

284. Corbel MJ. Recent advances in brucellosis. J Med Microbiol 1997;6:101–103.

285. Corboz L, Ossent P, Gruber H. Isolation and characterization of group EF-4 bacteria from various lesions in cat, dog, and badger. Int J Med Microbiol Virol Parasitol Infect Dis 1993;279:140–145.

286. Costas M, Owen RJ. Numerical analysis of electrophoretic protein patterns of *Streptobacillus moniliformis* strains from human, murine, and avian infections. J Med Microbiol 1987 ;23:393–311.

287. Courtney SE, Hall RT. *Haemophilus influenzae* sepsis in the premature infant. Am J Dis Child 1978;132:1039–1040.

288. Cox RA, Slack MP. Clinical and microbiological features of *Haemophilus influenzae* vulvovaginitis in young girls. J Clin Pathol 2002;55:961–964.

289. Craig-Mylius KA, Weiss AA. Antibacterial agents and release of periplasmic pertussis toxin from *Bordetella pertussis*. Antimicrob Agents Chemother 2000; 44:1383–1386.

290. Cross JT, Davidson KW, Bradsher RW Jr. *Haemophilus influenzae* epididymoorchitis and bacteremia in a man infected with the human immunodeficiency virus. Clin Infect Dis 1994;19:768–769.

291. Cross JT, Jacobs RF. Tularemia: treatment failures with outpatient use of ceftriaxone. Clin infect Dis 1993;17:976–980.

292. Cuadrado-Gomez LM, Arranz-Caso JA, Cuadros-Gonzalez J, Albarran-Hernandez F. *Pasteurella pneumotropica* pneumonia in a patient with AIDS. Clin Infect Dis 1995;21:445–446.

293. Cundell DR, Kanthakumar K, Taylor GW, et al. Effect of tracheal cytotoxin from *Bordetella pertussis* on human neutrophil function in vitro. Infect Immun 1994;62:639–643.

294. Cunningham BB, Paller As, Katz BZ. Rat bite fever in a pet lover. J Am Acad Dermatol 1998;38:330–332.

295. Currie PF, Codispoti M, Mankad PS, Goodman MJ. Late aortic homograft valve endocarditis caused by *Cardiobacterium hominis*: a case report and review of the literature. Heart 2000;83:579–581.

296. Cutter D, Mason KW, Howell AP, et al. Immunization with *Haemophilus influenzae* Hap adhesin protects against nasopharyngeal colonization in experimental mice. J Infect Dis 2002;186:1115–1121.

297. DaCosta M, Guillou J-P, Garin-Bastuji B, et al. Specificity of six genes sequences for the detection of the genus *Brucella* by DNA amplification. J Appl Bacteriol 1996 ;81:267–275.

298. Dalton MJ, Robinson LE, Cooper J, et al. Use of *Bartonella* antigens for sero-

logic diagnosis of cat-scratch disease at a national referral center. Arch Intern Med 1995;155:1670–1676.

299. Daly JS, Worthington MG, Brenner DJ, et al. *Rochalimaea elizabethae* sp. nov., isolated from a patient with endocarditis. J Clin Microbiol 1993;31:872–881.

300. Daneshvar MI, Hollis DG, Moss CW. Chemical characterization of clinical isolates which are similar to CDC group DF-3 bacteria. J Clin Microbiol 1991;29:2351–2353.

301. Das I, DeGiovanni JV, Gray J. Endocarditis caused by *Haemophilus parainfluenzae* identified by 16S ribosomal RNA sequencing. J Clin Pathol 1997;50:72–74.

302. Dauga C, Miras I, Grimont PAD. Identification of *Bartonella henselae* and *B. quintana* 16S rDNA sequences by branch-, genus-, and species-specific amplification. J Med Microbiol 1996;45:192–199.

303. Daum RS, Murphey-Corb M, Shapira E, et al. Epidemiology of ROB-1 β-lactamase among ampicillin-resistant *Haemophilus influenzae* isolates in the United States. J Infect Dis 1988;157:450–455.

304. Davies RL, Paster BJ, Dewhirst FE. Phylogenetic relationships and diversity within the *Pasteurella haemolytica* complex based on 16S rRNA sequence comparison and outer membrane protein and lipopolysaccharide analysis. Int J Syst Bacteriol 1996;46:736–744.

305. Decker MD. Principles of pediatric combination vaccines and practical issues related to use in clinical practice. Pediatr Infect Dis J 2001;20(Suppl 11):S10–S18.

306. Decker MD, Edwards KM. *Haemophilus influenzae* type b vaccines: history, comparisons, and choices. Pediatr Infect Dis J 1998;17:S113–S116.

307. Decker MD, Graham BS, Hunter EB, Liebowitz SM. Endocarditis and infections of intravascular devices due to *Eikenella corrodens*. Am J Med Sci 1986;292:209–212.

308. Dees SB, Karr DE, Hollis D. Cellular fatty acids of *Capnocytophaga* species. J Clin Microbiol 1982 ;16:779–783.

309. Dehio C, Lanz C, Pohl R, et al. *Bartonella schoenbuchii* sp. nov., isolated from the blood of wild roe deer. Int J Syst Evol Microbiol 2001;51:1557–1565.

310. De La Fuente A, Sanchez JR, Uriz J, et al. Infection of a pacemaker by *Brucella melitensis*. Tex Heart Inst J 1997;24:129–130.

311. De La Puente-Redondo VA, del Blanco NG, Gutierrez-Martin CB, et al. Comparison of different PCR approaches for typing of *Francisella tularensis* strains. J Clin Microbiol 2000;38:1016–1022.

312. De La Rosa GR, Barnett BJ, Ericsson CD, Turk JB. Native valve endocarditis due to *Bartonella henselae* in a middle-aged human immunodeficiency virus-negative woman. J Clin Microbiol 2001;39:3417–3419.

313. DeLey JW, Mannheim W, Mutters R, et al. Inter- and intrafamilial similarities of rRNA cistrons of the *Pasteurellaceae*. Int J Syst Bacteriol 1990;40:126–137.

314. De Ley J, Segers P, Kersters K, et al. Intra- and intergeneric similarities of the *Bordetella* ribosomal ribonucleic acid cistrons: proposal for a new family, *Alcaligenaceae*. Int J Syst Bacteriol 1986;26:405–414.

315. Del Vecchio VG, Kapatral V, Elzer P, et al. The genome of *Brucella melitensis*. Vet Microbiol 2002;90:587–592.

316. Del Vecchio VG, Kapatral V, Redkar RJ, et al. The genome sequence of the facultative intracellular pathogen *Brucella melitensis*. Proc Natl Acad Sci USA 2002;99:443–448.

317. DeMaria TF, Murwin DM, Leake ER. Immunization with outer membrane protein P6 from nontypeable *Haemophilus influenzae* induces bactericidal antibody and affords protection in the chinchilla model of otitis media. Infect Immun 1996;64:5187–5192.

318. De Melker HE, Versteegh FGA, Conyn-van Spaendonck MAE, et al. Specificity and sensitivity of high levels of immunoglobulin G antibodies against pertussis toxin in a single serum sample for diagnosis of infection with *Bordetella pertussis*. J Clin Microbiol 2000;38:800–806.

319. Demetrios P, Constantine B, Demetrios S, Nikolaos A. *Haemophilus influenzae* pyelonephritis in the elderly. Urol Nephrol 2002;34:23–24.

320. Demirkan F, Akalin HE, Simsek H, et al. Spontaneous peritonitis due to *Brucella melitensis* in a patient with cirrhosis. Eur J Clin Microbiol Infect Dis 1993;12:66–67.

321. Dennis DT, Inglesby TV, Henderson DA, et al. Tularemia as a biological weapon: medical and public health management. JAMA 2001;285:2763–2773.

322. Depres-Brummer P, Buijs J, van Engelenburg KC, Osten HR. *Capnocytophaga canimorsus* sepsis presenting as an acute abdomen in an asplenic patient. Neth J Med 200159:213–217.

323. Deshpande LM, Jones RN. Antimicrobial activity of advanced-spectrum fluoroquinolones tested against more than 2000 contemporary bacterial isolates of species causing community-acquired respiratory tract infections in the United States (1999). Diagn Microbiol Infect Dis 2000;37:139–142.

324. De Smet MD, Chan CC, Nussenblatt RB, et al. *Capnocytophaga canimorsus* as the cause of a chronic corneal infection. Am J Ophthalmol 1990;109:240–242.

325. Deulofeu F, Nava JM, Bella F, et al. Prospective epidemiological study of invasive *Haemophilus influenzae* disease in adults. Eur J Clin Microbiol Infect Dis 1994;13:633–638.

326. Dever LL, Shashikumar K, Johanson WG Jr. Antibiotics in the treatment of

acute exacerbations of chronic bronchitis. Expert Opin Investig Drugs 2002;11:911–925.

327. Deville JG, Cherry JD, Christenson PD, et al. Frequency of unrecognized *Bordetella pertussis* infections in adults. Clin Infect Dis 1995;21:639–642.

328. Dewhirst FE, Chen C-K, Paster BJ, Zambon JJ. Phylogeny of species in the Family *Neisseriaceae* isolated from human dental plaque and description of *Kingella orale* sp. nov. Int J Syst Bacteriol 1993;43:490–499.

329. Dewhirst FE, Paster BJ, Bright PL. *Chromobacterium*, *Eikenella*, *Kingella*, *Neisseria*, *Simonsiella*, and *Vitreoscilla* species comprise a major branch of the β-group Proteobacteria by 16S ribosomal ribonucleic acid sequence comparison: transfer of *Eikenella* and *Simonsiella* to the family *Neisseriaceae* (emend.). Int J Syst Bacteriol 1990;39:258–266.

330. Dewhirst FE, Paster BJ, La Fontaine S, et al. Transfer of *Kingella indologenes* (Snell and Lapage 1976) to the genus *Suttonella* gen. nov. as *Suttonella indologenes* comb. nov.; transfer of *Bacteroides nodosus* (Beveridge 1941) to the genus *Dichelobacter* gen. nov. as *Dichelobacter nodosus* comb. nov.; and assignment of the genera *Cardiobacterium*, *Dichelobacter*, and *Suttonella* to *Cardiobacteriaceae* fam. nov. in the γ-division of Proteobacteria on the basis of 16S rRNA sequence comparisons. Int J Syst Bacteriol 1990;40:426–433.

331. Dewhirst FE, Paster BJ, Olsen I, et al. Phylogeny of 54 representative strains of species in the Family *Pasteurellaceae* as determined by comparison of 16S rRNA sequences. J Bacteriol 1992;174:2002–2013.

332. Dewire P, McGrath BE, Brass C. *Haemophilus aphrophilus* osteomyelitis after dental prophylaxis: a case report. Clin Orthop 1999;363:196–202.

333. Dijkmans BAC, Thomeer RTWN, Vielvoye GJ, et al. Brain abscess due to *Streptobacillus moniliformis* and *Actinobacterium meyeri*. Infection 1984;12:262–264.

334. Di Mario A, Sica S, Zini G, et al. Microangiopathic hemolytic anemia and severe thrombocytopenia in *Brucella* infection. Ann Hematol 1995;70:59–60.

335. Dimmitt SB, Christiansen K, Newman M. *Haemophilus paraphrophilus:* an unusual cause of endocarditis. Aust NZ J Med 1994;24:581.

336. Dobrean V, Opris A, Daraban S. An epidemiological and surveillance overview of brucellosis in Romania. Vet Microbiol 2002;90:157–163.

337. Dobson SRM, Kroll JS, Moxon ER. Insertion sequence IS*1016* and absence of *Haemophilus* capsulation genes in the Brazilian purpuric fever clone of *Haemophilus influenzae* biogroup *aegyptius*. Infect Immun 1992;60:618–622.

338. Dockrell DH, Poland GA, Steckelberg JM, et al. Immunogenicity of three *Haemophilus influenzae* type b protein conjugate vaccines in HIV seropositive adults and analysis of predictors of vaccine response. Vaccine 1999;17:2779–2785.

339. Dodman T, Robson J, Pincus D. *Kingella kingae* infections in children. J Paediatr Child Health 2000;36:87–90.

340. Doebbeling BN, Feilmeier ML, Herwaldt LA. Pertussis in an adult man infected with the human immunodeficiency virus. J Infect Dis 1990;161:1296–1298.

341. Doern GV, Chapin KC. Laboratory identification of *Haemophilus influenzae*: effects of basal media on the results of the satellitism test and evaluation of the RapID NH system. J Clin Microbiol 1984;20:599–601.

342. Doern GV, Jones RN, Pfaller MA, et al. *Haemophilus influenzae* and *Moraxella catarrhalis* from patients with community-acquired respiratory tract infections: antimicrobial susceptibility patterns from the SENTRY antimicrobial surveillance program (United States and Canada, 1997). Antimicrob Agents Chemother 1999;43:385–389.

343. Dogan B, Asikainen S, Jousimies-Somer H. Evaluation of two commercial kits and arbitrarily primed PCR for identification and differentiation of *Actinobacillus actinomycetemcomitans*, *Haemophilus aphrophilus* and *Haemophilus paraphrophilus*. J Clin Microbiol 1999 ;37:742–747.

344. Dogan B, Saarela MH, Jousimies-Somer H, et al. *Actinobacillus actinomycetemcomitans* serotype e–biotypes, genetic diversity and distribution in relation to periodontal status. Oral Microbiol Immunol 1999 ;14:98–103.

345. Dolan MJ, Wong MT, Regnery RL, et al. Syndrome of *Rochalimaea henselae* suggesting cat scratch disease. Ann Intern Med 1993;118:331–336.

346. Dolan SA, Dommaraju CB, DeGuzman GB. Detection of *Francisella tularensis* in clinical specimens by use of polymerase chain reaction. Clin Infect Dis 1998;26:764–765.

347. Donnio PY, Allardet-Servent A, Perrin M, et al. Characterization of dermonecrotic toxin-producing strains of *Pasteurella multocida* subsp. *multocida* isolated from man and swine. J Med Microbiol 1999;48:125–131.

348. Dorittke C, Vandamme P, Hinz KH, et al. Isolation of a *Bordetella avium*-like organism from a human specimen. Eur J Clin Microbiol Infect Dis 1995;14:451–454.

349. Dougherty MJ, Spach DH, Larson AM, et al. Evaluation of an extended blood culture protocol to isolate fastidious organisms from patients with AIDS. J Clin Microbiol 1996;34:2444–2447.

350. Douglas E, Coote JG, Parton R, et al. Identification of *Bordetella pertussis* in nasopharyngeal swabs by PCR amplification of a region of the adenylate cyclase gene. J Mol Microbiol 1993;38:140–144.

351. Douglas W, Lundy MD, Kehl DK. Increasing prevalence of *Kingella kingae* in osteoarticular infections in young children. J Pediatr Orthop 1998;18:262–267.

352. Douvier S, Neuwirth C, Filipuzzi M, Kisterman J-P. Chorioamnionitis with intact membranes caused by *Capnocytophaga sputigena*. Eur J Obstet Gynecol Reprod Biol 1999;83:109–112.

353. Drancourt M, Birtles R, Chaumentin G, et al. New serotype of *Bartonella henselae* in endocarditis and cat-scratch disease. Lancet 1996;347:441–443.

354. Drancourt M, Mainardi JL, Brouqui P, et al. *Bartonella (Rochalimaea) henselae* endocarditis in three homeless men. N Engl J Med 1995;332:419–423.

355. Drancourt M, Moal V, Brunet P, et al. *Bartonella (Rochalimaea) quintana* infection in a seronegative hemodialyzed patient. J Clin Microbiol 1996 ;34: 1158–1160.

356. Drapkin MS, Wilson ME, Shrager SM, et al. Bacteremic *Haemophilus influenzae* type b cellulitis in the adult. Am J Med 1977;63:449–452.

357. Droz S, Chi B, Horn E, et al. *Bartonella koehlerae* sp. nov., isolated from cats. J Clin Microbiol 1999;37:1117–1122.

358. Duim B, Vogel L, Puijk W, et al. Fine mapping of outer membrane protein P2 antigenic sites which vary during persistent infection by *Haemophilus influenzae*. Infect Immun 1996;64:4673–4679.

359. Dul MJ, Shlaes DM, Lerner PI. EF-4 bacteremia in a patient with hepatic carcinoid. J Clin Microbiol 1983;18:1260–1261.

360. Duong M, Bescancenot JF, Neuwirth C, et al. Vertebral osteomyelitis due to *Capnocytophaga* species in immunocompetent patients: report of two cases and review. Clin Infect Dis 1996;22:1099–1101.

361. Durmaz G, Us T, Aydinli A, et al. Optimum detection times for bacteria and yeast species with the BACTEC 9120 aerobic blood culture system: evaluation for a 5-year period in a Turkish university hospital. J Clin Microbiol 2003;41: 819–821.

362. Dworkin MS, Sullivan PS, Buskin SE, et al. *Bordetella bronchiseptica* infection in human immunodeficiency virus-infected patients. Clin Infect Dis 1999;28: 1095–1099.

363. Ebinger M, Nichterlein T, Schumacher UK, et al. Isolation of *Capnocytophaga granulosa* from an abscess in an immunocompetent adolescent. Clin Infect Dis 2000;30:606–607.

364. Edwards KM, Decker MD, Graham BS, et al. Immunization of adults with acellular pertussis vaccine. JAMA 1993;269:53–56.

365. Edwards KM, Meade BD, Decker MD, et al. Comparison of 13 acellular pertussis vaccines: overview and serological response. Pediatrics 1995;96:548–557.

366. Edwards R, Finch RG. Characterization and antibiotic susceptibilities of *Streptobacillus moniliformis*. J Med Microbiol 1986;21:39–42.

367. Ehrbar H-U, Gubler J, Harbarth S, Hirschel B. *Capnocytophaga canimorsus* sepsis complicated by myocardial infarction in two patients with normal coronary arteries. Clin Infect Dis 1996;23:335–336.

368. Eigelsbach HT, McGann VG. Genus *Francisella* Dorofe'ev 1947m, 176[AL]. In: Krieg NR, Holt JG, eds. Bergey's Manual of Systematic Bacteriology. Vol. 1. Baltimore: Williams & Wilkins, 1984:394–399.

369. Ejlertsen T, Gahrn-Hansen B, Sogaard P, et al. *Pasteurella aerogenes* isolated from ulcers or wounds in humans with occupational exposure to pigs: a report of 7 Danish cases. Scand J Infect Dis 1996 ;28:567–570.

370. Elkins C. Identification and purification of a conserved heme-regulated hemoglobin- binding outer membrane protein from *Haemophilus ducreyi*. Infect Immun 1995;63:1241–1245.

371. Ellis BA, Regnery RL, Beati L, et al. Rats of the genus *Rattus* are reservoir hosts for pathogenic *Bartonella* species: an Old World origin for a New World disease? J Infect Dis 1999;180:220–224.

372. Ellis J, Oyston PC, Green M, Titball RW. Tularemia. Clin Microbiol Rev 2002; 15:631–646.

373. Elrazek MA. *Brucella* optic neuritis. Arch Intern Med 1991;151:776–778.

374. Elster AD, Macone AB, Kasser JR. Osteomyelitis caused by *Capnocytophaga ochracea*. J Pediatr Orthop 1983;3:613–615.

375. Emanuel PA, Bell R, Dang JL, et al. Detection of *Francisella tularensis* within infected mouse tissues by using a hand-held PCR thermocycler. J Clin Microbiol 2003;41:689–693.

376. Emmett L, Allman KC. *Eikenella corrodens* vertebral osteomyelitis. Clin Nucl Med 2000;25:1059–1069.

377. Enck RE, Bennett JM. Isolation of *Haemophilus aprophilus* from an adult with acute leukemia. J Clin Microbiol 1976;4:194–195.

378. Endara SA, Roati AA, Alizzi AM, et al. Aortic valve endocarditis caused by *Bartonella henselae*: a rare surgical entity. Heart Surg Forum 2001;4:359–360.

379. Enderlin G, Morales L, Jacobs RF, et al. Streptomycin and alternative agents for the treatment of tularemia: review of the literature. Clin Infect Dis 1994; 19:42–47.

380. English CK, Wear DJ, Margileth AM, et al. Cat-scratch disease: isolation and culture of the bacterial agent. JAMA 1988;259:1347–1352.

381. Ericsson M, Sandstrom G, Sjostedt A, et al. Persistence of cell-mediated immunity and decline of humoral immunity to the intracellular bacterium *Francisella tularensis* 25 years after natural infection. J Infect Dis 1994;170:110–114.

382. Eriksen N, Lemming L, Hojlyng N, Bruun B. Brucellosis in immigrants in Denmark. Scand J Infect Dis 2002;34:540–542.

383. Ertem M, Kurekci AE, Aysev D, et al. Brucellosis transmitted by bone marrow transplantation. Bone Marrow Transplant 2000;26:225–226.

384. Erwin AL, Munford RS, Brazilian Purpuric Fever Study Group. Comparison of lipopolysaccharides from Brazilian purpuric fever isolates and conjunctivitis isolates of *Haemophilus influenzae* biogroup Aegyptius. J Clin Microbiol 1989; 27:762–767.

385. Escande F, Bailly A, Bone S, Lemozy J. *Actinobacillus suis* infection after a pig bite. Lancet 1996;348:888.

386. Escande F, Grimont F, Grimont PAD, et al. Deoxyribonucleic acid relatedness among strains of *Actinobacillus* spp. and *Pasteurella ureae*. Int J Syst Bacteriol 1984;34:309–315.

387. Escande F, Vallee E, Aubart F. *Pasteurella caballi* infection following a horse bite. Zentralbl Bakteriol 1997;285:440–444.

388. Esteban J, Albalate M, Caramelo C, et al. Peritonitis involving a *Capnocytophaga* species in a patient undergoing continuous ambulatory peritoneal dialysis. J Clin Microbiol 1995;33:2471–2472.

389. Esteve V, Porcheret H, Clerc D, et al. Septic arthritis due to *Kingella kingae* in an adult. Joint Bone Spine 2001;68:85–86.

390. Ewalt DR, Bricker BJ. Validation of the abbreviated *Brucella* AMOS PCR as a rapid screening method for differentiation of *Brucella abortus* field strain isolates and the vaccine strains, 19 and RB51. J Clin Microbiol 2000;38: 3085–3086.

391. Fainstein V, Luna MA, Bodey GP. Endocarditis due to *Eikenella corrodens* in a patient with acute lymphocytic leukemia. Cancer 1981;48:40–42.

392. Fajfar-Whetstone CJ, Coleman L, Biggs DR, Fox BC. *Pasteurella multocida* septicemia and subsequent *Pasteurella dagmatis* septicemia in a diabetic patient. J Clin Microbiol 1995;33:202–204.

393. Fakih MG, Murphy TF, Pattoli MA, Berenson CS. Specific binding of *Haemophilus influenzae* to minor gangliosides of human respiratory epithelial cells. Infect Immun 1997;65:1695–1700.

394. Falla TJ, Crook DWM, Brophy LN, et al. PCR for capsular typing of *Haemophilus influenzae*. J Clin Microbiol 1994;32:2382–2386.

395. Falla TJ, Dobson SRM, Crook DWM, et al. Population-based study of nontypeable *Haemophilus influenzae* invasive disease in children and neonates. Lancet 1993;341:851–854.

396. Farfel Z, Konen S, Wiertz E, et al. Antibodies to *Bordetella pertussis* adenylate cyclase are produced in man during pertussis infection and after vaccination. J Med Microbiol 1990;32:173–177.

397. Farley MM, Stephens DS, Kaplan SL, et al. Pilus- and non-pilus-mediated interactions of *Haemophilus influenzae* type b with human erythrocytes and human nasopharyngeal mucosa. J Infect Dis 1990;161:274–280.

398. Farlow J, Smith KL, Wong J, et al. *Francisella tularensis* strain typing using multiple-locus, variable-number tandem repeat analysis. J Clin Microbiol 2001; 39:3186–3192.

399. Faro S, Walker C, Pierson RL. Amnionitis with intact amniotic membranes involving *Streptobacillus moniliformis*. Obstet Gynecol 1980;55(Suppl):9S–11S.

400. Feldman JD, Kontaxis EN, Sherman MP. Congenital bacteremia due to *Capnocytophaga*. Pediatr Infect Dis J 1985;4:415–416.

401. Feldman WE, Schwartz J. *Haemophilus influenzae* type b brain abscess complicating meningitis: a case report. Pediatrics 1983;72:473–475.

402. Fellows L, Boivin M, Kapusta M. *Pasteurella multocida* arthritis of the shoulder associated with postsurgical lymphedema. J Rheumatol 1996;23: 1824–1825.

403. Felmingham D, Gruneberg RN, Alexander Project Group. The Alexander Project 1996–1997: latest susceptibility data from this international study of bacterial pathogens from community-acquired lower respiratory tract infections. J Antimicrob Chemother 2000;45:191–203.

404. Fenichel S, Bodino C, Kocka F. Isolation of *Actinobacillus actinomycetemcomitans* from a skin lesion. Eur J Clin Microbiol 1985;4:428–429.

405. Ferber B, Bruckheimer E, Schlesinger Y, et al. *Kingella kingae* endocarditis in a child with hair-cartilage hypoplasia. Pediatr Cardiol 1997;18:445–446.

406. Fernandez-Esparrach G, Mascaro J, Rota R, et al. Septicemia, peritonitis, and empyema due to *Pasteurella multocida* in a cirrhotic patient. Clin Infect Dis 1994;18:486.

407. Ficht TA, Bearden SW, Sowa BA, Adams LG. DNA sequence and expression of the 36-kilodalton outer membrane protein gene of *Brucella abortus*. Infect Immun 1989;57:3281–3291.

408. Fink DL, Green BA, St Geme JW III. The *Haemophilus influenzae* Hap autotransporter binds to fibronectin, laminen, and collagen IV. Infect Immun 2002 ; 70:4902–4907.

409. Finkelstein JL, Brown TP, O'Reilly KL, et al. Studies on the growth of *Bartonella henselae* in the cat flea (Siphonaptera: *Pulicidae*). J Med Entomol 2002; 39:915–919.

410. Finlay FO, Witherow H, Rudd PT. Latex agglutination testing in bacterial meningitis. Arch Dis Child 1995;73:160–163.

411. Finn M, Dale B, Isles C. Beware of the dog! A syndrome resembling thrombotic

thrombocytopenic purpura associated with *Capnocytophaga canimorsus* septicaemia. Nephrol Dial Transplant 1996;11:1839–1840.

412. Fiori PL, Mastrandrea S, Rappelli P, Cappuccinelli P. *Brucella abortus* infection acquired in microbiology laboratories. J Clin Microbiol 2000;38:2005–2006.

413. Fischer LJ, Weyant RS, White EH, Quinn FD. Intracellular multiplication and toxic destruction of cultured macrophages by *Capnocytophaga canimorsus*. Infect Immun 1995;63:3483–3490.

414. Fisher RG, Benjamin DK Jr. Facial cellulitis in childhood: a changing spectrum. South Med J 2002;95:672–674.

415. Flemmig TF, Rudiger S, Hofman U, et al. Identification of *Actinobacillus actinomycetemcomitans* in subgingival plaque by PCR. J Clin Microbiol 33:3102–3105, 1995.

416. Flesher SA, Bottone EJ. *Eikenella corrodens* cellulitis and arthritis of the knee. J Clin Microbiol 1989;27:2606–2608.

417. Fordham JN, McKay-Ferguson E, Davies A, et al. Rat bite fever without the bite. Ann Rheum Dis 1992;51:411–412.

418. Forsman M, Sandstrom G, Jaurin B. Identification of *Francisella* species and discrimination of type A and type B strains of *F. tularensis* by 16S rRNA analysis. Appl Environ Microbiol 1990;56:949–955.

419. Forsman M, Sandstrom G, Sjostedt A. Analysis of 16S DNA sequence of *Francisella* strains and utilization for determination of the phylogeny of the genus and for identification of strains by PCR. Int J Syst Bacteriol 1994;44:38–46.

420. Fortier AH, Leiby DA, Narayanan RB, et al. Growth of *Francisella tularensis* LVS in macrophages: the acidic intracellular compartment provides essential iron required for growth. Infect Immun 1995;63:1478–1483.

421. Fortier AH, Slayter MV, Ziemba R, et al. Live vaccine strain of *Francisella tularensis*: infection and immunity in mice. Infect Immun 1999;59:2922–2928.

422. Foster G, Jahans KL, Reid RJ, Ross HM. Isolation of *Brucella* species from cetaceans, seals, and an otter. Vet Rec 1996;138:583–586.

423. Foster G, MacMillan AP, Godfroid J, et al. A review of *Brucella* sp. infection of sea mammals with particular emphasis on isolates from Scotland. Vet Microbiol 2002;90:563–580.

424. Foster G, Ross HM, Malnick H, et al. *Actinobacillus delphinicola* sp. nov., a new member of the family *Pasteurellaceae* Pohl (1979) 1981 isolated from sea mammals. Int J Syst Bacteriol 1996;46:648–652.

425. Foster G, Ross HM, Malnick H, et al. *Phocoenobacter uteri* gen. nov., sp. nov., a new member of the family *Pasteurellaceae* Pohl (1979) 1981 isolated from a harbor porpoise (*Phocoena phocoena*). Int J Syst Evol Microbiol 2000 50:135–139.

426. Foster G, Ross HM, Patterson IA, et al. *Actinobacillus scotiae* sp. nov., a new member of the family *Pasteurellaceae* Pohl (1979) 1981 isolated from porpoises (*Phocoena phocoena*). Int J Syst Bacteriol 1998;48:929–933.

427. Foucault C, Barrau K, Brouqui P, Raoult D. *Bartonella quintana* bacteremia among homeless people. Clin Infect Dis 2002;35:684–689.

428. Fournier PE, Bernabeu L, Schubert B, et al. Isolation of *Francisella tularensis* by centrifugation of shell vial cell culture from an inoculation eschar. J Clin Microbiol 1998;36:2782–2783.

429. Fournier PE, Lelievre H, Eykyn SJ, et al. Epidemiologic and clinical characteristics of *Bartonella quintana* and *Bartonella henselae* endocarditis: a study of 48 patients. Medicine (Baltimore) 2001;80:245–251.

430. Foweraker JE, Hawkey PM, Heritage J, et al. Novel β-lactamase from *Capnocytophaga* sp. Antimicrob Agents Chemother 1990;34:1501–1504.

431. Fox KF, Fox A, Nagpal M, et al. Identification of *Brucella* by ribosomal-spacer-region PCR and differentiation of *Brucella canis* from other *Brucella* spp. pathogenic for humans by carbohydrate profiles. J Clin Microbiol 1998;36:3217–3222.

432. Francioli PB, Foussianos D, Glauser MP. *Cardiobacterium hominis* endocarditis manifesting as bacterial meningitis. Arch Intern Med 1983;143:1483–1484.

433. Frandsen EVG, Reinholdt J, Kjeldsen M, et al. In vivo cleavage of immunoglobulin A1 by immunoglobulin A1 proteases from *Prevotella* and *Capnocytophaga* species. Oral Microbiol Immunol 1995;10:291–296.

434. Franz DR, Jahrling PB, Friedlander AM, et al. Clinical recognition and management of patients exposed to biological warfare agents. JAMA 1997;278:399–411.

435. Frazier JP, Cleary TG, Pickering LK. Meningitis due to *Haemophilus parainfluenzae*: report of three cases and review of the literature. Pediatr Infect Dis 1981;1:117–119.

436. Frebourg NB, Berthelot G, Hocq R, et al. Septicemia due to *Pasteurella pneumotropica*: 16S rRNA sequencing for diagnosis confirmation. J Clin Microbiol 2002;40:687–689.

437. Frederiksen W, Tonning B. Possible misidentification of *Haemophilus aphrophilus* as *Pasteurella gallinarum*. Clin Infect Dis 2001;32:987–989.

438. Friedl J, Stift A, Berlakovich GA, et al. *Haemophilus parainfluenzae* liver abscess after successful liver transplantation. J Clin Microbiol 1998;36:818–819.

439. Friedman RL, Paulaitis S, McMillan JW. Development of a rapid diagnostic test for pertussis: direct detection of pertussis toxin in respiratory secretions. J Clin Microbiol 1989;27:2466–2470.

440. Friesen CA, Cho CT. Characteristic features of neonatal sepsis due to *Haemophilus influenzae*. Rev Infect Dis 1986;8:777–780.

441. Friis-Moller A. A new *Actinobacillus* species from the human respiratory tract: *Actinobacillus hominis* nov. sp. In: Kilian M, Frederiksen W, Biberstein EL, eds. Haemophilus, Pasteurella, and Actinobacillus. London, Academic Press, 1981:151–160.

442. Friis-Moller A, Christensen JJ, Fussing V, et al. Clinical significance and taxonomy of *Actinobacillus hominis*. J Clin Microbiol 39:930–935, 2001.

443. Funke G, Hess T, von Graevenitz A, Vandamme P. Characteristics of *Bordetella hinzii* strains isolated from a cystic fibrosis patient over a 3-year period. J Clin Microbiol 1996;34:966–969.

444. Gadberry JL, Zipper R, Taylor JA, et al. *Pasteurella pneumotropica* isolated from bone and joint infections. J Clin Microbiol 1984;19:926–927.

445. Gadea I, Cuenca-Estrella M, Benito N, et al. *Bordetella hinzii*: a ''new'' opportunistic pathogen to think about. J Infect 2000;40:298–299.

446. Galle C, Streulens M, Liesnard C, et al. *Brucella melitensis* osteitis following craniotomy in a patient with AIDS. Clin Infect Dis 1997;24:1012.

447. Gan VN, Murphy TV. Pertussis in hospitalized children. Am J Dis Child 1990;144:1130–1134.

448. Gandara B, Merino AL, Rogel MA, Martinez-Romero E. Limited genetic diversity of *Brucella* spp. J Clin Microbiol 2001;39:235–240.

449. Garcia FU, Wojta J, Hoover RL. Interactions between live *Bartonella bacilliformis* and endothelial cells. J Infect Dis 1992;165:1138–1141.

450. Garcia del Blanco N, Dobson ME, Vela AI, et al. Genotyping of *Francisella tularensis* strains by pulsed-field gel electrophoresis, amplified fragment length polymorphism fingerprinting, and 16S rRNA sequencing. J Clin Microbiol 2002;40:2964–2972.

451. Garcia-Rodriguez JA, Baquero E, Garcia de Lomas J, et al. Antimicrobial susceptibility of 1,422 *Haemophilus influenzae* isolates from respiratory tract infections in Spain: results of a 1-year (1996–1997) multicenter surveillance study. Infection 1999;27:265–267.

452. Garcia San Miguel L, Quereda C, Martinez M, et al. *Bordetella bronchiseptica* cavitary pneumonia in a patient with AIDS. Eur J Clin Microbiol Infect Dis 1998;17:675–676.

453. Garin-Bastuiji B, Bowden RA, Dubray G, Limet JN. Sodium dodecyl sulfate-polyacrylamide gel electrophoresis and immunoblotting analysis of smooth-lipopolysaccharide heterogeneity among *Brucella* biovars related to A and M specificities. J Clin Microbiol 1990;28:2169–2174.

454. Garpenholdt O, Hugosson S, Fredlund H, et al. Epiglottitis in Sweden before and after introduction of vaccination against *Haemophilus influenzae* type b. Pediatr Infect Dis J 1999;18:490–493.

455. Garrity GM. Holt JG. Bergey's Manual of Systematic Bacteriology: an overview of the roadmap to the manual. New York: Bergey's Manual Trust/Springer, 2000.

456. Gasquet S, Maurin M, Brouqui P, et al. Bacillary angiomatosis in immunocompromised patients. AIDS 1998;12:1793–1803.

457. Gazi MI, Cox SW, Clark DT, Eley BM. Characterization of protease activities in *Capnocytophaga* spp., *Porphyromonas gingivalis*, *Prevotella* spp., *Treponema denticola*, and *Actinobacillus actinomycetemcomitans*. Oral Microbiol Immunol 199712:240–248.

458. Genne D, Siegrist HH, Monnier P, et al. *Pasteurella multocida* endocarditis: report of a case and review of the literature. Scand J Infect Dis 1996;28:95–97.

459. Georgilis K, Kontoyannis S, Prifti H, Petrocheilou-Paschou V. *Haemophilus influenzae* type b endocarditis in a woman with mitral valve prolapse. Clin Microbiol Infect 1998;4:115–116.

460. Gerber JE, Johnson JE, Scott MA, Madhusudhan KT. Fatal meningitis and encephalitis due to *Bartonella henselae* bacteria. J Forensic Sci 2002;47:640–644.

461. Ghez D, Bernard L, Bayou E, et al. *Bartonella henselae* infection mimicking a splenic lymphoma. Scand J Infect Dis 2001;33:935–936.

462. Giladi M, Avidor B, Kletter Y, et al. Cat scratch disease: the rare role of *Afipia felis*. J Clin Microbiol 1998;36:2499–2502.

463. Gill V, Cunha BA. Tularemia pneumonia. Semin Respir Infect 1997;12:61–67.

464. Gill VJ, Travis LB, Williams DY. Clinical and microbiological observations on CDC group DF-3, a gram-negative coccobacillus. J Clin Microbiol 1991;29:1589–1592.

465. Gilsdorf JR, Chang HY, McCrea KW, et al. Comparison of hemagglutinating pili of type b and nontypeable *Haemophilus influenzae*. J Infect Dis 1992;165(Suppl 1):S105–S106.

466. Gilsdorf JR, McCrea KW, Marrs CF. Role of pili in *Haemophilus influenzae* adherence and colonization. Infect Immun 1997;65:2997–3002.

467. Glare EM, Paton JC, Premier RR, et al. Analysis of a repetitive DNA sequence from *Bordetella pertussis* and its application to the diagnosis of pertussis using the polymerase chain reaction. J Clin Microbiol 1990;28:1982–1987.

468. Glasser DB. Angular blepharitis caused by gram-negative bacillus DF-2. Am J Ophthalmol 1986;102:119–120.

469. Glaus T, Greene R, Hofmann-Lehmann C, et al. Seroprevalence of *Bartonella henselae* infection and correlation with disease status in cats in Switzerland. J Clin Microbiol 1997;35:2883–2885.

470. Glickman M, Klein RS. Acute epiglottitis due to *Pasteurella multocida* in an adult without animal exposure. Emerg Infect Dis 1997;3:408–409.

471. Gmur R, McNabb H, van Steenbergen TJM, et al. Seroclassification of hitherto nontypeable *Actinobacillus actinomycetemcomitans* strains: evidence for a new serotype e. Oral Microbiol Immunol 8:116–120, 19.

472. Godfroid J, Kasbohrer A. Brucellosis in the European Union and Norway at the turn of the 21st century. Vet Microbiol 2002;90:135–145.

473. Goldbaum FA, Leoni J, Wallach JC, et al. Characterization of an 18-kilodalton *Brucella* cytoplasmic protein which appears to be a serological marker of active infection in both human and bovine brucellosis. J Clin Microbiol 1993;31:2141–2145.

474. Goldbaum FA, Velikovsky CA, Baldi P, et al. The 18-kDa cytoplasmic protein of *Brucella* species—an antigen useful in diagnosis—is a lumazine synthase. J Med Microbiol 1999;48:833–839.

475. Goldstein DA, Mouritsen L, Friedlander S, et al. Acute endogenous endophthalmitis due to *Bartonella henselae*. Clin Infect Dis 2001;33:718–721.

476. Goldstein EJC, Citron DM. Comparative activities of cefuroxime, amoxicillin-clavulanic acid, ciprofloxacin, enoxacin, and ofloxacin against aerobic and anaerobic bacteria isolated from bite wounds. Antimicrob Agents Chemother 1988;32:1143–1148.

477. Goldstein EJC, Citron DM. Comparative susceptibilities of 173 aerobic and anaerobic bite wound isolates to sparfloxacin, temafloxacin, clarithromycin, and older agents. Antimicrob Agents Chemother 1993;37:1150–1153.

478. Goldstein EJC, Citron DM, Gerardo SH, et al. Activities of HMR 3004 (RU 64004) and HMR 3647 (RU 66647) compared to those of erythromycin, azithromycin, clarithromycin, roxithromycin, and eight other antimicrobial agents against unusual aerobic and anaerobic human and animal bite pathogens isolated from skin and soft tissue infections in humans. Antimicrob Agents Chemother 199;42:1127–1132.

479. Goldstein EJC, Citron DM, Merriam CV. Linezolid activity compared to those of selected macrolides and other agents against aerobic and anaerobic pathogens isolated from soft tissue bite infections in humans. Antimicrob Agents Chemother 1999;43:1469–1474.

480. Goldstein EJC, Citron DM, Merriam CV, et al. Activity of gatifloxacin compared to those of five other quinolones versus aerobic and anaerobic isolates from skin and soft tissue samples of human and animal bite wound infections. Antimicrob Agents Chemother 1999;43:1475–1479.

481. Goldstein EJC, Sutter VL, Finegold SM. Susceptibility of *Eikenella corrodens* to ten cephalosporins. Antimicrob Agents Chemother 1978;14:639–641.

482. Golnik KC, Marotto ME, Fanous MM, et al. Ophthalmic manifestations of *Rochalimaea* species. Am J Ophthalmol 1994;118:145–151.

483. Gomez L, Grazziutti M, Sumoza D, et al. Bacterial pneumonia due to *Bordetella bronchiseptica* in a patient with acute leukemia. Clin Infect Dis 1998;26:1002–1003.

484. Gomez-Garces J-L, Alos J-I, Sanchez J, et al. Bacteremia by multidrug-resistant *Capnocytophaga sputigena*. J Clin Microbiol 1994;32:1067–1069.

485. Goncalves Da Costa PS, Gomes CA, Pinheiro Cangussu I, et al. *Pasteurella multocida* splenic abscess causing fever of unknown origin: report of one case. Braz J Infect Dis 1999;3:238–242.

486. Goncharoff P, Figurski DH, Stevens RH, et al. Identification of *Actinobacillus actinomycetemcomitans*: polymerase chain reaction amplification of *lktA*-specific sequences. Oral Microbiol Immunol 1993;8:105–110.

487. Gonin P, Lorange M, Delage G. Performance of a multiplex PCR for the determination of *Haemophilus influenzae* capsular types in the clinical microbiology laboratory. Diagn Microbiol Infect Dis 2000;37:1–4.

488. Gonzalez MH, Garst J, Nourbash P, et al. Abscesses of the upper extremity from drug abuse by injection. J Hand Surg Am 1993;18:868–870.

489. Goral S, Anderson B, Hager C, et al. Detection of *Rochalimaea henselae* DNA by polymerase chain reaction from suppurative nodes of children with cat-scratch disease. Pediatr Infect Dis J 1994;13:994–997.

490. Gotuzzo E, Carrillo C, Guerra J, et al. An evaluation of diagnostic methods for brucellosis: the value of bone marrow culture. J Infect Dis 1986;153:122–125.

491. Gousset N, Rosenau A, Sizaret P-Y, Quentin R. Nucleotide sequences of genes coding for fimbrial proteins in a cryptic genospecies of *Haemophilus* spp. isolated from neonatal and genital tract infections. Infect Immun 1999;67:8–15.

492. Gradus MS, Ng C, Pries R, et al. An unsuspected case of brucellosis mimicking appendicitis in a child. Clin Microbiol Newslett 1988;10:180–190.

493. Grahnquist L, Eriksson M. Pertussis and necrotizing enterocolitis in a previously healthy neonate. Pediatr Infect Dis J 1993;12:698–699.

494. Grando D, Sullivan LJ, Flexman JP, et al. *Bartonella henselae* associated with Parinaud's oculoglandular syndrome. Clin Infect Dis 1999;28:1156–1158.

495. Grasso RJ, West LA, Holbrook NJ, et al. Increased sensitivity of a new coagglutination test for rapid identification of *Haemophilus influenzae* type b. J Clin Microbiol 198113:1122–1124.

496. Gratten M. *Haemophilus influenzae* biotype VII. J Clin Microbiol 1983;13:1015–1016.

497. Graves MH, Janda JM. Rat-bite fever (*Streptobacillus moniliformis*): a potential emerging disease. Int J Infect Dis 2001 2001;5:151–155.

498. Gray CG, Cowley SC, Cheung KK, Nano FE. The identification of five genetic loci of *Francisella tularensis* associated with intracellular growth. FEMS Microbiol Lett 2002;215:53–56.

499. Greene BT, Ramsey KM, Nolan PE. *Pasteurella multocida* meningitis: case report and review of the last 11 years. Scand J Infect Dis 2002;34:213–217.

500. Greene JN, Sandin RL, Villanueva L, Sinnott JT. *Haemophilus parainfluenzae* endocarditis in a patient with mitral valve prolapse. Ann Clin Lab Sci 1993;23:203–206.

501. Gregory RL, Kim DE, Kindle JC, et al. Immunoglobulin-degrading enzymes in localized juvenile periodontitis. J Periodontal Res 1992;27:176–183.

502. Gruner E, Bernasconi E, Galeazzi L, et al. Brucellosis: an occupational hazard for medical laboratory personnel: report of five cases. Infection 1994;2:33–36.

503. Grunow R, Splettstoesser W, McDonald S, et al. Detection of *Francisella tularensis* in biological specimens using a capture enzyme-linked immunosorbent assay, an immunochromatographic handheld assay, and a PCR. Clin Diagn Lab Immunol 2000;7:86–90.

504. Gu K, Bainbridge B, Darveau RP, Page RC. Antigenic components of *Actinobacillus actinomycetemcomitans* lipopolysaccharide recognized by sera from patients with localized juvenile periodontitis. Oral Microbiol Immunol 1998;13:150–157.

505. Gu X-X, Rossau R, Jannes G, et al. The rrs (16S)-rrl (23S) ribosomal intergenic spacer region as a target for the detection of *Haemophilus ducreyi* by a heminested-PCR assay. Microbiology 1998 ;144:1013–1019.

506. Gu X-X, Sun J, Jin S, et al. Detoxified lipooligosaccharide from nontypeable *Haemophilus influenzae* conjugated to proteins confers protection against otitis media in chinchillas. Infect Immun 1997;65:4488–4493.

507. Gueirard P, Weber C, Le Coustumier A, Guiso N. Human *Bordetella bronchiseptica* infection related to contact with infected animals: persistence of bacteria in host. J Clin Microbiol 1995;33:2002–2006.

508. Guettler MV, Rumler D, Jain MK. *Actinobacillus succinogenes* sp. nov., a novel succinic acid-producing strain from the bovine rumen. Int J Syst Bacteriol 1999;49:207–216.

509. Guiso N, Grimprel E, Anjak I, et al. Western blot analysis of antibody responses of young infants to pertussis infection. Eur J Clin Microbiol Infect Dis 1993;12:506–600.

510. Gump DW, Holden RA. Endocarditis caused by a new species of *Pasteurella*. Ann Intern Med 1972;76:275–278.

511. Gurfield AN, Boulouis H-J, Chomel BB, et al. Coinfection with *Bartonella clarridgeiae* and *Bartonella henselae* and with different *Bartonella henselae* strains in domestic cats. J Clin Microbiol 1997;35:2120–2123.

512. Gurycova D. First isolation of *Francisella tularensis* subsp. *tularensis* in Europe. Eur J Epidemiol 1998;14:797–802.

513. Gustafsson B, Askelof P. Monoclonal antibody-based sandwich enzyme-linked immunosorbent assay for detection of *Bordetella pertussis* filamentous hemagglutinin. J Clin Microbiol 1988;26:2077–2082.

514. Gustafsson B, Lindquist U, Andersson M. Production and characterization of monoclonal antibodies directed against *Bordetella pertussis* lipopolysaccharide. J Clin Microbiol 1988;26:188–193.

515. Gustafsson L, Hallander HO, Olin P, et al. A controlled trial of a two-component acellular, a five-component acellular, and a whole-cell pertussis vaccine. N Engl J Med 1996;334:349–355.

516. Gustke CJ. A review of localized juvenile periodontitis (LJP). I. Clinical features, epidemiology, etiology, and pathogenesis. Gen Dent 1998;46:491–497.

517. Gustke CJ. A review of localized juvenile periodontitis (LJP). II. Clinical trials and treatment guidelines. Gen Dent 1998;46:580–587.

518. Guyot A, Bakhai A, Fry N, et al. Culture-positive *Bartonella quintana* endocarditis. Eur J Clin Microbiol Infect Dis 1999;18:145–147.

519. Habeeb YK, Al-Najdi AK, Sadek SA, Al-Onaizi E. Pediatric neurobrucellosis: case report and literature review. J Infect 199837:59–62.

520. Hadfield TL, Warren R, Kass M, et al. Endocarditis caused by *Rochalimaea henselae*. Hum Pathol 2001;24:1140–1141.

521. Hadjinikolaou L, Triposkiadis F, Zairis M, et al. Successful management of *Brucella melitensis* endocarditis with combined medical and surgical approach. Eur J Cardiothorac Surg 2001;19:806–810.

522. Hadley S, Albrecht MA, Tarsy D. Cat-scratch encephalopathy: a cause of status epilepticus and coma in a healthy young adult. Neurology 1995;45:196.

523. Hagelskjaer L, Sorensen I, Randers E. *Streptobacillus moniliformis* infection: 2 cases and a literature review. Scand J Infect Dis 1998;30:309–311.

524. Hallander HO. Microbiological and serological diagnosis of pertussis. Clin Infect Dis 1999;28(Suppl 2):S99–S106.

525. Hallander HO, Reizenstein E, Renemar B, et al. Comparison of nasopharyngeal aspirates with swabs for culture of *Bordetella pertussis*. J Clin Microbiol 1993;31:50–52.

526. Hallander HO, Storsaeter J, Mollby R. Evaluation of serology and nasopharyn-

geal cultures for diagnosis of pertussis in a vaccine efficacy trial. J Infect Dis 1991;163:1046–1054.

527. Halperin SA, Bortolussi R, Kasina A, et al. Use of a Chinese hamster ovary cell cytotoxicity assay for the rapid diagnosis of pertussis. J Clin Microbiol 1990;28:32–38.

528. Halperin SA, Bortolussi R, Wort J. Evaluation of culture, immunofluorescence, and serology for the diagnosis of pertussis. J Clin Microbiol 1989;27:752–757.

529. Halperin SA, King J, Law B, et al. Safety and immunogenicity of *Haemophilus influenzae*-tetanus toxoid conjugate vaccine given separately or in combination with a three-component acellular pertussis vaccine combined with diphtheria and tetanus toxoids and inactivated poliovirus vaccine for the first four doses. Clin Infect Dis 1999;28:995–1001.

530. Halperin SA, Marrie TJ. Pertussis encephalopathy in an adult: case report and review. Rev Infect Dis 1991;13:1043–1047.

531. Hamamoto Y, Soejima Y, Ogasawara M, et al. Necrotizing fasciitis due to *Pasteurella multocida* infection. Dermatology 1995 ;190:145–147.

532. Hamed KA, Dormitzer PR, Su CK, et al. *Haemophilus parainfluenzae* endocarditis: application of a molecular approach for identification of pathogenic bacterial species. Clin Infect Dis 1994;19:677–683.

533. Hammerberg O, Gregson DB, Gopaul D, et al. Recurrent cervical and submandibular lymphadenitis due to *Actinobacillus actinomycetemcomitans*. Clin Infect Dis 1998;17:1077–1078.

534. Han N, Hoover CI, Winkler JR, et al. Identification of genomic clonal types of *Actinobacillus actinomycetemcomitans* by restriction endonuclease analysis. J Clin Microbiol 29:1574–1578, 1991.

535. Handley SA, Regnery RL. Differentiation of pathogenic *Bartonella* species by infrequent restriction site PCR. J Clin Microbiol 2000;38:3010–3015.

536. Hannah P, Greenwood JR. Isolation and rapid identification of *Haemophilus ducreyi*. J Clin Microbiol 1982;7:39–43.

537. Hanner TL, Allen JW, Robertson-Byers A, Hurley SL. Characterization of eugonic fermenter group EF-4 by polyacrylamide gel electrophoresis and protein immunoblot analysis. Am J Vet Res 1991;52:1065–1068.

538. Hansen LM, Blanchard PC, Hirsh DC. Distribution of *tet(H)* among *Pasteurella* isolates from the United States and Canada. Antimicrob Agents Chemother 1996;40:1558–1560.

539. Hara H, Ochiai T, Morishima T, et al. *Pasteurella canis* osteomyelitis and cutaneous abscess after a domestic dog bite. J Am Acad Dermatol 2002;46(5 Suppl):S151–S152.

540. Haraszthy VI, Hariharan G, Tinoco EM, et al. Evidence for the role of highly leukotoxic *Actinobacillus actinomycetemcomitans* in the pathogenesis of localized juvenile and other forms of early-onset periodontitis. J Periodontol 2000; 71:912–922.

541. Harrison LH, deSilva GA, Pittman M, et al. Epidemiology and clinical spectrum of Brazilian purpuric fever. J Clin Microbiol 1989;27:599–604.

542. Hartley JW, Martin ED, Gothard WP, et al. Fulminant *Capnocytophaga canimorsus* (DF-2) septicaemia and diffuse intravascular coagulation in hairy cell leukemia with splenectomy. J Infect 1994;29:229–230.

543. Hassan IJ, Hayek L. Endocarditis caused by *Kingella denitrificans*. J Infect 1993;27:291–295.

544. Haubek D, Dirienzo JM, Tinoco EM, et al. Racial tropism of a highly toxic clone of *Actinobacillus actinomycetemcomitans* associated with juvenile periodontitis. J Clin Microbiol 1997;35:3037–3042.

545. He Q, Mertsola J, Himanen JP, et al. Evaluation of pooled and individual components of *Bordetella pertussis* as antigens in an enzyme immunoassay for diagnosis of pertussis. Eur J Clin Microbiol Infect Dis 1993;12:690–695.

546. He T, Nishihara T, Demuth DR, Ishikawa I. A novel insertion sequence increases the expression of leukotoxicity in *Actinobacillus actinomycetemcomitans* clinical isolates. J Periodontal 1999;70:1261–1268.

547. Heath PT. *Haemophilus influenzae* type b conjugate vaccines: a review of efficacy data. Pediatr Infect Dis J 1999;17:S117–S122.

548. Heath PT, Booy R, Azzopardi HJ, et al. Non-type b *Haemophilus influenzae* disease: clinical and epidemiologic characteristics in the *Haemophilus influenzae* type b vaccine era. Pediatr Infect Dis J 2001;20:300–305.

549. Heath TC, Hewitt MC, Jalaludin B, et al. Invasive *Haemophilus influenzae* type b disease in elderly nursing home residents: two related cases. Emerg Infect Dis 1997;3:179–182.

550. Hedegaard J, Okkels H, Bruun B, et al. Phylogeny of the genus *Haemophilus* as determined by comparison of partial *infB* sequences. Microbiology 2001; 147:2599–2609.

551. Heidemann DG, Pflugfelder SC, Kronish J, et al. Necrotizing keratitis caused by *Capnocytophaga ochracea*. Am J Ophthalmol 1988105:655–660.

552. Heiner AM, DiSario JA, Carroll K, et al. Dysgonic fermenter-3: a bacterium associated with diarrhea in immunocompromised host. Am J Gastroenterol 1992;87:1629–1630.

553. Heininger U, Stehr K, Schmitt-Grohe S, et al. Clinical characteristics of illness caused by *Bordetella parapertussis* compared with illness caused by *Bordetella pertussis*. Pediatr Infect Dis J 1994;13:306–309.

554. Heiro M, Nikoskelainen J, Engblom E, Kotilainen P. *Eikenella corrodens* pros-

555. Heiss LN, Flak TA, Lancaster JR Jr, et al. Nitric oxide mediates *Bordetella pertussis* tracheal cytotoxin damage to the respiratory epithelium. Infect Agents Dis 1994;2:173–177.

556. Heller R, Artois M, Xemar V, et al. Prevalence of *Bartonella henselae* and *Bartonella clarridgeiae* in stray cats. J Clin Microbiol 1997;35:1327–1331.

557. Heller R, Kubina M, Mariet P, et al. *Bartonella alsatica* sp nov., a new *Bartonella* species isolated from the blood of wild rabbits. Int J Syst Bacteriol 1999; 49:283–288.

558. Heller R, Riegel P, Hansmann Y, et al. *Bartonella tribocorum* sp. nov., a new *Bartonella* species isolated from the blood of wild rats. Int J Syst Bacteriol 1998;48:1333–1339.

559. Heltberg O, Busk HE, Bremmelgaard A, et al. The cultivation and rapid enzyme identification of DF-2. Eur J Clin Microbiol 1984;3:241–243.

560. Hemady R, Zimmerman A, Katzen BW, Karesh JW. Orbital cellulitis caused by *Eikenella corrodens*. Am J Ophthalmol 1992;114:584–588.

561. Hendolin PH, Karkkainen U, Himi T, et al. High incidence of *Alloiococcus otitidis* in otitis media with effusion. Pediatr Infect Dis J 1999;18:860–865.

562. Henriksen SD, Bovre K. Transfer of *Moraxella kingae* Henriksen and Bovre to the genus *Kingella* gen. nov. in the family *Neisseriaceae*. Int J Syst Bacteriol 1976;26:447–450.

563. Herman L, de Ridder H. Identification of *Brucella* spp. by using the polymerase chain reaction. Appl Env Microbiol 1992 ;58:2099–2101.

564. Hewlett EL. Pertussis: current concepts of pathogenesis and prevention. Pediatr Infect Dis J 1997;16(4 Suppl):S78–S84.

565. Hewlett EL. A commentary on the pathogenesis of pertussis. Clin Infect Dis 1999;28(Suppl 2):S94–S98.

566. Heymann WR, Drezner D. Submandibular abscess caused by *Eikenella corrodens*. Cutis 1997;60:101–102.

567. Hicklin H, Verghese A, Alvarez S. Dysgonic fermenter 2 septicemia. Rev Infect Dis 1987;9:884–890.

568. Higgins JA, Hubalek Z, Halouzka J, et al. Detection of *Francisella tularensis* in infected mammals and vectors using a probe-based polymerase chain reaction. Am J Trop Med Hyg 2000;62:310–318.

569. High NJ, Jennings MP, Moxon ER. Tandem repeats of the tetramer 5′-CAAT-3′ present in lic2A are required for phase variation but not lipopolysaccharide biosynthesis in *Haemophilus influenzae*. Mol Microbiol 1995;20:165–174.

570. Highlander SK. Molecular genetic analysis of virulence in *Mannheimia* (*Pasteurella*) *haemolytica*. Front Biosci 2001;6:D1128–D1150.

571. Highlander SK, Fedorova ND, Dusek DM, et al. Inactivation of *Pasteurella* (*Mannheimia*) *haemolytica* leukotoxin causes partial attenuation in virulence in a calf challenge model. Infect Immun 2000;68:3916–3922.

572. Hill BC, Baker CN, Tenover FC. A simplified method for testing *Bordetella pertussis* for resistance to erythromycin and other antimicrobial agents. J Clin Microbiol 2000;38:1151–1155.

573. Hill SL, Mitchell JL, Stockley RA, Wilson R. The role of *Haemophilus parainfluenzae* in COPD. Chest 2000;117(Suppl 1):293S.

574. Hiltke TJ, Sethi S, Murphy TF. Sequence stability of the gene encoding outer membrane protein P2 of nontypeable *Haemophilus influenzae* in the human respiratory tract. J Infect Dis 2002;185:627–631.

575. Hjelm E, McGill S, Blomqvist G. Prevalence of antibodies to *Bartonella henselae*, *B. elizabethae*, and *B. quintana* in Swedish domestic cats. Scand J Infect Dis 2002;34:192–196.

576. Hoberman A, Marchant CD, Kaplan SL, Feldman S. Treatment of acute otitis media: consensus recommendations. Clin Pediatr (Phila) 2002;41:373–390.

577. Hockman DE, Pence CD, Whittler RR, Smith LE. Septic arthritis of the hip secondary to rat-bite fever: a case report. Clin Orthop 2000;380:173–176.

578. Hodder SL, Cherry JD, Mortimer EA Jr, et al. Antibody responses to *Bordetella pertussis* antigens and clinical correlations in elderly community residents. Clin Infect Dis 2000;31:7–14.

579. Hoel T, Scheel O, Nordahl SHG, et al. Water- and airborne *Francisella tularensis* biovar *palaearctica* isolated from human blood. Infection 1991;19: 348–350.

580. Hoffman ME, Sorr EM, Barza M. *Pasteurella multocida* endophthalmitis. Br J Ophthalmol 1987;71:609–610.

581. Hofstad T, Olsen I, Eribe ER, et al. Dysgonomonas gen. nov. to accommodate *Dysgonomonas gadei*, sp. nov., an organism isolated from a human gall bladder, and *Dysgonomonas capnocytophagoides* (formerly CDC group DF-3). Int J Syst Evol Microbiol 2000;50:2189–2195.

582. Hoiseth SK, Corn PG, Anders J. Amplification status of capsule genes in *Haemophilus influenzae* type b clinical isolates. J Infect Dis 1992;165(Suppl 1):S114.

583. Hoiseth SK, Moxon ER, Silver RP. Genes involved in *Haemophilus influenzae* type b capsule expression are part of an 18-kilobase tandem duplication. Proc Natl Acad Sci USA 1986;83:1106–1110.

584. Holley HP. Successful treatment of cat-scratch disease with ciprofloxacin. JAMA 1991;265:1563–1565.

thetic valve endocarditis in a patient with ulcerative colitis. Scand J Infect Dis 2000;32:324–325.

585. Hollis DG, Weaver RE, Steigerwalt AG, et al. *Francisella philomiragia* comb. nov. (formerly *Yersinia philomiragia*) and *Francisella tularensis* biogroup Novicida (formerly *Francisella novicida*) associated with human disease. J Clin Microbiol 1989;27:1601–1608.

586. Hollis DG, Wiggins GL, Weaver RE. An unclassified gram-negative rod isolated from the pharynx on Thayer-Martin medium (selective agar). Appl Microbiol 24:772–777, 1972.

587. Holmberg M, McGill S, Ehrenborg C, et al. Evaluation of human seroreactivity to *Bartonella* species in Sweden. J Clin Microbiol 1999 ;37:1381–1384.

588. Holmes AH, Greenough TC, Balady GJ, et al. *Bartonella henselae* endocarditis in an immunocompetent adult. Clin Infect Dis 1995;21:1004–1007.

589. Holmes B, Popoff M, Kiredjian M, et al. *Ochrobactrum anthropi* gen. nov., sp. nov. from human clinical specimens and previously known as group Vd. Int J Syst Bacteriol 1988;38:406–416.

590. Holmes RL, Kozinin WP. Pneumonia and bacteremia associated with *Haemophilus influenzae* serotype d. J Clin Microbiol 1983;18:730–732.

591. Holroyd KJ, Reiner AP, Dick JD. *Streptobacillus moniliformis* polyarthritis mimicking rheumatoid arthritis: an urban case of rat-bite fever. Am J Med 1988 ;85:711–714.

592. Holst E, Rollof J, Larsson L, Nielsen JP, et al. Characterization and distribution of *Pasteurella* species recovered from infected humans. J Clin Microbiol 1992;30:2984–2987.

593. Holt SC, Leadbetter ER, Socransky SS. *Capnocytophaga*: a new genus of gram-negative gliding bacteria: II. Morphology and ultrastructure. Arch Microbiol 1979;122:17–27.

594. Honberg PZ, Fredricksen W. Isolation of *Pasteurella multocida* in a patient with spontaneous bacterial peritonitis and liver cirrhosis. Eur J Clin Microbiol Infect Dis 1986;5:340–342.

595. Hoppe JE. Update on respiratory infection caused by *Bordetella parapertussis*. Pediatr Infect Dis J 1999;18:375–381.

596. Hoppe JE, Bryskier A. In vitro susceptibilities of *Bordetella pertussis* and *Bordetella parapertussis* to two ketolides (HMR 3004 and HMR 3647) four macrolides (azithromycin, clarithromycin, erythromycin A and roxithromycin), and two ansamycins (rifampin and rifapentine). Antimicrob Agents Chemother 1998;42:965–966.

597. Hoppe JE, Dalhoff A, Pfrunder D. In vitro susceptibilities of *Bordetella pertussis* and *Bordetella parapertussis* to BAY 12-8039, trovafloxacin, and ciprofloxacin. Antimicrob Agents Chemother 1998;42:1868.

598. Hoppe JE, Halm U, Hagedorn HJ, Kraminer-Hagedorn A. Comparison of erythromycin ethylsuccinate and cotrimoxazole for treatment of pertussis. Infection 1989;17:227–231.

599. Hoppe JE, Paulus T. Comparison of three media for agar dilution testing of *Bordetella pertussis* using six antibiotics. Eur J Clin Microbiol Infect Dis 1998;17:391–393.

600. Hoppe JE, Rahimi-Galougahi E, Seibert G. In vitro susceptibilities of *Bordetella pertussis* and *Bordetella parapertussis* to four fluoroquinolones (levofloxacin, d-ofloxacin, ofloxacin, and ciprofloxacin), cefpirome, and meropenem. Antimicrob Agents Chemother 1996;40:807–808.

601. Hoppe JE, Schlagenhauf M. Comparison of three kinds of blood and two incubation atmospheres for cultivation of *Bordetella pertussis* on charcoal agar. J Clin Microbiol 1989;27:2115–2117.

602. Hoppe JE, Schwaderer J. Comparison of four charcoal media for the isolation of *Bordetella pertussis*. J Clin Microbiol 1989;27:1097–1098.

603. Hoppe JE, Simon CG. In vitro susceptibilities of *Bordetella pertussis* and *Bordetella parapertussis* to seven fluoroquinolones. Antimicrob Agents Chemother 1990;34:2287–2288.

604. Host B, Schumacher H, Prag J, Arpi M. Isolation of *Kingella kingae* from synovial fluids using four commercial blood culture bottles. Eur J Clin Microbiol Infect Dis 2000;19:608–611.

605. Houpikian P, Fournier PE, Raoult D. Phylogenetic position of *Bartonella vinsonii* subsp. *arupensis* based on 16S rRNA and *gltA* gene sequences. Int J Syst Evol Microbiol 2001;51:179–182.

606. Hovenga S, Tulleken JE, Moller LVM, et al. Dog-bite induced sepsis: a report of four cases. Intensive Care Med 1997;23:1179–1180.

607. Howard AW, Viskontas D, Sabbagh C. Reduction in osteomyelitis and septic arthritis related to *Haemophilus influenzae* type b vaccination. J Pediatr Orthop 1999;19:705–709.

608. Howell JM, Woodward GR. Precipitous hypotension in the emergency department caused by *Capnocytophaga canimorsus* sp. nov. sepsis. Am J Emerg Med 1990;8:312–314,.

609. Hoyler SL, Antony S. *Eikenella corrodens*: an unusual cause of severe parapneumonic infection and empyema in immunocompetent patients. J Natl Med Assoc 2001;93:224–229.

610. Hritz M, Fisher E, Demuth DR. Differential regulation of the leukotoxin operon in highly leukotoxic and minimally leukotoxic strains of *Actinobacillus actinomycetemcomitans*. Infect Immun 1996 ;64:2724–2729.

611. Huh Y, Rose S, Schoen R, et al. Colonic bacillary angiomatosis. Ann Intern Med 1996;124:735–737.

612. Hulzebos CV, Koetse HA, Kimpen JLL, Wolfs TFW. Vertebral osteomyelitis associated with cat-scratch disease. Clin Infect Dis 1999;28:1310–1312.

613. Hunt Gerardo S, Citron DM, Claros MC, et al. *Pasteurella multocida* subsp. *multocida* and *Pasteurella multocida* subsp. *septica* differentiation by PCR fingerprinting and α-glucosidase activity. J Clin Microbiol 2001;39:2558–2564.

614. Hussain S, Singh N. Pyomyositis associated with bacillary angiomatosis in a patient with HIV infection. Infection 2002;30:50–53.

615. Hutcheson KA, Magbalon M. Periocular abscess and cellulitis from *Pasteurella multocida* in a healthy child. Am J Ophthalmol 128:514–515, 1999.

616. Hwang JJ, Lau YJ, Hu BS, et al. *Haemophilus parainfluenzae* and *Fusobacterium necrophorum* liver abscess: a case report. J Microbiol Immunol Infect 2002;35:65–67.

617. Ikaheimo I, Syrjala H, Karhukorpi J, et al. In vitro antibiotic susceptibility of *Francisella tularensis* isolated from humans and animals. J Antimicrob Chemother 2000;46:287–290.

618. Inoue T, Ohta H, Kokeguchi S, et al. Colonial variation and fimbriation of *Actinobacillus actinomycetemcomitans*. FEMS Microbiol Lett 1990;57:13–17.

619. Ip M, Teo JG, Cheng AF. Waterhouse-Friderichsen syndrome complicating primary biliary sepsis due to *Pasteurella multocida* in a patient with cirrhosis. J Clin Pathol 1995;48:775–777.

620. Irono K, Grimont F, Casin I. rRNA gene restriction patterns of *Haemophilus influenzae* biogroup *aegyptius* strains associated with Brazilian purpuric fever. J Clin Microbiol 1988;26:1535–1538.

621. Ives TJ, Manzewitsch P, Regnery RL, et al. In vitro susceptibilities of *Bartonella henselae*, *B. quintana*, *B. elizabethae*, *Rickettsia rickettsii*, *R. conorii*, *R. akari*, and *R. prowazekii* to macrolide antibiotics as determined by immunofluorescent-antibody analysis of infected Vero cell monolayers. Antimicrob Agents Chemother 1997;41:578–582.

622. Ives TJ, Marston EL, Regnery RL, et al. In vitro susceptibilities of *Rickettsia* and *Bartonella* spp. to 14-hydroxy-clarithromycin as determined by immunofluorescent antibody analysis of infected Vero cell monolayers. J Antimicrob Chemother 2000;45:305–310.

623. Jackson LA, Cherry JD, Wang S-P, Grayston JT. Frequency of serological evidence of *Bordetella* infections and mixed infections with other respiratory pathogens in university students with cough illness. Clin Infect Dis 2000;31:3–6.

624. Jacobs RF, Condrey YM, Yamauchi T. Tularemia in adults and children: a changing presentation. Pediatrics 1985;76:818–822.

625. Jacobs RF, Schutze GE. *Bartonella henselae* as a cause of prolonged fever and fever of unknown origin in children. Clin Infect Dis 1998;26:80–84.

626. Jahans KL, Foster G, Broughton ES. The characteristics of *Brucella* strains isolated from marine mammals. Vet Microbiol 1997;57:373–382.

627. James EA, Hill J, Uppal R, Prentice MB. *Bartonella* infection: a significant cause of native valve endocarditis necessitating surgical management. J Thorac Cardiovasc Surg 2000;119:171–172.

628. Janda WM, Bradna JJ, Ruther P. Identification of *Neisseria* spp., *Haemophilus* spp, and other fastidious gram-negative bacteria with the MicroScan *Haemophilus-Neisseria* identification panel. J Clin Microbiol 1989;27:869–873.

629. Janda WM, Malloy PJ, Schreckenberger PC. Clinical evaluation of the Vitek *Neisseria-Haemophilus* identification card. J Clin Microbiol 1987;25:37–41.

630. Janda WM, Santos E, Stevens J, et al. Unexpected isolation of *Bordetella pertussis* from a blood culture. J Clin Microbiol 1994;32:2851–2853.

631. Jantzen E, Berdal BP, Omland T. Cellular fatty acid composition of *Francisella tularensis*. J Clin Microbiol 1979;10:928–930.

632. Jansen DL, Gray GC, Putnam SD, et al. Evaluation of pertussis infection among U.S. Marine Corps trainees. Clin Infect Dis 1997;25:1099–1107.

633. Jellicoe PA, Cohan A, Campbell P. *Haemophilus parainfluenzae* complicating total hip arthroplasty: a rapid failure. J Arthroplasty 2002;17:114–116.

634. Jenny DB, Letendre PW, Iverson G. Endocarditis caused by *Kingella indologenes*. Rev Infect Dis 1987;9:787–788.

635. Jensen AE, Cheville NF, Thoen CO, et al. Genomic fingerprinting and development of a dendrogram for *Brucella* spp. isolated from seals, porpoises, and dolphins. J Vet Diagn Invest 1999 ;11:152–157.

636. Jensen KT, Schonheyder H, Thomsen VF. In vitro activity of β-lactam and other antimicrobial agents against *Kingella kingae*. J Antimicrob Chemother 1994;33:635–640.

637. Jensen WA, Fall MZ, Rooney J, et al. Rapid identification and differentiation of *Bartonella* species using a single-step PCR assay. J Clin Microbiol 2000;38:1717–1722.

638. Jeppson KG, Reimer LG. *Eikenella corrodens* chorioamnionitis. Obstet Gynecol 1991;78:503–505.

639. Jepson PD, Brew S, MacMillan AP, et al. Antibodies to *Brucella* in marine animals around the coast of England and Wales. Vet Rec 1997;141:513–515.

640. Jimenez-Lucho V, Shulman M, Johnson J. *Bordetella bronchiseptica* in an AIDS patient cross-reacts with *Legionella* antisera. J Clin Microbiol 1994;32:3095–3096.

641. Joblet C, Roux V, Drancourt M, et al. Identification of *Bartonella* (*Rochali-*

maea) species among fastidious gram-negative bacteria on the basis of the partial sequence of the citrate-synthase gene. J Clin Microbiol 1995;33: 1879–1883.

642. Johansson A, Berglund L, Eriksson U, et al. Comparative analysis of PCR versus culture for diagnosis of ulceroglandular tularemia. J Clin Microbiol 2000;38:22–26.

643. Johansson A, Berglund L, Gothefors L, et al. Ciprofloxacin for treatment of tularemia in children. Pediatr Infect Dis J 2000;19:449–453.

644. Johansson A, Claesson R, Hanstrom L, et al. Polymorphonuclear leukocyte degranulation induced by leukotoxin from *Actinobacillus actinomycetemcomitans*. J Periodontal Res 2000;35:85–92.

645. Johansson A, Goransson I, Larsson P, Sjostedt A. Extensive allelic variation among *Francisella tularensis* strains in a short-sequence tandem repeat region. J Clin Microbiol 2001;39:3140–3146.

646. Johannson A, Ibrahim A, Goransson I, et al. Evaluation of PCR-based methods for discrimination of *Francisella* species and subspecies and development of specific PCR that distinguishes the two major subspecies of *Francisella tularensis*. J Clin Microbiol 2000;38:4180–4185.

647. Johansson A, Urich SK, Chu MC, et al. In vitro susceptibility to quinolones of *Francisella tularensis* subspecies *tularensis*. Scand J Infect Dis 2002;34: 327–330.

648. Johnson SR, Martin DH, Cammarata C, et al. Development of a polymerase chain reaction assay for detection of *Haemophilus ducreyi*. Sex Transm Dis 1994;21:13–23.

649. Jones ME, Karlowsky JA, Blosser-Middleton R, et al. Apparent plateau in β-lactamase production among clinical isolates of *Haemophilus influenzae* and *Moraxella catarrhalis* in the United States: results from the LIBRA surveillance initiative. Int J Antimicrob Agents 2002;19:119–123.

650. Jones RN, Slepak J, Bigelow J. Ampicillin-resistant *Haemophilus paraphrophilus* laryngo-epiglottitis. J Clin Microbiol 1976;4:405–407.

651. Jordens JZ, Leaves NI, Anderson EC, et al. Polymerase chain reaction-based strain characterization of noncapsulate *Haemophilus influenzae*. J Clin Microbiol 1993;31:2981–2987.

652. Jorgensen JH, Howell AW, Maher LA. Antimicrobial susceptibility testing of less commonly isolated *Haemophilus* species using *Haemophilus* test medium. J Clin Microbiol 1990;28:985–988.

653. Jorgensen JH, Redding JD, Maher LA, et al. Improved medium for antimicrobial susceptibility testing of *Haemophilus influenzae*. J Clin Microbiol 1987; 25:2105–2113.

654. Joseph A, Lobo DN, Gardner ID, Iftikhar SY. *Eikenella corrodens* liver abscess complicated by endophthalmitis. Eur J Gastroenterol Hepatol 1998;10: 709–711.

655. Joshi N, O'Bryan T, Appelbaum PC. Pleuropulmonary infections caused by *Eikenella corrodens*. Rev Infect Dis 1991;13:207–212.

656. Jumas-Bilak E, Michaus-Charachon, Bourg G, et al. Differences in chromosome number and genome rearrangements in the genus *Brucella*. Mol Microbiol 1998;27:99–106.

657. Junhui Z, Ruifu Y, Jianchun L, et al. Detection of *Francisella tularensis* by the polymerase chain reaction. J Med Microbiol 1996;45:477–482.

658. Kabeya H, Maruyama S, Irei M, et al. Genomic variation among *Bartonella henselae* isolates derived from naturally infected cats. Vet Microbiol 2002;89: 211–221.

659. Kadikoylu G, Tuncer G, Bolaman Z, Sina M. Brucellar orchitis in Innerwest Anatolia region of Turkey: a report of 12 cases. Urol Int 2002;69:33–35.

660. Kainz A, Lubitz W, Busse HJ. Genomic fingerprints, ARDRA profiles, and quinone systems for classification of *Pasteurella sensu stricto*. Syst Appl Microbiol 2000;23:292–503.

661. Kaka S, Lunz R, Klugman KP. *Actinobacillus* (*Pasteurella*) *ureae* meningitis in a HIV-positive patient. Diagn Microbiol Infect Dis 1994;20:105–107.

662. Kanaan N, Gavage P, Janssens M, et al. *Pasteurella multocida* in peritoneal dialysis: a rare case of peritonitis associated with exposure to domestic cats. Acta Clin Belg 2002;57:254–256.

663. Kao PT, Tseng HK, Su SC, Lee SM. *Haemophilus aphrophilus* brain abscess: a case report. J Microbiol Immunol Infect 2002;35:184–186.

664. Kaplan AH, Weber DJ, Oddone EZ, et al. Infection due to *Actinobacillus actinomycetemcomitans*: 15 cases and review. Rev Infect Dis 1989;11:46–63.

665. Kaplan JB, Schreiner HC, Furgang D, Fine DH. Population structure and genetic diversity of *Actinobacillus actinomycetemcomitans* strains isolated from localized juvenile periodontitis patients. J Clin Microbiol 2002;40:1181–1187.

666. Kaplan SL. Clinical presentations, diagnosis, and prognostic factors of bacterial meningitis. In: Schaad UB, ed. Infectious Disease Clinics of North America. Vol 13. Bacterial Meningitis. Philadelphia, Saunders, 1999:579–594.

667. Karhukorpi EK, Karhukorpi J. Rapid laboratory diagnosis of ulceroglandular tularemia with polymerase chain reaction. Scand J Infect Dis 2001;33:383–385.

668. Karlowsky JA, Critchley IA, Blosser-Middleton RS, et al. Antimicrobial surveillance of *Haemophilus influenzae* in the United States during 2000–2001 leads to detection of clonal dissemination of a β-lactamase-negative and ampicillin-resistant strain. J Clin Microbiol 2002;40:1063–1066.

669. Karlowsky JA, Jones ME, Mayfield DC, et al. Ceftriaxone activity against Gram-positive and Gram-negative pathogens isolated in U.S. clinical microbiology laboratories from 1996 to 2000: results from the Surveillance Network (TSN) Database-USA. Int J Antimicrob Agents 2002;19:413–426.

670. Kaslow HR, Platler BW, Blumberg DA, et al. Detection of antibodies inhibiting the ADP-ribosyltransferase activity of pertussis toxin in human serum. J Clin Microbiol 1992;30:1380–1387.

671. Kattar MM, Chavez JF, Limaye AP, et al. Application of 16S rRNA gene sequencing to identify *Bordetella hinzii* as the causative agent of fatal septicemia. J Clin Microbiol 2000;38:789–794.

672. Katti MK, Sarada C, Sivasankaran S, Shanmugham J. Serological diagnosis of human brucellosis: analysis of seven cases with neurological and cardiological manifestations. J Commun Dis 2001;33:36–43.

673. Katzko G, Hofmeister M, Church D. Extended incubation of culture plates improves recovery of *Bordetella* spp. J Clin Microbiol 1996;34:1563–1564.

674. Kaufmann AF, Meltzer MI, Schmid GP. The economic impact of a bioterrorist attack: are prevention and post-attack intervention programs justifiable? Emerg Infect Dis 1997;3:83–94.

675. Keitel WA. Cellular and acellular pertussis vaccines in adults. Clin Infect Dis 1999;28(Suppl 2):S118–S123.

676. Kemper CA, Lombard CM, Deresinski SC, et al. Visceral bacillary epithelioid angiomatosis: possible manifestations of disseminated cat scratch disease in the immunocompromised host: a report of two cases. Am J Med 1990;89: 216–222.

677. Kempf VA, Petzold H, Autenrieth IB. Cat scratch disease due to *Bartonella henselae* infection mimicking parotid malignancy. Eur J Clin Microbiol Infect Dis 2001;20:732–733.

678. Kennedy CA, Rosen H. *Kingella kingae* bacteremia and adult epiglottitis in a granulocytopenic host. Am J Med 1988;85:701–702.

679. Kerem E, Diav O, Navon P, et al. Pleural fluid characteristics in pulmonary brucellosis. Thorax 1994;49:89–90.

680. Kerkhoff FT, Bergmans AM, van Der Zee A, Rothova A. Demonstration of *Bartonella grahamii* DNA in ocular fluids of a patient with neuroretinitis. J Clin Microbiol 1999;37:4034–4038.

681. Kersters K, Hinz K-H, Hertle A, et al. *Bordetella avium* sp. nov., isolated from the respiratory tracts of turkeys and other birds. Int J Syst Bacteriol 1984;34: 56–70.

682. Khattak MN, Matthews RC. Genetic relatedness of *Bordetella* species as determined by macrorestriction digests resolved by pulsed-field gel electrophoresis. Int J Syst Bacteriol 1993;43:695–664.

683. Khelef N, Sakamoto H, Guiso N. Both adenylate cyclase and hemolytic activities are required by *Bordetella pertussis* to initiate infection. Microb Pathog 1992;12:227–235.

684. Kilian M. A rapid method for the differentiation of *Haemophilus* strains: the porphyrin test. Acta Pathol Microbiol Scand Sect B 1974;82:935–942.

685. Kilian M. A taxonomic study of the genus *Haemophilus* with the proposal of a new species. J Gen Microbiol 1976;93:9–62.

686. Kilian M, Biberstein EL. Genus II. Haemophilus. In: Krieg NR, Holt JG, eds. Bergey's Manual of Systematic Bacteriology. Vol. 1. Baltimore: Williams & Wilkins, 1984:558–559.

687. Kilian M, Poulsen K. Enzymatic, serologic, and genetic polymorphism of *Haemophilus influenzae* IgA1 proteases. J Infect Dis 1992;165(Suppl 1): S192–S193.

688. Killen JW, Swift GL, White RJ. Pleuropulmonary infection with chest wall infiltration by *Eikenella corrodens*. Thorax 1996;51:871–872.

689. Kilpi T, Herva E, Kaijalainen T, et al. Bacteriology of acute otitis media in a cohort of Finnish children followed for the first two years of life. Pediatr Infect Dis J 2001;20:654–662.

690. Kim JO, Ginsberg J, McGowan KL. *Capnocytophaga* meningitis in a cancer patient. Pediatr Infect Dis J 1996;15:636–637.

691. Kingsland RC, Guss DA. *Actinobacillus ureae* meningitis: case report and review of the literature. J Emerg Med 1995;13:623–627.

692. Kirchner BK, Lake SG, Wightman SR. Isolation of *Streptobacillus moniliformis* from a guinea pig with granulomatous pneumonia. Lab Anim Sci 42: 519–521, 1992.

693. Kirmani KI, Lofthus G, Pichichero ME, et al. Seven-year follow-up of vaccine response in extremely premature infants. Pediatrics 2002;109:498–504.

694. Kitzis M-D, Goldstein FW, Miegi M, Acar JF. In vitro activity of levofloxacin, a new fluoroquinolone: evaluation against *Haemophilus influenzae* and *Moraxella catarrhalis*. J Antimicrob Chemother 1999;43(Suppl C):21–26.

695. Klein B, Couch J, Thompson J. Ocular infections associated with *Eikenella corrodens*. Am J Ophthalmol 1990;109:127–131.

696. Klein JL, Nair SK, Harrison TG, et al. Prosthetic valve endocarditis caused by *Bartonella henselae*. Emerg Infect Dis 2002;8:202–203.

697. Kleinfelder JW, Mueller RF, Lange DE. Fluoroquinolones in the treatment of *Actinobacillus actinomycetemcomitans*-associated periodontitis. J Periodontol 2000;71:202–208.

698. Knapp JS, Back A, Babst AF, et al. In vitro susceptibilities of isolates of

Haemophilus ducreyi from Thailand and the United States to currently recommended and newer agents for treatment of chancroid. Antimicrob Agents Chemother 199337:1552–1555.

699. Knutsson N, Trollfors B, Taranger J, et al. Immunogenicity and reactogenicity of diphtheria, tetanus and pertussis toxoids combined with inactivated polio vaccine, when administered concomitantly with or as a diluent for a Hib conjugate vaccine. Vaccine 2001;19:4396–4403.

700. Kocagoz S, Akova M, Altun B, et al. In vitro activities of new quinolones against *Brucella melitensis* isolated in a tertiary care hospital in Turkey. Clin Microbiol Infect 2002;8:240–242.

701. Koch CA, Mabee CL, Robyn JA, et al. Exposure to domestic cats: risk factor for *Pasteurella multocida* peritonitis in liver cirrhosis? Am J Gastroenterol 1996;91:1447–1449.

702. Kodama S, Suenaga S, Hirano T, et al. Induction of specific immunoglobulin A and Th2 immune responses to P6 outer membrane protein of nontypeable *Haemophilus influenzae* in middle ear mucosa by intranasal immunization. Infect Immun 2000;68:2294–2300.

703. Koehler JE. Bacillary angiomatosis: investigation of the unusual interactions between *Rochalimaea* bacilli and endothelial cells. J Lab Clin Med 1994;124:475–477.

704. Koehler JE, Cederberg L. Intra-abdominal mass associated with gastrointestinal hemorrhage: a new manifestation of bacillary angiomatosis. Gastroenterology 1995;109:2011–2014.

705. Koehler JE, Glaser CA, Tappero JW. *Rochalimaea henselae* infection: a new zoonosis with the domestic cat as reservoir. JAMA 1994;271:531–535.

706. Koehler JE, LeBoit PE, Egbert BM, et al. Cutaneous vascular lesions and disseminated cat scratch disease in patients with the acquired immunodeficiency syndrome (AIDS) and AIDS-related complex. Ann Intern Med 1988;109:449–455.

707. Koehler JE, Quinn FD, Berger TG, et al. Isolation of *Rochalimaea* species from cutaneous and osseous lesions of bacillary angiomatosis. N Engl J Med 1992;325:1625–1631.

708. Koehler JE, Sanchez MA, Garrido CS, et al. Molecular epidemiology of *Bartonella* infections in patients with bacillary angiomatosis-peliosis. N Engl J Med 1997;337:1876–1883.

709. Kok RH, Wolfhagen MJ, Mooi BM, Offerman JJ. A patient with thrombotic thrombocytopenic purpura caused by *Capnocytophaga canimorsus* septicemia. Clin Microbiol Infect 1999;5:297–298.

710. Kolodrubetz D, Dailey T, Ebersole J, Craig E. Cloning and expression of the leukotoxin gene from *Actinobacillus actinomycetemcomitans*. Infect Immun 1989;57:1465–1469.

711. Kolodrubetz D, Spitznagel J, Wang B, et al. cis elements and trans factors are both important in strain-specific regulation of the leukotoxin gene in *Actinobacillus actinomycetemcomitans*. Infect Immun 1996;64:3451–3460.

712. Komiya A, Kato T, Nakagawa T, et al. A rapid DNA probe method for detection of *Porphyromonas gingivalis* and *Actinobacillus actinomycetemcomitans*. J Periodontol 71:760–767, 2000.

713. Koopman JP, Van den Brink, Vennix PPCA. Isolation of *Streptobacillus moniliformis* from the middle ear of rats. Lab Anim 1991;25:35–39.

714. Kooter AJ, Derks A, Vasmel WL. Rapidly progressive tricuspid valve endocarditis caused by *Capnocytophaga canimorsus* infection in an immunocompetent host. Clin Microbiol Infect 1999;5:173–175.

715. Kordick DL, Breitschwerdt EB. Persistent infection of pets within a household with three *Bartonella* species. Emerg Infect Dis 1998;4:325–328.

716. Kordick DL, Brown TT, Shin K, Breitschwerdt EB. Clinical and pathologic evaluation of chronic *Bartonella henselae* and *Bartonella clarridgeiae* infection in cats. J Clin Microbiol 1999;37:1536–1547.

717. Kordick DL, Hilyard EJ, Hadfield TL, et al. *Bartonella clarridgeiae*, a newly recognized zoonotic pathogen causing inoculation papules, fever, and lymphadenopathy (cat scratch disease). J Clin Microbiol 1997;35:1813–1818.

718. Kordick DL, Papich MG, Breitschwerdt EB. Efficacy of enrofloxacin and doxycycline for treatment of *Bartonella henselae* and *Bartonella clarridgeiae* infection in cats. Antimicrob Agents Chemother 1997;41:2448–2455.

719. Kordick DL, Swaminathan B, Greene CE, et al. *Bartonella vinsonii* subsp. *berkhoffii* subsp. nov., isolated from dogs; *Bartonella vinsonii* subsp. *vinsonii*; and emended description of *Bartonella vinsonii*. Int J Syst Bacteriol 1996;46:704–709.

720. Kordick DL, Wilson KH, Sexton DJ, et al. Prolonged *Bartonella* bacteremia in cats associated with cat-scratch disease patients. J Clin Microbiol 1995;33:3245–3251.

721. Korgenski EK, Daly JA. Surveillance and detection of erythromycin resistance in *Bordetella pertussis* isolates recovered from a pediatric population in the intermountain west region of the United States. J Clin Microbiol 1997;35:2989–2991.

722. Kosek M, Lavarello R, Gilman RH, et al. Natural history of infection with *Bartonella bacilliformis* in a nonendemic population. J Infect Dis 2000;182:865–872.

723. Koskela P, Salminen A. Humoral immunity against *Francisella tularensis* following natural infection. J Clin Microbiol 1985;22:973–979.

724. Kosoy MY, Regnery RL, Tzianabos T, et al. Distribution, diversity, and host specificity of *Bartonella* in rodents from the Southeastern United States. Am J Trop Med Hyg 1997;57:578–588.

725. Kostman JR, Sherry BL, Fligner CL, et al. Invasive *Haemophilus influenzae* infections in older children and adults in Seattle. Clin Infect Dis 1993;17:289–296.

726. Kragsbjerg P, Nilsson K, Persson L, et al. Deep obstetrical and gynecologic infections caused by non-typeable *Haemophilus influenzae*. Scand J Infect Dis 1993;25:341–346.

727. Krasan GP, Cutter D, Block SL, St Geme JW III. Adhesin expression in matched nasopharyngeal and middle ear isolates of nontypeable *Haemophilus influenzae* from children with acute otitis media. Infect Immun 1999;67:449–454.

728. Krause R, Wenisch C, Fladerer P, et al. Osteomyelitis of the hip joint associated with systemic cat scratch disease in an adult. Eur J Clin Microbiol Infect Dis 2000;19:781–783.

729. Kreiss JK, Koech D, Plummer FA, et al. AIDS virus infection in Nairobi prostitutes: spread of the epidemic to East Africa. N Engl J Med 1986;314:414–418.

730. Kreutzer DL, Robertson DC. Surface macromolecules and virulence in intracellular parasitism: comparison of the cell envelope components of smooth and rough strains of *Brucella abortus*. Infect Immun 1979;23:819–828.

731. Kristensen B, Schonheyder HC, Peterslund NA, et al. *Capnocytophaga* (*Capnocytophaga ochracea* group) bacteremia in hematological patients with profound granulocytopenia. Scand J Infect Dis 1995;27:153–155.

732. Kroll JS. The genetics of encapsulation in *Haemophilus influenzae*. J Infect Dis 1992;165(Suppl 1):S93–S96.

733. Kroll JS, Farrant JL, Tyler S, et al. Characterisation and genetic organisation of a 24-Mdal plasmid from the Brazilian purpuric fever clone of *Haemophilus influenzae* biogroup *aegyptius*. Plasmid 2002;48:38–48.

734. Kroll JS, Hopkins I, Moxon ER. Capsule loss in *H. influenzae* type b occurs by recombination-mediated disruption of a gene essential for polysaccharide export. Cell 1988;53:347–356.

735. Kubiet M, Ramphal E, Weber A, Smith A. Pilus-mediated adherence of *Haemophilus influenzae* to human respiratory mucins. Infect Immun 2000;68:3362–3367.

736. Kugler KC, Biedenbach DJ, Jones RN. Determination of the antimicrobial activity of 29 clinically important compounds tested against fastidious HACEK group organisms. Diagn Microbiol Infect Dis 1999;34:73–76.

737. Kuhnert P, Boerlin P, Emler S, et al. Phylogenetic analysis of *Pasteurella multocida* subspecies and molecular identification of feline *P. multocida* subsp. *septica* by 16S rRNA gene sequencing. Int J Med Microbiol 2000;290:599–604.

738. Kuijper EJ, Wiggerts HO, Jonker GJ, et al. Disseminated actinomycosis due to *Actinomyces meyeri* and *Actinobacillus actinomycetemcomitans*. Scand J Infect Dis 1992;24:667–672.

739. Kullberg B-J, Wastendorp RGJ, van't Wout JW, et al. Purpura fulminans and symmetrical peripheral gangrene caused by *Capnocytophaga canimorsus* (formerly S-2) septicemia: a complication of dogbite. Medicine (Baltimore) 1991;70:287–292.

740. Kurzynski TA, Boehm DM, Rott-Petri JA, et al. Antimicrobial susceptibilities of *Bordetella* species isolated in a multicenter pertussis surveillance project. Antimicrob Agents Chemother 1988;32:137–140.

741. Kurzynski TA, Boehm DM, Rott-Petri JA, et al. Comparison of modified Bordet-Gengou and modified Regan-Lowe media for the isolation of *Bordetella pertussis* and *Bordetella parapertussis*. J Clin Microbiol 1988;26:2661–2663.

742. Labrune P, Jabir B, Magny JF, et al. Recurrent enterocolitis-like symptoms as the possible presenting manifestations of neonatal *Brucella melitensis* infection. Acta Paediatr Scand 1990;79:707–709.

743. LaClaire LL, Tondella ML, Beall DS, et al. Identification of *Haemophilus influenzae* serotypes by standard slide agglutination serotyping and PCR-based capsule typing. J Clin Microbiol 2003;41:393–396.

744. Lacroix J-M, Walker C. Characterization of a β-lactamase found in *Eikenella corrodens*. Antimicrob Agents Chemother 1991;35:886–891.

745. Lambe DW. *Streptobacillus moniliformis* isolated from a case of Haverhill fever: biochemical characterization and inhibitory effect of sodium polyanethol sulfonate. Am J Clin Pathol 1973;60:854–860.

746. Lang R, Dagan R, Potasman I, et al. Failure of ceftriaxone in the treatment of acute brucellosis. Clin Infect Dis 1992;14:506–509.

747. Lang R, Raz R, Sacks T, et al. Failure of prolonged treatment with ciprofloxacin in acute infections due to *Brucella melitensis*. J Antimicrob Chemother 1990;26:841–846.

748. Larson AM, Dougherty MJ, Nowowifiski DJ, et al. Detection of *Bartonella* (*Rochalimaea*) *quintana* by routine acridine orange staining of broth blood cultures. J Clin Microbiol 1994;32:1492–1496.

749. Larson CL, Wicht W, Jellison WL. An organism resembling *P. tularensis* from water. Public Health Rep 1955;70:253–258.

750. LaScola B, Barrassi L, Raoult D. Isolation of new fastidious α-Proteobacteria and *Afipia felis* from hospital water supplies by direct plating and amoebal co-culture procedures. FEMS Microbiol Ecol 2000;34:129–137.

751. LaScola B, Iorgulescu I, Bollini G. Five cases of *Kingella kingae* skeletal infection in a French hospital. Eur J Clin Microbiol Infect Dis 1998 ;17: 512–515.

752. LaScola B, Mallet MN, Grimont PA, Raoult D. Description of *Afipia birgiae* sp. nov. and *Afipia massiliensis* sp. nov. and recognition of *Afipia felis* genospecies A. Int J Syst Evol Microbiol 2002;52:1773–1782.

753. LaScola B, Mezi L, Auffray JP, et al. Patients in the intensive care unit are exposed to amoeba-associated pathogens. Infect Control Hosp Epidemiol 2002; 23:462–465.

754. LaScola B, Raoult D. Serological cross-reactions between *Bartonella quintana*, *Bartonella henselae*, and *Coxiella burnetii*. J Clin Microbiol 1996;34: 2270–2274.

755. LaScola B, Raoult D. Culture of *Bartonella quintana* and *Bartonella henselae* from human samples: a 5-year experience (1993 to 1998). J Clin Microbiol 1999;37:1899–1905.

756. LaScola B, Raoult D. *Afipia felis* in hospital water supply in association with free-living amoebae. Lancet 1999;353:1330.

757. Lass JH, Varley MP, Frank KE, et al. *Actinobacillus actinomycetemcomitans* endophthalmitis with subacute endocarditis. Ann Ophthalmol 1984;16:54–61.

758. Lawson PA, Collins MD. Description of *Bartonella clarridgeiae* sp. nov., isolated from the cat of a patient with *Bartonella henselae* septicemia. Med Microbiol Lett 5:64–73.

759. Lawson PA, Falsen E, Inganas E, et al. *Dysgonomonas mossii* sp. nov., from human sources. Syst Appl Microbiol 2002;25:194–197.

760. Layton CT. *Pasteurella multocida* meningitis and septic arthritis secondary to a cat bite. J Emerg Med 1999;17:445–448.

761. Leadbetter ER, Holt SC, Socransky SS. *Capnocytophaga*: a new genus of gram-negative gliding bacteria. I. General characteristics, taxonomic considerations, and significance. Arch Microbiol 1979;122:9–16.

762. LeBoit PE, Berger TG, Egbert EM, et al. Epithelioid haemangioma-like vascular proliferation in AIDS: manifestation of cat scratch disease bacillus infection? Lancet 1988;2:960–963.

763. LeDoux MS. Tularemia presenting with ataxia. Clin Infect Dis 2000;30: 211–212.

764. Lehman CR, Deckley JE, Hu SS. *Eikenella corrodens* vertebral osteomyelitis secondary to direct inoculation: a case report. Spine 2000;25:1185–1187.

765. Lejbkowicz F, Cohn L, Hashman N, Kassis I. Recovery of *Kingella kingae* from blood and synovial fluid of two pediatric patients by using the BacT/Alert system. J Clin Microbiol 1999;37:878.

766. Le Moal G, Landron C, Grollier G, et al. Meningitis due to *Capnocytophaga canimorsus* after receipt of a dog bite: case report and review of the literature. Clin Infect Dis 2003;36:e42–e46.

767. Leonord A, Williams C. *Haemophilus influenzae* in acute exacerbations of chronic obstructive pulmonary disease. Int J Antimicrob Agents 2002;19: 371–375.

768. Lepine G, Caudry S, DiRenzo JM, Ellen RP. Epithelial cell invasion by *Actinobacillus actinomycetemcomitans* strains from restriction fragment-length polymorphism groups associated with juvenile periodontitis or carrier state. Oral Microbiol Immunol 1998;13:241–347.

769. Le Quellec A, Bessis D, Perez C, et al. Endocarditis due to a β-lactamase-producing *Cardiobacterium hominis*. Clin Infect Dis 1994;19:994–995.

770. Lesage V, Van Pee D, Luyx C, et al. Septic arthritis due to *Haemophilus influenzae* associated with endocarditis. Clin Rheumatol 1998;17:340–342.

771. Lesse AJ, Gheesling LL, Bittner WE, et al. Stable, conserved outer membrane epitope of strains of *Haemophilus influenzae* biogroup *aegyptius* associated with Brazilian purpuric fever. Infect Immun 1992;60:1351–1357.

772. Lev EI, Onn A, Levo Y, Giladi M. *Haemophilus influenzae* biotype III cellulitis in an adult. Infection 1999;27:42–43.

773. Lewis DA. Diagnostic tests for chancroid. Sex Transm Infect 2000;76: 137–141.

774. Lewis K, Saubolle MA, Tenover FC, et al. Pertussis caused by an erythromycin-resistant strain of *Bordetella pertussis*. Pediatr Infect Dis J 1995;14:388–391.

775. Li WC, Chiu NC, Hsu CH, et al. Pathogens in the middle ear effusion of children with persistent otitis media: implications of drug resistance and complications. J Microbiol Immunol Infect 2001;34:190–194.

776. Liang Z, Raoult D. Species-specific monoclonal antibodies for rapid identification of *Bartonella quintana*. Clin Diagn lab Immunol 2000;7:21–24.

777. Lichtensteiger CA, Steenbergen SM, Lee RM, et al. Direct PCR analysis for toxigenic *Pasteurella multocida*. J Clin Microbiol 1996;34:3035–3039.

778. Liese JG, Meschievitz CK, Harzer E, et al. Efficacy of a two-component acellular pertussis vaccine in infants. Pediatr Infect Dis J 1997;16:1038–1044.

779. Lim ME, Hoffman JA, Kim KS. Recurrent ventriculoperitoneal shunt infection due to nontypeable *Haemophilus influenzae*. Clin Infect Dis 1999;28:147–148.

780. Limaye AP, Hooper CJ. Treatment of tularemia with fluoroquinolones: two cases and review. Clin Infect Dis 1999;29:922–924.

781. Lin BH, Vieco PT. Intracranial mycotic aneurysm in a patient with endocarditis caused by *Cardiobacterium hominis*. Can Assoc Radiol J 1995;46:40–42.

782. Lindberg AA. Glycoprotein conjugate vaccines. Vaccine 1999;17:S28–S36.

783. Lind-Brandberg L, Welinder-Olsson C, Lagergard T, et al. Evaluation of PCR for diagnosis of *Bordetella pertussis* and *Bordetella parapertussis* infections. J Clin Microbiol 1998;36:679–683.

784. Lindquist SW, Weber DJ, Magnum ME, et al. *Bordetella holmesii* sepsis in an asplenic adolescent. Pediatr Infect Dis J 1995;14:813–815.

785. Lion C, Escande F, Burdin JC. *Capnocytophaga canimorsus* infections in humans: review of the literature and case reports. Eur J Epidemiol 1996;12: 521–533.

786. Lion C, Lozniewski A, Rosner V, Weber M. Lung abscess due to β-lactamase-producing *Pasteurella multocida*. Clin Infect Dis 29:1345–1346, 1999.

787. Lippke JA, Peros WJ, Keville MW, French CK. DNA probe detection of *Eikenella corrodens*, *Wolinella recta*, and *Fusobacterium nucleatum* in subgingival plaque. Oral Microbiol Immunol 1991;6:81–87.

788. LiPuma JJ, Richman H, Stull TL. Haemocin, a bacteriocin produced by *Haemophilus influenzae* type b: species distribution and role in colonization. Infect Immun 1990;58:1600–1605.

789. LiPuma JJ, Sharetzsky C, Edlind TD, et al. Haemocin production by encapsulated and nonencapsulated *Haemophilus influenzae*. J Infect Dis 1992; 165(Suppl 1):S118–S119.

790. Liu W, Chemaly RF, Tuohy MJ, et al. *Pasteurella multocida* urinary tract infection with molecular evidence of zoonotic transmission. Clin Infect Dis 2003;36:E58–E60.

791. Livrelli VO, Darfeuille-Richaud A, Rich CD, et al. Genetic determinant of the ROB-1 β-lactamase in bovine and porcine *Pasteurella* strains. Antimicrob Agents Chemother 1988;32:1282–1284.

792. Loe H, Brown LJ. Early-onset periodontitis in the United States of America. J Periodontol 1991;62:606–616.

793. Loeffelholz MJ, Thompson CJ, Long KS, Gilchrist MJ. Comparison of PCR, culture, and direct fluorescent antibody testing for detection of *Bordetella pertussis*. J Clin Microbiol 1999;37:2872–2876.

794. Loeffelholz MJ, Thompson CJ, Long KS, Gilchrist MJ. Detection of *Bordetella holmesii* using *Bordetella pertussis* IS481 PCR assay. J Clin Microbiol 2000; 38:467.

795. Loghman-Adham M. *Pasteurella multocida* peritonitis in patients undergoing peritoneal dialysis. Pediatr Nephrol 1997;11:353–354.

796. Loiez C, Wallet F, Husson MO, Courcol RJ. *Pasteurella multocida* and intrauterine device: a woman and her pets. Scand J Infect Dis 2002;34:473.

797. Lombardo J. Cat-scratch neuroretinitis. J Am Optom Assoc 1999;70:525–530.

798. Long GWE, Oprandy JJ, Narayanan RB, et al. Detection of *Francisella tularensis* in blood by polymerase chain reaction. J Clin Microbiol 1993;31: 152–154.

799. Lopez-Merino A, Monnet SL, Hernandez I, et al. Identification of *Brucella abortus*, *B. canis*, *B. melitensis*, and *B. suis* by carbon substrate assimilation tests. Vet Microbiol 2001;80:359–363.

800. Lozano Fm Corzo JE, Leon EM, et al. Massive hemoperitoneum: a new manifestation of bacillary peliosis in human immunodeficiency virus infection. Clin Infect Dis 1999;28:911–912.

801. Lu PL, Hsueh PR, Hung CC, et al. Infective endocarditis complicated with progressive heart failure due to β-lactamase-producing *Cardiobacterium hominis*. J Clin Microbiol 2000;38:2015–2016.

802. Lucey D, Dolan MJ, Moss CW, et al. Relapsing illness due to *Rochalimaea henselae* in immunocompetent hosts; implications for therapy and new epidemiological associations. Clin Infect Dis 1992;14:683–688.

803. Luhmann JD, Luhmann SJ. Etiology of septic arthritis in children: an update for the 1990's. Pediatr Emerg Care 1999;15:40–42.

804. Luong N, Tsai J, Chen C. Susceptibilities of *Eikenella corrodens*, *Prevotella intermedia*, and *Prevotella nigrescens* clinical isolates to amoxicillin and tetracycline. Antimicrob Agents Chemother 2001;45:3253–3255.

805. Maccato M, McLean W, Riddle G, Faro S. Isolation of *Kingella denitrificans* from amniotic fluid in a woman with chorioamnionitis. J Reprod Med 1991; 36:685–687.

806. Madhi SA, Petersen K, Khoosal M, et al. Reduced effectiveness of *Haemophilus influenzae* type b conjugate vaccine in children with a high prevalence of human immunodeficiency virus type 1 infection. Pediatr Infect Dis J 2002;21: 315–321.

807. Madinier IM, Fosse TB, Hitzig C, et al. Resistance profile survey of 50 periodontal strains of *Actinobacillus actinomycetemcomitans*. J Periodontol 1999; 70:888–892.

808. Maguina C, Garcia PJ, Gotuzzo E, et al. Bartonellosis (Carrion's disease) in the modern era. Clin Infect Dis 2001;33:772–779.

809. Maguina C, Gotuzzo E. Bartonellosis: new and old. Infect Dis Clin N Am 2000;14:1–22.

810. Mahrer S, Raik E. *Capnocytophaga canimorsus* septicemia associated with cat scratch. Pathology 1992;24;194–196.

811. Malavolta N, Frigato M, Zanardi M, et al. *Brucella* spondylitis was paravertebral abscess due to *Brucella melitensis* infection: a case report. Drugs Exp Clin Res 2002;28:95–98.

812. Maliszewski CR, Shuster CW, Badger SJ. A type-specific antigen of *Eikenella corrodens* is the major outer membrane protein. Infect Immun 1983;42: 208–213.

813. Malizos KN, Makris CA, Soucacos PN. Total knee arthroplasties infected by *Brucella melitensis*: a case report. Am J Orthop 1997;26:283–285.

814. Malone FD, Athanassiou A, Nores LA, Dalton ME. Poor perinatal outcome associated with maternal *Brucella abortus* infection. Obstet Gynecol 1997;90: 674–676.

815. Malonza IM, Tyndall MW, Ndinya-Achola JO, et al. A randomized, double-blind, placebo-controlled trial of single-dose ciprofloxacin versus erythromycin for the treatment of chancroid in Nairobi, Kenya. J Infect Dis 1999;180: 1886–1893.

816. Mangan DF, Taichman NS, Lally ET, et al. Lethal effects of *Actinobacillus actinomycetemcomitans* leukotoxin on human T lymphocytes. Infect Immun 1991;59:3267–3272.

817. Maradona JA, Asensi V, Carton JA, et al. Prosthetic joint infection by *Pasteurella multocida*. Eur J Clin Microbiol Infect Dis 1997;16:623–625.

818. Maranan RC, Schiff D, Johnson DC, et al. Pneumonic tularemia in a patient with chronic granulomatous disease. Clin Infect Dis 1997;25:630–633.

819. Marchette NJ, Nicholes PS. Virulence and citrulline ureidase activity of *Pasteurella tularensis*. J Bacteriol 82:26–32, 1961.

820. Marcon MJ, Hamoudi AC, Cannon HJ. Comparative laboratory evaluation of three antigen detection methods for diagnosis of *Haemophilus influenzae* type b disease. J Clin Microbiol 19:333–337, 1984.

821. Margileth AM, Baehren DF. Chest-wall abscess due to cat-scratch disease (CSD) in an adult with antibodies to *Bartonella clarridgeiae*: case report and review of the thoracopulmonary manifestations of CSD. Clin Infect Dis 1998; 27:353–357.

822. Markowitz SM. Isolation of an ampicillin-resistant, non-β-lactamase producing strain of *Haemophilus influenzae*. Antimicrob Agents Chemother 1980;17: 80–83.

823. Marston EL, Sumner JW, Regnery RL. Evaluation of intraspecies genetic variation within the 60 kDa heat-shock protein gene (*groEL*) of *Bartonella* species. Int J Syst Bacteriol 1999;49:1015–1023.

824. Martin DH, Sargent SJ, Wendel GD Jr, et al. Comparison of azithromycin and ceftriaxone for the treatment of chancroid. Clin Infect Dis 1995;21:409–414.

825. Martone WJ, Zuehl RW, Minson GE, et al. Postsplenectomy sepsis with DF-2: report of a case with isolation of the organism from the patient's dog. Ann Intern Med 1980;93:457–458.

826. Marullo S, Jaccard A, Roulot D, et al. Identification of the *Rochalimaea henselae* 16S rRNA sequence in the liver of a French patient with bacillary peliosis hepatis. J Infect Dis 1992;166:1462–1464.

827. Marx RE, Carlson ER, Smith BR, Toraya N. Isolation of *Actinomyces* species and *Eikenella corrodens* from patients with chronic diffuse sclerosing osteomyelitis. J Oral Maxillofac Surg 1994;52:26–33.

828. Mastrantonio P, Stefanelli P, Giuliano M, et al. *Bordetella parapertussis* infection in children: epidemiology, clinical symptoms, and molecular characterization of isolates. J Clin Microbiol1998; 36:999–1002.

829. Matar GM, Koehler JE, Malcolm G, et al. Identification of *Bartonella* species directly in clinical specimens by PCR-restriction fragment length polymorphism analysis of a 16S rRNA gene fragment. J Clin Microbiol 1999;37: 4045–4047.

830. Matar GM, Swaminathan B, Hunter SB, et al. Polymerase chain reaction-based restriction fragment length polymorphism analysis of a fragment of the ribosomal operon from *Rochalimaea* species for subtyping. J Clin Microbiol 1993; 31:1730–1734.

831. Matthews HW, Baker CN, Thornsberry C. Relationship between in vitro susceptibility test results for chloramphenicol and production of chloramphenicol acetyltransferase by *Haemophilus influenzae*, *Streptococcus pneumoniae* and *Aerococcus* species. J Clin Microbiol 1988;26:2387–2390.

832. Maurin M, Eb F, Etienne J, Raoult D. Serological cross-reactions between *Bartonella* and *Chlamydia* species: implications for diagnosis. J Clin Microbiol 1997;35:2283–2287.

833. Maurin M, Gasquet S, Ducco C, Raoult D. MICs of 28 antibiotic compounds for 14 *Bartonella* (formerly *Rochalimaea*) isolates. Antimicrob Agents Chemother 1995;39:2387–2391.

834. Maurin M, Lepocher H, Mallet D, et al. Antibiotic susceptibilities of *Afipia felis* in axenic medium and in cells. Antimicrob Agents Chemother 1993;37: 1410–1413.

835. Maurin M, Raoult D. Antimicrobial susceptibility of *Rochalimaea quintana*, *Rochalimaea vinsonii*, and the newly recognized *Rochalimaea henselae*. J Antimicrob Chemother 1993;32:587–594.

836. Maurin M, Rolain JM, Raoult D. Comparison of in-house and commercial

837. slides for detection by immunofluorescence of immunoglobulins G and M against *Bartonella henselae* and *Bartonella quintana*. Clin Diagn Lab Immunol 2002;9:1004–1009.

837. Maurin M, Roux V, Stein A, et al. Isolation and characterization by immunofluorescence, sodium dodecyl sulfate-polyacrylamide gel electrophoresis, Western blot, restriction fragment length polymorphism-PCR, 16S rRNA gene sequencing, and pulsed-field gel electrophoresis of *Rochalimaea quintana* from a patient with bacillary angiomatosis. J Clin Microbiol 1994;32:1166–1171.

838. Mayatepek E, Zilow E, Pohl S. Severe intrauterine infection due to *Capnocytophaga ochracea*. Biol Neonate 1991;60:184–186.

839. Mayer LW, Bibb WF, Birkness KA, et al. Distinguishing clonal characteristics of the Brazilian purpuric fever-producing strain. Pediatr Infect Dis 1989;J 8: 245–247.

840. Mayer MP, Bueno LC, Hansen EJ, DiRienzo JM. Identification of a cytolethal distending toxin gene locus and features of a virulence-associated region in *Actinobacillus actinomycetemcomitans*. Infect Immun 1999;67:1227–1237.

841. Mazengia E, Silva EA, Peppe JA, et al. Recovery of *Bordetella holmesii* from patients with pertussis-like symptoms: use of pulsed-field gel electrophoresis to characterize circulating strains. J Clin Microbiol 32000;8:2330–2333.

842. McAllister HA, Carter GR. An aerogenic *Pasteurella*-like organism recovered from swine. Am J Vet Res 1974;35:917–922.

843. McClain JB, Almazan RD, Keiser JF. *Haemophilus parainfluenzae* urethritis with accompanying bacteremia. Clin Microbiol Newslett 1983;5:31.

844. McCrary B, Cockerham W, Pierce P. Neuroretinitis in cat-scratch disease associated with the macular star. Pediatr Infect Dis J 1994;13:838–839.

845. McCrea KW, St Sauver J, Marrs CF, et al. Immunologic and structural relationships of the minor pilus subunits among *Haemophilus influenzae* isolates. Infect Immun 1998;66:4788–4796.

846. McDonald PJ, Pruul H. Phagocyte uptake and transport of azithromycin. Eur J Clin Microbiol Infect Dis 1991;10:828–833.

847. McIntyre P, Wheaton G, Erlich J. Brazilian purpuric fever in Central Australia. Lancet 1987;2:112.

848. McLaren BL. *Haemophilus parainfluenzae* endocarditis. NZ Med J 1993;106: 412.

849. Meade BD, Bollen A. Recommendations for use of the polymerase chain reaction in the diagnosis of *Bordetella pertussis* infections. J Med Microbiol 1994; 41:51–55.

850. Megraud F, Bebear C, Dabernat H, Delmas C. *Haemophilus* species in the human gastrointestinal tract. Eur J Clin Microbiol Infect Dis 1988;7:437–438.

851. Meininger GR, Nadasdy T, Hruban RH, et al. Chronic active myocarditis following acute *Bartonella henselae* infection (cat scratch disease). Am J Surg Pathol 2001;25:1211–1214.

852. Meis JF, Sauerwein RW, Gyssens IC, et al. *Kingella kingae* intervertebral diskitis in an adult. Clin Infect Dis 1992;15:530–532.

853. Melhus A. Isolation of dysgonic fermenter 3, a rare isolate associated with diarrhoea in immunocompromised patients. Scand J Infect Dis 1997;29: 195–196.

854. Memish ZA, Bannatyne RM, Alshaalan M. Endophlebitis of the leg caused by *Brucella* infection. J Infect 2001;42:281–283.

855. Memish ZA, Mah MW. Brucellosis in laboratory workers at a Saudi Arabian hospital. Am J Infect Control 2001;29:48–52.

856. Memish Z, Mah MW, Al-Mahmoud SA, et al. *Brucella* bacteraemia: clinical and laboratory observations in 160 patients. J Infect 2000;40:59–63.

857. Mendelman PM. Targets of the β-lactam antibiotics, penicillin binding proteins, in ampicillin-resistant, non-β-lactamase-producing *Haemophilus influenzae*. J Infect Dis 1992;165(Suppl 1):S107–S109.

858. Mendelman PM, Chaffin DO, Clausen C, et al. Failure to detect ampicillin-resistant, non-β-lactamase-producing *Haemophilus influenzae* by standard disk susceptibility testing. Antimicrob Agents Chemother 1986;30:274–280.

859. Mendelman PM, Chaffin DO, Stull TL, et al. Characterization of non-β-lactamase-mediated ampicillin resistance in *Haemophilus influenzae*. Antimicrob Agents Chemother 1984;26:235–244.

860. Mercer LJ. *Capnocytophaga* isolated from the endometrium as a cause of neonatal sepsis. J Reprod Med 1985;30:67–68.

861. Mesnard R, Guiso N, Michelet C, et al. Isolation of *Bordetella bronchiseptica* from a patient with AIDS. Eur J Clin Microbiol Infect Dis 1993;12:304–306.

862. Mexas AM, Hancock SI, Breitschwerdt EB. *Bartonella henselae* and *Bartonella elizabethae* as potential canine pathogens. J Clin Microbiol 2002;40: 4670–4674.

863. Meyer DH, Sreenivasan PK, Fives-Taylor PM. Evidence for invasion of a human oral cell line by *Actinobacillus actinomycetemcomitans*. Infect Immun 1991;59:2719–2726.

864. Michel F, Allaouchiche B, Chassard D. Postoperative adult respiratory distress syndrome (ARDS) due to *Pasteurella multocida*. J Infect 1999;38:133–134.

865. Miflin JK, Blackall PJ. Development of a 23S rRNA-based PCR assay for the identification of *Pasteurella multocida*. Lett Appl Microbiol 2001;33:216–221.

866. Milam MW, Balerdi MJ, Toney JF, et al. Epithelioid angiomatosis secondary to disseminated cat-scratch disease involving the bone marrow and skin of a

patient with acquired immunodeficiency syndrome. Am J Med 1989;88: 180–183.

867. Milionis H, Christou L, Elisaf M. Cutaneous manifestations in brucellosis: case report and review of the literature. Infection 1989;28:124–126.

868. Miller WG, Adams LG, Ficht TA, et al. *Brucella*-induced abortions and infection in bottlenose dolphins (*Tursiops truncatus*). J Zoo Wildl Med 1999;30: 100–110.

869. Min K-W, Reed JA, Welch DF, et al. Morphologically variable bacilli of cat scratch disease are identified by immunocytochemical labeling with antibodies to *Rochalimaea henselae*. Am J Clin Pathol 1994;101:607–610.

870. Minamoto GY, Sordillo EM. *Kingella denitrificans* as a cause of granulomatous disease in a patient with AIDS. Clin Infect Dis 1992;15:1052–1053.

871. Mink CM, Cherry JD, Christenson P, et al. A search for *Bordetella pertussis* infection in university students. Clin Infect Dis 1992;14:464–471.

872. Minton EJ. *Pasteurella pneumotropica*: meningitis following a dog bite. Postgrad Med J 1990;66:125–126.

873. Mintz KP, Fives-Taylor PM. Adhesion of *Actinobacillus actinomycetemcomitans* to a human oral cell line. Infect Immun 1994;62:3672–3678.

874. Mintz KP, Fives-Taylor PM. Identification of an immunoglobulin Fc receptor of *Actinobacillus actinomycetemcomitans*. Infect Immun 1994;62:4500–4505.

875. Miranda RT, Gimeno AE, Rodriguez TF, et al. Acute cholecystitis caused by *Brucella melitensis*: case report and review. J Infect 2001;42:77–78.

876. Miravitlles M, Espinosa C, Fernandez-Laso E, et al. Relationship between bacterial flora in sputum and functional impairment in patients with acute exacerbations of COPD. Chest 1999;116:40–46.

877. Mirza I, Wolk J, Toth L, et al. Waterhouse-Friderichsen syndrome secondary to *Capnocytophaga canimorsus* septicemia and demonstration of bacteremia by peripheral blood smear. Arch Pathol Lab Med 2000;124:859–863.

878. Modi SP, Eppes SC, Klein JD. Cat scratch disease presenting as multifocal osteomyelitis with thoracic abscess. Pediatr Infect Dis J 2001;20:1006–1007.

879. Mohle-Boetani J, Koehler J, Berger T, et al. Bacillary angiomatosis and bacillary peliosis in patients infected with human immunodeficiency virus: clinical characteristics in a case-control study. Clin Infect Dis 1996;22:794–800.

880. Molina F, Duran MT, Miguez E, et al. Isolation of *Haemophilus paraphrophilus* from an abdominal abscess. Eur J Clin Microbiol Infect Dis 1993;12:722–723.

881. Molina F, Echaniz A, Duran MT, et al. Infectious arthritis of the knee due to *Actinobacillus actinomycetemcomitans*. Eur J Clin Microbiol Infect Dis 1994; 13:687–689.

882. Molina R, Baro T, Torne J, et al. Empyema caused by *Kingella denitrificans* and *Peptostreptococcus* spp. in a patient with bronchogenic carcinoma. Eur Respir J 1988;1:870–871.

883. Mollee T, Kelly P, Tilee M. Isolation of *Kingella kingae* from a corneal ulcer. J Clin Microbiol 1992;30:2516–2517.

884. Moller K, Fussing V, Grimont PA, et al. *Actinobacillus minor* sp, nov., *Actinobacillus porcinus* sp. nov., and *Actinobacillus indolicus* sp. nov., three new V factor-dependent species from the respiratory tract of pigs. Int J Syst Bacteriol 1996;46:951–956.

885. Moncla BJ, Braham P, Hillier SL. Sialidase (neuraminidase) activity among gram-negative anaerobic and capnophilic bacteria. J Clin Microbiol 1990;28: 422–425.

886. Monkemuller KE, Bronze MS. Immunoblastic lymphadenopathy presenting as an acute abdomen and mixed bacteremia with *Eikenella corrodens* and group C streptococci. Am J Gastroenterol 1998;93:652–653.

887. Monso E, Ruiz J, Rozell A, et al. Bacterial infections in chronic obstructive pulmonary disease: a study of stable and exacerbated outpatients using the protected specimen brush. Am J Respir Crit Care Med 1995;152:1316–1320.

888. Montaraz JA, Winter AJ, Hunter DM, et al. Protection against *Brucella abortus* in mice with O-polysaccharide-specific monoclonal antibodies. Infect Immun 1986;51:961–963.

889. Mooi FR. Genes for the filamentous hemagglutinin and fimbriae of *Bordetella pertussis*: colocation, coregulation, and cooperation? In: Miller VL, Kaper JB, eds. Molecular Genetics of Bacterial Pathogenesis. Washington, DC: American Society for Microbiology, 1994:145–155.

890. Mooi FR, Hallander H, Wirsing von Konig CH, et al. Epidemiological typing of *Bordetella pertussis* isolates: recommendations for a standard methodology. Eur J Clin Microbiol Infect Dis 2000;19:174–181.

891. Moore CH, Foster L-A, Gerbig DG, et al. Identification of alcaligin as the siderophore produced by *Bordetella pertussis* and *B. bronchiseptica*. J Bacteriol 1995;177:1116–1118.

892. Moreno E. Brucellosis in Central America. Vet Microbiol 2002;90:31–38.

893. Moreno E, Cloeckaert A, Moriyon I. *Brucella* evolution and taxonomy. Vet Microbiol 2002;90:209–227.

894. Moreno E, Stackbrandt E, Dorsch M, et al. *Brucella abortus* 16S rRNA and lipid A reveal a phylogenetic relationship with members of the α-2 subgroup of the class *Proteobacter*. J Bacteriol 1990;172:3569–3576.

895. Morgan MG, Hamilton-Miller JMT. *Haemophilus influenzae* and *Haemophilus parainfluenzae* as urinary pathogens. J Infect 1990;20:143–145.

896. Moritz F, Martin E, Lemeland JF, et al. Fatal *Pasteurella bettyae* pleuropneumoniae in a patient infected with human immunodeficiency virus. Clin Infect Dis 1996;22:591–592.

897. Morris JF, Sewell DL. Necrotizing pneumonia caused by mixed infection with *Actinobacillus actinomycetemcomitans* and *Actinomyces israelii*: case report and review. Clin Infect Dis 1994;18:450–452.

898. Morris JT, Myers M. Bacteremia due to *Bordetella holmesii*. Clin Infect Dis 1998;27:912–913.

899. Mortensen JE, Giger O, Rodgers GL. In vitro activity of oral antimicrobial agents against clinical isolates of *Pasteurella multocida*. Diagn Microbiol Infect Dis 1998;30:99–102.

900. Moshal KL, Hodinka RL, McGowan KL. Concomitant viral and *Bordetella pertussis* infections in infants. Pediatr Infect Dis J 1998;17:353–354.

901. Moxon ER, Murphy TF. *Haemophilus influenzae*. In: Mandell GL, Bennett JE, Dolin R, eds. Mandell, Douglas, and Bennett's Principles and Practice of Infectious Diseases. 4th Ed. New York: Churchill-Livingstone, 2000: 2369–2378.

902. Moylett EH, Rossmann SN, Epps HR, Demmler GJ. Importance of *Kingella kingae* as a pediatric pathogen in the United States. Pediatr Infect Dis J 2000; 19:263–265.

903. Mueller NJ, Kaplan V, Zbinden R, Altwegg M. Diagnosis of *Cardiobacterium hominis* endocarditis by broad-range PCR from arterio-embolic tissue. Infection 1999;27:278–279.

904. Muhlemann K, Alexander ER, Pepe M, et al. Invasive *Haemophilus influenzae* disease and epiglottitis among Swiss children from 1980 to 1993: evidence for herd immunity among older age groups. The Swiss *Haemophilus influenzae* Study Group. Scand J Infect Dis 1996 ;28:265–268.

905. Mulder AH, Gerlag PG, Verhoef LH, van den Wall Bake AW. Hemolytic uremic syndrome after *Capnocytophaga canimorsus* (DF-2) septicemia. Clin Nephrol 2001;55:167–170.

906. Muller FM, Hoppe JE, Wirsing von Konig CH. Laboratory diagnosis of pertussis: state of the art in 1997. J Clin Microbiol 1997;35:2435–2443.

907. Muller HP, Holderrieth S, Burkhardt U, Hoffler U. In vitro antimicrobial susceptibility of oral strains of *Actinobacillus actinomycetemcomitans* to seven antibiotics. J Clin Periodontol 2002;29:736–742.

908. Mulvany NJ, Billson VR. Bacillary angiomatosis of the spleen. Pathology 1993; 25:398–401.

909. Munson E, Pfaller M, Koontz F, Doern G. Comparison of porphyrin-based, growth factor-based, and biochemical-based testing methods for identification of *Haemophilus influenzae*. Eur J Clin Microbiol Infect Dis 2002;21:196–203.

910. Murphy TF, Apicella MA. Nontypeable *Haemophilus influenzae*: a review of clinical aspects, surface antigens and human immune response to infection. Rev Infect Dis 1987;147:838–846.

911. Murphy TF, Bartos LC. Purification and analysis with monoclonal antibodies of P2, the major outer membrane protein of nontypeable *Haemophilus influenzae*. Infect Immun 1988;56:1084–1089.

912. Murphy TF, Bartos LC, Rice PA, et al. Identification of a 16,600-dalton outer membrane protein on nontypeable *Haemophilus influenzae* as a target for human bactericidal antibody. J Clin Invest 1986;78:1020–1027.

913. Murphy TF, Kirkham C, Sikkema DJ. Neonatal, urogenital isolates of biotype 4 nontypeable *Haemophilus influenzae* express a variant P6 outer membrane protein molecule. Infect Immun 1992;60:2016–2022.

914. Murphy TV, Pastor P, Medley F, et al. Decreased *Haemophilus* colonization in children vaccinated with *Haemophilus influenzae* type b conjugate vaccine. J Pediatr 1993;122:517–523.

915. Musio F, Tiu A. *Pasteurella multocida* peritonitis in peritoneal dialysis. Clin Nephrol 1998;49:258–261.

916. Musser JM, Selander RK. Brazilian purpuric fever: evolutionary genetic relationships of the case clone of *Haemophilus influenzae* biogroup *aegyptius* to encapsulated strains of *Haemophilus influenzae*. J Infect Dis 1990;161: 130–133.

917. Musso D, Drancourt M, Raoult D. Lack of bactericidal effect of antibiotics except aminoglycosides on *Bartonella* (*Rochalimaea*) *henselae*. J Antimicrob Chemother 1995;36:101–108.

918. Mutters R, Ihm P, Pohl S, et al. Reclassification of the genus *Pasteurella* Trevisan 1887 on the basis of deoxyribonucleic acid homology, with proposals for the new species *Pasteurella dagmatis*, *Pasteurella canis*, *Pasteurella stomatis*, *Pasteurella anatis*, and *Pasteurella langaa*. Int J Syst Bacteriol 1985; 35:309–322.

919. Mutters R, Peichulla K, Hinz K-H, et al. *Pasteurella avium* (Hinz and Kunjara) comb. nov. and *Pasteurella volantium* sp. nov. Int J Syst Bacteriol 1985;35: 509.

920. Mutters R, Peichulla K, Mannheim W. Phenotypic differentiation of *Pasteurella sensu stricto* and *Actinobacillus* group. Eur J Clin Microbiol 1984;3: 225–229.

921. Mutters R, Pohl S, Mannheim W. Transfer of *Pasteurella ureae* Jones 1962 to the genus *Actinobacillus* Brumpt 1910: *Actinobacillus ureae* comb. nov. Int J Syst Bacteriol 1986;36:343–344.

922. Naas T, Benaoudia F, Lebrun L, Nordmann P. Molecular identification of

TEM-1 β-lactamase in a *Pasteurella multocida* isolate of human origin. Eur J Clin Microbiol Infect Dis 2001;20:210–213.

923. Namiduru M, Gungor K, Dikensoy O, et al. Epidemiological, clinical and laboratory features of brucellosis: a prospective evaluation of 120 adult patients. Int J Clin Pract 2003 ;57:20–24.

924. Nashi M, Venkatachalam AK, Unsworth PF, Muddu BN. Diskitis caused by *Actinobacillus actinomycetemcomitans*. Orthopaedics 1998;21:714–716.

925. Naughton M, Brown R, Adkins D, DiPersio J. Tularemia: an unusual cause of a solitary pulmonary nodule in the post-transplant setting. Bone Marrow Transplant 1999;24:197–199.

926. Navarro E, Escribano J, Fernandez J, Solera J. Comparison of three different PCR methods for detection of *Brucella* spp. in human blood samples. FEMS Immunol Med Microbiol 2002 ;34:147–151.

927. Navarro V, Solera J, Martinez-Alfaro E, et al. Brucellar osteomyelitis involving prosthetic extra-articular hardware. J Infect 1997;35:192–194.

928. Navarro-Martinez A, Solera J, Corredoira J, et al. Epididymoorchitis due to *Brucella melitensis*: a retrospective study of 59 patients. Clin Infect Dis 2001; 33:2017–2022.

929. Neibylski ML, Peacock MG, Fischer ER, et al. Characterization of an endosymbiont infecting wood ticks, *Dermacentor andersoni*, as a member of the genus *Francisella*. Appl Environ Microbiol 1997;63:3933–3940.

930. Nelson MB, Apicella MA, Murphy TF, et al. Cloning and sequencing of *Haemophilus influenzae* outer membrane protein P6. Infect Immun 1988;56:128–134.

931. Nelson S, Matlow A, McDowell C, et al. Detection of *Bordetella pertussis* in clinical specimens by PCR and a microtiter plate-based DNA hybridization assay. J Clin Microbiol 1997;35:117–120.

932. Nettles RE, Sexton DJ. *Pasteurella multocida* prosthetic valve endocarditis: case report and review. Clin Infect Dis 1997;25:920–921.

933. Neuman HB, Wald ER. Bacterial meningitis in childhood at the Children's Hospital of Pittsburgh: 1988–1998. Clin Pediatr (Phila) 2001;40:595–600.

934. Newfield RS, Vargas I, Huma Z. *Eikenella corrodens* infections: case report in two adolescent females with IDDM. Diabetes Care 1996;19:1011–1013.

935. Newman MG, Sutter VL, Pickett MJ, et al. Detection, identification, and comparison of *Capnocytophaga*, *Bacteroides ochraceus*, and DF-1. J Clin Microbiol 1979;10:557–562.

936. Ng VL, Weir L, York MK, et al. *Bordetella pertussis* versus Non-*L. pneumophila Legionella* spp.: a continuing diagnostic challenge. J Clin Microbiol 1992;30:3300–3301.

937. Ng VL, York M, Hadley WK. Unexpected isolation of *Bordetella pertussis* from patients with acquired immunodeficiency syndrome. J Clin Microbiol 1989;27:337–338.

938. Ngaage DL, Kotidis KN, Sandoe JA, Unnikrishan Nair R. Do not snog the dog: infective endocarditis due to *Capnocytophaga canimorsus*. Eur J Cardiothorac Surg 1999;16:362–363.

939. Nikkari S, Gotoff R, Bourbeau PP, et al. Identification of *Cardiobacterium hominis* by broad-range bacterial polymerase chain reaction analysis in a case of culture-negative endocarditis. Arch Intern Med 2002;162:477–479.

940. Njankepo E, Delisle F, Hagege I, et al. *Bordetella holmesii* isolated from a patient with sickle cell anemia: analysis and comparison with other *Bordetella holmesii* isolates. Microbiol Infect 2000 ;6:131–136.

941. Noah DL, Bresee JS, Gorensek MJ, et al. Cluster of five children with acute encephalitis associated with cat-scratch disease in south Florida. Pediatr Infect Dis J 1995;14:866.

942. Noah DL, Kramer CM, Verbsky MP, et al. Survey of veterinary professionals and other veterinary conference attendees for antibodies to *Bartonella henselae* and *B. quintana*. J Am Vet Med Assoc 1997;210:342–344.

943. Noble RC, Marek BJ, Overman SB. Spontaneous bacterial peritonitis caused by *Pasteurella ureae*. J Clin Microbiol 1987;25:442–444.

944. Noele GL, Teele DW. In vitro activities of selected new and long-acting cephalosporins against *Pasteurella multocida*. Antimicrob Agents Chemother 1986; 29:344–345.

945. Nordahl SHG, Hoel T, Scheel O, et al. Tularemia: a differential diagnosis in oto-rhino-laryngology. J Laryngol Otol 1993;107:127–129.

946. Norman AF, Regnery R, Jameson P, et al. Differentiation of *Bartonella*-like isolates at the species level by PCR-restriction fragment length polymorphism in the citrate synthase gene. J Clin Microbiol 1995;33:1797–1803.

947. Novotny LA, Jurcisek JA, Pichichero ME, Bakaletz LO. Epitope mapping of the outer membrane protein P5-homologous fimbrin adhesin of nontypeable *Haemophilus influenzae*. Infect Immun 2000;68:2119–2128.

948. Nsanze H, Plummer FA, Maggwa ABN, et al. Comparison of media for the primary isolation of *Haemophilus ducreyi*. Sex Transm Dis 1984;11:6–9.

949. Nurnberger M, Treadwell T, Lin B, Weintraub A. Pacemaker lead infection and vertebral osteomyelitis presumed due to *Cardiobacterium hominis*. Clin Infect Dis 1998;27:890–891.

950. Nye KJ, Fallon D, Gee B, et al. A comparison of the performance of bacitracin-incorporated chocolate blood agar with a chocolate blood agar plus a bacitracin disk in the isolation of *Haemophilus influenzae* from sputum. J Med Microbiol 2001;50:472–475.

951. Nygren M, Reizenstein E, Ronaghi M, Lundeberg J. Polymorphism in the pertussis toxin promoter region affecting the DNA-based diagnosis of *Bordetella* infection. J Clin Microbiol 2000;38:55–60.

952. Oberhofer TR, Back AE. Biotypes of *Haemophilus influenzae* encountered in clinical laboratories. J Clin Microbiol 1979;10:168–174.

953. O'Bryan TA, Whitener CJ, Katzman M, et al. Hepatobiliary infections caused by *Haemophilus* species. Clin Infect Dis 1992;15:716–719.

954. Ochiai K, Senpuku H, Kurita-Ochiai T. Purification of an immunosuppressive factor from *Capnocytophaga ochracea*. J Med Microbiol 1998 ;47:1087–1095.

955. Ochiai T, Ochiai K, Saito N, et al. Adoptive transfer of suppressor T-cells induced by *Actinobacillus actinomycetemcomitans* regulates immune response. J Periodontol Res 29:1–8, 1994.

956. O'Connor SP, Dorsch M, Steigerwalt AG, et al. 16S rRNA sequences of *Bartonella bacilliformis* and cat-scratch disease bacillus reveal phylogenetic relationships with the α-2 subgroup of the class *Proteobacteria*. J Clin Microbiol 1991; 29:2144–2150.

957. Odeh M, Oliven A. Acute pancreatitis associated with brucellosis. J Gastroenterol Hepatol 1995;10:691–692.

958. Odeh M, Pick N, Oliven A. Deep venous thrombosis associated with acute brucellosis: a case report. Angiology 2000;1:253–256.

959. Ogilvie C, Omikunle A, Wang Y, et al. Capsulation loci of non-serotype b encapsulated *Haemophilus influenzae*. J Infect Dis 2001;184:144–149.

960. O'Halloran HS, Draud K, Minix M, et al. Leber's neuroretinitis in a patient with serologic evidence of *Bartonella elizabethae*. Retina 1998;18:276–278.

961. Ohl ME, Spach DH. *Bartonella quintana* and urban trench fever. Clin Infect Dis 2000;31:131–135.

962. Oill PA, Chow AW, Guze LB. Adult bacteremic *Haemophilus parainfluenzae* infections: seven reports of cases and a review of the literature. Arch Intern Med 1979;139:985–988.

963. Ojukwu IC, Chisty C. Rat bite fever in children: case report and review. Scand J Infect Dis 2002 ;34:474–477.

964. Okada K, Ueda K, Morokuma K, et al. Comparison of antibody titers in eleven-to twelve-year old Japanese school children six years after administration of acellular and whole cell pertussis vaccines combined with diphtheria-tetanus toxoids. Pediatr Infect Dis J 1998;17:1167–1168.

965. Olin P, Rasmussen F, Gustafsson L, et al. Randomised controlled trial of two-component, three-component, and five-component acellular pertussis vaccines compared with whole-cell pertussis vaccine. Lancet 1997;350:1569–1570.

966. Oliveira S, Splitter GA. Immunization of mice with recombinant L7/L12 ribosomal protein confers protection against *Brucella abortus* infection. Vaccine1996;14:959–962.

967. Olk DG, Hamill RJ, Procter RA. Case report: *Haemophilus parainfluenzae* vertebral osteomyelitis. Am J Med Sci 1987;294:114–116.

968. Olopoenia LA, Mody V, Reynolds M. *Eikenella corrodens* endocarditis in an intravenous drug user: case report and literature review. J Natl Med Assoc 1994;86:313–315.

969. Olsen I. Recent approaches to the chemotaxonomy of the *Actinobacillus-Haemophilus-Pasteurella* group (Family *Pasteurellaceae*). Oral Microbiol Immunol 1993;8:327–336.

970. Omikunle A, Takahashi S, Ogilvie CL, et al. Limited genetic diversity of recent invasive isolates of non-serotype b encapsulated *Haemophilus influenzae*. J Clin Microbiol 2002;40:1264–1270.

971. O'Reilly KL, Bauer RW, Freeland RL, et al. Acute clinical disease in cats following infection with a pathogenic strain of *Bartonella henselae* (LSU16). Infect Immun 1999;67:3066–3072.

972. Orenstein WA. Pertussis in adults: epidemiology, signs, symptoms, and implications for vaccination. Clin Infect Dis 1999;28(Suppl 2):S147–S150.

973. Orle KA, Gates CA, Martin DH, et al. Simultaneous PCR detection of *Haemophilus ducreyi*, *Treponema pallidum*, and herpes simplex virus types 1 and 2 from genital ulcers. J Clin Microbiol 1996;34:49–54.

974. Ory JM, Chuard C, Regamey C. *Pasteurella multocida* pneumonia with empyema. Scand J Infect Dis 1998;30:313–314.

975. Osawa R, Rainey F, Fujisawa T, et al. *Lonepinella koalarum* gen. nov., sp. nov., a new tannin-protein complex degrading bacterium. Syst Appl Microbiol 1995 ;18:368–373.

976. Oscherwitz SL. Brucellar bacteremia in pregnancy. Clin Infect Dis 1995;21:714–715.

977. Osoba AO, Balkhy H, Memish Z, et al. Diagnostic value of Brucella ELISA IgG and IgM in bacteremic and non-bacteremic patients with brucellosis. J Chemother 2001;13(Suppl 1):54–59.

978. Ozkurt Z, Erol Z, Tasyaran MA, Kaya A. Detection of *Brucella melitensis* by the BacT/Alert automated system and *Brucella* broth culture. Clin Microbiol Infect 2002;8:749–752.

979. Paavonen J, Lehtinen M, Teisala K, et al. *Haemophilus influenzae* causes purulent salpingitis. Am J Obstet Gynecol 1985;151:338–339.

980. Paju S, Carlson P, Jousimies-Somer H, Asikainen S. Heterogeneity of *Actino-*

bacillus actinomycetemcomitans strains in various human infections and relationships between serotype, genotype, and antimicrobial susceptibility. J Clin Microbiol 2000;38:79–84.

981. Pajukanta R, Asikainen S, Saarela M, et al. In vitro activity of azithromycin compared with that of erythromycin against *Actinobacillus actinomycetemcomitans*. Antimicrob Agents Chemother 36:1241–1243, 1992.

982. Pajukanta R, Asikainen S, Saarela M, et al. Evaluation of the E test for antimicrobial susceptibility testing of *Actinobacillus actinomycetemcomitans*. Oral Microbiol Immunol 1992;7:376–377.

983. Pajukanta R, Asikainen S, Saarela M, et al. In vitro antimicrobial susceptibility of different serotypes of *Actinobacillus actinomycetemcomitans*. Scand J Dent Res 1993;101:299–303.

984. Palanduz A, Palanduz S, Guler K, Guler N: Brucellosis in a mother and her young infant: probable transmission by breast milk. Int J Infect Dis 2000;4:55–56.

985. Parenti DM, Snydman DR. *Capnocytophaga* species: infections in nonimmunocompromised and immunocompromised hosts. J Infect Dis 1985;151:140–147.

986. Parsons LM, Shayegani M, Waring AL, et al. DNA probes for the identification of *Haemophilus ducreyi*. J Clin Microbiol 1989;27:1441–1445.

987. Patel A, Asirvatham S, Sebastian C, et al. Polymicrobial endocarditis with *Haemophilus parainfluenzae* in an intravenous drug user whose transesophageal echocardiogram appeared normal. Clin Infect Dis 1998;26:1245–1246.

988. Patel IS, Seemungal TA. Wilks M, et al. Relationship between bacterial colonization and the frequency, character, and severity of COPD exacerbations. Thorax 2002;57:759–764.

989. Paton BG, Ormerod LD, Peppe J, et al. Evidence for a feline reservoir for dysgonic fermenter 2 keratitis. J Clin Microbiol 1988;26:2439–2440.

990. Paul K, Patel SS. *Eikenella corrodens* infections in children and adolescents: case reports and review of the literature. Clin Infect Dis 2001;33:54–61.

991. Paul RV, Rostand SG. Cat bite peritonitis: *Pasteurella multocida* peritonitis following feline contamination of peritoneal dialysis tubing. Am J Kidney Dis 1987;10:318–319.

992. Paulsen IT, Seshadri R, Nelson KE, et al. The *Brucella suis* genome reveals fundamental similarities between animal and plant pathogens and symbionts. Proc Natl Acad Sci USA 2002;99:13148–13153.

993. Pavicic MJAMP, van Winkelhoff AJ, DeGraff J. In vitro susceptibilities of *Actinobacillus actinomycetemcomitans* to a number of antimicrobial combinations. Antimicrob Agents Chemother 1992;36:2634–2638.

994. Peake JE, Slaughter BD. Hemorrhagic conjunctivitis and invasive *Haemophilus influenzae* type b infection. Pediatr Infect Dis J 1994;13:230–231.

995. Peek RM, Truss C. Secretory diarrhea following a dog bite. Dig Dis Sci 36:1991;1151–1153.

996. Peel MM. Dog-associated bacterial infections in humans: isolates submitted to an Australian reference laboratory, 1981–1992. Pathology 1993;25:379–384.

997. Peel MM, Hornidge KA, Luppino M, et al. *Actinobacillus* spp. and related bacteria in infected wounds of humans bitten by horses and sheep. J Clin Microbiol 29:2535–2538, 1991.

998. Peltola H. Prophylaxis of bacterial meningitis. In: Schaad UB, ed. Infectious Disease Clinics of North America. Vol 13. Bacterial Meningitis. Philadelphia: Saunders, 1999:685–710.

999. Peltola H. Worldwide *Haemophilus influenzae* type b disease at the beginning of the 21st century: global analysis of the disease burden 25 years after the use of the polysaccharide vaccine and a decade after the advent of conjugates. Clin Microbiol Rev 2000;13:302–317.

1000. Perez-Calvo J, Matamala C, Sanjoaquin I, et al. Epidural abscess due to acute *Brucella melitensis* infection. Arch Intern Med 1994;154:1410–1411.

1001. Perkins MD, Mirrett S, Reller LB. Rapid bacterial antigen detection is not clinically useful. J Clin Microbiol 1995;33:1486–1491.

1002. Perkocha LA, Geaghan SM, Benedict TS, et al. Clinical and pathological features of bacillary peliosis hepatis in association with human immunodeficiency virus infection. N Engl J Med 1990;323:1581–1586.

1003. Pers C, Gahrn-Hansen B, Frederiksen W. *Capnocytophaga canimorsus* septicemia in Denmark, 1982–1995: review of 39 cases. Clin Infect Dis 1996 ;23:71–75.

1004. Peruski AH, Johnson LH III, Peruski LF Jr. Rapid and sensitive detection of biological warfare agents using time-resolved fluorescence assays. J Immunol Methods 2002;263:35–41.

1005. Peter G, Hall CB, Halsey NA, et al. *Haemophilus influenzae* infections. In: 1997 Red Book: Report of the Committee on Infectious Diseases. 24th ed. Elk Grove Village, IL: American Academy of Pediatrics, 1997:222–231.

1006. Peters VB, Sood S. Immunity to *Haemophilus influenzae* type b polysaccharide capsule in children with human immunodeficiency virus infection immunized with a single dose of *Haemophilus* vaccine. J Pediatr 1994;125:74–77.

1007. Petrocheilou-Pashou, Georgilis K, Kostis E, et al. Bronchitis caused by *Bordetella bronchiseptica* in an elderly woman. Clin Microbiol Infect 2000;6:147–148.

1008. Pettigrew MM, Foxman B, Marrs CF, Gilsdorf JR. Identification of the lipooligosaccharide biosynthesis gene *lic2B* as a putative virulence factor in strains of nontypeable *Haemophilus influenzae* that cause otitis media. Infect Immun 2002;70:3551–3556.

1009. Phillips JE. Genus III. *Actinobacillus* Brumpt 1910, 849AL. In: Krieg NR, Holt JG, eds. Bergey's Manual of Systematic Bacteriology. Vol. 1. Baltimore: Williams & Wilkins, 1984:570–575.

1010. Phipps SE, Tamblyn DM, Badenoch PR. *Capnocytophaga canimorsus* endophthalmitis following cataract surgery. Clin Exp Ophthalmol 2002 ;30:375–377.

1011. Pichichero ME, Casey JR. Otitis media. Expert Opin Pharmacother 2002;3:1073–1090.

1012. Pichichero ME, Deloria MA, Rennels MB, et al. A safety and immunogenicity comparison of 12 acellular pertussis vaccines and one whole-cell pertussis given as a fourth dose in 15- to 20-month old children. Pediatrics 1997;100:772–788.

1013. Pillai A, Mitchell JL, Hill SL, Stockley RA. A case of *Haemophilus parainfluenzae* pneumonia. Thorax 2000;55:623–624.

1014. Pins MR, Holden JM, Yang JM, et al. Isolation of presumptive *Streptobacillus moniliformis* from abscesses associated with the female genital tract. Clin Infect Dis 1996;22:471–476.

1015. Pittman M. Genus *Bordetella* Moreno-Lopez 1952, 178^AL. In: Krieg NR, Holt JG, eds. Bergey's Manual of Determinative Bacteriology. Vol. 1. Baltimore, Williams & Wilkins, 1984:388–393.

1016. Pittman T, Williams D, Friedman AD. A shunt infection caused by *Francisella tularensis*. Pediatr Neurosurg 1996;24:50–51.

1017. Plettenberg A, Lorenzen T, Burtsche BT, et al. Bacillary angiomatosis in HIV-infected patients: an epidemiological and clinical study. Dermatology 2000;201:326–331.

1018. Plourde PJ, Embree J, Friesen F, et al. Glandular tularemia with typhoidal features in a Manitoba child. Can Med Assoc J 1992 ;146:1953–1955.

1019. Pohl S, Bertschinger U, Frederiksen W, et al. Transfer of *Haemophilus pleuropneumoniae* and the *Pasteurella haemolytica*-like organism causing porcine necrotic pleuropneumonia in the genus *Actinobacillus* (*Actinobacillus pleuropneumoniae* comb. nov.) on the basis of phenotypic and deoxyribonucleic acid relatedness. Int J Syst Bacteriol 1983;33:510–514.

1020. Porter JF, Connor K, Donachie W. Isolation and characterization of *Bordetella parapertussis*-like bacteria from ovine lungs. Microbiology 1994;140:255–261.

1021. Portnoy BL, Satterwhite TK, Dyckman JK. Rat bite fever misdiagnosed as Rocky Mountain spotted fever. South Med J 1979;72:607–609.

1022. Porto MHO, Noel GJ, Edelson PJ, et al. Resistance to serum bactericidal activity distinguishes Brazilian purpuric fever (BPF) case strains of *Haemophilus influenzae* biogroup *aegyptius* (*H. aegyptius*) from non-BPF strains. J Clin Microbiol 1988;27:792–294.

1023. Postels-Multani S, Schmitt HJ, Wirsing von Konig CH, et al. Symptoms and complications of pertussis in adults. Infection 1995;23:139–142.

1024. Potts TV, Zambon JJ, Genco RJ. Reassignment of *Actinobacillus actinomycetemcomitans* to the genus *Haemophilus* as *Haemophilus actinomycetemcomitans* comb. nov. Int J Syst Bacteriol 1985;35:337–341.

1025. Pouedras P, Donnio PY, Le Tulzo Y, et al. *Pasteurella stomatis* infection following a dog bite. Eur J Clin Microbiol Infect Dis 1993;12:65.

1026. Prasadarao NV, Lysenko E, Wass CA, et al. Opacity-associated protein A contributes to the binding of *Haemophilus influenzae* to Chang epithelial cells. Infect Immun 1999;67:4153–4160.

1027. Pratt J, Cooley JD, Purdy CW, Straus DC. Lipase activity from strains of *Pasteurella multocida*. Curr Microbiol 2000;40:306–309.

1028. Preus HR, Sunday GJ, Haraszthy VI, et al. Rapid identification of *Actinobacillus actinomycetemcomitans* based on analysis of 23S ribosomal RNA. Oral Microbiol Immunol 1992;7:372–375.

1029. Prior RB, Spagna VA, Perkins RL. Endocarditis due to a strain of *Cardiobacterium hominis* resistant to erythromycin and vancomycin. Chest 1979;75:85–86.

1030. Pritchard TM, Foust RT, Cantey JR, et al. Prosthetic valve endocarditis due to *Cardiobacterium hominis* occurring after upper gastrointestinal endoscopy. Am J Med 1991;90:516–518.

1031. Privitera A, Licciardello L, Giannino V, et al. Molecular epidemiology and phylogenetic analysis of *Haemophilus parainfluenzae* from chronic obstructive pulmonary disease exacerbations. Eur J Epidemiol 1998;14:405–412.

1032. Progulske A, Mishell R, Trummel C, Holt SC. Biological activities of *Eikenella corrodens* outer membrane and lipopolysaccharide. Infect Immun 1984;43:178–182.

1033. Provenza JM, Klotz SA, Penn RL. Isolation of *Francisella tularensis* from blood. J Clin Microbiol 1986;24:453–455.

1034. Purdy D, Khandori N, Abbas F, et al. Postoperative pancreatic abscess due to *Haemophilus influenzae*. Clin Infect Dis 1993;17:49–51.

1035. Quentin R, Dubarry I, Martin C, et al. Evaluation of four commercial methods for identification and biotyping of genital and neonatal strains of *Haemophilus* species. Eur J Clin Microbiol Infect Dis 1992;11:546–549.

1036. Quentin R, Goudeau A, Wallace RJ Jr, et al. Urogenital, maternal, and neonatal isolates of *Haemophilus influenzae*: identification of unusually virulent serologically non-typeable clone families and evidence for a new *Haemophilus* species. J Gen Microbiol 1990;136:1203–1209.

1037. Quentin R, Martin C, Musser JM, et al. Genetic characterization of a cryptic genospecies of *Haemophilus* causing urogenital and neonatal infections. J Clin Microbiol 1993;31:1111–1116.

1038. Quentin R, Musser JM, Mellouett M, et al. Typing of urogenital, maternal, and neonatal isolates of *Haemophilus influenzae* and *Haemophilus parainfluenzae* in correlation with clinical course of isolation and evidence for a genital specificity of *Haemophilus influenzae* biotype IV. J Clin Microbiol 1989;27: 2286–2294.

1039. Quiles I, Blazquez JC, De Teresa L, et al. Vertebral osteomyelitis due to *Pasteurella aerogenes*. Scand J Infect Dis 2000;32:566–567.

1040. Raab MG, Lutz RA, Stauffer ES. *Eikenella corrodens* vertebral osteomyelitis: a case report and literature review. Clin Orthop 1993;293:144–147.

1041. Raad I, Rand K, Gaskins D. Buffered charcoal yeast extract medium for the isolation of brucellae. J Clin Microbiol 1990;28:1671–1672.

1042. Radolf JD. Brucellosis: don't let it get your goat. Am J Med Sci 1994;307: 64–75.

1043. Raffi F, Barner J, Baron D, et al. *Pasteurella multocida* bacteremia: report of 13 cases over 12 years and review of the literature. Scand J Infect Dis 1987; 19:385–393.

1044. Rahman A, Burma O, Felek S, Yekeler H. Atrial septal defect presenting with *Brucella* endocarditis. Scand J Infect Dis 2001;33:776–777.

1045. Ramdeen GD, Smith RJ, Smith EA, et al. *Pasteurella multocida* tonsillitis: case report and review. Clin Infect Dis 1995;20:1055–1057.

1046. Ramos JM, Pacho E, Garcia-Valle B, et al. Splenic abscess due to *Eikenella corrodens*. Postgrad Med J 1994;70:848–849.

1047. Rank EL, Mandour M, Zimmerman SE. Problems with species identification of *Pasteurella* sp., new species 1: two case reports. Clin Microbiol Newslett 1984;6:166–167.

1048. Raoult D, Birtles RJ, Montoya M, et al. Survey of three bacterial louse-associated diseases among rural Andean communities in Peru: prevalence of epidemic typhus, trench fever, and relapsing fever. Clin Infect Dis 1999;29:434–436.

1049. Raoult D, Drancourt M, Carta A, Gastaut JA. *Bartonella* (*Rochalimaea*) *quintana* isolation in a patient with chronic lymphadenopathy, lymphopenia, and a cat. Lancet 1994;343:977.

1050. Raoult D, Fournier PE, Drancourt M, et al. Diagnosis of 22 new cases of *Bartonella* endocarditis. Ann Intern Med 1996;125:646–652.

1051. Raucher B, Dobkin J, Mandel L, et al. Occult polymicrobial endocarditis with *Haemophilus parainfluenzae* in intravenous drug abusers. Am J Med 1989;86: 169–172.

1052. Rechtman DJ, Nadler JP. Abdominal abscess due to *Cardiobacterium hominis* and *Clostridium bifermentans*. Rev Infect Dis 1991;13:418–419.

1053. Redfield DC, Overturf GD, Ewing ND, et al. Bacteria, arthritis, and skin lesions due to *Kingella kingae*. Arch Dis Child 1980;55:411–414.

1054. Redkar R, Rose S, Bricker B, DelVecchio V. Real-time PCR detection of *Brucella abortus*, *Brucella melitensis*, and *Brucella suis*. Mol Cell Probes 2001; 15:43–52.

1055. Refai M. Incidence and control of brucellosis in the Near East region. Vet Microbiol 2002;90:81–110.

1056. Regan J, Lowe F. Enrichment medium for the isolation of *Bordetella pertussis*. J Clin Microbiol 1977;6:303–309.

1057. Regnery RL, Anderson BE, Clarridge JE, et al. Characterization of a novel *Rochalimaea* species, *R. henselae* sp. nov., isolated from blood of a febrile, human immunodeficiency virus-positive patient. J Clin Microbiol 1992;30: 265–274.

1058. Regnery RL, Martin M, Olson J. Naturally occurring "*Rochalimaea henselae*" infection in domestic cats. Lancet 1992;340:557–558.

1059. Regnery RL, Olson JG, Perkins BA, Bibb W. Serological response to "*Rochalimaea henselae*" antigen in suspected cat-scratch disease. Lancet 1992;339: 1443–1445.

1060. Reina J, Bassa A, Llompart I, et al. Pneumonia caused by *Bordetella bronchiseptica* in a patient with a thoracic trauma. Infection 1991;19:46–48.

1061. Reintjes R, Dedushaj I, Gjini A, et al. Tularemia outbreak investigation in Kosovo: case control and environmental studies. Emerg Infect Dis 2002;8: 69–73.

1062. Reitman CA, Watters WC III. Spinal brucellosis: case report in the United States. Spine 2002;27:E250–E252.

1063. Reizenstein E, Lindberg L, Mollby R, Hallander HO. Validation of nested *Bordetella* PCR in pertussis vaccine trial. J Clin Microbiol 1996;34:810–815.

1064. Relman DA, Domenighini M, Tuomanen E, et al. Filamentous hemagglutinin of *Bordetella pertussis*: nucleotide sequence and crucial role in adherence. Proc Natl Acad Sci USA 1989;86:2637–2641.

1065. Relman DA, Falkow S, LeBoit PE, et al. The organism causing bacillary angiomatosis, peliosis hepatis, and fever and bacteremia in immunocompromised patients. N Engl J Med 1991;324:1514.

1066. Relman DA, Loutit JS, Schmidt TM, et al. The agent of bacillary angiomatosis:

an approach to the identification of uncultured pathogens. N Engl J Med 1990; 323:1573–1580.

1067. Reyn A, Birch-Anderson A, Murray RGE. The fine structure of *Cardiobacterium hominis*. Acta Pathol Microbiol Scand 1971;79:51–60.

1068. Rhyan JC, Gidlewski T, Ewalt DR, et al. Seroconversion and abortion in cattle experimentally infected with *Brucella* sp. isolated from a Pacific harbor seal (*Phoca vitulina richardsi*). J Vet Diagn Invest 2001;13:379–382.

1069. Ribeiro GA, Carter GR, Frederiksen W, et al. *Pasteurella haemolytica*-like bacterium from a progressive granuloma of cattle in Brazil. J Clin Microbiol 1989;27:1401–1402.

1070. Ribeiro GS, Reis JN, Cordeiro SM, et al. Prevention of *Haemophilus influenzae* type b (Hib) meningitis and emergence of serotype replacement with type a strains after introduction of Hib immunization in Brazil. J Infect Dis 2003;187: 109–116.

1071. Riggio MP, Lennon A. Rapid identification of *Actinobacillus actinomycetemcomitans*, *Haemophilus aphrophilus*, and *Haemophilus paraphrophilus* by restriction enzyme analysis of PCR-amplified 16S rRNA genes. J Clin Microbiol 1997;35:1630–1632.

1072. Riley LK, Robertson DR. Ingestion and survival of *Brucella abortus* in human and bovine polymorphonuclear leukocytes. Infect Immun 1984;46:224–230.

1073. Riley UB, De P. *Pasteurella multocida*: an uncommon cause of obstetric and gynaecological sepsis. J Infect 1995 ;31:51–53.

1074. Risi GF, Plombo DJ. Relapse of tularemia after aminoglycoside therapy: case report and discussion of therapeutic options. Clin Infect Dis 1995;20:174–175.

1075. Ristic M, Kreier JP. Family II. *Bartonellaceae* Gieszczykiewicz 1939, 25^AL. In: Krieg NR, Holt JG, eds. Bergey's Manual of Systematic Bacteriology. Vol. 1. Baltimore: Williams & Wilkins, 1984:717–719.

1076. Rivera M, Hunter GC, Brooker J, et al. Aortic graft infection due to *Pasteurella haemolytica* and group C β-hemolytic streptococcus. Clin Infect Dis 1994;19: 941–943.

1077. Robinson-Dunne B. The microbiology laboratory's role in response to bioterrorism. Arch Pathol Lab Med 2002;126:291–294.

1078. Roblot P, Bazillou M, Grolier G, et al. Septicemia due to *Capnocytophaga canimorsus* after a dog bite in a cirrhotic patient. Eur J Clin Microbiol Infect Dis 1993;12:302–303.

1079. Rodgers BL, Duffield RP, Taylor T, et al. Tularemic meningitis. Pediatr Infect Dis J 1998;17:439–441.

1080. Rodriguez-Barradas MC, Hamill RJ, Houston ED, et al. Genomic fingerprinting of *Bartonella* species by repetitive element PCR for distinguishing species and isolates. J Clin Microbiol 33: 1995;1089–1093.

1081. Roe DE, Braham PH, Weinberg A, et al. Characterization of tetracycline resistance in *Actinobacillus actinomycetemcomitans*. Oral Microbiol Immunol 10: 227–232, 1995.

1082. Roebuck JD, Morris JT. Chronic otitis media due to EF-4 bacteria. Clin Infect Dis 29:1343–1344, 1999.

1083. Rogers BT, Anderson JC, Palmer CA, et al. Septicaemia due to *Pasteurella pneumotropica*. J Clin Pathol 1973;26:396–398.

1084. Roggen EL, Pansaerts R, Van Dyck E, et al. Antigen detection and immunological typing of *Haemophilus ducreyi* with a specific rabbit polyclonal serum. J Clin Microbiol 1993;31:1820–1825.

1085. Rohrbach BW, Westerman E, Istre GR. Epidemiology and clinical characteristics of tularemia in Oklahoma, 1979–1985. South Med J 1991;84:1091–1096.

1086. Roiz MP, Peralta FG, Arjona R. *Kingella kingae* bacteremia in an immunocompetent adult host. J Clin Microbiol 1997;35:1916.

1087. Rolle U, Schille R, Hormann D, et al. Soft tissue infection caused by *Kingella kingae* in a child. J Pediatr Surg 2001;36:946–947.

1088. Ronald AR, Albritton W. Chancroid and *Haemophilus ducreyi*. In: Holmes KK, Mardh P-A, Sparling PF, et al., eds. Sexually Transmitted Diseases., 3rd Ed. New York: McGraw-Hill, 1999:515–523.

1089. Ronnevik PK, Ness HC. Septicemia caused by *Cardiobacterium hominis*: a case report. Acta Pathol Microbiol Scand Sect B 1981;89:243–244.

1090. Rordorf T, Zuger C, Zbinden R, et al. *Streptobacillus moniliformis* endocarditis in an HIV-positive patient. Infection 2002;28:393–394.

1091. Roscoe DL, Zemcov SJV, Thornber D, et al. Antimicrobial susceptibilities and β-lactamase characterization of *Capnocytophaga* species. Antimicrob Agents Chemother 1992;36:2197–2200.

1092. Rosenau A, Cattier B, Gousset N, et al. *Capnocytophaga ochracea*: characterization of a plasmid-encoded extended spectrum TEM-17 β-lactamase in the phylum Flavobacter-Bacteroides. Antimicrob Agents Chemother 2000;44: 760–762.

1093. Rosenau A, Labigne A, Escande F, et al. Plasmid-mediated ROB-1 β-lactamase in *Pasteurella multocida* from a human specimen. Antimicrob Agents Chemother 1991;35:2419–2422.

1094. Rosenau A, Sizaret PY, Musser JM, et al. Adherence to human cells of a cryptic *Haemophilus* genospecies responsible for genital and neonatal infections. Infect Immun 1993;61:4112–4118.

1095. Rosenbach KA, Poblete J, Larkin I. Prosthetic valve endocarditis caused by *Pasteurella dagmatis*. South Med J 2001;94:1033–1035.

1096. Rosenbaum GS, Calubiran O, Cunha BA. *Haemophilus parainfluenzae* bacteremia associated with a pacemaker wire localized by gallium scan. Heart Lung 1990;19:271–273.

1097. Rosenfeld JA, Clarity G. Acute otitis media in children. Prim Care 1996;23: 677–686.

1098. Roson B, Carratala J, Verdaguer R, et al. Prospective study of the usefulness of the Gram stain in the initial approach to community-acquired pneumonia requiring hospitalization. Clin Infect Dis 2000;31:869–874.

1099. Rossau R, Duhamel M, Jannes G, et al. The development of specific rRNA-derived oligonucleotide probes for *Haemophilus ducreyi*, the causative agent of chancroid. J Gen Microbiol 1991;137:277–285.

1100. Rossau R, Vandenbussche G, Thielemans S, et al. Ribosomal ribonucleic acid cistron similarities and deoxyribonucleic acid homologies of *Neisseria*, *Kingella*, *Eikenella*, *Simonsiella*, *Alysiella*, and Centers for Disease Control Groups EF-4 and M-5 in the emended family *Neisseriaceae*. Int J Syst Bacteriol 1989;39:185–198.

1101. Rothstein EP, Anderson EL, Decker MD, et al. An acellular pertussis vaccine in healthy adults: safety and immunogenicity. Pennridge Pediatric Associates. Vaccine 1999;17:2999–3006.

1102. Roux V, Eykyn SJ, Wyllie S, Raoult D. *Bartonella vinsonii* subsp. *berkhoffii* as an agent of afebrile blood culture-negative endocarditis in a human. J Clin Microbiol 2000;38:1698–1700.

1103. Roux V, Raoult D. Body lice as tools for diagnosis and surveillance of reemerging diseases. J Clin Microbiol 1999;37:596–599.

1104. Rowbotham TJ. Rapid identification of *Streptobacillus moniliformis*. Lancet 1983;2:567.

1105. Rubin LG, Gloster ES, Carlone GM, et al. An infant rat model of bacteremia with Brazilian purpuric fever isolates of *Haemophilus influenzae* biogroup aegyptius. J Infect Dis 1989;160:476–482.

1106. Rubsamen PE, McLeish WM, Pflugfelder S, et al. *Capnocytophaga* endophthalmitis. Ophthalmology 100:456–459, 1993.

1107. Ruddock TL, Rindler JM, Bergfeld WF. *Capnocytophaga canimorsus* septicemia in an asplenic patient. Cutis 1997;60:95–97.

1108. Ruiz-Irastorza G, Garea C, Alonso JJ, et al. Septic shock due to *Pasteurella multocida* subspecies *multocida* in a previously healthy woman. Clin Infect Dis 1995;21:232–234.

1109. Rummens J-L, Gordts B, Van Landuyt HW. In vitro susceptibility of *Capnocytophaga* species to 29 antimicrobial agents. Antimicrob Agents Chemother 1986;30:739–742.

1110. Rupp ME. *Streptobacillus moniliformis* endocarditis: case report and review. Clin Infect Dis 1992;14:769–772.

1111. Rydkina EB, Roux V, Gagua EM, et al. *Bartonella quintana* in body lice collected from homeless persons in Russia. Emerg Infect Dis 1999;5:176–178.

1112. Rygg M, Bruun CF. Rat bite fever (*Streptobacillus moniliformis*) with septicemia in a child. Scand J Infect Dis 1992;24:535–540.

1113. Saab M, Corcoran JP, Southworth SA, Randell PE. Fatal septicemia in a previously healthy man following a dog bite. Int J Clin Pract 1998;52:205.

1114. Saadati M, Gibbs HA, Parton R, Coote JG. Characterisation of the leukotoxin produced by different strains of *Pasteurella haemolytica*. J Med Microbiol 1997;46:276–284.

1115. Saadeh AM, Abu-Farsakh NA, Omari HZ. Infective endocarditis and occult splenic abscess caused by *Brucella melitensis* infection: a case report and review of the literature. Acta Cardiol 1996;51:279–285.

1116. Saarela M, Asikainen S, Jousimies-Somer H, et al. Hybridization patterns of *Actinobacillus actinomycetemcomitans* serotypes a-e detected with an rRNA gene probe. Oral Microbiol Immunol 1993;8:111–115.

1117. Saarela M, Dogan B, Alaluusua S, et al. Persistence of oral colonization by the same *Actinobacillus actinomycetemcomitans* strain(s). J. Periodontol 1999; 70:504–509.

1118. Sacco RE, Register KB, Nordholm GE. Restriction enzyme analysis and ribotyping distinguish *Bordetella avium* and *Bordetella hinzii* isolates. Epidemiol Infect 2000;124:83–90.

1119. Saez-Llorens X, McCracken GH Jr. Antimicrobial and anti-inflammatory treatment of bacterial meningitis. In: Schaad UB, ed. Infectious Disease Clinics of North America. Vol. 13. Bacterial meningitis. Philadelphia: Saunders, 1999: 619–636.

1120. Saito A, Hosaka Y, Nakagawa T, et al. Significance of serum antibody against surface antigens of *Actinobacillus actinomycetemcomitans* in patients with adult periodontitis. Oral Microbiol Immunol 1993;8:146–153.

1121. Salgado F, Grana M, Ferrer V, et al. Splenic infarction associated with acute *Brucella melitensis* infection. Eur J Clin Microbiol Infect Dis 2002;21:63–64.

1122. Sanden GN, Cassiday PK, Barbaree JM. Rapid immunoblot technique for identifying *Bordetella pertussis*. J Clin Microbiol 1993;31:170–172.

1123. Sander A, Buhler C, Pelz K, et al. Detection and identification of two *Bartonella henselae* variants in domestic cats in Germany. J Clin Microbiol 1997;35: 584–587.

1124. Sander A, Penno S. Semiquantitative species-specific detection of *Bartonella*

1125. Sander A, Posselt M, Oberle K, Bredt W. Seroprevalence of antibodies to *Bartonella henselae* in patients with cat scratch disease and in healthy controls: evaluation and comparison of two commercial serological tests. Clin Diagn Lab Immunol 1998;5:486–490.

1126. Sander A, Zagrosek A, Bredt W, et al. Characterization of *Bartonella clarridgeiae* flagellin (FlaA) and detection of antiflagellin antibodies in patients with lymphadenopathy. J Clin Microbiol 2000;38:2943–2948.

1127. Sandstrom G, Lofgren S, Tarnvik A. A capsule-deficient mutant of *Francisella tularensis* LVS exhibits enhanced sensitivity to killing by serum but diminished sensitivity to killing by polymorphonuclear leukocytes. Infect Immun 1988; 56:1194–1202.

1128. Sandstrom G, Sjostedt A, Forsman M, et al. Characterization and classification of strains of *Francisella tularensis* isolated in the central Asian focus of the Soviet Union and Japan. J Clin Microbiol 1992;30:172–175.

1129. Sandstrom G, Sjostedt A, Johansson T, et al. Immunogenicity and toxicity of lipopolysaccharide from *Francisella tularensis* LVS. FEMS Microbiol Immunol 1993;5:201–210.

1130. Sane SM, Faerber RN, Belani KK. Respiratory foreign bodies and *Eikenella corrodens* brain abscess in two children. Pediatr Radiol 1999;29:327–330.

1131. Sanford JP. *Brucella* pneumonia. Semin Respir Infect 1997;12:24–27.

1132. Santini C, Baiocchi P, Berardelli A, et al. A case of brain abscess due to *Brucella melitensis*. Clin Infect Dis 1994;19:977–978.

1133. Santos R, Cardoso O, Rodrigues P, et al. Bacillary angiomatosis by *Bartonella quintana* in an HIV-infected patient. J Am Acad Dermatol 2000;42:299–301.

1134. Sarangi J, Cartwright K, Stuart J, et al. Invasive *Haemophilus influenzae* disease in adults. Epidemiol Infect 2000;124:441–447.

1135. Sari R, Buyukberber N, Sevinc A, et al. Brucellosis in the etiology of febrile neutropenia: case report. J Chemother 2002;14:88–91.

1136. Sarria JC, Vidal AM, Kimbrough RC III. *Haemophilus influenzae* osteomyelitis in adults: a report of 4 frontal bone infections and a review of the literature. Scand J Infect Dis 2001;33:263–265.

1137. Sarria C, Vidal M, Kimbrough C III, Figuroa E. Fatal infection caused by *Francisella tularensis* in a neutropenic bone marrow transplant recipient. Ann Hematol 2003;82:41–43.

1138. Sato T, Fujita H, Ohara Y, et al. Microagglutination test for early and specific serodiagnosis of tularemia. J Clin Microbiol 1990;28:2372–2374.

1139. Sawmiller CJ, Dudrick SJ, Hamzi M. Postsplenectomy *Capnocytophaga canimorsus* sepsis presenting as an acute abdomen. Arch Surg 1998;133: 1362–1365.

1140. Scannapieco FA, Millar SJ, Reynolds HS, et al. Effect of anaerobiosis on the surface ultrastructure and surface proteins of *Actinobacillus actinomycetemcomitans* (*Haemophilus actinomycetemcomitans*). Infect Immun 1987; 55:2320–2323.

1141. Schalla WO, Sanders LL, Schmid GP, et al. Use of dot immunobinding and fluorescence assays to investigate clinically suspected cases of chancroid. J Infect Dis 1986;153:879–887.

1142. Scheel O, Hoel T, Sandvik T, et al. Susceptibility pattern of Scandinavian *Francisella tularensis* isolated with regard to oral and parenteral antimicrobial agents. APMIS 1993;101:33–36.

1143. Scheel O, Reierson R, Hoel T. Treatment of tularemia with ciprofloxacin. Eur J Clin Microbiol Infect Dis 1992;11:447–448.

1144. Schlater LK, Brenner DJ, Steigerwalt AG, et al. *Pasteurella caballi*, a new species from equine clinical specimens. J Clin Microbiol 1989;27:2169–2174.

1145. Schlosser RJ, London SD, Gwaltney JM Jr, Gross CW. Microbiology of chronic frontal sinusitis. Laryngoscope 2001;111:1330–1332.

1146. Schmidt ME, Smith MA, Levy CS. Endophthalmitis caused by unusual gram-negative bacilli: three case reports and review. Clin Infect Dis 1993;17: 686–690.

1147. Schmitt HJ, Wirsing von Konig CH, Neiss A, et al. Efficacy of acellular pertussis vaccine in early childhood after household exposure. JAMA 1996;275: 37–41.

1148. Schmitt-Grohe S, Cherry JD, Heininger U, et al. Pertussis in German adults. Clin Infect Dis 1995;21:860–866.

1149. Schonheyder H, Ejlertson T, Frederiksen W. Isolation of a dysgonic fermenter (DF-3) from urine of a patient. Eur J Clin Microbiol Infect Dis 1991;10: 530–531.

1150. Schouls LM, van de Pol I, Rijpkema SGT, Schot CS. Detection and identification of *Ehrlichia*, *Borrelia burgdorferi* sensu lato, and *Bartonella* species in Dutch *Ixodes ricinus* ticks. J Clin Microbiol 1999;37:2215–2222.

1151. Schwartz RA, Gallardo MA, Kapila R, et al. Bacillary angiomatosis in an HIV seronegative patient on systemic steroid therapy. Br J Dermatol 1996;135: 982–987.

1152. Schwartzman WA, Patnaik M, Angulo FJ, et al. *Bartonella* (*Rochalimaea*) antibodies, dementia, and cat ownership among men infected with human immunodeficiency virus. Clin Infect Dis 1995;21:954–959.

henselae and *Bartonella quintana* by PCR-enzyme immunoassay. J Clin Microbiol 1999;37:3097–3101.

1153. Schwartzman WA, Patnaik M, Barka NE, et al. *Rochalimaea* antibodies in HIV-associated neurologic disease. Neurology 1994;44:1312–1316.

1154. Sedlacek I, Gerner-Smidt P, Schmidt J, et al. Genetic relationship of *Haemophilus aphrophilus*, *H. paraphrophilus*, and *Actinobacillus actinomycetemcomitans* studies by ribotyping. Int J Med Microbiol Virol Parasitol Infect Dis 1993; 279:51–59.

1155. Seger RA, Hollis DG, Weaver RE, Hitzig WH. Chronic granulomatous disease: fatal septicemia caused by an unnamed gram-negative bacterium. J. Clin Microbiol 1982;16:821–825.

1156. Seger RA, Kloeti J, Von Gravenitz A, et al. Cervical abscess due to *Capnocytophaga ochracea*. Pediatr Infect Dis 1982;1:170–172.

1157. Senol M, Ozcan A, Karincaoglu Y, et al. Tularemia: a case transmitted from a sheep. Cutis 1999;63:49–51.

1158. Sens MA, Brown EW, Wilson LR, Crocker TP. Fatal *Streptobacillus moniliformis* infection in a two-month-old infant. Am J Clin Pathol 1989;91:612–616.

1159. Sethi S, Murphy TF. Bacterial infection in chronic obstructive pulmonary disease in 2000: a state-of-the-art review. Clin Microbiol Rev 2001;14:336–363.

1160. Setta F, Baecke M, Jacquy J, et al. Cerebellar ataxia following whooping cough. Clin Neurol Neurosurg 1999;101:56–61.

1161. Severien C, Teig N, Riedal F, et al. Severe pneumonia and chronic lung disease in a young child with adenovirus and *Bordetella pertussis* infection. Pediatr Infect Dis J 1995;14:400–401.

1162. Sevinc A, Kutlu NO, Kuku I, et al. Severe epistaxis in brucellosis-induced isolated thrombocytopenia: a report of two cases. Clin Lab Haematol 2000;22: 373–375.

1163. Shah GM, Winer RL. Glomerulonephritis associated with endocarditis caused by *Actinobacillus actinomycetemcomitans*. Am J Kidney Dis 1981;1:113–115.

1164. Shanson DC, Gazzard BG. *Kingella kingae* septicaemia with a clinical presentation resembling disseminated gonococcal infection. BMJ 1984;289:730–731.

1165. Shanson DC, Gazzard BG, Midgley J, et al. *Streptobacillus moniliformis* isolated from blood in four cases of Haverhill fever: first outbreak in Britain. Lancet 1983;2:92–94.

1166. Shanson DC, Pratt J, Greene P. Comparison of media with and without "Panemede" for the isolation of *Streptobacillus moniliformis* from blood cultures and observations on the inhibitory effect of sodium polyanethol sulfonate. J Med Microbiol 1985;19:181–186.

1167. Shapira L, Soskolne WA, Sela MN, et al. The secretion of PGE2, IL-1β, IL-6, and TNF-α by adherent mononuclear cells from early onset periodontitis patients. J Periodontal 1994;65:139–146.

1168. Shapiro DS, Brooks PE, Coffey DM, Browne KF. Peripartum bacteremia with CDC group HB-5 (*Pasteurella bettyae*). Clin Infect Dis 1996;22:1125–1126.

1169. Shawar R, Sepulveda J, Clarridge JE. Use of the RapID-ANA system and sodium polyanetholsulfonate disk susceptibility testing in identifying *Haemophilus ducreyi*. J Clin Microbiol 1990;28:108–111.

1170. Sheng WS, Hsueh PR, Hung CC, et al. Clinical features of patients with invasive *Eikenella corrodens* infections and microbiological characteristics of the causative isolates. Eur J Clin Microbiol Infect Dis 2001;20:231–236.

1171. Shenoy S, Kavitha R, Laxmi V, et al. Septic arthritis due to *Actinobacillus actinomycetemcomitans*. Indian J Pediatr 1996;63:569–570.

1172. Shimshony A. Epidemiology of emerging zoonoses in Israel. Emerg Infect Dis 1997;3:229–238.

1173. Shoshan Y, Maayan S, Gomori MJ, Israel Z. Chronic subdural empyema: a new presentation of neurobrucellosis. Clin Infect Dis 2003;36:400–401.

1174. Shurin SB, Socransky SS, Sweeney E, et al. A neutrophil disorder induced by *Capnocytophaga*, a dental microorganism. N Engl J Med 1979;301:849–854.

1175. Sicherer SH, Asturias EJ, Winkelstein JA, et al. *Francisella philomiragia* sepsis in chronic granulomatous disease. Pediatr Infect Dis J 1997;16:420–422.

1176. Sikkema DJ, Murphy TF. Molecular analysis of the P2 porin protein of nontypeable *Haemophilus influenzae*. Infect Immun 1992;60:5204–5211.

1177. Simon MW, Mitchell BL, O'Connor WN, et al. Glomerulonephritis, pulmonary hemorrhage, and coagulopathy associated with *Haemophilus parainfluenzae* endocarditis. Pediatr Infect Dis J 1985;4:183–185.

1178. Simonsen JN, Cameron DW, Gakinya, MN, et al. Human immunodeficiency virus infection in men with sexually transmitted diseases: experience from a center in Africa. N Engl J Med 1988;319:274–278.

1179. Singhi SC, Mohankumar D, Singhi PD, et al. Evaluation of polymerase chain reaction (PCR) for diagnosing *Haemophilus influenzae* type b meningitis. Ann Trop Paediatr 1999;22:347–253.

1180. Sinnott JT, Blazejowski C, Bazzini MD. *Bordetella bronchiseptica* endocarditis: a tale of a boy and his dog. Clin Infect Dis Newslett 1989;11:111–112.

1181. Siverio CD Jr, Whitcher JP. *Haemophilus influenzae* corneal ulcer associated with atopic keratoconjunctivitis and herpes simplex keratitis (letter). Br J Ophthalmol 2002;86:478–479.

1182. Sjostedt A, Eriksson U, Berglund L, Tarnvik A. Detection of *Francisella tularensis* in ulcers of patients with tularemia by PCR. J Clin Microbiol 1997;35: 1045–1048.

1183. Sjostedt A, Sandstrom G, Tarnvik A. Several membrane polypeptides of the live vaccine strain *Francisella tularensis* LVS stimulate T cells from naturally infected individuals. J Clin Microbiol 1990;28:43–48.

1184. Slater LN, Coody DW, Woolridge LK, et al. Murine antibody responses distinguish *Rochalimaea henselae* from *Rochalimaea quintana*. J Clin Microbiol 1992;30:1722–1727.

1185. Slater LN, Min KW. Polypoid endobronchial lesions: a manifestation of bacillary angiomatosis. Chest 1992;102:972–974.

1186. Slater LN, Pitha JV, Herrera L, et al. *Rochalimaea henselae* infection in acquired immunodeficiency syndrome causing inflammatory disease without angiomatosis or peliosis. Arch Pathol Lab Med 1994;118:33–38.

1187. Slater LN, Welch DF, Hensel D, et al. A newly recognized fastidious gram-negative pathogen as a cause of fever and bacteremia. N Engl J Med 1990; 323:1587–1593.

1188. Slater LN, Welch DF, Min K-W. *Rochalimaea henselae* causes bacillary angiomatosis and peliosis hepatis. Arch Intern Med 1992;152:602–606.

1189. Slonim A, Walker ES, Mishori E, et al. Person-to-person transmission of *Kingella kingae* among day care center attendees. J Infect Dis 1998;178: 1843–1846.

1190. Slotnick IJ, Dougherty M. Further characterization of an unclassified group of bacteria causing endocarditis in man: *Cardiobacterium hominis* gen. et sp. nov. Antonie von Leeuwenhoek J Microbiol Serol 1964;30:261–272.

1191. Smith HM, Reporter R, Rood MP, et al. Prevalence study of antibody to ratborne pathogens and other agents among patients using a free clinic in downtown Los Angeles. J Infect 2002;186:1673–1676.

1192. Smith KJ, Skelton HG, Tuur S, et al. Bacillary angiomatosis in an immunocompetent child. Am J Dermatopathol 1996;18:597–600.

1193. Smith S, Tilton RC. Acute *Bordetella pertussis* infection in an adult. J Clin Microbiol 1996;34:429–430.

1194. Sneath PHA, Stevens M. *Actinobacillus rossii* sp. nov., *Actinobacillus seminis* sp. nov. nom. rev., *Pasteurella bettii* sp. nov., *Pasteurella lymphangitidis* sp. nov., *Pasteurella mairi* sp. nov., and *Pasteurella trehalosi* sp. nov. Int J Syst Bacteriol 40:148–153, 1990.

1195. Snell JJS. Genus IV. *Kingella* Henriksen and Bovre 1976, 449AL. In: Krieg NR, Holt JG, eds. Bergey's Manual of Systematic Bacteriology. Vol. 1. Baltimore: Williams & Wilkins, 1984:307–309.

1196. Snell JJS, LaPage SP. Transfer of some saccharolytic *Moraxella* species to *Kingella* Henriksen and Bovre 1976, with descriptions of *Kingella indologenes* sp. nov. and *Kingella denitrificans* sp. nov. Int J Syst Bacteriol 1976;26: 451–458.

1197. Snipes KP, Biberstein EL. *Pasteurella testudinis* sp. nov.: a parasite of desert tortoises (*Gopherus agassizi*). Int J Syst Bacteriol 1982;32:201–210.

1198. Sobraques M, Maurin M, Birtles RJ, Raoult D. In vitro susceptibilities of four *Bartonella bacilliformis* strains to 30 antibiotic compounds. Antimicrob Agents Chemother 1999;43:2090–2092.

1199. Socransky SS, Holt SC, Leadbetter EP, et al. *Capnocytophaga*: a new genus of gram-negative gliding bacteria. III. Physiological characterization. Arch Microbiol 1979;122:29–33.

1200. Sokol W. Epidemiology of sinusitis in the primary care setting: results from the 1999–2000 respiratory surveillance program. Am J Med 2001;111(Suppl 9A):19S–24S.

1201. Solera J, Lozano E, Martinez-Alfaro E, et al. Brucellar spondylitis: review of 35 cases and literature survey. Clin Infect Dis 1999;29:1440–1449.

1202. Sorbello AF, O'Donnell J, Kaiser-Smith J, et al. Infective endocarditis due to *Pasteurella dagmatis*: case report and review. Clin Infect Dis 199418:226–228.

1203. Sordillo EM, Rendel M, Sood R, et al. Septicemia due to β-lactamase-positive *Kingella kingae*. Clin Infect Dis 1993;17:818–819.

1204. Sottnek FO, Albritton WL. *Haemophilus influenzae* biotype VIII. J Clin Microbiol 1984;20:815–816.

1205. Spach DH, Callis KP, Paauw DS, et al. Endocarditis caused by *Rochalimaea quintana* in a patient infected with human immunodeficiency virus. J Clin Microbiol 1993;31:692–694.

1206. Spach DH, Kanter AS, Daniels NA, et al. *Bartonella* (*Rochalimaea*) species as a cause of apparent "culture-negative" endocarditis. Clin Infect Dis 1995; 20:1044–1047.

1207. Spach DH, Kanter AS, Doughertry MJ, et al. *Bartonella* (*Rochalimaea*) *quintana* bacteremia in inner-city patients with chronic alcoholism. N Engl J Med 1995;332:424–428.

1208. Spach DH, Koehler JE. *Bartonella*-associated infections. Infect Dis Clin N America 1998;12:137–155.

1209. Spach DH, Panther LA, Thorning DR, et al. Intracerebral bacillary angiomatosis in a patient infected with human immunodeficiency virus. Ann Intern Med 1992;116:740–742.

1210. Spagnuolo PJ, Ellner JJ, Lerner PI, et al. *Haemophilus influenzae* meningitis: the spectrum of disease in adults. Medicine (Baltimore) 1982;61:74–85.

1211. Spinola SM, Griffiths GE, Shanks KL, Blake MS. The major outer membrane protein of *Haemophilus ducreyi* is a member of the OmpA family of proteins. Infect Immun 1993;61:1326–1351.

1212. Spratt DA, Greenman J, Schaffer AG. *Capnocytophaga gingivalis* aminopeptidase: a potential virulence factor. Microbiology 1995;141:3087–3093.

1213. Stahelin J, Goldenberger D, Gnehm HE, Altwegg M. Polymerase chain reaction diagnosis of *Kingella kingae* arthritis in a young child. Clin Infect Dis 1998; 27:1328–1329.

1214. Steeper TA, Rosenstein H, Weiser J, et al. Bacillary angiomatosis involving the liver, spleen, and skin in an AIDS patient with concurrent Kaposi's sarcoma. Am J Clin Pathol 1992;97:713–718.

1215. Stefanelli P, Giuliano M, Bottone M, et al. Polymerase chain reaction for the identification of *Bordetella pertussis* and *Bordetella parapertussis*. Diagn Microbiol Infect Dis 1996;24:197–200.

1216. Stefanelli P, Mastrantonio P, Hausman SZ, et al. Molecular characterization of two *Bordetella bronchiseptica* strains isolated from children with coughs. J Clin Microbiol 1997;35:1550–1555.

1217. Steffens L, Franke S, Nickel S, et al. DNA fingerprinting of *Eikenella corrodens* by pulsed-field gel electrophoresis. Oral Microbiol Immunol 1994;9:95–108.

1218. Stein A, Teysseire N, Capobianco C, et al. *Eikenella corrodens*, a rare cause of pancreatic abscess: two case reports and review. Clin Infect Dis 1993;17: 273–275.

1219. Steinemann TL, Sheikholeslami MR, Brown HH, Bradsher RW. Oculoglandular tularemia. Arch Ophthalmol 1999;117:132–133.

1220. Steinhoff MC, Auerbach BS, Nelson KE, et al. Antibody responses to *Haemophilus influenzae* type b vaccines in men with human immunodeficiency virus infection. N Engl J Med 1991;325:1837–1842.

1221. Steitz A, Orth T, Feddersen A, et al. A case of endocarditis with vasculitis due to *Actinobacillus actinomycetemcomitans*: a 16S rDNA signature for distinction from related organisms. Clin Infect Dis 1998;27:224–225.

1222. Stevens PK, Czuprynski CJ. *Pasteurella haemolytica* leukotoxin induces bovine leukocytes to undergo morphologic changes consistent with apoptosis in vitro. Infect Immun 1996;64:2687–2694.

1223. Stevens-Krebbers AH, Schouten MA, Janssen J, Horrevorts AM. Nosocomial transmission of *Bordetella bronchiseptica*. J Hosp Infect 1999;43:323–324.

1224. St Geme JW III, Cutter D. Evidence that surface fibrils expressed by *Haemophilus influenzae* type b promote attachment to human epithelial cells. Mol Microbiol 1995;25:77–85.

1225. St Geme JW III, Cutter D. The *Haemophilus influenzae* Hia adhesin is an autotransporter protein that remains uncleaved at the C terminus and fully cell associated. J Bacteriol 2000;182:6005–6013.

1226. St Geme JW III, Cutter D, Barenkamp JS. Characterization of the genetic locus encoding *Haemophilus influenzae* type b surface fibrils. J Bacteriol 1996;178: 6281–6287.

1227. St Geme JW III, de la Morena ML, Falkow SA. *Haemophilus influenzae* IgA protease-like protein promotes intimate interaction with human epithelial cells. Mol Microbiol 1994;14:217–233.

1228. St Geme JW III, Falkow S. Capsule loss by *Haemophilus influenzae* type b results in enhanced adherence to and entry into human cells. J Infect Dis 1992; 165(Suppl 1):S117–S118.

1229. St Geme JW III, Falkow S. Isolation, expression, and nucleotide sequence of the pilin structural gene of the Brazilian purpuric fever clone of *Haemophilus influenzae* biogroup *aegyptius*. Infect Immun 1993;61:2233–2237.

1230. St Geme JW III, Falkow S, Barenkamp SJ. High-molecular-weight proteins of nontypeable *Haemophilus influenzae* mediate attachment to human epithelial cells. Proc Natl Acad Sci USA 1993;90:2875–2879.

1231. St Geme JW III, Gilsdorf JR, Falkow S. Surface structures and adherence properties of diverse strains of *Haemophilus influenzae* biogroup *aegyptius*. Infect Immun 1991;59:3366–3371.

1232. St Geme JW III, Pinkner JS, Krasan GP, et al. *Haemophilus influenzae* pili are composite structures assembled via the HifB chaperone. Proc Natl Acad Sci USA 1996;93:11913–11918.

1233. Strebel PM, Cochi SL, Farizo KM, et al. Pertussis in Missouri: evaluation of nasopharyngeal culture, direct fluorescent antibody testing, and clinical case definitions in the diagnosis of pertussis. Clin Infect Dis 1993;16:276–285.

1234. Sturm AW. *Haemophilus influenzae* and *Haemophilus parainfluenzae* in nongonococcal urethritis. J Infect Dis 1986;153:165–167.

1235. Sturm AW. Iron and virulence of *Haemophilus ducreyi* in a primate model. Sex Transm Dis 1997;24:64–68.

1236. Sturm AW, Zanen HC. Characteristics of *Haemophilus ducreyi* in culture. J Clin Microbiol 1984;19:672–674.

1237. Suda R, Lai CH, Yang HW, Hasegawa K. *Eikenella corrodens* in subgingival plaque: relationship to age and periodontal condition. J Periodontol 2002;73: 886–891.

1238. Sumerkan B, Gokahmetoglu S, Esel D. *Brucella* detection in blood: comparison of the BacT/Alert standard aerobic bottle, BacT/Alert FAN aerobic bottle and BacT/Alert enhanced FAN aerobic bottle in simulated blood culture. Clin Microbiol Infect 2001;7:369–372.

1239. Suzuki N, Nakano Y, Yoshida Y, et al. Identification of *Actinobacillus actinomycetemcomitans* serotypes by multiplex PCR. J Clin Microbiol 2001;39: 2002–2005.

1240. Sykes SO, Riemann C, Santos CI, et al. *Haemophilus influenzae* associated scleritis. Br J Ophthalmol 1999;83:410–413.

1241. Sylvester DA, Burnstine RA, Bower JR. Cat-inflicted corneal laceration: presentation of two cases and a discussion of infection-related management. J Pediatr Ophthalmol Strabismus 2002;39:114–117.

1242. Syrjala H, Koskela P, Ripatti T, et al. Agglutination and ELISA methods in the diagnosis of tularemia in different clinical forms and severities of the disease. J Infect Dis 1986;153:142–145.

1243. Syrjala H, Kujala P, Myllyla V, et al. Airborne transmission of tularemia in farmers. Scand J Infect Dis 1985;17:371–375.

1244. Syrjala H. Schildt R, Raisainen S. In vitro susceptibility of *Francisella tularensis* to fluoroquinolones and treatment of tularemia with norfloxacin and ciprofloxacin. Eur J Clin Microbiol Infect Dis 1991;10:68–70.

1245. Taichman NS, Dean RT, Sanderson CJ. Biochemical and morphological characterization of the killing of human monocytes by a leukotoxin derived from *Actinobacillus actinomycetemcomitans*. Infect Immun 1980;28:258–268.

1246. Takala AK, Eskola J, Leinonen M, et al. Reduction of oropharyngeal carriage of *Haemophilus influenzae* type b (Hib) in children immunized with an Hib conjugate vaccine. J Infect Dis 1991;164:982–986.

1247. Takala AK, Meurman O, Kleemola M, et al. Preceding respiratory infection predisposing for primary and secondary invasive *Haemophilus influenzae* type b disease. Pediatr Infect Dis J 1993;12:189–195.

1248. Takala AK, Peltola H, Eskola J. Disappearance of epiglottitis during large-scale vaccination with *Haemophilus influenzae* type b conjugate vaccine among children in Finland. Laryngoscope 1994;104:731–735.

1249. Takwale VJ, Wright ED, Bates J, Edge AJ. *Pasteurella multocida* infection of a total hip arthroplasty following a cat scratch. J Infect 1997;34:263–264.

1250. Talan DA, Citron DM, Abrahamian FM, et al. Bacteriologic analysis of infected dog and cat bites. N Engl J Med 1999;340:85–92.

1251. Talbodec N, Bottelin E, Boruchowicz A, et al. Splenic abscess associated with *Pasteurella multocida* in an immunocompetent patient. J Clin Gastroenterol 1995;21:76.

1252. Taleski V, Zerva L, Kantardjiev T, et al. An overview of the epidemiology and epizootiology of brucellosis in selected countries of Central and Southeast Europe. Vet Microbiol 2002;90:147–155.

1253. Tamion F, Girault C, Chevron V, et al. *Bordetella bronchiseptica* pneumonia with shock in an immunocompetent patient. Scand J Infect Dis 1996;28: 197–198.

1254. Tan KS, Song KP, Ong G. Cytolethal distending toxin of *Actinobacillus actinomycetemcomitans*: occurrence and association with periodontal disease. J Periodontal Res 2002;37:268–272.

1255. Tancik CA, Dillaha JA. *Francisella tularensis* endocarditis. Clin Infect Dis 2000;30:399–400.

1256. Tang CM, Conlon CP. Bronchitis and bronchiectasis. In: Root RK, Waldvodel F, Corey L, Stamm WE, eds. Clinical Infectious Diseases: A Practical Approach. New York: Oxford University Press, 1999:523–528.

1257. Tang YW, Hopkins MK, Kolbert CP, et al. *Bordetella holmesii*-like organisms associated with septicemia, endocarditis and respiratory failure. Clin Infect Dis 1998;26:389–392.

1258. Tanner ACR, Visconti RA, Socransky SS, et al. Classification and identification of *Actinobacillus actinomycetemcomitans* and *Haemophilus aphrophilus* by cluster analysis and deoxyribonucleic acid hybridizations. J Periodontal Res 1982;17:585–596.

1259. Tanner K, Fitzsimmons G, Carrol ED, et al. *Haemophilus influenzae* type b epiglottitis as a cause of acute airway obstruction in children. BMJ 2002;325: 1099–1100.

1260. Tappero JW, Koehler JE, Berger TG, et al. Bacillary angiomatosis and bacillary splenitis in immunocompetent adults. Ann Intern Med 1993;118:363–365.

1261. Taranger J, Trollfors B, Lagergard T, et al. Unchanged efficacy of a pertussis toxoid vaccine throughout the two years after the third vaccination of infants. Pediatr Infect Dis J 1997;16:180–184.

1262. Tarnvik A. Nature of protective immunity to *Francisella tularensis*. Rev Infect Dis 1989;11:440–451.

1263. Taskapan H, Oymak O, Sumerkan B, et al. *Brucella* peritonitis in a patient on continuous ambulatory peritoneal dialysis with acute brucellosis. Nephron 2002;91:156–158.

1264. Tatum FM, Briggs RE, Sreevatsan SS, et al. Construction of an isogenic leukotoxin mutant of *Pasteurella haemolytica* serotype 1: characterization and virulence. Microb Pathog 1998;24:37–46.

1265. Taveras JM III, Campo R, Segal N, et al. Apparent culture-negative endocarditis of the prosthetic valve caused by *Cardiobacterium hominis*. South Med J 1993; 86:1439–1440.

1266. Tay JS, Chusid MJ, Dunne WM Jr. *Capnocytophaga ochracea* pyonephrosis in an infant with obstructive nephropathy. Pediatr Infect Dis 1985;4:555–556.

1267. Taylor JP, Purdue JN. The changing epidemiology of human brucellosis in Texas, 1976–1986. Am J Epidemiol 1989;130:160–165.

1268. Tempro PJ, Slots J. Selective medium for the isolation of *Haemophilus aphrophilus* from the human periodontium and other oral sites and the low proportion of the organism in the oral flora. J Clin Microbiol 1986;23:777–782.

1269. Testillano Tarrero M, Montejo Baranda M, et al. Peritonitis involving *Capnocytophaga ochracea.* Am J Gastroenterol 1989;84:206–207.

1270. Thalhammer F, Ebert G, Kopetzki-Kogler U. Unusual route of transmission for *Brucella abortus.* Clin Infect Dis 1998;26:763–764.

1271. Tharmaseelan K, Morgan MS. *Pasteurella multocida* conjunctivitis. Br J Ophthalmol 77:815, 1993.

1272. Thomas R, Johansson A, Neeson B, et al. Discrimination of human pathogenic subspecies of *Francisella tularensis* by using restriction fragment length polymorphism. J Clin Microbiol 2003;41:50–57.

1273. Thornsberry C, Ogilvie PT, Holley HP Jr, Sahm DF. Survey of susceptibilities of *Streptococcus pneumoniae, Haemophilus influenzae,* and *Moraxella catarrhalis* isolates to 26 antimicrobial agents: a prospective U.S. study. Antimicrob Agents Chemother 1999;43:2612–2623.

1274. Thorsen P, Moller BR, Arpi M, et al. *Pasteurella aerogenes* isolated from stillbirth and mother. Lancet 1994;343:485–486.

1275. Tilley PAG, Kanchana MV, Knight I, et al. Detection of *Bordetella pertussis* in a clinical laboratory by culture, polymerase chain reaction, and the fluorescent antibody staining: accuracy and cost. Diagn Microbiol Infect Dis 2000;37:17–23.

1276. Tindberg Y, Blennow M, Granstrom M. A ten-year follow-up after immunization with a two-component acellular pertussis vaccine. Pediatr Infect Dis J 1999;18:361–365.

1277. Tison DL, Latimer JM. Lysis centrifugation-direct plating technique for isolation of group DF-2 from the blood of a dog bite victim. J Infect Dis 1986;153:1001–1002.

1278. Tobe TJ, Franssen CF, Zijlstra JG, et al. Hemolytic-uremic syndrome due to *Capnocytophaga canimorsus* bacteremia after a dog bite. Am J Kidney Dis 1999;33:e5.

1279. Tollo K, Helgeland K. Fc-binding components: a virulence factor in *Actinobacillus actinomycetemcomitans?* Oral Microbiol Immunol 1991;6:373–377.

1280. Tonjum T, Bukholm G, Bovre K. Identification of *Haemophilus aphrophilus* and *Actinobacillus actinomycetemcomitans* by DNA-DNA hybridization and genetic transformation. J Clin Microbiol 1990;28:1994–1998.

1281. Torok L, Viragh SZ, Borka I, et al. Bacillary angiomatosis in a patient with lymphocytic leukemia. Br J Dermatol 1994;130:665–668.

1282. Torres A, Cuende E, De Pablos M, et al. Remitting seronegative symmetrical synovitis with pitting edema associated with subcutaneous *Streptobacillus moniliformis* abscess. J Rheumatol 2001;28:1696–1698.

1283. Toshniwal R, Draghi TC, Kocka FE, Kallick CA. Manifestations of *Kingella kingae* infections in adults: resemblance to neisserial infections. Diagn Microbiol Infect Dis 1986;5:81–85.

1284. Totten PA, Norn SV, Stamm WE. Characterization of the hemolytic activity of *Haemophilus ducreyi.* Infect Immun 1995;63:4409–4416.

1285. Totten PA, Stamm WE. Clear broth and plate media for culture of *Haemophilus ducreyi.* J Clin Microbiol 1994;32:2019–2023.

1286. Townsend KM, Boyce JD, Chung JY, et al. Genetic organization of *Pasteurella multocida cap* loci and development of a multiplex capsular PCR typing system. J Clin Microbiol 2001;39:924–929.

1287. Tran SD, Rudney JD. Improved multiplex PCR using conserved and species-specific 16S rRNA gene primers for simultaneous detection of *Actinobacillus actinomycetemcomitans, Bacteroides forsythus,* and *Porphyromonas gingivalis.* J Clin Microbiol 1999;37:3504–3508.

1288. Trollfors B, Taranger J, Lagergard T, et al. A placebo-controlled trial of a pertussis toxoid vaccine. N Engl J Med 1995;333:1045–1050.

1289. Trollfors B, Taranger GJ, Lagergard T, et al. Serum IgG antibody responses to pertussis toxin and filamentous hemagglutinin in nonvaccinated and vaccinated children and adults with pertussis. Clin Infect Dis 1999;28:552–559.

1290. Trujillano-Martin I, Garcia-Sanchez E, Martinez IM, et al. In vitro activity of six new fluoroquinolones against *Brucella melitensis.* Antimicrob Agents Chemother 1999;43:194–195.

1291. Tryland M, Kleviane L, Alfredsson A, et al. Evidence of brucella infection in marine animals in the North Atlantic Ocean. Vet Rec 1999;144:588–592.

1292. Tsai PS, DeAngelis DD, Spencer WH, Seiff SR. Bacillary angiomatosis of the anterior orbit, eyelid, and conjunctiva. Am J Ophthalmol 2002;134:433–434.

1293. Tsukahara M, Tsuneoka H, Iino H, et al. *Bartonella henselae* infection as a cause of fever of unknown origin. J Clin Microbiol 2000;38:1990–1991.

1294. Tunkel AR, Scheld WM. Pathogenesis and pathophysiology of bacterial meningitis. Clin Microbiol Rev 1993;6:118–136.

1295. Tyndall MW, Agoki E, Plummer FA, et al. Single dose azithromycin for the treatment of chancroid: a randomized comparison with erythromycin. Sex Transm Dis 1994;21:231–234.

1296. Tyndall MW, Malisa M, Plummer FA, et al. Ceftriaxone no longer predictably cures chancroid in Kenya. J Infect Dis 1993;167:469–471.

1297. Ueda N, Nishihara T, Ishihara Y, et al. Role of prostaglandin in the formation of osteoclasts induced by capsular-like polysaccharide antigen of *Actinobacillus actinomycetemcomitans* strain Y4. Oral Microbiol Immunol 1995;10:69–75.

1298. Uhari M, Syrjala H, Salminen A. Tularemia in children caused by *Francisella tularensis* biovar *palaearctica.* Pediatr Infect Dis J 1990;9:80–83.

1299. United States Department of Health and Human Services, Centers for Disease Control and Prevention, National Institutes of Health. Appendix. 1. Biosafety in microbiological and biomedical laboratories (BMBL). In Fleming DO, Hunt DL, eds.: Biological Safety: Principals and Practices. 3rd Ed. Washington, DC: ASM Press, 2000:609–700.

1300. United States Department of Labor, Occupational Safety and Health. Occupational exposure to blood-borne pathogens; final rule (29 CFR Part 1910.1030). In: Fleming DO, Hunt DL, eds. Biological Safety: Principals and Practices. 3rd Ed. Washington, DC: ASM Press, 2000:701–712.

1301. Urs S, D'Silva BSV, Jeena CP, et al. *Kingella kingae* septicaemia in association with HIV disease. Trop Doct 1994;24:127.

1302. Valtonen M, Lauhio A, Carlson P, et al. *Capnocytophaga canimorsus* septicemia: fifth report of a cat-associated infection and five other cases. Eur J Clin Microbiol Infect Dis 1995;14:520–523.

1303. Vandamme P, Heyndrickx M, Vancanneyt M, et al. *Bordetella trematum* sp. nov., isolated from wounds and ear infections in humans, and reassessment of *Alcaligenes denitrificans* Ruger and Tan 1983. Int J Syst Bacteriol 1996;46:849–858.

1304. Vandamme P, Hommez J, Vancanneyt M, et al. *Bordetella hinzii* sp. nov., isolated from poultry and humans. Int J Syst Bacteriol 1995;45:37–45.

1305. Vandamme P, Vancanneyt M, Van Belkum A, et al. Polyphasic analysis of strains of the genus *Capnocytophaga* and Centers for Disease Control group DF-3. Int J Syst Bacteriol 1996;46:782–791.

1306. Van den Berg BM, Beekhuizen H, Willems RJ, et al. Role of *Bordetella pertussis* virulence factors in adherence to epithelial cell lines derived from the human respiratory tract. Infect Immun 1999;67:1056–1062.

1307. Van der Zee A, Agterberg C, Peeters M, et al. Polymerase chain reaction assay for pertussis: simultaneous detection and discrimination of *Bordetella pertussis* and *Bordetella parapertussis.* J Clin Microbiol 1993;31:2134–2140.

1308. Van der Zee A, Groenendijk H, Peeters M, Mooi FR. The differentiation of *Bordetella parapertussis* and *Bordetella bronchiseptica* from humans and animals as determined by DNA polymorphism mediated by two different insertion sequence elements suggests their phylogenetic relationship. Int J Syst Bacteriol 1996;46:640–647.

1309. Van Dyck E, Bogaerts J, Smet H, et al. Emergence of *Haemophilus ducreyi* resistance to trimethoprim-sulfamethoxazole in Rwanda. Antimicrob Agents Chemother 1994;38:1647–1648.

1310. Van Dyck E, Piot P. Enzyme profiles of *Haemophilus ducreyi* strains isolated on different continents. Eur J Clin Microbiol 1987; 6:40–43.

1311. Van Dyke TE, Bartholomew E, Genco RJ, et al. Inhibition of neutrophil chemotaxis by soluble bacterial products. J Periodontol 1982;53:502–508.

1312. Van Erps J, Schmedding E, Naessens A, Keymeulen B. *Kingella kingae,* a rare cause of meningitis. Clin Neurol Neurosurg 1992;94:173–175.

1313. Van Schilfgaarde M, van Ulsen P, Eikj P, et al. Characterization of adherence of nontypeable *Haemophilus influenzae* to human epithelial cells. Infect Immun 2000;68:4658–4665.

1314. Van Steenbergan TJM, Bosch-Tijhof CJ, van Winkelhoff AJ, et al. Comparison of six typing methods for *Actinobacillus actinomycetemcomitans.* J Clin Microbiol 1994;32:2769–2774.

1315. Van Winkelhoff AJ, Overbeek BP, Pavicic MJAMP, et al. Long-standing bacteremia caused by oral *Actinobacillus actinomycetemcomitans* in a patient with a pacemaker. Clin Infect Dis 1993;16:216–218.

1316. Van Winkelhoff AJ, Tijhof CJ, de Graff J. Microbiological and clinical results of metronidazole plus amoxicillin therapy in *Actinobacillus actinomycetemcomitans*-associated periodontitis. J Periodontol 1992;63:52–57.

1317. Vartian CV, Septimus E. Endophthalmitis due to *Pasteurella multocida* and CDC EF-4. J Infect Dis 1989;160:733.

1318. Vasquez JE, Ferguson SA Jr, Bin-Sagheer S, et al. *Pasteurella multocida* endocarditis: a molecular epidemiological study. Clin Infect Dis 1998;26:518–520.

1319. Vasseur E, Joly P, Nouvellon M, et al. Cutaneous abscess: a rare complication of *Streptobacillus moniliformis* infection. Br J Dermatol 1993;129:95–96.

1320. Velasco J, Romero C, Lopez-Goni I, et al. Evaluation of the relatedness of *Brucella* spp. and *Ochrobacterium anthropi* and description of *Ochrobacterium intermedium* sp. nov., a new species with a closer relationship to *Brucella* spp. Int J Syst Bacteriol 1998;48:759–768.

1321. Velazco CH, Coelho C, Salazar F, et al. Microbiological features of Papillon–Lefevre syndrome periodontitis. J Clin Periodontal 1999;26:622–627.

1322. Venkataramani A, Santo-Domingo NE, Main DM. *Actinobacillus actinomycetemcomitans* pneumonia with possible septic embolization. Chest 1994;105:645–646.

1323. Verdon R, Geffray L, Collet T, et al. Vertebral osteomyelitis due to *Bartonella henselae* in adults: a report of 2 cases. Clin Infect Dis 2002 ;35:141–144.

1324. Verger JM, Grayon M, Tibor A, et al. Differentiation of *Brucella melitensis, B. ovis,* and *B. suis* biovar 2 strains by use of membrane protein- or cytoplasmic protein-specific gene probes. Res Microbiol 1998;149:509–517.

1325. Verger JM, Grimont F, Grimont PAD, et al. *Brucella,* a monospecific genus as shown by deoxyribonucleic acid hybridization. Int J Syst Bacteriol 1985; 35:292–295.

1326. Verghese A, Hamati F, Berk S, et al. Susceptibility of dysgonic fermenter 2 to antimicrobial agents in vitro. Antimicrob Agents Chemother 1988;32:78–80.

1327. Viallard JF, Bonnet S, Couzi L, et al. Glomerulonephritis caused by *Actinobacillus actinomycetemcomitans* mimicking c-ANCA-positive vasculitis. Nephrol Dial Transplant 2002;17:663–665.

1328. Villar MT, Helber JT, Hood B, et al. *Eikenella corrodens* phase variation involves a posttranslational event in pilus formation. J Bacteriol 1999;181: 4154–4160.

1329. Villar MT, Hirschberg RL, Schaefer MR. Role of the *Eikenella corrodens* pilA locus in pilus formation and phase variation. J Bacteriol 2001;183:55–62.

1330. Vinogradov E, Perry MB, Conlan JW. Structural analysis of *Francisella tularensis* lipopolysaccharide. Eur J Biochem 2002;269:6112–6118.

1331. Virata M, Rosenstein NE, Hadler JL, et al. Suspected Brazilian purpuric fever in a toddler with overwhelming Epstein-Barr virus infection. Clin Infect Dis 1999;27:1238–1240.

1332. Visvanathan K, Jones PD. Ciprofloxacin treatment of *Haemophilus paraphrophilus* brain abscess. J Infect 1991;22:306–307.

1333. Vitovski S, Dunkin KT, Howard AJ, Sayers JR. Nontypeable *Haemophilus influenzae* in carriage and disease: difference in IgA1 protease activity levels. JAMA 2002;287:1699–1705.

1334. Vizcaino N, Fernandez-Lago L. A rapid and sensitive method for the identification of *Brucella* species with a monoclonal antibody. Res Microbiol 1992;143: 513–518.

1335. Vogt K, Klefisch F, Hahn H, Schmutzler H. Antibacterial efficacy of ciprofloxacin in a case of endocarditis due to *Cardiobacterium hominis*. Int J Med Microbiol Virol Parasitol Infect Dis 1994;281:80–84.

1336. Voss A, van Zwam YH, Meis JF, et al. Sepsis puerperalis caused by a genotypically proven cat-derived *Pasteurella multocida* strain. Eur J Obstet Gynecol Reprod Biol 1998;76:71–73.

1337. Wade NK, Levy L, Jones MR, et al. Optic disk edema associated with peripapillary serous retinal detachment: an early sign of systemic *Bartonella henselae* infection. Am J Ophthalmol 2000;130:327–334.

1338. Wade T, Booy R, Teare EL, Kroll S. *Pasteurella multocida* meningitis in infancy: a lick may be as bad as a bite. Eur J Paediatr 1999;158:875–878.

1339. Wadowsky RM, Laus S, Libert T, et al. Inhibition of PCR-based assay for *Bordetella pertussis* by using calcium alginate fiber and aluminum shaft components of a nasopharyngeal swab. J Clin Microbiol 1994;32:1054–1057.

1340. Wadowsky RM, Michaels RH, Libert T, et al. Multiplex PCR-based assay for detection of *Bordetella pertussis* in nasopharyngeal swab specimens. J Clin Microbiol 1996;34:2645–2649.

1341. Wagle A, Jones RM. Acute epiglottitis despite vaccination with *Haemophilus influenzae* type b vaccine. Paediatr Anaesth 1999;9:549–550.

1342. Wagner DK, Wright JJ, Ansher AF, Gill VJ. Dysgonic fermenter 3-associated gastrointestinal disease in a patient with common variable hypogammaglobulinemia. Am J Med 1988;84:315–318.

1343. Waldor M, Roberts D, Kazanjian P. In utero infection due to *Pasteurella multocida* in the first trimester of pregnancy: case report and review. Clin Infect Dis 1992;14:497–500.

1344. Wallace PL, Hollis DG, Weaver RE, Moss CW. Cellular fatty acid composition of *Kingella* species, *Cardiobacterium hominis*, and *Eikenella corrodens*. J Clin Microbiol 1988 ;26:1592–1594.

1345. Wallace PL, Hollis DG, Weaver RE, Moss CW. Characterization of CDC group DF-3 by cellular fatty acid analysis. J Clin Microbiol 1989;27:735–737.

1346. Wallace RJ, Baker CJ, Quinones FJ, et al. Nontypeable *Haemophilus influenzae* (biotype IV) as a neonatal, maternal, and genital pathogen. Rev Infect Dis 1983;5:123–136.

1347. Wallet F, Toure F, Devalckenaere A, et al. Molecular identification of *Pasteurella dagmatis* peritonitis in a patient undergoing peritoneal dialysis. J Clin Microbiol 2000;38:4681–4682.

1348. Wanager RA. Primary pneumonic tularemia with positive blood cultures. Clin Microbiol Newslett 1984;6:120–122.

1349. Warman ST, Reinitz E, Klein RS. *Haemophilus parainfluenzae* septic arthritis in an adult. JAMA 1981;246:868–869.

1350. Warren K, Goldstein E, Hung VS, et al. Use of retinal biopsy to diagnose *B. henselae* retinitis in an HIV-infected patient. Arch Ophthalmol 1998;116: 937–940.

1351. Washburn LK, O'Shea M, Gillis DC, et al. Response to *Haemophilus influenzae* type b conjugate vaccine in chronically ill premature infants. J Pediatr 1993; 123:791–794.

1352. Wasserman D, Asbell PA, Friedman AJ, Bottone EJ. *Capnocytophaga ochracea* chronic blepharoconjunctivitis. Cornea 1995;14:533–535.

1353. Watkin RW, Baker N, Lang S, Ment J. *Eikenella corrodens* infective endocarditis in a previously healthy non-drug user. Eur J Clin Microbiol Infect Dis 2002; 21:890–891.

1354. Weber G, Abu-Shakra M, Hertzanu Y, et al. Liver abscess caused by *Capnocytophaga* species. Clin Infect Dis 1997;25:152–153.

1355. Weiser JN, Chong STH, Creenberg D, Fong W. Identification and characterization of a cell-envelope protein of *Haemophilus influenzae* contributing to phase variation in colony opacity and nasopharyngeal colonization. Mol Microbiol 1995 ;17:555–564.

1356. Weiss E, Dasch GA. Differential characteristics of strains of *Rochalimaea*: *Rochalimaea vinsonii* sp nov., the Canadian vole agent. Int J Syst Bacteriol 1982;32:305–314.

1357. Weiss E, Moulder JW. Genus II. *Rochalimaea* (Macchiavello 1947) Krieg 1961. 162[AL]. In: Krieg NR, Holt JG, eds. Bergey's Manual of Systematic Bacteriology. Vol. 1. Baltimore: Williams & Wilkins, 1984:698–701.

1358. Welch DF, Carroll KC, Hofmeister EK, et al. Isolation of a new subspecies, *Bartonella vinsonii* subsp. *arupensis* from a cattle rancher: identity with isolates found in conjunction with *Borrelia burgdorferi* and *Babesia microti* among naturally infected mice. J Clin Microbiol 1999;37:2598–2601.

1359. Welch DF, Hensel D. Evaluation of Bactigen and Phadebact for detection of *Haemophilus influenzae* type b antigen in cerebrospinal fluid. J Clin Microbiol 1982;16:905–908.

1360. Welch DF, Hensel DM, Pickett DA, et al. Bacteremia due to *Rochalimaea henselae* in a child: practical identification of isolates in the clinical laboratory. J Clin Microbiol 1993;31:2381–2386.

1361. Welch DF, Pickett DA, Slater LN, et al. *Rochalimaea henselae* sp. nov., a cause of septicemia, bacillary angiomatosis, and parenchymal bacillary peliosis. J Clin Microbiol 1992;30:275–280.

1362. Welch DF, Southern PM, Schneider NR. Five cases of *Haemophilus segnis* appendicitis. J Clin Microbiol 1986;24:851–852.

1363. Wells L, Rutter N, Donald F. *Kingella kingae* endocarditis in a sixteen-month-old child. Pediatr Infect Dis J 2001;20:454–455.

1364. Wenger JD, Hollis DG, Weaver RE, et al. Infection caused by *Francisella philomiragia* (formerly *Yersinia philomiragia*), a newly recognized human pathogen. Ann Intern Med 1989;110:888–892.

1365. Westerman EL, McDonald J. Tularemia pneumonia mimicking legionnaires' disease: isolation of organism on CYE agar and successful treatment with erythromycin. South Med J 1983;76:1169–1170.

1366. Westling K, Bygdeman S, Engkvist O, Jorup-Ronstrom C. *Pasteurella multocida* infection following cat bites in humans. J Infect 2000;40:97–98.

1367. Weyant RS, Bibb WF, Stephens DS, et al. Purification and characterization of a pilin specific for Brazilian purpuric fever-associated *Haemophilus influenzae* biogroup *aegyptius* (*H. aegyptius*) strains. J Clin Microbiol 1990;28:756–763.

1368. Weyant RS, Burris JA, Nichols DK, et al. Epizootic feline pneumonia associated with Centers for Disease Control group EF-4 bacteria. Lab Anim Sci 1994; 44:180–183.

1369. Weyant RS, Hollis DG, Weaver RE, et al. *Bordetella holmesii* sp. nov., a new gram-negative species associated with septicemia. J Clin Microbiol 1995;33: 1–7.

1370. Weyant RS, Quinn FD, Utt EA, et al. Human microvascular endothelial cell toxicity caused by Brazilian purpuric fever-associated strains of *Haemophilus influenzae* biogroup *aegyptius*. J Infect Dis 1994;169:430–433.

1371. White CB, Lampe RM, Copeland RL, et al. Soft tissue infection associated with *Haemophilus aphrophilus*. Pediatrics 1981;67:434–435.

1372. Whitehouse RL, Jackson H, Jackson MC, Ramji MM. Isolation of *Simonsiella* sp. from a neonate. J Clin Microbiol 1987;25:522–525.

1373. Whitelaw AC, Shankland IM, Elisha BG. Use of 16S rRNA sequencing for identification of *Actinobacillus ureae* isolated from a cerebrospinal fluid sample. J Clin Microbiol 2002;40:666–668.

1374. Whitney AM, Farley MM. Cloning and sequence analysis of the structural pilin gene of Brazilian purpuric fever-associated *Haemophilus influenzae* biogroup aegyptius. Infect Immun 1993;61:1559–1562.

1375. Wild BE, Pearman JW, Campbell PB, et al. Brazilian purpuric fever in Western Australia. Med J Aust 1989;150:344–346.

1376. Willems A, Coopman R, Gillis M. Phylogenetic and DNA-DNA hybridization analyses of *Bradyrhizobium* species. Int J Syst Evol Microbiol 2001;51: 111–117.

1377. Williams BL, Hammond BF. *Capnocytophaga*: new genus of gram-negative gliding bacteria. IV. DNA base composition and sequence homology. Arch Microbiol 1979;122:35–39.

1378. Williams BL, Hollis D, Holdemann LV. Synonymy of strains of Centers for Disease Control group DF-1 with species of *Capnocytophaga*. J Clin Microbiol 1979;10:550–556.

1379. Wilson ME. Prosthetic valve endocarditis and paravalvular abscess caused by *Actinobacillus actinomycetemcomitans*. Rev Infect Dis 1989;11:665–667.

1380. Wilson ME, Jonak-Urbanczyk JT, Bronson PM, et al. *Capnocytophaga* species: increased resistance of clinical isolates to serum bactericidal action. J Infect Dis 1987;156:99–106.

1381. Wilson R. Evidence of bacterial infection in acute exacerbations of chronic bronchitis. Semin Respir Infect 215;2002 ;15:208.

1382. Wilson WR, Karchmer AW, Dajani AS, et al. Antibiotic treatment of adults with infective endocarditis due to streptococci, enterococci, staphylococci, and HACEK microorganisms. JAMA 1995;274:1706–1713.

1383. Wine N, Lim Y, Fierer J. *Pasteurella multocida* epiglottitis. Arch Otolaryngol Head Neck Surg 1997;123:759–761.

1384. Winn RE, Chase WF, Lauderdale PW, et al. Septic arthritis involving *Capnocytophaga ochracea*. J Clin Microbiol 1983;19:538–540.

1385. Wirsing von Konig CH, Finger H. Role of pertussis toxin in causing symptoms of *Bordetella parapertussis* infection. Eur J Clin Microbiol Infect Dis 1994; 13:455–458.

1386. Wirsing von Konig CH, Gounis D, Laukamp S, et al. Evaluation of a single-sample serological technique for diagnosing pertussis in unvaccinated children. Eur J Clin Microbiol 1999;18:341–345.

1387. Wolak T, Abu-Shakra M, Flusser D, et al. *Kingella* endocarditis and meningitis in a patient with SLE and associated antiphospholipid syndrome. Lupus 2000; 9:393–396.

1388. Wong DT, Thornton DC, Kennedy RC, Dolan MJ. A chemically-defined liquid medium that supports primary isolation of *Rochalimaea* (*Bartonella*) *henselae* from blood and tissue specimens. J Clin Microbiol 1995;33:742–744.

1389. Wong EY, Berkowitz RG. Acute epiglottitis in adults: the Royal Melbourne Hospital experience. ANZ J Surg 2001;71:740–743.

1390. Wong GWK, Oppenheimer SJ, Vaudry W. CSF shunt infection by unencapsulated *Haemophilus influenzae*. Clin Infect Dis 1993;17:519–520.

1391. Wong JD, Janda JM, Duffey PS. Preliminary studies on the use of carbon substrate utilization patterns for identification of *Brucella* species. Diagn Microbiol Infect Dis 1992;15:109–113.

1392. Wong MT, Dolan MJ, Lattuada CP Jr, et al. Neuroretinitis, aseptic meningitis, and lymphadenitis associated with *Bartonella* (*Rochalimaea*) *henselae* infection in immunocompetent patients and patients infected with human immunodeficiency type 1. Clin Infect Dis 1995;21:352–360.

1393. Wong R, Tappero J, Cockerell CJ. Bacillary angiomatosis and other *Bartonella* species infections. Semin Cutan Med Surg 1997;16:188–199.

1394. Wood GE, Dutro SM, Totten PA: Target cell range of *Haemophilus ducreyi* hemolysin and its involvement in invasion of human epithelial cells. Infect Immun 1999;67:3740–3749.

1395. Woolfrey RR, Moody JA. Human infections associated with *Bordetella bronchiseptica*. Clin Microbiol Rev 1991;4:243–255.

1396. World Health Organization. WHO meeting on case definitions of pertussis. Minutes/EPI/PERT91.1., January 10–11. Geneva: World Health Organization, 1991:4–5.

1397. Wormser GP, Bottone EJ. *Cardiobacterium hominis*: review of microbiologic and clinical features. Rev Infect Dis 1983;5:680–691.

1398. Wu T-H, Gu X-X. Outer membrane proteins as a carrier of detoxified lipooligosaccharide conjugate vaccines for nontypeable *Haemophilus influenzae*. Infect Immun 1999;67:5508–5513.

1399. Wullenweber M. *Streptobacillus moniliformis*: a zoonotic pathogen: taxonomic considerations, host species, diagnosis, therapy, geographical distribution. Lab Anim 1995;29:1–15.

1400. Wust J, Gubler J, Mannheim W, et al. *Actinobacillus hominis* as a causative agent of septicemia in hepatic failure. Eur J Clin Microbiol Infect Dis 1991; 10:693–694.

1401. Yaari E, Yafe-Zimerman Y, Schwartz SB, et al. Clinical manifestations of *Bordetella pertussis* infection in immunized children and young adults. Chest 1999;115:1254–1258.

1402. Yagupsky P. Detection of *Brucella melitensis* by BACTEC NR660 blood culture system. J Clin Microbiol 1994;32:1899–1901.

1403. Yagupsky P, Dagan R. *Kingella kingae*: an emerging cause of invasive infections in young children. Clin Infect Dis 1997;24:860–866.

1404. Yagupsky P, Dagan R. Population-based study of invasive *Kingella kingae* infections. Emerg Infect Dis 2000;6:85–87.

1405. Yagupsky P, Dagan R, Howard CW, et al. High prevalence of *Kingella kingae* in joint fluid from children with septic arthritis revealed by the BACTEC blood culture system. J Clin Microbiol 1992;30:1278–1281.

1406. Yagupsky P, Merires M, Bahar J, Dagan R. Evaluation of novel vancomycin-containing medium for primary isolation of *Kingella kingae* from upper respiratory tract specimens. J Clin Microbiol 1995;33:1426–1427.

1407. Yagupsky P, Peled N, Katz O. Epidemiological features of invasive *Kingella kingae* infections and respiratory carriage of the organism. J Clin Microbiol 2002;40:4180–4184.

1408. Yagupsky P, Peled N, Press J. Use of BACTEC 9240 blood culture system for detection of *Brucella melitensis* in synovial fluid. J Clin Microbiol 2001; 39:738–739.

1409. Yagupsky P, Peled N, Press J, et al. Rapid detection of *Brucella melitensis* from blood cultures by a commercial system. Eur J Clin Microbiol Infect Dis 1997;16:605–607.

1410. Yagupsky P, Peled N, Press J, et al. Comparison of BACTEC 9240 Peds Plus medium and Isolator 1.5 microbial tube for detection of *Brucella melitensis* from blood cultures. J Clin Microbiol 1997;35:1382–1384.

1411. Yagupsky P, Peled N, Riesenberg K, Banai M. Exposure of hospital personnel to *Brucella melitensis* and occurrence of laboratory-acquired disease in an endemic area. Scand J Infect Dis 2000;32:31–35.

1412. Yagupsky P, Press J. Use of the Isolator 1.5 microbial tube for culture of synovial fluid from patients with septic arthritis. J Clin Microbiol1997; 35: 2410–2412.

1413. Yamamoto T, Kajiura S, Hirai Y, Watanabe T. *Capnocytophaga haemolytica* sp. nov. and *Capnocytophaga granulosa* sp. nov., from human dental plaque. Int J Syst Bacteriol 1994;44:324–329.

1414. Yamazaki Y, Ebisu S, Okada H. Partial purification of a bacterial lectin-like substance from *Eikenella corrodens*. Infect Immun 1988;56:191–196.

1415. Yaneza AL, Jivan H, Kumari P, Togoo MS. *Pasteurella haemolytica* endocarditis. J Infect 1991;23:65–67.

1416. Yayli G, Isler M, Oyar O. Medically treated splenic abscess due to *Brucella melitensis*. Scand J Infect Dis 2002;34:133–135.

1417. Yi K, Murphy TF. Importance of an immunodominant surface-exposed loop on outer membrane protein P2 of nontypeable *Haemophilus influenzae*. Infect Immun 1997;65:150–155.

1418. Yih WK, Silva EA, Ida J, et al. *Bordetella holmesii*-like organisms isolated from Massachusetts patients with pertussis-like symptoms. Emerg Infect Dis 1999;5:441–443.

1419. Ying W, Nguyen MQ, Jahre JA. *Brucella canis* endocarditis: case report. Clin Infect Dis 1999;29:1593–1594.

1420. Young EJ. Serologic diagnosis of human brucellosis: analysis of 214 cases by agglutination tests and review of the literature. Rev Infect Dis 1991;13: 359–372.

1421. Young EJ. An overview of human brucellosis. Clin Infect Dis 1995;21: 283–290.

1422. Young EJ, Tarry A, Genta RM, et al. Thrombocytopenic purpura associated with brucellosis: report of 2 cases and literature review. Clin Infect Dis 2000; 31:904–909.

1423. Young SA, Anderson GL, Mitchell PD. Laboratory observations during an outbreak of pertussis. Clin Microbiol Newslett 1987;9:176–179.

1424. Yu GV, Boike AM, Hladik JR. An unusual case of diabetic cellulitis due to *Pasteurella multocida*. J Foot Ankle Surg 1995;34:91–95.

1425. Yuan A, Yang PCh, Lee LN, et al. *Actinobacillus actinomycetemcomitans* pneumonia with chest wall involvement and rib destruction. Chest 1992;101: 1450–1451.

1426. Zambon JJ, Haraszthy VI, Hariharan G, et al. The microbiology of early-onset periodontitis: association of highly toxic *Actinobacillus actinomycetemcomitans* with localized juvenile periodontitis. J Periodontol 1996;67:282–290.

1427. Zangwill KM, Hamilton DH, Perkins BA, et al. Cat scratch disease in Connecticut: epidemiology, risk factors, and evaluation of a new diagnostic test. N Engl J Med 1993;329:8–13.

1428. Zbinden R, Hochli M, Nadal D. Intracellular location of *Bartonella henselae* cocultivated with Vero cells and used in an indirect fluorescent antibody test. Clin Diagn Lab Immunol 1995;2:693–695.

1429. Zbinden R, Michael N, Sekulovski A, et al. Evaluation of commercial slides for detection of immunoglobulin G against *Bartonella henselae* by indirect immunofluorescence. Eur J Clin Microbiol 1997;16:648–652.

1430. Zbinden R, Sommerhalder P, von Wartburg U. Co-isolation of *Pasteurella dagmatis* and *Pasteurella multocida* from cat-bite wounds. Eur J Clin Microbiol Infect Dis 1988;7:203–204.

1431. Zeaiter Z, Liang Z, Raoult D. Genetic classification and differentiation of *Bartonella* species based on comparison of partial *ftsZ* gene sequences. J Clin Microbiol 2002;40:3641–3647.

1432. Zerva L, Bourantas K, Mitka S, et al. Serum is the preferred specimen for diagnosis of human brucellosis by PCR. J Clin Microbiol 2001;39:1661–1664.

1433. Zhao G, Galina L, Hanyanun W, et al. Human tonsillitis associated with porcine *Pasteurella multocida* ingestion. Lancet 1993;342:491.

1434. Zijlstra EE, Swart GR, Godfroy FJM, et al. Pericarditis, pneumonia, and brain abscess due to a combined *Actinomyces-Actinobacillus actinomycetemcomitans* infection. J Infect 1992;25:83–87.

1435. Zimmer-Galler IE, Pach JM. *Capnocytophaga canimorsus* endophthalmitis. Retina 1996;16:163–164.

1436. Zwahlen A, Winkelstein JA, Moxon ER. Surface determinants of *Haemophilus influenzae* pathogenicity: comparative virulence of capsular transformants in normal and complement-depleted rats. J Infect Dis 1983;148:385–394.

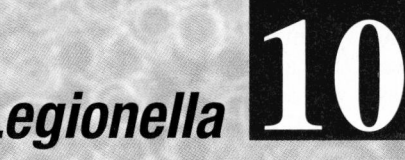

Legionella 10

Taxonomy and Characteristics of the Genus *Legionella*

Clinical and Pathologic Spectrum of Legionellosis

Predisposing Factors
Pathology and Pathogenesis

Epidemiologic and Ecologic Aspects of Legionellosis

Incidence
Legionellaceae in the Environment

Natural Habitats
Man-Made (Artificial) Aquatic Habitats

Legionellosis in Travelers
Nosocomial Outbreaks of Legionellosis

Laboratory Diagnosis

Selection, Collection, and Transport of Clinical Specimens
Direct Examination of Clinical Specimens

Gross Examination and Microscopic Examination of Stained Materials
Microscopic Examination of Stained Materials

Direct Fluorescent Antibody (DFA) Procedure
Antigen Detection in Urine and Body Fluids

Detection of *Legionella* in Clinical Specimens

Isolation of *Legionella* Species From Clinical Specimens

Biopsy, Surgical Removal, and Autopsy Tissue
Pleural Fluid and Transtracheal Aspirates
Acid-Wash Decontamination Procedure for Sputum and Other Contaminated Specimens
Blood Cultures

Identification of *Legionella* Species
Antimicrobial Susceptibility and Treatment
Serum Indirect Immunofluorescent Antibody Test
Molecular Diagnosis

Environmental Microbiology Studies

Isolation of *Legionella* from Environmental Samples
Typing of *Legionella* Isolates

uring the summer of 1976, an explosive outbreak of pneumonia of unknown etiology occurred among persons who attended an American Legion convention in Philadelphia.[63] Individuals in whom the multisystem illness (which included pneumonia) developed were said to have legionnaires' disease.[23] A total of 182 cases was documented; 29 of these patients died. By early January 1977, the etiologic agent had been isolated by Dr. Joseph McDade of the Centers for Disease Control (CDC).[104] Thus, within 6 months a major medical mystery was solved and a new family of bacteria, the *Legionellaceae,* was discovered. The history of legionnaires' disease was reviewed in 1988,[160] and several more recent reviews are available.[58,107,139] The availability of web sites has also been detailed.[10]

Taxonomy and Characteristics of the Genus Legionella

In 1979, Brenner, Steigerwalt, and McDade classified the bacterium that caused the Philadelphia outbreak of legionnaires' disease as *Legionella pneumophila,* in the family *Legionellaceae.*[20] At present, 50 validly published species and subspecies and a total of 71 serologic types of *Legionella* have been isolated from either human specimens, environmental sources, or both (Table 10-1).[78,162] Several recently described species are obligate intracellular parasites of free-living amoebae and can be isolated only by cocultivation with amoebae.[2,34] These amoeba pathogens were initially recognized by Rowbotham,[125] who called them *Legionella*-like amoeba pathogens (LLAPs). The most frequent of these species appears to be *L. lytica* (formerly called *Sarcobium lyticum*).

Legionella species are non–spore-forming, narrow, gram-negative rods, 0.3 μm to 0.9 μm in width. In length the bacteria vary from short forms, 1.5 to 2 μm in length, to longer filamentous forms. They are usually short and thin or coccobacillary when seen in direct smears of clinical specimens, but are more variable in length after growth in suboptimal culture media, when forms longer than 20 μm are not unusual. Legionellae stain much more readily with the Diff-Quik, Giemsa, or Gram-Weigert stains than they do with the traditional Gram stain in touch preparations of fresh tissue imprints, smears of bronchial alveolar lavage fluid, or sputum. Addition of 0.05% basic fuchsin to the safranin counterstain in the Gram procedure, however, yields far better staining of *Legionella* spp., as well as many other poorly staining gram-negative bacilli.

Except for three species that are nonmotile, *L. oakridgensis, L. nautarum,* and *L. londinensis,* the remainder of *Legionella* species are motile by means of one or more polar or subpolar flagella.[162] The Legionellaceae are aerobic and nutritionally fastidious. They require L-cysteine and iron salts for growth. R.E. Weaver first cultivated *L. pneumophila* on Mueller-Hinton agar supplemented with 1% IsoVitalex and 1% hemoglobin. Isolates may grow very slowly on the chocolate agar used for gonococcus isolation as well.[35] The optimal growth medium is a variation on the charcoal-yeast extract agar developed by the late James Feeley.[55] The yeast extract supplies the necessary nutrients. Activated charcoal

Table 10-1 Species of the Genus *Legionella* (Number of Serogroups)

SPECIES ISOLATED FROM HUMANS AND ENVIRONMENT	SPECIES ISOLATED FROM ENVIRONMENT ONLY
L. anisa	*L. adelaidensis*
L. bozemanii (2)	*L. beliardensis*
L. birminghamensis	*L. brunensis*
L. cincinnatiensis	*L. cherrii*
L. dumoffii	*L. drozanskii*
L. erythra (2)	*L. fairfieldensis*
L. feelei (2)	*L. fallonii*
L. gormanii	*L. geestiana*
L. hackeliae (2)	*L. gratiana*
L. jordanis	*L. gresilensis*
L. lansingensis	*L. israelensis*
L. longbeachae (2)	*L. jamestowniensis*
L. lytica	*L. londiniensis*
L. maceachernii	*L. moravica*
L. micdadei	*L. nautarum*
L. oakridgensis	*L. quateirensis*
L. parisiensis	*L. quinlivanii* (2)
L. pneumophila pneumophila (15)	*L. rowbothamii*
L. pneumophila fraseri	*L. rubrilucens*
L. pneumophila pascullei	*L. santicrucis*
L. sainthelensi (2)	*L. shakespearei*
L. tucsonensis	*L. spiritensis*
L. wadsworthii	*L. steigerwaltii*
	L. taurinensis
	L. waltersii
	L. worsleiensis
	Genomospecies

removes toxic oxygen radicals produced by exposure of many media to light.[77] ACES buffer has a pK of 6.9, the optimum for growth of *Legionella* spp. Addition of ACES buffer and α-ketoglutarate yields BCYEα agar.[38]

Growth on BCYEα agar with no growth on blood agar is one of the most useful **presumptive clues** that an isolate could be a species of *Legionella.* Another gram-negative organism that also grows on BCYE but not on ordinary blood agar is *Francisella tularensis.* In contrast to *Francisella* spp., which produce acid from carbohydrates, *Legionella* spp. neither ferment nor oxidize carbohydrates. Certain thermophilic spore-forming bacilli and *Bordetella pertussis* are also capable of growing on BCYEα agar; differences in morphology, serologic features, and cellular fatty acids aid in differentiating them. *Legionella* spp. produce characteristic branched-chain fatty acids in their cell walls.[162] Most species are weakly catalase- and peroxidase-positive. The sodium hippurate hydrolysis test, which is positive for *L. pneumophila* and negative for the majority of other *Legionella* species isolated from clinical materials, provides a useful presumptive procedure for differentiation between *L. pneumophila* and the other *Legionella* species. Phenotypic characterization of *Legionella* isolates using biochemical tests is of only limited value for presumptive identification of isolates to the species level. Serotyping of isolates using immunofluorescent antibody testing, however, is a practical way to differentiate isolates presumptively as species of *Legionella*. Definitive identification of *Legionella* species may require nucleic acid studies and other chemotaxonomic reference procedures.[46]

Clinical and Pathologic Spectrum of Legionellosis

Legionnaires' disease occurs both sporadically, in the form of community-acquired pneumonia, and in epidemics.[22,54,53] In addition to legionnaires' disease, a mild form of illness called Pontiac fever occurs.[69] Illness may also involve anatomic regions of the body outside the chest cavity. Thus, the term *legionellosis*, including legionnaires' disease, Pontiac fever, and extrapulmonary involvement with *Legionella* species, is used in this chapter to refer to any infection caused by bacteria of the family *Legionellaceae*. Approximately 85% of the documented cases of legionellosis have been caused by *L. pneumophila*. Serogroups 1 and 6 of *L. pneumophila* have, by themselves, accounted for up to 75% of the legionellae reported to cause human illness.[118] In addition to *L. pneumophila*, many other species have been isolated from clinical specimens collected from humans (see Table 10-1). In a recent international survey of culture-confirmed cases the most frequent nonpneumophila species were *L. longbeachae* and *L. bozemanii*.[163] *L. micdadei*[89,33] and *L. dumoffii*[145,82] have also been responsible for sporadic and epidemic

disease in certain locales. Multiple species and/or serogroups may be present in water systems, either environmental or potable, and the same patient may be infected with more than one serogroup or species at the same time.[96]

Legionellosis has most commonly been recognized as a form of pneumonia. The earliest symptoms typically include a run-down feeling, muscle aches, and a slight headache. During the first day, patients commonly experience a rapid onset of dry cough and elevated temperature (e.g., 102°F to 104°F or higher is not uncommon) with chills. Abdominal pain and gastrointestinal symptoms (e.g., nausea, vomiting, and diarrhea) occur in many patients. A summary of clinical manifestations is given in Table 10-2. Investigators have repeatedly demonstrated their inability to distinguish among the various etiologies of pneumonia based on clinical history, physical examination, or laboratory tests.[122]

At onset, chest roentgenograms typically show patchy infiltrates, which may progress to five-lobe consolidation.[142,51,106] Infiltrates are bilateral in two thirds of patients, and abscess cavities may be present, particularly in immunocompromised patients. Laboratory findings commonly include, in varying combinations, a moderate leukocytosis with a left shift, proteinuria, hyponatremia, azotemia, elevated serum glutamic oxaloacetic transaminase (also called aspartate aminotransferase, or AST), and a high erythrocyte sedimentation rate. As mentioned previously, legionellosis may also take the form of a mild, self-limited illness of short duration, known as Pontiac fever, with elevated temperature, myalgia, malaise, and headache, but with few or no respiratory findings and no pneumonia.[56,60] Table 10-2 provides a comparison of the clinical aspects of legionnaires' disease and Pontiac fever. Both pneumonic disease and nonpneumonic disease may result from exposure to the same environmental source.[68]

In recent years, the clinical spectrum of legionellosis has expanded. The illness may involve essentially any organ

Table 10-2 Clinical Manifestations in Two Kinds of Legionellosis

	LEGIONNAIRES' DISEASE	PONTIAC FEVER
Mortality	15%–30%	0%
Incubation period	2–10 days	1–2 days
Symptoms	Fever, chills, cough, myalgia, headache, chest pain, sputum and diarrhea (and confusion or other mental states in some)	Similar to influenza: fever, chills, and myalgia (and cough, chest pain, and confusion in some)
Lung	Pneumonia and pleural effusion (lung abscess in some)	Pleuritic pain; no pneumonia, no lung abscess
Kidney	Renal failure (proteinuria, azotemia, and hematuria in some)	No renal manifestations
Liver	Modest liver-function abnormalities	No liver-function abnormalities
Gastrointestinal tract	Watery diarrhea, abdominal pain, and nausea and vomiting	No abnormalities
Central nervous system	Somnolence, delirium, disorientation, confusion, and obtundation (seizure rarely documented)	No central nervous system manifestations

Modified from references[146,88].

system of the body, with or without pneumonia. Examples of selected manifestations of extrapulmonary involvement follow. Bacteremia has been reported, but data on its frequency are lacking.[40,121] Nearly half the patients with legionnaires' disease show central nervous system manifestations such as headache, lethargy, confusion, stupor, and other less frequent manifestations, including ataxia, coma, and seizures.[81] A painful, nonpruritic, macular rash, limited to the pretibial surfaces of the legs, has been reported; however, dermal manifestations are uncommon.[75] *L. pneumophila* serogroup 1 has been demonstrated in lymph nodes, spleen, kidney, and bone marrow and has been documented in acute myocarditis,[155,161] prosthetic valve endocarditis,[103] pericarditis,[102] and hemodialysis fistula infections.[86] Arnow and associates[7] reported the isolation of *L. pneumophila* serogroup 3, mixed with multiple species of anaerobic bacteria, from a perirectal abscess. *L. pneumophila* serogroup 4 was shown by direct immunofluorescence in lesions of acute pyelonephritis in a patient who had both pneumonia and pyelonephritis associated with this organism.[32] *L. micdadei* was the only organism isolated from a cutaneous leg abscess of a 62-year-old woman who had been receiving prednisone and cyclophosphamide for rapidly progressive glomerulonephritis.[4] In general, however, reports of extrapulmonary manifestations have been more commonly associated with *L. pneumophila* than with other species. Reviews of the manifestations of illness produced by *Legionella* species other than *L. pneumophila* have been presented by Fang[53,54] and Muder[106–108] and their colleagues.

The high prevalence of antibody to legionellae in some populations suggests that asymptomatic or subclinical infection may be common. This assumption is bolstered by the documentation of unrecognized infection (defined by seroconversion) that occurred even in a group of patients who had undergone renal transplantation.

Predisposing Factors

Three factors are required or enhance the likelihood of symptomatic infection:

1. The presence of virulent legionellae in an environmental source
2. An efficient mechanism for dissemination of bacteria from the environment to human subjects
3. Diminution of host defense mechanisms that are effective against this organism

Persons who have legionnaires' disease are usually middle-aged or older (mean age, about 55 years); however, the disease can occur in persons of any age, including children. Legionellosis must be included in the differential diagnosis of immunosuppressed patients in whom fever and pulmonary infiltrates develop; in patients in whom pneumonia not responsive to penicillins, cephalosporins, or aminoglycosides develops; or in any patient with severe pneumonia, especially when there is no other readily apparent alternative diagnosis. In individuals receiving hemodialysis, recipients of organ transplants, and other surgical patients, for example, legionnaires' disease has been a major cause of morbidity and mortality.[116,93]

Other potential predisposing conditions include diabetes mellitus, ethanolism, chronic obstructive pulmonary disease, and cardiovascular disease. Cigarette smoking was suggested as a predisposing factor in the Philadelphia outbreak and in some subsequent outbreaks. A prerequisite is exposure to concentrated virulent *Legionella* organisms in the environment. Thus, legionellosis has occurred with higher frequencies among travelers to a site with an ongoing hyperendemic (often unrecognized).[11] In recent years the site may be the travel vehicle, as epidemics have occurred repeatedly on cruise ships, usually associated with use of whirlpools or hot tubs.[80]

As a result of the prerequisites outlined above, sites where elderly or debilitated individuals congregate are most likely to be problems. Although there have been no studies that tried to correlate the "swinging singles" quotient of resorts with the frequency of legionellosis, it would not be surprising if there were such a correlation, given the frequency with which whirlpools and spas have been implicated as sources of infection. Certainly healthcare facilities have been a major problem, partially thanks to the unwitting collaboration of engineers who place cooling towers upwind from intake vents for fresh air—an undoubtedly fortuitous design that is distressing in its regularity.[31]

Pathology and Pathogenesis

Pathologic features of human infection with several species of *Legionella* other than *L. pneumophila* are similar to those found in *L. pneumophila* infections. A multifocal lobular pneumonia often becomes confluent and may assume a lobar appearance. Small abscesses are common; less frequently, large abscesses that can be visualized radiographically occur.

Histologically, neutrophils, macrophages, and large amounts of fibrin fill airspaces, and septic vasculitis of small blood vessels has been observed. Pulmonary fibrosis and decreased pulmonary function may occur as a long-term sequela.[26] Legionellae do not stain well with hematoxylin and eosin in formalin-fixed paraffin sections but may be visualized if large numbers are present. A silver impregnation method, such as the Dieterle, Steiner, or Warthin-Starry method will stain the organisms reliably.[148] Silver impregnation techniques are nonspecific and stain virtually all microorganisms present in addition to *Legionella*. The Brown-Hopps tissue Gram stain will also demonstrate the bacteria, but careful attention to detail and appropriate controls are essential.

Whenever possible, fresh imprints of lung biopsy material should be prepared, because visualization and analysis of all bacteria is easier in smears than in histologic sections. Legionellae can be demonstrated with Giemsa, Gram-Weigert, and Gram procedures, especially if 0.05% basic fuchsin is added to the traditional safranin counterstain in Gram's procedure (see Color Plate 10-1) The organisms are facultative intracellular pathogens and may be found within macrophages and neutrophils or extracellularly.

A distinctive characteristic of *L. micdadei* is the presence of acid-fastness in clinical material, a property that is lost after cultivation on agar. Modified decolorization, as used for *Nocardia* spp. may be necessary. Instances have been recorded in which *L. pneumophila* was isolated from a specimen in which acid-fast bacilli had been demonstrated.[12] It is difficult, however, to be certain that a coinfection with *L. micdadei* was not present, as this species is more difficult to isolate than is *L. pneumophila.*

Considerable progress has been made toward an understanding of the pathogenesis of legionellosis.[64,141,49,57,79] The bacteria are facultative intracellular pathogens and replicate predominantly within cells of the monocyte-macrophage system, including prominently pulmonary alveolar macrophages. In the natural environment a variety of free-living amoebae are nature's macrophages. Legionellae are often phagocytized by polymorphonuclear neutrophils, but they do not appear to replicate in these cells. Within macrophages, legionellae inhibit phagolysosomal fusion and acidification of the phagosome; they continue multiplying until the host cell ruptures, thus releasing the organisms, which can then infect other phagocytic cells. The detailed pathogenesis is a subject of intensive ongoing investigation. Cell-mediated immunity rather than humoral immunity appears to play the central role in the host's defense against legionellae.

Epidemiologic and Ecologic Aspects of Legionellosis

Legionella species are widespread in both natural and man-made environments. Legionnaires' disease and Pontiac fever may be contracted by exposure to a wide variety of environmental sources, but there is no convincing evidence of a carrier state in humans, or of person-to-person transmission. Thus, there is no evidence that patients who have or have had legionnaires' disease are "contagious." Furthermore, *Legionella* spp., once isolated in the laboratory, have not proven to be any more hazardous to laboratory personnel than bacteria routinely isolated in the clinical microbiology laboratory. Inhalation of aerosolized organisms from environmental sources or possibly the aspiration of organisms present in water or in oropharyngeal contents are the most likely routes of spread. An early review by Broome is still relevant.[22]

Incidence

Legionellosis has been documented in countries around the world, but the morbidity and mortality associated with both the epidemic and sporadic cases of legionellosis are underreported in public health statistics. Not only do most countries lack a disease-oriented surveillance system for tracking the disease, but clinicians and microbiology laboratories may overlook the infection because of lack of awareness on the part of clinicians and/or failure of laboratories to use proper diagnostic methods.[70]

In general, it has been estimated that less than 1–5% of cases of pneumonia are caused by *Legionella* species, but this is probably an oversimplification.[36] In outbreaks of legionnaires' disease (as opposed to Pontiac fever), attack rates for the exposed high-risk population are usually low, but have been reported to be as high as 30%.[6] *Legionella* species (6.7% of etiologic agents) ranked as the third most common etiologic agents (following *Streptococcus pneu-*

moniae, 15.3%, and *Haemophilus influenzae,* 10.9%) for community-acquired pneumonia among 359 patients admitted to university, community, and Veterans Affairs hospitals examined in a U.S. multicenter study.[53] In other countries, the frequency of sporadic cases of community-acquired pneumonias caused by *Legionella* species varied from 2% in the United Kingdom to 3–4% in Germany and 10% in France.[126] The incidence of Pontiac fever in the general population is not known. Outside an outbreak setting, sporadic cases of Pontiac fever are probably almost always unrecognized. In any event, the definition of Pontiac fever is partially epidemiologic; differentiation of sporadic nonpneumonic cases of "legionnaires' disease" and Pontiac fever is impossible clinically. Cases of pneumonic and nonpneumonic (i.e., Pontiac fever) have been reported from the same exposure to environmental bacteria, presumably reflecting differences in host defenses and/or number of bacteria inhaled.

When evaluating studies of incidence, it is important to recognize the inherent bias introduced by the methods chosen by the investigators, by the feasibility of diagnosing some causes of pneumonia, and probably also by the inherent interests of those collecting the data. In a recent comprehensive study of pneumonia acquired in the outpatient setting, *Legionella* spp. were far down the list of etiologic agents.[16] In all studies the most common etiologic agent has been "unknown."

Legionellaceae in the Environment

As mentioned earlier, species of the genus *Legionella* are present in diverse natural and man-made habitats. Numerous studies have been focused on the ecology of *Legionella* species in man-made habitats, such as cooling towers that use evaporation of water and potable (drinking) water systems within buildings. Man-made habitats probably serve as "amplifiers" or disseminators of legionellae that originated in natural environments.

NATURAL HABITATS

Legionella spp. have been found in natural waters from around the world, including ground water.[120] They are widespread in lakes, ponds, streams, and both cold and warm springs. They have been isolated from aquatic habitats with temperatures ranging from 5.7°C to 63°C[61] and in hot spring water used for hydrotherapy.[17] There appear to be higher concentrations of *Legionella* species in warmer waters (30°C to 45°C) than in water at cooler temperatures.[151] In Puerto Rico, legionellae were recovered from marine waters and from epiphytes in trees.[115]

Although soil (e.g., wind-blown dust from an excavation site) was implicated epidemiologically (but not studied microbiologically) as a source of *Legionella* in one of the early outbreaks of legionnaires' disease, there have been few reports of attempts to isolate *Legionella* spp. from soil. *L. pneumophila* and *L. bozemanii* were isolated from samples of wet soil soon after recognition of the organism.[105] More recently, Steele and colleagues isolated *L. pneumophila, L. longbeachae* serogroup 1, and *L. micdadei* from potting soils in Australia.[137] *L. longbeachae* serogroup 1 was also isolated from natural soil and from pine sawdust. Epidemiologic and microbiologic studies from South Australia in association with an outbreak of legionellosis due to *L. longbeachae* serogroup 1 suggested that soil, and not water, could be the natural habitat of *L. longbeachae* serogroup 1 and that soil could be the source of this organism in human disease. In this study, gardening in soil, rather than exposure to water contaminated with *L. longbeachae,* appeared to be the major environmental risk factor associated with legionellosis.[136] Much more work on the ecology of *Legionella* spp. in natural aquatic and terrestrial habitats is needed.

MAN-MADE (ARTIFICIAL) AQUATIC HABITATS

There have been numerous reports that associated the presence of *L. pneumophila* in institutional potable hot water with the occurrence of legionellosis. Legionellae appear to survive the usual chlorination procedures of municipal water treatment facilities, and thus, not unexpectedly, may be present in potable water supplied to homes, apartment buildings, hotels, hospitals, and other buildings.[3,140] Potable hot water, especially if it does not exceed 55°C, has contained heavy concentrations of *Legionella* in some instances. In addition to water temperature, the construction of the plumbing system also seems to play an important role; for example, the presence of certain kinds of resins in gaskets; the presence of dead ends or cul-de-sacs, where there is stasis, obstruction, or stagnation in water flow; and the presence of biofilms or slime layers on the surface of pipes containing other commensal bacteria, protozoa, and algae may favor the presence of legionellae.[94,135] Many of these studies were performed before the importance of environmental protozoa was realized, and it is not clear whether some of the associations may have been fortuitous rather than causal. Some of the factors associated with enhanced replication of the bacteria in homes have been defined,[28] but attacking the problem at the residential level will be all but impossible. It is worth noting that apparently nosocomially acquired infection may, in actuality, have been acquired in the patient's home.[129]

In modern society the mechanisms by which bacteria in water may be aerosolized and transmitted to unwitting respiratory tracts are legion. In 1990, the CDC reported an outbreak of community-acquired legionnaires' disease involving 33 persons that was associated with a grocery store mist machine.[97] The mist machine continuously generated a tap water aerosol (presumably containing *L. pneumophila*) in respirable (2–5 μm) droplets over the produce display. The system used ultrasonic transducers located in the humidifier's tap water reservoir to create the mist.

Other public sources of infection have included ornamental fountains.[76] Whirlpool spas have been implicated frequently in cases of legionellosis.[52,71] The popularity of these efficient disseminators of bacteria in water extends to the high seas, so landlubbers are not solely at risk. Dramatically, a large outbreak at a flower show in The Netherlands was traced to whirlpool spas used in the exhibits.[30] An isolate of *L. pneumophila* was also recovered from a sprinkler used in the exhibits, but the genotype of this strain was different from that of the two whirlpool spas and the infected patients. Such experiences emphasize the importance of bacterial culture and molecular analysis of clinical and environmental strains during the investigation of an epidemic.

Although legionellae have been isolated from shower heads and shower water on repeated occasions, the epidemiologic evidence that bathing or showering in such water leads to legionellosis has been rather weak.[62,108] Supportive evidence reported by Breiman and associates from an investigation of an outbreak of nosocomial legionnaires' disease at a hospital in South Dakota strengthened the hypothesis that aerosolized shower water can serve as the vehicle for spread of *Legionella pneumophila* to patients.[19] Perhaps the most bizarre case of water-associated legionnaires' disease was a neonatal infection that was acquired during a home birthing in a domestic spa bath.[112]

Factors that promote the growth of legionellae in plumbing systems are poorly known in spite of a large accumulation of literature. Legionellae are fastidious organisms that require enriched media for growth in the laboratory, and it is unlikely that drinking water supplies all their nutritional requirements for growth and energy. Rowbotham was the first to report that *Legionella* species multiply in close association with free-living aquatic and soil amebae of the genera *Acanthamoeba* and *Naegleria* (see Chapter 22).[124] Others have confirmed and extended these observations, not only with *Acanthamoeba* and *Naegleria,* but also with other amoebae, such as *Hartmannella* and the ciliate *Tetrahymena.*[59,113,150] Thus, amoebae or ciliates phagocytize legionellae, as they do other bacteria in nature, and the legionellae then survive and multiply within nutritionally deficient habitats by living parasitically within the protozoa. In addition, it has been suggested that the amoebae, which form cysts, might offer further protection to legionellae within the cysts against the effects of chlorine.[87,134] Scientists have taken advantage of this association to enhance recovery of legionellae from the environment, and one species, *L. lytica,* consists of strains that grow only intracellularly in amoebae.

Legionellosis in Travelers

Since the 1976 outbreak of legionnaires' disease, which occurred among travelers to Philadelphia, travel-associated epidemics and sporadic cases of legionnaires' disease have been recognized in many countries on all continents.[85,123] The true incidence of travel-associated disease is not clear. Cases are likely to be underreported not only because of underdiagnosis and lack of awareness of the epidemiologic significance, but also conceivably because of concerns about the effect of adverse publicity on tourism. Clusters and sporadic cases occur each year, nonetheless, associated especially with hotels and with hotel water systems contaminated with legionellae. Not surprisingly, the outbreaks may be recurrent and persistent until the nature of the problem is recognized and corrected. Clusters of cases have also been observed among travelers who have been on board cruise ships.

Cases and clusters of travel-associated *Legionella* infection should be reported to state and federal public health agencies and should lead to investigations of the source and magnitude of the outbreak to prevent further spread among the traveling public. As demonstrated first in the 1976 Philadelphia epidemic and confirmed repeatedly, it may only be the collection of multiple individual reports of disease by a central repository, such as a public health facility, that triggers the recognition of the problem.

Apparently sporadic disease that is not linked to travel may also be, in actuality, related to an unrecognized epidemic focus.[14] Bhopal has suggested approaches that may be useful for public health authorities to detect problems in their catchment areas.[13]

A recent twist on the theme of travel-associated infection has been the recognition that participants in holiday cruises are at risk of contracting this as well as other infections.[25] As has been true for resorts on dry land, these infections have been traced to contaminated water systems, such as whirlpool spas.

Nosocomial Outbreaks of Legionellosis

Within hospitalized populations are patients who may be compromised and are very susceptible to infections in general. These patients are at risk of acquiring legionellosis should they be exposed to virulent organisms.

The usual source of *Legionella* in hospitalized patients is water[131] (mainly the hot water system), especially from showers or baths.[50] In addition, patients may be infected from cooling towers that are part of or adjacent to the health care complex.[1,67] Other documented sources have included nasogastric tubes (with microaspiration of legionellae in contaminated water), humidifiers, respiratory therapy equipment (e.g., masks and hand-held nebulizers washed with contaminated tap water), whirlpools, and other less common sources. Early diagnosis of legionellosis and epidemiologic surveillance of cases within the hospital are needed not only for prompt and effective therapy but to aid in instituting control measures to prevent subsequent cases. With the high mortality rate for nosocomial legionnaires' disease (range, 30–50%) it would seem prudent that efforts be taken to prevent the spread of *Legionella* species from the hospital environment to patients who are likely to be most susceptible to infection.

Nosocomial legionnaires' disease has also been specifically linked to the use of tap water to clean nebulizers used for delivery of medication and to other respiratory therapy equipment. In a report by Mastro and colleagues, the use of tap water contaminated with *L. pneumophila* to wash medication nebulizers was a major factor that led to an outbreak of nosocomial legionnaires' disease in patients with chronic obstructive pulmonary disease.[101] In one particularly instructive cluster of infections, disease was more common in patients who were both receiving corticosteroids and exposed to nebulizer or room humidifiers filled with tap water.[8]

Of recent concern, some cases of nosocomial legionnaires' disease have been linked to microaspiration of water contaminated with *Legionella* species in patients with nasogastric tubes.[15,41,100,99] A different twist was documented at Stanford University Medical Center when wound infection caused by legionellae developed in postsurgical patients who had been bathed with tap water. The bacteria were clearly introduced directly into the wounds,[95] rather than into the respiratory tract with subsequent dissemination, a sequence of events that has also been documented.

Given all of these occurrences and the relative ease with which sterile water may be used in individuals at high risk, the continued use of tap water is difficult to justify or defend.[5]

Laboratory Diagnosis

The mainstay of diagnosis remains culture, which is absolutely specific and provides isolates for epidemiologic study and molecular typing. Detection of urinary antigen is a useful adjunctive technique, particularly in patients who do not produce adequate sputum for culture. Detection of nucleic acids has not yet reached the stage of widespread commercial availability and practicality, but will probably be a major diagnostic resource in the future.[110] Serologic diagnosis requires seroconversion and is, therefore, retrospective; it is useful for investigation of epidemics, but does not have a primary role in diagnosis of infections in individual patients. The limitations of current diagnostic tests have been discussed by Waterer and colleagues[153]; Marrie has made the case, however, for continuing to attempt laboratory confirmation of clinical suspicion.[98]

Selection, Collection, and Transport of Clinical Specimens

The broad clinical spectrum and severe morbidity and mortality of legionnaires' disease emphasize the need for rapid and accurate laboratory diagnosis. When legionellosis is suspected clinically, lower respiratory tract specimens should be collected for both culture and direct fluorescent antibody (DFA) testing. Appropriate specimens include expectorated sputum, materials collected using bronchoscopy (e.g., bronchial brush, biopsy, lavage, or washings), transtracheal aspirates, closed- and open-lung biopsy material, fine-needle aspirates of lung, and pleural fluid. In most situations it is appropriate to culture specimens for *Legionella* spp. only upon specific request. It would be appropriate, however, to include legionellae in the spectrum of pathogens sought when culturing lung tissue, in those collected both antemortem and postmortem. Such routine culture can serve as one part of the warning system that these water-associated pathogens are a problem in a particular institution.

Primary isolation of *Legionella* species on solid media has been successful from closed- and open-lung biopsy material, pleural fluid, and transtracheal aspirates, bronchial alveolar lavage samples, and sputum. A reasonably semieffective selective medium is available for the primary isolation of *L. pneumophila* from sputum and contaminated bronchial materials.[37,39,156]

Specimens should be collected carefully to avoid aerosols and transported to the laboratory at ambient temperature in sterile leakproof containers, preferably within 2 hours after collection. Specimens to be sent to a reference laboratory should be refrigerated or packed on wet ice if a delay of less than 2 days is anticipated. Specimens that are to be stored for days or weeks should be maintained at 70°C or colder. These may be shipped on dry ice. Specimens that must be shipped to a reference laboratory should be packaged and mailed in accordance with federal regulations (see Chapter 1). If specimens are being submitted only for pathological study and are to be fixed in buffered neutral formalin before shipment, they need not be refrigerated or frozen during transport.

L. pneumophila has been isolated from blood cultures on a few occasions using conventional media supplemented with L-cysteine and ferric pyrophosphate, or using BACTEC (Becton Dickinson Instrument Systems, Sparks, MD) radiometric aerobic and anaerobic media with no special supplements.[45] Blind subculture of the BACTEC aerobic and anaerobic bottles onto BCYEα appears to be necessary for isolation of legionellae. As mentioned previously, legionellae may also be encountered (rarely) in extrapulmonary sites. The practical value (or the clinical relevance) of seeking *Legionella* spp. in blood cultures or extrapulmonary sites, however, has not been established. In addition to the above specimens, urine (preferably an early morning sample) should be collected for detection of *Legionella* antigen.

An acute-phase serum sample should be collected early as an adjunct to other tests that may enable a more rapid diagnosis. A follow-up serum specimen should be collected within 2 to 6 weeks after collection of the acute-phase specimen, so that a fourfold rise in antibody titer against *Legionella* can be demonstrated. The diagnosis will, of necessity, be retrospective, but may be the only means of diagnosing the infection in some patients, particularly in those who produce minimal sputum.[156] Unfortunately, the development of a diagnostic fourfold rise in antibody titer can be slow and may occur in no more than 75–80% of patients who ultimately are shown to have legionnaires' disease.[156] In addition, some persons have seroconverted but remained asymptomatic (probably because of subclinical infection).

Direct Examination of Clinical Specimens
GROSS EXAMINATION AND MICROSCOPIC EXAMINATION OF STAINED MATERIALS

Gross examination of samples of lung may aid the pathologist in selecting the best areas for culture or histologic examination. Direct smears of exudates or touch preparations (dab smears) of fresh lung biopsy material should be prepared. Frozen sections of lung samples are also useful in diagnosis. Frozen sections and touch preparations should be placed in methanol for fixation if Gram's stain, hematoxylin and eosin, Giemsa's, "Diff-Quik," or modified-Kinyoun acid-fast stains are desired. The Giemsa stain is useful for demonstrating legionellae and other bacteria in fresh touch preparations of lung or bronchoscopic materials. Gram's stain should also be performed, however, because of the differential information it provides.

MICROSCOPIC EXAMINATION OF STAINED MATERIALS

Various specimens (e.g., transtracheal aspirates, pleural fluids, aspirates from thoracic empyema, fine-needle aspirates of lung, and touch preparations of lungs) can be stained with Gram's stain. Methanol fixation is better than heat fixation, and the intensity of staining can be improved by increasing the time of safranin staining to 10 minutes or longer. Alternatively, 0.05% carbolfuchsin has been added to the safranin by some workers to improve the intensity of staining with the counterstain. The Gram-Weigert, "Diff-Quik," or Giemsa stain may reveal more organisms than can be seen with routine Gram staining. In formalin-fixed, paraffin-embedded histologic sections, *Legionella* organisms cannot be readily seen in the hematoxylin and eosin (H&E), Gram, Brown-Brenn, Brown and Hopps, or MacCallum-Goodpasture stained preparations. The Gomori methenamine silver

(GMS) stain and periodic acid–Schiff stains are not useful for demonstrating legionellae. A modified acid-fast stain, as performed for *Nocardia* spp., is useful for demonstrating *L. micdadei*[111] and possibly some strains of *L. pneumophila*. All of these stains may be done on either impression smears or tissue sections but are most satisfactory on thin smears. A very sensitive histochemical method for demonstrating bacteria of all types is one of the silver impregnation stains, developed originally for spirochetes. A modified Dieterle stain was originally used; the organisms stain black to dark brown. Other silver impregnation techniques, such as the Steiner and Warthin-Starry methods, will also work. These silver stains are usually performed on histologic sections and are temperamental; the best choice is the stain that is done best by the local laboratory. Although sensitive, the deposited silver grains in these stains obscure the bacterial morphology and, of course, the Gram reaction cannot be determined. The morphology of *L. pneumophila* is shown in Color Plate 10-1 *A, B,* and *D.*

DIRECT FLUORESCENT ANTIBODY (DFA) PROCEDURE

Direct immunofluorescence assays, originally developed by Cherry and colleagues at the CDC,[27] have been used successfully for rapid detection of *Legionella* species in clinical specimens from the respiratory tract. Compared with cultures the DFA has a low sensitivity (25–70%).[162] The specificity has been high, but when there is a low prevalence of *Legionella* infection, false-positive results are unacceptably frequent. In addition to potential immunologic cross-reactions, contamination with environmental bacteria appears to have caused some false-positive results, even when scrupulous care is exercised when the test is performed. Use of immunofluorescence for diagnosis directly on patient specimens cannot, therefore, be recommended.

Immunofluorescence is a useful method, however, for identifying isolated bacteria. Several commercial suppliers market fluorescein isothiocyanate (FITC)-conjugated polyvalent antisera, as well as control sera and other reagents for *Legionella* DFA testing. Genetic Systems (Seattle, WA) offers a monoclonal antibody conjugate that has the advantage of decreasing the number of false-positive reactions while retaining the ability to react with most serotypes of *L. pneumophila*.[43] As a note of caution, the Genetic Systems monoclonal DFA conjugate failed to detect *L. pneumophila* in hot and cold storage tank water and in swab samples from showers and a water tap[149]; thus, it cannot be recommended for DFA studies of potable water or other samples from man-made water systems and its performance in natural habitat water studies is uncertain.

In performing the DFA test, specific antibody in the form of FITC-labeled polyvalent antiserum (conjugate) directed against the antigen(s) to be detected is usually purchased commercially. The directions of the manufacturer of the kit should be followed exactly. Antigen (present on or in *Legionella* organisms) is fixed on a slide, and then overlaid with FITC-labeled antibody. The antigen binds the globulin in the FITC-labeled antibody, forming an antigen-antibody complex (not washed away when gently rinsed with buffer) that is visible by the excitation of the FITC with ultraviolet light. When the antigen(s) of a *Legionella* species has reacted with FITC-conjugated antibody, exposure to ultraviolet light causes the FITC to emit longer wavelengths of light in the yellow-green region of the color spectrum, and the bacteria can be seen (using a fluorescence microscope) as brilliantly fluorescing yellow-green rods.

ANTIGEN DETECTION IN URINE AND BODY FLUIDS

Procedures for detecting *Legionella* antigens in urine, developed by Kohler and associates at the Indiana University Medical Center, include radioimmunoassay, enzyme-linked immunosorbent assay, and latex agglutination.[92] Commercially available immunoassays for detection of antigenuria caused by *L. pneumophila*, serogroup 1 have approximately specificity of 80–90% and specificity that approaches 100%. Radioimmunoassays, enzyme immunoassays, and particle agglutination assays have been used in the past. At present an immunochromographic strip assay (Binax NOW, Portland, Maine) is also available. This test is very useful, especially for patients who do not produce adequate sputum for culture. Limitations include restriction to a single serogroup, albeit the most common human pathogen in the genus, and prolonged excretion of antigen in some patients. In particular, immunosuppressed patients with delayed resolution of fever are likely to excrete antigen for more than 60 days.[133] Detection of urinary antigen must, therefore, be carefully correlated with the clinical history before ascribing the current infection to *Legionella*.[91] Occasional cross-reactions of among serogroups of *L. pneumophila* have also been described.[90]

Detection of *Legionella* in Clinical Specimens
Isolation of *Legionella* Species From Clinical Specimens

Bacteriologic culture of *Legionella* is the preferred (so-called gold standard) way to diagnose legionellosis.[165] According to Bridge and Edelstein, culture is one and one-half to three times more sensitive than the DFA test. *Legionella* species are not routinely isolated from the upper respiratory tract normal flora, although the DFA test for *L. pneumophila* was positive in a few healthy individuals,[21] although the specificity of the DFA reaction was not established.

The recommended nonselective solid medium for isolation of legionellae is buffered charcoal yeast extract agar (BCYEα), which contains L-cysteine, ferric pyrophosphate, ACES (*N*-[2-acetamido]-2-aminoethanesulfonic acid) buffer, α-ketoglutaric acid, and activated charcoal (BCYEα). The medium is available commercially from several manufacturers. In addition to BCYEα, it is recommended that one or more selective media be used to avoid overgrowth by normal flora and the possibility that other organisms may inhibit the growth of *Legionella*. Antibiotics have been added to the BCYEα base, resulting in reasonably effective selective media. One useful selective medium contains BCYEα base supplemented with cefamandole, polymyxin B, and anisomycin (BMPAα); a second contains glycine, vancomycin, polymyxin B, and anisomycin (referred to as "modified Wadowsky-Yee" or MWY medium). The cefamandole in BMPAα may inhibit *Legionella* species that do not produce β-lactamase, whereas the MWY medium is not as selective as BMPAα. BCYEα-based selective media are widely available commercially. Because the selective media may inhibit some legionellae, such media should be used in conjunction with nonselective BCYEα.

BIOPSY, SURGICAL REMOVAL, AND AUTOPSY TISSUE

To inoculate BCYEα or BMPAα media, the fresh-cut surface of lung should be gently dabbed in the first quadrant and a sterile inoculating loop used to transfer this inoculum to the other quadrants for primary isolation. Alternatively, a sterile tissue grinder can be used to homogenize 1- to 2-mm pieces of minced tissue in 0.5 to 1 mL of a sterile broth (such as trypticase soy broth or enriched thioglycolate medium). After homogenization, the plating medium is inoculated with approximately 0.1 mL of the homogenate and streaked for isolation. In addition, slides for Gram's stain should be prepared from the same specimen.

PLEURAL FLUID AND TRANSTRACHEAL ASPIRATES

Pleural fluid and transtracheal aspirates are inoculated directly onto the selective and nonselective media as for tissue homogenates. The BCYEα and BMPAα plates are incubated in a 5–10% CO_2 incubator at 35°C and examined daily for 5 days; they may be examined further every 2 to 3 days for up to 2 weeks. Other media for lower respiratory tract specimens (e.g., sheep blood agar, chocolate agar, and MacConkey agar) are inoculated and incubated in the usual way. The same specimen used for culture is further processed by making smears for Gram's stain.

ACID-WASH DECONTAMINATION PROCEDURE FOR SPUTUM AND OTHER CONTAMINATED SPECIMENS

The selective media currently available for primary isolation of legionellae are not completely selective, thus permitting breakthrough growth of certain unwanted organisms (e.g., *Bacillus* spp. or *Pseudomonas* spp.). In addition, growth of legionellae on BCYEα may be inhibited by other bacteria in clinical specimens, even when antibiotics are incorporated into the selective media. Treatment of contaminated respiratory specimens such as sputum, bronchial washings, bronchial lavages, and tracheal aspirates with an acid-wash solution before inoculation of BCYEα and BMPAα plates has been reported to improve isolation of *Legionella*.[24] The protocol outlined in Box 10-1 may be used for processing specimens that contain normal flora. It should be noted, however, that there are no other reports that either confirm or refute the efficacy of acid treatment, so the extra work involved must be evaluated in each laboratory. Heat treatment of specimens produced only a marginal increase in the yield of *Legionella* isolates and was not recommended for routine use.[48]

BLOOD CULTURES

Collection of blood for *Legionella* culture may occasionally be useful in certain clinical settings. Broth culture methods and lysis-centrifugation have both been used. Blind subculture or staining with a sensitive stain, such as acridine

Box 10-1 Protocol for Acid-Wash Decontamination of Sputum and Other Contaminated Specimens

1. Before performing the acid treatment of the specimen, prepare six smears for DFA testing.
2. Inoculate one BCYEα and one BMPAα plate with three to five drops of untreated respiratory specimen and streak for isolation.
3. Add 0.5 mL of respiratory specimen to 4.5 mL of acid solution (0.2 M KCl-HCl) in a screw-cap tube.
   a. Tightly seal the tube and thoroughly mix by vortexing under a safety hood.
   b. Allow the suspension to stand at room temperature for 5 minutes.
4. Inoculate a second set of BCYEα and BMPAα plates with three to five drops of the acid-specimen mixture prepared in step 3 and streak for isolation. Mark plates with an "A" to identify plates inoculated after acid treatment.
5. Place the four inoculated plates in CO_2-permeable plastic bags (two per bag) and incubate in CO_2 at 35°C for 2 weeks. Examine every 2 to 3 days for growth.

orange, of broth cultures must be performed, because legionellae do not regularly trigger indicators of growth in commercial systems. Patients with positive blood cultures had significantly higher concentrations of legionellae in respiratory specimens than those with negative blood cultures. The usefulness of routine blood cultures in less severely ill patients is not clear.

Identification of *Legionella* Species

Colonies of *Legionella* typically appear on BCYEα after 2 to 3 days of incubation in areas that have been heavily inoculated. If only a few organisms are present and if the plates have been lightly inoculated, however, isolated colonies may take several more days to develop. The colonies are variable in size (punctate or up to 3 to 4 mm). They are glistening, convex, circular, slightly irregular, and have an entire margin (see Color Plate 10-1*C*). When examined through a dissecting microscope (7X to 15X), *Legionella* colonies appear to have crystalline internal structures within the colonies or a speckled, opalescent appearance similar to that of *Fusobacterium nucleatum* (see Chapter 16, Color Plates 10-1*C* and *D*). Some species show a blue-white fluorescence under long-wave (366 nm) ultraviolet light (see Color Plate 10-1*E*); others exhibit a red fluorescence (Table 10-3). Colonies suspected of being *Legionella* should be subcultured onto an ordinary unsupplemented 5% sheep blood agar plate or BCYEα lacking L-cysteine and onto BCYEα medium that contains L-cysteine. Organisms that grow on 5% sheep blood, on BCYEα that lacks L-cysteine, or on other routine media (such as MacConkey agar) are probably not *Legionella*. Occasional isolates of *Legionella* spp. may be recovered on enriched chocolate agar. Isolates of gram-negative bacilli with typical colony characteristics of *Legionella* that grow on BCYEα or BMPAα medium after 48

hours or longer of incubation, but do not grow on BCYEα that lacks L-cysteine or on sheep blood agar should be characterized. Most such isolates belong to *L. pneumophila* serogroup 1, but there is geographic variation in the species and serogroups recovered. The most convenient laboratory test for confirming a suspected *Legionella* isolate is the DFA test. Colonies can be tested with the fluorescent-antibody conjugates mentioned previously to serogroup the isolate.

Occasionally organisms will be found that resemble *Legionella* but do not react with the serologic reagents used in the DFA test. Biochemical tests are unfortunately of limited use (Table 10-3); characterization of cellular fatty acids is useful if the laboratory has the capability of performing this analysis (Table 10-4). For most laboratories, however, the appropriate action will be submission of the isolate to a reference laboratory to determine if it represents a serogroup for which reagents were not available or even a previously unrecognized species or serogroup. It should be noted that there are non-*Legionella* species that require L-cysteine, fail to grow on blood agar, and may resemble *Legionella* in colony and microscopic morphology.[162] Tests used in definitive characterization of *Legionella* species in some reference or research laboratories include serologic tests, gas-liquid chromatography of cellular fatty acids, and nucleic acid genetic studies. As mentioned earlier, the commercially developed [152]I-labeled cDNA probe, designed to detect rRNA from legionellae, was shown to differentiate between the genus *Legionella* and non-*Legionella* organisms grown in culture.[44] Selected characteristics for laboratory recognition of *Legionella* species are shown in Color Plate 10-1.

Antimicrobial Susceptibility and Treatment

The mortality rate among patients with legionellosis caused by *L. pneumophila* has varied from 0% to 30%, depending on the clinical setting and patient population. Erythromycin has been effective in reducing the case-mortality rate and historically has been the drug of choice for legionellosis. Mortality from *Legionella* infection correlated both with delay in initiation of erythromycin therapy after admission to the hospital and with total delay in starting the antibiotic.[74]

Because *Legionella* spp. are facultative intracellular pathogens, which replicate inside monocytes and macrophages, antimicrobial agents that are concentrated within these cells are most likely to be successful in treatment. The newer macrolide antimicrobial agents (e.g., azithromycin and clarithromycin), and the fluoroquinolones (e.g., ciprofloxacin and perfloxacin) are more active in vitro and in experimental models than erythromycin, although clinical experience with these agents is still limited. Rifampin is known to be very active in vitro[144] and could be given in addition to erythromycin to some patients who are seriously ill or fail to respond to erythromycin alone, but rifampin should not be given alone. Alternatively, doxycycline in combination with rifampin has been recommended for moderately or severely ill patients. Trimethoprim-sulfamethoxazole with or without rifampin is another potential option. The penicillins (e.g., penicillin, carbenicillin, oxacillin), first- (e.g., cephalothin, cefazolin), second- (e.g., cefaman-

Table 10-3 Selected Characteristics of *Legionella* Species Implicated in Human Illnesses*

LEGIONELLA SPECIES	MODIFIED ACID-FASTNESS IN TISSUE	BROWNING OF TYROSINE-CONTAINING MEDIA	HIPPURATE HYDROLYSIS	GELATIN LIQUEFACTION	β-LACTAMASE PRODUCTION	OXIDASE	MOTILITY	AUTOFLUORESCENCE
L. anisa	−	+	−	+	+	+	+	BW
L. birminghamensis	−	−	−	+	+	+	+	−
L. bozemanii	−	+	−	+	±	±	+	BW
L. cincinnatiensis	−	+	−	+	+	−	+	−
L. dumoffii	−	+ᵃ	−	+	+	−	+	BW
L. feeleii	−	+(w)	±	±	−	−	+	−
L. gormanii	−	+	−	+	+	−	+	BW
L. hackelii	−	+	−	+	+	+	+	−
L. jordanis	−	+	−	+	+	+	+	−
L. lansingensis	−	−	−	−	±	+	+	−
L. longbeachae	−	+	−	−	±	+	+	NA
L. lytica	NA	NA	NA	NA	NA	NA	NA	NA
L. maceachernii	+	+	−	+	−	+	+	−
L. micdadei	+	−ᵇ	−	−	+	+	+	−
L. oakridgensis	−	+	−	+	+(w)	±	−	BW
L. parisiensis	−	+	−	+	+	+	+	BW
L. pneumophila spp. *pneumophila*	−ᶜ	+	+ᵈ	+	+	+/±	+	−
L. pneumophila spp. *fraseri*	−	+	±	+	+	+/±	+	−
L. pneumophila spp. *pascullei*	−	+	+	+	+	+/±	+	−
L. sainthelensi	−	+	−	+	+	+	+	−
L. tuconsensis	−	−	−	+	+	−	+	BW
L. wadsworthii	−	−	−	+	+	+	+	−

*All species are gram-negative, show no growth on unsupplemented blood agar, and require L-cysteine (present in BCYEα agar) for primary isolation (except for laboratory adapted strains of L. oakridgensis, which lose the requirement for L-cysteine). They are catalase- or peroxidase-positive. None reduce nitrate to nitrite, produce acid from D-glucose, or produce urease. +, positive; −, negative; +(w), weak reaction; w, weak reaction; NA, data not available; a, one strain negative; b, negative on initial isolation; may be positive after transfer on BCYE-α agar; c, rare strains have been isolated from cases with modified acid-fast bacilli in clinical specimens; these strains were not subspeciated; d, a few strains negative; BW, bluish-white autofluorescence. Adapted from reference[162].

Table 10-4 Major Cellular Fatty Acids of *Legionella* Species Isolated from Humans*

SPECIES	CELLULAR FATTY ACIDS†
L. anisa	a-$C_{15:0}$
L. birminghamensis	a-$C_{15:0}$, i-C_{14h}
L. bozemanii	a-$C_{15:0}$
L. cincinnatiensis	i-$C_{16:0}$, i-C_{16h}
L. dumoffii	a-$C_{15:0}$
L. feeleii	a-$C_{15:0}$, n-$C_{16:1}$
L. gormanii	a-$C_{15:0}$
L. hackeliae	a-$C_{15:0}$
L. jordanis	a-$C_{15:0}$
L. lansingensis	a-$C_{17:0}$, a-C_{15h}
L. longbeachae	i-$C_{16:0}$
L. maceachernii	a-$C_{15:0}$
L. micdadei	a-$C_{15:0}$
L. oakridgensis	i-$C_{16:0}$
L. pneumophila	i-$C_{16:0}$
L. sainthelensi	i-$C_{16:0}$
L. tucsonensis	a-$C_{15:0}$, n-C_{14h}
L. wadsworthii	a-$C_{15:0}$

* The major cellular fatty acids (determined by gas-liquid chromatography) of the Legionella species isolated from humans are listed. These bacteria are unusual compared with the other gram-negative bacteria because of their relatively large amounts of cellular branched-chain acids. The most abundant acid of L. pneumophila and some strains of L. longbeachae is i-$C_{16:0}$. However, strains of L. longbeachae may have either i-$C_{16:0}$ or $C_{16:1}$ as the major acid, or the two acids may be present in roughly equal amounts as the two most abundant acids. On the other hand, the major fatty acid of L. bozemanii, L. micdadei, L. dumoffii, L. gormanii, L. jordanis, and certain others is a saturated, branched-chain, 15-carbon acid (a-$C_{15:0}$).

† Numbers before the colon represent the number of carbon atoms contained in each of the different fatty acids; numbers after the colon are the number of double bonds; i_indicates a methyl ($-CH_3$) branch at the iso (next to last) carbon atom; a indicates a methyl branch at the anteiso (second from last) carbon atom.

Adapted from reference[162].

dole, cefoxitin), and presumably the third-generation cephalosporins, aminoglycosides (e.g., gentamicin, tobramycin, amikacin), and vancomycin are not effective in treatment. In vitro antimicrobial susceptibility testing of *Legionella* isolates has not been standardized and does not correlate with the clinical response to antibiotic therapy in patients. Therefore, performance of in vitro antimicrobial susceptibility testing on *Legionella* isolates in the hospital diagnostic laboratory is not recommended because the results are not readily interpretable by either the microbiologist or the clinician.

Serum Indirect Immunofluorescent Antibody Test

The serum indirect immunofluorescent antibody (IFA) test is recommended as an adjunct for diagnosis of legio-

nellosis, particularly for patients who do not or cannot provide adequate respiratory specimens (such as sputum) for culture. The sensitivity of the IFA test is 75–80%, and the specificity is 106%.[143,157,159] Clinicians must wait, however, 2 to 6 weeks for patients to develop a fourfold rise in antibody titer. Reagents for *Legionella* serodiagnostic tests should detect antibodies of IgG, IgM, and IgA classes. In some patients, a rise in IgM titer may occur without a detectable rise in IgG or IgA titers or may occur earlier in the course of illness than a rise in IgG titer.[164] IgM antibody may persist for as long as one year, so its presence cannot be used to diagnose a recent infection.

As documented by Wilkinson and colleagues, the serum IFA test using *Legionella* antigens may cross-react with the serum of patients who have certain other infections.[157,159] Sera of patients who had outbreak-associated *Mycoplasma pneumoniae* infections and patients with Q fever cross-reacted with *L. longbeachae* serogroup 2 and *L. jordanis*. Also, cross-reactions were noted between sera of patients who had outbreak-associated tularemia (*Francisella tularensis*) and *L. jordanis* antigen. In addition, false-positive cross-reactions have been observed in patients with *Bacteroides fragilis*, *Proteus vulgaris*, *Rickettsia* spp., and *Citrobacter* spp.[72] Some cross-reactions can be eliminated by absorption of antisera with *E. coli*, albeit with some diminution in the anti-*Legionella* titer.[158] Cross-reactions with *Campylobacter* spp. can be removed by absorption of sera with that bacterium.[18]

Seroconversions (fourfold increase in antibody titer) to reciprocal titers of 1:128 or greater are required for serodiagnosis of recent infection with *Legionella*. Single elevated reciprocal IFA titers of 256 or greater may be suggestive of *Legionella* infection during an outbreak. In sporadic cases of pneumonia, however, a 1:256 or higher titer does not necessarily indicate recent infection because such high titers can persist in healthy persons with no current clinical evidence of legionellosis. As a practical matter it is unlikely that the follow-up required to demonstrate seroconversion will happen in most sporadic cases.

Molecular Diagnosis

Given the necessity for laboratory confirmation of the diagnosis of legionnaires' disease and the inadequacy of traditional diagnostic methods, it is not surprising that molecular diagnosis has been much anticipated. As of yet this potential is unrealized, but development work continues. An early attempt to use DNA probes for clinical diagnosis was discontinued because of problems with sensitivity and specificity. Amplification methods have been successfully used to detect legionellae in environmental samples, and the commercially available method has been successfully applied to clinical specimens,[154] but the method has not been cleared by the Food and Drug Administration for human specimens. More recently, attention has been focused on the development of real- time amplification assays (RT-PCR)for use with clinical specimens.[117,119,73] These assays are still developmental, but hold promise for a rapid diagnostic tool. An indication of the developmental nature of amplification assays is the report that a commonly used commercial kit for extraction of DNA is not suitable for detection of *Legionella* spp. in clinical samples.[147]

Environmental Microbiology Studies
Isolation of *Legionella* From Environmental Samples

The widespread presence of *Legionella* spp. in both natural and man-made waters, in the absence of patients with clinical illness, has been observed repeatedly and argues against routine microbiologic culture of water. On the other hand, considerable evidence has accumulated that cites potable water as the source of the organism in many patients who have had infection with *L. pneumophila.* Institutional hot water has been implicated frequently in legionellosis; however, more studies are needed on the magnitude of *Legionella* contamination in home potable water and hot water systems and the frequency of association with legionellosis.[42] For instance, factors that increase the likelihood that *Legionella* spp. will colonize home water systems were defined, but these factors did not appear to increase the incidence of legionellosis acquired in the community. Given the high probability that large numbers of healthy persons are frequently exposed to these organisms in nature, in homes, in the workplace, and in private and public buildings of all sorts, it appears that many legionellae in natural and municipal waters are either not highly virulent, that exposure to the organism is minimal in extent, or that most persons are not susceptible hosts; or perhaps all are true. Thus, microbiologic enumeration of *Legionella* species in potable or other waters (such as cooling towers) has no clinical or epidemiologic relevance to disease in humans unless cases are documented clinically. Unfortunately, there are not sufficiently adequate markers of virulence to distinguish environmental isolates that are "pathogenic" from those that are unlikely to be pathogens, nor are there appropriate tests that predict in which human hosts legionellosis will develop versus who will be resistant when exposed to *Legionella* in the environment. Furthermore, the degree and extent of exposure to the organism cannot be measured accurately. Therefore, microbiologic surveillance of environmental waters is especially difficult to interpret in the absence of cases of the disease (and even in the presence of documented cases as well). On the other hand, the clinical and epidemiologic surveillance of patients (e.g., by hospital infection control nurses) is recommended as part of a program to prevent nosocomial legionellosis.

In outbreaks of nosocomial legionellosis, hyperchlorination of the hospital water to a level between 2 and 6 mg/L of free residual chlorine and raising the temperature of the hot water to more than 70°C or a combination of hyperchlorination and heat flushing are methods that have proven effective for suppressing the growth of *Legionella.*[109,132,134] To accomplish heat flushing or thermal eradication, the hot water is circulated throughout the building water system at a temperature of 70⁻75°C. All shower heads and faucets are flushed with hot water with the objective to kill the *Legionella* in these sites. Protocols for hyperchlorination and thermal eradication have been published elsewhere.[109,132,134] Unfortunately, there is a risk of scalding from the hot water, and precautions should be taken to minimize this possibility (e.g., warning signs, heating the water for relatively short periods of time when most patients are asleep). (Regulations in some states require that the water temperature in hospitals be less than 120°F [48.9°C] to prevent scalding of patients.) Continuous chlorination (i.e., to achieve 1.5 part per million free residual chlorine levels) may be unduly corrosive and destructive for some plumbing systems and equipment; there is also a potential risk of toxic exposure to trihalomethane. If the heat and/or chlorination treatments are not done continuously, treatment should be recurrent because recolonization of the water is highly predictable and tends to recur following cessation of either heat shock or chlorination. Other methods, including ultraviolet light sterilization, ozonation, addition of amebicidal agents, and addition of trace metal ions (e.g., silver, copper) are being investigated as alternative water system treatments.

If nosocomial cases of infection with *Legionella* are documented, a highly focused microbiologic investigation of environmental samples may be undertaken to aid in determining the most likely source of the *Legionella.* Control measures such as heat and/or chlorination may be designed in an effort to eliminate or suppress the organism, and follow-up environmental cultures may help determine the effectiveness of these measures. For hospitals with an outbreak or a hyperendemic *Legionella* problem, periodic microbiologic surveillance of the environment, combined with ongoing or repetitive control measures, should be considered unless it can be shown that no new cases of legionellosis have occurred.

The methods outlined in the protocol of Barbaree and coworkers[9] are recommended for persons who wish to isolate and identify *Legionella* species from environmental water. In this protocol, water samples (1 to 2 L) are collected and concentrated using 0.2-μm (pore size) polycarbonate filters. Viable counts are performed with and without prior acid treatment on BCYEα and medium that contains BCYEα base supplemented with glycine, polymyxin B, vancomycin, and anisomycin.

Typing of *Legionella* Isolates

Because of the widespread distribution of *L. pneumophila* serogroup 1 in the environment, serogrouping with the DFA reagents described previously has had only limited epidemiologic usefulness in investigating the source of different strains. A number of investigators have developed methods to type or subgroup strains of *L. pneumophila* serogroup 1. Analyses of subtypes within *L. pneumophila* serogroup 1 using panels of monoclonal antibodies,[84,83] genetic structural analysis of *L. pneumophila* using a multilocus enzyme electrophoresis technique,[47,130] and determination of plasmid contents[114] of different isolates from different sources have all been investigated. More recently developed techniques have included electrophoresis of *L. pneumophila* outer membrane proteins[138] and a typing method based on the use of cloned biotinylated DNA probes for analysis of restriction-fragment-length polymorphisms (RFLPs).[128] One of the more promising typing methods is random amplified polymorphic DNA (RAPD) profiling of *Legionella pneumophila* by PCR; this method appears to be faster and less costly than RFLP typing. RAPD profiling has been reported to be more discriminatory than RFLP typing of some *Legionella* isolates, and it is capable of detecting differences among isolates with identical RFLP types.[127] Investigation of an epidemic or analysis of apparently unrelated cases can be strengthened by comparison of the molecular pattern of strains isolated from patients and from the environment. Although sequencing of nucleic acid directly from specimens may prove feasible for epidemiologic studies eventually, at present isolated strains are required, emphasizing once again the importance of culture in the diagnosis of these infections. It is important to remember that demonstration of "identical" strains from patients and from an environmental site means that the environmental site is "in contention" as the source of the infections, but does not prove the association. Thorough epidemiologic analysis and consideration of all possibilities is essential. Unfortunately, some of those possible sources may not yet be apparent to anyone. The classic example of this phenomenon was the recognition that potable water was the source of infections at a Veterans Affairs Hospital after initial assumptions that cooling towers were the source proved to be unfounded.

In general, characterization of nucleic acids is more discriminatory than analysis of antigenic structure using monoclonal antibodies. Interestingly, antigenic types and genomic variants are not always concordant.[29] The ultimate test for any typing technique is discriminating strains into groups that make sense epidemiologically. The patterns must show enough differences to separate strains into related groups, but not so many that nonsensical groups of strains are discriminated. On the one hand, apparently similar strains might appear different if another typing tool was used. On the other hand, consensus agreement may be necessary to decide how many of what kind of differences actually define real-world differences with a particular technique. Whenever possible, it is optimal to analyze strains with more than one technique.

At its best, molecular or antigenic typing can rationalize an epidemic or endemic problem. Analysis of a group of clinical and environmental strains from one location over a period of years produced three clusters of strains, as summarized in Table 10-5. These strains were characterized with a panel of monoclonal antibodies, relatively nondiscriminatory reagents. Amplified-fragment-length polymorphism analysis has been used successfully by a group of European investigators.[66] The polymorphism types of *L. pneumophila* serogroup 1 have been defined and validated by proficiency testing.[65] The authors of a recent study of automated ribotyping, using reference strains, concluded that the procedure was useful for genomic analysis, but not sufficiently discrim-

inatory to be used for epidemic analysis. Clearly, more work needs to be done in this important area.

Table 10-5 Correlation of Monoclonal Antibody Patterns with Epidemiologic Analysis

MONOCLONAL ANTIBODY PATTERN	CLINICAL STRAINS	ENVIRONMENTAL STRAINS
A	Epidemic cases	Cooling tower
B	Sporadic nosocomial cases	Hospital potable water
C	Sporadic community case	–

Adapted from reference[82].

REFERENCES

1. Addiss DG, et al. Community-acquired Legionnaires' disease associated with a cooling tower: evidence for longer-distance transport of Legionella pneumophila. Am J Epidemiol 1989;130:557–568.
2. Adeleke AA, et al. Legionella drozanskii sp. nov., Legionella rowbothamii sp. nov. and Legionella fallonii sp. nov.: three unusual new Legionella species. Int J Syst Evol Microbiol 2001;51:1151–1160.
3. Alary M, Joly JR. Factors contributing to the contamination of hospital water distribution systems by legionellae. J Infect Dis 1992;165:565–569.
4. Ampel NM, et al. Cutaneous abscess caused by Legionella micdadei in an immunosuppressed patient. Ann Intern Med 1985;102:630–632.
5. Anaissie EJ, et al. The hospital water supply as a source of nosocomial infections: a plea for action. Arch Intern Med 2002;162:1483–1492.
6. Anonymous. Epidemiology, prevention and control of legionellosis: memorandum from a WHO meeting. Bull WHO 1990;68:155–164.
7. Arnow PM, et al. Perirectal abscess caused by Legionella pneumophila and mixed anaerobic bacteria. Ann Intern Med 1983;98:184–185.
8. Arnow PM, et al. Nosocomial Legionnaires' disease caused by aerosolized tap water from respiratory devices. J Infect Dis 1982;146:460–467.
9. Barbaree JM, et al. Protocol for sampling environmental sites for legionellae. Appl Environ Microbiol 1987;53:1454–1458.
10. Bassetti S, Widmer AF. Legionella resources on the world wide web. Clin Infect Dis 2002;34:1633–1640.
11. Benin AL, et al. An outbreak of travel-associated Legionnaires disease and Pontiac fever: the need for enhanced surveillance of travel-associated legionellosis in the United States. J Infect Dis 2002;185:237–243.
12. Bentz JS, et al. Acid-fast-positive Legionella pneumophila: a possible pitfall in the cytologic diagnosis of mycobacterial infection in pulmonary specimens. Diagn Cytopathol 2000;22:45–48.
13. Bhopal RS. A framework for investigating geographical variation in diseases, based on a study of Legionnaires' disease. J Public Health Med 1991;13:281–289.
14. Bhopal RS, et al. Pinpointing clusters of apparently sporadic cases of Legionnaires' disease. BMJ 1992;304:1022–1027.
15. Blatt SP, et al. Nosocomial Legionnaires' disease: aspiration as a primary mode of disease acquisition. Am J Med 1993;95:16–22.
16. Bochud PY, et al. Community-acquired pneumonia: a prospective outpatient study. Medicine (Baltimore) 2001;80:75–87.
17. Bornstein N, et al. Exposure to Legionellaceae at a hot spring spa: a prospective clinical and serological study. Epidemiol Infect 1989;102:31–36.
18. Boswell TC, Kudesia G. Serological cross-reaction between Legionella pneumophila and campylobacter in the indirect fluorescent antibody test. Epidemiol Infect 1992;109:291–295.
19. Breiman RF, et al. Association of shower use with Legionnaires' disease: possible role of amoebae. JAMA 1990;263:2924–2926.
20. Brenner DJ, et al. Classification of the legionnaires' disease bacterium: Legionella pneumophila, genus novum, species nova, of the family Legionellaceae, familia nova. Ann Intern Med 1979;90:656–658.
21. Bridge JA, Edelstein PH. Oropharyngeal colonization with Legionella pneumophila. J Clin Microbiol 1983;18:1108–1112.
22. Broome CV. Epidemiologic assessment of methods of transmission of legionellosis. Zentralbl Bakteriol Mikrobiol Hyg [A] 1983;255:52–57.
23. Broome CV, Fraser DW. Epidemiologic aspects of legionellosis. Epidemiol Rev 1979;1:1–16.
24. Buesching WJ, et al. Enhanced primary isolation of Legionella pneumophila from clinical specimens by low-pH treatment. J Clin Microbiol 1983;17:1153–1155.
25. Castellani PM, et al. Legionnaires' disease on a cruise ship linked to the water supply system: clinical and public health implications. Clin Infect Dis 1999;28:33–38.
26. Chastre J, et al. Pulmonary fibrosis following pneumonia due to acute Legionnaires' disease: clinical, ultrastructural, and immunofluorescent study. Chest 1987;91:57–62.
27. Cherry WB, et al. Detection of Legionnaires disease bacteria by direct immunofluorescent staining. J Clin Microbiol 1978;8:329–338.
28. Codony F, et al. Factors promoting colonization by legionellae in residential

water distribution systems: an environmental case-control survey. Eur J Clin Microbiol Infect Dis 2002;21:717–721.

29. Cordevant C, et al. Characterization of members of the legionellaceae family by automated ribotyping. J Clin Microbiol 2003;41:34–43.

30. Den Boer JW, et al. A large outbreak of Legionnaires' disease at a flower show, the Netherlands, 1999. Emerg Infect Dis 2002;8:37–43.

31. Dondero TJ, Jr., et al. An outbreak of Legionnaires' disease associated with a contaminated air-conditioning cooling tower. N Engl J Med 1980;302:365–370.

32. Dorman SA, et al. Pyelonephritis associated with *Legionella pneumophila,* serogroup 4. Ann Intern Med 1980;93:835–837.

33. Dowling JN, et al. Infections caused by *Legionella micdadei* and *Legionella pneumophila* among renal transplant recipients. J Infect Dis 1984;149:703–713.

34. Drozanski W. *Sarcobium lyticum* gen. nov., sp. nov., an obligate intracellular bacterial parasite of small, free-living amoebae. Int J Syst Bacteriol 1991;41:82–87.

35. Dumoff M. Direct in-vitro isolation of the legionnaires' disease bacterium in two fatal cases: cultural and staining characteristics. Ann Intern Med 1979;90:694–696.

36. Edelstein PH. Legionnaires' disease. Arthritis Rheum 1979;22:806–806.

37. Edelstein PH. Improved semiselective medium for isolation of *Legionella pneumophila* from contaminated clinical and environmental specimens. J Clin Microbiol 1981;14:298–303.

38. Edelstein PH. Comparative study of selective media for isolation of *Legionella pneumophila* from potable water. J Clin Microbiol 1982;16:697–699.

39. Edelstein PH. Laboratory diagnosis of infections caused by legionellae. Eur J Clin Microbiol 1987;6:4–10.

40. Edelstein PH. The laboratory diagnosis of Legionnaires' disease. Semin Respir Infect 1987;2:235–241.

41. Edelstein PH. Legionnaires' disease. Clin Infect Dis 1993;16:741–747.

42. Edelstein PH. Legionnaires' disease. N Engl J Med 1998;338:200–201.

43. Edelstein PH, et al. Clinical utility of a monoclonal direct fluorescent reagent specific for *Legionella pneumophila*: comparative study with other reagents. J Clin Microbiol 1985;22:419–421.

44. Edelstein PH, et al. Retrospective study of Gen-Probe rapid diagnostic system for detection of legionellae in frozen clinical respiratory tract samples. J Clin Microbiol 1987;25:1022–1026.

45. Edelstein PH, et al. Isolation of *Legionella pneumophila* from blood. Lancet 1979;1:750–751.

46. Edelstein PH, et al. Laboratory diagnosis of Legionnaires disease. Am Rev Respir Dis 1980;121:317–327.

47. Edelstein PH, et al. Paleoepidemiologic investigation of legionnaires' disease at Wadsworth Veterans Administration Hospital by using three typing methods for comparison of legionellae from clinical and environmental sources. J Clin Microbiol 1986;23:1121–1126.

48. Edelstein PH, et al. Enhancement of recovery of *Legionella pneumophila* from contaminated respiratory tract specimens by heat. J Clin Microbiol 1982;16:1061–1065.

49. Engleberg NC. Genetic studies of *Legionella* pathogenesis. In Barbaree JM, Breiman RF, Dufour AP (eds): Legionella: Current Status and Emerging Perspectives Washington, D.C., American Society for Microbiology, 63–68, 1993.

50. Ezzeddine H, et al. *Legionella* spp. in a hospital hot water system: effect of control measures. J Hosp Infect 1989;13:121–131.

51. Fairbank JT, et al. Legionnaires' disease. J Thorac Imaging 1991;6:6–13.

52. Fallon RJ, Rowbotham TJ. Microbiological investigations into an outbreak of Pontiac fever due to *Legionella micdadei* associated with use of a whirlpool. J Clin Pathol 1990;43:479–483.

53. Fang GD, et al. New and emerging etiologies for community-acquired pneumonia with implications for therapy: a prospective multicenter study of 359 cases. Medicine (Baltimore) 1990;69:307–316.

54. Fang GD, et al. Disease due to the *Legionellaceae* (other than *Legionella pneumophila*): historical, microbiological, clinical, and epidemiological review. Medicine (Baltimore) 1989;68:116–132.

55. Feeley JC, et al. Charcoal-yeast extract agar: primary isolation medium for *Legionella pneumophila*. J Clin Microbiol 1979;10:437–441.

56. Fenstersheib MD, et al. Outbreak of Pontiac fever due to *Legionella anisa*. Lancet 1990;336:35–37.

57. Fields BS. *Legionella* and protozoa: Interaction of a pathogen and its natural host. In Barbaree JM, Breiman RF, Dufour AP (eds): Legionella: Current Status and Emerging Perspectives Washington, D.C., American Society for Microbiology, 129–136, 1993.

58. Fields BS, et al. *Legionella* and Legionnaires' disease: 25 years of investigation. Clin Microbiol Rev 2002;15:506–526.

59. Fields BS, et al. Attachment and entry of *Legionella pneumophila* in Hartmannella vermiformis. J Infect Dis 1993;167:1146–1150.

60. Fields BS, et al. Pontiac fever due to *Legionella micdadei* from a whirlpool spa: possible role of bacterial endotoxin. J Infect Dis 2001;184:1289–1292.

61. Fliermans CB, et al. Ecological distribution of *Legionella pneumophila*. Appl Environ Microbiol 1981;41:9–16.

62. Fraser DW, Mcdade JE. Legionellosis. Sci Am 1979;241:82–99.

63. Fraser DW, et al. Legionnaires' disease: description of an epidemic of pneumonia. N Engl J Med 1977;297:1189–1197.

64. Friedman H, et al. *Legionella pneumophila* pathogenesis and immunity. Semin Pediatr Infect Dis 2002;13:273–279.

65. Fry NK, et al. Designation of the European Working Group on *Legionella* Infection (EWGLI) amplified fragment length polymorphism types of *Legionella pneumophila* serogroup 1 and results of intercentre proficiency testing using a standard protocol. Eur J Clin Microbiol Infect Dis 2002;21:722–728.

66. Fry NK, et al. Assessment of intercentre reproducibility and epidemiological concordance of *Legionella pneumophila* serogroup 1 genotyping by amplified fragment length polymorphism analysis. Eur J Clin Microbiol Infect Dis 2000;19:773–780.

67. Garbe PL, et al. Nosocomial Legionnaires' disease: epidemiologic demonstration of cooling towers as a source. JAMA 1985;254:521–524.

68. Girod JC, et al. Pneumonic and nonpneumonic forms of legionellosis: the result of a common-source exposure to *Legionella pneumophila*. Arch Intern Med 1982;142:545–547.

69. Glick TH, et al. Pontiac fever. An epidemic of unknown etiology in a health department: I. Clinical and epidemiologic aspects. Am J Epidemiol 1978;107:149–160.

70. Goetz AM, et al. Nosocomial legionnaires' disease discovered in community hospitals following cultures of the water system: seek and ye shall find. Am J Infect Control 1998;26:8–11.

71. Goldberg DJ, et al. Lochgoilhead fever: outbreak of non-pneumonic legionellosis due to *Legionella micdadei*. Lancet 1989;1:316–318.

72. Gray JJ, et al. Serological cross-reaction between *Legionella pneumophila* and *Citrobacter freundii* in indirect immunofluorescence and rapid microagglutination tests. J Clin Microbiol 1991;29:200–201.

73. Hayden RT, et al. Direct detection of *Legionella* species from bronchoalveolar lavage and open lung biopsy specimens: comparison of LightCycler PCR, in situ hybridization, direct fluorescence antigen detection, and culture. J Clin Microbiol 2001;39:2618–2626.

74. Heath CH, et al. Delay in appropriate therapy of *Legionella* pneumonia associated with increased mortality. Eur J Clin Microbiol Infect Dis 1996;15:286–290.

75. Helms CM, et al. Pretibial rash in *Legionella pneumophila* pneumonia. JAMA 1981;245:1758–1759.

76. Hlady WG, et al. Outbreak of Legionnaire's disease linked to a decorative fountain by molecular epidemiology. Am J Epidemiol 1993;138:555–562.

77. Hoffman PS, et al. Production of superoxide and hydrogen peroxide in medium used to culture *Legionella pneumophila*: catalytic decomposition by charcoal. Appl Environ Microbiol 1983;45:784–791.

78. Hookey JV, et al. Phylogeny of *Legionellaceae* based on small-subunit ribosomal DNA sequences and proposal of *Legionella lytica* comb. nov. for Legionella-like amoebal pathogens. Int J Syst Bacteriol 1996;46:526–531.

79. Horwitz MA. Toward an understanding of host and bacterial molecules mediating *Legionella pneumophila* pathogenesis. In Barbaree JM, Breiman RF, Dufour AP (eds): Legionella: Current Status and Emerging Perspectives Washington, D.C., American Society for Microbiology, 55–62, 1993.

80. Jernigan DB, et al. Outbreak of Legionnaires' disease among cruise ship passengers exposed to a contaminated whirlpool spa. Lancet 1996;347:494–499.

81. Johnson JD, et al. Neurologic manifestations of Legionnaires' disease. Medicine (Baltimore) 1984;63:303–310.

82. Joly JR, et al. Legionnaires' disease caused by *Legionella dumoffii* in distilled water. Can Med Assoc J 1986;135:1274–1277.

83. Joly JR, et al: Development of a standardized subgrouping scheme for *Legionella pneumophila* serogroup 1 using monoclonal antibodies. J Clin Microbiol 1986;23:768–771.

84. Joly JR, Winn WR. Correlation of subtypes of *Legionella pneumophila* defined by monoclonal antibodies with epidemiological classification of cases and environmental sources. J Infect Dis 1984;150:667–671.

85. Joseph C, et al. An international investigation of an outbreak of Legionnaires disease among UK and French tourists. Eur J Epidemiol 1996;12:215–219.

86. Kalweit WH, et al. Hemodialysis fistula infections caused by *Legionella pneumophila*. Ann Intern Med 1982;96:173–175.

87. King CH, et al. Survival of coliforms and bacterial pathogens within protozoa during chlorination. Appl Environ Microbiol 1988;54:3023–3033.

88. Kirby BD, et al. Legionnaires' disease: report of sixty-five nosocomially acquired cases of review of the literature. Medicine (Baltimore) 1980;59:188–205.

89. Knirsch CA, et al. An outbreak of *Legionella micdadei* pneumonia in transplant patients: evaluation, molecular epidemiology, and control. Am J Med 2000;108:290–295.

90. Kohler RB, et al. Cross-reactive urinary antigens among patients infected with *Legionella pneumophila* serogroups 1 and 4 and the Leiden 1 strain. J Infect Dis 1985;152:1007–1012.

91. Kohler RB, et al. Onset and duration of urinary antigen excretion in Legionnaires disease. J Clin Microbiol 1984;20:605–607.

92. Kohler RB, et al. Rapid radioimmunoassay diagnosis of Legionnaires' disease:

detection and partial characterization of urinary antigen. Ann Intern Med 1981; 94:601–605.

93. Korvick JA, Yu VL. Legionnaires' disease: an emerging surgical problem. Ann Thorac Surg 1987;43:341–347.

94. Lee TC, et al. Factors predisposing to *Legionella pneumophila* colonization in residential water systems. Arch Environ Health 1988;43:59–62.

95. Lowry PW, et al. A cluster of *Legionella* sternal-wound infections due to postoperative topical exposure to contaminated tap water. N Engl J Med 1991;324: 109–113.

96. Luck PC, et al. Nosocomial pneumonia caused by three genetically different strains of *Legionella pneumophila* and detection of these strains in the hospital water supply. J Clin Microbiol 1998;36:1160–1163.

97. Mahoney FJ, et al. Communitywide outbreak of Legionnaires' disease associated with a grocery store mist machine. J Infect Dis 1992;165:736–739.

98. Marrie TJ. Diagnosis of *Legionellaceae* as a cause of community-acquired pneumonia- ''. . . continue to treat first and not bother to ask questions later''—not a good idea. Am J Med 2001;110:73–75.

99. Marrie TJ, et al. Colonisation of the respiratory tract with *Legionella pneumophila* for 63 days before the onset of pneumonia. J Infect 1992;24:81–86.

100. Marrie TJ, et al. Control of endemic nosocomial legionnaires' disease by using sterile potable water for high risk patients. Epidemiol Infect 1991;107:591–605.

101. Mastro TD, et al. Nosocomial Legionnaires' disease and use of medication nebulizers. J Infect Dis 1991;163:667–671.

102. Mayock R, et al. *Legionella pneumophila* pericarditis proved by culture of pericardial fluid. Am J Med 1983;75:534–536.

103. McCabe RE, et al. Prosthetic valve endocarditis caused by *Legionella pneumophila*. Ann Intern Med 1984;100:525–527.

104. McDade JE, et al. Legionnaires' disease: isolation of a bacterium and demonstration of its role in other respiratory disease. N Engl J Med 1977;297:1197–1203.

105. Morris GK, et al. Isolation of the legionnaires' disease bacterium from environmental samples. Ann Intern Med 1979;90:664–666.

106. Muder RR, et al. Pneumonia caused by Pittsburgh pneumonia agent: radiologic manifestations. Radiology 1984;150:633–637.

107. Muder RR, Yu VL. Infection due to *Legionella* species other than *L. pneumophila*. Clin Infect Dis 2002;35:990–998.

108. Muder RR, et al. Mode of transmission of *Legionella pneumophila*: a critical review. Arch Intern Med 1986;146:1607–1612.

109. Muraca PW, et al. Disinfection of water distribution systems for *Legionella*: a review of application procedures and methodologies. Infect Control Hosp Epidemiol 1990;11:79–88.

110. Murdoch DR. Diagnosis of *Legionella* infection. Clin Infect Dis 2003;36:64–69.

111. Myerowitz RL, et al. Opportunistic lung infection due to ''Pittsburgh Pneumonia Agent.'' N Engl J Med 1979;301:953–958.

112. Nagai T, et al. Neonatal sudden death due to *Legionella* pneumonia associated with water birth in a domestic spa bath. J Clin Microbiol 2003;41:2227–2229.

113. Newsome AL, et al. Interactions between *Naegleria fowleri* and *Legionella pneumophila*. Infect Immun 1985;50:449–452.

114. Nolte FS, et al. Plasmids as epidemiological markers in nosocomial Legionnaires' disease. J Infect Dis 1984;149:251–256.

115. Ortiz-Roque CM, Hazen TC. Abundance and distribution of *Legionellaceae* in Puerto Rican waters. Appl Environ Microbiol 1987;53:2231–2236.

116. Patel R, Paya CV. Infections in solid-organ transplant recipients. Clin Microbiol Rev 1997;10:86–124.

117. Raggam RB, et al. Qualitative detection of *Legionella* species in bronchoalveolar lavages and induced sputa by automated DNA extraction and real-time polymerase chain reaction. Med Microbiol Immunol (Berl) 2002;191:119–125.

118. Reingold AL, et al. *Legionella* pneumonia in the United States: the distribution of serogroups and species causing human illness. J Infect Dis 1984;149:819–819.

119. Reischl U, et al. Direct detection and differentiation of *Legionella* spp. and *Legionella pneumophila* in clinical specimens by dual-color real-time PCR and melting curve analysis. J Clin Microbiol 2002;40:3814–3817.

120. Riffard S, et al. Occurrence of *Legionella* in groundwater: an ecological study. Water Sci Technol 2001;43:99–102.

121. Rihs JD, et al. Isolation of *Legionella pneumophila* from blood with the BACTEC system: a prospective study yielding positive results. J Clin Microbiol 1985; 22:422–424.

122. Roig J, et al. Comparative study of *Legionella pneumophila* and other nosocomial- acquired pneumonias. Chest 1991;99:344–350.

123. Rosmini F, et al. Febrile illness in successive cohorts of tourists at a hotel on the Italian Adriatic coast: evidence for a persistent focus of *Legionella* infection. Am J Epidemiol 1984;119:124–134.

124. Rowbotham TJ. Preliminary report on the pathogenicity of *Legionella pneumophila* for freshwater and soil amoebae. J Clin Pathol 1980;33:1179–1183.

125. Rowbotham TJ. Isolation of *Legionella pneumophila* from clinical specimens via amoebae, and the interaction of those and other isolates with amoebae. J Clin Pathol 1983;36:978–986.

126. Ruf B, et al. Prevalence and diagnosis of *Legionella* pneumonia: a 3-year prospective study with emphasis on application of urinary antigen detection. J Infect Dis 1990;162:1341–1348.

127. Sandery M, et al. Random amplified polymorphic DNA (RAPD) profiling of *Legionella pneumophila*. Lett Appl Microbiol 1994;19:184–187.

128. Saunders NA, et al. A method for typing strains of *Legionella pneumophila* serogroup 1 by analysis of restriction fragment length polymorphisms. J Med Microbiol 1990;31:45–55.

129. Sax H, et al. Legionnaires' disease in a renal transplant recipient: nosocomial or home-grown? Transplantation 2002;74:890–892.

130. Selander RK, et al. Genetic structure of populations of *Legionella pneumophila*. J Bacteriol 1985;163:1021–1037.

131. Shands KN, et al. Potable water as a source of Legionnaires' disease. JAMA 1985;253:1412–1416.

132. Snyder MB, et al. Reduction in *Legionella pneumophila* through heat flushing followed by continuous supplemental chlorination of hospital hot water. J Infect Dis 1990;162:127–132.

133. Sopena N, et al. Factors related to persistence of *Legionella* urinary antigen excretion in patients with legionnaires' disease. Eur J Clin Microbiol Infect Dis 2002;21:845–848.

134. States SJ, et al. Chlorine, pH, and control of *Legionella* in hospital plumbing systems. JAMA 1989;261:1882–1883.

135. States SJ, et al. Survival and multiplication of *Legionella pneumophila* in municipal drinking water systems. Appl Environ Microbiol 1987;53:979–986.

136. Steele TW, et al. Isolation of *Legionella longbeachae* serogroup 1 from potting mixes. Appl Environ Microbiol 1990;56:49–53.

137. Steele TW, et al. Distribution of *Legionella longbeachae* serogroup 1 and other legionellae in potting soils in Australia. Appl Environ Microbiol 1990;56: 2984–2988.

138. Stout JE, et al. Comparison of molecular methods for subtyping patients and epidemiologically linked environmental isolates of *Legionella pneumophila*. J Infect Dis 1988;157:486–495.

139. Stout JE, Yu VL. Legionellosis. N Engl J Med 1997;337:682–687.

140. Stout JE, et al. Potable water as a cause of sporadic cases of community-acquired legionnaires' disease. N Engl J Med 1992;326:151–155.

141. Swanson MS, Hammer BK. *Legionella pneumophila* pathogenesis: a fateful journey from amoebae to macrophages. Annu Rev Microbiol 2000;54:567–613.

142. Tan MJ, et al. The radiologic manifestations of Legionnaire's disease:. the Ohio Community-Based Pneumonia Incidence Study Group. Chest 2000;117: 398–403.

143. Thacker WL, et al. Comparison of slide agglutination test and direct immunofluorescence assay for identification of *Legionella* isolates. J Clin Microbiol 1983; 18:1113–1118.

144. Thornsberry C, et al. In vitro activity of antimicrobial agents on Legionnaires disease bacterium. Antimicrob Agents Chemother 1978;13:78–80.

145. Tompkins LS, et al. *Legionella* prosthetic-valve endocarditis. N Engl J Med 1988;318:530–535.

146. Tsai TF, et al. Legionnaires' disease: clinical features of the epidemic in Philadelphia. Ann Intern Med 1979;90:509–517.

147. van Der ZA, et al. Qiagen DNA extraction kits for sample preparation for legionella PCR are not suitable for diagnostic purposes. J Clin Microbiol 2002;40: 1126.

148. Van Orden AE, Greer PW. Modification of the Dieterle spirochete stain. Histotechnology 1977;1:51–53.

149. Vickers RM, et al. Failure of a diagnostic monoclonal immunofluorescent reagent to detect *Legionella pneumophila* in environmental samples. Appl Environ Microbiol 1990;56:2912–2914.

150. Wadowsky RM, et al. Growth-supporting activity for *Legionella pneumophila* in tap water cultures and implication of hartmannellid amoebae as growth factors. Appl Environ Microbiol 1988;54:2677–2682.

151. Wadowsky RM, et al. Effect of temperature, pH, and oxygen level on the multiplication of naturally occurring *Legionella pneumophila* in potable water. Appl Environ Microbiol 1985;49:1197–1205.

152. Wadowsky RM, et al. Hot water systems as sources of *Legionella pneumophila* in hospital and nonhospital plumbing fixtures. Appl Environ Microbiol 1982; 43:1104–1110.

153. Waterer GW, et al. *Legionella* and community-acquired pneumonia: a review of current diagnostic tests from a clinician's viewpoint. Am J Med 2001;110: 41–48.

154. Weir SC, et al. Detection of *Legionella* by PCR in respiratory specimens using a commercially available kit. Am J Clin Pathol 1998;110:295–300.

155. White HJ, et al. Extrapulmonary histopathologic manifestations of Legionnaires' disease: evidence for myocarditis and bacteremia. Arch Pathol Lab Med 1980; 104:287–289.

156. Wilkinson HW. Hospital-Laboratory Diagnosis of *Legionella* Infections. 2nd ed. Centers for Disease Control, Atlanta, GA, 1988.

157. Wilkinson HW, et al. Validation of *Legionella pneumophila* indirect immunofluorescence assay with epidemic sera. J Clin Microbiol 1981;13:139–146.

158. Wilkinson HW, et al. Measure of immunoglobulin G-, M-, and A-specific titers

against *Legionella pneumophila* and inhibition of titers against nonspecific, gram-negative bacterial antigens in the indirect immunofluorescence test for legionellosis. J Clin Microbiol 1979;10:685–689.

159. Wilkinson HW, et al. Reactivity of serum from patients with suspected legionellosis against 29 antigens of *Legionellaceae* and *Legionella*-like organisms by indirect immunofluorescence assay. J Infect Dis 1983;147:23–31.

160. Winn WC, Jr. Legionnaires disease: historical perspective. Clin Microbiol Rev 1988;1:60–81.

161. Winn WC, Jr., Myerowitz RL. The pathology of the *Legionella* pneumonias: a review of 74 cases and the literature. Hum Pathol 1981;12:401–422.

162. Winn WC, Jr: *Legionella*. In Garrity GM (ed). Bergey's Manual of Systematic Bacteriology. 2nd Ed. Baltimore: Williams & Wilkins, 2005.

163. Yu VL, et al. Distribution of *Legionella* species and serogroups isolated by culture in patients with sporadic community-acquired legionellosis: an international collaborative survey. J Infect Dis 2002;186:127–128.

164. Zimmerman SE, et al. Immunoglobulin M antibody titers in the diagnosis of Legionnaires disease. J Clin Microbiol 1982;16:1007–1011.

165. Zuravleff JJ, et al. Diagnosis of Legionnaires' disease. An update of laboratory methods with new emphasis on isolation by culture. JAMA 1983;250:1981–1985.

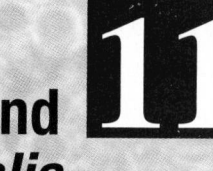
Neisseria Species and *Moraxella catarrhalis*

Taxonomy of the Family *Neisseriaceae* and the Family *Moraxellaceae*

General Characteristics of the Genus *Neisseria*

Clinical Significance of *Neisseria* Species

Neisseria gonorrhoeae

Epidemiology
Infections Caused by
N. gonorrhoeae

Neisseria meningitidis

Epidemiology
Infections Caused by
N. meningitidis
Meningococcal Prophylaxis and
Meningococcal Vaccines

Other *Neisseria* Species

Clinical Significance of *Moraxella catarrhalis*

Isolation of *Neisseria* Species

Neisseria gonorrhoeae

Direct Gram-Stained Smears
Specimen Collection
Specimen Transport
Selective Culture Media:
Inoculation and Incubation

Neisseria meningitidis

Laboratory Safety
Direct Gram-Stained Smears and
Direct Capsular Antigen Tests

Specimen Collection and
Transport
Isolation and Incubation

Identification of *Neisseria* Species

Colony Morphology
Gram Stain and Oxidase Test
Superoxol Test
Differentiation of Other
Organisms on Selective Media
Presumptive Criteria for
Identification of
N. gonorrhoeae
Identification Tests for *Neisseria*
Species
Carbohydrate-Utilization Tests

Conventional CTA Carbohydrates
Rapid Carbohydrate-Utilization
Test
RIM-Neisseria Test (Rapid
Identification Method-Neisseria)
Other Carbohydrate-Utilization
Methods

Chromogenic Enzyme Substrate
Tests

Gonochek II
BactiCard *Neisseria*

Immunologic Methods for
Culture Confirmation of
N. gonorrhoeae

Direct Fluorescent Monoclonal
Antibody Test
Coagglutination Tests
GonoGen II Test

Multitest Identification Systems
DNA Probe Test for Culture Confirmation of
 N. gonorrhoeae
Nucleic Acid Hybridization and Amplification Tests
 for *N. gonorrhoeae*
Molecular Methods for Detection of
 N. meningitidis

Cultural Characteristics of *Neisseria* Species

Neisseria gonorrhoeae
Neisseria meningitidis
Other *Neisseria* Species

 Neisseria lactamica
 Neisseria cinerea
 Neisseria flavescens

Neisseria subflava Biovars, *Neisseria mucosa*, and
 Neisseria sicca
Neisseria polysaccharea
Neisseria elongata Subspecies
Neisseria gonorrhoeae Subspecies *kochii* ("*Neisseria kochii*")
Atypical and Non-Human *Neisseria* Species

Cultural Characteristics and Identification of *Moraxella catarrhalis*

Antimicrobial Susceptibility of *Neisseria* Species

Neisseria gonorrhoeae
Neisseria meningitidis

Antimicrobial Susceptibility of *Moraxella catarrhalis*

Gonorrhea was recognized at least as early as the time of Galen (second century A.D.), who named the disease after the Greek words *gonor* ("seed") and *rhoia* ("flow"), suggesting that the disease was related to the flow of semen. References to this infection are also found in the Old Testament and in written histories of several cultures. Although well recognized as a sexually transmitted infection by the 13th century, gonorrhea was not distinguished from syphilis until the mid-19th century. In 1897, *Neisseria gonorrhoeae,* the etiologic agent of gonorrhea, was first observed in purulent exudates from the genital tract and conjunctiva by Albert Neisser at the University of Breslau in Germany. Subsequent isolation of the organism, inoculation into human volunteers, and reisolation of the organism by Bumm in 1885 proved the causal relationship between the organism and the disease (see Koch's postulates, Chapter 5).

Epidemic cerebrospinal meningitis was known early in the 19th century, but the etiologic agent was not described until 1884, when Marchiofava and Celli observed the organism in meningeal exudates. In 1887, Weichselbaum isolated the organism, now called *Neisseria meningitidis,* in pure culture and first described its characteristics and etiologic role in six patients with acute meningitis. Additional work by Kiefer in 1896 and Albrecht in 1901 established the existence of the meningococcal carrier state in healthy individuals.[97]

Over the period from 1929 through 1943, large outbreaks of meningococcal disease in Chile and U.S. cities (e.g., Detroit and Milwaukee) focused scientific attention on this organism. With subsequent outbreaks among military recruits in the U.S. and abroad, a better understanding of the epidemiology, pathogenesis, chemoprophylaxis, and prospects for vaccine development began to emerge.[680] During the late 1930s, sulfonamide agents were found to eradicate the meningococcal carrier state, thereby providing a means for prevention of disease spread. During the early 1960s, resistance to sulfonamides began to emerge among meningococci, along with the appearance of epidemic disease at two military installations in California. These outbreaks stimulated the development of effective polysaccharide vaccines against both serogroup A and C meningococci. At present, epidemic serogroup A *N. meningitidis* meningitis remains a serious problem in regions of Africa, and meningococcal disease is still seen among semiclosed military populations.[27,427,611] Epidemics of meningococcal disease have recently occurred in Norway, Canada, and the countries of the former Soviet Union, and disease associated with *N. meningitidis* serogroup W-135 has recently emerged in Saudi Arabia.[215,513,606] In both the U.S. and Europe, serogroup C meningococcal disease has increased in the community and on college and university campuses, resulting in marked increases in disease incidence among adolescents and young adults.[222,287,290,535] Molecular techniques have enabled researchers to examine possible meningococcal virulence factors and to understand the "molecular epidemiology" of meningococcal serogroups, serotypes, subserotypes, and clonal virulence.[427,513,535,611]

N. gonorrhoeae and *N. meningitidis* continue to be formidable and versatile pathogens that provide a challenge for both clinicians and clinical laboratorians. Although methods for isolation and identification of *Neisseria* species from clinical specimens have not changed significantly, new nucleic acid probe- and nucleic acid amplification-based techniques for direct detection of *N. gonorrhoeae* have greatly modified laboratory approaches to the diagnosis of gonococcal disease. The development of resistance to antimicrobial agents continues to be a major concern in the new millennium, particularly with the appearance of fluoroquinolone resistance among gonococci worldwide.[354] *N. meningitidis* has assumed additional prominence in recent years with the licensure of vaccines for other agents of meningitis (e.g., *Haemophilus influenzae* type b). Recognition, treatment, and management of meningococcal disease in a community require the cooperation of clinicians, clinical laboratories, and epidemiologists in order to formulate the most appropriate interventions. Like the gonococcus, rare *N. meningitidis* strains have acquired the genetic information to produce β-lactamase, while others have developed "decreased susceptibility" to some β-lactam agents because of acquisition of altered penicillin binding proteins.[189,482] On occasion, the recovery of "nonpathogenic" and newly recognized *Neisseria* species from immunocompromised patients must also be considered by the microbiologist in formulating an approach to the detection and identification of *Neisseria* species and "neisseria-like" bacteria in clinical specimens.

Taxonomy of the Family Neisseriaceae *and the* Family Moraxellaceae

In the 1984 edition of *Bergey's Manual of Systematic Bacteriology*, the family *Neisseriaceae* included four genera: *Neisseria, Moraxella, Kingella,* and *Acinetobacter.*[87] At that time, the genus *Neisseria* consisted of 11 species that were considered as "true neisseriae" and three animal species, collectively called the "false neisseriae" (*N. caviae, N. ovis,* and *N. cuniculi*), that were considered to be *species incertae sedis.*[691] The genus *Moraxella* was subdivided into two subgenera: the subgenus *Moraxella* and the subgenus *Branhamella.*[86] Six species—*M. (M.) lacunata, M. (M.) bovis, M. (M.) nonliquefaciens, M. (M.) atlantae, M. (M.) phenylpyruvica,* and *M. (M.) osloensis*—were placed into the genus *Moraxella* subgenus *Moraxella,* and four species—*M. (B.) catarrhalis, M. (B.) caviae, M. (B.) ovis,* and *M. (B.) cuniculi*—were placed in the subgenus *Branhamella.*[86,87] "*Moraxella urethralis*" was considered an organism of uncertain affiliation at that time. The family also included three *Kingella* species (*K. kingae, K. denitrificans,* and *K. indologenes*) and *Acinetobacter* phenotypic groups.[87] *Psychrobacter immobilis* was added to the family *Neisseriaceae* in 1986.[334]

In 1988, using several molecular techniques new to bacterial taxonomy, Stackebrandt and associates described the *Proteobacteria* and its phylogenetic RNA subgroups.[617] Application of molecular techniques (e.g., DNA-ribosomal RNA [rRNA] hybridization, DNA-DNA hybridization, 16S rRNA sequence analysis) resulted in several proposed changes in the taxonomy of the family *Neisseriaceae.*[186,554] The "true neisseriae," *Kingella* species and "*Moraxella urethralis,*" were assigned to the β-subgroup of the *Proteobacteria,* and recommendations were made to remove *Acinetobacter, Moraxella, Branhamella,* and the false neisseria from the family *Neisseriaceae.* Subsequently, "*M. urethralis*" was reclassified as *Oligella urethralis,* the type

strain of the genus *Oligella.*[553] Additional genetic work has also established that the genera *Eikenella, Simonsiella,* and *Alysiella* and the Centers for Disease Control and Prevention (CDC) groups EF-4A, EF-4B, M-5, and M-6 also belong in the emended family *Neisseriaceae.*[554] CDC groups M-5 and M-6, formerly considered as "moraxella-like" species, have been reclassified as *N. weaveri* and *N. elongata* subsp. *nitroreducens,* respectively.[25,268,299] The genus *Kingella* remains in the family *Neisseriaceae,* with *K. indologenes* now belonging to the genus *Suttonella* in the family *Cardiobacteriaceae* as *Suttonella indologenes* (see Chapter 9). *Psychrobacter immobilis* was also excluded from the family *Neisseriaceae* by the work of Rossau and colleagues.[554] In the next edition of *Bergey's Manual,* the *Neisseriaceae* is the only family in the proposed order "Neisseriales" within the β-subgroup of the *Proteobacteria,* along with *Eikenella, Kingella,* and several other genera of animal and environmental origin.[248]

The taxonomic status of *M. (B.) catarrhalis,* the other *Moraxella* species, and the false neisseriae have been the subjects of debate and disagreement among microbiologists and taxonomists for years.[88] In 1991, Rossau and colleagues delineated a new familial rRNA cluster within the γ-subgroup of the *Proteobacteria.*[555] This cluster contained the *Moraxella-Psychrobacter* group and the genus *Acinetobacter.* The former group was divided into the "*Moraxella lacunata* subgroup" (containing the classical moraxellae—*M. lacunata* subsp. *lacunata, M. lacunata* subsp. *liquefaciens, M. bovis, M. liquefaciens,* the false neisseriae, and *M. catarrhalis*), the "*Moraxella osloensis* subgroup," the "*Moraxella atlantae* subgroup," and the "*Psychrobacter-Moraxella phenylpyruvica* subgroup." These investigators proposed a new family—*Moraxellaceae*—for this rRNA cluster.[555] The same year, Catlin proposed the family *Branhamaceae* to accommodate genus *Branhamella* and genus *Moraxella.*[125] In this proposal, the genus *Branhamella* included *B. catarrhalis,* and the false neisseriae, whereas the genus *Moraxella* included all *Moraxella* species (*M. bovis, M. lacunata,* and *M. nonliquefaciens*) and moraxella-like species (*M. osloensis, M. phenylpyruvica,* and *M. atlantae*). The genus *Acinetobacter* was not accommodated in Catlin's proposal. (See Box 11-1).

The proposal of the family *Moraxellaceae* has garnered support with the application of 16S rDNA sequence analysis.[503] These data indicate that the members of the family *Moraxellaceae* constitute a monophyletic taxon forming a distinct line of descent within the γ-subgroup of the *Proteobacteria.* The genus *Moraxella* is comprised of four groups designated I through IV. Groups II through IV include *M. osloensis* and *M atlantae* (group II), *M. phenylpyruvica* and the genus *Psychrobacter* (group III), and the genus *Acinetobacter* (group IV). Group I is comprised of four "clusters," including the "*M. lacunata* cluster" (*M. lacunata* subspecies), the "*M. nonliquefaciens* cluster" (*M. nonliquefaciens*), the "*M. bovis* cluster" (*M. bovis* and *M ovis*), and the "*M. catarrhalis* cluster." The latter cluster includes the diplococcal *M. catarrhalis* and the former false neisseriae *M. cuniculi* and *M. caviae.* Despite the familiarity of the name "*Branhamella catarrhalis*" to clinical microbiologists, *Moraxella catarrhalis* has been accepted as the new

Box 11-1 Classification of Species Within the Family *Neisseriaceae* and the Family *Moraxellaceae* in Domain Bacteria[236,487]

Class	Order	Family	Genus	Species
β-Proteobacteria	"Neisseriales"	*Neisseriaceae*	*Neisseria*	*N. gonorrhoeae, N. meningitidis, N. lactamica, N. sicca, N. subflava biovars, N. mucosa, N. flavescens, N. cinerea, N. polysaccharea, N. elongata subspecies, N. weaveri, N. canis, N. macacae, N. denitrificans, N. iguanae, N. dentium*
γ-Proteobacteria	Pseudomonadales	*Moraxellaceae*	*Moraxella*	Group I — Four clusters: "*M. lacunata* cluster": *M. lacunata* subspecies,"*M. nonliquefaciens* cluster": *M. nonliquefaciens*, "*M. bovis* cluster": *M. bovis, M. ovis* "*M. catarrhalis* cluster": *M. catarrhalis, M. cuniculi, M. caviae* Group II—*M. osloensis, M. atlantae* Group III—*M. phenylpyruvica*

name for this organism. *M. catarrhalis* and the "coccal moraxellae" are discussed in this chapter along with the *Neisseria* species because of morphologic and biochemical similarities. The other *Moraxella* species are considered with the nonfermentative gram-negative bacilli in Chapter 5.

General Characteristics of the Genus Neisseria

Members of the genus *Neisseria* are coccal or rod-shaped gram-negative organisms that frequently occur in pairs or short chains. Diplococcal species have adjacent sides that are flattened, giving them a "coffee bean" appearance. All species in the genus *Neisseria* inhabit mucous membrane surfaces of warm-blooded hosts. These organisms are nonmotile, do not form spores, and most species grow optimally at 35 to 37°C. The organisms are capnophilic and grow best in a moist environment. *Neisseria* species produce acid from carbohydrates oxidatively, and acid production from various carbohydrates constitutes part of the reference identification of these species. Currently, *Neisseria* species (except for the three *N. elongata* subspecies and *N. weaveri*) are the only true coccal members of the family *Neisseriaceae*. *N. elongata* subspecies and *N. weaveri* are medium to large, plump rods that sometimes occur in pairs or short chains.[25,89,299] All species in the genus are oxidase-positive and (except for *N. elongata* subspecies *elongata* and *N. elongata* subspecies *nitroreducens*) are catalase-positive.[89,268] Members of the genus that are found in humans include *N. gonorrhoeae, N. meningitidis, N. lactamica, N. sicca, N. subflava* (including biovars *subflava, flava,* and *perflava*), *N. mucosa, N. flavescens, N. cinerea, N. polysaccharea,* and *N. elongata* subspecies. "*N. kochii*," a rare isolate that some consider a subspecies of *N. gonorrhoeae*, is both phenotypically and genetically related to *N. gonorrhoeae*.[426] Among animal species, *N. canis* and *N. weaveri* are found as part of the normal respiratory tract flora of dogs, *N. denitrificans* is present in the upper respiratory tract of guinea pigs, and *N. macacae, N. dentiae,* and *N. iguanae* are found in the mouths of rhesus monkeys, cows, and iguanid lizards, respectively.[25,51,]

[86,88,299,691] The clinical significance, cultural characteristics, and procedures for differentiating these organisms are discussed later in this chapter.

Most human *Neisseria* species are normal inhabitants of the upper respiratory tract and are not considered as pathogens, although on occasion these organisms may be isolated from infectious processes, particularly in the settings of underlying disease and immunosuppression. *N. gonorrhoeae* is always considered a pathogen, regardless of the site of isolation. *N. meningitidis* also causes significant and often severe disease but may also colonize the human nasopharynx without causing disease. Although most *Neisseria* species are not exacting in their nutritional requirements for growth, the pathogenic species, and *N. gonorrhoeae* in particular, are more nutritionally demanding. *N. gonorrhoeae* will not grow in the absence of the amino acid cysteine and a usable energy source (i.e., glucose, pyruvate, or lactate). Some strains display requirements for amino acids, pyrimidines, and purines as a result of defective or altered biosynthetic pathways.[599] Demonstration of these growth requirements forms the basis for a strain typing method for gonococcal isolates called *auxotyping* (discussed later in this chapter).[124] The neisseria are aerobic, but will grow under anaerobic conditions if low concentrations of an alternative electron acceptor (e.g., nitrites) are present.[352,353] Although the saprophytic *Neisseria* species can use amino acids for growth, glucose or another energy source is required by the pathogenic *Neisseria* for metabolism via the Krebs' cycle (see Chapter 5). The growth of *Neisseria* species is also stimulated by CO_2 and humidity. Atmospheric CO_2 shortens the lag phase by being rapidly assimilated for initial nucleic acid and protein biosynthesis. In the clinical laboratory use of enriched media and incubation of cultures in 5–7% CO_2 fulfills the requirements for recovery of these organisms from clinical specimens.

Both *N. gonorrhoeae* and *N. meningitidis* are able to exchange genetic information by transformation and conjugation (see Chapter 5). Neisseriae are competent for transformation by either chromosomal or plasmid DNA throughout their growth cycle and take up naked DNA with subsequent incorporation into the chromosome at regions of nucleotide sequence homology. Expression of functional PilE (major pilus protein) and PilC (minor pilus protein) are required for transformation to occur, along with the presence of a competence factor, suggesting that both are involved in recognition and/or uptake of transforming DNA (see Box 11-2).[216,557,558] *Neisseria* species probably exchange DNA in vivo by transformation from nucleic acid released from cells by autolytic mechanisms. Transformation may result in altered phenotypic characteristics. For example, transformational acquisition of a mutated dihydropteroate synthase gene has been suggested as the mechanism for the resistance of meningococci to sulfonamides.[520] Transfer of plasmid DNA but not chromosomal DNA also occurs by conjugation. Conjugation in gonococci and meningococci requires the presence of large 24.5- to 25.2-MDa conjugative plasmids for DNA mobilization to occur (see Box 11-2 and 11-3). These conjugative plasmids exist only in strains of *N. meningitidis*, *N. gonorrhoeae*, and *N. cinerea* and may be transferred to recipient cells along with genes coding for resistance to antimicrobial agents. Gonococcal or meningococcal bacteriophages have not been identified, so transfer of genetic elements by transduction does not occur.

The pathogenic *Neisseria* species possess several factors and characteristics that contribute to virulence. *N. meningitidis* strains isolated from serious infections usually possess polysaccharide capsules external to the outer membrane on the surface of the bacterial cells; 13 different capsular serogroups have been described (see discussion below). The capsules render the organisms resistant to phagocytosis, particularly in the absence of opsonizing antibodies.[33] Various outer-membrane protein antigens found in both *N. gonorrhoeae* and *N. meningitidis* also have functions associated with virulence (Fig. 11-1; see Boxes 11-2 and 11-3). Both gonococci and meningococci also produce an immunoglobulin A (IgA1) protease capable of splitting humoral and secretory IgA1 into Fab and Fc fragments, potentially neutralizing the effects of secretory IgA and abrogating mucosal resistance to infection.[457] Nutritional and atmospheric conditions also contribute to the virulence of both gonococci and meningococci. Colonization and subsequent infection of mucosal surfaces by these organisms require iron, and both of these organisms have genetically regulated enzymatic methods for releasing iron from transferrin and lactoferrin, making free iron available for bacterial metabolism (see Boxes 11-2 and 11-3). Requirements for individual amino acids or other trace nutrients may also restrict the abilities of different gonococcal and meningococcal strains to cause certain clinical syndromes. *N. gonorrhoeae* strains also have the ability to grow anaerobically in the presence of nitrite as an electron acceptor.[352,353] Under these conditions, new and different genetically regulated outer-membrane proteins are also expressed.[156] This property may contribute to gonococcal virulence by allowing the organism to proliferate in anaerobic milieus, such as the endocervix, the rectum, the genital tract, and the pharynx, and would also explain the pivotal role of this organism in pelvic inflammatory disease, in which the organism may be recovered in culture along with obligately anaerobic bacteria.

Clinical Significance of *Neisseria* Species
Neisseria gonorrhoeae

EPIDEMIOLOGY

N. gonorrhoeae is the causative agent of gonorrhea, a bacterial infection of great public health significance. In the U.S., the incidence of gonorrhea steadily increased during the 1960s and early 1970s, with the highest incidence—over 460 cases per 100,000 population—occurring in 1975.[614] The "gonorrhea epidemic" that occurred during that time was attributable to several factors, including an increasing at-risk population of young adults, importation of less susceptible gonococcal strains along with the return of servicemen from the Vietnam conflict, increasing use of nonbarrier contraceptive methods (i.e., the birth control pill and intrauterine devices), and improved screening, outreach, and contact tracing.[303,614] In the 1980s and 1990s, the incidence of gonorrhea steadily declined. This decline was largely due to changes in sexual behaviors, particularly among gay and bisexual men, in response to AIDS and to more effective case-finding and contact tracing among women. In 1994, reported cases of *Chlamydia trachomatis* infection exceeded those of gonococcal infection for the first time.[191] However, the downward trend in the incidence of gonococcal infections among homosexual and bisexual males has reversed in the past few years. Data from the CDC Gonococcal Isolate Surveillance Project has shown that the proportion of infections in gay/bisexual men increased from 4.5% in 1992 to 13.2% in 1999.[238] The incidence of gonorrhea is still high among sexually active teenagers (ages 10 through 19 years) and young adults (ages 20 through 24 years) of all races, with the highest attack rates being among 15- to 24-year-old men and women.[614] Disproportionately high rates of gonococcal infection are also found among urban-dwelling African Americans, particularly women 15 to 19 years of age. Transmission of gonorrhea is related to a social subset of "core" or "high-frequency transmitters," who serve as a reservoirs of infection.[101,612] Both social (i.e., low socioeconomic status, urban residence, lack of education, access to health care, unmarried status, race/ethnicity, male homosexuality, prostitution, histories of other sexually transmitted diseases [STDs]) and behavioral risk factors (i.e., unprotected intercourse, multiple partners, other high-risk partners, drug use) have been identified for targeting by outreach/intervention and STD control programs. In the U.S., gonococcal infection has increasingly become a disease of the poor and disenfranchised, and as with HIV infection, epidemiologic associations have been noted between gonorrhea, the use of crack cocaine and intravenous drugs, and the exchange of sex for money and drugs.[589] On a worldwide basis, the highest incidence of gonorrhea and its complications is found in developing countries, such as those in Africa and Latin America.

The risk of acquiring gonorrhea is multifactorial and is related to the frequency and sites of exposure. For heterosexual males, the risk of acquiring urethral infection from an infected female is about 20% for a single exposure and up to 80% for four exposures.[300] Because of anatomical considerations, the risk of infection of the female genital tract from a single exposure to an infected male is much higher. Trans-

Box 11-2 Virulence Factors and Virulence-Associated Antigens of *Neisseria gonorrhoeae*

Virulence Factors	Comments
Lipooligasaccharides	Like other gram-negative bacteria, *Neisseria* species possess an inner cytoplasmic membrane, a thin peptidoglycan layer, and an outer membrane containing lipopolysaccharide (LPS), proteins, and phospholipids (Fig. 11-1). Unlike many other gram-negative bacteria (e.g., the *Enterobacteriaceae*), gonococcal and meningococcal LPSs lack the repeatin "O" somatic antigen side chains external to the core polysaccharide; hence, these structures are more accurately called lipooligosaccharides (LOS).[272] Gonococcal LOS core polysaccharides undergo antigenic variation in molecular structure at a fairly high frequency (i.e., 10^{-2} to 10^{-3}), resulting in the cell surface exposure of different core LOS epitopes over time[34, 582] Terminal structures on the gonococcal LOS become sialylated in vivo by the addition of neuraminic acid from exogenous cytidine-5'-monophospho-*N*-acetyl-neuraminic acid (CMP-NANA).[493] LOS structural variation influences bacterial adherence and resistance to the bactericidal effects of normal human serum.[581] Gonococcal LOS also stimulates a brisk inflammatory response, activates complement, stimulates the production of cytokines, and induces lysis of polymorphonuclear neutrophils (PMNs) and epithelial cells.[468] Induction of tumor necrosis factor α (TNFα) by gonococcal LOS may cause some of the tissue damage seen in pelvic inflammatory disease (PID).[271] Gonococci also release peptidoglycan fragments upon autolysis in vivo and in vitro; these fragments are toxic to genital tract mucosa and other tissues and intensify the inflammatory response seen with gonococcal infections.[235]
Fimbriae (Pili)	Pili and other surface of *N. gonorrhoeae* have been investigated for years in attempts to identify immunogenic structures for the development of gonococcal vaccines[661] *N gonorrhoeae* and *N. meningitidis* possess fimbriae or pili, which partially mediate attachment of the organisms to mucosal surfaces (see Chapter 5).[292] Gonococcal pili are composed of pilin protein subunits that have a molecular weight of 16.5 to 21.5 kDa.[586] Gonococcal pili have three distinct regions: a conserved, 53-amino acid residue region adjacent to the outer membrane that functions in assembly, a central semivariable region, and a strain-variable carboxy-terminal region. Piliated gonococci adhere to susceptible cells to initiate infection; antibodies directed against gonococcal pili can inhibit adherence.[695] Gonococcal pili function during the part of a two-stage attachment process by helping to overcome electrostatic repulsion between the negatively charged mucosal surface and the similarly charged bacterial cells.[292] Pilus formation and pilus-mediated binding of *N. gonorrhoeae* are prerequisites for gonococcal infection in vivo.

Gonococcal pili undergo both **phase variation** and **antigenic variation.** In vitro, phase variation between the piliated (P^+ and $P++$) and nonpiliated (P^-) state occurs at a high frequency; in this situation the *pilE* genes (structural genes for pilus proteins) may not be expressed (i.e., pilus proteins are not produced) or the pilus proteins cannot be assembled into functional pili and are excreted into the medium. Reversible phase variation results from frame shifts in the signal peptide-coding region of *pilC1* and *pilC2*, genes that encode pilus assembly proteins.[330] Gonococcal pili also undergo antigenic variation. Most *N. gonorrhoeae* strains contain a single copy of *pilE*, which contains the expressed major pilin subunit gene and associated promoters, and at least 20 copies of *pilS*, transcriptionally silent, incomplete pilin genes that contain varying sequences and that lack the promoter region and 5'-coding sequences. Recombination between silent and expressed pili genes that contain varying sequences and that lack the promoter region and 5'-coding sequences. Recombination between silent and expressed pili genes results in new antigenic pilus types. In a single strain at any given time, only a single pilus gene is functional and only one pilus type is expressed. The total number of pilus types that can result from recombination among the 20 or so *pilS* genes suggests that the array of antigenic pilus types is theoretically large. Quantitative *pil* gene expression in gonococci also responds to transcriptional regulation by signal-transducing proteins that are coded by *pilA* and *pilB* and are formed in response to environmental stimuli, such as nitrogen levels. Other pilus-associated protein (e.g., PilV) are expressed at low levels relative to the major pilus structural protein (PilE) and interact with PilC pilus assembly proteins.[719] Studies in human volunteers have proven that pilus antigenic variation occurs during clinical infection, with several pilin variants being sequentially isolated during the course of infection.[596] Pili mediate gonococcal attachment to several cell types, including buccal and vaginal epithelial cells, erythrocytes, amniotic cells, neutrophils, and sperm cells. Pili also impede gonococcal phagocytosis by PMNs. |
| **Outer Membrane Proteins** PorI-PorA/PorB | *N. gonorrhoeae* cell walls contain proteins that reside on the outer membrane surface or that span the outer membrane (integral proteins) (Fig. 11-1). Gonococcal outer membrane proteins (OMPs) demonstrate or impart many biologic activities, including the elicitation of humoral and cell-mediated immune responses, |

(Continued)

Box 11-2 Continued

Virulence Factors	Comments
	decreased leukocyte association, and conference of resistance to the bactericidal effects of normal human serum.[613] Some of these proteins are species-, strain-, and type-specific and have been exploited as possible antigens for vaccine development.[661] Porin protein, or **protein I**, now termed **Por,** is a heatstable, LOS-associated, 34- to 36 kDa protein. Gonococci express one of two structurally related but chemically and immunologically distinct forms of this proteins, termed **PorA (PIA)** and **PorB (PIB).** A single copy of the structural gene for this protein exists in the chromosome, suggesting that the genes for PorA and PorB are alleles.[115] A strain of *N. gonorrhoeae* possesses either PorA or PorB, but never both. Por proteins are integral proteins and function as anion-specific channels though the gonococcal outer membrane.[613] Por protein may function in cell-cell interaction by collapsing the membrane potential on contact with epithelial cells and may influence intracellular killing of organisms in PMNs by preventing phagosome-lysosome fusion and diminishing the oxidative burst. Monoclonal antibodies directed against epitopes of Por are the basis for serologic gonococcal typing schemes.[360,573] Anti-Por antibodies are also used in commerically available coagglutination tests (i.e., GonoGen I and the Phadebact GC tests) for identification of *N. gonorrhoeae*. A system for typing the variable regions of the *porB* gene using oligonucleotide probes has been developed that can detect differences in *porB* among isolates belonging to the same serovar.
Opa Proteins (Protein II, P. II)	*N. gonorrhoeae* express outer membrane opacity (Opa) proteins that augment pilus mediated adherence to mucosal surfaces.[289] Certain Opa proteins also facilitate mucosal cell invasion by *N. gonorrhoeae*[233,370,440,468] These proteins are heat-labile and have molecular weights of 24 to 28 kDa.[633] *N. gonorrhoeae* strains possess 11 or 12 complete *Opa* genes in the chromosome; each has its own promoter region and is transcribed into mRNA continually.[63] A gonococcal strain may express four or five different *Opa* genes simultaneously, or may not express any. Regulation of *Opa* gene expression depends on the presence of a five-nucleotide sequence (CTCTT) occurring in triplicate (or multiples of three) at the 3′ end of the structural gene immediately adjacent to the ATG "start" codon.[626] Seven to 28 repeats of this pentameric sequence may be present in a gonococcal cell. When these repeats occur in triplicate (or multiples of three), the *Opa* genes are transcribed and translated in-frame, resulting in simultaneous expression of several different *Opa* genes. Other multiples of the pentameric repeat result in the transcription that is out-of-frame when translated, so Opa proteins are not produced. Copy number variability of this five-nucleotide sequence is generated during DNA replication.[160,161] In addition, hypervariable domains within each *Opa* gene can recombine with homologous domains at other *Opa* loci, leading to evolution of new *Opa* genes and protiens. Gonococcal colonies that express Opa proteins are opaque on certain transparent culture media, while Opa-negative strains produce clear colonies. Opa proteins also vary during uncomplicated urethral infection and are influenced by the menstrual cycle.[326] Endocervical isolates form menstruating women or from normally sterile sites (e.g., blood, joint fluids) often lack Opa proteins. Antigenic variation of Opa proteins during natural infections enables gonococci to circumvent effectors of the immune response.
Rmp Protein (Protein III, P.III)	A third gonococcal protein, called protein III or Rmp (reduction modifiable protein) has a molecular weight of 30 to 31 kDa, is closely associated with LOS and Por, shows little interstrain and intrastrain variation, and is homologous with an *Escherichia coli* outer membrane protein called OmpA (outer membrane protein A).[265,526] Antibodies directed against Rmp on the cell surface block binding of anti-LOS and anti-Por antibodies. The binding of these antibodies greatly diminishes the bactericidal effects of normal human serum on gonococci.[526]
H.8 Protein	*N. gonorrhoeae* strains also possess two H.8 proteins, named as such because they have epitopes that react with monoclonal antibody H.8.[112] Although the function of these copper-containing proteins is not known, similar proteins in other organisms are involved in electron transport.[343] H.8 proteins are present on all gonococci and meningococci, and on strains of *N. lactamica* and *N. cinerea*.[112] Interestingly, patients with DGI and with meningococcal infections demonstrate antibodies to these H.8 outer membrane antigens.[68]
Miscellaneous Outer Membrane Proteins	Many other outer membrane proteins have been described in *N. gonorrhoeae*. Unlike the ones discussed above, many of the others are produced only under conditions of iron starvation or anaerobiosis.[709] Several iron-repressible proteins (FRPs) have been described, including a 37-kDa ferric binding protein (Fbp), plus others ranging from 60 to over 100 kDa in molecular weight.[442] Similar 37 kDa Fbps have been described in both gonococci and meningococci.[441] Another protein, FrpB, is a 70-kDa iron transport protein that is also found in both *N. gonorrhoeae* and *N. meningitidis*.[61,69] These small iron-repressible outer-membrane proteins are receptors for transferrin, lactoferrin, or hemoglobin that bind their respective ligands and, through infection with integral proteins of the outer membrane, transport iron into the cell.[709]

Box 11-2 *Continued*

Virulence Factors	Comments
IgA1 Protease	All gonococci produce an IgA1 protease, which hydrolyzes IgA1 (but not IgA2) molecules at the hinge region (see Chapter 3). This enzyme acts as a virulence factor by inactivating IgA1 at mucosal surfaces, thereby enabling initial attachment and subsequent invasion.[457] IgA1 protease also promotes intracellular survival of gonococci by enzymatically modifying an intracellular protein called LAMP1 that is involved in phagosome/lysosome fusion.[43] Other research has documented that this exoenzyme can trigger the release of proinflammatory cytokines from human monocytes and can activate CD4(+) and CD8(+) T-lymphocytes, resulting in production of interferon gamma (IFN-γ) and TNF.[666] The protease is synthesized as a 169-kDa precursor protein that is enzymatically cleaved to form the mature 106-kDa IgA1 protease and a 45-kDa membrane-associated export protein.
Plasmids	Plasmid-borne virulence determinants in *N. gonorrhoeae* are associated with antimicrobial resistance. Although several others have been described, the two major plasmids that carry the structural genes for the TEM-1 β-lactamases have molecular weights of 3.2 MDa and 4.4 MDa.[29] The 3.2-MDa plasmid was imported from Africa around 1976 and was found primarily in Africa, Europe, and the eastern U.S., whereas the 4.4-MDa plasmid probably originated in Asia and was transported to large cities in the western U.S. in the late 1970s. Regions of the gene are homologous with TnA, an ampicillin-resistance transposon found in the *Enterobacteriaceae*. However, up to 60% of transposon sequences found in gonococcal plasmids are homologous with nucleotide sequences found in plasmids from *Haemophilus* species. Gonococcal β-lactamase plasmids may be transferred by conjugation if the donor cell also has the 24.5-MDa or the 25.2-MDa conjugative plasmid. The latter plasmid(s) also carries tetM, which phenotypically results in high-level resistance to tetracyclines (i.e., minimal inhibitory concentrations [MICs] ≥16 μ/ml). This self-mobilizing plasmid can be passed conjugatively to other gonococci, meningococci, saprophytic neisseriae, and some *Haemophilus* species. Most gonococcal strains also carry a 2.6-MDa "cryptic" plasmid that has no known function.

mission of rectal infection is also quite efficient, and recent studies among homosexual/bisexual men have demonstrated that urethral infection following fellatio from an infected partner may account for as much as 26% of urethral infections diagnosed in this population.[372] Among women, use of hormonal contraceptive methods is associated with an increased risk of gonococcal infection., while barrier method such as condoms and diaphragms used with spermicidal foams and gels (i.e., non-oxynol-9) exert a protective effect against infection.[403,404]

INFECTIONS CAUSED BY *N. GONORRHOEAE*

In males, *N. gonorrhoeae* causes an acute urethritis with dysuria and urethral discharge (Fig. 11-2).[303,614] The incubation period between acquisition of the organism and onset of symptoms ranges from 1 to 14 days or longer, with an average of 2 to 7 days. Infections in men are asymptomatic during the prodromal stages of infection, and conversely, 95–99% of men with urethral gonococcal infection will experience a discharge at some time. The discharge is purulent in 75% of cases, cloudy in 20%, and mucoid in about 5%; the consistency of the discharge at presentation is affected by the length of time that the infection has been incubating and whether the patient has recently urinated. About 2.5% of men presenting to sexually transmitted disease clinics are truly asymptomatic, and it is estimated that the prevalence of asymptomatic urogenital gonorrhea in men in the general population may be as high as 5%. This pattern of disease is often associated with infection by certain Por IA gonococcal

serovars and with arginine, hypoxanthine, and uracil (AHU) and certain other auxotypes of *N. gonorrhoeae* (see below).[102,356,360,453] If left untreated, most cases of gonorrhea in men resolve spontaneously, but in less than 10% of cases, ascending infection may result in gonococcal epididymitis, epididymo-orchitis, prostatitis, periurethral abscess, and urethral stricture. These complications are rarely seen in clinical practice in the U.S.

In females, the primary gonococcal infection is present in the endocervix, with concomitant urethral infection occurring in 70–90% of cases. After an incubation period of 8–10 days, patients may present with cervicovaginal discharge, abnormal or intermenstrual bleeding, and abdominal or pelvic pain; the latter suggests the presence of upper genital tract disease.[637] The presence of dysuria indicates significant urethral involvement. Gonococcal infection of the vaginal squamous epithelium of postpubertal women is uncommon, and in women who have had hysterectomies, the urethra is the most common primary site of infection. Although it has often been stated that most women with genital gonococcal infection are asymptomatic, this is probably not true. This assertion was based on the detection of infected women during widespread screening in locales such as family planning clinics, and did not account for women who presented to physicians or emergency rooms with a spectrum of symptoms referable to the genital tract (e.g., vaginal discharge, dyspareunia, menorrhagia) or the lower abdomen.[614] Symptoms of uncomplicated endocervical infection often resemble those of other conditions, such as cystitis or vaginal infections, and the symptomatology of gonococcal endo-

Box 11-3 Virulence Factors and Virulence-Associated Antigens of *Neisseria meningitidis*

Virulence Factors and Antigens	Comments
Capsular Polysaccharides	*N. meningitis* strains are frequently encapsulated, and 13 different capsular serogroups—designated serogroups A, B, C, D, H, I, K, L, W125, X, Y, Z, and 29E—have been described. With the exception of the serogroup A polysaccharide, these molecules are composed of *N*-acetyl-neuraminic acid (sialic acid) derivatives. The group A capsular polysaccharide is composed of repeating units of α-linked *N*-acetyl-mannosamine-1-phosphate. In the other major serogroups, cytosine-monophosphate-*N*-acetyl-neuraminic acid (CMP-NANA), a capsular polysaccharide precursor, is synthesized by the three-gene *sia* operon. A fourth gene of the capsule-biosynthesis operon is responsible for the polysialyltransferases that are unique to each meningococcal capsular serogroup.[635,636] Another conserved operon among the meningococcal serogroups—the four-gene *ctr* operon—encodes proteins required for capsular polysaccharide export from the cell.[634] Systemic isolates of *N. meningitidis* are usually heavily encapsulated, while carriage strains from the nasopharynx have less capsular material or are nonencapsulated (nongroupable). Non-groupable meningococci arise by downregulation of capsule production. This occurs by addition of an insertion sequence (e.g., IS*1301*) into the first gene of the *sia* operon or by genetic recombination/inactivation of serogroup-specific polysialyltransferase loci between meningococcal strains.[282,636] Capsular switching (i.e., changing from one serogroup to another) has also been demonstrated in vivo and in vitro and occurs by slipped-strand mispairing in the polysialyltransferase gene (*siaD*).[283] Meningococcal capsular polysaccharides prevent organism killing by phagocytic cells and enhance organism survival during bloodstream and CNS invasion. Meningococcal capsular polysaccharides do not mediate adherence to epithelial cells, and encapsulated cells adhere to mucosal cells less readily than nonencapsulated cells.[625]
Lipooligosaccharides	Like the gonococcal LOS, the LOS of *N. meningitidis* lacks the repeating O antigens and consists of a conserved inner core region composed of 3-deoxy-D-manno-2-octulosonic acid (KDO) and heptose attached to lipid A.[272] Variable outer-core carbohydrate residues (i.e., glucose, galactose, *N*-acetylglucosamine and *N*-acetylneuraminic acid) are attached to the heptoses of the inner core. In *N. meningitidis,* some of the heptose residues are attached to oligosaccharide chains of variable composition; these residues form the basis for immunotyping of meningococcal strains. At least 12 LOS immunotypes, designated L1 through L12, have been described.[412] The presence of the carbohydrate lacto-*N*-neotetrose in the LOS has been established as a meningococcal virulence determinant. Lacto-*N*-neotetrose moieties in terminal positions in the LOS mimic structural components of glycosphingolipids present on many types of human cells, including the human I erythrocyte antigen.[411] Eight of the 12 LOS immunotypes of *N. meningitidis* contain the lacto-*N*-neotetrose structure.[665] In animal models, isolates recovered from systemic infections express this determinant even when the strain originally used to establish infection did not. Systemic meningococcal isolates from humans also express this determinant, while the same strain isolated from the nasopharynx of the patient may not.[328] Terminal lacto-*N*-neotetrose moieties in LOS are also substrates for endogenous 2,3-sialyltransferases.[255] Sialylation of these residues masks their presence, resulting in downregulation of complement activation and inhibition of serum bactericidal activity. Meningococcal LOS also stimulates release of TNF-α, which results in further host-cell damage.
Fimbriae (Pili)	Freshly isolated meningococci are piliated; the pili mediate attachment of the organisms to the mucosal cells of the nasopharynx.[507] Organisms in the CSF are piliated in vivo, but whether pili play a role in the ability of meningococci to cross the blood-brain barrier or to interact with meningeal tissues is not known.[292] Pili of *N. meningitidis* are divided into class 1 and class 2 pili; class 1 pili resemble those of *N. gonorrhoeae* closely, while class 2 pili are composed of smaller subunit proteins that share conformational determinants with class 1 and gonococcal pili.[696] The pili are composed of 15- to 20-kDa pilin protein subunits that are encoded by the pilE locus. The C-terminal domain of pilE proteins contains variable regions that are responsible for pilin antigenic variation.[467] Stable piliation of meningococci requires the participation of two 110-kDa proteins, called PilC1 and PilC2, which are found at the tips of functional pili and on the surface of the outer membrane.[466,558] Expression of the PilC1 protein is necessary for adherence, as strains that lack the pilC1 locus and express only PilC2 do not adhere to epithelial cells despite having intact pili.[521] On contact with epithelial cells, *pilC1* gene expression is upregulated, leading to additional pilus synthesis.[639] Once pilus-mediated adherence occurs, another protein (PilT) initiates more intimate bacterium-cell surface contact.[518] Other loci (e.g., pilG, pilQ) encode proteins involved in pilin protein export and pilus assembly.[659,660] Membrane cofactor protein (CD46), a glycoprotein involved in complement regulation and found on many cell types, has been identified as a meningococcal pilus receptor.[336]

Box 11-3 *Continued*

Virulence Factors and Antigens	Comments
Outer Membrane Proteins	
PorA and PorB	The OMPs of *N. meningitidis* are divided into five classes based on molecular weight: class 1 (44 to 47 kDa), class 2 (40 to 42 kDa), class 3 (37 to 39 kDa), class 4 (33 to 34 kDa), and class 5 (26 to 30 kDa).[242] These proteins differ in their susceptibilities to enzymatic hydrolysis and thermal denaturation. All *N. meningitidis* strains possess either a class 2 or a class 3 OMP that constitutes the predominant outer-membrane protein. Class 1 and class 2 proteins are porins and are also responsible for serotype specificity. Class 1 and class 5 proteins are found in most meningococci, although qualitative and quantitative differences in their expression have been noted. The serologic typing system that is used for epidemiologic studies of meningococci is based on the polysaccharide grouping antigen along with antigenic differences between the class 2 or class 3 proteins and the LOS determinants present.[33,242] Antigenic determinants found on proteins 1 and 5, if present, are used to designate subserotypes. For example, a meningococcus of serotype C:2b:P1.3;P5.2;L3,7 is a serogroup C meningococcus expressing a serotype "b" class 2 protein, a serotype 3 class 1 protein, a serotype 2 class 5 protein, and LOS types 3 and 7.[242]
	Meningococcal porin proteins result from expression of two genes called *porA* and *porB*. PorA protein is produced by all meningococci and is a class 1 (cation-selective) porin; individual isolates may vary in the amounts PorA protein present in the outer membrane. PorB codes for either class 2 or class 3 PorB proteins. These are anion-selective porins that constitute the major porin constituent in the meningococcal outer membrane.. The class 2/class 3 proteins of *N. meningitidis* are analogous to the PorA(PIA)/PorB(PIB) proteins of *N. gonorrhoeae*. Por B proteins can insert themselves into membranes of target cells and phagolysosomes and induce apoptosis, thereby facilitating infection and invasion of the host.[458]
Opa and Opc proteins	Class 5 Opa proteins are also found in the outer membrane of *N. meningitidis*. However, instead of a 12-gene Opa repertoire as in gonococci, only three to four Opa genes have been identified in different isolates of meningococci.[440] Meningococcal Opa proteins also facilitate bacterial adherence to epithelial cells and neutrophils. Isolates from different anatomical sites (e.g., blood, CSF, nasopharynx) may also express different Opa proteins.[656] The human CD66 adhesion molecules are receptors for meningococcal Opa proteins.[697] Opc is another class 5 protein that is a heparin- and vitronectin-binding protein. Opc functions in mucosal adherence and invasion of endothelial cells and is also a target for bactericidal antibodies.[185]
Iron-Binding/ Acquisition Proteins	Like the gonococcus, *N. meningitidis* has evolved unique mechanisms for acquisition of iron. Three two-component transport systems, called TbpA/TbpB, LbpA/LbpB, and HpuA/HpuB are involved in the acquisition of iron from human transferrin, lactoferrin, and hemoglobin/haptoglobin, respectively.[387,388,502,546,627] The TbpA/TbpB system functions optimally during initial infection and invasion, since lactoferrin is the principal iron source at mucosal surfaces, while the HpuA/HpuB system is maximally expressed during bacteremia, when haptoglobin/hemoglobin complexes represent the most plentiful form of iron. Meningococci also have a surface protein called HmbR that can extract heme from surface-bound hemoglobin and transport it into the cell.[382] All of these proteins are integral OMPs.
IgA1 Protease	All meningococci produce an IgA1 protease similar to that found in *N. gonorrhoeae*. It is postulated to serve as a virulence factor by abrogating mucosal immunity. Antibodies against IgA1 protease are produced and detectable during meningococcal disease and also appear during asymptomatic nasopharyngeal carriage.[96]
Plasmids	Plasmids are not common in *N. meningitidis*. However, tetracycline-resistant *N. meningitidis* strains contain the same 25.2-Mda tetM-bearing plasmid that is found in tetracycline-resistant *N. gonorrhoeae*. The β-lactamase-encoding plasmids from *N. gonorrhoeae* can also be transferred to *N. meningitidis* in vitro by the 24.5- or the 25.2-Mda plasmid found in some gonococci.[542] Meningococcal acquisition of the β-lactamase gene is also likely to occur in vivo, especially when both organisms are present in the same site/specimen.[189] Backman and colleagues sequenced the plasmids from two β-lactamase-positive *N. meningitidis* strains recovered from patients in Spain.[44] The 5,597-base-pair plasmid was the same in both isolates and was virtually identical to a 5,597-base-pair β-lactamase plasmid found in *N. gonorrhoeae*.

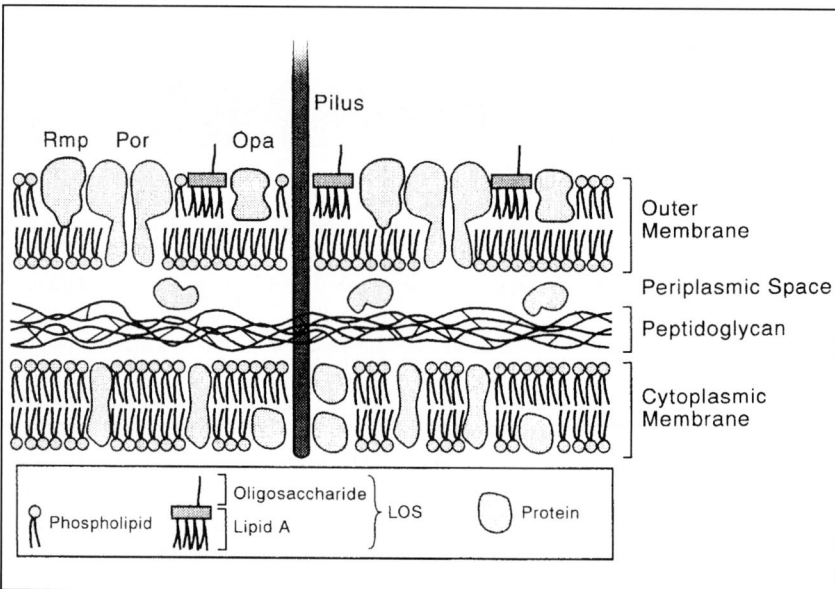

Figure 11-1 Schematic representation of the surface structure of *N. gonorrhoeae,* showing the major components that contribute to pathogenicity and antimicrobial resistance. Opa, Por, and Rmp are the designations of the major outer-membrane proteins (see text); LOS denotes lipooligosaccharide.

cervicitis is often clouded by coinfection with *Chlamydia trachomatis, Trichomonas vaginalis,* and/or *Candida albicans.* Although the genital tract may appear normal, careful endocervical examination often reveals areas of friable cervical mucosa that bleed on swabbing. Only 10–20% of infected women, however, will present with an obvious mucopurulent endocervical discharge. Infection of the Bartholin's and Skene's glands may be seen in about one third of women with genital tract infection. Careful manipulation of these areas can sometimes provide purulent material for direct examination and culture. Endocervical gonorrhea may also complicate pregnancy and is a recognized cofactor for spon-

taneous abortion, chorioamnionitis, premature rupture of membranes, and premature delivery.[303,637] Infants born to women with genital tract infection are at risk for gonococcal conjunctivitis (''ophthalmia neonatorum'') or pharyngeal gonococcal infection.

Ascending gonococcal infection may occur in 10–20% of infected women and can result in acute pelvic inflammatory disease (PID) that is manifested as salpingitis (infection of the fallopian tubes), endometritis, and tubo-ovarian abscess, all of which can lead to scarring of the fallopian tubes, ectopic pregnancies, sterility, and chronic pelvic pain.[303,614] Symptoms of gonococcal PID include bilateral lower abdominal pain, abnormal cervical discharge and bleeding, pain on motion, fever, and peripheral leukocytosis. PID caused by *N. gonorrhoeae* generally occurs early, rather than late, in infection and often during or shortly after the onset of menstruation. Fever, leukocytosis, elevated erythrocyte sedimentation rates, and C-reactive protein are seen in about two thirds of patients, while chills, nausea, and vomiting are variable features of PID. In women with salpingitis, a perihepatitis called the Fitz-Hugh-Curtis syndrome may also develop; it is characterized by direct extension of the organisms from the fallopian tube to the liver and peritoneum, resulting in right upper quadrant pain and the finding of adhesions between the liver and the anterior abdominal wall on laparoscopy.[614,637] The development of PID is influenced by many factors, including diagnosis and treatment for other genital tract infections (e.g., *C. trachomatis* infection, bacterial vaginosis), prior PID, the use of oral contraceptives, intrauterine devices, vaginal douching, characteristics of infecting strains, and the immune competence of the host. Obstruction of the fallopian tubes, leading to infertility, occurs in 10–20% of women following a single episode of acute gonococcal PID and in 50–80% after three or more episodes. Among women with ectopic pregnancies, up to 80% have a history of prior PID.[202] In pregnant women, gonococcal infection is associated with an increased risk of complications, including premature labor, premature rupture of the

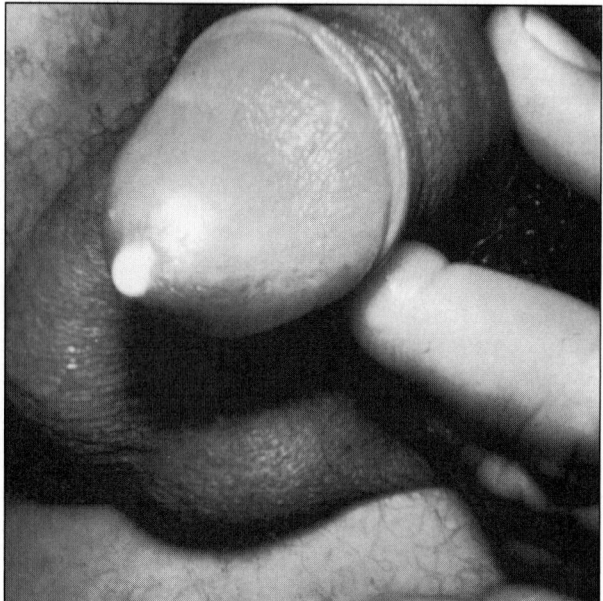

Figure 11-2 Male with purulent urethral discharge characteristic of *Neisseria gonorrhoeae* infection.

fetal membranes, spontaneous abortion, and infant mortality. Complications due to gonococcal infections are uncommon after the first trimester.

N. gonorrhoeae may also cause pharyngeal and anorectal infections. Oropharyngeal gonococcal infection is seen in homosexual and bisexual men and heterosexual women who acquire the infection by engaging in orogenital sexual contact with an infected partner. Pharyngeal gonorrhea may also be seen occasionally in heterosexual men, resulting from performing cunnilingus with an infected partner. Over 90% of oropharyngeal gonococcal infections are asymptomatic and are diagnosed by culture of the organism from the throat.[48] Anorectal infections occur in homosexual/bisexual men who practice unprotected receptive anal intercourse. Women may also acquire rectal infections by receptive anal intercourse, but most rectal infections in women are due to perianal contamination with infected cervicovaginal secretions. Rectal gonococcal infections are often asymptomatic, but some individuals may experience acute proctitis with mild anorectal pain and itching, a mucopurulent discharge, bleeding, tenesmus, and constipation 5 to 7 days after infection.[547] Anoscopic examination of the anal canal usually reveals an edematous and erythematous rectal mucosa and a purulent discharge associated with the anal crypts.[715] *Chlamydia* infection, herpes simplex virus infection, and other sexually transmitted infections are included in the differential diagnosis of anorectal gonococcal infection.

In a small percentage (approximately 0.5–3%) of infected individuals, gonococci may invade the bloodstream, resulting in disseminated gonococcal infection (DGI).[433,552] This infection is characterized by low-grade fever (rarely above 39°C), hemorrhagic skin lesions, tenosynovitis, migratory polyarthralgias, and frank arthritis. Women appear to be a greater risk for DGI, particularly during menstruation and during the second and third trimesters of pregnancy. The skin lesions are generally painful and appear as a papule that evolves into a necrotic pustule on an erythematous base (Fig. 11-3). Usually there are as few as 5 or up to 30 lesions present, and the majority of them are on the extremities (i.e., toes, fingers).[433] See Color Plate 11-1*B*. Cultures of skin lesions and synovial fluids from patients with DGI may be negative, suggesting that immune processes (e.g., antigen-antibody complex deposition) contribute to the pathogenesis of DGI. On occasion, extensive macular, papular, or petechial rashes may develop. Mastrolonardo and associates reported a DGI in a 24-year-old woman who presented with extensive vesicobullous, hemorrhagic, and necrotic lesions on the buttocks and lower limbs.[422] In 30–40% of cases, organisms from the bloodstream may localize in one or more joints to cause a purulent and destructive gonococcal arthritis.[170] Joint involvement is usually asymmetric and most commonly involves the knee, elbow, wrist, fingers, or ankle joints.[720] Occasionally, other joints may be involved.[381] Infected synovial fluid frequently contains 50,000 to 200,000 cells/mm³, with 90% being polymorphonuclear neutrophils.[170,235] Gram stain and culture of joint aspirates are positive in only 10–30% of cases. Polymerase chain reaction (PCR) has also been applied to the detection of gonococci in synovial fluid.[392,459]

Complications of DGI include permanent joint damage, endocarditis, and rarely, meningitis.[530,706] Gonococcal endo-

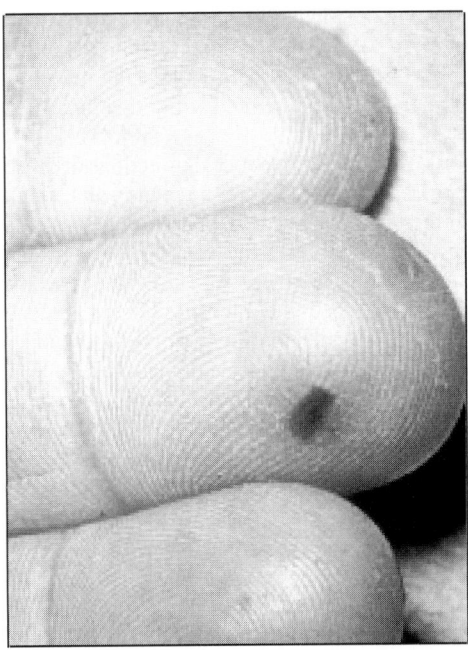

Figure 11-3 Characteristic skin lesion of disseminated gonococcal infection on finger. Skin lesions are usually located on the extremities.

carditis is a rare clinical entity, with fewer than 60 cases reported in the literature since 1938. Gonococcal endocarditis may develop in about 1–2% of patients with disseminated infection, usually involves the aortic valve, and follows a rapid and destructive course.[706] In 1996, Thompson and Brantley reported a case of gonococcal endocarditis in a 23-year-old man that required prosthetic-valve placement resulting from severe aortic insufficiency and a prolapsed aortic cusp.[652] In 1997, the first case of gonococcal endocarditis in association with systemic lupus erythematosus was diagnosed in a 24-year-old woman who presented with nonspecific symptoms of cough, chest pain, fever, and malaise without signs or symptoms of DGI.[655] Transthoracic and transesophageal echocardiograms showed a large vegetation on the pulmonary valve, and blood cultures were positive for *N. gonorrhoeae*. Pericarditis and pericardial effusions are also complications of DGI, and adult respiratory distress syndrome has been reported in association with gonococcal bacteremia.[56,159,717] Gonococcal meningitis is a rare complication of disseminated infection that has features typical of meningitides caused by other organisms.[530] Clinical entities that resemble DGI include Reiter's syndrome, pyogenic and crystal-induced arthritis, syphilitic and tuberculous arthritis, rheumatoid arthritis, Lyme disease, and rheumatic fever.[552] Repeated bouts of DGI have also been observed in individuals with certain complement deficiencies.[211,552] Disseminated disease may develop following infection at genital or extragenital sites. Studies of isolates recovered from cases of DGI have shown that these more invasive strains have unusual characteristics, including unique nutritional requirements (e.g., requirements for arginine, hypoxanthine, and uracil for growth [AHU strains]), defined PorIA serovar classification, resistance to the bactericidal action of normal human serum, and exquisite susceptibility to penicillin.[207,356,453,585] With the decline in the prevalence of AHU/Po IA serovars in recent years, increasing numbers of DGI infections have been associated with other auxotype/serovar classes.[102,645]

Reports of unusual gonococcal infections or presentations have appeared in the literature in recent years. Ocular gonococcal infections, once seen primarily among neonates who acquired the organism during passage through an infected birth canal (ophthalmia neonatorum), have been reported among adults who become infected via genital secretions.[704] Laboratory personnel working with cultures may also become accidentally infected if care is not taken to protect the eyes.[410] Infection of the eye results in periorbital cellulitis, a profuse purulent discharge, conjunctival injection, eyelid edema and erythema, and epithelial and stromal keratitis. Inadequate treatment of eye infections can lead to ulcerative keratitis, corneal perforation, and blindness.[704] Rare reports of primary cutaneous gonococcal infection, resulting from inoculation of a preexisting injury or lesion, have also appeared in the literature, including a case of gonococcal mastitis in a male.[74,592] Gonococcal scalp abscesses have been reported in neonates as a complication of intrauterine fetal monitoring.[40] Atypical presentations and clinical courses may be seen in patients with underlying diseases, including HIV infection. Jacoby and Mady described a case of acute gonococcal sepsis in a 35-year-old HIV-positive women that included profound hypotension and acidosis, findings that are usually not seen in patients with DGI.[316] Risher and McFadden reported a case of an *N. gonorrhoeae* mycotic aneurysm of the ascending aorta in a 38-year-old woman with systemic lupus erythematosus that required prolonged antimicrobial therapy and surgical resection of the affected valves.[540] Strongin and coworkers reported on a 27-year-old HIV-positive homosexual man who presented with gonococcal arthritis of the hip and a single sternoclavicular joint.[630] Brook and colleagues described a ''mini-outbreak'' of tissue-invasive *N. gonorrhoeae* among three female and two male sexual contacts that resulted in asymptomatic infection in one of the men, PID in one of the women, DGI in one other woman, and inguinal lymphadenopathy in two of the patients.[95] In 1994, Bodsworth and associates reported the first case of gonococcal infection of the ''neovagina'' of a male-to-female transexual.[73] Lastly, Burnett and colleagues reported a very unusual case of gonococcal ventriculoperitoneal shunt infection in a 17-year-old female.[103] The authors postulated that the peritoneal end of the shunt, which yielded the heaviest growth of the organism, may have become contaminated with gonococci during menstruation, when menstrual blood may reflux through the fallopian tubes and enter the peritoneal cavity.

Historically, gonococcal infections in children included only ophthalmia neonatorum, which is ocular gonorrhea transmitted to the infant during passage through the infected cervix.[389] Almost all cases of gonorrhea in children during the newborn period are the result of ocular contamination, although more serious infections with gonococci in newborns have been reported.[214] Transmission of gonorrhea from adults to children by fomites (e.g., shared towels) was proposed as a mode of transmission in older children. However, it is now recognized that gonococcal infections, includ-

ing conjunctivitis, and other sexually transmitted diseases in children beyond the immediate neonatal period are indicators of sexual abuse.[30,54,153,544] With a careful, multidisciplinary approach, histories of sexual contacts can usually be obtained from older children. When a child with gonorrhea is identified, investigation of both adult caretakers and other siblings frequently reveals infected adults and other infected children.[18] Gonococcal infections in children resemble those in adults, with some notable differences. *N. gonorrhoeae* causes a vaginitis, rather than a cervicitis, in prepubertal girls. The epithelium of the prepubertal vagina is composed of columnar epithelial cells, which are the cell types that *N. gonorrhoeae* preferentially infects. With the onset of puberty, these cells are replaced by a stratified squamous epithelium that is not susceptible to gonococcal infection. Female children with genital gonococcal infection generally present with a vaginal discharge. Urethral infection in male children, if present, resembles that seen in adults. Pharyngeal and rectal gonococcal infections, as in adults, are usually asymptomatic in children.

Neisseria meningitidis
EPIDEMIOLOGY

N. meningitidis is a primary pathogen that causes an array of infectious processes, ranging from occult sepsis with rapid recovery, to fulminant overwhelming fatal disease.[33] In some patients only limited aspects of this clinical spectrum may manifest, while in others it may progress across this spectrum with alarming rapidity. A major virulence factor of all disease-associated isolates of *N. meningitidis* is the polysaccharide capsule. Thirteen meningococcal capsular polysaccharide serogroups (A, B, C, D, H, I, K, L, X, Y, Z, W135, and 29E) have been recognized; most infections are caused by organisms belonging to serogroups A, B, C, Y, and W135. A variable percentage of strains recovered from nasopharyngeal carriers may not express a detectable capsular polysaccharide antigen (i.e., nongroupable). For example, in a recent study of meningococcal carriage among university students in the United Kingdom, 43.9% of 904 strains recovered from carriers were serologically nongroupable.[16] Meningococcal isolates can be further subdivided into 20 serotypes based on class 2 and 3 OMP (PorB) antigens, 10 subserotypes based on class 1 OMP (PorA) antigens, and 13 immunotypes based on lipooligosaccharide (LOS) structure (see Box 11-3). Although these serologic methods are helpful in determining the relatedness of strains locally and in defined clinical settings, none of them are able to discriminate and define the genetic relatedness of meningococcal strains for global epidemiologic purposes. Because of the high frequency of antigenic variation in outer-membrane proteins and the phenomenon of ''capsular switching,'' other methods have been developed to genetically define, identify, and track pathogenic *N. meningitidis* strains globally.[636] Techniques such as multilocus isoenzyme electrophoresis typing (ET typing) and multilocus sequence typing have helped scientists and epidemiologists identify a number of genetically defined clonal groups that are responsible for both epidemic and sporadic, endemic disease.[129,597] These **ET groups** may be further divided into **clonal subgroups.** For example, among over 500 epidemic serogroup A strains collected in Africa since the 1960s, 84 electrophoretic types

(ETs) have been recognized that are divisible into nine subgroups. Three of these subgroups have been responsible for all major epidemics that have occurred in the region.[278,427] Individual ET complexes will include strains bearing different serogroup antigens. For example, while the ET-37 complex includes mostly serogroup C strains and the ET-5 complex contains mostly serogroup B strains, both complexes include other serogroups as well. Molecular methods for meningococcal epidemiologic typing also have been described. For example, meningococcal serogroup antigen gene sequencing by sialyltransferase gene PCR can be used to confirm serologic grouping methods and to determine the genetic grouping of serologically "nongroupable" strains containing capsular genes that are "switched off."[81,222] Other molecular genetic methods (e.g., DNA fingerprinting, restriction-fragment-length polymorphisms, pulsed-field gel electrophoresis, ribotyping, repetitive element-based PCR analysis, random-amplified PCR, *porA* gene sequencing, and PCR-amplicon endonuclease analysis) have also been developed for monitoring the epidemiology of pathogenic *N. meningitidis* strains on a worldwide basis.[52,276,277,347,368,495,535,629,658,723,726]

Clonal analysis of *N. meningitidis* has revealed many interesting characteristics related to virulence and disease. Virulent clones are distinguished by having high transmission rates and causing high rates of disease upon introduction into a susceptible population. Avirulent clones are found in asymptomatic carriers and rarely cause disease, even when transmitted at rates similar to those of virulent clones.[671] The presence of virulent clones coupled with high transmission rates, a susceptible population, certain host factors (e.g., smoking, mucosal immunity, viral coinfections, congenital/acquired complement deficiencies), and environmental/behavioral factors (crowding, close contact, smoke exposure) leads to high carriage rates and the often explosive appearance of disease.[126,227,733] Eventually, circulating virulent clonal groups undergo genetic diversification via transformation and various selective environmental pressures; these clones may then disappear and/or reemerge at a later time.[126]

Worldwide, various pathogenic clones of *N. meningitidis* composed of different serogroups, serotypes, subserotypes, and immunotypes are responsible for both endemic and epidemic disease.[126] Endemic meningococcal disease occurs at rates of 1 to 3 cases per 100,000 persons in the United States, and in 10 to 25 cases per 100,000 persons in developing countries.[680] In the U.S. in recent years, the annual incidence of meningococcal disease has been 0.8 to 1 per 100,000 population, with infants, the elderly, and the immunocompromised being at greatest risk.[315] Attack rates are highest among children aged 3 months to 1 year and among older teenagers and young adults. In certain regions of sub-Saharan Africa that are referred to as the "meningitis belt," meningococcal disease caused primarily by serogroup A strains occurs annually, with incidences as high as 1,000 cases per 100,000 population.[278,534] Since the late 1960s, various clones of serogroup A *N. meningitidis* have spread throughout China, India, and the Middle East, culminating in a large outbreak of disease due to a clonal subgroup III-1 serogroup A strain among Moslems making the annual pilgrimage to Mecca (Hajj) in 1987.[451,478,534] During the

subsequent year and through 1996, this same clone spread and caused epidemics in the Sudan, Uganda, Kenya, Ethiopia, Saudi Arabia, Chad, Nigeria, Nepal, and South Africa.[275,427,449,451,506] Serogroup B strains belonging to the ET-5 complex have caused sporadic outbreaks in England, Denmark, Norway, and the Netherlands since the mid-1970s, and similar strains have been documented throughout the Far East (e.g., China, Japan, Thailand), South America (e.g., Brazil, Chile), the Caribbean (e.g., Cuba), Canada, and the U.S. (e.g., Oregon).[38,39,127,133,571,572,583,584,606] Serogroup B *N. meningitidis* strains belonging to other clonal types (i.e., ET-24 and ET-25) also emerged in Europe during the 1980s and spread to Finland, Norway, and Iceland during the 1990s, with outbreaks occurring in both the United Kingdom and Belgium.[690]

Certain clones, such as the ET-37 complex, have been the causes of sporadic outbreaks in Brazil, China, South Africa, and the U.S.[126] The ET-37 complex includes strains expressing serogroups B, C, Y, and W-135. During the 1980s, serogroup B strains belonging to this complex were recognized in China and South Africa, while serogroup C strains were isolated in other regions of Africa and Europe.[126] During the late 1980s and into the 1990s, serogroup C strains within the ET-37 complex became established in both the U.S., Canada, and overseas. These strains have been responsible for clusters of sporadic disease in Iowa, Illinois, Los Angeles, Ontario, and Saskatchewan, Canada, and have also been isolated in the United Kingdom, Italy, Denmark, and Brazil.[1,39,205,313,421,536,548,559,629] At the same time, a variant complex of ET-37, called complex ET-15, appeared, and group C strains within this variant complex emerged in the early 1990s as a major cause of sporadic disease in the U.S., Canada, England, Australia, and Eastern Europe.[39,290,313,536] In the U.S., these strains were associated with outbreaks in schools and correctional facilities.[98,642,735] Also during the early to mid-1990s, serogroup Y *N. meningitidis* strains appeared in the U.S. and certain clone complexes (e.g. ET-508 and others) bearing this serogroup antigen are now the cause of about 30% of endemic meningococcal disease in the U.S. In Chicago, the prevalence of serogroup Y strains increased from 6% in 1991 to 71% in 1995.[519] The balance of disease in the U.S. is caused by ET-37 and ET-15 serogroup C strains, ET-5 complex serogroup B strains, and serogroup W-135 strains.[126,519,657]

In the new millennium, meningococcal outbreaks continue to plague developing countries, and patterns of disease in the U.S. reflect significant changes in domestic meningococcal epidemiology. For the first time, pathogenic serogroup W-135 strains were isolated from over 300 Moslems who attended the year 2000 Hajj, which concluded in March of 2000.[137,572] An examination of four isolates from pilgrims who returned to the U.S. found that these meningococci belonged to ET-927, a cluster that is genetically closely related to the ET-37 complex.[513] These strains were also demonstrated in four additional French patients with epidemiologic links to the year 2000 Hajj.[572] These strains also showed similar pulsed-field gel electrophoretic patterns that were distinct from other serogroup W-135 strains.[513] In the U.S., changes in meningococcal epidemiology during the 1990s have included an increase in the incidence of community-acquired serogroup C infections, and an increase in disease among teenagers and young adults of both high school and college age.[135,288,550,735] Some outbreaks have occurred on college campuses and have been associated with patronage of bars and discos, drinking, cigarette smoking, and dormitory residence.[165,310,311] A recent collaborative study documented that first-year college students in the U.S. who resided in dormitories had an annual incidence rate of meningococcal disease of 5.4 per 100,000, which is five times the national rate and is exceeded in incidence only by the age group of children less than 2 years old.[99] Substantial amounts of disease have also been seen among non-first-year students and among students living in off-campus housing.[287,288] The reasons for the increasing incidence of group C disease among adolescents, and college dormitory residents in particular, are not known. In response to these changes in incidence patterns and the ability to prevent serious serogroup C disease with currently available vaccines, the Advisory Committee on Immunization Practices has recommended that meningococcal immunizations be offered to incoming college students who live in campus housing, while others have advocated making meningococcal vaccination available to all college undergraduate students.[134,136,243,287,288]

INFECTIONS CAUSED BY *N. MENINGITIDIS*

N. meningitidis may be carried asymptomatically in the oropharynx and nasopharynx of a variable percentage of individuals, and the rate of carriage is related to several factors, such as age, socioeconomic class, and the presence of actual disease in a community.[121] Carriage of meningococci in the nasopharynx may be transient, intermittent, or persistent.[16] In general, carriage rates tend to be about 8–20%, with older children and young adults having higher carriage rates (20–40%) than young children.[128,481] The duration of carriage may also vary with the individual and the serogroup of the colonizing strain. During periods when disease is present in a community, the carriage rates may not be very different from observed rates when no clinical disease is being reported, but the proportion of individuals carrying the more virulent strain has been noted to increase.[33] Contrary to what has been promulgated for years, the rate of meningococcal carriage does not appear to be seasonal, although most meningococcal disease in developed countries tends to occur during late winter and early spring. Crowded living conditions facilitate the respiratory spread of meningococci, and this crowding affects both the transmission of the organism and the occurrence of overt disease. This has been amply demonstrated by the large outbreaks that have occurred on military bases over the years, where large numbers of young, susceptible adults live together in close quarters for prolonged periods. Among such closed populations, carriage rates may approach 100%. Carriage strains may be encapsulated (groupable) or nonencapsulated (nongroupable) and result in the formation of serogroup-specific antibodies and broadly cross-reactive antibodies against several other outer membrane antigens. Even in individuals who are colonized with nongroupable strains high titers of antibodies develop against groupable strains, probably owing to the presence of shared antigenic determinants. In one study of 38 individuals who carried nongroupable strains in the nasopharynx, 2–52% of the men developed group-specific antibodies, de-

pending on the serogroup examined.[525] In most hosts, meningococcal colonization of the upper respiratory tract results in the formation of serogroup-specific serum bactericidal antibodies within 7 to 10 days.[33] This response does not eliminate the carriage state, but it may protect the host from overt disease.

In some individuals, the meningococcal strain that becomes established in the upper respiratory tract goes on to enter the bloodstream and initiate systemic disease. It appears that invasive *N. meningitidis* disease occurs in persons who are newly infected with a strain against which the individual lacks bactericidal meningococcal serogroup-specific antibodies. In a study among military personnel, Edwards and coworkers found that 86% of 31 patients had negative nasopharyngeal cultures during the 2 weeks before becoming ill and that four patients were culture-negative the day before disease onset.[206] However, in a recent report, a documented 7-week interval occurred between nasopharyngeal acquisition of the organism and onset of meningeal disease.[471] Concurrent viral or mycoplasmal infection of the upper respiratory tract may also facilitate systemic invasion by the organism because both sporadic and epidemic outbreaks of meningococcal disease have been associated with outbreaks of viral and mycoplasmal respiratory tract infections.[450] The risk of meningococcal disease is also higher among carriers with deficiencies in the terminal complement components (e.g., C5, C6, C7, C8, and C9) or the properdin system.[228,229,605] Other underlying conditions, such as hepatic failure, systemic lupus erythematosus, multiple myeloma, and asplenia may also predispose to serious meningococcal disease.[33]

The pathogenesis of meningococcal disease is poorly understood and, although much has been reported on the descriptive epidemiology of the organism and its disease states, very little is known about the dynamics of disease production.[439,671] Humans are the only natural host for *N. meningitidis,* and the organism is spread by respiratory droplets. Meningococci colonize the upper respiratory mucosa and may subsequently invade the bloodstream. Initial attachment to the nasopharyngeal mucosa is apparently mediated via interaction of pili with membrane cofactor protein (CD46).[336] Antigenic variation at the pilus level regulates the avoidance of nonspecific host factors during initial adherence to the epithelial mucosa.[467] Environmental factors such as smoking and concomitant viral upper respiratory tract infections increase the risk of colonization due to alterations in the mucosa or abrogation of local immunity.[450,619] Subsequently, class 5 outer-membrane proteins (OMPs) bind to the C46 receptor and Opa proteins bind the heparin sulfate proteoglycan receptors on endothelial and phagocytic cells, respectively.[439] This stimulates the release of cytokines by these cells, with subsequent endocytosis of the organisms by the epithelial cells.[624,671] PorB proteins subsequently become inserted into the membrane of the phagosome, preventing fusion with lysosomes.[439] In this way, meningococci can avoid humoral immune mechanisms and survive in mononuclear leukocytes in the subepithelium.[522] The principal meningococcal virulence factor associated with bloodstream invasion is the polysaccharide capsule. In the absence of opsonic antibodies, the capsule prevents phagocytosis of organisms and also protects against complement-mediated bacteriolysis. In addition, certain class 1 OMPs of *N. meningitidis* are able to downregulate the expression of various complement receptors on neutrophils, thereby inhibiting ingestion of the organisms.[66] Bloodstream invasion by meningococci also correlates with the systemic release of a variety of inflammatory cytokines (e.g., interleukin-1, interleukin-6, tumor necrosis factor-α) that contribute to the pathogenesis of meningococcemia and meningococcal septic shock.[93,94,680,699] Some of these cytokines may increase the permeability of the blood-brain barrier and allow entry of meningococci into the cerebrospinal fluid (CSF). In addition, meningococcal invasion of endothelial cells with resulting edema and induction of apoptosis may also release organisms into the CSF and other closed spaces.

Meningococci can cause epidemic and endemic meningitis, and serogroups A, B, and C are responsible for 90% of cases globally. At present, *N. meningitidis* is the second leading cause of community-acquired meningitis in the United States.[120,204] The most serious clinical manifestation of meningococcal disease is meningitis accompanied by acute meningococcal sepsis. Clinical presentations of disease may be quite varied and include meningoencephalitis, meningitis with or without meningococcemia, meningococcemia without meningitis, and bacteremia without septic complications.[33,120,340,570] The onset of acute meningococcal meningitis is sudden, with fever and chills, myalgias, and arthralgias.[120] The classic signs of meningitis, such as confusion, headache, fever, and nuchal rigidity, may be seen in only about half of the patients.[33] Vomiting may also be a part of the clinical presentation, particularly in children. Meningococcemia and widespread dissemination of the organism are heralded by the rapid development of a rash, which is seen in about 50–60% of patients. This rash starts as a pink, maculopapular eruption and then becomes petechial. Initially, these petechiae appear on the mucous membranes (e.g., the conjunctivae), and then spread to the trunk and the lower extremities. These lesions are indicators of bleeding complications and coagulopathies that are caused by the organism. Fulminant, rapidly progressive disease may result in formation of additional macules and papules that progress to form purpuric or ecchymotic areas of cutaneous hemorrhage and necrosis.[570] **Purpura fulminans** develops in about 10% of patients with meningococcemia, resulting in extensive areas of tissue destruction secondary to coagulopathy; aggressive monitoring of coagulation parameters and replacement of coagulation factors may benefit some of these patients.[516] Diffuse neurologic involvement, rather than focal signs and symptoms, and myocardial involvement are seen more frequently with meningococcal meningitis than with other types of bacterial meningitis. Cardiac abnormalities, including purulent pericarditis with tamponade, are complications of meningococcal disease that usually develop during convalescence.[306] In one case report, sepsis with a group B meningococcus triggered an acute myocardial infarction in a 42-year-old man with normal coronary arteries.[230]

Fulminant meningococcal shock often dominates the clinical picture of meningococcal meningitis and acute meningococcal sepsis.[33] The patient becomes unresponsive, with absence of superficial and deep tendon reflexes and a depressed sensorium. Because of peripheral vasoconstriction, gangrenous changes in the extremities may be noted. The presence of shock, a low white blood-cell count, a rash, and altered mental status on presentation are associated with a poor clinical outcome in these patients.[649] Mortality from meningococcal septic shock is also associated with low serum potassium and a negative base excess, reflecting generalized metabolic abnormalities, and low platelet and serum C-reactive protein levels, which are associated with durations of petechiae and purpura and are predictive of impending disseminated intravascular coagulation (DIC).[366] Death may supervene as a result of DIC. In these fatal cases, autopsies reveal terminal myocarditis and/or the lesions of DIC, with microthrombi and thromboses observed in many organs. Avascular necrosis of bone due to thrombosis in intraosseous blood vessels secondary to DIC has also been documented in severe meningococcal disease.[108] The classic finding of acute hemorrhagic necrosis of the adrenal glands represents the anatomic hallmark of the Waterhouse-Friderichsen syndrome.[9] Despite the availability of excellent therapeutic agents, meningitis with sepsis caused by *N. meningitidis* still may have a mortality rate of up to 30%. About 10% of survivors of infection will have sensorineural deafness.[425]

N. meningitidis may also cause bloodstream infection (meningococcemia) without meningitis.[33] Patients with meningococcal bacteremia without sepsis usually present with a fever, headache, malaise, and peripheral leukocytosis. Symptoms of a respiratory tract infection may also be present, but meningeal signs and symptoms are not. Meningococci are recovered from blood cultures, but the patient is usually clinically well by this time, and no therapy or a short course of therapy is administered. With chronic meningococcemia, the patient is generally symptomatic, with a low-grade fever, rash, and occasionally arthritis. This presentation is clinically very similar to the gonococcal arthritis-dermatitis syndrome. Unusual cutaneous manifestations, such as erythema nodosum, have also been described in association with chronic meningococcemia.[713] This form of meningococcal disease, with or without meningitis, has been noted to recur in some patients. Such individuals frequently have inherited underlying deficiencies in C3, properdin, C5, C8, and other late complement components.[146,228,229] Individuals with underlying conditions that are associated with hypocomplementemic states, such as systemic lupus erythematosus, are at risk for serious meningococcal disease, and chronic meningococcemia has also been documented in HIV-infected patients.[10,41,223] In one reported case, meningococcemia occurred as a complication of upper gastrointestinal endoscopy. The organism was probably introduced from the upper respiratory tract into the bloodstream by mucosal damage that occurred during passage of the endoscope through the mouth and down into the intestine.[19] *N. meningitidis* sepsis has also documented as a complication of preterm labor in a 19-year-old woman, although complement studies were not performed.[474]

N. meningitidis may also cause other infections, some of which result from hematogenous dissemination. Bloodborne spread of the organism may seed other internal organs, leading to complications such as osteomyelitis, arthritis, cellulitis; pericarditis, endophthalmitis, and spontaneous bacterial peritonitis.[32,252,306,383,409] Occasionally, *N. meningitidis* may be isolated from distant body sites without other clinical evidence of meningitis, meningococcemia, or other foci of meningococcal infection. For example, Baevsky reported a case of primary meningococcal pericarditis with tamponade in an 18-year-old male that was complicated by the development of DIC and both renal and hepatic injury due to cardiac tamponade-induced hypotension.[45] In another case report, *N. meningitidis* serogroup B was isolated from a knee-joint aspirate of an otherwise healthy 13-month-old boy with no other evidence of meningococcal infection.[171] Lastly, *N. meningitidis* is one of a long list of organisms that have been recovered from patients with peritonitis and bacteremia complicating continuous ambulatory peritoneal dialysis.[162]

Meningococcal pneumonia is infrequently seen, but presents primarily as a community-acquired pneumonia that is indistinguishable clinically from other acute bacterial pneumonias.[33,718] The pathogenesis of pneumonia may involve hematogenous dissemination or aspiration followed by direct invasion of the lung parenchyma. This infection occurs primarily in middle-aged to older persons with preexisting illnesses, including viral respiratory tract infections, chronic obstructive pulmonary disease, coronary artery disease, diabetes, HIV infection, and systemic lupus erythematosus.[524,718] In a study of 68 military recruits with meningococcal pneumonia proven by culture of transtracheal aspirates, fever, rales, and lobar infiltrates were common findings.[365] The patients were moderately ill, but there were no fatalities. In a review of 58 cases of community-acquired meningococcal pneumonia over 25 years, blood cultures were found to be positive in 79.3%, although symptoms and sequelae associated with meningococcemia failed to develop in these patients.[718] Sputum cultures were positive in 15 (83.3%) of 18 cases in which sputum specimens were collected, and 5 of the 58 patients died from their infection. The diagnosis of meningococcal pneumonia is complicated by the presence of the organism in the nasopharynx, resulting in oropharyngeal contamination of expectorated sputum specimens. In addition to pneumonia, fulminant bacteremic supraglottitis has been reported in association with serogroup B, C, and Y meningococcal infections.[424,472,588,604] These infections were characterized by sore throat, dysphagia, swollen supraglottic tissues, and cervical cellulitis. Five of the six patients described with this condition required intubation or emergency tracheostomy, indicating that meningococcal supraglottitis is a fulminant, potentially life-threatening infection.

Primary meningococcal conjunctivitis has also been recognized as a distinct clinical entity.[28,510] Most cases of meningococcal conjunctivitis occur as a part of systemic infection with *N. meningitidis,* and systemic meningococcal disease associated with conjunctival infection develops in 10–18% of patients.[50,210] Primary conjunctivitis caused by *N. meningitidis* has been reported in neonates, older children, and adults. In two thirds of cases, the infection is limited to only one eye. In a review of 84 cases of primary meningococcal conjunctivitis, systemic meningococcal disease (i.e., meningitis or meningococcemia) developed in 17.8%; among these patients; the mortality was 13.3%.[50] Systemic infection occurred more frequently among patients who received topical, rather than systemic, antimicrobial therapy; in fact, the risk of systemic disease was almost 20-fold greater for patients receiving topical therapy versus systemic therapy. Complications of the infection that were limited to

the eye included corneal ulcers, keratitis, subconjunctival hemorrhage, and iritis. In a report of three cases of primary meningococcal conjunctivitis in the United Kingdom, meningococcal meningitis developed in a younger sibling of the index case, prompting the authors of this report to suggest that prophylaxis for close contacts of cases of primary meningococcal conjunctivitis is warranted.[618] Saperstein and colleagues also reported a case of exogenous meningococcal endophthalmitis, in which the organism entered the eye via a leaky filtering bleb following cataract surgery instead of via bloodstream dissemination.[575] In addition to infection of the eye, either primarily or secondarily, the development of transient cataracts in conjunction with the onset of rash and fever has been reported in association with meningococcal disease.[286] In 1998, Garcia-Lechuz and colleagues reported the first case of primary meningococcal conjunctivitis in an HIV-1-infected patient.[247]

N. meningitidis may occasionally be isolated from the male urethra, the female genital tract, and the anal canal. In these sites, it may cause infections that are clinically indistinguishable from gonococcal infections, such as acute purulent urethritis, cervicitis, salpingitis, and proctitis.[149,172,317,348,714] Orogenital, anogenital, and oroanal sexual practices are believed to be responsible for the presence of meningococci in these anogenital sites.[291,317,716]

MENINGOCOCCAL PROPHYLAXIS AND MENINGOCOCCAL VACCINES

The risk of secondary meningococcal disease in close household contacts of a primary case of meningitis or meningococcemia is 500- to 800-fold greater than that of the general population.[436] Therefore, it is the standard of practice to provide chemoprophylactic antimicrobial therapy to these contacts as soon after exposure as possible. Secondary cases of meningococcal disease among close contacts of an index case usually occur within 10 days of exposure. Prophylaxis administered 2 weeks or more after exposure is not effective in preventing secondary cases. During the 1940s and 1950s, sulfonamides were effective in eradicating the meningococcal carrier state and in preventing disease. However, during the 1960s, resistance to the sulfonamides developed in *N. meningitidis* strains. High doses of penicillin transiently eliminate meningococci from the nasopharynx, but the organisms rapidly reestablish themselves after treatment is discontinued. Currently, oral rifampin (adults, 600 mg q12h for 2 days; children less than 1 month of age, 5 mg/kg for 2 days; children older than 1 month of age, 10 mg/kg for 2 days) is administered to eradicate carriage, although this drug may fail to eradicate the organisms in 10–20% of carriers.[496] Rapid emergence of rifampin resistance among meningococci has also been noted, even during the time of drug administration. In fact, a case of meningococcal meningitis caused by a rifampin-resistant strain was reported in a child who was receiving prophylactic rifampin at the time of disease onset.[166] Ciprofloxacin (adults, 500 mg single dose) and ofloxacin (400 mg single dose) have also been shown to eradicate nasopharyngeal meningococcal carriage for anywhere from 2 to 5 weeks.[249,256,517] Ceftriaxone, administered as a single intramuscular dose (children, 125 mg; adults, 250 mg) will also eradicate meningococcal carriage for about 2 weeks.[590,600] Azithromycin (500 mg, single dose) has also been shown to eradicate meningococcal carriage in adults.[232] Prophylaxis should be administered to household and day-care center contacts and to anyone intimately exposed to the patients' oral secretions. This may also include individuals who frequently sleep and/or eat in the same dwelling with an index case The latter also includes medical staff members who may have performed cardiopulmonary resuscitation or endotracheal intubation on the index patient. Intimate contacts within closed populations, such as college dormitories, military barracks, and long-term care facilities, should also receive prophylaxis.

Because the virulence of *N. meningitidis* is closely associated with the group-specific capsular polysaccharides of the organism, it has been possible to develop vaccines to protect against meningococcal disease. Univalent group A and group C polysaccharide vaccines have been developed, as has a quadrivalent vaccine incorporating group A, C, Y, and W135 capsular material. These vaccines are able to elicit an immune response in both older children and adults. However, the vaccines are generally poorly immunogenic in children younger than 2 to 3 years of age and induce only short-lived immune responses in older children.[262,344,384,498] In addition, the elicited antibody titer falls fairly rapidly over time.[344] Among infants less than 12 months of age who were vaccinated with group A polysaccharide, a detectable antibody response was maintained for only 12 months, and among children immunized at ages 12 to 17 months, titers were detectable for 2 years. In a recent study done in Montana, only 18% of 1-year-olds, 32% of 2-year-olds, and 50–60% of children aged 4 and 5 years produced bactericidal antibody titers in response to the serogroup C polysaccharide vaccine.[420] In addition, native serogroup C polysaccharide vaccines may induce immunologic hyporesponsiveness (tolerance) when two doses are given during the first 6 months of life.[262] Currently, the quadrivalent vaccine is recommended for individuals at high risk, including those with complement deficiencies or asplenia, travelers to areas that are highly endemic for meningococcal disease, military recruits and individuals living in outbreak situations. The vaccine may also be administered to control outbreaks and for prophylaxis of disease contacts, and it is now increasingly being offered to first-year college students residing in dormitories.[136] The CDC also recommends vaccination of research, industrial, and clinical laboratory personnel who are routinely exposed to meningococci that may become aerosolized. With recent reports of fatal *N. meningitidis* infections in hospital clinical laboratory workers who had handled cultures of meningococci from hospitalized patients, the CDC is considering whether to recommend vaccination for laboratory workers with occupational exposure to *N. meningitidis*.[21,141] In some institutions, the quadrivalent vaccine is being offered to laboratory employees on a voluntary basis. Because of the overall low risk for infection in the United States and the failure to provide lasting immunity, the vaccine is not recommended for use in children.

With the availability of relatively effective vaccines for meningococcal serogroups A, C, Y, and W135, and the conjugate vaccine against *H. influenzae* type b, serogroup B *N. meningitidis* has become the major cause of bacterial meningitis worldwide. Polysaccharide vaccines prepared from group B strains are poorly immunogenic both in children and adults. This lack of antigenicity results from the close resemblance of the group B capsular material to antigens found in human brain tissue; the capsule is recognized as "self" by the immune system, so there is no immune response to the group B organism's capsular material.[231] The immune response that does occur is transient and consists predominantly of IgM.[15] Efforts to develop group B vaccines have focused on the organism's OMP antigens. The OMPs of group B meningococci are immunogenic in both children and adults, but this immunity was demonstrated to be suboptimal in a double-blind placebo-controlled study.[241] To complicate matters, immunity to group B OMPs is type-specific rather than group-specific, so any potential vaccine would have to include the OMPs of several group B serotypes and subserotypes involved in disease production. Another approach is to modify the structure of the serogroup B capsular polysaccharide by replacing *N*-acetyl groups of the sialic acid material with *N*-propionyl groups before conjugation to protein. In this regard, a candidate serogroup B meningococcal vaccine (Npr-GBMP-rPorB) containing a modified polysaccharide (*N*-propionylated-polysialic acid-group B meningococcal polysaccharide, [NPr-GMBP]) conjugated to a recombinant class 3 carrier protein (rPorB) has been developed that is highly immunogenic and safe for human use.[244]

A few serogroup B meningococcal vaccines have been developed and field tested in parts of the world with high rates of both epidemic and endemic disease.[67,443,452] In an attempt to control an epidemic of group B disease in greater São Paolo State, Brazil, a Cuban-produced vaccine was given to over 2 million children aged 3 months to 6 years during 1989 and 1990. This vaccine, called the Cuban BC vaccine, consisted of purified, LOS-depleted, serogroup B OMPs of molecular weight 65 to 95 kDa. Purified group C polysaccharide was also included to provide protection against group C meningococci and to help solubilize the group B proteins. As reported with earlier group B vaccines, efficacy varied by age of the vaccinees. Among children 48 months and older, 74% had a protective immune response, whereas only 37% of children younger than 24 months of age had an effective immune response to the vaccine. In Norway, a group B vaccine efficacy trial was conducted using a vaccine containing group B polysaccharide, serotype (class 3) and subserotype (class 1) protein antigens, and LOS immunotype antigens.[67] Vaccine recipients were 171,800 persons 13 to 21 years of age. The vaccine demonstrated only 57.2% efficacy in preventing meningococcal disease.

In order to increase the immunogenicity of both the type B capsular antigens and OMPs and the native capsular polysaccharides of the other meningococcal serogroups, conjugate vaccines are being developed and investigated.[11,15,509] Some serogroup B conjugate vaccines either fail to induce an immune response or induce bactericidal antibodies that do not react with the native group polysaccharide.[324,325] However, when the polysaccharide is conjugated to a carrier protein via an adipic dihydrazide (ADH) linkage, an immune response can be detected against the group B polysaccharide, the carrier protein, and the epitope that is created by the ADH linkage.[53] Conjugate serogroup A and C meningococcal vaccines have also been developed and field tested. Conjugate vaccines prepared against serogroups A and C contain the polysaccharide conjugated to a protein like tetanus toxoid or CRM$_{197}$.[219,532,669] Serogroup C conjugate vaccines induced levels of bactericidal antibodies that were twofold higher in titer than those obtained with the native polysaccharide, while no differences in titers were observed between those engendered by the serogroup A conjugate vaccine and the native group A polysaccharide.[391] In addition, when children who were previously vaccinated with either the serogroup C conjugate or serogroup C native polysaccharide vaccine were revaccinated with the serogroup C conjugate vaccine, those who received the conjugate vaccine initially developed significantly higher anti–serogroup C antibody responses.[380] On the other hand, no difference in the anamnestic response on revaccination with a serogroup A conjugate vaccine was observed in children who had received either the native group A polysaccharide vaccine or the serogroup A polysaccharide conjugate vaccine.[497] A recent trial of a meningococcal capsular group C-CRM$_{197}$ (mutant diphtheria toxin) conjugate vaccine on 182 healthy infants found that the vaccine was safe, immunogenic, and resulted in immunologic memory when given along with other vaccines for infants at 2, 3 and 4 months of age.[408] Another approach to vaccine development involves the use of other antigens that are not part of the outer-membrane complex. For example, the meningococcal transferrin-binding proteins Tbp-1 and Tbp-2, which are expressed by meningococci during growth in vivo, are immunogenic in mice, and sera from eight patients convalescing from meningococcal disease caused by group A, B, and C *N. meningitidis* reacted immunologically with the Tbp-2 protein purified from both the homologous strain and representative heterologous strains.[17]

Other *Neisseria* Species

Neisseria lactamica is an organism that is of special concern because it is able to grow on selective media for gonococci and meningococci and must be differentiated from them. *N. lactamica* is found more frequently in the oropharynges of children than in adults. In a study of 2,969 infants and children, Gold and associates found that the carriage rates of *N. lactamica* increased from 3.8% at 3 months of age to a peak rate of 21% at 18 months of age, followed by a decrease to 1.8% by ages 14 to 17 years.[261] These same workers also demonstrated that carriage of *N. lactamica* may stimulate the production of bactericidal antibodies against *N. meningitidis* groups A, B, and C because of antigenic cross-reactivity between the two organisms.[261] *N. lactamica* has been isolated as a rare cause of meningitis and sepsis in both adults and children; the adult case was associated with a fracture of the cribriform plate.[181,376] This organism has been associated with recurrent otitis media and with septicemia in a 7-year-old child during immunosuppressive therapy for acute lymphocytic leukemia.[483,580] *N. lactamica* also has been recovered from the female genital tract in association with a persistent vaginal discharge.[647] Penicillin-resistant strains of *N. lactamica* contain an altered penicillin-binding protein (PBP 2) that is similar to the PBP 2 found in relatively penicillin-resistant strains of *N. meningitidis,* suggesting that commensal species like *N. lactamica* (and *N. polysaccharea*) are the source of genetic resistance determinants currently being found in meningococci.[405,565]

Neisseria subflava (biovars *flava, subflava,* and *perflava*), *N. mucosa, N. sicca,* and *N. flavescens* have been reported most frequently as uncommon causes of native and prosthetic-valve endocarditis.[22,31,176,293,393,400,602,676] With native-valve endocarditis, cardiac structural abnormalities caused by past infections (e.g., rheumatic fever) or prior surgery are frequently present. In some reports, the use of intravenous drugs was a significant risk factor for endocarditis, because oral secretions may be used to dissolve drugs or to clean the skin before injection.[176,676] In a recent case, *N. mucosa* endocarditis developed in a 20-year-old woman with no history of cardiac disease after having her tongue pierced one month prior to the onset of symptoms.[664] Myocardial abscess formation has also been documented as a complication of *N. mucosa* endocarditis.[226] In addition to endocarditis, these normally saprophytic organisms have been isolated from other significant infections. *N. subflava* has been isolated from joint fluid of a child with septic arthritis, from Bartholin's gland abscesses, and as a cause of bacteremia and meningitis primarily in compromised hosts.[46,180,199,479] At the University of Illinois, a *N. subflava* bv. *perflava* strain was repeatedly recovered from urine cultures of a 10-year-old boy with congenital structural abnormalities of the urinary bladder.[321] *N. subflava* bv. *perflava* peritonitis has also been reported as a complication of chronic ambulatory peritoneal dialysis.[692] *N. mucosa* has been isolated as an unusual cause of meningitis, pulmonary abscesses, ocular infections, arthritis, bursitis, crepitant cellulitis, dialysis-related bacteremia, and continuous ambulatory peritoneal dialysis-associated peritonitis.[4,118,259,307,395,407,628] *N. sicca* has been isolated as a rare cause of pneumonia, bronchiectasis, meningitis in compromised hosts, CSF shunt infection, sinusitis, osteomyelitis, septic arthritis/bursitis, Bartholin's gland abscess, and peritonitis in patients maintained on long-term peritoneal dialysis.[59,193,251,258,273,281,304,448,473,576] *N. subflava* bv. *perflava* and *N. sicca* have also been isolated from blood cultures of patients with end-stage HIV disease.[455] These organisms may present therapeutic dilemmas because some isolates may be penicillin-resistant because of elaboration of β-lactamase enzymes or altered penicillin binding proteins. In these cases, the isolates must be identified as to species, and antimicrobial susceptibility tests should be performed.

Neisseria cinerea is a saprophytic species of the upper respiratory tract that is of particular interest because of its cultural resemblance to *N. gonorrhoeae,* its occasional recovery from genital sites, and its association with syndromes similar to those caused by gonococci, such as ophthalmia neonatorum and proctitis.[42,85,91,201,357,361] *N cinerea* has also been recovered as the cause of nosocomial pneumonia in a patient with AIDS and as a cause of lymphadenitis.[92,157] *N. cinerea* bacteremia has been documented in a child with pneumonia and otitis media, in an alcoholic male with intra-abdominal disease, in a patient receiving hemodialysis, and in a 17-year-old male following a fist fight in which he suffered significant facial trauma.[327,349,610] In the latter case, the organism was also recovered from the CSF. *N. cinerea* has also been isolated from cases of purulent conjunctivitis, ophthalmia neonatorum, and peritonitis associated with chronic ambulatory peritoneal dialysis (CAPD).[40,85,198,253]

The ''species'' *N. gonorrhoeae* subspecies *kochii* (or *N. kochii*) has been isolated from patients with conjunctivitis in rural Egypt; no isolates have been described from the United States.[426] *N. polysaccharea* is found in the upper respiratory tract of about 0.5% of individuals and has not been described as part of a pathologic process.[84,111,538] *N. canis, N. denitrificans, N iguanae,* and *N. dentiae* are animal strains isolated from the oral cavity and upper respiratory tracts of cats, guinea pigs, iguanae, and cows, respectively.[51,608] *N. canis* has been recovered from human wounds resulting from cat bites.[279,566]

The rod-shaped members of the genus *Neisseria* include the three subspecies of *N. elongata* (subsp. *elongata,* subsp. *glycolytica,* and subsp. *nitroreducens*) and *N. weaveri.*[25,26,89,268,299] Up until 1990, *N. elongata* included only two subspecies, *N. elongata* subsp. *elongata* and *N. elongata* subsp. *glycolytica.* These organisms are normally found in the human upper respiratory tract. Neither of these subspecies had been implicated in human infections until 1995, when *N. elongata* subsp. *glycolytica* was isolated from wound specimens of three patients and from blood cultures of a 57-year-old man with subacute bacterial endocarditis and aortic insufficiency.[26] In 1996, Nawaz and colleagues reported another case of endocarditis caused by *N. elongata* subsp. *elongata* that was complicated by a ruptured mycotic aneurysm of the right brachial artery.[470] *N. elongata* subsp. *nitroreducens* was formerly called CDC group M-6.[268] This ''moraxella-like'' bacterium was shown to be related to the *Neisseria* species in general and to *N. elongata* subspecies in particular on the basis of genetic studies, cellular fatty acid composition, and phenotypic properties. *N. elongata* subsp. *nitroreducens* is found normally in the oropharynx of humans and has been reported as an opportunistic agent of bacteremia and endocarditis and as a cause of osteomyelitis following oral surgery.[200,268,295,437,631,721] This organism has also been isolated from urine and appendiceal tissue.[268] *N. weaveri,* a rod-shaped organism that was formerly called CDC group M-5, is part of the upper respiratory tract flora of dogs and cats and may be isolated from human wounds and blood cultures associated with animal bites.[25,116,299] In 2002, *N. weaveri* was isolated from bronchial washings and sputum of a 60-year-old male with bronchiectasis and from a wound infection in a 7-year-old girl following a tiger bite.[113,492]

Clinical Significance of Moraxella catarrhalis

During the past 10 years, the organism formerly called ''*Neisseria catarrhalis,*'' then ''*Branhamella catarrhalis,*'' and now *M. catarrhalis* has received a great deal of attention as an emerging human pathogen.[213,341] Prior to 1990, *M. catarrhalis* was thought to be a part of the normal human upper respiratory tract flora; over the years this assertion was made in many textbooks and case reports without any supporting evidence. Studies by Vaneechoutte and colleagues and Knapp and Hook have shown that the organism is found in the upper respiratory tracts of only about 1.5–5.4% of healthy adults and actually is more common in the respiratory tracts of healthy children (50.8%) and elderly adults (26.5%).[357,686] A subsequent study from Denmark also found that *M. catarrhalis* was not a significant member of the nasopharyngeal flora of adults and was rarely present

in children younger than 1 month of age.[209] However, 36% of children aged 1 to 48 months had *M. catarrhalis* as a part of their respiratory tract flora, and, in this same age group, the prevalence of *M. catarrhalis* in children with respiratory tract infections was 68%. A study of nasopharyngeal colonization with *M. catarrhalis* during the first 2 years of life showed that 66% of 120 serially cultured children become colonized during the first year and that 77.5% were colonized by the end of the second year.[217] This study also found that, in individual children, three to four different strains of *M. catarrhalis* were acquired and subsequently cleared during the first 2 years of life. Higher colonization rates have also been seen in preschool children with asthma (70%) than in healthy children (33%).[594] Among healthy adults, the colonization rate of *M. catarrhalis* is about 4%, which is indicative of the lower infection rates seen in adults compared with children.[332] When isolated from adults with respiratory tract disease, the organism is more frequently found in specimens judged to represent lower respiratory tract secretions than in those specimens determined to have large amounts of oropharyngeal contamination. Increased rates of respiratory tract colonization in adults are associated with chronic bronchitis, bronchiectasis, and chronic obstructive pulmonary disease.[461,734] Among adults with chronic airway disease who were followed over a 27-month period, Klingman and colleagues found that 42.9% were colonized with *M. catarrhalis* and that each patient was colonized with one to four different strains, each strain persisting for about 2.3 months.[351] Among patients with chronic bronchitis examined in Buffalo, New York, colonization rates for *M. catarrhalis* exceeded 10%.[461] The more frequent recovery of this organism from the respiratory tracts of children and elderly patients with chronic respiratory disease supports its role in certain childhood infections and in lower respiratory tract infections in older individuals.

Infections of the respiratory tract and adjacent anatomic areas account for the majority of clinical conditions involving *M. catarrhalis* as the etiologic agent. These infections include otitis media, sinusitis, bronchitis, and pneumonia.[213,341,367,414,688] Although otitis media caused by this organism may occur in any age group, most studies have centered on this organism's role in pediatric infection. In a study by Van Hare and coworkers, *M. catarrhalis* was the only bacterial pathogen isolated from middle ear fluid of 40 (11%) of 355 children with acute otitis media and was coisolated with either *H. influenzae* or *Streptococcus pneumoniae* in 21 (6%) of the patients.[688] In vitro studies have shown that *M. catarrhalis* strains demonstrate increased adherence to nasopharyngeal epithelial cells of otitis-prone children than to cells from non-otitis-prone children.[623] Serial culture studies of otitis-prone children over the first 2 years of life have also shown that these children have consistently higher rates of colonization with *M. catarrhalis* than other children.[217] In addition, serologic studies have indicated that children with otitis media due to *M. catarrhalis* produce antibodies against a variety of *M. catarrhalis* protein antigen (e.g. UspA, TpbB, and CopB) and LOS (Box 11-4).[423] These antigens are being investigated as candidates for vaccine development particularly for the pediatric age group. The bacteriologic findings with acute otitis media are mirrored in studies of acute sinusitis in the same age groups. In carefully

Box 11-4 Virulence Factors and Virulence-Associated Antigens of *Moraxella catarrhalis*

Virulence Factors and Antigens	Comments
Lipooligosaccharide	Studies using monoclonal antibodies have demonstrated that the LOS structure of *M. catarrhalis* is relatively conserved. Vaneechoutte and colleagues analyzed 302 *M. catarrhalis* strains and identified three LOS serotypes—designated A, B, and C—with LOS-directed monoclonal antibodies.[685] LOS serotypes A, B, and C accounted for 61.3%, 28.8%, and 5.3%, respectively, of the 302 strains examined. Gu and coworkers prepared a conjugate LOS vaccine by linking a serotype A LOS to either tetanus toxoid or to high-molecular-weight OMPs from nontypeable *H. influenzae* and tested these vaccines in mice.[274] Interestingly, antibodies having complement-dependent bactericidal activity developed in the mice. Theoretically, LOS conjugate vaccines prepared with the three LOS serotypes should provoke antibody responses that would have efficacy in preventing infections with at least 90% of strains. Potential problems with vaccines containing LOS components include the need for prior detoxification of the LOS and the development of a conjugative method that would not alter the necessary LOS antigenicity.
Fimbriae (Pili)	Fimbriae have been demonstrated in some strains of *M. catarrhalis*. Electron micrographs of piliated strains show surface fibrils that are 20 to 146 nm in length.[12] A gene probe directed against the type 4 pili of *Moraxella bovis* hybridized with genomic DNA of four *M. catarrhalis* strains, thereby reinforcing the close genetic relationship of *M. catarrhalis* to the other moraxellae.[415] Class 4 pili are also found on the pathogenic *Neisseria*, *Pseudomonas aeruginosa*, and *Vibrio cholerae*. Like the fimbriae of other organisms, those of *M. catarrhalis* apparently function as adhesins, and a specific glycosphingolipid fimbrial receptor has been identified on respiratory epithelial cells.[13]
Hemagglutinins	Hemagglutinins produced by *M. catarrhalis* are believed to contribute to adherence. The most well-defined hemagglutinin is a 200-kDa protein that binds to the glycolipid globotriaosylceramide.[234] This hemagglutinin is serologically variable, and little is known about its antigenicity or its potential for eliciting bactericidal or opsonizing antibodies. Hemagglutinins are not found on all strains. Isolates that express hemagglutinin are isolated more frequently from infected rather than from colonized patients, and there is a relationship between hemagglutinin expression and resistance to the bactericidal activity of normal human serum.[460]
Outer Membrane Proteins	
UspA proteins	Two bacterial surface proteins called UspA1 and UspA2 have been identified in *M. catarrhalis*. These proteins were initially thought to be a single protein because of the presence of a conserved domain in each that reacted with the same monoclonal antibody and comigration in sodium dodecyl sulfate–polyacrylamide-gel electrophoresis (SDS-PAGE).[432] *UspA1* and *UspA2* loci share a high degree of sequence homology and encode for proteins that have conserved and semiconserved domains.[167] The conserved N-terminal domains are recognized with the same monoclonal antibody, while the C-terminal domains set the two proteins apart and contain their unique functional regions. UspA proteins are found in all strains, although their molecular weights may vary from strain to strain. UspA1 is about 88 kDa in molecular weight and is an adhesin, since UspA1 mutants cannot adhere to epithelial cells, and anti-UspA1 antibodies block cellular adherence.[7,432] UspA1 also binds the host extracellular matrix protein, fibronectin. The UspA2 protein influences resistance to nonimmune sera, plays a role in mediating mucosal adherence, and binds to the host protein vitronectin, a regulator of the complement system.[373] Immunization of mice or guinea pigs with either protein results in the formation of antibodies that are bactericidal for both the homologous *M. catarrhalis* challenge strain and heterologous strains.[432] Sera from healthy adults contain high titers of bactericidal anti-UspA antibodies, whereas children ages 6 to 36 months have low titers.[147] These data, plus studies in animals, lend support to ongoing investigations of the UspA proteins as *M. catarrhalis* vaccine candidate antigens.[430,431]
CD protein	CD protein of *M. catarrhalis* is a conserved, 45-kDa integral OMP that functions as a porin protein.[462] CD may act as a virulence factor by specifically binding to nasal and middle ear mucins, but not to salivary mucins.[523] Mucins are complex glycoproteins, and binding of these molecules to the CD protein may facilitate attachment and transport of the microorganisms into the middle ear via the eustachian tube, where the organism can cause otitis media. Immunization of mice with purified or recombinant CD proteins engenders a strong antibody response that results in clearance of both homologous and heterologous *M. catarrhalis* organisms from the respiratory tract on challenge.[463] The immune mechanisms involved in organism clearance from the respiratory tract are not well understood since anti-CD antibodies lack complement-dependent bactericidal activity and are not opsonins. Clearance of the organisms may result from inhibition of mucin binding by the surface-associated CD protein.

Box 11-4 *Continued*

Virulence Factors and Antigens	Comments
LpbA and LpbB proteins	LpbA and LpbB are lactoferrin binding proteins of molecular weights 111 kDa and 99 kDa, respectively, that extract iron from lactoferrin when the organisms are grown under iron-limiting conditions.[76] These proteins are related to lactoferrin binding proteins of *Neisseria* species, and are highly conserved among different *M. catarrhalis* strains. Following human infection, antibodies against LbpB, but not LpbA, are detected, suggesting that the LpbA is not exposed on the organism surface.[732] LbpB is being further characterized as a possible vaccine antigen.
TbpA and TbpB proteins	TbpA and TbpB are transferrin binding proteins with molecular weights of 105 kDa and 74 kDa, respectively.[107,148,732] Like the lactoferrin binding proteins, these proteins have homology with similar proteins found in neisseriae, haemophili, and other bacteria. Purified or recombinant TbpA elicits bactericidal antibodies in animals, but only against the homologous strain. Antibodies against TbpA are not produced following natural infection in humans.[732] In mice, TbpB (also called B1 and 74K protein) stimulates production of antibodies that react with homologous and, to some extent, with heterologous strains, as evidenced by Western immunoblot analysis.[107,148] Sequencing of the TbpB protein from various strains has documented sequence identities ranging from 50 to 70%. Variations in immune responses to TbpB proteins from different *M. catarrhalis* strains is also evidenced by differences in complement-dependent bactericidal activity and in the efficacy of pulmonary clearance on respiratory challenge with *M. catarrhalis* in mice.[148,464] In humans, antibodies against TbpB react with both homologous and heterologous strains, but lack complement-dependent bactericidal activity.
CopB protein	The CopB protein is an 81-kDa, surface-exposed integral OMP that is conserved among strains of *M. catarrhalis* and is encoded by the *copB* gene.[8] This protein is homologous with the FrpB protein found in the neisseriae and functions in iron acquisition for growth and metabolism. Studies with monoclonal antibodies against different CopB epitopes of various *M. catarrhalis* strains indicate that there are at least two CopB serotypes.[6] Differences also exist in the bactericidal responses of mice immunized with monoclonal antibodies against the CopB protein from different *M. catarrhalis* strains.[598] This is surprising given that the CopB antigens from different strains have 97% homology in their amino acid sequences. Differences in antibody responses may be due to limited exposure of key antigen epitopes on the cell surface.[6]
E protein	E protein is a 47- to 50-kDa outer-membrane protein of uncertain function, although it may assist in the transport of fatty acids into the cell.[64] Using a specific anti-E monoclonal antibody called 1B3, at least two E protein serotypes have been defined, as evidenced by reactivity of 82% of strains with this reagent. E proteins from strains of *M. catarrhalis* that failed to react with 1B3 still have 97% sequence homology with 1B3-reactive strains, indicating that E protein serotypes are highly conserved. Infection with *M. catarrhalis* results in the formation of anti-E protein antibodies, but their biologic activity and functionality have not been investigated.

collected maxillary sinus aspirates from children with acute sinusitis, *M. catarrhalis* may be isolated in either pure or mixed cultures from 2–16% of patients.[414] Acute sinus infections in adults have also been associated with this organism but with less frequency than in children. Despite its involvement in otitis media and sinusitis in children, *M. catarrhalis* is an uncommon cause of community-acquired lower respiratory tract infection in this age group.[155] In children with pneumonia, *M. catarrhalis* may behave as a primary pathogen or as a secondary pathogen superimposed on an antecedent viral infection (e.g., respiratory syncytial virus).[225] On rare occasions, *M. catarrhalis* may cause fulminant tracheitis and lower respiratory tract disease in apparently healthy children.[601,603]

Lower respiratory tract infections due to *M. catarrhalis* in adults occur predominantly in elderly and immunocompromised patients, particularly those with chronic obstructive pulmonary disease, bronchiectasis, congestive heart fail-

ure, and predisposition to aspiration.[151,428,461] Immunologic abnormalities because of underlying diseases (e.g., diabetes, alcoholism, HIV infection, transplantation) are also important contributory factors.[413,595] In adults, *M. catarrhalis* is most often associated with clinical findings of acute bronchitis, with pneumonia being seen less often.[331] Patients with bronchitis present with increasing production of purulent sputum and mild respiratory distress without fever. Pneumonic involvement is heralded by the appearance of low-grade fever, dyspnea, and production of increasing amounts of purulent sputum. Progression to respiratory failure has been observed in some patients. Radiologically, the disease usually appears as patchy infiltrates in both lungs, although lobar involvement with and without subpleural abscess formation has also been documented.[208] Epiglottitis caused by *M. catarrhalis* has been reported as a complication of acute myeloid leukemia in a 65-year-old diabetic man.[693] *M. catarrhalis* bacteremia has been reported as a complication of respiratory tract infections. Most cases of pediatric *M. catarrhalis* bacteremia occur secondary to otitis media, sinusitis, or pneumonia in patients who are immunocompromised due to acute lymphoblastic leukemia, acute myeloid leukemia, lymphoma, AIDS, hypogammaglobulinemia, sickle cell disease, prematurity, and congenital neurologic abnormalities.[5,312,438,485] In a review of 53 cases of *M. catarrhalis* bacteremias, neutropenia and/or malignancy was present in 30.2% of patients and 24.5% had underlying respiratory tract disease.[312] However, 28.3% of the cases occurred in immunocompetent individuals. Bacteremia in adults may result from a primary focus, such as sinusitis or pneumonia, but in immunocompromised patients, the portal of entry may not be apparent.[485]

M. catarrhalis has also been isolated from patients with endocarditis, meningitis, eye infections, urogenital tract infections, wound infections, septic arthritis, nosocomial respiratory tract infections, and continuous ambulatory peritoneal dialysis-associated peritonitis.[105,163,194,269,406,434,475,531] Endocarditis has been reported in healthy individuals without prior valvular disease, in immunosuppressed patients with underlying conditions (e.g., leukemia, lymphoma, immunoglobulin deficiency states, AIDS), and following various types of invasive procedures (e.g., balloon angioplasty).[569,574,620,722] Rare cases of *M. catarrhalis* meningitis and ventriculitis have also occurred following surgical procedures involving the head and neck or from infected ventriculoperitoneal shunts or external ventricular drains.[164,465,556] Viagappan and colleagues reported an unusual case of *M. catarrhalis* brain abscess in a 36-year-old male following a penetrating orbital injury with a pool cue and fatal neonatal meningitis was described in a 26-day-old infant 2 weeks after undergoing abdominal surgery.[173,694] Conjunctival infections caused by *M. catarrhalis* have been documented in both the neonatal period and later in childhood. *M. catarrhalis* scleral buckle infections, endophthalmitis secondary to glaucoma filtering surgery, and periorbital cellulitis with sepsis have been documented in patients.[105,396,663] Ophthalmia neonatorum caused by *M. catarrhalis* results either from acquisition of the organism at birth from the mother's colonized genital tract or from respiratory tract secretions of the child's caretakers. Recovery of this organism from the male or female genital tract is rare, but *M. catarrhalis* has been reported as a cause of a gonorrhea-like urethritis in a few cases.[194] Nosocomially acquired pneumonia due to *M. catarrhalis* may occur in hospital respiratory units and pediatric intensive care units.[163,531]

Isolation of Neisseria *Species*
Neisseria gonorrhoeae

DIRECT GRAM-STAINED SMEARS

In sexually transmitted disease clinics the diagnosis of gonococcal urethritis in adult males is frequently made by the observation of gram-negative diplococci within or closely associated with polymorphonuclear leukocytes on a smear prepared from the urethral discharge (see Color Plate 11-1*A*). When properly performed, the Gram stain has a sensitivity of 90–95% and a specificity of 95–100% for diagnosing genital gonorrhea in symptomatic men.[350] In females, Gram stains of endocervical specimens collected

under direct visualization of the cervix (i.e., with a speculum in place) may also be very helpful in diagnosis (see section on "Specimen Collection"). Gram-stained smears of such specimens have a sensitivity of 50–70%, depending on the adequacy of the specimen and the patient population. An endocervical smear showing gram-negative intracellular diplococci, particularly from a woman with other signs and symptoms of gonococcal infection, is highly predictive.[401] In asymptomatic women, however, the predictive value of the Gram stain is much lower. In patients with symptomatic proctitis, smears collected under direct visualization through an anoscope may provide a diagnosis in 70–80% of such patients, as opposed to blind collection, where gram-stained smears have a sensitivity of only 40–60%.[715] Gram-stained smears have no value in the diagnosis of pharyngeal gonococcal infection. Gram-stained smears should not be relied on for diagnosis of gonorrhea and should be used adjunctively along with more specific tests.

Direct smears for Gram stain should be prepared from urethral and endocervical sites and should be collected with a separate swab. For smear preparation, the swab is rolled gently over the surface of a glass slide in one direction only. This technique minimizes distortion and breakage of polymorphonuclear (PMNs) leukocytes and preserves the characteristic appearance of the microorganisms (Color Plate 11-1*A*). Smears prepared from specimens submitted in transport media may be more difficult to interpret because of distortion of the PMNs or to interfering substances (e.g., charcoal). Smears from normally sterile or minimally contaminated sites (e.g., joint fluid, skin lesions) should also be prepared.

SPECIMEN COLLECTION

As with other pathogenic microorganisms, successful isolation depends on the collection of proper specimens, and this is particularly important for the recovery of *N. gonorrhoeae*. Because this organism can cause infection at a variety of body sites, collection of appropriate specimens for culture and diagnosis is dependent on the sex and sexual practices of the patient and on the clinical presentation. In all cases, specimens from genital sites (male urethra, female endocervix) should be collected. If the patient has a history of orogenital or anogenital sexual contacts, collection of oropharyngeal or anal canal specimens is also appropriate. In suspected cases of disseminated gonococcal infection, blood cultures and specimens from genital and extragenital sites should be obtained. Appropriate sites for culture are summarized in Table 11-1.

Specimens should be collected with Dacron or Rayon swabs. The calcium alginate used to prepare some swab lots may be toxic to gonococci.[377] Cotton swabs may also be used; however, some brands of cotton contain fatty acids that may be inhibitory for gonococci. Therefore, calcium alginate and cotton swabs should be used only if the specimens are inoculated directly onto growth media or are transported in nonnutritive transport media. Some transport medium formulations contain charcoal to inactivate toxic materials present in the swab material or in the specimen itself. Instruments used to aid in the proper collection of specimens (e.g., vaginal specula) should be lubricated with warm water or saline because various water- and oil-based

Table 11-1 Body Sites to Culture for *Neisseria gonorrhoeae*

PATIENT	PRIMARY SITE(S)	SECONDARY SITE(S)
Female	Endocervix	Rectum, urethra, pharynx
Male, heterosexual	Urethra	Pharynx
Male, homosexual/ bisexual	Urethra, rectum, pharynx	
Female, disseminated infection	Blood, endocervix, rectum	Pharynx, skin lesions,* joint fluid†
Male, disseminated infection	Blood, urethra	Pharynx, rectum, skin lesions, joint fluid†

* If present.
† Culture if arthritis present.

lubricants may also inhibit organism growth. Box 11-5 describes collection procedures for the recovery of *N. gonorrhoeae* from different anatomic sites.

The role of the clinical microbiology laboratory in diagnosing gonococcal infections in children is crucial and involves the proper handling of appropriately collected specimens and the accurate identification of isolated organisms.[30,153,712] In the case of prepubertal females, specimens should be obtained from the vagina or urethra, the oropharynx, and the rectum and inoculated onto media as described below. In male children, urethral, oropharyngeal and rectal swab specimens should be collected and inoculated onto growth media.

SPECIMEN TRANSPORT

Although maximal recovery of gonococci is obtained when specimens are plated directly onto growth medium after collection, this technique might not always be possible or practical, particularly in busy clinics or hospital emergency rooms.[398] For these situations, various transport systems are available:

Non-Nutritive Swab Transport Systems. Stuart's or Amies' buffered semisolid transport media are used for transport of swab specimens for *N. gonorrhoeae*. These media are readily available in most clinic and hospital settings and require no special equipment or storage conditions.[218] However, specimens sent to the laboratory in swab transport systems must be kept at room temperature and processed as soon after collection as possible. In 1997, Perry and colleagues performed a study on the quantitative recovery of *N. gonorrhoeae* using two swab transport systems—Copan swabs (Copan Diagnostics, Inc., Corona, CA; now marketed as BBL CultureSwab Plus, BD Biosciences, Sparks, MD) and Starswab swabs (Starplex Scientific, Etobicoke, Ontario, Canada)—containing liquid Stuart's transport medium.[501] In these systems, the swab is in contact with either a polyurethane (Copan) or a cellulose (Starplex) sponge that is soaked in Stuart's medium. These investigators found that quantitative recovery of *N. gonorrhoeae* decreased by 30% in the Copan system and by 100% in the Starswab system after 4 hours of incubation at room temperature. The authors pointed out that sponge materials in some swab transport systems may contain substances (e.g., sulfur, quaternary am-

Box 11-5 Specimen Collection Procedures for Diagnosis of Gonococcal Infections

Specimen	Collection Procedure
Male urethra	Purulent discharge may be expressed by stripping the penis anteriorly and collecting the material on a swab. Specimens from asymptomatic males are obtained by inserting a calcium alginate nasopharyngeal swab 2–3 cm into the urethra. The swab is gently rotated as it is withdrawn.
Endocervix	After the speculum is in place, remove any cervical mucus with cotton or gauze. Insert the swab and collect the specimen with a gentle side-to-side motion. Allow time for the organisms to adsorb onto the swab surface. Sample any cervical discharge present.
Rectum	Insert the swab 4–5 cm into the anal canal and gently move it from side to side to sample the anal crypts. Allow a few seconds for the organisms to adsorb onto the swab, and gently rotate the swab during withdrawal. If heavy fecal contamination is observed on the swab, collect another specimen with a fresh swab.
Oropharynx	With the aid of a tongue depressor, firmly swab the tonsillar areas and the posterior pharynx.
Blood	After venipuncture, inoculate suitable blood culture media (tryptic soy broth, Columbia broth) containing sodium polyanetholsulfonate (SPS). If SPS Vacutainer tubes are used for blood collection, transfer the blood specimen from the tube into blood culture medium as soon as possible, because exposure to high concentrations of SPS may be inhibitory to gonococci.
Joint fluid	Joint fluid should be aspirated with a needle and syringe and inoculated into an aerobic blood culture bottle.
Skin lesions	Punch biopsy specimens are collected and placed in a sterile container with a small amount of broth or sterile saline and hand-carried to the laboratory.
Conjunctivae	Collect conjunctival discharge from the inner aspect of the lower eyelid with a small nasopharyngeal swab. Prepare smears for Gram stains as described in the text.

monium compounds) that may inhibit or injure fastidious organisms. Although these problems have been addressed by the transport system manufacturer since publication of these studies, the importance of reliable collection devices for maintenance of organism viability has implications for other organisms and specimens beyond those collected for isolation of *N. gonorrhoeae.*

The nature of the transport medium is also central to the recovery of *N. gonorrhoeae* and other microorganisms. Thompson and French evaluated several commercially available Amies transport media for recovery of 30 fresh clinical isolates of *N. gonorrhoeae* and found that the Amies formulation without charcoal used in Copan Transystem devices (including CultureSwab, manufactured by Copan for Difco) were superior, preserving the viability of 29 of 30 *N. gonorrhoeae* isolates for up to 48 hours or longer.[651] Starswabs and BBL Culturette transport swabs (BD Biosciences) performed poorly, with major declines in organism viability between 24 and 48 hours. In another study, both Copan Amies gel transport media with and without charcoal detected 95% of *N. gonorrhoeae* isolates that were detected by direct specimen plating; Copan medium with charcoal detected 98% of isolates obtained by direct plating after being maintained in the transport medium for 6 hours.[480] Transport systems inoculated with specimens that may contain *N. gonorrhoeae* should be maintained at room temperature, since exposure to extremes in temperature (e.g., refrigeration) will compromise successful recovery of the organism.

Culture Media Transport Systems. Transport of specimens on culture media presents certain advantages, and several systems for this purpose are commercially available. These include JEMBEC (James E. Martin biological environmental chamber) plates containing various formulations of selective media, the Gono-Pak system (BD Biosciences), and the In-Tray GC system (BioMed Diagnostics, Inc., San Jose, CA).[62,184,417] While the Gono-Pak and JEMBEC systems require refrigerated storage prior to use, the sealed InTray system permits storage of the medium at room temperature for up to 1 year. With these systems, media are inoculated with the specimen and placed in an impermeable plastic bag with a bicarbonate-citric acid pellet. Contact of the pellet with moisture (via evaporation from the medium [JEMBEC] or via crushing an ampule of water adjacent to the pellet [Gono-Pak]) generates a CO_2-enriched environment within the bag. Incubation for at least 18 to 24 hours at 35°C prior to transport to a reference laboratory allows initial outgrowth of the organisms and minimizes the loss of viability that may be encountered with swab transport systems.

SELECTIVE CULTURE MEDIA: INOCULATION AND INCUBATION

A variety of enriched selective media for culture of *N. gonorrhoeae* are available and include modified Thayer-Martin (MTM) medium, Martin-Lewis (ML) medium, GC-Lect medium (BD Biosciences), and New York City (NYC) medium. MTM, ML, and GC-Lect are chocolate agar–based media that are supplemented with growth factors for fastidious microorganisms, whereas NYC medium is a clear peptone-cornstarch agar–based medium containing yeast di-

Table 11-2 Antimicrobial Agents in Selective *Neisseria* Media

ANTIMICROBIAL AGENT	MEDIA FORMULATION (μg/ml)			
	MTM	ML	NYC	GC-LECT
Vancomycin	3	4	2	2
Lincomycin	—	—	—	1
Colistin	7.5	7.5	5.5	7.5
Nystatin	12.5	—	—	—
Anisomycin	—	20	—	—
Amphotericin B	—	—	1.2	1.5
Trimethoprim	5	5	5	5

alysate, citrated horse plasma, and lysed horse erythrocytes.[221] These media contain antimicrobial agents that inhibit other microorganisms and allow the selective recovery of *N. gonorrhoeae, N. meningitidis,* and *N. lactamica* (Table 11-2). Vancomycin and colistin, antimicrobials present in all four formulations, inhibit gram-positive and gram-negative bacteria (including saprophytic *Neisseria* species), respectively. GC-Lect agar (BD Biosciences) also contains lincomycin. Trimethoprim is added to inhibit the swarming of *Proteus* species present in rectal and, occasionally, in cervicovaginal specimens. Nystatin, amphotericin B, or anisomycin is added to inhibit yeasts and molds. These media allow selective recovery of *N. gonorrhoeae* from body sites harboring a large endogenous bacterial flora. NYC medium will also support the growth of genital mycoplasmas and ureaplasmas. These media are commercially available in either Petri dishes or JEMBEC plates. The formulas for these media are available in general media references.

Commercially available selective media vary in their ability to support the growth of pathogenic *Neisseria* species and to inhibit growth of nonpathogenic neisseriae and other contaminants.[730] Failure of these various selective media to support gonococcal growth may also be due to the susceptibility of some *N. gonorrhoeae* strains to vancomycin. These strains account for a variable percentage of isolates depending on the geographic area.[730] Because of this, it is prudent to inoculate male and female genital specimens onto both selective (e.g., MTM) and nonselective (chocolate agar) media. Inoculation of nonselective media enable the recovery of other possible genital tract pathogens, such as *Haemophilus* species or *Pasteurella bettyae* (Chapter 9).

Media for isolation of *Neisseria* should be at room temperature before inoculation and should not be excessively dry or moist. If excessive moisture is present on the lid of the plates, place the plates upside down and slightly ajar in an air incubator at 35°C for 20 to 30 minutes. The "stacker plates" (BD Biosciences) tend to seal up if excessive moisture is present, and growth of the organisms is retarded. Specimens collected on swabs are firmly rolled in a "Z" pattern on selective media and cross-streaked with a bacteriologic loop. If nonselective media are also inoculated, these plates are streaked for isolation. The plates are incubated in a CO_2 incubator or a candle extinction jar at 35 to 37°C. The CO_2 level of the incubator should be 3–7%; higher CO_2 concentrations may actually inhibit growth of some strains.

Candle extinction jars achieve a CO_2 level of 3–4%. The atmosphere should be moist and, with candle jars, moisture evaporating from the medium during incubation is usually sufficient for organism growth. CO_2 incubators that are not equipped with humidifiers may be kept moist by placing a pan of water on the lower shelf. If candle jars are used, candles should be made of white wax or bees' wax; scented or colored candles release volatile products during burning and extinction that may inhibit the growth of the organisms. Plates are inspected at 24, 48, and 72 hours before a final report of "no growth" is issued. Suspect colonies are subcultured to chocolate agar, incubated, and used as an inoculum for identification procedures.

Neisseria meningitidis
LABORATORY SAFETY

N. meningitidis is classified as a BioSafety level 2 organism., which means that a biologic safety cabinet must be used for the manipulation of specimens that have a substantial risk for the generation of aerosols (e.g., grinding, centrifuging, vortex mixing). Reports of laboratory-acquired meningococcal infections suggest that manipulation of cultures, rather than specimens, increases the risk of infection for microbiology laboratory technologists and technicians.[21,141,674] Such manipulations include the preparation of heavy organism suspensions for inoculation of identification systems and for serogrouping of meningococcal isolates by slide agglutination. The use of a biologic safety cabinet when manipulating cultures for these purposes would ensure protection of the laboratory worker from aerosolized organisms. Alternative measures for protection (e.g., splash guards, masks) are currently being assessed. Education and adherence to established laboratory safety precautions should minimize the risk of meningococcal infections for clinical microbiology laboratory personnel. Laboratory policies should also be developed for situations that may require administration of prophylaxis to employees who are exposed to meningococci. Laboratory directors may also consider offering the quadrivalent meningococcal vaccine to microbiology laboratory staff. This measure would decrease but not eliminate the potential risk of laboratory-acquired meningococcal infections.

DIRECT GRAM-STAINED SMEARS AND DIRECT CAPSULAR ANTIGEN TESTS

On gram-stained smears prepared from clinical specimens, particularly CSF, meningococci appear as gram-negative diplococci both inside and outside PMNs. Organisms may display considerable size variation and tend to resist decolorization. Heavily encapsulated strains may have a distinct pink halo around the cells. Because the presence of inflammatory cells has prognostic value (e.g., with fulminant, rapidly fatal disease, many organisms and few inflammatory cells are present), the Gram stain report to the physician should include quantitation of both organisms and PMNs.

In addition to Gram stain and culture of the CSF, the laboratory may also perform direct antigen-detection tests for meningococcal capsular polysaccharides.[371] The direct antigen tests use antibody-sensitized latex agglutination or coagglutination to detect capsular antigens of groups A, B, C, Y, and W135. These reagents are available from several vendors (latex tests: Hynson, Westcott, and Dunning, Baltimore MD; Murex Diagnostics, Dartford, U.K.; Coagglutination tests: Boule Diagnostics AB, Huddinge, Sweden). Even though positive test results with these reagents are helpful for early diagnosis, a negative test does not rule out meningitis caused by any of the organisms that commonly occur. These tests should always be performed in conjunction with a Gram stain and culture on enriched agar media.

A recently developed modification of the manual latex agglutination test involves performance of these assays in the presence of an ultrasonic standing wave. Antibody-coated latex particles suspended in the wave are subjected to physical forces that increase particle-to-particle contact, and enhanced agglutination occurs in the presence of antigen, resulting in increased sensitivity. Ultrasound-enhanced latex agglutination for the detection of meningococcal serogroups A, B, C, Y, and W135 has demonstrated increased sensitivity with clinical specimens without any loss in specificity.[49,270] This assay has also been used to enhance the detection of meningococcal polysaccharides in serum and was used to quantitate blood antigen concentrations. In a study by Sobanski et al., as little as 0.05 μg/ml of antigen was detected with the ultrasound-enhanced assay compared with 1.98 μg/ml for the conventional latex agglutination assay, which represents a 30-fold improvement in test sensitivity.[609]

SPECIMEN COLLECTION AND TRANSPORT

Specimens helpful in the diagnosis of meningococcal disease include CSF, blood, aspirates and biopsy specimens, and nasopharyngeal and oropharyngeal swabs. Occasionally, meningococci may be sought in sputum and transtracheal aspirates. Procedures for collection and processing of specimens that may yield *N. meningitidis* are presented in Box 11-6. Genital, rectal, and oropharyngeal isolates of *N. meningitidis* may be recovered using the collection and inoculation procedures described for *N. gonorrhoeae* in Box 11-5. Incubation conditions for media inoculated with specimens are the same as those described for *N. gonorrhoeae* above. Meningococci grow well on all selective media for the pathogenic neisseriae, and vancomycin-susceptible strains have not been described. Contrary to widely held beliefs, most strains of *N. gonorrhoeae* will grow on commercially available sheep blood agar, albeit not as well as on chocolate agar. Recovery of both gonococci and meningococci from blood cultures may be adversely affected by the anticoagulant sodium polyanetholsulfonate (SPS) that is present in blood culture media. This effect may be neutralized by addition of sterile gelatin (1% final concentration) to the media or by processing the blood specimen by lysis-centrifugation (i.e., Isolator).[212,487,593]

ISOLATION AND INCUBATION

For recovery of *N. meningitidis,* CSF specimens should be cultured on nonselective chocolate agar and sheep blood agar as described in Box 11-6, whereas specimens that may harbor other organisms (e.g., oropharyngeal and nasopharyngeal swab specimens) should be inoculated onto both

Box 11-6 Specimen Collection Procedures for Isolation of *Neisseria meningitidis*

Specimen	Collection Procedure
CSF	In cases of suspected meningococcal meningitis, as much spinal fluid as possible (at least 1 mL) should be sent to the laboratory for culture, because small numbers of organisms may be present. The CSF specimen should be hand-carried to the laboratory after collection and must not be refrigerated. An aliquot of the CSF should be cyto-centrifuged for the Gram stain. If sufficient CSF is available, the specimen should be centrifuged and the pellet should be inoculated onto chocolate and blood agar media.
Blood	Blood should be cultured as described for gonococci in Box 11-5. Direct inoculation of blood culture bottles is preferred over SPS Vacutainer tubes owing to the recognized inhibitory effects of SPS on meningococci. This inhibition may be overcome by the addition of 1% (final volume) sterile gelatin to the blood culture media. Use of the Isolator system for blood cultures circumvents the SPS inhibition problem.
Petechiae	Specimens from petechial skin lesions may be collected by injection and aspiration of a small amount of sterile saline at the edge of the lesion, using a tuberculin syringe. Aspirates are cultured directly on chocolate and blood agars. Because some of the lesions are a result of immunologic phenomena, culture of skin lesions may be noncontributory for diagnosis.
Nasopharyngeal swabs	Nasopharyngeal swabs are particularly important for detecting colonization of individuals who are close contacts to cases of meningococcal disease and for carrier surveys. For these specimens, a fine swab on a flexible metal wire (e.g., a calcium alginate nasopharyngeal swab) is passed through to oropharynx and behind the uvula, where the nasopharynx is sampled. Usually, carefully collected throat swabs will provide the same information. These specimens are inoculated onto a selective medium such as MTM.
Biopsies	Biopsy specimens should be hand-carried to the laboratory in sterile containers. Specimens should be moistened with sterile saline or broth and should not be refrigerated. In the laboratory, the specimens should be aseptically teased apart and cultured on chocolate and blood agar.
Aspirates	Aspirates from closed spaces are collected with a needle and syringe. In the laboratory, these specimens are inoculated onto blood and chocolate agar media.

selective (e.g., MTM, Martin-Lewis, NYC, or GC Lect agar) and nonselective media. Plates are incubated in 5–7% CO_2 at 35°C (CO_2 incubator or candle extinction jar) and inspected after 24, 48, and 72 hours before a final report of "no growth" is issued. Suspicious colonies are subcultured to blood and chocolate agar for further identification.

Identification of Neisseria *Species*
Colony Morphology

Gonococci produce several colony types in culture. In Kellogg's scheme, these types are termed T1 through T5 and are described in terms of colony size and other colonial characteristics (coloration, topography of the colonies, reflection of light, and so forth).[345] On the individual cellular level, organisms comprising colony types P$^+$ and P^{++} (formerly T1 and T2, respectively) possess pili on the cell surface, whereas cells in colony type P$^+$ (T3, T4, and T5) lack pili. Isolates obtained on primary cultures are predominantly of the P$^+$ and P^{++} colony types. These colonies tend to be small, glistening, and raised (Color Plate 11-1C). With subculture of individual piliated colonies the culture can be maintained in this colonial type. Organism suspensions prepared from 18- to 24-hour cultures containing primarily P$^+$ and P^{++} colony types tend to be smooth and homogeneous. With nonselective subculture (i.e., a "sweep" of growth), the other colony types will become more evident, with all colonies eventually becoming the nonpiliated varieties.

These types are larger, flatter, and do not have the characteristic glistening highlights of the piliated colony types. Cultures containing predominantly the large colony types frequently do not form smooth suspensions, as the colonies become gummy owing to autolysis and release of cellular DNA. The presence of all of these colony types on a subculture from a primary plate may frequently give the appearance of a mixed culture. Careful scrutiny and subculture with the use of a dissecting microscope (10X) enables one to become familiar with these colony types (Color Plate 11-1D). Variation in colony type is invariably seen with fresh isolates of *N. gonorrhoeae*. Atypical gonococci (i.e., those with multiple nutritional requirements such as the AHU-requiring strains) also produce various colony types, but these develop more slowly and require the use of a dissecting microscope for detection and colony type characterization.[453]

Another descriptive system addresses colony opacity characteristics of gonococci as determined by examination of growth on a transparent medium using magnification and substage illumination. Opaque colonies, regardless of size, are termed O+ and O++, whereas transparent colonies are termed O$^+$. The colonial T types described by Kellogg and coworkers[345] can be recognized on routine MTM or chocolate agar cultures, but appropriate transparent medium for determining the opacity characteristics of the colonies is not routinely available.

Meningococci grow well on both blood and chocolate agars, as well as on the selective media for the pathogenic

Neisseria (Color Plate 11-1*F*). Heavily encapsulated strains of *N. meningitidis* may appear mucoid on agar media. Most meningococcal isolates are grayish and may show a diffuse greening reaction in areas of confluent growth. Some isolates may have a slight yellowish pigmentation. Variation in colony types may be observed with some fresh isolates.

Gram Stain and Oxidase Test

Primary plates for isolation of *N. gonorrhoeae* should be examined after 24, 48, and 72 hours of incubation using a hand lens or, preferably, a dissecting microscope. Smears prepared from suspicious colonies should be examined with the Gram stain, and an oxidase test should be performed. The Gram stain of the colony should show uniform, characteristic gram-negative diplococci. Some of the organisms may appear as tetrads, particularly on smears prepared from young colonies. Organisms on smears prepared from older cultures may appear swollen and display a wide variation in counter-staining intensity. Smears prepared from partially autolyzed colonies may be uninterpretable. Examination by Gram stain is essential for presumptive identification because other organisms may occasionally grow on selective media, particularly from oropharyngeal specimens (discussed below).

Oxidase test results are obtained with the tetramethyl derivative of the oxidase reagent (*N,N,N,N*-tetramethyl-1, 4-phenylenediamine, 1% aqueous solution). This solution is placed on a piece of filter paper and a portion of the colonial growth is rubbed onto the reagent with a platinum loop, a cotton swab, or a wooden applicator stick. With fresh cultures a dark purple color will appear within 10 seconds. Excellent results are obtained with the oxidase reagents that are packaged in crushable glass ampules. (e.g., BACTI-DROP Oxidase, Remel Laboratories).

Superoxol Test

Superoxol is another helpful test for the rapid presumptive identification of *N. gonorrhoeae*.[567] Superoxol is 30% hydrogen peroxide (not the 3% solution routinely used for the catalase test). *N. gonorrhoeae* strains produce immediate, brisk bubbling when some of the colony material is emulsified with the reagent on a glass slide. Both *N. meningitidis* and *N. lactamica,* the other species that grow on selective media, produce weak, delayed bubbling. In a study using this test on organisms recovered on selective media, all 201 gonococci tested produced immediate, vigorous bubbling in Superoxol, whereas 241 of 242 meningococci and one of two *N. lactamica* strains produced negative or delayed, weak positive reactions.[567]

Differentiation of Other Organisms on Selective Media

Both the presumptive and confirmatory identification of *Neisseria* species is dependent on the ability to differentiate these organisms from others that may also grow on selective media. These organisms include *Kingella denitrificans, Moraxella* species (other than *M. catarrhalis*), *Acineto-bacter* species, and *Capnocytophaga* species. *K. denitrificans* grows well on MTM medium and produces colony types that resemble those of *N. gonorrhoeae*.[298] The test that is useful in presumptively identifying gonococci and differentiating them from *K. denitrificans* is the **catalase test.** Gonococci will produce vigorous bubbling when growth from the plate is immersed in 3% hydrogen peroxide (H_2O_2): *K. denitrificans* produces a negative catalase reaction. *M. catarrhalis* and other *Moraxella* species, like gonococci, are oxidase-positive and catalase-positive. These organisms can be differentiated from *Neisseria* by the **penicillin disk test.**[123] The organism is subcultured to a trypticase-soy blood agar plate and streaked as a lawn to obtain confluent growth. A penicillin susceptibility disk (10 units) is then placed on the inoculum. After overnight incubation in CO_2, a Gram stain is prepared from growth at the edge of the zone of inhibition. *Neisseria* species and *M. catarrhalis* will retain their diplococcal morphology, although the cells may appear swollen. Coccobacillary *Moraxella* species will form long filaments or spindle-shaped cells under the influence of subinhibitory concentrations of penicillin. *Acinetobacter* species can be differentiated by their negative oxidase reaction. *Capnocytophaga* species appear as pale-staining, gram-negative, slightly curved, fusiform bacteria and are both oxidase- and catalase-negative. On prolonged incubation (i.e., longer than 48 hours) these organisms tend to spread owing to their gliding motility and may impede recovery of gonococci from oropharyngeal specimens.

Presumptive Criteria for Identification of *N. gonorrhoeae*

All isolates of oxidase-positive, gram-negative diplococci that are recovered from urogenital sites and that grow on selective media may be presumptively identified as *N. gonorrhoeae*. The Superoxol test described above provides an additional presumptive test for identifying these isolates. However, confirmatory identification tests are recommended for all isolates and are required for identification of isolates from extragenital sites (i.e., throat, rectum, blood, joint fluid, CSF). Furthermore, suspect gonococci isolated from children should also be confirmed by at least two different methods that involve different principles.[20,712] These may include carbohydrate-utilization tests, immunologic methods (e.g., monoclonal antibody fluorescence tests; coagglutination tests), enzymatic procedures (e.g., chromogenic detection of specific enzyme activities) or the DNA probe culture confirmation test (see below). This is extremely important because certain social and medical-legal issues are raised following release of the results.

Identification Tests for *Neisseria* Species

Confirmatory tests for gonococci, meningococci, and other *Neisseria* species include carbohydrate-utilization tests, chromogenic enzyme substrate tests, immunologic tests (e.g., fluorescent antibody, staphylococcal coagglutination, other tests), multitest identification systems, and DNA probe tests. Carbohydrate-utilization tests and the multitest identification systems can be used to identify *N. gonorrhoeae, N. meningitidis,* and the other *Neisseria* species. Chromogenic substrate identification procedures are limited to identifying isolates that are able to grow on selective media (i.e., *N. gonorrhoeae, N. meningitidis, N. lactamica,* and some strains of *M. catarrhalis*). Fluorescent antibodies, coagglutination, other immunologic tests, and the DNA probe culture confirmation test are available for identification of *N. gonorrhoeae* only. The newer nucleic acid hybridization and nucleic acid amplification procedures are approved for direct detection of *N. gonorrhoeae* in genital tract and urine specimens only.

Carbohydrate-Utilization Tests
CONVENTIONAL CTA CARBOHYDRATES

The conventional technique for the identification of *Neisseria* species uses cystine-tryptic digest semisolid agar-base (CTA) medium containing 1% carbohydrate and a phenol red pH indicator (Color Plate 11-1*E*). The usual test battery includes CTA-glucose, -maltose, -sucrose, and -lactose, plus a carbohydrate-free CTA control. The lactose structural analogue, *o*-nitrophenyl-β-D-galactopyranoside (ONPG), may be substituted for the lactose tube, and the addition of fructose to the test battery is helpful for identifying the various *N. subflava* biovars. Some commercial CTA formulations may be supplemented with ascitic fluid to support the growth of more fastidious organisms. CTA media are inoculated with a dense suspension of the organism to be identified from a pure 18- to 24-hour culture on chocolate agar. The inoculum is either prepared in 0.5 mL of saline and divided among the tubes, or each tube is individually inoculated with a loopful of the organism. The inoculum is restricted to the top 1/2 inch of the agar-deep tubes. The tubes are incubated in a non-CO_2 incubator at 35°C with the caps tightened firmly. With a heavy inoculum, most isolates produce a detectable change in the color of the phenol red indicator within 24 hours. If the inoculum is heavy enough, many strains will change the indicator within 4 hours. However, some fastidious gonococcal strains may require 24 to 72 hours to produce sufficient acid to change the indicator. Because CTA media containing 1% carbohydrate is used primarily for detection of acid by fermentative organisms, the small amounts of acid produced oxidatively by some strains of *Neisseria* species may not be detected.

RAPID CARBOHYDRATE-UTILIZATION TEST

This test is a non-growth-dependent method for the detection of acid production from carbohydrates. In this method, small volumes of a balanced salt solution (BSS; pH 7.0) with phenol red indicator are dispensed in nonsterile tubes to which single drops of 20% filter-sterilized carbohydrates are added (Color Plate 11-1*G*). A dense suspension of the organism is prepared in the BSS with a bacteriologic loop; this suspension may be mixed on a Vortex mixer to disperse clumps. One drop of this suspension is added to each of the carbohydrate-containing tubes. The tubes are incubated for 4 hours at 35°C in a non-CO_2 incubator or a water bath. This method is very economical, the reagents are easy to prepare and inoculate, and the results are clear-cut. Details for this method are presented in Chart 11-1. The key to this technique is the use of "reagent grade" carbohydrates. Maltose obtained from some bacteriologic media companies may produce positive or equivocal results for *N. gonorrhoeae* in the rapid carbohydrate degradation test, presumably owing

to the presence of contaminant glucose. Inocula for this procedure may be obtained from the primary culture if sufficient colonies are present and if the growth is less than 24 hours old. Because bacterial growth does not occur in the test medium, small numbers of contaminants that may be present do not interfere with results. However, incubation cannot be continued overnight.

RIM-NEISSERIA TEST (RAPID IDENTIFICATION METHOD-NEISSERIA)

In this kit system (Remel Laboratories), small quantities (two to three drops) of buffered, 2% carbohydrate-phenol red solutions (glucose, maltose, sucrose, lactose) and a buffer control lacking carbohydrate are added to five nonsterile, specially buffered microtubes included in the kit. Inocula from a pure 18- to 24-hour culture of oxidase-positive, gram-negative diplococci, growing on selective media or a chocolate agar subculture, are delivered into each of the tubes with small disposable plastic loops. After inoculation the tubes are agitated on a Vortex mixer for 10 seconds and incubated in air at 35°C for 1 hour. Acid production is indicated by a change in the phenol red indicator from red-pink to yellow or yellow-orange. Negative carbohydrate reactions remain red-pink or turn slightly pink-orange. In an evaluation of this system done at the University of Illinois, the RIM-Neisseria system identified 98% of 176 *N. gonorrhoeae,* 99% of 173 *N. meningitidis,* 94% of 48 *N. lactamica,* and 100% of 12 *M. catarrhalis* within 60 minutes.[322] Of the organisms correctly identified by the kit after 1 hour, 94% of the gonococci, 99% of the meningococci, and 84% of the *N. lactamica* strains were correctly identified after only 30 minutes. Other workers have also reported good agreement of the RIM-Neisseria test with conventional methods.[188,197,254,374,543] A similarly inoculated DNase test is also available separately for confirmation of *M. catarrhalis.*

OTHER CARBOHYDRATE-UTILIZATION METHODS

Neisseria-Kwik test kit (Micro-Biologics, St. Cloud MN), and the Gonobio Test (I.A.F. Production, Inc., Laval, Quebec, Canada) are also commercial modifications of the rapid carbohydrate test procedure. The *Neisseria*-Kwik uses a tray containing dehydrated carbohydrates in separate wells. Each well is inoculated with a heavy suspension of the organism prepared in buffer, and results are read after 3 to 4 hours by noting changes in the colors of indicators. The Gonobio Test is a 2-hour method that requires heavy inoculation of microtubes containing carbohydrate substrates. Both of these systems have been evaluated and compare well with conventional methods.[188]

Chromogenic Enzyme Substrate Tests

The enzymatic identification systems use specific biochemical substrates that, after hydrolysis by bacterial enzymes, yield a colored end product that is detected directly (e.g., a yellow nitrophenol or nitroaniline product) or after the addition of a diazo dye-coupling reagent (i.e., cinnamaldehyde reagent for detection of free β-naphthylamide). The use of these systems is restricted to species that are able to grow on selective media—*N. gonorrhoeae, N. meningitidis,* and *N. lactamica.* Because some strains of *M. catarrhalis* grow on selective media, these systems will also provide a presumptive identification of this organism. Chromogenic substrate-identification tests should not be used to identify suspected meningococci recovered on blood and chocolate agars without prior subculture of the isolate to selective media. The enzymatic activities that are detected in these systems include β-galactosidase, γ-glutamyl aminopeptidase, and prolyl-hydroxyprolyl aminopeptidase (Table 11-3). β-Galactosidase and γ-glutamyl aminopeptidase are specific for *N. lactamica* and *N. meningitidis,* respectively. Occasional isolates of *N. meningitidis* may lack γ-glutamyl aminopeptidase activity; in 2002, a meningococcal strain isolated from a carrier was found to lack this enzyme because of the presence of an insertional mutation in the *ggt* gene.[640] Absence of these activities and presence of prolyl-hydroxyprolyl aminopeptidase identifies an organism as *N. gonorrhoeae.* *M. catarrhalis* lacks all three of these enzymatic activities. The commercial systems that use this approach are the Gonochek II, the BactiCard *Neisseria,* and the Neisstrip.

GONOCHEK II

The Gonochek II (EY Laboratories, San Mateo, CA) is a single tube that contains the three dehydrated chromogenic substrates (Color Plate 11-1*H*). After rehydration with four drops of phosphate-buffered saline (pH 7.4), 5 to 10 colonies of oxidase-positive, gram-negative diplococci from a pure culture growing on selective medium, or a suitable subculture, are emulsified in the tube with a wooden applicator stick. The tube is capped with the stopper and incubated at 35°C for 30 minutes. Specific color reactions in the bacterial suspension confirm the isolate as *N. meningitidis* (hydrolysis of γ-glutamyl-*p*-nitroanilide; yellow) or *N. lactamica* (hydrolysis of 5-bromo-4-chloro-3-indoyl-β-D-galactopyranoside; blue). If the suspension is colorless at the end of the incubation period, the stopper is split apart and the top part of the stopper is inserted into the tube. The tube is inverted so that the bacterial suspension comes in contact with the diazo dye-coupler (*o*-aminoazotoluene diazonium salt [Fast Garnet]) present on the stopper. The detection of β-naphthylamine released by bacterial hydroxyprolyl aminopeptidase activity (red) identifies the isolate as *N. gonorrhoeae.* The absence of a colored product at the completion of the testing and reading steps provides a presumptive identification of *M. catarrhalis.* In a large evaluation of this system,

the Gonochek II identified 99% of 176 gonococci, 97% of 173 meningococci, and 100% of 48 *N. lactamica* and 10 *M. catarrhalis,* respectively.[322] Other investigators have also evaluated Gonochek II and have found it reliable for identifying these organisms.[188,707]

BACTICARD *NEISSERIA*

The BactiCard *Neisseria* (Remel Laboratories, Lenexa KA) uses four chromogenic substrates that are impregnated on four individual test circles within a cardboard holder (Color Plate 11-2*A*). After moistening each of the four circles with a single drop of rehydrating fluid, several colonies of the organism taken from selective media (or from a subculture from selective media) are rubbed onto each of the four test areas. After incubation on the bench top for 2 minutes, the indoxyl butyrate esterase substrate circle (IB; 5-bromo-4-chloro-3-indolyl butyrate) is inspected for the appearance of a blue to blue-green color. If this test is positive, the organism can be identified as *M. catarrhalis,* and no further testing is necessary. If the IB test is negative, the card is incubated on the bench for an additional 13 minutes (total test time, 15 minutes). After this time, the β-galactosidase substrate circle (BGAL; 5-bromo-4-chloro-3-indolyl-β-D-galactopyranoside) is inspected for the presence of a blue-green color. If this test is positive, the organism can be identified as *N. lactamica,* and no further testing is necessary. If the BGAL test is negative, a single drop of color developer reagent is placed on the prolyl amino-peptidase (PRO; L-proline-β-naphthylamide) and the γ-glutamyl aminopeptidase (GLUT; γ-glutamyl-β-naphthylamide) test circles. These two tests are read as positive if a definite pink or red develops within 30 seconds of reagent addition. A positive PRO reaction identifies the isolate as *N. gonorrhoeae,* whereas a positive GLUT reaction identifies the organism as *N. meningitidis.* The PRO reaction may also be positive for some *N. meningitidis* strains. At the University of Illinois, the BactiCard Neisseria test was compared with conventional identification procedures for 558 isolates. The BactiCard Neisseria identified 100% of 254 *N. gonorrhoeae,* 100% of 125 *N. meningitidis,* 98.2% of 54 *N. lactamica,* and 98.4% of 125 *M. catarrhalis* strains.[320] A third product, called Neisstrip (Lab M Ltd., Bury, United Kingdom) is very similar to the BactiCard-*Neisseria,* but does not have the indoxyl butyrate reagent for identifying *M. catarrhalis.* Dealler and colleagues reported that the Neisstrip

Table 11-3 Enzymatic Activities Used for Identification of the Pathogenic *Neisseria* Species

SPECIES	β-GALACTOSIDAS	γ-GLUTAMYL AMINOPEPTIDASE	HYDROXYPROLYL AMINOPEPTIDASE	BUTYRATE ESTERASE
N. lactamica	+	−	+	−
N. meningitidis	−	+	V	−
N. gonorrhoeae	−	−	+	−
M. catarrhalis	−	−	−	+

+, positive reaction; −, negative reaction; V, variable reaction.

identified 93 of 95 gonococcal strains; 2 of 400 nongono-coccal strains were misidentified with the strip.[178]

Immunologic Methods for Culture Confirmation of *N. gonorrhoeae*
DIRECT FLUORESCENT MONOCLONAL ANTIBODY TEST

The currently available direct fluorescence antibody (DFA) culture confirmation procedure uses monoclonal anti-bodies that recognize epitopes on the PorA outer-membrane protein (the old protein I), the principal outer-membrane pro-tein of *N. gonorrhoeae*.[378] The DFA test (*Neisseria gonorr-hoeae* Culture Confirmation Test; Wampole Laboratories, Cranberry, NJ) is performed by preparing a light suspension of the organism in 5 μL of water on a DFA slide, allowing the suspension to dry, heat-fixing the specimen, overlaying the smear with the DFA reagent, and incubating the smear for 15 minutes. The smear is rinsed, air-dried, mounted with a cover slip, and examined with a fluorescence microscope. Gonococci appear as apple-green fluorescent diplococci (Color Plate 11-2*B*).

When this test was originally marketed by Syva in 1986, sensitivities and specificities of 100% were reported.[197, 378,708] In 1989, Walton reported the isolation of two DFA-negative, β-lactamase-positive *N. gonorrhoeae* strains from two sexual partners.[703] Boehm and associates reported 100% sensitivity and specificity for the test but mentioned that a DFA-negative, β-lactamase-positive strain was isolated sub-sequent to the completion of their study.[75] In 1993, Janda and colleagues found that the DFA test correctly identified 95.4% of 151 β-lactamase negative strains but only 74.4% of 43 β-lactamase positive strains.[323] In another 1993 study, Beebe and coworkers found that 18 (4.6%) of 395 gonococ-cal strains isolated during 1991 and 1992 were DFA-nega-tive; 6 of these 18 strains were β-lactamase-positive.[55] Sero-typing and pulsed-field gel electrophoresis data indicate that β-lactamase-producing and non-β-lactamase-producing strains that are negative with the DFA reagent belong to a variety of serovars.[55,65,323,607] The current anti-Por mono-clonal antibody "cocktail" used in the original Syva product is manufactured by Trinity Biotech (Wicklow, Ireland) and has not been changed since the product was sold to Wampole Laboratories. In light of the studies cited above, package insert claims of 99.6% sensitivity and 100% specificity are no longer valid. Because of this, isolates that fail to stain with the DFA reagent must be identified by another method. This caveat limits the real advantages of the DFA procedure, which included its rapidity, the ability to test colonies di-rectly from primary cultures, and the small amount of growth required for test performance. The DFA test is not intended for direct detection and identification of organisms on smears from patient specimens.

COAGGLUTINATION TESTS

Coagglutination tests make use of the ability of protein A on *Staphylococcus aureus* cells to bind IgG molecules by their Fc region. Binding of antigonococcal antibody to killed *S. aureus* cells, and subsequent mixture with a suspension of gonococci causes visible agglutination of the suspension. Two coagglutination tests for the identification of *N. gonor-hoeae* are currently available—the Phadebact Monoclonal

GC Test and the GonoGen I test. The Phadebact monoclonal GC coagglutination test (Boule Diagnostics AB, Huddinge, Sweden) uses monoclonal antibodies to gonococcal Por (protein I). Unlike the GC OMNI test previously marketed by Boule Diagnostics, the monoclonal GC test contains one reagent that reacts with serogroup WI *N. gonorrhoeae* strains and a second reagent that reacts with serogroup WII/WIII strains. Because a negative control reagent is not included, gonococcal isolates will react with either the WI or the WII/WIII reagent, depending on the Por antigen composition of the individual isolate. Failure to agglutinate in either reagent constitutes a negative test. To perform the test, a suspension (0.5 McFarland standard) is prepared in buffered saline (pH 7.2 to 7.4) and is boiled for 5 minutes. After cooling, the suspension is mixed with test and control reagents on a card-board slide. Agglutination within 1 minute is a positive test result. A blue dye is incorporated in the reagents to help visualize agglutination against the white background of the card. Careful attention to procedural details are necessary in order to prevent false-positive and false-negative results. Evaluations of the previously available GC OMNI test reported sensitivities of 98–100% and specificities of 99–100%.[188,197,323] Organism suspensions heavier than the specified McFarland density, however, may yield false-positive results. In addition, the use of saline with a pH less than or greater than 7.4 has also been reported to produce false-positive results with some strains of *N. lactamica, N. cinerea,* and *M. catarrhalis*.[188,323]

The GonoGen I (New Horizons Diagnostics, Columbia MD) coagglutination test also uses staphylococcal cells coated with monoclonal antibodies directed against the Por outer-membrane protein of several gonococcal serovars.[444] The test is performed using a boiled suspension (McFarland no. 3) of the organism. Results are usually clear-cut and appear within 15 to 30 seconds of mixing the test reagent and suspension. The kit contains test and control coagglutination reagents, as well as both positive and negative gonococcal test control suspensions. Evaluations of this test have re-ported sensitivities of 86–100% and specificities of 99–100%.[24,323,346,379,444]

GONOGEN II TEST

The GonoGen II (New Horizons Diagnostics, Columbia MD) uses anti-Por monoclonal antibodies that are conju-gated to colloidal gold as the detection reagent. A suspension (McFarland no. 1) is prepared in 0.5 mL of an organism lysing solution, and one drop of the antibody reagent is added. After 5 minutes, two drops of the suspension are passed through a membrane filter that retains antigen-antibody complexes. Retention and concentration of the complex on the filter turns the filter red, identifying the or-ganism as *N. gonorrhoeae*. Nongonococcal isolates result in the filter remaining white or pale pink. Janda and associates found that the GonoGen II identified 91.8% of 194 *N. gonor-rhoeae* strains; five strains were negative and 11 strains pro-duced equivocal color reactions on the membrane. In addi-tion, a meningococcal strain and two *N. lactamica* isolates repeatedly produced false-positive test results.[323] Kellogg and Orwig found that the GonoGen II identified 99.6% of 248 gonococcal strains, but 7 of 22 *N. meningitidis* strains produced false-positive test results, leading these investigators to suggest that positive GonoGen II test results need to be confirmed by another method.[346]

Multitest Identification Systems

Four kit systems are available that can be used not only for identifying *Neisseria* species but also for identifying other fastidious gram-negative organisms. These systems are the RapID NH (*Neisseria-Haemophilus*) system (Remel Laboratories: Color Plate 11-2*C*) the Vitek NHI (*Neisseria-Haemophilus* Identification) card (bioMerieux, Inc., Hazelwood MO), the *Haemophilus-Neisseria* identification (HNID) panel (Dade/American Microscan, Sacramento CA; Color Plate 11-2*D*), and the API NH system (bioMerieux, Inc., La Balme-les-Grottes, France).[47,197,318,319] See Color Plates 11-2*E* and 11-2*F*. All of these systems use modified conventional tests (e.g., acid production from carbohydrates, urease, indole, ornithine decarboxylase) and chromogenic substrates to provide either 2- or 4-hour identifications of *Neisseria, Haemophilus,* and other fastidious gram-negative bacteria encountered in clinical specimens. The bioMerieux NHI card generally provides excellent results for the pathogenic *Neisseria* species, and is also able to identify *N. cinerea*.[319] However, *M. catarrhalis* strains cannot be differentiated from other *Moraxella* species with the tests currently present on the card. The MicroScan HNID panel does not include *N. cinerea* in its database, and these organisms are misidentified as either *N. gonorrhoeae* or as *M. catarrhalis* when tested on this system.[318] In addition, some *N. meningitidis* strains do not produce clear-cut reactions with key identification tests on the panel (i.e., acid production from maltose or γ-glutamyl aminopeptidase activity), resulting in misidentifications. The RapID NH contains tests (e.g., nitrite reduction and an esterase substrate) that will presumably allow reliable identification of both *N. cinerea* and *M. catarrhalis*. A single evaluation of this system indicated that the RapID NH was reliable for identifying *Neisseria* species, but that some reactions were difficult to interpret.[188] In the study by Barbe and coworkers, the API NH system was able to identify gonococci, meningococci, *N. lactamica,* and *M. catarrhalis* within 2 hours, whereas other *Neisseria* species required additional tests for correct species identification.[47]

DNA Probe Test for Culture Confirmation of *N. gonorrhoeae*

The Accuprobe *Neisseria gonorrhoeae* Culture Confirmation Test (Gen Probe) identifies the *N. gonorrhoeae* by the detection of species-specific rRNA sequences. In the test, organisms from growth on agar media are lysed and mixed with a chemiluminescent-labeled single-stranded DNA probe that is specifically complementary to gonococcal rRNA. After hybridization occurs, the DNA probe/rRNA double-stranded complex is selected by a chemical process, and the presence of the probe in the double-stranded material is detected by addition of detection reagents that hydrolyze the chemiluminescent tag on the probe, thereby releasing light energy. This energy is detected in a chemiluminometer instrument, and the result is reported as positive or negative. In an evaluation conducted at the University of Illinois examining monoclonal antibody coagglutination procedures, the direct fluorescent antibody test, and the AccuProbe for *N. gonorrhoeae* identification, the latter test was the only procedure that was 100% accurate in identifying *N. gonorrhoeae*.[323] Similar results for the AccuProbe test have been reported by others.[386,731] This test may be particularly useful for confirming those isolates that may not be easily identified by other confirmatory test procedures.

Nucleic Acid Hybridization and Amplification Tests for *N. gonorrhoeae*

Probe hybridization technology is also used in the currently available test for direct detection of *N. gonorrhoeae* in urogenital specimens. The PACE 2 (probe assay-chemiluminescence enhanced) system (GenProbe, San Diego, CA) is a nonisotopic chemiluminescent DNA probe that hybridizes specifically with multicopy gonococcal rRNA. Specimens are collected as for culture and are placed in a transport-lysing solution. A sample of the specimen is mixed with the acridinium ester-linked probe. Following incubation, hybridized nucleic acid is separated from nonhybridized material. The acridinium ester-labeled probe-rRNA complex is assayed in a semiautomated chemiluminometer by the addition of an alkaline hydrogen peroxide solution. This hydrolyzes the ester linkage of the probe label, causing a release of light, which is detected in a chemiluminometer instrument and reported as relative light units (RLUs). The amount of light released is directly proportional to the amount of gonococcal rRNA present in the specimen. The assay requires about 2 hours to perform.

Evaluations of the PACE 2 nucleic acid hybridization system indicate that the probe system may be more sensitive than culture, owing to the fastidious nature of the organisms.[145,280,394,698] This problem is more acute for laboratories that receive cultures of gonococci from remote sites, such as municipal sexually transmitted disease clinics. In all of the studies, probe competition assays were used to confirm whether culture-negative/probe-positive specimens were due to false-negative cultures or to false-positive probe results. Chapin-Robinson and coworkers compared the PACE 2 with culture on 795 endocervical specimens and found that the resolved sensitivity and specificity of the assay were 100% and 99.5%, respectively.[145] A similar study was conducted by Hale and associates in three public health laboratories on 271 endocervical and 165 male urethral specimens.[280] Twenty of 27 probe-positive/culture-negative specimens were resolved as false-negative cultures by probe competition; the resolved sensitivity and specificity of the PACE 2 were 99.4% and 99.6%, respectively. Finally, a large study of the PACE 2 direct detection system, conducted in the Netherlands on 1750 specimens, reported a sensitivity of 97.1% and a specificity of 99.1%.[698] In general, the sensitivities of the PACE 2 system have ranged from 85.5% to 100% for female endocervical specimens and from 91.5% to 100 for male urethral specimens.[368] Corresponding specificities have ranged from 93.5% to 99.7% for endocervical specimens and from 82.2% to 99.9% for male urethral specimens, respectively.[368] Several other studies on the PACE 2 system have reported similar sensitivities and specificities.[58,154,591] Hanks and coworkers evaluated the PACE 2 system as a test-of-cure and found that it was reliable for this application as soon as 6 days after treatment.[285] Koumans and coworkers reviewed several published evaluations of the PACE 2 system and found the aggregate sensitivities to be 92.1% and 96.4%, respectively, for endocervical and urethral specimens.[368] Some investigators have recommended that either all probe-positive specimens or specimens that yield RLU values within a certain range be confirmed with a probe competition assay.[725] For positive samples, reduction of 70% or more of the RLU signal in the PCA reaction tube compared with the signal generated in the standard tube with only the labeled probe constitutes a confirmed positive.

The PACE 2 system has also been evaluated for the detection of *N. gonorrhoeae* in pharyngeal and rectal specimens. Lewis and colleagues found that the overall accuracy of the PACE 2 system for evaluating these specimens was 99.4%, with a sensitivity of 87.5% and a specificity of 99.7%.[385] Young and colleagues found that the sensitivities of PACE 2 for detection of oropharyngeal and rectal gonococcal infections were 86.4% and 94.1%, with specificities of 100%.[729] Aggregate sensitivities of the PACE 2 system for detection of oropharyngeal and rectal gonococcal infections were 77.4% and 96.4%, respectively. At present, the PACE 2 system is not FDA-approved for the diagnosis of extragenital gonococcal infections.

In addition to direct probe detection, several nucleic acid amplification-based assays are now available for the direct detection of *N. gonorrhoeae* in clinical specimens. Currently available tests use various types of amplification approaches, including PCR (AMPLICOR *Neisseria gonorrhoeae* PCR and the COBAS AMPLICOR *Neisseria gonorrhoeae* PCR, Roche Diagnostic Systems, Branchburg, NJ), strand-displacement amplification (SDA) (BD ProbeTecET, BD Biosciences) and transcription-mediated amplification (AP-TIMA COMBO 2, Gen-Probe, San Diego). These methods amplify the target in some manner and are detected by chemiluminescence. The ligase chain reaction (LCR), another target-amplification approach, was used in the LCx *N. gonorrhoeae* and *C. trachomatis* assays.[302] Despite promising performances in clinical laboratories, this assay system was removed from the market after several reagent lots failed to meet the analytical claims made by the manufacturer.[143] Another method, the Digene Hybrid Capture test (Digene, Silver Spring, MD), is a chemiluminescent probe-based assay that uses hybridization and hybrid capture, followed by signal-amplification.[445] These tests are approved for testing of genital swab specimens and urine specimens from both men and women.

The AMPLICOR *N. gonorrhoeae* PCR assay and the automated COBAS AMPLICOR systems use conventional PCR-based amplification. The original nonautomated assay uses the PerkinElmer 9600 thermal cycler with subsequent enzyme immunoassay detection using microwell plates that are coated with an oligonucleotide to capture the biotinylated amplicon products. The COBAS AMPLICOR is a benchtop automated system in which target DNA is amplified by a conventional PCR reaction using thermal cyclers that are built into the instrument. For both AMPLICOR assays, the amplification target sequence in *N. gonorrhoeae* is a 201-base-pair fragment of the cytosine DNA methyltransferase gene. Biotinylated amplification products are captured with

magnetic particles that are coated with amplicon-specific oligonucleotide probes, and the products are detected colorimetrically using an avidin-horseradish peroxidase conjugate.[333]

Several studies have examined the performance of the AMPLICOR gonorrhea assay. Crotchfeldt and colleagues evaluated the Roche AMPLICOR microwell assay with 344 urine and urethral swab specimens from males and 192 urine and endocervical swab specimens from women. The sensitivity of the assay was 94.4% for male urine specimens and 97.3% for male urethral swab specimens. The sensitivities of the assay for urine and endocervical swab specimens from women were 90% and 100%, respectively. The specificity of the assay ranged from 95.9% to 98.5% for urine specimens and from 97.0% to 99.4% for swab specimens.[169] Palladino and coworkers evaluated the manual PCR assay with urine specimens from 73 males and found that the assay demonstrated 100% sensitivity and specificity compared with culture.[488] A large multicenter evaluation of both the semiautomated AMPLICOR microwell assay and automated COBAS AMPLICOR assay examined 2,192 matched endocervical swab and urine specimens from women and matched urine and urethral swab specimens from 1,981 men.[416] The AMPLICOR microwell assay and the COBAS AMPLICOR yielded concordant results on 98.8% of the specimens and exhibited virtually identical sensitivities of 99.5% and 99.8% for endocervical swab and urine specimens from women, respectively, and 98.9% and 99.9% for male urethral swab and urine specimens, respectively. Livengood and Wrenn found that the COBAS AMPLICOR system had an analytical sensitivity and specificity of 96.3% and 100%, respectively, in a study of 618 endocervical swab specimens.[399] In a study examining the specificity of the AMPLICOR microwell assay, Farrell found that 6 of 15 *N. subflava* strains produced positive results, including one that was isolated from a vaginal specimen.[220] Other studies, as well as the manufacturer, have also acknowledged that saprophytic neisseriae (e.g., *N. cinerea*, *N. subflava*, *N. sicca*, and *N. flavescens*) may produce cross-reactive results in the AMPLICOR microwell *N. gonorrhoeae* PCR assay.[491,545,678]

The BD ProbeTec ET system uses strand-displacement amplification rather than PCR for amplification, so all testing is performed isothermally without the need for a thermal cycler.[397] The system has a higher throughput than other amplification methods, with a capacity to perform 300 assays in an 8-hour shift. The system also has options for test performance and interpretation both with and without an amplification control, and uses reagents that can be stored at room temperature. In this assay, the amplification target is in the chromosomal pilin gene-inverting homolog, which is already present in multiple copies in the gonococcal cell.[117] Van Der Pol and associates evaluated the ProbeTec ET with both swab and urine specimens from men and women.[677] For swab and urine specimens from women, the sensitivities of the ProbeTec ET system were 96.6% and 84.9%, respectively. For swab and urine specimens from men, the sensitivities of the ProbeTec ET were 98.5% and 97.9%, respectively. Specificities ranged from 94.4% to 100% for urine specimens and from 94.8% to 99.6% for swab specimens. In another evaluation of the ProbeTec ET with 733 endocervical swab specimens from commercial sex workers in Belgium, the SDA procedure performed with a sensitivity of 90% and a specificity of 100% compared with culture.[681] In a study of 3,544 urine specimens submitted for *N. gonorrhoeae* testing, Akduman and colleagues found that the sensitivity and specificity of the ProbeTec ET were 99.2% and 99.3%, respectively, in a population with a prevalence of 3.6% by culture.[14] Another evaluation performed in Canada with urine specimens from 825 males and 399 females compared the ProbeTec ET with the Roche COBAS AMPLICOR PCR and found that the SDA procedure was 100% sensitive and 99.7% specific, while the PCR assay was 96.7% sensitive and 98.9% specific.[144] Like the AMPLICOR assays for *N. gonorrhoeae,* the BD ProbeTec ET also can yield false-positive reactions with several nongonococcal *Neisseria* species.[491]

The APTIMA Combo 2 assay is a newer assay that uses transcription-mediated amplification for detection of gonococci and chlamydiae in swab and urine specimens. Gaydos and colleagues evaluated this assay system with both endocervical swabs and urine specimens submitted for detection of *N. gonorrhoeae.*[250] The sensitivity and specificity of the APTIMA system were 99.2% and 98.7%, respectively, for endocervical swab specimens, and 91.3% and 99.3%, respectively, for first-collected urine specimens. This assay is undergoing further evaluations, including the use of physician- and self-collected vaginal swabs for organism detection. The APTIMA tests also appear to be less susceptible than other amplification assays to inhibitors of amplification that are usually found in urine specimens.[150]

The Digene hybrid capture assay, as mentioned, uses signal amplification instead of target amplification to increase its sensitivity of detection. In this assay, target DNA becomes hybridized to sequence-specific RNA probes provided with the assay. Hybrid products are transferred to wells of a microtiter tray, where they become immobilized by antibodies in a microtiter well. A detection reagent, consisting of an antibody conjugate that is specific for RNA/DNA hybrids, is then added to each microwell. Multiple enzymes are conjugated to each of these antibody molecules, and many antibody molecules bind to each RNA/DNA hybrid, resulting in marked signal amplification on addition of the chemiluminescent enzyme substrate. In a study performed with endocervical swab specimens from 1,370 women, the Digene assay demonstrated a sensitivity of 92.6% and a specificity of 98.5% compared with culture.[579] In an examination of 669 endocervical specimens, the Digene test performed with 92.2% sensitivity and greater than 99% specificity for detection of *N. gonorrhoeae* when compared with culture.[174] Van Der Pol and colleagues found that the Digene assay performed with a sensitivity of 100% and a specificity of 99% for detection of *N. gonorrhoeae* in endocervical swab specimens.[679]

In addition to the commercially available molecular-based amplification tests for *N. gonorrhoeae,* "real-time" PCR assays using the LightCycler platform have also been developed. In a study of 152 urine specimens, the LightCycler assay was compared with an in-house PCR assay for *N. gonorrhoeae.*[710] The LightCycler method was 94% sensitive and comparable to the in-house assay in specificity. Li and colleagues also devised a LightCycler assay that was able to detect both the organism and mutations in the *gyrA* gene that are responsible for quinolone resistance.[390]

The use of nucleic acid–based methods for detection of *N. gonorrhoeae* in clinical specimens has both advantages and disadvantages. The advantages include the ability to test easily collected specimens (i.e., urine), more rapid turnaround times, and the demonstrated increased sensitivity of these methods compared with culture. Disadvantages include the cost of the assays (including equipment and expendables), the need for separate, dedicated space for specimen processing and test performance, and modifications of laboratory workflow to prevent amplicon contamination of the instrumentation and the environment. A very real downside to the widespread use of these non-culture-based assays is the unavailability of gonococcal isolates for surveillance of emergent resistance to antimicrobial agents. Despite the high specificity of these assays, their performance in low-prevalence populations requires additional study; some workers have recommended confirmatory testing with more specific molecular methods (e.g., 16S rRNA PCR) for positive amplified test results obtained in populations with a low prevalence of gonorrhea.[187] Culture is still required for diagnosis of extragenital gonococcal infections and for documentation of genital, rectal, or oropharyngeal gonococcal infection in children.

Molecular Methods for Detection of *N. meningitidis*

Molecular methods for direct detection of *N. meningitidis* in clinical specimens have also been described, but none are commercially available. Lansac and colleagues described genus- and species-specific PCR identification assays using primer pairs derived from the aspartate β-semialdehyde gene (*asd*) of *Neisseria* species and a conserved outer-membrane protein gene (*ctrA*) of *N. meningitidis,* respectively.[375] The first assay was 100% specific for identification of 321 of 322 strains representing 13 *Neisseria* species, while the second assay amplified DNA from 256 *N. meningitidis* isolates belonging to nine different serogroups. Several PCR assays have also been described for direct detection of meningococci in clinical specimens. During an ongoing epidemic of serogroup B disease that began in Chile in 1987, Saunders and his research group developed a nested PCR assay that amplified the *porA* gene encoding the subserotype-specific protein.[578] Use of this assay on CSF specimens during the epidemic resulted in a test sensitivity of 96.7% and a specificity of 100%.[577] PCR methods that amplify multiple capsular polysaccharide genes (e.g., *ctrA* PCR assay) or that amplify serogroup-specific genes (e.g., the *siaD* PCR assay) have also been described.[81,82,335,514] Taha described a PCR assay performed directly on CSF for simultaneous meningococcal detection and serogrouping. The detection assay amplified a conserved gene involved in the regulation of meningococcal adherence to target cells (*crgA*), while a simultaneous multiplex PCR assay was performed with oligonucleotides in the *siaD* genes for serogroup B, C, Y, and W135 detection and in the *orf-2* gene cassette required for serogroup A capsular biosynthesis for serogroup A detection.[638] Orvelid and colleagues described a PCR-based method for detection of serogroup A meningococci in CSFs.[486] This assay used primers and probes specific for the gene cassette encoding the (α1-6)-linked *N*-acetyl-D-mannosamine comprising the serogroup A capsular polysaccharide.

LightCycler-based PCR assays also have been described that are able to detect, identify, and perform *porA* gene subserotyping of *N. meningitidis* directly from clinical specimens.[446]

Cultural Characteristics of Neisseria Species

The following sections present helpful features for the laboratory identification and characterization of the gram-negative cocci. Suggestions for the performance of differential and confirmatory tests described in detail in the previous section and additional test procedures are outlined. Characteristics for identification of *Neisseria* species and *M. catarrhalis* are shown in Table 11-4.

Neisseria gonorrhoeae

Although the identification systems discussed in the previous section of this chapter and the biochemical characteristics in Table 11-4 are reliable for the routine identification of *N. gonorrhoeae* in the clinical laboratory, other techniques have contributed greatly to our understanding of the biology and epidemiology of the gonococci. Techniques such as auxotyping and serotyping have been helpful in assessing the potential virulence, invasiveness, antimicrobial susceptibility, and genetic constitution of various strains of gonococci. Strains of gonococci that have specific requirements for certain nutritional growth factors are known as **auxotypes.**[124] Although as many as 15 different growth factors (such as requirements for valine, leucine, lysine, arginine, proline,

Table 11-4 Characteristics for Identification of *Neisseria* Species, *Moraxella catarrhalis*, and the "False *Neisseria*"

SPECIES	OXIDASE	CATALASE	Selective Media, 35°C	Chocolate Agar, 22°C	Nutrient Agar, 35°C	Glucose	Maltose	Fructose
				GROWTH		ACID PRODUCTION FROM		
N. gonorrhoeae	+	+	+	−	−	+	−	−
N. meningitidis	+	+	+	−	−	+	+	−
N. lactamica	+	+	+	−	−	+	+	−
N. cinerea	+	+	−†	−	−	−	−	−
N. polysaccharea	+	+	v	−	+	+	+	−
N. sicca	+	+	−	+	+	+	+	+
N. subflava								
bv. *subflava*	+	+	−	+	+	+	+	−
bv. *flava*	+	+	−	+	+	+	+	+
bv. *perflava*	+	+	−‡	+	+	+	+	+
N. mucosa	+	+	−	+	+	+	+	+
N. flavescens	+	+	−	−	+	−	−	−
"*N. kochii*"	+	+	+	−	−	+	−	−
N. elongata								
ssp. *elongata*	+	−	−	+	+	−	−	−
ssp. *glycolytica*	+	+	−	+	+	+w	−	−
ssp. *nitroreducens*	+	−	−	+	+	−/+w	−	−
N. weaveri	+	+	−	+	+	−	−	−
N. canis	+	+	NA	NA	NA	−	−	−
N. denitrificans	+	+	−	NA	NA	+	−	+
N. macacae	+	+	−	NA	NA	+	+	+
N. caviae	+	+	NA	NA	NA	−	−	−
N. ovis	+	+	NA	NA	NA	−	−	−
N. cuniculi	+	+	NA	NA	NA	−	−	−
N. iguanae	+	+	NA	NA	NA	v	−	NA
Moraxella catarrhalis	+	+	v	+	+	−	−	−

+, *positive reaction;* −, *negative reaction;* v, *variable reaction;* +w, *weak positive reaction;* −/+w, *negative to weakly positive reaction;* NA, *data not available.*
* *Reactions shown are for media with 0.1% nitrite, N. gonorrhoeae will reduce 0.01% nitrite.*
† *Some strains recovered on selective media.*
‡ *Some strains grow on selective media.*

hypoxanthine, citrulline, or others) may be assessed in auxo-typing studies, strains requiring the triad of arginine, hypoxanthine, and uracil (AHU strains) have been the most closely studied. These strains are of particular interest because they are commonly recovered from patients with disseminated gonococcal infection (DGI) and are highly susceptible to penicillin.[356,453] AHU strains that have been recovered from systemic infections are frequently resistant to the normal bactericidal action of human serum, which may partially explain their ability to enter the bloodstream.[585] AHU strains are also associated with asymptomatic urethral infections in men; in one study, 96% of asymptomatic men were infected with this auxotype.[168] AHU-requiring strains grow as atypical colonies on agar media; some may require 72 hours or more of incubation before visible growth is observed.[453] In addition to AHU strains,

proline-, citrulline-, and uracil-requiring auxotrophs have been associated with asymptomatic infections in men in the U.S., Canada, and Sweden.[102]

Studies of the immunologic characteristics of the gonococcus have included the characterization of the organism's outer-membrane proteins and the development of monoclonal antibodies against epitopes of Por protein (protein I), the principal outer-membrane protein of *N. gonorrhoeae*.[257,360] These antibodies can be adsorbed onto staphylococcal cells for use as coagglutination reagents. Differences in Por divide strains into three serogroups: serogroup WI contains Por IA, while serogroups WII and WIII contain Por IB. WI serotypes are associated with disseminated infections, asymptomatic infections in men, and complement-mediated resistance to the bactericidal activity of normal human serum. Exploration of various epitopes of Por IA and IB has

SPECIES	ACID PRODUCTION FROM		POLYSACCHA-RIDE FROM SUCROSE	REDUCTION OF		DNASE	TRIBUTYRIN HYDROLYSIS	HABITAT
	Sucrose	Lactose		NO_3	NO_2*			
N. gonorrhoeae	−	−	−	−	−	−	−	Humans
N. meningitidis	−	−	−	−	v	−	−	Humans
N. lactamica	−	+	−	−	v	−	−	Humans
N. cinerea	−	−	−	−	v	−	−	Humans
N. polysaccharea	−	−	+	−	v	−	−	Humans
N. sicca	+	−	+	−	+	−	−	Humans
N. subflava								
bv. *subflava*	−	−	−	−	+	−	−	Humans
bv. *flava*	−	−	−	−	+	−	−	Humans
bv. *perflava*	+	−	+	−	+	−	−	Humans
N. mucosa	+	−	+	+	+	−	−	Humans
N. flavescens	−	−	+	−	+	−	−	Humans
"*N. kochii*"	−	−	−	−	−	−	−	Humans (rare)
N. elongata								
ssp. *elongata*	−	−	−	−	+	−	−	Humans
ssp. *glycolytica*	−	−	−	−	+	−	−	Humans
ssp. *nitroreducens*	−	−	−	+	+	−	−	Humans
N. weaveri	−	−	−	−	+	−	−	Dogs
N. canis	−	−	−	+	−	NA	−	Dogs
N. denitrificans	+	−	+	−	+	NA	−	Guinea pigs
N. macacae	+	NA	+	−	+	NA	NA	Nonhuman primates
N. caviae	−	−	−	+	+	NA	+	Guinea pigs
N. ovis	−	−	−	+	−	NA	+	Sheep/cattle
N. cuniculi	−	−	−	−	−	NA	+	Rabbits
N. iguanae	v	NA	+	+	v	NA	NA	Iguanas
Moraxella catarrhalis	−	−	−	+	+	+	+	Humans

resulted in the subdivision of Por IA (serotype WI) into more than 18 serovars and of Por IB (serotype WII/WIII) into more than 28 serovars.[360] Serovar determinations are usually accomplished by coagglutination techniques, although the monoclonal typing reagents have also been adapted to an enzyme immunoassay format with less subjective and more reproducible results.[114] Applications of these typing schemes have included 1) the study of regional differences and temporal changes in gonococci nationwide and within communities, 2) the examination of serovar-auxotype relations, 3) the study of gonococcal serovars as indicators or predictors of virulence, 4) the use of serovar determinations to assess relapse versus reinfection in individual patients, and 5) the use of serovar determinations as a tool in forensic pathology relating to sexual assault and abuse.[257]

Newer molecular approaches have been developed to augment and extend the discriminatory power of auxotyping and serotyping. These techniques include antibiogram profiling, plasmid analysis, *Opa* typing, PorB gene sequencing, ribotyping, isoenzyme analysis, restriction endonuclease analysis, pulsed-field gel electrophoresis, arbitrarily primed PCR, amplified ribosomal RNA restriction analysis, and amplified fragment-length-polymorphism fingerprinting.[106,476,477,484,489,490,508,650,673] These novel typing methods have demonstrated the existence of "clusters" within existing auxotype(s)/serovar(s).[672,689]

Another typing system involves amplification and sequencing of the *lip* genes, which code for an outer-membrane lipoprotein of 18- to 30-Kda molecular weight that is found in all gonococci.[662] Three *lip* genes have been identified and sequenced. The nucleotide sequences of these genes predict peptides that consist of an amino acid pentamer that is repeated 13 to 19 times. Variations in the numbers of lip repeats in a sequence, and the nature of the sequences themselves, can be used along with auxotype, serovar, antimicrobial susceptibilities, and other characteristics to construct a highly discriminatory system for typing of individual isolates.

Because of the medical-legal issues that are raised after isolating *N. gonorrhoeae* from a child, and the recovery of gonococci from both genital and nongenital body sites, proper identification of isolates is imperative. Whittington and associates reported on 40 bacterial isolates from children younger than 15 years of age that had been identified as *N. gonorrhoeae* and that were referred to the CDC for confirmation.[712] Fourteen (35%) of these strains had been misidentified by the originating laboratory, including four *N. cinerea*, three *N. lactamica*, two *N. meningitidis*, three *M. catarrhalis*, one *K. denitrificans*, and an unidentified nongonococcal *Neisseria* species. In 10 of the 14 cases, the organisms were isolated from children for whom there was no supporting evidence of sexual abuse. In many instances, the laboratories reporting these isolates were using the commercial kits described above for identification of *N. gonorrhoeae*. As mentioned above, some commercial carbohydrate-utilization test systems may produce false-positive glucose reactions for *N. cinerea*, which could lead to the misidentification of this species as *N. gonorrhoeae*.[91,92] Coagglutination tests, although generally quite reliable, may produce false-negative results with some gonococcal strains and may also show false-positive results with some isolates of other *Neisseria* or related species, including *N. lactamica*, *N. cinerea*, and

M. catarrhalis. Procedural details for these tests (e.g., density of the test suspension, type and pH of the suspending fluid) differ among manufacturers, and package insert instructions must be followed closely. Enzymatic tests for detection of gonococcal prolyl aminopeptidase must be used only for neisserial isolates that are able to grow well on selective media. Some *N. cinerea* strains and occasional isolates of *N. subflava* bv. *perflava* may be recovered on selective media and may also be positive for prolyl aminopeptidase in commercial systems.[320] Isolates recovered from oropharyngeal sites may be particularly troublesome. *N. lactamica*, a species that grows well on selective media and that may be misidentified as *N. gonorrhoeae*, colonizes the oropharynges of almost 60% of children between the ages of 1 and 4 years.[261]

The Committee on Child Abuse and Neglect of the American Academy of Pediatrics recommends that presumptive isolates of *N. gonorrhoeae* from a child, regardless of the site of isolation, be confirmed by at least two methods.[20] Nonculture techniques, such as nucleic acid hybridization and amplification methods, are investigational tests in children, so positive results with these assays must be confirmed with a culture. If a laboratory is unable to establish a definitive identification, the isolate should be sent to a reference laboratory for further testing. If possible, the isolate should also be saved. This can be accomplished by removing the growth from a few chocolate agar plates, suspending the growth in 1 ml of decomplemented horse serum:brain-heart infusion broth (1:1), and storing at−70°C.

Neisseria meningitidis

Identification procedures for meningococci (and gonococci as well) produce the best results when inoculated from fresh 18- to 24-hour subcultures on chocolate or blood agar. In carbohydrate-utilization confirmatory tests, the acidic reaction in the maltose tube will frequently be stronger than that in the glucose tube because maltose is degraded by the organism to two glucose molecules, which are then metabolized. Glucose-negative, maltose-negative, and asaccharolytic *N. meningitidis* strains may also be isolated from time to time.[266,505,562,705] If such biochemically aberrant strains are recovered, chromogenic substrate confirmatory tests or serogrouping of the isolates should be performed.

Slide agglutination is the most commonly used technique for serogrouping meningococci. A dense suspension of the organism is prepared in 0.5 to 1.0 mL of phosphate-buffered saline (PBS), pH 7.2, from a 12- to 18-hour subculture on trypticase-soy blood agar. One drop of this suspension is mixed with one drop of meningococcal antisera on a sectored slide, and the slide is rotated for 2 to 4 minutes. Groupable strains will generally agglutinate strongly within this time. Although isolates from systemic infections will usually agglutinate rapidly, those from carriers may fail to agglutinate (nongroupable strains) or may autoagglutinate in the PBS. Use of younger cultures from blood agar (6 to 8 hours) or use of a serum-enriched media, such as trypticase-soy agar containing 10% decomplemented horse serum, may resolve these problems. Antisera for the major meningococcal serogroups is available from BD Biosciences. Some of these nongroupable strains may actually be *N. polysaccharea*; testing for production of polysaccharide from sucrose will help identify this species (see discussion below).[84] In addition to slide agglutination, serogrouping of meningococci may also be done by a whole-cell, indirect enzyme immunoassay and by a dot-blotting assay using monoclonal antibodies against serogroups A, B, C, Y, and W135. Rosenqvist and associates found that the latter two techniques were more sensitive, more specific, and easier to interpret than slide-agglutination tests, but their applicability was limited by the availability of monoclonal, serogroup-specific reagents.[549]

In addition to serogroup determinations, *N. meningitidis* isolates may also be serotyped and subserotyped on the basis of their outer membrane protein and LOS antigens (see Box 11-3). These techniques are used mainly for investigations of epidemics and sporadic outbreaks of disease and are not amenable for use in routine clinical microbiology laboratories. In addition to serologic techniques, several molecular techniques have been applied to investigations of meningococcal disease and to the epidemiology of *N. meningitidis* strains. These techniques include multilocus enzyme electrophoresis, restriction-fragment-length polymorphism analysis, rRNA probe technology (ribotyping), PCR amplicon restriction endonuclease analysis of the chromosomal *dhps* (dihydropteroate synthase) and *porA* genes of *N. meningitidis*, and pulsed-field gel electrophoresis.[276,277,347,369,495,629,658]

Other *Neisseria* Species
NEISSERIA LACTAMICA

N. lactamica resembles *N. meningitidis* in colony morphology and was initially thought to be a lactose-positive variant of *N. meningitidis*.[297] This species is resident in the throat and is found more frequently in children than in adults.[261] *N. lactamica* grows on selective media and produces acid from glucose, maltose, and lactose. ONPG is also hydrolyzed and can be used as a substitute for lactose in the test battery. Some strains of this organism have been reported to cause false-positive reactions with some commercial coagglutination tests.[322,323] Strains of *N. lactamica* have intermediate susceptibility to penicillin and ampicillin, but are susceptible to cefotaxime and ceftriaxone.[36]

NEISSERIA CINEREA

Colonies of *N. cinerea* resemble the large-colony types of *N. gonorrhoeae* and may yield results consistent with *N. gonorrhoeae* in some kit identification systems.[91] Although this organism is part of the commensal flora of the upper respiratory tract, it has been isolated from other sites, including the cervix, rectum, orbital cellulitis, conjunctivae, blood, and CSF.[42,85,198,201,361] *N. cinerea* grows on both blood and chocolate agar. On chocolate agar after 24 hours incubation, colonies are about 1 mm in diameter and are smooth with entire edges. The organism does not produce acid from carbohydrates in either CTA-based media or the rapid carbohydrate degradation test. Weak positive reactions with glucose after overnight incubation have been reported by some identification systems, and its positive hydroxyprolyl aminopeptidase reaction may also result in misidentifications of *N. cinerea* as *N. gonorrhoeae*. Most *N. cinerea* isolates, however, do not grow well on MTM or other selective media, which precludes testing of this organism on chromogenic substrate tests such as the Gonochek and the BactiCard-Neisseria. *N. cinerea* can be differentiated from the asaccharolytic species *N. flavescens* by its inability to produce

polysaccharide from sucrose (see discussion below) and the lack of a discernible yellow pigment. This species can also be separated from *M. catarrhalis,* another asaccharolytic species, by its negative nitrate reduction, DNase, and tributyrin hydrolysis reactions (see Table 11-4). A helpful test for differentiating *N. cinerea* from *N. gonorrhoeae* is the **colistin susceptibility test.** A suspension of the organism (0.5 MacFarland turbidity standard) is prepared in broth and is swabbed onto a chocolate or blood agar plate as for a disk diffusion susceptibility test. A 10 mg colistin disk is placed on the inoculum, and the plate is incubated in CO_2 for 18 to 24 hours. *N. cinerea* is colistin-susceptible and will have a zone that is ≥ 10 mm around the disk. Generally, *N. gonorrhoeae* will grow up to the edge of the disk.

NEISSERIA FLAVESCENS

N. flavescens is found in the respiratory tract and is rarely associated with infectious processes. This organism grows as smooth, yellowish colonies on both blood and chocolate agar. In addition to growth on nutrient agar at 35°C, most strains will also grow at room temperature on chocolate or blood agar. This organism is able to synthesize iodine-positive polysaccharides from sucrose (see discussion) and can be differentiated from *M. catarrhalis* by its inability to reduce nitrate and its negative DNase and tributyrin hydrolysis reactions.

NEISSERIA SUBFLAVA BIOVARS, NEISSERIA MUCOSA, AND NEISSERIA SICCA

Identification of the ''nonpathogenic'' *Neisseria* species is not generally necessary unless the organism is determined to be clinically significant or if the organism is isolated from a systemic site (e.g., blood, CSF) or in pure culture. Identification is based on colony morphology, growth on simple nutrient medium, inability to grow on selective media, acid production from carbohydrates, reduction of nitrate and nitrite, and synthesis of a starch-like, iodine-staining polysaccharide from sucrose. **Nitrate reduction** and **nitrite reduction** are determined in medium (tryptic-soy or heart infusion broth) containing 0.1% (w/v) KNO_3 and 0.01% (w/v) KNO_2, respectively. **Polysaccharide synthesis** is determined by inoculating the organism onto brain-heart infusion agar containing 5% sucrose. Medium lacking sucrose is inoculated as a negative control. After incubation at 35°C for 48 hours, the plates are flooded with Gram's or Lugol's iodine (1:4 dilution). A positive test is indicated by the development of a deep blue color in and around the colonies synthesizing the polysaccharide. We have also obtained excellent results by adding regular Gram's iodine (one to two drops) to the sucrose-containing tube in the rapid carbohydrate degradation technique after 4 hours of incubation. If positive, a deep blue color appears in the tube. This is compared with the tan color seen in the other carbohydrate tubes (e.g., the maltose tube) after addition of Gram's iodine.

Strains of *N. subflava* can be subdivided into three biovars (biovars *subflava, flava,* and *perflava*) on the basis of acid production from fructose and sucrose and synthesis of iodine-positive polysaccharide from sucrose (see Table 11-4). All three biovars reduce nitrite, but not nitrate. *N. mucosa* has a carbohydrate-utilization pattern similar to *N. subflava* bv. *perflava* and also produces the iodine-positive polysaccharide, but *N. mucosa* is able to reduce both nitrate and nitrite to N_2 gas (Color Plate 11-2*D*). All of these organisms also display varying degrees of yellow pigmentation. The *N. sicca* strains are biochemically identical with *N. subflava* bv. *perflava*, but they characteristically form dry (desiccated), adherent, leathery colonies on agar media that cannot be emulsified readily.

NEISSERIA POLYSACCHAREA

N. polysaccharea is found in the human oropharynx. This organism is an oxidase-positive, catalase-positive, gram-negative diplococcus that forms smooth yellow colonies.[538] In the original description of this organism, the ability to grow on selective media (e.g., MTM agar) was a key characteristic. Subsequent studies indicate, however, that growth on selective media for the pathogenic *Neisseria* is a variable characteristic of *N. polysaccharea* because of the colistin susceptibility of some strains.[23] Strains that are able to grow on selective media have colistin minimal inhibitory concentrations (MICs) of 64 μg/mL or greater, whereas strains that are inhibited have colistin MICs of 1 μg/mL or less. The organisms are resistant to vancomycin. After 24 hours of growth, *N. polysaccharea* forms colonies of about 2 mm in diameter on chocolate or blood agar. Acid is produced from glucose and maltose but not from fructose or lactose. Acid production from sucrose is variable and appears to depend on the types of media used to determine this characteristic. *N. polysaccharea* also possesses an amylosucrase that synthesizes an acidic extracellular polysaccharide from sucrose.[104,515] The polymer is composed mainly of α1,4-linked D-glucopyranosyl residues along with about 6% *O*-substituted α4,6-D-glucopyranosyl branch points.[539] Production of various amounts of the material by different strains may explain the variable nature of the sucrose reaction.[538,539] Nitrate is not reduced, whereas nitrite frequently is reduced. *N. polysaccharea* can be differentiated from *N. meningitidis* by polysaccharide synthesis and the γ-glutamyl aminopeptidase tests. *N. polysaccharea* produces iodine-positive polysaccharide from sucrose and is γ-glutamyl aminopeptidase-negative, whereas *N. meningitidis* does not produce iodine-positive polysaccharide from sucrose and is γ-glutamyl aminopeptidase-positive.[23,84] Like *N. gonorrhoeae*, *N. lactamica*, and some *N. meningitidis* strains, *N. polysaccharea* is prolyl aminopeptidase-positive. The organism requires cysteine for growth and does not grow on nutrient agar or on chocolate agar at 22°C. Although this organism's cultural characteristics resemble *N. meningitidis*, its outer-membrane protein profiles resemble *N. lactamica* more than the pathogenic species.[111]

NEISSERIA ELONGATA SUBSPECIES

N. elongata subspecies *elongata*, *glycolytica*, and nitroreducens are rod-shaped members of the genus *Neisseria*. The first two subspecies were recognized in the most recent edition of *Bergey's Manual of Systematic Bacteriology* as *Neisseria* species, whereas the last subspecies, formerly known as CDC group M-6, was recently reclassified in the genus.[89,268,721] All subspecies are members of the human upper respiratory tract flora and all have been isolated from infectious processes.[295,470,721] These subspecies can be differentiated on the basis of catalase reactivity, acid production from glucose, and reduction of nitrate (see Table 11-4).

NEISSERIA GONORRHOEAE SUBSPECIES KOCHII ("NEISSERIA KOCHII")

In 1986, seven isolates of an unusual *Neisseria* were recovered from conjunctival cultures of children in two rural villages in Egypt.[426] These isolates grew on chocolate agar and modified Thayer-Martin medium and produced large, smooth colonies resembling meningococci. Similar to gonococci, these organisms required the amino acid cysteine for growth. The isolates were oxidase-positive, produced acid from glucose only, and were γ-glutamyl aminopeptidase-negative. They did not react with fluorescent gonococcal monoclonal antibody reagents and failed to react with monoclonal coagglutination reagents used for serovar determinations for *N. gonorrhoeae*. On further analysis, these strains had different surface proteins than the gonococcal strains to which they were compared. However, plasmid analysis showed significant homology with the plasmids commonly found in gonococcal strains. The DNA homology experiments showed sufficient similarity to both *N. gonorrhoeae* and *N. meningitidis;* on this basis, the workers felt that these isolates did not represent a new species but rather a subspecies of *N. gonorrhoeae*. Because these isolates would probably be identified as *N. gonorrhoeae* in a clinical laboratory and because their site of isolation and carbohydrate-utilization pattern were similar to those associated with gonococci, these isolates have been named *N. gonorrhoeae* subsp. *kochii* or "*N. kochii*."[426] This species has not yet been formally adopted.

ATYPICAL AND NON-HUMAN NEISSERIA SPECIES

Neisseria species with atypical or unusual biochemical or serologic profiles are being increasingly recognized. Hodge and coworkers isolated an organism that was a meningococcus biochemically, yet reacted with monoclonal antibody immunofluorescence and coagglutination reagents for *N. gonorrhoeae*.[294] Janda and colleagues isolated *N. subflava* bv. *perflava* strains from oropharyngeal cultures of homosexual men that grew luxuriantly on selective media (modified Thayer-Martin agar).[320,322] In chromogenic enzyme substrate tests, these organisms were identified as *N. gonorrhoeae* based on positive hydroxyprolyl aminopeptidase reactions and negative β-galactosidase and γ-glutamyl aminopeptidase reactions. More complete characterization of neisserial isolates, particularly from immunocompromised patients, may uncover other aberrant and unusual isolates in the future.

On occasion, the clinical microbiology laboratory may recover *Neisseria* species of animal origin from human infections, such as bite wounds from animals. Isolates may include *N. weaveri*, *N. canis*, *N. denitrificans*, and members of the false neisseriae. All of these organisms exhibit typical gram-negative diplococcal morphology except for *N. weaveri*, which is a gram-negative rod. The biochemical reactions for these organisms are also presented in Table 11-4.

Cultural Characteristics and Identification of Moraxella catarrhalis

M. catarrhalis grows well on both blood and chocolate agars, and some strains will also grow well on MTM and other selective media. Colonies are generally gray-to-white, opaque, and smooth. A selective medium incorporating acetazolamide as an inhibitor of other respiratory tract flora has also been described.[684] The organism is asaccharolytic in carbohydrate degradation tests and may actually turn peptone-based identification media alkaline. Most strains reduce nitrate and nitrite and produce DNase.[192] The DNase activity is detected by heavily spot-inoculating a plate of DNase test medium containing toluidine blue 0 on an area the size of a dime (Color Plate 11-2*F*). After overnight incubation, hydrolysis of the DNA is detected by a change in the color of the media around and under the inoculum from blue to pink. *S. aureus* and *S. epidermidis* strains are also inoculated onto the plate as positive and negative, respectively, test controls.

M. catarrhalis may also be distinguished from *Neisseria* species by its ability to hydrolyze ester-linked butyrate groups (butyrate esterase).[615] See Color Plate 9-2*H*. This enzyme activity is detected with a substrate called tributyrin. A rapid fluorescent tributyrin hydrolysis test that uses 4-methylumbelliferyl butyrate as a substrate was reported by Vaneechoutte and coworkers.[683] In this study, all 62 *M. catarrhalis* strains were positive with this test within 5 minutes, whereas all other *Neisseria* species tested were negative. A very rapid (2.5 minute) and reliable indoxyl-butyrate hydrolysis spot test has also been described and is commercially available (Remel Laboratories; Carr-Scarbourough, Stone Mountain, GA; Color Plate 11-2*G*).[177,402] This same test is also included on the BactiCard-*Neisseria* along with the three other chromogenic substrates for *Neisseria* identification (see Color Plate 11-2*A*).[320] The RapID NH system also contains a fatty acid ester hydrolysis test to assist in the identification of *M. catarrhalis*. Indoxyl acetate, which is used for the identification of *Campylobacter* species, can also be used as a substrate for the esterase enzyme of *M. catarrhalis*.[320,615] In addition, most clinically significant *M. catarrhalis* strains also produce an inducible, cell-associated β-lactamase (see below).[196] Because of its inducible nature, rapid acidometric β-lactamase tests (i.e., those that rely on conversion of hydrolysis of penicillin to penicilloic acid) may yield false-negative results. Best results are obtained with the iodometric method or with the chromogenic cephalosporin test.[447]

With the recognition of *M. catarrhalis* as a primary pathogen in certain clinical settings and the suspicion that nosocomial infections with this organism may indeed occur, methods for strain typing have been investigated.[309,454] These methods include enzymatic biotyping, polyacrylamide gel electrophoresis of whole-cell proteins, immunoblotting, pulsed-field gel electrophoresis, and restriction-fragment-length polymorphism endonuclease analysis.[418,429,454] These techniques have been applied to investigations of outbreaks of respiratory tract disease in critical care units in the United States and abroad.[494,531] Two DNA typing methods, probe-generated restriction-fragment-length polymorphism analysis and single-adapter modified fragment polymorphism analysis, were recently used to demonstrate the existence of two subgroups within *M. catarrhalis* that may actually represent separate subspecies.[78]

Antimicrobial Susceptibility of *Neisseria* Species

Neisseria gonorrhoeae

Shortly after its discovery during the 1940s, penicillin rapidly became the treatment of choice for gonorrhea. Through the 1950s and into the mid-1970s, penicillin treatment schedules were regularly updated to keep up with increasing resistance to penicillin and other agents (e.g., tetracyclines and macrolides) that were used for treatment. This incremental resistance was due to mutations in several chromosomal genes such as *mtr* and *env*, which code for proteins involved in substrate efflux and membrane permeability, and *penA*, which codes for penicillin binding protein 2. In 1976, strains of *N. gonorrhoeae* with high-level resistance to penicillin were imported into the U.S. from West Africa, and the Far East. These isolates contained plasmids that carried genes for a β-lactamase enzyme and were given the moniker "PPNG" for penicillinase-producing *N. gonorrhoeae*.[301] Between 1976 and 1979, PPNG strains were associated with sporadic outbreaks in the U.S., and, between 1979 and 1982, the number of cases of gonorrhea caused by PPNG strains increased 15-fold, with large outbreaks occurring in New York City, Los Angeles, and Miami. During the mid- to late 1980s, PPNG strains became endemic in several metropolitan areas of the United States.[711] At that time, spectinomycin was recommended for the treatment of these infections. By 1981, however, four spectinomycin-resistant *N. gonorrhoeae* isolates had been reported, and subsequently, spectinomycin-resistant PPNG isolates also appeared.[37,511,736] Resistance to spectinomycin is due to a single-step mutation in 16S ribosomal RNA (rRNA) that results in high-level resistance (i.e., MICs of 256 μg/mL or higher).[245]

In 1983, a localized outbreak caused by penicillin-resistant, β-lactamase-negative gonococci was reported from North Carolina.[130] These strains lacked the β-lactamase plasmid and were negative with tests for β-lactamase detection. High-level resistance to penicillin in these strains was due to chromosomal mutations at loci known to contribute to antibiotic resistance; these strains were designated chromosomally mediated-resistant *N. gonorrhoeae* (CMRNG). By October 1984, 446 cases of CMRNG infection had been reported to the CDC from 23 states that had been screening for this type of resistance.[527] CMRNG strains have penicillin MICs higher than 1.0 μg/mL, with 75% of these having MICs higher than 2.0 μg/mL. CMRNGs are also moderately resistance to tetracycline (MICs ≥2 μg/mL), show decreased susceptibility to erythromycin, cefoxitin, and trimethoprim-sulfamethoxazole, and are usually susceptible to spectinomycin and ceftriaxone.

In 1985, the CDC reported on 12 *N. gonorrhoeae* strains isolated in Georgia, Pennsylvania, and New Hampshire from patients in whom tetracycline therapy had failed (tetracycline-resistant *N. gonorrhoeae* [TRNG]).[131] Agar dilution susceptibility testing showed high-level resistance to tetracycline (MICs of 16 to 32 μg/mL) and doxycycline (MICs of 8–32 μg/mL), but susceptibility to penicillin (MICs of 0.008 to 0.25 μg/mL), spectinomycin, and cefotaxime. These strains were also moderately resistant to cefoxitin. Studies have now determined that tetracycline-resistant *N. gonorrhoeae* (TRNG) harbor a 25.2-MDa plasmid constructed by the insertion of a tetracycline-resistance determinant (*tetM*) into the 24.5-MDa conjugative plasmid found in some gonococcal strains.[364,456] This transposon-associated gene has also been found in streptococci, *Mycoplasma hominis*, *Ureaplasma urealyticum*, *Gardnerella vaginalis*, *Kingella denitrificans*, *Eikenella corrodens*, and some *N. meningitidis*.[358,541,667] The conjugative plasmid carrying the *tetM* determinant can be transferred to recipient *N. gonorrhoeae* strains by transformation or conjugation.[541,542] The *tetM* determinant is believed to code for a protein or proteins that interact with the gonococcal ribosome to prevent inhibition of protein synthesis by tetracycline.

With the characterization of these resistant isolates, workers at the CDC have delineated five resistance phenotypes in *N. gonorrhoeae* strains.[528] These phenotypes include 1) penicillin-susceptible strains (MICs <2 μg/mL), 2) penicillinase-producing *N. gonorrhoeae* strains (PPNG, β-lactamase positive), 3) high-level, plasmid-mediated tetracycline-resistant strains (TRNG, MICs ≥2 μg/mL) possessing the *tetM* determinant, 4) strains with chromosomally mediated resistance to penicillin (CMRNG, MICs ≥2 μg/mL), and 5) strains with high-level, plasmid-mediated resistance to both penicillin and tetracycline (β-lactamase positive with the *tetM* determinant). The appearance and spread of other resistance determinants among these five phenotypes forms the basis of ongoing gonococcal surveillance conducted throughout the United States by the CDC.[139,140,264]

Because of increasing resistance of *N. gonorrhoeae* to previously recommended antimicrobial agents and based on several controlled clinical efficacy trials, the U.S. Public Health Service has recommended that all patients with uncomplicated gonococcal infection receive one of five single-dose treatment regimens.[142] These include ceftriaxone (125 mg IM), cefixime (400 mg PO), ciprofloxacin (500 mg PO), ofloxacin (400 mg PO), and levofloxacin (250 mg PO). Each of these therapies also includes azithromycin (1 g PO) or doxycycline (100 mg PO, twice a day for 7 days) for treatment of coinfecting *Chlamydia trachomatis*. Pregnant women should be treated with ceftriaxone (250 mg IM) followed by 7 to 10 days of erythromycin, because oral cephalosporins have not been studied in this population, and quinolones and tetracyclines are contraindicated in pregnant women. Additional regimens for inpatient and outpatient treatment of salpingitis and disseminated gonococcal infections are also included in the PHS Treatment Guidelines.[142] At the present time, no clinically significant resistance to the cephalosporins that are recommended for treatment of gonococcal infections has been identified.[239,342]

Even though resistance to the newer cephalosporins has not been seen, the emergence of *N. gonorrhoeae* strains with decreased susceptibility to the fluoroquinolones is a troublesome development.[240] In Europe, fluoroquinolone agents such as ciprofloxacin were being used for the treatment of gonococcal infections in the late 1980s and, beginning in 1990, treatment failures with ciprofloxacin were being seen in the U.K.[267] Subsequently, other failures were documented in patients treated with fluoroquinolones in the Far East, Canada, Australia, and the U.S.[132,138,338,643,644] Antimicrobial susceptibility testing of gonococcal strains from patients in whom therapy with 250 ciprofloxacin, PO, failed had ciprofloxacin MICs of ≥0.06 to 0.25 μg/mL, while strains from

infections treated with 500 mg ciprofloxacin, PO, or 400 mg ofloxacin, PO, had ciprofloxacin and ofloxacin MICs of ≥1.0 μg/mL and 2.0 μg/mL, respectively.[267,337,338,643,644] Based on achievable peak serum levels after oral administration, the CDC proposed criteria for the interpretation of in vitro susceptibilities to ciprofloxacin, ofloxacin, and other fluoroquinolone agents. Strains with intermediate resistance to ciprofloxacin and ofloxacin have MICs of 0.125 to 0.5 μg/mL and 0.5 to 1.0 μg/mL, respectively. Strains that are resistant to ciprofloxacin and ofloxacin have MICs of ≥1.0 μg/mL and ≥2.0 μg/mL, respectively.[355] *N. gonorrhoeae* strains that have decreased susceptibility or that are resistant to ciprofloxacin and ofloxacin have been documented in diverse geographical regions, including Canada, Australia, Hong Kong, Japan, Thailand, the Philippines, Spain, the U.K., and the U.S.[132,158,354,359,362,363,537,641,644] Some of these strains have ciprofloxacin MICs as high as 2.0 μg/mL.[354,359] Strains that were highly resistant to the fluoroquinolones were recovered from patients who had traveled to or were sexual contacts of individuals who had been in Southeast Asia. These strains were also resistant to penicillin and many were also resistant to tetracycline, but all strains were susceptible to ceftriaxone and cefixime. In almost all of these regions, the prevalence of strains with decreased susceptibility or resistance to the fluoroquinolones is increasing. Fluoroquinolone resistant isolates have gene mutations that result in amino acid substitutions in the A and B subunits (GyrA and GyrB, respectively) of DNA gyrase, and in the topoisomerase IV *parC*-encoded subunit.[57,179,621]

The emergence of decreased susceptibility and resistance to the fluoroquinolones in *N. gonorrhoeae* portend that the usefulness of these agents for treatment of gonorrhea will need to be reassessed in the near future.[240] Additional surveillance of gonococcal antimicrobial susceptibility in selected patient groups (e.g., women with pelvic inflammatory disease or other complications) who may receive other antimicrobial agents (e.g., cefoxitin, clindamycin, metronidazole, and gentamicin) is also necessary to prevent the emergence of clinically relevant resistance.[529] Although azithromycin is not a recommended treatment for gonorrhea, this agent may be useful in regions where quinolone resistance is prevalent. For azithromycin therapy, a regimen of 2 g PO is recommended over the 1-g-PO regimen used for treatment of chlamydia infections. Clinical failures following treatment with 1-g and 2-g azithromycin regimens have been associated with isolates having azithromycin MICs of 0.125–0.25 μg/mL and ≤0.5 μg/mL, respectively.[284,646] Gonococcal isolates with decreased susceptibility to azithromycin (MICs ≥ 1 μg/mL) have been reported in some regions of the U.S.[138,139]

The CDC has also made recommendations on indications and methods for antimicrobial susceptibility testing of *N. gonorrhoeae*. These recommendations relate more to ongoing surveillance of gonococcal resistance patterns than to individual patient management. In 1989, a multicenter study was published in which disk diffusion and agar dilution interpretive criteria for penicillin, tetracycline, spectinomycin, and ceftriaxone were determined.[329] Guidelines for antimicrobial susceptibility testing of *N. gonorrhoeae* have been published and are continually updated by the National Committee on Clinical Laboratory Standards (NCCLS).[469] At present, disk diffusion and agar dilution breakpoints of *N. gonorrhoeae* are available for penicillin, parenteral cephalosporins, oral cephems (e.g., cefixime), tetracycline, the fluoroquinolones, and spectinomycin.[469] In addition to disk diffusion and agar dilution, the E test (AB Biodisk, Solna, Norway) has also been used to determine antimicrobial susceptibilities of *N. gonorrhoeae*.[682,728]

Neisseria meningitidis

Despite the occasional recovery of *N. meningitidis* strains with decreased susceptibility to penicillin, penicillin G remains the drug of choice in the U.S. for treatment of meningococcal meningitis, since the vast majority of strains are susceptible to penicillin and ampicillin.[134] For treatment of serious meningococcal infections, parenteral penicillin G (300,000 U/kg/day) is administered for 10 to 14 days. Chloramphenicol (100/mg/kg/day up to 4 g/day) is an alternative in patients who are allergic to penicillin. The third-generation cephalosporins (i.e., cefotaxime, ceftriaxone, ceftizoxime, and ceftazidime) reach levels in the CSF that may be several-thousand times the MIC of the infecting isolate, and these agents have been used successfully in treating meningococcal disease; ceftriaxone (children, 50/mg/kg/day up to 4 g; adults, 2 g/day) is a currently recommended parenteral regimen. In addition to antimicrobial therapy, patients with serious meningococcal disease require intensive supportive care, including management of the shock state, and careful monitoring of vital signs for detection of complications (e.g., acute respiratory distress syndrome, neurologic sequelae, pericarditis) and disease progression (e.g., coagulation studies for DIC).[119,680] New adjunctive therapies, such as recombinant human bactericidal/permeability-increasing protein show promise in the prevention of multi-organ system failure due to endotoxemia.[260] Other biologic agents, such as monoclonal antibodies directed against endotoxin or against cytokines involved in meningococcal septic shock (e.g., IL-1, IL-6, TNF-α) may also play a role as adjunctive therapeutic interventions.[93,182,680,699]

Despite the fact that the vast majority of strains, particularly in the U.S., remain susceptible to penicillin, evidence is accumulating that the antimicrobial susceptibility profiles of *N. meningitidis* strains are also evolving. Historically, penicillin-susceptible strains of *N. meningitidis* have penicillin MICs of ≤0.06 μg/mL. In 1983, Dillon and associates in Canada isolated the first β-lactamase-producing meningococcal strain from a urogenital specimen.[189] This isolate harbored the gonococcal 4.5-Mda β-lactamase plasmid and the 24.5-Mda conjugative plasmid. Subsequently, only three additional β-lactamase-producing *N. meningitidis* isolates have been reported in the literature: two strains were isolated in 1988 from two patients with meningitis in South Africa, and the fourth was recovered in 1989 from a patient in Spain.[83,237,561] β-Lactamase-positive strains have penicillin MICs of >256 μg/mL. In 1987, an *N. meningitidis* isolate was recovered in Spain that had diminished susceptibility to penicillin (MIC >0.06 μg/mL) but was β-lactamase-negative.[563] These strains are referred to as relatively resistant, moderately susceptible, or having diminished susceptibility to penicillin. Since that time, additional isolates with similar characteristics have been reported in

United Kingdom, Europe, Greece, South Africa, and the U.S.[71,100,314,632,670,675,687,724] In Spain, the frequency of these isolates has increased from 0.4% in 1985 to 67% in 1994, while the frequency of these strains in the U.K. remains stable at about 9%.[35,236] In 1997, active surveillance by the CDC accumulated 90 isolates from 121 cases of reported meningococcal disease. Of these, three (<3%) were moderately susceptible to penicillin, with MICs of 0.12 μg/mL.[551] Of the remaining 87 penicillin-susceptible strains, 49 had MICs of 0.06 μg/mL. While penicillin-susceptible strains have MICs of ≤0.06 μg/mL, strains with decreased susceptibility have penicillin MICs ranging from 0.10 μg/mL to 1.0 μg/mL.[551,564] Resistant strains are defined as having penicillin MICs of ≥2 μg/mL. Most of the relatively resistant meningococci that have been reported have belonged to either serogroup B or C.[35,60,71,236] Penicillin/ampicillin resistance may also emerge during therapy with these agents. In an interesting case report, an ampicillin-resistant strain of serogroup W-135 *N. meningitidis* was isolated from blood cultures of an 82-year-old woman in fatal septic shock.[263] The initial blood and sputum isolates were susceptible to penicillin (MIC = 0.05 μg/mL) and ampicillin (0.016 μg/mL). Despite 7 days of high-dose ampicillin therapy, the patient died. The isolate recovered from the blood 7 days after admission had become moderately resistant to both penicillin (MIC = 1 μg/mL) and ampicillin (MIC = 1.2 μg/mL).

Diminished susceptibility to penicillin in moderately resistant *N. meningitidis* strains is apparently due to decreased binding of penicillin by altered meningococcal cell wall penicillin-binding proteins (PBP 2 and PBP 3).[435] In the case of the PBP 2 proteins, decreased binding of penicillin results from an altered nucleotide sequence of the PBP 2 gene, *penA*.[738] Similar low-affinity forms of PBP 2 are found in penicillin-resistant strains of other *Neisseria* species, including *N. lactamica, N. flavescens, N. polysaccharea,* and *N. gonorrhoeae*. The altered, low-affinity forms of PBP 2 in *N. meningitidis* strains apparently arose from recombination events that resulted in the replacement of sequences in the native meningococcal *penA* gene with corresponding genetic material from the commensal *Neisseria* species.[90,564,565,616]

The clinical significance of diminished penicillin susceptibility in *N. meningitidis* is unclear at present. Although both treatment failures and higher rates of complications have been observed in patients infected with relatively resistant strains, the administration of higher doses of penicillin has been clinically effective.[560,668] Certain third-generation cephalosporins, such as ceftriaxone and cefotaxime, are active against both susceptible and moderately susceptible *N. meningitidis* strains, but the MICs of some agents for moderately susceptible strains—particularly cefuroxime, aztreonam, and imipenem—may be significantly higher than those of susceptible strains.[499] Meropenem is highly active against meningococci, with more than 90% of strains inhibited by ≤1 μg/mL.[3,504]

N. meningitidis strains have also demonstrated resistance to other antimicrobial agents. High-level chloramphenicol resistance has been reported in isolates from France and Vietnam.[246] Fear of the spread of chloramphenicol resistance is justified since the drug is a mainstay of therapy for meningitis in sub-Saharan Africa.[611] High-level resistance to sulfonamides, the drug formerly used for prophylaxis, is now widespread and may be found commonly among certain epidemic clones of serogroup A *N. meningitidis*.[611] In a study conducted in Spain, 43.6% of 55 strains from both cases and carriers were resistant to trimethoprim-sulfamethoxazole.[236] The emergence of rifampin resistance has also been observed even during the administration of rifampin prophylaxis.[166] Rifampin resistance emerges either due to alterations in cell membrane permeability or to mutations in the *rpoB* gene that codes for the β-subunit of the meningococcal RNA polymerase.[2] In 2000, an *N. meningitidis* strain with decreased susceptibility to ciprofloxacin (MIC of 0.25 μg/mL) was isolated from a 19-year-old female in Australia who had invasive meningococcal disease.[587] Susceptible strains have ciprofloxacin MICs of ≤0.03 μg/mL. PCR amplification and sequencing of the *gyrA* gene of this isolate revealed a three-nucleotide difference from wild-type, ciprofloxacin-susceptible strains. The acquisition of the *tetM* tetracycline resistance determinant by *N. meningitidis* has already been mentioned.[667]

Antimicrobial susceptibility testing of *N. meningitidis* isolates is difficult, and MIC determinations are the methods of choice.[648] Accepted standards and susceptibility breakpoints for *N. meningitidis* are not available, and evaluations of disk diffusion methods using penicillin, oxacillin, ampicillin, and rifampin disks have produced disappointing results.[70,109,110,305,500] Currently, the NCCLS recommends either broth microdilution or agar dilution MIC testing of *N. meningitidis* using cation-supplemented Mueller-Hinton broth with 2–5% laked horse blood or Mueller-Hinton agar with 5% (v/v) sheep blood, respectively.[469] The E test may also prove valuable in determining the antimicrobial susceptibility of individual meningococcal isolates.[305,500] In some published reports on meningococcal susceptibilities to other agents, MIC breakpoints for *N. gonorrhoeae* are often used for interpretation.[35] Since most clinical microbiology laboratories are not equipped to perform agar-dilution tests, isolates from patients who are not responding to appropriate antimicrobial chemotherapy and any presumptively penicillin-resistant isolates should be tested for β-lactamase production with the chromogenic cephalosporin test (Nitrocefin, BD Biosciences) and forwarded to a reference laboratory for agar-dilution susceptibility testing.

Because zone size criteria for other *Neisseria* species have not been established, the method of choice for determining susceptibility to antimicrobial agents is the agar-dilution method. There are anecdotal reports that the disk diffusion procedure, agar-dilution procedure, and interpretive criteria published by NCCLS for gonococci also may be used for other *Neisseria* species.[469] Although these organisms will generally grow well on the blood-supplemented Mueller-Hinton agar recommended by NCCLS, some strains may require medium supplementation provided by additives such as IsoVitalex.

Antimicrobial Susceptibility of Moraxella catarrhalis

The appearance and spread of resistance to antimicrobial agents among the pathogenic *Neisseria* are also reflected in the antimicrobial susceptibility of *M. catarrhalis* isolates. Before the mid-1970s, this organism was broadly susceptible to antimicrobial agents. β-Lactamase-positive *M. catarrhalis* were first isolated in 1976; by the end of the 1970s, about 75% of strains produced β-lactamase enzymes. A study by Doern and Tubert demonstrated that the chromogenic cephalosporin (nitrocefin) disk and tube tests had superior sensitivity for detection of β-lactamase when compared with tests using pyridinium-2-azo-*p*-dimethylaniline cephalosporin (PADAC), tube and disk acidometric and iodometric procedures.[196] In the clinical laboratory, *M. catarrhalis* strains should be tested β-lactamase production, preferably with the chromogenic cephalosporin test.[447]

Broth-dilution ampicillin susceptibility tests on *M. catarrhalis* isolates may produce confusing results. Some β-lactamase-producing strains will have high ampicillin MICs (12.5 to 25.0 μg/mL), whereas others will have low ampicillin MICs (0.10 to 0.40 μg/mL). Ampicillin broth-dilution tests for the latter strains are inoculum-dependent.[727] With smaller inocula (10^4 cfu/mL), these strains appear susceptible to ampicillin and other β-lactam antibiotics. With higher inocula (10^7 cfu/mL), these strains have higher MICs and are resistant. This inoculum effect was observed for ampicillin, penicillin G, cephalothin, cefamandole, cefuroxime, and cefaclor.

Studies of *M. catarrhalis* β-lactamase enzymes have shown that two types of enzymes are found in strains of this organism.[701,702] These enzymes are called BRO-1 (or Ravisio-type) and BRO-2 (or 1908-type).[308,702] A third β-lactamase enzyme, named BRO-3, was described by Christensen and colleagues in 1991, but is now thought to be a membrane-bound precursor of the other BRO enzymes.[152,622] The "BRO" moniker is a contraction of "**BR**anhamella" and "m**O**raxella," since similar β-lactamases are found in rod-shaped moraxellae as well.[701] Strains of *M. catarrhalis* produce either BRO-1 or BRO-2, and these enzymes can be differentiated by isoelectric focusing. Strains that produce BRO-1 enzymes account for about 90% of the β-lactamase-producing *M. catarrhalis* isolated from clinical specimens, while BRO-2-producing strains account for the remaining 10%.[203,701] Molecular analysis of β-lactamase production indicates that the BRO-1 enzyme is encoded by a single chromosomal gene (*bla*) that encodes a 314-amino-acid polypeptide.[80] Sequence analysis of the *bla* genes from BRO-1- and BRO-2-producing isolates differ by five nucleotide bases that result in only a single amino acid residue difference in the amino acid sequences of the BRO-1 and BRO-2 enzymes. However, a 21-base-pair deletion was found in the promoter region of the BRO-2 gene. Differences in MICs of BRO-1- and BRO-2-producing *M. catarrhalis* strains may be explained by lower levels of BRO-2 production due to the deletion in the promoter region, while the structure and enzymatic activities of the two enzymes are similar.[80] Patients who have been infected with BRO-2 β-lactamase-producing *M. catarrhalis* strains have also responded clinically to ampicillin and penicillin. The BRO-1 has a molecular weight of about 32.5 kDa. Variations in the reported molecular weight of this enzyme, which range from 28 kDa to 41 kDa, are explained by the presence of free and lipid-associated forms of BRO-1.[77] The prevalence of strains that produce either BRO-1 or BRO-2 enzymes also differ. Among clinical isolates of *M. catarrhalis* collected during 1994–1995 and during 1997–1998 multicenter surveillance studies, the prevalence of BRO-1- and BRO-2-producing strains were 97.5% and 2.5%, respectively.[533] The *bla* gene may be transposon-associated and transferable by either transformational or conjugative mechanism.[79,339,702] In vitro studies indicate that the *M. catarrhalis* β-lactamases may indirectly function in virulence by inactivating penicillin or ampicillin given for other respiratory tract infections, such as pneumococcal pneumonia.[296]

Several studies conducted in the U.S. and abroad indicate that isolates of *M. catarrhalis* are generally susceptible to amoxicillin-clavulanate, second- and third-generation cephalosporins (i.e., cefuroxime, cefotaxime, ceftriaxone, cefpodoxime, ceftibuten, and the oral agents cefixime and cefaclor), macrolides (i.e., azithromycin, clarithromycin, erythromycin), tetracyclines, and rifampin.[72,99,195,224,568,653,654,700,737] While most isolates are susceptible to the fluoroquinolones (including ciprofloxacin, levofloxacin, sparfloxacin, grepafloxacin, trovafloxacin, and gemifloxacin), fluoroquinolone resistance has emerged in isolates recovered from patients who were on long-term therapy with such agents.[122,175,183,190,419,512] Other than variations in β-lactamase production, no notable differences in the antimicrobial susceptibilities of *M. catarrhalis* strains isolated from several countries (including Japan, the United Kingdom, Germany, Spain, France, Italy, and the U.S.) have been noted.[568] Rare strains of *M catarrhalis* may be resistant to tetracyclines, macrolides, or trimethoprim-sulfamethoxazole.[653,737]

More detailed information on antimicrobial susceptibility testing of these organisms is presented in Chapter 17.

References

1. Aakre RK, Jenkins A, Kristiansen B-E, Froholm LO. Clonal distribution of invasive *Neisseria meningitidis* isolates from the Norwegian county of Telemark, 1987–1995. J Clin Microbiol 1998;36:2623–2628.
2. Abadi FJR, Carter PE, Cash P, Pennington TH. Rifampin resistance in *Neisseria meningitidis* due to alterations in membrane permeability. Antimicrob Agents Chemother 1996;40:646–651.
3. Abadi FJR, Yakubu DE, Pennington TH. In vitro activities of meropenem and other antimicrobial agents against British meningococcal isolates. Chemotherapy 1999;45:253–257.
4. Abiteboul M, Mazieres, Causse B, et al. Septic arthritis of the knee due to *Neisseria mucosa*. Clin Rheumatol 1985;4:83–85.
5. Abuhammour WM, Abdel-Haq NM, Asmar BI, Dajani AS. *Moraxella catarrhalis* bacteremia: a 10-year experience. South Med J 1999;92:1071–1074.
6. Aeby C, Cope LD, Latimer JL, et al. Mapping of a protective epitope of the CopB outer membrane protein of *Moraxella catarrhalis*. Infect Immun 1998;66:540–548.
7. Aeby C, LaFontaine ER, Cope LD, et al. Phenotypic effect of isogenic *UspA1* and *UspA2* mutations on *Moraxella catarrhalis* strain O35E. Infect Immun 1998;66:3113–3119.
8. Aeby C, Stone B, Beucher M, et al. Expression of the CopB outer membrane protein by *Moraxella catarrhalis* is regulated by iron and affects iron acquisition from transferrin and lactoferrin. Infect Immun 1996;64:2024–2030.
9. Agraharkar M, Fahlen M, Siddiqui M, Rajaraman S. Waterhouse-Friderichsen syndrome and bilateral cortical necrosis in meningococcal sepsis. Am J Kidney Dis 2000;36:396–400.
10. Aguado JM, Vada J, Zuniga M. Meningococcemia: an undescribed cause of community-acquired bacteremia in patients with acquired immunodeficiency syndrome (AIDS) and AIDS-related complex. Am J Med 1990;88:314.
11. Ahmad H, Chapnick EK. Conjugated polysaccharide vaccines. In: Lutwick LI, ed.: Infectious Diseases Clinics of North America. Vol. 13. New vaccines and new vaccine technology, Philadelphia: WB Saunders, 1999:113–133.
12. Ahmed K. Fimbriae of *Branhamella catarrhalis* as possible mediators of adherence to pharyngeal epithelial cells. APMIS 1992;100:1066–1072.
13. Ahmed K, Matsumoto K, Rikitomi N, Nagatake T. Attachment of *Moraxella catarrhalis* to pharyngeal epithelial cells is mediated by a glycosphingolipid receptor. FEMS Microbiol Lett 1996;135:305–309.
14. Akduman D, Ehret JM, Messina K, et al. Evaluation of the strand displacement amplification assay (BD ProbeTec-SDA) for detection of *Neisseria gonorrhoeae* in urine specimens. J Clin Microbiol 2002;40:281–283.
15. Ala'aldeen DAA, Cartwright KCV. *Neisseria meningitidis*: vaccines and vaccine candidates. J Infect 1996;33:153–157.
16. Ala'aldeen DAA, Neal KR, Ait-Tahar K, et al. Dynamics of meningococcal long-term carriage among university students and their implications for mass vaccination. J Clin Microbiol 2000;38:2311–2316.
17. Ala'aldeen DAA, Stevenson P, Griffiths E, et al. Immune responses in humans and animals to meningococcal transferrin-binding proteins: implications for vaccine design. Infect Immun 1994;62:2984–2990.
18. Alexander WJ, Griffith H, Housch JG, et al. Infections in sexual contacts and associates of children with gonorrhea. Sex Transm Dis 1984;11:156–158.
19. Al-Zamil F, Al-Ballaa S, Nazer H, et al. Meningococcaemia: a life-threatening complication of upper gastrointestinal endoscopy. J Infect 1994;28:73–75.
20. American Academy of Pediatrics Committee on Child Abuse and Neglect. Gonorrhea in prepubertal children. Pediatrics 1998;101:134–135.
21. American Health Consultants. Vaccine could have saved lab workers from deadly meningitis infections. Hosp Infect Control 2001;28:45–60.
22. Amsel BJ, Moulijn AC. Nonfebrile mitral valve endocarditis due to *Neisseria subflava*. Chest 1996;109:280–282.
23. Anand CM, Ashton F, Shaw H, et al. Variability in growth of *Neisseria polysaccharea* on colistin-containing selective media for *Neisseria* spp. J Clin Microbiol 1991;29:2434–2437.
24. Anand CM, Gubash SM, Shaw H. Serologic confirmation of *Neisseria gonorrhoeae* by monoclonal antibody-based coagglutination reagents. J Clin Microbiol 1988;26:2283–2286.
25. Andersen BM, Steigerwalt AG, O'Connor SP, et al. *Neisseria weaveri* sp. nov., formerly CDC group M-5, a gram-negative bacterium associated with dog bite wounds. J Clin Microbiol 1993;31:2456–2466.
26. Andersen BM, Weyant RS, Steigerwalt AG, et al. Characterization of *Neisseria elongata* subsp. *glycolytica* isolates obtained from human wound specimens and blood cultures. J Clin Microbiol 1995;33:76–78.
27. Andersen J, Berthelsen L, Jensen BB, Lind I. Surveillance of cases of meningococcal disease associated with military recruits studied for meningococcal carriage. Scand J Infect Dis 2000;32:527–531.
28. Andersen J, Lind I. Characterization of *Neisseria meningitidis* isolates and clinical features of meningococcal conjunctivitis in ten patients. Eur J Clin Microbiol Infect Dis 1994;13:388–393.
29. Anderson B, Albritton WL, Biddle J, et al. Common β-lactamase specifying plasmid in *Haemophilus ducreyi* and *Neisseria gonorrhoeae*. Antimicrob Agents Chemother 1984;25:296–297.
30. Anderson C. Childhood sexually transmitted diseases: one consequence of sexual abuse. Publ Health Nursing 1995;12:41–46.
31. Anderson MD, Miller LK. Endocarditis due to *Neisseria mucosa*. Clin Infect Dis 1993;16:184.
32. Apfalter P, Horler R, Nehrer S. *Neisseria meningitidis* serogroup W-135 primary monoarthritis of the hip in an immunocompetent child. Eur J Clin Microbiol Infect Dis 2000;19:475–476.
33. Apicella MA. *Neisseria meningitidis*. In: Mandell GL, Bennett JE, Dolin R, eds.: Mandell, Douglas, and Bennett's Principles and Practice of Infectious Diseases. 5th Ed. New York:, Churchill Livingstone, 2000:2228–2241.
34. Apicella MA, Shero M, Jarvis GA, et al. Phenotypic variation in epitope expression of *Neisseria gonorrhoeae* lipooligosaccharide. Infect Immun 1987;55:1755–1751.
35. Arreaza L, de la Fuente L, Vazquez JA. Antibiotic susceptibility patterns of *Neisseria meningitidis* isolates from patients and asymptomatic carriers. Antimicrob Agents Chemother 2000;44:1705–1707.
36. Arreaza L, Salcedo C, Alcala B, Vazquez JA. What about antibiotic resistance in *Neisseria lactamica*. J Antimicrob Chemother 2002;49:545–547.
37. Ashford WA, Potts DW, Adams HJU, et al. Spectinomycin-resistant penicillinase-producing *Neisseria gonorrhoeae*. Lancet 1981;2:1035–1037.
38. Ashton FE, Mancino L, Ryan AJ, et al. Serotypes and subtypes of *Neisseria meningitidis* serogroup B strains associated with meningococcal disease in Canada, 1977–1989. Can J Microbiol 1991;37:613–617.
39. Ashton FE, Ryan JA, Borczyk A, et al. Emergence of a virulent clone of *Neisseria meningitidis* serotype 2a that is associated with meningococcal group C disease in Canada. J Clin Microbiol 1991;29:2489–2493.

40. Asnis DS, Brennessel DJ. Gonococcal scalp abscess: a risk of intrauterine monitoring. Clin Pediatr (Phila) 1992;31:316–317.

41. Assier H, Chosidow O, Rekacewicz I, et al. Chronic meningococcemia in acquired immunodeficiency infection. J Am Acad Dermatol 1993;29:793–794.

42. Au Y-K, Reynolds MD, Rambin ED, et al. *Neisseria cinerea* purulent conjunctivitis. Am J Ophthalmol 1990;109:96–97.

43. Ayala P, Vasquez B, Wetzler L, So M. *Neisseria gonorrhoeae* porin P1.B induces endosome exocytosis and a redistribution of Lamp1 to the plasma membrane. Infect Immun 2002;70:5965–5971.

44. Backman A, Orvelid P, Vazquez JA, et al. Complete sequence of a β-lactamase-encoding plasmid in *Neisseria meningitidis*. Antimicrob Agents Chemother 2000;44:210–212.

45. Baevski RH. Primary meningococcal pericarditis. Clin Infect Dis 1999;29:213–214.

46. Baraldes MA, Domingo P, Barrio JL, et al. Meningitis due to *Neisseria subflava*: case report and review. Clin Infect Dis 2000;30:615–617.

47. Barbe G, Babolat M, Boeufgras JM, et al. Evaluation of API NH, a new 2-hour system for identification of *Neisseria* and *Haemophilus* species and *Moraxella catarrhalis* in a routine clinical laboratory. J Clin Microbiol 1994;32:187–189.

48. Barlow D. The diagnosis of oropharyngeal gonorrhoea. Genitourin Med 1997;73:16–17

49. Barnes RA, Jenkins P, Coakley WT. Preliminary clinical evaluation of meningococcal disease and bacterial meningitis by ultrasonic enhancement. Arch Dis Child 1998;78:58–60.

50. Barquet N, Gasser I, Domingo P, et al. Primary meningococcal conjunctivitis: report of 21 patients and review. Rev Infect Dis 1990;12:838–847.

51. Barrett SJ, Schlater LK, et al. A new species of *Neisseria* from iguanid lizards, *Neisseria iguanae* sp. nov. Lett Appl Microbiol 1994;18:200–202.

52. Bart A, Schuurman IGA, Achtman M, et al. Randomly amplified polymorphic DNA genotyping of serogroup A meningococci yields results similar to those obtained by multilocus enzyme electrophoresis and reveals new genotypes. J Clin Microbiol 1998;36:1746–1749.

53. Bartoloni A, Norelli F, Ceccarini C, et al. Immunogenicity of the meningococcal B polysaccharide conjugated to tetanus toxoid or to CRM$_{197}$ via adipic acid dihydrazide. Vaccine 1995;13:463–470.

54. Beck-Sague CM, Solomon F. Sexually transmitted diseases in abused children and adolescent and adult victims of rape: review of selected literature. Clin Infect Dis 1999;28(Suppl 1):S74–S83.

55. Beebe JL, Rau MP, Flageolle S, et al. Incidence of *Neisseria gonorrhoeae* isolates negative by Syva direct fluorescent-antibody test but positive by Gen-Probe Accuprobe test in a sexually transmitted disease clinic population. J Clin Microbiol 1993;31:2535–2537.

56. Belding ME, Carbone J. Gonococcemia associated with adult respiratory distress syndrome. Rev Infect Dis 1991;13:1105–1107.

57. Belland RJ, Morrison SG, Ison C, Huang WM. *Neisseria gonorrhoeae* acquires mutations in analogous regions of *gryA* and *ParC* in fluoroquinolone-resistant isolates. Mol Microbiol 1994;14:371–380.

58. Beltrami JF, Farley TA, Hamrick JT, et al. Evaluation of the Gen-Probe PACE 2 assay for the detection of asymptomatic *Chlamydia trachomatis* and *Neisseria gonorrhoeae* infections in male arrestees. Sex Transm Dis 1998;25:501–504.

59. Berger SA, Gorea A, Peysser MR, et al. Bartholin's gland abscess caused by *Neisseria sicca*. J Clin Microbiol 1988;26:1589.

60. Berron S, Vazquez JA. Increase in moderate penicillin resistance and serogroup C in meningococcal strains isolated in Spain: is there any relationship? Clin Infect Dis 1994;18:161–165.

61. Beucher M, Sparling PF. Cloning, sequencing, and characterization of the gene encoding FrpB, a major iron-regulated, outer membrane protein of *Neisseria gonorrhoeae*. J Bacteriol 1995;177:2041–2049.

62. Beverly A, Bailey-Griffin JR, Schwebke JR. InTray GC medium versus modified Thayer-Martin agar plates for diagnosis of gonorrhea from endocervical specimens. J Clin Microbiol 2000;38:3825–3826.

63. Bhat KS, Gibbs CP, Barrera O, et al. The opacity proteins of *Neisseria gonorrhoeae* strain MS11 are encoded by a family of 11 complete genes. Mol Microbiol 1992;6:1073–1076.

64. Bhushan R, Craigie R, Murphy TF. Molecular cloning and characterization of outer membrane protein E of *Moraxella* (*Branhamella*) *catarrhalis*. J Bacteriol 1994;176:6636–6643.

65. Billings SD, Fuller DeAnna, LeMonte AM, et al. Characterization of DFA-negative, probe-positive *Neisseria gonorrhoeae* by pulsed field electrophoresis. Diagn Microbiol Infect Dis 1997;29:281–283.

66. Bjerknes R, Guttormsen H-K, Solberg SO, Wetzler LM. Neisserial porins inhibit human neutrophil actin polymerization, degranulation, opsonin receptor expression, and phagocytosis, but prime the neutrophils to increase their exudative burst. Infect Immun 1995;63:160–167.

67. Bjune G, Hoiby EA, Gronnesby JK, et al. Effect of outer membrane vesicle vaccine against group B meningococcal disease in Norway. Lancet 1991;338:1093–1096.

68. Black JR, Black WJ, Cannon JG. *Neisseria* antigen H.8 is immunogenic in

69. Black JR, Dyer DW, Thompson MK, Sparling PF. Human immune response to iron-repressible outer membrane proteins of *Neisseria meningitidis*. Infect Immun 1986;54:710–713.

70. Block C, Davidson Y, Keller N. Unreliability of disc diffusion test for screening for reduced penicillin susceptibility in *Neisseria meningitidis*. J Clin Microbiol 1998;36:3103–3104.

71. Blondeau JM, Ashton FE, Isaccson M, et al. *Neisseria meningitidis* with decreased susceptibility to penicillin in Saskatchewan, Canada. J Clin Microbiol 1995;33:1784–1786.

72. Blondeau JM, Suter M, Borsos S, Canadian Antimicrobial Study Group. Determination of the antimicrobial susceptibilities of Canadian isolates of *Haemophilus influenzae*, *Streptococcus pneumoniae*, and *Moraxella catarrhalis*. J Antimicrob Chemother 1999;43(Suppl A):25–30.

73. Bodsworth NJ, Price R, Davies SC. Gonococcal infection of the neovagina in a male-to-female transsexual. Sex Transm Dis 1994;21:211–212.

74. Bodsworth NJ, Price R, Nelson MJ. A case of gonococcal mastitis in a male. Genitourin Med 1993;69:222–223.

75. Boehm DM, Bernhardt M, Kurzynski TA, et al. Evaluation of two commercial procedures for rapid identification of *Neisseria gonorrhoeae* using a reference panel of antigenically diverse gonococci. J Clin Microbiol 1990;28:2099–2100.

76. Bonnah RA, Yu RH, Wong H, Schryvers AB. Biochemical and immunological properties of lactoferrin binding proteins from *Moraxella* (*Branhamella*) *catarrhalis*. Microb Pathog 1998;24:89–100.

77. Bootsma HJ, Aerts PC, Posthuma G, et al. *Moraxella* (*Branhamella*) catarrhalis BRO β-lactamase: a lipoprotein of gram-positive origin? J Bacteriol 1999;181:5090–5093.

78. Bootsma HJ, van der Heide HGJ, van de Pas S, et al. Analysis of *Moraxella catarrhalis* by DNA typing: evidence for a distinct subpopulation associated with virulence traits. J Infect Dis 2000;181:1376–1387.

79. Bootsma HJ, Van Dijk H, Vauterin P, et al. Genesis of BRO β-lactamase-producing *Moraxella catarrhalis*: evidence for transformation-mediated horizontal transfer. Mol Microbiol 2000;36:93–104.

80. Bootsma HJ, Van Dijk H, Verhoef J, et al. Molecular characterization of the BRO β-lactamase of *Moraxella* (*Branhamella*) *catarrhalis*. Antimicrob Agents Chemother 1996;40:966–972.

81. Borrow R, Claus H, Chaudhry U, et al. *siaD* PCR ELISA for the confirmation and identification of serogroup Y and W135 meningococcal infections. FEMS Microbiol Lett 1998;159:209–214.

82. Borrow R, Claus H, Guiver M, et al. Non-culture diagnosis and serogroup determination of meningococcal B and C infection by a sialyltransferase (*siaD*) PCR ELISA. Epidemiol Infect 1997;118:111–117.

83. Botha P. Penicillin-resistant *Neisseria meningitidis* in southern Africa. Lancet 1988;1:54.

84. Bouquete MT, Marcos C, Saez-Nieto JA. Characterization of *Neisseria polysaccharea* sp. nov. (Riou, 1983) in previously identified noncapsulated strains of *Neisseria meningitidis*. J Clin Microbiol 1986;23:973–975.

85. Bourbeau P, Holla V, Peimontese S. Ophthalmia neonatorum caused by *Neisseria cinerea*. J Clin Microbiol 1990;28:1640–1641.

86. Bovre K. Proposal to divide the genus *Moraxella* Lwoff 1939 emend. Henriksen and Bovre 1968 into two subgenera, subgenus *Moraxella* (Lwoff 1939) Bovre 1979 and subgenus *Branhamella* (Catlin 1970) Bovre 1979. Int J Syst Bacteriol 1979;29:403–406.

87. Bovre K. Family VIII. *Neisseriaceae* Prevot 1933, 119^{AL}. In: Krieg NR, Holt JG, eds.: Bergey's Manual of Systematic Bacteriology. Vol 1. Baltimore: Williams & Wilkins, 1984:288–290.

88. Bovre K. Genus II. *Moraxella* Lwoff 1939, 173 emend. Henriksen and Bovre 1968, 391. In Krieg NR, Holt JG. eds.: Bergey's Manual of Systematic Bacteriology. Vol 1. Baltimore: Williams & Wilkins, 1984:296–303.

89. Bovre K, Holten E. *Neisseria elongata* sp. nov., a rod-shaped member of the genus *Neisseria*: re-evaluation of cell shape as a criterion for classification. J Gen Microbiol 1970;60:67–75.

90. Bowler LD, Zhang Q-Y, Riou J-Y, et al. Interspecies recombination between the *penA* genes of *Neisseria meningitidis* and commensal *Neisseria* species during the emergence of penicillin resistance in *N. meningitidis*: natural events and laboratory simulation. J Bacteriol 1994;176:333–337.

91. Boyce JM, Mitchell EB. Difficulties in differentiating *Neisseria cinerea* from *Neisseria gonorrhoeae* in rapid systems used for identifying pathogenic *Neisseria* species. J Clin Microbiol 1985;22:731–734.

92. Boyce JM, Taylor MR, Mitchell EB, et al. Nosocomial pneumonia caused by a glucose-metabolizing strain of *Neisseria cinerea*. J Clin Microbiol 1985;21:1–3.

93. Brandtzaeg P, Halstensen A, Kierulf P, et al. Molecular mechanisms in the compartmentalized inflammatory response presenting as meningococcal meningitis or septic shock. Microb Pathog 1992;13:423–431.

94. Brandtzaeg P, Mollnes TE, Kierulf P. Complement activation and endotoxin levels in systemic meningococcal disease. J Infect Dis 1989;160:58–65.

patients with disseminated gonococcal and meningococcal infections. J Infect Dis 1985;151:650–657.

95. Brook MG, Clark S, Stirland A, et al. A case cluster of possible tissue invasive gonorrhoea. Genitourin Med 1995;71:126–128.

96. Brooks GF, Lammel CJ, Blake MS, et al. Antibodies against IgA$_1$ protease are stimulated both by clinical disease and asymptomatic carriage of serogroup A *Neisseria meningitidis*. J Infect Dis 1992;166:1316–1321.

97. Broome CV. The carrier state: *Neisseria meningitidis*. J Antimicrob Chemother 1986;18(Suppl A):25–34.

98. Bruce MG, Rosenstein NE, Capparella J, et al. Risk factors for meningococcal disease in college students (abstract). Clin Infect Dis 1999;29:973.

99. Brueggemann AB, Doern GV, Huynh HK, et al. In vitro activity of ABT, a new ketolide, against recent clinical isolates of *Streptococcus pneumoniae, Haemophilus influenzae,* and *Moraxella catarrhalis*. Antimicrob Agents Chemother 2000;44:447–449.

100. Brunen A, Peetermans W, Verhagen J, et al. Meningitis due to *Neisseria meningitidis* with intermediate susceptibility to penicillin. Eur J Clin Microbiol Infect Dis 1993;12:969–970.

101. Brunham RC. The concept of core and its relevance to the epidemiology and control of sexually transmitted diseases. Sex Transm Dis 2000;18:67–68.

102. Brunham RC, Plummer F, Slaney L, et al. Correlation of auxotype and protein I type with expression of disease due to *Neisseria gonorrhoeae*. J Infect Dis 1985;152:339–343.

103. Burnett IA, Denton K, Sutcliffe J. Cerebrospinal fluid shunt infection: an unusual case. J Infect 1990;22:205–206.

104. Buttcher V, Welsh T, Willmitzer L, Kossmann J. Cloning and characterization of the gene for amylosucrase from *Neisseria polysaccharea*: production of a linear α-1,4-glucan. J Bacteriol 1997;179:3324–3330.

105. Calanan D, Rubsamen PE. *Moraxella* infection of a scleral buckle. Am J Ophthalmol 1992;114:637–638.

106. Camarena JJ, Nogueira JM, Dasi MA, et al. DNA amplification fingerprinting for subtyping *Neisseria gonorrhoeae* strains. Sex Transm Dis 1995;22:128–136.

107. Campagnari AA, Ducey TF, Rebmann CA. Outer membrane protein B1, an iron-repressible protein conserved in the outer membrane of *Moraxella (Branhamella) catarrhalis*, binds human transferrin. Infect Immun 1996;64:3920–3924.

108. Campbell WN, Joshi M, Sileo D. Osteonecrosis following meningococcemia and disseminated intravascular coagulation in an adult: case report and review. Clin Infect Dis 1997;24:452–455.

109. Campos J. Disc testing of meningococci. J Clin Microbiol 37:879–880, 1999.

110. Campos J, Mendelman PM, Saku MU, et al. Detection of relatively penicillin G-resistant *Neisseria meningitidis* by disk susceptibility testing. Antimicrob Agents Chemother 1987;31:1478.

111. Cann KJ, Rogers TR. The phenotypic relationship of *Neisseria polysaccharea* to commensal and pathogenic *Neisseria* ssp. J Mol Microbiol 1989;39:351–354.

112. Cannon JG, Black WJ, Nachamkin I, Stewart PW. Monoclonal antibody that recognizes an outer membrane antigen common to the pathogenic *Neisseria* species but not to most nonpathogenic *Neisseria* species. Infect Immun 1984;43:994–999.

113. Capitini CM, Herrero IA, Patel R, et al. Wound infection with *Neisseria weaveri* and a novel subspecies of *Pasteurella multocida* in a child who sustained a tiger bite. Clin Infect Dis 2002;34:E74–E76.

114. Carballo M, Dillon JR. Evaluation of an enzyme immunoassay and a modified coagglutination assay for typing gonococcal isolates with monoclonal antibodies. Sex Transm Dis 1992;19:219–224.

115. Carbonetti NH, Sparling PF. Molecular cloning and characterization of the structural gene for protein I, the major outer membrane protein of *Neisseria gonorrhoeae*. Proc Natl Acad Sci USA 1987;84:9084–9088.

116. Carlson P, Kontiainen S, Anttila P, Eerola E. Septicemia caused by *Neisseria weaveri*. Clin Infect Dis 1997;24:739.

117. Carrick CS, Fyfer JAM, Davies JK. *Neisseria gonorrhoeae* contains multiple copies of a gene that may encode a site-specific recombinase and is associated with DNA rearrangements. Gene 1998;220:21–29.

118. Carter KD, Morgan CM, Otto MH. *Neisseria mucosa* endophthalmitis. Am J Ophthalmol 1987;104:663–664.

119. Cartwright KAV. Early management of meningococcal disease. In: Schhad UB, ed.: Infectious Disease Clinics of North America, Vol 13. Bacterial meningitis. Philadelphia: WB Saunders, 1999:661–684.

120. Cartwright KAV, Ala'aldeen DAA. *Neisseria meningitidis*: clinical aspects. J Infect 1997;34:15–19.

121. Cartwright KAV, Stuart JM, Robinson PM. Meningococcal carriage in close contacts of cases. Epidemiol Infect 1991;106:133–141.

122. Casellas JM, Gilardoni M, Tome G, et al. Comparative in-vitro activity of levofloxacin against isolates of bacteria from adult patients with community-acquired lower respiratory tract infections. J Antimicrob Chemother 1999;43(Suppl C):37–42.

123. Catlin BW. Cellular elongation under the influence of antibacterial agents: way to differentiate coccobacilli from cocci. J Clin Microbiol 1975;1:102–105.

124. Catlin BW. Nutritional profiles of *Neisseria gonorrhoeae, Neisseria meningitidis,* and *Neisseria lactamica* in chemically defined media and the use of growth requirements for gonococcal typing. J Infect Dis 1975;128:178–194.

125. Catlin BW. *Branhamaceae* fam. nov., a proposed family to accommodate the genera *Branhamella* and *Moraxella*. Int J Syst Bacteriol 1991;41:320–323.

126. Caugant DA. Population genetics and molecular epidemiology of *Neisseria meningitidis*. APMIS 1998;106:505–525.

127. Caugant DA, Bol P, Hoiby EA, et al. Clones of serogroup B *Neisseria meningitidis* causing systemic disease in the Netherlands, 1958–1986. J Infect Dis 1990;162:867–874.

128. Caugant DA, Hoiby EA, Magnus P, et al. Asymptomatic carriage of *Neisseria meningitidis* in a randomly sampled population. J Clin Microbiol 1994;32:323–330.

129. Caugant DA, Mocca LF, Frasch CE, et al. Genetic structure of *Neisseria meningitidis* populations in relation to serogroup, serotype, and outer membrane protein pattern. J Bacteriol 1987;169:2781–2792.

130. Centers for Disease Control. Chromosomally-mediated resistant *Neisseria gonorrhoeae*—United States. MMWR Morb Mortal Wkly Rep 1984;33:408–410.

131. Centers for Disease Control. Tetracycline-resistant *Neisseria gonorrhoeae*—Georgia, Pennsylvania, New Hampshire. MMWR Morb Mortal Wkly Rep 1985;34:563–570.

132. Centers for Disease Control and Prevention. Decreased susceptibility of *Neisseria gonorrhoeae* to fluoroquinolones—Ohio and Hawaii, 1992–1994. MMWR Morb Mortal Wkly Rep 1994;43:325–327.

133. Centers for Disease Control and Prevention. Serogroup B meningococcal disease—Oregon, 1994. MMWR Morb Mortal Wkly Rep 1995;44:121–134.

134. Centers for Disease Control and Prevention. Control and prevention of meningococcal disease and control and prevention of serogroup C meningococcal diseases: evaluation and management of suspected outbreaks. MMWR Morb Mortal Wkly Rep 1997;46(RR-5):1–22.

135. Centers for Disease Control and Prevention. Meningococcal disease—New England, 1993–1998. MMWR Morb Mortal Wkly Rep 1999;48:629–633.

136. Centers for Disease Control and Prevention. Meningococcal disease among college students. ACIP modifies recommendations for meningitis vaccination. (Accessed December 1999 at http://www.cdc.gov/ncidod/dbmd/diseaseinfo/meningococcal✂college.htm.).

137. Centers for Disease Control and Prevention. Serogroup W135 meningococcal disease among travelers returning from Saudi Arabia—United States, 2000. MMWR Morb Mortal Wkly Rep 2000;49:345–346.

138. Centers for Disease Control and Prevention. Fluoroquinolone resistance in *Neisseria gonorrhoeae*, Hawaii, 1999, and decreased susceptibility to azithromycin in *N. gonorrhoeae*, Missouri, 1999. MMWR Morb Mortal Wkly Rep 2000;49:844.

139. Centers for Disease Control and Prevention. Gonococcal Isolate Surveillance Project. Atlanta, GA: Centers for Disease Control and Prevention. Available at http://www.cdc.gov/ncidod/dastlr/gcdir/Resist/gisp.html.

140. Centers for Disease Control and Prevention. 2000 Sexually Transmitted Diseases Surveillance. Gonococcal Isolate Surveillance Project (GISP) Supplement. Atlanta, GA: Centers for Disease Control and Prevention. Available at http://www.cdc.gov/nchstp/dstd/Stats✂Trends/Stats✂and✂Trends.htm.

141. Centers for Disease Control and Prevention. Laboratory-acquired meningococcal disease—United States, 2000. MMWR Morb Mortal Wkly Rep 2002;71:141–144.

142. Centers for Disease Control and Prevention. Sexually transmitted diseases treatment guidelines 2002. MMWR 2002;51:RR-6.

143. Centers for Disease Control and Prevention. Recall of LCx *Neisseria gonorrhoeae* assay and implications for laboratory testing for *N. gonorrhoeae* and *C. trachomatis*. MMWR Morb Mortal Wkly Rep 200251:709.

144. Chan EL, Brandt K, Olienus K, et al. Performance characteristics of the Becton Dickinson ProbeTec system for direct detection of *Chlamydia trachomatis* and *Neisseria gonorrhoeae* in male and female urine specimens in comparison with the Roche COBAS system. Arch Pathol Lab Med 2000;124:1649–1652.

145. Chapin-Roberston K, Reece EA, Edberg SC. Evaluation of the Gen-Probe PACE II assay for the direct detection of *Neisseria gonorrhoeae* in endocervical specimens. Diagn Microbiol Infect Dis 1992;15:645–649.

146. Chaudhuri AKR, Banatvala, Caugant DA, et al. Phenotypically similar clones of serogroup B *Neisseria meningitidis* causing recurrent meningitis in a patient with total C5 deficiency. J Infect 1994;26:236–238.

147. Chen D, Barniak V, Van Der Meid KR, McMichael JC. The levels and bactericidal capacity of antibodies directed against the UspA1 and UsapA2 outer membrane proteins of *Moraxella (Branhamella) catarrhalis* in adults and children. Infect Immun 1999;67:1310–1316.

148. Chen D, McMichael JC, Van Der Meid KR, et al. Evaluation of a 74-kDa transferrin binding protein from *Moraxella (Branhamella) catarrhalis* as a vaccine candidate. Vaccine 1999;18:109–118.

149. Cher DJ, Maxwell WJ, Frusztajer N, et al. A case of pelvic inflammatory disease associated with *Neisseria meningitidis* bacteremia. Clin Infect Dis 1993;17:134–135.

150. Chong S, Jang D, Song X, et al. Specimen processing and concentration of *Chlamydia trachomatis* added can influence false-negative rates in the LCx assay

but not in the APTIMA Combo 2 assay when testing for inhibitors. J Clin Microbiol 2003;41:778–782.

151. Christensen JJ. *Moraxella (Branhamella) catarrhalis*: clinical, microbiological, and immunological features in lower respiratory tract infections. APMIS 1999; 88(Suppl):1–36.

152. Christensen JJ, Keiding J, Schumacher H, et al. Recognition of a new *Branhamella catarrhalis* β-lactamase—BRO 3. J Antimicrob Chemother 1991;28: 774–775.

153. Christian CW, Pinto-Martin JA, McGowan KL. The management of prepubertal children with gonorrhea. Clin Pediatr 1995;34:415–418.

154. Ciemins EL, Borenstein LA, Dyer IE, et al. Comparisons of cost and accuracy of DNA probe test and culture for the detection of *Neisseria gonorrhoeae* in patients attending public health sexually transmitted diseases clinics in Los Angeles County. Sex Transm Dis 1997;24:422–428.

155. Claesson BA, Leinonen M. *Moraxella catarrhalis*: an uncommon cause of community-acquired pneumonia in Swedish children. Scand J Infect Dis 1994;26: 399–402.

156. Clark VL, Campbell LA, Palermo DA, et al. Induction and repression of outer membrane proteins by anaerobic growth of *Neisseria gonorrhoeae*. Infect Immun 1987;55:1359–1364.

157. Clausen CR, Knapp JS, Totten PA. Lymphadenitis due to *Neisseria cinerea*. Lancet 1984;1:908.

158. Clendenning TE, Echeverria P, Saenguer S, et al. Antibiotic susceptibility survey of *Neisseria gonorrhoeae* in Thailand. Antimicrob Agents Chemother 1992;36: 1682–1687.

159. Coe MD, Hamer DH, Levy CS, et al. Gonococcal pericarditis with tamponade in a patient with systemic lupus erythematosus. Arthritis Rheum 1990;33: 1438–1441.

160. Connell TD, Black WJ, Kawula TH, et al. Recombination among protein II genes of *Neisseria gonorrhoeae* generates new coding sequences and increases structural variability in the protein II family. Mol Microbiol 1988;2:227–236.

161. Connell TD, Shaffer D, Cannon JG. Characterization of the repertoire of hypervariable regions in the protein II (*Opa*) gene family of *Neisseria gonorrhoeae*. Mol Microbiol 1990;4:439–449.

162. Conrads G, Haase G, Schnitzler N, et al. *Neisseria meningitidis* serogroup B peritonitis associated with continuous ambulatory peritoneal dialysis. Eur J Clin Microbiol Infect Dis 1998;17:341–343.

163. Cook PP, Hecht DW, Snydman DR. Nosocomial *Branhamella catarrhalis* in a paediatric intensive care unit: risk factors for disease. J Hosp Infect 1989;13: 299–307.

164. Cooke RP, Williams R, Bannister CM. Shunt-associated ventriculitis caused by *Branhamella catarrhalis*. J Hosp Infect 1990;15:197–198.

165. Cookson ST, Corrales JL, Lotero JO, et al. Disco fever: epidemic meningococcal disease in northeastern Argentina associated with disco patronage. J Infect Dis 1998;178:266–269.

166. Cooper ER, Ellison RT, Smith GS, et al. Rifampin-resistant meningococcal disease in a contact patient given prophylactic rifampin. J Pediatr 1985;107:93.

167. Cope LD, LaFontaine ER, Slaughter CA, et al. Characterization of the *Moraxella catarrhalis* UspA1 and UspA2 genes and their encoded products. J Bacteriol 1999;181:4026–4034.

168. Crawford G, Knapp JS, Hale J. Asymptomatic gonorrhea in men: caused by gonococci with unique nutritional requirements. Science 1977;196:1352–1353.

169. Crotchfelt KA, Welsh LE, DeBonville D, et al. Detection of *Neisseria gonorrhoeae* and *Chlamydia trachomatis* in genitourinary specimens from men and women by a coamplification PCR assay. J Clin Microbiol 1997;35:1536–1540.

170. Cucurull E, Espinoza LR. Gonococcal arthritis. In: Espinoza LR, ed.: Rheumatic Disease Clinics of North America. Vol. 24, Infectious arthritis. Philadelphia: WB Saunders, 1998:305–322.

171. Damany DS, Sherlock DA, Croall J. Primary meningococcal pyoarthrosis of the knee. J Infect 1997;35:320–321.

172. D'Antuono A, Andalo F, Varotti C. Acute urethritis due to *Neisseria meningitidis*. Sex Transm Dis 1999;75:362.

173. Daoud A, Abuekteish F, Masaadeh H. Neonatal meningitis due to *Moraxella catarrhalis* and review of the literature. Ann Trop Paediatr 1996;16:199–201.

174. Darwin LH, Cullen AP, Arthur PM, et al. Comparison of Digene hybrid capture 2 and conventional culture for detection of *Chlamydia trachomatis* and *Neisseria gonorrhoeae* in cervical specimens. J Clin Microbiol 2002;40:641–644.

175. Davies TA, Kelly LM, Hoellman DB, et al. Activities and postantibiotic effects of gemifloxacin compared to those of 11 other agents against *Haemophilus influenzae* and *Moraxella catarrhalis*. Antimicrob Agents Chemother 2000;44: 633–639.

176. Davis CL, Towns M, Henrich WL, et al. *Neisseria mucosa* endocarditis following drug abuse: case report and review of the literature. Arch Intern Med 1983; 143:583–385.

177. Dealler SF, Abbott M, Croughan MJ, et al. Identification of *Branhamella catarrhalis* in 2.5 min with an indoxyl butyrate strip test. J Clin Microbiol 1989;27: 1390–1391.

178. Dealler SF, Gough KR, Campbell L, et al. Identification of *Neisseria gonorrhoeae* using the Neisstrip rapid enzyme detection test. J Clin Pathol 1991;44: 376–379.

179. Deguchi T, Yasuda M, Nakano M, et al. Quinolone-resistant *Neisseria gonorrhoeae*: correlation of alterations in the GyrA subunit of DNA gyrase and the ParC subunit of topoisomerase IV with antimicrobial susceptibility profiles. Antimicrob Agents Chemother 1996;40:1020–1023.

180. Demmler GJ, Couch RS, Taber LH. *Neisseria subflava* bacteremia and meningitis in a child: report of a case and review of the literature. Pediatr Infect Dis 1985;4:286.

181. Denning DW, Gill SS. *Neisseria lactamica* meningitis following skull trauma. Rev Infect Dis 1991;13:216–218.

182. Derkx B, Wittes J, McCloskey R, et al. Randomized, placebo-controlled trial of HA-1A, a human monoclonal antibody to endotoxin, in children with meningococcal septic shock. Clin Infect Dis 1999;28:770–777.

183. Deshpande LM, Jones RN. Antimicrobial activity of advanced-spectrum fluoroquinolones tested against more than 2000 contemporary bacterial isolates of species causing community-acquired respiratory tract infections in the United States (1999). Diagn Microbiol Infect Dis 2000;37:139–142.

184. DeVaux DL, Evans GL, Arndt CW, et al. Comparison of the Gono-Pak system with the candle extinction jar for recovery of *Neisseria gonorrhoeae*. J Clin Microbiol 1987;25:571–572.

185. DeVries EP, Cole R, Dankert J, et al. *Neisseria meningitidis* producing the Opc adhesin binds epithelial cell proteoglycan receptors. Mol Microbiol 1998;27: 1203–1212.

186. Dewhirst FE, Paster BJ, Bright PL. *Chromobacterium*, *Eikenella*, *Kingella*, *Neisseria*, *Simonsiella*, and *Vitreoscilla* species comprise a major branch of the β-subgroup of the *Protobacteria* by 16S ribosomal nucleic acid sequence comparison: transfer of *Eikenella* and *Simonsiella* to the Family *Neisseriaceae* (emend.). Int J Syst Bacteriol 1989;39:258–266.

187. Diemert DJ, Libman MD, Lebel P. Confirmation by 16S rRNA PCR of the COBAS AMPLICOR CT/NG test for diagnosis of *Neisseria gonorrhoeae* infection in a low-prevalence population. J Clin Microbiol 2002;40:4056–4059.

188. Dillon JR, Carballo M, Pauze M. Evaluation of eight methods for identification of pathogenic *Neisseria* species: Neisseria-Kwik, RIM-N, Gonobio Test, Minitek, Gonochek II, GonoGen, Phadebact Monoclonal GC OMNI test, and Syva MicroTrak test. J Clin Microbiol 1988;26:493–497.

189. Dillon JR, Pauze M, Yeung K-H. Spread of penicillinase-producing and transfer plasmids from the gonococcus to *Neisseria meningitidis*. Lancet 1983;1:779–781.

190. DiPersio JR, Jones RN, Barrett T, et al. Fluoroquinolone-resistant *Moraxella catarrhalis* in a patient with pneumonia: report from the SENTRY antimicrobial surveillance program (1998). Diagn Microbiol Infect Dis 1998;32:131–135.

191. Division of STD Prevention. Sexually Transmitted Disease Surveillance, 1994. Atlanta: Department of Health and Human Services, Public Health Service, 1995.

192. Doern GV. *Branhamella catarrhalis*: phenotypic characteristics. Am J Med 1990;88(Suppl 5A):33S–35S.

193. Doern GV, Blacklow NR, Gantz NM, et al. *Neisseria sicca* osteomyelitis. J Clin Microbiol 1982;16:595–597.

194. Doern GV, Gantz NM. Isolation of *Branhamella (Neisseria) catarrhalis* from men with urethritis. Sex Transm Dis 1982;9:202–204.

195. Doern GV, Jones RN, Pfaller MA, et al. *Haemophilus influenzae* and *Moraxella catarrhalis* from patients with community-acquired respiratory tract infections: antimicrobial susceptibility patterns from the SENTRY antimicrobial surveillance program (United States and Canada, 1997). Antimicrob Agents Chemother 1999;43:385–389.

196. Doern GV, Tubert TA. Detection of β-lactamase activity among clinical isolates of *Branhamella catarrhalis* with six different β-lactamase assays. J Clin Microbiol 1987;25:1380–1383.

197. Dolter J, Bryant L, Janda JM. Evaluation of five rapid systems for the identification of *Neisseria gonorrhoeae*. Diagn Microbiol Infect Dis 1990;13:265–267.

198. Dolter J, Wong J, Janda JM. Association of *Neisseria cinerea* with ocular infections in paediatric patients. J Infect 1998;36:49–52.

199. Domingo P, Coll P, Maroto P, et al. *Neisseria subflava* bacteremia in a neutropenic patient. Arch Intern Med 1996;156:1762.

200. Dominguez EA, Smith TL. Endocarditis due to *Neisseria elongata* subspecies *nitroreducens*: case report and review. Clin Infect Dis 1998;26:1471–1473.

201. Dossett JH, Applebaum PC, Knapp JS, et al. Proctitis associated with *Neisseria cinerea* misidentified as *Neisseria gonorrhoeae* in a child. J Clin Microbiol 1985;21:575–577.

202. Doyle MB, DeCherney AH, Diamond MP. Epidemiology and etiology of ectopic pregnancy. Obstet Gynecol Clin North Am 1991;18:1–17.

203. Du Plessis M. Rapid discrimination between BRO β-lactamases from clinical isolates of *Moraxella catarrhalis* using restriction endonuclease analysis. Diag Microbiol Infect Dis 2001;39:65–67.

204. Durand ML, Calderwood SB, Weber DJ, et al. Acute bacterial meningitis in adults. N Engl J Med 1993;328:21–28.

205. Edmond MB, Hollis RJ, Houston AK, et al. Molecular epidemiology of an

outbreak of meningococcal disease in a university community. J Clin Microbiol 1995;33:2209–2211.

206. Edwards EA, Devine LF, Sengbusch CH, et al. Immunological investigations of meningococcal disease. III. Brevity of group C acquisition prior to disease occurrence. Scand J Infect Dis 1987;9:105–110.

207. Eisenstein BI, Lee TJ, Sparling PF. Penicillin sensitivity and serum resistance are independent attributes of strains of *Neisseria gonorrhoeae* causing disseminated gonococcal infections. Infect Immun 1977;5:834–841.

208. Ejlertsen T, Schonheuder HC. *Branhamella catarrhalis* as a cause of multiple subpleural abscess. Scand J Infect Dis 1991;23:117–118.

209. Ejlertsen T, Thisted E, Eddeson F, et al. *Branhamella catarrhalis* in children and adults: a study of prevalence, time of colonisation, and association with upper and lower respiratory tract infection. J Infect 1994;29:23–31.

210. Ellis M, Weindling AM, Davidson DC, et al. Neonatal meningococcal conjunctivitis associated with meningococcal meningitis. Arch Dis Child 1992;67:1219–1220.

211. Ellison RT III, Curd JG, Kohler PF, et al. Underlying complement deficiency in patients with disseminated gonococcal infection. Sex Transm Dis 1988;4:201–204.

212. Eng J, Holten E. Gelatin neutralization of the inhibitory effect of sodium polyanethol sulfonate on *Neisseria meningitidis* in blood culture media. J Clin Microbiol 1977;6:1–3.

213. Enright MC, McKenzie H. *Moraxella* (*Branhamella*) *catarrhalis*: clinical and molecular aspects of a rediscovered pathogen. J Med Microbiol 1997;46:360–371.

214. Erdem G, Schleiss MR. Gonococcal bacteremia in a neonate. Clin Pediatr 2000;39:43–44.

215. Erickson L, De Wals P. Complications and sequelae of meningococcal disease in Quebec, Canada. Clin Infect Dis 1998;26:1159–1164.

216. Facius D, Meyer TF. A novel determinant (comA) essential for natural transformation competence in *Neisseria gonorrhoeae* and the effect of a comA defect on pilin variation. Mol Microbiol 1993;10:699–712.

217. Faden H, Harabuchi Y, Hong JJ, et al. Epidemiology of *Moraxella catarrhalis* in children during the first two years of life: relationship to otitis media. J Infect Dis 1994;169:1312–1317.

218. Farhat SE, Thibault M, Devlin R. Efficacy of a swab transport system in maintaining the viability of *Neisseria gonorrhoeae* and *Streptococcus pneumoniae*. J Clin Microbiol 2001;39:2958–2960.

219. Fairley CK, Begg N, Borrow R, et al. Conjugate meningococcal serogroup A and C vaccine: reactogenicity and immunogenicity in United Kingdom infants. J Infect Dis 1996;174:1360–1363.

220. Farrell DJ. Evaluation of AMPLICOR *Neisseria gonorrhoeae* PCR using *cppB* nested PCR and 16S rRNA PCR. J Clin Microbiol 1999;37:386–399.

221. Faur YC, Weisburd MH, Wilson ME, et al. A new medium for the isolation of pathogenic *Neisseria* (NYC medium). Health Lab Sci 1973;10:44–54.

222. Feavers IM, Gray SJ, Urwin R, et al. Multilocus sequence typing and antigen gene sequencing in the investigation of a meningococcal disease outbreak. J Clin Microbiol 1999;37:3883–3887.

223. Feliciano R, Swedler W, Varga J. Infection with uncommon subgroup Y *Neisseria meningitidis* in patients with systemic lupus erythematosus. Clin Exp Rheumatol 1999;17:737–740.

224. Felmingham D, Gruneberg RN, Alexander Project Group. The Alexander project 1996–1997: latest susceptibility data from this international study of bacterial pathogens from community-acquired lower respiratory tract infections. J Antimicrob Chemother 2000;45:191–203.

225. Fenton AC, Foweraker JE, Pearson GA, et al. Bronchopulmonary infection with *Moraxella catarrhalis* in infants requiring extracorporeal membrane oxygenation. Pediatr Pulmonol 1994;17:393–395.

226. Fernandez-Guerrero ML, Barros C, Rodriguez Tedula JL. Endocarditis due to *Neisseria mucosa* complicated by myocardial abscess. J Infect 1989;18:294–295.

227. Figuroa J, Andreoni J, Densen P. Complement deficiency states and meningococcal disease. Immunol Res 1993;12:295–311.

228. Fijen CAP, Kuijper EJ, Te Bulte MT, et al. Assessment of complement deficiency in patients with meningococcal disease in the Netherlands. Clin Infect Dis 1999;28:98–105.

229. Fijen CAP, Kuijper EJ, Tjia HG, et al. Complement deficiency predisposes for meningitis due to nongroupable meningococci and *Neisseria*-related bacteria. Clin Infect Dis 1994;18:780–784.

230. Filippatos GS, Kardera D, Paramithiotou E, et al. Acute myocardial infarction with normal coronary arteries during septic shock from *Neisseria meningitidis*. Intensive Care Med 2000;26:252.

231. Finne J, Leinonen M, Makela PH. Antigenic similarities between brain components and bacteria causing meningitis: Implications for vaccine development and pathogenesis. Lancet 1983;2:355.

232. Firgis N, Sultan Y, Frenk RW Jr, et al. Azithromycin compared with rifampin for eradication of nasopharyngeal colonization by *Neisseria meningitidis*. Pediatr Infect Dis J 1998;17:816.

233. Fischer SH, Rest RF. Gonococci possessing only certain P.II outer membrane proteins interact with human neutrophils. Infect Immun 1988;56:1574–1579.

234. Fitzgerald M, Mulcahy R, Murphy S, et al. A 200 kDa protein is associated with haemagglutinating isolates of *Moraxella* (*Branhamella*) *catarrhalis*. FEMS Immunol Med Microbiol 1997;18:209–217.

235. Fleming TJ, Wallsmith DE, Rosenthal RS. Arthropathic properties of gonococcal peptidoglycan fragments: implications for the pathogenesis of disseminated gonococcal disease. Infect Immun 1986;52:600–608.

236. Florez C, Garcia-Lopez JL, Martin-Mazuelos E. Susceptibilities of 55 strains of *Neisseria meningitidis* isolated in Spain in 1993 and 1994. Chemotherapy 1997;43:168–170.

237. Fontanals D, Pineda V, Pons I, et al. Penicillin-resistant β-lactamase-producing *Neisseria meningitidis* in Spain. Eur J Clin Microbiol Infect Dis 1989;8:90–91.

238. Fox KK, del Rio C, Holmes KK, et al. Gonorrhea in the HIV era: a reversal in trends among men who have sex with men. Am J Public Health 2001;91:959–964.

239. Fox KK, Knapp JS. Antimicrobial resistance in *Neisseria gonorrhoeae*. Curr Opin Urol 1999;9:65–70.

240. Fox KK, Knapp JS, Holmes KK, et al. Antimicrobial resistance in *Neisseria gonorrhoeae* in the United States, 1988–1994: the emergence of decreased susceptibility to the fluoroquinolones. J Infect Dis 1997;175:1396–1403.

241. Frasch CE, Zahradnik JM, Wang LY, et al. Antibody response in adults to an aluminum hydroxide adsorbed *Neisseria meningitidis* serotype 2b protein group B-polysaccharide vaccine. J Infect Dis 1988;158:710–718.

242. Frasch CE, Zollinger WD, Poolman JT. Proposed scheme for identification of serotypes of *Neisseria meningitidis*. In: Schoolnik GK, ed.: The Pathogenic Neisseriae. Washington DC: American Society for Microbiology, 1985:519–524.

243. Froeschle JE. Meningococcal disease in college students. Clin Infect Dis 1999;29:215–216.

244. Fusco PC, Michon F, Tai JY, et al. Preclinical evaluation of a novel group B meningococcal conjugate vaccine conjugate vaccine that elicits bactericidal activity in both mice and nonhuman primates. J Infect Dis 1997;175:364–372.

245. Galimand M, Gerbaud G, Courvalin P. Spectinomycin resistance in *Neisseria* spp. due to mutations in 16S rRNA. Antimicrob Agents Chemother 2000;44:1365–1366.

246. Galimand M, Gerbaud G, Guibourdenche M, et al. High-level chloramphenicol resistance in *Neisseria meningitidis*. N Engl J Med 1998;339:868–874.

247. Garcia-Lechuz JM, Alcala L, Gijon P, et al. Primary meningococcal conjunctivitis in a human immunodeficiency virus-infected adult. Clin Infect Dis 1998;27:1556–1557.

248. Garrity GM, Holt JG. An overview of the road map to the manual. New York: Bergey's Trust/Springer, 2000.

249. Gaunt PN, Lambert PE. Single-dose ciprofloxacin for the eradication of pharyngeal carriage of *Neisseria meningitidis*. J Antimicrob Chemother 1988;21:489–496.

250. Gaydos CA, Quinn TC, Willis D, et al. Performance of the APTIMA Combo 2 assay for detection of *Chlamydia trachomatis* and *Neisseria gonorrhoeae* in female urine and endocervical swab specimens. J Clin Microbiol 2003;41:304–309.

251. Geisler WM, Markovitz DM. Septic arthritis caused by *Neisseria sicca*. J Rheumatol 1998;25:826–828.

252. Gelfand MS, Cleveland KO, Campagna C, Zolyomi A. Meningococcal cellulitis and sialadenitis. South Med J 1998;91:287–288.

253. George MJ, DeBin JA, Preston KE, et al. Recurrent bacterial peritonitis caused by *Neisseria cinerea* in a chronic ambulatory peritoneal dialysis (CAPD) patient. Diagn Microbiol Infect Dis 1996;26:91–93.

254. Germer JJ, Washington JA. Evaluation of a rapid identification method for *Neisseria* spp. J Clin Microbiol 1985;21:987–988.

255. Gilbert M, Watson DC, Cunningham AM, et al. Cloning of the lipooligosaccharide α-2,3 sialyltransferase from the bacterial pathogens *Neisseria meningitidis* and *Neisseria gonorrhoeae*. J Biol Chem 1996;271:28271–28276.

256. Gilja OH, Halstensen A, Digranes A, et al. Use of single-dose ofloxacin to eradicate tonsillopharyngeal carriage of *Neisseria meningitidis*. Antimicrob Agents Chemother 1993;37:2024–2026.

257. Gill MJ. Serotyping *Neisseria gonorrhoeae*: a report of the fourth international workshop. Genitourin Med 1991;67:53–57.

258. Gilrane T, Tracy JD, Greenlee RM, et al. *Neisseria sicca* pneumonia: report of two cases and review of the literature. Am J Med 1985;78:1038–1040.

259. Gini GA. Ocular infection in a newborn caused by *Neisseria mucosa*. J Clin Microbiol 1987;25:1574–1575.

260. Girior BP, Quint PA, Barton P, et al. Preliminary evaluation of recombinant amino-terminal fragment of human bactericidal/permeability-increasing protein in children with severe meningococcal sepsis. Lancet 1997;350:1439–1443.

261. Gold R, Goldschneider I, Lepow ML, et al. Carriage of *Neisseria meningitidis* and *Neisseria lactamica* in infants and children. J Infect Dis 1978;137:112–121.

262. Gold R, Lepow ML, Goldschneider I, Gotschlich ECL. Immune response of

human infants to polysaccharide vaccines of group A and group C *Neisseria meningitidis*. J Infect Dis 1977;136(Suppl):S31–S35.

263. Goldani LZ. Inducement of *Neisseria meningitidis* resistance to ampicillin and penicillin in a patient with meningococcemia treated with high doses of ampicillin. Clin Infect Dis 1998;26:772.

264. Gorwitz RJ, Nakashima AK, Moran JS, et al. Sentinel surveillance for antimicrobial resistance in *Neisseria gonorrhoeae*—United States, 1988–1991. MMWR Morb Mortal Wkly Rep 1993;42(Suppl):29–39.

265. Gotschlich EC, Seiff M, Blake MS. The DNA sequence of the structural gene of gonococcal protein III and the flanking region containing a repetitive sequence: homology of protein III with enterobacterial OmpA proteins. J Exp Med 1987; 165:471–481.

266. Granato PA, Howard R, Wilkinson B, et al. Meningitis caused by maltose-negative variant of *Neisseria meningitidis*. J Clin Microbiol 1980;11:270–273.

267. Gransden WR, Warren C, Phillips I. 4-Quinolone-resistant *Neisseria gonorrhoeae* in the United Kingdom. J Med Microbiol 1991;34:23–27.

268. Grant PE, Brenner DJ, Steigerwalt AG, et al. *Neisseria elongata* subsp. *nitroreducens* subsp. nov., formerly CDC group M-6, a gram-negative bacterium associated with endocarditis. J Clin Microbiol 1990;28:2591–2596.

269. Gray LD, Van Scoy RE, Anhalt JP, et al. Wound infection caused by *Branhamella catarrhalis*. J Clin Microbiol 1989;27:818–820.

270. Gray SJ, Sobanski MA, Kaczmarski EB, et al. Ultrasound-enhanced latex immunoagglutination and PCR as complementary methods for non-culture-based confirmation of meningococcal disease. J Clin Microbiol 1999;37:1797–1801.

271. Gregg CR, Melly MA, Hellguist CG, et al. Toxic activity of purified lipopolysaccharide of *Neisseria gonorrhoeae* for human Fallopian tube mucosa. J Infect Dis 1985;43:432–434.

272. Griffiss JM, Schneider H, Mandrell RE, et al. Lipooligosaccharides: the principal glycolipids of the neisserial outer membrane. Rev Infect Dis 1988;10:S87–S95.

273. Gris P, Vincke G, Delmez JP, et al. *Neisseria sicca* pneumonia and bronchiectasis. Eur Respir J 1989;2:685–687.

274. Gu XX, Chen J, Barenkamp SJ, et al. Synthesis and characterization of lipooligosaccharide-based conjugates as vaccine candidates for *Moraxella (Branhamella) catarrhalis*. Infect Immun 1998;66:1891–1897.

275. Guibourdenche M, Caugant DA, Herve V, et al. Characteristics of serogroup A *Neisseria meningitidis* strains isolated in the Central African Republic in February. Eur J Clin Microbiol Infect Dis 1994;13:174–177.

276. Guibourdenche M, Darchis J-P, Boisivon A, et al. Enzyme electrophoresis, sero- and subtyping, and outer membrane protein characterization of two *Neisseria meningitidis* strains involved in laboratory acquired infections. J Clin Microbiol 1994;32:701–704.

277. Guibourdenche M, Giorgini D, Gueye A, et al. Genetic analysis of a meningococcal population based on polymorphism of the *pilA-pilB* locus: a molecular approach for meningococcal epidemiology. J Clin Microbiol 1997;35:745–750.

278. Guibourdenche M, Hoiby EA, Riou JY, et al. Epidemics of serogroup A *Neisseria meningitidis* of subgroup III in Africa, 1989–1994. Epidemiol Infect 1996; 116:115–120.

279. Guibourdenche M, Lambert T, Riou JY. Isolation of *Neisseria canis* in mixed culture from a patient after a cat bite. J Clin Microbiol 1989;27:1673–1674.

280. Hale YM, Melton ME, Lewis JS, et al. Evaluation of the PACE 2 *Neisseria gonorrhoeae* assay by three public health laboratories. J Clin Microbiol 1993; 31:451–453.

281. Halla JT. Septic olecranon bursitis caused by *Neisseria sicca*. J Rheumatol 1990; 17:1240–1241.

282. Hammerschmidt S, Hilse R, Van Putten JP, et al. Modulation of cell surface sialic acid expression in *Neisseria meningitidis* via a transposable genetic element. EMBO J 1996;15:192–198.

283. Hammerschmidt S, Muller A, Sillman H, et al. Capsule phase variation in *Neisseria meningitidis* serogroup B by slipped strand mispairing in the polysialyltransferase gene (*siaD*): correlation with bacterial invasion and the outbreak of meningococcal disease. Mol Microbiol 1996;20:1211–1220.

284. Handsfield HH, Dalu ZA, Martin DH, et al. Multicenter trial of single-dose azithromycin vs. ceftriaxone in the treatment of uncomplicated gonorrhea. Sex Transm Dis 1994;21:107–111.

285. Hanks JW, Scott CT, Butler CE, et al. Evaluation of a DNA probe assay (Gen-Probe PACE 2) as the test of cure for *Neisseria gonorrhoeae* genital infections. J Pediatr 1994;125:161–162.

286. Hanna LS, Girgis NI, Farid Z, et al. Transient cataracts in a young child with meningococcal meningitis. Pediatr Infect Dis J 1989;8:802–803.

287. Harrison LH. Preventing meningococcal infection in college students. Clin Infect Dis 2000;30:648–651.

288. Harrison LH, Dwyer DM, Maples CT, Billiman L. The risk of meningococcal infection in college students. JAMA 1999;281:1906–1910.

289. Hauck CR, Meyer TF. "Small talk": Opa proteins as mediators of *Neisseria*-host cell communication. Curr Opin Microbiol 2003;6:43–49.

290. Hauri AM, Ehrhard I, Frank U, et al. Serogroup C meningococcal disease outbreak associated with discotheque attendance during carnival. Epidemiol Infect 2000;124:69–73.

291. Hay PE, Murphy SM, Chinn RJS. Acute urethritis due to *Neisseria meningitidis* group A acquired by oro-genital contact: case report. Genitourin Med 1989;65: 285–286.

292. Heckels JE. Structure and function of pili of pathogenic *Neisseria* species. Clin Microbiol Rev 1989;2(Suppl):S66–S73.

293. Heiddal S, Sverrisson JT, Yngvason FE, et al. Native valve endocarditis due to *Neisseria sicca:* case report and review. Clin Infect Dis 1993;16:667–670.

294. Hodge DS, Ashton FE, Terro R, et al. Organism resembling *Neisseria gonorrhoeae* and *Neisseria meningitidis*. J Clin Microbiol 1987;25:1546–1547.

295. Hofstad T, Hope O, Falsen E. Septicemia with *Neisseria elongata* ssp. *nitroreducens* in a patient with hypertrophic obstructive cardiomyopathy. Scand J Infect Dis 1998;30:200–201.

296. Hol C, Van Dijke EEM, Verduin CM, et al. Experimental evidence for *Moraxella*-induced penicillin neutralization in pneumococcal pneumonia. J Infect Dis 1994;170:1613–1616.

297. Hollis DG, Wiggins GL, Weaver RE. *Neisseria lactamica* sp. nov., a lactose-fermenting species resembling *Neisseria meningitidis*. Appl Microbiol 1969;17: 71–77.

298. Hollis DG, Wiggins WL, Weaver RE. An unclassified gram-negative rod isolated from the pharynx on Thayer-Martin medium (selective agar). Appl Microbiol 1972;24:772–777.

299. Holmes B, Costas M, On SLW, et al. *Neisseria weaveri* sp. nov. (formerly CDC group M-5), from dog bite wounds of humans. Int J Syst Bacteriol 1993;43: 687–693.

300. Holmes KK, Johnson DW, Trostle JH. An estimate of the risk of men acquiring gonorrhea by sexual contact with infected females. Am J Epidemiol 1970;91: 170–174.

301. Hook EW, Brady WE, Reichart CA, et al. Determinants of emergence of antibiotic-resistant *Neisseria gonorrhoeae*. J Infect Dis 1989;159:900–907.

302. Hook EW, Ching SF, Stephens J, et al. Diagnosis of *Neisseria gonorrhoeae* infections in women by using the ligase chain reaction on patient-obtained vaginal swabs. J Clin Microbiol 1997;35:2129–2132.

303. Hook EW III, Handsfield HH. Gonococcal infections in the adult. In: Holmes KK, Mardh P-A, Sparling PF, et al., eds.: Sexually Transmitted Diseases. 3rd Ed. New York: McGraw Hill, 1999:451–466.

304. Hornyik G, Piatt JH Jr. Cerebrospinal fluid shunt infection by *Neisseria sicca*. Pediatr Neurosurg 1994;21:189–191.

305. Hughes J, Biedenbach DJ, Erwin ME, et al. E test as susceptibility test and epidemiologic tool for evaluation of *Neisseria meningitidis* isolates. J Clin Microbiol 1993;31:3255–3259.

306. Hughes J, Goldsmith C, Shields MD, et al. Primary meningococcal pericarditis with tamponade in an infant. J Infect 1994;29:339–341.

307. Hussain Z, Lannigan R, Austin TW. Pulmonary cavitation due to *Neisseria mucosa* in a child with chronic neutropenia. Eur J Clin Microbiol Infect Dis 1988;7:175–176.

308. Ikeda F, Yokota Y, Mine Y, et al. Characterization of BRO enzymes and β-lactamase transfer of *Moraxella (Branhamella) catarrhalis* isolated in Japan. Chemotherapy 1993;39:88–95.

309. Ikram RB, Nixon M, Aitken J, et al. A prospective study of isolation of *Moraxella catarrhalis* in a hospital during the winter months. J Hosp Infect 1993;25:7–14.

310. Imrey PB, Jackson LA, Ludwinski PH, et al. Meningococcal carriage, alcohol consumption, and campus bar patronage in a serogroup C meningococcal disease outbreak. J Clin Microbiol 1995;33:3133–3137.

311. Imrey PB, Jackson LA, Ludwinski PH, et al. Outbreak of serogroup C meningococcal disease associated with campus bar patronage. Am J Epidemiol 1996; 143:624–630.

312. Ioannidis JPA, Worthington M, Griffiths JK, et al. Spectrum and significance of bacteremia due to *Moraxella catarrhalis*. Clin Infect Dis 1995;21:390–397.

313. Jackson LA, Schuchat A, Reeves MW, et al. Serogroup C meningococcal outbreaks in the United States: an emerging threat. JAMA 1995;273:383–389.

314. Jackson LA, Tenover FC, Baker C, et al. Prevalence of *Neisseria meningitidis* relatively resistant to penicillin in the United States, 1991. J Infect Dis 1994; 169:438–441.

315. Jackson LA, Wenger JD. Laboratory-based surveillance for meningococcal disease in selected areas, United States, 1989–1991. MMWR Morb Mortal Wkly Rep 1993;42:21–30.

316. Jacoby HM, Mady BJ. Acute gonococcal sepsis in an HIV-infected woman. Sex Transm Dis 1995;22:380–382.

317. Janda WM, Bohnhoff M, Morello JA, Lerner SA. Prevalence and site-pathogen studies of *Neisseria meningitidis* and *N. gonorrhoeae* in homosexual men. JAMA 1980;244:2060–2064.

318. Janda WM, Bradna JJ, Ruther P. Identification of *Neisseria* spp., *Haemophilus* spp., and other fastidious gram-negative bacteria with the MicroScan *Haemophilus-Neisseria* identification panel. J Clin Microbiol 1989;27:869–873.

319. Janda WM, Malloy PJ, Schreckenberger PC. Clinical evaluation of the Vitek *Neisseria-Haemophilus* identification card. J Clin Microbiol 1987;25:37–41.

320. Janda WM, Montero M, Wilcoski LM. Evaluation of the BactiCard *Neisseria*

for identification of pathogenic *Neisseria* species and *Moraxella catarrhalis.* Eur J Clin Microbiol Infect Dis 2002;21:875–879.

321. Janda WM, Sensung C, Todd KM, et al. Asymptomatic *Neisseria subflava* biovar. *perflava* bacteriuria in a child with obstructive uropathy. Eur J Clin Microbiol Infect Dis 1993;12:540–542.

322. Janda WM, Ulanday MG, Bohnhoff M, et al. Evaluation of the RIM-N, Gonochek II, and Phadebact systems for the identification of pathogenic *Neisseria* spp. and *Branhamella catarrhalis.* J Clin Microbiol 1985;21:734–737.

323. Janda WM, Wilcoski LM, Mandel KL, et al. Comparison of monoclonal antibody-based methods and a ribosomal ribonucleic acid probe test for *Neisseria gonorrhoeae* culture confirmation. Eur J Clin Microbiol Infect Dis 1993;12: 177–184.

324. Jennings HJ, Gamian A, Ashton FE. N-propionylated group B meningococcal polysaccharide mimics a unique epitope on group B *Neisseria meningitidis.* J Exp Med 1987;165:1207–1211.

325. Jennings HJ, Lugowski C. Immunochemistry of group A, B, and C meningococcal polysaccharide-tetanus toxoid conjugates. J Immunol 1981;127:1011–1018.

326. Jerse AE, Cohen MS, Drown PM, et al. Multiple gonococcal opacity proteins are expressed during experimental urethral infection in the male. J Exp Med 1994;179:911–920.

327. Johnson DH, Febre E, Schoch PE, et al. *Neisseria cinerea* bacteremia in a patient receiving hemodialysis. Clin Infect Dis 1994;19:990–991.

328. Jones DM, Borrow R, Fox AJ, et al. The lipooligosaccharide immunotype as a virulence determinant in *Neisseria meningitidis.* Microb Pathog 1992;13: 219–224.

329. Jones RN, Gavan TL, Thornsberry C, et al. Standardization of disk diffusion and agar dilution susceptibility tests for *Neisseria gonorrhoeae:* interpretive criteria and quality control guidelines for ceftriaxone, penicillin, spectinomycin, and tetracycline. J Clin Microbiol 1989;27:2758–2766.

330. Jonsson AB, Nyberg G, Normark S. Phase variation of gonococcal pili by frameshift mutation in *pilC,* a novel gene for pilus assembly. EMBO J 1991; 10:477–488.

331. Jonsson I, Holme T, Krook A. Significance of isolation of *Moraxella catarrhalis* in routine cultures from the respiratory tract in adults: antibody response studied in a whole cell EIA. Scand J Infect Dis 1994;26:553–558.

332. Jousimies-Somer HR, Savolainen S, Ylikoski JS. Comparison of the nasal bacterial floras in two groups of healthy subjects and in patients with acute maxillary sinusitis. J Clin Microbiol 1989;27:2836–2743.

333. Jungkind D, DiRenzo S, Beavis KG, Silverman NS. Evaluation of automated COBAS AMPLICOR PCR system for detection of several infectious agents and its impact on laboratory management. J Clin Microbiol 1996;34:2778–2783.

334. Juni E, Heym GA. *Psychrobacter immobilis* gen. nov., sp. nov.: genospecies composed of gram-negative, aerobic, oxidase-positive coccobacilli. Int J Syst Bacteriol 1986;36:366–391.

335. Kaczmarski EB, Ragunathan PL, Marsh J, et al. Creating a national service for the diagnosis of meningococcal disease by polymerase chain reaction. Commun Dis Public Health 1998;1:54–56.

336. Kallstrom H, Liszewski MK, Atkinson JP, Jonsson AB. Membrane cofactor protein (MCP or CD46) is a cellular pilus receptor for pathogenic *Neisseria.* Mol Microbiol 1997;25:639–647.

337. Kam KM, Lo KK, Chong LY, et al. Correlation between in vitro quinolone susceptibility of *Neisseria gonorrhoeae* and outcome of treatment of gonococcal urethritis with single-dose ofloxacin. Clin Infect Dis 1999;29:1165–1166.

338. Kam KM, Wong PW, Cheung MM, Ho NKY. Detection of fluoroquinolone-resistant *Neisseria gonorrhoeae.* J Clin Microbiol 1996;34:1462–1464.

339. Kamme C, Vang M, Stahl M. Intrageneric and intergeneric transfer of *Branhamella catarrhalis* β-lactamase production. Scand J Infect Dis 1984;16:153–155.

340. Kaplan SL. Clinical presentations, diagnosis, and prognostic factors of bacterial meningitis. In: Schaad UB, ed.: Infectious Disease Clinics of North America. Vol. 13. Bacterial meningitis. Philadelphia: WB Saunders, 1999;579–594.

341. Karalus R, Campagnari A. *Moraxella catarrhalis:* a review of an important human mucosal pathogen. Microbes Infect 2000;2:547–559.

342. Karlowsky JA, Jones ME, Mayfield DC, et al. Ceftriaxone activity against Gram-positive and Gram-negative pathogens isolated in U.S. clinical microbiology laboratories from 1996 to 2000: results from the Surveillance Network (TSN) database—USA. Int J Antimicrob Agents 2002;19:413–426.

343. Kawula TH, Spinola SM, Klapper DG, Cannon JG. Localization of a conserved epitope and azurin-like domain in the H.8 protein of pathogenic *Neisseria.* Mol Microbiol 1987;1:179–185.

344. Kayhty H, Karenko V, Peltola H, et al. Serum antibodies to capsular polysaccharide vaccine of group A *Neisseria meningitidis* followed for three years in infants and children. J Infect Dis 1980;142:861–868.

345. Kellogg DS, Peacock WL, Deacon WE, et al. *Neisseria gonorrhoeae.* I. Virulence genetically linked to clonal variation. J Bacteriol 1963;94:1274–1279.

346. Kellogg JA, Orwig LK. Comparison of GonoGen, GonoGen II, and MicroTrak direct fluorescent antibody test with carbohydrate fermentation for confirmation of culture isolates of *Neisseria gonorrhoeae.* J Clin Microbiol 1995;33:474–476.

347. Kertesz DA, Byrne SK, Chow AW. Characterization of *Neisseria meningitidis* by polymerase chain reaction and restriction endonuclease digestion of the *porA* gene. J Clin Microbiol 1993;31:2594–2598.

348. Keys TF, Hecht RH, Chow AW. Endocervical *Neisseria meningitidis* with meningococcemia. N Engl J Med 1971;285:505–506.

349. Kirchgesner V, Plesiat P, DuPont MJ, et al. Meningitis and septicemia due *to Neisseria cinerea.* Clin Infect Dis 1995;21:1351.

350. Kleris GS, Arnold AJ. Differential diagnosis of urethritis: predictive value and therapeutic implications of the urethral smear. Sex Transm Dis 1981;8:810–816.

351. Klingman KL, Pye A, Murphy TF, Hill SL. Dynamics of respiratory tract colonization by *Branhamella catarrhalis* in bronchiectasis. Am J Respir Crit Care Med 1995;152:1072–1078.

352. Knapp JS. Reduction of nitrite by *Neisseria gonorrhoeae.* Int J Syst Bacteriol 1984;34:376–377.

353. Knapp JS, Clark VL. Anaerobic growth of *Neisseria gonorrhoeae* coupled to nitrite reduction. Infect Immun 1984;46:176–181.

354. Knapp JS, Fox KK, Trees DL, Whittington WL. Fluoroquinolone resistance *in Neisseria gonorrhoeae.* Emerg Infect Dis 1997;3:33–39.

355. Knapp JS, Hale JA, Wintersheld K, et al. Proposed criteria for the interpretation of susceptibilities of strains of *Neisseria gonorrhoeae* to ciprofloxacin, ofloxacin, enoxacin, lomefloxacin, and norfloxacin. Antimicrob Agents Chemother 1995;39:2442–2445.

356. Knapp JS, Holmes KK. Disseminated gonococcal infections caused by *Neisseria gonorrhoeae* strains with unique nutritional requirements. J Infect Dis 1975; 132:204–208.

357. Knapp JS, Hook EW. Prevalence and persistence of *Neisseria cinerea* and other *Neisseria* spp. in adults. J Clin Microbiol 1988;26:896–900.

358. Knapp JS, Johnson SR, Zenilman JM, et al. High-level tetracycline resistance resulting from *TetM* in strains of *Neisseria* spp., *Kingella denitrificans,* and *Eikenella corrodens.* Antimicrob Agents Chemother 1988;32:765–767.

359. Knapp JS, Ohye R, Neal SW, et al. Emerging in vitro resistance to quinolones in penicillinase-producing *Neisseria gonorrhoeae* strains in Hawaii. Antimicrob Agents Chemother 1994;38:2200–2203.

360. Knapp JS, Tam MR, Nowinski RC, et al. Serological classification of *Neisseria gonorrhoeae* with use of monoclonal antibodies to gonococcal outer membrane protein I. J Infect Dis 150:44–48, 1984.

361. Knapp JS, Totten PA, Mulks MH, et al. Characterization of *Neisseria cinerea,* a non-pathogenic species isolated on Martin-Lewis medium selective for pathogenic *Neisseria* spp. J Clin Microbiol 1984;19:63–67.

362. Knapp JS, Washington JA, Doyle LJ, et al. Persistence of *Neisseria gonorrhoeae* strains with decreased susceptibilities to ciprofloxacin and ofloxacin in Cleveland, Ohio, from 1992 through 1993. Antimicrob Agents Chemother 1994;38: 2194–2196.

363. Knapp JS, Wongba C, Limpakarnjanarat K, et al. Antimicrobial susceptibilities of strains of *Neisseria gonorrhoeae* in Bangkok, Thailand: 1994–1995. Sex Transm Dis 1997;24:142–148.

364. Knapp JS, Zenilman JM, Biddle JW, et al. Frequency and distribution in the United States of strains of *Neisseria gonorrhoeae* with plasmid-mediated, high-level resistance to tetracycline. J Infect Dis 1987;155:819–822.

365. Koppes GM, Ellenbogen C, Gebhart RJ. Group Y meningococcal disease in United States Air Force recruits. Am J Med 1977;62:661–666.

366. Kornelisse RF, Hazelzet JA, Hop WCJ, et al. Meningococcal septic shock in children: clinical and laboratory features, outcome, and development of a prognostic score. Clin Infect Dis 1997;35:640–646.

367. Korppi M, Katila ML, Jaaskelainen J, et al. Role of *Moraxella (Branhamella) catarrhalis* as a respiratory pathogen in children. Acta Paediatr 1992;81:993–996.

368. Koumans EH, Johnson RE, Knapp JS, St. Louis ME. Laboratory testing for *Neisseria gonorrhoeae* by recently introduced nonculture tests: a performance review with clinical and public health considerations. Clin Infect Dis 1998;27: 1171–1180.

369. Kristiansen B-E, Fermer C, Jenkins A, et al. PCR amplicon restriction endonuclease analysis of the chromosomal *dhps* gene of *Neisseria meningitidis*: a method for studying spread of the disease-causing strain in contacts of patients with meningococcal disease. J Clin Microbiol 1995;33:1174–1179.

370. Kupsch E-M, Knepper B, Kuroki T, et al. Variable opacity (Opa) outer membrane proteins account for the cell tropisms displayed by *Neisseria gonorrhoeae* for human leukocytes and epithelial cells. EMBO J 1993;12:641–650.

371. Kurzynski TA, Kimball JL, Polyak MB. Evaluation of the Phadebact and Bactigen reagents for detection of *Neisseria meningitidis* in cerebrospinal fluid. J Clin Microbiol 1985;21:989–990.

372. Lafferty W, Hughes JP, Handsfield HH. Sexually transmitted diseases among men who have sex with men: acquisition of gonorrhea and non-gonococcal urethritis by fellatio and implications for STD/HIV prevention. Sex Transm Dis 1997;24:272–278.

373. LaFontaine ER, Cope LD, Aebi C, et al. The UspA1 protein and a second type of UspA2 protein mediate adherence of *Moraxella catarrhalis* to human epithelial cells in vitro. J Bacteriol 2000;182:1364–1373.

374. Lairscey RC, Kelly MT. Evaluation of a one-hour test for identification of *Neisseria* species. J Clin Microbiol 1985;22:238–240.

375. Lansac N, Picard FJ, Menard C, et al. Novel genus-specific PCR-based assays for rapid identification of *Neisseria* species and *Neisseria meningitidis*. Eur J Clin Microbiol Infect Dis 2000;19:443–451.

376. Lauer BA, Fisher E. *Neisseria lactamica* meningitis. Am J Dis Child 1976;130:198–199.

377. Lauer BA, Masters HB. Toxic effect of calcium alginate swabs on *Neisseria gonorrhoeae*. J Clin Microbiol 1988;26:54–56.

378. Laughon BE, Ehret JM, Tanino TT, et al. Fluorescent monoclonal antibody for confirmation of *Neisseria gonorrhoeae* cultures. J Clin Microbiol 1987;25:2388–2390.

379. Lawton WD, Battaglioli GJ. GonoGen coagglutination test for *Neisseria gonorrhoeae*. J Clin Microbiol 1983;18:1264–1265.

380. Leach A, Twumasi PA, Kumah S, et al. Induction of immunologic memory in Gambian children by vaccination in infancy with a group C meningococcal polysaccharide-protein conjugate vaccine. J Infect Dis 1997;175:200–204.

381. Lee AH, Chin AE, Ramanujam T, et al. Gonococcal septic arthritis of the hip. J Rheumatol 1991;18:1932–1933.

382. Lee BC, Hill P. Identification of an outer-membrane haemoglobin binding protein in *Neisseria meningitidis*. J Gen Microbiol 1992;138:2647–2656.

383. Leggiadro RJ, Lazar LF. Spontaneous bacterial peritonitis due to *Neisseria meningitidis* serogroup Z in an infant with liver failure. Clin Pediatr 1991;30:350–352.

384. Lepow ML, Beeler J, Randolph M, et al. Reactogenicity and immunogenicity of a quadrivalent combined meningococcal polysaccharide vaccine in children. J Infect Dis 1986;154:1033–1036.

385. Lewis JS, Fakile O, Foss E, et al. Direct DNA probe assay for *Neisseria gonorrhoeae* in pharyngeal and rectal specimens. J Clin Microbiol 1993;31:2783–2785.

386. Lewis JS, Kranig-Brown D, Trainor DA. DNA probe confirmatory test for *Neisseria gonorrhoeae*. J Clin Microbiol 1990;28:2349–2350.

387. Lewis LA, Gipson M, Hartman K, et al. Phase variation of HpuAB and HmbR, two distinct hemoglobin receptors of *Neisseria meningitidis* DNM2. Mol Microbiol 1999;32:977–989.

388. Lewis LA, Gray E, Wang YP, et al. Molecular characterization of *hpuAB*, the haemoglobin-haptoglobin utilization operon of *Neisseria meningitidis*. Mol Microbiol 1997;23:737–749.

389. Lewis LS, Glauser TA, Joffe MD. Gonococcal conjunctivitis in prepubertal children. Am J Dis Child 1990;144:546–548.

390. Li Z, Yokoi S, Kawamura Y, et al. Rapid detection of quinolone resistance-associated *gyrA* mutations in *Neisseria gonorrhoeae* with a LightCycler. J Infect Chemother 2002;8:145–150.

391. Lieberman JM, Chiu SS, Wong VK, et al. Safety and immunogenicity of a serogroups A/C *Neisseria meningitidis* oligosaccharide-protein conjugate vaccine in young children. A randomized controlled trial. JAMA 1996;275:1499–1503.

392. Liebling MR, Arkfeld DG, Michelini GA, et al. Identification of *Neisseria gonorrhoeae* in synovial fluid using the polymerase chain reaction. Arthritis Rheum 1994;37:702–709.

393. Lim YT, Lim MC, Choo MH, Gamini K. Severe aortic regurgitation due to *Neisseria mucosa* endocarditis. Singapore Med J 1994;35:650–652.

394. Limberger RJ, Biega R, Evancoe A, et al. Evaluation of culture and the Gen-Probe PACE 2 assay for detection of *Neisseria gonorrhoeae* and *Chlamydia trachomatis* in endocervical specimens transported to a state health laboratory. J Clin Microbiol 1992;30:1162–1166.

395. Linquist PR, Linquist JA. *Neisseria mucosa* bursitis: a rare case of gas in soft tissue. Clin Orthop 1988;231:222–224.

396. Lipman RM, Deutsch TA. Late-onset *Moraxella catarrhalis* endophthalmitis after filtering surgery. Can J Ophthalmol 1992;27:249–250.

397. Little MC, Andrews J, Moore R, et al. Strand displacement amplification and homogeneous real-time detection incorporated into a second-generation DNA probe system, BD DNA ProbeTec ET. Clin Chem 2000;45:777–784.

398. Littman H, Lazebnik R, Hall GS, et al. Isolation of *Neisseria gonorrhoeae*: directly plated cultures versus transport cultures. Clin Pediatr 1996;35:329–330.

399. Livengood CH III, Wrenn JW. Evaluation of COBAS AMPLICOR (Roche): accuracy in detecting *Chlamydia trachomatis* and *Neisseria gonorrhoeae* by coamplification of endocervical specimens. J Clin Microbiol 2001;39:2928–2932.

400. Lopez-Velez R, Fortun J, de Pablo C, et al.: Native valve endocarditis due to *Neisseria sicca*. Clin Infect Dis 1994;18:660–661.

401. Lossick JG, Smeltzer MP, Curran JW. The value of the cervical Gram stain in the diagnosis of gonorrhea in women in a sexually transmitted diseases clinic. Sex Transm Dis 1982;9:124–127.

402. Louie M, Ongsansoy EG, Forward KR. Rapid identification of *Branhamella catarrhalis*: a comparison of five rapid methods. Diagn Microbiol Infect Dis 1990;13:205–208.

403. Louv WC, Austin H, Alexander WJ, et al. A clinical trial of nonoxynol-9 for preventing gonococcal and chlamydial infections. J Infect Dis 1988;158:518–523.

404. Louv WC, Austin H, Perlman J, Alexander WJ. Oral contraceptive use and the risk of chlamydial and gonococcal infections. Am J Obstet Gynecol 1989;160:396–402.

405. Lujan R, Zhang Q-Y, Saez-Nieto JA, et al. Penicillin-resistant isolates of *Neisseria lactamica* produce altered forms of penicillin-binding protein 2 that arose by interspecies horizontal gene transfer. Antimicrob Agents Chemother 1991;35:300–304.

406. MacArthur RD. *Branhamella catarrhalis* peritonitis in two continuous ambulatory peritoneal dialysis patients. Perit Dial Int 1990;11:185.

407. Macia M, Vega N, Elcuaz R, et al. *Neisseria mucosa* peritonitis in CAPD: another case of ''non-pathogenic'' neisseriae infection. Perit Dial Int 1993;13:72–73.

408. MacLennan JM, Shackley F, Heath PT, et al. Safety, immunogenicity, and induction of immunologic memory by a serogroup C meningococcal conjugate vaccine in infants: a randomized controlled trial. JAMA 2000;283:2795–2801.

409. Malhotra A, Krilov LR. Isolated *Neisseria meningitidis* endophthalmitis. Pediatr Infect Dis J 1999;18:839–840.

410. Malhotra R, Karim QN, Acheson JF. Hospital-acquired adult gonococcal conjunctivitis. J Infect 1998;37:305–312.

411. Mandrell RE, Griffiss JM, Macher BA. Lipooligosaccharides (LOS) of *Neisseria gonorrhoeae* and *Neisseria meningitidis* have components that are immunochemically similar to precursors of human blood group antigens: carbohydrate sequence specificity of the mouse monoclonal antibodies that recognize crossreacting antigens on LOS and human erythrocytes. J Exp Med 1988;168:107–126.

412. Mandrell RE, Zollinger WD. Lipopolysaccharide serotyping of *Neisseria meningitidis* by hemagglutination inhibition. Infect Immun 1977;16:471–475.

413. Manfredi R, Nanetti A, Valentini R, Chiodo F. *Moraxella catarrhalis* pneumonia during HIV disease. J Chemother 2000;12:406–411.

414. Marchant CD: Spectrum of disease due to *Branhamella catarrhalis* in children with particular reference to acute otitis media. Am J Med 1990;88(Suppl 5A):15S–19S.

415. Marrs CF, Weir S. Pili (fimbriae) of *Branhamella* species. Am J Med 1990;88(Suppl 5A):36S–40S.

416. Martin DH, Cammarata C, Van der Pol B, et al. Multicenter study of AMPLICOR and automated COBAS AMPLICOR CT/NG tests for *Neisseria gonorrhoeae*. J Clin Microbiol 2000;38:3544–3549.

417. Martin JE, Jackson RL. A biological environmental chamber for the culture of *Neisseria gonorrhoeae*. J Am Vener Dis Assoc 1975;2:28–30.

418. Martinez G, Ahmed K, Zheng CH, et al. DNA restriction patterns produced by pulsed-field gel electrophoresis in *Moraxella catarrhalis* isolated from different geographical areas. Epidemiol Infect 1999;122:417–422.

419. Maskell JP, Whiley AC, Sefton AM. In vitro activity of grepafloxacin against *Haemophilus influenzae* and *Moraxella catarrhalis*. Eur J Clin Microbiol Infect Dis 1998;17:293–299.

420. Maslanka SE, Tappero JW, Plikaytis BD, et al. Age-dependent *Neisseria meningitidis* serogroup C class-specific antibody concentrations and bactericidal titers in sera from young children from Montana immunized with a licensed polysaccharide vaccine. Infect Immun 1998;66:2453–2459.

421. Mastrantonio P, Congiu ME, Selander RK, et al. Genetic relationships among strains of *Neisseria meningitidis* causing disease in Italy, 1984–1987. Epidemiol Infect 1991;106:143–150

422. Mastrolonardo M, Loconsole F, Conte A, et al. Cutaneous vasculitis as the sole manifestation of disseminated gonococcal infection: case report. Genitourin Med 1994;70:130–131.

423. Mathers K, Leinonen M, Goldblatt D. Antibody response to outer membrane proteins of *Moraxella catarrhalis* in children with otitis media. Pediatr Infect Dis J 1999;18:982–988.

424. Mattila PS, Carlson P. Pharyngolaryngitis caused by *Neisseria meningitidis*. Scand J Infect Dis 1998;30:198–200.

425. Mayatepek E, Grauer M, Hansch GM, et al. Deafness, complement deficiencies and immunoglobulin status in patients with meningococcal disease due to uncommon serogroups. Pediatr Infect Dis J 1993;12:808–811.

426. Mazloum H, Totten PA, Brooks GF, et al. An unusual *Neisseria* isolated from conjunctival cultures in rural Egypt. J Infect Dis 1986;154:212–224.

427. McGee L, Koornhof HJ, Caugant DA. Epidemic spread of subgroup III of *Neisseria meningitidis* serogroup A to South Africa in 1996. Clin Infect Dis 1998;27:1214–1220.

428. McGregor K, Chang BJ, Mee BJ, Riley TV. *Moraxella catarrhalis*: clinical significance, antimicrobial susceptibility, and BRO β-lactamases. Eur J Clin Microbiol Infect Dis 1998;17:219–234.

429. McKenzie H, Morgan MG, Jordens JZ, et al. Characterization of hospital isolates of *Moraxella (Branhamella) catarrhalis* by SDS-PAGE of whole cell proteins, immunoblotting and restriction endonuclease analysis. J Med Microbiol 1992;37:70–76.

430. McMichael JC. Progress toward the development of a vaccine to prevent *Moraxella (Branhamella) catarrhalis* infections. Microbes Infect 2000;2:561–568.

431. McMichael JC. Vaccines for *Moraxella catarrhalis*. Vaccine 2001;19:S101–S107.

432. McMichael JC, Fiske MJ, Fredenburg RA, et al. Isolation and characterization of two proteins from *Moraxella catarrhalis* that bear a common epitope. Infect Immun 1998 ;66:4374–4381.

433. Mehrany K, Kist JM, O'Connor WJ, DiCaudo DJ. Disseminated gonococcemia. Int J Dermatol 2003;42:208–209.

434. Melendez PR, Johnson RH: Bacteremia and septic arthritis caused by *Moraxella catarrhalis*. Rev Infect Dis 1991;13:428–429.

435. Mendelman PM, Campos J, Chaffin DO, et al. Relative penicillin G resistance in *Neisseria meningitidis* and reduced affinity of penicillin-binding protein 2. Antimicrob Agents Chemother 1988;32:706–709.

436. Meningococcal Disease Surveillance Group. Analysis of endemic meningococcal disease by serogroup and evaluation of chemoprophylaxis. J Infect Dis 1976; 134:201–204.

437. Meuleman P, Erard K, Herregods MC, et al. Bioprosthetic valve endocarditis caused by *Neisseria elongata* subspecies *nitroreducens*. Infection 1996;24:258–260.

438. Meyer GA, Shope TR, Waecker NJ Jr, Lanningham FH. *Moraxella (Branhamella) catarrhalis* bacteremia in children. Clin Pediatr 1995;34:146–150.

439. Meyer TF. Pathogenic neisseriae: complexity of pathogen-host cell interplay. Clin Infect Dis 1999;28:433–441.

440. Meyer TF, van Putten JPM. Genetic mechanisms and biological implications of phase variation in pathogenic neisseriae. Clin Micro Rev 1989;2(Suppl):S139–S145.

441. Mietzner TA, Bolan G, Schoolnik GK, Morse SA. Purification and characterization of the major iron-regulated protein expressed by pathogenic *Neisseria*. J Exp Med 1987;165:1041–1057.

442. Mietzner TA, Luginbuhl GH, Sandstrom E, Morse SA. Identification of an iron-regulated 37,000-dalton protein in the cell envelope of *Neisseria gonorrhoeae*. Infect Immun 1984;45:410–416.

443. Milagres LG, Ramos SR, Sacchi CT, et al. Immune response of Brazilian children to a *Neisseria meningitidis* serogroup b outer membrane protein vaccine: comparison with efficacy. Infect Immun 1994;62:4419–4424.

444. Minshew BH, Beardsley JL, Knapp JS. Evaluation of GonoGen coagglutination test for serodiagnosis of *Neisseria gonorrhoeae*: identification of problem isolates by auxotyping, serotyping, and with a fluorescent antibody reagent. Diagn Microbiol Infect Dis 1985;3:41–46.

445. Modarress KJ, Cullen AP, Jaffurs WJS, et al. Detection of *Chlamydia trachomatis* and *Neisseria gonorrhoeae* in swab specimen by the Hybrid Capture II and PACE 2 nucleic acid probe tests. Sex Transm Dis 1999;26:303–308.

446. Molling P, Jacobsson S, Backman A, Olcen P. Direct and rapid identification and genogrouping of meningococci and *porA* amplification by LightCycler PCR. J Clin Microbiol 2002;40:4531–4535.

447. Montgomery K, Raymundo L, Drew WL. Chromogenic cephalosporin spot test to detect β-lactamase in clinically significant bacteria. J Clin Microbiol 1979; 9:205–207.

448. Moon T, Lin RY, Jahn AF. Fatal frontal sinusitis due to *Neisseria sicca* and *Eubacterium lentum*. J Otolaryngol 1986;15:193–195.

449. Moore PS. Meningococcal meningitis in sub-Saharan Africa: a model for the epidemic process. Clin Infect Dis 1992;14:515–525.

450. Moore PS, Hierholzer J, DeWitt W, et al. Respiratory viruses and mycoplasma as cofactors for epidemic group A meningococcal meningitis. JAMA 1990;264:1271–1275.

451. Moore PS, Reeves MW, Schwartz B, et al. Intercontinental spread of an epidemic group A *Neisseria meningitidis* strain. Lancet 1989;2:260–263.

452. Moraes JC, Perkins BA, Camargo MCC, et al. Protective efficacy of a serogroup B meningococcal vaccine in Sao Paulo, Brazil. Lancet 1992;340:1074–1078.

453. Morello JA, Lerner SA, Bohnhoff M. Characteristics of atypical *Neisseria gonorrhoeae* from disseminated and localized infections. Infect Immun 1976;13:1510–1516.

454. Morgan MG, McKenzie H, Enright MC, et al. Use of molecular methods to characterize *Moraxella catarrhalis* strains in a suspected outbreak of nosocomial infection. Eur J Clin Microbiol Infect Dis 1992;11:305–312.

455. Morla N, Guibourdenche M, Riou J-Y. *Neisseria* spp. and AIDS. J Clin Microbiol 1992;30:2290–2294.

456. Morse SA, Johnson SR, Biddle JW, et al. High-level tetracycline resistance in *Neisseria gonorrhoeae* is a result of acquisition of streptococcal *tetM* determinant. Antimicrob Agents Chemother 1986;30:664–670.

457. Mulks MH, Plaut AG. IgA protease production as a characteristic distinguishing pathogenic from harmless *Neisseriaceae*. N Engl J Med 1978;299:973–976.

458. Muller A, Gunther D, Dux F, et al. Neisserial porin (PorB) causes rapid calcium influx in target cells and induces apoptosis by the activation of cysteine proteases. EMBO 1999;18:339–352.

459. Muralidhar B, Rumore PM, Steinman CR. Use of the polymerase chain reaction to study arthritis due to *Neisseria gonorrhoeae*. Arthritis Rheum 1994;37:710–717.

460. Murphy S, Fitzgerald M, Mulcahy R, et al. Studies on haemagglutination and serum resistance status of strains of *Moraxella catarrhalis* isolated from the elderly. Gerontology 1997;43:277–282.

461. Murphy TF. *Branhamella catarrhalis*: epidemiological and clinical aspects of a human respiratory tract pathogen. Thorax 1998;53:124–128.

462. Murphy TF, Kirkham C, Lesse AJ. The major heat-modifiable outer membrane protein CD is highly conserved among strains of *Moraxella catarrhalis*. Mol Microbiol 1993;10:87–97.

463. Murphy TF, Kyd JM, John A, et al. Enhancement of pulmonary clearance of *Moraxella (Branhamella) catarrhalis* following immunization with outer membrane protein CD in a mouse model. J Infect Dis 1998;178:1667–1675.

464. Myers LE, Yang YP, Du RP, et al. The transferrin binding protein B of *Moraxella catarrhalis* elicits bactericidal antibodies and is a potential vaccine antigen. Infect Immun 1998;66:4183–4192.

465. Naqvi SH, Kilpatrick B, Bouhasin J. *Branhamella catarrhalis* meningitis following otolaryngologic surgery. APMIS Suppl 1988;3:74–75.

466. Nassif X, Beretti JL, Lowy J, et al. Roles of pilin and PilC in adhesion of *Neisseria meningitidis* to human epithelial and endothelial cells. Proc Natl Acad Sci USA 1994;91:3769–3773.

467. Nassif X, Lowy J, Stenberg P, et al. Antigenic variation of pilin regulates adhesion of *Neisseria meningitidis* to human epithelial cells. Mol Microbiol 1993; 8:719–725.

468. Nassif X, So M. Interaction of pathogenic *Neisseria* with nonphagocytic cells. Clin Micro Rev 1995;8:376–388.

469. National Committee for Clinical Laboratory Standards. Performance standards for antimicrobial susceptibility testing; twelfth informational supplement. Wayne PA: author, 2002. NCCLS document M100-S12.

470. Nawaz T, Hardy DJ, Bonnez W. *Neisseria elongata* subsp. *elongata*: a case of human endocarditis complicated by pseudoaneurysm. J Clin Microbiol 1996; 34:756–758.

471. Neal KR, Hguyen-van-Tam JS, Slack RCB, et al. Seven-week interval between acquisition of a meningococcus and the onset of invasive disease: a case report. Epidemiol Infect 1999;123:507–509.

472. Nelson K, Watkins DA, Watanakunakorn C. Acute epiglottitis due to serogroup Y *Neisseria meningitidis* in an adult. Clin Infect Dis 1996;23:1192–1193.

473. Neu AM, Case B, Lederman HM, et al. *Neisseria sicca* peritonitis in a patient maintained on chronic peritoneal dialysis. Pediatr Nephrol 1994;8:601–602.

474. Neubert AG, Schwartz PA. *Neisseria meningitidis* sepsis as a complication of labor. J Reprod Med 1994;39:749–751.

475. Neumayer U, Schmidt HK, Mellwig KP, Kleikamp G. *Moraxella catarrhalis* endocarditis: report of a case and literature review. J Heart Valve Dis 1999;8:114–117.

476. Ng L-K, Carballo M, Dillon JR. Differentiation of *Neisseria gonorrhoeae* isolates requiring proline, citrulline, and uracil by plasmid content, serotyping, and pulsed-field gel electrophoresis. J Clin Microbiol 1995;33:1039–1041.

477. Ng L-K, Dillon JR. Typing by serovar, antibiogram, plasmid content, ribotyping, and isoenzyme typing to determine whether *Neisseria gonorrhoeae* isolates requiring proline, citrulline, and uracil for growth are clonal. J Clin Microbiol 1993;31:1555–1561.

478. Novelli VM, Lewis RG, Dawodd ST. Epidemic group A meningococcal disease in Haj pilgrims. Lancet 1987;2:863.

479. Obeid EMH. *Neisseria subflava* causing septic arthritis of the ankle of a child. J Infect 1993;27:100–101.

480. Olsen CC, Schwebke JR, Benjamin WH Jr, et al. Comparison of direct inoculation and Copan transport systems for isolation of *Neisseria gonorrhoeae* from endocervical specimens. J Clin Microbiol 1999;37:3583–3585.

481. Olsen SF, Djurhuus B, Rasmussen K, et al. Pharyngeal carriage of *Neisseria meningitidis* and *Neisseria lactamica* in households with infants within areas with high and low incidences of meningococcal disease. Epidemiol Infect 1991; 106:445–457.

482. Oppenheim BA. Antibiotic resistance in *Neisseria meningitidis*. Clin Infect Dis 1997;24(Suppl 1):S98–S101.

483. Orden B, Amerigo MA. Acute otitis media caused by *Neisseria lactamica*. Eur J Clin Microbiol Infect Dis 1991;10:986–987.

484. O'Rourke M, Ison CA, Renton AM, Spratt BG. Opa typing: a high resolution tool for studying the epidemiology of gonorrhea. Mol Microbiol 1995;17:865–875.

485. Orsson B, Haraldsdottir V, Kristjansson M. *Moraxella catarrhalis* bacteraemia: a report on 3 cases and a review of the literature. Scand J Infect Dis 1998;30:105–109.

486. Orvelid P, Backman A, Olcen P. PCR identification of the group A *Neisseria meningitidis* gene in cerebrospinal fluid. Scand J Infect Dis 1999;31:481–483.

487. Pai CH, Sorger S. Enhancement of recovery of *Neisseria meningitidis* by gelatin in blood culture media. J Clin Microbiol 1981;14:20–23.

488. Palladino S, Pearman JW, Kay ID, et al. Diagnosis of *Chlamydia trachomatis* and *Neisseria gonorrhoeae* genitourinary infections in males by the AMPLICOR PCR assay of urine. Diagn Microbiol Infect Dis 1999;33:141–146.

489. Palmer HM, Arnold C. Genotyping *Neisseria gonorrhoeae* using fluorescent amplified fragment length polymorphism analysis. J Clin Microbiol 2001;39:2325–2329.

490. Palmer HM, Leeming JP, Turner A. Investigation of an outbreak of ciprofloxacin-resistant *Neisseria gonorrhoeae* using a simplified Opa-typing method. Epidemiol Infect 2001;126:219–224.

491. Palmer HM, Mallinson H, Wood RL, Herring AJ. Evaluation of the specificities of five DNA amplification methods for the detection of *Neisseria gonorrhoeae*. J Clin Microbiol 2003;41:835–837.

492. Panagea S, Biboux R, Corkill JE, et al. A case of lower respiratory tract infection caused by *Neisseria weaveri* and review of the literature. J Infect 2002;44:96–98.

493. Parsons NJ Curry A, Fox AJ, et al. The serum resistance of gonococci in the majority of urethral exudates is due to sialylated lipooligosaccharide seen as a surface coat. FEMS Microbiol Lett 1992;90:295–300.

494. Patterson TF, Patterson EJ, Masecar BL, et al. A nosocomial outbreak of *Branhamella catarrhalis* confirmed by restriction endonuclease analysis. J Infect Dis 1988;157:996–1001.

495. Peixuan Z, Xujing H, Li X. Typing *Neisseria meningitidis* by analysis of restriction fragment length polymorphisms in the gene encoding the class 1 outer membrane protein: application to assessment of epidemics through the last four decades in China. J Clin Microbiol 1995;33:458–462.

496. Peltola H. Prophylaxis of bacterial meningitis. In: Schaad UB, ed.: Infectious Disease Clinics of North America. Vol 13. Bacterial meningitis. Philadelphia: WB Saunders, 1999:685–710.

497. Peltola H, Makela PH. Kayhty H, et al. Clinical efficacy of meningococcus group A capsular polysaccharide vaccine in children three months to five years of age. N Engl J Med 1977;297:686–691.

498. Peltola H, Safary A, Kayhty H, et al. Evaluation of 2 tetravalent (ACYW135) meningococcal vaccines in infants and small children: a clinical study comparing immunogenicity of *O*-acetyl-negative and *O*-acetyl-positive group C polysaccharides. Pediatrics 1985;76:91–96.

499. Perez-Trallero E, Garcia-Arenzana JM, Ayestaran I, et al. Comparative activity in vitro of 16 antimicrobial agents against penicillin-susceptible meningococci and meningococci with diminished susceptibility to penicillin. Antimicrob Agents Chemother 1989;33:1622–1623.

500. Perez-Trallero E, Gomez N, Garcia-Arenzana JM. E test as susceptibility test for evaluation of *Neisseria meningitidis* isolates. J Clin Microbiol 1994;32:2341–2342.

501. Perry JL, Ballou DR, Salyer JL. Inhibitory properties of a swab transport device. J Clin Microbiol 1997;35:3367–3368.

502. Pettersson A, Prinz T, Umar A, et al. Molecular characterization of LbpB, the second lactoferrin-binding protein of *Neisseria meningitidis*. Mol Microbiol 1998;27:599–610.

503. Pettersson B, Kodjo A, Ronaghi M, et al. Phylogeny of the family *Moraxellaceae* by 16S rDNA sequence analysis, with special emphasis on differentiation of *Moraxella* species. Int J Syst Evol Microbiol 1998;48:75–89.

504. Pfaller MA, Jones RN. A review of the in vitro activity of meropenem and comparative antimicrobial agents tested against 30,254 aerobic and anaerobic pathogens isolated worldwide. Diagn Microbiol Infect Dis 1997;28:157–163.

505. Phillips EA, Schultz TR, Tapsall JW, et al. Maltose-negative *Neisseria meningitidis* isolated from a case of male urethritis. J Clin Microbiol 1989;27:2851–2852.

506. Pinner R, Onyango F, Perkins BA, et al. Epidemic meningococcal disease in Nairobi, Kenya, 1989. J Infect Dis 1992;166:359–364.

507. Pinner R, Spellman P, Stephens DS. Evidence for functionally distinct pili expressed by *Neisseria meningitidis*. Infect Immun 1991;59:3169–3175.

508. Poh CL, Lau QC. Subtyping of *Neisseria gonorrhoeae* auxotype-serovar groups by pulsed-field gel electrophoresis. J Med Microbiol 1993;38:366–370.

509. Pollard AJ, Levin M. Vaccines for prevention of meningococcal disease. Pediatr Infect Dis J 2000;19:333–345.

510. Pomeranz HD, Storch GA, Lueder GT. Pediatric meningococcal conjunctivitis. J Pediatr Ophthalmol Strabismus 1999;36:161–163.

511. Pon E, Batchelor RA, Howell HB, et al. An unusual case of penicillinase-producing *Neisseria gonorrhoeae* resistant to spectinomycin in California. Sex Transm Dis 1986;13:47–49.

512. Pontani D, Washton H, Bouchillon S, Johnson J. Susceptibility of European respiratory tract isolates to trovafloxacin, ciprofloxacin, clarithromycin, azithromycin, and ampicillin. Eur J Clin Microbiol Infect Dis 1998;17:413–419.

513. Popovic T, Sacchi CT, Reeves MW, et al. *Neisseria meningitidis* serogroup W135 isolates associated with the ET-37 complex. Emerg Infect Dis 2000;6:428–429.

514. Porritt RJ, Mercer JL, Munro R. Detection and serogroup determination of *Neisseria meningitidis* in CSF by polymerase chain reaction. Pathology 2000;32:42–45.

515. Potocki de Montalk G, Remaud-Simeon M, Willemot RM, et al. Amylosucrase from *Neisseria polysaccharea*: novel catalytic properties. FEBS Lett 2000;471:219–223.

516. Powars D, Larsen R, Johnson J, et al. Epidemic meningococcemia and purpura fulminans with induced protein C deficiency. Clin Infect Dis 1993;17:254–261.

517. Pugsley PM, Dworzack DL, Horowitz EA, et al. Efficacy of ciprofloxacin in the treatment of nasopharyngeal carriers of *Neisseria meningitidis*. J Infect Dis 1987;156:211–213.

518. Pujol C, Eugene E, Marceau M, Nassif X. The meningococcal PilT protein is required for induction of intimate attachment to epithelial cells following pilus-mediated adhesion. Proc Natl Acad Sci USA 1999;96:4017–4022.

519. Racoosin JA, Whitney CG, Conover CS, Diaz PS. Serogroup Y meningococcal disease in Chicago, 1991–1997. JAMA 1998;280:2094–2098.

520. Radstrom P, Fermer C, Kristiansen B-E, et al. Transformational exchanges in the dihydropteroate synthase gene of *Neisseria meningitidis*: a novel mechanism of sulfonamide resistance. J Bacteriol 1992;174:6386–6393.

521. Rahman M, Kallstrom H, Normark S, Jonsson AB. PilC of pathogenic *Neisseria* is associated with the bacterial cell surface. Mol Microbiol 1997;25:11–25.

522. Read RC, Zimmerli S, Broaddus C, et al. The (α-8)-linked polysialic acid capsule of group B *Neisseria meningitidis* modifies multiple steps during interaction with human macrophages. Infect Immun 1996;64:3210–3217.

523. Reddy MS, Murphy TF, Faden HS, Bernstein JM. Middle ear mucin glycoprotein: purification and interaction with nontypeable *Haemophilus influenzae* and *Moraxella catarrhalis*. Otolaryngol Head Neck Surg 1997;116:175–180.

524. Reddy TS, Smith D, Roy TM. Primary meningococcal pneumonia in elderly patients. Am J Med Sci 2000;319:255–257.

525. Reller BL, MacGregor RR, Beaty HN. Bactericidal antibody after colonization with *Neisseria meningitidis*. J Infect Dis 1973;127:56–62.

526. Rice PA, Vayo HE, Tam MR, et al. Immunoglobulin G antibodies directed against protein III block killing of serum-resistant *Neisseria gonorrhoeae* by immune serum. J Exp Med 1986;164:1735–1748.

527. Rice RJ, Biddle JW, Jean-Louis YA, et al. Chromosomally-mediated resistance in *Neisseria gonorrhoeae* in the United States: results of surveillance and reporting, 1983–1984. J Infect Dis 1986;153:340–345.

528. Rice RJ, Knapp JS. Antimicrobial susceptibilities of *Neisseria gonorrhoeae* strains representing five distinct resistance phenotypes. Antimicrob Agents Chemother 1994;38:155–158.

529. Rice RJ, Knapp JS. Susceptibility of *Neisseria gonorrhoeae* associated with pelvic inflammatory disease to cefoxitin, ceftriaxone, clindamycin, gentamicin, doxycycline, azithromycin, and other antimicrobial agents. Antimicrob Agents Chemother 1994;38:1688–1691.

530. Rice RJ, Schalla WO, Whittington WL, et al. Phenotypic characteristics of *Neisseria gonorrhoeae* isolated from three cases of meningitis. J Infect Dis 1986;53:362–365.

531. Richards SJ, Greening AP, Enright MC, et al. Outbreak of *Moraxella catarrhalis* in a respiratory unit. Thorax 1993;48:91–92.

532. Richmond P, Goldblatt D, Fusco PC, et al. Safety and immunogenicity of a new *Neisseria meningitidis* serogroup C-tetanus toxoid conjugate vaccine in healthy adults. Vaccine 1999;18:641–646.

533. Richter SS, Winokur PL, Brueggemann AB, et al. Molecular characterization of the β-lactamases from clinical isolates of *Moraxella* (*Branhamella*) *catarrhalis* obtained from 24 U.S. medical centers during 1994–1995 and 1997–1998. Antimicrob Agents Chemother 2000;44:444–446.

534. Riedo FX, Plikaytis BD, Broome CV. Epidemiology and prevention of meningococcal disease. Pediatr Infect Dis J 1995;14:643–657.

535. Riesbeck K, Orvelid-Molling P, Fredlund H, Olcen P. Long-term persistence of a discotheque-associated invasive *Neisseria meningitidis* group C strain as proven by pulsed-field gel electrophoresis and *porA* gene sequencing. J Clin Microbiol 2000;38:1638–1640.

536. Ringuette L, Lorange M, Ryan A, et al. Meningococcal infections in the province of Quebec, Canada, during the period 1991 to 1992. J Clin Microbiol 1995;33:53–57.

537. Ringuette L, Trudeau T, Turcotte T, et al. Emergence of *Neisseria gonorrhoeae* strains with decreased susceptibility to ciprofloxacin—Quebec, 1994–1995. Can Commun Dis Rep 1996;22:121–125.

538. Riou JY, Guibourdenche M. *Neisseria polysaccharea* sp. nov. Int J Syst Bacteriol 1987;37:163–165.

539. Riou JY, Guibourdenche M, Perry MB, et al. Structure of the extracellular D-glucan produced by *Neisseria polysaccharea*. Can J Microbiol 1986;32:909–911.

540. Risher WH, McFadden PM. *Neisseria gonorrhoeae* mycotic ascending aortic aneurysm. Ann Thorac Surg 1994;57:748–750.

541. Roberts MC, Knapp JS. Host range of the conjugative 25.2 megadalton tetracycline resistance plasmid from *Neisseria gonorrhoeae* and related species. Antimicrob Agents Chemother 1988;32:488–491.

542. Roberts MC, Knapp JS. Transfer of β-lactamase plasmids from *Neisseria gonorrhoeae* to *Neisseria meningitidis* and commensal *Neisseria* species by the 25.2-megadalton conjugative plasmid. Antimicrob Agents Chemother 1988;32:1430–1432.

543. Robinson A, Griffith SB, Moore DG, et al. Evaluation of the RIM system and Gonogen test for identification of *Neisseria gonorrhoeae* from clinical specimens. Diagn Microbiol Infect Dis 1985;3:125–130.

544. Robinson AJ, Watkeys JEM, Ridgway GL. Sexually transmitted organisms in sexually abused children. Arch Dis Child 1998;79:356–358.

545. Roche Diagnostic Systems Inc. AMPLICOR™ *Chlamydia trachomatis/Neisseria*

gonorrhoeae (CT/NG) test package insert. Branchburg, NJ: Roche Diagnostic Systems, 1999.

546. Rokbi B, Mazarin V, Maitre-Wilmotte G, Quentin-Millet MJ. Identification of two major families of transferrin receptors among *Neisseria meningitidis* strains based on antigenic and genomic features. FEMS Microbiol Lett 1993;110: 51–57.

547. Rompalo AM. Diagnosis and treatment of sexually acquired proctitis and proctocolitis: an update. Clin Infect Dis 1999;28(Suppl):S84–S90.

548. Ronne T, Berthelsen L, Buhl L, et al. Comparative studies on pharyngeal carriage of *Neisseria meningitidis* during a localized outbreak of serogroup C meningococcal disease. Scand J Infect Dis 1993;25:331–339.

549. Rosenqvist E, Wedege E, Hoiby EA, et al. Serogroup determination of *Neisseria meningitidis* by whole-cell ELISA, dot-blotting, and agglutination. APMIS 1990; 98:501–506.

550. Rosenstein NE, Perkins BA, Stephens DS, et al. The changing epidemiology of meningococcal disease in the United States, 1992–1996. J Infect Dis 1999;180: 1894–1901.

551. Rosenstein NE, Stocker SA, Popovic T, et al. Antimicrobial resistance of *Neisseria meningitidis* in the United States, 1997. Clin Infect Dis 2000;30:212–213.

552. Ross JDC: Systemic gonococcal infection. Genitourin Med 1996;72:404–407.

553. Rossau R, Kersters K, Falsen E, et al. *Oligella*, a new genus including *Oligella urethralis* comb. nov. (formerly *Moraxella urethralis*) and *Oligella ureolytica* sp. nov. (formerly CDC group IVe): relationship to *Taylorella equigenitalis* and related taxa. Int J Syst Bacteriol 1987;37:198–210.

554. Rossau R, Vandenbussche G, Thielemans S, et al. Ribosomal ribonucleic acid cistron similarities and deoxyribonucleic acid homologies of *Neisseria, Kingella, Eikenella, Simonsiella, Alysiella,* and Centers for Disease Control groups EF-4 and M-5 in the emended Family *Neisseriaceae.* Int J Syst Bacteriol 1989;39: 185–198.

555. Rossau R, Van Landschoot A, Gillis M, et al. Taxonomy of *Moraxellaceae* fam. nov., a new bacterial family to accommodate the genera *Moraxella, Acinetobacter, Psychrobacter* and related organisms. Int J Syst Bacteriol 1991;41: 310–319.

556. Rotta AT, Asmar BI, Ballal N, et al. *Moraxella catarrhalis* ventriculitis in a child with hydrocephalus and an external ventricular drain. Pediatr Infect Dis J 1995;14:397–398.

557. Rudel T, Facius D, Barten R, et al. Role of pili and the phase-variable PilC protein in natural competence for transformation of *Neisseria gonorrhoeae.* Proc Natl Acad Sci USA 1995;92:7986–7990.

558. Rudel T, Scheurerpflug I, Meyer TF. *Neisseria* PilC protein identified as a type-4 pilus tip-located adhesin. Nature 1995;373:357–359.

559. Sacchi CT, Tondella MLC, de Lemos APS, et al. Characterization of epidemic *Neisseria meningitidis* serogroup C strains in several Brazilian states. J Clin Microbiol 1994;32:1783–787.

560. Saez-Llorens X, McCracken GH Jr. Antimicrobial and anti-inflammatory treatment of bacterial meningitis. In: Schaad UB, ed.: Infectious Diseases Clinics of North America. Vol. 13. Bacterial meningitis. Philadelphia: WB Saunders, 1999: 619–636.

561. Saez-Nieto JA, Campos J. Penicillin-resistant strains of *Neisseria meningitidis* in Spain. Lancet 1988;1:1452–1453.

562. Saez-Nieto JA, Fenoll A, Vasquez J, et al. Prevalence of maltose-negative *Neisseria meningitidis* variants during an epidemic period in Spain. J Clin Microbiol 1982;15:78–81.

563. Saez-Nieto JA, Fontanals D, Garcia De Jalon J, et al. Isolation of *Neisseria meningitidis* strains with increase of penicillin minimal inhibitory concentrations. Epidemiol Infect 1987;99:463–469.

564. Saez-Nieto JA, Lujan R, Berron S, et al. Epidemiology and molecular basis of penicillin-resistant *Neisseria meningitidis* in Spain: a 5-year history (1985–1989). Clin Infect Dis 1992;14:394–402.

565. Saez Nieto JA, Lujan R, Martinez-Suarez JV, et al. *Neisseria lactamica* and *Neisseria polysaccharea* as possible sources of meningococcal β-lactam resistance by genetic transformation. Antimicrob Agents Chemother 1990;34: 2269–2272.

566. Safton S, Cooper G, Harrison M, et al. *Neisseria canis* infection: a case report. Commun Dis Intell 1999;23:221.

567. Saginur R, Clecner B, Portnoy J, et al. Superoxol (catalase) test for identification of *Neisseria gonorrhoeae.* J Clin Microbiol 1982;15:475–477

568. Sahm DF, Jones ME, Hickey ML, et al. Resistance surveillance of *Streptococcus pneumoniae, Haemophilus influenzae,* and *Moraxella catarrhalis* isolated in Asia and Europe, 1997–1998. J Antimicrob Chemother 2000;45:457–466.

569. Saito H, Annaissie EJ, Khardori N, et al. *Branhamella catarrhalis* septicemia in patients with leukemia. Cancer 1988;61:3215–3217.

570. Salzman MB, Rubin LG. Meningococcemia. In: Litwick LI, ed.: Infectious Disease Clinics of North America. Vol. 10. Infectious disease emergencies. Philadelphia: WB Saunders, 1996:709–725.

571. Samuelsson S, Gustavsen S, Ronne T. Epidemiology of meningococcal disease in Denmark, 1980–1988. Scand J Infect Dis 1991;23:723–730.

572. Samuelsson S, Handysides S, Ramsay M, et al. Meningococcal infection in pilgrims returning from the Haj: update from Europe and beyond. Eurosurveill Wkly 2000;17:1–5.

573. Sandstrom EG, Ruden A-K. Markers of *Neisseria gonorrhoeae* for epidemiological studies. Scand J Infect Dis Suppl 1990;69:149–156.

574. Sanyal SK, Wilson N, Twum-Danso K, et al. *Moraxella* endocarditis following balloon angioplasty of aortic coarctation. Am Heart J 1991;119:1421–1423.

575. Saperstein DA, Bennett MD, Steinberg JP, et al. Exogenous *Neisseria meningitidis* endophthalmitis. Am J Ophthalmol 1997;123:135–136.

576. Sartin JS. *Neisseria sicca* meningitis in a woman with nascent pernicious anemia. Am J Med 2000;109:175–176.

577. Saunders NB, Shoemaker DR, Brandt BL, Zollinger WD. Confirmation of suspicious cases of meningococcal meningitis by PCR and enzyme-linked immunosorbent assay. J Clin Microbiol 1997;35:3215–3219.

578. Saunders NB, Zollinger WD, Rao VB. A rapid and sensitive PCR strategy employed for amplification and sequencing of *porA* from a single colony forming unit of *Neisseria meningitidis.* Gene 1993;137:153–162.

579. Schachter J, Hook EW, McCormack WM, et al. Ability of the Digene hybrid capture II test to identify *Chlamydia trachomatis* and *Neisseria gonorrhoeae* in cervical specimens. J Clin Microbiol 1999;37:3668–3671.

580. Schifman RB, Ryan KJ. *Neisseria lactamica* septicemia in an immunocompromised patient. J Clin Microbiol 1983;17:935–937.

581. Schneider H, Griffiss JM, Mandrell RE, et al. Elaboration of a 3.6-kilodalton lipooligosaccharide, antibody against which is absent from human sera, is associated with serum resistance of *Neisseria gonorrhoeae.* Infect Immun 1985;50: 672–677.

582. Schneider H, Hammack CA, Apicella MA, et al. Instability of expression of lipooligosaccharides and their epitopes in *Neisseria gonorrhoeae.* Infect Immun 1988;56:942–946.

583. Scholten RJPM, Bijlmer HA, Poolman JT, et al. Meningococcal disease in the Netherlands, 1958–1990: a steady increase in the incidence since 1982 partially caused by new serotypes and subtypes of *Neisseria meningitidis.* Clin Infect Dis 1993;16:237–246.

584. Scholten RJPM, Poolman JT, Valkenburg HA, et al. Phenotypic and genotypic changes in a new clone complex of *Neisseria meningitidis* causing disease in the Netherlands, 1958–1990. J Infect Dis 1994;169:673–676.

585. Schoolnik GK, Buchanen TM, Holmes KK. Gonococci causing disseminated gonococcal infections are resistant to the bactericidal action of normal human serum. J Clin Invest 1976;8:1163–1173.

586. Schoolnik GK, Fernandez R, Tai J-Y. Gonococcal pili: primary structure and receptor binding domain. J Exp Med 1984;159:1351–1370.

587. Schultz TR, Tapsall JW, White PA, Newton PJ. An invasive isolate of *Neisseria meningitidis* showing decreased susceptibility to the quinolones. Antimicrob Agents Chemother 2000;45:909–911.

588. Schwam E, Cox J. Fulminant meningococcal supraglottitis: an emerging infectious syndrome. Emerg Infect Dis 1999;5:464–467.

589. Schwarc SK, Bolan GA, Fullilove M, et al. Crack cocaine and the exchange of sex for money for drugs. Sex Transm Dis 1992;19:7–13.

590. Schwartz B, Al-Ruwais A, A'ashi J, et al. Comparative efficacy of ceftriaxone and rifampicin in eradicating pharyngeal carriage of group A *Neisseria meningitidis.* Lancet 1988;1:1239–1242.

591. Schwebke JR, Zajackowski ME. Comparison of DNA probe (Gen-Probe) with culture for the detection of *Neisseria gonorrhoeae* in an urban STD program. Genitourin Med 1996;72:108–110.

592. Scott MJ, Scott MJ. Primary cutaneous *Neisseria gonorrhoeae* infection. Arch Dermatol 1982;118:351–352.

593. Scribner RK. Neutralization of the inhibitory effect of sodium polyanethol sulfonate on *Neisseria meningitidis* in blood cultures processed with the DuPont Isolator system. J Clin Microbiol 20:40–42, 1984.

594. Seddon PC, Sunderland D, O'Halloran SM, et al. *Branhamella catarrhalis* colonization in pre-school asthmatics. Pediatr Pulmonol 1992;13:133–135.

595. Seidemann K, Lauten M, Gappa M, et al. Obstructive airway disease cause by *Moraxella catarrhalis* after renal transplantation. Pediatr Nephrol 2000;14: 707–709.

596. Seifert HS, Wright CJ, Jerse AE, et al. Multiple gonococcal pilin antigenic variants are produced during experimental human infections. J Clin Invest 1994; 93:2744–2749.

597. Selander RK, Caugant DA, Ochman H, et al. Methods of multilocus enzyme electrophoresis for bacterial population genetics and systematics. Appl Environ Microbiol 1986;51:873–884.

598. Sethi S, Surface JM, Murphy TF. Antigenic heterogeneity and molecular analysis of CopB of *Moraxella catarrhalis.* Infect Immun 1997;65:3666–3671.

599. Shinners EN, Catlin BW. Arginine and pyrimidine biosynthetic defects in *Neisseria gonorrhoeae* strains isolated from patients. J Bacteriol 1982;151:295–302.

600. Simmons G, Jones N, Calder L. Equivalence of ceftriaxone and rifampicin in eliminating nasopharyngeal carriage of serogroup B *Neisseria meningitidis.* J Antimicrob Chemother 2000;45:909–911.

601. Simmons WP. *Moraxella catarrhalis* pneumonia and bacteremia in an otherwise healthy child. Clin Pediatr 1999;38:560–561.

602. Sinave CP, Ratzan KR. Infective endocarditis caused by *Neisseria flavescens.* Am J Med 1987;82:163–164.

603. Singh RP, Marwaha RK. Fulminant *Branhamella catarrhalis* tracheitis. Ann Trop Paediatr 1990;10:221–222.

604. Sivalingam P, Tully AM. Acute meningococcal epiglottitis and septicaemia in a 65-year-old man. Scand J Infect Dis 1998;30:196–198.

605. Sjoholm AG, Kuijper EJ, Tijssen CC, et al. Dysfunctional properdin in a Dutch family with meningococcal disease. 1988;N Engl J Med 319:33–37.

606. Smith I, Lehmann AK, Lie L, et al. Outbreak of meningococcal disease in western Norway due to a new serogroup C variant of the ET-5 clone: effect of vaccination and selective carriage eradication. Epidemiol Infect 1999;123:373–382.

607. Smith KR, Fisher HC III, Hook EW III. Prevalence of fluorescent monoclonal antibody-nonreactive *Neisseria gonorrhoeae* in five North American sexually transmitted disease clinics. J Clin Microbiol 1996;34:1551–1552.

608. Sneath PH, Barrett SJ. A new species of *Neisseria* from the dental plaque of the domestic cow, *Neisseria dentiae* sp. nov. Lett Appl Microbiol 1996;23:355–358.

609. Sobanski MA, Barnes RA, Gray SJ, et al. Measurement of serum antigen concentration by ultrasound-enhanced immunoassay and correlation with clinical outcome in meningococcal disease. Eur J Clin Microbiol Infect Dis 2000;19:260–266.

610. Southern PM, Kutscher AE. Bacteremia due to *Neisseria cinerea:* report of two cases. Diagn Microbiol Infect Dis 1987l7:143–147.

611. Sow AI, Caugant DA, Cisse MF, et al. Molecular characteristics and susceptibility to antibiotics of serogroup A *Neisseria meningitidis* strains isolated in Senegal in 1999. Scand J Infect Dis 2000;32:185–187.

612. Spaargaren J, Stoof J, Fenema R, et al. Amplified fragment length polymorphism fingerprinting for identification of a core group of *Neisseria gonorrhoeae* transmitters in the population attending a clinic for sexually transmitted diseases in Amsterdam, the Netherlands. J Clin Microbiol 2001;39:2335–2337.

613. Sparling PF. Biology of *Neisseria gonorrhoeae.* In Holmes KK, Mardh P-A, Sparling PF et al., eds.: Sexually Transmitted Diseases. 3rd Ed. New York: McGraw-Hill, 1999:433–449.

614. Sparling PF, Handsfield HH. *Neisseria gonorrhoeae.* In: Mandell GL, Bennett JE, Dolin R, eds.: Mandell, Douglas, and Bennett's Principles and Practice of Infectious Diseases. 5th Ed. Philadelphia: Churchill-Livingstone, 2000:2242–2258.

615. Speeleveld E, Fossepre J-M, Gordts B, et al. Comparison of three rapid methods, tributyrine, 4-methylumbelliferyl butyrate, and indoxyl acetate, for rapid identification of *Moraxella catarrhalis.* J Clin Microbiol 1994;32:1362–1363.

616. Spratt BG, Zhang Q-Y, Jones DM, et al. Recruitment of a penicillin-binding protein gene from *Neisseria flavescens* during the emergence of penicillin resistance in *Neisseria meningitidis.* Proc Natl Acad Sci USA 1989;86:8988–8992.

617. Stackebrandt E, Murray RGE, Truper HG. *Proteobacteria* classis nov. a name for the phylogenetic taxon that includes the ''purple bacteria and their relatives.'' Int J Syst Bacteriol 1988;38:321–325.

618. Stansfield RE, Masterson RG, Dale BAS, et al. Primary meningococcal conjunctivitis and the need for prophylaxis in close contacts. J Infect 1994;29:211–214.

619. Stanwell-Smith RE, Stuart JM, Hughes AO, et al. Smoking, the environment, and meningococcal disease: a case-control study. Epidemiol Infect 1994;112:315–328.

620. Stefanou J, Agelopoulou AV, Sipsas NV, et al. *Moraxella catarrhalis* endocarditis: case report and review of the literature. Scand J Infect Dis 2000;32:217–218.

621. Stein DC, Danaher RJ, Cook TM. Characterization of a *gyrB* mutation responsible for low-level nalidixic acid resistance in *Neisseria gonorrhoeae.* Antimicrob Agents Chemother 1991;35:622–626.

622. Steingrube VA, Wallace RJ Jr, Beaulieu D. A membrane-bound precursor β-lactamase in strains of *Moraxella catarrhalis* and *Moraxella nonliquefaciens* that produce BRO-1 and BRO-2 β-lactamases. J Antimicrob Chemother 1993;31:237–244.

623. Stenfors L-E, Raisanen S. Abundant attachment of bacteria to nasopharyngeal epithelium in otitis-prone children. J Infect Dis 1992;165:1148–1150.

624. Stephens DS, Hoffman LH, McGee ZA. Interaction of *Neisseria meningitidis* with human nasopharyngeal mucosa: attachment and entry into columnar epithelial cells. J Infect Dis 1983;148:369–376.

625. Stephens DS, Spellman PA, Swartley JS. Effect of the (α2-8)-linked polysialic acid capsule on adherence of *Neisseria meningitidis* to human mucosal cells. J Infect Dis 1993;167:475–479.

626. Stern A, Brown M, Nickel P, et al. Opacity genes in *Neisseria gonorrhoeae:* control of phase and antigenic variation. Cell 1986;47:61–71.

627. Stojilkovic I, Larson J, Hwa V, et al. HmbR outer membrane receptors of pathogenic *Neisseria* spp.: iron-regulated, hemoglobin-binding proteins with a high level of primary structure conservation. J Bacteriol 1996;178:4670–4678.

628. Stotka JL, Rupp ME, Meier FA, et al. Meningitis due to *Neisseria mucosa:* case report and review. Rev Infect Dis 1991;13:837–841.

629. Strathdee CA, Tyler SD, Ryan JA, et al. Genomic fingerprinting of *Neisseria meningitidis* associated with group C meningococcal disease in Canada. J Clin Microbiol 1993;31:2506–2508.

630. Strongin IS, Kale SA, Raymond MK, et al. An unusual presentation of gonococcal arthritis in an HIV positive patient. Ann Rheum Dis 1991;50:572–573.

631. Struillou L, Raffi F, Barrier JH. Endocarditis caused by *Neisseria elongata* subspecies *nitroreducens:* case report and literature review. Eur J Clin Microbiol Infect Dis 1993;12:625–627.

632. Sutcliffe EM, Jones DM, El-Sheikh S, et al. Penicillin-insensitive meningococci in the U.K. Lancet 1988;1:657–658.

633. Swanson J. Colony opacity and protein II compositions of gonococci. Infect Immun 1982;37:359–368.

634. Swartley JS, Ahn JH, Liu LJ, et al. Expression of sialic acid and polysialic acid in serogroup B *Neisseria meningitidis:* divergent transcription of biosynthesis and transport operons through a common promoter region. J Bacteriol 1996;178:4052–4059.

635. Swartley JS, Liu LJ, Miller YK, et al. Characterization of the gene cassette required for biosynthesis of the (α1-6)-linked N-acetyl-D-mannosamine-1-phosphate capsule of serogroup A *Neisseria meningitidis.* J Bacteriol 1998;180:1533–1539.

636. Swartley JS, Marfin AA, Edupuganti S, et al. Capsule switching of *Neisseria meningitidis.* Proc Natl Acad Sci 1997;94:271–276.

637. Sweet RL. Pelvic inflammatory disease. Hosp Pract 1993;28(Suppl):S25–S30.

638. Taha M-K. Simultaneous approach for nonculture PCR-based identification and serogroup prediction of *Neisseria meningitidis.* J Clin Microbiol 2000;38:855–857.

639. Taha M-K, Morand PC, Pereira Y, et al. Pilus-mediated adhesion of *Neisseria meningitidis:* the essential role of cell contact-dependent upregulation of the PilC1 protein. Mol Microbiol 1998;28:1153–1163.

640. Takahashi H, Tanaka H, Inouye H, et al. Isolation from a healthy carrier and characterization of a *Neisseria meningitidis* strain that is deficient in γ-glutamyl aminopeptidase activity. J Clin Microbiol 2002;40:3035–3037.

641. Tanaka M, Matsumoto T, Kobayashi T, et al. Emergence of in vitro resistance to fluoroquinolones in *Neisseria gonorrhoeae* isolated in Japan. Antimicrob Agents Chemother 1995;39:2367–2370.

642. Tappero JW, Reporter R, Wenger JD, et al. Meningococcal disease in Los Angeles County, California, and among men in the county jails. N Engl J Med 1996;335:833–840.

643. Tapsall JW, Lovett R, Munro R. Failure of 500 mg ciprofloxacin therapy in male urethral gonorrhea. Med J Aust 1992;156:143.

644. Tapsall JW, Phillips EA, Schultz TR, Thacker CL. Quinolone-resistant *Neisseria gonorrhoeae* isolated in Sydney, Australia, 1991 to 1995. Sex Transm Dis 1996;23:425–428.

645. Tapsall JW, Phillips EA, Schultz TR, et al. Strain characteristics and antibiotic susceptibility of isolates of *Neisseria gonorrhoeae* causing disseminated gonococcal infection in Australia. Int J STD AIDS 1992:273–277.

646. Tapsall JW, Schultz TR, Limnios EA, et al. Failure of azithromycin therapy in gonorrhea and discorrelation with laboratory test parameters. Sex Transm Dis 1998;25:505–508.

647. Telfer Brunton WA, Young H, Fraser DR. Isolation of *Neisseria lactamica* from the female genital tract: a case report. Br J Vener Dis 1980;56:325–326.

648. Tenover FC. Antimicrobial susceptibility testing of *Neisseria meningitidis.* Clin Microbiol Newslett 1993;15:37–38.

649. Tesoro LJ, Selbst SM. Factors affecting outcome in meningococcal infections. Am J Dis Child 1991;145:218–220.

650. Thompson DK, Deal CD, Ison CA, et al. A typing system for *Neisseria gonorrhoeae* based on biotinylated oligonucleotide probes to PIB gene variable regions. J Infect Dis 2000;181:1652–1660.

651. Thompson DS, French SA. Comparison of commercial Amies transport systems with in-house Amies medium for recovery of *Neisseria gonorrhoeae.* J Clin Microbiol 1999;37:3020–3021.

652. Thompson EC, Brantley D. Gonococcal endocarditis. J Natl Med Assoc 1996;8:353–356.

653. Thornsberry C, Jones ME, Hickey ML, et al. Resistance surveillance of *Streptococcus pneumoniae, Haemophilus influenzae,* and *Moraxella catarrhalis* isolated in the United States. J Antimicrob Chemother 1999;44:749–759.

654. Thornsberry C, Ogilvie PT, Holley HP Jr, Sahm DF. Survey of susceptibilities of *Streptococcus pneumoniae, Haemophilus influenzae,* and *Moraxella catarrhalis* isolates to 26 antimicrobial agents: a prospective U.S. study. Antimicrob Agents Chemother 1999;43:2612–2623.

655. Tikly M, Diese M, Zannettou N, Essop R. Gonococcal endocarditis in a patient with systemic lupus erythematosus. Br J Rheumatol 1997;36:270–272.

656. Tinsley CR, Heckels JE. Variation in the expression of pili and outer membrane protein by *Neisseria meningitidis* during the course of meningococcal infection. J Gen Microbiol 1986;132:2483–2490.

657. Tondella ML, Popovic T, Rosenstein NE, et al. Distribution of *Neisseria meningitidis* serogroup B subserotypes and serotypes circulating in the United States. J Clin Microbiol 2000;38:3323–3328.

658. Tondella MLC, Sacchi CT, Neves BC. Ribotyping as an additional molecular

marker for studying *Neisseria meningitidis* serogroup B epidemic strains. J Clin Microbiol 1994;32:2745–2748.

659. Tonjum T, Caugant DA, Dunham SA, Koomey M. Structure and function of repetitive sequence elements associated with a highly polymorphic domain of the *Neisseria meningitidis* PilQ protein. Mol Microbiol 1998;29:111–124.

660. Tonjum T, Freitag NE, Namork E, Koomey M. Identification and characterization of *pilG*, a highly-conserved pilus assembly gene in pathogenic *Neisseria*. Mol Microbiol 1995;16:451–464.

661. Tramont EC. Gonococcal vaccines. Clin Microbiol Rev 1989;2(Suppl):S74–S77.

662. Trees DL, Schultz AJ, Knapp JS. Use of the neisserial lipoprotein (Lip) for subtyping *Neisseria gonorrhoeae*. J Clin Microbiol 2000;38:2914–2916.

663. Tritton D, Watts T, Sieratzki JS. Peri-orbital cellulitis and sepsis by *Branhamella catarrhalis*. Eur J Pediatr 1998;157:611–612.

664. Tronel H, Chaudemanche H, Pechier N, et al. Endocarditis due to *Neisseria mucosa* after tongue piercing. Clin Microbiol Infect 2001;7:275–276.

665. Tsai CM, Civin CI. Eight lipooligosaccharides of *Neisseria meningitidis* react with a monoclonal antibody which binds lacto-N-neotetrose (Gal β 1-4GlcNAc β 1-3Gal β 1-4Glc). Infect Immun 1991;59:3604–3609.

666. Tsirpouchtsidis A, Hurwitz R, Brinkman V, et al. Neisserial immunoglobulin A1 protease induces specific T-cell responses in humans. Infect Immun 2002; 70:335–344.

667. Turner A, Jephcott AE, Gough KR. Tetracycline-resistant meningococci. Lancet 1988;1:1454.

668. Turner PC, Southern KW, Spencer NJB, Pullen H. Treatment failure in meningococcal meningitis. Lancet 1990;335:732–733.

669. Twumasi PA Jr, Kumah S, Leach A, et al. A trial of a group A plus group C meningococcal polysaccharide-protein conjugate vaccine in African infants. J Infect Dis 1996;174:1360–1363.

670. Tzanakaki G, Blackwell CC, Kremastinou J, et al. Antibiotic sensitivities of *Neisseria meningitidis* isolates from patients and carriers in Greece. Epidemiol Infect 1992;108:449–455.

671. Tzeng Y-L, Stephens DS. Epidemiology and pathogenesis of *Neisseria meningitidis*. Microbes Infect 2000;2:687–700.

672. Unemo M, Berglund T, Olcen P, Fredlund H. Pulsed-field gel electrophoresis as an epidemiologic tool for *Neisseria gonorrhoeae*: identification of clusters within serovars. Sex Transm Dis 2002;29:25–31.

673. Unemo M, Olcen P, Berglund T, et al. Molecular epidemiology of *Neisseria gonorrhoeae*: sequence analysis of the porB gene confirms presence of two circulating strains. J Clin Microbiol 2002;40:3741–3749.

674. United States Department of Health and Human Services, Centers for Disease Control and Prevention, National Institutes of Health. Appendix 1. Biosafety in microbiological and biomedical laboratories (BM BL). In: Fleming DO, Hunt DL, eds.: Biological Safety: Principles and Practices. 3rd Ed. Washington, DC: ASM Press, 2000:609–700.

675. Uriz S, Pineda V, Grau M, et al. *Neisseria meningitidis* with reduced sensitivity to penicillin: observation in 10 children. Scand J Infect Dis 1991;23:171–174.

676. Valenzuela GA, Davis TD, Pizzani E, et al. Infective endocarditis due to *Neisseria sicca* and associated with intravenous drug abuse. South Med J 1992;85: 929.

677. Van Der Pol B, Ferrero DV, Buck-Barrington, et al. Multicenter evaluation of the BDProbeTec ET system for detection of *Chlamydia trachomatis* and *Neisseria gonorrhoeae* in urine specimens, female endocervical swabs, and male urethral swabs. J Clin Microbiol 2001;39:1008–1016.

678. Van Der Pol B, Martin DH, Schachter J, et al. Enhancing the specificity of the COBAS AMPLICOR CT/NG test for *Neisseria gonorrhoeae* by retesting specimens with equivocal results. J Clin Microbiol 2001;39:3092–3098.

679. Van Der Pol B, Williams JA, Smith NJ, et al. Evaluation of the Digene Hybrid Capture II assay with the rapid capture system for detection of *Chlamydia trachomatis* and *Neisseria gonorrhoeae*. J Clin Microbiol 2002;40:3558–3564.

680. Van Deuren M, Brandtzaeg P, van der Meer JWM. Update on meningococcal disease with emphasis on pathogenesis and clinical management. Clin Microbiol Rev 2000;12:144–166.

681. Van Dyck E, Ieven M, Pattyn S, et al. Detection of *Chlamydia trachomatis* and *Neisseria gonorrhoeae* by enzyme immunoassay, culture, and three nucleic acid amplification tests. J Clin Microbiol 2001;39:1751–1756.

682. Van Dyck E, Smet H, Piot P. Comparison of E test with agar dilution for antimicrobial susceptibility testing of *Neisseria gonorrhoeae*. J Clin Microbiol 1994;32:1586–1588.

683. Vaneechoutte M, Verschraegen G, Claeys G, Flamen P. Rapid identification of *Branhamella catarrhalis* with 4-methylumbelliferyl butyrate. J Clin Microbiol 1988;26:1227–1228.

684. Vaneechoutte M, Verschraegen G, Claeys G, Van Den Abeele AMD. Selective medium for *Branhamella catarrhalis* with acetazolamide as a specific inhibitor of *Neisseria* species. J Clin Microbiol 1988;26:2544–2548.

685. Vaneechoutte M, Verschraegen G, Claeys G, Van Den Abeele AMD. Serological typing of *Moraxella catarrhalis* strains on the basis of lipopolysaccharide antigens. J Clin Microbiol 1990;28:182–187.

686. Vaneechoutte M, Verschraegen G, Claeys G, et al. Respiratory tract carrier rates of *Moraxella (Branhamella) catarrhalis* in adults and children and interpretation of the isolation of *M. catarrhalis* from sputum. J Clin Microbiol 1990;28: 2674–2680.

687. Van Esso D, Fontanels D, Uriz S, et al. *Neisseria meningitidis* strains with decreased susceptibility to penicillin. Pediatr Infect Dis 1987;6:438–439.

688. Van Hare GF, Shurin PA, Marchant CD, et al. Acute otitis media caused by *Branhamella catarrhalis*: biology and therapy. Rev Infect Dis 1987;9:16–27.

689. Van Looveren M, Ison CA, Ieven M, et al. Evaluation of the discriminatory power of typing methods for *Neisseria gonorrhoeae*. J Clin Microbiol 1999;37: 2183–2188.

690. Van Looveren M, VanDamme P, Haucecorne M, et al. Molecular epidemiology of recent Belgian isolates of *Neisseria meningitidis* serogroup B. J Clin Microbiol 1998;36:2828–2834.

691. Vedros NA. Genus I. *Neisseria* Trevisan 1885, 105[AL]. In Krieg NR, Holt JG, eds.: *Bergey's Manual of Systematic Bacteriology*, Vol 1, Baltimore: Williams & Wilkins, 1984:190–196.

692. Vermeij CG, van Dam SW, Oosterkamp HM, Verburgh CA. *Neisseria subflava* biovar *perflava* peritonitis in a continuous cyclic peritoneal dialysis patient. Nephrol Dial Transplant 1999;14:1608.

693. Vernham GA, Crowther JA. Acute myeloid leukaemia presenting with acute *Branhamella catarrhalis* epiglottitis. J Infect 1993;26:93–95.

694. Viagappan GM, Cudlip S, Lee PYC, et al. Brain abscess caused by infection with *Moraxella catarrhalis* following a penetrating injury. J Infect 1998;36: 130–131.

695. Virji M, Heckels JE. The role of common and type-specific pilus antigenic domains in adhesion and virulence of gonococci for human epithelial cells. J Gen Microbiol 1984;130:1089–1095.

696. Virji MHJ, Potts WJ, Hart CA, Saunders JR. Identification of epitopes recognized by monoclonal antibodies SM1 and SM2 which react with all pili of *Neisseria gonorrhoeae* but which differentiate between two structural classes of pili expressed by *Neisseria meningitidis* and the distribution of their encoding sequences in the genomes of *Neisseria* species. J Gen Microbiol 1989;135: 3239–3251.

697. Virji M, Watt SM, Barker S, et al. The N-domain of the human CD66a adhesion molecule is a target for Opa proteins of *Neisseria meningitidis* and *Neisseria gonorrhoeae*. Mol Microbiol 1996;22:929–939.

698. Vlaspolder F, Mutsaers JAEM, Blog F, et al. Value of a DNA probe assay (Gen-Probe) compared with that of culture for diagnosis of gonococcal infection. J Clin Microbiol 1993;31:107–110.

699. Waage A, Brandtzaeg P, Halstensen A, et al. The complex pattern of cytokines in serum from patients with meningococcal septic shock. J Exp Med 1989;169: 333–338.

700. Walker ES, Neal CL, Laffan E, et al. Long-term trends in susceptibility of *Moraxella catarrhalis*: a population analysis. J Antimicrob Chemother 2000; 45:175–182.

701. Wallace RJ Jr, Nash DR, Steingrube VA. Antibiotic susceptibilities and drug resistance in *Moraxella (Branhamella) catarrhalis*. Am J Med 1990;88(Suppl 5A):46S–50S.

702. Wallace RJ Jr, Steingrube VA, Nash DR, et al. BRO β-lactamases of *Branhamella catarrhalis* and *Moraxella* subgenus *moraxella*, including evidence for chromosomal β-lactamase transfer by conjugation in *B. catarrhalis*, *M. nonliquefaciens*, and *M. lacunata*. Antimicrob Agents Chemother 1989;33:1845–1854.

703. Walton DT. Fluorescent antibody-negative penicillinase-producing *Neisseria gonorrhoeae*. J Clin Microbiol 1989;27:1885–1886.

704. Wan WL, Farkas GC, May WN, et al. The clinical characteristics and course of adult gonococcal conjunctivitis. Am J Ophthalmol 1986;102:575–583.

705. Watanakunakorn C, Thomson RB. Septicemia due to a maltose-positive, glucose-negative strain of group C *Neisseria meningitidis*. J Clin Microbiol 1983;18:436–437.

706. Weiss PJ, Kennedy CA, McCann DF, et al. Fulminant endocarditis due to infection with penicillinase-producing *Neisseria gonorrhoeae*. Sex Transm Dis 1992; 19:288–290.

707. Welborn PP, Uyeda CT, Ellison-Birang N. Evaluation of Gonochek II as a rapid identification system for pathogenic *Neisseria* species. J Clin Microbiol 1984; 20:680–683.

708. Welch WD, Cartwright G. Fluorescent monoclonal antibody compared with carbohydrate-utilization for rapid identification of *Neisseria gonorrhoeae*. J Clin Microbiol 1988;26:293–296.

709. West SE, Sparling PF. Response of *Neisseria gonorrhoeae* to iron limitation: alterations in expression of membrane proteins without apparent siderophore production. Infect Immun 1985;14:388–394.

710. Whiley DM, LeCornec GM, Mackay IM, et al. A real-time PCR assay for the detection of *Neisseria gonorrhoeae* by LightCycler. Diagn Microbiol Infect Dis 2002;42:85–89.

711. Whittington WL, Knapp JS. Trends in resistance of *Neisseria gonorrhoeae* to antimicrobial agents in the United States. Sex Transm Dis 1988;15:202–210.

712. Whittington WL, Rice RJ, Biddle JW, et al. Incorrect identification of *Neisseria gonorrhoeae* from infants and children. Pediatr Infect Dis J 1988;7:3–10

713. Whitton T, Smith AG. Erythema nodosum secondary to meningococcal septicaemia. Clin Exp Dermatol 1999;24:97–98.

714. William DC, Felman YM, Corsaro MC. *Neisseria meningitidis* probable pathogen in two related cases of urethritis, epididymitis, and acute pelvic inflammatory disease. JAMA 1979;242:1653–1654.

715. William DC, Felman YM, Riccardi NB, et al. The utility of anoscopy in the rapid diagnosis of symptomatic anorectal gonorrhea in men. Sex Transm Dis 1981;8:16–17.

716. Wilson APR, Wolff J, Atia W. Acute urethritis due to *Neisseria meningitidis* group A acquired by orogenital contact: a case report. Genitourin Med 1989; 65:122–123.

717. Wilson J, Zaman AG, Simmons AV. Gonococcal arthritis complicated by acute pericarditis and pericardial effusion. Br Heart J 1990;63:134–135.

718. Winstead JM, McKinsey DS, Tasker S, et al. Meningococcal pneumonia: characterization and review of cases seen over the past 25 years. Clin Infect Dis 2000; 30:87–94.

719. Winther-Larsen HC, Hegge FT, Wolfgang M, et al. *Neisseria gonorrhoeae* PilV, a type IV pilus-associated protein essential to human epithelial cell adherence. Proc Natl Acad Sci USA 2001;98:15276–15281.

720. Wise CM, Morris CR, Wausilauskas BL, et al. Gonococcal arthritis in an era of increasing penicillin resistance: presentations and outcomes in 41 recent cases (1985–1991). Arch Intern Med 1994;154:2690–2695.

721. Wong JD, Janda JM. Association of an important *Neisseria* species, *Neisseria elongata* subsp. *nitroreducens,* with bacteremia, endocarditis, and osteomyelitis. J Clin Microbiol 1992;30:719–720.

722. Wong VK, Ross LA. *Branhamella catarrhalis* septicemia in an infant with AIDS. Scand J Infect Dis 1988;20:559–560.

723. Woods CR, Koeuth T, Estabrook MM, Lupski JR. Rapid determination of outbreak-related strains of *Neisseria meningitidis* by repetitive element-based polymerase chain reaction. J Infect Dis 1996;174:760–767.

724. Woods CR, Smith AL Wasilauskas BL, et al. Invasive disease caused by *Neisseria meningitidis* relatively resistant to penicillin in North Carolina. J Infect Dis 1994;170:453–456.

725. Woods GL, Garza DM. Use of Gen-Probe competition assay as a supplement to probes for direct detection of *Chlamydia trachomatis* and *Neisseria gonorrhoeae* in urogenital specimens. J Clin Microbiol 1996;34:177–178.

726. Woods JP, Kersulyte D, Tolan RW, et al. Use of arbitrarily primed polymerase chain reaction analysis to type disease and carrier strains of *Neisseria meningitidis* during a university outbreak. J Infect Dis 1994;169:1384–1389.

727. Yeo SF, Livermore DM. Effect of inoculum size on the *in-vitro* susceptibility to β-lactam antibiotics of *Moraxella catarrhalis* isolates of different β-lactamase types. J Med Microbiol 1994;40:252–255.

728. Yeung K-H, Ng L-K, Dillon JR. Evaluation of E test for testing antimicrobial susceptibilities of *Neisseria gonorrhoeae* isolates with different growth media. J Clin Microbiol 1993;31:3053–3055.

729. Young H, Anderson J, Moyes A, McMillan A. Non-cultural detection of rectal and pharyngeal gonorrhoea by the Gen-Probe PACE 2 assay. Genitourin Med 1997;73:59–62.

730. Young H, Moyes A. An evaluation of pre-poured selective media for the isolation of *Neisseria gonorrhoeae.* J Med Microbiol 1996;44:253–260.

731. Young LS, Moyes A. Comparative evaluation of AccuProbe culture identification test for *Neisseria gonorrhoeae* and other rapid methods. J Clin Microbiol 1993;31:1996–1999.

732. Yu RH, Bonnah RA, Ainsworth S, Schryvers AB. Analysis of the immunological responses to transferrin and lactoferrin receptor proteins from *Moraxella catarrhalis.* Infect Immun 1999;67:3793–3799.

733. Yusuf HR, Rochat RW, Baughman WS, et al. Maternal cigarette smoking and invasive meningococcal disease: a cohort study among children in metropolitan Atlanta, 1989–1996. Am J Public Health 1999;89:712–717.

734. Zalacain R, Sobradillo V, Amilibia J, et al. Predisposing factors to bacterial colonization in chronic obstructive pulmonary disease. Eur Respir J 1999;13: 343–348

735. Zangwill KM, Schuchat A, Riedo FX. School-based clusters of meningococcal disease in the United States. Descriptive epidemiology and a case-control analysis. JAMA 1997;277:389–395.

736. Zenilman JM, Nims LJ, Menegus MA, et al. Spectinomycin-resistant gonococcal infections in the United States. J Infect Dis 1987;156:1002–1004.

737. Zhanel GG, Karlowsky JA, Low DE, et al. Antibiotic resistance in respiratory tract isolates of *Haemophilus influenzae* and *Moraxella catarrhalis* collected from across Canada from 1997–1998. J Antimicrob Chemother 2000;45:655–662.

738. Zhang QY, Jones DM, Saez-Nieto JA, et al. Genetic diversity of penicillin-binding protein 2 genes of penicillin-resistant strains of *Neisseria meningitidis* revealed by fingerprinting of amplified DNA. Antimicrob Agents Chemother 1990;34:1523–1528.

Gram-Positive Cocci
Part I: Staphylococci and Related Gram-Positive Cocci

Taxonomy of Staphylococci and Related Gram-Positive Cocci

Clinical Significance of Staphylococci and Related Gram-Positive Cocci

Staphylococcus aureus Subsp. *aureus*
Coagulase-Negative Staphylococci

Staphylococcus epidermidis
Staphylococcus saprophyticus
Subsp. *saprophyticus*
Other Coagulase-Negative Staphylococci

Micrococcus Species and Related Genera
Rothia mucilaginosa

Isolation and Preliminary Differentiation of Staphylococci and Related Gram-Positive Cocci

Direct Gram-Stained Smears
Isolation From Clinical Specimens
Colony Morphology
The Catalase Test
Methods for Differentiating Micrococci and Staphylococci

Fermentation of Glucose
Susceptibility to Lysostaphin

Production of Acid From Glycerol in the Presence of Erythromycin
Susceptibility to Furazolidone
Modified Oxidase Test
Susceptibility to Bacitracin

Identification of *Staphylococcus aureus*

Slide Coagulase Test
Tube Coagulase Test
Alternative Coagulase Test Procedures

Latex Agglutination
Passive Hemagglutination

Additional Confirmatory Tests

Deoxyribonuclease (DNase) Test
Thermostable Endonuclease Test
Mannitol Fermentation

Other Methods for Identification of *Staphylococcus aureus*
Rapid Tests for Detection of Methicillin Resistance
Differentiation of Coagulase-Positive Staphylococci of Veterinary Origin

Identification of Coagulase-Negative Staphylococci

Conventional Identification Methods

Production of Phosphatase for Identification of
   Staphylococcus epidermidis
Pyrrolidonyl Arylamidase Activity
Susceptibility to Polymyxin B
Ornithine Decarboxylase Test (ODC)
Urease Production
Acetoin Production
Susceptibility to Deferoxamine

Susceptibility to Novobiocin for Identification of *Staphylococcus saprophyticus*
Commercial Identification Systems

RapiDEC Staph
API Staph-IDENT
API Staph
API ID32 Staph

Vitek Gram-Positive Identification (GPI) Card
MicroScan Rapid Pos Combo Panel
MicroScan Pos ID Panel
BBL Crystal Gram-Positive (GP) Identification System
Staf-Sistem 18-R
Staph-Zym
Microbact Staphylococcal 12S
Microbial Identification System
   Biolog Microplate Identification System

Molecular Identification and Typing Methods for Staphylococci
Identification of *Micrococcus* and Related Species
Identification of *Rothia mucilaginosa*
Laboratory Approach to the Identification of Staphylococci

With the exception of the *Enterobacteriaceae*, gram-positive bacteria, particularly the cocci, are the microorganisms most frequently isolated from clinical specimens. These bacteria are widespread in nature and can be recovered from the environment or as commensal inhabitants of the skin, mucous membranes, and other body sites in humans and animals. The ubiquity of these gram-positive bacteria in nature makes the interpretation of their recovery from patient specimens occasionally difficult unless clinical manifestations of an infectious disease process are apparent. Recovery of these organisms from specimens should always be correlated with the clinical condition of the patient before their role in an infectious process can be established.

Although gram-positive bacteria may cause infection by multiplication both locally and systemically, some organisms may multiply at a localized site and exert their pathogenic effects by producing exotoxins or enzymes that act at distant sites. Staphylococcal toxins are responsible for food poisoning, scalded-skin syndrome, and toxic-shock syndrome. Streptococcal toxic shock syndrome (Chapter 13) is a clinical entity in which signs and symptoms of infection and pathologic features of disease are largely due to the effects of exotoxins. Gram-negative bacteria, on the other hand, possess endotoxin, which is the lipid portion of the outer membrane lipopolysaccharide. Systemic infections with gram-negative bacteria may lead to endotoxic shock, which is characterized by hypotension, vascular collapse, and sometimes death. This occurs most frequently when gram-negative organisms gain entrance to the bloodstream.

With the increasing numbers of staphylococcal species being recognized in human infections and the finding of resistance to multiple antimicrobial agents in both the common and the uncommon isolates, it is imperative that the clinical microbiologist be familiar with current methods for

characterizing these organisms. In this chapter, the clinical significance and laboratory procedures for isolation and identification of the staphylococci and related organisms will be presented. In Chapter 13, the streptococci and streptococcus-like bacteria will be discussed. Antimicrobial susceptibility testing of these bacterial groups will be addressed in Chapter 16.

Taxonomy of Staphylococci and Related Gram-Positive Cocci

In the 1986 edition of *Bergey's Manual of Systematic Bacteriology*, the Family *Micrococcaceae* included four genera: *Planococcus*, *Micrococcus*, *Stomatococcus*, and *Staphylococcus*.[29,30,225,232,233] Subsequent genetic studies (e.g., DNA-ribosomal RNA hybridization, 16S rRNA sequencing) and chemotaxonomic analyses (e.g., cell-wall composition, cellular fatty acids) documented the diversity of these microorganisms and established that these four genera should not be combined into a single family. Planococci and staphylococci belong to the *Bacillus/Lactobacillus/Streptococcus* phyletic line, while the micrococci and stomatococci are related to an assortment of amycelial actinomycetes. According to the "roadmap" of the new edition of *Bergey's Manual of Systematic Bacteriology*, the staphylococci are in the Phylum *Firmicutes* and comprise Genus I in Family V ("*Staphylococcaceae*"), Order I (*Bacillales*[AL]) in Class III "Bacilli." Family V also includes *Gemella* (see Chapter 13), *Macrococcus*, and *Salinicoccus*.[125] *Planococcus* species are marine cocci that are able to grow in media containing 15% NaCl. This genus currently includes nine species: *P. citreus*, *P. kocuri*, *P. antarcticus*, *P. psychrophilus*, *P. alkanoclasticus*, *P. lilacinus*, *P. rifietensis*, *P. maritimus*, *P. maitriensis*.[5,103,233,363,371,503] Two former *Plano-*

coccus species, *P. okeanokoites* and *P. mcmeekinii*, were recently reclassified in the new genus *Planomicrobium*.[198, 313,502] The planococci are now classified as Genus I in the Family *Planococcaceae* in Order I. *Bacillales*.

The genus *Micrococcus* was originally comprised of nine species: *M. luteus, M. lylae, M. varians, M. roseus, M. agilis, M. kristinae, M. nishinomiyaensis, M. sedentarius,* and *M. halobius*.[232] In 1995, Stackebrandt, Koch and associates performed 16S ribosomal DNA sequence analysis on these recognized species, resulting in the taxonomic dissection and reorganization of the genus.[231,423] *M. roseus, M. varians,* and *M. kristinae* now belong to the genus *Kocuria* as *K. rosea, K. varians,* and *K. kristinae,* respectively.[400] *M. halobius, M. nishinomiyaensis,* and *M. sedentarius* are now placed in three separate genera as *Nesterenkonia halobia, Kytococcus sedentarius,* and *Dermacoccus nishinomiyaensis,* respectively. *M. agilis* has been reclassified in the genus *Arthrobacter* as *A. agilis*.[231] In this new taxonomic scheme, *Micrococcus luteus* and *Micrococcus lylae* remain as the only species in the genus *Micrococcus*.[496] In 2000, a third *Micrococcus* species, *M. antarcticus* was described. This species is a psychrophile that was recovered from Antarctica.[269] Since 1995, three additional *Kocuria* species (*K. palustris, K. rhizophila, K. polaris*) and a new species of *Nesterenkonia* (*N. lacusekhoensis*) have been isolated from environmental sources, and a second *Kytococcus* species (*K. schroeteri*) was isolated from human blood.[25,80,237,364] These former *Micrococcus* species are now in a separate phylum and class from the staphylococci (Phylum Actinobacteria, Class Actinobacteria) and are in the same order as the actinomycetes (Order Actinomycetales). Within this order, former *Micrococcus* species reside in Family *Micrococcaceae* (*Micrococcus, Arthrobacter, Kocuria, Nesterenkonia*) and Family *Dermatophilaceae* (*Dermacoccus* and *Kytococcus*).[125] Micrococci and related species are gram-positive cocci that are slightly larger than staphylococcal cells. Micrococci are 1 to 1.8 μm in diameter, while staphylococci are 0.5 to 1.5 μm in diameter. The cells are arranged mostly as pairs, tetrads, and irregular clusters. In the rest of this chapter, these organisms will be referred to as micrococci and related species.

The newly described genus *Macrococcus* includes animal isolates that appear as large cocci (1.1–2.5 μm in diameter), hence the name ''macro''-coccus.[217] The genus differs from the staphylococci in having fewer 16S rRNA sequence similarities, higher DNA G+C content, lacking cell-wall teichoic acids, and having unique DNA restriction and ribotyping patterns. Members of the genus *Macrococcus* are clearly distinct from the genus *Staphylococcus*, but are closely related to the ''*S. sciuri* group,'' the only members of the staphylococci that are oxidase-positive.[244] Seven *Macrococcus* species have been described: *M. equipercicus* and *M. carouselicus* (both from horses), *M. bovicus* (isolated from cattle), *M. caseolyticus* (formerly *Staphylococcus caseolyticus*), isolated from dairy products, meats, and pilot whales, and *M. brunensis, M. hajekii,* and *M. lamae,* isolated from the skin of llamas.[217,280] Members of the genus *Macrococcus* have not been implicated in human infections.

Stomatococcus mucilaginosus, the only member of the former genus *Stomatococcus,* is an encapsulated gram-positive coccus that is a part of the normal human respiratory tract flora.[29,30] Based on 16S rDNA sequencing and chemotaxonomic data, stomatococci are most closely related to organisms in the genus *Rothia*. *S. mucilaginosus* has been transferred to the genus *Rothia* as *Rothia mucilaginosa* along with *R. dentocariosa* and a new species, *Rothia nasimurium,* an organism found in the nares of mice.[79] Although *R. mucilaginosa* and *R. nasimurium* are gram-positive cocci, *R. dentocariosa* is a gram-positive coryneform bacillus that shows rudimentary branching. Because of their coccal morphology, *R. mucilaginosa* will be described in this chapter; *R. dentocariosa* will be discussed in Chapter 14.

Clinical Significance of Staphylococci and Related Gram-Positive Cocci

The genus *Staphylococcus* is currently composed of several species, many of which may be encountered in human clinical specimens (Box 12-1). Staphylococci are nonmotile, non-spore-forming, catalase-positive, gram-positive cocci. These organisms are arranged as single cells, pairs, tetrads, and short chains, but appear predominantly in grape-like clusters. Most species are facultative anaerobes, except for *S. aureus* subsp. *anaerobius* and *S. saccharolyticus*. These two species grow anaerobically and, unlike the facultative species, are often catalase-negative. Staphylococci are generally found on the skin and mucous membranes of humans and other animals. In some cases, this association is amazingly specific. For example, *S. capitis* subsp. *capitis* is primarily found as a part of the human normal flora of the skin and sebaceous glands of the scalp, forehead, and neck, while *S. auricularis* is found primarily in the external auditory canal.[222,224] Some species are found only in animals and are recognized as veterinary pathogens. For example, *S. hyicus* causes an infectious dermatitis in swine, and *S. intermedius* has been isolated from several types of infections in dogs, including cutaneous infections, mastitis, wounds, and reproductive tract infections.[96,156,157] The latter species has also been isolated from dog-bite wounds in humans.[436,437] *S. delphini, S. felis, S. schleiferi* subsp. *coagulans,* and *S. lutrae* cause infectious processes in dolphins, domesticated cats, dogs, and sea otters, respectively.[111,190,191,469] Humans may become colonized or infected with these organisms by frequent or close contact with animals (e.g., veterinarians, zoo workers, farmers). Some of the pathogenic staphylococci in both humans and animals produce an enzyme called **coagulase,** and detection of this enzyme is used in the laboratory to identify these organisms (Box 12-2).[156,469] Among the staphylococci, the coagulase-positive species *S. aureus,* and two coagulase-negative species, *S. epidermidis* and *S. saprophyticus,* are seen frequently in human infections.

Staphylococcus aureus Subsp. aureus

S. aureus is by far the most important human pathogen among the staphylococci. It is found in the external environment and in the anterior nares of 20–40% of adults. Other sites of colonization include intertriginous skin folds, the perineum, the axillae, and the vagina. Although this organism is frequently a part of the normal human microflora,

Box 12-1 Human, Animal, and Environmental *Staphylococcus* Species

Species	Comments

STAPHYLOCOCCI FOUND IN HUMAN AND NONHUMAN PRIMATES

Species	Comments
S. aureus	See text
S. epididymidis	See text
S. saprophyticus	See text
S. haemolyticus[391]	*S. haemolyticus* is part of the human normal skin flora and is also found in nonhuman primates. This organism has been documented as a cause of primary and nosocomial bacteremia, wound and soft-tissue infections, urinary tract infections, and nosocomial pediatric and neonatal infections.[93,152,240,271,340,341,432] Strains of *S. haemolyticus* that have relatively high MICs (i.e., from 2 to ≥8 μg/mL) for vancomycin have been reported by several researchers in the clinical setting of prolonged vancomycin administration, suggesting selection of resistant clones arising from previously susceptible organism populations.[16,174,401,402,470] In this regard, strains of *S. haemolyticus* that are resistant to both glycopeptides (i.e., vancomycin and teicoplanin) and/or that are susceptible to vancomycin and resistant to teicoplanin have been described.[35,50,240] Glycopeptide resistance in *S. haemolyticus* and other coagulase-negative staphylococci is usually expressed heterogeneously, with both susceptible and resistant subpopulations existing within a single culture.[35,36] The emergence of glycopeptide resistance in *S. haemolyticus* has underscored the importance of correct identification and susceptibility testing of these isolates and monitoring of their spread within the hospital environment. Although phenotypic identification of *S. haemolyticus* is fairly straightforward, nucleic acid probes for specific identification of *S. haemolyticus* have been developed.[3] Studies on the mechanism of glycopeptide resistance suggest that the causes are multifactorial and may relate principally to cell-wall structure, where alterations in the cross-linkages within the peptidoglycan interfere with binding of glycopeptide dimers and, therefore, with the successful interaction of the antibiotic with its target.[37] In addition to glycopeptide resistance, methicillin- and quinolone-resistant isolates of *S. haemolyticus* have also been reported.[340,432,501] The presence of multiply-antibiotic-resistant *S. haemolyticus* in the hospital environment and transmission of resistant clones via the hands of health-care workers have been documented by several investigators using a variety of molecular methods (e.g., immunoblotting of staphylococcal polypeptides, plasmid analysis, restriction-length polymorphisms of chromosomal DNA, pulsed-field gel electrophoresis of total DNA).[93,340,432] *S. haemolyticus*, like *S. epidermidis*, *S. warneri*, *S. xylosus*, and *S. hyicus*, also produces an extracellular lipase that may function in virulence.[322,372]
S. warneri[222]	This species represents about 1% of the staphylococci normally found on human skin. *S. warneri* is now a well-recognized cause of catheter-related bacteremia, native-valve endocarditis, hematogenous vertebral osteomyelitis, and ventriculoperitoneal shunt–associated meningitis.[51,54,87,452,498] Isolates recovered from humans are now called *S. warneri* subsp. 1, while isolates from nonhuman primates are called *S. warneri* subsp 2. *S. warneri* strains produce an extracellular enzyme that has both lipase and phospholipase activity.[372,438,467]
S. hominis[220,222]	*S. hominis* is found on the skin of humans and has occasionally been isolated from infections as a low-grade pathogen, causing catheter-related sepsis in immunocompromised hosts.[45] *S. hominis* has also been reported as a cause of endocarditis in a patient as a complication of vasectomy.[214] In 1998, the species was divided into two subspecies: *S. hominis* subsp. *hominis*, and *S. hominis* subsp. *novobiosepticus*.[220] *S. hominis* subsp. *hominis* is found on the skin and is an infrequent isolate from infectious processes, while *S. hominis* subsp. *novobiosepticus* is recovered more frequently from blood cultures and bona fide infections. Subspecies *novobiosepticus* is novobiocin-resistant and does not produce acid from D-trehalose or *N*-acetyl-D-glucosamine, while the subspecies *hominis* is novobiocin-susceptible and produces acid aerobically from both D-trehalose and *N*-acetyl-D-glucosamine.[220] Subspecies *novobiosepticus* also tends to be more resistant to antimicrobial agents than subspecies *hominis*.
S. simulans[222]	*S. simulans* is found on the skin and in the urethras of healthy women. The organism has been isolated as a cause of septicemia, osteomyelitis, native-valve endocarditis, septic arthritis following open reduction of a fractured fibula, vertebral osteomyelitis, and prosthetic joint infection.[193,278,289,361,430] *S. simulans* possesses a capsule that inhibits phagocytosis *in vitro* and contributes to virulence *in vivo*.[323] As with certain other coagulase-negative staphylococci (i.e., *S. epidermidis*, *S. haemolyticus*, and *S. hominis*), methicillin-resistant strains of *S. simulans* possess an additional penicillin binding protein that exhibits a low affinity for methicillin, cephalothin, and cefamandole and has amino acid sequences analogous to the PBP2′ found in methicillin-resistant *S. aureus* isolates.[346]

Box 12-1 *Continued*

Species	Comments
S. lugdunensis[121]	This species, first described in 1988, has rapidly established itself as a significant human pathogen. *S. lugdunensis* colonizes the human inguinal area as established by inguinal fold culture sampling and the predominance of *S. lugdunensis* isolates obtained from abscesses in the pelvic girdle region.[27,326,465] *S. lugdunensis* has been associated with a wide variety of infections, including native- valve, prosthetic-valve, and pacemaker-associated endocarditis, meningitis, skin and soft-tissue abscesses, cellulitis, peritonitis, infected hip prostheses, osteomyelitis, vertebral diskitis, vascular line infections, oral infections, septic arthritis following arthroscopic surgery, urinary tract infections, and ventriculoperitoneal shunt infections.[42,53,57,64,101,107,155,197,200,203,238,264,312,329,332,383,399,421,461,485,504] A septic shock presentation similar to that seen with gram-negative bacteria has also been associated with *S. lugdunensis* bacteremia.[62] Oxacillin-resistant strains of *S. lugdunensis* carrying the *mecA* gene have also been characterized.[442] Examination of clinical isolates has demonstrated that *S. lugdunensis* produces a variety of potential virulence factors, including α- and δ-hemolysins, lipases, and esterases.[162,246]
S. schleiferi[121]	*S. schleiferi* was first described in 1988 and has been isolated from several human infections, including brain empyema, wound infections, bacteremia complicating vertebral osteitis, infection of a hip prosthesis, indwelling catheter infection, nosocomial urinary tract infections, prosthetic-valve endocarditis, osteomyelitis, and pacemaker infections.[56,65,172,229,261,328] In 1990, the species was divided into two subspecies; human and canine isolates (associated with pyoderma) have been designated *S. schleiferi* subsp. *schleiferi*, and isolates causing external otitis in dogs have been designated *S. schleiferi* subsp. *coagulans*.[119,191] The species produces a variety of putative virulence factors (e.g., glycocalyx, lipases, esterases, and hemolysins) that may contribute to pathogenicity.[162,246,336] When the subspecies were first described, it was thought that subspecies *schleiferi* isolates were clumping factor–positive and tube coagulase–negative, while subspecies *coagulans* isolates were clumping factor–negative and tube coagulase–positive.[191] Vandenesch and colleagues subsequently isolated three strains of *S. schleiferi* subsp. *schleiferi* that were both clumping factor– and tube coagulase–positive (Color Plates 12-3E–12-3H).[463]
S. capitis[222]	*S. capitis* is part of the normal human flora and is found surrounding the sebaceous glands on the scalp and forehead. In 1991, this species was divided into two subspecies, *S. capitis* subsp. *capitis* and *S. capitis* subsp. *ureolyticus*.[23] *S. capitis* subsp. *ureolyticus* can be differentiated from subsp. *capitis* by its positive urease activity, the ability to produce acid from maltose under aerobic conditions, and cellular fatty acid profiles. Since 1992, this species has been reported as a cause of native- and prosthetic-valve endocarditis (including aortic-valve endocarditis), endocarditis associated with upper endoscopy, and pacemaker implantation.[8,202,253,382,475] *S. capitis* was documented as the cause of 17 cases of sepsis in critically ill premature infants, including one case of meningitis.[483] In these cases, all of the isolates were resistant to oxacillin, erythromycin, and clindamycin. Strains of *S. capitis* isolated from neonatal intensive care units have also displayed heteroresistance to vancomycin.[466]
S. auricularis[224]	This species is found in the human external auditory canal and is rarely implicated in infections.
S. pasteuri[75]	*S. pasteuri* is a newly described species that is found in human and animal clinical specimens and in food. It has not yet been associated with infectious processes and is phenotypically similar to *S. warneri*. Oligonucleotide probes derived from randomly amplified DNA have been designed for differentiation and identification of *S. pasteuri*.[464]
S. caprae[97,210]	*S. caprae* was originally thought to be an animal species isolated from goats and goat milk. In 1991, *S. caprae* was cultured from an exudate from a patient with dermatitis and from the urine of a second patient.[204] Subsequently, *S. caprae* has been isolated from a patient with endocarditis, two patients with catheter-related bacteremia, two cases of urinary tract infection, and blood cultures of a neonate with congenital heart disease.[422,462] *S. caprae* has been reported primarily in association with bone and joint infections, including a case of intraarticular empyema following arthroscopic knee surgery, and as a cause of iatrogenic osteomyelitis following surgical implantation of orthopedic materials.[7,102,408] In a study of the distribution of *Staphylococcus* species among human clinical specimens, *S. caprae* comprised 10.7% of the 1,230 strains examined.[210] Similar ribotypes have been identified for *S. caprae* strains recovered from both goat milk and clinical specimens, even though phenotypic characteristics may vary among different isolates.[26] *S. caprae* is most closely related to *S. epidermidis* and *S. capitis* subspecies.[132] Strains of *S. caprae* from humans contain a five-gene *ica* operon that codes for gene products involved in biofilm formation.[6,7] The polypeptides deduced from the *ica* gene sequences exhibit 67% to 88% amino acid identity with similar *ica* gene operon products found in *S. aureus* and *S. epidermidis*.

(Continued)

Box 12-1 *Continued*

Species	Comments
S. cohnii[228,391]	*S. cohnii* was first described in 1975, and in 1991 it was divided into two subspecies designated *S. cohnii* subsp. *cohnii* and *S. cohnii* subsp. *urealyticum*.[228] Subspecies *cohnii* has only been isolated from humans, while the latter urease-positive subspecies *urealyticum* has been isolated from both human and nonhuman primates. Both are normal flora on the skin. *S. cohnii* is an emergent opportunistic agent, having been reported as a cause of community-acquired pneumonia, primary septic arthritis, and catheter-related sepsis in immunocompromised patients.[24,106,286,287] Chorioamnionitis and neonatal sepsis with meningitis due to *S. cohnii* have also been reported.[211,419]
S. xylosus[391]	*S. xylosus* is found in both human and nonhuman primates and has been reported as a cause of upper and lower urinary tract infections and endocarditis associated with intravenous drug use.[83,454] This organism was isolated from the blood and bile of an 11-year-old patient who had undergone cardiac and hepatic transplantation and from a pancreatic pseudocyst in an HIV-infected patient.[284,285] *S. xylosus* has also been isolated from goat milk and cheese.[297] Strains of *S. xylosus* also produce an extracellular lipase.[372]
S. saccharolyticus[215]	This anaerobic species was previously called *Peptococcus saccharolyticus* and was transferred to the genus *Staphylococcus* based on oligonucleotide analysis of 16S ribosomal RNA. The organism is found on human mucous membranes. Two cases of endocarditis (one involving a native heart valve, and the other a prosthetic heart valve) caused by this organism have been reported.[241,494]

STAPHYLOCOCCI FOUND IN OTHER ANIMALS

Species	Comments
S. intermedius[156]	This species is found as a part of the flora of dogs, minks, horses, and cats and may cause cutaneous, urinary tract, bone, and central nervous system infections in several animal species. *S. intermedius* is the predominant coagulase-positive staphylococcus recovered from normal and infected canine skin and from serious canine infections.[136] Human carriage of *S. intermedius* is rare even among individuals with frequent exposure to animals.[277,437] This organism has been isolated from humans with infected dog-bite wounds and has also been recovered from individuals with non-canine-inflicted injuries, including infections of varicose vein ulcers and suture incisions.[435,436] Minor infections (e.g., otitis externa) with this organism may also occur as a consequence of close, nontraumatic contact with the family canine.[441] *S. intermedius* catheter-related sepsis in a 63-year-old cancer patient and *S. intermedius* pneumonia following coronary-artery bypass surgery have also been reported.[134,460] *S. intermedius* is characterized by being tube coagulase–positive, but clumping factor–variable. The *S. intermedius* coagulase is a 64.6-kDa protein that induces clot formation in human and rabbit, but not in rat or guinea pig plasma.[234]
S. hyicus[96]	*S. hyicus* is found in cattle and in cow's milk and is associated with exudative epidermitis ("greasy pig syndrome"), an acute disease of suckling and weaned pigs. Strains of *S. hyicus* causing this skin infection produce three types of exfoliative toxins and a calcium-dependent extracellular lipase/phospholipase enzyme that contribute to the pathology of this syndrome.[10,372] Although not considered a pathogen of humans, a case of human wound infection caused by *S. sciuri* following a donkey bite was reported in 1997.[327]
S. sciuri[226]	*S. sciuri* is widely distributed in nature and has been isolated from foods, farm animals, rodents, marsupials, marine mammals, and occasionally from humans and their pets. Three subspecies are currently recognized.[218,283] *S. sciuri* subsp. *sciuri* is found in nature and as part of the transient skin flora in various mammalian and avian species; it is seldom found in humans or nonhuman primates. *S. sciuri* subsp. *carnaticus* is found mainly on bovine hosts and meat products derived from them. *S. sciuri* subsp. *rodentium* is found mainly in rodents. Human isolates have been recovered from wounds, skin, and soft-tissue infections, and, in 1998, a case of *S. sciuri* endocarditis was reported.[164,283,425] *S. sciuri* has also been isolated as a cause of peritonitis in a patient on dialysis.[480] An examination of 30 human clinical isolates of *S. sciuri* found that 70% were subsp. *sciuri*, 23% were subsp. *rodentium*, and 7% were subsp. *carnaticus*. All subspecies of *S. sciuri* have been found to harbor a homolog of the *S. aureus* methicillin resistance gene *mecA* and 46% of strains that have been examined also carry the *mecA* gene that is found in methicillin-resistant *S. aureus* strains.[84,500] These two *mecA* homologs have about 80% base-pair similarities. *S. sciuri* strains that carry their native *mecA* homolog express borderline resistance to methicillin, while the strains that carry the MRSA *mecA* gene express heterogeneous resistance to methicillin. *S. sciuri* produces a variety of putative virulence factors (e.g., biofilm formation, clumping factor, exotoxins, DNase and proteolytic activities) but their contributions to the pathogenicity of this organism have not been determined.[426]
S. chromogenes[96,157]	This species, formerly a subspecies of *S. hyicus*, causes cutaneous infections in cattle, swine, and goats.[11]
S. gallinarum[97]	This species is found in poultry and is nonpathogenic.
S. lentus[389]	*S. lentus*, formerly a subspecies of *S. sciuri* (i.e., *S. sciuri* subsp. *lentus*) is part of the normal skin flora of sheep and goats.

Box 12-1 *Continued*

Species	Comments
S. equorum[390]	*S. equorum* is a rare species of undetermined pathogenic significance. It has been recovered primarily from horses as well as from goat milk and cheese.[297]
S. delphini[469]	This coagulase-positive species causes purulent skin lesions in dolphins.
S. felis[189,190]	*S. felis* is the most commonly isolated *Staphylococcus* species in cats, causing otitis, cystitis, abscesses, wounds, and other cutaneous infections.
S. lutrae[111]	This species, described in 1997, was isolated during postmortem examinations of three sea otters (*Lutra lutra*) from the Inner Hebrides Islands west of the Scottish mainland. Isolates were obtained from liver tissue and spleen tissues and from a mammary gland and supramammary lymph node. *S. lutrae* is free coagulase–positive and clumping factor–negative, and is most closely related to *S. delphini, S. felis, S. intermedius, S. schleiferi,* and *S. muscae.*[111]
S. vitulinus[487]	This species was described in 1994 and is found as a part of the flora of horses, voles, and pilot whales. It has also been isolated from meat products, including lamb, chicken, ground beef, and veal. DNA hybridization studies show that this species is most closely related to *S. lentus* and *S. sciuri.*[487]
S. muscae[158]	This newly described species is found as a transient part of the body-surface flora of flies that inhabit cow barns, but it is not found on flies inhabiting human dwellings.
OTHER STAPHYLOCOCCI (MOSTLY ENVIRONMENTAL)	
S. carnosus[388]	This species is used as a starter culture in the processing of meats such as salami and sausage. At present, two subspecies are recognized: *S. carnosus* subsp. *carnosus* and *S. carnosus* subsp. *utilis.*[357]
S. kloosii[390]	This species is found in mammals and is of uncertain clinical significance and taxonomic status.
S. arlettae[390]	This species is found on mammals and birds and is of undetermined clinical significance and taxonomic status.
S. piscifermentans[440]	This species is found in fish, fermented fish products, and soy mash and is closely related to *S. carnosus* and *S.condomenti.*[330]
S. condimenti[357]	This species is found in soy sauce mash (as is *S. piscifermentans*) and is closely related to *S. carnosus* subspecies.
S. succinis[247]	This species, first described in 1998, was isolated from a fragment of 25- to 35-million-year-old Dominican amber. This species phenotypically resembles *S. xylosus* and is closely related to *S. xylosus, S. saprophyticus, S. equorum,* and other novobiocin-resistant staphylococci. A subspecies of *S. succinus, S. succinus* subsp. *casei,* has been proposed for isolates from Swiss surface-ripened cheese.[351]
S. fleurettii[471]	This species has been isolated from cheeses prepared from goats' milk.

it can cause significant opportunistic infections under the appropriate conditions.[478] Factors that may predispose an individual to serious *S. aureus* infections include:

- Defects in leukocyte chemotaxis, either congenital (e.g., Wiskott-Aldrich syndrome, Down's syndrome, Job's syndrome, and Chediak-Higashi syndrome) or acquired (e.g., diabetes mellitus, rheumatoid arthritis)
- Defects in opsonization by antibodies secondary to congenital or acquired hypogammaglobulinemias or complement component (especially C3 and C5) deficiencies and/or defects
- Defects in intracellular killing of bacteria following phagocytosis due to inability to activate the membrane-bound oxidase system, resulting in the absence of peroxides and superoxide from phagocytic vacuoles (e.g., chronic granulomatous disease, lymphoblastic leukemia, and both acute and chronic myelogenous leukemia)
- Skin injuries (e.g., burns, surgical incisions, eczema)
- Presence of foreign bodies (e.g., sutures, intravenous lines, prosthetic devices)

- Infection with other agents, particularly viruses (e.g., influenza)
- Chronic underlying diseases such as malignancy, alcoholism, and heart disease
- Therapeutic or prophylactic antimicrobial administration.

Under these circumstances, *S. aureus* may cause a variety of infectious processes ranging from relatively benign skin infections to life-threatening systemic illnesses (Box 12-3). Skin infections include simple folliculitis and impetigo (see Color Plate 12-1A), as well as furuncles and carbuncles involving subcutaneous tissues and causing systemic symptoms, such as fever. *S. aureus* is frequently isolated from postsurgical wound infections, which may serve as a nidus for the development of systemic infections. Community-acquired staphylococcal bronchopneumonia is usually seen in elderly individuals and is associated with viral pneumonia as a predisposing factor. Nosocomial pneumonia due to *S. aureus* occurs in the clinical settings of obstructive pulmonary disease, intubation, and aspiration. Underlying malignant diseases are recognized as important risk factors for the

Box 12-2 Virulence Factors of *Staphylococcus aureus*

Virulence Factor	Comments
Capsular polysaccharides	Some strains of *S. aureus* produce an exopolysaccharide that may prevent ingestion of the organism by polymorphonuclear cells. These exopolysaccharides have been observed by electron microscopic examination of *S. aureus*–infected pacemaker leads, peritoneal catheters, and intravenous lines and have been demonstrated immunologically in vitro.[178] This material may promote the adherence of the organisms to host cells and to prosthetic devices. Clinical isolates of *S. aureus* have been classified into 11 types based on capsular polysaccharide immunotyping, and 70–80% of significant clinical isolates belong to capsular serotype 5 or 8.[13,178] The production of capsular material by *S. aureus* is influenced by a variety of factors both in vitro and in vivo. In culture systems, the production of capsules is influenced by the composition of the growth medium and growth conditions (e.g., solid vs. liquid media, media complexity).[89,429] In vivo, the synthesis of high levels of type 8 polysaccharide has been demonstrated for *S. aureus* harvested from endocardial lesions in a rat model of endocarditis.[257] While earlier studies suggested that the capsule did not enhance virulence, subsequent studies have indicated that the *S. aureus* capsules do indeed contribute to staphylococcal pathogenicity and virulence. Karakawa et al. reported that capsules elaborated by type 5 and type 8 *S. aureus* strains were indeed antiphagocytic.[205] In a mouse model of bacteremia, optimal expression of type 5 capsular polysaccharide in *S. aureus* enhanced bacterial virulence by rendering the organisms resistant to opsonophagocytic killing by leukocytes.[446] Capsular type 5 has also been shown to be a virulence factor contributing to the development of staphylococcal bacteremia and arthritis in a mouse model, and antibodies elicited by immunization with a type 5 polysaccharide-protein "conjugate vaccine" were able to protect against infection with *S. aureus* expressing this capsular serotype in a rat model of endocarditis.[255,319] These two capsular types, particularly type 8, are also associated with other *S. aureus* virulence factors, such as the production of toxic shock syndrome toxin.[256] In addition, a predominant number of *S. aureus* strains that are resistant to oxacillin, the most widely used antistaphylococcal penicillin, express the serotype 5 capsular polysaccharide.[113] The capsular polysaccharides from *S. aureus* capsular serotypes 1, 2, 5, and 8 have been purified and characterized, and the genes encoding the type 1, type 5, and type 8 capsular polysaccharides have been cloned and sequenced.[115,263,308,387]
Peptidoglycan and teichoic acids	*S. aureus* cell walls contain peptidoglycans (cross-linked polymers of *N*-acetyl-glucosamine and *N*-acetyl-muramic acid), which are similar to those found in other gram-positive bacteria, and teichoic acids, which are unique ribitol (5-carbon monosaccharide)-phosphate polymers (see Chapter 5). Teichoic acids function in the specific adherence of gram-positive bacteria to mucosal surfaces. In addition to their role in providing rigidity and resilience to the staphylococcal cell wall, peptidoglycans and teichoic acids also have several biologic activities that are thought to contribute to virulence.[478] These properties include the ability to activate complement, enhancement of chemotaxis of polymorphonuclear cells, elicitation of interleukin-1 production by human monocytes, and stimulation of the production of opsonic antibodies. Serologic tests for the detection of antibodies to these molecules have been investigated for their possible diagnostic and/or prognostic value; results have been disappointing because of considerable overlap of antibody titers among infected and noninfected individuals, the wide spectrum of infection and disease caused by *S. aureus*, and the host-dependent variability of the immune response due to age, other infections, and general immunocompetence.[492] Several other proteins, including adhesins, fibronectin-binding proteins, collagen-binding proteins, and clumping factor, are covalently incorporated into the structure of the *S. aureus* peptidoglycan.
Protein A	*S. aureus* cell walls also contain a protein called protein A. Purified protein A has a molecular weight of 42 kDa and is found on both the cell surface and in the growth medium. This unique protein has the ability to bind the Fc region of all human IgG subclasses except IgG$_3$.[110] Protein A functions as a virulence factor by interfering with opsonization and ingestion of the organisms by polymorphonuclear cells, activating complement, and eliciting immediate and delayed-type hypersensitivity reactions.[478] Protein A is immunogenic, and antibodies against it are found in individuals with serious *S. aureus* infections. The presence of protein A on *S. aureus* provides the basis for coagglutination test procedures that are used in many clinical laboratories for organism identification (e.g., gonococci, streptococcal grouping) and for detection of bacterial antigens in body fluids.

Box 12-2 Continued

Virulence Factor	Comments
Enzymes	*S. aureus* produces several enzymes that contribute to its virulence. **Catalase** production by these organisms may function to inactivate toxic hydrogen peroxide and free radicals formed by the myeloperoxidase system within phagocytic cells after ingestion of the microorganisms.[279] **Clumping factor**, a cell-bound material that is able to bind fibrinogen, is responsible for the binding of *S. aureus* to both fibrin and fibrinogen. **Coagulase**, which can exist free in the medium or in a cell-bound form, binds to prothrombin and becomes enzymatically active, thereby catalyzing the conversion of fibrinogen to fibrin.[209] This enzymatic activity may act to coat the bacterial cells with fibrin, rendering them more resistant to opsonization and phagocytosis. **Fibrinolysins** break down fibrin clots and facilitate the spread of infection to contiguous tissues. Similarly, **hyaluronidase** hydrolyzes the intercellular matrix of acid mucopolysaccharides in tissue and, thus, may act to spread the organisms to adjacent areas in tissue. Strains of *S. aureus* causing chronic furunculosis have been found to be producers of potent **lipases** that may help to spread the organisms in cutaneous and subcutaneous tissues.[372] A **phosphatidylinositol-specific phospholipase C** has also been described that is associated with strains recovered from patients with adult respiratory distress syndrome and disseminated intravascular coagulation.[281] Tissues affected by this enzyme become more susceptible to damage and destruction by bioactive complement components and products during complement activation. *S. aureus* also produces a **nuclease** or **phosphodiesterase** having both exonuclease and endonuclease activities. Immunologic and substrate-specificity studies indicate that at least three different types of **β-lactamase enzymes** are produced by *S. aureus*. Production of these enzymes may be inducible (i.e., they are produced only in the presence of β-lactam antimicrobial agents) or constitutive (i.e., they are produced continually) and render these organisms resistant to penicillin and ampicillin. Genes coding for these enzymes usually reside on plasmids (extrachromosomal DNA) that also carry genes for resistance to several antibiotics, such as erythromycin and tetracycline.[478] These resistance genes may be transferred to other bacteria by transformation and transduction.
Hemolysins	*S. aureus* hemolysins have several biologic activities. **α-Hemolysin** has lethal effects on a wide variety of cell types, including human polymorphonuclear cells, and will lyse erythrocytes from several animal species. Rabbit erythrocytes are extremely susceptible to lysis by α-hemolysin, being 100 times more susceptible than other mammalian erythrocytes and over 1,000 times more susceptible than human erythrocytes.[34] The toxin is a protein with a molecular weight of 33 kDa and is secreted into the medium during late logarithmic growth.[146] Individual monomers interact on the target cell membrane to form cylindrical heptamers with a central pore.[458] The pores opened by these heptameric α-hemolysin aggregates allow rapid efflux of potassium ions and other small molecules and influx of sodium and calcium ions, leading to osmotic swelling and rupture of the cell. α-Hemolysin is also dermonecrotic on subcutaneous injection, and is lethal for animals when administered intravenously. These properties contribute to the belief that this toxin has an important role in the pathogenesis of *S. aureus* infections.[98] Neurotoxicity is also a property of α-hemolysin, causing demyelination of myelin sheaths in both rabbit and murine models of infection. This toxin is responsible for the zone of hemolyzed red blood cells observed around colonies of some *S. aureus* strains growing on sheep blood agar.

β-Hemolysin is a sphingomyelinase (acts on the complex lipocarbohydrate sphingomyelin) that is active on a variety of cells. However, it is not dermonecrotic in guinea pigs and is not lethal to mice.[98] β-Hemolysin is a protein exotoxin with a molecular weight of 35 kDa and is secreted into the medium toward the end of the logarithmic growth phase.[358] Hemolytic activity requires magnesium ions, and substrate specificity is restricted to sphingomyelin and lysophosphatidylcholine. The varying susceptibilities of erythrocytes from different animal species to β-hemolysin-mediated lysis is probably due to differences in membrane sphingomyelin content. The β-hemolysin is a "hot-cold" hemolysin; i.e., its hemolytic properties are enhanced by subsequent exposure of the red blood cells to cold temperatures. This property may be caused by initial disruption of cohesive forces within the membrane by the toxin and subsequent phase separation within the membrane itself as the temperature is lowered. The β-hemolysin, along with the CAMP factor produced by group B streptococci, is responsible for the synergistic hemolysis observed in a positive CAMP test for presumptive identification of group B streptococci. |

(Continued)

Box 12-2 *Continued*

Virulence Factor	Comments
Toxins	**δ-Hemolysin** and **γ-hemolysin** are found in some *S. aureus* strains and also cause lysis of a variety of cell types. δ-**Hemolysin** is a protein with a molecular weight of 3 kDa and is secreted into the medium toward the end of the exponential growth phase. This hemolysin is produced by over 97% of *S. aureus* strains and is also found in 50–70% of coagulase-negative staphylococci.[98]The δ-hemolysin acts primarily as a surfactant that disrupts the cell membrane, and may interact with the membrane to form channels that increase in size over time, resulting in leakage of cellular contents. The term "**γ-hemolysin**" actually describes three proteins that, along with the two proteins comprising the **Panton-Valentine leukocidin** (PV-leukocidin), constitute six "two component" toxins.[265,356,431] The three "γ-hemolysin" proteins, each of which have a molecular weight in the 32- to 35-kDa range, interact with one of the two PV-leukocidin proteins (with molecular weights of 32 and 34 kDa) to form six possible combinations, all of which have biologic activity. None of these five proteins have hemolytic or leukotoxic activity by themselves. While these six two-component toxins show varying degrees of hemolytic activity, all six are able to lyse leukocytes efficiently.[235] Leukocidal activity is exerted directly on human polymorphonuclear cell membranes, causing degranulation of the cytoplasm, cell swelling, and lysis. These toxins act by causing the formation of pores, thereby altering cellular permeability to potassium and other cations. **Exfoliatins** or **epidermolytic toxins** are produced by some staphylococcal strains and consist of two proteins, designated ET-A and ET-B, each with a molecular weight of 24 kDa.[478] The two molecules are biochemically and immunologically distinct, but they have similar biologic activities. ET-A is a thermostable protein for which the structural gene is chromosomal, while ET-B is heat-labile and of plasmid origin. These proteins have proteolytic activity and dissolve the mucopolysaccharide matrix of the epidermis, resulting in intraepithelial splitting of cellular linkages in the stratum granulosum.[433] Strains producing either one or both of these toxins are responsible for the "staphylococcal scalded skin syndrome". (See Color Plate 12-1*B*.) PCR approaches for the detection of exfoliatin toxin genes have been published.[294] **Enterotoxins A through E, H, and I** are heat-stable molecules that are responsible for the clinical features of staphylococcal food poisoning, which is probably the most common cause of food poisoning in the United States. The exact mode of action of these enterotoxins is unknown, but they have been shown to increase intestinal peristalsis. Ingestion of preformed enterotoxins in food supporting staphylococcal growth (e.g., bakery goods, custards, potato salad, processed meats, ice cream) results in vomiting with or without diarrhea within 2 to 8 hours. These toxic conditions are self-limited (24–48 hours) and require only supportive therapy. Inflammatory changes (e.g., a hyperemic mucosa, neutrophilic infiltrates, mucopurulent duodenal exudates, brush-border disruption) are seen throughout the gastrointestinal tract, with the more severe and extensive lesions being found in the stomach and the upper small intestine.[213] Immunologic detection methods and nucleic acid probes have been developed for the exfoliatins and the enterotoxins.[181,317] Immunologic methods detect the toxins directly, while the probes detect the structural genes within the bacterial cell that code for the toxins themselves. Multiplex PCR methods for detection of staphylococcal enterotoxins have been described.[396]
Superantigens	The **staphylococcal enterotoxins** belong to a group of toxins collectively known as pyrogenic toxin superantigens, which also includes the **toxic shock syndrome toxin-1** (TSST-1, see below), the streptococcal pyrogenic exotoxins (SPE A, B, C, F, G, H, and J), and the streptococcal superantigen.[44] All of these toxins share three biologic characteristics: pyrogenicity, superantigenicity, and the ability to enhance the lethal effects of minute amounts of endotoxin in rabbits up to 100,000-fold. Superantigenicity refers to the ability of these toxins to stimulate the proliferation of T lymphocytes without regard for their antigenic specificities. All of these toxins induce polyclonal T-cell proliferation through colligation between major histocompatibility complex class II molecules on antigen-presenting cells and the variable portion of the T-cell antigen receptor β-chain.[282] The role of these enterotoxins in conditions other than staphylococcal food poisoning has been confirmed by the documented involvement of enterotoxins A through D, H, and I with cases of non-menstrual-associated toxic shock syndrome (TSS) and two other TSS-like syndromes called staphylococcal scarlet fever and recalcitrant erythematous desquamating disorder, respectively.[195,259,393]

Box 12-2 *Continued*

Virulence Factor	Comments
	Soon after the illness was described, it was postulated that TSS was caused by a toxin. In 1981, two groups reported the isolation and characterization of unique toxins produced by *S. aureus* isolates from TSS patients.[31,32,394] These two proteins were designated pyrogenic exotoxin type C and staphylococcal enterotoxin F. Further studies indicated that these two were identical, and the toxin is now designated toxic shock syndrome toxin 1 (TSST-1). The mature toxin is a small protein with a molecular weight of 22 kDa that is resistant to inactivation by heat and proteolytic enzymes (e.g. trypsin). A different form of the toxin with a slightly different isoelectric point also has been described in some isolates, but is encoded by the same gene and has the same biologic effects.[40] Although this toxin has a broad range of biologic activity, its role in the pathogenesis of TSS is unclear. Like the enterotoxins, TSST-1 is a superantigen that is able to potentiate the lethal response to minute amounts of gram-negative endotoxin in animal models by bypassing the usual mononuclear cell antigen processing steps and binding directly to monocytes and lymphocytes, resulting in the release of lymphokines and monokines. The systemic release of these cytokines may explain the rapid appearance of multisystem involvement seen with TSS. Additional studies also suggested that some coagulase-negative staphylococci may also produce TSST-1, and cases of TSS due to these organisms have been reported.[85,201] A toxin similar to TSST-1 has also been identified in *S. aureus* strains isolated from sheep, goats, and cows.[177]
	A reverse passive latex agglutination test using latex beads sensitized with anti-TSST-1 antibodies has been described for detection of toxin production *in vitro*.[188] This test is performed on serial dilutions of culture filtrates from staphylococcal isolates. Miwa and associates developed an enzyme immunoassay for detection of TSST-1 in serum from patients with proven or suspected TSS.[304] Although the mean concentration of TSST-1 serum from healthy individuals was less than 30 pg/mL, the mean and maximum quantities detected in patients with TSS were 440 pg/mL and 5,450 pg/mL, respectively. Neill and coworkers described the synthesis and application of a radioactive oligonucleotide TSST-1 probe.[317] This probe hybridized with the bacterial structural genes that coded for TSST-1. Although methods for toxin detection (e.g., latex agglutination, colony immunoblot techniques, enzyme immunoassays) depend on the presence of TSST-1 at or above the level of detection for the assay and on the proper bacterial growth conditions for toxin production, the probe was able to detect the genetic capability of individual strains to produce TSST-1, regardless of the ability of the individual strains to produce toxin *in vitro*.[188,317] PCR-based methods for detection of TSST-1 have also been described.[294,305,396]

development of *S. aureus* bacteremia.[60] Bacteremia may also "seed" distant sites throughout the body, leading to endocarditis, osteomyelitis, pyoarthritis, and metastatic abscess formation, particularly in the skin, the subcutaneous tissues, lungs, liver, kidneys, and brain. *S. aureus* meningitis occurs in patients with central nervous system abnormalities related to trauma, surgery, malignancy, and hydrocephalus. *S. aureus* is also one of many microorganisms associated with peritonitis in patients receiving continuous ambulatory peritoneal dialysis.[347] Toxins produced by *S. aureus* are responsible for toxic epidermal necrolysis (staphylococcal scalded skin syndrome) and toxic shock syndrome (see Boxes 12-2, 12-3, and 12-4). *S. aureus* strains may also cause food poisoning due to the elaboration of exotoxins during growth in contaminated foods. *S. aureus* possesses several properties believed to contribute to their ability to cause disease (see Box 12-2). These virulence factors are not found in all strains of *S. aureus*, however, and this organism continues to be a constant source of surprise as new and different pathogenic properties are discovered. Virulence factors that are

produced by *S. aureus* are presented in Box 12-2 and details regarding infectious processes associated with *S. aureus* are presented in Box 12-3. The case definition of toxic shock syndrome is found in Box 12-4.

Originally, penicillin was the drug of choice for the treatment of serious *S. aureus* infections. The emergence of resistance to penicillin in *S. aureus* was due to the acquisition of plasmidborne genetic elements coding for β-lactamase production. Strains of *S. aureus* produce up to four different β-lactamase enzymes, as evidenced by molecular weights and substrate specificities. At present over 80% of *S. aureus* isolates are resistant to penicillin because of the action of these hydrolytic β-lactamase enzymes or penicillinases. Semisynthetic, penicillinase-resistant penicillins (i.e., oxacillin and methicillin) then became the drugs-of-choice for treatment of infections due to penicillin-resistant *S. aureus*. During the 1980s, resistance to the penicillinase-resistant penicillins emerged. The latter type of resistance is due to the presence of an altered penicillin-binding protein called PBP 2a (or PBP 2′) that results from acquisition of a chromo-

Box 12-3 Infections Associated With *Staphylococcus aureus*

Infection	Comments
Folliculitis	Folliculitis is a benign infection restricted to the ostia of the hair follicles and is characterized by the presence of small, reddish, painful lesions and the absence of systemic symptoms.
Furuncles and carbuncles	Furuncles are deep-seated pyodermas that present as painful, firm, raised lesions with necrotic centers containing purulent material. Carbuncles refer to even more deep-seated lesions that involve the subcutaneous tissues. Several lesions may be present and may coalescence via the formation of subcutaneous sinus tracts. Carbuncles are often associated with systemic signs of chills and fever.
Impetigo	Impetigo is a superficial staphylococcal infection that is seen mostly in children and usually presents on exposed areas, especially the face (Color Plate 12-1*B*). Lesions of impetigo begin as red macules that evolve into vesicles containing serosanguineous fluid. These lesions eventually rupture, becoming dry and crusted, with a honey-colored scab on an erythematous margin. *S. aureus* accounts for 80–90% of cases of impetigo, with the remaining being associated with group A β-hemolytic streptococci. Impetigo caused by these two organisms are indistinguishable clinically.
Hydradenitis suppurativa	This condition is characterized by the presence of multiple furuncle-like lesions associated with blocked and infected apocrine sweat glands. This cutaneous infection occurs predominantly in the intertriginous areas of the body (i.e., in the armpits, groin, and perineal areas). Although local pain, swelling and erythema are present, systemic symptoms such as fever are usually absent.
Mastitis	Mastitis refers to breast infections associated with childbirth and lactation and is characterized by edema, swelling, firmness and, occasionally, erythema of the breast tissues. Superficial abscesses may be drained by needle aspiration, while deeper, persistent lesions require incision and drainage for cure, often along with antibiotic therapy.
Wound infections	Most staphylococcal wound infections occur in the postsurgical setting and are recognized by redness, swelling, pain, and the presence of cloudy, serosanguineous drainage. The approach to wound care in patients with staphylococcal wound infection depends on the depth of the infection, the condition of the host, the presence and/or severity of clinical signs and symptoms, and the presence/absence of foreign bodies within the wound. These factors determine the extent of debridement necessary and the requirement for parenteral antimicrobial chemotherapy.
Bacteremia and endocarditis	Bacteremia with *S. aureus* usually occurs secondary to a localized infection elsewhere (e.g., abscesses, ulcers, burns, pneumonia) or by direct access of the organisms into the bloodstream via catheters, other indwelling devices, or syringes used for injection of recreational drugs.[60,143,424] Patients with staphylococcal bacteremia usually present with chills, rigors, and fever. Hemorrhagic skin lesions may be present and may evolve to form larger, necrotic ulcers. Endocarditis may present in a subtle manner, or with multiple signs and symptoms.[116,117] With infection of the heart valves, more subtle hemorrhagic manifestations (e.g., Janeway lesions, Roth spot, splinter hemorrhages) may be apparent. Heart murmurs, pericardial friction rubs, and pericardial effusions may be present and, depending on the type of murmur, often suggest the likely location(s) of bacterial involvement and valvular insufficiency. Transthoracic and transesophageal echocardiography aid in delineating the extent of cardiac involvement and help to determine the need for and immediacy of surgical interventions.[196] Thrombocytopenia is frequently present, and disseminated intravascular coagulation represents a rare but fatal complication occurring early in the clinical course. Hematogenous seeding of the kidney may result in renal insufficiency, renal abscesses and pyelonephritis.
Meningitis	Meningitis due to *S. aureus* may occur as a complication of bacteremia, local trauma due to surgery or injury, or colonization of intrathecal pump implants.[28] Although the signs and symptoms are similar to other meningeal infections, other cofactors (e.g., immunodeficiency, underlying disease) are present more frequently.[260]
Pericarditis	Pericarditis (infection of the membranes surrounding the heart) due to *S. aureus* may arise hematogenously or secondary to local infection from penetrating chest trauma.[376] Pericarditis may also occur as a complication of staphylococcal endocarditis. Patients present with chest pain, friction rubs, generalized heart failure, and/or mediastinitis.

Box 12-3 *Continued*

Infection	Comments
Pulmonary infections	Pulmonary infections caused by *S. aureus* may arise from aspiration or by hematogenous spread from another site. Aspiration pneumonia acquired in the community is usually seen in the elderly as a complication of influenza pneumonia, while that acquired in the hospital is usually secondary to intubation and ventilatory assistance. Chest x-ray films from these patients may show scattered, patchy infiltrates, defined abscesses or nodules, frank consolidation, or cavitation. In small children, thin-walled pneumatoceles with air-fluid levels may be seen. Hematogenous pulmonary infection occurs as a complication of right-sided endocarditis and is secondary to embolization from valvular lesions, resulting in pulmonary infarcts. In these patients, the chest radiograph usually shows discrete infiltrates along with emboli. Complications of both types of pulmonary infection include bacteremia, lung abscesses, and the development of pleural empyemas.[52,143]
Osteomyelitis/septic arthritis	*S. aureus* osteomyelitis most often occurs as a complication of local infection via direct extension, although hematogenous osteomyelitis may also occur. Hematogenous osteomyelitis usually involves the long bones in children, but osteomyelitis of the vertebral column accounts for over 60% of such infections in adults.[59] Various types of scans, including magnetic resonance imaging and computed tomography, are helpful in delineating the extent of vertebral involvement and the presence of paravertebral abscesses. Abscesses and lytic bone lesions must be aspirated and cultured to provide a definitive diagnosis. Osteomyelitis associated with contiguous infection is usually obvious because the bone infection is adjacent to a surgically induced or trauma-induced wound, and it is most serious when hip or knee prostheses become infected.[395] With the latter types of infection, the implanted materials often have to be removed and replaced following wide excision of involved or infected surrounding tissues. Septic arthritis due to *S. aureus* occurs primarily in prepubertal children and as a complication of bacteremia in adults. Usually the patient presents with a swollen, hot joint (most often involving the knee, hip, elbow, shoulder, or interphalangeal joints) that is painful on movement. Aspiration of the joint, and Gram stain and culture of the purulent exudate are required for management.
Pyomyositis	Pyomyositis is an infection of the skeletal muscles that usually occurs secondary to trauma, often in the neighborhood of an existing focus of infection (e.g., a furuncle).[333] Patients usually present with fever and muscle pain; aspiration and culture yield *S. aureus*. Cure is affected by incision and drainage under cover of an appropriate antimicrobial agent.
Staphylococcal food poisoning	Staphylococcal food poisoning results from ingestion of food contaminated with *S. aureus* strains that produce heat-stable enterotoxins. The implicated foodstuff usually becomes contaminated by a food handler, with subsequent organism growth and toxin production. Implicated foods include potato salads, ice cream, custards, bakery goods, canned foods, and processed meats. Symptoms, including nausea, vomiting, abdominal cramps, and diarrhea, usually begin 2 to 6 hours after ingestion and abate after 8 to 10 hours. Fever and neurologic signs are characteristically absent. Treatment involves replacement of fluids lost due to vomiting and diarrhea, and recovery is complete.
Staphylococcal scalded skin syndrome	In the staphylococcal scalded skin syndrome, bullous formations occur over large areas of the body, with subsequent sloughing of the superficial skin layers (Color Plate 12-1*C*). This results in the exposure of large areas of denuded and raw skin. The disease is usually seen in neonates and infants. The responsible toxins are antigenic and antibodies against them are protective (Box 12–2).
Staphylococcal toxic shock syndrome	Toxic shock syndrome (TSS), first described by Todd and associates in 1978, is a multisystem illness characterized by a clinical syndrome that includes fever, hypotension, orthostatic dizziness, erythroderma (blanching rash), and varying degrees of vomiting, diarrhea, renal failure, headache, chills, sore throat, and conjunctivitis.[160,449,478] Initially, the disease was noted most frequently in women, with onset occurring mainly during menstruation. Investigations of the initial cases noted an association between the onset of disease and the use of hyperabsorbable tampons. Subsequently non-menstrual-associated TSS has been reported in both males and females as a complication of staphylococcal abscesses, osteomyelitis, postsurgical wound infections, and postinfluenza pneumonia.[32]

(Continued)

Box 12-3 *Continued*

Infection	Comments
	The role of TSST-1 and other superantigens in the disease is also supported by the acute onset of symptoms, with vascular congestion developing over a 1- to 2-day period. With the increase in capillary leakage and the systemwide decrease in vascular resistance, there is loss of intravascular fluids into the interstitial spaces. Fluid loss is also exacerbated by the presence of diarrhea in some patients. Loss of intravascular volume leads to hypotension and tissue hypoxia. Acute respiratory distress syndrome and disseminated intravascular coagulation are common and life-threatening complications of TSS.[251] TSST-1 also appears to have some direct toxic effects on the myocardia, skeletal muscle, liver, and kidney tissue.[478] Other conditions that may be included in the differential diagnosis of TSS include other toxin-mediated infections, (e.g., scalded skin syndrome, gastroenteritis, scarlet fever), local infections with shock and/or acute abdominal pain (e.g., infectious gastroenteritis, salpingitis, septic abortion, acute urinary tract infections) and multisystem illnesses of infectious (e.g., septic shock associated with pneumococci, meningococci, or *Haemophilus influenzae* type b; rubeola, Rocky Mountain spotted fever, tickborne typhus, leptospirosis, *Legionella* infection; toxoplasmosis; and adenoviral or enteroviral syndromes) and noninfectious (Kawasaki's disease, systemic lupus erythematosus, acute rheumatic fever, rheumatoid arthritis, drug reactions) etiologies. Diagnosis of TSS is generally based on the clinical signs and symptoms according to the case definition (Box 12–4).

Box 12-4 Case Definition of Staphylococcal Toxic Shock Syndrome[331]

Feature	Comment
Fever	Temperature ≥38.9°C (102.0°F)
Rash	Diffuse macular erythroderma
Desquamation	1–2 weeks (usually 10–14 days) after onset of illness; particularly of palms, soles, fingers, and toes
Hypotension	Systolic blood pressure ≤90 mm Hg for adults or less than fifth percentile by age for children younger than 16 years of age. Orthostatic drop in diastolic pressure of ≥15 mm Hg from lying to sitting; orthostatic syncope or orthostatic dizziness

Involvement of Three or More Organ Systems

Gastrointestinal	Vomiting or diarrhea at onset of illness
Muscular	Severe myalgia or creatinine kinase greater than twice the upper limit of normal
Mucous membranes	Vaginal, oropharyngeal, or conjunctival hyperemia
Renal	Blood urea nitrogen (BUN) or serum creatinine greater than twice the upper limit of normal for laboratory *or* urinary sediment with pyuria (≥5 leukocytes per high-power field) in the absence of urinary tract infection
Hepatic	Total bilirubin, alanine aminotransferase, or aspartate aminotransferase levels at least twice the upper limit of normal for laboratory
Hematologic	Platelet count <100,000/mm³
CNS	Disorientation or alterations in consciousness without focal neurologic signs when fever and hypotension are absent

Laboratory Criteria

Negative Results on the Following Tests

Blood, throat, and spinal fluid cultures (blood cultures may be positive for *S. aureus*)
Serologic tests for Rocky Mountain spotted fever, leptospirosis, and measles

CASE CLASSIFICATION

Confirmed	A case in which all six of the clinical findings described above are present
Probable	A case in which five of the six clinical findings described above are present

Additional Laboratory Findings Pathognomic for TSS, But Presently Not Included in the Case Definition

Isolation of *S. aureus* from a mucosal or normally sterile body site
Production by an incriminated staphylococcal isolate of TSST-1 or an alternative toxin known to cause TSS
Serologic susceptibility to the relevant toxin at the time of acute illness
Development of antibody to the relevant toxin during convalescence

somal gene called *mecA*. PBP 2a has a low affinity for all β-lactam agents, including cephalosporins. Once the normally present PBPs have been inactivated by a β-lactam agent, PBP 2a continues to function and allows the synthesis of a stable peptidoglycan structure, thereby allowing the organism to grow and divide. *S. aureus* strains expressing the *mecA* determinant are termed MRSA (methicillin-resistant *S. aureus*). The *mecA* gene may be expressed by some or all of the cells in a given population, so resistance mediated by altered PBPs is termed **heteroresistance.** The *mecA* determinant of heteroresistant *S. aureus* is also found in methicillin-resistant coagulase-negative staphylococci and contains several other genetic elements involved in the expression and regulation of resistance to β-lactams and other classes of agents. Because of this, oxacillin-resistant staphylococci also tend to be resistant to other agents, such as clindamycin and erythromycin. Resistance to oxacillin and other penicillinase-resistant penicillins may also be seen in *S. aureus* strains that lack the *mecA* determinant. In these cases, resistance is due to "hyperproduction" of β-lactamase enzymes, resulting in slow hydrolysis of the semisynthetic penicillins and borderline methicillin/oxacillin resistance.

MRSA represents a challenge for virtually all healthcare institutions, and guidelines have been promulgated regarding how to manage and control the spread of MRSA within healthcare institutions.[46,490,491] Some hospitals have instituted routine nasal cultures of healthcare personnel to detect and treat MRSA carriers in order to reduce the number of patient exposures and, consequently, the in-house infection rates. Although MRSA initially was a nosocomial pathogen, it is now clear that individuals within the community and outside of healthcare institutions are also at risk for acquiring MSRA. Initial reports of community-acquired MRSA infections reflected certain circumstances and risk behaviors that were responsible for their MRSA infections, such as intravenous drug use, outpatient antimicrobial therapy, previous hospitalizations, and severe underlying diseases.[385] However, MRSA infections are now being seen in communities and populations that do not reflect these risk factors or behaviors. In a study conducted at Yale University School of Medicine, 41% of 87 patients with MRSA had acquired their infections in the community.[254] Organism acquisition was associated with the risk factors listed above, with residence in a nursing home being an additional identified risk factor; eight patients (22%) had no identifiable or discernible risk factors for their infections.

With the emergence of resistance to the penicillinase-resistant penicillins, the glycopeptide agent vancomycin became the treatment of choice for infections due to MRSA. However, in May 1996, the first documented infection caused by an *S. aureus* strain with intermediate resistance to vancomycin was reported from Japan.[66,175] Subsequently, *S. aureus* strains with diminished susceptibility to vancomycin were recovered from patients seen in Michigan, New York state, New Jersey, and Illinois.[67,68,374,417] These isolates have been given the mnemonic "GISA" for "glycopeptide-intermediate *S. aureus*" as these strains have diminished susceptibility to both vancomycin and teicoplanin glycopeptide antibiotics; VISA (vancomycin-intermediate *S. aureus*) is the moniker used mostly in the U.S.[444] These

strains have vancomycin minimal inhibitory concentrations (MICs) of 8 μg/mL. The CLSI (Clinical Laboratories Standards Institute, formerly NCCLS) defines staphylococci requiring concentrations of vancomycin of ≤4 μg/mL for growth inhibition as "susceptible," those requiring 8 to 16 μg/mL as intermediate, and those requiring ≥32 μg/mL as resistant.[316] In 2002, two strains of *S. aureus* that were resistant to vancomycin (MIC, ≥32 μg/mL) were reported from Michigan and Pennsylvania, and, in 2004, the third documented clinical isolate was reported from New York.[69–71] The reduced susceptibility to vancomycin found in these strains is not reliably detected by disk diffusion or automated, rapid susceptibility methods (e.g., Vitek, Microscan rapid panels).[445] The most accurate susceptibility testing method for detecting these strains is a nonautomated MIC method such as broth microdilution or agar dilution with incubation for a full 24 hours. The current recommendation for laboratories that use automated susceptibility methods is to inoculate the organism onto a vancomycin susceptibility screening plate, which contains brain heart infusion (BHI) agar and 6 μg/mL vancomycin, and inspection of the plate for growth after a full 24 hours of incubation. All isolates with vancomycin MICs of 8 μg/mL will grow on these screening plates. Isolates that grow on the screening plate should then be tested by a broth microdilution procedure. Based on a comparative study, an Etest (AB Biodisk, Piscataway, NJ) performed on Mueller-Hinton agar with an inoculum prepared from a no. 2 McFarland-equivalent suspension and incubated for a full 24 hours is also a very sensitive and specific method for detection of these strains; with Etest, VISA strains have vancomycin MICs of ≥6 μg/mL.[481] According to the Centers for Disease Control and Prevention (CDC), three criteria must be met to verify that a given strain is a VISA: broth microdilution vancomycin MICs of 8 to 16 μg/mL, Etest vancomycin MICs of ≥6 μg/mL, and growth within 24 hours on a BHI agar plate containing 6 μg/mL vancomycin.[444,445] Prompt and accurate detection and confirmation of these strains is necessary and critical for optimal treatment of individual patients and for prevention of transmission of these strains to other patients.[490]

The recovery of *S. aureus* with confirmed reduced susceptibility or frank resistance to vancomycin should be reported to infection control personnel within the institution, to both local and state health departments, and to the Centers for Disease Control and Prevention. The determination of optimal therapeutic approaches for individual patients may require additional laboratory testing (e.g., synergy studies, microdilution "checkerboard" studies, time-kill analysis, etc.), since there is evidence that MRSAs, VISAs, methicillin-resistant *S. epidermidis*, and vancomycin-resistant *S. haemolyticus* strains may respond synergistically to combinations of vancomycin and other β-lactam agents.[78] Additional information regarding other resistance mechanisms (e.g., erythromycin and clindamycin resistance) and antimicrobial susceptibility testing of staphylococci is found in Chapter 16.

S. aureus subsp. *anaerobius* causes abscess formation in sheep and has not been isolated from human infections or clinical specimens.[94]

Coagulase-Negative Staphylococci

In the past, coagulase-negative staphylococci were generally considered to be contaminants having little clinical significance. Over the past four decades, however, these organisms have become recognized as important agents of human disease. Although several different species of coagulase-negative staphylococci have been described (see Box 12-1), relatively few of them cause infections in humans. However, as more laboratories have attempted to identify the coagulase-negative staphylococci, infections caused by other species are being recognized more frequently. The types of infections associated with coagulase-negative staphylococci are listed and described in Box 12-5.

STAPHYLOCOCCUS EPIDERMIDIS

When clinical findings are correlated with the isolation of coagulase-negative staphylococci, *S. epidermidis* is by far the most frequently recovered organism, accounting for 50% to over 80% of isolates.[14] Almost all infections caused by *S. epidermidis* are nosocomially acquired, except for native-valve endocarditis and infections of semipermanent venous access devices. In addition to both native-valve and prosthetic-valve endocarditis, *S. epidermidis* has been isolated and documented as a pathogen in urinary tract infections, surgical wound infections, infections of various prosthetic devices, cerebrospinal fluid (CSF) shunt infections, peritoneal dialysis-related infections, and ophthalmic infections (see Box 12-5). Over the past several years, progress has been made in identifying several virulence factors in *S. epidermidis*. Scanning and transmission electron microscopic studies and immunologic examination of *S. epidermidis* strains from infections of indwelling medical devices have shown that these bacteria produce cell-surface and extracellular macromolecules that initiate and subsequently enhance bacterial adhesion to the plastic surfaces of foreign bodies to form a biofilm. Initial, specific adherence of most *S. epidermidis* strains to plastic surfaces appears to be largely mediated by a capsular polysaccharide-adhesin called **PS/A**.[310,450] PS/A is a high-molecular weight, variably *N*-succinylated, β-1,6-linked polyglucosamine molecule that is encoded by the *ica* locus of the *S. epidermidis* genome.[291] Purified PS/A can block adherence of PS/A-producing *S. epidermidis* to plastic catheters in vitro, and antibodies directed against PS/A also appear to block adherence to biomaterials. PS/A is also able to protect the organisms from complement-mediated phagocytic killing.[310,406,407] Other cell-surface polysaccharides have been described that may contribute to this process.[21] In addition, certain proteins may act to promote adherence to plastic in some *S. epidermidis* strains.[168,184,448] For example, Heilmann and coworkers identified an autolysin-adhesin coded for by a gene called *atlE* that works in concert with PS/A in initial adherence of *S. epidermidis* to biomaterials.[168]

Following initial adhesion to biomaterials, the pathogenesis of *S. epidermidis* infection apparently involves adhesion between cells that are adherent to the plastic surface, forming the rest of the bacterial cell/polysaccharide matrix biofilm.[15] Intercellular adhesion is mediated by a polysaccharide called **PIA** (polysaccharide intercellular adhesin) along with some other cell-associated proteins.[274] PIA is a linear polysaccharide composed of β-1,6-linked 2-deoxy-2-amino-D-glucopyranosyl residues, of which 80–85% are *N*-acetylated, with the rest being either non-*N*-acetylated and positively charged or modified with phosphate or succinate residues and negatively charged.[273] Like PS/A, the PIA structural genes also reside within the four-gene chromosomal operon called *ica*, with the four genes being designated *icaA*, *icaB*, *icaC*, and *icaD*.[133,169,291] PIA also appears to function as a hemagglutinin, in that anti-PIA antibodies and purified PIA are both able to inhibit hemagglutination. Furthermore, mutants that are impaired in PIA synthesis by genetic manipulations also lose the ability to agglutinate red blood cells from various species.[108,275] The role of *S. epidermidis* PS/A, PIA, and other putative virulence factors in the initiation and synthesis of biofilms on biomaterials is supported by studies with animal models using mutant strains that lack the capability to synthesize these molecules and by inhibition of these interactions by specific antibodies.[275,379,506] Using a mouse foreign body model and a rat central venous catheter–associated infection model, Rupp and coworkers showed that a wild-type *S. epidermidis* strain was significantly more likely to cause abscess formation, less likely to be eradicated by host defenses, and more adherent to implanted plastic than an isogenic, PIA-negative mutant strain.[379,380] Genetic studies also support the suggestion that the *ica* locus of *S. epidermidis* encodes proteins that can synthesize PS/A, which is chemically related to PIA, but distinguished from PIA by molecular size, biophysical properties, and the presence of succinate groups on the majority of the amino groups of the glucosamine residues that constitute the polymer. It is unlikely, however, that PS/A and PIA are the only factors involved in colonization and biofilm formation on biomaterials like catheter plastic. In fact, a 140-kDa extracellular protein has also been identified to have a role in biofilm accumulation, although this role has not been defined.[184]

Another attachment mechanism used by *S. epidermidis* involves specific interactions with various serum, plasma, and tissue components of the host, including connective-tissue proteins like collagen and laminin and serum-derived proteins like fibronectin and vitronectin.[173,307,335,505] Such interactions may constitute the initial steps in tissue colonization and establishment of infections in the absence of foreign bodies such as catheters or shunts. A fibrinogen-binding protein, called fbe, has also been detected on the surface of *S. epidermidis* isolates.[320] The purified fibrinogen-binding protein was able to completely inhibit the adherence of *S. epidermidis* to immobilized fibrinogen, and antibodies against the protein were also found to efficiently block adherence as well.[338] The gene coding for this protein (the *fbe* gene) has been cloned and sequenced; interestingly, this protein showed partial homology with two of the three types of clumping factor protein produced by *S. aureus*.[43,100,338]

Additional putative virulence factors have also been identified for other pathogenic capabilities ascribed to *S. epidermidis*. Some strains of *S. epidermidis* produce a fatty acid–modifying enzyme that inactivates bactericidal fatty acids by esterifying them to cholesterol, thereby inactivating the fatty acids and allowing *S. epidermidis* to live on or in the skin for long periods.[72,73] Some *S. epidermidis* strains

Box 12-5 Infections Associated With *Staphylococcus epidermidis* and Other Coagulase-Negative Staphylococci

Infection	Comments
Urinary tract infections	Among the coagulase-negative staphylococci, *S. saprophyticus* is a true urinary tract pathogen, causing both upper and lower urinary tract infections, primarily in young women. Several studies have found this organism to be the second most common cause of urinary tract infections after *Escherichia coli*, representing 11–32% of urinary tract infections in female outpatients.[182,252,378] Other coagulase-negative staphylococci are rare causes of urinary tract infections, and about 80–90% of these infections are caused by *S. epidermidis*.[262] Urinary tract infections due to *S. epidermidis* and other coagulase-negative staphylococci are usually catheter-associated and occur in elderly patients with prior urinary tract instrumentation or surgery, renal transplantation, urolithiasis, or other urologic abnormalities.[262] Pyuria and significant upper tract disease are usually seen in only about 10% of the latter group of patients. Coagulase-negative isolates from these patients are often nosocomially acquired and are multiply resistant.
Osteomyelitis	Osteomyelitis due to coagulase-negative staphylococci may occur as a complication of both cardiothoracic surgery and implantation of prosthetic materials, such as knee and hip prostheses. Cardiothoracic surgery can lead to sternal wound and bone infections that may require surgical debridement.[148,208] Prosthesis-associated infections are diagnosed by direct examination and culture of needle aspirates from the affected site, by bone biopsy, or by removal and culture of the implanted material. Hematogenous osteomyelitis may result from bacteremia with coagulase-negative staphylococci arising from infections of shunts or other prosthetic devices.
Native-valve endocarditis	Coagulase-negative staphylococci are rare causes of native-valve and pacemaker-related endocarditis, accounting for about 5% of all cases.[58] Pathogenesis involves seeding of previously damaged heart valves or endocardium during transient bacteremia. More than half of the patients with this infection manifest complications such as congestive heart failure or embolic phenomena. About half of these infections involve coagulase-negative staphylococci other than *S. epidermidis*. Certain other species, such as *S. lugdunensis*, have been reported to cause unusually severe endocarditis, with massive valve destruction.[461]
Prosthetic-valve endocarditis	In contrast to native-valve endocarditis, coagulase-negative staphylococci are the most common etiologic agents of prosthetic-valve endocarditis, with *S. epidermidis* being the most frequently isolated species, almost to the exclusion of all others.[14,206] In this infection, organisms infect the ring of sutures holding the valve in place, causing the formation of microabscesses that are relatively protected from antibiotics.[55] The patient usually presents with fever and evidence of valve dysfunction. Complications include dehiscence of the valve, obstruction of the valve due to the formation of bulky vegetations, and occasionally cardiac dysrhythmia. Since most of these infections are probably due to inoculation of small numbers of organisms into the site at the time of valve placement, the symptoms of endocarditis appear slowly over a period of several months.[55,206] In addition to prosthetic valves, staphylococci may also infect pacemaker wires and vascular grafts.[17]
Intravenous catheter infections	*S. epidermidis* is the most common isolate infecting intravenous catheters.[362] Implicated catheter types have included central and peripheral intravenous lines, central hyperalimentation catheters, subclavian hemodialysis catheters, Hickman and Broviac central lines, and Swan-Ganz catheters.[266,355] Infected catheters may be the source of bacteremias, which may seed distant sites to create additional infectious complications.[77] Infected catheters and catheter insertion sites often do not appear infected (e.g., erythema or purulence may not be present) and catheter-related bacteremia may be minimally symptomatic. Although assiduous care of catheters may decrease the incidence of these bacteremic episodes, other innovations, such as antibiotic (rifampin or minocycline)-impregnated catheters appear to significantly decrease the incidence of catheter-related infections.[88] Therapy for these infections includes removal of the catheter, if possible, along with systemic antimicrobial therapy. Documentation of intravenous catheter–related infections and bacteremias involves culture of peripheral blood, blood drawn through the catheter, and, often, culture of the catheter tip itself.[81,266]

(Continued)

Box 12-5 *Continued*

Infection	Comments
CSF shunt infections	*S. epidermidis* is the most common cause of infection associated with CSF shunts, indwelling CSF catheters, intrathecal pumps, and ventriculostomy sites.[288,478] These infections usually occur within a few weeks of shunt placement, but may also occur during other shunt manipulations.[249] Patients with CSF shunt infections may be relatively asymptomatic, although some may present with symptoms of meningitis. Examination of CSF aspirated from the shunt may show a mild pleocytosis, and the glucose levels may be normal or slightly low. Shunt removal is often necessary to effect cure, although some staphylococcal shunt infections have been effectively treated with antimicrobial agents alone.[118,482] These agents usually include vancomycin, rifampin, and an aminoglycoside administered intraventricularly, since these nosocomially acquired infections are often due to staphylococci that are resistant to the semisynthetic penicillins (e.g., oxacillin, methicillin).[142]
Peritoneal dialysis catheter–associated infections	*S. epidermidis* is the organism most frequently isolated from patients with continuous ambulatory peritoneal dialysis (CAPD)–associated peritonitis.[18,409,493] Peritonitis is characterized clinically by abdominal pain, nausea, vomiting, fever, and a cloudy effluent after dialysis, although many patients may have only a few or very mild symptoms. Peritoneal fluid may appear cloudy and may contain >100 leukocytes per milliliter. Gram stains of unconcentrated fluid may be negative, necessitating centrifugation or filtration for recovery of small numbers of organisms.[92] Antimicrobial therapy of CAPD-associated staphylococcal peritonitis may be administered parenterally, orally, and/or intraperitoneally and usually includes oxacillin or methicillin, cephalosporins, aminoglycosides, vancomycin, or trimethoprim-sulfamethoxazole.[242]
Vascular graft infections	Vascular graft infections are most often caused by *S. epidermidis*. Many of these grafts become seeded with small numbers of microorganisms at the time of graft placement, and infections may not become clinically apparent until months or even years later.[321,499] Staphylococcal isolates recovered from these infections are often multiply-resistant, suggesting that the infections are due to the presence of contaminating organisms in the grafts themselves.
Bacteremia	In most medical centers at present, *S. epidermidis* is the most common agent of bacteremia in immunocompromised patients.[77,109,353] These organism usually reach the bloodstream via infected vascular access devices.[362] Patients in whom catheter-related staphylococcal bacteremia develops usually have multiple access devices in place for treatment of hematologic malignancies or administration of chemotherapeutic agents for bone marrow transplantation.[477] Other species of coagulase-negative staphylococci have also been associated with bacteremia in compromised hosts.
Pediatric infections	Most pediatric infections are nosocomial staphylococcal bacteremias occurring in neonatal intensive care units.[9] These infections are associated with prematurity, the presence of indwelling peripheral and/or central lines, ventilatory assistance, and administration of total parenteral nutrition.[120] Although most staphylococcal agents in such infections are *S. epidermidis*, other species (e.g., *S. haemolyticus*) have also been involved.[271]
Ocular infections	*S. epidermidis* is the most frequently implicated pathogen causing postsurgical endophthalmitis. Surgical procedures associated with these infections include lens implantation and cataract surgeries.[486] The diagnosis is made by aspiration and culture of vitreous fluid. Treatment of *S. epidermidis* endophthalmitis requires both parenteral and intraorbital administration of antimicrobial agents (i.e., penicillins, cephalosporins, aminoglycosides, rifampin, and/or vancomycin. Other clinically significant ocular infections, including blepharitis, purulent conjunctivitis, and suppurative keratitis involving *S. epidermidis* and other coagulase-negative species (i.e., *S. warneri*, *S. capitis*, *S. hominis*, *S. simulans*, *S. lugdunensis*, and *S. xylosus*) have also been reported.[348]
Cutaneous infections	Coagulase-negative staphylococci may be recovered from a variety of cutaneous lesions (cysts, carbuncles, furuncles), both alone and along with other pyogenic bacteria, including *S. aureus* and β-hemolytic streptococci. The most commonly implicated species have included *S. epidermidis*, *S. haemolyticus*, *S. lugdunensis*, and *S. hominis*.[4] Unusual cutaneous infections involving *S. epidermidis* include malignant external otitis.[418]

also produce lipases, which may have a role in skin colonization, biofilm formation, and initiation of cutaneous infections.[411]

Although not generally considered a factor contributing to virulence, the recognition of increasing antimicrobial resistance among *S. epidermidis* isolates constitutes a potentially worrisome emerging characteristic.[360,416] Over the past several years, resistance of the coagulase-negative staphylococci to many classes of antimicrobial agents has emerged, including resistance to the penicillinase-resistant penicillins (i.e., oxacillin, methicillin). Increasing use of vancomycin has led to the emergence of coagulase-negative staphylococci with decreased susceptibility to vancomycin.[410] This has been seen primarily in *S. haemolyticus*, but has also occurred to a lesser extent among *S. epidermidis* clinical isolates.[409] Although reports of vancomycin-resistant *S. epidermidis* strains appeared in the mid to late 1980s, clinical information on these isolates was not provided.[402] However, in 1991, a vancomycin-resistant *S. epidermidis* strain was isolated from a patient with peritonitis in England.[384] Five years later, vancomycin-resistant *S. epidermidis* was reported in several patients in the Soviet Republic.[239] In 1999, the first case of bacteremia due to *S. epidermidis* with decreased susceptibility to vancomycin was reported in the United States.[124] The patient was a 49-year-old woman with carcinoma of the gallbladder who had received vancomycin and several other antimicrobial agents over her complicated clinical course. Two slightly different looking *S. epidermidis* isolates were recovered from both peripheral blood and from blood drawn through the central venous catheter. One isolate was vancomycin-susceptible (MIC, 4 μg/mL), while the other was vancomycin-intermediate (MIC, 8 μg/mL). Although both isolates tested as susceptible on disk diffusion testing (zone sizes, 16–17 mm), MIC testing with the MicroScan Pos Combo panel, E test, and broth dilution confirmed the elevated vancomycin MIC for the second isolate. The poor performance of the disk diffusion method led these investigators to recommend that MIC methods be used when testing staphylococci for susceptibility to vancomycin, particularly for isolates from body sites like blood and other normally sterile body fluids.[124]

STAPHYLOCOCCUS SAPROPHYTICUS SUBSP. SAPROPHYTICUS

The coagulase-negative species *S. saprophyticus* deserves special mention, since this species is a well-documented pathogen causing primarily acute urinary tract infections in young healthy, sexually active women.[182,252,398] In 1996, a new subspecies of *S. saprophyticus* was characterized among coagulase-negative, novobiocin-resistant strains recovered from 7% of nostril cultures from healthy cows.[159] Phenotypic characteristics, cell-wall and fatty acid analysis, and genetic relatedness studies showed that these isolates were similar to but distinct from *S. saprophyticus* isolates recovered from humans. These bovine strains have since been named *S. saprophyticus* subsp. *bovis*, while human isolates are now called *S. saprophyticus* subsp. *saprophyticus* (hereafter referred to as *S. saprophyticus*).

Among young women of college and child-bearing age, *S. saprophyticus* is the second most common cause of un-

complicated cystitis, after *Escherichia coli*.[153,293,398] In urine specimens from these patients, the organism is frequently present in quantities of less than 100,000 colony-forming units (cfu)/mL, but will be detected in sequential specimens from infected patients. Patients with this infection usually present with dysuria, pyuria, and hematuria. Upper urinary tract infections (i.e., pyelonephritis) may be seen in 41–86% of patients and, occasionally, *S. saprophyticus* bacteremia may be seen as a complication of upper urinary tract infection.[137,258] This organism has also been implicated as a cause of urinary tract infections and urethritis in men and women (i.e., the acute urethral syndrome), catheter-associated urinary tract infections, prostatitis in elderly men, and rarely, bacteremia, sepsis, and endocarditis.[33,137,207,315,412] *S. saprophyticus* has been demonstrated as a cause of acute, symptomatic urinary tract infections in both male and female children and teenagers in the absence of urinary tract structural abnormalities.[2,451] In 1999, Hell and colleagues reported the isolation of *S. saprophyticus* as a cause of nosocomially acquired pneumonia.[170]

The source of *S. saprophyticus* in the pathogenesis of urinary tract infections has also been investigated. Rupp and colleagues studied the prevalence of urogenital colonization in 276 women and found that the rectum was the most frequent site of colonization by *S. saprophyticus* (40%), followed by the urethra (30%), the urine (20%), and the cervix (10%).[378] In this study, follow-up of the colonized women for almost 7 months did not reveal any women with progression to symptomatic urinary tract infection with *S. saprophyticus*. In another study of 14 women with *S. saprophyticus* urinary tract infection, the same isolate was found in the stool of 6 women, suggesting that the rectal canal may be a principal reservoir for this organism.[167] *S. saprophyticus* has also been isolated from other animals (e.g., pigs), pasture grass and fodder, and there is evidence to suggest that food may be the ultimate source for the organism.[165,166] Hedman and colleagues found *S. saprophyticus* in 16.4% of 1,331 food specimens, with a prevalence of 34% in raw beef and pork.[165] These workers concluded that the organism originates from slaughtered animals, contaminates resulting foodstuffs, and subsequently colonizes the human gastrointestinal tract.

Several potential virulence factors of *S. saprophyticus* have been examined in recent years. In vitro studies on the adherence of this species to various cell types have shown that *S. saprophyticus* adheres to uroepithelial, urethral, and periurethral cells in greater numbers than other staphylococci, and does not adhere to other cell types, including skin and buccal mucosal cells.[293] This uroepithelial tissue tropism may partially explain the high frequency of urinary tract infections caused by this organism. Urease, a recognized virulence factor for other urogenital pathogens (e.g., *Proteus* spp., *Corynebacterium ureolyticum*) is also produced by *S. saprophyticus* and contributes to bladder tissue invasion in animal models of urinary tract infection.[176] Slime production has not been a consistent attribute of *S. saprophyticus* strains.[369] Hjelm and Lundell-Etherden found that, although only 9 of 30 *S. saprophyticus* strains produced slime in trypticase-soy broth, all 30 produced slime in urine.[176] These workers proposed that both the presence of urine and urease production were essential for slime production by this organism. A 95-kDa fibrillar protein associated with the surface of *S. saprophyticus* strains has also been identified as a putative virulence factor.[126] This protein, designated **Ssp** (for *S. saprophyticus* surface-associated protein) may be involved in initial interactions with and adherence to uroepithelial cells. A 160-kDa hemagglutinin has also been demonstrated on the surface of *S. saprophyticus* cells.[128] This hemagglutinin binds to a membrane protein or proteins present on the surface of sheep erythrocytes and has been shown to be a major adhesin for binding of organisms to uroepithelial cells.[299,300] This hemagglutinin is also able to bind to fibronection.[127] In addition to Ssp and hemagglutinin, another cell-surface protein that is able to bind both fibronectin and erythrocytes has recently been identified on the surface of *S. saprophyticus* cells.[171] This protein has both adhesive and autolytic properties, and the gene for this protein (called the *aas* gene) has been cloned and sequenced. Amino acid sequences for the autolysin functional domains code for *N*-acetylmuramyl-L-alanine amidase and endo-β-*N*-acetyl-D-glucosaminidase enzymes and are similar to autolysins identified in both *S. aureus* and *S. epidermidis*. The remaining sequences function as the adhesin and represent an apparently new class of staphylococcal virulence factors.[171] Lastly, Schneider and Riley reported that 79% of 100 urinary isolates of *S. saprophyticus* displayed strong cell-surface hydrophobicity in a two-phase aqueous:hydrocarbon partition assay.[397] Hydrophobicity was subsequently demonstrated to be independent of both Ssp and the hemagglutinin.[298] Because cell-surface hydrophobic interactions between bacteria and mammalian cells promote adherence, hydrophobic surface structures of *S. saprophyticus* may function in the initial interaction of these organisms with uroepithelial cells.

OTHER COAGULASE-NEGATIVE STAPHYLOCOCCI

Other staphylococcal species are found in both humans and animals as part of the normal flora and as causes of several types of infections (see Box 12-1). Some species are found in the environment and are used in various industries, including food processing. Although coagulase-negative species other than *S. epidermidis* and *S. saprophyticus* are frequently found as contaminants in clinical specimens, medical progress has created an important role for many of the other coagulase-negative staphylococci in human infections and disease. Several other species have now been reported as causes of human infections, principally in wounds, urinary tract infections, bacteremia, osteomyelitis, catheter-related sepsis, ventriculoperitoneal shunt infections, and both native-valve and prosthetic-valve endocarditis (Box 12-1 and Box 12-5). These agents are increasingly being recognized as important opportunistic pathogens in immunocompromised patients, including premature neonates, neutropenic cancer patients, elderly persons with serious underlying diseases, and hospitalized patients following invasive procedures and with indwelling plastic devices. Infections with many of these other species are acquired in the hospital setting. The more commonly implicated species include *S. haemolyticus*, *S. lugdunensis*, *S. schleiferi*, *S. warneri*, *S. hominis*, *S. simulans*, and *S. saccharolyticus*. Some of these agents, such as *S. schleiferi* and *S. warneri*, produce a variety of extracellular products (i.e., glycocalyx, DNase, lipase, es-

terase, protease, and α- and β-hemolysins) that contribute to virulence.[162] *S. haemolyticus* has demanded increased interest recently because of the emergence of glycopeptide resistance in this species.[271,401–403,470] The ecologic niches and clinical significance of staphylococci other than *S. aureus*, *S. epidermidis*, and *S. saprophyticus* are described in Box 12-1, while infectious processes associated with *S. epidermidis* and other coagulase-negative staphylococci are described in Box 12-5.

Micrococcus Species and Related Genera

Members of the former genus *Micrococcus* are more closely related to the gram-positive coryneform genus *Arthrobacter* than to the staphylococci. These organisms are found in the environment and as transient flora on the skin of humans and other mammals. Some species produce carotenoid pigments, resulting in growth of yellow or pink colonies on agar media. Micrococcal species have industrial uses as bioassay organisms for detection of antimicrobial agents in animal feeds, cosmetics, and body fluids. They are occasionally isolated from human clinical specimens, where they usually represent contaminants from the skin or mucous membrane surfaces or from the environment. These organisms may behave as opportunistic agents in immunocompromised patients, and they have been reported as causes of pneumonia, meningitis, septic arthritis, bacteremia, catheter-related sepsis, and peritonitis related to continuous ambulatory peritoneal dialysis.[61,276,337,381,474,495] *Kytococcus sedentarius* (formerly *Micrococcus sedentarius*) produces two enzyme capable of hydrolyzing keratin and is responsible for pitting of the human epidermis in the dermatologic condition called pitted keratolysis.[270]

Rothia mucilaginosa

The first human infection with *R. mucilaginosa* was reported in 1978 in a patient in whom endocarditis developed following cardiac catheterization.[377] Since then, several cases of native-valve and prosthetic-valve endocarditis caused by *R. mucilaginosa* have appeared in the literature. In some of these cases, cardiac infection was associated with the use of intravenous drugs.[82,349,365] *R. mucilaginosa* sepsis has been reported in association with head-and-neck trauma, central and peripheral access devices, cancer chemotherapy, cardiac catheterization following myocardial infarction, continuous ambulatory peritoneal dialysis, and extreme prematurity.[303,352,377] *R. mucilaginosa* also has emerged as a significant pathogen in both adults and children with underlying malignancies (e.g., leukemia, lymphoma, breast cancer, Hodgkin's disease, squamous-cell carcinoma, osteosarcoma, rhabdomyosarcoma, and AIDS) and in recipients of bone marrow transplants.[1,12,86,140,149,334,453,488] Infections have included transient and sustained bacteremias, peripheral and central line–associated sepsis, pneumonia, meningitis, vertebral osteomyelitis, and cholangitis.[1,12,86,140,161,318] Recovery of *R. mucilaginosa* from these patients was associated with severe neutropenia as a result of underlying disease, immunosuppression, or cytotoxic chemotherapy. Colonized indwelling access devices (e.g., intravenous or intraarterial lines, Brouviac and Hickman catheters) were the source of the organism in some patients, while mucosal or esophageal ulcerations secondary to cytotoxic chemotherapy, periodontal disease, or dental infections or procedures were believed to be possible sources in others. Severe *R. mucilaginosa* endophthalmitis following intraocular lens implantation that required evisceration of the eye has also been reported.[439]

Isolation and Preliminary Differentiation of Staphylococci and Related Gram-Positive Cocci
Direct Gram-Stained Smears

On direct Gram-stained smears from clinical specimens, staphylococci appear as gram-positive or gram-variable cocci ranging in diameter from 0.5 to about 1.5 μm. Larger cells are seen among members of the genus *Macrococcus*, but these species are not causes of human infections.[217] The organisms may appear singly, in pairs, in short chains, or in clusters, both within and outside of polymorphonuclear cells (PMNs) (Color Plates 12-1*D* and 12-1*F*). Variations in cell size and Gram reaction are probably due to the action of the inflammatory cells and their hydrolytic enzymes on the bacterial cells. On direct smears, pairs and short chains of organisms cannot be differentiated from streptococci, micrococci, or peptostreptococci, although streptococci frequently appear as chains of diplococci rather than as chains of discrete, individual cells. Reports of direct smears should include quantitation of cell types and microorganisms (e.g., "many PMNs, moderate gram-positive cocci"). If the Gram stain appearance is more typical, a report of "gram-positive cocci resembling staphylococci" can be issued, with culture confirmation to follow. Gram stain morphology cannot be used to differentiate staphylococci from micrococci and related genera or from planococci.

Isolation From Clinical Specimens

For recovery of staphylococci and related organisms, clinical specimens should be inoculated onto sheep blood agar (SBA) and other bacteriologic media. For isolation of organisms from heavily contaminated specimens, specimens can also be inoculated onto Columbia colistin-nalidixic acid (CNA) media or phenylethyl alcohol (PEA) agar, which inhibit the growth of gram-negative bacteria and allow the growth of gram-positive organisms. Mannitol-salts agar is a good selective medium for assessing the presence of *S. aureus* in specimens such as nasal cultures. On SBA, most staphylococci produce good growth within 24 hours, although micrococci may require 48 hours for the growth of sizable colonies. Some species of staphylococci may also require more than 24 to 48 hours of incubation in order to discern whether a specimen contains a pure or a mixed culture. Longer incubation—up to 72 hours—may be necessary to ensure that identification and susceptibility tests are being performed on a pure culture, especially if multiple colonies are being sampled to obtain a representative inoculum.

Colony Morphology

Micrococcus and *Staphylococcus* species form distinctive colonies on SBA. Colonies of most staphylococcal species grow more rapidly than micrococci, and are 1 to 3 mm in diameter after 24 hours of incubation, although some (e.g., *S. warneri*, *S. simulans*, *S. auricularis*, *S. vitulinus*, *S. lentus*) may form smaller colonies during this time. Strains of some staphylococcal species will show considerable variation in the size of colonies on the same culture plate, giving the appearance of a mixed culture. Staphylococcal colonies are usually smooth, butyrous, and have a low convex profile with an entire edge. Colonies of some *S. aureus* strains are usually large (4–6 mm in diameter) smooth, entire, and butyrous in consistency, although some strains may be wet-looking or "sticky." Some strains may be pigmented yellow or yellow-orange (hence the name "aureus," meaning "golden"), while other strains may produce off-white or gray colonies. The latter strains may resemble group D streptococci and enterococci (catalase-negative). Pigment production in both *S. aureus* and among the coagulase-negative staphylococci usually becomes more pronounced after incubation at room temperature for 2 to 3 days. Some *S. aureus* and some coagulase-negative species may have a distinct or hazy zone of β-hemolysis around the colonies; this hemolytic property may become apparent only after prolonged incubation (Color Plate 12-1*E*).

Isolates of *S. aureus* from patients who have been treated with antimicrobials for long periods or who have certain persistent underlying conditions such as cystic fibrosis may grow as small, atypical colonies that are known as **small colony variants**. These colonies are usually very small, nonpigmented, and grow better in the presence of CO_2. These isolates may also be difficult to test for antimicrobial susceptibility because of their poor growth. Broth used in microdilution susceptibility testing of these isolates may require supplementation, and agar dilution, disk diffusion, and Etest susceptibility methods should be performed on Mueller-Hinton agar containing 5% sheep blood.

Micrococci and related species generally grow more slowly, often requiring 48 hours of incubation before typical colony morphology can be discerned. After this time, micrococcal colonies are 1 to 2 mm in diameter, are dull or matte in textural appearance, and have a high convex profile with entire edges. The newly described species *M. antarctica* produces yellow-pigmented, mucoid colonies on agar.[269] Colonies of *Micrococcus*, *Nesterenkonia*, *Dermacoccus*, and *Kocuria* species, and *A. agilis* may be smooth or matte in appearance. Some species are nonpigmented (*M. lylae*, *N. halobia*), or may produce yellow (*M. luteus*, *K. sedentarius*, *K. varians*, *K. palustris*, *K. rhizophila*), orange (*D. nishinomiyaensis*, *K. kristinae*), or pink-to-red (*K. rosea*, *A. agilis*) colonies on agar media (Color Plate 12-1*H*). Pigmentation usually becomes more obvious or intense if plates are incubated at room temperature for several days. Colonies of *R. mucilaginosa* are grey to white and may be mucoid in appearance. They tend to adhere to the agar and, when removed from the media, are difficult to emulsify.

Recently, media containing chromogenic substrates have become available for the isolation and presumptive identification of *S. aureus*. Available formulations are CHROMagar Staph aureus (CHROMagar Microbiology, Paris, France) and S. aureus ID agar (bioMerieux, La Balme Les Grottes, France).[123,343] On CHROMagar Staph aureus, colonies of *S. aureus* are mauve in color, while *S. aureus* colonies on S.

aureus ID agar are green. Colored colonies develop on these media because of the production of α-glucosidase by the organisms during growth. Coagulase-negative staphylococci produce colonies on these media that are blue, white, or beige. In a comparative evaluation of CHROMagar Staph aureus and S. aureus ID agar, 96.8% of *S. aureus* strains produced green colonies on S. aureus ID agar after 18–20 hours of incubation, while 91.1% of strains formed mauve colonies on CHROMagar Staph aureus within the same period.[343] A total of 94.3% of the strains were recovered within 18–20 hours on conventional blood agar. The yields of growth on all media increased after an additional 20–24 hours of incubation. When the identities of the colored colonies were confirmed, 97.4% of the green colonies on S. aureus ID agar and 94.4% of mauve colonies on CHROMagar Staph. aureus agar were *S. aureus*. CHROMagar Staph aureus was shown to be more sensitive than routine blood agar media in detecting *S. aureus* when it was used as part of the primary specimen plating protocol.[123] Chromogenic agar media have also been exploited as a rapid method for simultaneously identifying *S. aureus* and determining methicillin-resistance by incorporating oxacillin or methicillin into the media.[230,296]

The Catalase Test

Staphylococci and micrococci are differentiated from the streptococci, enterococci, and "streptococcus-like" bacteria by the catalase test. This test detects the presence of cytochrome oxidase enzymes (Chart 12-1). The catalase test is performed with 3% hydrogen peroxide (H_2O_2) on a glass slide. Immediate and vigorous bubbling indicates conversion of the H_2O_2 to water and oxygen gas (Color Plate 12-1*G*).

Ideally, the catalase test should be performed from a medium that does not contain blood, since red blood cells themselves may produce a weakly positive catalase reaction. However, since most clinical laboratories recover staphylococci on either nonselective or selective blood-containing media (e.g., SBA and CNA agar, respectively), care should be taken to sample only the tops of colonies for the catalase test to avoid carryover of blood and possible false-positive reactions. This can be done most expeditiously with a wooden applicator stick. Rare strains of staphylococci may be catalase-negative, and some enterococci produce a "pseudocatalase" and are weakly reactive with H_2O_2.[455] *R. mucilaginosa* is usually catalase-negative or weakly positive.

Methods for Differentiating Micrococci and Staphylococci

Several methods are available for differentiating *Micrococcus* and *Staphylococcus* species, the two catalase-positive genera most frequently seen in the clinical laboratory, from other catalase-positive, gram-positive cocci. Some require special media and prolonged incubation, while others are commercially available and provide results within 18 to 24 hours or less. Table 12-1 lists the test methods and results for *Micrococcus*, *Macrococcus*, and *Staphylococcus* species. Although *Macrococcus* species are primarily equine isolates, reactions for these species are included for primary recognition of macrococcal isolates recovered in laboratories that provide services to veterinary practices.

FERMENTATION OF GLUCOSE

This test is performed in a manner similar to the oxidation-fermentation (OF) tests for nonfermentative gram-

Table 12-1 Phenotypic Characteristics for Differentiation of *Micrococcus*, *Macrococcus*, and *Staphylococcus*

CHARACTERISTIC	DESCRIPTION/REACTION FOR:		
	Micrococcus and Related Species[a]	*Macrococcus*	*Staphylococcus*
Colony size	1–1.8 μm	1.3–2.5 μm	0.6–1.5 μm
Colony orofile	Convex	Low convex, domed	Raised, low convex
Growth rate	Very slow	Slow	Slow to rapid
Acid production from glucose under anaerobic conditions	−	−	+
Lysostaphin	R	S	S
Production of acid from glycerol aerobically in the presence of 0.4 μg/mL erythromycin	−	NA	+
Furazolidone susceptibility (100 μg of furazolidone disk)	R	S	S
Bacitracin susceptibility (0.04 unit Taxo A disk)	S	R	R
Modified oxidase test	+	+	−[b]

[a] *Includes the genera Micrococcus, Kytococcus, Dermacoccus, Nesterenkonia, and Kocuria.*
[b] *All Staphylococcus species are modified oxidase-negative except for strains of S. sciuri, S. lentus, and S. vitulinus.*
+, positive reaction; −, negative reaction; S, susceptible; R, resistant; NA, data not available.

negative bacilli. The OF medium for staphylococci contains additional nutrients such as yeast extract to fulfill the more exacting growth requirements of staphylococci. This method, regarded as the reference procedure for differentiation of the *Micrococcaceae*, requires prolonged incubation and is not readily adaptable or amenable to routine laboratory use.[223]

SUSCEPTIBILITY TO LYSOSTAPHIN

Lysostaphin is an endopeptidase that cleaves the glycine-rich pentapeptide cross-bridges in the staphylococcal cell-wall peptidoglycan.[129] This activity renders the cells susceptible to osmotic lysis. Certain staphylococcal species (i.e., *S. aureus*, *S. simulans*, *S. cohnii*, and *S. xylosus*) are more susceptible to lysostaphin than others (e.g., *S. hominis*, *S. saprophyticus*, and *S. haemolyticus*), hence standardization and interpretation of this test are sometimes difficult. A tube test for lysostaphin susceptibility is commercially available from Remel (Lenexa, KA). A heavy suspension of the organism is prepared in 0.2 ml of sterile saline, after which 0.2 ml of the Remel lysostaphin solution is added. The suspension is incubated at 35°C for 2 hours. Clearing of the suspension indicates susceptibility to lysostaphin. Lysostaphin susceptibility can also be determined using a filter paper-disk diffusion method.[354] A plate of Mueller-Hinton agar is inoculated with the organism to be tested (0.5 McFarland turbidity standard) and a disk impregnated with 10 μg of lysostaphin filter-sterilized solution, 287 units/mL) is placed on the plate. The plate is incubated for 24 hours at 35°C. *Staphylococcus* species will generally show zones of inhibition of 10–16 mm in diameter. *Micrococcus* and related species will show no zones.

In order to obtain optimal results with the lysostaphin susceptibility test, the organism should be grown on a beef peptone–based medium rather than on a casein peptone–based medium. The crucial factor is the glycine content of the medium, since glycine is an important part of the staphylococcal cell wall and is essential for the action of lysostaphin.

PRODUCTION OF ACID FROM GLYCEROL IN THE PRESENCE OF ERYTHROMYCIN

In this test, medium containing glycerol (1%) and erythromycin (0.4 μg/mL) is prepared with an enriched agar base containing bromcresol purple indicator and poured into Petri plates.[392] Several colonies of the isolate are streaked as a single line on the medium and the plate is incubated for up to 3 days at 35°C. Staphylococci will produce acid on this medium, while micrococci will not.

SUSCEPTIBILITY TO FURAZOLIDONE[19,306,476]

This test is performed as a disk susceptibility procedure using commercially available disks (FX disks, 100 μg; BD Biosciences, Sparks, MD). The procedure for this test is described in detail in Chart 12-1 and in Color Plates 12-1*A* and 12-1*B*. Staphylococci are inhibited by furazolidone and show zones of 15 mm or more, while micrococci and related species are resistant and show zones of 6 mm (no zone) to

9 mm.[19] However, coagulase-negative staphylococci that are resistant to furazolidone may be seen occasionally.

MODIFIED OXIDASE TEST[19,105]

This test is also commercially available from Remel (Microdase Test Disks). Filter paper disks impregnated with tetramethyl-*p*-phenylenediamine dihydrochloride (oxidase reagent) in dimethyl sulfoxide (DMSO) are used. The DMSO renders the cells permeable to the reagent. A colony from the growth medium is removed with an applicator stick and rubbed onto the disk. The development of a blue-purple color within 30 seconds is a positive test (Color Plate 12-2*C*). No color development within this time is a negative test. *Micrococcus* species, *N. halobia*, *D. nishinomiyaensis*, *A. agilis*, *K. kristinae*, and *Macrococcus* species are modified oxidase-positive, while strains of *K. sedentarius*, *K. rosea*, *K. varians*. *K. palustris*, and *K. rhizophila* are modified oxidase-negative.[217,231,423] All *Staphylococcus* species are modified oxidase-negative except for strains of *S. sciuri*, *S. lentus*, and *S. vitulinus*.[218]

SUSCEPTIBILITY TO BACITRACIN[19,104]

This procedure uses the same bacitracin disk used for the presumptive identification of group A β-hemolytic streptococci. A lawn of growth is prepared on a Mueller-Hinton agar or a blood agar plate as described above for the FX disk test, and a bacitracin differential disk (Taxo A, 0.04 unit of bacitracin; BD Biosciences) is placed on the inoculum. After overnight incubation, zone sizes are measured. Staphylococci are resistant and grow to the edge of the disk, while micrococci and related species are susceptible, producing zones of 10 mm or greater.[19]

The choice of the method used in a given laboratory depends on the type of work performed (e.g., reference laboratory, environmental microbiology, clinical laboratory). In most clinical microbiology laboratories, the modified oxidase test, the furazolidone disk test, and the Taxo A bacitracin disk test are probably the most logical choices, since they are rapid, reliable, inexpensive, and commercially available.

Identification of *Staphylococcus aureus*

The single most reliable characteristic for identifying *S. aureus* is the coagulase test. The conventional coagulase test may be performed by the following slide or tube procedures.

Slide Coagulase Test

Most strains of *S. aureus* have a bound coagulase or "clumping factor" on the surface of the cell wall. This factor reacts directly with fibrinogen in plasma, causing rapid cell agglutination (Color Plate 12-2*D*). Performance of this test is described in detail in Chart 1-3. The test can be performed with growth from blood agar, CNA agar, or other nonselective nutrient medium, but should not be performed from media with a high salt content (e.g., mannitol salts agar) since the high salt content causes some strains of *S. aureus* to autoagglutinate. Any strain that is negative on the slide coagulase test must be confirmed with a tube coagulase test, because strains deficient in clumping factor will usually produce free coagulase. Some strains of the human coagulase–negative species *S. lugdunensis* and *S. schleiferi* subsp *schleiferi* also produce clumping factor and may be positive with the slide test.[121,162,463]

Tube Coagulase Test

The coagulase detected by this method is secreted extracellularly and reacts with a substance in the plasma called coagulase-reacting factor (CRF) to form a complex, which, in turn, reacts with fibrinogen to form fibrin (clot formation) (see Chart 1-3 and Color Plate 12-2*E*). Tests that are negative after 4 hours of incubation at 35°C should be held at room temperature and read again after 18 to 24 hours, because some strains will produce fibrinolysin on prolonged incubation at 35°C, causing dissolution of the clot during the incubation period.[248] Rare *S. aureus* strains may be coagulase-negative, and some animal isolates (*S. intermedius*, *S. hyicus*, *S. delphini*, and *S. schleiferi* subsp. *coagulans*) may be tube coagulase–positive.[96,156,157,463,469]

Recently, *S. schleiferi* subsp. *schleiferi* strains that were both clumping factor–and tube coagulase–positive have been recovered from human infections.[463] These isolates also produced a heat-stable DNase (see below) and, therefore could be misidentified as *S. aureus*. These strains can be differentiated from *S. aureus* by failure to produce acid from maltose, lactose, mannitol, sucrose and turanose. In addition, *S. schleiferi* subsp. *coagulans*, an organism that causes canine external otitis, has also been found in human infections and may also be misidentified as clumping factor–negative strains of *S. aureus*. This subspecies can also be differentiated from *S. aureus* by carbohydrate utilization tests.[463]

As mentioned above, the recommended medium for both the slide and the tube coagulase procedures is rabbit plasma with EDTA. Citrated plasma should not be used, because organisms that are able to use citrate (e.g., *Enterococcus* species) will yield positive results if they are inadvertently mistaken for staphylococci. This error can be avoided by always performing a catalase test first. Human plasma (e.g., outdated material from blood banks) contains variable amounts of CRF and antistaphylococcal antibodies and should not be used to perform coagulase tests.

The tube coagulase test is still the reference procedure for identification of *S. aureus*. Although it is generally performed with isolates taken from agar media, it may also be inoculated with positive blood culture broths or pelleted organisms centrifuged from positive blood culture broths. McDonald and Chapin reevaluated a 2-hour tube coagulase procedure for identification of *S. aureus* in positive blood cultures.[290] Inoculation of the coagulase test directly with positive culture media was compared with an inoculum obtained by centrifugation and resuspension of the organisms from the blood culture media. In addition, both the culture broth and the bacterial pellet were also tested with two commercial latex agglutination tests (see below). Using 180 clinical and seeded blood cultures, the 2-hour tube coagulase test showed sensitivities of 86.2% and 84.4% and 100% specificity when inoculated directly with positive blood culture broth and with a bacterial pellet, respectively. The latex

agglutination tests were 6.8–8.6% sensitive and only 95.9% specific when inoculated with positive blood culture broth or bacterial pellets, respectively.[290]

Alternative Coagulase Test Procedures
LATEX AGGLUTINATION

These procedures use latex beads coated with plasma. Fibrinogen bound to the latex detects clumping factor. In addition, immunoglobulin molecules also present on the beads detect protein A, the staphylococcal cell-wall protein that is able to bind immunoglobulin G molecules by the Fc region. Mixing of the test reagent with colony material from an agar plate results in rapid clumping of the latex-organism suspension (Color Plate 12-2*F*). Several products that use this approach are commercially available and include StaphAurex (Murex, Norcross, GA), Slidex Staph (bioMerieux, Hazelwood, MO), Staphylatex (Dade/MicroScan, West Sacramento, CA), Fastaph (Carr-Scarborough, Stone Mountain GA), Staph Rapid (Roche, Nutley, NJ), Staphylase (Oxoid Ltd., Basingstoke, England), Staphytect (Oxoid Unipath, Dardilly, France), and Veri-Staph (Zeus Technologies, Raritan, NJ). In addition, some strains of *S. lugdunensis* and *S. schleiferi* subsp. *schleiferi* produce clumping factor and may be positive with these rapid procedures.

PASSIVE HEMAGGLUTINATION

These test procedures use sheep red blood cells that are sensitized with fibrinogen to detect clumping factor on the surface of *S. aureus* cells (Color Plate 12-2*E*). Three commercial kits—Staphyloslide (BD Biosciences), Hemastaph (Remel Laboratories), and Staphyslide (bioMerieux, Marcy l'Etoile, France)—are available. Some workers prefer these tests to the latex agglutination tests because a nonsensitized red blood cell suspension is included as a negative control for each test. Some *S. saprophyticus* strains may also produce false-positive results with rapid latex or hemagglutination coagulase tests.[147] This can be explained by the presence of a hemagglutinin that is found on the surface of *S. saprophyticus* strains.[128]

Several evaluations have been published comparing latex and passive hemagglutination kits with the 4-hour and 24-hour tube coagulase tests. These kits have sensitivities and specificities of 94–100% and 93–100%, respectively.[20,199,339,373] Sensitivities ranging from as low as 6% to 62% have been observed when these tests have been used directly on blood cultures showing gram-positive cocci in clusters on Gram-stained smear.[290,414] Several investigators have reported that false-negative latex agglutination and passive hemagglutination results may be encountered when methicillin/oxacillin-resistant *S. aureus* are tested.[112,183,350,375,484] For example, Piper and coworkers found that only 82–86% of these strains were identified when tested with three of the latex agglutination and one of the hemagglutination procedures.[350] In another study that compared reactivity with the rapid coagulase tests to capsular serotype and oxacillin susceptibility, all isolates that were negative with the agglutination tests were capsular serotype 5, and all of these except one strain were oxacillin-resistant.[113] Failure of *S. aureus* strains to react with the rapid coagulase procedures was postulated to be related to the presence of the serotype

5 capsule on the cell surface. Interestingly, capsular serotype 5 strains are the predominant capsular serotype found among methicillin-resistant isolates.[113] The presence of this capsule may interfere with accessibility of the test reagents to the clumping factor and protein A present on the bacterial cell wall.

In 1993, Fournier and coworkers reported on a new latex agglutination test called "Pastorex Staph-Plus" (Sanofi-Diagnostics Pasteur, Marnes la Coquette, France).[114] This reagent consists of a 2:1 mixture of latex beads coated with fibrinogen for the detection of clumping factor and with IgG for the detection protein A, and latex beads coated with monoclonal antibodies directed against serotypes 5 and 8 capsular polysaccharides. The latter components of this reagent would presumably identify those strains not reliably identified by the regular latex agglutination reagents. In the study by Fournier and colleagues, this new reagent was compared with Staphyslide (a French hemagglutination reagent), StaphAurex (Murex), and Pastorex-Staph (a French equivalent of the StaphAurex).[114] Of 220 *S. aureus* strains (61 of which were oxacillin-resistant) and 128 coagulase-negative staphylococci tested, the Pastorex Staph-Plus identified 98.6% of the *S. aureus* strains, compared with 91.8%, 91.4%, and 84.5% for the Pastorex-Staph, the Staphyslide, and the StaphAurex tests, respectively. None of the coagulase-negative staphylococci reacted with the new reagents. When the 61 oxacillin-resistant strains were examined separately, the Pastorex Staph-Plus identified 95.1%, compared with 73.8%, 72.1%, and 49.2% obtained with the Pastorex Staph, the Staphyslide, and the StaphAurex tests, respectively. Because it is known that capsular types 5 and 8 predominate among clinical isolates, that capsular type 5 strains predominate among oxacillin-resistant strains, and that these latter strains may not be reliably identified by existing latex or passive hemagglutination tests, the incorporation of monoclonal antibodies against these capsular types in a latex preparation offers a theoretical and a real advantage in identifying methicillin-resistant *S. aureus*. In addition to Pastorex-Staph-Plus, the Slidex Staph-Kit (bioMerieux), and the Staphaurex-Plus (Murex Biotech, Chatillon, France) also are manufactured to include antibodies specific to type 5 and type 8 capsular polysaccharides. The Slidex Staph-Kit is a combined latex/hemagglutination product, while the StaphAurex-Plus is a latex agglutination test.[272,497] The Dryspot Staphylotec Plus (Oxoid, Hampshire, England) uses blue latex that is sensitized with porcine fibrinogen, rabbit IgG, and polyclonal anticapsular antibodies. The dried reagent is rehydrated with saline, mixed with colony material, and read within 20 seconds for agglutination. In a study of 202 isolates, Sariya and colleagues found the Dryspot test 99.1% sensitive and 93.1% specific for identification of *S. aureus*.[386] Another latex test, the Monostaph-Plus (Bionor, Skien, Norway) uses latex beads coated with fibrinogen, immunoglobulin G, and polyclonal antibodies against capsular polysaccharide type 5 only.[456] In a study comparing the Monostaph latex with the Monostaph-Plus latex reagent, Tveten found that the Monostaph identified only 79.5% of 78 oxacillin-resistant *S. aureus*, while the Monostaph-Plus identified 98.7%; both reagents correctly identified 50 isolates of oxacillin-susceptible *S. aureus*.[456]

Other studies have suggested that *S. aureus* strains that do not agglutinate with the latex reagents are genetically "deficient" with regard to both clumping factor and protein A. Schwarzkopf and coworkers examined 50 oxacillin-resistant, clumping factor–and protein A–negative strains in Germany, and found that all had similar antibiograms, were nontypeable with an international set of bacteriophages, and possessed a 30-kb plasmid that was similar for all strains on restriction enzyme analysis.[404] These data suggested that these deficient *S. aureus* strains belonged to a single clone. Amplification and restriction enzyme analysis of the coagulase genes of these strains revealed a single 650-bp product in the deficient strains, while similar analysis of coagulase-positive, oxacillin-resistant strains showed different restriction patterns, indicating substantial differences in coagulase gene loci.[404] PCR amplification of the protein A genes indicated that the protein A–negative strains possessed genes that coded for four IgG-binding domains, while wild-type strains possessed genes coding for five binding domains, suggesting that the missing protein A gene sequence is required for latex agglutination reactivity.[404]

A fluorogenic coagulase test is included as a test for *S. aureus* in the RapiDEC Staph (bioMerieux) identification system (see below). This test, which is performed by inoculating a small cupule containing the substrate, detects what the manufacturer calls "aurease" (coagulase). Aurease is a proteolytic enzyme of coagulation that reacts with prothrombin to form a complex called staphylothrombin. Staphylothrombin then enzymatically cleaves a fluorogenic peptide present in the test cupule, thereby releasing a peptide and a radical that fluoresces under ultraviolet light. Greater fluorescence in the test cupule relative to a control cupule lacking the substrate provides an identification of *S. aureus*. The "aurease" test on the RapiDEC Staph has been demonstrated to be highly sensitive and specific.[131,192,302] Mitchell et al. evaluated the RapIDEC aurease test for identifying *S. aureus* directly in blood cultures; 27 of 28 *S. aureus* were correctly identified within 2 hours using this test; none of the coagulase-negative staphylococci produced false-positive results when the aurease test was inoculated with bacterial suspensions from positive blood cultures.[302]

Additional Confirmatory Tests
DEOXYRIBONUCLEASE (DNASE) TEST

Some *S. aureus* strains may produce weak or equivocal tube coagulase reactions, and rare isolates may indeed be coagulase-negative. In these cases, it may be helpful to perform other tests that correlate highly with coagulase production. *S. aureus* produces both DNase and a thermostable nuclease having endonucleolytic and exonucleolytic activities.[151,250] Both of these enzymes hydrolyze nucleic acid (i.e., deoxyribonucleic acid, DNA). DNase can be detected by heavily spot-inoculating several colonies of the organism on DNase test medium containing the metachromatic dye toluidine blue O (commercially available from several vendors). After 24 hours of incubation at 35°C, the medium under and around the inoculum turns from azure blue to pink, indicating hydrolysis of the DNA (Color Plate 12-2*G*). The content of toluidine blue O in the medium should not exceed 0.005%, since the blue color imparted to the agar by higher concentrations may mask detection of DNase activity.[479] Spot inoculation is necessary because some *S. aureus* strains do not grow well on the media and growth is not required for detection of DNase activity. Although this test is helpful as an adjunctive test for identification of *S. aureus*, other staphylococci may also produce positive DNase reactions.

THERMOSTABLE ENDONUCLEASE TEST

For this test, the same DNase test medium is used, only 3 mm holes are cut into the agar with a sterile cork borer and the wells are filled with a 24-hour broth culture of the test organism that has been boiled in a water bath for 15 minutes. The plate is incubated overnight at 35°C. *S. aureus* strains will show a pink zone surrounding the well containing the boiled suspension. Certain animal isolates (e.g., *S. caprae*, *S. schleiferi*, *S. intermedius*, and *S. hyicus*) also produce a heat-stable thermonuclease, and some coagulase-negative staphylococci (i.e., *S. epidermidis*, *S. simulans*, *S. capitis*, and *S. carnosus*) may produce weakly positive reactions. Specificity of this assay for *S. aureus* thermostable endonuclease may be confirmed by seroinhibition of the reaction by polyclonal or monoclonal antibodies directed against the *S. aureus* enzyme, or by PCR amplification and sequencing of the *nuc* gene that encodes the *S. aureus* heat-stable endonuclease (see below).[48]

MANNITOL FERMENTATION

In addition to the above tests, *S. aureus*, unlike *S. epidermidis* and several other coagulase-negative species, is able to ferment mannitol. This property is exploited in epidemiologic studies to detect *S. aureus* in soil, feces, and in screening nasal carriers of *S. aureus*. The medium used is **mannitol salts agar**. This medium contains mannitol (1%), 7.5% NaCl, phenol red, and peptones. The high salt concentration discourages the growth of other organisms (except for enterococci) and selectively recovers staphylococci. *S. aureus* can be detected by the presence of a yellow zone around isolated colonies, indicating acid production from mannitol. However, other infrequently isolated staphylococcal species may also produce acid from mannitol, so mannitol-positive organisms recovered on this medium should be subcultured onto blood agar and checked for coagulase production.

Other Methods for Identification of *Staphylococcus aureus*

Detection of the presence of enzymes unique to *S. aureus* has also been exploited as a way to identify *S. aureus*. Guzman and colleagues developed an enzyme immunoassay for identifying *S. aureus* that uses simultaneous detection of protein A and *S. aureus* endo-β-*N*-acetylglucosaminidase (SaG), an enzyme produced by all isolates of this species.[154] By using a monoclonal capture antibody directed against SaG, this enzyme immunoassay could identify *S. aureus* strains by simultaneous detection of SaG (via binding of the bacterial enzyme to the Fab sites of the antibody) and protein A (via binding to the Fc region). This assay performed better than both latex agglutination and passive hemagglutination when compared with these commercially available products.[150] The test showed 100% sensitivity and specificity and was particularly helpful for identifying strains that lacked detectable clumping factor and/or protein A. Molecular biology techniques such as DNA probe methods and PCR have

also been used for identification of *S. aureus*. Davis and Fuller found that the AccuProbe for *S. aureus* culture confirmation (Gen-Probe, San Diego, CA) performed well for the direct identification of *S. aureus* in blood cultures that showed gram-positive cocci in clusters on Gram staining.[91] In a similar study, Skulnick reported a sensitivity of 95% and a specificity of 98.5% when the *S. aureus* AccuProbe test was performed directly on blood culture broths.[414] Primers and probes for amplification and detection of the *nuc* gene of *S. aureus* have also been synthesized and examined for their utility in culture confirmation and direct detection.[47] The *nuc* gene codes for the thermostable endonuclease of *S. aureus*. For identification, the lower limit of sensitivity of the PCR assay was 5–20 cfu of the organism. Using staphylococcus-free clinical specimens that were seeded with serial dilutions of *S. aureus*, the lower limit for direct detection of *S. aureus* by the PCR assay ranged from 10–20 cfu up to 1,000 cfu, depending on the type of clinical specimen. The PCR-based assay was 100% specific for *S. aureus*.[47]

Rapid Tests for Detection of Methicillin Resistance

Although not an identification method, the rapid detection of methicillin resistance in *S. aureus* is every bit as critical as the species identification. The *mecA* gene is the structural gene for a low-affinity penicillin-binding protein (PBP 2′ or PBP 2a) that is found in methicillin/oxacillin-resistant *S. aureus* (MRSA) strains.[405,457] Commercial detection methods using cycling probe amplification technology (Velogene Rapid MRSA identification assay, Alexon-Trend, Minneapolis), fluorescence technology (Crystal MRSA ID System, BD Biosciences), and latex agglutination (MRSA-Screen, Denka Seiken, Niigata, Japan; Oxoid Penicillin Binding Protein latex agglutination test, Oxoid) for detection of the PBP 2a (PBP 2′) of methicillin-resistant *S. aureus* strains are now available for use in clinical microbiology laboratories.[63,186, 314,359] These tests are accurate and results from them are available faster than conventional or automated antimicrobial susceptibility test results. Latex tests involve organism lysis/extraction, centrifugation to pellet cellular debris, and mixing of the supernatant with test and control latex reagents. In an evaluation of the MRSA-Screen, van Leeuwen and colleagues found that 97% of 90 methicillin-resistant *S. aureus* and none of 106 methicillin-susceptible *S. aureus* strains were detected by MRSA-Screen.[468] These tests are not substitutes for specific identification tests for *S. aureus*, since methicillin-susceptible *S. aureus* isolates will be MRSA-Screen test-negative, and methicillin-resistant coagulase-negative staphylococci that also carry the *mecA* gene will also be positive.[311,468] More information on methicillin resistance in staphylococci and the methods for its detection are available in Chapter 15.

Differentiation of Coagulase-Positive Staphylococci of Veterinary Origin

In veterinary medicine, three coagulase-positive cocci—*S. aureus* (both subsp. *aureus* and *anaerobius*), some *S. hyicus* strains, and *S. intermedius*—have been implicated as causes of bovine mastitis. These organisms produce free coagulase, as indicated by positive tube tests after 4 to 24 hours of incubation. Roberson et al. examined 80 strains of each of these species to investigate simple tests that could differentiate them.[370] *S. aureus* strains grew on P agar and on P agar with acriflavine (7 μg/mL), were VP-positive, and produced acid from mannitol under anaerobic conditions. *S. hyicus* and *S. intermedius* failed to grow on P agar or on P agar with acriflavine and did not produce acetoin or ferment mannitol. *S. intermedius* strains were β-galactosidase-positive, while *S. hyicus* strains were β-galactosidase-negative.

S. schleiferi subsp. *coagulans* causes infections in both dogs and humans; these strains are usually clumping factor–negative and tube coagulase–positive (the opposite reactions for these two tests are seen in strains of subspecies *schleiferi*). Both *S. schleiferi* subsp. *schleiferi* and subsp. *coagulans* can be differentiated from *S. aureus* by the lack of acid production from maltose and trehalose (see Table 12-3). *S. delphini* and *S. lutrae* are also coagulase-positive, but these species are associated only with marine environments and cutaneous infections in dolphins and sea otters, respectively.[111,469] Other species that are recovered from animals are coagulase-negative.

Identification of Coagulase-Negative Staphylococci

As described earlier, *S. epidermidis* and *S. saprophyticus* are the most frequently isolated and clinically significant coagulase-negative staphylococci in clinical laboratories working with specimens of human origin. Because of the recognized clinical significance of *S. saprophyticus* in urinary tract infections and the importance of *S. epidermidis* as an agent causing significant infections, it is advantageous for laboratories to use methods for confirmatory identification of these two species. In addition, kit systems are available that enable the laboratory to identify not only *S. epidermidis* and *S. saprophyticus*, but also several of the other human, animal, and environmental staphylococci. Although several coagulase-negative staphylococcal species have been described and many of them have been recovered from human clinical specimens, relatively few species are seen with any regularity in actual practice. In 1993, Kleeman and associates published the results of species identification on 500 coagulase-negative isolates recovered from specimens submitted to the microbiology laboratory of a 400-bed community hospital in Raleigh, NC.[216] *S. epidermidis* accounted for 64.5% of the isolates, followed in decreasing frequency by *S. haemolyticus* (13.4%), *S. hominis* (7.4%), *S. warneri* (4.0%), *S. lugdunensis* (2.8%), *S. simulans* (2.4%), *S. capitis* subsp *capitis* (2.0%), and *S. capitis* subsp. *ureolyticus* (1.6%). *S. saprophyticus*, *S. cohnii* (subsp. *urealyticum* and subsp. *cohnii*), and *S. auricularis* each accounted for less than 1% of significant isolates recovered in the laboratory (Color Plate 12-3*A*). A 1996 examination of 415 significant coagulase-negative staphylococci recovered from blood cultures in Denmark found that 68.7% were *S. epidermidis*, followed in frequency by *S. hominis* (14.7%), *S. haemolyticus* (10.4%), *S. warneri* (2.9%), and *S. cohnii* (1.7%), with *S. saprophyticus*, *S. capitis* and *S. lugdunensis* each account-

ing for 1% or less of the total.[194] The distribution of clinically significant species reported in these studies generally reflects the literature that has accumulated regarding the clinical significance of the individual species.

Conventional Identification Methods

In 1975, Kloos and Schleifer published a scheme for the biochemical identification of coagulase-negative staphylococci.[223] This scheme used the coagulase test for identifying *S. aureus*, and used a battery of physiologic and biochemical tests for differentiating the coagulase-negative species. This scheme was updated and expanded by Kloos and Lambe in 1991, but several new species have been described since that time.[221] In 1999, Freney and the members of the Subcommittee on the Taxonomy of Staphylococci and Streptococci of the International Committee on Systematic Bacteriology published a document setting forth the minimum standards for the genus *Staphylococcus* and for the description of new *Staphylococcus* species.[122] In this document, recommended minimal standards for new species designations are based on the results of phenotypic and genomic studies on at least five independently isolated strains. The phenotypic and genotypic criteria for genus-level and species-level identification are listed in Box 12-6.[122] Conventional procedures for the identification of staphylococci require a large battery of biochemical tests, are time-consuming and labor-intensive, and are not amenable to implementation as a routine procedure in a clinical laboratory. Fortunately, only a small number of staphylococcal species are recovered from significant human infections, and most of the commercially available kit systems described below will serve this purpose for most laboratories.[194,216] Reference laboratories wishing to use these procedures should consult several of the references at the end of the chapter for media formulations and inoculation procedures. Table 12-2 presents the phenotypic characteristics for identification of those staphylococci that are most commonly isolated from human clinical specimens, and Fig. 12-1 is a dichotomous key that will facilitate the identification of a majority of clinical isolates by conventional methods, although additional tests may be necessary on occasion. Table 12-3 includes the phenotypic criteria for identification of human, animal, and environmental species in the genus *Staphylococcus*.

In the conventional identification method, certain biochemical tests are performed using enteric media, such as nitrate broth, urease slants, and Moeller's arginine dihydrolase and ornithine decarboxylase broth media. Carbohydrate utilization tests are performed in purple broth agar containing 1% sterile carbohydrates, with incubation in ambient air at 35–37°C. Supplementation with yeast extract (1–2%) may be necessary to encourage growth of more fastidious strains. In addition to biochemical tests and acid production from carbohydrates, Hebert and associates have shown that susceptibility to polymyxin B (300 unit disk) and the pyrrolidonyl arylamidase (PYR) test (for identification of enterococci, Chapter 13), are also helpful for identifying coagulase-negative staphylococci.[163]

Rhoden and associates at the CDC formulated a modified conventional approach to identification of the catalase-positive, gram-positive cocci using conventional carbohy-

Box 12-6 Recommended Phenotypic and Genotypic Tests for Identification of Staphylococci at the Genus and Species Levels

Genus Level	Species Level
Phenotypic criteria:	**Phenotypic criteria:**
Gram reaction and general morphology	Growth requirements and characteristics
Catalase	Colony morphology
Oxidase	Pigmentation
Motility	Novobiocin susceptibility
Aerobic/fermentative metabolism	Fermentative/oxidative activity on carbohydrates
Cell wall structure	Enzymatic activities (nitrate reductase, ADH, ODC, urease)
Peptidoglycan type	
Presence of teichoic acids	Clumping factor
	Coagulase
Additional tests:	
Glycerol acidification	**Additional tests:**
Lysostaphin susceptibility	Additional carbohydrates
Lysozyme susceptibility	Fermentation end-product profiles
Furazolidone and bacitracin susceptibility	Acetoin production
Menaquinone pattern	Fosfomycin susceptibility
Cellular fatty acids	Enzymatic activities (e.g., β-GAL, β-GUR, lecithinase, etc.)
Fructose-1,6-bisphosphate ldolase class	
	Susceptibility to other antibiotics, antiseptics, etc.
Genotypic criteria:	Hemolysins
G+C content	Staphylolytic activities
rRNA oligonucleotide sequencing	Membrane analysis (teichoic acids, fatty acids, cytochromes, etc.)
	Protein A analysis
	Genotypic criteria:
	DNA-DNA hybridization
	DNA melting/annealing temperatures

drate utilization and biochemical tests along with selected chromogenic enzyme substrate tests from the API Staph-Ident system (see below).[367] This approach differed from previous reference identification methods in that a numerical coding system was designed for the conventional test batteries to generate a database similar to those for commercial systems, rather than using a "best fit" analysis based on reactions included in identification tables. Screening tests were used to identify morphology (Gram stain), family designation (catalase test), genus grouping (glucose fermentation), and presence of bound and free coagulase (slide and tube coagulase, StaphAurex latex agglutination test). A battery of 18 conventional primary tests were then inoculated for identification. A confirmatory battery of 11 additional tests was used to resolve the identity of problem isolates and rare or unusual biotypes that were generated from the primary test battery. Using 147 reference strains, 388 well-characterized control strains, and 289 clinical isolates, this method identified more than 95% of the *Staphylococcus*, *Micrococcus*, and *Stomatococcus* species tested.[367] Other workers have reported modified conventional identification schemes for staphylococci that rely on combinations of limited numbers of discriminatory tests for species identification of the more commonly isolated staphylococcal species.[187,306]

PRODUCTION OF PHOSPHATASE FOR IDENTIFICATION OF *STAPHYLOCOCCUS EPIDERMIDIS*

In traditional schemes for identifying coagulase-negative staphylococci, phosphatase activity was reported to be positive for *S. epidermidis* and *S. xylosus* strains and negative for other coagulase-negative staphylococci.[250,420] Subsequent studies have shown, however, that other staphylococcal species may also produce phosphatase enzymes. Using four different methods, Langlois and coworkers found phosphatase activity in all *S. aureus*, coagulase-positive *S. hyicus* and *S. intermedius* strains, and in most strains of *S. epidermidis*, *S. chromogenes*, coagulase-negative *S. hyicus*, *S. sciuri*, *S. simulans*, *S. xylosus*, and *S. warneri/hominis* after 24 and 48 hours of incubation.[250] Production of phosphatase activity was affected by pH and by the presence of inorganic phosphate (Pi) in the growth medium. Soro and associates found that all strains of various staphylococcal species were phosphatase-positive when testing was done at pH 8.0 and when the organisms were grown in the absence of Pi.[420] When grown on media supplemented with 0.3% Pi, only *S. aureus*, *S. epidermidis*, and *S. xylosus* strains were phosphatase-positive. These workers concluded that phosphatase activity was a more common property among human staphylococcal isolates than was previously thought and that this activity may be constitutive in some species and repressed by phosphates in others.[420]

At present, there are no commercially available standalone tests for detection of phosphatase activity in staphylococci, although several commercial kit systems (e.g., API Staph-IDENT, API Staph, ID32 Staph, and RapiDEC Staph) include a phosphatase test in the biochemical test battery. In these test systems, *S. aureus*, *S. schleiferi*, *S. intermedius*, *S. hyicus*, and most strains of *S. epidermidis* are phosphatase-positive. Geary and Stevens reported a simple agar method (PNP agar) that used Mueller-Hinton agar buffered at pH 5.6–5.8 and containing *p*-nitrophenyl-phosphate (0.495 mg/mL).[130] The medium is spot inoculated with the organism and is read after 18–24 hours of incubation. The presence of a bright yellow color under and around the inoculum is a positive test result. Geary and Stevens identified 305 coagulase-negative isolates to species and tested them with PNP agar.[130] They found that 83% of 170 *S. epidermidis*, 17% of 7 *S. cohnii*, and 75% of 4 *S. xylosus* strains were PNP positive, while 124 isolates representing six other species (including 38 *S. saprophyticus* strains) were PNP-negative.

PYRROLIDONYL ARYLAMIDASE ACTIVITY

The PYR test is also useful as a phenotypic test for identifying coagulase-negative staphylococci. As with the enterococci, L-pyrrolidonyl-β-naphthylamide is cleaved by the ary-

Table 12-2 Phenotypic Characteristics for Identification of Commonly Isolated *Staphylococcus* Species

TEST	S. AUREUS	S. EPIDERMIDIS	S. HAEMOLYTICUS	S. HOMINIS SUBSP. HOMINIS	S. HOMINIS SUBSP. NOVOBIOSEPTICUS	S. WARNERI	S. LUGDUNENSIS	S. SCHLEIFERI SUBSP. SCHLEIFERI	S. SAPROPHYTICUS SUBSP. SAPROPHYTICUS
Coagulase	+	−	−	−	−	−	−	−	−
Clumping factor	+	−	−	−	−	−	+^{sl}	+	−
Heat-stable nuclease	+	−	−	−	−	−	−	+	−
ODC	−	V−	−	−	−	−	+	−	−
PYR	−	−	+	−	−	−	+	+	−
Urease	V	+	−	+	+	+	V	−	+
Acetoin	+	+	+	V	V	+	+	+	+
Beta-galactosidase	−	−	−	−	−	−	−	+^{sl}	+
Alkaline phosphatase	+	+	−	−	−	−	−	+	−
Polymyxin B	R	R	S	S	NA	S	S/R	S	S
Novobiocin	S	S	S	S	R	S	S	S	R
Acid produced aerobically from:									
Glucose	+	+	+	+	+	+	+	+	+
Maltose	+	+	+	+	+	+^{sl}	+	−	+
Sucrose	+	+	+	+^{sl}	+^{sl}	+	+	−	+
Mannitol	+	−	V	−	−	V	−	−	V
Mannose	+	+^{sl}	−	−	−	−	+	+	−
Trehalose	+	−	+	V	−	+	+	V	+

ODC, ornithine decarboxylase; PAL, alkaline phosphatase; +, positive reaction; −, negative reaction; +^{sl}, slow positive reaction; V−, variable reaction, most strains negative; V, variable reaction; S, susceptible; R, resistant; NA, data not available.

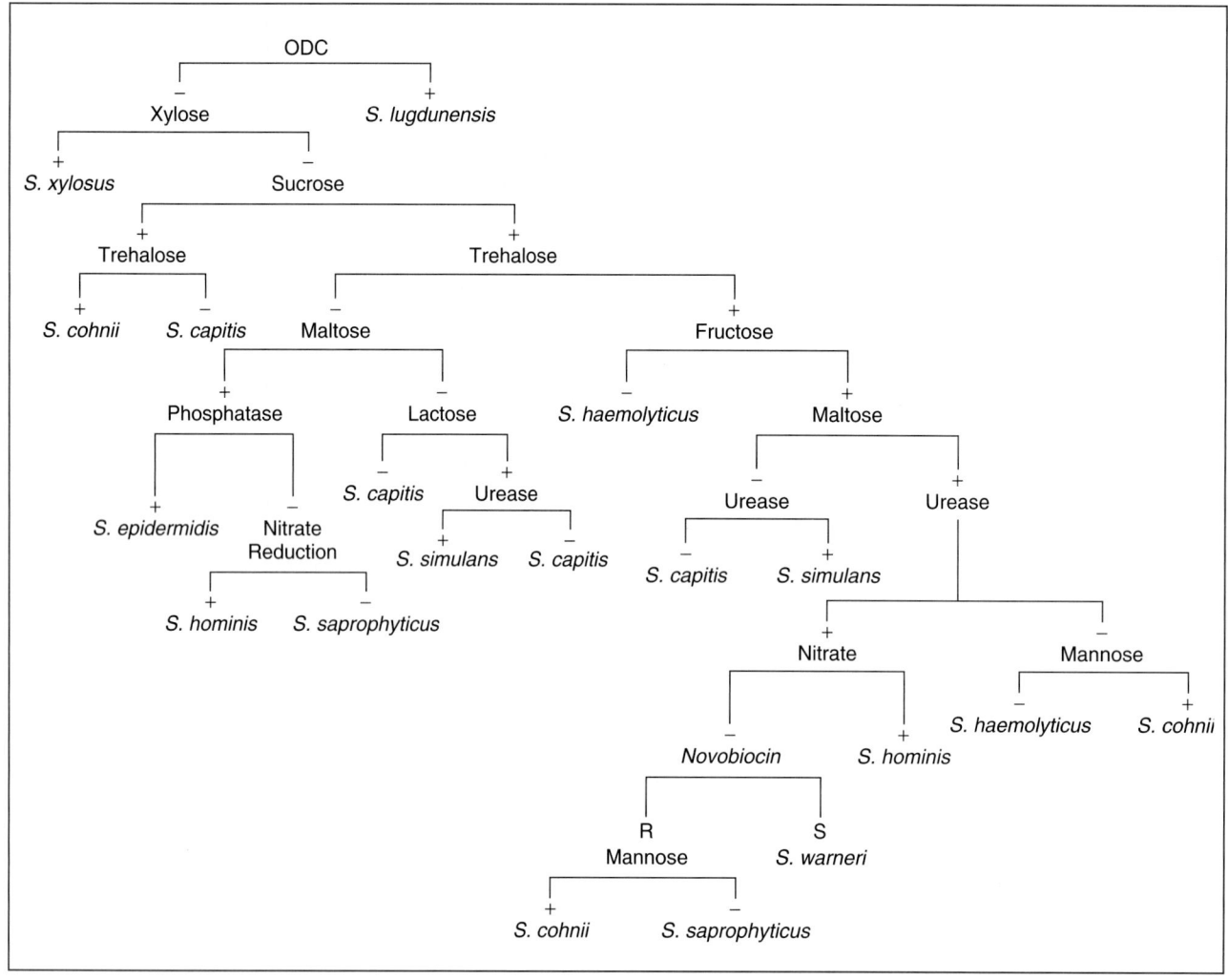

Figure 12-1 Dichotomous key for identification of the more common human coagulase-negative staphylococci.

lamidase to L-pyrrolidone and free β-naphthylamide, which combines with the PYR reagent (*p*-dimethylaminocinnamaldehyde) to produce a red color. The test is performed with PYR broth inoculated to approximate a no. 2 McFarland turbidity standard. After 2 hours of incubation at 35°C, the PYR reagent is added. The appearance of a red color within 2 minutes constitutes a positive test, with a yellow, orange, or pink color being negative. Alternatively, any of the commercial rapid PYR disk tests may be used. Hydrolysis of PYR is also found on some of the kit systems that are available for identifying staphylococci. Both *S. aureus* and *S. epidermidis* are PYR-negative, while *S. haemolyticus*, *S. intermedius*, *S. lugdunensis*, and *S. schleiferi* subsp. *schleiferi* are PYR-positive.

SUSCEPTIBILITY TO POLYMYXIN B

The disk diffusion test for susceptibility to polymyxin B is also helpful for identifying coagulase-negative staphylococci. The test can be done on SBA along with that for novobiocin susceptibility (see below). A suspension of the organism equivalent to a 0.5 McFarland turbidity standard is prepared in saline and swabbed onto a plate as for a Bauer-Kirby disk diffusion test. A polymyxin B disk (300 units; BD Biosciences) is applied to the inoculum and the plate is incubated overnight. Resistance is indicated by the presence of a zone of less than 10 mm. Susceptible strains have zones ≥10 mm. *S. aureus*, *S. epidermidis*, *S. hyicus*, and some *S. lugdunensis* strains are polymyxin resistant.

ORNITHINE DECARBOXYLASE TEST (ODC)

The ODC test is most useful for confirming the identity of *S. lugdunensis*, as this species is the only one that is consistently ornithine decarboxylase–positive. A tube of decarboxylase base and base with added ornithine (Remel) are inoculated heavily and overlaid with sterile mineral oil. On incubation at 35°C, both tubes will turn from pale-gray to yellow as glucose is fermented. Following this, the ornithine in the test tube will be decarboxylated, resulting in the ornithine broth turning a violet color. The base tube will turn and remain yellow, and the ornithine tube will remain yellow

Table 12-3 Phenotypic Characteristics for Identification of *Staphylococcus* Species

SPECIES	COAGULASE	CLUMPING FACTOR	ANAEROBIC GROWTH IN THIO	HEAT-STABLE ENDONUCLEASE	PAL	ADH	ODC	PYR	ACETOIN	NO₃ REDUCTION	UREASE	B-GLU	B-GAL	B-GUR	MODIFIED OXIDASE
S. aureus subsp. *aureus*	+	+	+	+	+	+	–	NA	+	+	V	+	–	–	–
S. aureus subsp. *anaerobius*	+	+	+sl	+	+	NA	NA	NA	–	–	NA	–	–	–	–
S. epidermidis	–	–	+	–	V⁺	V	V	–	+	+	+	V	–	–	–
S. saprophyticus subsp. *saprophyticus*	–	–	+sl	–	–	–	–	–	+	–	+	V	+	–	–
S. saprophyticus subsp. *bovis*	–	–	+sl	–	–	–	–	+	V	+	+	V	V	V	–
S. haemolyticus	–	–	+sl	–	–	–	–	+	+	+	+	+	–	V	–
S. warneri	–	–	+	–	–	V	–	–	V	V	+	+	–	V	–
S. hominis subsp. *hominis*	–	–	–	–	–	V	–	–	V	V	+	–	–	–	–
S. hominis subsp. *novobiosepticus*	–	–	+	–	–	–	–	–	V	V	+	–	+	V	+
S. simulans	–	+sl	+	–	Vsl	+	+	+	+	+	+	+	+	V	–
S. lugdunensis	–	+sl	+	–	–	–	+	+	+	+	V	+	–	+	–
S. schleiferi subsp. *schleiferi*	–	+	+	+	+	+	–	+	+	+	–	–	+	–	–
S. schleiferi subsp. *coagulans*	+	–	+	+	+	+	NA	NA	+	+	+	NA	NA	NA	NA
S. capitis subsp. *capitis*	–	–	+sl	–	+	V	–	–	V	V	–	–	–	+	–
S. capitis subsp. *urealyticus*	–	–	+sl	–	–	+	–	V	V	+	+	–	Vsl	+	–
S. auricularis	–	–	Vsl	–	–	+	–	V	–	Vsl	–	–	–	NA	–
S. pasteuri	–	–	+	–	–	V	–	+	V	V	+	+	–	+	–
S. caprae	–	–	+sl	–	+sl	V	–	V	+	+	+	–	–	–	+
S. cohnii subsp. *cohnii*	–	–	V	–	–	–	–	–	V	–	–	–	–	–	–
S. cohnii subsp. *urealyticum*	–	–	+sl	–	+	–	–	V	V	V	+	+	+	+	+
S. xylosus	–	–	V	–	V	–	–	V	V	V	+	+	+	+	–
S. saccharolyticus	–	–	+	–	V	+	NA	NA	NA	+	NA	NA	NA	NA	–
S. intermedius	+	V	+sl	+	+	V	–	+	–	+	+	V	+	–	+
S. hyicus	V	–	+sl	+	+	+	–	–	–	+	V	V	–	+	+
S. sciuri subsp. *sciuri*	–	–	+sl	–	+	–	–	–	+	+	+	+	–	V	+
S. sciuri subsp. *carnaticus*	–	V	Vsl	–	V	–	NA	NA	–	+	+	+	NA	NA	+
S. sciuri subsp. *rodentium*	–	+	Vsl	–	V	–	–	–	–	–	–	V	+	+	+
S. chromogenes	–	–	+sl	–	+	–	–	V	–	V	+	+	V	V	+
S. gallinarum	–	–	Vsl	–	V	+	–	+	V	+	V	+	+	V	+
S. lentus	–	–	Vsl	–	+sl	–	–	–	NA	–	+	+	–	+	+
S. equorum	–	–	–	–	+sl	–	–	–	–	+	+	NA	V	+	+
S. delphini	+	–	+sl	–	+	+	NA	NA	–	+	+	NA	NA	NA	+
S. felis	–	–	+	–	+	+	NA	NA	–	+	+	–	+	+	–
S. lutrae	+	–	+	V	+	–	NA	NA	–	+	+	NA	+	NA	+
S. vitulinus	–	–	–	–	–	–	–	–	–	+	–	V	+	–	+
S. muscae	–	–	+	–	+	–	–	NA	–	NA	NA	NA	–	NA	–
S. kloosii	–	–	–	–	V	–	–	V	V	–	V	V	V	V	–
S. arlettae	–	–	–	–	+sl	+	–	–	NA	+	+	+	+	+	–
S. piscifermentans	–	–	+	–	+	–	NA	NA	–	+	–	–	+	NA	–
S. condimenti	–	–	+	NA	+	+	NA	NA	NA	+	+	NA	+	NA	NA
S. succinus	–	–	–	NA	+	–	NA	NA	–	+	+	NA	NA	NA	–
S. fleuretii	–	–	+	–	V	V	–	+	+	+	–	NA	+	–	+
S. carnosus subsp. *carnosus*	–	–	+	–	–	–	–	+	+	+	–	–	–	–	–
S. carnosus subsp. *utilis*	–	–	+	NA	–	+	NA	NA	NA	V	–	NA	–	–	NA

(Continued)

Table 12-3 Continued

SPECIES	POLY-MYXIN B	NOVO-BIOCIN	GLUCOSE	MALTOSE	SUCROSE	LACTOSE	MANNITOL	MANNOSE	ARABINOSE	TREHALOSE	XYLOSE	RAFFINOSE	CELLO-BIOSE	N-ACETYL-GLUCOSAMINE
S. aureus subsp. *aureus*	R	S	+	+	+	+	+	+	-	+	-	-	-	+
S. aureus subsp. *anaerobius*	NA	S	+	+	+	-	NA	NA	-	-	-	-	-	-
S. epidermidis	R	S	+	+	+	V	-	+sl	-	-	-	-	-	-
S. saprophyticus subsp. *saprophyticus*	S	R	+	+	+	V	V	-	-	+	-	-	-	V
S. saprophyticus subsp. *bovis*	NA	R	+	+	+	+	+	-	-	+	-	-	-	+
S. haemolyticus	S	S	+	Vsl	+	V	V	-	-	+	-	-	-	-
S. warneri	S	S	+sl	Vsl	+	V	+	-	-	+	-	-	-	-
S. hominis subsp. *hominis*	S	S	+	Vsl	+sl	V	+	-	-	V	-	-	-	V
S. hominis subsp. *novobiosepticus*	NA	R	+	+	+sl	V	-	-	-	V	-	-	-	-
S. simulans	S	S	+	Vsl	+	+	+	V	-	V	-	-	-	+
S. lugdunensis	S/R	S	+	+	+	+	+	+	-	+	-	-	-	+
S. schleiferi subsp. *schleiferi*	S	S	+	-	-	V	+	+	-	V	-	-	-	+sl
S. schleiferi subsp. *coagulans*	NA	S	+	-	V	V	V	+	-	-	-	-	-	NA
S. capitis subsp. *capitis*	S	S	+	-	+sl	+	+	+	-	-	-	-	-	-
S. capitis subsp. *urealyticus*	NA	S	+	Vsl	V	Vsl	+	+	-	+	-	-	-	-
S. auricularis	NA	S	+sl	+sl	V	Vsl	+	-	-	+sl	-	-	-	NA
S. pasteuri	NA	S	+	Vsl	+	V	-	+	-	+sl	-	-	-	-
S. caprae	S	S	+	Vsl	-	+	V	Vsl	-	+sl	-	-	-	-
S. cohnii subsp. *cohnii*	S	R	+	Vsl	-	-	V	-	-	+	-	-	-	-
S. cohnii subsp. *urealyticum*	S	R	+	Vsl	-	V	+	+	-	+	-	-	V	V
S. xylosus	S	R	+	+	+	V	+	+	V	+	+	-	+	+
S. saccharolyticus	NA	S	+	+	-	-	+sl	+sl	-	+sl	-	-	NA	NA
S. intermedius	S	S	+	Vsl	+	V	Vsl	+	-	+	-	-	+	+
S. hyicus	R	S	+	-	+	-	-	+	-	+	-	-	-	-
S. sciuri subsp. *sciuri*	S	R	Vsl	Vsl	+	Vsl	+	Vsl	V	+	Vsl	-	+	-
S. sciuri subsp. *carnaticus*	S	R	Vsl	Vsl	+	Vsl	+	Vsl	V	+	+	-	+sl	-
S. sciuri subsp. *rodentium*	S	R	Vsl	Vsl	+	-	+	Vsl	Vsl	+sl	Vsl	-	V	-
S. chromogenes	R	S	+	V	+	+	V	+	-	+	-	-	V	V
S. gallinarum	S	R	+	+	+	V	+	+	+	+	+	+	+	+
S. lentus	S	R	+	V	Vsl	V	+sl	+	V	+	Vsl	+	+	V
S. equorum	NA	R	+	V	+	V	+	+	+	+	+	-	Vsl	V
S. delphini	NA	S	+	+	V	V	+sl	+sl	-	-	-	NA	NA	NA
S. felis	NA	S	+	-	V	V	V	+	-	+	-	-	-	+
S. lutrae	NA	S	+	+	NA	+	V	+	NA	+	+	NA	NA	NA
S. vitulinus	NA	R	+	-	+	-	V	-	-	Vsl	V	V	V	-
S. muscae	NA	NA	+	-	+	-	+	-	-	+	Vsl	-	+	NA
S. kloosii	S	S	V	V	Vsl	Vsl	+	-	V	+	Vsl	-	-	-
S. arlettae	NA	R	V	V	+sl	V	+	+	+	+	+	+	+	-
S. piscifermentans	NA	S	+	V	+	V	+	-	-	+	-	-	-	NA
S. condimenti	NA	NA	+	V	V	V	+	+	+	+	-	-	-	NA
S. succinus	NA	NA	+	-	NA	NA	+	+	NA	+	NA	NA	-	NA
S. fleurettii	NA	R	+	+	+	NA	-	V	V	+	V	Vsl	NA	NA
S. carnosus subsp. *carnosus*	S	S	+	-	-	V	V	+	-	V	Vsl	-	-	NA
S. carnosus subsp. *utilis*	NA	NA	+	-	-	-	-	-	-	V	NA	-	-	NA

+, positive reaction; −, negative reaction; V, variable reaction; V−, variable reaction, most strains negative; V+, variable reaction; +sl, slow or delayed positive reaction; but positive reactions are slow or delayed; NA, data not available; THIO, thioglycollate broth; PAL, alkaline phosphatase; ADH, arginine dihydrolase; ODC, ornithine decarboxylase; β-glucosidase; b-gal, beta-galactosidase; b-gut, beta-glucuronidase; S, susceptible; R, resistant.

if ODC is not produced. Although most positive tests may be detected within 6 to 8 hours, the test is read after 24 hours of incubation. The ODC test is not included in most of the kit systems for identifying staphylococci and must be set up as an additional test.

UREASE PRODUCTION

Some staphylococci are urease-positive, including *S. epidermidis*, *S. intermedius*, and most isolates of *S. saprophyticus*. Regular urease broth or urea agar slants can be used for this test. The slant or the broth is inoculated and incubated at 35°C for 18–24 hours. A change in the phenol red indicator from yellow to pink/red is a positive test.

ACETOIN PRODUCTION

Production of acetoin (the Voges-Proskauer test) is helpful in distinguishing *S. aureus* species, which are acetoin-positive, from other coagulase-positive species (*S. intermedius* and *S. hyicus*), which are both acetoin-negative. The conventional enteric acetoin production test (MR-VP broth) or the rapid disk method may be used with comparable results.[90]

SUSCEPTIBILITY TO DEFEROXAMINE

In 1991 and 1993, Lindsay and coworkers reported a new test for specific identification of *S. epidermidis* and *S. hominis*.[267,268] The test determines susceptibility to deferoxamine, which is a siderophore that is produced by *Streptomyces pilosus* and is used clinically to treat acute and chronic iron overload. The test is performed as a disk diffusion test like the furazolidone and bacitracin susceptibility tests. After preparing a suspension of the organism corresponding to a 0.5 McFarland turbidity standard, a plate of BHI agar is inoculated with the suspension and a 1 mg deferoxamine disk (Desferal; Ciba-Geigy, Switzerland) is placed on the inoculum. After overnight incubation at 35°C, the plate is inspected for a zone of growth inhibition around the disk. In their original study, Lindsay and Riley found that, among 95 coagulase-negative staphylococci, all 57 *S. epidermidis* and 4 *S. hominis* isolates were susceptible to deferoxamine, while all 34 other isolates were resistant.[268] In a subsequent study of 161 coagulase-negative staphylococci, all *S. epidermidis* and *S. hominis* strains were susceptible to deferoxamine, while all of the remaining staphylococci were resistant.[267] Mulder tested 670 *S. epidermidis*, 37 *S. hominis*, and 151 other coagulase-negative staphylococci for deferoxamine susceptibility using a disk test (50 μL per disk of a 2% deferoxamine stock solution) and found that all *S. epidermidis* and *S. hominis* isolates were deferoxamine-susceptible, while only 5 (3.3%) of 151 isolates identified as other staphylococcal species were deferoxamine-susceptible.[309] Monsen and colleagues also evaluated this test and found that all 139 *S. epidermidis* and all 18 *S. hominis* strains were deferoxamine-susceptible, showing zones of 28–31 mm and 15–41 mm, respectively.[306] All other coagulase-negative staphylococci tested in this study were highly resistant to deferoxamine. While deferoxamine is commercially available, standardized susceptibility test disks must be prepared in-house at the present time.

Susceptibility to Novobiocin for Identification of *Staphylococcus saprophyticus*

Four human staphylococcal species (*S. saprophyticus*, *S. cohnii* subspecies, *S. hominis* subsp. *novobiosepticus*, and *S. xylosus*), seven animal species (*S. sciuri*, *S. lentus*, *S. gallinarum*, *S. kloosii*, *S. equorum*, *S. arlettae*, and *S. vitulinus*) and one environmental species (*S. succinus*) are resistant to novobiocin, with minimal inhibitory concentrations (MICs) of ≥1.6 μg/mL.[220,226,228,247,389–391,487] Since novobiocin-resistant species other than *S. saprophyticus* are infrequently encountered in human clinical specimens, the novobiocin susceptibility test provides a useful method for *S. saprophyticus* identification. The novobiocin test is performed as a disk susceptibility test using a novobiocin disk (5 μg) and is described in detail in Chart 12-2 (Color Plates 12-3*B*, 12-3*C*, and 12-3*D*). Strains resistant to novobiocin will show zones measuring 6 mm (no zone) to 12 mm; susceptible strains will have zones of 16 mm to 27 mm. This test was originally described using a medium called P agar, which is not available commercially. However, studies with the routine media mentioned above have shown that comparable results are obtained.[141]

In an effort to assess the reliability and accuracy of the novobiocin susceptibility test, McTaggart and Elliott examined 36 presumptive *S. saprophyticus* strains (i.e., novobiocin-resistant organisms from urine specimens of patients with urinary tract infections) with a commercial identification system (API Staph-Ident, see below) and with expanded batteries of additional substrates, including carbohydrate utilization tests, 7-amino-4-methylumbelliferone derivatives of inorganic and organic esters and glycosides, and 7-amino-4-methylcoumarin derivatives of amino acids.[292] Of the 36 strains, 21 (58%) were identified as *S. saprophyticus*, 3 strains could not be identified, 9 strains had characteristics that were attributable to more than one novobiocin-resistant species, and 3 strains were identified as *S. epidermidis*, *S. hominis*, and *S. simulans*, respectively. Even strains that were identified as *S. saprophyticus* by the Staph-Ident produced a spectrum of reactivities with the other chromogenic substrates, illustrating the heterogeneity of organisms called "*S. saprophyticus*" and suggesting that organisms called *S. saprophyticus* may actually represent a heterogeneous group of novobiocin-resistant, genotypically and phenotypically related strains. These workers concluded that additional tests are needed for reliable presumptive identification of *S. saprophyticus* other than or in addition to the novobiocin susceptibility test. Occasional human isolates that are not *S. saprophyticus*, *S. cohnii* subspecies, *S. hominis* subsp. *novobiosepticus*, or *S. xylosus* may also be resistant to novobiocin. In an evaluation of the RapiDEC-Staph, Janda and colleagues found that, while all *S. saprophyticus* isolates were resistant to novobiocin, 5 (7%) of 74 *S. epidermidis* strains were also novobiocin-resistant.[192]

Commercial Identification Systems

Currently several commercial kits are available for the identification of coagulase-negative staphylococci. All of these kits use modified carbohydrate fermentation tests, adaptations of standard bacteriologic identification tests (e.g., nitrate reduction, urease, Voges-Proskauer), and chromogenic enzyme substrate tests for organism identification. These systems are adapted to the particular format used by the manufacturer (e.g., strip with small cupulae, microtiter trays, plastic cards, etc.).

RAPIDEC STAPH

RapiDEC Staph (bioMerieux) is a kit system that identifies *S. aureus*, *S. epidermidis*, and *S. saprophyticus* within 2 hours. The isolate to be identified is emulsified in water and the suspension is dispensed into four cupulae. The first cupule is a control, while the others contain a fluorescent coagulase substrate (see ''Aurease'' test above), an alkaline phosphatase substrate (PAL), and a β-galactosidase substrate (βGAL), respectively. After 2 hours of incubation, the cupulae are observed under an ultraviolet light (wavelength, 365 nm). If greater fluorescence is observed in the second cupule relative to the first control cupule, the isolate is identified as *S. aureus*. If this test is negative, the other two cupulae are read either directly (cupula 3) or after the addition of a detection reagent (cupula 4). A positive reaction in cupule 3 or cupule 4 identifies the isolate as *S. epidermidis* (alkaline phosphatase–positive) or *S. saprophyticus* (β-galactosidase-positive), respectively. Positive results in both the PAL and βGAL tests provide a presumptive identification of *S. xylosus/S. intermedius*. In one evaluation, RapIDEC Staph correctly identified 100% of 130 *S. aureus* strains, while only 70% of 74 *S. epidermidis* strains and 81% of 32 *S. saprophyticus* strains were correctly identified.[192] Among 62 other coagulase-negative isolates tested, 4 *S. sciuri* strains were misidentified as *S. epidermidis*, and 8 isolates (1 *S. hominis*, 3 *S. cohnii* subsp. *urealyticum*, 3 *S. simulans*, and 1 *S. kloosii*) were misidentified as *S. saprophyticus*. While the PAL test on the RapiDEC Staph appears to be relatively specific for detection of the phosphatase of *S. epidermidis*, strains of this species that are phosphatase-negative or that produce low levels of the enzyme will not be identified as *S. epidermidis* by RapiDEC Staph. Consequently, the sensitivity and performance of RapiDEC Staph for identifying *S. epidermidis* depends on the relative prevalence of PAL-positive and negative strains in a population.[192]

API STAPH-IDENT

The API Staph-IDENT (bioMerieux) product uses a battery of 10 miniaturized biochemical tests that are inoculated with a heavy suspension of the organism to be identified. Species identification is determined by the generation of a four-digit octal code derived from the positive tests on the strip and the database. Additional tests (e.g., acid from xylose, novobiocin susceptibility) may be required for identifying some strains. The database of the system includes several species or subspecies of staphylococci, micrococci, and *R. mucilaginosa*. Organisms that are called *R. mucilaginosa* on Staph-Ident require confirmation; recommendations include lysostaphin susceptibility to separate the organism from staphylococci, and catalase and growth in salt broth to separate the organism from *K. kristinae*. Staph-Ident has been extensively evaluated, and agreement with conventional procedures has ranged from 43% to 95% depending on the species tested.[99,135,145,185,227] Rhoden and Miller published a

four-year prospective study comparing the API Staph-Ident with reference methods on 1,106 isolates and found an overall agreement of 81.1%.[368] Agreement for the five most common isolates was 97.1% for *S. epidermidis*, 82.5% for *S. hominis*, 77.2% for *S. aureus*, 75.8% for *S. haemolyticus*, and 64.1% for *S. warneri*. These workers concluded that the database of the current Staph-Ident system is inadequate for identifying both common and uncommon species staphylococcal species.[368]

API STAPH

API Staph (formerly API Staph-Trac; bioMerieux) is an 18- to 24-hour identification system for both micrococci and staphylococci. This system contains 19 tests arranged in a strip format and is inoculated with a suspension of the organism prepared in a peptone-yeast extract broth medium provided with the kit. After reading the biochemical reactions, a seven-digit octal code is generated and identification of the organism is obtained with the computer assisted database (Color Plates 12-3*B*–12-3*H*). The database consists of 25 taxa and includes staphylococci of human and veterinary origin, *Micrococcus* species, and *R. mucilaginosa*. Although the database of this system is large, it has not been extensively evaluated.[135] A study by Perl and colleagues found that the API Staph system correctly identified 73% of 277 coagulase-negative staphylococci.[342] While 94% of 94 *S. epidermidis* isolates were correctly identified, the system performed poorly with less common isolates like *S. haemolyticus* (85% correct), *S. hominis* (75% correct), *S. simulans* (67% correct), and *S. warneri* (22% correct).

API ID32 STAPH

ID32 Staph (bioMerieux) is a 24-hour strip system for identifying staphylococci and related species. The panel contains 32 cupulae and currently has 26 biochemical tests, allowing room for expansion of the test battery. The system may be read manually to generate a profile number that is interpreted by a computer-assisted database (Color Plate 12-2*H*), or, alternatively, the strip can be used with the automated bioMerieux ATB system, which includes a densitometer, an inoculator, a reader, a microcomputer, and a printer. The ID32 Staph has the most extensive database of all the systems, with all human staphylococcal species (except *S. saccharolyticus*) and several animal and environmental species being included. The system also identifies six micrococcal species and *R. mucilaginosa*. An international collaborative evaluation with 792 strains conducted in eight laboratories found that the ID32 Staph correctly identified 95.5% of the isolates tested; 83.5% were identified without further testing, while, for an additional 12% of strains, the correct identification was among the proposed choices.[49] Only 1.2% of isolates were misidentified, and 3.3% were not identified by the ID32 Staph. In another study of 440 consecutive coagulase-negative staphylococcal isolates, Ieven and coworkers reported that the ID32 Staph panel identified 95.2%.[187] *S. epidermidis*, *S. haemolyticus*, *S. lugdunensis*, *S. schleiferi*, and *S. capitis* were identified with an accuracy of 98–100%.[187] Renneberg et al. found that the ID32 Staph panel identified 79.5% of 200 reference and clinical staphylococcal isolates.[366] Other European investigators challenged the system with a collection of 42 isolates that could not be classified by other available phenotypic procedures and found that only 22 (52%) could be identified by the ID32 Staph.[74]

VITEK GRAM-POSITIVE IDENTIFICATION (GPI) Card

The Vitek GPI card (bioMerieux) is a gram-positive organism identification card designed for use with the automated Vitek bacterial identification/susceptibility testing system. The card contains 30 microwells (28 test wells and 2 control wells) containing substrates for the identification of *Staphylococcus* species (11 human and 4 veterinary species), *Streptococcus* species, and several gram-positive bacillary species (e.g., *Corynebacterium* species, *Erysipelothrix rhusiopathiae*, and *Listeria monocytogenes*). A suspension of the organism is prepared in saline and the card is attached to the bacterial suspension via a transfer tube and placed in the filling module of the instrument. The card is inoculated by a vacuum/release method. The card is then placed in the reader/incubator module of the Vitek instrument, where it is optically scanned and read periodically. Identification of coagulase-negative staphylococci generally requires 10 to 13 hours. Bannerman et al. evaluated the updated GPI database with 500 clinical isolates.[22] The overall agreement between the GPI card and conventional methods was 89%. The card identified 92% of *S. epidermidis*, 95% of *S. haemolyticus*, 88% of *S. capitis* subsp. *capitis*, and 100% of *S. saprophyticus* strains tested. Organisms that are not currently in the database, like *S. lugdunensis*, were either misidentified or not identified by the GPI card. In the 1994 evaluation by Perl and associates, the GPI card correctly identified only 67% of 185 isolates.[342] These workers pointed out that the poorer performance of the GPI card in their study may have been due to the preponderance of ''non-*epidermidis*'' staphylococci among the 277 isolates tested. In 1996, Kellogg and colleagues challenged the GPI Card with 616 clinical isolates of coagulase-negative staphylococci.[212] The GPI card identified 100% of 12 *S. capitis* and 79 *S. saprophyticus* strains, 98.4% of 250 *S. epidermidis* strains, and 96% of 126 *S. haemolyticus* strains. Only 64.5% of the remaining 107 isolates were correctly identified.[212] All of these studies have concluded that the GPI card cannot reliably identify the less commonly encountered staphylococcal species and that the database for this product needs improvement. The GPI card for the Vitek 2 instrument awaits clinical evaluation.

MICROSCAN RAPID POS COMBO PANEL

The MicroScan Rapid Pos Combo Panel (Dade/MicroScan) is a microtiter-plate format system that uses fluorogenic substrates and a fluorescent pH indicator to detect various bacterial enzymatic activities.[219] The panel contains 42 tests for the identification of staphylococci, streptococci, and the listeriae. The tests are based on hydrolysis of fluorogenic substrates, pH changes following substrate utilization, and the production of specific metabolic products. The system is inoculated with a suspension of the organism and is incubated and read in the Microscan Walk/Away instrument. Identifications are available 2 hours after panel inoculation. In a Canadian evaluation of this system, the MicroScan Rapid Pos Combo panel correctly identified 91.6% of 239 staphylococcal isolates.[428] For an additional 3.8% of the isolates, the correct identification was listed among the species choices provided by the database. Another evaluation from Portland, Oregon, found that the Microscan Rapid Pos panel identified only 50.5% of 233 isolates, with an additional 24.9% having the correct identification among the possibilities generated by the database.[144] Weinstein and colleagues found that, while the system accurately identified *S. epidermidis* and several other coagulase-negative staphylococci, more than half of the *S. haemolyticus* and *S. hominis* isolates were misidentified.[489]

MICROSCAN POS ID PANEL

The MicroScan Pos ID panel (Dade/MicroScan) system offers combination identification and susceptibility testing capabilities for gram-positive organisms, including micrococci, staphylococci, streptococci, enterococci, and listeriae. The panel contains 27 miniaturized conventional biochemical identification tests, 18 of which are used for the identification of staphylococci and related species. The lyophilized panels are thawed, inoculated, incubated for 24 to 48 hours, and read manually or with the MicroScan Walk/Away automated system. The test results compute into a six-digit code, and the database of the MicroScan system provides an identification. In one evaluation, the panel provided accurate identification of *S. epidermidis* and *S. saprophyticus*, but only after 48 hours of incubation.[185] Other *Staphylococcus* species were identified less reliably within the same period. Skulnick et al. examined 163 staphylococcal isolates and found that the Microscan panel identified 96% of 163 staphylococcal isolates; organisms that were incorrectly identified included two strains of *S. haemolyticus* and a single strain each of *S. epidermidis*, *S. hominis*, *S. xylosus*, and *S. sciuri*.[413] Kloos and George also found that this system correctly identified most significant human staphylococcal isolates with greater than 80% accuracy.[219] A more recent MicroScan Pos ID panel evaluation reported that the system identified only 53.6% of 233 staphylococcal isolates, with an additional 24.9% of isolates having the correct identification listed among possible choices by the computer-assisted database.[144]

BBL CRYSTAL GRAM-POSITIVE (GP) IDENTIFICATION SYSTEM

The Crystal GP Identification System (BD Biosciences) is a miniaturized identification panel consisting of 29 fluorogenic, chromogenic, and modified conventional tests for the identification of gram-positive isolates belonging to several genera, including *Staphylococcus*, *Micrococcus*, *Stomatococcus*, *Streptococcus*, *Enterococcus*, *Aerococcus*, and *Lactococcus*. The system is inoculated with a suspension of organisms (0.5 McFarland turbidity standard), incubated for 18–24 hours at 35–37°C in an ambient atmosphere, and read with a special Crystal system panel viewer. von Baum and colleagues evaluated this system using 77 strains of *Staphylococcus* species, 5 *Micrococcus* species, and a single *R. mucilaginosa* isolate.[473] The BBL Crystal identified 100% of 22 *S. aureus* and 24 *S. epidermidis* isolates correctly. Among 31 strains representing 10 other coagulase-negative species, 29 were correctly identified. All micrococcal isolates and the *R. mucilaginosa* isolate were correctly identified. While the Crystal system appears to be useful for identification of clinically significant staphylococci, additional studies are needed because of the small number of challenge strains examined in the above evaluation and the failure to include certain other clinically significant species, such as *S. saprophyticus*, *S. schleiferi*, and *S. caprae*.

STAF-SISTEM 18-R

The Staf-Sistem 18-R (Liofilchem s.r.l. Roseto degli Abruzzi, Teramo, Italy) consists of a plastic tray containing 18 modified conventional substrates. The wells are inoculated with an organism suspension using a multichannel pipette and the panel is incubated and read after 18 to 24 hours. Piccolomini and colleagues evaluated this system with 523 strains belonging to 16 human *Staphylococcus* species and found that 491 strains (93.9%) were correctly identified, with another 28 strains (5.4%) requiring supplemental tests for complete identification.[344] As with many of these kit systems, the authors point out the need for database adjustment and more discriminating test selection to correctly identify important isolates like *S. lugdunensis* and *S. schleiferi*.

STAPH-ZYM

The Staph-Zym (ROSCO, Taastrup, Denmark) is a new Scandinavian identification system composed of a plastic strip of 10 minitubes that contain dehydrated chromogenic and modified conventional substrates. The individual microtubes are inoculated with an aliquot of a bacterial suspension prepared in saline, and the results are read after overnight incubation. Renneberg and colleagues challenged this system with 111 reference staphylococcal strains and 89 clinical isolates and found that the Staph-Zym system correctly identified 90–100% of the reference strains and 82.1% of the clinical isolates, for an accuracy of 91.5% compared with conventional identification methods.[366] In another evaluation, the Staph-Zym correctly identified 97.5% of 440 isolates when compared with reference identifications.[187] The Staph-Zym appears to be an accurate system for staphylococcal identification.

MICROBACT STAPHYLOCOCCAL 12S

The Microbact Staphylococcal 12S (Oxoid) is a 12-test identification system based on carbohydrate acidification and enzyme detection using chromogenic substrates. The wells of the strip are inoculated with a suspension of the organism and the strip is incubated overnight at 35°C. After addition of color development reagents to the enzymatic tests, the tests are read and interpreted according to the database included in the package insert. No evaluations of this new test system are available.

MICROBIAL IDENTIFICATION SYSTEM

The Microbial Identification System (MIS or MIDI; Microbial ID, Newark, DE) uses high-resolution gas-liquid chromatography (GLC) of cellular fatty acid derivatives for the identification of bacteria.[39] The database of the system is composed of libraries containing the analyses of cellular fatty acid profiles of various bacteria and compares the composition of individual isolates with those in the database using covariance matrix/pattern recognition software. A similarity index is used to express the relatedness of a profile of an unknown organism to representative profiles of known organisms. In a comparative evaluation of the MIS with conventional procedures for identifying staphylococci, the MIS system showed complete agreement with conventional methods for 87.8% of 470 isolates tested.[427] The system identified all strains of *S. epidermidis*, *S. intermedius*, *S. cohnii*, *S. lugdunensis*, *S. schleiferi*, *S. simulans*, *S. sciuri*, and *S. xylosus*. *S. hominis* and *S. saprophyticus* strains accounted for over half of the misidentifications obtained with the system. The GLC approach used in the MIS shows promise as an alternative method for species identification of the staphylococci.

BIOLOG MICROPLATE IDENTIFICATION SYSTEM

The Biolog Microplate Identification System (Biolog, Hayward, CA) identifies microorganisms on the basis of oxidation of a variety of substrates. The system uses a 96-well microtiter tray with 95 substrates plus a control well lacking substrate. The plate is inoculated with a suspension of the organism and is incubated for 4 or 24 hours. If the organism oxidizes a substrate in an individual well, the respiration of the organism during oxidative substrate assimilation causes the reduction of a tetrazolium indicator dye, turning the well from colorless to purple. At present, the Biolog MicroPlate System includes the GN MicroPlate for identifying 569 gram-negative species and the GP Biolog MicroPlate, which includes 225 gram-positive organisms in its database. Miller and Biddle at the CDC and Quenzer and McLaughlin at the University of New Mexico performed a joint evaluation of the GP Biolog MicroPlate for identification of 113 catalase-positive isolates, including 33 type strains of staphylococci, 5 strains of *Micrococcus* species, and 1 strain of *R. mucilaginosa*.[301] These workers found the overall accuracy of the system to be 69% and 73% at the CDC and the New Mexico laboratories, respectively. These results indicate that the Biolog system is not yet accurate enough to be used as a routine method for identifying the coagulase-negative staphylococci and related organisms.

Molecular Identification and Typing Methods for Staphylococci

Several approaches using both traditional and newly developed molecular methods have been used to identify staphylococci and to characterize strains in epidemiologic studies and in outbreaks of unusual or multiresistant strains. Formerly, epidemiologic studies were based on phenotypic markers such as unusual carbohydrate utilization and biochemical reactions, antimicrobial susceptibility patterns, serotyping, biotyping, and susceptibility to batteries of bacteriophages.[415,443] Other approaches, such as whole-cell protein analysis using sodium dodecyl sulfate–polyacrylamide gel electrophoresis (SDS-PAGE), gas-liquid chromatography, high-pressure liquid chromatography, mass spectrometry, and multilocus enzyme electrophoresis are more discriminating for recognizing similarities and differences among

Table 12-4 Phenotypic Characteristics for Identification of *Micrococcus* and Related Species

SPECIES	CELLULAR ARRANGEMENT				CATALASE	OXIDASE	PIGMENTATION	ADH	REDUCTION OF NITRATE
	Pairs	Tetrads	Cubes	Clusters					
Arthrobacter agilis	+	+	−	+	+	+	Rose-red	−	−
Dermacoccus nishinomiyaensis	+	+	−	+	+	+	Orange	−	V
Kocuria rosea	+	+	−	+	+	V−	Orange-to-pink-to-red	−	+
Kocuria varians	−	+	−	+	+	−	Dark yellow	−	+
Kocuria kristinae	−	+	−	+	+	+	Pale cream to pale orange	−	−
Kocuria palustris	+	+	+	−	+		Pale yellow	−	+
Kocuria rhizophila	+	+	+	−	+	−	Yellow	−	−
Kocuria polaris					+	+	Orange	−	+
Kytococcus sedentarius	−	+	+	−	+	−	Creamy white to deep buttercup yellow	+	V
Kytococcus schroeteri	+	+	−	−	+	−	Muddy yellow	+	−
Micrococcus luteus	+	+	+	+	+	+	Yellow or yellowish-green	−	−
Micrococcus lylae	+	+	+	+	+	+	White	−	−
Micrococcus antarcticus	+	−	+	+	+	+	Yellow, mucoid	−	+
Nesterenkonia halobia	+	+	−	+	+	+	Non-pigmented	−	−
Nesterenkonia lacusekhoensis[a]	NA	NA	NA	NA	+	−	Bright yellow	NA	−

(continued)

Table 12-4 *Continued*

SPECIES	MOTILITY	UREASE	HYDROLYSIS OF:			ACID AEROBICALLY FROM:					
			Esculin	Starch	Gelatin	Glucose	Glycerol	Lactose	Mannitol	Mannose	Xylose
Arthrobacter agilis	+	−	+	+	+	−	−	−	−	−	−
Dermacoccus nishinomiyaensis	−	V+	−	V	+	V	−	−	−	−	−
Kocuria rosea	−	−	−	+	−	−	−	−	−	−	−
Kocuria varians	−	+	−	−	+^w	+	NA	NA	−	−	+
Kocuria kristinae	−	V	+	−	−	+	NA	NA	−	+	−
Kocuria palustris	−	−	−	−	−	+	NA	NA	−	−	−
Kocuria rhizophila	−	−	−	−	+	+	NA	NA	−	+	−
Kocuria polaris	−	−	−	+	−	+	NA	NA	+	−	+
Kytococcus sedentarius	−	−	−	−	+	−	−	−	−	−	−
Kytococcus schroeteri	−	−	−	−	+	−	−	−	−	−	−
Micrococcus luteus	−	−	−	−	+	−	−	−	−	−	−
Micrococcus lylae	−	−	−	−	+	−	−	−	−	−	−
Micrococcus antarcticus	−	−	−	+	−	−	−	−	−	−	−
Nesterenkonia halobia	−	−	NA	+	NA	+	+	+	+	+	+
Nesterenkonia lacusekhoensis	−	NA	NA	−	NA	−	NA	−	−	NA	−

a Short rods with branching, cocci predominant in older cultures.
+, positive reaction; −, negative reaction; V, variable reaction; V+, variable reaction but most strains positive; V−, variable reaction but most strains negative; +^w, weak positive reaction.

strains, but are expensive and time-consuming to perform.[39,345,447] SDS-PAGE of total cell proteins and penicillin-binding proteins and gas-liquid chromatography of cellular fatty acids have shown 92% to over 95% agreement with phenotypic procedures for identification and typing coagulase-negative staphylococci.[236,345]

Newer molecular and genetic techniques have gained widespread popularity as highly discriminatory and relatively inexpensive methods for identification, epidemiologic typing, and characterization of *S. aureus* strains and for identification and molecular characterization of coagulase-negative staphylococci. These methods include restriction-fragment-length polymorphism analysis of plasmid, ribosomal, and chromosomal nucleic acids, pulsed-field gel electrophoresis of total DNA, ribotyping, polymerase chain reaction/nucleic acid probe hybridization procedures, PCR analysis of insertion elements and 16S–23S rRNA intergenic spacer regions, cloning/sequencing of heat-shock protein genes, restriction-fragment-length polymorphism analysis of *S. aureus* coagulase and protein A genes, 16S rRNA-directed *in situ* hybridization, and 16S sRNA sequencing.[38,41,76,95, 138,139,179,180,243,245,295,324,325,416,434,459,472]

These procedures have been used to investigate outbreaks of oxacillin-resistant *S. aureus* in neonatal and adult intensive-care units, the spread of vancomycin-resistant *S. haemolyticus* in patients and caregivers, and phenotypic variation and identification of other coagulase-negative staphylococci (e.g., *S. schleiferi*) recovered from serious infections. Such techniques have also been useful in studies designed to identify colonized individuals and to trace the sources of organisms responsible for infections, such as the relationship between carriage of a particular *S. aureus* strain in the nares of patients and caregivers and the subsequent development of CAPD-related peritonitis.[347] These methods are also being applied to taxonomic analysis of microorganisms and, in this regard, have already revolutionized our concepts of organism relatedness, classification, and identification.

Identification of *Micrococcus* and Related Species

Micrococci and related species are not generally identified to species level in clinical laboratories since they are rarely clinically significant. Using the tests described above and in Table 12-1, laboratories may issue reports of "*Micrococcus* species" without further testing. However, with the recognition of these agents as opportunistic pathogens, it may be necessary to identify these organisms to species on occasion. Identification criteria for the newly reclassified members of the former genus *Micrococcus* are presented in Table 12-4. As mentioned above, these organisms are also included in the databases of some of the commercial kit systems used in laboratories.

Identification of *Rothia mucilaginosa*

R. mucilaginosa colonies are sticky or mucoid, clear to white, and adherent to the agar surface. They appear on Gram-stained smears as large gram-positive cocci arranged in pairs or clusters. They are weakly catalase-positive, although some strains are catalase-negative. *R. mucilaginosa* can be differentiated from *Micrococcus* and *Staphylococcus* species by their failure to grow on nutrient agar medium containing 5% NaCl and by the presence of a capsule.[29,30] These organisms are also included in the database of the API Staph-Ident, the API Staph and ID32 Staph systems. Other biochemical characteristics are shown in Table 12-5. Medium used for enteric identification can be inoculated to determine biochemical reactions for this organism, and carbohydrate utilization tests may be performed with purple broth-based or cystine tryptic digest agar-based media containing 1% filter sterilized carbohydrates.

Laboratory Approach to the Identification of Staphylococci

Because staphylococci are among the most frequently isolated organisms in the clinical laboratory, decisions must be made on "how far to go" in identifying them. This is especially true regarding the coagulase-negative organisms. Many laboratories have adopted rapid coagulase procedures (i.e., latex or hemagglutination tests), so these tests may quickly be performed on colonies that "look like" staphylococci and are catalase-positive. If the colonies are coagulase-positive, the organism is identified as *S. aureus*. For isolates

---

Table 12-5 Phenotypic Characteristics for Identification of *Rothia mucilaginosa*

CHARACTERISTIC	REACTION	CHARACTERISTIC	REACTION
Catalase	V	Glucose	+
Acetoin (VP)	+	Sucrose	+
Gelatin hydrolysis	+	Fructose	+
Growth under anaerobic conditions	+	Salicin	+
Growth on nutrient agar with 5% NaCl	−	Mannose	V
Coagulase	−	Trehalose	V
Alkaline phosphatase	−	Mannitol	−
		Sorbitol	−

+, positive reaction; −, negative reaction; V, variable reaction.

that are coagulase-negative, a furazolidone or bacitracin disk test, or the modified oxidase test may be performed to differentiate coagulase-negative staphylococci from *Micrococcus* and related species. Significant staphylococcal isolates from urine cultures should also be tested for susceptibility to novobiocin for presumptive identification of *S. saprophyticus*. Complete species identification using a kit method or the reference procedure should be reserved for clinically significant isolates. These may include isolates that have been recovered from multiple sets of blood cultures, from infected intravenous catheters (where the patient may have the same isolate in multiple blood cultures), or from other normally sterile sites where the same coagulase-negative staphylococcus has been repeatedly isolated. Decisions involving further identification of these organisms should be made on a case-by-case basis with input from both the laboratory and the physicians caring for the patient.

REFERENCES

1. Abraham J, Bilgrami S, Dorsky D, et al. *Stomatococcus mucilaginosus* meningitis in a patient with multiple myeloma following autologous stem cell transplantation. Bone Marrow Transplant 1997;19:639–641.
2. Abrahamsson K, Hansson S, Jodal U, Lincoln K. *Staphylococcus saprophyticus* urinary tract infections in children. Eur J Pediatr 1993;152:69–71.
3. Akatova E, Schumacher-Perdreau F, Pulverer G. A DNA probe for the detection of the species *Staphylococcus haemolyticus*. FEMS Microbiol Lett 1992;15:93–96.
4. Akiyama H, Kanzaki H, Tada J, Arata J. Coagulase-negative staphylococci isolated from various skin lesions. J Dermatol 1998;25:563–568.
5. Alam SI, Singh L, Dube S, et al. Psychrophilic *Planococcus maitriensis* sp. nov. from Antarctica. Syst Appl Microbiol 2003;26:505–510.
6. Allignet J, Aubert S, Dyke KG, El Sohl N. *Staphylococcus caprae* strains carry determinants known to be involved in pathogenicity: a gene encoding an autolysin binding fibronectin and the *ica* operon involved in biofilm formation. Infect Immun 2001;69:712–718.
7. Allignet J, Galdbart JO, Morvan A, et al. Tracking adhesion factors in *Staphylococcus caprae* strains responsible for human bone infections following implantation of orthopaedic material. Microbiology 1999;145:2033–2042.
8. Al-Rashdan A, Bashir R, Khan FA. *Staphylococci capitis* causing aortic valve endocarditis. J Heart Valve Dis 1998;7:519–520.
9. Anday E, Talbot G. Coagulase-negative staphylococcal bacteremia: a rising threat in the newborn infant. Ann Clin Lab Sci 1985;13:246–251.
10. Andresen LO. Differentiation and distribution of three types of exfoliative toxin produced by *Staphylococcus hyicus* from pigs with exudative epidermitis. FEMS Immunol Med Microbiol 1998;20:301–310.
11. Andrews AH, Lamport A. Isolation of *Staphylococcus chromogenes* from an unusual case of impetigo in a goat. Vet Rec 1997;140:584.
12. Andstrom E, Bygdeman S, Ahlen S, et al. *Stomatococcus mucilaginosus* septicemia in two bone marrow transplanted patients. Scand J Infect Dis 1995;26:209–214.
13. Arbeit RD, Karakawa WW, Vann WF, et al. Predominance of two newly described capsular polysaccharide types among clinical isolates of *Staphylococcus aureus*. Diagn Microbiol Infect Dis 1984;2:85–91.
14. Archer GL. *Staphylococcus epidermidis* and other coagulase-negative staphylococci. In: Mandell GL, Bennett JE, Dolin R, eds. Mandell, Douglas, and Bennett's Principles and Practice of Infectious Diseases. 5th Ed. New York, Churchill-Livingstone, 2000:2092–2100.
15. Arciola CR, Montanaro L, Baldassarri L, et al. Slime production by staphylococci isolated from prosthesis-associated infections. New Microbiol 1999;22:337–341.
16. Aubert G, Passot S, Lucht F, Dorche G. Selection of vancomycin- and teicoplanin-resistant *Staphylococcus haemolyticus* during teicoplanin treatment of *S. epidermidis* infection. J Antimicrob Chemother 1990;25:491–493.
17. Baddour LM, Barker LP, Christensen GD, et al. Phenotypic variation of *Staphylococcus epidermidis* in infection of transvenous endocardial pacemaker electrodes. J Clin Microbiol 1990;28:676–679.
18. Baddour LM, Smalley DL, Kraus AP Jr, et al. Comparison of characteristics of pathogenic and saprophytic coagulase-negative staphylococci from patients on continuous ambulatory peritoneal dialysis. Diagn Microbiol Infect Dis 1986;5:197–205.
19. Baker JS. Comparison of various methods for differentiation of staphylococci and micrococci. J Clin Microbiol 1984;19:875–879.
20. Baker JS, Borman MA, Boudreau DH. Evaluation of various rapid agglutination methods for the identification of *Staphylococcus aureus*. J Clin Microbiol 1985;21:726–729.
21. Baldassarri L, Donelli G, Gelosia A, et al. Purification and characterization of the staphylococcal slime-associated antigen and its occurrence among *Staphylococcus epidermidis* clinical isolates. Infect Immun 1996;64:3410–3415.
22. Bannerman TL, Kleeman KT, Kloos WE. Evaluation of the Vitek Systems gram-positive identification card for species identification of coagulase-negative staphylococci. J Clin Microbiol 1993;31:1322–1325.
23. Bannerman TL, Kloos WE. *Staphylococcus capitis* subsp. *ureolyticus* subsp. nov. from human skin. Int J Syst Bacteriol 1991;41:144–147.
24. Basaglia G, Moras L, Bearz A, et al. *Staphylococcus cohnii* septicaemia in a patient with colon cancer. J Med Microbiol 2003;52:101–102.
25. Becker K, Schumann P, Wullenweber J, et al. *Kytococcus schroeteri* sp. nov., a novel gram-positive actinobacterium isolated from a human clinical source. Int J Syst Evol Microbiol 2002;52:1609–1614.
26. Bedidi-Madani N, Kodjo A, Villard L, Richard Y. Ribotyping of *Staphylococcus caprae* isolated from goat milk. Vet Res 1998;29:149–158.
27. Bellamy R, Barkham T. *Staphylococcus lugdunensis* infection sites: predominance of abscesses in the pelvic girdle region. Clin Infect Dis 2002;35:E32–E34.
28. Bennett MI, Tai YMA, Symonds JM. Staphylococcal meningitis following Synchromed intrathecal pump implant: a case report. Pain 1994;56:243–244.
29. Bergan T, Kocur M. *Stomatococcus mucilaginosus* gen. nov., sp. nov., emend. rev., a member of the family *Micrococcaceae*. Int J Syst Bacteriol 1982;32:374–377.
30. Bergan T, Kocur M. Genus II. Stomatococcus. In: Sneath PHA, Nair NS, Holt JG, eds. Bergey's Manual of Systematic Bacteriology. Vol. 2. Baltimore: Williams & Wilkins, 1986:1008–1010.
31. Bergdoll MS, Reiser RF, Crass BA, et al. A new staphylococcal enterotoxin, enterotoxin F, associated with toxic shock syndrome *Staphylococcus aureus* isolates. Lancet 1981;1:1017–1021.
32. Bergdoll MS, Schlievert PM. Toxic shock syndrome toxin. Lancet 1984;2:691.
33. Bergman B, Wedren H, Holm SE. *Staphylococcus saprophyticus* in males with symptoms of chronic prostatitis. Urology 1989;34:241–245.
34. Bhakdi S, Muhly M, Fussle R. Correlation between toxin binding and hemolytic activity in membrane damage by staphylococcal α-toxin. Infect Immun 1984;46:318–323.
35. Biavasco F, Vignaroli C, Lazzarini R, Varaldo PE. Glycopeptide susceptibility profiles of *Staphylococcus haemolyticus* bloodstream isolates. Antimicrob Agents Chemother 2000;44:3122–3126.
36. Biavasco F, Vignaroli C, Varaldo PE. Glycopeptide resistance in coagulase-negative staphylococci. Eur J Clin Microbiol Infect Dis 2000;19:403–417.
37. Billot-Klein D, Gutmann L, Bryant D, et al. Peptidoglycan synthesis and structure in *Staphylococcus haemolyticus* expressing increasing levels of resistance to glycopeptide antibiotics. J Bacteriol 1996;178:4696–4703.
38. Bingen E, Barc MC, Brahimi N, et al. Randomly amplified polymorphic DNA analysis provides rapid differentiation of methicillin-resistant coagulase-negative staphylococci. J Clin Microbiol 1995;32:2113–2119.
39. Birnbaum D, Herwaldt L, Low DE, et al. Efficacy of Microbial Identification System for epidemiologic typing of coagulase-negative staphylococci. J Clin Microbiol 1994;32:2113–2119.
40. Blomster-Hautamaa DA, Kreiswirth BN, Novick RP, Schlievert PM. The resolution of highly purified toxic shock syndrome toxin-1 (TSST-1) into two distinct proteins by isoelectric focusing. Biochemistry 1986;25:54–59.
41. Blumberg HM, Rimland D, Kiehlbauch JA, et al. Epidemiological typing of *Staphylococcus aureus* by DNA restriction fragment length polymorphisms of rRNA genes: elucidation of the clonal nature of a group of bacteriophage-nontypeable, ciprofloxacin-resistant, methicillin-susceptible *S. aureus* isolates. J Clin Microbiol 1992;30:362–369.
42. Bobin S, Durand-Dubief A, Bouhour D, et al. Pacemaker endocarditis due to *Staphylococcus lugdunensis*: report of two cases. Clin Infect Dis 1999;28:404–405.
43. Boden M, Flock J-L. Evidence for three different fibrinogen-binding proteins with unique properties from *Staphylococcus aureus* strain Newman. Microb Pathog 1992;12:289–298.
44. Bohach GA, Fast DJ, Nelson RD, Schlievert PM. Staphylococcal and streptococcal pyrogenic toxins involved in toxic shock syndrome and related illnesses. Crit Rev Microbiol 1990;17:251–272.
45. Bowman RA, Buck M. *Staphylococcus hominis* septicaemia in patients with cancer. Med J Aust 1984;140:26–27.

46. Boyce JM. Strategies for controlling methicillin-resistant *Staphylococcus aureus* in hospitals. J Chemother 1995;7(Suppl 3):81–85.

47. Brakstad OG, Aasbakk K, Maeland JA. Detection of *Staphylococcus aureus* by polymerase chain reaction amplification of the *nuc* gene. J Clin Microbiol 1992; 30:1654–1660.

48. Brakstad OG, Maeland JA, Chesneau O. Comparison of tests designed to identify *Staphylococcus aureus* thermostable endonuclease. APMIS 1995;103:219–224.

49. Brun Y, Bes M, Boeufgras JM, et al. International collaborative evaluation of the ATB 32 Staph gallery for identification of the *Staphylococcus* species. Zentralbl Bakteriol 1990;273:319–326.

50. Brunet F, Vedel G, Dreyfus F, et al. Failure of teicoplanin therapy in two neutropenic patients with staphylococcal septicemia who recovered after administration of vancomycin. Eur J Clin Microbiol Infect Dis 1990;9:145–147.

51. Bryan CS, Parisi JT, Strike DG. Vertebral osteomyelitis due to *Staphylococcus warneri* attributed to a Hickman catheter. Diagn Microbiol Infect Dis 1987;8: 57–59.

52. Bryant RE, Salmon CJ. Pleural empyema. Clin Infect Dis 1996;22:747–762.

53. Burgert SJ, LaRocco MT, Wilansky S. Destructive native valve endocarditis caused by *Staphylococcus lugdunensis*. South Med J 1999;92:812–814.

54. Buttery JP, Easton MN, Pearson SR, Hogg GG. Pediatric bacteremia due to *Staphylococcus warneri*: microbiological, epidemiological, and clinical features. J Clin Microbiol 1997;35:2174–2177.

55. Calderwood SB, Swinski LA, Waternaux CM, et al. Risk factors for the development of prosthetic valve endocarditis. Circulation 1985;72:31–37.

56. Calvo J, Hernandez JL, Farinas MC, et al. Osteomyelitis caused by *Staphylococcus schleiferi* and evidence of misidentification by an automated bacterial identification system. J Clin Microbiol 2000;38:3887–3889.

57. Camacho M, Guis S, Mattei JP, et al. Three-year outcome in a patient with *Staphylococcus lugdunensis* discitis. Joint Bone Spine 2002;69:85–87.

58. Caputo G, Archer G, Calderwood S, et al. Native valve endocarditis due to coagulase-negative staphylococci: clinical and microbiologic features. Am J Med 1987;83:619–625.

59. Caragee EJ. Pyogenic vertebral osteomyelitis. J Bone Joint Surg Am 1997;79: 874–880.

60. Carney DN, Fossieck BE, Parker RH, et al. Bacteremia due to *Staphylococcus aureus* in patients with cancer: report on 45 cases and a review of the literature. Rev Infect Dis 1982 ;4:1–12.

61. Cartwright MJ, King MH, Weinberg RS, Guerry RK. *Micrococcus* endophthalmitis. Arch Ophthalmol 1990;108:1523–1524.

62. Castro JG, Dowdy L. Septic shock caused by *Staphylococcus lugdunensis*. Clin Infect Dis 1999;28:681–682.

63. Cavassini N, Wenger A, Jaton K, et al. Evaluation of MRSA Screen, a simple anti-PBP 2a slide latex agglutination kit, for rapid detection of methicillin resistance in *Staphylococcus aureus*. J Clin Microbiol 1999;37:1591–1594.

64. Celard M, Lelievre H, Obadia JF, et al. Long-standing bacteremia and endocarditis caused by *Staphylococcus lugdunensis* in a patient with an implantable cardioverter defibrillator. Clin Microbiol Infect 1997;3:387–388.

65. Celard M, Vandenesch F, Darbas H, et al. Pacemaker infection caused by *Staphylococcus schleiferi*, a member of the human preaxillary flora: four case reports. Clin Infect Dis 1997;24:1014–1015.

66. Centers for Disease Control and Prevention. Reduced susceptibility of *Staphylococcus aureus* to vancomycin—Japan, 1996. MMWR Morb Mortal Wkly Rep 1997;46:624–626.

67. Centers for Disease Control and Prevention. *Staphylococcus aureus* with reduced susceptibility to vancomycin—United States, 1997. MMWR Morb Mortal Wkly Rep 1997;46:765–766.

68. Centers for Disease Control and Prevention. *Staphylococcus aureus* with reduced susceptibility to vancomycin—Illinois, 1999. MMWR Morb Mortal Wkly Rep 1999;48:1165–1167.

69. Centers for Disease Control and Prevention. *Staphylococcus aureus* resistant to vancomycin—United States, 2002. MMWR Morb Mortal Wkly Rep 2002;51: 565–567.

70. Centers for Disease Control and Prevention. Vancomycin-resistant *Staphylococcus aureus*—Pennsylvania, 2002. MMWR Morb Mortal Wkly Rep 2002;51: 902.

71. Centers for Disease Control and Prevention. Vancomycin-resistant *Staphylococcus aureus*—New York, 2004. MMWR Morb Mortal Wkly Rep 2004;53: 322–323.

72. Chamberlain NR. Identification and partial characterization of an extracellular activator of fatty acid modifying enzyme (FAME) expression in *Staphylococcus epidermidis*. J Med Microbiol 1999;48:245–252.

73. Chamberlain NR, Brueggemann SA. Characterisation and expression of fatty acid modifying enzyme produced by *Staphylococcus epidermidis*. J Med Microbiol 1997;46:693–697.

74. Chesneau O, Aubert S, Morvan A, et al. Usefulness of the ID32 Staph System and a method based on rRNA gene restriction site polymorphism analysis for species and subspecies identification of staphylococcal clinical isolates. J Clin Microbiol 1992;30:2346–2352.

75. Chesneau O, Morvan A, Grimont F, et al. *Staphylococcus pasteuri* sp. nov. isolated from human, animal, and food specimens. Int J Syst Bacteriol 1993; 43:237–244.

76. Chiou CS, Wei HL, Yang LC. Comparison of pulsed-field gel electrophoresis and coagulase gene restriction profile analysis techniques in the molecular typing of *Staphylococcus aureus*. J Clin Microbiol 2000;38:2186–2190.

77. Christensen GD, Bisno A, Parisi J, et al. Nosocomial septicemia due to multiply antibiotic resistant *Staphylococcus epidermidis*. Ann Intern Med 1992;96:1–10.

78. Climo MW, Patron RL, Archer GL. Combinations of vancomycin and β-lactams are synergistic against staphylococci with reduced susceptibilities to vancomycin. Antimicrob Agents Chemother 1999;43:1747–1753.

79. Collins MD, Hutson RA, Baverud V, Falsen E. Characterization of a *Rothia*-like organism from a mouse: description of *Rothia nasimurium* sp. nov. and reclassification of *Stomatococcus mucilaginosus* as *Rothia mucilaginosa* comb. nov. Int J Syst Evol Microbiol 2000;50:1247–1251.

80. Collins MD, Lawson PA, Labrenz M, et al. *Nesterenkonia lacusekhoensis* sp. nov., isolated from hypersaline Ekho Lake, East Antarctica, and emended description of the genus *Nesterenkonia*. Int J Syst Evol Microbiol 2002;52: 1145–1150.

81. Cooper GJ, Hopkins CC. Rapid diagnosis of intravascular catheter-associated infection by direct gram staining of catheter segments. N Engl J Med 1985;312: 1142–1147.

82. Coudron PE, Markowitz SM, Mohanty LB, et al. Isolation of *Stomatococcus mucilaginosus* from drug user with endocarditis. J Clin Microbiol 1987;25: 1359–1363.

83. Coural SA, SA, West BC. Endocarditis caused by *Staphylococcus xylosus* associated with intravenous drug abuse. J Infect Dis 1984;149:826–827.

84. Couto I, Sanches IS, Sa-Leao R, de Lencastre H. Molecular characterization of *Staphylococcus sciuri* strains isolated from humans. J Clin Microbiol 2000;38: 1136–1143.

85. Crass BA, Bergdoll MS. Involvement of coagulase-negative staphylococci in toxic shock syndrome. J Clin Microbiol 1986;23:43–45.

86. Cunniffe JG, Mallia C, Alcock PA. *Stomatococcus mucilaginosus* lower respiratory tract infection in a patient with AIDS. J Infect 1994;29:327–330.

87. Dan M, Marien G, Goldsand G. Endocarditis caused by *Staphylococcus warneri* on a normal aortic heart valve following vasectomy. Can Med Assoc J 1984; 131:211–213.

88. Darouche RO, Raad II, Heard SO, et al. A comparison of two antimicrobial-impregnated central venous catheters. N Engl J Med 1999;320:1–8.

89. Dassy B, Stringfellow WT, Lieb M, Fournier JM. Production of type 5 capsular polysaccharide by *Staphylococcus aureus* grown in a semi-synthetic medium. J Gen Microbiol 1991;137:1155–1162.

90. Davis GHG, Hoyling B. Use of a rapid acetoin test in the identification of staphylococci and micrococci. Int J Syst Bacteriol 1973;23:281–282.

91. Davis TE, Fuller DD. Direct identification of bacterial isolates in blood cultures by using a DNA probe. J Clin Microbiol 1991;29:2193–2196.

92. Dawson MS, Harford AM, Garner BK, et al. Total volume culture technique for the isolation of microorganisms from continuous ambulatory peritoneal dialysis patients with peritonitis. J Clin Microbiol 1985;22:391–394.

93. Degener JE, Heck MEO, van Leeuwen WJ, et al. Nosocomial infection by *Staphylococcus haemolyticus* and typing methods for epidemiological study. J Clin Microbiol 1994;32:2260–2265.

94. De La Fuente R, Suarez G, Schleifer JH. *Staphylococcus aureus* subsp. *anaerobius* subsp. nov., the causal agent of abscess disease of sheep. Int J Syst Bacteriol 1985;35:99–102.

95. Deplano A, Vaneechoutte M, Verschraegen G, Struelens MJ. Typing of *Staphylococcus aureus* and *Staphylococcus epidermidis* strains by PCR analysis of inter-*IS*256 spacer length polymorphisms. J Clin Microbiol 1997;35:2580–2587.

96. Devriese LA, Hajek V, Oeding P, et al. *Staphylococcus hyicus* (Sompolinsky 1953) comb. nov. and *Staphylococcus hyicus* subsp. *chromogenes* subsp. nov. Int J Syst Bacteriol 1978;28:482–490.

97. Devriese LA, Poutrel B, Kilpper-Balz R, et al. *Staphylococcus gallinarum* and *Staphylococcus caprae*, two new species from animals. Int J Syst Bacteriol 1983; 33:480–486.

98. Dinges MM, Orwin PM, Schlievert PM. Exotoxins of *Staphylococcus aureus*. Clin Microbiol Rev 2000;13:16–34.

99. Doern LK, Earls JE, Jeznach PA, et al. Species identification and biotyping of staphylococci by the API Staph-Ident system. J Clin Microbiol 1983;17: 260–263.

100. Eidhin DN, Perkins S, Francois P, et al. Clumping factor B (ClfB), a new surface-located fibrinogen binding adhesin of *Staphylococcus aureus*. Mol Microbiol 1998;30:245–257.

101. Elliott SP, Yogev R, Schulman ST. *Staphylococcus lugdunensis*: an emerging cause of ventriculoperitoneal shunt infections. Pediatr Neurosurg 2001;35: 128–130.

102. Elsner HA, Dahmen GP, Laufs R, Mack D. Intra-articular empyema due to *Staphylococcus caprae* following arthroscopic cruciate ligament repair. J Infect 1998;37:66–67.

103. Engelhardt MA, Daly K, Swannell RP, Head IM. Isolation and characterization of a novel hydrocarbon-degrading, gram-positive bacterium, isolated from intertidal beach sediment, and description of *Planococcus alkanoclasticus* sp. nov. J Appl Microbiol 2001;90:237–247.

104. Falk D, Guering SJ. Differentiation of *Staphylococcus* and *Micrococcus* spp. with the Taxo A bacitracin disk. J Clin Microbiol 1983;18:719–720.

105. Faller A, Schleifer KH. Modified oxidase and benzidine tests for separation of staphylococci and micrococci. J Clin Microbiol 1981;13:1031–1035.

106. Fernandes AP, Perl TM, Herwaldt LA. *Staphylococcus cohnii*: a case report on an unusual pathogen. Clin Perform Qual Health Care 1996;4:107–109.

107. Fervenza FC, Contreras GE, Garratt KN, Steckelberg JM. *Staphylococcus lugdunensis* endocarditis: a complication of vasectomy? Mayo Clin Proc 1999;74:1227–1230.

108. Fey PD, Ulphani JS, Gotz F, et al. Characterization of the relationship between polysaccharide intercellular adhesin and hemagglutination in *Staphylococcus epidermidis*. J Infect Dis 1999;179:1561–1564.

109. Fidalgo S, Vasquez F, Mendoza M, et al. Bacteremia due to *Staphylococcus epidermidis*: microbiologic, epidemiologic, clinical, and prognostic features. Rev Infect Dis 1990;12:520–528.

110. Forsgren A, Sjogulst J. "Protein A" from *Staphylococcus aureus* I. Pseudo immune reaction with human globulin. J. Immunol 1966;97:822.

111. Foster G, Ross HM, Hutson RA, Collins MD. *Staphylococcus lutrae* sp. nov., a new coagulase-positive species isolated from otters. Int J Syst Bacteriol 1997;47:724–726.

112. Fournier JM, Boutonnier A, Bouvet A. *Staphylococcus aureus* strains which are not identified by rapid agglutination procedures are of capsular serotype 5. J Clin Microbiol 1989;27:1372–1374.

113. Fournier JM, Bouvet A, Boutonnier A, et al. Predominance of capsular type 5 among oxacillin-resistant *Staphylococcus aureus*. J Clin Microbiol 1987;25:1932–1933.

114. Fournier JM, Bouvet A, Mathieu D, et al. New latex reagent using monoclonal antibodies to capsular polysaccharide for reliable identification of both oxacillin-susceptible and oxacillin-resistant *Staphylococcus aureus*. J Clin Microbiol 1993;31:1342–1344.

115. Fournier JM, Vann WF, Karakawa WW. Purification and characterization of *Staphylococcus aureus* type 8 capsular polysaccharide. Infect Immun 1984;45:87–93.

116. Fowler CG Jr, Sanders LL, Kong LK, et al. Infective endocarditis due to *Staphylococcus aureus*: 59 prospectively identified cases with follow-up. Clin Infect Dis 1999;28:106–114.

117. Fowler VG Jr, Sanders LL, Sexton DJ, et al. Outcome of *Staphylococcus aureus* bacteremia according to compliance with recommendations of infectious diseases specialists: experience with 244 patients. Clin Infect Dis 1998;27:478–486.

118. Frame PT, McLaurin RL. Treatment of CSF shunt infections with intrashunt plus oral antibiotic therapy. J Neurosurg 1984;60:354–360.

119. Frank LA, Kania SA, Hnilica KA, et al. Isolation of *Staphylococcus schleiferi* from dogs with pyoderma. J Am Vet Med Assoc 2003;222:451–454.

120. Freeman J, Goldmann DA, Smith NE, et al. Association of intravenous lipid emulsion and coagulase-negative staphylococcal bacteremia in neonatal intensive care units. N Engl J Med 1990;323:301–308.

121. Freney J, Brun Y, Bes M, et al. *Staphylococcus lugdunensis* sp. nov. and *Staphylococcus schleiferi* sp. nov., two species from human clinical specimens. Int J Syst Bacteriol 1988;38:168–172.

122. Freney J, Kloos WE, Hajek V, Webster JA. Recommended minimal standards for description of new staphylococcal species. Int J Syst Bacteriol 1999;49:489–501.

123. Gaillot O, Wetsch M, Fortineau N, Berche P. Evaluation of CHROMagar Staph. aureus, a new chromogenic medium, for isolation and presumptive identification of *Staphylococcus aureus* from human clinical specimens. J Clin Microbiol 2000;38:1587–1591.

124. Garrett DO, Jochimsen E, Murfitt K, et al. The emergence of decreased susceptibility to vancomycin in *Staphylococcus epidermidis*. Infect Control Hosp Epidemiol 1999;20:167–170.

125. Garrity G, Holt JG. Bergey's Manual of Systematic Bacteriology: an overview of the road map to the manual. New York: Bergey's Manual Trust, 2000.

126. Gatermann S, Kreft B, Marre R, et al. Identification and characterization of a surface-associated protein (Ssp) of *Staphylococcus saprophyticus*. Infect Immun 1992;60:1055–1060.

127. Gatermann SG, Meyer HG. *Staphylococcus saprophyticus* hemagglutinin binds fibronectin. Infect Immun 1994;62:4556–4563.

128. Gatermann S, Meyer HG, Wanner G. *Staphylococcus saprophyticus* hemagglutinin is a 160-kilodalton surface polypeptide. Infect Immun 1992;60:4127–4132.

129. Geary C, Stevens M. Rapid lysostaphin test to differentiate *Staphylococcus* and *Micrococcus* species. J Clin Microbiol 1986;23:1044–1045.

130. Geary C, Stevens M. Detection of phosphatase production by *Staphylococcus* species: a new method. Med Lab Sci 1989;46:291–294.

131. Geary C, Stevens M. A rapid test to detect the most clinically significant *Staphylococcus* species. Med Lab Sci 1991;48:99–105.

132. George CG, Kloos WE. Comparison of the SmaI-digested chromosomes of *Staphylococcus epidermidis* and the closely related species *Staphylococcus capitis* and *Staphylococcus caprae*. Int J Syst Bacteriol 1994;44:404–409.

133. Gerke C, Kraft A, Submuth R, et al. Characterization of *N*-acetyl-glucosaminyl-transferase activity in the biosynthesis of the *Staphylococcus epidermidis* polysaccharide intercellular adhesin. J Biol Chem 1998;273:18586–18593.

134. Gerstadt K, Daly JS, Mitchell M, et al. Methicillin-resistant *Staphylococcus intermedius* pneumonia following coronary artery bypass grafting. Clin Infect Dis 1999;29:218–219.

135. Giger P, Charilaou CC, Cundy KR. Comparison of the API Staph-Ident and the DMS Staph-Trac systems with conventional methods used for identification of coagulase-negative staphylococci. J Clin Microbiol 1984;19:68–72.

136. Girard C, Higgins R. *Staphylococcus intermedius* cellulitis and toxic shock in a dog. Can Vet J 1999;40:501–502.

137. Glimaker M, Granert C, Krook A. Septicemia caused by *Staphylococcus saprophyticus*. Scand J Infect Dis 1988;20:347–348.

138. Goh SH, Potter S, Wood JO, et al. *HSP60* gene sequences as universal targets for microbial species identification: studies with coagulase-negative staphylococci. J Clin Microbiol 1996;34:818–823.

139. Goh SH, Santucci Z, Kloos WE, et al. Identification of *Staphylococcus* species and subspecies by the chaperonin 60 gene identification method and reverse checkerboard hybridization. J Clin Microbiol 1997;35:3116–3121.

140. Goldman M, Chaudhary UB, Greist A, Fausel CA. Central nervous system infections due to *Stomatococcus mucilaginosus* in immunocompromised hosts. Clin Infect Dis 1998;27:1241–1246.

141. Goldstein J, Schulman R, Kelley E, et al. Effect of different media on determination of novobiocin resistance for differentiation of coagulase-negative staphylococci. J Clin Microbiol 1983;18:592–595.

142. Gombert ME, Landesman SH, Corrado ML, et al. Vancomycin and rifampin therapy for *Staphylococcus epidermidis* meningitis associated with CSF shunts: report of three cases. J Neurosurg 1981;55:633–636.

143. Gonzalez C, Rubio M, Romero-Vivas J, et al. Bacteremic pneumonia due to *Staphylococcus aureus*: a comparison of disease caused by methicillin-resistant and methicillin-susceptible organisms. Clin Infect Dis 1999;29:1171–1177.

144. Grant CE, Sewell DL, Pfaller M, et al. Evaluation of two commercial systems for identification of coagulase-negative staphylococci to species level. Diagn Microbiol Infect Dis 1994;18:1–5.

145. Grasmick AE, Naito N, Bruckner DA. Clinical comparison of the AutoMicrobic system gram-positive identification card, API Staph-Ident, and conventional methods in the identification of coagulase-negative *Staphylococcus* spp. J Clin Microbiol 1983;18:1323–1328.

146. Gray GS, Kehoe M. Primary sequence of the α-toxin gene from *Staphylococcus aureus* Wood 46. Infect Immun 1984;46:615–618.

147. Gregson DB, Low DE, Skulnick M, et al. Problems with rapid agglutination of *Staphylococcus aureus* when *Staphylococcus saprophyticus* is being tested. J Clin Microbiol 1988;26:1398–1399.

148. Grossi EA, Culliford AT, Krieger KH, et al. A survey of 77 major infectious complications of median sternotomy: a review of 7,949 consecutive operative procedures. Ann Thorac Surg 1985;40:224–228.

149. Gruson D, Hilbert G, Pigneux A, et al. Severe infection caused by *Stomatococcus mucilaginosus* in a neutropenic patient: case report and review of the literature. Hematol Cell Ther 1998;40:167–169.

150. Guardati MC, Guzman CA, Piatti G, et al. Rapid methods for identification of *Staphylococcus aureus* when both human and animal staphylococci are tested: comparison with a new immunoenzymatic assay. J Clin Microbiol 1993;31:1606–1608.

151. Gudding R. Differentiation of staphylococci on the basis of nuclease properties. J Clin Microbiol 1983;18:1098–1101.

152. Gunn BA, Davis CE Jr. *Staphylococcus haemolyticus* urinary tract infection in a male patient. J Clin Microbiol 1988;26:1055–1057.

153. Gupta K, Hooton TM, Wobbe CL, Stamm WE. The prevalence of antimicrobial resistance among uropathogens causing acute uncomplicated cystitis in young women. Int J Antimicrob Agents 1999;11:305–308.

154. Guzman CA, Guardati MC, Fenoglio D, et al. Novel immunoenzymatic assay for identification of coagulase- and protein A-negative *Staphylococcus aureus* strains. J Clin Microbiol 1992;30:1194–1197.

155. Haile DT, Hughes J, Vetter E, et al. Frequency of isolation of *Staphylococcus lugdunensis* in consecutive urine cultures and relationship to urinary tract infection. J Clin Microbiol 2002;40:654–656.

156. Hajek V. *Staphylococcus intermedius*, a new species isolated from animals. Int J Syst Bacteriol 1976;26:401–408.

157. Hajek V, Devreise LA, Mordarski M, et al. Elevation of *Staphylococcus hyicus* subsp. *chromogenes* (Devreise, et al., 1978) to species status: *Staphylococcus chromogenes* (Devreise, et al, 1978) comb. nov. Syst Appl Microbiol 1986;8:169–173.

158. Hajek V, Ludwig W, Schleifer KH, et al. *Staphylococcus muscae*, a new species isolated from flies. Int J Syst Bacteriol 1992;42:97–101.

159. Hajek V, Meugnier H, Bes M, et al. *Staphylococcus saprophyticus* subsp. *bovis* subsp. nov., isolated from bovine nostrils. Int J Syst Bacteriol 1996;46:792–796.

160. Hajjeh RA, Reingold A, Weil A, et al. Toxic shock syndrome in the United States: surveillance update, 1979–1996. Emerg Infect Dis 1999;5:807–810.

161. Harjola VP, Valtonen M, Sivonen A. Association of *Stomatococcus mucilaginosus* with cholangitis. Eur J Clin Microbiol Infect Dis 1994;13:606–608.

162. Hebert GA. Hemolysins and other characteristics that help differentiate and biotype *Staphylococcus lugdunensis* and *Staphylococcus schleiferi*. J Clin Microbiol 1990;28:2425–2431.

163. Hebert GA, Crowder CG, Hancock GA, et al. Characteristics of coagulase-negative staphylococci that help differentiate these species from other members of the Family Micrococcaceae. J Clin Microbiol 1988;26:1939–1946.

164. Hedin G, Wilderstrom M. Endocarditis due to *Staphylococcus sciuri*. Eur J Clin Microbiol Infect Dis 1998;17:673–675.

165. Hedman P, Ringertz O, Eriksson B, et al. *Staphylococcus saprophyticus* found to be a common contaminant of food. J Infect 1990;21:11–19.

166. Hedman P, Ringertz O, Lindstrom M, Olsson K. The origin of *Staphylococcus saprophyticus* from cattle and pigs. Scand J Infect Dis 1993;25:57–60.

167. Hedman P, Ringertz O, Olsson K, Wollin R. Plasmid-identified *Staphylococcus saprophyticus* isolated from the rectum of patients with urinary tract infections. Scand J Infect Dis 1991;23:569–572.

168. Heilmann C, Hussain M, Peter G, Gotz F. Evidence for autolysin-mediated primary attachment of *Staphylococcus epidermidis* to a polystyrene surface. Mol Microbiol 1997;24:1013–1024.

169. Heilmann, C, Schweitzer O, Gerke C, et al. Molecular basis of intercellular adhesion in the biofilm-forming *Staphylococcus epidermidis*. Mol Microbiol 1996;30:1083–1091.

170. Hell W, Kern T, Klouche M. *Staphylococcus saprophyticus* as an unusual cause of nosocomial pneumonia. Clin Infect Dis 1999;29:685–686.

171. Hell W, Meyer HG, Gatermann SG. Cloning of *aas*, a gene encoding a *Staphylococcus saprophyticus* surface protein with adhesive and autolytic properties. Mol Microbiol 1998;29:871–881.

172. Hernandez JL, Calvo J, Sota R, et al. Clinical and microbiological characteristics of 28 patients with *Staphylococcus schleiferi* infection. Eur J Clin Microbiol Infect Dis 2001;20:153–158.

173. Herrmann M, Vaudeaux PE, Pittet D, et al. Fibronectin, fibrinogen, and laminin act as mediators for adherence of clinical staphylococcal isolates to foreign materials. J Infect Dis 1988;158:693–701.

174. Herwaldt L, Boyken L, Pfaller M. *In vitro* selection of resistance to vancomycin in bloodstream isolates of *Staphylococcus haemolyticus* and *Staphylococcus epidermidis*. Eur J Clin Microbiol Infect Dis 1991;10:1007–1012.

175. Hiramatsu K, Hanaki H, Ino T, et al. Methicillin-resistant *Staphylococcus aureus* clinical strain with reduced vancomycin susceptibility. J Antimicrob Chemother 1997;40:135–136.

176. Hjelm E, Lundell-Etherden I. Slime production by *Staphylococcus saprophyticus*. Infect Immun 1991;59:445–448.

177. Ho G, Campbell WH, Bergdoll MS, et al. Production of a toxic shock syndrome toxin variant by *Staphylococcus aureus* strains associated with sheep, goats, and cows. J Clin Microbiol 1989;27:1946–1948.

178. Hochkeppel HK, Braun DG, Vischer W, et al. Serotyping and electron microscopy studies of *Staphylococcus aureus* clinical isolates with monoclonal antibodies to capsular serotypes 5 and 8. J Clin Microbiol 1987;25:526–530.

179. Hoefnagle-Schuermans A, Peetermans WE, Struelens MJ, et al. Clonal analysis and identification of epidemic strains of methicillin-resistant *Staphylococcus aureus* by antibiotyping and determination of protein A gene and coagulase gene polymorphisms. J Clin Microbiol 1997;35:2514–2520.

180. Hookey JV, Richardson JF, Cookson BD. Molecular typing based on PCR restriction fragment length polymorphism and DNA sequence analysis of the coagulase gene. J Clin Microbiol 1997;36:1083–1089.

181. Hosotsubo K, Hosotsubo H, Nishijima MK, et al. Rapid screening for *Staphylococcus aureus* infection by measuring enterotoxin B. J Clin Microbiol 1989;27:2794–2798.

182. Hovelius B, Mardh PA. *Staphylococcus saprophyticus* as a common cause of urinary tract infections. Rev Infect Dis 1984;6:328–337.

183. Hsueh P-R, Teng L-J, Yang P-C, et al. Dissemination of two methicillin-resistant *Staphylococcus aureus* clones exhibiting negative Staphylase reactions in intensive care units. J Clin Microbiol 1999;37:504–509.

184. Hussain M, Herrmann M, von Eiff C, et al. A 140 kilodalton extracellular protein is essential for the accumulation of *Staphylococcus epidermidis* strains on surfaces. Infect Immun 1997;65:519–524.

185. Hussain Z, Stoakes L, Stevens DL, et al. Comparison of the MicroScan system with the API Staph-Ident system for species identification of coagulase-negative staphylococci. J Clin Microbiol 1986;23:126–128.

186. Ieven M, Jansens H, Ursi D, et al. Rapid detection of methicillin resistance in coagulase-negative staphylococci by commercially available fluorescence test. J Clin Microbiol 1995;33:2183–2185.

187. Ieven M, Verhoeven J, Pattyn SR, Goossens H. Rapid and economical method for species identification of clinically significant coagulase-negative staphylococci. J Clin Microbiol 1995;33:1060–1063.

188. Igarashi MA, Fujikawa H, Shigaki M, et al. Latex agglutination test for staphylococcal toxic shock syndrome toxin. J Clin Microbiol 1986;23:509–512.

189. Igimi S, Atobe H, Tohya Y, et al. Characterization of the most frequently encountered *Staphylococcus* sp. in cats. Vet Microbiol 1994;39:255–260.

190. Igimi S, Kawamura S, Takahashi E, et al. *Staphylococcus felis*, a new species from clinical specimens from cats. Int J Syst Bacteriol 1989;39:373–377.

191. Igimi S, Takahashi E, Mitsuoka T. *Staphylococcus schleiferi* subsp. *coagulans* subsp. nov., isolated from the external auditory meatus of dogs with external ear otitis. Int J Syst Bacteriol 1990;40:409–411.

192. Janda WM, Ristow K, Novak D. Evaluation of RapiDEC Staph for identification of *Staphylococcus aureus*, *Staphylococcus epidermidis*, and *Staphylococcus saprophyticus*. J Clin Microbiol 1994;32:2056–2059.

193. Jansen B, Schumacher-Perdreau F, Peters G, et al. Native valve endocarditis caused by *Staphylococcus simulans*. Eur J Clin Microbiol Infect Dis 1992;11:268–269.

194. Jarlov JO, Hojbjerg T, Busch-Sorensen C, et al. Coagulase-negative staphylococci in Danish blood cultures: species distribution and antibiotic susceptibility. J Hosp Infect 1996;32:217–227.

195. Jarraud S, Cozon G, Vandenesch F, et al. Involvement of enterotoxins G and I in staphylococcal toxic shock syndrome and staphylococcal scarlet fever. J Clin Microbiol 1999;37:2446–2449.

196. John MDV, Hibberd PL, Karchmer AW, et al. *Staphylococcus aureus* prosthetic valve endocarditis: optimal management and risk factors for death. Clin Infect Dis 1998;26:1302–1309.

197. Jones RM, Jackson MA, Ong C, Lofland GK. Endocarditis caused by *Staphylococcus lugdunensis*. Pediatr Infect Dis J 2002;21:254–268.

198. Junge K, Gosink JJ, Hoppe HG, Staley JL. *Arthrobacter*, *Brachybacterium*, and *Planococcus* isolates identified from Antarctic sea brine. Description of *Planococcus mcmeekinii* sp. nov. Syst Appl Microbiol 1998;21:306–314.

199. Jungkind DJ, Torhan NJ, Korman KE, et al. Comparison of two commercially available test methods with conventional coagulase tests for identification of *Staphylococcus aureus*. J Clin Microbiol 1984;19:191–193.

200. Kaabia N, Scauarda D, Lena G, Drancourt M. Molecular identification of *Staphylococcus lugdunensis* in a patient with meningitis. J Clin Microbiol 2002;40:1824–1825.

201. Kahler RC, Boyce JM, Bergdoll MS, et al. Case report: toxic shock syndrome associated with TSST-1-producing coagulase-negative staphylococci. Am J Med Sci 1986;292:310–312.

202. Kamalesh M, Aslam S. Aortic valve endocarditis due to *Staphylococcus capitis*. Echocardiography 2000;17:685–687.

203. Kamaraju S, Nelson K, Williams DN, et al. *Staphylococcus lugdunensis* pulmonary valve endocarditis in a patient on chronic hemodialysis. Am J Nephrol 1999;19:605–608.

204. Kanda K, Suzuki E, Hiramatsu K, et al. Identification of a methicillin-resistant strain of *Staphylococcus caprae* from a human clinical specimen. Antimicrob Agents Chemother 1991;35:174–176.

205. Karakawa WW, Sutton A, Schneerson R, et al. Capsular antibodies induce type-specific phagocytosis of capsulated *Staphylococcus aureus* by human polymorphonuclear leukocytes. Infect Immun 1988;56:1090–1095.

206. Karchmer AW, Archer GL, Dismukes WE. *Staphylococcus epidermidis* causing prosthetic valve endocarditis: microbiologic and clinical observations as guides to therapy. Ann Intern Med 198;98:447–455.

207. Kauffman CA, Hertz CS, Sheagren JN. *Staphylococcus saprophyticus*: role in urinary tract infections in men. J Urol 1983;130:493–494.

208. Kauffman CA, Sheagren JN, Quie PG. *Staphylococcus epidermidis* mediastinitis and disseminated intravascular coagulation. Ann Intern Med 1984;100:60–61.

209. Kawabatta S, Morita T, Iwanaga S, et al. Enzymatic properties of staphylothrombin, an active molecular complex formed between staphylocoagulase and human prothrombin. J Biochem 1966;98:1603–1605.

210. Kawamura Y, Hou XG, Sultana F, et al. Distribution of *Staphylococcus* species among human clinical isolates and emended description of *Staphylococcus caprae*. J Clin Microbiol 1998;36:2038–2042.

211. Kaya IS, Gamberzade S, Toppare MF, et al. Neonatal sepsis and meningitis due to *Staphylococcus cohnii*. JPMA J Pak Med Assoc 1996;46:43–44.

212. Kellogg JA, Hanna MD, Nelsen SJ, et al. Predictive values of species identifications from the Vitek Gram-Positive Identification card using clinical isolates of coagulase-negative staphylococci. Am J Clin Pathol 1996;106:374–377.

213. Kent TH. Staphylococcal enterotoxin gastroenteritis in rhesus monkeys. Am J Pathol 1966;48:387–407.

214. Kessler RB, Kimbrough RC, Jones SR. Infective endocarditis caused by *Staphylococcus hominis* after vasectomy. Clin Infect Dis 1998;27:216–217.

215. Kilpper-Balz R, Schleifer KH. Transfer of *Peptococcus saccharolyticus* (Foubert and Douglas) to the genus *Staphylococcus*: *Staphylococcus saccharolyticus* (Foubert and Douglas) comb. nov. Zentralbl Bakteriol Parasitenkd Infektionskr Hyg Abt 1 Orig 1981;2:324–331.

216. Kleeman KT, Bannerman TL, Kloos WE. Species distribution of coagulase-negative staphylococcal isolates at a community hospital and implications for selection of staphylococcal identification procedures. J Clin Microbiol 1993;31:1318–1321.

217. Kloos WE, Ballard DN, George CG, et al. Delimiting the genus *Staphylococcus* through description of *Macrococcus caseolyticus* gen. nov., comb. nov., and *Macrococcus equipercicus* sp. nov., and *Macrococcus bovicus* sp. nov., and *Macrococcus carouselicus* sp. nov. Int J Syst Bacteriol 1998;48:859–877.

218. Kloos WE, Ballard DN, Webster JA, et al. Ribotype delineation and description of *Staphylococcus sciuri* subspecies and their potential as reservoirs of methicillin resistance and staphylolytic enzyme genes. Int J Syst Bacteriol 1997;47:313–323.

219. Kloos WE, George CG. Identification of *Staphylococcus* species and subspecies with the MicroScan Pos ID and Rapid Pos ID panel systems. J Clin Microbiol 1991;29:738–744.

220. Kloos WE, George CG, Oligiate JS, et al. *Staphylococcus hominis* subsp. *novobiosepticus* subsp. nov., a novel trehalose- and N-acetyl-D-glucosamine-negative, novobiocin- and multiple-antibiotic-resistant subspecies isolated from human blood cultures. Int J Syst Bacteriol 1998;48:799–812.

221. Kloos WE, Lambe DW Jr. Staphylococcus. In: Balows A, Hausler WJ Jr, Herrman KL, Isenberg HD, Shadomy HJ, eds. Manual of Clinical Microbiology. 5th Ed. Washington DC: American Society for Microbiology, 1991:222–237.

222. Kloos WE, Schleifer KH. Isolation and characterization of staphylococci from human skin: II. Description of four new species: *Staphylococcus warneri*, *Staphylococcus capitis*, *Staphylococcus hominis*, and *Staphylococcus simulans*. Int J Syst Bacteriol 1975;25:62–79.

223. Kloos WE, Schleifer KH. Simplified scheme for routine identification of human *Staphylococcus* species. J Clin Microbiol 1975;1:82–87.

224. Kloos WE, Schleifer KH. *Staphylococcus auricularis* sp. nov.: an inhabitant of the human external ear. Int J Syst Bacteriol 1983;33:9–14.

225. Kloos WE, Schleifer KH. Genus IV. *Staphylococcus* Rosenbach 1884, 19[AL] (Nom. Cons. Opin. 17 Jud. Comm. 1958, 163). In: Sneath PHA, Mair NS, Sharpe ME, Holt JG, eds. Bergey's Manual of Systematic Bacteriology. Vol. 2. Baltimore: Williams & Wilkins, 1986:1013–1035.

226. Kloos WE, Schleifer KH, Smith RF. Characterization of *Staphylococcus sciuri* sp. nov. and its subspecies. Int J Syst Bacteriol 1976;26:22–37.

227. Kloos WE, Wolfshohl JF. Identification of *Staphylococcus* species with the API Staph-Ident system. J Clin Microbiol 1982;16:509–516.

228. Kloos WE, Wolfsohl JF. *Staphylococcus cohnii* subspecies: *Staphylococcus cohnii* subsp. *cohnii* subsp. nov. and *Staphylococcus cohnii* subsp. *urealyticum* subsp. nov. Int J Syst Bacteriol 1991;41:284–289.

229. Kluytmans J, Berg H, Steegh P, et al. Outbreak of *Staphylococcus schleiferi* wound infections: strain characterization by randomly amplified polymorphic DNA analysis, PCR ribotyping, conventional ribotyping, and pulsed-field gel electrophoresis. J Clin Microbiol 1998;36:2214–2219.

230. Kluytmans J, Van Griethuysen A, Willemse P, Van Keulen P. Performance of CHROMagar selective medium with oxacillin-resistance screening agar base for identifying *Staphylococcus aureus* and detecting methicillin resistance. J Clin Microbiol 2002;40:2480–2482.

231. Koch C, Schumann P, Stackebrandt E. Reclassification of *Micrococcus agilis* (Ali-Cohen 1889) to the genus *Arthrobacter* as *Arthrobacter agilis* comb. nov. and emendation of the genus *Arthrobacter*. Int J Syst Bacteriol 1995;45:837–839.

232. Kocur M. Genus I. Micrococcus. In: Sneath PHA, Nair NS, Holt JG, eds. Bergey's Manual of Systematic Bacteriology. Vol. 2. Baltimore: Williams & Wilkins, 1986:1004–1008

233. Kocur M. Genus III. *Planococcus*. In: Sneath PHA, Nair NS, Holt JG, eds. Bergey's Manual of Systematic Bacteriology. Vol. 2. Baltimore: Williams & Wilkins, 1986:1011–1013.

234. Komori Y, Iimura N, Yamashita R, et al. Characterization of coagulase from *Staphylococcus intermedius*. J Nat Toxins 2001;10:111–118.

235. Konig B, Prevost G, Konig W. Composition of staphylococcal bi-component toxins determines pathophysiological reactions. J Med Microbiol 1993;46:479–485.

236. Kotilainen P, Huovinen P, Eerola E. Application of gas-liquid chromatographic analysis of cellular fatty acids for species identification and typing of coagulase-negative staphylococci. J Clin Microbiol 1991;29:315–322.

237. Kovacs G, Burghardt J, Pradella S, et al. *Kocuria palustris* sp. nov. and *Kocuria rhizophila* sp. nov., isolated from the rhizoplane of the narrow-leaved cattail (*Typha angustifolia*). Int J Syst Bacteriol 1999;49:167–173.

238. Kragsbjerg P, Bomfim-Loogna J, Tornqvist E, Soderqvist B. Development of antimicrobial resistance in *Staphylococcus lugdunensis* during treatment: report of a case of bacterial arthritis, vertebral osteomyelitis, and infective endocarditis. Clin Microbiol Infect 2000;6:496–499.

239. Kremery V Jr, Trupl J, Drgona L, et al. Nosocomial bacteremia due to vancomycin-resistant *Staphylococcus epidermidis* in four patients with cancer, neutropenia, and previous treatment with vancomycin. Eur J Clin Microbiol Infect Dis 1996;15:259–261.

240. Kremery V Jr, Trupl J, Spanik S. Bacteremia due to teicoplanin-resistant and vancomycin-susceptible *Staphylococcus haemolyticus* in seven patients with acute leukemia and neutropenia receiving prophylaxis with ofloxacin. Infection 1997;25:51–52.

241. Krishnan S, Haglund L, Ashfaq A, et al. Prosthetic valve endocarditis due to *Staphylococcus saccharolyticus*. Clin Infect Dis 1996;22:722–723.

242. Krothapalli RK, Senekjian HO, Ayus JC. Efficacy of intravenous vancomycin in the treatment of gram-positive peritonitis in long-term peritoneal dialysis. Am J Med 1983;75:345–348.

243. Kumari DN, Keer V, Hawkey PM, et al. Comparison and application of ribosomal spacer DNA amplicon polymorphisms and pulsed-field gel electrophoresis for differentiation of methicillin-resistant *Staphylococcus aureus* strains. J Clin Microbiol 1997;35:881–885.

244. Kwok AY, Chow AW. Phylogenetic study of *Staphylococcus* and *Macrococcus* species based on partial *hsp60* gene sequences. In J Syst Evol Microbiol 2003;53:87–92.

245. Kwok AY, Su SC, Reynolds RP, et al. Species identification and phylogenetic relationships based on partial *HSP*60 gene sequences within the genus *Staphylococcus*. Int J Syst Bacteriol 1999;49:1181–1192.

246. Lambe DW Jr, Ferguson KP, Keplinger JL, et al. Pathogenicity of *Staphylococcus lugdunensis*, *Staphylococcus schleiferi*, and three other coagulase-negative staphylococci in a mouse model and possible virulence factors. Can J Microbiol 1990;36:453–463.

247. Lambert LH, Cox T, Mitchell K, et al. *Staphylococcus succinus* sp. nov., isolated from Dominican amber. Int J Syst Bacteriol 1998;48:511–518.

248. Landau W, Kaplan RL. Room temperature coagulase production by *Staphylococcus aureus* strains. Clin Microbiol Newslett 1980;2:10.

249. Langbeg JM, LeBlarc JC, Drake J, Milner R. Efficacy of antimicrobial prophylaxis in placement of cerebrospinal fluid shunts: Meta-analysis. Clin Infect Dis 1993;17:98–103.

250. Langlois BE, Harmon RJ, Akers K, et al. Comparison of methods for determining DNase and phosphatase activities by staphylococci. J Clin Microbiol 1989;27:1127–1129.

251. Larkin SM, Williams DN, Osterholm MT, et al. Toxic shock syndrome: clinical, laboratory, and pathologic findings in nine fatal cases. Ann Intern Med 1982;96:858–864.

252. Latham RH, Running K, Stamm WE. Urinary tract infections in young adult women caused by *Staphylococcus saprophyticus*. JAMA 1983;250:3063–3066.

253. Latorre M, Rojo PM, Franco R, Cisterna R. Endocarditis due to *Staphylococcus capitis* subspecies *ureolyticus* (letter). Clin Infect Dis 1993;16:343–344.

254. Layton MC, Hierholzer WJ Jr, Patterson JE. The evolving epidemiology of methicillin-resistant *Staphylococcus aureus* at a university hospital. Infect Control Hosp Epidemiol 1995;16:12–17.

255. Lee JC, Park JS, Shepherd SE, et al. Protective efficacy of antibodies to the *Staphylococcus aureus* type 5 capsular polysaccharide in a modified model of endocarditis in rats. Infect Immun 1997;65:4146–4151.

256. Lee JC, Liu M-J, Parsonnet J, et al. Expression of type 8 capsular polysaccharide and production of toxic shock syndrome toxin 1 are associated among vaginal isolates of *Staphylococcus aureus*. J Clin Microbiol 1990;28:2612–2615.

257. Lee JC, Takeda S, Livolsi PJ, Paoletti LC. Effects of *in vivo* and *in vitro* growth conditions on expression of type-8 capsular polysaccharide by *Staphylococcus aureus*. Infect Immun 1993;61:1853–1858.

258. Lee W, Carpenter RJ, Phillips LE, Faro S. Pyelonephritis and sepsis due to *Staphylococcus saprophyticus*. J Infect Dis 1987;155:1079–1080.

259. Lee VT, Chang AH, Chow AW. Detection of staphylococcal enterotoxin B among toxic shock syndrome (TSS)- and non-TSS-associated *Staphylococcus aureus* isolates. J Infect Dis 1992;166:911–915.

260. Lerche A, Rasmussen N, Wandall JH, et al. *Staphylococcus aureus* meningitis: a review of 28 consecutive community-acquired cases. Scand J Infect Dis 1995;27:569–573.

261. Leung MJ, Nuttall N, Mazur M, et al. Case of *Staphylococcus schleiferi* endocarditis and a simple scheme to identify clumping factor-positive staphylococci. J Clin Microbiol 1999;37:3353–3356.

262. Lewis JF, Brake SR, Anderson DJ, et al. Urinary tract infection due to coagulase-negative staphylococci. Am J Clin Pathol 1992;77:736–739.

263. Lin WS, Cunneen T, Lee CY. Sequence analysis and molecular characterization of genes required for the biosynthesis of type 1 capsular polysaccharide in *Staphylococcus aureus*. J Bacteriol 1994;176:7005–7016.

264. Lina B, Vandenesch F, Reverdy ME, et al. Non-puerperal breast infection due to *Staphylococcus lugdunensis*. Eur J Clin Microbiol Infect Dis 1994;13:686–687.

265. Lina G, Piemont Y, Godall-Gamot F, et al. Involvement of Panton-Valentine leukocidin-producing *Staphylococcus aureus* in primary skin infections and pneumonia. Clin Infect Dis 1999;29:1128–1132.

266. Linares J, Stiges-Serra A, Garu J, et al. Pathogenesis of catheter sepsis: a prospective study with quantitative and semiquantitative cultures of catheter hub and segments. J Clin Microbiol 1985;21:357–360.

267. Lindsay JA, Aravena-Roman MA, Riley TV. Identification of *Staphylococcus*

epidermidis and *Staphylococcus hominis* from blood cultures by testing susceptibility to desferrioxamine. Eur J Clin Microbiol Infect Dis 1993;12:127–131.

268. Lindsay JA, Riley TV. Susceptibility to desferrioxamine: a new test for the identification of *Staphylococcus epidermidis*. J Med Microbiol 1991;35:45–48.

269. Liu H, Xu Y, Ma Y, Zhou P. Characterization of *Micrococcus antarcticus* sp. nov., a psychrophilic bacterium from Antarctica. Int J Syst Evol Microbiol 2000; 50:715–719.

270. Longshaw CM, Wright JD, Farrell AM, Holland KT. *Kytococcus sedentarius*, the organism associated with pitted keratolysis, produces two keratin-degrading enzymes. J Appl Microbiol 2002;93:810–816.

271. Low DE, Schmidt BK, Kirpalani HM, et al. An endemic strain of *Staphylococcus haemolyticus* colonizing and causing bacteremia in neonatal intensive care unit patients. Pediatrics 1992;89:696–700.

272. Luijendijk A, van Belkum A, Verbrugh H, Kluytmans J. Comparison of five tests for identification of *Staphylococcus aureus* from clinical samples. J Clin Microbiol 1996;34:2267–2269.

273. Mack D, Fischer W, Krotkotsch A, et al. The intercellular adhesin involved in biofilm accumulation of *Staphylococcus epidermidis* is a linear, β-1,6-linked glucosaminoglycan: purification and structural analysis. J Bacteriol 1996;178: 175–183.

274. Mack D, Haeder M, Siemssen N, Laufs R. Association of biofilm production of coagulase negative staphylococci with expression of a specific polysaccharide intercellular adhesin. J Infect Dis 1996;174:881–884.

275. Mack D, Riedewald J, Rohde H, et al. Essential functional role of the polysaccharide intercellular adhesin of *Staphylococcus epidermidis* in hemagglutination. Infect Immun 1999;67:1004–1008.

276. Magee JT, Burnett IA, Hindmarch JM, Spencer RC. *Micrococcus* and *Stomatococcus* spp. from human infections. J Hosp Infect 1990;16:67–73.

277. Mahoudeau I, Delabranche X, Prevost G, et al. Frequency of isolation of *Staphylococcus intermedius* from humans. J Clin Microbiol 1997;35:2153–2154.

278. Males BM, Bartholomew WR, Amsterdam D. *Staphylococcus simulans* septicemia in a patient with chronic osteomyelitis and pyoarthritis. J Clin Microbiol 1985;21:255–257.

279. Mandell GL. Catalase, superoxide dismutase, and virulence of *Staphylococcus aureus*. *In vitro* and *in vivo* studies with emphasis on staphylococcal-leukocyte interaction. J Clin Invest 1966;55:561–564.

280. Mannerova S, Pantucek R, Doskar J, et al. *Macrococcus brunensis* sp. nov., *Macrococcus hajekii* sp. nov., and *Macrococcus lamae* sp. nov., from the skin of llamas. Int J Syst Evol Microbiol 2003 ;53:1647–1654.

281. Marques MB, Weller PF, Parsonnet J, et al. Phosphatidylinositol-specific phospholipase C, a possible virulence factor of *Staphylococcus aureus*. J Clin Microbiol 1989;27:2451–2454.

282. Marrack P, Kappler J. The staphylococcal enterotoxins and their relatives. Science 1990;248:705–711.

283. Marsou R, Bes M, Boudouma M, et al. Distribution of *Staphylococcus sciuri* subspecies among human clinical specimens, and profile of antibiotic resistance. Res Microbiol 1999;150:531–541.

284. Martinez-Martinez L, Cuervez-Mons V, Alonso-Pulpon L, et al. *Staphylococcus xylosus* from a patient with cardiac and hepatic transplants. Clin Microbiol Newslett 1988;10:47–48.

285. Mastroianni A, Coronado O, Nanetti A, Chiodo F. *Staphylococcus xylosus* isolated from a pancreatic pseudocyst in a patient infected with human immunodeficiency virus. Clin Infect Dis 1994;19:1173–1174.

286. Mastroianni A, Coronado O, Nanetti A, et al. Community-acquired pneumonia due to *Staphylococcus cohnii* in an HIV-infected patient: case report and review. Eur J Clin Microbiol Infect Dis 1995;14:904–908.

287. Mastroianni A, Coronado O, Nanetti A, et al. *Staphylococcus cohnii*: an unusual cause of primary septic arthritis in a patient with AIDS. Clin Infect Dis 1996; 23:1312–1313.

288. Mayhall CG, Archer NH, Lamb A, et al. Ventriculostomy-related infections: a prospective epidemiologic study N Engl J Med 1984;310:553–550.

289. McCarthy JS, Stanley PA, Mayall B. A case of *Staphylococcus simulans* endocarditis affecting a native heart valve. J Infect 1991;22:211–212.

290. McDonald CL, Chapin K. Rapid identification of *Staphylococcus aureus* from blood culture bottles by a classic two-hour tube coagulase test. J Clin Microbiol 1995;33:50–52.

291. McKenney D, Hubner J, Muller E, et al. The *ica* locus of *Staphylococcus epidermidis* encodes production of capsular polysaccharide/adhesin. Infect Immun 1998;66:4711–4720.

292. McTaggart LA, Elliott TSJ. Is resistance to novobiocin a reliable test for confirmation of the identification of *Staphylococcus saprophyticus*? J Med Microbiol 1989;30:253–266.

293. McTaggart LA, Rigby RC, Elliott TSJ. The pathogenesis of urinary tract infections associated with *Escherichia coli*, *Staphylococcus saprophyticus*, and *S. epidermidis*. J Med Microbiol 1990;32:135–141.

294. Mehrotra M, Wang G, Johnson WM. Multiplex PCR for detection of genes for *Staphylococcus aureus* enterotoxins, exfoliative toxins, toxic shock syndrome toxin 1, and methicillin resistance. J Clin Microbiol 2000;38:1032–1035.

295. Mendoza M, Meugnier H, Bes M, et al. Identification of *Staphylococcus* species by 16S-23S rDNA intergenic spacer PCR analysis. Int J Syst Bacteriol 1998; 48:1039–1055.

296. Merlino J, Leroi M, Bradbury R, et al. New chromogenic identification and detection of *Staphylococcus aureus* and methicillin-resistant S. aureus. J Clin Microbiol 2000;38:2378–2380.

297. Meugnier H, Bes M, Vernozy-Rozand C, et al. Identification and ribotyping of *Staphylococcus xylosus* and *Staphylococcus equorum* strains isolated from goat milk and cheese. Int J Food Microbiol 1996;31:325–331.

298. Meyer HG, Gatermann S. Surface properties of *Staphylococcus saprophyticus*: hydrophobicity, haemagglutination, and *Staphylococcus saprophyticus* surface-associated protein (Ssp) represent distinct entities. APMIS 1994;102:538–544.

299. Meyer HG, Muthing J, Gatermann SG. The hemagglutinin of *Staphylococcus saprophyticus* binds to a protein receptor on sheep erythrocytes. Med Microbiol Immunol (Berl) 1997;186:37–43.

300. Meyer HG, Wengler-Becker U, Gatermann SG. The hemagglutinin of *Staphylococcus saprophyticus* is a major adhesin for uroepithelial cells. Infect Immun 1996;64:3893–3896.

301. Miller JM, Biddle JW, Quenzer VK, et al. Evaluation of the Biolog for identification of members of the Family *Micrococcaceae*. J Clin Microbiol 1993;31: 3170–3173.

302. Mitchell CJ, Geary C, Stevens M. Detection of *Staphylococcus aureus* in blood cultures: evaluation of a two-hour method. Med Lab Sci 1991;48:106–109.

303. Mitchell PS, Huston BJ, Jones RN, et al. *Stomatococcus mucilaginosus* bacteremias: typical case presentations, simplified diagnostic criteria, and a literature review. Diagn Microbiol Infect Dis 1990;13:521–525.

304. Miwa K, Fukuyama M, Kunitomo T, et al. Rapid assay for detection of toxic shock syndrome toxin 1 from human sera. J Clin Microbiol 199432:539–542.

305. Monday SR, Bohach GA. Use of multiplex PCR to detect classical and newly described pyrogenic toxin genes in staphylococcal isolates. J Clin Microbiol 1999;37:3411–3414.

306. Monson T, Ronnmark M, Olofsson C, Wistrom J. An inexpensive and reliable method for routine identification of staphylococcal species. Eur J Clin Microbiol Infect Dis 1998;17:327–335.

307. Montanaro L, Arciola CR, Borsetti E, et al. A polymerase chain reaction (PCR) method for the identification of collagen adhesin gene in *Staphylococcus*-induced prosthesis infection. New Microbiol 1998;21:359–263.

308. Moreau M, Richards JC, Fournier JM, et al. Structure of the type-5 capsular polysaccharide of *Staphylococcus aureus*. Carbohydr Res 1990;117:113–123.

309. Mulder JG. A simple and inexpensive method for the identification of *Staphylococcus epidermidis* and *Staphylococcus hominis*. Eur J Clin Microbiol Infect Dis 1995;14:1052–1056.

310. Muller E, Takeda H, Shiro D, et al. Occurrence of capsular polysaccharide-adhesin among clinical isolates of coagulase-negative staphylococci. J Infect Dis 1993;169:1211–1218.

311. Murakami K, Minamide W, Wada K, et al. Identification of methicillin-resistant strains of staphylococci by polymerase chain reaction. J Clin Microbiol 1991; 29:2240–2244.

312. Murdoch DR, Everts RJ, Chambers ST, Cowan IA. Vertebral osteomyelitis due to *Staphylococcus lugdunensis*. J Clin Microbiol 1996;34:993–994.

313. Nakagawa Y, Sakane T, Yokata A. Emendation of the genus *Planococcus* and transfer of *Flavobacterium okeanokoites* Zobell and Upham 1944 to the genus *Planococcus* as *Planococcus okeanokoites* comb. nov. Int J Syst Bacteriol 1996; 46:866–870.

314. Nakatomi Y, Sugiyama J. A rapid latex agglutination assay for the detection of penicillin binding protein 2′. Microbiol Immunol 1998;42:739–743.

315. Nataro JP, St Geme JW. Septicemia caused by *Staphylococcus saprophyticus* without associated urinary tract infection. Pediatr Infect Dis J 1988;7:601–602.

316. National Committee for Clinical Laboratory Standards. Methods for Dilution Antimicrobial Susceptibility Tests for Bacteria That Grow Aerobically. 6th Ed. Approved standard, M7-A6. Wayne, PA: National Committee for Laboratory Standards, 2003.

317. Neill RJ, Fanning GR, Delahoz F, et al. Oligonucleotide probes for detection and differentiation of *Staphylococcus aureus* strains containing genes for enterotoxins A, B, and C and toxic shock syndrome toxin 1. J Clin Microbiol 1990; 28:1514–1518.

318. Nielsen H. Vertebral osteomyelitis with *Stomatococcus mucilaginosus*. Eur J Clin Microbiol Infect Dis 1994;13:775–776.

319. Nilsson IM, Lee JC, Bremell T, et al. The role of staphylococcal polysaccharide microcapsule expression in septicemia and septic arthritis. Infect Immun 1997; 65:4216–4221.

320. Nilsson M, Frykberg L, Flock J-I, et al. A fibrinogen-binding protein of *Staphylococcus epidermidis*. Infect Immun 1998;66:2666–2673.

321. O'Brien T, Collin J. Prosthetic vascular graft infection. Br J Surg 1992;79: 1262–1267.

322. Oh B, Kim H, Lee J, et al. *Staphylococcus haemolyticus* lipase: biochemical properties, substrate specificity, and gene cloning. FEMS Microbiol Lett 1999; 179:385–392.

323. Ohshima Y, Schumacher-Perdreau F, Peters G, et al. Antiphagocytic effect of the capsule of *Staphylococcus simulans*. Infect Immun 1990;58:1350–1354.

324. Oliveira DC, Crisostomo I, Santos-Sanches P, et al. Comparison of DNA sequencing of the protein A gene polymorphic region with other molecular typing techniques for typing epidemiologically diverse collections of methicillin-resistant *Staphylococcus aureus*. J Clin Microbiol 2001;39:574–580.

325. Olmos A, Camarena JJ, Nogueira JM, et al. Application of an optimized and highly discriminatory method based on arbitrarily primed PCR for epidemiologic analysis of methicillin-resistant *Staphylococcus aureus* nosocomial infections. J Clin Microbiol 1998;36:1128–1134.

326. Ortiz de la Tabla V, Gutierrez-Rodero F, Martin C, et al. *Staphylococcus lugdunensis* as a cause of abscesses in the perineal area. Eur J Clin Microbiol Infect Dis 1996;15:405–407.

327. Osterlund A, Nordlund E. Wound infection caused by *Staphylococcus hyicus* subspecies *hyicus* after a donkey bite. Scand J Infect Dis 1997;29:95.

328. Ozturkeri H, Kocabeyoglu O, Yergok YZ, et al. Distribution of coagulase-negative staphylococci, including the newly described species *Staphylococcus schleiferi*, in nosocomial and community acquired urinary tract infections. Eur J Clin Microbiol Infect Dis 1994;13:1076–1079.

329. Palazzo E, Pierre J, Besbes N. *Staphylococcus lugdunensis* arthritis: a complication of arthroscopy. J Rheumatol 1992;19:327–328.

330. Pantucek R, Sedlacek I, Doskar J, Rosypal S. Complex genomic and phenotypic characterization of the related species *Staphylococcus carnosus* and *Staphylococcus piscifermentans*. Int J Syst Bacteriol 1999;49:941–951.

331. Parsonnet J. Case definition of staphylococcal TSS: A proposed revision incorporating laboratory findings. In: Arbuthnot J, Furman B, eds. European Conference on Toxic Shock Syndrome. International Conference and Symposium Series 229. New York: Royal Society of Medicine Press, 1998:15.

332. Patel R, Piper KE, Rouse MS, et al. Frequency of isolation of *Staphylococcus lugdunensis* among staphylococcal isolates causing endocarditis: a 20-year experience. J Clin Microbiol 2000;38:4262–4263.

333. Patel SR, Olenginski TP, Perrquet JL, et al. Pyomyositis: clinical features and predisposing conditions. J Rheumatol 1997;24:1734–1738.

334. Patey O, Malkin JE, Coutaux A, et al. AIDS-related *Stomatococcus mucilaginosus* infection. Lancet 1991;338:621–632.

335. Paulsson M, Ljungh A, Wadstrom T. Rapid identification of fibronectin, vitronectin, laminin, and collagen cell surface binding proteins in coagulase-negative staphylococci by particle agglutination assays. J Clin Microbiol 1992;30:2006–2012.

336. Peacock SJ, Lina G, Etienne J, Foster TJ. *Staphylococcus schleiferi* subsp. *schleiferi* expresses a fibronectin-binding protein. Infect Immun 1999;67:4272–4275.

337. Peces R, Gago E, Tejada F, et al. Relapsing bacteraemia due to *Micrococcus luteus* in a haemodialysis patient with a Perm-Cath catheter. Nephrol Dial Transplant 1997;12:2428–2429.

338. Pei L, Palma M, Nilsson M, et al. Functional studies of a fibrinogen binding protein from *Staphylococcus epidermidis*. Infect Immun 1999'67:4525–4530.

339. Pennell DR, Rott-Petri JA, Kurzynski TA. Evaluation of three commercial agglutination tests for the identification of *Staphylococcus aureus*. J Clin Microbiol 1984;20:614–617.

340. Perdeau-Remington F, Stefanik D, Peters G, et al. Methicillin-resistant *Staphylococcus haemolyticus* on the hands of health care workers: a route of transmission or a source? J Hosp Infect 1995;31:195–203.

341. Perl TM, Kruger WA, Houston A, et al. Investigation of suspected nosocomial clusters of *Staphylococcus haemolyticus* infections. Infect Contr Hosp Epidemiol 1999;20:128–131.

342. Perl TM, Rhomberg PR, Bale MJ, et al. Comparison of identification systems for *Staphylococcus epidermidis* and other coagulase-negative *Staphylococcus* species. Diagn Microbiol Infect Dis 1994;18:151–155.

343. Perry JD, Rennison C, Butterworth LA, et al. Evaluation of S. aureus ID, a new chromogenic agar medium for detection of *Staphylococcus aureus*. J Clin Microbiol 2003;41:5695–5698.

344. Piccolomini R, Catamo G, Picciani C, et al. Evaluation of Staf-Sistem 18-R for identification of staphylococcal clinical isolates to the species level. J Clin Microbiol 1994;32:649–653.

345. Pierre J, Gutmann L, Bornet M, et al. Identification of coagulase-negative staphylococci by electrophoretic profile of total proteins and analysis of penicillin-binding proteins. J Clin Microbiol 1990;28:443–446.

346. Pierre J, Williamson R, Bornet M, Gutmann L. Presence of an additional penicillin-binding protein in methicillin-resistant *Staphylococcus epidermidis*, *Staphylococcus haemolyticus*, *Staphylococcus hominis*, and *Staphylococcus simulans* with a low affinity for methicillin, cephalothin, and cefamandole. Antimicrob Agents Chemother 1990;34:1691–1694.

347. Pignatari A, Pfaller M, Hollis R, et al. *Staphylococcus aureus* colonization and infection in patients on continuous ambulatory peritoneal dialysis. J Clin Microbiol 1990;28:1898–1902.

348. Pinna A, Zanetti S, Sotgiu M, et al. Identification and antibiotic susceptibility of coagulase negative staphylococci isolated in corneal/external infections. Br J Ophthalmol 1999;83:771–773.

349. Pinsky RL, Piscitelli V, Patterson JE. Endocarditis caused by relatively penicillin-resistant *Stomatococcus mucilaginosus*. J Clin Microbiol 1989;27:215–216.

350. Piper J, Hadfield T, McClesky F, et al. Efficacies of rapid agglutination tests for identification of methicillin-resistant strains of *Staphylococcus aureus*. J Clin Microbiol 1988;26:1907–1909.

351. Place RB, Hiestand D, Burri S, Teuber M. *Staphylococcus succinus* subsp. *casei* subsp. nov., a dominant isolate from surface-ripened cheese. Syst Appl Microbiol 2002;25:353–359.

352. Poirier LP, Gaudreau CL. *Stomatococcus mucilaginosus* catheter-associated infection with septicemia. J Clin Microbiol 1989;27:1125–1126.

353. Ponce de leon S, Wenzel RP. Hospital-acquired bloodstream infections with *Staphylococcus epidermidis*: review of 100 cases. Am J Med 1984;77:639–644.

354. Poutrel B, Caffin JP. Lysostaphin disk test for routine presumptive identification of staphylococci. J Clin Microbiol 1981;13:1023–1025.

355. Press OW, Ramsey PG, Larson EB, et al. Hickman catheter infections in patients with malignancies. Medicine (Baltimore) 1984;63:189–200.

356. Prevost G, Cribier B, Couppie P, et al. Panton-Valentine leukocidin and γ-hemolysin from *Staphylococcus aureus* ATCC 49775 are encoded by distinct genetic loci and have different biological activities. Infect Immun 1995;63:4121–4129.

357. Probst AJ, Hertel C, Richter L, et al. *Staphylococcus condimenti* sp. nov., from soy sauce mash, and *Staphylococcus carnosus* (Schleifer and Fischer 1982) subsp. *utilis* subsp. nov. Int J Syst Bacteriol 1998;48:651–658.

358. Projan SJ, Kornblum J, Kreiswirth B, et al. Nucleotide sequence: the β-hemolysin gene of *Staphylococcus aureus*. Nucleic Acids Res 1989;17:3305.

359. Qadri SMH, Ueno Y, Imambaccus H, Almodovar E. Rapid detection of methicillin-resistant *Staphylococcus aureus* by Crystal MRSA ID System. J Clin Microbiol 1994;32:1830–1832.

360. Raad I, Alrahwan A, Rolston K. *Staphylococcus epidermidis*: emerging resistance and need for alternative agents. Clin Infect Dis 1998;26:1182–1187.

361. Razonable RR, Lewallen DG, Patel R, Osmon DR. Vertebral osteomyelitis and prosthetic joint infection due to *Staphylococcus simulans*. Mayo Clin Proc 2001;76:1067–1070.

362. Read II, Bodey GP. Infectious complications of indwelling vascular catheters. Clin Infect Dis 1992;15:197–210.

363. Reddy GS, Prakash JS, Prabahar V, et al. *Kocuria polaris* sp. nov., an orange-pigmented psychrophilic bacterium isolated from an Antarctic cyanobacterial mat sample. Int J Syst Evol Microbiol 2003;53:183–187.

364. Reddy GS, Prakash JS, Vairamani M, et al. *Planococcus antarcticus* and *Planococcus psychrophilus* spp. nov. isolated from cyanobacterial mat samples collected from ponds in Antarctica. Extremophiles 2002;6:253–261.

365. Relman DA, Ruoff K, Farraro MJ. *Stomatococcus mucilaginosus* endocarditis in an intravenous drug abuser. J Infect Dis 1987;5:1080–1082.

366. Renneberg J, Rieneck K, Gutschik E. Evaluation of Staph ID32 system and Staph-Zym system for identification of coagulase-negative staphylococci. J Clin Microbiol 1995;33:1150–1153.

367. Rhoden DL, Hancock GA, Miller JM. Numerical approach to reference identification of *Staphylococcus*, *Stomatococcus*, and *Micrococcus*. J Clin Microbiol 1993;31:490–493.

368. Rhoden DL, Miller JM. Four-year prospective study of Staph-Ident system and conventional method for reference identification of *Staphylococcus*, *Stomatococcus*, and *Micrococcus* spp. J Clin Microbiol 1995;33:96–98.

369. Riley TV, Schneider PF. Infrequency of slime production by urinary isolates of *Staphylococcus saprophyticus*. J Infect 1992;24:63–66.

370. Roberson JR, Fox LK, Hancock DD, et al. Evaluation of methods for differentiation of coagulase-positive staphylococci. J Clin Microbiol 1992;30:3217–3219.

371. Romano I, Giordano A, Lama L, et al. *Planococcus rifietensis* sp. nov., isolated from algal mat collected from a sulfurous spring in Campania (Italy). Syst Appl Microbiol 2003;26:357–366.

372. Rosenstein R, Gotz F. Staphylococcal lipases: biochemical and molecular characterization. Biochimie 2000;82:1005–1014.

373. Rossney AS, English LF, Keane CT. Coagulase testing compared with commercial kits for routinely identifying *Staphylococcus aureus*. J Clin Pathol 1990;43:246–252.

374. Rotun SS, McMath V, Schoonmaker DJ, et al. *Staphylococcus aureus* with reduced susceptibility to vancomycin isolated from a patient with bacteremia. Emerg Infect Dis 1999;5:147–149.

375. Ruane RJ, Morgan MM, Citron DM, et al. Failure of rapid agglutination methods to detect oxacillin-resistant *Staphylococcus aureus*. J Clin Microbiol 1986;24:490–491.

376. Rubin RH, Moellering RC Jr. Clinical, microbiologic, and therapeutic aspects of purulent pericarditis. Am J Med 1975;59:68–71.

377. Rubin SJ, Lyons RW, Murcia AJ. Endocarditis associated with cardiac catheterization due to gram-positive coccus designated *Micrococcus mucilaginosus incertae sedis*. J Clin Microbiol 1978;7:546–549.

378. Rupp ME, Soper DE, Archer GL. Colonization of the female genital tract with *Staphylococcus saprophyticus*. J Clin Microbiol 1992;30:2975–2979.

379. Rupp ME, Ulphani JS, Fey PD, et al. Characterization of the importance of polysaccharide intercellular adhesin/hemagglutinin of *Staphylococcus epidermidis* in the pathogenesis of biomaterial-based infection in a mouse foreign body model. Infect Immun 1999;67:2627–2632.

380. Rupp ME, Ulphani JS, Fey PD, Mack D. Characterization of *Staphylococcus epidermidis* polysaccharide intercellular adhesin/hemagglutinin in the pathogenesis of intravascular catheter-associated infection in a rat model. Infect Immun 1999;67:2656–2659.

381. Salar A, Carratala J, Fernandez-Sevilla A, et al. Pneumonia caused by *Micrococcus* species in a neutropenic patient with acute leukemia. Eur J Clin Microbiol Infect Dis 1997;16:546–548.

382. Sandoe JA, Kerr KG, Reynolds GW, Jain S. *Staphylococcus capitis* endocarditis: two cases and review of the literature. Heart (Br Card Soc Online) 1999;82:e1.

383. Sandoe JA, Longshaw CM. Ventriculoperitoneal shunt infection caused by *Staphylococcus lugdunensis*. Clin Microbiol Infect 2001;7:385–387.

384. Sanyal D, Johnson AP, George RC, et al. Peritonitis due to vancomycin-resistant *Staphylococcus epidermidis*. Lancet 1991;337:54.

385. Saravolatz LD, Pohlod DJ, Arking LM. Community-acquired methicillin-resistant *Staphylococcus aureus*: a new source for nosocomial outbreaks. Ann Intern Med 1982;97:325–329.

386. Sariya D, Hayden M, Verma P. Evaluation of Dryspot Staphytect Plus for the differentiation of Staphylococcus species. Abstracts of the 100th General Meeting of the American Society for Microbiology. Washington, DC: American Society for Microbiology, 2000:184.

387. Sau S, Sun J, Lee CY. Molecular characterization and transcriptional analysis of type 8 capsule genes in *Staphylococcus aureus*. J Bacteriol 1997;179:1614–1621.

388. Schleifer KH, Fischer U. Description of a new species in the genus *Staphylococcus*: *Staphylococcus carnosus*. Int J Syst Bacteriol 1982;32:153–156.

389. Schleifer KH, Geyer U, Kilpper-Balz R, et al. Elevation of *Staphylococcus sciuri* subsp. *lentus* (Kloos, et al.) to species status: *Staphylococcus lentus* (Kloos, et al.) comb. nov. Syst Appl Microbiol 1983;4:382–387.

390. Schleifer KH, Kilpper-Balz R, Devriese LA. *Staphylococcus arlettae* sp. nov., *S. equorum* sp. nov., and *S. kloosii* sp. nov.: three new coagulase-negative, novobiocin-resistant species from animals. Syst Appl Microbiol 1984;5:501–509.

391. Schleifer KH, Kloos WE. Isolation and characterization of staphylococci from human skin I. Amended descriptions of *Staphylococcus epidermidis* and *Staphylococcus saprophyticus* and descriptions of three new species: *Staphylococcus cohnii*, *Staphylococcus haemolyticus*, and *Staphylococcus xylosus*. Int J Syst Bacteriol 1975;25:50–61.

392. Schleifer KH, Kloos WE. A simple test system for the separation of staphylococci and micrococci. J Clin Microbiol 1975;1:337–338.

393. Schlievert PM. Staphylococcal enterotoxin B and toxic shock syndrome toxin-1 are significantly associated with non-menstrual TSS. Lancet 1986;1:1149–1150.

394. Schlievert PM, Shands KN, Dan BB, et al. Identification and characterization of an exotoxin from *Staphylococcus aureus* associated with toxic shock syndrome. J Infect Dis 1981;143:509–516.

395. Schmalzried TP, Amstutz HC, Au MK, et al. Etiology of deep sepsis in total hip arthroplasty. Clin Orthop 1992;280:200–202.

396. Schmitz FJ, Steiert M, Hofmann B, et al. Development of multiplex-PCR for direct detection of the genes for enterotoxin B and C, and toxic shock syndrome toxin 1 in *Staphylococcus aureus* isolates. J Med Microbiol 1998;47:335–340.

397. Schneider PF, Riley TV. Cell-surface hydrophobicity of *Staphylococcus saprophyticus*. Epidemiol Infect 1991;106:71–75.

398. Schneider PF, Riley TV. *Staphylococcus saprophyticus* urinary tract infections: epidemiological data from Western Australia. Eur J Epidemiol 1996;12:51–54.

399. Schnitzler N, Meilicke R, Conrads G, et al. *Staphylococcus lugdunensis*: report of a case of peritonitis and an easy-to-perform screening strategy. J Clin Microbiol 1998;36:812–813.

400. Schumann P, Sproer C, Burghardt J, et al. Reclassification of the species *Kocuria erythromyxa* (Brooks and Murray 1981) as *Kocuria rosea* (Flugge 1886). Int J Syst Bacteriol 1999;49:393–396.

401. Schwalbe RS, McIntosh AC, Qaiyumi S, et al. In vitro activity of LY333328, an investigational glycopeptide antibiotic, against enterococci and staphylococci. Antimicrob Agents Chemother 1996;40:2416–2419.

402. Schwalbe RS, Ritz WJ, Verma PR, et al. Selection for vancomycin resistance in clinical isolates of *Staphylococcus haemolyticus*. J Infect Dis 1990;161:45–561.

403. Schwalbe RS, Stapleton JT, Gilligan PH. Emergence of vancomycin resistance in coagulase-negative staphylococci. N Engl J Med 1987;316:927–931.

404. Schwarzkopf A, Karch H, Schmidt H, et al. Phenotypical and genotypical characterization of epidemic clumping factor-negative, oxacillin-resistant *Staphylococcus aureus*. J Clin Microbiol 1993;31:2281–2285.

405. Shimaoka M, Yoh M, Segawa A, et al. Development of enzyme-labeled oligonucleotide probe for detection of *mecA* gene in methicillin-resistant *Staphylococcus aureus*. J Clin Microbiol 1994;32:1866–1869.

406. Shiro H, Meluleni A, Groll A, et al. The pathogenic role of *Staphylococcus epidermidis* capsular polysaccharide/adhesin in a low-inoculum rabbit model of prosthetic valve endocarditis. Circulation 1995;92:2715–2722.

407. Shiro H, Muller E, Gutierrez N, et al. Transposon mutants of *Staphylococcus epidermidis* deficient in elaboration of capsular polysaccharide/adhesin and slime are avirulent in a rabbit model of endocarditis. J Infect Dis 1994;169:1042–1049.

408. Shuttleworth R, Behme RJ, McNabb A, Colby WD. Human isolates of *Staphylococcus caprae*: association with bone and joint infections. J Clin Microbiol 1997;35:2537–2541.

409. Sieradzki K, Roberts RB, Serur D, et al. Heterogeneously vancomycin-resistant *Staphylococcus epidermidis* strain causing recurrent peritonitis in a dialysis patient during vancomycin therapy. J Clin Microbiol 1999;37:39–44.

410. Sieradzki K, Villari P, Tomasz A. Decreased susceptibilities to teicoplanin and vancomycin among coagulase-negative methicillin-resistant clinical isolates of staphylococci. Antimicrob Agents Chemother 1998;42:100–107.

411. Simons JW, van Kampen MD, Riel S, et al. Cloning, purification and characterization of the lipase from *Staphylococcus epidermidis*—comparison with the substrate selectivity with those of other microbial lipases. Eur J Biochem 1998;253:675–683.

412. Singh VR, Raad I. Fatal *Staphylococcus saprophyticus* native valve endocarditis in an intravenous drug addict. J Infect Dis 1990;162:784–785.

413. Skulnick M, Patel MP, Low DE. Evaluation of five commercial systems for identification of staphylococci to species level. Eur J Clin Microbiol Infect Dis 1989;8:1001–1003.

414. Skulnick M, Simor AE, Patel MP, et al. Evaluation of three methods for the rapid identification of *Staphylococcus aureus* in blood cultures. Diagn Microbiol Infect Dis 1994;19:5–8.

415. Sloos JH, Horrevorts AM, Van Boven CP, Dijkshoorn L. Identification of multiresistant *Staphylococcus epidermidis* in neonates of a secondary care hospital using pulsed field gel electrophoresis and quantitative antibiogram typing. J Clin Pathol 1998;51:62–67.

416. Sloos JH, van de Klundert JA, Dijkshoorn L, van Boven CP. Changing susceptibilities of coagulase-negative staphylococci to teicoplanin in a teaching hospital. J Antimicrob Chemother 1998;42:787–791.

417. Smith TL, Pearson ML, Wilcox KR, et al. Emergence of vancomycin resistance in *Staphylococcus aureus*. N Engl J Med 1999;340:493–501.

418. Soldati D, Mudry A, Monnier P. Necrotizing otitis externa caused by *Staphylococcus epidermidis*. Eur Arch Otorhinolaryngol 1999;256:439–441.

419. Sorlin P, Maes N, Deplano A, et al. Chorioamnionitis as a apparent source of vertical transmission of *Staphylococcus cohnii* and *Ureaplasma urealyticum* to a neonate. Eur J Clin Microbiol Infect Dis 1998;17:807–808.

420. Soro O, Grazi G, Varaldo PE, et al. Phosphatase activity of staphylococci is constitutive in some species and repressed by phosphates in others. J Clin Microbiol 1990;28:2707–2710.

421. Sotutu V, Carapetis J, Wilkinson J, et al. The ''surreptitious *Staphylococcus*'': *Staphylococcus lugdunensis* endocarditis in a child. Pediatr Infect Dis J 2002;21:984–986.

422. Spellerberg B, Steidel K, Lutticken R, Haase G. Isolation of *Staphylococcus caprae* from blood cultures of a neonate with congenital heart disease. Eur J Clin Microbiol Infect Dis 1998;17:61–62.

423. Stackbrandt E, Koch C, Gvozdiak O, Schumann O. Taxonomic dissection of the genus *Micrococcus*: *Kocuria* gen. nov., *Nesterenkonia* gen. nov., *Kytococcus* gen. nov., *Dermacoccus* gen. nov., and *Micrococcus* Cohn 1872 gen. amend. Int J Syst Bacteriol 1995;45:682–692.

424. Steinberg JP, Clark CC, Hackman BO. Nosocomial and community-acquired *Staphylococcus aureus* bacteremias from 1980 to 1993: impact of intravascular devices and methicillin resistance. Clin Infect Dis 1996;23:255–259.

425. Stepanovic S, Dakic I, Djukic S, et al. Surgical wound infection associated with *Staphylococcus sciuri*. Scand J Infect Dis 2002;34:685–686.

426. Stepanovic S, Vukovicc D, Trajkovic V, et al. Possible virulence factors of *Staphylococcus sciuri*. FEMA Microbiol Lett 2001;15:47–53.

427. Stoakes L, John MA, Lannigan R, et al. Gas-liquid chromatography of cellular fatty acids for identification of staphylococci. J Clin Microbiol 1994;32:1908–1910.

428. Stoakes L, Schieven BC, Ofori E, et al. Evaluation of the MicroScan Rapid Pos Combo panels for identification of staphylococci. J Clin Microbiol 1992;30:93–95.

429. Stringfellow WT, Dassy B, Lieb M, Fournier JM. *Staphylococcus aureus* growth and type 5 capsular polysaccharide production in synthetic media. Appl Environ Microbiol 1991;57:618–621.

430. Sturgess I, Martin FC, Eykyn S. Pubic osteomyelitis caused by *Staphylococcus simulans*. Postgrad Med J 1993;69:927–929.

431. Supersac G, Prevost G, Piemont Y. Sequencing of leukocidin R from *Staphylococcus aureus* P83 suggests that staphylococcal leukocidins and γ-hemolysin are members of a single, two-component family of toxins. Infect Immun 1993;61:580–587.

432. Tabe Y, Nakamura A, Oguri T, Igari J. Molecular characterization of epidemic

multiresistant *Staphylococcus haemolyticus* isolates. Diagn Microbiol Infect Dis 1998;32:177–183.

433. Takagi Y, Futamura S, Asada Y. Action site of exfoliative toxin on keratinocytes. J Invest Dermatol 1990;94:52–543.

434. Takahashi T, Satoh I, Kikuchi N. Phylogenetic relationships of 38 taxa of the genus *Staphylococcus* based on 16S rRNA gene sequence analysis. Int J Syst Bacteriol 1999;49:725–728.

435. Talen DA, Goldstein EJC, Staatz D, et al. *Staphylococcus intermedius*: clinical presentation of a new human dog bite pathogen. Ann Emerg Med 1989;18:410–413.

436. Talen DA, Staatz, D, Staatz A, et al. *Staphylococcus intermedius* in canine gingiva and canine-inflicted wound infections: a newly recognized zoonotic pathogen. J Clin Microbiol 1989;27:78–81.

437. Talen DA, Staatz D, Staatz A, et al. Frequency of *Staphylococcus intermedius* as human nasopharyngeal flora. J Clin Microbiol 1989;27:2393.

438. Talon R, Dublet N, Montel MC, Cantonnet M. Purification and characterization of extracellular *Staphylococcus warneri* lipase. Curr Microbiol 1995;30:11–16.

439. Tan R, White V, Servais G, et al. Postoperative endophthalmitis caused by *Stomatococcus mucilaginosus*. Clin Infect Dis 1994;18:492–493.

440. Tanasupawat S, Hashimoto Y, Ezaki T, et al. *Staphylococcus piscifermentans* sp. nov. from fermented fish in Thailand. Int J Syst Bacteriol 1992;42:577–581.

441. Tanner MA, Everett CL, Youvan DC. Molecular phylogenetic evidence for non-invasive zoonotic transmission of *Staphylococcus intermedius* from a canine pet to a human. J Clin Microbiol 2000;38:1628–1631.

442. Tee WS, Soh SY, Lin R, Loo LH. *Staphylococcus lugdunensis* carrying the *mecA* gene causes catheter-associated bloodstream infection in premature neonate. J Clin Microbiol 2003;41:519–520.

443. Tenover FC, Arbeit R, Archer G, et al. Comparison of traditional and molecular methods of typing isolates of *Staphylococcus aureus*. J Clin Microbiol 1994;32:407–415.

444. Tenover FC, Biddle JW, Lancaster MV. Increasing resistance to vancomycin and other glycopeptides in *Staphylococcus aureus*. Emerg Infect Dis 2001;7:327–332.

445. Tenover FC, Lancaster MV, Hill BC, et al. Characterization of staphylococci with reduced susceptibilities to vancomycin and other glycopeptides. J Clin Microbiol 1998;36:1020–1027.

446. Thakker M, Park JS, Carey V, Lee JC. *Staphylococcus aureus* capsular serotype 5 capsular polysaccharide is antiphagocytic and enhances bacterial virulence in a murine bacteremia model. Infect Immun 1998;66:5183–5189.

447. Thomson-Carter FM, Pennington TH. Characterization of coagulase-negative staphylococci by sodium dodecyl sulfate-polyacrylamide gel electrophoresis and immunoblot analysis. J Clin Microbiol 1989;27:2199–2203.

448. Timmerman CP, Fleer A, Besnier JM, et al. Characterization of a proteinaceous adhesin of *Staphylococcus epidermidis* which mediates attachment to polystyrene. Infect Immun 1991;59:4187–4192.

449. Todd J, Fishaut M. Toxic shock syndrome associated with phage-group-1 staphylococci. Lancet 1978;2:1116–1118.

450. Tojo M, Yamashita N, Goldmann DA, et al. Isolation and characterization of a capsular polysaccharide adhesin from *Staphylococcus epidermidis*. J Infect Dis 1988;157:713–722.

451. Tolaymat A, Al-Jayousi Z. *Staphylococcus saprophyticus* urinary tract infection in male children. Child Nephrol Urol 1991;11:100–102.

452. Torre D, Ferraro G, Fiori GP, et al. Ventriculoatrial shunt infection caused by *Staphylococcus warneri*: case report and review. Clin Infect Dis 1992;14:49–52.

453. Trevino M, Garcia-Zabarte A, Quintas A, et al. *Stomatococcus mucilaginosus* septicemia in a patient with acute lymphoblastic leukaemia. Eur J Clin Microbiol Infect Dis 1998;17:505–507.

454. Tselenis-Kotsowilis AD, Koliomichalis MP, Papavasilov TT. Acute pyelonephritis caused by *Staphylococcus xylosus*. J Clin Microbiol 1982;16:593–594.

455. Tu KK, Palutke WA. Isolation and characterization of a catalase-negative strain of *Staphylococcus aureus*. J Clin Microbiol 1976;3:77–78.

456. Tveten Y. Evaluation of new agglutination test for identification of oxacillin-susceptible and oxacillin-resistant *Staphylococcus aureus*. J Clin Microbiol 1995;33:1333–1334.

457. Ubukata K, Nakagami S, Nitta A, et al. Rapid detection of the *mecA* gene in methicillin-resistant staphylococci by enzymatic detection of polymerase chain reaction products. J Clin Microbiol 1992;30:1728–1733.

458. Valeva A, Palmer M, Bhakdi S. Staphylococcal exotoxin: formation of the heptameric pore is cooperative and proceeds through multiple intermediate stages. Biochemistry 1997;36:13298–13304.

459. Van Belkum A, Kluytmans J, van Leeuwen W, et al. Multicenter evaluation of arbitrarily primed PCR for typing of *Staphylococcus aureus* strains. J Clin Microbiol 1995;33:1537–1547.

460. Vandenesch F, Celard M, Arpin D, et al. Catheter-related bacteremia associated with coagulase-positive *Staphylococcus intermedius*. J Clin Microbiol 1995;33:2508–2510.

461. Vandenesch F, Etienne J, Reverdy ME, et al. Endocarditis due to *Staphylococcus lugdunensis*: report of 11 cases and review. Clin Infect Dis 1993;17:871–876.

462. Vandenesch F, Eykyn SJ, Bes M, et al. Identification and ribotypes of *Staphylococcus caprae* isolated as human pathogens and from goat milk. J Clin Microbiol 1995;33:888–892.

463. Vandenesch F, LeBeau C, Bes M, et al. Clotting activity in *Staphylococcus schleiferi* subspecies from human patients. J Clin Microbiol 1994;32:388–392.

464. Vandenesch F, Perrier-Gros-Claude JD, Bes M, et al. *Staphylococcus pasteuri*-specific oligonucleotide probes derived from a randomly amplified DNA fragment. FEMS Microbiol Lett 1995;132:147–152.

465. Van Der Mee-Marquet N, Achard A, Mereghetti L, et al. *Staphylococcus lugdunensis* infections: high frequency of inguinal area carriage. J Clin Microbiol 2003;41:1404–1409.

466. Van Der Zwet WC, Debets-Ossenkopp YJ, Reinders E, et al. Nosocomial spread of a *Staphylococcus capitis* strain with heteroresistance to vancomycin in a neonatal intensive care unit. J Clin Microbiol 2002;40:2520–2525.

467. Van Kampen MD, Rosenstein R, Gotz F, Egmond MR. Cloning, purification, and characterization of *Staphylococcus warneri* lipase 2. Biochem Biophys Acta 2001;1544:229–241.

468. van Leeuwen WB, van Pelt C, Luijendijk A, et al. Rapid detection of methicillin resistance in *Staphylococcus aureus* isolates by the MRSA-Screen latex agglutination test. J Clin Microbiol 1999;37:3029–3030.

469. Varaldo PE, Kilpper-Balz R, Biavasco F, et al. *Staphylococcus delphini* sp. nov., a coagulase-positive species isolated from dolphins. Int J Syst Bacteriol 1988;38:436–439.

470. Veach LA, Pfaller MA, Barrett M, et al. Vancomycin resistance in *Staphylococcus haemolyticus* causing colonization and bloodstream infection. J Clin Microbiol 1990;28:2064–2068.

471. Vernozy-Rozand C, Mazuy C, Meugnier H, et al. *Staphylococcus fleurettii* sp. nov., isolated from goat's milk cheeses. Int J Syst Evol Microbiol 2000;50:1521–1527.

472. Villard L, Kodjo A, Borges E, et al. Ribotyping and rapid identification of *Staphylococcus xylosus* by 16-23S spacer amplification. FEMS Microbiol Lett 2000;185:83–87.

473. von Baum H, Klemme FR, Geiss HK, Sonntag H-G. Comparative evaluation of a commercial system for identification of gram-positive cocci. Eur J Clin Microbiol Infect Dis 1998;17:849–852.

474. von Eiff C, Kuhn N, Herrmann M, et al. *Micrococcus luteus* as a cause of recurrent bacteremia. Pediatr Infect Dis J 1996;15:711–713.

475. von Eiff C, Vaudaux P, Kahl BC, et al. Bloodstream infections caused by small-colony variants of coagulase-negative staphylococci following pacemaker implantation. Clin infect Dis 1999;29:932–934.

476. von Rheinbaben KE, Hadlock RM. Rapid distinction between micrococci and staphylococci with furazolidone agar. Antonie von Leeuwenhoek J Microbiol Serol 1981;47:41–51.

477. Wade JC, Schimpf SC, Newman KA. *Staphylococcus epidermidis*: an increasing cause of infection in patients with granulocytopenia. Ann Intern Med 1982;96:1–10.

478. Waldvogel FA. Chapter 183. *Staphylococcus aureus* (including toxic shock syndrome). In: Mandell GL, Bennett JE, Dolin R, eds. Mandell, Douglas, and Bennett's Principles and Practice of Infectious Diseases. 5th Ed. New York, Churchill-Livingstone, 2000:2069–2092.

479. Waller JR, Hodel SL, Nuti RN. Improvement of two toluidine blue O-mediated techniques for DNase detection. J Clin Microbiol 1985;21:195–199.

480. Wallet F, Stuit L, Boulanger E, et al. Peritonitis due to *Staphylococcus sciuri* in a patient on continuous ambulatory peritoneal dialysis. Scand J Infect Dis 2000;32:697–698.

481. Walsh TR, Bolmstrom A, Qwarnstrom A, et al. Evaluation of current methods for detection of staphylococci with reduced susceptibility to glycopeptides. J Clin Microbiol 2001;39:2439–2444.

482. Wang EEL, Prober CG, Hendrick BE, et al. Prophylactic sulfamethoxazole and trimethoprim in ventriculoperitoneal shunt surgery. JAMA 1984;251:1174–1177.

483. Wang SM, Liu CC, Tseng HW, et al. *Staphylococcus capitis* bacteremia of very low birth weight premature infants at neonatal intensive care units: clinical significance and antimicrobial susceptibility. J Microbiol Immunol Infect 1999;32:26–32.

484. Wanger AR, Morris SL, Ericsson C, et al. Latex agglutination-negative methicillin-resistant *Staphylococcus aureus* recovered from neonates: epidemiologic features and comparison of typing methods. J Clin Microbiol 1992;30:2583–2588.

485. Wasserman E, Lombard L, Walzi G. *Staphylococcus lugdunensis* endocarditis in a young, previously healthy female. Eur J Clin Microbiol Infect Dis 1999;18:289–291.

486. Weber DJ, Hoffman KL, Thoft RA, et al. Endophthalmitis following intraocular lens implantation: report of 30 cases and review of the literature. Rev Infect Dis 1986;8:12–20.

487. Webster JA, Bannerman TL, Hubner RJ, et al. Identification of the *Staphylococcus sciuri* species group with *Eco*R1 fragments containing rRNA sequences and description of *Staphylococcus vitulus* sp. nov. Int J Syst Bacteriol 1994;44:454–460.

488. Weinblatt ME, Sahdev I, Berman M. *Stomatococcus mucilaginosus* infections in children with leukemia. Pediatr Infect Dis J 1990;9:678–679.

489. Weinstein MP, Mirrett S, Van Pelt L, et al. Clinical importance of identifying coagulase-negative staphylococci isolated from blood cultures: evaluation of MicroScan Rapid and Dried Overnight Gram-Positive panels versus a conventional reference method. J Clin Microbiol 1998;36:2089–2092.

490. Wenzel RP, Edmond MB. Vancomycin-resistant *Staphylococcus aureus*: infection control considerations. Clin Infect Dis 1998;27:245–251.

491. Wenzel RP, Reagen DR, Bertino JS, et al. Methicillin-resistant *Staphylococcus aureus* outbreak: a consensus panel's definition and management guidelines. Am J Infect Control 1998;26:102–110.

492. Wergeland HI, Haaheim LR, Natas OB, et al. Antibodies to staphylococcal peptidoglycan and its peptide epitopes, teichoic acid, and lipoteichoic acid in sera from blood donors and patients with staphylococcal infections. J Clin Microbiol 1989;27:1286–1291.

493. West TE, Walshe JJ, Krol CP, et al. Staphylococcal peritonitis in patients on continuous peritoneal dialysis. J Clin Microbiol 1986;23:809–812.

494. Westblom TU, Gorse GJ, Milligan TW, et al. Anaerobic endocarditis caused by *Staphylococcus saccharolyticus*. J Clin Microbiol 1990;28:2818–2819.

495. Wharton M, Rice JR, McCallum R, et al. Septic arthritis due to *Micrococcus luteus*. J Rheumatol 1986;13:659–660.

496. Wieser M, Denner EBM, Kampfer P, et al. Emended descriptions of the genus *Micrococcus*, *Micrococcus luteus* (Cohn 1872) and *Micrococcus lylae* (Kloos, et al, 1974). Int J Syst Evol Microbiol 2002;52:629–637.

497. Wilkerson MS, McAllister S, Mill JM, et al. Comparison of five agglutination tests for identification of *Staphylococcus aureus*. J Clin Microbiol 1997;35:148–151.

498. Wood CA, Sewell DL, Strausbaugh LJ. Vertebral osteomyelitis and native valve endocarditis caused by *Staphylococcus warneri*. Diagn Microbiol Infect Dis 1989;12:261–263.

499. Wooster DL, Louch RE, Krajden S. Intraoperative bacterial contamination of vascular grafts: a prospective study. Can J Surg 1985;28:407–409.

500. Wu S, de Lencastre H, Tomasz A. Genetic organization of the *mecA* region in methicillin-susceptible and methicillin-resistant strains of *Staphylococcus sciuri*. J Bacteriol 1998;180:236–242.

501. Yonezawa M, Takahata M, Banzawa-Futakuchi N, et al. DNA gyrase *gryA* mutations in quinolone-resistant clinical isolates of *Staphylococcus haemolyticus*. Antimicrob Agents Chemother 1996;40:1065–1066.

502. Yoon JH, Kang SS, Lee KC, et al. *Planomicrobium koreense* gen. nov., sp. nov., a bacterium isolated from the Korean traditional fermented seafood jeotgal, and transfer of *Planococcus okeanokoites* (Nakagawa, et al. 1996) and *Planococcus mcmeekinii* (Junge et al. 1998) to the genus *Planobacterium*. Int J Syst Evol Microbiol 2001;51:1511–1520.

503. Yoon JH, Weiss N, Kang KH, et al. *Planococcus maritimus* sp. nov., isolated from sea water of a tidal flat in Korea. Int J Syst Evol Microbiol 2003;53:2013–2017.

504. You YO, Kim KJ, Min BM, Chung CP. *Staphylococcus lugdunensis*—a potential pathogen in oral infection. Oral Surg Oral Med Oral Pathol Oral Radiol Endod 1999;88:297–302.

505. Yu J, Montelius MN, Paulsson M, et al. Adhesion of coagulase-negative staphylococci and adsorption of plasma proteins to heparinized polymer surfaces. Biomaterials 1994;15:805–814.

506. Ziebuhr W, Krimmer V, Rachid S, et al. A novel mechanism of phase variation in virulence in *Staphylococcus epidermidis*: evidence for control of the polysaccharide intercellular adhesin synthesis by alternating insertion and excision of the insertion sequence element *IS*256. Mol Microbiol 1999;32:345–356.

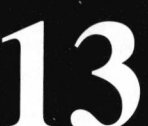
Gram-Positive Cocci
Part II: Streptococci, Enterococci, and the "Streptococcus-Like" Bacteria

General Characteristics of the Streptococci

Group A β-Hemolytic Streptococci (*Streptococcus pyogenes*)

Virulence Factors
Clinical Significance

Group B β-Hemolytic Streptococci (*Streptococcus agalactiae*)

Virulence Factors
Clinical Significance

Group C and Group G β-Hemolytic Streptococci

Group F β-Hemolytic Streptococci

Other Streptococci in the "Pyogenic Cocci" Group

Streptococcus pneumoniae

Virulence Factors
Pneumococcal Vaccines
Clinical Significance

Viridans Streptococci

The Anginosus Group: *Streptococcus anginosus*, *Streptococcus constellatus*, and *Streptococcus intermedius*

Group D Streptococci: The "*Streptococcus bovis/Streptococcus equinus* Complex" and Related Species

Streptococcus suis

Other Viridans Streptococci Isolated From Animals

Miscellaneous Streptococci

***Enterococcus* Species**

Taxonomy
Virulence Factors
Clinical Significance
Genus *Melissococcus*

The "Streptococcus-Like" Bacteria

Abiotrophia and *Granulicatella* Species
Aerococcus and *Helcococcus* Species

Leuconostoc Species
Pediococcus and *Tetragenococcus* Species
Gemella Species
Vagococcus Species
Alloiococcus Species
Globicatella Species
Facklamia Species
Dolosigranulum, *Ignavigranum*, and *Dolosicoccus* Species
Eremococcus Species
Genus *Lactococcus*

Isolation and Identification of Streptococci and "Streptococcus-Like" Bacteria

Direct Gram-Stained Smears
Culture Media
Hemolysis on Blood Agar
Nonculture, Direct Detection Techniques for Group A β-Hemolytic Streptococci in Pharyngeal Specimens
Nonculture, Direct Detection Techniques for Group B β-Hemolytic Streptococci and *Streptococcus pneumoniae*
Colony Morphology and Catalase Testing
Recognition and Preliminary Characterization of Streptococci and the "Streptococcus-Like" Bacteria
Presumptive Identification of Streptococci

Susceptibility to Bacitracin
Susceptibility to Sulfamethoxazole-Trimethoprim (SXT)
CAMP Test and Pigment Production
Hydrolysis of Sodium Hippurate
Bile-Esculin Test
Salt-Tolerance Test (6.5% NaCl Broth)
Leucine Aminopeptidase (LAP) Test
Pyrrolidonyl Arylamidase (PYR) Test
Susceptibility to Optochin
Bile Solubility Test

Commercial Presumptive Identification Tests

Serologic Identification of β-Hemolytic Streptococci

Capillary Precipitin Test
Coagglutination
Latex Agglutination

Serologic Identification of *Streptococcus pneumoniae*
Biochemical Characteristics for Identification of Groupable Streptococci
Identification of the Viridans Streptococci

Sanguis Group
Mitis Group
Mutans Group
Salivarius Group
Anginosus Group
Bovis Group

Identification of *Streptococcus suis* and Other Streptococci Isolated From Animals
Identification of *Enterococcus* Species
Identification of *Abiotrophia* and *Granulicatella* Species
Identification of *Aerococcus* and *Helcococcus* Species
Identification of *Leuconostoc*, *Pediococcus*, and *Tetragenococcus* Species
Identification of *Gemella* Species
Identification of *Vagococcus* Species
Identification of *Alloiococcus*, *Globicatella*, *Facklamia*, *Dolosigranulum*, *Ignavigranum*, and *Dolosicoccus* Species
Identification of *Lactococcus* Species
Commercially Available Systems for Identification of Streptococci, Enterococci, and Selected "Streptococcus-Like" Bacteria

API Rapid Strep
BBL Crystal Gram-Positive Identification System
Rapid ID 32 Strep
RapID STR
Vitek Gram-Positive Identification (GPI) Card
Microscan Gram-Positive Breakpoint Combo Panel

The streptococci, enterococci, and *Streptococcus*-like bacteria are gram-positive, catalase-negative bacteria that tend to grow in pairs and chains. The detection of cytochrome enzymes with the catalase test distinguishes members of the various micrococcal and staphylococcal species groups (catalase-positive) from the streptococci, enterococci, and ''*Streptococcus*-like'' bacteria, which are catalase-negative. As with other microbial groups, the classification and taxonomy of the streptococci and *Streptococcus*-like bacteria have changed radically with the descriptions of several new genera of catalase-negative cocci. These changes have more than academic significance for clinical microbiologists as we move into the 21st century because previously uncommon organisms belonging to these groups are being recovered from human infections with increasing regularity, and the pathogenic potentials of both old and newly described species are still not understood and are being actively investigated.

The application of molecular taxonomic methods and the description of several new genera of catalase-negative, gram-positive cocci has resulted in a complete reorganization of streptococcal taxonomy compared with that published in the 1984 edition of *Bergey's Manual of Systematic Bacteriology*. Molecular methods such as DNA-DNA hybridization, DNA-ribosomal RNA (rRNA) hybridization, and small-subunit (16S) rRNA sequencing were initially used to validate the division of the family *Streptococcaceae* into the genera *Streptococcus*, *Enterococcus*, and *Lactococcus*, and have now being applied to newly described viridans streptococci, enterococci, and other catalase-negative isolates to determine their relationships to these three genera.[79,80,558] In the upcoming edition of *Bergey's Manual*, catalase-negative, gram-positive cocci of human origin are now classified among six families in the proposed order ''Lactobacillales'' and one family in the order Bacillales, both of which are in the proposed class ''Bacilli'' in phylum *Firmicutes* (Box 13-1). The genus *Streptococcus*, which contains the most important human pathogens, can be operationally divided into seven groups, as shown in Box 13-2.

With the description of several new genera and species of catalase-negative, gram-positive cocci over the past decade, a note must be added regarding the bacterial names used in this chapter. Rules for naming bacteria as described in the International Code of Nomenclature of Bacteria are generally followed by bacterial taxonomists, but over the years, certain bacterial names that appear in the literature are grammatically incorrect according to the international code. For example, the species names in common use for four viridans streptococci—*S. sanguis*, *S. crista*, *S. parasanguis*, and *S. rattus*—are grammatically incorrect and should properly be changed to *S. sanguinis*, *S. cristatus*, *S. parasanguinis*, and *S. ratti*, respectively. However, another rule of the International Code states that the liberty to ''correct'' a bacterial name must be used with caution and reserve to avoid confusion. While proposals have been made to make these grammatical nomenclature changes, others have recommended conservation of the older, familiar ''grammatically incorrect'' names.[567,968] Therefore, the older, familiar names of these organisms are used in this chapter largely to avoid confusion.

General Characteristics of the Streptococci

Streptococci are facultative anaerobes, although some strains grow better under anaerobic conditions. Most species will grow in air; however, the growth of most species is stimulated by increased CO_2. Medically important streptococci, enterococci, and aerococci are **homofermentative,** meaning that the sole product of glucose fermentation is lactic acid with no gas formation. Streptococci are also catalase-negative and oxidase-negative, a property that, together with the Gram stain, differentiates streptococci from *Neisseria* species. Members of the genus *Streptococcus* characteristically grow in chains (or chains of diplococci) when grown in broth media. This characteristic is shared with the enterococci, the lactococci, and some of the newly recognized or proposed genera (i.e., *Leuconostoc* species, *Vagococcus* species, and *Globicatella* species). Other *Streptococcus*-like bacteria (i.e., aerococci, *Alloiococcus* species, *Gemella* species, *Pediococcus* species, *Tetragenococcus* species, and *Helcococcus* species) grow as pairs or tetrads in broth. Assessment of the cellular arrangement is best made by performing a Gram stain from a culture of the organism growing in thioglycolate broth. When thioglycolate broth is used, the smear preparation should be fixed in methanol after air-drying, rather than heat-fixed, to prevent the bacteria from ''washing off'' the slide during the staining process.

The cell wall composition of the streptococci is similar

Box 13-1 Classification of the Streptococci. Enterococci, and the "Streptococcus-Like" Bacteria Domain Bacteria, Phylum Firmicutes, Class "Bacilli"

Order	Family	Genera
Bacillales	"Staphylococcaceae"	*Gemella*
"Lactobacillales"	"Lactobacillaceae"	*Pediococcus*
	"Aerococcaceae"	*Aerococcus, Abiotrophia, Dolosicoccus, Eremococcus, Facklamia, Globicatella, Ignavigranum*
	"Carnobacteriaceae"	*Alloiococcus, Dolosigranulum*
	"Enterococcaceae"	*Enterococcus, Melissococcus, Tetragenococcus, Vagococcus*
	"Leuconostocaceae"	*Leuconostoc, Oenococcus, Weissella*
	Streptococcaceae	*Streptococcus, Lactococcus*

Box 13-2 Streptococcal Species Groups Based on Small-Subunit rRNA Sequence Analysis

Group	Group Name	Group Members (Lancefield group[s])	Habitats
I	Pyogenic group	*S. pyogenes* (Group A β-hemolytic streptococci)	Humans
		S. agalactiae (Group B β-hemolytic streptococci)	Humans
		S. equi subsp. *equi* (Group C β-hemolytic streptococci)	Horses, donkeys
		S. equi subsp. *zooepidemicus* (Group C β-hemolytic streptococci)	Many animals
		S. dysgalactiae subsp. *dysgalactiae* (Groups C and L β hemolytic streptococci)	Pigs, cattle
		S. dysgalactiae subsp. *equisimilis* (Groups C and G β-hemolytic streptococci)	Humans
		S. canis (Groups G, L, and M streptococci)	Many animals
		S. iniae (non–Lancefield group designation)	Freshwater dolphins
		S. porcinus (Groups E, P, U, and V streptococci)	Swine, humans
		S. phocae (Group C, F, or nongroupable streptococci)	Seals
		S. didelphis (no group)	Opossums
		S. urinalis (no group)	Humans
II	Sanguis group	*S. sanguis* (*S. sanguinis*) (3 biotypes)	Humans
		S. parasanguis (*S. parasanguinis*)	Humans
		S. gordonii	Humans
		S. sinensis	Humans
III	Mitis group	*S. mitis*	Humans
		S. oralis	Humans
		S. crista (*S. cristatus*)	Humans
		S. peroris	Humans
		S. infantis	Humans
		S. australis	Humans
		S. oligofermentans	Humans
IV	Mutans group	*S. mutans*	Humans
		S. sobrinus	Humans
		S. cricetus	Hamsters, rats, (humans)
		S. downei	Monkeys
		S. rattus (*S. ratti*)	Rats, humans
		S. macacae	Monkeys
		S. ferus	Rats
V	Salivarius group	*S. salivarius*	Humans
		S. vestibularis	Humans
		S. infantarius	Humans
		S. thermophilus	Dairy products
		S. hyointestinalis	Sows
VI	Anginosus group	*S. constellatus* subsp.	Humans
		S. anginosus	Humans
		S. intermedius	Humans
VII	Bovis group	*S. bovis/S. equinus*	Cattle, horses
		S. gallolyticus subsp *gallolyticus* (*S. bovis* I)	Humans, cattle, koala bears
		S. gallolyticus subsp. *pasteurianus* (*S. bovis* II.2) ("*S. pasteurianus*")	Humans
		S. gallolyticus subsp. *macedonicus* (*S. macedonicus, S. waius*)	Environmental (cheeses)
		S. infantarius subsp *infantarius* (*S. bovis* II.1)	Humans, cattle
		S. infantarius subsp *coli* ("*S. lutetiensis*")	Humans
		S. alactolyticus	Swine, dogs, chickens
		S. suis (Groups R, S, T)	Pigs, cattle, humans

(Continued)

Box 13-2 *Continued*

Group	Group Name	Group Members (Lancefield group[s])	Habitats
VII	Other	*S. uberis/parauberis* (Group E or nongroupable)	Cattle
		S. hyointestinalis	Swine
		S. hyovaginalis	Swine
		S. thoraltensis	Swine
		S. pluranimalium	Cattle, sheep, cats, canaries
		S. uberis/parauberis (Group E or nongroupable)	Cattle
		S. entericus	Cattle
		S. ovis	Sheep
		S. gallinaceus	Chickens
		S. minor	Dogs, cats, cattle

to that of other gram-positive bacteria, being composed primarily of peptidoglycan, in which are embedded a variety of carbohydrates, teichoic acids, lipoproteins, and surface protein antigens (see Chapter 5). Some streptococcal species may be serologically classified on the basis of cell-surface carbohydrate antigens. The pioneering work of Rebecca Lancefield established the Lancefield grouping system for the β-hemolytic streptococci.[596] The antigens detected in the Lancefield grouping system are either cell wall polysaccharides (as in the human groups A, B, C, F, and G streptococci) or are cell wall lipoteichoic acids (group D streptococci and *Enterococcus* species). Originally, these cell wall grouping antigens were extracted with dilute hydrochloric or nitrous acid, formamide, or by autoclaving, and groups were determined by capillary precipitin reactions. Commercially available streptococcal-grouping kits use enzymatic extraction techniques and either coagglutination or latex particle agglutination for antigen detection. Other streptococci, particularly members of the viridans streptococcal groups, do not possess any of the recognized Lancefield cell wall grouping antigens, although some strains may possess similar antigens that will cross-react with β-hemolytic streptococcal group-specific antisera. Well-studied viridans streptococci, such as the cariogenic organism *S. mutans*, have been divided into serotypes based on their own cell wall carbohydrate antigens. The various serotypes of *S. mutans* have subsequently been elevated to species status and now comprise the ''mutans group'' of oral streptococci.

Group A β-Hemolytic Streptococci (Streptococcus pyogenes)
Virulence Factors

The pathogenic streptococci have several characteristics that contribute to their virulence. The virulence mechanisms of the group A β-hemolytic streptococci (*S. pyogenes*), in particular, have been studied most extensively. This organism remains an extremely important human pathogen, and the only known reservoirs of group A streptococci in nature are the skin and mucous membranes of humans. In the U.S.,

group A streptococcal infections occur at an annual rate of about 3.5 cases per 100,000 population, resulting in over 9,600 cases and 1,100 to 1,300 fatalities per year.[734] In addition to acute infections, the group A *Streptococcus* is also associated with two nonsuppurative sequelae—acute rheumatic fever and acute poststreptococcal glomerulonephritis—that continue to occur, particular in developing countries.

The cell wall of group A β-hemolytic streptococci consists of a thick peptidoglycan along with integral lipoteichoic acids (LTAs) and other surface-associated molecules, as described in Chapter 5. Lipoteichoic acids are believed to play a central role in promoting initial adherence of the group A streptococci to pharyngeal epithelial cells.[66,737] In addition to LTAs, several other group A streptococcal adhesins have been described, including several fibronectin-binding proteins (FBPs) such as protein F1 (SfbI, streptococcal fibronectin-binding protein), protein F2 (SbfII), FPB54, and PFBP.[239,459,529,588,817] These latter proteins promote adherence to both pharyngeal and cutaneous cell types. M proteins are also believed to play a role in adherence, particularly adherence to keratinocytes in skin via interaction with the keratinocyte membrane cofactor CD46.[739] The major group A cell wall antigen is a complex polysaccharide consisting of L-rhamnose and *N*-acetyl-D-glucosamine in a 2:1 ratio.[100] The antigen is covalently attached to the peptidoglycan. The role of the cell wall grouping antigen as a virulence factor is not known, although the peptidoglycan material itself has biologic activity, including the induction of fever, dermal and cardiac necrosis in animals, lysis of erythrocytes and platelets, and enhancement of nonspecific resistance.

Some group A strains possess a **capsule** composed of hyaluronic acid, which is a high-molecular-weight linear polymer composed of β(1-4)-linked disaccharide repeating units of D-glucuronic acid and (1-3)-β-D-*N*-acetylglucosamine.[1038] This material is the product of enzymes encoded by a three-gene cluster consisting of *hasA*, *hasB*, and *hasC*.[242] These three genes encode a hyaluronic acid synthase, a UDP-glucose dehydrogenase, and a glucose pyrophosphorylase, respectively.[17] These genes are highly conserved among group A streptococcal strains, and variations in the degree of capsular gene expression likely reflect differences in regulation of gene transcription. Strains that maximally express these genes appear mucoid when grown on sheep blood agar.[1041] Two gene products, **CrsS** and **CrsR**, appear to function as a two-component regulatory system that is able to increase or decrease the degree of encapsulation by upregulation or downregulation of *has* gene expression.[621] Chemically, this capsular material is indistinguishable from the ground substance of connective tissue, which may explain the lack of immunogenicity of this substance in the infected host. In vitro, capsule production is maximal during logarithmic growth, and the organisms shed their capsules as they enter the stationary phase of growth; this loss is probably due to the elaboration of **hyaluronidase** during the latter stages of the logarithmic growth phase. The hyaluronic acid capsule functions to help the organisms resist complement-dependent killing by phagocytic cells. In animal models, the hyaluronic acid capsule has been shown to contribute to the capacity of group A streptococci to produce invasive soft-tissue infections.[40] The capsule also influences the ability of group A streptococci to adhere to epithelial cells by modulating the interaction of M protein and other surface molecules and by serving as a ligand for binding to the CD44 receptor on epithelial cell surfaces.[864,1038]

The major virulence factor of the group A *Streptococcus* is a cell-surface antigen designated **M protein**.[100] M proteins are acid- and heat-stable, trypsin-labile, fibrillar proteins associated with the outer surface of the cell wall. M proteins are composed of two polypeptide chains complexed together in an α-helical coiled-coil configuration.[363] The M protein is anchored in the cell membrane, extends through the peptidoglycan layer, and projects from the surface of the bacterial cell (Fig. 13-1).[774] The amino acid sequence and structure of the carboxy-terminal end of the molecule is located within the cell membrane and cell wall of the organism and is highly conserved among group A strains. The N-terminus extends beyond the cell surface and terminates with a sequence of about 11 amino acid residues. This terminal sequence varies among clinical isolates and constitutes the basis for the Lancefield serologic classification of group A streptococci. Strains that are rich in M protein are resistant to phagocytosis and intracellular killing by polymorphonuclear (PMN) cells; cells lacking demonstrable M protein are readily phagocytosed and killed.[597] M protein apparently exerts its antiphagocytic effects by interfering with opsonization of the bacterial cells via the alternative complement pathway.[95] M proteins are also able to form complexes with fibrinogen that consequently bind to β$_2$ integrins of neutrophils. This binding causes the release of inflammatory mediators that induce vascular leakage, a pathologic component of streptococcal toxic shock.[481] Serologic M typing is usually performed on hot acid extracts of group A streptococci using capillary precipitin or agarose gel immunodiffusion techniques. Only a single M-type antigen is expressed by group A strains, and 93 different M serotypes have been identified using these methods.[334,543] Unfortunately, many strains of group A streptococci are serologically nontypeable; either appropriate M antiserum is not available, or the M protein of a given strain may not be optimally expressed under the conditions of cultivation.[809] The genes encoding various M proteins have also been identified using oligonucleotide probes corresponding to the NH$_2$-terminal sequences of specific M types.[555] These probes were able to hybridize to dot-blotted genomic DNA from group A streptococcal strains and were able to identify several M types more readily than conventional serologic M-typing procedures. In addition to M protein, some streptococci have other "M-like" proteins (e.g., the Spa protein of M type 18 group A streptococci) that have been shown to contribute to and augment virulence.[678]

Cloning of the M protein gene, called the *emm* gene, has resulted in the expansion and standardization of *emm* typing to replace the conventional serologic method. The *emm* typing system is performed by sequence analysis of the NH$_2$-terminal nucleotide residues and has resulted in the identifi-

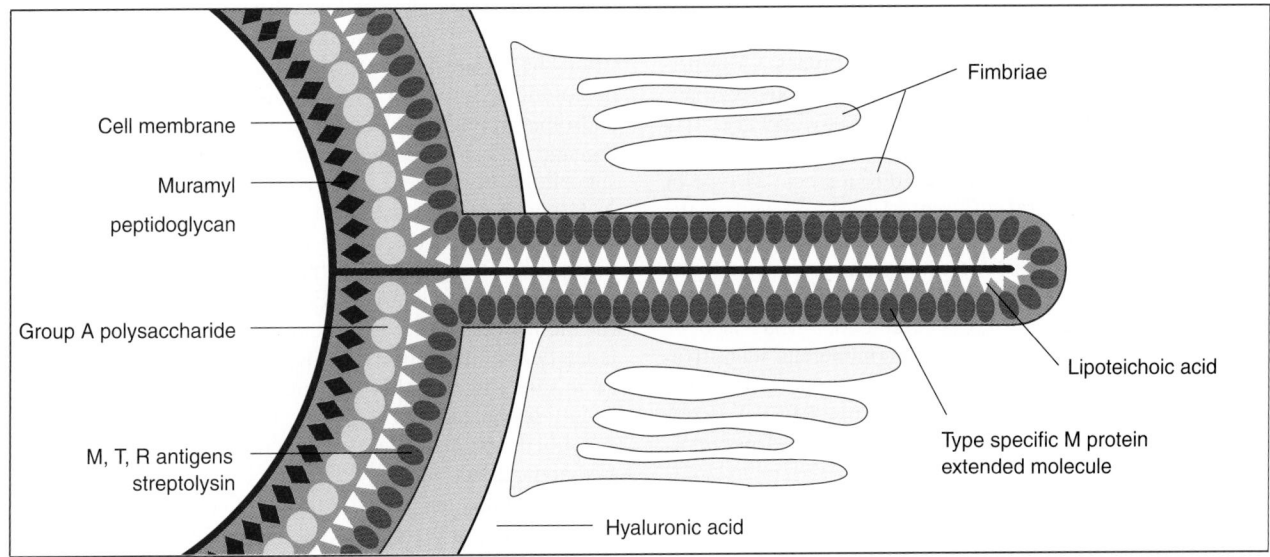

Figure 13-1 The major known antigenic determinants on the surface of virulent, encapsulated group A streptococci.

cation of over 124 recognized *emm* genotypes.[340,848] The definition of a new *emm* type sequence is based on the identification of more than 160 nucleotide bases at the 5′ terminus of the hypervariable region. Different *emm* types will have less than 80% sequence homology with other *emm* types.[67,334] Amino acid sequence analysis of M proteins of many types has also identified portions of the M protein molecule that are common among several M protein types; that is, this sequence of amino acids is highly conserved.[791] Sera from individuals living in different geographic areas with high rates of streptococcal infection reacted with this conserved M peptide in an enzyme-linked immunosorbent assay (ELISA). Furthermore, antibodies directed against this peptide were able to opsonize streptococci belonging to a variety of M types. This highly conserved part of the M protein molecule is being investigated further as a possible candidate vaccine antigen against group A streptococcal infection and rheumatic fever. In addition to M protein, several other M-related cell-surface proteins have been identified on group A streptococci, and the genes encoding these molecules (e.g., *enn*, *mrp*, *arp*, *fcrA*, *protH*) have been grouped together as members of the *emm* gene superfamily.[539] These molecules apparently work in concert with M proteins to help the organisms resist phagocytosis. These M-protein-like molecules are also able to bind to several host proteins such as plasminogen and fibrinogen, and, via this interaction, also exert antiopsonic effects. The sequences of the recognized *emm* types may be found online at http://www.cdc.gov/nci-dod/biotech/infotech_hp.html.

Opacity factor (OF) describes another M-protein-associated cell-surface antigen of group A streptococci that is a putative virulence factor.[806] OF is an α-lipoproteinase that is able to opacify (render opaque) media containing mammalian serum.[543] Antibodies directed against OF are specific in inhibiting the opacity reaction of the M type producing it, so OF typing can be used as a supplementary or complementary typing reaction. OF is produced by strains that belong to 29 different M types and can be detected in those M types even if M-type-specific reactivity is lost or undetectable (i.e., the presence of OF is associated only with specific M types). Therefore, OF-positive and OF-negative reactions are consistently associated with specific M types. OF is primarily associated with strains of group A streptococci isolated from skin infections.[91] Group A streptococci also may possess T and R antigens. T antigens are acid- and heat-stable antigens that may be restricted to a single M type or may be shared by several different M types.[100] Neither the T nor the R antigen is associated with virulence, and these antigens are rarely used in current typing systems since the description of *emm* and OF typing. In addition to these serologic typing methods, group A streptococci may also be typed by phenotypic biotyping with commercial identification systems, multilocus enzyme electrophoresis, DNA restriction-fragment-length polymorphisms (RFLPs), rRNA gene RFLPs (ribotyping), and random amplified polymorphic DNA analysis.[124,133,440,713,877]

Group A streptococci produce two hemolysins: streptolysin O and streptolysin S. **Streptolysin O (SLO)** is oxygen-labile, antigenic, inhibited by cholesterol, and toxic to a variety of cell types, including leukocytes, monocytes, and cultured cells. Because of its oxygen lability, SLO is primarily responsible for the β-hemolysis seen around subsurface colonies of group A streptococci in pour plates or in the stabbed regions of surface-inoculated sheep blood agar plates. SLO is also produced by some group C and group G streptococci. It appears to exist in two active forms, with molecular weights of between 50 and 70 kDa; cleavage of these molecules during secretion results in the fully-active form of SLO having a molecular weight of about 57 kDa.[93] SLO causes the formation of pores in the membrane of susceptible cells by initial binding of SLO monomers to cholesterol in the cell membrane. This binding results in a conformational change in the molecule that causes the coaggregation of additional SLO monomers on the membrane.[876] These aggregates initially form arc-shaped structures on the membrane that eventually become fully formed pores, resulting in osmotic lysis of the affected cell. SLO also induces degranulation and lysis of PMNs, inhibits phagocytosis by macrophages, and impairs the response of lymphocytes to mitogens. SLO may also stimulate the production of cytokines.[447] Measurement of antibodies against streptolysin O (antistreptolysin O [ASO] titers) in serum is useful for retrospective diagnosis of recent pharyngeal streptococcal infections. The ASO response following skin infections is poor, presumably because of inactivation of the antigen by cholesterol present in skin. In such cases, anti-DNaseB titers are more reliable (see later discussion).

Streptolysin S (SLS) is oxygen-stable, non-antigenic, and, like SLO, is toxic to a variety of cell types. SLS exists in intracellular, cell-surface bound, and intracellular forms and is usually associated with some type of carrier molecule, such as serum albumin, RNA, or α-lipoprotein. SLS, a small molecule having a molecular weight of about 1,800 daltons, is maximally produced during the late logarithmic and early stationary phases of growth, and requires iron for maximal production.[19,439] SLS is believed to interact with membrane phospholipids in exerting its toxic effects. Erythrocytes exposed to SLS undergo swelling, followed by lysis due to the disruption of the osmotic barrier and the leakage of ions from the cell.[19] Unlike SLO, no slits or pores are observed on affected erythrocyte cell membranes by electron microscopy. SLS is active in both surface and subsurface hemolysis when the organisms are grown on sheep blood agar. The hemolytic activity of SLS is inhibited by serum lipoproteins and other simple phospholipids. Like SLO, SLS is able to damage the membranes of PMN cells, platelets, and internal subcellular organelles.

Group A streptococci also produce several extracellular products; many of these play a real or theoretical role in the virulence of the organism. **Streptococcal pyrogenic exotoxins (SPEs)** (particularly SPE A and SPE B) are responsible for the rash of scarlet fever and are also the principal virulence determinants in the pathogenesis of the streptococcal toxic shock-like syndrome. Three immunologically distinct SPEs, designated SPE types A, B, and C, have been well described, and the genes that encode them have been identified and characterized.[417,418,468,729,1033] The genes for streptococcal pyrogenic exotoxins A and C (*speA* and *speC*) are encoded on a streptococcal lysogenic bacteriophage, whereas the gene for the type B exotoxin (*speB*) is chromosomal. The *speB* gene is found in all group A streptococci, whereas the other two genes may or may not be present.

SPE B, the product of the *speB* gene, is actually a **cysteine protease** enzyme that is able to cleave human immunoglobulin, fibronectin, vitronectin, and other host cell proteins, resulting in the formation of small, biologically active peptides, including interleukin-1, histamine, and kinins.[480,1026] Pyrogenic exotoxins like SPE A and SPE C not only induce fever, as their name implies, but they also function as superantigens. **Superantigens** are molecules that are able to induce proliferation of host T-lymphocytes, regardless of their antigenic specificity, by binding to class II major histocompatibility complex (MHC) molecules.[630,790] Activation of T-cells by superantigens results in the massive release of various cytokines by human monocytes and lymphocytes, including tumor necrosis factor-α (TNFα), interleukin 1β, and T-cell mediators such as interleukin-2 and interferon-γ.[447,448] These cytokines activate the complement, coagulation, and fibrinolytic cascades and cause leakage from the capillaries with resulting hypotension and shock, which are the most severe manifestations of streptococcal toxic shock syndrome. These superantigens also potentiate the host response to minute amounts of Gram-negative endotoxin by a factor greater than 100,000-fold, and have direct toxic effects on endothelial cells lining the capillaries. Streptococcal pyrogenic exotoxins have molecular weights of about 25 to 28 kDa and contain T-cell receptor binding and class II MHC binding sites, plus a zinc binding site that functions in mediating the binding of the class II molecules to the exotoxin. In addition to SPEs A, B, and C, several other pyrogenic exotoxins (e.g., SSA [streptococcal superantigen], SPE D, SPE F MF [mitogenic factor], SMEZ-1, SMEZ-2, SpeG-SpeL) and their genetic loci (e.g., *speG*, *speH*, *speJ*) have been identified from sequencing studies of various group A streptococcal isolates.[693,730,789,802,909,982] Production of these superantigens varies among streptococcal strains belonging to different M or *emm* types. In addition to group A streptococci, various streptococcal superantigen genes (e.g., *ssa*, *speM*, *smeZ*) are also found in some group C and G β-hemolytic streptococci (*S. dysgalactiae* subsp. *equisimilis* and *S. canis*).[509]

Group A β-hemolytic streptococci also produce several other products that contribute to virulence. As mentioned, SPE B is actually a **C5a peptidase** that is bound to the cell surface. The current thought is that this molecule contributes to disease largely because of its peptidase activity rather than as a functioning superantigen. C5a peptidase cleaves and inactivates C5a, the chemotactic complement component, resulting in limiting the recruitment and chemotaxis of polymorphonuclear leukocytes.[736] These organisms also produce four immunologically and electrophoretically distinct **deoxyribonucleases**, designated DNase A, B, C, and D. Antibodies against DNase B (anti-DNase B) are helpful, along with ASO titers, for serologic documentation of prior group A streptococcal pharyngeal or skin infections. **Hyaluronidase** produced by group A streptococci depolymerizes the ground substance of connective tissue, resulting in contiguous spread of the organism. **Streptokinases** produced by group A streptococci hydrolyze fibrin clots and may function in virulence by preventing the formation of fibrin barriers at the periphery of spreading streptococcal lesions. The contribution of these enzymes and toxins to infection is

uncertain. Many of these factors are produced by other β-hemolytic streptococci as well. Strains of group A *Streptococcus* M-1 and certain other M-types produce a protein called **SIC** that inhibits complement by becoming incorporated into the membrane-attack complex of complement (C5b-C9), thereby inhibiting lysis of the target cell.[14] Polymorphism in the *sic* gene can be used to characterize M-1 strains that may be epidemiologically linked.[486]

Clinical Significance

Humans are the natural reservoir for group A, β-hemolytic streptococci, and the organism is transmitted from person to person by the respiratory route. The most common infection caused by group A streptococci is **streptococcal pharyngitis**. Most cases of pharyngitis are seen in school-aged children (5 to 15 years old) during the winter or spring. Following an initial incubation period of 2 to 4 days, onset is generally abrupt, with fever, sore throat, headache, malaise, and abdominal pain. The posterior pharynx is usually inflamed and swollen, and a grayish-white exudate may be present on the tonsils. The anterior cervical lymph nodes are usually tender and swollen. The presence of rhinorrhea, hoarseness, cough, or diarrhea speaks against group A streptococcal infection, instead suggesting a viral or mycoplasmal etiology.[98,890] Infection with strains that elaborate pyrogenic exotoxins A, B, or C may also cause a scarlatiniform rash (i.e., classic scarlet fever). Complications of group A streptococcal pharyngitis may be suppurative (i.e., peritonsillar abscess, retropharyngeal abscess, suppurative cervical adenitis, otitis media, sinusitis, mastoiditis, bacteremia), nonsuppurative (i.e., acute and chronic rheumatic fever, glomerulonephritis), or toxin-mediated (streptococcal toxic shock-like syndrome).[889,890] In the absence of complications, streptococcal pharyngitis is self-limited. However, treatment (ideally, culture followed by antimicrobial therapy) is usually sought. About 15% of individuals with streptococcal pharyngitis may become asymptomatic carriers of the organisms following treatment.[100] Currently, recommendations for treatment of streptococcal pharyngitis include oral penicillin V (children, 250 mg b.i.d. or t.i.d.; adolescents and adults, 250 mg t.i.d. or q.i.d.; adolescents and adults, 500 mg b.i.d.) for 10 days, or intramuscular benzathine penicillin G (600,000 to 1.2 million units).[98] Erythromycin (dosage dependent on the formulation used) is a suitable alternative for those patients who are allergic to penicillin. Although significant resistance to macrolides among group A streptococci has been reported in several countries (e.g., Australia, Finland, Canada, Hawaii, Japan, Italy, Finland, Greece, the Philippines, Sweden), less than 5% of group A streptococcal isolates in the U.S. have been demonstrated to be resistant to erythromycin.[231,235,531,549,552,878,879,1035,1089] Group A β-hemolytic streptococci remain highly susceptible to penicillin G. For those patients who are infected with erythromycin-resistant group A streptococci and are unable to tolerate β-lactam agents, clindamycin may also be used.[98]

In addition to pharyngitis, Group A β-hemolytic streptococci cause of variety of superficial cutaneous infections, including impetigo, erysipelas, cellulitis, puerperal sepsis, and post-partum infections. **Impetigo** usually occurs in children ages 5 to 15 years and is characterized by the development of vesicular lesions that evolve into pustules.[132] These pustules break down over the next 5 to 7 days to form thick scabs. Impetigo lesions are usually on the lower extremities and may also involve other pathogens, such as *Staphylococcus aureus*. As mentioned, cutaneous infection with nephritogenic group A streptococcal strains may give rise to poststreptococcal glomerulonephritis (see below). **Erysipelas** is an acute infection that is associated with involvement of the soft tissues and cutaneous lymphatics and results in systemic evidence of infection, including fever. The lesions present as areas of edema and erythema that spread rapidly and have a raised, well-demarcated margin. Lesions of erysipelas are often on the face, and patients often have accompanying streptococcal pharyngitis (see Color Plate 13-1*A*).[113] **Cellulitis** usually results from streptococcal infection of previous lesions, such as wounds, burns, or surgical incisions. This infection presents as a spreading inflammatory process that may involve large areas of the skin and subcutaneous tissues, along with fever, chills, lymphangitis and, occasionally, bacteremia. This infection is often seen in intravenous drug users.[313] **Puerperal sepsis** is seen in women following delivery or abortion. Organisms colonizing the genital tract or from obstetrical personnel invade the upper genital tract, causing endometritis, lymphangitis, bacteremia, necrotizing fasciitis, and streptococcal toxic shock syndrome.[56,406] Genital tract infection may be complicated by pelvic cellulitis, peritonitis, and abscess formation. Intrapartum transmission of group A streptococci, leading to severe and often fatal group A streptococcal disease in the neonate has also been observed.[753] Manifestations in the neonate include stillbirth, septicemia, jaundice, and cellulitis.

Of concern in the management of group A streptococcal pharyngitis are the well-studied ''nonsuppurative'' complications of group A streptococcal infections, acute rheumatic fever and glomerulonephritis.[96,655,932] **Acute rheumatic fever (ARF)** is associated with prior group A streptococcal pharyngitis, whereas glomerulonephritis is associated with prior pharyngeal or skin infection with the organism. ARF is a delayed, multisystem collagen-vascular disease characterized by the major manifestations of carditis, polyarthritis, subcutaneous nodules, erythema marginatum, and chorea. Onset of acute rheumatic fever occurs from 2 to 5 weeks after streptococcal pharyngitis.[96] Cutaneous group A streptococcal infections do not initiate ARF. Cardiac pathology usually involves the endocardium, myocardium, pericardium and, most frequently, the mitral valve; clinically this pathologic manifestation appears as characteristic heart murmurs, cardiac enlargement, congestive heart failure, or, rarely, intractable cardiac arrest and death. The arthritis is usually migratory, involves multiple joints (especially the knees, elbows, ankles, and wrists), and resolves spontaneously. Subcutaneous, firm, painless nodules appear at the same time as carditis and are usually found on the extremities near the bony areas of the feet and hands. Erythema marginatum lesions are erythematous eruptions with red, raised, serpiginous borders and central areas of clearing that usually appear on the trunk, arms, and legs. Chorea is a neurologic manifestation that is characterized by muscular spasms, incoordination, and muscle weakness that develop during ARF or after several months. Attacks

of ARF generally last 3 to 6 months. The differential diagnosis of this illness is broad owing to the protean manifestations of the syndrome and includes rheumatoid arthritis, systemic lupus erythematosus, sickle cell disease, rubella, septic arthritis, disseminated gonococcal infection, Lyme disease, bacterial endocarditis, and myocarditis. Laboratory findings associated with ARF include elevated sedimentation rate, elevated C-reactive protein, and the occurrence of an antecedent streptococcal infection, as evidenced by a positive throat culture or a positive direct antigen test for group A streptococci, or by elevated or rising streptococcal antibody titers (e.g., ASO, anti-DNaseB, anti-hyaluronidase).[248] A single positive antistreptococcal antibody test is not diagnostic of ARF, so it is recommended that all three specific antibody tests be performed if ARF is highly suspected. Therapy for ARF includes analgesics, salicylates, and corticosteroids for treatment of fever and inflammation, plus supportive therapy to prevent cardiac failure.[96]

Acute glomerulonephritis is an inflammatory disease of the renal glomerulus that is associated with diffuse glomerular lesions, hypertension, hematuria, and proteinuria.[96] Glomerular lesions can be demonstrated to contain depositions of complement components (especially C3), properdin, and immunoglobulin by immunofluorescence techniques.[599,683] While rheumatic fever may appear 1 to 5 weeks following streptococcal pharyngitis, glomerulonephritis may occur as soon as 10 days following pharyngitis or 3 to 6 weeks following skin infections.[31] Clinically, the disease is characterized by malaise, weakness, anorexia, headache, edema, and circulatory congestion, as evidenced by hypertension and encephalopathy. Laboratory findings include anemia, an elevated sedimentation rate, decreased C3 and total complement, hematuria, and proteinuria. Urinalysis reveals red blood cells, leukocytes, and casts. Antecedent group A streptococcal infection is usually demonstrable by recovery of organisms from the throat or from skin lesions or by elevation of antistreptococcal antibodies. ASO responses following streptococcal skin infections are not reliably elevated, and titers for anti-DNaseB and anti-hyaluronidase should be performed.[96]

Several theories have been advanced concerning the mechanism by which group A streptococci induce ARF and glomerulonephritis.[44,491] The most tenable theory is that the streptococci induce the formation of antistreptococcal antibodies against capsular (hyaluronic acid), cell wall (anti-group-carbohydrate, anti-M, and other associated proteins), and cell membrane antigens that cross-react with various antigenic moieties in myocardial, endocardial, and valvular heart tissue, the myocardial sarcolemma, skeletal muscle, and the joints. Group A streptococci vary in their abilities to trigger ARF or AGN, and certain streptococcal M types have now been identified as being ''rheumatogenic'' or ''nephritogenic'' Strains of group A β-hemolytic strains that are responsible for ARF are usually rich in M protein, display a mucoid colony morphology due to heavy encapsulation, are usually OF negative, and are primarily associated with pharyngeal infections. These strains also evoke a strong type-specific immune response. Group A streptococcal M types, including types M1, M3, M5, M16, M18, M-19, M-24, and a few others have been shown to be ''rheumatogenic.''[931,932] Antigenic epitopes of some of these M types have been demonstrated to share determinants with human cardiac muscle, sarcolemma membrane proteins, and synovial membranes.[46,249,250,267] Other workers have shown similar immunologic cross-reactions between the polysaccharide antigen of group A streptococci and certain heart valve glycoproteins, between streptococcal hyaluronic acid (i.e., the capsular material) and human hyaluronic acid, and between streptococcal cell membranes and the caudate and subthalamic neuronal nuclei in the human central nervous system.[360,409,503,870] The latter may explain the role of antecedent streptococcal infection in the neurologic components of ARF. Similarly, "nephritogenic" group A streptococcal strains belonging to certain M types have also been identified. M types M-2, M-49, M-55, M-57, M59, M-60, and M-61 have been associated with glomerulonephritis following skin infections, whereas types M-1, M-4, M-12, and M-25 are most frequently implicated following pharyngeal infections. Although cross-reactions between nephritogenic streptococcal strains and renal tissues have been demonstrated, the pathologic abnormalities of nephritis may actually be due to the deposition of preformed immune complexes containing streptococcal antigens and host antibodies in the glomerular tissues or to renal binding of streptococcal products followed by deposition of antibodies to create immune complexes.[101,416,491,972,996]

Since the end of World War II, the incidence of streptococcal pharyngitis in North America and Western Europe has remained fairly stable, while the incidence of acute rheumatic fever and acute post-streptococcal glomerulonephritis has decreased dramatically.[794] Beginning in the mid-80's, however, "outbreaks" of rheumatic fever were reported in the Salt Lake City area, Colorado, California, Pennsylvania, North Carolina, Tennessee, Missouri, West Virginia, Texas, Ohio, and New York.[141,164,165,438,616,666,1004,1023,1044,1045] In these outbreaks, many individuals did not recall having had a streptococcal infection. In such cases, and in the diagnosis of the nonsuppurative sequelae, serologic studies (serum antibodies to streptolysin O, serum antibodies to DNase B, serum antibodies to hyaluronidase) must be performed for retrospective documentation of previous group A streptococcal infections. Among the strains of group A streptococci recovered from patients who had positive pharyngeal cultures during these various outbreaks, it was noted that many were mucoid strains belonging to M types 1, 3, 5, 6, and 18; these strains had not been recovered with any great frequency before 1985.

Shortly after reports of resurgent rheumatic fever caused by these recognized rheumatogenic M serotypes appeared in the literature, severe invasive group A streptococcal infections associated with a toxic shock-like syndrome (TSLS) were reported from European and American medical centers.[62,136,176,183,230,369] In one of the initial publications, Stevens and coworkers reported on 20 patients from the Rocky Mountain region of the United States who presented with various types of group A streptococcal soft-tissue infections (pharyngitis, cellulitis, suppurative thrombophlebitis, peritonitis, necrotizing fasciitis, postpartum myometritis, localized wound infection) and went on to develop additional symptoms that were similar to those found in patients with classic staphylococcal toxic shock syndrome.[924,928] These clinical characteristics included hypotension, renal dysfunction, hypoalbuminuria, thrombocytopenia, hypocalcemia, and respi-

ratory failure. All of the patients had positive cultures for group A streptococci, including 12 patients with positive blood cultures. Of the 20 patients, 19 developed shock, and six died as a result of their infections. Interestingly, eight of the 10 group A streptococcal strains that were available for subsequent study produced streptococcal pyrogenic exotoxin A (SPE A), the toxin associated with scarlet fever. This was of particular interest because strains that produce SPE A had been infrequently isolated in the United States since 1976. Active laboratory, and population based surveillance from July of 1995 through December 1999 in five U.S. states found that M types 1, 3, 11, 12 and 28 accounted for 49.2% of isolates from invasive infections, with newly characterized *emm* types accounting for 8.9% of strains.[734]

The group A streptococcal toxic shock-like syndrome (TSLS) is now a well-recognized clinical entity.[927] In the U.S., the attack rate has been estimated by the CDC to be approximately 1 case per 100,000 population, although higher rates may be observed regionally and among the very young and very old.[924,925] Patients who develop invasive group A streptococcal infections often have co-morbid diseases, especially diabetes mellitus, congestive heart failure, malignancies, and immunosuppression.[76] About 20% of patients with TSLS present with a viral-like prodrome of fever, chills, and myalgias. Signs of soft tissue infection, such as swelling, tenderness, erythema or pain may be evident if the primary infection is cutaneous. Patients with necrotizing fasciitis or myositis appear toxic and may rapidly develop violaceous bullous lesions. Patients may go on to develop a wide variety of clinical manifestations of disease, including, myocarditis, hepatitis, peritonitis, myocarditis, septic arthritis, endophthalmitis, puerperal sepsis, meningitis, and overwhelming toxemia.[538] Pulmonary pathology associated with the infection includes cyanosis, tachypnea, and respiratory failure. Renal involvement occurs early in the clinical course in over 80% of patients, as evidenced by high serum creatinine levels and hemoglobinuria. Renal impairment often persists in patients despite aggressive treatment with antibiotics and intravenous fluids, and dialysis may be necessary. Patients may rapidly become hypotensive, and most patients do not respond to albumin and electrolyte fluid. The acute respiratory distress syndrome develops in more than half of the patients, requiring intubation and mechanical ventilation. In fulminant, ultimately fatal infections, the Waterhouse-Friederichsen syndrome and disseminated intravascular coagulation may be seen.[371,550] Bacteremia with group A streptococci occurs in about 70% of patients. If soft tissue infection is present, surgical procedures may be necessary to remove infected, de-vitalized and necrotic tissues. This syndrome characteristically results in shock and multi-organ system failure shortly after the onset of symptoms and may have a mortality rate of from 30% to over 80%.[65] Management requires antibiotic therapy, volume resuscitation, and intensive supportive care. Clindamycin has greater efficacy than penicillin, and this drug is often used for therapy along with pencillin.[53] Clindamycin has been shown to inhibit the expression of M proteins and the synthesis and export of toxins (including the pyrogenic exotoxins SPE A and SPE B), enzymes (e.g., DNase, SLO and SLS), and capsular material.[131,665,916] There is also some evidence to indicate that intravenous immunoglobulin infusions may also be beneficial.[731]

Streptococcal pyrogenic exotoxins (SPEs) have been shown to play a major role in the pathogenesis of TSLS. Hauser and colleagues examined 34 TSLS group A streptococcal isolates and found that 74% were either type M1 or M3. Although 53% produced SPE A, 85% contained the *speA* gene that codes for SPE A.[469] All strains contained the gene coding for SPE B (*speB*), and 21% contained the gene coding for SPE C (*speC*). These workers concluded that SPE A was strongly associated with group A streptococci that were capable of causing TSLS, although they postulated that other factors may also be involved since not all strains recovered from patients with TSLS contained the *speA* gene. Musser and coworkers examined the M types and the presence of genes coding for SPE A (*speA* genotype) and SPE C (*speC* genotype) in a collection of group A streptococcal isolates from cases of pharyngitis occurring in nine different states.[714] More than 50% of the isolates that expressed the M1 or M3 serotype hybridized specifically with a probe for *speA*, indicating that strains with the potential for causing severe streptococcal disease were well represented among those causing community-acquired pharyngitis. Others have now shown that SPE A and other pyrogenic exotoxins are similar to the staphylococcal enterotoxins and are superantigens that are capable of inducing the release of various cytokines and lymphokines.[97,353,448] These molecules, in turn, mediate the profound systemic effects that promote rapid systemic invasion by the organisms and precipitate the multiorgan system involvement that characterizes the syndrome.[630,790] As mentioned, treatment of patients with clindamycin and penicillin is recommended, since clindamycin is much more potent at inhibiting the synthesis of pyrogenic exotoxins (particularly SPE A and SPE B) than penicillin.[665]

At the same time that TSLS was being recognized, increases in the incidence of other group A streptococcal infections, especially bacteremias, necrotizing fasciitis, and myositis, were being observed in both adult and pediatric populations in the United States and abroad.[247,926] Initially, these severe streptococcal infections were reported among intravenous drug users in Philadelphia, adults in the Denver and Los Angeles areas, and children in Winston-Salem, North Carolina and Denver, Colorado.[166,619,1045] Familial clusters and outbreaks centered in hospitals and nursing homes were also reported.[872] Besides bacteremia, many patients developed streptococcal necrotizing fasciitis. Necrotizing fasciitis is an infection of the deep subcutaneous tissues that results in progressive devitalization and destruction of the fascia.[874] This infection presents with erythema initially at the site of apparent or trivial trauma, although hematogenous seeding of subcutaneous muscle and soft tissue also occurs. In children, this infection is often associated with streptococcal infection of varicella lesions in previously well children.[517] The infection rapidly develops and spreads so that, over the next 24 to 72 hours, the tissues change in color from an erythematous red hue to deep blue or purple, with the formation of bullous lesions containing serosanguineous fluid. At this point, the tissues become gangrenous, with devitalized tissue being sloughed to reveal extensive subcutaneous tissue necrosis.[371] The infection rapidly spreads along the fascial planes to involve soft tissues and the muscles, resulting in myositis and myonecrosis.[721,936,1031] Magnetic resonance imaging studies are useful in identifying the extent of fasciitis and soft-tissue edema infiltrating the fascial planes prior to necrosis presenting clinically. The patient becomes increasingly obtunded and stuporous due to overwhelming intoxication and, even with appropriate antimicrobial coverage and extensive surgical debridement of devitalized tissues, mortality rates may be 30% to 60%, with some deaths occurring as rapidly as 48 hours after the onset of signs and symptoms. Extensive muscle involvement predicts an even more dire prognosis, with fatality rates between 80% and 100%. Because of the severity of these infections and the high mortality associated with them, aggressive medical and surgical interventions have been necessary and lifesaving in many patients.[371,1076] With the recognition of these severe streptococcal infections and the emergence of TSLS, the group A *Streptococcus* has reestablished itself as an organism to be reckoned with in the 21st century.

Group A β-hemolytic streptococci also may cause a variety of other infections, including pneumonia, meningitis, osteomyelitis, endocarditis, peritonitis, and nosocomial infections. Pneumonia due to group A streptococci usually occurs in debilitated hosts with other conditions, including influenza or other intercurrent respiratory virus infections, chronic obstructive pulmonary disease, alcoholism, and neoplastic disease.[57] Pneumonia may also be a part of the clinical presentation of invasive group A streptococcal diseases, such as streptococcal toxic shock syndrome. Streptococcal pneumonia often presents with an abrupt onset of fever, chills, malaise, and dyspnea, and chest pain. Chest films usually show basilar infiltrates with pleural effusions. Diagnosis is usually made by culture of sputum, pleural fluid, empyema fluid, and/or blood.[702,826] Sputum is usually purulent and streaked with blood. Complications of pulmonary group A streptococcal infections include sepsis, pleural effusions, empyema, pneumothorax, pericarditis, mediastinitis, shock, pulmonary cavitation, bronchiectasis, metastatic abscesses, and osteomyelitis.[57,718] Osteomyelitis due to group A streptococci is often seen as a complication of varicella infections in children; in adults, streptococcal osteomyelitis usually occurs as a complication of bacteremia.[13] Meningitis due to group A streptococci occurs in about 2% of all patients with systemic group A streptococcal infection and accounts for anywhere from 0.2% to 1% of all cases of meningitis.[187] This infection is similar in presentation to other acute bacterial meningitides, with headache, fever, nuchal rigidity, and focal neurological deficits.[538,709] Patients with meningitis may also have a focus of infection that results in bacteremia, with subsequent invasion of the meninges.[912] In a review of 41 adult patients with this infection, 60% had a history of otitis media, sinusitis, pneumonia, recent head injury, recent neurosurgery, or the presence of a neurosurgical device.[994] Group A streptococcal endocarditis is a rare infection that occurs in infants, children, and adults. Pediatric endocarditis may be associated with bacteremia and varicella infection.[691,1065] Endocarditis in adults usually occurs in patients with no antecedent cardiac abnormalities and is associated with a high rate of complications, including cerebral or other systemic emboli, arthritis, diskitis, and osteomyelitis.[45] Nosocomial group A streptococcal infections have also been reported, usually in association with the presence of catheters and other indwelling medical devices.[660] Group A streptococci have also joined the growing list of other microorganisms implicated in continuous ambulatory peritoneal dialysis-associated peritonitis.[163]

Group B β-Hemolytic Streptococci (*Streptococcus agalactiae*)
Virulence Factors

The group B β-hemolytic *Streptococcus* (*S. agalactiae*) contains a Lancefield-grouping antigen, a type-specific cell-surface polysaccharide and protein antigens. The group B antigen is composed of a rhamnose-glucosamine polymer attached to the peptidoglycan layer. Type specificity is provided by both capsular polysaccharide and protein antigens. Group B streptococci are invariable encapsulated and belong to one of nine recognized capsular serotypes. The nine capsular types are composed of glucose, galactose, N-acetylglucosamine, and N-acetyl-neuraminic acid (sialic acid); serotype specificity is determined by differing arrangements of these four components in each of the nine capsular types. The **polysaccharide capsular antigens** are designated Ia, Ib, II, III, IV, V, VI, VII, and VIII.[533,582,1018,1019,1039] The **protein antigen** is designated by the single letter c, which exists in two forms, designated cα and cβ. This c antigen is found in all Ib strains (type Ia strains lack the c protein), in 60% of type II strains, and is rarely found in type III strains (not enough serotype IV-VIII strains have been examined for the presence of the c antigen). Therefore, serotype designations for c-antigen-containing strains are expressed as Ib/c and II/c. The importance of these capsular components as virulence factors is demonstrated by both in vitro and in vitro data. Opsonizing antibodies against group B streptococci are serotype-specific as demonstrated by studies using PMN cells and macrophages, and lack of maternal antibodies to these type-specific antigens is a recognized risk factor for development of group B streptococcal disease in the neonate.[358]

Although serologic techniques are the reference methods for determinations of serotypes, molecular-based methods have also been developed for both serotyping and subserotyping of isolates. Kong and colleagues developed primers and polymerase chain reaction (PCR)–based sequencing assays for the capsular *cps* genes of all serotypes that correlated 100% with serologic approaches.[583] Further subtyping was achieved by amplification and sequencing of the genes for cα (*bca* gene), cα-like (*alp2*, *alp3*, and *alp4* genes), Rib (*rib* gene), and cβ (*bac* gene) cell-surface proteins.[583,584] Bohnsack and colleagues used DNA restriction digest patterns of the group B streptococcal hyaluronate lyase gene (*hylB*) to subdivide serotype III strains, one of which (III-3) correlated with clones having increased virulence.[111] Molecular serotyping methods have also been described for use in clinical laboratories. Borchardt and coinvestigators designed primers to amplify the *cps* capsular gene sequences and then applied *cps* type-specific probes in a dot-blot format to determine the serotype.[114] Using this approach, 99% of 306 isolates were assigned to a serotype, compared with 89% that were typeable by the capillary precipitin reference

method. Other molecular methods have also been used to further characterize isolates of group B streptococci.[1093]

The prevalence of the various group B capsular serotypes varies over time and may differ from place to place. Prior to the 1990s, most group B streptococcal disease was caused by serotypes Ia, Ib, II, III, and V; serotypes IV and VI through VIII were relatively uncommon. During the early to mid-1990s, serotype V strains began to emerge, with the percentage of isolates in this group increasing from 2.6% in 1992 to 20% in 1994.[324,436] Studies conducted in the U.S. and abroad indicate that serotypes Ia, Ib, II, III, and V now predominate among vaginal isolates and clinical isolates from patients.[82,106,628] Recently, serotypes VI and VIII have appeared as the predominant serotypes in Japan.[591] In a study of 73 vaginal isolates from pregnant women attending an urban obstetrics clinic in Kawasaki, Japan, 35.6% of isolates were serotype VIII and 24.7% were serotype VI. Neonatal early-onset disease due to serotype VIII has also been reported in Japan.[669] Type III strains of group B streptococci account for 60% of isolates from cases of neonatal sepsis and over 80% of isolates from infants with meningitis, suggesting that this group B streptococcal serotype possesses enhanced virulence.[286,628] The type III capsular polysaccharide is composed of a repeating structural backbone consisting of galactose, glucose, and *N*-acetyl-glucosamine with side chains consisting of galactose and a terminal *N*-acetyl-neuraminic acid moiety. The structural component of the type III capsule that appears to be associated with augmented virulence is the presence of *N*-acetyl-neuraminic acid (sialic acid). The presence of this molecule on the surface of the organism inhibits activation of the alternative complement cascade and prevents phagocytosis. Removal of sialic acid residues with neuraminidase leads to complement activation, phagocytosis, and intracellular killing of the organisms and diminished virulence on intravenous challenge in a rat model.[311,312,1040] Similar results have been obtained with isogenic serotype III group B streptococcal capsule-deficient mutants that lack the terminal sialic acid residues. When compared with the parent strains, these mutants are opsonized and killed in the presence of complement and PMN cells.[827,1042] These mutants also bind the active complement factor C3b more efficiently than the wild type. In the wild type, sialic acid residues block the binding of C3 and promote the inactivation of C3b.[656] These type III capsular mutants are also less virulent in neonatal rat models of group B streptococcal bacteremia and pneumonia than isogenic type III parent strains.[661,1042] Molecular analysis of virulent subtypes of serotype III strains (serotype III-3) identified regions of genomic DNA that encoded a surface protein (Spb 1) that mediates internalization and invasion of epithelial cells by serotype III organisms.[3]

Group B streptococci also produce a variety of other potential virulence determinants. Like the group A streptococci, Group B streptococci also produce **C5a peptidase.** C5a is a complement component cleavage product that is produced by alveolar epithelial cells, acts as an attractant for inflammatory cells, and is involved in the process of pulmonary inflammation.[933] The C5a peptidase produced by the streptococci cleaves C5a at the C-terminus, thereby interfering with C5a-mediated neutrophil chemotaxis.[110] New information indicates that this peptidase also binds to fibronectin and serves as a bacterial adhesin and invasin.[69,182] This enzyme exists in a cell-associated form and also requires the presence of the group B capsule for maximal activity. Opsonization of Group B streptococci belonging to serotypes Ia, Ib, II, III, and V with anti-C5a peptidase antibodies results in increased killing by both macrophages and PMN cells.[180] Immunization of mice with purified streptococcal C5a peptidase elicits an antibody response that protects them from infection with encapsulated group B organisms independent of serotype, suggesting that C5a peptidase may be a strong vaccine candidate antigen.[181] C5a peptidase is also produced by group A and group G β-hemolytic streptococci, and the genes encoding the C5a peptidase in group B (*scpB*) and group A strains (*scpA*) demonstrate 98% sequence homology with each other. The **β-hemolysin/cytolysin** of group B streptococci may act as a virulence factor particularly in pulmonary infections.[397,723] This pore-forming β-hemolysin is able to lyse pulmonary alveolar epithelial and endothelial cells in vitro, suggesting a role for the hemolysin as a virulence factor in neonatal lung infections.[724] The β-hemolysin may also augment the ability of the organisms to invade endothelial cells in the central nervous system (CNS).[725] In vivo and in vitro studies also indicate that β-hemolysin contributes to bacteremia and bacterial invasion of the liver and activates apoptotic pathways in hepatocytes, resulting in liver necrosis.[814] **Lipoteichoic acid** is also found in group B streptococci and may participate in facilitating adherence as a first step in infection.[720] Purified group B streptococcal lipoteichoic acid also is cytotoxic for human embryonic brain and amniotic cells grown in tissue culture.[407] Several **cell-surface proteins** (e.g., c, R, BPS, and Rib antigens) are also found in various combinations in different group B streptococcal serotypes.[328] The **c antigen,** in particular, may act to mediate internalization of organisms within human cervical epithelial cells following attachment and to protect organisms from intracellular killing following phagocytosis.[112,763] These molecules are antigenic, and antibodies directed against them are protective against microbial challenge in animal models. Recently, Jones and colleagues identified a **cell-surface penicillin-binding protein** (PBP1a) that enabled streptococcal cells to resist intracellular killing by phagocytic cells.[544] Group B streptococci also produce a **hyaluronic acid lyase,** which may act to spread infection by breakdown of hyaluronic acid in the extracellular matrix, and may also act on the hyaluronic acid present in high concentrations in placental tissues, fetal tissues, and amniotic fluids.[788] The presence of CAMP factor, protease enzymes, and various nucleases have also been identified in some group B streptococci, but the role of these molecules in disease pathogenesis is uncertain.

Clinical Significance

Group B β-hemolytic streptococci are a major cause of disease in the neonatal and perinatal periods. Women become colonized with the organism in the vagina and the rectum, and vaginal colonization is found in 10–35% of pregnant women; up to 60% of the colonized women will carry the organism intermittently.[458,805] Colonization of the vagina may actually reflect contamination from the rectum, with the gastrointestinal tract being the principal reservoir of the organisms. Vaginal colonization with group B streptococci is usually asymptomatic, although reports have appeared that document vaginitis associated with heavy colonization and resolution of vaginal symptoms with treatment.[493,494] Vaginal colonization generates a serotype-specific immune response, with cumulative increases of antibodies with increasing age; lower antibody levels in teenaged girls may translate to increased risk of group B streptococcal disease in babies born to these younger women.[149] The sexual transmission of group B streptococci is controversial. Some studies have documented higher colonization rates among attendees at sexually transmitted disease clinics and in patients with gonorrhea.[824] Higher rates of colonization have also been documented in women with more prolific sexual experience and greater numbers of sexual partners.[515] However, other studies have documented no correlation between group B streptococcal colonization, sexual experience, or the presence of other sexually transmitted diseases.[494] Group B streptococci have also been recovered from throat and genital cultures of men.

The presence of group B streptococci in the female genital tract at the time of birth can lead to infection of the neonate. One in two infants born to colonized mothers become colonized on the skin or mucosal surfaces by vertical transmission from the colonized mother, either in utero or during delivery. In addition, the neonate may become colonized by nosocomial exposure to the organism after birth. Among colonized infants, disease may occur in 1 to 4 infants per 1,000 live births.[311,915] Neonatal disease with group B streptococci follows two patterns, termed early-onset disease and late-onset disease.

Early-onset disease occurs with an incidence of 0.7 in 1,000 to 3.7 in 1,000 live births and is associated with in utero or perinatal organism acquisition.[311] This incidence is probably an underestimate; a study of early-onset disease conducted in the United Kingdom reported an incidence of 3 to 6 infections per 1,000 live births based on the number of neonates requiring screening for possible sepsis during the first 72 hours of life.[639] The organism is acquired either by ascending infection in utero before delivery, through ruptured fetal membranes, or during passage through a birth canal that is colonized with group B streptococci. Although a substantial proportion of these infants (approximately 50%) will be colonized with group B streptococci, only 1–2% of them become infected.[311,359] Onset of disease occurs during the first 5 days of life; in more than half the cases, infants become ill within the first 12 to 20 hours after birth.[374] The disease spectrum includes bacteremia, pneumonia, meningitis, septic shock, and neutropenia. Although more than 50% of cases occur in full-term infants, a higher attack rate and greater morbidity are associated with preterm infants.[359] Mortality owing to early-onset disease in full-term infants ranges from 2% to 8%; higher mortality rates are seen in premature infants and are inversely proportional to the birth weight of the neonate.[866,1081] Maternal factors that increase the risk for early-onset infection of the neonate include premature labor, prolonged rupture of the fetal membranes, postpartum bacteremia, maternal amnionitis, heavy vaginal colonization with group B streptococci, and group B streptococcal bacteriuria.[24,286,331,374] During the 1970s, about half of the infants in whom early onset disease developed died of the infection, and many patients who survived group B streptococcal meningitis had permanent neurologic sequelae.

Late-Onset disease occurs with an incidence of 0.5 in 1,000 to 1.8 in 1,000 live births.[311] Disease becomes clinically evident 7 days to 3 months (average, 3 to 4 weeks) after birth. Whereas about half of the late-onset infections are acquired from the birth canal of colonized mothers, the remaining cases result from postnatal organism acquisition from the mother or other caregivers or nosocomially.[755] Bacteremia with accompanying meningitis is the predominant clinical presentation.[574] Mortality associated with late-onset disease is about 10–15%. Up to 50% of children with late-onset meningitis will have permanent neurologic complications and sequelae.[1022] The distribution of group B streptococcal serotypes also varies according to whether it is early-onset or late-onset disease.[311] Among neonates with early-onset disease without meningitis, the serotype distribution is equally divided among types Ic, II, and III. Among similarly infected neonates with meningitis, serotype III strains predominate. In late-onset disease, in which meningitis is the common clinical presentation, serotype III strains account for over 90% of the isolates. On the other hand, group B streptococcal meningitis in adults is associated primarily with serotype II organisms.

By the mid-1980s, increased knowledge regarding group B streptococcal infections and the recognition of the symptoms in at-risk patients led to improvements in neonatal care that resulted in reduction of the fatality rate to about 15%. Since infants born to heavily colonized mothers are more likely to have early-onset disease and because infants who acquire a large bacterial inoculum during birth have significantly increased likelihoods of having both early- and late-onset disease, the identification of colonized mothers became a central focus for prevention strategies. Investigators examined possible interventions to prevent group B streptococcal disease, and several clinical trials demonstrated that intrapartum administration of antimicrobial agents interrupted the transmission of group B streptococci from the mother to the neonate and reduced the incidence of early-onset infections.[128,387,624,697,976] This chemoprophylactic approach prevented about 70–75% of early-onset disease, but it had no effect on the development of late-onset disease. At that time, several manufacturers of microbiology products started to develop direct detection methods for group B streptococci in vaginal swab specimens similar to those used for direct detection of group A streptococci in throat swab specimens. These tests used anti–group B streptococcal antibodies to detect organisms directly by latex agglutination or rapid visual or colorimetric immunoassay formats. Theoretically, these rapid tests could be performed in the immediate prepartum period to determine colonization status, and antimicrobial chemoprophylaxis could be administered prior to and during delivery if the antepartum assays were positive. These commercial rapid tests for direct detection of group B streptococci in vaginal swab specimens varied significantly in sensitivity (i.e., 11–88%) when compared with overnight broth techniques and, in general, identified only women who were heavily colonized.[47,297,625,913,1084] The validity of the premise that the risk of neonatal infection is greater for infants born to heavily colonized women was

confounded by a few clinical reports. In an evaluation of a rapid enzyme immunoassay (EIA) kit for direct detection of group B streptococci in vaginal specimens, Towers and coworkers reported that fatal early-onset disease developed in two of nine infants born to mothers with light colonization and negative rapid EIA results.[959] In another study of a rapid detection method for group B streptococcal colonization, Morales and Lim reported that, among 37 women with light colonization and negative rapid screening tests, 6 delivered babies with early-onset sepsis.[697] In addition, the timing of antepartum testing for group B streptococcal colonization is also an issue. About 60–70% of women with positive vaginal cultures for group B streptococci in the second trimester will be colonized at term, but up to 30% of women with negative cultures during the second trimester will be culture-positive at delivery. Therefore, the development of accurate methods for rapid, sensitive, and specific detection of group B streptococcal colonization in women at or near the time of delivery became a central focus of clinical microbiologic research.

In 1996, the Centers for Disease Control and Prevention (CDC), together with the American Academy of Pediatrics (AAP) and the American College of Obstetrics and Gynecology (ACOG) issued consensus recommendations on a prevention strategy for group B streptococcal disease.[21,22,167] These guidelines recommended that obstetrical healthcare providers adopt either a culture-based or a risk-based strategy for the prevention of early-onset group B streptococcal disease. Subsequent implementation of and compliance with these guidelines has resulted in a significant decrease in the incidence of early-onset neonatal group B streptococcal disease.[863] A critical component of these guidelines is the use of maternal antimicrobial prophylaxis during labor and delivery. This raised concerns regarding the adverse effects of increased antibiotic usage and the increased risk of anaphylactic reactions to penicillin, the drug of choice for chemoprophylaxis. Another concern has been the potential emergence of antimicrobial resistance in group B streptococci. To date, no penicillin-resistant strains of group B streptococci have been isolated, although clindamycin and erythromycin resistance has become relatively common. A third concern was that increased penicillin administration in the newborn period may provide sufficient selective pressure to result in neonatal infections due to penicillin-resistant organisms like *Escherichia coli*, which is the second most common agent of sepsis in the newborn period. This scenario has not developed to date, and continued surveillance will be required to detect and contain this possibility. In 2002, the Committee on Obstetrical Practice issued a statement supporting the use of culture-based prevention strategies based on data from the Active Bacterial Core Surveillance/ Emerging Infections Program network suggesting that the culture-based approach was superior to the risk-based approach.[23] New guidelines were issued by the CDC in 2002, replacing the 1996 guidelines and recommending universal, prenatal, culture-based screening for vaginal and rectal colonization of all pregnant women at 35–37 weeks of gestation (Box 13-3).[170]

The culture protocol recommended by the CDC, ACOG, and the FDA involves collection of vaginal and rectal swab specimens during the 35th to 37th week of gestation.[167,170,]

Box 13-3 Procedures for Collecting and Processing Clinical Specimens for Group B Streptococcal Culture and Performing Susceptibility Testing for Clindamycin and Erythromycin[170]

Procedure for collecting clinical specimens for culture of group B streptococci (GBS) at 35–37 weeks of gestation

- Swab the lower vagina (vaginal introitus) followed by the rectum (i.e., insert swab through the anal sphincter) using the same swab or two different swabs. Culture should be collected in the outpatient setting by the healthcare provider or the patient herself, with appropriate instruction. Cervical cultures are not recommended and a speculum should not be used for culture collection.
- Place the swab(s) into a nonnutritive transport medium. Appropriate transport systems (e.g., Amie's or Stuart's without charcoal) are commercially available. If vaginal and rectal swabs are collected separately, both swabs can be placed in the same container of medium. Transport media will maintain GBS viability for up to 4 days at room temperature or under refrigeration.
- Specimen labels should clearly identify that specimens are for group B streptococcal culture. If susceptibility testing is ordered for penicillin-allergic women, specimen labels should also identify the patient as penicillin-allergic and should specify that susceptibility testing for clindamycin and erythromycin should be performed if GBS are isolated.

Procedure for processing clinical specimens for culture of GBS

- Remove swab(s) from transport medium.[a] Inoculate swab(s) into a recommended selective broth medium, such as Todd-Hewitt broth supplemented with either gentamicin (8 μg/mL) and nalidixic acid (15 μg/mL), or with colistin (10 μg/mL) and nalidixic acid (15 μg/mL). Examples of appropriate commercially available options include Trans-Vag broth supplemented with 5% defibrinated sheep blood or LIM broth.[b]
- Incubate inoculated selective broth for 18–24 hours at 35–37°C in ambient air or 5% CO_2. Subculture the broth to a sheep blood agar plate (e.g., tryptic soy agar with 5% defibrinated sheep blood).
- Inspect and identify organisms suggestive of GBS (i.e., narrow zone of β-hemolysis, gram-positive cocci, catalase-negative). Note that hemolysis may be difficult to observe, so typical colonies without hemolysis should also be further tested. If GBS is not identified after incubation for 18–24 hours, reincubate and inspect at 48 hours to identify suspected organisms.
- Various *Streptococcus* grouping latex tests or other tests for GBS antigen detection (e.g., genetic probe) may be used for specific identification, or the CAMP test may be used for presumptive identification.

Procedure for clindamycin and erythromycin disk susceptibility testing of isolates, when ordered for allergic-allergic patients[c]

- Use a cotton swab to make a suspension from 18–24-hour growth of the organism in saline or Mueller-Hinton broth to match a 0.5 McFarland turbidity standard.
- Within 15 minutes of adjusting the turbidity, dip a sterile cotton swab into the adjusted suspension. The swab should be rotated several times and pressed firmly onto the side wall of the tube above the fluid level. Use the swab to inoculate the entire surface of a Mueller-Hinton sheep blood agar plate. After the plate is dry, use sterile forceps to place a clindamycin (2 μg) disk onto half of the plate and an erythromycin (15 μg) disk onto the other half.
- Incubate at 35°C in 5% CO_2 for 20–24 hours.
- Measure the diameter of the zone of inhibition using a ruler or calipers. Interpret according to NCCLS guidelines for *Streptococcus* species other than *S. pneumoniae* (2002 breakpoints[c]: clindamycin: $\geq$19 mm = susceptible, 16–18 mm = intermediate, $\leq$15mm = resistant; erythromycin: $\geq$21 mm = susceptible, 16–20 mm = intermediate, $\leq$15 mm = resistant).

[a] *Before inoculation step, some laboratories may choose to roll swab(s) on a single sheep blood agar plate or colistin-nalidixic acid (CAN) sheep blood agar plate. This should be done only in addition to, not instead of, inoculation into selective broth. The plate should be streaked for isolation, incubated at 35–37°C in ambient air or 5% CO_2 for 18–24 hours and inspected for organisms suggestive of GBS as described above. If suspected colonies are confirmed as GBS, the broth can be discarded, thus shortening the time to obtaining culture results.*

[b] *Fenton LJ, Harper MH. Evaluation of colistin and nalidixic acid in Todd-Hewitt broth for selective recovery of group B streptococci. J Clin Microbiol 1979;9:167-169. Although Trans-Vag medium is often available without sheep blood, direct comparison of medium with and without sheep blood has shown higher yield when blood is added. LIM broth may also benefit from the addition of sheep blood, although the improvement in yield is smaller and sufficient data are not yet available to support a recommendation.*

[c] *National Committee for Clinical Laboratory Standards. Performance standard for antimicrobial susceptibility testing. M100-S12, Table 2H, Wayne, PA.:NCCLS, 2002. NCCLS recommends disk diffusion (M-2) or broth microdilution testing (M-7) for susceptibility testing of GBS. Commercial systems that have been cleared or approved for testing of streptococci other than S. pneumoniae may also be used. Penicillin susceptibility testing is not routinely recommended for GBS because resistant-resistant isolates have not been confirmed to date.*

[367,865] Vaginal swab specimens are collected from the lower third of the vagina and from the anal canal (a single swab from the vagina then the anal canal, or a swab collected from each site). The swabs are placed in Trans-Vag or LIM broth (Todd-Hewitt broth with 10 μg/mL nalidixic acid, 15 μg/mL colistin, and 10 mg/mL yeast extract) and incubated for 18 to 24 hours.[625] After incubation, the broth is subcultured to sheep blood agar and incubated for 18–24 hours. Plates are reincubated for an additional day if no group B streptococci are found. Group B streptococci are then identified by biochemical (e.g., CAMP test, hippurate hydrolysis, API Rapid Strep), serologic (i.e., serogrouping by coagglutination or latex agglutination), or chemiluminescent hybridiza-

tion (i.e., Gen-Probe AccuProbe) methods. The entire screening procedure may take 2 to 3 days. Direct detection of group B streptococci in the LIM broth following incubation may also be of value in shortening the time to detection, but this method needs further evaluation. Guerrero and colleagues examined 551 rectovaginal cultures for group B streptococci, and 101 were positive by the subculture method.[442] Of these 101 specimens, 99 (98%) of the broth cultures were agglutination-positive with the group B latex reagent. The AccuProbe Group B Streptococcus Culture Identification test (Gen-Probe, San Diego, CA), a chemiluminescent nucleic acid probe culture-confirmation assay, was also evaluated for detection of group B streptococci in LIM broth specimens containing vaginal-anorectal swabs after incubation for 18 to 24 hours. Sensitivities of 94.7–95.6% and specificities of 98.4–99.5% were obtained when the AccuProbe test was compared with LIM broth incubation with subculture and identification.[122,1063] The AccuProbe chemiluminescent DNA probe can also be used to identify isolates from culture media or from bacterial pellets obtained by centrifugation of positive blood culture broths.[251,257] Occasionally, screening cultures will yield other agents of infection. Stefonek and colleagues reported the isolation of group A β-hemolytic streptococci from rectovaginal screening cultures of two patients in who group A streptococcal puerperal sepsis developed.[919]

In 2002, the Food and Drug Administration approved a new product called the IDI-Strep B assay (Infection Diagnostic, Sainte Foy, Quebec, Canada) as a new test for detection of group B streptococci in rectovaginal swabs collected from pregnant women. This is a real-time PCR assay that uses the Cepheid Smart Cycler instrument to detect group B streptococcal DNA. The test can provide results within 1 hour and is the first nonculture test that meets the performance criteria recommended by the CDC guidelines in Box 13-3. This method is at least 85% sensitive compared with the broth amplification-culture method. Like the standard method, the specimen is collected from a patient who is in her 35th to 37th week of pregnancy, or when labor begins. This test needs to be performed so that the results are available early enough for the woman to receive 4 hours of antimicrobial therapy prior to delivery. Even though this test can be performed as a stand-alone test, culture of the specimens is still necessary in order to perform antimicrobial susceptibility testing for clindamycin and erythromycin if the patient is allergic to penicillin. Because of the 4-hour treatment window, this test is useful only if the results are available at least 4 hours before delivery. For patients who present during labor or who have had no prenatal care, the IDI-Strep B assay can be performed if 5 to 6 hours is available for testing and administration of antimicrobial therapy.

While group B streptococci are associated with about 20% of postpartum endometritis, 25% of bacteremias following cesarean section, and 25–30% of cases of asymptomatic bacteriuria during and after pregnancy, they are also associated with a variety of infections in nonpregnant adults.[344] With the decline in neonatal group B streptococcal disease, over two-thirds of infections now occur in adults and are not associated with pregnancy. Adults with group B disease usually have significant underlying disease, including diabetes, liver cirrhosis, stroke, neoplasia, or urinary tract dysfunction.[516] Skin and soft-tissue infections are the most common clinical entities associated with invasive group B streptococci and include cellulitis, abscesses, infected decubitus ulcers, and invasive wound infections following surgical procedures.[99,146] Osteomyelitis may occur as a complication of cellulitis by contiguous spread, particularly in association with decubitus ulcers, or as a result of hematogenous seeding from another site of infection.[385,414] Antimicrobial therapy with aspiration or open drainage of infected joints and removal of prosthetic devices, if present, are necessary to effect cure. Group B streptococci are also the major cause of osteomyelitis in infants, with hematogenous seeding of bone being the source of the organism.[940]

Vertebral osteomyelitis caused by group B streptococci is rare and usually results from hematogenous spread from another focus or from the gastrointestinal tract.[320,352] Vertebral osteomyelitis has also been reported as a rare complication of postpartum bacteremia and urinary tract infections.[64,629] Septic arthritis with group B streptococci usually presents with fever and joint pain following or concomitant with bacteremia.[384] Patients with arthritis are usually elderly, have diabetes or malignancy as risk factors, and will have positive blood and synovial fluid cultures.[851] Rare cases of necrotizing fasciitis due to group B streptococci have also been reported.[812,937] Group B streptococcal pneumonia usually occurs in older debilitated hosts, often results from aspiration of oropharyngeal contents, and may be complicated by the development of empyema.[392,1007] Group B streptococcal conjunctivitis, keratitis, and hematogenous endophthalmitis are severe, albeit rare, infections that occur in previously damaged eyes and result in significant pathology, leading to decreased visual acuity or even blindness.[747]

Group B streptococcal bacteremia from a distant focus of infection can lead to meningitis and endocarditis. Meningitis is rare, accounts for about 4% of bacterial meningitis in adults, and occurs most frequently in postpartum women and older adults with chronic underlying diseases, such as diabetes, cirrhosis, neurologic impairment, malignancy, renal failure, cardiovascular/pulmonary disease, and HIV infection.[295,441,635] Group B streptococcal meningitis following severe head trauma or associated with cerebrospinal rhinorrhea has also been reported.[1002] Endocarditis occurs in both men and women, may present acutely or subacutely, and accounts for 2–18% of invasive group B disease in adults.[45,345] Preexisting cardiac abnormalities are usually present before disease onset and, once established, large vegetations usually develop, with the mitral valve being the most commonly affected. Complications caused by embolic phenomena or rapid destruction of valvular tissue may necessitate valve replacement.[382,873] Endocarditis in neonates and infants occurs rarely but resembles adult cases, with extensive valvular destruction and the occurrence of embolic phenomena.[20,901] Group B streptococcal bacteremia, endocarditis, and meningitis in patients with gastrointestinal, colonic, and pancreatic malignancies have suggested an association similar to that between *S. bovis* and colonic pathology and malignancy.[390,1066]

Bacteriuria with group B streptococci has been associated with adverse pregnancy outcome, increased rates of premature labor, and premature rupture of fetal membranes.[692,1074] Besides being a well-recognized cause of urinary tract infection in pregnant women, this organism is also a cause of cystitis and pyelonephritis in men, nonpregnant women, and children.[704] Anywhere from 5% to over 20% of nonpregnant adults with bacteremia will have group B streptococcal urinary tract infection.[516,705] Risk factors for urinary tract infection caused by group B streptococci include advanced age, underlying disease (especially diabetes), presence of an indwelling urinary catheter, prior urinary tract infections, structural abnormalities of the urinary tract, and other comorbid conditions (e.g., prostatic disease).[345,704] Pyelonephritis and renal abscess are potential complications of both ascending infection and hematogenous dissemination of group B streptococci.[1079]

Group B streptococci may also be capable of causing the toxic shock–like syndrome (TSLS) that is associated with group A streptococci.[386,860] Schlievert and colleagues reported a case of a 27-year-old woman who presented with a toxic shock–like illness consisting of fever, hypotension, an erythematous rash, desquamation, and multiorgan system involvement.[860] Although her blood cultures were negative, group B β-hemolytic streptococci were isolated from urine and vaginal cultures. Further study of these isolates demonstrated that they produced a toxic substance that had the properties associated with pyrogenic exotoxins; the substance caused fever, enhanced susceptibility to endotoxin in experimental animals, and acted as a potent lymphocyte mitogen.

Like the group A streptococci, isolates of group B streptococci remain susceptible to penicillin G, the drug of choice for treatment of infections and for perinatal chemoprophylaxis of women who are vaginal carriers of group B streptococci.[708] Ampicillin, cefotaxime, ceftriaxone, cefazolin, quinupristin-dalfopristin, and meropenem are also highly active, with most strains having minimal inhibitory concentrations (MICs) of ≤0.06 μg/mL.[27,551,668,708] Some group B streptococci demonstrate resistance to erythromycin and clindamycin, and the proportion of resistant strains varies with geographic locale. In a survey of 119 invasive and 227 colonizing strains of group B β-hemolytic streptococci isolated from neonates at six academic centers in the U.S., 20.2% and 6.9% were resistant to erythromycin and clindamycin, respectively.[627] Among strains isolated in California, 32% and 12% were resistant to erythromycin and clindamycin, respectively, while the corresponding figures for strains isolated in Florida were 8.5% and 2.1%. National susceptibility data on bloodstream isolates from centers participating in the SENTRY surveillance program reported that 25.4% of U.S. isolates and 14.3% of Canadian isolates were resistant to erythromycin, and 7% of isolates from both the U.S. and Canada were resistant to clindamycin.[27] Macrolide-lincosamide resistance genotypes that have been detected in group B streptococci include *ermA* (erythromycin-resistant, clindamycin-susceptible), *ermB* (erythromycin resistant, clindamycin-resistant), and *mef* (erythromycin-resistant, clindamycin-susceptible).[285] All group B streptococcal strains tested to date have been susceptible to vancomycin.

Group C and Group G β-Hemolytic Streptococci

The group C β-hemolytic streptococci currently include *S. dysgalactiae* subsp. *equisimilis*, *S. dysgalactiae* subsp. *dysgalactiae*, *S. equi* subsp. *equi*, and *S. equi* subsp. *zooepidemicus*. Former *S. equisimilis* strains isolated from humans have been shown to carry the group C or group G Lancefield antigens and are genetically similar enough to animal group C strains (subsp. *dysgalactiae*) to be placed in the same species, but different subspecies.[89,992,1011] *S. dysgalactiae* subsp. *equisimilis* grows as large colonies on sheep blood agar (SBA) and is usually β-hemolytic. Related strains that carry the C or the L grouping antigen and are isolated primarily from animals are now named *S. dysgalactiae* subsp. *dysgalactiae*.[992] Isolates of this subspecies may be α-hemolytic, β-hemolytic, or nonhemolytic. In addition, molecular genetic studies have demonstrated extensive similarities between the former species *S. equi* and *S. zooepidemicus;* these species have now been reclassified as *S. equi* subsp. *equi* and *S. equi* subsp. *zooepidemicus*.[348] These subspecies carry the Lancefield group C carbohydrate antigen in their cell wall and produce hemolysins that are similar to those of group A streptococci. *S. equi* and *S. dysgalactiae* subspecies form large colonies on SBA, which differentiates them from the "minute" or "small-colony" α-hemolytic, β-hemolytic, or nonhemolytic streptococci of the anginosus group of viridans streptococci, which also may carry the group C polysaccharide antigen.[987] The anginosus group organisms also differ from the "large-colony" group C organisms genetically and phenotypically.[332,604] Case-control studies indicate that large-colony group C organisms may cause pharyngitis, whereas the anginosus group organisms carrying the group C (or A, G, or F) antigen do not.[198] Recent studies, however, have made an association between pharyngitis and a newly described subspecies of *S. constellatus*, *S. constellatus* subsp. *pharyngis*.[1051]

S. dysgalactiae subsp. *equisimilis*, the most common human isolate, has been recovered from the pharynges of carriers and from those with exudative pharyngitis and tonsillitis.[236,370,681,977,978,1090] This organism has also been recovered from several other infections in both children and adults, including sepsis in neutropenic hosts, puerperal sepsis, cellulitis, necrotizing fasciitis, pneumonia, epiglottitis, empyema, bacteremia, meningitis, brain abscess, osteomyelitis, septic arthritis, endocarditis, endophthalmitis, intraabdominal abscess, catheter-related sepsis, and meningitis.[35,39,81,157,732,757,796,840,892,895,911,1062] Most of the patients with these infections have underlying diseases, including chronic cardiopulmonary disease, diabetes, immunosuppression, dermatologic conditions, neoplasms, HIV infection, and alcoholism.[840,892,922] β-Hemolytic streptococci bearing the group C and group G antigens have also been associated with streptococcal toxic chock syndrome, necrotizing fasciitis, and acute rheumatic fever.[466,562,1062] Screening of group C and group G streptococcal isolates for streptococcal pyrogenic exotoxins has identified only the gene for SPE G (*speG*), with all other SPEs and their respective structural genes being absent.[466,836] However, Igwe and colleagues examined 21 group C and group G β-hemolytic streptococcal isolates and found that 11 strains were PCR-positive for at least one of the *speM*, *ssa*, or *smeZ*, genes, which are members of the group A streptococcal superantigen family.[509]

S. equi subsp. *zooepidemicus* causes various types of diseases in animals, including bovine mastitis, respiratory infections in horses, purulent arthritis in lambs and goats, and genital tract infections in poultry. *S. equis* subsp. *zooepidemicus* has also been implicated in human infections, including pneumonia, bacteremia, endocarditis, meningitis, septic arthritis, abdominal aortic aneurysm, deep-vein thrombosis, nephritis, and cervical lymphadenitis.[54,55,204,601,1088] Outbreaks of human pharyngitis caused by *S. equi* subsp. *zooepidemicus* have been traced to consumption of unpasteurized cows' milk and homemade cheese that contained the organisms.[310,375] In some of the affected individuals, poststreptococcal glomerulonephritis was also observed.[375] *S. equi* subsp. *equi* is the cause of a respiratory tract infection in horses called "strangles," which is characterized by a high fever, a mucopurulent nasal discharge, and abscesses in the submandibular and retropharyngeal lymph nodes that eventually rupture and drain into the respiratory tract of the infected animal.[957] This organism is extremely rare in humans, and has been isolated from cases of bacteremia and meningitis.[81,326]

Group G β-hemolytic streptococci constitute a part of the normal human gastrointestinal, vaginal, oropharyngeal, and skin flora. Human isolates that carry the group G antigen are also named *S. dysgalactiae* subspecies *equisimilis*, and animal isolates with this antigen correspond to *S. canis*.[277,1010] Infections caused by human-associated group G strains include pharyngitis, otitis media, pleuropulmonary infections, cellulitis, septic thrombophlebitis, bacteremia, endocarditis, and meningitis.[519,644,1001,1032,1069,1072] Severe infections of bone and joint prostheses caused by these organisms have also been reported.[139] Group G streptococcal cellulitis and septic arthritis at or near sites of parenteral injection, with bacteremia and subsequent hematogenous complications, have been reported in intravenous drug users.[243,408] Bacteremia with this organism is also seen in the clinical settings of underlying malignancies, puerperal sepsis, septic abortion, chronic pulmonary disease, and congestive heart failure. Group G streptococcal meningitis and sepsis have also been reported in a patient with AIDS.[800] *S. canis*, the group G *Streptococcus* isolated from dogs, was isolated from a human with sepsis in 1997.[90]

Group C and group G β-hemolytic streptococci are generally susceptible to penicillin, ampicillin, and third-generation cephalosporins like ceftriaxone.[52,159,961] Occasional isolates may show intermediate susceptibility to penicillin G, but these are susceptible to the third- and fourth-generation cephalosporins. Some strains may be resistant to erythromycin and other macrolides (e.g., clindamycin, clarithromycin, and azithromycin). All strains tested to date have been susceptible to vancomycin.

Group F β-Hemolytic Streptococci

Organisms of this group have been called *S. milleri* in the British taxonomic scheme and the **anginosus group** (i.e., *S. anginosus*, *S. constellatus*, and *S. intermedius*) in American taxonomic schemes. These organisms may be α-hemolytic, β-hemolytic, or nonhemolytic and may possess the group F, C, or G antigen or may be nongroupable. These streptococci characteristically grow as minute colonies on agar media. The colonies are pinpoints after 24 hours and, if β-hemolytic, have a large zone of hemolysis that extends well beyond the margin of the colony. Group F β-hemolytic streptococci are recognized causes of severe suppurative infections, including cellulitis, deep-tissue abscesses, bacteremia, osteomyelitis, and endocarditis (see the section on "The Anginosus Group" below). The anginosus group will be discussed under the viridans streptococci.

Other Streptococci in the "Pyogenic Cocci" Group

Other pyogenic β-hemolytic streptococci have been described that carry other Lancefield cell wall antigens and that cause infections in animals other than humans. These include *S. porcinus*, *S. iniae* (*S. shiloi*), *S. phocae*, and *S. didelphis*. *S. porcinus* strains belong to Lancefield group E, P, U, or V and cause infections in swine. In 1995, Facklam and colleagues reported on 13 isolates of *S. porcinus* that had been recovered from humans and forwarded to the CDC over the previous 10 years.[337] Of these 13 isolates, 5 were from the female genital tract (vagina, cervix), 3 were from placental tissues, 2 were recovered from blood, and 1 isolate each was recovered from skin, urine, and an infected wound. Nine of these 13 isolates reacted with the new provisional group antigen C1, 3 reacted with Lancefield group P antiserum, and 1 isolate was nongroupable. *S. iniae* is a pathogen of certain fish, such as tilapia, but it can cause bacteremia, meningitis, and endocarditis in individuals who handle contaminated fish.[1034] *S. shiloi*, a β-hemolytic streptococcal species that causes meningoencephalitis in trout, is identical biochemically and genetically to *S. iniae*.[317] *S. phocae* is a β-hemolytic *Streptococcus* that causes pleuropulmonary infections in harbor seals and gray seals. In the original description of this species, 22 strains were characterized.[898] Five of the 22 strains reacted with Lancefield group C antisera, but the remaining 17 were nongroupable. The same 5 strains reacted with the Streptex group C latex reagent, 13 reacted with the Streptex group F latex reagent, and 4 failed to react with any Streptex reagent. *S. didelphis* is a β-hemolytic *Streptococcus* that has been isolated from skin lesions, liver, spleen, and lungs of oppossums.[835] This species is unusual in that the catalase test is strongly positive until the organism has been subcultured several times.

S. urinalis is a previously undescribed *Streptococcus* that was isolated from a urine specimen of a male patient with cystitis.[212] Comparative 16S ribosomal RNA (rRNA) gene sequencing shows that this organism belongs to the pyogenic cocci subgroup of the streptococci, and has close phylogenetic affinities to group A β-hemolytic streptococci and *S. canis* (group G). Unlike most members of the pyogenic subgroup, this species is α-hemolytic on SBA.

Streptococcus pneumoniae
Virulence Factors

The virulence of *S. pneumoniae* is attributable primarily to its ability to resist opsonization, phagocytosis, and intracellular killing by phagocytic cells.[711] This resistance is related primarily to the **polysaccharide capsule** of the organism. Inhibition of capsule production by genetic techniques (i.e., transposon mutagenesis) renders these organisms avirulent in animal models. There are at least 90 capsular types of *S. pneumoniae;* 23 of these types account for over 88% of pneumococcal bacteremia and meningitis.[711] Capsular polysaccharides in *S. pneumoniae* are comprised of long polymers of repeating units comprised of two to seven monosaccharides, some of which may be in long or branching chains.[988] These polymers are synthesized by the addition of carbohydrate moieties to the proximal end of the chain, and most types are anchored to the peptidoglycan and the C-polysaccharide of the cell wall. Certain pneumococcal capsular types (e.g., type 3) have biologic properties that render these organisms more virulent than others, and pneumococci that belong to different capsular serotypes vary in their ability to elicit humoral antibody responses.[988] These characteristics may account for the greater virulence associated with some capsular types over others. Initial adherence of pneumococci to the nasopharyngeal mucosa apparently is not mediated by capsular material but is related to bacterial adhesins that interact with receptors on pharyngeal epithelial cell surfaces. Interaction may occur with mucosal sialic acid via pneumococcal neuraminidase or via pneumococcal cell-surface ligands that bind to *N*-acetyl-D-galactosamine-galactose disaccharide residues on respiratory tract cell surfaces.[26] Pneumococci also possess both teichoic acids and lipoteichoic acids. **Teichoic acids** are covalently linked to the peptidoglycan of the cell wall by phosphodiester linkages, while the **lipoteichoic acids** are linked to the cell membrane. These molecules are structurally similar and are composed of repeating units containing glucose, 2-acetamido-4-amino-2,4,6-trideoxy-D-galactose, *N*-acetyl-glucosamine, phosphocholine, and ribitol-5-phosphate. Repeating units are linked to each other by phosphodiester bonds. Teichoic acids and lipoteichoic acids of *S. pneumoniae* are also called C polysaccharide and F antigen, respectively, and all pneumococcal serotypes possess both of these antigens.

Other cellular products of *S. pneumoniae*, such as the pneumolysin, autolysin, and cell-surface molecules, may also play a role in pneumococcal virulence. Mutants that are defective in the production of these various components have diminished virulence in animal models, and immunization with purified products results in the production of specific antibodies that confer partial resistance to challenge infection.[120] **Pneumolysin** is a 53-kDa thiol-activated cytotoxin protein that accumulates within the cells during growth and is released on cell lysis by the autolysin.[121] Pneumolysin interacts with cholesterol in the cell membranes of a variety of host cells, forms oligomers on and in the membrane that evolve into pores, and ultimately lyses the cells. Pneumolysin inhibits the bactericidal activity of phagocytic cells, arrests ciliary motility, stimulates cytokine production by macrophages (especially interleukin [IL]-1, IL-8 and tumor necrosis factor [TNF]), and activates the classical complement pathway.[202,203,828] Mutants that lack the ability to produce pneumolysin have diminished virulence in animal models, and immunization with purified pneumolysin provides partial protection on challenge with virulent, pneumolysin-producing strains.[87,761] **Autolysin** is an *N*-acetyl-muramoyl-L-alanine amidase that, along with a glycosidase enzyme, functions during cell division to separate daughter cells, and at the end of exponential growth to break down the organisms, causing lytic dispersal of both pneumolysin and α-hemolysin.[85] Virulence is reduced in autolysin-negative mutants as compared with wild-type strains.[151] Reduced virulence is likely due to failure to release toxic cell wall components and pneumolysin and, hence, the generation of a greatly reduced inflammatory response. *S. pneumoniae* strains also produce two different **neuraminidase enzymes (NanA and NanB)**, which cleave terminal sialic acid from cell surfaces to expose *N*-acetyl-glucosamine-galactose moieties that mediate bacterial cell adherence.[148] It has been proposed that the neuraminidases released into the central nervous system (CNS) by pneumococci in vivo may desialylate the sialylated gp120 of HIV and the HIV target

lymphocyte/microglial cell CD4/chemokine receptors, resulting in the progression of HIV infection to full-blown HIV encephalitis.[822] Pneumococcal strains also produce **hyaluronidase** and **IgA₁ proteases**. The former enzyme facilitates the spread of the organisms in tissue, while the latter inactivates secretory IgA to facilitate pneumococcal colonization and subsequent invasion of mucosal surfaces.[86] A surface protein called **PspA** (pneumococcal surface protein A) has also been described that is important for pneumococcal virulence, although its function is unknown.[241,674] PspA is the immunodominant antigenic protein on the surface of pneumococcal cells, and antibodies directed against PspA from a given pneumococcal strain protect experimental animals against challenge with both the homologous strain and heterologous strains. Mutants that are defective in PspA production are avirulent. Intranasal inoculation of mice with PspA prevents both respiratory-tract colonization and the development of invasive disease.[1080] For this reason, PspA has potential for use as a vaccine candidate antigen.[130]

Pneumococcal Vaccines

Two types of vaccines are now available for the prevention of disease due to *S. pneumoniae*: pure polysaccharide vaccines and polysaccharide-protein conjugate vaccines. The **pneumococcal polysaccharide vaccines**—Pneumovax23 (Merck and Company, Whitehouse Station, NJ) and Pneu-Imune23 (Lederle, Wyeth-Lederle, Inc., Pearl River, NY)—are composed of a mixture of 23 pneumococcal capsular polysaccharides.[712] The 23 capsular serotypes included in these vaccines are 1, 2, 3, 4, 5, 6B, 7F, 8, 9N, 9V, 10A, 11A, 12F, 14, 15B, 17F, 18C, 19A, 19F, 20, 22F, 23F, and 33F. These capsular types represent at least 85–90% of the serotypes that cause invasive pneumococcal infections in adults and children in the U.S., and all six serotypes that most frequently cause drug-resistant pneumococcal infections in the U.S. (serotypes 6B, 9V, 14, 19A, 19F, and 23F).[733] The Immunization Practices Advisory Committee of the CDC recommends vaccination of: 1) persons 65 years of age or older; 2) persons 2–64 years of age who have chronic illness (e.g., chronic cardiovascular disease, cardiomyopathies), chronic pulmonary disease (e.g., chronic obstructive pulmonary disease [COPD], emphysema, but not asthma), diabetes mellitus, alcoholism, liver disease (e.g., cirrhosis), or cerebrospinal fluid (CSF) leaks; 3) those who have functional or anatomic asplenia (e.g., sickle cell disease, splenectomy); 4) persons 2–64 years of age who live in environments or settings that render them at risk for invasive pneumococcal disease (i.e., Alaskan Natives, certain American Indian populations, residents of nursing homes and other long-term care facilities); and 5) individuals 2 years of age or older who are immuno-compromised, including individuals with HIV infection, leukemia, lymphoma, Hodgkin's disease, multiple myeloma, malignancies, chronic renal failure, nephritic syndrome, and other conditions associated with immunosuppression (e.g., bone marrow transplantation) and persons receiving immunosuppressive chemotherapy.[143,168] These vaccines have been demonstrated to be safe and efficacious and are relatively inexpensive. These pure polysaccharide vaccines provoke a B-cell antibody response but are T-cell-independent antigens, so a protective immune response is not seen in children less than 2 years old.[772] Other drawbacks to the pneumococcal polysaccharide vaccines include its inability to affect nasopharyngeal pneumococcal carriage and, therefore, the spread of organisms from person to person, and its limited efficacy in patients with underlying hematologic malignancies or immunodeficiency states.

In February 2000, PCV7 (Pneumococcal Conjugate Vaccine 7), a new 7-valent pneumococcal conjugate vaccine (Prevnar; Wyeth Lederle Vaccines, Pearl River, NY) was licensed for use in infants and children.[169] PCV7 is composed of an inert diphtheria toxin carrier protein (CRM_{197}) that is covalently linked to the capsular polysaccharide antigens of seven serotypes of *S. pneumoniae*. The seven serotypes included in the vaccine are serotypes 4, 6B, 9V, 14, 18C, 19F, and 23F, which are associated with about 80% of pneumococcal disease occurring in children less than 6 years of age.[169,772] This new vaccine is given via intramuscular injection and can be administered simultaneously with other childhood immunizations. PCV7 is recommended for children 2 years of age and under and is administered at 2, 4, and 6 months of age, with a booster immunization at 12 to 15 months of age. Initial immunization with PCV7 can start as early as 6 weeks of age. For children 2 to 5 years of age, the Advisory Committee on Immunization Practices has recommended that children at high risk for pneumococcal disease (i.e., children with sickle cell hemoglobinopathies, congenital/acquired/functional asplenia, congenital or acquired immunodeficiencies, immunosuppressive therapies, chronic illnesses) receive both PCV7 and the polysaccharide vaccine to enhance the immune response by administration of a T-cell-dependent antigen and to expand antibody coverage beyond the seven serotypes included in PCV7. The PCV7 conjugate vaccine provokes a brisk T-cell-dependent antibody response, which is required for optimal antibody production and ability to mount an anamnestic response via immunologic memory.[169,733,886] Large studies have demonstrated that the new pneumococcal heptavalent conjugate vaccine is efficacious in preventing invasive disease in young children due to vaccine serotypes of *S. pneumoniae*.[547,810] These studies indicate that more than 90% of invasive pneumococcal disease due to vaccine serotypes were prevented in immunized children. Interestingly, no increases in infections due to nonvaccine serotypes were observed during the clinical efficacy trials, and the rates of nasopharyngeal carriage of *S. pneumoniae* were found to be decreased in vaccinated children, a phenomenon not seen in polysaccharide vaccine recipients. A small efficacy study found that PCV7 provoked protective antibody responses in children with sickle cell disease as well.[735]

Clinical Significance

S. pneumoniae is the major cause of community-acquired bacterial pneumonia. The organism may be harbored in the upper respiratory tract of 5–10% of adults, although carriage rates higher than 60% have been reported in closed populations.[711] Infants usually become colonized at about 3 to 4 months of age and remain colonized for about 4 months with a given serotype; the peak incidence of pneumococcal colonization occurs by age 2 to 3 years when the rate may be 40–60%.[109,430] In adults, colonization and carriage persist from 2 to 4 weeks but may remain much longer, and carriage rates among adults usually range from 5% to 10%.[316] The duration of carriage decreases with age, and, therefore, tends to be longer in children than in adults. Colonization of infants with pneumococci is related to the absence of specific anticapsular antibody and the poorly immunogenic serotypes that are common in this age group.[432] The susceptibility of elderly persons to pneumococcal disease reflects aging of the immune system and consequent diminished production of antibodies, along with general changes in levels of activity, compromised mucociliary clearance mechanisms, malnutrition, or debilitation owing to other underlying chronic diseases such as diabetes and alcoholism.[140]

Most serious infections with *S. pneumoniae* occur in infants younger than 3 years of age and in adults older than 65 years of age.[686,711] Attack rates are four to five times greater among blacks than among whites.[78] This difference appears to be real, although several other factors (e.g., access to health care, other underlying biologic or environmental conditions) may also influence these rates. Attack rates are also higher among native Alaskan populations, native American Indian populations, and Australian Aborigines.[256,964] Patients with underlying abrogations of various host defense mechanisms such as hypogammaglobulinemia, complement component deficiencies, and sickle cell disease, are at increased risk for invasive pneumococcal disease.[5,431,1068] Persons with functional asplenia or those who have had surgical splenectomies are at particularly high risk for the development of invasive, often fatal, pneumococcal bactermia.[934] Among children, infections are usually associated with serotypes 6, 14, 18, 19, and 23. In a 15-year pediatric study conducted in Birmingham, Alabama, these serotypes were responsible for 70% of cases of meningitis and bacteremia.[432,745] Among adults, serotypes 1, 3, 4, 7, 8, and 12 predominate.

In the appropriate host, *S. pneumoniae* gains access to the alveolar spaces by aspiration or inhalation and eventually may cause a lobar pneumonia, with consolidation and bacteremia.[711] Conditions that are recognized to predispose adults to pneumococcal disease include underlying bronchopulmonary disease and compromised humoral immunity.[140] Conditions that abrogate the humoral immune response (e.g., myeloma, lymphoma, chronic lymphocytic leukemia, hepatic cirrhosis, complement component deficiencies) probably have the greatest influence on individual susceptibility to pneumococcal infection. The incidence and severity of pneumococcal disease are also increased among persons with defects in upper respiratory tract clearance mechanisms, including smokers, and individuals with asthma, chronic bronchitis, COPD, or bronchogenic and squamous-cell carcinoma of the lung. Viral respiratory tract infections also predispose to pneumococcal infection of the respiratory tract because these agents also damage the bronchial clearance mechanisms. The onset of pneumococcal pneumonia is generally abrupt, even in patients in whom a prior respiratory viral infection is the principal predisposing factor. In older children and young adults, symptoms include shaking chills, followed by sustained fever, cough, and production of purulent, often blood-tinged, sputum In elderly patients, the infection may present insidiously over several days.[631] Symptoms may vary from a minimal cough, with an actual decrease in temperature, to a fulminant presentation, leading rapidly to shock and death. Blood cultures are positive in 20–30% of patients with pneumococcal pneumonia. Older adults usually have additional conditions that put them at higher risk for serious disease, including malignancies, alcoholism, heart disease, COPD, and diabetes.[658,711] Chest x-ray films from patients with pneumococcal pneumonia demonstrate lobar consolidation in about 40–50%, with the remaining showing a patchy bronchopneumonic pattern. Infiltrates due to pneumococcal disease tend to be unilateral, involving the alveoli, rather than the bronchioles and interstitial tissues. Complications of pneumococcal pneumonia include lung abscess, pericardial infections, empyema, pleural effusions, and endocarditis.[134,1086] Pleural effusions and empyemas may be visualized on chest films, but they are more accurately delineated by computed tomography (CT) and ultrasound diagnostic approaches.[134] If these fluid collections are sufficiently large, drainage via chest tube placement may be necessary to effect cure, along with antimicrobial therapy. CT scans and ultrasound are also helpful for diagnosing necrotizing pneumonias and deep lung abscesses due to *S. pneumoniae*. The case fatality rate for pneumococcal pneumonia is about 5%, but it may approach 20–30% when accompanied by bacteremia. Pneumococcal bacteremia without pulmonary involvement is an entity that occurs in immunologically compromised hosts. Underlying diseases or conditions that predispose patients to recurrent or relapsing pneumococcal bacteremia include splenectomy, acute myelogenous leukemia, bone marrow transplantation, sickle cell disease, HIV infection, and short bowel syndrome.[395,404,589,743,803,808,1068]

S. pneumoniae is also a leading cause of bacteremia and sepsis in both children and adults. In otherwise normal children with bacteremia, about 25% are associated with coexisting pneumococcal otitis media, 30–40% are linked to pneumonia or focal pneumococcal infections, and the remainder have no identifiable focus.[246,431,745] On the other hand, over 90% of bacteremias in adults result from pneumonia.[5] As mentioned, other comorbid conditions—asplenia, malignancy, sickle cell disease, and HIV infection—contribute to the development of bacteremia and also affect the ultimate response to antimicrobial agents and supportive therapy. Although the mortality rate for pneumococcal bacteremia and sepsis is fairly low in children, adults with bacteremia have fatality rates approaching 35–40%. *S. pneumoniae* has also emerged as a significant cause of disease in HIV-infected patients.[803] These infections tend to occur early in the course of HIV infection (often before a diagnosis of HIV infection has even been considered), are unusually severe, and may have unusual clinical presentations along with bacteremia.[770] Rodriguez-Barradas reported five cases of severe pneumococcal infections in HIV-infected patients; presentations included pneumonia with recurrent pleural effusions, pyopneumothorax complicated by a bronchopleural fistula, purpura fulminans with peripheral gangrene of the extremities, pneumococcal mediastinitis with adjacent chest-wall soft-tissue infection, and pneumococcal brain abscess.[819]

S. pneumoniae is also the most common cause of bacterial meningitis in adults; with the increasing use of the conjugate vaccines for *Haemophilus influenzae* type b, the pneumococcus is now also the most common agent in infants and toddlers.[711] In adults, the pneumococcus accounts for about one third of community-acquired meningitis in the United States and has an associated mortality of 20–25%.[304] *S. pneumoniae* meningitis usually occurs as a result of seeding of the meninges during bacteremia, with the organisms probably entering via the choroid plexus. The presenting symptoms in about 60–70% of adults are fever, nuchal rigidity, and mental status changes.[973] In infants, crying, irritability, malaise, failure to feed, vomiting, and seizures may dominate the clinical picture; a bulging fontanelle will develop in only about one third of these babies. In elderly and/or compromised adults, the presentation may be insidious, with lethargy, obtundation, and little or no fever being the norm. However, meningitis, along with ultimately fatal septic shock may occur in patients who are profoundly immunosuppressed (e.g., patients who have undergone bone marrow transplantation).[449] *S. pneumoniae* is also the leading cause of meningitis following skull fractures. Head trauma resulting in basilar skull fracture with leakage of CSF interrupts the integrity of the dura mater and may allow direct entry of organisms into the CNS from an adjacent site of infection (e.g., sinusitis, mastoiditis, otitis media).[711]

In pediatric populations, *S. pneumoniae* accounts for 40–50% of cases of acute otitis media and has been associated with sinusitis and mastoiditis.[105,577] In patients with otitis media, the tympanic membrane appears inflamed, immobile, and bulging on examination with an otoscope. Complications of acute pneumococcal otitis media include tympanic membrane perforation, mastoiditis, facial-nerve paralysis, bacteremia, and septic arthritis.[586] Specimens for diagnosis are best obtained via myringotomy or tympanocentesis. Pneumococci, along with *H. influenzae*, are also responsible for about 70% of acute and subacute sinus infections.

S. pneumoniae is an infrequent cause of endocarditis, pericarditis, osteomyelitis, septic arthritis, peritonitis, female pelvic infections, neonatal infections, and skin/soft-tissue infections. Most patients have underlying disease, such as diabetes, malignancies, alcoholism, systemic lupus erythematosus, or HIV infection and have other foci of pneumococcal disease, such as meningitis or pneumonia. Pneumococci account for less than 3% of cases of bacterial endocarditis and 3–7% of all cases of pediatric endocarditis.[403] Pneumococcal endocarditis follows an acute course, is associated with valve destruction and formation of aortic perivalvular abscesses, and has a mortality rate of about 24% to over 50%.[391,615,783,893] Treatment of pneumococcal endocarditis with medical therapy alone is associated with poor outcomes. Usually patients have preexisting heart disease, and, in one study of pneumococcal endocarditis in children, congenital heart disease was the only identifiable risk factor.[186] Primary peritonitis caused by the pneumococci was once a frequently seen clinical entity in children in association with nephrotic syndrome, but is now occurs primarily in adults with cirrhosis and other liver diseases along with enteric gram-negative bacilli. Osteomyelitis and septic arthritis caused by *S. pneumoniae* often occurs in children with sickle cell disease.[942] In adults, pneumococcal septic arthritis usually occurs in patients with bacteremia and involves more than one joint in about one third of patients.[825] Most cases can be managed with appropriate antimicrobial coverage and arthrocentesis. In some women, *S. pneumoniae* may be a transient part of the vaginal flora, and pelvic, obstetric, and gynecologic infections may occur, particularly with predisposing conditions such as the presence of an intrauterine device or recent gynecologic surgery.[303,1043] Tuboovarian abscesses due to *S. pneumoniae* may also be a source of pneumococcal peritoneal infections.[897] Neonatal pneumococcal infections have also been reported and represent 1–11% of cases of neonatal sepsis.[488] These babies present with meningitis, bacteremia, pneumonia, septic arthritis/osteomyelitis, or otitis media, are usually born at full term, and are 2 to 3 weeks of age at presentation. The likely source of infection in these babies is the mothers' genital tract. *S. pneumoniae* has also been recognized as a significant cause of soft-tissue infections, including facial and periorbital cellulitis, fasciitis, rhabdomyolysis, and abscesses.[104,428,603,758, 765,771,786,914,920] These infections occur in hosts with underlying conditions, such as systemic lupus erythematosus, end-stage renal disease, rheumatoid arthritis, type 2 diabetes, or HIV infection. An association with connective-tissue disorders has been noted by some investigators as well.[287]

A major concern surrounding *S. pneumoniae* is the emergence of resistance to antimicrobial agents, especially penicillin.[33,153,579] Pneumococci with decreased resistance to penicillin were first reported in the 1960s. During the 1970s and 1980s, penicillin-resistance among *S. pneumoniae* isolates was rare in the U.S., with only 0.2% of strains being resistant. However, by the mid-1990s, 35% of the aggregate pneumococcal isolates from the U.S. demonstrated reduced susceptibility to penicillin.[49,867] More recent studies among populations in the CDC national surveillance system indicate that decreased susceptibility to penicillin among *S. pneumoniae* isolates ranges from 15% to 35%, depending on the geographic region.[1056] Among 10,103 community-acquired respiratory tract isolates of *S. pneumoniae* collected in 2000–2001 from 206 centers in 154 regions of the U.S., 38.9% showed decreased susceptibility to penicillin.[291] Decreased susceptibility to penicillin has also been documented in foreign isolates of *S. pneumoniae*. In a 2003 study, the percent of strains with diminished susceptibility to penicillin was 6.5% in the U.K., 9.1% in Germany, 12.4% in Italy, 36.4% in Greece, 54.5% in Spain, and 56.7% in France.[545] Penicillin resistance in *S. pneumoniae* is associated with altered penicillin-binding proteins (PBPs) that have a decreased affinity for binding penicillin to the bacterial cell wall.[527] PBPs are actually transpeptidase enzymes that are involved in peptidoglycan synthesis, and six PBPs—designated 1A, 1B, 2A, 2B, 2X, and 3—have been identified in *S. pneumoniae*. Mutations in the genes coding for PBP 2B account for low-level penicillin resistance, while mutations in the gene for PBP 2X are associated with high-level penicillin resistance.[903,904] Strains with penicillin MICs of 0.06 μg/mL or less are considered susceptible, those with MICs of 0.1 to 1 μg/mL are considered intermediately resistant (having decreased susceptibility to penicillin), and those with MICs greater than 1 μg/mL are considered resistant.[526] Strains with high-level penicillin resistance have penicillin MIC of ≥2 μg/mL. Isolates of *S. pneumoniae* that show decreased susceptibility or frank resistance to penicillin G are also less susceptible to other penicillins and cephalosporins of all generations, and treatment failures for serious pneumococcal infections have been reported with previously useful agents such as cefotaxime, cefuroxime, and ceftriaxone.[153,162,526,542] Besides the penicillins and cephalosporins, pneumococcal coresistance to several other antimicrobial agents, including macrolides, sulfonamides, and tetracyclines, has been reported.[293,294,546,1056] In an international study published in 2004, macrolide resistance among *S. pneumoniae* isolates was highest in Asia (51.7% resistant), followed by Europe (26.0% resistant), North America (21.6% resistant), the Middle East (13.7% resistant), the South Pacific (10.6% resistant), and Africa (10% resistant).[119] A particularly alarming trend has been the development of pneumococcal resistance to fluoroquinolone antimicrobial agents.[415,1056] Additional information regarding antimicrobial susceptibility of *S. pneumoniae* and methods for antimicrobial susceptibility testing are found in Chapter 15.

Viridans Streptococci

The viridans group includes several species of α-hemolytic and nonhemolytic streptococci, most of which constitute part of the normal upper respiratory tract and urogenital tract flora.[376] Viridans streptococci cause 30–40% of cases of subacute bacterial endocarditis, and in this setting cause a sustained bacteremia, leading to their recovery from multiple sets of blood cultures.[1027] Viridans streptococcal endocarditis occurs most frequently in individuals with preexisting native-valve disease; they may also be associated with infection of prosthetic valves. Viridans streptococcal endocarditis presents insidiously, with fever, fatigue, and weight loss being the most common findings. Heart murmurs, peripheral stigmata of endocarditis (e.g., splinter and conjunctival hemorrhages, petechiae), and vegetations on echocardiograms are also frequently present. Complications of viridans streptococcal endocarditis include multivalvular disease, mitral-valve aneurysms, paravalvular abscesses and glomerulonephritis associated with circulating immune complexes.[746,799] In a recent study of 77 patients with endocarditis, 18% had multivalve involvement, and 36% of these infections were due to viridans streptococci.[573] Reference identifications of viridans streptococcal species associated with subacute bacterial endocarditis indicate that *S. mitis*, *S. sanguis*, *S. oralis*, *S. gordonii*, *S. mutans*, *S. salivarius*, *S. vestibularis*, and *S. sinensis*, a new α-hemolytic species, are the viridans streptococci most frequently associated with endocarditis.[301,302,523, 622,1027,1071] The oropharynx is the probable source of bacteria in most of these infections; poor oral hygiene and periodontal disease are often noted in these patients. Other procedures, such as fiberoptic sigmoidoscopy and upper gastrointestinal endoscopy, may also cause a transient bacteremia that may infect previously damaged heart valves.[695,727] Recent reports of endocarditis due to penicillin-resistant viridans streptococci have occurred in patients who received penicillin prophylaxis for dental procedures.[450,500]

Although transient bacteremias with these organisms are generally cleared in the normal host without any adverse sequelae, prolonged bacteremia with viridans streptococci, particularly in neutropenic pediatric and adult patients undergoing cancer chemotherapy, has become recognized as a distinct clinical entity.[12,107,108,253,752,974,1096] Bacteremia in these patients is associated with aggressive cytotoxic chemotherapy administered for the treatment of leukemias, lymphomas, or solid tumors and for bone marrow transplantation.[12,43,138,921] Risk factors for the development of viridans streptococcal bacteremia in these immunocompromised patients include the administration of high doses of cytotoxic agents (e.g., cytarabine), the presence of oral mucosal ulcerations secondary to cytotoxic chemotherapy or radiation, the absence of previous antimicrobial therapy, and severe neutropenia.[12,108,752] Oral mucositis probably serves as the portal of entry for these organisms into the bloodstream.[253] In this regard, poor underlying dental health and periodontal disease are also risk factors for the development of viridans streptococcal bacteremia in neutropenic hosts.[426] Certain antimicrobial agents used for prophylaxis in neutropenic hosts are also associated with viridans streptococcal bacteremia. In one study of 38 children with neutropenia, 60% were receiving prophylactic trimethoprim-sulfamethoxazole at the time the first blood culture become positive.[12] Prophylactic use of fluoroquinolones has also been identified as a potential risk factor for development of bacteremia in patients with acute myeloid leukemia.[769] Viridans streptococcal bacteremia in these patients may be complicated by the development of adult respiratory distress syndrome (ARDS), hypotension, shock, and bacterial endocarditis.[12,107,108,741] Viridans streptococcal species that have been associated with neutropenic bacteremia primarily include *S. mitis, S. oralis, S. salivarius,* and *S. sanguis.*[12,70,107,108,138,921] Bacteremic infections with viridans streptococci have also been reported in low-birth-weight full-term and preterm neonates.[2] The mothers of these neonates frequently have several risk factors that adversely affect pregnancy outcome, including chorioamnionitis, premature rupture of fetal membranes, premature onset of labor, and urinary tract infection at the time of delivery.

Viridans streptococci may also be isolated on rare occasions from other serious infections, such as meningitis and pneumonia, particularly in compromised hosts. Meningitis caused by viridans streptococci may occur in both adults and children, and the clinical presentation differs little from that of the other pyogenic meningitides (i.e., nuchal rigidity, seizures, meningeal inflammation, and altered mental status).[244,636] The source of the organism is usually endogenous; congenital structural abnormalities of the head and neck, head and neck infections, endocarditis, extracranial infections, and previous head trauma or neurosurgical procedures (e.g., craniotomy) have been associated with the development of meningitis, but definite sources of infection may not be pinpointed in up to a third of cases.[585] Recurrent viridans streptococcal meningitis has been documented in children with structural abnormalities of the inner ear and mastoid sinuses.[684] Complications of meningitis include intracranial suppuration and cerebral vasulitis.[636] Meningitis and bacteremia caused by *S. mitis* and *S. salivarius* have also been reported following lumbar puncture, upper gastrointestinal endoscopy, and cauterization for a gastric bleed.[156,1085] Similarly, recurrent *S. sanguis* meningitis was reported in a 15-year-old boy with a ventriculoperitoneal shunt.[16] Colville and associates reported the first case of meningitis caused by *S. oralis* in a healthy 12-year-old girl

following extraction of a deciduous canine tooth as part of her orthodontic treatments.[229] *S. salivarius* was isolated as a cause of meningitis in a previously healthy 73-year-old woman who was subsequently found to have an asymptomatic colonic adenocarcinoma, suggesting an association of this ''*S. bovis*–like'' species with occult neoplastic disease.[617] Other CNS infections such as brain abscess may occur following cranial trauma or surgery, or secondary to a primary focus of infection elsewhere via direct extension from a contiguous site or via the hematogenous route.[237,637] Direct extension may occur from dental infections (e.g., root abscesses, periodontitis), paranasal sinus infections, or otogenic sources.[637] Brain abscesses are usually singular, are located in the frontal or temporal lobes, and may be polymicrobial. Predisposing conditions for viridans streptococcal brain abscess include congestive heart failure, chronic otitis media, head injuries with CSF rhinorrhea, sinusectomy, and craniotomy followed by ventriculoperitoneal shunt placement.[935]

Bacteremic viridans streptococcal pneumonia has also been reported but is rare. Marrie reported on seven patients with community-acquired viridans streptococcal pneumonia.[657] All patients were older (49 to 80 years), had several predisposing conditions (including alcoholism, resected carcinoma of the lung, hypothyroidism, and diabetes mellitus), and were bacteremic. Viridans streptococcal isolates from these patients included *S. mitis, S. sanguis,* and *S. intermedius.* Sarker and colleagues reported three cases of community-acquired viridans streptococcal pneumonia with concomitant positive blood cultures in previously healthy adults.[843] Viridans streptococcal pneumonia occurs in older patients in the setting of oropharyngeal aspiration.[954] Complications of pneumonia, including empyema and lung abscesses associated with viridans streptococcal pneumonia, are relatively rare clinical entities.[158,535] Miscellaneous infections caused by various species of viridans streptococci have included epiglottitis, septic arthritis, vertebral osteomyelitis secondary to bacteremia/endocarditis, pericarditis, Lemierre's syndrome, and infectious crystalline keratitis.[117,309,512,611,676,969,980] In 2003, an outbreak of a toxic shock–like syndrome was reported in immunocompetent patients residing in the YangZi River Delta in Jiangsu Province, China.[638] This outbreak, which occurred during 1990–1991, was due to a clone of *S. mitis.* This same clone, as judged by pulsed-field gel electrophoretic patterns, was subsequently found in other patients with the syndrome from 1991 through 1995. This strain produced a 34-kDa protein that was pyrogenic in rabbits, mitogenic in cultured splenocytes, and enhanced the susceptibility of rabbits to endotoxin challenge. Sequencing of this protein showed that it was unrelated to known pyrogenic exotoxins produced by group A or other β-hemolytic streptococci.

Some viridans streptococci inhabiting the oral cavity have emerged as significant pathogens associated predominantly with the initiation and pathogenesis of dental caries. *S. mutans, S. sobrinus,* and other members of the ''mutans group'' of oral streptococci are able to produce enzymes called **glucosyltransferases,** which hydrolyze dietary sucrose (a disaccharide of glucose and fructose) and connect the glucose moieties together in α1,6 and α1,4 glycosidic linkages to form insoluble glucans.[1083] These glucans enable these organisms to adhere to the smooth surfaces of the teeth and form the matrix of dental plaque. Specific and nonspecific attachment of *S. mutans* and other organisms to the insoluble, adherent glucans and subsequent formation of acid leads to demineralization of the tooth enamel and the initiation of carious lesions.[50] Other oral streptococci, including *S. sanguis*, *S. salivarius*, and possibly *S. gordonii*, are also able to synthesize these polysaccharides, but only the "mutans strep" display sucrose-induced enhancement of oral colonization.[632,983,1009] In addition, the mutans streptococci also appear to produce a greater amount of acid from carbohydrates than other oral bacteria because they are able to ferment a wide variety of sugars, and they are more acid-tolerant than other oral streptococci.[465,632] These organisms also synthesize intracellular polysaccharides that can be metabolized to acid in the absence of exogenous fermentable carbohydrates, enabling them to produce significant amounts of acid even "between meals."[632] The mutans streptococci originally described a single species—*S. mutans*—that was divided into eight serotypes designated a through h based on the serologic specificity of cell wall carbohydrate antigens. Subsequently, these various serotypes were assigned separate species status.[240] *S. mutans* (serotypes c, e, and f) and *S. sobrinus* (serotypes d and g) are the species that predominate in humans, with the other species being found in various animals.[240] Molecular approaches for direct detection of *S. mutans* in plaque and gingival samples have been developed, and monoclonal antibodies against *S. mutans* that are used along with colony immunoblot techniques have been developed by workers in dental microbiology for the identification and enumeration of these organisms in saliva and dental plaque specimens.[271]

Before the 1980s, the various species of viridans streptococci were described entirely in terms of their phenotypic characteristics. Analysis of the viridans streptococci by molecular and genetic techniques and with expanded batteries of phenotypic tests has considerably altered the taxonomy of these organisms. Major changes that have occurred as a result of these analyses include emended descriptions of well-recognized species such as *S. mitis* and *S. sanguis*, the discovery and description of several new species of oral viridans streptococci (e.g., *S. vestibularis*, *S. gordonii*, *S. parasanguis*, *S. oralis*, *S. crista*, *S. sinensis*, and *S. oligofermentans*), the division of the various serotypes of the *S. mutans* group into distinct species, and the taxonomic reassignment of the viridans "*Streptococcus*" *S. morbillorum* as a second species in the genus *Gemella*.[240,456,568,571,958,1049,1052,1071] The frequency of some of the newly described species in clinical specimens is not known and awaits further investigations as more reliable methods for their identification become more widely available to clinical microbiology laboratories. Although reported from human specimens, *S. uberis* and *S. parauberis* are primarily animal isolates; they cause bovine mastitis.[484,532,1059]

In the past, the viridans streptococci were generally susceptible to penicillin, ampicillin, and most other antimicrobial agents. However, over the past two decades, antimicrobial susceptibility surveys of viridans streptococci have clearly shown that resistance to penicillins, cephalosporins, aminoglycosides, and other classes of antimicrobial agents is increasing, particularly among strains of *S. mitis*. In 1992,

Potgieter and colleagues reported the antimicrobial susceptibilities of 211 viridans streptococci recovered from blood cultures.[782] Although all isolates were susceptible to cefotaxime, ceftriaxone, imipenem, and vancomycin, 38% were resistant to penicillin (MICs, ≥0.25 µg/mL), 41% were resistant to erythromycin, and 7% were resistant to both erythromycin and tetracycline. Five *S. mitis* strains were resistant to penicillin (MICs, 16 to 32 µg/mL) and also showed increased resistance (MICs, 64 to 128 µg/mL) or high-level resistance (MICs, ≥500 µg/mL) to gentamicin and tobramycin. Kaufhold and Potgieter reported on four blood culture isolates of *S. mitis* that were resistant to penicillin (MICs, 16 to 32 µg/mL); two of these were resistant to gentamicin (MIC, 128 µg/mL), and two demonstrated high-level gentamicin resistance (MIC, >1,000 µg/mL l).[556] In a study of 352 viridans streptococcal isolates from 43 U.S. medical centers, 13% showed high-level resistance to penicillin (MIC ≥4 µg/mL) and 43% had intermediate resistance (MIC, 0.25–2.0 µg/mL) to penicillin, with *S. mitis* and *S. salivarius* comprising the highly penicillin resistant isolates.[292] Similarly, among 50 blood isolates from Memorial Sloan-Kettering Cancer Center, 44% were penicillin-resistant.[974] In 2001, Levy and colleagues reported two patients with endocarditis caused by penicillin- resistant strains of *S. mitis* and *S. sanguis*, respectively.[622] Both isolates were also resistant to ceftriaxone and susceptible to clindamycin and vancomycin. A study published in 2004 from Finland found that *S. mitis* constituted 82% of the viridans streptococci isolated from patients with neutropenia, and that 5% and 4% of these *S. mitis* isolates exhibited high-level resistance to penicillin (MIC, ≥4 µg/mL) and cefotaxime (MIC, ≥4 µg/mL), respectively.[645] To date, viridans streptococci that are resistant to vancomycin have not been described.

The Anginosus Group: *Streptococcus anginosus, Streptococcus constellatus, and Streptococcus intermedius*

Among the viridans streptococci, a group of organisms that has gone through repeated taxonomic revisions is the "anginosus group," which is also known as the "*Streptococcus milleri* group" in British taxonomic literature. The anginosus group of viridans streptococci corresponds to three species—*S. intermedius*, *S. constellatus*, and *S. anginosus*—that form minute colonies on agar media. These organisms may or may not carry Lancefield group antigens (group A, C, F, or G) and may or may not be hemolytic on sheep blood agar.[1046] Most *S. anginosus* isolates are nonhemolytic, while more than half of *S. constellatus* strains may be β-hemolytic; isolates of *S. intermedius* are rarely β-hemolytic.[521,1046,1050] These organisms are part of the human oropharyngeal flora and may be cultivated from the throat, the nasopharynx, and the gingival crevices. They are also found normally in the gastrointestinal tract and in the vagina. The virulence of this group may be related to the presence of a capsule on some strains, production of a partially characterized immunosuppressive protein, and the production of a variety of hydrolytic and glycosaminoglycan-degrading enzymes (e.g., neuraminidase, DNase, chondroitin sulfate depolymerase, and hyaluronidase).[34,74,492,524,834] Some isolates belonging to the anginosus group also are able to bind fibronectin and to produce thrombin-like activity.[1057] In addition, in vitro studies have shown that the anginosus group streptococci inhibit polymorphonuclear leukocyte chemotaxis and are ingested by PMN cells more readily than *S. aureus;* once ingested, however, they are killed more slowly than *S. aureus.*[1025] *S. intermedius* strains also produce a staphylococcal leukocidin-like toxin, called **intermedilysin,** that may be virulence-associated, although neither the toxin nor its genes are found in *S. constellatus* or *S. anginosus.*[647] Study of anginosus group isolates from the human throat has resulted in the description of a new subspecies of *S. constellatus—S. constellatus* subsp. *pharyngis—*that expresses the group C carbohydrate and is associated with phayngitis.[1051] In addition, five 16S rRNA ''ribogroups'' were recently delineated among strains of *S. anginosus* that differ somewhat in their phenotypic characteristics and pathogenic potential.[522]

S. intermedius, S. constellatus, and *S. anginosus* are recognized for their propensity to cause purulent, deep-tissue abscesses, bacteremia, endocarditis, intraabdominal infections, pulmonary infections, CNS infections, and oral infections.[88,365,520] Bacteremia with these organisms is usually attributable to a focus of infection elsewhere, with the gastrointestinal and the upper respiratory tracts being the most common sources. Suppurative metastatic abscesses are a significant complication of bacteremia. Isolates of *S. intermedius* and *S. constellatus* are more often associated with abscess formation than *S. anginosus.*[199] *S. constellatus* is isolated from odontogenic, pleuropulmonary, and intraabdominal infections. *S. intermedius* is also recovered from pulmonary infections, but it is associated more frequently with deep soft-tissue abscesses, liver abscesses, and CNS infections (e.g., brain abscesses).[199,1048] *S. anginosus* is often involved in mixed infections having gastrointestinal or genitourinary sources.[411,1048] In addition, these bacteria are the causative agents in from 8% to over 30% of all skin and subcutaneous infections, and may cause severe soft-tissue infections, particularly in patients with underlying conditions such as uncontrolled diabetes and intravenous-drug use.[885,930] Like other viridans streptococci, anginosus group streptococci cause bacteremia in patients with neutropenia and underlying diseases who are being treated with cytotoxic regimens, although fulminant bacteremia in previously healthy individuals may also occur.[365,521] The anginosus group streptococci are rare isolates from individuals with endocarditis.[614] Woo and colleagues reported six cases of anginosus group endocarditis out of 377 cases of endocarditis that occurred in Hong Kong over a 5-year period.[1073] Five patients had underlying diseases (i.e., rheumatic heart disease, ischemic heart disease, chronic obstructive pulmonary disease, supraventricular tachycardia) and one was an IV-drug user. All isolates from these patients were identified as *S. anginosus.*

Pleuropulmonary and head and neck infections caused by anginosus group streptococci usually occur as mixed-flora abscesses, which also serve as sources for hematogenous dissemination. Pulmonary infections often result from aspiration of oropharyngeal contents, leading to pneumonia. Pneumonia may be complicated by empyema and the formation of lung abscesses.[780,888] Anginosus group organisms resident in the oral cavity may cause periodontal and periapi-

cal abscesses and other suppurative maxillofacial infections.[51] Fisher and Russell isolated anginosus group streptococci from 37% of 45 patients with dentoalveolar periapical abscesses; all but one of these isolates was *S. anginosus.*[364] Organisms from infected dental sites, paranasal sinuses, soft tissues, and peritonsillar regions may spread by direct extension to involve the cranium, orbit, deep-tissue spaces in the neck, and the CNS.[455,1030] Consequently, anginosus group organisms may be recovered in pure or mixed culture from cases of chronic sinusitis, brain abscesses, submandibular abscesses, middle and inner ear fluid, cervical abscesses, epidural abscesses, and subdural empyema fluid.[282,478,504,1082]

Up to 40% of infections associated with the anginosus group are intraabdominal infections that develop following appendectomy or other surgery or as a result of colonic perforation caused by trauma or other gastrointestinal lesions (e.g., colonic carcinoma). Intraabdominal anginosus group infections are associated with peritonitis and the formation of appendicular, hepatic, subphrenic, and pancreatic abscesses.[299,463] Mucosal bowel trauma and disease apparently facilitate the invasion of the bloodstream by the organisms. Intraabdominal abscesses usually yield mixed aerobes and anaerobes on culture, and evidence from animal models suggests that the pathogenic potential of these streptococci is enhanced by synergistic growth with anaerobic bacteria.[887] Tresadern and associates reported on anginosus group infections in 23 general surgery patients, many of whom had undergone colorectal procedures, and concluded that the use of preoperative antibiotics, such as gentamicin and metronidazole, may actually promote the emergence of these organisms as pathogens in this anatomic sight.[962] Anginosus group streptococci are occasionally recovered from gynecologic, obstetric, urogenital, and neonatal infections, including pelvic abscesses, colorectal carcinoma, tubo-ovarian abscesses, intrauterine infections, and lesions of the external genitalia.[675,801]

Members of the anginosus group have generally been considered susceptible to a variety of antimicrobial agents, but there are indications that antibiotic resistance may be increasing in these organisms. In a 1999 examination of 180 anginosus group isolates, 94.4%, 92.8%, 87.1%, 97.3%, and 97.3% of isolates were susceptible to penicillin, ampicillin, cefuroxime, cefazolin, and cefotaxime, respectively.[626] A more recent examination of 44 genotypically characterized strains found no penicillin resistance among 12 *S. intermedius,* 16 *S. constellatus,* and 16 *S. anginosus* isolates, although 4 isolates showed decreased susceptibility to penicillin and 4 were intermediate to ampicillin; all isolates were ceftriaxone-susceptible.[960] MLS (macrolide-lincosamide-streptogramin) resistance is also emerging among these organisms. In the study by Limia et al., 17.7% and 18.3% of the 180 strains tested were resistant to erythromycin and clindamycin, respectively.[626] Antimicrobial susceptibility surveillance studies indicate that erythromycin resistance may be found in 3.2–17.7% of isolates, depending on geographic location, and only slight differences have been noted in MLS resistance among the three anginosus group species.[525,960] Genetic analysis of some MLS-resistant strains has documented the presence of *erm*(B), *erm*(TR), and *mef*(A)-*mef*(E) genes that result in constitutive erythromycin resistance, inducible erythromycin resistance, and macrolide efflux-mediated resistance, respectively. Even though most anginosus group isolates are relatively resistant to aminoglycosides (i.e., gentamicin), synergy with β-lactam agents can usually be demonstrated. Anginosus group organisms are susceptible to vancomycin.[626]

Group D Streptococci: The "Streptococcus bovis/Streptococcus equinus *Complex" and Related Species*

Group D streptococci, which are commonly found among the intestinal flora of vertebrates, were first identified by their biochemical and antigenic features. These streptococci possess the group D lipoteichoic acid antigen in their cell walls. Some former group D species are predominant normal inhabitants of the human gastrointestinal tract and were termed "enterococci," whereas other species that possess the group D antigen and compose only a small part of the normal enteric flora were termed "nonenterococci." The practical consideration behind the division of these organisms into two groups was that the enterococci are generally more resistant to penicillins, cephalosporins, and the aminoglycosides than the nonenterococcal group D streptococci. The application of molecular genetic techniques during the mid- to late 1980s led to the division of the group D streptococci into two groups. Enterococcal species were placed in the genus *Enterococcus*, whereas the group D nonenterococcal species remained in the genus *Streptococcus*.

The nonenterococcal group D streptococci were designated as *S. bovis* or *S. equinus* based on their phenotypic characteristics and their origin. *S. bovis* strains were divided into two biotypes based on mannitol fermentation: *S. bovis* biotype I strains were mannitol-positive, while biotype II (or *S. bovis* variant) strains were mannitol-negative. Biotype two strains were phenotypically divided based on the β-glucuronidase (β-GUR) activity: *S. bovis* biotype II.1 were β-GUR-negative, while *S. bovis* biotype II.2 were β-GUR-positive. In 1984, Farrow and colleagues delineated six different DNA homology groups among the group D streptococci.[351] The *S. equinus* type strain and *S. bovis* biotype II.1 (mannitol-negative, β-GUR-negative) strains from cattle belonged to genomic group 1. Genomic group 2 included strains identified as *S. bovis* biotype I (mannitol-positive) and included human isolates from blood and cases of endocarditis; these strains were subsequently reclassified as the new species *S. gallolyticus*, because these strains also hydrolyzed gallate.[750] Group 3 was comprised of atypical, mannitol-variable strains of *S. bovis* and *S. equinus*, while group 4 was comprised of a heterogenous collection of esculin hydrolysis–positive and–negative strains. DNA group 4 strains were classified as the new species *Streptococcus infantarius*.[125] Subsequently, analysis of *S. infantarius* delineated two subspecies within this group: *S. infantarius* subsp. *infantarius* and *S. infantarius* subsp. *coli*.[853] Groups 5 and 6 were comprised of organisms now classified as *Enterococcus saccharolyticus* and *Streptococcus alactolyticus*, respectively. At the same time, two other new streptococcal isolates were described that were related to the *S. bovis* group: *S. macedonicus*, an α-hemolytic species originally isolated

from Greek cheese, and *S. waius*, an α-hemolytic species recovered from skimmed milk biofilms.[366,970] *S. waius* was subsequently found to be identical to *S. macedonicus*, so the species epithet was retained as *S. macedonicus*.[651] Similarly *S. caprinus* was also found to be a later subjective synonym for *S. gallolyticus*, so the name *S. gallolyticus* was retained.[902]

In 2001, Clarridge and colleagues examined 22 clinical strains of *S. bovis* and the related species described above by phenotypic and genotypic methods and suggested that *S. bovis* biotype II.2 strains constituted a separate genospecies distinct from *S. bovis*, *S. gallolyticus*, and *S. infantarius*.[200] Because the 16S rDNA sequences of these species exhibit 97.1–99.8% identity with one another, alternative gene sequences were sought to genotypically discriminate among these closely related species. To this end, Poyart and colleagues amplified and sequenced an internal portion of the *sodA* gene, which codes for a manganese-dependent superoxide dismutase, to create a *sodA* sequence-based data base for examining these organisms.[784] Based on these sequences, five clusters corresponding to five distinct species were delineated. Three of the five clusters corresponded to *S. equinus*, *S. gallolyticus*, and *S. infantarius*. The fourth cluster was comprised of strains phenotypically identified as *S. bovis* biotype II.2, and the fifth cluster corresponded to strains identified as *S. infantarius* subsp. *coli*. These workers proposed that *S. bovis* biotype II.2 strains be assigned to the new species, *S. pasteurianus*, and that *S. infantarius* subsp. *coli* strains be renamed *Streptococcus lutetiensis*.[784]

In 2003, a further reappraisal of the taxonomy of the *S. bovis/S. equinus* group was done in an effort to improve physiologic differentiation among these species and to clarify their phylogenetic positions.[852] Using DNA-DNA hybridization and 16S rDNA sequence analysis, these workers showed that many of these new "species" (e.g. "*S. pasteurianus*," "*S. lutetiensis*") did not show sufficient sequence divergence to assign them separate species status. Since the species epithet "*Streptococcus gallolyticus*" had taxonomic precedence, Schlegel and colleagues proposed that the names *S. gallolyticus* subsp. *gallolyticus*, *S. gallolyticus* subsp. *pasteurianus*, and *S. gallolyticus* subsp. *macedonicus* be adopted for *S. bovis* biotype I, *S. bovis* biotype II.2 ("*S. pasteurianus*"), and *S. macedonicus*, respectively. Furthermore, hybridization studies did not support the assignment of *S. infantarius* subsp. *coli* strains to the proposed species "*S. lutetiensis*," so retention of the two *S. infantarius* subspecies was proposed. If the proposed nomenclature changes are accepted, *S. bovis* I, *S. bovis* II.1, and *S. bovis* II.2 correspond to *S. gallolyticus* subsp. *gallolyticus*, *S. infantarius* subsp. *coli* (*S. lutetiensis*), and *S. gallolyticus* subsp. *pasteurianus* ("*S. pasteurianus*"), respectively.[854] These taxonomic studies also established that *S. bovis* and *S. equinus* are the same species, suggesting that strains of "*S. equinus*" isolated from human clinical specimens were probably misidentified.[325,401,854] These studies confirmed that *S. alactolyticus* and *S. intestinalis* are identical as well.

S. bovis causes bacteremia, meningitis, and both native- and prosthetic-valve endocarditis; isolation of this organism from the blood is also associated with carcinoma of the colon.[307,464,487,1021] In a study of 16 evaluable patients with *S. bovis* endocarditis, 11 (69%) had colonic tumors.[307] *S.*

bovis is found significantly more often in the stool of patients with colorectal malignancies than in that of healthy controls or in those with benign intestinal polyps. A bacteriologic survey of patients with colon cancer and other bowel diseases showed that 56% of patients with colon cancer had *S. bovis* in their feces, compared with 10% of control patients with no bowel disorders.[578] Zarkin and coworkers found that *S. bovis* bacteremia was also associated with hepatic disease and dysfunction.[1091] In this study, 58% percent of patients with *S. bovis* endocarditis and 46% of those with bacteremia had colonic disease; liver disease was found in 52% of the patients with endocarditis and 57% of those with bacteremia. Both colon and liver disease were found in 27% of the patients in whom endocarditis developed. Gonzalez-Quintela and associates also found that 55% of 22 patients with *S. bovis* bacteremia had underlying liver disease, including cirrhosis and hepatitis C infection.[412] Wilson and others have also reported an association between *S. bovis* endocarditis and diseases of the colon other than carcinoma.[464,1064] Among 21 patients with *S. bovis* endocarditis, 62% had colonic disease that was not restricted to carcinoma; 24% had inflammatory bowel disease, 14% had diverticulitis, 10% had colonic polyps, 10% had colonic villous adenomas, and 5% had colonic carcinoma.[1064] An association between disseminated *S. bovis* infections and both idiopathic ulcerative colitis and chronic radiation enterocolitis has also been found.[528,700] Osada and colleagues reported a case in which *S. bovis* was isolated from thoracic empyema in a patient undergoing therapy for recurrent colon cancer.[749] A mechanism has been postulated that either the underlying colonic disease or changes in hepatic secretion of bile or immunoglobulins into the intestinal lumen may promote the overgrowth of *S. bovis* and the movement of the organisms from the intestine into the portal venous circulation. Failure of the compromised reticuloendothelial system of the liver to contain the organisms results in bacteremia and endocarditis. Patients with *S. bovis* bacteremia, endocarditis, or meningitis should have a complete colonoscopy to detect occult gastrointestinal lesions.[653]

Bacteremia and hematogenous dissemination of *S. bovis* may result in a variety of other clinical presentations. Despite the frequent association with colonic carcinoma, *S. bovis* meningitis and bacteremia have been reported in patients with no underlying malignancies.[356,389,792] Jain and associates reported an unusual case of *S. bovis* meningitis in an HIV-infected patient, who also had severe colitis and gastrointestinal bleeding secondary to *Strongyloides stercoralis* infection.[530] Presumably, the mucosal ulcerations created by the migration of strongyloides organisms allowed the *S. bovis* organisms access to the bloodstream. Some reports have also established *S. bovis* as an occasional cause of spontaneous bacterial peritonitis.[319,1012] White and colleagues reported a case of fatal intraamniotic infection of a 24-week-old fetus in which *S. bovis* was recovered from maternal blood and fetal tissues.[1054] In 2002, the first case of *S. bovis* bacteremia due to luminal colonization of a venous access port was reported in a patient with advanced HIV disease and hepatitis B; the patient had no gastrointestinal or liver disease and the bacteremia resolved with removal of the catheter.[28] Other infections associated with *S. bovis* have included pneumonia, acute spondylodiscitis, septic arthritis,

brain abscess, continuous ambulatory peritoneal dialysis–associated peritonitis, ileal and vertebral osteomyelitis, and arthroplasty infection secondary to bacteremia in association with colonic carcinoma.[327,471,618,659,716,773,1014,1067] Penicillin remains highly active against most strains of *S. bovis*, although occasional isolates that are relatively resistant to penicillin have been reported. Similarly, clindamycin is also active against most strains, but resistance to this agent appears to be emerging.[894]

S. bovis is also found in several animal species, in which it is generally considered to be a harmless inhabitant of the gastrointestinal tract. In fact, the type strain of *S. bovis* was originally recovered from cow dung and differs from human clinical isolates in several physiologic tests.[580] Some strains appear to be important causes of septicemia in pigeons.[264] *S. bovis*–like strains have also been isolated from the gastrointestinal tracts of pigs and chickens and have been identified as *S. alactolyticus*.[351] Chemotaxonomic studies with isolates from animals and humans also support the newer taxonomic literature, indicating that *S. gallolyticus* subsp. *gallolyticus* is more likely to be involved in human infections than *S. bovis sensu sritcto*.[281]

Streptococcus suis

Streptococcus suis deserves special mention because of its economic importance as an important swine and an occasional human pathogen. Infections caused by *S. suis* represent significant sanitary and economic problems in countries with intensive swine industries, such as Spain, Australia, Germany, Belgium, the Netherlands, and the United Kingdom. *S. suis* causes a wide spectrum of severe disease in piglets and pigs, including pneumonia, meningitis, septicemia, and purulent arthritis.[483] Piglets become colonized in the tonsils and nasal passages between 5 and 10 weeks of age; carriage rates among healthy animals may be as high as 80%.[37] Studies performed in Australia showed that over 70% of pigs slaughtered for human consumption in that country were carriers of *S. suis*.[816] In infected animals, *S. suis* initially causes fever, anorexia, and other constitutional symptoms, with meningeal involvement being manifested by the rapid onset of seizures, paralysis, and death.[642] The organisms can be readily recovered from the cerebral ventricles and from the regional lymph nodes of the upper respiratory tract, while isolation from splenic or liver tissue is uncommon.[648] Although disease in swine in the U.S. is not common, *S. suis* has been isolated from swine herds in Minnesota and Nebraska.[329]

The first human cases of *S. suis* infection were reported in 1968 from Denmark, and by 1989, 108 human cases of *S. suis* infection had been reported in the literature. Human infections have been reported from Hong Kong, the Netherlands, Denmark, Great Britain, France, Belgium, Germany, and Sweden.[917,947] The first case of a human infection reported in North America was a case of *S. suis* endocarditis in a patient in Canada.[965] Human infections with *S. suis* occur mostly in individuals who work directly with swine (e.g., abattoir and slaughterhouse workers, pig farmers, meat inspectors, veterinarians) or in the industrial processing and manufacture of pork products.[137,1029] In fact, some human cases reported from Hong Kong have been attributed to the popularity and consumption of large amounts of pork in China.[179] *S. suis* is believed to enter the host percutaneously through cuts, scratches, or abrasions in the skin. Entry via the nasopharynx and the gastrointestinal tract has also been proposed, and acute gastroenteritis may be a prominent part of the septic presentation.[649] After infection, disease onset is heralded by an "influenza-like" prodrome, followed by the rapid development of bacteremia and meningitis.[38,298,643] Overwhelming bacteremia without the development of meningitis may also occur.[137] The most common sequela of meningeal infection is cochlear-vestibular involvement resulting in ataxia and dizziness.[298] Involvement of the eighth cranial nerve is also commonly seen, and results in unilateral or bilateral hearing loss.[862] Complications result from seeding of distant sites during bacteremia and may include arthritis, spondylodiscitis, endophthalmitis, peritonitis, and pneumonia.[36,679,1013] Several cases of *S. suis* endocarditis have also been reported.[485,766,965]

Studies have also been performed in several countries on the antimicrobial susceptibility of *S. suis* type 2 isolates and other serotypes obtained from both animals and humans. In a study of 110 strains from pigs and 25 strains from humans conducted in France, nearly all strains were susceptible to penicillin, amoxicillin, and gentamicin; the least active agents were the macrolides, lincosamides, and doxycycline.[654] A survey of 689 porcine strains collected in Japan from 1987 through 1996 found that *S. suis* type 2 strains were highly susceptible to the penicillins, cefazolin, ofloxacin, and trimethoprim-sulfamethoxazole.[553] Almost 87% of strains were resistant to tetracyclines, and 71.4% and 29.5% were resistant to kanamycin and streptomycin, respectively. Studies conducted on strains isolated in Sweden and Denmark from 1967 through 1981 and from 1992 through 1997 reported that all isolates were susceptible to penicillin, ampicillin, vancomycin, and trimethoprim. Among isolates collected in Denmark from 1992 through 1997, 20.4% of serotype 2 strains and 44.8% of serotype 7 strains were macrolide (erythromycin, clindamycin)-resistant.[1] Tetracycline resistance was also observed in 43.9% of serotype 2 and 15.5% of serotype 7 strains collected during the same time period. Less than 5% of the isolates collected from 1967 through 1981 were resistant to these agents. Among the contemporary isolates, 15.4% of the serotype 2 strains from Sweden, 57.1% of the serotype 2 strains from Denmark, and 91.4% of the serotype 7 strains from Sweden were resistant to sulfamethoxazole. Penicillin is considered the drug of choice for treating systemic *S. suis* infection. However, non-β-lactamase-mediated resistance to penicillin has been reported among *S. suis* isolates from pigs in Spain, and in an isolate from a case of human meningitis.[787,862]

S. suis was officially recognized as an extant *Streptococcus* species in 1987.[569] Strains are groupable by Lancefield antisera into groups R, S, RS, and T or are ungroupable.[270] Some strains also react with group D streptococcal antiserum, suggesting possession of the group D lipoteichoic antigen. For this reason, this organism was initially thought to be a group D *Streptococcus* or an *Enterococcus* species. This observation was not substantiated by molecular techniques, and reactivity with group D antisera is due to spurious cross-reactions between groups D and R. *S. suis* strains

are also encapsulated, and 35 different capsular serotypes, designated 1 through 35, have been described.[421–423,482,767] *S. suis* serotype 1 causes meningitis in piglets younger than 6 weeks of age. This serotype includes strains belonging to Lancefield group S. *S. suis* capsular serotype 2 is also associated with systemic disease in pigs 3 to 20 weeks of age, and it is the only serotype that has been reported to cause systemic disease in humans. In the series of human cases reported in 1988 by Arends and Zanen from the Netherlands, 28 of 30 strains recovered from human infections were capsular serotype 2, one was serotype 4, and one was nontypeable.[38] This serotype encompasses the Lancefield group R streptococci. Other serotypes having Lancefield groups RS (reacts with both R and S antisera) and T reactivity may be found in both asymptomatic and diseased pigs. Serotypes can be determined by slide agglutination, immunodiffusion, or coagglutination.[420] Despite the fact that the majority of disease is caused by a small number of different serotypes, capsular serotype is not a predictor of virulence. Several genomic fingerprinting methods, including pulsed-field gel electrophoresis, ribotyping, random amplification polymorphic DNA analysis, and multilocus sequence typing have demonstrated considerable genetic heterogeneity among *S. suis* strains that belong to the same capsular serotype or to different capsular serotypes.[177,178,576,798,1006] Ribotyping methods have been able to identify two major clusters among porcine *S. suis* type 2 isolates in Demark.[797] Strains in one cluster were associated with meningitis, while those in the second cluster were associated with pneumonia, sepsis, and endocarditis. Meningitis strains in the first cluster were sulfamethoxazole-resistant, while strains in the second cluster were tetracycline-resistant.

S. suis serotype 2 produces a variety of factors that are associated with virulence, although the pathogenesis of infection in animals and humans is currently unclear.[425] The capsule of serotype 2 strains is a virulence factor composed of glucose, galactose, rhamnose, *N*-acetyl-glucosamine, and sialic acid.[906] The *cps* gene locus of *S. suis* type 2 has been cloned, characterized, and manipulated by insertional mutagenesis to produce capsule-deficient mutants.[905] These nonencapsulated strains were very sensitive to ingestion and killing by porcine lung alveolar macrophages in vitro and were avirulent in germ-free pigs following intranasal challenge. *S. suis* also produces a thiol-activate, pore-forming, cholesterol-binding cytolysin/hemolysin called suilysin.[518] The gene for suilysin (*sly*) has been sequenced and is structurally similar to the pneumolysin produced by *S. pneumoniae*.[875] This hemolysin/cytolysin is responsible for direct toxic effects on epithelial cells.[595] Mutants lacking suilysin were nonhemolytic, noncytotoxic for cultured macrophages, and avirulent in mice when inoculated via the intraperitoneal route, but these mutants were only slightly attenuated in a porcine model of systemic infection.[18] Using PCR approaches, the *sly* gene was found in more than 80% of strains associated with cases of meningitis, septicemia, and arthritis, and in more than 90% of strains from the tonsils of healthy pigs, but in only 44% of strains associated with porcine pneumonia.[575] Encapsulated type 2 strains also produce two proteins—muramidase-released protein (MRP) and extracellular protein factor (EF)—that are associated with virulence, but their role in disease pathogenesis is unclear since isogenic mutants lacking these proteins behave no differently than wild-type strains in mouse infection models.[425,918] Four distinct cell-associated and extracellular proteases have been described in virulent *S. suis* type 2 strains.[541] These proteases may function to obtain nutrients, to neutralize host defense mechanisms, and to assist in tissue invasion and destruction. *S. suis* type 2 strains produce an 18-kDa hemagglutinin adhesin that binds to galactose and galactose-*N*-acetylglucosamine moieties, a 39-kDa albumin-binding protein, and a 60-kDa IgG-binding protein have also been described. Since these adhesins have been found in both virulent and avirulent strains, their roles in disease pathogenesis, if any, are unclear.[77,424,793]

Other Viridans Streptococci Isolated From Animals

Several other ''species'' of α-hemolytic and nonhemolytic streptococci have been described in the medical, veterinary, and taxonomy literature. These species include *S. thoraltensis*, *S. hyovaginalis*, *S. hyointestinalis*, *S. pluranimalium*, *S. uberis*, *S. parauberis*, *S. entericus*, *S. ovis*, *S. gallinaceus*, and *S. minor*. *S. thoraltensis* and *S. hyovaginalis* are α-hemolytic streptococcal species that have been isolated from the genital tract of sows, while *S. hyointestinalis* is found in the porcine gastrointestinal tract.[278,279] *S. pluranimalium* is a new species that resembles strains of the former species *S. acidominimus* (see below). *S. pluranimalium* is an α-hemolytic species that is found in the genital tract and tonsils of cattle, ovine and feline tonsillar tissues, and the crop and respiratory tract of canaries.[280] This species has also been isolated from subclinical mastitis in cattle. *S. uberis* and *S. parauberis* are causes of bovine mastitis and have not been isolated from humans. These two species are indistinguishable from one another using phenotypic criteria, and species-specific molecular probes for these two organisms have been developed. Human isolates that were phenotypically identified as *S. uberis* have been reidentified as *Globicatella sanguinis*.[80] *S. entericus* is a new α-hemolytic *Streptococcus* that is found in the bovine intestine.[1005] *S. ovis* and *S. gallinaceus* are α-hemolytic species that have been isolated from infections (including bacteremia) in sheep and chickens, respectively.[216a,217] *S. minor* was described in 2004 and has been isolated from tonsils, anal swabs, and feces of dogs, and from the tonsils of calves and cats.[985]

Eremococcus coleocola is an α-hemolytic *Streptococcus*-like organism that is isolated from the reproductive tract of horses.[222] This species is most closely related to the *Streptococcus*-like organisms in the genera *Abiotrophia*, *Ignavigranum*, *Facklamia*, and *Globicatella*, which have been isolated from human clinical specimens.

Miscellaneous Streptococci

S. acidominimus strains have been poorly characterized since the original species description in 1922.[80] Reexamination of *S. acidominimus* strains recovered from humans established the true identity of these isolates as *Facklamia*

sourekii.[213] *S. thermophilus* and *S. macedonicus* are found in cheeses and other dairy products. *S. thermophilus* is related to *S. salivarius*, and may be incorporated as a subspecies of *S. salivarius* or may be a distinct species.[347,856] *S. macedonicus* has been reclassified as *S. gallolyticus* subsp. *macedonicus*, which is a part of the *S. bovis/S. equinus* complex. *S. caprinus* is a later subjective synonym of *S. gallolyticus* and *S. intestinalis* is a junior synonym of *S. alactolyticus*.[902,989] *S. difficile* was found to correspond to nonhemolytic strains of group B streptococci (*S. agalactiae*).[990]

Enterococcus *Species*
Taxonomy

The genus *Enterococcus* includes the enterococcal members previously classified with the group D streptococci.[857,858] These organisms are normal residents of the gastrointestinal and biliary tracts and, in lower numbers, of the vagina and male urethra. They are becoming increasingly important agents of human disease, largely because of their resistance to antimicrobial agents to which other streptococci are generally susceptible. In vitro, enterococci have penicillin MICs that are 10- to 100-fold higher than for other streptococci. Enterococci are the second most common cause of nosocomial urinary tract and wound infections and the third most common cause of nosocomial bacteremias.[354,690] Because of their resistance to penicillins and cephalosporins of several generations, the acquisition of high-level resistance to aminoglycosides, and now the emergence of vancomycin resistance, these bacteria are often involved in serious superinfections among patients receiving broad-spectrum antimicrobial chemotherapy.

The taxonomy of *Enterococcus* species has undergone considerable change since the mid-1980s. Before the advent and widespread use of genetic techniques for taxonomic analysis, enterococci were distinguished from streptococci and related taxa by their ability to grow at 10°C and 45°C, growth in the presence of 6.5% NaCl, growth at pH 9.6, ability to hydrolyze esculin in the presence of 40% bile, and production of pyrrolidonyl arylamidase (PYR). More than 90% of strains also possessed the Lancefield group D lipoteichoic antigen in their cell walls. Current taxonomic studies have subsequently revealed several species that are members of the genus *Enterococcus* by genetic criteria, but that lack many of the phenotypic characteristics typical of the genus.[1061] Fortunately, most of these species are not commonly found in human clinical specimens. *E. faecalis* is the most common isolate, being associated with 80–90% of human enterococcal infections. *E. faecium* ranks second and is isolated from 10–15% of infections.[833] Other enterococcal species, including *E. avium*, *E. casseliflavus*, *E. cecorum*, *E. durans*, *E. gallinarum*, *E. hirae*, *E. raffinosus*, *E. malodoratus*, *E. dispar*, *E. raffinosus*, and *E. mundtii* are infrequently isolated from human infections (see Box 13-4). The remaining species are found primarily in the gastrointestinal tracts of various animals and are rarely, if ever, recovered from significant human infections (see Box 13-4). Over the past few years, several new enterococcal species have been described from human clinical sources (i.e., *E. gilvus*, *E.*

pallens, CDC PNS [for probable new species]-E1, CDC PNS-E2, CDC PNS-E3), animals (i.e., *E. canis*, *E. villorum* [same as *E. porcinus*], *E. ratti*, *E. asini*, *E. phoeniculicola*), and the environment (i.e., *E. haemoperoxidus*, *E. moraviensis*) (Box 13-4). With the help of molecular taxonomic techniques, some former *Enterococcus* species have been reclassified or found to be the same as previously recognized species. For example, *E. seriolicida* was found to be identical to *Lactococcus garvieae*, *E. flavescens* was shown to be the same as *E. casseliflavus*, and *E. solitarius* was found to be identical to *Tetragenococcus halophilus*.[318,590,951,952,1061] Reports of unusual or uncommon *Enterococcus* species isolated from human infections will be seen from time to time in the literature. In the era of the compromised host, the clinical microbiologist should be aware of these other species and the methods for their identification. Members of the genus *Enterococcus* are described in Box 13-4.

Virulence Factors

Unlike several of the streptococcal species discussed thus far, the factors that determine the virulence of the enterococci are not well understood.[536,703] Some strains of *E. faecalis* produce a **cytolysin/hemolysin** that acts on human, rabbit, equine, and bovine erythrocytes (but not sheep erythrocytes) and has demonstrated significant toxicity in rabbit endophthalmitis and endocarditis models.[188,537] **Aggregation substance** is a surface-bound, plasmid-encoded protein that promotes clumping of the organisms to facilitate the plasmid exchange.[188,201] This substance also functions in facilitating enterococcal adherence to cultured intestinal and renal epithelial cells and promotes growth of cardiac vegetations in the rabbit endocarditis model.[188,383,587] Other studies suggest that aggregation substance may be involved in binding of *E. faecalis* to neutrophils and cultured intestinal epithelial cells and in subsequent internalization and intracellular survival of these organisms.[742,795,998] About 40% of blood and endocarditis isolates of *E. faecalis* produce a unique surface protein called **Esp (extracellular surface protein)** that functions to help the organism evade antibodies by its ability to be retracted away from the cell surface.[880] Most *E. faecalis* and some *E. faecium* isolates from bacteremias produce large amounts of extracellular superoxide that may enhance enterococcal virulence in mixed-flora abscesses.[505] **Lipoteichoic acids** constitute the group D antigen of enterococci and may also function in virulence by inducing the production of tumor necrosis factor (TNF) and interferon, leading to modulation of the immune response.[971] Lastly, 50–65% of *E. faecalis* strains produce **coccolysin,** an extracellular metalloendopeptidase, which may play a role in virulence by inactivating endothelin, a vasoactive peptide.[650]

Clinical Significance

Enterococcus species cause complicated urinary tract infections (UTIs), bacteremia, endocarditis, intraabdominal and pelvic infections, wound and soft-tissue infections, neonatal sepsis, and, rarely, meningitis.[690] UTIs are the most commonly encountered enterococcal infection, and include cystitis, pyelonephritis, prostatitis, perinephric abscesses,

and complicated infections with bacteremia. Most of these are nosocomial in origin or are associated with structural abnormalities or instrumentation of the urinary tract.[699,850] Enterococcal bacteremias usually result from infection at other sites (e.g., UTIs, biliary tract infection, gastrointestinal/genitourinary infections) and are most often hospital-acquired. Risk factors for the development of bacteremia include advanced age, immunosuppression, underlying diseases and conditions (e.g., prematurity, diabetes, malignancy, congestive heart failure, renal insufficiency, deep-seated infections), prior gastrointestinal, genitourinary, or respiratory tract instrumentation, long-term hospitalization, and the use of broad-spectrum antibiotics having little or no antienterococcal activity (e.g., cephalosporins).[427,443,1028] The organisms generally gain entry into the bloodstream through the urinary tract, intraabdominal or pelvic abscesses, wounds, decubitus ulcers, or intravenous access devices. Enterococci also cause 5–20% of cases of endocarditis, and they are a common cause of prosthetic-valve endocarditis.[680] Endocarditis usually occurs in older patients with underlying valvular disease or with prosthetic valves and is generally subacute in clinical presentation.[25,811]

In intraabdominal and pelvic infections, enterococci usually are found admixed with other indigenous aerobic and anaerobic organisms; pure spontaneous enterococcal peritonitis and enterococcal peritonitis associated with continuous ambulatory peritoneal dialysis have also been reported.[300,722] Though many invasive enterococcal infections originate in intraabdominal sites, controversy exists regarding the organisms' role in the pathogenesis of intraabdominal infections and peritonitis.[722] Studies have shown that empiric antienterococcal antimicrobial coverage is beneficial for immunocompromised patients with nosocomially acquired postoperative peritonitis, patients with abdominal sepsis who have received antimicrobials that select for enterococci, and patients with peritonitis and coexisting heart disease or prostheses who are at risk for enterococcal endocarditis.[460] Enterococci are often found in wound and soft-tissue infections (e.g., burns, decubitus ulcers) with other facultative and anaerobic bacteria, and complications associated with such infections (e.g., enterococcal osteomyelitis) are rarely due to enterococci unless they are present as superinfecting agents. Neonatal enterococcal sepsis has an acute, early-onset presentation, characterized by fever, lethargy and respiratory distress accompanied by bacteremia and meningitis.[290] Premature neonates are at greater risk of serious nosocomial enterococcal infections, particularly if peripheral access devices or feeding tubes are in place.[641] Enterococcal meningitis is a rare enterococcal infection that may be seen in both adults and children.[634,777,929] Enterococcal meningitis may develop spontaneously or as a postoperative infection. Individuals with spontaneous enterococcal meningitis usually have enterococcal infection at other sites, have severe underlying disease, and have concomitant enterococcal bacteremia more frequently than those with postoperative infections. Underlying disease in patients with spontaneous meningitis include malignancy, diabetes, renal failure, and treatment with immunosuppressive agents. Patients with postsurgical enterococcal meningitis usually have an antecedent history of trauma to the CNS (e.g., accidents, shunt placement).[634] In a recent review of enterococcal men-

Box 13-4 Members of the Genus *Enterococcus*

GROUP/Species	Comments
GROUP 1	
E. avium[218]	Isolated from avian, canine, and human gastrointestinal tracts; strains may carry both Lancefield group D and group Q carbohydrate antigens; this species (and *E. malodoratus*) are the two enterococcal species that produce H_2S. *E. avium* has been isolated from cases of bacteremia and osteomyelitis.[238,258,435,682,759]
E. gilvus[979]	New species described in 2002; originally isolated from a bile specimen of a patient with cholecystitis
E. malodoratus[218]	Isolated from Gouda cheese and unpasteurized milk products; name means "ill smelling"; also produces H_2S
E. pallens[979]	New species described in 2002; isolated from a peritoneal dialysate specimen of a patient in whom peritonitis developed from a perforated intestine
E. pseudoavium[207]	Genetic relatedness studies and certain phenotypic characteristics differentiate this species from *E. avium*; type strain isolated from a case of bovine mastitis
E. raffinosus[207]	Originally considered to be related to *E. avium* (along with *E. solitarius* and *E. pseudoavium*); named for its ability to produce acid from raffinose; recovered from human infections, including blood cultures, urine, abscesses, and vertebral osteomyelitis.[185,842]
E. saccharolyticus[818]	Originally called *S. saccharolyticus*; described a group of *S. bovis*–like strains recovered from cows; genetic analysis showed that this organisms is more closely related to the enterococci than the streptococci; has certain phenotypic characteristics that are similar to *Enterococcus* species (e.g., growth at 10°C and 45°C, growth in 6.5% NaCl), but does not react with group D antisera; proposed that this species be moved from the viridans *Streptococcus* group to the genus *Enterococcus* as *E. saccharolyticus*
Enterococcus sp. CDC PNS-E-3[161]	CDC "proposed new species," isolated from brain tissue obtained from an 11-month-old patient in Honolulu, Hawaii, in 2001
GROUP 2	
E. faecalis	Most frequent isolate from human clinical specimens and from the human gastrointestinal tract; also found in the intestinal tracts of poultry, cattle, pigs, dogs, horses, sheep, and goats
E. faecium	Found in human clinical specimens; generally more resistant to antimicrobial agents than *E. faecalis*; also found in the gastrointestinal tracts of various species of animals
E.casseliflavus[218]	Recovered from plants, soil, and rarely, from the feces of chickens; originally classified as a subspecies of *E. faecium*; produces a yellow pigment and is also motile. This organism is an opportunistic agent in human infections and has been isolated from patients with bacteremia.[754,779,807,832,999]
E. gallinarum[218]	Isolated from chicken feces; originally classified as *Streptococcus gallinarum* "chicken group D"; one of the two motile *Enterococcus* species; has also been isolated from an infection in a hemodialysis patient, as a cause of native-valve endocarditis, and from blood cultures.[254,807]
E. mundtii[211]	Yellow-pigmented, nonmotile organism; isolated from plants, soil, and the gastrointestinal tracts of cattle, pigs, and horses; named after J.O. Mundt, an American microbiologist. This species has been isolated from a human thigh abscess and from an operatively obtained sinus mucosal specimen.[554]
E. haemoperoxidus[938]	New environmental enterococcal species described in 2001; isolated from surface waters, swimming pools, and drinking water in the North Moravia region of the Czech Republic
Enterococcus sp. CDC PNS-E2[161]	CDC "proposed new species," isolated from blood cultures of a patient in Los Angeles in 1997
GROUP 3	
E. dispar[226]	Species originally thought to be a biochemical variant of *E. hirae*, but analysis of 16S rRNA indicated that this organism is indeed a previously undescribed species; recovered from human specimens, including stool and synovial fluid.[226]
E. durans[218]	This species is found mainly in milk and other dairy products and is a rare clinical isolate. In 2004, *E. durans* was isolated as a cause of native-valve endocarditis.[923]
E. hirae[349]	Causes growth depression in chickens; isolated from chicken crops and feces, and the gastrointestinal tracts of cattle, pigs, dogs, horses, sheep, goats, and rabbits; type strain (*E. hirae* ATCC 8043) has complex nutritional requirements and is used in the food industry as a bioassay organism for amino acids and vitamins. *E. hirae* was isolated from the blood of a 49-year-old patient with end-stage renal disease who was undergoing hemodialysis.[399]
E. ratti[949]	Described in 2001, this new species was originally isolated from the intestines and feces of rats with diarrhea.
E. villorum[263,949,986]	Isolated from the gastrointestinal tract of dogs; phenotypically identical with *E. porcinus*, which is considered as a junior synonym of *E. villorum* and was originally isolated from the intestines and feces of pigs with diarrhea.

Box 13-4 *Continued*

GROUP/Species	Comments
GROUP 4	
E. asini[272]	Described in 1998, this species is found in the cecum of donkeys; most closely related to *E. avium*, *E. pseudoavium*, and *E. faecium*
E. cecorum[276]	Newly reclassified streptococcal species found in the intestines of chickens; lacks the group D antigen, is PYR-negative and is unable to grow in 6.5% NaCl broth; similar to *E. columbae*, it may be confused with *E. avium* and with *S. bovis*.[274,276,1060] *E. cecorum* has been isolated as a cause of peritoneal dialysis–associated peritonitis, recurrent bacteremic peritonitis, and spontaneous bacterial peritonitis with empyema, and has been isolated from blood cultures of a patient with severe malnutrition.[260,437,499,1070]
E. sulfureus[663]	Newly described, yellow-pigmented species; recovered from plants; has not yet been isolated from humans.
E. phoeniculicola[602]	Described in 2003, this species is found in the preen glands of wild red-billed Woodhoopoes; does not grow on BE agar or in 6.5% NaCl broth
Enterococcus sp.[161] CDC PNS-E1	CDC "proposed new species" isolated from the blood of a patient in Evanston, Illinois, in 1991
GROUP 5	
E. columbae[275]	Newly reclassified streptococcal species isolated from the intestinal tract of pigeons; closely related to *E. cecorum* and *E. avium;* characterized by being PYR-negative and unable to grow in 6.5% NaCl broth
E. canis[263]	Originally isolated from a dog with chronic otitis externa; probably a resident of the canine gut; grows on BE agar, grows in 6.5% NaCl broth, and is PYR-positive
E. moraviensis[938]	New environmental enterococcal species described in 2001; isolated from surface and drinking water in the North Moravia region of the Czech Republic

ingitis, *E. faecalis* accounted for 76% of isolates, and 15 of the 25 cases that were due to *E. faecium* were caused by vancomycin-resistant strains.[777] Respiratory-tract infection caused by enterococci are rare and are seen only in severely debilitated patients.[84]

The resistance of enterococci to a variety of antimicrobial agents does indeed contribute to their pathogenicity. These organisms display intrinsic, low-level resistance to the aminoglycosides and lincosamides, have relatively high MICs for penicillins and cephalosporins, and are resistant to the action of sulfonamide agents in vitro. The higher MICs for the β-lactam agents are due to diminished affinity of cell wall penicillin-binding proteins (PBPs) for these agents. Low-level aminoglycoside resistance is due to decreased penetrability of the enterococcal cell wall.[321] Although enterococci appear susceptible to sulfonamides in vitro, they are able to circumvent the block in folate synthesis in vitro. Serious infections associated with enterococci are usually treated with a combination of penicillin or ampicillin with an aminoglycoside. The emergence of high-level resistance to aminoglycosides (i.e., streptomycin MICs >2,000 μg/mL; gentamicin MICs >500 μg/mL) in enterococci, particularly *E. faecalis* and *E. faecium*, seriously affected the therapeutic approach to and clinical response of patients with bacteremia, endocarditis, and other serious infections.[30,142] High-level aminoglycoside resistance has disseminated among several enterococcal species and has been documented in strains of *E. avium*, *E. casseliflavus*, *E. gallinarum*, *E. raffinosus*, and *E. mundtii*.[837] Strains displaying high-level resistance to aminoglycosides are not killed by the synergistic activity of the β-lactam agent along with an aminoglycoside. This high-level resistance is transposon-mediated and can be transferred to other organisms.[321] Bactericidal synergism between penicillin and aminoglycosides

requires that the organism not only have MICs for aminoglycosides lower than the values cited in the foregoing, but that the serum concentration of penicillin be near or exceed the MIC; increasing β-lactam resistance among enterococci along with high aminoglycoside MICs further abrogate synergism. Because of the lack of reliable penicillin-aminoglycoside synergism among high-level aminoglycoside-resistant enterococci and the emergence of methicillin-resistant *S. aureus*, vancomycin became a first-line drug effective against both staphylococci and enterococci.

Until the early 1980s, the susceptibility of enterococci to ampicillin and vancomycin remained fairly predictable. Since that time, *Enterococcus* species resistant to ampicillin and vancomycin have been reported with increasing frequency. Resistance to ampicillin in some *E. faecalis* strains was demonstrated to be due to production of β-lactamase enzymes.[762] Subsequently, ampicillin resistance in strains of *E. faecium*, *E. gallinarum*, and *E. raffinosus* was reported; with these organisms, resistance was due to decreased penicillin-binding affinity of the cell wall penicillin-binding proteins.[185,321,673] The appearance of vancomycin-resistant strains of *E. faecalis* and *E. faecium* heralded a major change in the enterococci.

Acquired glycopeptide (i.e., vancomycin and teicoplanin) resistance in *Enterococcus* species corresponds to five different phenotypes, designated VanA, VanB, VanD, VanE and VanG, with VanA and VanB phenotypes being the most prevalent and important clinically.[396,405,1077] These phenotypes correspond to genotypes that are designated *vanA*, *vanB*, *vanD*, *vanE*, and *vanG*, respectively. These genotypes actually describe gene clusters that code for enzymes that create the structural components that result in phenotypic resistance. This resistance to glycopeptides results from the synthesis of different peptidoglycan precursors that become incorporated into the cell wall and have decreased binding affinity for vancomycin, teicoplanin, or both. Normally, vancomycin-susceptible strains have peptidoglycan side chains that terminate with the depsipeptide ''D-alanyl-D-alanine,'' and the glycopeptide antibiotic binds to this depsipeptide. In glycopeptide-resistant strains, the depsipeptide is replaced by ''D-alanyl-D-lactate'' (VanA, VanB, and VanD phenotypes) or by ''D-alanyl-D-serine'' (VanE and VanG phenotypes). *E. faecium* and *E. faecalis* isolates that have the *vanA* genotype characteristically display inducible, transposon-mediated, high-level resistance to both vancomycin (MIC, 64–1000 μg/mL) and teicoplanin (MIC, 16-512 μg/mL, both of which are glycopeptide-class antimicrobial agents.[1077] Strains with the *vanB* genotype have acquired inducible resistance to various concentrations of vancomycin (MIC, 4–1000 μg/mL) but remain susceptible to teicoplanin (MIC, 0.5–1 μg/mL), although rare *vanB* strains may also be resistant to the latter antibiotic.[396,1077] Isolates expressing the *vanB* genotype also include *E. faecalis* and *E. faecium* strains. Some *E. faecium* strains express the *vanD* genotype; these strains are constitutively resistant to both vancomycin (MIC, 64–28 μg/mL) and teicoplanin (MIC, 4–64 μg/mL) and resistance is not transferable to other enterococci.[768] Rare *E. faecalis* strains expressing the *vanE* genotype express inducible, low-level resistance to vancomycin (MIC, 16 μg/mL), yet remain susceptible to teicoplanin (MIC, 0.5 μg/mL).[361] The VanG phenotype is associated with low-level resistance to vancomycin (MIC, 16 μg/mL) but susceptibility to teicoplanin (MIC, 0.5 μg/mL) and was initially found in *E. faecalis* isolates from Australia.[677] Isolates that have the *vanC* genotype display intrinsic, constitutive, low-level resistance to vancomycin (MIC, 2–32 μg/mL) and are susceptible to teicoplanin (MIC, 0.5–1 μg/mL). The *vanC* genotype corresponds to the intrinsic glycopeptide resistance seen in *E. gallinarum*, *E. casseliflavus*, and *E. flavescens*. This *vanC* gene cluster is not transferred by conjugation to other organisms, is generally constitutively expressed, and is chromosomal in origin.[610,719] The *vanF* genotype refers to the glycopeptide-resistance gene cluster found in the former *Bacillus* species, *Paenibacillus popillae*.[760] Enterococci with the VanA phenotype are most worrisome because these strains are able to transfer *vanA* resistance markers by a conjugative mechanism to other enterococci and other gram-positive organisms, including *Staphylococcus aureus*.[726] However, in 1994, strains with the *vanB* class genotype were shown to be able to transfer their vancomycin resistance genes as well.[127] Epidemiologic investigations of nosocomial outbreaks caused by vancomycin-resistant enterococci (VRE) have been aided by the development of DNA probes for direct detection of resistance loci.[1078]

Another enterococcal phenomenon is that of vancomycin dependence. This refers to strains of enterococci that grow only in the presence of vancomycin. Vancomycin-dependent enterococci (VDE) were first described in 1994, when these organisms were cultured from the urine of a patient receiving long-term therapy with vancomycin.[372,373] Since that time, other isolations of VDE have been reported.[273] Patients exposed to vancomycin and other agents (e.g., extended-spectrum cephalosporins) are at risk for colonization with VRE, and this exposure also places them at risk for becoming

colonized with VDE as well. VRE and VDE have the ability to use cell wall ligases to make an alternative cell wall depsipeptide (D-alanine-D-lactate), which replaces the normally found D-alanine-D-alanine. If vancomycin is not present in the milieu, VRE retain their ability to make the D-alanine-D-alanine depsipeptide and proceed to grow normally. Because of mutations in the ligase genes that result in amino acid deletions/substitutions in the ligase enzyme, VDE strains are unable to make the original D-alanine-D-alanine depsipeptide. The presence of vancomycin enables these strains to use the D-alanine-D-lactate as a cell wall constituent, so their growth is actually dependent on vancomycin. These VDE strains are relatively uncommon. VDE strains derived from both *E. faecalis* and *E. faecium* have been described.[273,373]

Identification of *Enterococcus* species is discussed later in this chapter. Additional information on antimicrobial resistance and methods for antimicrobial susceptibility testing are discussed in detail in Chapter 17.

Genus *Melissococcus*

The genus *Melissococcus* contains a single species, *M. pluton*. This organism causes a disease of bees called ''European foulbrood.'' In 1994, using 16S rRNA sequence data, Cai and Collins demonstrated that *M. pluton* was most closely related to the genus *Enterococcus*.[145] Since the naming of this organism in the genus *Melissococcus* predated the description of the genus *Enterococcus*, incorporation of *M. pluton* among the enterococci would, according to the rules of nomenclature, necessitate that all of the enterococcal species be transferred to the genus *Melissococcus*. Because of the familiarity of the enterococci to both clinicians and microbiologists, Cai and Collins recommended that *M. pluton* remain as the only species in the genus *Melissococcus*.[145]

The ''Streptococcus-Like'' Bacteria
Abiotrophia and *Granulicatella* Species

The ''nutritionally variant streptococci'' were originally thought to be viridans streptococci that required thiol compounds (e.g., cysteine) or the active form of vitamin B_6 (i.e., pyridoxal or pyridoxamine) for growth on bacteriologic media.[155] These organisms have also been called nutritionally deficient, thiol-requiring, pyridoxal-requiring, and ''satelliting'' streptococci. DNA relatedness studies comparing nutritionally variant streptococci with other viridans streptococci identified two DNA hybridization groups that corresponded to two species, which were named *Streptococcus defectivus* and *Streptococcus adjacens*.[126] In 1995, Kawamura and associates in Japan performed 16S rRNA sequence analysis of these two species and found that they were not related to any species belonging to the genus *Streptococcus*. The new genus *Abiotrophia* was proposed to accommodate these ''streptococci,'' with the new species names being *Abiotrophia adiacens* and *Abiotrophia defectiva*.[557] In 1998 and 1999, two additional members of this genus were characterized: *Abiotrophia elegans*, from a human patient with endocarditis, and *Abiotrophia balaenopterae*, isolated from a minke whale (*Balaenoptera acutorostrata*).[609,820] In 2000,

Kanamoto and colleagues identified and characterized another new *Abiotrophia* species using genetic and phenotypic criteria that was closely related to *A. adiacens* and proposed the species name *Abiotrophia para-adiacens* for this new isolate.[548] These new species were subsequently demonstrated to have a closer phylogenetic affinity with *A. adiacens* than with *A. defectiva*. The latter species is phylogenetically more closely related to several non-*Abiotrophia* "*Streptococcus*-like" species, including *Globicatella sanguinis*, *Facklamia* species, *Eremococcus* species, and *Ignavigranum* species. Several studies have now demonstrated the polyphyletic nature of the genus *Abiotrophia* and the close affinity between *A. adiacens*, *A. elegans*, *A. para-adiacens*, and *A. balaenopterae*. Based on these studies, these three organisms have been reclassified in the new genus *Granulicatella* as *Granulicatella adiacens*, *Granulicatella para-adiacens*, *Granulicatella elegans*, and *Granulicatella balaenopterae*.[223] *A. defectiva* is retained as the sole species in the genus *Abiotrophia*.

A. defectiva, *G. adiacens*, and *G. elegans* are part of the normal flora of the upper respiratory, urogenital, and gastrointestinal tracts.[687,845] *Abiotrophia* and *Granulicatella* species cause sepsis and bacteremia and are the cause of 5–6% of cases of infective endocarditis and bacteremic complications associated with endocarditis.[123,173,189,190,710,820,823] Since 1999, *A defectiva*, and *G. adiacens* have been documented as causes of CNS infections, including meningitis and brain and epidural abscesses.[94,171,685,855] In almost all cases, infection was associated with prior neurosurgical procedures, including craniotomy, ventriculoperitoneal shunt placement, CT-guided myelography, and tumor resection. These organisms have also been isolated from significant ocular infections, including conjunctivitis, endophthalmitis following cataract surgery, and keratitis associated with extended-wear hydrogel contact lenses.[58,561,715,748] Other infections involving *Abiotrophia* and *Granulicatella* species include pneumonia, scrotal abscess, sinusitis, septic arthritis, vertebral osteomyelitis, arthroplasty infection, and bone marrow infection.[189,470,479,510,823] These organisms produce a variety of extracellular factors in vitro, including neuraminidase and several aminopeptidases, that may contribute to their virulence; they are also able to bind to fibronectin and other extracellular matrix proteins.[72,740] Because of their clinical significance and their exacting cultural requirements, it is essential that the clinical microbiologist be familiar with the clinical settings in which they occur and the laboratory methods that are necessary for their isolation from patient specimens.

Abiotrophia and *Granulicatella* species are more resistant to antimicrobial agents than the viridans streptococci. Although most strains are susceptible to clindamycin, erythromycin, rifampin, and vancomycin, studies have demonstrated decreased susceptibility to penicillin and variable susceptibility to cephalosporins and aminoglycosides.[710] In a study by Tuohy and colleagues, 41% of 27 *G. adiacens* isolates and 12 *A. defectiva* isolates were penicillin-susceptible (MIC, ≤0.12 µg/mL), 51% were intermediate (MIC, 0.25–2 µg/mL), and 8% were penicillin-resistant (MIC, ≥4 µg/mL).[975] Strains of *G. adiacens* were more susceptible to penicillin and cefazolin (55% susceptible to penicillin, 52% susceptible to cefazolin) than *A. defectiva* strains (8% sus-

ceptible to penicillin, 0% susceptible to cefazolin). For ceftriaxone, 83% of *A. defectiva* strains and 63% of *G. adiacens* were susceptible at the Clinical Laboratory Standards Institute (CLSI) breakpoint. In this study, all isolates were susceptible to clindamycin, rifampin, ofloxacin, levofloxacin, quinupristin-dalfopristin, and vancomycin and no high-level aminoglycoside resistance was detected. Since these organisms require pyridoxal for growth, antimicrobial susceptibility testing media must be supplemented with pyridoxal hydrochloride (0.001% final concentration) for test performance.[956]

Aerococcus and *Helcococcus* Species

Aerococci are *Streptococcus*-like organisms that are found in the environment, usually in association with water, and they may be recovered from air, dust, soil, vegetation, meat products, and the hospital environment.[564] *Aerococcus viridans*, the oldest species in the genus, causes a fatal disease called gaffkemia in lobsters, but in humans they are primarily opportunists.[63,756] Aerococci have been isolated from patients with a number of clinical conditions, including endocarditis, bacteremia, meningitis, septic arthritis, osteomyelitis, and wound infections.[565,717,775,939,948] Aerococci are included occasionally in proficiency surveys and can easily be confused with the viridans streptococci and enterococci. Aerococci have a characteristic tendency to form tetrads when grown in broth media. The organisms are microaerophilic, and sparse or no growth is observed under anaerobic conditions. Isolates that were previously assigned to the genus *Pediococcus* as *P. urinae-equi* have been shown to be closely related phylogenetically to *A. viridans*.[228] Strains of *A. viridans* are usually susceptible to penicillin, macrolides, sulfonamides, and trimethoprim.

In 1989, Christensen and colleagues in Copenhagen reported on a group of 29 patients with suspected urinary tract infections from whom "*Aerococcus*-like organisms" (ALOs) were recovered from urine specimens.[193,194] In 11 of these patients, this organism was isolated in pure culture (>10[6] colony-forming units [CFU]/mL). The patients (20 women and 9 men) ranged in age from 49 to 88 years, and half of them had either local or systemic conditions (e.g., diabetes, urinary-tract and non-urinary-tract malignancies, urolithiasis) that may have predisposed them to infection with opportunistic organisms. Patients with septicemia and endocarditis caused by these organisms were elderly, had some type of underlying disease (e.g., myocardial infarction, prostate cancer, diabetes), and had ALOs recovered from both blood and urine specimens.[191,192] Phenotypic characterization of these ALO strains demonstrated that they differed from *A. viridans* strains in several respects.[8,194] On the basis of differing phenotypic criteria and phylogenetic analysis of 16S rRNA sequence data from reference strains of *A. viridans*, Aguirre and Collins proposed that ALOs be classified as the new species *Aerococcus urinae*.[8] The inclusion of *A. urinae* in the genus *Aerococcus* is supported by results of 16S rRNA sequencing, and these data also support the inclusion of both esculin-positive and esculin-negative biotypes within the same species.[195] Since the naming of this new species, *A. urinae* has been reported as a cause of urinary-tract infections, septicemia, endocarditis, soft-tissue infections, spondylodiscitis, and lymphadenitis.[308,473,868,869,900,1092,1094] Isolates of *A. urinae* are usually susceptible to penicillin, amoxicillin, piperacillin, cefepime, rifampin, and vancomycin.[193,899] The quinolones, tetracyclines, and erythromycin show moderate to good activity, and most isolates have elevated MICs for certain cephalosporins and reduced susceptibility to the aminoglycosides. Time-kill studies indicate that penicillin or vancomycin combined with gentamicin show bactericidal synergy, suggesting that combination therapy is the therapy of choice for endocarditis caused by this organism.[899]

Since the description of *A. urinae*, three additional *Aerococcus* species have been described: *Aerococcus christensenii*, *Aerococcus urinaehominis*, and *Aerococcus sanguinicola*.[221,606,607] *A. christensenii* was isolated from vaginal specimens at the University of Washington in Seattle and had been tentatively identified as *Streptococcus acidominimus*.[221] The description of *A. sanguinicola* is based on a single human blood culture isolate, but this species has been isolated from both urine and blood cultures (including endocarditis) since its initial description in 2001.[339,607] Isolates of *A. sanguinicola* are susceptible to penicillin, amoxicillin, cefotaxime, cefuroxime, erythromycin, vancomycin, quinupristin-dalfopristin, rifampin, linezolid, and tetracyclines, and variably susceptible to the quinolones; some strains are resistant to clindamycin, meropenem, and trimethoprim-sulfamethoxazole.[339] Similarly, the description of *A. urinaehominis* is based on a single isolate from a human urine specimen.[606] Information on the antimicrobial susceptibility of *A. urinaehominis* is not available.

During an examination of several *Streptococcus*-like isolates from human clinical sources, Collins and coworkers encountered nine strains of facultative, gram-positive, catalase-negative cocci that resembled aerococci but produced variable growth in 6.5% NaCl broth.[208] Seven of the nine strains were recovered from wounds on the feet or legs, and two isolates were from cultures of breast masses. The other unusual feature of these organisms was that they were lipophilic; growth on agar media and in broth was enhanced by the presence of serum or Tween 80. These organisms were shown to belong a new genus and species of gram-positive cocci by genetic analysis and phenotypic criteria and have been assigned to the new genus *Helcococcus* as *Helcococcus kunzii*. Additional studies on the ecology of this new organism suggest an association with the bacterial flora of the lower extremities and a propensity to be isolated from wound infections and cellulitis along with more virulent organisms, such as *Staphylococcus aureus*.[147,445] Since its description, *H. kunzii* has been isolated in pure culture from an infected sebaceous cyst, a breast abscess, and a postsurgical foot abscess.[172,764,813] In 1999, a second *Helcococcus* species, *Helcococcus ovis*, was described.[209] This organism is found in sheep.

Leuconostoc Species

Leuconostoc species are gram-positive, nonmotile, nonspore-forming, heterofermentative, facultative cocci that are found in the environment (i.e., on plants and in soil). These organisms have economic importance because of their use in the dairy and pickling industries and in wine making.

These organisms have been isolated from human infections, most of them occurring in immunocompromised hosts.[434,457,513,694] *Leuconostoc* species have been isolated from blood cultures of patients with underlying malignancies and indwelling intravenous catheters and have also been isolated from hepatic and intraabdominal abscesses, gastrostomy and tracheostomy sites, odontogenic abscesses, breast abscesses, osteomyelitis, pleural empyema, dialysis-related and spontaneous bacterial peritonitis, and draining fistulas.[59,116,400,462,696,701,953,984,1037] *Leuconostoc* species have been recovered as opportunistic agents causing bacteremia and pulmonary infections in bone marrow recipients, solid-organ transplant recipients, gastroenterology patients, burn patients, and AIDS patients.[330,357,402,433,540,694] A *Leuconostoc* species was also isolated from the CSF of a previously healthy 16-year-old girl, in whom the organism caused a purulent meningeal infection.[233] Friedland and colleagues also reported a case of purulent meningitis due to *L. mesenteroides* in a 1-month-old girl.[380] Carapetis and coworkers described two cases of bacteremia caused by *Leuconostoc* species (specifically, *L. lactis* and *L. pseudomesenteroides*) in children with necrotizing enterocolitis who were receiving long-term parenteral nutrition.[154] In one of these cases, the same *L. lactis* strain was recovered from the patient's gastrostomy tube site. Bacteremia caused by *L. mesenteroides* and *Enterobacter sakazakii* was also reported in association with contaminated infant formula.[728] *Leuconostoc* species have also been documented as causes of nosocomially acquired infections.[152,849]

Leuconostoc species may be misidentified as pneumococci, viridans streptococci, or lactobacilli. Similar to pediococci and certain lactobacilli, but unlike most other gram-positive bacteria, *Leuconostoc* species are intrinsically resistant to vancomycin.[646] In some case reports, patients were being treated with vancomycin when infections with these organisms became clinically apparent. The characteristics of *Leuconostoc* species that help to differentiate them from the other *Streptococcus*-like bacteria are their resistance to vancomycin and the formation of gas from glucose during growth in MRS broth (discussed below). Therapy for serious *Leuconostoc* infections includes penicillin and aminoglycosides; most isolates are susceptible to tetracyclines, imipenem, clindamycin, and gentamicin.

Pediococcus and *Tetragenococcus* Species

Pediococcus species are gram-positive cocci that, like the streptococci, produce lactic acid as the sole product of glucose fermentation. These organisms are found naturally on plants and are important in the brewing and food industries. Pediococci may be found in beers and ales and are also used in foods for processing and preservation. They are included as flavor enhancers in processed vegetables and soy products and are used in biotechnology as indicator strains for vitamin bioassays. The genus *Pediococcus* includes seven species: *P. acidilactici*, *P. damnosus*, *P. dextrinicus*, *P. inopinatus*, *P. parvulus*, *P. pentosaceus*, and *P. claussenii*.[289] Isolates of *P. urinae-equi*, a former *Pediococcus* species, phenotypically resemble *A. viridans*, and a DNA probe specific for *A. viridans* also reacts with *P. urinae-equi*, indicating that these two organisms are the same.[228,429] In addition, genetic studies using 16S rRNA and DNA-DNA hybridization indicate that the former species *Pediococcus halophilus* represents a line of descent that is separate from both pediococci and aerococci, and more closely related to the enterococci. Because of these genetic data, isolates that were previously called *P. halophilus* have been placed in the new genus *Tetragenococcus*, with the type species being *Tetragenococcus halophilus*.[228] *T. halophilus* has also been found to be identical to *Enterococcus solitarius*. In 1997, Satomi and colleagues described another *Tetragenococcus* species, *T. muriaticus*, that was isolated from squid liver sauce, a traditional Japanese fermented seafood.[847] This species can grow in NaCl concentrations as high as 25%.

The Bacterial Reference Laboratory of the Respiratory Diseases Branch at the CDC has received isolates of pediococci from a variety of human clinical specimens, including saliva, stool, urine, wounds, abscesses, and blood.[667] Pediococci have usually been isolated from patients with various underlying conditions, including hematologic malignancies, cardiovascular disease, chronic lung disease, gastroschisis, pancreatitis, and diabetes.[42,61,234,474,844,896] Many patients with these infections had had previous abdominal surgery or had nasogastric tubes or central venous catheters in place for total parenteral nutrition for prolonged periods. Pediococci recovered from blood cultures were usually single, positive cultures among several cultures positive with other organisms. In a study of 26 patients who were undergoing total bowel decontamination with gentamicin-vancomycin-colimycin preparatory to remission induction therapy or bone marrow transplantation, Maugein and colleagues found *Pediococcus* species in 89% of the stool specimens collected from these patients.[670] Like *Leuconostoc* species, these organisms are resistant to vancomycin; many patients first manifest symptoms of infection while being treated with this antimicrobial agent.[667,941] In one report, *P. acidilactici* was identified in multiple blood cultures from a 53-year-old man with acute myeloblastic leukemia.[410] At the time of the first positive blood culture, this patient had been receiving vancomycin for 14 days, along with ceftazidime, metronidazole, and cancer chemotherapy. Isolates of pediococci from clinical specimens have been identified as either *P. acidilactici* or *P. pentosaceus*. Pediococci are generally susceptible to penicillin G, erythromycin, clindamycin, gentamicin, and imipenem.[941,944]

Gemella Species

At present, the genus *Gemella* includes six species: *G. haemolysans*, *G. morbillorum*, *G. bergeriae*, *G. sanguinis*, *G. palaticanis*, and *G. cuniculi*.[215,216,219,496,570] *G. haemolysans*, the type species of the genus, is an easily decolorized gram-positive coccus that characteristically appears as diplococci with adjacent sides flattened. Because of these properties, it was previously included with the gram-negative cocci in the genus *Neisseria*. Cell wall analysis demonstrated that the organism did have a gram-positive type cell wall, although it is much thinner than that of other gram-positive organisms. Nucleic-acid hybridization studies showed no relatedness to members of the family *Neisseriaceae*. These data, along with the negative catalase reaction, relegated this species to the family *Streptococcaceae*. Unlike the strepto-

cocci, however, growth is poor under anaerobic conditions. *G. morbillorum* was previously classified with the streptococci as *Streptococcus morbillorum* and was originally included among the viridans streptococci. Genetic analysis of *S. morbillorum* strains indicated that the organism was more closely related to *G. haemolysans* than to the streptococci and peptostreptococci.[570,640,1055] Gas-liquid chromatography studies showed that, in addition to lactic acid, some strains also produced acetic, formic, succinic, and pyruvic acids, plus traces of ethanol, therefore supporting the transfer of *S. morbillorum* to the genus *Gemella* as *Gemella morbillorum*. In 1998, two new *Gemella* species—*Gemella bergeriae* and *Gemella sanguinis*—were characterized and described.[215,216] These isolates (six strains of each species) were recovered from blood and were distinct from the previously described *Gemella* species by biochemical and molecular characterization. Subsequently, two additional species—*Gemella palaticanis* and *Gemella cuniculi*—were described.[219,496] *G. palaticanis* was isolated from a vesicle in the oral cavity of a Labrador retriever, and *G. cuniculi* was recovered from a submandibular abscess of a lop-eared pet rabbit. At present, the habitat of *G. bergeriae* and *G. sanguinis* in humans is not known, and, other than recovery from blood cultures, no specific infections have been associated with these new species.

Members of the genus *Gemella* are infrequently isolated from clinical specimens. However, their similarity to the viridans streptococci has probably resulted in their being underrecognized and misidentified. *G. haemolysans* is part of the upper respiratory tract flora, whereas *G. morbillorum* can be found in the human respiratory and gastrointestinal tracts. Both *G. haemolysans* and *G. morbillorum* have been isolated as occasional causes of bacteremia and endocarditis involving both native and prosthetic heart valves.[75,346,379,490,600,698,744] Cases of meningitis, meningoencephalitis, septic arthritis, osteomyelitis, spondylodiscitis, keratitis with endophthalmitis, retropharyngeal abscess, thoracic empyema with lung abscess, septic shock, and an infected knee arthroplasty associated with *Gemella* species have also been reported.[41,245,261,314,315,671,689,744,785,815,997,1003,1008,1017] Like *S. bovis* infections, an association has also been made between endocarditis due to *Gemella* species and the presence of adenomatous polyps and colon carcinoma.[477,633] *Gemella* species are usually susceptible to a wide variety of antimicrobial agents, including penicillin, ampicillin, rifampin, and vancomycin, but low-level resistance to aminoglycosides and trimethoprim may be observed in some isolates.[144] In 1993, a strain of *G. haemolysans* that was recovered from a blood culture was found to have decreased susceptibility to penicillin and frank resistance to vancomycin, teicoplanin, erythromycin, and tetracycline.[804]

Vagococcus Species

The genus *Vagococcus* was proposed in 1989 to accommodate a group of motile gram-positive, catalase-negative cocci that resembled lactococci.[206] These motile organisms had been recovered from chicken feces and river water. Using 16S rRNA sequencing data, it was shown that these motile "*Lactococcus*-like" strains formed a distinct line of descent within the lactic acid–producing bacteria and were clearly separate from the streptococci, enterococci, and *Lactococcus* species *sensu stricto*. Furthermore, these strains were also found to be phenotypically distinct. Collins and associates placed these organisms into the new genus *Vagococcus* ("wandering coccus").[206] The motile group N *Lactococcus*-like isolates in the genus *Vagococcus* are now named *Vagococcus fluvialis* ("belonging to a river"). Strains of *V. fluvialis* have also been recovered from cutaneous lesions and tonsils of pigs, cattle, horses, and domestic cats.[781] The CDC has reported receipt of two *V. fluvialis* strains, one from a blood culture and the other from the peritoneal fluid of a renal dialysis patient.[336] Additional isolates of *V. fluvialis* have been recovered from human clinical sources (i.e., blood cultures, peritoneal fluid, wounds), animals (i.e., pigs), and the environment (i.e., well water).[950]

During a genetic study of atypical lactobacilli isolated from various meat products (members of the genus *Carnobacterium*), two isolates from adult rainbow trout were described that were distinct from the poultry isolates.[1024] These two strains showed the highest degree of 16S rRNA sequence homology with strains of *V. fluvialis*, forming a genetic cluster that was phylogenetically close to, but distinct from, the carnobacteria, the streptococci, the lactococci, and the enterococci. These two salmonid isolates have been assigned to the genus *Vagococcus* as *Vagococcus salmoninarum*. Subsequently, this organism was shown to cause peritoneal infections in salmon and brown trout.[861] In 1999, a third *Vagococcus* species was described that was isolated from blood, liver, lung, and spleen specimens of a common otter (*Lutra lutra*). This isolate was characterized genetically and was named *Vagococcus lutrae*.[608] In 2000, a fourth *Vagococcus* species was isolated during postmortem examinations of a seal and a harbor porpoise. This isolate was found in pure culture in the liver and kidney tissues from the seal, and heavy growth was found in peritoneal, spleen, kidney, liver, lung, brain, placenta, and intestinal tissues of the harbor porpoise. Based on both phylogenetic and phenotypic data, this isolate was named *Vagococcus fessus*.[498] *V. salmoninarum*, *V. lutrae*, and *V. fessus* have not been isolated from clinical specimens obtained from humans.

Alloiococcus Species

In 1989, Faden and Dryja reported on the recovery of a slow-growing, large, gram-positive coccus from 10 children with chronic otitis media with effusion.[343] The children ranged in age from 10 months to almost 3 years, and each child had a history of two to five previous episodes of otitis media. Middle ear aspirates from these children consisted of serous, mucoid, or frankly purulent fluid; inflammatory cells were observed in all specimens. In most cases, large, gram-positive, coccal organisms could also be seen on Gram-stained smears of these fluids. A novel organism was recovered in pure culture from 11 ear aspirates and in mixed culture with nontypeable *Haemophilus influenzae*, diphtheroids, micrococci, or coagulase-negative staphylococci in five specimens. One of the children examined in the study had the same organism isolated from three separate middle ear specimens collected over an 8-month period. On culture, the organisms grew extremely slowly, leading the authors to suggest that perhaps they had been missed in the past

because culture plates had not been incubated long enough. Because of the association of this slow-growing gram-positive coccus with chronic otitis media, Faden and Dryja recommended that middle ear aspirates submitted for culture should be incubated for at least 5 days to facilitate detection of these bacteria.[343] Aguirre and Collins subsequently characterized this unusual coccus and named it *Alloiococcus otitis*.[6] A revision of the name of this organism from *A. otitis* to *A. otitidis* was subsequently suggested and approved in keeping with the rules of binomial nomenclature. In addition to isolates from middle ear fluids, the CDC has received strains of *A. otitidis* that were isolated from blood cultures and sputum.[336] Isolates of *A. otitidis* are susceptible or intermediately resistant to penicillin, ampicillin, and the expanded-spectrum cephalosporins (i.e., cefixime, ceftriaxone), and are resistant to erythromycin and trimethoprim-sulfamethoxazole.[118] Because of its slow growth, several workers have developed molecular amplification methods for detection of this organism is middle ear effusions.[7,92,620] These highly sensitive techniques have also enabled the detection of this organism in the nasopharynx and the outer ear canal, suggesting that these sites are the natural habitat of *A. otitidis*.[305]

Globicatella Species

In 1992, Collins and associates described nine unique human clinical isolates (five from blood cultures, three from urine cultures, and one from CSF).[205] Phenotypic traits indicated that these strains were not members of the *Streptococcus*, *Lactococcus*, *Enterococcus*, or *Aerococcus* groups. Furthermore, genetic investigations clearly showed a distinct line of descent for these isolates within the "lactic acid group" of bacteria. These strains have been assigned to the new genus *Globicatella* (meaning a short chain composed of spherical cells). All of these strains were phenotypically similar and have been given the species name *Globicatella sanguinis* (formerly *G. sanguis*). Isolates of *G. sanguinis* that have been submitted to the CDC have been from blood cultures, urine cultures, and wound cultures and from a CSF specimen obtained during an autopsy.[336] In 2001, Shewmaker and colleagues reported on 28 strains of *G. sanguinis* that had been isolated from urine cultures and from blood cultures of patients with diagnoses of endocarditis, sepsis, and bacteremia.[884] Vandamme and colleagues in Belgium characterized a second *Globicatella* species that was isolated from respiratory tract and septic joint infections in calves, sheep, and swine.[991] This isolate was named *Globicatella sulfidifaciens* because of its ability to produce H_2S.

Facklamia Species

In 1997, Collins and associates characterized five human isolates of catalase-negative, gram-positive cocci from urine, vaginal, blood, and abscess specimens.[210] Comparative 16S rRNA gene-sequencing studies demonstrated that these unknown strains were genealogically homogeneous and constituted a new phylogenetic line that was closely related to but distinct from the genus *Globicatella*. These isolates also differed from *G. sanguinis* in their peptidoglycan murein structure. Even though these isolates were most closely related to *G. sanguinis* phylogenetically, phenotypically they were quite different. *G. sanguinis* produced acid from several carbohydrates, while the new isolates were totally asaccharolytic. These strains also had some characteristics that resembled salt-tolerant *Gemella*-like organisms like *D. pigrum* (see below). These isolates were placed in the new genus *Facklamia* as *Facklamia hominis*.[210]

Several additional *Facklamia* species have been described in the taxonomy and microbiology literature in subsequent years. Collins and his associates characterized two human blood isolates as a second asaccharolytic species, *Facklamia ignava*.[224] The next year, the same group described *Facklamia sourekii* in their characterization of another two isolates recovered from human blood cultures.[213] This new species differed from *F. hominis* and *F. ignava* in being an active fermenter. *Facklamia languida* was proposed as a new *Facklamia* species to describe three human isolates from blood and CSF specimens.[605] This species is asaccharolytic, but differs phenotypically from the other species in several enzymatic reactions. *Facklamia tabacinalis* was also described in 1999 and named to describe an isolate recovered as a contaminant from snuff.[214] Its 16S rRNA gene sequence most closely resembled *F. ignava*. *Facklamia miroungae* was described in 2001 and was isolated from a nasal swab of a juvenile elephant seal (*Mirounga leonina*).[497]

The various *Facklamia* species appear to have slightly different antimicrobial susceptibility profiles. LaClaire and Facklam determined the susceptibilities of *F. hominis* (four strains), *F. ignava* (five strains), *F. languida* (six strains), *F. sourekii* (three strains), and *F. tabacinalis* (one strain), and found that one *F. hominis* and two *F. ignava* strains had penicillin MICs that fell in the intermediate range, while all other strains were penicillin-susceptible.[593] One strain of *F. ignava*, one of *F. sourekii*, and all six *F. languida* strains were resistant to cefotaxime; five of the six latter strains were also resistant to cefuroxime. Although most isolates were susceptible to erythromycin, three *F. ignava* strains and two *F. languida* strains were erythromycin-resistant. Five of the six *F. languida* strains and one of the five *F. ignava* strains were resistant to clindamycin. All isolates were either intermediate or resistant to trimethoprim-sulfamethoxazole, and none of the isolates were resistant to levofloxacin or vancomycin.

Dolosigranulum, *Ignavigranum*, and *Dolosicoccus* Species

The genera *Dolosigranulum* and *Ignavigranum* describe *Gemella*-like bacteria that are able to grow in 6.5% NaCl. *Dolosigranulum pigrum*, the sole species in the genus, was described in 1993, and the CDC Streptococcus Laboratory has characterized several isolates from blood cultures, eye specimens, nasopharyngeal swabs, sputum, urine, gastric and sinus aspirates, and autopsy spinal cord specimens.[11] *D. pigrum* has also been isolated from blood cultures of a 64-year-old male patient with synovitis.[451] LaClaire and Facklam performed susceptibility tests on 27 clinical isolates of *D. pigrum* and found that all were susceptible to penicillin, amoxicillin, cephalosporins (i.e., cefotaxime, cefuroxime), clindamycin, levofloxacin, meropenem, rifampin, tetracy-

cline, and vancomycin; 15 of the isolates were resistant to erythromycin.[592]

Ignavigranum ruoffiae is the name given to two strains of catalase-negative gram-positive cocci that were isolated from a wound and an ear abscess.[225] These salt-tolerant strains were phylogenetically related to *Globicatella* and *Facklamia* species and phenotypically resemble the asaccharolytic *Facklamia* species. Antimicrobial susceptibility data on these strains are not available.

The genus *Dolosicoccus* was created to accommodate another unique catalase-negative gram-positive coccus that was isolated from a blood culture.[220] This isolate was phylogenetically related to *G. sanguinis* and the *Facklamia* species cluster and phenotypically resembles *F. hominis* and *F. ignava*. The sole species in the genus is *Dolosicoccus paucivorans*.

Eremococcus Species

The genus *Eremococcus* was created to accommodate two phylogenetically and phenotypically unique cocci recovered from the genital tracts of thoroughbred mares.[222] Comparative 16S rRNA sequencing demonstrated that these strains were related to *A. defectiva* and *G. sanguinis* and more distantly related to *Facklamia* species and *I. ruoffiae*. The single species in the genus is *Eremococcus coleocola*.

Genus *Lactococcus*

The genus *Lactococcus* consists of the "lactic acid streptococci" or "milk streptococci." Historically, these organisms carry the Lancefield group N antigen, although only about 80% of lactococcal isolates carry extractable antigen in their cell walls. Lactococci are rare clinical isolates that have been recovered from blood, urine, and wound specimens.[322,652,859,1075] Lactococci should be considered opportunistic pathogens of low virulence.[10] Members of the genus *Lactococcus* include *L. lactis* subsp. *lactis*, *L. lactis* subsp. *cremoris*, *L. lactis* subsp. *hordniae*, *L. garveiae*, *L. plantarum*, *L. raffinolactis*, and *L. xylosus*. *L. lactis* subsp. *lactis* and *L. garveiae* are the lactococcal species most frequently recovered from human clinical specimens.

Isolation and Identification of Streptococci and "Streptococcus-Like" Bacteria
Direct Gram-Stained Smears

Gram-stained smears of clinical specimens that yield streptococci on culture will generally show gram-positive or gram-variable cocci arranged in pairs and chains (see Color Plate 13-1*B*). Chains of cells in both specimens and broth cultures tend to appear as chains of pairs of cells rather than as chains of individual cells. Individual cell shapes range from those that resemble diplococci to those that appear coccobacillary or coryneform. This morphology is often observed on smears from broth cultures and from solid media as well. Viridans streptococci, in particular, tend to have cells that appear more elongated. *S. pneumoniae* will most often appear as pairs of lanceolate cells (see Color Plate 13-1*C*). On smears of specimens yielding mucoid, heavily encapsulated strains, the capsule may appear as a pink halo or as a nonstaining area surrounding the cells in relief against a pink background surrounding the organism.

A rapid diagnosis of group B streptococcal and pneumococcal meningitis can be made by examination of a Gram-stained smear of CSF. If sufficient CSF is submitted (i.e., more than 1–2 mL), the specimen should be centrifuged to obtain a pellet for examination and culture. Cytocentrifugation of CSF specimens enhances the detection of small numbers of organisms and increases the sensitivity of the Gram stain in comparison with conventionally centrifuged or uncentrifuged specimens.[175] Use of cytocentrifugation circumvents the need for the performance of latex or coagglutination tests for detection of group B streptococcal or pneumococcal capsular antigens (see section on "Direct Detection," below).

Culture Media

Specimens that may be expected to yield streptococci on culture should be plated onto a suitable blood-containing medium that has a peptone base rich enough to support these fastidious organisms. The agar base medium should be a peptone infusion medium (e.g., tryptic-soy, proteose-peptone, Todd-Hewitt) without added carbohydrates. Although the colonies will generally be larger on glucose-containing media (e.g., Columbia base medium) after 24 hours, acid produced from glucose utilization inactivates the streptolysin S (SLS) of group A β-hemolytic streptococci and may interfere with the interpretation of the hemolytic qualities of the organism. Sheep blood is added to the basal medium at a 5% concentration as the indicator cells for hemolysis. Lower concentrations of blood in the media make the hemolytic reaction difficult to discern, whereas higher concentrations may obscure hemolysis entirely. On sheep blood agar, streptococci belonging to groups A, B, C, F, and G are β-hemolytic (to be described below), whereas the majority of *Enterococcus* species and group D streptococci are α-hemolytic or nonhemolytic. Except for group D and occasional group B strains, nonhemolytic groupable streptococci are rare. Sheep blood agar does not support the growth of *Haemophilus haemolyticus* or *Haemophilus parahaemolyticus;* hence small, β-hemolytic colonies recovered from specimens on sheep blood agar are usually streptococci. The growing literature on *Arcanobacterium haemolyticum* as a cause of pharyngitis may require changes in the laboratory approach to throat cultures, for this organism is β-hemolytic and catalase-negative but is a Gram-positive rod (Chapter 14).

Selective agar may also enhance the recovery of group A streptococci from throat cultures. The formulations that are most often used and that are commercially available use a tryptic-soy agar base containing 5% sheep blood and sulfamethoxazole (23.75 μg/mL)-trimethoprim (1.25 μg/mL).[1036] Much of the normal oropharyngeal flora (e.g., viridans streptococci, micrococci, staphylococci, and neisseriae) will be inhibited on this medium. Use of this selective medium enhances recovery of group A and B streptococci and allows visualization of β-hemolysis without the "background" of other organism growth. Commercially available selective media include Group A Selective Strep A with 5% sheep blood (ssA; BD Diagnostic Systems, Sparks, MD),

and Strep A Isolation Agar (Remel Laboratories, Lenexa KS). In a side-by-side evaluation, Pacifico and coworkers compared the recovery of group A streptococci on selective streptococcal media (ssA) and regular sheep blood agar incubated under different incubation conditions (in air, in CO₂, and in anaerobic atmosphere).[751] The highest yield of positive cultures in this study was obtained using the selective *Streptococcus* medium incubated under anaerobic conditions for 48 hours. Most laboratories incubate media for isolation of group A β-hemolytic streptococci for 48 hours in a CO₂-enriched environment, assuming that only cultures from patients with small numbers of organisms or from those who are group A streptococcal carriers will grow under anaerobic conditions.[29] However, even patients with small numbers of organisms may have an immune response, suggesting that they are infected and not merely carrying the organism.[751] Small numbers of organisms on a culture plate in a patient with clinical streptococcal pharyngitis may also reflect inadequate specimen collection.

Streptococci recovered from human clinical specimens are identified on the basis of their hemolytic qualities, serologic tests for the detection of cell wall or capsular antigens, and physiologic and biochemical tests. Some of the tests performed in the laboratory for identification of these organisms provide presumptive results, whereas others provide definitive results. Before proceeding with identification tests, however, one must be sure that the gram-positive cocci under consideration are **catalase-negative** using 3% H_2O_2, placing them in the *Streptococcus* and *Streptococcus*-like bacterial groups. The catalase test is discussed in detail in Chapter 12.

Hemolysis on Blood Agar

Four types of hemolysis may be produced by streptococci on sheep blood agar (Box 13-5). Observation and correct interpretation of the hemolytic properties of streptococci are very important because the performance of subsequent tests is predicated on this initial evaluation. Hemolysis is best observed by examining colonies grown under anaerobic conditions or by inspecting subsurface colonies in pour plates or streak-stab plates because, for group A streptococci, maximal activity of both the oxygen-labile (SLO) and oxygen-stable (SLS) hemolysins is observed only under anaerobic conditions. Oxygen-labile hemolysins are also produced by group C and some group G strains, so detection of hemolysis by these organisms is also enhanced by anaerobic incubation. Although routine anaerobic incubation of specimens expected to yield streptococci is not recommended, steps can be taken to maximize detection of hemolysis under aerobic or capnophilic incubation. This is the point of the "streak-and-stab" technique that is used for inoculating throat swab specimens on blood agar for diagnosis of streptococcal pharyngitis (Fig. 13-2; see Color Plates 13-1*D* and 13-1*F*). This technique forces some of the inoculum under the agar, thereby creating a relatively anaerobic environment. Areas of the plate not inoculated with specimen should also be stabbed. Plates should be incubated at 35°C in air or in 5–7% CO₂. Although some laboratorians advocate one incubation environment over the other for throat cultures, the recovery of β-hemolytic streptococci from patients with

Box 13-5 Identification of Hemolysis

Type of Hemolysis	Comments
α-Hemolysis	Partial lysis of the erythrocytes surrounding a colony, causing a greenish-gray or brownish discoloration in the medium (Color Plate 13-1*E*).
β-Hemolysis	Complete lysis of the red blood cells, causing a clearing of blood from the medium under and surrounding the colonies (Color Plates 13-1*D* and 13-1*F*).
γ-Hemolysis	No hemolysis and, consequently, no change of the medium under and surrounding the colonies. Organisms showing no hemolysis are said to be γ-hemolytic or nonhemolytic.
α-Prime or "wide-zone" α-hemolysis	A small zone of intact erythrocytes immediately adjacent to the colony, with a zone of complete red-cell hemolysis surrounding the zone of intact erythrocytes. This type of hemolysis may be confused with β-hemolysis.

streptococcal pharyngitis will not generally be compromised under either environmental condition.[1036]

Nonculture, Direct Detection Techniques for Group A β-Hemolytic Streptococci in Pharyngeal Specimens

Nonculture techniques for direct detection of group A streptococci on throat swab specimens have been in wide use in clinical laboratories since the early 1980s. In these kits, the streptococcal-grouping antigen is extracted from the swab using nitrous acid or an enzymatic extraction step, followed by detection of the extracted antigen. In the initially marketed kits, latex agglutination or enzyme immunoassay (EIA) formats were the approaches used for antigen detection (see Color Plate 13-1*G*). The sensitivities of these assays for detecting group A streptococcal antigen ranged from 62% up to 96%; specificities in most cases exceeded 97%.[150,288,333,393,489,871,1087] Liposome immunoassay techniques such as the Q Test Strep kit (BD Diagnostic Systems) were also introduced in which, instead of using anti-group-

A streptococcal antibodies conjugated to an enzyme, the antibodies were conjugated to a liposome (an artificial phospholipid "sphere") containing the dye rhodamine sulfate. Reaction of the antigen with the antibodies lysed the liposome and released the rhodamine sulfate dye. The liposome method has been evaluated; the sensitivity and specificity were 91% and 83%, respectively.[394,501]

The "Strep A OIA" (for optical immunoassay) (Biostar, Boulder CO) is a direct "optical immunoassay" test that is performed on a slide. The end point is visualized by a physical change in the thickness of thin films resulting from binding reactions between the group A antigen and anti–group A antibodies (see Color Plate 13-1*H*). The antigen is extracted from the swab with acetic acid (0.3 M), and a horseradish peroxidase–labeled rabbit anti–group A streptococcal antibody is added to the extract. This mixture is deposited on the OIA slide, where the antigen binds to the anti–group A streptococcal antibodies fixed on the slide. The slide is washed and an enzyme substrate (tetramethyl benzidine containing hydrogen peroxide) is applied and allowed to react for 4 minutes. After washing, the reaction is read by examining the hue of light reflected from the reaction spot on the slide; if group A streptococcal antigen is present in the original swab specimen, the reaction area on the slide appears as a purple spot. If antigen is not present, the slide surface retains its golden color. The sensitivities and specificities of the Strep OIA have ranged from 81.0% to 98.9% and 95.0% to 100%, respectively.[174,252,268,461,476]

DNA probe and amplified probe technologies have also been used for direct detection of group A streptococci in throat swab specimens. The Group A Streptococcus Direct Test (Gen-Probe, San Diego CA) is a nonisotopic chemiluminescent method that uses a DNA probe to detect the complementary rRNA sequences of group A streptococci directly in an extract from a throat swab. This test has been evaluated by several groups; sensitivities of 88.6% to 94.8% and specificities of 98.0% to 99.7% have been reported.[174,472,475,778] A drawback of the Gen-Probe Group A Strep Direct test is that the swab used to collect the specimen must be composed of rayon or Dacron fibers that are sterilized by ethylene oxide or Dacron swabs that are sterilized by γ-irradiation. Swabs composed of rayon fibers that are sterilized by γ-irradiation cause elevated background chemiluminescence. For this reason, the CulturettePlus (irradiated

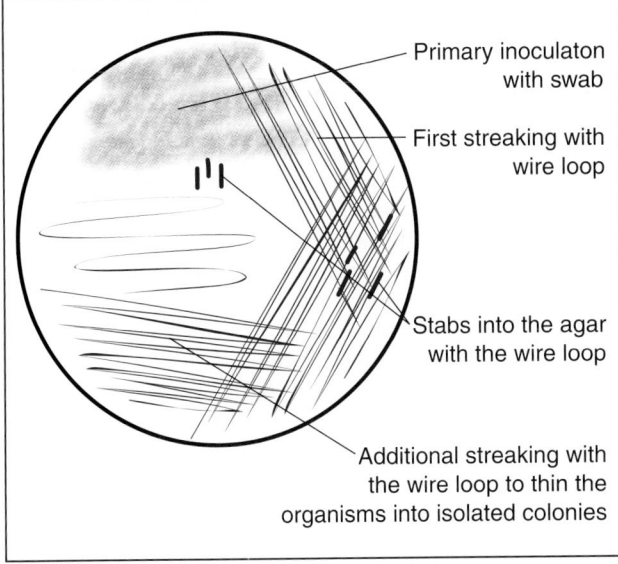

Primary inoculaton with swab

First streaking with wire loop

Stabs into the agar with the wire loop

Additional streaking with the wire loop to thin the organisms into isolated colonies

Figure 13-2 Streak–stab technique for isolation of β-hemolytic streptococci.

rayon) swabs (BD Biosciences) should not be used with this test. Recently, the LightCycler Strep-A assay (Roche Applied Science, Indianapolis, IN), an amplified probe test using real-time PCR, has been marketed for use in clinical laboratories. This method uses the LightCycler instrument and can test up to 32 specimens in a 1.5-our run time. Uhl and colleagues at the Mayo Clinic evaluated this assay and found a sensitivity and specificity of 93% and 98%, respectively.[981] The sensitivity of this assay was probably greater than 93%, given that seven specimens in the evaluation were LightCycler assay–positive and culture-negative. Further study of this new assay will likely clarify the performance characteristics of this new approach to the diagnosis of streptococcal pharyngitis.

Many of the immunoassay-based tests for direct detection of group A streptococci have been granted Clinical Laboratory Improvement Act-waived status by the FDA based on their complexity and are in use in physicians' office laboratories. Some of these waived tests include the BD Link2 Strep A (BD Diagnostic Systems), the QuickVue Dipstick Strep A test (Quidel, San Diego, CA), and the ImmunoCard STAT Strep A test (Meridian Bioscience, Cincinnati, OH). Although the specificity of both latex agglutination and EIA kits is quite high (usually more than 97%), the sensitivities of the various kits for group A streptococcal antigen detection vary widely (between 62% and 95%). Although the American College of Physicians and the American Society of Internal Medicine recently proposed practice guidelines for treatment of adults with pharyngitis that relied on clinical criteria alone (without even using rapid antigen tests) for diagnosis, this approach is considered to be controversial by other professional societies, including the Infectious Diseases Society of America, the American Heart Association, and the American Academy of Pediatrics.[98,232,398,910] The American Heart Association, package inserts for many of the rapid antigen test kits, and most clinical microbiologists recommend that all specimens that yield negative rapid antigen results be confirmed by culture. Regardless of the test kits' assay method or the manufacturers' claims for a given test kit or technique, it is recommended that two throat swabs be collected. A standard throat culture should be performed with the second swab for specimens that yield negative rapid antigen detection results with the first swab. Some laboratories have substituted the Gen-Probe Group A Strep Direct test in place of culture for confirmation of negative direct antigen results.[475]

Nonculture, Direct Detection Techniques for Group B β-Hemolytic Streptococci and *Streptococcus pneumoniae*

Diagnosis of systemic group B streptococcal disease is best accomplished by culture of the organisms from appropriately collected specimens. Methods are also available for direct detection of group B streptococcal capsular antigen in CSF, serum, and urine. Latex agglutination (LA) and coagglutination (COA) tests have been used in many laboratories for rapid diagnosis of systemic group B streptococcal infections, particularly meningitis during the newborn period. Currently available LA tests include the Directogen Meningitis Combo Test kit (BD Biosciences Microbiology Products, Sparks, MD), and the Wellcogen Bacterial Antigen kit (Murex Diagnostics, Dartford, UK). The commercial

COA test kit is the Phadebact CSF test (Boule Diagnostics, Huddinge, Sweden). Sensitivities of the latex agglutination products for detection of group B streptococcal antigens range from mid-80% to 100%, although some studies have reported sensitivities as low as 27% to 54%.[48,68,381,446,454,511] Corresponding specificities of the latex agglutination tests range from 80% to 100%.[48,381,446,511] Despite the performance of these tests in clinical trials that led to their approval for use, many laboratories have discontinued offering these tests routinely. Aside from their relatively high cost, the diagnostic and prognostic utility of these tests has not been borne out after years of experience. These tests may be most useful in cases of suspected meningitis in which the Gram stain is negative and/or when CSF cultures are negative after 48 hours.[362] At present, the recommended method for optimal direct detection of group B streptococci in CSF depends on careful inspection of a Gram-stained smear of a cytocentrifuged specimen.[175]

Direct detection methods for group B streptococci in rectovaginal specimens are relatively insensitive compared with the broth amplification method recommended by the CDC (Box 13-3). Rapid latex agglutination- or EIA-format assays should not be used for screening of rectovaginal swab specimens for group B β-hemolytic streptococci (see the "Clinical Significance" section under "Group B β-Hemolytic Streptococci," above, for a discussion of screening methods).[367]

As an adjunct to cultural diagnosis of respiratory tract infection by *S. pneumoniae*, methods are now available for detection of pneumococcal antigen in urine in patients with pneumococcal pneumonia. The Binax NOW *Streptococcus pneumoniae* urinary antigen test (Binax, Portland, ME) is a rapid immunochromatographic assay that allows a presumptive diagnosis of pneumococcal pneumonia by detection of specific soluble capsular antigens in urine specimens. The pneumococcal antigens detected by this test account for more than 90% of invasive disease occurring in the U.S. and worldwide. In a study conducted in the U.K., the NOW assay was positive in 82% of 107 urine specimens from patients with bacteremic pneumococcal pneumonia; 3 of 106 patients with pneumonia and bacteremia due to other organisms were also NOW test–positive, giving a specificity of 97%.[908] In a prospective, population-based study of adults with pneumonia in Spain, the test was positive in 70.4% of 27 patients with culture-documented pneumococcal pneumonia; the corresponding specificity of the test in this study was 89.7%.[444] In another study, the urinary antigen was detected in 80% of 20 patients with pneumococcal bacteremia and in 52% of 54 patients with *S. pneumoniae* isolated from sputum.[707] Samra and coworkers evaluated the NOW test with both CSF and urine specimens from 22 patients with culture-documented pneumococcal meningitis.[841] For CSF specimens, 21 of 22 were positive (95.4% sensitivity) with the rapid test; only 12 of 21 urine specimens were positive (57.1% sensitivity). Testing of CSF specimens that were culture-negative for *S. pneumoniae* or positive for other organisms were all negative, for a specificity of 100% for CSF specimens. However, 5 (18.5%) of 27 urine specimens from patients with CSF cultures positive with other bacteria, and 63 (13.4%) of 470 urine specimens from patients with negative CSF cultures were positive with the NOW test. A potential drawback of the NOW urine test is that healthy nasopharyngeal carriers of *S. pneumoniae* may also have positive tests. A study conducted in the Gambia, where the carriage rate among evaluated children was 87%, reported that 55% of urine specimens from healthy children who were pneumococcal carriers were Binax NOW test–positive.[4] Another study conducted in Ecuador found that 21.7% of children who carried nasopharyngeal *S. pneumoniae* were NOW test–positive and 4.2% of noncarriers had false-positive urine antigen tests.[452] These workers postulated that the Binax NOW urine assay may be most useful for the diagnosis of pneumococcal pneumonia and bacteremia in populations with low rates of nasopharyngeal pneumococcal carriage.

In addition to urinary antigen detection, several PCR-based molecular methods have been developed for direct detection, identification, and typing of *S. pneumoniae*.[467,613, 831,1015] Real-time PCR techniques using the LightCycler and involving amplification of pneumolysin or autolysin genes have also been described for direct detection of pneumococci in clinical samples, such as blood and CSF.[672,883,1000]

Colony Morphology and Catalase Testing

After 18 to 24 hours of incubation on blood agar, colonies of group A β-hemolytic *Streptococcus* are about 0.5 mm in diameter, translucent or transparent, and have a smooth or matte surface. The zone of β-hemolysis is usually two to four times the diameter of the colony. The colonies are domed and have an entire edge. Occasional strains of group A streptococci will be mucoid because of the presence of large amounts of capsular material. Groups C and G also have a similar appearance, although colonies of some group G strains may have a golden cast on close inspection and the hemolytic zones are usually very large. Group B β-hemolytic streptococci form larger colonies on agar medium, the margin of hemolysis around the colony is comparatively smaller for group B streptococci than for the other β-hemolytic streptococci, and the hemolysis is generally "softer" and less obvious. A significant proportion of group B streptococci (up to 11%) may be nonhemolytic. Group D streptococcal colonies tend to be larger than those of group A streptococci, being 0.5 to 1.0 mm after overnight incubation. Group D isolates are α-hemolytic or nonhemolytic on sheep blood agar (see Color Plate 13-4*C*). The colonies are usually gray, smooth, and have an entire edge. Group F streptococci form very small, pinpoint colonies with a large zone of β-hemolysis. These extremely small colonies are called "minute colonies" and they are characteristic of the anginosus group of streptococci—*S. anginosus*, *S. constellatus*, and *S. intermedius*. Minute β-hemolytic colonies are generally pinpoint after 24 hours of incubation, yet will have a rather large, florid zone of β-hemolysis. The anginosus group organisms growing on solid media also have a distinct sweet, caramel ("butterscotch") or honeysuckle odor owing to the production of diacetyl.[184] This characteristic may be noted with α-hemolytic, β-hemolytic, and nonhemolytic members of this group.

S. pneumoniae displays a spectrum of colony types, the appearance of which depends on the degree of encapsulation. These colonies are generally surrounded by a large zone of intense green α-hemolysis. Colonies of heavily encapsulated strains may be several millimeters in diameter, are very mucoid, appear gray, and may resemble drops of oil on the agar surface. Colonies of the less heavily encapsulated strains are smaller (see Color Plate 13-2*H*). On prolonged incubation, the central portion of the colony may collapse, giving the characteristic "checker piece" appearance. Some colonies may collapse altogether, giving the appearance of a flat nailhead on the surface of the agar.

Other species of viridans streptococci form colonies of various sizes and textures (see Color Plate 13-1*E*). Some may be smooth and have an entire edge, whereas others may appear rough, with the formation of scalloped edges on prolonged incubation. Colonies of *Aerococcus, Pediococcus, Gemella, Leuconostoc, Tetragenococcus, Vagococcus, Globicatella, Helcococcus, Facklamia, Dolosicoccus, Dolosigranulum, Ignavigranum,* and the facultative *Lactobacillus* species strongly resemble viridans streptococci or group D streptococci in their appearance, and they are either α-hemolytic or nonhemolytic.

Members of the streptococci and *Streptococcus*-like bacterial groups are catalase-negative, except for *A. otitidis*. This organism is *Streptococcus*-like in its colony morphology but is catalase-positive. Some enterococcal strains (particularly *E. faecalis* strains) produce a "pseudocatalase" that is responsible for the weak-positive catalase reaction that is seen with some strains, particularly on primary isolation. The strength of this reaction may diminish after a few serial subcultures.

Recognition and Preliminary Characterization of Streptococci and the "Streptococcus-Like" Bacteria

The determination of hemolysis and the performance of a catalase test were once the only requirements to preliminarily characterize streptococci. However, with the recognition of several groups of *Streptococcus*-like bacteria in human infections, it is also necessary to perform additional tests, particularly for isolates recovered from sterile body fluids. Some of these organisms (i.e., *Leuconostoc* and *Pediococcus* species) are intrinsically resistant to vancomycin and related cyclic glycopeptide antibiotics (e.g., ristocetin, Aricidin, and teicoplanin). The apparent increase in the recognition and isolation of these organisms may be partly related to the emergence of methicillin-resistant *S. aureus* and the consequent use of vancomycin as a first-line antibiotic, particularly in severely debilitated hosts. These and other "lookalike" organisms may be preliminarily differentiated from *Streptococcus* and *Enterococcus* species and from one another with the tests shown in Table 13-1.

On sheep blood agar, these organisms resemble viridans streptococci or enterococci; all of them are α-hemolytic or nonhemolytic. The characteristic streptococcal morphology—chains of cocci—is seen with the streptococci, enterococci, lactococci, *Leuconostoc/Weissella* species, *Vagococcus* species, *Abiotrophia/Granulicatella* species, *Dolosicoccus* species, *Ignavigranum* species, *Globicatella* species, and *Lactococcus* species on Gram-stained smears prepared from thioglycolate broth cultures. Gram-positive cocci arranged predominantly in pairs, tetrads, and or clusters are more characteristic of the aerococci, *Alloiococcus* species, *Gemella* species, *Pediococcus* species *Helcococcus* species, and *Tetragenococcus* species. Some of

Table 13-1 Phenotypic Characteristics for Presumptive Identification of Catalase-Negative, Gram-Positive Cocci

GENUS	GROWTH, 35–37°C, CA	GROWTH, 35–37°C, SBA	GRAM STAIN MORPHOLOGY	HEMOLYSIS, SBA	CAT	LAP	PYR	SUSCEPTIBILITY TO VANCOMYCIN	GAS, MRS BROTH	MOT	GROWTH, 6.5% NaCl BROTH	GROWTH, 10°C	GROWTH, 45°C
Streptococcus	+	+	Chains	α, β, γ	–	+	–	S	–	–	V	–	V
Enterococcus	+	+	Chains	α, γ	–	+	+	S/R	–	V	+	+	+
Abiotrophia	+	–	Chains	α, γ	–	+	+	S	–	–	–	–	V
Granulicatella	+	–	Chains	α, γ	–	+	+	S	–	–	–	–	V
Aerococcus	+	+	Tetrads, clusters	α	–	V	V	S	–	–	+	–	–
Helcococcus	+	+	Tetrads, clusters	γ	–	–	+	S	–	–	+	–	–
Leuconostoc	+	+	Chains	α, γ	–	–	–	R	+	–	V	+	+
Weisella	+	+	Chains	α, γ	–	–	–	R	+	–	+	V	V
Pediococcus	+	+	Tetrads, clusters	α	–	+	–	R	–	–	V	–	+
Tetragenococcus	+	+	Tetrads, clusters	α	–	+	–	S	–	–	+	–	+
Gemella	+	+	Tetrads, clusters, chains	α, γ	–	V	+	S	–	–	–	–	–
Vagococcus	+	+	Chains	α, γ	–	+	+	S	–	+	+	+	–
Alloiococcus	+	+	Clusters, tetrads	α	+	+	+	S	–	–	+	–	–
Globicatella	+	+	Chains	α	–	–	+	S	–	–	+	–	–
Facklamia	+	+	Clusters, chains	α	–	+	+	S	–	–	+	–	–
Dolosigranulum	+	+	Clusters, tetrads	α	–	+	+	S	–	–	+	–	–
Ignavigranum	+	+	Clusters, chains	α	–	+	+	S	–	–	+	–	–
Dolosicoccus	+	+	Chains	α	–	–	+	S	–	–	–	–	–
Eremococcus	+	+	Chains	α	–	+	NA	S	–	–	+ʷ	–	+
Lactococcus	+	+	Chains	α, γ	–	+	+	S	–	–	V	+	V

+, positive reaction; –, negative reaction; V, variable reaction; NA, data not available; CA, chocolate agar; Hemolysis SBA, hemolysis on sheep blood agar; CAT, catalase; LAP, leucine aminopeptidase; PYR, pyrrolidonyl arylamidase; MOT, motility; $+^w$, weak positive reaction.

the recently described *Streptococcus*-like bacteria (e.g., *Facklamia* species, *Tetragenococcus* species) often form pairs or short chains. Facultative lactobacilli will generally show the typical rod-shaped morphology, whereas other species will appear coccal. Observation of gram-positive cocci in short chains in blood culture media and growth of organisms on subculture to chocolate agar with no growth on a corresponding SBA subculture suggests *Abiotrophia/Granulicatella* species. On media containing blood, some isolates may produce a weak catalase reaction with 3% H_2O_2; therefore, strains showing this reaction should be subcultured onto blood-free medium and retested for catalase activity. It is noteworthy that the only species among the *Streptococcus*-like bacteria that is truly catalase-positive is *Alloiococcus otitidis*.

Viridans or nonhemolytic streptococci from sterile body fluids can be screened for susceptibility to vancomycin using the regular 30-mg disk on a sheep blood agar plate incubated at 35°C for 18 to 24 hours. Occasional isolates may require prolonged incubation (i.e., up to 72 hours) for test interpretation. Organisms that are resistant to vancomycin (i.e., *Pediococcus* species, *Leuconostoc* species) generally have MICs higher than 250 μg/mL and will grow right up to the edge of the disk. The presence of any zone around the disk indicates susceptibility to vancomycin. Production of gas from glucose, a helpful test for differentiation of *Leuconostoc* species from the other organisms, is best determined in *Lactobacillus*. Mann, Rogosa, and Sharpe (MRS) broth (Difco Laboratories, Detroit MI) overlaid with petrolatum.[269] The formation of bubbles under the petrolatum seal indicates gas production and the heterofermentative nature of their metabolism. The MRS broth is incubated for up to 7 days. Other tests that are helpful for preliminary characterization of the *Streptococcus*-like organisms include pyrrolidonyl arylamidase (PYR), leucine aminopeptidase (LAP), and salt-tolerance tests. The latter test is performed in heart infusion broth containing 6.5% NaCl and is incubated up to 14 days before being called negative. The presence of growth is the end point, as in the salt-tolerance test for identification of enterococci. The PYR and LAP tests are available as rapid disk tests from several manufacturers (e.g., Remel; Carr-Scarborough, Decatur, GA) and are also on some of the kit systems (e.g., API Rapid STREP). The BactiCard *Streptococcus test* (Remel) includes PYR, LAP, and an esculin hydrolysis test. This card, when used with vancomycin susceptibility results, can provide preliminary characterization of *Enterococcus, Lactococcus, Aerococcus, Gemella, Leuconostoc, Pediococcus,* and *Globicatella* species.

Occasionally, more uncommon tests may be helpful to augment traditional tests or to confirm identifications obtained with kit systems. For the growth temperature tests, a water bath set at 45°C and a 10°C refrigerator are recommended. Growth, if any, is observed after 24 to 48 hours of incubation. Motility is determined in regular semisolid motility agar medium, with or without the addition of tetrazolium. This test should be incubated for up to 48 hours at room temperature. The Voges-Proskauer (VP) test for acetylmethyl carbinol that is used for streptococci is performed in heavily inoculated VP broth incubated overnight. After addition of α-naphthol and sodium hydroxide reagents, the tube is shaken or vortexed and incubated at room tempera-

ture for 30 minutes. Red, pink, and colorless reactions at this time correspond to positive, weakly positive, and negative reactions, respectively.

Presumptive Identification of Streptococci

β-Hemolytic streptococci, pneumococci, group D streptococci, and enterococci are definitively identified using serologic procedures (discussed later) that detect either the Lancefield group antigens (groups A, B, C, D, F, and G) or the capsular polysaccharide antigens (*S. pneumoniae*) of the organisms. Species identification of group D streptococci, *Enterococcus* species, and the viridans streptococci is accomplished primarily by biochemical, physiologic, and enzymatic tests. Many laboratories, however, use a handful of presumptive tests that correlate highly with the serologic methods, yet are less expensive to perform. Results of presumptive tests for the major streptococcal groups are summarized in Table 13-2. Detailed procedures for performance and interpretation of the more commonly used presumptive tests are described in Charts 1-2, 1-6, 8-1, and 13-1 to 13-4.

SUSCEPTIBILITY TO BACITRACIN

The bacitracin susceptibility test is used for the presumptive identification of group A β-hemolytic streptococci. The test is performed on a blood agar medium with a bacitracin differential disk (e.g., TAXO A Bacitracin Disk, 0.04 unit, BD Microbiology Systems, Cockeysville, MD; Bacitracin Differentiation disks, 0.04 unit, Remel). The procedure is described in detail in Chart 13-1. Any zone of inhibition around the disk is considered a positive test (see Color Plates 13-2B and 13-2C). Although this test is simple, inexpensive, and fairly accurate for presumptive identification of group A streptococci, it is not highly specific. Over 10% of group C and G streptococcal strains are also susceptible to bacitracin, as are about 5% of group B strains. Consequently, this test is often performed along with the sulfamethoxazole-trimethoprim (SXT) susceptibility test because groups C and G streptococci are usually susceptible to SXT, whereas groups A and B streptococci are resistant. Some workers have advocated the use of bacitracin disks directly on primary, nonselective blood agar for rapid detection and identification of group A streptococci in throat cultures. However, this method will identify only 50–60% of isolates. Placement of bacitracin disks on primary plates containing selective media is considerably more sensitive. The laboratory report should reflect the use of a presumptive method: "β-hemolytic streptococci, presumptively group A by bacitracin" or "β-hemolytic streptococci, presumptively not group A by bacitracin."

SUSCEPTIBILITY TO SULFAMETHOXAZOLE-TRIMETHOPRIM (SXT)

The SXT susceptibility test presumptively distinguishes groups A and B streptococci from other β-hemolytic streptococci. When used in conjunction with the bacitracin test, the SXT susceptibility test helps screen out those non-A, non-B streptococci that may be susceptible to bacitracin because

Table 13-2 Phenotypic Criteria for Presumptive Identification of Clinically Significant Streptococci and Enterococci

ORGANISM	HEMOLYSIS	BACITRACIN	SXT	CAMP TEST	HIPPURATE HYDROLYSIS	LAP	PYR	BILE ESCULIN	GROWTH, 6.5% NaCl BROTH	OPTOCHIN	BILE SOLUBILITY
Group A streptococci	β	S	R	−	−	+	+	−	−	R	−
Group B streptococci	β, none	R	R	+	+	+	−	−	V	R	−
Groups C, F, and G streptococci	β,	V	S	−	−	+	−	−	−	R	−
Group D enterococci	α, β, none	R	R	−	V	+	+	+	+	R	−
Group D streptococci, not enterococci	α, none	R	S	−	−	+	−	+	−	R	−
Viridans streptococci	α, none	V	S	−	V	+	−	V	−	R	−
Pneumococci	α	V	S	−	−	+	−	−	−	S	+

+, positive reaction; −, negative reaction; S, susceptible; R, resistant; SXT, sulfamethoxazole-trimethoprim; LAP, leucine aminopeptidase; PYR, pyrrolidonyl arylamidase.

both group A and B strains are SXT-resistant, whereas groups C, F, and G are SXT-susceptible (see Color Plate 13-2C). The test is performed in the same way as the bacitracin test, except that a commercial disk containing 1.25 µg trimethoprim and 23.75 µg of sulfamethoxazole is used. Any zone of inhibition indicates susceptibility to SXT (see Chart 13-1).

CAMP TEST AND PIGMENT PRODUCTION

The CAMP test (named for Christie, Atkins, and Munch-Petersen) is used to presumptively identify group B streptococci (see Chart 8-1) and is performed using a β-hemolysin-producing strain of *S. aureus* (ATCC [American Type Culture Collection] 25923).[196] Group B streptococci secrete a protein called "CAMP factor" that interacts with the β-hemolysin produced and secreted by *S. aureus* to cause enhanced or synergistic hemolysis. This appears as an arrowhead-shaped area of increased hemolysis in the area where the two streaks of growth are closest (see Color Plate 13-2D).[255] This test is highly sensitive, and even nonhemolytic group B strains will be CAMP-positive. A small percentage of group A streptococci will also be CAMP-positive, as will some *Listeria monocytogenes* strains. This test is frequently used in conjunction with the bacitracin and SXT tests on the same blood agar plate to presumptively identify these organisms (Table 13-2). Reports should state "presumptive β-hemolytic group B streptococci by CAMP test."

The CAMP test is still widely used for presumptive identification of group B streptococci, but other physiologic characteristics of the organism have been exploited as possible identification methods. Group B streptococci produce a red-orange carotenoid pigment in certain types of culture media. This property has been exploited for presumptive identification of group B streptococci, and several workers have published media formulations for this purpose.[266,945] De la Rosa and his colleagues in Spain reported on a medium called NGM (new Granada medium).[265] This medium contains proteose peptone, soluble starch, glucose, pyruvate, and agar as the basal medium, with sodium methotrexate as a pigment enhancer and colistin as a selective agent. When female genital tract specimens were plated on NGM and incubated anaerobically, 95% of the group B streptococci were detected by the growth of red-orange colonies after 18 hours of incubation. Dispensing the NGM in agar deep tubes detected 98% of the group B streptococci within 12 hours. Pigmentation was less obvious or intense when plates were incubated aerobically, but this difference was not noted with tubed NGM. Agar and broth Granada media have been used for vaginal screening for group B streptococci in prepartum women and have yielded results similar to those obtained with selective LIM broth.[103,1020] Granada media is used mostly in European centers and is not commercially available in the U.S.

A commercially available adaptation of Granada medium has recently been marketed for detection of group B streptococci in rectovaginal specimens. The Strep B Carrot Broth kit (Hardy Diagnostics, Santa Maria, CA) consists of a tube of liquid medium containing proteose peptone, starch, and buffers. Supplemental enrichments necessary for growth of group B streptococci are provided on a filter-paper disk that is aseptically dropped into the broth medium prior to inoculation. A rectovaginal swab from the patient is placed into the medium after collection and the tube is tightly sealed with the screw-cap. The broth is then incubated for 6 to 24 hours at 35°C. Group B β-hemolytic streptococci turn the Strep B Carrot broth orange to red within 6 to 24 hours, thereby confirming the presence of group B streptococci in the specimen. Broth tests that turn red or orange do not need to be subcultured to confirm the presence of group B streptococci; tubes that fail to turn orange or red after incubation must be subcultured to blood agar. Only group B streptococci that are β-hemolytic will turn the Carrot broth orange to red; a color change does not reliably occur with nonhemolytic strains. This new test is currently undergoing evaluations to determine if the Strep B Carrot Broth kit is equivalent to the method that uses LIM broth with blood agar plate subcultures.

HYDROLYSIS OF SODIUM HIPPURATE

Group B streptococci are also able to hydrolyze hippurate to its components, glycine and benzoic acid. To perform the test, broth containing sodium hippurate is inoculated with the organism and incubated overnight at 35°C. The cells are centrifuged and the supernatant is removed. Ferric chloride reagent (0.2 mL; $FeCl_3 \cdot 6H_2O$, 12 g, in 100 mL 2% aqueous HCl) is then added to the supernatant (0.8 mL), with the formation of a heavy precipitate. If the precipitate remains after 10 minutes, benzoic acid is present and the test is positive for hippurate hydrolysis. Alternatively, Ninhydrin reagent may be added to the supernatant to detect free glycine.[506] In this method, the formation of a deep-blue color is positive. Hippurate-positive, β-hemolytic streptococci are reported as "presumptive group B streptococci by hippurate hydrolysis."

BILE-ESCULIN TEST

This test is used for the presumptive identification of *Enterococcus* species and group D streptococci. It is generally performed on an agar slant or in a plate (Chart 13-2). Organisms that are bile-esculin-positive are able to grow in the presence of 40% bile and to hydrolyze esculin. Most *Enterococcus* species and group D streptococci will blacken bile-esculin medium within 24 hours (see Color Plate 13-2F); rare strains may require a 48-hour incubation before hydrolysis is apparent.[197] Care should be taken to use bile-esculin agar formulations that contain the requisite 40% bile; some manufacturers' products contain less bile than this amount, resulting in misidentification of some viridans streptococci as group D streptococci or enterococci.

SALT-TOLERANCE TEST (6.5% NaCl BROTH)

The salt-tolerance test (6.5% NaCl broth) separates *Enterococcus* species from the group D nonenterococcal streptococci *S. bovis* and *S. equinus* (see Chart 13-4). The organism to be identified is inoculated into an infusion-based agar or broth containing 6.5% NaCl. After overnight incubation, the medium is observed for the presence of growth, indicating tolerance to 6.5% salt. *Enterococcus* species will be salt-tolerant (see Color Plate 13-2D); *S. bovis* will not grow.

LEUCINE AMINOPEPTIDASE (LAP) TEST

Production of leucine aminopeptidase (LAP), along with PYR, is helpful for identifying streptococci, enterococci, and some of the *Streptococcus*-like organisms. This test is available as a disk spot test (Remel; Carr-Scarborough), as a part of a three-test presumptive identification system (Remel BactiCard Strep) or on 4-hour or overnight panels for streptococcal identification (the API Rapid Strep).[341] Disks are moistened and heavily inoculated with colony material from an agar plate (this may require that plates of very slow-growing isolates be incubated 2 to 3 days before sufficient inoculum is available for testing). After 10 minutes, a drop of the detection reagent is added to the disk. Development of a red color on the disk after 3 minutes indicates a positive LAP reaction; a yellow color indicates a negative test; and a pink color is coded as a weakly positive test. The LAP test is positive for all streptococci and enterococci, the latter also being PYR-positive.

PYRROLIDONYL ARYLAMIDASE (PYR) TEST

The PYR hydrolysis test (Chart 1-6) is a presumptive test for both group A and group D enterococcal streptococci.[342] It replaces the bacitracin test and the salt-tolerance test for group A streptococci and *Enterococcus* species, respectively. The enzyme that is detected is called pyrrolidonyl arylamidase. Broth containing PYR (L-pyrrolidonyl-β-naphthylamide) is inoculated with the organism and incubated at 35°C for 4 hours. During this time PYR is hydrolyzed. Free β-naphthylamide is then detected by addition of the diazo dye coupler, *N,N*-dimethylaminocinnamaldehyde. A red color develops if PYR has been hydrolyzed (see Color Plate 13-2*G*). This test is highly sensitive and specific for group A streptococci and most *Enterococcus* species. Several adaptations of the PYR hydrolysis test are commercially available and provide rapid results (15 minutes or less). Other organisms (e.g., most lactococci, *A. viridans*, *G. haemolysans*, the nutritionally variant streptococci, and some staphylococci) are also PYR-positive. This test is included along with esculin hydrolysis and leucine aminopeptidase on the BactiCard Strep system (Remel)

SUSCEPTIBILITY TO OPTOCHIN

Susceptibility to Optochin (ethyl hydrocupreine hydrochloride) is used to differentiate *S. pneumoniae* from the other viridans streptococci (see Chart 13-3). As with the bacitracin and SXT tests, the Optochin susceptibility test is performed on blood agar media. Unlike the former two tests, however, zones of inhibition must be measured before interpretation. A zone of 14 mm or wider around the 6-mm disk indicates susceptibility to Optochin and identifies the organism as a pneumococcus (see Color Plate 13-2*E*). If the zone is smaller than 14 mm, an alternative identification test (e.g., serology or bile solubility) should be performed because some nonpneumococcal viridans streptococci and aerococci may show small zones of inhibition. Viridans streptococci and group D enterococci are generally Optochin-resistant. A recent evaluation of the Optochin test with 99 clinical isolates of *S. pneumoniae* and 101 viridans streptococci reported sensitivity and specificity of 99% and 98%, respectively.[563] Optochin-resistant *S. pneumoniae* isolates have

been reported but are rarely encountered.[355,706] Borek and colleagues also reported isolation of a viridans *Streptococcus* with an 18 mm zone of inhibition around the Optochin disk.[115] Characterization of Optochin-susceptible strains of *S. mitis* revealed acquisition of genes from *S. pneumoniae* that encode subunits of the H+ ATPase, which is the target of Optochin.[664] Strains of *S. pneumoniae* that are Optochin-resistant have point mutations in either the a- or c-subunit of the H+ ATPase and have Optochin MICs that are 4- to 30-fold higher than those of susceptible strains.[776]

BILE-SOLUBILITY TEST

The bile-solubility test is another test for identification of *S. pneumoniae*. The test can be performed on a broth or saline suspension of the organism or directly on a plate. Both procedures are described in Chart 1-2. Deoxycholate, the "bile" reagent used in these procedures, activates the autolytic enzymes of the organism.

Commercial Presumptive Identification Tests

Commercially produced triplates are available for the presumptive identification of β-hemolytic streptococcal groups A and B, the group D streptococci, and *Enterococcus* species. The Strep-ID Tri-Plate (Remel) contains three compartments: a sheep blood agar quadrant for assessment of hemolysis and performance of the CAMP and SXT tests, a bile-esculin agar quadrant, and a PYR-medium quadrant. After inoculation and overnight incubation, the tests are interpreted as shown in Table 13-2 and in Color Plate 13-2*H*.

Serologic Identification of β-Hemolytic Streptococci

The pioneering work of Rebecca Lancefield set the stage for the serologic classification of human streptococci. This classification is based on the detection of the group-specific carbohydrate antigen from the cell wall of the organism. Groupable streptococci that cause disease in humans belong to Lancefield groups A, B, C, D, F, and G. Only β-hemolytic streptococci and the α-hemolytic or nonhemolytic group D organisms can be classified with this scheme. To detect the cell wall antigens of these organisms, the antigen must first be extracted from the cell wall and solubilized. This may be accomplished by acid extraction (e.g., nitrous acid), autoclave extraction (Rantz-Randall method), or by enzymatic extraction. Once extracted, the antigen may be detected by a variety of methods.

CAPILLARY PRECIPITIN TEST

In this method used by Lancefield, the extracted antigen is layered over group-specific antisera in a capillary tube.[596] The formation of a precipitin reaction at the extract-antiserum interface provides the group designation of the organism.

COAGGLUTINATION

In this technique, the antigen extract is reacted with *S. aureus* cells sensitized with group-specific antisera. Visible agglutination of the staphylococcal cells coated with a specific antiserum provides the group designation of the organism. Commercial coagglutination test kits are available (Phadebact Streptococcus, Boule Diagnostics, Huddinge, Sweden; Meritec Strep, Meridian Diagnostics, Cincinnati OH).

LATEX AGGLUTINATION

The latex agglutination tests use polystyrene latex beads as the carriers for the group-specific antisera that are reacted with the organism extract. Commercial kits for this method are widely used as well (Patho-D$_X$ Strep Grouping Kit, Diagnostic Products, Los Angeles CA; Slidex Strep, BioMérieux, Hazelwood MO; Meritec-Strep, Meridian Diagnostics, Cincinnati, OH).[453] Latex agglutination procedures have essentially replaced the Lancefield extraction-capillary precipitin technique as the reference method for serogrouping of β-hemolytic streptococci (see Color Plate 13-3A). The proper assessment of hemolysis is essential for test reliability, and cross-reactions with other organisms have been reported. For example, Lee and Wetherall demonstrated that some S. pneumoniae strains may cross-react with the group C streptococcal latex reagent.[612] This error may occur when organisms are tested directly from blood culture bottles without first determining the hemolytic character of the isolate. Some of the commercial reagents may also have difficulty detecting the group D antigen in Enterococcus species.[966] Thompson and Facklam also reported that the group B reagent in latex agglutination reagent kits from several manufacturers cross-reacts with S. porcinus strains, which may be isolated from both humans and swine.[337,955] At the University of Illinois, we have isolated S. porcinus from several rectovaginal swab specimens submitted for group B streptococcal screening. Although these strains react with the group B latex reagents, the organisms form small colonies with very large, clear zones of β-hemolysis, which is very different from the soft, marginal β-hemolysis associated with group B streptococci.

Serologic Identification of *Streptococcus pneumoniae*

Definitive identification of S. pneumoniae involves the serologic detection of pneumococcal capsular polysaccharides using specific antisera. This is complicated because there are more than 83 different capsular serotypes. Omniserum, a Scandinavian product, is capable of detecting all pneumococcal serotypes. Such antiserum pools have been used to develop commercial coagglutination (Phadebact Pneumococcus, Boule Diagnostics) and latex agglutination tests (Pneumoslide, BD Microbiology Systems; Slidex Pneumo, BioMérieux) for rapid serologic identification of S. pneumoniae (see Color Plate 13-3C). In a recent reevaluation of these test kits, sensitivities and specificities were 99–100% and 85.1–98%, respectively.[563] Specific identification and assignment to an individual capsular serotype is accomplished with the Quellung test.

The Quellung test may use a serum pool, as well as type-specific antisera (Pneumotest, Statens Serum Institut, Copenhagen, Denmark). A light suspension of the organism is prepared in saline, and a loopful of this suspension is mixed with a loopful of antiserum and a loopful of methylene blue on a glass slide. A glass coverslip is applied, and the slide

is incubated at room temperature for 10 minutes. The slide is examined under the high dry objective and under oil immersion, with decreased light. Because of a microprecipitin reaction occurring on the surface of the organism, the refractive index of the capsule changes and takes on a "swollen," more visible appearance as a halo around the blue-stained bacterial cells (see Color Plate 13-3B). Microscopic organism agglutination may also be observed, particularly with heavily encapsulated strains. Quellung results must be compared microscopically with a similar preparation made with saline instead of antisera.

A commercially available slide agglutination test for pneumococcal serotyping is also available from Denka Seiken (Tokyo, Japan). This test uses eight polyvalent reagents, each of which contain antisera to four to seven different serotypes and is performed on a suspension of the organisms prepared in phosphate-buffered saline. If agglutination is observed with one of the pools, the individual serotypes within the pool are tested to determine the serotype of the isolate. In a recent comparison of the Denka Seiken test with the Pneumotest Quellung technique, there was 95.7% agreement between the two methods; the authors also noted that the slide agglutination test was easier to perform and interpret.[891]

Biochemical Characteristics for Identification of Groupable Streptococci

The groupable streptococci can be identified to species on the basis of physiologic characteristics. Several of these reactions are used in the various kit systems for identifying the β-hemolytic streptococci. Biochemical identification methods may also enable detection of aberrant strains of β-hemolytic streptococci. For example, Brandt and colleagues isolated three strains of β-hemolytic streptococci from blood cultures that possessed the group A antigen but were identified as S. dysgalactiae subsp. equisimilis by phenotypic testing and 16S rDNA sequencing.[129] These strains were acetoin-negative and PYR-negative, unlike group A streptococci. Although most clinical laboratories dealing with specimens from humans use serologic methods for identification of these organisms, workers in veterinary microbiology may find these tests helpful because Lancefield antisera for groups other than A, B, C, F, and G are not readily available. Phenotypic characteristics for the identification of groupable streptococci are presented in Table 13-3.

Identification of the Viridans Streptococci

The viridans streptococci other than S. pneumoniae encompass several species of α-hemolytic and nonhemolytic organisms (see Table 13-4; see Color Plate 13-4F). Unlike the human β-hemolytic streptococci, these organisms, with the exception of members of the bovis group, lack specific Lancefield serologic group antigens, although some may carry antigens that cross-react with these antisera. Unlike the pneumococci, they are Optochin-resistant and bile-insoluble. Under certain circumstances, such as in cases of endocarditis and bacteremia in patients with neutropenia, it may be clinically helpful to identify these organisms. Indi-

Table 13-3 Phenotypic Characteristics for the Identification of the β-Hemolytic Streptococci

SPECIES	LANCEFIELD GROUP	BAC	SXT	CAMP TEST	LAP	PYR	ADH	ESC	HIPP	ACETOIN	STA HYDR	PAL	α-GAL	β-GUR	ACID PRODUCED FROM GLU	LAC	MNTL	RAFF	RIB	SAL	SORB	TRE
S. pyogenes	A	S	R	−	+	+	+	V	−	−	−	+	−	V	+	+	−	−	−	+	−	+
S. agalactiae	B	R	R/S	+	+	−	+	−	+	−	−	+	V	V	+	V	−	−	+	V	−	+
S. dysgalactiae subsp. dysgalactiae	C	R	S	−	+	−	+	V	−	−	−	+	−	+	+	+	−	−	+	V	V	+
S. dysgalactiae subsp. equisimilis	A, C, G, L	R	S	−	+	−	+	+	−	−	−	+	−	+	+	+	−	−	+	V	−	+
S. equi subsp. equi	C	R	S	−	+	−	+	V	−	−	+	+	−	+	+	−	−	−	−	+	−	−
S. equi subsp. zooepidemicus	C	R	S	−	+	−	+	V	−	−	+	+	−	+	+	−	−	−	−	+	+	V
S. canis	G	R	S	+	+	−	+	+	−	−	−	−	−	+	+	+	−	−	+	NA	−	+
S. phocae	C, F	S	S	−	+	−	−	−	−	−	−	+	−	−	+	−	−	−	+	−	−	−
S. porcinus	E, P, U, V, none	R	S	+	+	+	+	+	V	+	−	+	−	+	+	V	+	−	+	+	+	+
S. iniae	None	R	S	+	+	+	−	+	−	−	+	NA	−	NA	+	+	+	−	+	+	−	+
S. didelphis	None	R	S	−	+	−	+	−	+	−	−	+	V	+	+	V	−	V	+	−	−	+
S. urinalis	None	R	S	−	+	+	+	+	−	+	−	+	−	−	+	+	NA	NA	+	NA	−	+

+, positive reaction; −, negative reaction; NA, data not available; BAC, bacitracin, 0.04-unit disk; SXT, sulfamethoxazole-trimethoprim; LAP, leucine aminopeptidase; PYR, pyrrolidonyl arylamidase; ADH, arginine dihydrolase; ESC, esculin hydrolysis; HIPP, hippurate hydrolysis; STA HYDR, starch hydrolysis; β-GUR, β-glucuronidase; PAL, alkaline phosphatase; α-GAL, α-galactosidase; Glu, glucose; Lac, lactose; Mnl, mannitol; Raff, raffinose; Rib, ribose; Sal, salicin; Sorb, sorbitol; Tre, trehalose; R, resistant; S, susceptible.

Table 13-4 Phenotypic Differentiation of Viridans Streptococcal Groups Found in Humans

VIRIDANS GROUP	ADH	ESCULIN HYDROLYSIS	ACETOIN (VP)	MANNITOL	SORBITOL	UREASE	GROUP MEMBERS
Sanguis group	+	+	–	–	–	–	*S. sanguis* (*S. sanguinis*), *S. parasanguis* (*S. parasanguinis*), *S. gordonii, S. sinensis* (VP+)
Mitis group	–	–	–	–	–	–	*S. mitis, S. oralis, S. crista* (*S. cristatus*), *S. peroris, S. infantis, S. australis, S. oligofermentans*
Mutans group	–	+	+	+	+	–	*S. mutans, S. sobrinus, S. cricetus, S. ratti, S. macacae, S. downei, S. ferus,* and *S. hyovaginalis*
Salivarius group	–	V	V	–	–	V	*S. salivarius, S. vestibularis, S. infantarius, S. alactolyticus, S. hyointestinalis,* and *S. thermophilus*
Anginosus group	+	+	+	–	–	–	*S. intermedius, S. constellatus* subspecies, *S. anginosus*
Bovis group	–	+	+	V	–	–	*S. bovis/S. equinus, S. gallolyticus* subspecies, *S. infantarius* subspecies, *S. alactolyticus*

+, positive reaction; –, negative reaction; V, variable reaction.

viduals with preexisting valvular damage may have recurrent episodes of endocarditis or experience relapse following inadequate treatment. A knowledge of the identity and the antimicrobial susceptibility of these isolates may help sort out problems such as treatment failures, reinfections, and antimicrobial tolerance.

The application of molecular and chemotaxonomic techniques has resulted in significant modifications in viridans streptococcal taxonomy and approaches to identification. Because of the large number of recognized viridans streptococci, phenotypic identification methods involve the performance of a number of biochemical and enzymatic tests.[1047] Most laboratories that attempt to identify these organism use one or more commercial kits for this purpose (see Color Plates 13-4F, 13-4G and 13-4H). Unfortunately, the databases of the various kit systems are not updated frequently enough to reliably identify newer species, and additional tests are often required for species identification. These kits use modified conventional tests and novel chromogenic and fluorogenic substrates for the detection of preformed enzyme activities, and these approaches have become a standard part of the test batteries used for identification of these bacteria.[378,566,1047] Nonphenotypic methods for characterizing these organisms, such as pyrolysis-gas chromatography and Fourier-transform infrared spectroscopy, have shown promise as adjunct methods for identification.[377,995] Other molecular and chemotaxonomic approaches for species identification of the viridans streptococci include PCR-mediated amplification and detection of species-specific nucleic acid sequences, restriction-fragment-length polymorphism analysis of 16S rRNA genes, analysis of the electrophoretic patterns of whole-cell proteins, and mass spectrometry.[15,60,262,508,560,623,829,830,846,967,993] None of these methods, however, lend themselves to routine use in busy hospital laboratories. Therefore, identification of these organisms in clinical laboratories still relies on the use of key phenotypic features.

For convenience, the viridans streptococci can be placed in groups based on common biochemical features. These groups include the **sanguis group**, the **mitis group**, the **mutans group**, the **salivarius group**, the **anginosus group**, and the **bovis group**. Organisms can be assigned to these groups based on arginine dihydrolase, esculin hydrolysis, production of acetoin (VP test), acid production from mannitol and sorbitol, and the presence of urease. (Table 13-4).

In 1991 and 1998, Beighton and coworkers in the Department of Oral Microbiology at London Hospital Medical College published comprehensive schemes for phenotypic identification of the currently recognized members of the viridans streptococci.[71,1047] This scheme uses conventional 24-hour carbohydrate fermentation tests plus a battery of 4-methylumbelliferyl-linked substrates for the rapid (3-hour) determination of glycosidic enzymes. Table 13-5 is based on the taxonomic descriptions of viridans species presented by Beighton and others.[71,376,1047] The dichotomous key in Figure 13-3 incorporates the ''grouping'' tests from Table 13-4 and additional tests from Table 13-5 for identifying the ''typical'' individual species within a group. Until commercial vendors update the databases of individual commercial systems to include the newer species and phenotypic tests, microbiologists will have to use a ''best fit'' approach to species-level identification of the viridans streptococci.

SANGUIS GROUP

This viridans streptococcal group includes three species that are found in the human oral cavity: *S. sanguis*, *S. parasanguis*, *S. gordonii*, and *S. sinensis*. Although some investigators considers these species to be part of the mitis group based on 16S rRNA sequence studies, they can easily be phenotypically differentiated from the mitis group by their positive reactions for arginine dihydrolase and esculin hydrolysis.[558] *S. parasanguis* was described in 1990 and has been isolated from human throat cultures, blood, and urine specimens.[1049] *S. sanguis* can be divided into three biotypes based on phenotypic tests (Table 13-5). *S. sinensis* is a new α-hemolytic *Streptococcus* that was isolated from the blood of a patient with endocarditis in 2002.[1071] This organism is most closely related to *S. gordonii*.

MITIS GROUP

These α-hemolytic streptococci are found in the oral cavity. *S. mitis* is one of the species more frequently isolated from blood cultures and is of some importance because of its emerging resistance to penicillin and other β-lactam agents. Analysis of *S. sanguis*–like strains by several researchers resulted in the description of *S. gordonii* and *S. oralis*.[568] Although related genotypically to other mitis group organisms, *S. gordonii* phenotypically resembles the sanguis group organisms (i.e., arginine dihydrolase-positive and often esculin hydrolysis–positive). *S. crista* is a fairly new species that has been isolated from the human oral cavity.[456] *S. crista* is unusual in possessing tufts of short fibrils located in a lateral position on the cell surface that help the organism to coaggregate with other organisms in dental plaque. *S. peroris*, *S. australis*, *S. infantis*, and *S. oligofermentans* are new members of the mitis group and are found on the teeth and in the nasopharynx.[559,1058] *S. orisratti* is found in the oral cavity of Sprague-Dawley rats because of its biochemical consistency with other mitis group members. This species is unusual because it possesses the Lancefield group A carbohydrate antigen.[1095]

MUTANS GROUP

The mutans group includes oral streptococci found in humans and various animal species (Box 13-2). As mentioned previously, species in the mutans group were originally serotypes of *S. mutans* that were subsequently elevated to species status. *S. mutans* and *S. sobrinus* are the species most commonly isolated from humans.[73] *S. hyovaginalis* is also included in the mutans group because of its biochemical consistency with other mutans group streptococci, but this species is part of the normal flora in the genital tracts of swine.[279]

SALIVARIUS GROUP

Among the species in the salivarius, only *S. salivarius*, *S. vestibularis*, and *S. infantarius* have been recovered from human clinical specimens. *S. salivarius* and *S. vestibularis* are found in the human oral cavity, while *S. infantarius* has been isolated from humans and food products.[853,1052] *S. infantarius* strains are also included in the bovis group because some strains are bile-esculin– and esculin hydrolysis–positive. *S. alactolyticus* is also closely related to the bovis group

Table 13-5 Phenotypic Characteristics for Identification of the Mitis Group, Mutans Group, and Salivarius Group Species of the Viridans Streptococci Isolated From Humans

GROUP/SPECIES	HEM SBA	ESC	ADH	VP	URE	GLU	MAL	SUC	LAC	MNTL	MANN	SORB	ARAB	INU	MEL	RAFF	RIB	SAL	TRE	STA	GLYC	GLYG	AMGD
												ACID PRODUCED FROM:											
Sanguis Group																							
S. sanguis bio. 1	α	+	+	–	–	+	+	NA	+	–	NA	V–	NA	V–	+	+	–	+	+	NA	–	NA	–
S. sanguis bio. 2	α	+	+	–	–	+	+	NA	+	–	NA	V+	NA	–	V+	+	–	+	+	NA	–	NA	+
S. sanguis bio. 3	α	–	+	–	–	+	+	NA	+	–	NA	–	NA	+	–	V–	–	+	+	NA	–	NA	–
S. parasanguis	α	V–	+	–	–	+	+	NA	+	–	NA	V–	NA	–	V+	V+	NA	V+	V+	NA	NA	NA	V–
S. gordonii	α	+	+	–	–	+	+	NA	+	–	NA	–	NA	+	V–	V–	–	+	+	+	–	NA	+
S. sinensis	α	+	+	+	–	+	+	+	+	–	+	–	–	–	–	–	–	+	+	+	NA	–	NA
Mitis Group																							
S. mitis	α	–	–	–	–	+	+	NA	V+	–	NA	V–	NA	V–	V+	V+	V–	V–	V–	NA	NA	+	–
S. oralis	α	V–	–	–	–	+	+	NA	+	–	NA	–	NA	–	V+	V+	V+	–	V–	NA	NA	NA	–
S. crista	α	–	V+	–	–	+	+	NA	V+	–	NA	–	–	–	–	–	+	NA	+	NA	NA	NA	–
S. peroris	α	–	–	–	–	+	+	+	+	–	NA	–	–	–	V–	–	–	NA	–	NA	NA	–	–
S. infantis	α	–	–	–	–	+	+	+	V+	–	NA	–	–	–	V–	–	–	NA	–	NA	NA	–	NA
S. australis	α	NA	+	–	–	+	+	+	+	–	NA	–	NA	–	NA	–	–	NA	–	+	NA	–	NA
S. oligofermentans	α	–	+	+	–	+	+	+	V	–	+	V–	–	–	–	–	V	–	–	V	–	NA	–
Mutans Group																							
S. mutans	α, γ	+	–	V+	–	+	+	+	+	+	NA	+	NA	+	V+	V+	–	+	+	NA	NA	–	+
S. sobrinus	γ, α	V+	–	V+	–	+	+	+	V+	V+	NA	V–	NA	+	–	–	–	–	+	–	NA	–	–
Salivarius Group																							
S. salivarius	γ, α	+	–	V+	V+	+	NA	NA	+	–	NA	–	–	V+	V–	V+	NA	+	V	NA	–	NA	V
S. vestibularis	α	V+	–	+	+	+	+	NA	V+	–	NA	–	NA	–	–	–	–	+	V	–	NA	NA	V+

(Continued)

Table 13-5 *Continued*

GROUP/SPECIES	PRODUCTION OF										
	α-GAL	β-GAL	α-GLU	β-GLU	β-GUR	NAGA	α-ARAB	α-FUC	β-FUC	NAGALA	PAL
Sanguis Group											
S. sanguis bio. 1	V+	−	−	V	−	−	−	−	−	−	−
S. sanguis bio. 2	+	V−	−	+	−	V−	−	−	+	−	−
S. sanguis bio. 3	−	+	−	V	−	+	−	−	V+	−	−
S. parasanguis	+	+	+	V−	−	+	−	V−	V−	+	+
S. gordonii	V−	V−	V−	+	−	+	V−	+	−	V+	+
S. sinensis	−	−	NA	+	−	NA	NA	NA	NA	NA	−
Mitis Group											
S. mitis	V+	V−	V+	V+	−	−	−	−	V+	−	V+
S. oralis	V−	+	+	−	−	+	−	−	−	+	+
S. crista	−	V−	−	−	NA	+	−	+	−	+	−
S. peroris	−	−	NA	−	−	−	NA	−	−	NA	V
S. infantis	−	+	NA	−	−	V+	NA	V	V	NA	−
S. australis	−	−	NA	−	−	−	NA	NA	NA	NA	+
S. oligofermentans	V−	−	NA	NA	NA	NA	NA	NA	NA	NA	−
Mutans Group											
S. mutans	+	−	+	+	−	−	−	−	−	−	
S. sobrinus	−	−	+	−	−	−	−	−	−	−	
Salivarius Group											
S. salivarius	V−	+	V+	V+	NA	−	+	V+	V+	−	V+
S. vestibularis	+	+	V+	−	NA	−	+	−	−	−	−

+, positive reaction; −, negative reaction; V, variable reaction; V+, variable reaction, most strains positive; V−, variable reaction, most strains negative; NA, data not available; Hem SBA, hemolysis on sheep blood agar; ESC, esculin hydrolysis; ADH, arginine dihydrolase; VP, acetoin production; URE, urease; GLU, glucose; MAL, maltose; SUC, sucrose; LAC, lactose; MNTL, mannitol; MANN, mannose; SORB, sorbitol; ARAB, arabinose; INU, inulin; MEL, melibiose; RAFF, raffinose; RIB, ribose; SAL, salicin; TRE, trehalose; STA, starch; GLY, glycerol; GLYC, glycogen; AMGD, amygdalin; α-GAL, α-galactosidase; β-GAL, β-galactosidase; α-GLU, α-glucosidase; β-GLU, β-glucosidase; β-GUR, β-glucuronidase; NAGA, N-acetyl-β-D-glucosaminidase; α-ARAB, α-arabinosidase; α-FUC, α-fucosidase; β-FUC, β-fucosidase; NAGALA, N-acetyl-β-D-galactosaminidase; PAL, alkaline phosphatase.

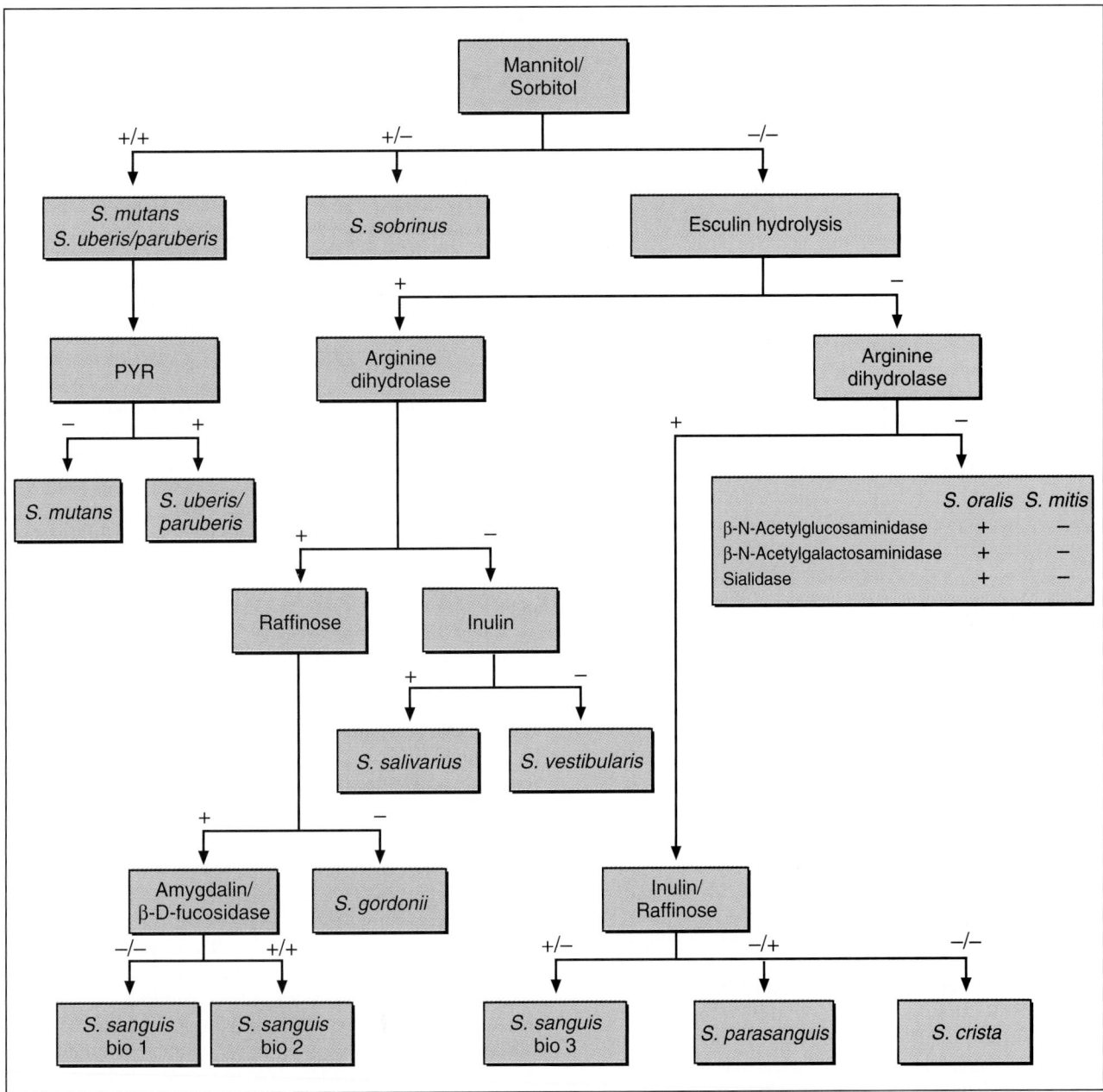

Figure 13-3 Flow chart for identification of viridans streptococci.

organisms and is found in various avian species and in swine. *S. hyointestinalis* is a salivarius group species that is found in the gut of swine, and *S. thermophilus* is isolated from dairy products.[278] In the salivarius group, all strains of *S. vestibularis* and some *S. salivarius* strains produce urease.

ANGINOSUS GROUP

The three species that compose the anginosus group of streptococci—*S. anginosus*, *S. constellatus* subspecies, and *S. intermedius*—produce "pinpoint" colonies on blood agar and may be β-hemolytic, α-hemolytic, or nonhemolytic. A greater proportion of *S. intermedius* strains are nonhemolytic, and *S. constellatus* strains are often β-hemolytic. For

β-hemolytic strains, the size of the hemolytic zone is several times the diameter of the colony. Besides the size of the colony, another clue that an isolate may be a member of this group is the presence of a sweet odor that has been described as "caramel," "butterscotch," or "honeysuckle." This odor is due to the production of the metabolite diacetyl.[184] Isolates may carry group A, C, F, or G antigens or may be nongroupable. The growth of these organisms is enhanced by incubation in a CO_2-enriched environment, and some strains may require anaerobic incubation for optimal growth. As with all streptococci, these organisms are LAP-positive. All species in the anginosus group are positive for esculin hydrolysis, arginine dihydrolase, and production of acetoin and alkaline phosphatase, and all are negative for hippurate hydrolysis, urease, and PYR. The individual species may be differentiated by the biochemical and enzymatic tests shown in Table 13-6.[1046,1050,1053] Many of the tests shown in Table 13-6 are found in the commercially available kit systems. These organisms are included in the databases of commercial kits (e.g., API Rapid Strep, RapID STR, and the API ID32 kits), although additional tests may need to be performed along with serogrouping of β-hemolytic strains. Recently, *S. constellatus* has been divided into two subspecies—*S. constellatus* subsp. *constellatus* and *S. constellatus* subsp. *pharyngis*.[1051] In addition to phenotypic identification, molecular-based assays have also been developed for identifying these organsism.[419,943]

S. anginosus strains have been shown to encompass five distinct ribogroups that are closely related at the 16S rRNA level and show greater than 97% sequence similarity with each other.[522] These five groups have been designated ''ATCC-like'' strains, motile strains, and ribogroups I, II, and III. The ATCC-like strains hybridized with oligonucleotide probes prepared from *S. anginosus* ATCC 33397. The motile group represented 37.8% of the *S. anginosus* strains examined, and 83% of these were recovered from the urogenital tract as part of the normal urogenital flora. These motile *S. anginosus* isolates fermented mannitol and raffinose, while isolates in the other groups did not. Often, ribogroup I *S. anginosus* carried the Lancefield group C antigen. Ribogroup II strains were associated with abdominal infections, and ribogroup III isolates were recovered from abdominal, soft-tissue, head and neck, and urinary-tract infections. At present, there are no easily determined phenotypic criteria available to separate these five ribogroups from one another.

BOVIS GROUP

As discussed previously, the *S. bovis* group has undergone significant taxonomic revision. Like the enterococci, the group D streptococci possess the group D antigen, hydrolyze esculin in the presence of 40% bile, and grow at 45°C. They do not grow in 6.5% NaCl broth, do not hydrolyze PYR, and do not grow at 10°C. Most isolates are LAP-positive, produce acetoin, do not produce arginine dihydrolase or urease, and acidify lactose but not sorbitol. On the basis of phenotypic criteria, the API Rapid Strep identification system splits *S. bovis* strains into *S. bovis* I, *S. bovis* II.1, and *S. bovis* II.2. *S. bovis* I strains (i.e., *S. gallolyticus* subsp. *gallolyticus*) are mannitol-, raffinose-, glycogen-, amygdalin-, and α-GAL-positive, and are β-GUR-negative (see Color Plates 13-4D and 13-4E). *S. bovis* II.1 (*S. infantarius* subsp. *infantarius*) and *S. bovis* II.2 (*S. gallolyticus* subsp. *pasteurianus*) are mannitol-negative, with *S. bovis* II.1 strains being β-GUR-negative and *S. bovis* II.2 strains being β-GUR-positive. These characteristics are presented in Table 13-7. Strains of *S. bovis* I (*S. gallolyticus* subsp. *gallolyticus*) also produce extracellular dextrans from sucrose and are able to hydrolyze starch. Starch hydrolysis can be detected with Mueller-Hinton agar plates that are streaked with the organism and incubated for 48 hours. The plates are then flooded with Gram's iodine. Colorless areas under and surrounding organism growth indicate hydrolysis of starch, whereas the maintenance of the blue or purple color

around the colonies indicates no hydrolysis of starch. Alternatively, starch plates (various manufacturers) can be used.

Identification of *Streptococcus suis* and Other Streptococci Isolated From Animals

S. suis should be suspected in patients with systemic signs of sepsis and meningitis who have had contact with pigs or porcine products. The organism is a typical-looking, catalase-negative, nonmotile, gram-positive coccus that occurs singly, in pairs, or in short chains. *S. suis* is α-hemolytic on sheep blood agar (β-hemolytic on horse blood agar), resistant to Optochin, and does not grow in 6.5% NaCl broth. Some strains will grow in the presence of 40% bile, and all strains are able to hydrolyze esculin. *S. suis* phenotypically resembles certain viridans streptococci, particularly *S. gordonii*, *S. sanguinis*, and *S. parasanguinis*. Human isolates are usually capsular serotype 2 strains that react with Lancefield group R antisera (Statens Serum Institute, Copenhagen, Denmark). Capsular typing may also be accomplished using molecular methods by sequence analysis of capsular *cps* genes.[907] Additional characteristics that are helpful for identification of *S. suis* are presented in Table 13-8.[946] This important animal pathogen is included in the database of the API Rapid Strep system (see discussion below).

Table 13-8 also presents the phenotypic characteristics of α-hemolytic and nonhemolytic streptococci and related isolates from various animal species. These species include *S. entericus*, *S. pluranimalium*, *S. uberis/parauberis*, *S. thoraltensis*, *S. hyovaginalis*, *S. hyointestinalis*, *S. ovis*, *S. minor*, *S. gallinaceus*, and *Eremococcus coleocola*. The ''mutans group'' species from animals are not included in this table since they constitute part of the animals' normal oral flora and are not likely to be seen in either human or animal infections.

Identification of *Enterococcus* Species

Enterococcus species grow well on most bacteriologic media, including 5% sheep blood colistin-nalidixic acid (CNA), and chocolate agars (see Color Plate 13-3E). On SBA, most strains are nonhemolytic or α-hemolytic. Most strains are able to grow at 35–37°C in ambient air, although incubation in a CO_2-enriched environment stimulates growth of most isolates. Specimens containing enterococci that are heavily contaminated with gram-negative bacilli may be easily isolated on media containing sodium azide (e.g., Pfizer selective enterococcus agar, bile-esculin-azide agar). Ford and colleagues described a medium called cephalexin-aztreonam-arabinose agar that can be used for epidemiologic studies to detect the presence of *E. faecium* in stools of hospitalized patients who are at risk for serious enterococcal infections.[368] This medium contains arabinose (10 g/L), aztreonam (75 mg/L), cephalexin (50 mg/L), and phenol-red indicator (2%) in a Columbia agar base (40 g/L). *E. faecium* grows on this media as white colonies with yellow haloes, indicating acid production from arabinose, while *E. faecalis* grows as clear colonies with no haloes, indicating lack of arabinose utilization.

Identification of enterococci to species level is often helpful and sometimes crucial for proper patient treatment and for epidemiologic and infection-control purposes. Iso-

Table 13-6 Phenotypic Characteristics for Identification of the Anginosus Group: *Streptococcus anginosus*, *Streptococcus constellatus*, and *Streptococcus intermedius*

SPECIES	HEMO-LYSIS	LANCEFIELD GROUPS	ACID PRODUCTION FROM:					PRODUCTION OF:			
			Glucose	Lactose	Mannitol	Raffinose	Amygdalin	β-GAL	α-GLU	β-GLU	NAGA
S. anginosus	β	A,C,F,G, none	+	+	−	−	+	+	−	+	V
	Non-β	C,F,G, none[a]	+	+	−	−	+	−	V	+	−
S. constellatus subsp. *constellatus*	β	F, none	+	V	−	−	V	−	+	−	−
	Non-β	F, none	+	V	−	−	V	−	+	−	−
S. constellatus subsp. *pharyngis*	β	C	+	+	−	−	+	+	+	+	+
S. intermedius	β	None	+	+	−	−	+	+	+	V	+
	Non-β	None	+	+	−	−	+	+	+	V	+

[a] A motile nonhemolytic *S. anginosus* variant was described in 1995 that fermented lactose, mannitol, raffinose, and amygdalin and produced both α- and β-glucosidase.[83]

+, positive reaction; −, negative reaction; V, variable reaction; β-GAL, β-galactosidase; α-GLU, α-glucosidase; β-GLU, β-glucosidase; NAGA, β-N-acetyl-glucosaminidase.

Table 13-7 Phenotypic Characteristics for Identification of Members of the "Streptococcus bovis/Streptococcus equinus" Group

TEST	S. BOVIS/S. EQUINUS	S. GALLOLYTICUS SUBSP. GALLOLYTICUS	S. GALLOLYTICUS SUBSP. PASTEURIANUS	S. GALLOLYTICUS SUBSP. MACEDONICUS	S. INFANTARIUS SUBSP. INFANTARIUS	S. INFANTARIUS SUBSP. COLI	S. ALACTOLYTICUS
Esculin hydrolysis	+	+	+	−	V	+	+
Gallate hydrolysis	−	+	−	−	−	−	−
Acid produced from:							
Glucose	+/+	+	+	+	+	+	+
Lactose	−/+	+	+	+	+	+	−
Mannitol	−	+	−	−	−	−	−
Raffinose	−/+	+	V	−	+	−	−
Trehalose	V	+	+	−	−	−	−
Inulin	−/+	+	−	−	−	−	−
Starch	−/+	+	−	+	+	V	−
Glycogen	−/+	+	−	+	+	V	−
Production of:							
α-GAL	−/+	+	V	V	+	+	+
β-GAL	−	−	V	V+	−	−	−
β-GLU	+	+	+	−	V	+	+
β-GUR	−	−	+	−	−	−	−
Comments (new proposed names, etc.)	S. bovis type strain/isolates of S. equinus (91–100% sequence homology). Strains represented are primarily bovine and equine in origin.	S. bovis I; includes strains isolated from humans, cattle, and koala bears	S. bovis II.2; includes human strains.	S. macedonicus, S. waius	S. bovis II.1; includes human and bovine stains	"S. lutetiensis"	S. intestinalis

+, positive reaction; −, negative reaction; V, variable reaction; V+, variable reaction, but most strains positive; α-GAL, α-galactosidase; β-GAL, β-galactosidase; β-GLU, β-glucosidase; β-GUR, β-glucuronidase.

Table 13-8 Biochemical Characteristics for Identification of *Streptococcus suis*, *Eremococcus coleocola*, and Other α- and Nonhemolytic Streptococci Isolated From Animals

CHARACTERISTIC	S. SUIS	S. ENTERICUS	S. PLURANIMALIUM	S. UBERIS/PARAUBERIS	S. THORALTENSIS	S. HYOVAGINALIS	S. HYOINTESTINALIS	S. OVIS	S. MINOR	S. GALLINACEUS	E. COLEOCOLA
Hemolysis, SBA	α	α	α	α, none	α	α	α	α	α	α	α
Growth, 10°C	–	–	–	NA	–	–	NA	NA	NA	NA	–
Growth, 45°C	–	–	+	NA	–	–	NA	NA	NA	NA	+
LAP	+	+	+	+	+	+w	+	+	+	NA	–
PYR	NA	NA	–	+	–	–	–	NA	–	NA	NA
Growth, BE agar	V	–	+	–/+w	+	–	–	NA	+	NA	–
Growth, 6.5% NaCl	–	–	V	+	+	–	–	NA	NA	NA	+w
Esculin hydrolysis	+	+	+	+	+	NA	+	+	+	+	–
ADH	+	–	–	+	+	–	–	V+	+	+	+
Hippurate hydrolysis	–	–	+	+	V	+	–	–	–	–	+
Urease	–	–	–	–	–	–	–	–	–	–	V
Acetoin	–	–	–	V	+	+	+	–	NA	–	–
Motility	–	–	–	–	–	–	–	–	–	–	–
Acid produced from:											
Glucose	+	+	+	+	+	+	+	+	+	+	+
Maltose	+	+	NA	+	+	+	+	+	+	+	–
Sucrose	+	+	NA	+	+	+	+	+	+	+	–
Lactose	+	+	NA	+	+	+	+	+	+	+	–
Mannitol	–	–	V+	+	+	+	–	+	+w	+	–
Melibiose	V	–	NA	NA	V	–	NA	–	–	+	NA
Inulin	+	–	–	V	+	–	–	NA	V	–	NA
Arabinose	–	–	–	–	+	–	–	–	–	–	–
Sorbitol	–	–	–	+	V	+	–	+	V	–	–
Starch	NA	+	–	NA	+	+	+	NA	V	NA	NA
Raffinose	V	–	NA	–	V	–	NA	+	V	+	NA
Ribose	–	–	V	+	+	V	–	–	–	+	NA
Trehalose	NA	+	+	+	+	+	+	+	+	+	–
Glycogen	NA	+	–	NA	–	–	–	+	+	–	–

(Continued)

Table 13-8 *Continued*

CHARAC-TERISTIC	S. SUIS	S. ENTE-RICUS	S. PLURANI-MALIUM	S. UBERIS/PARAUBERIS	S. THORAL-TENSIS	S. HYOVA-GINALIS	S. HYOINTES-TINALIS	S. OVIS	S. MINOR	S. GALLI-NACEUS	E. COLEO-COLA
Production of:											
α-GAL	+	−	NA	NA	V	−	V	V	V+ʷ	+	NA
β-GAL	V	+	NA	NA	−	+	−	−	−	+	−
α-GLU	NA	NA	NA	NA	NA	NA	NA	+	NA	+	−
β-GLU	NA	+	V	NA	+	V	+	+	NA	+	−
β-GUR	+	−	V+	+	+	+	−	−	−	−	−
NAGA	NA	−	NA	NA	−	+	NA	−	NA	−/+ʷ	NA
PAL	NA	−	V+	NA	+ʷ	+	+	−	NA	NA	NA
Habitat	Infections in piglets; serotype 2 causes meningitis in humans	Intestinal tract of cattle	Cattle (mastitis, genital tract (tonsils), goats (tonsils), cats (tonsils), canaries (crop, respiratory tract)	Cattle (mastitis)	Genital and intestinal tract of sows	Genital tract of sows	Intestinal tract of pigs	Clinical specimens from sheep	Tonsils and feces of dogs, bovine and feline tonsils	Chickens	Horses

+, *positive reaction;* −, *negative reaction;* V, *variable reaction;* V+ʷ, *variable reaction, but delayed or weak when positive;* +ʷ, *weak or delayed positive reaction;* −/+ʷ, *negative or weak or delayed positive reaction;* NA, *data not available:* α-GAL, α-*galactosidase;* β-GAL, β-*galactosidase;* α-GLU, α-*glucosidase;* β-GLU, β-*glucosidase;* β-GUR, β-*glucuronidase;* NAGA, N-*acetyl-*β-D-*glucosaminidase;* AL, *alkaline phosphatase.*

lates of *E. faecium* tend to be more resistant to penicillin and ampicillin than *E. faecalis* isolates, and the vast majority of vancomycin-resistant enterococci (VRE) are strains of *E. faecium*. Early detection of VRE in at-risk patients enables the timely institution of infection-control practices that are known to limit the spread of these opportunistic agents.[495] To this end, several agar and broth media formulations have been used for rapid detection of VRE in anatomic sites that harbor enterococci (i.e., stool specimens, rectal swabs) (see Color Plate 13-3*H*).[507,598,838] Broth for growth enrichment of VRE is made semiselective by addition of vancomycin to the media, usually at a concentration of 6 μg/mL; other selective agents (e.g., clindamycin, aztreonam) may also be added. Because some VRE strains may be inhibited by these combinations of antimicrobial agents, subculture from selective broth medium to both selective and nonselective agar media is suggested in order to optimize recovery of VRE.

Identification of *Enterococcus* species is accomplished by biochemical and physiologic tests (Table 13-9). Most (about 80%) *Enterococcus* species react with antiserum against Lancefield group D by capillary precipitin or latex agglutination; the group D antigen cannot be demonstrated in strains of *E. pseudoavium*, *E. dispar*, *E. cecorum*, *E. sulfureus*, *E. columbae*, and *E. saccharolyticus*. Most species of enterococci are able to grow within 48 hours in brain-heart infusion (BHI) broth incubated at both 10 and 45°C; however *E. cecorum* and *E. columbae* fail to grow at 10°C and *E. sulfureus*, *E. malodoratus*, and *E. dispar* do not grow at 45°C. Most *Enterococcus* species hydrolyze esculin in the presence of 40% bile (BE test), grow in broth containing 6.5% NaCl, and are PYR-positive, although some species are negative in these tests as well (Table 13-9). Although *E. faecalis* and *E. faecium* are the species most commonly recovered from clinical specimens, the incidence of the other species and their roles in specific disease processes are unknown. Facklam and Collins have proposed a stepwise method for identifying *Enterococcus* species.[335] Isolates that fit the criteria listed above are inoculated into several test media and are divided into five groups based on those reactions. Individual species within each group are further differentiated into separate species on the basis of additional tests or characteristics. In 1992, Knudtson and Hartman at Iowa State University examined 59 strains of 13 *Enterococcus* species with conventional methods and two kit systems (including the API Rapid Strep system and the MicroScan Pos ID panel) (see Color Plates 13-3*F* and 13-3*G*).[581] These workers found several discrepancies between published reactions for individual tests, reactions in their own conventional tests, and individual test results obtained with the two kit systems. By using combinations of various conventional and kit-based tests, these workers also published multiphasic dichotomous keys for identifying these organisms. A flow chart for identifying the clinically significant *Enterococcus* species is presented in Figure 13-4.

For identification of enterococci by conventional procedures, carbohydrate fermentation tests and pyruvate utilization are determined in heart infusion broth base media containing bromcresol purple and 1% filter-sterilized carbohydrates or 1% pyruvate. Deamination of arginine is determined using Moeller's decarboxylase broth, and motility is determined in semisolid motility medium (see Color Plate 13-4*B*). Detection of the yellow pigment produced by *E. casseliflavus*, *E. gallinarum*, and *E. mundtii* is achieved by sweeping up some of the growth on a white Dacron swab and observing the colonial material on the swab for a yellow or yellow-orange color (see Color Plate 13-4*B*). Cartwright and coworkers found that the use of both motility and pigment detection tests together with a commercial test system greatly improved the reliability and accuracy of enterococcal identification in the clinical laboratory.[160]

Many laboratories rely on kit systems for identifying enterococci. Most of the kit systems described later in this chapter also perform very well for identifying the more common species. Enterococci can also be accurately identified to the genus level with the AccuProbe *Enterococcus* test (Gen-Probe), which uses a acridinium ester–labeled chemiluminescent oligomeric DNA probe to detect the rRNA of the target organism.[251,257] This test can be performed on isolates growing on agar media or from pellets obtained by centrifugation of blood culture broth.[257] Genetic and molecular methods for identification of *Enterococcus* species and for genotypic characterization of phenotypically derived antimicrobial susceptibilities have also been developed and include DNA hybridization methods, contour-clamped homogeneous electric field electrophoresis, ribotyping, pulsed-field gel electrophoresis, and PCR.[296,306,413]

Identification of *Abiotrophia* and *Granulicatella* Species

A. defectiva and *Granulicatella* species should be suspected when direct Gram stains of specimens or of positive blood cultures show streptococcal organisms that fail to grow on subsequent culture or subculture. Commercial blood culture media contain pyridoxal and will support the growth of these organisms. Subculture onto blood agar and the placement of a staphylococcal streak as is done in the satellite test for *Haemophilus* spp. will ensure growth of the nutritionally variant streptococci adjacent to the staph streak (see Color Plate 13-3*D*). Alternatively, disks impregnated with pyridoxal may also be placed on the subculture plate, with subsequent growth of the organisms appearing as satellite colonies surrounding the disk. Commercially available chocolate agar contains pyridoxal, so these organisms will grow on chocolate agar.

When grown on pyridoxal-supplemented (10-mg pyridoxal hydrochloride per liter) or cysteine-supplemented (100 mg L-cysteine per liter) media, these organisms can be identified with the biochemical tests shown in Table 13-10. Many of these tests are found on commercial kit systems (e.g., API Rapid Strep). Like the streptococci, these two species are LAP-positive, but unlike the streptococci, *A. defectiva* and *Granulicatella* species are PYR-positive. These organisms are homofermentative, with lactic acid as the sole end product of glucose fermentation. They are also Optochin-resistant and vancomycin-susceptible. It should also be kept in mind that occasional isolates of other viridans streptococci (e.g., *S. mitis*) may also display nutritional variance.[882] Molecular approaches to the identification of these nutritionally variant species have also been described.[738,821]

Identification of *Aerococcus* and *Helcococcus* Species

The genus *Aerococcus* contains five species: *A. viridans*, *A. urinae*, *A. sanguinicola*, *A. christensenii*, and *A. urinae-*

Table 13-9 Phenotypic Characteristics for Identification of *Enterococcus* and Related Species

GROUP/SPECIES	GROUP D ANTIGEN	GROWTH, BE AGAR	GROWTH, 6.5% NACL	GROWTH, 10°C	GROWTH, 45°C	LAP	PYR	MOT	YELLOW PIGM	ADH	HIP	ACID PRODUCED FROM:								
												GLU	MNTL	SORB	ARAB	SBTL	RAFF	SUC	PYRV	MGP
Group I																				
E avium	+	+	+	NA	+	+	+	–	–	–	V	+	+	+	+	+	–	+	+	V
E. gilvus	+	+	+	+	+	+	+	–	+	–	–	+	+	+	–	+	+	+	+	–
E. maldoratus	+	+	+	NA	–	+	+	–	–	–	V	+	+	+	–	+	+	+	+	V
E. pallens	+	+	+	+	+	+	–	–	+	–	+	+	+	+	+	+	+	+	+	–
E. pseudoavium	–	+	–	+	+	+	+	–	–	–	+	+	+	+	+	+	+	+	+	+
E. raffinosus	+	+	+	NA	+	+	+	–	–	–	V	+	+	+	+	+	+	+	+	V
E. saccharolyticus	–	NA	+	NA	NA	+	–	–	–	–	+	+	+	+	–	+	+	–	–	+
Enterococcus sp. CDC PNS-E3	–	–	+	+	–	+^w	–	–	–	–	–	+	+	+	–	+	–	–	+	–
Group II																				
E. faecalis	+	+	+	+	+	+	+	–	–	+	–	+	+	–	–	–	–	+	+	+
E. faecium	+	+	+	+	+	+	+	–	–	+	–	+	+	–	+	V	V	+	–	–
E. casseliflavus	+	+	+	NA	+	+	+	+	+	+	–	+	+	–	+	V	+	+	V	+
E. gallinarum	+	+	+	+	+	+	+	+	–	+	–	+	+	–	+	–	+	+	+	+
E. mundtii	+	+	+	+	+	+	+	–	+^w	+	–	+	+	+	+	V	+	+	+	+
E. haemoperoxidus	+	+	+	+	–	+	+	–	+^w	+	–	+	+	–	–	–	+	+	+	+
Enterococcus sp. CDC PNS-E2	+	+	+	+	+	+	+	–	–	+	–	+	+	–	–	–	–	+	+	–
Lactococcus spp.	–	–	V	+	–	V	V	–	V	V+	V	+	+	–	–	–	–	V	+	–
Group III																				
E. dispar	–	+	+	+	–	+	+	–	–	+	V	+	–	–	–	–	+	+	+	+
E. durans	+	NA	+	NA	+	+	+	–	–	+	V	+	–	–	+	–	V	–	–	–
E. hirae	+	+	+	+	+	+	+	–	–	+	–	+	–	–	+	–	+	+	+	+
E. ratti	+^w	+	+	+	+	NA	NA	–	–	+	V	+	–	+	–	–	+	–	NA	+
E. villorum	+	+	+	+	+	+	+	–	–	+	–	+	–	–	–	–	–	–	+	+
Group IV																				
E. asini	+	+	–	V	V	+	+	–	–	–	+	+	–	–	+	–	+	–	–	V
E. cecorum	NA	NA	–	–	+	+	+	–	–	–	–	+	–	–	+	+	+	+	+	+
E. sulfureus	–	+	+	–	–	+	+	–	+	–	–	+	–	+	+	+	+	–	+	+
E. phoeniculicola	NA	–	–	–	–	NA	NA	–	–	–	NA	+	–	–	–	–	–	–	+	+
Enterococcus sp. CDC PNS-E1	+	+	+	+	+	+	+	–	–	–	+	+	–	–	–	–	+	+	+	+
Group V																				
E. columbae	–	+	–	NA	NA	+	–	–	–	–	–	+	+	–	+	+	+	+	+	–
E. canis	NA	+	+	NA	NA	+	+	–	–	–	–	+	+	–	+	–	–	V	+	+
E. moraviensis	+	+	+	+	–	+	V	–	–	V–	+	+	+	–	+	+	+	+	+	+
Vagococcus spp.	–	NA	+	+	–	+	+	+	–	V–	+	+	–	–	–	+	–	–	+	+

BE agar, bile-esculin agar; LAP, leucine aminopeptidase; PYR, pyrrolidonyl arylamidase; MOT, motility; PIGM, pigment; ADH, arginine dihydrolase; HIP, hippurate hydrolysis; GLU, glucose; MNTL, mannitol; SORB, sorbitol; ARAB, arabinose, SBTL, sorbitol; RAFF, raffinose; SUC, sucrose; PYRV, pyruvate; MGP, methyl-α-D-glucopyranoside.

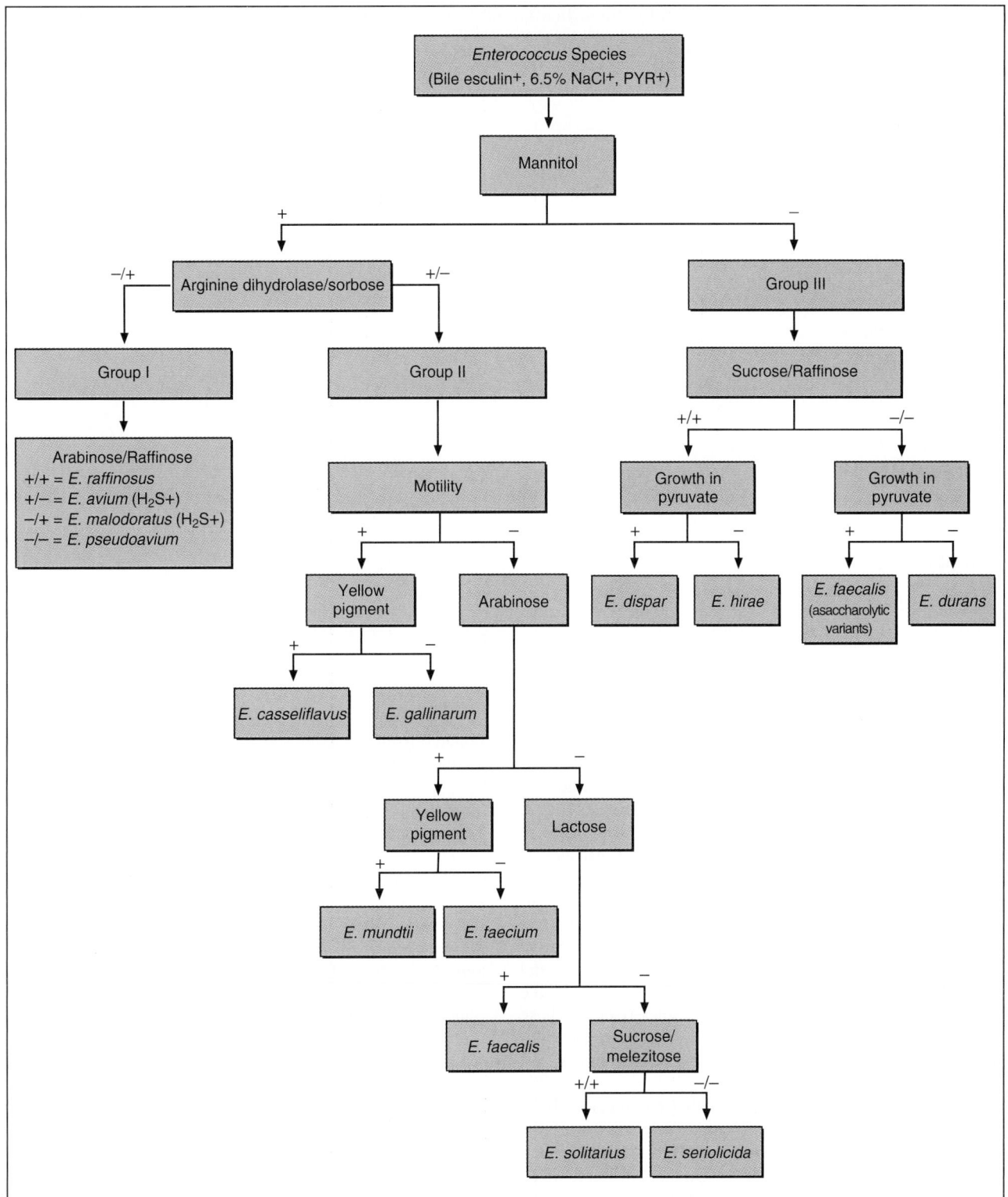

Figure 13-4 Flow chart for identification of *Enterococcus* species (adapted from reference [335]).

Table 13-10 Phenotypic Characteristics for Identification of *Abiotrophia defectiva* and *Granulicatella* Species

CHARACTERISTIC	A. DEFECTIVA	G. ADIACENS	G. PARA-ADIACENS	G. ELEGANS	G. BALAENOPTERAE
Requirement for pyridoxal	+	+	+	+	+
Growth, 10°C	−	−	−	−	−
Growth, 45°C	−	−	−	−	−
Gas, MRS broth	−	−	−	−	−
Growth, BE agar	−	−	−	−	−
Growth, 6.5% NaCl broth	−	−	−	−	−
Arginine dihydrolase	−	−	−	+	+
Hippurate hydrolysis	−	−	−	+	−
Acid produced from:					
Glucose	+	+	+	+	+
Sucrose	+	+	+	+	−
Trehalose	+	−	−	−	+
Production of:					
α-GAL	+	−	−	−	−
β-GAL	+	−	−	−	−
β-GLU	−	+	−	−	−
Habitat	Humans	Humans	Humans	Humans	Cetaceans

+, *positive reaction;* −, *negative reaction;* α-GAL, α-*galactosidase;* β-GAL, β-*galactosidase;* β-GLU, β-*glucosidase;* MRS, Mann-Rugosa–Sharpe Lactobacillus broth; BE agar, bile-esculin agar.

hominis. All species are α-hemolytic on SBA and grow in broth cultures as pairs, tetrads, and small clusters. Strains of *A. viridans* characteristically appear mostly as tetrads on Gram-stained smears, whereas *A. urinae* isolates occur mostly in clusters. On agar media, strains of *A. viridans* form large colonies that resemble those of enterococci. All species except *A. christensenii* grow in 6.5% NaCl; *A. sanginicola* and some *A. viridans* grow as black colonies on BE agar. Isolates of *A. viridans* are PYR-positive and LAP-negative, but *A. urinae* and *A. christensenii* strains are PYR-negative and LAP-positive. *A. sanguinicola* is positive for LAP and PYR, while *A. urinaehominis* is negative in both tests. Table 13-11 provides additional phenotypic characteristics of these species. PCR- and DNA probe–based assays have been developed for identification of both *A. viridans* and *A. urinae.*[9,429]

Another *Aerococcus*-like species that has recently been described is *Helcococcus kunzii.* Unlike most aerococci, this species produces variable growth in 6.5% NaCl, and growth is stimulated by serum or Tween 80. On the API Rapid Strep system, *H. kunzii* produces a profile that corresponds to a "doubtful" identification of *A. viridans* (API profile 4100413). Isolates of *H. kunzii* are nonhemolytic and do not grow at either 10°C or 45°C. The organism is esculin- and PYR-positive and LAP-negative, produces acid from glucose, maltose, lactose, trehalose, and glycogen, and does not produce β-galactosidase or β-glucuronidase. These organisms are commonly penicillin-, ampicillin-, and vancomycin-susceptible. The human isolate *H. kunzii* is easily differ-

entiated from the ovine species *H. ovis* by biochemical tests (Table 13-11).

Identification of *Leuconostoc, Pediococcus,* and *Tetragenococcus* Species

The genus *Leuconostoc* contains several species: *L. mesenteroides* subsp. *mesenteroides, L. mesenteroides* subsp. *cremoris, L. mesenteroides* subsp. *dextranicum, L. pseudomesenteroides, L. lactis, L. citreum, L. gelidum, L. carnosum, L. fallax, L. argentinum, L. gasicomitatum, L. kimchii, L. ficulneum,* and *L. fructosum.*[32,102,284,350,572,662,881] The organisms formerly designated *L. cremoris* and *L. dextranicum* are now included as subspecies of *L. mesenteroides.* Organisms belonging to the former species *L. paramesenteroides* have been reclassified in the new genus *Weissella* as *Weissella paramesenteroides.*[227] Similarly, genetic sequencing and hybridization studies and electrophoretic analysis of enzyme activities of the former *Leuconostoc* species *L. oenos* have demonstrated that this organism forms a distinct branch away from the other *Leuconostoc* species, so this organism has been placed in the genus *Oenococcus* as *Oenococcus oeni.*[283,388] *L. mesenteroides* subspecies and *L. lactis* are found primarily in milk and milk products, whereas *O. oenos* is isolated only from wine and related habitats. *L. pseudomesenteroides, L. citreum,* and *L. kimchii* are found on plants and vegetables and in dairy products. *L. gelidum, L. carnosum,* and *L. gasicomitatum* are found in meats (beef, pork, bacon, ham). *L. fallax* is found in pickled cabbage (sauer-

Table 13-11 Biochemical Characteristics for Identification of *Aerococcus* and *Helcococcus* Species

CHARACTERISTIC	A. VIRIDANS	A. URINAE	A. SANGUINICOLA	A. CHRISTENSENII	A. URINAEHOMINIS	H. KUNZII	H. OVIS
Cellular arrangement	Pairs, tetrads, clusters	Pairs, tetrads, clusters	Pairs, tetrads, clusters	Pairs, tetrads, clusters	Pairs, tetrads, clusters	Pairs, clusters	Pairs, clusters
Hemolysis	α	α	α	α	α	None, α	None
Growth, 10°C	NA	NA	NA	NA	NA	−	NA
Growth, 45°C	NA	NA	NA	NA	NA	−	NA
PYR	+	−	+	−	−	+	NA
LAP	−	+	+	+	−	−	+
Motility	−	−	−	−	−	−	−
Growth, BE agar	V	−	+	−	−	−	NA
Growth, 6.5% NaCl	+	+	+	−	+	V	NA
Esculin hydrolysis	+	V	+	−	+	+	−
Starch hydrolysis	NA	NA	NA	NA	NA	V	−
Hippurate hydrolysis	V	+	+	+	+	−	−
Arginine dihydrolase	−	−	−	−	−	−	−
Urease	−	−	−	−	−	−	−
Alkaline phosphatase	NA	−	NA	−	+^{w}	−	+
Acetoin	−	−	−	−	−	−	−
Acid from:							
Glucose	+	+	+	+	+	+	+
Maltose	V+	−	+	−	+	+	V
Sucrose	+	+	+	−	+	+	−
Lactose	V+	−	V−	−	−	+	−
Mannitol	V	+	+	−	−	−	−
Ribose	V	+	+	−	+	+	−
Trehalose	+	−	+	−	−	+	−
Arabinose	NA	−	−	−	−	−	−
Raffinose	NA	NA	−	−	−	−	−
Sorbitol	−	+	+	−	+	−	−
Glycogen	+	−	−	−	−	V	V
α-GAL	NA	−	−	−	−	−	NA
β-GAL	+	−	−	−	−	−	V
β-GUR	−	+	+	−	+	−	NA
α-GLU	NA	NA	−	NA	−	NA	NA
β-GLU	NA	−	−	−	V	+	−
NAGA	NA	NA	−	−	−	+	−

+, positive reaction; −, negative reaction; V, variable reaction; V+, variable, but most strains positive; V−, variable, but most strains negative; +^{w}, weak positive reaction; NA, data not available; PYR, pyrrolidonyl arylamidase; LAP, leucine aminopeptidase; α-GAL, α-galactosidase; β-GAL, β-galactosidase; β-GUR, β-glucuronidase; α-GLU, α-glucosidase; β-GLU, β-glucosidase; NAGA, N-acetyl-β-D-glucosaminidase.

kraut), and *L. argentinum* has been isolated from raw Argentinian milk.[284]

Leuconostoc species are gram-positive, catalase-negative, lactic acid-producing cocci that are resistant to vancomycin and produce CO_2 gas from glucose.[338] These bacteria may be differentiated from the gas-producing lactobacilli by careful scrutiny of Gram-stained smears made from thioglycolate broth (see Color Plates 13-3*E* and 13-3*F*). *Leuconostoc* species do not grow at 45°C and are arginine dihydrolase–negative, PYR-negative, and LAP-negative. Production of gas from glucose is best determined in *Lactobacillus* MRS (Mann-Rogosa-Sharpe) broth (Difco Laboratories, Detroit, MI) overlaid with sterile petrolatum. The formation of bubbles under the petrolatum seal indicates gas production and confirms their heterofermentative metabolism. *Leuconostoc* species are further identified by a battery of biochemical tests (Table 13-12). *Leuconostoc* species have also been identified by sodium dodecyl sulfate–polyacrylamide gel electrophoresis (SDS-PAGE) analysis of soluble whole-cell proteins.[323] Table 13-12 shows the phenotypic characteristics of *L. mesenteroides* subsp. *mesenteroides*, *L. mesenteroides* subsp. *dextranicum*, *L. mesenteroides* subsp. *cremoris*, *L. pseudomesenteroides*, *L. citreum*, *L. lactis*, and *Weissella paramesenteroides* (formerly *L. paramesenteroides*), which are the *Leuconostoc/ Weissella* species that have been isolated from human clinical specimens.

Pediococcus species are also intrinsically vancomycin-resistant gram-positive cocci. However, they are generally homofermentative, similar to the streptococci and, unlike *Leuconostoc* species, they do not produce gas from glucose in MRS broth.[338] The organisms appear as gram-positive cocci in pairs, clusters, and tetrads, and they are catalase-negative. Growth occurs over a temperature range of 25 to 50°C. On plates, they resemble viridans streptococci in their colony morphology. They may be confused with group D streptococci or enterococci because they are bile-esculin–positive, they possess the Lancefield group D antigen, and some strains grow in the presence of 6.5% NaCl. Pediococci are PYR-negative and LAP-positive. The species that have been recovered from human infections include *P. acidilactici* and *P. pentosaceus*. These organisms may be difficult to differentiate from one another, with maltose fermentation—positive for *P. pentosaceus* and negative for *P. acidilactici*—being the most reliable test for separation of the two. Tankovic and associates noted, however, that the two species could be separated by susceptibility to novobiocin.[944] All 25 *P. acidilactici* strains were susceptible to novobiocin (5-mg disk zone diameters, ≥16 mm), whereas all nine *P. pentosaceus* strains were resistant to novobiocin (zone diameters, ≤10 mm). Both of these species are susceptible to β-lactams, clindamycin, rifampin, erythromycin, gentamicin, and imipenem and are resistant to vancomycin, teicoplanin, and the fluoroquinolones.[944]

As mentioned, *P. halophilus* is phylogenetically closer to the enterococci and has been reclassified in the genus *Tetragenococcus* as *T. halophilus*. From data given in the original description of this species, *T. halophilus* characteristically grows as pairs or tetrads (hence, the name) and, occasionally, as clusters, does not grow at 10°C or at 45°C, is nonmotile, grows in 6.5% NaCl (actually will grow in up to 10% NaCl) and on BE agar, and is arginine dihydrolase–negative. Most strains produce acid from arabinose, glucose, glycerol, maltose, ribose, sucrose, and trehalose, and do not produce acid from lactose, mannose, mannitol, and sorbitol (see Table 13-13). Unlike the other pediococci, *T. halophilus* is susceptible to vancomycin. *T. muriaticus* is not associated with human infections.

Identification of *Gemella* Species

Of the six *Gemella* species that have been described, four—*G. haemolysans*, *G. morbillorum*, *G. bergeriae*, and *G sanguinis*—have been isolated from human clinical specimens. The two remaining species—*G. palaticanis* and *G. cuniculi*—are found in dogs and rabbits, respectively. *Gemella* species are catalase-negative, gram-positive cocci that characteristically grow as pinpoint colonies on SBA, often requiring 48 hours or more for distinct colonies to grow. Incubation in a CO_2-enriched atmosphere stimulates growth. They are α-hemolytic or nonhemolytic, except for the animal species *G. cuniculi*, which is β-hemolytic. On Gram-stained smears from broth cultures, the organisms appear as single cells, pairs, or short chains. All *Gemella* species are PYR-positive, LAP-positive, nonmotile, and fail to grow at 10°C or 45°C. They do not grow on BE agar, do not hydrolyze esculin, urea, starch, or gelatin, and do not grow in 6.5% NaCl broth. *Gemella* species can be differentiated on the basis of acid formation from maltose, sucrose, lactose, mannitol, sorbitol, and trehalose. *G. haemolysans* and *G. morbillorum*, the most common clinical isolates, can also be differentiated by reduction of nitrite. Because of their thin cell walls, *G. haemolysans* and *G. morbillorum* easily decolorize on Gram staining and may appear as gram-negative cocci in pairs, clusters, and short chains. Growth of some strains is enhanced by the presence of fermentable carbohydrates and by the addition of Tween 80 to the growth media. Because of limited numbers of clinical isolates, the performance of kit systems for identifying these bacteria cannot be assessed critically. Only *G. haemolysans* and *G. morbillorum* are included in the databases of the various kit systems at this time. Phenotypic characteristics for identification of *Gemella* species are found in Table 13-14.

Identification of *Vagococcus* Species

The genus *Vagococcus* includes the human and animal isolate, *V. fluvialis*, plus the animal isolates *V. salmoninarum*, *V. lutre*, and *V. fessus*. The genus *Vagococcus* was initially described as motile, group N lactococci, with the type strain being *V. fluvialis*. *V. fluvialis* is *Streptococcus*-like in its colony morphology and is α-hemolytic or nonhemolytic, facultative and homofermentative in its metabolism, and catalase-negative. On Gram stains, the organisms appear as spherical to ovoid cells, arranged in pairs or chains. According to the original description by Collins and coauthors, *V. fluvialis* are motile cocci that produce peritrichous flagella. Motility can be demonstrated with motility medium incubated at room temperature. *V. fluvialis* is PYR-positive, LAP-positive, and hydrolyzes esculin in the presence of 40%

Table 13-12 Phenotypic Characteristics for Identification of *Leuconostoc* Species Isolated From Human Clinical Specimens

CHARACTERISTIC	*L. MESENTEROIDES* SUBSP. *MESENTEROIDES*	*L. MESENTEROIDES* SUBSP. *DEXTRANICUM*	*L. MESENTEROIDES* SUBSP. *CREMORIS*	*L. PSEUDOMESENTEROIDES*	*L. CITREUM*	*L. LACTIS*	*WEISSELLA PARAMESENTEROIDES*
Hemolysis, SBA	–	–	–	–	–	–	–
Yellow pigment	–	–	–	–	+	–	–
Growth 10°C	NA	NA	NA	–	+	NA	NA
Growth, 37°C	V+	+	+	+	–	+	+
Growth, 45°C	–	–	–	–	–	–	–
LAP	–	–	–	–	–	–	–
PYR	–	–	–	–	–	–	–
Esculin hydrolysis	+	V+	–	+	+	V–	V+
Dextran from sucrose	+	+	–	NA	NA	–	–
Acid produced from:							
Amygdalin	V	V	–	V–	V+	–	–
Arabinose	V+	–	–	V+	+	–	+
Cellobiose	V+	V	–	V+	+	+	V
Fructose	+	+	V	+	+	+	+
Galactose	V+	V	+	V+	V–	+	+
Glucose	+	+	+	+	+	+	+
Lactose	V	+	V	V	–	+	–
Maltose	+	+	V–	+	+	+	+
Mannitol	+	V	–	V–	V	–	+
Mannose	+	V	V	+	+	+	+
Melibiose	+	V	V–	V+	–	V+	+
Raffinose	V+	V	V–	V+	–	V+	V–
Ribose	V+	NA	V–	+	–	–	+
Salicin	+	V	–	V	+	–	V–
Starch	–	–	–	+	–	–	–
Sucrose	+	+	V	V+	+	+	+
Trehalose	+	+	V	+	+	V	+
Xylose	+	V	V–	+	V–	–	+
Habitat	Dairy products, vegetation	Dairy products	Dairy products	Plants, vegetation, dairy products	Plants	Dairy products	Dairy products

+, positive reaction; –, negative reaction; V+, most strains positive; V–, most strains negative; rare strains positive; V, variable reaction; NA, data not available; LAP, leucine aminopeptidase; PYR, pyrrolidonyl arylamidase.

Table 13-13 Characteristics for Identification of *Pediococcus* Species and *Tetragenococcus halophilus*

CHARACTERISTIC	P. ACIDILACTICI	P. PENTOSACEUS	P. DEXTRINICUS	P. DAMNOSUS	P. PARVULUS	P. INOPINATUS	T. HALOPHILUS
Growth, 45°C	+	V	−	−	−	−	−
Acid produced from:							
Glucose	+	+	+	+	+	+	+
Maltose	−	+	+	V	+	+	+
Arabinose	V	+	−	−	−	−	+
Starch	−	−	+	−	−	−	−
Glycerol	−	−	−	−	−	−	+
Melezitose	−	−	−	V	−	−	+
Dextrin	−	−	+	−	−	V	−
Xylose	+	V	−	−	−	−	−
Novobiocin	S	R	NA	NA	NA	NA	NA

+, positive reaction; −, negative reaction; V, variable reaction; NA, data not available; S, susceptible to novobiocin (5-mg disk zone, ≥16 mm); R, resistant to novobiocin (5-mg disk zone, ≤10 mm).

bile (Table 13-15).[950] Most strains grow at 10°C, but growth at 45°C is variable. Most strains also grow in 6.5% NaCl, and some strains produce acetoin.[336,950] *V. fluvialis* produces acid from glucose, maltose, mannitol, sorbitol, ribose and trehalose, but not from arabinose, inulin, melibiose, or raffinose (Table 13-15).[950] Strains of *V. fluvialis* have been recovered from pigs, cats, and horses; these strains were VP-, alkaline phosphatase- and LAP-positive, and some of the strains were nonmotile.[781] Isolates of *V. fluvialis* recovered from human clinical specimens are susceptible to ampicillin, cefotaxime, trimethoprim-sulfamethoxazole, and vancomycin and are resistant to clindamycin and oflaxacin.[950]

V. salmoninarum, V. lutre, and *V. fessus* are found in diseased fish, the common otter, and seals and porpoises, respectively, so their isolation from human clinical specimens is unlikely. All three species are α-hemolytic cocci that appear as single cells, pairs, or chains on Gram-stained smears from broth cultures. Unlike *V. fluvialis* and *V. lutre,* *V. salmoninarum* is nonmotile and produces H₂S. *V. fluvialis* also produces acid from glycerol and sorbitol, while *V. salmoninarum* does not. *V. lutre* is motile, but it can be differentiated from *V. fluvialis* by its positive reactions for α-galactosidase and β-galactosidase.[608] Although the motility of *V. fessus* has not been described, this species can be differentiated from *V. fluvialis, V. lutre,* and *V. salmoninarum* by its inability to produce acid from maltose, ribose, sucrose, or trehalose. Both *V. salmoninarum* and *V. fluvialis* produce positive reactions with the AccuProbe *Enterococcus* test (Gen-Probe). Members of the genus *Vagococcus* are not included in the databases of any of the commercial identification systems.

Identification of *Alloiococcus, Globicatella, Facklamia, Dolosigranulum, Ignavigranum,* and *Dolosicoccus* Species

The organisms included in the genus *Alloiococcus* and the genera *Globicatella, Facklamia, Dolosigranulum,* and *Ignavigranum* are *Gemella*-like species that are able to grow

in 6.5% NaCl (Table 13-16). *A. otitidis,* the sole member of the genus *Alloiococcus,* is isolated from tympanocentesis specimens obtained from the middle ear of children with chronic otitis media, from blood cultures, and from sputum.[6,620] The organism grows slowly on agar media, with visible colonies apparent only after 2 to 3 days, and it does not grow in thioglycolate broth. Gram-stained smears from agar media show cocci arranged in pairs, tetrads, and sometimes clusters. Optimal growth occurs at 35 to 37°C and requires CO₂, and no growth occurs at either 10°C or 45°C.[688] Colonies appear off-white, pinpoint, and nonhemolytic, although α-hemolysis and slightly yellow pigmentation may be observed after several days of incubation.[118] Fresh clinical isolates of *A. otitidis* will grow on blood agar but may not grow on chocolate agar. Luxuriant growth in broth containing 0.5% Tween or 0.07% lecithin suggests that the organism may require lipid for optimal growth. Unlike the other organisms considered in this chapter, *A. otitidis* is catalase-positive; this reaction may be quite weak or delayed. The organism is aerobic rather than facultative and does not produce acid from any carbohydrates. *A. otitidis* grows on bile-esculin agar but does not hydrolyze esculin, and grows slowly in 6.5% NaCl broth. PYR, LAP, and β-galactosidase are produced, and hippurate is hydrolyzed by some isolates. Bosley and colleagues performed antimicrobial susceptibility studies on 19 *A. otitidis* strains and found that all 19 were resistant to trimethoprim-sulfamethoxazole and 18 were resistant to erythromycin.[118] The MICs for penicillin and ampicillin ranged from susceptible to intermediately resistant (MIC range for penicillin, 0.06 to 0.12 μg/mL; ampicillin MIC range, 0.12 to 0.5 μg/mL), with the same degree of relative resistance being seen for ceftriaxone and cefixime. None of the strains they examined produced β-lactamase enzymes.[118]

G. sanguinis has been recovered from human specimens, including blood, CSF, and urine. On Gram-stained smears from broth cultures, these organisms appear as gram-positive cocci in pairs and short chains. Colonies on sheep blood

Table 13-14 Phenotypic Characteristics for Identification of Gemella Species

CHARACTERISTIC	G. HAEMOLYSANS	G. MORBILLORUM	G. BERGERIAE	G. SANGUINIS	G. PALATICANIS	G. CUNICULI
Hemolysis	None, α	None, α	None, α	None, β	None	β
Growth, 10°C	-	-	-	-	NA	NA
Growth, 45°C	-	-	-	-	NA	NA
PYR	+	+	+	+	NA	NA
LAP	+	+	+	+	NA	NA
Motility	-	-	-	-	-	-
Bile-esculin	-	-	-	-	NA	NA
Growth, 6.5% NaCl	-	-	-	-	NA	NA
Esculin hydrolysis	-	-	-	-	-	-
Hippurate hydrolysis	-	-	-	-	-	NA
Starch hydrolysis	-	-	-	-	NA	NA
Arginine dihydrolase	-	-	-	-	-	-
Urease	-	-	-	-	-	-
Alkaline phosphatase	V+	-	-	+	-	+
Acetoin (VP)	-	-	-	V	-	-
Production of:						
α-GAL	-	-	-	-	-	-
β-GAL	-	-	-	-	-	-
α-GLU	NA	NA	NA	NA	NA	-
β-GLU	-	-	NA	NA	NA	-
β-GUR	-	-	-	-	NA	-
NAGA	NA	-	-	-	NA	-
NO₃ reduction	-	-	-	-	-	-
NO₂ reduction	+	-	NA	NA	NA	NA
Acid from:						
Glucose	+	+	+	+	+	+
Maltose	+	+	-/+ʷ	+	+	-
Sucrose	V	+	-	+	+w	-
Lactose	-	-	-	V-	+	-
Mannitol	-	V+	V-	+	-	+
Sorbitol	-	V+	-	+	-	+
Trehalose	-	-	-	-	+	-
Habitat	Humans	Humans	Humans	Humans	Canines	Rabbits

+, positive reaction; − negative reaction; V, variable reaction; V+, variable but most strains negative; positive strains produce weak reactions; −/+ʷ, most strains negative, positive strains produce weak reactions; NA, data not available; PYR, pyrrolidonyl arylamidase; LAP, leucine aminopeptidase; α-GAL, α-galactosidase; β-GAL, β-galactosidase; α-GLU, α-glucosidase; β-GLU, β-glucosidase; β-GUR, β-glucuronidase; NAGA, N-acetyl-β-D-glucosaminidase.

Table 13-15 Biochemical Characteristics for Identification of *Vagococcus* Species

CHARACTERISTIC	V. FLUVIALIS	V. SALMONINARUM	V. LUTRE	V. FESSUS
Cellular arrangement	Single, pairs, short chains	Single, pairs, short chains	Single, pairs, short chains	Single, pairs, short chains
Hemolysis, SBA	α, γ	α, γ	NA	α
Growth, 10°C	V+	+	NA	NA
Growth, 45°C	V−	−	NA	NA
Motility	+	−	+	−
Catalase	−	−	−	−
LAP	+	NA	NA	+
PYR	+	NA	NA	NA
Esculin hydrolysis	+	+	+	NA
Growth, 6.5% NaCl	+	+	NA	NA
Arginine dihydrolase	V	−	−	−
Hippurate hydrolysis	−	−	−	−
Urease	−	−	−	−
Growth, BE agar	+	NA	NA	NA
H$_2$S in KIA	−	+	NA	NA
Acetoin	V	−	−	−
Alkaline phosphatase	NA	NA	NA	V
Vancomycin	S	S	S	S
Acid produced from:				
Glucose/gas	+/−	+/−	+	+
Maltose	+	+	+	−
Sucrose	V	+	+	−
Lactose	−	−	−	−
Mannitol	+	−	−	−
Sorbitol	+	−	+	−
Arabinose	−	−	−	−
Melibiose	−	−	−	−
Raffinose	−	−	−	−
Ribose	+	+	+	−
Trehalose	+	+	+	−
Glycogen	NA	−	−	−
Hydrolysis of:				
α-GAL	−	NA	+	−
β-GAL	V	NA	−/+^{w}	V
α-GLU	NA	NA	+	−
β-GLU	NA	NA	+	V
β-GUR	−	NA	−	−
NAGA	NA	NA	+	−
Habitat	Water, human clinical specimens	Salmonid fish	Otters	Seals, harbor porpoises

+, positive reaction; −, negative reaction; +^{w}, weak positive reaction; NA, data not available; LAP, leucine aminopeptidase; PYR, pyrrolidonyl arylamidase; α-GAL, α-galactosidase; β-GAL, β-galactosidase; α-GLU, α-glucosidase; β-GLU, β-glucosidase; β-GUR, β-glucuronidase; NAGA, N-acetyl-β-D-glucosaminidase.

Table 13-16 Phenotypic Characteristics for Identification of *Globicatella, Alloiococcus, Facklamia, Ignavigranulum, Dolosigranulum,* and *Dolosicoccus* Species

CHARACTERISTIC	G. SANGUINIS	G. SULFIDIFACIENS	A. OTITIDIS	F. HOMINIS	F. IGNAVA	F. SOUREKII	F. LANGUIDA	F. TABACINALIS	F. MIROUNGAE	I. RUOFFIAE	D. PIGRUM	D. PAUCIVORANS
Cellular arrangement	Short chains, pairs	Singly, pairs, short chains	Pairs, tetrads, Clusters	Clusters, pairs	Pairs, short chains	Pairs, short chains	Pairs, short chains	Pairs, single cells, short chains	Pairs, short chains	Single cells, pairs, clusters	Clusters, tetrads	Pairs, short chains
Hemolysis, SBA	α	α	γ	α	γ	α	γ	α	α	γ	α	α
Growth, 10°C	-	NA	-	-	-	-	-	-	NA	-	-	-
Growth, 45°C	+	NA	-	-	-	-	-	-	NA	-	-	-
Motility	-	-	-	-	-	-	-	-	-	-	-	-
Catalase	-	-	+	-	-	-	-	-	-	-	-	-
LAP	-	NA	+	+	+	+	+	+	+	+	+	+
PYR	V+	-	+	V+	+	+	+	+	+	+	+	+
Esculin hydrolysis	+	NA	-	-	-	-	-	-	-	-	+	-
Growth, 6.5% broth	+	+	+	+	+	+	+	+	+	+	+	-
Arginine dihydrolase	-	-	-	+	-	-	-	-	+	+	-	NA
Hippurate hydrolysis	+	-	V	+	+	+	-	-	-	-	-	-
Urease	-	-	-	V	+	+	-	-	+	+	-	-
Growth, BE agar	+	+	+	NA	NA	NA	NA	NA	NA	NA	+	+
H₂S in KIA	-	+	NA	NA	NA	NA	NA	NA	NA	NA	NA	NA
Acetoin (VP)	-	-	NA	-	-	-	-	-	-	-	-	-
Alkaline phosphatase	NA	-	NA	-	-	V	+	-	V	-	-	-
Vancomycin	S	S	S	S	S	S	S	S	S	S	S	S
Acid produced from:												
Glucose	+	+	-	-	+ʷ	+	+	+	+	+	+	+
Maltose	+	+	-	-	-	+	+	-	+	-	+	+ʷ
Sucrose	+	+	-	-	-	+	-	+	-	+	-	+
Lactose	V+	-	-	-	-	-	-	-	-	-	-	+ʷ
Mannitol	+	-	-	-	-	+	-	+	-	V	V	+ʷ
Sorbitol	V	-	-	-	-	+	-	+	-	-	-	-
Arabinose	V	-	-	-	-	-	-	-	-	-	V	-
Melibiose	+	-	-	-	-	-	-	-	-	-	NA	-
Raffinose	+	+	-	-	-	-	-	-	-	-	+	+
Ribose	V+	-	-	-	-	-	-	-	-	-	NA	+
Trehalose	+	+	-	-	-	+	+	-	+	-	NA	-
Glycogen	+	NA	-	-	-	-	-	-	-	-	NA	-
Production of:												
α-GAL	NA	+	-	+	-	-	-	+	-	+	+	-
β-GAL	+	-	+	+	-	-	-	-	-	-	V	-
α-GLU	NA	NA	NA	NA	-	-	-	-	-	-	NA	-
β-GLU	V	NA	NA	-	-	-	-	-	-	-	NA	-
β-GUR	NA	NA	NA	-	-	-	-	-	-	-	NA	-
NAGA	NA	NA	NA	NA	-	-	-	-	V+	-	V	-

+, positive reaction; −, negative reaction; V, variable reaction; V+, variable but most strains positive; +ʷ, weak positive reaction; V−, variable but most strains negative; NA, data not available; LAP, leucine aminopeptidase; PYR, pyrrolidonyl arylamidase; α-GAL, α-galactosidase; β-GAL, β-galactosidase; α-GLU, α-glucosidase; β-GLU, β-glucosidase; β-GUR, β-glucuronidase; NAGA, N-acetyl-β-D-glucosaminidase.

agar are *Streptococcus*-like and are α-hemolytic. Like the enterococci, *G. sanguinis* is bile-esculin–positive, grows in 6.5% NaCl, and produces PYR; unlike both the enterococci and the streptococci, LAP is not produced. *G. sanguinis* grows at 45°C but not at 10°C.[884] These reactions also differentiate *G. sanguinis* from other viridans streptococci in that the latter species are PYR-negative and LAP-positive and do not grow in 6.5% NaCl broth. The BactiCard STREP (Remel), which includes rapid PYR, LAP, and esculin hydrolysis tests in a card format, can be used for these determinations. Unlike the aerococci, *G. sanguinis* produces distinct chains in broth media instead of tetrads. This growth characteristic must be determined to differentiate *G. sanguinis* from *A. viridans*, which, like *G. sanguinis*, is LAP-negative, PYR-positive, and hippurate hydrolysis-positive. *G. sanguinis* produces acid from several carbohydrates, including glucose, maltose, sucrose, lactose, mannitol, raffinose, and trehalose; acid production from arabinose, ribose, and sorbitol is variable (Table 13-16). *G. sanguinis* is in the database of the BBL Crystal Gram-Positive ID kit, but not in the databases of the API Rapid Strep, the RapID STR, or the ID32 identification systems.[884] Using CLSI breakpoints for *Streptococcus* species other than *S. pneumoniae*, Shewmaker and colleagues determined the antimicrobial susceptibility of 28 strains of *G. sanguinis* and found that all strains were susceptible to amoxicillin and vancomycin, and some strains had penicillin MICs that fell in the intermediate range.[884] Variable susceptibility was observed for other agents, including cefotaxime (52% susceptible), cefuroxime (26% susceptible), meropenem (63% susceptible), erythromycin (52% susceptible), trimethoprim-sulfamethoxazole (48% susceptible), clindamycin (70% susceptible), and tetracycline (48% susceptible).

The bovine/ovine pathogen, *G. sulfidifaciens*, can easily be differentiated from *G. sanguinis*.[991] *G. sulfidifaciens* produces H₂S and β-glucuronidase, while *G. sanguinis* does not. *G. sanguinis* also produces β-galactosidase, ferments mannitol, and hydrolyzes hippurate; *G. sulfidifaciens* produces negative reactions in these three tests.

Members of the genus *Facklamia* are catalase-negative, gram-positive cocci that are related to but phylogenetically distinct from *Globicatella* species. Species isolated from human clinical specimens are *F. hominis*, *F. sourekii*, *F. ignava*, and *F. languida*. *F. miroungae* and *F. tabacinalis* have been isolated from elephant seals and powdered tobacco, respectively. On Gram-stained smears from thioglycolate broth, *Facklamia* species appear as gram-positive cocci arranged in pairs or short chains, except for *F. hominus*, which usually forms clusters. On SBA, colonies are usually α-hemolytic and similar to viridans streptococci. *Facklamia* species do not grow on bile-esculin media, but do grow in 6.5% NaCl. *Facklamia* species do not grow at either 10°C or 45°C and are LAP- and PYR-positive (Table 13-16).

The genus *Ignavigranum*, with its single species, *I. ruoffiae*, was first described in 1999. This species grows primarily as chains in thioglycolate broth and is closely related phylogenetically to both *F. hominis* and *G. sanguinis*. *I. ruoffiae* is PYR- and LAP-positive, grows in 6.5% NaCl broth, and does not hydrolyze esculin. Some strains are arginine dihydrolase–positive. Although most strains of *F. hominis*

are also arginine dihydrolase–positive, this species is hippurate hydrolysis-positive, while *I. ruoffiae* is hippurate-negative (Table 13-16). A distinctive feature of *I. ruoffiae* is the "sauerkraut" odor produced by the organism when grown on SBA.

The genus *Dolosigranulum* contains a single species, *D. pigrum*. On SBA, this organism grows as small, grayish-white, α-hemolytic colonies. On Gram stains from broth (both thioglycolate, and, in one case report, Organon-Teknika BacT/Alert FAN blood culture medium), this organism appears in pairs, *Gemella*-like tetrads, and clusters.[451] Like *Facklamia* species, *D. pigrum* is PYR- and LAP-positive and grows in 6.5% salt. This organism is esculin hydrolysis–positive, but this reaction may take several days to develop. No growth is observed at 10 or 45°C or on BE agar (Table 13-16).

The genus *Dolosicoccus*, with its single member, *Dolosicoccus paucivorans*, is a new group that is based on two isolates recovered from human blood cultures. This organism is distinct from, but phylogenetically related to the *Facklamia* and *Globicatella* genera. Like the organism discussed above, *D. paucivorans* is PYR-positive, but unlike these others, it is LAP-negative, does not grow in 6.5% NaCl broth, and appears on broth Gram-stained smears as single cells, pairs, and short chains. Like *D. pigrum*, *D. paucivorans* does not grow on BE medium, and does not grow at 10 or 45°C (Table 13-16).

Identification of *Lactococcus* Species

Because of the superficial resemblance to enterococci or the viridans streptococci, these organisms have been misidentified as atypical streptococci or enterococci in the clinical laboratory. The lactococci show many of the characteristics of both streptococci and enterococci; many strains are PYR-, LAP-, BE-, and 6.5% NaCl-positive, and are able to grow at 10°C. Lactococci, unlike enterococci, do not grow at 45°C. A tip-off to the possibility that an isolate is a *Lactococcus* species is the generation of a list of characteristics that do not fit either streptococci or enterococci.[336] Most clinical isolates of lactococci submitted to the CDC have been either *L. lactis* subsp. *lactis* or *L. garvieae*. These two species can be differentiated from common *Enterococcus* species in that both species produce acid from mannitol but do not produce acid from raffinose, sorbitol, or arabinose. *L. garvieae*, *L. lactis* subsp. *cremoris*, *L. lactis* subsp. *lactis*, and *L. raffinolactis* are included in the database of the ID32 Strep, API Rapid Strep, and BBL Crystal identification kits, respectively (see the following section). Oligonucleotide probe methods and genus-specific PCR techniques for separating enterococci and lactococci have also been described.[259,839] Biochemical characteristics for identifying *Lactococcus* species are presented in Table 13-17.

Commercially Available Systems for Identification of Streptococci, Enterococci, and Selected "Streptococcus-Like" Bacteria

The development of kit systems that incorporate similar types of physiologic and enzymatic tests for streptococcal identification have been of great help in species identifica-

Table 13-17 Phenotypic Characteristics for Identification of *Lactococcus* Species

TEST	L. LACTIS SUBSP. LACTIS	L. LACTIS SUBSP. CREMORIS	L. LACTIS SUBSP. HORDNIAE	L. GAR-VEIAE	L. PLAN-TARUM	L. RAFFINO-LACTIS	L. XY-LOSUS
Arginine dihydrolase	+	−	+	+	−	−	+
Hippurate hydrolysis	−	+	−	−	−	−	−
PYR	V	−	−	+	−	−	−
Acetoin (VP)	+	+	+	+	+	+	+
Acid produced from:							
Glucose	+	+	+	+	+	+	+
Maltose	+	−	−	+	+	+	+
Sucrose	+	−	+	V	+	−	+
Lactose	+	+	−	V	−	+	−
Mannitol	+	−	−	+	+	V	+
Sorbitol	−	−	−	−	+	−	−
Raffinose	−	−	−	−	−	+	−
Trehalose	+	−	+	+	+	−	+

+, positive reaction; −, negative reaction; V, variable reaction; PYR, pyrrolidonyl arylamidase.

tion of the viridans streptococci, *Enterococcus* species, and the group D streptococci. The biochemical reactions included in the kit systems are used to generate an organism biotype number that corresponds to the organism's identity. Although these systems include the β-hemolytic streptococci in their databases, these organisms are best handled using other methods, such as the presumptive tests described earlier or the rapid streptococcal-grouping kits that are available. However, caution should also be exercised with the commercial identification kits. For example, the API Rapid Strep will misidentify *Leuconostoc* organisms as species of viridans streptococci, so vancomycin resistance and other preliminary test results must be considered along with the biochemical reactions that are observed on the strip. Commercial systems for the identification of streptococci include the following.

API RAPID STREP

This strip format system (BioMérieux) includes 20 tests, including physiologic tests, chromogenic enzyme substrate tests, and carbohydrate-utilization tests. The unique thing about this system is that the strip can be read twice. If an identification is not obtained after 4 hours of incubation using the physiologic and chromogenic substrates, the strip can be reincubated and read after overnight incubation to include acid production from 10 carbohydrates (see Color Plate 13-3*C*). The database includes groupable β-hemolytic streptococci, *Enterococcus* species (*E. faecalis*, *E. faecium*, *E. gallinarum*, *E. avium*, and *E. durans*), viridans streptococci, lactococci, aerococci, *Gemella* species, *S. bovis* strains, and *Listeria monocytogenes*. The API Rapid Strep is now the most widely available commercial system for identifying the streptococci and *Streptococcus*-like bacteria. Identification of strains that have been completely characterized by conventional biochemical tests and genetic analysis

(e.g., DNA relatedness, 16S rRNA sequencing) indicate that the API Rapid Strep system is reproducible and complements existing genetic studies. In some cases, tests on the strip actually revealed phenotypic differences not seen with conventional methods. In other instances, the presence of phenotypic differences between strains on the Rapid Strep system could be demonstrated to be genotypically distinct when nucleic-acid studies were performed. The biochemical reactions for many organisms shown in the tables of this chapter reflect the recent studies during which genetic analysis and the description of new species were performed along with the API Rapid Strep characterization. However, the database for this system has not been updated or expanded to include newer streptococcal species (e.g., *S. vestibularis*, *S. gordonii*, *S. crista*).

BBL CRYSTAL GRAM-POSITIVE IDENTIFICATION SYSTEM

The Crystal Gram-Positive identification system contains 29 dried biochemical and enzymatic substrates plus a fluorescence-negative control. The inoculum is prepared by suspending colonies of the pure isolate in the fluid provided with the kit to a turbidity equivalent to a 0.5 McFarland standard. The suspension is then poured into a specific area of the base of the panel, which is then manipulated to distribute the inoculum. The panel lid, which contains the test substrates, is then snapped onto the base, with consequent hydration of the substrates with the inoculum. After incubation, tests are read for fluorescence or for changes in the colors of pH indicators using a special panel viewer. The resulting pattern of the 29 reactions is converted into a 10-digit profile number that correlates with an identification provided by the Crystal Electronic Code book. The panel can be interpreted using a 4-hour or an 18–24-hour incubation database.

In an evaluation of this system, the Crystal Gram-Positive identified all strains of groupable β-hemolytic streptococci and *S. pneumoniae*, but only identified 25 of 37 strains of viridans streptococci to the species level. The system correctly identified all of 23 *E. faecalis*, 2 of 2 *E. avium*, and all of 14 *E. faecium*.[1016] Hudson and coworkers challenged the system with genotypically defined veterinary strains of enterococci and found that repeated testing of the same strains resulted in different profile numbers, some of which resulted in different identifications.[502] In fact, 19 of the 50 strains tested were identified at different times as both *E. faecalis* and *E. faecium*. When this system was challenged with 55 isolates that belong to the *Streptococcus*-like genera (i.e., *Alloiococcus otitidis*, *Facklamia* species, *D. pigrum*, and *I. ruoffiae*) that are not in the current database, the system produced "unacceptable identification" results for 14 isolates, and misidentified the others as *Micrococcus* species.[594]

RAPID ID 32 STREP

This system (BioMérieux) is a 32-test strip format identification system for the streptococci and *Streptococcus*-like bacteria. The database of this system is extensive and includes the groupable streptococci, several *Enterococcus* species, and the viridans streptococci (including newly described species such as the "mutans group" oral streptococci, *S. oralis*, *S. gordonii*, and *S. vestibularis*). A suspension of the organism is prepared in sterile water to a turbidity equivalent of a McFarland 4 standard and 55 μL of the suspension is placed into each of the 32 cupules. The strip is incubated at 35 to 37°C for 4 hours and either read manually using a code book or with the automated reader (ATB 1520 Reader linked with an ATB 1545 computer, BioMérieux; see Color Plate 13-3*G*). In an evaluation of the Rapid ID 32 Strep system with 433 strains belonging to the genera *Streptococcus*, *Enterococcus*, *Lactococcus*, *Aerococcus*, *Gemella*, *Leuconostoc*, *Erysipelothrix*, *Gardnerella*, and *Listeria*, 95.3% of strains were correctly identified.[378] Additional tests were required for identification of 25.1% of the strains. Only 16 isolates (3.7%) were not identified, and only four isolates (1.0%) were misidentified. Another evaluation by Kikuchi and coworkers reported that the ID32 Strep system identified 87% of 156 viridans streptococcal strains and that most misidentification involved strains of *S. oralis*, *S. mitis*, and *S. gordonii*.[566] Jensen and colleagues tested 122 streptococcal and enterococcal isolates on the ID 32 Strep system and found that, regardless of whether reaction interpretations were obtained by automated or manual reading, 75–77% of the 122 strains were identified correctly, 7% were misidentified, and 16–18% were not identified.[534] Most of the pyogenic cocci and enterococci and only two thirds of the viridans streptococci were correctly identified. When tested with 55 isolates of "*Streptococcus*-like" organisms not included in the current database, the ID 32 Strep correctly provided no identifications for all of 27 *D. pigrum*, 6 of 18 *Facklamia* species, and 2 of 3 *I. ruoffiae* isolates as "unacceptable identifications."[594] The most common misidentifications of *Facklamia* species provided by the ID 32 were as various *Streptococcus* and *Gemella* species.

RapID STR

The RapID STR system (Remel) uses a small cuvette containing 10 wells, 4 of which are bifunctional, resulting in a total of 14 biochemical tests (used in conjunction with the hemolytic reaction of the isolate). Tests include physiologic determinations (arginine dihydrolase, esculin hydrolysis), carbohydrate-utilization tests, and chromogenic enzyme substrate hydrolysis (see Color Plate 13-3*H*). The system is inoculated with a suspension of the organism (McFarland 1 turbidity standard) prepared in a fluid purchased with the kit, and the tests are read after 4-hour incubation at 35°C in a non-CO$_2$ incubator. The database of this system includes the β-hemolytic streptococci groups A, B, and C/G, group D streptococci (*S. bovis*, *S. bovis* variant, *S. equinus*), the *S. milleri* group (*S. anginosus*, *S. constellatus*, *S. intermedius*), *Enterococcus* species (*E. faecalis*, *E. faecium*, *E. avium*, *E. cassiliflavus/mundtii*, *E. durans/hirae*, *E. gallinarum*, *E. raffinosus*, and *E. malodoratus*), viridans streptococcal species (*S. mitis*, *S. mutans*, *S. salivarius/vestibularis*, *S. sanguinis/gordonii*), *S. pneumoniae*, *Aerococcus* species, *Gemella morbillorum*, *Leuconostoc* species, *Lactococcus* species (*L. lactis*, *L. mesenteroides* group), and *Pediococcus* species (*P. acidilactici*, *P. pentosaceus*). The recently described viridans streptococci, enterococci, and *Streptococcus*-like bacteria are not included in the database at this time. In a recent study by Shewmaker et al. on phenotypic characterization of 28 *G. sanguinis* strains, the RapID STR misidentified 7 strains: 5 as *S. mutans*, 1 as *E. casseliflavus*, and 1 as *E. malodoratus*, while the remaining strains gave inadequate profiles for identification.[884] At present, the newly described *Streptococcus*-like genera are not part of the RapID Strep database. LaClaire and Facklam tested 27 *D. pigrum* isolates on the RapID Strep; only one of 27 *D. pigrum* strains provided a "no choice" identification, 2 produced a "questionable biocode," and the remainder were identified as "inadequate ID, *E. faecalis* 90%." Two of 18 *Facklamia* species and all 3 *I. ruoffiae* isolates tested were correctly identified as "no choice" by the RapID Strep system.[594] *A. otitidis* isolates were misidentified as *G. morbillorum*, *A. viridans*, *S. mitis*, or *S. acidominimus*.

VITEK GRAM-POSITIVE IDENTIFICATION (GPI) CARD

The GPI card (BioMérieux) is the same one used for identifying the coagulase-negative staphylococci and certain non-spore-forming facultative gram-positive bacilli. The card contains 30 wells, 29 of which contain biochemical identification substrates, with the remaining well being a negative control. The card provides automated identifications in from 2 to 15 hours. This card has been modified slightly since its initial release, and the database has been updated. The database for streptococcal identification includes the β-hemolytic streptococci (groups A, B, C, and G), group D streptococci (*S. bovis*, *S. bovis* variant, and *S. equinus*), *S. pneumoniae*, seven *Enterococcus* species (*E. faecalis*, *E. faecium*, *E. avium*, *E. durans*, *E. casseliflavus*, *E. gallinarum*, and *E. hirae*), some species of viridans streptococci (*S. mitis*, *S. mutans*, *S. oralis*, *S. salivarius*, *S. sanguinis/gordonii*, and *S. uberis*), the anginosus group (*S. anginosus*, *S. constellatus*, and *S. intermedius*), *Aerococcus* species, and *Gemella morbillorum*. As with the other systems, the more recently described viridans streptococcal species are not yet included in the database. The GPI card database also includes some *Staphylococcus*, *Corynebacterium*,

Arcanobacterium, *Listeria*, and *Erysipelothrix* species. The modified card with the expanded database has not been recently evaluated for its ability to correctly identify the viridans streptococci. The GPI card is able to correctly identify *E. faecalis* and *E. faecium*, but it performs less well for identifying other *Enterococcus* species.[135]

MICROSCAN GRAM-POSITIVE BREAKPOINT COMBO PANEL

The MicroScan identification panels (Dade MicroScan, West Sacramento, CA) provide simultaneous identification and antimicrobial susceptibility results in a microtiter format. Tritz and colleagues evaluated this system for its ability to identify enterococci and found that both *E. faecalis* and *E. faecium* were reliably identified, but less common enterococcal species were misidentified.[963] Iwen and colleagues evaluated the revised MicroScan Dried Overnight Gram-Positive Identification panel for its ability to identify 8 different *Enterococcus* species and found that the system identified 98.5% of isolates tested; resolution of low-probability identifications with additional tests (i.e., motility and pigmentation) was only necessary for *E. gallinarum/casseliflavus* isolates.[514]

Other microtiter format systems for streptococcal identification are available from American MicroScan (Sacramento, CA) and from MicroMedia (San Jose, CA), but these have not been evaluated.

REFERENCES

1. Aarestrup FM, Rasmussen SR, Artursson K, Jensen NE. Trends in the resistance to antimicrobial agents of *Streptococcus suis* isolates from Denmark and Sweden. Vet Microbiol 1998;63:71–80.
2. Adams JT, Faix RG. *Streptococcus mitis* infection in newborns. J Perinatol 1994;14:473–478.
3. Adderson EE, Takahashi S, Wang Y, et al. Subtractive hybridization identifies a novel predicted protein mediating epithelial cell invasion by virulent serotype III group B *Streptococcus agalactiae*. Infect Immun 2003;71:6857–6863.
4. Adegbola RA, Obaro SK, Biney E, Greenwood BM. Evaluation of Binax NOW *Streptococcus pneumoniae* urinary antigen test in children in a community with a high carriage rate of pneumococcus. Pediatr Infect Dis J 2001;20:718–719.
5. Afessa B, Greaves WL, Frederick WR. Pneumococcal bacteremia in adults: a 14-year experience in an inner-city university hospital. Clin Infect Dis 1995; 21:345–351.
6. Aguirre M, Collins MD. Phylogenetic analysis of *Alloiococcus otitis* gen. nov. sp. nov., an organism from human middle ear fluid. Int J Syst Bacteriol 1992; 42:79–83.
7. Aguirre M, Collins MD. Development of a polymerase chain reaction-probe test for identification of *Alloiococcus otitis*. J Clin Microbiol 1992;30:2177–2180.
8. Aguirre M, Collins MD. Phylogenetic analysis of some *Aerococcus*-like organisms from urinary tract infections: description of *Aerococcus urinae* sp. nov. J Gen Microbiol 1992;138:401–405.
9. Aguirre M, Collins MD. Development of polymerase chain reaction test for specific identification of the urinary tract pathogen *Aerococcus urinae*. J Clin Microbiol 1993;31:1350–1353.
10. Aguirre M, Collins MD. Lactic acid bacteria and human clinical infection. J Appl Microbiol 1993;75:95–107.
11. Aguirre M, Morrison D, Cookson BD, et al. Phenotypic and phylogenetic characterization of some *Gemella*-like organisms from human infections: description of *Dolosigranulum pigrum* gen. nov., sp. nov. J Appl Microbiol 1993;75: 608–612.
12. Ahmed R, Hassall T, Morland B, Gray J. Viridans streptococcal bacteremia in children on chemotherapy for cancer: as underestimated problem. Pediatr Hematol Oncol 2003;20:439–444.
13. Akesson P, Linder A, Cronqvist J Christensson B. Group A streptococcus bacteraemia complicated by osteomyelitis in an immunocompetent adult. Scand J Infect Dis 2004;36:63–65.
14. Akesson P, Sjoholm AG, Bjorck L. Protein SIC, a novel extracellular protein of *Streptococcus pyogenes* interfering with complement function. J Biol Chem 1996;271:1081–1088.
15. Alam S, Brailsford SR, Whiley RA, Beighton D. PCR-based methods for genotyping viridans group streptococci. J Clin Microbiol 1999;37:2772–2776.
16. Alba D, Zapater P, Torres E. Recurrent *Streptococcus sanguis* meningitis in a patient with a ventriculoperitoneal shunt. Clin Infect Dis 1994;19:808.
17. Alberti S, Ashbaugh CD, Wessels M. Structure of the *has* operon promoter and regulation of hyaluronic acid capsule expression in group A streptococci. Mol Microbiol 1998;28:343–353.
18. Allen AG, Bolitho S, Lindsay H, et al. Generation and characterization of a defined mutant of *Streptococcus suis* lacking suilysin. Infect Immun 2001;69: 2732–2735.
19. Alouf JE, Loridan C. Production, purification, and assay of streptolysin S. Methods Enzymol 1988;165:59–64.
20. Al-Shahrani DA, Al-Mohsen IZ, Al-Jumaah SA, Al-Oufi SH. Group B streptococcal endocarditis. Saudi Med J 2002;23:1127–1129.
21. American Academy of Pediatrics Committee on Infectious Diseases and Committee on Fetus and Newborn: Revised guidelines for prevention of early onset group B streptococcal (GBS) infections. Pediatrics 1997;99:489–496.
22. American College of Obstetricians and Gynecologists. ACOG Committee Opinion: number 279, December 2002. Prevention of early-onset group B streptococcal disease in newborns. Obstet Gynecol 2002;100:1405–1412.
23. American College of Obstetricians and Gynecologists Committee on Obstetric Practice (ACOG). Prevention of early-onset group B streptococcal disease in newborns [ACOG committee opinion]. Washington, DC: ACOG, 1996.
24. Ancona RJ, Ferrieri P, Williams PP. Maternal factors that enhance the acquisition of group B streptococci by newborn infants. J Med Microbiol 1980;13: 273–280.
25. Anderson DJ, Murdoch DR, Sexton DJ, et al. Risk factors for infective endocarditis in patients with enterococcal bacteremia: a case-control study. Infection 2004;32:72–77.
26. Andersson B, Dahmen J, Frejd T, et al. Identification of an active disaccharide unit of a glycoconjugate receptor for pneumococci attaching to human pharyngeal epithelial cells. J Exp Med 1983;158:559–569.
27. Andrews JI, Diekema DJ, Hunter SK, et al. Group B streptococci causing neonatal bloodstream infection: antimicrobial susceptibility and serotyping results from SENTRY centers in the western hemisphere. Am J Obstet Gynecol 2000;183:859–862.
28. Angel-Moreno A, Bolanos M, Buceta E, et al. *Streptococcus bovis* bacteremia from a venous access port in a patient with AIDS. Scand J Infect Dis 2002; 34:764–766.
29. Anhalt JP, Heiter BJ, Naumovitz DW, et al. Comparison of three methods for detection of group A streptococci in throat swabs. J Clin Microbiol 1992;30: 2135–2138.
30. Antalek MD, Mylotte JM, Lesse AJ, et al. Clinical and molecular epidemiology of *Enterococcus faecalis* bacteremia, with special reference to strains with high-level resistance to gentamicin. Clin Infect Dis 1995;20:103–109.
31. Anthony BF, Kaplan EL, Wannamaker LW, et al. Attack rates of acute nephritis after type 49 streptococcal infection of the skin and the respiratory tract. J Clin Invest 1969;48:1697–1704.
32. Antunes A, Rainey FA, Fernanda-Nobre M, et al. *Leuconostoc ficulneum* sp. nov., a novel lactic acid bacterium isolated from a ripe fig, and reclassification of *Lactobacillus fructosus* as *Leuconostoc fructosum* comb. nov. Int J Syst Evol Microbiol 2002;52:647–655.
33. Appelbaum PC. Antimicrobial resistance in *Streptococcus pneumoniae*: an overview. Clin Infect Dis 1992;15:77–83.
34. Arala-Chaves MP, Ribeiro AS, Santarem MMG, et al. Strong mitogenic effect for murine B lymphocytes of an immunosuppressor substance released by *Streptococcus intermedius*. Infect Immun 1986;54:543–548.
35. Arditi M, Shulman ST, Davis AT, et al. Group C β-hemolytic streptococcal infections in children: nine pediatric cases and review. Rev Infect Dis 1989; 11:34–45.
36. Arend SM, Van Buchem MA, van Ogtrop ML, et al. Septicaemia, meningitis, and spondylodiscitis caused by *Streptococcus suis* type 2. Infection 1995;23: 128.
37. Arends JP, Hartwig N, Rudolphy M, et al. Carrier rate of *Streptococcus suis* capsular type 2 in palatine tonsils of slaughtered pigs. J Clin Microbiol 1984; 20:945–947.
38. Arends JP, Zanen HC. Meningitis caused by *Streptococcus suis* in humans. Rev Infect Dis 1988;10:131–137.
39. Asciutto R, Drennan J, Fitzgerald V, et al. Group C streptococcal arthritis and

osteomyelitis in an adolescent with a hereditary sensory neuropathy. Pediatr Infect Dis J 1985;4:553–554.

40. Ashbaugh CD, Warren HB, Carey VJ, Wessels MR. Molecular analysis of the role of the group A streptococcal cysteine protease, hyaluronic acid capsule, and M protein in a murine model of human invasive soft-tissue infection. J Clin Invest 1998;102:550–560.

41. Aspevall O, Hillebrant E, Linderoth B, et al. Meningitis due to *Gemella haemolysans* after neurosurgical treatment of trigeminal neuralgia. Scand J Infect Dis 1991;23:503–505.

42. Atkins JT, Tillman J, Tan TQ, et al. *Pediococcus pentosaceus* catheter-associated infection in an infant with gastroschisis. Pediatr Infect Dis 1994;J 13:75–76.

43. Awada A, van der Auwera P, Meunier F, et al. Streptococcal and enterococcal bacteremia in patients with cancer. Clin Infect Dis 1992;15:33–48.

44. Ayoub EM, Kotb M, Cunningham MW. Rheumatic fever pathogenesis. In: Stevens DL, Kaplan EL, eds. Streptococcal Infections: Clinical Aspects, Microbiology, and Molecular Pathogenesis. New York: Oxford University Press, 2000:102–132.

45. Baddour LM. Infective endocarditis caused by β-hemolytic streptococci: the Infectious Diseases Society of America's Emerging Infections Network. Clin Infect Dis 1998;26:66–71.

46. Baird RW, Bronze MS, Kraus W, et al. Epitopes of group A streptococcal M proteins shared with antigens of articular cartilage and synovium. J Immunol 1991;146:3132–3137.

47. Baker CJ. Inadequacy of rapid immunoassays for intrapartum detection of group B streptococcal carriers. Obstet Gynecol 1996;88:51–55.

48. Baker CJ, Rench MA. Commercial latex agglutination for detection of group B streptococcal antigen in body fluids. J Pediatr 1983;102:393–395.

49. Ballow CH, Jones RN, Johnson DM, et al. Comparative in vitro assessment of sparfloxacion activity and spectrum using results from over 14,000 pathogens isolated at 190 medical centers in the U.S.A. Diagnb Microbiol Infect Dis 1997;29:173–186.

50. Banas JA, Vickerman MM. Glucan-binding proteins of the oral streptococci. Crit Rev Oral Biol Med 2003;14:89–99.

51. Bancescu G, Dumitriu S, Bancescu A, Skaug N. Streptococci species of anginosus group isolated from oral and maxillofacial infections. Roum Arch Microbiol Immunol 1999;58:49–55.

52. Baquero F, Garcia-Rodriguez JA, DeLomas JG, et al. Antimicrobial susceptibility of 914 β-hemolytic streptococci isolated from pharyngeal swabs in Spain: results of a 1-year (1996–1997) multicenter surveillance study. Antimicrob Agents Chemother 1999;43:178–180.

53. Baraco GJ, Bisno AL. Therapeutic approaches to streptococcal toxic shock syndrome. Curr Infect Dis Rep 1999;1:230–237.

54. Barnham M, Ljunggren A, McIntyre M. Human infection with *Streptococcus zooepidemicus* (Lancefield group C): three case reports. Epidemiol Infect 1987;98:183–190.

55. Barnham M, Thornton TJ, Lange K. Nephritis caused by *Streptococcus zooepidemicus* (Lancefield group C). Lancet 1983;1:45–946.

56. Barnham MR, Weightman NC. Bacteraemic *Streptococcus pyogenes* infection in the peri-partum period: now a rare disease and prior carriage by the patient may be important. J Infect 2001;43:173–176.

57. Barnham MR, Weightman N, Anderson A, et al. Review of 17 cases of pneumonia caused by *Streptococcus pyogenes*. Eur J Clin Microbiol Infect Dis 1999;18:506–509.

58. Barrios H, Bump CM. Conjunctivitis caused by a nutritionally variant *Streptococcus*. J Clin Microbiol 1986;23:379–380.

59. Barry H, Clancy MT, Brady A, et al. Isolation of a *Leuconostoc* species from a retroareolar breast abscess. J Infect 1993;27:208–210.

60. Barsotti O, Decoret D, Renaud FN. Identification of the streptococcus mitis group species by RFLP of the PCR-amplified 16S–23S rDNA intergenic spacer. Res Microbiol 2002;153:687–691.

61. Barton LL, Rider ED, Coen RW. Bacteremic infection with *Pediococcus*: vancomycin-resistant opportunists. Pediatrics 2001;107:775–776.

62. Bartter T, Dascal A, Carroll K, et al. "Toxic strep syndrome": manifestation of group A streptococcal infection. Arch Intern Med 1988;148:1421–1424.

63. Battison A, Cawthorn R, Horney B. Classification of *Homarus americanus* hemocytes and the use of differential hemocyte counts in lobsters infected with *Aerococcus viridans* var. *homari* (gaffemia). J Invertebr Pathol 2003;84:177–197.

64. Bauer TM, Pippert H, Zimmerli W. Vertebral osteomyelitis cause by group B streptococci (*Streptococcus agalactiae*) secondary to urinary tract infection. Eur J Clin Microbiol Infect Dis 1997;16:244–246.

65. Baxter F, McChesney J. Severe group A streptococcal infection and streptococcal toxic shock syndrome. Can J Anaesth 2000;47:1129–1140.

66. Beachey EH, Simpson WA. The adherence of group A streptococci to oropharyngeal cells: the lipoteichoic acid adhesin and fibronectin receptor. Infection 1982;10:107–111.

67. Beal B, Facklam R, Thompson T. Sequencing *emm*-specific PCR products for routine and accurate typing of group A streptococci. J Clin Microbiol 1996;34:953–958.

68. Becker JA, Ascher DP, Mendiola J, et al. False-negative urine latex particle agglutination testing in neonates with group B streptococcal bacteremia. Clin Pediatr 1993;32:467–471.

69. Beckmann C, Waggoner JD, Harris TO, et al. Identification of novel adhesins from group B streptococci by use of phage display reveals the C5a peptidase mediates fibronectin binding. Infect Immun 2002;70:2869–2876.

70. Beighton D, Carr AD, Oppenheim BA. Identification of viridans streptococci associated with bacteremia in neutropenic cancer patients. J Med Microbiol 1994;40:202–204.

71. Beighton D, Hardie JM, Whiley RA. A scheme for the identification of viridans streptococci. J Med Microbiol 1991;35:367–372.

72. Beighton D, Homer KA, Bouvet A, et al. Analysis of enzymatic activities for differentiation of two species of nutritionally variant streptococci, *Streptococcus defectivus* and *Streptococcus adjacens*. J Clin Microbiol 1995;33:1584–1587.

73. Beighton D, Russell RRB, Whiley RA. A simple scheme biochemical for the differentiation of *Streptococcus mutans* and *Streptococcus sobrinus*. Caries Res 1991;25:174–178.

74. Beighton D, Whiley RA. Sialidase activity of the "*Streptococcus milleri* group" and other viridans group streptococci. J Clin Microbiol 1990;28:1431–1433.

75. Bell E, McCartney AC. *Gemella morbillorum* endocarditis in an intravenous drug abuser. J Infect 1992;25:110–112.

76. Ben-Abraham R, Keller N, Vered R, et al. Invasive group A streptococcal infections in a large tertiary center: epidemiology, characteristics, and outcome. Infection 30:81–85, 2002.

77. Benkirane R, Gottschalk M, Jacques M, Dubreuil JD. Immunochemical characterization of a IgG-binding protein of *Streptococcus suis*. FEMS Immunol Med Microbiol 1998;20:121–127.

78. Bennett NM, Buffington J, LaForce FM. Pneumococcal bacteremia in Monroe County, New York. Am J Public Health 1992;82:1513–1516.

79. Bentley RW, Leigh JA. Development of PCR-based hybridization protocol for identification of streptococcal species. J Clin Microbiol 1995;33:1296–1301.

80. Bentley RW, Leigh JA, Collins MD. Intrageneric structure of *Streptococcus* based on comparative analysis of small-subunit rRNA sequences. Int J Syst Bacteriol 1991;41:487–494.

81. Berenguer J, Sampedro I, Cercenado E, et al. Group C β-hemolytic streptococcus bacteremia. Diagn Microbiol Infect Dis 1992;15:151–155.

82. Berg S, Trollfors B, Lagergard T, et al. Serotypes and clinical manifestation of group B streptococcal infections in western Sweden. Clin Microbiol Infect 2000 ;6:9–13.

83. Bergman S, Selig M, Collins MD, et al. "*Streptococcus milleri*" strains displaying a gliding type of motility. Int J Syst Bacteriol 1995;45:235–239.

84. Berk SL, Verghese A, Holtzclaw SA, et al. Enterococcal pneumonia. Occurrence in patients receiving broad-spectrum antibiotic regimens and enteral feeding. Am J Med 1983;74:153–154.

85. Berry AM, Lock RA, Hansman D, et al. Contribution of autolysin to virulence of *Streptococcus pneumoniae*. Infect Immun 1989;57:2324–2330.

86. Berry AM, Lock RA, Thomas SM, et al. Cloning and nucleotide sequence of the *Streptococcus pneumoniae* hyaluronidase gene and purification of the enzyme from recombinant *Escherichia coli*. Infect Immun 1994;62:1101–1108.

87. Berry AM, Yother J, Briles DE, et al. Reduced virulence of a defined pneumolysin-negative mutant of *Streptococcus pneumoniae*. Infect Immun 1989;57:2037–2042.

88. Bert F, Bariou-Lancelin M, Lambert-Zechovsky N. Clinical significance of bacteremia involving the "*Streptococcus milleri*" group: 51 cases and review. Clin Infect Dis 1998;27:385–387.

89. Bert F, Branger C, Poutrel B, Lambert-Zechovsky N. Differentiation of human and animal strains of *Streptococcus dysgalactiae* by pulsed-field gel electrophoresis. FEMS Microbiol Lett 1997;150:107–112.

90. Bert F, Lambert-Zechovsky N. Septicemia caused by *Streptococcus canis* in a human. J Clin Microbiol 1997;35:777–779.

91. Bessen DE, Sotir CM, Readdy T, Hollingshead SK. Genetic correlates of throat and skin isolates of group A streptococci. J Infect Dis 1996;173:896–900.

92. Beswick AJ, Lawley B, Fraise AP, et al. Detection of *Alloiococcus otitidis* in mixed bacterial populations from middle-ear effusions of patients with otitis media. Lancet 1999;354:386–389.

93. Bhakdi S, Roth M, Sziegoleit A, Tranum-Jensen J. Isolation and identification of two hemolytic forms of streptolysin O. Infect Immun 1984;46:394–400.

94. Biermann C, Fries G, Jehnichen P, et al. Isolation of *Abiotrophia adiacens* from a brain abscess which developed in a patient after neurosurgery. J Clin Microbiol 1999;37:769–771.

95. Bisno AL. Alternate complement pathway activation by group A streptococci: role of M protein. Infect Immun 1979;26:1172–1176.

96. Bisno AL. Nonsuppurative poststreptococcal sequelae: rheumatic fever and glomerulonephritis. In: Mandell GL, Bennett JE, Dolin R, eds. Mandell, Doug-

las, and Bennett's Principles and Practice of Infectious Diseases. 5th Ed. New York, Churchill-Livingstone, 2000:2117–2128.

97. Bisno AL, Brito MO, Collins CM. Molecular basis of group A streptococcal virulence. Lancet Infect Dis 2003;3:191–200.

98. Bisno AL, Gerber MA, Gwaltney JM Jr, et al. Practice guidelines for the diagnosis and management of group A streptococcal pharyngitis. Clin Infect Dis 2002;35:113–125.

99. Bisno AL, Stevens DL. Streptococcal infections of skin and soft tissue. N Engl J Med 1995;334:240–245.

100. Bisno AL, Stevens DL. *Streptococcus pyogenes* (including streptococcal toxic shock syndrome and necrotizing fasciitis). In: Mandell GL, Bennett JE, Dolin R, eds. Mandell, Douglas, and Bennett's Principles and Practice of Infectious Diseases. 5th Ed. New York: Churchill Livingstone, 2000:2101–2117.

101. Bisno AL, Wood JW, Lawson J, et al. Antigens in urine of patients with glomerulonephritis and in normal human serum which cross-react with group A streptococci: identification and partial characterization. J Lab Clin Med 1978; 91:500–513.

102. Bjorkroth KJ, Geisen R, Schillinger U, et al. Characterization of *Leuconostoc gasicomitatum* sp., nov., associated with spoiled raw tomato-marinated broiler meat strips packaged under modified-atmosphere conditions. Appl Environ Microbiol 2000;66:3764–3772.

103. Blanckaert H, Frans J, Bosteels J, et al. Optimization of prenatal group B streptococcal screening. Eur J Clin Microbiol Infect Dis 2003;22:619–621.

104. Blanco JR, Zabalza M, Salcedo J, San Roman J. Rhabdomyolysis as a result of *Streptococcus pneumoniae*: case report and review. Clin Microbiol Infect 2003;9:944–948.

105. Bluestone CD, Stephenson JS, Martin LM. Ten-year review of otitis media pathogens. Pediatr Infect Dis J 1992;11:S7–S11.

106. Blumberg HM, Stephens DS, Modanski M, et al. Invasive group B streptococcal disease: the emergence of serotype V. J Infect Dis 1996;173:365–373.

107. Bochud P-Y, Calandra T, Francioli P. Bacteremia due to viridans streptococci in neutropenic patients: a review. Am J Med 1994;97:256–264.

108. Bochud P-Y, Eggiman P, Calandra T, et al. Bacteremia due to viridans streptococcus in neutropenic patients with cancer: clinical spectrum and risk factors. Clin Infect Dis 1994;18:25–31.

109. Bogaerts D, de Groot R, Hermans PWM. *Streptococcus pneumoniae* colonization: the key to pneumococcal disease. Lancet 2004;4:144–154.

110. Bohnsack JF, Mollison KW, Buko AM, et al. Group B streptococci inactivate complement component C5a by enzymatic cleavage at the C-terminus. Biochem J 1991;273:635–640.

111. Bohnsack JF, Takahashi S, Detrick SR, et al. Phylogenetic classification of serotype III group B streptococci on the basis of *hylB* gene analysis and DNA sequences specific to restriction digest pattern type III-3. J Infect Dis 2001; 183:1694–1697.

112. Bolduc GR, Baron MJ, Gravekamp C, et al. The αC protein mediates internalization of group B streptococcus within human cervical epithelial cells. Cell Microbiol 2002;4:751–758.

113. Bonnetblanc JM, Bedane C. Erysipelas: recognition and management. Am J Clin Dermatol 2003;4:157–163.

114. Borchardt SM, Foxman B, Chaffin DO, et al. Comparison of DNA dot blot hybridization and lancefield capillary precipitin methods for group B streptococcal capsular typing. J Clin Microbiol 2004;42:146–150.

115. Borek AP, Dressel DC, Hussong J, Peterson LR. Evolving clinical problems with *Streptococcus pneumoniae*: increasing resistance to antimicrobial agents and failure of traditional Optochin identification in Chicago, Illinois, between 1993 and 1996. Diagn Microbiol Infect Dis 1997;29:209–214.

116. Borer A, Weber G, Avnon LS, et al. Pleural empyema caused by *Leuconostoc* spp. Scand J Infect Dis 1997;29:311–312.

117. Bos AP, Fetter WPF, Baerts W, et al. Streptococcal pharyngitis and epiglottitis in a newborn infant. Eur J Pediatr 1992;151:874–875.

118. Bosley GS, Whitney AM, Pruckler JM, et al. Characterization of ear fluid isolates of *Alloiococcus otitidis* from patients with recurrent otitis media. J Clin Microbiol 1995;33:2876–2880.

119. Bouchillon SK, Hoban DJ, Johnson JL, et al. In vitro activity of gemifloxacin and contemporary oral antimicrobial agents against 27,247 gram-positive and gram-negative aerobic isolates: a global surveillance study. Int J Antimicrob Agents 2004;23:181–196.

120. Boulnois GJ. Pneumococcal proteins and the pathogenesis of disease caused by *Streptococcus pneumoniae*. J Gen Microbiol 1992;138:249–259.

121. Boulnois GJ, Paton JC, Mitchell TJ, Andrew PW. Structure and function of pneumolysin, the multifunctional, thiol-activated toxin of *Streptococcus pneumoniae*. Mol Microbiol 1991;5:2611–2616.

122. Bourbeau PP, Heiter BJ, Figdore M. Use of Gen-Probe AccuProbe group B streptococcus test to detect group B streptococci in broth cultures of vaginal-anorectal specimens from pregnant women: comparison with traditional culture method. J Clin Microbiol 1997;35:144–147.

123. Bouvet A. Human endocarditis due to nutritionally variant streptococci: *Strep-*

tococcus adjacens and *Streptococcus defectivus*. Eur Heart J 1995;16(Suppl B):24–27.

124. Bouvet A, Geslin P, Kriz-Kuzemenska P, et al. Restricted association between biotypes and serotypes with group A streptococci. J Clin Microbiol 1994;32: 1312–1317.

125. Bouvet A, Grimont F, Collins MD, et al. *Streptococcus infantarius* sp. nov. related to *Streptococcus bovis* and *Streptococcus equinus*. Adv Exp Med Biol 1997;418:393–395.

126. Bouvet A, Grimont F, Grimont PAD. *Streptococcus defectivus* sp. nov. and *Streptococcus adjacens* sp. nov., nutritionally variant streptococci from human clinical specimens. Int J Syst Bacteriol 1989;39:290–294.

127. Boyce JM, Opal DSM, Chow JW, et al. Outbreak of multidrug-resistant *Enterococcus faecium* with transferable *vanB* class vancomycin resistance. J Clin Microbiol 1994;32:1148–1153.

128. Boyer KM, Gotoff SP. Prevention of early-onset neonatal group B streptococcal disease with selective intrapartum chemoprophylaxis. N Engl J Med 1986;314: 1665–1669.

129. Brandt CM, Haase G, Schnitzler N, et al. Characterization of blood culture isolates of *Streptococcus dysgalactiae* subsp. *equisimilis* possessing Lancefield's group A antigen. J Clin Microbiol 1999;37:4194–4197.

130. Briles DE, Hollingshead SK, Swiatlo E, et al. PspA and PspC: their potential for use as pneumococcal vaccines. Microb Drug Resist 1997;3:401–408.

131. Brook I, Gober AE, Leyva F. In vitro and in vitro effects of penicillin and clindamycin on expression of group A β-hemolytic streptococcal capsule. Antimicrob Agents Chemother 1995;39:1565–1568.

132. Brown J, Shriner DL, Schwartz RA, Janniger CK. Impetigo: an update. Int J Dermatol 2003;42:251–255.

133. Bruneau S, de Montclos H, Drouet E, et al. rRNA gene restriction patterns of *Streptococcus pyogenes*: epidemiological applications and relation to serotypes. J Clin Microbiol 1994;32:2953–2958.

134. Bryant ER, Salmon CJ. Pleural empyema. Clin Infect Dis 1996;22:747–764.

135. Bryce EA, Zemcov SJ, Clarke AM. Species identification and antibiotic resistance patterns of the enterococci. Eur J Clin Microbiol Infect Dis 1991;10: 745–747.

136. Bucher A, Martin PR, Hoiby EA, et al. Spectrum of disease in bacteremic patients during a *Streptococcus pyogenes* serotype M-1 epidemic in Norway in 1988. Eur J Clin Microbiol Infect Dis 1992;11:416–426.

137. Bungener W, Bialek R. Fatal *Streptococcus suis* septicemia in an abattoir worker. Eur J Clin Microbiol Infect Dis 1989;8:306–308.

138. Burden AD, Oppenheim BA, Crowther D, et al. Viridans streptococcal bacteraemia in patients with haematological and solid malignancies. Eur J Cancer 1991;27:409–411.

139. Burkert T, Watanakunakorn C. Group G streptococcus septic arthritis and osteomyelitis: report and literature review. J Rheumatol 1991;18:904–907.

140. Burman LA, Norrby R, Trollfors B. Invasive pneumococcal infections: incidence, predisposing factors, and prognosis. Rev Infect Dis 1985;7:133–142.

141. Burns DL, Ginsburg CM. Recrudescence of acute rheumatic fever in Dallas, Texas. Pediatr Res 1987;21(Suppl):256A.

142. Buschelman BJ, Bale MJ, Jones RN. Species identification and determination of high-level aminoglycoside resistance among enterococci: comparison study of sterile body fluid isolates, 1985-1991. Diagn Microbiol Infect Dis 1993;16: 119–122.

143. Butler JC, Breiman RF, Campbell JF, et al. Pneumococcal polysaccharide vaccine efficacy: an evaluation of current recommendations. JAMA 1993;270: 1826–1831.

144. Buu-Hoi A, Sapoetra A, Branger C, et al. Antimicrobial susceptibility of *Gemella hemolysans* isolated from patients with subacute endocarditis. Eur J Clin Microbiol 1982;1:102–106.

145. Cai J, Collins MD. Evidence for a close phylogenetic relationship between *Melissococcus pluton*, the causative agent of European foulbrood disease, and the genus *Enterococcus*. Int J Syst Bacteriol 1994;44:365–367.

146. Cainzos M, Hindi EY, Fernandez F, et al. Wound erysipelas following appendectomy caused by Group B β-hemolytic *Streptococcus* (*Streptococcus agalactiae*). Surg Infect 2001;2:37–40.

147. Caliendo AM, Jordan CD, Ruoff KL. *Helcococcus*: a new genus of catalase-negative, gram-positive cocci isolated from clinical specimens. J Clin Microbiol 1995;33:1638–1639.

148. Camara M, Mitchell TJ, Andrew PW, Boulnois GJ. *Streptococcus pneumoniae* produces at least two distinct enzymes with neuraminidase activity: cloning and expression of a second neuraminidase gene in *Escherichia coli*. Infect Immun 1991;59:2856–2858.

149. Campbell JR, Hillier SL, Krohn MA, et al. Group B streptococcal colonization and serotype-specific immunity in pregnant women at delivery. Obstet Gynecol 2000;96:498–503.

150. Campos JM, Charilaou CC. Evaluation of Detect-A-Strep and the Culturette Ten-Minute Strep ID kits for detection of group A streptococcal antigen in oropharyngeal swabs from children. J Clin Microbiol 1985;22:145–148.

151. Canvin JR, Marvin AP, Sivakumaran M, et al. The role of pneumolysin and

autolysin in the pathology of pneumonia and septicemia in mice infected with type 2 pneumococcus. J Infect Dis 1995;172:119–123.

152. Cappelli EA, Barros RR, Camello TC, et al. *Leuconostoc pseudomesenteroides* as a cause of nosocomial urinary tract infections. J Clin Microbiol 1999;37: 4124–4126.

153. Caputo GM, Appelbaum PC, Liu HH. Infections due to penicillin-resistant pneumococci: clinical, epidemiologic, and microbiologic features. Arch Intern Med 1993;153:1301–1310.

154. Carapetis J, Bishop S, Davis J, et al. *Leuconostoc* sepsis in association with continuous enteral feeding: two case reports and a review. Pediatr Infect Dis J 1994;13:816–823.

155. Carey RB, Gross KC, Roberts RB. Vitamin B$_6$ dependent *Streptococcus mitior* (*mitis*) isolated from patients with systemic infections. J Infect Dis 1975;131: 722–726.

156. Carley NH. *Streptococcus salivarius* bacteremia and meningitis following upper gastrointestinal endoscopy and cauterization for gastric bleeding. Clin Infect Dis 1992;14:947–948.

157. Carmeli Y, Ruoff KL. Report of cases of and taxonomic considerations for large-colony-forming Lancefield group C streptococcal bacteremia. J Clin Microbiol 1995;33:2114–2117.

158. Carrascosa M, Perez-Castrillon JL, Sampedro I, et al. Lung abscess due to *Streptococcus mitis*: case report and review. Clin Infect Dis 1994;19:781–783.

159. Carroll KC, Monroe P, Cohen S, et al. Susceptibility of β-hemolytic streptococci to nine antimicrobial agents among four medical centers in Salt Lake City, Utah, USA. Diagn Microbiol Infect Dis 1997;27:123–128.

160. Cartwright CP, Stock F, Fahle GA, et al. Comparison of pigment production and motility tests with PCR for reliable identification of intrinsically vancomycin-resistant enterococci. J Clin Microbiol 1995;33:1931–1933.

161. Carvalho MS, Steigerwalt AG, Morey RE, et al. Characterization of three new enterococcal species, *Enterococcus* sp. nov. CDC PNS-E1, *Enterococcus* sp. nov. CDC PNS-E2, and *Enterococcus* sp. nov. CDC PNS-E3, isolated from human clinical specimens. J Clin Microbiol 2004;42:1192–1198.

162. Catalan MJ, Fernandez JM, Vazquez A, et al. Failure of cefotaxime in the treatment of meningitis due to relatively resistant *Streptococcus pneumoniae*. Clin Infect Dis 1994;18:766–769.

163. Cavalieri SJ, Allais JM, Schlievert PM, et al. Group A streptococcal peritonitis in a patient undergoing continuous ambulatory peritoneal dialysis. Am J Med 1989;86:249–250.

164. Centers for Disease Control and Prevention. Acute rheumatic fever at a Navy training center—San Diego. MMWR Morb Mortal Wkly Rep 1988;37: 101–104.

165. Centers for Disease Control and Prevention. Acute rheumatic fever among Army trainees—Fort Leonard Wood, Missouri, 1987-1988. MMWR Morb Mortal Wkly Rep 1988;37:519–522.

166. Centers for Disease Control and Prevention. Group A β-hemolytic streptococcal bacteremia—Colorado, 1989. MMWR Morb Mortal Wkly Rep 39:3–11, 1990.

167. Centers for Disease Control and Prevention. Prevention of perinatal group B streptococcal disease: a public health perspective. MMWR Morb Mortal Wkly Rep 1996;45(RR-7):1–24.

168. Centers for Disease Control and Prevention. Prevention of pneumococcal disease: recommendations of the Advisory Committee on Immunization Practices (ACIP). MMWR Morb Mortal Wkly Rep 1997;46(RR-8):1–24.

169. Centers for Disease Control and Prevention. Preventing pneumococcal disease among infants and young children: recommendations of the Advisory Committee on Immunization Practices (ACIP). MMWR Morb Mortal Wkly Rep 2000; 49(RR-9):1–35.

170. Centers for Disease Control and Prevention. Prevention of perinatal group B streptococcal disease. MMWR Morb Mortal Wkly Rep 2002;51:1–22.

171. Cerceo E, Christie JD, Nachamkin I, Lautenbach E. Central nervous system infections due to *Abiotrophia* and *Granulicatella* species: an emerging challenge? Diagn Microbiol Infect Dis 2004;48:161–165.

172. Chagla AH, Borczyk AA, Facklam RR, Lovgren M. Breast abscess associated with *Helcococcus kunzii*. J Clin Microbiol 1998;36:2377–2379.

173. Chang HH, Lu CY, Hsueh PR, et al. Endocarditis caused by *Abiotrophia defectiva* in children. Pediatr Infect Dis J 2002;21:697–700.

174. Chapin KC, Blake P, Wilson CD. Performance characteristics and utilization of rapid antigen test, DNA probe, and culture for detection of group A streptococci in an acute care clinic. J Clin Microbiol 2002;40:4207–4210.

175. Chapin-Robertson C, Dahlberg SE, Edberg SC. Clinical and laboratory analyses of cytospin-prepared Gram stains for recovery and diagnosis of bacteria from sterile body fluids. J Clin Microbiol 1992;30:377–380.

176. Chapnick EK, Gradon JD, Lutwick LI, et al. Streptococcal toxic shock syndrome due to noninvasive pharyngitis. Clin Infect Dis 1992;14:1074–1077.

177. Chatellier S, Gottschalk M, Higgins R, et al. Relatedness of *Streptococcus suis* serotype 2 isolates from different geographic origins as evaluated by molecular fingerprinting and phenotyping. J Clin Microbiol 1999;37:362–366.

178. Chatellier S, Harel J, Zhang Y, et al. Phylogenetic diversity of *Streptococcus*

suis strains of various serotypes as revealed by 16S rRNA gene sequence comparison. Int J Syst Bacteriol 1998;48:581–589.

179. Chau PY, Huang CY, Kay R. *Streptococcus suis* meningitis: an important underdiagnosed disease in Hong Kong. Med J Aust 1983;1:414–417.

180. Cheng Q, Carlson B, Pillai S, et al. Antibody against surface-bound C5a peptidase is opsonic and initiates macrophage killing of group B streptococci. Infect Immun 2001;69:2302–2308.

181. Cheng Q, Debol S, Lam H, et al. Immunization with C5a peptidase or peptidase-type III polysaccharide conjugate vaccines enhances clearance of group B streptococci from lungs of infected mice. Infect Immun 2002;70:6409–6415.

182. Cheng Q, Stafslien D, Purushothamen SS, Cleary P. The group B streptococcal C5a peptidase is both a specific protease and an invasin. Infect Immun 2002; 70:2408–2413.

183. Cherchi GB, Kaplan EL, Schlievert PM, et al. First reported case of *Streptococcus pyogenes* infection with toxic shock-like syndrome in Italy. Eur J Clin Microbiol Infect Dis 1992;11:836–838.

184. Chew TA, Smith JMB. Detection of diacetyl (caramel odor) in presumptive identification of the "*Streptococcus milleri*" group. J Clin Microbiol 1992;30: 3028–3029.

185. Chirurgi VA, Oster SE, Goldberg AA, et al. Ampicillin-resistant *Enterococcus raffinosus* in an acute-care hospital: case-control study and antimicrobial susceptibilities. J Clin Microbiol 1991;29:2663–2665.

186. Choi KC, Mailman TL. Pneumococcal endocarditis in infants and children. Pediatr Infect Dis J 2004;23:166–171.

187. Chow JW, Muder RR. Group A streptococcal meningitis. Clin Infect Dis 1992; 14:418–421.

188. Chow JW, Thal LA, Perri MB, et al. Plasmid-associated hemolysin and aggregation substance production contributes to virulence in experimental enterococcal endocarditis. Antimicrob Agents Chemother 1993;37:2472–2477.

189. Christensen JJ, Facklam RR. *Granulicatella* and *Abiotrophia* species from human clinical specimens. J Clin Microbiol 2001;39:3520–3523.

190. Christensen JJ, Gruhn N, Facklam RR. Endocarditis caused by *Abiotrophia* species. Scand J Infect Dis 1999;31:210–212.

191. Christensen JJ, Gutschik E, Friss-Moller A, et al. Urosepticemia and fatal endocarditis caused by *Aerococcus*-like organisms. Scand J Infect Dis 1991;23: 717–721.

192. Christensen JJ, Jensen IP, Faerk J, et al. Bacteremia/septicemia due to *Aerococcus*-like organisms: report of seventeen cases. Clin Infect Dis 1995;21: 943–947.

193. Christensen JJ, Korner B, Kjaergaard H. *Aerococcus*-like organism—an unnoticed urinary tract pathogen. APMIS 1989;97:539–546.

194. Christensen JJ, Vibits H, Ursing J, et al. *Aerococcus*-like organism, a newly recognized urinary tract pathogen. J Clin Microbiol 1991;29:1049–1053.

195. Christensen JJ, Whitney AM, Teixeira LM, et al. *Aerococcus urinae*: intraspecies genetic and phenotypic relatedness. Int J Syst Bacteriol 1997;47:28–32.

196. Christie R, Atkins NE, Munch-Petersen E. A note on a lytic phenomenon shown by group B streptococci. Aust J Exp Biol Med Sci 1944;22:197–200.

197. Chuard C, Reller LB. Bile-esculin test for presumptive identification of enterococci and streptococci: effects of bile concentration, inoculation technique, and incubation time. J Clin Microbiol 1998;36:1135–1136.

198. Cimolai N, Morrison BJ, MacCulloch L, et al. β-Haemolytic non-group A streptococci and pharyngitis: a case-control study. Eur J Pediatr 1991;150: 776–779.

199. Clarridge JE III, Attorri SM, Musher DM, et al. *Streptococcus intermedius*, *Streptococcus constellatus*, and *Streptococcus anginosus* ("*Streptococcus milleri* group") are of different clinical importance and are not equally associated with abscess. Clin Infect Dis 2001;32:1511–1515.

200. Clarridge JE III, Attorri SM, Zhang Q, Bartell J. 16S Ribosomal DNA sequence analysis distinguishes biotypes of *Streptococcus bovis*: *Streptococcus bovis* biotype II/2 is a separate genospecies and the predominant clinical isolate in adult males. J Clin Microbiol 2001;39:1549–1552.

201. Clewell DB. Bacterial sex pheromone-induced plasmid transfer. Cell 1993;73: 9–12.

202. Cockeran R, Anderson R, Feldman C. The role of pneumolysin in the pathogenesis of *Streptococcus pneumoniae* infection. Curr Opin Infect Dis 2002;15: 235–239.

203. Cockeran R, Durandt C, Feldman C, et al. Pneumolysin activates the synthesis and release of interleukin-8 by human neutrophils in vitro. J Infect Dis 2002; 186:562–565.

204. Collazos J, Echevarria MJ, Ayarza R, et al. *Streptococcus zooepidemicus* septic arthritis: case report and review of group C streptococcal arthritis. Clin Infect Dis 1992;15:744–746.

205. Collins MD, Aguirre M, Facklam RR, et al. *Globicatella sanguis* gen. nov., sp. nov., a new gram-positive, catalase-negative bacterium from human sources. J Appl Microbiol 1992;73:433–437.

206. Collins MD, Ash C, Farrow JAE, et al. 16S ribosomal ribonucleic acid sequence analysis of lactococci and related taxa: description of *Vagococcus fluvialis* gen. nov. sp. nov. J Appl Microbiol 1989;67:453–460.

207. Collins MD, Facklam RR, Farrow JAE, et al. *Enterococcus raffinosus* sp. nov., *Enterococcus solitarius* sp. nov., and *Enterococcus pseudoavium* sp. nov. FEMS Microbiol Lett 1989;57:283–288.

208. Collins MD, Facklam RR, Rodrigues UM, et al. Phylogenetic analysis of some *Aerococcus*-like organisms from clinical sources: description of *Helcococcus kunzii* gen. nov. sp. nov. Int J Syst Bacteriol 1993;43:425–429.

209. Collins MD, Falsen E, Foster G, et al. *Helcococcus ovis* sp. nov., a gram-positive organism from sheep. Int J Syst Bacteriol 1999;49:1429–1432.

210. Collins MD, Falsen E, Lemozy J, et al. Phenotypic and phylogenetic characterization of some *Globicatella*-like organisms from human sources: description of *Facklamia hominis* gen. nov., sp. nov. Int J Syst Bacteriol 1997;47:880–882.

211. Collins MD, Farrow JAE, Jones D. *Enterococcus mundtii* sp. nov. Int J Syst Bacteriol 1986;36:8–12.

212. Collins MD, Hutson RA, Falsen E, et al. An unusual *Streptococcus* from human urine, *Streptococcus urinalis* sp. nov. Int J Syst Evol Microbiol 2000;50:1173–1178.

213. Collins MD, Hutson RA, Falsen E, Sjoden B. *Facklamia sourekii* sp. nov., isolated from human sources. Int J Syst Bacteriol 1999;49:635–638.

214. Collins MD, Hutson RA, Falsen E, Sjoden B. *Facklamia tabacinalis* sp. nov., from powdered tobacco. Int J Syst Bacteriol 1999;49:1247–1250.

215. Collins MD, Hutson RA, Falsen E, et al. *Gemella bergeriae* sp. nov., isolated from human clinical specimens. J Clin Microbiol 1998;36:1290–1293.

216. Collins MD, Hutson RA, Falsen E, et al. Description of *Gemella sanguinis* sp. nov., isolated from human clinical specimens. J Clin Microbiol 1998;36:3090–3093.

216a. Collins MD, Hutson RA, Falsen E, et al. *Streptococcus gallinaceus* sp. nov., from chickens. Int J Syst Evol Microbiol 2002;52:1161–1164.

217. Collins MD, Hutson RA, Hoyles L, et al. *Streptococcus ovis* sp. nov., isolated from sheep. Int J Syst Evol Microbiol 2001;51:1147–1150.

218. Collins MD, Jones D, Farrow JAE, et al. *Enterococcus avium* nom. rev., comb. nov.; *E. casseliflavus* nom. rev., comb. nov.; *E. durans* nom. rev., comb. nov.; *E. gallinarum* nom. rev., comb. nov., and *E. malodoratus* sp. nov. Int J Syst Bacteriol 1984;34:220–223.

219. Collins MD, Jovita MR, Foster G, et al. Characterization of a *Gemella*-like organism from the oral cavity of a dog: description of *Gemella palaticanis* sp. nov. Int J Syst Bacteriol 1999;49:1523–1526.

220. Collins MD, Jovita MR, Hutson RA, et al. *Dolosicoccus paucivorans* gen. nov. sp. nov., isolated from human blood. Int J Syst Bacteriol 1999;49:1439–1442.

221. Collins MD, Jovita MR, Hutson RA, et al. *Aerococcus christensenii* sp. nov., from the human vagina. Int J Syst Bacteriol 1999;49:1125–1128.

222. Collins MD, Jovita MR, Lawson PA, et al. Characterization of a novel catalase-negative coccus from humans: description of *Eremococcus coleocola* gen. nov., sp. nov. Int J Syst Bacteriol 1999;49:1381–1385.

223. Collins MD, Lawson PA. The genus *Abiotrophia* (Kawamura et al) is not monophyletic: proposal of *Granulicatella* gen. nov., *Granulicatella adiacens* comb. nov., *Granulicatella elegans* comb. nov., and *Granulicatella balaenopterae* comb. nov. Int J Syst Evol Microbiol 2000;50:365–369.

224. Collins MD, Lawson PA, Monasterio R, et al. *Facklamia ignava* sp. nov., isolated from human clinical specimens. J Clin Microbiol 1998;36:2146–2148.

225. Collins MD, Lawson PA, Monasterio R, et al. *Ignavigranum ruoffiae* sp. nov., isolated from human clinical specimens. Int J Syst Bacteriol 1999;49:97–101.

226. Collins MD, Rodrigues UM, Piggott NE, et al. *Enterococcus dispar* sp. nov., a new *Enterococcus* species from human sources. Lett Appl Microbiol 1991;12:95–98.

227. Collins MD, Samelis J, Metazopoulos J, et al. Taxonomic studies of some *Leuconostoc*-like organisms from fermented sausages: description of a new genus *Weissella* for the *Leuconostoc paramesenteroides* group of species. J Appl Microbiol 1993;75:595–603.

228. Collins MD, Williams AM, Wallbanks S. The phylogeny of *Aerococcus* and *Pediococcus* as determined by 16S rRNA sequence analysis: description of *Tetragenococcus* gen. nov. FEMS Microbiol Lett 1990;70:255–262.

229. Colville A, Davies W, Heneghan M, et al. A rare complication of dental treatment: *Streptococcus oralis* meningitis. Br Dent J 1993;175:133–134.

230. Cone LA, Woodard DR, Schlievert PM, et al. Clinical and bacteriologic observations of a toxic shock-like syndrome due to *Streptococcus pyogenes*. N Engl J Med 1987;317:146–149.

231. Coonan KM, Kaplan EL. In vitro susceptibility of recent North American group A streptococcal isolates to eleven oral antibiotics. Pediatr Infect Dis J 1994;13:630–635.

232. Cooper RJ, Hoffman JR, Bartlett JG, et al. Principles of appropriate antibiotic use for acute pharyngitis in adults: background. Ann Inter Med 2001;134:509–517.

233. Coovadia YM, Solwa Z, van den Ende J. Meningitis caused by vancomycin-resistant *Leuconostoc* sp. J Clin Microbiol 1987;25:1784–1785.

234. Corcoran GD, Gibbons N, Mulvihill TE. Septicaemia caused by *Pediococcus pentosaceus*: a new opportunistic pathogen. J Infect 1991;23:179–182.

235. Cornaglia G, Ligozzi M, Mazzariol A, et al. Resistance of *Streptococcus pyogenes* to erythromycin and related antibiotics in Italy. Clin Infect Dis 1998;27(Suppl 1):S87–S82.

236. Corson AP, Garigusa VF, Chretien JH. Group C β-hemolytic streptococci causing pharyngitis and scarlet fever. South Med J 1989;82:1119–1121.

237. Corson MA, Postlethwaite KP, Seymour RA. Are dental infections a cause of brain abscess? Case report and review of the literature. Oral Diseases 2001;7:61–65.

238. Cottagnoud P, Rossi M. *Enterococcus avium* osteomyelitis. Clin Microbiol Infect 1998;4:290.

239. Courtney HS, Hasty DL, Dale JB. Molecular mechanisms of adhesion, colonization, and invasion of group A streptococci. Ann Med 2002;34:77–87.

240. Coykendall AL. Classification and identification of the viridans streptococci. Clin Microbiol Rev 1989;2:315–328.

241. Crain MJ, Waltman WD, Turner JS, et al. Pneumococcal surface protein A (PspA) is serologically highly variable and is expressed by all clinically important capsular serotypes of *Streptococcus pneumoniae*. Infect Immun 1990;58:3293–3299.

242. Crater DL, van de Rijn I. Hyaluronic acid synthesis operon (*has*) expression in group A streptococci. J Biol Chem 1995;270:18452–18458.

243. Craven DE, Rixinger AI, Bisno AL, et al. Bacteremia caused by group G streptococci in parenteral drug abusers: epidemiological and clinical aspects. J Infect Dis 1986;153:988–992.

244. Cunney RJ, Fenton S, Fielding JF, et al. *Streptococcus mitis* meningitis in an adult. J Infect 1993;27:96–97.

245. Da Costa CT, Porter C, Parry K, et al. Empyema thoracis and lung abscess due to *Gemella morbillorum*. Eur J Clin Microbiol Infect Dis 1996;15:75–77.

246. Dagan R, Englehard D, Piccard E. Epidemiology of invasive childhood pneumococcal infections in Israel. JAMA 1992;268:3328–3332.

247. Dahl PR, Perniciaro C, Holmkvist KA, et al. Fulminant group A streptococcal necrotizing fasciitis: clinical and pathological findings in 7 patients. J Am Acad Dermatol 2002;47:489–492.

248. Dajani AS, Ayoub E, Bierman FZ, et al. Guidelines for the diagnosis of rheumatic fever: Jones criteria, updated 1992. Circulation 1993;87:302–307.

249. Dale JB, Beachey EH. Protective antigenic determinant of streptococcal M protein shared with sarcolemmal membrane protein of human heart. J Exp Med 1982;156:1165–1176.

250. Dale JB, Beachey EH. Epitopes of streptococcal M proteins shared with cardiac myosin. J Exp Med 1985;162:583–591.

251. Daly JA, Clifton NL, Seskin KC, Gooch WM III. Use of rapid, nonradioactive DNA probes in culture confirmation tests to detect *Streptococcus agalactiae*, *Haemophilus influenzae*, and *Enterococcus* spp. from pediatric patients with significant infections. J Clin Microbiol 1991;29:80–82.

252. Daly JA, Korgenski EK, Munson AC, et al. Optical immunoassay for streptococcal pharyngitis: evaluation of accuracy with routine and mucoid strains associated with acute rheumatic fever outbreak in the intermountain area of the United States. J Clin Microbiol 1994;32:531–532.

253. Danilitou V, Mantadakis E, Galanakis E, et al. Three cases of viridans group streptococcal bacteremia in children with febrile neutropenia and literature review. Scand J Infect Dis 2003;35:873–876.

254. Dargere S, Vergnaud M, Verdon R, et al. *Enterococcus gallinarum* endocarditis occurring on native heart valves. J Clin Microbiol 2002;40:2308–2310.

255. Darling CL. Standardization and evaluation of the CAMP reaction for the prompt, presumptive identification of *Streptococcus agalactiae* (Lancefield group B) in clinical material. J Clin Microbiol 1975;1:171–174.

256. Davidson M, Parkinson AJ, Bulkow LR, et al. The epidemiology of invasive pneumococcal disease in Alaska, 1986–1990—ethnic differences and opportunities for prevention. J Infect Dis 1994;170:368–376.

257. Davis TE, Fuller DD. Direct identification of bacterial isolates in blood cultures by using a DNA probe. J Clin Microbiol 1991;29:2193–2196.

258. Dealler SF, Grace RJ, Norfolk DR. *Enterococcus avium* septicemia in an immunocompromised patient. Eur J Clin Microbiol Infect Dis 1990;9:367–368.

259. Deasy BM, Rea MC, Fitzgerald GF, et al. A rapid PCR based method to distinguish between *Lactococcus* and *Enterococcus*. Syst Appl Microbiol 2000;23:510–522.

260. DeBaere T, Claeys G, Verschraegen G, et al. Continuous ambulatory peritoneal dialysis peritonitis due to *Enterococcus cecorum*. J Clin Microbiol 2000;38:3511–3512.

261. Debast SB, Koot R, Meis JFGM. Infections caused by *Gemella morbillorum*. Lancet 1993;342:560.

262. De Gheldre Y, Vandamme P, Goossens H, Struelens MJ. Identification of clinically relevant viridans streptococci by analysis of transfer RNA intergenic spacer length polymorphism. Int J Syst Bacteriol 1999;49:1591–1598.

263. De Graef EM, Devriese LA, Vancanneyt M, et al. Description of *Enterococcus canis* sp. nov. from dogs and reclassification of *Enterococcus porcinus* Teixeira et al 2001 as a junior synonym of *Enterococcus villorum* Vancanneyt et al 2001. Int J Syst Evol Microbiol 2003;53:1069–1074.

264. De Herdt P, Haesebrouck F, Devriese LA, et al. Biochemical and antigenic

properties of *Streptococcus bovis* isolated from pigeons. J Clin Microbiol 1992; 30:2432–2434.

265. De la Rosa M, Perez M, Carazo C, et al. New Granada medium for detection and identification of group B streptococci. J Clin Microbiol 1992;30:1019–1021.

266. De la Rosa M, Villarreal R, Vega D, et al. Granada medium for detection and identification of group B streptococci. J Clin Microbiol 1983;18:779–785.

267. Dell A, Antone SM, Gauntt CJ, et al. Autoimmune determinants of rheumatic carditis: Localization of epitopes in human cardiac myosin. Eur Heart J 1991; 12(Suppl D):158–162.

268. Della-Latta P, Whittier S, Hosmer M, et al. Rapid detection of group A streptococcal pharyngitis in a pediatric population with optical immunoassay. Pediatr Infect Dis J 1994;13:742–743.

269. DeMan JC, Rogosa M, Sharpe ME. A medium for the cultivation of lactobacilli. J Appl Microbiol 1960;23:130–135.

270. De Moor CE. Septicaemic infections in pigs caused by haemolytic streptococci of new Lancefield groups designated R, S, and T. Antonie Leeuwenhoek J Microbiol Serol 1963;29:272–280.

271. De Soet JJ, De Graf J. Monoclonal antibodies for enumeration and identification of mutans streptococci in epidemiological studies. Arch Oral Biol 1990;35:165S–168S.

272. De Vaux A, Laguerre G, Divies C, Prevost H. *Enterococcus asini* sp. nov. isolated from the caecum of donkeys (*Equus asinus*). Int J Syst Evol Microbiol 1998;48:383–387.

273. Dever LL, Smith SM, Handwerger S, Eng RHK. Vancomycin-dependent *Enterococcus faecium* isolated from stool following oral vancomycin therapy. J Clin Microbiol 1995;33:2770–2773.

274. Devriese LA, Ceyssens K, Haesebrouck F. Characteristics of *Enterococcus cecorum* strains from the intestines of different animal species. Lett Appl Microbiol 1991;12:137–139.

275. Devriese LA, Ceyssens K, Rodrigues UM, et al. *Enterococcus columbae*, a species from pigeon intestines. FEMS Microbiol Lett 1990;71:247–252.

276. Devriese LA, Dutta GN, Farrow JAE, et al. *Streptococcus cecorum*, a new species isolated from chickens. Int J Syst Bacteriol 1983;33:772–776.

277. Devriese LA, Hommez J, Kilpper-Balz R, Schleifer KH. *Streptococcus canis* sp. nov.: a species of group G streptococci from animals. Int J Syst Bacteriol 1986;36:422–425.

278. Devriese LA, Kilpper-Balz R, Schleifer KH. *Streptococcus hyointestinalis* sp. nov. from the gut of swine. Int J Syst Bacteriol 1988;38:440–441.

279. Devriese LA, Pot B, Vandamme P, et al. *Streptococcus hyovaginalis* sp. nov., and *Streptococcus thoraltensis* sp. nov. from the genital tract of sows. Int J Syst Bacteriol 1997;47:1073–1077.

280. Devriese LA, Vandamme P, Collins MD, et al. *Streptococcus pluranimalium* sp. nov., from cattle and other animals. Int J Syst Bacteriol 1999;49:1221–1226.

281. Devriese LA, Vandamme P, Pot B, et al. Differentiation between *Streptococcus gallolyticus* strains of human clinical and veterinary origins and *Streptococcus bovis* strains from the intestinal tracts of ruminants. J Clin Microbiol 1998;36:3520–2523.

282. Dhariwal DK, Patton DW, Gregory MC. Epidural spinal abscess following dental extraction: a rare and potentially fatal complication. Br J Oral Maxillofac Surg 2003;41:56–58.

283. Dicks LMT, Dellaglio F, Collins MD. Proposal to reclassify *Leuconostoc oenos* as *Oenococcus oeni* [corrig.] gen. nov. comb. nov. Int J Syst Bacteriol 1995; 45:395–397.

284. Dicks LMT, Fantuzzi L, Gonzales FC, et al. *Leuconostoc argentinum* sp. nov., isolated from Argentine raw milk. Int J Syst Bacteriol 1993;43:347–351.

285. Diekema DJ, Andrews JI, Huynh H, et al. Molecular epidemiology of macrolide resistance in neonatal bloodstream isolates of group B streptococci. J Clin Microbiol 2003;41:2659–2661.

286. Dillon HC Jr, Khare S, Gray BM. Group B streptococcal carriage and disease: a 6-year prospective study. J Pediatr 1987;110:31–36.

287. DiNubile MJ, Albornoz MA, Stumacher RJ, et al. Pneumococcal soft-tissue infections: possible association with connective tissue diseases. J Infect Dis 1991;163:897–900.

288. Dobkin D, Shulman ST. Evaluation of an ELISA for group A streptococcal antigen for diagnosis of pharyngitis. J Pediatr 1987;110:566–568.

289. Dobson CM, Deneer H, Lee S, et al. Phylogenetic analysis of the genus *Pediococcus*, including *Pediococcus claussenii* sp. nov., a novel lactic acid bacterium isolated from beer. Int J Syst Evol Microbiol 2002;52:2003–2010.

290. Dobson SRM, Baker CJ. Enterococcal sepsis in neonates: features by age at onset and occurrence of focal infections. Pediatrics 1990;85:165–171.

291. Doern GV, Brown SD. Antimicrobial susceptibility among community-acquired respiratory tract pathogens in the U.S.A.: data from PROTEKT US 2000-01. J Infect 2004;48:56–65.

292. Doern GV, Ferraro J, Brueggemann AB, Ruoff KL. Emergence of high rates of antimicrobial resistance among viridans group streptococci in the United States. Antimicrob Agents Chemother 1996;40:891–894.

293. Doern GV, Heilmann KP, Huynh HK, et al. Antimicrobial resistance among clinical isolates of *Streptococcus pneumoniae* in the United States during 1999–2000, including a comparison of resistance rates since 1994–1995. Antimicrob Agents Chemother 2001;45:1721–1729.

294. Doern GV, Pfaller MA, Kugler K, et al. Prevalence of antimicrobial resistance among respiratory tract isolates of *Streptococcus pneumoniae* in North America: 1997 results from the SENTRY Antimicrobial Surveillance Program. Clin Infect Dis 1998;27:764–770.

295. Domingo P, Barquet N, Alvarez M, et al. Group B streptococcal meningitis in adults: report of twelve cases and review. Clin Infect Dis 1997;25:1180–1187.

296. Donabedian S, Chow JW, Shlaes DM, et al. DNA hybridization and contour-clamped homogeneous electric field electrophoresis for identification of enterococci to the species level. J Clin Microbiol 1995;33:141–145.

297. Donders GG, Vereecken A, Salembier G, Spitz B. Accuracy of rapid antigen detection test for group B streptococci in the indigenous vaginal bacterial flora. Arch Gynecol Obstet 1999;263:34–36.

298. Donsakul K, Dejthevaporn C, Witoonpanich R. *Streptococccus suis* infection: clinical features and diagnostic pitfalls. Southeast Asian J Trop Med Public Health 2003;34:154–158.

299. Dorvilus P, Edoo-Sowah R. *Streptococcus milleri*: a cause of pyogenic liver abscess. J Natl Med Assoc 2001;93:276–277.

300. Dougherty SH. Role of enterococcus in intraabdominal sepsis. Am J Surg 1984; 148:308–312.

301. Douglas CWI, Heath J, Hampton KK, et al. Identity of viridans streptococci isolated from cases of infective endocarditis. J Med Microbiol 1993;39:179–182.

302. Doyuk E, Ormerod OJ, Bowler ICJW. Native valve endocarditis due to *Streptococcus vestibularis* and *Streptococcus oralis*. J Infect 2002;45:39–41.

303. Duff P, Gibbs RS. Acute intraamniotic infection due to *Streptococcus pneumoniae*. Obstet Gynecol 1983;61(Suppl):25S–27S.

304. Durand ML, Calderwood SB, Weber DJ, et al. Acute bacterial meningitis in adults. N Engl J Med 1993;328:21–28.

305. Durmaz R, Ozerol IH, Kalcioglu MT, et al. Detection of *Alloiococcus otitidis* in the nasopharynx and in the outer ear canal. New Microbiol 2002;25:265–268.

306. Dutka-Malen S, Evers S, Courvalin P. Detection of glycopeptide resistance genotypes and identification to the species level of clinically relevant enterococci by PCR. J Clin Microbiol 1995;33:24–27.

307. Duval X, Papastamopoulos V, Longuet P, et al. Definite *Streptococcus bovis* endocarditis: characteristics in 20 patients. Clin Microbiol Infect 2001;7:3–10.

308. Ebnother C, Altwegg M, Gottschalk J, et al. *Aerococcus urinae* endocarditis: case report and review of the literature. Infection 2002;30:310–313.

309. Edson RS, Osmon DR, Berry DJ. Septic arthritis due to *Streptococcus sanguis*. Mayo Clin Proc 2002;77:709–710.

310. Edwards AT, Roulson M. A milk-borne outbreak of serious infection due to *Streptococcus zooepidemicus* (Lancefield group C). Epidemiol Infect 1988; 101:43–51.

311. Edwards MS, Baker CJ. *Streptococcus agalactiae* (group B streptococcus). In: Mandell GL, Bennett JE, Dolin R, eds. Mandell, Douglas, and Bennett's Principles and Practice of Infectious Diseases. Vol. 2, 5th Ed. New York: Churchill Livingstone, 2000:2156–2167.

312. Edwards MS, Kasper DL, Jennings HJ, et al. Capsular sialic acid prevents activation of the alternative complement pathway by type III, group B streptococci. J Immunol 1982;128:1278–1283.

313. Efstratiou A, Emery M, Lamagni TL, et al. Increasing incidence of group A streptococcal infections amongst injecting drug users in England and Wales. J Med Microbiol 2003;52:525–526.

314. Eggelmeijer F, Petit P, Dijkmans BA. Total knee arthroplasty infection due to *Gemella haemolysans*. Br J Rheumatol 1992;31:67–69.

315. Eisenberger U, Brunkhorst R, Perharic L, et al. *Gemella morbillorum*—spondylodiscitis in a patient with a renal graft. Nephrol Dial Transplant 1998;13:1565–1567.

316. Ekdahl K, Ahlinder I, Hansson H, et al. Duration of nasopharyngeal carriage of penicillin-resistant *Streptococcus pneumoniae*: experience from the South Swedish pneumococcal intervention project. Clin Infect Dis 1997;25:1113–1117.

317. Eldar A, Frelier PF, Assenta L, et al. *Streptococcus shiloi*, the name for an agent causing septicemic infection in fish, is a junior synonym of *Streptococcus iniae*. Int J Syst Bacteriol 1995;45:840–842.

318. Eldar A, Ghittino C, Asanta L, et al. *Enterococcus seriolicida* is a junior synonym of *Lactococcus garvieae*, a causative agent of septicemia and meningoencephalitis in fish. Curr Microbiol 1996;32:85–88.

319. Eledrisi MS, Zuckerman MJ, Ho H. Spontaneous bacterial peritonitis caused by *Streptococcus bovis*. Am J Gastroenterol 2000;95:1110–1111.

320. Elhanen G, Raz R. Group B streptococcal vertebral osteomyelitis in an adult. Infection 1993;21:397–399.

321. Eliopoulos GM. Increasing problems in the therapy of enterococcal infections. Eur J Clin Microbiol Infect Dis 1993;12:409–412.

322. Elliott JA, Collins MD, Pigott NE, Facklam RR. Differentiation of *Lactococcus lactis* and *Lactococcus garvieae* from humans by comparison of whole-cell protein patterns. J Clin Microbiol 1991;29:2731–2734.

323. Elliott JA, Facklam RR. Identification of *Leuconostoc* spp. by analysis of soluble whole cell protein patterns. J Clin Microbiol 1993;31:1030–1033.

324. Elliott JA, Farmer KD, Facklam RR. Sudden increase in isolation of group B streptococci, serotype V, is not due to emergence of a new pulsed-field gel electrophoresis type. J Clin Microbiol 1998;36:2115–2116.

325. Elliott PM, Williams H, Brooksby IAB. A case of infective endocarditis in a farmer caused by *Streptococcus equinus*. Eur Heart J 1993;14:1291–1293.

326. Elsayed S, Hammerberg O, Massey V, Hussain Z. *Streptococcus equi* subspecies *equi* (Lancefield group C) meningitis in a child. Clin Microbiol Infect 2003;9:869–872.

327. Emiliani VJ, Chodos JE, Comer GM, et al. *Streptococcus bovis* brain abscess associated with an occult colonic villous adenoma. Am J Gastroenterol 1990;85:78–80.

328. Erdogan S, Fagan PK, Talay SR, et al. Molecular analysis of group B protective surface protein, a new cell surface protective antigen of group B streptococci. Infect Immun 2002;70:803–811.

329. Erickson D, Doster AR, Pokorny TS. Isolation of *Streptococcus suis* from swine in Nebraska. J Am Vet Assoc 1984;185:666–668.

330. Espinoza R, Kusne S, Pasculle AW, et al. *Leuconostoc* bacteremia after liver transplantation: another cause of vancomycin-resistant gram-positive infection. Clin Transplant 1997;11:322–324.

331. Evaldson GR, Malmborg A-S, Nord CE. Premature rupture of the membranes and ascending infection. Br J Obstet Gynaecol 1982;89:793–801.

332. Ezaki T, Facklam RR, Takeuchi N, et al. Genetic relatedness between the type strain of *Streptococcus anginosus* and minute-colony-forming β-hemolytic streptococci carrying different Lancefield grouping antigens. Int J Syst Bacteriol 1986;36:345–347.

333. Facklam RR. Specificity study of kits for detection of group A streptococci directly from throat swabs. J Clin Microbiol 1987;25:504–508.

334. Facklam R, Beall B, Efstratiou A, et al. *emm* typing and validation of provisional M types for group A streptococci. Emerg Infect Dis 1999;5:247–253.

335. Facklam RR, Collins MD. Identification of *Enterococcus* species isolated from human infections by a conventional test scheme. J Clin Microbiol 1989;27:731–734.

336. Facklam R, Elliott JA. Identification, classification, and clinical relevance of catalase-negative, gram-positive cocci, excluding streptococci and enterococci. Clin Microbiol Rev 1995;8:479–495.

337. Facklam R, Elliott J, Pigott N, Franklin AR. Identification of *Streptococcus porcinus* from human sources. J Clin Microbiol 1995;33:385–388.

338. Facklam R, Hollis D, Collins MD. Identification of gram-positive coccal and coccobacillary vancomycin-resistant bacteria. J Clin Microbiol 1989;27:724–730.

339. Facklam R, Lovgren M, Shewmaker PL, Tyrrell G. Phenotypic description and antimicrobial susceptibilities of *Aerococcus sanguinicola* isolates from human clinical samples. J Clin Microbiol 2003;41:2587–2592.

340. Facklam RR, Martin DR, Lovgren M, et al. Extension of the Lancefield classification for group A streptococci by addition of 22 new M protein gene sequence types from clinical isolates: *emm*103 to *emm*124. Clin Infect Dis 2002;34:28–38.

341. Facklam R, Pigott N, Franklin R, et al. Evaluation of three disk tests for identification of enterococci, leuconostocs, and pediococci. J Clin Microbiol 1995;33:885–887.

342. Facklam RR, Thacker LG, Fox B, et al. Presumptive identification of streptococci with a new test system. J Clin Microbiol 1982;15:987–990.

343. Faden H, Dryja D. Recovery of a unique bacterial organism in human middle ear fluid and its possible role in chronic otitis media. J Clin Microbiol 1989;27:2488–2491.

344. Farley MM. Group B streptococcal disease in nonpregnant adults. Clin Infect Dis 2001;33:556–561.

345. Farley MM, Harvey C, Stull T, et al. A population-based assessment of invasive disease due to group B streptococcus in non-pregnant adults. N Engl J Med 1993;328:1807–1811.

346. Farmaki E, Roilides E, Darilis E, et al. *Gemella morbillorum* endocarditis in a child. Pediatr Infect Dis J 2000;19:751–753.

347. Farrow JAE, Collins MD. DNA base composition, DNA-DNA homology, and long-chain fatty acid studies on *Streptococcus thermophilus* and *Streptococcus salivarius*. J Gen Microbiol 1984;130:357–362.

348. Farrow JAE, Collins MD. Taxonomic studies on streptococci of serological groups C, G, and L and possibly related taxa. Syst Appl Microbiol 1984;5:483–493.

349. Farrow JAE, Collins MD. *Enterococcus hirae*, a new species that includes amino acid assay strain NCDO 1258 and strains causing growth depression in young chickens. Int J Syst Bacteriol 1985;35:73–75.

350. Farrow JAE, Facklam RR, Collins MD. Nucleic acid homologies of some vancomycin-resistant leuconostocs and description of *Leuconostoc citreum* sp. nov. and *Leuconostoc pseudomesenteroides* sp. nov. Int J Syst Bacteriol 1989;39:279–283.

351. Farrow JAE, Kruze J, Phillips BA, et al. Taxonomic studies on *Streptococcus bovis* and *Streptococcus equinus*: description of *Streptococcus alactolyticus* sp. nov. and *Streptococcus saccharolyticus* sp. nov. Syst Appl Microbiol 1984;5:467–483.

352. Fasano FJ, Graham DR, Stauffer ES. Vertebral osteomyelitis secondary to *Streptococcus agalactiae*. Clin Orthop 1990;256:101–104.

353. Fast DJ, Schlievert PM, Nelson RD. Toxic shock syndrome-associated staphylococcal and streptococcal pyrogenic toxins are potent inducers of tumor necrosis factor production. Infect Immun 1989;57:291–294.

354. Felmingham D, Wilson APR, Quintana AI, Gruneberg RN. *Enterococcus* species in urinary tract infection. Clin Infect Dis 1992;15:295–301.

355. Fenoll A, Martinez-Suarez JV, Munoz R, et al. Identification of atypical strains of *Streptococcus pneumoniae* by a specific DNA probe. Eur J Clin Microbiol Infect Dis 1990;9:396–401.

356. Ferrer JC, Padilla JJV, Igual RI, et al. *Streptococcus bovis* meningitis: no association with colonic malignancy. Clin Infect Dis 1993;17:527–528.

357. Ferrer S, deMiguel G, Domingo P, et al. Pulmonary infection due to *Leuconostoc* species in a patient with AIDS. Clin Infect Dis 1995;21:225–226.

358. Ferrieri P. Neonatal susceptibility and immunity to major bacterial pathogens. Rev Infect Dis 1990;12(Suppl 4):S394–S400.

359. Ferrieri P, Cleary PP, Seeds SE. Epidemiology of group B streptococcal carriage in pregnant women and newborn infants. J Med Microbiol 1976;13:273–280.

360. Fillit HM, McCarty M, Blake M. Induction of antibodies to hyaluronic acid by immunization of rabbits with encapsulated streptococci. J Exp Med 1986;164:762–776.

361. Fines M, Perichon B, Reynolds PE, et al. VanE, a new type of acquired glycopeptide resistance in *Enterococcus faecalis* BM4405. Antimicrob Agents Chemother 1999;43:2161–2164.

362. Finlay FO, Witherow H, Rudd PT. Latex agglutination testing in bacterial meningitis. Arch Dis Child 1995;73:160–163.

363. Fischetti VA. Streptococcal M protein: molecular design and biological behavior. Clin Microbiol Rev 1989;2:285–314.

364. Fisher LE, Russell RRB. The isolation and characterization of milleri group streptococci from dental periapical abscesses. J Dent Res 1993;72:1191–1193.

365. Flanagan PG, Mills RG. Fulminant septicaemia due to *Streptococcus milleri* infection in a previously healthy adult. Eur J Clin Microbiol Infect Dis 1994;13:247–248.

366. Flint SH, Ward LJH, Brooks JD. *Streptococcus waius* sp. nov., a thermophilic streptococcus from a biofilm. Int J Syst Bacteriol 1999;49:759–767.

367. Food and Drug Administration. Risks of devices for direct detection of group B streptococcal antigen. J Nurse Midwifery 1997;42:408–409.

368. Ford M, Perry JD, Gould FK. Use of cephalexin-aztreonam-arabinose agar for selective isolation of *Enterococcus faecium*. J Clin Microbiol 1994;32:2999–3001.

369. Forni AL, Kaplan EL, Schlievert PM, et al. Clinical and microbiological characteristics of severe group A streptococcus infections and streptococcal toxic shock syndrome. Clin Infect Dis 1995;21:333–340.

370. Fox K, Turner J, Fox A. Role of β-hemolytic group C streptococci in pharyngitis: incidence and biochemical characteristics of *Streptococcus equisimilis* and *Streptococcus anginosus* in patients and healthy controls. J Clin Microbiol 1993;31:804–807.

371. Fox KL, Born MW, Cohen MA. Fulminant infection and toxic shock syndrome caused by *Streptococcus pyogenes*. J Emerg Med 2002;22:357–366.

372. Fraimow HS, Jungkind DL. Vancomycin-dependent enterococci: a clinical and laboratory assessment. Adv Exp Med Biol 1995;390:97–107.

373. Fraimow HS, Jungkind DL, Lander DW, et al. Urinary tract infection with an *Enterococcus faecalis* isolate that requires vancomycin for growth. Ann Intern Med 1994;121:22–26.

374. Franciosi RA, Knostman JD, Zimmerman RA. Group B streptococcal neonatal and infant infections. J Pediatr 1973;82:707–718.

375. Francis AJ, Nimmo GR, Efstratiou A, et al. Investigation of milk-borne *Streptococcus zooepidemicus* infection associated with glomerulonephritis in Australia. J Infect 1993;27:317–323.

376. Frandsen EVG, Pedrazzol V, Kilian M. Ecology of viridans streptococci in the oral cavity and pharynx. Oral Microbiol Immunol 1991;6:129–133.

377. French GL, Talsania H, Phillips I. Identification of viridans streptococci by pyrolysis-gas chromatography. J Med Microbiol 1989;29:19–27.

378. Freney J, Bland S, Etienne J, et al. Description and evaluation of the semi-automated 4-hour rapid ID 32 Strep method for identification of streptococci and members of related genera. J Clin Microbiol 1992;30:2657–2661.

379. Fresard S, Michel VP, Rueda X, et al. *Gemella hemolysans* endocarditis. Clin Infect Dis 1993;16:586–587.

380. Friedland IR, Snipelisky M, Khoosal M. Meningitis in a neonate caused by *Leuconostoc* sp. J Clin Microbiol 1990;28:2125–2126.

381. Friedman CA, Wender DF, Rawson JE. Rapid diagnosis of group B streptococcal infection utilizing a commercially available latex agglutination assay. Pediatrics 1984;73:27–30.

382. Gallagher PG, Watanakunakorn C. Group B streptococcal endocarditis: report

of seven cases and review of the literature, 1962–1985. Rev Infect Dis 1986; 8:175–188.

383. Galli D, Wirth R. Comparative analysis of *Enterococcus faecalis* sex phero-mone plasmids identifies a single homologous DNA region which codes for aggregation substance. J Bacteriol 1991;173:3029–3033.

384. Garcia S, Combalia A, Segur JM. Septic arthritis of the shoulder due to *Streptococcus agalactiae*. Acta Orthop Belg 1996;62:66–68.

385. Garcia-Lechuz JM, Bachiller P, Vasallo FJ, et al. Group B streptococcal osteo-myelitis in adults. Medicine (Baltimore) 1999;78:191–199.

386. Gardam MA, Low DE, Saginur R, Miller MA. Group B streptococcal necrotiz-ing fasciitis and streptococcal toxic shock syndrome in adults. Arch Intern Med 1998;158:1704–1708.

387. Garland SM, Fliegner JR. Group B streptococcus and neonatal infections: the case for intrapartum prophylaxis. Aust NZ J Obstet Gynecol 1991;31:119–122.

388. Garvie EI. *Leuconostoc oenos* sp. nov. J Gen Microbiol 1967;48:431–438.

389. Gavin PJ, Thomson RB Jr, Horng S-J, Yogev R. Neonatal sepsis caused by *Streptococcus bovis* variant (biotype II/2): report of a case and review. J Clin Microbiol 2003;41:3433–3435.

390. Gelfand MS, Hughey JR, Sloas DD. Group B streptococcal bacteremia associ-ated with adenocarcinoma of the stomach. Clin Infect Dis 1994;19:364.

391. Gelfand MS, Threlkeld MG. Subacute bacterial endocarditis secondary to *Streptococcus pneumoniae*. Am J Med 1992;93:91.

392. George AL Jr, Savage AM. Fatal group B streptococcal empyema in an adult. South Med J 1987;80:1436–1438.

393. Gerber MA. Comparison of throat cultures and rapid strep tests for diagnosis of streptococcal pharyngitis. Pediatr Infect Dis 1989;8:820–824.

394. Gerber MA, Randolph MF, DeMeo KK. Liposome immunoassay for rapid identification of group A streptococci directly from throat swabs. J Clin Micro-biol 1990;28:1463–1464.

395. Gesner M, Desiderio D, Kim M, et al. *Streptococcus pneumoniae* in human immunodeficiency virus type 1-infected children. Pediatr Infect Dis J 1994; 13:697–703.

396. Gholizadeh Y, Courvalin P. Acquired and intrinsic glycopeptide resistance in enterococci. Int J Antimicrob Agents 2000;16:S11–S17.

397. Gibson RL, Nizet V, Rubens CE. Group B streptococcal β-hemolysin promotes injury of lung microvascular endothelial cells. Pediatr Res 1999;45:626–634.

398. Gieseker KE, Roe MH, MacKenzie T, Todd JK. Evaluating the American Academy of Pediatrics diagnostic standard for *Streptococcus pyogenes* pharyn-gitis: backup culture versus repeat rapid antigen testing. Pediatrics 2003;111: e666–e670.

399. Gilad J, Borer A, Riesenberg K, et al. *Enterococcus hirae* septicemia in a patient with end-stage renal disease undergoing hemodialysis. Eur J Clin Micro-biol Infect Dis 1998;17:576–577.

400. Gillespie RS, Symons JM, McDonald RA. Peritonitis due to *Leuconostoc* spe-cies in a child receiving peritoneal dialysis. Pediatr Nephrol 2002;17:966–968.

401. Gilon D, Moses A. Carcinoma of the colon presenting as *Streptococcus equinus* bacteremia. Am J Med 1989;86:135–136.

402. Giraud P, Attal M, Lemouzy J, et al. *Leuconostoc*: a potential pathogen in bone marrow transplantation. Lancet 1993;341:1481–1482.

403. Givner LB, Mason EO Jr, Tan TQ, et al. Pneumococcal endocarditis in children. Clin Infect Dis 2004;38:1273–1278.

404. Godeau B, Bachir D, Schaeffer A, et al. Severe pneumococcal sepsis and menin-gitis in human immunodeficiency virus-infected adults with sickle cell disease. Clin Infect Dis 1992;15:327–329.

405. Gold HS. Vancomycin-resistant enterococci: mechanisms and clinical observa-tions. Clin Infect Dis 2001;33:210–219.

406. Golden S. Group A streptococcus and streptococcal toxic shock syndrome: a post-partum case report. J Midwifery Womens Health 2003;48:357–359.

407. Goldschmidt JC, Panos C. Teichoic acids of *Streptococcus agalactiae*: chemis-try, cytotoxicity, and effect on bacterial adherence. Infect Immun 1984;43: 670–677.

408. Goldshlack P, Blackburn G. Lancefield group G streptococcus septic arthritis in a heroin user: report of a case. J Am Osteopath Assoc 1984;84:60–61.

409. Goldstein I, Rebeyrotte P, Parlebas J, et al. Isolation from heart valves of glycopeptides which share immunological properties with *Streptococcus haemolyticus* group A polysaccharides. Nature 1968;219:866–868.

410. Golledge CL, Stringemore N, Aravena M, et al. Septicemia caused by vancomy-cin-resistant *Pediococcus acidilactici*. J Clin Microbiol 1990;28:1678–1679.

411. Gomez-Garces J-L, Alos J-I, Cogollos R. Bacteriological characteristics and antimicrobial susceptibility of 70 clinically significant isolates of the *Strepto-coccus milleri* group. Diagn Microbiol Infect Dis 1994;19:69–73.

412. Gonzalez-Quintela A, Marinez-Rey C, Castroagudin JF, et al. Prevalence of liver disease in patients with *Streptococcus bovis* bacteremia. J Infect 2001; 42:116–119.

413. Gordillo ME, Singh KV, Murray BE. Comparison of ribotyping and pulsed-field gel electrophoresis for subspecies differentiation of strains of *Enterococ-cus faecalis*. J Clin Microbiol 1993;31:1570–1574.

414. Gordon DM, Oster CN. Hematogenous group B streptococcal osteomyelitis in an adult. South Med J 1984;77:643–645.

415. Gordon KA, Biedenbach DJ, Jones RN. Comparison of *Streptococcus pneu-moniae* and *Haemophilus influenzae* susceptibilities from community-acquired respiratory tract infections and hospitalized patients with pneumonia: five-year results for the SENTRY Antimicrobial Surveillance Program. Diagn Microbiol Infect Dis 2003;46:285–289.

416. Goroncy-Bermes P, Dale JB, Beachey EH, et al. Monoclonal antibody to human renal glomeruli cross-reacts with streptococcal M-protein. Infect Immun 1987; 55:2416–2419.

417. Goshorn SC, Bohach GA, Schlievert PM. Cloning and characterization of the gene, *speC*, for pyrogenic exotoxin type C from *Streptococcus pyogenes*. Mol Gen Genet 1988;212:66–70.

418. Goshorn SC, Schlievert PM. Nucleotide sequence of streptococcal pyrogenic exotoxin type C. Infect Immun 1988;56:2518.

419. Goto T, Nagamune H, Miyazaki A, et al. Rapid identification of *Streptococcus intermedius* by PCR with the *ily* gene as a species marker gene. J Med Microbiol 2002;51:178–186.

420. Gottschalk M, Higgins R, Boudreau M. Use of polyvalent coagglutination re-agents for serotyping of *Streptococcus suis*. J Clin Microbiol 1993;31: 2192–2194.

421. Gottschalk M, Higgins R, Jacques M, et al. Isolation and characterization of *Streptococcus suis* capsular types 9-22. J Vet Diagn Investig 1991;3:60–65.

422. Gottschalk M, Higgins R, Jacques M, et al. Characterization of six new capsular types (23 through 28) of *Streptococcus suis*. J Clin Microbiol 1991;29: 2590–2594.

423. Gottschalk M, Higgins R, Jacques M, et al. Description of 14 new capsular types of *Streptococcus suis*. J Clin Microbiol 1989;27:2633–2636.

424. Gottschalk M, LeBrun A, Jacques M, et al. Hemagglutination properties of *Streptococcus suis*. J Clin Microbiol 1990;28:2156–2158.

425. Gottschalk M, Sequra M. The pathogenesis of the meningitis caused by *Strepto-coccus suis*: the unsolved questions. Vet Microbiol 2000;76:259–270.

426. Graber CJ, de Almeida KN, Atkinson JC, et al. Dental health and viridans streptococcal bacteremia in allogeneic hematopoietic stem cell transplant recip-ients. Bone Marrow Transplant 2001;27:537–542.

427. Graninger W, Ragette R. Nosocomial bacteremia due to *Enterococcus faecalis* without endocarditis. Clin Infect Dis 1992;15:49–57.

428. Granowitz EV, Donaldson WR, Skolnick PR. Gas-forming soft tissue abscess caused by *Streptococcus pneumoniae*. Am J Med 1992;93:105–107.

429. Grant KA, Dickinson JH, Collins MD, et al. Rapid identification of *Aerococcus viridans* using the polymerase chain reaction and an oligonucleotide probe. FEMS Microbiol Lett 1992;95:63–68.

430. Gray BM, Converse GM III, Dillon HC Jr. Epidemiologic studies of *Streptococ-cus pneumoniae* in infants: acquisition, carriage, and infection during the first 24 months of life. J Infect Dis 1980;142:923–933.

431. Gray BM, Dillon HC Jr. Clinical and epidemiologic studies of pneumococcal infection in children. Pediatr Infect Dis J 1986;5:201–207.

432. Gray BM, Dillon HC Jr. Epidemiological studies of *Streptococcus pneumoniae* in infants: antibody to types 3, 6, 14, and 23 in the first two years of life. J Infect Dis 1988;158:948–955.

433. Green M, Barbadora K, Michaels M. Recovery of vancomycin-resistant gram-positive cocci from pediatric liver transplant recipients. J Clin Microbiol 1991; 29:2503–2506.

434. Green M, Wadowsky RW, Barbadora K. Recovery of vancomycin-resistant gram-positive cocci from children. J Clin Microbiol 1990;28:484–488.

435. Green PA, Campbell JR. Transient, asymptomatic bacteremia due to *Enterococ-cus avium* in a 33-month-old child. Clin Infect Dis 1994;19:561.

436. Greenberg DN, Ascher DP, Yoder BA, et al. Group B streptococcus serotype V. J Pediatr 1993;123:494–495.

437. Greub G, Devriese LA, Pot B, et al. *Enterococcus cecorum* septicemia in a malnourished adult patient. Eur J Clin Microbiol Infect Dis 1997;16:594–598.

438. Griffith SP, Gersony WM. Acute rheumatic fever in New York City (1969–1988): a comparative study of two decades. J Pediatr 1990;116: 882–887.

439. Griffiths BB, McClain O. The role of iron in the growth and hemolysin (strepto-lysin S) production in *Streptococcus pyogenes*. J Basic Microbiol 1988;28: 427–436.

440. Gruteke P, van Belkum A, Schouls LM, et al. Outbreak of group A streptococci in a burn center: use of pheno- and genotypic procedures for strain tracking. J Clin Microbiol 1996;34:114–118.

441. Guerin JM, Mofredj A, Leibinger F, et al. Group B streptococcal meningitis in an HIV-positive adult: case report and review. Scand J Infect Dis 2000;32: 215–217.

442. Guerrero C, Martinez J, Menasalvas A, et al. Use of direct latex agglutination testing of selective broth in the detection of group B streptococcal carriage in pregnant women. Eur J Clin Microbiol Infect Dis 2004;23:61–62.

443. Gullberg RM, Homann SR, Phair JP. Enterococcal bacteremia: analysis of 75 episodes. Rev Infect Dis 1989;11:74–85.

444. Gutierrez F, Masia M, Rodriguez JC, et al. Evaluation of the immunochromatographic Binax NOW assay for detection of *Streptococcus pneumoniae* urinary antigen in a prospective study of community-acquired pneumonia in Spain. Clin Infect Dis 2003;36:286–292.

445. Haas J, Jernick SL, Scardina RJ, et al. Colonization of skin by *Helcococcus kunzii*. J Clin Microbiol 1997;35:2759–2761.

446. Hachey WE, Wiswell TE. Limitations in the usefulness of urine latex particle agglutination and hematologic measurements in diagnosing neonatal sepsis during the first week of life. J Perinatol 1992;12:240–245.

447. Hackett SP, Stevens DL. Streptococcal toxic shock syndrome: synthesis of tumor necrosis factor and interleukin-1 by monocytes stimulated with pyrogenic exotoxin A and streptolysin O. J Infect Dis 1992;165:879–885.

448. Hackett SP, Stevens DL. Superantigens associated with staphylococcal and streptococcal toxic shock syndrome are potent inducers of tumor necrosis factor-β synthesis. J Infect Dis 1993;168:232–235.

449. Haddad PA, Repka TL, Weisdorf D. Penicillin-resistant *Streptococcus pneumoniae* septic shock and meningitis complicating chronic graft versus host disease: a case report and review of the literature. Am J Med 2002;113: 152–155.

450. Hall GE, Baddour LM. Apparent failure of endocarditis prophylaxis caused by penicillin-resistant *Streptococcus mitis*. Am J Med Sci 2002;324:51–53.

451. Hall GS, Gordon S, Schroeder S, et al. Case of synovitis potentially caused by *Dolosigranulum pigrum*. J Clin Microbiol 2001;39:1202–1203.

452. Hamer DH, Egas J, Estrella B, et al. Assessment of the Binax NOW *Streptococcus pneumoniae* urinary antigen test in children with nasopharyngeal pneumococcal carriage. Clin Infect Dis 2002;34:1025–1028.

453. Hamilton JR. Comparison of Meritec-Strep with Streptex for direct colony grouping of β-hemolytic streptococci from primary isolation and subculture plates. J Clin Microbiol 1988;26:692–695.

454. Hamoudi AC, Marcon MJ, Cannon HJ, et al. Comparison of three major antigen detection methods for the diagnosis of group B streptococcal sepsis in neonates. Pediatr Infect Dis 1983;2:432–435.

455. Han JK, Kerschner JE. *Streptococcus milleri*: an organism for head and neck infections and abscess. Arch Otolaryngol Head Neck Surg 2001;127:650–654.

456. Handley P, Coykendall A, Beighton D, et al. *Streptococcus crista* sp. nov., a viridans streptococcus with tufted fibrils, isolated from the human oral cavity and throat. Int J Syst Bacteriol 1991;41:543–547.

457. Handwerger S, Horowitz H, Coburn K, et al. Infection due to *Leuconostoc* species: six cases and review. Rev Infect Dis 1990;12:602–610.

458. Hansen SM, Uldbjerg N, Kilian M, Sorensen UB. Dynamics of *Streptococcus agalactiae* colonization in women during and after pregnancy and in their infants. J Clin Microbiol 2004;42:83–89.

459. Hanski E, Caparon M. Protein F, a fibronectin-binding protein, is an adhesin of the group A streptococcus, *Streptococcus pyogenes*. Proc Natl Acad Sci USA 1992;89:6172–6176.

460. Harbarth S, Uckay I. Are there patients with peritonitis who require empiric therapy for enterococcus? Eur J Clin Microbiol Infect Dis 2004;23:73–77.

461. Harbeck RJ, Teague J, Crossen GR, et al. Novel, rapid optical immunoassay technique for detection of group A streptococci from pharyngeal specimens: comparison with standard culture methods. J Clin Microbiol 1993;31:839–844.

462. Hardy S, Ruoff KL, Catlin EA, et al. Catheter-associated infection with a vancomycin-resistant gram-positive coccus of the *Leuconostoc* sp. Pediatr Infect Dis J 1988;7:519–520.

463. Hardwick RH, Taylor A, Thompson MH, et al. Association between *Streptococcus milleri* and abscess formation after appendicitis. Ann R Coll Surg Engl 2000;82:24–26.

464. Harley WB, Gibbs C, Horton JM. *Streptococcus bovis* meningitis associated with a colonic villous adenoma. Clin Infect Dis 1992;14:979–980.

465. Harper DS, Loesche WJ. Growth and acid tolerance of human dental plaque bacteria. Arch Oral Biol 1984;29:843–848.

466. Hashikawa S, Iinuma Y, Furushita M, et al. Characterization of group C and group G streptococcal strains that cause streptococcal toxic shock syndrome. J Clin Microbiol 2004;42:186–192.

467. Hassan-King M, Baldeh I, Secka O, et al. Detection of *Streptococcus pneumoniae* DNA in blood cultures by PCR. J Clin Microbiol 1994;32:1721–1724.

468. Hauser AR, Schlievert PM. Nucleotide sequence of the streptococcal pyrogenic exotoxin type B gene and relationship between toxin and the streptococcal proteinase precursor. J Bacteriol 1990;172:4536–4542.

469. Hauser AR, Stevens DL, Kaplan EL, et al. Molecular analysis of pyrogenic exotoxins from *Streptococcus pyogenes* isolates associated with toxic shock-like syndrome. J Clin Microbiol 1991;29:1562–1567.

470. Heath CH, Bowen SF, McCarthy JS, Dwyer B. Vertebral osteomyelitis and discitis associated with *Abiotrophia adiacens* (nutritionally variant streptococcus) infection. Aust NZ Med J 1998;28:663.

471. Hechmann-Wittrup I, Chenoufi-Schaadt ML, Arpi M, Danneskiold-Samsoe B. Bacteremia complicated by vertebral osteomyelitis due to *Streptococcus bovis*. Eur J Clin Microbiol Infect Dis 1999;18:365–367.

472. Heelan JS, Wilbur S, Depetris G, Letourneau C. Rapid antigen testing for group A streptococcus by DNA probe. Diagn Microbiol Infect Dis 1996;24:65–69.

473. Heilesen AM. Septicaemia due to *Aerococcus urinae*. Scand J Infect Dis 1994; 26:759–760.

474. Heinz M, von Wintzingerode F, Moter A, et al. A case of septicemia with *Pediococcus acidilactici* after long-term antibiotic treatment. Eur J Clin Microbiol Infect Dis 2000;19:946–948.

475. Heiter BJ, Bourbeau PP. Comparison of the Gen-Probe group A streptococcus direct test with culture and a rapid streptococcal antigen assay for diagnosis of streptococcal pharyngitis. J Clin Microbiol 1993;31:2070–2073.

476. Heiter BJ, Bourbeau PP. Comparison of two rapid streptococcal antigen detection assay with culture for diagnosis of streptococcal pharyngitis. J Clin Microbiol 1995;33:1408–1410.

477. Helft G, Tabone X, Metzger JP, Vacheron A. *Gemella haemolysans* endocarditis with colonic carcinoma. Eur J Med 1993;2:369–370.

478. Hendrickx B, Vandepitte J, DeWit P, Van den Bergh R. Brain abscess associated with *Streptococcus milleri*. A report of eight cases. Acta Clin Belg 1982; 37:307–313.

479. Hepburn MJ, Fraser SL, Rennie TA, et al. Septic arthritis caused by *Granulicatella adiacens*: diagnosis by inoculation of synovial fluid into blood culture bottles. Rheumatol Int 2003;23:255–257.

480. Herwald H, Collin M, Muller-Esterl W, Bjorck L. Streptococcal cysteine protease releases kinins: a novel virulence mechanism. J Exp Med 1996;184: 665–673.

481. Herwald H, Cramer H, Morgelin M, et al. M protein, a classical bacterial virulence determinant, forms complexes with fibrinogen that induce vascular leakage. Cell 2004;116:367–379.

482. Higgins R, Gottschalk M, Boudreau M, et al. Description of six new capsular types (29-34) of *Streptococcus suis*. J Vet Diagn Invest 1995;7:405–406.

483. Higgins R, Gottschalk M, Mittal MK, et al. *Streptococcus suis* infections in swine: a 16-month study. Can J Vet Res 1990;54:170–173.

484. Hill AW, Leigh JA. DNA fingerprinting of *Streptococcus uberis*: a useful tool for epidemiology of bovine mastitis. Epidemiol Infect 1989;103:165–271.

485. Ho AKC, Woo KS, Tse KK, et al. Infective endocarditis caused by *Streptococcus suis* serotype 2. J Infect 1990;21:209–211.

486. Hoe N, Nakashima K, Grigsby D, et al. Rapid molecular genetic subtyping of serotype M-1 group A streptococcus strains. Emerg Infect Dis 1999;5:254–263.

487. Hoen B, Briancon S, Delahaye F, et al. Tumors of the colon increase the risk of developing *Streptococcus bovis* endocarditis: case-control study. Clin Infect Dis 1994;19:361–362.

488. Hoffman JA, Mason EO, Schutze GE, et al. *Streptococcus pneumoniae* infections in the neonate. Pediatrics 2003;112:1095–1102.

489. Hoffmann S. Detection of group A streptococcal antigen from throat swabs with five diagnostic kits in general practice. Diagn Microbiol Infect Dis 1990; 13:209–215.

490. Holland J, Wilson R, Cumpston N. *Gemella morbillorum* prosthetic valve endocarditis. NZ Med J 1996;109:367.

491. Holm SE, Nordstrand A, Stevens DL, Norgren M. Acute poststreptococcal glomerulonephritis. In: Stevens DL, Kaplan EL, eds. Streptococcal Infections: Clinical Aspects, Microbiology, and Molecular Pathogenesis. New York: Oxford University Press, 2000:152–162.

492. Homer KA, Denbow L, Whiley RA, et al. Chondroitin sulfate depolymerase and hyaluronidase activities of viridans streptococci determined by a sensitive spectrophotometric assay. J Clin Microbiol 1993;31:1648–1651.

493. Honig E, Mouton JW, van der Meijden WI. Can group B streptococci cause symptomatic vaginitis? Infect Dis Obstet Gynecol 1999;7:206–209.

494. Honig E, Mouton JW, van der Meijden WI. The epidemiology of vaginal colonization with group B streptococci in a sexually transmitted disease clinic. Eur J Obstet Gynecol 2002;105:177–180.

495. Hospital Infection Control Practices Advisory Committee. Recommendations for preventing the spread of vancomycin resistance. Infect Control Hosp Epidemiol 1995;16:105–113.

496. Hoyles L, Foster G, Falsen E, Collins MD. Characterization of a *Gemella*-like organism isolates from an abscess of a rabbit: description of *Gemella cuniculi* sp. nov. Int J Syst Evol Microbiol 2000; 50:2037–2041.

497. Hoyles L, Foster G, Falsen E, et al. *Facklamia miroungae* sp. nov., from a juvenile southern elephant seal (*Mirounga leonina*). Int J Syst Evol Microbiol 2001;51:1401–1403.

498. Hoyles L, Lawson PA, Foster G, et al. *Vagococcus fessus* sp. nov., isolated from a seal and a harbor porpoise. Int J Syst Evol Microbiol 2000;50:1151–1154.

499. Hsueh P-R, Teng L-J, Chen Y-C, et al. Recurrent bacteremic peritonitis caused by *Enterococcus cecorum* in a patient with liver cirrhosis. J Clin Microbiol 2000;38:2450–2452.

500. Huang IF, Chiou CC, Liu YC, Hsieh KS. Endocarditis caused by penicillin-resistant *Streptococcus mitis* in a 12-year-old boy. J Microbiol Immunol Infect 2002;35:129–132.

501. Huck W, Reed BD, French T, et al. Comparison of the Directigen 1-2-3 Group

A Strep Test with culture for detection of group A β-hemolytic streptococci. J Clin Microbiol 1989;27:1715–1718.

502. Hudson CR, Fedorka-Cray PJ, Jackson-Hall MC, Hiott LM. Anomalies in species identification of enterococci from veterinary sources using a commercial biochemical identification system. Lett Appl Microbiol 2003;36:245–250.

503. Husby G, van de Rijn I, Zabriskie JB, et al. Antibodies reacting with cytoplasm of subthalamic and caudate nuclei neurons in chorea and rheumatic fever. J Exp Med 1976;144:1094–1100.

504. Hutchin ME, Shores CG, Bauer MS, Yarbrough WG. Sinogenic subdural empyema and *Streptococcus anginosus.* Arch Otolaryngol Head Neck Surg 1999; 125:1262–1266.

505. Huycke M, Gilmore M. In vitro survival of *Enterococcus faecalis* is enhanced by extracellular superoxide production. Adv Exp Med Biol 1997;418:781–784.

506. Hwang M, Ederer GM. Rapid hippurate hydrolysis method for presumptive identification of group B streptococci. J Clin Microbiol 1975;1:114–115.

507. Ieven M, Vercauteren E, Descheemaeker P, et al. Comparison of direct plating and broth enrichment culture for the detection of intestinal colonization by glycopeptide-resistant enterococci among hospitalized patients. J Clin Microbiol 1999;37:1436–1440.

508. Igarishi T, Ichikawa K, Yamamoto A, Goto N. Identification of mutans streptococcal species by the PCR products of the dex genes. J Microbiol Meth 2001; 46:99–105.

509. Igwe EI, Shewmaker PL, Facklam RR, et al. Identification of superantigen genes *speM, ssa,* and *smeZ* in invasive strains of β-hemolytic group C and G streptococci recovered from humans. FEMS Microbiol Lett 2003;229:259–264.

510. Ince A, Tiemer B, Gille J, et al. Total knee arthroplasty infection due to *Abiotrophia defectiva.* J Med Microbiol 2002;51:899–902.

511. Ingram DL, Suggs DM, Pearson AW. Detection of group B streptococcal antigen in early-onset and late-onset group B streptococcal disease with the Wellcogen Strep B latex agglutination test. J Clin Microbiol 1982;16:656–658.

512. Irvine MCG, Solomons NB. Atypical supraglottitis caused by *Streptococcus sanguis.* J Laryngol Otol 1990;104:430–431.

513. Isenberg HD, Vellozi EM, Shapiro J, et al. Clinical laboratory challenges in the recognition of *Leuconostoc* spp. J Clin Microbiol 1988;26:479–484.

514. Iwen PC, Rupp ME, Schreckenberger PC, Hinrichs SH. Evaluation of the revised MicroScan dried overnight Gram-Positive identification panel to identify *Enterococcus* species. J Clin Microbiol 1999;37:3756–3758.

515. Jackson DH, Hinder SM, Stringer J, Easmon CSF. Carriage and transmission of group B streptococci among STD clinic patients. Br J Vener Dis 1982;58:334–337.

516. Jackson LA, Hilsdon R, Farley MM, et al. Risk factors for group B streptococcal disease in adults. Ann Intern Med 1995;123:415–420.

517. Jackson MA, Columbo J, Boldrey A. Streptococcal fasciitis with toxic shock syndrome in the pediatric patient. Orthop Nurs 2003;22:4–8.

518. Jacobs AAC, Loeffen PLW, van den Berg AJG, et al. Identification, purification, and characterization of a thiol-activated hemolysin (suilysin) of *Streptococcus suis.* Infect Immun 1994;62:1742–1748.

519. Jacobs JA, de Krom MCT, Kellens JTC, et al. Meningitis and sepsis due to group G streptococcus. Eur J Clin Microbiol Infect Dis 1993;12:224–225.

520. Jacobs JA, Pietersen HG, Stobberingh EE, Soeters PB. Bacteremia involving the "*Streptococcus milleri*" group: analysis of 19 cases. Clin Infect Dis 1994; 19:704–713.

521. Jacobs JA, Pietersen HG, Stobberingh EE, Soeters PB. *Streptococcus anginosus, Streptococcus constellatus* and *Streptococcus intermedius.* Clinical relevance, hemolytic and serologic characteristics. Am J Clin Pathol 1995;104:547–553.

522. Jacobs JA, Schot CS, Schouls LM. The *Streptococcus anginosus* species comprises five 16S rRNA ribotypes with different phenotypic characteristics and clinical relevance. Int J Syst Evol Microbiol 2000;50:1073–1079.

523. Jacobs JA, Stappers JLN, Sels JP. Endocarditis due to *Streptococcus oralis* in a patient with a colon tumour. Eur J Clin Microbiol Infect Dis 1995;14:557–558.

524. Jacobs JA, Stobberingh EE. Hydrolytic enzymes of *Streptococcus anginosus, Streptococcus constellatus,* and *Streptococcus intermedius* in relation to infection. Eur J Clin Microbiol Infect Dis 1995;14:818–820.

525. Jacobs JA, van Baar G, London NHHJ, et al. Prevalence of macrolide resistance genes in clinical isolates of the *Streptococcus anginosus* ("*S. milleri*") group. Antimicrob Agents Chemother 2001;45:2375–2377.

526. Jacobs MR. Treatment and diagnosis of infections caused by drug-resistant *Streptococcus pneumoniae.* Clin Infect Dis 1992;15:119–127.

527. Jacoby GA. Prevalence and resistance mechanisms of common bacterial respiratory pathogens. Clin Infect Dis 1994;18:951–957.

528. Jadeja L, Kantarjian H, Bolivar R. *Streptococcus bovis* bacteremia and meningitis associated with chronic radiation enterocolitis. South Med J 1983;76:1588–1589.

529. Jaffe J, Natanson-Yaron S, Caparon MG, Hanski E. Protein F2, a novel fibronectin-binding protein from *Streptococcus pyogenes,* possesses two binding domains. Mol Microbiol 1996;21:373–384.

530. Jain AK, Agarwal SK, El-Sadr W. *Streptococcus bovis* bacteremia and meningitis associated with *Strongyloides stercoralis* colitis in a patient infected with human immunodeficiency virus. Clin Infect Dis 1994;18:253–254.

531. Jasir A, Tanna A, Efstratiou A, Schalen C. Unusual occurrence of M type 77, antibiotic-resistant group A streptococci in southern Sweden. J Clin Microbiol 2001;39:586–590.

532. Jayarao BM, Dore JJ, Jr, Baumbach GA, et al. Differentiation of *Streptococcus uberis* from *Streptococcus paruberis* by polymerase chain reaction and restriction fragment length polymorphism analysis of 16S ribosomal DNA. J Clin Microbiol 1991;29:2774–2778.

533. Jelinkova J, Motlova J. Worldwide distribution of two new serotypes of group B streptococci: type IV and provisional type V. J Clin Microbiol 1985;21:361–362.

534. Jensen TG, Konradsen HB, Bruun B. Evaluation of the Rapid ID 32 Strep system. Clin Microbiol Infect 1999;5:417–423.

535. Jerng J-S, Hsueh P-R, Teng L-J, et al. Empyema thoracis and lung abscess caused by viridans streptococci. Am J Respir Crit Care Med 1997;156:1508–1514.

536. Jett BD, Huycke MM, Gilmore MS. Virulence of enterococci. Clin Microbiol Rev 1994;7:462–478.

537. Jett BD, Jensen HG, Atkuri V, Gilmore MS. Evaluation of therapeutic measures for treating endophthalmitis caused by isogenic toxin-producing and toxin-nonproducing *Enterococcus faecalis* strains. Invest Ophthalmol Vis Sci 1995; 36:9–16.

538. Jevon GP, Dunne WM, Jr, Hawkins HK, et al. Fatal group A streptococcal meningitis and toxic shock-like syndrome: case report. Clin Infect Dis 1994; 18:91–93.

539. Ji Y, Schnitzler N, DeMaster E, Cleary P. Impact of M49, Mrp, Enn, and C5a peptidase proteins on colonization of the mouse oral mucosa by *Streptococcus pyogenes.* Infect Immun 1998;66:5399–5405.

540. Jimenez-Mejias ME, Becerril B, Gomez-Cia T, et al. Bacteremia caused by *Leuconostoc cremoris* in a patient with severe burn injuries. Eur J Clin Microbiol Infect Dis 1997;16:533–535.

541. Jobin M-C, Grenier D. Identification and characterization of four proteases produced by *Streptococcus suis.* FEMS Microbiol Lett 2003;220:113–119.

542. John CC. Treatment failure with use of third-generation cephalosporin for penicillin-resistant pneumococcal meningitis: case report and review. Clin Infect Dis 1994;18:188–193.

543. Johnson DR, Kaplan EL. A review of the correlation of T-agglutination patterns and M-protein typing and opacity factor production in the identification of group A streptococci. J Med Microbiol 1993;38:311–315.

544. Jones AL, Needham RHV, Clancy A, et al. Penicillin binding proteins in *Streptococcus agalactiae*: a novel mechanism for evasion of immune clearance. Mol Microbiol 2003;47:247–256.

545. Jones ME, Blosser-Middleton RS, Critchley IA, et al. In vitro susceptibility of *Streptococcus pneumoniae, Haemophilus influenzae,* and *Moraxella catarrhalis*: a European multicenter study during 2000–2001. Clin Microbiol Infect 2003;9:590–599.

546. Jones RN, Pfaller MA. In vitro activity of newer fluoroquinolones for respiratory tract infections and emerging patterns of antimicrobial resistance. Data from the SENTRY Antimicrobial Surveillance Program. Clin Infect Dis 2000; 31(Suppl 2):S16–S23.

547. Kaiser Permanente Vaccine Study Center Group. Efficacy, safety, and immunogenicity of heptavalent pneumococcal conjugate vaccine in children. Pediatr Infect Dis J 2000;19:187–195.

548. Kanamoto T, Sato S, Inoue M. Genetic heterogeneities and phenotypic characteristics of strains of the genus *Abiotrophia* and proposal of *Abiotrophia para-adiacens* sp. nov. J Clin Microbiol 2000;38:492–498.

549. Kaplan EL, Johnson DR, Del Rosario MC, Horn DL. Susceptibility of group A β-hemolytic streptococci to thirteen antibiotics: examination of 301 strains isolated in the United States between 1994 and 1997. Pediatr Infect Dis J 1999; 18:1069–1072.

550. Karakousis PC, Page KR, Varello MA, et al. Waterhouse-Friderichsen syndrome after infection with group A streptococcus. May Clin Proc 2001;76:1167–1170.

551. Karlowsky JA, Jones ME, Mayfield DC, et al. Ceftriaxone activity against Gram-positive and Gram-negative pathogens isolated in U.S. clinical microbiology laboratories from 1996 to 2000: results from The Surveillance Network (TSN) database-USA. Int J Antimicrob Agents 2002;19:413–426.

552. Kataja J, Huovinen P, Skurnik M, et al. Erythromycin resistance genes in group A streptococci in Finland. Antimicrob Agents Chemother 1999;43:48–52.

553. Kataoka Y, Yoshida T, Sawada T. A 10-year survey of antimicrobial susceptibility of *Streptococcus suis* isolates from swine in Japan. J Vet Med Sci 2000; 62:1053–1057.

554. Kaufhold A, Ferrieri P. Isolation of *Enterococcus mundtii* from normally sterile body sites in two patients. J Clin Microbiol 1991;29:1075–1077.

555. Kaufhold A, Podbielski A, Baumgarten G, et al. Rapid typing of group A

streptococci by the use of DNA amplification and non-radioactive allele-specific oligonucleotide probes. FEMS Microbiol Lett 1994;119:19–25.

556. Kaufhold A, Potgieter E. Chromosomally mediated high-level gentamicin-resistance in *Streptococcus mitis*. Antimicrob Agents Chemother 1993;37:2740–2742.

557. Kawamura Y, Hou X-G, Sultana F, et al. Transfer of *Streptococcus adjacens* and *Streptococcus defectivus* to *Abiotrophia* gen. nov. and *Abiotrophia adiacens* comb. nov. and *Abiotrophia defectiva* comb. nov. Int J Syst Bacteriol 1995;45:798–803.

558. Kawamura Y, Hou X-C, Sultana F, et al. Determination of 16S rRNA sequences of *Streptococcus mitis* and *Streptococcus gordonii* and phylogenetic relationships among members of the genus *Streptococcus*. Int J Syst Bacteriol 1995;45:406–408.

559. Kawamura Y, Hou X-G, Todome Y, et al. *Streptococcus peroris* sp. nov. and *Streptococcus infantis* sp. nov., new members of the *Streptococcus mitis* group, isolated from human clinical specimens. Int J Syst Bacteriol 1998;48:921–927.

560. Kawamura Y, Whiley RA, Shu S-E, et al. Genetic approaches to the identification of the mitis group within the genus *Streptococcus*. Microbiology 1999;145:2605–2613.

561. Keay L, Harmis N, Corrigan K, et al. Infiltrative keratitis associated with extended wear of hydrogel lenses and *Abiotrophia defectiva*. Cornea 2000;19:864–869.

562. Keiser P, Campbell W. ''Toxic strep syndrome'' associated with group C streptococcus. Arch Intern Med 1992;152:882–884.

563. Kellogg JA, Bankert DA, Elder CJ, et al. Identification of *Streptococcus pneumoniae* revisited. J Clin Microbiol 2001;39:3373–3375.

564. Kerbaugh MA, Evans JB. *Aerococcus viridans* in the hospital environment. Appl Microbiol 1968;16:519–523.

565. Kern W, Vanek E. *Aerococcus* bacteremia associated with granulocytopenia. Eur J Clin Microbiol 1987;6:670–673.

566. Kikuchi K, Enari T, Totsuka K-I, Shimizu K. Comparison of phenotypic characteristics, DNA-DNA hybridization results, and results with a commercial rapid biochemical and enzymatic reaction system for identification of viridans group streptococci. J Clin Microbiol 1995;33:1215–1222.

567. Kilian M. Recommended conservation of the names *Streptococcus sanguis*, *Streptococcus rattus*, *Streptococcus cricetus*, and seven other names included in the Approved Lists of Bacterial Names. Request for an opinion. Int J Syst Evol Microbiol 2001;51:723–724.

568. Kilian M, Mikkelson L, Henrichsen J. Taxonomic study of viridans streptococci: description of *Streptococcus gordonii* sp. nov. and emended descriptions of *Streptococcus sanguis* (White and Niven 1946), *Streptococcus oralis* (Bridge and Sneath 1982), and *Streptococcus mitis* (Andrewes and Horder 1906). Int J Syst Bacteriol 1989;39:471–484.

569. Kilpper-Balz R, Schleifer KH. *Streptococcus suis* sp. nov. nom. rev. Int J Syst Bacteriol 1987;37:160–162.

570. Kilpper-Balz R, Schleifer KH. Transfer of *Streptococcus morbillorum* to the genus *Gemella* as *Gemella morbillorum* comb. nov. Int J Syst Bacteriol 1988;38:442–443.

571. Kilpper-Balz R, Wenzig P, Schleifer KH. Molecular relationships and classification of some viridans streptococci as *Streptococcus oralis* and emended description of *Streptococcus oralis* (Bridge and Sneath 1982). Int J Syst Bacteriol 1985;35:482–488.

572. Kim J, Chun J, Han H-U. *Leuconostoc kimchii* sp. nov., a new species from kimchi. Int J Syst Evol Microbiol 2000;50:1915–1919.

573. Kim N, Lazar JM, Cunha BA, et al. Multi-valvular endocarditis. Clin Microbiol Infect 2000;6:207–212.

574. Kimberlin DW. Meningitis in the neonate. Curr Treat Options Neurol 2002;4:239–248.

575. King SJ, Heath PJ, Luque I, et al. Distribution and genetic diversity of suilysin in *Streptococcus suis* isolated from different diseases of pigs and characterization of the genetic basis of suilysin absence. Infect Immun 2001;69:7572–7582.

576. King SJ, Leigh JA, Heath PJ, et al. Development of a multilocus sequence typing scheme for the pig pathogen *Streptococcus suis*: identification of virulent clones and potential capsular serotype exchange. J Clin Microbiol 2002;40:3671–3680.

577. Klein JO. Otitis media. Clin Infect Dis 1994;19:823–833.

578. Klein RS, Recca RA, Catalano MT, et al. Association of *Streptococcus bovis* with carcinoma of the colon. N Engl J Med 1977;296:800–802.

579. Klugman KP. Pneumococcal resistance to antibiotics. Clin Microbiol Rev 1990;3:171–196.

580. Knight RG, Shlaes DM. Physiological characteristics and deoxyribonucleic acid relatedness of *Streptococcus bovis* and *Streptococcus bovis* (var.). Int J Syst Bacteriol 1985;35:357–361.

581. Knudtson LM, Hartman PA. Routine procedures for isolation and identification of enterococci and fecal streptococci. Appl Env Microbiol 1992;58:3027–3031.

582. Kogan G, Uhrin D, Brisson J-R, et al. Structure and immunochemical characterization of the type VIII group B *Streptococcus* capsular polysaccharide. J Biol Chem 1996;271:8786–8796.

583. Kong F, Gowan S, Martin D, et al. Serotype identification of group B streptococci by PCR and sequencing. J Clin Microbiol 2002;40:216–226.

584. Kong F, Gowan S, Martin D, et al. Molecular profiles of group B streptococcal surface protein antigen genes: relationship to molecular serotypes. J Clin Microbiol 2002;40:620–626.

585. Koorevaar CT, Scherpenzeel PGN, Neijens HJ, et al. Childhood meningitis caused by enterococci and viridans streptococci. Infection 1992;20:118–121.

586. Kouppari G, Zaphiropoulou A, Stamos G, et al. Pneumococcal acute otitis media in children. Clin Microbiol Infect 2000;6:69–73.

587. Kreft B, Marre R, Schramm U, et al. Aggregation substance of *Enterococcus faecalis* mediates adhesion to cultured renal tubular cells. Infect Immun 1992;60:25–30.

588. Kreikemeyer B, Talay SR, Chhatwal GS. Characterization of a novel fibronectin-binding surface protein in group A streptococci. Mol Microbiol 1995;17:137–145.

589. Kuhls TL, Viering TP, Leach CT, et al. Relapsing pneumococcal bacteremia in immunocompromised patients. Clin Infect Dis 1992;14:1050–1054.

590. Kusuda R, Kawai K, Salati F, et al. *Enterococcus seriolicida* sp. nov., a fish pathogen. Int J Syst Bacteriol 1991;41:406–409.

591. Lachnauer CS, Kasper DL, Shimada J, et al. Serotypes VI and VIII predominate among group B streptococci isolated from pregnant Japanese women. J Infect Dis 1999;179:1030–1033.

592. LaClaire L, Facklam R. Antimicrobial susceptibility and clinical sources of *Dolosigranulum pigrum* cultures. Antimicrob Agents Chemother 2000;44:2001–2003.

593. LaClaire L, Facklam R. Antimicrobial susceptibilities and clinical sources of *Facklamia* species. Antimicrob Agents Chemother 2000;44:2130–2132.

594. LaClaire LL, Facklam RR. Comparison of three commercial rapid identification systems for the unusual Gram-positive cocci *Dolosigranulum pigrum*, *Ignavigranum ruoffiae*, and *Facklamia* species. J Clin Microbiol 2000;38:2037–2042.

595. Lalonde M, Segura M, Lacouture S, Gottschalk M. Interactions between *Streptococcus suis* serotype 2 and different epithelial cell lines. Microbiology 2000;146:1913–1921.

596. Lancefield RC. A serological differentiation of human and other groups of β-hemolytic streptococci. J Exp Med 1933;57:571–595.

597. Lancefield RC. Current knowledge of type-specific M antigens of group A streptococci. J Immunol 1962;89:307–313.

598. Landman D, Quale JM, Odyna E, et al. Comparison of five selective media for identifying fecal carriage of vancomycin-resistant enterococci. J Clin Microbiol 1996;34:751–752.

599. Lang MM, Towers C. Identifying poststreptococcal glomerulonephritis. Nurse Pract 2001;26:34, 37–47.

600. LaScola B, Raoult D. Molecular identification of *Gemella* species from three patients with endocarditis. J Clin Microbiol 1998;36:866–871.

601. Lattore M, Alvarez M, Fernandez JM, et al. A case of meningitis due to ''*Streptococcus zooepidemicus*.'' Clin Infect Dis 1993;17:932–933.

602. Law-Brown J, Meyers PR. *Enterococcus phoeniculicola* sp. nov., a novel member of the enterococci isolated from the uropygial gland of the red-billed woodhoopoe, *Phoeniculus purpureus*. Int J Syst Evol Microbiol 2003;53:683–685.

603. Lawlor MT, Crowe HM, Quintiliani R. Cellulitis due to *Streptococcus pneumoniae*: case report and review. Clin Infect Dis 1992;14:247–250.

604. Lawrence J, Yajko DM, Hadley WK. Incidence and characterization of β-hemolytic *Streptococcus milleri* and differentiation from *S. pyogenes* (group A), *S. equisimilis* (group C), and large colony group G streptococci. J Clin Microbiol 1985;22:772–777.

605. Lawson PA, Collins MD, Falsen E, et al. *Facklamia languida* sp. nov., isolated from human clinical specimens. J Clin Microbiol 1999;37:1161–1164.

606. Lawson PA, Falsen E, Ohlen M, Collins MD. *Aerococcus urinaehominis* sp. nov., isolated from human urine. Int J Syst Evol Microbiol 2001;51:683–686.

607. Lawson PA, Falsen E, Truberg-Jensen K, Collins MD. *Aerococcus sanguicola* sp. nov., isolated from a human clinical source. Int J Syst Evol Microbiol 2001;51:475–479.

608. Lawson PA, Foster G, Falsen E, et al. *Vagococcus lutrae* sp. nov., isolated from the common otter (*Lutra lutra*). Int J Syst Bacteriol 1999;49:1251–1254.

609. Lawson PA, Foster G, Falsen E, et al. *Abiotrophia balaenopterae* sp. nov., isolated from the minke whale (*Balaenoptera acutorostrata*). Int J Syst Bacteriol 1999;49:503–506.

610. Leclercq R, Dutka-Malen S, Duval J, Courvalin P. Vancomycin resistance gene *vanC* is specific to *Enterococcus gallinarum*. Antimicrob Agents Chemother 1992;36:2005–2008.

611. Lee KC, Tsai YT, Lin CY, Tsai CS. Vertebral osteomyelitis combined streptococcal viridans endocarditis. Eur J Cardiothorac Surg 2003;23:125–127.

612. Lee P-C, Wetherall BL. Cross-reaction between *Streptococcus pneumoniae* and group C streptococcal latex reagent. J Clin Microbiol 1987;25:152–153.

613. Lefevre JC, Faucon G, Sicard AM, et al. DNA fingerprinting of *Streptococcus pneumoniae* strains by pulsed-field gel electrophoresis. J Clin Microbiol 1993;31:2724–2728.

614. LeFort A, Lortholary O, Casassus P, et al. Comparison between adult endocar-

ditis due to β-hemolytic streptococci (serogroups A, B, C, and G) and *Strepto-coccus milleri:* a multicenter study in France. Arch Intern Med 2002;162: 2450–2456.

615. Lefort A, Mainardi JL, Selton-Suty C, et al. *Streptococcus pneumoniae* endo-carditis in adults: a multicenter study in France in the era of penicillin resistance (1991–1998). Medicine (Baltimore) 2000;79:327–337.

616. Leggiadro RJ, Birnbaum SE, Chase NA, et al. A resurgence of acute rheumatic fever in a mid-South children's hospital. South Med J 1990;83:1418–1420.

617. Legier JF. *Streptococcus salivarius* meningitis and colonic carcinoma. South Med J 1991;84:1058–1059.

618. Leibovitch G, Maaravi Y, Shalev O. Multiple brain abscesses caused by *Strepto-coccus bovis.* J Infect 1991;23:195–196.

619. Lentnek AL, Giger O, O'Rourke E. Group A β-hemolytic streptococcal bacter-emia and intravenous drug abuse: a growing clinical problem? Arch Intern Med 1990;150:89–93.

620. Leskinen K, Hendolin P, Virolainen-Julkunen A, et al. *Alloiococcus otitidis* in acute otitis media. Int J Pediatr Otorhinolaryngol 2004;68:51–56.

621. Levin JC, Wessels MR. Identification of *csrR/csrS,* a genetic locus that regu-lates hyaluronic acid capsule synthesis in group A *Streptococcus.* Mol Micro-biol 1998;30:209–219.

622. Levy CS, Kogulan P, Gill VJ, et al. Endocarditis caused by penicillin-resistant viridans streptococci: two cases and controversies in therapy. Clin Infect Dis 2001;33:577–579.

623. Li Y, Pan Y, Qi F, Caulfield PW. Identification of *Streptococcus sanguinis* with a PCR-generated species-specific DNA probe. J Clin Microbiol 2003;41: 3481–3486.

624. Lim DV, Morales WJ, Walsh AF. Reduction of morbidity and mortality rates for neonatal group B streptococcal disease through early diagnosis and chemo-prophylaxis. J Clin Microbiol 1986;23:489–492.

625. Lim DV, Morales WJ, Walsh AF. Lim group B strep broth and coagglutination for rapid identification of group B streptococci in preterm pregnant women. J Clin Microbiol 1987;25:452–453.

626. Limia A, Jimenez ML, Alarcon T, Lopez-Brea M. Five-year analysis of antimi-crobial susceptibility of the *Streptococcus milleri* group. Eur J Clin Microbiol Infect Dis 1999;18:440–444.

627. Lin FY, Azimi PH, Weisman LE, et al. Antibiotic susceptibility profiles for group B streptococci isolated from neonates, 1995–1998. Clin Infect Dis 2000; 31:76–79.

628. Lin FY, Clemens JD, Azimi PH, et al. Capsular polysaccharide types of group B streptococcal isolates from neonates with early-onset systemic infection. J Infect Dis 1998;177:790–792.

629. Lischke JH, McCreight PHB. Maternal group B streptococcal vertebral osteo-myelitis: an unusual complication of vaginal delivery. Obstet Gynecol 1990; 76:489–491.

630. Llewelyn M, Cohen J. Superantigens: microbial agents that corrupt immunity. Lancet Infect Dis 2001;2:156–162.

631. Loeb M. Pneumonia in older persons. Clin Infect Dis 2003;37:1335–1339.

632. Loesche WJ. Role of *Streptococcus mutans* in human dental decay. Microbiol Rev 1986;50:353–380.

633. Lopez-Dupla M, Creus M, Navarro O, Raga X. Association of *Gemella morbil-lorum* endocarditis with adenomatous polyps and carcinoma of the colon: case report and review. Clin Infect Dis 1996;22:379–380.

634. Losonsky GA, Wolf A, Schwalbe RS, et al. Successful treatment of meningitis due to multiply resistant *Enterococcus faecium* with a combination of intrathe-cal teicoplanin and intravenous antimicrobial agents. Clin Infect Dis 1994;19: 163–165.

635. Lu C-H, Chang W-N, Chang H-W. Streptococcal meningitis in adults: therapeu-tic outcomes and prognostic factors. Clin Neurol Neurosurg 2001;103: 137–142.

636. Lu C-H, Chang W-N, Chang H-W. Adults with meningitis caused by viridans streptococci. Infection 2001;29:305–309.

637. Lu C-H, Chang W-N, Lin Y-C, et al. Bacterial brain abscess: microbiological features, epidemiological trends, and therapeutic outcomes. QJ Med 2002;95: 501–509.

638. Lu H-Z, Weng X-H, Zhu B, et al. Major outbreak of toxic shock-like syndrome caused by *Streptococcus mitis.* J Clin Microbiol 2003;41:3051–3055.

639. Luck S, Torny M, d'Agapeyeff K, et al. Estimated early-onset group B strepto-coccal neonatal disease. Lancet 2003;361:1953–1954.

640. Ludwig W, Weizenegger M, Kilpper-Balz R, et al. Phylogenetic relationships of anaerobic streptococci. Int J Syst Bacteriol 1988;38:15–18.

641. Luginbuhl LM, Rotbart HA, Facklam RR, et al. Neonatal enterococcal sepsis: case-control study and description of an outbreak. Pediatr Infect Dis 1987;6: 1022–1030.

642. Luque L, Tarradas C, Arenas A, et al. *Streptococcus suis* serotypes associated with different disease conditions in pigs. Vet Rec 1998;142:726–727.

643. Lutticken R, Temme N, Hahn G, Bartelheimer EW. Meningitis caused by *Streptococcus suis:* case report and review of the literature. Infection 1986;14: 181–185.

644. Luyx C, Vanpee D, Glupczynski Y, et al. Delayed diagnosis of meningitis caused by β-haemolytic group G streptococcus in an older woman. J Emerg Med 2001;21:393–396.

645. Lyytikainen O, Rautio M, Carlson P, et al. Nosocomial bloodstream infections due to viridans streptococci in haematological and non-haematological patients: species distribution and antimicrobial resistance. J Antimicrob Chemother 2004;53:631–634.

646. Mackey T, Lejeune V, Janssens M, et al. Identification of vancomycin-resistant lactic acid bacteria isolated from humans. J Clin Microbiol 1993;31: 2499–2501.

647. Macy MG, Whiley RA, Miller L, Nagamune H. Effect on polymorphonuclear cell function of a specific cytotoxin, intermedilysin, expressed by *Streptococcus intermedius.* Infect Immun 2001;69:6102–6109.

648. Madsen LW, Svensmark B, Elvestad K, et al. *Streptococcus suis* serotype 2 infection in pigs: new diagnostic and pathogenetic aspects. J Comp Pathol 2002;126:57–65.

649. Maher D. *Streptococcus suis* septicaemia presenting as severe, acute gastroen-teritis. J Infect 1990;21:303–304.

650. Makinen P-L, Makinen KK. The *Enterococcus faecalis* extracellular metalloen-dopeptidase (EC3.4.24.30; Coccolysin) inactivates human endothelin and bonds involving hydrophobic amino acid residues. Biochem Biophys Res Com-mun 1994;200:981–985.

651. Manachini PL, Flint SH, Ward LJH, et al. Comparison between *Streptococcus macedonicus* and *Streptococcus waius* strains and reclassification of *Strepto-coccus waius* (Flint et al. 1999) as *Streptococcus macedonicus* (Tsakalidou et al. 1998). Int J Syst Evol Microbiol 2002;52:945–951.

652. Mannion PT, Rothburn MM. Diagnosis of bacterial endocarditis caused by *Streptococcus lactis* assisted by immunoblotting of serum antibodies. J Infect 1990;21:317–326.

653. Manzella JP. *Streptococcus bovis* bacteremia: diagnosis of neoplasms by colon-oscopy. South Med J 1981;74:999–1000.

654. Marie J, Morvan H, Berthelot-Herault F, et al. Antimicrobial susceptibility of *Streptococcus suis* isolated from swine in France and from humans in different countries between 1996 and 2000. J Antimicrob Chemother 2002;50:201–209.

655. Markowitz M, Kaplan EL. Rheumatic fever. In: Stevens DL, Kaplan EL, eds. Streptococcal Infections: Clinical Aspects, Microbiology, and Molecular Patho-genesis. New York: Oxford University Press, 2000:133–143.

656. Marques MB, Kasper DL, Pangburn MK, Wessels MR. Prevention of C3 depo-sition by capsular polysaccharide is a virulence mechanism of type III group B streptococci. Infect Immun 1992;60:3986–3993.

657. Marrie TJ. Bacteremic community-acquired pneumonia due to viridans group streptococci. Clin Invest Med 1993;16:38–44.

658. Marrie TJ. Community acquired pneumonia. Clin Infect Dis 1994;18:501–515.

659. Marsal S, Castro-Guardiola A, Clemente C, et al. *Streptococcus bovis* endocar-ditis presenting as acute spondylodiscitis. Br J Rheumatol 1994;33:403–404.

660. Martin MA, Hebden JN, Bustamante CI, et al. Group A streptococcal bacter-emias associated with intravenous catheters. Infect Control Hosp Epidemiol 1990;11:542–544.

661. Martin TR, Ruzinski JT, Rubens CE, et al. The effect of type-specific polysac-charide capsule on the clearance of group B streptococci from the lungs of infant and adult rats. J Infect Dis 1992;165:306–314.

662. Martinez-Murcia AJ, Collins MD. A phylogenetic analysis of an atypical leuco-nostoc: description of *Leuconostoc fallax* sp. nov. FEMS Microbiol Lett 1991; 82:55–60.

663. Martinez-Murcia AJ, Collins MD. *Enterococcus sulfureus,* a new yellow-pigmented *Enterococcus* species. FEMS Microbiol Lett 1991;80:69–74.

664. Martin-Galiano AJ, Balsalobre L, Fenoll A, de la Campa AG. Genetic charac-terization of Optochin-susceptible viridans group streptococci. Antimicrob Agents Chemother 2003;47:3187–3194.

665. Mascini EM, Jansze M, Schouls LM, et al. Penicillin and clindamycin differen-tially inhibit the production of pyrogenic exotoxins A and B by group A strepto-cocci. Int J Antimicrob Agents 2001;18:395–398.

666. Mason T, Fisher M, Kujala G. Acute rheumatic fever in West Virginia: not just a disease of children. Arch Intern Med 1991;151:133–136.

667. Mastro TD, Spika JS, Lozano P, et al. Vancomycin-resistant *Pediococcus acidi-lactici:* nine cases of bacteremia. J Infect Dis 1990;161:956–960.

668. Matsubara K, Nishiyama Y, Katayama K, et al. Change of antimicrobial suscep-tibility of group B streptococci over 15 years in Japan. J Antimicrob Chemother 2001;48:579–582.

669. Matsubara K, Sugiyama M, Hoshina K, et al. Early onset neonatal sepsis caused by serotype VIII group B streptococci. Pediatr Infect Dis J 2000;19:359–360.

670. Maugein J, Crouzit P, Cony Makhoul P, et al. Characterization and antibiotic susceptibility of *Pediococcus acidilactici* strains isolated from neutropenic pa-tients. Eur J Clin Microbiol Infect Dis 1992;11:383–385.

671. May T, Amiel C, Lion C, et al. Meningitis due to *Gemella haemolysans.* Eur J Clin Microbiol Infect Dis 1993;12:644–645.

672. McAvin JC, Reilly PA, Roudabush RM, et al. Sensitive and specific method for

rapid identification of *Streptococcus pneumoniae* using real-time fluorescence PCR. J Clin Microbiol 2001;39:3446–3451.

673. McCarthy AE, Victor G, Ramotar K, et al. Risk factors for acquiring ampicillin-resistant enterococci and clinical outcomes at a Canadian tertiary-care hospital. J Clin Microbiol 1994;32:2671–2676.

674. McDaniel LS, Sheffield JS, Delucchi P, et al. PspA, a surface protein of *Streptococcus pneumoniae*, is capable of eliciting protection against pneumococci of more than one serotype. Infect Immun 1991;59:222–228.

675. McDonald HM, Chambers HM. Intrauterine infection and spontaneous midgestation preterm abortion: is the spectrum of microorganisms similar to that in preterm labor? Infect Dis Obstet Gynecol 2000;8:220–227.

676. McDonnell PJ, Kwitko S, McDonnell JM, et al. Characterization of infectious crystalline keratitis caused by a human isolate of *Streptococcus mitis*. Arch Ophthalmol 1991;109:1147–1151.

677. McKessar SJ, Berry AM, Bell JM, et al. Genetic characterization of *vanG*, a novel vancomycin resistance locus in *Enterococcus faecalis*. Antimicrob Agents Chemother 2000;44:3224–3228.

678. McLellan DG, Chiang EY, Courtney HS, et al. Spa contributes to the virulence of type 18 group A streptococci. Infect Immun 2001;69:2943–2949.

679. McLendon BF, Bron AJ, Mitchell CJ. *Streptococcus suis* type II (group R) as a cause of endophthalmitis. Br J Ophthalmol 1978;62:729–731.

680. Megran DW. Enterococcal endocarditis. Clin Infect Dis 1992;15:63–71.

681. Meier FA, Centor RM, Graham L, et al. Clinical and microbiologic evidence for endemic pharyngitis among adults due to group C streptococci. Arch Intern Med 1990;150:825–829.

682. Mellman RL, Spisak GM, Burakoff R. *Enterococcus avium* bacteremia in association with ulcerative colitis. Am J Gastroenterol 1992;87:375–378.

683. Michael AF, Drummond KN, Good RA, et al. Acute poststreptococcal glomerulonephritis: immune deposit disease. J Clin Invest 1966;45:237–248.

684. Michel RS, DeFlora E, Jefferies J, et al. Recurrent meningitis in a child with inner ear dysplasia. Pediatr Infect Dis J 1992;11:336–338.

685. Michelow IC, McCracken G, Luckett PM, Krisher K. *Abiotrophia* spp. brain abscess in a child with Down's syndrome. Pediatr Infect Dis J 2000;19:760–762.

686. Michelow IC, Olsen K, Lozano J, et al. Epidemiology and clinical characteristics of community-acquired pneumonia in hospitalized children. Pediatrics 2004;113:701–707.

687. Mikkelsen L, Theilade E, Poulsen K. *Abiotrophia* species in early dental plaque. Oral Microbiol Immunol 2000;15:263–268.

688. Miller PH, Facklam RR, Miller JM. Atmospheric growth requirements for *Alloiococcus* species and related Gram-positive cocci. J Clin Microbiol 1996;34:1027–1028.

689. Mitchell RG, Teddy PJ. Meningitis due to *Gemella haemolysans* after radiofrequency trigeminal rhizotomy. J Clin Pathol 1985;38:558–560.

690. Moellering RC Jr. Emergence of *Enterococcus* as a significant pathogen. Clin Infect Dis 1992;14:1173–1178.

691. Mohan UR, Walters S, Kroll JS. Endocarditis due to group A β-hemolytic streptococcus in children with potentially lethal sequelae: two cases and review. Clin Infect Dis 2000;30:624–625.

692. Moller M, Thomsen AC, Borch K, et al. Rupture of fetal membranes and premature delivery associated with group B streptococci in urine of pregnant women. Lancet 19842:69–70.

693. Mollick JA, Miller GG, Musser JM, et al. A novel superantigen isolated from pathogenic strains of *Streptococcus pyogenes* with aminoterminal homology to staphylococcal enterotoxins B and C. J Clin Invest 1993;92:710–719.

694. Monsen T, Granlund M, Olofsson K, Olsen B. *Leuconostoc* spp. septicaemia in a child with short bowel syndrome. Scand J Infect Dis 1997;29:310–311.

695. Montalto M, La Regina M, Gemelli P, et al. Mitral valve endocarditis caused by *Streptococcus oralis* occurring after upper gastrointestinal endoscopy. Am J Gastroenterol 2002;97:49–50.

696. Montejo M, Grande C, Valdivieso A, et al. Abdominal abscess due to *Leuconostoc* species in a liver transplant recipient. J Infect 2000;41:197–198.

697. Morales WJ, Lim DV. Reduction in group B streptococcal maternal and neonatal infections in preterm pregnancies with premature rupture of membranes through a rapid identification test. Am J Obstet Gynecol 1987;157:13–16.

698. Morea P, Toni M, Bressan M, et al. Prosthetic valve endocarditis caused by *Gemella haemolysans*. Infection 1991;19:446.

699. Morrison AJ Jr, Wenzel RP. Nosocomial urinary tract infections due to enterococcus; ten years' experience at a university hospital. Arch Intern Med 1986;146:1549–1551.

700. Moshkowitz M, Arber N, Wajsman R, et al. *Streptococcus bovis* endocarditis as a presenting manifestation of idiopathic ulcerative colitis. Postgrad Med J 1992;68:930–931.

701. Mulford JS, Mills J. Osteomyelitis caused by *Leuconostoc* species. Aust NZ J Surg 1999;69:541–542.

702. Muller MP, Low DE, Green KA, et al. Clinical and epidemiologic features of group A streptococcal pneumonia in Ontario, Canada. Arch Intern Med 2003;163:467–472.

703. Mundy LM, Sahm DF, Gilmore M. Relationships between enterococcal resistance and virulence. Clin Microbiol Rev 2000;13:513–522.

704. Munoz P, Coque T, Creixems MR, et al. Group B *Streptococcus*: a cause of urinary tract infection in non-pregnant adults. Clin Infect Dis 1992;14:492–496.

705. Munoz P, Llancaqueo A, Rodriguez-Creixems M, et al. Group B streptococcus bacteremia in nonpregnant adults. Arch Intern Med 1997;157:213–216.

706. Munoz R, Fenoll A, Vicioso D, et al. Optochin-resistant variants of *Streptococcus pneumoniae*. Diagn Microbiol Infect Dis 1989;13:63–66.

707. Murdoch DR, Laing RTR, Mills GD, et al. Evaluation of a rapid immunochromatographic test for detection of *Streptococcus pneumoniae* antigen in urine samples from adults with community acquired pneumonia. J Clin Microbiol 2001;39:3495–3498.

708. Murdoch DR, Reller LB. Antimicrobial susceptibilities of group B streptococci isolated from patients with invasive disease: 10-year perspective. Antimicrob Agents Chemother 2001;45:3623–3624.

709. Murphy DJ Jr. Group A streptococcal meningitis. Pediatrics 1983;71:1–5.

710. Murray CK, Walter EA, Crawford S, et al. *Abiotrophia* bacteremia in a patient with neutropenic fever and antimicrobial susceptibility testing of *Abiotrophia* isolates. Clin Infect Dis 2001;32:E140–E142.

711. Musher DM. *Streptococcus pneumoniae*. In: Mandell GL, Bennett JE, Dolin R, eds. Mandell, Douglas, and Bennett's Principles and Practice of Infectious Diseases. 5th ed. New York: Churchill Livingstone, 2000:2128–2147.

712. Musher DM, Groover JE, Rowland JM, et al. Antibody to capsular polysaccharides of *Streptococcus pneumoniae*: prevalence, persistence, and response to revaccination. Clin Infect Dis 1993;17:66–73.

713. Musser JM, Gray BM, Schlievert M, et al. *Streptococcus pyogenes* pharyngitis: characterization of strains by multilocus enzyme genotype, M and T protein serotype, and pyrogenic exotoxin gene probing. J Clin Microbiol 1992;30:600–603.

714. Musser JM, Hauser AR, Kim MH, et al. *Streptococcus pyogenes* causing toxic shock-like syndrome and other invasive diseases: clonal diversity and pyrogenic exotoxin expression. Proc Natl Acad Sci USA 1991;88:2668–2672.

715. Namdari H, Kintner K, Jackson BA, et al. *Abiotrophia* species as a cause of endophthalmitis following cataract extraction. J Clin Microbiol 1999;37:1564–1566.

716. Namiduru M, Karaoglan I, Aktaran S, et al. A case of septicaemia, meningitis, and pneumonia caused by *Streptococcus bovis* type II. Int J Clin Pract 2003;57:735–736.

717. Nathavitharana KA, Arseculeratne SN, Aponso HA, et al. Acute meningitis in early childhood caused by *Aerococcus viridans*. BMJ 1983;286:1248.

718. Nathavitharana KA, Watkinson M. Neonatal pleural empyema caused by group A streptococcus. Pediatr Infect Dis J 1994;13:671–672.

719. Navarro F. Courvalin P. Analysis of genes encoding D-alanine:D-alanine ligase-related enzymes in *Enterococcus casseliflavus* and *Enterococcus flavescens*. Antimicrob Agents Chemother 1994;38:1788–1793.

720. Nealon TJ, Mattingly SJ. Kinetic and chemical analysis of the biological significance of lipoteichoic acids in mediating adherence of serotype III group B streptococci. Infect Immun 1985;50:107–115.

721. Nichol P, Rod R, Corliss RF, Schurr M. Central myonecrosis in a patient with group A β-hemolytic streptococcus toxic shock syndrome. J Trauma 2003;55:994–996.

722. Nichols RL, Muzik AC. Enterococcal infections in surgical patients: the mystery continues. Clin Infect Dis 1992;15:72–76.

723. Nizet V, Gibson RL, Chi EY, et al. Group B streptococcal β-hemolysin expression is associated with injury of lung epithelial cells. Infect Immun 1996;64:3818–3826.

724. Nizet V, Gibson RL, Rubens CE. The role of group B streptococci β-hemolysin expression in newborn lung injury. Adv Exp Med Biol 1997;418:627–630.

725. Nizet V, Kims KS, Stins M, et al. Invasion of brain microvascular endothelial cells by group B streptococci. Infect Immun 1997;65:5074–7081.

726. Noble WC, Virani Z, Cree RGA. Co-transfer of vancomycin and other resistance genes from *Enterococcus faecalis* NCTC 12201 to *Staphylococcus aureus*. FEMS Microbiol Lett 1992;93:195–198.

727. Norfleet RG. Infectious endocarditis after fiberoptic sigmoidoscopy. J Clin Gastroenterol 1991;13:448–451.

728. Noriega FR, Kotloff KL, Martin MA, et al. Nosocomial bacteremia caused by *Enterobacter sakazakii* and *Leuconostoc mesenteroides* resulting from extrinsic contamination of infant formula. Pediatr Infect Dis J 1990;9:447–449.

729. Norrby-Teglund A, Holm SE, Norgren M. Detection and nucleotide sequence analysis of the *speC* gene in Swedish clinical group A streptococcal isolates. J Clin Microbiol 1994;32:705–709.

730. Norrby-Teglund A, Newton D, Kotb M, et al. Superantigenic properties of the group A streptococcal exotoxin SPE F (MF). Infect Immun 1994;62:5227–5233.

731. Norrby-Teglund A, Norrby SR, Low DE. The treatment of severe group A streptococcal infections. Curr Infect Dis Rep 2003;5:28–37.

732. Obando I, Garcia-Navarrete A, Moreno MJ, Chileme A. Catheter-related *Strep-*

tococcus equisimilis bacteremia in a four-month old infant with congenital CMV infection. Pediatr Infect Dis J 1997;16:910–911.

733. Obaro SK. The new pneumococcal vaccine. Clin Microbiol Infect 2002;8: 623–633.

734. O'Brien KL, Beall B, Barrett NL, et al. Epidemiology of invasive group A streptococcus disease in the United States, 1995–1999. Clin Infect Dis 2002; 35:268–276.

735. O'Brien KL, Swift AJ, Winkelstea JA. Safety and immunogenicity of heptavalent pneumococcal vaccine conjugated to CRM$_{197}$ among infants with sickle cell disease. Pediatrics 2000;106:965–972.

736. O'Connor AP, Cleary PP. Localization of the streptococcal C5a peptidase to the surface of group A streptococci. Infect Immun 1986;53:432–434.

737. Ofek I, Beachey EH, Jefferson W, Campbell GL. Cell-membrane binding properties of group A streptococcal lipoteichoic acid. J Exp Med 1975;187: 1161–1167.

738. Ohara-Nemoto Y, Tajika S, Sasaki M, Kaneko M. Identification of *Abiotrophia adiacens* and *Abiotrophia defectiva* by 16S rRNA gene PCR and restriction fragment length polymorphism analysis. J Clin Microbiol 1997;35:2458–2463.

739. Okada N, Liszewski MK, Atkinson JP, Caparon M. Membrane cofactor protein (CD46) is a keratinocyte receptor for the M protein of the group A streptococcus. Proc Natl Acad Sci USA 1995;92:2489–2493.

740. Okada Y, Kitada K, Takagaki M, et al. Endocardiac infectivity and binding to extracellular matrix proteins of oral *Abiotrophia* species. FEMS Immunol Med Microbiol 2000;27:257–261.

741. Okamoto Y, Ribeiro RC, Srivastava DK, et al. Viridans streptococcal sepsis: clinical features and complications in childhood acute myeloid leukemia. J Pediatr Hematol Oncol 2003;25:696–703.

742. Olmested S, Dunny G, Erlandsen S, Wells C. A plasmid-encoded surface protein on *Enterococcus faecalis* augments its internalization by cultured intestinal epithelial cells. J Infect Dis 1994;170:1549–1556.

743. Olopoenia L, Frederick W, Greaves W, et al. Pneumococcal sepsis and meningitis in adults with sickle cell disease. South Med J 1990;83:1002–1004.

744. Omran Y, Wood CA. Endovascular infection and septic arthritis caused by *Gemella morbillorum*. Diagn Microbiol Infect Dis 1993;16:131–134.

745. Orange M, Gray BM. Pneumococcal serotypes causing disease in children in Alabama. Pediatr Infect Dis J 1993;12:244–246.

746. Orfila C, Lepert J-C, Modesto A, et al. Rapidly progressive glomerulonephritis associated with bacterial endocarditis: efficacy of antibiotic therapy alone. Am J Nephrol 1993;13:218–222.

747. Ormerod LD, Paton BG. Severe group B streptococcal eye infections in adults. J Infect 1989;18:29–34.

748. Ormerod LD, Ruoff KL, Meisler DM, et al. Infectious crystalline keratopathy: role of nutritionally variant streptococci and other bacterial factors. Ophthalmology 1991;98:159–169.

749. Osada T, Nagawa H, Masaki T, et al. Thoracic empyema associated with recurrent colon cancer: report of a case and review of the literature. Dis Colon Rectum 2001;44:291–294.

750. Osawa R, Fujisawa T, Sly LI. *Streptococcus gallolyticus* sp. nov.; gallate-degrading organisms formerly assigned to *Streptococcus bovis*. Syst Appl Microbiol 1995;18:74–78.

751. Pacifico L, Ranucci A, Ravagnan G, et al. Relative value of selective group A streptococcal agar incubated under different atmospheres. J Clin Microbiol 1995;33:2480–2482.

752. Paganini H, Staffolani V, Zubizarreta P, et al. Viridans streptococci bacteremia in children with fever and neutropenia: a case-control study of predisposing factors. Eur J Cancer 2003;39:1284–1289.

753. Panaro NR, Lutwick LI, Chapnick EK. Intrapartum transmission of group A *Streptococcus*. Clin Infect Dis 1993;17:79–81.

754. Pappas G, Liberopoulos E, Tsianos E, Elisaf M. *Enterococcus casseliflavus* bacteremia. Case report and review. J Infect 2004;48:206–208.

755. Paredes A, Wong P, Mason EO Jr, et al. Nosocomial transmission of group B streptococci in a newborn nursery. Pediatrics 1976;59:679–682.

756. Park JW, Grossman O. *Aerococcus viridans* infection: case report and review. Clin Pediatr 1990;29:525–526.

757. Parola P, Brouqui P, Maurin M, Bourgeade A. A new case of *Streptococcus equisimilis* septic arthritis. Clin Rheumatol 1998;17:71–72.

758. Patel M, Ahrens JC, Moyer DV, et al. Pneumococcal soft-tissue infections: a problem deserving more recognition. Clin Infect Dis 1994;19:149–151.

759. Patel R, Keating MR, Cockerill FR III, et al. Bacteremia due to *Enterococcus avium*. Clin Infect Dis 1993;17:1006–1011.

760. Patel R, Piper K, Cockerill FRI, et al. The biopesticide *Paenibacillus popilliae* has a vancomycin resistance gene cluster homologous to the enterococcal VanA vancomycin resistance gene cluster. Antimicrob Agents Chemother 2000;44: 705–709.

761. Paton JC, Lock RA, Lee C-J, et al. Purification and immunogenicity of genetically toxoided derivatives of pneumolysin and their conjugation to *Streptococcus pneumoniae* type 19F polysaccharide. Infect Immun 1991;59:2297–2304.

762. Patterson JE, Masecar BL, Zervos MJ. Characterization and comparison of

763. Payne NR, Kim YK, Ferrieri P. Effect of differences in antibody and complement requirements on phagocytic uptake and intracellular killing of "c" protein-positive and -negative strains of type II group B streptococci. Infect Immun 1987;55:1243–1251.

764. Peel MM, Davis JM, Griffin KJ, Freedman DL. *Helcococcus kunzii* as sole isolate from an infected sebaceous cyst. J Clin Microbiol 1997;35:328–329.

765. Peetermans WE, Buyse B, Vanhoof J. Pyogenic abscess of the gluteal muscle due to *Streptococcus pneumoniae*. Clin Infect Dis 1993;17:939.

766. Peetermans WEC, Moffie BG, Thompson J. Bacterial endocarditis caused by *Streptococcus suis* type 2. J Infect Dis 1989;159:595–596.

767. Perch B, Pedersen KB, Henrichsen J. Serology of encapsulated streptococci pathogenic for pigs: six new serotypes of *Streptococcus suis*. J Clin Microbiol 1983;17:993–996.

768. Perichon B, Reynolds P, Courvalin P. VanD-type glycopeptide-resistant *Enterococcus faecium* BM4339. Antimicrob Agents Chemother 1997;43: 2161–2164.

769. Persson L, Vickerfors T, Sjoberg L, et al. Increased incidence of bacteraemia due to viridans streptococci in an unselected population of patients with acute myeloid leukemia. Scand J Infect Dis 2000;32:615–521.

770. Pesanti EL, Lyons RW, Verilli M, et al. Infection with the human immunodeficiency virus (HIV) as a risk factor for bacteremic illness due to *Streptococcus pneumoniae*. Conn Med 1988;52:703–704.

771. Peters NS, Eykyn SJ, Rudd SG. Pneumococcal cellulitis: a rare manifestation of pneumococcaemia in adults. J Infect 1989;19:57–59.

772. Peters TR, Edwards KM. The pneumococcal protein conjugate vaccines. J Pediatr 2000;137:416–420.

773. Peyser A, Liebergall M, Bar-On E, et al. *Streptococcus bovis* osteomyelitis of the ileum. Clin Infect Dis 1994;19:205–206.

774. Phillips GN Jr, Flicker PF, Cohen C, et al. Streptococcal M protein: α-helical coiled-coil structure and arrangement on the cell surface. Proc Natl Acad Sci USA 1981;78:4689–4693.

775. Pien FD, Wilson WR, Kunz K, et al. *Aerococcus viridans* endocarditis. Mayo Clin Proc 1984;59:47–48.

776. Pikis A, Campos JM, Rodriguez WJ, Keith JM. Optochin resistance in *Streptococcus pneumoniae*: mechanism, significance, and clinical implications. J Infect Dis 2001;184:582–590.

777. Pintado V, Cabellos C, Moreno S, et al. Enterococcal meningitis: a clinical study of 39 cases and review of the literature. Medicine (Baltimore) 2003;82: 346–364.

778. Pokorski SJ, Vetter EA, Wollan PC, et al. Comparison of Gen-Probe group A streptococcus direct test with culture for diagnosing streptococcal pharyngitis. J Clin Microbiol 1994;32:1440–1443.

779. Pompei R, Lampis G, Berlutti F, et al. Characterization of yellow-pigmented enterococci from severe human infections. J Clin Microbiol 1991;29: 2884–2886.

780. Porta G, Rodriguez-Carballeira M, Gomez L, et al. Thoracic infection caused by *Streptococcus milleri*. Eur Respir J 1998;12:357–362.

781. Pot B, Devriese LA, Hommez J, et al. Characterization and identification of *Vagococcus fluvialis* strains isolated from domestic animals. J Appl Bacteriol 1994;77:362–369.

782. Potgieter E, Carmichael M, Koornhof HJ, et al. In vitro antimicrobial susceptibility of viridans streptococci isolated from blood cultures. Eur J Clin Microbiol Infect Dis 1992;11:543–546.

783. Powderly WG, Stanley SL Jr, Medoff G. Pneumococcal endocarditis: report of a series and review of the literature. Rev Infect Dis 1986;8:786–791.

784. Poyart C, Quesne G, Trieu-Cuot P. Taxonomic dissection of the *Streptococcus bovis* group by analysis of manganese-dependent superoxide dismutase gene (*sodA*) sequences: reclassification of "*Streptococcus infantarius* subsp. *coli*" as *Streptococcus lutetiensis* and of *Streptococcus bovis* biotype II.2 as *Streptococcus pasteurianus* sp. nov. Int J Syst Evol Microbiol 2002;52:1247–1255.

785. Pradeep R, Ali M, Encarnacion CF. Retropharyngeal abscess due to *Gemella morbillorum*. Clin Infect Dis 1997;24:284–285.

786. Prakash PK, Biswas M, El Bouri K, et al. Pneumococcal necrotizing fasciitis in a patient with type 2 diabetes. Diabet Med 2003;20:899–903.

787. Prieto C, Garcia FJ, Suarez P, et al. Biochemical traits and antimicrobial susceptibility of *Streptococcus suis* isolated from slaughtered pigs. Zentralbl Veterinarmedizin Reihe B 1994;41:608–617.

788. Pritchard DG, Lin B, Willingham TR, Baker JR. Characterization of the group B streptococcal hyaluronate lyase. Arch Biochem Biophys 1994;315:431–437.

789. Proft T, Louise-Moffatt S, Berkahn CJ, Fraser JD. Identification and characterization of novel superantigens from *Streptococcus pyogenes*. J Exp Med 1999; 189:89–102.

790. Proft T, Sriskandan S, Yang L, Fraser JD. Superantigens and streptococcal toxic shock syndrome. Emerg Infect Dis 2003;9:1211–1218.

791. Prusakorn S, Currie B, Brandt E, et al. Towards a vaccine for rheumatic fever:

identification of a conserved target epitope on M protein of group A streptococci. Lancet 1994;344:639–642.

792. Purdy RA, Cassidy B, Marrie TJ. *Streptococcus bovis* meningitis: report of two cases. Neurology 1990;40:1782–1784.

793. Quessy S, Busque P, Higgins R, et al. Description of an albumin-binding activity for *Streptococcus suis* serotype 2. FEMS Microbiol Lett 1997;147:245–250.

794. Quinn RW. Comprehensive review of morbidity and mortality trends for rheumatic fever, streptococcal disease, and scarlet fever: the decline of rheumatic fever. Rev Infect Dis 1989;11:928–953.

795. Rakita RM, Vanek NN, Jacques-Palaz K, et al. *Enterococcus faecalis* bearing aggregation substance is resistant to killing by human neutrophils despite phagocytosis and neutrophil activation. Infect Immun 1999;67:6067–6075.

796. Ramaswamy G, Ng A, Quinlan L, et al. *Streptococcus equisimilis* (group C) as a cause of ophthalmic infection. Am J Clin Pathol 1983;79:385–387.

797. Rasmussen SR, Aarestrup FM, Jensen NE, Jorsal SE. Associations of *Streptococcus suis* serotype 2 ribotype profiles with clinical disease and antimicrobial resistance. J Clin Microbiol 1999;37:404–408.

798. Rasmussen SR, Andresen LO. 16S rDNA sequence variations of some *Streptococcus suis* serotypes. Int J Syst Bacteriol 1998;48:1063–1065.

799. Raval AN, Menkis AH, Boughner DR. Mitral valve aneurysm associated with aortic valve endocarditis and regurgitation. Heart Surg Forum 2002;5:298–299.

800. Raviglione MC, Tierno PM, Ottuso P, et al. Group G streptococcal meningitis and sepsis in a patient with AIDS. Diagn Microbiol Infect Dis 1990;13:261–264.

801. Raymond J, Bergeret M, Francoual C, et al. Neonatal infection with *Streptococcus milleri*. Eur J Clin Microbiol Infect Dis 1995;14:799–801.

802. Reda KB, Kapur V, Mollick J, et al. Molecular characterization and phylogenetic distribution of the streptococcus superantigen (ssa) from *Streptococcus pyogenes*. Infect Immun 1994;62:1867–1874.

803. Redd SC, Rutherford GW III, Sande MA, et al. The role of human immunodeficiency virus infection in pneumococcal bacteremia in San Francisco residents. J Infect Dis 1990;162:1012–1017.

804. Reed C, Efstratiou A, Morrison D, et al. Glycopeptide-resistant *Gemella haemolysans* from blood. Lancet 1993;342:927–928.

805. Regan JA, Klebanoff MA, Nugent RP. The epidemiology of group B streptococci in pregnancy. Vaginal Infections and Prematurity Study Group. Obstet Gynecol 1991;77:604–610.

806. Rehder CD, Johnson DR, Kaplan EL. Comparison of methods for obtaining serum opacity factor from group A streptococci. J Clin Microbiol 1995;33:2963–2967.

807. Reid KC, Cockerill FR, Patel R. Clinical and epidemiological features of *Enterococcus casseliflavus/flavescens* and *Enterococcus gallinarum* bacteremia: a report of 20 cases. Clin Infect Dis 2001;32:1540–1546.

808. Reinert RR, Bussing A, Kierdorf H, et al. Recurrent systemic pneumococcal infection in an immunocompromised patient. Eur J Clin Microbiol Infect Dis 1994;13:304–307.

809. Relf WA, Martin DR, Sriprakash KS. Identification of sequence types among the M-nontypeable group A streptococci. J Clin Microbiol 1992;30:3190–3194.

810. Rennels MB, Edwards KM, Keyserling HL, et al. Safety and immunogenicity of heptavalent pneumococcal vaccine conjugated to CRM$_{197}$ in United States infants. Pediatrics 1998;101:604–611.

811. Rice LB, Calderwood SB, Eliopoulos GM, et al. Enterococcal endocarditis: a comparison of prosthetic and native valve disease. Rev Infect Dis 1991;13:1–7.

812. Riefler J, Molavi A, Schwartz D, et al. Necrotizing fasciitis in adults due to group B *Streptococcus*. Arch Intern Med 1988;148:727–729.

813. Riegel P, Lepargneur JP. Isolation of *Helcococcus kunzii* from a post-surgical foot abscess. Int J Med Microbiol 2003;293:437–439.

814. Ring A, Braun JS, Pohl J, et al. Group B streptococcal β-hemolysin induces mortality and liver injury in experimental sepsis. J Infect Dis 2002;185:1745–1753.

815. Ritterband D, Shah M, Kresloff M, et al. *Gemella hemolysans* keratitis and consecutive endophthalmitis. Am J Ophthalmol 2002;133:268–269.

816. Robertson ID, Blackmore DK. Prevalence of *Streptococcus suis* types 1 and 2 in domestic pigs in Australia and New Zealand. Vet Rec 1989;124:391–394.

817. Rocha CL, Fischetti VA. Identification and characterization of a novel fibronectin-binding protein on the surface of group A streptococci. Infect Immun 1999;67:2720–2728.

818. Rodrigues U, Collins MD. Phylogenetic analysis of *Streptococcus saccharolyticus* based on 16S rRNA sequencing. FEMS Microbiol Lett 1990;71:231–234.

819. Rodriguez-Barradas MC, Musher DM, Hamill RJ, et al. Unusual manifestations of pneumococcal infection in human immunodeficiency virus-infected individuals: the past revisited. Clin Infect Dis 1992;14:192–199.

820. Roggenkamp A, Abele-Horn M, Trebesius K-H, et al. *Abiotrophia elegans* sp. nov., a possible pathogen in patients with culture-negative endocarditis. J Clin Microbiol 1998;36:100–104.

821. Roggenkamp A, Leitritz L, Baus K, et al. PCR for detection and identification of *Abiotrophia* spp. J Clin Microbiol 1998;36:2844–2846.

822. Rosenberg A. Pneumococcus virulence factor sialidase: a new direction in neuro-AIDS research? J Neuroimmunol 2004;147:33–34.

823. Rosenthal O, Woywodt A, Kirschner P, Haller H. Vertebral osteomyelitis and endocarditis of a pacemaker lead due to *Granulicatella* (*Abiotrophia*) *adiacens*. Infection 2002;30:317–319.

824. Ross PW, Cumming CG. Group B streptococci in women attending a sexually transmitted disease clinic. J Infect 1982;4:161–166.

825. Ross SS, Saltzman CL, Carling P, Shapiro DS. Pneumococcal septic arthritis: review of 100 cases. Clin Infect Dis 2003;36:319–327.

826. Roy S, Kaplan EL, Rodriguez B, et al. A family cluster of five cases of group A streptococcal pneumonia. Pediatrics 2003;112:e61–e65.

827. Rubens CE, Wessels MR, Heggen LM, Kasper DL. Transposon mutagenesis of type III group B streptococcus: correlation of capsule expression with virulence. Proc Natl Acad Sci USA 1987;84:7208–7212.

828. Rubins J, Charboneau D, Fasching C, et al. Distinct role for pneumolysin's cytotoxic and complement activities in the pathogenesis of pneumococcal pneumonia. Am J Crit Care Med 1996;153:1339–1346.

829. Rudney JD, Larson CJ. Species identification of oral viridans streptococci by restriction fragment polymorphism analysis of rRNA genes. J Clin Microbiol 1993;31:2467–2473.

830. Rudney JD, Larson CJ. Use of restriction fragment polymorphism analysis of rRNA genes to assign species to unknown clinical isolates of oral viridans streptococci. J Clin Microbiol 1994;32:437–443.

831. Rudolph KM, Parkinson AJ, Black CM, et al. Evaluation of polymerase chain reaction for diagnosis of pneumococcal pneumonia. J Clin Microbiol 1993;31:2661–2666.

832. Ruess M, Sander A, Hentschel R, Berner R. *Enterococcus casseliflavus* septicaemia in a preterm neonate. Scand J Infect Dis 2002;34:471–472.

833. Ruoff KL, de la Maza L, Murtaugh MJ, et al. Species identities of enterococci from clinical specimens. J Clin Microbiol 1990;28:435–437.

834. Ruoff KL, Ferraro MJ. Hydrolytic enzymes of ''*Streptococcus milleri.*'' J Clin Microbiol 1987;25:1645–1647.

835. Rurangirwa FR, Teitzel CA, Cui J, et al. *Streptococcus didelphis* sp. nov., a streptococcus with marked catalase activity isolated from opossums (*Didelphis virginiana*) with suppurative dermatitis and liver fibrosis. Int J Syst Evol Microbiol 2000;50:759–765.

836. Sachse S, Seidel P, Gerlach D, et al. Superantigen-like gene(s) in human pathogenic *Streptococcus dysgalactiae* subsp. *equisimilis*: genomic localization of the gene encoding streptococcal pyrogenic exotoxin G (*speG^{dys}*). FEMS Immunol Med Microbiol 2002;34:159–167.

837. Sahm DF, Boonlayangoor S, Schulz JE. Detection of high-level aminoglycoside resistance in enterococci other than *Enterococcus faecalis*. J Clin Microbiol 1991;29:2595–2598.

838. Sahm DF, Free L, Smith C, et al. Rapid characterization schemes for surveillance isolates of vancomycin-resistant enterococci. J Clin Microbiol 1997;35:2026–2030.

839. Salama M, Sandine W, Giovannoni S. Development and application of oligonucleotide probes for identification of *Lactococcus lactis* subsp. *cremoris*. Appl Environ Microbiol 1991;57:1313–1318.

840. Salata RA, Lerner PI, Shlaes DM, et al. Infections due to Lancefield group C streptococci. Medicine (Baltimore) 1989;68:225–239.

841. Samra Z, Shmuely H, Nahum E, et al. Use of the NOW *Streptococcus pneumoniae* urinary antigen test in cerebrospinal fluid for rapid diagnosis of pneumococcal meningitis. Diagn Microbiol Infect Dis 2003;45:237–240.

842. Sandoe JAT, Witherden IR, Settle C. Vertebral osteomyelitis caused by *Enterococcus raffinosus*. J Clin Microbiol 2001;39:1678–1679.

843. Sarker TK, Murarka RS, Gilardi GL. Primary *Streptococcus viridans* pneumonia. Chest 1989;96:831–834.

844. Sarma PS, Mohanty S. *Pediococcus acidilactici* pneumonitis and bacteremia in a pregnant woman. J Clin Microbiol 1998;36:2392–2393.

845. Sato S, Kanamoto T, Inoue M. *Abiotrophia elegans* strains comprise 8% of the nutritionally variant streptococci isolated from the human mouth. J Clin Microbiol 1999;37:2553–2556.

846. Sato T, Hu JP, Ohki K, et al. Identification of mutans streptococci by restriction fragment length polymorphism analysis of polymerase chain reaction-amplified 16S ribosomal RNA genes. Oral Microbiol Immunol 2003;18:323–326.

847. Satomi M, Kimura B, Mizoi T, et al. *Tetragenococcus muriaticus* sp. nov., a new moderately halophilic lactic acid bacterium isolated from fermented squid liver sauce. Int J Syst Bacteriol 1997;47:832–836.

848. Saunders NA, Hallas G, Gaworzewska ET, et al. PCR-enzyme linked immunosorbent assay and sequencing as an alternative to serology for M-antigen typing of *Streptococcus pyogenes*. J Clin Microbiol 1997;35:2689–2691.

849. Scano F, Rossi L, Cattelan A, et al. *Leuconostoc* species: a case-cluster hospital infection. Scand J Infect Dis 1999;31:371–373.

850. Schaberg DR, Culver DH, Gaynes RP. Major trends in the microbial etiology of nosocomial infections. Am J Med 1991;91(Suppl 3B):72S–75S.

851. Schattner A, Vosti KL. Bacterial arthritis due to β-hemolytic streptococci of

serogroups A, B, C, F, and G. Analysis of 23 cases and a review of the literature. Medicine (Baltimore) 1998;77:122–139.

852. Schlegel L, Grimont F, Ageron E, et al. Reappraisal of the taxonomy of the *Streptococcus bovis/Streptococcus equinus* complex and related species: description of *Streptococcus gallolyticus* subsp. *gallolyticus* subsp. nov., *S. gallolyticus* subsp. *macedonicus* subsp. nov., and *S. gallolyticus* subsp. *pasteurianus* subsp. nov. Int J Syst Evol Microbiol 2003;53:631–645.

853. Schlegel L, Grimont F, Collins MD, et al. *Streptococcus infantarius* sp. nov., *Streptococcus infantarius* subsp. *infantarius* subsp. nov., and *Streptococcus infantarius* subsp. *coli* subsp. nov., isolated from humans and food. Int J Syst Evol Microbiol 2000;50:1425–1434.

854. Schlegel L, Grimont F, Grimont PA, Bouvet A. New group D streptococcal species. Ind J Med Res 2004;119(Suppl):252–256.

855. Schlegel L, Merlet C, Laroche JM, et al. Iatrogenic meningitis due to *Abiotrophia defectiva* after myelography. Clin Infect Dis 1999;28:155–156.

856. Schleifer KH, Ehrmann M, Krusch U, et al. Revival of the species *Streptococcus thermophilus* (ex. Orla-Jensen, 1919) nom. rev. Syst Appl Microbiol 1991; 14:386–388.

857. Schleifer KH, Kilpper-Balz R. Transfer of *Streptococcus faecalis* and *Streptococcus faecium* to the genus *Enterococcus* nom. rev. as *Enterococcus faecalis* comb. nov. and *Enterococcus faecium* comb. nov. Int J Syst Bacteriol 1984; 34:31–34.

858. Schleifer KH, Kilpper-Balz R. Molecular and chemotaxonomic approaches to the classification of streptococci, enterococci, and lactococci: a review. Syst Appl Microbiol 1987;10:1–9.

859. Schleifer KH, Kraus J, Dvorak C, et al. Transfer of *Streptococcus lactis* and related streptococci to the genus *Lactococcus* gen nov. Syst Appl Microbiol 1985;6:183–195.

860. Schlievert PM, Gocke JA, Deringer JR. Group B streptococcal toxic shock-like syndrome: report of a case and purification of an associated pyrogenic toxin. Clin Infect Dis 1993;17:26–31.

861. Schmidtke LM, Carson J. Characteristics of *Vagococcus salmoninarum* isolated from diseased salmonid fish. J Appl Bacteriol 1994;77:229–236.

862. Schneerson JM, Chattopadhyay B, Murphy MFG, et al. Permanent perceptive deafness due to *Streptococcus suis* type II infection. J Laryngol Otol 1980;94: 425–427.

863. Schrag S, Zywicki S, Farley MM, et al. Group B streptococcal disease in the era of intrapartum antibiotic prophylaxis. N Engl J Med 2000;342:15–20.

864. Schrager HM, Alberti S, Cywes C, et al. Hyaluronic acid capsule modulates M protein-mediated adherence and acts as a ligand for attachment of group A *Streptococcus* to CD44 on human keratinocytes. J Clin Invest 1998;101: 1708–1716.

865. Schuchat A. Neonatal group B streptococcal disease–screening and prevention. N Engl J Med 2000;343:209–210.

866. Schuchat A, Oxtoby M, Cochi S, et al. Population-based risk factors for neonatal group B streptococcal disease: results of a cohort study in metropolitan Atlanta. J Infect Dis 1990;162:672–677.

867. Schutze GE, Kaplan SL, Jacob RF. Resistant pneumococcus: a worldwide problem. Infection 1994;22:233–237.

868. Schuur PM, Kasteren ME, Sabbe L, et al. Urinary tract infections with *Aerococcus urinae* in the south of the Netherlands. Eur J Clin Microbiol Infect Dis 1997;16:871–875.

869. Schuur PM, Sabbe L, van der Wouw AJ, et al. Three cases of serious infection caused by *Aerococcus urinae*. Eur J Clin Microbiol Infect Dis 1999;18: 368–371.

870. Schwab JH, Cromartie WJ. Immunological studies on a C polysaccharide complex of group A streptococci having a direct toxic effect on connective tissue. J Exp Med 1960;111:295–307.

871. Schwabe LD, Small MT, Randall EL. Comparison of TestPack Strep A test kit and culture technique for detection of group A streptococci. J Clin Microbiol 1987;25:309–311.

872. Schwartz B, Elliott JA, Butler JC, et al. Clusters of invasive group A streptococcal infections in family, hospital, and nursing home settings. Clin Infect Dis 1992;15:277–284.

873. Scully BE, Spriggs D, Neu HC. *Streptococcus agalactiae* (group B) endocarditis: a description of twelve cases and review of the literature. Infection 1987; 15:169–176.

874. Seal DV. Necrotizing fasciitis. Curr Opin Infect Dis 2001;14:127–132.

875. Segers RP, Kenter L, De Haan A, Jacobs AA. Characterisation of the gene encoding suilysin from *Streptococcus suis* and expression in field strains. FEMS Microbiol Lett 1998;167:255–261.

876. Sekiya K, Datoh R, Danbara H, Futaesaku Y. A ring-shaped structure with a crown formed by streptolysin O on the erythrocyte membrane. J Bacteriol 1993; 175:5953–5961.

877. Seppala H, He Q, Osterblad M, et al. Typing of group A streptococci by random amplified polymorphic DNA analysis. J Clin Microbiol 1994;32:1945–1948.

878. Seppala H, Klaukka T, Vuopio-Varkila J, et al. The effect of changes in the consumption of macrolide antibiotics on erythromycin resistance in group A streptococci in Finland. N Engl J Med 1997;337:441–446.

879. Seppala H, Nissinen A, Jarvinen H, et al. Resistance to erythromycin in group A streptococci. N Engl J Med 1992;326:292–297.

880. Shankar V, Baghdayan A, Huycke M, et al. Infection-derived *Enterococcus faecalis* strains are enriched in *esp*, a gene encoding a novel surface protein. Infect Immun 1999;67:193–200.

881. Shaw BG, Harding CD. *Leuconostoc gelidum* sp nov. and *Leuconostoc carnosum* sp. nov. from chill-stored meats. Int J Syst Bacteriol 1989;39:217–223.

882. Shea KW, Schoch PE, Klein NC, et al. Liver abscess due to pyridoxal-dependent *Streptococcus mitis*. Clin Infect Dis 1995;21:238–289.

883. Sheppard CL, Harrison TG, Morris R, et al. Autolysin targeted LightCycler assay including internal process control for detection of *Streptococcus pneumoniae* DNA in clinical samples. J Med Microbiol 2004;53:189–195.

884. Shewmaker PL, Steigerwalt AG, Shealey L, et al. DNA relatedness, phenotypic characteristics, and antimicrobial susceptibility of *Globicatella sanguinis* strains. J Clin Microbiol 2001;39:4052–4057.

885. Shimizu T, Harada M, Zempo N, et al. Nonclostridial gas gangrene due to *Streptococcus anginosus* in a diabetic patient. J Am Acad Dermatol 1999;40: 347–349.

886. Shinefield HR, Black S, Ray P, et al. Safety and immunogenicity of heptavalent pneumococcal CRM 197 conjugate vaccine in infants and toddlers. Pediatr Infect Dis J 1999;18:757–763.

887. Shinzato T, Saito A. A mechanism of pathogenicity of "*Streptococcus milleri* group" in pulmonary infection: synergy with an anaerobe. J Med Microbiol 1994;40:118–123.

888. Shinzato T, Saito A. The *Streptococcus milleri* group as a cause of pulmonary infections. Clin Infect Dis 1995;21(Suppl 3):S238–S243.

889. Shulman ST. Complications of streptococcal pharyngitis. Pediatr Infect Dis J 1994;13:S70–S74.

890. Shulman ST. Acute streptococcal pharyngitis in pediatric medicine: current issues in diagnosis and treatment. Paediatr Drugs 2003;5(Suppl 1):13–23.

891. Shutt CK, Samore M, Carroll KC. Comparison of the Denka Seiken slide agglutination method to the quelling test for serogrouping of *Streptococcus pneumoniae* isolates. J Clin Microbiol 2004;42:1274–1276.

892. Siefkin AD, Peterson DL, Hansen B. *Streptococcus equisimilis* pneumonia in a compromised host. J Clin Microbiol 1983;17:306–308.

893. Siegel M, Timpone J. Penicillin-resistant *Streptococcus pneumoniae* endocarditis: a case report and review. Clin Infect Dis 2001;15:972–974.

894. Siegman-Igra Y, Schwartz D. *Streptococcus bovis* revisited: a clinical review of 81 bacteremic episodes paying special attention to emerging antibiotic resistance. Scand J Infect Dis 2003;35:90–93.

895. Sing A, Trebesius K, Heesemann J. Diagnosis of *Streptococcus dysgalactiae* subspecies *equisimilis* (group C streptococci) associated with deep soft tissue infection using fluorescent *in situ* hybridization. Eur J Clin Microbiol Infect Dis 2001;20:146–149.

896. Sire JM, Donnio PY, Mesnard R, et al. Septicemia and hepatic abscess caused by *Pediococcus acidilactici*. Eur J Clin Microbiol Infect Dis 1992;11:623–625.

897. Sirotnak AP, Eppes SC, Klein JD. Tuboovarian abscess and peritonitis caused by *Streptococcus pneumoniae* serotype 1 in young girls. Clin Infect Dis 1996; 22:993–996.

898. Skaar I, Gaustad P, Tonjum T, et al. *Streptococcus phocae* sp. nov., a new species isolated from clinical specimens from seals. Int J Syst Bacteriol 1994; 44:646–650.

899. Skov R, Christensen JJ, Korner B, et al. In vitro antimicrobial susceptibility of *Aerococcus urinae* to 14 antibiotics, and time-kill curves for penicillin, gentamicin, and vancomycin. J Antimicrob Chemother 2001;48:653–658.

900. Skov RL, Klarlund M, Thorsen S. Fatal endocarditis due to *Aerococcus urinae*. Diagn Microbiol Infect Dis 1995;21:219–221.

901. Sledge D, Austin E, Sobczyk W, et al. Group B streptococcal endocarditis involving the tricuspid valve in a 7-month-old infant. Clin Infect Dis 1994;19: 166–168.

902. Sly LI, Cahill MM, Osawa R, Fujisawa T. The tannin-degrading species *Streptococcus gallolyticus* and *Streptococcus caprinus* are subjective synonyms. Int J Syst Bacteriol 1997;47:893–894.

903. Smith AM, Klugman KP. Alterations in penicillin-binding protein 2B from penicillin-resistant wild-type strains of *Streptococcus pneumoniae*. Antimicrob Agents Chemother 1995;39:859–867.

904. Smith AM, Klugman KP, Coffey TJ, Spratt BG. Genetic diversity of penicillin binding protein 2B and 2X from *Streptococcus pneumoniae* in South Africa. Antimicrob Agents Chemother 1993;37:1938–1944.

905. Smith HE, Damman M, van der Velde J, et al. Identification and characterization of the *cps* locus of *Streptococcus suis* serotype 2: the capsule protects against phagocytosis and is an important virulence factor. Infect Immun 1999; 67:1750–1756.

906. Smith HE, DeVries R, van't Slot R, Smits MA. The *cps* locus of *Streptococcus suis* serotype 2: genetic determinant of the synthesis of sialic acid. Microb Pathog 2000;29:127–134.

907. Smith HE, Veenbergen V, van der Velde J, et al. The *cps* genes of *Streptococcus suis* serotypes 1, 2, and 9: development of rapid serotype-specific PCR assays. J Clin Microbiol 1999;37:3146–3152.

908. Smith MD, Derrington P, Evans R, et al. Rapid diagnosis of bacteremia pneumococcal infections in adults by using the Binax NOW *Streptococcus pneumoniae* urinary antigen test: a prospective, controlled clinical evaluation. J Clin Microbiol 2003;41:2810–2813.

909. Smoot LM, McCormick JK, Smoot JC, et al. Characterization of two novel pyrogenic toxin superantigens made by an acute rheumatic fever clone of *Streptococcus pyogenes* associated with multiple disease outbreaks. Infect Immun 2002;70:7095–7104.

910. Snow V, Mottur-Pilson C, Cooper RJ, et al. Principles of appropriate antibiotic use for acute pharyngitis in adults. Ann Intern Med 2001;134:506–508.

911. Sobrino J, Bosch X, Wennberg P, et al. Septic arthritis secondary to group C streptococcus typed as *Streptococcus equisimilis*. J Rheumatol 1991;18:485–486.

912. Sommer R, Rohner P, Garbino J, et al. Group A β-hemolytic streptococcus meningitis: clinical and microbiological features of nine cases. Clin Infect Dis 1999;29:929–931.

913. Song JY, Lin LL, Schott S, et al. Evaluation of the Strep B OIA test compared to standard culture methods for detection of group B streptococci. Infect Dis Obstet Gynecol 1999;7:202–205.

914. Spataro V, Marone C. Rhabdomyolysis associated with bacteremia due to *Streptococcus pneumoniae*: case report and review. Clin Infect Dis 1993;17:1063–1064.

915. Spellerberg B. Pathogenesis of neonatal *Streptococcus agalactiae* infection. Microb Infect 2000;2:1733–1742.

916. Sriskandan S, McKee A, Hall L, Cohen J. Comparative effects of clindamycin and ampicillin on superantigenic activity of *Streptococcus pyogenes*. J Antimicrob Chemother 1997;40:275–277.

917. Staats JJ, Feder I, Okwumabua O, Chengappa MM. *Streptococcus suis*: past and present. Vet Res Commun 1997;21:381–407.

918. Staats JJ, Plattner BL, Stewart GC, Changappa MM. Presence of the *Streptococcus suis* suilysin gene and expression of MRP and RF correlates with high virulence in *Streptococcus suis* type 2 isolates. Vet Microbiol 1999;70:201–211.

919. Stefonek KR, Maerz LL, Nielsen MP, et al. Group A streptococcal puerperal sepsis preceded by positive surveillance cultures. Obstet Gynecol 2001;98:846–848.

920. Steiner JL, Septimus EJ, Vartian CV. Infection of the psoas muscle secondary to *Streptococcus pneumoniae* infection. Clin Infect Dis 1992;15:1047–1048.

921. Steiner M, Villablanca J, Kersey J, et al. Viridans streptococcal shock in bone marrow transplantation patients. Am J Hematol 1993;42:354–358.

922. Steinfield S, Galle C, Struelens M, et al. Pyogenic arthritis caused by *Streptococcus equisimilis* (group C streptococcus) in a patient with AIDS. Clin Rheumatol 1997;16:314–316.

923. Stepanovic S, Jovanovic M, Lavadinovic L, et al. *Enterococcus durans* endocarditis in a patient with transposition of the great vessels. J Med Microbiol 2004;53:259–261.

924. Stevens DL. Invasive group A streptococcus infections. Clin Infect Dis 1992;14:2–13.

925. Stevens DL. Invasive group A streptococcal infections: the past, present, and future. Pediatr Infect Dis J 1994;13:561–566.

926. Stevens DL. Streptococcal toxic shock syndrome associated with necrotizing fasciitis. Ann Rev Med 2000;51:271–288.

927. Stevens DL. Streptococcal toxic shock syndrome. Clin Microbiol Infect 2002;8:133–136.

928. Stevens DL, Tanner MH, Winship J, et al. Severe group A streptococcal infections associated with a toxic shock-like syndrome and scarlet fever toxin A. N Engl J Med 1989;321:1–7.

929. Stevenson KB, Murray EW, Sarubbi FA. Enterococcal meningitis: report of four cases and review. Clin Infect Dis 1994;18:233–239.

930. Stocker E, Cortes E, Pema K, et al. *Streptococcus milleri* as a cause of antecubital abscess and bacteremia in intravenous drug abusers. South Med J 1994;87:95–96.

931. Stollerman GH. Rheumatogenic streptococci and autoimmunity. Clin Immunol Immunopathol 1991;61:131–142.

932. Stollerman GH. Rheumatic fever in the 21st century. Clin Infect Dis 2001;33:806–814.

933. Strunk RC, Eidlen DM, Mason RJ. Pulmonary alveolar type II epithelial cells synthesize and secrete proteins of the classical and alternative complement pathways. J Clin Invest 1988;81:1419–1426.

934. Stryt B. Infection associated with asplenia: risks, mechanism, and prevention. Am J Med 1990;88(5N):33N–42N.

935. Su T-M, Lin Y-C, Lu C-H, et al. Streptococcal brain abscess: analysis of clinical features in 20 patients. Surg Neurol 2001;56:189–194.

936. Subramanian KN, Lam KS. Malignant necrotizing streptococcal myositis: a rare and fatal condition. J Bone Joint Surg Br 2003;85:277–278.

937. Sutton GP, Smirz LR, Clark DH, et al. Group B streptococcal necrotizing fasciitis arising from an episiotomy. Obstet Gynecol 1985;66:733–736.

938. Svec P, Devriese LA, Sedlacek I, et al. *Enterococcus haemoperoxidus* sp. nov. and *Enterococcus moraviensis* sp. nov., isolated from water. Int J Syst Evol Microbiol 2001;51:1567–1674.

939. Swanson H, Cutts E, Lepow M. Penicillin-resistant *Aerococcus viridans* bacteremia in a child receiving prophylaxis for sickle-cell disease. Clin Infect Dis 1996;22:387–388.

940. Swarztrauber K, Cohen I. Nonhemolytic group B streptococcal osteomyelitis: identification and treatment in a five-week-old infant. J La State Med Soc 1991;143:29–32.

941. Swenson JM, Facklam RR, Thornsberry C. Antimicrobial susceptibility of vancomycin-resistant *Leuconostoc*, *Pediococcus*, and *Lactobacillus* species. Antimicrob Agents Chemother 1990;34:543–549.

942. Syrogiannopoulos GA, McCraken GH Jr, Nelson JD. Osteoarticular infections in children with sickle cell disease. Pediatrics 1986;78:1090–1096.

943. Takao A, Nagamune H, Maeda N. Identification of the anginosus group within the genus *Streptococcus* using polymerase chain reaction. FEMS Microbiol Lett 2004;233:83–89.

944. Tankovic J, Leclercq R, Duval J. Antimicrobial susceptibility of *Pediococcus* spp. and genetic basis of macrolide resistance in *Pediococcus acidilactici* HM3020. Antimicrob Agents Chemother 1993;37:789–792.

945. Tapsall JW. Pigment production by Lancefield group B streptococci (*Streptococcus agalactiae*). J Med Microbiol 1986;21:75–81.

946. Tarradas C, Arenas A, Maldonado A, et al. Identification of *Streptococcus suis* isolated from swine: proposal for biochemical parameters. J Clin Microbiol 1994;32:578–580.

947. Tarradas C, Luque I, DeAndres D, et al. Epidemiological relationship of human and swine *Streptococcus suis* isolates. J Vet Med B 2001;48:347–355.

948. Taylor PW, Trueblood MC. Septic arthritis due to *Aerococcus viridans*. J Rheumatol 1985;12:1004–1005.

949. Teixeira LM, Carvalho MGS, Espinola MMB, et al. *Enterococcus porcinus* sp. nov., and *Enterococcus ratti* sp. nov. associated with enteric disorders in animals. Int J Syst Evol Microbiol 2001;51:1737–1743.

950. Teixeira LM, Carvalho MGS, Merquior VLC, et al. Phenotypic and genotypic characterization of *Vagococcus fluvialis*, including strains isolated from human sources. J Clin Microbiol 1997;35:2778–2781.

951. Teixeira LM, Carvalho MGS, Merquior VLC, et al. Recent approaches on the taxonomy of the enterococci and some related microorganisms. Adv Exp Med 1997;418:397–400.

952. Teixeira LM, Merquior VLC, Vianni MCE, et al. Phenotypic and genotypic characterization of atypical *Lactococcus garvieae* strains isolated from water buffalos with subclinical mastitis and confirmation of *L. garvieae* as a senior subjective synonym of *Enterococcus seriolicida*. Int J Syst Bacteriol 1996;46:664–668.

953. Templin KS, Crook T, Riley T, et al. Spontaneous bacterial peritonitis and bacteremia due to *Leuconostoc* species in a patient with end-stage renal disease: a case report. J Infect 2001;43:155–157.

954. Terpenning MS, Taylor GW, Lopatin DE, et al. Aspiration pneumonia: dental and oral risk factors in an older veteran population. J Am Geriatr Soc 2001;49:557–563.

955. Thompson T, Facklam R. Cross reactions of reagents from streptococcal grouping kits with *Streptococcus porcinus*. J Clin Microbiol 1997;35:1885–1886.

956. Thornsberry C, Swenson JM, Baker CN, et al. Methods for determining susceptibility of fastidious and unusual pathogens to selected antimicrobial agents. Diagn Microbiol Infect Dis 1988;9:139–153.

957. Timoney JF. Strangles. Vet Clin North Am Equine Pract 1993;9:365–74.

958. Tong H, Gao X, Dong X. *Streptococcus oligofermentans* sp. nov., a novel oral isolate from caries-free humans. Int J Syst Evol Microbiol 2003';53:1101–1104.

959. Towers CV, Garite TJ, Friedman WW, et al. Comparison of a rapid enzyme-linked immunosorbent assay test and the Gram stain for detection of group B *Streptococcus* in high-risk antepartum patients. Am J Obstet Gynecol 1990;163:965–967.

960. Tracy M, Wanahita A, Shuhatovich Y, et al. Antibiotic susceptibilities of genetically characterized *Streptococcus milleri* group strains. Antimicrob Agents Chemother 2001;45:1511–1514.

961. Traub WH, Leonard B. Comparative susceptibility of clinical group A, B, C, F, and G β-hemolytic streptococcal isolates to 24 antimicrobial agents. Chemotherapy 1997;43:10–20.

962. Tresadern JC, Farrand RJ, Irving MH. *Streptococcus milleri* and surgical sepsis. Annu Rev Coll Surg (Engl) 1983;65:78–79.

963. Tritz DM, Iwen PC, Woods GL. Evaluation of MicroScan for identification of *Enterococcus* species. J Clin Microbiol 1990;28:1477–1478.

964. Trotman J, Highes B, Mollison L. Invasive pneumococcal disease in central Australia. Clin Invest Dis 1994;20:1553–1556.

965. Trottier S, Higgins R, Brochu G, et al. A case of human endocarditis due to *Streptococcus suis* in North America. Rev Infect Dis 1991;13:1251–1252.

966. Truant AL, Satishchandran V. Comparison of Streptex versus PathoDx for group D typing of vancomycin-resistant *Enterococcus*. Diagn Microbiol Infect Dis 1993;16:89–91.

967. Truong TL, Menard C, Mouton C, Trahan L. Identification of mutans and other oral streptococci by random amplified polymorphic DNA analysis. J Med Microbiol 2000;49:63–71.

968. Truper HG, de Clari L. Taxonomic note: necessary correction of specific epithets formed as substantives (nouns) "in apposition." Int J Syst Bacteriol 1997;47:908–909.

969. Tsai MS, Huang TC, Liu JW. Lemierre's syndrome caused by viridans streptococci: a case report. J Microbiol Immunol Infect 1999;32:126–128.

970. Tsakalidou E, Zoidou E, Pot B, et al. Identification of streptococci from Greek Kasseri cheese and description of *Streptococcus macedonicus* sp. nov. Int J Syst Bacteriol 1998;48:519–527.

971. Tsutsui O, Kokeguchi S, Matsumura T, et al. Relationship of the chemical structure and immunobiological activities of lipoteichoic acid from *Streptococcus faecalis* (*Enterococcus hirae*) ATCC 9790. FEMS Microbiol Immunol 1991;3:211–218.

972. Tung KSK, Woodroffe AJ, Ahlin TD, et al. Application of the solid phase C1q and Raji cell radioimmune assays for the detection of circulating immune complexes in glomerulonephritis. J Clin Invest 1978;62:61–72.

973. Tunkel AR, Scheld MW. Acute bacterial meningitis. Lancet 1995;346:1675–1680.

974. Tunkel AR, Sepkowitz KA. Infections caused by viridans streptococci in patients with neutropenia. Clin Infect Dis 2002;34:1524–1529.

975. Tuohy MJ, Procop GW, Washington JA. Antimicrobial susceptibility of *Abiotrophia adiacens* and *Abiotrophia defectiva*. Diagn Microbiol Infect Dis 2000;38:189–191.

976. Tupperainen N, Hallman M. Prevention of neonatal group B streptococcal disease: intrapartum detection and chemoprophylaxis of heavily colonized parturients. Obstet Gynecol 1989;73:583–587.

977. Turner JC, Fox A, Fox K, et al. Role of group C β-hemolytic streptococci in pharyngitis: epidemiologic study of clinical features associated with isolation of group C streptococci. J Clin Microbiol 1993;31:808–811.

978. Turner JC, Hayden GF, Kiselica D, et al. Association of group C β-hemolytic streptococci with endemic pharyngitis among college students. JAMA 1990;264:2644–2647.

979. Tyrrell GJ, Turnbull L, Teixeira LM, et al. *Enterococcus gilvus* and *Enterococcus pallens* sp. nov. isolated from human clinical specimens. J Clin Microbiol 2002;40:1140–1145.

980. Udayaraj UP, Gendi NS, Osman EM. Septic discitis as a complication of infective endocarditis caused by *Streptococcus oralis*. J Rheumatol 2003;30:632–633.

981. Uhl JR, Adamson SC, Vetter EA, et al. Comparison of LightCycler PCR, rapid antigen immunoassay, and culture for detection of group A streptococci from throat swabs. J Clin Microbiol 2003;41:242–249.

982. Unnikrishnan M, Altmann DM, Proft T, et al. The bacterial superantigen streptococcal mitogenic exotoxin Z is the major immunoactive agent of *Streptococcus pyogenes*. J Immunol 2002;169:2561–2569.

983. Vacca-Smith AM, Jones CA, Levine MJ, et al. Glucosyltransferase mediates adhesion of *Streptococcus gordonii* to human epithelial cells in vitro. Infect Immun 1994;62:2187–2194.

984. Vagiakou-Voudris E, Mylona-Petropoulou D, Kalogeropoulou E, et al. Multiple liver abscesses associated with bacteremia due to *Leuconostoc lactis*. Scand J Infect Dis 2002;34:766–767.

985. Vancanneyt M, Devriese LA, DeGraef EM, et al. *Streptococcus minor* sp. nov. from faecal samples and tonsils of domestic animals. Int J Syst Evol Microbiol 2004;54:449–452.

986. Vancanneyt M, Snauwaert C, Cleenwerck I, et al. *Enterococcus villorum* sp. nov., an enteroadherent bacterium associated with diarrhoea in piglets. Int J Syst Evol Microbiol 2001;51:393–400.

987. Vance DW Jr. Group C streptococci: "*Streptococcus equisimilis*" or *Streptococcus anginosus*. Clin Infect Dis 1992;14:616.

988. Van Dam JEG, Fleer A, Snippe H. Immunogenicity and immunochemistry of *Streptococcus pneumoniae* capsular polysaccharides. Antonie von Leeuwenkoek 1990;58:1–47.

989. Vandamme P, Devriese LA, Haesebrouck F, Kersters K. *Streptococcus intestinalis* Robinson et al 1988 and *Streptococcus alactolyticus* Farrow et al 1984 are phenotypically indistinguishable. Int J Syst Bacteriol 1999;49:737–741.

990. Vandamme P, Devriese LA, Pot B, et al. *Streptococcus difficile* is a nonhemolytic group B type Ib streptococcus. Int J Syst Bacteriol 1997;47:81–85.

991. Vandamme P, Hommez J, Snauwaert C, et al. *Globicatella sulfidifaciens* sp. nov., isolated from purulent infections in domestic animals. Int J Syst Evol Microbiol 2001;51:1745–1749.

992. Vandamme P, Pot B, Falsen E, et al. Taxonomic study of Lancefield streptococcal groups C, G, and L (*Streptococcus dysgalactiae*) and proposal of *S. dysgalactiae* subsp. *equisimilis* subsp. nov. Int J Syst Bacteriol 1996;46:774–781.

993. Vandamme P, Torck U, Falsen E, et al. Whole-cell protein electrophoretic analysis of viridans streptococci: evidence for heterogeneity among *Streptococcus mitis* biovars. Int J Syst Bacteriol 1998;48:117–125.

994. Van de Beek D, de Gans J, Spanjaard L, et al. Group A streptococcal meningitis in adults: report of 41 cases and a review of the literature. Clin Infect Dis 2004;34:e32–e36.

995. Van der Mei, Naumann D, Busscher HJ. Grouping of oral streptococcal species using Fourier-transform infrared spectroscopy in comparison with classical microbiological identification. Arch Oral Biol 1993;38:1013–1019.

996. Van de Tijn I, Fillit H, Brandeis WE, et al. Serial studies on circulating immune complexes in post-streptococcal sequelae. Clin Exp Immunol 1978;34:318–325.

997. van Dijk M, van Toyen BJ, Wuisman PI, et al. Trochanter osteomyelitis and ipsilateral arthritis due to *Gemella morbillorum*. Eur J Clin Microbiol Infect Dis 1999;18:600–602.

998. Vanek NN, Simon SI, Jacques-Palaz K, et al. *Enterococcus faecalis* aggregation substance promotes opsonin-independent binding to human neutrophils via a complement receptor type 3-mediated mechanism. FEMS Immunol Med Microbiol 1999;26:49–60.

999. Van Goethem GF, Louwagie BM, Simoens MJ, et al. *Enterococcus casseliflavus* septicaemia in a patient with acute myeloid leukemia. Eur J Clin Microbiol Infect Dis 1994;13:519–520.

1000. Van Haeften R, Palladino S, Kay I, et al. A quantitative LightCycler PCR to detect *Streptococcus pneumoniae* in blood and CSF. Diagn Microbiol Infect Dis 2003;47:407–414.

1001. Vartian C, Lerner PI, Shlaes DM, et al. Infections due to Lancefield group G streptococci. Medicine (Baltimore) 1985;64:75–88.

1002. Vartian CV, Septimus EJ. Meningitis caused by group B *Streptococcus* in association with cerebrospinal rhinorrhea. Clin Infect Dis 1992;14:1261–1262.

1003. Vasishtha S, Isenberg HD, Sood SK. *Gemella morbillorum* as a cause of septic shock. Clin Infect Dis 1996;22:1084–1086.

1004. Veasy LG, Wiedmeier SE, Orsmond GS. Resurgence of acute rheumatic fever in the intermountain area of the United States. N Engl J Med 1987;316:421–427.

1005. Vela AI, Fernandez E, Lawson PA, et al. *Streptococcus entericus* sp. nov., isolated from cattle intestines. Int J Syst Evol Microbiol 2002;52:665–669.

1006. Vela AI, Goyache J, Tarradas C, et al. Analysis of genetic diversity of *Streptococcus suis* clinical isolates from pigs in Spain by pulsed-field gel electrophoresis. J Clin Microbiol 2003;41:2498–2502.

1007. Verghese A, Berk SL, Boelen LJ, et al. Group B streptococcal pneumonia in the elderly. Arch Intern Med 1982;142:1642–1645.

1008. Veziris N, Fuhrman C, Chouaid C, et al. Empyema of the thorax due to *Gemella haemolysans*. J Infect 1999;39:245–246.

1009. Vickerman MM, Clewell DB, Jones GW. Sucrose-promoted accumulation of growing glucosyltransferase variants of *Streptococcus gordonii* on hydroxyapatite surfaces. Infect Immun 1991;59:3523–3530.

1010. Vieira VV, Castro ACD. Biochemical properties and whole cell protein profiles of group G streptococci isolated from dogs. J Appl Bacteriol 1994;77:408–411.

1011. Vieira VV, Teixeira LM, Zahner V, et al. Genetic relationships among the different phenotypes of *Streptococcus dysgalactiae* strains. Int J Syst Bacteriol 1998;48:1231–1243.

1012. Vilaichone RK, Mahachai V, Kullavanijaya P, Nunthapisud P. Spontaneous bacterial peritonitis caused by *Streptococcus bovis*: case series and review of the literature. Am J Gastroenterol 2002;97:1476–1479.

1013. Vilaichone RK, Mahachai V, Nunthapisud P. *Streptococcus suis* peritonitis: case report. J Med Assoc Thai 2000;83:1274–1277.

1014. Vince KG, Kantor SR, Descalzi J. Late infection of a total knee arthroplasty with *Streptococcus bovis* in association with carcinoma of the large intestine. J Arthroplasty 2003;18:813–815.

1015. Virolainen A, Salo P, Jero J, et al. Comparison of PCR assay with bacterial culture for detecting *Streptococcus pneumoniae* in middle ear fluid of children with acute otitis media. J Clin Microbiol 1994;32:2667–2670.

1016. Von Baum H, Klemme FR, Geiss HK, Sonntag H-G. Comparative evaluation of a commercial system for identification of Gram-positive cocci. Eur J Clin Microbiol Infect Dis 1998;17:849–852.

1017. von Essen R, Ikavalko M, Forsblom B. Isolation of *Gemella morbillorum* from joint fluid. Lancet 1993;342:177–178.

1018. von Hunolstein C, D'Ascenzi S, Wagner B, et al. Immunochemistry of capsular type polysaccharide and virulence properties of type VI *Streptococcus agalactiae* (group B streptococci). Infect Immun 1993;61:1272–1280.

1019. von Hunolstein C, Parisi L, Tissi L, et al. Virulence properties of the type VII *Streptococcus agalactiae* (group B streptococci) and immunochemical analysis of capsular type polysaccharide. J Med Microbiol 1999;48:983–990.

1020. Votava M, Tejkalova M, Drabkova M, et al. Use of GBS media for rapid detection of group B streptococci in vaginal and rectal swabs from women in labor. Eur J Clin Microbiol Infect Dis 2001;20:120–122.

1021. Waisberg J, Matheus CO, Pimenta J. Infectious endocarditis from *Streptococcus bovis* associated with colonic carcinoma: case report and literature review. Arq Gastroenterol 2002;39:177–180.

1022. Wald ER, Bergman I, Taylor HG, et al. Long-term outcome of group B streptococcal meningitis. Pediatrics 1986;77:217–221.

1023. Wald ER, Dashefsky B, Feidt C, et al. Acute rheumatic fever in western Pennsylvania and the tri-state area. Pediatrics 1987;80:371–374.

1024. Wallbanks S, Martinez-Murcia AJ, Fryer JL, et al. 16S rRNA sequence determination for members of the genus *Carnobacterium* and related lactic acid bacteria and description of *Vagococcus salmoninarum*. Int J Syst Bacteriol 1990;40:224–230.

1025. Wanahita A, Goldsmith EA, Musher DM, et al. Interaction between human polymorphonuclear leukocytes and *Streptococccus milleri* group bacteria. J Infect Dis 2002;185:85–90.

1026. Watanabe Y, Todome Y, Ohkuni H, et al. Cysteine protease activity and histamine release from the human mast cell line HMC-1 stimulated by recombinant streptococcal pyrogenic exotoxin B/streptococcal cysteine protease. Infect Immun 2002;70:3944–3947.

1027. Watanakunikorn C, Pantelakis J. α-Hemolytic streptococcal bacteremia: a review of 203 episodes during 1980–1991. Scand J Infect Dis 1993;25:403–408.

1028. Watanakunikorn C, Patel R. Comparison of patients with enterococcal bacteremia due to strains with and without high-level resistance to gentamicin. Clin Infect Dis 1993;17:74–78.

1029. Watkins EJ, Brooksby P, Schweiger MS, Enright SM. Septicaemia in a pig-farm worker. Lancet 2001;357:1147–1148.

1030. Watkins LM, Pasternack MS, Banks M, et al. Bilateral cavernous sinus thromboses and intraorbital abscesses secondary to *Streptococcus milleri*. Ophthalmology 2003;110:569–574.

1031. Watkins R, Vyas H. Toxic shock syndrome and streptococcal myositis: three case reports. Eur J Pediatr 2002;161:497–498.

1032. Watsky KL, Kollisch N, Densen P. Group G streptococcal bacteremia: the clinical experience at Boston University Medical Center and a critical review of the literature. Arch Intern Med 1985;145:58–61.

1033. Weeks CR, Ferretti JJ. Nucleotide sequence of the type A streptococcal exotoxin (erythrogenic toxin) gene from *Streptococcus pyogenes* bacteriophage T12. Infect Immun 1986;52:144.

1034. Weinstein MR, Litt M, Kertesz DA, et al. Invasive infections due to a fish pathogen, *Streptococcus iniae*. N Engl J Med 1997;337:589–594.

1035. Weiss K, DeAzavedo J, Restieri C, et al. Phenotypic and genotypic characterization of macrolide-resistant group A *Streptococcus* strains in the province of Quebec, Canada. J Antimicrob Chemother 2001;47:345–348.

1036. Welch DF, Hensel D, Pickett D, et al. Comparative evaluation of selective and nonselective culture techniques for isolation of group A β-hemolytic streptococci. Am J Clin Pathol 1991;95:587–590.

1037. Wenocur HS, Smith MA, Vellozi EM, et al. Odontogenic infection secondary to *Leuconostoc* species. J Clin Microbiol 1988;26:1893–1894.

1038. Wessels MR. Capsular polysaccharide of group A *Streptococcus*. In: Fischetti VA, Novick RP, Ferretti JJ et al., eds. Gram-Positive Pathogens. Washington, DC: ASM Press, 2000:34–42.

1039. Wessels MR, DiFabio JL, Benedi V-J, et al. Structural determination and immunochemical characterization of the type V group B *Streptococcus* capsular polysaccharide. J Biol Chem 1991;266:6714–6719.

1040. Wessels MR, Haft R, Heggen LM, et al. Identification of a genetic locus essential for capsule sialylation in type III group B streptococci. Infect Immun 1992;60:392–400.

1041. Wessels MR, Moses AE, Goldberg JB, DiCesare TJ. Hyaluronic acid capsule is a virulence factor for mucoid group A streptococci. Proc Natl Acad Sci USA 1991;88:8317–8321.

1042. Wessels MR, Rubens CE, Benedi VJ, Kasper DL. Definition of a bacterial virulence factor: sialylation of the group B streptococcal capsule. Proc Natl Acad Sci USA 1989;86:8983–8987.

1043. Westh H, Skibsted L, Korner B. *Streptococcus pneumoniae* infections of the female genital tract and the newborn child. Rev Infect Dis 1990;12:416–422.

1044. Westlake RM, Graham TP, Edwards KM. An outbreak of acute rheumatic fever in Tennessee. Pediatr Infect Dis J 1990;9:97–100.

1045. Wheeler MC, Roe MH, Kaplan EL, et al. Outbreak of group A streptococcal septicemia in children: clinical, epidemiologic, and microbiological correlates. JAMA 1991;266:533–537.

1046. Whiley RA, Beighton D. Emended descriptions and recognition of *Streptococcus constellatus*, *Streptococcus intermedius*, and *Streptococcus anginosus* as distinct species. Int J Syst Bacteriol 1991;41:1–5.

1047. Whiley RA, Beighton D. Current classification of the oral streptococci. Oral Microbiol Immunol 1998;13:195–216.

1048. Whiley RA, Beighton D, Winstanley TG, et al. *Streptococcus intermedius*, *Streptococcus constellatus*, and *Streptococcus anginosus* (the *Streptococcus milleri* group): association with different body sites and clinical infections. J Clin Microbiol 1992;30:243–244.

1049. Whiley RA, Fraser HY, Douglas CWI, et al. *Streptococcus parasanguis* sp. nov., an atypical viridans streptococcus from human clinical specimens. FEMS Microbiol Lett 1990;68:115–122.

1050. Whiley RA, Fraser H, Hardie JM, Beighton D. Phenotypic differentiation of *Streptococcus intermedius*, *Streptococcus constellatus*, and *Streptococcus anginosus* strains within the "*Streptococcus milleri*" group. J Clin Microbiol 1990;28:1497–1501.

1051. Whiley RA, Hall LMC, Hardie JM, Brighton D. A study of small-colony, β-haemolytic, Lancefield group C streptococci within the anginosus group: description of *Streptococcus constellatus* subsp. *pharyngis* subsp. nov., associated with the human throat and pharyngitis. Int J Syst Bacteriol 1999;49:1443–1449.

1052. Whiley RA, Hardie JM. *Streptococcus vestibularis* sp. nov. from the human oral cavity. Int J Syst Bacteriol 1988;38:335–339.

1053. Whiley RA, Hardie JM. DNA-DNA hybridization studies and phenotypic characteristics of strains within the "*Streptococcus milleri*" group." J Gen Microbiol 1989;135:2623–2633.

1054. White BA, Labhsetwar SA, Mian AN. *Streptococcus bovis* bacteremia and fetal death. Obstet Gynecol 2002;100:1126–1129.

1055. Whitney AM, O'Connor SP. Phylogenetic relationship of *Gemella morbillorum* to *Gemella haemolysans*. Int J Syst Bacteriol 1993;43:832–838.

1056. Whitney CG, Farley MM, Hadler J, et al. Increasing prevalence of multi-drug resistant *Streptococcus pneumoniae* in the United States. N Engl J Med 2000;343:1917–1924.

1057. Willcox MD. Potential pathogenic properties of members of the "*Streptococcus milleri*" group in relation to the production of endocarditis and abscesses. J Med Microbiol 1995;43:405–410.

1058. Willcox MDP, Zhu H, Knox KW. *Streptococcus australis* sp. nov., a novel oral streptococcus. Int J Syst Evol Microbiol 2001;51:1277–1281.

1059. Williams AM, Collins MD. Molecular taxonomic studies on *Streptococcus uberis* types I and II. Description of *Streptococcus parauberis* sp. nov. J Appl Bacteriol 1990;68:485–490.

1060. Williams AM, Farrow JAE, Collins MD. Reverse transcriptase sequencing of 16S ribosomal RNA from *Streptococcus cecorum*. Lett Appl Microbiol 1989;8:185–189.

1061. Williams AM, Rodrigues UM, Collins MD. Intrageneric relationships of enterococci as determined by reverse transcriptase sequencing of small subunit rRNA. Res Microbiol 1990;142:67–74.

1062. Williams GS. Group C and group G streptococci infections: emerging challenges. Clin Lab Sci 2003;16:209–213.

1063. Williams-Bouyer N, Reisner BS, Woods GL. Comparison of Gen-Probe Accu-Probe Group B streptococcus culture identification test with conventional culture for the detection of group B streptococci in broth cultures of vaginal-anorectal specimens from pregnant women. Diagn Microbiol Infect Dis 2000;36:159–162.

1064. Wilson WR, Thompson RL, Wilkowske CJ, et al. Short-term therapy for streptococcal infective endocarditis. JAMA 1981;245:360–363.

1065. Winterbotham A, Riley S, Kavanaugh-McHugh A, Dermody TS. Endocarditis caused by group A β-hemolytic streptococci in an infant: case report and review. Clin Infect Dis 1999;29:196–198.

1066. Wiseman A, Rene P, Crelinsten GL. *Streptococcus agalactiae* endocarditis: an association with villous adenomas of the large intestine. Ann Intern Med 1985;103:893–894.

1067. Wong SS, Woo PC, Ho PL, Wang TK. Continuous ambulatory peritoneal dialysis-related peritonitis caused by *Streptococcus bovis*. Eur J Clin Microbiol Infect Dis 2003;22:424–426.

1068. Wong WY, Overturf GD, Powars DR. Infection caused by *Streptococcus pneumoniae* in children with sickle cell disease: epidemiology, immunologic mechanisms, prophylaxis, and vaccination. Clin Infect Dis 1992;14:1124–1136.

1069. Woo PCY, Fung AMY, Lau SKP, et al. Group G β-hemolytic streptococcal bacteremia characterized by 16S ribosomal RNA gene sequencing. J Clin Microbiol 2001;39:3147–3155.

1070. Woo PCY, Tam DM, Lau SK, et al. *Enterococcus cecorum* empyema thoracis successfully treated with cefotaxime. J Clin Microbiol 2004;42:919–922.

1071. Woo PCY, Tam DMW, Leung K-W, et al. *Streptococcus sinensis* sp. nov., a novel species isolated from a patient with infective endocarditis. J Clin Microbiol 2002;40:805–810.

1072. Woo PCY, To AP, Tse H, et al. Clinical and molecular epidemiology of erythromycin-resistant β-hemolytic lancefield group G streptococci causing bacteremia. J Clin Microbiol 2003;41:5188–5191.

1073. Woo PCY, Tse H, Chan K, et al. "*Streptococcus milleri*" endocarditis caused by *Streptococcus anginosus*. Diagn Microbiol Infect Dis 2004;48:81–88.

1074. Wood EG, Dillon HC. A prospective study of group B streptococcal bacteriuria in pregnancy. Am J Obstet Gynecol 1981;140:515–520.

1075. Wood HF, Jacobs K, McCarty M. *Streptococcus lactis* isolated from a patient with subacute bacterial endocarditis. Am J Med 1985;18:345–347.

1076. Wood TF, Potter MA, Jonasson O. Streptococcal toxic shock-like syndrome: the importance of surgical intervention. Ann Surg 1993;217:109–114.

1077. Woodford N. Epidemiology of genetic elements responsible for acquired glycopeptide resistance in enterococci. Microb Drug Resist 2001;7:229–236.

1078. Woodford N, Morrison D, Johnson AP, et al. Application of DNA probes for rRNA and *vanA* genes to investigation of a nosocomial cluster of vancomycin-resistant enterococci. J Clin Microbiol 1993;31:653–658.

1079. Woods CR, Edwards MS. Renal abscess caused by group B *Streptococcus*. Clin Infect Dis 1994;18:662–663.

1080. Wu HY, Nahm MH, Guo Y, et al. Intranasal immunization with PspA (Pneumococcal surface protein A) can prevent carriage and infection with *Streptococcus pneumoniae*. J Infect Dis 1997;175:839–846.

1081. Yagupsky P, Menegus MA, Powell KR. The changing spectrum of group B streptococcal disease in infants: an eleven-year experience in a tertiary care hospital. Pediatr Infect Dis J 1991;10:801–808.

1082. Yamamoto M, Fukushima T, Ohshiro S, et al. Brain abscess caused by *Streptococcus intermedius*: two case reports. Surg Neurol 1999;51:219–222.

1083. Yamashita Y, Bowen WE, Burne RA, Kuramitsu HK. Role of *Streptococcus mutans gtf* genes in caries induction in the specific-pathogen free rat model. Infect Immun 1997;61:3811–3817.

1084. Yancey MK, Armer T, Clark P, Duff P. Assessment of rapid identification tests for genital carriage of group B streptococci. Obstet Gynecol 1992;80:1038–1047.

1085. Yaniv LG, Potasman I. Iatrogenic meningitis: an increasing role for resistant viridans streptococci? Case report and review of the last 20 years. Scand J Infect Dis 2000;32:693–696.

1086. Yen CC, Tang RB, Chen SJ, Chin TW. Pediatric lung abscess: a retrospective review of 23 cases. J Microbiol Immunol Infect 2004;37:45–49.

1087. Yu PKW, Germer JJ, Torgerson CA, Anhalt JP. Evaluation of TestPack Strep A for the detection of group A streptococci in throat swabs. Mayo Clin Proc 1988;63:33–36.

1088. Yuen KY, Sato WH, Choi CH, et al. *Streptococcus zooepidemicus* (Lancefield group C) septicaemia in Hong Kong. J Infect 1990;21:241–250.

1089. Zachariadou L, Papaparaskevas J, Paraskakis I, et al. Predominance of two M-types among erythromycin-resistant group A streptococci from Greek children. Clin Microbiol Infect 2003;9:310–314.

1090. Zaoutis T, Attia M, Gross R, Klein J. The role of group C and group G streptococci in acute pharyngitis in children. Clin Microbiol Infect 2004;10:37–40.

1091. Zarkin BA, Lillemore KD, Cameron JL, et al. The triad of *Streptococcus bovis* bacteremia, colonic pathology, and liver disease. Ann Surg 1990;211:786–791.

1092. Zbinden R, Satanam P, Hunziker L, et al. Endocarditis due to *Aerococcus urinae*: diagnostic tests, fatty acid composition, and killing kinetics. Infection 1999;27:122–124.

1093. Zhang GW, Kotiw M, Daggard G. A RAPD-PCR genotyping assay which correlates with serotypes of group B streptococci. Lett Appl Microbiol 2002;35:247–250.

1094. Zhang Q, Kwoh C, Attorri S, Clarridge JE III. *Aerococcus urinae* in urinary tract infections. J Clin Microbiol 2000;38:1703–1705.

1095. Zhu H, Willcox MDP, Knox KW. A new species of oral *Streptococcus* isolated from Sprague-Dawley rats, *Streptococcus orisratti* sp. nov. Int J Syst Evol Microbiol 2000;50:55–61.

1096. Zinner SH. Changing epidemiology of infections in patients with neutropenia and cancer with an emphasis on gram-positive and resistant bacteria. Clin Infect Dis 1999;29:490–494.

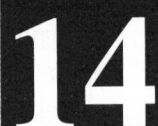

Aerobic and Facultative Gram-Positive Bacilli

Listeria Species and Listeria monocytogenes

Taxonomy of the Genus *Listeria*
Virulence Factors of
   L. monocytogenes
Epidemiology of
   L. monocytogenes
Clinical Significance of
   L. monocytogenes
Isolation of *L. monocytogenes*
   From Clinical Specimens
Identification of *Listeria* Species
Antimicrobial Susceptibility and
   Treatment of *Listeria*
   Infections
Pathogenicity of Other *Listeria*
   Species

Erysipelothrix Species: Erysipelothrix rhusiopathiae and Erysipelothrix tonsillarum

Taxonomy of the Genus
   Erysipelothrix
Virulence Factors of
   E. rhusiopathiae
Clinical Significance of
   E. rhusiopathiae
Isolation and Identification of
   E. rhusiopathiae
Antimicrobial Susceptibility of
   E. rhusiopathiae

Bacillus Species and Related Genera

Taxonomy and the Taxonomic
   Dissection of the Genus
   Bacillus
Bacillus anthracis

   Epidemiology of Anthrax
   Virulence Factors of *B. anthracis*
   Clinical Presentations of Anthrax
   Treatment of Anthrax
   Prevention of Anthrax

Bacillus cereus

   Virulence Factors of *B. cereus*
   B. cereus Gastroenteritis

Opportunistic *Bacillus* Species
Infections

   Bacteremia and Endocarditis
   Infections in Compromised Hosts
   Ocular Infections
   Musculoskeletal Infections
   Nosocomial Infections

Laboratory Safety, Specimen
   Collection, and Processing
Isolation and Identification of
   Bacillus Species: The
   "*Bacillus cereus* Group":
   B. anthracis, *B. cereus*,
   B. thuringiensis, and
   B. mycoides
Antimicrobial Susceptibility of
   Bacillus Species

Corynebacterium Species

Introduction and Taxonomy

Identification of *Corynebacterium* Species and the Coryneform Bacteria
Antimicrobial Susceptibility Testing of *Corynebacterium* Species and the Coryneform Bacteria
Members of the Genus *Corynebacterium* Isolated From Humans

Corynebacterium amycolatum
Corynebacterium diphtheriae
Corynebacterium jeikeium
Corynebacterium pseudodiphtheriticum
Corynebacterium striatum
Corynebacterium urealyticum

Corynebacterium Species Associated With Animals
Corynebacterium Species Isolated From Foods and the Environment

Other Coryneform Bacteria

Actinobaculum Species
Actinomyces Species Isolated From Humans
Actinomyces Species Isolated From Animals

Arcanobacterium Species
Arthrobacter Species
Brevibacterium Species
Cellulomonas, Cellulosimicrobium, and *Oerskovia* Species
Dermabacter Species
Exiguobacterium Species
Leifsonia Species
Microbacterium (*Aureobacterium*) Species
Rothia and "Rothia-Like" Species (CDC Group 4)
Turicella Species

Gardinerella vaginalis

Taxonomy and Cellular Morphology
Virulence Factors of *G. vaginalis*
Clinical Significance of *G. vaginalis*
Isolation and Identification
Antimicrobial Susceptibility

Lactobacillus Species

Taxonomy and Epidemiology
Clinical Significance
Isolation and Identification
Antimicrobial Susceptibility

The aerobic/facultative gram-positive bacilli include a wide variety of organisms that are responsible for "classical" diseases such as listeriosis, anthrax, and diphtheria, and also for newer disease syndromes, particularly in immunocompromised hosts. The aerobic/facultative gram-positive bacilli also include several newly recognized genera that are environmental or veterinary organisms not previously associated with humans or human infections. The use of molecular techniques for characterization of many new species has required reexamination of classical pathogens as well. For example, the recognition of several new facultative species in the genus *Actinomyces* has enabled recognition of the facultative nature of classical pathogens such as *A. israelii* that were previously considered to be obligately anaerobic organisms. These new techniques have also permitted the classification of previously unnamed bacteria, such as the CDC (Centers for Disease Control and Prevention) coryneform groups, into new or existing genera, and has led to the taxonomic dissection of genera known to contain many unrelated species (e.g., the genus *Bacillus*). The classification scheme presented in the forthcoming edition of *Bergey's Manual of Systematic Bacteriology* now reflects the genotypic relationships rather than phenotypic similarities among these organism. Box 14-1 presents the classification of the organisms to be discussed in this chapter.

Listeria *Species and* Listeria monocytogenes
Taxonomy of the Genus *Listeria*

The genus *Listeria* consists of gram-positive, non–spore-forming, facultatively anaerobic, regular rod-shaped bacteria (see Color Plate 14-1A). The genus is defined by a G + C DNA content of 36–38%, a typical gram-positive cell wall with a peptidoglycan murein layer containing *meso*-diaminopimelic acid (*meso*-DAP) attached to the cell membrane by lipoteichoic acid, and membrane-associated polyribitol teichoic acids.[272] Genetic studies indicate that *Listeria* organisms exhibit the closest phylogenetic relationship to the genus *Brochothrix* (an environmental organism) and are more distantly related to organisms in genus *Bacillus*, related spore-forming genera, and the genus *Lactobacillus*, rather than to organisms in the genera *Streptococcus, Enterococcus,* and *Lactococcus*.[460,738] The relationship between *Listeria* and *Brochothrix* species is also supported by chemotaxonomic data.[176] Although some taxonomists have favored the inclusion of *Listeria* species in the Family *Lactobacillaceae*, Collins[176] and other workers believe that *Listeria* species merit inclusion in a new family. In the upcoming edition of *Bergey's Manual of Systematic Bacteriology*, *Listeria* and *Brochothrix* species are included in the proposed family "*Listeriaceae*" in the order *Bacillales*, class "*Bacilli*" in the phylum *Firmicutes*.[329] The genus *Erysipelothrix* is in-

Box 14-1 Classification of the Aerobic/Facultative Gram-Positive Bacilli in the Domain Bacteria[329]

Phylum	Class/Subclass	Order/Suborder	Family	Genera
Firmicutes	Mollicutes "Bacilli"	Incertae sedis Bacillales	*"Erysipelotrichaceae"* *Bacillaceae*	*Erysipelothrix* *Bacillus, Amphibacillus, Exiguobacterium, Gracilibacillus, Halobacillus, Salibacillus, Virgibacillus*
			"Listeriaceae"	*Listeria, Brochothrix*
			"Sporolactobacillaceae"	*Sporolactobacillus*
			"Paenibacillaceae"	*Paenibacillus, Aneurinibacillus, Brevibacillus, Thermobacillus*
			"Alicyclobacillaceae"	*Alicyclobacillus, Sulfobacillus*
		"Lactobacillales"	*Lactobacillaceae*	*Lactobacillus*
Actinobacteria	Actinobacteria/ Actinobacteridae	Actinomycetales/ Actinomycineae	*Actinomycetaceae*	*Actinomyces, Actinobaculum, Arcanobacterium, Mobiluncus*
		Actinomycetales/ Micrococcineae	*Micrococcaceae*	*Rothia*
			Brevibacteriaceae	*Brevibacterium*
			Cellulomonadaceae	*Cellulomonas, Cellulosimicrobium, Oerskovia*
			Dermabacteriaceae	*Dermabacter*
			Intrasporangiaceae	*Sanguibacter*
			Jonesiaceae	*Jonesia*
			Microbacteriaceae	*Microbacterium (Aureobacterium), Leifsonia*
		Actinomycetales/ Corynebacterineae	*Corynebacteriaceae*	*Corynebacterium*
		Bifidobacteriales	*Bifidobacteriaceae*	*Gardnerella*
			"Unknown affiliation"	*Turicella*

cluded in the phylum *Firmicutes* along with *Listeria* species, but is in a different class, order, and family (Box 14-1). Table 14-1 presents the major characteristics that differentiate *Listeria, Erysipelothrix, Lactobacillus,* and *Brochothrix* from one another.

For many years, the genus *Listeria* consisted of eight species—*L. monocytogenes, L. grayi, L. innocua, L. ivanovii, L. murrayi, L. seeligeri, L. welshimeri,* and *L. denitrificans.*[787] Based on sequencing of the 16S rRNA of *L. denitrificans,* this organism has been excluded from the genus *Listeria* and

placed in the genus *Jonesia* as *Jonesia denitrificans,* which is now in its own family (*Jonesiaceae*) in the Order Actinomycetales, Class Actinobacteria, phylum Actinobacteria (Box 14-1).[329,703,740] Additional sequencing data on the other members of the genus *Listeria* have identified two closely related but distinct lines of descent: the "*L. monocytogenes* group" (consisting of *L. monocytogenes, L. innocua, L. ivanovii, L. seeligeri,* and *L. welshimeri*), and the "*L. grayi/L. murrayi* group." *L. grayi* and *L. murrayi* have since been combined into a single species, *L. grayi.*[739] In addition,

Table 14-1 Characteristics for Differentiation of *Listeria, Erysipelothrix, Lactobacillus,* and *Brochothrix*

GENUS	RELATION- SHIP TO O$_2$	GROWTH, 35°C	CATA- LASE	PRODUC- TION OF H$_2$S IN KIA/TSI	MOTI- LITY	ACID FROM GLU- COSE	PEPTIDO- GLYCAN DI-AMINO ACID	MOL% G+C
Listeria	Facultative	+	+	−	+[a]	+	*meso*-DAP	36–38
Erysipelothrix	Facultative	+	−	+	−	+	L-lysine	36–40
Lactobacillus	Facultative	+	−	−	−[b]	+	L-lysine, or *meso*-DAP or L-ornithine	34–53
Brochothrix	Facultative	−	+	−	−	+	*meso*-DAP	35.6–36.1

[a] All strains motile at 20–25°C. Poorly motile or nonmotile at 35–37°C

[b] Most species nonmotile, but a few motile species have been described.

KIA, Kligler's iron agar; +, positive reaction; −, negative reaction.

multilocus enzyme electrophoretic studies of *L. ivanovii* strains suggested that this species could also be divided into two genomic groups.[95] Subsequently, DNA homology studies have shown that these two groups represented two subspecies: *L. ivanovii* subsp. *ivanovii* and *L. ivanovii* subsp. *londoniensis*.[94] Therefore, at present, the genus *Listeria* includes six species *L. monocytogenes*, *L. ivanovii* subsp. *ivanovii*, *L. ivanovii* subsp. *londoniensis*, *L. seeligeri*, *L. innocua*, *L. grayi*, and *L. welshimeri*. *L. monocytogenes* can be divided into 13 serotypes based on somatic (S) and flagellar (H) antigens. Among the 13 serotypes (1/2a, 1/2b, 1/2c, 3a, 3b, 3c, 4a, 4ab, 4b, 4c, 4d, 4e, and 7), most disease is due to types 4b, 1/2a, and 1/2b.[553]

Virulence Factors of *L. monocytogenes*

L. monocytogenes is a facultative intracellular pathogen that is able to invade and survive within mammalian cells, including macrophages and several human tissue culture cell lines. These organisms possess an 80-kDa surface protein called **internalin**.[320,525,659] Internalin interacts with a cell adhesion receptor called **E-cadherin** on human epithelial cells, resulting in the induction of phagocytosis.[602] Cadherins are 110-kDa transmembrane glycoproteins that are structurally related and tissue specific. Experiments using several different cell lines have established that the internalin/E-cadherin interaction promotes both specific binding and entry of *L. monocytogenes* into epithelial cells.[602] The presence of internalin alone is sufficient for entry of the organism into epithelial cells if the cells have the appropriate receptor. Other surface proteins in the internalin family have been described (e.g., inlB, inlC), and appear to mediate invasion of other cell types, such as endothelial cells and hepatocytes.[231,321,659] Once sequestered within the phagosomes, the organisms produce **listeriolysin O** and several phospholipases that enable the organism to escape from the phagosome before lysosomal fusion, thereby avoiding intracellular killing. Listeriolysin O is encoded by the *hly* gene and is a pore-forming hemolysin that is similar to streptolysin O of group A streptococci.[689] Listeriolysin O acts by binding to membrane cholesterol and then inserting itself into the target membrane, resulting in the formation of transmembrane pores. Mutants that lack the *hly* gene are avirulent and unable to escape from the internalized vacuole.[689] In addition, expression of this gene in avirulent bacteria (e.g., *B. subtilis*) promotes the escape of these organisms into the cytosol.[690] Similarly, mutants lacking broad-range phospholipase (PlcB) and phosphatidylinositol-specific phospholipase (PlcA) demonstrate about half the efficiency in escape from macrophage phagosomes as wild-type strains.[818] Once within the cytosol, another listerial surface protein, **ActA**, causes intracellular polymerization of actin.[497] This results in translocation of the bacteria toward the surface of the target cell membrane to form pseudopodlike projections that bud off and are ingested by macrophages and other cells, such as hepatocytes and enterocytes. Both of the bacterial phospholipases and an additional metalloprotease enzyme also function in facilitating cell-to-cell spread of the bacteria following actin-mediated translocation to the cell surface.[694,818] These mechanisms enable the organism to move directly from cell to cell without exposure to soluble immune factors like antibodies and complement.

Epidemiology of *L. monocytogenes*

While all *Listeria* species may be isolated from the environment and from a wide variety of animals, both as pathogens and as commensals, only *L. monocytogenes* is a well-recognized animal and human pathogen. This organism can be isolated from soil, water, sewage, and vegetation and as a part of the fecal flora of a wide variety of animals.[783] *L. monocytogenes* can infect a wide variety of domesticated animals, including rodents, rabbits, sheep, and ruminants. These animals become infected from their environment, where the organism contaminates vegetation and soil. Infections in these animals include sepsis, rhombencephalitis, prematurity, and abortion.[515] *L. monocytogenes* is also a common contaminant in food products. *L. monocytogenes* is able to grow in biofilms on the surface of various foods, and refrigeration actually augments further organism growth because of the ability of the organisms to grow at 4°C. Because of their ubiquity in foods, humans probably have contact with these organisms on a daily basis, and, as a result, some individuals become fecal carriers of *L. monocytogenes*.[587] The organism is a transient constituent of the human intestinal flora and may be excreted in the feces by 1–10% of healthy humans.[780,783] Human listeriosis occurs mostly in the spring and summer months, and sporadic cases (outside of foodborne outbreaks) occur at annualized rates of less than 1 case per 100,000 population, although the infection is more common in infants (10 cases per 100,000 population) and the elderly (1.4 cases/100,000 population).[334] While symptomatic infection is relatively rare, it should always be suspected in infections of immunocompromised hosts.

Clinical Significance of *L. monocytogenes*

L. monocytogenes is associated with a spectrum of clinical syndromes.[553,599,600,621,669] The most common result of organism acquisition is a transient asymptomatic gastrointestinal carrier state that usually results from ingestion of contaminated food. During this time the organism may be excreted in the feces. Acute symptomatic infection with this organism often occurs during pregnancy, usually during the last half of pregnancy (second or third trimester), and the illness presents with influenzalike symptoms of fever, sore throat, myalgia, malaise, lower abdominal pain, and back pain.[856] Occasionally, a vaginal discharge, diarrhea, and urinary tract symptoms are noted. Peripheral leukocytosis may be present, and blood cultures collected during the acute phase of this transient illness may be positive. During maternal infection, occult bacteremia and transplacental transmission of the organism may occur, leading to intrauterine infection of the fetus.[856] Infection in utero may induce labor, resulting in premature birth of an infected or stillborn fetus. Symptoms in the mother usually subside following the delivery of the infected infant and the placenta. Fetal survival is partly determined by the length of gestation, with spontaneous abortion occurring when the infection is acquired early in pregnancy, and neonatal infection resulting when the infection is acquired later.[281,564]

Neonates can be categorized as having "early-onset" or "late-onset" disease. Newborns who are infected in utero generally present with acute sepsis, have disseminated disease, with pustular skin lesions and granulomas containing *L. monocytogenes* being found in the brain, liver, kidneys, lung, and spleen (early-onset disease). The placental tissues usually show evidence of acute chorioamnionitis. The mortality rate of early-onset listeriosis is high, but fatal neonatal infections are more common among immunocompromised children.[588] Listeriosis in infants may also present as late-onset infections, in which the neonate becomes infected through maternal gastrointestinal carriage of the organism. The infant is exposed to the organisms during vaginal delivery through the birth canal; swallowing or aspiration of the organisms in this milieu is the likely mode of organism acquisition and infection. Infants presenting with this clinical picture are usually more than 3 to 5 days of age, with disease appearing 7 to 14 days after birth.[553,599] Late-onset listeriosis usually presents as neonatal meningitis, with signs and symptoms of fever, irritability, and bulging fontanelles being present. In these infants, Gram staining of cerebrospinal fluid (CSF) will show polymorphonuclear leukocytes along with high protein and low glucose indexes; the gram-positive rods of *L. monocytogenes* will usually be seen in over 50% of cases. In cases of late-onset disease, the mother has usually had an uncomplicated pregnancy, with no signs of infection (e.g., fever) or sepsis (e.g., positive blood cultures) being present

Nonpregnant adults may also become infected with *L. monocytogenes*, and these patients present with acute sepsis, subacute meningitis, meningoencephalitis, or rhombencephalitis.[600] Adults with acute listerial sepsis usually have underlying malignancies or are immunocompromised (e.g., lymphoma, organ transplantation, diabetes, chronic liver/renal disease, collagen-vascular disease). Positive blood cultures and a clinical picture similar to sepsis associated with gram-negative bacteremia are usually observed. In some patients, the organisms cross the blood-brain barrier, resulting in infection of the meninges and the brain itself.[857] Subacute meningitis develops over several days and is characterized by low-grade fever, headaches, and nuchal rigidity. In the subacute presentation, CSF cell counts are generally lower and the organisms are often not observed on Gram stains of the CSF. Meningoencephalitis caused by *L. monocytogenes* is associated with several unique features. Nuchal rigidity is less common, being found in 80–85% of adults. Motor disorders, such as ataxia, tremors, cranial-nerve palsies, and seizure activity, are more common with listerial infection than with other etiologic agents of meningoencephalitis.[35,790] Fluctuating mental status is another clinical feature in these patients. In some cases, central nervous system listerial infection may progress to include brainstem involvement (i.e., rhombencephalitis), and imaging studies usually show microabscesses in the diencephalon and cerebellum.[790] Brain abscesses, both solitary and multiple, may occur as complications of listerial meningoencephalitis.[210,920] Diagnosis of meningoencephalitis and rhombencephalitis is established by culture of CSF and blood specimens.

Focal infections caused by *L. monocytogenes* include cutaneous infections, abscesses, arthritis, peritonitis (including spontaneous bacterial peritonitis), liver and splenic abscesses, cholecystitis, endophthalmitis, prosthetic joint/vascular graft infections, osteomyelitis, myocarditis, and endocarditis.[108,149,217,241,332,351,452,453,472,544,812,837,844,915] Most of these complications are associated with hematogenous dissemination and usually occur in immunocompromised hosts. Cases have been reported in patients who are immunocompromised because of underlying acute or chronic diseases characterized by cellular and/or humoral immunodeficiency (i.e., malignancies, systemic lupus erythematosus, rheumatoid arthritis, organ transplantation, ulcerative colitis, diabetes, renal disease, alcoholic cirrhosis, and HIV infection) and in those being treated with cytotoxic chemotherapeutic agents or steroids for their underlying conditions.[24,73,147,343,393,540,551,594] Cutaneous infections have been observed in previously healthy individuals who have had direct contact with infected animals or animal tissues (i.e., placental tissues, amniotic fluids). These infections occur in veterinarians, individuals with occupations associated with animals, and occasionally laboratory workers. Cutaneous infections are characterized by papular or pustular lesions, and disseminated infections have occurred following primary cutaneous inoculation.[125,819] *L. monocytogenes* endocarditis results from bacteremia and usually involves damaged native aortic/mitral valves or prosthetic valves. Septic embolization and consequent abscess formation at distant sites is common. Hepatic and splenic abscesses, hepatitis, hepatic granulomas, and spontaneous peritonitis caused by disseminated *L. monocytogenes* is seen in transplant patients, diabetics, and individuals with cirrhosis or other hepatic diseases.[102] Pleural fluid infections with *L. monocytogenes* have been documented in patients with malignancies, in whom pleural infection occurred by hematogenous seeding of malignant pleural effusions rather than secondary to a parapneumonic process.[591] *L. monocytogenes* is also capable of causing infections in patients on continuous ambulatory peritoneal dialysis and in those with ventriculoperitoneal shunts.[228,558,812,956] Studies have shown that individuals with HIV infection have a 500- to 1,000-fold increased risk of developing *L. monocytogenes* infection over the general population.[470] Listerial infections in HIV-infected individuals typically present as meningitis or as bacteremia without an identifiable source.[73,209,252,475]

L. monocytogenes is present as a contaminant in many kinds of foodstuffs, including raw milk, raw vegetables, fish, poultry, and both fresh and processed meats.[683,775,781] In contaminated food, colony counts of the organism may exceed 10^9 colony-forming unit (CFU)/g of food. In recent years, foodborne outbreaks of febrile gastroenteritis due to *L. monocytogenes* have been recognized with increasing frequency.[44,120,141,142,198,724,759] In dairy cattle *L. monocytogenes* can cause encephalitis, meningitis, septicemia, and mastitis. Shedding of the organisms from the udder or contamination from the environment can lead to the presence of *L. monocytogenes* in raw milk.[198] Surveys have indicated that *L. monocytogenes* may be present in approximately 4% of raw milk samples examined in the U.S.[781] The organism has also been recovered from unpasteurized milk and cheeses prepared from unpasteurized dairy products. Another outbreak was traced to contaminated cabbage and cole slaw.[775] The cabbage implicated in these outbreaks was grown in soil contaminated with fecal droppings from infected sheep. In 1985, a large outbreak in Los Angeles County, California, involved over 181 people, including 93 perinatal cases, and resulted in a 33% fatality rate.[141] The implicated food was a soft Mexican-style cheese that had been prepared from unpasteurized milk. Contaminated ice cream has also been implicated in some outbreaks, and raw meats and processed products prepared from meats and fish may also harbor the organisms.[142] In 1994, a foodborne outbreak occurred in 10 of 36 people (including two pregnant women) attending a party in New York City.[724] In this outbreak, shrimp were implicated as the contaminated food. Another outbreak among 45 people who had attended a picnic in Illinois was traced to contaminated chocolate milk.[198,774] As a corollary to the recognition of foodborne outbreaks of listeriosis, a syndrome of febrile gastroenteritis caused by *L. monocytogenes* has also been described. This syndrome includes nonbloody diarrhea, nausea, and vomiting accompanied by fever, fatigue, chills, and myalgias.[724,759,774] Retrospective serologic analysis of patients with febrile gastroenteritis has been able to demonstrate immune responses to listeriolysin, a putative virulence factor of *L. monocytogenes*.[198] Febrile gastroenteritis due to *L. monocytogenes* is usually self-limited, but invasive disease may occur in immunocompromised patients and those with other underlying bacterial or viral gastrointestinal infections.[552]

Along with the recognition and documentation of foodborne outbreaks due to *L. monocytogenes*, the CDC has promulgated guidelines for the prevention of foodborne listeriosis.[143] Guidelines that apply to all individuals include thoroughly cooking raw food from animal sources, thoroughly washing raw vegetables before eating; keeping uncooked meats separate from vegetables, cooked foods, and "ready-to-eat foods"; and avoiding the consumption of raw (unpasteurized) milk or foods made from raw milk. Hands, knives, and cutting boards should be thoroughly washed after handling uncooked foods. For persons at high risk for listeriosis (i.e., immunocompromised persons, pregnant women, elderly individuals), soft cheeses (e.g., Mexican-style, feta, Brie, Camembert and blue-veined cheese) should be avoided, although there is no need to avoid hard cheeses (e.g., Swiss cheese, Colby cheese), cream cheese, cottage cheese, or yogurt.[339] Leftover foods or "ready-to-eat" foods (e.g., hot dogs) should be reheated until steaming hot before eating. "Delicatessen counter" food (e.g., cold cuts, salami) should be avoided or thoroughly heated before eating. During the mid-1990s, the food industry introduced an initiative called Hazard Analysis at Critical Control Points (HACCP) to improve the surveillance and control of *L. monocytogenes* and other foodborne pathogens in the food-processing plant environment, and the Food and Drug Administration (FDA) has mandated a "zero-tolerance" approach to the control of listeriosis, with increases in both the numbers of FDA inspections of food-processing centers and recalls of foods suspected of harboring pathogens.[873]

Nosocomially acquired listerial infections have also been documented. In June 1989, an outbreak of nosocomial listeriosis occurred in Costa Rica among nine infants 4 to 8 days of age following the delivery of an infant with early-onset listerial infection.[782] Investigation of possible sources of the organism for the nine cases revealed that all of the infants had been bathed with mineral oil from a multidose container.

An *L. monocytogenes* strain that was identical to the isolates from the infants by multilocus enzyme electrophoresis was recovered from the multidose mineral oil vial by cold enrichment. Another outbreak of nosocomial listeriosis among neonates was traced to common use of an improperly cleaned rectal thermometer.[674] Clusters of nosocomial infections with *L. monocytogenes* among immunosuppressed adults have also occurred in several hospitals. In many cases, the sources of the organisms involved in these outbreaks were never determined.

Isolation of *L. monocytogenes* From Clinical Specimens

L. monocytogenes may be isolated from the blood, CSF, genital tract specimens, amniotic fluid, and biopsy specimens derived from maternal/fetal tissues. Direct inoculation of both agar and broth media with overnight incubation will usually yield the organism. On Gram stains of clinical specimens and from blood cultures, the organism may appear as regular, gram-positive bacilli or as short, plump coccobacilli. If polymorphonuclear or mononuclear cells are present, organisms are found both intracellularly and extracellularly. Because of variations in Gram stain morphology that are observed with this organism, *L. monocytogenes* morphotypes may be mistaken for diphtheroids or for certain streptococci, particularly *Streptococcus pneumoniae*, enterococci, and some viridans streptococci.

Methods for the recovery of *L. monocytogenes* from foods differ significantly from those used for isolation from human clinical specimens. These methods involve broth enrichment and subculture to various types of selective media, including Chromagar (Paris, France). Recognition of *L. monocytogenes* is enabled by the presence of chemicals in the media that result in colored colonies. These methods can be found in publications from the U.S. Department of Agriculture and the Netherlands Government Food Inspection Service.[401,914]

Identification of *Listeria* Species

L. monocytogenes grows well on sheep blood agar (SBA), producing gray-white colonies that closely resemble those of group B β-hemolytic streptococci. After 18–24 hours of incubation, colonies may show a narrow zone of β-hemolysis that does not extend very far beyond the edge of the colony (see Color Plates 14-1*B* and 14-1*C*). Before this time, β-hemolysis may only be noted directly under the colony after removal of the colonial growth from the agar surface with a swab. On longer incubation, or in areas of the plate that have been stab-inoculated, the β-hemolysis of the organism becomes more obvious. Among the other species, *L. ivanovii* subspecies produce wide zones or even multiple zones of β-hemolysis on sheep blood- or horse blood-containing media, while *L. seeligeri* produces hemolytic zones that are narrower than those of *L. monocytogenes*. Fujisawa and Mori evaluated several basal media and blood from different animal species for the detection of β-hemolysis produced by *L. monocytogenes* and found that blood agar base no. 2 (Oxoid, Basingstoke, England) supplemented with 5% defibrinated horse blood provided the clearest detection of hemolysin activity.[287] Because of the resemblance of the colonies of *L. monocytogenes* to those of enterococci and group B β-hemolytic streptococci, shortcuts in laboratory identification are to be discouraged. Gram stains and catalase tests should always be performed.

L. monocytogenes is a catalase-positive, facultative, gram-positive bacillus (Table 14-2). The organism is motile, showing "tumbling motility" particularly in hanging-drop preparations prepared from overnight broth cultures incubated at 25°C. This greater motility following room temperature incubation is also apparent in semisolid motility medium, where the organism displays a characteristic "umbrella" of motility near the surface of semisolid motility medium containing 0.2–0.4% agar after incubation at 25°C (see Color Plate 14-1*E*).[17] The organism also grows in the presence of 40% bile and hydrolyzes esculin; therefore, bile-esculin agar slants used for presumptive identification of group D streptococci (i.e., *Streptococcus bovis*) and enterococci may be used to demonstrate esculin hydrolysis. The organism is fermentative, producing acid from glucose, and produces acetoin, resulting in a positive Voges-Proskauer reaction. All strains of *L. monocytogenes* ferment α-methyl-D-mannoside and do not ferment D-xylose. The β-hemolytic reaction, positive catalase test, lack of H_2S production in triple sugar iron (TSI) agar, room temperature motility, and esculin hydrolysis differentiate *L. monocytogenes* from *Erysipelothrix rhusiopathiae*. Motility differentiates this organism from all *Corynebacterium* species. *Leifsonia aquatica*, the former "*Corynebacterium aquaticum*" is also a motile, catalase-positive, gram-positive bacillus, but this organism is nonhemolytic, grows as yellow-pigmented colonies, and is Voges-Proskauer-negative (see section on *Leifsonia* species). Although the biochemical characteristics of *L. monocytogenes* are usually uniform and unambiguous, aberrant strains lacking catalase activity have been isolated from patients with typical listerial sepsis and meningitis.[119,242,857] Biochemical characteristics for identification of *Listeria* species are presented in Table 14-2.

The CAMP test has also been used to identify *L. monocytogenes*.[17] With *Listeria* species, the CAMP test is performed with a β-lysin-producing *S. aureus* strain and with a strain of *Rhodococcus equi*. Synergistic hemolysis is seen between *S. aureus* and putative *L. monocytogenes* and *L. seeligeri* strains, while enhanced hemolysis is seen between *R. equi* and putative *L. ivanovii* strains. With *L. monocytogenes*, a positive CAMP test with *S. aureus* is indicated by enhanced hemolysis in the region between the two nonintersecting streaks of growth at right angle to one another, while that seen between *R. equi* and *L. ivanovii* appears as a area of shovel-shaped enhanced hemolysis. This test may be difficult to interpret, as some investigators have reported synergistic hemolytic reactions between *L. monocytogenes* and *R. equi*.[17]

Kit systems are also available for identifying *Listeria* species. The API Coryne (BioMérieux, Marcy l'Etoile, France) and the RapID CB-Plus systems (Remel, Lenexa, KS) contain *Listeria* species in their databases and have been shown to reliably identify these organisms to at least the genus level. In an evaluation of this system for identification of *Listeria* species, the API Coryne identified all 72 *L. monocytogenes* strains that were tested as *L. monocytogenes/innocua*, with definitive species identification being dependent

on the presence of β-hemolysis and a positive CAMP reaction (see Color Plate 14-1*F*).[485] Similar results have been reported by other investigators for both the API Coryne and the RapID CB-Plus.[283,305,310,333,438,833] The API *Listeria* (BioMérieux) and the Micro-ID *Listeria* (Remel, Lenexa, KS) are identification systems designed specifically for identification of *Listeria* species. The API *Listeria* is a 10-test, chromogenic enzyme substrate system that has been shown to reliably identify several species in the genus, including *L. monocytogenes*, within 24 hours.[84,287,671] This identification panel includes a test for glycyl arylamidase (DIM test) that differentiates *L. monocytogenes* (DIM test–negative) from *L. innocua* (DIM test–positive) without the need for assessing hemolytic activity on SBA. Stand-alone tests for detection of alanyl arylamidase using either D,L-alanine-β-naphthylamide or D,L-alanine-p-nitroanilide can also be used to identify *Listeria* species.[160] *L. monocytogenes* does not hydrolyze these compounds because of absence of specific arylamidases, while all other species, including *L. innocua*, are alanyl or glycyl arylamidase–positive. This test is particularly helpful in identifying *L. monocytogenes* strains that are poorly hemolytic or nonhemolytic. The 15-test Micro-ID *Listeria* also identifies these organisms correctly, but, like the API Coryne, requires an assessment of hemolysis for differentiation of *L. monocytogenes* and *L. innocua*.[54] Certain substrates on the API 50CH (BioMérieux) carbohydrate assimilation panel have also used for identification of *Listeria* species.[486]

Molecular approaches to the identification of *Listeria* species have also been developed. A highly sensitive and specific chemiluminescent DNA probe assay—the AccuProbe *Listeria* (Gen-Probe, San Diego, CA) and a spectrophotometric DNA probe assay—the GeneTrak *Listeria* (GeneTrak Systems, Framingham MA)—are also available for rapid identification of *L. monocytogenes* from colonies grown on primary isolation media.[638,651] The latter test was developed and is used primarily for the detection of *L. monocytogenes* in foods. Volohov and colleagues at the Food and Drug Administration developed a molecular microarray assay for identification of all six *Listeria* species.[924] This assay involved multiplex polymerase-chain-reaction (PCR) amplification of six target genes and hybridization of fluorescently labeled single-stranded DNA probes specific for each of the six species.

Several methods have been used for molecular characterization of *L. monocytogenes* isolates from the environment and from both human and animal infections. Multilocus enzyme electrophoretic methods have been useful in taxonomic studies of listeriae, but are not sufficiently discriminatory for epidemiologic purposes.[93,95,358] Ribotyping, PCR-based DNA fingerprinting, restriction-fragment-length polymorphism (RFLP), pulsed-field gel electrophoresis (PFGE), and arbitrarily primed PCR have been particularly useful for the identification of *Listeria* species, in investigations of foodborne outbreaks of listerial disease, in the differentiation of relapse from reinfection, and in the determination of strain difference between environmental isolates and those from animals with listeriosis.[195,338,518,534,554,640,655,901,909] Similar methods have been used for *Listeria* surveillance in slaughterhouses and for characterization of isolates from various food products.[342,692] PFGE appears to be the most robust

Table 14-2 Phenotypic Characteristics for Identification of *Listeria* Species

SPECIES	HEMOLYSIS, SBA	NO₃ REDUCTION	HIPPURATE HYDROLYSIS	CAMP TEST S. AUREUS	CAMP TEST R. EQUI	ACID PRODUCTION FROM:						
						Mannitol	α-Methyl-D-mannoside	L-Rhamnose	D-Xylose	Ribose	N-Acetyl-β-D-mannosamine	Soluble Starch
L. monocytogenes	β	−	+	+	V	−	+	+	−	−	NA	−
L. ivanovii subsp. *ivanovii*	β^a	−	+	−	+	−	−	−	+	+	V	−
L. ivanovii subsp. *londoniensis*	β^a	−	+	−	+	−	−	−	+	−	+	−
L. innocua	None	−	+	−	−	−	+	V	−	−	NA	−
L. grayi	None	V	−	−	−	+	+	V	−	V	NA	+
L. seeligeri	β	NA	NA	+	−	−	−	−	+	−	NA	NA
L. welshimeri	None	NA	NA	−	−	−	+	V	+	−	NA	NA

a Wide zones or multiple zones of β-hemolysis.
+, positive reaction; −, negative reaction; V, variable reaction; NA, data not available.

method for subtyping of some listerial serotypes such as those in serotype 4b, which are not reliably subtyped by other molecular approaches like ribotyping and RFLP. The automated RiboPrinter system (Qualicon, Wilmington, DE) facilitates the rapid (8-hour) recognition of related strains and may be helpful as a first step in characterizing strains recovered during outbreaks, with other methods (PFGE) being used for further characterization. Cai and colleagues have described a typing method involving multilocus sequencing of specific genes (i.e., housekeeping genes, virulence-associated genes) and intergenic spacer regions that was found to be reproducible and highly discriminatory for differentiating human, animal, and foodborne strains of *L. monocytogenes*.[124] Serotyping, the classical method for strain characterization, has not been particularly useful, since only a small number of serotypes (specifically serotypes 1/2a, 1/2b, and 4b) have been involved in outbreaks and as causes of disease. Furthermore, some *L. monocytogenes* antigens used in the typing scheme are shared with *L. innocua*, *L. seeligeri*, and *L. welshimeri*. Sets of bacteriophages for phage-typing of *L. monocytogenes* also exist and are used by many food processing plants in Europe. Phage typing is not very efficient because some strains are nontypeable with existing phage sets. Studies have demonstrated that strains of the same serotype from different geographic areas may not be equally susceptible to lysis by the same set of bacteriophages.[128]

Antimicrobial Susceptibility and Treatment of *Listeria* Infections

Except for women who deliver infants with early-onset disease, infection with *L. monocytogenes* is usually fatal if left untreated. *L. monocytogenes* is generally susceptible to penicillin, ampicillin, the aminoglycosides, erythromycin, tetracycline, trimethoprim-sulfamethoxazole, and imipenem.[582] Cephalosporins (first, second, and third generations) and the fluoroquinolones are not active against *L. monocytogenes*.[254,421] Ampicillin with or without an aminoglycoside (e.g., gentamicin) is considered the therapy of choice for systemic infections.[421,463,553] For patients with penicillin allergy, trimethoprim-sulfamethoxazole with or without rifampin is believed to be the best alternative agent for treating *L. monocytogenes* infections.[603,835,955] Amoxicillin with trimethoprim-sulfamethoxazole was also found to be an effective therapeutic regimen in one retrospective study.[603] Patients should be treated for at least 3 weeks, depending on their immune status. Patients with advanced HIV disease may require life-long therapy to prevent relapses. Interestingly, the use of trimethoprim-sulfamethoxazole as a prophylactic agent for *Pneumocystis jiroveci* infection in HIV-positive patients may be partially responsible for protecting these individuals from *Listeria* infections, although widely promulgated dietary guidelines may also have some impact on disease incidence in this population.[252] Vancomycin is an appropriate therapeutic agent for primary *L. monocytogenes* bacteremia, but it does not cross the blood-brain barrier sufficiently well to be useful in treating meningitis. Naturally occurring, high-level resistance to vancomycin among the listeriae has never been reported, but the *vanA* genes that code for vancomycin resistance in *Enterococcus*

faecium (VRE) have been transferred to *L. monocytogenes* and four other *Listeria* species in the research laboratory.[82] For antimicrobial susceptibility testing of *Listeria* species, the Clinical Laboratory Standards Institute (CLSI) recommends using a broth microdilution method with cation-supplemented Mueller-Hinton broth with 2–5% lysed horse blood for testing of penicillin and ampicillin only.[626]

Pathogenicity of Other *Listeria* Species

In both mouse and tissue culture models, only *L. monocytogenes* and *L. ivanovii* demonstrate pathogenic properties, while the other species in the genus are considered to be nonpathogenic.[420] Gouin et al. demonstrated that the gene cluster associated with virulence of *L. monocytogenes* is also found in *L. ivanovii* and *L. seeligeri*.[353] Although both *L. monocytogenes* and *L. ivanovii* are able to invade mammalian cells in tissue culture and to spread from cell to cell, the latter species lacks the cytotoxin associated with *L. monocytogenes*, suggesting that lack of cytotoxin may account for the lower virulence of *L. ivanovii*.[481] *L. ivanovii* is a cause of contagious abortion in both sheep and cattle.[15,788] Cummins and colleagues isolated *L. ivanovii* from blood cultures of a patient with AIDS complicated by non-Hodgkin's lymphoma.[193] Lessing and coworkers also recovered *L. ivanovii* from a blood culture of an alcoholic 26-year-old intravenous-drug user.[533] In 2003, *L. innocua* was reported for the first time as a cause of fatal bacteremia in a nonimmunocompromised 62-year-old patient with cholangitis and septic shock.[678] The organism was identified by conventional methods and confirmed by the API *Listeria* and sequencing of the 16S rDNA.

Erysipelothrix Species: *Erysipelothrix rhusiopathiae* and *Erysipelothrix tonsillarum*
Taxonomy of the Genus *Erysipelothrix*

In the 1984 edition of *Bergey's Manual*, the genus *Erysipelothrix* is included with the regular, non–spore-forming, gram-positive rods of uncertain familial status.[459] Sequencing studies of 16S rRNA indicate that this genus is closely related to the mycoplasmas, while cell-wall analysis suggests an affiliation with clostridia and the actinomycetes. In the next edition of *Bergey's Manual*, the genus *Erysipelothrix* is classified in the new Phylum Firmicutes in the Class Mollicutes (Box 14-1). Within this class, orders I through IV include the mycoplasmas and related organisms, while order V (*incertae sedis*) includes the genus *Erysipelothrix* and the genus *Holdemania* within the proposed family "Erysipelotrichaceae."[329] *Erysipelothrix* strains may be subdivided serologically into serotypes, the most recently described of these being serotype 26. These are also some strains, termed "N strains," that do not produce any precipitating antibodies against homologous or heterologous heat-stable extracts in rabbits. DNA-DNA hybridization studies performed with these various serotypes indicate that the genus *Erysipelothrix* contains two species: *E. rhusiopathiae* (composed of serotypes 1a, 1b, 2a, 2b, 4–6, 8, 9, 11, 12, 15–17, 19, 21, and type N) and *E. tonsillarum* (composed of serotypes 3, 7, 10,

14, 20, 22, and 23).[864,870] Strains representing the first group of serotypes exhibited more than 73% hybridization with the type strain of *E. rhusiopathiae* but less than 24% hybridization with the type strain of *E. tonsillarum*.[861] Conversely, strains belonging to the second group of serotypes exhibited more than 66% hybridization with the *E. tonsillarum* type strain and less than 27% with the *E. rhusiopathiae* type strain.[861] These genetic data have also been supported by examinations of whole cell protein patterns on SDS-PAGE.[152,870] Isolates of *E. tonsillarum* are phenotypically identical to *E. rhusiopathiae*, except that the former species is able to ferment sucrose (Table 14-3). Studies of the 16S rRNA genes of *E. rhusiopathiae* and *E. tonsillarum* have shown that the nucleotides sequences are 99.8% concordant, with only a three-nucleotide difference between the two sequences.[490] Two serotypes (13 and 18) are distinct from the others by DNA hybridization and may represent separate, unnamed genomic species. *E. tonsillarum* has been isolated from porcine tonsillar tissue and from the blood of dogs with endocarditis; it has not been isolated from human infections.[860-862] Strains belonging to the same serotype have been shown to represent diverse strains, as demonstrated by ribotyping and sequencing of 16S rDNA.[11] PCR-based methods have been developed for the direct detection of the organism in tissues from slaughter-bound pigs.[572,798,865]

Virulence Factors of *E. rhusiopathiae*

E. rhusiopathiae produces several factors that may function in enhancing the virulence of these organsims.[796] Neuraminidase, an enzyme that releases terminal sialic acid residues from glycolipids and glycoproteins, apparently functions in promoting bacterial attachment and subsequent cellular invasion of *E. rhusiopathiae*.[624] Further spread of the organism in tissues may be due to the production of hyaluronidase by *E. rhusiopathiae*, although the role of this enzyme in disease pathogenesis is not entirely clear.[796] *E. rhusiopathiae* also produces a polysaccharide capsule. The capsule has a molecular weight of 14 to 22 kDa and has been demonstrated to function by helping the organism resist phagocytosis by polymorphonuclear leukocytes.[800] In the presence of normal serum, macrophages are able to phagocytize these organisms, but the capsule enables the organisms to survive and reproduce intracellularly by inhibition of the oxidative burst within the macrophages and reduced production of reactive oxidative metabolites.[799] Opsonization with anticapsular antibodies and complement promotes phagocytosis and intracellular killing of the organisms. Cell surface structures other than the capsule have also been shown to influence the induction of protective immunity to *E. rhusiopathiae* infection. Antisera directed against purified SpaA, a 69-kDa surface protein that extends from the cell surface through the capsule, can protect mice from challenge with a virulent *E. rhusiopathiae* strain, and administration of purified SpaA to guinea pigs induces the formation of protective, opsonic antibodies.[442,797] A similar role has also been suggested for a 64–66-kDa surface protein, although this protein, and perhaps others, may be responsible for the induction of cell-mediated rather than humoral immunity.[368]

Clinical Significance of *E. rhusiopathiae*

E. rhusiopathiae is widely distributed in nature, where it is found in various species of animals, mainly swine and cattle. It is also found in fish, birds, and other wild and domestic mammals.[737] In swine and cattle, the organism causes the economically important disease known as **erysipelas**, but may cause significant illness in other species of wild and domesticated animals. Swine erysipelas results from the ingestion of contaminated food and water. The organisms multiply in the tonsils and lymphoid tissues in the gut and gain access to the bloodstream. In these animals, *E. rhusiopathiae* causes acute septicemia or a chronic illness with the development of polyarthritis and endocarditis. The organism is also commonly found in decomposing organic matter and may be isolated from the soil. Humans generally acquire the organism through contact with the tissues of infected animals or animal products. Hence, infection is usually, but not always, limited to individuals in certain occupations, such as butchers, veterinarians, farmers, and fishermen.[182,413,709]

In humans, *E. rhusiopathiae* may cause a mild, localized cutaneous infection, or infrequently, a systemic infection

Table 14-3 Phenotypic Characteristics for Identification of *Erysipelothrix* Species		
CHARACTERISTIC	*E. RHUSIOPATHIAE*	*E. TONSILLARUM*
Hemolysis, SBA	None, α	None, α
Catalase	−	−
Nitrate reduction	−	−
H$_2$S in Kligler's iron agar (KIA)	+	+
Acetoin	+	+
Acid production from glucose	+	+
Acid production from sucrose	−	+
Serotypes included[a]	1a, 1b,2a,2b,4–6,8,9,11, 12,15–17,19,21, type N	3,7,10,14,20,22,23

[a] *Serotypes 13 and 18 are distinct from the others by DNA hybridization and may represent another, separate genomic species.*

with septicemia.[115,709] The first form, called **erysipeloid**, develops following cutaneous inoculation of the organism, and is usually found on the fingers or hand.[708] Localized pain, swelling, and purplish erythema typically develop and may spread to the wrist and forearm. Lesions appear 2 to 7 days after organism acquisition and are characterized by an elevated, erythematous, advancing border and a faded central area. A more severe, cutaneous manifestation includes the formation of hemorrhagic bullae along with regional lymphadenitis or lymphangitis. Since the organism is located in the perivascular regions of the dermis, biopsy specimens of the advancing margin of the lesion are required to isolate the organism from localized infections. This form of infection is usually self-limited and heals in 2 to 4 weeks.

Systemic infections occur infrequently and are characterized by sepsis and bacteremia.[115,324,464,785] In these patients, *E. rhusiopathiae* endocarditis (particularly left-sided) is common, causes extensive damage to healthy heart valves and cardiac tissues, and has a high mortality rate.[115,413,565,899,916] Both native-valve endocarditis and prosthetic-valve endocarditis (including both Starr-Edwards prosthetic valves and porcine xenograft valves) caused by *E. rhusiopathiae* have been reported.[400] Individuals with systemic infections frequently have no prior history of primary cutaneous infection.[899] Patients with systemic involvement are usually debilitated by immunosuppressive therapy (e.g., corticosteroid administration) or underlying conditions that result in immunocompromised states, such as cancer, diabetes, alcoholism, or systemic lupus erythematosus.[324,793,890] Multisystem disease evidenced by shock and renal failure has also been reported, particularly among those with endocarditis.[264,340,916] Unusual manifestations and complications of sepsis and bacteremia with this organisms include paravalvular and myocardial abscesses, septic arthritis, necrotizing fasciitis, and intracranial infarcts.[38,496,750,808]

Isolation and Identification of *E. rhusiopathiae*

E. rhusiopathiae may be isolated from biopsy specimens of erysipeloid lesions and occasionally from blood cultures. The specimen of choice for isolation of the organism from skin lesions is an aspirate obtained by injection and aspiration of sterile saline from the leading edge of the cellulitis or a punch biopsy from the same area. The organism grows well in commercially available blood culture media. *E. rhusiopathiae* grows adequately on SBA, forming small (0.1–0.5 mm in diameter), circular, convex, smooth colonies (see Color Plate 14-1*H*). A weak α-hemolytic reaction may be noted in the media, particularly in areas where the growth is more confluent. On Gram-stained smears, the organisms appear as slender rods; chains of nonbranching bacilli may also be observed (see Color Plate 14-1*G*). *E. rhusiopathiae* is catalase-negative and nonmotile (Table 14-3). The most useful property for identifying this organism is the production of H_2S in the butt of a TSI agar or Kligler's iron agar (KIA) slant. Failure to look for H_2S production by suspect isolates may result in misidentification of theses organisms as *Lactobacillus* species.[235] A properly streaked and stabbed KIA slant will show an acid slant and acid butt, due to acid production from glucose and lactose; H_2S may be noted throughout the butt or only along the streak line in the butt

(see Color Plate 14-2*A*). This reaction helps to differentiate *E. rhusiopathiae* from other catalase-negative bacilli such as *Arcanobacterium haemolyticum;* this latter species is also β-hemolytic on SBA. The negative catalase reaction, lack of hemolysis or weak α-hemolysis on SBA, and production of H_2S in KIA or TSI agar also help to differentiate *E. rhusiopathiae* from *L. monocytogenes*. Stab inoculation of a tube of gelatin agar and incubation at 22°C results in the production of ''bottle brush'' or ''pipe cleaner'' growth, where the organisms grow out in straight lines perpendicular to the stab inoculation, giving the appearance of ''bristles'' (see Color Plate 14-1*G*). It has been reported that *E. rhusiopathiae* produces a coagulase enzyme that is able to clot bovine and rabbit plasma.[881] This trait, however, was found to be due to utilization of citrate that was present in the plasma; no coagulase activity was observed when oxalate-, EDTA-, or heparin-containing plasma preparations were used.[863]

E. rhusiopathiae is weakly fermentative, producing acid from glucose, galactose, fructose, lactose, maltose, and *N*-acetyl-glucosamine. No acid is produced from glycerol, arabinose, xylose, adonitol, inositol, mannitol, sorbitol, amygdalin, melibiose, trehalose, cellobiose, inulin, melezitose, raffinose, and glycogen.[459] Acetoin and indole are not produced and nitrate is not reduced to nitrite. *E. rhusiopathiae* is included in the databases of both the API Coryne and the RapID CB-Plus identification systems. Isolates of *E. tonsillarum* are phenotypically identical to *E. rhusiopathiae*, except that the former species also produces acid from sucrose. Biochemical characteristics for identification of *Erysipelothrix* species are shown in Table 14-3.

Antimicrobial Susceptibility of *E. rhusiopathiae*

E. rhusiopathiae strains are generally susceptible to penicillin, cefotaxime, imipenem, piperacillin, clindamycin, and ciprofloxacin.[271,565,917] Variable susceptibilities have been reported for erythromycin, tetracycline, and chloramphenicol. Trimethoprim-sulfamethoxazole, gentamicin, and netilmicin show poor activity against isolates of *E. rhusiopathiae*. Of considerable therapeutic importance is the fact that *E. rhusiopathiae* strains are intrinsically resistant to vancomycin, teicoplanin, and other glycopeptide drugs.[271,666] Penicillin, imipenem, and the fluoroquinolones have been found to be the most active agents against this organism. Even with appropriate antimicrobial therapy, the mortality associated with disseminated disease may be as high as 35–40%. This high mortality rate is largely attributable to complications resulting from endocarditis.

Bacillus *Species and Related Genera*
Taxonomy and the Taxonomic Dissection of the Genus *Bacillus*

The genus *Bacillus* is comprised of a large group of aerobic and facultative, catalase-positive, gram-positive rods that are characterized by the ability to form spores under aerobic conditions (see Color Plate 14-2*B*). A second spore-forming genus, *Sporolactobacillus*, was also described in the 1986 edition of *Bergey's Manual of Systematic Bacteriology*.[163] This genus contains a single species—*S. inulinus*—a gram-positive, spore-forming bacillus that is catalase-negative, lacks cytochromes, and possesses menaquinones. In 1990, a third endospore-forming genus, *Amphibacillus*, containing the species *A. xylanus*, was described by Nimura and co-workers.[637] The genus *Amphibacillus* includes facultative bacilli that form endospores under either aerobic or anaerobic conditions and lack cytochromes, menaquinones, and catalase activity.

Because the description of the genus *Bacillus* placed particular emphasis on endospore formation as a taxonomic criterion, an extremely diverse collection of species has been assigned to this genus over several decades. Even within this criterion, endospore shape (i.e., spherical, oval, ellipsoidal, cylindrical), spore location within the cell (i.e., central, subterminal, terminal), and spore-induced changes in cell shape (i.e., cells swollen or not swollen by the intracellular spore) are also used as taxonomic descriptors. Until recently, members of genus *Bacillus* included aerobic and facultative organisms that were also acidophiles, alcaliphiles, psychrophiles, mesophiles, and thermophiles, reflecting growth and metabolism over wide temperature and pH ranges. Some species are able to metabolize a wide assortment of carbon sources, including methanol, cellulose, and chitin. Significant variation also is found in the amino acids comprising the cross-linkages within the cell wall peptidoglycan. At the genetic level, diversity within the genus is exemplified by $G + C$ contents, which range from 33 to 69 mol%. Such genetic heterogeneity is incompatible with inclusion in a single genus as defined by current bacterial taxonomic methods. Not surprisingly, 16S rRNA sequencing studies demonstrated that extant ''genus *Bacillus*'' was phylogenetically heterogeneous, with at least eight highly divergent phyletic lines being represented.[41,42,632,702,745]

Polyphasic taxonomic dissection of the genus *Bacillus* has resulted in the description of many new genera since 1990. In 1992, *Bacillus* species that were acidophilic thermophiles and that contained unique cycloheptane/cyclohexane cell membrane fatty acids (i.e., *B. acidoterrestris*, *B. cycloheptanicus*, and *B. acidocaldarius*) were placed in the new genus *Alicyclobacillus* (as *A. acidoterrestris*, *A. cycloheptanicus*, and *A. acidocaldarius*) in the Family *Bacillaceae*; additional *Alicyclobacillus* species were described in 2000 and 2002.[14,352,590,895,957] In 1993–1994, the genus *Paenibacillus* was proposed to accommodate certain facultative *Bacillus* species, with the subsequent transfer of several other *Bacillus* and ''presumptive *Bacillus*'' species to the genus *Paenibacillus* since that time.[42,409–411,795] In 1996, Shida and colleagues demonstrated that two related groups within genus *Bacillus*—the ''*Bacillus brevis* group'' (10 extant *Bacillus* species) and the ''*Bacillus aneurolyticus* group'' (2 *Bacillus* species)—represented taxa phylogenetically distinct from one another and from other genera, including *Bacillus*, *Sporolactobacillus*, *Paenibacillus*, *Amphibacillus*, and *Alicyclobacillus*.[794] These two ''*Bacillus* groups'' became genus *Brevibacillus* (containing 10 species) and genus *Aneurinibacillus* (containing 3 species), respectively. Since 1996, genetic examination and reevaluation of other aerobic spore-forming isolates has resulted in the creation of additional genera, including *Virgibacillus*, *Ureibacillus*, *Thermobacillus*, *Halobacillus*, *Gracilibacillus*, *Filobacillus*, *Geobacillus*, *Sulfobacillus*, *Paraliobacillus*, *Salibacillus*, and *Lentibacillus*.[33,234,279,280,318,349,408,412,445,627,642,688,777,836,854,892,932,981]

Phenotypic characterization of these new genera are methodologically complex and not amenable to routine identification techniques. Several familiar species remain in the genus *Bacillus*, including *B. anthracis*, *B. cereus*, *B. subtilis*, *B. thuringiensis*, *B. licheniformis*, *B. pumilus*, *B. sphaericus*, and *B. circulans*. In all likelihood, the genus *Bacillus* will continue to undergo systematic dissection, resulting in new genera and species of spore-forming bacteria (see Color Plate 14-1*I*).

The genus *Bacillus sensu stricto* is composed of aerobic gram-positive rods that produced endospores under aerobic conditions. All species in the genus are aerobic or facultative except for *B. infernos*, which is a strictly anaerobic species found in soil.[97] With rare exceptions, *Bacillus* species are mesophilic. The primary pathogen in this group is *Bacillus anthracis*, the causative agent of anthrax. These organisms are catalase-positive, and, with the exception of *B. anthracis* and *B. mycoides*, almost all of the other species are motile via peritrichous flagella (H antigens). Most non-*anthracis Bacillus* species are ubiquitous in the environment (dust, soil, water, materials of both plant and animal origin). Some species are recognized pathogens in animals and insects. Some *Bacillus* species are used in antibiotic and vitamin manufacturing and production, in bioassays, and as indicator organisms for monitoring the efficacy of disinfectants and sterilization procedures (e.g., autoclaving, heat and radiation sterilization). Various species within this group, particularly *B. cereus*, are being increasingly recognized for their potential to cause significant human infections, particularly among immunocompromised hosts. *B. anthracis* belongs to the ''*B. cereus* group,'' which includes *B. cereus*, *B. thuringiensis*, and *B. mycoides*, but is most closely related to *B. cereus* based on DNA hybridization, 16S and 23S rRNA sequence analysis, and the presence of certain intergenic DNA sequences.[40,394]

Bacillus anthracis
EPIDEMIOLOGY OF ANTHRAX

Anthrax, the classical disease caused by *B. anthracis*, is primarily a disease of herbivorous animals; humans become infected by having contact with infected animals and animal products.[877] In the U.S., this disease has been essentially eradicated because of the widespread use of effective human and animal vaccines since the late 1930s, improvements in hygienic procedures used in factories processing animal products, and increased use of synthetic fibers as alternatives to animal hides, fur, and hair. However, because the spores of *B. anthracis* are highly resistant to adverse environmental conditions and because it is exceedingly difficult to be sure that the organism has been truly eradicated from formerly endemic regions, a high index of suspicion should be maintained if a clinically compatible illness suddenly appears. The causative agent, *B. anthracis*, is maintained in the soil as resistant endospores and, in this form, may remain infective for years. Traditionally, anthrax is usually defined in terms of its mode of acquisition. **Industrial anthrax** refers to acquisition of the organism by individuals employed in the processing of leather hides, wool, hair, or bone from various animals. **Nonindustrial anthrax** refers to the acquisition of the organisms from close contact with infected animals or with their carcasses. Industrial acquisition is associated with the cutaneous and pulmonary forms of the disease, while nonindustrial acquisition is associated with oropharyngeal and gastrointestinal anthrax as well as with cutaneous anthrax.

B. anthracis has also been exploited and developed as an agent of biological warfare by several countries, including Japan, the former Soviet Union, the United Kingdom, Iraq, and the United States.[156,514] In 1992, the Soviets admitted their ongoing efforts in the weaponization of anthrax over the previous few decades, and divulged that in 1979 an accidental release of anthrax spores from a Soviet military laboratory in Sverdlovsk resulted in over 77 cases of inhalational anthrax, with more than 66 fatalities.[146] The potential for bioterrorism associated with *B. anthracis* was brought into sharp focus in the U.S. during the last four months of 2001, when spores of *B. anthracis* were delivered in mailed letters and packages to locales within the continental U.S. These incidents resulted in 11 cases of inhalational anthrax and 11 cases of cutaneous anthrax.

These incidents resulted in the passage of antiterrorism legislation in the United States and the development of the Bioterrorism Preparedness Initiative. Through this initiative, the CDC, along with the Association of Public Health Laboratories (APHL), various federal agencies (i.e., the Federal Bureau of Investigation [FBI], and the Department of Defense [DOD]), and the various states' public health laboratories, established the Laboratory Response Network (LRN). In the LRN, clinical microbiology laboratories throughout the country are integrated into a four-tier network—from Level A to Level D—based on the laboratories' diagnostic testing capabilities and safety facilities. Most hospital-based clinical laboratories with microbiology capabilities are Level A members of the LRN.[145] At this level, laboratories are involved in the early detection of microbial agents of bioterrorism and are capable of performing and interpreting observational and simple biochemical tests to rule out potential agents of bioterrorism. If the screening tests suggest that a given isolate is a potential bioterrorism pathogen, that isolate would then be forwarded to a Level B or higher laboratory in the LRN.[146] The Level A screening tests for detection of possible *B. anthracis* are found in Table 14-5 and will be addressed in the "Isolation and Identification" section later in this chapter.

VIRULENCE FACTORS OF *B. ANTHRACIS*

B. anthracis produces toxins that are composed of three distinct proteins: protective antigen (PA), edema factor (EF), and lethal factor (LF). Virulent strains also are encapsulated. The structural genes for PA, EF, and LF—*pagA*, *cya*, and *lef*, respectively—reside on a plasmid termed pXO1. These genes are noncontiguous within a 30-kb area on the pXO1 plasmid. Another pXO1 gene called *atxA* encodes a *trans*-acting regulatory protein that activates the transcription of *pagA*, *cya*, and *lef*.[196,612] PA is synthesized and secreted by the organism and binds to unidentified receptors on target cells, where it undergoes proteolytic cleavage. A 20-kDa amino-terminal fragment is released, and the remaining 63-kDa fragment polymerizes with other similar fragments to form a ring-shaped heptamer, which forms a pore through the cell membrane.[257,948] Each monomer in the heptamer binds EF or LF, enabling them to enter the target cell. These three proteins subsequently act in binary combinations; none have any toxic activities by themselves. Each 63-kDa PA monomer is able to bind one molecule of EF or LF.[391] EF and PA form a complex called **edema toxin (ET)**, which has adenylate cyclase activity. LF and PA form a complex called **lethal toxin (LT)**, which is the principal virulence factor of *B. anthracis*. Together, ET and LT increase intracellular cyclic adenosine monophosphate (cAMP) levels, inhibit bacterial phagocytosis, and block the oxidative burst of polymorphonuclear leukocytes. In macrophages, LT inhibits macromolecular synthesis, promotes apoptosis, and acts as a protease by hydrolyzing protein kinases involved in intracellular signal transduction. Interruption of this signaling pathway results in the inactivation of transcriptional factors in the cell nucleus. Toxin gene expression and toxin production are specifically enhanced at the genetic level by CO_2 and growth at 35–37°C.[498] Organism growth under these conditions results in fourfold to sixfold enhancements in the transcription of toxin genes and in toxin synthesis.[612,811]

Virulent strains of *B. anthracis* are also encapsulated. The genes for capsule production reside on a second plasmid termed pXO2 and consist of three genes that code for three proteins involved in capsular synthesis (*capB*, *capC*, *capA*) and a fourth regulatory gene (*acpA*). The proteins have molecular weights of 44, 16, and 46 kDa, respectively, and are membrane-associated. A fifth pXO2 gene, *dep*, codes for another 51-kDa protein that hydrolyzes the capsular material, generating lower molecular weight peptides.[898] The capsule itself is a polymer of γ-linked α-peptide chains of 50–100 D-glutamic acid residues and contributes to virulence by inhibiting phagocytosis of the organisms.[573,612] Like toxin production, synthesis of capsular material in *B. anthracis* is enhanced by the elevated levels of atmospheric CO_2 and bicarbonate both in vivo and in vitro.[612]

CLINICAL PRESENTATIONS OF ANTHRAX

Human anthrax may be divided into four clinical forms, depending on the mode of organism acquisition.[510,612] **Cutaneous anthrax** accounts for 95–99% of cases worldwide and results from direct mucosal contact with infected animals, animal products (e.g., hair or animal hides), soil containing the organism, or exposure to spores. Lesions of cutaneous anthrax usually occur on exposed areas of the skin (e.g., hands, arms, neck, and face). After an incubation period of 2 to 5 days, an initial papule develops at the site of inoculation. This lesion is surrounded by an area of edema and erythema due to growth of the organism and elaboration of edema toxin locally.[575] The lesion rapidly evolves into a vesicle or bullus that is 1 to 3 cm in diameter, and the fluid within the vesicle becomes black from hemorrhage into the area. This lesion eventually ulcerates and develops a black-bottomed, central eschar with surrounding edema. Frequently, small, pearl-like satellite lesions may appear surrounding the central eschar. Eschars of cutaneous anthrax are characteristically painless, although the surrounding edematous reaction may be painful. Localized or generalized painful lymphadenopathy may be observed, depending on the extent and severity of the initial infection, and constitutional symptoms (e.g., fever, malaise, headache) may also be present. The mortality rate associated with untreated cutaneous anthrax is about 10–20%.

Pulmonary or inhalational anthrax results from inhalation of endospores. The spores reach the lungs, where they are cleared by macrophages of the reticuloendothelial system that are found in the hilar and mediastinal lymph nodes. Active infection occurs in the lymph nodes draining the lungs rather than in the lungs themselves.[676] The spores germinate to form vegetative bacterial cells within the macrophages. This results in edema and hemorrhagic necrosis of the mediastinum, which is evident on chest films as marked mediastinal widening. From the substernal area, the organisms invade the pleural space, resulting in hemorrhagic pleural effusions. The macrophages harboring the organisms are killed and the vegetative bacteria escape into the general circulation, where they continue to multiply. Hematogenous dissemination seeds distant sites in the body, leading to metastatic lesions throughout the body, including the gastrointestinal tract and central nervous system. Most patients do not survive long enough to manifest signs and symptoms of meningitis; patients are usually lucid until systemic shock supervenes, resulting in coma and death.[508,859] The incubation period for inhalational anthrax is 1 to 3 days, followed by the sudden onset of symptoms. Symptoms of the illness include fever and chills, a dry, nonproductive cough, substernal pain, dyspnea, and nausea with vomiting. On chest x-ray films, infiltrates, pleural effusions, and widening of the mediastinum may be noted. Gastrointestinal involvement results in abdominal pain, hematemesis, and melena. The mortality associated with this form of the disease exceeds 80–90% if left untreated.

Oropharyngeal anthrax and **gastrointestinal anthrax** are acquired by ingestion of inadequately cooked foods containing either spores or vegetative bacilli. Both of these forms of infection may become systemic and, like the pulmonary form, have a high mortality rate if untreated. The incubation period of gastrointestinal anthrax is 2 to 7 days. Symptoms begin with fever and nausea with bloody vomiting. Subsequently, abdominal pain and bloody diarrhea appear, followed by overwhelming toxemia, cyanosis, shock, and death (see Color Plate 14-2*C*). In fatal cases, death usually ensues within 2 to 5 days after onset. Oropharyngeal involvement is suggested by cervical and oral pain and edema. Eschars may be noted on the posterior pharynx, tonsillar areas, or the hard palate. Progression of the infection results in dysphagia, severe sore throat, and cervical lymphadenopathy. Death results from overwhelming sepsis.

TREATMENT OF ANTHRAX

A variety of agents may be used for the treatment of anthrax. High-dose penicillin G (4 million units every 4–6 hours) is the drug of choice. In penicillin-allergic patients, ciprofloxacin (400 mg IV every 8 to 12 hours) or doxycycline (200 mg IV every 8–12 hours) may be used. In outbreak situations, and during the recent bioterrorism-related events of 2001, prophylaxis with ciprofloxacin (500 mg PO, bid) or doxycycline (100 mg PO, bid) was given to potentially exposed individuals for 6 weeks. While most cases of inhalational anthrax are fatal, treatment of cutaneous infections is almost always efficacious.

PREVENTION OF ANTHRAX

Both animal and human vaccines for anthrax are available.[260,388] The animal vaccine is actually a spore preparation from an attenuated strain of *B. anthracis* that produces all three toxin proteins, but lacks the capsule because of the absence of the pXO2 plasmid. The human vaccine licensed for use in the U.S. is BioThrax (formerly Anthrax Vaccine Adsorbed [AVA], Bioport, Lansing, MI), an acellular formulation prepared from a culture filtrate of a toxigenic, nonencapsulated, avirulent strain of *B. anthracis* (strain V770-NP-1-R). This culture filtrate contains PA, LF, and EF, with PA being the major component. Protection of humans against anthrax by this vaccine requires multiple initial doses (i.e., three subcutaneous inoculations at 2-week intervals followed by additional injections at 6, 12, and 18 months) followed by annual booster immunizations to maintain a protective level of antibodies. In general, the animal vaccine produces higher, longer-lasting titers of protective antibodies than the human vaccine. This may be due to augmentation of the immune response by continuous production of PA and other protective antigens by the attenuated strain or by involvement of cellular immunity in the response to the attenuated organisms but not to the purified PA found in the human vaccine.[592] The AVA vaccine is recommended for those who work directly with *B. anthracis* in the laboratory, those who work with animal products (e.g., hides and furs) imported from areas of anthrax endemicity, those who work with animals and animal products within endemic regions, and military personnel who are deployed to high-risk regions of the world. In addition, anthrax vaccine may be used as preexposure prophylaxis for individuals with quantifiable risks of exposure to anthrax. These individuals would include laboratory personnel handling environmental specimens such as powders, those performing confirmatory tests for *B. anthracis* in LRN Level B and above laboratories, and individuals working in contaminated areas following a terrorist attack.[146]

Bacillus cereus
VIRULENCE FACTORS OF *B. CEREUS*

Like other *Bacillus* species. *B. cereus* is commonly found in soil and may also be isolated from straw and rice. This species is phenotypically and genotypically similar to related *Bacillus* species, including *B. anthracis*, *B. mycoides*, and *B. thuringiensis*. Genetic and chemotaxonomic studies have suggested that *B. cereus*, *B. thuringiensis*, and *B. anthracis* belong to the same species, with the distinguishing characteristics that functionally set them apart from one another being primarily plasmidborne and transmissible.[39,40,402] For example, the only difference between *B. cereus* and *B. thuringiensis* is the presence of plasmids coding for insecticidal toxins in the latter. *B. cereus* produces several potential virulence factors in addition to the toxins associated with gastrointestinal infections (see below), and these factors are thought to play a role in nongastrointestinal infections. These virulence factors include three hemolysins and three phospholipases.[48,356,801] The hemolysins are called cereolysin, hemolysin II, and hemolysin III, respectively. **Cereolysin** is similar to streptolysin O (SLO) in being a heat-labile protein that is activated by thiols and inhibited by cholesterol. **Hemolysin II** is a hemolytic toxin that is also a lethal toxin in mice, and **hemolysin III** causes osmotic lysis of erythrocytes by transmembrane pore formation. Phospholipases include phosphatidylinositol hydrolase, phosphatidylcholine hydrolase, and a sphingomyelinase. The phospholipases cleave lipid moieties that serve to anchor cell surface proteins, compromise cell membrane integrity, and abrogate regenerative capacities of injured cells. *B. cereus* strains also produce three different β-lactamases, extracellular collagenases, and membrane-bound proteases.[569,571,653,806]

B. CEREUS GASTROENTERITIS

B. cereus is responsible for foodborne disease because of the formation of exotoxins. Since foodborne illness due to this organism is not reportable, exact figures on incidence and prevalence are not available for most parts of the world. Between 1973 and 1985, the percentages of foodborne illness associated with *B. cereus* ranged from 0.7% in England and Wales to 17.8% in Finland.[500] The incidence in the U.S. appears to be much lower, with only 1.3% of bacterial food poisoning cases being attributable to *B. cereus* between 1972 and 1982. Foodstuffs become contaminated from the environment, and the highly resistant spores can withstand pasteurization and exposure to γ-radiation. The ability of some strains of *B. cereus* to grow at low temperatures (i.e., 4–7°C) partially explains the presence of *B. cereus* in pasteurized and refrigerated dairy products. Several different food items may become contaminated with vegetative cells or spores of *B. cereus,* including pastas, rice, milk products, grains, spices, vegetables, meat, chicken, and seafoods. Contaminated foods, dairy products, and hospital- or pharmacy-prepared supplements and infant formulas represent potential risks for hospitalized patients, particularly children and immunosuppressed patients.

Enterotoxin-producing strains of *B. cereus* are known to cause acute, self-limited gastroenteritis in humans, usually following ingestion of contaminated foods.[500] This syndrome follows two clinical forms, depending on the type of toxin produced by the organisms present in the suspect food. Short-incubation illness (or emetic illness) is characterized by the onset of symptoms within 1 to 6 hours after ingestion of contaminated foods, with the predominant symptoms being vomiting and abdominal cramping. Symptoms generally abate within 10–24 hours of onset. The responsible heat-stable exotoxin produced by these *B. cereus* strains is a cyclic dodecadepsipeptide called **cereulide**, which has a molecular weight of about 5 kDa.[4,6,7] This molecule is stable in the presence of acids, alkalis, proteases and heat, and is nonantigenic, necessitating the use of bioassays or mass spectrometry for detection of the toxin.[27,380] Cereulide is produced during the stationary phase of growth and is associated primarily with flagellar serotype H-1.[6] Cereulide causes swelling of the mitochondria and uncoupling of oxidative phosphorylation.[607] Incriminated foods associated with the emetic type of illness include fried Oriental rice dishes, cream and milk products, pastas, and reconstituted infant formula.

Long-incubation *B. cereus* food poisoning occurs 8 to 16 hours following ingestion, and is characterized predominantly by the onset of profuse watery diarrhea, nausea, tenesmus, and lower abdominal cramps. Symptoms usually abate after 12 to 36 hours. Four different heat-labile enterotoxins are associated with this clinical presentation, including two protein complexes (hemolysin BL [HBL] and nonhemolytic enterotoxin [NHE]), and two enterotoxic proteins (enterotoxin T and cytotoxin K).[5,70,357,560,752] HBL and NHE are composed of three proteins each, and the genetic loci encoding for either HBL or NHE are organized in discreet and separate operons. HBL is an exotoxin that has hemolytic activity (H) and is composed of three proteins: a 35-kDa binding component (B) and two proteins (L1, 36 kDa, and L2, 45 kDa) that have cytolytic and dermonecrotic properties.[69] The principal component of NHE is a 45-kDa antigenic protein that is associated with 39- and 105-kDa proteins. This tripartite toxin is dermonecrotic and cytotoxic, and it alters membrane permeability.[561] Other workers have characterized and reported on other enterotoxins from various *B. cereus* strains, but HBL and NHE are considered to be the toxins responsible for *B. cereus* diarrheal illness resulting from food poisoning.[802] Foods associated with this type of illness include meat and vegetable dishes, cakes, sauces, and dairy products. Some isolates of *B. cereus* may produce both the emetic toxin and the enterotoxin complexes. Intoxication associated with *B. cereus* and its toxins may be avoided by adequate cooking of foods, particularly meats, and proper refrigerated storage. *B. thuringiensis* has also been isolated in association with gastroenteritis outbreaks and has demonstrated cytotoxicity that is similar to that caused by enterotoxigenic *B. cereus*.[448] On rare occasions, other *Bacillus* species (e.g., *B. subtilis, B. licheniformis*) may also cause gastroenteritis and food poisoning.[559]

Opportunistic *Bacillus* Species Infections

Because of their ubiquity in the environment, the recovery of *Bacillus* species from clinical specimens has most frequently been considered as nuisance contamination. However, the increasing frequency of reports in the literature of *Bacillus* species as agents of disease in compromised hosts suggests that these organisms should not be dismissed as contaminants in all cases. Serious *Bacillus* species infections have been associated with operative procedures, immunosuppression, traumatic wounds, burns, hemodialysis, and parenteral drug abuse. Isolates recovered from nongastrointestinal infections produce a variety of putative virulence factors, including hemolysins, necrotizing exotoxins, and phospholipases. Analyses of large series of cases involving significant *Bacillus* infections indicate their involvement in the clinical syndromes discussed below.

BACTEREMIA AND ENDOCARDITIS

Many of the patients in these studies were intravenous-drug users, had indwelling central or peripheral vascular catheters in place, or were immunosuppressed because of cancer or chemotherapy.[52,330,620] Endocarditis caused by *Bacillus* species is a rare event, but in the setting of parenteral (usually heroin) drug abuse, it is a well-recognized complication.[134,815,845] In these cases, organisms likely originated from contaminated needles and syringes or from the heroin itself. In these patients, infection usually involves the tricuspid valve, with septic emboli to the lungs being noted on chest films. Drug users with *Bacillus* endocarditis will have compatible clinical findings and multiple positive blood cultures with *Bacillus* species a short time after parenteral-drug administration. Endocarditis with *Bacillus* species also may occur in patients with prosthetic heart valves or pacemakers.[134] *Bacillus* bacteremia may also reflect nosocomial contamination of implanted intravascular catheters.[91,406] In these cases, removal of the catheter hardware usually will result in clearance of the organisms from the bloodstream. Bacteremia with *Bacillus* species also may occur in patients with profound neutropenia.

INFECTIONS IN COMPROMISED HOSTS

Serious *Bacillus* infections have occurred in immunocompromised patients and have included central nervous system infections (meningitis, meningoencephalitis, brain abscess), lower respiratory tract infections with empyema, primary bacteremia, penetrating wound infections, postsurgical infections, refractory sepsis, and burns.[13,36,155,157,331,414,579,617,695,757,888,896] Central nervous system infections may occur as a result of spinal anesthesia, fistula repair, spread from a contiguous focus of infection (e.g., otitis media, mastoiditis), or from contaminated ventriculoperitoneal shunts.[580] Pulmonary infections, including necrotizing pneumonitis, pseudomembranous tracheobronchitis, pneumonia, and acute respiratory failure with sepsis have occurred primarily in patients with leukemias and liver cancers and in premature neonates.[71,186,454,847] Cutaneous non-*anthracis Bacillus* infections have also been reported in immunocompromised patients.[566] Reasons for immunosuppression in these patients have included severe alcohol abuse, leukemia, lymphoma, induction chemotherapy, meningioma, rheumatoid arthritis, systemic lupus erythematosus, severe burns, diabetes, severe combined immunodeficiency disease, and AIDS.[132,341,654,847] Outcomes in patients with systemic *Bacillus* infections are usually poor and reflect generalized immunosuppression resulting from underlying disease and the cytotoxic chemotherapies used for treatment. *Bacillus* infections in immunocompetent individuals are rare. For example, Latsios and colleagues have described a case of peritonitis due to *Bacillus cereus* as a result of a ruptured liver abscess in a previously healthy 72-year-old woman.[519]

OCULAR INFECTIONS

Endophthalmitis (an infection of the aqueous and vitreous chambers of the eye) with *Bacillus* species occurs following penetrating eye injuries or as a consequence of bacterial seeding during bacteremic episodes.[16,90,205,404,772,885] In those with penetrating injuries and/or retained foreign bodies within the orbit, periorbital edema and corneal inflammation lead to vitreal infection that spreads to the retina, resulting in lose of visual acuity within 12 to 24 hours after the injury. Fever and leukocytosis are usually present. Endophthalmitis due to *Bacillus* species may be complicated by spread of the organisms to contiguous anatomic sites, including the brain

and central nervous system.[80] Patients with endophthalmitis of hematogenous origin often have a history of parenteral-drug use. Rare cases of *Bacillus* endophthalmitis have also been reported following cataract surgery.[747] This syndrome follows a rapid clinical course resulting in loss of vision and enucleation of the eye. Because these infections are rapidly destructive, a high index of suspicion and aggressive therapy (e.g., clindamycin and gentamicin administered systemically and intraocularly) is required. In the clinical laboratory, Gram stains of material aspirated from specimens of aqueous and vitreous humor should be interpreted carefully, and the isolation of a *Bacillus* species from these specimens must be reported to the physician and not dismissed as a contaminant. In addition to endophthalmitis, other ocular infections (e.g., keratitis) associated with *Bacillus* species have also been reported in association with the use of contact lenses.[230,682] The rapidly destructive course of intraocular *Bacillus* infections has been attributed to the production of toxins and destructive enzymes by the causative organisms.[126]

MUSCULOSKELETAL INFECTIONS

Bacillus species may also cause various musculoskeletal infections, including acute and chronic osteomyelitis, necrotizing fasciitis, and crepitant cellulitis.[201,617,779] Again, infected individuals have often been intravenous-drug users, had underlying hematologic malignancies, or were being treated with immunosuppressive therapies. In intravenous-drug users, acute vertebral osteomyelitis has been reported as a result of hematogenous spread, with contaminated drugs or syringes being the likely sources of the organisms. Necrotizing fasciitis has been reported in patients with leukemia, sickle cell disease, and myelodysplastic syndrome.[617,815] This infection may be quite destructive to tissues, resembling clostridial gas gangrene and often requiring amputation of affected limbs. Severe infections (posttraumatic and postoperative wound infection, soft-tissue infection, necrotizing fasciitis, osteomyelitis) caused by *Bacillus* species have been documented in individuals who had sustained severe trauma from automobile and motorcycle accidents or gunshot wounds.[502,960] *Bacillus* species may also cause significant infections in burn patients. The tissue destruction that is seen with severe wound infections caused by *Bacillus* species may be partially related to the production of a variety of noxious extracellular enzymes having histolytic and histotoxic properties (e.g., hemolysins, phospholipases, proteases).

NOSOCOMIAL INFECTIONS

Outbreaks of *Bacillus* gastroenteritis have been reported in healthcare facilities and in other institutional settings. In these cases, implicated foods have been beef stews, fried rice, chicken, and processed turkey. Other nosocomial outbreaks of *Bacillus* infections have involved common-source spread from contaminated reservoirs in the environment.[884] These sources have included contaminated hemodialyzers, bronchoscopes, Ommaya reservoirs, manual ventilation balloons, multiple-unit injectables, and contaminated diapers, gloves, and surgical bandages.[194,323,346,723,908,983] In 2001, pseudobacteremia in a neonatal intensive care unit caused by

Paenibacillus macerans was traced to contaminated blood culture bottles.[643] *Bacillus* species have also been isolated from peritoneal fluids in cases of nosocomial peritoneal dialysis-associated peritonitis.[681] Pseudobacteremias caused by *Bacillus* species have also been traced to contaminated needles of radiometric blood culture instruments and have been temporally related to environmental disruption, such as hospital contruction.[548]

Laboratory Safety, Specimen Collection, and Processing

If anthrax is suspected, the states' public health laboratory and the CDC should be notified immediately. Specimens that may be collected include material from cutaneous lesions, blood cultures, and any other potentially infected tissues. Laboratory safety is of utmost importance when working with any materials thought to contain *B. anthracis*. All specimens and cultures must be examined and carefully processed in a biologic safety cabinet (Table 14-5). All precautions should be taken to minimize the formation of aerosols from the potentially infected material. Laboratory personnel must wear protective coats or gowns, masks, and gloves when manipulating the specimens. This apparel must be discarded or autoclaved before reuse. After completion of specimen processing and inoculation of plated and tubed media, all surfaces in the biologic safety cabinet and the open benchtops must be disinfected with 5% sodium hypochlorite and all instruments used for specimen processing must be autoclaved. In addition, laboratory personnel who work with spore suspensions or contaminated animal carcasses and tissues must be appropriately immunized.

Specimens for isolation of *B. anthracis* should reflect the mode of acquisition and the consequent pathology of the infection. For diagnosis of cutaneous anthrax, swab specimens of serous fluids obtained from beneath the surface of the eschar must be collected along with blood cultures. Diagnosis of suspected inhalational anthrax necessitates collection of sputum specimens and blood cultures. Gastric aspirates and fecal specimens may be submitted to aid in the diagnosis of gastrointestinal anthrax, along with blood cultures.

For suspected *B. cereus* gastroenteritis, food that is epidemiologically linked to the illness should be collected. Since *B. cereus* may be present in the stool of healthy individuals and since there is no typing system for this organism readily available to clinical laboratories, the recovery of *B. cereus* from the stools of ill patients does not provide sufficient evidence to ascribe an etiologic role to the isolates. It may be worthwhile, however, to recover the organism from the feces of individuals in an outbreak situation provided similar specimens from appropriately matched controls are demonstrated not to contain the organism. Isolates from implicated foods and from the stool of patients can then be sent to a reference laboratory (e.g., the state health department laboratory or the CDC) for identity confirmation and strain typing. A stool specimen of sufficient volume (25–50 g) should be collected in a sterile, leakproof container. Shipment of the food, stool specimens, and/or isolates to the state health department or the CDC should be undertaken after prior notification and after discussion of the outbreak situation with these agencies.

Isolation and Identification of *Bacillus* Species: The "*Bacillus cereus* Group": *B. anthracis*, *B. cereus*, *B. thuringiensis*, and *B. mycoides*

Members of the genus *Bacillus* that are recovered from clinical specimens usually grow well and sporulate on sheep blood and chocolate agars incubated at 37°C under aerobic conditions. Sporulation may be stimulated by subculture onto nutrient agar supplemented with $MnSO_4$ (5 µg/mL final concentration) and subsequent incubation. On Gram stains from blood cultures, other broth media, and occasionally solid media, *Bacillus* and related species may appear as Gram-negative bacilli, resulting in the mistaken impression that the organism is a gram-negative, nonfermentative bacillus.[89] Inoculation of broth media and preparation of a Gram-stained smear after a few hours of growth may reveal the Gram-positive nature of the organisms. Intracellular and cell-free spores do not stain by the Gram technique but may be visualized with the malachite green stain. A smear of the organism is made on a slide, heat-fixed, and stained with 10% malachite green for 45 minutes. The smear is washed, counterstained with safranin for 30 seconds, and observed under oil immersion. The spores will appear green, while vegetative cells are stained pink to red (see Color Plate 14-2D).

On SBA, colonies of *B. cereus* and *B. thuringiensis* are usually large, with a matte or granular texture, and most strains are β-hemolytic (see Color Plate 14-2H). These colonies have a butyrous consistency with entire, crenated or fimbriated edges. In contrast, colonies of *B. anthracis* are usually smaller, gray-white, rough-surfaced, nonhemolytic, and have a tenacious consistency such that when the colonies are touched with an inoculating loop, they form standing peaks resembling beaten egg whites (see Color Plates 14-2E, 14-2F, and 14-2G). Under the dissecting microscope, numerous undulated outgrowths consisting of filamentous chains of bacilli surround the *B. anthracis* colony, giving the appearance of a "Medusa head" from Greek mythology. Colonies of *B. mycoides* are flat, nonhemolytic, and have a sinuous or rhizoid appearance that resembles some clostridia. On Gram-stained smears, cells of the *B. cereus* group (including *B. anthracis*) are 1.2 to 1.4 µm wide, gram-positive bacilli that occur singly or in chains. Individual cells have squared-off or concave ends. Oval spores may be observed centrally or subterminally, and the cells are not swollen in the areas where the spore is located. Phase-contrast microscopy of smears of *B. thuringiensis* may show crystals adjacent to the spore (parasporal crystals). These crystals, which consist of the naturally produced insecticidal toxin, may also be observed by staining a smear of the organism with malachite green. All members of the *B. cereus* group produce lecithinase on egg-yolk agar and hydrolyze casein, starch, and gelatin. *B. thuringiensis* and some *B. cereus* and *B. mycoides* strains are arginine dihydrolase-positive; *B. anthracis* is arginine dihydrolase–negative. Indole is not produced, and most strains reduce nitrate to nitrite. *B. anthracis* is also nonmotile in hanging-drop preparations or in semisolid motility medium, while *B. cereus*, *B. thuringiensis*, and *B. mycoides* are motile. In addition, *B. anthracis* strains are often encapsulated in infected tissues, as demonstrated with an India ink wet preparation or with the M'Fadyean capsule stain. Formation of capsular material can be stimulated by subculture of the organism on nutrient agar containing 0.7% NaHCO$_3$ and incubation at 37°C overnight. *B. anthracis* may also be definitively identified and differentiated from the other *Bacillus* species by gas chromatographic whole-cell fatty acid analysis or by susceptibility to the γ-bacteriophage.[521] Biochemical characteristics for identification of *B. anthracis*, *B. cereus*, and *B. thuringiensis* are presented in Table 14-4.

As mentioned previously, *B. anthracis* is one of several potential agents of bioterrorism. The CDC and members of the LRN have determined that all *Bacillus* species recovered in the clinical laboratory be screened for detection of possible *B. anthracis*. Agents that fit the screening criteria are forwarded to state public health laboratories for definitive identification. In general, these characteristics include Gram stain and colony morphology, presence or absence of hemolysis, production of catalase, and determination of motility. At the referral laboratories, the identity of presumptive *B. anthracis* strains is confirmed by whole-cell fatty acid analysis, susceptibility to γ-bacteriophage, or real-time PCR methods. The Level A laboratory characteristics for screening of *Bacillus* isolates for possible *B. anthracis* are presented in Table 14-5. Additional characteristics that may be helpful include the capsule stain (performed directly in

clinical material) and a β-lactamase test. Most nonanthrax *Bacillus* species are nonencapsulated and resistant to penicillin because of production of β-lactamase enzymes. The chromogenic cephalosporin disk test (Nitrocefin; BD Microbiology Systems, Franklin Lakes, NJ) can be used for the latter test.

Identification of *Bacillus* species in the non–*B. cereus* groups and related species in the newly described genera can be accomplished by observation of cellular morphology; the shape, position, and appearance of endospores; and the determination of biochemical characteristics using conventional tests (Table 14-6) (see Color Plate 14-1*J*).[719] Spore shapes and locations are usually determined by Gram stain or a spore stain, and cell motility is determined by stab inoculation of semisolid motility medium. Carbohydrate acidification can be assessed with semisolid CTA (cystine tryptic digest agar) medium containing 1% carbohydrates. Nitrate reduction and production of indole are detected by inoculation of indole nitrate broth and development with the appropriate reagents, respectively. Gelatin, casein, and starch hydrolysis are determined by inoculation of tubed or plated conventional media. Miniaturized kit systems like API 20E (includes cupules for arginine dihydrolase [ADH], indole, nitrate reduction, and gelatin hydrolysis) and the API 50CHB may also be helpful for differentiation of *B. an-*

Table 14-4 Identification of the *"Bacillus cereus* Group*"*—*B. anthracis, B. cereus, B. thuringiensis,* and *B. mycoides*

CHARACTERISTIC	B. ANTHRACIS	B. CEREUS	B. THURINGIENSIS	B. MYCOIDES
Cell diameter	1.3 μm	1.4 μm	1.4 μm	1.3 μm
Cells in chains	+	+	+	+
Spore shape	Oval	Oval, cylindrical	Oval, cylindrical	Oval
Spore location	Subterminal	Subterminal, central	Subterminal	Subterminal
Spores swells cell	−	−	−	−
Anaerobic growth	+	+	+	+
Motility	−	+	+	−
Lecithinase (egg yolk agar)	+	+	+	+
Arginine dihydrolase[a]	−	V	+	V
Nitrate reduction[a]	+	V+	+	V+
Gelatin hydrolysis[a]	V+	+	+	+
Starch hydrolysis	+	+	+	+
Casein hydrolysis	+	+	+	+
Production of acid from:[b]				
Arabinose	−	−	−	−
Mannitol	−	−	−	−
Salicin	−	+	V+	V+
Trehalose	+	+	+	+
Inulin	−	−	−	−
Glycerol	−	+	+	+
Glycogen	+	+	+	+
β-lactamase production	−	+	+	NA

[a] *Reaction determined with API 20E.*
[b] *Reaction determined with API 50CHB.*
+, *positive reaction;* −, *negative reaction; V+, variable reaction, most strains positive; NA, data not available.*

Table 14-5 Level A Laboratory Guide for Identification of *Bacillus anthracis*

CATEGORY	CHARACTERISTICS
Safety	Biosafety level 2 for processing of clinical specimens
	Biosafety level 3 laboratory safety practices for all culture manipulations that might produce aerosols (cutting, mincing, vortexing, etc.)
	Perform all work in a biologic safety cabinet.
Colony characteristics	Rapidly growing colonies, 2–5 mm in diameter after overnight incubation at 35–37°C
	Nonpigmented, dry, "ground-glass" surface, flat or slightly convex
	Irregular edges with "comma-shaped" projections (Medusa head colony)
	Sticky, tenacious consistency; when colonies are touched with a loop, the colonial growth will stand up like beaten egg whites.
	Nonhemolytic on SBA
Microscopic characteristics	Large gram-positive bacilli, single and/or in chains. May become gram-variable after 72 hours
	May be encapsulated in clinical material and in blood culture media
	Terminal/subterminal spores doe not swell the vegetative cell (spores may be seen on the Gram strain, the malachite green stain, or by phase-contrast microscopy).
	Spores are not present in clinical material unless exposed to low CO_2 levels, such as those found in the atmosphere.
	Higher CO_2 levels will inhibit sporulation.
Key characteristics	Gram positive bacilli
	Nonhemolytic
	Nonmotile
	Catalase-positive
	Spores present when cultured aerobically without CO_2

thracis from other *B. cereus*–group organisms, and for identifying other *Bacillus* and related species (Table 14-5 and Table 14-6).[549] The Vitek system (BioMérieux, Marcy l'Etoile, France) has a stand-alone *Bacillus* identification card, and the Biolog system (Biolog, Hayward, CA) also has a robust database of *Bacillus* species.[49] Fatty-acid methylester analysis using the Microbial Identification System (MIDI) (Microbial ID, Newark, DE) is also available for identification of these organisms. *Bacillus* species have also been identified using a variety of chemotaxonomic methods, including pyrolysis mass spectroscopy, Fourier-transform infrared spectroscopy, and polyacrylamide gel electrophoresis. Molecular methods have also been used for identification and for strain typing of *B. cereus* isolates associated with foodborne outbreaks and clusters of apparent nosocomially transmitted infections.[546,589,878]

Antimicrobial Susceptibility of *Bacillus* Species

While most *Bacillus* species are penicillin-resistant because of production of a broad-spectrum β-lactamase enzyme, *B. anthracis* is virtually always susceptible to penicillin.[720] In addition, most *B. anthracis* isolates are also susceptible to the fluoroquinolones, tetracyclines, erythromycin, gentamicin, and chloramphenicol.[227,943] Interestingly, most strains of *B. anthracis* are resistant to the cephalosporins. *B. cereus* and *B. thuringiensis* produce a β-lactamase enzyme that hydrolyzes penicillin, ampicillin, and cephalosporins, but most strains of these species are susceptible to clindamycin, erythromycin, chloramphenicol, the aminoglycosides, and vancomycin.

Corynebacterium *Species*
Introduction and Taxonomy

The genus *Corynebacterium* is composed of many species, including the classical pathogen *C. diphtheriae*, the causative agent of diphtheria. Although diphtheria is relatively uncommon in developed countries because of the widespread vaccination of susceptible individuals, it is a cause of significant morbidity and mortality in developing countries, and sporadic outbreaks are occasionally reported in the U.S. Many of the organisms in the genus *Corynebacterium* constitute part of the normal flora of the skin and the upper respiratory tract.[928] These same species, as well as other *Corynebacterium* species and related coryneform bacteria, have become recognized as

Table 14-6 Biochemical Characteristics of *Aneurinibacillus*, Non–*Bacillus cereus* Group *Bacillus*, *Brevibacillus*, *Geobacillus*, and *Paenibacillus* Species Isolated From Human Clinical Specimens

SPECIES	SPORE SHAPE	SPORE LOCATION	SPORE SWELLS CELL	MOTILITY	LECITHINASE, EYA	ADH	INDOLE	NITRATE REDUCTION	GELATIN HYDROL	CASEIN HYDROL	STARCH HYDROL	GAS FROM GLUCOSE	ACID PRODUCTION FROM: ARAB	GLY	GLYC	INU	MNTL	SAL	TRE
Aneurinibacillus aneurinilyticus	Oval	C/ST	+	+	NA	NA	NA	+	−	+	NA	NA	NA	+	NA	NA	−	NA	−
Bacillus amyloliquefaciens	Oval	C/T	−	+	−	−	−	+	+	+	+	−	−	+	+	−	+	+	+
Bacillus badius	Oval	C/ST/T	−	+	NA	NA	NA	−	+	−	NA	NA	NA	−	NA	NA	−	NA	−
Bacillus circulans	Oval	ST/T	+	+	−	V−	−	V	−	−	+	−	V	+	−	V+	−	+	+
Bacillus coagulans	Oval	ST/T	+	+	−	V	−	V−	−	V	+	−	+	−	−	−	V	+	V
Bacillus firmus	Oval	ST	V	+	−	−	−	V+	V	+	+	−	−	−	−	V−	V	−	V+
Bacillus lentus	Oval	ST/C	V	+	−	−	−	V+	V	V	+	−	−	V	V	V−	V+	+	V+
Bacillus licheniformis	Oval	ST/C	−	+	−	+	−	+	+	+	+	−	+	+	+	V	+	+	+
Bacillus megaterium	Oval/Spherical	ST/C	−	+	−	−	−	−	+	+	+	−	−	+	+	+	+	+	+
Bacillus pumilis	Spherical/Oval	ST/C	−	+	−	−	−	−	+	+	−	−	+	+	+	+	+	+	+
Bacillus sphaericus	Spherical/Oval	ST/T	+	+	NA	NA	NA	+	−	V	NA	NA	−	−	−	NA	−	NA	−
Bacillus subtilis	Oval	ST/C	−	+	−	−	−	+	+	+	+	−	+	+	+	V+	+	+	V
Brevibacillus agri	Oval	ST/C	+	+	NA	NA	NA	−	+	+	NA	NA	−	−	NA	NA	+	NA	V
Brevibacillus brevis	Oval	ST/C	+	+	NA	NA	NA	+	+	+	NA	NA	NA	V	NA	NA	V	NA	−
Brevibacillus laterosporus	Oval	ST/C	+	+	NA	NA	NA	+	+	+	NA	NA	NA	+	NA	NA	+	NA	+
Geobacillus stearothermophilus	Oval	ST/T	+	+	−	−	−	V	+	V+	+	−	−	V+	+	−	−	V−	+
Geobacillus thermodenitrificans	Oval	ST	−	−	−	−	−	V	+	V−	+	−	−	V	−	−	V	V	+
Paenibacillus alvei	Oval	ST/C	+	+	−	−	+	+	+	+	+	−	−	+	V	−	−	V	V
Paenibacillus macerans	Oval	ST/T	+	+	−	−	−	+	V	−	+	+	+	+	+	+	+	+	+
Paenibacillus polymyxa	Oval	ST/C	+	+	−	−	−	V	+	+	+	+	+	+	+	+	+	+	+
Paenibacillus validus	Oval	ST/T	+	+	−	−	−	V	−	+	+	−	+	+	V	V	+	−	V+
Virgibacillus pantothenticus	Oval/spherical	ST/T	+	+	−	V−	−	V	+	+	+	−	+	+	−	−	+	+	+

C, spore located centrally; ST, spore located subterminally; T, spore located terminally; +, positive; −, negative; V, variable reaction; V+, variable, most strains positive; V−, variable, most strains negative; NA, data not available; EYA, egg yolk agar; ADH, arginine dihydrolase; Gelatin Hydrol, hydrolysis of gelatin; Casein Hydrol, hydrolysis of casein; Starch Hydrol, hydrolysis of starch; Arab, arabinose; Gly, glycerol; Mntl, mannitol; Sal, salicin; Tre, trehalose.

significant agents of human disease, particularly in compromised hosts.[315,925] The application of molecular techniques to the characterization of gram-positive bacilli has resulted in the description of several new *Corynebacterium* species isolated from human clinical specimens. These methods include genetic analyses (i.e., 16S rRNA and rDNA sequencing, nucleic acid hybridization, etc.), chemotaxonomic methods (i.e., detection of mycolic acids, peptidoglycan analysis, cellular fatty acid studies, menaquinone characterization, Fourier-transform infrared spectroscopy), and phenotypic techniques (i.e., conventional phenotypic tests, kit identification systems, organic compound assimilation tests, detection of preformed glycosidase or aminopeptidase enzymes).[75,207,646,665,706,749,872,911,926,927,973] Analysis of several unnamed coryneform isolates has resulted in their assignment to previously described genera (e.g., *Corynebacterium*, *Arcanobacterium*, and *Actinomyces*) and to new genera (e.g., *Turicella*, *Cellulosimicrobium*, and *Dermabacter*). New and previously recognized CDC coryneform group isolates have been found to belong to genera that were previously believed not to harbor human pathogens (e.g., *Arthrobacter*, *Brevibacterium*, *Cellulomonas*, *Microbacterium*). Genera that are related to *Corynebacterium* species include the nocardioform organisms (*Nocardia*, *Streptomyces*, *Oerskovia*, *Rhodococcus*, *Rothia*, *Gordona*, *Dietzia*, *Tsukamurella*), the facultative and anaerobic actinomycetes (*Actinomyces*, *Arachnia*), anaerobic ''diphtheroids'' (*Propionibacterium*, *Propioniferax*), and the acid-fast bacilli (*Mycobacterium*). Chemotaxonomic and phenotypic descriptions of the genus *Corynebacterium* and related coryneform genera found in human clinical specimens are presented in Table 14-7. Some of these genera will be discussed in this chapter, while others (e.g., *Propionibacterium* species) are described in subsequent chapters.

The genus *Corynebacterium* is composed of pleomorphic, club-shaped, gram-positive bacilli that are catalase-positive, nonmotile, non–spore-forming, and non–acid-fast. Most *Corynebacterium* species contain mycolic acids, arabinose, and galactose in their cell walls.[973] The peptidoglycan of *Corynebacterium* species contains **meso-diaminopimelic acid** (*meso*-DAP) as the constituent diamino acid. Distinctive cellular fatty acids and menaquinones are also found in the cell membranes of these organisms (Table 14-5). Classical descriptions of this genus include their tendency to form ''picket fence'' and ''Chinese letters'' arrangements on Gram-stained smears (Color Plate 14-3*A*). Most species are facultative and are fermentative in their metabolism of carbohydrates, although a few species are nonfermentative and/or use carbohydrates oxidatively. Some species also require lipids for optimal growth (lipophilism). This requirement is suggested by growth on lipid-containing media (e.g., SBA) and either poor or no growth on commercially available chocolate agar, which contains hemin powder instead of lysed erythrocytes. Lipophilism is best demonstrated by enhanced growth of these species on medium containing 0.1–1% Tween 80 in comparison with the same medium lacking Tween-80.

The application of ''research'' techniques to the characterization of coryneform organisms has also created problems for the clinical laboratory, where resources for genetic and chemotaxonomic identification methods are limited

and phenotypic identification is the norm. Two clinical isolates may produce identical results on phenotypic testing (e.g., an API Coryne), but when genetic and chemotaxonomic methods are applied, these isolates may be different (e.g., different cellular fatty acids, different diamino acids in the peptidoglycan, etc.) Because of limited phenotypic characterization of many environmental genera (e.g., *Microbacterium* species), the assignment of clinical isolates to these genera is more difficult and, unfortunately, less accurate. As a result of scientific progress, the interpretation of clinical case reports regarding individual *Corynebacterium* or coryneform species has become problematic because isolates described in these reports have not been rigorously characterized.

Identification of *Corynebacterium* Species and the Coryneform Bacteria

Identification of *Corynebacterium* species and other coryneform bacteria was originally performed with phenotypic tests in the same manner as for other facultative bacteria. With the application of molecular methods, the number of species in the genus *Corynebacterium* and related genera has expanded greatly. By necessity, the number of phenotypic tests required for identification increased as well. Conventional tests are performed as for other organisms (e.g., enteric gram-negative bacilli), with some modifications. Requirements for lipid are determined by inoculating the organism as a lawn onto a non–lipid-containing medium (e.g., Mueller-Hinton agar, BHI agar, Tryptic soy agar) and placing a drop of 0.1% Tween 80 onto the inoculum. After incubation, lipophilic strains will show enhance growth in the area of Tween deposition and poor or no growth in areas away from the lipid. Nonlipophilic strains will grow over the entire agar surface (see Color Plate 14-3*B*). Conventional identification media (i.e., carbohydrate utilization tests) may also require supplementation with three to four drops of 0.1–1% Tween 80 (per 5 mL of broth media) for identification of lipophilic strains.

Gas-liquid chromatography (GLC) for the detection of volatile and nonvolatile products of glucose fermentation is also helpful for identifying *Corynebacterium* species. All taxa produce small to moderate amounts of acetic, lactic, and succinic acids from glucose, but some species also produce major amount of propionic acid from glucose. This characteristic is often helpful in separating strains that have very similar biochemical profiles (e.g., separation of *C. amycolatum* [propionate-positive] from *C. striatum* [propionate-negative]). Species that produce and do not produce propionic acid from glucose as determined by GLC are listed in Box 14-2.

Two kit systems that address the identification of coryneform gram-positive bacilli are the **API Coryne** (BioMérieux, La-Balme-les-Grottes, France) and the **RapID CB Plus** (Remel Laboratories, Lenexa, KS). The API Coryne is a microcupule gallery identification kit comprised of 11 enzymatic tests, 8 carbohydrate fermentation tests, and a fermentation control cupule. A heavy organism suspension (#6 or greater McFarland standard) is prepared in water and placed

Table 14-7 Characteristics of the Genus *Corynebacterium* and Other Coryneform Gram-Positive Bacilli

GENUS	CELL MORPHOLOGY	CATALASE	MOTILITY	PIGMENT	GROWTH	CHO METABOLISM	MYCOLIC ACIDS	PEPTIDOGLYCAN DI-AMINO ACID	MENAQUINONES	CELLULAR FATTY ACIDS	COMMENTS
Actinobaculum	Straight to slightly curved slender rods; may show some branching	–	–	None	Fac/Ana	Ferm	Absent	L-Lysine, L-Ornithine	MK-10(H4)	C16:0, C18:1ω9C, cycl), C18:0	Four species, including former *Actinomyces suis*
Actinomyces	Rods, filamentous, branching	V	–	None; occasionally pink/red	Fac/Ana	Ferm	Absent	L-Lysine, L-Ornithine	MK-10(H4)	C16:0, C18:1ω9C, cycl), C18:0	CDC group 1, group 2, "group 1-like", and group E strains, plus other previously described *Actinomyces* species
Arcanobacterium	Short, irregular rods	V	–	None	Fac	Ferm	Absent	L-Lysine	MK-9(H4)	C16:0, C18:1ω9C, cycl), C18:0	Five species, including former *Actinomyces bernardiae*
Arthrobacter	Rod-to-coccus cycle	+	V	Variable	Aer	Oxid	Absent	L-Lysine	MK-8, MK-9, MK-9(H2)	C15:0ai, C17:0ai, C15:0i	Some CDC group B-1 and B-3 strains
Brevibacterium	Rod-to-coccus cycle	+	–	Dirty white, yellow, orange, purple	Aer	Oxid (inert)	Absent	*meso*-DAP	MK-8(H2), MK-7(H2)	C15:0ai, C17:0ai, C16:0i	Some CDC group B1 and B-3 strains
Cellulomonas	Irregular rods; coccal forms	+	V	Yellow	Fac	Ferm/Oxid	Absent	L-Ornithine	MK-9(H4)	C15:0ai, C16:0	CDC group A-3 (*C. hominis*); classification of *O. turbata* as *C. cellulans* unclear at present
Cellulosimicrobium	Irregular rods; rod-to-coccus cycle	+	–	Yellowish white	Fac	Ferm	Absent	L-Lysine	MK-9(H4)	C15:0ai, C16:0i, C16:0, C16:0i	Includes *Cellulosimicrobium cellulans*, formerly *Oerskovia xanthineolytica*
Corynebacterium	Rods, club-shaped bacilli	+	–	None, gray/white	Fac	Ferm/inert	V (C22–C38)	*meso*-DAP	MK-9(H2), MK-8(H2)	C18:1, C16:0, C18:0	*Corynebacterium* species
Dermabacter	Short bacilli or coccobacilli	+	–	None	Fac	Ferm	Absent	*meso*-DAP	MK-9, MK-8, MK-7	C17:0ai, C15:0ai, C16:0i	CDC groups 3 and 5
Exiguobacterium	Short, irregular rods with rod-to-coccus cycle	+	+	Pale orange, yellow	Fac	Ferm	Absent	L-Lysine	MK-7	C17:0i, C15:0i, C16:0	Includes *E. acetylicum*; resembles some CDC group A-4 strains

Genus	Morphology			Pigment	O₂ relation	Metabolism	Spores	Cell wall	Menaquinones	Fatty acids	Comments
Leifsonia	Pleomorphic rods that fragment into shorter rods and cocci; motile via peritrichous flagella	+	+	Yellowish to deep yellow with age	Aer	Oxid, ferm (so CHO's)	Absent	DL-Diaminobutyric acid	MK-11, MK-10	C15:0ai, C17:0ai, C16:0i	Includes *L. aquatica* (former "*Corynebacterium aquaticum*" and other environmental bacteria
Microbacterium	Irregular, thin rods; some coccal forms	+	V	None-to-yellow	Aer	Oxid/weakly ferm	Absent	L-Lysine	MK-12, MK-11, MK-10	C15:0ai, C17:0ai, C16:0i	Some CDC group A-4 and A-5 strains; includes former *Aureobacterium* species
Oerskovia	Coccoid to rudimentary filaments; vegetative but no aerial "hyphae"	+	V	Yellow	Fac/Aer	Ferm	Absent	L-Lysine	MK-9(H₄)	C15:0, C16:0, C15:0i, C17:0ai	Includes *Oerskovia turbata* (*Cellulomonas cellulans*); *O. jenensis* (from insects) and *O. paurometabola* (from soil)
Propionibacterium	Irregular rods with branching or "bifid" ends; some coccoid forms	V	−	White/gray-white	Ana/Fac	Ferm	Absent	LL-DAP	MK-9(H₄)	C15:0, C15:0ai, C17:0ai	Usually grow better under anaerobic conditions, especially on primary isolation; produce major amount of lactic acid from glucose
Propioniferax	Irregular rods	+	−	None	Aer	Ferm	Absent	LL-A₂pm	MK-9(H₄)	C15:0ai, C16:0i	Includes single species *Propioniferax innocua* (formerly *Propionibacterium innocuum*)
Rothia	Irregular rods with rudimentary branching	+	−	White, gray-white	Fac	Ferm	Absent	L-Lysine	MK-7	C15:0ai, C17:0ai, C16:0	Includes white and black colony variants and "*Rothia*-like" CDC fermentative coryneform group 4; other human isolate in the genus is *R. mucilaginosa*
Turicella	Irregular rods	+	−	None	Aer	Inert	Absent	*meso*-DAP	MK-10(H₂), MK-11(H₂)	C18:1, C16:0, C18:0	Single species (*T. otitidis*) phenotypically similar to *C. auris* and *C. afermentans*

Box 14-2 **Members of the Genus *Corynebacterium***

Species	Clinical Significance and Identification
Corynebacterium accolens	*C. accolens*, described by Neubauer and colleagues in 1991, has been isolated from human clinical specimens, including wound drainage, endocervical specimens, sputum, and throat swabs.[629] Similar strains submitted to the CDC from clinical specimens were previously called CDC coryneform group 6. This organism was originally noted for its satellite growth around a *Staphylococcus aureus* streak on blood agar, but repeated subculture of the organism resulted in adaptation to growth away from the staphylococcal streak. No growth was observed around or between factor X– or factor V–impregnated disks. Satellite growth was probably due to fulfillment of the lipid requirement by the action of the staphylococci on the erythrocytes in SBA. A single case of native mitral- and aortic-valve endocarditis caused by *C. accolens* has been reported.[159] *C. accolens* is a lipophilic species that forms small (i.e., <0.5 mm in diameter), gray, smooth, transparent, nonhemolytic colonies on SBA after 48 hours of incubation. It reduces nitrate but does not hydrolyze esculin or produce urease. Like most other corynebacteria, most *C. accolens* strains are pyrazina-midase-positive; however alkaline phosphatase is not produced. Glucose and ribose are fermented, and some strains will also produce acid from sucrose and/or mannitol. Isolates of this species are susceptible to penicillin, cephalosporins, erythromycin, clindamycin, tetracycline, and the amino-glycosides, and are resistant to sulfamethoxazole.[159,629]
Corynebacterium afermentans subsp. *afermentans,* *Corynebacterium afermentans* subsp. *lipophilum*	Organisms belonging to CDC group ANF-1 were first described in 1981. These organisms are pleomorphic gram-positive bacilli that do not produce acid from any carbohydrates, hence the name ANF, meaning "absolute non-fermenter." These organisms have been isolated from blood cultures and ear specimens; however, their clinical significance is not clear. Riegel and coworkers examined the genetic and biochemical characteristics of 11 ANF-1 strains and proposed a new species, *Corynebacterium afermentans*, containing two subspecies, *C. afermentans* subsp. *afermentans* and *C. afermentans* subsp. *lipophilum*.[726] The former subspecies grows equally well in both the absence or presence of 1% Tween 80, although the colonies acquire a beige pigmentation on Tween-containing media. The latter subspecies forms very small colonies on SBA after 24 hours, but produces large, beige colonies on Tween 80–supplemented SBA. Other than the lipid requirement, these organisms are biochemically inert except for positive pyrazinamidase (PYZ) and alkaline phosphatase (PAL) reactions. Phenotypically, *C. afermentans* subsp. *afermentans* resembles two other coryneform species—*Corynebacterium auris* and *Turicella otitidis*–both of which are associated with otitis media. All produce the same biocode on the API Coryne (biocode 2100004). These three organisms can be differentiated on the basis of colony morphology, the CAMP test, DNase, and leucine arylamidase (LAP) activities. *C. afermentans* subsp. *lipophilum* also produces the same API biocode and is the only lipophilic species that may be CAMP test–positive. Sewell and colleagues reported the first case of *C. afermentans* subsp. *lipophilum* prosthetic-valve endocarditis in a 76-year-old man.[789] The organism was recovered from 5 of 15 BACTEC blood cultures and from a perivalvular abscess. The isolate was susceptible to penicillin, ampicillin, vancomycin, cefazolin, ceftriaxone, gentamicin, erythromycin, ciprofloxacin, and imipenem, and was resistant to clindamycin, and trimethoprim-sulfamethoxazole. *C. afermentans* subsp. *lipophilum* has also been described as the cause of a brain and a liver abscess in a previously healthy 39-year-old man.[237] *C. afermentans* subsp. *afermentans* has also been documented as a cause of sepsis following neurosurgery.[505] See text.
Corynebacterium amycolatum *Corynebacterium appendicis*	*C. appendicis* is a recently described species that was isolated from a postsurgical wound in a patient with appendicitis.[977] Genotypically, this new species is most closely related to *C. afermentans*, *C. coyleae*, and *C. lipophiloflavum*. This lipophilic species is pyrazinamidase-, alkaline phosphatase– and urease-positive and produces acid from glucose and maltose only within 7 days (API Coryne reactions). Lactate is the major product from glucose fermentation.
Corynebacterium argentoratense	*C. argentoratense* was named after Argentoratum, the Latin name of Strasbourg, France, where this organism was isolated.[732] The original four isolates were recovered from human throat cultures patients with tonsillitis, but the role of these bacteria in disease is not known. This species is closely related to members of the "*C. diphtheriae* group" (i.e., *C. diphtheriae*, *C. pseudotuberculosis*, and *C. ulcerans*) and to *C. kutscheri*. Because of the genetic similarity to the "*C. diphtheriae* group," these strains were examined for the presence of the *tox* gene of the β-corynephage, but this gene was not detected in any of the strains. *C. argentoratense* is nonlipophilic, forms creamy gray-white, nonhemolytic colonies on SBA, and rapidly produces acid from glucose, fructose, and occasionally ribose.[732] Nitrate is not reduced, and urea, esculin, and gelatin are not hydrolyzed. Pyrazinamidase is produced, but most strains are alkaline phosphatase–negative. This organism resembles *C. coyleae* except that *C. coyleae* is strongly CAMP test–positive and acidifies ribose, while *C. argentoratense* is CAMP test–negative and is ribose fermentation–variable. Like *C. amycolatum*, *C. argentoratense* produces propionic acid from glucose fermentation.

Box 14-2 *Continued*

Species	Clinical Significance and Identification
Corynebacterium atypicum	The description of *C. atypicum* corresponds to a single isolate obtained from an undisclosed human source.[385] The isolate was nonlipophilic, nonhemolytic, and did not hydrolyze esculin, gelatin, or starch, and was leucine aminopeptidase–positive. Unlike most *Corynebacterium* species, both pyrazinamidase and alkaline phosphatase tests are negative. Acid is produced from glucose, maltose, sucrose, and ribose. This new species, like *C. amycolatum* and *C. kroppenstedtii*, lacks cell wall mycolic acids. Like *C. glucuronolyticum*, this species produces β-glucuronidase (β-GUR), with other enzymatic tests on the API Coryne being negative. The unique API code for this atypical species is 0200365.
Corynebacterium aurimucosum	This species has been isolated from human clinical specimens, including blood cultures from a patient with bronchitis.[976] The organism grows as sticky, slightly yellow colonies on SBA. On the API Coryne, the pyrazinamidase and alkaline phosphatase tests are positive and acid is produced from glucose, maltose, and sucrose, resulting in API Coryne biocode 2100125. Lactic acid is the principle product of glucose fermentation. Genotypically and phenotypically, *C. aurimucosum* closely resembles *C. minutissimum*. The API Coryne profile, 2100125, is the same for both species, except that *C. aurimucosum* produces yellow colonies and is hippurate hydrolysis–positive, while *C. minutissimum* grows as moist, gray-white colonies and is hippurate-negative. In 2004, Daneshvar et al. reported on several charcoal-black–pigmented isolates from female genital tract specimens that were provisionally designated as CDC fermentative coryneform group 4.[202] These isolates were related at the species level to *C. aurimucosum* and *C. nigricans*, which was originally isolated from female genital tract specimens. Because of these isolates and their close relationship to *C. aurimucosum*, the description of this organism has been amended to include not only the original colony types ("sticky, slightly yellow") but also these charcoal-black pigmented variants. *C. nigricans* is now considered a "pro synonym" of *C. nigricans*.
Corynebacterium auris	Some CDC group ANF-1 bacteria recovered from pediatric patients with ear infections have been characterized and assigned to the genus *Corynebacterium* as *C. afermentans* subspecies (see above).[726] Other coryneform isolates recovered from ear specimens that phenotypically resemble CDC group ANF-1 organisms but are genetically and chemotaxonomically distinct (i.e. "ANF-1-like" bacteria), have been given the name *Turicella otitidis*.[298,809] Funke and coworkers also reported isolation of 10 strains that were identified as CDC group "ANF-1-like," but were distinct from both *C. afermentans* subspecies and *T. otitidis* by cellular morphology and colonial appearance.[298] Colonies of these isolates were dry, weakly adherent to the agar, and became slightly yellow with time, while colonies of both *C. afermentans* and *T. otitidis* were creamy, smooth, and gray-white. These strains were phenotypically similar to both *C. afermentans* subsp. *afermentans* and *T. otitidis* using common biochemical tests. However, they could be differentiated by various substrates in the BIOLOG identification system. Genetic analysis confirmed that the 10 strains were a new *Corynebacterium* species, and the name *Corynebacterium auris* ("auris" referring to the ear) was proposed. *C. auris* grows as nonlipophilic, nonhemolytic, dry, adherent, yellowish colonies on SBA and, as mentioned, produces reactions in common phenotypic tests that are identical to *C. afermentans* subsp. *afermentans* and *T. otitidis*. However, both *C. auris* and *T. otitidis* are strongly CAMP test–positive, while *C. afermentans* is CAMP test–variable.[298] In addition, *C. afermentans* subspecies and *C. auris* are DNase-negative, while *T. otitidis* is DNase-positive. Leucine arylamidase (LAP) activity can be detected in *T. otitidis* and *C. auris*, while *C. afermentans* subsp. *afermentans* is LAP-negative.[718] On the API Coryne, the numerical biocode for *C. auris* is 2100004. A study of 48 *C. auris* strains showed that all were resistant to penicillin, with the MIC50% being 1 μg/mL.[306] These strains were also more susceptible to cephalothin than to ceftriaxone. All *C. auris* strains were susceptible to chloramphenicol, ciprofloxacin, gentamicin, rifampin, and tetracycline. Clindamycin and tetracycline coresistance was found in 30% of the isolates.
Corynebacterium bovis	This lipophilic species is associated mainly with cattle, although rare human infections have been documented.[77,315] *C. bovis* is a lipophilic species that is pyrazinamidase-negative, alkaline phosphatase– and urease-positive, and produces acid from glucose only. Rare strains are also weakly maltose-positive, although this reaction is negative on the API Coryne. The API Coryne profile for *C. bovis* is 0101104.[77]
Corynebacterium confusum	*C. confusum* is a new species that has been isolated from a plantar abscess, calcaneal osteomyelitis, and from blood.[302] The blood culture isolate was recovered from a 20-year-old nonimmunocompromised man during a febrile episode following back surgery. This organism is nonlipophilic and produces a delayed acidic reaction from glucose (i.e., the GLU cupule on the API Coryne was positive only after 48–72 hours of incubation). Failure to prolong incubation of

(Continued)

Box 14-2 *Continued*

Species	Clinical Significance and Identification
	the API Coryne strip past 24 hours resulted in identification of these strains as *C. propinquum* (see below), but these strains did not hydrolyze tyrosine (*C. propinquum* is tyrosine hydrolysis–positive). *C. confusum* reduces nitrate to nitrite, produces pyrazinamidase and alkaline phosphatase, does not hydrolyze esculin or urea, and is CAMP test–negative. All API enzymatic tests are negative. On the API Coryne, codes generated by this organism are 3100304 or 3100104, indicating that some strains are also ribose-positive. In the original report, strains of *C. confusum* were susceptible to the penicillins, cephalosporins, aminoglycosides, tetracyclines, quinolones, and glycopeptides, and were variably susceptible to rifampin, and the macrolides.[302] All strains were resistant to aztreonam.
Corynebacterium coyleae	*C. coyleae* has been recovered from pleural fluid specimens, breast abscesses, genitourinary tract specimens, and blood cultures of patients with fevers of unknown origin secondary to underlying conditions (i.e., AIDS, surgery).[308] Colonies of *C. coyleae* are nonlipophilic, nonhemolytic on SBA, creamy to sticky in consistency, and about 1 mm in diameter after 24 hours of incubation. The organism is pyrazinamidase-, alkaline phosphatase–, and CAMP test–positive, and produces acid from glucose, ribose, fructose, and mannose. Most strains produce API Coryne biocode numbers 2100304 or 6100304. The latter biocode is the same as that for *C. jeikeium*, but *C. coyleae* is nonlipophilic and does not display multiple resistance to antimicrobial agents. The six strains of *C. coyleae* described in the original report were susceptible to ampicillin, amoxicillin clavulanate, cephalothin, ceftriaxone, cefuroxime, ciprofloxacin, erythromycin, gentamicin, imipenem, penicillin G, rifampin, tetracycline, vancomycin, and teicoplanin. Four of the six strains were susceptible to clindamycin.
Corynebacterium diphtheriae	See text.
Corynebacterium durum	*C. durum* is a newly described species that has been recovered from throat cultures of healthy individuals and from sputum and lavage specimens of immunocompromised hosts (i.e., neoplasms, leukemia, renal failure).[728,928] On culture, this nonlipophilic organism produces small, beige colonies that are adherent to the agar, although not all isolates have this appearance. On Gram stains, the cells are long, pleomorphic, and sometimes filamentous, somewhat resembling the cellular morphology of *C. matruchotii*, but lacking the characteristic "whip handle" of the latter species. Most strains of *C. durum* are alkaline phosphatase– and PYR-negative. Esculin is hydrolyzed weakly and urea hydrolysis is slowly positive or negative. *C. durum* is also one of the few *Corynebacterium* species that strongly ferments both mannitol and galactose, which helps to differentiate this organism from *C. matruchotii*, which does not ferment these carbohydrates. On the API Coryne strip, *C. durum* produces unique numerical profiles (i.e., 3000135, 3001135, 3040135, 3400115, 3400135, 3400305, 3400325, 3400335, 3040325, 3040335, 3440335, 3441335) even though this organism is not included in the database of that system.[61] Data on the antimicrobial susceptibility of this new species are not available.
Corynebacterium falsenii	*C. falsenii* was described in 1998 by Sjoden and colleagues at the University of Goteborg, Sweden.[813] Isolates were obtained from blood (three isolates) and cerebrospinal fluid (one isolate) cultures. Two of the blood culture isolates were from patients with malignant lymphoma and lymphatic leukemia, respectively. These isolates were nonlipophilic and developed a distinct yellow pigmentation after 72 hours; prolonged incubation beyond this time resulted in more intense pigmentation. The isolates did not reduce nitrate and did not hydrolyze esculin. All four strains fermented glucose slowly, while a single strain also produced a slow acidic reaction with maltose. Conventional urea was hydrolyzed after overnight incubation, and the urease cupule of the API Coryne became positive only after 48 hours of incubation. These fermentative, nonlipophilic strains were genetically and chemotaxonomically distinct, and the name *C. falsenii* was proposed. Since the description of *C. falsenii* from human clinical specimens, similar strains also have been isolated from the mouths of eagles, along with a second nonlipophilic isolate (*C. aquilae*).[267] On the API Coryne, the biocodes for *C. falsenii* include 2101104 and 2101304. Some API Coryne biocodes for this organism are identical to those for *C. jeikeium* (2100304, 2100324), but *C. falsenii* strains will be yellowish and nonlipophilic. *C. falsenii* isolates are susceptible to cephalothin, ciprofloxacin, erythromycin, gentamicin, imipenem, rifampin, tetracycline, cefetamet, and ceftibuten and resistant to aztreonam. MICs for penicillin ranged from 0.25 to 0.50 µg/mL.
Corynebacterium freneyi	This new species encompasses five clinical isolates from, blood, wounds, abscesses, and a sperm specimen.[46,716] *C. freneyi* strains are genotypically related to *C. xerosis* and *C. amycolatum* and can be phenotypically differentiated from them by carbon source assimilations and certain biochemical characteristics. Colonies of this organism are white, dry, 0.5 to 1 mm in diameter after 24 hours of growth, nonhemolytic, and nonlipophilic. Like *C. xerosis*, isolates of *C. freneyi* are α-glucosidase-positive. *C. freneyi* is able to grow at 20°C, ferments glucose at 42°C, and does not acidify ethylene glycol, while *C. xerosis* strains do not grow at 20°C and do not ferment glucose at 42°C;

Box 14-2 *Continued*

Species	Clinical Significance and Identification
	some strains acidify ethylene glycol. The ability of *C. freneyi* to grow at 20°C also helps differentiate it from *C. amycolatum*, which is not able to grow at 20°C. *C. striatum* and *C. minutissimum* may also resemble *C. freneyi*, but *C. striatum* grows at 20°C, ferments glucose at 42°C, and acidifies ethylene glycol. *C. minutissimum* ferments glucose at 42°C, but does not grow at 20°C and does not acidify ethylene glycol. On the API Coryne, *C. freneyi* yields a biocode of 3110325, which corresponds to a *C. striatum/C. amycolatum* cross-call; these species can be separated by the tests described above.
Corynebacterium glucuronolyticum ("*Corynebacterium seminale*")	This species is a nonlipophilic coryneform that has been isolated from male patients with genitourinary tract infections and from semen specimens of patients with prostatitis.[289,733] This organism has also been found in the semen of boars and in uterine and vaginal secretions of sows.[218] Phylogenetic analysis of these strains defined a distinct taxon that is closely related to *T. otitidis*. This organism produces gray-white to slightly yellow, nonhemolytic colonies on SBA (see Color Plates 14-4*G* and 14-4*H*). While some phenotypic test results are variable (i.e., nitrate reduction, esculin hydrolysis, urease), most isolates are strongly CAMP test–positive and β-glucuronidase (β-GUR)–positive (see Color Plates 14-5*A* and 14-5*B*). On GLC of spent culture media, this species also produces propionic, lactic, and succinic acids from glucose. Strains of this organism are usually susceptible to β-lactams, aminoglycosides, rifampin, and vancomycin; some strains are resistant to tetracycline, doxycycline, erythromycin, clindamycin, and certain quinolones (e.g., ciprofloxacin, norfloxacin).[289,396,733] Another group of investigators also have described this organism and named it "*Corynebacterium seminale*," but the name *C. glucuronolyticum* has been given precedence.[733]
Corynebacterium imitans	*C. imitans* has been recovered from pharyngeal cultures of patients with suspected diphtheria in Poland.[291] In addition to the index case, a 5-month-old boy, seven additional cases were subsequently reported, all of whom had contact with the index case. A "*C. diphtheriae*–like" organism was recovered from the index case and three of the other cases. All strains were negative for diphtheria toxin by both animal challenge and the Elek method. Two independent PCR methods also failed to demonstrate the presence of any portion of the *tox* gene in any of the isolates. Because the isolates did not produce diphtheria toxin, the authors felt that they were not the cause of the patients' illness and that they had been misdiagnosed, although person-to-person transmission of the organisms had likely occurred. *C. imitans* is a nonlipophilic species that can easily be distinguished from *C. diphtheriae*. Unlike *C. diphtheriae*, *C. imitans* is weakly pyrazinamidase-positive, α-glucosidase negative, and CAMP test–positive, while *C. diphtheriae* strains are pyrazinamidase-negative, α-glucosidase-positive, and CAMP test–negative. All four isolates in the initial report produced identical profile numbers on the API Coryne (2100324).[291] *C. imitans* could be differentiated from *C. striatum* and from *C. minutissimum/C. amycolatum* by maltose fermentation and the CAMP test, respectively. Lactate and succinate are the sole products of glucose fermentation by *C. imitans*, while both *C. amycolatum* and *C. diphtheriae* produce mostly propionic acid. All four of the isolates described in the original report were susceptible to antimicrobial agents except aztreonam, clindamycin, erythromycin, and azithromycin.[291]
Corynebacterium jeikeium	See text.
Corynebacterium kroppenstedtii	The description of *C. kroppenstedtii* is based on a single human isolate that was recovered from the sputum of an 82-year-old woman with pulmonary disease.[167] Cell wall analysis revealed the presence of *meso*-DAP and arabinogalactan, and 16S rRNA sequence analysis supported the inclusion of this organism in the genus *Corynebacterium*. However, this species lacks cell wall mycolic acids, making this organism and *C. amycolatum* the only two members of the genus that lack cell wall mycolic acids. Recent studies suggest a role for this organism in the pathogenesis of granulomatous mastitis in women.[670,876] *C. kroppenstedtii* is a lipophilic species that produces gray, nonpigmented, slightly dry or smooth colonies on blood agar. Colonies are usually less than 0.5mm in diameter after 24 hours of incubation. This organism is esculin-positive, urease- and nitrate reductase-negative, and CAMP test–negative. Acid is produced from glucose, sucrose, and maltose (weak reaction). API Coryne biocodes for this strain are 2040105 or 2040125, depending on the interpretation of the maltose reaction. *C. kroppenstedtii* does not grow at 42°C. In vitro testing of the single isolate demonstrated susceptibility to penicillin, cefuroxime, clindamycin, erythromycin, and vancomycin.[167]
Corynebacterium lipophiloflavum	During a search for microorganisms involved in the pathogenesis of bacterial vaginosis, Funke and colleagues isolated a previously undescribed coryneform organism from the vagina of a 32-year-old woman with this clinical diagnosis.[296] This isolate fulfilled the initial criteria for being a member of the genus *Corynebacterium*, was intensely yellow-pigmented, and displayed a lipid requirement for growth. The organism was oxidative in its metabolism, did not produce acid from carbohydrates, and was urease-positive after 24 hours in urease broth. The API Coryne produced the same profile number as *C. urealyticum* (profile #2101004). However, *C. urealyticum* is rapidly urease-positive

Box 14-2 *Continued*

Species	Clinical Significance and Identification
	(i.e., Christianson's urea slants become noticeably positive within minutes) and is not pigmented. In addition, this new isolate was broadly susceptible to β-lactams, macrolides, clindamycin, and aminoglycosides, while *C. urealyticum* is usually multiply resistant to these antimicrobial agents. The role of this isolate, if any, in the pathogenesis of bacterial vaginosis is unclear. The name *C. lipophiloflavum* has been proposed for this atypical corynebacterium.
Corynebacterium macginleyi	This species was proposed following a genetic examination of 51 lipophilic coryneform isolates (13 reference strains and 38 clinical isolates) that exhibited heterogeneous biochemical patterns.[731] Isolates of *C. macginleyi* have been recovered mostly from ocular specimens of patients with conjunctivitis or corneal ulcers.[303,335,468] This organism has also been isolated from the urine of a patient with a long-term indwelling catheter and from blood cultures obtained from a patient with catheter related sepsis.[226,918] Strains of *C. macginleyi* are similar to some lipophilic CDC coryneform group G-1 strains. On SBA, the organism forms pinpoint colonies after 48 hours; on SBA supplemented with 0.1% Tween 80, large, reddish beige colonies are produced. Higher concentrations of Tween 80 (i.e., 1% vs. 0.1%) may be somewhat inhibitory to the growth of some strains. *C. macginleyi* is alkaline phosphatase–positive, but is pyrazinamidase-negative (like *C. diphtheriae*, *C. pseudotuberculosis,* and *C. ulcerans*). Acid is produced from glucose, sucrose, and mannitol and propionic acid is not produced from glucose fermentation. *C. macginleyi* isolates are usually susceptible to a broad range of antimicrobial agents.
Corynebacterium matruchotii	This organism was previously called *Bacterionema matruchotii* and was transferred into the genus *Corynebacterium* in 1983.[164] *C. matruchotii* is a part of the oral flora of humans and animals and has been isolated on rare occasions from cases of endophthalmitis and corneal ulcers in compromised patients.[950] Although this organism may appear on Gram stain as typical coryneform bacteria, they may also appear as a "whip and handle" form on staining and may also show rudimentary branching.[188] Colonies of *C. matruchotii* are also atypical compared with other coryneforms, being small and flat. *C. matruchotii* is nonlipophilic, produces pyrazinamidase but not alkaline phosphatase, reduces nitrate to nitrite, and is usually esculin-positive. Acid is produced from glucose, maltose, sucrose, and ribose. Recent analysis of several ATCC strains of *C. matruchotii* revealed that some were actually members of the recently described species *C. durum*.[61] Although they are not included in the API Coryne database, bona fide *C. matruchotii* strains produce API Coryne biocodes 7000325, 7010325, or 7050325. The original ATCC strain of *C. matruchotii* (ATCC #43833) has also been found to be distinct from true *C. matruchotii* strains by 16S rDNA sequence analysis. This strain is now called "*C. matruchotii*–like strain" and yields biocode 2140325 on the API Coryne.[61]
Corynebacterium minutissimum	*C. minutissimum* is a nonlipophilic species of uncertain clinical significance because most case reports do not contain sufficient phenotypic data to rule out other species, particularly *C. amycolatum*.[940] Historically, *C. minutissimum* is associated with erythrasma, which is a superficial skin infection characterized by small, brownish-red macular patches, generally in the intertriginous areas. Lesions may be pruritic and scaly or the infection may be asymptomatic. Case reports implicating "*C. minutissimum*" as an etiologic agent include recurrent deep tissue breast abscesses, bacteremia associated with multiple myeloma, postdiskectomy/postvertebral fusion surgical wound infection, pediatric pyelonephritis, costochondral abscess, polymicrobial central venous catheter-related sepsis, and continuous ambulatory peritoneal dialysis (CAPD)–associated peritonitis.[53,74,140,189,268,348,751] Van Bosterhaut and colleagues reported the isolation of multiply resistant strains of "*C. minutissimum*" from blood cultures in a 60-year-old man undergoing treatment for lymphocytic leukemia, a 50-year-old hemodialysis patient, and a 77-year-old women on peritoneal dialysis for chronic renal failure.[904] These isolates were very likely to be *C. amycolatum*, since propionic acid was produced from glucose fermentation and the organism was multiply resistant to antimicrobial agents. True *C. minutissimum* strains grow as smooth, moist, gray-white, nonhemolytic colonies on SBA, unlike the waxy colonies of *C. amycolatum*.[988] Phenotypically, this organism closely resembles *C. aurimucosum*.[976] Acid is produced from glucose and maltose; most strains also acidify sucrose. No acid is produced from glycogen, inulin, lactose, mannose, ribose, sorbitol, trehalose, or xylose. Pyrazinamidase, alkaline phosphatase, and leucine arylamidase are positive. *C. minutissimum* strains also produce acetoin, are PYR-negative, and are rarely CAMP test–positive. *C. minutissimum* strains are also DNase positive and produce lactic and succinic acid from glucose, while *C. amycolatum* strains are DNase-negative and produce lactic and propionic acid from glucose.[940,988]
Corynebacterium mucifaciens	*C. mucifaciens* has been recovered from human blood, wound, and joint fluid specimens.[299] Colonies of this species are unusual in that they are nonlipophilic, glistening, slightly yellowish, and very mucoid, a characteristic that is uncommon among the corynebacteria but is seen among members of the genus *Rhodococcus*. On the API Coryne, these organisms produce profile numbers that

Box 14-2 *Continued*

Species	Clinical Significance and Identification
	correspond to several lipophilic species (i.e., *C. jeikeium*, *C. bovis*, CDC group G) or the nonlipophilic fermentative species *C. striatum* (Table 14–10). *C. mucifaciens* produces pyrazinamidase and alkaline phosphatase and does not hydrolyze esculin, urea, or gelatin. The oxidative metabolism displayed by this species is likely responsible for failure to rapidly acidify carbohydrates present on the API Coryne gallery. *C. mucifaciens* produces acid oxidatively from glucose and occasionally from sucrose; acid production from fructose, mannose, and glycerol help differentiate this species from *R. equi*. Cell wall analysis confirmed the relationship to the genus *Corynebacterium* and indicated that the organism did not belong to the genus *Rhodococcus*. The eight strains of *C. mucifaciens* described in the original report were also examined for antimicrobial susceptibility.[299] Seven of the eight isolates were susceptible to β-lactams (cefazolin, penicillin), and all were susceptible to the glycopeptides (teicoplanin and vancomycin) and aminoglycosides. The susceptibilities of these strains to the tetracyclines, the macrolides (erythromycin, azithromycin, clarithromycin), clindamycin, and the quinolones were variable. All eight strains were resistant to aztreonam, cefetamet, ceftibuten, and fosfomycin.
Corynebacterium nigricans	*C. nigricans* is an unusual black-pigmented *Corynebacterium* species that has been isolated from the human female genital tract. These isolates have been associated with complications of pregnancy, including spontaneous abortion and preterm labor.[803,804] Morphologically, colonies of *C. nigricans* are black, adherent and tend to "dig into" the agar. This organism must be differentiated from gray-black pigmented strains of CDC group 4, which resemble *Rothia* species more closely than corynebacteria. Colonies of *C. nigricans* are about 2–3 mm in diameter after 48 hours of incubation and are nonlipophilic. This species ferments glucose, maltose, and sucrose; glycogen and/or ribose are fermented by some strains. While pyrazinamidase and alkaline phosphatase reactions are variable, the reduction of nitrate and hydrolysis of esculin, urea, and gelatin are negative. On the API Coryne, *C. nigricans* produces biocodes 0000125, 2000125, and 2100327. These codes correspond to low-confidence identifications for *C. striatum*, *C. amycolatum*, *C. minutissimum*, and CDC groups G and F-1, but the colony morphology of *C. nigricans* is distinctive enough that identification is not a problem. Strains of CDC group 4 bacteria reduce nitrate and hydrolyze both esculin and gelatin.[803] *C. nigricans* is also related at the species level to black-pigmented variants of *C. aurimucosum*.[202]
Corynebacterium propinquum	This new species includes strains formerly belonging to CDC group ANF-3.[725] These nonlipophilic isolates have all been recovered from human respiratory tract or blood specimens, including a case of native-aortic-valve endocarditis.[679] The organism is phylogenetically related to *C. pseudodiphtheriticum*. Colonies on SBA are 1–2 mm in diameter after 24 hours of incubation and are off-white and dry, with entire edges. Esculin and urea are not hydrolyzed, and strains variably produce pyrazinamidase and alkaline phosphatase. Like *C. pseudodiphtheriticum*, *C. propinquum* is asaccharolytic, but the two may be differentiated by the production of urease by *C. pseudodiphtheriticum*. Furthermore, *C. propinquum* can be differentiated from *C. afermentans* subsp. *afermentans* by the ability of the former to reduce nitrate and from *C. afermentans* subsp. *lipophilum* by both nitrate reduction and the lack of a lipid requirement. Data on the antimicrobial susceptibility of this species are not available.
Corynebacterium pseudodiphtheriticum	See text.
Corynebacterium pseudotuberculosis	*C. pseudotuberculosis* (formerly called *Corynebacterium ovis*) causes caseous lymphadenitis (CLA or "cheesy gland") in sheep, cattle, and other small ruminants.[951] The organism has also been shown to cause abortion or stillbirth in experimentally infected ewes and folliculitis in horses. Most of the human infections associated with *C. pseudotuberculosis* have been reported among rural sheepherders in Australia or in butchers, and, as in the animal infections, have presented as either acute or chronic lymphadenitis.[110,608,672] A single case of suppurative, granulomatous cervical lymphadenopathy due to *C. pseudotuberculosis* has been described in an urban-dwelling (Seattle) male who had a history of ingesting raw cow and goat milk.[345] In these human infections, surgical drainage and excision of the affected lymph node(s) was necessary, and most of the patients had persistent or recurrent drainage from the wound site for prolonged periods. Because of the slow healing process, most of the patients were treated with several antibiotics, including penicillin G, tetracycline, erythromycin, sulfisoxazole, and antistaphylococcal penicillins. An unusual case of pneumonia in a 28-year-old veterinary medical student caused by *C. pseudotuberculosis* was reported in 1978.[487] This patient had worked with the organism in his veterinary microbiology class during the 4 weeks prior to onset of pulmonary symptoms, and he had also been exposed to "sick" horses in practice. *C. pseudotuberculosis* is a member of the "*C. diphtheriae* group," which also includes *C. diphtheriae* and *C. ulcerans*. *C. pseudotuberculosis*

(Continued)

Box 14-2 *Continued*

Species	Clinical Significance and Identification
	has also been transformed into a diphtheria toxin–producing species by experimental infection and lysogenization with the β-corynephage, but naturally occurring lysogenized strains have not been isolated. All of these organisms are pyrazinamidase-negative (unlike the vast majority of *Corynebacterium* species) and produce cystinase activity, as evidenced by the production of brown haloes around colonies on modified Tinsdale medium.[616,853] *C. pseudotuberculosis* is urease-positive and nitrate reductase– and alkaline phosphatase–variable and differs from *C. ulcerans* in that it does not produce acid from glycogen or trehalose and does not hydrolyze gelatin. Like *C. ulcerans* and *A. haemolyticum*, *C. pseudotuberculosis* is reverse CAMP test–positive. In the report on 10 cases of human lymphadenitis due to *C. pseudotuberculosis* published by Peel and colleagues, all isolates produced API Coryne profile #0111324, indicating positive reactions for alkaline phosphatase, α-glucosidase, urease, glucose, maltose, and ribose.[672] Much of the research concerning *C. pseudotuberculosis* in recent years has focused on the development of diagnostic tests for CLA and a vaccine to prevent CLA in sheepherders and goatherds.[215,684] These organisms are generally susceptible to penicillins, macrolides, tetracyclines, cephalosporins, quinolones and rifampin; most are resistant to aminoglycosides, nitrofurans, and polymyxin.[469]
Corynebacterium riegelii	This newly described species has been recovered in urine specimens from women with symptoms of urinary tract infection and from blood cultures.[300] Urine isolates were recovered from women aged 21 to 62 years with no underlying diseases. The organisms were present in significant numbers (i.e., >100,000 CFU/mL). Isolates of *C. riegelii* are nonlipophilic and produce white, glistening sticky colonies on SBA (see Color Plate 14-5*E*). Isolates are strongly urease-positive (like *C. urealyticum*), with positive reactions on Christensen's urea slants being noted within 5 minutes after inoculation (see Color Plate 14-5*F*). An unusual characteristic of this species is that strains produce acid slowly from maltose, but no acid is formed from glucose. These atypical reactions occur with conventional media (e.g., CTA-based carbohydrates) and with the API Coryne strip. API Coryne profile numbers for *C. riegelii* are 0101224, 2001224, and 2101224 (see Color Plates 14-5*G* and 15-5 *H*). Strains of *C. riegelii* are susceptible to penicillin, cephalothin, chloramphenicol, ciprofloxacin, gentamicin, rifampin, tetracycline, and vancomycin and are resistant to cefetamet, ceftibuten, and fosfomycin.[300]
Corynebacterium sanguinis	To date, this new nonlipophilic species has been recovered only from blood cultures.[294] Colonies of this organism on SBA are 1–2 mm in diameter after 48 hours of incubation, smooth, dry, and yellowish. Pyrazinamidase, alkaline phosphatase, and PYR tests are positive, and the CAMP test is negative. The organism slowly ferments glucose and ribose (on the API Coryne) but no other carbohydrates. *C. sanguinis* is nitrate-, urease-, esculin-, and CAMP test–negative. On the API Coryne, all isolates produced the biocode number 6100304.
Corynebacterium simulans	*C. simulans* is a new species that has been isolated from a foot abscess, a lymph node biopsy, and a boil.[936] This organism is a nonlipophilic fermentative species that is phenotypically similar to *C. minutissimum* and *C. striatum*, but phylogenetically distinct based on 16S rRNA sequences. *C. simulans* strains grow as nonlipophilic, gray-white, glistening, creamy colonies that are 1–2 mm in diameter after 48 hours. *C. simulans* is nitrate-positive and maltose-negative (*C. minutissimum* is nitrate-negative and maltose-positive) and does not ferment ethylene glycol or grow at 20°C (*C. striatum* ferments ethylene glycol and grows at 20°C). This is the only *Corynebacterium* species that is able to reduce nitrate to nitrite and then further reduce nitrite to nitrogen gas, so a negative nitrate test must be challenged with zinc to confirm this reaction. In addition, some strains may be catalase-negative. On the API Coryne, *C. simulans* produces several biocodes (Table 14–10). Data on the antimicrobial susceptibility of *C. simulans* are not available.
Corynebacterium singulare	The description of *C. singulare* is based on two human isolates (one from semen, the other from blood).[734] These two isolates possessed all the key chemotaxonomic characteristics of the genus *Corynebacterium* and resembled *C. minutissimum* by both morphologic and biochemical characteristics. Colonies of *C. singulare* are convex, entire, creamy, and white-gray. Unlike *C. minutissimum*, however, the two isolates were urease-positive. Examination of other urease-positive taxa within the genus confirmed that the two isolates were indeed distinct from them by several characteristics, including increased fermentative ability, failure to reduce nitrate, and the absence of β-glucuronidase. The organism can be differentiated from *C. amycolatum* by its failure to produce propionic acid from glucose. On the API Coryne, the organism generates a unique octal code (biocode 6101125). Based on these criteria, the name *C. singulare* has been proposed for these isolates.[734] Antimicrobial susceptibility data for this species are not available.
Corynebacterium striatum	See text.
Corynebacterium sundsvallense	*C. sundsvallense* has been recovered from blood cultures, a vaginal specimen, and a groin wound culture.[165] The Gram stain appearance of this organism is unique in that knobs or "bulges" may

Box 14-2 *Continued*

Species	Clinical Significance and Identification
	be noted on the ends of some of the bacilli. The organism is nonlipophilic, and produces buff-to-yellow, sticky, adherent colonies on SBA. The organism slowly ferments glucose, maltose, and sucrose, but not lactose, mannitol, ribose, xylose, or amygdalin. Nitrate is not reduced and esculin is not hydrolyzed, but urease is produced and the α-glucosidase reaction is positive (Table 14–9 and 14–10). Lactic and succinic acids are the major products of glucose fermentation. Antimicrobial susceptibility data on this organism are not available.[x-refs]
Corynebacterium thomssenii	The species description of this organism is based on two similar isolates that were recovered from pleural fluid specimens of a 56-year-old man with chronic renal failure, stroke, and pneumonia.[987] *C. thomssenii* is a slow-growing, nonlipophilic organism that produces sticky, adherent colonies that are less than 0.5 mm in diameter even after 48 hours of incubation. The organism is urease-positive, DNase-positive, and both nitrate- and esculin hydrolysis-negative. Acid is slowly produced from glucose, maltose, and sucrose. Unlike all other *Corynebacterium* species, isolates of this species are strongly N-acetyl-β-glucosaminidase-positive, producing the API Coryne profile number 2121125. Isolates of *C. thomssenii* are susceptible to penicillin, ampicillin, cefazolin, gentamicin, erythromycin, clindamycin, tetracycline, ciprofloxacin, rifampin, and vancomycin and resistant to aztreonam, cefetamet, ceftibuten, and fosfomycin.[987]
Corynebacterium ulcerans	*C. ulcerans* is a nonlipophilic member of the "*C. diphtheriae* group," along with *C. diphtheriae* and *C. pseudotuberculosis*. In years past, the validity of *C. ulcerans* as a separate *Corynebacterium* species has been controversial. However, in 1995, the species status of this organism was reaffirmed by Riegel and coworkers.[730] They found that the three organisms comprising the "*C. diphtheriae* group" were separate taxa and that biotypes and biovars within each species were closely related genomically. Analyses of 16S rRNA sequences showed that *C. ulcerans* forms a tight relatedness cluster with *C. pseudotuberculosis* and is indeed a separate species. In addition, it has been shown that most *C. ulcerans* isolates (and some isolates of *C. pseudotuberculosis*) produce diphtheria toxin. In one study, 25 of 37 *C. ulcerans* strains and 1 of 14 *C. pseudotuberculosis* strains produced positive Elek tests for diphtheria toxin.[367] In addition, all the Elek test–positive strains and two Elek test–negative strains produced positive signals when hybridized with a DNA probe for the *tox* structural gene for diphtheria toxin. Restriction endonuclease fragment analyses have shown that *C. diphtheriae* and *C. ulcerans* strains share considerable homology on Southern blots; these homologous fragments include the integration site for the β family of corynephages. Wong and Groman also demonstrated that the diphtheria toxins produced by strains of *C. ulcerans* and *C. pseudotuberculosis* were similar in molecular weight and immunologic structure, in enzymatic ADP-ribosylating activity, and in the regulation of their synthesis by iron.[961] Strains of *C. ulcerans* may also produce a second toxin—phospholipase D—that is identical to that produced by *C. pseudotuberculosis*.[57] This toxin affects sphingomyelin and alters target cell membrane permeability. *C. ulcerans* is a rare cause of infections in both animals and man. It causes mastitis in cattle, nonhuman primates, and other animals and has also been recovered from unpasteurized cow milk and other dairy products.[100] The organism has also been recovered from wild ground squirrels, in which it causes gangrenous dermatitis, toxemia, and sepsis.[652] Human infections have generally occurred in rural areas in individuals with histories of animal exposure or ingestion of raw dairy products.[100] *C. ulcerans* has been isolated from patients with illnesses indistinguishable from classical diphtheria, with and without the presence of both cardiac and neurologic sequelae.[208,396,482] In 1985, a case of ultimately fatal *C. ulcerans* pneumonia was reported in a 78-year-old Baltimore man who 1 year earlier had received radiation therapy to the right upper chest for treatment of squamous-cell lung carcinoma with metastasis to the ribs.[805] In this case, the organism was susceptible to penicillin, ampicillin, cephalothin, erythromycin, clindamycin, tetracycline, and gentamicin. Another case of pulmonary *C. ulcerans* infection was reported in a 53-year-old man who presented with multiple, bilateral pulmonary nodules suggestive of metastatic carcinoma.[216] Histopathologic examination of these nodules revealed granulomatous necrotizing inflammation, and culture grew a non-diphtheria toxin–producing strain of *C. ulcerans*. In 1996, a case of respiratory diphtheria due to toxigenic *C. ulcerans* was reported in a 54-year-old woman from Terre Haute, Indiana.[144] The patient, who had never been immunized against diphtheria, was treated with ceftriaxone, erythromycin, and 40,000 international units (IU) of equine diphtheria antitoxin, and had a rapid clinical response. Culture of clinical specimens (throat swabs and fragments of diphtheritic pseudomembrane) confirmed the presence of *C. ulcerans* and toxigenicity of this isolate was demonstrated by both the Elek immunoprecipitation assay and by a PCR assay for diphtheria toxin. Toxin-producing isolates of *C. ulcerans* have also caused cases of cutaneous "diphtheria."[931] In 2002, Wellinghausen and colleagues described a fatal case of necrotizing sinusitis in an elderly man due to toxigenic *C. ulcerans*.[947] Colonies of *C. ulcerans* are gray-

(Continued)

Box 14-2 *Continued*

Species	Clinical Significance and Identification
	white, dry, and waxy-appearing, with a slight diffusely β-hemolytic area under and surrounding individual colonies. The organism is nonlipophilic and colonies are 1–2 mm in diameter after 24 hours of incubation. *C. ulcerans* is pyrazinamidase-negative and alkaline phosphatase– and urease-positive. Acid is produced from glucose, maltose, mannose, arabinose, ribose, and glycogen. Like *C. pseudotuberculosis*, *C. ulcerans* is reverse CAMP test–positive and produces propionic acid as a product of glucose fermentation.
Corynebacterium urealyticum	See text.
Corynebacterium xerosis	Until recently, *C. xerosis* was believed to be the most common coryneform on the skin and, consequently, the most common clinical isolate belonging to the genus *Corynebacterium*. Substantial data now indicate that most clinical isolates of "*C. xerosis*" are actually *C. amycolatum* (see discussion of this organism above).[297] True *C. xerosis* produce granular, yellowish colonies, contain mycolic acids in their cell walls, are LAP- and α-glucosidase-positive, and produce lactic acid from glucose fermentation, while strains of *C. amycolatum* produce dry, waxy, whitish-gray colonies; lack mycolic acids; are negative or weakly-positive for LAP; are α-glucosidase-negative; and produce propionic acid from glucose fermentation.[297,315,940] Unlike *C. striatum*, true *C. xerosis* isolates do not hydrolyze tyrosine and ferment sugars slowly (72–96 hours). The literature contains several case reports regarding *C. xerosis* as the etiologic agent in a variety of types of human infections. In these reports, the isolates were often found to be multiply resistant to antimicrobial agents. These multiply resistant strains were actually *C. amycolatum* and not *C. xerosis*, since bona fide strains of the latter species are quite rare and are known to be broadly susceptible. Because of its infrequent isolation in the clinical laboratory, *C. xerosis* was deleted from version 2 of the API Coryne database. However, certain biocodes—2110325 and 3110325—do correspond to true isolates of *C. xerosis*.
Corynebacterium group F1	CDC coryneform group F1 is a lipophilic, fermentative coryneform that can be separated into two phenotypically indistinguishable DNA homology groups. As a urease-positive, lipid-requiring coryneform, CDC group F1 closely resembles the newly named lipid-requiring species *C. macginleyi*.[731] However, CDC group F1 strains are pyrazinamidase-positive, alkaline phosphatase–negative, and ferment glucose, maltose, and sucrose, while *C. macginleyi* strains are pyrazinamidase-negative, alkaline phosphatase–positive, and ferment glucose and sucrose but not maltose. CDC coryneform group F1 has been recovered most frequently from the urogenital tract. In 1992, a case of struvite stone formation in a 40-year-old male patient associated with CDC group F1 was reported.[224] The organism was present in the urine in significant numbers ($>10^8$ CFU/mL) and was susceptible to tetracycline. Treatment of the patient with doxycycline resulted in resolution of the infection and cessation of stone formation.
Corynebacterium group G	CDC coryneform group G has been isolated from vitreous humor specimens, blood, cerebrospinal fluid, and the genitourinary tract (see Color Plates 14-6*C* and 14-6*D*).[700,731] Growth of isolates belonging to group G are lipophilic, and growth is stimulated by Tween-80. In 1983, Austin and Hill reported a case of fatal prosthetic-valve endocarditis associated with CDC group G in a 40-year-old male.[45] The isolate was susceptible to ampicillin, cephalothin, cefamandole, cefoxitin, gentamicin, and vancomycin. Group G coryneforms were also isolated from blood cultures of a 74-year-old male patient undergoing maintenance hemodialysis due to chronic renal failure.[484] This isolate was also uniformly susceptible to antimicrobial agents.
Corynebacterium groups F2 and I	CDC groups F2 and I have been shown to correspond to strains of *C. amycolatum*.[261,574,940]

in the enzyme test cupules (nitrate [NIT] through gelatin [GEL]). A 0.5-mL aliquot of this suspension is then placed in the GP medium (enriched medium with phenol-red indicator) provided; this is used to fill the carbohydrate control and test cupules (O through GLYG). Each of the latter cupules are overlaid with sterile mineral oil. The strip is incubated for 24–48 hours in a non-CO$_2$ incubator. Reagents A and B are added to the nitrate cupule and ZYM A and ZYM B reagents are added to the enzyme cupules (pyrazinamidase [PYZ] through β-N-acetylglucosminidase [β-NAG]); these reactions are read after 10 minutes. Esculin (ESC), urease (URE), GEL, and the carbohydrate tests are read directly without the addition of reagents. From the pattern of reactions on the strip, a biocode is generated and interpreted by consulting the API Coryne Analytical Profile Index or calling in the biocode to the API Computer Service by phone.

Evaluations of the API Coryne version 1 in 1991 found that from 65% to 86.5% of *Corynebacterium* species were correctly identified by the kit alone. From 21.8% to 31.8% of isolates were identified with additional tests (e.g., pigment production, motility, growth in 6.5% NaCl, CAMP test, hemolysis, growth at 42°C).[283,833] This version identified only 36.4% of 22 characterized CDC coryneform bacteria without additional testing.[333] The API Coryne database was updated in 1997 to accommodate some newly described taxa and to reflect changes in taxonomy. Funke et al. evaluated the API Coryne version 2.0 with 390 strains representing all 49 taxa included in the new database plus 17 strains belonging to taxa not included in the database.[310] The kit identified 90.5% of the strains belonging to included taxa, with additional tests being required for correct identification of 55.1% of all strains tested. Only 5.6% of isolates were not identified and 3.8% were misidentified. The API Coryne requires a heavy inoculum to prevent false-negative reactions, and longer incubation may be necessary to detect carbohydrate fermentation reactions of some species (e.g., *Arthrobacter* species).[304]

In several of the reports on new species of *Corynebacterium*, the API Coryne was used to phenotypically characterize the new isolates and biocodes were generated from the patterns of positive and negative reactions. Some biocodes for new species give identifications for species already included in the database. In these cases, additional tests must be performed to arrive at the correct identification. However, some new species do generate biocodes that are unique.

The RapID CB-Plus uses the cuvette format similar to other Remel identification kits and includes 18 single-test wells. To inoculate the system, a suspension of the organism grown on 5% SBA (tryptic soy, Columbia, or BHI base) equivalent to a #4 McFarland turbidity standard is prepared in 2 mL of RapID inoculation fluid. The suspension is poured or pipetted into the cuvette, and all 18 wells are simultaneously inoculated by manual manipulations of the cuvette. The system is incubated for 4–6 hours at 35–37°C in a non-CO_2 incubator. Nitrate reagents A and B are added to the NIT well, and a second reagent (RapID CB Plus Reagent) is added to the arylamidase test wells. Thirty seconds to 1 minute after reagent addition, the color reactions in the wells are read and a numeric microcode is generated. The RapID CB Plus Code Compendium is consulted for the identification. Evaluations of RapID CB-Plus have reported that the kit correctly identifies 88.5–95% of *Corynebacterium* species, particularly the species commonly encountered in the clinical laboratory (i.e., *C. amycolatum*, *C. jeikeium*, *C. striatum*, *C. urealyticum*, *C. minutissimum*, *C. pseudodiphtheriticum*, and CDC group G).[305,438] Isolates of some newly described taxa (e.g., *Dermabacter hominis*, *Microbacterium* species, *Turicella otitidis*, *Cellulomonas* species, *Brevibacterium casei*, and *Arthrobacter cumminsii*) were also correctly identified. Difficulties with this system were related to the interpretation of some of the carbohydrate acidification and aminopeptidase reactions.

Antimicrobial Susceptibility Testing of *Corynebacterium* Species and the Coryneform Bacteria

Antimicrobial susceptibilities of many of the newly described coryneforms have been reported in several publications. In these reports, both agar dilution and microbroth dilution procedures have been used.[306,347,583,584,832] Both Soriano and coworkers and Funke and coworkers used an agar dilution procedure with Mueller-Hinton agar supplemented with 5% sheep blood and an inoculum of 10^4 CFU per organism.[306,832] Martinez-Martinez and colleagues used a broth microdilution procedure with cation-supplemented Mueller-Hinton broth containing 0.5% Tween 80 and an inoculum of 5×10^4 CFU per microtiter well.[583,584] Plates or trays were incubated at 35°C for 18–24 hours under aerobic conditions. Because there are no CLSI-determined breakpoints for susceptibility testing of *Corynebacterium* species or other coryneforms, "breakpoints" for interpretation of MICs obtained by the above methods were defined by the investigators in these studies. In the case of penicillin, ampicillin, amoxicillin-clavulanate, and oxacillin, CLSI-determined breakpoints for the staphylococci have been used. Table 14-8 lists the breakpoints used for the determination of antimicrobial susceptibilities of corynebacteria and other coryneforms from the literature.[306,832] Some workers have also used Etest methods for determining the antimicrobial susceptibility of *Corynebacterium* species and coryneforms like *Arcanobacterium haemolyticum*.[129,583] Using Etest, agreement with broth dilution MICs varied with the agent being tested. Agreement between methods ranged from 88.2% for cephalothin and rifampin to 65.4% for amikacin and 31.1% for vancomycin.[583] At present, the CLSI has convened a new subcommittee to prepare recommendations for clinical laboratories for testing of coryneform gram-positive bacilli as well as fastidious gram-negative bacteria. These recommendations will address the most appropriate methods to use, the media and incubation conditions, and breakpoints for determining the antimicrobial susceptibility of these organisms.

Members of the Genus *Corynebacterium* Isolated From Humans

The Genus *Corynebacterium* contains a large number of species that have been isolated from human clinical specimens, animals, and the environment. *C. diphtheriae*, a classical pathogen, is the cause of diphtheria. Other species, such as *C. jeikeium*, *C. striatum*, *C. pseudodiphtheriticum*, and *C. urealyticum*, are isolated more frequently than the other *Corynebacterium* species and behave primarily as opportunistic agents in immunocompromised and/or debilitated patients. *C. amycolatum* is the most commonly isolated species in the clinical laboratory and may represent a skin contaminant or a significant agent of infection. This species is also difficult to differentiate from other species that have similar biochemical characteristics.

C. amycolatum, *C.*, *diphtheriae*, *C. jeikeium*, *C. pseudodiphtheriticum*, *C. striatum*, and *C. urealyticum* are discussed below. Box 14-2 lists the other *Corynebacterium* species, describes their clinical significance, and includes additional helpful information on identification of these organisms. Table 14-9 presents the phenotypic biochemical characteristics of *Corynebacterium* species isolated from human clinical specimens. Table 14-10 is a compendium of API Coryne biocodes for those *Corynebacterium* species not

Table 14-8 Breakpoints Used for Determining the Antimicrobial Susceptibility of *Corynebacterium* Species and Other Coryneform Bacteria[306,832]

ANTIMICROBIAL AGENT	SUSCEPTIBLE, μG/ML	RESISTANT, μG/ML
Penicillin	≤0.12	>0.12
Ampicillin	≤0.25	>0.25
Amoxicillin/clavulanate	≤4/2	>4/2
Oxacillin	≤2	>2
Cephalothin	≤8	>8
Ceftriaxone	≤8	>8
Cefuroxime	≤8	>8
Chloramphenicol	≤8	>8
Clindamycin	≤0.5	>0.5
Erythromycin	≤0.5	>0.5
Ciprofloxacin	≤1	>1
Gentamicin	≤4	>4
Rifampin	≤1	>1
Imipenem	≤4	>4
Tetracycline	≤4	>4
Vancomycin	≤4	>4
Teicoplanin	≤8	>8
Nitrofurantoin	≤1	>1

yet included in the API Coryne database. These biocodes have been obtained from the original descriptions of the various species if the API Coryne was included as a part of the organisms' characterization.

CORYNEBACTERIUM AMYCOLATUM

In 1988, Collins and associates reported a new species of *Corynebacterium* isolated from human skin.[166] Although *meso*-DAP, arabinose, and galactose were present in the cell wall, this new organism lacked the corynemycolic acids that are found in all other *Corynebacterium* species. Despite this departure from an important criterion used to assign gram-positive bacilli to the genus *Corynebacterium*, 16S rRNA sequence analysis supported the inclusion of this organism. This organism was named *Corynebacterium amycolatum* ("without mycolic acids") and accepted as a valid *Corynebacterium* species in 1988.

Several studies indicate that *C. amycolatum* has probably been misidentified by clinical laboratories for many years as *C. striatum*, *C. xerosis*, *C. minutissimum*, and CDC group I-1.[60,297,940,988] *C. amycolatum* characteristically produces flat, dry, whitish-gray, matte or waxy colonies on SBA (see Color Plate 14-3*C*). Confluent areas of growth on agar media may become wrinkled-looking on prolonged incubation. This colony morphology is easily differentiated from those of either *C. minutissimum* or *C. striatum*, which always produce gray-white, moist colonies. *C. amycolatum* is pyrazinamidase- and alkaline phosphatase–positive, and most strains also reduce nitrate to nitrite. *C. amycolatum* produces acid from glucose and ribose,

and most strains also ferment maltose and sucrose. Some isolates may be urease-positive and PYR-positive. All *C. amycolatum* strains produce propionic acid as the major end product of glucose metabolism. Table 14-9 shows the additional tests that can be used to differentiate *C. amycolatum*, *C. striatum*, *C. minutissimum*, and *C. xerosis*.[60,717,940,942,988] Common API Coryne profile numbers are 3100325, 3100125, 7100125, 3100365, 4100325, and 3040121 (see Color Plates 14-3*D* and 14-3*E*); these numbers usually identify the organisms as *C. amycolatum*/*C. striatum*, necessitating these additional tests for definitive identification. Chemotaxonomic approaches may also be used to resolve these species identifications.[923]

C. amycolatum has been isolated from significant human infections. A chemotaxonomically confirmed strain of *C. amycolatum* has been reported as the cause of fatal sepsis in a premature infant.[79] Since then, *C. amycolatum* has been isolated from catheter-related infections, surgical wound infections, pilonidal cysts, mastitis, native-valve and nosocomial endocarditis, cardioverter lead–electrode infection, and septic arthritis following vascular graft sepsis.[161,202,250,494,670,910] Isolates of *C. amycolatum* are frequently multiply resistant to antimicrobial agents, including β-lactams, macrolides, clindamycin, aminoglycosides, quinolones, and rifampin.[729,826,832] About 40% of 101 *C. amycolatum* strains tested in a recent study were resistant to β-lactam antimicrobial agents (MICs >64 μg/mL).[306] In addition, the MICs of ciprofloxacin, chloramphenicol, clindamycin, and erythromycin at which 50% of the isolates were inhibited were all greater than the susceptibility breakpoints for staphylococci. Resistance to gentamicin

Table 14-9 Biochemical Characteristics for Identification of *Corynebacterium* Species Isolated From Humans

SPECIES	LIPID REQ	HEMOL SBA	NO₃ RED	PYZ	AP	ESC	URE	GEL	CAMP TEST	GLU	MAL	SUC	MNTL	XYL
C. accolens	+	−	+	V+	−	−	−	−	−	+	−	V	−	−
C. afermentans subsp. *afermentans*	−	−	−	+	+	−	−	−	V	−	−	−	−	−
C. afermentans subsp. *lipophilum*	+	−	−	+	+	−	−	−	V	−	−	−	−	−
C. amycolatum	−	−	V+	+	+	−	V−	−	−	+	V+	V+	−	−
C. appendices	+	−	−	+	+	−	+	−	NA	+sl	+sl	−	−	−
C. argentoratense	−	−	−	+	V−	−	−	−	−	+	−	−	−	−
C. atypicum	−	−	−	−	−	−	−	−	NA	+	+	+	−	−
C. aurimucosum	−	−	−	+	+	V	V−	V−	NA	+	+	+	−	−
C. auris	−	−	−	+	+	−	−	NA	+	−	−	−	−	−
C. confusum	−	−	+	+	+	−	−	−	−	+	−	−	−	−
C. coyleae	−	−	−	+	+	−	−	NA	+	+	−	−	−	−
C. diphtheriae gravis	−	−	+	−	−	−	−	V−	−	+	+	−	−	−
C. diphtheriae intermedius	+	−	+	−	−	−	−	V−	−	+	+	−	−	−
C. diphtheriae mitis	−	−	+	−	−	−	−	V−	−	+	+	−	−	−
C. diphtheriae belfanti	−	−	−	−	−	−	−	V−	−	+	+	−	−	−
C. durum	−	−	+	+	−	+	V+	−	NA	+	+	+	+⁻	−
C. falsenii	−	−	−	+w	+	−	+sl	−	−	+sl	V+	−	−	−
C. freneyi	−	−	V	+	+	−	−	−	NA	+	+	+	−	−
C. glucuronolyticum	−	−	V	+	V−	V	V+	V−	+	+	V	+	−	V
C. imitans	−	−	−	+w	+	−	−	−	+	+	+	+w	−	−
C. jeikeium	+	−	−	+	+	−	−	−	−	+	V	−	−	−
C. kroppenstedtii	−	−	−	+	−	+	−	−	NA	+	+w	+	−	−
C. lipophiloflavum	+	−	−	+	+	−	+24h	NA	NA	−	−	−	−	−
C. macginleyi	+	−	+	−	+	−	−	−	NA	+	−	+	−	−
C. matruchotii	−	−	+	+	+	−	−	−	−	+	+	+	−	−
C. minutissimum	−	−	−	+	+	+	−	−	−	+	+	+	−	−
C. mucifaciens	−	−	−	+	+	−	−	−	−	+	−	V	−	−
C. nigricans	−	−	−	V	V	−	−	−	−	+	+	+	NA	−
C. propinquum	−	−	V	V	V	−	−	−	−	−	−	−	−	−

(Continued)

Table 14-9 *Continued*

SPECIES	LAC	MNE	ARA	SOR	RIB	GLYG	AMYG	α-GAL	β-GAL	α-GLU	β-GLU	β-GUR	NAGA	PYR	LAP
C. accolens	-	+	-	-	+	-	NA	NA	-	-	-	-	-	V	NA
C. afermentans subsp. afermentans	-	-	NA	-	-	-	NA	-	-	-	-	-	-	-	-
C. afermentans subsp. lipophilum	-	-	NA	-	-	-	NA	-	-	-	-	-	-	-	-
C. amycolatum	-	NA	NA	NA	+	-	NA	-	-	-	-	-	-	V–	NA
C. appendices	-	NA	-	-	-	NA	-	-	-	-	-	-	-	-	-
C. argentoratense	-	NA	NA	NA	V	-	NA	NA	-	-	-	-	-	-	V
C. atypicum	-	NA	NA	NA	+	-	NA	-	-	-	-	+	-	-	+
C. aurimucosum	-	-	-	-	-	-	-	-	-	-	-	-	-	-	+
C. auris	-	NA	NA	NA	-	-	NA	NA	-	-	-	-	-	-	NA
C. confusum	-	NA	-	-	+	-	-	-	-	-	-	-	-	-	V
C. coyleae	-	+	-	NA	+	-	-	-	-	-	-	-	-	V	+
C. diphtheriae gravis	-	NA	NA	NA	+	+	NA	-	-	+	-	-	-	-	NA
C. diphtheriae intermedius	-	NA	NA	NA	+	-	NA	-	-	+	-	-	-	-	NA
C. diphtheriae mitis	-	NA	NA	NA	+	-	NA	-	-	+	-	-	-	-	NA
C. diphtheriae belfanti	-	NA	NA	NA	+	-	NA	-	-	+	-	-	-	-	NA
C. durum	-	NA	NA	NA	+	-	-	NA	V	-	NA	-	-	-	NA
C. falsenii	V	NA	-	-	+	-	-	-	-	-	-	-	-	-	V
C. freneyi	-	NA	NA	NA	+sl	-	NA	NA	-	+	-	-	-	-	NA
C. glucuronolyticum	NA	NA	NA	NA	+	-	-	-	-	-	-	+	-	-	+
C. imitans	-	+	+	-	+	-	-	-	-	-	-	-	-	-	-
C. jeikeium	-	NA	NA	NA	V–	-	-	-	-	-	-	-	-	-	NA
C. kroppenstedtii	-	NA	NA	NA	-	-	NA	-	-	-	-	-	-	-	+
C. lipophiloflavum	-	NA	NA	NA	-	-	NA	-	-	-	-	-	-	-	+
C. macginleyi	-	NA	NA	NA	+	-	NA	NA	-	V	-	-	-	-	NA
C. matruchotii	-	NA	NA	NA	+	-	NA	NA	-	-	-	-	-	+	NA
C. minutissimum	-	-	-	-	-	-	-	-	-	-	-	-	-	-	+
C. mucifaciens	-	+	-	-	V	-	-	-	-	-	-	-	-	V	-
C. nigricans	-	+	NA	NA	V	V	NA	NA	-	-	-	-	-	-	NA
C. propinquum	-	NA	NA	NA	-	-	NA	NA	-	-	-	-	-	V	NA

Table 14-9 *Continued*

SPECIES	LIPID REQ	HEMOL SBA	NO₃ RED	PYZ	AP	ESC	URE	GEL	CAMP TEST	GLU	MAL	SUC	MNTL	XYL
C. pseudodiphthericum	–	–	+	+	V	–	+	V	–	–	–	–	–	–
C. pseudotuberculosis	–	β	–	–	V	–	+	V	Rev+	+	+	–	–	–
C. riegelii	–	–	–	V	V	–	Rapid+	–	–	–	+sl	–	–	–
C. sanguinis	–	–	–	+	+	–	–	–	–	+sl	–	–	–	–
C. simulans	–	–	+	V	+	–	–	–	–	+	–	+	–	–
C. singulare	–	–	–	+	+	–	+	–	NA	+	+	+	–	–
C. striatum	–	–	+	+	+	–	–	–	V	+	–	V+	–	–
C. sundsvallense	–	–	–	V	V	–	+	–	–	+	+	+	–	–
C. thomssenii	–	–	–	+	+	–	+	–	–	+sl	+sl	+sl	–	–
C. ulcerans	–	β	–	–	+	–	+	+	Rev+	+	+	–	–	–
C. urealyticum	+	–	–	+	V	–	Rapid+	–	–	–	–	–	–	–
C. xerosis	–	–	V	+	+	–	–	–	–	+	+	+	–	–
Corynebacterium group F1	+	–	V+	+	–	–	+	–	–	+	+	+	–	–
Corynebacterium group G	+	–	V	+	+	–	–	–	–	+	V	V	–	–

Table 14-9 *Continued*

SPECIES	LAC	MNE	ARA	SOR	RIB	GLYG	AMYG	α-GAL	β-GAL	α-GLU	β-GLU	β-GUR	NAGA	PYR	LAP
C. pseudodiphthericum	–	NA	NA	NA	–	–	NA	NA	–	–	–	–	–	V	NA
C. pseudotuberculosis	–	+	NA	NA	+	–	NA	NA	–	V	–	–	–	–	NA
C. riegelii	–	–	–	–	+	–	–	–	–	–	–	–	–	–	+
C. sanguinis	–	NA	NA	NA	+	–	NA	–	–	–	–	–	–	+	NA
C. simulans	–	+	–	–	V	–	–	–	–	–	–	–	–	–	+
C. singulare	–	NA	NA	NA	–	–	NA	NA	–	–	–	–	–	+	NA
C. striatum	–	NA	NA	NA	–	–	NA	–	–	–	–	–	–	–	NA
C. sundsvallense	–	NA	NA	NA	–	–	–	–	–	+	–	–	NA	–	V
C. thomssenii	–	+	–	–	–	–	–	–	–	–	–	–	+	–	+
C. ulcerans	–	+	+	NA	+	+	NA	NA	–	+	–	–	–	–	NA
C. urealyticum	–	NA	NA	NA	–	–	NA	–	–	–	–	–	–	–	NA
C. xerosis	–	NA	NA	NA	+	–	NA	NA	–	+	–	–	–	–	NA
Corynebacterium group F1	–	NA	NA	NA	V–	–	NA	NA	–	–	–	–	–	–	NA
Corynebacterium group G	–	NA	NA	NA	+	–	NA	NA	–	–	–	–	–	V	NA

+, *positive reaction;* –, *negative reaction;* V, *variable reaction;* +sl, *delayed positive reaction;* +w, *weak reaction;* V+, *variable reaction, most strains positive;* V–, *variable reaction, most strains negative;* R+, *rapid positive reaction;* Rev+, *reverse CAMP test positive;* NA, *data not available*

Legend: Lipid Req, *requirement for lipids for growth;* Hemol SBA, *hemolysis, sheep blood agar;* NO3 Red, *Reduction of nitrate;* PYZ, *pyrazinamidase;* AP, *alkaline phosphatase;* ESC, *esculin hydrolysis;* URE, *urease;* Glu, *acid from glucose;* Mal, *acid from maltose;* Suc, *acid from sucrose;* Mntl, *acid from mannitol;* Xyl, *acid from xylose;* Lac, *acid from lactose;* Mne, *acid from mannose;* Ara, *acid from arabinose;* Sor, *acid from sorbitol;* Rib, *acid from ribose;* Glyg, *acid from glycogen;* Amyg, *acid from amygdalin;* α-GAL, *α-galactosidase;* β-GAL, *β-galactosidase;* α-GLU, *α-glucosidase;* β-GLU, *β-glucosidase;* β-GUR, *β-glucuronidase;* NAGA, *N-acetyl-β-D-glucosaminidase;* PYR, *pyrrolidonyl arylamidase;* LAP, *leucine aminopeptidase.*

Table 14-10 API Coryne Biocodes for *Corynebacterium* Species Not Included in the Current Database

SPECIES	API CORYNE BIOCODES	SPECIES	API CORYNE BIOCODES
C. appendicis	2101124	*C. matruchotii*	7000325, 7010325, 7050325
C. argentoratense	2000104	"*C. matruchotii*-like"	2140325
C. atypicum	0200365	*C. mucifaciens*	2000004, 2000104, 2000105, 2100104, 2100105, 2100004, 6000004, 6100104, 6100105, 0000004, 6100125
C. aurimusocum	2100125		
C. auris	2100004		
C. bovis	0101104	*C. nigricans*	0000125, 2000125, 2100327
C. confusum	3100304, 3100104	*C. riegelii*	0101224, 2001224, 2101224
C. coyleae	2100104, 6100304, 2100304, 4100304, 6100004	*C. sanguinis*	6100304
		C. simulans	0100305, 2100105, 2100301, 2100305, 3000125
C. durum	3000135, 3001135, 3040135, 3400115, 3400135, 3400305, 3400325, 3400335, 3040325, 3040335, 3440335, 3441335, 3440125, 3441125		
		C. singulare	6101125
		C. sundsvallense	0011125, 0111125, 2011125, 2111125, 2001004, 2101125
C. falsenii	2101104, 2101304, 2100304, 2100324		
C. freneyi	3110325	*C. thomssenii*	2121125, 0101004
C. imitans	2100324	*C. xerosis*	2110325, 3110325
C. kroppenstedtii	2040105, 2040125		
C. lipophiloflavum	2101004		

was also seen in some isolates. All strains of *C. amycola-tum* were susceptible to tetracycline and vancomycin.[306]

CORYNEBACTERIUM DIPHTHERIAE

C. diphtheriae is the cause of the classic disease diphtheria. This infection is relatively uncommon in the U.S., although it is still seen in developing countries.[31,921] The infection is prevented by widespread immunization of at-risk populations with diphtheria toxoid; use of this material in other countries has resulted in dramatic decreases in the incidence of diphtheria in those locales as well. Despite the success of widespread immunization in many countries, diphtheria continues to be a lethal, resurgent infectious agent, particularly within certain parts of the world, including Eastern Europe, Southeast Asia, South America, and the Indian subcontinent.[473] The importation of toxigenic *C. diphtheriae* from developing countries where diphtheria remains endemic poses a constant threat and has accounted for most cases of diphtheria in recent years in industrialized countries. For example, in a 1993 case-control study of the first case of fatal respiratory diphtheria to occur in Dade County, Florida, in over 20 years, recent travel to Haiti among contacts to the index case suggested that the organism may have been imported.[259] In addition, several reports have now documented the clinical importance of nontoxigenic strains of *C. diphtheriae*.[370,374,426,952,990] These organisms have been isolated from pharyngeal cultures and skin lesions of homeless, intravenous-drug users, and bacteremia and endocarditis due to nontoxigenic strains of *C. diphtheriae* have also been reported in these patients. Currently, the Immunization Practices Advisory Committee of the Public Health Service recommends that three intra-muscular doses of DPT (diphtheria toxoid, pertussis acellular vaccine, and tetanus toxoid) be given at 4- to 8-week intervals to all children beginning at 6–8 weeks of age, with a fourth dose being given 6–12 months after the third dose. Children who have completed the primary series of immunizations should receive a booster dose at the time of entry into school. For children 7 years of age and older, diphtheria toxoid alone should be given two times at a 4- to 8-week interval, with a third dose given 6 to 12 months later. Older individuals should receive a booster of diphtheria toxoid at 10-year intervals. Travelers to diphtheria-endemic areas should also receive booster inoculations. In addition, persons convalescing from clinical diphtheria should also receive toxoid immunization, since clinical infection does not necessarily induce protective levels of antitoxin. With the reporting of new cases of respiratory diphtheria in the U.S., it is imperative that the public health response include both case management and the identification of close contacts. Because of the failure of most adults to receive booster injections, a susceptible adult population currently exists; 10–60% of individuals more than 30 years of age have inadequate levels of circulating antibodies against diphtheria toxin. Because of this, outbreaks of diphtheria continue to be reported.

C. diphtheriae is the classical prototype of the toxigenic organism. Virulence of the organism is related almost entirely to the production of diphtheria toxin.[424] Diphtheria toxin is a 58,342-Da polypeptide containing 535 amino acid residues. The toxin is composed of two fragments: fragment A is 21,500 Da, and fragment B is 37,200 Da. Fragment B, containing the receptor binding/translocation domains, allows the passage of the toxin molecule through the cell membrane of the target cells. Fragment A, the biologically active part of the molecule, catalyzes the transfer of the adenosine diphosphate ribose (ADPR) moiety from nicotinamide adenine dinucleotide (NAD) to elongation factor 2 (EF-2), a soluble protein that is required for the translocation of peptidyl-transfer RNA from the acceptor to the donor site on the eukaryotic ribosome. This adenoribosylation inactivates EF-2, and protein synthesis in the affected cell is inhibited. The structural gene (*tox* gene) that codes for diphtheria toxin resides on the DNA of a corynephage (bacteriophage) called the β-corynephage.[424] On infection of a *C. diphtheriae* strain with the *tox*[+] corynephage, the nucleic acid containing the *tox* gene becomes integrated into the bacterial chromosome (lysogeny) and replicates along with it. Most nontoxigenic isolates of *C. diphtheriae* and most *tox*[-] corynephages do not contain any detectable *tox*-related DNA sequences. Only *C. diphtheriae* strains that are lysogenized by a β-phage containing the *tox* gene are capable of producing diphtheria toxin. *C. ulcerans* and *C. pseudotuberculosis* (the "*C. diphtheriae* group" organisms) are also capable of carrying the β corynephage and producing diphtheria toxin.

Respiratory tract diphtheria is primarily transmitted among humans via direct contact or by sneezing or coughing.[379] Carriage of the organism on the skin and asymptomatic carriage of the organisms in the upper respiratory tract are common sources of transmission to other susceptible individuals.[78] During an incubation period of 2–7 days, the organism multiplies locally in the posterior nasopharynx and oropharynx. During this time, there is an accumulation of organisms, fibrin, and inflammatory cells to produce the characteristic **diphtheritic pseudomembrane**, which may eventually cover the tonsils, pharynx, larynx, and posterior nasal passages (see Color Plate 14-3*F*). Extension of the pseudomembrane anteriorly may lead to involvement of the soft palate and the uvula. In severe cases, the pseudomembrane may extend into the trachea and bronchi, resulting in airway obstruction. Cervical and submandibular lymphadenopathy is also usually present. Further extension of the pseudomembrane into the posterior nasopharynx and nasal passages is associated with a serosanguineous or purulent discharge from the nose that is highly infectious. Middle-ear involvement may result from contiguous extension of the infectious process. Extension of respiratory tract infections to the skin of the face (i.e., nose, ears, cheeks) and neck also occurs occasionally. Inoculation of the organisms into the eyes may lead to conjunctivitis with or without involvement of the cornea. Satellite lesions may also occur in the esophagus, stomach, or lower airways.

C. diphtheriae may also cause a primary cutaneous infection, in which toxin is also absorbed systemically. Skin lesions may resemble several other skin conditions, including folliculitis, impetigo, pyoderma, or seborrheic dermatitis. Other pyogenic organisms, such as *Streptococcus pyogenes*, may be coisolated with *C. diphtheriae*. Cutaneous diphtheria has also been reported following the bites of insects, such as spiders, and infection of preexisting wounds (e.g., surgical wounds, pyoderma, eczema, impetigo, dermatitis) has also been documented.[31,379] An ulcerative lesion called **ecthyma diphtheriticum** is the initial lesion. This lesion begins as a vesicle or pustule containing a straw-colored or serosanguineous fluid. After this material drains, the lesion becomes a punched-out ulcer a few millimeters to a few centimeters in size. The margins of the lesion are elevated and undermined. Diphtheritic skin lesions are usually painful and subsequently become covered with a dark, adherent pseudomembranous eschar or scab. This pseudomembrane eventually falls off, leaving a beefy, hemorrhagic base that oozes serosanguineous fluid. As the initial lesion develops, the surrounding skin becomes red and edematous, with the formation of satellite bullae surrounding the ecthyma diphtheriticum lesion. Most of the cutaneous lesions are on the arms, hands, feet, or lower legs. Although cutaneous lesions are much less likely to cause serious systemic toxicity, they do pose a significant risk of spread to the environment and to other individuals.

Locally multiplying bacteria synthesize and release diphtheria toxin, which is absorbed systemically. The toxin has direct toxic effects on the heart, the central and peripheral nervous system, liver, and kidneys.[379] A diffuse myocardiopathy may result in 20–70% of patients. These symptoms may appear insidiously or cataclysmically, resulting in circulatory collapse and acute congestive heart failure. Neurologic complications and neuropathies may appear in 20–75% of patients and usually correlate with the severity of the illness. These complications may initially include paralysis of the soft palate and posterior pharyngeal wall, followed by oculomotor and ciliary paralysis. The latter contributes to the risk of oropharyngeal aspiration and pneumonia. Fatty degenerative changes and focal necrosis in the kidneys, liver, and adrenals may also complicate severe infections. In general, the myocardiopathy and neuropathy occur later and are less severe following cutaneous diphtheritic infections than those following respiratory tract infection. Death may ensue from cardiac failure or paralysis of the diaphragm.

Infections other than classical diphtheria have also been associated with *C. diphtheriae;* some of these severe infections have been due to nontoxigenic strains.[668] Several reports of infective endocarditis due to both toxigenic and nontoxigenic strains and involving both native and prosthetic heart valves have appeared in the literature in recent years. In 1993, Tiley and colleagues reported on seven cases of endocarditis due to nontoxigenic strains that occurred in New South Wales, Australia, over a 12-month period.[886] The patients ranged in age from 12 to 49 years. Three of the seven had preexisting cardiac abnormalities and only one was an intravenous-drug user. The patients presented with a prodromal illness (headache, malaise, fever, myalgias) of 4 to 10 days' duration; five had a nonexudative pharyngitis on presentation as well. Echocardiography demonstrated large valvular vegetations in five patients. Widespread septic emboli to small blood vessels developed in four patients, while emboli to the brain, spleen, and kidneys developed in the fifth, resulting in the patient's death. Mycotic aneurysms complicated two cases, and septic arthritis developed in four of the seven patients. The pathogenesis of severe infections due to nontoxigenic *C. diphtheriae* is not understood at present.

The organism is able to actively invade tissue, causing a fulminant disease involving the cardiac, endothelial, and synovial tissues. Endocarditis with a nontoxigenic *C. diphtheriae* strain has also been reported in a 20-year-old male student in whom cerebral emboli and severe rhabdomyolysis developed, requiring mitral and aortic valve replacement.[98]

The capacity of *C. diphtheriae* to infect a wide variety of cell types may be responsible for some of the unusual presentations of diphtheria. Havaldar and Shanthala reported a case in an 11-year-old girl who presented with abdominal pain of 2 weeks' duration.[398] Bilateral, conjunctival pseudomembranes that were culture-positive for *C. diphtheriae* subsequently developed. Intestinal involvement became apparent with the passage of bloody stools and casts of sloughed intestinal tissue. Other infections associated with *C. diphtheriae* (e.g., septic arthritis, osteomyelitis) have been reported but are rare.[56,687]

In spite of immunization practices and an apparently low risk of indigenously acquired diphtheria in the U.S., large subgroups of susceptible individuals currently exist. Surveys conducted in the U.S. suggest that only 40–60% of children at least 2 years of age have received all of the routinely recommended childhood vaccinations. Similar studies have also shown that as many as 20% of preschool-aged children lack protective immunity to diphtheria toxin. In addition, serosurveys of adolescents and adults in the U.S. have shown that 20% to more than 50% of these individuals lacked immunity to diphtheria toxin. Levels of immunity in elderly individuals were particularly low, probably as a result of lack of natural exposure during the early vaccine era, low rates of vaccination, and waning or absent vaccine-induced immunity.

Treatment of diphtheria involves the administration of equine antitoxin to neutralize toxin not already bound to target cells. There is no effective therapy for reversal of cardiac or neurologic involvement that might have occurred prior to specific diagnosis. Supportive care (tracheostomy or intubation, airway clearance, monitoring of cardiac function) is necessary and of extreme importance. Penicillin or erythromycin may also be administered to speed the eradication of the organisms from the respiratory tract of the patient.[493] Both rifampin and erythromycin have been used to eradicate carriage of *C. diphtheriae* in exposed individuals. In vitro antimicrobial susceptibility testing has shown that *C. diphtheriae* strains are generally susceptible to penicillin, ampicillin, cefuroxime, erythromycin, tetracycline, ciprofloxacin, gentamicin, trimethoprim, and rifampin.[578]

For the isolation of *C. diphtheriae*, swab specimens are obtained from the oropharynx, nasopharynx, or cutaneous lesions. Swabs should be made of Dacron and should be used to sample multiple, inflamed areas of the nasopharynx. If a pseudomembrane is present, swab specimens from beneath the membrane should be collected. Swab specimens may be sent to the laboratory in a routine semisolid transport medium such as Amies. These swabs are inoculated onto a sheep blood plate and/or a Columbia colistin-nalidixic acid (CNA) agar plate, and an agar medium containing cystine and potassium tellurite. For the cystine-tellurite medium,

laboratories should use cystine-tellurite blood agar or modified Tinsdale agar for the recovery of *C. diphtheriae*. Although not routinely done, some laboratories will also inoculate a slant of Loeffler medium, which contains coagulated beef serum and egg. Methylene blue staining of smears prepared from 8- to 18-hour growth on Loeffler medium may provide a preliminary diagnosis of diphtheria, since these organisms grow rapidly on this medium and produce distinctive, club-shaped, diphtheroid cells containing metachromatic granules (see Color Plate 14-3*H*). However, since other coryneforms may also have this appearance on Loeffler medium, results should only be reported as presumptive and must be correlated with the clinical presentation of the patient. SBA and CNA are used to screen for β-hemolytic streptococci, *Staphylococcus aureus,* and *Arcanobacterium haemolyticum. S. aureus* may be coisolated with *C. diphtheriae* and will also grow as black colonies on Tinsdale medium, so the blood agar plate or CNA plate will help to assess the extent of staphylococcal growth on the tellurite-containing medium. Since some laboratories may not stock tellurite-containing medium because of infrequent requests, the inoculation of blood and/or CNA agar will still enable the recovery of *C. diphtheriae* and other pathogenic organisms, enabling suspected coryneform isolates to be subcultured and examined further should the clinical presentation and history of the patient (e.g., presence of a characteristic pseudomembranous oropharyngeal lesion, lack of immunizations, outbreak settings) strongly suggest *C. diphtheriae* infection. (See Charts 14-1 and 14-2 for descriptions of preparing Loeffler's methylene blue stain and serum medium.)

C. diphtheriae, C. ulcerans, and *C. pseudotuberculosis* produce black colonies that are surrounded by brown halos on modified Tinsdale medium (see Color Plate 14-3*G*).[616] Black coloration of the colonies results from tellurite reductase activity, resulting in the reduction of tellurium, while the brown haloes indicate cystinase activity.[853] Other diphtheroids, staphylococci, and some streptococci may also reduce tellurite (although halos around the colonies generally are not present), so Gram stains and catalase tests should be performed on all suspicious colonies. *C. diphtheriae* does not produce urease, so this test may be used to distinguish this organism from *C. ulcerans* and *C. pseudotuberculosis* (both urease-positive). The latter two organisms can be separated from one another by the production of acid from starch or glycogen. Deamidation of pyrazinamide to pyrazinoic acid by pyrazinamidase, a test used in mycobacteriology, is also helpful for distinguishing the ''*C. diphtheriae*'' organisms (pyrazinamidase-negative) from other *Corynebacterium* species (mostly pyrazinamidase-positive). A flow chart for detecting and presumptively identifying isolates recovered on Tinsdale medium is presented in Figure 14-1.

C. diphtheriae may appear as four distinct colony types (biotypes) designated *gravis, mitis, intermedius,* and *belfanti.* These biotypes also differ slightly in Gram stain morphology, certain biochemical reactions, and historically, in the severity of the disease processes they produce. *C. diphtheriae* biotype *gravis* and biotype *mitis* strains produce fairly large (1–2 mm in diameter at 24 hours), convex colonies with entire edges, while biotype *intermedius* strains produce

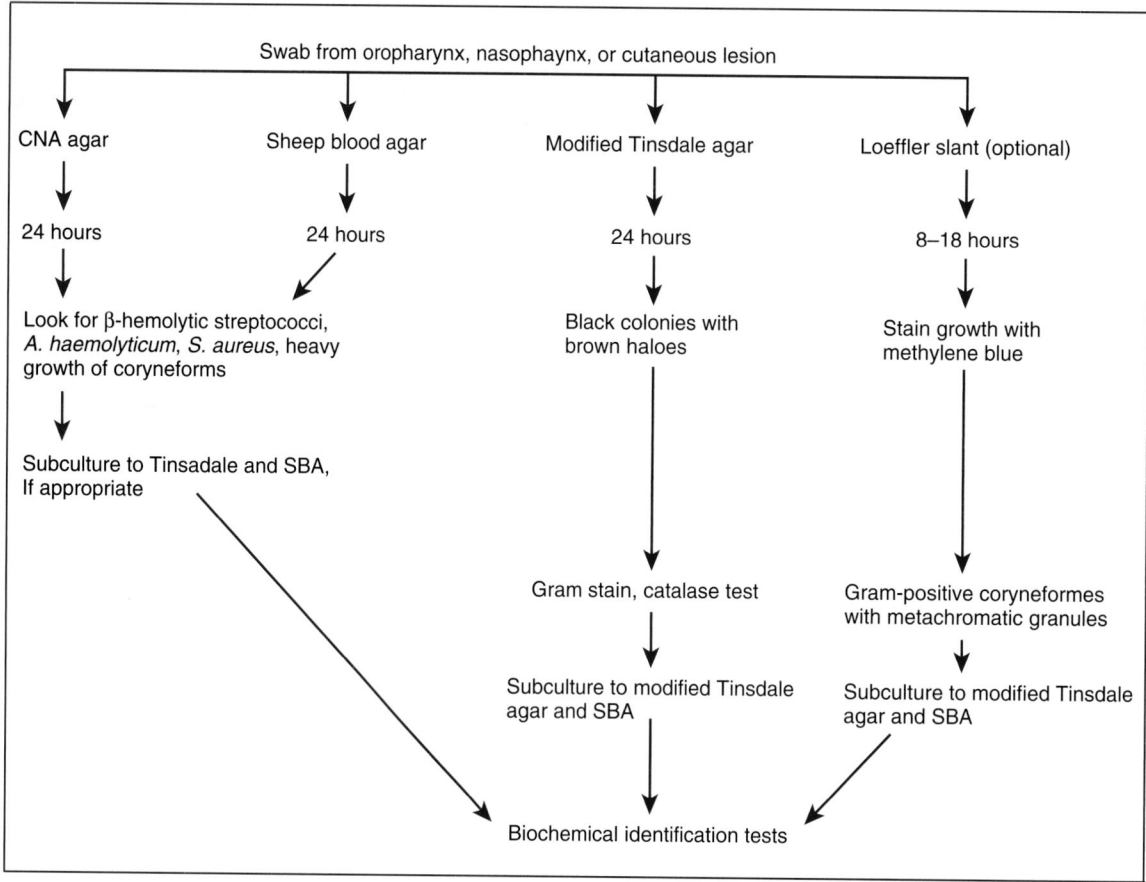

Figure 14-1 Flowchart for identification of *Corynebacterium Diphtheriae.*

small (<1 mm at 24 hours), blacker, dense colonies on tellurite-containing agar. Most *mitis* and some *gravis* strains are weakly β-hemolytic on SBA (see Color Plate 14-4*A*). All four biotypes grow as black colonies surrounded by brown halos on modified Tinsdale medium, and all form gray-white, smooth, nonhemolytic colonies on SBA. All biotypes lack pyrazinamidase activity, do not produce alkaline phosphatase, and do not hydrolyze esculin or urea. Acid is produced from glucose and maltose, but not from sucrose, mannitol, or xylose; rare sucrose-fermenting strains have been reported (see Color Plates 14-4*B* and 14-4*C*).[211] (The preparation and use of Tinsdale medium is presented in Chart 14-3, and the preparation and use of cystine-tellurite blood agar is presented in Chart 14-4.)

Once an organism is biochemically identified as a possible *C. diphtheriae*, the isolate must be tested for the ability to produce diphtheria toxin. Many laboratories that perform toxigenicity tests use the modified Elek immunoprecipitation procedure—an immunodiffusion method similar to the classical Ouchterlony test. The test uses KL Virulence agar (Difco, Franklin Lakes, NJ), a proteose peptone-based agar, supplemented with sterile rabbit serum or with KL Virulence enrichment (a nonserous enrichment designed for use with KL Virulence agar by Difco) and with 0.03% potassium

tellurite (supplied as Bacto-Chapman tellurite solution, 1%; Difco) as the basal medium. This medium is poured into a sterile 150-mm Petri plate. Before the medium solidifies, a 1 cm × 8 cm strip of filter paper that is saturated with diphtheria antitoxin (Bacto-KL antitoxin strips; Difco) is submerged in the medium and oriented across the diameter of the plate. After cooling, the isolate to be tested for toxin production is streaked perpendicularly to the submerged antitoxin strip. Equidistant from either side of this streak, a known toxigenic *C. diphtheriae* strain and a known nontoxigenic *C. diphtheriae* strain are also streaked for control of the test. The plate is then incubated at 35°C and examined every 24 hours for 3 days. If the unknown strain is toxigenic, precipitin lines will form at 45-degree angles between the inoculum and the antitoxin strip. These lines will show identity with the toxigenic control *C. diphtheriae* strain. A modified Elek immunodiffusion procedure uses a centrally placed disk containing antitoxin with the test organisms being spot inoculated 7 to 9 mm away from the central antitoxin disk.[246] Such modifications enable simultaneous testing of multiple isolates and are adaptable to outbreak situations. High-quality antitoxin can be obtained from several sources (Pasteur-Merieux, Lyon, France; CNG, Peyrm, Russia; Wyeth Laboratories, Marietta, PA; Connaught Laboratories, Swiftwater, PA).

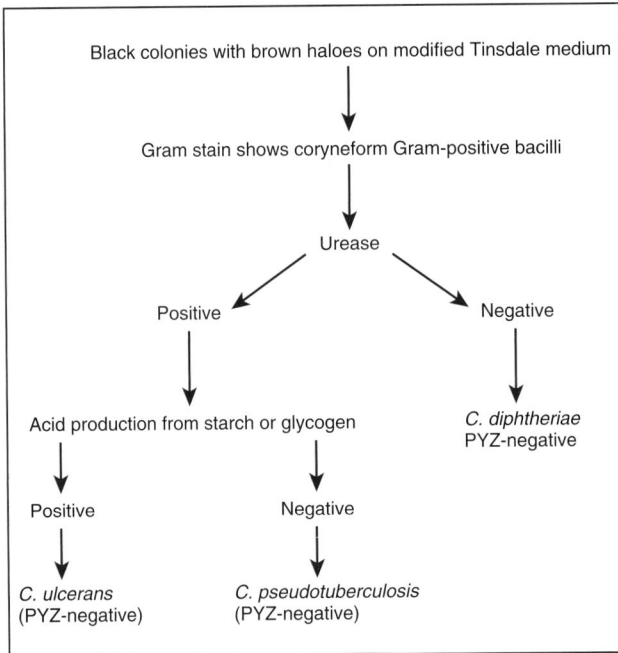

Black colonies with brown haloes on modified Tinsdale medium

↓

Gram stain shows coryneform Gram-positive bacilli

↓

Urease

↙ ↘

Positive   Negative

↓   ↓

Acid production from starch or glycogen   C. diphtheriae
                                                 PYZ-negative

↓   ↓

Positive   Negative

↓   ↓

C. ulcerans   C. pseudotuberculosis
(PYZ-negative) (PYZ-negative)

Figure 14-2 Flowchart for isolation of *C. diphtheriae*.

Several other methods, including enzyme immunoassays and reverse passive latex agglutination tests have also been developed for the detection of toxin production by *C. diphtheriae*.[244,245,633,889] The rapid EIA developed by Engler and Efstratiou used equine polyclonal antitoxin as the capture antibody, and an alkaline phosphatase–labeled monoclonal antibody directed against fragment A of diphtheria toxin as the detection antibody. This method detected 87 toxigenic stains among 245 *C. diphtheriae* isolates and was completely concordant with the results from the modified Elek method.[244] In 2002, an immunochromatographic strip (ICS) assay was developed and marketed by the World Health Organization and the Program for Appropriate Technology in Health (Seattle, WA).[245] For this test, a suspension of the organism is prepared in an enrichment broth and incubated for 3 hours. An ICS strip is placed in the tube. After 10 minutes, the strip is examined for the presence of a band that is parallel to an internal positive control present on the strip. This assay can detect as little as 0.5 ng/mL of diphtheria toxin and is 10 times more sensitive than EIA methods and 20 times more sensitive than agglutination assays.[245]

Molecular methods have also been developed for detection of toxin production by *C. diphtheriae*. Most PCR methods have been directed at the *tox* gene, using primers that flank sequences corresponding to the biologically active toxin fragment A.[34,606,622,656] These assays have been used for toxin detection in pure cultures of *C. diphtheriae* and directly in clinical specimens. Some studies have noted a 100% correlation between molecular-based techniques and phenotypic methods for detection of toxin production (e.g., the Elek test).[606] However, PCR methods may also detect toxin gene sequences in isolates that do not produce biologi-

cally active toxin.[619,656] In one study, 6 of 55 *C. diphtheriae* isolates did not produce toxin but possessed the *tox* gene, in whole or in part.[238] Therefore, negative PCR tests on suspected isolates are helpful for excluding the diagnosis of diphtheria but may not predict phenotypic expression of toxin production. Molecular methods have also been used for typing both toxigenic and nontoxigenic *C. diphtheriae* isolates from outbreaks. These methods have included ribotyping, amplified fragment-length-polymorphism analysis, pulsed-field gel electrophoresis, and random amplified polymorphic DNA analysis.[219–221,581,623,887,929]

CORYNEBACTERIUM JEIKEIUM

C. jeikeium is one of the *Corynebacterium* species most commonly isolated from human infections.[315] This lipophilic species colonizes the skin of hospitalized patients and may also be recovered from inanimate objects in the hospital environment.[199,831,879] Infections with *C. jeikeium* are seen predominantly in immunocompromised hosts with malignancies and other underlying diseases (including AIDS), indwelling medical devices, integumentary barrier breaks, neutropenia, and therapy with broad-spectrum antimicrobial agents.[828,834,907,934] This organism is a well-documented cause of many serious infections, including community-acquired and nosocomially acquired bacteremia and sepsis, native- and prosthetic-valve endocarditis, meningitis, ventriculitis, pneumonia, pyelonephritis, osteomyelitis, peritonitis, otitis media, and cutaneous/soft-tissue infections.[92,188,212,360,447,456,495,744,905,946,978]

After 24 hours of incubation, colonies of *C. jeikeium* on SBA are small (0.5–1 mm in diameter), nonhemolytic, and gray-white (see Color Plate 14-4*D*). Growth on commercially available chocolate agar is usually scant because of the absence of lipids in current chocolate agar formulations. Unlike several other species, this organism is strictly aerobic. In the absence of supplementation of the growth media with Tween 80, acidification of the glucose and ribose test cupules in the API Coryne is often weak after 24 hours (see Color Plate 14-2*F*). The organism is pyrazinamidase- and alkaline phosphatase–positive, and acidifies glucose, ribose, and galactose, and some strains also acidify maltose. All of the enzymatic tests on the API Coryne are negative for *C. jeikeium* (see Color Plates 14-4*E* and 14-4*F*).

C. jeikeium was the first *Corynebacterium* species documented as being multiresistant to antimicrobial agents.[447] Isolates of this species often show resistance to β-lactams (penicillins, cephalosporins, imipenem) and aminoglycosides (gentamicin, tobramycin), variable susceptibility to the macrolides, tetracyclines, rifampin, and the quinolones (i.e., ciprofloxacin), and susceptibility to the glycopeptides (e.g., vancomycin and teicoplanin) and quinupristin-dalfopristin.[51,457,511,584,615,677,680,764,832,893] *C. jeikeium* is also resistant to many of the newer fluoroquinolone (i.e., gemifloxacin, trovafloxacin) and macrolide (i.e., azithromycin) antiinfectives.[285] Multiple antibiotic resistance in *C. jeikeium* is believed to be chromosomal rather than plasmid-associated. However, inducible, transposon-associated macrolide-lincosamide-streptogramin (MLS) resistance has been demonstrated in *C. jeikeium*.[742]

CORYNEBACTERIUM PSEUDODIPHTHERITICUM

Although not a newly described species, increasing numbers of case reports suggest that *C. pseudodiphtheriticum* may be an important emerging pathogen, particularly among immunocompromised hosts. Although this organism is considered a member of the normal human oropharyngeal flora, respiratory tract infections associated with it include exudative pharyngitis, bronchitis, bronchiolitis, necrotizing tracheitis, tracheobronchitis, pneumonia, and lung abscess.[10,25,121,148,178,190,282,378,577] In compromised hosts with these infections, underlying diseases or predisposing factors have included permanent tracheostomy secondary to laryngeal carcinoma, chronic obstructive pulmonary disease, diabetes mellitus, coronary artery disease, intubation and mechanical ventilation secondary to a motor vehicle accident, and HIV infection. In some cases, respiratory tract infection with *C. pseudodiphtheriticum* may mimic respiratory diphtheria.[446] Cases of both native-valve and prosthetic-valve endocarditis caused by *C. pseudodiphtheriticum* have also been reported. Most of the cases of native-valve endocarditis have occurred in patients with preexisting valve damage.[139,618,954] In one report, the large vegetation in the area around the mitral valve completely occluded the inlet from the left atrium and extended down into the left ventricle.[618] Suppurative *C. pseudodiphtheriticum* cervical lymphadenitis in a 3½-year-old child and a case of vertebral diskitis due to *C. pseudodiphtheriticum* have also been reported.[516,966] In the latter case, the infection was preceded by nasal turbinate surgery; it was postulated that this procedure may have caused a bacteremia that seeded the vertebral disk. In addition, both cutaneous wound and eye infections (i.e., keratitis and conjunctivitis) caused by *C. pseudodiphtheriticum* have been reported.[405,536]

C. pseudodiphtheriticum is nonlipophilic and grows as smooth, white colonies on SBA (see Color Plate 14-5*C*). Pyrazinamidase and nitrate reductase reactions are positive, and the alkaline phosphatase reaction is variable. This organism is urease-positive after 24 hours and does not ferment or oxidize carbohydrates. *C. pseudodiphtheriticum* isolates are generally susceptible to β-lactam agents, vancomycin, and aminoglycosides, but strains that are resistant to clindamycin, erythromycin, tetracycline, and the quinolones have been found. Like *C. afermentans* subspecies and *C. auris*, *C. pseudodiphtheriticum* does not produce acid from carbohydrates, but it is easily differentiated from these species by its positive urease and nitrate reductase reactions (see Color Plate 14-5*D*).

CORYNEBACTERIUM STRIATUM

C. striatum has been found in cattle, as part of the normal flora of the human nasal passages, and on human skin. In 1980, the first case of human pleuropulmonary infection with *C. striatum* was reported in a 79-year-old man with chronic lymphocytic leukemia.[104] The organism was isolated from the sputum, two sets of blood cultures, and a pleural fluid culture. This organism was also recovered, along with group B streptococci and peptostreptococci, from the sputum and tracheal secretions of a 22-year-old male who had sustained a severe skull fracture

in an automobile accident and from blood cultures collected from a 64-year-old female with metastatic endometrial carcinoma.[59,197]

Since 1993, several additional case reports have appeared regarding *C. striatum* that further support the role of this organism as an emerging pathogen in compromised individuals.[187] Watkins and colleagues at Case Western Reserve University reported on the recovery of *C. striatum* from six patients.[935] These patients ranged from 19 to 78 years of age and had various underlying diseases, including lymphoblastic lymphoma with autologous bone marrow transplantation, myelodysplasia with allogeneic bone marrow transplantation, amyotrophic lateral sclerosis, colorectal cancer, diabetes, purulent conjunctivitis, and premature rupture of amniotic membranes. Sources of the *C. striatum* isolates included blood, catheter tips, peritoneal fluids, finger-wound granuloma, conjunctiva, uterine/placental tissues, and urine. Peiris and associates in the United Kingdom isolated pure cultures of *C. striatum* from sputum, amniotic membranes, and a deep elbow wound in three patients.[673] In 1994, Wolde Rufael and Cohn reported the first case of native-valve endocarditis caused by *C. striatum* and Tumbarello and associates reported the first case of *C. striatum* bacteremia in a patient with HIV infection.[897,959] Evidence from studies conducted in intensive-care units suggests that *C. striatum* may occasionally be transmitted nosocomially.[107,529] Since the mid-1990s, significant isolates of *C. striatum* have been recovered from patients with vertebral osteomyelitis, septic arthritis and synovitis, pulmonary abscesses, breast abscess, meningitis, CSF shunt infections, and CAPD-associated peritonitis.[64,81,179,263,585,846,945] Several additional cases of *C. striatum* endocarditis, including pacemaker-associated endocarditis and the first case of prosthetic-valve endocarditis, have been reported since 1994.[206,471,601,748,875]

C. striatum isolates are nonlipophilic and grow as gray-white, moist, smooth, nonhemolytic colonies with entire edges on SBA (see Color Plate 14-6*A*). Colonies are about 1–2 mm in diameter after 24 hours of incubation. Pyrazinamidase and alkaline phosphatase are produced, and urea, esculin, and gelatin are not hydrolyzed. Most strains reduce nitrate and produce acid from glucose, sucrose, fructose, and galactose only (see Color Plate 14-6*B*).[586] *C. striatum* strains produce lactic and succinic acids from glucose, which is helpful in differentiating isolates from *C. amycolatum*. A 1995 examination of 31 clinical isolates found that all strains were susceptible to both imipenem and vancomycin; most strains were susceptible to ampicillin, cephalosporins, and aminoglycosides, and most were resistant to clindamycin, erythromycin, and tetracycline.[586] In the report from Tumbarello et al., the *C. striatum* isolate was susceptible to vancomycin, teicoplanin, rifampin, and tetracycline, but was resistant to all β-lactam antibiotics (including imipenem), all the aminoglycosides, the fluoroquinolones, erythromycin, and clindamycin.[897]

CORYNEBACTERIUM UREALYTICUM

C. urealyticum was formerly called CDC coryneform group D-2; in 1992, the name *Corynebacterium urealyticum* was formally proposed and adopted.[8,9,686] DNA restriction digestion of clinical and reference strains and rRNA gene probe studies have shown that this species represents a unique taxon among the coryneforms.[727] Normally a saprophytic organism found on the skin, this species has been associated with acute and chronic urinary tract infections, urolithiasis, renal cysts, and ureteral stenosis.[229,628,649,810,824,825,830] This organism causes similar infections in dogs as well.[239,851] *C. urealyticum* is highly associated with a clinical condition called **alkaline encrusted cystitis.** The latter is a chronic condition seen in compromised hosts with preexisting bladder injury, where ulcerative inflammation results from the deposition of ammonium-magnesium phosphate crystals (struvite; $MgNH_4PO_4 \cdot 6H_2O$) and apatite crystals ($Ca[OH][PO_4]_3$) on the bladder wall.[336] This condition is caused by organisms that are able to rapidly split urea, such as *Proteus* species. Pyelonephritis caused by *C. urealyticum* is seen primarily in immunocompromised patients and in patients who have undergone kidney transplantation and have had postsurgical complications.[8,229] In addition to its role as a urinary tract pathogen, *C. urealyticum* has also been isolated occasionally from blood cultures and as a cause of bacteremia, endocarditis, pericarditis, osteomyelitis, and wound/soft-tissue infections.[150,243,269,650,753,829,964]

C. urealyticum is a lipophilic coryneform that grows slowly on SBA, producing small (<0.5 mm in diameter after 24 hours of incubation) gray, nonhemolytic colonies on SBA. It is pyrazinamidase- and alkaline phosphatase–positive, asaccharolytic, and rapidly urease-positive. Urea agar slants begin to turn positive immediately on inoculation. *C. urealyticum* strains are usually multiply resistant to β-lactam, aminoglycoside, and macrolide antimicrobial agents; occasional strains may be β-lactam-susceptible.[325,634,986] Fluoroquinolones show irregular activity, with ofloxacin being the most active agent.[827] Doxycycline, rifampin, and the glycopeptide antibiotics vancomycin and teicoplanin are the most active agents against this bacterial species. Isolates that are resistant to the quinolones and rifampin may be selected during therapy with these drugs. PCR approaches for identification of *C. urealyticum* have also been described.[810] Ribotyping appears to be the most useful tool for strain characterization of *C. urealyticum* isolates.[634]

Corynebacterium Species Associated With Animals

Some *Corynebacterium* species have been isolated from animals, in which they may constitute part of the normal flora or be a cause of an infectious process. As mentioned previously, *C. pseudotuberculosis* is primarily an animal isolate that may occasionally cause disease in humans who have contact with infected animals or animal products (e.g., unpasteurized milk).[608,672] *C. bovis* is a part of the normal flora of the bovine udder and has also been implicated as a cause of mastitis in these animals. This organism is a rare cause of human infections (see above). *C. kutscheri* is a known pathogen of experimental rats and mice, in which it may cause rapidly progressive and fatal illnesses.[117] In these animals, the organism may be recovered

from the oral cavity and from the regional lymph nodes. In order to ascertain the presence of this organism in colonies of experimental rodents, nucleic acid probes have been developed to detect the organism in touch blots prepared from lymph node biopsy specimens of the animals.[763] Although two reports of *C. kutscheri* infections in humans have appeared in the literature (chorioamnionitis and septic arthritis), the organisms were incompletely characterized so there is doubt about the validity of the identifications.[276,604] *C. vitaruman* was originally isolated from the rumen of a cow and was first called *Flavobacterium vitaruman*. This organism is believed to participate in the synthesis of the vitamin B complex, especially production of riboflavin, in the rumen. It has not been isolated from humans.

The "*C. renale* group," which includes *C. renale, C. cystiditis,* and *C. pilosum,* causes genitourinary tract disease in cattle and other animals.[506,974] No cases of human infections due to either *C. renale* or *C. cystiditis* have been reported. *C. pilosum* has been described in a human perirectal abscess and as a cause of prosthetic-valve endocarditis in a 79-year-old woman 8 years after aortic-valve replacement with a bovine pericardial bioprosthesis.[315,822] In these case reports, however, the descriptions of the colony morphology of these isolates did not correspond to that of the *C. pilosum* type strain, and the biochemical characteristics that were used for identifications were incomplete. The colonial morphologies described in these reports, and the fact that the isolates were often multiply resistant, suggest that *C. amycolatum* was the true isolate from these patients.

In recent years, several new *Corynebacterium* species that are found in animals have been described. *C. auriscanis* has been isolated from external otitis, pyoderma, and interdigital wounds of dogs.[171] This species is most closely related to *C. falsenii, C. jeikeium,* and *C. urealyticum,* and is both phylogenetically and phenotypically distinct. *C. mastiditis* and *C. camporealensis* were first described as causes of subclinical mastitis in sheep.[265,266] Both organisms have been isolated from milk specimens in Spain. *C. mastiditis* is a lipophilic species that is similar biochemically to *C. urealyticum* and *C. afermentans* subsp. *lipophilum* but is distinct from them based on chemotaxonomic characteristics and 16S rRNA gene sequence studies. *C. camporealensis* is nonlipophilic and most closely related phylogenetically to *C. striatum. C. capitovis* is a nonlipophilic species that was isolated from skin lesions on the head of a sheep.[168] *C. testudinoris* and *C. felinum* are new nonlipophilic species that have been isolated from necrotic lesions in the mouth of a tortoise and from lung tissue of a Scottish wildcat, respectively.[169] *C. phocae* is a nonlipophilic species that has been isolated from *Phoca vitulina,* the common seal.[663] Phylogenetically, this species is most closely related to *C. striatum, C. vitarumen,* and *C. flavescens. C. spheniscorum* and *C. sphenisci* are newly described nonlipophilic species that were isolated from the cloacae of wild penguins.[354,355] Lastly, *C. aquilae* is a new species that was isolated from the mouths of adult and juvenile Spanish Imperial eagles (*Aquila adalberti*) along with strains of *C. falsenii*.[267] The phenotypic properties for the identification of the more recently identified and

Table 14-11 Biochemical Characteristics of *Corynebacterium* Species Isolated From Animals

SPECIES	LIP REQ	HEMOL, SBA	NO3 RED	PYZ	AP	ESC	URE	GEL	CAMP TEST	GLU	MAL	SUC	MNTL	XYL
C. aquilae	−	−	−	+	+	−	−	−	−	+	−	−	−	−
C. auriscanis	−	−	−	−	+	V	−	−	−	+	−	−	−	−
C. bovis	+	−	−	V	+	−	−	−	−	+	−	−	−	−
C. camporealensis	−	−	−	+	+	−	−	−	+	+	−	−	−	−
C. capitovis	−	−	−	−	+	−	−	−	NA	+	−	−	−	−
C. felinum	−	−	−	+	−	−	−	−	NA	+	+	−	−	−
C. mastiditis	+	−	−	+	+	−	V	−	NA	−	−	−	−	−
C. phocae	−	−	−	+	+	−	V	−	NA	+	+	V	−	−
C. sphensci	−	−	+	+	−	−	−	−	−	+	+	−	−	−
C. spheniscorum	−	−	−	+	−	−	−	−	+	+	+	−	−	−
C. testudinoris	−	−	+	−	−	+	−	−	NA	+	+	+	−	−

See Table 14–9 for legend.

characterized *Corynebacterium* species from animals are found in Table 14-11.

Corynebacterium Species Isolated From Foods and the Environment

Several new and previously described *Corynebacterium* species are found in various food products and in the environment, but have not been isolated from human clinical specimens. *C. flavescens* was originally called *Microbacterium flavus* when described in 1919 and was formally transferred to the genus *Corynebacterium* in 1979. This organism has been isolated from cheese and other dairy products. *C. mooreparkense* and *C. casei* are new species that are found on the surfaces of smear-ripened cheese such as Limburger and Tilsit.[111] *C. ammoniagenes* is also found in foods, particularly as part of the microflora of brick cheeses.[900] *C. terpenotabidum* is an environmental species that is able to degrade the linear triterpene (C_{30}) squalene.[867] *C. glutamicum* (also called *C. lillium*), *C. callunae*, and *C. efficiens* are environmental corynebacteria that are used in industry because of their ability to produce large amounts of L-glutamic acid in the culture medium during aerobic growth.[286] The new species *C. glaucum* was isolated from a cosmetic dye specimen.[975]

Other Coryneform Bacteria

Other coryneform bacteria that have been isolated from human clinical specimens include pleomorphic gram-positive bacilli that form characteristic Chinese letters, V forms, and occasional coccoid forms on Gram staining. These species differ from recognized *Corynebacterium* species in several respects. Most of them lack *meso*-DAP as the diamino acid comprising the cross-linkages in the peptidoglycan structure and have other amino acids (e.g., L-lysine, L-ornithine) instead (Table 14-7).[315] Other components nor-

mally found in the corynebacterial cell wall, such as arabinose, galactose, and short chain mycolic acids may also be absent. The menaquinones present as part of the electron transport system also vary from group to group. In addition, some of the coryneform organisms are oxidative rather than fermentative with respect to carbohydrate metabolism. These bacteria have been recovered from several types of human clinical specimens, including blood, cerebrospinal fluid, urine, and other normally sterile body sites and fluids.[315]

Although some of the former CDC coryneform groups have been formally reclassified in the genus *Corynebacterium*, others have been found to belong to genera not previously associated with human pathology. Several research groups in the U.S. and Europe are currently working to unravel the complex taxonomic relationships among these disparate organisms using both genetic (e.g., DNA-DNA hybridization, 16S and 5S ribosomal RNA [rRNA]sequencing) and chemotaxonomic (e.g., cell wall, cellular fatty acid, cellular menaquinone analyses) approaches.[60,75,207,706] These methods have established that reliance on phenotypic characteristics alone may not be sufficient for identification of these organisms, and that molecular and chemotaxonomic analyses of subcellular components may be necessary to differentiate among organisms that have identical or similar phenotypic characteristics. Although these organisms are relatively uncommon isolates in the clinical laboratory, they are increasingly being recovered as nosocomial colonizers and occasional pathogens, particularly in immunocompromised patients.

Actinobaculum Species

Intensive examination of other ''*Actinomyces*-like'' strains from human clinical specimens has also resulted in the description of totally new genera and reclassification of existing *Actinomyces* species. Lawson and associates examined five strains of an unknown *Actinomyces*-like

LAC	MNE	ARAB	SORB	RIB	GLYG	AMYG	α-GAL	β-GAL	α-GLU	β-GLU	β-GUR	NAGA	PYR	LAP
–	+	–	–	+	–	–	–	–	–	–	–	–	–	+
–	NA	NA	NA	–	–	NA	–	–	–	–	–	–	+	+
–	NA	NA	NA	–	–	NA	–	V	–	–	–	–	NA	NA
–	NA	NA	NA	–	–	NA	–	–	–	–	–	–	–	+
–	NA	NA	NA	–	NA	NA	–	–	–	–	–	–	–	+
–	NA	NA	NA	+	NA	NA	–	–	+	–	–	NA	+	+
–	NA	NA	NA	–	–	NA	–	–	–	–	–	–	–	+
V	+	–	–	NA	–	–	–	–	+	–	–	–	NA	V
–	+	–	–	–	–	–	–	–	–	–	–	–	–	+
–	+	NA	NA	+	–	NA	–	–	–	–	–	NA	–	+w
–	NA	NA	NA	+	–	NA	–	–	V	+	–	–	–	+

organism that were recovered from human specimens (including blood) and found that they were distinct from previously described *Actinomyces* species.[522] The most closely related organism to these unknown strains was *Actinomyces suis*, and even this organism was phylogenetically divergent from other *Actinomyces* species that were examined.[556] Based on their genetic, chemotaxonomic, and biochemical data, these workers proposed a new genus, *Actinobaculum*, and species name, *Actinobaculum schaalii*, for the five previously undescribed human isolates from blood and urinary tract specimens and proposed that *Actinomyces suis* be reclassified as *Actinobaculum suis*.[522] *Actinobaculum* species are anaerobic or facultatively anaerobic, catalase-negative, gram-positive bacilli. Individual cells may be slightly curved or may exhibit branching. The principal products of glucose or maltose fermentation are lactic and acetic acids; *A. schaalii* produces succinate as well, and *A. suis* produces acetic and formic acids plus some ethanol from maltose fermentation (glucose is not fermented). Members of the genus do not reduce nitrate to nitrite, and esculin and gelatin are not hydrolyzed. Since the description of *A. schaalii* and the reclassification of *A. suis*, two additional *Actinobaculum* species—"*A. massiliae*" and *A. urinale*—have been isolated from urine specimens from patients with chronic urinary tract infections.[365,382] Phenotypic characteristics for identification of *Actinobaculum* species are included in Table 14-12.

Actinomyces Species Isolated From Humans

The genus *Actinomyces* is composed of a heterogeneous group of gram-positive, facultatively anaerobic or microaerophilic, non-spore-forming, non-acid-fast nonmotile bacilli. Some isolates display rudimentary branching. Many *Actinomyces* species are part of the oral microflora of humans and various animals. Some species, such as *A. israelii*, *A. gerencseriae*, *A. georgiae*, *A. odontolyticus*, and *A. naeslundii* are highly prevalent in both supragingival and subgingival plaque specimens from patients with adult periodontitis and

gingivitis. These same organisms also play a significant role in the development of root-surface caries.[106] *Actinomyces* species may cause classical actinomycosis, wound infections, abscesses, genital tract infections, and urinary tract infections. Genital tract infections, particular with *A. israelii*, are often associated with the presence of intrauterine contraceptive devices.[274,982] In the new *Bergey's Manual*, the genus *Actinomyces* is included in the new phylum Actinobacteria, class Actinobacteria, order Actinomycetales, family Actinomycetaceae along with *Actinobaculum*, *Arcanobacterium*, and *Mobiluncus* genera (Box 14-1).[329]

The genus *Actinomyces* has undergone rapid expansion over the past several years, with the description of several new species from both humans and animals. In the past, clinical laboratories have relied on conventional aerobic identification techniques and anaerobic bacteriology methods for identification, such as those presented in the *VPI Anaerobe Manual*, *Bergey's Manual of Systematic Bacteriology*, and the *Wadsworth Anaerobic Bacteriology Manual*.[422,467,767,771] Many laboratories use rapid enzymatic anaerobe identification kits (e.g., RapID ANA system) for identification of *Actinomyces* species, but these system do not perform well for identifying these organisms.[609] Santala and colleagues recently evaluated the RapID ANA II (Remel), the RapID CB-Plus (Remel), the BBL Crystal ANR ID (BD Microbiology Systems, Cockeysville, MD) and the RapID 32A (BioMerieux, Inc.) for their ability to identify "classical" and newly described *Actinomyces* species.[765] These kits correctly identified only 26% to 65% of the "classical" *Actinomyces* strains to the species level, and only 13% to 49% of newly described species to the genus level, indicating that the data bases of these systems need to be updated. The facultative nature of most *Actinomyces* species has resulted in the inclusion of some species in the databases of identification systems for facultative and anaerobic bacteria, such as the API Coryne, the API Rapid ID32A, and the API Rapid ID32 Strep (all from BioMérieux). Some of the descriptions of new *Actinomyces* species are based on biochemical reactions obtained with

Table 14-12 Biochemical Characteristics for Identification of *Actinobaculum* Species

CHARACTERISTIC	A. SCHAALII	A. SUIS	A. MASSILIAE	A. URINALE
Colony morphology/ pigment	Small, gray-white	White, granular, entire or irregular edges, raised center	Small, gray, entire	Small, gray-white, convex, entire, smooth
Hemolysis, SBA	−	−	−	β
Pyrazinamidase	V	NA	+	−
Alkaline phosphatase	−	+	−	−
Urease	−	+	−	V+
Arginine dihydrolase	−	NA	−	−
Hippurate hydrolysis	+	NA	+	+
Acetoin (VP)	−	−	NA	−
LAP	NA	NA	−	−
CAMP test	+w	NA	NA	NA
PYR	V	NA		NA
α-GAL	−	NA	−	−
β-GAL	−	+	−	−
α-GLU	+	+	+	
β-GLU	−	NA	NA	−
β-GUR	−	+	−	+
NAGA	−	NA	−	−
Acid produced from:				
Glucose	+	−	+	+
Maltose	+	V	+	V
Sucrose	V	−	NA	V
Mannitol	−	−	−	−
Xylose	+	−	+	
Lactose	−	−	NA	−
Mannose	V	−	−	−
Arabinose	V	−	NA	
Sorbitol	−	−	−	−
Raffinose	−	−	+w	−
Ribose	+	NA	+	+
Trehalose	V	−	+	−
Glycogen	−	+	+	−
Melibiose	−	−	NA	−
Melezitose	−	−	NA	−
Products, glucose fermentation	A, S	A, f, EtOH (from maltose)	NA	L, a

these systems, and the resulting biocodes are included as part of the phenotypic descriptions in the publications. Gas-liquid chromatography for detection of volatile and nonvolatile products of glucose fermentation is extremely helpful for identification, since Gram-positive, non-spore-forming bacilli that produce major amounts of succinic acid can be placed in the genus *Actinomyces* without further testing. Since new species are now validated by genotypic, molecular approaches, GLC data are not available for many recently described species. Because of the

difficulties with phenotypic identification, genus- and species-specific DNA probes have been developed by many researchers, particularly for investigating the role of these bacteria in periodontal disease.[871,972] *Actinomyces* species can also be identified by molecular methods such as 16S rDNA PCR and restriction-fragment-length polymorphism analysis.[387,768] However, none of these molecular techniques are available to the routine clinical laboratory. Box 14-3 describe the *Actinomyces* species that have been isolated from humans, while those species isolated from

Box 14-3 **Members of the Genus _Actinomyces_**

Species	Clinical Significance and Identification
Actinomyces bovis	_A. bovis_ causes actinomycosis in cattle and other animals. This organism has not been isolated from human infections, however, a recent case of _A. bovis_ bacteremia in a human was reported by Bernard et al. (in press). This organism was confirmed with phenotypic, chemotaxonomic, and genotypic approaches. On the API Coryne, this isolate produced biocode number 0101104, indicating positive reactions for alkaline phosphatase, urease, glucose, and catalase.
Actinomyces cardiffensis	This new species has been isolated from human pleural fluid, a paracolonic abscess, a jaw abscess, a postmastoidectomy ear abscess, a sinus washout, and intrauterine devices.[381] On Gram stains, the organisms appear as slender, slightly curved rods with beaded, branching filaments. After 48 hours of incubation, colonies are small, convex, entire, and may be creamy to pinkish. _A. cardiffensis_ a facultative anaerobe that is catalase-negative and produces major amounts of succinic and lactic acids and small amounts of acetic acid from glucose fermentation. Esculin, urea, and gelatin are not hydrolyzed.
Actinomyces europaeus	This new species was described in 1997, when it was isolated as the sole organism or as the only aerobic organism recovered from human abscess material.[288] This organism has also been recovered from skin-related infections (e.g., pilonidal sinus infection, perianal abscesses, decubitus ulcers) and urinary tract infections.[754] On Gram-stained smears, this organism appears as short, gram-positive rods arranged in small clusters with no discernible branching. Colonies on SBA are small ($<$0.5 mm after 48 hours of incubation in CO_2), gray, and translucent. This organism is catalase-negative, nonmotile, and ferments glucose and maltose but not mannitol or xylose. Some strains of this organism also hydrolyze esculin and gelatin, but these reactions are delayed. Nitrate is not reduced to nitrite and urease is not produced. As with other _Actinomyces_ species, succinic acid is produced as the major product of glucose fermentation.
Actinomyces funkei	This recently described species was originally recovered from blood cultures, a sternal wound culture, and a human abdominal incision, and was recently reported as a cause of native tricuspid-valve endocarditis.[524,949] These isolates were originally identified as strains of _A. turicensis_, but certain phenotypic traits and 16S rRNA sequencing showed that this organism was closely related to but not identical with _A. turicensis_. Cells of _A. funkei_ are gram-positive, slender, slightly curved, and exhibit some branching. Growth occurs under both aerobic and anaerobic conditions. On SBA, colonies are small, nonhemolytic, and gray after 24 hours of incubation. Acid is produced from glucose, sucrose, and xylose, but not from arabinose, mannitol, glycogen, raffinose, sorbitol, or trehalose. Hippurate is hydrolyzed, but esculin and gelatin are not. On the API Coryne system, the original isolate produced biocode numbers 0130761 or 3530761, indicating the variability of the pyrazinamidase, nitrate reductase, and β-galactosidase reactions on the strip.
Actinomyces georgiae	_A. georgiae_ was described in 1990 and is found as a part of the normal flora of the gingival crevices of adults and children. Strains of this species are facultatively anaerobic. On Gram stains, this species appears as rods that occur in pairs or short chains; cells may also have swellings along their length and branching is seldom seen.[458] In older broth cultures, cells may have a coccoid appearance. After 48 hours of anaerobic incubation, colonies are 1 mm in diameter, circular, entire, shiny, and smooth with entire edges. Colonies may be white, tan, or beige. The organism is catalase-negative, and succinic, acetic, formic, and small amounts of lactic acid are produced from glucose fermentation. Acid is produced from a variety of carbohydrates, including glucose, maltose, sucrose, xylose, trehalose, and glycogen. The majority of strains hydrolyze esculin and do not reduce nitrate to nitrite.
Actinomyces gerencseriae	This species was described in 1990 and was formerly called _A. israelii_ serotype II.[458] However, it is genetically unrelated to the type strain of _A. israelii_. _A. gerencseriae_ is found in the human oral cavity and in the gingival crevices. About 12% of isolates are obligately anaerobic, while the remainder produce scant to moderate growth on blood agar incubated in 5–7% CO_2. On Gram stains, the organisms appear as filamentous cells with occasional swellings and branching. After 48 hours of incubation under anaerobic conditions, colonies are about 0.2 mm in diameter, white, opaque, nonhemolytic, and may have a "lumpy" topography. This species is catalase-negative, esculin hydrolysis–positive, gelatin hydrolysis–negative, and produces acid from a variety of carbohydrates, including glucose, maltose, mannose, sucrose, and trehalose. Lactic, succinic, formic, and acetic acids are produced by glucose fermentation.

(Continued)

Box 14-3 *Continued*

Species	Clinical Significance and Identification
Actinomyces graevenitzii	The original report of this new species described four human isolates, three of which were from respiratory tract specimens, while the fourth was isolated from the jaw of a patient with osteitis.[704] These isolates were gram-positive, nonmotile, slightly curved rods with some branching and occasional swollen ends. Colonies on SBA are very small (0.2 mm in diameter after 24 hours of incubation) and are adherent to the agar, particular on primary isolation. This species is catalase-negative, does not hydrolyze esculin, urea, or hippurate, and does not reduce nitrate to nitrite. This species is also strongly N-acetyl-β-D-glucosaminidase-positive on the API Coryne strip, which helps to differentiate it from the other closely related *Actinomyces* species. Succinic and lactic acids constitute the end products of glucose fermentation.
Actinomyces hongkongensis	This novel species, described in 2003, was isolated from purulent material of a patient with pelvic actinomycosis.[962] This species is strictly anaerobic, grows on SBA as pinpoint, non-hemolytic colonies, and is catalase-negative. By 16S rRNA gene sequencing, this species is most closely related to *A. maramammalium*, which has been isolated from seals and porpoises.
Actinomyces houstonensis	This human species originated with three isolates from serious subcutaneous abscesses that required drainage.[162] *A. houstonensis* is a facultative anaerobe, producing α-hemolytic, gray colonies that are about 0.2 mm in diameter after 48 hours of incubation at 35–37°C. The cells are pleomorphic gram-positive rods that tend to form half-circles. The organism is catalase-negative and does not hydrolyze esculin, urea, or gelatin. Nitrate is reduced to nitrite and acid is produced from glucose and sucrose, but not from xylose.
Actinomyces israelii	*A. israelii* is the actinomycotic agent most frequently associated with classical cervicofacial actinomycosis. This organism can also cause musculoskeletal infections associated with adjacent soft-tissue infections, trauma, and hematogenous dissemination.[535] Infections of prosthetic joints following bacteremia with *A. israelii* have also been reported.[985] This organism is primarily anaerobic, with facultative growth in a CO_2-enriched atmosphere only occurring after repeated subcultures. Colonies of *A. israelii* may resemble a molar tooth, are nonhemolytic on SBA, and are not pigmented. This species is catalase-negative, esculin hydrolysis–positive, and most strains reduce nitrate to nitrite. Acid is produced from glucose, maltose, sucrose, raffinose, xylose, lactose, and trehalose.
Actinomyces meyeri	*A. meyeri* is an obligately anaerobic species that has been associated with a variety of human infections, including thoracic and disseminated actinomycosis; pneumonia; brain, cutaneous and splenic abscesses; endocarditis; funisitis; chorioamnionitis; and osteomyelitis.[32,177,327,437,537,657,913,967] Colonies on blood agar are white and nonpigmented. Strains of *A. meyeri* are catalase-negative, do not hydrolyze esculin, and do not reduce nitrate. The CAMP test is positive, and some strains also produce urease. Acid is produced from glucose, maltose, sucrose, and xylose, and some strains will also ferment glycerol and glycogen. Mannitol, trehalose, raffinose, and mannose are not fermented.
Actinomyces naeslundii	*A. naeslundii* is found in the human oropharynx and is a rare cause of cervicofacial actinomycosis, intrauterine device (IUD)–associated endocervical actinomycosis, septic arthritis, periodontal disease, and other infections.[387,532,971] *A. naeslundii* strains are divided into genospecies I and II, both of which are facultative anaerobes. Group I strains are usually catalase-negative, may or may not reduce nitrate to nitrite, and are CAMP test–negative, while group II strains are usually catalase-positive, reduce nitrate to nitrite, and are CAMP test–positive. Both groups hydrolyze esculin, ferment a variety of carbohydrates, and are urease-positive. Colonies on blood agar are nonpigmented.
Actinomyces nasicola	This species was originally isolated from pus that was aspirated from the antrum of a patient undergoing a routine nasal polypectomy.[386] On Gram stains, this organism appears as coryneform gram-positive bacilli, with some branching and coccoid forms being evident as well. The organism is facultatively anaerobic and catalase-negative; acetic, lactic and succinic acid are produced as products of glucose fermentation. Esculin, gelatin, and starch are not hydrolyzed and urease is not produced. Acid is produced from fructose and cellobiose, but not from glucose, maltose, sucrose, ribose, xylose, lactose, mannitol, or amygdalin.

Box 14-3 *Continued*

Species	Clinical Significance and Identification
Actinomyces neuii subsp. *neuii* and *Actinomyces neuii* subsp. *anitratus*	These *Actinomyces* species were described in 1994 and encompass former members of CDC coryneform group 1 and "group 1–like" strains that were recovered from a variety of clinical specimens, including cerebrospinal shunt fluid, ear cultures, vitreous fluids, mammary gland abscesses, furuncles, and blood.[301] Group 1 strains were α-hemolytic on human blood agar, reduced nitrate to nitrite, were unable to ferment adonitol, and were alkaline phosphatase–negative, while the group 1–like strains were nonhemolytic, failed to reduce nitrate to nitrite, fermented adonitol, and were alkaline phosphatase-positive. Both groups of organisms grew under both aerobic and strictly anaerobic conditions. Cell wall analysis showed that these isolates lacked *meso*-DAP and mycolic acids in their cell walls. Analysis of volatile and nonvolatile fatty acids showed that succinic acid was the major end product of glucose fermentation for both groups of organisms, and examination of fatty acid methyl esters revealed that the cell walls contained C16:0, C18:1cis-9, and C18:0 fatty acid methyl esters as their major cell wall constituents. These data suggested a phylogenetic relationship between CDC group 1 and group 1-like strains and *Actinomyces* species.[301,771] Subsequently, 16S rRNA gene sequences of these organisms were determined and found to support the inclusion of CDC group 1 and group 1–like isolates in the genus *Actinomyces*. In 1994, CDC group 1 and group 1–like strains were formally proposed as *Actinomyces neuii* subsp. *neuii* and *Actinomyces neuii* subsp. *anitratus*, respectively.[313] Since the deposition of this coryneform in the genus *Actinomyces*, this species has been associated with chorioamnionitis and neonatal sepsis, fatal bacteremia in a nonimmunocompromised host, postoperative endophthalmitis, and infection of a mammary prosthesis.[118,314,328,576] Both *A. neuii* subsp. *neuii* and *A. neuii* subsp. *nitratus* are catalase-positive, nonhemolytic gram-positive bacilli. Colonies are circular, smooth, convex, and white with entire edges; subsp. *neuii* is α-hemolytic on SBA, while subsp. *anitratus* is nonhemolytic. These organisms are very active fermenters and produce acid from glucose, maltose, sucrose, mannitol, lactose, mannose, trehalose, and xylose. Both species produce leucine arylamidase, α-galactosidase, β-galactosidase, and α-glucosidase, and both are CAMP test–positive. *A. neuii* subsp. *neuii* reduces nitrate to nitrite, while subsp. *anitratus* is negative for this characteristic. Rare strains of *A. neuii* may be catalase-negative.[118]
Actinomyces odontolyticus	This species is found in the human oropharynx in association with the gingival crevices and deep carious lesions. This organism is also a rare cause of bacteremia, thoracopulmonary infections, lung abscesses, soft-tissue infections, and IUD-associated pelvic actinomycosis.[62,180,545,823,869,962] This species is catalase-negative, produces pinkish colonies on SBA, and forms red colonies on brain-heart infusion agar. Nitrate is reduced to nitrite, and urease is not produced. Acid is produced from glucose, maltose, and sucrose, and some strains also ferment glycerol, glycogen, and xylose.
Actinomyces oricola	This new species, like *A. radicidentis* (see below), was isolated originally from a dental abscess.[384] This species includes gram-positive rods that display both branching and filament formation. The organism is facultatively anaerobic, catalase-negative, and produces pinpoint colonies on SBA after 48 hours of incubation. GLC analysis of spent glucose broth cultures reveals the formation of acetic, lactic, and succinic acids. On the API Coryne strip, acid is produced from glucose, maltose, and sucrose only and produced a biocode number of 2550121, indicating positive reactions for pyrazinamidase, alkaline phosphatase, esculin hydrolysis, α-glucosidase, and β-galactosidase.
Actinomyces radicidentis	*A. radicidentis* is a new species that has been isolated in pure cultures from infected root canals in humans.[170,476] These isolates were gram-positive, catalase-positive, coccoid to coccobacillary in morphology, and grew under both aerobic and anaerobic conditions. Colonies on SBA may produce a pink pigment. This species is fermentatively active, producing acid from glucose, maltose, mannitol, lactose, ribose, and sucrose on the API Coryne. This species hydrolyzes esculin, and reduction of nitrate and production of urease are variable characteristics. Sequencing

(Continued)

Box 14-3 *Continued*

Species	Clinical Significance and Identification
	of the 16S rRNA of this organism confirmed close relatedness to *A. slackii*, *A. bovis*, *A. bowdenii*, *A. naeslundii*, and *A. viscosus*.[170] This organism is probably a previously unrecognized member of the normal indigenous oral microflora of humans.
Actinomyces radingae	CDC group E organisms were originally described as "*A. pyogenes*-like" bacteria that have been recovered from a variety of human clinical sources including middle ear specimens, empyema fluid, pilonidal cysts, perianal abscesses, blood cultures, urine cultures, and decubitus ulcers.[969] Initially it was thought that these organisms were aerotolerant strains of the anaerobic organism *Bifidobacterium adolescentis* that differed in their aerobic growth and in the volatile and nonvolatile end products produced from glucose fermentation.[375] Using genetic and chemotaxonomic approaches, Wust and colleagues found that these strains were closely related to *Actinomyces* species and proposed two new species in the genus *Actinomyces: Actinomyces radingae* and *Actinomyces turicensis*.[970] Vandamme and associates subsequently used whole-cell protein electrophoresis, fatty acid analysis, biochemical phenotypic tests (i.e., API Coryne and the IDS Rapid ANA panel) and species-specific oligonucleotide probes to characterize a group of unidentified, catalase-negative coryneform bacteria.[906] These workers found that the organisms formed two clusters that corresponded to *A. turicensis* and *A. radingae*, respectively. These analyses enabled the publication of emended descriptions of these *A. pyogenes*-like isolates from human clinical specimens.[906] Using species-specific oligonucleotide probes for *A. turicensis* and *A. radingae*, Sabbe and colleagues examined 294 "actinomyces-like" isolates from human clinical specimens collected over a 7-year period and found that *A. radingae* is primarily associated with skin-related infections (e.g., skin abscesses, pilonidal cysts, perianal abscesses).[754] Isolates of *A. radingae* are facultative, catalase-negative, gram-positive bacilli. After 48 hours of incubation, colonies on SBA are small, gray, convex, and circular with a butyrous consistency. Most strains are α-hemolytic. Esculin is hydrolyzed, but gelatin and urea are not. Nitrate is not reduced to nitrite and the CAMP test is negative. Acid is produced from glucose, maltose, sucrose, lactose, xylose and ribose, but not from mannitol or glycogen. With enzymatic tests on the API Coryne, *A. radingae* produces α-glucosidase, β-glucosidase, α-galactosidase, β-galactosidase, and *N*-acetyl-β-D-glucosaminidase, but does not produce leucine arylamidase, pyrrolidonyl arylamidase, alkaline phosphatase, or β-glucuronidase. *A. radingae* isolates are susceptible to penicillin, cephalosporins, erythromycin, and tetracyclines.[906]
Actinomyces turicensis	*A. turicensis* is found mainly in genital tract infections, skin-related infections, and urinary tract infections, and some isolates have been recovered from appendiceal tissue, hepatic abscess, head/neck infections, and blood.[735,754] On Gram stain, cells of *A. turicensis* are straight, slightly curved, or club-shaped. Colonies on SBA are small, gray, convex, and entire after 48 hours of incubation in a CO_2 atmosphere. The organism is catalase-negative, does not hydrolyze esculin, urea, or gelatin, does not reduce nitrate to nitrite, and is CAMP test–negative. Acid is produced from glucose, maltose, sucrose, xylose, ribose, and trehalose, but lactose and mannitol are not fermented. On the API Coryne, α-glucosidase is detected, but the other enzymatic tests are negative. *A. turicensis* is broadly susceptible to a variety of agents, including penicillin, cephalosporins, erythromycin, and doxycycline.[906]
Actinomyces urogenitalis	Isolates of this new species were originally recovered from urine, vaginal discharge, and urethral cultures.[636] These organisms are facultative, regular gram-positive, catalase-negative rods. This species produces acid from glucose, maltose, sucrose, lactose, and xylose, and some strains also ferment mannitol and ribose. Nitrate is reduced to nitrite and esculin is hydrolyzed, but gelatin, urea, and hippurate are not. This species is believed to be a commensal of the human vagina and it is not yet recognized as a cause of urogenital tract disease.
Actinomyces viscosus	*A. viscosus* is found in the oral cavity of human and animals. This species is a catalase-positive, gram-positive rod. Colonies on SBA are small and nonhemolytic after growth for 48 hours. Esculin and urea are hydrolyzed, and nitrate is reduced to nitrite. Acid is produced from glucose and sucrose, and some strains produce acid from xylose as well.

animals are described briefly below. The phenotypic data presented in Table 14-13 include both humans and animal isolates and represent a synthesis of phenotypic characteristics and descriptions from several sources.[422,467,771] Sarconeme and coworkers also published a dichotomous flow chart for assistance in identifying *Actinomyces, Arcanobacterium*, and *Actinobaculum* species using readily available reagents (e.g., Rosco reagent tablets, Rosco, Taastrup, Denmark).[767] These flow charts are presented in Fig. 14-3.

A. israelii is the most common cause of actinomycosis in humans, although other species (i.e., *A. meyeri, A. naeslundii, A. odontolyticus, A. gerencseriae*, and *A. viscosus*) may also occasionally cause this infection.[697] Actinomycosis is a chronic infection characterized by abscess formation, draining sinus tracts, and tissue fibrosis. Because of their chronic nature, actinomycotic infections frequently mimic carcinomas.[223,436] Clinical forms of actinomycosis include cervicofacial actinomycosis, thoracic actinomycosis, abdominal/pelvic actinomycosis, and central nervous system (CNS) actinomycosis.[816] **Cervicofacial actinomycosis** is associated with poor dentition, dental manipulations, and other head-and-neck infections (e.g., otitis, mastoiditis).[12] At least nine different *Actinomyces* species can cause this infection, although *A. israelii* and *A. gerencseriae* predominate.[697] In most cases, endogenous oral *Actinomyces* are introduced by some sort of trauma and begin to grow in the head and neck tissues to form an acute, pyogenic abscess that may evolve into an indurated submandibular mass with one or more draining sinus tracts. Microcolonies of the organisms called sulfur granules are discharged from these sinus tracts. **Thoracic actinomycosis** occurs as an extension of cervicofacial infection into the chest and mediastinal region, as a result of aspiration of oropharyngeal contents, or as an extension of an abdominal/pelvic infection that has spread retroperitoneally or transdiaphragmatically.[874] The infection presents initially as an aspiration pneumonitis, with the eventual development of cavitations or lung masses. Symptoms include cough, chest pain, and low-grade fever, and chest x-ray films may reveal fibronodular or cavitary lesions with accompanying pleural effusions or empyema.[489] Pulmonary infection may also extend to involve the bones (i.e., ribs, sternum, shoulder girdle), chest wall muscles, and soft tissues.[62] **Abdominal actinomycosis** results from penetrating trauma, colonic perforation, or following gastrointestinal tract surgery. Usually, the ileocecal region of the colon is involved, and the infection may remain localized or may spread hematogenously or by direct extension.[158] Anorectal actinomycosis may originate in an infected anal crypt, fissure, or abscess or by direct extension from an intraabdominal location. Infection of the kidney, liver, and spleen may rarely occur via direct extension from an abdominal focus or via the bloodstream. **Pelvic actinomycosis** may result from contiguous spread of abdominal actinomycosis or may originate in the pelvis itself. This infection is associated with intrauterine contraceptive devices that become colonized with actinomyces organisms.[274,962] This leads to endometrial infection with extension to the ovaries. **CNS actinomycosis** occurs as a result of hematogenous dissemination or by direct extension from actinomycotic infections in the head/neck areas.[816] Patients usually present with a chronic meningitis or meningoencephalitis complicated by the development of subdural empyema, epidural and spinal abscesses, and cranial osteo-

myelitis. In 75% of cases, CNS actinomycosis presents with single or multiple brain abscesses, usually in the temporal or frontal lobes.[816,817] Patients may have a chronic meningitis picture that resembles tuberculous meningitis. CSF usually shows a mononuclear pleocytosis, elevated protein, and normal or low glucose concentrations. Interestingly, fever is usually present in only about half of patients with CNS actinomycosis.

Actinomyces Species Isolated From Animals

Many *Actinomyces* species, including several recently described genera, are animal pathogens. As mentioned above, *A. bovis* is a cause of bovine actinomycosis. *A. hordeovulneris, A. canis, A. catuli*, and *A. coleocanis* are found in the vaginas of dogs, and *A. bowdenii* has been isolated from cutaneous infections of both dogs and cats.[429,430,433,664] *A. hordeovulneris* and *A. denticolens* are also found in the gingival crevices of cats.[555] *A. hordeovulneris* has been associated with canine actinomycosis, pyogranulomatous pleuritis, peritonitis, pericarditis, and septic arthritis.[675] *A. hyovaginalis* is found in the genital tract of pigs and has been recovered from purulent genital tract and pulmonary lesions in these animals.[1,175] The new species *A. suimastiditis* was originally isolated from a pig with mastitis.[432] *A. howellii, A. denticolens, A. slackii*, and *A. vaccimaxillae* are found in the oropharynges of cows; the latter species was originally recovered from a jaw lesion of a cow.[214,383,698] *A. marimammalium* has been isolated from marine mammals, including seals and porpoises.[434] Table 14-13 contains the phenotypic characteristics for all of the *Actinomyces* species.

Arcanobacterium Species

Arcanobacterium species are facultative gram-positive bacilli that may be slightly curved and may show rudimentary branching along with Chinese letter and V forms. Unlike *Corynebacterium* species, these organisms are catalase-negative, do not possess cell wall mycolic acids, and contain L-lysine and L-ornithine rather than *meso*-DAP as the peptidoglycan diamino acid. The genus *Arcanobacterium* currently includes six species: *A. haemolyticum, A. pyogenes, A. bernardiae, A. phocae, A. pluranimalium*, and *A. hippocoleae*.[174,431,523,705] *A. haemolyticum, A. pyogenes*, and *A. bernardiae* were formerly members of the genus *Corynebacterium* and subsequently the genus *Actinomyces* before 16S rRNA sequence analysis established their membership in the genus *Arcanobacterium*.[174,705,710] *A. phocae* has been isolated from seals and other marine animals, while *A. pluranimalium* has been recovered from porpoises and deer.[523,705] The newest member of the genus, *A. hippocoleae*, has only been isolated from the vaginal secretions of a horse.[431]

A. haemolyticum is associated with acute pharyngitis in humans.[480,930] Cervical lymphadenopathy, tonsillitis, and rash frequently may accompany the infection.[567] Because of the rash, patients may be thought to have scarlet fever. Extensive pharyngeal "pseudomembranes" resembling those seen with diphtheria have also been noted in some patients.[359] *A. haemolyticum* pharyngitis usually occurs in children and young adults (i.e., 10- to 30-year-old age group). *A. haemolyticum* has also been recovered from

Table 14-13A Biochemical Characteristics for Identification of *Actinomyces* Species Isolated From Humans and Animals

SPECIES	CAT	COLONY MORPHOLOGY PIGMENTATION	HEMOL SBA	NO₃ RED	PYZ	AP	ESC	URE	ADH
A. bovis	−	Smooth or granular with dark centers, white, entire	−/β	−	NA	−	V+	−	NA
A. bowdenii	+	Small, grayish-white	−	+	+	V	+	−	−
A. canis	+	Not given	−	−	+^w	−	−	−	−
A. cardiffensis	−	Small, convex, entire, cream-to-pink		V					
A. catuli	V	Small, convex, white, adherent	−	+	+	−	+	−	V
A. coleocanis	−	Not given	−	−	+^w	−	−	−	−
A. denticolens	−	Entire, convex or umbonate, smooth, slight pink pigment	−	+	NA	−	+	NA	NA
A. europaeus	−	Small, grayish, translucent	−/β^w	−	−	−	V	−	NA
A. funkei	−	Small, gray	−	V	V	+	−	−	−
A. georgiae	−	Small, circular, entire, convex	−	V−	NA	NA	+^−	−	NA
A. gerencseriae	−	Small, circular, convex	V	V−	NA	NA	+	−	NA
A. graevenitzii	−	Small, adherent, slightly pink on SBA	−	−	NA	NA			NA
A. hongkongensis	−	Small, pinpoint	−	−	NA	+	−	−	+
A. hordeovulneris	+^w	White, adherent, domed, butter consistency	−	−	V	−	+	−	NA
A. howellii	+	White, smooth, convex, entire	NA	−	+	+	+	−	+
A. hyovaginalis	−	Flat with outrunning edges	−	V	−	+	+	−	−
A. houstoniensis	−	Small, gray, convex	−	+	NA	−	−	−	NA
A. israelii	−	Rough, heaped, "molar tooth," white to gray white	−	V+	NA	NA	+	−	NA
A. marimammalium	−	Small, gray, entire, convex	−	−	−	V	−	−	−
A. meyeri	−	Small, flat to convex, white, shiny, smooth	−	V−	NA	−	−	V	NA
A. naeslundii genospecies 1	V−	Smooth, circular, convex, umbonate	−	V+	+	−	+	+	−
A. naeslundii genospecies 2	V+	Smooth, circular, convex, umbonate	−	+	+	+^w	+	+	−
A. nasicola	−	Pinpoint, gray-white, opaque, entire	−	−	NA	−	V	−	V
A. neuii subsp. neuii	+	Circular, small, convex, opaque	α	+	+	−	−	−	NA
A. neuii subsp. anitratus	+	Circular, small, convex, opaque	−	−	+	V	−	−	NA
A. odontolyticus	−	Small, pink pigment on SBA, red on BHI	−	+	NA	−	V	−	−
A. oricola	−	Pinpoint, bread-crumb-like, white	−	−	+	V	+	−	−
A. radicidentis	+	Pink pigment, small entire	−	V	+	−	+^w	V	−
A. radingae	−	Small, gray, convex, circular, opaque	α/β^w	−	V	−	+	−	NA
A. slackii	+	Small, gray, opaque	−	+	V	−	+	V−	
A. suimastitidis	−	Not described	−	−	+^w	V	+	−	−
A. turicensis	−	Small, gray, opaque, entire	β^w	−	−	−	−	−	NA
A. urogenitalis	−	Not described	−	+	−	V	+	−	−
A. vaccimaxillae	−	Small, white, opaque, entire	−	−	+	+	+	−	−
A. viscosus serotype 1	+	Small, entire smooth, circular	−	V	−	−	+	+	−
A. viscosus serotype 2	+	Small, smooth, circular entite	−	V	+	−	V	V	V

+, positive reaction; −, negative reaction; +w, weak or delayed positive reaction; V, variable reaction; V+, variable, most strains positive; V−, variable, NO₃ Red, reduction of nitrate to nitrite; PYZ, pyrazinamidase; AP, alkaline phosphatase; ESC, esculin hydrolysis; URE, urea hydrolysis; ADH, arginine producing S. aureus; α-GAL, α-galactosidase; β-GAL, β-galactosidase; α-GLU, α-glucosidase; β-GLU, β-glucosidase; β-GUR, β-glucuronidase; Mne, mannose; Arab, arabinose; Sorb, sorbitol; Raff, raffinose; Tre, trehalose; Glycg, glycogen; Amyg, amygdalin; Meli, melibose; Melez, melezitose;

GEL	LAP	PYR	CAMP TEST	α-GAL	β-GAL	α-GLU	β-GLU	β-GUR	NAGA	HIPP	ACETOIN
−	+	NA	NA	−	−	−	−	−	+	−	−
−	+	NA	NA	+	+	V	+	−	−	−	−
−	+	−	NA	+	+	+	−	−	+	−	−
	+	−	NA	−	−	+	−	−	−	−	−
−	+	+	NA	V	+	+	+	+	V	−	−
−	NA	−	NA	−	+	+	−	−	−	−	NA
NA	+	NA	NA	V	+	+	V	−	−	−	NA
+sl	+	−	−	+	+	+	−	−	−	NA	NA
−	+	−	+	−	V	+	−	−	V	+	−
V	NA	NA	−	NA	+	+	NA	NA	−	NA	NA
V−	NA	NA	−	NA	+	+	NA	NA	−	NA	NA
−	+	−	−	−	+	−	−	−	+	−	NA
−	+	NA	NA	−	−	−	−	−	−	NA	NA
+w	NA	V	NA	+	NA	+	V	−	+	NA	NA
−	NA	NA	NA	NA	NA	NA	+	−	+	NA	NA
−	+	−	NA	V	+	+	+	−	NA	−	−
−	NA	−	NA	NA	NA	+	NA	NA	NA	NA	NA
−	NA	NA	−	NA	+	+	NA	NA	−	NA	NA
−	+	−	NA	−	+	−	−	−	+	−	NA
−	+	NA	+	−	V	+	−	−	V	−	−
−	+	NA	−	V	+	+	+	−	−	−	−
−	+	NA	+	V	V	+	+	−	−	NA	NA
−	+	−	NA	−	+	+	V	−	+	NA	−
−	+	NA	+	+	+	+	−	−	−	NA	NA
−	+	NA	+	+	+	+	−	−	−	NA	NA
−	V	NA	−	−	+	V	V	−	−	−	−
−	−	NA	NA	+	V	+	+	−	−	−	−
+w	+	NA	−	+	+	+	+	−	−	−	+w
−/+w	−	−	−	+	+	+	+	−	+	NA	NA
V	NA	+	NA	+	NA	+	+	−	−	NA	NA
−	NA	NA	NA	+	+	+	+	−	V	−	+w
−	+	−	−	−	−	+	−	−	−	NA	NA
−	+	+	NA	+	+	+	+	−	+	NA	V
−	+	−	NA	−	−	+	−	−	−	−	−
−	+	NA	NA	−	V	V	+	−	−	−	−
−	+	NA	NA	−	V	V	+	−	−	−	−

most strains negative; NA, data not available; Cat, catalase; Fac, facultative; Ana, anaerobic; Cat, catalase; Hemol SBA, hemolysis on sheep blood agar; dihydrolase; MOT, motility; GEL, gelatin hydrolysis; LAP, leucine arylamidase; PYR, pyrrolidonyl arylamidase; CAMP Test, CAMP test with β-hemolysin NAGA, N-acetyl-β-D-glucosaminidase; Hipp, hippurate hydrolysis; Glu, glucose; Mal, maltose; Suc, sucrose; Mntl, mannitol; Xyl, xylose; Lac, lactose, S, major amounts of succinic acid from glucose; l, minor amounts of lactic acid from glucose; f, minor amount of formic acid from glucose.

(Continued)

Table 14-13B Biochemical Characteristics for Identification of *Actinomyces* Species Isolated From Humans and Animals

SPECIES	RELATIONSHIP TO O₂	GLU	MAL	SUC	MNTL	XYL	LAC	MNE	ARAB	SORB	RAFF
A. bovis	Ana/Fac	+	+	+	−	−	+	V	−	−	−
A. bowdenii	Fac	+	+	+	−	−	+	NA	−	−	+
A. canis	Fac	+	+	V	−	+	+	NA	+	−	V
A. cardiffensis	Fac	+	V	V	−	−	−	V	−	−	V
A. catuli	Fac	+	+	+	−	+	+	NA	V	−	+
A. coleocanis	Fac	+	+	−	−	−	+	NA	−	−	−
A. denticolens	Fac	+	+	+	V	−	+	V	−	−	+
A. europaeus	Fac	+	+	V	−	−	−	V	−	−	−
A. funkei	Fac	+	V	+	−	+	V	NA	−	−	−
A. georgiae	Fac	+	+	+	V−	+	V+	V−	V−	V−	V−
A. gerencseriae	Ana/Fac	+	+	V	+	+	+	+	−	V	+
A. graevenitzii	Fac	+	+	+	−	−	+	NA	−	−	−
A. hongkongensis	Ana	−	NA	NA	NA	−	NA	−	−	NA	−
A. hordeovulneris	Ana/Fac	+	+	+	−	+	+	+ʷ	V	NA	+ʷ
A. howellii	Ana/Fac	+	+	+	−	+	V	V	−	NA	+ʷ
A. hyovaginalis	Fac	+	+	+	−	+	V	+	+	−	−
A. houstoniensis	Fac	+	NA	+	NA	−	NA	NA	NA	NA	NA
A. israelii	Ana/Fac	+	+	+	V+	+	+	+	V+	V−	+
A. marimammalium	Fac	+	+	−	−	−	+	NA	−	−	−
A. meyeri	Ana/Fac	+	+	+	−	+	V+	−	V−	−	−
A. naeslundii genospecies 1	Fac	+	+	V+	−	V−	V	+	−	−	+
A. naeslundii genospecies 2	Fac	+	+	V+	+	V+	V	+	−	V	+
A. nasicola	Fac	−	−	−	−	−	−	−	−	−	−
A. neuii subsp. neuii	Fac	+	+	+	V	+	+	+	V+	NA	+
A. neuii subsp anitratus	Fac	+	+	+	V+	+	+	+	−	NA	+
A. odontolyticus	Ana/Fac	+	V+	+	−	V	V	−	V	−	−
A. oricola	Fac	+	V+	+	−	−	−	NA	−	−	+
A. radicidentis	Fac	+	+	+	+	−	+	NA	−	−	+
A. radingae	Fac	+	+	+	−	+	V+	NA	NA	NA	V
A. slackii	Fac	+	NA	V	−	+	NA	NA	−	NA	NA
A. suimastiditis	Fac	+	V	+	−	+	−	NA	+ʷ	−	+
A. turicensis	Fac	+	+	+	−	+	−	NA	NA	NA	−
A. urogenitalis	Fac	+	+	+	V	+	+	NA	V	−	+
A. vaccimaxillae	Fac	+	−	V	V	+	+	NA	+	−	−
A. viscosus serotype 1	Fac	+	V	+	−	V−	V+	V	−	−	+
A. viscosus serotype 2	Fac	+	V	+	−	−	V+	V	−	−	+

+, *positive reaction;* −, *negative reaction;* +w, *weak or delayed positive reaction;* V, *variable reaction;* V+, *variable, most strains positive;* V−, *variable,* NO₃ Red, *reduction of nitrate to nitrite;* PYZ, *pyrazinamidase;* AP, *alkaline phosphatase;* ESC, *esculin hydrolysis;* URE, *urea hydrolysis;* ADH, *arginine producing* S. *aureus;* α-GAL, *α-galactosidase;* β-GAL, *β-galactosidase;* α-GLU, *α-glucosidase;* β-GLU, *β-glucosidase;* β-GUR, *β-glucuronidase;* Mne, *mannose;* Arab, *arabinose;* Sorb, *sorbitol;* Raff, *raffinose;* Tre, *trehalose;* Glycg, *glycogen;* Amyg, *amygdalin;* Meli, *melibose;* Melez, *melezitose;*

chronic skin ulcers, soft-tissue infections, deep-tissue abscesses (including brain, peritonsillar, paravertebral, and intraabdominal abscesses), and joint-space infection, and has been associated with sinusitis, orbital cellulites, pneumonia, osteomyelitis, endocarditis, and meningitis.[21,225,278,541,814] A. haemolyticum was also involved in a case of Lemierre's disease associated with *Fusobacterium necrophorum*.[984] A. haemolyticum is usually susceptible to all classes of antimicrobial agents, including penicillins, cephalosporins, macrolides, and vancomycin, with resistance to trimethoprim-sulfamethoxazole being a consistent finding.[19,129–131] Occasional isolates may be resistant to tetracyclines, the macrolides, clindamycin, and ciprofloxacin.[131]

Arcanobacterium bernardiae is a newly described species that includes isolates formerly called CDC coryneform group 2.[309] This organism has been recovered from various human clinical sources, including blood, wounds, and urine. In 1995, Funke and colleagues proposed the inclusion of

RIB	TRE	GLY	GLYCG	AMYG	MELI	MELEZ	FERMENTATION (GLC)	PRODUCTS OF GLUCOSE COMMON API BIOCODES
–	–	–	+	–	V	–	S, A, L, f	0101104
+	+	NA	NA	NA	+	+	S, L, A	3410365, 3400365, 3510365, 3500365
+	–	NA	+	NA	–	–	NA	2430766, 2430767
V	–	NA	–	–	–	–	L, S, a	0010121, 0010321, 1010121, 1010321
+	+	NA	–	NA	V	–	S, L, a	7650761, 7650765, 7670761, 7670765
–	–	NA	+	NA	–	–	S, L	2410162
V	–	–	NA	–	NA	–	S, A, L	NA
V	V	NA	V	–	V	V	S	04 (1/5) 0 (1/3) 2 (0/1/2/3); GEL+ after 5 days
V	–	NA	–	NA	–	–	NA	0130761, 3530761
–	+	V	+	V–	–	V–	S, l, a, f	NA
V+	+	–	V–	V+	V	V	S, L,a, f	NA
+	–	+	–	–	–	–	L, S	(0,2)(0,4)20361
–	–	NA	NA	NA	NA	NA	NA	NA
V	V	–	V	NA	–	–	L, S	NA
–	V+	–	–	–	V	V	NA	NA
V	–	V	–	+	–	–	NA	0570721, 0170721
NA	NA	NA	NA	NA	NA	NA	NA	NA
V+	+	–	–	V+	V+	V	S, A, L, f	NA
–	–	NA	V	NA	–	–	S, A, L	0520162, 0420160, 0520160
+	–	V	V	V+	–	–	S, a, l, f	NA
V	V+	V	–	V	V	–	L, s, a, f	NA
V	V+	V	V	V	V	V	L, s, a, f	NA
–	–	–	–	–	–	–	S, a, l	NA
+	+	+	V+	NA	V+	+	S, L	Included in API Coryne database
+	+	+	V	NA	+	+	S, L	Included in API Coryne database
V	V	V	V	–	–	–	S, A, f	NA
V	+	NA	NA	+w	–	–	S, A, L	NA
+	+	NA	–	NA	+	+	NA	NA
+	NA	NA	–	NA	NA	NA	NA	Include in API Coryne database
–	+	NA	–	NA	+	NA	NA	NA
+w	–	NA	NA	NA	+	–	NA	NA
+	+	+	–	NA	NA	NA	NA	0010721, 0010701, 0010723, 1010701; included in API Coryne database
V	+	NA	–	NA	+	+	NA	NA
+	+	NA	+	–	–	–	S, L, a	NA
–	V–	–	V	–	–	–	S, A, L, f	NA
+	V	V	V	–	V	–	S, A, L, f	NA

most strains negative; NA, data not available; Cat, catalase; Fac, facultative; Ana, anaerobic; Cat, catalase; Hemol SBA, hemolysis on sheep blood agar; dihydrolase; MOT, motility; GEL, gelatin hydrolysis; LAP, leucine arylamidase; PYR, pyrrolidonyl arylamidase; CAMP Test, CAMP test with β-hemolysin NAGA, N-acetyl-β-D-glucosaminidase; Hipp, hippurate hydrolysis; Glu, glucose; Mal, maltose; Suc, sucrose; Mntl, mannitol; Xyl, xylose; Lac, lactose; S, major amounts of succinic acid from glucose; l, minor amounts of lactic acid from glucose; f, minor amount of formic acid from glucose.

CDC group 2 organisms in the genus *Actinomyces* as *Actinomyces bernardiae*.[309] Sequence analysis of the 16S rRNA of these isolates resulted in a subsequent proposal to transfer this species to the genus *Arcanobacterium* as *Arcanobacterium bernardiae*.[705] Two cases of complicated urinary tract infections and one case of septic arthritis due to *A. bernardiae* have been reported.[3,441,530] In one of these cases, the patient had long-standing bladder dysfunction and devel-

oped hydroureteronephrosis, renal stones, perirenal abscesses, and septicemia with *A. bernardiae*.[441]

A. pyogenes is recognized as a veterinary pathogen, causing infections in pigs, cattle, sheep, goats, and domesticated companion animals (i.e., dogs and cats).[85] In this regard, the organism and its infections have significant economic importance. It may also be recovered from milk and other dairy products produced from infected animals. Although human

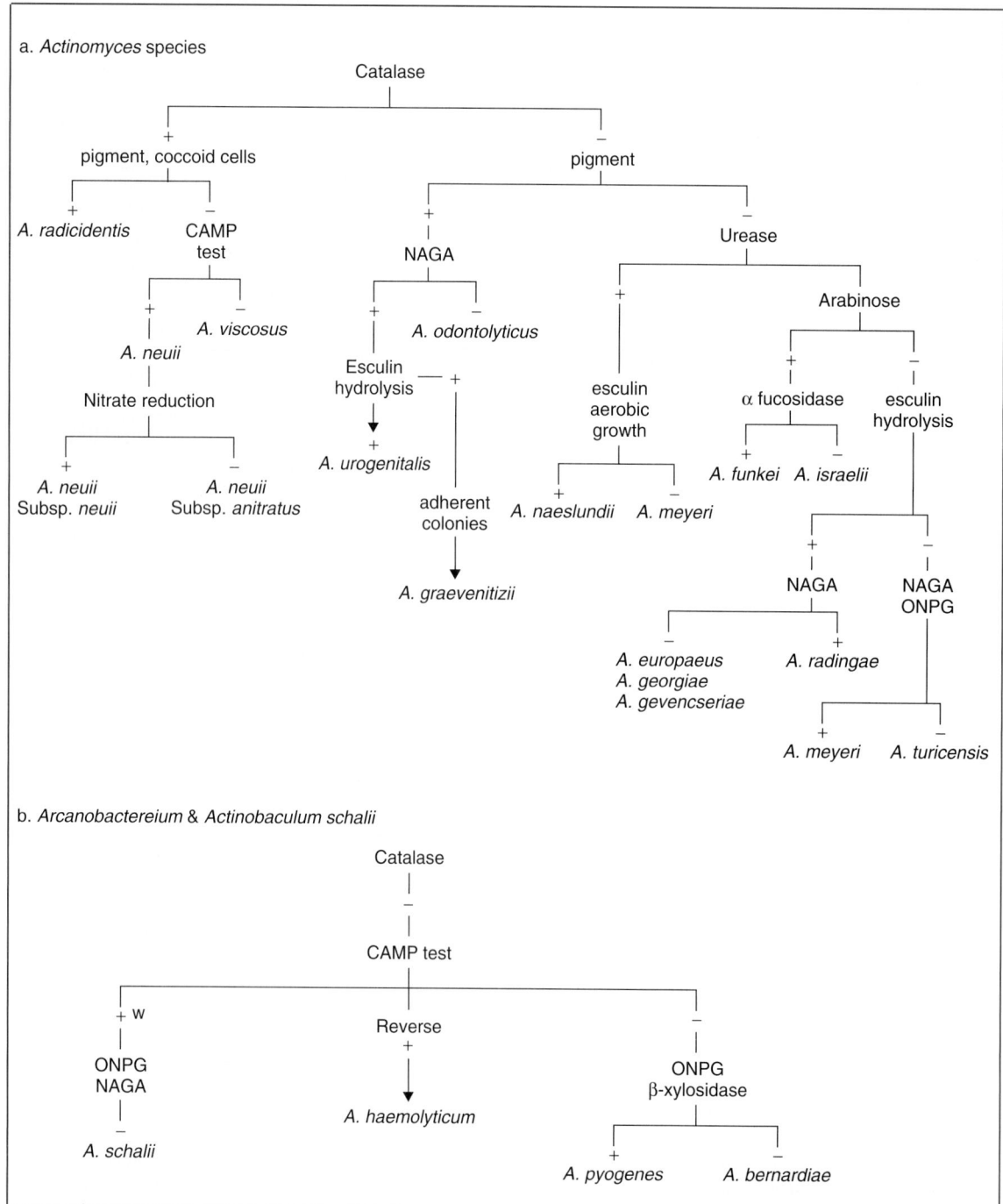

Figure 14-3 Flowchart for identification of *Actinomyces, Actinobaculum,* and *Arcanobacterium* species from human clinical specimens.

infections caused by this organism have been reported since 1940, the validity of these reports is questionable because of a lack of microbiologic data ensuring a definite distinction of this agent from closely related bacteria like *A. haemolyticum* (see Color Plate 14-2G). Bacteriologically confirmed human *A. pyogenes* infections have included bacteremia in a patient with colon cancer, five patients with intraabdominal infections (including one with cervical cancer), two with otitis media, one with mastoiditis, two with cystitis (including one

with prostatic carcinoma), two with skin abscesses, and one patient with diabetes and a mixed wound infection and positive blood cultures containing *A. pyogenes*.[58,232,319,563] The organism was also isolated as a cause of leg ulcers among a group of children in rural Thailand.[501]

A. haemolyticum, A. bernardiae, and *A. pyogenes* are the species that may be encountered in clinical specimens from humans. On SBA, *A. haemolyticum* grows as small, dull, matte colonies that are β-hemolytic (see Color Plate 14-6E).

Hemolysis may first be noted in areas of confluent growth after 24 hours of incubation; isolated colonies will be β-hemolytic after 48 hours of incubation. *A. haemolyticum* is also catalase-negative and does not hydrolyze esculin or urea. Most strains are pyrazinamidase-, alkaline phosphatase-, β-galactosidase-, α-glucosidase-, and *N*-acetyl-β-D-glucosaminidase-positive and gelatin hydrolysis- and β-glucuronidase-negative. Most strains ferment glucose, maltose, lactose, and ribose and do not ferment mannitol, xylose, or glycogen (see Color Plate 14-6*F*). *A. haemolyticum* is the only *Arcanobacterium* species that is reverse CAMP test–positive (or CAMP test inhibition–positive). In this test, the effect of the β-hemolysin of *S. aureus* on sheep red blood cells is inhibited by the phospholipase of *A. haemolyticum*. This appears on the SBA plate as an arrowhead-shaped nonhemolyzed area between *S. aureus* and the *A. haemolyticum* streaked at right angles to the staph streak. *A. bernardiae* forms small, smooth, glassy colonies on SBA that may or may not be β-hemolytic on SBA. This organism is catalase-negative, and produces acid from glucose and maltose, but not from sucrose, mannitol, xylose, and lactose. Unlike *A. haemolyticum*, glucose is more readily fermented than maltose, and glycogen is readily fermented. *A. pyogenes*, the species isolated most infrequently from humans, is also β-hemolytic and catalase-negative. This species is easily differentiated from *A. haemolyticum* and *A. bernardiae* because it is obviously β-hemolytic at 24 hours, is gelatin hydrolysis–positive, ferments xylose, and is β-glucuronidase (β-GUR)-positive. All three species are readily identified with the API Coryne. The phenotypic characteristics of *Arcanobacterium* species are found in Table 14-14.

Arthrobacter Species

During their examination of various CDC group B-1 and B-3 strains, Funke and colleagues encountered 11 human clinical isolates (from urine, skin infection, blood cultures, and endophthalmitis) that displayed a marked rod-to-coccus cycle. Cell wall analysis revealed lysine as the principal cell wall diamino acid and the presence of different cellular fatty acid.[295] These data were consistent with members of the genus *Arthrobacter*. Members of the genus *Arthrobacter* are found in the environment and are also isolated from animals; they are rarely isolated from human clinical specimens.[249,435] Chemotaxonomic and genetic comparisons of these strains with existing environmental *Arthrobacter* species resulted in the proposal of two new *Arthrobacter* species—*A. cumminsii* and *A. woluwensis*—for some CDC group B-1 and B-3 strains.[295] A 1998 analysis of 15 clinical isolates of *A. cumminsii* from the urinary tract, middle ear, amniotic fluid, vagina, calcaneal osteomyelitis, deep-tissue cellulitis, cervix, blood, and wounds revealed unique cellular fatty acid patterns, with the consistent presence of C14:0i and C14:0, and unusually high amounts of C16:0 and C16:0i fatty acids, which are not found in other *Arthrobacter* species.[304] When these isolates were tested on the API Coryne, numerous biotype numbers were observed after 24 hours, 48 hours, and 7 days of incubation. (See Table 14-13.)

A. cumminsii is the *Arthrobacter* species isolated most frequently from human clinical specimens. This organism is catalase-positive, LAP-positive, nonmotile, and both nitrate re-

ductase–and esculin hydrolysis–negative. Some strains produce urease, and both DNase and gelatinase activity are produced by most isolates. Although most strains produce acid from ribose, acid production from glucose is variable, and no acid is produced from maltose, sucrose, mannitol, xylose, lactose, or glycogen.[304] *A. woluwensis* hydrolyzes esculin, urea, gelatin, and DNA, and unlike *A. cumminsii*, produces several enzymatic activities, including β-galactosidase (β-GAL), α-glucosidase (α-GLU), β-glucosidase (β-GLU), and *N*-acetyl-β-D-glucosaminidase (NAGA). In most reports on these organisms, the API CHO (BioMérieux), a carbohydrate assimilation (not fermentation) panel was used for characterization, but this system is not usually used in clinical laboratories. Since *A. cumminsii* and *A. woluwensis* were described, another previously described *Arthrobacter* species (*A. oxydans*) and three new *Arthrobacter* species (*A. creatinolyticus, A. luteolus,* and *A. albus*) have been recovered from human clinical specimens, including blood, surgical wounds, and urine.[428,938] *A. creatinolyticus* hydrolyzes creatine, xanthine, and gelatin but does not hydrolyze starch. This species also produces acid from glycerol, but the original description did not describe the acidification of carbohydrates. *Arthrobacter* species are included in the API Coryne database, however, the carbohydrate fermentation cupules will usually be negative after 24 hours. Prolonged incubation of the identification panels (up to 5 to 7 days) may result in slow oxidative utilization of some carbohydrates. Phenotypic and biochemical characteristics of *Arthrobacter* species isolated from clinical species are presented in Table 14-15.

Brevibacterium Species

Brevibacterium species are irregular, slender, rod-shaped bacteria that display a marked rod-to-coccus cycle. Fresh subcultures (<3 days) stain as bacilli, but as the culture ages (4–7 days), the cells may appear coccal in morphology. Both organism forms are gram-positive, but may be easily decolorized. The rod-shaped cells show diphtheroid morphology and are non-acid-fast. *Brevibacterium* species are obligately aerobic and are oxidative in their metabolism. They are nonmotile and salt-tolerant (>6.5% NaCl), produce catalase and proteinases, do not possess urease, and do not produce acid from glucose or other carbohydrates in peptone media. Brevibacteria also characteristically produce methanethiol (CH₃SH) from L-methionine. The peptidoglycan contains *meso*-DAP as the principal diamino acid, but does not contain arabinose, lysine, or mycolic acids (galactose may or may not be present).[123,462]

At present, the genus *Brevibacterium* is composed of nine species: *B. linens, B. iodinum, B. casei, B. epidermidis, B. mcbrellneri, B. otitidis, B. paucivorans, B. lutescens,* and *B. avium*. In the 1986 edition of *Bergey's Manual*, four species—*B. linens, B. iodinum, B. casei,* and *B. epidermidis*—were described.[462] *B. casei* and *B. epidermidis* grow optimally at 30–37°C, while *B. linens* and *B. iodinum* prefer to grow at 20–30°C. Colonies of these organisms are grayish-white, yellowish-white, yellow, or tan and have an intense "cheesy" odor (see Color Plate 14-6*G*). The habitat of the brevibacteria is primarily milk products, in which the bacteria contribute to the aroma and the color (e.g., orange-pigmented *B. linens*) of surface-ripened cheeses (e.g., Lim-

Table 14-14 Biochemical Characteristics for Identification of *Arcanobacterium* Species

TEST	A. BERNARDIAE	A. HAEMOLYTICUM	A. HIPPOCOLEAE	A. PHOCAE	A. PLURANIMALIUM	A. PYOGENES
Catalase	−	−	−	V	+	−
Hemolysis, SBA	V	β	β	β	α	β
NO$_3$ reduction	−	−	−	−	−	V
Pyrazinamidase	+	+	−	+	V	V−
Alkaline phosphatase	−	V+	V	+	−	V
Esculin hydrolysis	−	−	+w	−	+w	−
Arginine dihydrolase	NA	NA	−	NA	−	NA
Hippurate hydrolysis	NA	NA	+	NA	+	NA
Acetoin production	NA	NA	−	NA	−	NA
Gelatin hydrolysis	−	NA	−	−	+	+
Acid produced from:						
Glucose	+	+	+	+	+	+
Maltose	+	+	V	+	V	+
Sucrose	−	V	−	+	−	V
Mannitol	−	−	−	V−	−	V
Xylose	−	−	−	−	−	+
Lactose	−	+	+	+	−	+
Mannose	NA	NA	NA	V+	NA	+
Arabinose	NA	NA	−	−	−	V
Sorbitol	NA	NA	−	−	−	V
Raffinose	NA	NA	−	−	−	−
Ribose	V+	V+	−	+	+	NA
Trehalose	NA	NA	−	V+	−	+
Glycerol	+	−	NA	+	NA	NA
Glycogen	V+	NA	−	+	−	+
Amygdalin	−	NA	NA	NA	NA	−
Melibiose	NA	NA	−	−	−	−
Melezitose	NA	NA	−	V+	−	+
LAP	+	NA	+	+	NA	NA
PYR	V	V	−	−	NA	+
α-GAL	−	NA	−	+	−	−
β-GAL	−	V+	+	+	−	+
α-GLU	+	+	+	+	−	+
β-GLU	−	−	−	−	−	−
β-GUR	−	V	+	−	+	+
NAGA	−	V+	V	−	−	V

+, *positive reaction;* −, *negative reaction;* V, *variable reaction;* V+, *variable reaction, most strains positive;* V−, *variable reaction, most strains negative;* +w, *weak positive reaction.*

burger cheese). They are also found on human skin surfaces. When resident on human skin under moist, macerating conditions (e.g., between the toes and other intertriginous areas), these organisms are believed to contribute to body odor. *B. mcbrellneri,* described in 1993, was isolated from human genital hairs that were coinfected with *Trichosporon* *beigelii.*[593] *Brevibacterium otitidis,* a species recovered from humans with bilateral otorrhea, was described in 1996.[662] *B. paucivorans,* which was described in 2001, has been isolated from CSF, abscesses, wounds, blood, ear discharge, and intravascular catheters.[939] *B. lutescens* is a *B. otitidis*–like species that was isolated from human peritoneal dialysis fluid

Table 14-15 Biochemical Characteristics for Identification of *Arthrobacter* Species

CHARACTERISTIC	A. ALBUS	A. CITREUS	A. CREATINOLYTICUS	A. CUMMINSII	A. LUTEOLUS	A. OXYDANS	A. WOLUWENSIS
Catalase	+	+	+	+	+	+	+
Hemolysis, SBA	−	NA	−	−	−	−	−
Growth, 20°C	−	+	NA	V	+	+	+
Growth, 42°C	+	−	NA	+	+	V	+
NO$_3$ reduction	−	+	+	−	+	+	−
Pyrazinamidase	+	NA	NA	V	+	NA	NA
Alkaline phosphatase	+	NA	NA	V	NA	NA	+
Esculin hydrolysis	−	NA	NA	−	−	−	+3 days
Urease	−	NA	NA	V	−	−	+3 days
Motility	−	+sl	−	−	+	−	−
Gelatin hydrolysis	+sl	+	+	+10 days	+	+	+24 hours
DNase	−	+	NA	+10 days	+	+	+24 hours
LAP	+	NA	NA	+	+	NA	+
PYR	+	−	NA	+	−	−	+
α-GAL	−	NA	NA	−	−	NA	−
β-GAL	−	+	NA	−	−	+	+
α-GLU	−	+	NA	−	+	+	+
β-GLU	−	NA	NA	−	−	NA	+
α-GUR	−	NA	NA	−	−	NA	−
NAGA	−	+	NA	−	−	−	+
Acid oxidatively from:							
Glucose	−	+	−	V	+	+	+
Maltose	−	NA	NA	−	+	−	NA
Sucrose	−	NA	NA	−	+	+	NA
Mannitol	−	+	NA	−	−	+	+
Xylose	−	NA	−	−	+	−	NA
Lactose	NA	NA	NA	−	−	NA	NA
Common API Coryne biocodes	6102004, 6100004	NA	NA	Varies (depends on length of incubation)	3110004	3750004	NA

+, positive reaction; −, negative reaction; V, variable reaction; +sl, slow positive reaction; NA, data not available.

and infected ear drainage in 2003.[937] *B. avium* has been isolated from granulomatous lesions of poultry.[661]

Brevibacteria are rare causes of human infections, and examination of strains previously classified as CDC groups B-1 and B-3 established that some of these isolates were, in fact, *Brevibacterium* species. In 1991, McCaughey reported the first documented case of a central venous line infection caused by *B. epidermidis* in a 40-year-old man.[595] In 1993, Gruner et al. isolated nine *Brevibacterium* strains; these organisms were recovered from dialysate fluids of patients on continuous ambulatory peritoneal dialysis, blood cultures, sputum, CSF, pleural fluid, and a miscellaneous body fluid.[371] Comparison of their biochemical characteristics with reference *Brevibacterium* strains indicated that these organisms were either *B. casei* or *B. epidermidis*. These researchers suggested that aerobic, gram-positive and catalase-positive bacilli that are nonmotile and fail to ferment sugars may be identified as presumptive *Brevibacterium* species

based on colony pigmentation and morphology (gray-white to yellow, opaque, convex, and smooth) and an intensive "cheesy" or "stinky feet" odor. These same workers subsequently examined 41 clinical strains of CDC groups B-1 and B-3 and found that 22 were identical to *B. casei*, with 5 additional isolates forming another phenotypic cluster within the genus *Brevibacterium*.[372] Funke and Carlotti also examined 43 *Brevibacterium* strains recovered from clinical specimens over the past 20 years and compared them to reference *Brevibacterium* strains.[290] Using chemotaxonomic analysis and carbohydrate assimilation tests with the API 50CH carbohydrate assimilation panel, 41 were identified as *B. casei* and 2 as *B. epidermidis*. Colonies of *B. casei* are usually whitish-gray, while *B. epidermidis* strains develop yellowish colonies with time. Detection of methanethiol and cellular fatty acid analysis can be used to confirm the assignment of the isolate to the genus *Brevibacterium*, and carbohydrate assimilations can be used to identify the isolate to species.

Brevibacteria are also included in the databases of the API Coryne and the RapID CB-Plus (see Color Plate 14-6*H*). Biochemical characteristics of *Brevibacterium* species are shown in Table 14-16.

Several case reports have now been published documenting *Brevibacterium* species as opportunistic agents. Brevibacteria have been reported as a cause of persistent bacteremia in patients with underlying diseases such as lymphoblastic leukemia, non-Hodgkin's lymphoma, and testicular cancer.[483,543,648,714] A *Brevibacterium* species was also isolated as a cause of sternal osteomyelitis in a 4-week-old male.[630] Both *B. iodinum* and *B. otitidis* have been reported as causes of peritonitis in patients undergoing continuous ambulatory peritoneal dialysis.[29,941] In 2000, Brazzola and colleagues isolated *B. casei* from both peripheral blood and blood collected through a Porto-Cath (Xxxxx, Xxxxx, XX) from an 18-year-old female with AIDS, and in 2002, Janda and colleagues isolated *B. casei* from the blood of a 34-year-old male patient with AIDS and line sepsis.[109,451] Prosthetic-valve endocarditis due to *B. otitidis* has been described in a patient at the National Institutes of Health.[204]

Cellulomonas, *Cellulosimicrobium*, and *Oerskovia* and Species

Cellulomonas species are principally environmental organisms that appear as slender, irregular coryneform rods that may appear more coccoid in older cultures. They are gram-positive (although easily decolorized), non-acid-fast, and may be nonmotile or motile because of single polar or sparse lateral flagella. Colonies of these organisms are usually opaque, convex, and yellow-pigmented. The cell wall peptidoglycan contains L-ornithine and does not contain *meso*-DAP, glycine, lysine, or homoserine.[841] These organisms are either oxidative or fermentative in their metabolism; most strains produce acid from glucose both aerobically and anaerobically. *Cellulomonas* species are catalase-positive, hydrolyze cellulose, starch, and gelatin (weak reaction), reduce nitrate to nitrite, and produce DNase. The genus *Cellulomonas* includes over eight valid species that are isolated from various environments.[307]

Some isolates of CDC coryneform groups A-3 and A-4 are now recognized as *Cellulomonas* species that have been isolated from human clinical specimens.[307,315,397] Funke et al. examined clinical isolates from CSF (two isolates) and blood (2 isolates); both of the CSF isolates had been phenotypically identified as CDC group A-3, while the blood culture isolates were identified as CDC group A-4.[307] These isolates were compared to type strains of the characterized environmental *Cellulomonas* species using peptidoglycan and cellular fatty acid analysis in addition to the phenotypic tests used for characterization of coryneforms. Phenotypic test results for these isolates did not correspond to any of the extant *Cellulomonas* species. The four clinical isolates contained L-ornithine as the peptidoglycan diamino acid, thereby reinforcing affinity with *Cellulomonas* species. Partial sequencing of the 16S rRNAs of these organisms further validated the similarities with *Cellulomonas* species, and Funke and coworkers formally proposed that CDC group A-3 and some group A-4 strains be assigned to a new genus, *Cellulomonas hominis*. These organisms have been isolated

from vitreous humor specimens following penetrating injuries or intraocular lens transplantations, blood cultures associated with catheter-related sepsis, native-valve endocarditis, and cerebrospinal fluid.[88,185,392,539]

Isolates of *C. hominis* are short, thin, motile gram-positive rods. Colonies on SBA are smooth, circular, convex, and white; a yellowish pigmentation develops after about 3 days. Esculin, gelatin, and DNA are hydrolyzed and nitrate is reduced to nitrite, but urease is not produced. This organism is fermentative, producing acid from glucose, maltose, sucrose, xylose, and lactose, but not from mannitol. Unlike environmental *Cellulomonas* species, *C. hominis* does not hydrolyze cellulose. *Cellulomonas* species are included in the API Coryne database, but these organisms will usually give a cross-call with *Microbacterium* species. *Cellulomonas turbata* is the same organism as *Oerskovia turbata* (see below).

Coryneform rods assigned to genus *Oerskovia*—*O. turbata* and *O. xanthineolytica*—were originally designated CDC coryneform groups A-1 and A-2, respectively, and were related to groups A-3, A-4, and A-5. However, early genetic and chemotaxonomic evidence suggested that the two *Oerskovia* species were not closely related. In 1982 Stackbrandt et al. proposed the union of the genera *Oerskovia* and *Cellulomonas* based on phylogenetic evidence, with the genus epithet *Cellulomonas* having precedence.[840,842] The name *Cellulomonas cellulans* was proposed for *O. xanthineolytica*, and *O. turbata* became *Cellulomonas turbata*. However, this name change did not address the apparent unrelatedness of "*C. cellulans*" and "*C. turbata*." Analysis of 16S rDNA dendrograms provided evidence that "*C. cellulans*" branched outside of the phylogenetic confines of the genus *Cellulomonas* and was a phylogenetic "nearest neighbor" of the genus *Promicromonospora*. In addition, chemotaxonomic analysis of the cell wall of "*C. cellulans*" has shown that the type strain and other strains of this species possess a "type A4α" peptidoglycan, a characteristic not found among members of the genus *Cellulomonas*, including "*C. turbata*." L-Lysine was found to be the principal cell wall diamino acid of "*C. cellulans*," while other *Cellulomonas* species contain L-ornithine. The agreement between the phylogenetically distinct position of this organism in the 16S rDNA dendrogram, and the different chemotaxonomic properties exhibited by this organism justified the assignment of "*C. cellulans*" to the new genus *Cellulosimicrobium*, with the type species being *Cellulosimicrobium cellulans* ("*Oerskovia xanthineolytica*").[784] In 2002, a second *Cellulosimicrobium* species (*C. variabile*) was isolated from the termite hindgut.[50] Taxonomists also disagree on the status of *Oerskovia turbata* as a *Cellulomonas* species. Recent studies using 16S DNA sequencing and cell wall structural analysis also suggest that transfer of *O. turbata* to the genus *Cellulomonas* may not be valid.[839]

Members of the emended genus *Oerskovia* demonstrate branching vegetative hyphae that penetrate into the agar and fragment into motile rodlike elements.[839] On smears, the organisms appear as coryneform bacilli. Organisms may or may not be motile. They are catalase- and oxidase-positive and facultative with respect to oxygen, although some strains may be strictly aerobic. Major fatty acids, isoprenoid quinone composition, and other characteristics of the genus are

Table 14-16 Biochemical Characteristics for Identification of *Brevibacterium* Species

CHARACTERISTIC	B. AVIUM	B. CASEI	B. EPIDERMIDIS	B. IODINUM	B. LINENS	B. LUTESCENS	B. MCBRELLNERI	B. OTITIDIS	B. PAUCIVORANS
Catalase	+	+	+	+	+	+	+	+	+
Hemolysis, SBA	−	−	−	−	−	−	−	−	−
NO₃ reduction	+	V−	V+	+	NA	−	−	−	−
Pyrazinamidase	NA	+	+	+	+	+	−	+	−
Alkaline phosphatase	+	+	NA	NA	NA	V	NA	+	
Esculin hydrolysis	−	−	NA	NA	NA	−	NA	−	−
Urease	−	−	NA	NA	NA	−	NA	−	−
Growth, 6.5% NaCl	NA	+	+	NA	NA	+	NA	NA	NA
DNase	+	+	NA	NA	NA	NA	NA	+	NA
Hydrolysis of:									
Gelatin	+	+	+	+	+	+	+sl	+	+sl
Casein	+	+	+	+	+	+	+	+	−
Xanthine	+	+	+	+	+	−	V	−	−
Acid from carbohydrates	−	−	−	−	−	−	−	−	−
LAP	+	+	NA	NA	NA	+	NA	+	+
PYR	NA	V+	−	−	−	+	−	+	−
α-GAL	−	−	NA	NA	NA	−	NA	−	−
β-GAL	−	−	NA	NA	NA	−	NA	−	−
α-GLU	−	V+	−	−	−	−	−	−	−
β-GLU	−	−	NA	NA	NA	−	NA	−	−
β-GUR	−	−	NA	NA	NA	−	NA	−	−
NAGA	−	−	+	−	−	+	+	−	V−
Common API Coryne biocodes	NA	6112004, 4112004	NA	NA	NA	6002004, 6102004	NA	6002004	0000004

+, positive reaction; −, negative reaction; +sl, slow positive reaction; V, variable reaction; V+, variable reaction, most strains positive; V−, variable reaction, most strains negative; NA, data not available.

shown in Table 14-7. In addition to the type strain, *O. turbata*, three other species have been described. *O. enterophila* is recovered from insects and was formerly a *Promicromonospora* species, while *O. jenensis* and *O. paurometabola* are soil isolates.[839] The biochemical characteristics that are helpful for identifying *Cellulomonas* species, *C. hominis*, *C. (O.) turbata*, and *C. cellulans* are shown in Table 14-17.

Cellulosimicrobium cellulans produces smooth, glistening, entire colonies that are strongly yellow-pigmented (see Color Plate 14-7*C*). The organism's actinomycetes affinities are manifested by the production of a substrate "mycelium" that fragments into irregular, curved and club-shaped rods arranged in V-forms and "Chinese letters." After exhaustion of fermentable carbohydrate from broth media, these rod-shaped organisms are transformed into even shorter rods or coccal forms. These organisms are biochemically active and are included in the databases of both the API Coryne and the IDS RapID CB plus systems for the identification of coryneform bacteria. The common API Coryne biocodes for *C. cellulans* are 3552727, 7552727, 3572727, or 7572727 (see Color Plate 14-7*D*). Both *O. turbata* and *Cellulosimicrobium cellulans* hydrolyze casein, but only the latter species hydrolyzes xanthine. In addition, *Cellulosimicrobium cellulans* grows at 42°C, while *O. turbata* does not.

Cellulosimicrobium cellulans and *O. turbata* are rare causes of opportunistic infections in immunocompromised hosts. *O. turbata* has been isolated as the cause of Broviac catheter–related bacteremia in a 3-year-old male and as a cause of endocarditis in a 68-year-old man whose aortic valve had been replaced with a homograft heart valve because of severe aortic insufficiency related to ankylosing spondylitis.[531,715] In 1996, this organism was reported as a cause of bacteremia (along with *Comomonas acidovorans*) in a patient with AIDS.[512] *C. cellulans* has been reported as a rare cause of keratitis, endophthalmitis, pneumonia, prosthetic joint–related infection, catheter-related bacteremia, ventriculoperitoneal shunt–associated meningitis, and peritonitis in patients receiving chronic ambulatory peritoneal dialysis.[99,395,440,474,557,596,631,736,791] *C. cellulans* bacteremia has also been documented in recipients of bone marrow transplants, in patients with AIDS, and in patients with underlying liver disease.[240,570] These organisms have also been isolated as contaminants in total parenteral nutrition solutions; this was discovered only after signs and symptoms of bacteremia developed in a patient immediately following parenteral infusion, with recovery of the organisms from blood cultures, from the patient's central venous catheter, and from the nutritional supplement itself.[377]

O. turbata and *C. cellulans* are variable in their susceptibility to antimicrobial agents. While many isolates have been reported as susceptible to penicillin, ampicillin, cephalothin, tetracycline, clindamycin, erythromycin, gentamicin, trimethoprim-sulfamethoxazole, ciprofloxacin, and vancomycin, strains that are resistant to these agents have also been reported.[377,440,596,736,894] High-level vancomycin and teicoplanin resistance have also been reported in a clinical isolate of *O. turbata*.[693] This glycopeptide resistance was shown to be due to modified cell wall peptidoglycan structure related to the presence of *vanA* gene sequences similar to those found in vancomycin-resistant strains of *Enterococcus faecium*.

Dermabacter Species

In 1988, Jones and Collins described four strains of coryneform bacteria that were isolated exclusively from human skin.[461] The cell walls of these isolates contained *meso*-DAP, alanine, and glutamic acid, but lacked cell wall mycolic acids.[123] These bacteria also contained predominantly branched-carbon cellular fatty acids, a characteristic found only in *Brevibacterium* species and the environmental organism *Brachybacterium faecium*.[123] The organisms were fermentative (not oxidative like *Brevibacterium* and *Brachybacterium* species) and produced acid from several carbohydrates. The name *Dermabacter hominis* was proposed for these strains. Subsequent examination of CDC group 3 and group 5 isolates recovered from a variety of human clinical specimens by Gruner et al., Bernard et al., and Funke et al. established that these two CDC groups were identical to the type strain of *Dermabacter hominis* described by Jones and Collins.[76,312,373,461] *D. hominis* has been recovered from a variety of clinical specimens, including blood, lung tissue, abscesses, CSF, peritoneal fluid, conjunctivae, calcaneal osteomyelitis, and infected vascular grafts.[350,903] In 1998, Bavbek and colleagues described a case of *D. hominis* cerebral abscess in the recipient of a renal transplant that presented as a contrast-enhancing brain mass.[65] *D. hominis* has also been recovered as a cause of peritonitis from a patient on continuous ambulatory peritoneal dialysis.[701]

D. hominis strains are catalase-positive, nonhemolytic, nonmotile coryneforms. On Gram-stained smears, the organisms appear coccobacillary or coccoid. Colonies are usually white, convex, and have a creamy or slightly sticky consistency. After 48 hours of incubation, colonies are usually about 1.5 mm in diameter. They do not reduce nitrate or produce pyrazinamidase, but they hydrolyze esculin and produce alkaline phosphatase, pyrrolidonyl arylamidase, leucine aminopeptidase, and DNase. They also produce both lysine and ornithine decarboxylases. Acid is produced from glucose, maltose, sucrose, and lactose; former CDC group 3 *D. hominis* strains also ferment xylose, while former CDC group 5 strains do not. This organism is included in the API Coryne database.[76] Additional phenotypic characteristics are presented in Table 14-17.

Exiguobacterium Species

Exiguobacterium species are short, irregular coryneform bacilli that demonstrate a marked rod-to-coccus cycle in their growth. They characteristically produce yellow or pale orange colonies on agar media and are facultative and fermentative in their metabolism. Mycolic acids are absent and L-lysine is the peptidoglycan diamino acid. *Exiguobacterium* species are catalase-positive, motile, and resemble *Microbacterium* and *Oerskovia* species, although they differ in their cell wall fatty acids. *E. acetylicum*, a former *Brevibacterium* species, has been isolated from wounds and cerebrospinal fluid. *E. acetylicum* produces light yellow, intense yellow, or orange colonies on SBA. This catalase-positive organism is rapidly fermentative, producing acid from glucose, maltose, sucrose, and mannitol but not from xylose.

Table 14-17 Biochemical Characteristics for Identification of Cellulomonas Species, Cellulomonas hominis, Cellulomonas turbata, Cellulosimicrobium cellulans, and Dermabacter hominis

CHARACTERISTIC	CELLULOMONAS SPP.	C. HOMINIS	C. (O.) TURBATA	CELLULOSIMICROBIUM CELLULANS	DERMABACTER HOMINIS
Catalase	+	+	+	+	+
Hemolysis, SBA	-	-	-	-	-
Motility	V+	+	+	+	-
NO₃ reduction	+	+	+	+	-
Pyrazinamidase	NA	NA	-	NA	-
Alkaline phosphatase	V	-	NA	NA	+
Esculin hydrolysis	+	+	+	+	+
Urease	-	-	-	-	-
DNase	V	+	+	+	+
Hydrolysis of:					
Gelatin	+	+	+	+sl	V+
Starch	NA	NA	NA	+	+
Casein	NA	NA	+	+	NA
Xanthine	NA	NA	-	+	NA
Tyrosine	NA	NA	-	-	NA
Acid produced fermentatively from:					
Glucose	+	+	+	+	+
Maltose	+	+	+	+	+
Sucrose	+	+	+	+	+
Mannitol	V	-	-	-	-
Xylose	+	+	+	+	V
Lactose	NA	+	NA	+	+
Arabinose	NA	+	NA	NA	NA
LAP	+	+	NA	NA	+
PYR	NA	NA	-	NA	+
α-GAL	NA	NA	NA	NA	V+
β-GAL	NA	NA	+	NA	+
α-GLU	+	+	+	NA	+
β-GLU	NA	NA	+	NA	+
β-GUR	NA	-	-	NA	-
NAGA	NA	NA	+	NA	+

+, positive reaction; -, negative reaction; +w, weak or delayed positive reaction; V, variable reaction; V+, variable, most strains positive; V-, variable, most strains negative; NA, data not available; Cat, catalase; Fac, facultative; Ana, anaerobic; Cat, catalase; Hemol SBA, hemolysis on sheep blood agar; NO₃ Red, reduction of nitrate to nitrite; PYZ, pyrazinamidase; AP, alkaline phosphatase; ESC, esculin hydrolysis; URE, urea hydrolysis; ADH, arginine dihydrolase; MOT, motility; GEL, gelatin hydrolysis; LAP, leucine arylamidase; PYR, pyrrolidonyl arylamidase; CAMP Test, CAMP test with β-hemolysin producing S. aureus; α-GAL, α-galactosidase; β-GAL, β-galactosidase; β-GUR, β-glucuronidase; NAGA, N-acetyl-β-D-glucosaminidase; Hipp, hippurate hydrolysis; Glu, glucose; Mal, maltose; Suc, sucrose; Mnt, mannitol; Xyl, xylose; Lac, lactose; Mne, mannose; Arab, arabinose; Sorb, sorbitol; Raff, raffinose; Tre, trehalose; Glycg, glycogen; Amyg, amygdalin; Meli, melibiose; Melez, melezitose; S, major amounts of succinic acid from glucose; A, major amounts of acetic acid from glucose; L, major amounts of lactic acid from glucose; a, minor amounts of acetic acid from glucose; l, minor amounts of lactic acid from glucose; f, minor amount of formic acid from glucose.

Esculin is hydrolyzed, but urease is not produced. Some strains reduce nitrate to nitrite. (See Table 14-18.)

Leifsonia Species

During a taxonomic investigation of microbes isolated from grass-root galls induced by a free-living nematode, Evtushenko and colleagues recognized a group of coryneform bacteria that were phenotypically similar to the motile coryneform that has historically been called "*C. aquaticum.*"[251] Although long considered a *Corynebacterium* species, certain properties (e.g., motility and oxidative carbohydrate metabolism) serve to exclude this organism from the genus *Corynebacterium*. Strains previously called "*C. aquaticum*" also contained DL-2,4-diaminobutyric acid in the cell wall, as did the grass-root gall isolates. This unusual diamino acid is found in the cell walls of *Clavibacter* species. Further analysis of the grass-root gall isolates, reference strains of "*C. aquaticum,*" and existing *Clavibacter* species isolates established that these organisms were chemotaxonomically and phylogenetically related. The genus *Leifsonia* was created to accommodate previously described *Clavibacter* species, the isolate from grass-root galls, and "*C. aquaticum.*" Therefore, the genus *Leifsonia* is comprised of *L. xyli* subsp. *xyli* and *L. xyli* subsp. *cynodontis* (former *Clavibacter* species), *L. poae* (the isolate from *Poa annua* root galls induced by the nematode *Subanguina radicola*), and *L. aquatica* ("*C. aquaticum*").[855]

L. aquatica has been described as a rare cause of infections in humans, including bacteremia, endocarditis, access-device infection, meningitis, chronic ambulatory peritoneal dialysis–associated peritonitis, wound infections, and urinary tract infections.[68,133,275,479,507,517,614,880] Colonies of *L. aquatica* are opaque, butyrous, and yellow-pigmented. This pigmentation increases with the age of the culture. The cells are motile at 35–37° C and at room temperature via long, peritrichous flagella. The organism demonstrates a rod-to-coccus cycle, so in older cultures, coccoid cells predominate. *L. aquatica* is aerobic and catalase- and oxidase-positive (see Table 14-18). Acid is produced oxidatively from glucose, sucrose, fructose, arabinose, galactose, and mannose. The organism is urease-negative and esculin is not hydrolyzed, but H₂S is produced. In the past, some *Microbacterium* species recovered from human clinical specimens have been misidentified as "*C. aquaticum.*"[316,369] Hydrolysis of casein and gelatin are helpful for separating possible *Microbacterium* species (gelatin hydrolysis– and casein hydrolysis–positive) from "*C. aquaticum*" (gelatin hydrolysis– and casein hydrolysis–negative). *L. aquaticum* also produces strong DNase activity. Additional *Leifsonia* species (i.e., *L. cynodontis*, *L. rubra*, *L. aurea*, *L. shinshuensis*, *C. naganoensis*) are environmental isolates and have not been isolated from human clinical specimens.[711,855]

Microbacterium (Aureobacterium) Species

Microbacterium species are small, irregularly shaped, gram-positive, catalase-positive bacilli that grow with typical "diphtheroid" morphology. They may be nonmotile or motile, with one to three flagella and are oxidative and aerobic in their metabolism, although some species may be fermentative. Instead of *meso*-DAP, these organisms contain lysine as the diamino acid in their cell walls and have "glycine-glycine-lysine" or "glycine-lysine" as the interpeptide cross-linkage in the cell wall peptidoglycan.[292,866,979] Unlike *Corynebacterium* species, arabinose, galactose, and mycolic acids are not components of the cell wall. Prior to 1998, the genus *Microbacterium* contained six valid species isolated from soil, sewage, and dairy products.[868] In 1998, Takeuchi and Hitano analyzed extant *Microbacterium* and *Aureobacterium* species using 16S rRNA sequencing and found that the species in these two genera formed a monophyletic intermixed association. This and additional physiologic and chemotaxonomic features resulted in the unification of these genera in a redefined genus *Microbacterium* containing the 13 former *Aureobacterium* species.[173,979,980]

Members of the genus *Microbacterium* are composed of irregular, short, catalase-positive, obligately aerobic gram-positive bacilli. Production of acid from carbohydrates results from oxidation rather than fermentation. Unlike *Cellulomonas* species, *Microbacterium* do not hydrolyze cellulose. Members of this genus contain ornithine in the cell wall peptidoglycan along with glycine residues within the interpeptide bridge.[173] *Microbacterium* species also contain high concentrations of glycolate in the peptidoglycan, suggesting that the muramic acid in the cell wall occurs in the N-glycolyl form rather than the usual N-acetyl form. In addition to D-ornithine and glycine, the cell wall also contains alanine, glutamic acid, and homoserine. Since 1998, over 15 other *Microbacterium* species have been isolated from foods, plants, soil, sewage, and insects.

Microbacterium species have been isolated from human clinical specimens and some former CDC coryneform group A-4 and group A-5 isolates have been assigned to the genus *Microbacterium* based on phenotypic, chemotaxonomic, and genotypic analyses. Funke and colleagues examined 22 strains of yellow- and orange-pigmented, gram-positive bacilli by a variety of chemotaxonomic and phenotypic techniques.[292] These strains included *Microbacterium*-type strains, environmental isolates, and 13 clinical isolates, 10 of which were recovered from blood cultures. All were *Microbacterium* species by cell wall analysis; three clinical isolates were phenotypically identical to *M. imperiale* and two others were identical to the *M. arborescens* type strain. The remaining clinical isolates did not resemble any other recognized *Microbacterium* species phenotypically, although they were *Microbacterium* species based on chemotaxonomic analysis.

Microbacterium species have been associated with severe human infections, including a fatal disseminated infection in a 75-year-old man and persistent bacteremia from cellulitis in a 39-year-old man with acute myelogenous leukemia and porphyria cutanea tarda.[641,769] In the latter case, the isolate was vancomycin-resistant. These organisms have also been associated with nosocomial and catheter-related bacteremias in patients with leukemia, and with contamination of peripheral blood stem cell products infused into stem-cell transplant recipients.[20,127,418,520] In a recent case report, a yellow-pigmented coryneform isolate was recovered from blood cultures of a child with leukemia. Genetic and chemotaxonomic comparisons with existing *Microbacterium* spe-

Table 14-18 Biochemical Characteristics for Identification of *Exiguobacterium acetylicum*, *Leifsonia aquatica*, and *Microbacterium* Species

CHARACTERISTIC	EXIGUOBACTERIUM ACETYLICUM	LEIFSONIA AQUATICA	MICROBACTERIUM SPP.	MICROBACTERIUM ARBORESCENS	MICROBACTERIUM IMPERIALE	MICROBACTERIUM PARAOXYDANS
Pigment	Yellow, pale orange	Yellow, smooth	Yellow-white, yellow	Orange, intense yellow	Orange, intense yellow	Bright yellow, sticky, smooth
Catalase	+	+	+	+	+	+
Hemolysis, SBA	−	−	−	−	−	−
NO$_3$ reduction	V	V	V	−	−	−
Pyrazinamidase	NA	+	V+	NA	NA	NA
Alkaline phosphatase	NA	V	NA	NA	NA	NA
Esculin hydrolysis	+	V	V	+	+	+sl
Urease	−	−	V	−	−	−
Motility	+	+	V+	+	+	+
DNase	+	−	NA	NA	NA	+
Hydrolysis of:						
Gelatin	+	−	+	NA	NA	+
Casein	+	−	V	NA	NA	+
Xanthine	NA	−	NA	NA	NA	NA
Tyrosine	NA	−	NA	NA	NA	−
Starch	+	+	NA	NA	NA	NA
Ferm/Oxid	Ferm	Oxid	Oxid	Ferm	Ferm	Oxid
Acid from:						
Glucose	+	+	+	+	+	+
Maltose	+	V	+	+	+	+
Sucrose	+	V	V	+	+	+
Mannitol	+	+	V+	+	+	+
Xylose	−	NA	V	+	+	NA
Lactose	−	+	V	NA	NA	NA
Arabinose	−	+	−	+	+	NA
Raffinose	−	NA	−	−	+	NA
LAP	NA	NA	NA	NA	NA	+
PYR	NA	V−	NA	NA	NA	NA
β-GAL	NA	NA	V+	+	+	V
α-GLU	NA	+	V+	NA	NA	+
β-GLU	NA	NA	V	+	+	−
β-GUR	NA	−	NA	NA	NA	−
NAGA	NA	V+	V	+	+	V
Common API biocode numbers	NA	CHO's usually negative due to oxidative metabolism	Isolates that fail to ferment CHO's may represent former *Aureobacterium* species, which have oxidative CHO metabolism			NA

+, positive reaction; −, negative reaction; V, variable reaction; V+, variable reaction, most strains positive; V−, variable reaction, most strains negative; +sl, delayed or weak positive reaction; NA, data not available; Oxid, oxidative utilization of carbohydrates (CHO's); Ferm, fermentative utilization of carbohydrates.

cies resulted in the characterization of *M. paraoxydans*, another new *Microbacterium* species.[509] Funke and colleagues in Switzerland and Germany reported a case of endophthalmitis due to a *Microbacterium* species following a penetrating eye injury.[293] Phylogenetically, the organism clustered with recognized *Microbacterium* species, suggesting that the isolate may actually represent yet another new *Microbacterium* species.[293] The isolate was susceptible to cefazolin, cefotetan, ciprofloxacin, clindamycin, imipenem, piperacillin, teicoplanin, and vancomycin and was resistant to gentamicin and tobramycin.

Microbacterium species form whitish-yellow-, yellow-, or orange-pigmented colonies on SBA (see Color Plate 14-6E). All species are catalase-positive, and a some species (*M. arborescens*, *M. imperiale*, *M paraoxydans*) are motile. Most species hydrolyze esculin and do not hydrolyze urea. Acid is produced oxidatively from a variety of carbohydrates. The original members of the genus *Microbacterium* species tend to be fermentative, while the former *Aureobacterium* species that were transferred into the genus *Microbacterium* are oxidative in their utilization of carbohydrates. *Microbacterium* species are included in the API Coryne data base, but additional tests are required to separate them from *Cellulomonas* species and ''*C. aquaticum*'' (see Color Plate 14-6F). Because some microbacteria produce acid from carbohydrates oxidatively rather than fermentatively, acidification of carbohydrates may not be apparent after 24 hours incubation. API Coryne biocodes (0470004, 0452004, 0472004, 0570004, 0572004) included in the data base usually give cross calls with ''*C. aquaticum*,'' and incubation of the API Coryne galleries beyond 24 hours may be necessary to determine acidification of carbohydrates. Those species that are fermentative may produce some positive acidification reactions on the API Coryne, but incubation beyond 24 hours may be necessary. Additional phenotypic data is found in Table 14-18.

Rothia and ''Rothia-Like Species'' (CDC Group 4)

Rothia species are members of the newly described phylum Actinobacteria, subclass Actinobacteridae, order Actinomycetales. In the upcoming edition of *Bergey's Manual of Systematic Bacteriology*, the genus *Rothia* is included in the family *Micrococcaceae*, which also includes the *Micrococcus*, *Arthrobacter*, *Kocuria*, *Nesterenkonia*, and *Stomatococcus* genera.[329] Historically, the genus *Rothia* included a single species, *Rothia dentocariosa*. Based on 16S rDNA sequencing and chemotaxonomic data, the genus *Rothia* has been expanded. *Stomatococcus mucilaginosus*, the catalase-variable gram-positive coccus found in the human oropharynx, is closely related to organisms in the genus *Rothia* and has been transferred to the genus *Rothia* as *Rothia mucilaginosa*.[172] A third species in the genus, *Rothia nasimurium*, has been described; this species is found in the anterior nares of mice. Whereas *R. mucilaginosa* and *R. nasimurium* are gram-positive cocci, *R. dentocariosa* is a gram-positive coryneform bacillus that shows rudimentary branching, although, in older broth cultures, coccoid cells may predominate. *R. dentocariosa* does not produce major amounts of succinic acid from glucose, a characteristic that distinguishes this organism from facultative *Actinomyces* species. Like the corynebacteria and aerobic actinomycetes, these organisms are catalase-positive

and tend to grow better under aerobic conditions. However, unlike *Nocardia* species, these organisms are fermentative and lend themselves to identification by phenotypic tests routinely used for *Corynebacterium* species and the coryneform groups described above.

Rothia dentocariosa is part of the normal human oropharyngeal and gingival flora and may be isolated from saliva and supragingival plaque. During the 1950s and 1960s, the Special Bacteriology Branch at the CDC collected several isolates, most of which were from abscesses, respiratory tract specimens, pilonidal cysts, cerebrospinal fluid, urine, and blood.[562,610,773,933] Since 1979, several reports of *R. dentocariosa* endocarditis involving both native valves and prosthetic valves have appeared in the medical literature.[26,87,101,105,499,944] In several cases, this infection was associated with severe, life-threatening complications, including the involvement of multiple cardiac valves and the development of aortic-root paravalvular abscesses.[270,852] Valvular infections often result in the formation of large vegetations, which may lead to the development of pulmonary infarcts, intercranial hemorrhages, and brain abscesses.[444,722] Bacteremia without endocarditis has also been reported.[758] And *R. dentocariosa* has been isolated from drainage at the site of an arteriovenous fistula in a 46-year-old diabetic man with renal failure.[639] Recent case reports have documented *R. dentocariosa* as a cause of endophthalmitis, vertebral osteomyelitis with paraspinal abscess, and peritonitis associated with chronic ambulatory peritoneal dialysis.[83,547,568] Although rare, *R. dentocariosa* has also been recognized as a cause of pneumonia in patients with severe underlying diseases, including acute myelocytic leukemia and adenocarcinoma of the lung.

The affinities of *R. dentocariosa* with other aerobic actinomycetes are apparent on examination of colony morphology. After 72 hours of incubation at 35–37°C in CO_2, colonies are usually dry, rough, and bone-white. The colonies often appear heaped and cerebriform, particularly in areas of confluent growth (see Color Plate 14-7A). Inspection of the edges of colonies reveals that the colonies tend to ''dig into'' the agar surface like those of *Nocardia* species. Strains of *R. dentocariosa* also have relatively uniform phenotypic characteristics and are quite biochemically active. *R. dentocariosa* is catalase-positive, reduces nitrate to nitrite and produces pyrazinamidase and pyrrolidonyl arylamidase (see Table 14-19). The organism hydrolyzes esculin but does not hydrolyze urea or gelatin, and acid is produced fermentatively from glucose, maltose, and sucrose. Acetic and lactic acids with trace amount of pyruvic acid and *R. dentocariosa* are included in the databases of both the API Coryne and the RapID CB-Plus. On the API Coryne, most strains produce the biocodes 7050125, 7052125, 7050165, or 7052165 (see Color Plate 14-7B). Although these organisms are usually uniformly susceptible to all classes of antimicrobial agents, strains that are resistant to β-lactams because of β-lactamase production have been isolated.[610] The latter strains contain plasmids bearing the β-lactamase structural genes.

CDC fermentative coryneform group 4 organisms are closely related to *R. dentocariosa*. These organisms have been recovered mostly from female genitourinary tract specimens, although no specific human infections with CDC group 4 isolates have been reported. Morphologically, some

Table 14-19 Biochemical Characteristics for Identification of *Rothia dentocariosa*, "Rothia-Like" CDC Fermentative Coryneform Group 4, *Corynebacterium aurimucosum*, and *Corynebacterium nigricans*

CHARACTERISTIC	*ROTHIA DENTOCARIOSA*	"ROTHIA-LIKE" CDC FERMENTATIVE CORYNEFORM GROUP 4	*C. AURIMUCOSUM*	*C. NIGRICANS*
Lipophilic	–	–	–	–
Colony morphology	Bone white, off-white, dry, rough, adherent or convex, smooth or charcoal-black, entire, and soft in texture	Charcoal-black, circular, convex, entire, smooth or rough and adherent	Sticky, white-to yellowish or charcoal-black	Charcoal-black, adherent
Hemolysis, SBA	–	–	–	–
Catalase	V	V	+	+
Pyrazinamidase	+	NA	+	+
Alkaline phosphatase	V	NA	+	+
Motility	–	–	–	–
NO₃ reduction	+	+	–	–
Esculin hydrolysis	+	+	V	–
Urease	–	–	V–	–
Hippurate hydrolysis	NA	NA	+	NA
Acetoin	+	NA	+	NA
H₂S (lead acetate paper)	+	+	NA	NA
Hydrolysis of:				
Gelatin	V	+	V–	–
Starch	–	NA	–	–
Casein	–	NA	NA	–
Acid produced from:				
Glucose	+	+	+	+
Maltose	+	+	+	+
Sucrose	+	+	+	+
Mannitol	–	–	V	–
Lactose	–	–	–	–
Xylose	–	–	–	–
LAP	NA	NA	+	NA
PYR	+	NA	–	–
α-GAL	–	NA	–	NA
β-GAL	–	NA	–	–
α-GLU	+	NA	–	–
β-GLU	+	NA	–	–
α-GUR	–	NA	–	–
NAGA	–	NA	–	NA

+, *positive reaction;* –, *negative reaction;* V, *variable reaction;* V+, *variable reaction, most strains positive;* V–, *variable reaction, most strains negative;* +sl, *delayed or weak positive reaction;* NA, *data not available;* Oxid, *oxidative utilization of carbohydrates (CHO's);* Ferm, *fermentative utilization of carbohydrates.*

of these isolates form charcoal-black colonies on agar media, resembling those of *C. nigricans* (see Box 14-2) Recently, Daaneshvar and colleagues at the CDC investigated several black colony-forming isolates that were provisionally categorized as group 4 bacteria.[202] These organism segregated into two groups by molecular genetic analysis. One group (including only one genital tract isolate) was most closely related to *R. dentocariosa*, while the other group, which included isolates that were mainly recovered from female genital tract specimens, were most closely related to *C. aurimucosum*, a recently described *Corynebacterium* species isolated predominantly from the female genital tract (see Box 14-2). This work resulted in emendations of the species descriptions of both *R. dentocariosa* and *C. aurimucosum* to include variants that formed charcoal-black colonies on agar media. Table 14-19 presents the phenotypic characteristics of *R. dentocariosa* and CDC fermentative coryneform group 4. The phenotypic characteristics of *C. aurimucosum* and *C. nigricans* are also included in Table 14-19 for comparison to aid in the identification of coryneforms that produce charcoal-black pigmented colonies.

Turicella Species

In 1993, Simonet and colleagues in France reported the recovery of a coryneform isolate in pure culture from middle ear fluids collected by tympanocentesis from children with acute otitis media.[809] These isolates contained *meso*-DAP, arabinose, and galactose in their cell walls, but corynemycolic acids were absent. The isolate grew as convex, whitish, creamy, nonhemolytic colonies on blood agar that became yellowish with age. This colony morphology was distinctly different from the flat, gray-white, nonhemolytic colonies produced by *C. afermentans* subspecies or the convex dry, adherent, slightly yellowish colonies of *C. auris*, coryneforms that have both been associated with acute and chronic otitis media.[298,726] On chemotaxonomic analysis, the cellular menaquinone patterns of this middle-ear isolate were also different from the two *Corynebacterium* species. Even though these organisms displayed markedly different colony morphologies, the two *Corynebacterium* species and the third isolate had identical phenotypic characteristics. These middle-ear isolates have now been assigned to the new genus *Turicella* (referring to *Turicum,* the Latin name for Zurich,

Switzerland, where the first isolates were collected) as *Turicella otitidis*.[311] Since its description, *T. otitidis* has been recovered from other head and neck infections (e.g., posterior auricular abscess) and from blood cultures.[200,550,721]

On Gram stains, *T. otitidis* appear as long rods, and, in culture, colonies of the organism are white-gray, convex, and have entire edges. Colonies on SBA are 1.5 to 2 mm in diameter after 48 hours of incubation. All *T. otitidis* isolates produce the biocode number 2100004 on the API Coryne system, indicating positive test results for pyrazinamidase, alkaline phosphatase, and catalase, and negative tests for glucose, ribose, xylose, mannitol, maltose, lactose, sucrose, and glycogen fermentation, nitrate reductase, urease, esculin hydrolysis, β-glucuronidase, β-galactosidase, α-glucosidase, esculin hydrolysis, urease, and gelatin hydrolysis. These phenotypic characteristics are similar to those of both *C. afermentans* subsp. afermentans and *C. auris*. *T. otitidis*, *C. afermentans* subspecies, and *C. auris* can be differentiated most efficiently by genetic and chemotaxonomic analyses. However, Renaud et al. have shown that colony morphology, the CAMP test, certain enzymatic activities (e.g., LAP, DNase), and carbon substrate assimilations are useful for separating these species, as shown in Table 14-20.[718] Isolates of *T. otitidis* are susceptible to ampicillin, cephalosporins, ciprofloxacin, gentamicin, rifampin, tetracyclines, and chloramphenicol; some strains are resistant to clindamycin and erythromycin.[306,729]

Gardnerella vaginalis
Taxonomy and Cellular Morphology

Gardnerella vaginalis was first described in 1953 by Leopold and was subsequently named *Haemophilus vaginalis* by Gardner and Dukes in 1955.[326,362] In 1963, Zinnemann and Turner proposed the name *Corynebacterium vaginale* for this organism because of its tendency to stain gram-positive and the lack of requirements for factor X and/or factor V.[989] In 1980, this organism was formally placed in the new genus, *Gardnerella*, by Greenwood, Pickett, and others based on electron microscopic, biochemical and chemotaxonomic data, and DNA-DNA hybridization studies.[361,362] Ultrastructural studies of *G. vaginalis* indicate that this organism has a gram-positive type of cell wall, but the

Table 14-20 Differentiation of *Turicella otitidis, Corynebacterium afermentans* Subsp. *afermentans*, and *Corynebacterium auris*

CHARACTERISTIC	T. OTITIDIS	C. AFERMENTANS SUBSP. AFERMENTANS	C. AURIS
Colony morphology	Creamy, convex, circular	Flat, smooth	Circular, convex, dry, slightly adherent
Colony pigmentation	Pale yellow with prolonged incubation	Grayish-white	Slightly yellowish
CAMP test	+	V	+
DNase	+	−	−
Leucine arylamidase	+	−	+

+, positive reaction; −, negative reaction; V, variable reaction.

peptidoglycan layer is much thinner than that found in the cell walls of *Corynebacterium*, *Lactobacillus*, or *Staphylococcus* species. The peptidoglycan content of the *G. vaginalis* cell wall constitutes about 20% of the total cell wall weight, which is similar to that found in gram-negative enterics such as *Escherichia coli*, in which the peptidoglycan constitutes about 23% of the cell wall weight.[192] Consequently, different strains of *G. vaginalis* may appear predominantly gram-positive, gram-negative, or gram-variable.[755] Cell wall extracts of *G. vaginalis* do not contain compounds normally present in gram-negative cell wall lipopolysaccharides (e.g., *meso*-DAP, 2-keto-3-deoxy-D-manno-2-octonoic acid, hydroxy fatty acids). The absence of *meso*-DAP, arabinogalactans, and mycolic acids confirms that the *G. vaginalis* cell wall is also distinct from the gram-positive cell wall type found in *Corynebacterium* species. Digests of *G. vaginalis* cell walls contain the amino acids alanine, glutamic acid, glycine, and lysine and the carbohydrates glucose, galactose, and 6-deoxytalose.[647,755]

Nucleic acid hybridization studies have shown that *G. vaginalis* is not genetically related to *Corynebacterium*, *Haemophilus*, *Streptococcus*, *Lactobacillus*, or *Propionibacterium* species. In a recent study using 16S rRNA gene sequence analysis to examine the type strains of 21 *Bifidobacterium* species, Miyake and associates showed that *G. vaginalis* clustered together with 19 of the 21 *Bifidobacterium* species.[611] Another study, by van Esbroeck and colleagues in Belgium, used phenotypic, chemotaxonomic (e.g., whole-cell protein and fatty acid analysis), and 16S rRNA sequence analysis to characterize *G. vaginalis* and ''*G. vaginalis*–like'' strains.[912] Chemotaxonomic methods resulted in the recognition of two major ''clusters'' that were shown by sequence analysis to represent different genera. These different genera, in turn, could be distinguished by phenotypic methods. In their study, cluster I strains represented *G. vaginalis*, with its closest relative being members of the genus *Bifidobacterium*. *G. vaginalis* strains demonstrated a level of similarity of 93.1% to *Bifidobacterium bifidum*.[912] However, these investigators felt that the G + C contents of the *G. vaginalis* and *Bifidobacterium* species were different enough that *G. vaginalis* cannot be considered a member of the genus *Bifidobacterium*. Analysis of heat-shock protein gene sequences also suggested a phylogenetic relationship between *G. vaginalis* and bifidobacteria, but this relationship was more distant than suggested by 16S rRNA analysis and confirmed the genus status of *Gardnerella*.[455] At present, this genus contains a single species and is not assigned to any existing bacterial family. In addition to biotypes, which are determined by phenotypic tests, amplified ribosomal DNA restriction analysis has shown that *G. vaginalis* strains are fairly heterogeneous and may be divided into at least three or four genotypes depending on the restriction enzymes used.[443] In culture, it may be difficult to differentiate some *G. vaginalis* strains from ''look-alike'' organisms, which are termed ''unclassified, catalase-negative coryneform'' bacteria.

Virulence Factors of *G. vaginalis*

Apart from its unique cell wall structure, *G. vaginalis* possesses several other properties that may contribute to its ability to cause infectious processes. These organisms possess a fibrillar exopolysaccharide that has been observed by electron microscopy and has been shown to function in adherence of the organism to vaginal epithelial cells.[755,786] Pili have also been demonstrated on the *G. vaginalis* cell surface and are believed to contribute to mucosal adherence.[103] In 1990, Rottini and coworkers described an extracellular cytolysin (hemolysin) produced by *G. vaginalis*.[746] This cytolysin is a protein with a molecular weight of 59 to 63 kDa that has a specificity for human red blood cells; 100-fold higher concentrations of this cytolysin are required for lysis of other animal erythrocytes. This cytolysin is also able to lyse other human cells, including endothelial cells and polymorphonuclear leukocytes.[746] The cytolysin causes the formation of small pores in the erythrocyte membrane; formation of these pores is competitively inhibited by cholesterol complexed with negatively charged phospholipids.[137] Evidence that this cytolysin may play a role in organism pathogenicity is supported by the finding of cytolysin-specific IgA in the vaginal fluids of women with bacterial vaginosis, an infection in which *G. vaginalis* plays a significant but heretofore-undefined role.[135,136,138] Some *G. vaginalis* strains may also produce phospholipase C, an enzyme that hydrolyzes lecithin into phosphorylcholine and 1,2-diglyceride.[598] Phospholipase C is known to damage reproductive tract tissues by both direct and indirect mechanisms. *G. vaginalis* strains apparently do not produce sialidases (neuraminidases), which are recognized virulence factors in other organisms.[114]

Clinical Significance of *G. vaginalis*

G. vaginalis is associated with the clinical syndrome called **bacterial vaginosis**.[821] This condition is termed bacterial vaginosis because no single organism is solely responsible for the condition and inflammatory cells (seen with both *Candida* and *Trichomonas* vaginal infections) are not observed on Gram-stained smears of the vaginal discharge (see Color Plate 14-8*C*). Bacterial vaginosis is characterized clinically by a malodorous vaginal discharge associated with a significant increase in the numbers of *G. vaginalis* and various obligate anaerobes (e.g., including *Prevotella bivia*, *Prevotella disiens*, *Mycoplasma* species, peptostreptococci, and *Mobiluncus* species) with a concomitant decrease in the numbers of normal vaginal lactobacilli.[403,415,821] Bacterial vaginosis is a risk factor for obstetrical infections, various types of adverse pregnancy outcomes, and pelvic inflammatory disease.[248,415] When this condition was originally described by Gardner and Dukes, *G. vaginalis* was hypothesized to be the etiologic agent.[326] Subsequent studies determined that other organisms were also involved, and that, while *G. vaginalis* was invariably present in the vaginas of women with bacterial vaginosis, it was also present in more than 50% of women without bacterial vaginosis.[605] Using semiselective media, *G. vaginalis* may be found in 14–70% of healthy women without bacterial vaginosis.[191,891] It does appear, however, that the presence of large numbers of these organisms in the vagina are indicative of bacterial vaginosis. Using a radiolabeled oligonucleotide probe specific for *G. vaginalis* 16S rRNA, Sheiness and coworkers in Seattle showed that the presence of these bacteria at concentrations of $\geq 2 \times 10^7$ CFU/mL of vaginal fluid, along with a vaginal pH greater than 4.5, had a sensitivity and specificity of 95% and 99%, respectively, in classifying women with and without bacterial vaginosis when compared with strictly clinical diagnostic criteria.[792] Immunofluorescence techniques have demonstrated that the predominant organisms adherent on classical "clue cells" suggestive of bacterial vaginosis are indeed *G. vaginalis*.[183] Between 93% and 100% of women with bacterial vaginosis are heavily colonized with *G. vaginalis*, with the number of CFUs per milliliter of vaginal fluid being much higher in specimens from infected women than in similar specimens from healthy women.[23,248,415,425,891]

Diagnosis of bacterial vaginosis is best accomplished with clinical criteria along with a Gram stain of the vaginal discharge.[415,644] Routine culture of vaginal specimens for *G. vaginalis* for diagnosis of bacterial vaginosis is not recommended since culture does not provide decisive evidence of infection due to the presence of *G. vaginalis* as part of the resident vaginal microflora. *G. vaginalis* has been isolated from rectal specimens of 56% of 148 women with bacterial vaginosis, 12% of 69 healthy women, 9% of 83 male sexual partners of women with bacterial vaginosis, and 6% of 49 male sexual partners of healthy women.[425,919] These latter data suggest that *G. vaginalis* is not sexually transmitted, but probably colonizes the vagina endogenously from the intestinal tract.[425] On the other hand, Villegas and colleagues recently performed an ultrastructural study of the vaginal secretions from 10 women with bacterial vaginosis and semen samples from their asymptomatic sexual partners using optical and electron microscopy.[919] *G. vaginalis* was isolated from semen specimens of 50% of the men. Electron microscopy showed that the organisms adhered to the cell membranes and penetrated into the cytoplasm of both vaginal and male urethral epithelial cells. These workers suggested that asymptomatic colonization of the male lower genital tract by *G. vaginalis* may have some relevance regarding the role of the male partner in "recolonization" ("reinfection"?) of the female vagina.

In addition to its role in bacterial vaginosis, *G. vaginalis* has also been recovered from female genital tract infections associated with complications of pregnancy and from infants born to mothers with such complications, particularly during and after delivery. These complications include intrauterine infections, intraamniotic infections, chorioamnionitis, post-abortal pelvic inflammatory disease, and postpartum endometritis after cesarean delivery.[337,417,504,526,743] Tissues obtained surgically from these infections may yield *G. vaginalis* in pure or mixed culture with other facultative and/or obligately anaerobic organisms. Postpartum and post-abortal bacteremia with *G. vaginalis* and other genital tract microorganisms may also occur in these clinical settings.[96,277,712] Bacteremia with genital tract microflora occurs when these organisms gain access to venous channels of the placental bed, which is disrupted prior to and during both vaginal and cesarean deliveries. Systemic and localized infections with *G. vaginalis* have also been reported in neonates born to mothers with these complications. These infections have included amnionitis, episiotomy wound infection, neonatal bacteremias, meningitis, cellulitis, conjunctivitis, and osteomyelitis from an infected hematoma caused by a fetal scalp monitor.[22,72,153,154,528,635,850] Oropharyngeal cultures, gastric aspirates, and tracheal suction specimens from neonates have also yielded *G. vaginalis*, presumably ac-

quired during passage through a heavily colonized birth canal.[317] In both pregnant and nonpregnant women, *G. vaginalis* has been isolated, in either pure or mixed culture, from Bartholin's gland abscesses and from surgical wound infections following cesarean sections, abdominal surgeries, hysterectomies, and episiotomies.[153,503,850]

G. vaginalis has also been a cause of infections in males. Bacteremia with *G. vaginalis* has been reported in men following transurethral prostatectomy, and surgical correction of urethral strictures.[63,953] This organism was also recovered from blood cultures of a 65-year-old man with urinary retention due to an adenoma of the prostate.[213] Unusual extragenital infections with *G. vaginalis* have included a pyogenic liver abscess in a 23-year-old woman following a cesarean section, bacteremia with lung abscess and empyema in a alcoholic man with aspiration pneumonia, vertebral disk space infection in a 50-year-old postmenopausal woman, and joint space infections.[253,419,527]

G. vaginalis may also play a role in urinary tract infections in both men and women.[466] Given its normal ecosystem as part of the normal vaginal flora, it is not surprising that *G. vaginalis* has been recovered from urinary tract specimens from women more frequently than from men.[466,513] *G. vaginalis* has been isolated from both the upper (i.e., ureters, renal pelvis, and calyx) and the lower urinary tracts (i.e., bladder) of both symptomatic and asymptomatic patients.[255,597] Isolation rates from urine specimens are greater among pregnant women than among nonpregnant women, and many of these patients are asymptomatic.[597] Pyuria appears to be infrequently associated with *G. vaginalis* urinary tract infection and may be absent even in the presence of serious upper urinary tract disease.[255,256,466] In a study of the role of *G. vaginalis* in urinary tract infections in men, two thirds of 15 men with significant numbers of *G. vaginalis* in the urine had signs and symptoms referable to the urinary tract (i.e., urgency, frequency, hematuria).[820] Most of these patients also had underlying diseases, including diabetes, hypertension, spinal cord injuries, prior urinary tract infections, and cardiovascular accidents. As in previous studies of *G. vaginalis* and the urinary tract, pyuria was present in only 7 of the 15 males evaluated. Significant numbers (i.e., $>10^4$ CFU/mL) of *G. vaginalis* in urine specimen from men are difficult to evaluate because such numbers may be seen in cultures from asymptomatic males and from men with underlying renal diseases such as ureteral obstruction, chronic prostatitis, and end-stage renal disease.[466,849] Rarely, *G. vaginalis* may cause complicated ascending urinary tract infection in healthy males, although such scenarios are more likely in compromised hosts, such as recipients of renal transplants.[273,953] The consensus is that *G. vaginalis* may play an important role in complicated and uncomplicated urinary tract infections in both men and women and, if present in significant numbers, the organism should be identified and reported. *G. vaginalis* and other organisms that are closely related to it may also be isolated from animals (e.g., mares).[762] It is not known currently whether these organisms cause pathology in these animals, or whether the bacteria are a part of the resident equine genital tract flora.

Isolation and Identification

Recovery of *G. vaginalis* from clinical specimens is best accomplished using semiselective media, although the organism does grow on routine SBA, CNA, and chocolate agars used in clinical laboratories (see Color Plate 14-8*D*). Semiselective media include human blood bilayer-Tween agar (HBT agar) or V agar.[891] HBT agar consists of a bottom layer of Columbia colistin-nalidixic acid agar base supplemented with Proteose Peptone no. 3 (BD Microbiology Systems, Sparks, MD), amphotericin B (2.0 μg/mL), and 0.0075% Tween 80, overlaid with a top layer of the same composition, except that 5% human blood is added. The Tween 80 in the medium improves the growth and enhances the β-hemolysis produced by strains of *G. vaginalis*. V agar contains Columbia agar base with 1% Proteose Peptone and 5% human blood. As far as routine media are concerned, *G. vaginalis* grows better on CNA agar containing sheep blood than on blood agar prepared with a tryptic soy base.[344] *G. vaginalis* is β-hemolytic on media containing human blood, but not on media containing sheep blood. Cultures of *G. vaginalis* growing on CNA agar with sheep blood may show a subtle, ''diffuse'' hemolysis surrounding the colonies, particularly after prolonged incubation (i.e., >72 hours). The organism grows best at 35–37°C in a 5–7% CO_2 atmosphere (i.e., a CO_2 incubator or a candle jar). Cultures usually take longer than 24 hours to grow, with most isolates being recovered after 48 to 72 hours of incubation. The organism will also grow in most blood culture media, however the anticoagulant additive sodium polyanethol sulfonate (SPS) is inhibitory to *G. vaginalis* and may compromise the recovery of this organism from blood cultures.[712,713] As with the pathogenic *Neisseria*, this growth inhibition by SPS may be overcome by adding gelatin (1% v/v) to the blood culture bottles.[713]

Presumptive identification of *G. vaginalis* is based on typical cellular morphology on Gram-stained smears (small gram-positive, gram-negative, or gram-variable coccobacilli), characteristic growth and hemolysis on HBT agar (small, clear zones of β-hemolytic colonies surrounding colonies with diffuse edges, colonies 0.3–0.5 mm in diameter after 48 hours of incubation), and negative oxidase and catalase tests (see Color Plate 14-8*E*). Definitive identification of *G. vaginalis* can be made based on the reactions shown in Table 14-21. Other characteristics that confirm the identification of *G. vaginalis* and help to separate it from other so-called unclassified, catalase-negative coryneform (UCNC) organisms include the presence of α-glucosidase, the absence of β-glucosidase, and positive starch and hippurate hydrolysis reactions.[361] Carbohydrate utilization tests are best performed in a medium containing Proteose Peptone No. 3, phenol red indicator, and 1% filter-sterilized carbohydrate. This medium may be supplemented with 0.5% agar or 5% horse serum. Such media should be heavily inoculated with organisms grown for 18–24 hours and incubated for 5 days. Acid is produced from glucose, maltose, and starch, but not from mannitol, sorbitol, raffinose, rhamnose, or salicin (see Color Plate 14-8*F*).[236,362] The organism does not possess lysine or ornithine decarboxylases or arginine dihydrolase, does not reduce nitrate, and does not produce indole, urease, or acetoin. *G. vaginalis* strains will show zones of inhibition around disks containing metronidazole (50 μg) and trimethoprim (5 μg).

Other rapid, modified conventional methods and kit systems can be used to identify *G. vaginalis*. Greenwood et al. described an identification method using a buffered salts-

Table 14-21 Biochemical Characteristics for the Identification of *Gardnerella vaginalis*

CHARACTERISTIC	REACTION
Hemolysis on human blood bilayer Tween (HBT) agar	β
Oxidase	−
Catalase	−
Hippurate hydrolysis	+
Acid production from:	
Glucose	+
Maltose	+
Sucrose	+
Mannitol	−
Starch	+
Zone of growth inhibition with:	
Metronidazole (50 ug disk)	+
Trimethoprim	+
Sulfonamide	+

+, *positive reaction;* −, *negative reaction.*

phenol red solution, filter sterilized carbohydrates, and a heavy inoculum.[363] At the University of Illinois, we have used this method for identification of *G. vaginalis* using a test battery consisting of glucose (positive reaction), maltose (positive reaction), mannitol (negative reaction), and soluble starch (positive reaction) along with a 4-hour hippurate hydrolysis test developed with Ninhydrin (positive reaction). The enhanced rapid identification method (RIM) system (Austin Biologicals, Austin, TX) is a commercial system that uses starch and raffinose fermentation and hippurate hydrolysis to identify *G. vaginalis*. In one study, this method correctly identified 91.4% of 105 *G. vaginalis* isolates.[538] *G. vaginalis* is also included in the database of the API Coryne system (BioMérieux, Hazelwood, MO) for the identification of gram-positive bacilli and in the databases of two kits—the *Haemophilus-Neisseria* Identification (HNID) Panel (American MicroScan, West Sacramento, CA) and the Vitek Neisseria-*Haemophilus* Identification (NHI) card (BioMérieux, Hazelwood, MO)—for the identification of fastidious gram-negative bacilli.[310,449,450]

G. vaginalis strains may also be divided into biotypes based on reactions for lipase, hippurate hydrolysis, and β-galactosidase production.[685] Using these three reactions, eight different biotypes (all combinations of positive and negative reactions) have been described. In their study, the most common biotypes were those in which the hippurate reaction was positive and the other two reactions were positive and/or negative. Piot and coworkers found no correlation between vaginal biotypes and the presence or absence of bacterial vaginosis.[685] Identical biotypes were isolated before and after treatment for bacterial vaginosis when the time interval between vaginal specimen collections was less than 1 week. In addition, similar biotypes were recovered from the vaginas of women with bacterial vaginosis and the urethras of their sexual partners. On the other hand, Briselden and Hillier found that the distribution of *G. vaginalis* biotypes from women with and without bacterial vaginosis were different, with lipase-positive biotypes (e.g., biotypes 1, 2, 3, and 4) being more predominant in women with bacterial vaginosis.[112] Wu et al. examined 20 biotype 1 isolates (which are positive for hippurate hydrolysis, lipase, and β-galactosidase [ONPG]) and found these strains to be genetically heterogeneous; no discrimination could be made between biotype 1 strains isolated from women with bacterial vaginosis and from women without bacterial vaginosis.[968] These workers did not investigate other lipase-positive or lipase-negative biotypes in this study. Results from the latter study suggest that genomic fingerprinting of other *G. vaginalis* biotypes will probably not offer any additional insights into the recognition of strains that are more "virulent" than others.

Nucleic acid probe and amplification technology have also been used to detect and identify *G. vaginalis* in clinical specimens, including vaginal specimens and amniotic fluids.[122,542,645,902] Van Belkum and colleagues sequenced the region between the 16S and 23S rRNA genes of *G. vaginalis* and developed a specific, probe-confirmable PCR-based assay for this organism.[902] Using this PCR method, *G. vaginalis* was detected in 40% of vaginal specimens from women regardless of their clinical status. Of 11 patients diagnosed clinically with bacterial vaginosis, 10 were positive for *G. vaginalis* using the PCR/probe-based assay. Pao and coworkers used cloned, labeled, restriction endonuclease–digested *G. vaginalis* DNA as a probe in a slot-blot assay for detection of *G. vaginalis* in vaginal specimens and found that the probe could detect as few as 10^4 organisms.[658] The Affirm VP Microbial Identification Test (Becton-Dickinson, Sparks, MD), a commercially available system, uses synthetic, oligonucleotide probes for the simultaneous detection of *G. vaginalis*, *Trichomonas vaginalis* and *Candida* species from a single vaginal swab.[113] When compared to routine wet preparations for detection of clue cells, the Affirm VP test showed a sensitivity and specificity of 90% and 97%, respectively, suggesting that the test could be used as a replacement for wet-mount microscopy for the detection of clue cells. Since the probe was more sensitive than culture of *G. vaginalis* on HBT medium, it was suggested that the test could be made more specific by using it in conjunction with other diagnostic criteria (i.e., vaginal pH, presence of amine odor with KOH ["whiff test"]) for bacterial vaginosis. Overall, Briselden and Hillier found that the Affirm VP test for *G. vaginalis* was positive for 97% of women who had bacterial vaginosis based on clinical criteria and had a specificity of 71%.[113] Witt and colleagues found that the Affirm VP III had a specificity of more than 97% when compared with Gram-stained smears.[958] The sensitivity of the assay varied depending on the score given the Gram-stained smear by established scoring criteria and ranged from 73.2% to 89.5%.[644,958]

Antimicrobial Susceptibility

Strains of *G. vaginalis* are generally susceptible to penicillin, ampicillin, erythromycin, clindamycin, trimethoprim, and vancomycin.[488] Ciprofloxacin and imipenem show variable activity against *G. vaginalis*. Some strains are resistant to tetracycline and minocycline, and marked resistance to

amikacin, aztreonam, and sulfamethoxazole is seen in most strains. Because of resistance to sulfamethoxazole, no synergistic activity against *G. vaginalis* is seen with cotrimoxazole (i.e., sulfamethoxazole and trimethoprim in a 19:1 ratio).

As mentioned, *G. vaginalis* is associated with bacterial vaginosis, which is known to have a polymicrobial etiology, but can also be isolated from the vaginas of normal, healthy women. Because of this, culture of vaginal specimens for *G. vaginalis* should be discouraged. Routine use of semiselective media such as HBT and V agars for culture of vaginal specimens represents an unnecessary expense that contributes little useful information, given that the laboratory diagnosis of bacterial vaginosis rests on careful clinical examination and the interpretation of a properly collected Gram-stained smear of vaginal discharge.[415,644,821] *G. vaginalis* can be recovered on regular CNA agar medium after prolonged incubation, and presumptive identification will usually suffice in these circumstances.[344] However, isolates from systemic body sites (e.g., blood, joint fluid, etc.) should be confirmed with additional biochemical tests as described above.

Lactobacillus *Species*
Taxonomy and Epidemiology

Lactobacilli are gram-positive bacilli that are part of the normal flora of the human vagina, gastrointestinal tract, and oropharynx. They are widely distributed in nature (i.e., water, sewage, and silage), and comprise part of the normal flora of many other animal species. Lactobacilli are also found in various foods (e.g., dairy products, grains, meats, fish, sauerkraut) largely because of their wide range of fermentative capabilities. Certain *Lactobacillus* species are now commonly added to foods as probiotics, presumably for their beneficial health effects. Individual cells of *Lactobacillus* species are often long and slender, although smaller "coryneform" bacilli or "coccobacilli" may be observed. Some *Lactobacillus* species may form long chains of bacilli (see Color Plates 14-2*H* and *I*). Most species are nonmotile; the rare motile species having peritrichous flagella.[478] Most species are facultative, although certain species grow best under either anaerobic or microaerophilic conditions, particularly on primary isolation. Lactobacilli are so named because over half of the end products from glucose fermentation is lactic acid; some species may also produce acetic, formic, and succinic acids, along with CO_2. Lactobacilli are uniformly catalase-negative and oxidase-negative, do not reduce nitrate, do not produce indole or H_2S, do not liquefy gelatin, and do not form spores. The cell walls of *Lactobacillus* species contain a thick peptidoglycan and membrane-bound teichoic acids. Lysine, *meso*-DAP, and ornithine are the diamino acids comprising the peptidoglycan cross-linkages. Electron transport menaquinones are absent. A few species (e.g., *L. confusus*) produce extracellular "slime" from sucrose. Over 45 *Lactobacillus* or *Lactobacillus*-like species are listed in the 1986 edition of *Bergey's Manual of Systematic Bacteriology,* and several more have been described since then. In the forthcoming edition of *Bergey's Manual*, the lactobacilli are classified in phylum Firmicutes in the class Bacilli, proposed order Lactobacillales. In this order, genus *Lactobacillus* and genus *Pediococcus* are included in the Family *Lactobacillaceae*.[329]

Clinical Significance

Although inherently of low virulence, lactobacilli cause rare opportunistic infections primarily in compromised hosts. *Lactobacillus* species have been reported to cause endocarditis in patients with congenital heart defects (e.g., ventral septal defect, bicuspid-aortic valve defects), acquired native-valve defects (e.g., prior endocarditis, rheumatic heart disease), vascular grafts, and prosthetic valves.[43,322,366,439,696,778,882,922] Transient bacteremia originating from localized abscesses (e.g., periapical tooth abscesses), dental manipulations (e.g., extractions, root canal), postpartum endometritis, neonatal periomphalitis, and gastrointestinal endoscopy can seed the abnormal valves and initiate endocardial lesions. In those with native-valve disease, large vegetations containing the lactobacilli may be noted by echocardiograms on aortic, mitral, tricuspid, and pulmonic valves.[696] These cardiac vegetations have a marked propensity to embolize to the brain. In the series of patients reviewed by Gallemore and colleagues, septic emboli to the brain developed in 14 of 35 patients; 5 of these patients died and 9 required surgery.[322] For patients with endocarditis due to *Lactobacillus* species, synergistic therapy with a β-lactam agent plus an aminoglycoside for at least 4 to 6 weeks appears to be the optimal therapy. However, medical cure without relapse or the necessity for valve replacement is often difficult. In one series, cure with antimicrobials alone was achieved in only 39% of patients.[366]

Lactobacillus bacteremia without concomitant endocarditis is relatively uncommon and occurs primarily in patients with underlying conditions, including cancer with chemotherapy, bone marrow and organ (particularly liver) transplantation, diabetes, kidney disease, and gynecologic surgery.[28,30,37,667,770,776] The portals of entry for septic episodes with lactobacilli reflect the normal habitats of these organisms within the oropharynx, the genitourinary tract, and the gastrointestinal tract. These organism are not part of the resident skin flora and have not been shown to cause intravenous catheter–related infections.[30] Risk factors for the development of *Lactobacillus* bacteremia include persistent neutropenia, use of broad-spectrum antibiotics, allograft transplantation with immunosuppressive therapy, chemotherapy for cancer, and invasive gastrointestinal or respiratory tract instrumentation and procedures.[151,184,284,477,770] *Lactobacillus* bacteremia has also been associated with HIV infection and AIDS.[2,427,741] In profoundly immunosuppressed patients, bacteremia with vancomycin-resistant *Lactobacillus* strains may occur during or shortly after administration of vancomycin (and other broad-spectrum agents).

Lactobacillus bacteremia is also associated with gynecologic and pleuropulmonary infections. Women with lactobacillemia usually have underlying disease or abnormalities or have undergone invasive gynecologic or obstetrical procedures. These have included endometritis following dilation-and-curettage procedures, pelvic abscesses, and neoplasms of the female genitourinary tract (e.g., ovarian cancer with large-bowel invasion, choriocarcinoma).[28,66,181] In these

cases, the source of the organism is usually the patients' own vaginal microflora. Pleuropulmonary infections and lung abscesses due to *Lactobacillus* species have also been reported in compromised patients. These infections have included necrotizing pneumonia secondary to a tracheoesophageal fistula in a patient with esophageal cancer, pleural empyema secondary to a pleuroesophageal fistula in a patient with squamous-cell carcinoma of the esophagus, pleural empyema due to bleeding esophageal varices, community-acquired lung abscess, and aspiration pneumonias in patients with AIDS.[625,699,741] Sriskanden et al. also documented pneumonia due to *Lactobacillus* species in three patients with profound neutropenia secondary to immunosuppression from AIDS and from cytotoxic chemotherapy for vasculitis and subsequent bone marrow transplantation.[838] A single case report described *Lactobacillus* pneumonia in a 52-year-old man in whom the organism was apparently transmitted to the patient by the transplanted lung itself.[465] In 2002, Wood and colleagues reported the first case of ventilator-associated pneumonia in a critically ill immunocompetent patient.[965]

Lactobacillus infections have also been reported in neonates. Broughton and colleagues reported a case of meningitis due to lactobacilli that occurred in an immunologically normal newborn infant.[116] In this case, vertical transmission of the organism from the mother to the infant during passage through the birth canal was believed to be the source of the organism isolated from the neonate's cerebrospinal fluid. Thompson and colleagues reported a case of *L. acidophilus* sepsis in a 2-month-old infant in whom the source of the organism was an infected central venous catheter.[883]

Several case reports have documented lactobacilli as etiologic agents in a variety of other types of infections. Uncommon clinical presentations have included abscesses associated with retained foreign bodies (e.g., splinters), endophthalmitis following penetrating eye injuries, chondritis following ear piercing, empyema of the gallbladder, splenic abscess with empyema, bacteremic cholecystitis, intravascular infection following intrasplenic rupture of a mycotic aneurysm, and primary peritonitis.[18,55,222,364,707,756,848,963] *Lactobacillus* sepsis was also documented in a patient with ulcerative colitis, in which the physiologic ultrastructure of the intestinal mucosa had been disrupted by endoscopic and surgical procedures.[258] Like many other opportunistic agents, lactobacilli have also been recovered from peritoneal infections in patients on continuous ambulatory peritoneal dialysis.[492,766] Despite the increasing and widespread use of lactobacilli in various foods as probiotics (i.e., *L. acidophilus*, *L. rhamnosus* GG), the incidence of *Lactobacillus* infections or the proportion of bacteremic lactobacillus infections have not increased.[760,761]

In their normal ecologic niche in the human vagina, lactobacilli may play a key role in defense against the development of *Candida* vaginitis, bacterial vaginosis, urinary tract infections, and sexually transmitted infections such as gonorrhea (see Color Plate 14-8*B*).[247,376,416,843] Facultative lactobacilli constitute the predominant normal flora of the healthy vagina, while the anaerobic species of lactobacilli are more often isolated from women with the clinical diagnosis of bacterial vaginosis. The facultative species produce large amounts of hydrogen peroxide, while the anaerobic species do not. It is postulated that colonization of the vagina with facultative, hydrogen peroxide–producing organisms may represent a nonspecific antimicrobial defense mechanism for the normal vagina and may prevent the development of bacterial vaginosis and *Candida* vaginitis by the direct toxic effect of peroxide free radicals on the facultative and obligately anaerobic organisms associated with vaginal infections.[399,416,491]

Isolation and Identification

After growth for 24 hours on SBA, colonies of *Lactobacillus* species are usually small (2–5 mm), convex, and smooth with entire edges; some α-hemolysis or "graying" of the media may also be observed (see Color Plates 14-6*G* and 14-6*H*). Because of the large number of *Lactobacillus* species that have been described, isolates are not generally identified to the species level.[478] In reports in which species identifications were performed, most workers have used the phenotypic methods described by Holdeman and Moore in the *Virginia Polytechnic Institute (VPI) Anaerobe Manual*, cross-referenced with species descriptions in *Bergey's Manual of Systematic Bacteriology*.[422,478] In addition to conventional, phenotypic methods, highly standardized whole-cell protein patterns obtained by sodium dodecyl sulfate-polyacrylamide gel electrophoresis (SDS-PAGE) have proved helpful for identifying *Lactobacillus* species.[613,691] Oligonucleotide hybridization and molecular taxonomic methods (PCR, 16S rRNA sequencing) have also been developed for both genus- and species-level identification of lactobacilli.[47,233,660,807,963]

Recognition and confirmation of lactobacilli in the clinical microbiology laboratory can be accurately obtained with a handful of phenotypic tests. Some species of *Lactobacillus* are intrinsically resistant to vancomycin, and this characteristic is often helpful in identifying these organisms.[423] Resistant isolates will generally grow right up to the edge of a vancomycin test in a disk diffusion test (see Color Plate 14-7*A*). Vancomycin-resistant isolates must be differentiated from *Leuconostoc* and *Pediococcus* species, which are both vancomycin-resistant and can look coccobacillary on Gram stains. *Leuconostoc* species produced gas from glucose in Mann-Rugosa-Sharp (MRS) broth, while the majority of *Lactobacillus* species isolated in the clinical laboratory do not produce gas. Lactobacilli are also PYR-positive, while both *Leuconostoc* and *Pediococcus* species are PYR-negative. Lactobacilli are also LAP-negative, while *Streptococcus*, *Enterococcus*, *Pediococcus*, and *Lactococcus* species are LAP-positive. Of course, gas-liquid chromatography from glucose broth cultures can be used to obtain accurate genus-level identification of isolates, because of the formation of large amounts of lactic acid by these organisms. *Lactobacillus* species that have been identified in association with human infections include *L. rhamnosus*, *L. plantarum*, *L. leishmanii*, *L. fermentum*, *L. casei* subsp. *casei*, *L. paracasei*, *L. confusus*, and the *L. acidophilus* group. Strains of *L. rhamnosus*, *L. casei*, and *L. plantarum*, in particular, may be intrinsically resistant to vancomycin and teicoplanin.[858]

Antimicrobial Susceptibility

Lactobacilli are usually susceptible to penicillin G, ampicillin, the cephalosporins, and clindamycin.[389,407] However, it has been shown that several *Lactobacillus* species are tolerant to the penicillins and cephalosporins. Ratios of minimal bactericidal concentration to minimal inhibitory concentration (MBC:MIC) from 30:1 for cephalothin up to 266:1 for ampicillin have been demonstrated for several clinically significant isolates.[66,67] These in vitro data correlate with the dilemma of antibiotic therapy for patients with *Lactobacillus* endocarditis caused by penicillin/ampicillin-tolerant strains. In a study of nine patients with endocarditis, all nine strains of lactobacilli had MICs for penicillin and cephalothin that were in the susceptible range, but only 52% had MBCs for these agents that were achievable in serum by standard dosing regimens.[43,66] A similar situation was observed for clindamycin in these isolates. Eight of the nine strains had MICs for clindamycin that were in the susceptible range, yet all nine had MBCs that far exceeded achievable serum levels for clindamycin.

As mentioned above, combination therapy with penicillin and an aminoglycoside appears to be the therapeutic approach of choice for the treatment of serious *Lactobacillus* infections such as endocarditis and deep-seated infections (e.g., intrauterine infection). Bayer and colleagues demonstrated synergistic activity with penicillin/ampicillin and either gentamicin or streptomycin.[66] Furthermore, neither cephalosporins nor vancomycin can be assumed to be acceptable alternatives to penicillin/ampicillin.[366] *Lactobacillus* strains that are resistant to penicillin and ampicillin also tend to be resistant to or have elevated MICs for both cephalosporins (e.g., cephalothin, ceftazidime, cefuroxime, cefotaxime) and cephamycins (i.e., cefoxitin).[55] Lactobacilli are almost uniformly resistant to the fluoroquinolones and trimethoprim-sulfamethoxazole, while most strains are susceptible to gentamicin, tobramycin, and chloramphenicol.[30,66,67,203] MICs of lactobacilli for imipenem and macrolide antimicrobial agents generally fall within the susceptible range and appear to be effective in patients with allergy to pencillins.[30,151,858]

In addition to penicillins and cephalosporins, some species of lactobacilli are resistant to the glycopeptide antibiotics vancomycin and teicoplanin (see above). The susceptibilities of various species of lactobacilli to these agents is related to their cell wall structure. Analysis of the cell walls of vancomycin-resistant strains (e.g., *L. rhamnosus*) reveals that the peptidoglycan precursors for these species have a terminal depsipeptide "D-alanine-D-lactate," while species that are vancomycin-susceptible (e.g., the *L. acidophilus* group) have a terminal "D-alanine-D-alanine" structure.[86,390] This single amino-acid difference in the peptidoglycan structure effectively alters the target site for vancomycin, allowing peptidoglycan synthesis to occur in the presence of vancomycin. Interestingly, glycopeptide susceptibility has been shown to be species-related.[262] For example, *L. rhamnosus* (formerly *L. casei* subsp. *rhamnosus*), a species that has been associated with severe infections in compromised hosts, and *L. paracasei* subsp. *paracasei*, are intrinsically resistant to glycopeptides, with vancomycin MICs in excess of 256 μg/mL.[151,262] Other species isolated from serious infections have been susceptible to vancomycin by MIC testing, but, as with the MBCs for the penicillins and clindamycin, the MBCs of vancomycin may be several two-fold dilutions higher than the MIC.[366]

REFERENCES

1. Aalbaek B, Christensen H, Bisgaard M, et al. *Actinomyces hyovaginalis* associated with disseminated necrotic lung lesions in slaughter pigs. J Comp Pathol 2003;129:70–77.

2. Abgrall S, Joly V, Derkinderen P, et al. *Lactobacillus casei* infection in an AIDS patient. Eur J Clin Microbiol Infect Dis 1997;16:180–182.

3. Adderson EE, Croft A, Leonard R, Carroll K. Septic arthritis due to *Arcanobacterium bernardiae* in an immunocompromised patient. Clin Infect Dis 1998;27:211–212.

4. Agata N, Mori M, Ohta M, et al. A novel dodecadepsipeptide, cereulide, isolated from *Bacillus cereus* causes vacuole formation in Hep-2 cells. FEMS Microbiol Lett 1994;121:31–34.

5. Agata N, Ohta M, Arakawa Y, Mori M. The *bceT* gene of *Bacillus cereus* encodes an enterotoxic protein. Microbiology 1995;1431:983–988.

6. Agata N, Ohta M, Mori M. Production of an emetic toxin, cereulide, is associated with a specific class of *Bacillus cereus*. Curr Microbiol 1996;33:67–69.

7. Agata N, Ohta M, Mori M, Isobe M. A novel dodecadepsipeptide, creulide, is an emetic toxin of *Bacillus cereus*. FEMS Microbiol Lett 1995;129:17–20.

8. Aguado JM, Morales JM, Saito E, et al. Encrusted pyelitis and cystitis by *Corynebacterium urealyticum* (CDC group D2): a new and threatening complication following renal transplant. Transplantation 1993;56:617–622.

9. Aguado JM, Ponte C, Soriano F. Bacteriuria with a multiply resistant species of *Corynebacterium* (*Corynebacterium* group D2): an unnoticed cause of urinary tract infection. J Infect Dis 1987;156:144–150.

10. Ahmed K, Kawakami K, Watanabe K, et al. *Corynebacterium pseudodiphtheriticum*: a respiratory tract pathogen. Clin Infect Dis 1995;20:41–46.

11. Ahrne S, Stenstrom I-M, Jensen NE, et al. Classification of *Erysipelothrix* strains on the basis of restriction fragment length polymorphisms. Int J Syst Bacteriol 1995;45:382–385.

12. Ajal M, Turner J, Fagan P, Walker P: Actinomycosis oto-mastoiditis. J Laryngol Otol 1997;111:1069–1071.

13. Akesson A, Hedstrom SA, Ripa T. *Bacillus cereus*: a significant pathogen in postoperative and post-traumatic wounds in orthopaedic wards. Scand J Infect Dis 1991;23:71–77.

14. Albuquerque L, Rainey FA, Chung AP, et al. *Alicyclobacillus hesperidum* sp. nov. and a related genomic species from solfataric soils of Sao Miguel in the Azores. Int J Syst Evol Microbiol 2000;50:451–457.

15. Alexander AV, Walker RL, Johnson BJ, et al. Bovine abortion attributable to *Listeria ivanovii*: four cases (1988–1990). J Am Vet Med Assoc 1993;200:711–714.

16. Alfaro DV, Roth D, Liggett PE. Posttraumatic endophthalmitis. Causative organisms, treatment, and prevention. Retina 1994;14:201–211.

17. Allerberger F. *Listeria*: growth, phenotypic differentiation and molecular microbiology. FEMS Immunol Med Microbiol 2003;35:183–189.

18. Allison D, Galloway A. Empyema of the gall-bladder due to *Lactobacillus casei*. J Infect 1988;17:191.

19. Almuzara MN, De Mier C, Barberis CM, et al. *Arcanobacterium haemolyticum*: identification and susceptibility to nine antimicrobial agents. Clin Microbiol Infect 2002;8:828–829.

20. Alonso-Echanove J, Shah SS, Valenti AJ, et al. Nosocomial outbreak of *Microbacterium* species bacteremia among cancer patients. J Infect Dis 2001;184:754–760.

21. Alos JI, Barros C, Gomez-Garces JL. Endocarditis caused by *Arcanobacterium haremolyticum*. Eur J Clin Microbiol Infect Dis 199514:1085–1088.

22. Amaya RA, Al-Dossary F, Demmler GJ. *Gardnerella vaginalis* bacteremia in a premature neonate. J Perinatol 2002;22:585–587.

23. Amsel R, Totten PA, Spiegel CA, et al. Nonspecific vaginitis: diagnostic criteria and microbial and epidemiological associations. Am J Med 1983;74:14–22.

24. Anaissie E, Kontoyiannis DP, Kantarjian H, et al. Listeriosis in patients with chronic lymphocytic leukemia who were treated with fludarabine and prednisone. Ann Intern Med 1992;117:466–459.

25. Andavolu RH, Jagadha V, Lue Y, McLean T. Lung abscess involving *Corynebacterium pseudodiphtheriticum* in a patient with AIDS-related complex. NY State J Med 1986;86:594–596.

26. Anderson MD, Kennedy CA, Walsh TP, Bowler WA. Prosthetic valve endocarditis due to *Rothia dentocariosa*. Clin Infect Dis 1993;17:945–946.

27. Andersson MA, Mikkola R, Helin J, et al. A novel sensitive bioassay for detection of *Bacillus cereus* emetic toxin and related depsipeptide ionophores. Appl Environ Microbiol 1998;64:1338–1343.

28. Andriessen MP, Mulder JG, Sleijfer DT. *Lactobacillus* septicemia, an unusual complication during the treatment of choriocarcinoma. Gynecol Oncol 1991;40:87–89.

29. Antoniou S, Dimitriadis A, Polydorou F, Malaka E. *Brevibacterium iodinum* peritonitis associated with acute urticaria in a CAPD patient. Perit Dial Int 1997;17:614–615.

30. Antony SJ, Stratton CW, Dummer JS. *Lactobacillus* bacteremia: description of the clinical course in patients without endocarditis. Clin Infect Dis 1996;23:773–778.

31. Antos H, Mollison LC, Richards MC, et al. Diphtheria: another risk of travel. J Infect 1992;25:307–310.

32. Apotheloz C, Regamey C. Disseminated infection due to *Actinomyces meyeri*: case report and review. Clin Infect Dis 1996;22:621–625.

33. Arahal DR, Marquez MC, Volcani BE, et al. Reclassification of *Bacillus marismortui* as *Salibacillus marismortui* comb. nov. Int J Syst Evol Microbiol 2000;50:1501–1503.

34. Aravena-Roman M, Bowman R, O'Neill G. Polymerase chain reaction for the detection of toxigenic *Corynebacterium diphtheriae*. Pathology 1995;27:71–73.

35. Armstrong RW, Fung PC. Brainstem encephalitis (rhombencephalitis) due to *Listeria monocytogenes*: case report and review. Clin Infect Dis 1993;16:689–702.

36. Arnaout MK, Tamburro RF, Bodner SM, et al. *Bacillus cereus* causing fulminant sepsis and hemolysis in two patients with acute leukemia. J Pediatr Hematol Oncol 1999;21:431–435.

37. Arpi M, Vancanneyt M, Swings J, Leisner JJ. Six cases of *Lactobacillus* bacteraemia: identification of organisms and antibiotic susceptibility and therapy. Scand J Infect Dis 2003;35:404–408.

38. Artz AL, Szabo S, Zabel LT, Hoffmeister HM. Aortic valve endocarditis with paravalvular abscesses caused by *Erysipelothrix rhusiopathiae*. Eur J Clin Microbiol Infect Dis 2001;20:587–588.

39. Ash C, Collins MD. Comparative analysis of 23s ribosomal RNA gene sequences of *Bacillus anthracis* and emetic *Bacillus cereus* determined by PCR-direct sequencing. FEMS Microbiol Lett 1992;73:75–80.

40. Ash C, Farrow JA, Dorsch M, et al. Comparative analysis of *Bacillus anthracis*, *Bacillus cereus*, and related species on the basis of reverse transcriptase sequencing of 16S rRNA. Int J Syst Bacteriol 1991;41:242–246.

41. Ash C, Farrow JAE, Wallbanks S, Collins MD. Phylogenetic heterogeneity of the genus *Bacillus* revealed by comparative analysis of small subunit-ribosomal RNA sequences. Lett Appl Microbiol 1991;13:202–206.

42. Ash C, Priest FG, Collins MD. Molecular identification of rRNA group 3 bacillus (Ash, Farrow, Wallbanks, Collins) using a PCR probe test. Proposal for the creation of a new genus *Paenibacillus*. Antonie Van Leeuwenhoek 1993/1994;64:253–260.

43. Atkins MC, Nicolson L, Harrison GAJ, et al. *Lactobacillus jensenii* prosthetic valve endocarditis. J Infect 1990;21:322–324.

44. Aureli P, Fiorucci GC, Caroli D, et al. An outbreak of febrile gastroenteritis associated with corn contaminated by *Listeria monocytogenes*. N Engl J Med 2000;342:1236–1241.

45. Austin G, Hill E. Endocarditis due to Corynebacterium CDC group G-2. J Infect Dis 1983;147:1106.

46. Auzias A, Bollet C, Ayari R, et al. *Corynebacterium freneyi* bacteremia. J Clin Microbiol 2003;41:2777–2778.

47. Baele M, Vaneechoutte M, Verhelst R, et al. Identification of *Lactobacillus* species using tDNA-PCR. J Microbiol Meth 2002;50:263–271.

48. Baida GE, Kuzmin NP. Mechanism of action of hemolysin III from *Bacillus cereus*. Biochem Biophy Acta 1996;1284:122–124.

49. Baillie LW, Jones MN, Turnbull PC, Manchee RJ. Evaluation of the Biolog system for the identification of *Bacillus anthracis*. Lett Appl Microbiol 1995;20:209–211.

50. Bakalidou A, Kampfer P, Berchtold M, et al. *Cellulosimicrobium variabile* sp. nov., a cellulolytic bacterium from the hindgut of the termite *Mastotermes darwiniensis*. Int J Syst Evol Microbiol 2002;52:1185–1192.

51. Balci I, Eksi F, Bayram A. Coryneform bacteria isolated from blood cultures and their antibiotic susceptibilities. J Int Med Res 2002;30:422–427.

52. Ball SC, Sepkowitz K. Infection due to *Bacillus cereus* in an injection drug user with AIDS: bacteremia without morbidity. Clin Infect Dis 1994;19:216–217.

53. Bandera A, Gori A, Rossi MC, et al. A case of costochondral abscess due to *Corynebacterium minutissimum* in an HIV-infected patient. J Infect 2000;41:103–105.

54. Bannerman E, Yersin M-N, Bille J. Evaluation of the Organon-Teknika Micro-ID *Listeria* system. Appl Environ Microbiol 1992;58:2011–2015.

55. Bantar CE, Relloso S, Castell FR, et al. Abscess caused by vancomycin-resistant *Lactobacillus confusus*. J Clin Microbiol 1991;29:2063–2064.

56. Barakett V, Morel G, Lesage G, Petit JC. Septic arthritis due to non-toxigenic strain of *Corynebacterium diphtheriae* subspecies *mitis*. Clin Infect Dis 1993;17:520–521.

57. Barksdale I, Linder R, Sulea T, Pollice M. Phospholipase D activity of *Corynebacterium pseudotuberculosis* (*Corynebacterium ovis*) and *Corynebacterium ulcerans*, a distinctive marker within the genus *Corynebacterium*. J Clin Microbiol 1981;13:335–343.

58. Barnham M. *Actinomyces pyogenes* bacteraemia in a patient with carcinoma of the colon. J Infect 1988;17:231–234.

59. Barr JG, Murphy PG. *Corynebacterium striatum*: an unusual organism isolated in pure culture from sputum. J Infect 1986;13:297–315.

60. Barreau C, Bimet F, Kiredjian M, et al. Comparative chemotaxonomic studies

of mycolic acid-free coryneform bacteria of human origin. J Clin Microbiol 1993;31:2085–2090.

61. Barrett SLR, Cookson BT, Carlson, LC, et al. Diversity within reference strains of *Corynebacterium matruchotii* includes *Corynebacterium durum* and a novel organism. J Clin Microbiol 2001;39:943–948.

62. Bassiri AG, Girgis RE, Theodore J. *Actinomyces odontolyticus* thoracopulmonary infections. Two cases in lung and heart-lung transplant recipients. Chest 1996;109:1109–1111.

63. Bastida-Vila MT, Lopez-Onrubia P, Rovira-Lledos J, et al. *Gardnerella vaginalis* bacteremia. Eur J Clin Microbiol Infect Dis 1997;16:400–401.

64. Batson JH, Mukkamala R, Byrd RP Jr, Roy TM. Pulmonary abscess due to *Corynebacterium striatum*. J Tenn Med Assoc 1996;89:115–116.

65. Bavbek M, Caner H, Atslan H, et al. Cerebral *Dermabacter hominis* abscess. Infection 1998;26:181–183.

66. Bayer AS, Chow AW, Betts D, Guze LB. Lactobacillemia: report of nine cases: important clinical and therapeutic considerations. Am J Med 1978;64:808–813.

67. Bayer AS, Chow AW, Concepcion N, Guze LB: Susceptibility of 40 lactobacilli to six antimicrobial agents with broad gram-positive anaerobic spectra. Antimicrob Agents Chemother 1978;14:720–722.

68. Beckwith DG, Jahre JA, Haggerty S. Isolation of *Corynebacterium aquaticum* from spinal fluid of an infant with meningitis. J Clin Microbiol 1986;23:375–376.

69. Beecher DJ, Schoeni JL, Wong AC. Enterotoxic activity of hemolysin BL from *Bacillus cereus*. Infect Immun 1995;63:4423–4428.

70. Beecher DJ, Wong AC. Improved purification and characterization of hemolysin BL, a hemolytic dermonecrotic vascular permeability factor from *Bacillus cereus*. Infect Immun 1994;62:980–986.

71. Bekemeyer WB, Zimmerman GA. Life threatening complications associated with pneumonia due to *Bacillus cereus*. Am Rev Respir Dis 1985;131:466–469.

72. Berardi-Grassias L, Roy O, Berardi JC, Furioli J. Neonatal meningitis due to *Gardnerella vaginalis*. Eur J Clin Microbiol 1988;7:406–407.

73. Berenguer, Solera J, Diaz MD, et al. Listeriosis in patients infected with human immunodeficiency virus. Rev Infect Dis 1991;13:115–119.

74. Berger SA, Gorea A, Stadler J, et al. Recurrent breast abscess caused by *Corynebacterium minutissimum*. J Clin Microbiol 1984;20:1219–1220.

75. Bernard KA, Bellefeuille M, Ewan EP. Cellular fatty acid composition as an adjunct to the identification of asporogenous, aerobic gram-positive rods. J Clin Microbiol 1991;29:83–89.

76. Bernard K, Bellefeuille M, Hollis DG, et al. Cellular fatty acid composition and phenotypic and cultural characterization of CDC fermentative coryneform groups 3 and 5. J Clin Microbiol 1994;32:1217–1222.

77. Bernard KA, Munro C, Weibe D, Ongsansoy E. Characteristics of rare or recently described *Corynebacterium* species recovered from human clinical material in Canada. J Clin Microbiol 2002;40:4375–4381.

78. Berner R, Leititis JU, Furste HO, Brandis M. Bacterial tracheitis caused by *Corynebacterium diphtheriae*. Eur J Pediatr 1997;156:207–2081.

79. Berner R, Pelz K, Wilhelm C, et al. Fatal sepsis caused by *Corynebacterium amycolatum* in a premature infant. J Clin Microbiol 1997;35:1011–1012.

80. Bert F, Ouahes O, Lambert-Zechovsky N. Brain abscess due to *Bacillus macerans* following a penetrating periorbital injury. J Clin Microbiol 1995;33:1950–1953.

81. Bhandari S, Meigh JA, Sellars L. CAPD peritonitis due to *Corynebacterium striatum*. Perit Dial Int 1995;15:88–89.

82. Biavasco F, Giovanetti E, Miele A. *In vitro* co-transfer of *vanA* vancomycin resistance between enterococci and listeria of different species. Eur J Clin Microbiol Infect Dis 1996;15:50–59.

83. Bibashi E, Kokolina E, Mitsopoulos E, et al. Peritonitis due to *Rothia dentocariosa* in a patient receiving continuous ambulatory peritoneal dialysis. Clin Infect Dis 1999;28:696.

84. Bille J, Catimel B, Bannerman E, et al. API *Listeria*, a new and promising one-day system to identify *Listeria* isolates. Appl Environ Microbiol 1992;59:1857–1860.

85. Billington SJ, Post KW, Jjost BH. Isolation of *Arcanobacterium* (*Actinomyces*) *pyogenes* from cases of feline otitis externa and canine cystitis. J Vet Diagn Invest 2002;14:159–162.

86. Billot-Klein D, Gutmann L, Sable S, et al. Modification of peptidoglycan precursors is a common feature of the low-level vancomycin resistant VanB type *Enterococcus* D366 and of the naturally vancomycin-resistant species *Lactobacillus casei*, *Pediococcus pentosaceus*, *Leuconostoc mesenteroides*, and *Enterococcus gallinarum*. J Bacteriol 1994;176:2398–2405.

87. Binder D, Zbinden R, Widmer U, et al. Native and prosthetic valve endocarditis caused by *Rothia dentocariosa*. Infection 1997;25:22–26.

88. Bizette GA, Kemmerly SA, Cole JT, et al. Sepsis due to coryneform group A-4 in an immunocompromised host. Clin Infect Dis 1995;21:1334–1336.

89. Blachman U, Gilardi GL, Pickett MJ. *Bacillus* species strains posing as nonfermentative gram-negative rods. Clin Microbiol Newslett 1980;2:8.

90. Blackmon DM, Calvert HM, Henry PM, Westfall CT. *Bacillus cereus* endoph-

thalmitis secondary to self-inflicted periocular injection. Arch Ophthalmol 2000;118:1585–1586.

91. Blue SR, Singh VR, Sauboulle MA: *Bacillus licheniformis* bacteremia: five cases associated with central venous catheters. Clin Infect Dis 1995;20:629–633.

92. Boc SF, Martone JD. Osteomyelitis caused by *Corynebacterium jeikeium*. J Am Podiatr Med Assoc 1995;85:338–339.

93. Boerlin P, Piffaretti J-C. Typing of human, animal, food, and environmental isolates of *Listeria monocytogenes* by multilocus enzyme electrophoresis. Int J Syst Bacteriol 1991;41:59–64.

94. Boerlin P, Rocourt J, Grimont F, et al. *Listeria ivanovii* subsp. *londoniensis* subsp. nov. Int J Syst Bacteriol 1992;42:69–73.

95. Boerlin P, Rocourt J, Piffaretti J-C. Taxonomy of the genus *Listeria* by using multilocus enzyme electrophoresis. Int J Syst Bacteriol 1991;41:59–64.

96. Boggess JA, Watts DH, Hillier SL, et al. Bacteremia shortly after placental separation during cesarean delivery. Obstet Gynecol 1996;87:779–784.

97. Boone DR, Liu Y, Zhao Z-J, et al. *Bacillus infernus* sp. nov., an Fe(III)- and Mn(IV)-reducing anaerobe from the deep terrestrial subsurface. Int J Syst Bacteriol 1995;45:441–448.

98. Booth LV, Ellis C, Wale MC, et al. An atypical case of *Corynebacterium diphtheriae* endocarditis and subsequent outbreak control measures. J Infect 1995;31:63–65.

99. Borra S, Kleinfeld M. Peritonitis caused by *Oerskovia xanthineolytica* in a patient on chronic ambulatory peritoneal dialysis (letter). Am J Kidney Dis 1996;27:458.

100. Bostock AD, Gilbert FR, Lewis D, Smith DC: *Corynebacterium ulcerans* infection associated with untreated milk. J Infect 1984;9:286–288.

101. Boudewijns M, Magerman J, Verhaegen J, et al. *Rothia dentocariosa* endocarditis and mycotic aneurysms: case report and review of the literature. Clin Microbiol Infect 2003;9:222–229.

102. Bourgeois N, Jacobs F, Tavares ML, et al. *Listeria monocytogenes* hepatitis in a liver transplant recipient: a case report and review of the literature. J Hepatol 1993;18:284–289.

103. Boustouller YL, Johnson AP, Taylor-Robinson D. Pili on *Gardnerella vaginalis* studied by electron microscopy. J Med Microbiol 1987;23:327–329.

104. Bowstead TT, Santiago SM Jr: Pleuropulmonary infection due to *Corynebacterium striatum*. Br J Dis Chest 1980;74:198–200.

105. Braden DS, Feldman S, Palmer AL: *Rothia* endocarditis in a child. South Med J 1999;92:815–816.

106. Brailsford SR, Tregaskis RB, Leftwich HS, Beighton D. The predominant *Actinomyces* spp. isolated from infected dentin of active root caries lesions. J Dent Res 1999;78:1525–1534.

107. Brandenburg AH, van Belkum A, van Pelt C, et al. Patient-to-patient spread of a single strain of *Corynebacterium striatum* causing infections in a surgical intensive care unit. J Clin Microbiol 1996;34:2089–2094.

108. Braun TI, Travis D, Dee RR, Nieman RE. Liver abscess due to *Listeria monocytogenes*: case report and review. Clin Infect Dis 1993;17:267–269.

109. Brazzola P, Zbinden R, Rudin C, et al. *Brevibacterium casei* sepsis in an 18-year-old female with AIDS. J Clin Microbiol 2000;38:3513–3514.

110. Bregenzer T, Frei R, Ohnacker H, Zimmerli W. *Corynebacterium pseudotuberculosis* infection in a butcher. Clin Microbiol Infect 1997;3:696–698.

111. Brennan NM, Brown R, Goodfellow M, et al. *Corynebacterium mooreparkense* sp. nov. and *Corynebacterium casei* sp. nov., isolated from the surface of smear-ripened cheese. Int J Syst Evol Microbiol 2001;51:843–852.

112. Briselden AM, Hillier SL. Longitudinal study of the biotypes of *Gardnerella vaginalis*. J Clin Microbiol 1990;28:2761–2764.

113. Briselden AM, Hillier SL. Evaluation of Affirm VP microbial identification test for *Gardnerella vaginalis* and *Trichomonas vaginalis*. J Clin Microbiol 1994;32:148–152.

114. Briselden AM, Moncla BJ, Stevens CE, Hillier SL: Sialidases (neuraminidases) in bacterial vaginosis and bacterial vaginosis-associated microflora. J Clin Microbiol 1992;30:663–666.

115. Brooke CJ, Riley TV. *Erysipelothrix rhusiopathiae*: bacteriology, epidemiology, and clinical manifestations of an occupational pathogen. J Med Microbiol 1999;48:789–799.

116. Broughton RA, Gruber WC, Hafar AAM, Baker CJ. Neonatal meningitis due to *Lactobacillus*. Pediatr Infect Dis 1983;2:382–384.

117. Brownstein DG, Barthold SW, Adams RL, et al. Experimental *Corynebacterium kutscheri* infection in rats: bacteriology and serology. Lab Anim Sci 1985;35:135–138.

118. Brunner S, Graf S, Riegel P, Altweg M. Catalase-negative *Actinomyces neuii* subsp. *neuii* isolated from an infected mammary prosthesis. Int J Med Microbiol 2000;290:285–287.

119. Bubert A, Riebe J, Schnitzler N, et al. Isolation of catalase-negative *Listeria monocytogenes* strains from listeriosis patients and their rapid identification by anti-p60 antibodies and/or PCR. J Clin Microbiol 1997;35:179–183.

120. Bula CJ, Bille J, Glauser MP. An epidemic of food-borne listeriosis in Western Switzerland: description of 57 cases involving adults. Clin Infect Dis 1995;20:66–72.

121. Burke GJ, Malouf MA, Glanville AR. Opportunistic lung infection with *Corynebacterium pseudodiphtheriticum* after lung and heart transplantation. Med J Aust 1997;166:362–364.

122. Burton JP, Dixon JL, Reid G. Detection of *Bifidobacterium* species and *Gardnerella vaginalis* in the vagina using PCR and denaturing gradient gel electrophoresis (DGGE). Int J Obstet Gynecol 2003;81:61–63.

123. Cai J, Collins MD. Phylogenetic analysis of species of the *meso*-diaminopimelic acid-containing genera *Brevibacterium* and *Dermabacter*. Int J Syst Bacteriol 1994;44:583–585.

124. Cai S, Kabuki DY, Kuaye AY, et al. Rational design of DNA sequence-based strategies for subtyping *Listeria monocytogenes*. J Clin Microbiol 2002;40: 3319–3324.

125. Cain DB, McCann VL. An unusual case of cutaneous listeriosis. J Clin Microbiol 1996;23:976–977.

126. Callegan MC, Kane ST, Cochran DC, et al. Relationship of *plcR*-regulated factors to *Bacillus* endophthalmitis virulence. Infect Immun 2003;71:3116–3124.

127. Campbell PB, Palladino S, Flexman JP. Catheter-related septicemia caused by a vancomycin-resistant coryneform CDC group A-5. Pathology 1994;26:56–58.

128. Capita R, Alonso-Calleja C, Mereghetti L, et al. Evaluation of the international phage typing set and some experimental phages for typing of *Listeria monocytogenes* from poultry in Spain. J Appl Microbiol 2002;92:90–96.

129. Carlson P. Comparison of the E test and agar dilution methods for susceptibility testing of *Arcanobacterium haemolyticum*. Eur J Clin Microbiol Infect Dis 2000; 19:891–893.

130. Carlson P, Kontiainen S, Renkonen OV. Antimicrobial susceptibility of *Arcanobacterium haemolyticum*. Antimicrob Agents Chemother 1994;38:142–143.

131. Carlson P, Korpela J, Walder M, Nyman M. Antimicrobial susceptibilities and biotypes of *Arcanobacterium haemolyticum* blood isolates. Eur J Clin Microbiol Infect Dis 1999;18:915–917.

132. Carretto E, Barbarini D, Poletti F, et al. *Bacillus cereus* fatal bacteremia and apparent association with nosocomial transmission in an intensive care unit. Scand J Infect Dis 2000;32:98–100.

133. Casella P, Bosoni MA, Tommasi A. Recurrent *Corynebacterium aquaticum* peritonitis in a patient undergoing continuous ambulatory peritoneal dialysis. Clin Microbiol Newslett 1988;10:62–63.

134. Castedo E, Castro A, Martin P, et al. *Bacillus cereus* prosthetic valve endocarditis. Ann Thorac Surg 1999;68:2351–23452.

135. Cauci S, Driussi S, Monte R, et al. Immunoglobulin A response against *Gardnerella vaginalis* hemolysin and sialidase activity in bacterial vaginosis. Am J Obstet Gynecol 1998;178:511–515.

136. Cauci S, Hitti J, Noonan C, et al. Vaginal hydrolytic enzymes, immunoglobulin A against *Gardnerella vaginalis* toxin, and risk of early preterm birth among women in preterm labor with bacterial vaginosis or intermediate flora. Am J Obstet Gynecol 2002;187:877–881.

137. Cauci S, Monte R, Ropele M, et al. Pore-forming and haemolytic properties of the *Gardnerella vaginalis* cytolysin. Mol Microbiol 1993;9:1143–1155.

138. Cauci S, Scrimin F, Driussi S, et al. Specific immune response against *Gardnerella vaginalis* hemolysin in patients with bacterial vaginosis. Am J Obstet Gynecol 1996;175:1601–1605.

139. Cauda R, Tamburrini E, Ventura G, Ortona L. Effective vancomycin therapy for *Corynebacterium pseudodiphtheriticum* endocarditis. South Med J 1987;80: 1598.

140. Cavendish J, Cole JB, Ohl CA: Polymicrobial central venous catheter sepsis involving a multiantibiotic-resistant strain of *Corynebacterium minutissimum*. Clin Infect Dis 1994;19:204–205.

141. Centers for Disease Control. Listeriosis outbreak associated with Mexican-style cheese—California. MMWR Morbid Mortal Wkly Rep 1985;34:357–359.

142. Centers for Disease Control: Listeriosis associated with consumption of turkey franks. MMWR Morbid Mortal Wkly Rep 38:267–268, 1989.

143. Centers for Disease Control and Prevention. Update: foodborne listeriosis—United States, 1988–1990. MMWR Morbid Mortal Wkly Rep 1992;41: 251.

144. Centers for Disease Control and Prevention. Respiratory diphtheria caused by *Corynebacterium ulcerans*—- Terre Haute, Indiana, 1996. MMWR Morbid Mortal Wkly Rep 1997;46:330–332.

145. Centers for Disease Control and Prevention: *Bioterrorism Response Guide for Clinical Laboratories*. Atlanta: Department of Health and Human Services, Public Health Service, 2002.

146. Centers for Disease Control and Prevention. Use of anthrax vaccine in response to terrorism: supplemental recommendations of the Advisory Committee on Immunization practices. MMWR Morbid Mortal Wkly Rep 2002;51: 1024–1026.

147. Chang J, Powles R, Mehta J, et al. Listeriosis in bone marrow transplant recipients: incidence, clinical features, and treatment. Clin Infect Dis 1995;21: 1289–1290.

148. Chiner E, Arriero JM, Signes-Costa J, et al. *Corynebacterium pseudodiphtheriticum* pneumonia in an immunocompetent patient. Monaldi Arch Chest Dis 1999; 54:325–327.

149. Chirgwin K, Gleich S. *Listeria monocytogenes* osteomyelitis. Arch Intern Med 1989;149:931–932.

150. Chomarat M, Breton P, Dubost J. Osteomyelitis due to Corynebacterium D2. Eur J Clin Microbiol Infect Dis 1991;10:43.

151. Chomarat M, Espinouse D. *Lactobacillus rhamnosus* septicemia in patients with prolonged aplasia receiving ceftazidime-vancomycin. Eur J Clin Microbiol Infect Dis 1991;10:44.

152. Chooromoney KN, Hampson DJ, Eamens JG, Turner MJ. Analysis of *Erysipelothrix rhusiopathiae* and *Erysipelothrix tonsillarum* by multilocus enzyme electrophoresis. J Clin Microbiol 1994;32:371–376.

153. Chowdhury MNH, Desilva SK. Episiotomy wound infection due to *Gardnerella vaginalis*. Eur J Clin Microbiol 1986;5:164–165.

154. Chowdhury MNH, Kambal AM. A case of conjunctivitis in a neonate due to *Gardnerella vaginalis*. Trop Geogr Med 1985;37:365–366.

155. Christenson JC, Byington C, Korgenski WK, et al. *Bacillus cereus* infections among oncology patients at a children's hospital. Am J Infect Control 1999;27: 543–546.

156. Christopher GW, Cieslak TJ, Pavlin JA, Eitzen EM Jr. Biological warfare: a historical perspective. JAMA 1997;278:412–417.

157. Chu WP, Que TL, Lee WK, Wong SN. Meningoencephalitis caused by *Bacillus cereus* in a neonate. Hong Kong Med J 2001;7:89–92.

158. Cintron JR, Del Pino A, Duarte B, Wood D. Abdominal actinomycosis, Report of two cases and review of the literature. Dis Colon Rectum 1996;39:103–108.

159. Claeys G, Vanhouteghem H, Riegel P, et al. Endocarditis of native aortic and mitral valves due to *Corynebacterium accolens*: report of a case and application of phenotypic and genotypic techniques for identification. J Clin Microbiol 1996; 34:1290–1292.

160. Clark AG, McLauchlin J. A simple colour test based on an alanyl peptidase reaction which differentiates *Listeria monocytogenes* from other *Listeria* species. J Clin Microbiol 1997;35:2155–2156.

161. Clarke R, Qamruddin A, Taylor M, Panigrahi H: Septic arthritis caused by *Corynebacterium amycolatum* following vascular graft sepsis. J Infect 1999;38: 126–127.

162. Clarridge JE III, Zhang Q. Genotypic diversity of clinical *Actinomyces* species: phenotype, source, and disease correlation among genospecies. J Clin Microbiol 2002;40:3442–3448.

163. Claus D, Berkeley RCW. Genus *Bacillus* Cohn 1872, 174. In: Sneath PHA, Mair NS, Sharpe ME, eds. Bergey's Manual of Systematic Bacteriology. Vol. 2. Baltimore: Williams & Wilkins, 1986:1105–1139.

164. Collins MD. Reclassification of *Bacterionema matruchotii* (Mendal) in the genus *Corynebacterium* as *Corynebacterium matruchotii* comb. nov. Zentralbl Bakteriol Mikrobiolm Hyg 1 Abt Orig C 1983;3:399–400.

165. Collins MD, Bernard KA, Hutson A, et al. *Corynebacterium sundsvallense* sp. nov., from human clinical specimens. Int J Syst Bacteriol 1999;49:361–366.

166. Collins MD, Burton RA, Jones D. *Corynebacterium amycolatum* sp. nov., a new mycolic acid-less *Corynebacterium* species from human skin. FEMS Microbiol. Lett. 1988;49:349–352.

167. Collins MD, Falsen E, Akervall E, et al. *Corynebacterium kroppenstedtii* sp. nov., a novel corynebacterium that does not contain mycolic acids. Int J Syst Bacteriol 1998;48:1449–1454.

168. Collins MD, Hoyles L, Foster G, et al. *Corynebacterium capitovis* sp. nov., from a sheep. Int J Syst Evol Microbiol 2001;51:857–860.

169. Collins MD, Hoyles L, Hutson RA, et al. *Corynebacterium testudinoris* sp. nov., from a tortoise, and *Corynebacterium felinum* sp. nov., from a Scottish wild cat. Int J Syst Evol Microbiol 2001;51:1349–1352.

170. Collins MD, Hoyles L, Kalfas S, et al. Characterization of *Actinomyces* isolates from infected root canals of teeth: description of *Actinomyces radicidentis*. J Clin Microbiol 2000;38:3399–3403.

171. Collins MD, Hoyles L, Lawson PA, et al. Phenotypic and phylogenetic characterization of a new *Corynebacterium* species from dogs: description of *Corynebacterium auriscanis* sp. nov. J Clin Microbiol 1999;37:3443–3447.

172. Collins MD, Hutson RA, Baverud V, Falsen E. Characterization of a *Rothia*-like organism from a mouse: description of *Rothia nasimurium* sp. nov. and reclassification of *Stomatococcus mucilaginosus* as *Rothia mucilaginosa* comb. nov. Int J Syst Evol Microbiol 2000;50:1247–1251.

173. Collins MD, Jones D, Keddie RM, et al. Classification of some coryneform bacteria in a new genus *Aureobacterium*. Syst Appl Microbiol 1983;4:236–252.

174. Collins MD, Jones D, Schofield GM. Reclassification of ''*Corynebacterium haemolyticum*'' (MacLean, Liebow, and Rosenberg) in the genus *Arcanobacterium* gen. nov. as *Arcanobacterium haemolyticum* nom. rev., comb. nov. J Gen Microbiol 1982;128:1279–1281.

175. Collins MD, Stubbs S, Hommez J, Devriese LA. Molecular taxonomic studies of *Actinomyces*-like bacteria isolated from purulent lesions in pigs and description of *Actinomyces hyovaginalis* sp. nov. Int J Syst Bacteriol 1993;43:471–473.

176. Collins MD, Wallbanks S, Lane D, et al. Phylogenetic analysis of the genus *Listeria* based on reverse transcriptase sequencing of 16S rRNA. Int J Syst Bacteriol 1991;41:240–246.

177. Colmegna I, Rodriguez-Barradas M, Rauch M, et al. Disseminated *Actinomyces*

meyeri infection resembling lung cancer with brain metastases. Am J Med Sci 2003;326:152–155.

178. Colt HG, Morris JF, Marston BJ, Sewell DL. Necrotizing tracheitis caused by *Corynebacterium pseudodiphtheriticum*: unique case and review. Rev Infect Dis 1991;13:73–76.

179. Cone LA, Curry N, Wuestoff MA, et al. Septic synovitis and arthritis due to *Corynebacterium striatum* following an accidental scalpel injury. Clin Infect Dis 1998;27:1532–1533.

180. Come LA, Leung MM, Hirschberg J. *Actinomyces odontolyticus* bacteremia. Emerg Infect Dis 2003;9:1629–1632.

181. Connor JP, Buller RE: *Lactobacillus* sepsis with pelvic abscess. Gynecol Oncol 1994;54:99–100.

182. Connor MP, Green AD. Erysipeloid infection in a sheep farmer with coexisting orf. J Infect 1995;30:161–163.

183. Cook RL, Reid G, Pond DG, et al. Clue cells in bacterial vaginosis: immunofluorescent identification of the adherent gram-negative bacteria as *Gardnerella vaginalis*. J Infect Dis 1989;160:490–496.

184. Cooper CD, Vincent A, Greene JN, et al. *Lactobacillus* bacteremia in febrile neutropenic patients in a cancer hospital. Clin Infect Dis 1998;26:1247–1248.

185. Coudron PE, Harris RC, Vaughan MG, Dalton HP. Two similar but atypical strains of coryneform group A-4 isolated from patients with endophthalmitis. J Clin Microbiol 1985;22:475–477.

186. Coudron PE, Payne JM, Markowitz SM. Pneumonia and empyema infection associated with a *Bacillus* species that resembles *B. alvei*. J Clin Microbiol 1991; 29:1777–1779.

187. Cowling P, Hall L. *Corynebacterium striatum*: a clinically significant isolate from sputum in chronic obstructive airways disease. J Infect 1993;26:335–336.

188. Coyle MB, Lipsky BA. Coryneform bacteria in infectious diseases: clinical and laboratory aspects. Clin Microbiol Rev 1990;3:227–246.

189. Craig J, Grigor W, Doyle B, Arnold D: Pyelonephritis caused by *Corynebacterium minutissimum*. Pediatr Infect Dis J 1994;13:1151–1152.

190. Craig TJ, Maguire FE, Wallace MR: Tracheobronchitis due to *Corynebacterium pseudodiphtheriticum*. South Med J 1991;84:504–506.

191. Cristiano L, Coffetti N, Dalvai G, et al. Bacterial vaginosis; prevalence in outpatients, association with some microorganisms, and laboratory indices. Genitourin Med 1989;65:382–387.

192. Criswell BS, Stenback WA, Black SH, Gardner HL. Fine structure of *Haemophilus vaginalis*. J Bacteriol 1972;109:930–932.

193. Cummins AJ, Fielding AK, McLauchin J. *Listeria ivanovii* infection in a patient with AIDS. J Infect 1994;28:89–91.

194. Curtis JR, Wing AJ, Coleman JC. *Bacillus cereus* bacteremia: a complication of intermittent haemodialysis. Lancet 1967;1:136–138.

195. Czajka J, Batt CA. Verification of causal relationships between *Listeria monocytogenes* isolates implicated in food-borne outbreaks of listeriosis by randomly amplified polymorphic DNA patterns. J Clin Microbiol 1994;32:1280–1287.

196. Dai Z, Sirard J-C, Mock M, Koehler TM. The *atxA* gene product activates transcription of anthrax toxin genes and is essential for virulence. Mol Microbiol 1995;16:1171–1181.

197. Dall L, Barnes WG, Hurdford D. Septicaemia in a granulocytopenic patient caused by *Corynebacterium striatum*. Postgrad Med J 1989;65:247–248.

198. Dalton SB, Austin CA, Sobel J, et al. An outbreak of gastroenteritis and fever due to *Listeria monocytogenes* in milk. N Engl J Med 1997;336:100–105.

199. Dan M, Somer I, Knobel B, Gutman R. Cutaneous manifestations of infection with *Corynebacterium* group JK. Rev Infect Dis 1988;10:1204–1207.

200. Dana A, Fader R, Sterken D. *Turicella otitidis* mastoiditis in a healthy child. Pediatr Infect Dis J 2001;20:84–85.

201. Dancer SJ, McNair D, Finn P, Kolsto AB. *Bacillus cereus* cellulitis from contaminated heroin. J Med Microbiol 2002;51:278–281.

202. Daneshvar MI, Hollis DG, Weyant RS et al. Identification of some charcoal-black-pigmented CDC fermentative coryneform group 4 isolates as *Rothia dentocariosa* and some as *Corynebacterium aurimucosum*: proposal of *Rothia dentocariosa* emend. Georg and Brown 1967, *Corynebacterium aurimucosum* emend. Yassin et al. 2002, and *Corynebacterium nigricans* Shukla et al. 2003 pro synon. *Corynebacterium aurimucosum*. J Clin Microbiol 2004;42:4189–4198

203. Danielsen M, Wind A. Susceptibility of lactobacillus spp. to antimicrobial agents. Int J Food Microbiol 2003;82:1–11.

204. Dass KN, Smith MA, Gill VJ, et al. *Brevibacterium* endocarditis: a first report. Clin Infect Dis 2002;35:e20–e21.

205. Davey RT, Tauber WB. Posttraumatic endophthalmitis: the emerging role of *Bacillus cereus* infection. Rev Infect Dis 1987;9:110–123.

206. de Arriba JJ, Blanch JJ, Mateos F, et al. *Corynebacterium striatum* first reported case of prosthetic valve endocarditis. J Infect 2002;44:193.

207. DeBriel D, Couderc F, Riegel P, et al. High-performance liquid chromatography of corynemycolic acids as a tool in identification of *Corynebacterium* species and related microorganisms. J Clin Microbiol 1992;30:1407–1417.

208. de Carpentier JP, Flanagan PM, Singh IP, et al. Nasopharyngeal *Corynebacterium ulcerans*: a different diphtheria. J Laryngol Otol 1992;106:824–826.

209. Decker CF, Simon GL, DiGioia RA, Tuazon CU. *Listeria monocytogenes* infec-

tions in patients with AIDS: report of five cases and review. Rev Infect Dis 1991;13:413–417.

210. Dee RR, Lorber B. Brain abscess due to *Listeria monocytogenes*: case report and literature review. Rev Infect Dis 1986;8:968–977.

211. de Mattos-Guaraldi AL, Formiga LC. Bacteriological properties of a sucrose-fermenting *Corynebacterium diphtheriae* strain isolated from a case of endocarditis. Curr Microbiol 1998;37:156–158.

212. de Miguel-Martinez I, Ramos-Macias A, Martin-Sanchez AM. Otitis media due to *Corynebacterium jeikeium*. Eur J Clin Microbiol Infect Dis 1999;18:231–232.

213. Denoyal G-A, Drouert EB, De Montclos HP, et al. *Gardnerella vaginalis* bacteremia in a man with prostatic adenoma. J Infect Dis 1990;161:367–368.

214. Dent VE, Williams RA. *Actinomyces denticolens* Dent and Williams sp. nov.: a new species from the dental plaque of cattle. J Appl Microbiol 1984;56:183–192.

215. Dercksen DP, Brinkhof JM, Decker-Nooren T, et al. A comparison of four serological tests for the diagnosis of caseous lymphadenitis in sheep and goats. Vet Microbiol 2000;75:167–175.

216. Dessau RB, Brandt-Christensen M, Jensen OJ, Tonnesen P. Pulmonary nodules due to *Corynebacterium ulcerans*. Eur Respir J 1995;8:651–653.

217. DeVega T, Echevarria S, Crespo J, et al. Acute hepatitis by *Listeria monocytogenes* in an HIV patient with chronic HBV hepatitis. J Clin Gastroenterol 1992; 15:251–255.

218. Devriese LA, Riegel P, Hommez J, et al. Identification of *Corynebacterium glucuronolyticum* strains from the urogenital tracts of humans and pigs. J Clin Microbiol 2000;38:4657–4659.

219. DeZoysa A, Efstratiou A. Use of amplified fragment length polymorphisms for typing *Corynebacterium diphtheriae*. J Clin Microbiol 2000;38:3843–3845.

220. DeZoysa AS, Efstratiou A. PCR typing of *Corynebacterium diphtheriae* by random amplification of polymorphic DNA. J Med Microbiol 1999;48:335–340.

221. DeZoysa A, Efstratiou A, George RC, et al. Molecular epidemiology of *Corynebacterium diphtheriae* from northwestern Russia and surrounding countries studied by ribotyping and pulsed-field gel electrophoresis. J Clin Microbiol 1995; 33:1080–1083.

222. Dickens A, Greven CM. Posttraumatic endophthalmitis caused by *Lactobacillus*. Arch Ophthalmol 1993;111:1169.

223. Dieckmann K-P, Henke R-P, Ovenbeck R. Renal actinomycosis mimicking renal carcinoma. Eur Urol 2001;39:357–359.

224. Digenis G, Dombros N, Devlin R, et al. Struvite stone formation by Corynebacterium group F1: a case report. J Urol 1992;147:169–170.

225. Dobinsky S, Noesselt T, Rucker A, et al. Three cases of *Arcanobacterium haemolyticum* associated with abscess formation and cellulitis. Eur J Clin Microbiol Infect Dis 1999;18:804–806.

226. Dobler G, Braveny I. Highly resistant *Corynebacterium macginleyi* as a cause of intravenous catheter-related infection. Eur J Clin Microbiol Infect Dis 2003; 22:72–73.

227. Doganay M, Aydin N. Antimicrobial susceptibility of *Bacillus anthracis*. Scand J Infect Dis 1991;23:333–335.

228. Dominguez EA, Patil AA, Johnson WM: Ventriculoperitoneal shunt infection due to *Listeria monocytogenes*. Clin Infect Dis 1994;19:223–224.

229. Dominguez-Gil B, Herrero JC, Carreno A, et al. Ureteral stenosis secondary to encrustation by urea-splitting *Corynebacterium urealyticum* in a kidney transplant patient. Nephrol Dial Transplant 14:977–978, 1999.

230. Donzis PB, Mondino BJ, Weissman BA. *Bacillus* keratitis associated with contaminated contact lens care systems. Am J Ophthalmol 1988;105:195–197.

231. Dramsi S, Dehoux P, Lebrun M, et al. Identification of four new members of the internalin multigene family in *Listeria monocytogenes* strain EGD. Infect Immun 1997;65:1615–1625.

232. Drancourt M, Oules O, Bouche V, Peloux Y. Two cases of *Actinomyces pyogenes* infection in humans. Eur J Clin Microbiol Infect Dis 1993;12:55–57.

233. Dubernet S, Desmasures N, Gueguen M. A PCR-based method for identification of lactobacilli at the genus level. FEMS Microbiol Lett 2002;214:271–275.

234. Dufresne S, Bousquet J, Boissinot M, Guay R. *Sulfobacillus disulfidooxidans* sp. nov., a new acidophilic disulfide-oxidizing, gram-positive, spore-forming bacterium. Int J Syst Bacteriol 1996;46:1056–1064.

235. Dunbar SA, Clarridge JE. Potential errors in recognition of *Erysipelothrix rhusiopathiae*. J Clin Microbiol 2000;38:1302–1304.

236. Dunkelberg WE, Skaggs R, Kellogg DS Jr. Method for isolation and identification of *Corynebacterium vaginale* (*Haemophilus vaginalis*). Appl Microbiol 1970;19:47–52.

237. Dykhuizen RS, Douglas G, Weir J, Gould IM. *Corynebacterium afermentans* subsp. *lipophilum*: multiple abscess formation in brain and liver. Scand J Infect Dis 1995;27:637–639.

238. Efstratiou A, Engler KH, Dawes CS, Sesardic D. Comparison of phenotypic and genotypic methods for detection of diphtheria toxin among isolates of pathogenic corynebacteria. J Clin Microbiol 1998;36:3173–3177.

239. Elad D, Aizenberg I, Soriano F, Shlomovitz S. Isolation of *Corynebacterium* group D2 from two dogs with urinary tract infections. J Clin Microbiol 1992; 30:1167–1169.

240. Ellerbroek P, Kuipers S, Rozenberg-Arska M, et al. *Oerskovia xanthineolytica*: a

new pathogen in bone marrow transplantation. Bone Marrow Transplant 199822:
503–505.

241. Ellis LC, Segreti J, Gitelis S, Huber JF. Joint infections due to *Listeria monocytogenes*: case report and review. Clin Infect Dis 1995;20:1548–1550.

242. Elsner H-A, Sobottka I, Bubert A, et al. Catalase-negative *Listeria monocytogenes* causing lethal sepsis and meningitis in an adult hematologic patient. Eur J Clin Microbiol Infect Dis 1996;15:965–967.

243. Ena J, Berenguer J, Palaez T, Bouza E. Endocarditis caused by *Corynebacterium* group D2. J Infect 1991;22:95–111.

244. Engler KH, Efstratiou A. Rapid enzyme immunoassay for determination of toxigenicity among clinical isolates of corynebacteria. J Clin Microbiol 2000;38:1385–1389.

245. Engler KH, Efstratiou A, Norn D, et al. Immunochromatographic strip test for rapid detection of diphtheria toxin: description and multicenter evaluation in areas of low and high prevalence of diphtheria. J Clin Microbiol 2002;40:80–83.

246. Engler KH, Glushkevich T, Mazurova IK, et al. A modified Elek test for detection of toxigenic corynebacteria in the diagnostic laboratory. J Clin Microbiol 1997;35:495–498.

247. Eschenbach DA, Davick PR, Williams BL, et al. Prevalence of hydrogen peroxide-producing *Lactobacillus* species in normal women and women with bacterial vaginosis. J Clin Microbiol 1989;27:251–256.

248. Eschenbach DA, Hillier S, Critchlow C, et al. Diagnosis and clinical manifestations of bacterial vaginosis. Am J Obstet Gynecol 1988;158:819–828.

249. Esteban J, Bueno J, Perez-Santonja JJ, Soriano F. Endophthalmitis involving an *Arthrobacter*-like organism following intraocular lens implantation. Clin Infect Dis 1996;23:1180–1181,.

250. Esteban J, Nieto E, Calvo R, et al. Microbiological characterization and clinical significance of *Corynebacterium amycolatum* strains. Eur J Clin Microbiol Infect Dis 1999;18:518–521.

251. Evtushenko LI, Dorofeeva LV, Subbotin SA, et al. *Leifsonia poae* gen. nov., sp. nov., isolated from nematode galls on *Poa annua*, and reclassification of ''*Corynebacterium aquaticum*'' Leifson 1962 as *Leifsonia aquatica* (ex Leifson 1962) gen. nov., nom. rev., comb. nov. and *Clavibacter xyli* Davis et al. 1984 with two subspecies as *Leifsonia xyli* (Davis et al. 1984) gen. nov., comb. nov. Int J Syst Evol Microbiol 2000;50:371–380.

252. Ewert DP, Lieb L, Hayes PS, et al. *Listeria monocytogenes* infection and serotype distribution among HIV-infected persons in Los Angeles County, 1985–1992. J Acquir Immune Defic Syndr and Human Retrovirol 1995;8:461–465.

253. Ezzell JH Jr, Many WJ Jr. *Gardnerella vaginalis*: an unusual case of pyogenic liver abscess. Am J Gastroenterol 1988;83:1409–1411.

254. Facinella B, Magi G, Prenna M, et al. *In vitro* extracellular and intracellular activity of two newer and two earlier fluoroquinolones against *Listeria monocytogenes*. Eur J Clin Microbiol Infect Dis 1997;16:827–833.

255. Fairley KF, Birch DF. Unconventional bacteria in urinary tract disease: *Gardnerella vaginalis*. Kidney Int 1989;23:862–865.

256. Fairley KF, Birch DF. Detection of bladder bacteriuria in patients with acute urinary symptoms. J Infect Dis 1989;159:226–231.

257. Farchaus JW, Ribot WJ, Jendrek S, Little SF. Fermentation, purification, and characterization of protective antigen from a recombinant, avirulent strain of *Bacillus anthracis*. Appl Environ Microbiol 1998;64:982–991.

258. Farina C, Arosio M, Mangia M, Moioli F. *Lactobacillus casei* subsp. *rhamnosus* sepsis in a patient with ulcerative colitis. J Clin Gastroenterol 2001;33:251–252.

259. Farizo KM, Strebel PM, Chen RT, et al. Fatal respiratory disease due to *Corynebacterium diphtheriae*: case report and review of guidelines for management, investigation, and control. Clin Infect Dis 1993;16:59–68.

260. Farrar WE. Anthrax: virulence and vaccines. Ann Intern Med 1994;121:379–380.

261. Farrer W. Four-valve endocarditis caused by Corynebacterium CDC group I1. South Med J 1987;80:923–925.

262. Felten A, Barreau C, Bizet C, et al. *Lactobacillus* species identification, H_2O_2 production, and antibiotic resistance, and correlation with human clinical status. J Clin Microbiol 1999;37:729–733.

263. Fernandez-Ayala M, Nan DN, Farinas MC. Vertebral osteomyelitis due to *Corynebacterium striatum* (letter). Am J Med 2001;111:1676.

264. Fernandez-Crespo P, Serra A, Bonet J, Gimenez M. Acute oliguric renal failure in a patient with an *Erysipelothrix rhusiopathiae* bacteremia and endocarditis. Nephron 1996;74:231.

265. Fernandez-Garayzabal JF, Collins MD, Hutson RA, et al. *Corynebacterium mastiditis* sp. nov., isolated from milk of sheep with subclinical mastitis. Int J Syst Bacteriol 1997;47:1082–1085.

266. Fernandez-Garayzabal JF, Collins MD, Hutson RA, et al. *Corynebacterium camporealensis* sp. nov., associated with subclinical mastitis in sheep. Int J Syst Bacteriol 1998;48:463–468.

267. Fernandez-Garayzabal JF, Eguido R, Vela AI, et al. Isolation of *Corynebacterium falsenii* and description of *Corynebacterium aquilae* sp. nov., from eagles. Int J Syst Evol Microbiol 2003;53:1135–1138.

268. Fernandez-Giron F, Saavedra-Martin JM, Benitez-Sanchez M, et al. *Corynebac-

terium minutissimum* peritonitis in a CAPD patient. Perit Dial Int 1998;18:345–346.

269. Fernandez-Natal I, Guerra J, Alcoba M, et al. Bacteremia caused by multiply resistant *Corynebacterium urealyticum:* six case reports and review. Eur J Clin Microbiol Infect Dis 2001;20:514–517.

270. Ferraz V, McCarthy K, Smith D, Koornhof HJ. Rothia dentocariosa endocarditis and aortic root abscess. J Infect 1998;37:292–295.

271. Fidalgo SG, Longbottom CJ, Riley TV. Susceptibility of *Erysipelothrix rhusiopathiae* to antimicrobial agents and home disinfectants. Pathology 2002;34:462–263.

272. Fiedler F. Biochemistry of the cell surface of *Listeria* strains: a locating general view. Infection 1988;16(Suppl 2):S92–S97.

273. Finkelhor RS, Wolinsky E, Kim CH, et al. *Gardnerella vaginalis* perinephric abscess in a transplanted kidney. N Engl J Med 1981;304:346.

274. Fiorino A-S. Intrauterine contraceptive device-associated actinomycotic abscess and *Actinomyces* detection on cervical smear. Obstet Gynecol 1996;87:142–149.

275. Fischer RA, Peters G, Gehrmann J, Jurgens H. *Corynebacterium aquaticum* septicemia with acute lymphoblastic leukemia (letter). Pediatr Infect Dis J 1994;13:836–837.

276. Fitter WF, DeSa DJ, Richardson H. Chorioamnionitis and funisitis due to *Corynebacterium kutscheri*. Arch Dis Child 1979;55:710–712.

277. Florez C, Muchada B, Nogales MC, et al. Bacteremia due to *Gardnerella vaginalis*: report of two cases. Clin Infect Dis 1994;18:125.

278. Ford JG, Yeatts RP, Givner LB. Orbital cellulitis, subperiosteal abscess, sinusitis, and septicemia caused by *Arcanobacterium haemolyticum*. Am J Ophthalmol 1995;120:261–262.

279. Fortina MG, Mora D, Schumann P, et al. Reclassification of *Saccharococcus caldoxylosilyticus* as *Geobacillus caldoxylosilyticus* (Ahmad et al. 2000) comb. nov. Int J Syst Evol Microbiol 2001;51:2063–2071.

280. Fortina MG, Pukall R, Schumann P, et al. *Ureibacillius* gen. nov., a new genus to accommodate *Bacillus thermosphaericus* (Andersson et al. 1995), emendation of *Ureibacillus thermosphaericus* and description of *Ureibacillus terrenus* sp. nov. Int J Syst Evol Microbiol 2001;51:447–455.

281. Frederiksen B. Maternal septicemia with *Listeria monocytogenes* in second trimester without infection of the fetus. Acta Obstet Gynecol Scand 1992;71:313–315.

282. Freeman JD, Smith HG, Haines HG, Hellyar AG. Seven patient with respiratory infections due to *Corynebacterium pseudodiphtheriticum*. Pathology 1994;26:311–314.

283. Freney J, Duperron MT, Courtier C, et al. Evaluation of API Coryne in comparison with conventional methods for identifying coryneform bacteria. J Clin Microbiol 1991;29:38–71.

284. Fruchart C, Salah A, Gray C, et al. *Lactobacillus* species as emerging pathogens in neutropenic patients. Eur J Clin Microbiol Infect Dis 1997;16:681–684.

285. Fuchs PC, Barry AL, Brown SD. *In vitro* activity of gemifloxacin against contemporary clinical bacterial isolates from eleven North American medical centers, and assessment of disk diffusion test interpretive criteria. Diagn Microbiol Infect Dis 2000;38:243–253.

286. Fudou R, Jojima Y, Seto A, et al. *Corynebacterium efficiens* sp. nov., a glutamic-acid-producing species from soil and vegetables. Int J Syst Evol Microbiol 2002;52:1127–1131.

287. Fujisawa T, Mori M. Evaluation of media for determining hemolytic activity and that of API *Listeria* system for identifying strains of *Listeria monocytogenes*. J Clin Microbiol 1994;32:1127–1129.

288. Funke G, Alvarez N, Pascual C, et al. *Actinomyces europaeus* sp. nov., isolated from human clinical specimens. Int J Syst Bacteriol 1997;47:687–692.

289. Funke G, Bernard KA, Bucher C, et al. *Corynebacterium glucuronolyticum* sp. nov. isolated from male patients with genitourinary infections. Med Microbiol Lett 1995;4:205–215.

290. Funke G, Carlotti A. Differentiation of *Brevibacterium* spp. encountered in clinical specimens. J Clin Microbiol 1994;32:1729–1732.

291. Funke G, Efstratiou A, Kuklinska D, et al. *Corynebacterium imitans* sp. nov. isolated from patients with suspected diphtheria. J Clin Microbiol 1997;35:1978–1983.

292. Funke G, Falsen E, Barrreau C. Primary identification of *Microbacterium* spp. encountered in clinical specimens as CDC coryneform group A-4 and A-5 bacteria. J Clin Microbiol 1995;33:188–192.

293. Funke G, Haase G, Schnitzler N, et al. Endophthalmitis due to *Microbacterium* species: case report and review of microbacterium infections. Clin Infect Dis 1997;24:713–716.

294. Funke G, Hoyles L, Collins MD. *Corynebacterium sanguinis* sp. nov., isolated from human blood cultures. In press.

295. Funke G, Hutson RA, Bernard KA, et al. Isolation of *Arthrobacter* spp. from clinical specimens and description of *Arthrobacter cumminsii* sp. nov. and *Arthrobacter woluwensis* sp. nov. J Clin Microbiol 1996;34:2356–2363.

296. Funke G, Hutson RA, Hilleringmann M, et al. *Corynebacterium lipophiloflavum* sp. nov. isolated from a patient with bacterial vaginosis. FEMS Microbiol Lett 1997;15:219–224.

297. Funke G, Lawson PA, Bernard KA, Collins MD. Most *Corynebacterium xerosis* strains identified in the routine clinical laboratory correspond to *Corynebacterium amycolatum*. J Clin Microbiol 1996;34:1124–1128.

298. Funke G, Lawson PA, Collins MD. Heterogeneity within human-derived Centers for Disease Control and Prevention (CDC) coryneform group ANF-1-like bacteria and description of *Corynebacterium auris* sp. nov. Int J Syst Bacteriol 1995; 45:735–739.

299. Funke G, Lawson PA, Collins MD. *Corynebacterium mucifaciens* sp. nov., an unusual species from human clinical material. Int J Syst Bacteriol 1997;47: 952–957.

300. Funke G, Lawson PA, Collins MD. *Corynebacterium riegelii* sp. nov., an unusual species isolated from female patients with urinary tract infections. J Clin Microbiol 1998;36:624–627.

301. Funke G, Lucchini GM, Pfyffer GE, et al. Characteristics of CDC group 1 and group 1-like coryneform bacteria isolated from clinical specimens. J Clin Microbiol 1993;31:2907–2912.

302. Funke G, Osorio CR, Frei R, et al. *Corynebacterium confusum* sp. nov., isolated from human clinical specimens. Int J Syst Bacteriol 1998;48:1291–1296.

303. Funke G, Pagano-Niederer M, Bernauer W. *Corynebacterium macginleyi* has to date been isolated exclusively from conjunctival swabs. J Clin Microbiol 1998;36:3670–3673.

304. Funke G, Pagano-Niederer M, Sjoden B, Falsen E. Characteristics of *Arthrobacter cumminsii*, the most frequently encountered *Arthrobacter* species in human clinical specimens. J Clin Microbiol 1998;36:1539–1543.

305. Funke G, Peters K, Aravena-Roman M. Evaluation of the RapID CB plus system for identification of coryneform bacteria and *Listeria* spp. J Clin Microbiol 1998; 36:2439–2442.

306. Funke G, Punter V, von Graevenitz A. Antimicrobial susceptibility patterns of some recently established coryneform bacteria. Antimicrob Agents Chemother 1996;40:2874–2878.

307. Funke G, Ramos C, Collins MD. Identification of some clinical strains of CDC coryneform group A-3 and A-4 bacteria as *Cellulomonas* species and proposal of *Cellulomonas hominis* sp. nov. for some group A-3 strains. Int J Syst Bacteriol 1995;33:2091–2097.

308. Funke G, Ramos CP, Collins MD. *Corynebacterium coyleae* sp. nov., isolated from human clinical specimens. Int J Syst Bacteriol 1997;47:92–96.

309. Funke G, Ramos CP, Fernandez-Garayzabal JF, et al. Description of human-derived Centers for Disease Control coryneform group 2 bacteria as *Actinomyces bernardiae* sp. nov. Int J Syst Bacteriol 1995;45:57–60.

310. Funke G, Renaud FN, Freney J, Riegel P. Multicenter evaluation of the updated and extended API (RAPID) Coryne database 2.0. J Clin Microbiol 1997;35: 3122–3126.

311. Funke G, Stubbs S, Altweg M, et al. *Turicella otitidis* gen. nov., sp. nov., a coryneform bacterium isolated from patients with otitis media. Int J Syst Bacteriol 1994;44:270–273.

312. Funke G, Stubbs S, Pfyffer GE, et al. Characteristics of CDC group 3 and group 5 coryneform bacteria isolated from clinical specimens and assignment to the genus *Dermabacter*. J Clin Microbiol 1994;32:1223–1228.

313. Funke G, Stubbs S, von Graevenitz A, Collins MD. Assignment of human-derived CDC group 1 coryneform bacteria and CDC group 1-like coryneform bacteria to the genus *Actinomyces* as *Actinomyces neuii* subsp. *neuii* sp. nov., subsp. nov., and *Actinomyces neuii* subsp. *anitratus* subsp. nov. Int J Syst Bacteriol 1994;44:167–171.

314. Funke G, von Graevenitz A. Infections due to *Actinomyces neuii* (former "CDC coryneform group 1" bacteria). Infection 1995;23:73–75.

315. Funke G, von Graevenitz A, Clarridge JE III, Bernard KA. Clinical microbiology of coryneform bacteria. Clin Microbiol Rev 1997;10:125–159.

316. Funke, G, von Graevenitz A, Weiss N. Primary identification of *Aureobacterium* spp. isolated from clinical specimens as "*Corynebacterium aquaticum*." J Clin Microbiol 1994;32:2686–2691.

317. Furman LM. Neonatal *Gardnerella vaginalis* infection. Pediatr Infect Dis J 1988; 7:890.

318. Gagne A, Chicoine M, Morin A, Houde A. Phenotypic and genotypic characterization of esterase-producing *Ureibacillus thermosphaericus* isolated from an aerobic digestor of swine waste. Can J Microbiol 2001;47:908–915.

319. Gahrn-Hansen B, Frederiksen W. Human infections with *Actinomyces pyogenes* (*Corynebacterium pyogenes*). Diagn Microbiol Infect Dis 1992;15:349–354.

320. Gaillard JL, Berche P, Frehel C, et al. Entry of *L. monocytogenes* into cells is mediated by Internalin, a repeat protein reminiscent of surface antigens from gram-positive cocci. Cell 1991;65:1127–1141.

321. Gaillard JL, Jaubert F, Berche P. The *inlAB* locus mediates the entry of *Listeria monocytogenes* into hepatocytes *in vivo*. J Exp Med 1996 ;183:359–369.

322. Gallemore GH, Mohon RT, Ferguson DA. *Lactobacillus fermentum* endocarditis involving a native mitral valve. J Tenn Med Assoc 1995;88:306–308.

323. Garcia I., Fainstein V, McLaughlin P. *Bacillus cereus* meningitis and bacteremia associated with an Ommaya reservoir in a patient with lymphoma. South Med J 1984;77:928–929.

324. Garcia-Restoy E, Espejo E, Bella F, Llebot J. Bacteremia due to *Erysipelothrix*

325. Garcia-Rodriguez JA, Garcia Sanchez JE, Munoz Bellido L, et al. In vitro activity of 79 antimicrobial agents against *Corynebacterium* group D2. Antimicrob Agents Chemother 1991;35:2140–2143.

326. Gardner HL, Dukes CD. *Haemophilus vaginalis* vaginitis: a newly defined specific infection previously classified as "nonspecific vaginitis." Am J Obstet Gynecol 1955;69:962–965.

327. Garduno E, Rebollo M, Asencio MA, et al. Splenic abscess caused by *Actinomyces meyeri* in a patient with autoimmune hepatitis. Diagn Microbiol Infect Dis 2000;37:213–214.

328. Garelick JM, Khodabakhsh AJ, Josephberg RG. Acute postoperative endophthalmitis caused by *Actinomyces neuii*. Am J Ophthalmol 2002;133:145–147.

329. Garrity GM, Holt JG. An overview of the road map to the manual. New York: Bergey's Manual Trust, 2000.

330. Gatermann S, Mitusch R, Djonlagic H, et al. Endocarditis caused by *Bacillus circulans*. Infection 1991;19:445.

331. Gaur AH, Patrick CC, McCullers JA, et al. *Bacillus cereus* bacteremia and meningitis in immunocompromised children. Clin Infect Dis 2001;32: 1456–1462.

332. Gauto AR, Cone LA, Woodard DR, et al. Arterial infections due to *Listeria monocytogenes*: report of four cases and review of world literature. Clin Infect Dis 1992;14:23–28.

333. Gavin SE, Leonard RB, Briselden AM, Coyle MB. Evaluation of the Rapid Coryne identification system for *Corynebacterium* species and other coryneforms. J Clin Microbiol 1992;30:1692–1695.

334. Gellin BG, Broome CV, Bibb WF, et al. The epidemiology of listeriosis in the United States, 1986. Am J Epidemiol 1991;133:392.

335. Giammanco GM, Di Marco V, Priolo I, et al. *Corynebacterium macginleyi* isolation from conjunctival swab in Italy. Diagn Microbiol Infect Dis 2002;44: 205–207,.

336. Giannakopoulos S, Alivizatos G, Deliveliotis C, et al. Encrusted cystitis and pyelitis. Eur Urol 2001;39:4476–448.

337. Gibbs RS, Weiner MH, Walmer K, St. Clair PJ. Microbiologic and serologic studies of *Gardnerella vaginalis* in intra-amniotic infection. Obstet Gynecol 1987;70:187–190.

338. Gilot P, Genicot A, Andre P. Serotyping and esterase typing for analysis of *Listeria monocytogenes* populations recovered from foodstuffs and from human patients with listeriosis in Belgium. J Clin Microbiol 1996;34:1007–1010.

339. Gilot P, Hermans C, Yde M, et al. Sporadic case of listeriosis associated with the consumption of a *Listeria monocytogenes*-contaminated 'Camembert' cheese. J Infect 1997;35:195–197.

340. Gimenez M, Fernandez P, Padilla E, et al. Endocarditis and acute renal failure due to *Erysipelothrix rhusiopathiae*. Eur J Clin Microbiol Infect Dis 1996;5: 347–348.

341. Ginsburg AS, Salazar LG, True LD, Disis ML. Fatal *Bacillus cereus* sepsis following resolving neutropenic enterocolitis during the treatment of acute leukemia. Am J Hematol 2003;2:204–208.

342. Giovannaci I, Ragimbeau C, Queguiner S, et al. *Listeria monocytogenes* in pork slaughtering and cutting plants: use of RAPD, PFGE, and PCR-REA for tracing and molecular epidemiology. Int J Food Microbiol 1999;53:127–140.

343. Girmenia C, Mauro FR, Rahimi S. Late listeriosis after fludarabine plus prednisone treatment. Br J Haematol 1994;87:407–408.

344. Golberg RL, Washington JA. Comparison of isolation of *Haemophilus vaginalis* (*Corynebacterium vaginale*) from peptone-starch-dextrose agar and Columbia colistin-nalidixic acid agar. J Clin Microbiol 1976;4:245–247.

345. Goldberger AC, Lipsky BA, Plorde JJ. Suppurative granulomatous lymphadenitis caused by *Corynebacterium ovis* (*pseudotuberculosis*). Am J Clin Pathol 1981;76:486–490.

346. Goldstein B, Abrutyn E. Pseudo-outbreak of *Bacillus* species: related to fibreoptic bronchoscopy. J Hosp Infect 1985;6:194–200.

347. Goldstein EJ, Citron DM, Merriam CV, et al. In vitro activities of daptomycin, vancomycin, quinupristin-dalfopristin, linezolid, and five other antimicrobials against 307 gram-positive anaerobic and 31 corynebacterium clinical isolates. Antimicrob Agents Chemother 2003;47:337–341.

348. Golledge CL, Phillips G. *Corynebacterium minutissimum* infection. J Infect 1991;23:73–76.

349. Golovacheva RS, Karavaiko GL. *Sulfobacillus*, a new genus of thermophilic sporulating bacteria. Mikrobiologiia 1978;8:15–22.

350. Gomez-Garces JL, Oteo J, Garcia G, et al. Bacteremia by *Dermabacter hominis*, a rare pathogen. J Clin Microbiol 2001;39:2356–2357.

351. Gordon S, Singer C. *Listeria monocytogenes* cholecystitis. J Infect Dis 1986; 154:918.

352. Goto K, Matsubara H, Mochida K, et al. *Alicyclobacillus herbarius* sp. nov., a novel bacterium containing o-cycloheptane fatty acids, isolated from herbal tea. Int J Syst Evol Microbiol 2002;52:109–113.

353. Gouin E, Mengaud J, Cossart P. The virulence gene cluster of *Listeria monocyto-*

rhusiopathiae in immunocompromised hosts without endocarditis. Rev Infect Dis 1991;13:1252–1253.

genes is also present in *Listeria ivanovii*, an animal pathogen, and *Listeria seeligeri*, a nonpathogenic species. Infect Immun 1994;62:3550–3553.

354. Goyache J, Ballesteros C, Vela AI, et al. *Corynebacterium sphenisci* sp. nov., isolated from wild penguins. Int J Syst Evol Microbiol 2003;53:1009–1012.

355. Goyache J, Vela AI, Collins MD, et al. *Corynebacterium spheniscorum* sp. nov., isolated from the cloacae of wild penguins. Int J Syst Evol Microbiol 2003;53: 43–46.

356. Granum PE. *Bacillus cereus* and its toxins. J Appl Bacteriol Symp Suppl 1996; 76:61S–66S.

357. Granum PE, O'Sullivan K, Lund T. The sequence of the non-haemolytic enterotoxin operon from *Bacillus cereus*. FEMS Microbiol Lett 1999;177:225–229.

358. Graves LM, Swaminathan B, Reeves MW, et al. Comparison of ribotyping and multilocus enzyme electrophoresis for subtyping of *Listeria monocytogenes* isolates. J Clin Microbiol 1994;32:2936–2943.

359. Green SL, LaPeter KS. Pseudodiphtheritic membranous pharyngitis caused by *Corynebacterium haemolyticum*. JAMA 1981;245:2330–2331.

360. Greene KA, Clark RJ, Zabransky JM. Ventricular CSF shunt infections associated with *Corynebacterium jeikeium*: report of three cases and review. Clin Infect Dis 1993;16:139–141.

361. Greenwood JR, Pickett MJ. Transfer of *Haemophilus vaginalis* Gardner and Dukes to a new genus, *Gardnerella*: *G. vaginalis* (Gardner and Dukes) comb. nov. Int J Syst Bacteriol 1980;30:170–178.

362. Greenwood JR, Pickett MJ. Genus *Gardnerella* Greenwood and Pickett 1980, 170. In: Sneath MHA, Mair NS, Sharpe ME, eds. Bergey's Manual of Systematic Bacteriology. Vol. 2. Baltimore: Williams & Wilkins, 1986:1283–1286.

363. Greenwood JR, Pickett MJ, Martin WJ, Mack EG. *Haemophilus vaginalis* (*Corynebacterium vaginale*): method for isolation and rapid biochemical identification. Health Lab Sci 1977;14:102–106.

364. Greig JR, Eltringham IJ, Birthistle K. Primary peritonitis due to *Lactobacillus fermentum*. J Infect 1998;36:242–243.

365. Greub G, Raoult D. ''*Actinobaculum massiliae*,'' a new species causing chronic urinary tract infection. J Clin Microbiol 2002;40:3938–3941.

366. Griffiths JK, Daly JS, Dodge RA. Two cases of endocarditis due to *Lactobacillus* species: antimicrobial susceptibility, review, and discussion of therapy. Clin Infect Dis 1992;15:250–255.

367. Groman N, Schiller J, Russell J. *Corynebacterium ulcerans* and *Corynebacterium pseudotuberculosis* responses to DNA probes derived from corynephage β and *Corynebacterium diphtheriae*. Infect Immun 1984;45:511–517.

368. Groschup MH, Cussler K, Weiss R, Timoney JF. Characterization of a protective protein antigen of *Erysipelothrix rhusiopathiae*. Epidemiol Infect 1991;107: 637–649.

369. Grove DI, Der-Haroutian V, Ratcliff RM. *Aureobacterium* masquerading as ''*Corynebacterium aquaticum*'' infection: case report and review of the literature. J Med Microbiol 1999;48:965–970.

370. Gruner E, Opravil M, Altwegg M, von Graevenitz A. Non-toxigenic *Corynebacterium diphtheriae* isolated from intravenous drug users. Clin Infect Dis 1994; 18:94–96.

371. Gruner E, Pfyffer GE, von Graevenitz A. Characterization of *Brevibacterium* spp. from clinical specimens. J Clin Microbiol 1993;31:1408–1412.

372. Gruner E, Steigerwalt AG, Hollis DG, et al. Human infections caused by *Brevibacterium casei*, formerly CDC groups B-1 and B-3. J Clin Microbiol 1994;32: 1511–1518.

373. Gruner E, Steigerwalt AG, Hollis DG, et al. Recognition of *Dermabacter hominis*, formerly CDC fermentative coryneform group 3 and group 5, as a potential human pathogen. J Clin Microbiol 1994;32:1918–1922.

374. Gubler J, Huber-Schneider C, Gruner E, Altwegg M. An outbreak of non-toxigenic *Corynebacterium diphtheriae* infection: single bacterial clone causing invasive infection among Swiss drug users. Clin Infect Dis 1998;27:1295–1298.

375. Guillard F, Appelbaum PC, Sparrow FB. Pyelonephritis and septicemia due to gram-positive rods similar to *Corynebacterium* group E (aerotolerant *Bifidobacterium adolescentis*). Ann Intern Med 1980;92:635–636.

376. Gupta K, Stapleton AE, Hooton TM, et al. Inverse association of H_2O_2-producing lactobacilli and vaginal *Escherichia coli* colonization in women with recurrent urinary tract infections. J Infect Dis 1998;178:446–450.

377. Guss WJ, Ament ME. *Oerskovia* infection caused by contaminated home parenteral nutrition solution. Arch Intern Med 1989;149:1457–1458.

378. Gutierrez-Rodero F, Ortiz de la Tabla V, Martinez C, et al. *Corynebacterium pseudodiphtheriticum*: an easily missed respiratory pathogen in HIV-infected patients. Diagn Microbiol Infect Dis 1999;33:209–216.

379. Hadfield TL, McEvoy P, Polotsky Y, et al. The pathology of diphtheria. J Infect Dis 2000;181(Suppl):S116–S120.

380. Haggblom MM, Apetroaie C, Andersson MA, Salkinoja-Salonen MS. Quantitative analysis of cereulide, the emetic toxin of *Bacillus cereus*, produced under various conditions. Appl Env Microbiol 2002;68:2479–2483.

381. Hall V, Collins MD, Hutson R, Falsen E, Duerden BI. *Actinomyces cardiffensis* sp. nov. from human clinical sources. J Clin Microbiol 2002;40:3427–3431.

382. Hall V, Collins MD, Hutson RA, et al. *Actinobaculum urinale* sp. nov., from human urine. Int J Syst Evol Microbiol 2003;53:679–682.

383. Hall V, Collins MD, Hutson R, et al. *Actinomyces vaccimaxillae* sp. nov., from the jaw of a cow. Int J Syst Evol Microbiol 2003;53:603–606.

384. Hall V, Collins MD, Hutson RA, et al. *Actinomyces oricola* sp. nov., from a human dental abscess. Int J Syst Evol Microbiol 2003;53:1515–1518.

385. Hall V, Collins MD, Hutson R, et al. *Corynebacterium atypicum* sp. nov., from a human clinical source, does not contain corynomycolic acids. Int J Syst Evol Microbiol 2003;53:1065–1068.

386. Hall V, Collins MD, Lawson PA, et al. *Actinomyces nasicola* sp. nov., isolated from a human nose. Int J Syst Evol Microbiol 2003;53:1445–1448.

387. Hall V, Talbot PR, Stubbs SL, Duerden BI. Identification of clinical isolates of *Actinomyces* species by amplified 16S ribosomal DNA restriction analysis. J Clin Microbiol 2001;39:3555–3562.

388. Hambleton P, Turnbull PC. Anthrax vaccine development: a continuing story. Adv Biotechnol Processes 1990;13:105–122.

389. Hamilton-Miller JMT, Shah S. Susceptibility patterns of vaginal lactobacilli to eleven oral antibiotics. J Antimicrob Chemother 1994;33:1059–1060.

390. Handwerger S, Pucci MJ, Volk KJ, et al. Vancomycin resistant *Leuconostoc mesenteroides* and *Lactobacillus casei* synthesize peptidoglycan precursors that terminate in lactate. J. Bacteriol. 1994;176:260–264.

391. Hanna P. Anthrax pathogenesis and host response. Curr Top Microbiol Immunol 1998;225:13–35.

392. Hanscom T, Maxwell WA. *Corynebacterium* endophthalmitis: laboratory studies and report of a case treated by vitrectomy. Arch Ophthalmol 1979;97:500–502.

393. Harisdangkul V, Songcharoen S, Lin AC. Listerial infections in patients with systemic lupus erythematosus. South Med J 1992;85:957–960.

394. Harrell LJ, Andersen GL, Wilson KH. Genetic variability of *Bacillus anthracis* and related species. J Clin Microbiol 1995;33:1847–1850.

395. Harrington RD, Lewis CG, Aslanzadeh J, et al. *Oerskovia xanthineolytica* infection of a prosthetic joint: case report and review. J Clin Microbiol 1996;34: 1821–1824.

396. Hatanaka A, Tsunoda A, Okamoto M, et al. *Corynebacterium ulcerans* diphtheria in Japan. Emerg Infect Dis 2003;9:1–4.

397. Haupert CL, Postel EA, Khawly JA. Posttraumatic endophthalmitis due to CDC coryneform group A-3 bacteria. Retina 2000;20:412–413.

398. Havaldar PV, Shanthala CC. Diphtheria presenting as abdominal pain and arthralgia. Pediatr Infect Dis J 1993;12:538–539.

399. Hawes SE, Hillier Sl, Benedetti J, et al. Hydrogen peroxide-producing lactobacilli and acquisition of vaginal infections. J Infect Dis 1996;74:1058–1063.

400. Hayek LJ. *Erysipelothrix* endocarditis affecting a porcine xenograft heart valve. J Infect 1993;7:203–204.

401. Hayes PS, Graves LM, Swaminathan B, et al. Comparison of three selective enrichment methods for the isolation of *Listeria monocytogenes* from naturally contaminated foods. J Food Prot 1992;55:952–959.

402. Helgason E, Okstad OA, Caugant DA, et al. *Bacillus anthracis, Bacillus cereus,* and *Bacillus thuringiensis:* one species on the basis of genetic evidence. Appl Environ Microbiol 2000;6:2627–2630.

403. Hellberg D, Nilsson S, Mardh PA. The diagnosis of bacterial vaginosis and vaginal flora changes. Arch Gynecol Obstet 2001;265:11–15.

404. Hemady R, Zaltas M, Paton B, et al. *Bacillus*-induced endophthalmitis: new series of 10 cases and review of the literature. Br J Ophthalmol 1990;74:26–29.

405. Hemsley C, Abraham S, Rowland-Jones S. *Corynebacterium pseudodiphtheriticum*: a skin pathogen. Clin Infect Dis 1999;29:938–939.

406. Hernaiz C, Picardo A, Alos JI, Gomez-Garces JL. Nosocomial bacteremia and catheter infection by *Bacillus cereus* in an immunocompetent patient. Clin Microbiol Infect 2003;9:973–975.

407. Herra CM, McCafferkey MT, Keane CT. The *in-vitro* susceptibilities of vaginal lactobacilli to four broad spectrum antibiotics as determined by agar dilution and E-test methods. J Antimicrob Chemother 1995;35:775–783.

408. Heyndrickx M, Lebbe L, Kersters K, et al. Proposal of *Virgibacillus proomii* sp. nov., and emended description of *Virgibacillus pantothenticus* (Proom and Knight 1950) Heyndrickx et al. 1998. Int J Syst Bacteriol 1999;49:1083–1090.

409. Heyndrickx M, Vandemeulbroecke K, Hoste B, et al. Reclassification of *Paenibacillus* (formerly *Bacillus*) *pulvifaciens* (Nakamura 1984) Ash, et al. 1994, a later subjective synonym of *Paenibacillus* (formerly *Bacillus*) *larvae* (White 1906) Ash, et al. 1994, as a subspecies of *P. larvae*, with emended descriptions of *P. larvae* as *P. larvae* subsp. *larvae* and *P. larvae* subsp. *pulvifaciens*. Int J Syst Bacteriol 1996;46:270–279.

410. Heyndrickx M, Vandemeulbroecke K, Scheldeman P, et al. *Paenibacillus* (formerly *Bacillus*) *gordonae* (Pichinoty, et al. 1986) Ash et al., 1994 is a later subjective synonym of *Paenibacillus* (formerly *Bacillus*) *validus* (Nakamura 1984) Ash, et al. 1994: emended description of *P. validus*. Int J Syst Bacteriol 1995;45:661–669.

411. Heyndrickx M, Vandemeulbroecke K, Scheldeman P, et al. A polyphasic reassessment of the genus *Paenibacillus*, reclassification of *Bacillus lautus* (Nakamura 1984) as *Paenibacillus lautus* comb. nov. and of *Bacillus peoriae* (Montefusco, et al. 1993) as *Paenibacillus peoriae* comb. nov., and emended descriptions of *P. lautus* and *P. peoriae*. Int J Syst Bacteriol 1996;46:988–1003.

412. Heyrman J, Logan NA, Busse HJ, et al. *Virgibacillus carmonensis* sp. nov.,

Virgibacillus necropolis sp. nov., and *Virgibacillus picturae* sp. nov., three novel species isolated from deteriorated mural paintings, transfer of the species of the genus *Salibacillus* to *Virgibacillus* as *Virgibacillus marismortui* comb. nov., and *Virgibacillus salexigens* comb. nov., and emended description of the genus *Virgibacillus*. Int J Syst Evol Microbiol 2003;53:501–511.

413. Hill DC, Ghassemian JN. *Erysipelothrix rhusiopathiae* endocarditis: clinical features of an occupational disease. South Med J 1997;90:1147–1148.

414. Hilliard NJ, Schelonka RL, Waites KB. *Bacillus cereus* bacteremia in a preterm neonate. J Clin Microbiol 2003;41:3441–3444.

415. Hillier SL. Diagnostic microbiology of bacterial vaginosis. Am J Obstet Gynecol 1993;169:455–459.

416. Hillier SL, Krohn MA, Rabe LK, et al. The normal vaginal flora, H$_2$O$_2$-producing lactobacilli, and bacterial vaginosis in pregnant women. Clin Infect Dis 1993;16(Suppl 4):S273–S281.

417. Hillier SL, Martius J, Frohn M, et al. A case-control study of chorioamnionic infection and histologic chorioamnionitis in prematurity. N Engl J Med 1988;319:972–978.

418. Hirji Z, Saragosa R, Dedier H, et al. Contamination of bone marrow products with an actinomycete resembling *Microbacterium* species and reinfusion into autologous stem cell and bone marrow transplant recipients. Clin Infect Dis 2003;36:e115–e121.

419. Hodge TW Jr, Levy CS, Smith MA. Disk space infection due to *Gardnerella vaginalis*. Clin Infect Dis 1995;21:443–445.

420. Hof H, Hefner P. Pathogenicity of *Listeria monocytogenes* in comparison to other *Listeria* species. Infection 198816(Suppl. 2):S141–S144.

421. Hof N, Nichterlein T, Kretschmar M. Management of listeriosis. Clin Microbiol Rev 1997;10:345–357.

422. Holdeman LV, Cato EP, Moore WEC. Anaerobe Laboratory Manual. 4th Ed. Blacksburg, VA: Virginia Polytechnic Institute and State University, 1977.

423. Holliman RE, Bone GP. Vancomycin resistance of clinical isolates of lactobacilli. J Infect 1988;16:279–283.

424. Holmes RK. Biology and molecular epidemiology of diphtheria toxin and the *tox* gene. J Infect Dis 2000;181(Suppl):S156–S167.

425. Holst E. Reservoir of four organisms associated with bacterial vaginosis suggests lack of sexual transmission. J Clin Microbiol 1990;28:2035–2039.

426. Holthouse DJ, Power B, Kermode A, Golledge C. Non-toxigenic *Corynebacterium diphtheriae*: two cases and review of the literature. J Infect 1998;37:62–66.

427. Horwitch CA, Furseth HA, Larson AM, et al. Lactobacillemia in three patients with AIDS. Clin Infect Dis 1995;21:1460–1462.

428. Hou XG, Kawamura Y, Sultana F, et al. Description of *Arthrobacter creatinolyticus* sp. nov., isolated from human urine. Int J Syst Bacteriol 1998;48:423–429.

429. Hoyles L, Falsen E, Foster G, Collins MD. *Actinomyces coleocanis* sp. nov., from the vagina of a dog. Int J Syst Evol Microbiol 2002;52:1201–1203.

430. Hoyles L, Falsen E, Foster G, et al. *Actinomyces canis* sp. nov., isolated from dogs. Int J Syst Evol Microbiol 2000;50:1547–1551.

431. Hoyles L, Falsen E, Foster G, et al. *Arcanobacterium hippocoleae* sp. nov., from the vagina of a horse. Int J Syst Evol Microbiol 2002;52:617–619.

432. Hoyles L, Falsen E, Holmstrom G, et al. *Actinomyces suimastitidis* sp. nov., isolated from pig mastitis. Int J Syst Evol Microbiol 2001;51:1323–1326.

433. Hoyles L, Falsen E, Pascual C, et al. *Actinomyces catuli* sp. nov., from dogs. Int J Syst Evol Microbiol 2001;51:679–682.

434. Hoyles L, Pascual C, Falsen E, et al. *Actinomyces marimammalium* sp. nov., from marine mammals. Int J Syst Evol Microbiol 2001;51:151–156.

435. Hsu CL, Shih LY, Leu HS, et al. Septicemia due to *Arthrobacter* species in a neutropenic patient with acutelymphoblastic leukemia. Clin Infect Dis 1998;27:1334–1335.

436. Huang CJ, Huang TJ, Hsieh JS. Pseudo-colonic carcinoma caused by abdominal actinomycosis: report of two cases. Int J Colorectal Dis 2004;19:286–286.

437. Huang KL, Beutler SM, Wang C: Endocarditis due to *Actinomyces meyeri*. Clin Infect Dis 1998;27:909–910.

438. Hudspeth MK, Gerardo SH, Citron DM, Goldstein EJ. Evaluation of the RapID CB Plus system for identification of *Corynebacterium* species and other gram-positive rods. J Clin Microbiol 1998;36:543–547.

439. Husni RN, Gordon SM, Washington JA, Longworth DL. *Lactobacillus* bacteremia and endocarditis: review of 45 cases. Clin Infect Dis 1997;25:1048–1055.

440. Hussain Z, Gonder JR, Lannigan R, Stoakes L. Endophthalmitis due to *Oerskovia xanthineolytica*. Can J Ophthalmol 1987;22:234–236.

441. Ieven M, Verhoeven J, Gentens P, Goossens H. Severe infection due to *Actinomyces bernardiae*: case report. Clin Infect Dis 1996;22:157–158.

442. Imada Y, Goji N, Ishikawa H, et al. Truncated surface protective antigen (SpaA) of *Erysipelothrix rhusiopathiae* serotype 1a elicits protection against challenge with serotypes 1a and 2b in pigs. Infect Immun 1999;57:4376–4382.

443. Ingianni A, Petruzzelli S, Morandotti G, Pompei R. Genotypic differentiation of *Gardnerella vaginalis* by amplified ribosomal DNA restriction analysis (ARDRA). FEMS Immunol Med Microbiol 1997;18:61–66.

444. Isaacson JH, Grenko RT. *Rothia dentocariosa* endocarditis complicated by brain abscess. Am J Med 1988;84:352–354.

445. Ishikawa M, Ishizaki S, Yamamoto Y, Yamasato K. *Paraliobacillus ryukyuensis*

gen. nov., sp. nov., a new Gram-positive, slightly halophilic, extremely halotolerant, facultative anaerobe isolated from a decomposing marine alga. J Gen Appl Microbiol 2002;48:269–279.

446. Izurieta HS, Strebel PM, Youngblood T, et al. Exudative pharyngitis possibly due to *Corynebacterium pseudodiphtheriticum*, a new challenge in the differential diagnosis of diphtheria. Emerg Infect Dis 1997;3:65–68.

447. Jackman PHG, Pitcher DG, Pelczynska S, Borman P. Classification of corynebacteria associated with endocarditis (group JK) as *Corynebacterium jeikeium* sp. nov. Syst Appl Microbiol 1987;9:83–90.

448. Jackson SG, Goodbrand RB, Ahmed R, Kasatiya S. *Bacillus cereus* and *Bacillus thuringiensis* isolated in a gastroenteritis outbreak investigation. Lett Appl Microbiol 1995;21:103–105.

449. Janda WM, Bradna JJ, Ruther P. Identification of *Neisseria* spp., *Haemophilus* spp., and other fastidious gram-negative bacteria with the MicroScan Haemophilus-*Neisseria* identification panel. J Clin Microbiol 1989;27:869–873.

450. Janda WM, Malloy PJ, Schreckenberger PC. Clinical evaluation of the Vitek *Neisseria-Haemophilus* identification card. J Clin Microbiol 1987;25:37–41.

451. Janda WM, Tipirneni P, Novak RM. *Brevibacterium casei* bacteremia and line sepsis in an AIDS patient. J Infect 2003;46:61–64.

452. Janssen TL, van Heereveld HA, Laan RF, et al. Septic arthritis with *Listeria monocytogenes* during low-dose methotrexate. J Intern Med 1998;244:87–90.

453. Jayaraj K, Bisceglie AM, Gibson S. Spontaneous bacterial peritonitis caused by infection with *Listeria monocytogenes*: a case report and review of the literature. Am J Gastroenterol 1998;93:1556–1558.

454. Jevon GP, Dunne WM, Hicks MJ, et al. *Bacillus cereus* pneumonia in premature neonates: a report of two cases. Pediatr Infect Dis J 1993;12:251–253.

455. Jian W, Zhu L, Dong X. New approach to phylogenetic analysis of the genus *Bifidobacterium* based on partial HSP gene sequences. Int J Syst Evol Microbiol 2001;51:1633–1638.

456. Johnson A, Hulse P, Oppenheim BA. *Corynebacterium jeikeium* meningitis and transverse myelitis in a neutropenic patient. Eur J Clin Microbiol Infect Dis 1992;11:473–479.

457. Johnson AP, Warner M, Malnick H, Livermore DM. Activity of the oxazolidinones AZD2563 and linezolid against *Corynebacterium jeikeium* and other *Corynebacterium* spp. J Antimicrob Chemother 2003;51:745–747.

458. Johnson JL, Moore LVH, Kaneko B, Moore WEC. *Actinomyces georgiae* sp. nov., *Actinomyces gerencseriae* sp. nov., designation of two genospecies of *Actinomyces naeslundii*, and inclusion of A. *naeslundii* serotypes II and III and *Actinomyces viscosus* serotype II in A. *naeslundii* genospecies 2. Int J Syst Bacteriol 1990;40:273–286.

459. Jones D. Genus *Erysipelothrix* Rosenback 1909, 367. In: Sneath PHA, Mair NS, Sharpe ME, eds. Bergey's Manual of Systematic Bacteriology. Vol. 2. Baltimore: Williams & Wilkins, 1986:1245–1249.

460. Jones D. The place of *Listeria* among gram-positive bacteria. Infection 1988;16(Suppl 2):S85–S88.

461. Jones D, Collins MD. Taxonomic studies on some human cutaneous coryneform bacteria: description of *Dermabacter hominis* gen. nov., sp. nov. FEMS Microbiol Lett 1988;51:51–56.

462. Jones D, Keddie RM. Genus *Brevibacterium*. In: Sneath PHA, Mair NS, Sharpe ME, Holt JG, eds., Bergey's Manual of Systematic Bacteriology. Vol. 2. Baltimore: Williams & Wilkins, 1986:1301–1313.

463. Jones EM, MacGowan AP. Antimicrobial chemotherapy of human infection due to *Listeria monocytogenes*. Eur J Clin Microbiol Infect Dis 1995;14:165–175.

464. Jones N, Khoosal M. *Erysipelothrix rhusiopathiae* septicemia in a neonate. Clin Infect Dis 1997;24:511.

465. Jones SD, Fullerton DA, Zamora MR, et al. Transmission of *Lactobacillus* pneumonia by a transplanted lung. Ann Thorac Surg 1994;58:887–889.

466. Josephson S, Thomason JL, Sturino K, et al. *Gardnerella vaginalis* in the urinary tract: incidence and significance in a hospital population. Obstet Gynecol 1988;71:245–250.

467. Jousimies-Somer H, Summanen P, Citron DM, et al. Wadsworth-KTL Anaerobic Bacteriology Manual. 6th Ed. Belmont, CA: Starr Publishing Company, 2002.

468. Joussen AM, Funke G, Joussen F, Herbertz G. Corynebacterium macginleyi: a conjunctiva-specific pathogen. J Ophthalmol 2000;84:1420–1422.

469. Judson R, Songer JG. *Corynebacterium pseudotuberculosis*: in vitro susceptibility to 39 antimicrobial agents. Vet Microbiol 1991;27:145–150.

470. Jurado RL, Farley MM, Pereira E, et al. Increased risk of meningitis and bacteremia due to *Listeria monocytogenes* in patients with human immunodeficiency virus infection. Clin Infect Dis 1993;17:224–227.

471. Juurlink DN, Borczyk A, Simor AE. Native valve endocarditis due to *Corynebacterium striatum*. Eur J Clin Microbiol Infect Dis 1996;15:963–965.

472. Kabel PJ, Lorie CAM, Vos MC, Buiting AGM. Prosthetic hip-joint infection due to *Listeria monocytogenes*. Clin Infect Dis 1995;20:1080–1081.

473. Kadirova R, Kartoglu HU, Strebel PM. Clinical characteristics and management of 676 hospitalized diphtheria cases, Kyrgyz Republic, 1995. J Infect Dis 2000;181(Suppl):S110–S115.

474. Kailath EJ, Goldstein E, Wagner FH. Meningitis caused by *Oerskovia xanthineolyica*. Am J Med Sci 1988;295:216–217.

475. Kales CP, Holzman RS. Listeriosis in patients with HIV infection: clinical manifestations and response to therapy. J Acquir Immune Defic Syndr 1990;3:139–143.

476. Kalfas S, Figdor D, Sundqvist G. A new bacterial species associated with failed endodontic treatment: identification and description of *Actinomyces radicidentis*. Oral Surg Oral Med Oral Pathol Oral Radiol Endod 2001;92:208–214.

477. Kalima P, Masterton RG, Roddie PH, Thomas AE. *Lactobacillus rhamnosus* infection in a child following bone marrow transplantation. J Infect 1996;32:165–167.

478. Kandler O, Weiss N. Genus *Lactobacillus* Beijerinck 1901, 212. In: Sneath PHA, Mair NS, Sharpe ME, eds. Bergey's Manual of Systematic Bacteriology. Vol. 2. Baltimore: Williams & Wilkins, 1986:1209–1234.

479. Kaplan A, Israel F. *Corynebacterium aquaticum* infection in a patient with chronic granulomatous disease. Am J Med Sci 1988;296:57–58.

480. Karpathios T, Drakonaki S, Zervoudaki A, et al. *Arcanobacterium haemolyticum* in children with presumed streptococcal pharyngotonsillitis or scarlet fever. J Pediatr 1992;121:735–737.

481. Karunasagar I, Krohne G, Goebel W. *Listeria ivanovii* is capable of cell-to-cell spread involving actin polymerization. Infect Immun 1993;61:162–169.

482. Kaufmann D, Ott P, Ruegg C. Laryngopharyngitis by *Corynebacterium ulcerans*. Infection 2002;30:168–170.

483. Kaukoranta-Tolvanen SSE, Sivonen A, Kostiala AAI, et al. Bacteremia caused by *Brevibacterium* species in an immunocompromised patient. Eur J Clin Microbiol Infect Dis 1995;14:801–804.

484. Kerr JR, Murphy PG, Doherty CC. Corynebacterium CDC group G1 infection in a patient receiving maintenance haemodialysis. Nephrol Dial Transplant 1995;10:559.

485. Kerr KG, Hawkey PM, Lacey RW. Evaluation of the API Coryne system for identification of *Listeria* species. J Clin Microbiol 1993;31:749–750.

486. Kerr KG, Rotowa NA, Hawkey PM, Lacey RW. Evaluation of the Mast ID and API 50CH systems for identification of *Listeria* species. Appl Environ Microbiol 1990;56:657–660.

487. Keslin MH, McCoy EL, McCusker JJ, Lutch JS. *Corynebacterium pseudotuberculosis*: a new cause of infectious and eosinophilic pneumonia. Am J Med 1978;87:228–231.

488. Kharsany ABM, Hoosen AA, Van Den Ende J. Antimicrobial susceptibilities of *Gardnerella vaginalis*. Antimicrob Agents Chemother 1993;37:2733–2735.

489. Kinnear W, MacFarlane J. A survey of thoracic actinomycosis. Respir Med 1990;84:57–59.

490. Kiuchi A, Hara M, Pham HS, et al. Phylogenetic analysis of *Erysipelothrix rhusiopathiae* and *Erysipelothrix tonsillarum* based upon 16S rRNA. DNA Seq 2000;11:257–260.

491. Klebanoff SJ, Hillier SL, Eschenbach DA, Waltersdorph AM. Control of the microbial flora of the vagina by H_2O_2-generating lactobacilli. J Infect Dis 1991;164:94–100.

492. Klein G, Zill E, Schindler R, Louwers J. Peritonitis associated with vancomycin-resistant *Lactobacillus rhamnosus* in a continuous ambulatory peritoneal dialysis patient: organism identification, antibiotic therapy, and case report. J Clin Microbiol 1998;36:1781–1783.

493. Kneen R, Phan NG, Solomon T, et al. Penicillin vs. erythromycin in the treatment of diphtheria. Clin Infect Dis 1998;27:845–850.

494. Knox KL, Holmes AH. Nosocomial endocarditis caused by *Corynebacterium amycolatum* and other nondiphtheriae corynebacteria. Emerg Infect Dis 2002;8:97–99.

495. Knudsen JD, Nielsen CJ, Espersen F. Treatment of shunt-related cerebral ventriculitis due to *Corynebacterium jeikeium* with vancomycin administered intraventricularly. APMIS 1994;102:317–320.

496. Ko S-B, Kim D-E, Kwon H-M, Roh J-K. A case of multiple brain infarctions associated with *Erysipelothrix rhusiopathiae* endocarditis. Arch Neurol 2003;60:434–436.

497. Kocks C, Gouin E, Tabouret M, et al. *L. monocytogenes*-induced actin assembly requires the *actA* gene product, a surface protein. Cell 1992;68:521–531.

498. Koehler TM, Dai Z, Kaufman-Yarbray M. Regulation of the *Bacillus anthracis* protective antigen gene: CO_2 and a *trans*-acting element activate transcription from one of two promoters. J Bacteriol 1994;176:586–595.

499. Kong R, Mebazaa A, Heitz B, et al. Case of triple endocarditis caused by *Rothia dentocariosa* and results of a survey in France. J Clin Microbiol 1998;36:309–310.

500. Kotiranta A, Lounatmaa K, Haapasalo M. Epidemiology and pathogenesis of *Bacillus cereus* infections. Microbes Infect 20002:189–198.

501. Kotrajaras R, Togami H: *Corynebacterium pyogenes*: its pathogenic mechanism in epidemic leg ulcers in Thailand. Int J Dermatol 1987;26:45–50.

502. Krause A, Freeman R, Sisson PR, Murphy OM. Infection with *Bacillus cereus* after close-range gunshot injuries. J Trauma 1996;41:546–548.

503. Kristiansen FV, Frost L, Korsager B, Moller R. *Gardnerella vaginalis* in posthysterectomy infection. Eur J Obstet Gynecol Reprod Biol 1990;35:69–73.

504. Kristiansen FV, Oster S, Frost L, et al. Isolation of *Gardnerella vaginalis* in pure culture from the uterine cavity of patients with irregular bleedings. Br J Obstet Gynaecol 1987;94:978–984.

505. Kumari P, Tyagi A, Marks P, Kerr KG. *Corynebacterium afermentans* spp. *afermentans* sepsis in a neurosurgical patient. J Infect 1997;35:201–202.

506. Kumazawa N, Yanagawa R. DNA base composition of the three types of *Corynebacterium renale*. Infect Immun 1969;5:27–30.

507. Kwon YJ, Lee DY. *Corynebacterium aquaticum* peritonitis in a patient on CAPD. Perit Dial Int 1997;17:98–99.

508. Kwong KL, Que TL, Wong SN, So KT. Fatal meningoencephalitis due to *Bacillus anthracis*. J Paediatr Child Health 1997;33:539–541.

509. Laffineur K, Avesani V, Cornu G, et al. Bacteremia due to a novel *Microbacterium* species in a patient with leukemia and description of *Microbacterium paraoxydans* sp. nov. J Clin Microbiol 2003;41:2242–2246.

510. LaForce FM. Anthrax. Clin Infect Dis 1994;19:1009–1013.

511. Lagrou K, Verhaegen J, Janssens M, et al. Prospective study of catalase-positive coryneform organisms in clinical specimens: identification, clinical relevance, and antibiotic susceptibility. Diagn Microbiol Infect Dis 1998;30:7–15.

512. Lair MI, Bentolila S, Grenet D, et al. *Oerskovia turbata* and *Comamonas acidovorans* bacteremia in a patient with AIDS. Eur J Clin Microbiol Infect Dis 1996;15:424–426.

513. Lam MH, Birch DF, Fairley KF. Prevalence of *Gardnerella vaginalis* in the urinary tract. J Clin Microbiol 1988;26:1130–1133.

514. Lane HC, Fauci AS. Bioterrorism on the home front: a new challenge for American medicine. JAMA 2001;286:2595–2597.

515. Lanmerding AM, Glass KA, Gendron-Fitzpatrick, Doyle MP. Determination of virulence of different strains of *Listeria monocytogenes* and *Listeria innocua* by oral inoculation of pregnant mice. Appl Environ Microbiol 1992;58:3991–4000.

516. LaRocco M, Robinson C, Robinson A. *Corynebacterium pseudodiphtheriticum* associated with suppurative lymphadenitis. Eur J Clin Microbiol 1987;6:79.

517. Larsson P, Lundin O, Falsen E: ''*Corynebacterium aquaticum*'' wound infection after high-pressure water injection into the foot. Scand J Infect Dis 1996;28:635–535.

518. LaScola B, Fournier PE, Musso D, Tissot-Dupont H. Pseudo-outbreak of listeriosis elucidated by pulsed-field gel electrophoresis. Eur J Clin Microbiol Infect Dis 1997;16:756–760.

519. Latsios G, Petrogiannopoulos C, Hartzoulakis G, et al. Liver abscess due to *Bacillus cereus*: a case report. Clin Microbiol Infect 2003;9:1234–1237.

520. Lau SK, Woo PC, Woo GK, Yuen KY. Catheter-related *Microbacterium* bacteremia identified by 16S rRNA gene sequencing. J Clin Microbiol 2002;40:2681–2685.

521. Lawrence D, Heitefuss S, Seifert HS: Differentiation of *Bacillus anthracis* from *Bacillus cereus* by gas chromatographic whole-cell fatty acid analysis. J Clin Microbiol 1991;29:1508–1512.

522. Lawson PA, Falsen E, Akervall E, et al. Characterization of some *Actinomyces*-like isolates from human clinical specimens: reclassification of *Actinomyces suis* (Soltys and Spratling) as *Actinobaculum suis* comb. nov. and description of *Actinobaculum schaalii* sp. nov. Int J Syst Bacteriol 1997;47:899–903.

523. Lawson PA, Falsen E, Foster G, et al. *Arcanobacterium pluranimalium* sp. nov., isolated from porpoise and deer. Int J Syst Evol Microbiol 2001;51:55–59.

524. Lawson PA, Nikolaitchouk N, Falsen E, et al. *Actinomyces funkei* sp. nov., isolated from human clinical specimens. Int J Syst Evol Microbiol 2001;51:853–855.

525. Lecuit M, Ohayon H, Braun L, et al. Internalin of *Listeria monocytogenes* with an intact leucine-rich repeat region is sufficient to promote internalization. Infect Immun 1997;65:5309–5319.

526. Lee W, Phillips LE, Carpenter RJ, et al. *Gardnerella vaginalis* chorioamnionitis: a report of two cases and a review of the pathogenic role of *G. vaginalis* in obstetrics. Diagn Microbiol Infect Dis 1987;8:107–111.

527. Legrand JC, Alewaeters A, Leenaerts L, et al. *Gardnerella vaginalis* bacteremia from pulmonary abscess in a male alcohol abuser. J Clin Microbiol 1989;27:1132–1134.

528. Leighton PM, Bulleid B, Taylor R. Neonatal cellulitis due to *Gardnerella vaginalis*. Pediatr Infect Dis J 1982;1:339–340.

529. Leonard RB, Nowowiejski DJ, Warren JJ, et al. Molecular evidence of person-to-person transmission of a pigmented strain of *Corynebacterium striatum* in intensive care units. J Clin Microbiol 1994;32:164–169.

530. Lepargneur JP, Heller R, Soulie R, Riegel P. Urinary tract infection due to *Arcanobacterium bernardiae* in a patient with urinary tract diversion. Eur J Clin Microbiol Infect Dis 1998;17:399–401.

531. LeProwse CR, McNeil MM, McCarty JM. Catheter-related bacteremia caused by *Oerskovia turbata*. J Clin Microbiol 1989;27:571–572.

532. Lequerre T, Nouvellon M, Kraznowska K, et al. Septic arthritis due to *Actinomyces naeslundii*: report of a case. Joint Bone Spine 2002;69:499–501.

533. Lessing MP, Curtis GD, Bowler JC. *Listeria ivanovii* infection. J. Infect. 1994;29:230–231.

534. Levett PN, Bennett P, O'Donaghue K, et al. Relapsed infection due to *Listeria monocytogenes* confirmed by random amplified polymorphic DNA (RAPD) analysis. J Infect 1994;27:205–207.

535. Lewis RP, Sutter VL, Finegold SM. Bone infections involving anaerobic bacteria. Medicine (Baltimore) 1978 ;57:278–305.

536. Li A, Lal S. *Corynebacterium pseudodiphtheriticum* keratitis and conjunctivitis: a case report. Clin Experiment Ophthalmol 2000;28:60–61.

537. Liaudet L, Erard P, Kaeser P. Cutaneous and muscular abscesses secondary to *Actinomyces meyeri* pneumonia. Clin Infect Dis 1996;22:185–186.

538. Lien EA, Hillier SL. Evaluation of the enhanced rapid identification method for *Gardnerella vaginalis*. J Clin Microbiol 1989;27:566–567.

539. Lifshitz A, Arber N, Pras E, et al. *Corynebacterium* CDC group A-4 native valve endocarditis. Eur J Clin Microbiol Infect Dis 1991;10:1056–1057.

540. Limaye AP, Perkins JD, Kowdley KV. Listeria infection after liver transplantation: report of a case and review of the literature. Am J Gastroenterol 1998;93:1942–1944.

541. Limjoco-Antonio AD, Janda WM, Schreckenberger PC. *Arcanobacterium haemolyticum* sinusitis and orbital cellulitis. Pediatr Infect Dis J 2003;22:465–467.

542. Lin HM, Tsui MS, Tu FC. Detection of *Gardnerella vaginalis* in the vagina and amniotic fluid using the polymerase chain reaction. In J Obstet Gynecol 2000;71:221–222.

543. Lina B, Carlotti A, Lesaint V, et al. Persistent bacteremia due to *Brevibacterium* species in an immunocompromised patient. Clin Infect Dis 1994;18:487–488.

544. Lindgren P, Pla JC, Hogberg U, Tarnvik A. *Listeria monocytogenes*-induced liver abscess in pregnancy. Acta Obstet Gynecol Scand 1997;76:486–488.

545. Litwin KA, Jadbabaie F, Villanueva M. Case of pleuropericardial disease caused by *Actinomyces odontolyticus* that resulted in cardiac tamponade. Clin Infect Dis 1999;29:219–220.

546. Liu PY, Ke SC, Chen SL. Use of pulsed-field gel electrophoresis to investigate a pseudo-outbreak of *Bacillus cereus* in a pediatric unit. J Clin Microbiol 1997;35:1533–1535.

547. Llopis F, Carratala J. Vertebral osteomyelitis complicating Rothia dentocariosa endocarditis. Eur J Clin Microbiol Infect Dis 2000;19:562–5673,.

548. Loeb M, Wilcox L, Thornley D, et al. *Bacillus* species pseudobacteremia following hospital construction. Can J Infect Contr 1995;10:37–40.

549. Logan NA, Berkeley RCW. Identification of *Bacillus* strains using the API system. J Gen Microbiol 1984;130:1871–1882.

550. Loiez C, Wallet F, Fruchart A, et al. Turicella otitidis in a bacteremic child with acute lymphoblastic leukemia. Clin Microbiol Infect 2002;8:758–759.

551. Lopez R, Martino R, Brunet S, et al. Infection by *Listeria monocytogenes* in the early period post-bone marrow transplantation. Eur J Haematol 1994;53:251–252.

552. Lorber B. Listeriosis following shigellosis. Rev Infect Dis 1991;13:865–866.

553. Lorber B. Listeriosis. Clin Infect Dis 1997;24:1–11.

554. Louie M, Jayaratne P, Luchsinger I, et al. Comparison of ribotyping, arbitrarily primed PCR, and pulsed-field gel electrophoresis for molecular typing of *Listeria monocytogenes*. J Clin Microbiol 1996;34:15–19.

555. Love DN, Vekselstein R, Collings S. The obligate and facultatively anaerobic bacterial flora of the normal feline gingival margin. Vet Microbiol 1990;22:267–275.

556. Ludwig W, Kirchhof G, Weizenegger M, Weiss N. Phylogenetic evidence for the transfer of *Eubacterium suis* to the genus *Actinomyces* as *Actinomyces suis* comb. nov. Int J Syst Bacteriol 1992;42:161–165.

557. Lujan-Zilbermann J, Jones D, DeVincenzo J. *Oerskovia xanthineolytica* peritonitis: case report and review. Pediatr Infect Dis J 1999;18:738–739.

558. Lund NM, Messana JM, Swartz RD. Unusual causes of peritonitis in patients undergoing continuous peritoneal dialysis with emphasis on *Listeria monocytogenes*. J Am Soc Nephrol 1992;3:1092–1097.

559. Lund T. Foodborne disease due to *Bacillus* and *Clostridium* species. Lancet 1990;336:982–986.

560. Lund T, DeBuyser ML, Granum PE. A new cytotoxin from *Bacillus cereus* that may cause necrotic enteritis. Mol Microbiol 2000;38:254–261.

561. Lund T, Granum PE. Characterization of a non-haemolytic enterotoxin complex from *Bacillus cereus* isolated after a foodborne outbreak. FEMS Microbiol Lett 1996;141:151–156.

562. Lutwick LI, Rockhill RC. Abscess associated with *Rothia dentocariosa*. J Clin Microbiol 1978;8:612–613.

563. Lynch M, O'Leary J, Murnaghan ZD, Cryan B. Actinomyces pyogenes septic arthritis in a diabetic farmer. J Infect 1998;37:71–73.

564. MacGowan AP, Cartlidge PHT, MacLeod F, McLaughlin J. Maternal listeriosis in pregnancy without fetal or neonatal infection. J Infect 1991;22:53–57.

565. MacGowan AP, Reeves DS, Wright C, Glover SC. Tricuspid valve infective endocarditis and pulmonary sepsis due to *Erysipelothrix rhusiopathiae* successfully treated with high doses of ciprofloxacin but complicated by gynaecomastia. J Infect 1991;22:100–101.

566. Machado LS, Sleasman JW, Ford MJ. *Bacillus* species infection of the skin as a presentation of severe combined immunodeficiency disease. J Am Acad Dermatol 1998;39:285–287.

567. Mackenzie A, Fuite LA, Chan FTH, et al. Incidence and pathogenicity of *Arca-*

nobacterium haemolyticum during a 2-year study in Ottawa. Clin Infect Dis 1995;21:177–181.

568. Mackinnon MM, Amezaga MR, Mackinnon JR. A case of *Rothia dentocariosa* endophthalmitis. Eur J Clin Microbiol Infect Dis 2001;20:756–757.

569. Madgwick PJ, Waley SG. β-Lactamase I from *Bacillus cereus*. Biochem J 1987;37:10173–10180.

570. Maguire JD, McCarthy MC, Decker CF. *Oerskovia xanthineolytica* bacteremia in an immunocompromised host: case report and review. Clin Infect Dis 1996;22:554–556.

571. Makinen KK, Makinen PL. Purification and properties of an extracellular collagenolytic protease produced by human oral bacterium *Bacillus cereus* (strain Soc 67). J Biol Chem 1998;262:12488–12495.

572. Makino S, Okada Y, Maruyama T, et al. Direct and rapid detection of *Erysipelothrix rhusiopathiae* DNA in animals by PCR. J Clin Microbiol 1994;32:1526–1531.

573. Makino S-I, Uchida I, Terakado N, et al. Molecular characterization and protein analysis of the *cap* region, which is essential for encapsulation in *Bacillus anthracis*. J Bacteriol 1989;171:722–730.

574. Malanoski GJ, Parker R, Eliopoulos GM. Antimicrobial susceptibilities of a *Corynebacterium* CDC group I2 strain isolated from a patient with endocarditis. Antimicrob Agents Chemother 1992;36:1329–1331.

575. Mallon E, McKee PH. Extraordinary case report: cutaneous anthrax. Am J Dermatopathol 1997;19:79–82.

576. Mann C, Dertinger S, Hartmann G, et al. *Actinomyces neuii* and neonatal sepsis. Infection 2002;30:178–180.

577. Manzella JP, Kellogg JA, Parsey KS. *Corynebacterium pseudodiphtheriticum*: a respiratory tract pathogen in adults. Clin Infect Dis 1995;20:37–40.

578. Maple PAC, Efstratiou A, Tseneva G, et al. The *in-vitro* susceptibilities of toxigenic strains of *Corynebacterium diphtheriae* isolated in northwestern Russia and surrounding areas to ten antibiotics. J Antimicrob Chemother 1994;34:1037–1040.

579. Marley EF, Saini NK, Venkatraman C, Orenstein JM. Fatal *Bacillus cereus* meningoencephalitis in an adult with acute myelogenous leukemia. South Med J 1995;88:969–972.

580. Marshman LA, Hardwidge C, Donaldson PM. *Bacillus cereus* meningitis complicating cerebrospinal fluid fistula repair and spinal drainage. Br J Neurosurg 2000;14:580–582.

581. Marston CK, Jamieson F, Cahoon F, et al. Persistence of a distinct *Corynebacterium diphtheriae* clonal group within two communities in the United States and Canada where diphtheria is endemic. J Clin Microbiol 2001;39:1586–1590.

582. Martinez-Martinez L, Joyanes P, Suarez AI, Perea EJ. Activities of gemifloxacin and five other antimicrobial agents against *Listeria monocytogenes* and coryneform bacteria isolated from clinical samples. Antimicrob Agents Chemother 2001;45:2390–2392.

583. Martinez-Martinez L, Ortega MC, Suarez AI. Comparison of E-test with broth microdilution and disk diffusion for susceptibility testing of coryneform bacteria. J Clin Microbiol 1995;33:1318–1321.

584. Martinez-Martinez L, Pascual A, Suarez AI, Perea EJ. In vitro activity of levofloxacin, ofloxacin, and D-ofloxacin against coryneform bacteria and *Listeria monocytogenes*. J Antimicrob Chemother 1999;43(Suppl C):27–32.

585. Martinez-Martinez L, Suarez AI, Rodriguez-Bano J, et al. Clinical significance of *Corynebacterium striatum* isolated from human samples. Clin Microbiol Infect 1997;3:634–639.

586. Martinez-Martinez L, Suarez AI, Winstanley J, et al. Phenotypic characteristics of 31 strains of *Corynebacterium striatum* isolated from clinical samples. J Clin Microbiol 1995;33:2458–2461.

587. Mascola L, Sorvillo F, Goulet V, et al. Fecal carriage of *Listeria monocytogenes*: observations during a community-wide, common-source outbreak. Clin Infect Dis 1992;15:557–558.

588. Mascola L, Sorvillo F, Lashley N, Steinberg E. Fatal listeria meningitis in an immunocompromised infant: therapeutic implications. J Infect 1991;23:287–291.

589. Matar GM, Slieman TA, Nabbut NH. Subtyping of *Bacillus cereus* by total cell protein patterns and arbitrary primer polymerase chain reaction. Eur J Epidemiol 1996;12:309–314.

590. Matsubara H, Goto K, Matsumura T, et al. *Alicyclobacillus acidophilus* sp. nov., a novel thermoacidophilic o-alicyclic fatty acid-containing bacterium isolated from acidic beverages. Int J Syst Evol Microbiol 2002;52:1681–1685.

591. Mazzulli T, Salit IE. Pleural fluid infection caused by *Listeria monocytogenes*: case report and review. Rev Infect Dis 1991;13:564–570.

592. McBride BW, Moggs A, Telfer JL, et al. Protective efficacy of a recombinant protective antigen against *Bacillus anthracis* challenge and assessment of immunological markers. Vaccine 1998;16:810–817.

593. McBride ME, Ellner KM, Black HS, et al. A new *Brevibacterium* sp. isolated from infected genital hair of patients with white piedra. J Med Microbiol 1993;39:255–261.

594. McCambridge MM, Vogelgesang SA, Ockenhouse CF, et al. *Listeria monocyto-*

genes infection in a patient treated with methotrexate for rheumatoid arthritis. J Rheumatol 1995;22:786–787.

595. McCaughey C, Damani NN. Central venous line infection caused by *Brevibacterium epidermidis*. J Infect 1991;23:211–212.

596. McDonald CL, Chapin-Robertson K, Dill SR, Martino RL. *Oerskovia xanthineolytica* bacteremia in an immunocompromised patient with pneumonia. Diagn Microbiol Infect Dis 1994;18:259–261.

597. McDowell DRM, Buchanan JD, Fairley KF, Gilbert GL. Anaerobic and other fastidious microorganisms in asymptomatic bacteriuria in pregnant women. J Infect Dis 1982;44:114–122.

598. McGregor JA, Lawellin D, Franco-Buff A, Todd JK. Phospholipase C activity in microorganisms associated with reproductive tract infection. Am J Obstet Gynecol 1991;164:682–686.

599. McLauchlin J.: Human listeriosis in Britain, 1967–1985: a summary of 722 cases. 1. Listeriosis during pregnancy and in the newborn. Epidemiol Infect 1990;104:181–189.

600. McLauchlin J. Human listeriosis in Britain, 1967–1985: a summary of 722 cases. 2. Listeriosis in non-pregnant individuals, a changing pattern of infection and seasonal incidence. Epidemiol Infect 1990;104:191–201.

601. Melero-Bascones M, Munoz P, Rodriguez-Creixems M, Bouza E. *Corynebacterium striatum*: an undescribed agent of pacemaker-related endocarditis. Clin Infect Dis 1996;22:576–577.

602. Mengaud H, Ohayon H, Gounon P, et al. E-cadherin is the receptor for internalin, a surface protein required for entry of *Listeria monocytogenes* into epithelial cells. Cell 1996;84:923–932.

603. Merle-Melet M, Dossou-Glete L, Maurer P, et al. Is amoxicillin-cotrimoxazole the most appropriate antibiotic regimen for listeria meningoencephalitis? Review of 22 cases and the literature. J Infect 1996;33:79–85.

604. Messina OD, Maldonado-Cocco JA, Pescio A, et al. *Corynebacterium kutscheri* septic arthritis. Arthritis Rheum 1989;32:1053.

605. Mikamo H, Sato Y, Hayasaki, et al. Vaginal microflora in healthy women with *Gardnerella vaginalis*. J Infect Chemother 2000;6:173–177.

606. Mikhailovich VM, Melnikov G, Mazurova IK, et al. Application of PCR for detection of toxigenic *Corynebacterium diphtheriae* strains isolated during the Russian diphtheria epidemic, 1990 through 1994. J Clin Microbiol 1995;33:3061–3063.

607. Mikkola R, Saris NEL, Grigoriev PA, et al. Iontophoretic properties and mitochondrial effects of cereulide, the emetic toxin of *B. cereus*. Eur J Biochem 1999;263:112–117.

608. Mills AE, Mitchell RD, Lim EK. *Corynebacterium pseudotuberculosis* is a cause of human necrotizing granulomatous lymphadenitis. Pathology 1997;29:231–233.

609. Miller PH, Wiggs LS, Miller JM. Evaluation of API An-IDENT and RapID ANA II systems for identification of *Actinomyces* species from clinical specimens. J. Clin Microbiol 1995;33:329–330.

610. Minato K, Abiko Y. β-lactam antibiotic-resistant *Rothia dentocariosa* from infected postoperative maxillary cyst: studies on R-plasmid and β-lactamase. Gen Pharmacol 1984;15:287–292.

611. Miyake T, Watanabe K, Watanabe T, Oyaizu H. Phylogenetic analysis of the genus *Bifidobacterium* and related genera based on 16S rDNA sequences. Microbiol Immunol 1998;42:661–667.

612. Mock M, Fouet A. Anthrax. Annu Rev Microbiol 200155:647–671.

613. Molin G, Jeppsson B, Johansson ML, et al. Numerical taxonomy of *Lactobacillus* spp. associated with healthy and diseased mucosa of the human intestines. J Appl Bacteriol 1993;74:314–323.

614. Moore C, Norton R. *Corynebacterium aquaticum* septicaemia in a neutropenic patient. J Clin Pathol 1995;48:971–972.

615. Moore LS, Schneider B, Holloway WJ. Minimal inhibitory concentrations and minimal bactericidal concentrations of quinupristin/dalfopristin against clinical isolates of *Corynebacterium jeikeium* and *Listeria monocytogenes*. J Antimicrob Chemother 1997;39(Suppl A):67–68.

616. Moore MS, Parsons EI. A study of modified Tinsdale medium for the primary isolation of *Corynebacterium diphtheriae*. J Infect Dis 1958;102:88–93.

617. Mori T, Tokuhira M, Takae Y, et al. Successful non-surgical treatment of brain abscess and necrotizing fasciitis caused by *Bacillus cereus*. Intern Med 2002;41:671–673.

618. Morris A, Guild I. Endocarditis due to *Corynebacterium pseudodiphtheriticum*: five case reports, review, and antibiotic susceptibilities of nine strains. Rev Infect Dis 1991;13:887–892.

619. Mothershed EA, Cassiday PK, Pierson K, et al. Development of a real-time fluorescence PCR assay for rapid detection of the diphtheria toxin gene. J Clin Microbiol 2002;40:2713–4719.

620. Musa MO, Al Douri M, Khan S, et al. Fulminant septicaemic syndrome of *Bacillus cereus*: three cases. J Infect 1999;39:154–156.

621. Mylonakis E, Hohmann EL, Calderwood SB. Central nervous system infection with *Listeria monocytogenes*. 33 years' experience at a general hospital and review of 776 episodes from the literature. Medicine (Baltimore) 1998;77:313–336.

622. Nakao H, Popovic T. Development of a direct PCR assay for detection of diphtheria toxin gene. J Clin Microbiol 1997;35:1651–1655.

623. Nakao H, Popovic T. Use of random amplified polymorphic DNA for rapid molecular typing of *Corynebacterium diphtheriae*. Diagn Microbiol Infect Dis 1998;30:167–172.

624. Nakato H, Shinomiya K, Mikawa H. Adhesion of *Erysipelothrix rhusiopathiae* to cultured rat aortic endothelial cells: role of bacterial neuraminidase in the induction of arteritis. Pathol Res Pract 1987;182:255–260.

625. Namnyak SS, Blair AL, Hughes DF, et al. Fatal lung abscess due to *Lactobacillus casei* subsp. *rhamnosus*. Thorax 1992;47:666–667.

626. National Committee for Clinical Laboratory Standards. MIC Testing Supplemental Tables M100–S13 (M7). Wayne, PA: NCCLS, 2003.

627. Nazina TN, Tourova TP, Poltaraus AB, et al. Taxonomic study of aerobic thermophilic bacilli: descriptions of *Geobacillus subterraneus* gen. nov., sp. nov. and *Geobacillus uzenensis* sp. nov. from petroleum reservoirs and transfer of *Bacillus stearothermophilus*, *Bacillus thermocatenulatus*, *Bacillus thermoleovorans*, *Bacillus kaustophilus*, *Bacillus thermodenitrificans* to *Geobacillus* as the new combinations *G. stearothermophilus*, *G. thermocatenulatus*, *G. thermoleovorans*, *G. kaustophilus*, and *G. thermodenitrificans*. Int J Syst Evol Microbiol 2001;51:433–446.

628. Nebreda-Mayoral T, Munoz-Bellido JL, Garcia-Rodriguez JA. Incidence and characteristics of urinary tract infections caused by *Corynebacterium urealyticum*. Eur J Clin Microbiol Infect Dis 1994;13:600–604.

629. Neubauer M, Sourek J, Ryc M, et al. *Corynebacterium accolens* sp. nov., a gram-positive rod exhibiting satellitism, from clinical material. Syst Appl Microbiol 1991;14:46–51.

630. Neumeister B, Mandel T, Gruner E, Pfyffer GE. *Brevibacterium* species as a cause of osteomyelitis in a neonate. Infection 1993;21:177–178.

631. Niamut SM, van der Vorm ER, van Luyn-Wiegers CG, Gokemeijer JD. *Oerskovia xanthineolytica* bacteremia in an immunocompromised patient without a foreign body. Eur J Clin Microbiol Infect Dis 2003;22:274–275.

632. Nielsen P, Rainey FA, Outtrup FA, et al. Comparative 16S rDNA sequence analysis of some alkaliphilic bacilli and the establishment of a sixth rRNA group within the genus *Bacillus*. FEMS Microbiol Lett 1994;117:61–66.

633. Nielsen PB, Koch C, Friss H, et al. Double-sandwich enzyme-linked immunosorbent assay for rapid detection of toxin-producing *Corynebacterium diphtheriae*. J Clin Microbiol 1987;25:1280–1284.

634. Nieto E, Vindel A, Valero-Guillen PL, et al. Biochemical, antimicrobial susceptibility, and genotyping studies on *Corynebacterium urealyticum* isolates from diverse sources. J Med Microbiol 2000;49:759–763.

635. Nightingale LM, Eaton CB, Fruehan AE, et al. Cephalohematoma complicated by osteomyelitis presumed due to *Gardnerella vaginalis*. JAMA 1996;256:1936–1937.

636. Nikolaitchouk N, Hoyles L, Falsen E, et al. Characterization of *Actinomyces* isolates from samples from the human urogenital tract: description of *Actinomyces urogenitalis* sp. nov. Int J Syst Evol Microbiol 2000;50:1649–1654.

637. Nimura Y, Koh E, Yanagida F, et al. *Amphibacillus xylanus* gen. nov., sp. nov., a facultatively anaerobic sporeforming xylan-digesting bacterium which lacks cytochrome, quinones, and catalase. Int J Syst Bacteriol 1990;40:297–301.

638. Ninet B, Bannerman E, Bille J. Assessment of the AccuProbe *Listeria monocytogenes* culture identification reagent kit for rapid colony confirmation and its application in various enrichment broths. Appl Environ Microbiol 1992;58:4055–4059.

639. Nivar-Aristy RA, Krajewski LP, Washington JA. Infection of an arteriovenous fistula with *Rothia dentocariosa*. Diagn Microbiol Infect Dis 1991;14:167–169.

640. Nocera D, Altwegg M, Martinetti-Lucchini G, et al. Characterization of *Listeria* strains from a foodborne listeriosis outbreak by rDNA gene restriction patterns compared to four other typing methods. Eur J Clin Microbiol Infect Dis 1993;12:162–169.

641. Nolte FS, Arnold KE, Sweat H, et al. Vancomycin-resistant *Aureobacterium* species cellulitis and bacteremia in a patient with acute myelogenous leukemia. J Clin Microbiol 1996;34:1992–1994.

642. Norris PR, Clark DA, Owen JP, Waterhouse SW. Characteristics of *Sulfobacillus acidophilus* sp. nov. and other moderately thermophilic mineral-sulphide-oxidizing bacteria. Microbiology 1996;142:775–783.

643. Noskin GA, Suriano T, Collins S, et al. *Paenibacillus macerans* pseudobacteremia resulting from contaminated blood culture bottles in a neonatal intensive care unit. Am J Infect Control 2001;29:126–129.

644. Nugent RP, Krohn MA, Hillier SL. Reliability of diagnosing bacterial vaginosis is improved by a standardized method of Gram stain interpretation. J Clin Microbiol 1991;29:297–301.

645. Obata-Yasuoka M, Ba-Thein W, Hamada HG, Hayashi H. A multiplex polymerase chain reaction-based diagnostic method for bacterial vaginosis. Obstet Gynecol 2002;100:759–764.

646. Oberreuter H, Seiler H, Scherer S. Identification of coryneform bacteria and related taxa by Fourier-transform infrared (Ft-IR) spectroscopy. Int J Syst Evol Microbiol 2002;52:91–100.

647. O'Donnell AG, Minnikin DE, Goodfellow M, Piot P. Fatty acid, polar lipid and

wall amino acid composition of *Gardnerella vaginalis*. Arch Microbiol 1984; 138:68–71.

648. Ogunc D, Gultekin M, Colak D, et al. Bacteremia caused by *Brevibacterium* species in a patient with chronic lymphocytic leukemia. Haematologia 2002;32: 151–153.

649. Ohl C, Tribble DR. *Corynebacterium* group D2 infection of a complex renal cyst in a debilitated patient. Clin Infect Dis 1992;14:1160–1161.

650. Ojeda-Vargas M, Gonzalez-Fernandez MA, Romero D, et al. Pericarditis caused by *Corynebacterium urealyticum*. Clin Microbiol Infect 2000;6:560–561.

651. Okwumabua O, Swaminathan B, Edmonds P, et al. Evaluation of a chemiluminescent DNA probe assay for the rapid confirmation of *Listeria monocytogenes*. Res Microbiol 1992;143:183–189.

652. Olson ME, Goemans I, Bolingbroke D, Lundberg S. Gangrenous dermatitis caused by *Corynebacterium ulcerans* in Richardson ground squirrels. J Am Vet Med Assoc 1993;193:367–368.

653. Orellano EG, Girardini JE, Cricco JA, et al. Spectroscopic characterization of a bionuclear metal site in *Bacillus cereus* β-lactamase II. Biochemistry 1998; 27:10173–10180.

654. Orrett FA. Fatal *Bacillus cereus* bacteremia in a patient with diabetes. J Natl Med Assoc 2000;2:206–208.

655. Paillard D, Dubois V, Duran R, et al. Rapid identification of *Listeria* species by using restriction fragment length polymorphism of PCR-amplified 23S rRNA gene fragments. Appl Environ Microbiol 2003;69:6386–6392.

656. Pallen MJ, Hay AJ, Puckey LH, Efstratiou A. Polymerase chain reaction for screening clinical isolates of corynebacteria for the production of diphtheria toxin. J Clin Pathol 1994;47:353–356.

657. Pang DK, Abdalla M. Osteomyelitis of the foot due to *Actinomyces meyeri*: a case report. Foot Ankle 1987;8:169–171.

658. Pao CC, Lin SS, Hsieh TT. The detection of *Gardnerella vaginalis* DNA sequences in uncultured specimens with cloned *G. vaginalis* DNA as probes. Mol Cell Probes 1990;4:367–373.

659. Parida SK, Domann E, Rohde M, et al. Internalin B is essential for adhesion and mediates the invasion of *Listeria monocytogenes* into human endothelial cells. Mol Microbiol 1998;28:81–93.

660. Parola P, Maurin M, Alimi Y, et al. Use of 16S rRNA gene sequencing to identify *Lactobacillus casei* in septicaemia secondary to a paraprosthetic enteric fistula. Eur J Clin Microbiol Infect Dis 1998;17:203–205,.

661. Pascual C, Collins MD. *Brevibacterium avium* sp. nov., isolated from poultry. Int J Syst Bacteriol 1999;49:1527–1530.

662. Pascual C, Collins MD, Funke G, Pitcher DG. Phenotypic and genotypic characterization of two *Brevibacterium* strains from the human ear: description of *Brevibacterium otitidis* sp. nov. Med Microbiol Lett 1996;5:113–123.

663. Pascual C, Foster G, Alvarez N, Collins MD. *Corynebacterium phocae* sp. nov., isolated from the common seal (*Phoca vitulina*). Int J Syst Bacteriol 1998;48: 601–604.

664. Pascual C, Foster G, Falsen E, et al. *Actinomyces bowdenii* sp. nov., isolated from canine and feline clinical specimens. Int J Syst Evol Microbiol 1999;49: 1873–1877.

665. Pascual C, Lawson PA, Farrow JA, et al. Phylogenetic analysis of the genus *Corynebacterium* based on 16S rRNA gene sequences. Int J Syst Bacteriol 1995; 45:724–728.

666. Patel R. Enterococcal-type glycopeptide resistance genes in non-enterococcal organisms. FEMS Microbiol Lett 2000;185:1–7.

667. Patel R, Cockerill FR, Porayko MK, et al. Lactobacillemia in liver transplant patients. Clin Infect Dis 1994;18:207–212.

668. Patey O, Bimet F, Riegel P, et al. Clinical and molecular study of *Corynebacterium diphtheriae* systemic infections in France. Coryne Study Group. J Clin Microbiol 1997;35:441–445.

669. Paul ML, Dwyer DE, Chow C, et al. Listeriosis: a review of eighty-four cases. Med J Aust 1994;160:489–493.

670. Paviour S, Musaad S, Roberts S, et al. *Corynebacterium* species isolated from patients with mastitis. Clin Infect Dis 2002;35:1434–1440.

671. Paziak-Domanska B, Boguslawska E, Wieckowska-Szakiel M, et al. Evaluation of the API test, phosphatidylinositol-specific phospholipase C activity and PCR method in identification of *Listeria monocytogenes* in meat foods. FEMS Microbiol Lett 1999;171:209–214.

672. Peel MM, Palmer GG, Stacpoole AM, Kerr TG. Human lymphadenitis due to *Corynebacterium pseudotuberculosis*: report of ten cases from Australia and review. Clin Infect Dis 1997;24:185–191.

673. Peiris V, Fraser S, Knowles C, et al. Isolation of *Corynebacterium striatum* from three hospitalized patients (letter). Eur J Clin Microbiol Infect Dis 1994;13: 36–38.

674. Pejaver RK, Watson AH, Mucklow ES. Neonatal cross-infection with *Listeria monocytogenes*. J Infect 1993;26:301–303.

675. Pelle G, Makrai L, Fodor L, et al. Actinomycosis in dogs caused by *Actinomyces hordeovulneris*. J Comp Pathol 2000;123:72–76.

676. Penn CC, Klotz SA. Anthrax pneumonia. Semin Respir Infect 1997;12:28–30.

677. Pennekamp A, Punter V, Zbinden R. Disk diffusion, agar dilution, and the E-test for susceptibility testing of *Corynebacterium jeikeium*. Clin Microbiol Infect 1996;2:209–213.

678. Perrin M, Bemer M, Delamare C. Fatal case of *Listeria innocua* bacteremia. J Clin Microbiol 2003;41:5308–5309.

679. Petit PLC, Bok W, Thompson J, et al. Native-valve endocarditis due to CDC coryneform group ANF-3: report of a case and review of corynebacterial endocarditis. Clin Infect Dis 1994;19:897–901.

680. Philippon P, Bimet F. *In vitro* susceptibility of *Corynebacterium* group D2 and *Corynebacterium jeikeium* to twelve antibiotics. Eur J Clin Microbiol Infect Dis 1990;9:892–895.

681. Pinedo S, Bos AJ, Siegert CE. Relapsing *Bacillus cereus* peritonitis in two patients on peritoneal dialysis. Perit Dial Int 2002;22:424–426.

682. Pinna A, Sechi LA, Zanetti S, et al. *Bacillus cereus* keratitis associated with contact lens wear. Ophthalmology 2001;108:1830–1834.

683. Pinner RW, Schuchat A, Swaminathan B, et al. Role of food in sporadic listeriosis: II. Microbiologic and epidemiologic investigation. JAMA 1992;267: 2046–2050.

684. Piontkowski MD, Shivvers DW. Evaluation of a commercially available vaccine against *Corynebacterium pseudotuberculosis* for use in sheep. J Am Vet Med Assoc 1998;212:1765–1768.

685. Piot P, Van Dyck E, Peeters M, et al. Biotypes of *Gardnerella vaginalis*. J Clin Microbiol 1984;20:677–679.

686. Pitcher D, Soto A, Soriano F, Valero-Guillen P. Classification of coryneform bacteria associated with human urinary tract infection (group D2) as *Corynebacterium urealyticum* sp. nov. Int J Syst Bacteriol 1992;42:178–181.

687. Poilane I, Fawaz F, Nathanson M, et al. *Corynebacterium diphtheriae* osteomyelitis in an immunocompetent child: a case report. Eur J Pediatr 1995;154: 381–383.

688. Popova NA, Nikolaev IA, Turova TP, et al. *Geobacillus uralicus*, a new species of thermophilic bacteria. Mikrobiologiia 2002;71:391–398.

689. Portnoy DA, Chakraborty T, Goebel W, Cossart P. Molecular determinants of *Listeria monocytogenes* pathogenesis. Infect Immun 1992 ;60:1263–1267.

690. Portnoy DA, Tweten RK, Kehoe M, Bielecki J. Capacity of listeriolysin O, streptolysin O, and perfringolysin O to mediate growth of *Bacillus subtilis* within mammalian cells. Infect Immun 1992 ;60:2710–2717.

691. Pot B, Hertel C, Ludwig W, et al. Identification and classification of *Lactobacillus acidophilus*, *L. gasseri*, and *L. johnsonii* strains by SDS-PAGE and rRNA targeted oligonucleotide probe hybridization. J Gen Microbiol 1993;139: 513–517.

692. Pourshaban M, Gianfranceschi M, Gattuso A, et al. Identification of *Listeria monocytogenes* contamination sources in two fresh sauce production plants by pulsed-field gel electrophoresis. Food Microbiol 2000;17:393–400.

693. Power EG, Abdulla YH, Talsania HG, et al. VanA genes in vancomycin-resistant clinical isolates of *Oerskovia turbata* and *Arcanobacterium* (*Corynebacterium*) *haemolyticum*. J Antimicrob Chemother 1995;36:595–606.

694. Poyart C, Abachin E, Razafimanantsoa I, Berche P. The zinc metalloprotease of *Listeria monocytogenes* is required for maturation of phosphatidylcholine phospholipase C: direct evidence obtained by gene complementation. Infect Immun 1993;61:1576–1580.

695. Psiachou-Leonard E, Sidi V, Tsivitanidou M, et al. Brain abscesses resulting from *Bacillus cereus* and an *Aspergillus*-like mold. J Pediatr Hematol Oncol 2002;24:569–571.

696. Puleo JA, Shammas NW, Kelly P, Allen M. *Lactobacillus* isolated pulmonic valve endocarditis with ventricular septal defect detected by transesophageal echocardiography. Am Heart J 1994;128:1248–1250.

697. Pulverer G, Schutt-Gerowitt H, Schaal KP. Human cervicofacial actinomycoses: microbiological data for 1997. Clin Infect Dis 2003;37:490–497.

698. Putnins EE, Bowden GH. Antigenic relationships among oral *Actinomyces* isolates, *Actinomyces naeslundii* genospecies 1 and 2, *Actinomyces howellii*, *Actinomyces denticolens*, and *Actinomyces slackii*. J Dent Res 1993;72:1374–1385.

699. Querol-Borras JM, Manresa F, Barbe F, Cisnal M. Lactobacilli and pleuropulmonary infection. Eur Resp J 1989;2:1021.

700. Quinn AG, Comaish JS, Pedler SJ. Septic arthritis and endocarditis due to group G-2 coryneform organism. Lancet 1991;338:62–63.

701. Radtke A, Bergh K, Oien CM, Bevanger LS. Peritoneal dialysis-associated peritonitis caused by *Dermabacter hominis*. J Clin Microbiol 2001;39:3420–3421.

702. Rainey FA, Fritze D, Stackebrandt E. The phylogenetic diversity of thermophilic members of the genus *Bacillus* as revealed by 16S rDNA analysis. FEMS Microbiol Lett 1994;115:205–212.

703. Rainey FA, Weiss N, Stackebrandt E. Phylogenetic analysis of the genera *Cellulomonas*, *Promicromonospora*, and *Jonesia* and proposal to exclude the genus *Jonesia* from the family *Cellulomonadaceae*. Int J Syst Bacteriol 1996;45: 649–652.

704. Ramos CP, Falsen E, Alvarez N, et al. *Actinomyces graevenitzii* sp. nov., isolated from human clinical specimens. Int J Syst Bacteriol 1997;47:885–888.

705. Ramos CP, Foster G, Collins MD. Phylogenetic analysis of the genus *Actinomyces* based on 16S rRNA gene sequences: description of *Arcanobacterium phocae*

sp. nov., *Arcanobacterium bernardiae* comb. nov., and *Arcanobacterium pyogenes* comb. nov. Int J Syst Bacteriol 1997;47:46–53.

706. Ramos CP, Lawson PA, Farrow JAE, et al. Phylogenetic analysis of the genus *Corynebacterium* based on 16S rRNA gene sequences. Int J Syst Bacteriol 1995; 45:724–728.

707. Razavi B, Schilling M. Chondritis attributable to *Lactobacillus* after ear piercing. Diagn Microbiol Infect Dis 2000;37:75–76.

708. Razsi L, Sanchez MR. Progressively enlarging painful annular plaque on the hand. Erysipeloid. Arch Dermatol 1994;130:1314–1315.

709. Reboli AC, Farrar WE. *Erysipelothrix rhusiopathiae*: an occupational pathogen. Clin Microbiol Rev 1989;2:354–359.

710. Reddy CA, Cornell CP, Fraga AM. Transfer of *Corynebacterium pyogenes* (Glage) Eberson to the genus *Actinomyces* as *Actinomyces pyogenes* (Glage) comb. nov. Int J Syst Bacteriol 1982;32:419–429.

711. Reddy GS, Prakash JS, Srinivas R, et al. *Leifsonia rubra* sp. nov. and *Leifsonia aurea* species nov., psychrophiles from a pond in Antarctica. Int J Syst Evol Microbiol 2003;53:977–984.

712. Reimer LG, Reller LB. *Gardnerella vaginalis* bacteremia: a review of thirty cases. Obstet Gynecol 1984;64:170–172.

713. Reimer LG, Reller LB. Effect of sodium polyanethol sulfonate and gelatin on the recovery of *Gardnerella vaginalis* from blood culture media. J Clin Microbiol 1985;21:686–688.

714. Reinert RR, Schnitzler N, Haase G, et al. Recurrent bacteremia due to *Brevibacterium casei* in an immunocompromised patient. Eur J Clin Microbiol Infect Dis 1995;14:1082–1085.

715. Reller LB, Maddoux GL, Eckman MR, Pappas G. Bacterial endocarditis caused by *Oerskovia turbata*. Ann Intern Med 1975;83:664–666.

716. Renaud FN, Aubel D, Riegel P, et al. *Corynebacterium freneyi* sp. nov., α-glucosidase-positive strains related to *Corynebacterium xerosis*. Int J Syst Evol Microbiol 2001;51:1723–1728.

717. Renaud FN, Dutaur M, Daoud S, et al. Differentiation of *Corynebacterium amycolatum*, *C. minutissimum*, and *C. striatum* by carbon substrate assimilation tests. J Clin Microbiol 1998;36:3698–3702.

718. Renaud FNR, Gregory A, Barreau C, et al. Identification of *Turicella otitidis* isolated from a patient with otorrhea associated with surgery: differentiation from *Corynebacterium afermentans* and *Corynebacterium auris*. J Clin Microbiol 1996;34:2625–2627.

719. Reva ON, Sorokulova IB, Smirnov VV. Simplified technique for identification of the aerobic spore-forming bacteria by phenotype. Int J Syst Evol Microbiol 2001;51:1361–1371.

720. Reva ON, Vyunitskaya VA, Resnick SR, et al. Antibiotic susceptibility as a taxonomic characteristic of the genus *Bacillus*. Int J Syst Bacteriol 1995;45: 409–411.

721. Reynolds SJ, Behr M, McDonald J: *Turicella otitidis* as a unusual agent causing a posterior auricular abscess. J Clin Microbiol 2001;39:1672–1673.

722. Ricaurte JC, Klein O, LaBombardi V, et al. *Rothia dentocariosa* endocarditis complicated by multiple intracranial hemorrhages. South Med J 2001;94: 438–440.

723. Richardson AJ, Rothburn MM, Roberts C. Pseudo-outbreak of *Bacillus* species: related to fibreoptic bronchoscopy. J Hosp Infect 1986;7:208–210.

724. Riedo FX, Pinner RW, Tosca MD, et al. A point-source foodborne listeriosis outbreak: documented incubation period and possible mild illness. J Infect Dis 1994;170:693–696.

725. Riegel P, DeBriel D, Prevost G, et al. Proposal of *Corynebacterium propinquum* sp. nov. for *Corynebacterium* group ANF-3 strains. FEMS Microbiol Lett 1993; 113:229–234.

726. Riegel P, DeBriel D, Prevost G, Jehl F, Monteil H, Minck R, et al. Taxonomic study of *Corynebacterium* group ANF-1 strains: proposal of *Corynebacterium afermentans* sp. nov. containing the subspecies *C. afermentans* subspecies *afermentans* subsp. nov. and *C. afermentans* subsp. *lipophilum* subsp. nov. Int J Syst Bacteriol 1993;43:287–292.

727. Riegel P, Grimont PAD, DeBriel D, et al. Corynebacterium group D2 ("*Corynebacterium urealyticum*") constitutes a new genomic species. Res Microbiol 1992;143:307–313.

728. Riegel P, Heller R, Prevost G, et al. *Corynebacterium durum* sp. nov., from human clinical specimens. Int J Syst Bacteriol 1997;47:1107–1111.

729. Riegel P, Ruimy R, Christen R, Monteil H. Species identification and antimicrobial susceptibilities of corynebacteria isolated from various clinical sources. Eur J Clin Microbiol Infect Dis 1996;15:657–662.

730. Riegel P, Ruimy R, De Briel D, et al. Taxonomy of *Corynebacterium diphtheriae* and related taxa, with recognition of *Corynebacterium ulcerans* sp. nov., nom. rev. FEMS Microbiol Lett 1995;126:271–276.

731. Riegel P, Ruimy R, DeBriel D, et al. Genomic diversity and phylogenetic relationships among lipid-requiring diphtheroids from humans and characterization of *Corynebacterium macginleyi* sp. nov. Int J Syst Bacteriol 1995;45:128–133.

732. Riegel P, Ruimy R, DeBriel D, et al. *Corynebacterium argentoratense* sp. nov., from the human throat. Int J Syst Bacteriol 1995;45:533–537.

733. Riegel P, Ruimy R, DeBriel D, et al. *Corynebacterium seminale* sp. nov., a new species associated with genital infections in male patients. J Clin Microbiol 1995;33:2244–2249.

734. Riegel P, Ruimy R, Renaud FNR, et al. *Corynebacterium singulare* sp. nov., a new species for urease-positive strains related to *Corynebacterium minutissimum*. Int J Syst Bacteriol 1997;47:1092–1096.

735. Riegert-Johnson DL, Sandhu N, Rajkumar SV, Patel R. Thrombotic thrombocytopenic purpura associated with a hepatic abscess due to *Actinomyces turicensis*. Clin Infect Dis 2002;35:636–637.

736. Rihs JD, McNeil MM, Brown JM, Yu VL. *Oerskovia xanthineolytica* implicated in peritonitis associated with peritoneal dialysis and review of *Oerskovia* infections in humans. J Clin Microbiol 1990;28:1934–1937.

737. Robson JM, McDougall R, van der Valk S, et al. *Erysipelothrix rhusiopathiae*: an uncommon but ever present zoonoses. Pathology 1998;30:391–394.

738. Rocourt J. Taxonomy of the genus *Listeria*. Infection 1988;16(Suppl 2): S89–S91.

739. Rocourt J, Boerlin P, Grimont F, et al. Assignment of *Listeria grayi* and *Listeria murrayi* to a single species, *Listeria grayi*, with a revised description of *Listeria grayi*. Int J Syst Bacteriol 1992;42:171–174.

740. Rocourt J, Wehmeyer U, Stackebrandt E. Transfer of *Listeria denitrificans* to a new genus, *Jonesia* gen. nov. as *Jonesia denitrificans* comb. nov. Int J Syst Bacteriol 1987;37:266–270.

741. Rogasi PG, Vigano S, Pecile P, Leoncini F. *Lactobacillus casei* pneumonia and sepsis in a patient with AIDS. Case report and review of the literature. Ann Ital Med Int 1998;13:180–182.

742. Rosato AE, Lee BS, Nash KA. Inducible macrolide resistance in *Corynebacterium jeikeium*. Antimicrob Agents Chemother 2001;45:1982–1989.

743. Rosene K, Eschenbach DA, Tompkins LS, et al. Polymicrobial early postpartum endometritis with facultative and anaerobic bacteria, genital mycoplasmas, and *Chlamydia trachomatis*: treatment with piperacillin or cefoxitin. J Infect Dis 1986;153:1028–1037.

744. Ross MJ, Sakoulas G, Manning WJ, et al. *Corynebacterium jeikeium* native valve endocarditis following femoral access for coronary angiography. Clin Infect Dis 2001;32:E120–E121.

745. Rossler D, Ludwig W, Schleifer KH, et al. Phylogenetic diversity in the genus *Bacillus* as seen by 16S rRNA sequencing studies. Syst Appl Microbiol 1991; 14:266–269.

746. Rottini G, Dobrina A, Forgiarini O, et al. Identification and partial characterization of a cytolytic toxin produced by *Gardnerella vaginalis*. Infect Immun 1990; 58:3751–3758.

747. Roy M, Chen JC, Miller M, et al. Epidemic *Bacillus* endophthalmitis after cataract surgery: I. Acute presentation and outcome. Ophthalmology 1997;104: 1768–1772.

748. Rufael DW, Cohn SE. Native valve endocarditis due to *Corynebacterium striatum*. Clin Infect Dis 1994;19:1054–1061.

749. Ruimy R, Riegel P, Boiron P, et al. Phylogeny of the genus *Corynebacterium* deduced from analyses of small-subunit ribosomal RNA sequences. Int J Syst Bacteriol 1995;45:740–746.

750. Ruiz ME, Richards JS, Kerr GS, Kan VL. *Erysipelothrix rhusiopathiae* septic arthritis. Arthritis Rheum 2003;48:1156–1157.

751. Rupp ME, Stiles KG, Tarantolo S, Goering RV. Central venous catheter-related *Corynebacterium minutissimum* bacteremia. Infect Control Hosp Epidemiol 1998;19:786–789.

752. Ryan PA, MacMillan JD, Zilinskas BA. Molecular cloning and characterization of the genes encoding the L1 and L2 components of hemolysin BL from *Bacillus cereus*. J Bacteriol 1997;179:2551–2556.

753. Saavedra J, Rodriguez JN, Fernandez-Jurado A, et al. A necrotic soft-tissue lesion due to *Corynebacterium urealyticum* in a neutropenic child. Clin Infect Dis 1996;22:851–852.

754. Sabbe LJM, Van De Merwe D, Schouls L, et al. Clinical spectrum of infections due to the newly described *Actinomyces* species A. turicensis, A. radingae, and A. europaeus. J Clin Microbiol 1999;37:8–13.

755. Sadhu K, Domingue PA, Chow AW, et al. *Gardnerella vaginalis* has a gram-positive cell-wall ultrastructure and lacks classical cell-wall lipopolysaccharide. J Med Microbiol 1989;29:229–235.

756. Saez Roca G, Fernandez E, Diez JM, et al. Splenic abscess and empyema due to *Lactobacillus* species in an immunocompetent host. Clin Infect Dis 1998;26: 498–499.

757. Sakai C, Iuchi T, Ishii A, et al. *Bacillus cereus* brain abscesses occurring in a severely neutropenic patient: successful treatment with antimicrobial agents, granulocyte colony-stimulating factor, and surgical drainage. Intern Med 2001; 40:654–657.

758. Salaman SA, Prag J. Three cases of *Rothia dentocariosa* bacteraemia: frequency in Denmark and a review. Scand J Infect Dis 2002;34:153–157.

759. Salamina G, Dalle Donne E, Niccolini A, et al. A foodborne outbreak of gastroenteritis involving *Listeria monocytogenes*. Epidemiol Infect 1996;117: 429–436.

760. Salminen MK, Rautelin H, Tynkkynen S, et al. *Lactobacillus* bacteremia, clinical

significance, and patient outcome, with special emphasis on probiotic *L. rhamnosus* GG. Clin Infect Dis 2004;38:62–69.

761. Salminen MK, Tynkkynen S, Rautelin H, et al. *Lactobacillus* bacteremia during a rapid increase in probiotic use of *Lactobacillus rhamnosus* GG in Finland. Clin Infect Dis 2002;35:1155–1160.

762. Salmon SA, Walker RD, Carleton CL, et al. Characterization of *Gardnerella vaginalis* and *G. vaginalis*-like organisms from the reproductive tract of the mare. J Clin Microbiol 1991;29:1157–1161.

763. Saltzgaber-Muller J, Stone BA. Detection of *Corynebacterium kutscheri* in animal tissues by DNA-DNA hybridization. J Clin Microbiol 1986;24:759–763.

764. Sanchez Hernandez J, Mora Peris B, Yague Guirao N, et al. *In vitro* activity of newer antibiotics against *Corynebacterium jeikeium*, *Corynebacterium amycolatum*, and *Corynebacterium urealyticum*. Int J Antimicrob Agents 2003;22:492–496.

765. Santos MR, Gandhi S, Vogler M, et al. Suspected diphtheria in an Uzbek national: isolation of *Corynebacterium pseudodiphtheriticum* resulted in a false-positive presumptive diagnosis. Clin Infect Dis 1999;22:735.

766. Sanyal D, Bhandari S. CAPD peritonitis caused by *Lactobacillus rhamnosus*. J Hosp Infect 1992;22:325–327.

767. Sarkonen N, Kononen E, Summanen P, et al. Phenotypic differentiation of *Actinomyces* and related species isolated from human sources. J Clin Microbiol 2001;39:3955–3961.

768. Sato T, Matsuyama J, Takahashi N, et al. Differentiation of oral *Actinomyces* species by 16S ribosomal DNA polymerase chain reaction-restriction fragment length polymorphism. Arch Oral Biol 1998;43:247–252.

769. Saweljew P, Kunkel J, Feddersen A, et al. Case of fatal systemic infection with an *Aureobacterium* sp.: identification of isolate by 16S rRNA gene analysis. J Clin Microbiol 1996;34:1540–1541.

770. Saxelin M, Chuang NH, Chassy B, et al. Lactobacilli and bacteremia in southern Finland, 1989–1992. Clin Infect Dis 1996;22:564–566.

771. Schaal KP. Genus *Actinomyces*. In: Sneath PHA, Mair NS, Sharpe ME, Holt JG, eds. Bergey's Manual of Systematic Bacteriology. Vol. 2. Baltimore: Williams & Wilkins, 1986:1383–1418.

772. Schemmer GB, Driebe WT Jr. Posttraumatic *Bacillus cereus* endophthalmitis. Arch Ophthalmol 1987;105:342–344.

773. Schiff MJ, Kaplan MH. *Rothia dentocariosa* pneumonia in an immunocompromised patient. Lung 1987;165:279–282.

774. Schlech WF. Listeria gastroenteritis: old syndrome, new pathogen. N Engl J Med 1997;336:130–132.

775. Schlech WF. Foodborne listeriosis. Clin Infect Dis 2000;31:770–775.

776. Schlegel L, Lemerle S, Geslin P. *Lactobacillus* species as opportunistic pathogens in immunocompromised patients. Eur J Clin Microbiol Infect Dis 1998;17:887–888.

777. Schlesner H, Lawson PA, Collins MD, et al. *Filobacillus milensis* gen. nov., sp. nov., a new halophilic spore-forming bacterium with orn-D-glu-type peptidoglycan. Int J Syst Evol Microbiol 2001;51:425–431.

778. Schoon Y, Schuurman, Buiting AG, et al. Aortic graft infection by *Lactobacillus casei*: a case report. Neth J Med 1998;52:71–74.

779. Schricker ME, Thompson GH, Schreiber JR. Osteomyelitis due to *Bacillus cereus* in an adolescent: case report and review. Clin Infect Dis 1994;18:863–867.

780. Schuchat A, Deaver K, Hayes PS, et al. Gastrointestinal carriage of *Listeria monocytogenes* in household contacts of patients with listeriosis. J Infect Dis 1993;167:1261–1262.

781. Schuchat A, Deaver KA, Wenger JD, et al. Role of foods in sporadic listeriosis: I. Case-control study of dietary risk factors. JAMA 1992;267:169–183.

782. Schuchat A, Lizano C, Broome CV, et al. Outbreak of neonatal listeriosis associated with mineral oil. Pediatr Infect Dis J 1991;10:183–189.

783. Schuchat A, Swaminathan B, Broome CV. Epidemiology of human listeriosis. Clin Microbiol Rev 1991;4:169–183.

784. Schumann P, Weiss N, Stackebrandt E. Reclassification of *Cellulomonas cellulans* (Stackbrandt and Keddie 1986) as *Cellulosimicrobium cellulans* gen. nov., com. nov. Int J Syst Evol Microbiol 2001;51:1007–1010.

785. Schuster MG, Brennan PJ, Edelstein P.: Persistent bacteremia with *Erysipelothrix rhusiopathiae* in a hospitalized patient. Clin Infect Dis 1993;17:783–784.

786. Scott TG, Curran B, Smith CJ. Electron microscopy of adhesive interactions between *Gardnerella vaginalis* and vaginal epithelial cells, McCoy cells, and human red blood cells. J Gen Microbiol 1989;135:475–480.

787. Seeliger HPR, Jones D. Genus *Listeria* Pirie 1940, 383. In: Sneath PHA, Mair NS, Sharpe ME, eds. Bergey's Manual of Systematic Bacteriology. Vol. 2. Baltimore: Williams & Wilkins, 1986:1235–1245.

788. Sergeant ES, Love SC, McInnes A. Abortions in sheep due to *Listeria ivanovii*. Aust Vet J 1991;68:39.

789. Sewell DL, Coyle MB, Funke G. Prosthetic valve endocarditis caused by *Corynebacterium afermentans* subsp. *lipophilum* (CDC coryneform group ANF-1). J Clin Microbiol 1995;33:759–761.

790. Shaffer DN, Drevets DA, Farr RW. *Listeria monocytogenes* rhombencephalitis with cranial nerve palsies. WV Med J 1999;94:80–83.

791. Shah M, Gentile RC, McCormick SA, Rogers SH. *Oerskovia xanthineolytica* keratitis. CLAO J 1996;22:96.

792. Sheiness D, Dix K, Watanabe S, Hillier SL. High levels of *Gardnerella vaginalis* detected with an oligonucleotide probe combined with elevated pH as a diagnostic indicator of bacterial vaginosis. J Clin Microbiol 1992;30:642–648.

793. Sheng WH, Hsueh PR, Hung CC, et al. Fatal outcome of *Erysipelothrix rhusiopathiae* bacteremia in a patient with oropharyngeal cancer. J Formos Med Assoc 2000;99:431–434.

794. Shida O, Takagi H, Kadowaki K, Komagata K. Proposal for two new genera, *Brevibacillus* gen. nov. and *Aneurinibacillus* gen. nov. Int J Syst Bacteriol 1996;46:939–946.

795. Shida O, Takagi H, Kadowaki K, et al. Transfer of *Bacillus alginolyticus*, *Bacillus chondroitinus*, *Bacillus curdlanolyticus*, *Bacillus glucanolyticus*, *Bacillus kobensis*, and *Bacillus thiaminolyticus* to the genus *Paenibacillus* and emended description of the genus *Paenibacillus*. Int J Syst Bacteriol 1997;47:289–298.

796. Shimoji Y. Pathogenicity of *Erysipelothrix rhusiopathiae*: virulence factors and protective immunity. Microbes Infect 2000;2:965–972.

797. Shimoji Y, Mori Y, Fischetti VA. Immunological characterization of a protective antigen of *Erysipelothrix rhusiopathiae*: identification of the region responsible for protective immunity. Infect Immun 1999;67:1646–1651.

798. Shimoji Y, Mori Y, Hyakutake K, et al. Use of an enrichment broth cultivation-PCR combination assay for rapid diagnosis of swine erysipelas. J Clin Microbiol 1998;36:86–89.

799. Shimoji Y, Yokomizo Y, Mori Y. Intracellular survival and replication of *Erysipelothrix rhusiopathiae* within murine macrophages: failure of induction of the oxidative burst of macrophages. Infect Immun 1996;64:1789–1793.

800. Shimoji Y, Yokomizo Y, Sekizaki T, et al. Presence of a capsule in *Erysipelothrix rhusiopathiae* and its relationship to virulence for mice. Infect Immun 1994;62:2806–2810.

801. Shinagawa K, Ichikawa K, Matsusaka N, Sugii S. Purification and some properties of a *Bacillus cereus* mouse lethal toxin. J Vet Med Sci 1991;53:469–474.

802. Shinagawa K, Ueno S, Konuma H, et al. Purification and characterization of the vascular permeability factor produced by *Bacillus cereus*. J Vet Med Sci 1991;53:281–286.

803. Shukla SK, Bernard KA, Harney M, et al. *Corynebacterium nigricans* sp. nov.: proposed name for a black-pigmented *Corynebacterium* species recovered from the human female genital tract. J Clin Microbiol 2003;41:4353–4358.

804. Shukla SK, Vevea DN, Frank DN, et al. Isolation and characterization of a black-pigmented *Corynebacterium* sp. from a woman with spontaneous abortion. J Clin Microbiol 2001;39:1109–1113.

805. Siegel SM, Haile CA. *Corynebacterium ulcerans* pneumonia. South Med J 1985;78:1267–1268.

806. Sierecka JK. Purification and partial characterization of a neutral protease from a virulent strain of *Bacillus cereus*. J Biochem Cell Biol 1998;30:579–595.

807. Silvester ME, Dicks LMT. Identification of lactic acid bacteria isolated from human vaginal secretions. Antonie van Leeuwenhoek 2003;83:117–123.

808. Simionescu R, Grover S, Shekar R, West BC. Necrotizing fasciitis caused by *Erysipelothrix rhusiopathiae*. South Med J 2003;96:937–939.

809. Simonet M, DeBriel D, Boucot I, et al. Coryneform bacteria isolated from middle ear fluid. J Clin Microbiol 1993;31:1667–1668.

810. Simoons-Smit AM, Savelkoul PH, Newling DW, Vandenbrouche-Grauls CM. Chronic cystitis caused by Corynebacterium urealyticum detected by polymerase chain reaction. Eur J Clin Microbiol Infect Dis 2000;19:949–952.

811. Sirard JC, Mock M, Fouet A. The three *Bacillus anthracis* toxin genes are coordinately regulated by bicarbonate and temperature. J Bacteriol 1994;176:5188–5192.

812. Sivalingam JJ, Martin P, Fraimow HS, et al. *Listeria monocytogenes* peritonitis: case report and literature review. Am J Gastroenterol 1992;87:1839–1845.

813. Sjoden B, Funke G, Izquierdo A, et al. Description of some coryneform bacteria isolated from human clinical specimens as *Corynebacterium falsenii* sp. nov. Int J Syst Bacteriol 1998;48:69–74.

814. Skov RL, Sanden AK, Danchell VH, et al. Systemic and deep-seated infections caused by *Arcanobacterium haemolyticum*. Eur J Clin Microbiol infect Dis 1998;17:578–582.

815. Sliman R, Rehm S, Shlaes DM. Serious infections caused by *Bacillus* species. Medicine (Baltimore) 1987;66:218–223.

816. Smego RA Jr. Actinomycosis of the central nervous system. Rev Infect Dis 1987;9:855–865.

817. Smego RA Jr, Foglia G. Actinomycosis. Clin Infect Dis 1998;26:1255–1263.

818. Smith GA, Marquis H, Jones S, et al. The two distinct phospholipases C of *Listeria monocytogenes* have overlapping roles in escape from a vacuole and cell-to-cell spread. Infect Immun 1995;63:4231–4237.

819. Smith KJ, Skelton HG III, Angritt P, et al. Cutaneous lesions of listeriosis in a newborn. J Cutan Pathol 1991;18:474–476.

820. Smith SM, Ogbara T, Eng RHK. Involvement of *Gardnerella vaginalis* in urinary tract infections in men. J Clin Microbiol 1991;30:1575–1577.

821. Sobel JD. Bacterial vaginosis. Annu Rev Med 2000;51:349–356.

822. Sobrino J, Marco F, Miro JM, et al. Prosthetic valve endocarditis caused by *Corynebacterium pilosum*. Infection 1991;19:247–249.

823. Sofianou D, Avgoustinakis E, Dilopoulou A, et al. Soft-tissue abscess involving *Actinomyces odontolyticus* and two *Prevotella* species in an intravenous drug abuser. Comp Immunol Microbiol Infect Dis 2004;27:75–79.

824. Soriano F, Aguado JM, Ponte C, et al. Urinary tract infection caused by *Corynebacterium* group D2: report of 82 cases and review. Rev Infect Dis 1990;12:1019–1034.

825. Soriano F, Fernandez-Roblas R. Infections caused by antibiotic-resistant *Corynebacterium* group D2. Eur J Clin Microbiol Infect Dis 1988;7:337–341.

826. Soriano F, Fernandez-Roblas R, Calvo R, Garcia-Calvo G. In vitro susceptibilities of aerobic and facultative non-spore-forming gram-positive bacilli to HMR 3647 (RU 66647) and 14 other antimicrobials. Antimicrob Agents Chemother 1998;42:1028–1033.

827. Soriano F, Fernandez-Roblas R, Zapardiel J, et al. Increasing incidence of *Corynebacterium* group D2 strains resistant to norfloxacin and ciprofloxacin. Eur J Clin Microbiol Infect Dis 1989;8:1117–1118.

828. Soriano F, Ponte C, Galliano MJ. Adherence of *Corynebacterium urealyticum* (CDC group D2) and *Corynebacterium jeikeium* to intravenous and urinary catheters. Eur J Clin Microbiol Infect Dis 1993;12:453–456.

829. Soriano F, Ponte C, Ruiz P, Zapardiel J. Non-urinary tract infections caused by multiply antibiotic-resistant *Corynebacterium urealyticum*. Clin Infect Dis 1993;17:890–891.

830. Soriano F, Ponte C, Santamaria M, et al. *Corynebacterium* group D2 as a cause of alkaline-encrusted cystitis: report of four cases and characterization of the organisms. J Clin Microbiol 1985;21:788–792.

831. Soriano F, Rodriguez-Tudela JL, Fernandez-Roblas R, et al. Skin colonization by Corynebacterium groups D2 and JK in hospitalized patients. J Clin Microbiol 1988;26:1878–1880.

832. Soriano F, Zapardiel J, Nieto E. Antimicrobial susceptibilities of *Corynebacterium* species and other non-spore-forming gram-positive bacilli to 18 antimicrobial agents. Antimicrob Agents Chemother 1995;39:208–214.

833. Soto A, Zapardiel J, Soriano F. Evaluation of the API Coryne system for identifying coryneform bacteria. J Clin Pathol 1994;47:756–759.

834. Spach DH, Opp DR, Gabre-Kidan T. Bacteremia due to *Corynebacterium jeikeium* in a patient with AIDS. Rev Infect Dis 1991;13:342–343.

835. Spitzer PG, Hammer SM, Karchmer AW. Treatment of *Listeria monocytogenes* infection with trimethoprim-sulfamethoxazole: case report and review of the literature. Rev Infect Dis 1986;8:427–430.

836. Spring S, Ludwig W, Marquez MC, et al. *Halobacillus* gen. nov., with descriptions of *Halobacillus litoralis* sp. nov. and *Halobacillus trueperi* sp. nov., and transfer of *Sporosarcina halophila* to *Halobacillus halophilus* comb. nov. Int J Syst Bacteriol 1996;46:492–496.

837. Spyrou N, Anderson M, Foale R. *Listeria* endocarditis: current management and patient outcome: world literature review. Heart 1997;77:380–383.

838. Sriskandan S, Lacey S, Fischer L. Isolation of vancomycin-resistant lactobacilli from three neutropenic patients with pneumonia. Eur J Clin Microbiol Infect Dis 1993;12:649–650.

839. Stackebrandt E, Breymann S, Steiner U, et al. Re-evaluation of the status of the genus *Oerskovia*, reclassification of *Promicromonospora enterophila* (Jager et al. 1983) as *Oerskovia enterophila* comb. nov. and description of *Oerskovia jenensis* sp. nov. and *Oerskovia paurometabola* sp. nov. Int J Syst Evol Microbiol 2002;52:1105–1111.

840. Stackebrandt E, Haringer M, Schleifer K-H. Molecular evidence for the transfer of *Oerskovia* species into the genus *Cellulomonas*. Arch Microbiol 1980;127:179–185.

841. Stackebrandt E, Keddie RM. Genus *Cellulomonas* Bergey et al. 1923, 154, emend. mut. char. Clark 1952, 50^{AL}. In: Sneath PHA, Mair NS, Sharpe ME, Holt JG, eds. Bergey's Manual of Systematic Bacteriology. Vol. 2. Baltimore: Williams & Wilkins, 1986:1325–1329.

842. Stackebrandt E, Seiler H, Schleifer K-H. Union of the genera *Cellulomonas* Bergey et al. and *Oerskovia* Prauser et al. in a redefined genus. Zentralbl Bakteriol Parasitenkd Infektkrankh Hyg Abt 1 Orig 1982;C3:401–409.

843. St Amant DC, Valentin-Bon IE, Jerse AE. Inhibition of Neisseria gonorrhoeae by Lactobacillus species that are commonly isolated from the female genital tract Infect Immun 2002;70:7169–7171.

844. Stamm AM, Smith SH, Kirklin JK, McGiffin DC. Listerial myocarditis in cardiac transplantation. Rev Infect Dis 1990;12:820–823.

845. Steen MK, Bruno-Murtha LA, Chaux G, et al. *Bacillus cereus* endocarditis: report of a case and review. Clin Infect Dis 1992;14:945–946.

846. Stone N, Gillett P, Burge S. Breast abscess due to *Corynebacterium striatum*. Br J Dermatol 1997;137:623–625.

847. Strauss R, Mueller A, Wehler M, et al. Pseudomembranous tracheobronchitis due to *Bacillus cereus*. Clin Infect Dis 2001;33:e39–e41.

848. Sturdee S, Bainton R, Barnham M. Intravascular infection with *Lactobacillus paracasei*. J Infect 1998;37:184–186.

849. Sturm AW. *Gardnerella vaginalis* in infections of the urinary tract. J Infect 1989;18:45–49.

850. Sturm AW, de Leeuw JHA, dePree NTCM. Postoperative wound infection with *Gardnerella vaginalis*. J Infect 1983;7:264–266.

851. Suarez ML, Espino L, Vila M, Santamarina G. Urinary tract infection caused by *Corynebacterium urealyticum* in a dog. J Small Anim Pract 2002;43:299–302.

852. Sudduth EJ, Rozich JD, Farrar WE. *Rothia dentocariosa* endocarditis complicated by perivalvular abscess. Clin Infect Dis 1993;17:772–775.

853. Sulea IT, Pollice MC, Barksdale L. Pyrazine carboxylamidase activity in *Corynebacterium*. Int J Syst Bacteriol 1980;30:466–472.

854. Sung MH, Kim H, Bae JW, et al. *Geobacillus toebii* sp. nov., a novel thermophilic bacterium isolated from hay compost. Int J Syst Evol Microbiol 2002;52:2251–2255.

855. Suzuki KI, Suzuki M, Sasaki J, et al. *Leifsonia* gen. nov., a genus for 2,4-diaminobutyric acid-containing actinomycetes to accommodate "*Corynebacterium aquaticum*" Leifson 1962 and *Clavibacter xyli* subspecies *cynodontis* Davis et al. 1984. J Gen Appl Microbiol 1999;45:253–262.

856. Svare J, Andersen LF, Langhoff-Roos J, et al. Maternal-fetal listeriosis: two case reports. Gynecol Obstet Invest 1991;31:179–181.

857. Swartz MA, Welch DF, Narayanan RP, Greenfield RA. Catalase-negative *Listeria monocytogenes* causing meningitis in an adult. Am J Clin Pathol 1991;96:130–133.

858. Swenson JM, Facklam RR, Thornsberry C. Antimicrobial susceptibility of vancomycin-resistant *Leuconostoc*, *Pediococcus*, and *Lactobacillus* species. Antimicrob Agents Chemother 1990;34:543–547.

859. Tabatabaie P, Syadati A. *Bacillus anthracis* as a cause of bacterial meningitis. Pediatr Infect Dis J 1993;12:1035–1037.

860. Takahashi T, Fujisawa T, Benno Y, et al. *Erysipelothrix tonsillarum* sp. nov. isolated from tonsils of apparently healthy pigs. Int J Syst Bacteriol 1987;37:166–168.

861. Takahashi T, Fujisawa T, Tamura Y, et al. DNA relatedness among *Erysipelothrix rhusiopathiae* strains representing all twenty-three serovars and *Erysipelothrix tonsillarum*. Int J Syst Bacteriol 1992;42:469–473.

862. Takahashi T, Fujisawa T, Yamamoto K, et al. Taxonomic evidence that serovar 7 of *Erysipelothrix rhusiopathiae* isolated from dogs with endocarditis are *Erysipelothrix tonsillarum*. J Vet Med B Infect Dis Vet Public Health 2000;47:311–312.

863. Takahashi T, Takahashi I, Tamura Y, et al. Mechanism of plasma clotting by *Erysipelothrix rhusiopathiae*. J Clin Microbiol 1990;28:2161–2164.

864. Takahashi T, Tamura Y, Yoshimura H, et al. *Erysipelothrix tonsillarum* isolated from dogs with endocarditis in Belgium. Res Vet Sci 1993;54:264–265.

865. Takeshi K, Makino S, Ikeda T, et al. Direct and rapid detection by PCR of *Erysipelothrix* sp. DNAs prepared from bacterial strains and animal tissues. J Clin Microbiol 1999;37:4093–4098.

866. Takeuchi M, Hatano K. Union of the genera *Microbacterium* Orla-Jensen and *Aureobacterium* Collins, et al. in a redefined genus *Microbacterium*. Int J Syst Bacteriol 1998;48:739–747.

867. Takeuchi M, Sakane T, Nihira T, et al. *Corynebacterium terpenotabidum* sp. nov., a bacterium capable of degrading squalene. Int J Syst Bacteriol 199949:223–229.

868. Takeuchi M, Yokota A. Phylogenetic analysis of the genus *Microbacterium* based on 16S rRNA gene sequences. FEMS Microbiol Lett 1994;124:11–16.

869. Takiguchi Y, Terano T, Hirai A. Lung abscess caused by *Actinomyces odontolyticus*. Intern Med 2003;42:723–725.

870. Tamura Y, Takahashi T, Zarkasie K, et al. Differentiation of *Erysipelothrix rhusiopathiae* and *Erysipelothrix tonsillarum* by sodium dodecyl sulfate-polyacrylamide gel electrophoresis of cell proteins. Int J Syst Bacteriol 1993;43:111–114.

871. Tang G, Yip H-K, Luo G, et al. Development of novel oligonucleotide probes for seven *Actinomyces* species and their utility in supragingival plaque analysis. Oral Diseases 2003;9:203–209.

872. Tang YW, von Graevenitz A, Waddington MG, et al. Identification of coryneform bacterial isolates by ribosomal DNA sequence analysis. J Clin Microbiol 2000;38:1676–1678.

873. Tappero JW, Schuchat A, Deaver KS, et al. Reduction in the incidence of human listeriosis in the United States: effectiveness of prevention efforts? JAMA 1995;273:1118–1122.

874. Tastepe AI, Ulasan NG, Liman ST, et al. Thoracic actinomycosis. Eur J Cardiothorac Surg 1998;14:578–583.

875. Tattevin P, Bremieux AC, Muller-Serieys C, Carbon C. Native valve endocarditis due to *Corynebacterium striatum*: first reported case of medical treatment alone. Clin Infect Dis 1996;23:1330–1331.

876. Taylor GB, Paviour SD, Musaad S, et al. A clinicopathological review of 34 cases of inflammatory breast disease showing an association between corynebacteria infection and granulomatous mastitis. Pathology 2003;35:109–119.

877. Taylor JP, Dimmitt DC, Ezzell JW, Whitford H. Indigenous human cutaneous anthrax in Texas. South Med J 1993;86:1–4.

878. Te Giffel MC, Beumer RR, Klijn N, et al. Discrimination between *Bacillus cereus* and *Bacillus thuringiensis* using specific DNA probes based on variable regions of 16S rRNA. FEMS Microbiol Lett 1997;146:47–51.

879. Telander B, Lerner R, Palmblad J, Ringertz O. *Corynebacterium* group JK in a hematological ward: infections, colonization, and environmental contamination. Scand. J Infect Dis 1988;20:55–61.

880. Tendler C, Bottone EJ. *Corynebacterium aquaticum* urinary tract infection in a neonate and concepts regarding the role of the organism as a neonatal pathogen. J Clin Microbiol 1989;27:343–345.

881. Tesh MJ, Wood RL. Detection of coagulase activity in *Erysipelothrix rhusiopathiae*. J Clin Microbiol 1988;26:1058–1060.

882. Thangkhiew I, Gunstone RF. Association of *Lactobacillus plantarum* with endocarditis. J Infect 1998;16:304–305.

883. Thompson C, McCarter YS, Krause PJ, Herson VC. *Lactobacillus acidophilus* sepsis in a neonate. J Perinatol 2001;21:258–260.

884. Thuler LC, Velasco E, de Souza Martins CA, et al. An outbreak of *Bacillus* species in a cancer hospital. Infect Control Hosp Epidemiol 1998;19:856–858.

885. Thurn JR, Goodman JL. Post-traumatic ophthalmitis due to *Bacillus licheniformis*. Am J Med 1988;85:708–709.

886. Tiley SM, Kociuba KR, Heron LG, Munro R. Infective endocarditis due to nontoxigenic *Corynebacterium diphtheriae*: report of seven cases and review. Clin Infect Dis 1993;16:271–275.

887. Titov L, Kolodkina V, Dronina A, et al. Genotypic and phenotypic characteristics of *Corynebacterium diphtheriae* strains isolated from patients in Belarus during an epidemic period. J Clin Microbiol 2003;41:1285–1288.

888. Tokieda K, Morikawa Y, Maeyama K, et al. Clinical manifestations of *Bacillus cereus* meningitis in newborn infants. J Paediatr Child Health 1999;35:582–584.

889. Toma C, Sisavath L, Iwanga M. Reversed passive latex agglutination assay for detection of toxigenic *Corynebacterium diphtheriae*. J Clin Microbiol 1997;35:3147–3149.

890. Totemchokchyakarn K, Janwityanujit S, Sathapatayavongs B, Puavilai S. *Erysipelothrix rhusiopathiae* septicemia in systemic lupus erythematosus. Int J Dermatol 1996;35:818–820.

891. Totten PA, Amsel R, Hale J, et al. Selective differential human blood bilayer media for isolation of *Gardnerella (Haemophilus) vaginalis*. J Clin Microbiol 1982;15:141–147.

892. Touzel JP, O'Donohue M, Debeire P, et al. *Thermobacillus xylanilyticus* gen. nov., sp. nov., a new aerobic thermophilic xylan-degrading bacterium isolated from farm soil. Int J Syst Evol Microbiol 2000;50:315–320.

893. Traub WH, Geipel U, Leonhard B, Bauer D. Antibiotic susceptibility testing (agar disk diffusion and agar dilution) of clinical isolates of *Corynebacterium jeikeium*. Chemotherapy 1998;44:230–237.

894. Truant AL, Satishchandran V, Eisenstaedt R, et al. *Oerskovia xanthineolytica* and methicillin-resistant *Staphylococcus aureus* in a patient with cirrhosis and variceal hemorrhage. Eur J Clin Microbiol Infect Dis 1992;11:950–951.

895. Tsuruoka N, Nakayama T, Ashida M, et al. Collagenolytic serine carboxyl proteinase from *Alicyclobacillus sendaiensis* strain NTAP-1: purification, characterization, gene cloning, and heterologous expression. Appl Environ Microbiol 2003;69:162–169.

896. Tuladhar R, Patole SK, Koh TH, et al. Refractory *Bacillus cereus* infection in a neonate. Int J Clin Pract 2000;54:345–347.

897. Tumbarello M, Tacconelli E, Del Forno A, et al. *Corynebacterium striatum* bacteremia in a patient with AIDS (letter). Clin Infect Dis 1994;18:1007–1008.

898. Uchida I, Makino S, Sasakawa C, et al. Identification of a novel gene, *dep*, associated with depolymerization of the capsular polymer in *Bacillus anthracis*. Mol Microbiol 1993;9:487–496.

899. Umana E. *Erysipelothrix rhusiopathiae*: an unusual pathogen of infective endocarditis. Int J Cardiol 2003;88:297–299.

900. Valdes-Stauber N, Scherer S, Seiler H. Identification of yeasts and coryneform bacteria from the surface microflora of brick cheeses. Int J Food Microbiol 1997;34:115–129.

901. Van J-C, Nguyen L, Guillemain R, et al. Relapse of infection or reinfection with *Listeria monocytogenes* in a patient with a heart transplant: usefulness of pulsed-field gel electrophoresis for diagnosis. Clin Infect Dis 1994;19:208–209.

902. Van Belkum A, Koeken A, Vandamme P, et al. Development of a species-specific polymerase chain reaction assay for *Gardnerella vaginalis*. Mol Cell Probes 1995;9:167–174.

903. Van Bosterhaut B, Boucquey P, Janssens M, et al. Chronic osteomyelitis due to *Actinomyces neuii* subspecies *neuii* and *Dermabacter hominis*. Eur J Clin Microbiol Infect Dis 2002;21:486–487.

904. Van Bosterhaut B, Cuvelier R, Serruys E, et al. Three cases of opportunistic infection caused by propionic acid producing *Corynebacterium minutissimum*. Eur J Clin Microbiol Infect Dis 1992;11:628–631.

905. Van Bosterhaut B, Surmont I, Vandeven J, et al. *Corynebacterium jeikeium* (group JK diphtheroids) endocarditis: a report of five cases. Diagn Microbiol Infect Dis 1989;12:265–268.

906. Vandamme P, Falsen E, Vancanneyt M, et al. Characterization of *Actinomyces turicensis* and *Actinomyces radingae* strains from human clinical samples. Int J Syst Bacteriol 1998;48:503–510.

907. van der Lelie H, Leverstein-van Hall M, Mertens M, et al. *Corynebacterium* CDC group JK (*Corynebacterium jeikeium*) sepsis in haematological patients:

908. Van der Zwet WC, Parlevliet GA, Savelkoul PH, et al. Outbreak of *Bacillus cereus* infection in a neonatal intensive care unit traced to balloons used in manual ventilation. J Clin Microbiol 2000;38:4131–4136.

909. Vaneechoutte M, Boerlin P, Tichy HV, et al. Comparison of PCR-based DNA fingerprinting techniques for the identification of *Listeria* species and their use for atypical *Listeria* isolates. Int J Syst Bacteriol 1998;48:127–139.

910. Vaneechoutte M, DeBleser D, Claeys G, et al. Cardioverter-lead electrode infection due to *Corynebacterium amycolatum*. Clin Infect Dis 1998;27:1553–1554.

911. Vaneechoutte M, Riegel R, DeBriel D, et al. Evaluation of the applicability of amplified rDNA-restriction analysis (ARDRA) to identification of species in the genus *Corynebacterium*. Res Microbiol 1995;146:633–641.

912. Van Esbroeck M, Vandamme P, Falsen E, et al. Polyphasic approach to the classification and identification of *Gardnerella vaginalis* and unidentified *Gardnerella vaginalis*-like coryneforms present in bacterial vaginosis. Int J Syst Bacteriol 1996;46:675–682.

913. Van Mook WN, Simonis FS, Schneeberger PM, van Opstal JL. A rare case of disseminated actinomycosis caused by *Actinomyces meyeri*. Neth J Med 1997;51:39–45.

914. Van Netten P, Perales I, van de Moosdijk A, et al. Liquid and solid differential media for the detection and enumeration of *Listeria monocytogenes* and other *Listeria* species. Int J Food Microbiol 1989;8:299–316.

915. Van Noyen R, Reybrouck R, Peeters P, et al. *Listeria monocytogenes* infection of a prosthetic vascular graft. Infection 1993;21:125–126.

916. Venditti M, Gelfusa V, Castelli F, et al. *Erysipelothrix rhusiopathiae* endocarditis. Eur J Clin Microbiol Infect Dis 1990;9:50–52.

917. Venditti M, Gelfusa V, Tarasi A, et al. Antimicrobial susceptibilities of *Erysipelothrix rhusiopathiae*. Antimicrob Agents Chemother 1990;34:2038–2040.

918. Villanueva JL, Dominguez A, Rios MJ, Iglesias C. *Corynebacterium macginleyi* isolated from urine in a patient with a permanent bladder catheter. Scand J Infect Dis 2002;34:699–700.

919. Villegas H, Arias F, Flores E, et al. Ultrastructural characteristics of *Gardnerella vaginalis* infection in the heterosexual couple. Arch Androl 1997;39:147–153.

920. Viscoli C, Garaventa A, Ferrea G, et al. *Listeria monocytogenes* brain abscesses in a girl with acute lymphoblastic leukaemia after late central nervous system relapse. Eur J Cancer 1991;27:435–437.

921. Vitek CR, Wharton M. Diphtheria in the former Soviet Union: reemergence of a pandemic disease. Emerg Infect Dis 1998;4:539–550.

922. Vogt HB, Hoffman WW. A case of *Lactobacillus acidophilus* endocarditis successfully treated with cefazolin and gentamicin. SDJ Med 1998;51:153–156.

923. Voisin S, Deruaz D, Freney J, Renaud FN. Differentiation of *Corynebacterium amycolatum*, *C. miniutissimum*, *C. striatum*, and related species by pyrolysis-gas-liquid chromatography with atomic emission detection. Res Microbiol 2002;153:307–311.

924. Volokhov D, Rasooly A, Chumakov K, Chizhikov V. Identification of *Listeria* species by microarray-based assay. J Clin Microbiol 2002;40:4720–4728.

925. von Graevenitz A, Frommelt L, Punter-Streit V, Funke G. Diversity of coryneforms found in infections following prosthetic joint insertion and open fractures. Infection 1998;26:36–38.

926. von Graevenitz A, Osterhout G, Dick J. Grouping of some clinically relevant Gram-positive rods by automated fatty acid analysis. APMIS 1991;99:147–154.

927. von Graevenitz A, Punter V, Gruner E, et al. Identification of coryneform and other Gram-positive rods with several methods. APMIS 1994;120:381–389.

928. von Graevenitz, A., Punter-Streit V, Riegel P, Funke G. Coryneform bacteria in throat cultures of healthy individuals. J Clin Microbiol 1998;36:2087–2088.

929. Von Hunolstein C, Alfarone G, Scopetti F, et al. Molecular epidemiology and characteristics of *Corynebacterium diphtheriae* and *Corynebacterium ulcerans* strains isolated in Italy during the 1990's. J Med Microbiol 2003;52:181–188.

930. Waagner DC. *Arcanobacterium haemolyticum*: biology of the organism and diseases in man. Pediatr Infect Dis J 1991;10:933–939.

931. Wagner J, Ignatius R, Voss S, et al. Infection of the skin caused by *Corynebacterium ulcerans* and mimicking classical cutaneous diphtheria. Clin Infect Dis 2001;33:1598–1600.

932. Waino M, Tindall BJ, Schumann P, Ingvorsen K. *Gracilibacillus* gen. nov., with description of *Gracilibacillus halotolerans* gen. nov., sp. nov., transfer of *Bacillus dipsosauri* to *Gracilibacillus dipsosauri* comb. nov., and *Bacillus salexigens* to the genus *Salibacillus* gen. nov., as *Salibacillus salexigens* comb. nov. Int J Syst Bacteriol 1999;49:821–831.

933. Wallet F, Perez T, Roussel-Delvallez M, et al. *Rothia dentocariosa*: two new cases of pneumonia revealing lung cancer. Scand J Infect Dis 1997;29:419–520.

934. Wang CC, Mattson D, Wald A. *Corynebacterium jeikeium* bacteremia in bone marrow transplant patients with Hickman catheters. Bone Marrow Transplant 2001;27:445–449.

935. Watkins DA, Chachine A, Creger RG, et al. *Corynebacterium striatum*: a diphtheroid with pathogenic potential. Clin Infect Dis 1993;17:21–25.

936. Wattiau P, Janssens M, Wauters G. *Corynebacterium simulans* sp. nov., a non-

a report of three cases and a systematic literature review. Scand J Infect Dis 1995;27:581–584.

lipophilic, fermentative *Corynebacterium*. Int J Syst Evol Microbiol 2000;50: 347–353.

937. Wauters G, Avesani V, Laffineur K, et al. *Brevibacterium lutescens* sp. nov., from human and environmental samples. Int J Syst Evol Microbiol 2003;53: 1321–1325.

938. Wauters G, Charlier J, Janssens M, Delmee M. Identification of *Arthrobacter oxydans, Arthrobacter luteus* sp. nov., and *Arthrobacter albus* sp. nov., isolated from human clinical specimens. J Clin Microbiol 2000;38:2412–2415.

939. Wauters G, Charlier J, Janssens M, Delmee M. *Brevibacterium paucivorans* sp. nov., from human clinical specimens. Int J Syst Evol Microbiol 2001;51: 1703–1707.

940. Wauters G, Driessen A, Ageron E, et al. Propionic acid-producing strains previously designated as *Corynebacterium xerosis, C. minutissimum, C. striatum,* and CDC group I-2 and group F-2 coryneforms belong to the species *Corynebacterium amycolatum*. Int J Syst Bacteriol 1996;46:653–657.

941. Wauters G, Van Bosterhaut B, Avesani V, et al. Peritonitis due to *Brevibacterium otitidis* in a patient undergoing continuous ambulatory peritoneal dialysis. J Clin Microbiol 2000;38:4292–4293.

942. Wauters G, Van Bosterhaut B, Janssens M, Verhaegen J. Identification of *Corynebacterium amycolatum* and other nonlipophilic fermentative corynebacteria of human origin. J Clin Microbiol 1998;36:1430–1432.

943. Weber DJ, Saviteer SM, Rutala WA, Thomann CA. In vitro susceptibility of *Bacillus* spp. to selected antimicrobial agents. Antimicrob Agents Chemother 1988;32:642–645.

944. Weersink AJL, Rozenberg-Arska M, Westerhof PW, Verhoef J. *Rothia dentocariosa* endocarditis complicated by an abdominal aneurysm. Clin Infect Dis 1994; 18:489–490.

945. Weiss K, Labbe AC, Laverdiere M. *Corynebacterium striatum* meningitis: case report and review of an increasingly important *Corynebacterium* species. Clin Infect Dis 1996;23:1246–1248.

946. Weller TMA, McLardy-Smith P, Crook DW. *Corynebacterium jeikeium* osteomyelitis following total hip joint replacement. J Infect 1994;29:113–114.

947. Wellinghausen N, Sing A, Kern WW, et al. A fatal case of necrotizing sinusitis due to toxigenic *Corynebacterium ulcerans*. Int J Med Microbiol 2002;292: 59–63.

948. Wesche J, Elliott JL, Falnes S, et al. Characterization of membrane translocation by anthrax protective antigen. Biochemistry 1998;37:15737–15746.

949. Westling K, Lidman C, Thalme A. Tricuspid valve endocarditis caused by a new species of actinomyces: *Actinomyces funkei*. Scand J Infect Dis 2002;34: 206–207.

950. Wilhelmus KR, Robinson NM, Jones DB. *Bacterionema matruchotii* ocular infections. Am J Ophthalmol 1979;87:143–147.

951. Williamson LH. Caseous lymphadenitis in small ruminants. Vet Clin North Am Food Anim Pract 2001;17:359–371.

952. Wilson APR. The return of *Corynebacterium diphtheriae*: the rise of non-toxigenic strains. J Hosp Infect 1995;30(Suppl):306–312.

953. Wilson JA, Barratt AJ. An unusual case of *Gardnerella vaginalis* septicaemia. Br Med J 1986;293:309.

954. Wilson ME, Shapiro DS. Native valve endocarditis due to *Corynebacterium pseudodiphtheriticum*. Clin Infect Dis 1992;15:1059–1060.

955. Winslow DL, Pankey GA. *In vitro* activities of trimethoprim and sulfamethoxazole against *Listeria monocytogenes*. Antimicrob Agents Chemother 1982;22: 51–54.

956. Winslow DL, Steele-Moore L. Ventriculoperitoneal shunt infection due to *Listeria monocytogenes*. Clin Infect Dis 1995;20:1437.

957. Wisotzkey JD, Jurtshuk P Jr, Fox GE, et al. Comparative sequence analyses on the 16S rRNA (rDNA) of *Bacillus acidocaldarius, Bacillus acidoterrestris,* and *Bacillus cycloheptanicus* and proposal for creation of a new genus, *Alicyclobacillus* gen. nov. Int J Syst Bacteriol 1992;42:263–269.

958. Witt A, Petricevic L, Kaufmann U, et al. DNA hybridization test: rapid diagnostic tool for excluding bacterial vaginosis in pregnant women with symptoms suggestive of infection. J Clin Microbiol 2002;40:3057–3059.

959. Wolde Rufael D, Cohn SE. Native valve endocarditis due to *Corynebacterium striatum*: case report and review. Clin Infect Dis 1994;19:1054–1061.

960. Wong MT, Dolan MJ. Significant infections due to *Bacillus* species following abrasions associated with motor vehicle-related trauma. Clin Infect Dis 1992; 15:855–857.

961. Wong TP, Groman H. Production of diphtheria toxin by selected isolates of *Corynebacterium ulcerans* and *Corynebacterium pseudotuberculosis*. Infect Immun 1984;43:1114–1116.

962. Woo PCY, Fung AMY, Lau SKP, et al. Diagnosis of pelvic actinomycosis by 16S ribosomal RNA gene sequencing and its clinical significance. Diagn Microbiol Infect Dis 2002;43:113–118.

963. Woo PCY, Fung AMY, Lau SKP, Yuen K-Y. Identification by 16S rRNA sequencing of *Lactobacillus salivarius* bacteremic cholecystitis. J Clin Microbiol 2002;40:265–267.

964. Wood CA, Pepe R. Bacteremia in a patient with non-urinary tract infection due to *Corynebacterium urealyticum*. Clin Infect Dis 1994;19:367–368.

965. Wood GC, Boucher BA, Croce MA, Fabian TC. *Lactobacillus* species as the cause of ventilator-associated pneumonia in a critically ill trauma patient. Pharmacotherapy 2002;22:1180–1182.

966. Wright ED, Richards AJ, Edge AJ. Discitis caused by *Corynebacterium pseudodiphtheriticum* following ear, nose, and throat surgery. Br J Rheumatol 1994; 34:585–586.

967. Wright JR Jr, Stinson D, Wade A, et al. Necrotizing funisitis associated with *Actinomyces meyeri* infection: a case report. Pediatr Pathol 1994;14:927–934.

968. Wu S-R, Hillier SL, Nath K. Genomic fingerprint analysis of biotype 1 *Gardnerella vaginalis* from patients with and without bacterial vaginosis. J Clin Microbiol 1996;34:192–195.

969. Wust J, Martinetti Lucchini G, Luthy-Hottenstein J, et al. Isolation of gram-positive rods that resemble but are clearly distinct from *Actinomyces pyogenes* from mixed wound infections. J Clin Microbiol 1993;31:1127–1145.

970. Wust J, Stubbs S, Weiss N, et al. Assignment of *Actinomyces pyogenes*-like (CDC coryneform group E) bacteria to the genus *Actinomyces* as *Actinomyces radingae* sp. nov., and *Actinomyces turicensis* sp. nov. Lett Appl Microbiol 1995;20:76–81.

971. Xia T, Baumgartner JC. Occurrence of *Actinomyces* in infections of endodontic origin. J Endod 2003;29:549–552.

972. Ximenez-Fyvie LA, Haffajee AD, Martin L, et al. Identification of oral *Actinomyces* species using DNA probes. Oral Microbiol Immunol 1999;14:257–265.

973. Yague G, Segovia M, Valero-Guillen PL. Detection of mycoloylglycerol by thin-layer chromatography as a tool for the rapid inclusion of corynebacteria of clinical origin in the genus *Corynebacterium*. J Chromatogr B Biomed Sci Appl 2000;738:181–185.

974. Yanagawa R, Honda E. *Corynebacterium pilosum* and *Corynebacterium cystiditis*, two new species from cows. Int J Syst Bacteriol 1978;28:209–216.

975. Yassin AF, Kroppenstedt RM, Ludwig W. *Corynebacterium glaucum* sp. nov. Int J Syst Evol Microbiol 2003;53:705–709.

976. Yassin AF, Steiner U, Ludwig W. *Corynebacterium aurimucosum* sp. nov. and emended description of *Corynebacterium minutissimum* Collins and Jones (1983). Int J Syst Evol Microbiol 2002;52:1001–1005.

977. Yassin AF, Steiner U, Ludwig W. *Corynebacterium appendicis* sp. nov. Int J Syst Evol Microbiol 2003;52:1165–1169.

978. Yildiz S, Yildiz HY, Cetin I, Ucar DH. Total knee arthroplasty complicated by *Corynebacterium jeikeium* infection. Scand J Infect Dis 1995;27:635–636.

979. Yokota A, Takeguchi M, Weiss N. Proposal of two new species in the genus *Microbacterium*: *Microbacterium dextranolyticum* sp. nov. and *Microbacterium aurum* sp. nov. Int J Syst Bacteriol 1993;43:549–554.

980. Yokota A, Takeuchi M, Sakane T, Weiss N. Proposal of six new species in the genus *Aureobacterium* and transfer of *Flavobacterium esteraromaticum* Omelianski to the genus *Aureobacterium* as Aureobacterium esteraromaticum comb. nov. Int J Syst Bacteriol 1993;43:555–564.

981. Yoon JH, Kang PH, Park YH. *Lentibacillus salicampi* gen. nov., sp. nov., a moderately halophilic bacterium isolated from a salt field in Korea. Int J Syst Evol Microbiol 2002;52:2043–2048.

982. Yoonessi M, Crickard K, Cellino IS, et al. Association of *Actinomyces* and intrauterine contraceptive devices. J Reprod Med 1985;30:48–52.

983. York M. *Bacillus* species pseudobacteremia traced to contaminated gloves used in collection of blood from patients with acquired immunodeficiency syndrome. J Clin Microbiol 1990;28:2114–2116.

984. Younus F, Chua A, Tortura G, Jimenez VE. Lemierre's disease caused by co-infection of *Arcanobacterium haemolyticum* and *Fusobacterium necrophorum*: a case report. J Infect 2002;45:114–117.

985. Zaman R, Abbas M, Burd E. Late prosthetic hip joint infection with *Actinomyces israelii* in an intravenous drug user: case report and literature review. J Clin Microbiol 2002;40:4391–4392.

986. Zapardiel J, Nieto E, Soriano F. Urinary tract infections caused by β-lactam-sensitive *Corynebacterium urealyticum* strains. Eur J Cin Microbiol Infect Dis 1997;16:174–176.

987. Zimmerman O, Sproer C, Kroppenstedt RM, et al. *Corynebacterium thomssenii* sp. nov., a *Corynebacterium* with *N*-acetyl-β-glucosaminidase activity from human clinical specimens. Int J Syst Bacteriol 1998;48:489–494.

988. Zinkernagal AS, von Graevenitz A, Funke G. Heterogeneity within *Corynebacterium minutissimum* strains is explained by misidentified *Corynebacterium amycolatum* strains. Am J Clin Pathol 1996;106:378–383.

989. Zinnemann K, Turner GC. The taxonomic position of ''*Haemophilus vaginalis*'' (*Corynebacterium vaginale*). J Pathol Bacteriol 1963;85:213–219.

990. Zuber PLF, Gruner E, Altwegg M, von Graevenitz A. Invasive infection with non-toxigenic *Corynebacterium diphtheriae* among drug users. Lancet 1992; 330:1359.

Aerobic Actinomycetes

Introduction, Classification, and Taxonomy

The Nocardioform Group

Nocardia

Epidemiology, Pathology, and Pathogenesis

Clinical Disease

Rhodococcus

Epidemiology, Pathology, and Pathogenesis

Clinical Disease

Other Nocardioform Bacteria

The Maduromycetes and Thermonosporas

Actinomadura

Epidemiology

Clinical Disease and Pathology

Nocardiopsis

The Streptomycetes

Streptomyces

Thermophilic Actinomycetes

Miscellaneous Actinomycetes

Oerskovia

Dermatophilus

Tropheryma whipplei

History and Taxonomy

Ecology

Clinical Disease and Pathology

Laboratory Diagnosis of Infections Caused by Aerobic Actinomycetes

Primary Isolation

Differentiation of *Nocardia* From Other Genera of Aerobic Actinomycetes

Identification of Thermophilic Actinomycetes

Identification of *Tropheryma whipplei*

In Vitro Susceptibility of *Nocardia* and Related Bacteria to Antimicrobial Agents and Therapy of Infections

---

Introduction, Classification, and Taxonomy

The aerobic actinomycetes are gram-positive bacteria that are usually more filamentous and branched than the bacteria discussed in previous chapters, commonly producing a funguslike mycelium that fragments or breaks up into rod-shaped and short coccoid forms. These organisms, when isolated in many clinical laboratories, are referred for identification to the ''mycology section'' or the ''mycobacteriology section,'' rather than to the routine bacteriology laboratory.

The reasons are that most species grow more slowly than other aerobic and facultatively anaerobic bacteria and they can be isolated on commonly used fungus media (e.g., Sabouraud dextrose agar) or mycobacteria isolation media (e.g., Middlebrook synthetic agars and Lowenstein-Jensen medium). These aerobic, branching, filamentous gram-positive rods are, nonetheless, bacteria, not fungi. True fungi have a eukaryotic cellular organization. In contrast to the fungi, the prokaryotic aerobic actinomycetes do not have a membrane-enclosed nucleus; they lack the intracellular organelles possessed by eukaryotic organisms (e.g., no mitochondria); their cell walls contain muramic acid, diaminopimelic acid, or lysine (which fungi lack); they are inhibited by antibacterial antibiotics, but not by antifungal agents; and they differ in other fundamental characteristics. The branching hyphae of the aerobic actinomycetes are more narrow than fungal hyphae, measuring 0.5 to 1.2 μm in diameter.

Modern chemical and genetic techniques have established the great diversity of this group, but the phenotypic characteristics described above remain an important part of the microbiologic definition (Table 15-1).[10] The aerobic actinomycetes as a whole are placed taxonomically in the class *Actinobacteria*, order *Actinomycetales*, suborder *Corynebacterineae*. The flowchart in Figure 15-1 depicts the relationships among these bacteria. Although the taxonomy and nomenclature of these bacteria are still in flux, a provisional, ad hoc phenotypic characterization of the group remains useful (Table 15-1).[10,30,58]

The scheme outlined in Figure 15-1 uses tests that are commonly performed in clinical microbiology laboratories when possible. The non–acid-fast genera present the greatest

Table 15-1 Phenotypic Grouping of Aerobic Actinomycetes

PHENOTYPIC GROUP	REPRESENTATIVE GENERA AND SPECIES
Maduromycetes	*Actinomadura pusilla* group
Nocardioforms[a]	*Nocardia* spp.
	Rhodococcus spp.
	Gordonia spp.
	Tsukamurella spp.
	Dietzia spp.
	Mycobacterium spp.
Nocardioides	*Nocardioides* spp.
Streptomycetes	*Streptomyces* spp.
Micropolysporas	*Faenia* spp. (*Micropolyspora* spp.)[b]
	Saccharomonospora spp.[b]
	Saccharopolyspora spp.[b]
Thermomonosporas	*Actinomadura madurae* group
	Nocardiopsis
Other actinomycetes	*Thermoactinomyces* spp.[b]
	Tropheryma whipplei
	Oerskovia spp.
	Dermatophilus spp.

[a] *The Nocardioform group contains mycolic acids in the cell walls, as do Corynebacterium spp.*
[b] *Thermophilic species that grow at temperatures above 50°C.*

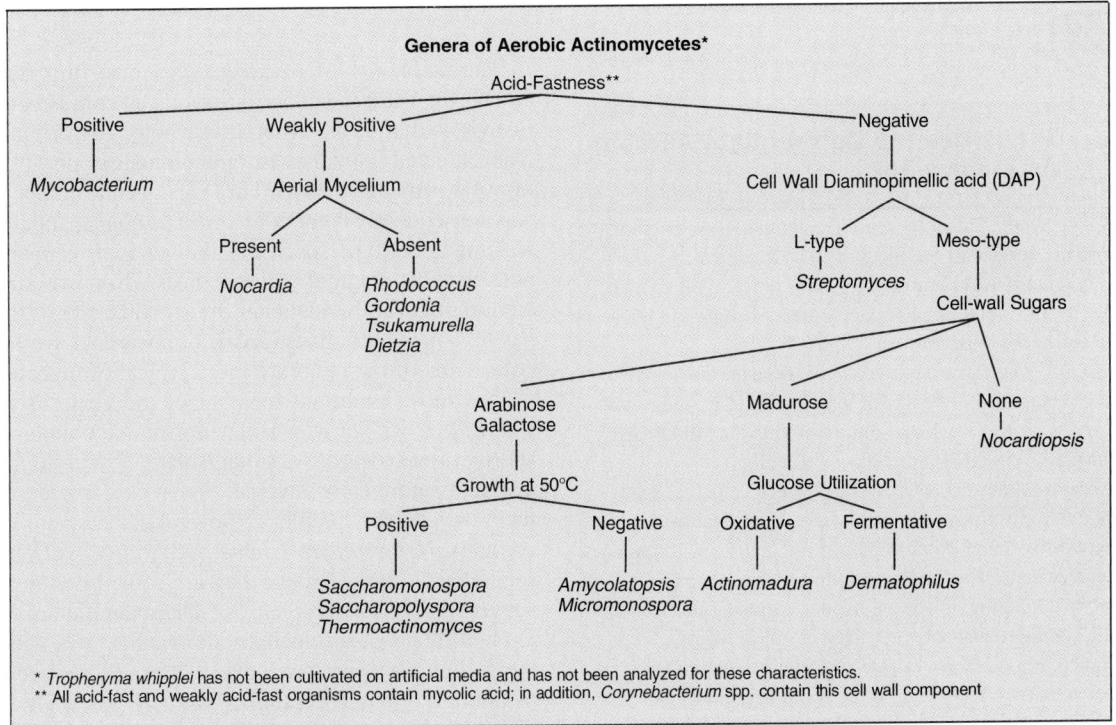

Figure 15-1 Classification of aerobic actinomycetes associated with human disease.

problem, because the cell wall analyses required for their identification are beyond the capacity of most clinical laboratories. The most common saprophytes isolated in daily practice are *Streptomyces* spp. If the isolate is from a patient who has a clinically compatible illness, it should be referred to a reference laboratory for complete identification. Even within the acid-fast group the increasing complexity of the required testing will encourage the referral of many clinically significant isolates. The presence of a *Mycobacterium* species is usually evident from the full acid-fastness, the absence of filamentous bacilli, and the associated clinical condition (see Chapter 19).

A different diagnostic flowchart, based on growth in lysozyme, is provided by Brown and McNeil,[10] while Kiska and colleagues have presented a simplified battery of tests for the identification of *Nocardia* spp.[43] The terms defined in Box 15-1 are used in differentiating these bacteria.

The aerobic actinomycetes are widely distributed in nature, where they participate in the decomposition of organic plant material.[33,80] Isolates of various species are made regularly from soil and marine sediments, as well as from the feces of a variety of animals. They should be considered opportunistic pathogens, causing infection primarily in individuals whose defense mechanisms have been compromised. In addition, however, these bacteria have provided some of our most important antibiotics: streptomycin (*Streptomyces* spp.), vancomycin (*Amycolatopsis orientalis*), macrolides (*Micromonospora* spp.), and aminoglycosides (*Micromonospora* spp.). By far the most important pathogens are in the genus *Nocardia*, which will be considered in detail. Other genera will be discussed more briefly.

From a practical standpoint these organisms can be recognized in the laboratory because they form glabrous, tough, adherent, waxy, or dry chalky colonies that grow after 3 days to 2 weeks of incubation. Tan, pink, orange, or gray

pigments may be observed. The odor of a musty basement or freshly turned soil is an important clue by which they can be recognized. The optimal temperature for growth is 30 to 36°C, both in the CO_2 incubator (as for the culture of mycobacteria) or in ambient air (as in the incubator used for fungal cultures). They grow well on culture media such as Lowenstein-Jensen egg-based medium or Middlebrook synthetic agar and on most fungal recovery media that are free of cycloheximide. Most routine bacterial cultures are retained for only 48 hours, so isolates are often made in the mycobacteriology or mycology laboratory.

All species are gram-positive, although *Nocardia* spp., in particular, tend to stain with a beaded, gram-variable pattern. Thus, the finding of gram-positive or gram-variable, beaded, delicate (1 μm in diameter), branching organisms should alert one to the possibility of an aerobic actinomycete; isolation plates should be held for 2 to 4 weeks to ensure recovery. The practical characteristics by which *Nocardia* spp. are most commonly separated from *Mycobacterium* species in clinical laboratories are the branching of the bacterial cells, their "partial" acid-fastness (acid-fast reaction only when a low-concentration, inorganic acid instead of acid alcohol is used as the decolorizer) and the detection of a musty odor produced by the mature colonies. These properties are variable, however, and not always reliable. In problem cases, analysis of the cell wall or genome is required, but these techniques are unfortunately available only in reference laboratories at this point.[17,67,80] The cell wall composition of the aerobic actinomycetes, useful both taxonomically and diagnostically, is detailed in Table 15-2.

The Nocardioform Group
Nocardia

The taxonomy of *Nocardia*, the most important genus among the aerobic actinomycetes, is as confused (and confusing) as that of the group as a whole. The original isolate from infected animals with granulomatous disease (bovine farcy) was made by Nocard in 1888 on Guadeloupe Island. It was subsequently named *Nocardia farcinica*, and this isolate was made the type species of the genus. It is instructive to note that the original isolate consisted of two strains that were thought to be identical. In actuality one of the strains has mycolic acids characteristic of nocardiae, while the mycolic acids of the other are more typical of mycobacteria.[51]

The most important member of the genus is *Nocardia asteroides*, which was isolated from a human infection shortly after Nocard's original isolate. *N. asteroides* is once again taxonomically diverse, and it is often described as the *N. asteroides* complex.[78] Several named members of the complex, *N. farcinica*, *N. nova*, and *N. abscessus*, have been separated from the group; they are sometimes described as subgroups of *N. asteroides*.[58,80] The separation of *N. farcinica* and *N. nova*, originally controversial, was validated by the recognition that they have a markedly different profile of antimicrobial susceptibility from *N. asteroides*.[58] These differences in antimicrobial susceptibility have practical clinical significance, as well as taxonomic import. Some ex-

---

Box 15-1 Terms Used to Differentiate Aerobic Actinomycetes

Substrate mycelium: This refers to the cells that grow on and then into the surface of the medium. These organisms characteristically form branching cells ("hyphae") that grow together to form tough, leathery colonies. This growth may also be called the vegetative mycelium.

Fragmentation: The substrate mycelia of these organisms are generally composed of chains of long bacilli that, on growth and aging, start to "break up" into individual bacilli-shaped (bacillary) and coccus-shaped (coccoid) cells.

Aerial hyphae: Some species actually produce cells that grow upright and away from the agar surface. More mature aerial hyphae will be found in the center of the colony, with more rudimentary aerial hyphae being found on the periphery of the colony. On aging, the aerial hyphae fragment into coccoid "spores," giving older colonies a velvety or powdery appearance. For one species (*Dermatophilus congoliensis*), the spores that are produced on the aerial mycelium are motile.

Table 15-2 Cell Wall Composition of Aerobic Actinomycetes

CELL WALL CHEMOTYPE[a]	COMPOSITION	GENERA
I	l-DAP and no diagnostic sugars	Streptomyces
III	meso-DAP and no diagnostic sugars	Thermoactinomyces, Nocardiopsis
III	meso-DAP and madurose	Dermatophilus, Actinomadura
IV	meso-DAP, arabinose, and galactose	Faenia (Micropolyspora), Nocardia,[b] Rhodococcus,[b] Gordonia,[b] Tsukamurella,[b] Dietzia,[b] Saccaromonospora, Saccaropolyspora, Mycobacterium
VI	No DAP, aspartic acid and galactose (variable)	Oerskovia
NA	No DAP and madurose	Actinomadura
NA	Information not available	Tropheryma

[a] Cell walls of all genera contain major amounts of alanine, glutamic acid, glucosamine, and muramic acid. No major human pathogens have the characteristics of type I, V, VII, or VIII cell walls. For more details see references[10, 30, 50, 58].
[b] Nocardomycolic acid present.
NA, not applicable.
Data from reference[101].

perts suggest that patients should not be treated with cephalosporins, to which *N. farcinica* is resistant, until susceptibility testing has been performed.

Initially Steingrube and associates defined four separate unnamed groups, designated type I, type II, type IV, and type VI.[88] They used DNA amplification and restriction-fragment-length polymorphism (RFLP) to characterize products derived from the 65-kDa heat-shock protein gene of strains. The various groups show differences in antimicrobial susceptibility profiles. The type IV and *N. transvalensis* isolates studied were resistant to aminoglycosides. All but types II and IV have been named. Strains that match the classical description may be designated *Nocardia asteroides sensu stricto* type VI (referred to hereafter as *N. asteroides*). It should be noted that ''type VI'' in this context refers to the antimicrobial susceptibility profile, not to the components of the cell wall. It has been proposed that the isolates with a type VI susceptibility pattern should

be named *N. cyriacigeorgica*.[78] The antimicrobial susceptibility profiles of the members of the *Nocardia asteroides* complex are detailed in Table 15-3, which includes current nomenclature. Many early reports did not distinguish these pathogens.

Many cases of invasive infection that were attributed to *N. brasiliensis* are now ascribed to a related species, *N. pseudobrasiliensis*.[79,98] Other species that are pathogenic for or have been isolated from humans include *N. otitidiscaviarum*,[1,14,16,69] *N. transvalensis*,[28,59] *N. africana*,[37] *N. veterana*,[18,71] *N. paucivorans*,[23,109] *N. brevicatena*,[78] *N. arthritidis*,[41] *N. cyriacigeorgici*,[112] *N. abscessus*,[111] *N. punis*,[113] and possibly other named and unnamed species.[43]

EPIDEMIOLOGY, PATHOLOGY, AND PATHOGENESIS

N. asteroides, which is the most frequently isolated pathogen, is distributed widely throughout the United States.[80] *N. farcinica*, which is less prevalent, is also widely distributed throughout the country. *N. nova* appears to be less common in southwestern states.

N. brasiliensis is a common cause of subcutaneous infections and mycetoma in South America, much of Latin America, and Mexico. In the 1960s, 85–95% of reported mycetomas in Mexico were caused by *N. brasiliensis*.[29] Castro and associates noted that *N. brasiliensis* was by far the most common actinomycete isolated from 41 patients seen in Sao Paulo, Brazil, between 1978 and 1989.[13] Most patients were from rural areas in the northeast regions of the country, and the majority were field laborers. Significant infection of skin and soft tissues with *N. brasiliensis* was also found in patients from Queensland, Australia, who had nocardiosis.[28] Although primarily found in tropical countries, *N. brasiliensis* is, nonetheless, the second most common isolate in the United States, where it is most prevalent in southwestern and southeastern states.[84]

N. otitidiscaviarum (formerly *N. caviae*) has been isolated from soil widely throughout the world. The distribution of other rarely isolated species is less clear. It has been estimated that 500 to 1,000 cases of nocardiosis occur in the United States each year,[5] but that figure is likely to be an underestimate.[4]

Nocardiae are opportunistic pathogens, producing infections in patients who are immunocompromised or have debilitating diseases. A combination of long-term corticosteroid therapy and chronic lung disease has been suggested as a particularly important combination of risks.[80] Approximately 10% of patients with nocardiosis have no demonstrable underlying defect. Significantly, nocardiae may colonize the skin and respiratory tract. In one Australian study 20% of isolates were not associated with clinical disease.[28] Even the recovery of *Nocardia* species from blood cultures may not be significant. Of eight patients with *Nocardia* bacteremia reported by Esteban and associates, *N. asteroides* was thought to be clinically relevant in only two; the remaining isolates were considered insignificant or of uncertain significance.[24] All patients were cured. These authors conclude that *Nocardia* spp. may be a contaminant and the significance of any given isolate remains a matter of clinical judgment.

Table 15-3 Antimicrobial Susceptibility Profiles of 78 Isolates of the *Nocardia asteroides* Complex

TYPE	% ISOLATES	SUSCEPTIBLE	RESISTANT	SPECIES CORRELATION
I	20	Ampicillin, carbenicillin, broad-spectrum cephalosporins, imipenem (50%)	Imipenem (50%)	*Nocardia abscessus*
II	0	Same as type I, but kanamycin- and ciprofloxacin-susceptible		
III	18	Ampicillin, erythromycin	Carbenicillin	*Nocardia nova*
IV	5	Ciprofloxacin	All aminoglycosides, including amikacin	
V	17	Ciprofloxacin, imipenem	All penicillins and broad-spectrum cephalosporins, all aminoglycosides except amikacin	*Nocardia farcinica*
VI	35	Broad-spectrum cephalosporins	Penicillins	*Nocardia asteroides sensu stricto*, *Nocardia cyriacigeorgica*

The most serious form of nocardiosis is chronic pulmonary infection, with or without dissemination to other organs. The pathogenesis of infection with the *Nocardia* asteroides complex is probably inhalation of airborne bacteria, which perhaps explains the frequency of infection in the dry southwestern states, analogous to *Coccidioides immitis*.[80] Cutaneous disease, including actinomycotic mycetoma, probably results from direct introduction of bacteria after trauma, including walking barefoot.[80] Although most infections are acquired from the environment, nosocomial acquisition has been described.[103]

Nocardia spp. are facultative intracellular pathogens. Their ability to grow in macrophages and probably also polymorphonuclear neutrophils is undoubtedly important for their ability to produce infection. The organisms are capable of living inside macrophages by inhibiting phagosome-lysosome fusion and by their ability to produce catalase and superoxide dismutase, which inactivate the myeloperoxidase system of these phagocytic cells. Patients with chronic granulomatous disease are at risk of serious nocardial infection, as they are for other bacteria that produce catalase.[20] The cellular immune response is critical for control of the infection, as suggested by experimental studies and the occurrence of disease in patients with compromise of cellular immunity.[4] Some clinicians have expressed the opinion that nocardial infection is underrepresented in patients who are infected with human immunodeficiency virus (HIV). Beaman, however, notes the accumulating number of case reports and unreported infections, and that the geographic variations in environmental nocardiae, which do not match

centers of HIV infection, may partially explain the discrepancy.[4] A similar situation probably obtains with *Legionella pneumophila*, another pathogen for which cell-mediated immunity is critical. In both cases a susceptible population of patients must be in proximity to environmental sites that harbor the bacteria (see Chapter 10).

The bacterial cells of *Nocardia* spp. are not usually seen in hematoxylin and eosin–stained sections, and may not be seen in periodic acid–Schiff stains. They are quite readily observed in Gomori methenamine–silver, Gram-Weigert, Giemsa, or tissue Gram stains (e.g., Brown and Brenn, or Brown-Hopps stains). In a tissue Gram stain, the organisms are usually thin, beaded, branched filamentous rods. The modified Kinyoun acid-fast stain (in which destaining is done with 1% aqueous H_2SO_4 instead of the usual acid alcohol that is used in the Ziehl-Neelsen method) is useful for direct smears and frozen sections, whereas the Fite-Ferraco acid-fast stain is recommended for paraffin sections.[45,106,107] With these stains, *Nocardia* spp. are acid-fast (or "partially acid-fast"), *Mycobacterium* spp. are strongly acid-fast, whereas *Actinomyces israelii* and the other anaerobic actinomycetes are not acid-fast.

CLINICAL DISEASE

The clinical disease produced by all species of the genus, termed nocardiosis, is similar. Visceral infection is an acute, subacute, or chronic disease, which usually begins in the respiratory tract.[58] Manifestations include fever, a cough productive of mucopurulent sputum, and nonresolving infiltrates of varying appearance on chest radiographs. There may be progressive bronchopneumonia, localized or diffuse infiltrates, extensive consolidation, single or multiple abscesses, pleural effusions, empyema, and sinus tracts with involvement of the chest wall. Granuloma formation and presence of giant cells has been described with *Nocardia* spp., but in our experience granulomas are not typical of pulmonary involvement with these bacteria.

Disseminated infection usually originates from a pulmonary focus, but it may also occur after a primary cutaneous infection. Bacteremic spread results in multiorgan infection, especially in the brain and skin.[19] Approximately 45% of patients with disseminated nocardiosis have infections of the central nervous system.[54] The prognosis is poor with a fatality rate of 7–44% overall and up to 85% in severely immunosuppressed patients.[58] Serious infection with *Nocardia* spp. has been documented in patients who have neoplastic disease[94] or acquired immunodeficiency syndrome[40] and in recipients of renal transplants,[104] among others. Metastatic brain abscesses, which develop in about one third of patients, produce headaches, changing mental status, seizures, focal neurologic deficits, or other neurologic abnormalities. Blood cultures (in spite of hematogenous spread of the organism) and CSF cultures almost invariably fail to demonstrate the bacteria.

Cutaneous infections are probably underdiagnosed because they are often self-limited and adequate microbiologic studies may not be done on superficial infections.[54] Pustules, abscesses, cellulitis, and paronychia may all result from traumatic introduction of nocardiae into the skin. The inflammation resembles that seen in other bacterial infections, except that it tends to be more indolent. When the process extends to the regional lymph nodes, it may resemble sporotrichosis, referred to as sporotrichoid nocardiosis.[83] If the bacteria are introduced into the eye by penetrating trauma, keratitis or endophthalmitis may result.

A classic cutaneous lesion, mycetoma, may be caused by true fungi (eumycotic mycetoma) or by aerobic actinomycetes (actinomycotic mycetoma). (See discussion in the section on ''*Actinomadura*,'' below.)

Although the disease produced by various species is similar, there are distinguishing features. Members of the *N. asteroides* complex produce pulmonary and disseminated disease, but *N. farcinica* is particularly likely to disseminate and *N. nova* does so rather rarely.[58] *N. brasiliensis* produces cutaneous infections most often, whereas the more recently delineated *N. pseudobrasiliensis* tends to produce disseminated disease. Clinical information on other nocardial species is less extensive.

Rhodococcus

Rhodococcus equi is the most important human pathogen in the genus. The other human pathogens, *R. erythropolis*, *R. rhodnii*, and *R. rhodochrous* are rarely recovered from clinical specimens. *R. equi* was previously known as *Corynebacterium equi*. It has also been called ''*Mycobacterium rhodochrous*'' and has been referred to as the ''rhodochrous'' complex.[32]

EPIDEMIOLOGY, PATHOLOGY, AND PATHOGENESIS

R. equi is the cause of pulmonary disease in foals and other domestic animals.[72] Between 1967 and the early 1980s, only a handful of human infections were reported. Human infections are believed to result from contact with animal carriers (e.g., cattle, pig, horses, or cattle manure), presumably by a respiratory route.[97] Rhodococci are widely distributed in soil, perhaps accounting for infection in persons who do not recall contact with animals. Takai and associates noted the association of virulent rhodococci in the soil of a horse-breeding farm with clinical disease in foals on that farm, in contrast to another farm that lacked equine disease and had fewer isolates from soil.[92]

Human infections most commonly occur in immunocompromised individuals, primarily those with defects in cell-mediated immunity—e.g., patients with lymphoma, Hodgkin's disease, leukemia, or acquired immune deficiency syndrome (AIDS), and following transplantation.[9,55,97] McNeil and Brown cite over 100 cases of *R. equi* infections in patients with AIDS.[58]

The histopathology of *Rhodococcus* infection resembles that of *Nocardia* spp. There is chronic inflammation (primarily of macrophages) and fibrosis, interspersed with microabscesses.[58] Well-formed caseating granulomas, as seen in tuberculosis, are not typically present. Malacoplakia, a distinctive histologic reaction in which laminated basophilic concretions (Michaelis-Gutmann bodies) are found amid the macrophages, has been described in cases of pulmonary *Rhodococcus equi* infection.[35]

CLINICAL DISEASE

Pulmonary infections may mimic tuberculosis, become slowly progressive, and cavitate.[48,81,97] Invasive pneumonia with cavity formation is noted particularly in patients with AIDS, in whom there is a high propensity for the infection to disseminate to the brain, liver, spleen, and other organs.[58] Other forms of infection include endophthalmitis, osteomyelitis, pleurisy with effusion, and wound infection.

Other Nocardioform Bacteria

Gordonia spp. (originally *Gordona* spp.) consists of species that were once classified in the genus *Rhodococcus*. Members of this genus are difficult to identify and to separate from one another and from related genera, so evaluation of the clinical literature is difficult.[10] *Gordonia aurantiaca* (formerly *R. aurantiacus*) has been isolated from the sputum of patients with chronic pulmonary disease,[96] from the cerebrospinal fluid (CSF) of a patient with hairy-cell leukemia, and from a severe gangrenous tenosynovitis lesion with multiple subcutaneous abscesses in a woman with de Quervain disease.[95]

Tsukamurella spp. were first described in Japan as agents of chronic pulmonary disease that resembled tuberculosis.[10] Infections have been reported rarely as opportunistic disease in patients who are immunocompromised or have foreign bodies.

Dietzia spp. were defined more frequently. The type species, *D. maris* (formerly *Rhodococcus maris*) has been isolated from the bloodstream of an immunosuppressed patient who had an indwelling intravascular catheter.[7]

The Maduromycetes and Thermomonosporas
Actinomadura

The genus *Actinomadura* is genetically diverse, falling into two suprageneric groups.[30,58] Once again the terminology is confusing and in transition. Goodfellow suggests that *Actinomadura* spp. should be reserved for *A. madurae* and related species (including *A. pelletieri*), which are genetically most closely related to the *Thermomonospora* group.[31] In contrast, "maduromycetes" is reserved for a natural group of bacteria that includes *A. pusilla* and related organisms.[31] From a practical standpoint, the major human pathogens, *A. madurae* and *A. pelletieri* fall into the former group. Members of the genus *Actinomadura* contain *meso*-DAP in their cell walls (cell wall type IIIB; madurose is a major carbohydrate component).[31]

EPIDEMIOLOGY

Actinomadura spp. are soil organisms that are introduced through the skin by trauma, which may be minor. The infections are found primarily in tropical and subtropical countries, which may, in part, reflect the greater propensity for people who live in warmer climes to walk barefoot.[58]

CLINICAL DISEASE AND PATHOLOGY

Mycetomas are chronic, penetrating, progressively destructive lesions that destroy skin, subcutaneous tissue, and underlying structures, such as bone, muscle, and fascia. Not surprisingly for infections caused by soil organisms, they tend to occur on the extremities, with the foot being a particularly common site. The chronic, granulomatous inflammation often results in multiple draining sinuses, from which granules (or grains) are extruded. Bone is commonly involved. These granules, which usually measure less than 1

mm in diameter, represent colonies of the infectious agent. They vary in color depending on the nature of the infecting agent—e.g., white grain mycetoma.[54] Microscopically, granules consist of masses of filamentous bacteria or hyphae embedded in a cementlike matrix, which imparts the color that is seen macroscopically. An immunologic reaction, known as the Splendore-Hoeppli phenomenon, may be present. Fibrosis is often the end result of mycetoma, although not to the extent seen in actinomycosis caused by *Actinomyces israelii* (see Chapters 14 and 16).

Mycetomas are caused by true fungi (eumycotic mycetoma) and by aerobic actinomycetes (actinomycotic mycetoma). Colloquially, actinomycotic mycetoma is sometimes called "Madura foot." The most common etiologic agents and their associated granules are summarized in Table 15-4. In a study of 366 isolates of aerobic actinomycetes from mycetomas submitted to the Centers for Disease Control (now, the Centers for Disease Control and Prevention [CDC]) in the late 1980s, *A. madurae* was second in incidence only to *N. asteroides* (11.5% vs. 26%).[60] Most infections occur in tropical countries, particularly in India and Tunisia (*A. madurae*) or in Senegal, Chad, and Somalia (*A. pelletieri*). As noted above, *Nocardia asteroides* causes infections worldwide, whereas *N. brasiliensis* is limited to South America, Central America, and Mexico. Twenty-three of 28 culture-proven cases of actinomycotic mycetoma in the United States were from southern and western states, including 11 from Texas, and 3 each from California and Florida.[93]

Although the vast majority of *A. madurae* infections are superficial, systemic infections have been reported in patients with compromised host defenses. A case of *A. madurae* peritonitis in a patient undergoing continuous peritoneal dialysis has been recorded.[108] Disseminated *A. madurae* infection occurred in a patient with AIDS who was also a habitual user of heroin.[62]

Nocardiopsis

Nocardiopsis dassonvillei, the most important species in the genus, forms zigzag chains of spores within a

---

Table 15-4 Etiologic Agents of Mycetomas

WHITE GRAIN MYCETOMA (EUMYCOTIC)	BLACK GRAIN MYCETOMA (EUMYCOTIC)	WHITE/YELLOW GRAIN MYCETOMAS (ACTINOMYCOTIC)	BROWN/RED GRAIN MYCETOMAS (ACTINOMYCOTIC)
Acremonium spp.	*Curvularia* spp.	*Actinomadura madurae*	*Actinomadura pelletieri*
Aspergillus spp.	*Exophiala jeanselmei*	*Nocardia asteroides*	*Streptomyces somaliensis*
Corynespora cassicola	*Leptosphaeris* spp.	*Nocardia brasiliensis*	
Fusarium spp.	*Madurella* spp.		
Neotestudina rosatii	*Phialophora cyanescens*		
Pseudallescheria boydii	*Plenodomas arramii*		
Pseudochaetoapheronema larense	*Pyrenochaeta* spp.		

Adapted from reference[15].

sheathlike structure and has a type III cell wall (*meso*-DAP) with no diagnostic sugars. The genus *Nocardiopsis* was split off from the genus *Actinomadura* to accommodate related organisms that lack the unique cell wall carbohydrate madurose. *N. dassonvillei*, ordinarily a soil saprophyte, has been recovered from animals and rarely from human infections, primarily mycetoma.[10] In 1997 Yassin and colleagues reported the isolation of a new species, *N. synnemataformans* from the sputum of a renal transplant recipient[110]; the role of this new species in human disease is unclear.

The Streptomycetes
Streptomyces

Streptomyces spp. are soil organisms that have considerable importance in the industrial and pharmaceutical fields. A few species that cause human infections have been isolated from sputum, other respiratory specimens, superficial wounds, skin, and other specimens. In a study of 366 aerobic actinomyces isolates from clinical mycetomas submitted for study at the CDC in the late 1980s, only *N. asteroides* and *A. madurae* were recovered more frequently than *Streptomyces* species.[60] *S. somaliensis*, which causes actinomycotic mycetoma, has virtually a worldwide distribution, having been recovered from cases of mycetoma in Saudi Arabia, Nigeria, Niger, Sudan, Somalia, South Africa, Venezuela, India, and Mexico.[58] A high proportion of these cases involved the head and neck, producing what is known as "Madura skull." As of 1981, streptomycetes had not been isolated from mycetomas in the United States.[93] Grains from streptomycete mycetomas are large (2 to 4 mm) and yellow-brown. *Streptomyces anulatus* (formerly *S. griseus*), an organism that causes subcutaneous mycetomas in felines and dolphin, also has been recovered from human mycetomas.

Thermophilic Actinomycetes

Thermophilic actinomycetes cause human disease, but they are rarely encountered in the clinical microbiology laboratory, because they produce allergic reactions rather than productive infections. In 1963 Pepys and colleagues defined the antigen present in moldy hay as *Saccharopolyspora rectivirgula*.[68] Subsequently, *Thermoactinomyces vulgaris* was recognized as an additional allergen. The clinical disease, farmer's lung, is an example of hypersensitivity pneumonitis or extrinsic allergic pneumonitis. The illness can be chronic and disabling, with deterioration of lung function until the offending antigen is removed or avoided. Other similar situations occur after exposure to moldy compost, sugar cane (bagassosis), air conditioners, or ventilation ducts.[10] Various members of the *Saccharopolyspora*, *Micropolyspora* (*Faenia*), and *Thermoactinomyces* genera are responsible. The taxonomy of these organisms has undergone multiple changes over the years.

Miscellaneous Actinomycetes
Oerskovia

The two most important species of *Oerskovia* are *O. turbata* and *O. xanthineolytica*. After some taxonomic controversy concerning the relationship of these organisms to the genus *Cellulomonas*, the genus *Oerskovia* has been reconstituted with *O. turbata* as the type species.[87] These bacteria were previously classified as CDC Coryneform Groups A-3 and A-4 (*O. turbata*) and A-1 and A-2 (*O. xanthineolytica*).[86] They are aerobic, gram-positive bacilli that are found in the soil. Sottnek and coauthors described the characteristics of 57 clinical isolates, belonging to the genus *Oerskovia*, that had been referred to the CDC from hospital and public health laboratories throughout the country.[86] Five of these isolates were from heart valves or cardiac isolates, nine were from blood, one was from the CSF, and the remainder were from sites such as urine, traumatic and surgical wounds, eye drainage, pleural fluids, and pilonidal cysts. *Oerskovia* spp. have caused nosocomial infection after contamination of home parenteral nutrition fluids[36] and have been responsible for bacterial endocarditis,[76] catheter-associated bacteremia,[53] infection of prosthetic joints,[38] and peritoneal dialysis infection.[77]

Dermatophilus

Dermatophilus congolensis is an interesting actinomycete that causes a pustular, exudative dermatitis known as dermatophilosis (also called foot rot, pitted keratolysis, or streptotrichosis) in many species of animals (including cattle, sheep, horses, goats, deer, swine, squirrels, and domestic cats). It infrequently produces disease in humans. The exact mode of transmission is unknown, although most infections occur following direct contact with infected materials, and possibly from the bites of ectoparasites and flying insects. Occupations and avocations that appear at particular risk are primarily those that involve extensive contact with animals, such as veterinarians, abattoir workers, and hunters.[10] Pathologists may encounter these organisms within hair follicles or keratin layers of the soles of the feet in the forms of masses of non-acid-fast, branching, septate filaments.

Tropheryma whipplei
HISTORY AND TAXONOMY

This bacterium is the latest addition to the aerobic actinomycetes, but the associated disease, intestinal lipodystrophy (Whipple's disease), was first described in 1907 by George Whipple. Bacteria had been identified in affected tissues by light and electron microscopy, but the nature of the etiologic agent remained a mystery until 1991, when Wilson and colleagues used nucleic acid amplification and sequencing of 16S RNA in a duodenal biopsy from a patient with Whipple's disease to delineate the nature of the etiologic agent.[57] The morphologic appearance of the bacteria in tissue was not considered typical for either gram-positive or gram-negative bacilli, perhaps because of the intracellular location of the organisms.[57] By molecular analysis, however, the organism fits into the gram-positive family—most closely related to

Rothia,[57] *Rhodococcus, Arthrobacter,* and *Streptomyces,* less closely related to the mycobacteria.[105] Less than a decade later the bacterium was cultivated in human fibroblasts[74] and named *Tropheryma whipplei* (an emended designation from the original *T. whippelii*).[46] The genome of *T. whipplei* has now been sequenced completely, providing useful insights into its nature.[8] It has a surprisingly small genome, demonstrating characteristics of other intracellular bacteria that require external amino acids and are deficient in energy metabolism. The amount of genetic material devoted to coding surface structures is, nonetheless, relatively large, suggesting that interactions between the outside of the bacteria and the host are critical to its survival. Finally, there is considerable genetic variability (including phase variation), which may be advantageous for adapting to changing intracellular environments.[8]

ECOLOGY

The place of *T. whipplei* in nature is unknown. It has been detected in human feces and in sewage, but it is unclear whether the nucleic acid was a source of infection for humans or a result of excretion by infected individuals.[57] Amplification of nucleic acid from human saliva[91] and gastric secretions[22] has been reported. It has been detected in duodenal biopsy specimens from patients who do not have Whipple's disease,[22] although other investigators have found DNA only rarely in the absence of clinical evidence of the disease.[56] It is possible, therefore, that humans are reservoirs for the bacteria, but the jury is still out. Potential problems with the specificity of amplification procedures and the presence of extraintestinal Whipple's disease without overt involvement of the bowel[34] complicate the analysis.

CLINICAL DISEASE AND PATHOLOGY

Whipple's disease is a rare, chronic, multisystem disease.[21,57] The classic triad of diarrhea, weight loss, and malabsorption reflects the frequency with which the gastrointestinal tract is affected. Other organ systems are also involved, particularly joints and the nervous system (Box 15-2). The heart may also be affected, and *T. whipplei* is a cause of culture-negative bacterial endocarditis.[25,34]

The pathogenesis of Whipple's disease is poorly understood. It is likely that defects in cellular immunity and/or

macrophage function are important, but they appear to be specific to this agent, as patients are not usually infected with other opportunistic pathogens.

T. whipplei is a facultative intracellular pathogen. As is true for other bacteria that fall into this category, the pathologic hallmark of infection is the macrophage. Foamy macrophages, which contain numerous bacteria within vacuoles, were responsible for the yellow lacteals that George Whipple observed in the small bowel. The bacteria in these cells can be stained by the periodic acid–Schiff method, but this technique is not specific. Other bacteria, particularly *Mycobacterium avium* complex and *Rhodococcus equi* can present a similar picture. Acid-fast stains can help with the differentiation, as *T. whipplei* is not acid-fast. Ultimately, immunologic staining of tissues, culture, or nucleic acid amplification is required for problem cases. In extraintestinal tissues noncaseating, sarcoidlike granulomas may be observed.[57]

Laboratory Diagnosis of Infections Caused by Aerobic Actinomycetes
Primary Isolation

N. asteroides and other aerobic actinomycetes are aerobic organisms that grow on a variety of bacteriologic media, including blood agar, brain-heart infusion agar, or Sabouraud's dextrose agar without antibiotics (they are inhibited by chloramphenicol, penicillin, and streptomycin), and on media designed for the recovery of mycobacteria. *N. asteroides* grows well at 25°C, at 35 to 37°C, and at 42 to 45°C. Incubation at the higher temperature permits growth of *N. asteroides*, whereas many other bacteria will be inhibited. Growth may take from 4 days to 6 weeks of incubation and is enhanced by incubation in 10% CO_2. Isolates are often made in the mycology or mycobacteriology laboratories, because the cultures have been incubated for a sufficiently long time.

Nocardia species can be recovered from contaminated specimens using modified Thayer-Martin (MTM) medium.[65] Shawar and associates took advantage of the peculiar ability to grow with paraffin as a sole source of carbon to develop a selective, chemically defined medium that contained paraffin (paraffin-baiting technique).[82] By this technique, a paraffin-coated glass rod is inserted into a carbon-free broth mixed with the sputum specimen. In positive cultures, growth appears on the rod just above the surface of the broth. Similarly, Ayyar and colleagues found paraffin agar an inexpensive selective medium for *Nocardia* spp, being superior to either MTM or the paraffin bait technique.[2]

Selective buffered charcoal yeast extract agar (BCYE, commonly used for the recovery of *Legionella* spp. from respiratory specimens) also facilitates the recovery of *Nocardia* spp. from sputum and other specimens that may be contaminated with mixed bacteria.[27,42] The use of selective BCYE agar, to which polymyxin B, anisomycin, and vancomycin have been added, and pretreatment of the specimen by an acid wash improved recovery of *Nocardia* spp. from 8% to 33% for the former and to 67% for the latter.[42]

N. asteroides survives the usual *N*-acetyl-L-cysteine digestion procedure (without NaOH) that is used for recov-

Box 15-2 Extraintestinal Sites of Whipple's Disease: An Analysis of 52 Cases[a]	
Extraintestinal Site	No. (%) of Cases
Joints	43 (83)
Nervous system	11 (21)
Skin and mucous membranes	9 (17)
Heart and blood vessels	9 (17)
Lung and pleura	7 (13)
Eye	5 (10)

[a] Multiple sites affected in some patients.

Adapted from reference[21].

ery of mycobacteria from sputum or bronchial washings.[64] It has been recommended that cultures of sputum and bronchial washings for isolation of *Nocardia* spp. be done both before and after the digestion procedure, although this approach doubles the work. Colonies on Löwenstein-Jensen (LJ) media often develop within 1 to 2 weeks. They may be similar in appearance to atypical mycobacteria (see Chapter 19). *Mycobacterium* spp., however, do not produce aerial hyphae and differ biochemically from nocardiae. The branched hyphae of *Nocardia* that may not always be seen in smears prepared from growth on solid media can sometimes be demonstrated from growth in broth cultures, whereas mycobacteria do not usually branch (even though the rods may be elongated). One noteworthy exception is *Mycobacterium fortuitum*, which has been observed to produce branching filaments in smears of pus and may produce filamentous colonies.

Differentiation of *Nocardia* From Other Genera of Aerobic Actinomycetes

Infections of humans with the genera *Streptomyces*, *Nocardiopsis*, *Rhodococcus*, *Actinomadura*, *Gordonia*, *Tsukamurella*, *Oerskovia*, and *Dermatophilus* appear to be rare in the United States, although good incidence data are lacking. Some differential characteristics that may aid in differentiating among and within genera of aerobic actinomycetes and other related bacteria are given in Tables 15-5 and 15-6. A brief glossary of terms used in the differentiation of actinomycetes is provided in Box 15-1.

The presence of *Nocardia* and *Streptomyces* spp. can be suspected on the basis of a few simple characteristics. The typical colonies of *Nocardia* and *Streptomyces* spp. are dry to chalky in consistency, usually heaped or folded, and range in color from yellow to gray-white (see Color Plate 15-1*A*). *Nocardia* spp. are commonly some shade of yellow, whereas *Streptomyces* spp. are most frequently gray-white. Both groups produce colonies with a pungent musty-basement odor (probably because your basement is a *Streptomyces* factory). The colonies of *Rhodococcus equi* lack the musty odor and often have a pink or salmon color on agar media (Color Plate 15-1*B*).

Typically, Gram's stain of material from a colony will show delicate, branching filaments no more than 1 μm in diameter (see Color Plate 15-1*C*). *Nocardia* spp. are partially acid-fast (i.e., they do not decolorize when treated with 1% H_2SO_4 or 3% HCl, but will decolorize when the more active acid-alcohol decolorizer used in the Ziehl-Neelsen or Kinyoun stains is applied) (Box 15-3). *Streptomyces* spp., in contrast, are not partially acid-fast. Acid-fastness may be enhanced by growing the organism on certain media, such as Middlebrook 7H11 agar or casein agar (see discussion of identification techniques below). If the unknown organism is not acid-fast, a report of ''non-acid-fast aerobic actinomycete'' can be made, but such a report should be delayed until adequate attempts to boost the acid-fastness have been made.

Rhodococcus spp. do not form the long filaments seen in isolates of *Nocardia* and *Streptomyces*. They are gram-positive bacilli that may cluster like Chinese characters, reflecting their former taxonomic home in the genus *Corynebacterium* (Color Plate 15-1*D*). Isolates are often partially acid-fast (Color Plate 1-*E*).

Growth in the presence of lysozyme is useful for identifying *Nocardia* spp. (see Table 15-5), particularly those strains that are not acid-fast. All *Nocardia* species are resistant to lysozyme and will grow in its presence within 5 to 20 days. A control tube of glycerol broth without lysozyme and both positive and negative controls should be performed with each test. The test is performed as outlined in Box 15-4.

The differential ability of the various nocardiae and related aerobic actinomyces, to hydrolyze casein, tyrosine, xanthine, and hypoxanthine is one of the mainstays of identification protocols in most clinical laboratories. The procedure is described in Chart 15-1, and the patterns of reaction are shown in Table 15-5. The differential plates are inoculated with the unknown organism for up to 3 weeks at 30°C and observed for hydrolysis (clearing of the medium around the colonies). An example of casein hydrolysis by a colony of *Streptomyces* spp. is shown in Figure 15-2. Differentiation of certain species cannot be accomplished solely with the analysis of hydrolysis. Characterization of the ability to decompose carbohydrates or use them as a sole carbon source may be necessary.[10,63] Differentiation of *Nocardia farcinica* from *N. asteroides* is facilitated by analysis of the temperature of growth,[12] by the ability to opacify Middlebrook 7H10 or 7H11 media (Table 15-5),[12,26,43] and by the antimicrobial susceptibility profile (see Table 15-10).[85] A polymerase chain reaction, in which a species-specific DNA sequence that is specific for *N. farcinica* is amplified, has been described.[11]

Mishra and colleagues have devised a key for more detailed differentiation of the nocardiae and the streptomycetes than is presented in Table 15-5.[63] Their differential table is particularly useful in that it lists percentages of strains positive for a large battery of biochemical tests, morphologic features, and various physiologic characteristics. More recently, Kiska and associates have suggested tests that are of particular use for differentiation of the *Nocardia* spp (Table 15-7).[43] They developed an effective algorithm that uses antimicrobial suscepitility patterns, citrate utilization, acetamide utilization, and assimilation of two sugars (inositol and adonitol).

For many laboratories the API 20C AUX strips (BioMeriéux, Hazelwood, MO) will provide an expeditious tool for identification of *Nocardia* spp. (Table 15-8).[43] In some cases supplemental tests may be required to resolve duplicate patterns of carbohydrate assimilation (Table 15-9).

If the results of these tests are equivocal, thin-layer chromatography may be helpful. Differences in the cell wall composition are used in some research laboratories or reference laboratories for taxonomic purposes. The primary constituents of the cell walls are summarized in Table 15-2 (see also, Figure 15-1). Most of the nocardioform organisms, including *Nocardia* and *Rhodococcus*, have a type IV cell wall composition (the significant constituents are *meso*-diaminopimelic acid [DAP], arabinose, and galactose, with mycolic acids present). *Streptomyces* species have type I cell walls (no L-DAP and no diagnostic carbohydrates). *Oerskovia* species have type VI cell walls (no DAP and no diagnostic carbohydrates). Other chemotaxonomic tests, in addition to determining cell wall type, include analyses of menaquinones, long-chain fatty acids, phospholipids, and mycolic acids. These studies are not practical, nor are they

Table 15-5 Biochemical and Physiologic Tests for the Identification of Selected Medically Important Aerobic Actinomycetes

ORGANISM	MODIFIED ACID-FAST	GROWTH IN LYSOZYME	OPACIFICATION OF MIDDLEBROOK	GROWTH AT 45°C IN 3 DAYS	DECOMPOSITION OF				UREASE	GELATIN HYDROLYSIS
					Casein	Tyrosine	Xanthine	Hypoxanthine		
Nocardia asteroides	+	+	−	V	−	−	−	−	+	−
Nocardia brasiliensis	+	+	−	−	+	+	−	+	+	+
Nocardia otitidiscaviarum (N. caviae)	+	+	−	V	−	−	+	+	+	−
Nocardia transvalensis	+	+	−	−	−	−	+	+	+	+
Nocardia farcinica	+	+	+	+	−	−	−	−	+	−
Nocardia nova	+	+	−	−	−	−	−	−	V	−
Nocardia pseudobrasiliensis	+	+	−	−	+	+	−	+		+
Rhodococcus equi	+	−	NA	NA	NA	−	−	−	NA	NA
Rhodococcus erythropolis	+	+	NA	NA	NA	−	−	−	NA	NA
Rhodococcus rhodnii	+	+	NA	NA	NA	+	−	−	NA	NA
Rhodococcus rhodochrous	+	−	NA	NA	NA	−	−	−	NA	NA
Gordonia bronchialis	+	+	NA	NA	−	−	−	−	NA	NA
Gordonia rubropertincta	+	−	NA	NA	NA	NA	NA	NA	NA	NA
Gordonia sputi	+	−	NA	NA	NA	NA	NA	NA	NA	NA
Gordonia terrae	+	−	NA	NA	NA	NA	NA	NA	NA	NA
Tsukamurella inchonensis	+	+	NA	NA	+	−	−	+	NA	NA
Tsukamurella paurometabola (Rhodococcus aurantiacus)	+	+	NA	NA	−	−	−	−	+	NA
Tsukamurella pulmonis	+	+	NA	NA	−	−	−	−	NA	NA
Tsukamurella strandjordae	+	+	NA	NA	−	−	−	+	NA	NA
Tsukamurella tyrosinosolvens	+	+	NA	NA	−	+	+	+	NA	+
Tsukamurella wratislaviensis	+	+	NA	NA	NA	+	+	+	NA	+
Dietzia (Rhodococcus) maris	−	−	NA	NA	NA	−	−	NA	+	NA
Dermatophilus spp.	NA	NA	NA	NA	+	+	−	NA	+	+
Oerskovia turbata	−	−	NA	−	+	−	−	−	+	+
Oerskovia xanthineolytica	−	−	NA	V	+	−	+	+	NA	NA
Actinomadura madurae	−	−	NA	NA	+	+	−	+	−	NA
Actinomadura pelletieri	−	−	NA	NA	+	+	−	+	−	+
Streptomyces somaliensis	−	−	NA	NA	+	+	−	−	−	+
Streptomyces griseus	−	−	NA	NA	+	+	+	+	V	+
Nocardiopsis dassonvillei	−	−	NA	NA	+	+	+	+	+	+

Table 15-5 Continued

ORGANISM	UTILIZATION AS A SOLE SOURCE OF CARBON OF										
	Adonitol (ribitol)	L-Arabinose	Citrate	i-Erythritol	D-Galactose	D-Glucose	i-Myoinositol	D-Mannitol	L-Rhamnose	D-Sorbitol	D-Trehalose
Nocardia asteroides	–	–	V	–	V	+	–	–	V	–	V
Nocardia brasiliensis	–	–	+	–	+	+	+	+	–	–	+
Nocardia otitidiscaviarum (N. caviae)	–	V	–	–	–	+	+	V	–	–	V
Nocardia transvalensis	V	–	+	V	V	V	V	V	–	V	+
Nocardia farcinica	–	–	–	+	–	+	–	–	+	–	–
Nocardia nova	–	–	–	–	–	+	+	–	–	–	V
Nocardia pseudobrasiliensis	–	–	+	–	+	+	+	+	–	–	+
Rhodococcus equi	NA	NA	–	NA	+	NA	–	–	V	–	NA
Rhodococcus erythropolis	NA	NA	+	NA	V	NA	+	+	–	+	NA
Rhodococcus rhodnii	NA	NA	V	NA	+	NA	–	+	–	–	NA
Rhodococcus rhodochrous	NA	NA	V	NA	V	NA	+	+	–	+	NA
Gordonia bronchialis	NA	NA	–	NA	–	NA	+	+	–	–	NA
Gordonia rubropertincta	NA	NA	+	NA	+	NA	–	+	–	+	NA
Gordonia sputi	NA	NA	–	NA	+	NA	–	+	–	+	NA
Gordonia terrae	NA	NA	+	NA	+	NA	–	+	+	+	NA
Tsukamurella inchonensis	NA	NA	+	NA	NA	NA	+	+	NA	+	NA
Tsukamurella paurometabola (Rhodococcus aurantiacus)	NA	NA	+	NA	NA	NA	–	–	NA	–	NA
Tsukamurella pulmonis	NA	NA	–	NA	NA	NA	–	+	NA	+	NA
Tsukamurella strandjordae	NA	NA	+	NA	NA	NA	+	+	NA	+	NA
Tsukamurella tyrosinosolvens	NA	NA	V	NA	NA	NA	+	+	NA	+	NA
Tsukamurella wratislaviensis	NA	NA	–	NA	NA	NA	+	+	NA	+	NA
Dietzia (Rhodococcus) maris	NA	NA	NA	NA	NA	NA	NA	NA	NA	NA	NA
Dermatophilus spp.	NA	NA	NA	NA	NA	NA	NA	NA	NA	NA	NA
Oerskovia turbata	NA	NA	–	NA	NA	NA	NA	NA	NA	NA	NA
Oerskovia xanthineolytica	NA	NA	NA	NA	NA	NA	NA	NA	NA	NA	NA
Actinomadura madurae	NA	NA	NA	NA	NA	NA	+	+	+	+	+
Actinomadura pelletieri	NA	NA	NA	NA	NA	NA	+	—	–	–	+
Streptomyces somaliensis	NA	NA	NA	NA	NA	NA	+	–	–	–	–
Streptomyces griseus	NA	NA	NA	NA	NA	NA	+	–	–	–	–
Nocardiopsis dassonvillei	NA	NA	NA	NA	NA	NA	+	–	+	+	+

+, positive; −, negative; V, variable; R, resistant; S, susceptible; NA, not available.

Table 15-6 Additional Differential Characteristics: *Nocardia*, Other Actinomycetes, and Related Genera That May Be Encountered in the Clinical Laboratory

GENUS	RELATION TO OXYGEN[a]	AERIAL MYCELIUM[b]	CONIDIA	BRANCHING FILAMENTS (MICROSCOPIC)	FRAGMENTATION OF MYCELIA IN OLDER[d] CULTURES	CATALASE	STRONGLY ACID-FAST[e]	BOTH PARTIALLY ACID-FAST[f] AND ARYLSULFATASE[g]- POSITIVE	MOTILITY[b]
Actinomadura	A	+	+	+	−	+	−	−	−
Actinomyces	OA, F, M	−	−	+	−	D[g]	−	−	−
Arcanobacterium	A, F	−	−	−	−	−	−	−	−
Bacterionema	A, F	−	−	+	−	+	−	−	−
Bifidobacterium	OA	−	−	+[c]	−	−	−	−	−
Corynebacterium	A, F	−	−	−	−	+	−	−	−
Dermatophilus	A, M	−	−	+	−[i]	+	−	−	+
Mycobacterium	A	−	−	+[c]	−	+	+	+	−
Nocardia	A	+	+	+	+	+	−	−	−
Nocardiopsis	A	+	+	+	D	+	−	−	−
Oerskovia	A, F	−	−	+	+	D	−	−	+
Propionibacterium	OA, F, M	−	−	+[c]	−	D	−	−	−
Rhodococcus	A	−	−	+	+	+	−	+	−
Rothia	A, M	−	−	+	+	+	−	−	−
Streptomyces	A	+	+	+	−	+	−	−	−

[a] Relation to oxygen: A, aerobic; F, facultative anaerobe; M, microaerophilic; OA, obligate anaerobe.

[b] Aerial mycelium: +, produced either persistently or transiently; −, not produced.

[c] Branching filaments (microscopic): The bifurcated cells ordinarily produced by *Bifidobacterium* are not considered to be true branches. Most strains of *Propionibacterium* isolated clinically do not branch; the occasional strains that branch might be confused with *Actinomyces* or *Arachnia*. Most clinically encountered *Mycobacterium* do not branch. However, *M. fortuitum*, a rapid grower, may form branching hyphae and resemble *Nocardia*.

[d] Fragmentation of mycelium in older cultures; the filaments tend to break up into short rod or coccoid elements. *Dermatophilus congolensis*, a skin parasite and agent of exudative dermatitis in animals (rarely in humans), forms mycelial filaments that divide both transversely and longitudinally to form packets of up to eight motile coccoid cells.

[e] *Mycobacterium* spp. are strongly acid-fast when stained with Ziehl-Neelsen, auramine-rhodamine, or modified Kinyoun stains. In contrast, *Nocardia* spp. and *Rhodococcus* spp. are only weakly or partially acid-fast and stain only with a modified acid-fast stain (see text).

[f] Partially acid fast: Positive only when a low concentration of inorganic acid (e.g., 1% sulfuric acid) is used instead of acid alcohol; staining of bacteria is often irregular with unstained segments.

[g] Arylsulfatase test (3 day). See Chapter 19.

[h] D, *Actinomyces viscosus* and two species of nonmedical importance, *A. howelii* and *A. hordeovulneris*, are the only species of *Actinomyces* that are catalase positive.

−, 90% or more of strains negative; +, 90% or more of strains are positive; D, 11–89% of strains are positive

Data from Sneath PHA, Mair NS, Sharpe ME, Holt G. Bergey's Manual of Systematic Bacteriology. Vol. 2. Baltimore: Williams & Wilkins, 1986; Buchanan RE, Gibbons NE.: Bergey's Manual of Determinative Bacteriology. Ed. 8. Baltimore: Williams & Wilkins, 1974; and Rippon JW. Medical Mycology. Ed. 2. Philadelphia: Saunders, 1982.

Box 15-3 Modified Acid-Fast Stain for *Nocardia* Species

1. Make a smear of the organism from growth media and heat-fix.
2. Flood the slide with Kinyoun carbolfuchsin for 5 minutes.
3. Pour off the excess stain.
4. Decolorized with a 1% aqueous solution of sulfuric acid.
5. Wash with tap water.
6. Counterstain with methylene blue for 1 minute.
7. Rinse with water and dry. Examine under oil-immersion optics.

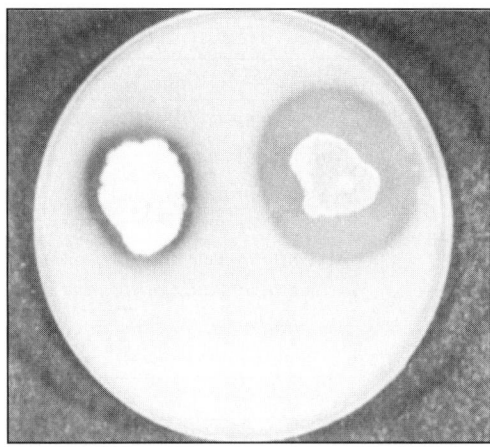

Figure 15-2 Casein agar plate illustrating the hydrolytic action of two species of *Streptomyces*.

necessary for differentiation of most isolates of *Nocardia* and *Rhodococcus* in the clinical microbiology laboratory. If definitive identification is necessary, microbiologists may wish to send isolates to a reference laboratory.

Increasingly, molecular amplification and sequencing procedures are useful both for direct detection of aerobic actinomycetes in clinical specimens and for identification of isolated bacteria.[6,47,49,67,70,90] Cloud and colleagues have suggested that sequencing of 16S ribosomal RNA is more accurate than a combination of conventional biochemical tests and antimicrobial susceptibility profiles for identification of *Nocardia* spp.[17] In the case of *Tropheryma whipplei*, molecular approaches are the primary diagnostic method. These techniques are currently used primarily in research or large reference laboratories; microbiologists must remain

alert to the future availability of commercial products. The issues are sufficiently complex that even some molecular analyses may not differentiate between certain species.[18]

Identification of Thermophilic Actinomycetes

The thermophilic actinomycetes are rarely encountered in the clinical laboratory because they are environmental organisms that produce disease in humans by an allergic reaction, rather than productive infection.[68] Their ability to grow at elevated temperatures provides a useful means by which to evaluate their presence in environmental specimens, if desired. Protocols for identification of these bacteria have been suggested.[39,44]

Identification of *Tropheryma whipplei*

This actinomycete can be cultured, but only with difficulty.[75] In most cases the diagnosis will be made by clinical and histologic criteria. Immunohistochemical identification of the organism in sectioned tissue has been recorded.[3,52,75] Alternatively, the organism can be recognized by nucleic acid amplification techniques.[73] Although experience is limited, it has been suggested that molecular amplification may be more useful than histology for monitoring the course of patients with Whipple's disease.[73] It is important to recognize that *T. whipplei* DNA can be detected in the absence of overt clinical disease.[22,91] The significance of these results is unclear, but the diagnosis of Whipple's disease should not be based solely on molecular detection of bacterial DNA.

In Vitro Susceptibility of *Nocardia* and Related Bacteria to Antimicrobial Agents and Therapy of Infections

The antimicrobial susceptibility patterns of aerobic actinomycetes are useful for taxonomists, clinical microbiologists (as a clue to the identification of an isolate), and clinicians for treatment of infected patients. The pattern of susceptibility is summarized in Table 15-10. Standardization of susceptibility testing for clinical use is a recent phenome-

Box 15-4 Lysozyme Test for the Identification of *Nocardia* Species

1. Prepare glycerol broth by adding 5 g of peptone and 70 mL of glycerol to 1,000 mL of distilled water (reduce amounts proportionately if smaller quantities are desired). Sterilize by autoclaving at 15 psi for 15 minutes.
2. Prepare lysozyme solution by dissolving 100 mg of lysozyme powder in 100 mL of 0.01 N HCl.
3. Combine 95 mL of glycerol broth with 5 mL of lysozyme solution and dispense in 5-mL aliquots into screw-capped tubes. Use 5-mL aliquots of glycerol broth without lysozyme for the growth control.
4. Prepare a light suspension of the unknown organism in sterile saline. Using a Pasteur pipette, inoculate 1 or 2 drops into the lysozyme and control tube (keep the inoculum light).
5. Incubate at 25°C. Examine each tube for growth in 7 to 14 days. Growth will appear as a pellicle on the surface, as a sediment, or as both. The tubes can be gently shaken to observe bread crumb–like particles in the tubes showing positive growth.
6. An organism resistant to lysozyme will grow in both the lysozyme tube and the control; an organism that is susceptible will grow only in the control tube.

Table 15-7 Key Tests for Differentiation Among *Nocardia* Species

ORGANISM	TEST OR CHARACTERISTIC
Nocardia nova	Positive for arylsulfatase
Nocardia farcinica	Opacification of Middlebrook agar
Nocardia brasiliensis and *Nocardia pseudobrasiliensis*	Liquefaction of gelatin
Nocardia transvalensis, Nocardia asteroides type IV, *Nocardia brevicatena*	API 20C yeast sugar assimilation pattern
Nocardia nova, Nocardia farcinica, Nocardia brevicatena	Susceptibility pattern to gentamicin, tobramycin, amikacin, and erythromycin

From reference[43].

non.[66] For laboratories that perform these tests rarely, it is judicious to send isolates to a reference laboratory that has considerable experience with aerobic actinomycetes.

Part of the resistance of *Nocardia* spp. may be mediated by β-lactamases. Those that have been characterized are primarily penicillinases with considerably less activity against cephalosporins. The enzymes found in *N. farcinica* are relatively homogeneous and are distinct from the enzymes found in other species.[89] In contrast, there is considerable diversity in the enzymes of *N. brasiliensis*, although the substrate profile is uniform.[99] The β-lactamases are inhibited by clavulanic acid, suggesting that combinations of penicillins and β-lactamase inhibitors (some of which can be administered orally) might be useful.[99] In one study (performed before the delineation of the components of the *N. asteroides* group) almost all isolates contained β-lactamases.[102] The best correlation between the presence of a β-lactamase and resistance to penicillins in vitro was the presence of extracellular enzyme in addition to cell-associated or cryptic β-lactamase. The clinical importance of enzymatic inactivation of penicillins is not clear.

The drugs of choice for treatment of nocardiosis, even in immunosuppressed patients, are still the sulfonamides (e.g., sulfadiazine, sulfisoxazole, and triple-sulfonamide combinations). The combination of trimethoprim and sulfamethoxazole (TMP-SMX) is preferred by most clinicians,[85] but the question of whether the combination is more effective than a sulfa drug alone remains open.[85,100] In vitro studies may be needed to aid in the selection of antimicrobial agents for patients who are hypersensitive to sulfonamides or who are infected with *N. otitidiscaviarum*, which demonstrates inconsistent susceptibility to sulfonamides. Imipenem, minocycline, and amikacin are potential choices, based on in vitro studies and limited clinical trials. Alternatively, desensitization to sulfonamides may be considered.[85] For mycetomas, a combination of surgical and pharmacologic approaches is indicated.

The recommended therapy for Whipple's disease is prolonged (at least 1 year) treatment with trimethoprim-sulfamethoxazole.[57] Tetracycline therapy, previously used commonly, is associated with an unacceptably high frequency of relapses. Especially in seriously ill patients, an initial course of parenteral therapy with ceftriaxone or a combination of penicillin and streptomycin is administered before long-term oral trimethoprim-sulfamethoxazole therapy is begun.[57]

Rhodococcus equi is susceptible to vancomycin, which is considered the therapy of choice, and most isolates are susceptible to erythromycin, aminoglycosides, rifampin, and chloramphenicol.[85] Experience with treatment is very lim-

Table 15-8 Use of API 20C AUX Strips for Identification of *Nocardia* Species[a]

SPECIES (NO. OF STRAINS)	GLUCOSE	GLYCINE	GALACTOSE	N-ACETYLGLUCOSAMINE	INOSITOL	ADONITOL	TREHALOSE
N. asteroides type I (8)	+	+	−	+ (63)	−	−	−
N. asteroides type IV (1)	+	+	+	−	−	−	+
N. asteroides type VI (10)	+	+ (90)	−	− (90)	−	−	− (80)
N. farcinica (16)	+	+[w]	+[w] (63)	−	−	−	− (94)
N. nova (19)	+	−	−	−	−	−	−
N. brasiliensis (6)	+	+	+	+	+	−	+
N. pseudobrasiliensis (5)	+	+	+	+	+	−	+
N. otitidiscaviarum (8)	+	+	− (75)	+	+	−	+ (50)
N. transvalensis	+	+	+	+	−	+	+ (90)[c]

[a] Assimilation tests incubated for 4 to 7 days at 35°C. Numbers in parentheses indicate the percentage of strains with the indicated reaction.
w, weak reactions may be observed; c, result based on reported clinical strains.
Adapted from Reference[43].

Table 15-9 Supplemental Tests Required to Resolve Patterns Carbohydrate Utilization by *Nocardia* Species Using API 20C AUX[a]

SPECIES 1	SPECIES 2	SUSCEPTIBILITY PATTERN[b]	ARYLSULFATASE (7 DAYS)	GELATIN (7 DAYS)	ACETAMIDE (3 DAYS)	OPACIFICATION OF 7H11	YELLOW COLONIES ON MUELLER–HINTON AGAR
N. nova	*N. asteroides* type VI	SSSS, SRSS, or RRSS / SSSR	+ (89)		−	−	
	N. farcinica	RRSS or RRSR	−		+	+	
N. farcinica	*N. asteroides* type IV	RRSS or RRSR	−		+	+	
	N. asteroides type IV	RRSR, SRSR, RRRR, or SRRR			−	−	
	N. asteroides type I	SSSR or SRSR				−	
	N. asteroides type VI	SSSR				−	
N. otitidiscaviarum	*N. brasiliensis*			−			−
				+ (83)			+
	N. pseudobrasiliensis			+			+

[a] Any one or more of the differentiating characteristics may be used. Numbers in parentheses indicate the percentage of strains with the indicated reaction.
[b] Disk diffusion (Kirby-Bauer) susceptibility tests performed at 35°C; antibiotics in order are gentamicin, tobramycin, amikacin, and erythromycin.
Adapted from reference[43].

Table 15-10 In Vitro Antimicrobial Susceptibility Profiles of Aerobic Actinomycetes (% Susceptible)

ORGANISM	SULFAME-THOXAZOLE	ERYTHRO-MYCIN	MINO-CYCLINE	DOXY-CYCLINE	CIPRO-FLOXACIN	GENTA-MICIN	KANA-MYCIN	AMIKA-CIN	AMPI-CILLIN	AMOXICILLIN-CLAVULANATE	CEFO-TAXIME	CEFTRIA-XONE	IMIPENEM
Nocardia asteroides complex (all types)	91–100[a]	22–35[a]	94–100[a]	NA	29–50[a]	67[b]	55[b]	95[b]	18–40[a]	41–58[a]	79–82[a]	79–82[a]	71–100[a]
Nocardia asteroides sensu stricto type VI	96–99[a]	23–93[a]	78–94[a]	48–88[a]	38–98[a]	NA	NA	100[a]	40–93[a]	53–67[a]	94–100[a]	94–100[a]	77–98[a]
Nocardia farcinica	89–100[a]	0–3[a]	20–96[a]	0–14[a]	68–88[a]	0[d]	0[d]	100[a,d]	0–5[a]	47–71[a]	0–7[a]	0–73[a]	64–87[a]
Nocardia nova	89–97[a]	100[a]	89–100[a]	19–94[a]	0[a]	NA	NA	100[a]	100[a]	3–6[a]	87–100[a]	100[a]	100[a]
N. transvalensis	90[a]	50[a]	54[a]	36[e]	60[a]	NA	NA	28[a]	10[a]	30[a]	50[a]	50[a]	90[a]
N. otitidiscaviarum	V[a]	NA	S[a]	NA	R[a]	NA	NA	S[a]	NA	R[a]	R[a]	R[a]	R[a]
Rhodococcus equi	NA	97[c]	NA	NA	82[c]	100[c]	NA	NA	32[c]	100[c]	NA	NA	100[c]
Actinomadura madurae	84[d]	93[d]	90[d]	93[d]	97[d]	NA	NA	NA	37[d]	81[d]	90[d]	100[d]	100[d]
Streptomyces anulatus (griseus)	57[d]	86[d]	90[d]	81[d]	43[d]	NA	NA	NA	20[d]	57[d]	48[d]	80[d]	81[d]

[a] From reference 85.
[b] From reference 101.
[c] From reference 58.
[d] From reference 61.
[e] From reference 59.
V, variable; S, susceptible; R, resistant.

ited, however. Even less information is available for other aerobic actinomycetes.

REFERENCES

1. Arroyo JC, et al. Disseminated *Nocardia caviae* infection. Am J Med 1977;62:409–412.
2. Ayyar S, et al. A comparison of three media for isolation of *Nocardia* species from clinical specimens. J Postgrad Med 1992;38:70–72.
3. Baisden BL, et al. Diagnosis of Whipple disease by immunohistochemical analysis: a sensitive and specific method for the detection of *Tropheryma whipplei* (the Whipple bacillus) in paraffin-embedded tissue. Am J Clin Pathol 2002;118:742–748.
4. Beaman BL, Beaman L. *Nocardia* species: host-parasite relationships. Clin Microbiol Rev 1994;7:213–264.
5. Beaman BL, et al. *Nocardia* infections in the United States, 1972–1974. J Infect Dis 1976;134:286–289.
6. Beau F, et al. Molecular identification of a *Nocardiopsis dassonvillei* blood isolate. J Clin Microbiol 1999;37:3366–3368.
7. Bemer-Melchior P, et al. Bacteremia due to *Dietzia maris* in an immunocompromised patient. Clin Infect Dis 1999;29:1338–1340.
8. Bentley SD, et al. Sequencing and analysis of the genome of the Whipple's disease bacterium *Tropheryma whipplei*. Lancet 2003;361:637–644.
9. Berg R, et al. *Corynebacterium equi* infection complicating neoplastic disease. Am J Clin Pathol 1977;68:73–77.
10. Brown JM, McNeil MM. *Nocardia, Rhodococcus, Gordonia, Actinomadura, Streptomyces*, and other aerobic actinomycetes. In: Murray PR, Baron EJ, Jorgensen JH, Pfaller MA, Yolken RH, eds. Manual of Clinical Microbiology. Ed. 8. Washington, DC: ASM Press, 2004:502–531.
11. Browns JM, et al. Rapid identification of *Nocardia farcinica* clinical isolates by a PCR assay targeting a 314-base-pair species-specific DNA fragment. J Clin Microbiol 2004;42:3655–3660.
12. Carson M, Hellyar A. Opacification of Middlebrook agar as an aid in distinguishing *Nocardia farcinica* within the *Nocardia asteroides* complex. J Clin Microbiol 1994;32:2270–2271.
13. Castro LG, et al. Mycetoma: a retrospective study of 41 cases seen in Sao Paulo, Brazil, from 1978 to 1989. Mycoses 1993;36:89–95.
14. Causey WA. *Nocardia caviae*: a report of 13 new isolations with clinical correlation. Appl Microbiol 1974;28:193–198.
15. Chandler FW, Watts JC. Pathologic Diagnosis of Fungal Infections. Chicago, ASCP Press, 1987.
16. Clark NM, et al. Primary cutaneous *Nocardia otitidiscaviarum* infection: case report and review. Clin Infect Dis 1995;20:1266–1270.
17. Cloud JL, et al. Evaluation of partial 16S ribosomal DNA sequencing for identification of *Nocardia* species by using the MicroSeq 500 system with an expanded database. J Clin Microbiol 2004;42:578–584.
18. Conville PS, et al. *Nocardia veterana* as a pathogen in North American patients. J Clin Microbiol 2003;41:2560–2568.
19. Curry WA.s Human nocardiosis: a clinical review with selected case reports. Arch Intern Med 1980;140:818–826.
20. Dorman SE, et al. *Nocardia* infection in chronic granulomatous disease. Clin Infect Dis 2002;35:390–394.
21. Durand DV, et al. Whipple disease: clinical review of 52 cases: the SNFMI Research Group on Whipple Disease. Societe Nationale Francaise de Medecine Interne. Medicine (Baltimore) 1997;76:170–184.
22. Ehrbar HU, et al. PCR-positive tests for *Tropheryma whippelii* in patients without Whipple's disease. Lancet 1999;353:2214.
23. Eisenblatter M, et al. Isolation of *Nocardia paucivorans* from the cerebrospinal fluid of a patient with relapse of cerebral nocardiosis. J Clin Microbiol 2002;40:3532–3534.
24. Esteban J, et al. Isolation of *Nocardia* sp. from blood cultures in a teaching hospital. Scand J Infect Dis 1994;26:693–696.
25. Fenollar F, et al. Whipple's endocarditis: review of the literature and comparisons with Q fever, *Bartonella* infection, and blood culture-positive endocarditis. Clin Infect Dis 2001;33:1309–1316.
26. Flores M, Desmond E. Opacification of Middlebrook agar as an aid in identification of *Nocardia farcinica*. J Clin Microbiol 1993;31:3040–3041.
27. Garrett MA, et al. Selective buffered charcoal-yeast extract medium for isolation of nocardiae from mixed cultures. J Clin Microbiol 1992;30:1891–1892.
28. Georghiou PR, Blacklock ZM. Infection with *Nocardia* species in Queensland: a review of 102 clinical isolates. Med J Aust 1992;156:692–697.
29. Gonzalez Ochoa A. Mycetoma caused by *Nocardia braziliensis* with a note on the isolation of the causative organism from soil. Lab Invest 1962;11:1123.
30. Goodfellow M. Suprageneric classification of actinomycetes. In: Holt JG, Williams ST, Sharpe ME, ed. Bergey's Manual of Systematic Bacteriology. Baltimore: Williams & Wilkins,1989:2333–2339.
31. Goodfellow M. Maduromycetes. In: Holt JG, Williams ST, Sharpe ME, eds. Bergey's Manual of Systematic Bacteriology. Baltimore: Williams & Wilkins,1989:2509–2551.
32. Goodfellow M, Alderson G. The actinomycete-genus *Rhodococcus*: a home for the ''rhodochrous'' complex. J Gen Microbiol 1977;100:99–122.
33. Goodfellow M, Williams ST. Ecology of actinomycetes. Annu Rev Microbiol 1983;37:189–216.
34. Gubler JG, et al. Whipple endocarditis without overt gastrointestinal disease: report of four cases. Ann Intern Med 1999;l131:112–116.
35. Guerrero MF, et al. Pulmonary malacoplakia associated with *Rhodococcus equi* infection in patients with AIDS: case report and review. Clin Infect Dis 1999;28:1334–1336.
36. Guss WJ, Ament ME. *Oerskovia* infection caused by contaminated home parenteral nutrition solution. Arch Intern Med 1989;149:1457–1458.
37. Hamid ME, et al. *Nocardia africana* sp. nov., a new pathogen isolated from patients with pulmonary infections. J Clin Microbiol 2001;39:625–630.
38. Harrington RD, et al. *Oerskovia xanthineolytica* infection of a prosthetic joint: case report and review. J Clin Microbiol 1996;34:1821–1824.
39. Hollick GE, Kurups VP. Isolation and identification of thermophilic actinomycetes associated with hypersensitivity pneumonitis. Lab Med 1983;14:39–44.
40. Javaly K, et al. Nocardiosis in patients with human immunodeficiency virus infection: report of 2 cases and review of the literature. Medicine (Baltimore) 1992;71:128–138.
41. Kageyama A, et al. *Nocardia arthritidis* sp. nov., a new pathogen isolated from a patient with rheumatoid arthritis in Japan. J Clin Microbiol 2004;42:2366–2371.
42. Kerr E, et al. Isolation of *Nocardia asteroides* from respiratory specimens by using selective buffered charcoal-yeast extract agar. J Clin Microbiol 1992;30:1320–1322.
43. Kiska DL, et al. Identification of medically relevant *Nocardia* species with an abbreviated battery of tests. J Clin Microbiol 2002;40:1346–1351.
44. Kurup VP, Fink, JN. A scheme for the identification of thermophilic actinomycetes associated with hypersensitivity pneumonitis. J Clin Microbiol 1975;2:55–61.
45. Kwon-Chung KJ, Bennett JE. Medical Mycology. Philadelphia: Lea & Febiger,1992.
46. La Scola B, et al. Description of *Tropheryma whipplei* gen. nov., sp. nov., the Whipple's disease bacillus. Int J Syst Evol Microbiol 2001;51:1471–1479.
47. Ladron N, et al. Rapid identification of *Rhodococcus equi* by a PCR assay targeting the choE gene. J Clin Microbiol 2003;41:3241–3245.
48. Lasky JA, et al. *Rhodococcus equi* causing human pulmonary infection: review of 29 cases. South Med J 1991;84:1217–1220.
49. Laurent FJ, et al. Rapid identification of clinically relevant *Nocardia* species to genus level by 16S rRNA gene PCR. J Clin Microbiol 1999;37:99–102.
50. Lechevalier HA. A practical guide to generic identification of actinomycetes. In: Holt JG, Williams ST, Sharpe ME, eds. Bergey's Manual of Systematic Bacteriology. Baltimore: Williams & Wilkins,1989:2344–2347.
51. Lechevalier HA. Nocardioform actinomycetes. In: Holt JG, Williams ST, Sharpe ME, eds. Bergey's Manual of Systematic Bacteriology. Baltimore: Williams & Wilkins,1989:2348–2404.
52. Lepidi H, et al. Immunohistological detection of *Tropheryma whipplei* (Whipple bacillus) in lymph nodes. Am J Med 2002;113:334–336.
53. LeProwse CR, et al. Catheter-related bacteremia caused by *Oerskovia turbata*. J Clin Microbiol 1989;27:571–572.
54. Lerner PI. Nocardiosis. Clin Infect Dis 1996;22:891–903.
55. MacGregor JH, et al. Opportunistic lung infection caused by *Rhodococcus (Corynebacterium) equi*. Radiology 1986;160:83–84.
56. Maiwald M, et al. *Tropheryma whippelii* DNA is rare in the intestinal mucosa of patients without other evidence of Whipple disease. Ann Intern Med 2001;134:115–119.
57. Marth T, Raoult D. Whipple's disease. Lancet 2003;361:239–246.
58. McNeil MM, Brown JM. The medically important aerobic actinomycetes: epidemiology and microbiology. Clin Microbiol Rev 1994;7:357–417.
59. McNeil MM, et al. Infections due to *Nocardia transvalensis*: clinical spectrum and antimicrobial therapy. Clin Infect Dis 1992;15:453–463.
60. McNeil MM, et al. Comparison of species distribution and antimicrobial susceptibility of aerobic actinomycetes from clinical specimens. Rev Infect Dis 1990;12:778–783.
61. McNeil MM, et al. Comparison of species distribution and antimicrobial susceptibility of aerobic actinomycetes from clinical specimens. Rev Infect Dis 1990;12:778–783.

62. McNeil MM, et al. Nonmycetomic *Actinomadura madurae* infection in a patient with AIDS. J Clin Microbiol 1992;30:1008–1010.

63. Mishra SK, et al. Identification of nocardiae and streptomycetes of medical importance. J Clin Microbiol 1980;11:728–736.

64. Murray PR, et al. Effect of decontamination procedures on recovery of *Nocardia* spp. J Clin Microbiol 1987;25:2010–2011.

65. Murray PR, et al. Modified Thayer-Martin medium for recovery of *Nocardia* species from contaminated specimens. J Clin Microbiol 1988;26:1219–1220.

66. National Committee for Clinical Laboratory Standards. Susceptibility testing of mycobacteria, nocardiae, and other aerobic actinomycetes; approved standard (M24-A). Wayne, PA: National Committee for Clinical Laboratory Standards, 2003.

67. Patel JB, et al. Sequence-based identification of aerobic actinomycetes. J Clin Microbiol 2004;42:2530–2540.

68. Pepys J, et al. Farmer's lung: thermophilic actinomycetes as a source of ''farmer's lung hay'' antigen. Lancet 1963;41:607–611.

69. Petersen DL, et al. Disseminated *Nocardia caviae* with positive blood cultures. Arch Intern Med 1978;138:1164–1165.

70. Pidoux O, et al. Molecular identification of a *Dietzia maris* hip prosthesis infection isolate. J Clin Microbiol 2001;39:2634–2636.

71. Pottumarthy S, et al. *Nocardia veterana*, a new emerging pathogen. J Clin Microbiol 2003;41:1705–1709.

72. Prescott JF. *Rhodococcus equi*: an animal and human pathogen. Clin Microbiol Rev 1991;4:20–34.

73. Ramzan NN, et al. Diagnosis and monitoring of Whipple disease by polymerase chain reaction. Ann Intern Med 1997;126:520–527.

74. Raoult D, et al. Cultivation of the bacillus of Whipple's disease. N Engl J Med 2000;342:620–625.

75. Raoult D, et al. Culture and immunological detection of *Tropheryma whippelii* from the duodenum of a patient with Whipple disease. JAMA 2001;285:1039–1043.

76. Reller LB, et al. Bacterial endocarditis caused by *Oerskovia turbata*. Ann Intern Med 1975;83:664–666.

77. Rihs JD, et al. *Oerskovia xanthineolytica* implicated in peritonitis associated with peritoneal dialysis: case report and review of Oerskovia infections in humans. J Clin Microbiol 1990;28:1934–1937.

78. Roth A, et al. Phylogeny of the genus *Nocardia* based on reassessed 16S rRNA gene sequences reveals underspeciation and division of strains classified as *Nocardia asteroides* into three established species and two unnamed taxons. J Clin Microbiol 2003;41:851–856.

79. Ruimy R, et al. *Nocardia pseudobrasiliensis* sp. nov., a new species of *Nocardia* which groups bacterial strains previously identified as *Nocardia brasiliensis* and associated with invasive diseases. Int J Syst Bacteriol 1996;46:259–264.

80. Saubolle MA, Sussland D. Nocardiosis: review of clinical and laboratory experience. J Clin Microbiol 2003;41:4497–4501.

81. Scott MA, et al. *Rhodococcus equi*: an increasingly recognized opportunistic pathogen: report of 12 cases and review of 65 cases in the literature. Am J Clin Pathol 1995;103:649–655.

82. Shawar RM, et al. Cultivation of *Nocardia* spp. on chemically defined media for selective recovery of isolates from clinical specimens. J Clin Microbiol 1990;28:508–512.

83. Smego RA Jr, et al. Lymphocutaneous syndrome: a review of non-sporothrix causes. Medicine (Baltimore) 1999;78:38–63.

84. Smego RA Jr, Gallis HA. The clinical spectrum of *Nocardia brasiliensis* infection in the United States. Rev Infect Dis 1984;6:164–180.

85. Sorrell TC, Iredell JR, Mitchell DH. *Nocardia* species. In: Mandell GL, Bennett JE, Dolin R, ed. Mandell, Douglas, and Bennett's Principles and Practice of Infectious Diseases. Ed. 5. New York: Churchill Livingstone, 2000:2637–2645.

86. Sottnek FO, et al. Recognition of *Oerskovia* species in the clinical laboratory: characterization of 35 isolates. Int J Syst Bacteriol 1977;27:263–270.

87. Stackebrandt E, et al. Re-evaluation of the status of the genus *Oerskovia*, reclassification of *Promicromonospora enterophila* (Jager et al. 1983) as *Oerskovia enterophila* comb. nov. and description of *Oerskovia jenensis* sp. nov. and *Oerskovia paurometabola* sp. nov. Int J Syst Evol Microbiol 2002;52:1105–1111.

88. Steingrube VA, et al. DNA amplification and restriction endonuclease analysis for differentiation of 12 species and taxa of *Nocardia*, including recognition of four new taxa within the *Nocardia asteroides* complex. J Clin Microbiol 1995; 33:3096–3101.

89. Steingrube VA, et al. Partial characterization of *Nocardia farcinica* beta-lactamases. Antimicrob Agents Chemother 1993;37:1850–1855.

90. Steingrube VA, et al. Rapid identification of clinically significant species and taxa of aerobic actinomycetes, including *Actinomadura*, *Gordona*, *Nocardia*, *Rhodococcus*, *Streptomyces*, and *Tsukamurella* isolates, by DNA amplification and restriction endonuclease analysis. J Clin Microbiol 1997;35:817–822.

91. Street S, et al. *Tropheryma whippelii* DNA in saliva of healthy people. Lancet 1999;354:1178–1179.

92. Takai S, et al. Prevalence of virulent *Rhodococcus equi* in isolates from soil and feces of horses from horse-breeding farms with and without endemic infections. J Clin Microbiol 1991;29:2887–2889.

93. Tight RR, Bartlett MS. Actinomycetoma in the United States. Rev Infect Dis 1981;3:1139–1150.

94. Torres HA, et al. Nocardiosis in cancer patients. Medicine (Baltimore) 2002; 81:388–397.

95. Tsukamura M, et al. Severe progressive subcutaneous abscesses and necrotizing tenosynovitis caused by *Rhodococcus aurantiacus*. J Clin Microbiol 1988;26: 201–205.

96. Tsukamura M, Kawakami K. Lung infection caused by *Gordona aurantiaca* (*Rhodococcus aurantiacus*). J Clin Microbiol 1982;16:604–607.

97. van Etta LL, et al. *Corynebacterium equi*: a review of 12 cases of human infection. Rev Infect Dis 1983;5:1012–1018.

98. Wallace RJ Jr, et al. New *Nocardia* taxon among isolates of *Nocardia brasiliensis* associated with invasive disease. J Clin Microbiol 1995;33:1528–1533.

99. Wallace RJ Jr, et al. Beta-lactam resistance in *Nocardia brasiliensis* is mediated by beta-lactamase and reversed in the presence of clavulanic acid. J Infect Dis 1987;156:959–966.

100. Wallace RJ Jr, et al. Use of trimethoprim-sulfamethoxazole for treatment of infections due to *Nocardia*. Rev Infect Dis 1982;4:315–325.

101. Wallace RJ Jr, et al. Antimicrobial susceptibility patterns of *Nocardia asteroides*. Antimicrob Agents Chemother 1988;32:1776–1779.

102. Wallace RJ Jr, et al. Beta-lactamase production and resistance to beta-lactam antibiotics in *Nocardia*. Antimicrob Agents Chemother 1978;14:704–709.

103. Wenger PN, et al. *Nocardia farcinica* sternotomy site infections in patients following open heart surgery. J Infect Dis 1998;178:1539–1543.

104. Wilson JP, et al. Nocardial infections in renal transplant recipients. Medicine (Baltimore) 1989;68:38–57.

105. Wilson KH. Detection of culture-resistant bacterial pathogens by amplification and sequencing of ribosomal DNA. Clin Infect Dis 1994;18:958–962.

106. Winn WC Jr., Frable WJ. Infectious Diseases. In: Silverberg SG, DeLellis RA, Frable WJ, eds. Principles and Practice of Surgical Pathology and Cytopathology. Ed. 3. New York: Churchill Livingstone, 1997:155–226.

107. Winn WC Jr, Kissane JM. Bacterial infections. In: Damjanov I, Linder J, ed. Anderson's Textbook of Pathology. Ed.10. St. Louis: Mosby, 1995: 747–865.

108. Wust J, et al. Peritonitis caused by *Actinomadura madurae* in a patient on CAPD. Eur J Clin Microbiol Infect Dis 1990;9:700–701.

109. Yassin AF, et al. *Nocardia paucivorans* sp. nov. Int J Syst Evol Microbiol 2000; 50(Pt 2):803–809.

110. Yassin AF, et al. Description of *Nocardiopsis synnemataformans* sp. nov., elevation of *Nocardiopsis alba* subsp. *prasina* to *Nocardiopsis prasina* comb. nov., and designation of *Nocardiopsis antarctica* and *Nocardiopsis alborubida* as later subjective synonyms of *Nocardiopsis dassonvillei*. Int J Syst Bacteriol 1997;47: 983–988.

111. Yassin AF, et al. *Nocardia abscessus* sp. nov. Int J Syst Evol Microbiol 2000; 50(Pt 4):1487–1493.

112. Yassin AF, et al. *Nocardia cyriacigeorgici* sp. nov. Int J Syst Evol Microbiol 2001;51:1419–1423.

113. Yassins AF, et al. *Nocardia puris* sp. nov. Int J Syst Evol Microbiol 2003;53: 1595–1599.

The Anaerobic Bacteria **16**

Relationships of Bacteria to Oxygen
Oxygen Tolerance
Oxidation-Reduction Potential

Habitats

Taxonomic Classification and Nomenclature

Human Infections

Isolation of Anaerobic Bacteria
Selection of Specimens for Culture
Collection and Transport of Specimens
Anaerobic Blood Culture (Summary of Guidelines for Traditional Broth and Instrumented Systems)
Direct Examination of Clinical Materials
Selection and Use of Media

Anaerobic Systems for the Cultivation of Anaerobic Bacteria
Anaerobic Jar Techniques
Use of the Anaerobic Glove Box
The Roll-Streak System
Anaerobic Disposable Plastic Bags
Use of the Anaerobic Holding Jar

Incubation of Cultures

Inspection and Subculture of Colonies

Aerotolerance Tests

Preliminary Reporting of Results

Determination of Cultural and Biochemical Characteristics for Differentiation of Anaerobic Isolates
Presumptive Identification
Use of Differential Agar Media
Presumpto Plates
Antimicrobial Susceptibility Plates
Characterization of Anaerobes Using Conventional Biochemical Tests in Large Tubes
Alternative Procedures
The Nagler Test and the CAMP Test for *C. perfringens*
Packaged Microsystems
Commercial Packaged Kits for Identification of Anaerobes After 4 Hours of Aerobic Incubation

Determination of Metabolic Products By Gas-Liquid Chromatography
Identification of Volatile Fatty Acids

Analysis of Nonvolatile Acids
Gas-Liquid Chromatography Controls

Identification of Anaerobic Bacteria

Anaerobic Gram-Negative Non–Spore-Forming
  Bacilli

  Classification and Nomenclature
  Presumptive or Preliminary Group Identification of
    Bacteroides, Prevotella, Porphyromonas, and
    Fusobacterium
Identification of the Anaerobic Cocci
Identification of the Anaerobic Non–Spore-
  Forming Gram-Positive Bacilli

  Propionibacterium Species
  Bifidobacterium Species
  Lactobacillus Species

Actinomyces Species
Eubacterium Species
Mobiluncus and Bacterial Vaginosis
Additional Genera and Species of Anaerobic
  Non–Spore-Forming Gram-Positive Bacilli

Identification of *Clostridium* Species

  Histotoxic Clostridia Involved in Clostridial
    Myonecrosis or Gas Gangrene
  Miscellaneous Clostridia in Other Clinical Settings
  Clostridium difficile–Associated Intestinal Disease
  Botulism
  Tetanus

Antimicrobial Susceptibility Testing of Anaerobic Bacteria

Methods for Antimicrobial Susceptibility Testing of
  Anaerobes

Relationships of Bacteria to Oxygen

Although defined in various ways by different authors, a practical working definition is that the *obligately anaerobic bacteria* are those bacteria that grow in the absence of free oxygen but fail to multiply in the presence of oxygen on the surface of nutritionally adequate solid media incubated in room air or in a CO_2 incubator (containing 5–10% CO_2 in air). The amount of O_2 in a CO_2 incubator, or in a candle extinction jar, is considerable (about 18–19%). In practice, anaerobic bacteria are most often recognized in the clinical laboratory following aerotolerance tests of colonies that grew on primary isolation plates incubated anaerobically (see below). Thus, most anaerobes identified in the clinical laboratory grow initially on anaerobic blood agar, or on one of the selective anaerobic media, or in an enrichment broth incubated anaerobically, but not on blood agar or chocolate agar plates incubated aerobically or in a CO_2 incubator.

It is an oversimplification to discuss the anaerobes as if they fit uniformly in one large group, just as it is an oversimplification (and incorrect) to refer to all bacteria that grow in room air as aerobes. Thus, several terms, including *obligate aerobe, facultative anaerobe, microaerophile, aerotolerant anaerobe* and *obligate anaerobe* (strict and moderate), have been used to subdivide bacteria based on their relationships to oxygen. These terms reflect a continuous spectrum of bacteria that cannot tolerate oxygen to those that require it for growth.

Obligate aerobes, including species of *Micrococcus* and *Pseudomonas*, require molecular oxygen as a terminal electron acceptor, resulting in the formation of water, and do not obtain energy by fermentative pathways. However, it is not uncommon to find *P. aeruginosa* growing scantily on anaerobically incubated media in the clinical laboratory, since these bacteria can use nitrate in the medium as a terminal electron acceptor (through anaerobic respiration) in place of O_2. In contrast, molecular oxygen varies in its toxicity to different species of anaerobic bacteria and is not a terminal electron acceptor for the anaerobic bacteria. In general, the clinically important anaerobes obtain their energy through fermentative pathways, in which organic compounds such as organic acids, alcohols, and other products serve as final electron acceptors.

Anaerobes, on the other hand, are divided into two major groups: the obligate anaerobes (defined previously) and the aerotolerant anaerobes. The obligate anaerobes have been further subdivided into two groups based on their ability to grow in the presence of or to tolerate oxygen. Strict obligate anaerobes are not capable of growth on agar surfaces exposed to O_2 levels above 0.5%. Atmospheric oxygen is highly toxic for these microorganisms for reasons that are not entirely known. Examples of these bacteria include *Clostridium haemolyticum, C. novyi* type B, *Selenomonas ruminatium,* and *Treponema denticola.* The second group of obligate anaerobes, the moderate obligate anaerobes, are bacteria that can grow when exposed to oxygen levels ranging from about 2% to 8% (average, 3%). Examples of these bacteria include members of the *Bacteroides fragilis* and the pigmented *Prevotella-Porphyromonas* groups (or formerly called the pigmented *Bacteroides* group), *Fusobacterium nucleatum,* and *C. perfringens.*[151]

The term *aerotolerant anaerobe* is used by some microbiologists to describe anaerobic bacteria that will show limited or scant growth on agar in room air or in a 5–10% CO_2

incubator, but show good growth under anaerobic conditions. Examples of these bacteria include *Clostridium carnis, C. histolyticum,* and *C. tertium.* Most of the anaerobes isolated from properly selected and collected specimens in the clinical laboratory fit into the moderate obligate anaerobe category. These organisms are more tolerant to the toxic effects of oxygen than the strict obligate anaerobes, but are still killed by oxygen, unless anaerobic conditions are maintained properly during specimen collection and transport to the laboratory and during the steps required for processing of specimens and isolation and identification, as discussed in later sections of the chapter. Strict obligate anaerobes are rare in infections of humans, but both the moderate and the strict obligate anaerobes are found in a variety of nonpathogenic habitats (e.g., feces and the oropharynx), as part of the normal flora.

The facultative anaerobes (e.g., *Escherichia coli* and *Staphylococcus aureus*) grow under either aerobic or anaerobic conditions. They use oxygen as a terminal electron acceptor or, less efficiently, can obtain their energy through fermentation reactions under anaerobic conditions. Grown aerobically, facultative anaerobes obtain much more energy (38 ATP) when they completely catabolize a molecule of glucose to CO_2 and H_2O, than when grown anaerobically. Under anaerobic conditions, fermentative metabolism of the glucose molecule yields only 2–3 ATP.[163]

The microaerophiles require oxygen as a terminal electron acceptor, yet these bacteria do not grow on the surface of solid media in an aerobic incubator (21% O_2) and grow minimally if at all under anaerobic conditions. An example of a microaerophile is *Campylobacter jejuni,* which grows optimally in 5% O_2 (the gas mixture of the incubation environment commonly used for recovering this organism in clinical laboratories is 5% O_2, 10% CO_2, and 85% N_2).

Through the years, bacteriologists working on the development of improved media and systems for cultivation of anaerobes have focused on two fundamental limiting factors that may affect the growth of anaerobes. The first and most important of these are the inhibitory effects of atmospheric oxygen and its toxic derivatives. The second limiting factor of concern is the oxidation-reduction potential (Eh) of the culture medium.

Oxygen Tolerance

Some of the strictest obligate anaerobes (e.g., *Clostridium haemolyticum* and *C. novyi* type B) are killed when exposed to atmospheric oxygen on the open laboratory bench for 10 minutes or longer. On the other hand, most of the moderate obligate anaerobes encountered in human infections tolerate exposure to oxygen for longer times. The reasons why anaerobes vary in their tolerance to oxygen are probably multiple, but one idea is that the oxygen tolerance of many moderate obligate anaerobes depends on their production of superoxide dismutase, catalases, and possibly peroxidase enzymes, which are protective against toxic oxygen reduction products.[23,87,101,163,235]

A popular notion is that exposure to atmospheric O_2 results in a series of reactions within the bacterial cells, possibly reactions mediated by flavoproteins, which result in production of the negatively charged superoxide radical (O_2^-), hydrogen peroxide (H_2O_2), and other toxic oxygen reduction products.[23,172] The superoxide anion and H_2O_2 may react together to produce free hydroxyl radicals (OH·), the most powerful biologic oxidants known, and there may also be the production of toxic singlet oxygen ($^1O_2$) through the reaction of superoxide anions with free hydroxyl radicals. Superoxide dismutase catalyzes the conversion of superoxide radicals to less toxic hydrogen peroxide and molecular oxygen. Catalase catalyzes the conversion of hydrogen peroxide to form water and oxygen. Several species of oxygen tolerant moderate obligate anaerobes were shown to produce superoxide dismutase (SOD) and the level of SOD produced correlated with the level of oxygen tolerance and virulence of the organism.[235] In another study, several strains of the genus *Bacteroides,* several anaerobic cocci, anaerobic non–spore-forming Gram-positive rods, and clostridia produced SOD, but no correlation was found between the source of the organism, the presumed level of pathogenicity, and the SOD level produced.[87] Several species of anaerobes have been shown to produce catalase (e.g., members of the *Bacteroides fragilis* group, *Propionibacterium acnes,* and others), as well as SOD, but some anaerobes that are relatively oxygen-tolerant or aerotolerant (e.g. *Clostridium tertium*), produce neither SOD nor catalase. Rolfe et al., observed that the degree of oxygen tolerance of anaerobic bacteria is related to the proportion of the bacterial cells in the population that survive following exposure to oxygen.[200] In practice, it is often essential to use large inocula when inoculating or subculturing anaerobic culture media, which probably serves to minimize the harmful effects of multiple toxic oxygen growth limiting factors. Clearly, much more work is needed on the mechanisms of oxygen tolerance and intolerance of anaerobic bacteria.

Oxidation-Reduction Potential

The oxidation-reduction potential (abbreviated "redox" potential or Eh) of a culture medium, expressed in volts or millivolts, can be measured by using a platinum wire electrode, along with a standard reference electrode connected to a pH meter. Eh is affected by pH (or the hydrogen ion concentration); thus, redox potential is commonly expressed at neutral pH (pH 7) as Eh. Reducing agents, such as thioglycolate and L-cysteine may be added to anaerobic transport media and to certain culture media to help maintain reduced conditions (or a low Eh) in the medium. A positive oxidation-reduction potential (e.g., as indicated by pink color of resazurin indicator in certain media, or a blue color of methylene blue indicator in other media) means that the medium is oxidized. In nature, the upper limit of Eh is +820 mV, which might be found in some environments that have considerable oxygenation. Oxidizing conditions prevail in healthy human tissue that is well-oxygenated and has an intact blood supply (e.g., the Eh is about +150 mV). In contrast, the lower limit of Eh in nature is about −420 mV. An anaerobic environment (e.g., an abscess or necrotic tissue) or a culture medium rich in hydrogen might have such a low Eh. The large bowel of humans, containing enormous numbers of strict obligate anaerobes, has an Eh of about −250 mV.[163]

What is the relative significance of the oxidation-reduction potential versus atmospheric oxygen in relation to survival and growth of anaerobic bacteria? As reviewed several years ago by Hentges and Maier,[101] there are older reports indicating that certain anaerobes would not grow above a certain low Eh level and that some obligate anaerobes would grow in room air if the Eh of the medium was kept sufficiently low. In an excellent study reported by Walden and Hentges,[248] some of the misconceptions about Eh effects on anaerobic bacteria were dispelled. These workers studied the differential effects of O_2 and redox potential on the growth of *C. perfringens*, *B. fragilis*, and *P. magnus*. Oxygen inhibited multiplication of these three anaerobes whether the medium was at a negative redox potential (Eh = −50 mV), poised by the addition of dithiothreitol ([DTT] a reducing agent), or at a positive redox potential (Eh near +500 mV) in aerated medium without DTT. In the absence of O_2, these organisms were able to multiply even when the Eh was maintained at +325 mV, by the addition of potassium ferricyanide (an oxidizing agent). From their work, a practical conclusion was drawn that the purging of oxygen from the cultural environment, to avoid oxygen toxicity, is probably more important than the establishment of a low Eh.[248] Thus, the rapid achievement and maintenance of a low oxygen tension, or the absence of oxygen, is an essential requirement for the successful cultivation of anaerobes in modern anaerobic systems (e.g., anaerobic jars and glove boxes used for incubation of anaerobes in the clinical laboratory).

Habitats

Anaerobic bacteria are widespread in soil, marshes, lake and river sediments, the oceans, sewage, foods, and animals. In humans, anaerobic bacteria normally are prevalent in the oral cavity around the teeth, in the gastrointestinal tract, especially in the colon, where they outnumber coliforms by at least 1,000:1, and in the orifices of the genitourinary tract, and on the skin.[69,100] Most of these anaerobic habitats have both a low oxygen tension and reduced oxidation-reduction potential (Eh) resulting from the metabolic activity of microorganisms that consume oxygen through respiration.[163] If the oxygen is not replaced, anaerobic conditions are maintained in the environment.

A brief summary of commonly encountered anaerobes in the normal flora of the human body is given in Box 16-1.

Taxonomic Classification and Nomenclature

The anaerobes include essentially all morphologic forms of bacteria; gram-negative rods, curved, spiral-shaped, and spirochete forms, gram-positive and gram-negative cocci, gram-positive non–spore-forming rods, and spore-formers.[8] Based on their morphologic features as observed in Gram-stained preparations and the absence or presence of spores, the anaerobic bacteria are broadly classified as shown in Table 16-1. Several of the genera in this list have been found only in nonpathogenic habitats (e.g., sites harboring normal flora such as the oral cavity, lower intestinal tract, genitouri-

nary tract, and skin of humans or various animals) and have not been reported to occur in diseases of humans. Most of these genera will not be discussed further.

There have been many recent developments in the taxonomic classification and nomenclature of anaerobes since the fifth edition of this book was published. Genetic studies utilizing PCR and 16S ribosomal (r) RNA, 16S rDNA sequencing, 16S-23S rRNA spacer-region (SR)-PCR, and other molecular methods have placed the classification of anaerobes on much more solid ground scientifically than

---

Box 16-1 Anaerobes Found in Normal Human Flora

Oral cavity and upper respiratory passages

Pigmented *Prevotella* species; *Porphyromonas* species
Nonpigmented *Prevotella* species (e.g., *P. oralis*)
Bacteroides species (e.g., *B. ureolyticus*)
Fusobacterium species (e.g., *F. nucleatum*)
Anaerobic cocci
Veillonella species
Actinomyces species and *Propionibacterium* species

Stomach (during fasting)

Lactobacilli

Small intestine (proximal portion)

Streptococci
Lactobacilli

Large bowel (and terminal ileum)

Bacteroides fragilis group
Porphyromonas species
Fusobacterium species
Anaerobic cocci—many species
Clostridium species
Eubacterium species
Bifidobacterium species
Propionibacterium species

Genitourinary tract; vagina and cervix

Pigmented *Prevotella* species; *Porphyromonas* species
Nonpigmented *Prevotella*
Bacteroides species
Anaerobic cocci
Clostridium species
Veillonella species
Lactobacillus species
Eubacterium species
Propionibacterium species

Urethra (male and female)

Propionibacterium species
Anaerobic cocci
Bacteroides (*Prevotella*) species
Fusobacterium species

Skin

Propionibacterium species
Anaerobic cocci

Table 16-1 Classification of the Genera of Anaerobic Bacteria

Gram-negative bacilli (curved, spiral, and spirochete forms are included)	*Megamonas*	*Micromonas[a]*	*Eggerthella[a]*
	Mitsuokella	*Peptococcus*	*Eubacterium[a]*
	Pectinatus	*Peptostreptococcus[a]*	*Holdemania*
	Porphyromonas[a]	*Ruminococcus*	*Lachnospira*
	Prevotella[a]	*Sarcina*	*Lactobacillus[a]*
Alistipes	*Propionigenium*	*Peptoniphilus[a]*	*Methanobacterium*
Anaerobacter	*Propionispira*	*Staphylococcus[a]*	*Mobiluncus[a]*
Anaerobiospirillum	*Rikenella*	*Streptococcus[a]*	*Mogibacterium*
Anaerorhabdus	*Ruminobacter*	*Gemella[a]*	*Propionibacterium[a]*
Bacteroides[a]	*Sebaldella*		*Roseburia*
Bilophila[a]	*Selenomonas*	**Gram-negative cocci**	*Shuttleworthia*
Borrelia	*Serpula*	*Acidaminococcus*	*Slackia[a]*
Butyrivibrio[c]	*Spirochaeta*	*Anaeroglobus*	*Varibaculum*
Capnocytophaga	*Succinimonas*	*Anaerosphaera*	
Capsularis	*Succinivibrio*	*Megasphaera*	**Spores formed**
Campylobacter[a]	*Sutterella[a]*	*Veillonella[a]*	**Gram-positive bacilli**
Catonella[a]	*Tannerella[a]*		*Clostridium[a,b]*
Centipeda	*Tissierella*	**Spores not formed**	*Desulfotomaculum*
Cetobacterium	*Treponema*	**Gram-positive bacilli**	*Desulfosporosinus*
Desulfuromonas	*Wolinella*	*Actinobaculum*	*Caloramator[b]*
Desulfovibrio		*Actinomyces[a]*	*Filifactor[b]*
Dialister[a]	**Gram-positive cocci**	*Arcanobacterium[a]*	*Moorella[b]*
Dichelobacter	*Anaerococcus[a]*	*Atopobium[a]*	*Oxobacter[b]*
Faecalibacterium	*Atopobium[a]*	*Bifidobacterium[a]*	*Oxalophagus[b]*
Fibrobacter	*Coprococcus*	*Bulleidia*	
Fusobacterium[a]	*Finegoldia[a]*	*Catenibacterium*	
Johnsonella[a]	*Gallicola*	*Cryptobacterium*	
Leptotrichia	*Gemmiger*	*Collinsella*	

[a] In the majority of properly collected clinical specimens, only these genera will need to be considered by the clinical microbiologist. However, on rare occasions, serious illness may involve Anaerobiospirillum,[191] Leptotrichia,[144] Selenomonas,[256] Desulfovibrio,[85] or one of the other genera that is not listed above.

[b] The genus Clostridium continues to be under major taxonomic revision. Thus, in 1994, five new genera of spore-forming anaerobes were proposed by Collins et al.[44] With a single exception, none of these is known to be pathogenic for humans. Filifactor alocis has been isolated from patients with endodontic infections.[218]

[c] Butyrivibrio is discussed with the gram-negative bacilli in Vol. 1 and with the irregular non–spore-forming gram-positive anaerobic rods in Vol. 2 of Bergey's Manual.[141,223] Although they are gram-negative with the Gram stain, some strains have atypical gram-positive cell wall features by electron microscopy.

Adapted and modified from Bergey's Manual of Systematic Bacteriology[141,223] and from very recent volumes of the International Journal of Systematic and Evolutionary Microbiology that contain numerous publications related to recent changes in anaerobe taxonomy.

was possible using phenotypic characterization and the older, less sophisticated genetic methods available in the past.[226,227] These studies have resulted in the descriptions of many new species and other taxa. Fortunately, some excellent taxonomic updates have simplified the task of keeping up with ongoing changes in nomenclature.[67,71,121–123] Table 16-2 provides a compendium of changes, compiled over the past two decades, in the taxo-nomic designations of clinically significant anaerobic bacteria. Table 16-3 lists the anaerobes that are most important clinically and/or the anaerobes most commonly encountered in properly selected and collected specimens from humans. Up-to-date, correct species identifications can have important implications related to prognosis, treatment, and clinical outcomes of patients with anaerobic infectious diseases.[15,69]

Table 16-2 Present and Former Names of Anaerobic Bacteria

PRESENT NAME	FORMER NAME/COMMENT	PRESENT NAME	FORMER NAME/COMMENT
Anaerobic Gram-Negative Rods		*P. disiens*	*Bacteroides disiens*—genitourinary tract infections
Genus *Bacteroides*—*Bacteroides fragilis* Group		*P. enoeca*	Human oral cavity; not pigmented
Bacteroides caccae	"3452A"—human fecal flora	*P. heparinolytica*	*Bacteroides heparinolyticus*
B. distasonis	Human infections infrequently—related to *Tannerella forsythensis* (formerly *B. forsythus*)	*P. intermedia*	*Bacteroides intermedius*—common in humans; head and neck, abdominal, pelvic sites; pigmented
B. eggerthii	Fecal flora—not common in infections	*P. loescheii*	*Bacteroides loescheii*—humans; pigmented
B. fragilis	The most common anaerobe in human infections	*P. melaninogenica*	*Bacteroides melaninogenicus*—various human infection sites; pigmented
B. merdae	"T4-1"—human fecal flora—related to *T. forsythensis* (formerly *B. forsythus*)	*P. nigrescens*	Formerly genotype II of *P. intermedia*—humans; pigmented
B. ovatus	Human fecal flora—occasionally infections	*P. oralis*	*Bacteroides oralis*
B. stercoris	"Subsp. A"—human fecal flora	*P. oris*	*Bacteroides oris*
B. thetaiotaomicron	The second most common *Bacteroides* spp. in human infections	*P. oulorum*	*B. oulorum; Prevotella oulora*
B. uniformis	Occasional isolates in human infections	*P. pallens*	New species
		P. salivae	New species—human saliva
B. vulgatus	Common in human fecal flora—occasional isolates in infections	*P. shahii*	New species—human saliva
		P. tannerae	New species—humans; ~40% of strains pigmented
Other species remaining in the genus *Bacteroides*, but not of the *Bacteroides fragilis* Group		*P. uenoni*	*Fusobacterium uenonas* (New species; Finegold SM: personal communication)
B. capillosus	Rare in clinical specimens	*P. veroralis*	*Bacteroides veroralis*
B. coagulans	Rare in clinical specimens	*P. zoogleoformans*	*Bacteroides zoogleoformis*
B. forsythus	New genus—*Tannerella forsythensis* human oral cavity	**Genus *Porphyromonas***	
B. galacturonicus	Human fecal flora	*P. asaccharolytica*	*Bacteroides asaccharolyticus*—various clinical infections of humans; pigmented
B. heparinolyticus	*P. heparinolytica*, but inhibited by bile, human fecal flora	*P. cangingivalis*	Dogs
B. pectinophilus	Human fecal flora	*P. canoris*	Dogs
B. splanchnicus	Resembles *B. fragilis* group but probably represents a new genus	*P. cansulci*	Dogs
B. tectus	*B. tectum*—cats and dogs	*P. catoniae*	*Oribaculum catoniae*—human oral cavity; the only nonpigmented *Porphyromonas*
B. ureolyticus	*Bacteroides corrodens*—related to genus *Campylobacter*	*P. circumdentaria*	Cats
B. zoogleoformans	*P. zoogleoformans*—related to *B. fragilis* group, but inhibited by bile	*P. crevioricanis*	Dogs
Genus *Prevotella*		*P. endodontalis*	*Bacteroides endodontalis*—humans; pigmented
P. bivia	*Bacteroides bivius*—genitourinary tract infections	*P. gingivalis*	*Bacteroides gingivalis*—human root canal and other dental/oral infections; pigmented
P. buccae	*Bacteroides buccae*—head and neck, chest infections	*P. gingivicanis*	Dogs
P. buccalis	*Bacteroides buccalis*	*P. gulae*	Gingival crevices—various animals
P. corporis	*Bacteroides corporis*—humans; pigmented	*P. levii*	*Bacteroides levii*—cattle
P. dentalis	*Mistuokella dentalis* and *Hallela seregens*	*P. macacae*	*Bacteroides macacae*—monkeys; *Porphyromonas salivosa*—cats; *Bacteroides salivosus*—cats
P. denticola	*Bacteroides denticola*—humans; pigmented		

Table 16-2 *Continued*

PRESENT NAME	FORMER NAME/COMMENT	PRESENT NAME	FORMER NAME/COMMENT
Genus *Fusobacterium*		*C. rectus*	*Wolinella recta*
F. gonidiaformans	Human infections	*C. showae*	Human oral cavity
F. mortiferum	Human infections; resembles *F. varium* and *F. ulcerans*	*C. sputorum*	
F. naviforme	Human infections	**Genus *Capnocytophaga***	
F. necrogenes	Human feces—animals	*C. canimorsus*	CDC group DF-2; Human infection after dog bites
F. necrophorum subsp. *funduli-forme*	*F. necrophorum* Biovar B—lipase-negative; less virulent than subsp. *necrophorum*	*C. cynodegmi*	Human infection after dog bites
		C. gingivalis	
F. necrophorum subsp. *necropho-rum*	*F. necrophorum* Biovar A—lipase-positive; the most virulent subspecies	*C. granulosa*	Dental plaque
		C. haemolytica	Dental plaque
		C. ochracea	*Bacteroides ocharaceus*
F. nucleatum—currently with the following five subspecies:	*animalis*	*C. sputigena*	
	fusiforme	**More genera of Gram-negative rods**	
	nucleatum	*Catonella morbi*	Related to *Clostridium* subphylum of gram-positive bacteria, cluster XIVa
	polymorphum		
	vincentii		
F. periodonticum	Related to *F. nucleatum*	*Centipeda periodontii*	Related to *Clostridium* subphylum of gram-positive bacteria, cluster XIVa
F. russii	Human feces		
F. ulcerans	New species—cutaneous ulcers		
F. varium	Various human infections	*Cetobacterium somerae*	New species—human feces
Other *Fusobacterium* species—encountered in animals		*Desulfovibrio piger*	*Desulfomonas pigra*
F. equinum	Oral cavities of horses	*Dialister pneumosintes*	*Bacteroides pneumosintes;* related to *Sporomusa* branch of *Clostridium* subphylum, cluster IX
F. perfoetans	Pig feces		
F. russii	Canine and feline oral flora		
F. simiae	Mouth of stump-tailed macaque	*Dichelobacter nodosus*	*Bacteroides nodosus*—foot rot in sheep and cattle
Other genera of anaerobic Gram-negative rods			
Alistipes finegoldii	New species—human appendicitis	*Faecalibacterium prausnitzii*	*Fusobacterium prausnitzii*—human feces; related to *Clostridium* subphylum, cluster IV
A. putredinis	*Bacteroides putredinis,* New genus; rare—human intraabdominal infections		
		Fibrobacter intestinalis	New species
Anaerobiospirillum succinicipro-ducens	Bacteremia of humans; feces of humans, cats, and dogs	*F. succinogenes*	*Bacteroides succinogenes*
		Filifactor alocis	*Fusobacterium alocis,* human gingi-val sulci
Anaerobiospirillum thomasii	New species; feces of humans, cats, and dogs	*Johnsonella ignava*	Related to *Clostridium* subphylum of gram-positive bacteria, cluster XIVa
Anaerostipes caccae	New species—human feces		
Anaerorhabdus furcosa	*Bacteroides furcosus; Anaerohabdus furcosus*	**Genus *Leptotrichia***	In *Fusobacterium* phylum
		L. amnionii	New species—amniotic fluid; related to *Sneathia* spp.
Bilophila wadswor-thia	Human infections		
Genus *Campylobacter*		*L. buccalis*	"*Leptothrix buccalis*"
C. concisus		*L. goodfellowii*	New species—blood
C. curvus	*Wolinella curva*	*L. hofstadii*	New species—saliva
C. gracilis	*Bacteroides gracilis*	*L. shahii*	New species—gingivitis
C. hominis	New species—human gastrointestinal tract	*L. trevisanii*	New species—bacteremia
		L. wadeii	New species—saliva

(Continued)

Table 16-2 *Continued*

PRESENT NAME	FORMER NAME/COMMENT	PRESENT NAME	FORMER NAME/COMMENT
Mitsuokella multiacida	*Bacteroides multiacidus*; related to *Sporomusa* branch of *Clostridium* subphylum cluster IX	*Finegoldia magna*	*Peptostreptococcus magnus*—human soft tissue, bone and joint infections; fecal and vaginal flora
Oxalobacter formigenes	Human colon—degrades calcium oxalate	*Gallicola barnesae*	*Peptostreptococcus barnesae*—isolated from chicken feces
Rikenella microfusus	*Bacteroides microfusus*	*Micromonas micros*	*Peptostreptococcus micros*—human specimens including mouth; flora of mouth, feces, vagina
Ruminobacter amylophilus	*Bacteroides amylophilus*	*Peptoniphilus asaccharolyticus*	*Peptostreptococcus asaccharolyticus*—vaginal discharges, ovarian, peritoneal, and other abscesses; does not produce acid from carbohydrates
Sebaldella termitidis	*Bacteroides termitidis*		
Genus *Selenomonas*			
S. artemidis		*P. harei*	*Peptostreptococcus harei*—human sacral ulcer pus
S. dianae	Human gingival crevice		
S. flueggei	Human oral flora	*P. indolicus*	*Peptostreptococcus indolicus*—cattle (mastitis); indole-positive, coagulase-positive
S. infelix	Human gingival crevice		
S. noxia	Human gingival crevice		
Sneathia sanguinegens	*Leptotrichia sanguinegens*—bacteremia in humans	*P. ivorii*	*Peptostreptococcus ivorii*—human leg ulcer
Sutterella wadsworthensis	*Campylobacter* (*Bacteroides*) *gracilis*—in part	*P. lacrimalis*	*Peptostreptococcus lacrimalis*—human lachrymal gland abscess
Tannerella forsythensis	*Bacteroides forsythus*	**Other anaerobic Gram-positive cocci**	
Tissierella praeacuta	*Bacteroides praeacutus*—Related to *Clostridium* subphylum of gram-positive bacteria, cluster XII	*Atopobium minutum*	*Lactobacillus minutus*—human abdominal wounds, pelvic abscesses
Anaerobic Cocci		*Atopobium parvulum*	*Streptococcus parvulus*—dental abscesses; gingival crevice flora
Gram-positive cocci			
Peptococcus niger	Only remaining species in this genus	*Atopobium rimae*	*Lactobacillus rimae*—dental abscesses; gingival crevice flora
Peptostreptococcus anaerobius	Only remaining species in this genus	*Atopobium vaginae*	New species—human vaginal flora
Reclassified anaerobic cocci		*Coprococcus catus*	Human feces
Anaerococcus prevotii	*Peptostreptococcus prevotii*—vaginal discharges, ovarian and peritoneal abscesses	*Coprococcus comes*	Human feces
		Coprococcus eutactus	Human feces
A. tetradius	*Peptostreptococcus tetradius*—vaginal discharges, ovarian abscesses	*Gemella morbillorum*	*Streptococcus morbillorum*
A. hydrogenalis	*Peptostreptococcus hydrogenalis*—vaginal discharges, ovarian abscesses	*Ruminococcus hansenii*	*Streptococcus hansenii*
A. vaginalis	*Peptostreptococcus vaginalis*—vaginal discharges, ovarian abscesses	*Ruminococcus productus*	*Streptococcus productus*
		Sarcina ventriculi	Diseased stomach, colon of humans
A. lactolyticus	*Peptostreptococcus lactolyticus*—vaginal discharges, ovarian abscesses	**Gram-positive cocci not considered true anaerobes—may appear initially as anaerobes on primary isolation but on subculture, grow aerobically in 10% CO2 atmosphere**	
A. octavius	*Peptostreptococcus octavius*—human nasal cavity, skin, vagina	*Staphylococcus saccharolyticus*	*Peptococcus saccharolyticus*
		Streptococcus. anginosus	"*S. milleri*" group

Table 16-2 *Continued*

PRESENT NAME	FORMER NAME/COMMENT	PRESENT NAME	FORMER NAME/COMMENT
S. constellatus	"*S. milleri*" group	*A. odontolyticus*	Human oral cavity—rare cause of actinomycosis
S. intermedius	"*S. MG-intermedius*," "*S. MG*"	*A. oricola*	New species—human dental abscess
Gram-negative cocci		*A. radicidentis*	New species—infected root canals of teeth
Acidaminococcus fermentans	Human clinical specimens; also feces of humans and hogs	*A. radingae*	New species—human clinical samples
Anaeroglobus geminatus	New species—human mouth, gastrointestinal tract; clinical material	*A. turicensis*	New species—human clinical samples
Megasphaera elsdenii	Human feces and clinical specimens; rumen of cattle and sheep, cecum of hogs	*A. urogenitalis*	New species—human urogenital tract
		A. viscosus	Human oral cavity and cervicovaginal sources; actinomycosis occasionally
Megasphaera micronuciformis	New species—human clinical specimens	**Other genera closely related to *Actinomyces***	
Megasphaera cerevisiae	New species—spoiled beer	*Actinobaculum schaalii*	New species—human blood; habitat not known
Veillonella. atypica	Human flora or from clinical samples during infectious processes	*Actinobaculum urinale*	New species—human urine
V. dispar	Human flora or from clinical samples during infectious processes	*Arcanobacterium bernardiae*	*Actinomyces* (CDC coryneform group 2) *bernardiae*—human sources
V. parvula	Human flora or from clinical samples during infectious processes	*Arcanobacterium pyogenes*	*Actinomyces* (*Corynebacterium*) *pyogenes*—human sources
V. ratti	Human semen	**Genus *Bifidobacterium***	
V. montpellierensis	New species—human clinical samples	*B. breve*	
Anaerobic Gram-positive, Non–spore-forming Rods		*B. denticolens*	No longer *Bifidobacterium*—now *Parascardovia denticolens*
Genus *Actinomyces*		*B. dentium*	*Bifidobacterium ericksonii*
A. cardiffensis	New species—human clinical sources including abscesses from various sites	*B. gallicum*	Human feces
		B. inopinatum	No longer *Bifidobacterium*—now *Scardovia inopinata*—human feces
A. europaeus	New species—human clinical specimens	*B. longum*	Human dental caries; now with three biotypes: *B. longum*, *B. infantis*, and *B. suis*
A. funkei	New species—human clinical specimens		
A. georgiae	Human gingival crevice	**Genus *Eubacterium***	
A. gerencseriae	Human periodontal flora	*E. biforme*	Human fecal flora
A. graevenitzii	New species—human clinical specimens	*E. brachy*	Human periodontitis
A. hongkongensis	New species—human clinical specimen	*E. infirmum*	New oral, asaccharolytic species
A. israelii	Major cause of human actinomycosis	*E. minutum*	*Eubacterium tardum*—a later synonym (does not have priority)
A. meyeri	Human periodontal sulcus—abscesses of brain; head and neck infections	*E. saphenum*	Human dental
		E. sulci	*Fusobacterium sulci*
A. naeslundii	A cause of human actinomycosis	*E. yurii* subsp. *margaretiae*	Human dental plaque
A. nasicola	New species—human nose		
A. neuii subsp. *neuii*	CDC coryneform group 1; from human sources	*E. yurii* subsp. *schtitka*	Human dental plaque
A. neuii subsp. *anitratus*	CDC coryneform group 1-"like," from human sources	*E. yurii* subsp. *yurii*	Human dental plaque

(Continued)

Table 16-2 *Continued*

PRESENT NAME	FORMER NAME/COMMENT	PRESENT NAME	FORMER NAME/COMMENT
Genus *Lactobacillus*		*Mogibacterium diversum*	New species—human oral cavities
L. coleohominis	New species—human clinical specimens	*Mogibacterium neglectum*	New species—human oral cavities
L. oris	Human saliva	*Olsenella profusa*	New species—human oral cavity
L. paraplantarum	New species—human feces	*Propionibacterium propionicum*	*Arachnia propionica*
L. rimae	Human gingival crevices		
L. uli	Human gingival crevices	*Pseudoramibacter alactolyticus*	*New genus—Eubacterium alactolyticum*
Other Recent Changes in the Gram-positive, Non–spore-forming Rods		*Roseburia intestinalis*	*New species—human feces*
Anaerofustis stercorihominis	New genus and species—human feces; related to rRNA cluster XV of the *Clostridium* subphylum of gram-positive bacteria	*Shuttleworthia satelles*	*New genus and species—human oral cavity*
		Slackia exigua	New genus; *Eubacterium exiguum*
		Slackia helion-trinireducens	*Peptostreptococcus heliontrinireducens*
Anaerotruncus colihominis	New genus and species—human feces; related to the *Clostridium leptum* rRNA cluster of bacteria	*Varibaculum cambriensis*	New genus and species—Actinomyces-like bacteria from human clinical specimens
Atopobium species	New genus; coccoid bacteria; listed elsewhere with the anaerobic gram-positive cocci	**Gram-positive Spore-forming Rods**	
		***Clostridium*: Human**	
Bulleidia extructa	New genus and species—human oral cavity	*C. argentinense*	*C. botulinum* type G and some non-toxigenic *C. hastiforme* and *C. subterminale*
Catenibacterium mitsuokai	New genus and species—human feces	*C. baratii*	*C. baratii*, *C. paraperfringens*, *C. perenne*
Collinsella aerofaciens	New genus; *Eubacterium aerofaciens*—human fecal flora	*Clostridium bartlettii*	New species—isolated from human feces
Collinsella stercoris	New species—human fecal flora	*Clostridium bolteae*	New species—isolated from human feces, especially children with autism
Collinsella intestinalis	New species—human fecal flora	*Clostridium botulinum*	Conservation of *Clostridium botulinum* (toxigenic) and *C. sporogenes* (nontoxigenic) which are genetically related at species level; rejection of *C. putrificum* (an earlier synonym)
Cryptobacterium curtum	New genus and species—human oral cavities		
Dorea formicigenerans	New genus; *Eubacterium formicigenerans*—human feces		
Dorea longicatena	New species—human feces		
Eggerthella lenta	New genus; *Eubacterium lentum*—human feces	*C. butyricum*	*C. pseudotetanicum*
Holdemania filiformis	New genus and species—human feces	*Clostridium clostridioforme*	Human strains identified phenotypically as *C. clostridioforme* were recently found to be *C. bolteae*, *C. clostridioforme* or *Clostridium hathewayi*
Mobiluncus curtisii	Proposal to emend *M. curtisii* (i.e., to include those formerly called *Falcivibrio vaginalis*; also included are the former subspecies of *Mobiluncus curtisii*)		
		Clostridium hathewayi	New species—isolated from human feces
Mogibacterium pumilum	New genus and species—human oral cavities	*Clostridium hiranonis*	New species—isolated from human feces
Mogibacterium vescum	New genus and species—human oral cavities	*Clostridium hylemonae*	New species—isolated from human feces
Mogibacterium timidum	New genus; *Eubacterium timidum*		

Table 16-2 *Continued*

PRESENT NAME	FORMER NAME/COMMENT	PRESENT NAME	FORMER NAME/COMMENT
C. methylpentosum	Human fecal flora	*C. ramosum*	*Eubacterium filamentosum, Ramibacterium ramosum, Actinomyces ramosus, Eubacterium ramosus*
C. orbiscindens	Human fecal flora		
Clostridium neonatale	New species—isolated from feces and blood of infant with neonatal necrotizing enterocolitis		
		C. scindens	New species—human fecal flora
C. orbiscindens	Human fecal flora	*C. symbiosum*	*Fusobacterium symbiosum*
C. perfringens	*C. welchii*	*C. tetanomorphorum*	Revived name—human infections

This is not intended to be an all-inclusive list. A number of species of no or doubtful clinical relevance have not been included, especially in the genera Bacteroides, Eubacterium, Lactobacillus, and Clostridium.
Based on information compiled from 1) references[7,71,122,125,177] and 2) numerous taxa published in the International Journal of Systematic and Evolutionary Microbiology, Volumes 47–54; 1997–2004.

Human Infections

Anaerobic bacteria have been encountered in infections involving virtually every organ and anatomic region of the body.[19,69] Some of the more commonly involved sites are illustrated in Figure 16-1.

Based on other reports in the literature, the relative incidence of anaerobes in infections is summarized in Table 16-4.[19,69,70]

Most deep-seated abscesses and necrotizing lesions involving anaerobes are polymicrobial, and may include obligate aerobes, facultative anaerobes, or microaerophiles as concomitant microorganisms.[69,70] These microorganisms, acting in concert with trauma, vascular stasis, or tissue necrosis, lower the oxygen tension and the oxidation-reduction potential in tissues, and provide favorable conditions for obligate anaerobes to multiply. Historically, infections and diseases involving anaerobes from exogenous sources are the ones that have been best known (Box 16-2).

Within the past few decades, however, endogenous anaerobic infections have become far more common. There are two probable explanations. One is that laboratory recovery of anaerobic bacteria has improved so that endogenous infections are no longer misdiagnosed or overlooked as they were in the past. The other is that a larger proportion of the patient population is receiving immunosuppressive drugs for malignancy and other disorders, resulting in compromised host resistance.[9,69,70] Primary anaerobic infections easily become established in areas of tissue damage, and bacteremia, metastatic spread of bacteria with formation of distant abscesses, and a progressive chain of events, sometimes resulting in a fatal outcome, may occur. The more common endogenous anaerobic infections are listed in Box 16-3.

It is essential to isolate and identify anaerobic bacteria because (1) these infections are associated with high morbidity and mortality and (2) the treatment of the infection varies with the bacterial species involved. Antibiotic therapy for certain anaerobic infections is different from that used for many infections caused by aerobic or facultatively anaerobic bacteria.[19,69] Prompt surgical intervention, including debridement of necrotic tissue or amputation of a limb, may be of extreme importance, particularly in cases of clostridial gas gangrene or in loculated abscesses in which antibiotics may be ineffective until the exudate is drained.

Prior to the mid-1960s, clostridial infections predominated. In recent years, however, <15% of all anaerobes isolated from such specimens were species of *Clostridium*.[135] Currently, more than three fourths of anaerobes isolated from properly selected clinical specimens are accounted for by the *Bacteroides fragilis* group, *Prevotella*, *Porphyromonas*, *Fusobacterium*, the anaerobic cocci, and the anaerobic gram-positive, non–spore-forming rods (see Table 16-3).

The most common disease-producing, anaerobic gram-negative, non–spore-forming rods isolated from clinical specimens are the *Bacteroides fragilis* and pigmented *Prevotella-Porphyromonas* (formerly the pigmented *Bacteroides*) groups and *Fusobacterium nucleatum*. *B. fragilis*, *B. thetaiotaomicron*, and other species of the *B. fragilis* group are especially common. They are particularly important not only because they may be isolated from a variety of life-threatening infections, but also because of their resistance to the action of penicillin and its analogues; their resistance to many cephalosporins, including the third-generation cephalosporins; the tetracyclines; the aminoglycosides; the emergence of resistance to several of the newer quinolones, and increasing resistance to clindamycin.[48,58,64,84,186,188,224]

Penicillin G was historically the antibiotic of choice for clinical infections caused by most anaerobic bacteria. Now, in addition to the *B. fragilis* group, *Fusobacterium mortiferum*, *F. varium*, members of the pigmented *Prevotella-Porphyromonas* group, *Prevotella bivia*, *P. disiens*, and some *Clostridium* species are resistant to penicillin G, some of its analogues, and many of the cephalosporins. Although the clostridia are recovered from anaerobic infections less frequently than *Bacteroides* species, *Fusobacterium* species, and the anaerobic cocci, they can be responsible for life-threatening illness.

The more common species of *Clostridium* isolated from clinical sources include *C. perfringens*, the *C. clostridioforme* group *C. ramosum*, *C. difficile*, *C. innocuum*, *C. septicum*, *C. sordellii*, and *C. bifermentans* (see Table 16-3).[7] Many *Clostridium* species are of unknown clinical impor-

Table 16-3 Anaerobes Most Important Clinically and/or Those Most Frequently Encountered in Clinical Specimens

Gram-negative rods

Bacteroides fragilis group (especially *B. fragilis, B. thetaiotaomicron, B. vulgatus, B. distasonis,* and *B. ovatus*)

Other *Bacteroides* (*B. ureolyticus*)

Porphyromonas (especially *P. asaccharolytica, P. gingivalis,* and *P. endodontalis*)

Pigmented *Prevotella* (*P. melaninogenica, P. loescheii, P. denticola, P. tannerae, P. intermedia, P. nigrescens,* and *P. corporis*)

Nonpigmented *Prevotella* (*P. oralis* group, *P. oris/buccae, P. bivia, P. disiens*)

Fusobacterium (especially *F. nucleatum, F. necrophorum, F. mortiferum,* and *F. varium*)

Bilophila wadsworthia

Anaerobic cocci

Gram-positive cocci (especially *Peptostreptococcus anaerobius, Finegoldia magna, Micromonas micros, Peptoniphilus asaccharolyticus, Anaerococcus prevotii,* and the microaerophilic streptococci, including *Streptococcus intermedius*)

Gram-negative cocci (*Veillonella* spp.)

Anaerobic Gram-positive, non–spore-forming rods

Actinomyces (especially *A. israelii, A. meyeri, A. naeslundii, A. odontolyticus,* and *A. viscosus*)

Propionibacterium (*P. acnes,* and *P. propionicum*)

Bifidobacterium dentium

Eubacterium (*E. limosum,* and *Eggerthella lenta* [*Eubacterium lentum*])

Gram-positive, spore-forming rods

Clostridium

   C. perfringens

   C. clostridioforme group (especially *C. clostridioforme, C. hathewayi,* and *C. bolteae*)

   C. innocuum

   C. ramosum

   C. difficile

   C. bifermentans

   C. sporogenes

   C. septicum

   C. sordellii

   C. novyi

   C. histolyticum

   C. botulinum

   C. tetani

tance; in most cases, their significance varies with the clinical setting.

Isolation of a *Clostridium* species from a wound, blood culture, or other body fluid does not necessarily have clinical significance. *C. perfringens*, the most frequently isolated *Clostridium* species, is a common inhabitant of the large bowel; it and other clostridia transiently contaminate the skin of the perianal area and other skin surfaces. *C. perfringens* is not always pathogenic. However, it, along with *C. difficile, C. septicum, C. botulinum, C. tetani,* and a few other clostridia are associated with major diseases and are discussed later in this chapter.

Actinomyces israelii is the major cause of actinomycosis. Other species that are established causes of actinomycosis, though less frequently encountered in this condition than *A. israelii,* are *A. naeslundii, A. odontolyticus, A. meyeri, A. viscosus, A. gerencseriae,* and *Propionibacterium propionicum* (formerly *Arachnia propionica*). Although encountered in relatively low frequency in routine specimens, these species are well-documented pathogens. Actinomycosis is an acute and chronic infectious disease characterized by suppurative lesions, abscesses, and draining sinus tracts. The disease most often presents as cervicofacial, thoracic, abdominal, or pelvic actinomycosis, but it can occur in other regions of the body.[6,202]

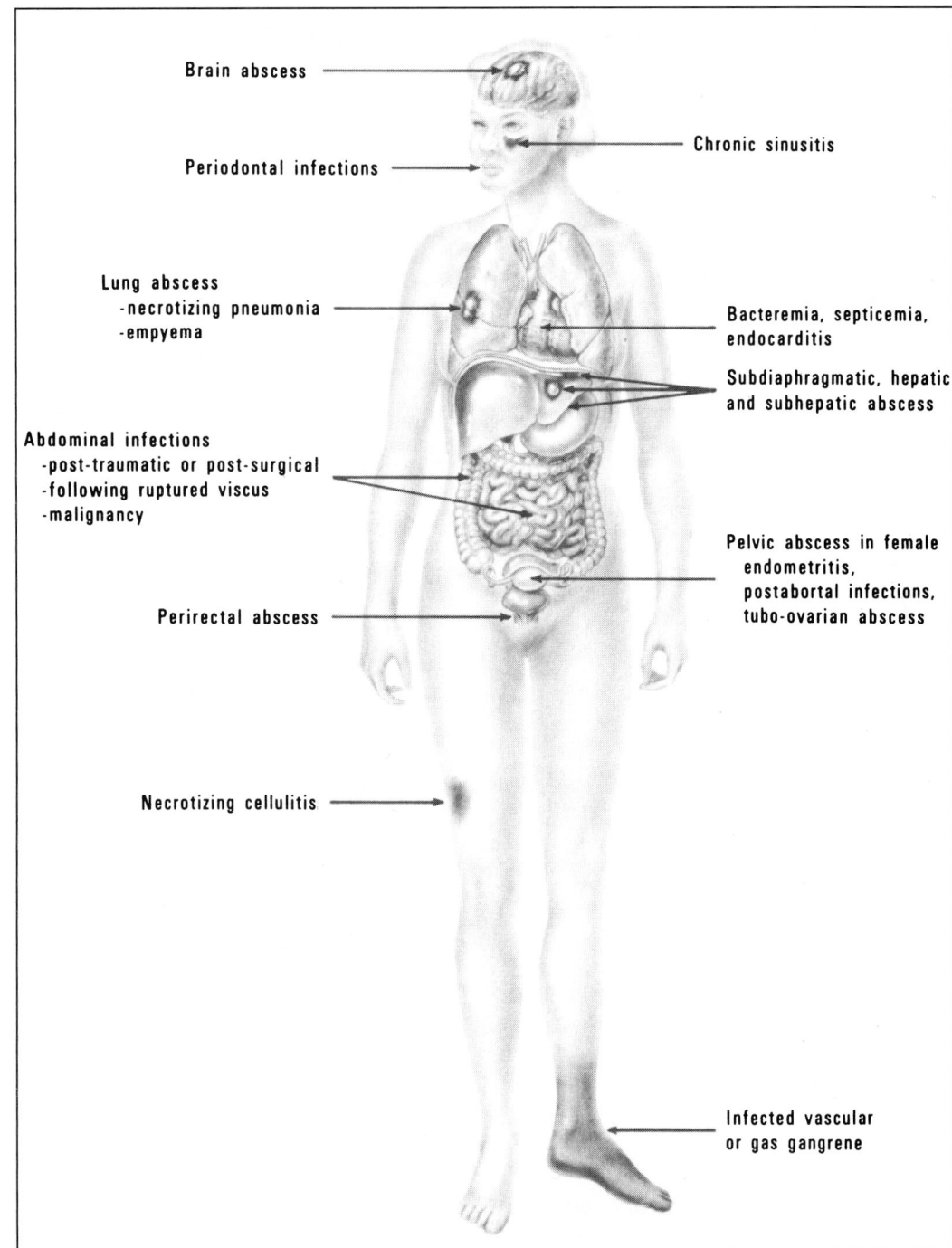

Figure 16-1 Common locations of infections involving anaerobic bacteria.

Bifidobacterium eriksonii (previously *Actinomyces eriksonii*, but now called *Bifidobacterium dentium*), a potential cause of pulmonary and genital tract infections, is the only documented pathogenic species of this genus.[34,70,72] Other bifidobacteria (e.g., *B. longum* and *B. breve*) are isolated rarely from clinical materials,[177] but are not known to have clinical significance. *Propionibacterium acnes*, usually a contaminant in clinical specimens, has been recovered from cases of endocarditis and other diseases, frequently those associated with implanted prosthetic devices.

The anaerobic cocci most commonly encountered in clinical specimens include *Finegoldia magna* (formerly *Peptostreptococcus magnus*), *Peptostreptococcus anaerobius*, *Peptoniphilus asaccharolyticus* (formerly *Peptostreptococcus asaccharolyticus*), *Anaerococcus prevotii* (formerly *Peptostreptococcus prevotii*), *Micromonas micros* (formerly *Peptostreptococcus micros*), and *Streptococcus intermedius*.[135] Current nomenclature changes for the anaerobic cocci are listed in Table 16-2. There is little doubt that some of the anaerobic cocci are pathogenic for humans in certain

Table 16-4 Incidence of Anaerobes in Infections

TYPE OF INFECTION	INCIDENCE (%)
Aspiration pneumonia, lung abscess, necrotizing pneumonia	62–93
Bacteremia	6–10
Brain abscess	60–89
Chronic sinusitis	52
Dental/oral	90–100
Empyema (thoracic)	76
Intraabdominal/pelvic sepsis	60–100
Miscellaneous soft-tissue infections:	53–83
Breast abscess	79–95
Postappendectomy and elective colon surgery	40
Osteomyelitis	77
Wounds	60–62
Perirectal abscess	75
Soft-tissue and cutaneous abscesses	100
Nonclostridial crepitant cellulitis	88
Gas gangrene (clostridial myonecrosis)	85–95
Pilonidal abscess	≤1
Diabetic foot ulcers, infected diabetic gangrene	
Urinary tract infection	

Modified from references[19,69,70].

Box 16-3 Anaerobic Infections of Endogenous Origin

Abscess of any organ
Actinomycosis
Antibiotic-associated diarrhea and colitis
Aspiration pneumonia
Complications of appendicitis or cholecystitis
Crepitant and noncrepitant cellulitis
Clostridial myonecrosis
Dental and periodontal infections
Endocarditis
Meningitis, usually following brain abscess
Necrotizing pneumonia
Osteomyelitis
Otitis media
Peritonitis
Septic arthritis
Sinusitis
Subdural empyema
Tetanus
Thoracic empyema

Anaerobic and microaerophilic cocci are also important in brain abscess, chronic maxillary sinusitis, anaerobic pleuropulmonary, and pelvic infections. While most first-line antimicrobial agents used in empirical treatment of anaerobic infections (in general) are active against the majority of these bacteria, resistance to clindamycin, metronidazole, ciprofloxacin, penicillin G, other penicillins, and certain cephalosporins has been reported among occasional strains of anaerobic cocci.[2,181]

Isolation of Anaerobic Bacteria

The steps involved in the laboratory diagnosis of anaerobic bacterial infections are similar to those for bacterial infections not involving anaerobes, as described in Chapters 1 and 2 of this book. It is particularly important that attention be paid to the proper selection, collection, and transport of clinical specimens for recovering anaerobic bacteria. The processing of specimens, selection of media, inoculation and incubation methods, and inspection of positive cultures are laboratory procedures that must be carefully quality-controlled. Performing any one step incorrectly may lead to erroneous results, thus creating the potential to supply misinformation to the physician.

Since Chapters 1 and 2 cover each of these steps in detail, with the exception of anaerobic blood cultures, only a few comments pertaining specifically to the anaerobic bacteria are included here.

Selection of Specimens for Culture

With few exceptions, all materials collected from sites not harboring an indigenous flora, such as body fluids other than urine, exudates from deep abscesses, fine-needle aspi-

clinical settings. At the Mayo Clinic, *F. magna* was recovered from 10% of anaerobic cultures collected from patients with suspected infections and was the anaerobic grampositive coccus isolated most frequently.[31] It was usually involved in bone and joint, soft-tissue, foot ulcer, and abdominal infections.

Box 16-2 Anaerobic Infections of Exogenous Origin

Clostridium difficile hospital-acquired (nosocomial) diarrhea
Foodborne botulism
Infant botulism
Wound botulism
Clostridium perfringens gastroenteritis
Myonecrosis (gas gangrene)
Tetanus
Crepitant cellulitis
Benign superficial infections
Infections following animal or human bites
Infections of injection-drug abusers
Septic abortion

Table 16-5 Specimens That Should Not Be Cultured for Anaerobic Bacteria

THROAT OR NASOPHARYNGEAL SWABS

Gingival swabs

Sputum or bronchoscopic specimens

Gastric contents, small-bowel contents, feces, rectal swabs, colocutaneous fistulae, colostomy stomata[a]

Surfaces of decubitus ulcers, swab samples of encrusted walls of abscesses, mucosal linings, and eschars

Material adjacent to skin or mucous membranes other than the above that have not been properly decontaminated

Voided urine

Vaginal or cervical swabs

[a] *When indicated clinically, specimens from these sources can aid in the diagnosis of botulism and for intestinal disease caused by Clostridium difficile and C. perfringens.*

rates, and tissue biopsies, should be cultured for anaerobic bacteria. However, since anaerobes normally inhabit the skin and mucous membranes as part of the normal indigenous flora, the specimens in the list in Table 16-5 are virtually always unacceptable for anaerobic culture because the results cannot be interpreted.

Collection and Transport of Specimens

When collecting specimens through the skin or mucous membranes, stringent precautions must be taken to decontaminate the surface properly. A surgical soap scrub should be used, followed by application of 70% ethyl or isopropyl alcohol, then tincture of iodine for 1 minute (in concentric circles starting from the center). Because some patients are sensitive or allergic to tincture of iodine, it is important to remove the iodine with alcohol after collecting the specimen.

Alternatively, an alcohol scrub followed by 10% povidone-iodine (Betadine) is also satisfactory provided the Betadine is allowed to remain on the skin for at least 2 minutes before the specimen is collected.

A needle and syringe should be used whenever possible for collecting specimens for anaerobic culture. Collection of swab specimens should be discouraged because they dry out and also because they expose anaerobes, if present, to ambient oxygen. Once the specimens are collected, particular precautions should be taken to protect them from oxygen exposure and to deliver them to the laboratory promptly.

Anaerobic Blood Culture (Summary of Guidelines for Traditional Broth and Instrumented Systems)

Blood-culture techniques should permit optimal recovery of obligate anaerobes as well as aerobes and facultative anaerobes. For many years, anaerobes were encountered in about 9–20% of all positive blood-culture sets at a number of medical centers.[68] In the late 1980s through the early 1990s, the percentage of gram-positive cocci (e.g., staphylococci, enterococci, streptococci) and Enterobacteriaceae in-

creased at Indiana University Medical Center and elsewhere, probably as a result of shifting antimicrobial treatments and greater proportions of immunocompromised patients in tertiary care. During the past two decades, anaerobes were widely reported to account for only about 2–5% of bacteremias.[47,51,140,153,184] Interestingly, a relative increase in numbers of patients with bacteremia involving species of the *Bacteroides fragilis* group that were less common during the 1970s and 1980s, and are now more resistant to antibiotics, has been documented recently at Indiana University Medical Center.[5] In addition, increased numbers of *Fusobacterium mortiferum, Clostridium* species, *Leptotrichia buccalis, Lactobacillus* species, and *Actinomyces* species are now being encountered, reflecting the emergence of anaerobes now resistant to a number of widely used antimicrobial agents. A recent report documented adverse outcomes in patients with antibiotic-resistant *Bacteroides* bacteremia,[186] stimulating renewed interest in the laboratory diagnosis of anaerobic bacteremia and the need for antimicrobial susceptibility testing of these bacteria.[98]

Similar to the collection of other specimens, the importance of decontaminating the skin at the venipuncture site cannot be overemphasized. For many years it was recommended that prior to venipuncture, the skin be prepared using alcohol and povidone-iodine.[197] Alternatively, chlorhexidine appears to be comparable to alcohol and povidone-iodine or alcohol and tincture of iodine,[14,175] and is now being used for skin antisepsis in a number of medical centers. It has long been recommended that skin flora contaminants (especially *Propionibacterium acnes* and coagulase-negative Staphylococci) should be in less than 3% of all blood specimens cultured, although there is wide variability between institutions.[207] Also, blood for culture should not be drawn through indwelling venous or arterial catheter lines unless it cannot be obtained by venipuncture.[197] To optimize recovery of microorganisms from patients with bloodstream infections, the blood specimen volume from adult patients should be 20 to 30 mL per venipuncture.[252] If the Bactec (Becton Dickinson Microbiology Systems, Sparks, MD) system is used, a 20-mL blood sample can be divided into three standard anaerobic and aerobic bottles (~7 mL/bottle). One or two of these bottles could be for anaerobic culture and the remainder for aerobic incubation. Alternatively, 8–10 mL blood can be inoculated into each Bactec Plus (Anaerobic/F and Aerobic/F) or 8–10 mL blood into a Bactec Lytic/10 Anaerobic F bottle. For neonates and older children, smaller volumes must be collected (e.g., ≤0.5 mL for an infant; 2–5 mL for an older child). Collection of more than two to three blood specimens per 24-hour period to diagnose a suspected episode of bacteremia is not required and is not recommended.[197,255]

Several traditional broth media formulations, available in unvented bottles under vacuum with CO_2, appear to be satisfactory for isolation of anaerobes (e.g., enriched thioglycolate medium, trypticase-soy broth, supplemented peptone broth, brain-heart infusion broth, *Brucella* broth, Columbia broth, and others).[197,250,251] These media are usually dispensed in volumes of about 40 to 100 mL per bottle.

For instrumented blood-culture systems, bottles currently available that support growth of obligately anaerobic bacteria, as well as facultatively anaerobic bacteria, are listed below.

Bactec Plus Anaerobic/F (resin, anaerobic; 3–10 mL of blood)

Bactec Lytic/10 Anaerobic F (lytic agent, anaerobic; 3–10 mL of blood)

Bactec Anaerobic F (standard anaerobic; 3–7 mL of blood)

BacT/Alert FN (FAN, anaerobic with activated charcoal; up to 10 mL of blood)

BacT/Alert (standard anaerobic; up to 10 mL of blood)

ESP 80N Anaerobic Broth (standard anaerobic; up to 10 mL of blood)

ESP 40N Anaerobic Broth (anaerobic broth inoculated with only 5 mL of blood)

The recommended blood to broth volume ratio for traditional blood culture bottles is 1:5 to 1:10.[197] However, the volume of medium was decreased in the Bactec resin–containing bottles to accommodate a higher blood volume. Thus, the inoculation of 10 mL into a Bactec Plus Anaerobic/F bottle creates a dilution factor of only 1:3.5; the resins in the medium offset the problem of residual antimicrobial activity that might be present in patients' blood.[137]

Although the addition of sodium polyanethol sulfonate (SPS) to blood-culture media enhances the recovery of most bacteria, including anaerobes, it may be inhibitory to some bacteria, such as the pathogenic *Neisseria* species. *Peptostreptococcus anaerobius* is the only anaerobe known to be inhibited by SPS in blood-culture media. *P. anaerobius* is so uncommon in blood cultures that special attempts to isolate it using special supplemented media (e.g., by adding 1.2% gelatin to overcome the SPS effect) may not be very cost-effective. The atmospheres of incubation for broth blood cultures should include at least one anaerobic bottle incubated unvented, and at least one aerobic bottle should be transiently vented per blood-culture set (if a traditional broth system is used). Instrumented blood culture systems have special head space anaerobic atmospheres containing nitrogen and carbon dioxide without oxygen. Both the aerobic and anaerobic bottles should be shaken during incubation and should be incubated at 35°C for 5 to 7 days. Traditional broth bottles should be inspected visually for growth (e.g., for turbidity, gas production, hemolysis, colonies in the sediment, etc.) twice daily during the first 72 hours and once daily thereafter. Gram stains and blind subcultures of traditional blood cultures should be performed aerobically during the first 6–12 hours of incubation, regardless of whether macroscopic evidence of growth is seen.[197] Blind anaerobic subcultures are not currently recommended for macroscopically negative traditional blood cultures. Negative cultures should be held for 5 to 7 days before they are finally reported as negative.

Blind subcultures are not required for the aerobic or anaerobic bottles in the Bactec, BacT/Alert, or ESP instrumented systems. When either the aerobic or anaerobic bottles show macroscopic evidence of growth, they should be subcultured onto chocolate agar (incubated in a 5–10% CO_2-air incubator) and anaerobe blood agar (incubated anaerobically). Also, the use of selective plating media for anaerobic subculture (such as phenylethyl alcohol anaerobe blood agar

or kanamycin-vancomycin blood agar), in addition to nonselective anaerobe blood agar, is recommended to aid in recovery of anaerobes in the setting of polymicrobial bacteremia. Anaerobes are isolated on occasion from the aerobic bottles (as well as from anaerobic bottles). Failure to perform anaerobic subcultures of macroscopically positive aerobic bottles is an unacceptable practice. With regard to recovering anaerobic bacteria, the lysis/centrifugation (Isolator; Wampole, Cranbury, NJ) system[250] and the Septichek (Roche, Indianapolis, IN) blood culture system[264] (discussed in Chapters 1 and 2), thus far, have performed only suboptimally compared with the traditional and Bactec broth systems for anaerobic blood culture. It is recommended that laboratories using either of these systems also use a traditional or an instrumented broth culture system (in addition) for anaerobic blood cultures.[129,254]

Direct Examination of Clinical Materials

Gross examination of specimens is particularly valuable in bringing to light the possible presence of anaerobes. A foul odor, purulent appearance of fluid specimens, and the presence of necrotic tissue and gas or sulfur granules are all valuable clues.

The importance of microscopic examination of clinical specimens has been emphasized by several authors, and the information derived may give immediate presumptive evidence that anaerobes are present.[125,166] In preparing slides for Gram-staining, methanol fixation is much better than traditional heat fixation. The background and cellular characteristics of the smear should be observed; and the Gram reaction; the size, shape, and arrangement of bacteria; and the relative number of organisms present should be recorded. The presence of spores, their shape and position in the bacterial cell, and other distinctive morphologic features such as branching, filaments with spherical bodies, pointed ends, and granular forms should be noted. Although the Gram stain is ordinarily satisfactory for determining cellular characteristics, the Giemsa and Wright's stains may occasionally reveal valuable additional information. Acridine orange stains are most worthwhile for detecting bacteria in blood cultures, cerebrospinal fluid (CSF), pleural fluid, joint fluid, and exudates.[142] The morphology of several anaerobes in stained preparations examined microscopically is illustrated in the photomicrographs included in Color Plates 16-1, 16-2, and 16-3 and in the color plates of Chapter 1.

The presence of numerous squamous epithelial cells without inflammatory cells in skin wounds and in respiratory and urogenital tract specimens usually indicates poor quality, superficially collected material that probably will yield mixtures of insignificant organisms from the normal flora or contaminants. It is worthwhile to limit the extent of identifications when the direct microscopic examinations reveal samples of poor quality. Of course, clinicians should be notified of the direct examination results and the problem of specimen quality discussed in a timely fashion prior to discarding the primary culture plates. Microbiologists should work closely with clinicians in an effort to enhance the quality and the clinical relevance of the specimens processed and the results reported.

Immunologic tests for the direct detection of anaerobic

antigens have had only limited successful applications. Fluorescent antibody products to detect *Clostridium chauvoei*, *C. novyi*, *C. septicum*, and *C. sordellii* are currently available for use in veterinary medicine (VMRD, Pullman, WA; www.vmrd.com). Fluorescent antibodies in kits developed commercially for *Bacteroides* species several years ago were hampered in general by nonspecificity and cross-reactions, with insufficient sensitivity to aid in direct identification of organisms in fresh specimens.

A number of procedures other than culture (discussed later in the chapter) can aid in the diagnosis of *Clostridium difficile*–associated disease (CDAD).[7,8] These include a latex agglutination test and an immunoassay for the glutamate dehydrogenase common antigen,[232] and gas-liquid chromatography to detect isocaproic acid.[119] Specificity has been an issue for these methods. Polymerase chain reaction (PCR) amplification procedures appear promising,[24,88,148] but are not commercially available. A *Clostridium difficile* cytotoxin B neutralization test, based on the use of antisera specific for toxin B, coupled with clinical findings, is considered to be the gold standard procedure against which other *C. difficile* diagnostic tests should be compared. There are problems with the cytotoxin B assay, however, including a relatively poor sensitivity, a turnaround time of 1 to 4 days, the requirement for tissue culture facilities, and lack of standardization among laboratories.[8,239]

Alternative immunologic procedures for the direct detection of *C. difficile* toxin(s) in fecal samples include several commercially available enzyme immunoassays (EIAs), which have been reviewed in detail elsewhere.[8] Commercial products recently evaluated in a major study by Turgeon et al.[239] include the Prima System *Clostridium difficile* Tox A (Trinity Biotech, Bray, Ireland) and the VIDAS *Clostridium difficile* Tox A II (BioMérieux-Vitek, Hazelwood, MO), both of which detect *C. difficile* toxin A. The Premier Cytoclone A/B (Meridian Diagnostics, Cincinnati, OH) and the *Clostridium difficile* Tox A/B (Techlab, Blacksburg, VA) detect both toxins A and B. The ImmunoCard *Clostridium difficile* (ICard; Meridian Diagnostics) and the Triage Micro *C. difficile* (Triage; Biosite Diagnostics, San Diego, CA) panels detect both the glutamate dehydrogenase common antigen and toxin A. All of these EIAs, and others reviewed by Allen et al.,[8] are rapid (e.g., 1-to-3-hour turnaround time), easy to use, and have offered promising alternatives to the traditional cytotoxin neutralization assays. Theoretically, both the sensitivity and specificity of direct *C. difficile* toxin testing in feces should be greatly improved using an EIA to detect the enterotoxin (toxin A) or the cytotoxin (toxin B), or both, produced by the organism in feces. Although a number of these EIAs appear to be very specific (e.g., 98% to >99% specificity), most are less sensitive than the cytotoxin B assays to which they have been compared (e.g., 56–82% sensitivity).[8,239]

It was once believed that both toxin A and toxin B of *C. difficile* were required for CDAD to be produced. It is now clear that severe illness may be caused by toxin A–negative/toxin B–positive strains of *C. difficile*, which could be missed if the EIA is designed to detect only toxin A.[1,120,149,260] New cases and outbreaks of toxin A–negative/toxin B–positive CDAD are being reported with increasing frequency worldwide. Thus, in addition to, or instead of an EIA for toxin A, a cytotoxin assay for toxin B and/or culture for toxigenic *C. difficile* can be recommended.[7]

Use of gas-liquid chromatography (GLC) to detect anaerobes in exudates and body fluids has been described but has not been widely popular.[86] The value of this procedure is increased by careful direct microscopic examination of material from the same specimens. A major amount of butyric acid in a specimen that contains only thin, pointed, gram-negative rods would suggest *Fusobacterium* species. A major peak of succinate and the presence of only gram-negative rods would suggest *Bacteroides* species, *Prevotella* species, or *Porphyromonas* species. A major propionate peak in a positive blood culture containing pleomorphic, non–spore-forming gram-positive rods (so-called diphtheroids) would be most consistent with *Propionibacterium* species. However, direct GLC provides only presumptive clues, and should be interpreted cautiously in polymicrobial infections.

Selection and Use of Media

The media used for recovering anaerobes from specimens should include nonselective, selective, and enrichment types, as illustrated in Table 16-6. Other media may also be included or substituted for those listed in Table 16-6. For example, chopped-meat glucose medium is commonly used instead of enriched thioglycolate medium; colistin nalidixic acid (CNA) agar may be used instead of phenylethyl alcohol (PEA) agar.

Either paromomycin-vancomycin blood agar or kanamycin-vancomycin blood agar can be used for the selective isolation of the gram-negative non–spore-forming anaerobes. Bacteroides bile esculin agar is recommended in the Wadsworth Anaerobic Bacteriology manual for the selection and presumptive identification of the *Bacteroides fragilis* group[125] and has also been found useful as a selective medium for *Bilophila wadsworthia*.[16] Results obtained with plating media formulations such as Schaedler, Columbia, Brucella, or others may not be entirely comparable to the morphology and growth characteristics of anaerobes seen on the Centers for Disease Control and Prevention (CDC) anaerobe blood agar base media formulations (see Color Plates 16-1 through 16-4).

The anaerobe blood agar used at the CDC and at Indiana University is recommended as a nonselective medium. It contains 5% defibrinated rabbit or sheep blood added to trypticase-soy agar (Becton Dickinson Microbiology Systems; BDMS, Cockeysville, MD), with L-cystine, yeast extract (Difco, Detroit, MI), vitamin K_2, and hemin added.[56] The formula is found in Box 16-4.

Plates of this medium are commercially available from Becton Dickinson Microbiology Systems and Remel (Lenexa, KS). Provided they do not dry out, commercially prepared anaerobe blood agar plates can be stored in the refrigerator in cellophane bags for at least 6 weeks.

Prior to use, the plates are held for 4 to 16 hours in an anaerobic jar or an anaerobic glove box in an atmosphere of 85% N_2, 10% H_2, and 5% CO_2. An added benefit of the CDC anaerobe blood agar described above is that the added L-cystine in the medium permits growth of certain thiol-dependent or sulfur-containing amino-acid–requiring bacteria such as *Fusobacterium necrophorum* and fastidious,

Table 16-6 Representative Media for Primary Isolation of Anaerobes From Clinical Specimens[a]

MEDIUM	MAJOR INGREDIENTS AND COMMENTS	PURPOSE
CDC anaerobe blood agar (AnBAP)	Trypticase soy agar base with 5% sheep blood; supplemented with yeast extract, hemin, vitamin K_1 and L-cystine for anaerobes requiring additional growth factors (e.g., *Prevotella melaninogenica, Fusobacterium necrophorum,* and others). Additional media bases, including Brucella, brain-heart infusion, Schaedler, and Columbia blood agar support excellent growth of many anaerobes, but morphology and other characteristics tend to differ on these media.	Nonselective blood agar–plating medium for primary isolation of essentially all types of anaerobes found in clinical materials (see text and Color Plates 16–1 through 16–4).
Anaerobe phenylethyl alcohol blood agar (PEA)	In addition to containing the same ingredients as the CDC anaerobe blood agar formulation above, this medium has phenylethyl alcohol (2.5 g/L). PEA inhibits the swarming of *Proteus* spp. and inhibits the growth of many other gram-negative facultatively anaerobic bacteria, including most *Enterobacteriaceae.* PEA is volatile. Plates should be tightly sealed in cellophane or plastic bags and stored at 4°C. A batch of plates that no longer inhibits the swarming of *Proteus* should be discarded, regardless of the expiration date.	PEA medium aids in selective isolation of anaerobes from infected materials containing a mixture of bacteria. It should support good growth of most gram-positive and gram-negative obligately anaerobic bacteria. Facultatively anaerobic gram-positive bacteria such as staphylococci, streptococci, *Bacillus* spp., and coryneform bacteria also grow well on it.
Anaerobe kanamycin-vancomycin blood agar (KV)	Contains the same CDC anaerobe blood agar formulation as AnBAP above, but in addition, contains 100 mg/L of kanamycin and 7.5 mg/L of vancomycin. The kanamycin inhibits many (but not all) facultatively anaerobic gram-negative rods and the vancomycin inhibits gram-positive bacteria in general (including most gram-positive anaerobes and nonanaerobes). Vancomycin in this concentration can also inhibit the *Porphyromonas* spp.	KV medium is useful for selective isolation of most *Bacteroides* spp., *Prevotella* spp., *Fusobacterium* spp., and *Veillonella* spp. from clinical specimens containing mixed aerobic and anaerobic bacteria.
Anaerobe laked paromomycin-vancomycin blood agar (PV)	Laked PV medium is similar to the formulation above, except that 100 mg/L of paromomycin is substituted for the kanamycin. Also in PV, the blood is laked before it is added (by freezing and thawing the blood). Performance is similar to KV, except that the paromomycin may inhibit some additional facultative anaerobes that are resistant to kanamycin, such as some strains of *Klebsiella* spp. Similar to KV agar, laked PV should inhibit growth of gram-positive organisms in general. The laked blood may aid in early recognition of pigmented *Prevotella.*	Laked PV is an excellent medium for selective primary isolation of organisms in the *Bacteroides fragilis* group, the pigmented and nonpigmented *Prevotella* spp., *Fusobacterium nucleatum, F. necrophorum, F. mortiferum, Veillonella,* and other obligately anaerobic gram-negative non–spore-forming anaerobes. It is not necessary to use both KV and PV; rather, it is reasonable to select one or the other of these media, based on preferences of the microbiologist.
Cycloserine-cefoxitin fructose agar (CCFA)	Trypticase-soy or proteose peptone base containing fructose and neutral red indicator. In addition, cycloserine (500 mg/L) and cefoxitin (16 mg/L) are added to inhibit intestinal flora. *C. difficile,* at 48 hours of incubation, forms 4 mm or larger yellowish rhizoid colonies that have birefringent crystalline internal structures ("speckled opalescence"). *C. difficile* colonies show yellow-green fluorescence under long-wave UV light (their odor is reminiscent of horse manure). *C. difficile* is negative for both lipase and lecithinase activity.	CCFA is for selective isolation of *C. difficile* from stool specimens or other intestinal materials. However, growth on CCFA is not specific for only *C. difficile;* therefore, identification of pure culture isolates is still required. (It is common to find breakthrough growth on the medium of unwanted *Enterobacteriaceae, Bacillus* spp., staphylococci, and other clostridia).
Enriched thioglycolate medium (THIO)	THIO is an enriched liquid medium prepared by supplementing the BBL-0135C formula thioglycolate medium (without indicator) with hemin and vitamin K_1.	This is a noninhibitory broth that is especially useful for primary isolation of actinomycetes. THIO is also an excellent supplement or backup to solid plating media for isolation of slow-growing or fastidious organisms. It should support good growth of essentially all anaerobes commonly found in clinical materials.

[a] *All the media in this table are available in prepared form from several manufacturers (see text). All but CCFA were originally described by Dowell, Lombard, and colleagues in a CDC manual.*[56] *For more information on CCFA, publications by George et al.,*[77] *Bartley and Dowell,*[22] *and Marler et al.*[167] *are recommended.*

Box 16-4 CDC Anaerobe Blood Agar

INGREDIENT	AMOUNT
Trypticase-soy agar (BDMS)	15 g
Phytone (BDMS)	5 g
Sodium chloride	5 g
Agar	20 g
Yeast extract (Difco)	5 g
Hemin	5 mg
Vitamin K_1 (3-phytylmenadione)	10 mg
L-Cystine	400 mg
Demineralized water	1 L
Blood (sheep or rabbit), defibrinated	50 mL

Box 16-5 Principles for Optimal Recovery of Anaerobes

1. Proper collection and transport of the clinical specimens
2. Processing of specimens with minimal exposure to atmospheric oxygen
3. Use of fresh or prereduced media
4. Proper use of an anaerobic system, with inclusion of an active catalyst to allow removal of oxygen (from jar or glove box system)

thiol-dependent streptococci that have been isolated from patients with endocarditis.[9] This medium also supports excellent growth of the strict anaerobes *Clostridium novyi* type B, and *Clostridium haemolyticum*.

The phenylethyl alcohol blood agar is prepared by supplementing the anaerobe blood agar described above with 0.25% phenylethyl alcohol. Similarly, the kanamycin-vancomycin or the paromomycin-vancomycin blood agar is prepared by adding 100 μg of kanamycin or paromomycin and 7.5 μg of vancomycin per milliliter of the blood agar medium.

The enriched thioglycolate medium (BBL-135C with hemin and vitamin K_1 supplement) is primarily recommended as a backup to the plating media.[56] This medium is particularly helpful for cultivating slow-growing species of *Actinomyces*. Chopped-meat glucose broth, a good alternative to enriched thioglycolate medium, is useful for isolation of *Clostridium* species by the spore selection technique and as a holding medium for anaerobic cultures in general.

Other special purpose selective media for primary isolation of anaerobes in normal flora studies have been described in detail in the Wadsworth Manual.[125] In addition, Smith and Moore described selective media and a cold enrichment technique to aid in isolation of *Mobiluncus* species from vaginal specimens.[220] Eley et al. reported on a selective and differential medium for isolation of *Bacteroides ureolyticus*.[59] Lee and coworkers developed a new selective medium for *Bacteroides gracilis*.[147] Malnick and associates formulated a new selective medium for isolating *Anaerobiospirillum* spp. from feces.[164] Additional special-purpose selective media and isolation procedures have been developed for the isolation and enumeration of *Clostridium difficile*, *C. perfringens*, and *C. botulinum* from feces (and/or food samples).[7,22,125]

Anaerobic Systems for the Cultivation of Anaerobic Bacteria

Comparative studies have shown that the following systems are satisfactory for the cultivation of anaerobic bacteria commonly associated with human disease if used properly[130,201]: evacuation-replacement jars; anaerobic jars with disposable gas generators; anaerobic glove box techniques;

roll tube and roll-streak tube with prereduced anaerobically sterilized (PRAS) media. To ensure optimal results, the general principles listed in Box 16-5 must be followed.

Anaerobic Jar Techniques

Anaerobic jars are commonly used for cultivating anaerobic bacteria on primary plating media or on subculture plates. The GasPak jar (Becton Dickinson), illustrated in Figure 16-2, has long been used in clinical laboratories in the United States.

The Oxoid anaerobic jar (Fig. 16-3) has a metal lid, Schrader valves and a pressure gauge. Like the GasPak jar, the Oxoid jar can be used either as an evacuation-replacement jar, or it can be used with a disposable gas generator. Other commercially available sources of anaerobic jars in-

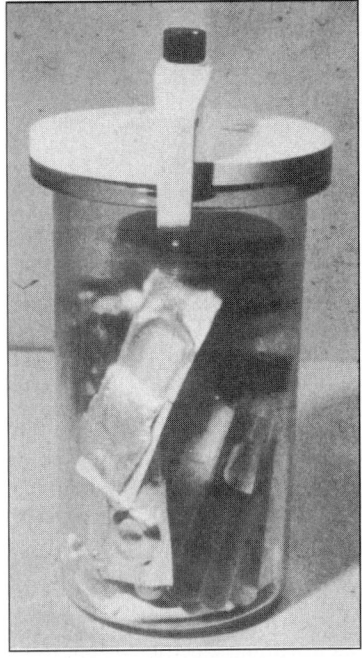

Figure 16-2 The GasPak (Becton Dickinson Microbiology Systems, Cockeysville, MD) anaerobic system: The jar contains inoculated plates, broth tubes, a GasPak hydrogen and carbon dioxide generator envelope, a disposable methylene blue indicator strip, and a catalyst basket in the lid.

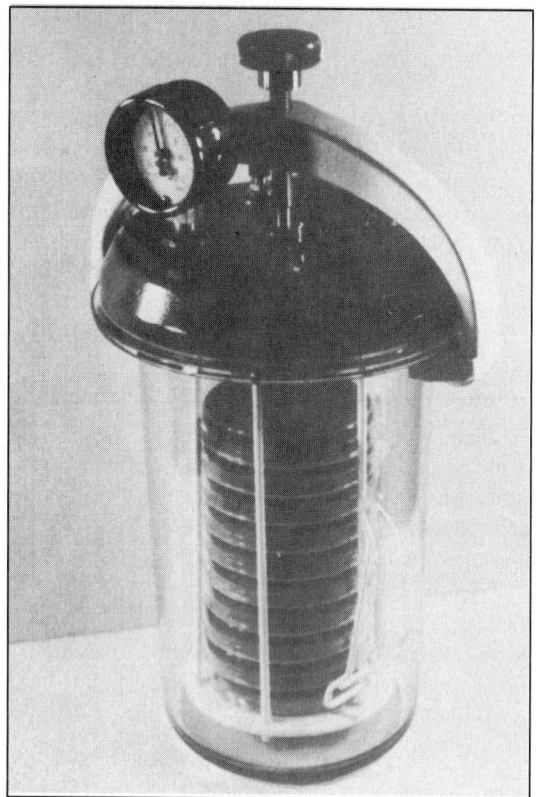

Figure 16-3 The Oxoid anaerobic jar (Oxoid USA, Columbia, MD) contains a 3.5-L polycarbonate jar closed by a heavy-duty metal lid and metal clamp. The lid center has two Schrader valves and a plus-or-minus pressure gauge, with two valves to facilitate the evacuation/replacement (E/R) technique. There is also a safety valve in the lid to prevent extra gas pressure caused by incorrect use of the E/R technique. A sachet containing a low-temperature catalyst is clipped to the undersurface of the lid. In lieu of using the E/R technique, the jar can be used with the Oxoid generating kit available from the manufacturer.

clude Almoore (Hardy Diagnostics, Santa Maria, CA), Key Scientific Products, Rockville, MD), Mitsubishi Gas Chemical America (New York, NY) and EM Science (Darmstadt, Germany).

The basic principle of the jars that require catalyst (e.g., GasPak) is the removal of oxygen from the chamber by reaction with hydrogen added to the system in the presence of the catalyst. Oxygen is reduced to water as follows:

$$2H_2 + O_2 \xrightleftharpoons{\text{catalyst}} 2H_2O$$

The older Brewer jar technique used a palladium catalyst in the lid of the jar (a modified McIntosh-Fildes jar), which had to be heated with an electric current to be fully active. The GasPak jar uses a "cold" catalyst, composed of palladium-coated aluminum pellets, which does not require heating. The cold catalyst is more convenient to use and has no explosion hazard. The cold palladium catalyst can be inactivated in the jar by the production of hydrogen sulfide

or other volatile metabolic products of the bacteria. It is recommended that the catalyst pellets be replaced with new or rejuvenated pellets each time the jar is used. The pellets can be rejuvenated or restored to full activity by heating them in a dry-heat oven at 160 to 170°C for 2 hours. After heating, the pellets are stored at room temperature in a clean, dry container or in a desiccator until the time of use.

Anaerobic conditions can be produced in jar systems with either the disposable hydrogen-carbon dioxide generator (GasPak, Oxoid) or by the evacuation/replacement procedure. The evacuation/replacement procedure, in which the air in the jar is removed and replaced with a mixture of 85% N_2, 10% H_2, and 5% CO_2 is more economical than gas generators and allows anaerobic conditions to be established more rapidly. Any airtight container can be used, including a GasPak jar with a vented lid, a Brewer jar, an Oxoid jar, or even a modified pressure cooker.

Whaley and Gorman described an inexpensive device for evacuating and gassing jars or other systems.[258] This device can be used with an in-house vacuum, thereby eliminating the need for a vacuum pump when the evacuation/replacement procedure is used. Air is evacuated from the jar by drawing a vacuum of 20 to 24 inches of mercury. This procedure is repeated three times. The jar is then filled with N_2 after the first two evacuations and the final replacement is made with the 85% N_2, 10% H_2, and 5% CO_2 gas mixture.

The Anoxomat (Mart Microbiology, Lichtenvoorde, The Netherlands) is an automated evacuation/replacement system. Although it is similar in principle to the procedure described above, studies have shown somewhat better growth using the Anoxomat than with the other anaerobic systems with which it was compared.[32,215]

The GasPak disposable H_2 and CO_2 generators are used by opening the generator envelope and placing it into the jar to be used. Approximately 10 mL of water is added to allow the generation of hydrogen and carbon dioxide, and the lid is tightly sealed. If the lid is not warm to the touch within 40 minutes after it is sealed, or if condensation does not appear on the inner surface of the glass within 25 minutes, the jar should be opened and the generator envelope discarded and replaced with a new generator. A defective gasket in the lid that allows escape of gas or inactivated catalyst pellets are the two most common causes of failure of this system.

Anaerobic conditions should always be monitored when using either of the two jar techniques by including an oxidation-reduction indicator. Methylene blue strips are available commercially for this purpose (BD Microbiology Systems). Alternatively, a 13-mm × 100-mm test tube containing a few milliliters of methylene blue-$NaHCO_3$-glucose mixture can be placed in the jar.[53] Methylene blue is blue when oxidized, clear when reduced. The color changes at about +11.0 mV. Thus, if anaerobic conditions are achieved, the methylene blue indicator solution will gradually turn colorless and will remain that way if there are no leaks that allow additional oxygen to enter the system. If the solution turns blue after being colorless, this indicates that anaerobic conditions were not maintained and that the culture results may not be valid.

The GasPak 100 Anaerobic system has been analyzed with respect to O_2 and CO_2 concentrations, time of appearance of water condensate, catalyst temperature and Eh of commercially prepared plated media at various time intervals at 20 to 25°C.[208] The O_2 concentration was 0.2–0.6% within 60 minutes after activating the generator and less than 0.2% at 100 minutes. The CO_2 concentration was 4.6–6.2% at 60 minutes after activation. The Eh of the three different media tested varied from $+60$ mV (Columbia agar with 5% sheep blood) to $+500$ mV (Schaedler agar with 5% sheep blood) at zero time. The Eh ranged from -30 mV to -229 mV after 60 minutes and ranged from -115 mV to -300 mV after 100 minutes. This indicates rapid reduction of the media, even though the methylene blue indicator did not become decolorized in less than 6 hours at 25°C. At 35°C, the methylene blue usually becomes reduced in about 5 hours, and it is likely that the media is reduced more rapidly at 35°C than at 25°C. However, if ambient air enters the system, the methylene blue indicator changes to blue within minutes.

Relatively recently, anaerobic gas-generating systems have been introduced that do not require either catalyst or the addition of water to activate these systems. The AnaeroPack (Mitsubishi Gas Chemical America, New York, NY), for example, absorbs oxygen and generates carbon dioxide, but does not generate hydrogen. It appears to be an excellent alternative to the GasPak and other established anaerobic incubation systems.[49] Another type of commercially available catalyst-free system makes use of iron filings in a sachet to which water is added (Anaerocult, Merck, Darmstadt, Germany), producing an oxygen-free, carbon dioxide–rich atmosphere.[125]

Use of the Anaerobic Glove Box

An anaerobic glove box (or anaerobic chamber) is a self-contained anaerobic system that allows the microbiologist to process specimens and perform most bacteriologic techniques for isolation and identification of anaerobic bacteria without exposure to air. Glove boxes suitable for cultivation of anaerobes can be constructed from various materials, including steel, acrylic plastic, or fiberglass (Fig. 16-4). The flexible vinyl plastic anaerobic chamber developed at the University of Michigan has enjoyed wide popularity,[11] and a modification of this design is available in varying sizes from Coy Manufacturing (Ann Arbor, MI). A glove box of different design is shown in Figure 16-5. Other manufacturers of anaerobic glove boxes include Forma Scientific (Marietta, OH), and Toucan Technologies (Cincinnati, OH). Rigid, "gloveless," glove boxes are marketed by Anaerobe Systems (Bactron Anaerobe Chamber; Sheldon Manufacturing, Cornelius, OR) and by Russkinn Technology and Don Whitley (Shipley, West Yorkshire, England).

An anaerobic glove box, if properly constructed, is economical to operate because it permits the use of conventional plating media and the cost of gases for operation of the system is minimal. Once set up, the major expense is for the 85% nitrogen–10% hydrogen–5% carbon dioxide gas mixture used to replace the air in the entry lock when materials are passed into the glove box chamber.

The Roll-Streak System

The roll-streak system, developed by W.E.C. Moore and associates of the VPI Anaerobe Laboratory[107], is a modification of the roll-tube technique developed by Hungate and associates for culturing anaerobic bacteria from the rumen of cows and other herbivorous animals. Equipment for the VPI anaerobic culture system (including Hungate tubes) is available commercially from Bellco Glass (Vineland, NJ).

The roll-streak system uses PRAS media prepared in tubes with rubber stoppers. After autoclaving, the tubes of agar media are cooled in a rolling machine, which results in a thin coating of the inner surfaces of the tubes with solidified medium. Both the roll-streak tubes and the PRAS liquid media require the addition of a reducing agent, such as L-cysteine-hydrochloride, which is added just before autoclaving to help maintain a low oxidation-reduction potential

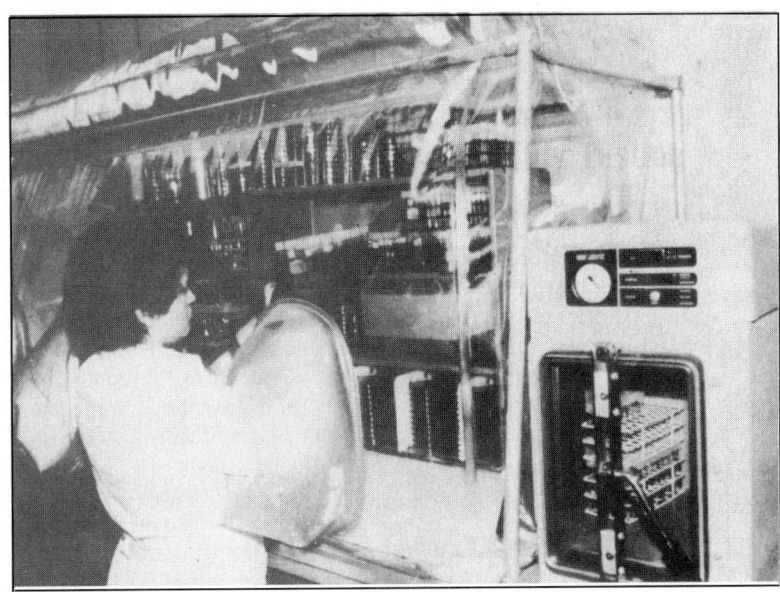

Figure 16-4 The anaerobic glove box (Coy Laboratory Products, Ann Arbor, MI). Materials are passed in and out of the large, flexible plastic chamber through an automatic entry lock. Anaerobic conditions are maintained by constant recirculation of the atmosphere within the plastic chamber (85% N_2, 10% H_2, and 5% CO_2) through a palladium catalyst. Cultures are incubated either within a separate incubator inside the glove box, or by maintaining the entire chamber at 35°C through use of heated catalyst boxes.

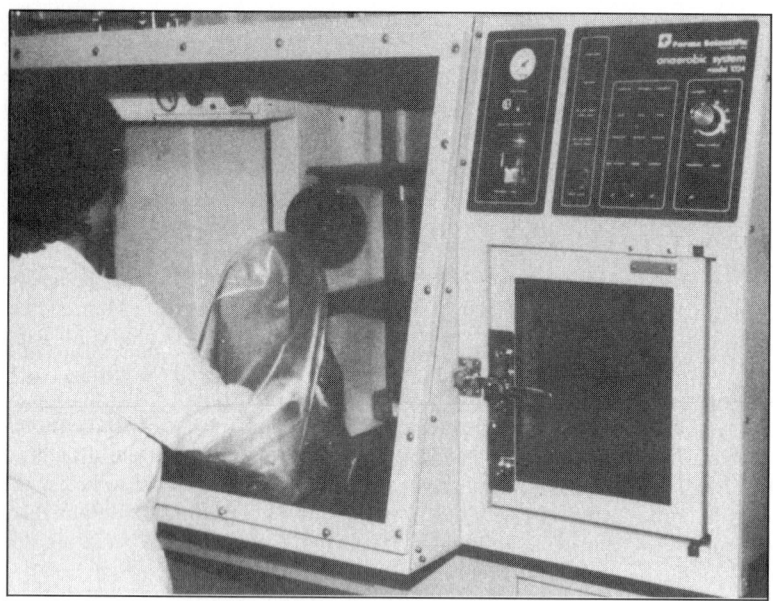

Figure 16-5 The Forma Model 1024 anaerobic glove box (Forma Scientific, Marietta, OH). This system has an automatic entry lock. During routine daily operation, atmospheric air is bubbled through a methylene blue–glucose–HEPES buffer solution, which aids in monitoring O_2 leaks or determining if the catalyst is not working properly.

within the system. All inoculating and subculturing of the PRAS solid and liquid media are performed under a stream of oxygen-free carbon dioxide, which minimizes exposure to air and helps to maintain a reduced oxidation-reduction potential in the media before and after growth of the obligate anaerobes. The Hungate technique requires less equipment than the roll-streak technique for inoculating liquid media. A needle and syringe are used to inoculate PRAS media in Hungate tubes through a rubber stopper–screw cap closure assembly.

Anaerobic Disposable Plastic Bags

The Anaerobic Bag system is available from BD Microbiology Systems (Sparks, MD). A second system called the AnaeroPouch is available from Mitsubishi (New York, NY). A third anaerobic disposable bag system, called the Anaerocult P, is manufactured in Germany (Merck, Darmstadt, Germany). Additional bag systems are the Anaerogen (Oxoid) and the Anabag (Hardy Diagnostics).

The Anaerobic Bag (BD) consists of a clear-plastic bag (sold in varying sizes capable of holding one to three, 100-mm-diameter Petri dishes), an H_2-CO_2 gas generator that generates an atmosphere when water is added to it (analogous to the generator used in a GasPak jar), cold palladium catalyst pellets, and a resazurin indicator. The bag is heat-sealed following activation of the generator to permit maintenance of anaerobic conditions according to the same principle as described for the GasPak jar system.

On the other hand, the AnaeroPouch and the Anaerocult both achieve anaerobic conditions differently, without catalyst, to remove oxygen from the atmosphere and generate CO_2. Oxygen is removed from within the sealed Anaerocult pouch by combining with iron powder to produce iron oxides. These anaerobic bag systems appear to be practical alternatives to anaerobic jar or glove box systems for the incubation of anaerobes when only a few plates are to be incubated.

Use of the Anaerobic Holding Jar

A modification of the Martin holding jar procedure is a convenient and inexpensive adjunct to the jar and glove box anaerobic systems that allows primary plating, inspection of cultures, and subculture of colonies at the bench with only minimal exposure of anaerobic bacteria to atmospheric oxygen.[9,168]

The holding jar assembly is illustrated in Figure 16-6, and its use is briefly described in Box 16-6.

Inexpensive, commercial-grade N_2 can be used in the holding jar system. Open the small needle valve on the gas manifold (Fig. 16-7) and set the gas-tank regulator to 4 lb/in² for 20 to 30 seconds to rapidly purge the jar of air. Then turn the regulator pressure down to about ½ to 1 lb/in² and regulate the flow to each jar at 50 to 100 mL/min, using the small needle valve on the manifold. This is equivalent to a flow rate of one to two bubbles per second when the rubber tubing in the jar is placed just beneath the surface of water in a beaker. Alternatively, CO_2 passed through a tube of heated copper catalyst (Sargent furnace) can be used in the holding jars instead of N_2.

Incubation of Cultures

In most instances, 35 to 37°C is the temperature most satisfactory for primary isolation of anaerobic bacteria from clinical specimens. Plates inoculated at the bench and placed in anaerobic jars should be incubated for at least 48 hours, and reincubated for another 2–4 days to allow slow-growing organisms to form colonies; some anaerobes, such as certain species of *Actinomyces* and *Eubacterium*, grow rather slowly, and colonies may not be detected if jars are opened sooner. Also, if the jar is opened too soon, some of the slow-growing organisms may be killed owing to oxygen exposure. In emergency situations, duplicate sets of plating media can be incubated in two different jars, one set incubated for 18

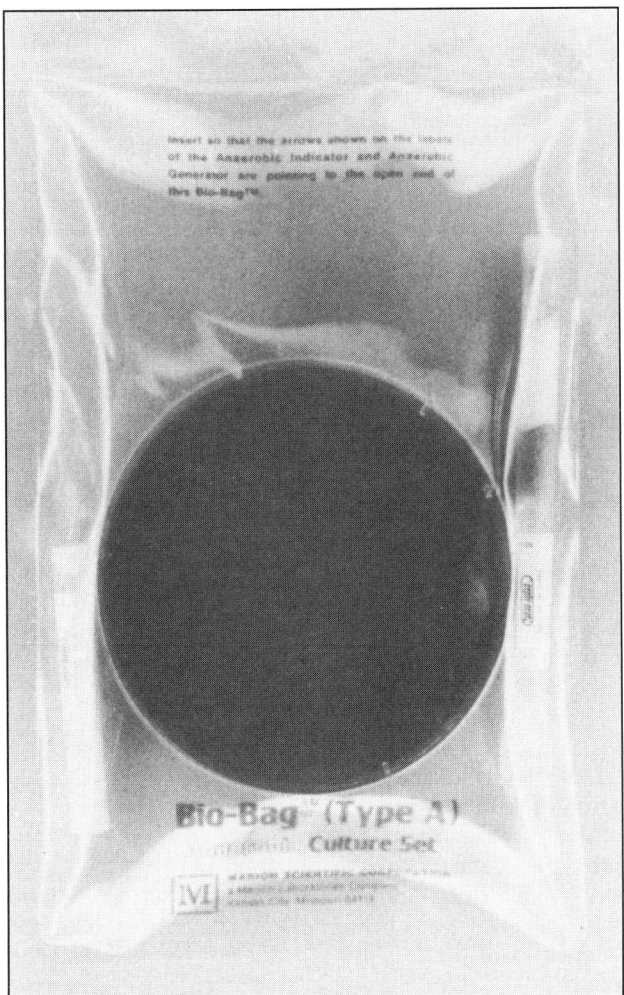

Figure 16-6 The Anaerobic Bag Culture Set (Becton Dickinson Microbiology Systems, Sparks, MD). This culture set includes a plate of CDC–anaerobic blood agar contained within an oxygen-impermeable bag. The system contains its own gas-generating kit and cold catalyst.

<table>
<tr><td colspan="2">

Box 16-6 Anaerobic Holding Jar Procedure

</td></tr>
</table>

1. Three holding jars are used, the first to hold uninoculated media, the second for plates on which colonies to be subcultured are growing, and the third to receive freshly inoculated plates of media.
2. Commercially prepared agar plates or agar media freshly prepared in the laboratory can be used. These may be held in a refrigerator for up to 6 weeks if bagged in cellophane.
3. The plates to be used on any given day should first be placed in an anaerobic glove box or an anaerobic jar for 4 to 15 hours before use to reduce the media.
4. As needed, the reduced media are placed in the first holding jar and continuously flushed with a gentle stream of N2.
5. The plates of reduced media are surface-inoculated, one at a time, in ambient air and immediately placed in the third holding jar, which is also flushed with N2. The second holding jar is used to hold any plates removed from the GasPak jar that require subculture.
6. After the jar containing the newly inoculated plates is filled, the plates can be transferred to a conventional anaerobic system, such as a GasPak jar, or into an anaerobic glove box for incubation at 35°C.

obes. PRAS media in rubber-stoppered tubes can also be used. It is not necessary to boil the tubes of enriched thioglycolate or chopped-meat glucose broth if they are prepared in tight-fitting screw-capped tubes and gassed in a glove box after autoclaving. Unless growth is apparent visually, broth cultures should be held a minimum of 5 to 7 days before discarding them as negative.

to 24 hours and the other for 3 to 5 days. This procedure allows rapid isolation of fast-growing anaerobes in the 18- to 24-hour jar and the later recovery of slow growers in the jars left for delayed incubation. If clostridial myonecrosis is suspected clinically, plates can be inspected as early as 6 to 12 hours after inoculation.

Prolonged exposure of freshly inoculated plates to ambient air must be avoided. Certain anaerobes commonly encountered in clinical specimens, such as *Peptostreptococcus anaerobius*, may either fail to grow or may exhibit a prolonged lag in growth when freshly inoculated plates are held in ambient air for as short a time as 2 hours. Thus, if a holding jar procedure is not used, inoculated plates must be immediately placed in an anaerobic system (anaerobic jar or anaerobic glove box) to allow for effective cultivation of these anaerobes.

Enriched thioglycolate and chopped-meat glucose media should also be inoculated with clinical materials incubated in an anaerobic system to allow maximum recovery of anaer-

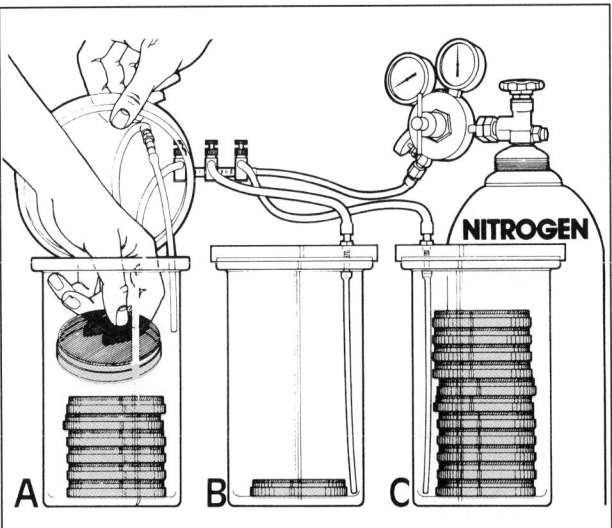

Figure 16-7 Schematic of the anaerobic-holding jar system. The flow rate of nitrogen to each jar is regulated by the needle valves on the manifold (three-gang valve, available where aquarium supplies are sold). Jars *A, B,* and *C* contain uninoculated plates, plates with colonies to be subcultured, and freshly inoculated plates, respectively.

Inspection and Subculture of Colonies

After incubation, plates incubated in 5–10% CO_2 atmospheres should be examined with a hand lens or, preferably, a dissecting microscope. If anaerobic jars are used, a holding jar system should be used at the time of colony examination and subculture to minimize exposure of oxygen-sensitive isolates to air. The anaerobic glove box and the anaerobic disposable bag systems (Fig. 16-6), allow inspection of colonies in the absence of air.

Use of the stereoscopic dissecting microscope during examination of colonies is extremely helpful because a number of anaerobes have distinctive colonial features. The dissecting microscope is also a valuable aid during the subculture of colonies to obtain pure culture isolates.

During the inspection of colonies, any action on the medium, such as hemolysis of blood agar or clearing of egg yolk agar, as well as the size and distinctive features of the colonies should be recorded. A number of characteristic colonies of anaerobes are illustrated in Color Plates 16-1, 16-2, and 16-3. When recording colony characteristics, the following should be noted: the age of the culture and the name of the medium, the diameter in millimeters of each colony in addition to its color, surface features (glistening, dull), density (opaque, translucent), consistency (butyrous, viscid, membranous, brittle), and other descriptive features (see Chapters 1 and 2).

Gram-stained smears of colonies from the anaerobic and CO_2-incubated plates should also be examined. Do not assume on the basis of colony and microscopic features only that colonies on plates that have been incubated in an anaerobic system are obligate anaerobes. Although the morphology and colony characteristics of certain anaerobes are distinctive, it is often impossible to distinguish some facultative anaerobes from obligate anaerobes without aerotolerance tests, even when the CO_2 incubated plates show no growth.

The number of different colony types on the anaerobe plates should be determined and a semiquantitative estimate of the number of each type should be recorded (light, moderate, or heavy growth). Using a needle or a sterile Pasteur capillary pipette, transfer each different colony to another anaerobe blood agar plate to obtain a pure culture and an aerobic blood agar plate for aerotolerance testing (described below). If colonies are well separated on the primary isolation plate, a tube of enrichment broth, such as enriched thioglycolate or chopped-meat glucose medium, should be inoculated to provide a source of inoculum for differential tests.

After incubation, Gram-stain the enriched thioglycolate and chopped-meat glucose subcultures. If the organisms appear to be in pure culture, they can be used to inoculate appropriate differential media for identification of isolates.

Examine enriched thioglycolate and chopped-meat glucose cultures that were inoculated with the original specimen along with all primary isolation plates. If no growth is evident on the primary anaerobic plates, or if the colonies isolated fail to account for all the morphologic types found in the direct Gram-stained smear of the specimen, each broth medium should be subcultured to two anaerobe blood agar plates, one for anaerobic incubation and the other incubated in a 5–10% CO_2 air incubator. Alternatively, a chocolate agar plate can be used for the subculture plate to be incubated in the 5–10% CO_2-air incubator. These subculture plates should then be examined as described above.

Aerotolerance Tests

Each colony type from the anaerobic isolation plate is subcultured to an aerobic (5–10% CO_2, or candle jar) and anaerobic blood agar plate for overnight incubation.

Haemophilus influenzae, which grows on anaerobic blood agar anaerobically but not on ordinary blood agar aerobically, can be mistaken for an anaerobe. This can be avoided by inoculating a chocolate agar plate (in place of the aerobic blood agar plate) for incubation in a 5–10% CO_2-air incubator. It may be expedient to inoculate quadrants or sixths of the chocolate agar plate for testing the aerotolerance of four to six colonies from a primary isolation plate (Fig. 16-8). However, this should be done only if colonies are well separated or were picked from a purity plate. Otherwise, single

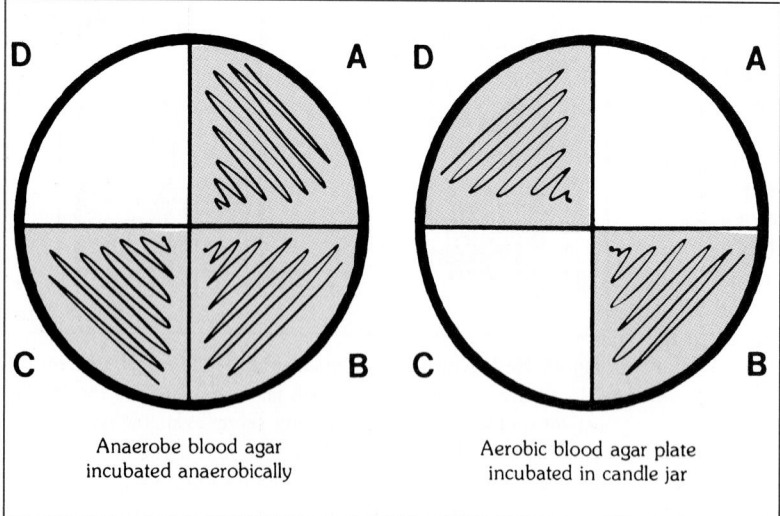

Anaerobe blood agar incubated anaerobically

Aerobic blood agar plate incubated in candle jar

Figure 16-8 Quadrant plating technique used for aerotolerance testing of four anaerobe isolates. The *left plate* has been incubated in an anaerobe jar for 18 to 24 hours, whereas the plate on the *right* was incubated in a candle jar. Isolates *A* and *C* are obligate anaerobes. Isolate *B* is facultatively anaerobic. Isolate *D* is either a microaerophile or an obligate anaerobe and should be further tested for its ability to grow in ambient air, compared with the environment containing increased CO_2. A candle jar is not adequate for testing *Campylobacter jejuni;* this species grows optimally in 5–10% CO_2, 10% CO_2, and 85% N_2.

plates should be streaked with each isolate in order to transfer a pure culture and avoid contamination.

Preliminary Reporting of Results

Organisms that are shown to be obligate anaerobes should be reported to the clinician immediately, together with the results from observing a Gram-stained preparation and characteristics of colonies. However, it is not justified to report the presence of an obligate anaerobe until aerotolerance studies have been completed.

Unfortunately, a period of 3 days or longer often is required for these studies to be completed. Clinicians should be made aware that this lengthy time cannot be avoided with some slow-growing anaerobes (e.g., some species of *Actinomyces* and *Propionibacterium*). Fortunately, the colonial and microscopic morphology of certain anaerobic bacteria is often so distinctive that *preliminary* or *presumptive* reports of these isolates can be made prior to aerotolerance studies. Examples include *Clostridium perfringens*, members of the *Bacteroides fragilis* group, the pigmenting *Prevotella* and *Porphyromonas* group, and others.

Determination of Cultural and Biochemical Characteristics for Differentiation of Anaerobic Isolates

Once the presence of anaerobes has been confirmed by aerotolerance tests and a description of morphologic features has been reported, the next priority is to identify the pure-culture isolates as rapidly and as accurately as possible and to report the results to the clinician within a relevant time. Although several hundred species of anaerobes are currently recognized by taxonomists, the task of identifying anaerobes for the clinical microbiologist is not nearly as formidable as it might seem because only a relatively small number is involved in anaerobic infections with any frequency.[69,125]

Presumptive Identification

Nearly all clinically significant isolates are moderate obligate or aerotolerant anaerobes, and with practice are not particularly difficult to isolate and identify. In addition to organisms of the *Bacteroides fragilis* group, the pigmented *Prevotella-Porphyromonas* group, *F. nucleatum,* and the anaerobic cocci that are quite frequently isolated, certain other, less common, anaerobes nonetheless have major pathogenic potential. Consequently, it is important to be familiar with and be able to recognize *Actinomyces israelii, A. naeslundii, A. meyeri, Propionibacterium propionicum,* and *Bifidobacterium dentium* (formerly *B. eriksonii*), all of which may cause serious acute suppurative and chronic inflammatory disease; *Prevotella bivia* and *P. disiens*, which are commonly resistant to various penicillins and cephalosporins; *Fusobacterium necrophorum* (which may be highly virulent); *F. mortiferum* and *F. varium*, which vary in susceptibility to certain penicillins, cephalosporins, and clindamycin; *C. septicum*, an organism frequently associated with

carcinoma of the colon or hematopoietic malignancy when isolated from patients' blood; the "histotoxic" clostridia in addition to *C. perfringens*, which can cause gas gangrene and various wound infections; *C. difficile*, a major cause of antibiotic-associated diarrhea and colitis; and *C. tetani* and *C. botulinum* because of the diseases they cause.[7,10,69,125]

Reference laboratories commonly use large batteries of tests in characterizing anaerobe isolates referred to them for identification or confirmation. These are listed in Box 16-7. In addition, new species are being recognized based on use of chemotaxonomic methods and molecular genetic studies. The data derived from the characterization of cultures with large numbers of tests has provided valuable databases for compiling tables of differential characteristics such as those published by the CDC, Virginia Polytechnic Institute (VPI) and State University, and Wadsworth Anaerobe Laboratories.[53,107,125,259] However, in most clinical diagnostic laboratories it is not practical or economically feasible to use such a large number of differential media and biochemical determinations to identify isolates from clinical specimens.

Fortunately, certain characteristics (Box 16-8) are especially useful in the identification of anaerobes. These characteristics form the basis of a practical approach for identifying anaerobic isolates that are commonly encountered in the clinical laboratory and additional species that either are less common or are potential major pathogens, even if they are rare.

Use of Differential Agar Media

Several important characteristics for identifying anaerobic bacteria can be obtained with pure cultures on CDC anaerobic blood agar and in enriched thioglycolate medium. These characteristics, outlined in Table 16-7, provide important clues for differentiating anaerobes in general. Additional characteristics are determined by use of differential disks, which are added to freshly inoculated anaerobe blood agar plates. A 2-U penicillin disk, 1000-μg kanamycin disk and 15-μg revamping disk (available from Becton Dickinson Microbiology Systems) aid in the differentiation

---

Box 16-7 Characterization of Anaerobic Bacteria

Relation to O_2
Colony morphology
Gram stain reaction
Microscopic features
Motility
Growth in liquid media
Biochemical tests
Metabolic products (GLC)
Antibiotic susceptibility
Serologic tests
Toxicity, toxin neutralization, pathogenicity in animals
Polyacrylamide gel electrophoresis of soluble proteins
Cell-wall long-chain fatty acids; menaquinones

Box 16-8 Some Cardinal Identifying Characteristics of Anaerobes

Relation to O_2
Colonial characteristics
Pigment
Hemolysis
Pitting of medium
Gram stain reaction
Morphology
Spores
Motility
Flagella
Miscellaneous
Growth in thioglycolate broth, catalase, lecithinase, lipase; reactions on milk medium; production of indole; hydrolysis of starch, esculin, and gelatin; reduction of nitrate; fermentation of key carbohydrates (e.g., glucose, mannitol, lactose, rhamnose); growth in presence of bile, penicillin, rifampin, and kanamycin; inhibition by sodium polyanetholsulfonate; production of toxins; metabolic products

of anaerobic, non–spore-forming, gram-negative bacilli. Colistin and vancomycin disks may also be extremely useful, as described elsewhere.[125] A sodium polyanetholsulfonate disk test is a practical way to separate *Peptostreptococcus anaerobius* from other anaerobic cocci. A nitrate disk test is a convenient method to demonstrate nitrate reduction during the workup of anaerobic bacteria (in general).

PRESUMPTO PLATES

Three types of quadrant plates (Presumpto 1, 2, and 3) containing 12 differential agar media were developed by Dowell, Lombard, and associates into a system that allows determination of 20 different characteristics (Table 16-7) of anaerobic isolates at a minimal cost.[55] The information derived from using the three-quadrant plates, along with the other characteristics obtained from anaerobe blood agar and enriched thioglycolate medium plus metabolic product analysis using GLC, permits definitive identification of many clinically significant anaerobic bacteria that are encountered in the laboratory. In addition, the quadrant plates, especially the Presumpto 1 and 2 plates, can be used to supplement several of the commercial packaged kit systems, as well as traditional broth identification systems, with important tests or characteristics these non-agar systems lack.

The basal medium in the Presumpto quadrant plate system is Lombard-Dowell (LD) medium. LD agar is a specially designed medium that supports growth of a wide variety of anaerobes, including fastidious ones. It is noteworthy that LD broth (the same medium without agar or with only a small amount) is the inoculum broth for both the Minitek (Becton Dickinson Microbiology Systems) and API systems (BioMérieux-Vitek).[8]

The Presumpto 1 plate is a four-quadrant Petri dish containing the following media: LD agar, LD esculin agar, LD. egg yolk agar, and LD bile agar. Details on the use of the Presumpto 1 plate were first published by Dowell and Lombard of the CDC.[54] It was first used for presumptive identification of *Bacteroides* and *Fusobacterium* (without Presumpto plates 2 and 3) but since has been useful for identifying other anaerobic bacteria.

The Presumpto 2 plate contains LD glucose agar, LD DNA agar, LD milk agar, and LD starch agar. It is useful for characterization of clostridia, the anaerobic, non–spore-forming gram-negative and gram-positive bacilli, and the anaerobic cocci. Like the Presumpto 1 plate, it can be used along with packaged micromethod kits that lack the tests it contains, or along with conventional tube tests.

The Presumpto 3 plate contains LD gelatin agar, LD mannitol agar, LD lactose agar, and LD rhamnose agar. Use of LD gelatin agar and the use of the carbohydrates in this quadrant plate has been described.[55]

Characteristics that can be determined with each of the three-quadrant plates are shown in Table 16-7. Formulations and preparation of the media and reagents used in the quadrant plate system are given in detail elsewhere.[8,259]

Inoculation and Reading of Presumpto Plates. The procedures for inoculation of the media in the Presumpto quadrant plates, the method of incubation, and the use of differential inhibitory and antibiotic disk tests are outlined in Box 16-9.

Observation and Interpretation of Results. After incubation, examine the quadrant plates and the anaerobic blood agar plates containing the antibiotic disks and the SPS and nitrate differentiation disks.

Presumpto Quadrant Plate I (Color Plate 16-5).

LD Agar Note and record the degree of growth on LD agar (light, moderate, heavy). Test for indole by adding two drops of para-dimethylaminocinnamaldehyde reagent to the paper disk on the medium. Observe for the development of a blue or bluish-green color in the disk within 30 seconds, which is a positive reaction for indole. Development of another color (pink, red, violet) or no color is negative for indole. A lavender to violet color indicates a positive reaction for indole derivative(s).

LD Egg Yolk Agar Formation of a zone of insoluble precipitate in the medium surrounding the bacterial colonies indicates a positive reaction for lecithinase production. This is best seen with transmitted light.

The presence of an iridescent sheen (a pearly layer on the surface of colonies and on the medium immediately surrounding the bacterial growth, best demonstrated with reflected light) indicates lipase production. If the reaction is questionable, add a few drops of water and look for a film that floats on top of water.

Clearing of the medium in the vicinity of the bacterial growth indicates proteolysis, as exhibited by certain proteolytic clostridia.

LD Esculin Agar A positive test for esculin hydrolysis is indicated by the development of a reddish brown to dark brown color in the esculin agar surrounding the bacterial growth after exposure of the quadrant plate cultures to air for at least 15 minutes. Additional evidence for esculin hy-

Table 16-7 Media and Characteristics of Cultures That Can Be Determined Using the Differential Agar Media System for Identifying Anaerobes

MEDIA	CHARACTERISTICS
Blood agar	Relation to O_2[a], colony characteristics, hemolysis, pigment, fluorescence with UV light (Wood's lamp), pitting of agar, cellular morphology, Gram stain reaction, spores, motility (wet mount); inhibition by penicillin, rifampin, and kanamycin
Enriched thioglycolate medium	Appearance of growth, rapidity of growth, gas production, odor, cellular morphology
Presumpto 1 plate	
LD agar	Indole, growth on LD medium, catalase[b]
LD esculin agar	Esculin hydrolysis, H2S, catalase
LD egg yolk agar	Lipase, lecithinase, proteolysis
LD bile agar	Growth in presence of 20% bile (2% oxgall), insoluble precipitate under and immediately surrounding growth
Presumpto 2 plate	
LD glucose agar	Glucose fermentation; stimulation of growth by fermentable carbohydrate
LD starch agar	Starch hydrolysis
LD milk agar	Casein hydrolysis
LD DNA agar	Deoxyribonuclease activity
Presumpto 3 plate	
LD mannitol agar	Mannitol fermentation
LD lactose agar	Lactose fermentation
LD rhamnose agar	Rhamnose fermentation
LD gelatin	Gelatin hydrolysis

[a] *By comparing growth on anaerobe plate with blood agar (or chocolate agar) incubated in 5–10% CO_2 incubator (or candle jar) or in room air.*
[b] *The catalase test can be performed by adding 3% hydrogen peroxide to the growth on LD agar, but the reactions of catalase-positive cultures are more vigorous on LD esculin agar.*

drolysis can be obtained by examining the esculin agar quadrant under a Wood's lamp. Esculin agar exhibits a bright blue fluorescence under the ultraviolet light that is not present after the esculin is hydrolyzed.

Blackening of the bacterial colonies on the esculin agar indicates H2S production. The blackening dissipates very rapidly after exposure to air. Therefore, the bacterial growth should be observed for blackening under anaerobic conditions (anaerobic glove box) or immediately after opening anaerobic jars to air. To test for hydrogen peroxide degradation as an indication of catalase, expose the plates to air for at least 30 minutes and then flood the esculin agar quadrant with a few drops of fresh 3% H_2O_2. Sustained bubbling after addition of the H_2O_2 is a positive reaction for catalase. In some cases, rapid bubbling may not be evident until after 30 seconds to a minute.

LD Bile Agar Compare the degree of bacterial growth on the LD bile agar with that on the plain LD agar and record as I (growth less than on the LD agar control) or E (growth equal to or greater than on the LD agar control). Using trans-

mitted light, look for the presence or lack of an insoluble white precipitate underneath or immediately surrounding the bacterial growth. If in doubt, inspect under a stereomicroscope using transmitted light.

Presumpto Quadrant Plate 2 (Color Plate 16-5).

LD Glucose Agar Fermentation of glucose is indicated by acid production or a yellow color in and around the growth in the medium. A blue color around the growth is a negative reaction. Some bacteria reduce the indicator; therefore, it is sometimes necessary to flood the quadrant with dilute bromthymol blue reagent to see whether acid has been produced.

Glucose stimulation can be observed by comparing the amount of bacterial growth on LD glucose agar with that on plain LD agar.

LD Starch Agar To detect hydrolysis of starch, flood the quadrant with Gram's iodine solution; clearing around the growth indicates a positive reaction. A brownish color indicates unhydrolyzed starch and a negative reaction.

LD Milk Agar A clear zone around the growth in the quadrant indicates hydrolysis of casein (i.e., digestion of

---

Box 16-9 Use of Presumpto Quadrant Plates

1. Prepare the inoculum from fresh growth of a pure culture of the anaerobic isolate. Use either a turbid cell suspension (McFarland 3) in LD broth prepared from isolated colonies or a 24- to 48-hour enriched thioglycolate medium subculture from an isolated colony (alternatively, a 24-to 48-hour chopped-meat glucose broth subculture can be used).
2. Inoculate the quadrant plates as follows:
   a. Saturate one sterile swab (for each quadrant plate to be inoculated) in either the cell suspension or broth culture.
   b. Streak the middle portion of each quadrant with the swab containing bacteria.
3. Place a sterile, blank, 1/2-in.-diameter paper disk on the LD agar near the outer periphery of the quadrant. This disk is used in the test for indole after incubation of the plates.

In addition to setting up the Presumpto plates, also:

1. Inoculate the surface of an anaerobic blood agar plate evenly with a sterile swab that has been dipped in the cell suspension or broth culture.
2. Place the antibiotic disks (penicillin, 2 U; rifampin, 15 μg; kanamycin, 1,000 μg) on the blood agar with sterile forceps. Space the disks evenly such that overlapping zones of inhibition will not be a problem.
3. Place the sodium polyanetholsulfonate (SPS) and nitrate disks on a second anaerobic blood agar plate, if they are used in addition to the antibiotic disks. To prepare the SPS disk, pipette 20 μL of 5% SPS (available from Anaerobe Systems [Morgan Hill, CA] and Remel [Lenexa, KS]) onto 1/4-in. (0.635-cm) sterile blank disks (Becton Dickinson [BD], Sparks, MD) and dry. SPS disks are stable at room temperature for 6 months. To prepare the nitrate disk, dissolve 30 g KNO_3 and 0.1 g sodium molybdate ($Na_2MoO_4 \cdot 2H_2O$) in 100 mL distilled water and filter-sterilize the solution using a 0.45-μm membrane filter. Then add 20 μL of this reagent to 1/4-in. (0.635-cm) sterile blank disks and dry at room temperature for at least 72 hours.

---

milk proteins) and a positive reaction. If casein is unhydrolyzed, the medium remains cloudy (a negative reaction).

LD DNA Agar A pink to reddish zone around the growth on the quadrant indicates a positive reaction for the degradation of DNA (i.e., deoxyribonuclease activity). If the medium remains blue around the growth, DNA was not degraded and the reaction is negative.

Presumpto Quadrant Plate 3

LD Gelatin Agar To detect the hydrolysis of gelatin, flood the quadrant with acidified mercuric chloride reagent. This reagent binds to unhydrolyzed gelatin. A zone of complete clearing around the growth on the quadrant indicates that gelatin has been hydrolyzed and is recorded as a positive test.

LD Mannitol Agar, LD Lactose Agar, and LD Rhamnose Agar Examine and interpret these quadrants as described for LD glucose agar.

ANTIMICROBIAL SUSCEPTIBILITY PLATES

Growth Inhibition on Anaerobe Blood Agar Using Antibiotic Disk TEST.
Zones of inhibition around the antibiotic disks are observed and recorded as follows:

Penicillin, 2-U disk: sensitive (S) if zone of growth inhibition is ≥12 mm in diameter; and resistant (R) if the zone is <12 mm.

Rifampin, 15-μg disk: sensitive (S) if zone of growth inhibition is ≥15 mm; and resistant (R) if zone is <12 mm.

Kanamycin, 1,000-μg disk: sensitive (S) if zone of growth inhibition is ≥12 mm; and resistant (R) if zone is <12 mm.

Use of SPS and Nitrate Disk Tests

SPS Disk Test Measure the zone of inhibition around the 1/4-in. disk. A ≥12-mm zone of inhibition is recorded as sensitive (S).

Nitrate Disk Test Test for nitrate reduction by adding one drop of nitrate A reagent (sulfanilic acid) and one drop of nitrate B reagent (1,6 Cleave's acid) to the disk.[125] A pink or red color indicates that nitrate has been reduced to nitrite. If the disk was colorless after the addition of reagents A and B, sprinkle zinc dust on the disk to confirm a negative reaction. The development of a red color after zinc dust is added confirms that nitrate is still present in the disk (a negative reaction).

For summaries of characteristics for the identification of various species of anaerobes using differential tests in/on agar media are found in Tables 16-14 to 16-16 and 16-18 to 16-25.

The anaerobe blood agar, Presumpto quadrant plates and other media described in this section are available commercially (Remel) or can be prepared in the laboratory. Details for preparation of the media and reagents may be found in previous editions of this textbook and elsewhere.[53,55,56] If prepared in one's own laboratory, there is the option of putting a single differential medium in a plate and not using quadrant Petri dishes. This approach increases the flexibility of the system for microbiologists who would prefer to use other combinations of tests.

Characterization of Anaerobes Using Conventional Biochemical Tests in Large Tubes

It is not possible in this textbook to discuss all the procedures that are available for biochemical characterization of anaerobes. Conventional tube culture procedures are covered briefly below. For further details, refer to the laboratory manuals on anaerobic bacteriology.[53,107,125,179]

Instead of the differential tests in agar media described, one may use PRAS media in large test tubes for determining biochemical characteristics. These are inoculated either through a rubber diaphragm in Hungate tubes or with a special gassing device according to procedures of the VPI manual.[107,179] PRAS media can be prepared in the laboratory or can be obtained commercially. If PRAS media are used for characterization of isolates, the identification tables of Holdeman, Moore, and associates should also be used.[107,109,112,179]

The pH of PRAS peptone yeast-extract (PY)-based carbohydrate fermentation tests is determined directly by using a pH meter; a long, thin, combination electrode is inserted into each culture tube. According to the VPI manual, pH 5.5 to 6.0 is recorded as weakly acid, whereas pH below 5.5 is strongly acid. Note that the pH of PY carbohydrate cultures should be compared with that of plain PY cultures (without carbohydrate). The pH of PY broth ranges between 6.2 and 6.4 when inoculated under CO_2. Also, some organisms apparently may produce acid from peptones in plain PY medium.[107] Furthermore, the pH of uninoculated PRAS PY-arabinose, PY-ribose, or PY-xylose may be as low as 5.9 after the medium has been held for 1 to 2 days under a CO_2 atmosphere; thus, the pH of cultures in these media is not interpreted as acid unless it is below 5.7.[107]

The conventional media of Dowell et al. are commercially available in 15-mm × 90-mm screw-capped tubes (Remel, Lenexa, KS). Details on preparation and use of these media are published elsewhere.[53] If these differential media are used, one should refer to the identification tables of Dowell and Hawkins.[53] With either the VPI or CDC conventional system, biochemicals can be read after overnight incubation of certain rapid-growing cultures of anaerobes (e.g., some *B. fragilis* and clostridia), or after good growth is seen (usually 48 hours, but longer for slow-growing species). The fermentation tests are read by using bromthymol blue (yellow at pH 6.0) or can be read using a pH meter (a pH below 6.0 is considered acid). In our experience, some of the so-called rapid micromethod systems are not really more rapid.

Alternative Procedures

Use of conventional media in Hungate or other large tubes is relatively time-consuming, and the media are costly to prepare or purchase. As alternatives to conventional media and methods, as well as to the Presumpto Quadrant Plate system, a variety of other procedures for characterizing and identifying isolates and alternative identification schemas have been described.[8,10] A number of these contain smaller volumes of media in containers that can be manipulated with reasonable speed at the bench. One of the more popular alternative approaches has been to test for certain key characteristics of isolates on differential agar media (e.g., Bacteroides bile esculin agar; Anaerobe Systems, Morgan Hill, CA). Another has been to use disks impregnated with antibiotics or various other chemicals to test for growth inhibition or growth stimulation. Another excellent approach has been to use small tablets (e.g., WEE-TABS, Key Scientific Products, Round Rock, TX) for determining certain enzyme-chromogenic substrate reactions. WEE-TABS have been used both as supplemental or stand-alone tests for differentiating various anaerobes. Details for their use and descriptions of several other tests for characterization of anaerobe isolates are given in the Wadsworth Anaerobic Bacteriology Manual[125] and reviewed elsewhere.[8]

THE NAGLER TEST AND THE CAMP TEST FOR *C. PERFRINGENS*

Historically, the Nagler test has been used for the presumptive identification of *Clostridium perfringens*. Although most of the clostridia isolated in the clinical laboratory that give a positive reaction are *C. perfringens*, the antitoxin used in the test is not specific. *C. bifermentans*, *C. sordellii*, and *C. barattii* (formerly *C. paraperfringens*) are also known to be Nagler-positive and additional tests are still necessary to separate them. During the past few years, popularity of the Nagler test has waned because the antitoxin has not been widely available. Additional details describing the Nagler test are given in previous editions of this textbook.

An alternative to the Nagler test, used in some laboratories, is the so-called reverse CAMP test.[35] To perform the test, inoculate an anaerobe blood agar plate with a single streak of an unknown organism that is possibly a *C. perfringens* isolate. Next, make a single streak at a 90-degree angle to within 1–2 mm of the first streak, using an inoculum of a group B β-hemolytic *Streptococcus*. An arrowhead of synergistic hemolysis, with the tip of the arrow pointing from the *Streptococcus* toward the *C. perfringens*, is a positive test. Both false—positive and false negative results may occur. Additional data on the specificity of this test for clinical isolates of *C. perfringens* are needed. In our view, most laboratories experienced in anaerobic bacteriology and the additional morphologic and cultural characteristics of *C. perfringens* may find the Nagler test and the reverse CAMP test, while perhaps ''novel,'' to be unnecessary.

Packaged Microsystems

Historically, two commercial packaged micromethod kits developed in the 1970s have continued to be used through the years in clinical microbiology laboratories for identification of anaerobes, namely the API-20A (BioMérieux-Vitek) and the Minitek (Becton Dickinson Microbiology Systems). The construction and use of these systems have been reviewed by Stargel et al.[233]

Commercial Packaged Kits for Aerobic Identification of Anaerobes After 4 Hours of Incubation

Several manufacturers have marketed packaged kits that test for preformed enzymes. Most of these systems utilize a battery of chromogenic substrates to rapidly test for a number of amino peptidases and glycosidases. Each system requires the preparation of a heavy cell suspension from the surface of a purity plate culture. These packaged kits enable the microbiologist to determine multiple enzymatic characteristics of a pure culture isolate after 4 hours or less of aerobic incubation. Except for the API-ZYM kit,[8,233] all of these packaged systems provide numerical codes, computerized databases and identification tables to aid in identification once an isolate has been characterized using the system. The list of products includes the following:

API An-Ident (BioMerieux-Vitek)
API-ZYM (BioMerieux-Vitek)
Crystal Anaerobe Identification System (Becton Dickinson Microbiology Systems)
MicroScan Rapid Anaerobe Panel (Dade Behring Microscan)
RapID-ANA II (Remel)
Rapid ID 32A (BioMerieux-Vitek)
Vitek Anaerobe Identification (ANI) Card (BioMerieux-Vitek).

These kits are popular with microbiologists and are being used widely in diagnostic microbiology laboratories. In general, they are simple to use and less time-consuming than conventional methods. A detailed description of each of the systems, including the substrates, procedures for use, interpretation of test results, and a discussion of performance evaluations is available elsewhere.[8] All of the packaged microsystems listed above must be supplemented with additional tests for accurate and definitive identification of selected groups of anaerobes (e.g., use of egg yolk agar and GLC for clostridia other than *C. perfringens;* the use of rapidity of growth and growth appearance in liquid as well as solid media, several additional supplemental tests, plus GLC for the anaerobic gram-positive non–spore-forming rods; the use of 20% bile, esculin, selected conventional carbohydrate tests for *Bacteroides* spp., the use of GLC and egg yolk reactions for differentiation of *Fusobacterium* spp., as well as additional tests for other anaerobes). Of course, it is still necessary to observe and correctly interpret Gram reactions, microscopic and colony morphology and the results of aerotolerance tests and to always use pure cultures when attempting to differentiate anaerobes with the commercial packaged systems.

When a kit produces an identification of a rare species, one should not accept this identification without repeat testing with alternative procedures, or perhaps confirmation from a reference laboratory when relevant clinically.

Determination of Metabolic Products by Gas-Liquid Chromatography

Analysis of metabolic products by GLC is a practical, inexpensive procedure that is easily performed by personnel in the clinical laboratory.[217] Metabolic products, released into broth culture media during anaerobic growth, are key characteristics of anaerobic bacteria and many facultatively anaerobic bacteria. Together with determining the relationship to oxygen, most anaerobic bacteria can be identified to the genus level based on presence or lack of spores, Gram reaction, cellular morphology, and results of GLC analysis. This technique improves the speed and accuracy of identification; cost actually decreases because of the time saved.[180]

As mentioned previously, facultative anaerobes use aerobic respiration in their production of energy from glucose, but in addition they are capable of obtaining energy by fermentation reactions. Obligate anaerobes are similar to facultative anaerobes in terms of the pathways used for fermentation reactions. Like the obligate aerobes and facultative anaerobes, some obligate anaerobes also use anaerobic respiration as a means of obtaining energy, but the obligate anaerobes do not use aerobic respiration, and oxygen is not a terminal electron acceptor for them. When grown in a liquid medium containing glucose, many of the obligate anaerobes isolated in the clinical laboratory produce pyruvate from glucose by way of the Embden-Meyerhof and other pathways. However, many anaerobic bacteria obtain energy in media that are deficient in glucose or other carbohydrates by fermenting one or more amino acids. For example, *Clostridium sporogenes* ferments ala-

nine and glycine (the Strickland reaction) to produce acetate, CO_2, and NH_3.[163] There is a direct relationship between the amounts of peptone and glucose in a medium and the production of branched, short-chain, fatty acids (e.g., isobutyrate, isovalerate, isocaproate) by certain anaerobes.[152] Fermentation products produced by bacteria from organic compounds such as pyruvic acid vary among different genera and species of obligate anaerobes and among facultatively anaerobic microorganisms.

The fermentation patterns of microorganisms have long been used for taxonomic groupings.[163] Certain yeasts such as *Saccharomyces* carry out an alcoholic fermentation in which the metabolic products consist mainly of ethanol and CO_2. The lactic acid bacteria, which include the genera *Lactobacillus* and *Streptococcus*, are well known for their characteristic pattern of fermentation in which lactic acid accumulates as the major product. *Escherichia coli* and certain other Enterobacteriaceae are metabolically characterized by their mixed-acid fermentation in which acetate, lactate, and succinate are formed in significant amounts along with ethanol, CO_2, and H_2. Other members of the Enterobacteriaceae, for example, *Enterobacter aerogenes*, produce a butanediol type of fermentation; major products include 2,3-butanediol, ethanol, CO_2, and H_2, and smaller amounts of acetate, lactate, and succinate are formed. The presence of this type of fermentation is ordinarily determined in the clinical laboratory by the Voges-Proskauer test (see Chapter 6). The butyric acid fermentation, in which butyric acid, limited amounts of acetic acid, CO_2, and H_2 are produced, is carried out by certain species of *Clostridium* (e.g., *C. butyricum*). The butyric acid fermentation pattern is one of about 14 groupings or subdivisions that can be made of this genus based on metabolic product analysis alone. On the other hand, many of the other genera of anaerobes have long been defined based on a single major metabolic pattern (e.g., propionic acid for the genus *Propionibacterium*).

Definitions of genera based on metabolic pathways has held up scientifically because metabolic pathways represent genetically stable or conserved traits of bacteria.[180] The schemas in Tables 16-8 and 16-9 illustrate the value of acid metabolic product analysis for differentiating genera of anaerobic bacteria.

Although GLC analysis is not mandatory for presumptive identification of the *B. fragilis* group, the pigmenting anaerobic gram-negative bacilli, *F. nucleatum, C. perfringens, P. anaerobius,* and a few other anaerobes commonly recovered from clinical specimens, it is necessary for definitive identification of many species of *Bacteroides* and *Fusobacterium,* for most *Actinomyces, Bifidobacterium, Clostridium, Eubacterium, Lactobacillus, Propionibacterium,* and for nearly all of the anaerobic cocci.[217]

Gas chromatographs are now relatively inexpensive, safe, simple to operate, and reliable, and are commercially available from various scientific instrument manufacturing companies. Equipment and procedures for determining metabolic products by GLC are described in more detail elsewhere.[53,107,125,152,180,217]

Identification of Volatile Fatty Acids

GLC is used for identifying short-chain, volatile fatty acids that are soluble in ether. The acids detected with this

Table 16-8 Differentiation of Anaerobic, Gram-Negative, Non–Spore-Forming Rods to the Genus Level

I. Nonmotile or motile with peritrichous flagella; straight or coccobacillary rods

    A. Proposal by Shah and Collins[210] to include only the highly fermentative and bile-resistant species resembling *B. fragilis* (i.e., *B. distasonis, B. caccae, B. ovatus, B. thetaiotaomicron, B. merdae, B. vulgatus, B. uniformis, B. eggerthii,* and *B. stercoris*). Several other species remain in this genus; further studies are needed to determine their correct place (e.g., *B. capillosus, B. coagulans, B. cellulosolvens, B. pectinophilus, B. tectum, B. ureolyticus,* and others).   *Bacteroides*[a]

        Until the latter group is moved this genus remains heterogeneous.

    B. Most often black-pigmented colonies; produces acetic, butyric, and succinic acids, with minor amounts of propionic, isobutyric, and isovaleric acids. All are asaccharolytic and indole-positive.   *Porphyromonas*[b]

    C. Nonpigmented to pigmented colonies; bile-inhibited and saccharolytic; usually oral microbiota   *Prevotella*[a]

    D. Bile-resistant, catalase-positive, nitrate-reduced, and urease-positive   *Bilophila*[b]

    E. Found as a part of the human normal microbiota, but rarely encountered in properly selected clinical specimens   *Alistipes*[c]
Anaerostipes[c]
Anaerorhabdus[c]
Catonella[c]
Cetobacterium[c]
Dialister[c]
Faecalibacter[c]
Fibrobacter[c]
Johnsonella
Megamonas[c]
Mitsuokella[c]
Oxalobacter[c]
Sneathia[c]
Sutterella[c]
Tannerella[c]
Tissierella[c]

    F. Found in animals and nature.   *Dichelobacter*[c]
Pectinatus[c]
Rikenella[c]
Roseburia[c]
Ruminobacter[c]
Sebaldella[c]

    G. Produces major amounts of butyric acid (but little or no isoacids) as the major metabolic product; succinic acid is not produced; all species are nonmotile   *Fusobacterium*[a]

    H. Lactic acid is the only major product; *L. buccalis,* the only species, is nonmotile.   *Leptotrichia*[b]

    I. Acetic acid is the major acid metabolic product; produces hydrogen sulfide; reduces sulfate; *D. pigra,* the only species, is nonmotile.   *Desulfomonas*[c]

II. Motile, peritrichous flagella not produced

    A. Curved rods with monotrichous or lophotrichous polar flagella or subpolar flagella; butyric acid is a major product of fermentation.   *Butyrivibrio*[b]

    B. Succinic and acetic acids are major products of fermentation.   *Succinimonas*[c]

        1. Short, straight rods to coccobacilli; a single polar flagellum; found only in bovine rumen.   *Succinivibrio*[b]

        2. Curved, helically twisted rods with pointed ends; vibrating-type motility by a single polar flagellum   *Anaerobiospirillum*[b]

        3. Helical, curved rods; bipolar tufts of flagella   *Campylobacter*[d]

    C. Microaerophilic; oxidase-positive, curved and spiral rods; single polar flagellum, with absence of a flagellar sheath; carbohydrates not fermented; produce succinic acid from fumaric acid   *Wollinella*[e]

    D. Propionic and acetic acids are major fermentation products

        1. Tufts of flagella on concave side of crescent-shaped cells   *Selenomonas*[b]

        2. Single polar flagellum; lipolytic; curved rods   *Anaerovibrio*[b]

        3. Flagella are inserted in a spiral along the cell   *Centipeda*[c]

[a] *Commonly found in clinical specimens.*
[b] *Rarely found in clinical specimens.*
[c] *Normal flora of humans or other animals only.*
[d] *Campylobacter gracilis is oxidase-negative and lacks flagella, but has "twitching motility"; it differs from other Campylobacter species in these two respects.*
[e] *Wolinella succinogenes, isolated from the bovine rumen and now the only species remaining in Wolinella, is difficult to differentiate from species of the genus Campylobacter.*
Modified from Koneman et. al.[135] and other references cited elsewhere in the text.

Table 16-9 Differentiation of Anaerobic, Gram-Positive Rods Encountered in Human Specimens to the Genus Level

I. Bacterial endospores not produced	
A. Produce major amounts of propionic and acetic acids; catalase usually produced; irregular- or regular-shaped rods, coccoid cells; occasional branching	*Propionibacterium*
B. Produce acetic and lactic acids (>1 : 1 ratio); very irregular rods with bifid forms and branching.	*Bifidobacterium*
C. Produce lactic acid as sole major product	
1. Short to long and slender rods; chain formation common; irregular rods uncommon; usually grow on tomato juice agar at pH ≤4.5 (see Chapter 14).	*Lactobacillus*
2. Small, elongated cocci that occur singly, in pairs, or in short chains	*Atopobium*
D. Produce moderate acetic, lactic and major succinic acids; irregular rods predominant; filamentous forms with branching.	*Actinomyces*
E. Produce mixtures of acetic, butyric, lactic and sometimes formic acids; pleomorphic diphtheroid rods; saccharolytic	*Eubacterium*
F. Produces minor amounts of acetic acid and traces of lactic and succinic acids; asaccharolytic	*Eggerthella*
G. Produces major amounts of acetic acid and a small amount of succinate; straight to curved rods with some branching ("*Actinomyces*-like")	*Actinobaculum*
H. Acetate and butyrate are the only acid metabolic products; saccharolytic; thin rods	*Anaerotruncus*
I. Produces major amount of lactate with variable amounts of formic, acetic and succinic acids; coccobacilli, pleomorphic, short diphtheroidal rods; facultatively anaerobic; saccharolytic; *A. pyogenes* is β-hemolytic on sheep blood agar	*Arcanobacterium*
J. Produces moderate amount of acetate and lactate and trace amount of succinic acid; saccharolytic; short rods	*Bulleidia*
K. Acetic, butyric, isobutyric, and lactic acids produced; saccharolytic; occur as short rods in tangled chains	*Catenibacterium*
L. No metabolic products detected in peptone yeast-extract glucose broth; asaccharolytic; very short rods	*Cryptobacterium*
M. Produces acetic, formic, and lactic acids, sometimes with a trace of succinic acid; abundant ethanol; saccharolytic; often in the form of pleomorphic cocci to short rods; may be confused with streptococci or lactobacilli but is distinguished by producing abundant H_2	*Collinsella*
N. Acetate and lactate are major products with a small amount of succinate; saccharolytic (weakly); short to long rods occur in pairs and short chains	*Holdemania*
O. Phenylacetic acid produced as sole metabolic product in peptone yeast-extract glucose broth; asaccharolytic; short rods occur singly, in short chains, or clumps	*Mogibacterium*
P. Succinic and acetic acids are major fermentation products, with or without lactic acid; oxidase-negative, curved rods, motile with multiple subterminal flagella; fermentative in peptone yeast glycogen broth, supplemented with rabbit serum	*Mobiluncus*
Q. Produces formate, acetate, butyrate, caproate, and H_2; pleomorphic rods occur in pairs resembling birds in flight, clumps, or Chinese letters (formerly *Eubacterium alactolyticum*)	*Pseudoramibacter*
R. Produce only acetic acid or no acid metabolic products; occur in rods, cocci, or coccobacilli in chains and clumps	*Slackia*
II. Bacterial endospores produced	*Clostridium*

Adapted from Koneman et al.[135] and other references cited elsewhere in the text.

procedure include acetic, propionic, isobutyric, butyric iso-valeric, valeric, isocaproic, and caproic. The procedure is explained in Box 16-10.

Volatile fatty acids can be identified by comparing elution times of products in extracts with those of a known acid mixture (volatile fatty acid standard) chromatographed under the same conditions on the same day. A representative standard tracing is shown in Figure 16-9, and examples of the GLC results for three anaerobe isolates are shown in Figures 16-10, 16-11, and 16-12.

Analysis of Nonvolatile Acids

Pyruvic, lactic, fumaric, succinic, hydrocinnamic, and phenylacetic acids are not detected with the ether extraction procedure for volatile fatty acids (above). These nonvolatile acids are identified after preparation of methylated derivatives. The procedure is outlined in Box 16-11.

Analysis of chloroform extracts is performed using the same chromatographic conditions as for the volatile acids. Identify nonvolatile or methylated acids by comparing elu-

Box 16-10 Identifying Volatile Fatty Acids

1. Inoculate tubes containing 7 to 8 mL of prereduced peptone–yeast extract–glucose (PYG) broth with a few drops (0.05 to 0.1 mL) of an actively growing culture.
2. Incubate under anaerobic conditions for 48 hours, or until adequate growth is obtained.
3. Transfer 2 mL of the culture to a clean, 13- by 100-mm screw-capped tube.
4. Acidify the culture to pH 2.0 or lower by adding 0.2 mL of 50% (v/v) aqueous H_2SO_4.
5. Add 1 mL of ethyl ether, tighten the cap, and mix by gently inverting the tube about 20 times.
6. Centrifuge briefly in a clinical centrifuge (1,500 to 2,000 rpm) to break the ether–culture emulsion.
7. Place the ether–culture mixture in a freezer at $-20\,^\circ C$ or lower or in an alcohol-dry ice bath until the aqueous portion (bottom) is frozen.
8. Rapidly pour off the ether layer into a clean screw-capped tube. If desired, add one or two anhydrous $CaCl_2$ pellets to the ether extract to allow removal of residual water.
9. Inject 14 μL of the extract into the column of a gas chromatograph packed with SP-1220.

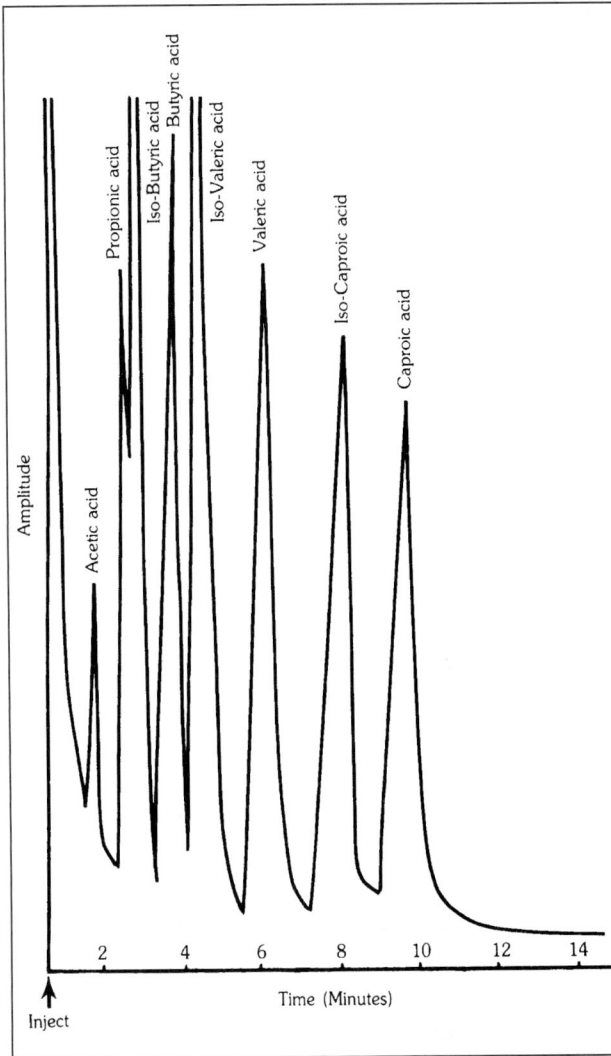

Figure 16-9 A typical volatile acid standard chromatogram. The time elapsed between the injection of an ether extract of the standard solution and the peak for each acid (retention time) is used to identify the acids. Note, for example, that the retention time for acetic acid is 1.8 minutes and for valeric acid is 6 minutes (instrument used: Dohrmann Anabac, Clinical Analysis Products, Sunnyvale CA; Detector: thermal conductivity; column packing: 15%, SP–1220/1% H_3PO_4 on 100/120 Chromasorb W/AW from Supelco, Bellefonte, PA)

tion times of products in extracts with those of known acids chromatographed on the same day. After testing approximately 20 methylated samples, recondition the packing material by injecting 14 μL of methanol into the gas chromatograph.

Gas-Liquid Chromatography Controls

Standard solutions containing 1 mEq/100 mL of each volatile acid and nonvolatile acid should be examined each time unknowns are tested. The volatile acid standard should contain at least the following acids: acetic, propionic, isobutyric, butyric, isovaleric, valeric, isocaproic, and caproic acids. The nonvolatile acid standard should contain at least pyruvic, lactic, fumaric, succinic, hydrocinnamic, and phenylacetic acids. A tube of uninoculated medium should be examined in the same manner, since various lots of PYG broth may contain significant quantities of these acids.

Lombard and associates have found that several other liquid media as well as PYG broth can be used for analysis of acid metabolic products.[152] These media include enriched thioglycolate broth, chopped-meat glucose, Lombard-Dowell glucose broth, and modified Schaedler broth (BD Microbiology Systems). When grown in these other broth media, however, results for a given organism may differ from those attained in PYG. Thus, caution should be exercised in interpreting products from different media when the identification tables have been prepared from a PYG database. A further note of caution is warranted; the amount of acetic, lactic, and other acids present in certain liquid media such as chopped-meat glucose broth may make it difficult or at times impossible to determine if the acetic or lactic acid peak was produced by the unknown isolate or simply by the uninoculated medium.[152]

Chromatographic tracings of a volatile acid standard; PYG broth cultures of *Fusobacterium mortiferum*, *Clostridium difficile*, and *Peptostreptococcus anaerobius*; and a nonvolatile acid standard are shown in Figures 16-9 through 16-13. The metabolic products of common species of anaerobic gram-negative rods are listed in Table 16-11.

Identification of Anaerobic Bacteria

An extensive update on the nomenclature (current names and former names) of the anaerobic bacteria is provided in Table 16-2. Fortunately, the anaerobes most important clini-

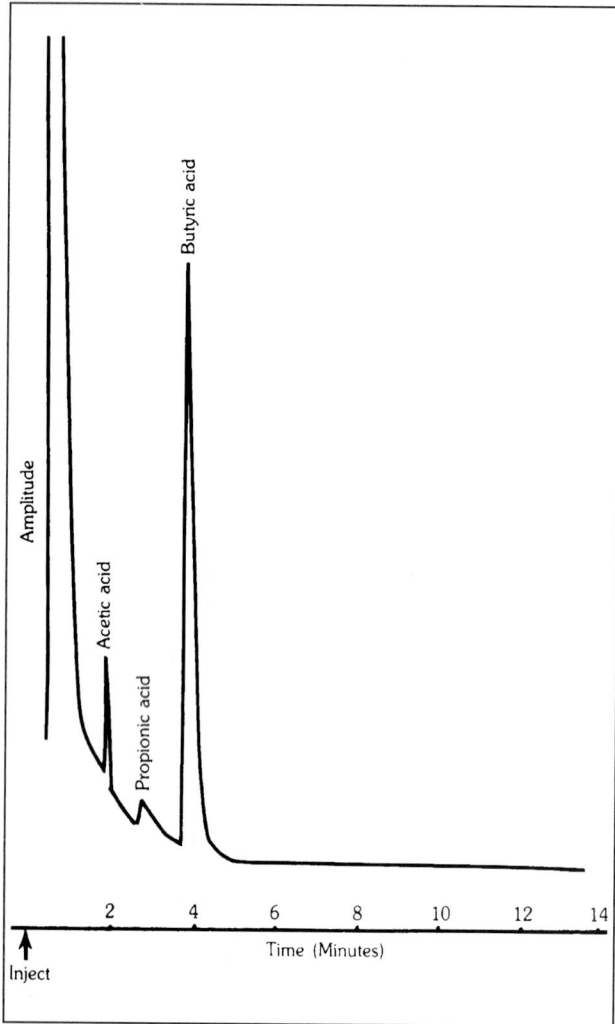

Figure 16-10 Volatile acid chromatogram of a 48-hour peptone–yeast extract–glucose broth culture of *Fusobacterium mortiferum.* The retention times of the products in the broth culture are compared with those of the standard tracing (see Fig. 16-9) to identify the unknown acids. The peaks indicate major amounts of butyric and acetic acids, but only a minor amount of propionate for this culture. The same instrument and operating conditions were used as for the tracing in Figure 16-9.

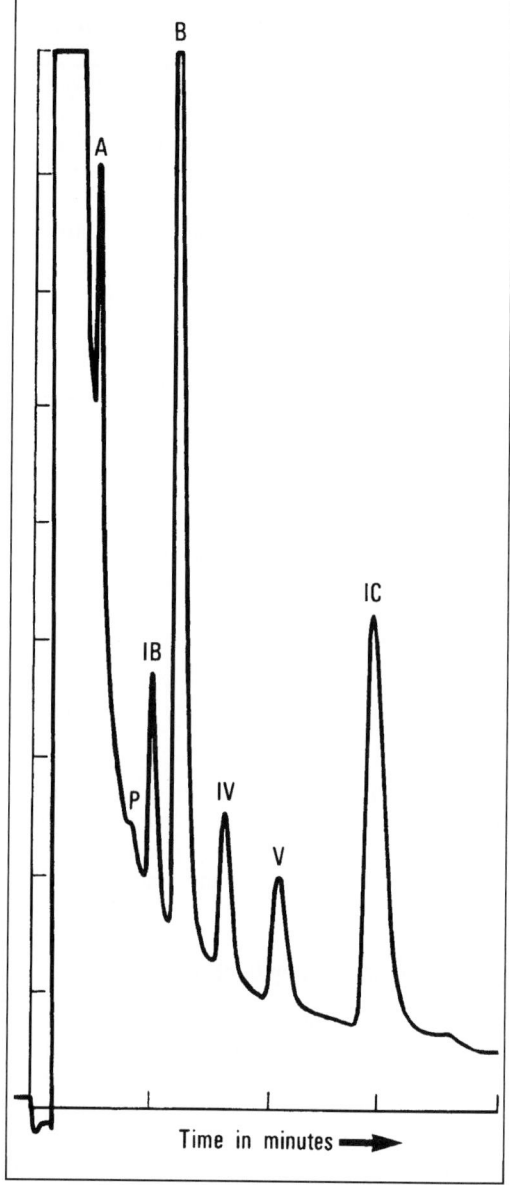

Figure 16-11 Example of a volatile acid chromatograph of a 48-hour peptone–yeast extract–glucose broth culture of *Clostridium difficile. A,* acetic acid; *P,* propionic acid; *IB,* isobutyric acid; *B,* butyric acid; *IV,* isovaleric acid; *V,* valeric acid; *IC,* isocaproic acid.

cally and/or those most frequently isolated from properly selected and collected clinical specimens comprise a much smaller list (Table 16-3). Only about 12–15 groups or species account for about 75% or more of the isolates from properly collected species. These include the *Bacteroides fragilis* group, the pigmented *Prevotella-Porphyromonas* group, *Fusobacterium nucleatum, Peptostreptococcus anaerobius, Finegoldia magna* (and a few other species of anaerobic cocci), *Propionibacterium acnes, Clostridium perfringens, C. ramosum,* and *Veillonella* spp. Laboratory personnel should be familiar with these species, because they are so common and often clinically significant. It is also especially important that clinical microbiologists know about and be able to recognize *Fusobacterium necrophorum, Actinomyces israelii, Propionibacterium propionicum,* the

C. clostridioforme group, *C. septicum, C. difficile, C. botulinum, C. tetani* and a few other species (discussed later in the text) because these organisms may be highly pathogenic for patients (even though they are not so common).

Beyond considerations of the need to be familiar with the common and/or medically significant anaerobes, it has been proposed that microbiologists in clinical laboratories may wish to limit the extent of anaerobe identification, based on levels of capability.[8,10] As proposed previously, laboratories with limited capability (level 1 or extent 1) should be able to isolate anaerobes in pure culture and to evaluate microscopic and colony morphology. Together with results of aer-

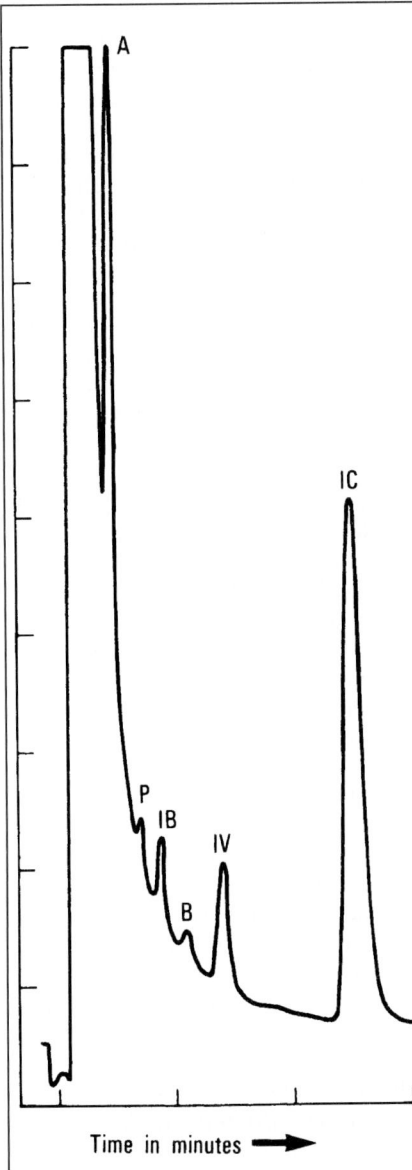

Figure 16-12 Example of a volatile acid chromatograph tracing of a 48-hour peptone–yeast extract–glucose broth culture of *Peptostreptococcus anaerobius.: A*, acetic acid; *P*, propionic acid; *IB*, isobutyric acid; *B*, butyric acid; *IV*, isovaleric acid; *IC*, isocaproic acid.

otolerance testing, this information would then be reported to the clinician (as a preliminary report). If clinically relevant, based on 1) the clinical situation as viewed by the clinician; 2) a direct Gram-stained smear of a wound or abscess, peritoneal fluid, or other specimen, showing evidence of acute inflammation (such as numerous polymorphonuclear leukocytes, but a lack of squamous epithelial cells) or necrosis; 3) microscopic evidence of clostridial myonecrosis (Plate 16-3*D*); 4) sulfur granules suggestive of actinomycetes (Color Plate 16-2*C* and *D*); 5) positive blood cultures or other positive body fluid cultures (e.g., pleural fluid, spinal fluid, joint fluid), the isolates, together with direct smears,

Box 16-11 Identifying Nonvolatile Fatty Acids

1. Transfer 1 mL of the original PYG culture to a clean 13- by 100-mm screw-capped tube.
2. Add 0.4 mL of H_2SO_4 (v/v) and 2 mL of methanol.
3. Place the tube in a 55°C water bath for 1 hour or overnight.
4. Add 1 mL of distilled water and 0.5 mL of chloroform, and centrifuge briefly to break any emulsion in the chloroform layer (chloroform will be in the bottom of the tube).
5. Fill a syringe with the chloroform extract after placing the tip of the needle beneath the aqueous layer.
6. Wipe off the outside of the needle with a clean tissue and inject 14 μL into a GLC column packed with SP-1000.

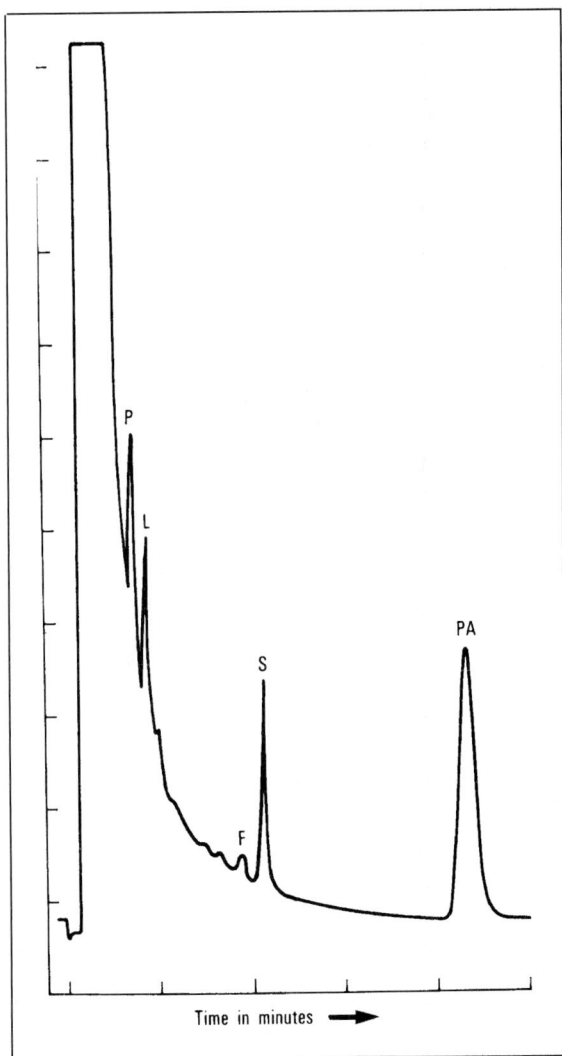

Figure 16-13 A typical nonvolatile acid standard chromatogram. The column was packed with 10% SP. 1000/1% H_3PO_4 on 100/120 chromasorb W/AW (Supelco, Bellefonte, PA). *P*, pyruvic acid; *L*, lactic acid; *F*, fumaric acid; *S*, succinic acid; *PA*, phenylacetic acid.

should be transported to a reference laboratory and processed further. Alternatively, laboratories with even the capability of definitive identification (level 4) of anaerobic isolates may wish to limit the extent of processing to level 1 when there is no clinical reason to take the identification further. One example would be of a peritoneal swab sample obtained at operation from a patient within hours of a penetrating knife or gunshot wound to the abdomen. Predictably, perforation of the large bowel or distal small intestine results in fecal spillage into the abdomen. Samples obtained at this time will probably show many mixed bacterial morphologic forms and few polymorphonuclear leukocytes in Gram-stained smears and will grow a mixture of normal bowel flora. Identification of these organisms would have no clinical usefulness and would be inordinately expensive.

The second level of capability that was proposed would require, in addition to level 1, some identification capability.[8,10] Specifically, the differentiation of the *B. fragilis* group from the other gram-negative anaerobes and identification of *C. perfringens* would be performed. Similar to the first level of identification, isolates and direct smears from clinically relevant cases would be transported to a reference laboratory for further identification of isolates.

The third level of capability that was proposed would require the presumptive identification of most of the twelve or so common anaerobe groups and species mentioned previously. This third category or extent of identification can be accomplished without the use of gas chromatography. As mentioned in the discussion of GLC procedures, the common and clinically important anaerobes that can be presumptively identified, using a few simple rapid tests, include the *B. fragilis* group, the pigmented *Prevotella-Porphyromonas* groups (when pigment is formed), *F. nucleatum*, *P. anaerobius*, *F. magna*, *P. acnes*, *C. perfringens*, *C. ramosum*, *A. israelii*, and several not-so-common species. Details of how morphology, growth characteristics, aerotolerance, some rapid spot tests, the Presumpto plate system, and other practical methods permit recognition and separation of these groups and species are given in the text that follows. It was pointed out previously that isolates requiring GLC and further characterization to permit accurate identification include most *Clostridium* species other than *C. perfringens* or *C. ramosum*, most species of *Fusobacterium*, most genera and species of anaerobic gram-negative non–spore-forming bacilli other than the *B. fragilis* group, some of the anaerobic cocci, and most of the anaerobic non–spore-forming gram-positive rods. This is mentioned again because the fourth level of identification (or definitive identification), including the tests done in the previous levels, also includes GLC for organisms that require it. In addition to determining morphology, growth characteristics, relationships to oxygen, preliminary spot tests, use of the Presumpto system, and GLC, definitive identification (level 4) includes determining whatever additional characteristics are needed (within reason) to arrive at an accurate identification to species (including those species that are not frequently isolated). Thus, additional characteristics might be obtained by traditional broth biochemical tests, the use of certain rapid enzyme tests (e.g., available in the API-ZYM (BioMérieux Vitek, Inc., Hazelwood, MO), RapID-ANA II (Remel, Leneka, KS), or in one of the other packaged kits), toxicity testing, slab gel polyacrylamide electrophoresis of soluble whole-cell pro-

teins, long-chain fatty acid analysis, 16S rRNA-DNA sequencing, or other procedures (e.g., through referral of isolates to a research laboratory for more extensive molecular testing) as necessary. Laboratories capable of definitive identification have the choice of limiting identifications to the preliminary or presumptive levels described previously. Laboratories capable of performing definitive or level 4 identification might include those at large university medical centers, many of the larger community and private hospitals, and state and federal public health laboratories.

Definitive identification is required to better define the role of anaerobic bacteria in diseases, to provide an accurate microbiologic diagnosis that can aid in the optimal choice of antibiotics and clinical treatment of the patient, for public health purposes (e.g., nosocomial diarrhea caused by *C. difficile*), and to help educate both clinicians and clinical microbiologists. How far one should go with anaerobe identification depends on several considerations that will differ among laboratories. Not all laboratories can be expected to perform the same levels of anaerobic bacteriologic studies. Factors that influence decision-making for the extent of identification include the technical competence and experience of the people who work in the laboratory, the number of personnel available, supplies and capital equipment budgeted (as well as other considerations), the patient population being served, and the needs of the clinicians who have responsibility for their patients.[8,10] Clinical microbiologists must be competent in the work that they do and should not hesitate to use the services of reference laboratories for aid in definitive identification or for reference confirmation of isolates, as well as antimicrobial susceptibility testing, toxigenicity testing, nucleic-acid studies, or other procedures when relevant clinically, if the referring laboratory lacks this capability. Additional approaches and current information on anaerobe identification, based on various combinations of tests at different levels, is given elsewhere.[60,125]

Anaerobic Gram-Negative Non–Spore-Forming Bacilli
CLASSIFICATION AND NOMENCLATURE

The anaerobic, gram-negative, non–spore-forming bacteria are now classified in the genera listed in Table 16-1. Key characteristics for differentiation of these are given in Table 16-8. The anaerobic gram-negative bacilli are among the normal flora of the oropharynx, lower digestive tract, vagina, cervix, urethra, and external genitalia. Only *Bacteroides, Prevotella, Porphyromonas, Fusobacterium,* and *Bilophila* among these genera are commonly isolated from properly selected and collected specimens (i.e., specimens without contamination with normal flora) from humans with significant infections.

As reviewed recently by others, the names of the anaerobic gram-negative bacilli continue to change (Table 16-2), largely as a result of taxonomic studies in which molecular procedures such as 16S rDNA sequencing are used.[67,123,124] Anaerobic bacteria are now being classified and reclassified based on phylogenetic relatedness, and the results of these molecular taxonomic investigations may not relate to Gram reaction, rod or coccus morphology, the ability to form spores, relationships to oxygen, or other phenotypic characteristics traditionally used to classify anaerobes. According to current phylogenetic studies, many species of anaerobic gram-negative rods cluster within the *Clostridium* subphylum of the gram-positive bacteria; these include a large number of bacteria that are among the indigenous microflora of humans and various other animals, and either are rare in clinical specimens or have not yet been isolated from clinical specimens (e.g., *Leptotrichia* spp., *Butyrivibrio fibrisolvens*, *Catonella morbi*, *Centipeda periodontii*, *Dialister pneumosintes*, *Johnsonella ignava*, *Mitsuokella multiacida*, *Selenomonas* spp., *Tissierella* spp., and others).[44,67,123,124]

In spite of many exciting new taxonomic breakthroughs based on molecular genetic research methods, phenotypic tests are still important for clinical diagnostic purposes, and must be relied on in hospital laboratories to identify anaerobes until simple, user-friendly, low-cost molecular identification procedures become available for these bacteria.[67] Thus, for identification of isolates in diagnostic laboratories, clinical microbiologists continue to depend on key morphologic features, biochemical and physiological characteristics, and in many instances, susceptibility or resistance to certain antimicrobial agents.

PRESUMPTIVE OR PRELIMINARY GROUP IDENTIFICATION OF *BACTEROIDES, PREVOTELLA, PORPHYROMONAS,* AND *FUSOBACTERIUM*

As previously indicated, the first major goal of identification should be to determine whether anaerobic bacteria are present and to isolate them in pure culture.[10] The presence of anaerobic gram-negative rods suggestive of *Bacteroides, Prevotella, Porphyromonas,* or *Fusobacterium* spp. (based on determining relationships to oxygen), together with the Gram stain results and colony observations, should be promptly reported to the clinician. Presumptive or preliminary identification of the *B. fragilis* group, and the *Prevotella-Porphyromonas* group, along with other obligately anaerobic, gram-negative rods, can easily be done using differential characteristics obtained with the Presumpto 1 plate and anaerobe blood agar (Tables 16-10 and 16-11). Additional clues for group identification along with key characteristics for various species are provided in Tables 16-12 through 16-16. Note that the common anaerobic gram-negative, non–spore-forming bacilli encountered clinically (Tables 16-10 and 16-11) are all nonmotile. In practice it is not practical or necessary to determine motility and perform flagella stains to differentiate the other genera of anaerobic Gram-negative bacilli (Table 16-8), unless the differential characteristics of an isolate (in pure culture) do not clearly fit those of species listed in Tables 16-10 through 16-16.

Identification of Bacteroides: The Bacteroides fragilis Group. As mentioned previously, organisms of the *B. fragilis* group are the anaerobic bacteria most often isolated from infections of humans, and these bacteria are particularly important clinically (Table 16-10). They are a part of the indigenous microbiota of the intestinal tract of most persons but are seldom found in the mouth. Through the years, numerous species names have been used for this group (e.g., *convexus, convexa, pseudoinsolita, inequalis, incommunis, uncata*), and likewise, several genus names, but now the group includes only those listed in Table 16-2.

The previously unnamed DNA homology group VPI "3452A," which closely resembles *B. distasonis* phenotypically, was given the name *B. caccae*.[118] Most strains of *B. caccae* have been isolated from feces; they are not common

in properly collected human clinical specimens. Two other DNA homology groups, VPI "T4-1" and "B5-21," were named *B. merdae* and *B. stercoralis*, respectively. These species also bear a close phenotypic similarity to *B. fragilis* and all the other species of the *B. fragilis* group. *B. merdae* and *B. stercoralis* have both been isolated from fecal samples and have been isolated rarely from clinical samples contaminated with feces or intestinal contents (unpublished data, Allen SD and Siders JA).

B. fragilis is the most common species of the group found in clinical specimens, but it is not often isolated from feces during studies of the intestinal flora. On the other hand, *B. ovatus* is not as frequently isolated from properly collected specimens, but is common in fecal materials. However, *B. ovatus* is occasionally isolated from the blood of compromised patients with polymicrobial bacteremia secondary to massive trauma or necrosis of the bowel. The chances of isolating *B. ovatus, B. caccae, B. merdae,* or *B. stercoralis* from properly collected, nonintestinal specimens are so low that isolates believed to show the differential characteristics of these species should be brought to the attention of the laboratory supervisor and/or director. *B. thetaiotaomicron* is the second most common species of the *B. fragilis* group in clinical infections (Table 16-2). For more information on the pathogenic properties and infections caused by the *B. fragilis* group, the reader is referred elsewhere.[6,70,155,222]

Organisms of the *B. fragilis* group are nonmotile, gram-negative rods with rounded ends, and are 0.5–0.8 μm in diameter $\times$ 1.5–9 μm long.[222] Cells from broth culture tend to be pleomorphic, often with vacuoles. Many strains are encapsulated; the pathogenic significance of their capsules is not clear. Colonies of *B. fragilis* on CDC anaerobe blood agar are 1 mm to 4 mm in diameter, nonhemolytic, gray, entire, and semiopaque with concentric whorls or ringlike structures inside the colonies (Color Plate 16-1). Colonies of other species of the group are similar in size and shape, but differ with regard to their internal structures. A key characteristic of species of the *B. fragilis* group is that their growth is enhanced by bile (Tables 16-10 and 16-12). They are all resistant to penicillin, kanamycin, colistin, and vancomycin, but sensitive to rifampin by the disk technique (Table 16-10). All are saccharolytic and their carbohydrate fermentation patterns (along with indole) help to differentiate between the species (Table 16-12). Detailed characteristics of the species are given in Tables 16-10 through 16-15. There are two species of *Bacteroides* in Table 16-12 that do not ferment sucrose, *B. eggerthii* and *B. splanchnicus*, and these share several phenotypic characteristics. In their proposal to restrict the genus *Bacteroides* to *Bacteroides fragilis* and closely related species, Shah and Collins included *B. eggerthii*, but not *B. splanchnicus*, in the *B. fragilis* group.[210] For practical purposes, both species are rare in properly selected and collected clinical materials. Thus, the differentiation between *B. eggerthii* and *B. splanchnicus* is seldom an issue in the clinical laboratory. For additional detailed characteristics of *B. splanchnicus*, see Table 16-14. For more information on *B. splanchnicus* and *B. eggerthii*, the chapter in Bergey's Manual by Holdeman and colleagues is recommended[110].

Pigmenting Anaerobic Gram-Negative Bacilli. As mentioned previously, Shah and Collins proposed that the genus

Table 16-10 Presumptive or Preliminary Identification of Obligately Anaerobic Gram-Negative Bacilli

GROUPS OR SPECIES	ANAEROBE BLOOD AGAR							PRESUMPTO 1 QUADRANT PLATE					
	Red Fluorescence (UV Light)	Brown-Black Colonies	Colonies <1 mm in Diameter	Agar Pitted	Penicillin (2-U Disk)	Rifampin (15-μg Disk)	Kanamycin 1-μg Disk	Indole	Lipase	Esculin	H$_2$S	Catalase (LD Esculin Agar)	Growth on Bile Agar
B. fragilis group	–	–	–	–	R	S	R	V	–	+/–	–	V	E
Pigmenting													
Porphyromonas–Prevotella	+	+	–	–	S or R	S	R	+	–/+	–	–	–	I or E
B. ureolyticus	–	–	+	+	S	S	S	–	–	–	–	–	I
Fusobacterium mortiferum	–	–	–	–	R or S	R	S	–	–	+	+	–	E
F. necrophorum	–	–	–	–	S	S	S	+	+	–	+	–	I
F. nucleatum	–	–	–	–	S	S	S	+	–	–	–	–	I
F. varium	–	–	–	–	R or S	R	S	+	–	–	+	–	E

R, growth not inhibited; S, growth inhibited; LD, Lombard-Dowell; V, variable reaction; +, positive reaction of 90–100% of strains tested; –, negative reaction strains tested; E, growth ≥ growth on LD agar; I, growth inhibited (compared with LD agar).

Table 16-11 Some Key Differential Characteristics of Commonly Isolated *Bacteroides* and *Fusobacterium* Species Available on CDC Anaerobe Blood Agar

SPECIES	RELATION TO O₂	COLONY CHARACTERISTICS	HEMOLYSIS OF SHEEP BLOOD	BRICK-RED FLUORESCENCE	BLACK PIGMENT	PITTING OF AGAR	CELLULAR MORPHOLOGY	GRAM-NEGATIVE SPORE MOTILITY	PENICILLIN (2-U DISK)	RIFAMPIN (15-µG DISK)	KANAMYCIN (1-µG DISK)	NITRATE REDUCTION
B. distasonis	OA	Small to medium, convex, semiopaque, entire edge	–	–	–	–	Small rods, variable length	–	R	S	R	–
B. fragilis	OA	Small to medium, convex, mottled surface, concentric rings, entire edge	–	–	–	–	Small rods, variable length	–	R	S	R	–
B. ovatus	OA	Small to medium, convex, opaque, entire edge	–	–	–	–	Small rods, variable length	–	R	S	R	–
B. thetaiotaomicron	OA	Small to medium, convex, opaque, entire edge	–	–	–	–	Small rods, variable length	–	R	S	R	–
B. uniformis	OA	Small to medium, convex, opaque, entire edge	–	–	–	–	Small rods, variable length	–	R	S	R	–
B. ureolyticus	OA	Pinpoint, convex, irregular edge	–	–	–	+	Small, slim rods, variable length	–	S	S	S	+
B. vulgatus	OA	Small to medium, convex, semiopaque, entire edge	–	–	–	–	Small rods, variable length	–	R	S	R	–
Porphyromonas as asaccharolytic a–P. gingivalis group	OA	Small to medium, convex, entire edge	+	+	+	–	Tiny coccoid rods	–	S	S	S	–
Prevotella bivia	OA	Small to medium, convex, entire edge	–	–	–	–	Tiny coccoid rods, vary in length	–	R	S	R	–
P. disiens	OA	Small to medium, convex, entire edge	–	–	–	–	Tiny coccoid rods, vary in length	–	R	S	R	–
P. intermedia	OA	Small to medium, convex, entire edge	+	+	+	–	Tiny coccoid rods	–	S or R	S	R	–
Fusobacterium F. mortiferum	OA	Small to medium, fried egg[a]	–	–	–	–	Highly pleomorphic rods, filaments, large round bodies	–	R or S	R	S	–
F. naviforme	OA	Small, low-convex, mottled, entire	–	–	–	–	Pleomorphic slim rods, some with pointed ends	–	S	S	S	–
F. necrophorum	OA	Small to medium, raised with opaque centers	–[b]	–	–	–	Highly variable in length and width	–	S	S	S	–
F. nucleatum	OA	Small to medium, speckled opalescence.[c] Occasionally colonies will resemble bread crumbs (rough colony form)	Green	–	–	–	Slim filamentous rods, even diameter, usually with pointed ends	–	S	S	S	–
F. varium	OA	Small to medium, fried egg[a]	–	–	–	–	Small rods, variable length, rounded ends	–	R or S	R	S	–

[a] Fried egg: raised opaque center with translucent, entire edge.
[b] F. necrophorum hemolyzes rabbit, but not sheep, red cells.
[c] Speckled opalescence: colonies of F. nucleatum show flecking (in the colonies) when viewed through the dissecting microscope with reflected light; they usually are not hemolytic, but may cause greenish discoloration of the blood agar on exposure to oxygen.
OA, obligate anaerobe; +, positive reaction in 90% of strains tested; –, negative reaction in 90% of strains tested; R, resistant; S, sensitive.
After Dowell VR, Allen SD. Anaerobic bacterial infections. In: Balows A, Hausler WJ Jr, eds. Diagnostic Procedures for Bacterial, Mycotic, and Parasitic Infections. Ed. 6. Washington, DC:174–219.

Table 16-12 Some Key Characteristics of Commonly Isolated Anaerobic, Gram-Negative Rods on CDC Differential Agar Media

SPECIES	NO. OF STRAINS EXAMINED	PRESUMPTO 1 PLATE								PRESUMPTO 2 PLATE					PRESUMPTO 3 PLATE		
		Indole	Indole Derivative	Esculin Hydrolysis	H₂S	Catalase	Lecithinase	Lipase	Growth on Bile Agar	Glucose Fermentation	Starch Hydrolysis	Milk Proteolysis	DNase	Gelatin Hydrolysis	Mannitol Fermentation	Lactose Fermentation	Rhamnose Fermentation
B. distasonis	21	−	−	+	−	+/−	−	−	E	+	+	−/+	−	−	−	+	+
B. fragilis	135	−	−	+	−	+	−	−	E-ppt	+	−/+	−/+	−	−/+	−	+	+
B. ovatus	5	+/−	−	+	−	V	−	−	E-ppt	+	V	V	V	−	+/−	+	−
B. thetaiotaomicron	71	+	−	+	−	+	−	−	E	+	−/+	−/+	+/−	−	−	+	+
B. uniformis	5	+	−	+/−	−	−	−	−	E	+	V	V	V	−	−	+	−/+
B. vulgatus	23	−	−	−/+	−	−	−	−	E	+	−	−	−	−	−	+	+
B. splanchnicus	2	+	−	+	V	−	−	−	E	+	−	−	−	V	−	+	−
B. ureolyticus	1	−	−	−	−	−	−	−	V	−	−	−/+	−	−/+	−	−	−
Campylobacter gracilis	10	−	−	−	−	−	−	−	V	−	−	−	−	−	−	−	−
Porphyromonas asaccharolytica	6	+/−	−	−	−	−	−	−/+	NG	−	−	+/−	−/+	V	−	−	−
P. gingivalis	13	+	−	−	V	−	−	−	NG	−	−/+	+	−/+	+	−	−	−
Prevotella bivia	14	−	−	−	−	−	−	−	NG	+	−/+	+/−	+/−	V	−/+	+	−/+
P. disiens	3	−	−	−	−	−	−	−	V	+/−	−	+	V	+	−	−	−
P. denticola	5	−	−	−/+	−	−	−	−	NG	+	+	+	+/−	−/+	−	+	−
P. intermedia/nigrescens	16	+	−	−	−	−	−	+	NG	+/−	+/−	+	+	+	−	+	−/+
P. melaninogenica	10	−	−	−	−	−	−	−	NG	+	+	−	+/−	V	−	+	−
P. oralis	2	−	−	+	−	−	−	−	NG	V	V	−	V	−	−	V	V
P. oris/buccae	9	−	−	+	−	−	−	−	NG	+	+	+/−	+	+	−	+	−/+
P. veroralis	2	−	−	V	−	−	−	−	NG	+	+	−	V	V	−	+	V
Fusobacterium gonidiaformans	6	+/−	−	−	−/+	−	−	−	NG	−/+	−	−	−	−	−	−	−
F. mortiferum	5	−/+	−	+	−	−	−	−	E	+	+	−	+	+	−	V	−
F. naviforme	6	+	−	−	−	−	−	−	NG	−/+	−	−	−	−	−	−	−
F. necrophorum	18	+	−	−	V	−	−	+	NG	V	V	+	V	V	−/+	−	−
F. nucleatum	31	+	−	−	V	−	−	−	NG	V	−	−	−/+	−	−	−	−
F. varium	6	V	−	−	V	−	−	−	E	−	−	−	−	−	−	−	−

+, positive reaction in <90% strains; −, negative reaction in <90% strains; +/−, most strains positive, occasional strain negative; −/+, most strains negative, occasional strain positive; V, variable; I, growth inhibited; E, growth equal to control without bile; E¹, equal growth with an occasional strain inhibited; E-ppt, equal growth with a precipitate adjacent to or under growth; NG, no growth. *Use of Presumpto plates to identify anaerobic bacteria.*
Adapted from Whaley DN, Wiggs LS, Miller PH, Srivastava PU, Miller JM. *J Clin Microbiol 33: 1196–1202, 1995; and previous editions of this book.*

Table 16-13 Characteristics Helpful in Differentiation of *Bacteroides fragilis* Group and Closely Related Species That Grow Well in 20% Bile

SPECIES	PRODUCTION OF		FERMENTATION OF										
	Indole	Catalase	Arabinose	Cellobiose	Glucose	Melezitose	Rhamnose	Ribose	Salicin	Sucrose	Trehalose	Xylan
B. fragilis group												
A. Indole-negative subgroup												
B. caccae	–	–	+	+	+	+	+/–	+	+	+	+	–
B. distasonis	–	+	–	+	+	+	+/–	+/–	+	+	+	–
B. fragilis	–	+	–	–/w	+	–	–	–	+	+	–	–
B. merdae	–	–	–/+	–	+	+	–/+	–	w	+	+	–
B. vulgatus	–	V	+	–	+	–	+	–/+	–	+	–	–/+
B. Indole-positive subgroup												
B. ovatus	+	+	+	+	+	+/–	+	+	+	+	+	+
B. stercoris	+	–	–/+	–	+	–	+	–/w	–	+	–	–
B. thetaiotaomicron	+	+	+	+	+	V	+	+	–/+	+	+	–
B. uniformis	+	–	+	+	+	–	–/+	–/+	+/–	+	–	ND
B. eggerthii	+	V	+	–/w	+	–	w/–	–	–	–	–	+
Other Related *Bacteroides* spp.												
B. splanchnicus	+	–	+	–	+	–	–	–	–	–	–	ND

+, Positive reaction for 90% or more of strains (includes weak and strong reactions); +/–, 51–89% strains positive; –/+, 10–50% strains positive; –, less than 10% strains positive; V, variable reactions; w, weak reactions; ND, data not available. After Holdeman et al[105]; Johnson et al[116]; and Allen and Siders, unpublished data.

Table 16-14 Characteristics of Glucose-Fermenting, Bile-Sensitive, Pigmented and Nonpigmented *Prevotella* Spp. Isolated From Clinical Specimens[a]

	FERMENTATION OF									ESCULIN HYDROLYSIS	INDOLE
	Amygdalin	Arabinose	Cellobiose	Lactose	Melibiose	Raffinose	Salicin	Sucrose	Xylose		
May be pigmented											
P. corporis	–	–	–	–	–	–	–	–	–	–	–
P. denticola	–	–	V	+	–	+	V	+	–	+	–
P. intermedia	–	–	–	–	–	V	–	+	–	–	+
P. loescheii	–	–	+	+	V	+	V	+	–	+	–/+
P. melaninogenica	–	–	V	+	–/+	NT	–	+	–	V	–
P. nigrescens	–	–	–	–	–	–	–	+	–	–	+
P. tannerae	–	–	–	V	–	V	–	V	–	V	–
Not pigmented											
P. bivia	–	–	–	+	–	–	–	–	–	–	–
P. buccae	+/–	+	+	+	+	+	+	+	+	+	–
P. buccalis	NT	–	+	+	+	+	+	+	–	+	–
P. dentalis	NT	+	+	+	W	+	–	W	–	–	–
P. disiens	–	–	–	–	–	–	–	–	–	–	–
P. enoeca	–	–	–	+	–	–	–	–	V	V	–
P. heparinolytica[b]	NT	+	+	+	NT	–	+	+	+	+	+
P. oralis	+	–	+	+	+	+	+	+	+	+	–
P. oris	+/–	+	+	+	V	+	+	+	–	+	–
P. oulora	NT	–	–	+	w/+	+	–	+	–	+	–
P. veroralis	–	–	V	+	w	+	V	+	V	V	–
P. zoogleoformans[b]	–/w	V	V	V	V	V	V	+	V	V	+/–

[a] Biochemical features modified from Holdeman, Kelly, and Moore (*Bergey's Manual of Systematic Bacteriology*; 1984), Shah and Collins (*Int J System Bacteriol* 1990;40:205–208), Shah and Gharbia (*Int J Syst Bacteriol* 1992;42:542–546), Moore and Moore (*Int J System Bacteriol* 1994;44:599–602), and Williams and Collins (*Int J System Bacteriol* 1995;45:832–836).
[b] Broth cultures have a glutinous or sticky sediment.
–, negative reaction; +, positive reaction; V, variable; +/–, most strains positive; –/+, most strains negative; NT, not tested; +/w, most strains positive, some weakly positive; w/+, most weakly positive; w, weak reaction.

Table 16-15 Metabolic Products of *Bacteroides, Porphyromonas, Prevotella,* and *Fusobacterium* Species in Peptone-Yeast Extract-Glucose Broth Cultures After 48 Hours at 35°C[a]

SPECIES OR GROUP	A	P	IB	B	IV	V	IC	C	L	S	PA[S]	PROPIONATE FROM THREONINE
Bacteroides												
B. capillosus	+	V	−	−	−	−	−	−	−	+		
B. distasonis	+	+/−	−	−	V	−	−	−	+/−	+	+	
B. fragilis	+	+/−	V	−	V	−	−	−	+	+	+	
B. ovatus	+	+	V	−	V	−	−	−	V	+	+	
B. splanchnicus	+	+	+	+	V	−	−	−	V	S		
B. thetaiotaomicron	+	+/−	V	−	V	−	−	−	V	+	+	
B. uniformis	+	+/−	V	−	V	−	−	−	+	+		
B. ureolyticus	+	−	−	−	−	−	−	−	−	+		
B. vulgatus	+	+	V	−	−	V	−	−	+	+	−	
Porphyromonas												
P. asaccharolytica[b]	+	+	+	+	+	−	−	−	−	+	−	
P. gingivalis	+	+	+	+	+	−	−	−	−	+	+	
Prevotella												
P. bivia	+	−	V	−	+/−	−	−	−	−	+		
P. disiens	+	V	V	−	V	−	−	−	−	+		
P. intermedia	+	V	V	−	+	−	−	−	−	+	−	
Fusobacterium												
F. gonidiaformans	+	+	−	+	−	−	−	−	−	−		+
F. mortiferum	+	+/−	−	+	−	−/+	−	−	−	−		+
F. naviforme	+	V	−	+	−	−	−	−	−	−		−
F. necrophorum	+	+	−	+	−	−	−	−	−	−		+
F. nucleatum	+	+	−	+	−	−	−	−	−	−/+		+
F. varium	+	+	−	+	−	−	−	−	+	−/+		+

[a] *The species listed in this table are those that can be differentiated using the differential agar media system (see Tables 16–10, 16–11, and 16–12). The asaccharolytic, black-pigmented Porphyromonas, P. asaccharolyticus and P. gingivalis, can be presumptively differentiated by the presence or lack of phenylacetic (PA) acid and additional tests described in the text.*

[b] *Data on differentiation of certain Bacteroides fragilis group organisms and black pigmented species using PA acid is from Mayrand and Shah and Collins, as cited in the 5th edition of this book.*

A, acetic; P, propionic; IB, isobutyric; B, butyric; IV, isovaleric; IC, isocaproic; C, caproic; L, lactic; PA, phenylacetic acid; S, succinic acid; +, major peak; −, no major peak; +/−, usually a major peak, but may be negative; −/+, usually negative, but may be present; V, variable.

After Dowell VR, Lombard GL. Presumptive Identification of Anaerobic Non-spore-forming Gram-negative Bacilli. Atlanta: Centers for Disease Control, 1977: 13.

Bacteroides be restricted to the *Bacteroides fragilis* group and related species, which actively ferment glucose (pH ≤5.4) (highly saccharolytic), grow in the presence of 20% bile, and hydrolyze esculin.[210] Their major acid metabolic products from glucose metabolism are acetic and succinic acids, and smaller amounts of other short-chain fatty acids may be produced.[210] Thus, the pigmenting anaerobic gram-negative bacilli are no longer classified in the genus *Bacteroides*. The moderately saccharolytic, pigmenting species were placed in the genus *Prevotella*. In 1988, the asaccharolytic, pigmented *Bacteroides*, all isolated from humans, were reclassified in the genus *Porphyromonas* as *P. asaccharolytica, P. gingivalis,* and *P. endodontalis*.[209] Additional *Porphyromonas* species of human origin now include *P. catoniae* (nonpigmented), and those considered to be *P. levii*-like.[124]

The following pigmenting, saccharolytic species are encountered in clinical specimens from humans: *Prevotella melaninogenica, P. corporis, P. denticola, P. intermedia, P. nigrescens, P. loescheii, P. tannerae,* and *P. pallens, P. shahii,* and *P. salivae*.[136,178,204,211,213,214,261] Many species of *Prevotella* are commonly isolated from the oral cavity, from infections involving the head and neck and lower respiratory tract, and from the urogenital tract.

A large proportion, if not most, *Porphyromonas* strains isolated from the oral cavity probably are *Porphyromonas gingivalis*[244]; most of the nonoral clinical isolates of *Porphyromonas* isolated from other anatomic regions of humans are probably *Porphyromonas asaccharolytica,* whereas *Porphyromonas endodontalis* strains have been isolated from infected root canals.[209]

Box 16-12 Characteristics for Identification of *Porphyromonas* Spp.

1. *P. gingivalis*: Produces phenylacetic acid (see Table 16–11) and agglutinates sheep red blood cells[173]; produces β-galactose-6-phosphatase, and *N*-acetyl-β-glucosaminidase, but not α-fucosidase; can be tested in the Rapid ID 32A system (BioMérieux-Vitek).[204,206]
2. *P. asaccharolytica:* not as the foregoing species; produces α-fucosidase; as tested in the Rapid ID 32A system.[204,206]
3. *P. endodontalis:* not as either of the foregoing species.

Since 1992, the genus *Porphyromonas* has changed markedly with a grand total now of 13 species (Tables 16-2). Five of these species were isolated from oral cavities of dogs only (*P. cangingivalis, P. canoris, P. cansulci, P. crevioricanis,* and *P. gingivicanis*),[45,105,159] one has been isolated from the oral cavities of cats only (*P. circumdentaria*),[157] another has been isolated from both monkeys and cats (*P. macacae,* which includes those previously called *P. salivosa*),[156-158] another is from cattle (*P. levii*),[212] one species was isolated from the human oral cavity (*P. catoniae*),[262] and *P. gulae,* described in 2001, was isolated from various animals (i.e., including bear, cat, coyote, dog, wolf and monkey). Presumably, although their clinical importance in humans is unknown, the species isolated from the mouths of animals could be encountered in bite-wound infections.

In 1995, not only did Willems and Collins reclassify *Oribaculum catoniae* as *Porphyromonas catoniae,* but they emended the genus *Porphyromonas* as well. In accordance with their emended description, some species are now included that are saccharolytic (*P. levii, P. macacae,* and *P. catoniae*), and *P. catoniae* does not form pigment.[262]

Presumptive clues for the recognition of anaerobic gram-negative bacilli that belong to the genus *Porphyromonas* include the formation of tan to buff colonies that fluoresce brick-red under long-wave ultraviolet light or brown-black colonies (most species), inhibition of growth in the presence of vancomycin (i.e., failure to grow on kanamycin-vancomycin blood agar), inhibition by bile, inhibition by penicillin and rifampin, but resistance to kanamycin, formation of indole, and failure of most species to ferment glucose or other carbohydrates. Definitive identification of *Porphyromonas* to the species level based on phenotypic characteristics is difficult. Some key differential characteristics of the asaccharolytic, pigmented, and catalase negative species encountered in human illnesses are listed in Box 16-12.

Thus, the determination of enzyme activities through the use of a rapid, 4-hour test system (*i.e.,* the Rapid ID 32A system or RapID ANA II) is a practical aid to identify *Porphyromonas* species encountered in humans.[50,243,244] Additional characteristics of *Porphyromonas* species are given in Table 16-16.

In contrast to *Porphyromonas,* all of the pigmented species of *Prevotella* ferment glucose and other carbohydrates (Tables 16-14 and 16-16). It is emphasized that the "pigmenting" *Prevotella* group described in Table 16-16 may take from 2 days to 3 weeks to form pigment on CDC anaerobic blood agar or may even fail to produce pigmented colonies. *Prevotella intermedia* is distinctive in that it forms black colonies, produces indole, is lipase-positive on egg yolk agar, and ferments sucrose. *Prevotella nigrescens* is a species derived from a genetically distinct group of strains formerly included in *Prevotella intermedia.*[213] Some of these strains were from patients with periodontitis; others were

---

Table 16-16 Characteristics That Are Especially Useful for Identifying Commonly Encountered *Bacteroides, Porphyromonas, Prevotella,* and *Fusobacterium* Species

CHARACTERISTIC	SPECIES
Brick-red fluorescence (with long-wave UV light) or brown-black pigment	*Prevotella melaninogenica* group[a], *Porphyromonas* spp.
Good growth on 20% bile; resistant to penicillin (2-U disk), kanamycin (1-μg disk); and inhibited by rifampin (15-μg disk)	*Bacteroides fragilis* group[a]
Catalase produced on LD esculin agar	*B. fragilis, B. thetaiotaomicron, B. distasonis, B. ovatus*
Lipase produced on LD egg yolk agar	*Prevotella intermedia, F. necrophorum*
Asaccharolytic (glucose or other carbohydrates not fermented)	*Bacteroides* CDC group F$_2$, *Porphyromonas asaccharolytica, P. gingivalis, B. capillosis* (this species is rare), *B. ureolyticus, F. gonidiaformans* (rare), *F. naviforme, F. nucleatum*
Agar pitted; urease-positive	*B. ureolyticus*
Gelatin hydrolyzed; milk digested	*Prevotella bivia, P. disiens, P. intermedia*
DNase-positive; enhanced growth on 20% bile	*B. thetaiotaomicron, B. uniformis, B. ovatus*
Resistant to rifampin; esculin hydrolyzed	*F. mortiferum*
Resistant to rifampin; esculin not hydrolyzed	*F. varium*
Long, thin, filamentous rods; internal speckling of colonies; propionate produced from threonine	*F. nucleatum*

[a] See text for listing of species included.

from healthy individuals. Whereas both *P. nigrescens* and *P. intermedia* form brown to black colonies on blood agar, produce indole, and ferment sucrose, only *P. intermedia* produces lipase. *Prevotella corporis*, formerly classified as *Bacteroides melaninogenicus* subsp. *intermedius*, differs from *P. intermedia* in that *P. corporis* does not produce indole, is lipase-negative, and does not ferment sucrose (Table 16-16). *Prevotella bivia* and *Prevotella disiens* are very similar phenotypically to *P. intermedius* and *P. corporis*. *Prevotella bivia* is found in the urogenital tract and mouth, and *P. disiens* is commonly isolated from the urogenital tract. They are saccharolytic, and can easily be confused when *P. intermedia* and *P. corporis* fail to produce pigment. In addition, it has been reported by Ueno (personal communication) that *P. bivia* may produce pigment under certain conditions. Four other species of saccharolytic, pigmenting *Prevotella* that may be isolated from humans (*Prevotella melaninogenica*, *P. loescheii*, *P. denticola.*, and *P. tannerae*) usually ferment lactose, in contrast to *P. intermedia*, *P. nigrescens* and *P. corporis*, which are lactose-negative. *P. denticola* is slow to produce pigment; some strains may not produce pigment even after 3 weeks of incubation. *P. denticola* ferments esculin (acid produced) and ribose, characteristics that help to separate it from *P. melaninogenica* (which is negative for these characteristics).[109] *P. loescheii* also does not ferment esculin, in contrast to both *P. denticola* and *P. melaninogenica*, and is cellobiose-positive. Most strains of *P. tannerae* do not hydrolyze esculin (86% of strains negative for esculin), and most (69%) do not ferment sucrose. Another pigmented organism, *Porphyromonas levii*, has been isolated only from ruminants and will not be discussed further.[212]

A major problem in identifying the pigmented group to species is that they are often fastidious and slow-growing, and they may require anywhere from 2 days to a full 3 weeks to form pigment (on laked rabbit blood or on sheep blood agar). The pigmented *Prevotella-Porphyromonas* groups are part of the normal flora of the oropharynx, nose, and gastrointestinal and genitourinary tracts. They are the second most common group of anaerobic bacteria encountered in human infections (Table 16-3). In some clinical situations—for example, orofacial lesions and anaerobic pleuropulmonary infections—they are more common than the *B. fragilis* group. Certain species, in particular *Prevotella intermedia* (and possibly *P. nigrescens*), are of special clinical interest because they commonly produce β-lactamase and may be resistant in vitro to penicillin G and other antibiotics.[69] Prior to pigmentation, young colonies often exhibit a brick-red fluorescence when examined under long-wave (365 nm) ultraviolet light. In Gram-stained preparations, the cells are short, coccoid, gram-negative rods, usually 0.3–0.4 μm in diameter × 0.6–1 μm long (Color Plate 16-1). In the Presumptoplate system, these species are inhibited by bile, usually (but not always) sensitive by the 2-U penicillin disk test, sensitive to rifampin, and resistant to kanamycin. Further characteristics for differentiation include those given in Table 16-16, or may be determined using tests for enzymatic activities.[50,178,214,242,244]

Other Species of **Prevotella.** As mentioned previously, *Prevotella bivia* and *P. disiens* are species that phenotypically resemble *P. intermedia*, *P. nigrescins*, and *P. corporis*. They are inhibited by bile, usually resistant to penicillin, susceptible to rifampin, and resistant to kanamycin. Acetate and suc-

cinate are major metabolic products. Besides their usual lack of pigment on CDC anaerobic blood agar held for 5 to 7 days, *P. bivia* and *P. disiens* differ from *P. intermedia-nigrescens* in being indole-negative and lipase-negative. In addition, *P. bivia* ferments lactose, whereas neither *P. disiens* nor *P. intermedia-nigrescens* ferments lactose.[108] A nonpigmented *P. corporis* would appear virtually identical to *P. disiens* (Table 16-16). Like the *B. fragilis* and pigmented *Prevotella-Porphyromonas* groups, strains of *P. bivia* and *P. disiens* produce β-lactamase and may be resistant to several β-lactam antibiotics.[69] They have been isolated from blood, head and neck infections, genitourinary tract infections in both males and females, and other infection sites. Characteristics useful for separating *P. bivia* and *P. disiens* from phenotypically similar *P. oralis* and related species are given in Table 16-16. In addition to *Prevotella tannerae*, described above, Moore and associates described another species that inhabits the human gingival crevice, *Prevotella enoeca*, and emended the description of *Prevotella zoogleoformans*.[178] Both species have been isolated from patients with periodontitis, neither forms pigment on blood agar, and both ferment a variety of carbohydrates. Key features that aid in distinguishing *P. enoeca* from other species of *Prevotella* are its inability to digest gelatin, its failure to ferment sucrose, and its cellular fatty acid profile. Fermentation of cellobiose and lactose, lack of pigment, and its cellular fatty acid profile, are key characteristics that aid in differentiating *P. zoogleoformans* from other indole-positive *Prevotella* species, especially *P. intermedia* and *P. nigrescens*, with which it shares phenotypic characteristics.[178] An additional taxonomic change in 1995 was the reclassification of *Hallella seregens* and *Mitsuokella dentalis* as *Prevotella dentalis*.[261] Isolated from dental root canals, the colonies of *P. dentalis* are not pigmented; they differ from those of other *Prevotella* species by having a "characteristic water drop appearance."

Prevotella oralis *and Related Species.* Major changes in the taxonomic classification of organisms previously called *Bacteroides oralis* and *B. ruminicola* (human strains) were made on the basis of DNA-homology studies.[106] Some of the isolates identified as "*B. oralis*" in the past undoubtedly were members of the *B. melaninogenicus* group that had not formed pigment, especially *Prevotella denticola* (discussed previously). *Prevotella buccalis*, *P. veroralis*, and *B. oralis* were all previously called *B. oralis*. They are all inhibited in 20% bile medium, are indole-negative and positive for esculin hydrolysis, and ferment several carbohydrates.[109] Differential tests that aid in separating these species include fermentation of salicin, amygdalin, and xylan and hydrolysis of starch (Table 16-16). If they fail to produce pigment, *P. denticola* and *P. melaninogenica* can be easily confused with *P. buccalis*, *P. veroralis*, and *P. oralis*. However, the latter three species ferment cellobiose; *P. denticola* and *P. melaninogenica* are cellobiose-negative. *P. oris* and *P. buccae* have been isolated from periodontal infections and various other infection sites in humans.[113] Many strains of these species were previously called *B. ruminicola* (human strains). Like *P. buccalis*, *P. veroralis* and *P. oralis*, *P. oris* and *P. buccae* are inhibited by bile, are indole-negative and positive for esculin hydrolysis, and ferment glucose plus additional carbohydrates. The production of acid from either arabinose or xylose separates *P. oris* and *P. buccae* from *P.*

oralis.[113] The fermentation of salicin helps to separate *P. buccae* and *P. oris* from *P. buccalis* and *P. veroralis*, which are salicin-negative. A test that is positive for β-glucosidase activity by *P. buccae* but negative for *P. oris* aids in separating these species.[109] Reactions obtained using the RapID-ANA II system may also be useful as a supplement to the tests in Table 16-16, to help differentiate these species.[50]

Bacteroides ureolyticus *and Other Asaccharolytic Nitrate-Positive Species.*

Bacteroides ureolyticus (formerly *B. corrodens*), is a microaerophilic (but previously thought to be anaerobic), fastidious, relatively small gram-negative rod (about 0.5 μm in diameter by 1.5 to 2 μm in length) that produces pitting of anaerobic blood agar. This species is in need of reclassification. The cells do not produce flagella and are nonmotile. Characteristically, the colonies may be of two types: 1) 0.5–1 mm diameter after 2 or more days incubation, circular, convex, and translucent with entire or erose margins, or 2) thin, flat, spreading, irregular translucent colonies that extend out from a slightly raised central area. These latter colony types produce depressions or "pits" within the surface of agar, perhaps resembling the "corrosion" of pitted sheet metal. *B. ureolyticus* is inhibited by penicillin (2-U disk), rifampin (15-μg disk), and kanamycin (1-μg disk) and does not grow in the presence of 20% bile, nor does it ferment any carbohydrates (i.e., it is asaccharolytic). *Campylobacter gracilis*, formerly called *Bacteroides gracilis*,[245] is also microaerophilic, and has growth characteristics similar to those of *B. ureolyticus*. A positive test for urease activity separates *B. ureolyticus* from *C. gracilis* and phenotypically similar species of *Campylobacter* and *Wollinella succinogenes* (the only remaining species after *W. curva* and *W. rectus* were reclassified as *Campylobacter curvus* and *C. rectus*), which are all urease-negative. *C. gracilis* (*B. gracilis*) does not form flagella and is nonmotile, in contradistinction to *C. curvus*, *C. rectus*, and *W. succinogenes*. *C. rectus*, for example, is actively motile (by means of a single polar flagellum).[125] According to one report,[116] *B. ureolyticus* was most frequently isolated from superficial soft-tissue or bone infections that tended to be mild. *C. gracilis* (*B. gracilis*), in contrast, was commonly isolated from "serious" deep-seated infections, including head and neck infections, pleuropulmonary infections and infected sites within the abdomen and pelvis. *B. ureolyticus* was uniformly susceptible to the various penicillins, cephalosporins, and other antimicrobial agents tested (included clindamycin, chloramphenicol, metronidazole, and even aminoglycosides), whereas the *C. gracilis* isolates were commonly resistant to the penicillins, cephalosporins, and clindamycin.[116] Thus, *C. gracilis* is probably a more virulent organism for humans than *B. ureolyticus*, and its frequent resistance to antimicrobial agents may contribute to its clinical significance. The clinical importance of *C. concisus* and *C. recta*, which share some features with *B. ureolyticus* and *C. gracilis*, has not been established.

Examples of other *Bacteroides* spp. or former *Bacteroides* species whose clinical significance is not well known or established include *B. amylophilus*, *B. coagulans*, *B. eggerthii*, *B. hypermegas* (now called *Megamonas hypermegas*), *B. multiacidus* (now called *Mitsuokella multiacidus*), *B. nodosus*, *B. pneumosintes*, *B. praeacutus* (now called *Tissierella praeacuta*), *B. putredinis*, *B. splanchnicus*, and others. Most of these species are encountered only rarely

in human clinical specimens. Detailed characteristics of these and other little-known species of *Bacteroides* are given in the *VPI Manual*[107] and in *Bergey's Manual*.[109] For an excellent review of their role in infections and their susceptibility to antimicrobial agents, see Kirby et al.[133]

Bilophila *Species.*

During a study of bacteria isolated from appendicitis specimens and human feces, a unique new anaerobic gram-negative bacillus was isolated on *Bacteroides* bile-esculin agar by Baron and associates.[17] This new species was reported to show the characteristics listed in Box 16-13.

Although *Bilophila wadsworthia* is similar to species of the *B. fragilis* group and to certain *Fusobacterium* species that grow in the presence of 20% bile, several of the phenotypic properties of *Bilophila wadsworthia* are different from those of the *Bacteroides fragilis* group and *Fusobacterium* spp. *Bilophila wadsworthia* differs from the *B. fragilis* group by its failure to ferment carbohydrates, its production of urease, and its failure to produce a major amount of succinic acid. The production of strong catalase activity and its lack of butyric acid production are key characteristics that separate *B. wadsworthia* from *Fusobacterium* species.

Fusobacterium.

The genus *Fusobacterium* includes several species of anaerobic, gram-negative, non–spore-forming rods that can be differentiated from species of *Bacteroides, Prevotella, Porphyromonas,* and *Leptotrichia* by their production of major amounts of butyric acid but no isobutyric or isovaleric acid (Fig. 16-10 and Table 16-15). The species of *Bacteroides* and *Porphyromonas* that produce butyric acid also produce isobutyric and isovaleric acids. Historically, *Fusobacterium* species have had many other genus names,

---

Box 16-13 Characteristics of *Bilophila* Spp.

Gram-negative, non–spore-forming, nonmotile, pleomorphic rods; 0.7–1.1 μm in width by 1–10 μm in length

Growth enhanced by 20% bile and by 1% pyruvate; grow slowly on bacteroides bile esculin (BBE); colonies on BBE after 4 days of incubation were described as 1- to 2-mm (diameter), either as circular, erose, umbonate, and translucent with dark black centers, or as irregular, low convex, opaque black colonies

Colonies on *Brucella* agar formed slowly (4 to 7 days), were punctate, less than 1-mm in diameter, circular, erose, translucent, and gray

Strongly catalase-positive (using 15% H_2O_2)

Asaccharolytic

Urease-positive

H_2S-positive, desulfoviridin-positive

Nitrate-positive

Negative for the hydrolysis of esculin or starch

Indole-negative; gelatin not liquefied; no reactions produced in milk or on egg-yolk agar; oxidase-negative

β-lactamase-negative (nitrocefin test), but nonetheless, resistant to β-lactam antibiotics

Acetate is the major metabolic product; lactate not detected; minor or trace amounts of succinate produced in peptone–yeast glucose (supplemented by pyruvate)

including *Sphaerophorus*, *Fusiformis*, *Pseudobacterium, Ristella, Necrobacterium,* and *Zuberella*.[222]

Although their name would seem to suggest that the fusobacteria are "fusiform" or "spindle-shaped," only a few of them are—the majority are not; rather, they are rod-shaped with parallel sides and rounded (not pointed) ends. While they grow well on anaerobic blood agar under anaerobic conditions, they are readily killed by exposure to ambient air. Most species are either nonfermentative or only weakly fermentative.[222]

Fusobacterium species are normally found in the upper respiratory, gastrointestinal, and genitourinary tracts of humans. They are commonly involved in serious infections in various body sites.[6,155] They are especially associated with infections of the mouth, bite wounds, and respiratory tract, which should not be surprising, since the mouth is a major habitat. In some hospital settings, fusobacteria are not uncommon in blood cultures.[5] Felner and Dowell[66] described 55 patients with *Fusobacterium* bacteremia (compared to 196 cases of *Bacteroides* bacteremia). An additional series of 26 cases of *Fusobacterium* bacteremia was published by Henry et. al.[99] Bourgault and colleagues reported significant mortality with *Fusobacterium* bacteremia; 13 of 40 (32.5%) patients whose blood cultures yielded fusobacteria died.[30] In the latter study, 36 isolates were identified to the species level: these included *F. nucleatum* (17 isolates), *F. necrophorum* (8 isolates), *F. mortiferum* (5), *F. varium* (3), and *F. gonidiaformans* (3). The following antimicrobial agents were active against all 36 isolates: penicillin, piperacillin, cefoxitin, clindamycin, metronidazole, and imipenem.[30]

F. nucleatum and members of the *Prevotella-Porphyromonas* group are the organisms most frequently involved in anaerobic pleuropulmonary infections (e.g., aspiration pneumonia, lung abscess, necrotizing pneumonia, thoracic empyema). Fusobacteria are also fairly common pathogens in brain abscess, chronic sinusitis, metastatic osteomyelitis, septic arthritis, liver abscess, and other intraabdominal infections.[6]

F. nucleatum is the species most commonly found in clinical materials. Recent attention has been called to severe systemic infections caused by *F. nucleatum* in patients with neutropenia and mucositis following chemotherapy.[36,65,143] Early recognition of *F. nucleatum* in clinical materials, particularly during direct microscopic examination of body fluids or exudates, can be important. The spindle-shaped cells are long, slender filaments with tapered ends (Color Plate 16-1).[166] Sometimes there are spherical swellings. Cells are usually 5 μm to 10 μm long, but shorter forms are often seen. Colonies on anaerobe blood agar are 1 mm to 2 mm in diameter, slightly convex with slightly irregular margins, and have a characteristic internal flecking referred to as "crystalline internal structures" (CIS) by J.A. Siders, and also called "speckled opalescence" by the late G.L. Lombard (Color Plate 16-1). Biochemically, *F. nucleatum* is relatively inactive (Table 16-12). Based on electrophoretic patterns of whole-cell proteins and DNA homology studies, it was proposed in 1990 that *F. nucleatum* be subdivided into three subspecies: *F. nucleatum* subsp. *nucleatum, F. nucleatum* subsp. *polymorphum,* and *F. nucleatum* subsp. *vincentii.*[57] In 1992, Gharbia and Shah proposed that two additional subspecies should be recognized, *F. nucleatum* subsp. *fusiforme* and *F. nucleatum* subsp. *animalis.*[82] At

present, traditional phenotypic methods do not differentiate between these subspecies, and it is not clinically relevant to distinguish them.

F. necrophorum has the ability to cause serious infections (e.g., liver abscess), and it is not unusual to isolate it alone (in pure culture) from soft-tissue lesions.[6,222] Several recent reports have drawn attention to the life-threatening Lemierre's syndrome, or postanginal septicemia, which is a severe suppurative illness caused by this organism.[25,194,198,237] Lemierre's syndrome, also referred to as "necrobacillosis," occurs mostly in people between the ages of 12 and 25 years. Most patients with this syndrome are without predisposing factors and were previously healthy. The condition is characterized by oropharyngeal infection (e.g., tonsillitis, peritonsillar abscess, or pharyngeal abscess) followed by anaerobic septicemia, and subsequent metastatic complications, frequently involving the lungs, and/or large joints, and less frequently the meninges.[89] Common findings with metastatic spread to the lungs are lung abscesses and thoracic empyema. This syndrome should especially be suspected in young patients in whom septic thrombophlebitis of the internal jugular vein develops. Since 1980, the mortality rate in treated patients has been about 18%, but without antibiotics it is >50%. Fortunately, *F. necrophorum* is susceptible in vitro to metronidazole, clindamycin, chloramphenicol, imipenem, and to nearly all of the β-lactam agents, including penicillin G and the newer penicillins, as well as the third generation cephalosporins. However, erythromycin is only moderately active, many strains are resistant to the tetracyclines, and it is resistant to aztreonam, trimethoprim-sulfamethoxazole, and the aminoglycosides.[40,89]

The cells of *F. necrophorum* measure about 0.6 μm × 5 μm and are pleomorphic, often with curved forms and spherical areas within cells (Color Plate 16-1). Like *F. mortiferum* (discussed below), they also produce free coccoid bodies which, on direct examination, sometimes resemble degenerated leukocytes. Most strains produce lipase on LD egg yolk agar. *F. necrophorum* has been divided into three varieties (or "biovars" A, B, and C). A new species, *Fusobacterium pseudonecrophorum* was proposed for *F. necrophorum* biovar C in 1990.[216] *F. necrophorum* is pathogenic, producing liver abscesses in mice, and is susceptible to penicillin (500 U/mL), whereas the new species does not produce abscesses in mice and is highly resistant to penicillin (500 U/mL).

F. mortiferum and *F. varium* isolates are often resistant to clindamycin,[6,135] and they may produce β-lactamase.[70] The cells are 0.5–2 μm wide by 2–10 μm long, highly pleomorphic, coccoid to filamentous, with spherical swellings near the center or one end of unevenly stained rods. Colonies on blood agar are 1 mm to 2 mm in diameter and have a distinctive fried-egg appearance, with raised, opaque centers and a flat, translucent margin. *F. mortiferum* and *F. varium* are resistant to rifampin (15-μg disk), which helps separate them from other *Fusobacterium, Bacteroides, Porphyromonas,* and *Prevotella* species. These two *Fusobacterium* species can be differentiated with tests for esculin hydrolysis and lactose fermentation (Table 16-12).

Other *Fusobacterium* species may be encountered rarely in infections. The characteristics of *F. gonidiaformans* and *F. naviforme* obtained using the Presumpto plate system are shown in Table 16-12. For additional characteristics of these and other species, the following references are recommended.[6,41,124,125,155]

Identification of the Anaerobic Cocci

The anaerobic cocci are the second most common group of anaerobes encountered in human infections, the first being the anaerobic gram-negative bacilli (Table 16-3). Like the anaerobic gram-negative rods, they are frequently encountered in the clinical laboratory in blood cultures, in other body fluids, and in a wide variety of wound and abscess specimens. In the eighth edition of *Bergey's Manual of Determinative Bacteriology*, anaerobic gram-positive cocci were classified in the family *Peptococcaceae* in the following genera: *Peptococcus, Peptostreptococcus, Ruminococcus*, and *Sarcina*.[134] The gram-negative anaerobic cocci were listed in three genera in the family *Veillonellaceae* as follows: *Veillonella, Acidaminococcus,* and *Megasphaera*. Later, in 1974, Holdeman and Moore proposed that a new genus, *Coprococcus*, be added to the family *Peptococcaceae*.[111] They also proposed two new *Ruminococcus* species and a new *Streptococcus* species. They recommended the transfer of *Peptostreptococcus intermedius, Peptostreptococcus morbillorum*, and *Peptococcus constellatus* to the genus *Streptococcus*, since these species produce lactic acid as the only major metabolic product. In 1981, *Peptococcus saccharolyticus* was transferred to the genus *Staphylococcus*.[131] Thus, *S. saccharolyticus* is considered to be an anaerobic species of the genus *Staphylococcus*. In 1983, far-ranging changes in the taxonomic classification of the anaerobic cocci were made, based on the percentage guanine plus cytosine (G + C) data and DNA homology studies of Ezaki and colleagues.[63] Except for *Peptococcus niger*, all former species of the genus *Peptococcus* were transferred to the genus *Peptostreptococcus*. Subsequently in 1994, Ezaki et al. determined the 16S rDNA sequences of all species of *Peptostreptococcus*, reported that the members of the genus could be divided into five different phylogenetic groups, and transferred the species formerly called *Peptostreptococcus productus* and *Streptococcus hansenii* to the genus *Ruminococcus* in 1994.[62] Both are members of the human fecal microbiota but are rare in properly collected clinical specimens.

Since 1999, many additional changes have been made to the genus *Peptostreptococcus*, including the transfer of all but one species to five new genera (Table 16-2).[61,182] As of this writing, the only remaining species of *Peptostreptococcus* is *P. anaerobius*.[183] Those formerly called *P. magnus* and *P. micros*[61] are now *Finegoldia magna* and *Micromonas micros*, respectively.[182] Those formerly called *Peptostreptococcus hydrogenalis, P. lactolyticus, P. octavius, P. prevotii, P. tetradius*, and *P. vaginalis* still have the same species names, but are now members of the genus *Anaerococcus*.[61] Other species formerly called *Peptostreptococcus asaccharolyticus, P. harei, P. indolicus, P. ivorii*, and *P. lacramaris* retained their species names, but were moved to the new genus *Peptoniphilus*.[61]

Another new genus with a single new species was proposed, *Gallicola barnesae;* it has been isolated from chicken feces, but will not be discussed further because it has not been reported from human sources.[61] Likewise, a species isolated from the rumen of sheep, *Slackia heliotriniredcens*

(formerly called *Peptostreptococcus heliotrinreducens*), will not be discussed further.[247]

In addition, the former *Peptostreptococcus parvulus* is now *Atopobium parvulum*.[46] This species has been isolated from human gingival crevices. Little is known about the clinical significance of this and the other *Atopobium* species (Table 16-2). Other microaerophilic or anaerobic streptococci are *Streptococcus intermedius*, and *S. pleomorphus*. Those formerly called *Streptococcus morbillorum* are now *Gemella morbillorum*.[132]

The anaerobic gram-negative cocci are classified in the family *Veillonellaceae*.[199] Three genera—*Veillonella, Acidaminococcus*, and *Megasphaera*—had long been the members of the family, but in 2002 a fourth genus (*Anaeroglobus germinatus*) was described.[37] Prior to 1982, *V. parvula* was the only species of *Veillonella* recognized. In 1982, six additional species, *V. dispar, V. atypica, V. rodentium, V. ratti, V. criceti*, and *V. caviaei*, were proposed.[171] In 2004, a new species of *Veillonella* was isolated from human samples, *V. montpellierensis*.[126] Information on its clinical significance is lacking.

Veillonella species are part of the microbiota of the mouth, upper respiratory tract, intestine, and genitourinary tract. *Acidaminococcus* inhabits the large bowel of humans. The principal habitats of *Megasphaera* species apparently are the human large bowel and genitourinary tract, as well as the rumen of cattle.[222] The single strain of *Anaeroglobus geminatus* described thus far was isolated with a mixture of other bacteria from postoperative fluid collected 27 days after a gastrectomy and esophagojejunal anastomosis in a 70-year-old woman.[37] Neither its habitat nor its clinical significance are known.

Veillonella parvula remains as the most common species of all the anaerobic gram-negative cocci in properly collected specimens from humans. It has been encountered as a causative agent in life-threatening endocarditis,[26,192] bacteremia,[73,150] and in polymicrobial infections in which its pathogenetic role is uncertain.[6]

Although representatives of the above genera of anaerobic gram-positive and gram-negative cocci may be part of the normal microbiota of various sites in humans and other animals, only the species listed in Table 16-3 are encountered with any significant frequency from properly collected and processed clinical specimens. Identifying characteristics of the most commonly encountered species are given in Tables 16-17 and 16-18. For additional information, the following references recommended.[37,61,107,125,199,222] A typical volatile acid chromatogram tracing of *Peptostreptococcus anaerobius* is shown in Figure 16-12.

The *in vitro* susceptibility of the anaerobic cocci to antimicrobial agents has been described elsewhere.[135,181] According to recent guidelines, the antimicrobial agents of choice for the empirical treatment of patients with infections involving anaerobic cocci are penicillin (e.g., penicillin G, ampicillin, amoxicillin) and clindamycin.[18,169] Unfortunately, several *P. anaerobius* isolates are resistant to penicillin G. Metronidazole is active against >90% of the obligately anaerobic cocci, but is not active against most strains of the microaerophilic streptococci (e.g., *Streptococcus intermedius*).[135] Other compounds that are active in vitro against most of the anaerobic cocci include chloramphenicol, imipenem, ampicillin/sulbactam, piperacillin/tazobactam,

Table 16-17 Some Key Characteristics of Anaerobic Cocci Commonly Isolated From Clinical Specimens

SPECIES	GRAM REACTION	BLACK PIGMENT	INDOLE	NITRATE	COAGULASE	UREASE	INHIBITED BY SPS	ALKALINE PHOSPHATASE	FERMENTATION OF			ACID METABOLIC PRODUCTS IN PYG, 48 HOURS AT 35°C
									Glucose	Lactose	Maltose	
Anaerococcus hydrogenalis	+	−	+	−	−	−	−	+	+	NT	−	A, B
A. prevotii	+	−	−	−/+	−	−/+	−	+	−	−	−	A, (P), B
A. tetradius	+	−	−	−	−	+	−	−	+^{a}	−	+	A, B
Finegoldia magna	+	−	−	−	−	−	−	−	−	−	−	A
Gemella morbillorum	+	−	−	−	−	−	−	NT	+	−	w	A, L
Micromonas. micros^b	+	−	−	−	−	−	−	+	−	−	−	A
Peptoniphilus asaccharolyticus	+	−	+	−	−	−	−	−	−	−	−	A, (P), B
P. indolicus	+	−	+	+	+	−	−	+	−	−	−	A, (P), B
Peptococcus niger	+	+	−	−	−	−	−	NT	−	−	−	A, (P), IB, B, IV, (V), C
Peptostreptococcus anaerobius	+	−	−	−	−	−	+	−	w/−	−	w/−	A, (IB), (B), (IV), IC
Ruminococcus productus	+	−	−	+	−	−	−	NT	+	+	+	A
Staphylococcus saccharolyticus	+	−	−	−	−	−	−	NT	+	+	+	A
Streptococcus intermedius	+	−	−	−	−	−	−	NT	+	+	+	A, L
Veillonella spp.	−	−	−	+	−	−	−	NT	−	−	−	A, P

^{a} *A. tetradius* strains lose their ability to ferment sugars rapidly after subculturing so it is not uncommon for these reactions to be negative.
^{b} Most strains of *M. micros* will produce a very slight β-hemolysis on CDC anaerobe blood agar (Remel, Lenexa, KS), which helps distinguish it from *F. magna* (Allen and Siders: unpublished data).
SPS, sodium polyanethol sulfonate; +, positive reaction; w, weakly fermentative; −, negative reaction; −/+, occasional strains positive; w/−, most strains weakly fermentative, but occasional strains negative; A, acetic acid; P, propionic acid; IB, isobutyric acid; B, butyric acid; IV, isovaleric acid; V, valeric acid; IC, isocaproic acid; C, caproic acid; L, lactic acid; ( ), variable acid; NT, not tested.

Table 16-18 Reactions of Anaerobic Cocci on CDC Differential Agar Media

SPECIES	NO. OF STRAINS EXAMINED	PRESUMPTO 1 PLATE							PRESUMPTO 2 PLATE				PRESUMPTO 3 PLATE			
		Indole	Esculin Hydrolysis	H_2S	Catalase	Lecithinase	Lipase	Growth on Bile Agar	Glucose Fermentation	Starch Hydrolysis	Milk Proteolysis	DNase	Gelatin Hydrolysis	Mannitol Fermentation	Lactose Fermentation	Rhamnose Fermentation
Anaerococcus prevotii	15	–	–	–	–	–	–	V	–	–	–	–	–	–	–	–
Finegoldia magna	21	–	–	–	–/+	–	–	I	–	–	–	–	–	–	–	–
Micromonas micros	1	–	–	–	–	–	–	NG	–	–	–	–	–	–	–	–
Peptoniphilus asaccharolyticus	22	+	–	–	–	–	–	V	–	–	–	–	–	–	–	–
Peptostreptococcus anaerobius	21	–	–	V	–	–	–	V	V	–	–	–	–	–	–	–
Staphylococcus saccharolyticus	2	–	–	–	+	–	–	V	+	–	–	–	–	–	–	–
Streptococcus intermedius	9	–	+	–	–	–	–	I	+	–	–	–	–	–	+	–
Veillonella spp.	6	–	–	–	–/+	–	–	I	–	–	–	–	–	–	–	–

+, positive reaction in >90% of strains; –, negative reaction in >90% of strains; –/+, most strains negative, occasional strain positive; I, growth inhibited; V, variable; NG, no growth.
Adapted from Whaley DN, Wiggs LS, Miller PH, Srivastava PU, Miller JM. Use of Presumpto plates to identify anaerobic bacteria. J Clin Microbiol 1995;33:1196–1202, and previous editions of this book.

and cefoxitin, but not cefoperazone, cefotaxime, or cefotetan.[135] Compounds that show promise against the gram-positive anaerobic cocci include some of the newer fluoroquinolones (e.g., moxifloxacin, gatifloxacin), quinupristin/dalfopristin, and linezolid.[18,169] *Veillonella* species are resistant to vancomycin and some of the quinolones. Antimicrobial agents not active against the anaerobic cocci include the aminoglycosides, aztreonam, and trimethoprim-sulfamethoxazole.[18,169]

Identification of the Anaerobic Non–Spore-Forming Gram-Positive Bacilli

Included in this group of anaerobes are species of the genera *Actinomyces, Arcanobacterium, Bifidobacterium, Eggerthella, Eubacterium, Lactobacillus, Propionibacterium, Pseudoramibacter,* and many others.[6,67,125,177] An extensive list of recent changes in the taxonomy of these bacteria is provided in Table 16-2. Some key differential characteristics of species of non–spore-forming, gram-positive bacilli are given in Tables 16-19 and 16-20. The microscopic morphology and colonial characteristics of *Actinomyces israelii* and *Eggerthella lenta* (formerly *Eubacterium lentum*) are shown in Color Plate 16-2.

Identification of the anaerobic, gram-positive, non–spore-forming bacilli requires the use of GLC for metabolic product analysis. Cellular morphology of many of these organisms tends to vary with the type of culture medium and growth conditions. On morphologic grounds alone, they can sometimes be confused with several other genera, including *Clostridium, Corynebacterium, Lactobacillus, Leptotrichia, Listeria, Nocardia, Peptostreptococcus,* and *Streptococcus.* Thus, GLC results and morphologic characteristics, considered together, aid in practical differentiation (Table 16-9 and 16-19).

At times some strains of anaerobic bacilli resemble cocci, particularly in Gram-stained preparations of young colonies on blood agar. In addition, some streptococci, such as *S. mutans, S. intermedius, S. constellatus,* and *Gemella morbillorum* and certain peptostreptococci, may appear rod-shaped when cells from colonies on blood agar are examined microscopically. On the other hand, these bacteria usually form long chains of cells in enriched thioglycolate broth and other liquid media. It should be remembered that many gram-positive bacteria tend to become gram-negative as they age. Also, some clostridia (e.g., *C. perfringens, C. ramosum,* and *C. clostridioforme*) fail to produce spores in media routinely used in the clinical laboratory, whereas other clostridia do so as they age. Thus, Gram-stained preparations of very young cultures may aid in demonstration of Gram-variability, and observation of smears from older cultures may aid in demonstrating spores of clostridia.

PROPIONIBACTERIUM SPECIES

Propionibacterium acnes is by far the most common gram-positive, non–spore-forming anaerobic rod encountered in clinical specimens. It is part of the normal flora of the skin, nasopharynx, oral cavity, and gastrointestinal and genitourinary tracts. As a predominant member of the skin microbiota and an inhabitant of the hair follicle/sebaceous gland apparatus, *P. acnes* is frequently a contaminant of blood cultures. However, it occasionally causes endocarditis,

central nervous system shunt infections, and other infections. *P. avidum* and *P. granulosum* are seldom encountered in the clinical laboratory, and usually are not clinically significant. The cells of *P. acnes* usually measure 0.3–1.3 μm in diameter × 1–10 μm in length.[222] Their morphology has often been described as diphtheroid in appearance. The cells are markedly pleomorphic and occur in varying shapes and sizes, ranging from coccoid to definite rods. Cells are often unevenly stained by Gram's procedure. Like the corynebacteria, the cells reveal Chinese letters, birds-in-flight, and picket-fence arrangements, presumably because of ''snapping'' after they divide. *P. acnes* typically grows as an obligate anaerobe; however, some strains show sparse growth in a candle jar (but better growth anaerobically), and have been described as aerotolerant or microaerophilic. Colonies of *P. acnes* on anaerobe blood agar are 1 mm to 2 mm in diameter, circular, entire, convex, glistening, and opaque. Some strains produce a narrow zone of hemolysis. Analysis of short-chain acid metabolic products by GLC reveals the production of a major amount of propionic acid, a smaller amount of acetic acid, and only a minor amount of isovaleric acid [abbreviated aP(iv)]. *P. acnes* can be recognized without the use of GLC when it produces both indole and catalase. However, not all strains produce indole; nor do all strains produce catalase. In addition, *Actinomyces viscosus,* which has a similar morphology on some media, produces catalase.

Propionibacterium propionicum. In 1988, *Arachnia propionica* was reclassified as *Propionibacterium propionicum.*[39] Previously, the name *Arachnia propionica* had been created to accommodate the bacteria once called *Actinomyces propionicus.* This species, while its pathogenicity and morphologic characteristics resemble those of certain species of *Actinomyces,* differs from *Actinomyces* spp. by producing propionic acid as a major metabolic product and by its cell wall murein content and menaquinone composition that resemble those of *Propionibacterium* spp. *Propionibacterium propionicum* should still be considered as a potential etiologic agent of human actinomycosis. The organisms have been incriminated in cases involving cervicofacial ''actinomycosis,'' pulmonary abscess formation with or without thoracic empyema, a neck abscess, a finger wound infection following a human bite, a renal abscess, and a few cases of lacrimal canaliculitis.[33] *Propionibacterium propionicum* is morphologically indistinguishable, in tissue and in culture, from *Actinomyces israelii.* Both *P. propionicum* and *A. israelii* form pleomorphic ''diphtheroidal'' rods and long, branched, filaments (described in more detail in the section on *Actinomyces* spp.). Both species are microaerophilic to anaerobic and grow optimally under anaerobic conditions.

BIFIDOBACTERIUM SPECIES

Currently, more than 30 species of the genus *Bifidobacterium* are recognized taxonomically and most inhabit the intestines of humans and other animals.[114] Recent changes in this group include the transfer of *B. inopinatum* to *Scardovia* as *Scardovia inopinata,* and the transfer of *B. denticolens* to *Parascardovia* as *Parascardovia denticolens.*[115] With the exception of *Bifidobacterium dentium,* all of the species of the genus *Bifidobacterium* appear to be nonpathogenic for humans.[6] *Bifidobacterium dentium* now includes

Table 16-19 Some Key Differential Characteristics of Anaerobic, Gram-Positive Non-Spore-Forming Bacilli

SPECIES	RELATION TO OXYGEN	RAPIDITY OF GROWTH	COLONIES ON BLOOD AGAR	RED PIGMENT ON BLOOD AGAR	APPEARANCE IN ENRICHED THIOGLYCOLATE BROTH	CELLULAR MORPHOLOGY IN ENRICHED THIOGLYCOLATE BROTH	NITRATE REDUCTION	METABOLIC PRODUCTS IN PYG BROTH, 48 HOURS AT 35°C
Actinomyces israelii	M or OA	Slow	Rough	–	Granular or diffuse	Branching filaments or diphtheroidal	V	A, L, S
A. naeslundii	F	Moderate	Smooth	+	Diffuse	Diphtheroidal, branching	+/–	A, L, S
A. odontolyticus	M or OA	Moderate	Smooth	+	Diffuse	Diphtheroidal, branching	+	A, L, S
A. viscosus	F	Rapid	Smooth	–	Diffuse	Diphtheroidal, branching	+	A, L, S
A. meyeri	OA, F		Smooth	–	Diffuse	Diphtheroidal, branching	–	A, L, S
Arcanobacterium pyogenes	F		Smooth	–	Diffuse	Diphtheroidal, coccoidal	–	A, L, S
Bifidobacterium dentium	OA	Rapid	Smooth	–	Diffuse	Thin rods, bifid ends, bulbous ends	–	A, L
Eggerthella lenta	OA	Moderate	Smooth	–	Diffuse	Short coccoidal rods, diphtheroidal	V	A
Eubacterium limosum	OA	Rapid	Smooth	–	Diffuse	Plump rods, bulbous and bifid formsucts	V	A, B (acid prod from a non–glucose-containing broth are A, IB, B, IV)
Lactobacillus catenaformis	OA	Rapid	Smooth	–	Diffuse (granular)	Short rods in chains or singly	–	A, L
Propionibacterium avidum	F	Rapid	Smooth	–	Diffuse	Diphtheroidal	V	A, P
P. acnes	OA^F	Moderate	Smooth	–	Diffuse (granular)	Diphtheroidal	+	A, P
P. granulosum	F	Rapid	Smooth	–	Diffuse	Diphtheroidal	–	A, P
P. propionicum	M or OA	Slow	Rough	–	Granular or diffuse	Branching filaments or diphtheroidal	+	A, P
Pseudoramibacter alactolyticum	OA	Slow	Smooth	–	Diffuse	Thin rods, V-forms, cross-stick arrangements	–	A, B, C

+, positive reaction for 90–100% of strains tested; –, negative reaction for 90–100% of strains tested; superscript, reaction shown with 11–25% of strains tested; V, variable reaction; parentheses, variable; F, facultatively anaerobic; M, microaerophilic; OA, obligately anaerobic; A, acetic acid, B, butyric acid; C, caproic acid; L, lactic acid; P, propionic acid; S, succinic acid; IB, isobutyric acid; IC, isocaproic acid.

Modified from Dowell VR. Clinical Veterinary Anaerobic Bacteriology. Atlanta: Centers for Disease Control. 1977 : 1–25; and adapted from the following references: Allen SD. Gram-positive, non-spore-forming anaerobic bacilli. In: Lennette EH, Balows A, Hausler WJ Jr, Shadomy EJ, eds. Manual of Clinical Microbiology. Ed. 4. Washington, DC: American Society for Microbiology. 1985 : 461–472; Jones D, Collins MD. Irregular, nonsporing gram-positive rods. In: Sneath PHA, Mair NS, Sharpe MG, Holt JG, eds. Bergey's Manual of Systematic Bacteriology. Baltimore: Williams & Wilkins. 1986 : 1261–1434.

Table 16-20 Reactions of Gram-Positive, Non-Spore-Forming Bacilli on CDC Differential Agar Media

SPECIES	NO. OF STRAINS EXAMINED	PRESUMPTO 1 PLATE								PRESUMPTO 2 PLATE				PRESUMPTO 3 PLATE			
		Indole	Indole Derivative	Esculin Hydrolysis	H₂S	Catalase	Lecithinase	Lipase	Growth on Bile Agar	Glucose Fermentation	Starch Hydrolysis	Milk Proteolysis	DNase	Gelatin Hydrolysis	Mannitol Fermentation	Lactose Fermentation	Rhamnose Fermentation
Actinomyces																	
A. israelii	12	–	–	+	–	–	–	–	V	+	–	–/+	–/+	–	V	–/+	–/+
A. meyeri	39	–	–	–	–	–	–	–	I^{NG}	+/–	–	–	–/+	–	–	V	–
A. naeslundii	31	–	–	+/–	–	–	–	–	V	+	–	–	–	–	–/+	+/–	–
A. odontolyticus	56	–	–	V	–	–	–	–	V	+	–	–	–	–	–/+	V	–/+
A. viscosus	25	–	–	V	–	+/–	–	–	NG^I	+	–	–	–	–	–	V	–
Arcanobacterium																	
A. pyogenes	12	–	–	–	–	–	–	–	I^{NG}	+	–	+	–/+	+/–	–/+	–/+	–
Bifidobacterium																	
B. adolescentis	8	–	–	V	–	–	–	–	E	+	–/+	–	–	–	–/+	+	–
B. bifidum	4	–	–	–	–	–	–	–	E	+	–	–	–	–	–	+	–
B. breve	4	–	–	+/–	–	–	–	–	E	+	–/+	–	–	–	V	+	–
B. dentium^a	3	–	–	–	–/+	–	–	–	E	+	V	–	–	–	+	+/–	–
B. infantis/longum	3	–	–	–	–	–	–	–	E	+	V	–	–	–	–	+	–
Collinsella																	
C. aerofaciens	3	–	–	–/+	–	–	–	–	E	+	–	+/–	–	–	–	+	–
Eggerthella																	
E. lenta	33	–	–	–	–/+	V	–	–	E^I	–	–	–	–	–	–	–	–
Eubacterium																	
E. brachy	2	–	–	–	–	–	–	–	NG	–	–	–	–	–	–	–	–
E. limosum	8	–	–	–	+	–	–	–	E	+	V	–	–	–	+	–	–
E. nodatum	3	–	–	–	–	–	–	–	NG	–	–	–	–	–	–	–	–
E. saburreum	2	V	–	V	–	–	–	–	NG	–	–	–	–	–	–	V	–
E. timidum	3	–	–	–	–	–	–	–	NG	–	–	–	–	–	–	–	–
Propionibacterium																	
P. acnes	144	+/–	–	–	–	+	–	–/+	V	+	–	+/–	–	V	–	–	–
P. avidum	5	–	–	+/–	–	+	–	+/–	E	+	–	V	–	+/–	–	–	–
P. granulosum	7	–	–	–	–	+	–	–/+	V	+	–	V	–/+	–/+	–/+	–/+	–
P. propionicum	10	–	–	–	–	–	–	–	I	V	–	–	–	–	V	V	–
Pseudoramibacter																	
P. alactolyticum	4	–	–	–	–	–	–	–	I	V	–	–	–	–	–	–	–

^a Formerly called B. eriksonii.

+, positive reaction in >90% of strains; –, negative reaction in >90% of strains; +/–, most strains positive, occasional strain negative; –/+, most strains negative, occasional strain positive; I, growth inhibited; V, variable; E, growth equal to control without bile; E^I, equal growth with an occasional strain inhibited; I^{NG}, inhibited growth with occasional strains not growing; NG^I, growth equal to control with an occasional strain inhibited; NG, growth not inhibited.

Adapted from Whaley DN, Wiggs LS, Miller PH, Srivastava PU, Miller JM. Use of Presumpto plates to identify anaerobic bacteria. J Clin Microbiol 1995;33:1196–1202, and previous editions of this book.

those formerly called *Actinomyces eriksonii* and later *Bifidobacterium eriksonii*. It is part of the normal microbiota of the mouth and gastrointestinal tract, and has been found in polymicrobial infections of the lower respiratory tract. The morphology of *B. dentium* is somewhat similar to that of *Actinomyces*, but it differs in not producing branched filaments in thioglycolate medium. Gram-stained smears prepared from solid media or broth cultures show Gram-positive diphtheroidal forms that are much more variable in size and shape than *P. acnes*. Cells vary from coccoid forms to long, often curved forms, with characteristic swollen ends and/or bifid forms that are regularly produced by *B. dentium*. On GLC analysis of short-chain acid metabolic products, the bifidobacteria produce major amounts of acetic and lactic acids.

LACTOBACILLUS SPECIES

Lactobacillus species are part of the microbiota of the human oral cavity, pharynx, intestinal tract, and genitourinary tract (especially the vagina); they are sometimes encountered in clinical specimens. It is often difficult to ascribe pathogenic significance to most isolates recovered in the laboratory, but *Lactobacillus* species have been reported in several cases of bacterial endocarditis, meningitis, clinically significant bacteremia, peritonitis, abscesses and other life-threatening infections. Although the majority of *Lactobacillus* isolates are not strictly anaerobic, many grow better anaerobically. Clues that aid in the recognition of lactobacilli include their growth on Rogosa's selective tomato juice agar at relatively low pH (Becton Dickinson Microbiology Systems), their negative catalase reaction, their tendency to form chains of relatively uniform gram-positive rods, and their production of lactic acid as a major product with only a small amount of acetate (detected using GLC). Identification of the lactobacilli beyond a presumptive level is difficult and beyond the scope of this textbook. It is noteworthy that the lactobacilli are resistant to vancomycin. For additional information on identification and the susceptibility of *Lactobacillus* species to antimicrobial agents, see Chapter 14.

ACTINOMYCES SPECIES

In recent years, abundant taxonomic revisions have been made within the genus *Actinomyces* (Table 16-2). These changes have included the designation of several new or additional species including *A. cardiffensis*,[90] *A. europaeus*,[74,203] *A. funkei*,[146] *A. georgiae*,[117] *A. gerencseriae*,[117] *A. graevenitzii*,[195] *A. hongkongensis*,[265] *A. nasicola*,[93] *A. neuii*,[75,76,165] *A. oricola*,[92] *A. radicidentis*,[43,128,219] *A. radingae*,[266] *A. turicensis*,[203,246] and *A. urogenitalis*.[187] Other genera closely related to the genus *Actinomyces* are *Actinobaculum* (e.g., *Actinobaculum schaalii* and *A. urinale*)[91,145] and *Arcanobacterium* (e.g., *Arcanobacterium bernardiae* and *A. pyogenes*),[196] The report by Clarridge and colleagues aids in assessing the significance of several recently described species.[42] Although the new species listed in Table 16-2 have been isolated from various human clinical sources, information still is lacking for many of them as to their clinical importance.[170]

The bacteria that have been reported to cause actinomycosis in humans include *Actinomyces israelii*, *A. naeslundii*,

A. odontolyticus, *A. gerencseriae*, *A. viscosus*, *A. meyeri*, *A. georgiae*, *A. neuii* subsp. *neuii*, *P. propionicum* and *B. dentium* (includes those formerly called *B. eriksonii*, in part).[193,206,222] These bacteria are part of the normal flora of the mouth, and many of them can be found in the genitourinary tract. *A. israelii* is the most common species in clinical infections. However, actinomycosis (with lesions in tissue) is currently rare. In Gram-stained smears prepared from lesions, one may observe characteristic sulfur granules, which are granular microcolonies of the organism surrounded by purulent exudate. The cells of *A. israelii* are gram-positive rods, usually 1 μm in diameter, but they are extremely variable in length. The cells may be short diphtheroid rods, club-shaped, branched, or unbranched filaments (Color Plate 16-2). Rough colonies composed of branched rods or filaments usually develop slowly on blood agar. Young colonies (2 to 3 days old), when viewed with the dissecting microscope, appear as thin radiating filaments known as spider colonies. When the colonies get to be about 7 to 14 days old, they are often raised, heaped-up, white, opaque, and glistening; have irregular or lobate margins; and are called molar tooth colonies (Color Plate 16-2). However, smooth strains (about one third of *A. israelii*) produce colonies more rapidly than rough strains. Smooth strains may produce 1-mm to 2-mm, circular, slightly raised white, opaque, smooth, glistening colonies after only 2 to 3 days of incubation. *A. naeslundii* may also produce smooth or rough colonies. Colonies of *A. viscosus* are most often 0.5 mm to 2 mm in diameter, entire, convex, grayish, and translucent. In *A. odontolyticus* colonies, a red color may develop on blood agar after 7 to 14 days of anaerobic incubation or after the plates have been left out in room air at ambient temperature for several days. As mentioned previously, cellular and colony characteristics of *Propionibacterium propionicum* are similar to those of the other *Actinomyces*.

Besides morphology, colony characteristics, and metabolic products, characteristics useful for identification of the actinomycetes include relationship to oxygen, appearance and rapidity of growth in enriched thioglycolate medium, indole production, esculin and gelatin hydrolysis, fermentation of certain carbohydrates, results of testing with several rapid enzyme tests, 16S rRNA sequencing and other molecular methods. For further information relative to characterization and identification of isolates beyond that given in Tables 16-19 and 16-20, the following references are recommended.[42,125,177,205]

EUBACTERIUM SPECIES

Eubacterium species are relatively common in wounds and abscesses, in which they are usually mixed with other bacteria. Their pathogenic significance in clinical specimens is often uncertain.[222] However, as reviewed by Mascini and Verhoef,[170] *Eubacterium* species have been reported, though rarely, to cause bacteremia, endocarditis, and other life-threatening infections. The species isolated most often from nonoral clinical specimens have long been *E. lentum* (now *Eggerthella lenta*) and *E. limosum*. Tables 16-19 and 16-20 provide information for the presumptive identification of the more commonly encountered *Eubacterium* species.

As noted by Wade and colleagues, for many years by default, the genus *Eubacterium* was regarded as heterogeneous, containing many unrelated species.[247] Based on the results of 16S rRNA gene-sequence determinations and other data, the genus is currently undergoing major taxonomic revision. Thus, *E. lentum* was transferred to the genus *Eggerthella* as *Eggerthella lenta*, while *E. limosum* remained the type species of the genus *Eubacterium*.[247] Table 16-2 lists many additional changes, including the transfer of *Eubacterium aerofaciens* to the genus *Collinsella* as *Collinsella aerofaciens*.[127] In addition, the organism previously called *Eubacterium formicigenerans* is now *Doria formicigenerans*,[236] the species previously called *E. timidum* is now *Mogibacterium timidum*,[94] and the species formerly known as *E. alactolyticum* is now *Pseudoramibacter alactolyticus*.[263]

Other genera of non–spore-forming gram-positive rods, including *Cryptobacterium, Bulleidia, Atopobium, Slackia, Holdemania*, and *Catenibacterium,* have been described, but their clinical significance remains poorly understood.[170,176]

MOBILUNCUS AND BACTERIAL VAGINOSIS

Mobiluncus, along with other anaerobes, is present in vaginal samples of women with nonspecific vaginitis (or bacterial vaginosis).[104,177,230] In 1984, Spiegel and Roberts proposed the name *Mobiluncus* for a new genus of gram-variable or gram-negative, motile, curved, non–spore-forming anaerobic rods, which occur singly or in pairs and with a "gull wing" appearance.[231] Electron micrographs revealed multilayered cell walls lacking an outer membrane that were probably more typical of gram-positive than gram-negative cell walls; nonetheless, the organisms tend to stain gram-variable in young culture and gram-negative in older culture. The name *Mobiluncus* was derived from the Latin words *mobilis* (meaning capable of movement) and *uncus* (which means hook).[231] The pathogenic potential of *Mobiluncus* spp., if any, is still not clear. It has been isolated from patients with extragenital infections on a few occasions, and there is a case report of its isolation from a patient with severe sepsis.[83,102] The organism is one of many genera of anaerobes that colonizes the vagina in both health and disease.[177]

Bacterial vaginosis involves an overgrowth of multiple bacteria, including *Gardnerella vaginalis, Mycoplasma hominis, Mobiluncus* spp., *Prevotella bivia, Prevotella disiens,* other *Prevotella* spp., *Peptostreptococcus anaerobius, P. asaccharolyticus, P. magnus,* and other anaerobic cocci, plus anaerobic gram-positive rods including *Propionibacterium* spp.[103,104,230] Therefore, vaginosis is probably a synergistic infection in which many organisms play a role. As reviewed elsewhere,[225] the diagnosis of bacterial vaginosis is based on demonstrating three of the following four criteria: 1) a "thin" (but profuse) vaginal discharge, 2) a pH greater than 4.5, 3) an odor usually described as "fishy" (especially with the addition of 10% potassium hydroxide), and d) the demonstration of "clue cells" by microscopic examination. "Clue cells" are squamous epithelial cells of the vagina with myriad small rods adherent to their surfaces. "Clue cells" may be observed in wet-mounts or in Gram-stained smears (or in Papanicalaou-stained preparations).

Mobiluncus spp. grow on several kinds of nonselective plating media, including anaerobe blood agar (e.g., brain-heart infusion, *Brucella,* and CDC-anaerobe blood-agar–based media) and chocolate agar. After 3 to 5 days of incubation, colonies are 2 to 4 mm in diameter, colorless, translucent, smooth, and flat, sometimes with a spreading appearance. The cells are less than $0.5~\mu m$ in width by about 1.5 to $3~\mu m$ in length. Succinate and acetate are major products (with or without minor amounts of lactate) after growth in peptone yeast-extract broth supplemented with glycogen and 2% rabbit serum. Differentiation between the two currently recognized species, *M. curtisii* and *M. mulieris,*[238] based on differences in morphology, negative reactions for indole and catalase, growth in the presence of arginine, hippurate hydrolysis, variable nitrate reduction, and other characteristics is difficult.[125,177,231]

ADDITIONAL GENERA AND SPECIES OF ANAEROBIC NON–SPORE-FORMING GRAM-POSITIVE BACILLI

Finegold has provided an update on changes in the taxonomy of anaerobes associated with humans, including information on additional genera and species not mentioned in this textbook.[67] For those interested in definitive identification of the anaerobic non–spore-forming gram-positive bacilli, which requires resources beyond those available in many (if not most) clinical microbiology laboratories, the following references are recommended.[42,125,177]

Identification of *Clostridium* Species

The anaerobic gram-positive, spore-forming bacilli encountered in human clinical materials are members of the genus *Clostridium*. In 1994, Collins and associates,[44] on the basis of 16S rRNA gene sequences determined by PCR direct sequencing, found that the genus *Clostridium* is extremely heterogeneous. Thus, Collins et al. named five new genera of spore-forming rods.[44] Included were the following: *Caloramator, Filifactor, Moorella, Oxobacter,* and *Oxalophagus* species. In addition, 11 new species combinations were proposed. None of these new generic and species designations were relevant to infectious diseases of humans. Newly created species at the time of this writing include *Clostridium bartlettii,*[229] *C. bolteae,*[228] *C. hathewayi,*[234] and *C. neonatale.*[3a] The original papers should be consulted for information on their clinical significance.

Currently, species of *Clostridium* encountered clinically vary in their relationships to oxygen and in their anabolic and catabolic physiologic activities. Certain clostridia, for example *C. haemolyticum* and *C. novyi* type B, are among the strictest of obligate anaerobes. At the other end of the spectrum, *C. histolyticum, C. tertium,* and *C. carnis* are aerotolerant, and form colonies on anaerobe blood agar plates incubated in a candle jar or in a 5–10% CO_2 incubator. In the clinical laboratory the problem sometimes arises of determining whether an isolate is an aerotolerant *Clostridium* or a facultatively anaerobic *Bacillus*. Aerotolerant clostridia rarely form spores when grown aerobically and are catalase-negative, whereas species of the genus *Bacillus* rarely form spores when grown under anaerobic conditions, and they produce catalase.[222]

Although the clostridia are considered gram-positive, many are gram-negative by the time smears of growing cultures are prepared. For example, *Clostridium ramosum* and *C. clostridioforme* are usually gram-negative.

The demonstration of spores is frequently difficult with some species, for example, *C. perfringens, C. ramosum,* and

C. clostridioforme. Demonstration of spore production is not necessary for identifying these three species. They have several other distinctive properties. To demonstrate spores, Gram-stained preparations are usually sufficient; special spore stains generally offer no particular advantage. However, examination of wet mounts with a phase contrast microscope is useful when spores are mature and refractile. In our experience, the best way to demonstrate production of spores is to inoculate a cooked-meat agar slant and incubate anaerobically for 5 to 7 days at 30°C. The cells from the growth on the slant are then observed in a Gram-stained preparation or in a wet mount by phase contrast microscopy. In addition, a heat-shock or alcohol spore selection technique may be used.[138] Identifying characteristics for most of the clostridia encountered in human infections are given in Tables 16-21, 16-22 and 16-23.

Some of the key reactions for identifying *C. perfringens* are illustrated in Color Plate 16-3. The double zone of hemolysis on blood agar, production of lecithinase on egg-yolk agar, and stormy fermentation of litmus milk (or proteolysis of milk agar) are characteristic of this species. The cells of *C. perfringens* are usually 0.8–1.5 µm in diameter × 2–4 µm long and have blunt ends. They are often described as boxcar-shaped. However, cells examined during early growth in broth culture tend to be short and coccoid, while older cultures contain longer cells that may be almost filamentous. After overnight incubation on blood agar, colonies are usually 1 mm to 3 mm in diameter, but may reach a diameter of 4 mm to 15 mm after prolonged incubation. Colonies are usually flat, somewhat rhizoid, and raised centrally. Some colonies tend to spread, but they do not swarm. *C. perfringens* is nonmotile.

C. perfringens is by far the most commonly isolated species of *Clostridium* from human sources. However, clostridia account for only about 10–12% of the anaerobic bacteria isolated from properly selected and collected clinical specimens. *C. perfringens* and other clostridia are commonly found among the normal flora of the gastrointestinal tract. They also transiently inhabit the skin. Many clostridia isolated from clinical specimens, even blood cultures, are accidental contaminants and may have no clinical significance. In other circumstances, the presence of certain clostridia in a lesion can have dire consequences to the host. Thus, the pathogenic properties of clostridia may be manifested only in special circumstances, and communication between the microbiologist and the attending physician is usually necessary to assess the significance of a given isolate. *C. perfringens* is also encountered in myonecrosis (gas gangrene), gangrenous cholecystitis, septicemia, and intravascular hemolysis following abortion and anaerobic pleuropulmonary infections; it is a major cause of food poisoning in the United States and is also one cause of antibiotic-associated diarrhea and a major worldwide cause of necrotizing enterocolitis involving children and adults.[4,7,28,81,189,222,253]

HISTOTOXIC CLOSTRIDIA INVOLVED IN CLOSTRIDIAL MYONECROSIS OR GAS GANGRENE

The clostridia most often involved in gas gangrene are *C. perfringens* (80%), *C. novyi* (40%), and *C. septicum* (20%), followed occasionally by *C. histolyticum* and *C. sordellii.*[222] Clostridial myonecrosis (gas gangrene) is a clinical entity that involves rapid invasion and liquefactive necrosis of muscle with gas formation and clinical signs of toxicity. Nonetheless, close cooperation between the microbiology laboratory and clinical staff is often an urgent necessity for confirmation of the clinical diagnosis. Gram-stained smears of aspirated material from myonecrosis reveal a necrotic background with a lack of inflammatory cells and presence of morphologic forms resembling *C. perfringens* or other clostridia. In other conditions, such as simple wound infection or anaerobic cellulitis (in which there may also be gas in tissue), muscle cell outlines or presence of granulocytes and mixed morphologic forms of bacteria in Gram-stained smears of lesions would be evidence against clostridial myonecrosis.

For further details on the histotoxic clostridia, several references are available.[7,70,154,222]

***Intestinal Diseases Involving* C. perfringens.** *C. perfringens*, ranking behind *Salmonella* spp. and *Staphylococcus aureus*, has been the third most common etiologic agent of foodborne disease in the United States for many years.[38] Most of the *C. perfringens* foodborne outbreaks in the United States have involved strains of toxin type A.[7,38] *C. perfringens* food poisoning results from eating contaminated beef, turkey, chicken, pork, gravy, and other foods containing large numbers of the organism. Crampy abdominal pain develops, usually within 7 to 15 hours after eating the suspected food. In most cases, there is diarrhea, with foamy, "foul-smelling" stools, but there is little vomiting or fever. Illness occurs after about 10^8 viable vegetative *C. perfringens* cells reach the small intestine and undergo sporulation. A potent enterotoxin (a protein of about 34 kDa), produced in the gut while the spores are being formed, causes the diarrhea. The illness tends to be mild and self-limited, and patients usually recover in 2 to 3 days from the onset. Quantitative anaerobic cultures on selective plating media, demonstrating at least 10^5 *C. perfringens* organisms in the epidemiologically implicated food, and spore counts showing 10^6 or more *C. perfringens* spores per gram of feces collected within 24 hours of onset of symptoms, are done to confirm the diagnosis in an outbreak investigation. In addition, serotyping of the isolates is done to demonstrate that the same serotype of *C. perfringens* is present in epidemiologically implicated food and in the feces of ill persons, but not in controls. Serologic typing must be done in established laboratories that are satisfactorily equipped to perform this service (such as at the Centers for Disease Control and Prevention [CDC]).[7,53]

A kit for the detection of *C. perfringens* enterotoxin has been marketed by Oxoid (Basingstoke, England). Supernatant of a saline homogenate of feces is tested for enterotoxin using a reversed passive latex agglutination procedure, according to directions provided by the manufacturer. Data are lacking with regard to the sensitivity, specificity, and accuracy of the test.

Necrotizing bowel disease (NBD), caused by *Clostridium perfringens*, is much more serious than the foodborne illness described above. NBD is characterized by the sudden onset of abdominal cramps and abdominal distention, vomiting, bloody diarrhea, and shock related to fluid and electrolyte problems, and acute inflammation and focal or widespread necrosis of the intestinal mucosa. The disease, recognized in post-war Germany, called "Darmbrand" (meaning "fire

Table 16-21 Some Key Characteristics of *Clostridium* Species Associated with Disease in Humans

SPECIES[a]	AEROTOLERANT	DOUBLE ZONE HEMOLYSIS	TERMINAL SPORES	MOTILITY	VOLATILE METABOLIC PRODUCTS (GLC) IN PYG, 48 HOURS AT 35°C	OTHER
C. bifermentans	–	–	–	+	A, IC, (P), (IB), (B), (IV)	Urease-negative; indole-positive
C. botulinum[b]	–	–	–	+	A, (P), (IB), B, IV, (V), (IC)	Lipase-positive
C. butyricum	–	–	–	+	A, B	Very saccharolytic
C. difficile	–	–	–	+	A, IB, B, IV, IC	
C. innocuum	–	–	+	–	A, B	Lactose- and maltose-negative
C. limosum	–	–	–	+	A	Asaccharolytic; gelatin-positive
C. novyi type A	–	–	–	+	A, P, B	Rarely encountered in clinical species
C. perfringens	–	+	–	–	A, B, (P)	Spores seldom observed
C. ramosum	–	–	+	–	A	Spores seldom observed; frequently gram-negative
C. septicum	–	–	–	+	A, B	Saccharolytic, but sucrose-negative
C. sordellii	–	–	–	+	A, IC, (P), (IB), (IV)	Urease-positive; indole-positive
C. sporogenes[b]	–	–	–	+	A, P, IB, B, IB, V, IC	Lipase-positive
C. subterminale	–	–	–	+	A, IB, B, IV, (P)	Asaccharolytic; gelatin-positive
C. tetani	–	–	+	+	A, (P), B	May appear gram-negative
C. tertium	+	–	+	+	A, B	No spores under aerobic conditions

[a] For additional information on definitive identification of these species and other clostridia that may be encountered in clinical specimens is available elsewhere.[7,53,107,112,125]

[b] Toxin neutralization tests required for definitive identification.

+, positive reaction for 90–100% of strains tested; –, negative reaction for 90–100% of strains tested; V, variable reaction; parentheses, variable; A, acetic acid; P, propionic acid; IB, isobutyric acid; IV, isovaleric acid; V, valeric acid; IC, isocaproic acid.

Table 16-22 Reactions of *Clostridium* Species on CDC Differential Agar Media

SPECIES	NO. OF STRAINS EXAMINED	PRESUMPTO 1 PLATE							Growth on Bile Agar	PRESUMPTO 2 PLATE				PRESUMPTO 3 PLATE			
		Indole	Indole Derivative	Esculin Hydrolysis	H_2S	Catalase	Lecithinase	Lipase		Glucose Fermentation	Starch Hydrolysis	Milk Proteolysis	DNase	Gelatin Hydrolysis	Mannitol Fermentation	Lactose Fermentation	Rhamnose Fermentation
C. baratii	8	−	−	+	−	−	+	−	E	+	V	V	−	−	−	+/−	−
C. bifermentans	16	+	−	+	−	−	+	−	E	+	+/−	+/−	−	+	−	−	−
C. butyricum	31	−	−	+	−	−	−	−	I	+	+/−	−	−	−	−	+	−
C. cadaveris	6	+/−	−/+	−	V	−	−	−	E^{NG}	+	+/−	−	+	−/+	−	−	−
C. clostridioforme	18	−/+	−	V	−	−	−	−	V	+/−	−	−	−/+	−	−	+/−	V
C. difficile	490	−	−	+	−	−	−	−	E	+	−	−	−	−	+	−	−
C. histolyticum	5	−	−	−	−	−	−	−	V	−	−	+	+	+/−	−	−	−
C. innocuum	18	−	−	+	−	−	−	−	E	+	−	−	−	−	+/−	−	−
C. limosum	2	−	−	−	−	−	−	−	NG	V	V	V	V	−	−	−	−
C. malenominatum	7	+	−	−	V	−	−	−	I^{E}	−	−	−	−/+	−	−	−	−
C. paraputrificum	13	−	−	+	−	−	−	−	E	+	−/+	−	−	−	−	+	−
C. perfringens	79	−	−	V	−/+	−	+	−	E	+	+/−	V	+	+	−	+	−
C. ramosum	16	−	−	+	−	−	−	−	E	+	−	−	−	−	V	+	V
C. septicum	56	−	−	+/−	+/−	−	−	−	E	+	+/−	−	+	+/−	−	+/−	−
C. sordellii	32	+	−	−	V	−	+/−	−	E	+	−	+	−	+	−	−	−
C. sphenoides	8	+/−	−	V	−	−	−	−	V	+	V	−	V	−	V	V	V
C. sporogenes	52	−	+	+	−	−	−/+	+	E	+	−	+	−/+	+	−	−	V
C. subterminale	7	−	−	−	V	−	−	−	V	−	−/+	V	−/+	+/−	−	−	−
C. symbosium	2	−	−	+	−	−	−	−	V	V	−	−	−	−	V	−	−
C. tertium	44	−	−	+	−	−	−	−	E	+	V	−	+/−	−	+	+	−
C. tetani	27	+/−	−	+	V	−	−	−/+	E^{I}	−	−	V	V	+	−	−	−

+, positive reaction in >90% of strains; −, negative reaction in >90% of strains; +/−, most strains positive, occasional strain negative; −/+, most strains negative, occasional strain positive; V, variable; E, growth equal to control without bile; E^{I}, growth inhibited; E^{NG}, equal growth with occasional strains not growing; NG, no growth; I^{E}, most strains inhibited with equal growth for occasional strains.

Adapted from reference 259 by Whaley DN, Wiggs LS, Miller PH, Srivastava PU, Miller JM. Use of Presumpto plates to identify anaerobic bacteria. J Clin Microbiol 1995;33: 1196–1202, and previous editions of this book.

Table 16-23 Characteristics Especially Useful for Identifying Some *Clostridium* Species

CHARACTERISTIC	SPECIES
Aerotolerant	*C. carnis, C. histolyticum, C. tertium,*
Nonmotile	*C. innocuum, C. perfringens, C. ramosum*
Terminal spores	*C. baratii, C. cadaveris, C. innocuum, C. ramosum, C. tertium, C. tetani*
Lecithinase produced on egg-yolk agar	*C. bifermentans, C. limosum, C. novyi, C. perfringens, C. sordellii, C. subterminale, C. baratii, C. haemolyticum*
Lipase produced on egg-yolk agar	*C. botulinum, C. novyi* type A, *C. sporogenes*
Asaccharolytic and proteolytic (i.e., gelatin-positive)	*C. histolyticum, C. limosum, C. subterminale, C. tetani, C. malenominatum* (weak to negative gelatin)
Urease-positive	*C. sordellii* (*C. bifermentans,* which it resembles, is urease-negative)
Do not hydrolyze gelatin	*C. butyricum, C. clostridioforme, C. malenominatum, C. paraputrificum, C. baratii, C. ramosum*
Mannitol fermented	*C. difficile, C. innocuum, C. ramosum, C. sphenoides, C. symbiosum, C. tertium*
Rhamnose fermented	*C. clostridioforme, C. ramosum, C. sporogenes*
Saccharolytic and proteolytic	*C. bifermentans, C. botulinum, C. cadaveris, C. difficile, C. haemolyticum, C. novyi, C. perfringens, C. putrificum, C. septicum, C. sordellii, C. sporogenes*
Saccharolytic and nonproteolytic	*C. baratii, C. beijerinckii, C. butyricum, C. clostridioforme, C. glycolicum, C. innocuum, C. paraputrificum, C. ramosum, C. tertium*

bowels'') was a severe form of necrotizing enterocolitis with an associated mortality of approximately 40%. ''Pig bel,'' a form of necrotizing enteritis seen mainly in children in the highlands of Papua New Guinea, has been associated with a mortality rate of about 30–60%.[174,249] Sporadic cases of *C. perfringens* NBD have been reported from many countries around the world, including Europe and the United States.[4] Factors believed to be important predisposing conditions to NBD include the consumption of excessive amounts of rich food or foods containing trypsin inhibitors (e.g., sweet potatoes, peanuts) by malnourished individuals. As reviewed elsewhere, *C. perfringens* type C has been implicated in both Darmbrand and the pig bel syndrome and in NBD in Western countries during recent times.[4] It has been suggested that *C. perfringens* type A also plays a role in some cases of NBD, particularly in Western countries.[241] In the native highlanders of Papua New Guinea, the disease typically develops after the consumption of large amounts of poorly cooked pork at a pig feast. A heavy inoculum of *C. perfringens* type C is ingested with the meal, the organism proliferates in the small intestine, where it produces β-toxin. Low levels of pancreatic proteolytic enzymes, associated with the usual low-protein diet of the highlanders, but a diet rich in sweet potatoes, may permit the β-toxin of *C. perfringens* to act on the small intestine without the β-toxin being destroyed by pancreatic trypsin or other proteases. There is both a clinical and pathological spectrum in terms of the severity of NBD. Some patients may survive with supportive care and decompression of the bowel; others may require resection of the involved intestinal segment; still others are inoperable and die with extensive gangrenous necrosis of the small and large bowel. The differential diagnosis includes pseudomembranous colitis (whether or not associated with *Clostridium difficile*), acute shigellosis, foodborne illness caused by various agents (including *Escherichia coli, Campylo-*

bacter jejuni, and others), acute ulcerative colitis, and obstruction of the bowel (due to adhesions, volvulus, etc.). In suspected cases, efforts to culture *C. perfringens* type A and C (e.g., blood cultures, peritoneal cultures if there is peritonitis, and intestinal contents of surgical removal or necropsy specimens) should be made. A reference laboratory (such as the CDC), where typing of isolates can be accomplished, should be consulted. Paired sera should be obtained for serologic studies (e.g., to attempt to show a rise in serum antibody titer to β-toxin). A rise in antibody titer would be consistent with either type B or type C *C. perfringens* disease.[249]

MISCELLANEOUS CLOSTRIDIA IN OTHER CLINICAL SETTINGS

Clostridium ramosum. *Clostridium ramosum* has in the past been called *Eubacterium filamentosum, Catenabacterium filamentosum, Actinomyces ramosus, Fusiformis ramosus, Ramibacterium ramosus,* and other names.[222] In 1971, as referred to previously, it was found to produce terminal spores and was placed in the genus *Clostridium.*[135] It is a prominent member of the large bowel flora and is the second most common *Clostridium* isolated from properly collected clinical specimens. It is particularly common in intraabdominal infections following trauma. *Clostridium ramosum* is especially important clinically because of its resistance to penicillin G, clindamycin, and other antibiotics. Although it has been found in severe infections from virtually all body sites, *C. ramosum* can easily be misidentified or overlooked, since it usually stains as a gram-negative rod and its terminal spores are frequently hard to demonstrate.

Cells of *C. ramosum* are usually less than 0.6 μm in diameter × 2–5 μm long, but are extremely pleomorphic, sometimes producing short chains or long filaments. On blood agar, colonies are often 1 mm to 2 mm in diameter, usually nonhemolytic, slightly irregular or circular, entire, low convex, and translucent. Isolates of *C. ramosum* are characteristically resistant to rifampin by the 15-μg disk method discussed above, but inhibited by the 2-U penicillin disk and the 1-mg kanamycin disk (similar to *F. mortiferum* and *F. varium*). *C. ramosum* is indole-negative (*F. mortiferum* and *F. varium* are indole-positive); shows enhanced growth on bile agar; hydrolyzes esculin; and is negative for catalase, lipase, and lecithinase. It is among the few clostridia that ferment mannitol (Table 16-23). Acetic, lactic, and succinic acids are the major metabolic products.

Clostridium septicum. Although *Clostridium septicum* is not nearly as common as *C. perfringens* and *C. ramosum*, it is especially important to recognize in the clinical laboratory. *C. septicum* is usually isolated from serious, often fatal infections. *C. septicum* bacteremia, for unknown reasons, is often associated with underlying malignancy, particularly carcinoma of the colon or cecum, carcinoma of the breast, and hematologic malignancies (e.g., leukemia-lymphoma).[139] The cells are usually about 0.6 μm wide and 3 μm to 6 μm long. It tends to be pleomorphic, sometimes producing long, thin filaments. Chain formation is common, as are intensely staining citron (lemon-shaped) forms. Spores are oval and subterminal, and distend the organism. After 48 hours of incubation on blood agar, colonies are 2 mm to 5 mm in diameter, surrounded by a 1-mm to 4-mm zone of complete hemolysis; they are flat, slightly raised, gray, glistening, and semitranslucent, and have markedly irregular to rhizoid margins, often surrounded by a zone of swarming. Extremely motile strains may swarm across a wide area of the plate. Stiff blood agar, which contains 4–6% instead of the usual 1.5% agar, is sometimes used in plating media to minimize swarming. Some key characteristics of *C. septicum* are that it hydrolyzes gelatin; does not produce indole, lipase, or lecithinase; and ferments lactose but not mannitol, rhamnose, or sucrose. Acetic and butyric acids are the major metabolic products.

CLOSTRIDIUM DIFFICILE–ASSOCIATED INTESTINAL DISEASE

C. difficile, first isolated in 1935, was believed to be nonpathogenic for humans until the late 1970s, when it was implicated as a causative agent in antibiotic-associated diarrhea (AAD) and pseudomembranous colitis (PMC).[7,21] Benign, self-limited diarrhea frequently develops in hospitalized patients who are being treated with antibiotics. The mild diarrhea often subsides following discontinuation of the antibiotic, and the cause of the diarrhea is not determined. In other patients, the intestinal symptoms may be more severe, and the diarrhea may persist. These patients may have antibiotic-associated colitis (AAC) or life-threatening PMC.[7,20,21] *C. difficile* probably causes most cases of PMC; however, it is infrequently caused by *Staphylococcus aureus* or by *C. perfringens*.[7] As reviewed elsewhere, Borriello and associates have seen an association between enterotoxigenic *C. perfringens* and antibiotic-associated diarrhea in the United Kingdom.[28,29] In addition to PMC, *C. difficile* has been estimated to cause some "60 to 75% of antibiotic-associated cases of colitis, and 11–33% of cases of AAD."[173] Whether or not *C. perfringens* causes AAD in the United States, with any frequency, has not been established. The severity of illness, as well as pathologic findings, are highly variable,

depending on whether the patient has PMC, AAC, AAD without anatomic evidence of colitis, or is simply colonized with *C. difficile* (or is an asymptomatic carrier). The pathologic findings in PMC and AAC have been adequately reviewed elsewhere.[27]

As reviewed elsewhere, factors involved in *C. difficile*–associated disease include: 1) toxin A, which is an enterotoxin capable of producing fluid accumulation in rabbit ligated ileal loop assays, 2) toxin B, which is a potent cytotoxin capable of producing cytopathogenic effects in several tissue culture cell lines, and 3) a "motility-altering factor," which stimulates smooth muscle contractions of intestine and is distinct from toxins A and B.[7] Toxin A is also cytotoxic in certain cell lines, but is not as cytotoxic as toxin B in the cell lines that have long been used for toxin B testing.[160,162] For additional information on *C. difficile* and its toxins, the following references are recommended.[3,7,20,21,81,161]

C. difficile is ubiquitous in nature, and has been isolated from soil, water, intestinal contents of various animals, the vagina and urethra of humans, and feces of many healthy infants, but from the stools of only about 3% of healthy adult volunteers. However, the organism is more prevalent in the feces of some hospitalized adults who do not have diarrhea or colitis. It has been found in the feces of about 13–30% of hospitalized adults who were colonized but had no evidence of disease caused by *C. difficile* or antecedent antibiotic treatment. However, *C. difficile* is also implicated frequently as the causative agent of hospital-acquired diarrhea and colitis.[81,173] Although *C. difficile* is commonly found in the feces of many healthy infants, some infants with severe and protracted diarrhea, associated with antecedent antibiotic therapy, have had pseudomembranous colitis and at the same time, *C. difficile* cytotoxin present in their feces without any other putative etiologic agent. These patients have often responded clinically to oral vancomycin treatment (Schaeffer J: personal communication, 1986).

Antimicrobial agents implicated in *C. difficile*–associated gastrointestinal illness have included numerous aminoglycosides, penicillins, cephalosporins, second- and third-generation β-lactam compounds, clindamycin, erythromycin, lincomycin, metronidazole, rifampin, trimethoprim-sulfamethoxazole, amphotericin B, and the fluoroquinolones.[80,81]

In addition, *C. difficile* has been involved in the following clinical settings with no association with antimicrobial therapy: 1) pseudomembranous colitis; 2) diarrhea associated with methotrexate treatment and other anticancer chemotherapeutic agents; 3) relapses of nonspecific inflammatory bowel disease (e.g., Crohn's disease; ulcerative colitis); 4) obstruction or strangulation of the bowel; and in 5) a few cases of sudden infant death syndrome.[70] However, the role of *C. difficile* in these conditions, if any, has not been clarified. For more information on the clinical findings and clinical diagnosis of AAD, AAC, and PMC, the reader is referred to other sources.[20,21,78,79,81]

Collection and Transport of Specimens Containing C. difficile. Ordinarily, passed liquid or semisolid, unformed fecal specimens (about 5–50 g or 5–50 mL, if liquid) are the preferred specimens for laboratory diagnosis. Swab specimens, because of the small volume obtained, are inadequate. Formed stool specimens are inappropriate unless an epidemiologic study of stool carriage is being conducted. Other suitable specimens include biopsy material or lumen contents obtained by colonoscopy and involved bowel (surgical removal; autopsy). However, lumen contents or biopsy material from colonoscopic procedures may excessively dilute the sample, or the quantity obtained by biopsy may be insufficient for the laboratory work required. Leakproof plastic containers should be used for transport of specimens. If specimens are to be processed by the laboratory on the same day they are collected, transportation at room temperature will suffice. If a specimen arrives late in the day and cannot be processed until the following day, it can be held in the refrigerator without demonstrable loss of cytotoxic activity. Optimally, specimens should not remain at room temperature longer than 2 hours before either being processed or refrigerated. However, for shipment of specimens to a reference laboratory for a toxin assay, we recommend they be shipped on dry ice. On the other hand, an anaerobic transport container (transported at 25°C) should be used for specimens to be processed for isolation and identification of *C. difficile*. Specimens to be processed for the *C. difficile* latex agglutination test (Culturette Brand *CDT C. difficile* test; Becton Dickinson Microbiology Systems, Sparks, MD) should not be frozen, because the antigen detected is unstable on freezing.

***Laboratory Diagnosis of* C. difficile.** As discussed in the "Direct Examination" section of this chapter, diagnostic testing in cases of suspected *C. difficile*–associated disease can be accomplished in the laboratory either by demonstrating the cytotoxin, by isolation and identification of toxin producing *C. difficile* from stool specimens, by performing a latex agglutination test or an enzyme immunoassay (EIA) for the glutamate dehydrogenase of *C. difficile,* by an EIA test for the enterotoxin and/or cytotoxin produced by the organism in feces, or by a combination of methods. A brief description of a practical procedure for detection of the cytotoxin of *C. difficile* is described in Box 16-14.

C. difficile can be isolated by the use of a spore selection technique (i.e., heat shock or alcohol spore selection procedures) and by use of selective plating media such as phenylethyl alcohol (PEA) blood agar (Remel, Lenexa, KS; or BD Microbiology Systems) or cycloserine-cefoxitin, egg yolk, fructose agar (CCFA) plus nonselective CDC-anaerobe blood agar.[7,167] Detailed descriptions of the alcohol- and heat-treatment spore-selection procedures are given elsewhere.[7] If either of these procedures is used, the alcohol- or heat-treated sample is inoculated onto CDC anaerobe blood agar (AnBAP) (and/or on egg yolk agar) after the treatment. Following 48 hours of incubation anaerobically, colonies of *C. difficile* on AnBAP are non-hemolytic, about 2 to 4 mm in diameter, grayish-translucent, slightly raised, flat, and spreading, with rhizoid margins. As seen through a dissecting microscope, the colonies show an iridescent, "speckled-opalescent" appearance. *C. difficile* is negative for lipase and lecithinase on egg yolk agar.

In addition to the spore-selection procedure, a plate of PEA medium and a CCFA plate should be inoculated with untreated stool (or stool suspension prepared in buffered gelatin diluent). After 48 hours of incubation, colonies of *C. difficile* on PEA medium will be virtually identical to those on AnBAP (described above). The appearance of *C. difficile* colonies on CCFA medium is described in Table 16-6. Previ-

---

Box 16-14 Assay for Toxin in Feces by Tissue Culture Cytotoxicity Procedure[a]

1. Centrifuge liquid stool or extract of formed stool (2,000 *g* for 20 minutes or 10,000 *g* for 10 minutes).
2. Filter through 0.45-μm membrane filter.
3. Add 0.1 mL of cell-free supernatant plus 0.1 mL buffered gelatin diluent (pH 7.0 to 7.2) or phosphate-buffered saline (PBS) to a tissue culture tube. Commercially available human diploid lung fibroblasts (WI-38 cells) are convenient to use.
4. Observe the tissue culture cells for cytotoxicity at 4, 24, and 48 hours (most are positive at 24 hours).
5. For the antitoxin neutralization test, add 0.1 mL of *C. difficile* antitoxin (TechLab, Blacksburg, VA) to 0.1 mL cell-free supernatant and carry out steps 1 and 4. Rounding of WI-38 cells (so-called actinomorphic change) or other cytopathic effects should not be seen if toxin that is present in the stool is neutralized.
6. The toxin titer is determined using serial twofold or tenfold dilutions of the filtered fecal sample in buffered gelatin diluent (pH 7.0 to 7.2) or PBS. Correlation between the toxin titers and severity of illness is very crude.

---

[a] *Commercial kits for performing C. difficile cytotoxin neutralization assays are available from at least two manufacturers (Bartels Diagnostics; Bio-Whittaker/Wampole). The kits can be purchased complete with human foreskin fibroblasts in microbroth dilution trays, and they provide the necessary antitoxin and other reagents to accomplish the cytotoxin neutralization assay.*

ously, Marler and colleagues found major differences in the performance of CCFA medium that had been prepared by three different manufacturers.[167] Bartley and Dowell evaluated additional selective media formulations for the primary isolation of *C. difficile*.[22]

Identification of *C. difficile* is described by several authors.[7,125,189,190] In addition to the colony characteristics already described, there is a distinctive odor. The gram-positive to gram-variable rods have subterminal spores and, in early broth culture, are motile. Metabolic product analysis reveals acetic, propionic, isobutyric, butyric, isovaleric, valeric, and isocaproic acids (Table 16-21). Esculin and gelatin are hydrolyzed. Indole, nitrate, and urease are negative. Most strains ferment glucose, mannitol and mannose. Salicin and xylose are variable (Tables 16-22 and 16-23).

BOTULISM

Botulism is a life-threatening neuroparalytic disease caused by antigenically distinct, heat-labile, protein toxins of *C. botulinum*.[52,221] Although seven toxin types (A, B, C, D, E, F, G) are produced by different strains of *C. botulinum*, most cases of botulism in humans are caused by types A, B, E, and F. Of these, type F is the least common. Types C and D are associated with botulism in birds and mammals, but not in humans. Type C can be subdivided into two types, C_1 and C_2.[95] Although type G organisms, now called *Clostridium argentinense*—as referred to by Hatheway,[96] have been isolated from autopsy samples of a few individuals who died suddenly, it is not clear whether type G organisms cause botulism in humans. Regardless of which antigenic type (i.e. A, B, D, or E), botulinum toxin acts primarily by binding to synaptic vesicles of cholinergic nerves, thereby preventing the release of acetylcholine at the peripheral nerve endings (including neuromuscular junctions), and acute, flaccid, descending paralysis develops.[52] The paralysis begins with bilateral impairment of cranial nerves resulting in paralysis of muscles of the face (including eyelids), head, and throat. The paralysis then descends symmetrically to involve the muscles of the thorax, diaphragm, and extremities. Patients may die of respiratory paralysis unless they have proper respiratory intensive care, including mechanical ventilation; death may also result from secondary pneumonia (caused by nonbotulinum organisms).[68,221]

Four different categories of botulism are recognized by the CDC. The first of these is classical foodborne botulism, typically seen in adults, resulting from the ingestion of preformed toxin in contaminated food. The second category, wound botulism, is the rarest form; it results from production of botulinum toxin in vivo after *C. botulinum* has multiplied in an infected wound. The third category, infant botulism, is the most common; it results from in vivo multiplication of *C. botulinum* with production of the neurotoxin within the infant gut. The fourth category, "classification undetermined," is for cases of botulism in individuals who are older than 12 months in whom no food or wound source of *C. botulinum* can be implicated.[52] Home-processed foods, rather than commercially processed foods, have been involved in most of the outbreaks of foodborne botulism. The foods most often implicated have been vegetables (e.g., home-canned tomatoes, tomato juice, green beans, greens, peppers, corn, beets, spinach), fish (e.g., home-processed tuna fish, smoked salmon, fish eggs, commercially processed tuna, smoked whitefish, etc.), fruits (home-canned apple butter, blackberries, etc.), and miscellaneous foods (e.g., beef stew, chili, spaghetti sauce, luncheon meats, etc.).

Infant botulism was recognized as a distinct clinical entity in 1976.[12,13] From 1976 to 1988, 760 cases were diagnosed.[135] Infant botulism has been reported from many different states, with the greatest number of cases in California.[95] Most cases reported west of the Mississippi River have been type A; the majority of those east of it have been type B. Affected infants have ranged from 6 days to 11.7 months in age, and both sexes have been affected equally.[95] Almost all racial and ethnic groups have been affected. The infants ingest spores, but not preformed toxin (preformed toxin is ingested in foodborne botulism), from soil, household dust, honey, or another source. Within the gut, *C. botulinum* multiplies and elaborates toxin. Clinical features include constipation (usually the first sign), listlessness, difficulty in sucking and swallowing, an altered cry, hypotonia, and muscle weakness. Eventually the baby appears "floppy" and loses head control, and ptosis, ophthalmoplegia, flaccid facial expression, dysphagia, and other neurologic signs may develop. Respiratory arrest or respiratory insufficiency necessitating respiratory therapy occur. A small number of infants with laboratory-confirmed infant botulism have died. Infant botulism has accounted for a small number of cases of sudden infant death syndrome.[12]

The diagnosis of classical foodborne botulism is con-

firmed in reference laboratories such as the CDC by demonstrating botulinum toxin in serum, feces, gastric contents, or vomitus. Also, the organism may be isolated from the patient's feces.[52] The detection of botulinum toxin in epidemiologically implicated food, with or without isolating the organism, is useful for ascertaining what food was involved in the outbreak. About 15 to 20 mL of serum and 25 to 50 g of feces should be collected for shipment to the appropriate reference laboratory (as directed by the appropriate state or federal public health official who is capable of providing epidemiologic and laboratory aid in the investigation). In suspected wound botulism, serum, exudate, or swab samples from the wound should be collected, along with tissue (e.g., at autopsy), and feces should also be collected.

When infant botulism is suspected, serum (2–3 mL) and as much stool as possible (ideally, 25–50 g) should be collected in a leakproof plastic container and refrigerated or placed on ice for shipment. However, many, if not most, of these infants are constipated early in the illness, and stool may not be available. Therefore, the clinician must decide whether the risk of obtaining an anorectal swab specimen is clinically warranted for the laboratory to isolate *C. botulinum* from this source.

Some, but not all, state health department laboratories provide diagnostic services for botulism. With prior approval of the CDC (Tel. 770-488-7100 or 770-488-4819; website www.cdc.gov/ncidod/hip or www.bt.cdc.gov), and the local state health department laboratory, specimens may be submitted to the CDC for laboratory diagnosis. Confirmation of the clinical diagnosis of botulism requires demonstration of botulinum toxin (mouse neutralization test) in serum or feces, and/or *C. botulinum* in feces.[7,52,97] Isolation and identification of the organism is by conventional cultural biochemical procedures and the toxin neutralization test. Toxin has only rarely been detected in serum from an affected infant. It is recommended that culture and toxin testing for *C. botulinum* be done only by properly equipped reference laboratories for this specialized testing. For further details, the interested reader is referred to the following references.[7,52,97]

TETANUS

Tetanus is an infectious disease, caused by *C. tetani*, that largely involves unimmunized persons in the United States—mostly of the rural South.[7,52] It is a dramatic illness characterized by spastic contractions of voluntary muscles and hyperreflexia, caused by a protoplasmic, heat-labile protein toxin (tetanospasmin) elaborated by *C. tetani*.[7,52,68] Tetanus shares some similarity to diphtheria, in that the infection (and the organism) remains localized (usually a minor penetrating wound), and the toxin is absorbed, producing major systemic effects. The spores of *C. tetani*, like those of *C. botulinum*, are widely distributed in the soil, as well as in aquatic environments. Tetanus usually results from spore contamination of puncture wounds, lacerations, or even crush injuries.[7,52,68] Fecal contamination of the umbilical cord has been the source of *C. tetani* in some cases of neonatal tetanus. Following a localized penetrating injury, there may be a deep-seated mixed infection involving anaerobes plus nonanaerobes in devitalized tissue, resulting in a low oxygen tension and low oxidation reduction potential, thus providing favorable conditions for *C. tetani* spores to germinate, for the vegetative cells to multiply and release the tetanospasmin on autolysis of the bacterial cells.[52] Tetanospasmin attaches to peripheral motor nerve endings, and it travels along nerves to the central nervous system (CNS). The toxin binds to gangliosides in the CNS, and blocks inhibitory impulses to the motor neurons. Patients have prolonged muscle spasms of both flexor and extensor muscles. Tetanospasmin attaches to binding sites at myoneural junctions, thus inhibiting the release of acetylcholine. This is like the attachment of botulinum toxin to myoneural junctions, except that the binding sites for tetanospasmin and for botulinum toxin are different.[52] As indicated previously, patients with tetanus have spastic muscle contractions, difficulty opening the jaw (called lockjaw, "trismus"), a characteristic smile called "risus sardonicus," and contractions of back muscles resulting in backward arching. Patients are extremely irritable, and tetanic seizures develop, brought about by violent, painful muscle contractions following some minor stimulus such as a noise. Diagnosis of tetanus is based largely on the clinical findings, not on laboratory studies. The antecedent wound is often minor or trivial. Direct Gram-stained smears and anaerobic cultures of the wound site are often negative, failing to reveal the organism. *C. tetani* forms round, terminal spores, produces spreading or swarming growth on anaerobe blood agar, produces major amounts of acetate and butyrate, with only a minor amount of propionate, is lipase- and lecithinase-negative on egg yolk agar, and is asaccharolytic. For more information on *C. tetani*, the books by Finegold and George[70] and Smith and Williams[222] and the review articles by Dowell[52] and Hatheway[96] are recommended.

Antimicrobial Susceptibility Testing of Anaerobic Bacteria

Successful management of diseases involving anaerobic bacteria requires selection and treatment with appropriate antimicrobial agents, often in conjunction with removal of bacteria by drainage of abscesses, elimination of foreign bodies, and debridement of necrotic tissue and other surgical measures. It was once believed that most anaerobes had predictable antimicrobial susceptibility patterns and that accurate identification of isolates was all that was necessary for one to predict the susceptibility of individual isolates to various antibiotics. This is an oversimplification. While some antimicrobial agents are active against nearly all (e.g., >95%) anaerobic bacteria (e.g., imipenem, meropenem, piperacillin-tazobactam, and chloramphenicol), several other antimicrobial agents that might be selected for use in treatment are not nearly as predictable in their activities against selected genera and species of anaerobes. For example, metronidazole is highly active against most gram-negative anaerobic bacteria tested in the United States, but resistance to metronidazole has emerged in *B. fragilis* strains in other countries.[98] In addition, metronidazole resistance frequently occurs in *Actinomyces* species, *Propionibacterium* species, *Lactobacillus* species, the anaerobic cocci, and other gram-positive anaerobes.[6] Although some of the fluoroquinolones showed good activity against anaerobes initially, resistance

to these agents has developed rapidly.[98] The penicillins and ureidopenicillins, the second- and third-generation cephalosporins and clindamycin may or may not be active against certain commonly encountered species of anaerobic gram-negative bacilli and clostridia.[2] Resistance to these agents is variable.[98,240,257] Nonetheless, it is usually necessary for the attending physician to start antimicrobial therapy empirically, before results of identification and susceptibility testing are available. Therefore, tabulated susceptibility and treatment results reported in the literature or in the local hospital, and clinical experience of the physician may of necessity be the basis for the initial choice of antibiotics. Excellent sources of additional information relative to selection of antimicrobial agents for treatment purposes have been published recently elsewhere.[98,155,240] However, there is enough variability in the susceptibility patterns of clinically significant anaerobes that in vitro susceptibility testing of individual isolates is indicated at times to aid clinicians with the management of serious infections and those that require prolonged therapy such as brain abscess, endocarditis, lung abscess, infections involving joints, osteomyelitis, infections involving prosthetic devices, vascular grafts, recurrent or refractory bacteremia, or when infection does not respond to empirical therapy.[185]

Another indication for testing is the setting in which there has not been a clear-cut clinical precedent on which to base treatment decisions. In addition, clinical microbiologists experienced with work with anaerobes are encouraged to investigate the activities of newly marketed and/or investigational antimicrobial agents on anaerobes isolated in their hospital laboratory. Also, there is a need to monitor susceptibility patterns of anaerobes at the local community and hospital levels and in multiple medical centers around the United States and in various countries around the world.[135]

Organisms to be considered for antimicrobial susceptibility testing, because of their virulence, or because they are commonly resistant to certain antimicrobial agents include species of the *Bacteroides fragilis* group, species of the pigmented *Prevotella-Porphyromonas* group, other *Prevotella*, *Fusobacterium mortiferum, F. varium,* and *F. necrophorum, Bilophila, Sutterrella,* and some *Clostridium* species.

Methods for Antimicrobial Susceptibility Testing of Anaerobes

At present, no automated procedures are recommended for antimicrobial susceptibility testing of anaerobes. As reviewed elsewhere, reproducible results can be obtained by one of three methods.[98,185] The agar dilution method for antimicrobial susceptibility testing is particularly useful for batch testing 30 or more isolates of any anaerobe. The medium used is *Brucella* blood agar supplemented with hemin, vitamin K_1, and laked sheep blood. The use of broth microdilution panels is a less labor-intensive alternative to the agar dilution procedure, and it is considered equivalent to the agar dilution procedure for antimicrobial susceptibility testing *Bacteroides fragilis* group isolates.[98,185] The recommended medium for the broth microdilution procedure is *Brucella* broth supplemented with hemin, vitamin K_1, and lysed horse blood. It supports the growth of most anaerobes. However, the Clinical Laboratory Standards Institute (formerly, the National Committee for Clinical Laboratory Standards) does not currently recommend the broth microdilution procedure for testing nonbacteroides anaerobes. The third recommended way to test anaerobes (which also is user-friendly), is the Etest (AB Biodisk North America, Piscataway, NJ) gradient test strip method. Both the Etest procedure and the broth microdilution procedure are practical ways for testing individual isolates against a limited number of antimicrobial agents, as reviewed in detail elsewhere.[98,185]

Broth disk elution and disk agar diffusion techniques have been used in the past but should not be used for anaerobe testing despite their convenience. Most anaerobes other than *Bacteroides* spp. grow too slowly for the disk diffusion procedure to work; the Bauer-Kirby interpretive charts were not designed for anaerobes, and interpretive charts based on standardized media and methods for disk-diffusion testing of anaerobes are lacking; also, there has been poor correlation between zone size measurements and the results from minimal inhibitory concentration dilution tests. For details of the recommended procedures, the reader is referred to the most current Clinical Laboratory Standards Institute document.[98,185]

REFERENCES

1. al-Barrak A, Embil J, Dyck B, et al. An outbreak of toxin A negative, toxin B positive *Clostridium difficile*-associated diarrhea in a Canadian tertiary-care hospital. Can Commun Dis Rep 1999;25:65–69.
2. Aldridge KE, Ashcraft D, Cambre K, et al. Multicenter survey of the changing in vitro antimicrobial susceptibilities of clinical isolates of *Bacteroides fragilis* group, *Prevotella, Fusobacterium, Porphyromonas,* and *Peptostreptococcus* species. Antimicrob Agents Chemother 2001;45:1238–1243.
3. Alfa MJ, Kabani A, Lyerly D, et al. Characterization of a toxin A-negative, toxin B-positive strain of *Clostridium difficile* responsible for a nosocomial outbreak of *Clostridium difficile*-associated diarrhea. J Clin Microbiol 2000;38:2706–2714.
3a. Alfa MJ, Robson D, Davi M, et al. An outbreak of necrotizing enterocolitis associated with a novel *Clostridium* species in a neonatal intensive care unit. Clin Infect Dis 2002;35:S101–105.
4. Allen SD. Pig-bel and other necrotizing disorders of the gut involving *Clostridium perfringens*. In: Connor DH, Chandler FW, Schwartz DA et al., eds. Pathology of Infectious Diseases. Norwalk, CT, Appleton & Lange, 1997:717–724.
5. Allen SD, Blue-Hnidy DE, Tibbs ME, et al. Anaerobic bacteremia: three decades of experience at a university medical center with projections for the 21st century. Paper presented at the Anaerobe Olympiad 2002: The 6th Biennial Congress of the Anaerobe Society of the Americas, 2002.
6. Allen SD, Duerden BI. Infections due to non-sporing anaerobic bacilli and cocci. In: Hausler WJJ, Sussman M, eds. Bacterial Infections. Vol 3. Ed. 9. London: Edward Arnold, 1998:743–776.
7. Allen SD, Emery CL, Lyerly DM. *Clostridium.* In: Murray PR, Baron EJ, Pfaller MA, et al., eds. Manual of Clinical Microbiology. Vol 1. Ed. 8. Washington, ASM Press, 2003:835–856.
8. Allen SD, Emery CL, Siders JA. Anaerobic Bacteriology. In: Truant AL, ed. Manual of Commercial Methods in Clinical Microbiology. Washington, D. C., ASM Press, 2002:50–81.
9. Allen SD, Lombard GL, Armfield AY, et al. Development and evaluation of an improved anaerobic holding jar procedure. Abstr Ann Meet Am Soc Microbiol Abstr C142, 1977:59.
10. Allen SD, Siders JA, Marler LM. Current issues and problems in dealing with anaerobes in the clinical laboratory. Clin Lab Med 1995;15:333–364.
11. Aranki A, Freter R. Use of anaerobic glove boxes for the cultivation of strictly anaerobic bacteria. Am J Clin Nutr 1972;25:1329–1334.
12. Arnon SS. Infant botulism. In: Finegold SM, George WL, eds. Anaerobic infections in humans. New York, NY, Academic Press, 1989:601–609.
13. Arnon SS. Human tetanus and human botulism. In: Rood JI, McClane BA,

14. Songer JG et al., eds. The Clostridia: Molecular Biology and Pathogenesis. New York, NY, Academic Press, 1997:95–115.
14. Barenfanger J, Drake C, Lawhorn J, et al. Comparison of chlorhexidine and tincture of iodine for skin antisepsis in preparation for blood sample collection. J Clin Microbiol 2004;42:2216–2217.
15. Baron EJ, Allen SD. Should clinical laboratories adopt new taxonomic changes? If so, when? Clin Infect Dis 1993;16:S449–S450.
16. Baron EJ, Curren M, Henderson G, et al. *Bilophila wadsworthia* isolates from clinical specimens. J Clin Microbiol 1992;30:1882–1884.
17. Baron EJ, Summanen P, Downes J, et al. *Bilophila wadsworthia,* gen. nov. and sp. nov., a unique gram-negative anaerobic rod recovered from appendicitis specimens and human faeces. J Gen Microbiol 1989;135(Pt 12):3405–3411.
18. Bartlett GL. Pocket Book of Infectious Disease Therapy. Philadelphia, Lippincott Williams & Wilkins, 2004.
19. Bartlett JG. Anaerobic bacteria. In: Gorbach SL, Bartlett JG, Blacklow NR, eds. Infectious Diseases. Ed. 2. Philadelphia, W. B. Saunders Company, 1998:1888–1901.
20. Bartlett JG. Antibiotic-associated diarrhea. N Engl J Med 2002;346:334–339.
21. Bartlett JG. *Clostridium difficile*-associated enteric disease. Curr Infect Dis Rep 2002;4:477–483.
22. Bartley SL, Dowell VR Jr. Comparison of media for the isolation of *Clostridium difficile* from fecal specimens. Lab Med 1991;22:335–338.
23. Beaman L, Beaman BL. The role of oxygen and its derivatives in microbial pathogenesis and host defense. Annu Rev Microbiol 1984;38:27–48.
24. Belanger SD, Boissinot M, Clairoux N, et al. Rapid detection of *Clostridium difficile* in feces by real-time PCR. J Clin Microbiol 2003;41:730–734.
25. Bentham JR, Pollard AJ, Milford CA, et al. Cerebral infarct and meningitis secondary to Lemierre's syndrome. Pediatr Neurol 2004;30:281–283.
26. Boo TW, Cryan B, O'Donnell A, et al. Prosthetic valve endocarditis caused by *Veillonella parvula.* J Infect 2005;50:81–83.
27. Borriello SP. Clostridia in gastrointestinal disease. Boca Raton, CRC Press, 1985:1–239.
28. Borriello SP. Clostridial disease of the gut. Clin Infect Dis 1995;20:Suppl 2:S242–S250.
29. Borriello SP, Barclay FE, Welch AR, et al. Epidemiology of diarrhoea caused by enterotoxigenic *Clostridium perfringens.* J Med Microbiol 1985;20:363–372.
30. Bourgault AM, Lamothe F, Dolce P, et al. *Fusobacterium* bacteremia. clinical experience with 40 cases. Clin Infect Dis 1997;25:Suppl 2:S181–S183.
31. Bourgault AM, Rosenblatt JE, Fitzgerald RH. *Peptococcus magnus*: a significant human pathogen. Ann Intern Med 1980;93:244–248.
32. Brazier JS, Smith SA. Evaluation of the Anoxomat: a new technique for anaerobic and microaerophilic clinical bacteriology. J Clin Pathol 1989;42:640–644.
33. Brock DW, Georg LK, Brown JM, et al. Actinomycosis caused by *Arachnia propionica*: report of 11 cases. Am J Clin Pathol 1973;59:66–77.
34. Brook I, Frazier EH. Significant recovery of nonsporulating anaerobic rods from clinical specimens. Clin Infect Dis 1993;16:476–480.
35. Buchanan AG. Clinical laboratory evaluation of a reverse CAMP test for presumptive identification of *Clostridium perfringens.* J Clin Microbiol 1982;16:761–762.
36. Candoni A, Fili C, Trevisan R, et al. *Fusobacterium nucleatum*: a rare cause of bacteremia in neutropenic patients with leukemia and lymphoma. Clin Microbiol Infect 2003;9:1112–1115.
37. Carlier JP, Marchandin H, Jumas-Bilak E, et al. *Anaeroglobus geminatus* gen. nov., sp. nov., a novel member of the family *Veillonellaceae.* Int J Syst Evol Microbiol 2002;52:983–986.
38. Centers for Disease Control and Prevention. Foodborne disease outbreaks, annual summary, 1982. CDC Surveill Summ 1986;35:7SS–16SS.
39. Charfreitag O, Collins MD, Stackebrandt E. Reclassification of *Arachnia propionica* as *Propionibacterium propionicus* comb. nov. Int J Syst Bacteriol 1988;38:354–357.
40. Chirinos JA, Lichtstein DM, Garcia J, et al. The evolution of Lemierre syndrome: report of 2 cases and review of the literature. Medicine (Baltimore) 2002;81:458–465.
41. Citron DM. Update on the taxonomy and clinical aspects of the genus *Fusobacterium.* Clin Infect Dis 2002;35:S22–27.
42. Clarridge JE III, Zhang Q. Genotypic diversity of clinical *Actinomyces* species: phenotype, source, and disease correlation among genospecies. J Clin Microbiol 2002;40:3442–3448.
43. Collins MD, Hoyles L, Kalfas S, et al. Characterization of *Actinomyces* isolates from infected root canals of teeth: description of *Actinomyces radicidentis* sp. nov. J Clin Microbiol 2000;38:3399–3403.
44. Collins MD, Lawson PA, Willems A, et al. The phylogeny of the genus *Clostridium*: proposal of five new genera and eleven new species combinations. Int J Syst Bacteriol 1994;44:812–826.
45. Collins MD, Love DN, Karjalainen J, et al. Phylogenetic analysis of members of the genus *Porphyromonas* and description of *Porphyromonas cangingivalis* sp. nov. and *Porphyromonas cansulci* sp. nov. Int J Syst Bacteriol 1994;44:674–679.

46. Collins MD, Wallbanks S. Comparative sequence analyses of the 16S rRNA genes of *Lactobacillus minutus*, *Lactobacillus rimae* and *Streptococcus parvulus*: proposal for the creation of a new genus *Atopobium*. FEMS Microbiol Lett 1992;74:235–240.

47. Cregan P, Fiss EH, Sullivan A, et al. Comparison of two BACTEC anaerobic culture media for recovery of anaerobic bacteria. Diagn Microbiol Infect Dis 1993;17:239–242.

48. Dalmau D, Cayouette M, Lamothe F, et al. Clindamycin resistance in the *Bacteroides fragilis* group: association with hospital-acquired infections. Clin Infect Dis 1997;24:874–877.

49. Delaney ML, Onderdonk AB. Evaluation of the AnaeroPack system for growth of clinically significant anaerobes. J Clin Microbiol 1997;35:558–562.

50. Dellinger CA, Moore LV. Use of the RapID-ANA System to screen for enzyme activities that differ among species of bile-inhibited *Bacteroides*. J Clin Microbiol 1986;23:289–293.

51. Dorsher CW, Rosenblatt JE, Wilson WR, et al. Anaerobic bacteremia: decreasing rate over a 15-year period. Rev Infect Dis 1991;13:633–636.

52. Dowell VR Jr. Botulism and tetanus: selected epidemiologic and microbiologic aspects. Reviews of Infectious Diseases 1984;6:S202–S207.

53. Dowell VR Jr, Hawkins TM. Laboratory Methods in Anaerobic Bacteriology, CDC Laboratory Manual. Washington, DC: Government Printing Office, 1981. DHHS publication no. (CDC) 81–8272.

54. Dowell VR Jr, Lombard GL. Presumptive identification of anaerobic non–spore-forming gram-negative bacilli. Atlanta: Centers for Disease Control, 1977.

55. Dowell VR Jr, Lombard GL. Differential agar media for identification of anaerobic bacteria. In: Tilton RC, ed. Rapid methods and automation in microbiology. Washington, DC, American Society for Microbiology, 1982:258–262.

56. Dowell VR Jr, Lombard GL, Thompson FS, et al. Media for isolation, characterization, and identification of obligately anaerobic bacteria. Atlanta: Centers for Disease Control, 1977.

57. Dzink JL, Sheenan MT, Socransky SS. Proposal of three subspecies of *Fusobacterium nucleatum* Knorr 1922: *Fusobacterium nucleatum* subsp. *nucleatum* subsp. nov., comb. nov.; *Fusobacterium nucleatum* subsp. *polymorphum* subsp. nov., nom. rev., comb. nov.; and *Fusobacterium nucleatum* subsp. *vincentii* subsp. nov., nom. rev., comb. nov. Int J Syst Bacteriol 1990;40:74–78.

58. Edwards R. Resistance to beta-lactam antibiotics in *Bacteroides* spp. J Med Microbiol 1997;46:979–986.

59. Eley A, Clarry T, Bennett KW. Selective and differential medium for isolation of *Bacteroides ureolyticus* from clinical specimens. Eur J Clin Microbiol Infect Dis 1989;8:83–85.

60. Engelkirk PG, Duben-Engelkirk J, Dowell VR Jr. Principles and practice of clinical anaerobic bacteriology. Belmont, CA: Star, 1992.

61. Ezaki T, Kawamura Y, Li N, et al. Proposal of the genera *Anaerococcus* gen. nov., *Peptoniphilus* gen. nov. and *Gallicola* gen. nov. for members of the genus *Peptostreptococcus*. Int J Syst Evol Microbiol 2001;51:1521–1528.

62. Ezaki T, Li N, Hashimoto Y, et al. 16S ribosomal DNA sequences of anaerobic cocci and proposal of *Ruminococcus hansenii* comb. nov. and *Ruminococcus productus* comb. nov. Int J Syst Bacteriol 1994;44:130–136.

63. Ezaki T, Yamamoto N, Ninomiya K, et al. Transfer of *Peptococcus indolicus*, *Peptococcus asaccharolyticus*, *Peptococcus prevotii* and *Peptococcus magnus* to the genus *Peptostreptococcus* and proposal of *Peptostreptococcus tetradius* sp. nov. International Journal of Systemic Bacteriology 1983;33:683–698.

64. Falagas ME, Siakavellas E. *Bacteroides*, *Prevotella*, and *Porphyromonas* species: a review of antibiotic resistance and therapeutic options. Int J Antimicrob Agents 2000;15:1–9.

65. Fanourgiakis P, Vekemans M, Georgala A, et al. Febrile neutropenia and *Fusobacterium* bacteremia: clinical experience with 13 cases. Support Care Cancer 2003;11:332–335.

66. Felner JM, Dowell VR Jr. "*Bacteroides*" bacteremia. Am J Med 1971;50:787–796.

67. Finegold S. Changes in taxonomy, anaerobes associated with humans, 2001–2004. Anaerobe 2004;10:309–312.

68. Finegold SM. Anaerobic bacteria in human disease. New York, Academic Press, 1977.

69. Finegold SM. Anaerobic bacteria: general concepts. In: Mandell GL, Bennett JE, Dolin R, eds. Mandell, Douglas, and Bennett's Principles and Practice of Infectious Diseases. Vol. 2. Ed. 5. Philadelphia, Churchill Livingstone, 2000:2519–2537.

70. Finegold SM, George WL. Anaerobic infections in humans. San Diego, CA: Academic Press, 1989.

71. Finegold SM, Song Y, Liu C. Taxonomy: general comments and update on taxonomy of Clostridia and anaerobic cocci. Anaerobe 2002;8:283–285.

72. Finegold SM, Sutter VL, Sugihara PT, et al. Fecal microbial flora in Seventh Day Adventist populations and control subjects. Am J Clin Nutr 1977;30:1781–1792.

73. Fisher RG, Denison MR. *Veillonella parvula* bacteremia without an underlying source. J Clin Microbiol 1996;34:3235–3236.

74. Funke G, Alvarez N, Pascual C, et al. *Actinomyces europaeus* sp. nov., isolated from human clinical specimens. Int J Syst Bacteriol 1997;47:687–692.

75. Funke G, Stubbs S, von Graevenitz A, et al. Assignment of human-derived CDC group 1 coryneform bacteria and CDC group 1-like coryneform bacteria to the genus *Actinomyces* as *Actinomyces neuii* subsp. *neuii* sp. nov., subsp. nov., and *Actinomyces neuii* subsp. *anitratus* subsp. nov. Int J Syst Bacteriol 1994;44:167–171.

76. Funke G, von Graevenitz A. Infections due to *Actinomyces neuii* (former "CDC coryneform group 1" bacteria). Infection 1995;23:73–75.

77. George WL, Sutter VL, Citron D, et al. Selective and differential medium for isolation of *Clostridium difficile*. J Clin Microbiol 1979;9:214–219.

78. Gerding DN. Diagnosis of *Clostridium difficile*–associated disease: patient selection and test perfection. Am J Med 1996;100:485–486.

79. Gerding DN. Treatment of *Clostridium difficile*-associated diarrhea and colitis. Curr Top Microbiol Immunol 2000;250:127–139.

80. Gerding DN. Clindamycin, cephalosporins, fluoroquinolones, and *Clostridium difficile*-associated diarrhea: this is an antimicrobial resistance problem. Clin Infect Dis 2004;38:646–648.

81. Gerding DN, Johnson S, Peterson LR, et al. *Clostridium difficile*-associated diarrhea and colitis. Infect Control Hosp Epidemiol 1995;16:459–477.

82. Gharbia SE, Shah HN. *Fusobacterium nucleatum* subsp. *fusiforme* subsp. nov. and *Fusobacterium nucleatum* subsp. *animalis* subsp. nov. as additional subspecies within *Fusobacterium nucleatum*. Int J Syst Bacteriol 1992;42:296–298.

83. Glupczynski Y, Labbe M, Crokaert F, et al. Isolation of *Mobiluncus* in four cases of extragenital infections in adult women. Eur J Clin Microbiol 1984;3:433–435.

84. Golan Y, McDermott LA, Jacobus NV, et al. Emergence of fluoroquinolone resistance among *Bacteroides* species. J Antimicrob Chemother 2003;52:208–213.

85. Goldstein EJ, Citron DM, Peraino VA, et al. *Desulfovibrio desulfuricans* bacteremia and review of human *Desulfovibrio* infections. J Clin Microbiol 2003;41:2752–2754.

86. Gorbach SL, Mayhew JW, Bartlett JG, et al. Rapid diagnosis of anaerobic infections by direct gas-liquid chromatography of clinical specimens. J Clin Invest 1976;57:478–484.

87. Gregory EM, Moore WE, Holdeman LV. Superoxide dismutase in anaerobes: survey. Appl Environ Microbiol 1978;35:988–991.

88. Guilbault C, Labbe AC, Poirier L, et al. Development and evaluation of a PCR method for detection of the *Clostridium difficile* toxin B gene in stool specimens. J Clin Microbiol 2002;40:2288–2290.

89. Hagelskjaer Kristensen L, Prag J. Human necrobacillosis, with emphasis on Lemierre's syndrome. Clin Infect Dis 2000;31:524–532.

90. Hall V, Collins MD, Hutson R, et al. *Actinomyces cardiffensis* sp. nov. from human clinical sources. J Clin Microbiol 2002;40:3427–3431.

91. Hall V, Collins MD, Hutson RA, et al. *Actinobaculum urinale* sp. nov., from human urine. Int J Syst Evol Microbiol 2003;53:679–682.

92. Hall V, Collins MD, Hutson RA, et al. *Actinomyces oricola* sp. nov., from a human dental abscess. Int J Syst Evol Microbiol 2003;53:1515–1518.

93. Hall V, Collins MD, Lawson PA, et al. *Actinomyces nasicola* sp. nov., isolated from a human nose. Int J Syst Evol Microbiol 2003;53:1445–1448.

94. Hashimura T, Sato M, Hoshino E. Detection of *Slackia exigua*, *Mogibacterium timidum* and *Eubacterium saphenum* from pulpal and periradicular samples using the polymerase chain reaction (PCR) method. Int Endod J 2001;34:463–470.

95. Hatheway CL. Botulism. In: Balows A, Hausler WJ Jr, Ohashi M, et al., eds. Laboratory diagnosis of infectious diseases: principles and practice. Vol. 1 New York: Springer, 1988:111–133.

96. Hatheway CL. Toxigenic clostridia. Clin Microbiol Rev 1990;3:66–98.

97. Hatheway CL. Botulism: the present status of the disease. Curr Top Microbiol Immunol 1995;195:55–75.

98. Hecht DW. Prevalence of antibiotic resistance in anaerobic bacteria: worrisome developments. Clin Infect Dis 2004;39:92–97.

99. Henry S, DeMaria A Jr, McCabe WR. Bacteremia due to *Fusobacterium* species. Am J Med 1983;75:225–231.

100. Hentges DJ. The anaerobic microflora of the human body. Clin Infect Dis 16: Suppl 1993;4:S175–S180.

101. Hentges DJ, Maier BR. Theoretical basis for anaerobic methodology. Am J Clin Nutr 1972;25:1299–1305.

102. Hill DA, Seaton RA, Cameron FM, et al. Severe sepsis caused by *Mobiluncus curtisii* subsp. *curtisii* in a previously healthy female: case report and review. J Infect 1998;37:194–196.

103. Hill GB. The microbiology of bacterial vaginosis. Am J Obstet Gynecol 1993;169:450–454.

104. Hillier SL. Diagnostic microbiology of bacterial vaginosis. Am J Obstet Gynecol 1993;169:455–459.

105. Hirasawa M, Takada K. *Porphyromonas gingivicanis* sp. nov. and *Porphyromonas crevioricanis* sp. nov., isolated from beagles. Int J Syst Bacteriol 1994;44:637–640.

106. Holdeman LV, Cato EP, Moore WE. Taxonomy of anaerobes: present state of the art. Rev Infect Dis 1984;6:Suppl 1:S3–S10.

107. Holdeman LV, Cato EP, Moore WEC. Anaerobe laboratory manual. Blacksburg, VA: Virginia Polytechnic Institute and State University, 1977.

108. Holdeman LV, Johnson JL. *Bacteroides disiens* sp. nov. and *Bacteroides bivius* sp. nov. from human clinical infections. Int J Syst Bacteriol 1977;27:337–345.

109. Holdeman LV, Kelley RW, Moore WEC. Anaerobic gram-negative straight, curved, and helical rods. Family 1. *Bacteroidaceae* Pribram 1933, 10^{AL}. In: Krieg NR, Holt JG, eds. Bergey's Manual of Systematic Bacteriology. Baltimore: Williams & Wilkins, 1984:602–662.

110. Holdeman LV, Kelley RW, Moore WEC. *Bacteroidaceae*. In: Krieg NR, Holt JG, eds. Bergey's Manual of Systemica Bacteriology. Baltimore: Williams and Wilkins, 1984:602–662.

111. Holdeman LV, Moore WEC. New genus *Coprococcus*: Twelve new species and emended descriptions of four previously described species of bacteria from human species. Int J Syst Bacteriol 1974;24:260–277.

112. Holdeman LV, Moore WEC. Anaerobe laboratory manual. Ed. 4 (Supplement). Blacksburg, VA: Virginia Polytechnic Institute and State University, 1987.

113. Holdeman LV, Moore WEC, Churn PJ, et al. *Bacteroides oris* and *Bacteroides buccae*: new species from human periodontitis and other human infections. Int J Syst Bacteriol 1982;32:125–131.

114. Hoyles L, Inganas E, Falsen E, et al. *Bifidobacterium scardovii* sp. nov., from human sources. Int J Syst Evol Microbiol 2002;52:995–999.

115. Jian W, Dong X. Transfer of *Bifidobacterium inopinatum* and *Bifidobacterium denticolens* to *Scardovia inopinata* gen. nov., comb. nov., and *Parascardovia denticolens* gen. nov., comb. nov., respectively. Int J Syst Evol Microbiol 2002; 52:809–812.

116. Johnson CC, Reinhardt JF, Edelstein MA, et al. *Bacteroides gracilis*, an important anaerobic bacterial pathogen. J Clin Microbiol 1985;22:799–802.

117. Johnson JL, Moore LV, Kaneko B, et al. *Actinomyces georgiae* sp. nov., *Actinomyces gerencseriae* sp. nov., designation of two genospecies of *Actinomyces naeslundii*, and inclusion of *A. naeslundii* serotypes II and III and *Actinomyces viscosus* serotype II in *A. naeslundii* genospecies 2. Int J Syst Bacteriol 1990; 40:273–286.

118. Johnson JL, Moore WEC, Moore LVH. *Bacteroides caccae* sp. nov., *Bacteroides merdae* sp. nov., and *Bacteroides stercoris* sp. nov. isolated from human feces. Int J Syst Bacteriol 1986;36:499–501.

119. Johnson LL, McFarland LV, Dearing P, et al. Identification of *Clostridium difficile* in stool specimens by culture-enhanced gas-liquid chromatography. J Clin Microbiol 1989;27:2218–2221.

120. Johnson S, Kent SA, O'Leary KJ, et al. Fatal pseudomembranous colitis associated with a variant *Clostridium difficile* strain not detected by toxin A immunoassay. Ann Intern Med 2001;135:434–438.

121. Jousimies-Somer H, Summanen P. Microbiology terminology update: clinically significant anaerobic gram-positive and gram-negative bacteria (excluding spirochetes). Clin Infect Dis 1997;25:11–14.

122. Jousimies-Somer H, Summanen P. Microbiology terminology update: clinically significant anaerobic gram-positive and gram-negative bacteria (excluding spirochetes). Clin Infect Dis 1999;29:724–727.

123. Jousimies-Somer H, Summanen P. Recent taxonomic changes and terminology update of clinically significant anaerobic gram-negative bacteria (excluding spirochetes). Clin Infect Dis 2002;35:S17–S21.

124. Jousimies-Somer H, Summanen PH, Wexler H, et al. *Bacteroides, Porphyromonas, Prevotella, Fusobacterium*, and other anaerobic gram-negative bacteria. In: Murray PR, Baron EJ, Pfaller MA et al., eds. Manual of Clinical Microbiology. Washington, ASM Press, 2003:880–901.

125. Jousimies-Somer HR, Summanen P, Citron DM, et al. Wadsworth-KTL anaerobic Bacteriology Manual. Ed. 6. Belmont, CA: Star, 2002.

126. Jumas-Bilak E, Carlier JP, Jean-Pierre H, et al. *Veillonella montpellierensis* sp. nov., a novel, anaerobic, gram-negative coccus isolated from human clinical samples. Int J Syst Evol Microbiol 2004;54:1311–1316.

127. Kageyama A, Benno Y, Nakase T. Phylogenetic and phenotypic evidence for the transfer of *Eubacterium aerofaciens* to the genus *Collinsella* as *Collinsella aerofaciens* gen. nov., comb. nov. Int J Syst Bacteriol 1999;49:Pt 2:557–565.

128. Kalfas S, Figdor D, Sundqvist G. A new bacterial species associated with failed endodontic treatment: identification and description of *Actinomyces radicidentis*. Oral Surg Oral Med Oral Pathol Oral Radiol Endod 2001;92:208–214.

129. Kelly MT, Fojtasek MF, Abbott TM, et al. Clinical evaluation of a lysis-centrifugation technique for the detection of septicemia. JAMA 1983;250:2185–2188.

130. Killgore GE, Starr SE, Del Bene VE, et al. Comparison of three anaerobic systems for the isolation of anaerobic bacteria from clinical specimens. Am J Clin Pathol 1973;59:552–559.

131. Kilpper-Balz R, Schleifer KH. Transfer of *Peptococcus saccharolyticus* Foubert and Douglas to the genus *Staphylococcus*: *Staphylococcus saccharolyticus* (Foubert and Douglas) comb. nov. Zentralbl Baketeriol Parasitenkd Infektionskr Hyg 1981;2:324–331.

132. Kilpper-Balz R, Schleifer KH. Transfer of *Streptococcus morbillorum* to the genus *Gemella* as *Gemella morbillorum* comb. nov. Int J Syst Bacteriol 1988; 38:442–443.

133. Kirby BD, George WL, Sutter VL, et al. Gram-negative anaerobic bacilli: their role in infection and patterns of susceptibility to antimicrobial agents. I. Little-known *Bacteroides* species. Rev Infect Dis 1980;2:914–951.

134. Koneman EW, Allen SD, Janda WM, et al. Color Atlas and Textbook of Diagnostic Microbiology. Ed. 4. Philadelphia: Lippincott, 1992.

135. Koneman EW, Allen SD, Janda WM, et al. Color Atlas and Textbook of Diagnostic Microbiology. Ed. 5. Philadelphia: Lippincott-Raven, 1997.

136. Kononen E, Eerola E, Frandsen EV, et al. Phylogenetic characterization and proposal of a new pigmented species to the genus *Prevotella*: *Prevotella pallens* sp. nov. Int J Syst Bacteriol 1998;48:Pt 1:47–51.

137. Koontz FP, Flint KK, Reynolds JK, et al. Multicenter comparison of the high volume (10 ml) NR BACTEC PLUS system and the standard (5 ml) NR BACTEC system. Diagn Microbiol Infect Dis 1991;14:111–118.

138. Koransky JR, Allen SD, Dowell VR Jr. Use of ethanol for selective isolation of spore-forming microorganisms. Appl Environ Microbiol 1978;35:762–765.

139. Koransky JR, Stargel MD, Dowell VR Jr. *Clostridium septicum* bacteremia: its clinical significance. Am J Med 1979;66:63–66.

140. Kornowski R, Schwartz D, Averbuch M, et al. Anaerobic bacteremia: a retrospective four-year analysis in general medicine and cancer patients. Infection 1993;21:241–244.

141. In: Krieg NR, Holt JG, eds. Bergey's Manual of Systematic Bacteriology. Vol. 1. Baltimore: Williams & Wilkins, 1984.

142. Kronvall G, Myhre E. Differential staining of bacteria in clinical specimens using acridine orange buffered at low pH. Acta Pathol Microbiol Scand B Microbiol 1977;85:249–254.

143. Landsaat PM, van der Lelie H, Bongaerts G, et al. *Fusobacterium nucleatum*, a new invasive pathogen in neutropenic patients? Scand J Infect Dis 1995;27: 83–84.

144. Lark RL, McNeil SA, VanderHyde K, et al. Risk factors for anaerobic bloodstream infections in bone marrow transplant recipients. Clin Infect Dis 2001; 33:338–343.

145. Lawson PA, Falsen E, Akervall E, et al. Characterization of some *Actinomyces*-like isolates from human clinical specimens. reclassification of *Actinomyces suis* (Soltys and Spratling) as *Actinobaculum suis* comb. nov. and description of *Actinobaculum schaalii* sp. nov. Int J Syst Bacteriol 1997;47:899–903.

146. Lawson PA, Nikolaitchouk N, Falsen E, et al. *Actinomyces funkei* sp. nov., isolated from human clinical specimens. Int J Syst Evol Microbiol 2001;51: 853–855.

147. Lee K, Baron EJ, Summanen P, et al. Selective medium for isolation of *Bacteroides gracilis*. J Clin Microbiol 1990;28:1747–1750.

148. Lemee L, Dhalluin A, Testelin S, et al. Multiplex PCR targeting tpi (triose phosphate isomerase), tcdA (Toxin A), and tcdB (Toxin B) genes for toxigenic culture of *Clostridium difficile*. J Clin Microbiol 2004;42:5710–5714.

149. Limaye AP, Turgeon DK, Cookson BT, et al. Pseudomembranous colitis caused by a toxin A(-) B(+) strain of *Clostridium difficile*. J Clin Microbiol 2000;38: 1696–1697.

150. Liu JW, Wu JJ, Wang LR, et al. Two fatal cases of *Veillonella* bacteremia. Eur J Clin Microbiol Infect Dis 1998;17:62–64.

151. Loesche WJ. Oxygen sensitivity of various anaerobic bacteria. Appl Microbiol 1969;18:723–727.

152. Lombard GL, Dowell VR Jr. Gas liquid chromatography: analysis of acid products of bacteria. Atlanta: Centers for Disease Control, 1982.

153. Lombardi DP, Engleberg NC. Anaerobic bacteremia: incidence, patient characteristics, and clinical significance. Am J Med 1992;92:53–60.

154. Lorber B. Gas gangrene and other clostridium-associated diseases. In: Mandell GL, Bennett JE, Dolin R, eds. Mandell, Douglas and Bennett's Principles and Practice of Infectious Diseases. Vol. 2. Ed. 5. Philadelphia: Churchill Livingstone, 2000:2549–2561.

155. Lorber B. *Bacteroides, Prevotella, Porphyromonas*, and *Fusobacterium* species (and other medically important anaerobic gram-negative bacilli). In: Mandell GL, Bennett JE, Dolin R, eds. Mandell, Douglas, and Bennett's Principles and Practice of Infectious Diseases. Vol. 2. Ed. 6. Philadelphia: Elsevier, Churchill Livingstone2005:2838–2846.

156. Love DN. *Porphyromonas macacae* comb. nov., a consequence of *Bacteroides macacae* being a senior synonym of *Porphyromonas salivosa*. Int J Syst Bacteriol 1995;45:90–92.

157. Love DN, Bailey GD, Collings S, et al. Description of *Porphyromonas circumdentaria* sp. nov. and reassignment of *Bacteroides salivosus* (Love, Johnson, Jones, and Calverley 1987) as *Porphyromonas* (Shah and Collins 1988) salivosa comb. nov [published errata appear in Int J Syst Bacteriol 1992;42(4):660 and 1993; 43(3):630]. Int J Syst Bacteriol 1992;42:434–438.

158. Love DN, Johnson JL, Jones RF, et al. *Bacteroides salivosus* sp. nov., an asaccharolytic, black-pigmented species from cats. Int J Syst Bacteriol 1987;37: 307–309.

159. Love DN, Karjalainen J, Kanervo A, et al. *Porphyromonas canoris* sp. nov., an asaccharolytic, black-pigmented species from the gingival sulcus of dogs. Int J Syst Bacteriol 1994;44:204–208.

160. Lyerly DM. *Clostridium difficile* testing. Clin Microbiol Newslett 1995;17:17.

161. Lyerly DM, Allen SD. The Clostridia. In: Emmerson AM, Hawkey P, Gillespie

S, eds. Principles and Practice of Clinical Bacteriology. New York: Wiley, 1997: 559–623.

162. Lyerly DM, Krivan HC, Wilkins TD. *Clostridium difficile*: its disease and toxins. Clin Microbiol Rev 1988;1:1–18.

163. Madigan M, Martinko J, Parker J. Brock Biology of Microorganisms. Ed. 8. Upper Saddle River, NJ: Prentice Hall, 1997.

164. Malnick H, Williams K, Phil-Ebosie J, et al. Description of a medium for isolating *Anaerobiospirillum* spp., a possible cause of zoonotic disease, from diarrheal feces and blood of humans and use of the medium in a survey of human, canine, and feline feces. J Clin Microbiol 1990;28:1380–1384.

165. Mann C, Dertinger S, Hartmann G, et al. *Actinomyces neuii* and neonatal sepsis. Infection 2002;30:178–180.

166. Marler LM, Siders JA, Allen SD. Direct Smear Atlas: A Monograph of Gram-Stained Preparations of Clinical Specimens. Philadelphia: Lippincott Williams & Wilkins, 2001.

167. Marler LM, Siders JA, Wolters LC, et al. Comparison of five cultural procedures for isolation of *Clostridium difficile* from stools. J Clin Microbiol 1992;30: 514–516.

168. Martin WJ. Practical method for isolation of anaerobic bacteria in the clinical laboratory. Appl Microbiol 1971;22.

169. Mascini EM, Verhoef J. Anaerobic cocci. In: Mandell GL, Bennett JE, Dolin R, eds. Mandell, Douglas, and Bennett's Principles and Practice of Infectious Diseases. Vol. 2. Philadelphia, Elsevier, Churchill, Livingstone, 2005: 2847–2849.

170. Mascini EM, Verhoef J. Anaerobic gram-positive nonsporulating bacilli. In: Mandell GL, Bennett JE, Dolin R, eds. Mandell, Douglas, and Bennett's Principles and Practice of Infectious Diseases. Vol. 2. Philadelphia: Elsevier, Churchill Livingstone2005:2849–2852.

171. Mays TD, Holdeman LV, Moore WEC. Taxonomy of the genus *Veillonella* Prevot. Int J Syst Bacteriol 1982;32:28–36.

172. McCord JM, Keele BB Jr, Fridovich I. An enzyme-based theory of obligate anaerobiosis: the physiological function of superoxide dismutase. Proc Natl Acad Sci USA 1971;68:1024–1027.

173. McFarland LV, Mulligan ME, Kwok RY, et al. Nosocomial acquisition of *Clostridium difficile* infection. N Engl J Med 1989;320:204–210.

174. Millar JS. Enteritis necroticans: a review. Trop Gastroenterol 1989;10:3–8.

175. Mimoz O, Karim A, Mercat A, et al. Chlorhexidine compared with povidone-iodine as skin preparation before blood culture: a randomized, controlled trial. Ann Intern Med 1999;131:834–837.

176. Monciardini P, Sosio M. Reclassification as a Nonomuraea sp. of the strain ATCC 39727, producing the glycopeptide antibiotic A40926. J Antibiot (Tokyo) 2004;57:68–70.

177. Moncla BJ, Hillier SL. *Peptostreptococcus, Propionibacterium, Lactobacillus, Actinomyces*, and other non–spore-forming anaerobic gram-positive bacteria. In: Murray PR, Baron EJ, Pfaller MA et al., eds. Manual of Clinical Microbiology. Vol. 1. Ed. 8. Washington, DC: ASM Press, 2003:857–879.

178. Moore LV, Johnson JL, Moore WE. Descriptions of *Prevotella tannerae* sp. nov. and *Prevotella enoeca* sp. nov. from the human gingival crevice and emendation of the description of *Prevotella zoogleoformans*. Int J Syst Bacteriol 1994; 44:599–602.

179. Moore LVH, Cato EP, Moore WEC. Anaerobe laboratory manual update: supplements to the VPI anaerobe laboratory manual. Ed. 4. Blacksburg, VA: Virginia Polytechnic Institute and State University, 1987.

180. Moore WEC. Chromatography for the clinical laboratory: all you wanted to know (and possibly more). API Species 1980;4:21–28.

181. Murdoch DA. Gram-positive anaerobic cocci. Clin Microbiol Rev 1998;11: 81–120.

182. Murdoch DA. Reclassification of *Peptostreptococcus magnus* (Prevot 1933) Holdeman and Moore 1972 as *Finegoldia magna* comb. nov. and *Peptostreptococcus micros* (Prevot 1933) Smith 1957 as *Micromonas micros* comb. nov. Anaerobe 1999;5:555–559.

183. Murdoch DA, Shah HN, Gharbia SE, et al. Proposal to restrict the genus *Peptostreptococcus* (Kluyver & van Niel 1936) to *Peptostreptococcus anaerobius*. Anaerobe 2000;6:257–260.

184. Murray PR, Traynor P, Hopson D. Critical assessment of blood culture techniques: analysis of recovery of obligate and facultative anaerobes, strict aerobic bacteria, and fungi in aerobic and anaerobic blood culture bottles. J Clin Microbiol 1992;30:1462–1468.

185. National Committee for Clinical Laboratory Standards. Methods for antimicrobial susceptibility testing of anaerobic bacteria; approved standard. Ed. 6. Villanova, PA: NCCLS, 2004.

186. Nguyen MH, Yu VL, Morris AJ, et al. Antimicrobial resistance and clinical outcome of *Bacteroides* bacteremia: findings of a multicenter prospective observational trial. Clin Infect Dis 2000;30:870–876.

187. Nikolaitchouk N, Hoyles L, Falsen E, et al. Characterization of *Actinomyces* isolates from samples from the human urogenital tract: description of *Actinomyces urogenitalis* sp. nov. Int J Syst Evol Microbiol 2000;50 Pt 4:1649–1654.

188. Oteo J, Aracil B, Alos JI, et al. High prevalence of resistance to clindamycin in *Bacteroides fragilis* group isolates. J Antimicrob Chemother 2000;45:691–693.

189. Peterson LR, Kelly PJ. The role of the clinical microbiology laboratory in the management of *Clostridium difficile*-associated diarrhea. Infect Dis Clin North Am 1993;7:277–293.

190. Peterson LR, Kelly PJ, Nordbrock HA. Role of culture and toxin detection in laboratory testing for diagnosis of *Clostridium difficile*-associated diarrhea. Eur J Clin Microbiol Infect Dis 1996;15:330–336.

191. Pienaar C, Kruger AJ, Venter EC, et al. *Anaerobiospirillum succiniciproducens* bacteraemia. J Clin Pathol 2003;56:316–318.

192. Prpic-Mehicic G, Marsan T, Miletic I, et al. Infective endocarditis caused by *Veillonella* of dental origin. Coll Antropol 1998;22:Suppl:39–43.

193. Pulverer G, Schutt-Gerowitt H, Schaal KP. Human cervicofacial actinomycoses: microbiological data for 1997 cases. Clin Infect Dis 2003;37:490–497.

194. Ramirez S, Hild TG, Rudolph CN, et al. Increased diagnosis of Lemierre syndrome and other *Fusobacterium necrophorum* infections at a Children's Hospital. Pediatrics 2003;112:e380.

195. Ramos CP, Falsen E, Alvarez N, et al. *Actinomyces graevenitzii* sp. nov., isolated from human clinical specimens. Int J Syst Bacteriol 1997;47:885–888.

196. Ramos CP, Foster G, Collins MD. Phylogenetic analysis of the genus *Actinomyces* based on 16S rRNA gene sequences: description of *Arcanobacterium phocae* sp. nov., *Arcanobacterium bernardiae* comb. nov., and *Arcanobacterium pyogenes* comb. nov. Int J Syst Bacteriol 1997;47:46–53.

197. Reller LB, Murray PR, MacLowry JD. Cumitech IA, Blood Cultures II. Washington, DC: American Society for Microbiology, 1982.

198. Riordan T, Wilson M. Lemierre's syndrome: more than a historical curiosa. Postgrad Med J 2004;80:328–334.

199. Rogosa M. Family I. *Veillonellaceae* Rogosa 1971. In: Krieg NR, Holt JG, eds. In: Krieg NR, Holt JG, eds. Bergey's Manual of Systematic Bacteriology. Vol. 1. Baltimore: Williams and Wilkins, 1984:680–685.

200. Rolfe RD, Hentges DJ, Campbell BJ, et al. Factors related to the oxygen tolerance of anaerobic bacteria. Appl Environ Microbiol 1978;36:306–313.

201. Rosenblatt JE, Fallon A, Finegold SM. Comparison of methods for isolation of anaerobic bacteria from clinical specimens. Appl Microbiol 1973;25:77–85.

202. Russo TA. Agents of actinomycosis. In: Mandell GL, Bennett JE, Dolin R, eds. Mandell, Douglas, and Bennett's Principles and Practice of Infectious Diseases. Vol. 2. Philadelphia, Churchill Livingstone, 2000:2645–2654.

203. Sabbe LJ, Van De Merwe D, Schouls L, et al. Clinical spectrum of infections due to the newly described *Actinomyces* species *A. turicensis, A. radingae*, and *A. europaeus*. J Clin Microbiol 1999;37:8–13.

204. Sakamoto M, Suzuki M, Huang Y, et al. *Prevotella shahii* sp. nov. and *Prevotella salivae* sp. nov., isolated from the human oral cavity. Int J Syst Evol Microbiol 2004;54:877–883.

205. Sarkonen N, Kononen E, Summanen P, et al. Phenotypic identification of *Actinomyces* and related species isolated from human sources. J Clin Microbiol 2001; 39:3955–3961.

206. Schaal KP. Actinomycosis, actinobacillosis and related diseases. In: Hausler WJJ, ed. Bacterial Infections. Vol. 3. Ed. 9. London: Arnold, 1998:777–798.

207. Schifman RB, Strand CL, Meier FA, et al. Blood culture contamination: a College of American Pathologists Q-Probes study involving 640 institutions and 497134 specimens from adult patients. Arch Pathol Lab Med 1998;122:216–221.

208. Seip WF, Evans GL. Atmospheric analysis and redox potentials of culture media in the GasPak System. J Clin Microbiol 1980;11:226–233.

209. Shah HN, Collins DM. Proposal for re-classification of *Bacteroides asaccharolyticus, Bacteroides gingivalis*, and *Bacteroides endodontalis* in a new genus, *Porphyromonas*. Int J System Bacteriol 1988;38:128–131.

210. Shah HN, Collins DM. Proposal to restrict the genus *Bacteroides*(Castellani and Chalmers) to *Bacteroides fragilis* and closely related species. Int J Syst Bacteriol 1989;39:85–87.

211. Shah HN, Collins DM. *Prevotella*, a new genus to include *Bacteroides melaninogenicus* and related species formerly classified in the genus *Bacteroides*. Int J Syst Bacteriol 1990;40:205–208.

212. Shah HN, Collins MD, Olsen I, et al. Reclassification of *Bacteroides levii* (Holdeman, Cato, and Moore) in the genus *Porphyromonas*, as *Porphyromonas levii* comb. nov. Int J Syst Bacteriol 1995;45:586–588.

213. Shah HN, Gharbia SE. Biochemical and chemical studies on strains designated *Prevotella intermedia* and proposal of a new pigmented species, *Prevotella nigrescens* sp. nov. Int J Syst Bacteriol 1992;42:542–546.

214. Shah HN, Gharbia SE. Proposal of a new species Prevotella nigrescens sp. nov. among strains previously classified as Pr. intermedia. FEMS Immunol Med Microbiol 1993;6:97.

215. Shahin M, Jamal W, Verghese T, et al. Comparative evaluation of anoxomat and conventional anaerobic GasPak jar systems for the isolation of anaerobic bacteria. Med Princ Pract 2003;12:81–86.

216. Shinjo T, Hiraiwa K, Miyazato S. Recognition of biovar C of *Fusobacterium necrophorum* (Flugge) Moore and Holdeman as *Fusobacterium pseudonecrophorum* sp. nov., nom. rev. (ex Prevot 1940). Int J Syst Bacteriol 1990;40:71–73.

217. Siders JA. Gas-liquid chromatography. In: Isenberg HD, ed. Clinical Microbiol-

ogy Procedures Handbook. Washington, DC, American Society for Clinical Microbiology, 1992:2–6.

218. Siqueira JF Jr, Rocas IN. Detection of *Filifactor alocis* in endodontic infections associated with different forms of periradicular diseases. Oral Microbiol Immunol 2003;18:263–265.

219. Siqueira JF Jr, Rocas IN. Polymerase chain reaction detection of *Propionibacterium propionicus* and *Actinomyces radicidentis* in primary and persistent endodontic infections. Oral Surg Oral Med Oral Pathol Oral Radiol Endodont 2003; 96:215–222.

220. Smith HJ, Moore HB. Isolation of *Mobiluncus* species from clinical specimens by using cold enrichment and selective media. J Clin Microbiol 1988;26: 1134–1137.

221. Smith LDS. Botulism: the Organism, Its Toxins, The Disease. Springfield, IL: Charles C Thomas, 1977.

222. Smith LDS, Williams BL. The pathogenic anaerobic bacteria. Ed. 3. Springfield, IL: Charles C Thomas, 1984.

223. Sneath PHA, Mair NS, Sharpe ME, et al. Bergey's Manual of Systematic Bacteriology. Vol. 2. Baltimore: Williams & Wilkins, 1986.

224. Snydman DR, Jacobus NV, McDermott LA, et al. National survey on the susceptibility of *Bacteroides fragilis* Group: report and analysis of trends for 1997–2000. Clin Infect Dis 2002;35:S126–S134.

225. Sobel JD. Bacterial vaginosis. Annu Rev Med 2000;51:349–356.

226. Song Y, Liu C, McTeague M, et al. 16S ribosomal DNA sequence-based analysis of clinically significant gram-positive anaerobic cocci. J Clin Microbiol 2003; 41:1363–1369.

227. Song Y, Liu C, Molitoris D, et al. Use of 16S-23S rRNA spacer-region (SR)-PCR for identification of intestinal clostridia. Syst Appl Microbiol 2002;25: 528–535.

228. Song Y, Liu C, Molitoris DR, et al. *Clostridium bolteae* sp. nov., isolated from human sources. Syst Appl Microbiol 2003;26:84–89.

229. Song YL, Liu CX, McTeague M, et al. *Clostridium bartlettii* sp. nov., isolated from human faeces. Anaerobe 2004;10:179–184.

230. Spiegel CA. Bacterial vaginosis. Clin Microbiol Rev 1991;4:485–502.

231. Spiegel CA, Roberts M. *Mobiluncus* gen. nov., *Mobiluncus cutisii* subsp. *curtisii* sp. nov., and *Mobiluncus mulieris* sp. nov., curved rods from the human vagina. Int J Syst Bacteriol 1984;34:177–184.

232. Staneck JL, Weckbach LS, Allen SD, et al. Multicenter evaluation of four methods for *Clostridium difficile* detection: ImmunoCard *C. difficile*, cytotoxin assay, culture, and latex agglutination. J Clin Microbiol 1996;34:2718–2721.

233. Stargel MD, Lombard GL, Dowell VR Jr. Alternative procedures for identification of anaerobic bacteria. Am J Med Technol 1978;44:709–722.

234. Steer T, Collins MD, Gibson GR, et al. *Clostridium hathewayi* sp. nov., from human faeces. Syst Appl Microbiol 2001;24:353–357.

235. Tally FP, Goldin BR, Jacobus NV, et al. Superoxide dismutase in anaerobic bacteria of clinical significance. Infect Immun 1977;16:20–25.

236. Taras D, Simmering R, Collins MD, et al. Reclassification of *Eubacterium formicigenerans* Holdeman and Moore 1974 as *Dorea formicigenerans* gen. nov., comb. nov., and description of *Dorea longicatena* sp. nov., isolated from human faeces. Int J Syst Evol Microbiol 2002;52:423–428.

237. Thatcher P. Hepatic abscesses caused by *Fusobacterium necrophorum* as part of the Lemierre syndrome. J Clin Gastroenterol 2003;37:196–197.

238. Tiveljung A, Forsum U, Monstein HJ. Classification of the genus *Mobiluncus* based on comparative partial 16S rRNA gene analysis. Int J Syst Bacteriol 1996; 46:332–336.

239. Turgeon DK, Novicki TJ, Quick J, et al. Six rapid tests for direct detection of *Clostridium difficile* and its toxins in fecal samples compared with the fibroblast cytotoxicity assay. J Clin Microbiol 2003;41:667–670.

240. Tzianabos AO, Kasper DL. Anaerobic infections: general concepts. In: Mandell GL, Bennett JE, Dolin R, eds. Mandell, Douglas, and Bennett's Principles and Practice of Infectious Diseases. Vol. 2. Philadelphia: Elsevier Churchill Livingstone, 2005:2810–2816.

241. Van Kessel LJ, Verbrugh HA, Stringer MF, et al. Necrotizing enteritis associated with toxigenic type A *Clostridium perfringens*. J Infect Dis 1985;151:974–975.

242. van Winkelhoff AJ, Clement M, de Graaff J. Rapid characterization of oral and nonoral pigmented *Bacteroides* species with the ATB Anaerobes ID system. J Clin Microbiol 1988;26:1063–1065.

243. van Winkelhoff AJ, van Steenbergen TJ, Kippuw N, et al. Further characteriza-

tion of *Bacteroides endodontalis*, an asaccharolytic black-pigmented *Bacteroides* species from the oral S cavity. J Clin Microbiol 1985;22:75–79.

244. van Winkelhoff AJ, van Steenbergen TJ, Kippuw N, et al. Enzymatic characterization of oral and non-oral black-pigmented *Bacteroides* species. Antonie van Leeuwenhoek 1986;52:163–171.

245. Vandamme P, Daneshvar MI, Dewhirst FE, et al. Chemotaxonomic analyses of *Bacteroides gracilis* and *Bacteroides ureolyticus* and reclassification of *B. gracilis* as *Campylobacter gracilis* comb. nov. Int J Syst Bacteriol 1995;45:145–152.

246. Vandamme P, Falsen E, Vancanneyt M, et al. Characterization of *Actinomyces turicensis* and *Actinomyces radingae* strains from human clinical samples. Int J Syst Bacteriol 1998;48 Pt 2:503–510.

247. Wade WG, Downes J, Dymock D, et al. The family *Coriobacteriaceae*: reclassification of *Eubacterium exiguum* (Poco et al. 1996) and *Peptostreptococcus heliotrinreducens* (Lanigan 1976) as *Slackia exigua* gen. nov., comb. nov. and *Slackia heliotrinireducens* gen. nov., comb. nov., and *Eubacterium lentum* (Prevot 1938) as *Eggerthella lenta* gen. nov., comb. nov. Int J Syst Bacteriol 1999; 49 Pt 2:595–600.

248. Walden WC, Hentges DJ. Differential effects of oxygen and oxidation-reduction potential on the multiplication of three species of anaerobic intestinal bacteria. Appl Microbiol 1975;30:781–785.

249. Walker PD. Pig-Bel. In: Borriello SP, ed. Clostridia in Gastrointestinal Disease. Boca Raton, CRC Press, 1985:94–115.

250. Washington JA. Evolving concepts on the laboratory diagnosis of septicemia. Infect Dis Clin Pract 1993;2:65.

251. Washington JA. Collection, transport, and processing of blood cultures. Clin Lab Med 1994;14:59–68.

252. Washington JA II, Ilstrup DM. Blood cultures: issues and controversies. Rev Infect Dis 1986;8:792–802.

253. Watson DA, Andrew JH, Banting S, et al. Pig-bel but no pig: enteritis necroticans acquired in Australia. Med J Aust 1991;155:47–50.

254. Weinstein MP, Reller LB, Mirrett S, et al. Controlled evaluation of Trypticase soy broth in agar slide and conventional blood culture systems. J Clin Microbiol 1985;21:626–629.

255. Weinstein MP, Reller LB, Murphy JR, et al. The clinical significance of positive blood cultures: a comprehensive analysis of 500 episodes of bacteremia and fungemia in adults. I. Laboratory and epidemiologic observations. Rev Infect Dis 1983;5:35–53.

256. Westh H, Christensen JJ, Blom J, et al. Fatal septicaemia with *Selenomonas sputigena* and *Acinetobacter calcoaceticus*: a case report. APMIS 1991;99: 75–77.

257. Wexler HM. Susceptibility testing of anaerobic bacteria: the state of the art. Clin Infect Dis 1993;16:S328–333.

258. Whaley DN, Gorman GW. An inexpensive device for evacuating and gassing anaerobic systems with in-house vacuum. J Clin Microbiol 1977;5:668–669.

259. Whaley DN, Wiggs LS, Miller PH, et al. Use of Presumpto Plates to identify anaerobic bacteria. J Clin Microbiol 1995;33:1196–1202.

260. Wilcox MH, Fawley WN. Virulence of *Clostridium difficile* toxin A negative strains. J Hosp Infect 2001;48:81.

261. Willems A, Collins MD. 16S rRNA gene similarities indicate that *Hallella seregens* (Moore and Moore) and *Mitsuokella dentalis* (Haapsalo et al.) are genealogically highly related and are members of the genus *Prevotella*: emended description of the genus *Prevotella* (Shah and Collins) and description of *Prevotella dentalis* comb. nov. Int J Syst Bacteriol 1995;45:832–836.

262. Willems A, Collins MD. Reclassification of *Oribaculum catoniae* (Moore and Moore 1994) as *Porphyromonas catoniae* comb. nov. and emendation of the genus *Porphyromonas*. Int J Syst Bacteriol 1995;45:578–581.

263. Willems A, Collins MD. Phylogenetic relationships of the genera *Acetobacterium* and *Eubacterium* sensu stricto and reclassification of *Eubacterium alactolyticum* as *Pseudoramibacter alactolyticus* gen. nov., comb. nov. Int J Syst Bacteriol 1996;46:1083–1087.

264. Wilson ML, Harrell LJ, Mirrett S, et al. Controlled evaluation of BACTEC PLUS 27 and Roche Septi-Chek anaerobic blood culture bottles. J Clin Microbiol 1992;30:63–66.

265. Woo PC, Fung AM, Lau SK, et al. *Actinomyces hongkongensis* sp. nov. a novel *Actinomyces* species isolated from a patient with pelvic actinomycosis. Syst Appl Microbiol 2003;26:518–522.

266. Wust J, Stubbs S, Weiss N, et al. Assignment of *Actinomyces pyogenes*-like (CDC coryneform group E) bacteria to the genus *Actinomyces* as *Actinomyces radingae* sp. nov. and *Actinomyces turicensis* sp. nov. Lett Appl Microbiol 1995; 20:76–81.

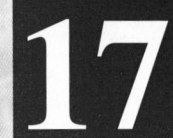
Antimicrobial Susceptibility Testing

Historical Introduction

Bacterial Resistance to Antimicrobial Agents

Mechanistic Variables

Mechanisms of Resistance

    Transport of Antimicrobial Agents Across the Cell Wall and Cell Membranes

    Antibiotics That Interfere With Formation of Bacterial Cell Walls: The β-Lactam and Glycopeptide Antibiotics

    Antimicrobial Agents That Do Not Exert Their Effect on Cell Walls

    Interactions Among Resistance Mechanisms

Laboratory Guidance of Antimicrobial Therapy

Tests for Determining Inhibitory Activity of Antimicrobial Agents

    Indications

    Choice of Test

    Selection of Antimicrobial Agents

    Standardization

        Growth Medium

        pH

        Serum

        Cation Concentration

        Atmosphere

        Temperature

        Inoculum

        Antimicrobial Agents

        Quality Control

Quality Assurance

Interpretation of Results

Selection of Antimicrobial Agents To Be Reported

Macrodilution Broth Susceptibility Test

Agar Dilution Susceptibility Test

Disk Diffusion Susceptibility Test

    Development of a Standardized Disk Diffusion Procedure

    Interpretation of Results

    Quality Control

    Limitations

Microbroth Dilution Susceptibility Test

Commercial Systems

    Vitek and MicroScan

    Epsilometer Test

Special Issues in Susceptibility Testing

    β-Lactamases

        Staphylococcus Species

        Haemophilus Species

        Neisseria gonorrhoeae

        Moraxella (*Branhamella*) *catarrhalis*

Enterococcus Species
Extended-Spectrum β-Lactamases

Staphylococcus Species

β-Lactam Antibiotics (Oxacillin-Resistant
   Staphylococcus Species)
Vancomycin
Macrolides, Lincosamides, and Streptogramins
Fluoroquinolones

Haemophilus Species

Penicillin Antibiotics
Chloramphenicol
Cephalosporins
Trimethoprim-Sulfamethoxazole

Streptococcus pneumoniae

Penicillin and Other β-Lactam Antibiotics
Multiple Resistance
Macrolides and Lincosamides

Neisseria gonorrhoeae

Neisseria meningitidis
Enterococcus Species

Aminoglycoside Antibiotics
β-Lactam Antibiotics
Vancomycin

Listeria monocytogenes
Streptococcus pyogenes (Group A β-Hemolytic *Streptococcus*)

Penicillin
Erythromycin
Fluoroquinolones

Streptococcus agalactiae (Group B β-Hemolytic *Streptococcus*)
Viridans Streptococci
Other Gram-Positive Bacteria
Pseudomonas aeruginosa, Burkholderia cepacia, and *Stenotrophomonas maltophilia* in Patients With Cystic Fibrosis
Direct Susceptibility Testing

Historical Introduction

The primary role of clinical microbiology laboratory personnel is to provide information with which physicians can diagnose and treat infectious diseases. If a communicable disease is present, the identification of a specific pathogen is of utmost importance to a hospital epidemiologist or public healthcare worker. Identification of a microbe that has been recovered from a clinical specimen often benefits the patient by definitively identifying a puzzling disease and assisting in the provisional selection of chemotherapy. However, the two most important pieces of information for a clinician are 1) whether an infectious agent is present and 2) which antimicrobial agent should provide adequate therapy.

These priorities were dependent on one of the great medical advances of the 20th century—the discovery of penicillin.[88] In 1928, Alexander Fleming observed that a contaminant mold was growing in a culture dish that had been carelessly left open to the air. In addition, bacterial colonies growing adjacent to the mold were undergoing lysis (Fig. 17-1). Fleming correctly concluded that the mold, later identified as a strain of *Penicillium notatum*, was producing a diffusible bacteriolytic substance capable of killing bacteria. Fleming's unknown antibiotic, which was later named penicillin, heralded the advent of the modern antibiotic era. The practical application of Fleming's discovery did not begin until 1939, when Florey and Chain developed a practical technique by which the antimicrobial extract of *Penicillium* could be obtained in sufficient purity and quantity for use in humans.

The need for antimicrobial susceptibility testing became evident soon after antibiotics became commercially available. Before World War II, penicillin production was limited and extremely expensive. During World War II, additional antibiotics were discovered and patterns of susceptibility against various organisms were established. Through his long-time interest in soil microbes Waksman discovered streptomycin in 1943, and Dubos discovered gramicidin and tyrocidin soon thereafter. Duggar's research resulted in the discovery of chlortetracycline (aureomycin) by Lederle Laboratories (Pearl River, NY) in 1944. Although these new antibiotics were truly "wonder drugs" at the time of their introduction, it was not long before resistant bacterial strains emerged. Susceptibility testing became a practical necessity.

Initial optimism that antimicrobial agents would put an end to bacterial infection has given way to reluctant acceptance that chemotherapeutic resources must be managed wisely to control disease.[221] A few bacteria, such as *Streptococcus pyogenes* (group A β-hemolytic streptococci), have maintained their predictable susceptibility to penicillin. This persistent susceptibility is, unfortunately, the exception rather than the rule. Bacteria have been so inventive that strains have been isolated that require the presence of a therapeutic antibiotic for growth![92,166] The ingenuity of the chemists in the pharmaceutical industry has also been great and

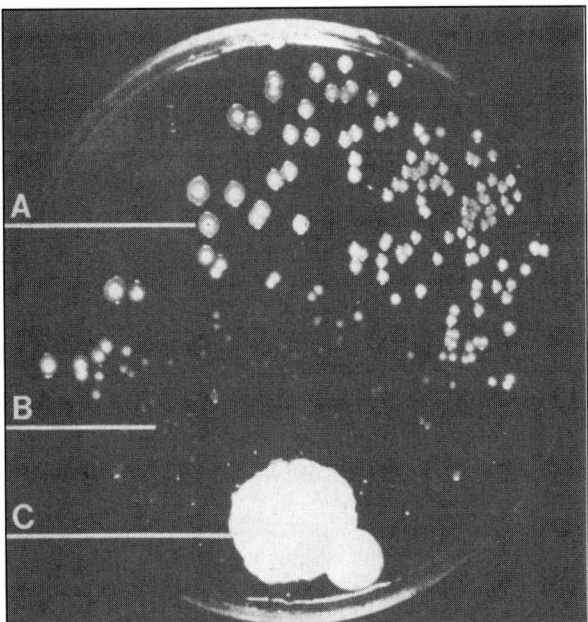

Figure 17-1 Reconstruction of Fleming's discovery of the antibiotic action of *Penicillium*. In Fleming's laboratory, colonies of *Bacillus* (*Haemophilus*) *influenzae* were inhibited by the "contaminating" mold. In this reconstruction, colonies of *Staphylococcus* are seen growing at *A;* a contaminating colony of *Penicillium* is growing at *C.* The *Staphylococcus* colonies around the fungus colony in area *B* are poorly developed and are undergoing lysis caused by an antibiotic substance produced by the mold. This unknown substance was later called penicillin.

is reflected in the large number of antimicrobial agents available to physicians (Table 17-1).

Bacterial Resistance to Antimicrobial Agents

The mechanisms of bacterial resistance are complex, varied, and not completely understood. Interested readers should consult an excellent discussion in Mandell's *Principles and Practice of Infectious Diseases*[235] and several comprehensive reviews of the major resistance mechanisms found in the most important human pathogens.[89,104,248] The tools of molecular biology have added greatly to our understanding of resistance mechanisms. For the clinical microbiologist the result can sometimes be intimidating: unfriendly terminology and extremely complex ideas. It is worth taking the time to understand at least the basics, however, because of the beauty of the biologic systems and also because of the increased sophistication with which day-to-day clinical decisions can be made. Individual mechanisms and organisms will be discussed in detail below.

Mechanistic Variables

To understand the mechanisms of bacterial resistance it is necessary to understand bacterial physiology, the pharmacology of antimicrobial drugs, and the molecular biology of infectious agents. Some of the important variables needed

to understand resistance mechanisms are listed in Table 17-2.

The genes for the resistance mechanism may be located either on the chromosome or on an extrachromosomal element called a plasmid. Plasmids are circularized pieces of DNA that act independently of the chromosome. The practical significance of the difference is that the chromosomal DNA is relatively stable, whereas the plasmid DNA is easily mobilized from one strain to another, one species to another, or even one genus to another. In addition, the linking of resistance genes for multiple antimicrobial agents on a plasmid allows the bulk transfer of resistance that characterizes many newly resistant organisms.[274]

The most common mechanism by which resistance genes are transferred is conjugation. An additional genetic transfer factor is necessary before a plasmid that carries a resistance gene can move from one organism to another. The most recently delineated transfer mechanism is the transposon (transposable genetic element).[283] Transposons can carry portions of plasmids. More importantly, they can also carry a piece of the chromosome from one bacterium to another by conjugal transfer (conjugative transposon or "jumping gene"). The result may be a mosaic of genetic material from the donor and recipient bacteria.[189] Transfer of antibiotic resistance across a major barrier between gram-positive and gram-negative bacteria has been documented.[51] It is impossible to overstate the importance of horizontal transfer of resistance to antimicrobial agents for the present and future infectious disease.

A resistance mechanism may be expressed continuously whether an inciting challenge is present or not. This state is referred to as constitutive expression. In contrast, some genes must be "induced" by exposure to the challenge substance before they produce the induced gene product. Staphylococcal β-lactamase (penicillinase) is an example of an inducible enzyme. It is present on a plasmid and is not produced unless the bacteria are exposed to a β-lactam antibiotic, such as penicillin, after which production of the enzyme is turned on. Many β-lactamases of gram-negative bacteria are present on the chromosome and are produced constitutively, but may be induced to produce even greater levels of the enzyme.

Some enzymes are secreted actively into the extracellular environment, where they can exert their antibacterial action. The β-lactamases of staphylococci are secreted. In contrast, most of the enzymes of gram-negative bacteria are cell-bound so that they exert their effects only if the antimicrobial agent enters the bacterial cell wall.

Finally, some resistance mechanisms are expressed homogeneously, while others are expressed heterogeneously. Homogeneous or uniform expression of a factor facilitates detection of the factor in the laboratory. If only a small fraction of the bacteria expresses the resistance mechanism (heterogeneous expression or heteroresistance), sampling error may compromise detection of the resistance in the laboratory.

A fascinating, but disturbing finding is the documentation that some antibiotics elicit a transient increase in the mutation rate of bacteria.[20] Thus, antibiotics may not only serve as selectors of antibiotic-resistant clones, but also as primary promoters of de novo resistance.

Table 17-1 **Classification of Antimicrobial Agents**

CLASS	GROUP	EXAMPLES
β-Lactams	Natural penicillins	Penicillin G, penicillin V
	Penicillinase-resistant penicillins (PRP)	Methicillin, nafcillin
	PRP: isoxazolyl penicillins	Cloxacillin, dicloxacillin, ofloxacin
	Aminopenicillins	Amoxicillin, ampicillin
	Carboxypenicillins	Carbenicillin, ticarcillin
	Ureidopenicillins	Azlocillin, mezlocillin, piperacillin
	First-generation cephalosporins	Cefazolin, cephalothin, cephapirin, cephradine
	Second-generation cephalosporins	Cefamandole, cefonicid, cefuroxime
	Cephamycins	Cefmetazole, cefotetan, cefoxitin
	Third-generation cephalosporins	Cefoperazone, cefotaxime, ceftazidime, ceftizoxime, ceftriaxone
	Fourth-generation cephalosporins	Cefipime
	Cephalosporins available for oral use	Cefaclor, cefadroxil, cefdinir, cefditoren, cefetamet, cefixime, cefpodoxime, cefprozil, ceftibuten, cefuroxime (axetil), cephalexin, cephradine
	Carbacephem	Loracarbef
	Monobactams	Aztreonam
	Carbapenems	Ertapenem, imipenem, meropenem
	β-Lactamase–β-lactamase- inhibitor combinations	Amoxicillin-clavulanic acid, ampicillin-sulbactam, piperacillin-tazobactam, ticarcillin-clavulanic acid
Aminocyclitols		Spectinomycin, trospectinomycin
Aminoglycosides		Amikacin, gentamicin, kanamycin, netilmicin, streptomycin, tobramycin
Ansamycins		Rifampin
Macrolides		Azithromycin, clarithromycin, dirithromycin, erythromycin
Lincosamides		Clindamycin
Glycopeptides	Glycopeptide	Vancomycin
	Lipopeptide	Teicoplanin
Quinolones	Quinolones	Cinoxacin, garenoxacin, nalidixic acid
	Fluoroquinolones	Ciprofloxacin, clinafloxacin, enoxacin, fleroxacin, gatifloxacin, gemifloxacin, grepafloxacin, levofloxacin, lomefloxacin, moxifloxacin, norfloxacin, ofloxacin, sparfloxacin, trovafloxacin
Oxazolidinones		Linezolid
Streptogramins		Quinupristin-dalfopristin
Folate pathway inhibitors		Sulfonamides, trimethoprim, trimethoprim-sulfamethoxazole
Fosfomycins		Fosfomycin
Ketolides		Telithromycin
Lipopeptides		Daptomycin
Nitrofurans		Nitrofurantoin
Nitroimidazoles		Metronidazole
Phenicols		Chloramphenicol
Tetracyclines		Doxycycline, minocycline, tetracycline

Adapted from Glossary I, MIC Testing, Supplementary Tables, NCCLS.[218]

Table 17-2 Variables in the Expression and Transfer of Bacterial Resistance

CHARACTERISTIC	VARIABLE	COMMENTS
Location	Chromosomal	Genetic stability; expression often constitutive
	Extrachromosomal	Plasmids easily mobilized for transfer from bacterial cell to cell
	Transposon	Can move genetic material between chromosome and plasmid or between bacterial cells
Transfer	Conjugation	Either plasmids (R-factor) or transposons
	Transduction	Transfer by bacteriophage
	Transformation	Direct transfer of DNA between compatible species
Expression	Constitutive	Produced with or without exposure to a stimulus
	Inducible	Produced only after exposure to a stimulus
	Constitutive-inducible	Produced at low level without stimulus; production greatly increased after stimulation

Mechanisms of Resistance

The mechanisms by which resistance is expressed in bacteria are summarized in Table 17-3 and Figure 17-2.

Transport of antimicrobial agents to their site of action in the bacterial cell will be considered first, because it is important for all compounds and all bacteria. Other mechanisms of resistance will be considered separately for antimicrobial agents that are active against cell walls (the β-lactam antibiotics, the single most important group of antimicrobial agents, and the glycopeptides) and for antimicrobial agents that work by other mechanisms. It should be emphasized at the outset that virtually any resistance mechanism may be found in most bacteria and that multiple mechanisms are often found in a single organism (Table 17-4).

It is impossible to overestimate the importance of multiple, often complementary mechanisms of resistance in bacterial species. When a pharmaceutical representative boasts that the antimicrobial agent from his company should be used because of its effectiveness against prevalent resistant strains, be assured that it will only be a matter of time before the bacteria develop resistance to this product also.

TRANSPORT OF ANTIMICROBIAL AGENTS ACROSS THE CELL WALL AND CELL MEMBRANES

Accumulation of antimicrobial agents at their site of action in the bacterial cell is the sum of transport into the cell, inactivation during the transport process, and clearance of antimicrobial agent from the cell. The process of forward movement across the membrane(s) will be considered first. To understand transport of molecules to the active site it is necessary to consider the structural differences between gram-positive and gram-negative bacteria. Bacteria are prokaryotic organisms, and both gram-positive and gram-negative species contain a mixture of nucleic acids, ribosomes, and other cellular machinery in their cytoplasm (Fig. 17-3). Gram-positive bacteria have a single cell membrane with a generous external layer of peptidoglycan (Fig. 17-3A and Fig. 17-4). For β-lactam and glycopeptide antibiotics, which probably do not have to traverse the plasma membrane to exert their antimicrobial

Table 17-3 Mechanisms of Bacterial Resistance to Antimicrobial Agents

MECHANISM	ANTIMICROBIAL AGENT GROUP	EXAMPLES
Enzymatic inactivation	β-Lactams	β-Lactamases: penicillinases; cephalosporinases; carbapenemases
	Aminoglycosides	Aminoglycoside-modifying enzymes of gram-negative and gram-positive bacteria
Altered receptors	β-Lactams	Altered penicillin-binding proteins of gram-negative and gram-positive bacteria
	Ribosomal alterations	Tetracycline; erythromycin; aminoglycosides
	DNA gyrase alterations	Quinolones
	Altered bacterial enzymes	Sulfamethoxazole; trimethoprim
Altered antibiotic transport	Alterations in outer membrane proteins (porins)	Gram-negative bacteria; decreased influx
	Reduced protein motive force	Aminoglycosides and gram-negative bacteria; decreased influx
	Active transport from bacterial cells	Tetracycline; erythromycin; active efflux

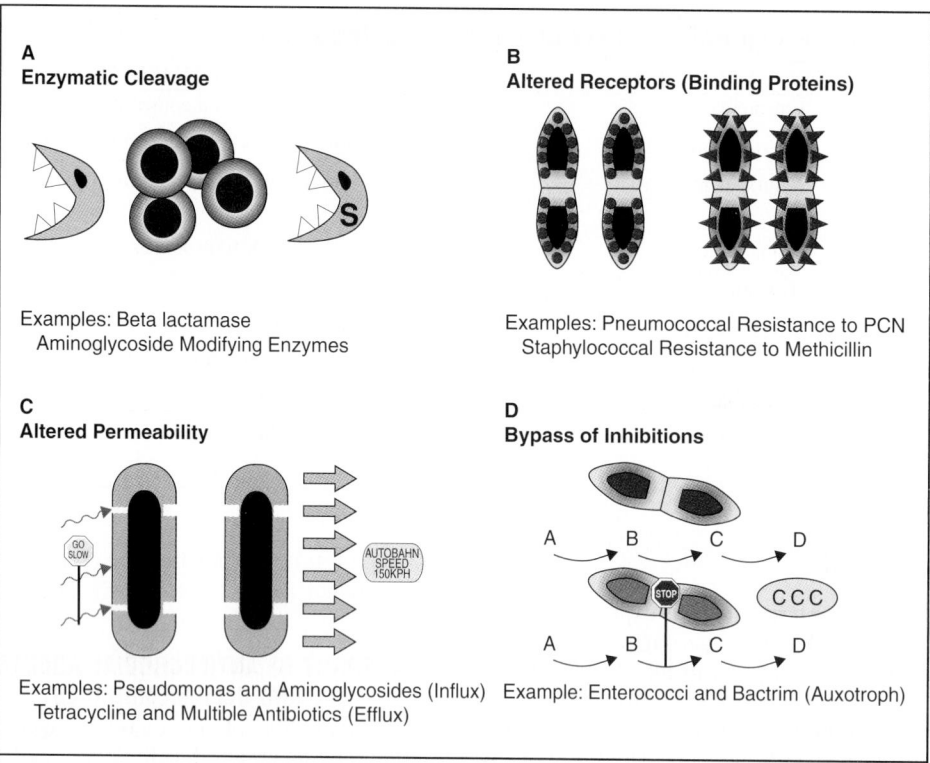

Figure 17-2 The four most important classes of antimicrobial resistance to antibiotics are illustrated. (**A**) Enzymatic inactivation of antimicrobial agents is represented by the voracious sharks of β-lactamase (*S*) released from staphylococcal cells. Other classes of antibiotics are degraded by other enzymes, such as the aminoglycoside-modifying enzymes or chloramphenicol acetyltransferase. (**B**) The second most important mechanism is the change in receptors for antibiotic attachment to critical structures, here represented by alteration of normal binding proteins (*circles*) on the cell membranes of gram-positive bacteria to binding proteins with reduced affinity for antibiotics (*triangles*). Changes in the affinity of receptors for other antibiotics, such as DNA gyrase and quinolones or ribosomes and aminoglycosides, are also important. (**C**) A third class of mechanism is represented by the effect of membrane permeability on resistance to several classes of antibiotics in gram-negative bacteria. The gram-negative bacillus on the left restricts entry of antibiotics by changes in transport proteins, such as porins. The bacillus on the right is pumping antibiotics out of the cell so fast that they cannot accumulate in the cytoplasm. (**D**) Lastly, bypass of a metabolic block imposed by antimicrobial agents is illustrated by trimethoprim-sulfamethoxazole and enterococci. The metabolic block produced by the antibiotics between steps **B** and **C** is obviated when the bacteria obtain preformed compound C in vivo.

activity, transport across membranes of gram-positive bacteria is not an issue.

Gram-negative bacteria possess an inner plasma membrane and an outer cell membrane, between which is an attenuated peptidoglycan layer (Fig. 17-3*B* and Fig. 17-5). Permeability of membranes to antimicrobial agents and transport of the molecules across the barriers are most important for gram-negative bacteria, which have two membrane hurdles for antimicrobial agents that have targets inside the cell.

The outer cell membrane, which is a crucial barrier for all antimicrobial agents, will be considered first. Several excellent reviews of the subject have been published.[180,226,229] The simplest method for entry of drugs into the cell is direct diffusion across the lipid membrane, but even very hydrophobic substances do not cross the lipid

bilayer efficiently. The reason for this block to diffusion is in part the asymmetric, polarized nature of the bacterial outer cell membrane, which has lipopolysaccharide with lipid A and an attached oligosaccharide on the outer aspect of the membrane only.

Porin Proteins and Diffusion Through the Outer Membrane.
For many antimicrobial agents, including the β-lactam group, the primary means of transport across the outer membrane of enteric bacteria are a remarkable group of membrane proteins, called porins (Fig. 17-5).[228,229,346] Two major porin proteins have been identified in *E. coli*, the most extensively studied species: a large porin channel designated Omp F (outer-membrane-protein F) and a small channel porin named Omp C.[346] A third channel called PhoE is produced in mutants that lack both Omp F and Omp C, but this channel does not appear to be important for movement of antimicro-

Table 17-4 Mechanisms of Antimicrobial Resistance in Clinically Important Bacteria

BACTERIAL TYPE	ANTIBIOTIC GROUP	COMMON MECHANISM(S)	OTHER MECHANISM(S)
Staphylococcus spp.	Penicillins	β-Lactamase (penicillinase)	Altered penicillin-binding proteins
	Penicillinase-resistant penicillins	Altered penicillin-binding proteins	Borderline: Altered penicillin-binding proteins; methicillinase; hyperproduction of β-lactamase
	Quinolones	Active efflux; altered DNA gyrase	Poor transport across membrane
	Erythromycin	Altered ribosomal targets	Active efflux of antibiotic
Streptococcus pneumoniae	β-Lactams	Altered penicillin-binding proteins	
	Erythromycin	Altered ribosomal targets	Active efflux of antibiotic
Enterococcus spp.	β-Lactams	Low-affinity penicillin-binding proteins	β-Lactamase
	Aminoglycosides	Low level: Poor transport across membrane	Altered ribosomal binding sites
		High level: Aminoglycoside-modifying enzymes	
	Glycopeptides	Altered binding proteins	
Haemophilus influenzae	Penicillins	β-Lactamase (penicillinase)	Altered penicillin-binding proteins
	Chloramphenicol	Chloramphenicol acetyltransferase	Altered membrane transport
Neisseria gonorrhoeae	Penicillins	β-Lactamase (penicillinase)	Altered penicillin-binding proteins
Neisseria meningitidis	Penicillins		β-Lactamase (penicillinase); altered penicillin-binding proteins
	β-Lactans	Poor diffusion or altered porins; β-lactamases	Altered penicillin-binding proteins; low protein motive force; extended-spectrum β-lactamases
	Aminoglycosides	Poor diffusion or altered porins; aminoglycoside-modifying enzymes	
	Quinolones	Altered DNA gyrase	Altered transport through outer membrane
	Tetracyclines	Active efflux	
	Trimethoprim-sulfamethoxazole	Altered enzyme targets	
Pseudomonads	β-Lactams	Poor diffusion or altered porins; β-lactamases	Altered penicillin-binding proteins; low protein motive force; extended-spectrum b-lactamases
	Aminoglycosides	Poor diffusion or altered porins; aminoglycoside-modifying enzymes	
	Quinolones	Altered DNA gyrase	Altered transport through outer membrane

bial agents.[228] Factors such as the charge on the molecule and the hydrophobicity of the compound play an important role (Fig. 17-6). Negatively charged molecules move more slowly across the membrane than do more positively charged molecules or zwitterions (compounds with balanced positive and negative charges). Presumably, the negative charges cause the antibiotic to ''hang up'' as it crosses the negatively charged porin channel. The exclusion of hydrophobic compounds from the aqueous environment of the porin may explain the lack of efficacy of the hydrophobic compound methicillin against gram-negative bacteria. Likewise, β-lactam antibiotics with large bulky side chains, such as mez-

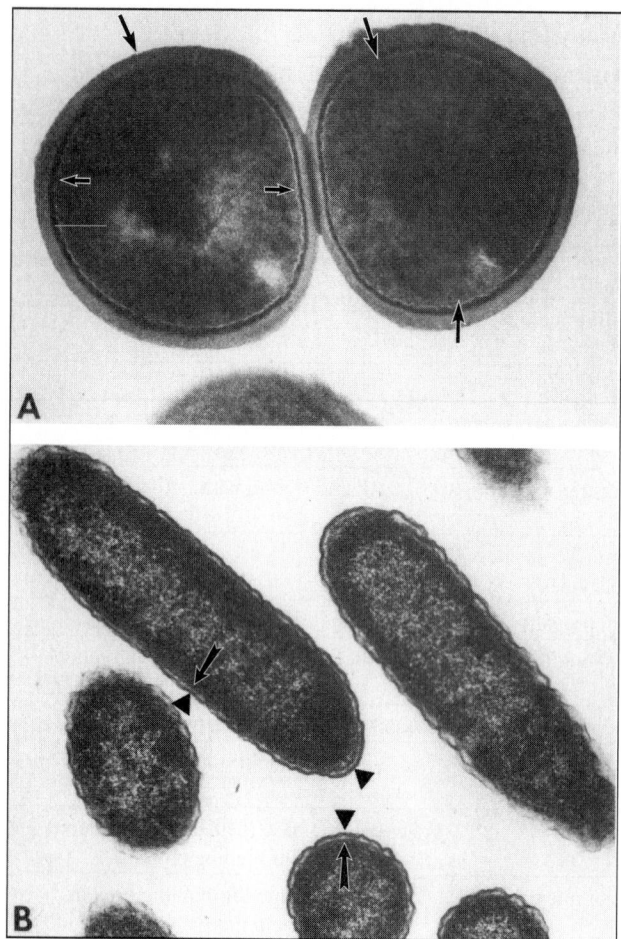

Figure 17-3 Ultrastructure of bacteria. (**A**) *Staphylococcus aureus.* Two gram-positive cocci are in the final stages of division. The bacterial cell membrane (arrows) is surrounded by a thick peptidoglycan layer that is freely accessible to antibiotics (30,000×). (**B**) *Pseudomonas aeruginosa.* These gram-negative bacilli have an internal cytoplasmic membrane (arrows) and an outer cell membrane (arrowheads). Between these two membranes lies the periplasmic space that contains the peptidoglycan. β-Lactam antibiotics must cross the cell membrane before they reach the peptidoglycan (35,000×).

whereas strain 2 produced only protein F, the large-channel porin. Under conditions of high osmolality, such as might occur in the patient's tissues, synthesis of the OmpF protein was repressed in both strains. On closure of the OmpF porin, expression of OmpC continued in strain 1, while in strain 2 there were no remaining transport channels (porins), so transport of the antibiotic across the membrane ceased and bacterial resistance resulted.

The porin proteins of other enteric gram-negative bacteria appear to behave in a similar fashion to those of *E. coli.* The porins of *Pseudomonas aeruginosa,* however, do not behave in the same way.[184] The only antimicrobial agent for which resistance in *P. aeruginosa* by means of altered membrane transport is clearly explained is imipenem. In some situations this antimicrobial agent gains entry, not through the main porin protein, but through a specific transport protein, designated D2.[261] It appears, however, that the presence of a chromosomal Class C β-lactamase is necessary for resistance in addition to the altered porin protein.[181]

Antimicrobial agents other than β-lactam compounds may also depend on porin channels for access to the cell. Resistance to chloramphenicol, which is usually caused by enzymatic degradation, may also be mediated by altered porin proteins in enteric bacteria[324] and *Haemophilus influenzae.*[30] Similarly, resistance to aminoglycosides may be mediated by alterations in porin proteins, although the primary mechanism for resistance is enzymatic degradation.[106] Resistance to quinolones, which is principally mediated by changes in the structure of the target enzyme, may also be caused by alterations in membrane proteins.[278]

Specific transport proteins have evolved in bacteria for transport of large molecules, such as vitamins, across the cell membrane. If antimicrobial agents could be devised that availed themselves of this ready-made superhighway into the bacterial cell, they would have a major competitive advantage. Unfortunately, it has been difficult to develop such compounds that are also clinically useful.

For some bacteria that must gain entrance to the bacterial cytoplasm, a second barrier may exist at the inner plasma membrane. Crossing the second membrane is accomplished by a process that requires expenditure of energy and a minimal negative charge in the cytoplasm, the proton motive force, in order to "pull" aminoglycoside antibiotics into the cytoplasm. This transport mechanism has been demonstrated in both gram-positive[196] and gram-negative bacteria.[29] Mutant *Enterobacteriaceae* have been described that are resistant to antimicrobial agents in vitro because of deficiencies in this transport mechanism, but their clinical significance is unclear.[275] These variants appear as small colonies on agar media, but they may revert to normal colony morphology.

Active Transport of Antimicrobial Agents out of the Bacterial Cell. For some bacteria, an important mechanism of resistance is active removal of antimicrobial agents from the bacterial cell, so that the intracellular concentrations of antimicrobial agents never reach a sufficiently high level to exert effective antimicrobial activity.

Active transport mechanisms are teleologically useful for removal of a variety of potentially toxic substances, of which antimicrobial agents may not even be the most important. The energy-dependent efflux mechanism is a prime defense for bacteria against tetracyclines[199] and macrolides,[105] two

locillin, piperacillin, and cefoperazone, also cross the membrane poorly. In one study the "best performer" among the β-lactam antibiotics was imipenem, which is a zwitterionic, hydrophilic compound with a very compact structure.[346] It has been proposed that the explanation for susceptibility of *Enterobacter cloacae* to imipenem in the presence of resistance to third-generation cephalosporins is the greater accessibility of imipenem to targets, mediated by rapid transit probably through several porin channels.[246]

The influence of porins on susceptibility is well illustrated by an interesting case reported by Medeiros and colleagues (Fig. 17-7).[201] These researchers isolated a strain of *Salmonella typhimurium* that contained two porin proteins, OmpF and OmpC (isolate 1). A variant strain isolated from the same patient produced only the OmpF protein (isolate 2). The two strains produced a similar β-lactamase. In low-osmolality media, strain 1 produced proteins F and C,

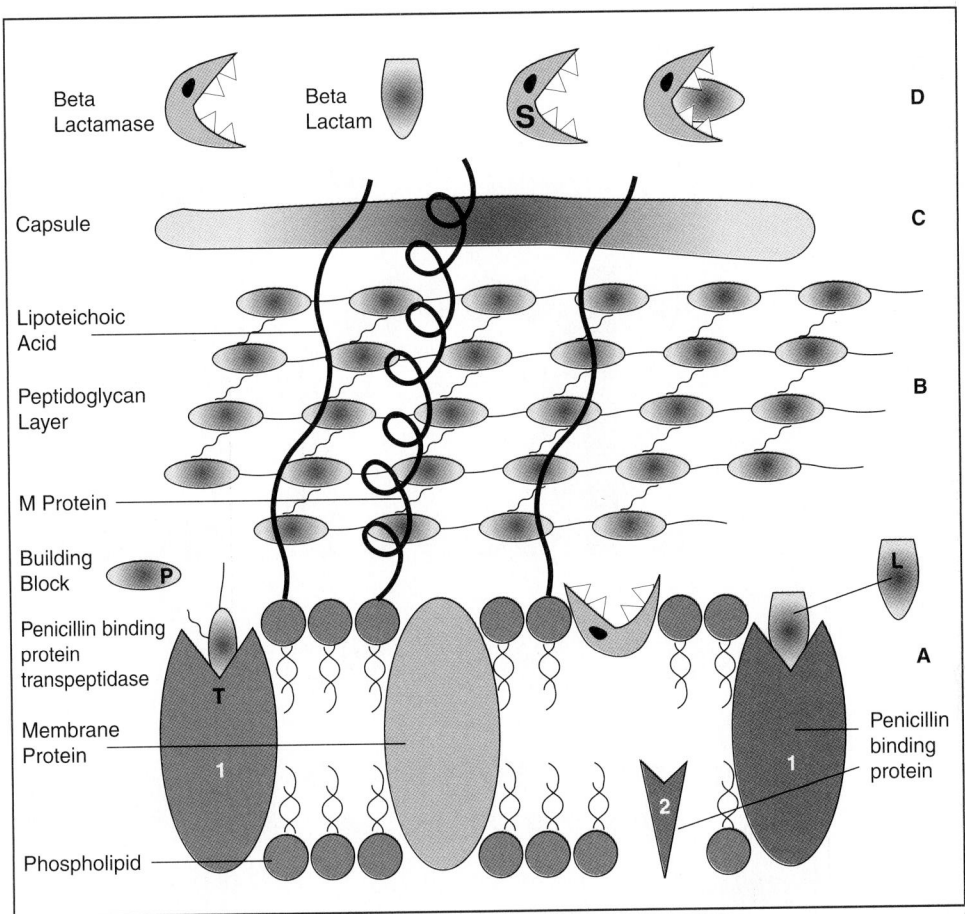

Figure 17-4 The cell wall of gram-positive bacteria consists, from inside out, of *(A)* a lipoprotein cell membrane, *(B)* a peptidoglycan cell wall, *(C)* a polysaccharide capsule (in some strains of some species, such as *Streptococcus pneumoniae*), and *(D)* the extracellular environment. The cell membrane *A* contains phospholipid, membrane proteins (including M protein in *Streptococcus pyogenes*), lipoteichoic acid in staphylococci, and a variety of penicillin-binding proteins, including β-lactamase, illustrated by the pac-men with shark's teeth *(S)*. In gram-positive bacteria the β-lactamases are secreted into the extracellular environment *(D)*, where they can inactivate β-lactam antibiotics. The peptidoglycan building blocks *(P)* in the cell wall *(B)* are integrated into the peptidoglycan by penicillin-binding transpeptidase in the membrane *(A)*. β-Lactam antibiotics *(L)* also interact with these proteins in the membrane *(A)* and interfere with the process.

groups of antibiotics that interfere with protein synthesis at the ribosomal level. Similarly, removal of the antibiotic is a resistance mechanism of staphylococci against the quinolones, which interfere with DNA gyrase.[223] The transporter may effectively remove multiple types of antibiotic, as in the case of an outer membrane protein (OprK) that is involved in secretion of siderophores in *Pseudomonas aeruginosa*.[257] Mutant strains that overproduced the protein demonstrated resistance to multiple antimicrobial agents, including ciprofloxacin, nalidixic acid, tetracycline, and chloramphenicol. Strains that had lost the ability to produce the transporter protein showed enhanced susceptibility to the antimicrobial agents.[227]

Among gram-positive bacteria there are two classes of multidrug efflux pumps within the major facilitator (MF) group of transporters, which depend on protein motive force for energy: 1) the Bmr/NorA transporters, which pump out cationic dyes, membrane-permeable cations, and quinolones and 2) the quaternary ammonium compound group, which rids the cell of disinfectants and cationic dyes. In contrast to the mef transporter found in many gram-positive bacteria (including staphylococci), the msr transporter found only in staphylococci also confers resistance to streptogramin B antibiotics.[271]

There are also two classes of multidrug pumps among gram-negative bacteria. The first, which is related to the Smr family, may confer a slight increase in resistance to some antibiotics, but is not considered clinically significant; the compounds are apparently exported into the periplasmic space. The second group, which is more complicated, is very important clinically and has a broad spectrum of specificity; it contains transporters of the MF family or of the resistance-

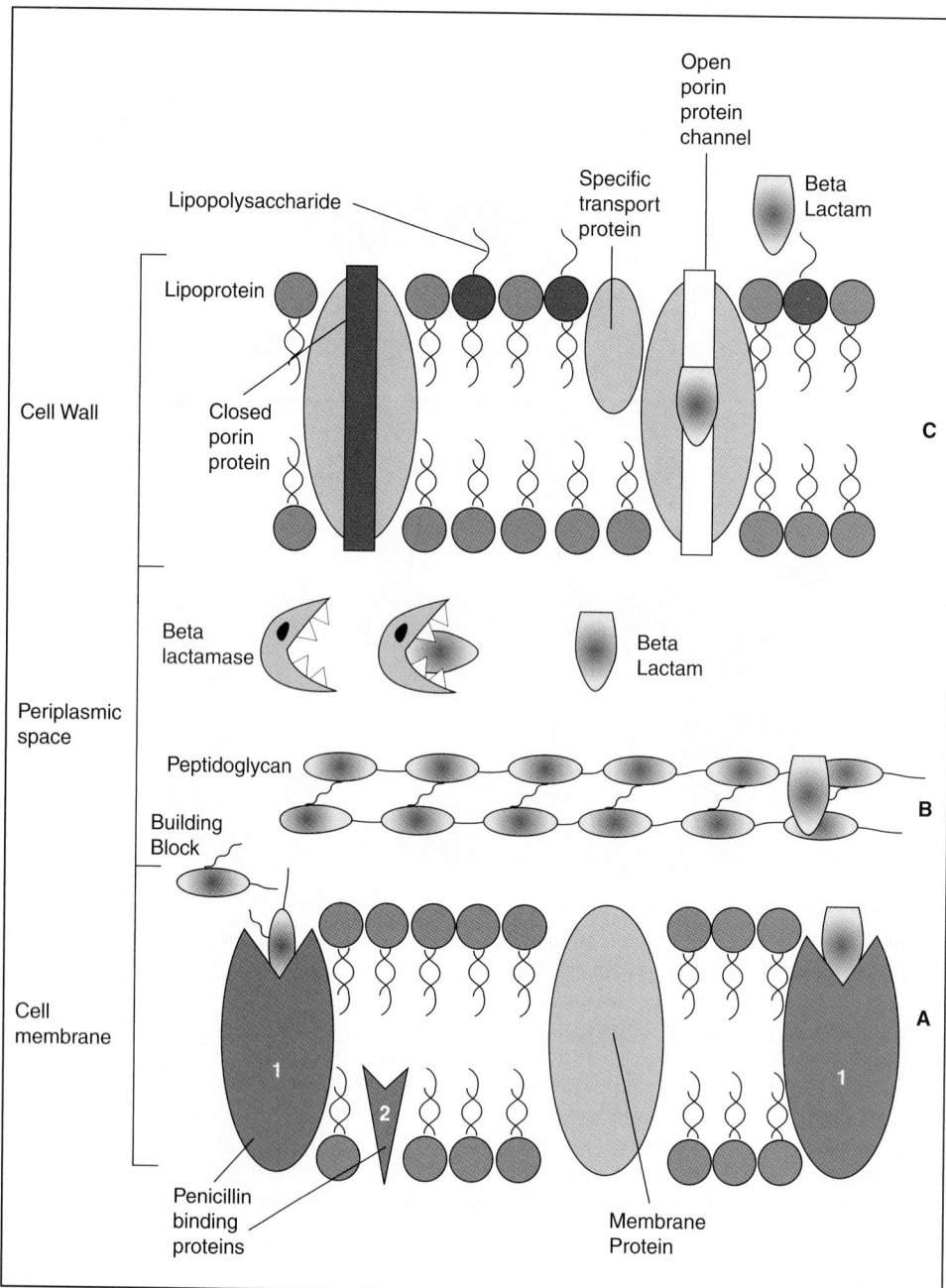

Figure 17-5 Gram-negative bacteria consist of an inner plasma membrane *(A)*, a periplasmic space with a loose arrangement of peptidoglycan *(B)*, and an outer cell membrane *(C)*. The two cell membranes consist of asymmetric lipoprotein bilayers with phospholipids and protein moieties. The plasma membrane *(A)* contains a variety of penicillin-binding proteins, which participate in the process of peptidoglycan formation and are inhibited by β-lactam antibiotics. The outer cell membrane *(C)* includes lipopolysaccharide, which consists of lipid A (endotoxin), a covalently bound core, and a polysaccharide chain that determines the O somatic antigen used in many serologic typing schemes. The outer membrane also includes important transport proteins, including specific transporters and the important porin proteins of several sizes and types. β-Lactamase in gram-negative bacteria is limited to the periplasmic space, where it can inactivate antibiotics as they pass through; the β-lactamase is not secreted into the external environment.

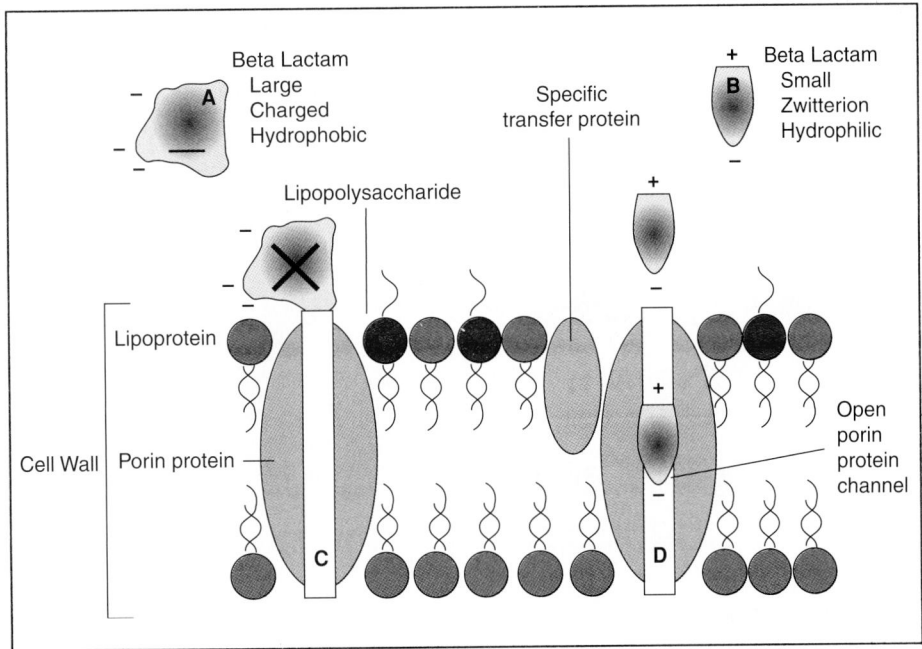

Figure 17-6 Factors influencing movement of antibiotics through the porin proteins of gram-negative bacteria: The outer cell membrane (see Fig. 17-5C) is depicted. Two antibiotics with different characteristics are depicted. Antibiotic A, which is large, hydrophobic, and has multiple negative charges, is excluded by the porin channel (C). Antibiotic (B), which is compact, has balanced charges (zwitterionic) and is hydrophilic, moves through porin channel D without any difficulty.

nodulation-division (RND) family. In this group the transporter is composed of three components: 1) a transporter protein in the cytoplasmic membrane, 2) a membrane pore, and 3) a periplasmic "linker" protein that connects the other two components.

The resistance of gram-negative bacilli to many antibiotics was originally attributed to poor entry of the antibiotic into the bacterial cell because of size, hydrophobicity, or charge. It is now thought that active efflux of these antibiotics from the bacterial cell is at least equally important, because the pumps can excrete chemical compounds, including antimicrobial agents, directly into the extracellular medium, where their reentry is restricted.[227]

ANTIBIOTICS THAT INTERFERE WITH FORMATION OF BACTERIAL CELL WALLS: THE β-LACTAM AND GLYCOPEPTIDE ANTIBIOTICS

The Superfamily of Penicillin-Recognizing Enzymes and Antibiotics Active at Cell Membranes. Before trying to understand individual mechanisms of resistance it is important to consider the evolving concept of a superfamily of penicillin-recognizing enzymes and their relationship to the structure of bacterial cells. These interactions are integral to understanding the most important group of antimicrobial agents, the β-lactam family of antibiotics. As often happens in biology, the complexity of the processes and interactions become more evident as we learn more about them. What appears at first glance to be an isolated process may eventually be seen as part of a much larger and more complex biologic system, much as a single dot in a Seurat painting can be appreciated as part of a beautiful work of art when one backs away and looks at the whole canvas.

The Penicillin and Vancomycin-Binding Proteins Peptidoglycan, which provides rigidity and functional stability to the bacterial cell, consists of strands of alternating amino sugars, *N*-acetylglucosamine and *N*-acetylmuramic acid, cross-linked by peptides. As discussed above, the peptidoglycan layer of gram-positive bacteria is a thick layer external to the single cell membrane (Fig. 17-3A and Fig. 17-4), whereas the peptidoglycan layer of gram-negative bacteria, which is attenuated, is located between the plasma membrane and the outer cell membrane (Fig. 17-3B and Fig. 17-5). The biosynthesis of peptidoglycan consists of many steps that begin in the cytoplasm and end outside the cell membrane. The final stage in the process is the transpeptidation of the developing peptidoglycan molecule, in which a terminal glycine residue on a pentaglycine side chain is linked to D-alanine on an adjacent strand, releasing a second D-alanine molecule in the process. A glycosylase and carboxylase also appear to be involved in the process, but their roles are less clear.[191] The transpeptidase, which is bound to the cell membrane, is one of a family of enzymes known as penicillin-binding proteins, which in turn are part of the superfamily of penicillin-recognizing enzymes.[200] In addition to the transpeptidases, other penicillin-binding proteins participate in the formation of the bacterial cell wall. These binding proteins are attached to the cell membrane in gram-positive bacteria and to the inner plasma membrane in gram-negative species. The distinct function of different penicillin-binding proteins has been illustrated dramatically in *Escherichia coli*, in which interference with different proteins produces different morphologic effects as the synthesis of cell walls is impaired (Fig. 17-8).[291] In bacillary organisms, different

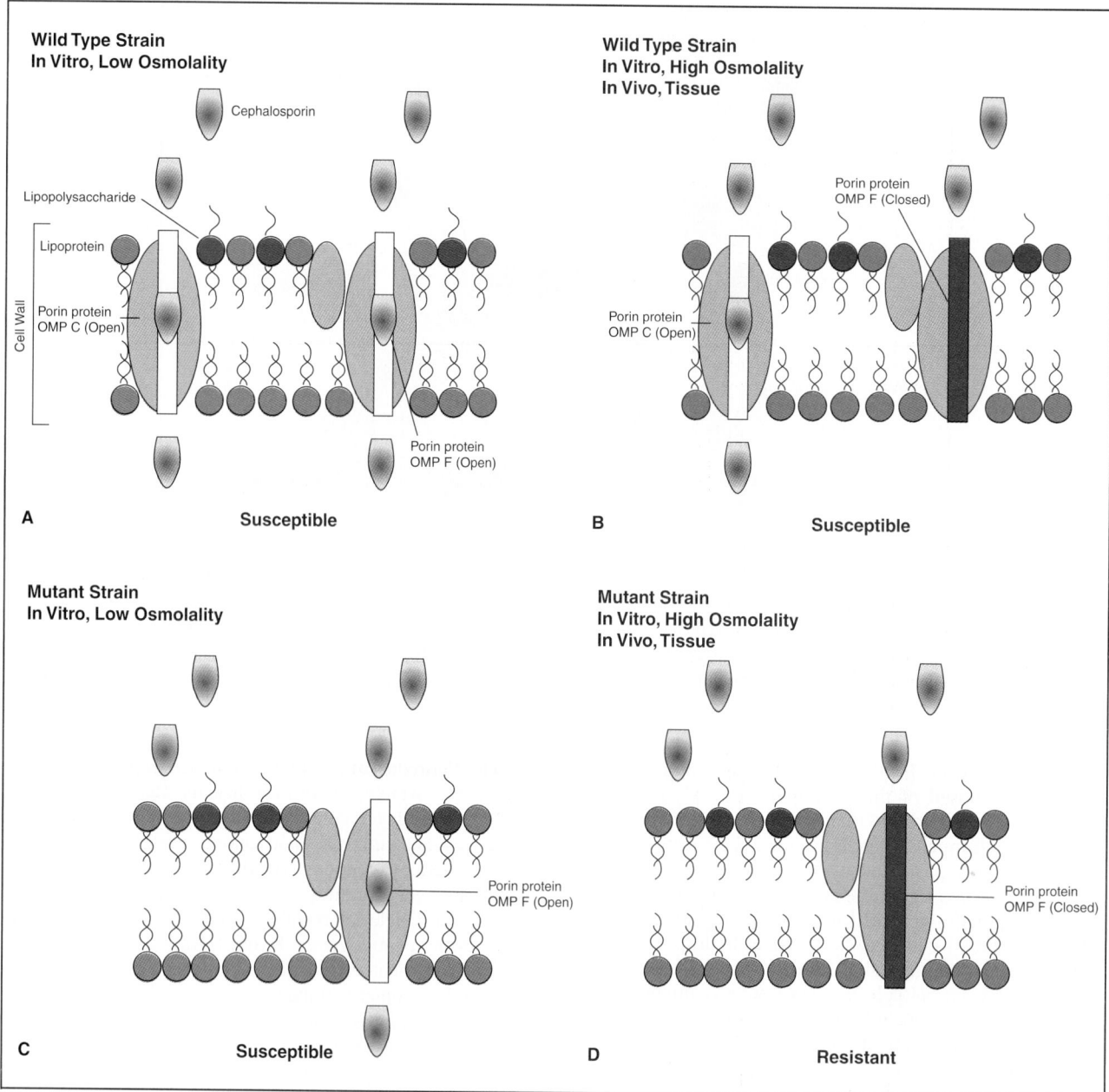

Figure 17-7 The critical importance of porin proteins in antimicrobial resistance as illustrated by a mutant strain of *Salmonella typhimurium*:[201] The outer cell membrane is illustrated for four combinations of bacterium and environment. (**A**) The wild-type strain grown in low-osmolality medium in the laboratory has a small channel porin (OmpC) and a large-channel porin (OmpF). The cephalosporin has free access to its binding sites on the inner plasma membrane (not shown) and the strain is susceptible. (**B**) The wild-type strain has been grown in high-osmolality medium in the laboratory, mimicking the conditions in vivo. The large-channel porin (OmpF) has closed down, but the small-channel porin is still available for the cephalosporin, and the strain remains susceptible. (**C**) A mutant strain has lost its small-channel porin (OmpC), but it still has the OmpF porin when grown in low-osmolality medium in the laboratory. The cephalosporin can traverse the membrane through OmpF, and the mutant strain is susceptible in vitro. (**D**) The mutant strain in high-osmolality media or in vivo. The OmpF protein shuts down, as it did in the wild-type strain under similar conditions, but there is now no OmpC porin available for the antibiotic. With no means for entering the cell the cephalosporin is ineffective and the mutant strain is now resistant.

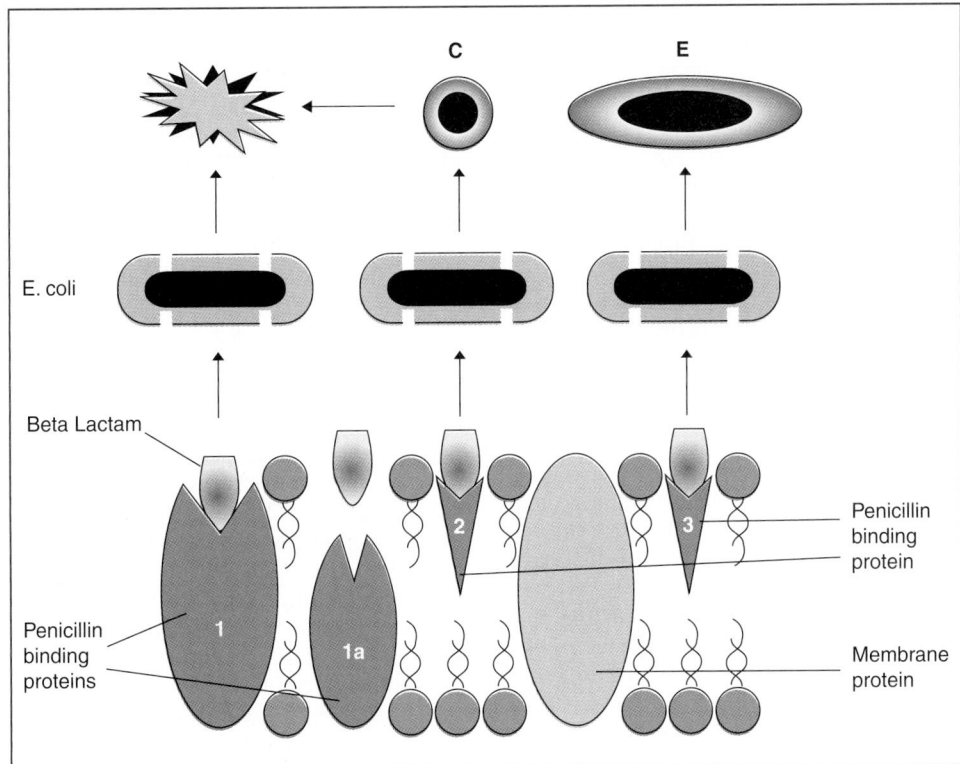

Figure 17-8 Effects of three penicillin-binding proteins on the structure of *Escherichia coli:* The inner plasma membrane of *E. coli* (corresponding to layer *A* in Figure 17-5) is depicted. Three different penicillin-binding proteins are numbered 1 through 3, in order of decreasing molecular weight. A variant of protein 1 (1a) is also present. β-Lactam antibiotics that interact with protein 1 cause the bacillus to lyse rapidly. Interaction with protein 2 causes formation of coccal cells (*C*), which eventually progress to lysis. Antibiotics that interact with protein 3 do not cause lysis, but cause a defect in information of cross-walls so that the bacterial cells elongate and assume bizarre shapes (*E*). Penicillin-binding proteins 4 through 6 (not shown) are not essential and do not produce obvious changes when antibiotics interact with them.[291]

binding proteins appear to function in the formation of cross-walls at cell division (protein 2 in *E. coli*) and in elongation of the cells after division (protein 3 in *E. coli*).[291] Penicillin-binding proteins are numbered according to their molecular weight, with protein 1 having the highest molecular weight. The numbering system is specific for each species, so that penicillin-binding protein 1 in *Escherichia coli* is not the same as protein 1 in *Klebsiella pneumoniae* or *Streptococcus pneumoniae*. The high-molecular-weight compounds function as the transpeptidases that are essential for formation of peptidoglycan.[96,293] The low-molecular-weight compounds appear to function as D-alanine carboxypeptidases, and their biologic significance is unclear.

β-Lactam antibiotics exert their effects by interfering with the formation of peptidoglycan, a mechanism that is shared with the glycopeptide agents, such as vancomycin.[321,335] Many years ago it was recognized that a structural similarity between the penicillin molecule and the D-alanine–D-alanine terminus of the peptidoglycan chain was integral to the antibacterial action of the compound.[320] Kelly and colleagues have elucidated the three-dimensional structure of the transpeptidase penicillin-binding protein and observed directly its interaction with penicillins and cephalosporins, definitively establishing the identity of the

penicillin-binding site and the transpeptidase enzyme.[162] In essence, penicillin fools the penicillin-binding protein into thinking it is the next building block to be added to the peptidoglycan chain. Once inserted, the penicillin molecule abrogates further elongation of the peptidoglycan. Various members of the large β-lactam group of antibiotics have differing affinities for individual penicillin-binding proteins. The efficacy of compounds against bacteria is, in part, determined by the degree to which they are bound. Aztreonam, which is a β-lactam antibiotic, does not interact with the binding proteins of gram-positive bacteria and is the only member of the group that is ineffective against these organisms. Bactericidal activity may require the interaction of a β-lactam antibiotic with more than one penicillin-binding protein.[112] Satta and colleagues demonstrated that resistance to *E. coli* increased as more critical binding proteins were saturated. Saturation of nonessential binding proteins had no effect on antimicrobial susceptibility.[279] The action of autolytic enzymes may also be important for the bactericidal activity of β-lactam antibiotics.[90]

The other major class of antibiotics that actively interferes with the synthesis of bacterial cell walls is the glycopeptide group, represented by vancomycin and teicoplanin. In contrast to β-lactam antibiotics, which block the activity of the cell membrane–bound peptidases, the glycopeptides bind noncovalently to the D-alanyl-D-alanyl terminus of a pentapeptide peptidoglycan precursor.[215] The antibiotic has structural and functional similarities to a D-alanyl-D-alanyl peptidase that participates in the elongation of the peptidoglycan chain.[169] Binding of the antibiotic to the precursor protein may block access of the crucial building block to the peptidase by steric interference.

Modification of Target Enzymes: Binding Proteins and Antibiotic Resistance An important mechanism for resistance of bacteria to β-lactam antibiotics is an alteration of penicillin-binding proteins so that the antibiotic no longer has access to the enlarging peptidoglycan chain. Altered proteins are indicated by addition of a suffix, which may either be a letter or a prime designation, to the numbering scheme. For instance, the mechanism for high-level resistance of *Staphylococcus aureus* to penicillinase-resistant penicillins is the production of a variant of penicillin-binding protein 2 (PBP 2) to a variant that is designated PBP 2a. Alternatively, there may be a loss of the binding proteins that have the highest affinity for the antibiotic.

The evidence supporting the role of altered binding proteins comes from two sources. First, the presence of the altered proteins is associated with the appearance of resistance. Exposure of staphylococci to methicillin induced an alteration of penicillin-binding protein 2 (PBP 2) to a variant (PBP 2a).[119,326] Variants that lost resistance did not contain the variant binding protein.[119,326] Similarly, isolates of *Streptococcus pneumoniae* that were resistant to penicillin exhibited decreased affinity of penicillin for whole bacterial cells, membrane preparations, and two major penicillin-binding proteins.[115] Similar results have been reported for viridans streptococci in South Africa.[80] Conversely, the transition from resistance to hypersusceptibility was associated with the loss of a low-affinity binding protein. The resulting binding protein of high affinity was then associated with susceptibility to the bound antibiotic.

The alterations in binding proteins may be a one-step process, controlled by a single gene, such as the *MecA* gene, which codes for variant PBP 2a in *Staphylococcus aureus*.[326] In the case of *Streptococcus pneumoniae*, however, alterations of multiple binding proteins result in a multistep process of increasing resistance.[137]

Alterations in binding proteins are more important for resistance of gram-positive bacteria to β-lactam antibiotics than for enteric gram-negative bacteria and *Pseudomonas* spp. Changes in binding proteins do have major effects on some gram-negative bacteria and some β-lactam antibiotics, however. The mechanism by which *Haemophilus influenzae* and *Neisseria gonorrhoeae* that do not produce β-lactamase are resistant to β-lactam antibiotics is the alteration of binding proteins.[72,239] Even *N. meningitidis*, which for so many years remained uniformly susceptible to penicillin, has developed altered binding proteins that have produced resistance to penicillin.[349] The clinical importance of these binding proteins is well illustrated by a patient in whom nontypeable *H. influenzae* produced meningitis. The patient was treated unsuccessfully with cefuroxime. The isolate did not produce β-lactamase and did not contain permeability barriers, but it did contain proteins that bound cefuroxime poorly.[202] Even among the *Enterobacteriaceae* changes in binding proteins may be important. Changes in PBP 3 of

Escherichia coli were associated with resistance to cephalexin and some other cephalosporin antibiotics.[123] Similarly, resistance to imipenem may be mediated by changes in binding proteins, both among enteric bacteria, such as *Enterobacter aerogenes*, or *Acinetobacter baumanii*.[45,100] In the case of the *Enterobacter* strain, the binding protein was in the outer membrane rather than at the cytoplasmic membrane, and it may have been important in transport of the antibiotic across the membrane.

The second line of evidence supporting the role of binding proteins comes from the observation that loss of the variant protein results in the restoration of susceptibility or even the hypersusceptible state.[80,91,119,326]

Similar events occur during the development of resistance to vancomycin. The *vanA* gene of enterococci encodes depsipeptide precursor proteins for peptidoglycan that bypass the interaction of vancomycin with the D-alanyl-D-alanyl terminus of peptides.[169,174] Resistance of *Staphylococcus aureus* to glycopeptides was presaged by the development of mutants with decreased susceptibility in the laboratory. The decrease in susceptibility was associated with the appearance of a new 39-kDa protein in the cytoplasm and in some membrane fractions along with considerable disorganization of the peptidoglycan layer.[53]

Several useful reviews of penicillin-binding proteins as resistance mechanisms are available.[42,190,292]

Antibiotic-Modifying Enzymes: The β-Lactamases Another major group of penicillin-recognizing proteins is the class of enzymes known as β-lactamases. It is now clear that the β-lactamases and the penicillin-binding proteins have a common, although distant evolutionary origin.[293] Both classes of compound must interact with β-lactam antibiotics in order to perform their function. Similar amino acid sequences have been demonstrated in penicillin-binding proteins of high and low molecular weight and certain types of β-lactamase. In addition, similarities in conformation and three-dimensional structure have been documented. Interestingly, some penicillin-binding proteins can function as a β-lactamase, albeit not as efficiently or with as great clinical importance as "professional" β-lactamases.[200,225] Furthermore, the mechanism of action of both β-lactamases and the transpeptidase penicillin-binding protein is cleavage of an amide bond by an acyl-enzyme mechanism.[19]

β-lactamases are a family of enzymes that range in importance from the almost exclusive mechanism of staphylococcal resistance to penicillin at one extreme to clinically insignificant constituents of the cell wall in some enteric bacteria. Any β-lactam antibiotic or group of antibiotics may be inactivated by these enzymes. The number of different enzymes now exceeds 340, and the growth spurt shows no signs of slowing.[25,35,200] Just as the specificity of penicillin-binding proteins for β-lactam antibiotics is a factor in determining the susceptibility of the bacterium to the antibiotic, so the specificity of the β-lactamase for a β-lactam antibiotic is an important determinant in the efficiency with which the enzyme hydrolyzes the antibiotic. A point mutation in one or more amino acids can change the specificity of the molecule if it occurs in a structurally critical area of the enzyme,[21,36] causing the lamentation that bacteria can with one stroke undo millions of dollars of pharmaceutical research and development.

There is evidence that the microbial sources of antibiotics (such as *Streptomyces* spp.) produce the antibiotic and also modifying enzymes that protect the producer against self-destruction. It is interesting that Abraham and Chain, two of the scientists who were instrumental in the development of penicillin, reported the presence of penicillinase in a strain of *Bacillus (Escherichia) coli* before the introduction of the antibiotic into clinical use.[3] Examples exist of β-lactamase enzymes being documented before local introduction of the relevant antibiotic substrate.[25] Clearly nature did not invent β-lactamases solely to bedevil infectious disease physicians and pharmaceutical companies. Two groups of investigators have presented evidence to support the concept that the physiologic role of β-lactamases is to restructure the peptidoglycan during bacterial cell growth.[19,325] They found that synthesis of β-lactamase was induced both by the presence of β-lactam antibiotics and cell-wall precursors in the extracellular environment, recalling the structural similarity of penicillin and the D-alanine-d-alanine dipeptide terminus of peptidoglycan chains.

A variety of classification schemes has been developed, leading to some confusion in nomenclature. A useful early classification scheme was provided by Richmond and Sykes,[268] but the number and variety of enzymes have proliferated beyond the boundaries of their scheme. A more modern scheme, based on molecular structure proposed by Ambler[6] includes, of necessity, only enzymes that have been characterized. Subsequently, a classification of β-lactamases, the Bush-Jacoby-Medeiros scheme has been developed to integrate functional and molecular characteristics.[36] The Bush-Jacoby-Medeiros classification is summarized in Table 17-5, which also includes the corresponding Ambler class for each of the groups.

The most important group consists of serine proteases that have either preference for penicillins or have broad-spectrum activity (Ambler A; Bush-Jacoby-Medeiros Group 2). They are found either on chromosomes or on plasmids and may be, therefore, easily transferable from one bacterium to another. They may also be located on transposons that contain genes for resistance to other classes of antibiotics, resulting in multiply resistant bacterial strains.[35] These Class A/Group 2 β-lactamases may be produced constitutively or may require induction. Most of them are blocked by β-lactamase inhibitors. In this group are the staphylococcal enzymes and many of the most important β-lactamases of gram-negative bacteria.

Ambler Class C/Bush-Jacoby-Medeiros Group 1 enzymes are primarily cephalosporinases, either constitutive or inducible, that are found on the chromosomes of gram-negative bacteria. Characteristics of these ''wide-spectrum β-lactamases'' are summarized in Table 17-6.

More recently and ominously the Class C enzymes have found their way on to plasmids, by means of which they have been disseminated among bacterial strains.[233,262,316] Ambler Class B/Bush-Jacoby-Medeiros Group 3 enzymes (metalloenzymes) and Ambler Class D/Bush-Jacoby-Medeiros Group 2d enzymes (oxacillinases) have been generally considered less important clinically, but the role of metalloenzymes is increasingly emphasized.[34,183]

Some β-lactamases, such as those produced by *Staphylococcus aureus*, have been stable over several decades. These enzymes have a rather narrow spectrum of activity aimed at penicillin molecules. The broader-spectrum, plasmid-mediated β-lactamases of gram-negative bacteria, such as TEM-1 and SHV-1, were also stable for many years. Beginning in the early 1980s, however, a series of enzymatic variants appeared that had a broadened spectrum of activity against many of the newly developed β-lactam antibiotics. These extended-spectrum β-lactamases (ESBLs) were first found in Europe, most commonly in isolates of *Klebsiella* spp., less commonly in *Escherichia coli*.[252] The number of enzymes continues to increase.[139] These enzymes have now been demonstrated in many species within the *Enterobacteriaceae* (including *Enterobacter* spp., *Serratia* spp., and *Proteus mirabilis*) and more recently in other genera, such as *Pseudomonas aeruginosa*.[340] The new enzymes and their precursors, such as TEM-1 and SHV-1, are located on plasmids, but may have been derived originally from a chromosomal enzyme. Many of the new β-lactamases differ from each other only in a single amino acid substitution, but the changes have profound implications for clinical management of infectious diseases.[46,200] The characteristics of the extended-spectrum enzymes are summarized in Table 17-6. They have assumed special importance for several reasons: 1) they have become prevalent in some medical centers in Europe and the United States,[345,259] 2) they confer resistance to virtually all β-lactam antibiotics with the major exception of carbapenems, such as imipenem, 3) resistance to many antibiotics is not easily detectable by commonly used laboratory techniques[160] (see discussion of detection below), and 4) in some instances clinical failures have resulted from therapy with β-lactam antibiotics that appeared to be effective in vitro.[241] Recognition of an epidemic of infection caused by extended-spectrum β-lactamases was delayed because disk diffusion susceptibility tests produced false reports of susceptibility.[204]

β-Lactamase Inhibitors The final piece in the penicillin-recognizing protein puzzle is the introduction of β-lactamase inhibitors.[33,182] These compounds resemble β-lactam antibiotics sufficiently well that they can bind to the β-lactamase, either reversibly or irreversibly, protecting the antibiotic from destruction. When they are most effective, they serve as suicide bombers, sopping up all available enzyme.[182] It should not be surprising that these compounds, which must mimic β-lactams in order to function, also have limited antibacterial activity in their own right. In fact, aztreonam, which was developed as a β-lactam antibiotic was later discovered to have additional activity as an inhibitor of β-lactamase.[33] The three inhibitors of β-lactamase activity that have found a place in clinical medicine are clavulanic acid, sulbactam, and tazobactam. All three inhibitors are effective against staphylococcal penicillinase and have variable effectiveness against the chromosomal enzymes of gram-negative bacteria. Clavulanate and tazobactam are superior to sulbactam in activity against plasmid-mediated β-lactamases of gram-negative organisms, including the extended-spectrum β-lactamases.[244] There is no significant difference between the inhibitory activities of clavulanate and tazobactam, although the spectrum of their activity is different. Some extended-spectrum enzymes are resistant to the activity of all three compounds. Clavulanate is a more efficient inducer of Class C/Group 1 AmpC β-lactamases than is either tazobactam or sulbactam.

Table 17-5 Bush-Jacoby-Medeiros Functional Classification Scheme for β-Lactamases (With Correlation to the Ambler Molecular Classification Scheme)

GROUP	ENZYME TYPE	INHIBITION BY CLAVULANATE	MOLECULAR CLASS (AMBLER)	NUMBER OF ENZYMES (MINIMUM)	PREDOMINANT LOCATION OF ENZYME	PREDOMINANT EXPRESSION	EXAMPLES
1	Cephalosporinase	No	C	53	Chromosomal or plasmid	Chromosomal enzymes usually inducible; plasmid enzymes usually constitutive	Resistance to all β-lactams except carbapenems (unless combined with porin changes)
2a	Penicillinase	Yes	A	23	Plasmid or transposon	Inducible in *S. aureus*	*Staphylococcus aureus; S. epidermidis; Enterococcus* spp.; predominantly penicillins
2b	Broad-spectrum	Yes	A	16	Chromosomal or plasmid	Inducible or constitutive	TEM-1, SHV-1; penicillins and cephalosporins
2be	Extended-spectrum	Yes	A	119	Plasmid	Constitutive	TEM-3; SHV-2; *Klebsiella oxytoca* K-1; Penicillins and cephalosporins
2br	Inhibitor-resistant	Diminished	A	24			Primarily derived from TEM type
2c	Carbenicillinase	Yes	A	19			PSE-1; CARB-3; BRO-1; Carbenicillin
2d	Cloxacillinase	Yes	D or A	31			OXA-1; PSE-2; *Streptomyces cacaoi;* cloxacillin/oxacillin
2e	Cephalosporinase	Yes		20			*Proteus vulgaris; Bacteroides fragilis* CepA; Cephalosporins
2f	Carbapenemase	Yes	A	4			*Enterobacter cloacae* IMI-1; NMC-A; carbapenems
3	Metalloenzyme	No	B	24			*Stenotrophomonas maltophilia L1;* all β-lactam classes except monobactams
4	Penicillinase	No		9			*Burkholderia cepacia;* miscellaneous unsequenced enzymes that do not fit into other groups

Adapted from references[25,35,200,218,231,316].

Table 17-6 Characteristics of the Most Common Plasmid-Mediated "Wide-Spectrum" β-Lactamases

PARAMETER	EXTENDED-SPECTRUM β-LACTAMASES	AMPC β-LACTAMASES
Year first reported	1983	1988
Bacterial species affected	*Escherichia coli; Klebsiella pneumoniae; Enterobacter* spp.; *Salmonella* spp.; *Proteus* spp.; *Citrobacter* spp.; *Morganella morganii; Serratia marcescens; Shigella dysenteriae; Pseudomonas aeruginosa; Burkholderia cepacia; Capnocytophaga ochracea*; and others	*Escherichia coli; Klebsiella pneumoniae; Salmonella* spp.; *Citrobacter freundii; Enterobacter aerogenes; Proteus mirabilis*
Inhibition by inhibitors of β-lactamases (e.g., clavulanate)	Yes	No
Location of enzyme	Plasmid	Plasmid (derived from inducible chromosomal enzyme)
Expression	Constitutive	Constitutive (one exception)
Indicator antibiotics	Aztreonam, ceftazidime, ceftriaxone, cefotaxime, cefpodoxime	Possibly cefoxitin or cefotetan
Detection mechanism (screening)	Indicator antibiotic with and without β-lactamase inhibitor	Problematic; Use *K. pneumoniae* (no chromosomal AmpC enzyme) as an "institutional screen"
Associated problems	Presence of an ESBL may be masked by coincident AmpC enzyme	Difficult to differentiate plasmid from chromosomal enzyme
Inoculum effect	Yes	Yes
Efficacy of apparently susceptible β-lactams in the presence of enzyme	No	Probably no
Therapy with β-lactam/β-lactamase inhibitor combinations	Controversial	No

Adapted from references[25,35,200,218,231,316].

β-Lactamases and Antimicrobial Resistance β-lactamases of gram-positive bacteria, represented predominantly by the staphylococci, are for the most part inducible Class A enzymes that are formed at the cell membrane, but are also secreted extracellularly (Fig. 17-4). The practical implications of these characteristics are twofold. First, the bacteria must be exposed to the β-lactam antibiotic before the enzyme is produced in large quantities. In the laboratory it is possible to kill the bacteria with large quantities of antibiotic before enzymatic induction occurs, producing a false impression of susceptibility. Theoretically, small numbers of staphylococci might also be killed in vivo before induction of β-lactamase, but this eventuality has not been documented. Second, the extracellular production of β-lactamase could protect coinfecting bacteria that do not produce the enzyme. It has been hypothesized that relapses of streptococcal pharyngitis after treatment with penicillin might be caused by this mechanism,[27] but other investigators have not been able to document a relationship between the presence of bacteria that produce β-lactamase and the outcome of treatment.[306]

The β-lactamases of gram-negative bacteria are more complicated and the increasing level of complexity shows no signs of decreasing (Table 17-5). The chromosomal enzymes that were expressed constitutively at a low level in many enteric species (Class C/Group 1) were augmented first by

inducible broad-spectrum enzymes encoded on plasmids or transposons (Class A/Group 2), later by mutations to the plasmid-mediated extended-spectrum enzymes (also Class A/Group 2), and more recently by the appearance of the Class C/Group 1 enzymes on plasmids. The complexity is accentuated by several factors, which are summarized in Box 17-1.

ANTIMICROBIAL AGENTS THAT DO NOT EXERT THEIR EFFECT ON CELL WALLS

Production of Modifying Enzymes. Modifying enzymes are also important for some antimicrobial agents that exert their effects within the cytoplasm of the bacterial cells. The primary mechanism for resistance to aminoglycosides is modifying enzymes. There are three general types of processes: 1) phosphorylation, 2) acetylation, and 3) adenylation. All aminoglycoside antibiotics are at risk to inactivation by one of these enzymes.[197,253] Although all three types of enzymes are found in all types of bacteria, the enzymes of gram-positive and gram-negative organisms are different. The enzymes in gram-negative bacteria that inactivate streptomycin and kanamycin have become so widely distributed that these antibiotics have fallen out of common clinical use. Amikacin is least vulnerable to these inactivating enzymes but may be

Box 17-1 Selected Characteristics of β-Lactamases

1. Multiple β-lactamases of different types may be expressed in the same strain of bacteria. The different enzymes may have different clinical implications and it is becoming increasingly difficult to dissect the enzymatic profiles in all but the most sophisticated clinical laboratories. For instance, the presence of a Class A/Group 2 extended-spectrum β-lactamase may be masked by the presence of a Class C/Group 1 β-lactamase[25,316] (see discussion of detection below).

2. Inoculum effects may make detection of clinically relevant resistance diffcult.[316] The organisms that produce extended-spectrum β-lactamases demonstrate increasing resistance to third-generation cephalosporins with increasing bacterial inoculum (inoculum effect),[139] a phenomenon that is probably caused by the inability of the antibiotics to kill the bacteria as well as inhibit them.[204] The cephamycins, which often appear susceptible in vitro, also fail to exert bactericidal activity,[204] and the place of these antibiotics in therapy is unclear. Imipenem, which has bacteriostatic and bactericidal activity, appears effective in vitro and is therapeutically active against strains that do not have other mechanisms for resistance. Although inhibitors of β-lactamase inhibit ESBLs, the role of these agents in therapy of human infections is also controversial. In one study, use of β-lactamase inhibitors did appear to decrease spread of ESBL-producing strains, but use of these agents is not generally recommended and handwashing remains the cornerstone of measures to control the spread of nosocomial infections.[255] When rats were infected experimentally with a strain of *Klebsiella pneumoniae* that produced a TEM-26 β-lactamase, the combinations of ampicillin-sulbactam and piperacillin-tazobactam were effective in reducing bacterial colony counts in intra-abdominal abscesses, but imipenem provided the most effective therapy.[266]

3. Each enzyme has different affinities for various β-lactam antibiotics, but hyperproduction of an enzyme may render a normally effective antibiotic inactive.[122,249]

4. Enzymes have been characterized that are active against virtually every β-lactam antibiotic, even those (such as the carbapenems) that are not usually affected by the common enzymes.[232,334]

5. It is not uncommon for redundant mechanisms of resistance to be present in the same bacterial strain. For instance, a Class A/Group 2 β-lactamase that is inhibited by clavulanic acid (and might be treated with a β-lactam-β-lactamase-inhibitor combination theoretically) may also contain a porin mutation that renders the bacterium resistant to multiple antibiotics with or without the presence of β-lactamase inhibitors.[25] Resistance to ceftazidime and piperacillin-tazobactam (not usually inactivated in vitro by ESBL) in an isolate of *Klebsiella pneumoniae* was ascribed to the combination of a SHV-1 β-lactamase (Class A; Group 2) and an alteration in outer membrane proteins.[265] Similarly, Imipenem (not affected by ESBL) was inactivated by a combination of a plasmid-mediated AmpC β-lactamase (Class C; Group 1) and the loss of an outer membrane protein.[26]

6. Finally, transposons may carry genes for resistance to multiple antibiotics other than β-lactam agents, such as fluoroquinolones, trimethoprim-sulfamethoxazole, or aminoglycosides.[111,231]

rendered ineffective by other mechanisms, particularly in *Pseudomonas aeruginosa*. Aminoglycoside resistance has developed in epidemic proportions at hospitals around the world.[197] Miller and colleagues, who summarized the results of multiple studies, found variations over time and among geographic areas.[206] There appeared to be a correlation of resistance with patterns of antibiotic use. Notably, the presence of an enzyme that acetylates amikacin but not gentamicin was noted, another illustration of the inventiveness of bacteria.

Erythromycin and chloramphenicol may also be inactivated enzymatically. In the case of chloramphenicol, the acetyltransferase enzyme is responsible for most clinical resistance.[97] A minor mechanism for resistance to tetracyclines is enzymatic inactivation.[307]

In gram-positive bacteria, resistance to macrolides and lincosamides may be produced by several methods alone or in combination—enzymatic inactivation, alteration of ribosomal targets, or active efflux.[172] Many rRNA methylase genes (erm) have been identified.[271] These genes are particularly important because they produce the MLS$_B$ phenotype, which confers resistance to all macrolides (including clarithromycin and azithromycin), lincosamides (clindamycin), and streptogramins (quinupristin-dalfopristin).

Alteration of Targets. Changes in affinity of ribosomal targets for enzymes are important for resistance to some antimicrobial agents, particularly tetracycline, erythromycin, quinolones, aminoglycosides, trimethoprim, and sulfamethoxazole. Although the primary resistance mechanism for tetracyclines is the efflux mechanism, protection of ribosomes by a soluble protein has also been described as an important secondary mechanism.[307] Alterations in the ribosomal site of action of macrolides and lincosamides, such as erythromycin and clindamycin, are important mechanisms for resistance to this group of antibiotics.[172,338] Mutation in the DNA gyrase target of quinolone antibiotics is the most important mechanism for resistance to this important group of antibiotics in both gram-positive and gram-negative bacteria,[126,127] although resistance may also be mediated by barriers in diffusion through the cell wall. In some genera (e.g., *Staphylococcus aureus* or *Pseudomonas aeruginosa*) a single mutation is sufficient to confer resistance; in others (e.g. *Campylobacter jejuni, Escherichia coli*, or *Neisseria gonorrhoeae*) multiple mutations are required.[127] Aminoglycoside resistance may be mediated by alterations in ribosomal targets as well as by enzymatic inactivation. When this mechanism is operative, there may actually be an accumulation of (ineffective) antibiotic within the bacterial cell.[4] A major mechanism for resistance to both sulfamethoxazole and trimethoprim is alteration of the sequential target enzymes in the biochemical pathway for formation of nucleic acids, dihydropteroate synthetase for sulfonamides, and dihydrofolate reductase for trimethoprim.[132]

Bypass as a Resistance Mechanism. Auxotrophic mutants that require thymine for growth may be able to circumvent the activity of trimethoprim and sulfamethoxazole in vitro by using available substrates and alternative pathways.[245] The most clinically important example of a bypass mechanism is the ability of naturally occurring strains of *Enterococcus* sp. to use compounds such as folinic acid for growth in vivo in the presence of trimethoprim-sulfamethoxazole.[108,348] Strains may appear susceptible in vitro, although they do not respond to chemotherapy in vivo. The in vitro result can be converted from susceptible to resistant by the addition of folinic acid to the testing medium. Enterococci should not, therefore, be tested against trimethoprim-sulfamethoxazole.

INTERACTIONS AMONG RESISTANCE MECHANISMS

Many bacteria have developed multiple resistance mechanisms, and they are often complementary. The presence of multiple, different β-lactamase enzymes in the same bacterium has already been mentioned. A classic case study for resistance problems is *Pseudomonas aeruginosa*, which combines an accumulating list of resistance mechanisms with the ability to cause serious infections in seriously ill patients.[183]

The best example of synergistic defenses is the combination of barriers to diffusion of β-lactam antibiotics through the outer cell membrane of gram-negative bacteria and production of β-lactamases in the confined space of the peptidoglycan layer between the two membranes (Fig. 17-5). As a result the effectiveness with which the enzymes can degrade the antibiotic is considerably enhanced. A military analogy can be used to illustrate the utility of the bacterial strategy. Gram-positive bacteria that allow relatively free access to the inner cell membrane, but can secrete enzyme into the extracellular environment (Fig. 17-4) are analogous to defenders that have heavy-duty long-range artillery, but face an opposing army arrayed on an open plain. In contrast, gram-negative bacteria have only single-shot rifles, but they have positioned their sharpshooters to pick off the enemy soldiers as they march single-file through the mountain pass of the porin channels and peptidoglycan layer. The effect of the combined strategy is well-illustrated by *Serratia marcescens*, which is usually susceptible to third-generation cephalosporins and carbapenems.[122] An isolate that produced large amounts of a chromosomal β-lactamase possessed low-level resistance to these antibiotics. When barriers to passage of antibiotic through the outer membrane were added to the β-lactamase, however, the isolate became highly resistant to the antibiotics.

The complementation phenomenon can also be illustrated by looking at inoculum effects in the interaction between various gram-negative bacteria and β-lactam antibiotics (Fig. 17-9). A β-lactamase producing strain of *Haemophilus influenzae*, which has minimal barriers to transport of ampicillin across the membrane, is effectively killed if the ratio of bacteria to antibiotic molecules is small. If the ratio is increased, however, antibiotic molecules are not able to reach all the bacteria, so that some organisms escape damage and are able to multiply. This phenomenon is known as an inoculum effect, which has potential important implications for testing in the laboratory. In contrast, enteric bacteria that have significant barriers to passage of the antibiotic across the membrane are resistant to bactericidal activity even when few bacteria are present. There is no inoculum effect.

On the other hand, scientists have used their knowledge of the mechanisms of action of antimicrobial agents to construct synergistic combinations that can defeat bacterial resistance mechanisms. The combination of sulfamethoxazole and trimethoprim is a good example of the efficacy of using two drugs that act at different points in an important bacterial biochemical pathway. Similarly, combination of β-lactam antibiotics and inhibitors of β-lactamase has obvious logic as a therapeutic strategy. Finally, the combination of aminoglycoside and β-lactam antibiotics for serious enterococcal infection, which was used initially empirically,[131] has a rational basis once one understands the mechanisms of action of antibiotics and bacterial resistance (Fig. 17-10). Enterococci are intrinsically resistant to aminoglycoside antibiotics, which do not cross the bacterial cell wall efficiently. The addition of β-lactam antibiotics, however, sufficiently disorganizes the cell-wall peptidoglycan that the aminoglycosides can penetrate into the cytoplasm and gain access to their ribosomal targets. The enterococci have, in turn, responded by developing several mechanisms for resistance to the synergistic combination: binding protein alterations and β-lactamase for the penicillins and high-level resistance to the aminoglycosides by enzymatic degradation or ribosomal alterations.

Laboratory Guidance of Antimicrobial Therapy

A chemotherapeutic drug is a chemical compound that is used in the treatment of a disease. The compound may come from natural sources or may have been synthesized by a chemist in the laboratory. The disease may be of any type, including infectious and neoplastic processes. An antibiotic is an antimicrobial agent that is derived from a microorganism; an antimicrobial agent is a drug that acts primarily against infectious organisms.

Microbiologists can be of great assistance to clinicians. They can evaluate the in vitro interactions between an isolated microbe and antimicrobial agents that would be appropriate for treatment of an infection in vivo. Their work in the laboratory can provide data to help the clinician decide whether the selected doses of an antimicrobial agents are adequate.

Several of the commercially available susceptibility systems can provide expedited results, allowing microbiologists to report identification and susceptibility results on the same day that the strain is recovered in culture. Doern and colleagues carefully assessed the clinical impact of ''rapid'' reporting.[70] For 1 year bacterial isolates were tested using an expedited commercial method (rapid group) or traditional overnight methods (conventional group). The mean time to reporting results was 11.3 hours and 19.6 hours in the rapid and conventional groups, respectively. The length of hospitalization was comparable in the two groups, but there were significant improvements in the rapid group for the factors listed in Box 17-2.

A subsequent study of isolates from blood cultures demonstrated a statistical correlation of increased time from collection of blood cultures to initial reporting of results with increased length of hospital stay.[16] In this case more rapid detection of bacteremic isolates with instruments that continuously evaluate growth in blood culture bottles was responsible for the effect. Presumably, more rapid detection and more rapid reporting of susceptibility results could produce additive, if not synergistic, results.

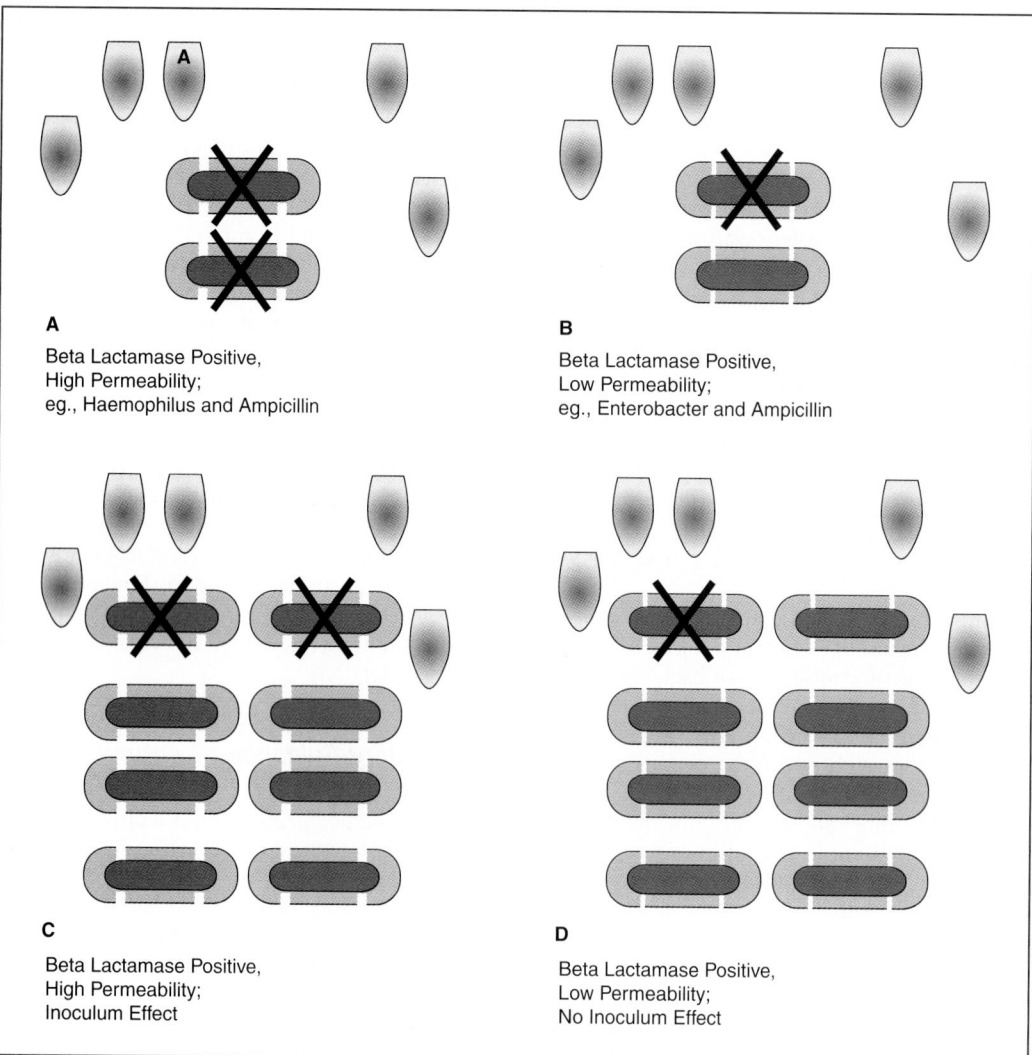

A
Beta Lactamase Positive,
High Permeability;
eg., Haemophilus and Ampicillin

B
Beta Lactamase Positive,
Low Permeability;
eg., Enterobacter and Ampicillin

C
Beta Lactamase Positive,
High Permeability;
Inoculum Effect

D
Beta Lactamase Positive,
Low Permeability;
No Inoculum Effect

Figure 17-9 Complementary activity of β-lactamase and barriers to diffusion through outer membranes, as illustrated by inoculum effects in gram-negative bacteria (**A**) A β-lactamase-producing strain of *Haemophilus influenzae* allows free diffusion of ampicillin (*A*) across the cell wall. Despite the presence of the enzyme the antibiotic is able to kill a small number of bacteria (*X*). (**C**) The presence of a large number of bacteria overcomes the effect of the antibiotic; a portion of the bacterial population escapes injury and is able to replicate. (**B** and **D**) In contrast, a strain of *Enterobacter cloacae* also produces β-lactamase, but in addition restricts entry of the antibiotic to its site of action on the inner plasma membrane. As a result, a portion of the bacterial population is able to escape antibiotic killing and replicate, whether the inoculum is large or small. There is an inoculum effect with *H. influenzae* and ampicillin, but not with *Enterobacter* and ampicillin. The importance of combining two resistance mechanisms—production of inactivating enzymes and restriction of antibiotic transport across the outer cell membrane—is critical for the dichotomous result. Other causes of inoculum effects are discussed in the text.

Figure 17-10 The microbial response of enterococci to the synergistic activity of aminoglycoside and β-lactam antibiotics. In each panel the single-cell membrane and surrounding peptidoglycan cell wall (compare Figure 17-4) of an enterococcus surrounds a cytoplasm that contains ribosomes. (**A**) The intrinsic resistance of enterococci to gentamicin, which does not cross the cell membrane efficiently and thus never reaches its target, the bacterial ribosome. (**B**) A β-lactam antibiotic has disorganized the cell membrane, ''poking holes'' in the membrane so that the aminoglycoside can pour through to reach its ribosomal target. The combination of β-lactam and aminoglycoside, neither of which is fully effective alone, produces a synergistic antimicrobial action. (**C**) The resilient enterococcus has produced β-lactamase, negating the effect of the β-lactam antibiotic and reproducing the situation found in **A.** Once again the

(continued)

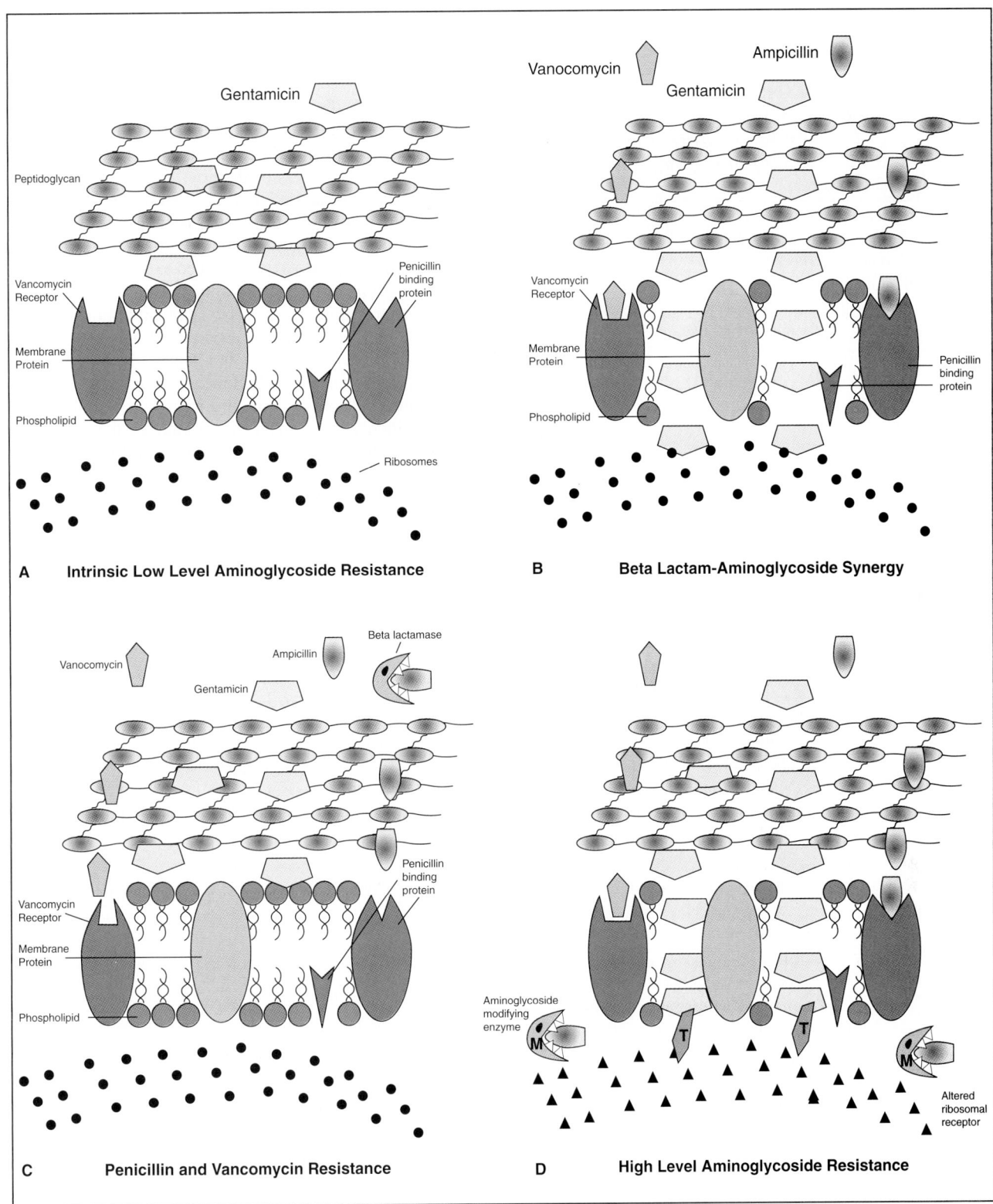

Figure 17-10 (*continued*) aminoglycoside is unable to reach the ribosomal target. **(D)** Another microbial strategy: In this case the β-lactam is still effective and the aminoglycoside is able to reach its ribosomal target. Altered ribosomes, however, block the antibacterial activity of the aminoglycoside (*T*) once it reaches the target. Synergistic activity is no longer present. Alternatively, aminoglycoside-modifying enzymes (*M*) inactivate the antibiotic before it reaches the ribosome. Synergistic activity is again lost, because the bacteria have acquired high-level resistance to the aminoglycoside. Obviously, the bacterial resistance mechanisms depicted in **C** and **D** could both be operative in the same strain, producing a double whammy.

> **Box 17-2 Factors Positively Affected by Rapid Determination of Antimicrobial Susceptibility in Pathogenic Bacteria**
>
> 1. Mortality rate
> 2. Number of laboratory studies performed
> 3. Number of imaging procedures
> 4. Days of intubation
> 5. Days spent in an intensive or intermediate care area
> 6. Time to alteration of antimicrobial therapy
> 7. Total costs of hospitalization

In this chapter, the evaluation of antimicrobial agents that are active against aerobic and facultatively anaerobic bacteria is discussed. Testing of anaerobic bacteria, mycobacteria, and fungi is discussed in Chapters 16, 19, and 21, respectively.

Antimicrobial test procedures are summarized in Table 17-7, which includes a brief description of each test and a list of specimens that the laboratory must have in hand. The tests may be divided conveniently into two groups: (1) tests that *predict* the effectiveness of therapy and (2) tests that *monitor* the effectiveness of therapy.

Several types of antimicrobial susceptibility (preferred to the term "sensitivity") tests have been devised. The two reference tests are the macroscopic broth dilution and agar dilution procedures. Both are designed to quantitate the lowest concentration of an antimicrobial agent that inhibits visible in vitro growth of the microbe—the minimum inhibitory concentration (MIC). The test used most frequently to guide antimicrobial agent therapy is the disk diffusion procedure (Bauer-Kirby test), in which clinical interpretations are derived from correlations with the reference test. In recent years, an increasing number of laboratories have routinely used a miniaturized broth test (microbroth dilution test) or an automated commercial system. The broth-microdilution test has become so prevalent and so well studied that it has become the reference standard for many investigators.

A variety of options for antimicrobial susceptibility studies are now commercially available, including commercially available MIC plates (both frozen and dehydrated),

Table 17-7 Guidance of Antimicrobial Therapy

PROCEDURE	DEFINITION	SPECIMENS	INDICATIONS
Minimum inhibitory concentration (MIC, broth or agar)	Lowest concentration of antimicrobial agent that inhibits visible growth	Microbial isolate	Antimicrobial susceptibility of isolates if etiologic role is established and susceptibility (or resistance) is not predictable
Disk diffusion	Diameter of inhibition of growth around paper disk impregnated with antimicrobial agent	Microbial isolate	Simplified method to approximate MIC with interpretive correlates
Growth curve calculation	Calculated MIC based on effect of antimicrobial agent on the particular species	Microbial isolate	Computer-generated MIC calculation integrated with identification (e.g. Vitek)
Gradient diffusion	MIC determined by intersection of bacterial growth with graded concentrations of antimicrobial agent in paper strip	Microbial isolate	Commercial method (Etest) valuable in selected situations
Molecular detection	Molecular demonstration of gene(s) or gene product(s) responsible for resistance	Microbial isolate	Most useful when a single resistance gene is present, e.g. alterations in PBP 2 in staphylococci; also used for characterization of β-lactamases
Minimum bactericidal concentrations	Lowest concentration of antimicrobial agent that kills 99.9% of the inoculum	Microbial isolate	Rarely indicated; possibly streptococcal endocarditis; potentially for osteomyelitis; potentially tolerant isolates if unresponsive to therapy
Antimicrobial levels	Concentration (μg/mL) of antimicrobial agent in serum	Peak serum, Trough serum	Unpredictability of peak levels or potential for toxicity; may be incorporated in a management algorithm
Serum bactericidal titers	Dilution of serum that kills 99.9% of the inoculum	Peak serum, Trough serum, Microbial isolate	Rarely indicated; possibly bacterial endocarditis, osteomyelitis, gram-negative sepsis in immunocompromised patients
Synergy tests	Synergistic activity of multiple antimicrobial agents	Microbial isolate	Research procedure for development of therapeutic regimens; rarely, confirmation of synergy against individual isolates, most commonly in respiratory isolates from patients with cystic fibrosis

computer-assisted growth analysis, and gradient diffusion. For the purposes of discussion in this chapter these approaches will be included in the designation "dilution tests" or "MIC tests."

The remaining antimicrobial agent test procedures are rarely used or are usually performed in clinical chemistry laboratories. These supplemental test procedures are listed in Box 17-3. The interested reader can consult the previous edition of this book.

The most useful means for assessing the adequacy of antimicrobial therapy in many infections are the clinical response of the patient to treatment and, if needed, the demonstration by repeated culture that the infecting organism either has been eliminated (bacterial cure) or persists (bacterial failure). Unfortunately, a bacterial cure does not always ensure a successful clinical outcome.

It is important to emphasize that antimicrobial agent susceptibility tests are intended to be a guide for the clinician, not a guarantee that an antimicrobial agent will be effective in therapy. A goal of microbiologists has been, and should continue to be, the provision of standardized in vitro tests that can be reproduced from day to day and from laboratory to laboratory. Without reproducibility there is no scientific basis for therapy. In striving for standardization, however, it is possible that the variability of each infection and each patient is not addressed. The factors that determine the outcome of an infectious process are complex and, in many instances, are incompletely addressed by in vitro tests.[332] The examples that follow may clarify the elusiveness of an absolute correlation between laboratory interactions and clinical outcome.

pH: Microbial susceptibility tests are standardized at physiologic pH (7.2 to 7.4), yet unphysiologic levels of pH often develop at the sites of purulent infections (such as bacterial meningitis[298] or abscesses[121]). Some antimicrobial agents, such as the penicillins and cephalosporins, function well at a wide range of pH. Tetracyclines function better in more acidic environments and might actually perform better in an acidic inflammatory exudate than in laboratory culture media. In contrast, aminoglycosides and macrolides, such as erythromycin, are less effective in acidic environments than at neutral pH. Although high concentrations of aminoglycosides may be achieved in the urinary tract, the drugs will not function optimally if the pH of the urine is low.

Box 17-3 Miscellaneous Antimicrobial Agent Test Procedures

1. Determination of bactericidal activity as well as inhibitory activity of antimicrobial agents against bacterial isolates
2. Measurement of antibacterial activity of drugs in combination, also known as synergy testing
3. Quantitation of antimicrobial agent levels in body fluids, especially serum
4. Determination of serum bactericidal activity, sometimes referred to as the Schlichter test

---

Cations: With certain combinations of bacterium and antimicrobial agent, most notably *Pseudomonas aeruginosa* and aminoglycosides, the concentration of divalent cations, particularly calcium (Ca^{2+}) and magnesium (Mg^{2+}), has a dramatic effect on the apparent in vitro susceptibility. A result that ranges from susceptible to resistant can be achieved by varying the cation concentration,[264] because of changes in transport of the antimicrobial agent across the cell membrane. Agar and broth media vary greatly in the concentration of divalent cations. By convention, testing is done under physiologic conditions.

Inoculum: For some combinations of bacterium and antimicrobial agent, the inoculum is of great importance in determining the in vitro susceptibility.[79] Enzymatic inactivation of β-lactam antibiotics, such as the penicillins and cephalosporins, is an important mechanism of bacterial resistance. These enzymes are always expressed in some bacteria but must be induced by the presence of the antibiotic in other bacteria. If small numbers of *Staphylococcus aureus*, which contains an inducible β-lactamase, are incubated in vitro with penicillin, the bacteria may be killed before the enzyme can be produced in effective quantities. In contrast, large numbers of bacteria in an active, clinical infection may survive to produce the inactivating enzyme and destroy the antibiotic. In this case, a false impression of bacterial susceptibility and false sense of security might be produced by the laboratory test.

When staphylococci and β-lactamase-resistant penicillins, such as methicillin, interact, only a small fraction of bacteria express resistance (heteroresistance). Therefore, if the inoculum is small, the resistant bacterial cells may not be included. The number of bacteria in infected patients varies greatly, so the standardized inocula used in the laboratory represent a reasonable compromise rather than a reproduction of in vivo conditions.

Finally, the interaction between β-lactamases and the membranes of gram-negative bacteria may result in inoculum effects, as illustrated in Figure 17-9.

Clinical pharmacology: The penetration of antimicrobial agents into sites of infection is another important variable that cannot be addressed in vitro. High concentrations of antimicrobial agents may be achieved in sites where they are excreted from the body, usually the urine or the bile. In contrast, low concentrations relative to serum may be found in tissues such as prostatic fluid, bone, or cerebrospinal fluid. In the case of chloramphenicol, excretion is via the biliary tract, and the drug does not appear in the urine. The reverse holds for certain antimicrobial agents, such as nitrofurantoin and norfloxacin, which do not achieve effective levels in sites other than the urinary tract.

The ineffectiveness of many antimicrobial agents, such as the aminoglycosides, in the treatment of *Legionella* infections, despite their excellent activity in vitro, is probably caused by the poor penetration of the antibiotics into macrophages where the bacteria are growing.[205] In other situations, bacterial physiology is a significant determinant (e.g., bypass of trimethoprim and sulfonamide effects by enterococci; see section on enterococci below).

Some interactions favor resolution of infection, even if the antimicrobial therapy is suboptimal. The inflammatory and immune defenses of the patient are essential to a successful clinical outcome. It is clear that low concentrations of antimicrobial agents, below the concentration necessary to kill the bacterium, may enhance the ability of phagocytic cells to ingest and kill an infecting microorganism.[128]

Many infections, particularly those caused by obligately anaerobic bacteria, are synergistic; that is, the bacteria depend on each other for survival. Such an infection may be cured by drugs that are ineffective against some of the infecting bacteria if the essential participants are eliminated.[273] Considering all the factors that influence the outcome of an infection, it is imperative that the laboratory provide physicians with the ''track record'' of the antimicrobial agent to guide them in the selection of appropriate antimicrobial agent therapy. Well-designed clinical studies have demonstrated a correlation of outcome with the appropriateness of therapy.[337] Physicians must, therefore, correlate the results of antimicrobial agent susceptibility tests and clinical experience when selecting therapeutic regimens for patients with similar infections.

Tests for Determining Inhibitory Activity of Antimicrobial Agents
Indications

Tests of inhibitory activity of antimicrobial agents are designed for bacteria that grow well after overnight incubation in air and have unpredictable susceptibilities. Fastidious bacteria, which grow more slowly or require nutritional or atmospheric supplements, should be tested with a dilution test only if careful use of control bacterial strains demonstrates the absence of inhibitory effects on the interactions. The disk diffusion test may be modified for such organisms if the procedure has been validated by comparison to reference tests and to clinical experience.[222]

Microbiologists should resist pressure from clinicians to extend the procedures beyond their established limits. Many mistakes were made by participants in the proficiency testing surveys of the College of American Pathologists in the determination of the susceptibility of *Listeria monocytogenes* to penicillin and ampicillin because the published guidelines were not designed for this bacterium.[144] Further studies made it possible to establish valid guidelines for *Listeria* species, and results of the surveys have improved.

The list of bacteria that have consistently predictable susceptibilities is, unfortunately, becoming shorter. The prevalence of β-lactamase–producing strains of *Haemophilus influenzae* and *Neisseria gonorrhoeae* is sufficiently high that susceptibility to penicillin analogues can no longer be assumed.[66] Pneumococci that are relatively resistant to penicillin (MIC, 0.12–1.0 µg/mL) or have high-level resistance (MIC, >1.0 µg/mL) are increasingly common in the United States, and pneumococcal strains isolated from serious infections should be tested for resistance.[63] Even vancomycin, the bastion of antibiotic therapy for infections caused by gram-positive bacteria, has developed chinks in its armor against enterococci[103] and staphylococci.[94] Almost alone, *Streptococcus pyogenes* remains susceptible to penicillin,

although resistance to macrolide antibiotics has become a fact of life in several important genera of gram-positive cocci.[39,63,172]

In a variety of situations, summarized in Table 17-8, susceptibility tests should not be performed and/or the results should not be reported to clinicians. Some of these issues are considered more completely in appropriate sections of this chapter.

In some cases susceptibility or resistance is still predictable and routine testing is not indicated. Testing may be indicated when the clinical response is not as expected. It should be remembered, however, that there may be alternative explanations for the lack of a clinical response. Most commonly, patients with *Streptococcus pyogenes* pharyngitis suffer clinical and/or bacteriologic relapses, after which clinicians suspect resistance to penicillin. As mentioned, resistance of *S. pyogenes* to penicillin has not yet been detected; of the possible alternative explanations for the relapse the most likely is inadequate penetration of orally administered antibiotic into the crypts of the tonsils and adenoids where the bacteria lurk. Microbiologists must of course be ready to revise the list when appropriate.

Only isolates producing an infection should be tested. Bacteria recovered from a normally sterile body fluid are usually pathogenic. If the potentially pathogenic bacterium is isolated from a site that contains colonizing flora, such as the upper respiratory tract or the skin, the culture should be scrutinized more closely before a susceptibility test is performed, particularly if multiple species of organisms are present. Examination of a Gram-stained smear may document the inclusion of squamous epithelial cells, which suggests contamination by colonized secretions, or the absence of segmented neutrophils, which indicates the lack of an inflammatory response. In situations in which the microbiologist cannot determine the suitability of a susceptibility test, consultation with the clinician is appropriate.

Choice of Test

In most situations either a disk diffusion (Chart 17-1) or a microbroth dilution (Chart 17-2) test is adequate to guide clinical therapy. A more recent alternative is the gradient diffusion test (Etest, AB Biodisk, Solna, Sweden) (Chart 17-3). Advantages of dilution tests are that they provide more quantitative information and may be applied to a wider range of isolates than the diffusion test. There is definite potential, however, for misinterpretation of a quantitative result if physicians do not understand how to use the information and the laboratory fails to provide sufficient guidance in interpretation. The disk diffusion test has a long and successful track record. The choice of which method to use will depend on local needs and resources. For evaluation of susceptibility tests, most investigators use the following convention:

- Very major error: characterization of a resistant isolate as susceptible
- Major error: characterization of a susceptible isolate as resistant
- Minor error: characterization of a susceptible or resistant isolate as intermediate, or characterization of an intermediate isolate as susceptible or resistant.

Table 17-8 Situations in Which Antimicrobial Testing Should Not Be Performed and/or the Results Not Reported

CATEGORY	ANTIMICROBIAL AGENT(S)	ORGANISM(S)	SITE	ACTION	RATIONALE
Susceptibility predictable	Penicillins	*Streptococcus pyogenes; Streptococcus agalactiae*	All	Do not test routinely; send resistant isolates to a reference laboratory	Testing not indicated
	Nitrofurantoin; trimethoprim-sulfamethoxazole;	*Staphylococcus saprophyticus*	Urine	Testing not necessary	Susceptibility predictable
Resistance predictable	Trimethoprim-sulfamethoxazole	fluoroquinolones *Streptococcus pyogenes*	All	Do not test routinely	Testing not indicated
Antimicrobial agent does not accumulate at site of infection	First- and second-generation cephalosporins; clindamycin; macrolides; tetracyclines; fluoroquinolones; antibiotics administered orally	All	CSF	Do not test	Antimicrobial agents do not penetrate into CSF or do not accumulate in therapeutic concentrations
	Various	*Streptococcus pneumoniae*	CSF	Test and report only penicillin, cefotaxime, ceftriaxone, meropenem, and/or vancomycin	Clinical efficacy not clearly established at concentrations achieved in CSF
	Chloramphenicol	All	Urinary tract	Do not test	Antibiotic excreted through biliary tract; not excreted in urine
	Norfloxacin; Nitrofurantoin	All	Non-urine sites	Do not test	Antibiotic excreted in urine; urine; does not reach therapeutic concentrations in other sites
In vitro testing does not predict resistance reliably	Cephalosporins	*Enterococcus* spp.; *Listeria monocytogenes*	All	Do not test	Testing not indicated and susceptibility results may be misleading
	Aminoglycosides (low dose)	*Enterococcus* spp.	All	Do not test	Testing not indicated except high dose testing for determination of synergy; susceptible results may be misleading
	Clindamycin; trimethoprim; trimethoprim-sulfamethoxazole	*Enterococcus* spp.	All	Do not test	Testing not indicated and susceptibility results may be misleading
	All β-lactam antibiotics	*Staphylococcus* spp. resistant to oxacillin	All	Report as resistant	Susceptibility results do not predict clinical efficacy and will be misleading
	First- and second-generation cephalosporins; aminoglycosides	*Salmonella* spp.; *Shigella* spp.	All	Do not test or report as resistant	Susceptibility results do not predict clinical efficacy and wil be misleading
	β-Lactam antibiotics except carbapenems (imipenem and meropenem)	*Escherichia coli* and *Klebsiella pneumoniae* that produce extended-spectrum β-lactamases	All	Do not report or report as resistant	Susceptibility results do not predict clinical efficacy and will be misleading

Adapted from references[217,218].

Selection of Antimicrobial Agents

The final selection of antimicrobial agents for the hospital formulary should be decided in consultation with members of the medical staff. Lists of antimicrobial agents that have been suggested by the Clinical and Laboratory Standards Institute (CLSI) (formerly the National Committee for Clinical Laboratory Standards) are detailed in Tables 17-9 and 17-10.[1]

Note that many antimicrobial agents are grouped by class because the spectrum of activity is similar. The recent recommendations of the CLSI address selective testing and selective reporting, recognizing that the issues are complex and vary from institution to institution. Washington has provided a guide to the antimicrobial groupings (Table 17-11).[333] It is not necessary to test each antimicrobial agent in the list. Patterns of antimicrobial agent usage and bacterial resistance in each community should be known and considered when selecting antimicrobial agents for testing. Distinctions may be made between antimicrobial agents that are tested routinely and those for which results are reported routinely to physicians.

Tables 17-9 and 17-10 offer choices of antimicrobial agents for testing. In some cases several antimicrobial agents may be therapeutically equivalent—i.e., they provide a similar spectrum of antimicrobial activity. The results of in vitro testing of a specific isolate for one agent, however, may not predict the in vitro result for other antimicrobial agents in the group; in effect, these antimicrobial agents are equivalent but not necessarily equally effective against every isolate. Each agent in the group that is considered for therapeutic use must be tested.

In contrast the results of in vitro testing of some antimicrobial agents may be applied to close relatives. It is not necessary to test each agent in the group. Some of these situations are detailed in Table 17-12.[217,218]

Standardization

The major improvement in laboratory guidance of susceptibility testing over the past several decades has come from the development of standardized procedures that have been widely adopted. It is extremely important to adhere to the recommended protocols if reproducible results are to be achieved. The CLSI publishes standards for these and other tests on a continuing basis. (Copies of the *Performance Standards for Antimicrobial Disk Susceptibility Tests* and the *Methods for Dilution Antimicrobial Susceptibility Tests for Bacteria that Grow Aerobically* may be obtained on request by writing the CLSI at 940 West Valley Road, Suite 1400, Wayne, PA 19087-1898).[217–220] It is important that revised

procedures and current recommendations be promptly promulgated in all clinical laboratories. An institutional membership in the CLSI ensures the timely receipt of all new and revised recommendations. Washington has summarized the resources and processes of this national consensus organization that affect clinical microbiologists.[333]

The following parameters are some of the important facets of susceptibility testing that have been standardized.

GROWTH MEDIUM

Mueller-Hinton broth and agar have been selected for testing aerobic and facultatively anaerobic bacterial isolates. These formulations most closely approximate the criteria for a reproducible medium. They contain dehydrated beef infusion, acid digest of casein, and cornstarch. Most pathogens grow satisfactorily, and the media have minimal inhibitory effect on sulfonamides, trimethoprim, and tetracycline.[10] Large quantities of thymidine are present in some lots of media. Some organisms can use the thymidine to bypass the mechanism of action of trimethoprim and grow, even though they are innately resistant to the antibiotic. Enterococci are particularly affected; isolated colonies may appear within the established zone of inhibition around disks that contain trimethoprim.

It is obvious from examining the formula that even Mueller-Hinton medium is not chemically defined.[171] Agar is a natural compound that is prepared from red seaweed. Variation occurs in the composition of agar among manufacturers and even among lots produced by a single company, depending on the source of the seaweed. Attempts to minimize the variation among lots of Mueller-Hinton agar continue. A reference standard for manufacturers may provide greater reproducibility.[256] A specially formulated medium for testing of *Haemophilus influenzae* has been developed and recommended by the CLSI for routine use.[154] This *Haemophilus* test medium can also be used for *Haemophilus* spp., as described below.[151]

pH

The pH of the medium should be between 7.2 and 7.4 at room temperature. The pH of broth media may be tested directly with a pH electrode, and agar media may be tested by macerating enough agar so that the tip of the electrode can be submerged, by allowing a portion of agar to solidify around the electrode, or by using a properly calibrated surface electrode.

SERUM

Antibiotics differ greatly in the degree to which they bind to proteins. In the bloodstream, free antibiotic is in equilibrium with serum protein-bound antibiotic. Free and protein-bound antibiotic can be measured, but it is not clear which is the more useful result. In the laboratory, different values can be obtained for highly protein-bound antibiotics if serum is added to the medium. The CLSI method does not include added serum because of the difficulty in standardization of the product and uncertainty about how to interpret the results. Perl and colleagues studied the effect of serum on 11 broad-spectrum antibiotics used to treat nosocomial gram-

---

[1] Permission to use portions of M100-S7 (MIC Testing. Supplemental Tables, January 2003) and M100-S13 (Disk Diffusion: Supplemental Tables, January 2003) has been granted by the NCCLS. The interpretive data are valid only if the methods in M7-A6 (Methods for dilution antimicrobial susceptibility tests for bacteria that grow aerobically; Approved standard. 6th Ed.) and M2-A8 (Performance standards for antimicrobial disk susceptibility tests; Approved standard. 8th Ed.) are followed. The NCCLS periodically updates the M2 and M7 tables through new editions of the standards and supplements. Users should refer to the most recent editions. The current standards may be obtained from NCCLS, 940 West Valley Road, Suite 1400, Wayne, PA 19087, or from their web site (http://www.nccls.org/).

Table 17-9 **Suggested Groupings of FDA-Approved Antimicrobial Agents That Should Be Considered for Routine Testing and Reporting on Nonfastidious Organisms by Clinical Microbiology Laboratories**

	ENTEROBACTERIACEAE[g]	PSEUDOMONAS AERUGINOSA AND OTHER NON-ENTEROBACTERIACEAE[j]	STAPHYLOCOCCUS SPP.	ENTEROCOCCUS SPP.[n]
GROUP A PRIMARY TEST AND REPORT	Ampicillin[g] Cefazolin[a] Cephalothin[a] Gentamicin	Ceftazidime Gentamicin Mezlocillin or ticarcillin Piperacillin	Oxacillin[l] Penicillin[l]	Penicillin[o] or ampicillin
GROUP B[e] PRIMARY TEST REPORT SELECTIVELY	Amikacin Amoxicillin-clavulanic acid or ampicillin-sulbactam Piperacillin-tazobactam Ticarcillin-clavulanic acid Cefamandole or cefonicid or cefuroxime Cefepime Cefmetazole Cefoperazone[g] Cefotetan Cefoxitin Cefotaxime[g,h,i] or ceftizoxime[g,i] or ceftriaxone[g,h,i] Ciprofloxacin[g] or levofloxacin[g] Ertapenem Imipenem or meropenem Mezlocillin or piperacillin Ticarcillin Trimethoprim-sulfamethoxazole[g]	Amikacin Cefepime Cefoperazone Aztreonam Ciprofloxacin Imipenem Meropenem Ticarcillin-clavulanic acid[k] Tobramycin Trimethoprim-sulfamethoxazole[k]	Azithromycin[d] or clarithromycin[d] or erythromycin[d] Clindamycin[d] Linezolid Trimethoprim-sulfamethoxazole Vancomycin	Linezolid Quinupristin-dalfopristin[r] Vancomycin[p]
GROUP C[f] SUPPLEMENTAL REPORT SELECTIVELY	Aztreonam Ceftazidime (Both are helpful indicators of extended-spectrum β-lactamases.)[i] Chloramphenicol[d,g] Kanamycin Netilmicin Tetracycline[b] Tobramycin	Cefotaxime or ceftriaxone Chloramphenicol[d,k] Netilmicin	Chloramphenicol[d] Ciprofloxacin or levofloxacin or ofloxacin Gatifloxacin Gentamicin Quinupristin-dalfopristin[m] Rifampin[c] Tetracycline[b]	Gentamicin (high-level resistance screen only) Streptomycin (high-level resistance screen only) Chloramphenicol[d] Erythromycin[d] Rifampin[c] Tetracycline[b] (These agents may be tested for VRE.)[q]
GROUP U SUPPLEMENTAL FOR URINE ONLY	Carbenicillin Cinoxacin Lomefloxacin or norfloxacin or ofloxacin Gatifloxacin Loracarbef Nitrofurantoin Sulfisoxazole Trimethoprim	Carbenicillin Ceftizoxime Levofloxacin or lomefloxacin or norfloxacin or ofloxacin Sulfisoxazole Tetracycline[b,k]	Lomefloxacin or norfloxacin Nitrofurantoin Sulfisoxazole Trimethoprim	Ciprofloxacin Levofloxacin Norfloxacin Nitrofurantoin Tetracycline[b]

(Continued)

Table 17-9 *Continued*

Warning: The following antimicrobial agents should not be routinely reported for bacteria isolated from the CSF and which are included in this document. These antimicrobial agents are not the drugs of choice and may not be effective for treating CSF infections caused by these organisms (i.e., the bacteria included in Tables 2A to 2J):

agents administered by oral route only
first- and second-generation cephalosporins (except cefuroxime sodium)
clindamycin
macrolides
tetracyclines

fluoroquinolones

Note 1: Selection of the most appropriate antimicrobial agents to test and to report is a decision made best by each clinical laboratory in consultation with the infectious-disease practitioners and the pharmacy, as well as the pharmacy and therapeutics and infection control committees of the medical staff. The lists for each organism group comprise agents of proven efficacy that show acceptable in vitro test performance. Considerations in the assignment of agents to Groups A, B, C, and U include clinical efficacy, prevalence of resistance, minimizing emergence of resistance, cost, and current consensus recommendations for first-choice and alternative drugs, in addition to the specific comments in footnotes f and g. Tests of selected agents may be useful for infection control purposes.

Note 2: The boxes in the table designate clusters of comparable agents that need not be duplicated in testing, because interpretive results are usually similar and clinical efficacy comparable. In addition, "or" designates a related group of agents that has an almost identical spectrum of activity and interpretive results, and for which cross-resistance and susceptibility are nearly complete. Therefore, usually only one of the agents within each selection box (cluster or related group) need be selected for testing. Agents that are reported must be tested, unless reporting based on testing another agent provides a more accurate result (e.g., susceptibility of staphylococci to cefazolin or cephalothin based on oxacillin testing), and they usually should match those included in the hospital formulary; or else the report should include footnotes indicating the agents that usually have comparable interpretive results. Finally, unexpected results should be considered for reporting (e.g., resistance of *Enterobacteriaceae* to third-generation cephalosporins or imipenem).

Note 3: Information in boldface type in considered tentative for 1 year.

General Comments

[a] *Cephalothin can be used to represent cephalothin, cephapirin, cephradine, cephalexin, cefaclor, and cefadroxil. Cefazolin, cefuroxime, cefpodoxime, cefprozil, and loracarbef (urinary isolates only) may be tested individually, because some isolates may be susceptible to these agents when resistant to cephalothin.*

[b] *Organisms that are susceptible to tetracycline are also considered susceptible to doxycycline and minocycline. However, some organisms that are intermediate or resistant to tetracycline may be susceptible to doxycycline or minocycline or both.*

[c] ***Rx:*** *Rifampin should not be used alone for chemotherapy.*

[d] *Not routinely reported on organisms isolated from the urinary tract.*

[e] *Group B represents agents that may warrant primary testing but which should be reported only selectively, such as when the organism is resistant to agents of the same family in Group A. Other indications for reporting the result might include selected specimen sources (e.g., selected third-generation cephalosporins for isolates of enteric bacteria from CSF or trimethoprim-sulfamethoxazole for urinary tract isolates); stated allergy or intolerance, or failure to respond to an agent in Group A; polymicrobial infections; infections involving multiple sites with different microorganisms; or reports to infection control for epidemiologic aid.*

[f] *Group C represents alternative or supplemental antimicrobial agents that may require testing in institutions that harbor endemic or epidemic strains resistant to one or more of the primary drugs (especially in the same family, e.g., β-lactams or aminoglycosides), or for treatment of unusual organisms (e.g., chloramphenicol for some Pseudomonas spp., and chloramphenicol, erythromycin, rifampin, and tetracycline for some vancomycin-resistant enterococci), or reporting to infection control as an epidemiologic aid.*

Enterobacteriaceae

[g] *For fecal isolates of Salmonella and Shigella spp., only ampicillin, a fluoroquinolone, and trimethoprim-sulfamethoxazole should be tested and reported routinely. In addition, chloramphenicol and a third-generation cephalosporin should be tested and reported for extraintestinal isolates of Salmonella spp.*

[h] *Cefotaxime and ceftriaxone should be tested and reported on isolates from CSF in place of cephalothin and cefazolin.*

[i] *Strains of Klebsiella spp. and E. coli that produce ESBLs may be clinically resistant to therapy with penicillins, cephalosporins, or aztreonam, despite apparent in vitro susceptibility to some of these agents. Some of these strains will show MICs above the normal susceptible population but below the standard breakpoints for certain extended-spectrum cephalosporins or aztreonam; such strains may be screened for potential ESBL production by using the screening breakpoints listed at the end of Table 2A, **Initial Screen Test.** Other strains may test intermediate or resistant by standard breakpoints to one or more of these agents. In all strains with ESBLs, the MICs for one or more of the extended-spectrum cephalosporins or aztreonam should decrease in the presence of clavulanic acid **as described at the end of Table 2A, Phenotypic Confirmatory Test.** For all confirmed ESBL-producing strains, the test interpretation should be reported as resistant for all penicillins, cephalosporins, and aztreonam. (See Glossary I for specific agents included in the antimicrobial class, penicillins, and antimicrobial subclass, cephalosporins.)*

Pseudomonas aeruginosa and Other Non-Enterobacteriaceae

[j] *Non-Enterobacteriaceae include Acinetobacter spp., Stenotrophomonas maltophilia, Pseudomonas spp., and other nonfastidious, glucose-nonfermenting, gram-negative bacilli.*

[k] *May be indicated for primary testing of some Pseudomonas spp. (other than P. aeruginosa), S. maltophilia (moxalactam may also be tested), and Acinetobacter spp. (ampicillin-sulbactam may be tested and reported for Acinetobacter spp. resistant to other agents).*

Staphylococcus spp.

[l] *Penicillin-susceptible staphylococci are also susceptible to other penicillins, cephems, and carbapenems approved for use by the FDA for staphylococcal infections. Penicillin-resistant, oxacillin-susceptible strains are resistant to **penicillinase-**labile penicillins but susceptible to other **penicillinase-**stable penicillins, β-lactam/β-lactamase inhibitor combinations, relevant cephems, and carbapenems. (See Glossary I for specific agents included in the antimicrobial class or antimicrobial subclass indicated Oxacillin-resistant staphylococci are resistant to all currently available β-lactam antibiotics. Thus, susceptibility or resistance to a wide array of β-lactam antibiotics may be deduced from testing only penicillin and oxacillin. Routine testing of other penicillins, β-lactamase inhibitor combinations, cephems, and carbapenems is not advised.*

[m] *For reporting against methicillin-susceptible Staphylococcus aureus.*

Enterococcus spp.

[n] ***Warning:*** *For Enterococcus spp., cephalosporins, aminoglycosides (except for high-level resistance screening), clindamycin, and trimethoprim- sulfamethoxazole may appear active in vitro but are not effective clinically and should not be reported as susceptible.*

[o] *Penicillin susceptibility may be used to predict the susceptibility to ampicillin, amoxicillin, ampicillin-sulbactam, amoxicillin-clavulanic acid, piperacillin, and piperacillin-tazobactam for non-β-lactamase-producing enterococci. For blood and CSF isolates, a β-lactamase test is also recommended. **Rx:** Combination therapy of penicillin or ampicillin, plus an aminoglycoside, is usually indicated for serious enterococcal infections, such as endocarditis.*

Table 17-10 Suggested Groupings of FDA-Approved Antimicrobial Agents That Should Be Considered for Routine Testing and Reporting on Fastidious Organisms by Clinical Microbiology Laboratories

	HAEMOPHILUS SPP.[e]	*NEISSERIA GONORRHOEAE*[i]	*STREPTOCOCCUS PNEUMONIAE*	*STREPTOCOCCUS* SPP. OTHER THAN *S. PNEUMONIAE*
GROUP A PRIMARY TEST AND REPORT	Ampicillin[e,g] Trimethoprim-sulfamethoxazole		Erythromycin[a] Penicillin[j] Trimethoprim-sulfamethoxazole	Erythromycin[a,m] Penicillin[l,n] or ampicillin[l,n]
GROUP B[b] PRIMARY TEST	Cefuroxime sodium (parenteral) Cefotaxime[e] or ceftazidime or ceftizoxime[e] or ceftriaxone[e] Chloramphenicol[e] Meropenem[e,h]		Cefepime Cefotaxime[j] or ceftriaxone[j] Clindamycin Gatifloxacin, levofloxacin, moxifloxcin, sparfloxacin Ofloxacin, Gemifloxacin Tetracycline[d] Vancomycin[j]	Chloramphenicol[m] Clindamycin[m] Vancomycin
GROUP C[c] SUPPLEMENTAL REPORT SELECTIVELY	Azithromycin[f] or clarithromycin[f] Aztreonam Amoxicillin-clavulanic acid[f] Cefaclor[f] or cefprozil[f] or loracarbef[f] Cefdinir[f] or cefixime[f] or cefpodoxime[f] Cefonicid Cefuroxime axetil[f] (oral) Ciprofloxacin or gatifloxacin or levofloxacin or lomefloxacin or moxifloxacin or ofloxacin or sparfloxacin Ertapenem or imipenem Rifampin Tetracycline[d]	Cefixime or cefotaxime or cefpodoxime or ceftizoxime or ceftriaxone Cefmetazole Cefotetan Cefoxitin Cefuroxime Ciprofloxacin or gatifloxacin or ofloxacin Penicillin Spectinomycin Tetracycline[d]	Amoxicillin or amoxicillin-clavulanic acid Cefuroxime Chloramphenicol Ertapenem Imipenem Linezolid Rifampin[k]	Cefepime or cefotaxime or ceftriaxone Levofloxacin Ofloxacin Linezolid Quinupristin-dalfopristin[o]

Warning: The following antimicrobial agents should not be routinely reported for bacteria isolated from the CSF and which are included in this document. These antimicrobial agents are not the drugs of choice and may not be effective for treating CSF infections caused by these organisms (i.e., the bacteria included in Tables 2A to 2J:

agents administered by oral route only
first- and second-generation cephalosporins (except cefuroxime sodium)
clindamycin
macrolides
tetracyclines
fluoroquinolones

Table 17-10 *Continued*

NOTE 1: Selection of the most appropriate antimicrobial agents to test and to report is a decision made best by each clinical laboratory in consultation with the infectious-disease practitioners and the pharmacy, as well as the pharmacy and therapeutics and infection control committees of the medical staff. The lists for each organism group comprise agents of proven efficacy that show acceptable in vitro test performance. Considerations in the assignment of agents to Groups A, B, and C include clinical efficacy, prevalence of resistance, minimizing emergence of resistance, cost, and current consensus recommendations for first-choice and alternative drugs, in addition to the specific comments in footnotes b and c. Tests on selected agents may be useful for infection-control purposes.

NOTE 2: The boxes in the table designate clusters of comparable agents that need not be duplicated in testing, because interpretive results are usually similar and clinical efficacy comparable. In addition, "or" designates a related group of agents that has an almost identical spectrum of activity and interpretive results, and for which cross-resistance and susceptibility are nearly complete. Therefore, usually only one of the agents within each selection box (cluster or related group) need be selected for testing. Agents that are reported must be tested, unless reporting based on testing another agent provides a more accurate result, and usually, they should match those included in the hospital formulary; or else the report should include footnotes indicating the agents that usually show comparable interpretive results. Lastly, unexpected results should be considered for reporting.

NOTE 3: Information in boldface type is considered tentative for 1 year.

General Comments

[a] *Susceptibility and resistance to azithromycin, clarithromycin, and dirithromycin can be predicted by testing erythromycin.*

[b] *Group B represents agents that may warrant primary testing but which should be reported only selectively, such as when the organism is resistant to agents of the same class in Group A. Other indications for reporting the result might include selected specimen sources (e.g., third-generation cephalosporin for isolates of H. influenzae from CSF); stated allergy or intolerance, or failure to respond to an agent in Group A; polymicrobial infections; infections involving multiple sites with different microorganisms; or reports to infection control for epidemiologic acid.*

[c] *Group C represents alternative or supplemental antimicrobial agents that may require testing in institutions that harbor endemic or epidemic strains resistant to one or more of the primary drugs (especially in the same class, e.g., β-lactams), or for treatment of unusual organisms, or reporting to infection control as an epidemiologic aid.*

[d] **Organisms that are susceptible to tetracycline are also considered susceptible to doxycycline and minocycline.**
Haemophilus spp.

[e] *Only results of testing with ampicillin, one of the third-generation cephalosporins, chloramphenicol, and meropenem should be reported routinely with CSF isolates with Haemophilus influenzae.*

[f] *Amoxicillin-clavulanic acid, azithromycin, clarithromycin, cefaclor, cefprozil, loracarbef, cefdinir, cefixime, cefpodoxime, and cefuroxime axetil are oral agents that may be used by empiric therapy for respiratory tract infections due to Haemophilus spp. The results of susceptibility test with these antimicrobial agents are often not useful for treatment of individual patients. However, susceptibility testing of Haemophilus spp. with these compounds may be appropriate for surveillance or epidemiologic studies.*

[g] *The results of ampicillin susceptibility tests should be used to predict the activity of amoxicillin. The majority of isolates of H. influenzae that are resistant to ampicillin and amoxicillin produce a TEM-type β-lactamase. In most cases, a direct β-lactamase test can provide a rapid means of detecting ampicillin and amoxicillin resistance.*

[h] *Clinical indications and relevant pathogens include bacterial meningitis and concurrent bacteremia in association with meningitis caused by Haemophilus influenzae (β-lactamase- and non-β-lactamase producing strains.)*
Neisseria gonorrhoeae

[i] *A β-lactamase test will detect one form of penicillin resistance in N. gonorrhoeae and also may be used to provide epidemiologic information. Strains with chromosomally mediated resistance can be detected only by additional susceptibility testing, such as the disk diffusion method or the agar dilution MIC method.*
Streptococcus pneumoniae

[j] *Only results of testing with penicillin, cefotaxime, ceftriaxone, meropenem, and vancomycin should be reported routinely for CSF isolates of S. pneumoniae.*

[k] **Rx:** *Rifampin should not be used alone for chemotherapy.*
Streptococcus spp.

[l] **Rx:** *Penicillin or ampicillin intermediate isolates may require combined therapy with an aminoglycoside for bactericidal action.*

[m] *Not routinely reported for organisms isolated from the urinary tract.*

[n] *Susceptibility testing of penicillins and other β-lactams approved by FDA for treatment of Streptococcus pyogenes or Streptococcus agalactiae is not necessary for clinical purposes and need not be done routinely, since as with vancomycin, resistant strains have not been recognized. Interpretive criteria are provided for pharmaceutical development, epidemiology, or monitoring for emerging resistance. Any strains found to be intermediate or resistant should be referred to a reference laboratory for confirmation.*

[o] *Report against Streptococcus pyogenes.*

Table 17-11	**Grouping of Recommended Antimicrobial Agents for Testing and Reporting**	
GROUP	CATEGORY	TYPE OF ANTIMICROBIAL AGENT
A	Primary test and report	Include in routine panel and report routinely
B	Primary test, report selectively	Second-line or backup antimicrobial agents for Group A, because of greater expense or toxicity, appropriateness for a specific site, or clinical failure with a Group A antimicrobial agent.
C	Supplemental testing; selective reporting	Testing in institutions with specific bacterial resistance problems, or in patients who are allergic to other antimicrobial agents, or in unusual infections
D	Supplemental	Testing of lower urinary tract infections only

Adapted from reference[333].

negative bacillary infections.[247] The results were identical with 9 of the 11 antibiotics. Only in the case of ceftriaxone (>95% protein-bound) and cefoperazone (90% protein-bound) were there substantial differences when serum was incorporated into the reference procedure.

CATION CONCENTRATION

As previously discussed, the concentration of the divalent cations Ca^{2+} and Mg^{2+} affects the susceptibility results when certain combinations of bacterial species and antibiotic are tested.[264] Barry has postulated that the mechanism by which cation concentration affects the activity of *Pseudomonas aeruginosa*, for example, involves the permeability of the bacterial cell wall.[10] The lipopolysaccharides in the cell wall of *P. aeruginosa* are cross-linked with divalent cations, providing stability. When the organisms are grown in media deficient in cations, cell-wall permeability to the aminoglycoside antibiotics and other compounds is increased. The organisms, therefore, are more sensitive to the action of the aminoglycosides, producing falsely low MIC results or large inhibitory zone sizes. Mueller-Hinton broth has very low concentrations of divalent cations and should be supplemented to physiologic concentrations (20 to 35 μg/L Mg^{2+} and 50–100 μg/L Ca^{2+}). Some batches of Mueller-Hinton agar may actually have an abnormally high concentration of these cations, so that small inhibitory zones are produced when *P. aeruginosa* is tested against aminoglycosides. Such lots, which can be identified by testing with reference strains of known reactivity, should be discarded.

Detection of resistance of certain strains of staphylococci to semisynthetic penicillins is improved by including 2% NaCl in the media for dilution susceptibility tests.[218]

ATMOSPHERE

Agar or broth is incubated in an ambient-air incubator. A CO_2 incubator should not be used for routine tests. The carbonic acid formed on the surface of the agar or in the broth can cause a decrease in pH, which can affect the antibacterial activity of certain antibiotics, as previously discussed. In laboratories with a small workload and where only a CO_2 incubator is available, it is acceptable to place the susceptibility plates or tubes in a sealed jar to prevent access of the CO_2 from the incubator.

TEMPERATURE

Plates and tubes should be incubated routinely at 35°C. At higher temperatures, the detection of oxacillin-resistant staphylococci is compromised. If oxacillin resistance is suspected and not manifested at 35°C, the plates or tubes may be incubated at 30°C.

INOCULUM

The inoculum is usually prepared from a broth culture that has been incubated for 4 to 6 hours, when growth is considered to be in the logarithmic phase. Several similar-appearing colonies should be sampled to minimize variation in the bacterial population. The density of the suspension is adjusted to approximately 10^8 colony-forming units (CFUs) per milliliter by comparing its turbidity to a McFarland 0.5 $BaSO_4$ standard. The standard is prepared by adding 0.5 mL of 0.048 M $BaCl_2$ (1.175% w/v $BaCl_2 \bullet H_2O$) to 99.5 mL of 0.36 N H_2SO_4. Aliquots of 4 to 6 mL of the barium sulfate turbidity standard are distributed to screw-capped tubes of the same size, sealed tightly, and stored in the dark at room temperature. Nephelometers may be used to determine turbidity. Commonly, the degree of cloudiness in the broth is compared with the standard, visualizing the two against a white background on which black lines have been drawn. Further adjustments to the inoculum depend on the type of test used. Alternatively, commercially available devices for preparing a standardized inoculum have worked well.[11]

If time does not permit incubation for 4 to 6 hours, young colonies may be removed from the surface of an agar plate that has been incubated overnight and diluted to the proper density (the direct colony suspension method). This method is recommended when staphylococci are tested for resistance to methicillin and when testing isolates of *Streptococcus pneumoniae* and *Haemophilus influenzae*.

If a McFarland standard is used to prepare the inoculum, the density of the standard should be checked, using a spectrophotometer with a 1-cm light path and matched cuvettes. The absorbance at 625 nm should be 0.08 to 0.10 for the 0.5 McFarland standard. The standard should be replaced or checked for adequacy monthly.[219] It is useful, but not essential, to document the number of organisms in the inoculum periodically by inoculating serial dilutions of the suspension onto agar plates.

ANTIMICROBIAL AGENTS

Reference antimicrobial agent powders for use in dilution tests should be obtained from the manufacturer or from the U.S. Pharmacopeia in Rockville, Md. These reference pow-

Table 17-12 Situations in Which a Surrogate Antibiotic Can Be Used to Predict Results of In Vitro Susceptibility Tests

ORGANISM(S)	SURROGATE ANTIBIOTIC	ANTIBIOTICS IN SURROGATE GROUP	COMMENTS
Staphylococci	Penicillin	Penicillinase-labile agents, penicillinase-stable agents, penicillinase-β-lactamase inhibitor combinations	Susceptibility (including β-lactamase testing after induction) predicts susceptibility to all agents; resistance predicts resistance to penicillinase-labile agents, but other antibiotics will be effective unless isolate is resistant to oxacillin also.
Staphylococci	Oxacillin	Nafcillin, methicillin, oxacillin, dicloxacillin, aztreonam, all cephems, all carbapenems	Susceptibility or resistance predicts result for penicillinase-labile agents and combinations with β-lactamase inhibitors; testing of surrogate antibiotics is not recommended.
Streptococci	Penicillin	All β-lactam antibiotics; including penicillins, cephems, carbapenems, monobactams, and these agents in combination with inhibitors of β-lactamase	Susceptibility indicates susceptibility to all agents in surrogate group; resistance does not predict resistance of other agents.
All organisms	Tetracycline	Tetracycline, minocycline, doxycycline	Susceptibility predicts result for surrogate group; resistance does not predict resistance in surrogate group.
All organisms	Erythromycin	Erythromycin, azithromycin, clarithromycin, dirithromycin	Susceptibility predicts result for surrogate group; resistance does not predict resistance in surrogate group.
Enterobacteriaceae	Cephalothin	Cephalothin, cephapirin, cephradine, cephalexin, cefaclor, cefadroxil	Note that results for other cephalosporins are not predicted by cephalothin.
Enterococci that do not produce β-lactamase	Penicillin	All penicillins, with or without inhibitors of β-lactamase	
Agents for which oral therapy is appropriate	Ampicillin	Ampicillin, amoxicillin	

Adapted from references[217,218].

ders are documented with an assay of antimicrobial activity. For example, the label may indicate that the powder contains 1,075 μg of active chemical in each 1,000 μg of powder. The amount of powder weighed must be adjusted for the activity of each lot. Vials should not be obtained from the hospital pharmacy because they may contain fillers and are not assayed for biologic activity. The antimicrobial agents should be stored in a desiccator as indicated for each agent. Many antimicrobial agents, especially those of the β-lactam class, are more stable at temperatures below −20°C. Suspensions of antimicrobial agent should be stored at −20°C or less, preferably at −70°C; they should not be refrozen after dispensing. Imipenem, which is particularly affected by freezing and thawing,[343] should be reconstituted each time a batch of plates or tubes is prepared. A frost-free freezer should not be used because repeated cycles of freezing and thawing occur.

Antimicrobial-impregnated disks should be stored at −20°C or lower in an anhydrous condition. Under guidelines established by the U.S. Food and Drug Administration, manufacturers of antimicrobial agent disks must carefully control the concentration of antimicrobial agents in the disks

to within 60–120% of the stated content; the actual variation is usually considerably less. A small working supply may be maintained at refrigerator temperatures in a desiccator. Disks should always be allowed to warm to room temperature before opening the desiccator, so that condensation of moisture from the air does not partially rehydrate the disks. Spurious resistance of *Staphylococcus aureus* to oxacillin has resulted from use of a defective lot of disks.[24]

QUALITY CONTROL

Rigorous quality control is important for antimicrobial susceptibility testing because of the large numbers of variables that may affect the results. Some of the physical and chemical characteristics of the media, such as pH and depth of agar, may be monitored, but the final control is provided by a series of reference bacterial strains (Table 17-13).[217–220] The ideal control strains have susceptibility end points in the midrange of antimicrobial concentrations tested and have minimal tendencies to change susceptibility patterns over time.

These reference strains must be stored in a condition

Table 17-13 Quality Control Strains for Susceptibility Testing

TYPE OF TEST	STRAIN	COMMENTS
Dilution and disk diffusion	*Enterococcus faecalis* (ATCC 29212)	Vancomycin- and high-dose aminoglycoside–susceptible; for general use
Dilution and disk diffusion	*Enterococcus faecalis* (ATCC 51299)	Vancomycin- and high-dose aminoglycoside–resistant; for high-dose aminoglycoside testing and for vancomycin screen agar
Dilution and disk diffusion	*Escherichia coli* (ATCC 25922)	General quality control, including β-lactam antibiotics
Dilution and disk diffusion	*Escherichia coli* (ATCC 35218)	Control of β-lactamase inhibitors; may be used in conjunction with *E. coli* ATCC 25922 for β-lactam-β-lactamase-inhibitor combinations
		ATCC 25922 for β-lactam-β-lactamase-inhibitor combinations
Dilution and disk diffusion	*Haemophilus influenzae* (ATCC 49247)	Ampicillin-resistant; β-lactamase-negative
Dilution and disk diffusion	*Haemophilus influenzae* (ATCC 49766)	Ampicillin-susceptible; more reproducible than *H. influenzae* (ATCC 49247) for selected β-lactams
Dilution	*Helicobacter pylori* (ATCC 43504)	For specialized laboratories
Dilution and disk diffusion	*Klebsiella pneumoniae* (ATCC 700603)	Control for extended-spectrum β-lactamase tests
Agar dilution and disk diffusion	*Neisseria gonorrhoeae* (ATCC 49226)	
Dilution and disk diffusion	*Pseudomonas aeruginosa* (ATCC 27853)	General testing
Dilution	*Staphylococcus aureus* (ATCC 29213)	General testing
Dilution	*Staphylococcus aureus* (ATCC 43300)	Used in conjunction with *S. aureus* (ATCC 29213) to control oxacillin salt agar screening tests
Disk diffusion	*Staphylococcus aureus* (ATCC 25923)	General testing; susceptible strain for vancomycin screen agar
Disk diffusion	*Enterococcus faecalis* (ATCC 29212 or ATCC© 33186)	Monitoring batches of Mueller-Hinton agar for unsatisfactory levels of compounds inhibitory to sulfonamides, trimethoprim, or trimethoprim-sulfamethoxazole
Dilution and disk diffusion	*Streptococcus pneumoniae* (ATCC 49619)	General testing

ATCC, American Type Culture Collection.
Adapted from references[217,218].

that minimizes the possibility of mutation. They may be stored frozen (below −20°C or preferably below −60°C) after suspension in a stabilizer, such as defibrinated whole blood, 50% fetal-calf serum in bacteriologic broth, or 10% glycerol in broth. Alternatively, the strains may be lyophilized. For short-term storage, the bacteria may be grown on soybean-casein digest agar and stored at 2–8°C. Fresh slants should be prepared every 2 weeks, and a new stock culture should be obtained when aberrant results are noted. A fresh subculture should be prepared each day the control strain is used.

Rules for the frequency of susceptibility testing have been established by the CLSI (Table 17-14). Similarly, CLSI has defined the appropriate corrective actions to take when quality control parameters are not met (Table 17-15).

Quality Assurance

In addition to traditional quality control, participation in a proficiency testing program, now mandated by federal law, improves performance and provides useful aggregate data for evaluating the status of susceptibility testing on a national basis.[61,65,142,145] Targeted proficiency programs have also been implemented successfully.[311]

Interpretation of Results

A clinician who receives the results of a dilution susceptibility test knows the concentrations of a group of drugs that inhibited growth of the pathogen under carefully defined conditions in the laboratory. To make a rational selection of the most appropriate antimicrobial agent for a patient, the

Table 17-14 Frequency of Quality Control (QC) for Antimicrobial Susceptibility Testing

TYPE OF TEST	APPROACH	FREQUENCY	INITIAL VALIDATION TESTING	CRITERIA FOR CORRECTIVE ACTION	COMMENTS
Disk diffusion or dilution	Daily QC	Daily	None	>1 result in 20 consecutive tests out of control	Conversion to weekly testing if <2 of 20 or <4 of 30 consecutive tests for each antimicrobial agent is out of control
Disk diffusion or dilution	Weekly	Weekly or when there is a change in a reagent component (e.g.., new lot of disks or trays) or of method	Test all applicable control strains for 20 or 30 consecutive test days; weekly testing can be implemented if <2 of 20 or <4 of 30 consecutive tests for each antimicrobial agent is out of control	Any result out of control	If a new antimicrobial agent is added, it must be validated. Weekly testing is appropriate only for routinely tested antimicrobial agents. Infrequently tested antimicrobial agents must be tested on the day of use.
Agar screen tests	Daily	Daily	None	>1 result in 20 consecutive tests out of control	Daily testing must be performed if the screen test is performed less frequently than weekly or if the antimicrobial agent is labile (e.g., oxacillin screen test for *S. aureus*)
Agar screen tests	Weekly	Weekly or when there is a change in a reagent component (e.g.., new lot of disks or trays) or change of method	Test all applicable control strains for 20 or 30 consecutive test days; weekly testing can be implemented if <2 of 20 or <4 of 30 consecutive tests for each antimicrobial agent is out of control	Any result out of control	If a new antimicrobial agent is added, it must be validated; weekly testing is appropriate only for routinely tested antimicrobial agents; infrequently tested antimicrobial agents must be tested on the day of use

Adapted from references[219,220].

Table 17-15 Corrective Action for Antimicrobial Tests That Are Out of Control

SOURCE OF ERROR	CORRECTIVE ACTION	ADDITIONAL CORRECTIVE ACTION
Obvious (e.g., wrong control strain, wrong temperature, contamination)	Retest on day quality control failure is noted; continue testing if new result is in control	Proceed as for unknown error
Unknown	1. Test the failed antimicrobial agent for five consecutive test days 2. If all results are in control, proceed with weekly testing 3. If any results are out of control, proceed with additional testing 4. Suppress reporting of any antimicrobial agents that are out of control until the problem is resolved	1. Possible explanations for the continued failure are summarized in Table 17–23 2. After implementing possible problems (e.g., new reagents), proceed with validation testing 3. Continue daily testing until the problem is resolved 4. Suppress reporting of any antimicrobial agents that are out of control until the problem is resolved

Adapted from references[219,220].

physician needs at least three other pieces of information: 1) the pharmacokinetics of the antimicrobial agent, including the peak level that can be expected at the site of infection and the rapidity with which that level will decrease, that is, the half-life; 2) how the isolated bacterium compares to other isolates of the same species; and 3) any available clinical data on the in vivo response of similar isolates in similar situations.

Without complete knowledge of these factors, it is easy to misinterpret the raw data. For instance, a β-lactam antibiotic such as ampicillin, with a minimal inhibitory concentration (MIC) of 2 μg/mL for an isolate of *E. coli*, might be considered less effective than an aminoglycoside antibiotic, such as gentamicin, with a MIC of 0.5 μg/mL. In fact, the achievable levels of drug in serum are far greater for ampicillin than for gentamicin and the risk of toxicity is much lower in the absence of a history of allergic reactions to the drug. The appropriate choice of therapy would, therefore, be ampicillin, and not the antimicrobial agent with the lowest MIC.

The laboratory must assist the clinician in making a rational selection of therapy by providing suggested interpretations of the quantitative results. The recommendations address the expected response in serum and in body fluids or tissues where concentrations similar to serum accumulate. The physician must remember that higher levels of certain drugs accumulate in certain sites, such as urine or bile; an organism that is classified as "resistant" by the criteria for serum may well be treatable if it is in the lower urinary tract. For example, an isolate of *E. coli* with a MIC of 32 μg/mL for ampicillin would be considered resistant in serum in which relatively low concentrations of drug are present. In contrast, concentrations of ampicillin in the hundreds of micrograms per milliliter would be expected in the urine; one would expect to use ampicillin successfully for an infection of the lower urinary tract, even though the isolate is intrinsically rather resistant. Assuming that ampicillin is the least costly and least toxic antimicrobial agent available, the clinician must decide whether the patient has an infection that involves the parenchyma of the kidney (pyelonephritis), in which case ampicillin would be inappropriate, or whether the infection is in the urinary bladder, in which case ampicillin may well be effective even against this resistant organism. Obviously, the severity of the infection and the potential damage to the patient if a miscalculation is made also have an impact on the decision.

Similarly, an isolate of *E. coli* with an MIC of 8 μg/mL to cefazolin would be considered susceptible in serum or most tissues. Cefazolin penetrates through the meninges very poorly, however, and this antibiotic should not be used to treat a patient with meningitis, no matter what the MIC. In fact, if the isolate comes from the cerebrospinal fluid, the laboratory should not even report results with this antibiotic.

Three categories of antimicrobial agent susceptibility are recognized by the NCCLS for dilution tests (Table 17-16) (Charts 17-2 and 17-3). "Susceptible" implies that the organism should respond to usual doses of the antimicrobial agent administered by an appropriate route, includ-ing orally. "Intermediate" implies that the isolate may be inhibited by concentrations of drug that are achieved when the maximum parenteral doses are given; the antimicrobial agent may be selected, but consideration should be given to other choices that may provide more optimal therapy. "Resistant" indicates that the bacterium is not inhibited by achievable concentrations of drug and, therefore, the drug should not be selected for therapy, except in certain body fluids, in which high concentrations of the antimicrobial agent may accumulate. The number of "major and very major errors"—those that transpose susceptible and resistant—should be kept to the absolute minimum.

If the laboratory performs a disk diffusion test, the standardized method and interpretations suggested by the CLSI should be reported (Table 17-17) (Chart 17-1).[217,220] Occasionally, a physician may derive useful information from the closeness of the actual zone size to the MIC breakpoints, but this information is rarely reported.

A laboratory that performs dilution susceptibility tests may report the interpretive correlate alone—that is, susceptible, intermediate, or resistant—or may report the MIC value along with the interpretive correlate. Increasingly, many institutions have chosen to report only the interpretation, although they actually determine a MIC, because of the potential for misunderstanding of the numerical value by clinicians. The MIC values are reserved for knowledgeable users, such as infectious-disease physicians. If the MIC is included in the report, the clinicians must be educated about its purpose.

Often clinicians must make decisions about antimicrobial therapy empirically, because the decision cannot await isolation and testing of a bacterium. To make those decisions, knowledge of local susceptibility patterns is essential. It is part of the duty of each microbiology laboratory to provide that information. The CLSI has published recommendations for the format of susceptibility summaries.[216] Selected parameters and the rationale for their inclusion are summarized in Table 17-18. Several additional factors worth noting are summarized in Box 17-4.

A sample of the yearly antimicrobial summary from one institution, along with the accompanying instructions, is presented in Table 17-19.

If a local web site or shared access to an electronic file is available, posting of the spreadsheet is a convenient way to provide general access. It may be possible to download the information into personal data assistants (PDAs). In addition, it may be useful to provide a hard copy to clinicians; a useful format is a card that will fit into a pocket for easy access.

In addition to local data there are several regional or national databases for tracking of antimicrobial susceptibility profiles.[116] These resources may also be useful, but cannot replace local data.

The mark of a true microbiologist, as opposed to a microbial technocrat, is the ability to synthesize data from multiple sources and draw inferences that may alert laboratory workers and/or clinicians to a potential problem with the data. In the case of antimicrobial susceptibility testing, comparison

Table 17-16 MIC Interpretive Standards (μg/mL) for *Enterobacteriaceae*[a]

TESTING CONDITIONS

Medium:	Broth dilution: cation-adjusted Mueller-Hinton broth (CAMHB)
	Agar dilution: Mueller Hinton agar (MHA)
Inoculum:	Growth method or direct colony suspension, **equivalent to a 0.5 McFarland standard**
Incubation:	35°C; ambient air; 16 to 20 hours, **24 hours for *Yersinia pestis***

Minimal QC Recommendations (See Table 17–3 for acceptable QC ranges).

Escherichia coli ATCC 25922
Escherichia coli ATCC 35218 (for β-lactam/β-lactamase inhibitor combinations)

General Comments

(1) For fecal isolates of *Salmonella* and *Shigella* spp., only ampicillin, a fluoroquinolone, and trimethoprim-sulfamethoxazole should be tested and reported routinely. In addition, chloramphenicol and a third-generation cephalosporin should be tested and reported for extraintestinal isolates of *Salmonella* spp.

NOTE: Information in boldface type is considered tentative for 1 year.

TEST/REPORT GROUP	ANTIMICROBIAL AGENT	MIC (μG/ML) INTERPRETIVE STANDARD			COMMENTS
		S	I	R	
PENICILLINS					
A	Ampicillin	≤8	16	≥32	(2) Class representative for ampicillin and amoxicillin.
B	Mezlocillin or piperacillin	≤16	32–64	≥128	
B		≤16	32–64	≥128	
B	Ticarcillin	≤16	32–64	≥128	
U	Carbenicillin	≤16	32	≥64	
U/Inv.	Mecillinam	≤8		≥32	(3) For use against *E. coli* for urinary tract isolates only.
β-LACTAM/β-LACTAMASE INHIBITOR COMBINATIONS					
B	Amoxicillin-clavulanic acid or	≤8/4	16/8	≥32/16	
B	ampicillin-sulbactam	≤8/4	16/8	≥32/16	
B	Piperacillin-tazobactam	≤16/4	32/4–64/4	≥128/4	
B	Ticarcillin-clavulanic acid	≤16/2	32/2–64/2	≥128/2	

CEPHEMS (PARENTERAL) (Including cephalosporins I, II, III, and IV. Please refer to Glossary I.

(4) **WARNING:** For *Salmonella* spp. and *Shigella* spp., first- and second-generation cephalosporins may appear active *in vitro* but are not effective clinically and should not be reported as susceptible.

(5) **WARNING: For *Yersinia pestis*, studies have demonstrated that although β-lactam antimicrobial agents may appear active in vitro they lack efficacy in animal models of infection. These antimicrobial agents should not be reported as susceptible.**

(6) Strains of *Klebsiella spp.* and *E. coli* that produce extended-spectrum beta-lactamase (ESBLs) may be clinically resistant to therapy with penicillins, cephalosporins, or aztreonam, despite apparent in vitro susceptibility to some of these agents. Some of these strains will show MICs above the normal susceptible population but below the standard breakpoints for certain extended-spectrum cephalosporins or aztreonam. Such strains should be screened for potential ESBL production by using the ESBL screening breakpoints listed at the end of the table before reporting results for penicillins, extended-spectrum cephalosporins, or aztreonam. Other strains may test intermediate or resistant by standard breakpoints to one or more of these agents. In all strains with ESBLs, the MICs for one or more of the extended-spectrum cephalosporins or aztreonam should decrease in the presence of clavulanic acid as determined in phenotypic confirmatory testing. For all confirmed ESBL-producing strains, the test interpretation should be reported as resistant for all penicillins, cephalosporins, and aztreonam. (See table located at the end of the table for ESBL screening and confirmatory tests. Refer to the glossary for definitions of penicillins and cephalosporins.) The decision to perform ESBL screening tests on all urine isolates should be made on an institutional basis, considering prevalence, therapy, and infection control issues.

R, resistant; I, intermediate; S, susceptible.
[a] Callouts are to CLSI documents.

Table 17-17 **Zone Diameter Interpretive Standards and Equivalent MIC Breakpoints for *Enterobacteriaceae*[a]**

TESTING CONDITIONS

Medium:	Mueller-Hinton agar	
Inoculum:	Growth method or direct colony suspension, **equivalent to a 0.5 McFarland standard**	
Incubation:	35°C; ambient air; 16 to 18 hours	

Minimal QC Recommendations (See Table 17–3 for acceptable QC ranges.)

Escherichia coli ATCC 25922
Escherichia coli ATCC 35218 (for β-lactam/β-lactamase inhibitor combinations)

General Comments

(1) For fecal isolates of *Salmonella* and *Shigella* spp. only ampicillin, a quinolone, and trimethoprim-sulfamethoxazole should be tested and reported routinely. In addition, chloramphenicol and a third-generation cephalosporin should be tested and reported for extraintestinal isolates of *Salmonella* spp.

NOTE: Information in boldface type is considered tentative for 1 year.

TEST/REPORT GROUP	ANTIMICROBIAL AGENT	DISK CONTENT	ZONE DIAMETER (NEAREST WHOLE MM) R	I	S	EQUIVALENT MIC BREAK-POINTS (μG/ML) R	S	COMMENT
PENICILLINS								
A	Ampicillin	10 μg	≤13	14–16	≥17	≥32	≤8	(2) Class representative for ampicillin and amoxicillin.
B	Mezlocillin or piperacillin	75 μg	≤17	18–20	≥21	≥128	≤16	
B		100 μg	≤17	18–20	≥21	≥128	≤16	
B	Ticarcillin	75 μg	≤14	15–19	≥20	≥128	≤16	
U	Carbenicillin	100 μg	≤19	20–22	≥23	≥64	≤16	
U	Mecillinam	10 μg	≤11	12–14	≥15	≥32	≤8	(3) For use against *E. coli* urinary tract isolates only.
β-LACTAM/β-LACTAMASE INHIBITOR COMBINATIONS								
B	Amoxicillin-clavulanic acid or	20/10 μg	≤13	14–17	≥18	≥32/16	≤8/4	
B	ampicillin-sulbactam	10/10 μg	≤11	12–14	≥15	≥32/16	≤8/4	
B	Piperacillin-tazobactam	100/10 μg	≤17	18–20	≥21	≥128/4	≤16/4	
B	Ticarcillin-clavulanic acid	75/10 μg	≤14	15–19	≥20	≥128/2	≤16/2	

R, resistant; I, intermediate; S, susceptible.
[a] *Callouts are to CLSI documents.*

of the results with the putative identification of the organism may alert the microbiologist to a potential problem with one or both pieces of data. Some of these clues are summarized in Table 17-20. In addition to erroneous susceptibility results or organism identifications, inadvertent testing of mixed cultures is a frequent cause of mistakes; inclusion of a "purity" plate with the susceptibility test is essential, but apparent purity of the tested isolate is not an absolute guarantee of purity.

Selection of Antimicrobial Agents To Be Reported

Only antimicrobial agents appropriate for the infection should be included in a report. Drugs that are active only in the urinary tract should not be reported if the isolate comes from another site. Antimicrobial agents that do not penetrate into a site, such as cefazolin or cephalothin in the meninges, should not be reported for organisms isolated from that site. Use of chloramphenicol for urinary tract infections is inappropriate because it is not excreted in the urine; microbiologists should not encourage inappropriate use by including the susceptibility results in a laboratory report. Similarly, isolates of *Streptococcus pneumoniae* from cerebrospinal fluid (CSF) should be tested against only one or more of the following antibiotics: penicillin, cefotaxime, ceftriaxone, meropenem, and vancomycin.[218] There are unfortunately very few of these absolute prohibitions. Most of the decisions should be made in consultation

Table 17-18 Recommendations for Production of Institutional Antimicrobial Susceptibility Summaries

PARAMETER	RECOMMENDED ACTION	JUSTIFICATION
Facility	Separate data from each facility served by the laboratory; indicate name of facility on report.	In a system that includes multiple institutions results may vary greatly among units.
Frequency	At least yearly; indicate time frame on report.	Increases likelihood that an adequate number of strains will be included; avoids potential seasonal variation in resistance.
Duplicate testing	Include only the first isolate (see Box 17-4 for discussion of the definition of duplicate).	Frequent culturing of problem patients may result in overrepresentation of these strains in the data.
Source of strains	Include only isolates submitted for diagnostic purposes.	Isolates submitted as part of a protocol may not be representative; isolates recovered from the environment may not be clinically relevant.
Number of isolates	Include only bacterial species for which at least 10 strains were tested; results based on intermediate numbers (e.g., <25 or <50 strains may be indicated with an asterisk).	Smaller numbers of strains may not yield statistically significant results.
Antimicrobial agents that are reported selectively by "cascade" method	Include all results in summary, not just those that were reported.	Excluding unreported antimicrobial agents potentially introduces bias.
Antimicrobial agents that are tested or reported selectively (see Box 17-4)	Do not include results in summary (or indicate the parameters of testing).	The nonrandom nature of the testing potentially introduces bias into the results.
"Calculated" interpretations	Include the clinically relevant result.	Results that are modified by protocol; e.g., staphylococci and β-lactam antibiotics based on oxacillin results; or modification of β-lactam results for ESBL producers.
Supplemental analysis (see text)	Include additional factors.	Decisions based on local parameters and needs.

Adapted from reference[216].

with members of the medical staff and pharmacy. All accredited hospitals have pharmacy and therapeutics committees (or the equivalent) that provide a useful forum for coordinated effort. Several reasonable strategies, depending on local policy, needs, and resources, are listed in Box 17-5.

Macrodilution Broth Susceptibility Test

The macrodilution broth susceptibility test was among the first to be developed and still serves as a reference method. Serial dilutions of antimicrobial agent are made in broth or in agar, after which a standardized bacterial suspension is added. Figure 17-11 shows 10 test tubes that contain cation-supplemented Mueller-Hinton broth. Quantities of antimicrobial agent are serially diluted from 100 µg/mL to 0.4 µg/mL. Tube number 10 is free of antimicrobial agent and serves as a growth control. Each of the 10 tubes is inoculated with a calibrated suspension of the microorganism to be tested and incubated at 35°C for 18 hours. At the end of the incubation period, the tubes are visually examined for turbidity. Note in Figure

17-11 that the five tubes to the left are clear and the five to the right appear cloudy. Cloudiness indicates that bacterial growth has not been inhibited by the concentration of antimicrobial agent contained in the medium.

Figure 17-12 illustrates that the breakpoint of growth inhibition in Figure 17-11 is between tubes 5 and 6, or between 6.25 µg/mL and 3.12 µg/mL of antimicrobial agent. This breakpoint represents the MIC, defined as the lowest concentration of antimicrobial agent in micrograms per milliliter that prevents the in vitro growth of bacteria. Thus, in the example shown in Figures 17-11 and 17-12, the MIC lies somewhere between 6.25 µg/mL and 3.12 µg/mL. However, by convention, the MIC is interpreted as the concentration of the antimicrobial agent, contained in the first tube in the series, that inhibits visible growth. Therefore, in this example, the MIC is 6.25 µg/mL.

The adaptation of this test to small volumes for routine testing is described in a later section.

Agar Dilution Susceptibility Test

The agar dilution procedure, which is the second reference method, has been successfully adapted for routine use in large laboratories by testing only selected concentrations of antimicrobial agent. A standardized suspension of

---

Box 17-4 Recommendations for Formatting Summaries of Antimicrobial Susceptibility Tests

1. Interested parties in each institution must decide how they wish to present the data. Some laboratory and/or institutional information systems may not allow adherence to all recommendations.
2. Duplicate results should clearly be excluded, so as not to bias the results toward patients in whom cultures are performed more frequently. The definition of "duplicate" is susceptible to several interpretations, however. For instance, NCCLS recommends that only the first isolate of a particular bacterium from a particular patient in a given time period (e.g., 1 year) be included in the analysis, regardless of other characteristics of the isolates. It will be practically impossible for most institutions to track duplicate status for a year. More importantly, this recommendation would exclude from view multiple strains of important pathogens that cocirculate in an institution and would certainly decrease the likelihood that a burgeoning outbreak of resistant infection would be detected.
3. Antimicrobial agents that are tested and reported selectively should be excluded, because they have not been tested randomly. For instance, if third-generation cephalosporins are tested only against isolates of *S. pneumoniae* that are not susceptible to penicillin, using an oxacillin disk screen, the results will not be representative of all pneumococci in the institution; in this case, the results can be adjusted by assuming that all pneumococci that are clearly susceptible to penicillin by the disk screen are also susceptible to the third-generation cephalosporin. Conversely, if isolates of *H. influenzae* are tested against ampicillin only if they do not produce β-lactamase, the results will be biased toward susceptibility of the remaining isolates to ampicillin. In certain instances, specific requests for susceptibility testing may indicate a bias toward resistance.
4. Supplemental analysis may be appropriate in several clinical or microbiologic situations:
   a. Although it is recommended that the "intermediate" category not be included for most combinations, it is appropriate to report this category for *S. pneumoniae* and for viridans streptococci isolated from sterile sites.
   b. For most combinations the reported interpretation is based on achievable serum levels of antimicrobial agents. In the case of *S. pneumoniae*, however, it is recommended that the data for cefotaxime and ceftriaxone (and for Cefipime in countries where there is both a meningitis and nonmeningitis indication for use of this antibiotic) be reported using the interpretive breakpoints both for blood and for CSF isolates.
   c. The results for coagulase-positive staphylococcus, *S. aureus*, may be analyzed separately for isolates that are sensitive and resistant to oxacillin. The general patterns for these two groups are very different and may be lost by merging the data.
   d. If the number of isolates permits, it may be useful to differentiate populations of patients (inpatient vs. outpatient, intensive care units, children vs. adults), body sites (urinary tract, respiratory tract, blood, etc.), source of infection (nosocomial vs. community-acquired), or specific clinical situations in which special problems exist (cystic fibrosis).

---

bacteria is inoculated onto a series of agar plates, each containing a different concentration of antimicrobial agent, encompassing the therapeutic range of the drug. For example, if the therapeutic range for a given antimicrobial agent is 2 to 12 μg/mL, a series of agar plates containing 1, 4, 8, 16, and 32 μg/mL of antimicrobial agent might be used to determine the susceptibility of the organism being tested. If the organism grows on the first three plates but not in the plate containing 16 μg/mL of antimicrobial agent, a MIC value of 16 μg/mL can be established, similar to the interpretation of the end point in the broth dilution technique.

Agar dilution plates ready for interpretation are shown in Figure 17-13. Note that microorganisms that are sensitive to the concentration of antimicrobial agent contained in any given agar plate do not produce a circle of growth at the inoculum site, whereas those that are resistant appear as circular colonies. The agar plates are marked with a grid so that each microorganism can be identified by a number and the results entered on the worksheet.

To facilitate testing of a large volume of cultures, an instrument known as the Steers replicator is used (Fig. 17-14). The main feature of the instrument is a spring-loaded head that is fitted with 32 to 36 flat-surfaced inoculating pins, each about 3 mm in diameter. The head is attached to a piston and spring-loaded cylinder mecha-

nism by which it can be moved up and down in a vertical plane. The counterpart is an aluminum seed plate containing 32 to 36 wells. These wells are tooled in such a manner that when the seed plate is properly aligned within the guide at the base of the replicator, each of the inoculating pins on the movable head fits exactly into the wells. Each well in the seed plate provides a receptacle into which different bacterial suspensions can be placed.

The agar dilution susceptibility plate is inoculated by placing the seed tray with its multiple suspensions directly under the inoculating head. The head is lowered so that the pins extend fully into each of the wells, thus sampling approximately 0.003 mL of each bacterial suspension on the surface of each inoculating pin. Next, the head is raised and an agar plate is moved into position under the prongs, which in turn are lowered so that the flat surface of each inoculating pin just touches the agar surface. The head is again raised, and the seed plate is moved back into position for inoculation of the next agar plate. The procedure is repeated for all of the antimicrobial agent plates to be tested. After all the plates have been inoculated, they are incubated at 35°C for 18 hours.

Disk Diffusion Susceptibility Test

Figure 17-15 illustrates the basic principle of the disk diffusion method of antimicrobial susceptibility testing.[10] As

Table 17-19 Sample Antimicrobial Susceptibility Summary Report

ANTIMICROBIAL SUSCEPTIBILITY RESULTS

July 1, 2003 through June 30, 2004

	ESCHE-RICHIA SPP.	ENTERO-BACTER SPP.	KLEBSIELLA SPP.	PROTEUS MIRABILIS	PROTEUS SPP.	SERRATIA SPP.	ACINETO-BACTER SPP.	CITROBACTER FREUNDII	CITROBACTER KOSERI	PSEUDOMONAS AERUGINOSA	STAPHYLOCOCCUS COAGULASE-POSITIVE	STAPHYLOCOCCUS COAGULASE-NEGATIVE	ENTEROCOCCUS[A]	STREPTOCOCCUS PNEUMONIAE
Maximum strains tested	3497	312	748	269	106	107	45	89	24	1333	2174	894	1234	148
% Susceptible														
Ampicillin	71	1	1	93	14	11	7[b]	11[b]	0[b]	1	c	c	94	—
Ampicillin-sulbactam	78	23	75	100[b]	54[b]	20	100[b]	50[b]	60[b]	4	—	—	—	—
Ampicillin	—	—	—	—	—	—	—	—	—	—	—	—	—	—
Amikacin	99+	99	99+	99+	100	97[b]	100[b]	100	100[b]	89	—	—	—	—
Aztreonam	99	82	99	99	94	100[b]	11[b]	67	100[b]	71	—	—	—	—
Ceftazidime	99	82	98	99+	92	96	97[b]	65	100[b]	80	—	—	—	—
Cefotaxime	99+	85	100	99+	97	96[b]	80[b]	74	100[b]	17	—	—	—	—
Ceftriaxone	98	75	100	100	90[b]	97	31[b]	—	—	21	—	—	—	—
Clindamycin	—	—	—	—	—	—	—	—	—	—	54	37	—	—
Ciprofloxacin	98	95	99	92	95	99	100[b]	95	100[b]	68	66	51	—	—
Cefotetan	97	61	98	96	100[b]	99	3[b]	57[b]	100[b]	1	—	—	—	—
Cefazolin	97	7	95	97	15	0	0[b]	2	100[b]	0	67	34	—	—
Cephalothin[d]	89	1	84	97[b]	0	0	0[b]	14[b]	60[b]	0	67	34	—	—
Cotrimoxazole	87	93	93	84	83	98	93[b]	86	100[b]	5	—	—	—	—
Erythromycin	—	—	—	—	—	—	—	—	—	—	54	37	—	—
Gentamicin	98	97	98	95	96	98	98[b]	98	100[b]	75	—	—	—	—
Imipenem	100	100	100	99+	96	99	100[b]	100	100[b]	78	—	—	—	—
Meropenem	—	—	—	—	—	—	—	—	—	—	—	—	—	—

Table 17-19 Continued

ANTIMICROBIAL SUSCEPTIBILITY RESULTS
July 1, 2003, through June 30, 2004

	ESCHERICHIA SPP.	ENTEROBACTER SPP.	KLEBSIELLA SPP.	PROTEUS MIRABILIS	PROTEUS SPP.	SERRATIA SPP.	ACINETOBACTER SPP.	CITROBACTER FREUNDII	CITROBACTER KOSERI	PSEUDOMONAS AERUGINOSA	STAPHYLOCOCCUS COAGULASE-POSITIVE	STAPHYLOCOCCUS COAGULASE-NEGATIVE	ENTEROCOCCUS[a]	STREPTOCOCCUS PNEUMONIAE
Oxacillin-nafcillin	—	—	—	—	—	—	—	—	—	—	67	—	—	—
Oxacillin-nafcillin	—	—	—	—	—	—	—	—	—	—	—	34	—	—
Piperacillin	74	79	92	97	90	94	75[b]	67	95[b]	—	—	—	—	—
Piperacillin	—	—	—	—	—	—	—	—	—	90	—	—	—	—
Piperacillin-tazobactam	97	62[b]	100[b]	—	—	—	100[b]	—	—	—	—	—	—	—
Piperacillin-tazobactam	—	—	—	—	—	—	—	—	—	84	—	—	—	—
Tobramycin	99	99	98	96	100	96	100[b]	100	100[b]	87	—	—	—	—
Vancomycin	—	—	—	—	—	—	—	—	—	—	100	100	97	—
Penicillin	—	—	—	—	—	—	—	—	—	—	—	—	—	76% susceptible; 14% intermediate
Ceftriaxone (CSF criteria)	—	—	—	—	—	—	—	—	—	—	—	—	—	NA
Ceftriaxone (serum criteria)	—	—	—	—	—	—	—	—	—	—	—	—	—	NA
For urinary tract infections only														
Nitrofurantoin	99	67	68	1	19	0[b]	0[b]	96	94[b]	1	100	99+	98	—

[a] For serious enterococcal infections combination therapy with a b-lactam and an aminoglycoside antibiotic should be used.

[b] <50 strains tested.

[c] >90% of Staphylococcus spp. are resistant to penicillin and ampicillin.

[d] Cephalothin should be used as the class drug for determining susceptibility to oral first generation cephalosporins.

[e] 69 pneumococcal strains tested against ceftriaxone; only strains NOT susceptible to penicillin in a screening procedure tested against ceftriaxone.

NA, not available.

Table 17-20 Flags That Suggest the Need to Verify the Antimicrobial Susceptibility Profile and/or the Identification of the Bacterial Isolate[a]

ORGANISM	PHENOTYPES THAT ARE RARE OR MAY RESULT FROM TECHNICAL ERRORS	PHENOTYPES THAT MAY BE RARE IN CERTAIN INSTITUTIONS
Enterobacteriaceae (any)	I or R to carbapenems	R to amikacin or fluoroquinolones
Citrobacter freundii *Enterobacter* spp., *Serratia marcescens*	S to ampicillin, cefazolin, or cephalothin	
Proteus vulgaris *Providencia* spp.	S to ampicillin	
Pseudomonas aeruginosa		R to gentamicin, tobramycin, and amikacin concurrently
Stenotrophomonas maltophilia	S to carbapenems	R to trimethoprim-sulfamethoxazole
Proteus mirabilis	S to nitrofurantoin	
Enterococcus faecalis	R to penicillin or ampicillin; S to quinupristin-dalfopristin; R to linezolid	R to high-level aminoglycosides (sterile body sites)
Enterococcus faecium	R to linezolid	R to high-level aminoglycosides (sterile body sites); R to quinupristin-dalfopristin
Staphylococcus aureus	I or R to linezolid; I or R to quinupristin-dalfopristin; I or R to vancomycin	R to oxacillin
Staphylococcus, coagulase-negative	I or R to linezolid; I or R to vancomycin	
Streptococcus pneumoniae	R to fluoroquinolone; I or R to linezolid; I or R to vancomycin	R to penicillin; R to third-generation cephalosporins
Streptococcus, viridians group	I or R to linezolid; I or R to vancomycin	I or R to penicillin
Streptococcus, β-hemolytic	I or R to penicillin or ampicillin; I or R to third-generation cephalosporins; I or R to linezolid; I or R to vancomycin	
Any organisms	Resistant of all agents tested	

[a] *All of these situations are subject to change as new mechanisms of antimicrobial resistance develop and spread.*
Adapted from references[217,218].
R, resistant; I, intermediate; S, susceptible.

soon as the antimicrobial agent–impregnated disk comes in contact with the moist agar surface, water is absorbed into the filter paper and the antimicrobial agent diffuses into the surrounding medium. The rate of extraction of the antimicrobial agent out of the disk is greater than its outward diffusion into the medium, so that the concentration immediately adjacent to the disk may exceed that in the disk itself. As the distance from the disk increases, however, there is a logarithmic reduction in the antimicrobial agent concentration. If the plate has been previously inoculated with a bacterial suspension, simultaneous growth of bacteria occurs on the surface of the agar. When a critical cell mass of bacteria is reached, the inhibitory activity of the antimicrobial agent is overcome and bacterial growth occurs. The time required to reach the critical cell mass (critical time; 4 to 10 hours for commonly tested bacteria) is characteristic of each species but is influenced by the composition of the medium and temperature of incubation. The lateral extent of antimicrobial diffusion before the critical time is reached will be affected by the depth of the agar because diffusion occurs in three dimensions. The points at which the critical cell mass is reached appear as a sharply marginated circle of bacterial growth, with the middle of the disk forming the center of the circle if the test has been performed properly (Fig. 17-16). The concentration of diffused antimicrobial agent at this interface of growing and inhibited bacteria is known as the critical concentration and approximates the MIC obtained in dilution tests. Although direct calculation of the inhibitory concentration is not done in practice, the MIC can actually be calculated with reasonable accuracy if the characteristics of antimicrobial diffusion and bacterial growth are known.[10]

DEVELOPMENT OF A STANDARDIZED DISK DIFFUSION PROCEDURE

By the end of the 1950s, the status of antimicrobial susceptibility testing in microbiology laboratories throughout the world was in chaos, primarily because of the lack of

1. If use of more expensive or toxic agents is controlled by the pharmacy personnel or medical consultants, the laboratory may report the results of all drugs tested. The check on inappropriate use will come at the time the drug is ordered.

2. The laboratory may report the results of the most appropriate antimicrobial agents and report other drugs only if there is resistance to a preferred agent or if a physician specifically requests the result. For instance, susceptibility results for third-generation cephalosporins are reported only if the isolate is resistant to the first-generation antimicrobial agents.

3. If resources are limited, the most appropriate antimicrobial agents may be tested and reported first, followed by other antimicrobial agents if requested by the physician. The medical staff should be kept informed of additional antimicrobial agents that are not tested routinely, but are available in the laboratory for testing.

4. Some laboratories publish the cost of the antimicrobial agent beside the susceptibility result. The impetus for such a policy is obvious, but the efficacy of displaying costs has not been documented. The constant repetition of cost data might imprint the information on the mind of the viewing physician, but it might also have the usefulness of often-repeated parental advice.

5. The decision about what cost to include on the report is not straightforward: cost to the pharmacy? charge to the patient? per dose? per day? include ancillary charges such as administration and laboratory tests for monitoring? The cost data may appear greatly different depending on the approach taken.

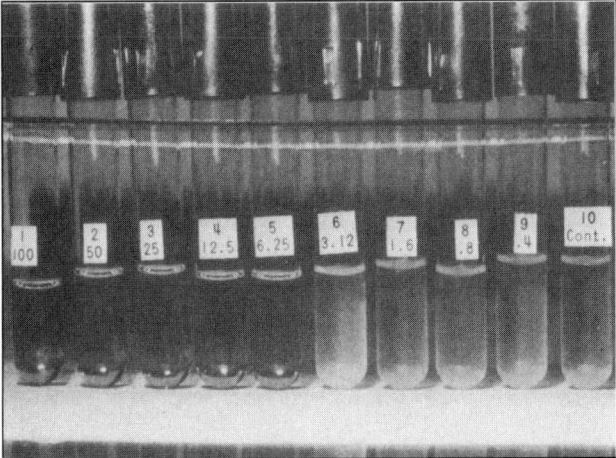

Figure 17-11 Illustration of broth dilution antibiotic susceptibility test in which the antibiotic to be tested is serially diluted in a range between 100 μg/mL and 0.4 μg/mL. Tube number 10 serves as a positive control.

an acceptable standard procedure. The antimicrobial agent concentrations in disks varied considerably, a wide variety of media was being used, methods of inoculation differed from laboratory to laboratory, the length of incubation time was not uniform, and results were being interpreted by several criteria. A World Health Organization committee was formed to investigate this problem, and the deliberation of this committee provided the groundwork that led to the development of several standardized procedures (Chart 17-1).[1] The test that has become standard in the United States is based on the work of Bauer, Kirby, and coworkers.[13,14]

If the test is properly performed, the edges of the inhibitory zones should be clear and easy to measure. Situations in which the technologist must learn to interpret unclear results correctly are listed in Box 17-6.

INTERPRETATION OF RESULTS

The zone size observed in a disk diffusion test has no meaning in and of itself. The interpretive standards provided by the CLSI are derived from a correlation between zone sizes and MICs of the species that can be tested by the disk diffusion method. A prototype of a regression curve providing such a correlation is illustrated in Figure 17-21. Multiple strains have been tested against a single antimicrobial agent both by the disk diffusion technique and by a dilution method. Each triangle represents the results of both tests for a single strain. A regression line has been drawn through the many individual points. Once the regression line is established, an approximate MIC result can be inferred from any zone diameter. In this example, a zone size of 18 mm corresponds to a MIC of 6.25 μg/mL—the breakpoint of the broth dilution test illustrated in Figure 17-11.

Thus, an antimicrobial agent that produces a zone diameter greater than 18 mm would theoretically have a MIC less than 6.25 μg/mL, and the organism would be considered susceptible; one producing a zone size less than 18 mm would, conversely, be considered resistant. In actual practice, regression curves are not that clearly defined, and a 2- to 4-mm zone may be established where it is not possible to determine whether the organism is susceptible or resistant (see Table 17-17). Isolates that produce an inhibitory zone in this range are characterized as intermediate in susceptibility. In studies conducted late in the 1950s, Bauer, Perry, and Kirby first demonstrated that bacterial strains tested against a given antimicrobial agent tend to fall either into the resistant or susceptible categories; only a small percentage (5% or less) fall into the intermediate range.[14] Thus, if a high percentage of intermediate reports is issued by a certain laboratory, a reexamination of the procedure is indicated.

The interpretive guidelines for the disk diffusion test (see Table 17-17) permit the user to make approximations of the MIC for each of the antimicrobial agents listed (last two columns), with zone diameters as determined by the disk diffusion technique. These correlates are not intended to match the breakpoints for susceptibility and resistance established for the dilution tests, but they do give the user an appreciation of the meaning of the report. For example, a microorganism showing an 11-mm zone of inhibition against

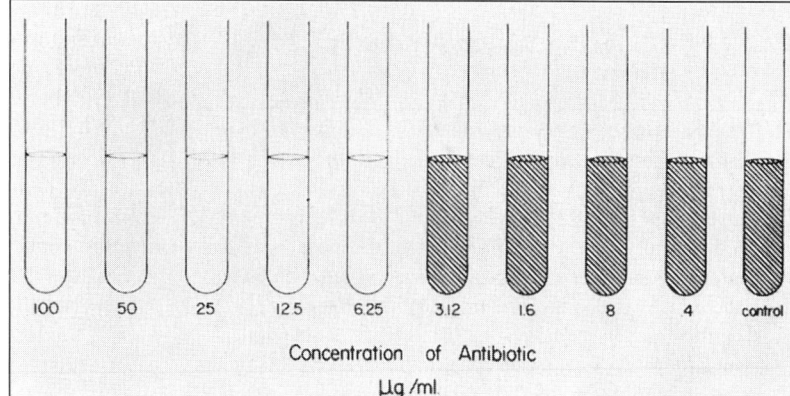

Figure 17-12 Line drawing of the broth dilution susceptibility test shown in Figure 17-11. The MIC for the test illustrated here is 6.25 μg/mL.

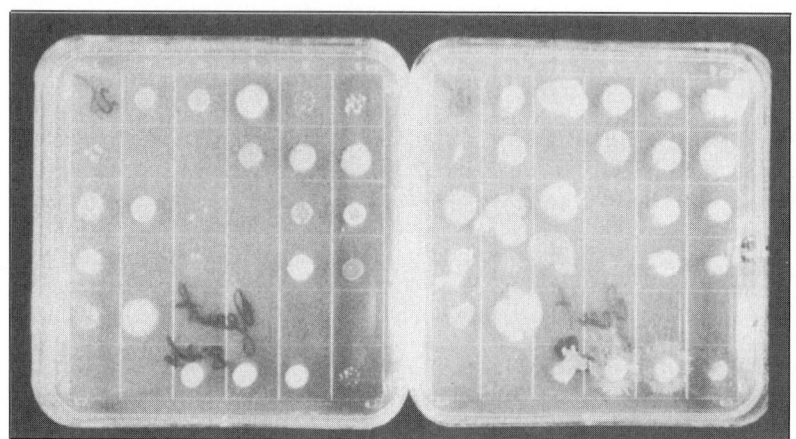

Figure 17-13 Agar dilution antimicrobial susceptibility plates that have been inoculated with several species of bacteria from a Steers replicator. Sensitive organisms are inhibited by the concentration of antibiotic contained in the plate, and no growth is evident at the points of inoculation; resistant organisms appear as distinct colonies of bacterial growth.

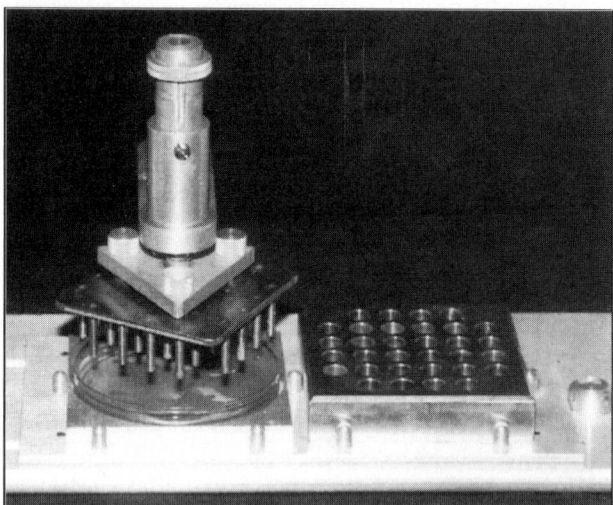

Figure 17-14 Steers replicator: The inoculating head and prongs are fixed. A sliding tray alternately positions a template containing the inoculum and an agar plate under the head. The parts can be disassembled for autoclaving.

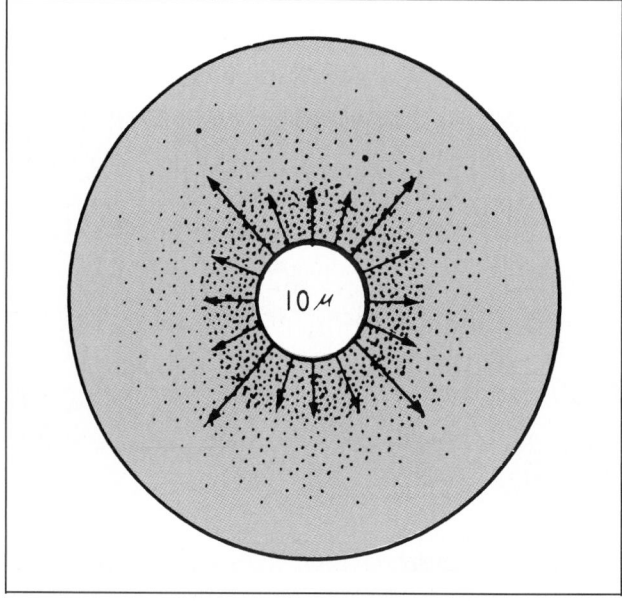

Figure 17-15 The principle of antibiotic diffusion in agar. The concentration of antibiotic decreases as the distance from the disk increases.

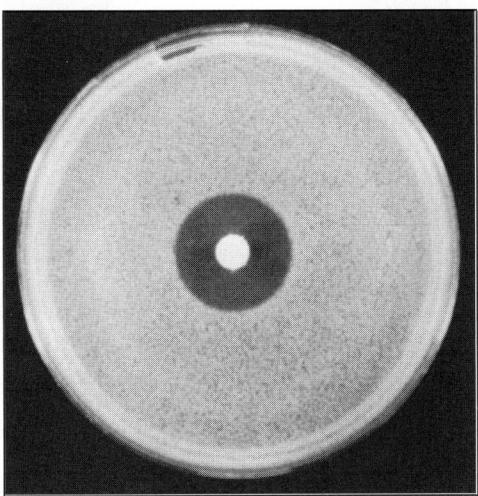

Figure 17-16 Disk antibiotic susceptibility plate showing the same principle as in Figure 17-15. At the area where the concentration of antibiotic is insufficient to prevent bacterial growth, a distinct margin can be seen.

ampicillin would be considered resistant at a level of greater than 32 μg/mL.

If the infection is in the lower urinary tract, however, very high concentrations of ampicillin are achieved, and the organism might be treatable even in the presence of an apparently resistant result. It may be necessary to perform a dilution test to obtain a more precise result.

QUALITY CONTROL

Quality control should be performed each time a new lot of disks or agar is used. In the interim, controls should be tested each day the procedure is performed unless stringent criteria for weekly testing are met. The CLSI has established limits on zone sizes that are acceptable for the quality control strains (Table 17-21); these limits provide a means by which to measure the accuracy of testing.

LIMITATIONS

The Bauer-Kirby test, as modified by the CLSI, has been accepted in the United States as the standard technique for performing disk diffusion susceptibility tests, giving useful information in most instances. There are, however, a few distinct limitations. The test should be applied only to bacterial species that have been thoroughly evaluated. Bacteria that grow slowly, need special nutrients, or require CO_2 or anaerobic conditions for growth should not be tested, unless the validity of the procedure has been documented.[144]

Microbroth Dilution Susceptibility Test

Concurrent with the development of a usable disk diffusion test, other investigators attempted to simplify the broth dilution test. The microtube dilution procedure is similar in principle to the macrotube method, except that the susceptibility of microorganisms to antimicrobial agents

---

Box 17-6 **Correctly Interpreting Antimicrobial Agents: Special Situations**

1. Motile organisms such as *Proteus mirabilis* or *P. vulgaris* may swarm when growing on agar surfaces, resulting in a thin veil that may penetrate into the zones of inhibition around antimicrobial agent susceptibility disks (Fig. 17–17). This zone of swarming should be ignored; the outer margin, which is usually clearly outlined, should be measured. Similarly, with sulfonamide disks, growth may not be completely inhibited at the outer margin, resulting in a faint veil, where 80% or more of the organisms are inhibited. The clear zone of ~80% inhibition should be read as the zone diameter.

2. The phenomenon shown in Figure 17–18 must be interpreted differently from that shown in Figure 17–17. Note that distinct colonies are present within the zone of inhibition. This does not represent swarming. Rather, these colonies are either mutants that are more resistant to the antimicrobial agent than the major portion of the bacterial strain being tested or the culture is not pure and the separate colonies are of a different species. Isolation, identification, and susceptibility testing of the resistant colonies may be required to resolve this problem. If it is determined that the separate colonies represent a variant of a mutant strain, the bacterial species being tested must be considered resistant, even though a wide zone of inhibition may be present for the remainder of the growth.

3. Figure 17–19 demonstrates the difficulty in measuring one zone diameter when there is overlapping with adjacent antimicrobial agent zones, or when the zone extends beyond the margin of the Petri dish. Oval or elliptical zones may occur, and it is difficult to determine whether to measure the short or long diameters. Unless the zones are very wide and the organism being tested is obviously susceptible, the test must be repeated with more careful placement of the antimicrobial agent disks so that overlapping will not occur.

4. Figure 17–20 illustrates a poorly prepared plate. The lines of streaking are irregular, leaving spaces between adjacent colonies. The margins of the zones are indistinct, making it difficult to pick the exact points at which to make the measurements. Readings should not be attempted on a poorly inoculated plate such as this, and the test should be repeated.

---

is determined in a series of microtube wells that are molded into a plastic plate. Each plate may contain 80, 96, or more wells, depending on the number and concentration of antimicrobial agents that are to be included in the susceptibility test panel.

The advantages of the microtube method are that small volumes of reagents are used and that large numbers of bacteria can be tested simply and inexpensively against a panel of antimicrobial agents (Chart 17-2). The intensive labor involved in preparing the multiwell plates was a major impediment to their routine use.

A major advance in microbroth dilution testing came

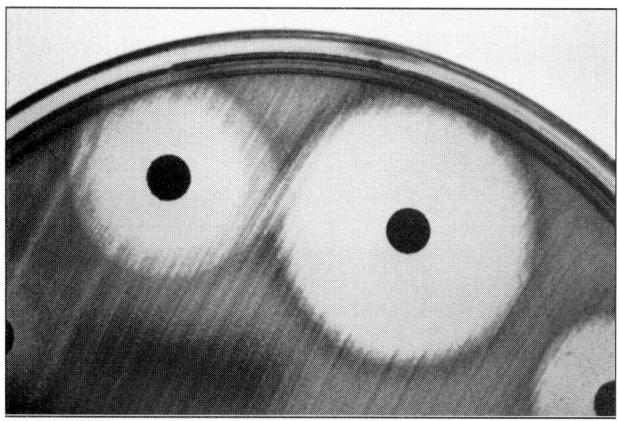

Figure 17-17 Photograph of an antibiotic susceptibility plate using a species of *Proteus* as the test organism. Note the swarming into the zone of inhibition at the peripheral margins. The second outer zone of growth inhibition should be used when measuring the width of the zone.

from the development of instruments that dispensed replicate aliquots from tubes in which large volumes of antimicrobial agent had been prepared. The precision of dilution in large volumes was combined with the ease of testing in microtiter plates. The Autospense (Sandy Spring Technologies, Gaithersburg, MD) (formerly Quickspense) instrument is commercially available and is used in some hospital laboratories. If the resources are available, local production of plates allows the use of a tailored panel of antimicrobial agents; users can change the panel at will. In Figure 17-22, an early version of the Quickspense instrument is demonstrated. Dilutions are prepared in large volumes, after which the fluid is dispensed mechanically into the microtiter trays. After preparation of the dilutions

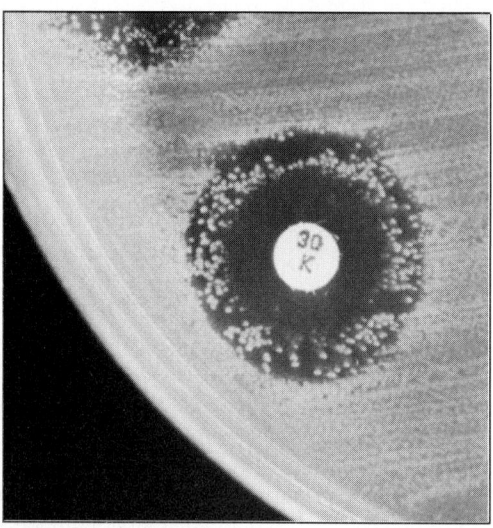

Figure 17-18 An antibiotic susceptibility plate in which colonies resistant to kanamycin are growing within the zone of inhibition: Biochemical tests must be performed to determine if the resistant strain is a mutant of the organisms being tested or represents a second species growing in mixed culture.

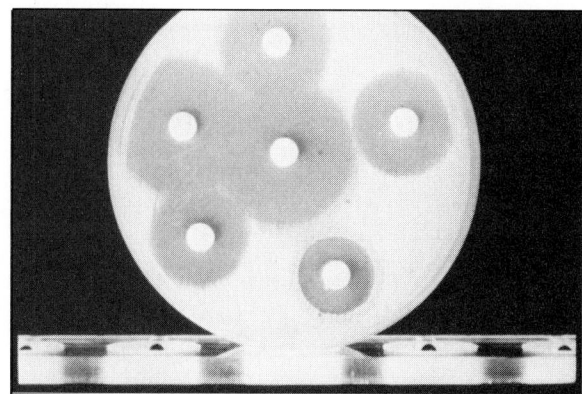

Figure 17-19 A poorly prepared antibiotic susceptibility plate showing objectionable overlapping of the zones of growth inhibition from adjacent disks.

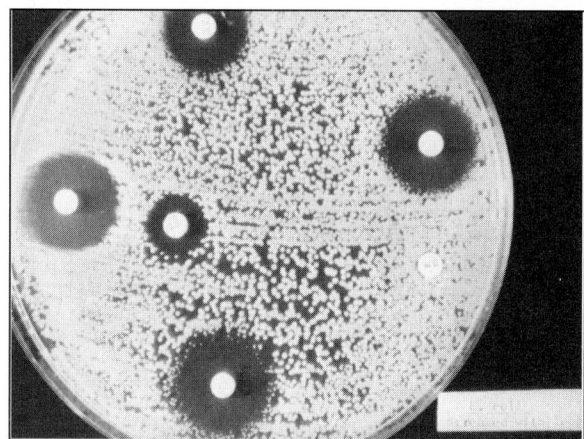

Figure 17-20 A poorly streaked antimicrobial susceptibility plate showing uneven growth. The zone margins are indistinct, compromising accurate measurement.

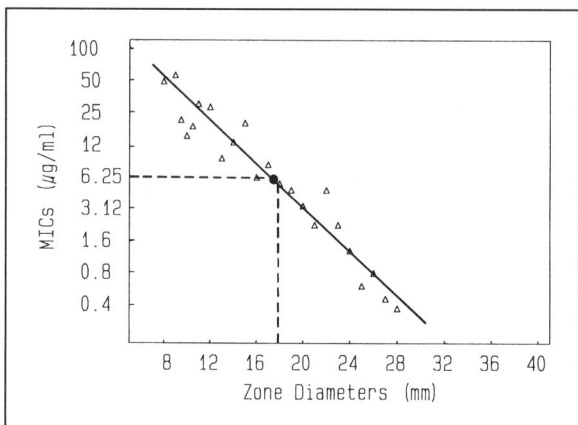

Figure 17-21 Prototype regression curve comparing MICs in micrograms per milliliter with zone size in millimeters. Each triangle represents the MIC (vertical axis) and inhibitory zone (horizontal axis) of a single isolate. A zone diameter of 18 mm corresponds with the MIC breakpoint of 6.25 μg/mL, a correlation that, theoretically, could be made for the test illustrated in Figures 17-11 and 17-12.

Table 17-21 Quality Control Limits for Disk Diffusion Tests

ANTIMICROBIAL AGENT	DISK CONTENT	ESCHERICHIA COLI (ATCC 25922)[b]	STAPHYLOCOCCUS AUREUS (ATCC 25923)	PSEUDOMONAS AERUGINOSA (ATCC 27853)	ESCHERICHIA COLI (ATCC 35218)[f]
Amikacin	30 µg	19–26	20–26	18–26	–
Amoxicillin-clavulanic acid	20/10 µg	18–24	28–36	–	17–22
Ampicillin	10 µg	16–22	27–35	–	6
Ampicillin-sulbactam	10/10 µg	19–24	29–37	–	13–19
Azithromycin	15 µg	–	21–26	–	–
Azlocillin	75 µg	–	–	24–30	–
Aztreonam	30 µg	28–36	–	23–29	–
Carbenicillin	100 µg	23–29	–	18–24	–
Cefaclor	30 µg	23–27	27–31	–	–
Cefamandole	30 µg	26–32	26–34	–	–
Cefazolin	30 µg	21–27	29–35	–	–
Cefdinir	5 µg	24–28	25–32	–	–
Cefditoren	5 µg	22–28	20–28	–	–
Cefepime	30 µg	31–37	23–29	24–30	–
Cefetamet	10 µg	24–29	–	–	–
Cefixime	5 µg	23–27	–	–	–
Cefmetazole	30 µg	26–32	25–34	–	–
Cefonicid	30 µg	25–29	22–28	–	–
Cefoperazone	75 µg	28–34	24–33	23–29	–
Cefotaxime	30 µg	29–35	25–31	18–22	–
Cefotetan	30 µg	28–34	17–23	–	–
Cefoxitin	30 µg	23–29	23–29	–	–
Cefpodoxime	10 µg	23–28	19–25	–	–
Cefprozil	30 µg	21–27	27–33	–	–
Ceftazidime	30 µg	25–32	16–20	22–29	–
Ceftibuten	30 µg	27–35	–	–	–
Ceftizoxime	30 µg	30–36	27–35	12–17	–
Ceftriaxone	30 µg	29–35	22–28	17–23	–
Cefuroxime	30 µg	20–26	27–35	–	–
Cephalothin	30 µg	15–21	29–37	–	–
Chloramphenicol	30 µg	21–27	19–26	–	–

(Continued)

Table 17-21 *Continued*

ANTIMICROBIAL AGENT	DISK CONTENT	ESCHERICHIA COLI (ATCC 25922)[b]	STAPHYLOCOCCUS AUREUS (ATCC 25923)	PSEUDOMONAS AERUGINOSA (ATCC 27853)	ESCHERICHIA COLI (ATCC 35218)[f]
Cinoxacin	100 µg	26–32	–	–	–
Ciprofloxacin	5 µg	30–40	22–30	25–33	–
Clarithromycin	15 µg	–	26–32	–	–
Clinafloxacin	5 µg	31–40	28–37	27–35	–
Clindamycin	2 µg	–	24–30	–	–
Daptomycin[d]	30 µg	–	18–23	–	–
Dirithromycin	15 µg	–	18–26	–	–
Doxycycline	30 µg	18–24	23–29	–	–
Enoxacin	10 µg	28–36	22–28	22–28	–
Ertapenem	10 µg	29–36	24–31	13–21	–
Erythromycin	15 µg	–	22–30	–	–
Fleroxacin	5 µg	28–34	21–27	12–20	–
Fosfomycin[c]	200 µg	22–30	25–33	–	–
Garenoxacin	**5 µg**	**28–35**	**30–36**	**19–25**	**–**
Gatifloxacin	5 µg	30–37	27–33	20–28	–
Gemifloxacin	5 µg	29–36	27–33	19–25	–
Gentamicin[a]	10 µg	19–26	19–27	16–21	–
Grepafloxacin	5 µg	28–36	26–31	20–27	–
Imipenem	10 µg	26–32	–	20–28	–
Kanamycin	30 µg	17–25	19–26	–	–
Levofloxacin	5 µg	29–37	25–30	19–26	–
Linezolid	30 µg	–	25–32	–	–
Lomefloxacin	10 µg	27–33	23–29	22–28	–
Loracarbef	30 µg	23–29	23–31	–	–
Mecillinam	10 µg	24–30	–	–	–

ATCC, American Type Culture Collection.

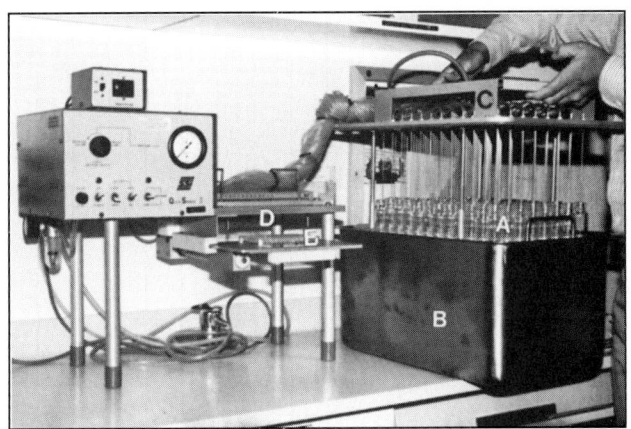

Figure 17-22 Quickspense instrument for dispensing fluid into microtiter plates. Dilutions of antibiotics are prepared in large volumes, using a set of 96 calibrated macrotubes *(A)*. The tubes are placed in an air-tight dispensing chamber *(B)*, the top of which contains a cannula for each macrotube *(C)*. These cannulae are connected by plastic tubing to a set of 96 needles *(D)*, through which antibiotic solutions are dropped into a microtiter plate *(E)*. A measured volume is dispensed by introduction of pressure into the dispensing chamber.

is complete, antimicrobial agent solutions can be dispensed into a large number of plates quickly. Such instruments combine the accuracy of preparing dilutions in large volumes with the convenience and economy of microtiter systems.

The antimicrobial agent-containing plates must be frozen at −20°C or lower until used. Frozen prepared plates can be obtained from several commercial sources. Storage of large numbers of frozen microplates may be difficult in some laboratories. In this case, plates that contain lyophilized antimicrobial agent solutions—the laboratory equivalent of instant coffee—may be purchased. Rehydration of the wells adds another step to the procedure, but the extended shelf-life of the freeze-dried plates is valuable, especially for laboratories in which small numbers of tests are performed. Both the frozen and lyophilized broth dilution systems have performed well in comparison to reference methods.[99,250,280] As might be expected, the interlaboratory reproducibility of the commercial systems that use standardized batches of very large volume has been greater than that for homemade plates, even when the plates were prepared for investigational use.[99] Some of the commercial systems have not performed well in certain special situations, as discussed below.

The interpretive guidelines suggested by the CLSI, which should be reported along with or in place of the actual MIC values, are listed in Table 17-16. Separate guidelines for interpreting *Haemophilus* species, *Streptococcus pneumoniae*, and *Neisseria gonorrhoeae* have been published by the CLSI. The guidelines for quality control are similar to those for the disk diffusion test (Table 17-22).

End points are usually easily defined (Fig. 17-23). Examination of the microplates is facilitated by use of a viewing mirror (Fig. 17-24). Occasionally, growth may be inhibited in a well that is adjacent to wells with uninhibited growth

(skipped well). If a single well is skipped and the interpretation of the result is not affected, the skipped well may be ignored. If multiple wells are skipped, if the skipped well occurs at a dilution that is critical for determining susceptibility of the isolate, or if multiple isolates demonstrate the phenomenon, the problem should be investigated and the test repeated.

The results of quality control testing may give clues to the nature of the problem. Certain errors are particularly common. Some of the possible problems and explanations are summarized in Table 17-23. The CLSI has provided guidelines for testing in special clinical situations, which are illustrated in Table 17-24.

Commercial Systems
VITEK (BIOMÉRIEUX VITEK, HAZELWOOD, MO) AND MICROSCAN (DADE INTERNATIONAL, WEST SACRAMENTO, CA)

The Vitek instrument uses a computer-assisted analysis of growth in plastic cards to calculate a MIC. In some instances the calculation of the MIC depends on the bacterial identification. The additional accuracy provided by the computer-driven correlation of growth pattern and identification is counterbalanced by the uncertainty about the susceptibility result if the identification is not yet known or cannot be provided with adequate certainty by the system.

The MicroScan products are based on traditional MIC methods. The line runs the gamut from plates—either frozen or lyophilized—that are interpreted manually at one extreme to a semiautomated instrument, the "Walkaway" at the other. Biochemical reagents for bacterial identification are incorporated into the same microtiter plates. Traditional overnight incubation is used for most of the MicroScan products. The Walkaway system, however, incorporates a fluorescence detection system that will provide same-day identification and susceptibility testing for some organisms. A variety of other semiautomated systems is available, as well as several choices for purchase of commercially prepared microdilution plates, either frozen or lyophilized. In general the systems work well. The two major systems have generally performed well in comparisons against reference methods,[175,179,250] although a troubling number of minor errors was noted in one report.[297] Furthermore, the Vitek instrument proved to be as accurate as the microdilution procedure when direct susceptibility tests were performed on material removed from positive blood culture bottles.[258]

From time to time problems are reported with each of these systems. The formulations or systems that produce the most rapid results appear to be most prone to error. As an example of current problems, the Vitek instrument produced more than expected errors when isolates of *Pseudomonas aeruginosa* from patients with cystic fibrosis were tested[143] and when this species was tested against carbapenems (imipenem and meropenem).[295] History indicates that all of the companies monitor such reports carefully and move quickly to address the problems.

Quality control of the automated results has been difficult and largely unsatisfactory. For most drug-organism combinations, the standard control strains produce results that are

Table 17-22 Quality Control Limits for Dilution Susceptibility Tests

ANTIMICROBIAL AGENT	STAPHYLOCOCCUS AUREUS (ATCC 29213)[a]	ENTEROCOCCUS FAECALIS (ATCC 29212)	ESCHERICHIA COLI (ATCC 25922)	PSEUDOMONAS AERUGINOSA (ATCC 27853)	ESCHERICHIA COLI (ATCC 35218)[b]
Amikacin	1–4	64–256	0.5–4	1–4	–
Amoxicillin-clavulanic acid	0.12/0.06–0.5/0.25	0.25/0.12–1.0/0.5	2/1–8/4	–	4/2–16/8
Ampicillin	0.5–2	0.5–2	2–8	–	–
Ampicillin-sulbactam	–	–	2/1	–	8/4–32/16
Azithromycin	0.5–2	–	–	–	–
Azlocillin	2–8	1–4	8–32	2–8	–
Aztreonam	–	–	0.06–0.25	2–8	–
Carbenicillin	2–8	16–64	4–16	16–64	–
Cefaclor	1–4	–	1–4	–	–
Cefamandole	0.25–1	–	0.25–1	–	–
Cefazolin	0.25–1	–	4	–	–
Cefdinir	0.12–0.5	–	0.12–0.5	–	–
Cefditoren	0.25–2	–	0.12–1	–	–
Cefepime	1–4	–	0.016–0.12	1–8	–
Cefetamet	–	–	0.25–1	–	–
Cefixime	8–32	–	0.25–1	–	–
Cefmetazole	0.5–2	–	0.25–2	>32	–
Cefonicid	1–4	–	0.25–1	–	–
Cefoperazone	1–4	–	0.12–0.5	2–8	–
Cefotaxime	1–4	–	0.03–0.12	8–32	–
Cefotetan	4–16	–	0.06–0.25	–	–
Cefoxitin	1–4	–	2–8	–	–
Cefpodoxime	1–8	–	0.25–1	–	–
Cefprozil	0.25–1	–	1–4	–	–
Ceftazidime	4–16	–	0.06–0.5	1–4	–
Ceftibuten	–	–	0.12–0.5	–	–

Ceftizoxime	2–8	—	0.03–0.12	16–64
Ceftriaxone	1–8	—	0.03–0.12	8–64
Cefuroxime	0.5–2	—	2–8	—
Cephalothin	0.12–0.5	—	4–16	—
Chloramphenicol	2–8	4–16	2–8	—
Cinoxacin	—	—	2–8	—
Ciprofloxacin	0.12–0.5	0.25–2	0.004–0.016	0.25–1
Clarithromycin	0.12–0.5	—	—	—
Clinafloxacin	0.008–0.06	0.03–0.25	0.002–0.016	0.06–0.5
Clindamycin	0.06	4–16	—	—
Daptomycin[c]	0.25–1	1–8	—	—
Dirithromycin	1–4	—	—	—
Doxycycline	—	—	0.5–2	—
Enoxacin	0.5–2	2–16	0.06–0.25	2–8
Ertapenem	0.06–0.25	4–16	0.004–0.016	2–8
Erythromycin	0.25–1	1–4	—	—
Fleroxacin	0.25–1	2–8	0.03–0.12	1–4
Fosfomycin[d]	0.5–4	32–128	0.5–2	2–8
Garenoxacin	**0.004–0.03**	**0.03–0.25**	**0.004–0.03**	**0.5–2**
Gatifloxacin	0.03–0.12	0.12–1.0	0.008–0.03	0.5–2
Gemifloxacin	0.008–0.03	0.016–0.12	0.004–0.016	0.25–1
Gentamicin[e]	0.12–1	4–16	0.25–1	0.5–2
Grepafloxacin	0.03–0.12	0.12–0.5	0.004–0.03	0.25–2.0
Imipenem	0.016–0.06	0.5–2	0.06–0.25	1–4
Kanamycin	1–4	16–64	1–4	—
Levofloxacin	0.06–0.5	0.25–2	0.008–0.06	0.5–4
Linezolid	1–4	1–4	—	—

ATCC, American Type Culture Collection.

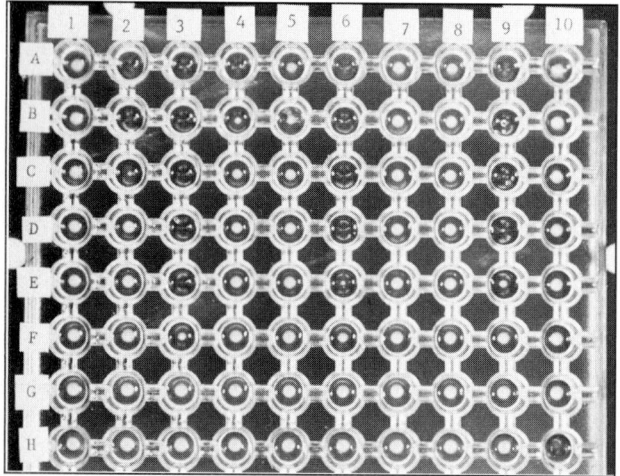

Figure 17-23 Microtube broth dilution antibiotic susceptibility plate. The numbers across the top indicate the different antibiotics being tested within each vertical column; the letters along the left border reflect the concentration of antibiotics contained within each well. The appearance of a button of bacterial growth in any well indicates resistance to that concentration of antibiotic.

at the extremes of the parameter measured and cannot be quantitated precisely.[161]

Epsilometer Test (Etest; AB Biodisk, Sweden)

A useful addition to the diagnostic armamentarium is the Etest, which consists of antimicrobial agent–impregnated strips that are placed on the surface of agar (Chart 17-3). The principle is an expansion of the disk diffusion method, and the protocol for preparing the inoculum is the same. The antimicrobial agent content of the strips is graded, and the concentration is printed linearly along the strip (Fig. 17-25). After incubation the MIC is read from the point on the strip where the zone of growth inhibition passes. If the strips are placed on the agar upside down (impregnated side not in contact with the agar), erroneous determinations of the MIC will likely result.[117] The manufacturer indicates, however, that an upside-down strip can be repositioned without problems if the mistake is recognized immediately.

The same factors that influence the disk diffusion susceptibility test apply to its stepchild, the Etest. Diffusion of antimicrobial agents begins immediately after placement of the strip, which cannot, therefore, be moved once the impregnated surface has touched the agar. A poorly streaked plate may produce an irregular zone of inhibition at the MIC point. Swarming of *Proteus* spp. and mutant colonies within the zone of inhibition may be challenges with the Etest, as with disk diffusion.

The Etest has proven to be effective for general use.[8] The expense of this approach makes it difficult to justify for testing multiple antimicrobial agents against organisms that grow well in one of the dilution or disk diffusion procedures. It is invaluable, however, for testing highly selected antimicrobial agents against fastidious organisms that do not grow well in the other tests (e.g., *Streptococcus pneumoniae*[163] or viridans streptococci[272]).

The procedure for performing a susceptibility test with the Etest strips is summarized in Chart 17-3. In addition to the general issues common to all susceptibility tests, specific suggestions for trouble-shooting the Etest are summarized in Box 17-7.

Special Issues in Susceptibility Testing
β-Lactamases

β-Lactamases are heterogeneous bacterial enzymes that cleave the β-lactam ring of penicillins and cephalosporins to inactivate the antibiotic. β-Lactamases are found in a wide variety of gram-positive and gram-negative bacterial species. The enzymes produced by *Staphylococcus* species, *Haemophilus* species, *Moraxella* (*Branhamella*) *catarrhalis*, and *Neisseria gonorrhoeae* have been the most important clinically. The significance of the conventional enzymes produced by many enteric bacteria is less clear, and these bacteria should not be tested for β-lactamase. The appearance of β-lactamases with a broad spectrum in gram-negative bacteria, however, has focused increased attention on this resistance mechanism.

The presence of many β-lactamases may be detected quickly and reliably, providing an early clue that an isolate will not respond to the β-lactam antibiotics in question. Staphylococcal enzymes and the broad/extended-spectrum enzymes of gram-negative bacteria, however, present special problems, as discussed below.

The chromogenic cephalosporin test, using Nitrocefin (Cefinase; BD Diagnostic Systems, Sparks, MD), is the most sensitive. Filter-paper disks impregnated with Nitrocefin are commercially available. A loopful of a colony is smeared

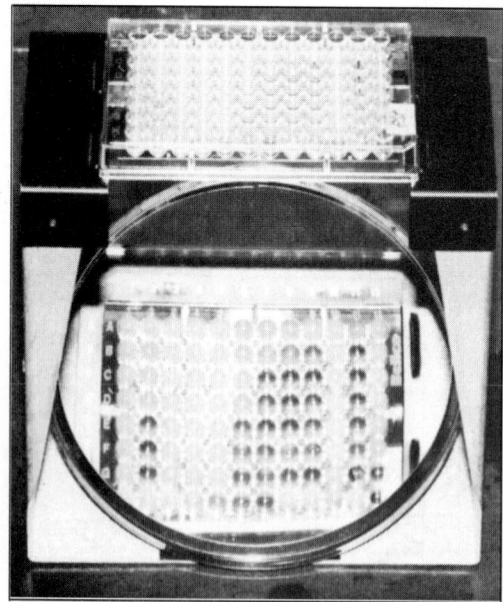

Figure 17-24 Viewing mirror for visualization of bacterial growth in broth microdilution test.

Table 17-23 Trouble-Shooting Quality Control Problems in Susceptibility Tests*

OBSERVATION	DIAGNOSIS	CORRECTIVE TESTS*
MICs too large or zone sizes too small (isolates too resistant)	1. Inoculum too high	1. Check and adjust inoculum if necessary
	2. Deterioration of antimicrobial agent	2. Check potency of disks or powder; try new lot
	3. Change in quality control (QC) strain	3. Test new stock of QC strain
	4. Agar too deep	4. Check depth of agar
	5. Incorrect reading of results	5. Repeat with multiple observers
MICs too small or zone sizes too large (isolates too susceptible)	1. Inoculum too low	1. Check and adjust inoculum if necessary
	2. Antimicrobial agent too potent	2. Check potency of disks or powder; try new lots
	3. Change in QC strain	3. Test new stock of QC strain
	4. Agar too thin	4. Check depth of agar
	5. Incorrect reading of results	5. Repeat with multiple observers
Results for *Pseudomonas* and aminoglycosides out of control	Cation content incorrect	Use cation-supplemented broth or try different lot of agar
Aminoglycosides and macrolides too resistant; tetracycline too susceptible	Medium too acid	Check pH of media
Aminoglycosides and macrolides too susceptible; tetracycline too resistant	Medium too alkaline	Check pH of media
Trimethoprim MICs too large or zone sizes too small; results difficult to read	Excess thymidine in medium	Test medium with *Enterococcus faecalis* (ATCC 29212); add thymidine phosphorylase or lysed horse blood
General	1. Turbidity standard expired, stored improperly, not made to standard, or inadequately mixed before testing	1. Check turbidity standard; prepare new standard if necessary
	2. Materials and reagents used after expiration date or improperly stored	2. Check expiration date and storage temperature of media and reagents
	3. Incubator temperature and/or atmosphere improperly set	3. Check incubator records
	4. Other equipment (e.g., pipettes) functioning improperly	4. Check equipment; revalidate if necessary
	5. Plates stored at wrong temperature	5. Check storage of plates and temperature records of storage location
	6. Control strain mutated or contaminated	6. Obtain fresh control strain and retest
	7. Inoculum suspensions adjusted incorrectly	7. Review preparation of suspensions with staff
	8. Inoculum prepared from a plate that was >24 hours old	8. Review standards for sources of inoculum

*In addition to actions suggested in table, results that are out of control will require retesting and withholding of results until QC is back in control (see Table 17-15).[217-220] ATCC, American Type Culture Collection.

Table 17-24 Summary of Testing Methods for Selected Organisms

ORGANISM	METHOD	MEDIUM	INOCULUM	INCUBATION	COMMENTS
Staphylococcus spp.	Broth microdilution; agar dilution	Cation-adjusted Mueller-Hinton broth (CAMHB) or Mueller-Hinton agar (MHA); CAMHB or MHA plus 2% NaCl for oxacillin, methicillin, and nafcillin	Direct colony suspension, equivalent to 0.5 McFarland standard (DCS)	35°C; ambient air; 16 to 20 hr; 24 hr for oxacillin, nafcillin, and methicillin	Consider molecular testing for *mecA* gene and/or multiple phenotypic tests; consider vancomycin agar screen if automated commercial systems used; confirm vancomycin intermediate or resistant strains
	Oxacillin-salt agar screening test	Mueller-Hinton agar (MHA) with 4% NaCl	DCS	35°C; ambient air; 24 hr	
	Disk diffusion	MHA	DCS	35°C; ambient air; 16 to 20 hr; 24 hr for oxacillin, nafcillin, methicillin, and vancomycin	Consider confirming vancomycin results with a MIC test, especially for oxacillin-resistant strains; low-level resistance not well detected
	Gradient diffusion (Etest)	MHA; MHA with 2% NaCl for oxacillin, methicillin, and nafcillin	DCS in broth	35°C; ambient air; 16 to 20 hr.; 24 hours for oxacillin, nafcillin, and methicillin and vancomycin	Incubate plate for 48 hr to detect oxacillin resistant coagulase negative staphylococci
Enterococcus spp.	Broth microdilution; Agar dilution	CAMHB; MHA	Growth method or DCS	35°C; ambient air; 16 to 20 hr.; 24 hours for vancomycin	Confirm vancomycin resistant strains; perform β-lactamase test
	Disk diffusion	MHA	Growth method or DCS	35°C; ambient air; 16 to 18 hr; 24 hr for vancomycin	
	Gradient diffusion	MHA	DCS in broth	35°C; ambient air; 16 to 18 hr; 24 hr for vancomycin	
Enterococcus spp. high-level gentamicin resistance	Broth microdilution; agar dilution	Brain-heart infusion (BHI) broth or agar; gentamicin 500 µg/mL	Growth method or DCS; standard microdilution inoculum; 10 µL spotted on agar surface	35°C; ambient air; 24 hours	Perform on isolates from serious systemic infections only
Enterococcus spp. High-level streptomycin resistance	Broth microdilution; agar dilution	BHI broth or agar; streptomycin 1000 µg/mL (broth) or 2000 µg/mL (agar)	Growth method or DCS; standard microdilution inoculum; 10 µl spotted on agar surface	35°C; ambient air; 24 hours; reincubate an additional 24 hours if susceptible	Perform on isolates from serious systemic infections only

Organism	Method	Medium	Growth method or DCS	Incubation	Comments
Enterococcus spp. High-level aminoglycoside resistance	Disk diffusion	MHA; 120 μg disk (gentamicin); 300 μg disk (streptomycin)	DCS	35°C; ambient air; 16 to 18 hr	Confirm intermediate results with an MIC test
Enterococcus spp. high-level aminoglycoside resistance	Gradient diffusion	MHA; gentamicin and streptomycin high-dose strips	Suspension in broth to 0.5–1.0 McFarland standard	35°C; ambient air; 48 hr	
Enterococcus spp. vancomycin resistance	Agar dilution	BHI agar; vancomycin 6 μg/mL	Growth method or DCS; standard microdilution inoculum; 1–10 μL spotted on agar surface	35°C; ambient air; 24 hours	
Haemophilus spp.	Broth microdilution	Haemophilus test medium (HTM) broth	DCS	35°C; 5% CO_2; 20 to 24 hr.	
	Disk diffusion	Haemophilus test medium (HTM)	DCS	35°C; 5% CO_2; 20 to 24 hr.	
	Gradient diffusion	HTM or MHA with 1% hemoglobin and 1% Isovitalex (BBL) if validated against NCCLS	DCS in broth	35°C; ambient air; 24 hr	
Neisseria gonorrhoeae	Agar dilution	GC agar base and 1% defined growth supplement (see text)	DCS	35°C; 5% CO_2; 20–24 hr	Perform β-lactamase test
	Disk diffusion	GC agar base with 1% defined growth supplement (see text)	DCS	35°C; 5% CO_2; 20–24 hr	Cysteine-free medium not required; perform β-lactamase test
	Gradient diffusion	GC agar base with 1% defined growth supplement (see text)	DCS in broth	35°C; 5% CO_2; 20 to 24 hr	
Neisseria meningitidis	Broth microdilution	CAMHB plus 2–5% v/v lysed horse blood	DCS	35°C; ambient air; 16–20 hr.	
	Agar dilution	MHA plus 5% v/v sheep blood	DCS	35°C; ambient air; 16–20 hr	Use 2–5% v/v lysed horse blood instead of sheep blood if sulfonamides are tested
	Disk diffusion	Not validated			
	Gradient diffusion	MHA plus 5% sheep blood or MHA plus 1% hemoglobin and 1% Isovitalex (BBL)	DCS in broth	35°C; 5% CO_2; 18–24 hr	
Streptococcus pneumoniae	Broth microdilution	CAMHB with 2–5% (v/v) lysed horse blood	DCS	35°C; ambient air; 20 to 24 hr.	May perform oxacillin disk screen for penicillin susceptibility as a preliminary test

(Continued)

Table 17-24 *Continued*

ORGANISM	METHOD	MEDIUM	INOCULUM	INCUBATION	COMMENTS
	Disk diffusion	MHA with 5% sheep blood	DCS	35°C; 5% CO_2; 20–24 hr	Reliable disk tests not available for some antimicrobial agents; MIC test recommended for CSF isolates
	Gradient diffusion	MHA with 5% sheep blood	DCS in broth	35°C; 5% CO_2; 20–24 hr	If the bacterial lawn is too sparse, repeat using a 1.0 McFarland standard
Streptococcus spp. other than *S. pneumoniae*	Broth microdilution	CAMHB with 2–5% v/v lysed horse blood	DCS	35°C; ambient air; 20–24 hr	
	Agar dilution	MHA with 5% v/v sheep blood	DCS	35°C; ambient air; 20–24 hr; CO_2 if necessary for growth	Use lysed horse blood instead of sheep blood if testing a sulfonamide
	Disk diffusion	Not validated			
	Gradient diffusion	MHA with 5% sheep blood	DCS	35°C; 5% CO_2; 20–24 hr	Match inoculum to a 1.0 McFarland standard for mucoid strains
Vibrio cholerae	Broth microdilution; agar dilution	CAMHB; MHA	Growth method or DCS	35°C; ambient air; 16–20 hr	
	Disk diffusion	MHA	Growth method or DCS	35°C; ambient air; 16–18 hr	
Listeria spp.	Broth microdilution	CMHB plus 2–5% lysed horse blood	DCS	35°C; ambient air; 16–20 hr	For ampicillin and penicillin ≤2 µg/mL = susceptible (resistant strains not characterized)

Adapted from Etest application sheets, AB Biodisk, Solna, Sweden; and from references[217,218].

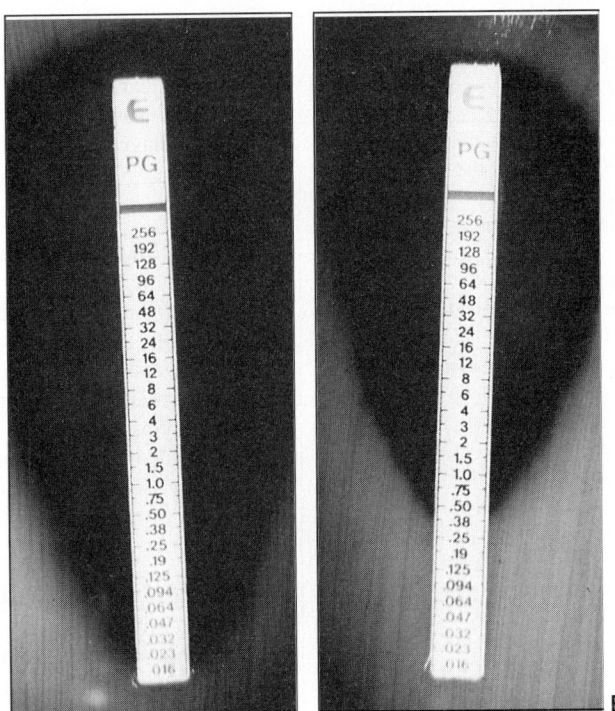

Figure 17-25 Etest for *Streptococcus pneumoniae* on Mueller-Hinton agar with blood. The plates have been prepared as for the disk diffusion test, after which the test strips have been applied. The MIC of the isolate is read where the line of growth inhibition crosses the strip. (**A**) Fully susceptible strain with a MIC of 0.016 μg/mL. (**B**) Strain with intermediate susceptibility and an MIC of 0.38 μg/mL.

on the disk and placed in a closed Petri dish to prevent rapid desiccation. Organisms that contain β-lactamase will change the color of the disk from yellow to red. The reaction usually occurs within 30 seconds, but tests are read finally after 15 minutes.

Acidimetric tests are less expensive to perform but are less sensitive than the Nitrocefin assay. Opening of the β-lactam ring produces penicilloic acid, which is more acid than penicillin. The change in pH is detected by visual observation of an indicator dye, phenol red. A suspension of phenol red and penicillin G is adjusted with NaOH to pH 8.5 (the point at which the color changes to purple) and stored at −20°C for up to 1 week.[7] At the time of testing, a capillary tube is dipped into the phenol red solution until 1 cm of the tube is filled. The filled end of the tube is scraped across a bacterial colony to plug the tube, then incubated at room temperature for 60 minutes. A change in the phenol red indicator to yellow indicates the presence of β-lactamase.

In every case the Nitrocefin test has been the most sensitive and the most specific method for measuring β-lactamases. It must be used when testing *Moraxella catarrhalis*. There is little reason to use one of the other methods when the Nitrocefin test serves all purposes.

STAPHYLOCOCCUS SPECIES

The β-lactamases of staphylococci are induced by exposure to penicillins. They are responsible for most of the resistance to penicillin G and related compounds but are not ac-

tive against the cephalosporins or the penicillinase-resistant penicillins, such as methicillin and nafcillin, unless produced in large amounts. Detection of these enzymes is particularly difficult with the microbroth dilution test, because the bacteria in the relatively small inoculum used in this test may be killed before the enzyme is induced.

If the MIC of a staphylococcal strain to penicillin is greater than 0.25 μg/mL, the presence of a β-lactamase can be inferred. Isolates with penicillin MICs less than 0.03 μg/mL are considered nonproducers and susceptible. Isolates for which the MIC falls between these limits (0.06 or 0.12 μg/mL) should be tested for the presence of β-lactamase before the results are reported. Use of bacterial growth from a well that contains a penicillin-class drug or from the edge of a zone of inhibition around a disk that contains a penicillin compound may induce activity and enhance detection of the enzyme. The results from the testing of penicillin can be extrapolated to ampicillin.

β-Lactam antibiotics, such as first-generation cephalosporins and penicillinase-resistant penicillins (methicillin, nafcillin, oxacillin, dicloxacillin, etc.) have a modified β-lactam ring that resists enzymatic digestion by staphylococcal β-lactamases. If a strain produces a large quantity of enzyme, however, it can inactivate these antibiotics in vitro. These strains usually exhibit borderline resistance to oxacillin (MIC, 4 μg/mL) and susceptibility to other commonly used antimicrobial agents. In contrast, strains that are resistant to oxacillin by means of altered penicillin-binding proteins usually have higher levels of oxacillin resistance and

Box 17-7 Trouble-Shooting Etest Susceptibility Assays

1. Place Etest on the surface of the agar, which has been streaked with the inoculum. Do not move the strip once the antibiotic-impregnated surface has touched the agar. If the strip is accidentally placed upside down (non-antibiotic-impregnated side in contact with the agar), it is permissible to remove the strip and position it properly.

2. If growth is insufficient to see a clearly defined ellipse of inhibition after initial incubation, continue incubation within the limits defined in the procedure. If incubation must be prolonged beyond the recommended limits, the published breakpoints cannot be used without qualification.

3. Read the MIC where the ellipse intersects the scale on the strip. The point of intersection is complete inhibition of all growth, including hazes and isolated colonies.
   a. If microcolonies are present in the zone of inhibition, check the purity of the culture (as for the disk diffusion test); do not ignore these colonies in determining the MIC.
   b. Tilt the plate to visualize pinpoint colonies and hazes, especially for enterococci, pneumococci, and *Stenotrophomonas* spp. Alternatively, a magnifying glass may be used to detect microcolonies (in contradistinction to the rules for the disk diffusion test).
   c. Include a haze as growth when determining inhibition, but ignore the swarming of *Proteus* spp.
   d. When testing β-hemolytic bacteria, assess the zone of inhibition and ignore the hemolysis.
   e. If a paradoxical effect (inhibition at low MIC and regrowth at higher MICs), read the MIC as the zone of final, complete inhibition.
   f. Bacteriostatic drugs, such as trimethoprim-sulfamethoxazole may produce growth with a diffuse, fuzzy edge; read the MIC at 80% inhibition (as for the disk diffusion test).
   g. When testing combinations of β-lactams and β-lactamase inhibitors, the inhibitor may have intrinsic activity, producing an extended ellipse at the lowest MICs. Extrapolate the upper ellipse of inhibition to determine the MIC.
   h. A "dip" effect at the lowest MIC may be seen when inducible macrolide resistance is present, producing an ellipse with an elongated nipple at the end. Extrapolate the curvature of the primary ellipse to determine the MIC.
   i. Ignore a thin line of growth along the lower portion of the strip, a phenomenon caused by organisms growing in a tunnel of water along the strip.

4. If the zone of inhibition intersects the strip between two markings, read the higher value. Similarly, if the zone intersects the strip slightly differently on the two sides, read the higher value.

5. If the MIC produced by the strip is between numbers in the classic twofold-dilution scheme (on which all standard recommendations are based), round the "answer" up to the next twofold dilution. For instance, a MIC of 1.5 μg/mL would be reported as 2.0 μg/mL.

Adapted from Etest Technical Guide: Etest for MIC determination, AB Biodisk, Solna, Sweden.

resistance to multiple other antimicrobial agents, as discussed below. The clinical significance of these strains has been unclear. Kernodle and colleagues, however, have described a group of such strains of *Staphylococcus aureus* of a certain phage type that produced clinically significant wound infections.[164]

HAEMOPHILUS SPECIES

As many as 20–40% of type B *Haemophilus influenzae* isolates from serious infections produce β-lactamases.[66] Detection of the enzymes should be performed on any isolate that is considered a pathogen. A few strains have demonstrated resistance to ampicillin by other mechanisms, so a non-enzyme-producing strain should also be tested against ampicillin by a diffusion or dilution susceptibility test, at least for isolates that have been isolated from sterile sites and are producing clinically significant infections.[17]

NEISSERIA GONORRHOEAE

Penicillinase-producing gonococci were detected initially in the Far East but are now widely distributed. All isolates should be tested for β-lactamase. As with *Haemophilus* species, some strains that are resistant to penicillin by nonenzymatic means have now been identified,[267] so that a susceptibility test should also be performed if the treatment fails or if the frequency of resistance is high in the population served.

MORAXELLA (BRANHAMELLA) CATARRHALIS

Moraxella (Branhamella) catarrhalis has been recognized in recent years as an important cause of upper respiratory tract infection and of nosocomial lower respiratory tract infection. Most strains produce β-lactamases, which are of two types. The most common enzyme (Ravasio type) is chromosomal, constitutive, tightly cell-associated, and blocked by β-lactamase inhibitors such as clavulanate and sulbactam.[60,81] A second, less common enzyme (1908 type) differs in several important respects. It is produced in 10- to 100-fold lower amounts than the Ravasio type. As a result, the quantitative susceptibility result may be in the susceptible range in the presence of a positive β-lactamase test. In the absence of good clinical data, these strains should probably be considered resistant. There is little reason to perform any test routinely other than β-lactamase on *Moraxella (Branhamella) catarrhalis* because the susceptibility of the organism to other antimicrobial agents is predictable.[69] Doern and colleagues found that the Nitrocefin tube or disk test was the most effective means of detecting β-lactamase.[64,68] The subject has been reviewed by Doern and Jones.[64]

ENTEROCOCCUS SPECIES

Isolates of enterococci that produce β-lactamase have been identified.[213] This high-level resistance to penicillin can be detected by the Nitrocefin test. The β-lactamase, which resembles that of staphylococci, is carried on a plasmid,[214] but the enterococcal and staphylococcal plasmids themselves are not homologous.[331] Strains of *Enterococcus faecalis* that produce β-lactamase and also exhibit high-level resistance to aminoglycosides have become epidemic in some institutions.[341] If the Nitrocefin disk test is not performed on isolates, resistance to β-lactam antibiotics may not be recognized. In a survey of New Jersey laboratories by Tenover and colleagues a β-lactamase producing strain of *E. faecalis* was recognized as resistant to penicillin by only 66% of 76 participants and to ampicillin by a startling 8% of laboratories. Only 3 of the 76 laboratories recognized that the strain produced β-lactamase, emphasizing the importance of performing a β-lactamase test on enterococci, especially if they have been isolated from sterile sites.[314] A combination of piperacillin and tazobactam is effective against β-lactamase-producing enterococci,[234] and it is possible that this combination will provide synergy with aminoglycosides for such strains.

EXTENDED-SPECTRUM β-LACTAMASES

The presence of extended-spectrum β-lactamases (ESBLs) can be suspected if an isolate of *Klebsiella pneumoniae* or *Escherichia coli* demonstrates resistance to one or more of the indicator β-lactam antibiotics but susceptibility to other third-generation cephalosporins. Unfortunately, there is no single indicator antibiotic that works in all situations. ESBLs occur in other *Enterobacteriaceae*, such as *Enterobacter* spp. and *Citrobacter* spp., but detection is more difficult because of the frequent occurrence of other types of β-lactamases, especially AmpC enzymes, in these species. The CLSI has provided recommendations, which are summarized in Table 17-25, only for *Klebsiella pneumoniae* and *Escherichia coli*.

Once the possibility of an ESBL has been suggested by the initial testing, it is necessary to perform a confirmatory test, based on the fact that these enzymes are almost always blocked by inhibitors of β-lactamase. The tests that are currently available are summarized in Table 17-26.

The CLSI criteria for screening and confirming ESBL production in *Escherichia coli* and *Klebsiella* spp. have proven reliable, although there is a possibility of missing some strains if the inoculum is too low.[260] Although ESBLs are found in other species, at this juncture it is not useful to apply the CLSI criteria to these organisms.[281]

These enzymes are carried on plasmids that often mediate resistance to other antimicrobial agents, such as aminoglycosides, tetracycline, and sulfonamides, so the appearance of unusual resistance patterns can also serve as a clue that the extended-spectrum enzymes are present.[84,160] Several methods have been suggested to augment the detection of this resistance mechanism. A double-disk synergy test with disks of cetotaxime and Augmentin placed 30 mm apart from center to center was effective at detecting resistance mediated by EBS-Bla type enzymes.[141] Thomson and Sanders evaluated two methods for detecting resistance.[317] A double-disk test was performed with ampicillin-clavulanate disks surrounded by aztreonam and third-generation cephalosporin disks (separated by 30 mm center-to-center). Distortion of the zone sizes in a synergistic fashion (Fig. 17-29C) indicated production of enzyme. This method detected true resistance in 22 of 28 strains (79%). The second method was a three-dimensional test in which a circular hole in the agar was cut just inside the eventual position of antimicrobial disks. The hole was filled with bacterial inoculum. Otherwise the procedure followed the standard disk-diffusion pro-

---

Table 17-25 Screening Tests for Extended-Spectrum β-Lactamases

ANTIBIOTIC[a]	MIC BREAKPOINT	DISK AND ZONE BREAKPOINT	COMMENTS[b]
Cefpodoxime	4 μg/mL	10 μg; ≤17 mm	Appears to be most sensitive general indicator[318]; not useful for *K. oxytoca*[316]; may give false-positive results with *E. coli*[312]
Ceftazidime	1 μg/mL	30 μg; ≤22 mm	Strains with high-level resistance cannot be tested in the ceftazidime confirmatory assay[296]; may not detect resistance in *K. pneumoniae* and *E. coli*
Aztreonam	1 μg/mL	30 μg; ≤27 mm	
Cefotaxime	1 μg/mL	30 μg; ≤27 mm	
Ceftriaxone	1 μg/mL	30 μg; ≤25 mm	Very sensitive strains cannot be tested in the ceftriaxone confirmatory assay[296]
Cefipime	1 μg/mL	NA	Not included in CLSI documents; may be useful for differentiating AmpC enzymes of *Enterobacter* spp. and *Serratia* spp.[296,316]
Cefoxitin	NCCLS breakpoints	NCCLS breakpoints	Not included in the CLSI documents; resistance may indicate AmpC producer[50] or differentiate among non-ESBL resistance mechanisms[296]

[a] *Sensitivity of detection and ease of interpretation is increased if more than one indicator antibiotic is used.*
[b] *Note that the current CLSI recommendations may differ from those in force at the time the referenced studies were performed.*
NA, not available.
Adapted from references[217,218].

Table 17-26 Confirmatory Tests for Extended-Spectrum β-Lactamases

METHOD	CRITERIA FOR ESBL	COMMENTS	ILLUSTRATION
Double-disk test	Enhancement of inhibition zone facing disk that contains β-lactamase inhibitor	Placement of disks is critical; separation of disk centers by both 20 mm and 30 mm may be necessary	Figure 17–26
Comparison of MIC or inhibitory zone around disk in presence or absence of β-lactamase inhibitor	Decrease in MIC of ≥8-fold (three doubling dilutions) or ≥5 mm increase in zone size in the presence of the β-lactamase inhibitor	CLSI recommends use of both ceftazidime and cefotaxime with and without clavulanic acid	Figure 17–27
Vitek ESBL test	Decrease in calculated MIC in the presence of β-lactamase inhibitor	Result calculated by software	Not pictured
Etest	Double-ended strip with β-lactam on one end and combination of β-lactam and β-lactamase inhibitor on the other	Reduction in MIC by ≥8-fold in the presence of β-lactamase inhibitor	Figure 17–28
Three-dimensional test	Circular hole cut in agar between position of disks, then filled with bacterial inoculum; distortion of zone size at the point of cut indicates ESBL	Most sensitive method, but technically very demanding to perform	Not pictured

tocol. Distortion of the zone sizes at the point of the cut in the agar indicated the presence of enzyme. The three-dimensional test detected resistance in 26 of 28 isolates (93%), but the technique and interpretation are exacting.

Staphylococcus Species
β-LACTAM ANTIBIOTICS (OXACILLIN-RESISTANT *STAPHYLOCOCCUS* SPECIES)

For several decades the penicillin antibiotics that are stable to β-lactamase (penicillinase) were the mainstay of antimicrobial therapy for *Staphylococcus aureus;* in contrast, the vast majority of the coagulase-negative staphylococci

have always been resistant to these compounds. Clinically, methicillin and nafcillin are the most commonly used drugs of this class, and the isolates are usually described as methicillin-resistant *S. aureus* (MRSA) or methicillin-resistant *Staphylococcus epidermidis* (MRSE). This resistance is particularly difficult to detect in the laboratory. Staphylococci are heteroresistant; that is, only a small fraction of the bacteria in a culture express resistance, a characteristic that is chromosomally mediated. Binding of methicillin to penicillin binding protein 2a correlates with resistance to the antibiotic.[43] The resistant cells grow more slowly than the susceptible bacteria, unless incubated at reduced temper-

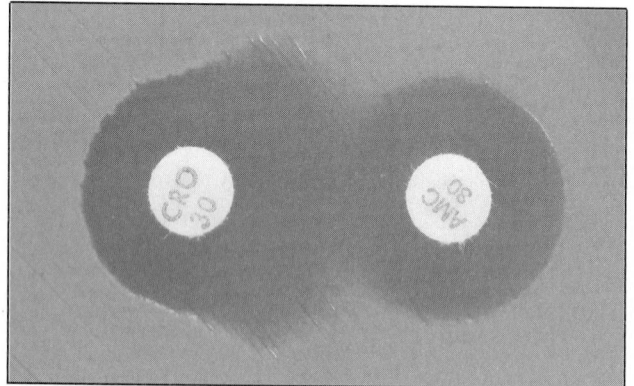
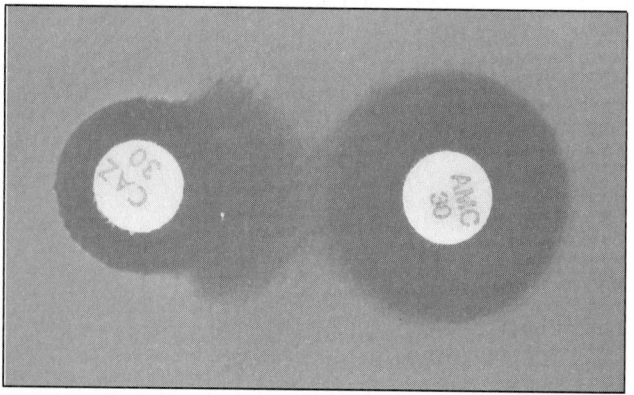

A   B

Figure 17-26 Double-disk test for ESBL production in an isolate of *Klebsiella pneumoniae.* **(A)** The zone around a ceftriaxone disk (CRO) is distorted and enlarged on the side facing a disk that contains clavulanic acid (AMC). **(B)** A similar phenomenon is demonstrated with a disk containing ceftazidime (CAZ) adjacent to a disk that contains clavulanic acid (AMC).

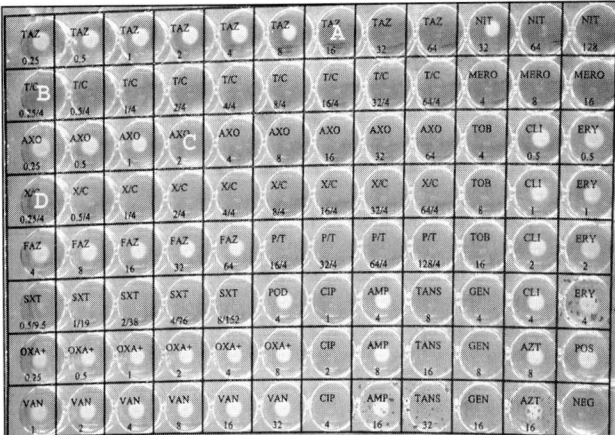

Figure 17-27 MIC test for ESBL production in an isolate of *Escherichia coli*. The MIC of this isolate for ceftazidime is 16 μg/mL *(A)*; when combined with clavulanic acid the MIC is ≤0.25 μg/mL *(B)*. The MIC of the isolate for ceftriaxone is 2 μg/mL *(C)*; in the presence of clavulanic acid the MIC is ≤0.25 μg/mL *(D)*. Thus, in each case there is a >4-fold reduction of the MIC in the presence of clavulanic acid, demonstrating the presence of an ESBL.

ature. The relatively low inoculum used in the microbroth dilution test may compromise detection of the small fraction of resistant cells. Variations in the ability of different lots of Mueller-Hinton agar to detect heteroresistance have been reported.[125] These isolates, which express PBP 2a, are clinically resistant to all β-lactam antibiotics, but the resistance is most readily detected with oxacillin in the laboratory. They will be referred to as oxacillin-resistant staphylococci,

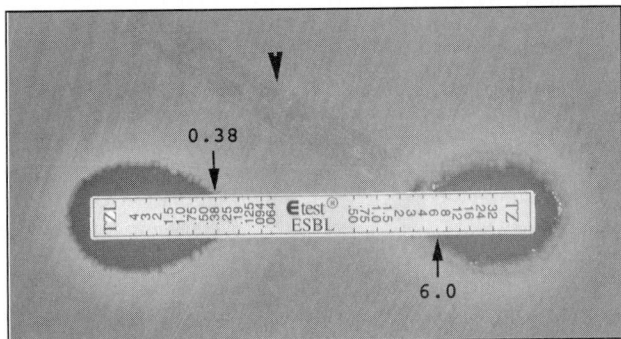

Figure 17-28 Etest strip for demonstration of ESBL production in an isolate of *Klebsiella pneumoniae*. The MIC of the isolate for ceftazidime (TZ) is 6 μg/mL. (Note that the zone of inhibition intersects the strip closer to 4 μg/mL on the lower side, but the intersection is at 6 μg/mL on the upper side; the higher value is recorded.) At the other end of the strip the MIC of the isolate for ceftazidime in the presence of clavulanic acid is 0.38 μg/mL. The reduction of the MIC is >4-fold, indicating the presence of an ESBL enzyme in the strain. Note the impression on the lawn of bacteria of the strip (arrowhead), which was initially dropped upside down on the plate; because the side that was impregnated with antibiotic did not touch the agar, it was acceptable to reposition the strip and continue the test.

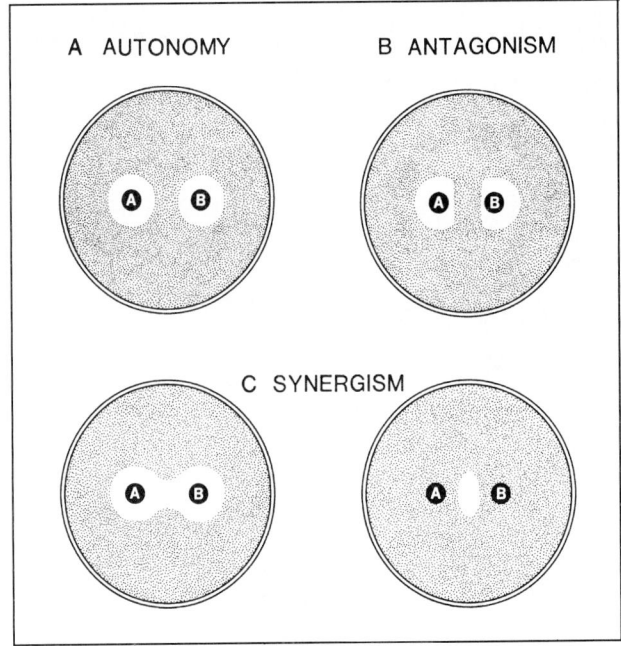

Figure 17-29 Diagram of potential interactions in disk-diffusion test for bacterial synergy: Disks containing antibiotics A and B have been placed on Mueller-Hinton agar plates that have been inoculated with a bacterial isolate. **(A)** Additive or indifferent effects; each antibiotic produces a zone of inhibition that is not affected by the adjacent antibiotic. **(B)** Antagonistic effects, in which the inhibitory zones of each antibiotic are diminished in the presence of the other antibiotic. **(C)** Two possible manifestations of the synergistic interactions. On the left, an enlarged inhibitory zone occurs where the two antibiotics meet. On the right, neither antibiotic is inhibitory in its own right, but bacterial growth is inhibited where the two antibiotics diffuse together.

but all penicillin, cephalosporin, and carbapenem antibiotics should be reported as resistant (Table 17-12).

In a study of 975 clinical isolates, Varaldo and colleagues found 122 strains of *S. aureus* (12.5%) that had borderline susceptibility to β-lactamase-resistant penicillins.[329] There are four potential mechanisms for this result. Initially, McDougal and Thornsberry reported that hyperproduction of β-lactamase is the mechanism by which some borderline-susceptible strains of *S. aureus* express resistance to oxacillin, and this appears to be the most common explanation.[198] The hyperproducing strains can be detected by performing an MIC test with a combination of β-lactamase inhibitor and a β-lactam antibiotic (Fig. 17-30). Chang and colleagues found that in *S. aureus* strains with a MIC of <64 μg/mL, the MIC was reduced by 4-fold to 32-fold if either 4 μg/mL of sulbactam or 8 μg/mL of tazobactam was added.[44] Addition of inhibitor to strains with an oxacillin MIC >64 μg/mL did not alter the MIC, although these strains also produced β-lactamase. The mechanism for borderline susceptibility is not always hyperproduction of conventional β-lactamase.[9] A β-lactamase that specifically hydrolyzes methicillin has been described.[194] A third mechanism is modification of the binding of antibiotic to normal penicillin

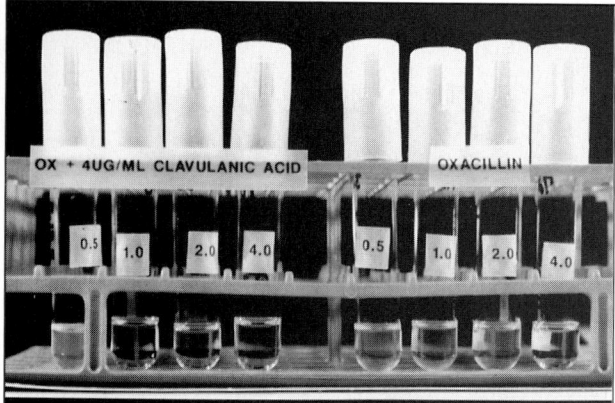

Figure 17-30 An isolate of *Staphylococcus aureus* with borderline susceptibility to oxacillin has been tested with and without the addition of clavulanic acid, an inhibitor of β-lactamase. In the absence of the inhibitor, the MIC of the strain is 4 μg/mL. After the addition of clavulanic acid the MIC is 1 μg/mL. The resistance of this strain is derived from the hyperproduction of β-lactamase.

binding proteins.[322] Finally, some strains with borderline susceptibility possess the *mecA* gene and produce penicillin binding protein 2a at a low level.[101] For these borderline strains a variant of the disk diffusion test or demonstration of the altered binding protein may be useful.[83]

The hyperproducing borderline strains usually have an MIC of 4 or 8 μg/mL. In contrast to the heteroresistant strains, which demonstrate multiple drug resistance, these strains are usually susceptible to other antimicrobial agents. Experimental evidence from an animal model of endocarditis suggests that these borderline susceptible strains should respond to treatment with oxacillin just as do fully susceptible strains.[315] Limited clinical studies suggest the same.[118,193] If there is any question about clinical response, administration of vancomycin is the appropriate conservative treatment.

It is probable that no single phenotypic procedure detects staphylococcal resistance to oxacillin with absolute reliability. Certain manipulations will enhance the likelihood that resistance will be demonstrated (Box 17-8). It is also probable, however, that false estimates of resistance can be generated by some manipulations, such as prolonged incubation of susceptibility tests.[49] The most reliable of the phenotypic methods is probably the agar dilution screen with 6 μg/mL of oxacillin. Swenson and colleagues have investigated the optimal conditions for this phenotypic approach.[303] The gold standard, not yet widely available, is detection of the *mecA* gene by nucleic acid amplification.

Detection of resistance is particularly acute with coagulase-negative staphylococci. In an attempt to correct the inappropriate characterization of strains as susceptible to oxacillin, the CLSI has changed the susceptible breakpoint for coagulase-negative strains from 2 μg/mL to 0.25 μg/mL.[217,218] This manipulation improved the situation for *S. epidermidis*, the most commonly isolated species, but in the process, strains of some less commonly isolated species, such as *S. lugdunensis* and *S. saprophyticus*, were inappro-

Box 17-8 Maximizing Detection of Methicillin-Resistant Staphylococci

1. For *S. aureus*, oxacillin is more likely to detect cross-resistance among penicillinase-resistant penicillins than other compounds. Cloxacillin and dicloxacillin should not be used, because they may not detect oxacillin resistance.[217] Coudron and colleagues have suggested that methicillin may detect resistance in *S. epidermidis* better than oxacillin.[49]
2. Addition of 2% NaCl to broth or agar for dilution tests enhances detection of resistance.[218]
3. The inoculum should be prepared by the alternative direct method, using colonies from fresh overnight plate (see Chart 17-1).
4. The cultures should be incubated at 35°C for a full 24 hr.
5. If the disk diffusion procedure is used, the edge of the apparent zone of inhibition should be examined closely. The border is sharp and clear when oxacillin-susceptible organisms are tested. Growth of oxacillin-resistant organisms "feathers" or "trails" as the disk is approached so that the inside edge of growth may be difficult to detect (Fig. 17-31).
6. If the susceptibility of an *S. aureus* strain to oxacillin is not clear, perform a test for the *mecA* gene (see text) and/or an oxacillin-salt agar screening test. For the screen, use Mueller-Hinton agar with 4% w/v NaCl and 6 μg/mL oxacillin per milliliter. Make a direct suspension of colonies to a density comparable to a 0.5 McFarland standard. Using a 1-μl loop, spot the suspension onto an area that is 10 to 1 mm in diameter. Alternatively, spot a similar area or streak a quadrant with a swab that has been dipped into the suspension. Incubate the plate at 35°C in ambient air for 24 hr. Examine with transmitted light for >1 colony or a light film of growth.[218]

priately classified as resistant when they lacked the *mecA* gene.[85,110]

Fortunately, the only mechanism for true resistance among staphylococci to oxacillin is alteration of PBP 2. Given the vagaries of phenotypic characterization, genotypic detection of resistance is the obvious solution. The gold standard is, in fact, detection of the gene for the altered protein by an amplification method, such as PCR.[186,188] At this point, these tests are limited to specialty laboratories, but it is likely that the technique will become more widely available in the near future. In the meantime, simplified tests for detection of the gene or the gene product, which are commercially available, serve a useful purpose.[129,140] Although theoretically more desirable than phenotypic tests, the current crop of genotypic assays also present methodologic difficulties, so use of a combination of tests, either routinely or selectively, is probably wise.[304] For antimicrobial agents other than β-lactams it is still necessary to use phenotypic tests.

As mentioned above, resistance to cephalosporins among staphylococci is difficult to detect. There is clinical evidence that isolates of *S. aureus* that are resistant to oxacillin do

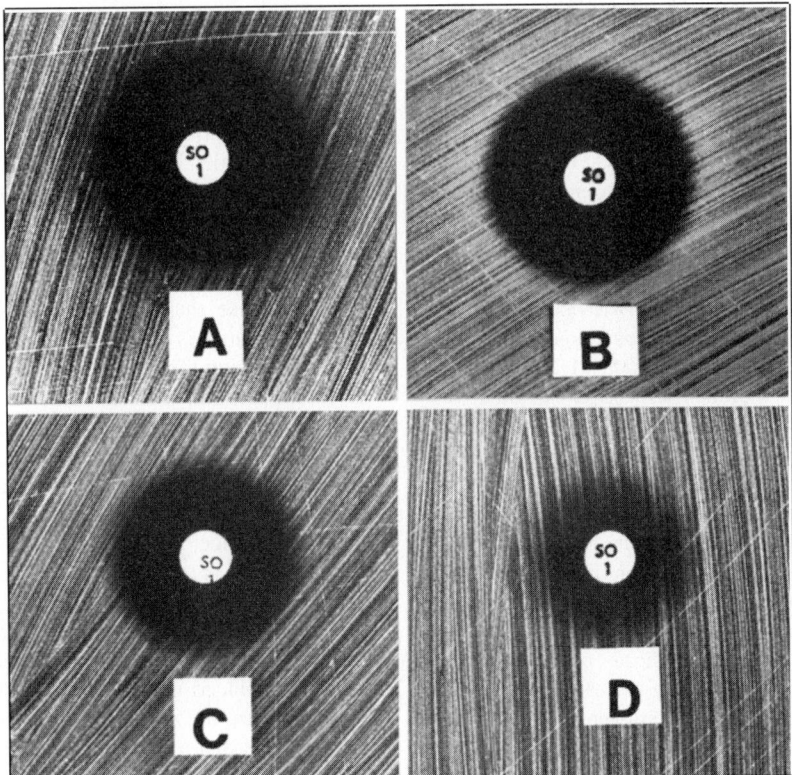

Figure 17-31 The effect of salt on the expression of methicillin resistance to staphylococci is shown. A susceptible strain was tested against a 1-µg oxacillin disk on Mueller-Hinton agar that had no supplemental salt (**A**) or that contained 4% NaCl (**B**). The zone of bacterial inhibition was unaffected by addition of the salt. A methicillin-resistant strain was also tested against oxacillin on Mueller-Hinton agar without (**C**) and with (**D**) the addition of 4% NaCl. Without salt, a clear zone of inhibition was produced (**C**), and the isolate would be considered susceptible. In the presence of salt there was a gradually decreasing growth or "feathering" right up to the disk; this organism should be considered resistant to oxacillin and other penicillinase-resistant penicillins.

not respond in vivo to cephalosporin therapy; the same phenomenon has also been suggested for *S. epidermidis*.[218,219] If resistance to nafcillin, oxacillin, or methicillin is demonstrated, the bacterial strain should be reported as resistant to other β-lactam antibiotics, including all cephalosporins, such as cefazolin or cephalothin, and the carbapenem antibiotic imipenem (see Table 17-12).

VANCOMYCIN

A strain of *S. haemolyticus* that developed resistance to vancomycin during treatment of a patient with recurrent episodes of peritonitis described in 1987[282] was the harbinger of everyone's nightmare—development of similar resistance in *S. aureus*. Production in the laboratory of isolates of *S. aureus* with a fourfold decrease in susceptibility to vancomycin was a warning that it was only a matter of time.[53] The change in susceptibility was correlated with the presence of a 39-kDa cytoplasmic protein. Furthermore, the enterococcal genes for resistance to vancomycin could be transferred in the laboratory to *S. aureus*.[230]

Fortunately, it took a decade for clinical strains to express resistance. The first isolate, which expressed reduced sus-

ceptibility rather than complete resistance to vancomycin, was recorded in Japan,[2] but soon similar strains were recovered from patients in the other parts of the world, including the United States.[310] The acronyms VISA and VRSA are commonly used to describe strains of *S. aureus* that are intermediate or resistant to vancomycin.[294] Although vancomycin is the only glycopeptide antibiotic commonly used in the United States, other glycopeptides are also affected, so the terms GISA (or by extension GRSA) are also used synonymously.[308]

Vancomycin resistance may be expressed homogeneously in staphylococci, but, as with oxacillin, the strains may be heteroresistant (expressed in a small portion of the bacterial cells).[294] Detection of heteroresistant strains can be problematic, and the CDC has promulgated recommendations for laboratory testing (Box 17-9). Disk diffusion and methods in which incubation time is reduced are problematic.

Clinically, the problem of resistance is compounded by three factors: 1) staphylococci, particularly *S. aureus*, are major pathogens; 2) vancomycin has been the therapeutic safety net for many years; and 3) strains often express resis-

---

Box 17-9 Detection of Vancomycin Resistance in Staphylococci

1. Quantitative (MIC) methods have been validated by the CDC for the detection of VISA and VRSA. Both microdilution and agar dilution methods were evaluated. The commercial systems studied included MicroScan Conventional MIC panels (Dade MicroScan, West Sacramento, CA), Vitek and Vitek 2 systems (BioMérieux, Hazelwood, MO), Sensititer System (TREK Diagnostic Systems, Cleveland, OH), Pasco Microdilution panels (BD, Franklin Lakes, NJ), and Etest using a 0.5 McFarland standard to prepare the inoculum suspension (AB Biodisk, Piscataway, NJ). Some automated systems failed to detect all VRSA strains, so additional testing with an agar screen plate is recommended.

2. The vancomycin agar screen test uses brain heart infusion agar containing 6 μg/mL of vancomycin. An inoculum of 1 to 10 μL of a 0.5 McFarland suspension (final concentration of bacteria, 10^5 to 10^6 CFUs/mL) is streaked or spotted onto the surface of the agar. Growth of >1 colony after incubation for 24 hr indicates resistance. Control strains, which should be used on each day of testing, are *S. aureus* (ATCC 25923, susceptible) and *E. faecalis* (ATCC 51299, resistant).

3. An insufficient number of nonsusceptible strains has been accumulated to set breakpoint zone sizes for the disk diffusion test. A zone of at least 15 mm is considered susceptible; if zones are smaller, a dilution susceptibility test should be performed and/or the isolate should be sent to a reference laboratory.

4. Isolates with a MIC of 4 μg/mL or 8 μg/mL (VISA or GISA) are not detected reliably by the disk diffusion test. If this method is used, therefore, an additional procedure, such as the vancomycin agar screen test, should be used. Testing may be performed on all isolates; alternatively, strains that are resistant to oxacillin may be selected, as most strains that are resistant to vancomycin are also resistant to oxacillin.

5. Plates or trays for determination of vancomycin susceptibility in staphylococci should be incubated in ambient air for a full 24 hr at 37°C.

6. Strains of staphylococci that appear to be intermediate or resistant to vancomycin should be referred to a reference laboratory and/or a public health laboratory for further analysis.

Reference found at http://www.cdc.gov/ncidod/hip/lab/FactSheet/vrsa.htm.

---

tance to multiple antimicrobial agents, including oxacillin and quinupristin-dalfopristin (a recently developed antistaphylococcal antibiotic).[342]

MACROLIDES, LINCOSAMIDES, AND STREPTOGRAMINS

Resistance to macrolides among staphylococci is mediated either by active efflux of antibiotics from the bacterial cells (*msrA*) or by modification of ribosomal targets (usually *ermA* or *ermC*).[176] Ribosomal modification may be expressed constitutively or it may be inducible.[271] Resistance to erythromycin is more easily detected than is resistance to clindamycin. Strains that are susceptible to erythromycin are reliably susceptible to clindamycin, but the opposite is not necessarily true. Nomenclature for resistance mechanisms for this group of antibiotics has been reviewed by Roberts and colleagues.[271]

Strains of staphylococci that express constitutive resistance to erythromycin and clindamycin present little difficulty, because they will be detected as resistant in vitro. When resistance is inducible, however, there may be a dissociation between the results. Resistance to 14-membered and 15-membered macrolides, such as erythromycin, is more readily induced than is resistance to 16-membered macrolides and lincosamides, such as clindamycin. There is evidence that inducible resistance to clindamycin is clinically significant.[237,288] If an isolate of *S. aureus* expresses dissociated resistance, an induction test should be performed before the strain is reported as susceptible to clindamycin. The simplest method is to take advantage of the propensity for erythromycin to induce resistance by performing a double-disk test.[86,237] If disks containing erythromycin and clindamycin are placed in proximity and resistance is induced by erythromycin, the zone of inhibition around the clindamycin disk will be distorted. The resultant flattening of the zone of inhibition produces a D-shape that is similar to that produced by antagonistic antibiotics in Figure 17-29*B*. This pattern indicates inducible resistance; the isolate should be reported as resistant to clindamycin. In the absence of resistance—either intrinsic or inducible—the isolate may be reported as susceptible to clindamycin.

Although most attention has been focused on staphylococci, inducible clindamycin resistance may also be found in streptococci and more rarely among enterococci. It appears that the double-disk test will detect this phenomenon in streptococci as well as staphylococci. (See the discussion of a case of group B streptococcal infection at the CDC web site—https://www.phppo.cdc.gov/dls/master/view_document.aspx?id=2.)

FLUOROQUINOLONES

The fluoroquinolones, initially a potentially important therapeutic alternative for methicillin-resistant staphylococci, have become increasingly compromised by burgeoning resistance. Two mechanisms are operative: 1) a mutation in the gyrase that is the target of this antibiotic class[109] and 2) and an active efflux pump mediated by NorA, a multidrug transporter protein.[223] Fluoroquinolone resistance is more common in stains that are resistant to methicillin (oxacillin) than in susceptible strains; it can develop with distressing rapidity when this class of antibiotic is used without restriction in hospitals.[5]

Haemophilus Species

Haemophilus organisms require hemin (factor X) and/or nicotinamide adenine dinucleotide (NAD) (factor V) for growth. The validity of adding supplements both to dilution and also to diffusion susceptibility media has been established. A supplement for susceptibility testing of *Haemophilus* has been suggested by Jorgensen and colleagues.[154] The NCCLS has adopted the *Haemophilus* test medium, which may contain cation supplements if appropriate. The advantages of the medium include visual clarity and reliability of testing with trimethoprim-sulfamethoxazole.[154] Some investigators, however, have experienced problems with the performance of both homemade and commercially prepared *Haemophilus* test medium.[203]

Proper preparation of the inoculum is very important for testing *Haemophilus* species. The alternative direct method of standardizing the bacterial suspension from an overnight culture should be used (see Chart 17-1).

Jorgensen and colleagues found a good correlation of the Etest and standardized microdilution tests for *Haemophilus influenzae*.[151] A recent study of susceptibility-testing methods for *H. influenzae* documented a generally acceptable performance among commonly used methods.[102] The procedures and interpretations that have been developed for *H. influenzae* can be applied also to other *Haemophilus* spp.[150,151]

Antimicrobial susceptibility testing of *H. influenzae* has been reviewed by Doern and Jones.[64]

PENICILLIN ANTIBIOTICS

Doern and colleagues documented a prevalence of 15.2% for β-lactamase production in *Haemophilus influenzae*. The frequency of enzymatic degradation of ampicillin was 21% for encapsulated strains of *H. influenzae* type b and 12% for nonencapsulated strains of *H. influenzae*.[64,66] Isolates were more likely to produce β-lactamase if they were recovered from infants and young children rather than from adults and if they were recovered from blood and cerebrospinal fluid rather than from other fluids or tissues.

The incidence of β-lactamase production in a national collaborative survey was 20%, but once again there was a dichotomy between encapsulated and nonencapsulated strains.[67] The prevalence of the β-lactamase enzyme was 31.7% in type b strains and 15.6% in nonencapsulated strains of *H. influenzae*. Intrinsic resistance to ampicillin, not mediated by β-lactamase, was detected in only 0.1% of strains.

A repeat survey a few years later, limited to respiratory isolates, documented a prevalence of 16.5% for production of β-lactamase by *H. influenzae*. The frequency of resistance in encapsulated type b strains and in nonencapsulated strains was 29.5% and 15%, respectively.[147]

All isolates of *Haemophilus* species that are etiologic agents of serious infections should be tested for production of β-lactamase, preferably by the Nitrocefin procedure. Isolates from sterile body sites that do not produce the enzyme should be tested for intrinsic resistance if possible. Although intrinsic resistance has been rare, there is evidence of clonal dissemination of such strains in certain hospitals.[156] In any event, isolates should be referred to a reference laboratory if there is any question about correlation of the laboratory and clinical results.

CHLORAMPHENICOL

For years the backup drug for serious *Haemophilus* infections was chloramphenicol. Although infrequent, resistance to this antibiotic has also developed. The frequency of resistance to chloramphenicol among isolates of *H. influenzae* was 0.5% in a national collaborative study.[67] In almost all instances resistance is mediated by enzymatic degradation.[97] Doern and colleagues have found the tube test significantly more accurate than a disk modification of the rapid assay for chloramphenicol acetyltransferase.[62]

CEPHALOSPORINS

The first-generation cephalosporins are poorly effective against *Haemophilus influenzae* and need not be tested. Second-generation cephalosporins, such as cefamandole and cefuroxime, are effective against *Haemophilus* species in vitro, but are least effective where they are needed most—for isolates that produce β-lactamase.[148] Therapeutic failures have been described with second-generation cephalosporin antibiotics. Third-generation cephalosporins, such as ceftriaxone, are uniformly effective against *H. influenzae*.

TRIMETHOPRIM-SULFAMETHOXAZOLE

Resistance of *Haemophilus influenzae* to trimethoprim-sulfamethoxazole can be detected in less than 1% of strains.[147] Although not the drug of choice for serious systemic disease, therapy with trimethoprim-sulfamethoxazole has been successful in treating pulmonary infections.

Streptococcus pneumoniae
PENICILLIN AND OTHER β-LACTAM ANTIBIOTICS

For many years, penicillin was the standard treatment for pneumococcal infections and susceptibility testing was not indicated. The emergence of strains that are resistant to multiple antibiotics, including penicillin, has breached even this bastion of antimicrobial therapy. Strains that have MICs between 0.1 and 1.0 μg/mL are considered relatively resistant to penicillin; those with MICs greater than 1.0 μg/mL are designated as resistant. Unfortunately, the frequency of strains that are relatively or completely resistant to penicillin is increasing in the United States.[63,319,344] There remains, however, considerable geographic variation in the frequency of resistance.[319] Part of the reason for this irregular geographic distribution may be the apparent dissemination of a small number of resistant pneumococcal clones.[270]

The mechanism of pneumococcal resistance to penicillin is the alteration of penicillin-binding proteins.[42] *Streptococcus pneumoniae* does not produce β-lactamases. Multiple binding-proteins are involved in the acquisition of resistance, producing a stepwise decrease in susceptibility. It is interesting to note that 70% of clinical pneumococcal isolates that are resistant to penicillin also show defective lysis, a property that would also enhance their survival.[208] Two kinds of antibiotic pressure on pneumococci are hypothesized as explanations for the concordant phenomena. Pneumococcal strains resistant to penicillin may be clonal, but multiple pathways to resistance are possible, and resistant strains have emerged independently in diverse geographic locations. Penicillin resistance can be transferred horizontally from one pneumococcal strain to another, apparently by transformation.[189] Considerable variation in the genes for the altered proteins occurs from mismatch repair after the transfer. Penicillin resistance occurs with a variety of serogroups and among diverse strains that can be differentiated by molecular typing,[74] but it does appear that a relatively few clones are the dominant source of multiply resistant strains.[270] Unfortunately, many of the resistant strains belong to serotypes that are included in the commonly used pneumococcal vaccines.[130]

Risk factors for serious infection with resistant strains include prior use of β-lactam antibiotics, age less than 15 years, infection in the upper respiratory tract, and nosocomial origin of infection.[15] In addition, the frequency with which β-lactam antibiotics are used in the community may have an effect on the occurrence of resistant pneumococcal strains.[98,58]

Pneumococci that are resistant to penicillin also have decreased susceptibility to other β-lactam antibiotics.[177] Imipenem, meropenem, cefotaxime, ceftriaxone, and cefpirome are more active in vitro than penicillin. Ampicillin, cefdinir, cefuroxime, cefoperazone, azlocillin, mezlocillin, piperacillin, cephalothin, and cefamandole demonstrate slightly less activity than penicillin. Oxacillin, cefixime, ceftizoxime, cefetamet, cefaclor, ceftazidime, cefoxitin, cefonicid, and latamoxef show very poor activity against resistant strains. It has been suggested that penicillin can be used to predict the susceptibility of other β-lactam antibiotics, because the relationships of the minimal inhibitory concentrations are consistent.[28,58] The mechanism for resistance to these other β-lactam antibiotics is also an alteration in penicillin-binding proteins.[210]

Five percent sheep blood may be added to Mueller-Hinton agar and 2–5% lysed horse blood may be added to broth media for growth of *S. pneumoniae*. Quality control of these tests should include known resistant pneumococcal strains in addition to standard control organisms. Incubation in CO_2 is acceptable if necessary for growth of the strain. The *Haemophilus* test medium described earlier has been reported to work well for support of pneumococcal growth in broth microdilution tests,[152] although it has not worked well in all laboratories.

In most laboratories, the simplest screening test for resistance is a variation of the disk diffusion test. Although penicillin disks have been used in some studies, the procedure recommended by the NCCLS for detection of resistance to penicillin incorporates a 1-µg disk of oxacillin. Strains that have a zone diameter less than or equal to 19 mm should be reported as provisionally nonsusceptible to penicillin (Fig 17-32); confirmation by a dilution susceptibility test should be arranged. Swenson and colleagues found that oxacillin was a better predictor of penicillin susceptibility than was methicillin.[302] The disk diffusion test does not differentiate strains that are relatively resistant (MIC, 0.1 to 1.0 µg/mL) from strains that are resistant (MIC, ≥ 2.0 µg/mL). A strain of *S. pneumoniae* that is presumptively resistant to penicillin should be tested in a reliable broth dilution test.

Commercial susceptibility testing systems perform variably for detection of penicillin resistance in pneumococci. The Pasco system and the Etest performed best, producing results that were comparable to the reference methods for all antimicrobial agents except for the combination of Etest and trimethoprim-sulfamethoxazole. Other systems, including the MicroScan rapid panels, performed less well or

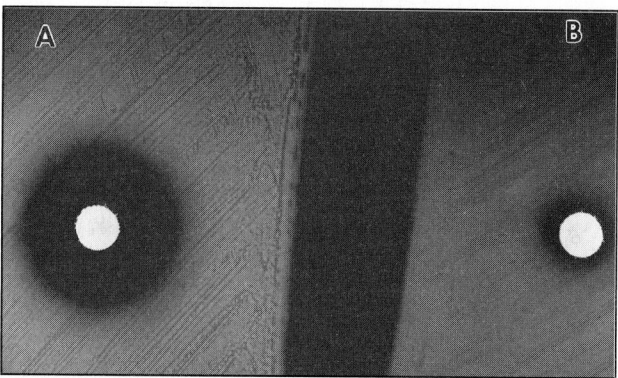

Figure 17-32 Screening test for resistance of pneumococci to penicillin, using a 1-µg oxacillin disk on Mueller-Hinton agar with sheep blood. A susceptible strain (**A**) shows a large zone of inhibition and can be reported as susceptible without further testing. The second strain (**B**) demonstrates a very small zone of inhibition. This strain could be susceptible, intermediate, or resistant (although the very small zone suggests that it will not be susceptible). In order to determine the correct interpretation, a MIC test must be performed.

poorly.[309] Subsequent evaluations, however, have documented better performance of several of the systems, including MicroScan MICroSTREP panels.[113,153]

The Etest has been evaluated independently in a collaborative study, which documented low minor error rates with penicillin (9.5%) and cefotaxime (5.4%) (see Fig. 17-25).[149] Vancomycin is the standard of therapy for resistant strains causing serious systemic infection. Hashemi and colleagues have noted that the Etest produces higher MIC results than does the microbroth dilution test, raising concern that reports of false resistance might result.[120]

Although relatively resistant strains have responded to penicillin therapy in pneumococcal pneumonia,[87] meningitis may not be treated successfully because concentrations of antimicrobial agent are lower in cerebrospinal fluid.[238] Strains that have a MIC greater than 4.0 µg/mL are unlikely to respond to penicillin therapy in any clinical situation. The NCCLS has differentiated breakpoints for potentially effective cephalosporin antibiotics depending on whether the strains were isolated from cerebrospinal fluid or from other sites.[217,218]

MULTIPLE RESISTANCE

Unfortunately, many of the pneumococcal strains that are resistant to β-lactam antibiotics are also resistant to other classes of antimicrobial agents (multiply resistant strains).[63,319] Macrolides, tetracyclines, chloramphenicol, trimethoprim-sulfamethoxazole, and to a lesser extent fluoroquinolones have been affected.[167,339]

MACROLIDES AND LINCOSAMIDES

Resistance of *S. pneumoniae* to macrolides has been increasing for many years. An association between antimicrobial resistance and antimicrobial agent use has been documented.[98,254] There are two classes of resistance mechanisms: 1) antimicrobial inactivation at the ribosomal level by a methylase (Erm) and 2) active pumping of antibiotic out of the bacterial cell by an efflux system (Mef).[287] The efflux pump is the most common mechanism in strains isolated in the United States.[287] Resistance produced by this mechanism is less extensive that that produced by ribosomal inactivation; in addition, strains that are ribosomally resistant often express resistance to clindamycin also.[135] Several investigators have described double-disk tests for evaluating inducible resistance to clindamycin in pneumococcal strains.[207,330] As for staphylococci, pneumococcal strains that exhibit inducible resistance to clindamycin should be reported as resistant; strains that lack both intrinsic and inducible resistance to clindamycin may be reported as susceptible.

Resistance to other macrolides can be inferred from the erythromycin result.[218] It has been suggested that the lower level of resistance to erythromycin conferred by the Mef mechanism may not be clinically significant, but several reports have documented therapeutic failures with such strains.[138,185]

Neisseria gonorrhoeae

For many years the gonococcus was uniformly susceptible to penicillin and the therapeutic approach to gonococcal infection was relatively straightforward. In the mid-1970s strains of *Neisseria gonorrhoeae* that produced β-lactamase appeared[78] and spread rapidly.[289] This β-lactamase resembles the TEM enzyme found in enteric bacilli and *Haemophilus influenzae*. A second mechanism of resistance appeared a few years later when Dougherty and colleagues described resistant strains that lacked β-lactamase but contained altered penicillin-binding proteins.[72] These strains have produced epidemic as well as sporadic infection.[82]

A second weapon in the antigonococcal armamentarium was removed when a plasmid that mediated high-level resistance to tetracycline appeared in *N. gonorrhoeae*.[168] Resistance to quinolones has been documented in many areas and resistance to azithromycin has also developed.[40,305]

The tests recommended by the NCCLS for detection of chromosomally mediated resistance in *N. gonorrhoeae* are agar dilution and agar diffusion. The subject has been reviewed by Doern and Jones.[64] The recommended medium for agar dilution tests is GC agar with the addition after autoclaving of a 1% defined growth supplement (1.1 g L-cysteine, 0.03 g guanine HCl, 3 mg thiamine HCl, 13 mg para-aminobenzoic acid [PABA], 0.01 g vitamin B_{12}, 0.1 g cocarboxylase, 0.25 g NAD, 1.0 g adenine, 10 g L-glutamine, 100 g glucose, 0.02 g ferric nitrate in 1 L H_2O). Cysteine must be omitted if carbapenems or clavulanate are to be tested.[219]

Agar diffusion tests are performed on GC agar base with addition of the defined growth supplement. Cysteine-free medium is not required for disk testing; enriched chocolate agar is not recommended.[220] Susceptibility plates for testing *N. gonorrhoeae* must be incubated at 35°C in CO_2. A zone of less than or equal to 26 mm in the disk diffusion test for penicillin (10-μg disk) indicates resistance. A zone size of less than or equal to 19 mm usually indicates production of β-lactamase, but the β-lactamase test is preferred for assessing this mechanism of resistance. Criteria for interpretation of spectinomycin and tetracycline have been developed by the NCCLS. An isolate with a zone size of less than or equal to 19 mm around a 30-μg tetracycline disk is likely to have a plasmid-mediated resistance mechanism; such strains should be evaluated by a dilution test. There have been no gonococcal strains resistant to certain cephalosporins, so the resistant breakpoint has not been set.[220]

All isolates of *N. gonorrhoeae* should be tested for β-lactamase production, preferably using the Nitrocefin method. An agar dilution or disk diffusion test should be performed on β-lactamase-negative isolates if the frequency of intrinsic resistance to penicillin or the prevalence of tetracycline resistance in the population is high. Any isolates from treatment failures should be tested locally or referred to a reference laboratory. The Etest has shown good correlation with agar dilution techniques for non-β-lactamase-producing strains,[328] but resistance may not be detected in strains that produce β-lactamase,[347] emphasizing the necessity for performing a test for β-lactamase production in all strains.

Neisseria meningitidis

Plasmid-mediated transfer of β-lactamase to *Neisseria meningitidis* has been documented.[59] In addition, strains have been described that are resistant on the basis of altered penicillin-binding proteins.[349] It appears that the altered membrane proteins were transferred to *N. meningitidis* from commensal *Neisseria* spp.[23] The Etest has been evaluated for testing of *N. meningitidis* with mixed results. Pascual and colleagues have reported that this method overstates the degree of resistance and suggest that further evaluation of appropriate media is necessary.[240] Marshall and colleagues, however, found a good correlation between the Etest and reference methods, using criteria of the Food and Drug Administration.[192] The disk diffusion test has not proved reliable for testing this organism.[22,220]

Susceptibility testing of meningococci to rifampin may occasionally be requested for epidemiologic purposes.[222] It is often difficult for the laboratory to generate a result in time to guide prophylaxis, which must start at the time the clinical diagnosis of meningococcal infection is made.

Enterococcus Species

The mainstay of antimicrobial therapy of serious enterococcal infections has been the use of combinations of β-lactam and aminoglycoside antibiotics.[131,323] The underpinnings of this approach have been seriously undermined in recent years.[187] The subject has been reviewed by several authors.[124,174,276] The interactions among antibiotics and resistance mechanisms in enterococci are illustrated in Figure 17-10. More recently, resistance has also been detected in the "antibiotics of last resort," especially in strains of *E. faecium*.[134] Standard procedures have been applied with success to enterococci, although there were some difficulties with a few antibiotics when the disk diffusion test was used.[48] Problems with commercial systems have been promptly addressed by the manufacturers.

AMINOGLYCOSIDE ANTIBIOTICS

There are three mechanisms for enterococcal resistance to aminoglycosides. Aminoglycoside-modifying enzymes, which include phosphotransferases, nucleotidyltransferases, and an acetyltransferase, are produced constitutively on plasmids.[174] They resemble the enzymes found in staphylococci rather than those produced in gram-negative bacilli. Additional mechanisms include modification of the ribosomal target[77] and interference with transport of the antibiotic. There is evidence for transmission of strains that are resistant to gentamicin from animals to humans through the food supply.[71]

Detection of high-level resistance of enterococci to aminoglycosides is important because these strains are not inhibited synergistically by combination therapy with β-lactam antibiotics. Resistance of *E. faecium* to kanamycin, amikacin, netilmicin, and tobramycin can be assumed. Resistance of this species to gentamicin and streptomycin and of *E. faecalis* to all of the aminoglycosides can be predicted by in vitro testing with large concentrations of antibiotic in a dilution test or by disks with a high antibiotic content. Concentrations of 1,000 μg/mL of streptomycin by microdilution, 2,000 μg/mL of streptomycin by agar dilution, and 500 μg/mL of gentamicin by either method are recommended as break points.[301,218] Growth of a single colony on agar dilution plates indicates resistance. Disks with 120 μg of gentamicin or 300 μg of streptomycin are recommended for the disk diffusion test. Resistance is indicated by ≤6 mm (no zone) and susceptibility by a zone of ≥10 mm. Strains with zones of 7 to 9 mm should be tested by dilution methods.[220] Problems with detection of this resistance by commercial susceptibility systems have been addressed by the manufacturers. A recent study found virtually complete agreement among high-potency disks, commercially available microdilution panels, and a commercial agar dilution "synergy" plate.[211]

β-LACTAM ANTIBIOTICS

Many strains of enterococci, particularly *Enterococcus faecium*, are intrinsically resistant to β-lactam antibiotics because they possess binding proteins with low affinity for these drugs. In particular, the cephalosporins are uniformly ineffective against enterococci and should not be tested. In general, ampicillin is more effective than penicillin in vitro. In at least one study strains of *E. faecium* that were resistant to ampicillin were distinct by molecular analysis from susceptible strains.[155] The recent emergence of enterococcal strains that produce β-lactamase has been discussed previously.

VANCOMYCIN

The last therapeutic resort for enterococci was vancomycin until Leclercq and colleagues described strains of *E. faecium* that contained a plasmid mediating resistance to the glycopeptide antibiotics vancomycin and teicoplanin.[173] Vancomycin-resistant isolates of *E. faecalis* have also been described.[224] Resistance to glycopeptides appears to be transferred by dissemination of a gene rather than a plasmid.[75] Three genetic mechanisms for resistance of enterococci to glycopeptides have been described.[276] The *vanA* gene complex is inducible and is carried on a family of plasmids in *E. faecium* and *E. faecalis*. It encodes high-level resistance to both vancomycin and teicoplanin. *VanB* is an inducible gene in *E. faecium* that mediates low-level resistance only to vancomycin by means of a carboxypeptidase. *VanC* is a constitutive chromosomal gene that mediates low-level resistance in *E. gallinarum*, an unusual clinical isolate. Resistance to vancomycin, particularly that mediated by the *vanB* gene, is not reliably detected by all methods.

Unfortunately, vancomycin-resistant enterococci have taken a firm hold and have become epidemic in some hospitals and regions.[95,209] The characteristics of resistant strains vary over time and with geographic location. In a group of Connecticut hospitals, the mean rate of high-level resistance to gentamicin was 29%; to ampicillin, 10% (all being isolates of *E. faecium*); and to vancomycin, 8%, but no isolates produced β-lactamase.[242] Enterococci are pathogens-in-training in comparison to staphylococci and streptococci, but they can produce serious, life-threatening infections in hospitalized patients whose feces are colonized by resistant strains. Risk factors for colonization and invasive disease include serious illness and prior receipt of antibiotics, including vancomycin and drugs active against anaerobic bacteria.[37] Vancomycin resistance in enterococci has been associated with more frequent episodes of recurrent bacteremia, persistent isolation of enterococci from primary sites of infection, increased frequency of endovascular infection, and increased mortality.[178]

Detection of enterococcal resistance to vancomycin, particularly the *vanB* phenotype, in clinical laboratories is not optimal, primarily because commercially available testing systems, including the two most commonly used methods—Vitek and various MicroScan systems—do not pick up the moderate- and low-level resistance efficiently.[313] In a survey of New Jersey laboratories, 96% of 76 clinical laboratories were able to recognize resistance in a strain of *E. faecium* with high-level resistance to vancomycin (MIC, 512 μg/mL), but only 27% of laboratories reported an *E. faecium* strain with moderate resistance (MIC, 64 μg/mL) as resistant.[314] A strain of *E. faecalis* with low-level resistance (MIC, 32 μg/mL), a typical *vanB* phenotype, was recognized as resistant by only 16% of laboratories, and a strain of *E. gallinarum* with a typical *vanC* phenotype (MIC, 8 μg/mL) was correctly characterized by 74% of participants. In a comparative study from the Centers for Disease Control and Prevention, Tenover and colleagues evaluated 10 commercial systems for detection of vancomycin resistance in enterococci.[313] A reference microdilution method was used as the standard for evaluation of 50 reference strains. An agar dilution screening test, the Etest, and some commercial microdilution systems performed well. Increased numbers of minor errors were seen with the disk diffusion test and other commercial microdilution systems. Very major error rates were produced by the Vitek system (10.3%) and the MicroScan Rapid system (20.7%), which was the only system to produce major errors (13.3%). On repeat testing with the Vitek very major errors were reduced to 3.4%, whereas the errors with the MicroScan Rapid system increased to 27.6%. A recent report confirms the ability of MicroScan conventional Positive Breakpoint Combo Type 6 panels to detect resistance among enterococci to ampicillin and vancomycin.[136]

Fourteen of the 15 incorrect results with vancomycin were in motile enterococci, which are less frequently isolated from serious infections than *E. faecium* and *E. faecalis*. There were no β-lactamase-producing strains among the 132 isolates studied. The initial problems with the Vitek system were corrected with modifications of the software, and the new Vitek 2 system has proven reliable.[175,327]

A commercial version of the agar screen test, the Remel Synergy Quad Plate, compares well to the reference test.[93] It incorporates 6 μg/mL of vancomycin into brain-heart infusion agar as recommended by Swenson and colleagues.[299]

Clinical microbiologists may be asked to screen feces for vancomycin-resistant enterococci to determine the prevalence of resistant organisms in an institution or to pinpoint patients at increased risk of invasive enterococcal infection. Several methods have been recommended. Barton and Doern found that bile esculin azide agar supplemented with 8 μg/mL of vancomycin was a useful screening medium.[12] Landman and colleagues compared five selective media, and found that Enterococcosel broth (BD Diagnostics, Franklin Lakes, NJ) supplemented with 64 μg/mL of vancomycin and 60 μg/mL of aztreonam, was the most sensitive method.[170] Use of bile esculin azide agar with a 30-μg vancomycin disk was less sensitive, but would be easy to implement in most laboratories. Swabs collected from the rectum and the perirectal area provide equivalent results.[336] For laboratories with molecular capability, nucleic acid amplification provides a more sensitive method than culture to detect colonization.[243]

The risk factors for colonization by vancomycin-resistant enterococci are similar to those for acquisition of *Clostridium difficile*. It is not surprising, therefore, that evaluation of patients with *C. difficile* toxin in their stools is a useful technique for targeted surveillance of vancomycin-resistant enterococci in the feces.[114] This approach will not replace systematic surveillance, because all colonized patients will not have been tested for *C. difficile*.

Should screening of enterococcal isolates from primary plates for vancomycin resistance without performing susceptibility tests be desired, CAMPY agar may be used.[286] The media from different manufacturers and perhaps from different lots should be evaluated for adequate performance.

The battle between the chemists and bacteria continues. New agents for treating gram-positive bacteria have been developed. In addition to teicoplanin (another glycopeptide), linezolid (an oxazolidinone antibiotic), and quinupristin-dalfopristin (a streptogramin combination) have been brought to market[76]; although largely effective against enterococci, reports of resistance are beginning to appear. Not surprisingly, an increased risk of acquiring a strain resistant to linezolid was associated with the use of the antibiotic and with the duration of therapy.[236]

The subject of vancomycin resistance in enterococci has been reviewed extensively.[41,103,212] It is important to remember that inanimate surfaces in the microbiology laboratory may be contaminated with resistant bacteria, including vancomycin-resistant enterococci, just as surfaces in clinical areas are.[47]

Listeria monocytogenes

Microbroth dilution tests may be performed in cation-supplemented Mueller-Hinton broth with 2–5% lysed horse blood. *Listeria monocytogenes* provides a good example of the care needed in extrapolating the zone size criteria in the disk diffusion test to bacteria that have not been evaluated. The diffusion test appears to be satisfactory for evaluation of *L. monocytogenes*, but susceptibilities to penicillin and ampicillin were not adequately determined by participants in proficiency test programs until the NCCLS clarified the zone sizes to be used for establishing breakpoints.[144]

Streptococcus pyogenes (Group A β-Hemolytic Streptococcus)
PENICILLIN

Occasionally the laboratory may receive a request to perform a susceptibility test on an isolate of group A β-hemolytic *Streptococcus*. Such testing is appropriate for alternative drugs, such as erythromycin, if the patient is allergic to penicillin. To date there have been no strains of *Streptococcus pyogenes* resistant to penicillin in vitro. Therapeutic failures result from inadequate penetration of antibiotic into the crypts of the tonsils and adenoidal tissue, where the bacteria may hide. In the absence of documented resistance and without a standardized, validated method for testing, acquiescence to such a test is more likely to cause problems than to solve them. If testing is believed to be indicated, any resistant results should be validated by a reference laboratory.

If testing is performed by the disk diffusion procedure, penicillin or ampicillin disks may be used to predict susceptibility; use of oxacillin disks, as for pneumococci, is not recommended.[220]

ERYTHROMYCIN

Although penicillin remains uniformly effective,[263] resistance to erythromycin and tetracycline has steadily increased globally.[18,133] Resistance to erythromycin is mediated by both the M macrolide phenotype (an efflux mechanism)[18] and by a newly described mechanism, termed the NR phenotype (also an efflux mechanism).[158] Less frequently the MLS$_B$ mechanism was responsible for resistance. In a series of 573 strains from Sweden the NR phenotype was found in 82%; an inducible MLS$_B$ phenotype, in 17%; and a constitutive MLS$_B$ phenotype, in 0.4%.[158] Strains that contain an inducible MLS$_B$ mechanism and are susceptible to clindamycin may be tested for inducible clindamycin resistance by the double-disk test (D test), as described for staphylococci (earlier in this chapter). If neither intrinsic nor inducible resistance is documented, the strain may be reported as susceptible to clindamycin.

There are many different clones of strains that are resistant to erythromycin and they are not restricted to specific geographic locations.[157,159] The likelihood of resistance to erythromycin in strains recovered from children with pharyngitis is inversely related to the age of the child.[285]

FLUOROQUINOLONES

In addition, isolates with high-level resistance to fluoroquinolones have been described.[269] For patients who are allergic to penicillin, therefore, the therapeutic choices may become increasingly limited. Resistance to vancomycin has not been described.

Streptococcus agalactiae (Group B β-Hemolytic Streptococcus)

As for *Streptococcus pyogenes*, reduced susceptibility to penicillin has not been demonstrated,[263] but resistance to macrolides is extant. The most common mechanism of resistance is by a ribosomal methylase (ermA or ermB), but a minority of strains may express resistance through an active efflux mechanism, either alone or in combination with the methylase.[54,57] Resistance to vancomycin has not been described.

If testing is performed by the disk diffusion procedure, penicillin or ampicillin disks may be used to predict susceptibility; use of oxacillin disks, as for pneumococci, is not recommended.[220]

It has been recommended that a comment be appended to the report when *S. agalactiae* is isolated from clinically significant sites (including rectal-vaginal cultures in pregnant women) to indicate that susceptibility to β-lactam antibiotics can be assumed, but that the laboratory should be consulted for testing of erythromycin and clindamycin if the patient has high-level allergy to penicillin. As is true for staphylococci and other streptococci, some strains may have inducible resistance to clindamycin. In this case an induction test must be performed.

Viridans Streptococci

Although they are less frequent pathogens than pneumococci, viridans streptococci cause endocarditis and other serious infections. Alterations in penicillin-binding proteins have produced resistance to multiple β-lactam antibiotics among several of the species, including *S. mitis*,[80] *S. sanguis*,[350] and *S. oralis*.[263]

It appears that the resistance in viridans streptococci originated in penicillin-resistant pneumococcal strains.[73] Reduced susceptibility to penicillin may be found in as many as 25% of strains.[146] As for pneumococci, these strains are usually more susceptible to third- and fourth-generation cephalosporins.[251] Disk diffusion tests for viridans streptococci are not recommended; a MIC determination should be made using a dilution method or gradient diffusion.[220]

In a study of viridans streptococci recovered from the normal oropharynx, resistance to erythromycin, tetracycline, and quinupristin-dalfopristin was documented frequently; strains expressed resistance to levofloxacin and moxifloxacin much less commonly.[284] The distribution of phenotypes for erythromycin resistance resembled that found in *S. pyogenes* and *S. agalactiae*.

So far these resistant isolates have remained susceptible to vancomycin. In the laboratory, susceptibility results obtained with the Etest have correlated well with agar dilution for penicillin and the cephalosporins, but somewhat less well with vancomycin.[272] In any event, a strain determined to be resistant to vancomycin should be referred to a reference laboratory for confirmation.

Other Gram-Positive Bacteria

Vancomycin resistance is commonly found in strains of *Leuconostoc*, *Pediococcus*, and *Lactobacillus*.[300] These genera are infrequently pathogens, but on occasion they do produce bacteremia[195] and septicemia.[107] Resistance to vancomycin may be a useful clue to the correct identification, because streptococci, with which these genera may be confused, are uniformly susceptible to vancomycin.

Pseudomonas aeruginosa, Burkholderia cepacia, and Stenotrophomonas maltophilia in Patients With Cystic Fibrosis

Isolates of this species are a particular challenge both for clinicians and for microbiology laboratories, particularly those strains that express a mucoid phenotype. The mucoid isolates frequently grow insufficiently to determine a valid result. When the disk diffusion test was compared to a reference method, poor correlation was observed when mucoid strains were tested against some antibiotics. The interpretive category, however, agreed well between the two methods.[32] The Etest (AB Biodisk, Solna, Sweden) correlated well with the reference method, both for mucoid and nonmucoid isolates.[32] In contrast, the two dominant commercial systems, Vitek and MicroScan WalkAway produced an unacceptably high frequency of erroneous results when compared to a reference method.[31]

It should be noted that patients with cystic fibrosis present a problem even for reference methods. Smith and colleagues were unable to find a correlation between susceptibility results for tobramycin and ceftazidime, using a reference dilution method, and clinical response.[290] Although broth microdilution compared well with a reference agar dilution technique for *Pseudomonas aeruginosa*, discordant results were found significantly more frequently in isolates from patients with cystic fibrosis than in other patients.[277]

Many laboratories do not routinely test isolates of *Burkholderia cepacia* and *Stenotrophomonas maltophilia* for susceptibility to antimicrobial agents. Both organisms remain largely susceptible to trimethoprim-sulfamethoxazole, which is the clinical therapy of choice.[38,56] In addition, the correlation of clinical results with in vitro susceptibility results is inadequate, and the results of testing may actually be misleading.[218] The disk diffusion method is not recommended for testing either of these organisms. If testing is not performed, a note should be appended indicating that in vitro testing may be unhelpful or misleading and that therapy with trimethoprim-sulfamethoxazole should be considered.

Direct Susceptibility Testing

Direct susceptibility testing of clinical specimens is not generally recommended because the inoculum is not standardized and mixed bacterial species are often present. Direct susceptibility testing of broth from positive blood culture bottles has correlated well with standard tests from isolated colonies. The tests have been performed both with unadjusted broth from the bottles[52] and after adjustment of the density of the culture by comparison to a 0.5 McFarland standard.[165] In addition, urine from patients with urinary tract infections may be tested directly if a single bacterial strain is present.[55]

Chapter Update: The most recent CLSI informational supplement (M100-S15, January, 2005) includes 1) expanded recommendations for non-fermenting gram-negative bacilli (to cover *Acinetobacter* spp.; *Burkholderia cepacia*, and *Stenotrophomonas maltophilia*); 2) revised criteria for testing staphylococci, especially coagulase-negative species, including seperate criteria for *Staphylococcus lugdunensis* and suggestions for use of a 30 μg cefoxitin disk as an alternative to oxacillin in the disk diffusion test; 3) interpretive breakpoints for dilution testing of polymyxin B (results applicable to colistin also); 4) suggestions for ESBL testing of *Proteus mirabilis*; and 5) recommendations for quality assessment of the inducible clindamycin resistance test.

REFERENCES

1. World Health Organization: Standardization of methods for conducting microbic sensitivity tests. World Health Organization Tech Rep Ser 1961;210.
2. Reduced susceptibility of *Staphylococcus aureus* to vancomycin-Japan, 1996. MMWR Morb Mortal Wkly Rep 1997;46:624–626.
3. Abraham EP, Chain E. An enzyme from bacteria able to destroy penicillin. Nature 1940;146:837–837.
4. Ahmad MH, et al. Interaction between aminoglycoside uptake and ribosomal resistance mutations. Antimicrob Agents Chemother 1980;18:798–806.
5. Aldridge, KE et al. The rapid emergence of fluoroquinolone-methicillin-resistant *Staphylococcus aureus* infections in a community hospital: an in vitro look at alternative antimicrobial agents. Diagn Microbiol Infect Dis 1992;15:601–608.
6. Ambler RP. The structure of beta-lactamases. Phil Trans R Soc Lond B 1980; 289:321–331.
7. Anhalt JP, Washington JA II. Laboratory Procedures in Clinical Microbiology. 2nd Ed. New York: Springer-Verlag,1985.
8. Baker CN, et al. Comparison of the E test to agar dilution, broth microdilution, and agar diffusion susceptibility testing techniques by using a special challenge set of bacteria. J Clin Microbiol 1991;29:533–538.
9. Barg N, et al. Borderline susceptibility to antistaphylococcal penicillins is not conferred exclusively by the hyperproduction of beta-lactamase. Antimicrob Agents Chemother 1991;35:1975–1979.
10. Barry AL. Procedure for testing antimicrobial agents in agar medium: theoretical considerations. In: Lorian, V, ed. Antibiotics in Laboratory Medicine. 2nd Ed. Baltimore: Williams & Wilkins,1986:1–26.
11. Barry AL, et al. Influence of inoculum growth phase on microdilution susceptibility tests. J Clin Microbiol 1983;18:645–651.
12. Barton AL, Doern GV. Selective media for detecting gastrointestinal carriage of vancomycin-resistant enterococci. Diagn Microbiol Infect Dis 1995;23: 119–122.
13. Bauer AW, et al. Antibiotic susceptibility testing by a standardized single disk method. Am J Clin Pathol 1966;45:493–496.
14. Bauer AW, et al. Single-disk antibiotic-sensitivity testing of staphylococci. A M A Arch Intern Med 1959;104:208–216.
15. Bedos JP, et al. Epidemiological features of and risk factors for infection by *Streptococcus pneumoniae* strains with diminished susceptibility to penicillin: findings of a French survey. Clin Infect Dis 1996;22:63–72.
16. Beekmann SE, et al. Effects of rapid detection of bloodstream infections on length of hospitalization and hospital charges. J Clin Microbiol 2003;41: 3119–3125.
17. Bell SM, Plowman D. Mechanisms of ampicillin resistance in *Haemophilus influenzae* from respiratory tract. Lancet 1980;1:279–280.
18. Betriu C, et al. Incidence of erythromycin resistance in *Streptococcus pyogenes*: a 10-year study. Diagn Microbiol Infect Dis 1999;33:255–260.
19. Bishop RE, Weiner JH. Hypothesis: coordinate regulation of murein peptidase activity and AmpC beta-lactamase synthesis in *Escherichia coli*. FEBS Lett 1992;304:103–108.
20. Blazquez J. Hypermutation as a factor contributing to the acquisition of antimicrobial resistance. Clin Infect Dis 2003;37:1201–1209.
21. Blazquez J, et al. Single amino acid replacements at positions altered in naturally occurring extended-spectrum TEM beta-lactamases. Antimicrob Agents Chemother 1995;39:145–149.
22. Block C, et al. Unreliability of disc diffusion test for screening for reduced penicillin susceptibility in *Neisseria meningitidis*. J Clin Microbiol 1998;36: 3103–3104.
23. Bowler LD, et al. Interspecies recombination between the penA genes of *Neisseria meningitidis* and commensal *Neisseria* species during the emergence of penicillin resistance in *N. meningitidis*: natural events and laboratory simulation. J Bacteriol 1994;176:333–337.
24. Boyce JM, et al. Spurious oxacillin resistance in *Staphylococcus aureus* because of defective oxacillin disks. J Clin Microbiol 1988;26:1425–1427.
25. Bradford PA. Extended-spectrum beta-lactamases in the 21st century: characterization, epidemiology, and detection of this important resistance threat. Clin Microbiol Rev 2001;14:933–951.
26. Bradford, PA et al. Imipenem resistance in *Klebsiella pneumoniae* is associated with the combination of ACT-1, a plasmid-mediated AmpC b-lactamase, and the loss of an outer membrane protein. Antimicrob Agents Chemother 41: 563–569, 1997
27. Brook I. Penicillin failure and copathogenicity in streptococcal pharyngotonsillitis. J Fam Pract 1994;38:175–179.
28. Brueggemann, AB et al. Use of penicillin MICs to predict In vitro activity of other beta-lactam antimicrobial agents against *Streptococcus pneumoniae*. J Clin Microbiol 39:367–369, 2001
29. Bryan LE, Kwan S. Roles of ribosomal binding, membrane potential, and electron transport in bacterial uptake of streptomycin and gentamicin. Antimicrob Agents Chemother 1983;23:835–845.
30. Burns JL, et al. A permeability barrier as a mechanism of chloramphenicol resistance in *Haemophilus influenzae*. Antimicrob Agents Chemother 1985;27: 46–54.
31. Burns JL, et al. Comparison of two commercial systems (Vitek and MicroScan-WalkAway) for antimicrobial susceptibility testing of *Pseudomonas aeruginosa* isolates from cystic fibrosis patients. Diagn Microbiol Infect Dis 39:257–260, 2001
32. Burns JL, et al. Comparison of agar diffusion methodologies for antimicrobial susceptibility testing of *Pseudomonas aeruginosa* isolates from cystic fibrosis patients. J Clin Microbiol 38:1818–1822, 2000
33. Bush K. β-lactamase inhibitors from laboratory to clinic. Clin Microbiol Rev 1988;1:109–123.
34. Bush K, Metallo-beta-lactamases: a class apart. Clin Infect Dis 1998;27:Suppl 53.
35. Bush K. New beta-lactamases in Gram-negative bacteria: diversity and impact on the selection of antimicrobial therapy. Clin Infect Dis 2001;32:1085–1089.
36. Bush K, et al. A functional classification scheme for beta-lactamase and its correlation with molecular structure. Antimicrob Agents Chemother 1995;39: 1211–1233.
37. Carmeli Y, et al. Antecedent treatment with different antibiotic agents as a risk factor for vancomycin-resistant *Enterococcus*. Emerg Infect Dis 2002;8: 802–807.
38. Carroll, KC et al. Comparison of various in vitro susceptibility methods for testing *Stenotrophomonas maltophilia*. Diagn Microbiol Infect Dis 32:229–235, 1998
39. Carroll KC, et al. Susceptibility of beta-hemolytic streptococci to nine antimicrobial agents among four medical centers in Salt Lake City, Utah, USA. Diagn Microbiol Infect Dis 1997;27:123–128.
40. Center for Disease Control and Prevention. Fluoroquinolone-resistance in *Neisseria gonorrhoeae*, Hawaii, 1999, and decreased susceptibility to azithromycin in *N. gonorrhoeae*-Missouri, 1999. MMWR Morb Mortal Wkly Rep 2000;49: 833–837.
41. Cetinkaya Y, et al. Vancomycin-resistant enterococci. Clin Microbiol Rev 2000; 13:686–707.
42. Chambers HF. Penicillin-binding protein-mediated resistance in pneumococci and staphylococci. J Infect Dis 1999;179:Suppl 9.
43. Chambers HF, Sachdeva M. Binding of beta-lactam antibiotics to penicillin-binding proteins in methicillin-resistant *Staphylococcus aureus*. J Infect Dis 1990;161:1170–1176.
44. Chang SC, et al. Influence of beta-lactamase inhibitors on the activity of oxacillin against methicillin-resistant *Staphylococcus aureus*. Diagn Microbiol Infect Dis 1995;21:81–84.
45. Chow JW, Shlaes DM. Imipenem resistance associated with the loss of a 40 kDa outer membrane protein in *Enterobacter aerogenes*. J Antimicrob Chemother 1991;28:499–504.
46. Collatz E, et al. Molecular evolution of ubiquitous beta-lactamases towards extended-spectrum enzymes active against newer beta-lactam antibiotics. Mol Microbiol 1990;4:1615–1620.
47. Collins SM, et al. Contamination of the clinical microbiology laboratory with

vancomycin-resistant enterococci and multidrug-resistant *Enterobacteriaceae:* implications for hospital and laboratory workers. J Clin Microbiol 2001;39: 3772–3774.

48. Cotter G, Adley CC. Comparison and evaluation of antimicrobial susceptibility testing of enterococci performed in accordance with six national committee standardized disk diffusion procedures. J Clin Microbiol 2001;39:3753–3756.

49. Coudron PE, et al. Evaluation of laboratory tests for detection of methicillin-resistant *Staphylococcus aureus* and *Staphylococcus epidermidis.* J Clin Microbiol 1986;24:764–769.

50. Coudron PE, et al. Occurrence and detection of AmpC beta-lactamases among *Escherichia coli, Klebsiella pneumoniae,* and *Proteus mirabilis* isolates at a veterans medical center. J Clin Microbiol 2000;38:1791–1796.

51. Courvalin P. Transfer of antibiotic resistance genes between gram-positive and gram-negative bacteria. Antimicrob Agents Chemother 1994;38:1447–1451.

52. Coyle, MB et al. Rapid antimicrobial susceptibility testing of isolates from blood cultures by direct inoculation and early reading of disk diffusion tests. J Clin Microbiol 20:473–477, 1984.

53. Daum RS, et al. Characterization of *Staphylococcus aureus* isolates with decreased susceptibility to vancomycin and teicoplanin: isolation and purification of a constitutively produced protein associated with decreased susceptibility. J Infect Dis 1992;166:1066–1072.

54. De Mouy D, et al. Antibiotic susceptibility and mechanisms of erythromycin resistance in clinical isolates of *Streptococcus agalactiae*: French multicenter study. Antimicrob Agents Chemother 2001;45:2400–2402.

55. Dennstedt, FE et al. Rapid method for identification and susceptibility testing of *Escherichia coli* bacteriuria. J Clin Microbiol 18:150–153, 1983

56. Denton, M, Kerr, KG: Microbiological and clinical aspects of infection associated with *Stenotrophomonas maltophilia.* Clin Microbiol Rev 11:57–80, 1998

57. Diekema DJ, et al. Molecular epidemiology of macrolide resistance in neonatal bloodstream isolates of group B streptococci. J Clin Microbiol 2003;41: 2659–2661.

58. Diekema DJ, et al. Antimicrobial-drug use and changes in resistance in *Streptococcus pneumoniae.* Emerg Infect Dis 2000;6:552–556.

59. Dillon JR, et al. Spread of penicillinase-producing and transfer plasmids from the gonococcus to *Neisseria meningitidis.* Lancet 1983;1:779–781.

60. Doern GV. Antimicrobial resistance among clinical isolates of *Haemophilus influenzae* and *Branhamella catarrhalis.* Clin Microbiol Newsletter 1988;10: 1185–1187.

61. Doern GV, et al. Assessment of laboratory performance with *Streptococcus pneumoniae* antimicrobial susceptibility testing in the United States: a report from the College of American Pathologists Microbiology Proficiency Survey Program. Arch Pathol Lab Med 1999;123:285–289.

62. Doern GV, et al. In vitro chloramphenicol susceptibility testing of *Haemophilus influenzae*: Disk diffusion procedures and assays for chloramphenicol acetyltransferase. J Clin Microbiol 1987;25:1453–1455.

63. Doern GV, et al. Antimicrobial resistance among clinical isolates of *Streptococcus pneumoniae* in the United States during 1999–2000, including a comparison of resistance rates since 1994–1995. Antimicrob Agents Chemother 2001;45: 1721–1729.

64. Doern GV, Jones RN. Antimicrobial susceptibility testing of *Haemophilus influenzae, Branhamella catarrhalis,* and *Neisseria gonorrhoeae.* Antimicrob Agents Chemother 1988;32:1747–1753.

65. Doern GV, Jones RN. In vitro susceptibility test practices with *Haemophilus influenzae* among College of American Pathologists survey participants in the United States. Diagn Microbiol Infect Dis 1993;17:61–65.

66. Doern GV, et al. Prevalence of antimicrobial resistance among clinical isolates of *Haemophilus influenzae*: a collaborative study. Diagn Microbiol Infect Dis 1986;4:95–107.

67. Doern GV, et al. National collaborative study of the prevalence of antimicrobial resistance among clinical isolates of *Haemophilus influenzae.* Antimicrob Agents Chemother 1988;32:180–185.

68. Doern GV, Tubert TA. Detection of beta-lactamase activity among clinical isolates of *Branhamella catarrhalis* with six different beta-lactamase assays. J Clin Microbiol 1987;25:1380–1383.

69. Doern GV, Tubert TA. In vitro activities of 39 antimicrobial agents for *Branhamella catarrhalis* and comparison of results with different quantitative susceptibility test methods. Antimicrob Agents Chemother 1988;32:259–261.

70. Doern GV, et al. Clinical impact of rapid in vitro susceptibility testing and bacterial identification. J Clin Microbiol 1994;32:1757–1762.

71. Donabedian SM, et al. Molecular characterization of gentamicin-resistant enterococci in the United States: evidence of spread from animals to humans through food. J Clin Microbiol 2003;41:1109–1113.

72. Dougherty TJ, et al. Penicillin-binding proteins of penicillin-susceptible and intrinsically resistant *Neisseria gonorrhoeae.* Antimicrob Agents Chemother 1980;18:730–737.

73. Dowson, CG et al. Penicillin-resistant viridans streptococci have obtained altered penicillin-binding protein genes from penicillin-resistant strains of *Streptococcus pneumoniae.* Proc Natl Acad Sci USA 87:5858–5862, 1990

74. Dunne WM Jr, et al. Comparison of results generated by serotyping, pulsed-field restriction analysis, ribotyping, and repetitive-sequence PCR used to characterize penicillin-resistant pneumococci from the United States. J Clin Microbiol 2001; 39:1791–1795.

75. Dutka-Malen S, et al. Phenotypic and genotypic heterogeneity of glycopeptide resistance determinants in gram-positive bacteria. Antimicrob Agents Chemother 1990;34:1875–1879.

76. Eliopoulos GM. Quinupristin-dalfopristin and linezolid: evidence and opinion. Clin Infect Dis 2003;36:473–481.

77. Eliopoulos GM, et al. Ribosomal resistance of clinical enterococcal to streptomycin isolates. Antimicrob Agents Chemother 1984;25:398–399.

78. Elwell LP, et al. Plasmid-mediated beta-lactamase production in *Neisseria gonorrhoeae.* Antimicrob Agents Chemother 1977;11:528–533.

79. Eng RHK, et al. Inoculum effect of new beta-lactam antibiotics on *Pseudomonas aeruginosa.* Antimicrob Agents Chemother 1984;26:42–47.

80. Farber BF, et al. Multiply resistant viridans streptococci: susceptibility to b-lactam antibiotics and comparison of penicillin-binding protein patterns. Antimicrob Agents Chemother 1983;24:702–705.

81. Farmer TA, Reading C. Beta-lactamases of *Branhamella catarrhalis* and their inhibition of clavulanic acid. Antimicrob Agents Chemother 1982;21:506–508.

82. Faruki H, et al. A community-based outbreak of infection with penicillin- resistant *Neisseria gonorrhoeae* not producing penicillinase (chromosomally mediated resistance). N Engl J Med 1985;313:607–611.

83. Felten A, et al. Evaluation of three techniques for detection of low-level methicillin-resistant *Staphylococcus aureus* (MRSA): a disk diffusion method with cefoxitin and moxalactam, the Vitek 2 system, and the MRSA-screen latex agglutination test. J Clin Microbiol 2002;40:2766–2771.

84. Fernandez-Rodriguez A, et al. Aminoglycoside-modifying enzymes in clinical isolates harboring extended-spectrum beta-lactamases. Antimicrob Agents Chemother 1992;36:2536–2538,.

85. Ferreira RB, et al. Coagulase-negative staphylococci: comparison of phenotypic and genotypic oxacillin susceptibility tests and evaluation of the agar screening test by using different concentrations of oxacillin. J Clin Microbiol 2003;41: 3609–3614.

86. Fiebelkorn KR, et al. Practical disk diffusion method for detection of inducible clindamycin resistance in *Staphylococcus aureus* and coagulase-negative staphylococci. J Clin Microbiol 2003;41:4740–4744.

87. File TM Jr. Appropriate use of antimicrobials for drug-resistant pneumonia: focus on the significance of beta-lactam-resistant *Streptococcus pneumoniae.* Clin Infect Dis 2002;34:Suppl 26.

88. Fleming A. On the antibacterial action of cultures of a penicillium with special reference to their use in isolation of *B. influenzae.* Br J Exp Pathol 1929;110: 226–236.

89. Fluit AC, et al. Molecular detection of antimicrobial resistance. Clin Microbiol Rev 2001;14:836–871.

90. Fontana R, et al. Mechanisms of resistance to growth inhibition and killing by beta-lactam antibiotics in enterococci. Clin Infect Dis 1992;15:486–489.

91. Fontana R, et al. Transition from resistance to hypersusceptibility to β-lactam antibiotics associated with loss of a low-affinity penicillin-binding protein in a *Streptococcus faecium* mutant highly resistant to penicillin. Antimicrob Agents Chemother 1985;28:678–683.

92. Fraimow HS, et al. Urinary tract infection with an *Enterococcus faecalis* isolate that requires vancomycin for growth. Ann Intern Med 1994;121:22–26.

93. Free L, Sahm DF. Investigation of the reformulated Remel Synergy Quad plate for detection of high-level aminoglycoside and vancomycin resistance among enterococci. J Clin Microbiol 1995;33:1643–1645.

94. Fridkin SK, et al. Epidemiological and microbiological characterization of infections caused by *Staphylococcus aureus* with reduced susceptibility to vancomycin, United States, 1997–2001. Clin Infect Dis 2003;36:429–439.

95. Frieden TR, et al. Emergence of vancomycin-resistant enterococci in New York City. Lancet 1993;342:76–79.

96. Frere JM, Joris B. Penicillin-sensitive enzymes in peptidoglycan biosynthesis. CRC Crit Rev Microbiol 1985;11:299–396.

97. Gaffney DF, Foster TJ. Chloramphenicol acetyltransferases determined by R plasmids from gram-negative bacteria. J Gen Microbiol 1978;109:351–358.

98. Garcia-Rey C, et al. Importance of local variations in antibiotic consumption and geographical differences of erythromycin and penicillin resistance in *Streptococcus pneumoniae.* J Clin Microbiol 2002;40:159–164.

99. Gavan TL, et al. Evaluation of the Sensititre System for quantitative antimicrobial drug susceptibility testing: a collaborative study. Antimicrob Agents Chemother 1980;17:464–469.

100. Gehrlein M, et al. Imipenem resistance in *Acinetobacter baumanii* is due to altered penicillin-binding proteins. Chemotherapy 1991;37:405–412.

101. Gerberding JL, et al. Comparison of conventional susceptibility tests with direct detection of penicillin-binding protein 2a in borderline oxacillin-resistant strains of *Staphylococcus aureus.* Antimicrob Agents Chemother 1991;35:2574–2579.

102. Giger O, et al. Comparison of five different susceptibility test methods for detect-

ing antimicrobial agent resistance among *Haemophilus influenzae* isolates. Diagn Microbiol Infect Dis 1996;24:143–153.

103. Gold HS. Vancomycin-resistant enterococci: mechanisms and clinical observations. Clin Infect Dis 2001;33:210–219.

104. Gold HS, Moellering RC. Antimicrobial-drug resistance. N Engl J Med 1996; 335:1445–1453.

105. Goldman RC, Capobianco JO. Role of an energy-dependent efflux pump in plasmid pNE24-mediated resistance to 14- and 15-membered macrolides in *Staphylococcus epidermidis*. Antimicrob Agents Chemother 1990;34:1973–1980.

106. Goldstein FW, et al. In vivo and in vitro emergence of simultaneous resistance to both beta lactam and aminoglycoside antibiotics in a strain of *Serratia marcescens*. Ann Inst Pasteur Microbiol 1983;134A:329–337.

107. Golledge CL, et al. Septicemia caused by vancomycin-resistant *Pediococcus acidilactici*. J Clin Microbiol 1990;28:1678–1679.

108. Goodhart GL. In vivo v in vitro susceptibility of enterococcus to trimethoprim-sulfamethoxazole. JAMA 1984;252:2748–2749.

109. Goswitz JJ, et al. Detection of gyrA gene mutations associated with ciprofloxacin resistance in methicillin-resistant *Staphylococcus aureus*: analysis by polymerase chain reaction and automated direct DNA sequencing. Antimicrob Agents Chemother 1992;36:1166–1169.

110. Gradelski E, et al. Correlation between genotype and phenotypic categorization of staphylococci based on methicillin susceptibility and resistance. J Clin Microbiol 2001;39:2961–2963.

111. Gruteke, P et al. Patterns of resistance associated with integrons, the extended-spectrum beta-lactamase SHV-5 gene, and a multidrug efflux pump of *Klebsiella pneumoniae* causing a nosocomial outbreak. J Clin Microbiol 41:1161–1166, 2003

112. Gunkel AG, et al. State of penicillin-binding proteins and requirements for their bactericidal interaction with beta-lactam antibiotics in *Serratia marcescens* highly resistant to extended-spectrum beta-lactams. J Gen Microbiol 1991;137:243–252.

113. Guthrie LL, et al. Comparison of MicroScan MICroSTREP, PASCO, and Sensititre MIC panels for determining antimicrobial susceptibilities of *Streptococcus pneumoniae*. Diagn Microbiol Infect Dis 1999;33:267–273.

114. Hacek DM, et al. Yield of vancomycin-resistant enterococci and multidrug-resistant *Enterobacteriaceae* from stools submitted for *Clostridium difficile* testing compared to results from a focused surveillance program. J Clin Microbiol 2001;39:1152–1154.

115. Hackenbeck R, et al. Penicillin-binding proteins of penicillin-susceptible and -resistant pneumococci: immunological relatedness of altered proteins and changes in peptides carrying the beta-lactam binding site. Antimicrob Agents Chemother 1986;30:553–558.

116. Halstead DC, et al. Reality of developing a community-wide antibiogram. J Clin Microbiol 2004;42:1–6.

117. Hamilton-Miller JMT, et al. Errors arising from incorrect orientation of E test strips. J Clin Microbiol 1995;33:1966–1967.

118. Hansen SL, Walsh TJ. Detection of intrinsically resistant (heteroresistant) *Staphylococcus aureus* with the Sceptor and AutoMicrobic systems. J Clin Microbiol 1987;25:412–415.

119. Hartman BJ, Tomasz A. Low-affinity penicillin-binding protein associated with b-lactam resistance in *Staphylococcus aureus*. J Bacteriol 1984;158:513–516.

120. Hashemi FB, et al. Discrepancies between results of E-test and standard microbroth dilution testing of *Streptococcus pneumoniae* for susceptibility to vancomycin. J Clin Microbiol 1996;34:1546–1547.

121. Hays RC, Mandell GL. pO2, pH, and redox potential of experimental abscesses. Proc Soc Exp Biol Med 1974;147:29–30.

122. Hechler U, et al. Overproduced beta-lactamase and the outer-membrane barrier as resistance factors in *Serratia marcescens* highly resistant to beta-lactamase-stable beta-lactam antibiotics. J Gen Microbiol 1989'135:1275–1290.

123. Hedge PJ, Spratt BG. Amino acid substitutions that reduce the affinity of penicillin-binding protein 3 of *Escherichia coli* for cephalexin. Eur J Biochem 1985; 151:111–121.

124. Herman DJ, Gerding DN. Antimicrobial resistance among enterococci. Antimicrob Agents Chemother 1991;35:1–4.

125. Hindler JA, Inderlied CB. Effect of the source of Mueller-Hinton agar and resistance frequency on the detection of methicillin-resistant Staphylococcus aureus. J Clin Microbiol 1985;21:205–210.

126. Hooper DC. Mechanisms of action and resistance of older and newer fluoroquinolones. Clin Infect Dis 2000;31:Suppl 8.

127. Hooper DC. Emerging mechanisms of fluoroquinolone resistance. Emerg Infect Dis 2001;7:337–341.

128. Horne D, Tomasz A. Hypersusceptibility of penicillin-treated group B streptococci to bactericidal activity of human polymorphonuclear leukocytes. Antimicrob Agents Chemother 1981;19:745–753.

129. Horstkotte MA, et al. Rapid detection of methicillin resistance in coagulase-negative staphylococci by a penicillin-binding protein 2a-specific latex agglutination test. J Clin Microbiol 2001;39:3700–3702.

130. Hudspeth MK, et al. National Department of Defense surveillance for invasive *Streptococcus pneumoniae*: antibiotic resistance, serotype distribution, and arbitrarily primed polymerase chain reaction analyses. J Infect Dis 2001;184:591–596.

131. Hunter TH. Use of streptomycin in treatment of bacterial endocarditis. Am J Med 1947;2:436–442.

132. Huovinen P. Trimethoprim resistance. Antimicrob Agents Chemother 1987;31:1451–1456.

133. Huovinen P. Macrolide-resistant group A streptococcus-now in the United States. N Engl J Med 2002;346:1243–1245.

134. Huycke MM, et al. Multiple-drug resistant enterococci: the nature of the problem and an agenda for the future. Emerg Infect Dis 1998;4:239–249.

135. Hyde TB, et al. Macrolide resistance among invasive *Streptococcus pneumoniae* isolates. JAMA 2001;286:1857–1862.

136. Iwen PC, et al. Revised approach for identification and detection of ampicillin and vancomycin resistance in *Enterococcus* species by using MicroScan panels. J Clin Microbiol 1996;34:1779–1783

137. Jabes D, et al. Penicillin-binding protein families: evidence for the clonal nature of penicillin resistance in clinical isolates of pneumococci. J Infect Dis 1989; 159:16–24.

138. Jacobs MR. In vivo veritas: in vitro macrolide resistance in systemic *Streptococcus pneumoniae* infections does result in clinical failure. Clin Infect Dis 2002; 35:565–569.

139. Jacoby GA, Medeiros AA. More extended-spectrum beta-lactamases. Antimicrob Agents Chemother 1991;35:1697–1704.

140. Jafri AK, et al. Evaluation of a latex agglutination assay for rapid detection of oxacillin resistant *Staphylococcus aureus*. Diagn Microbiol Infect Dis 36:57–59, 2000

141. Jarlier V, et al. Extended broad-spectrum beta-lactamases conferring transferable resistance to newer beta-lactam agents in *Enterobacteriaceae*: hospital prevalence and susceptibility patterns. Rev Infect Dis 1988;10:867–878.

142. Jones RN.: Method preferences and test accuracy of antimicrobial susceptibility testing: updates from the College of American Pathologists Microbiology Surveys Program. Arch Pathol Lab Med 2001;125:1285–1289.

143. Jones RN, et al. Evaluation of the Vitek system to accurately test the susceptibility of *Pseudomonas aeruginosa* clinical isolates against cefepime. Diagn Microbiol Infect Dis 1998;32:107–110.

144. Jones RN, Edson DC. Antibiotic susceptibility testing accuracy: Review of the College of American Pathologists Microbiology Survey, 1972–1983. Arch Pathol Lab Med 1985;109:595–601.

145. Jones RN, Edson DC Antimicrobial susceptibility testing trends and accuracy in the United States: a review of the College of American Pathologists Microbiology Surveys, 1972–1989. Microbiology Resource Committee of the College of American Pathologists. Arch Pathol Lab Med 1991;115:429–436.

146. Jones, RN, Wilson, WR: Epidemiology, laboratory detection, and therapy of penicillin-resistant streptococcal infections. Diagn Microbiol Infect Dis 31:453–459, 1998

147. Jorgensen JH, et al. Antimicrobial resistance among respiratory isolates of *Haemophilus influenzae*, *Moraxella catarrhalis*, and *Streptococcus pneumoniae* in the United States. Antimicrob Agents Chemother 1990;34:2075–2080.

148. Jorgensen JH, et al. Susceptibility of multiply resistant *Haemophilus influenzae* to newer antimicrobial agents. Diagn Microbiol Infect Dis 1988;9:27–32.

149. Jorgensen JH, et al. Detection of penicillin and extended-spectrum cephalosporin resistance among *Streptococcus pneumoniae* clinical isolates by use of the E test. J Clin Microbiol 1994;32:159–163.

150. Jorgensen JH, et al. Antimicrobial susceptibility testing of less commonly isolated *Haemophilus* species using *Haemophilus* test medium. J Clin Microbiol 1990;28:985–988.

151. Jorgensen JH et al. Quantitative antimicrobial susceptibility testing of *Haemophilus influenzae* and *Streptococcus pneumoniae* by using the E-test. J Clin Microbiol 1991;29:109–114.

152. Jorgensen JH, et al. Use of *Haemophilus* test medium for broth microdilution antimicrobial susceptibility testing of *Streptococcus pneumoniae*. J Clin Microbiol 1990;28:430–434.

153. Jorgensen JH, et al. Evaluation of the Dade MicroScan MICroSTREP antimicrobial susceptibility testing panel with selected *Streptococcus pneumoniae* challenge strains and recent clinical isolates. J Clin Microbiol 1998;36:788–791.

154. Jorgensen JH, et al. Improved medium for antimicrobial susceptibility testing of *Haemophilus influenzae*. J Clin Microbiol 1987;25:2105–2113.

155. Jureen R, et al. Molecular characterization of ampicillin-resistant *Enterococcus faecium* isolates from hospitalized patients in Norway. J Clin Microbiol 2003; 41:2330–2336.

156. Karlowsky JA, et al. Antimicrobial surveillance of *Haemophilus influenzae* in the United States during 2000–2001 leads to detection of clonal dissemination of a beta-lactamase-negative and ampicillin-resistant strain. J Clin Microbiol 2002;40:1063–1066.

157. Kataja J, et al. Clonal relationships among isolates of erythromycin-resistant

Streptococcus pyogenes of different geographical origin. Eur J Clin Microbiol Infect Dis 2002;21:589–595.

158. Kataja J, et al. Clonal spread of group A streptococcus with the new type of erythromycin resistance: Finnish Study Group for Antimicrobial Resistance. J Infect Dis 1998;177:786–789.

159. Kataja J, et al. Erythromycin resistance genes in group A streptococci of different geographical origins: the Macrolide Resistance Study Group. J Antimicrob Chemother 2000;46:789–792.

160. Katsanis GP, et al. Detection of *Klebsiella pneumoniae* and *Escherichia coli* strains producing extended-spectrum beta-lactamases. J Clin Microbiol 1994;32:691–696.

161. Kellogg JA. Inability to adequately control antimicrobial agents on automicrobic system gram-positive and gram-negative susceptibility cards. J Clin Microbiol 1985;21:454–456.

162. Kelly JA, et al. Penicillin target enzyme and the antibiotic binding site. Science 1982;218:479–481.

163. Kelly LM, et al. Comparison of agar dilution, microdilution, E-test, and disk diffusion methods for testing activity of cefditoren against *Streptococcus pneumoniae*. J Clin Microbiol 1999;37:3296–3299.

164. Kernodle DS, et al. Association of borderline oxacillin-susceptible strains of *Staphylococcus aureus* with surgical wound infections. J Clin Microbiol 1998;36:219–222.

165. Kiehn, TE et al. Comparison of direct and standard microtiter broth dilution susceptibility testing of blood culture isolates. J Clin Microbiol 16:96–98, 1982

166. Kirkpatrick BD, et al. An outbreak of vancomycin-dependent Enterococcus faecium in a bone marrow transplant unit. Clin Infect Dis 1999;29:1268–1273.

167. Klugman KP. Pneumococcal resistance to antibiotics. Clin Microbiol Rev 1990;3:171–196.

168. Knapp JS et al. Frequency and distribution in the United States of strains of *Neisseria gonorrhoeae* with plasmid-mediated, high-level resistance to tetracycline. J Infect Dis 1987;155:819–822.

169. Knox JR Pratt, RF: Different modes of vancomycin and D-alanyl-D-alanine peptidase binding to cell wall peptide and a possible role for the vancomycin resistance protein. Antimicrob Agents Chemother 1990;34:1342–1347.

170. Landman D, et al. Comparison of five selective media for identifying fecal carriage of vancomycin-resistant enterococci. J Clin Microbiol 1996;34:751–752.

171. Lawrence RM, Hoeprich PD. Totally synthetic medium for susceptibility testing. Antimicrob Agents Chemother 1978;13:394–398.

172. Leclercq R. Mechanisms of resistance to macrolides and lincosamides: nature of the resistance elements and their clinical implications. Clin Infect Dis 2002;34:482–492.

173. Leclercq R, et al. Plasmid-mediated resistance to vancomycin and teicoplanin in *Enterococcus faecium*. N Engl J Med 1988;319:157–161.

174. Leclercq R, et al. Resistance of enterococci to aminoglycosides and glycopeptides. Clin Infect Dis 1992;15:495–501.

175. Ligozzi M, et al. Evaluation of the VITEK 2 system for identification and antimicrobial susceptibility testing of medically relevant gram-positive cocci. J Clin Microbiol 2002;40:1681–1686.

176. Lina G, et al. Distribution of genes encoding resistance to macrolides, lincosamides, and streptogramins among staphylococci. Antimicrob Agents Chemother 1999;43:1062–1066.

177. Linares J, et al. Decreased susceptibility of penicillin-resistant pneumococci to twenty-four beta-lactam antibiotics. J Antimicrob Chemother 1992;30:279–288.

178. Linden PK, et al. Differences in outcomes for patients with bacteriemia due to vancomycin-resistant *Enterococcus faecium* or vancomycin-susceptible E. faecium. Clin Infect Dis 1995;22:663–670.

179. Ling TK, et al. Evaluation of VITEK 2 rapid identification and susceptibility testing system against gram-negative clinical isolates. J Clin Microbiol 2001;39:2964–2966.

180. Livermore DM. Permeation of beta-lactam antibiotics into *Escherichia coli*, *Pseudomonas aeruginosa*, and other gram-negative bacteria. Rev Infect Dis 1988;10:691–698,

181. Livermore DM. Interplay of impermeability and chromosomal beta-lactamase activity in imipenem-resistant *Pseudomonas aeruginosa*. Antimicrob Agents Chemother 1992;36:2046–2048.

182. Livermore DM. Determinants of the activity of beta-lactamase inhibitor combinations. J Antimicrob Ther 1993;31:9–21.

183. Livermore, DM: Multiple mechanisms of antimicrobial resistance in *Pseudomonas aeruginosa*: our worst nightmare? Clin Infect Dis 2002;34:634–640.

184. Livermore DM, Davy KW. Invalidity for *Pseudomonas aeruginosa* of an accepted model of bacterial permeability to beta-lactam antibiotics. Antimicrob Agents Chemother 1991;35:916–921.

185. Lonks JR, et al. Failure of macrolide antibiotic treatment in patients with bacteremia due to erythromycin-resistant *Streptococcus pneumoniae*. Clin Infect Dis 2002;35:556–564.

186. Louie L, et al. Rapid detection of methicillin-resistant staphylococci from blood culture bottles by using a multiplex PCR assay. J Clin Microbiol 2002;40:2786–2790.

187. Low DE, et al. Clinical prevalence, antimicrobial susceptibility, and geographic resistance patterns of enterococci: results from the sentry antimicrobial surveillance program, 1997–1999. Clin Infect Dis 2001;32:Suppl 45.

188. Maes N, et al. Evaluation of a triplex PCR assay to discriminate *Staphylococcus aureus* from coagulase-negative staphylococci and determine methicillin resistance from blood cultures. J Clin Microbiol 2002;40:1514–1517.

189. Maiden MC. Horizontal genetic exchange, evolution, and spread of antibiotic resistance in bacteria. Clin Infect Dis 1998;27:Suppl 20.

190. Malquin F, Bryan LE. Modification of penicillin-binding proteins as mechanisms of β-lactam resistance. Antimicrob Agents Chemother 1986;30:1–5.

191. Mandell GL, Petri WA Jr. Antimicrobial agents: penicillins, cephalosporins, and other beta-lactam antibiotics. In: Hardman JG, Limbird LE, ed. The Pharmacological Basis of Therapeutics. 9th Ed. New York: McGraw-Hill,1996:1073–1101.

192. Marshall SA, et al. Comparative evaluation of E-test for susceptibility testing *Neisseria meningitidis* with eight antimicrobial agents: an investigation using U.S. Food and Drug Administration regulatory criteria. Diagn Microbiol Infect Dis 1997;27:93–97.

193. Massanari RM, et al. Implications of acquired oxacillin resistance in the management and control of *Staphylococcus aureus* infections. J Infect Dis 1988;158:702–709.

194. Massidda O, et al. Evidence for a methicillin-hydrolyzing beta-lactamase in *Staphylococcus aureus* strains with borderline susceptibility to this drug. FEMS Microbiol Lett 1992;92:223–227.

195. Mastro TD, et al. Vancomycin-resistant *Pediococcus acidilactici*: Nine cases of bacteremia. J Infect Dis 161:956–960, 1990

196. Mates SM, et al. Membrane potential and gentamicin uptake in *Staphylococcus aureus*. Proc Natl Acad Sci USA 1982;79:6693–6697.

197. Mayer KH. Review of epidemic aminoglycoside resistance worldwide. Am J Med 1986;80:56–64.

198. McDougal LK, Thornsberry C. The role of β-lactamase in staphylococcal resistance to penicillinase-resistant penicillins and cephalosporins. J Clin Microbiol 1986;23:832–839.

199. McMurry L, et al. Active efflux of tetracycline encoded by four genetically different tetracycline resistance determinants in *Escherichia coli*. Proc Natl Acad Sci USA 1980;71:3974–3977.

200. Medeiros AA. Evolution and dissemination of beta-lactamases accelerated by generation of beta-lactam antibiotics. Clin Infect Dis 1997;24:S19–S45.

201. Medeiros AA, et al. Loss of OmpC porin in a strain of *Salmonella typhimurium* causes increased resistance to cephalosporins during therapy. J Infect Dis 1987;156:751–757.

202. Mendelman PM, et al. Cefuroxime treatment failure of nontypeable *Haemophilus influenzae* meningitis associated with alteration of penicillin- binding proteins. J Infect Dis 1990;162:1118–1123.

203. Mendelman PM, et al. Problems with current recommendations for susceptibility testing of *Haemophilus influenzae*. Antimicrob Agents Chemother 1990;34:1480–1484.

204. Meyer KS, et al. Nosocomial outbreak of *Klebsiella* infection resistant to late-generation cephalosporins. Ann Intern Med 1993;119:353–358.

205. Meyer RD. *Legionella* infections: a review of five years of research. Rev Infect Dis 1983;5:258–278.

206. Miller GH, et al. The most frequent aminoglycoside resistance mechanisms: changes with time and geographic area: a reflection of aminoglycoside usage patterns? Clin Infect Dis 1997;24:S46–S62.

207. Montanari MP, et al. Differentiation of resistance phenotypes among erythromycin-resistant pneumococci. J Clin Microbiol 2001;39:1311–1315.

208. Moreillon P, Tomasz A. Penicillin resistance and defective lysis in clinical isolates of pneumococci: evidence for two kinds of antibiotic pressure operating in the clinical environment. J Infect Dis 1988;157:1150–1157.

209. Morris JG Jr, et al. Enterococci resistant to multiple antimicrobial agents, including vancomycin. Establishment of endemicity in a university medical center. Ann Intern Med 1995;123:250–259.

210. Munoz R, et al. Genetics of resistance to third-generation cephalosporins in clinical isolates of *Streptococcus pneumoniae*. Mol Microbiol 1992;6:2461–2465.

211. Murdoch DR, et al. Comparison of microscan broth microdilution, synergy quad plate agar dilution, and disk diffusion screening methods for detection of high-level aminoglycoside resistance in *Enterococcus* species. J Clin Microbiol 2003;41:2703–2705.

212. Murray BE. Vancomycin-resistant enterococcal infections. N Engl J Med 2000;342:710–721.

213. Murray BE, et al. Comparison of two b-lactamase-producing strains of *Streptococcus faecalis*. Antimicrob Agents Chemother 1986;30:861–864.

214. Murray BE, et al. In vitro studies of plasmid-mediated penicillinase from streptococcus faecalis suggest a staphylococcal origin. J Clin Invest 1986;77:289–293.

215. Nagarajan R. Antibacterial activities and modes of action of vancomycin and related glycopeptides. Antimicrob Agents Chemother 1991;35:605–609.

216. National Committee for Clinical Laboratory Standards. Analysis and presentation of cumulative antimicrobial susceptibility test data: approved guideline M39-A. Wayne, PA: NCCLS, 2002.

217. National Committee for Clinical Laboratory Standards. Disk diffusion: supplemental tables, M100-S13 (M2). Wayne, PA: NCCLS, 2003.

218. National Committee for Clinical Laboratory Standards: M100-S13 (M7) MIC testing: supplemental tables. Wayne, PA: NCCLS, 2003.

219. National Committee for Clinical Laboratory Standards: M7-A6 Methods for dilution antimicrobial susceptibility tests for bacteria that grow aerobically: approved standard. 6th Ed. Wayne, PA: NCCLS, 2003

220. National Committee for Clinical Laboratory Standards. Performance standards for antimicrobial disk susceptibility tests: approved standard (M2-A8). Wayne, PA: NCCLS, 2003.

221. Neu HC. The emergence of bacterial resistance and its influence on empiric therapy. Rev Infect Dis 19835:S9–S20.

222. Neumann MA, et al. New developments in antimicrobial agent susceptibility testing: a practical guide. Cumitech 1991;6A:1–26.

223. Neyfakh AA, et al. Fluoroquinolone resistance protein NorA of Staphylococcus aureus is a multidrug efflux transporter. Antimicrob Agents Chemother 1993; 37:128–129.

224. Nicas TI, et al. Activity of glycopeptides against vancomycin-resistant gram-positive bacteria. Antimicrob Agents Chemother 1989;33:1477–1481.

225. Nicholas RA, Strominger JL. Relations between beta-lactamases and penicillin-binding proteins: beta-lactamase activity of penicillin-binding protein 5 from Escherichia coli. Rev Infect Dis 1988;10:733–738.

226. Nikaido H. Outer membrane barrier as a mechanism of antimicrobial resistance. Antimicrob Agents Chemother 1989;33:1831–1836.

227. Nikaido H. Antibiotic resistance caused by gram-negative multidrug efflux pumps. Clin Infect Dis 1998;27:Suppl 41.

228. Nikaido H, et al. Porin channels in Escherichia coli: studies with beta-lactams in intact cells. J Bacteriol 1983;153:232–240.

229. Nikaido H, Vaara M. Molecular basis of bacterial outer membrane permeability. Microbiol Rev 1985;49:1–32.

230. Noble WC, et al. Co-transfer of vancomycin and other resistance genes from Enterococcus faecalis NCTC 12201 to Staphylococcus aureus. FEMS Microbiol Lett 1992;72:195–198.

231. Nordmann P. Trends in beta-lactam resistance among Enterobacteriaceae. Clin Infect Dis 1998;27:Suppl 6.

232. Nordmann P, et al. Biochemical properties of a carbapenem-hydrolyzing beta-lactamase from Enterobacter cloacae and cloning of the gene into Escherichia coli. Antimicrob Agents Chemother 1993;37:939–946.

233. Odeh R, et al. Broad resistance due to plasmid-mediated AmpC beta-lactamases in clinical isolates of Escherichia coli. Clin Infect Dis 200235:140–145.

234. Okhuysen PC, et al. Susceptibility of beta-lactamase-producing enterococci to piperacillin with tazobactam. Diagn Microbiol Infect Dis 1993;17:219–224.

235. Opal SM, Mayer KH, Medeiros AA. Mechanisms of bacterial antibiotic resistance. In: Mandell GL, Bennett JE, Dolin R, eds. Principles and Practice of Infectious Diseases. 5th Ed. Philadelphia: Churchill Livingstone, 2000:236–253.

236. Pai MP, et al. Risk factors associated with the development of infection with linezolid- and vancomycin-resistant Enterococcus faecium. Clin Infect Dis 2002; 35:1269–1272.

237. Panagea S, et al. Should clindamycin be used as treatment of patients with infections caused by erythromycin-resistant staphylococci? J Antimicrob Chemother 1999;44:577–582.

238. Paredes A, et al. Prolonged pneumococcal meningitis due to an organism with increased resistance to penicillin. Pediatrics 1976;58:378–381.

239. Parr TR Jr, Bryan LE. Mechanism of resistance of an ampicillin-resistant, β-lactamase- negative clinical isolate of Haemophilus influenzae type b to β-lactam antibiotics. Antimicrob Agents Chemother 1984;25:747–753.

240. Pascual A, et al. Comparison of broth microdilution and E-test for susceptibility of Neisseria meningitidis. J Clin Microbiol 1996;34:588–591.

241. Paterson DL, et al. Outcome of cephalosporin treatment for serious infections due to apparently susceptible organisms producing extended-spectrum beta-lactamases: implications for the clinical microbiology laboratory. J Clin Microbiol 2001;39:2206–2212.

242. Patterson JE, et al. An analysis of 110 serious enterococcal infections: epidemiology, antibiotic susceptibility, and outcome. Medicine (Baltimore) 1995;74: 191–200.

243. Paule SM, et al. Comparison of PCR assay to culture for surveillance detection of vancomycin-resistant enterococci. J Clin Microbiol 2003;41:4805–4807.

244. Payne DJ, et al. Comparative activities of clavulanic acid, sulbactam, and tazobactam against clinically important beta-lactamases. Antimicrob Agents Chemother 1994;38:767–772.

245. Maskell R, Okubadejo OA, Payne RH, Pead L. Human infections with thymine-requiring bacteria. J Med Microbiol 1978;11:33–42.

246. Pechere JC. Why are carbapenems active against Enterobacter cloacae resistant to third generation cephalosporins? Scand J Infect Dis Suppl 1991;78:17–21.

247. Perl TM, et al. Effect of serum on the in vitro activities of 11 broad-spectrum antibiotics. Antimicrob Agents Chemother 199032:2234–2239.

248. Persing DH, Relman DA, Tenover FC. Genotypic detection of antimicrobial resistance. In: Persing DH, ed. PCR Protocols for Emerging Infectious Diseases. Washington, DC: American Society for Microbiology,1996:33–58.

249. Peter K, et al. Impact of the ampD gene and its product on beta-lactamase production in Enterobacter cloacae. Rev Infect Dis 1988;10:800–805.

250. Peterson EM, et al. Evaluation of four anti-microbic susceptibility testing systems for gram-negative bacilli. Am J Clin Pathol 1986;86:619–623.

251. Pfaller, MA, Jones, RN: In vitro evaluation of contemporary beta-lactam drugs tested against viridans group and beta-haemolytic streptococci. Diagn Microbiol Infect Dis 27:151–154, 1997

252. Philippon A, et al. Extended-spectrum beta-lactamases. Antimicrob Agents Chemother 1989;33:1131–1136.

253. Phillips I, et al. Prevalence and mechanisms of aminoglycoside resistance. A ten- year study. Am J Med 1986;80:48–55.

254. Pihlajamaki M, et al. Macrolide-resistant Streptococcus pneumoniae and use of antimicrobial agents. Clin Infect Dis 2001;33:483–488.

255. Piroth L, et al. Spread of extended-spectrum beta-lactamase-producing Klebsiella pneumoniae: are beta-lactamase inhibitors of therapeutic value? Clin Infect Dis 1998;27:76–80.

256. Pollock HM, et al. Selection of a reference lot of Mueller-Hinton agar. J Clin Microbiol 1986;24:1–6.

257. Poole K, et al. Multiple antibiotic resistance in Pseudomonas aeruginosa: evidence for involvement of an efflux operon. J Bacteriol 1993;175:7363–7372.

258. Putnam LR, et al. Accuracy of the Vitek system for antimicrobial susceptibility testing Enterobacteriaceae bloodstream infection isolates: use of ''direct'' inoculation from Bactec 9240 blood culture bottles. Diagn Microbiol Infect Dis 1997; 28:101–104.

259. Quale JM, et al. Molecular epidemiology of a citywide outbreak of extended-spectrum beta-lactamase-producing Klebsiella pneumoniae infection. Clin Infect Dis 2002;35:834–841.

260. Queenan AM, et al. Effects of inoculum and beta-lactamase activity in AmpC- and extended-spectrum beta-lactamase (ESBL)-producing Escherichia coli and Klebsiella pneumoniae clinical isolates tested by using NCCLS ESBL methodology. J Clin Microbiol 2004;42:269–275.

261. Quinn JP, et al. Emergence of resistance to imipenem during therapy for Pseudomonas aeruginosa infections. J Infect Dis 1986;154:289–294.

262. Raimondi A, et al. Mutation in Serratia marcescens AmpC beta-lactamase producing high-level resistance to ceftazidime and cefpirome. Antimicrob Agents Chemother 2001;45:2331–2339.

263. Reinert RR, et al. Nationwide German multicenter study on the prevalence of antibiotic resistance in streptococcal blood isolates from neutropenic patients and comparative in vitro activities of quinupristin-dalfopristin and eight other antimicrobials. J Clin Microbiol 2001;39:1928–1931.

264. Reller LB, et al. Antibiotic susceptibility testing of Pseudomonas aeruginosa: selection of a control strain and criteria for magnesium and calcium content in media. J Infect Dis 1974;130:454–462.

265. Rice LB, et al. High-level expression of chromosomally encoded SHV-1 b-lactamase and an outer membrane protein change confer resistance to ceftazidime and piperacillin-tazobactamin a clinical isolate of Klebsiella pneumoniae. Antimicrob Agents Chemother 2000;44:362–367.

266. Rice LB, et al. In vivo efficacies of beta-lactam-beta-lactamase inhibitor combinations against a TEM-26-producing strain of Klebsiella pneumoniae. Antimicrob Agents Chemother 1994;38:2663–2664.

267. Rice RJ, et al. Chromosomally mediated resistance in Neisseria gonorrhoeae in the United States: results of surveillance and reporting, 1983–1984. J Infect Dis 1986;153:340–345.

268. Richmond MH, Sykes RB. The beta-lactamases of gram negative bacteria and their possible physiological role. Adv Microb Physiol 1973;9:31–88.

269. Richter SS, et al. Fluoroquinolone resistance in Streptococcus pyogenes. Clin Infect Dis 2003;36:380–383.

270. Richter SS, et al. The molecular epidemiology of penicillin-resistant Streptococcus pneumoniae in the United States, 1994–2000. Clin Infect Dis 2002;34: 330–339.

271. Roberts MC, et al. Nomenclature for macrolide and macrolide-lincosamide-streptogramin B resistance determinants. Antimicrob Agents Chemother 1999; 43:2823–2830.

272. Rosser SJ, et al. E test versus agar dilution for antimicrobial susceptibility testing of viridans group streptococci. J Clin Microbiol 1999;37:26–30.

273. Rotstein OD, et al. Mechanisms of microbial synergy in polymicrobial surgical infections. Rev Infect Dis 1985;7:151–170.

274. Rubens CE, et al. Evolution of multiple-antibiotic-resistance plasmids mediated by transposable plasmid deoxyribonucleic acid sequences. J Bacteriol 1979;140: 713–719,.

275. Rusthoven JJ, et al. Clinical isolation and characterization of aminoglycoside-

resistant small colony variants of *Enterobacter aerogenes*. Am J Med 1979;67: 702–706.

276. Saha V, et al. Occurrence and mechanisms of glycopeptide resistance in gram-positive cocci. Infect Agents Dis 1992;1:310–318.

277. Saiman L, et al. Evaluation of reference dilution test methods for antimicrobial susceptibility testing of *Pseudomonas aeruginosa* strains isolated from patients with cystic fibrosis. J Clin Microbiol 37:2987–2991, 1999

278. Sanders CC, et al. Selection of multiple antibiotic resistance by quinolones, b-lactams, and aminoglycosides with special reference to cross-resistance between unrelated drug classes. Antimicrob Agents Chemother 1984;26:797–801.

279. Satta G, et al. Target for bacteriostatic and bactericidal activities of beta-lactam antibiotics against *Escherichia coli* resides in different penicillin binding proteins (dag). Antimicrob Agents Chemother 1995;39:812–818.

280. Schieven BC, et al. Comparison of America MICroScan dry and frozen microdilution trays. J Clin Microbiol 1985;22:495–496.

281. Schwaber MJ, et al. Utility of NCCLS guidelines for identifying extended-spectrum beta-lactamases in non-*Escherichia coli* and non-*Klebsiella* spp. of Enterobacteriaceae. J Clin Microbiol 2004;42:294–298.

282. Schwalbe, RS et al. Emergence of vancomycin resistance in coagulase-negative staphylococci. N Engl J Med 316:927–931, 1987

283. Scott JR. Sex and the single circle: conjugative transposition. J Bacteriol 1992; 174:6005–6010.

284. Seppala H, et al. Antimicrobial susceptibility patterns and macrolide resistance genes of viridans group streptococci from normal flora. J Antimicrob Chemother 52:636–644, 2003

285. Seppala H, et al. Erythromycin resistance of group A streptococci from throat samples is related to age. Pediatr Infect Dis J 1997;16:651–656.

286. Shigei J, et al. Comparison of two commercially available selective media to screen for vancomycin-resistant enterococci. Am J Clin Pathol 2002;117: 152–155.

287. Shortridge VD, et al. Prevalence of macrolide resistance mechanisms in *Streptococcus pneumoniae* isolates from a multicenter antibiotic resistance surveillance study conducted in the United States in 1994–1995. Clin Infect Dis 1999;29: 1186–1188.

288. Siberry GK, et al. Failure of clindamycin treatment of methicillin-resistant *Staphylococcus aureus* expressing inducible clindamycin resistance in vitro. Clin Infect Dis 2003;37:1257–1260.

289. Siegel MS, et al. Penicillinase-producing Neisseria gonorrhoeae: results of surveillance in the United States. J Infect Dis 1978;137:170–175.

290. Smith AL, et al. Susceptibility testing of *Pseudomonas aeruginosa* isolates and clinical response to parenteral antibiotic administration: lack of association in cystic fibrosis. Chest 123:1495–1502, 2003

291. Spratt BG. Distinct penicillin binding proteins involved in the division, elongation, and shape of *Escherichia coli* K12. Proc Natl Acad Sci USA 1975;72: 2999–3003.

292. Spratt BG. Resistance to antibiotics mediated by target alterations. Science 1994; 264:388–393.

293. Spratt BG, Cromie KD. Penicillin-binding proteins of gram-negative bacteria. Rev Infect Dis 1988;10:699–711.

294. Srinivasan A, et al. Vancomycin resistance in staphylococci. Clin Microbiol Rev 2002;15:430–438.

295. Steward CD, et al. Antimicrobial susceptibility testing of carbapenems: multicenter validity testing and accuracy levels of five antimicrobial test methods for detecting resistance in *Enterobacteriaceae* and *Pseudomonas aeruginosa* isolates. J Clin Microbiol 2003;41:351–358.

296. Steward CD, et al. Characterization of clinical isolates of *Klebsiella pneumoniae* from 19 laboratories using the National Committee for Clinical Laboratory Standards extended-spectrum beta-lactamase detection methods. J Clin Microbiol 2001;39:2864–2872.

297. Steward CD, et al. Comparison of agar dilution, disk diffusion, MicroScan, and Vitek antimicrobial susceptibility testing methods to broth microdilution for detection of fluoroquinolone-resistant isolates of the family *Enterobacteriaceae*. J Clin Microbiol 1999;37:544–547.

298. Strausbaugh LJ, Sande MA. Factors influencing the therapy of experimental *Proteus mirabilis* meningitis in rabbits. J Infect Dis 1978;137:251–260.

299. Swenson JM, et al. Development of a standardized screening method for detection of vancomycin-resistant enterococci. J Clin Microbiol 1994;32:1700–1704.

300. Swenson, JM et al. Antimicrobial susceptibility of vancomycin-resistant *Leuconostoc, Pediococcus, and Lactobacillus* species. Antimicrob Agents Chemother 34:543–549, 1990

301. Swenson JM, et al. Multilaboratory evaluation of screening methods for detection of high-level aminoglycoside resistance in enterococci. J Clin Microbiol 1995;33:3008–3018.

302. Swenson JM, et al. Screening pneumococci for penicillin resistance. J Clin Microbiol 1986;24:749–752.

303. Swenson JM, et al. Optimal inoculation methods and quality control for the NCCLS oxacillin agar screen test for detection of oxacillin resistance in *Staphylococcus aureus*. J Clin Microbiol 2001;39:3781–3784.

304. Swenson JM, et al. Performance of eight methods, including two new rapid methods, for detection of oxacillin resistance in a challenge set of *Staphylococcus aureus* organisms. J Clin Microbiol 2001;39:3785–3788.

305. Tanaka M, et al. Antimicrobial resistance of *Neisseria gonorrhoeae* and high prevalence of ciprofloxacin-resistant isolates in Japan, 1993 to 1998. J Clin Microbiol 2000;38:521–525.

306. Tanz RR, et al. Lack of influence of beta-lactamase-producing flora on recovery of group A streptococci after treatment of acute pharyngitis. J Pediatr 1990;117: 859–863.

307. Taylor DE, Chau A. Tetracycline resistance mediated by ribosomal protection. Antimicrob Agents Chemother 1996;40:1–5.

308. Tenover FC. VRSA, VISA, and GISA: the dilemma behind the name game. Clin Microbiol Newslett 2000;22:49–53.

309. Tenover FC, et al. Evaluation of commercial methods for determining antimicrobial susceptibility of *Streptococcus pneumoniae*. J Clin Microbiol 1996;34: 10–14.

310. Tenover FC, et al. Characterization of staphylococci with reduced susceptibilities to vancomycin and other glycopeptides. J Clin Microbiol 1998;36:1020–1027.

311. Tenover FC, et al. Ability of laboratories to detect emerging antimicrobial resistance: proficiency testing and quality control results from the World Health Organization's external quality assurance system for antimicrobial susceptibility testing. J Clin Microbiol 2001;39:241–250.

312. Tenover FC, et al. Evaluation of the NCCLS extended-spectrum beta-lactamase confirmation methods for *Escherichia coli* with isolates collected during Project ICARE. J Clin Microbiol 2003;41:3142–3146.

313. Tenover FC, et al. Ability of commercial and reference antimicrobial susceptibility testing methods to detect vancomycin resistance in enterococci. J Clin Microbiol 1995;33:1524–1527.

314. Tenover FC, et al. Ability of clinical laboratories to detect antimicrobial agent-resistant enterococci. J Clin Microbiol 1993;31:1695–1699.

315. Thauvin-Eliopoulos C, et al. Efficacy of oxacillin and ampicillin-sulbactam combination in experimental endocarditis caused by b-lactamase-hyperproducing *Staphylococcus aureus*. Antimicrob Agents Chemother 1990;34:702–705.

316. Thomson KS. Controversies about extended-spectrum and AmpC beta-lactamases. Emerg Infect Dis 2001;7:333–336.

317. Thomson KS, Sanders CC. Detection of extended-spectrum beta-lactamases in members of the family *Enterobacteriaceae*: comparison of the double-disk and three-dimensional tests. Antimicrob Agents Chemother 1992;36:1877–1882.

318. Thomson KS, et al. Use of microdilution panels with and without β-lactamase inhibitors as a phenotypic test for β-lactamase production among *Escherichia coli, Klebsiella* spp., *Enterobacter* spp., *Citrobacter freundii*, and *Serratia marcescens*. Antimicrob Agents Chemother 1999;43:1393–1400.

319. Thornsberry C, et al. Regional trends in antimicrobial resistance among clinical isolates of *Streptococcus pneumoniae, Haemophilus influenzae*, and *Moraxella catarrhalis* in the United States: results from the TRUST Surveillance Program, 1999–2000. Clin Infect Dis 2002;34:Suppl S16.

320. Tipper DJ, Strominger JL. Mechanism of action of penicillins: a proposal based on their structural similarity to acyl-D-alanine-D-alanine. Proc Natl Acad Sci USA 1965;54:1133–1141.

321. Tomasz A. The mechanism of the irreversible antimicrobial effects of penicillin: how the beta-lactam antibiotics kill and lyse bacteria. Annu Rev Microbiol 1979; 33:113–137.

322. Tomasz A, et al. New mechanism for methicillin resistance in *Staphylococcus aureus*: clinical isolates that lack the PBP 2a gene and contain normal penicillin-binding proteins with modified penicillin-binding capacity. Antimicrob Agents Chemother 1989;33:1869–1874.

323. Tompsett R, McDermott W. Recent advances in streptomycin therapy. Am J Med 1949;7:371–381.

324. Toro CS, et al. Clinical isolate of a porinless *Salmonella typhi* resistant to high levels of chloramphenicol. Antimicrob Agents Chemother 1990;34:1715–1719.

325. Tuomanen E, et al. Coordinate regulation of beta-lactamase induction and peptidoglycan composition by the amp operon. Science 1991;251:201–204.

326. Ubukata K, et al. Expression and inducibility in *Staphylococcus aureus* of the mecA gene, which encodes a methicillin-resistant *S. aureus*-specific penicillin-binding protein. J Bacteriol 1989;171:2882–2885.

327. van den Braak N, et al. Accuracy of the VITEK 2 system to detect glycopeptide resistance in enterococci. J Clin Microbiol 2001;39:351–353.

328. Van Dyck E, et al. Comparison of E test with agar dilution for antimicrobial susceptibility testing of *Neisseria gonorrhoeae*. J Clin Microbiol 1994;32: 1586–1588.

329. Varaldo PE, et al. Survey of clinical isolates of *Staphylococcus aureus* for borderline susceptibility to antistaphylococcal penicillins. Eur J Clin Microbiol Infect Dis 1993;12:677–682.

330. Waites K, et al. Use of clindamycin disks to detect macrolide resistance mediated by ermB and mefE in *Streptococcus pneumoniae* isolates from adults and children. J Clin Microbiol 2000;38:1731–1734.

331. Wanger AR, Murray BE. Comparison of enterococcal and staphylococcal beta-lactamase plasmids. J Infect Dis 1990;161:54–58.

332. Washington JA. Discrepancies between in vitro activity of and in vivo response to antimicrobial agents. Diagn Microbiol Infect Dis 1983;1:25–31.

333. Washington JA. Functions and activities of the area committee on microbiology of the National Committee for Clinical Laboratory Standards. Clin Microbiol Rev 1991;4:150–155.

334. Watanabe M, et al. Transferable imipenem resistance in *Pseudomonas aeruginosa*. Antimicrob Agents Chemother 1991;35:147–151.

335. Waxman DJ, Strominger JL. Penicillin-binding proteins and the mechanism of action of β-lactam antibiotics. Annu Rev Biochem 1983;52:825–869.

336. Weinstein JW, et al. Comparison of rectal and perirectal swabs for detection of colonization with vancomycin-resistant enterococci. J Clin Microbiol 1996;34:210–212.

337. Weinstein MP, et al. The clinical significance of positive blood cultures: a comprehensive analysis of 500 episodes of bacteremia and fungemia in adults: II. Clinical observations, with special reference to factors influencing prognosis. Rev Infect Dis 1983;5:54–70.

338. Weisblum B. Erythromycin resistance by ribosome modification. Antimicrob Agents Chemother 1995;39:577–585.

339. Weiss K, et al. A nosocomial outbreak of fluoroquinolone-resistant *Streptococcus pneumoniae*. Clin Infect Dis 2001;33:517–522.

340. Weldhagen GF, et al. Ambler class A extended-spectrum b-lactamase in *Pseudomonas aeruginosa*: novel developments and clinical impact. Antimicrob Agents Chemother 2003;47:2385–2392.

341. Wells VD, et al. Infections due to beta-lactamase-producing, high-level gentamicin-resistant *Enterococcus faecalis*. Ann Intern Med 1992;116:285–292.

342. Werner G, et al. Methicillin-resistant, quinupristin-dalfopristin-resistant *Staphylococcus aureus* with reduced sensitivity to glycopeptides. J Clin Microbiol 2001;39:3586–3590.

343. White RL, et al. Pseudoresistance of *Pseudomonas aeruginosa* resulting from degradation of imipenem in an automated susceptibility testing system with predried panels. J Clin Microbiol 1991;29:398–400.

344. Whitney CG, et al. Increasing prevalence of multidrug resistant *Streptococcus pneumoniae* in the United States: the Active Bacterial Core Surveillance Program of the Emerging Infections Program Network. N Engl J Med 2000;343:1917–1924.

345. Wiener J, et al. Multiple antibiotic-resistant *Klebsiella* and *Escherichia coli* in nursing homes. JAMA 1999;281:517–523.

346. Yoshimura F, Nikaido H. Diffusion of b-lactam antibiotics through the porin channels of *Escherichia coli* K-12. Antimicrob Agents Chemother 1985;27:84–92.

347. Young H, et al. Penicillin susceptibility testing of penicillinase producing *Neisseria gonorrhoeae* by the E test: a need for caution. J Antimicrob Chemother 1994;34:585–588.

348. Zervos MJ, Schaberg DR. Reversal of the in vitro susceptibility of enterococci to trimethoprim-sulfamethoxazole by folinic acid. Antimicrob Agents Chemother 1985;28:446–448.

349. Zhang Q, et al. Genetic diversity of penicillin-binding protein 2 genes of penicillin-resistant strains of *Neisseria meningitidis* revealed by fingerprinting of amplified DNA. Antimicrob Agents Chemother 1990;34:1523–1528.

350. Zito ET, Daneo Moore L. Transformation of *Streptococcus sanguis* to intrinsic penicillin resistance. J Gen Microbiol 134:1237–1249.

Mycoplasmas and Ureaplasmas

Taxonomy of Mycoplasmas and Ureaplasmas

Virulence Factors of Human Mycoplasmas

Clinical Significance of the Human Mycoplasmas

Mycoplasma pneumoniae
Mycoplasma hominis and *Ureaplasma urealyticum*
Mycoplasma genitalium
Mycoplasma fermentans
Mycoplasma penetrans
Mycoplasma pirum
Mycoplasma primatum
Mycoplasma spermatophilum
Human Infections Due to *Mycoplasma* Species of Animal Origin
Hemotrophic *Mycoplasma* Species

Culture of Human Mycoplasmas From Clinical Specimens

General Considerations
Specimen Collection
Transport Media

Media for Culture of Mycoplasmas
Isolation and Identification of *Mycoplasma pneumoniae*
Noncultural Detection of *Mycoplasma pneumoniae*
Isolation and Identification of the Genital Mycoplasmas
Noncultural Detection of the Genital Mycoplasmas
Commercial Mycoplasma Culture Systems
Isolation of Mycoplasmas on Routine Culture Media

Serologic Tests for Diagnosis of *Mycoplasma pneumoniae* Infections

Serologic Tests for Genital Mycoplasmas

Antimicrobial Susceptibility and Treatment of *Mycoplasma* Infections

Diagnosis and Treatment of Hemotrophic *Mycoplasma* Infections in Animals ycoplasmas and ureaplasmas are organisms that differ from other bacteria in that they lack a rigid cell wall. Individual cells are bound only by a trilaminar unit membrane. In addition, the amount of genetic material comprising the genome of these organisms is quite small (molecular weight, 4.5×10^8 to 1×10^9 Da). Because of their lower genetic "IQ," these organisms have limited biosynthetic capabilities. Consequently, the cultivation of mycoplasmas and ureaplasmas requires an enriched medium containing precursors for nucleic acid, protein, and lipid biosynthesis. Precursors for nucleic acids and proteins are provided principally by the enriched basal peptone medium and yeast extract, while lipids are provided by the inclusion of serum. In fact, one of the principal criteria used in the taxonomic classification of these organisms is the requirement for the complex lipid cholesterol in the growth medium by certain mycoplasma and mycoplasma-like organisms.[427,454] All *Mycoplasma* species produce adenosine triphosphate (ATP) by substrate-level phosphorylation effected by phosphoglyceric acid kinase and pyruvate kinase, two enzymes of the glycolytic pathway from glucose to pyruvate.[350] These two enzymes appear to be the major source of most of the ATP synthesized by organisms in the class *Mollicutes*. These organisms are also much smaller than most bacteria, measuring 0.2 to 0.3 μm; hence, they are able to pass through bacteriologic filters. The lack of a typical bacterial cell wall containing peptidoglycan renders these organisms insensitive to cell wall–active antimicrobial agents, such as penicillins and cephalosporins. Because of this, the recovery of these organisms from clinical specimens may have significant therapeutic implications.

Mycoplasmas and ureaplasmas have been recovered from humans, animals, birds, insects, and plants, and new species are being continually identified and reported in the taxonomic literature.[454] Some species also have a free-living existence in soil and water. The human mycoplasmas belong to the genus *Mycoplasma* and to the genus *Ureaplasma*, which contains those mycoplasmas that are able to hydrolyze urea. Several species in the genus *Mycoplasma* and two species in the genus *Ureaplasma*, *U. urealyticum* and *U. parvum*, are found in human clinical specimens.

With the exception of *M. pneumoniae*, the role of other mycoplasmas—specifically *M. hominis*, *U. urealyticum*, and *U. parvum*—in human disease is controversial. *M. pneumoniae* is the well-recognized cause of atypical pneumonia, whereas *M. hominis*, *U. urealyticum*, and *U. parvum* are associated primarily with genital tract colonization and infection in adults and respiratory tract colonization and disease in newborns.[111,391] These species are associated with and implicated as causative agents in a wide variety of pathologic conditions. However, these same species may also be isolated from asymptomatic individuals, suggesting that they may behave principally as opportunistic pathogens.[289,291,292] *M. genitalium* has been isolated from both the genital and respiratory tracts, and its role as a sexually transmitted agent causing nongonococcal, nonchlamydial urethritis (NGNCU) and other genital tract infections is currently being elucidated.[20,458] However, its presence and behavior in the respiratory tract is not clear. Other *Mycoplasma* species are found as part of the normal flora of the mouth, particularly in the gingival areas surrounding the teeth. In the late 1980s, an-

other "new" mycoplasma, termed "*M. incognitus*" at that time, was detected in autopsy specimens from AIDS patients, suggesting that this organism may be either another opportunistic infection or a sexually transmissible cofactor that influenced disease progression.[264,309] This organism was subsequently identified as a strain of the fastidious mycoplasma *M. fermentans*. Several other newly described mycoplasmas have been isolated from HIV-infected patients, and these discoveries have spurred a renewed interest in virulence factors of mycoplasmas and in methods for their detection and identification.[491] In this chapter, the human mycoplasmas will be addressed, with emphasis on the clinical significance of *M. pneumoniae* and the genital mycoplasmas (*M. hominis* and *U. urealyticum*) and the methods used for the isolation and identification of these bacteria in the clinical laboratory.

Taxonomy of Mycoplasmas and Ureaplasmas

Mycoplasmas and ureaplasmas are classified in the class *Mollicutes* (Box 18-1). The name mollicutes means "soft skin," referring to the lack of a rigid bacterial cell wall. Analysis of ribosomal RNA (rRNA) sequences have revealed that the mollicutes are most closely related to the bacillus–lactobacillus–streptococcus subdivision of the eubacteria, with the closest bacterial relatives being members of the clostridia, lactobacilli, streptococci, and the genus *Erysipelothrix*.[343,371,495] The class *Mollicutes* contains four orders: *Mycoplasmatales*, *Entomoplasmatales*, *Acholeplasmatales*, and *Anaeroplasmatales* (Box 18-1). The order *Entomoplasmatales* was created to accommodate the families *Entomoplasmataceae* and *Spiroplasmataceae*. The genera *Entomoplasma* and *Mesoplasma* in the family *Entomoplasmataceae* are found in insects and plants.[455] The genus *Entomoplasma* contains sterol-requiring species that grow optimally at 30°C, whereas the genus *Mesoplasma* contains species that do not require cholesterol but grow best at 30°C in cholesterol- or serum-free media supplemented with Tween 80 (0.04%). The family *Spiroplasmataceae* includes the single genus *Spiroplasma*, which are spiral-shaped mollicutes that require cholesterol for growth and are found in plants and insects. Members of the order *Acholeplasmatales* do not require sterols for growth and are found predominantly in plants, animals, and insects.[2,13,460] The presence of these organisms in animal tissues is documented by the occurrence of acholeplasmas as contaminants in tissue culture media that are supplemented with animal serum.[13] Two species, *Acholeplasma laidlawii* and *Acholeplasma oculi*, have been isolated from humans.[282,358,481] *A. laidlawii* is immunologically related to both *M. pneumoniae* and *M. genitalium*.[65] Because sterol compounds are not required for growth, acholeplasmas may be cultivated in medium lacking exogenous serum. The order *Anaeroplasmatales* is composed of a single family (*Anaeroplasmataceae*) containing two species, *Anaeroplasma* and *Asteroleplasma*.[455] These two species are strictly anaerobic in their metabolism. *Anaeroplasma* species require cholesterol for growth, whereas members of the genus *Asteroleplasma* do not. Both of these species are found in the rumens of cattle and sheep. The family *Mycoplasmataceae* now includes the hemotrophic mycoplasmas that were previously classified in the genus *Eperythrozoon* and the genus *Haemobartonella* (Box 18-1). These organisms parasitize the erythrocyte surfaces of various animals.

Members of the order *Mycoplasmatales* require sterols, such as cholesterol, for cultivation *in vitro*. The sole family in the order—*Mycoplasmataceae*—contains two genera: *Mycoplasma* and *Ureaplasma*. The genus *Mycoplasma* contains over 100 species that inhabit a wide variety of plants and animals, including mammals, insects, birds, and reptiles, and may exist as commensals, parasites, and pathogens.[288,360,454,467] The *Mycoplasma* species that have been isolated from humans are listed in Box 18-2. *M. hominis*, *M. genitalium*, *M. fermentans*, *M. primatum*, *M. spermatophilum*, and *M. penetrans* are isolated primarily from the human genital tract, whereas *M. pneumoniae*, *M. salivarium*, *M. orale*, *M. buccale*, *M. faucium*, and *M. lipophilum* may be recovered from the human respiratory tract. *M. salivarium* is found in the gingival crevices and may play a role in certain types of periodontal disease. *M. orale*, *M. faucium*, *M. buccale*, and *M. lipophilum* are considered part of the normal upper respiratory tract flora and are nonpathogenic. *M. genitalium* has garnered much scientific interest in recent years as the etiologic agent of acute and chronic nongonococcal urethritis and a host of other genital tract infections.[467] *M. fermentans* was first isolated from the human

urogenital tract and is postulated to play roles in urethritis, rheumatoid arthritis, and progressive HIV-related disease. This species is the same as ''*M. incognitus*,'' recovered from AIDS patients (see discussion below).[376] *M. penetrans*, a relatively new addition to the genus, has been isolated from the urine of AIDS patients and, like *M. fermentans*, may act primarily as an opportunistic infectious agent in immunocompromised hosts. The ecologic niche of *M. pirum* in humans is uncertain.

As with other bacteria, the human mycoplasmas recovered from clinical material differ in certain phenotypic characteristics that are exploited for their isolation and identification (Table 18-1). *M. pneumoniae* ferments glucose with the production of acidic end products, whereas *M. hominis* uses arginine, with the formation of basic end products. Cultivation of these organisms is dependent on the use of special agar and broth media that are enriched with factors required for mycoplasmal growth in addition to specific growth substrates, such as glucose and arginine. *M. pneumoniae* strains are antigenically homogeneous, with only one recognized serovar. The number of different *M. hominis* serovars is unknown. Genetic hybridization studies using rRNA probes have supported the serologic studies, with *M. pneumoniae* strains collected over many years displaying similar rRNA composition and *M. hominis* strains showing heterogeneous rRNA patterns.[34,64,503] In addition to certain ultra-

Box 18-1 Taxonomy of the Phylum Firmicutes, Class Mollicutes

Order	Family	Genus	Sterols Required for Growth	Habitat	Comments
Mycoplasmatales	*Mycoplasmatacea*	*Mycoplamsa*	Yes	Humans, animals	Optimal growth at 35–37°C; metabolize glucose or arginine or both
		Ureaplasma	Yes	Humans, animals	Optimal growth at 35–37°C; metabolize urea
		"*Eperythrozoon*" (now members of the genus *Mycoplasma*)		Animals, including primates	Noncultivable, cell wall-less, parasitic bacteria found on the membrane surfaces of red blood cells
		"*Haemobartonella*" (now members of the genus *Mycoplasma*)		Animals, humans (?)	Noncultivable, cell wall-less, parasitic bacteria found on the membrane surfaces of red blood cells
Entomoplasmatales	*Entomoplasmataceae*	*Entomoplasma*	Yes	Insects, plants	Optimal growth at 30°C
		Mesoplasma	No	Insects, plants	Optimal growth at 30°C; grow in serum-free medium with 0.04% Tween 80
	Spiroplasmataceae	*Spiroplasma*	Yes	Insects, plants	Optimal growth at 30–37°C
Acholeplasmatales	*Acholeplasmataceae*	*Acholeplasma*	No	Animals, insects, plants	Optimal growth at 30–37°C
Anaeroplasmatales	*Anaeroplasmataceae*	*Anaeroplasma*	Yes	Rumen of cattle, sheep	Anaerobic
		Asteroleplasma	No	Rumen of cattle, sheep	Anaerobic

Box 18-2 Mycoplasmas and Ureaplasmas Isolated From Humans

Species	Common Site(s) of Isolation	Comments (i.e., other sites of isolation, associated diseases)
Mycoplasma pneumoniae	Respiratory tract, genital tract (very rare), joint fluid aspirates (very rare)	Pneumonia, bronchitis, bronchiolitis, pharyngitis, croup; rare isolate from genital tract and joint fluid aspirates
Mycoplasma orale	Oropharynx and nasopharynx	No disease association; has been isolated from leukemic bone marrow and lymph nodes
Mycoplasma salivarium	Oropharynx and nasopharynx	No disease association, questionable role in periodontal disease; rare isolates from cervix/vagina and arthritic joints
Mycoplasma buccale	Oropharynx and nasopharynx	No disease association
Mycoplasma faucium	Oropharynx and nasopharynx	No disease association
Mycoplasma lipophilum	Oropharynx and nasopharynx	No disease association
Mycoplasma spermatophilum	Cervix, sperm	No disease association
Mycoplasma primatum	Oropharynx and nasopharynx; female urethra	No disease association; recovered from umbilicus site
Mycoplasma hominis	Female genitourinary tract, oropharynx	Blood cultures (postpartum septicemia), bacterial vaginosis and other genital tract infections, lung and pleural effusion specimens; organ and tissue transplant infections; surgical wound infections; prostheses-associated infections; neonatal infections; amnionitis
Mycoplasma genitalium	Genitourinary tract, oropharynx	Some cases of nongonococcal, nonchlamydial urethritis; role in respiratory tract infection unknown, presence in joint fluid (rare) probably results from bacteremia and seeding of joint spaces
Mycoplasma fermentans	Genitourinary tract, respiratory tract	Peripheral blood lymphocytes and urine in AIDS patients; arthritic joints; bone marrow; possible role in pathogenesis of HIV infection
Mycoplasma penetrans	Genitourinary tract, urine	Urine in AIDS patients; possible role in HIV pathogenesis; opportunistic infectious agent
Mycoplasma pirum	Blood (rare)	Peripheral blood lymphocytes; a contaminant in tissue culture cells of human origin; ? role in HIV pathogenesis
Ureaplasma urealyticum	Genitourinary tract; oropharynx, lower respiratory tract, placental tissues	Lower respiratory tract, blood (neonatal sepsis); cerebrospinal fluid; surgical sites, possible role in nongonococcal urethritis, genital tract infections, neonatal infections
Ureaplasma parvum	Genitourinary tract	Genital tract infections

Table 18-1 Characteristics for the Identification of Human Mycoplasma and Ureaplasma Species

SITE OF ISOLATION SPECIES	UTILIZATION OF			OPTIMAL PH	TIME TO RECOVERY	GROWTH IN			SEROVARS
	Glucose	Arginine	Urea			Air	CO$_2$	Anaerobic	
Respiratory tract									
Mycoplasma pneumoniae	+	−	−	6.5–7.5	4–21 days	4+	4+	1+	1
Mycoplasma salivarium	−	+	−	6.0–7.0	2–5 days	2+	NA	4+	1
Mycoplasma orale	−	+	−	7.0	4–10 days	2+	NA	4+	1
Genital tract									
Mycoplasma hominis	−	+	−	5.5–8.0	1–5 days	4+	4+	4+	Unknown
Ureaplasma urealyticum/ U. parvum	−	−	+	5.5–6.5	1–4 days	4+	4+	4+	14
Mycoplasma fermentans	+	+	−	7.0	4–21 days	2+	NA	4+	1
Respiratory/genital tracts									
Mycoplasma genitalium	+	−	−	7.0	SLOW	2+	3–4+	1+	Unknown
Acholeplasma laidlawii	+	−	−	6.0–8.0	1–5 days	4+	4+	4+	1

+, positive; −, negative; NA, data not available.

structural similarities, both serologic cross-reactivities and genetic homologies have been described between *M. pneumoniae* and *M. genitalium*.[65,254,504]

The genus *Ureaplasma* includes mycoplasmal organisms that are specifically able to hydrolyze urea. The genus currently contains seven species: *U. urealyticum*, *U. parvum*, *U. diversum*, *U. gallorale*, *U. felinum*, *U. cati*, and *U. canigenitalium*.[16,148,149,173,228,394] *Ureaplasma* used to be called "T-strain" mycoplasmas because of the small ("T" for "tiny") size of their colonies on solid media.[394] Prior to 1999, 14 serotypes of *U. urealyticum* had been described in humans, nonhuman primates, and other animals. These 14 serotypes were defined by reactivity with a panel of polyclonal antisera.[16,369] These serotypes clustered into two biovars: biovar 1 was composed of serotypes 1, 3, 6, and 14, and biovar 2 included serotypes 2, 4, 5, and 7 through 13.[147] Members of these two biovars also demonstrated differences in other properties, including restriction-fragment-length polymorphisms, whole-cell protein patterns on polyacrylamide gel electrophoresis, and sensitivity to manganese salts.[16,147,357,369,420] Additional studies using cellular protein analysis and DNA restriction endonuclease patterns supported the serologic grouping of distinct biovars as well.[359] Organisms belonging to biovar 1 also were shown to have smaller genomes than those in biovar 2, so biovar 1 organisms were dubbed the "parvo" (small) biovar.[204] Within biovars, analysis of rRNA with nucleic acid probes demonstrated significant nucleotide sequence homology among constituent serotypes. The percent of DNA-DNA hybridization among serotypes 1, 3, and 6 in biovar 1 was 91% to 92%, whereas that among serotypes 2, 4, 5, 7, and 8 in biovar 2 ranged from 69% to 97%. However, monoclonal antibodies developed against biovar 1 serotypes also reacted on Western immunoblots with clinical biovar 2 isolates, indicating considerable antigenic cross-reactivity within the polyclonally defined serotypes.[58] Immunoblot analyses of clinical biovar 1 isolates with monoclonal antibodies showed highly variable patterns compared with each other and with specific reference serotype strains, suggesting that a high degree of antigenic variation exists within and among the various serotypes. Polymerase chain reaction (PCR) techniques that detect biovar-specific 16S rRNA were developed and have been used to examine reference strains and clinical isolates to determine relationships between biovars and specific disease entities associated with *U. urealyticum*.[370,444] In 1998, *U. urealyticum* biovars 1 and 2 were formally classified as *Ureaplasma parvum* and *Ureaplasma urealyticum*, respectively.[227]

The other *Ureaplasma* species are found exclusively in animals. *U. diversum* (three serovars) is found in the bovine and ovine respiratory and genital tracts; it is the etiologic agent of maternal and fetal infections, including amnionitis, abortion, low birth weight, infant pneumonia, and neonatal death.[173] *U. gallorale* (one serovar) is a nonpathogenic species found in the respiratory tract of chickens and other fowl.[16,228] Two species—*U. felinum* and *U. cati*—have been recovered from the respiratory tracts of healthy domestic cats.[148] *U. canigenitalium*, the most recently described species, was isolated from oral, nasal, and prepuce cultures of dogs and includes four serovars.[149] In addition to these seven formally described species, genetically and antigenically distinct avian, porcine, simian, bovine, and caprine/ovine ureaplasmas have also been described but have not been assigned definitive species status or epithets.[16,150]

Virulence Factors of Human Mycoplasmas

Potential virulence factors in human pathogenic mycoplasmas have not been studied extensively, but a few candidate factors have been described. *M. pneumoniae* possesses an attachment organelle, which is a tapered extension at one pole of the cell that has an electron dense core and a terminal "button."[235,236,389] These structures make up part of the mycoplasmal cytoskeleton, which is comprised of a network of various proteins. Clustered at the tip of the attachment organelle is a membrane-associated, 169-kDa protein called P1, which is the major cytadhesin that mediates the adherence of *M. pneumoniae* to host cells.[19,185] Studies on noncytadherent mutants of *M. pneumoniae* have identified several additional accessory proteins (HMW1, HMW2, HMW3, HMW4, P90, P65, P40, P30, P116) that are essential for adherence to target tissues and are localized and clustered within the attachment organelle along with P1.[19,116,174,201,411,412,418,494] Because cytadherence is a necessary first step for infection of susceptible mucosal surfaces, these proteins represent true virulence factors in this organism. Individuals infected with *M. pneumoniae* produce a vigorous antibody response against the P1 adhesin, suggesting that purified adhesin proteins may be useful in serologic tests for diagnosis of *M. pneumoniae* infections.[102,184,185] Substantial literature also exists on the induction of various cytokines resulting from infection with *M. pneumoniae* and the role of these cytokines in the pathogenesis of mycoplasmal disease.[501]

Cytadherence proteins responsible for the initiation of colonization and infection have also been demonstrated in *M. hominis*. P50 and P100, two surface-localized polypeptides of *M. hominis*, function in adherence of this species to eukaryotic cells.[157] *M. hominis* also binds sulfated glycolipids in a time-, temperature-, and dose-dependent manner that can be inhibited by preincubation of the organisms with high-molecular-weight dextran sulfate.[329] Binding of recombinant P50 protein to HeLa cells is also inhibited by high-molecular-weight dextrans, indicating that P50 cytadherence protein binds to sulfatides on the host-cell membrane.[223] Sulfated glycolipids and other glycoconjugates are present in high concentrations in the male and female urogenital tracts, and specific interaction of *M. hominis* with these molecules may help explain the urogenital tissue tropism of *M. hominis*. The P100 cytadherence lipoprotein of *M. hominis* also possesses a substrate-binding domain for peptide transport across the cell membrane.[158] *M. hominis* strains also possess another surface-exposed, adherence-associated protein called Vaa (variable adherence-associated) antigen, which is encoded by six distinct *vaa* gene types.[38,39] Expression of these genes can be switched on and off; this ability has been postulated to promote spread of the organisms from one cell to another.[509]

U. urealyticum also produces a variety of virulence-associated factors. Isolates of *U. urealyticum* produce three phospholipase enzymes (A$_1$, A$_2$, and C) that are localized in the plasma membrane.[97] These enzymes hydrolyze phospholipids, with the release of arachidonic acid. Because *U. urealyticum* is associated with amnionitis and perinatal morbidity and mortality (i.e., spontaneous abortions, prematurity, stillbirth), it has been postulated that infection of the female genital tract may initiate a sequence of pathologic events related to phospholipase production.[111] Release of arachidonic acids from amniotic membranes may lead to production of prostaglandins, which can trigger premature labor.[26] *U. urealyticum* has also been shown to induce the production of inflammatory cytokines (i.e., tumor necrosis factor-α [TNF-α], interleukin-6 [IL-6]) in both human and rat macrophage cell lines, and to stimulate the release of nitric oxide by cultured alveolar macrophage.[248,250] The extensive release of these cytokines may contribute to the inflammatory response and to the pathology of chronic lung disease seen in very-low-birth-weight premature infants. *U. urealyticum* has also been demonstrated to induce apoptosis in human lung epithelial cells and macrophages; cell death was abrogated by anti-TNF-α monoclonal antibodies.[249] These data suggest that *U. urealyticum* lung infection in these neonates may be involved in the chronic impairment of lung tissues both directly and indirectly by the production of inflammatory cytokines that are known to play roles in chronic lung disease of premature infants.[230,453] The three phospholipases described above may also contribute to fetal lung disease related to respiratory tract infection with *U. urealyticum*.[379] Both *M. hominis* and *U. urealyticum* also produce immunoglobulin A proteases, which may facilitate mucosal invasion by hydrolyzing mucosal IgA.[206]

M. fermentans (including the "incognitus" strain [see below]) *M. penetrans*, and *M. pirum*, have been associated with disease in both healthy individuals and patients with AIDS. These organisms have been implicated as opportunistic agents or cofactors that contribute to the pathology and pathogenesis of HIV-related disease.[309] The mechanisms involved in these postulated roles include specific activation of the cellular immune system, production of superantigens that stimulate the release of various immunomodulating lymphokines and cytokines, and the generation of free radicals that contribute to oxidative stress observed in HIV infection. All of these "AIDS-associated" mycoplasmas use glucose and hydrolyze arginine. Mycoplasmal arginine deaminase may cause depletion of arginine in infected macrophages. Arginine is a precursor for a molecule that is directly involved in macrophage-mediated cytotoxicity; therefore, depletion of arginine by mycoplasmal infection may result in diminished macrophage cytotoxicity. Mycoplasmas also release into the growth medium nucleases that degrade host-cell nucleic acids to generate precursors for synthesis of their own nucleic acids. *M. fermentans*, *M. penetrans*, and *M. pirum* are also able to invade cells and survive as intracellular pathogens.[76] The association of these organisms with intracellular locations in lymphocytes and macrophages helps explain the recovery of these organisms, especially, *M. fermentans* from the blood of AIDS and non-AIDS patients.

Clinical Significance of the Human Mycoplasmas
Mycoplasma pneumoniae

M. pneumoniae is one of many causes of a pneumonic process called atypical pneumonia, along with several viral (e.g., influenza, respiratory syncytial virus, adenoviruses), fungal (e.g., *Pneumocystis carinii*), and bacterial (e.g., *Chlamydia pneumoniae*, *Legionella pneumophila*) agents.[37,69,121,252] *M. pneumoniae* is transmitted by airborne transfer of droplets containing the organisms and is highly communicable. About 10–30% of community-acquired pneumonias are caused by *M. pneumoniae*, however, these cases represent only 3–10% of *M. pneumoniae* infections, since tracheobronchitis or minor upper respiratory tract infections develop in most infected individuals, or they remain asymptomatic.[69,121] In closed populations (e.g., summer camps, military bases, schools), *M. pneumoniae* may cause 25% to over 75% of pneumonic infections. Disease is generally not seasonal and may occur year-round, but the incidence of overt disease is usually highest in late fall and winter, when young people are going back to school. Infection occurs in school-age children older than 5 years, adolescents, and young adults. However, both endemic and epidemic disease may occur in younger children and in older adults.[178] Upper respiratory tract infections tend to develop in children younger than 3 years of age, whereas tracheobronchitis or pneumonia more often develops in older children and adults. Interestingly, studies in pediatric populations have not demonstrated a role for *M. pneumoniae* in acute myringitis or otitis media with effusion.[231,415] Most infections caused by *M. pneumoniae* are relatively minor and include pharyngitis, tracheobronchitis, bronchiolitis, and croup; up to one fifth of infections are actually asymptomatic and may represent reinfection.[69,121] Severe infections requiring hospitalization may develop in elderly and immunocompromised patients, and death may result from some of these.[284,341]

After exposure in susceptible hosts, the organism attaches to epithelial cells in the respiratory tract and multiplies. The organisms do not penetrate the epithelial cells of the respiratory tract but remain localized. Organisms may be recovered on culture during the incubation period and for several weeks during and after clinical illness, even in the presence of specific antibodies. Following a 2- to 3-week incubation period, the clinical presentation of mycoplasmal pneumonia is usually insidious, rather than abrupt, with the gradual onset of constitutional and pneumonic symptoms that mimic influenza.[69] Fevers of 101 to 102°F will develop over a few days in most patients, with chills, malaise, headache, sore throat, nasal congestion, and a dry, nonproductive cough appearing early in the clinical course. The leukocyte count is often normal or only slightly elevated. In 5–10% of patients, progressive lower respiratory tract symptoms develop; the sputum becomes more mucoid or mucopurulent and blood may be noted in the sputum occasionally.[69] Gram-stained smears of sputum at this point usually show few to moderate amounts of polymorphonuclear inflammatory cells and no organisms. With the onset of pneumonic symptoms, patients may feel as if they have a severe cold or the "flu," yet will continue to function relatively normally; hence, the application of the term "walking pneumonia" to this disease. On chest examination, localized rhonchi and scattered rales are usually detected, and findings on chest roentgenograms are consistent with a diffuse bronchopneumonia, generally involving multiple lobes of the lung without consolidation. With *M. pneumoniae* pneumonia, x-ray patterns vary widely and may show peribronchial pneumonic infiltrates, atelectasis, nodules, and hilar lymphadenopathy.[69] Radiologic findings usually appear more extensive than the physical examination of the patient would suggest. Pleural effusions are relatively rare in mycoplasmal pneumonia, occurring in up to 20% of patients. Other pleuropulmonary complications, such as pneumothorax and lung abscess, are also uncommon.

M. pneumoniae pneumonia is generally self-limited, with resolution of most constitutional symptoms in 3 to 10 days without antimicrobial therapy.[69] Abnormalities on chest films generally resolve more slowly, and complete resolution may take anywhere from 10 days to 6 weeks. Although antimicrobial therapy with tetracycline or erythromycin significantly reduces the duration of signs and symptoms and hastens resolution of abnormalities seen on chest films, the organism is generally not eradicated from the respiratory tract by chemotherapy.[69] In one study, throat cultures for *M. pneumoniae* were still positive 4 months after resolution of the infection.[121] Recurrences and relapses of pneumonia despite appropriate antimicrobial therapy may also occur. Using serologic methods and molecular detection techniques, several studies have now shown that *M. pneumoniae* may play significant roles in acute and chronic asthma is children and adults, exacerbations of chronic obstructive pulmonary disease particularly among older adults, and adult respiratory distress syndrome.[30,120,234,297] Recent data also suggest that *M. pneumoniae* may be implicated in acute chest syndrome, a pneumonia-like disease seen in patients with sickle-cell disease.[322]

Complications caused by *M. pneumoniae* infection are rare but protean in the numbers of organ systems that may be involved. Complications may be dermatologic, cardiovascular, musculoskeletal, neurologic, urologic, hepatobiliary, or ocular. Dermatologic complications include erythema multiforme major (Stevens-Johnson syndrome); various types of cutaneous macular, morbilliform, and vesicular eruptions; and erythema nodosum.[60,246] Erythema multiforme major, the cutaneous manifestation that is linked most frequently with mycoplasma infection, presents as vesicular lesions in mucocutaneous areas of the body.[246,375] Cardiovascular manifestations may occur in as many as 10% of cases and include conduction defects, cardiac arrhythmia, pericarditis, tamponade, and congestive heart failure.[212,300,380] Although arthralgias are a common manifestation of mycoplasma infection, frank arthritis, with positive cultures from joint fluids, has been reported but is very uncommon.[56,81] Neurologic complications may result from direct mycoplasmal invasion of the nervous system (i.e., septic meningitis, meningoencephalitis, transverse myelitis, acute disseminated encephalomyelitis), whereas postinfectious neurologic syndromes probably occur via an autoimmune mechanism induced by mycoplasma infection and/or via thromboembolic events leading to microangiopathy, cerebral vasculitis, and demyelination in perivascular areas in the central nervous system (CNS).[28,31,316,344,363,405] Severe CNS complications of the latter type have been associated with strokes following acute *M. pneumoniae* infection.[331,406] Urologic and hepatobiliary complications are manifested as acute nephritis and cholestatic hepatitis, respectively.[140,401] Ocular complications, including optic disk swelling, optic nerve atrophy, optic papillitis, retinal exudation, and hemorrhage, have also been reported in association with *M. pneu-*

moniae infection.[305,377] Various type of hematologic complications (i.e., hemolytic anemia secondary to the formation of cold agglutinins, intravascular coagulopathy, neutropenia, thrombocytopenia, paroxysmal cold hemoglobinuria) may result from the generation of specific antibodies and autoantibodies directed against lung, tissue, cardiolipin, and muscle tissues.[57,59,85]

Humoral and cellular immunodeficiency states also predispose individuals to more serious disease with *M. pneumoniae* as well as other mycoplasmas.[121,334,372] Individuals with hypogammaglobulinemia may suffer repeated bouts of *M. pneumoniae* pneumonia and have difficulty eliminating the organism from the respiratory tract despite adequate therapy. These patients often have severe upper and lower respiratory tract symptoms, with few or no infiltrates observed on chest radiography, and have significant complications, including rashes, joint pain, septic arthritis, and osteomyelitis.[200,240,440,442] *M. pneumoniae* may also cause severe disease in patients with conditions that abrogate cellular immunity, including HIV infection and sickle cell disease.[194,222,322,334]

Fulminant, disseminated *M. pneumoniae* infection with multisystem involvement is rare, but it has been reported. Kountouras and colleagues reported on a previously healthy 50-year-old male who presented with progressive respiratory distress, aseptic meningitis, cholestatic hepatitis, renal failure, and disseminated intravascular coagulation.[232] *M. pneumoniae* infection was diagnosed serologically; the patient was treated with erythromycin and experienced an uneventful recovery. Takiguchi and colleagues reported on a previously healthy 64-year-old woman in whom progressive respiratory distress developed, with widespread bilateral alveolar infiltrates on chest radiographs.[423] Acute respiratory distress syndrome and disseminated intravascular coagulation then developed. *M. pneumoniae* infection was diagnosed serologically. Despite intensive antimicrobial and corticosteroid therapy, mechanical ventilation, hemodialysis, and plasma exchanges, the patient died of multiple organ system failure. Koletsky and Weinstein reported a case of rapidly fatal, disseminated *M. pneumoniae* infection during which severe respiratory disease, pneumonia, cardiovascular collapse, and renal failure developed in a 30-year-old female patient after a 9-day clinical course.[225] The patient died within 24 hours of admission to the hospital. On autopsy, the organism was recovered from the lungs, kidneys, and brain. Tissue sections revealed bilateral consolidated pneumonia and disseminated intravascular coagulation.

M. pneumoniae may occasionally be isolated from unusual extrapulmonary sites other than joint fluids and the CNS. Goulet and coworkers isolated *M. pneumoniae* from urogenital tract specimens of 22 female patients over a 2-year period.[132] In addition, the organism was recovered from the urethra of one of three male sexual partners of a female patient who harbored the organism in her genital tract. *M. pneumoniae* has also been isolated from a tubo-ovarian abscess.[448]

Mycoplasma hominis and *Ureaplasma urealyticum*

Both *M. hominis* and *U. urealyticum* may be isolated from the genital tracts of asymptomatic men and women.[289,291,292]

McCormack and colleagues demonstrated that rates of colonization with *M. hominis* and *U. urealyticum* in men varied from zero to 13% and 3% to 56%, respectively.[289,290] Similar data on women have shown that vaginal colonization rates for *M. hominis* and *U. urealyticum* range from zero to 31% and 8.5% to 77.5%, respectively, depending on age, race, sexual experience, and socioeconomic status.[289,290,292] Rates of genital tract colonization in both men and women are related to sexual activity, and individuals with multiple sexual partners are more likely to be colonized. Therefore, the epidemiology of organism acquisition suggests that these mycoplasmas are indeed sexually transmitted. Additional evidence for sexual acquisition is suggested by much lower isolation rates among women who use barrier contraceptives.[292] Given these data, it is clear that these organisms are exceedingly prevalent, particularly in the lower genital tracts of sexually active women.

Over the past several years, both *U. urealyticum* and *M. hominis* have been implicated in a variety of clinical conditions primarily related to lower genital tract colonization and infection, upper genital tract infections in women, and, rarely, upper genital tract infection and prostatitis in men.[111,151,188,339] Both organisms have been postulated to play roles in early and late endometritis, chorioamnionitis, and premature rupture of membranes.[99,111,137] The presence of *U. urealyticum* in the genital tract, in particular, has been associated statistically with prematurity, low-birth-weight infants, and infertility.[113,137,151,207] Controlled studies on the pathogenicity of the genital mycoplasmas are complicated because both organisms are highly prevalent in sexually active asymptomatic adults. To further confound issues of etiology, genital mycoplasmas are often recovered in culture along with other recognized genital tract pathogens, such as *Chlamydia trachomatis*, *Neisseria gonorrhoeae*, and group B streptococci.[8] These associations make it difficult to determine whether a pathologic condition is attributable solely to the presence of genital mycoplasmas per se. An excellent example of this dilemma is the clinical condition bacterial vaginosis. *M. hominis* is associated with bacterial vaginosis and is often isolated from women with this infection.[160,211,238] However, bacterial vaginosis is now known to result from a complex interaction among aerobic and anaerobic bacterial organisms. The roles of genital mycoplasmas in this condition have not been elucidated or defined, but a causal relationship between *M. hominis* and bacterial vaginosis has not been proven. Studies on the pathogenicity of the genital mycoplasmas are further confounded by recovery of the organisms during or after the administration of antimicrobial agents for other genital tract pathogens.[73] Antimicrobial therapy for these other organisms may act to select for mycoplasmas that are resistant to the agents being used (e.g., penicillins and cephalosporins). After their recovery from a genital culture or a site of pathology, it becomes difficult to ascribe an etiologic role for the organisms in light of previous or ongoing antibiotic administration.

M. hominis and *U. urealyticum* have been isolated from blood cultures of women with postpartum fever.[88,111,112,239, 293,315] About 10% of women with fever post partum or post abortion will have either *M. hominis* or *U. urealyticum* isolated from blood cultures. In some cases, either mycoplasma or both may be recovered from blood cultures, along with other genital tract microorganisms, again confounding the etiologic role of the mycoplasmas. Postpartum bacteremia results from the ascension of the organisms from the vagina into the endometrium, where the organisms apparently cause an endometritis. Infection of the placental membranes and amniotic fluid with mycoplasmas most frequently occurs in colonized women with premature rupture of the fetal membranes and preterm or prolonged labor.[125] From these sites, the organisms enter the bloodstream during and after labor and delivery or after a cesarean section. *U. urealyticum* bacteremia has also been documented as a complication in women undergoing hysterectomy.[83]

Isolation of mycoplasmas from the lower genital tracts of pregnant women is associated with several adverse outcomes of pregnancy, including the delivery of low-birth-weight infants. In a study conducted by Kass and coworkers, women whose genital tracts were colonized with *U. urealyticum* and who demonstrated a fourfold or greater antibody response to the organism showed a rate of 30% of having low-birth-weight infants, whereas colonized women who did mount this antibody response had a rate of 7.3% of having low-birth-weight infants.[207] Furthermore, this antibody response was serotype-specific, suggesting that the additional rate of low birth weight was related to recent infection with a new serotype of *U. urealyticum* that differed from the serotype or serotypes already present in the vagina. A study that examined the relationship between the two *U. urealyticum* biovars and pregnancy outcomes found that the *urealyticum* biovar was associated with more adverse outcomes with regard to birth weight, gestational age, and preterm delivery than the *parvo* biovar.[1] Studies of treatment with either tetracycline or erythromycin have resulted in decreases in rates of low birth weight, implying that eradication of mycoplasmas (or other organisms) from the genital tract may have a direct, beneficial effect on certain adverse outcomes of pregnancy.[207]

Amniotic infections with *U. urealyticum* may be demonstrated in asymptomatic women with intact fetal membranes, and these infections are frequently associated with adverse pregnancy outcomes.[52,138,171,505] *U. urealyticum* is capable of initiating an intense inflammatory tissue response, with no associated symptoms and serologic evidence of an antibody response to these organisms and simultaneous recovery of ureaplasmas from the blood appear to confirm the possibility of silent amniotic infections.[52,127] Gray and associates studied two groups of asymptomatic pregnant women who were matched for maternal age, gestational age, and indications for amniocentesis.[138] Transabdominal amniocentesis specimens were cultured for mycoplasmas. Among the 86 women in the ureaplasma-negative group, there was a 1.2% incidence of spontaneous second trimester abortion and a prematurity rate of 9.3%, for an overall adverse outcome rate of 10.5%. However, the rate of adverse outcomes among the eight ureaplasma-positive women was 100%, representing an 8.6-fold greater risk of adverse outcome. Adverse outcomes in these eight pregnancies included spontaneous abortion (75%), premature deliveries with a 50% mortality rate (25%), and hyaline membrane disease (seen in the single surviving infant). Introduction of the organisms into the amniotic fluid is also a crucial step in the development of chorioamnionitis and endometritis. Histologic examination of placental tissues from the eight infected women revealed chorioamnionitis in all of them, and all seven lung tissue specimens from the infants showed pneumonia.[138] Four of five placentas and three of five fetal lung tissue specimens that were cultured grew *U. urealyticum*. Horowitz and colleagues also showed that 50% of six women with positive midtrimester amniotic cultures for *U. urealyticum* had adverse pregnancy outcomes, as compared with 12% of 123 women with negative amniotic fluid cultures.[171] Eschenbach reviewed the lines of evidence relative to the contribution of *U. urealyticum* to adverse outcomes of pregnancy and concluded that, although the presence of *U. urealyticum* in the lower genital tract was not associated with premature birth, the presence of the organism in the chorioamnion was strongly associated with histologic evidence of chorioamnionitis and weakly associated with premature birth as an outcome.[113] In another study that examined endocervical colonization with and serologic responses to *U. urealyticum*, Horowitz and colleagues found that cervical colonization, when associated with increased titers to *U. urealyticum*, identified a population of women who were at risk for complications of pregnancy.[169,170] Although it has been well established that healthy women who are colonized with *M. hominis* in the genital tract usually deliver healthy colonized infants, *M. hominis* has also occasionally been associated with chorioamnionitis, abortion, stillbirth, and intrauterine fetal death.[296]

In some cases, placental infection with ureaplasmas has been shown to contribute a priori to subsequent endometritis, premature rupture of membranes, and premature labor. Colonization of the placenta permits infection of the endometrium, from which the organisms can gain access to the bloodstream. The recovery of *U. urealyticum* and *M. hominis* from endometrial tissue sometime after delivery has established that mycoplasmas and ureaplasmas, in particular, are the probable causes of early- and late-onset endometritis in some cases. Postpartum endometritis is a major complication of pregnancy and occurs more frequently after cesarean section than after vaginal delivery. In one study, endometritis occurred in 28% of women with *U. urealyticum* present in the chorioamnion at cesarean delivery, compared with only 8.4% if the culture was negative and 8.8% if only bacteria other than *U. urealyticum* were present.[12] These workers concluded that chorioamniotic colonization with *U. urealyticum* in women with intact membranes being delivered by cesarean section was an independent predictor of subsequent endometritis. A subsequent randomized clinical trial of extended-spectrum antimicrobial prophylaxis using agents active against *U. urealyticum* in women undergoing cesarean delivery was found to reduce the frequency of postdelivery endometritis.[11] Although it has been suggested by some studies, a definite causal relation between genital mycoplasmas and pelvic inflammatory disease (salpingitis) has not been unequivocally demonstrated.[41,111,253,391,419]

Because of the high colonization rates of genital mycoplasmas in both men and women, these organisms have also been evaluated for relationships with involuntary infertility. Again, although some studies suggest a possible role for these organisms in this condition, there is no proof indicating that these organisms cause either male or female infertility.[426] In a 2002 study of 50 infertile women and 46 fertile

women, *M. hominis* was isolated from the genital tracts of 8% of the infertile women and was not isolated from any of the controls.[118] *U. urealyticum* was isolated from 56% of the infertile women and from 39% of the control women; this difference was not statistically significant, but the authors suggested that an association between infertility and *U. urealyticum* may exist. In a study of 92 asymptomatic male partners of infertile couples, 12 (13%) men had *U. urealyticum* in their ejaculates. Again, these workers suggested that *U. urealyticum* may play a role in infertility in the absence of other conditions.[247] In vitro, *U. urealyticum* has been shown to adhere to sperm cells, resulting in significant reductions in sperm motility and alterations in cell membranes.[325] Scanning electron micrographic pictures of these cells reveal spermatozoa with masses of *U. urealyticum* organisms adherent to the sperm head along with other structural abnormalities. Consequently, these investigators also suggested a possible role of *U. urealyticum* in infertility due to alterations in structure and motility of the spermatozoa.[325] However, another study found no difference in sperm quality in men with and without positive cultures for *M. hominis* or *U. ureaplasma*, as assessed by sperm density, vitality, motility and morphology.[10]

U. urealyticum may play a role in spontaneous abortion that is related to its ability to cause chorioamnionitis but, like the other conditions described above, definitive proof has not been obtained. Joste and associates examined 42 first trimester spontaneous abortions and 21 elective first-trimester abortions and compared them histologically and culturally with 32 third-trimester, preterm deliveries, 11 of which were culture-positive for *U. urealyticum*.[203] Among specimens obtained from first-trimester spontaneous abortions, 26% grew ureaplasmas, compared with none of the 21 elective abortion specimens. Histologic evidence of chorioamnionitis did not correlate with culture positivity for the spontaneous abortion specimens. However, evidence of chorioamnionitis did correlate with positive ureaplasma cultures for the 11 third-trimester, preterm deliveries. These workers postulated that early changes caused by *U. urealyticum* infection other than histologically evident chorioamnionitis may be responsible for the pathogenesis of spontaneous abortions related to ureaplasmal infection.[203] A study conducted from 1989 to 1994 in Belgium examined the possible links between a diagnosis of bacterial vaginosis during the first trimester and spontaneous abortion at less than 20 weeks' gestation. A strong association was noted between bacterial vaginosis and miscarriage.[100] On multivariate analysis, *M. hominis* and *U. urealyticum*, but no other microorganisms, remained significantly associated with increased risk of miscarriage. However, another study published in 2004 found no association between first-trimester miscarriages and the presence of mycoplasmas or ureaplasmas in expelled placental specimens.[287] A study that examined specimens for specific *U. urealyticum* biovars found that biovar *urealyticum* was found more frequently in patients with pelvic inflammatory disease and those who had miscarriage.[1]

Urinary tract infections caused by mycoplasmas have also been reported, and, again, most work in this area has been in pregnant women. Determination of the significance of mycoplasmas in clean-catch urine specimens from women is difficult, owing to the likely contamination of the specimen from organisms colonizing the vagina and the distal urethra. Because of the recognized association between bacteriuria during pregnancy and the increased incidence of premature delivery and preeclampsia, Savige and coworkers collected suprapubic bladder aspirates from 72 healthy pregnant women and 51 women with preeclampsia and cultured the urine specimens for mycoplasmas.[386] *U. urealyticum* was isolated from the urine of 7% of the healthy women and from 20% of those with preeclampsia. In a subsequent study of bacteriuria in 340 pregnant women, the presence of *U. urealyticum* in the urine during the first trimester correlated with the development of preeclampsia during the third trimester of pregnancy.[129] Among the 21 women in whom preeclampsia developed, 29% had ureaplasmas present in urine during the first trimester, compared with only 10% of the patients in whom preeclampsia did not develop. Therefore, the development of preeclampsia was three times more likely in women who had ureaplasmas in the urine at the start of pregnancy than in women who were culture-negative. Although the mechanisms involved in the pathogenesis of preeclampsia are unclear, it is suggested that ureaplasmas, similar to other bacteria involved in bacteriuria, may also contribute to adverse pregnancy outcome. In another study of mycoplasmas in 48 women with chronic symptoms of urinary tract infection, 23 (48%) had positive cultures; 22 had *U. urealyticum* and 1 had *M. hominis*.[351] After targeted therapy, cultures from all the women were negative and 21 of the 23 infected women experienced alleviation of their chronic symptoms. These investigators concluded that, following exclusion of common agents of urologic infections, anatomic abnormalities, and neurologic dysfunctions, culture for mycoplasmas and subsequent targeted antimycoplasmal chemotherapy is warranted before other diagnostic procedures are entertained.[351]

In men, *M. hominis* is relatively uncommon as a cause of clinical disease, and most research on mycoplasmas has concentrated on the association of *U. urealyticum* with nongonococcal, nonchlamydial urethritis (NGNCU). *Chlamydia trachomatis* is well established as the etiologic agent responsible for 30–50% of acute urethritis not attributable to *N. gonorrhoeae*, and a significant association has been made between NGNCU and *Mycoplasma genitalium*, which may account for 15–25% of cases of acute NGNCU.[90,91,164] Although several studies have been done, the role of *U. urealyticum* in male urethritis is not entirely clear. Although earlier data suggested that *U. urealyticum* is the cause of some NGNCU, it is not known what proportion of infections are due to the organism, and, even if the organism is present in the urethras of symptomatic men, its role as the causative agent may not be established. Studies of symptomatic men treated with antibiotics having differential activity between *Chlamydia trachomatis* and *U. urealyticum*, and cultures performed on men with persistent symptoms of urethritis following antigonococcal and antichlamydial therapies indeed suggested that some cases of nongonococcal urethritis are caused by *U. urealyticum*.[73,431] Use of highly sensitive molecular approaches along with serologic responses has already provided more complete information regarding the role of *U. urealyticum* in nongonococcal urethritis. A study conducted by Horner and colleagues found that *U. urealyticum* was not associated with acute NGNCU in multivariate

analysis, but was associated with chronic NGNCU, which was defined for the study as urethritis occurring 30 to 92 days after commencement of treatment.[165,166] These workers concluded that ureaplasmas were a probable cause of chronic NGNCU occurring after treatment. A 2004 study conducted in Japan reported a significant association between *U. urealyticum* and NGNCU and suggested that the presence of *U. parvum* in the urethra may reflect colonization and not infection.[93] Other recent studies using sensitive molecular techniques have established that *U. urealyticum* is associated with some cases of NGNCU and that *U. parvum* is seen more often in asymptomatic infections, although some patients with *U. parvum* may be symptomatic.[353,507]

Ureaplasmas may also be involved in the etiology of chronic prostatitis. Using classical techniques for localizing infections to the prostate, several investigators have documented *U. urealyticum* as being responsible for a small proportion of cases of chronic prostatitis.[326,327,339,402] In a 2002 study from Croatia, *U. urealyticum* was the sole agent isolated from the prostatic fluids of 2.54% of 276 patients with chronic prostatic infection.[402] In a study from Japan, *U. urealyticum* was recovered from prostatic fluid secretions of 18 of 143 patients with prostatitis.[327] Targeted anti-ureaplasma treatment eradicated the organisms along with resolution of symptoms, suggesting that *U. urealyticum* was the causative agent in these patients. *U. urealyticum* is rare as a cause of epididymitis; a single case has been reported from whom the organisms were isolated from an epididymal aspirate in association with a significant rise in antibodies to the organism.[188]

Infants born to mothers who are colonized with genital mycoplasmas are also frequently colonized themselves. In survey studies, 18–45% of neonates delivered to colonized mothers were also colonized with *M. hominis*, with positive cultures being obtained from the throat, the genital tract, or the urine.[99,111] The rate of vertical transmission of *U. urealyticum* ranges from 18% to 55% among full-term infants and from 29% to 55% among preterm infants.[378] Syrogiannopoulos and associates cultured the throat, eyes, and vaginas of 193 full-term infants born to women colonized vaginally with *U. urealyticum*.[422] Of these, 107 (55%) had *U. urealyticum* present in at least one culture site. Colonization may persist in these babies for prolonged periods with no ill effects to the child. In the latter study, 68%, 33%, and 37% of the infants who had colonization at birth in the throat, eyes, and vagina, respectively, still had colonization on follow-up at 3 months of age. Among the children who had colonization in the respiratory tract, there was no increased incidence of respiratory tract illnesses when compared with children who did not have colonization in this area. In a study performed in Israel, 24% of 99 preterm infants were colonized with mycoplasmas; *U. urealyticum* was isolated from 21 infants, and *M. hominis* was isolated from three infants.[181] In this study, the colonization rate was inversely correlated with gestational age, with 80% of infants younger than 28 weeks of gestation having colonization as opposed to 17.9% of infants at 28 to 36 weeks of gestation.[181] Of the 27 infants requiring ventilatory assistance in this study, 22% had *U. urealyticum* isolated from lower respiratory tract secretions.

Several studies have suggested that *U. urealyticum* is

associated with chronic lung disease, bronchopulmonary dysplasia, persistent pulmonary hypertension, and systemic infection in premature infants.[29,51,53,142,338,476,478,482] Prospective studies and animal model studies have now shown a significant relation between *U. urealyticum* respiratory tract infection and the development of chronic lung disease of the newborn.[74,373,482] Cassell and others found that the recovery of *U. urealyticum* from the tracheas of infants weighing less than 1,000 g, who also required ventilatory assistance, was associated with the development of bronchopulmonary dysplasia and associated conditions (e.g., hyaline membrane disease, patent ductus arteriosus, and pneumonia).[51] A subsequent study by Crouse and associates showed that low-birth-weight infants with respiratory distress who had *U. urealyticum* recovered from tracheal cultures were more likely to show dysplasia and evidence of pneumonia on chest radiography than those without *U. urealyticum*.[74] Nasopharyngeal or tracheal colonization of preterm infants with *U. urealyticum* is also associated with an elevated peripheral white blood cell count.[328] Sanchez and Regan found that, among infants colonized with ureaplasmas in the respiratory tract, chronic lung disease requiring mechanical ventilatory assistance developed in 30%, whereas respiratory tract illness developed in only 8% of noncolonized neonates.[379] Bloodstream infection with *U. urealyticum* has been documented in newborn infants, and these infections are often associated with coexisting respiratory tract infections.[45,29,476] These systemic infections are associated with urinary tract infection, preterm or prolonged membrane rupture, preterm labor, and chorioamnionitis in the mother, and with low birth weight, presence of congenital anomalies, and perinatal asphyxia in the newborn.[476] The pathogenesis of this syndrome in the neonate has been supported by animal models and reflects both the nature of these bacteria as opportunistic agents and the immunocompromised status of the premature infant. Studies with neonatal lung fibroblast cultures have demonstrated induction of cytokine release from these cells by infection with *U. urealyticum* in vitro, suggesting a role for cytokines in the pathogenesis of bronchopulmonary dysplasia in prematurity.[409] Serologic studies indicate that the neonate or fetus systemically infected with *U. urealyticum* mounts serovar-specific anti-ureaplasma IgM and IgG responses, providing additional evidence for the pathogenic potential of these organisms.[356]

Several reports and studies have also shown that both *U. urealyticum* and *M. hominis* may be recovered infrequently from the CNS as a cause of silent or clinically symptomatic meningitis in the newborn period.[468] Several cases of *M. hominis* CNS infections in the neonate have been described; most of these occurred in premature infants for whom prolonged rupture of membranes had been documented, although cases have also been described in full-term infants.[9,294,496] In a prospective study of 100 preterm infants, Waites and coworkers isolated *U. urealyticum* from the cerebrospinal fluid (CSF) of eight babies and *M. hominis* from the CSF of five babies.[479] Among the babies with *U. urealyticum* infection, six had intraventricular hemorrhage, three had hydrocephalus, and three died. None of the infants with *M. hominis* infections died, and only one had neurologic signs of meningitis. Gilbert and Drew, however, reported a case of meningitis in a premature infant caused by *M. hom-*

inis that ran a chronic course, with the development of intraventricular hemorrhage.[128] In all of these infants, eradication of the organisms with antimicrobial therapy proved difficult. In a study of 318 predominantly full-term infants with signs of suspected sepsis or meningitis born to primarily low-risk women, *M. hominis* was isolated from the CSF of 9 infants and *U. urealyticum* was recovered from the CSF of 5 infants.[476] Of these 14 infected infants, 12 recovered without therapy and 2 died. Of these 2 infants, 1 with *M. hominis* died of *Haemophilus influenzae* sepsis, whereas the other, infected with *U. urealyticum*, had intraventricular hemorrhage. This study suggested that mycoplasmas are more common in neonatal CNS infections than had been appreciated previously. Although CNS infections with *M. hominis* usually resolve spontaneously, ureaplasmas apparently can elicit an inflammatory response that is associated with intraventricular hemorrhage.[156]

In addition to CNS infections, mycoplasmas, particularly *M. hominis*, have also been isolated from other extragenital infections in both children and adults. Perinatally acquired *M. hominis* has been recovered from subcutaneous scalp abscesses at the site of forceps or monitor injuries, conjunctival infections, and submandibular lymph nodes in the newborn.[43,131,354] *M. hominis* was also isolated in multiple blood cultures from a 10-month-old child who had suffered severe burns.[79] In adults, *M. hominis* has been cultured from a wide variety of infections, including bacteremia, postoperative and posthysterectomy wound infections, hematomas, septic arthritis, aspiration-associated empyema, septic thrombophlebitis, peritonitis, periorbital abscesses, intraabdominal and retroperitoneal abscesses, and brain abscesses.[44,68,126,221,245,278,285,295,306,307,337,362] *M. hominis* bacteremia and postoperative sternal wound infection have occurred in patients following cardiothoracic surgery.[311,404] In another case report of *M. hominis* sternal wound infection, *U. urealyticum* was also recovered.[348] *M. hominis* prosthetic valve endocarditis has been reported, and both *M. hominis* and *U. urealyticum* have been isolated from pericardial tissues or fluids of patients with pericardial effusions.[35,212] Patients with these infections had histories of recent cardiac surgery (e.g., coronary artery bypass surgery, aortic valve replacement, heart transplantation secondary to idiopathic dilated cardiomyopathy) or were immunocompromised (e.g., systemic lupus erythematosus, chronic obstructive pulmonary disease).[212] *M. hominis* was also isolated from a surgical wound infection following insertion of a silicone breast prosthesis.[381]

M. hominis and *U. urealyticum* can behave as opportunistic infectious agents in those with underlying diseases or conditions, such as hypogammaglobulinemia, Hodgkin's disease, systemic lupus erythematosus, renal transplantation, heart disease, leukemia, lymphoma, rheumatoid arthritis, and severe trauma.[68,205,276,304,307,330,336,435,449] *M. hominis* and *U. urealyticum* septic arthritis has been reported in patients with hypogammaglobulinemia, hematologic malignancies, massive trauma, postpartum bacteremia, lupus erythematosus, and common variable immunodeficiency; this clinical entity likely occurs following hematologic seeding of the joint spaces.[47,68,202,449] In 1994, Kane and associates reported the first case of respiratory tract infection with diffuse alveolar hemorrhage caused by *M. hominis* in the recipient of a bone marrow tranplant.[205] *M. hominis* was isolated from postoperative perihepatic hematomas that developed in the abdomen of the recipient of a liver transplant a month after the transplant surgery.[187] Both *M. hominis* and *U. urealyticum* were isolated from a retroperitoneal hematoma 12 days after liver transplantation in a 45-year-old woman with fulminant hepatic failure.[141] Infections of prosthetic joints by *M. hominis* have also occurred, and *M. hominis* wound infections following open reduction of fractured mandibles and after cesarean sections have been reported as well.[346,404] Infections in the head, neck, and chest areas and in tissue contiguous with the genital tract may reflect the presence of these organisms in the adjacent respiratory and urogenital tracts, respectively.[306,362] For example, Kayser and Bhend reported a case of paraspinal, intervertebral soft-tissue infection in a 45-year-old woman that developed 16 days after the patient underwent an abdominal hysterectomy.[210]

M. hominis has also been isolated from the urine of patients with HIV infection. In a study by Chirgwin and colleagues at the State University of New York in Brooklyn, *M. hominis* was isolated from 18% of the urine specimens obtained from 180 HIV-positive individuals and from 21% of urine specimens from 38 HIV-negative individuals.[62] In this study, an additional 30 glucose-using mycoplasmas were recovered only from the HIV-positive individuals.[62] Growth inhibition with species-specific antisera allowed identification of 18 of these isolates: 14 were identified as *M. fermentans* and four were identified as *M. pirum*. The remaining 12 isolates were nonviable on subculture.

Mycoplasma genitalium

In 1981, Tully and coworkers isolated a previously undescribed and unusually fastidious mycoplasma from urethral specimens of two of 13 homosexual men with NGNCU.[458] Although several subsequent attempts to isolate this new organism failed, several isolates of the same organism were recovered from urogenital specimens in China.[275] In 1983, this new species was named *M. genitalium*.[459] Ultrastructural analysis of these isolates indicated that the new organism shared several characteristics with *M. pneumoniae*. These characteristics included the tapering flasklike shape of the individual cells and the presence of a specialized apical structure that facilitated the adherence of the organisms to tissue cells, erythrocytes, and inert material such as plastic and glass.[459] *M. genitalium* possesses a species-specific, 140-kDa protein called P140 that is a structural and functional counterpart of the 170-kDa P1 cytadhesin protein of *M. pneumoniae*.[310] Nonadherent variants of *M. genitalium* have an altered P140 adhesin or have lost the membrane-associated adhesin molecule.[299] *M. genitalium* and *M. pneumoniae* contain a 43-kDa cross-reactive protein that is also detectable on isolates of *Acholeplasma laidlawii*.[65] These shared antigenic epitopes are likely to be responsible for the serologic cross-reactions observed with *M. genitalium* in most tests for *M. pneumoniae* antibodies, including complement fixation, indirect immunofluorescence assays, and metabolic inhibition and growth inhibition tests using heterologous antisera.[77,78,254] DNA hybridization studies have shown that the two organisms have 6.5–8.1% nucleotide sequence homology, the latter probably reflecting those

genes that code for the antigenically cross-reactive proteins.[254,504] Other gene sequences are indeed unique for the two species, providing evidence that *M. pneumoniae* and *M. genitalium* are distinct species.[459]

Initially, epidemiologic studies using both culture and serology established a link between this fastidious *Mycoplasma* species and NGNCU. In a study by Taylor-Robinson and colleagues, rises in antibody titers to *M. genitalium* were detected in 4 of 14 patients with NGU and in 2 of 17 patients without urethritis, but only 1 of the 4 patients who seroconverted had a positive culture.[433] Failure to isolate the organisms in studies on urethritis probably reflected the lack of adequate techniques for reliable culture of this fastidious species. To circumvent the inherent problems of culture, Hooton and coworkers investigated the occurrence of *M. genitalium* in men using a species-specific nucleic acid probe prepared from genomic DNA of *M. genitalium*.[163] These workers detected the organism in 14% of 21 men with gonococcal urethritis, 10% of 30 men with chlamydial urethritis, 13% of 31 men with NGNCU, and 27% of 37 men with recurrent or persistent urethritis. However, the organism was also detected in 12% of 84 men who had no genitourinary tract symptoms. In 1996, Jensen and colleagues succeeded in isolating four strains of *M. genitalium* from urethral specimens of male patients with NGNCU; these patients were also PCR-positive.[193] By using a PCR probe-based technique that detected the nucleotide sequence specific for the *M. genitalium* 140-kDa adhesin gene, Jensen and associates found *M. genitalium* DNA in 17% of urethral specimens from 99 men; 20% of specimens from symptomatic men were positive, whereas only 9% of specimens from asymptomatic men were positive.[195,196] In this study, all attempts to culture the organism from PCR-positive specimens were unsuccessful. Horner and coworkers also used PCR probe technology for detection of *M. genitalium* and found that 23% of 103 men with signs or symptoms of acute NGNCU and 6% of 53 men without NGNCU were positive.[164] The presence of this organism in the male urogenital tract was independent of the presence of *Chlamydia trachomatis*. Using PCR techniques, the same research group failed to detect *M. fermentans*, *M. penetrans*, or *M. pirum* in urethral specimens from patients with NGNCU.[89] These workers concluded that *M. genitalium* was the etiologic agent in many cases of NGNCU; this was also supported by the clinical response of the infected men to treatment with doxycycline.[164]

Several studies using molecular techniques have now established that *M. genitalium* is the cause of 18.4–45.5% of all cases of NGNCU in men and that persistence of the organisms in the urethra after antimicrobial therapy is associated with persistent or recurrent nongonococcal urethritis.[91,190,279,298,439,452] Molecular approaches for the detection of *M. genitalium* include conventional and real-time PCR assays that amplify the *M. genitalium*–specific adhesin (MgPa) gene or species-specific regions of the 16S rRNA gene.[94,109,192,506] The use of real-time assays for detection of *M. genitalium* in first-pass urine specimens has resulted in quantitative results showing that the organism loads of *M. genitalium* in first-pass urine specimens of symptomatic men are much higher than those seen in asymptomatic men. Organism loads in men with *M. genitalium*–positive nongonococcal urethritis were suppressed during levofloxacin therapy, and the patients became asymptomatic. Following treatment, symptoms often disappeared, but the organisms remained detectable in the urethra. The reappearance of symptoms was associated with an increase in organism load in patients in whom treatment failed. These studies have suggested that antimicrobial therapy that results in the elimination of the organisms from the genital tract are required for the management of *M. genitalium*–associated urethritis to prevent subsequent recurrence of NGNCU.[94]

In 1988, Baseman and coworkers recovered *M. genitalium* along with *M. pneumoniae* from 4 of 16 frozen specimens collected from the upper respiratory tracts of military recruits during an *M. pneumoniae* vaccine trial in 1974 and 1975.[20] The role of *M. genitalium* in respiratory tract disease is not clear, but it has been suggested that the association with *M. pneumoniae* may result in a synergistic infection that causes more severe pneumonic disease or may contribute to the pathogenesis of extrapulmonary complications of *M. pneumoniae* infection.[190] The presence of *M. genitalium* in the respiratory tract, with or without *M. pneumoniae*, and the immunologic cross-reactivity between the two organisms may not only complicate the infectious process in coinfected individuals but may also affect the immunologic response to infection. Such interactions, consequently, may interfere with the interpretation of serologic tests that are frequently used to diagnose *M. pneumoniae* infections. The use of PCR primers and nucleic acid probes that are specific for *M. pneumoniae* and *M. genitalium* may provide a solution to clinical and diagnostic problems by circumventing the need to cultivate these agents and clarifying the immune responses and consequent serologic cross-reactions that occur with these organisms.[177]

A few studies have addressed the detection and significance of *M. genitalium* in the female genital tract.[18,436] In a study performed in a sexually transmitted disease clinic in London, *M. genitalium* was detected by PCR in genital tract specimens from 18% of 57 female patients.[333] Another study, done in Copenhagen, reported finding *M. genitalium* in endocervical specimens from 5 of 74 women.[196] Neither of these studies addressed the association of these isolates with the presence of disease or pathology. Although definitive data on the pathogenicity of *M. genitalium* in the female genital tract are lacking, indirect evidence suggests that it may also be involved in both lower and upper genital tract infection. A study conducted in Japan found *M. genitalium* in 7.8% of 64 women with purulent cervicitis, and studies conducted in the U.S. found that, once gonococcal and chlamydial infections were excluded, patients with purulent cervicitis were more than three times as likely to have *M. genitalium* in the cervix than those without purulent cervicitis.[281,463] On the other hand, Casin and colleagues examined 170 women with genital tract symptoms attending a sexually transmitted disease (STD) clinic in Paris and found no correlation between mucopurulent cervicitis and the presence of *M. genitalium*, despite the fact that 38% of the women had positive PCR results for *M. genitalium* at one or more genital sites (usually vaginal).[50] Evidence also exists for *M. genitalium* being involved in endometritis and acute pelvic inflammatory disease. A study conducted in Nairobi, Kenya, on 115 women who presented with persistent pelvic pain found that 16% of 58 women with histologi-

cally confirmed endometritis were PCR-positive for *M. genitalium* in the cervix, the endometrium, or both.[70] In another study conducted in London, 13% of 45 women with pelvic inflammatory disease had PCR-based evidence of *M. genitalium* in the endocervix, compared with none of the control patients.[400] Serologic studies have also documented elevated antibody titers to *M. genitalium* in some women with pelvic inflammatory disease that was not attributable to gonococci, chlamydia, or *M. hominis*, and upper and lower genital tract disease has developed in chimpanzees experimentally inoculated with *M. genitalium*.[308,434] Serologic studies also suggest that *M. genitalium* infection may be an independent risk factor in the pathogenesis of an inflammatory process that may lead to scarring of the uterine tissues, resulting in infertility.[67]

Besides the respiratory and genital tracts, *M. genitalium* has also been recovered from joint fluid aspirates of patients with arthritis. In a report on two such cases, *M. genitalium* was detected by PCR analysis in the knee joint of a 25-year-old man with Reiter's syndrome and in the knee joint of a 58-year-old man with seronegative rheumatoid arthritis.[437] Both *M. pneumoniae* and *M. genitalium* were detected in a specimen of knee joint fluid from a patient with hypogammaglobulinemia, mycoplasma pneumonia, and polyarthritis following a bout of pneumonia.[456]

M. genitalium has also been associated with HIV infection, although not to the extent that other species, like *M. fermentans* and *M. penetrans,* have been. Montagnier and Blanchard detected *M. genitalium* by PCR in the blood of a patient with AIDS in 1993.[309] However, a 1996 search for the presence of six *Mycoplasma* species in peripheral blood mononuclear cells of 154 HIV-seropositive patients, 40 HIV-seronegative STD clinic patients, and 40 HIV-seronegative blood donors failed to detect *M. genitalium* by PCR in any of them.[233] Another search for mycoplasmas in the urine of 15 HIV-seropositive children conducted in 1999 found only a single specimen positive for *M. genitalium* in 1 of 9 HIV-infected children classified as having severe HIV disease.[176] *M. genitalium* was also detected by PCR in urethral and rectal specimens from homosexual men with and without NGNCU.[438]

Mycoplasma fermentans

M. fermentans is a fastidious human mycoplasma species that has been recognized as a tissue culture contaminant for many years.[464] The increased usage of human-derived lymphocytes and macrophages in immunologic and viral research was likely responsible for recognition of this agent as a tissue culture contaminant. *M. fermentans* has been detected by PCR in salivary samples of healthy individuals and has also been detected in the genitourinary and respiratory tracts of humans.[61,395] In a study conducted in London, a PCR assay was used to detect *M. fermentans* in throat swabs and urine specimens from healthy university students and from patients with congenital immunodeficiencies.[5] Of 45 students who submitted both throat and urine specimens, 12 (27%) students had *M. fermentans* present in at least one of their specimens. Among 19 patients with congenital immunodeficiencies, one throat swab specimen and three urine specimens were *M. fermentans* PCR-positive.

In 1986, interest in *M. fermentans* as a human pathogen was stimulated when Lo and coworkers at the AFIP and the National Institutes of Health (NIH) reported the isolation of a novel mycoplasma from Kaposi's sarcoma tissues of patients with AIDS.[255,265] This mycoplasma was given the provisional name *Mycoplasma incognitus*.[264] Using immunohistochemical techniques employing monoclonal antibodies against this new agent, Lo and coworkers detected *M. incognitus* antigens in thymus, liver, spleen, lymph nodes, and brain tissue of patients with AIDS, and in placental tissues delivered by pregnant women with AIDS.[258] The histopathology of the infected tissues showed a range of responses; in some tissues no histologic changes were observed, whereas in others fulminant necrosis with inflammation was noted. Intraperitoneal inoculation of four silver leaf monkeys with this agent resulted in a wasting syndrome and death within 7 to 9 months.[268,270] These same workers also reported on six patients, from six different geographic areas, who presented with an acute flulike illness and a syndrome of persistent fevers, lymphadenopathy, diarrhea, and multiple-organ failure, resulting in death within 1 to 7 weeks. Autopsies revealed fulminant necrosis of lymph node, lungs, liver, adrenal gland, heart, and brain tissues. Immunohistochemical techniques and electron microscopy revealed mycoplasmal antigens in the areas of necrosis, and a labeled, specific DNA probe detected the genetic material of the agent in the infected tissues.[257] None of these patients were infected with HIV-1 or HIV-2. Nucleic acid hybridization profiles, restriction endonuclease mapping, and antigenic analyses indicated that *M. incognitus* was not a new mycoplasma but a strain of *M. fermentans*, a fastidious, "nonpathogenic" mycoplasma found in the genital tract.[49,376,383]

The "incognitus" strain of *M. fermentans* was subsequently found to be associated with other pathology in patients with AIDS. Bauer and colleagues examined kidney tissues of 15 patients with AIDS with light-microscopic evidence of AIDS-associated nephropathy.[21] Tissues from these patients showed immunofluorescence reactions with *M. fermentans* incognitus strain-specific monoclonal antibodies in glomerular endothelial and epithelial cells, glomerular basement membranes, tubular epithelial cells and casts, and mononuclear interstitial cells. Mycoplasmal structures were also seen by immunoelectron microscopy in kidney tissues of these patients. Renal tissues from AIDS patients without renal involvement and from non-AIDS patients with and without nephropathy did not reveal any organisms on histopathologic examination.[21] Ainsworth and associates also reported a patient with HIV-associated nephropathy in whom *M. fermentans* was detected in renal tissues by PCR when nephropathy first became clinically apparent; 18 months later, as the patient's disease progressed and renal function deteriorated, PCR detected *M. fermentans* in the patient's urine, throat, and peripheral blood.[6] *M. fermentans* DNA was also detected in lymph node specimens from four of seven AIDS patients.[384] Lo and colleagues reported three non-AIDS patients in whom fulminant adult respiratory distress syndrome associated with *M. fermentans* developed; immunohistochemical and electron microscopic studies revealed the organisms in the patients' lungs and liver.[269] Disseminated *M. fermentans* infection has also been documented in HIV-positive patients with non-Hodgkin's lymphoma.[3]

Others also reported on the association of the *M. fermentans* incognitus strain with ultimately fatal disease in non-AIDS patients. Macon and colleagues described a 35-year-old homosexual man with Kaposi's sarcoma and T-cell lymphoma with a peripheral CD4 cell count of 43 per cubic millimeter.[277] Fatal pneumocystis pneumonia and disseminated cryptococcal infection subsequently developed. Multiple enzyme immunoassays and Western immunoblots for HIV-1, HIV-2, human T-cell lymphotropic virus (HTLV)-I, and HTLV-II antibodies were negative, as were retroviral cultures and PCR studies. Systemic *M. fermentans* infection was documented by immunohistochemical and PCR methods in premortem and postmortem tissue specimens. Beecham and coworkers reported a similar case in a previously healthy 28-year-old nonimmunocompromised man who presented with a 7-day history of fever, abdominal pain, diarrhea, rash, and shortness of breath. *M. fermentans* was detected in bone marrow biopsy specimens by PCR and electron microscopy.[25] In another report of a previously healthy HIV-seronegative man with AIDS-like symptoms of fever, malaise, weight loss, diarrhea, and extensive liver and spleen necrosis, treatment with doxycycline (300 mg/day, orally for 6 weeks) resulted in resolution of the patient's symptoms and full recovery.[256] These studies suggested that *M. fermentans*, or a specific strain of this species, may be a systemic pathogen in non-HIV-infected patients.

The application of molecular methods to detection of *M. fermentans* has resulted in several reports documenting the presence of this organism in various body sites of both HIV-positive and HIV-negative individuals. Although cultural isolation of *M. fermentans* is quite difficult, it has been attempted in some studies. Using PCR technology, Dawson and associates detected *M. fermentans* in 23% of 43 urine sediment specimens from patients with AIDS-associated nephropathy.[82] Three urine specimens from two patients were culture-positive for *M. fermentans* in modified SP-4, A-7, and Hayflick's media. Among these same patients, four cultures grew *U. urealyticum* and two grew *M. hominis*. None of 50 urine sediment specimens from 50 HIV-negative, healthy patients was culture- or PCR-positive for *M. fermentans*, although 23 specimens grew *U. urealyticum* and one specimen grew *M. hominis*. Katseni and coworkers examined blood, throat, and urine specimens from 117 HIV-positive patients, 114 of whom were homosexual men, and from 73 HIV-seronegative patients attending an STD clinic in London.[208] *M. fermentans* was detected by PCR in 10% of 117 peripheral blood mononuclear specimens, 23% of 65 throat specimens, and 8% of 55 urine specimens from the HIV-positive subjects. Among the 73 HIV-seronegative patients, *M. fermentans* was detected in peripheral blood mononuclear cells, throat, and urine specimens of 9%, 20%, and 6%, respectively. Hawkins and colleagues at the NIH detected *M. fermentans* DNA sequences in 11% of blood specimens from 55 HIV-seropositive patients but detected none in 26 HIV-seronegative, low-risk individuals.[152] In France, Bebear and coworkers performed culture and PCR on throat, endocervical, urethral, urine, and peripheral blood mononuclear cell specimens from 105 HIV-positive individuals.[22] Although culture and PCR assays for *M. pneumoniae* and *M. geni-*

talium were negative, *M. fermentans* was detected by PCR in a least one specimen site in 26.7% of the 105 patients. The presence of *M. fermentans* in these patients was not associated with the stage of HIV disease, the viral load, or the CD4 count.

M. fermentans is able to actively invade cultured cells, a property not previously associated with *Mycoplasma* species. Although an *M. fermentans* reference strain and the incognitus strain were able to invade HeLa cells, *M. fermentans* incognitus strains were more invasive when tested in tracheal explant cell cultures. Incognitus strain organisms could be observed intracellularly, whereas the reference strain was observed only between and adherent to cells.[408,441] Intranasal infection of rats and subsequent explant culture of the tracheal tissues of these animals also revealed intracellular localization of the organisms within the cultured cells.[408] *M. fermentans* incognitus strain and the other *M. fermentans* strains cause ciliostasis and cytopathology in tracheal explant cultures, but the extent and severity of the cytopathology varied considerably from strain to strain. Studies in animals also indicated that immunosuppression may allow *M. fermentans* to grow and flourish. Intravenous administration of *M. fermentans* incognitus strain killed BALB/c nude mice but did not kill immunocompetent BALB/c mice.[432]

Although some investigators have noted differences between the *M. fermentans* incognitus strain and other *M. fermentans* strains, others have noted no differences. Sasaki and coworkers compared the original incognitus strain with three other reference and clinical isolates of *M. fermentans*.[383] Restriction-fragment-length polymorphism analysis of the DNA from these strains showed similar patterns on gel and immunoblot profiles of cellular proteins, indicating a high degree of antigenic homogeneity among the four strains examined. Exposure of peripheral blood mononuclear cells (PBMCs) to these mycoplasmas resulted in significant increases in the production of IL-1β, IL-6, and TNF-α; these increases were observed after exposure to all four *M. fermentans* strains and were not restricted to the incognitus strain alone. Lastly, exposure of HIV-infected PBMCs to any of the *M. fermentans* strains resulted in a 1.8- to 4.3-fold enhancement of reverse transcriptase activity and a 3.3- to 7.0-fold increase in the production of p24 antigen in the culture. These workers concluded that the incognitus strain of *M. fermentans* was not unique when compared with other *M. fermentans* strains.[383]

Several investigators are currently examining the role of *M. fermentans* and other mycoplasmas as cofactors affecting progression of HIV-associated disease.[4,168] *In vitro* studies on HIV-infected CEM cells (a CD4-enriched T-lymphoblastoid tumor cell line) showed that treatment of the cells with tetracycline analogues or fluoroquinolones was able to inhibit the production of virus-induced cytopathic effects without inhibiting the replication and production of progeny virus.[243,324] Subsequent studies have indeed shown that *M. fermentans* acts synergistically with HIV-1 in lymphoblastoid and promonocytic cells to produce cell death; this ability has also been demonstrated to occur with other *Mycoplasma* species, including *M. penetrans*, *M. pirum*, and *M. arginini*.[244,266] Phillips and associates showed that mycoplasmal attachment to HIV-infected lymphocytes was associated

with sites of viral budding, leading these investigators to surmise that attachment of mycoplasmas may trigger or enhance production of progeny virus by infected cells.[345]

Several mechanisms have been proposed whereby mycoplasmas such as *M. fermentans* may act as cofactors or immunomodulators in the production of HIV-associated disease.[309] Lymphocyte activation stimulates the replication of HIV, and *Mycoplasma* species, including *M. fermentans* and *M. penetrans*, have the capacity to behave as polyclonal activators of both B and T lymphocytes.[117,180,416] *M. fermentans* is able to induce the production of lymphokines (i.e., TNF-α, IL-1, and IL-6) in various cell types (i.e., monocytes, macrophages, astrocytes, and glial cells) in vitro.[123,313,314] Muhlradt and Frisch isolated and partially purified a substance, which they termed MDHM (mycoplasma-derived high-molecular-weight material), that was membrane-associated, contained lipid, and existed in an aggregated form when purified.[312] The presence of MDHM in nanogram-per-milliliter amounts activates macrophages to release nitric oxide, IL-6, and TNF. Another group identified a 48-kDa, hydrophobic, membrane-associated *M. fermentans* antigen, distinct from MDHM, that also stimulates the secretion of both TNF and IL-1 from cultured monocytes.[229] *M. fermentans* may also produce superantigens that bind directly to the major histocompatibility complex (MHC) proteins, thereby stimulating T-lymphocyte activation. Another *M. fermentans*–derived lipoprotein called MALP-2 (macrophage-activating lipopeptide 2) has also been shown to induce the release of proinflammatory cytokines, chemokines, and nitric oxide by mouse peritoneal macrophages.[209] *M. fermentans* also enhances concanavalin A–induced apoptosis of T cells.[397] Some investigators have proposed that the production of peroxides and free radicals by mycoplasmas or the production of enzymes that inactivate the normal intracellular catalase may induce HIV gene expression and activate viral replication. Peroxides and other reactive oxygen species induce HIV gene expression *in vitro* by *trans*-activation of viral promoter regions and contribute to programmed cell death.[241] *M. fermentans* incognitus strain is able to fuse with both T cells and peripheral blood lymphocytes.[98] The delivery of mycoplasmal components into these cells may directly affect normal lymphocyte functions. In addition, the fusion of mycoplasmal and lymphocyte membranes may significantly change the structure or orientation of various receptors on the lymphocyte surface, thereby altering the binding, induction, or production of various lymphokines. These fundamental alterations in lymphocyte structure and function may influence attachment, integration, and gene expression of HIV. Both *M. fermentans* and *M. penetrans* also possess membrane-associated phospholipase C, which can induce an inflammatory response, cause membrane damage to host cells, and activate the arachidonic acid cascade.[396]

M. fermentans may also play a role in genital tract infection. In 1989, *M. fermentans* was detected in the placental tissues of two women with AIDS.[258] Blanchard and coworkers used culture and PCR methods to examine the presence of both *M. genitalium* and *M. fermentans* in the genital tracts of sexually active adults and in the amniotic fluids of women with intact fetal membrane who were undergoing cesarean deliveries.[32] *M. genitalium* was detected by PCR, but not by culture, in 11% of 94 men and 87 women with clinical symptoms of nongonococcal urethritis or cervicitis and was not detected by either method in any of 232 amniotic fluid specimens. On the other hand, *M. fermentans* was not detected by either method in any of the urogenital specimens but was detected by PCR in four of the 232 amniotic fluid specimens, suggesting that the organism may be transmitted transplacentally. Interestingly, two of the four patients with positive *M. fermentans* PCR results had histologic evidence of chorioamnionitis, implying that *M. fermentans* may also be a genital tract pathogen.[32]

M. fermentans is also a cause of some cases of rheumatoid arthritis and other rheumatic disorders.[167,199] In a 1996 study conducted in London, *M. fermentans* was detected by PCR in synovial fluid specimens from 21% of 38 patients with rheumatoid arthritis, 20% of 10 patients with spondyloarthropathy, 20% of 5 patients with psoriatic arthritis, and 13% of 31 patients with unclassified arthritic condtions.[388] Genotypic characterization of isolates from synovia of patients with arthritis revealed no unique characteristics; some were related to the *M. fermentans* American Type Culture Collection (ATCC) type strain, while others were related to strains isolated from tissue cultures as contaminants.[387] *M. fermentans*, *M. salivarium*, or both were detected by PCR in synovial fluid specimens from the temporomandibular joint of patients with destructive osteoarthritis of the jaw.[489] This condition is thought to result from the action of proteases and cytokines on the articular cartilage of the mandibular joint. Watanabe and coworkers suggested that mycoplasmas present in the mandibular joints damage the synovium and cartilage by their enzymatic activities plus the recognized ability of mycoplasmas to stimulate release of cytokines from immune effector cells.[489] In a 2000 study, *M. fermentans* was detected by PCR in the synovial fluid of 88% of 26 rheumatoid arthritis patients. Seven of eight patients with a variety of other inflammatory arthritides were also positive for *M. fermentans*.[167] Finally, a study published in 2001 also found *M. fermentans* DNA in synovial fluids of 17% of 35 patients with rheumatoid arthritis, 25% of 44 patients with undifferentiated seronegative arthritis, and 17% of 24 patients with psoriatic arthritis.[130]

M. fermentans infection has been investigated for its relationship to chronic fatigue syndrome. Using PCR-based assays for *M. fermentans*, *M. hominis*, and *M. penetrans*, Choppa and colleagues examined PBMCs from 100 patients with chronic fatigue syndrome (CFS).[63] *M. fermentans*, *M. hominis*, and *M. penetrans* were detected in the PBMCs of 32%, 9%, and 6% of the 100 patients with CFS, respectively, whereas they were detected in 8%, 3%, and 2% of healthy controls, respectively. A subsequent study by the same research group detected *M. fermentans* in PBMCs of 36% of 50 patients with typical CFS as defined by the Centers for Disease Control and Prevention (CDC), 32% of 50 patients with atypical CFS, and in 8% of 50 healthy control subjects.[470] Nasralla, Haier, and Nicolson used PCR methods to detect *M. fermentans*, *M, pneumoniae*, *M. penetrans*, and *M. hominis* in blood specimens of 91 patients with CFS and/or fibromyalgia syndromes.[317] Among the 91 subjects, 59%, 48%, 31%, and 20% were positive for *M. pneumoniae*, *M. fermentans*, *M. hominis*, and *M. penetrans*, respectively. Of the 91 subjects, 53% had molecular evidence of bloodstream

infection with multiple *Mycoplasma* species. In a survey of 261 patients with CFS and 36 healthy volunteers, bloodstream infection by at least one *Mycoplasma* species was detected by a forensic PCR test in 68.6% of the patients with CFS and in 5.6% of healthy volunteers.[323] *M. hominis* was detected in 36.8%, followed by *M. fermentans* and *M. pneumoniae* in 25.7% and 25.7%, respectively. Infection with multiple *Mycoplasma* species was detected in 17% of the patients with CFS. Although these studies show that high rates of infection with *Mycoplasma* species are found in patients with CFS, there is no evidence that these mycoplasmas are the causative agents of CFS. The development of sensitive assays and improvements in culture techniques for these organisms will hopefully enable natural history and treatment studies to be undertaken.

M. fermentans was also postulated to play a role in the illness observed among veterans of Operation Desert Storm. A serologic survey study was conducted among Persian Gulf War veterans and nondeployed servicemen using both prewar and postwar serum specimens. *M. fermentans* infections were documented to have occurred in this military population both before and after service in the war, but these infections were independent of deployment to the Persian Gulf, indicating that epidemiologic and serologic data did not support a role for *M. fermentans* in the illness seen in Gulf War vetereans.[139] A similar study conducted by the Armed Forces Institute of Pathology (AFIP) also concluded that there was no serologic evidence for an association between *M. fermentans* infection and the "Gulf War illness."[263]

Even with its relatively short but fascinating epidemiologic history and the intensity of investigations by several research groups, the role of *M. fermentans* in HIV pathogenesis, sexually transmitted diseases, rheumatoid arthritis, chronic fatigue syndrome, and other conditions is not known. Although molecular methods facilitate the detection of specific gene sequences of the organisms, the lack of reliable culture techniques complicates studies that may include various treatment methods. *M. fermentans* has been recovered in culture from joint fluid specimens, but it is often not known whether molecular assays are detecting viable or nonviable organisms. Molecular studies have shown that *M. fermentans* is genotypically heterogeneous, as evidenced by the presence of insertion sequence-like elements at various locations in the DNA, resulting in interstrain and intrastrain variation.[349] In studies in which the organism has been successfully grown in SP-4 medium, biochemical testing has delineated four phenotypic clusters based on the utilization of arginine, glucose, fructose, and *N*-acetyl-glucosamine.[332] Systematic phenotypic and genotypic analysis of *M. fermentans* isolates from a variety of clinical specimens and conditions may help to define the pathogenicity and pathogenesis of *M. fermentans* infections and the role this organism plays in various clinical settings.

Mycoplasma penetrans

In 1991, Lo and colleagues at the AFIP in Washington, D.C., reported the isolation of a new *Mycoplasma* species from the urogenital tracts of homosexual men with HIV infection.[261] This organism exhibited unique morphologic characteristics, including a flask-shaped cell body composed of two compartments: one containing loosely packed, coarse granules consistent with ribosomal structures, and the other a tapered, smaller compartment containing densely packed fine granules.[260] This organism fermented glucose, hydrolyzed arginine but not urea, required cholesterol for growth, and could be cultivated in SP-4 medium. It was also able to adhere to and actively invade mammalian cells.[259] Intracellular organisms were observed to be inside membrane-bound vesicles, with subsequent cell disruption and necrosis. This new species was given the name *Mycoplasma penetrans*.[260,385]

Seroepidemiologic studies have documented a high frequency of antibodies against *M. penetrans* in HIV-infected individuals.[87,135,461,485] Wang and associates found that 35.4% of serum samples from 444 HIV-1-infected patients were positive for antibodies against *M. penetrans*.[485] Among 234 men with AIDS, 41.5% were seropositive; 20.3% of 118 asymptomatic, HIV-1-infected individuals were also seropositive. Only one of 384 HIV-negative blood donors had antibodies against *M. penetrans*. Interestingly, 40% of 85 serum samples archived from patients with ''GRID'' (gay-related immunodeficiency), a term used in the early 1980s to describe AIDS, were also positive for anti–*M. penetrans* antibodies. Among 336 serum specimens from STD clinics in southern California, Brooklyn, and Milwaukee, only three were positive for *M. penetrans* antibodies. None of the 178 serum specimens obtained from HIV-1-seronegative individuals with other diseases or immunologic disorders (e.g., patients on dialysis, or patients with systemic lupus erythematosus, rheumatoid arthritis, multiple sclerosis, leukemia, lymphoma or other cancers) was positive for antibodies against *M. penetrans*.[485] Additional seroepidemiologic studies by the same research group found high rates of mycoplasmal antibodies in both symptomatic and asymptomatic HIV-1-positive homosexual men but only 1% of 308 specimens from intravenous drug users and only 0.6% of 165 specimens from patients with hemophilia with or without HIV-1 infection, suggesting that *M. penetrans* may be sexually transmitted.[486] Grau and coauthors reported very similar findings on the presence of *M. penetrans* antibodies in a study conducted in France.[135] These workers found that positive *M. penetrans* serology was associated with both HIV-1 infection and with high-risk sexual practices among homosexual men and that the seroprevalence increased with progression of AIDS-related disease. During the early 1990s, some researchers reported an epidemiologic relationship between the presence of *M. penetrans* antibodies and the development of Kaposi's sarcoma (KS). Lo and colleagues examined *M. penetrans* seroprevalence in a cohort of 33 HIV-seropositive and 31 HIV-seronegative homosexual men who were enrolled in an AIDS natural history study in New York City in 1984.[262] Testing of archived serum specimens from 1984 to 1985 revealed that 45.5% of the HIV-positive men and 22.5% of the HIV-negative men had antibodies against *M. penetrans*, suggesting that *M. penetrans* was circulating as a probable sexually transmissible agent early in the AIDS epidemic and was not necessarily associated with HIV infection. Over the subsequent 8 years, Kaposi's sarcoma (KS) developed in nine men; seven men were *M. penetrans* antibody-positive and two were *M. penetrans* antibody-negative. Baseline seropositivity to *M. penetrans* was statistically as-

sociated with the subsequent development of KS, and, among the HIV-positive men, KS was more likely to occur among men who had positive baseline serologies for *M. penetrans*. These workers concluded that *M. penetrans* infection may act as a cofactor with HIV in the subsequent development of KS.[262,486] However, others have found no association between *M. penetrans* infection and Kaposi's sarcoma, which is now known to be associated with human herpesvirus type 8 infection.[135]

The use of sensitive molecular techniques for direct detection of *M. penetrans* has shown that this organism may be involved in chronic infections of cells and/or tissues other than blood mononuclear cells. Kovacic and colleagues used specific PCR assays for *M. pneumoniae*, *M. fermentans*, *M. genitalium*, *M. pirum*, *M. penetrans*, and *M. hominis* to investigate the presence of these organisms in peripheral blood mononuclear cells from subjects infected or not infected with HIV-1.[233] Only *M. fermentans* was detected in 5.8% of 154 HIV-seropositive and 11.1% of HIV-seronegative patients. These investigators suggested that the urogenital tract is the probable ecologic niche of this organism, since it was originally isolated from urine specimens and has been detected by PCR in urine specimens from patients who are seropositive for *M. penetrans* antibodies.[135,260,261] *M. penetrans* bacteremia has also been reported in non-HIV-infected patients with antiphospholipid syndrome.[500]

The exact role of *M. penetrans* in the pathogenesis of HIV infection is not known. Most work has centered on its putative role as a cofactor in HIV-associated disease progression. Sasaki and colleagues at the Institut Pasteur demonstrated that *M. penetrans* was able to activate human T lymphocytes to undergo blastogenesis followed by cell proliferation and expression of cell surface markers of activation.[382] These phenomena were observed with lymphocytes from healthy donors and from both symptomatic and asymptomatic HIV-infected patients. Characterization of the lymphocytes activated by exposure to *M. penetrans* showed that lymphocytes expressing either CD4 or CD8 underwent blastogenesis as a result of this expression. Activation activity was associated exclusively with cells of *M. penetrans* and not with culture supernatants. In cultured lymphoid cells, infection with M. penetrans stimulates the release of TNF-α and enhances replication of coinfecting HIV-1.[180] Longitudinal serologic studies have also demonstrated higher HIV viral loads and more rapid declines in CD4 cell counts in patients with persistently high or increasing anti–*M. penetrans* antibody titers, suggesting an association between active *M. penetrans* infection and progression of HIV disease.[136]

Mycoplasma pirum

Although originally described in 1985, *M. pirum* has attracted some attention recently because it is another of the AIDS-associated mycoplasmas, along with *M. fermentans* and *M. penetrans*. Before this association, *M. pirum* had been isolated only from cell cultures as a presumed contaminant, but the cell lines from which it was isolated were of human origin; it is now thought that these mycoplasmas may have been in the cultured tissues naturally.[96] *M. pirum* has been isolated from peripheral blood mononuclear cells of a patient with HIV infection and has been detected by PCR in blood mononuclear cells of HIV-seropositive individuals.[133] Similar to *M. fermentans*, HIV-associated cytopathic effects *in vitro* are also enhanced by the presence of *M. pirum*, leading to the suggestion that, similar to *M. fermentans*, *M. pirum* may act as a cofactor in the pathogenesis of HIV-related conditions.[309]

M. pirum is closely related to *M. penetrans* and *M. pneumoniae* and, similar to these two other mycoplasmas, has a flask-shaped morphology and a "tip" by which the organism is able to attach to glass or plastic. The P1-like adhesin protein of *M. pirum* and the gene coding for it have been characterized.[447] Following attachment, *M. pirum*, as do *M. fermentans* and *M. penetrans*, is able to actively invade cells.[430] Research is underway to further define the interaction of *M. pirum* and other mycoplasmas with human cells and to investigate the role of these organisms, if any, in the pathogenesis of HIV-associated disease.

Mycoplasma primatum

M. primatum is a common inhabitant of the oral and urogenital tracts of cercopithecine monkeys, and was first isolated from these animals in 1971.[95] The strains isolated from monkey tissues in 1971 were found to be similar to unclassified mycoplasmas that had been isolated from an infected umbilicus and from the vagina of a human patient in 1955.[374] Reexamination of the monkey isolates and the unclassified human isolates found them to be all the same. This mycoplasma used arginine, required serum or cholesterol for growth, and was negative for glucose fermentation, urease, hemolysis, hemadsorption activity, and tetrazolium reduction. These human/primate isolates were given the name *M. primatum*. To date, this mycoplasma has not been associated with infections or clinical disease.

Mycoplasma spermatophilum

M. spermatophilum is a newly described anaerobic *Mycoplasma* species that has been isolated from five sperm specimens and from a single endocervical specimen obtained from six patients who were attending an infertility clinic.[159] In culture, this obligate anaerobic species grows best at 35 to 37°C and produces a hemolysin that lyses guinea pig, sheep, and human erythrocytes. Colonies have the typical fried-egg appearance on agar media. This species requires sterols for growth and does not use glucose or hydrolyze either arginine or urea; it is not yet thought to be a pathogen.

Human Infections Due to Mycoplasmas of Animal Origin

M. arginini is one of the few mycoplasmas found in a number of animal hosts, including sheep and goats (respiratory and ocular tissues), cattle (respiratory tract, blood, udder, eyes, urogenital tract), and felines (respiratory tract). These animals may or may not exhibit pathologic symptoms, and the role of this organism in animal diseases is still unknown. Yechouran and colleagues reported a case of pneumonia complicated by fatal septicemia caused by *M. arginini* in a 64-year-old man with stage IVB non-Hodgkin's lym-

phoma, who had hypogammaglobulinemia and had been receiving prednisone.[502] Before his admission to the hospital, the patient had worked in a slaughterhouse, where he slaughtered sheep, cows, and chickens. *M. arginini* grew from three blood cultures: a bronchial brush specimen, a bronchoalveolar lavage specimen, and a Swan-Ganz catheter tip. Susceptibility testing of the isolate using a broth dilution procedure found that it was susceptible to tetracycline, doxycycline, and ciprofloxacin and resistant to erythromycin and streptomycin. This susceptibility pattern has also been found in *M. arginini* isolates recovered from animals. The authors of this case report suggested that the patient acquired his infection by inhalation of contaminated aerosols in the slaughterhouse setting.

Armstrong and colleagues reported a case of pulmonary infection caused by *M. canis* in a female patient who was receiving antineoplastic therapy for metastatic carcinoma of the cervix.[14] The same organism was isolated from the respiratory tract of other family members and from the family dog, all of whom had upper respiratory tract infections at the same time. Bonilla and colleagues also reported a case of septic arthritis of the left hip and right knee due to *M. canis* in a woman with common variable immunodeficiency.[40] The patient had a history of exposure to cats. Despite surgical debridement and treatment with doxycycline, widespread chronic osteomyelitis of the hip was noted, necessitating hip arthroplasty.

Hemotrophic *Mycoplasma* Species

Haemobartonella and *Eperythrozoon* species are mycoplasma-like bacteria that adhere to and grow on the surfaces of red blood cells of several vertebrate species.[237] Until recently, these organisms were classified in the Order Rickettsiales, since they resemble the rickettsias with respect to their size, staining properties, tropism for erythrocytes, and transmission from animal to animal by arthropod vectors. On the red blood cell surface, these bacteria appear as small, blue-to-purple, coccoid, rod- or ring-shaped structures when stained by the Wright-Giemsa method or by acridine orange.[36] Phenotypically *Eperythrozoon* species form ring-shaped structures on the surface of red cells and often may appear unattached to red cells and free in the plasma. *Haemobartonella* species, on the other hand, do not form ring-shaped structures and are rarely seen in the free unattached state. The arbitrariness of the phenotypic differentiation of these two species has been recognized for some time and has led to their recent reclassification (see below). These bacteria are noncultivable in bacteriologic media and are maintained in research laboratories by serial passage in their animal hosts. Infections in animals caused by *Eperythrozoon* and *Haemobartonella* species are usually asymptomatic and may persist in a latent form for years, and it is thought that the organisms are cleared from the circulation by the spleen.[280] Because of predisposing factors that are not completely understood (i.e., stress etc.), large numbers of organisms may reappear in the bloodstream. In some animals a subtle, chronic anemia develops or an overt, severe, and often fatal hemolytic anemia may develop.[301,302] For example, the well-studied feline hemotrophic mycoplasmas ordinarily do not cause disease in naturally infected animals, but may cause anemia in feline leukemia virus (FeLV)–infected cats and may accelerate the development of FeLV-induced myeloproliferative diseases.[421] Hemotrophic mycoplasmas are transmitted from animal to animal by various blood-feeding arthropods, including lice, ticks, flies, fleas, and mosquitoes.

As they were discovered, the various species of *Haemobartonella* and *Eperythrozoon* were named after the host that they primarily infected, although the host ranges of the various species were really not known. As of the mid-1990s, the recognized species of *Haemobartonella* and *Eperythrozoon* were *H. canis* (canines), *H. felis* (cats), *H. muris* (rodents), *E. coccoides* (mice), *E. ovis* (sheep), *E. suis* (swine), *E. parvum* (pigs), and *E. wenyonii* (cattle). In 1997, the 16S rRNA gene sequences of *H. felis*, *H. muris*, *E. suis*, and *E. wenyonii* were investigated, and it was demonstrated that these bacteria were not phylogenetically related to the rickettsiae but were most closely related to members of the genus *Mycoplasma*.[321,364] In 2001, these four species organisms were removed from the Order Rickettsiales, Family Anaplasmatales, and were given "candidatus" status in the genus *Mycoplasma* as "*Candidatus* Mycoplasma hemofelis," "*Candidatus* Mycoplasma haemomuris," "*Candidatus* Mycoplasma haemosuis," and "*Candidatus* Mycoplasma wenyonii."[198,319,424] "Candidatus" status is usually reserved for new, incompletely described taxa. Because of this, the Judicial Commission of the International Committee on the Systematics of the Prokaryotes ruled that, by changing validly published organism names to the taxonomically demoted "candidatus" status, the original names would lose standing because there would be no new or replacement names to add to the Approved List of Bacterial Names. As a result, all the species that had been renamed under "candidatus" status were revised by eliminating the "candidatus" status and renaming them as new species in the genus *Mycoplasma*.[320] At the same time this opinion was published, three additional "candidatus" species—"candidatus Mycoplasma haemodidelphidis," "candidatus Mycoplasma haemolamae," and "candidatus Mycoplasma haemominutum"—were described as hemotrophic bacteria from naturally infected opossums, alpacas, and cats, respectively.[303] As a result, the former *Eperythrozoon* and *Haemobartonella* species are now classified in the genus *Mycoplasma* as *M. hemofelis* (cats), *M. haemomuris* (mice), *M. haemosuis* (pigs), *M. wenyonii* (cattle), *M. ovis* (sheep and goats), *M. haemolamae* (lamas), *M. haemocanis* (canines), *M. haemodidelphidis* (opossums), and "candidatus *M. haemominutum*."[318,319,425] Together, these hemophilic mycoplasma have been given the trivial name "hemoplasmas."

Culture of Human Mycoplasmas From Clinical Specimens
General Considerations

Human mycoplasmas can be divided into three groups on the basis of the utilization of three substrates: glucose, arginine, and urea (see Table 18-1). Depending on the species of mycoplasma that is being sought, an enriched peptone basal medium, containing yeast extract and serum, is supplemented with one of these three substrates and a pH indicator

(usually phenol red) is added. *M. pneumoniae* metabolizes glucose to produce lactic acid, resulting in a shift to an acidic pH. *M. hominis* metabolizes arginine with the production of ammonia and a shift in pH from neutral to alkaline. Similarly, *U. urealyticum* produces urease enzymes that hydrolyze urea to ammonia, again resulting in an alkaline pH shift. *M. fermentans* produces acid from glucose and also metabolizes arginine.

Specimens for the isolation of mycoplasmas, particularly the more rapidly growing genital mycoplasmas, are routinely inoculated onto both solid agar media and into some type of selective/differential broth enrichment media. Many broth media formulations used for isolation of mycoplasmas are diphasic, with medium containing agar in the butt of a tube overlaid with broth of similar composition but without added agar. Media for isolation of mycoplasmas also contain antibiotics (e.g., ampicillin, penicillin, polymyxin B, and amphotericin) to inhibit contaminant bacteria and fungi. Thallium acetate was formerly commonly included as an antibacterial agent in media as well, but this compound is inhibitory for *U. urealyticum* and *M. genitalium* and is also highly poisonous for humans.

Human mycoplasmas differ in their optimal pH for growth and in the atmospheric conditions that are required for successful recovery from clinical specimens (see Table 18-1). Media for the isolation of *M. pneumoniae* are buffered at an initial pH of about 7.8, whereas the growth medium for *M. hominis* is buffered initially at an neutral pH (7.0). *U. urealyticum* grows optimally in an environment with a slightly acid pH, so a primary isolation medium for this species is buffered at about pH 6.0. The optimal temperature for mycoplasmal growth is 35 to 37°C. *M. pneumoniae* and *M. hominis* grow well in air or in an atmosphere of 95% nitrogen and 5% carbon dioxide. *U. urealyticum* tends to be capnophilic, with optimal growth occurring in an atmosphere of 10–20% carbon dioxide and 80–90% nitrogen. An agar medium inoculated directly with specimens or subcultures from broths should be incubated under the appropriate conditions described in the foregoing; a broth medium can always be incubated under aerobic conditions.

Broth media are generally inoculated with 0.1 to 0.2 ml of the specimen contained in a transport fluid. Agar plates are inoculated with a similar amount, and the inoculum is spread over the surface of the agar with a sterile bent glass rod. Agar plates are sealed with air-permeable cellophane tape to prevent the agar from drying out. Media for isolation of *M. pneumoniae* should be incubated for up to 4 weeks before a final culture report is made. Cultures for genital mycoplasmas should be incubated for 7 to 8 days; most positive broth cultures will be detected after 5 days of incubation. Diphasic media are compared with coincubated tubes of the same media inoculated with sterile transport medium and with tubes inoculated with control mycoplasma strains to detect subtle differences in color or turbidity. Cultures should be inspected daily for subtle changes because the organisms die rapidly once growth occurs and the substrates are exhausted. If a potentially positive culture is detected visually in diphasic medium, the broth is subcultured onto a solid agar medium, such as SP-4 agar or A7 differential agar (see discussion below).

Identification of the mycoplasmas requires the recognition of typical colonies on solid media directly inoculated with the specimen or with a loopful of broth medium from a presumptively positive diphasic broth medium. Colonies on agar media can be directly examined under 30× to 100× magnification with peripherally incident light to ascertain morphology and growth characteristics. Supravital dyes, such as Diene's stain, can be used to further characterize colonies and to differentiate them from artifacts. Various identification tests may be performed directly on solid medium, such as the hemadsorption test for presumptive identification of *M. pneumoniae*, or substrates such as arginine or urea, plus a phenol red indicator, may be incorporated into the agar to provide a direct assessment of substrate utilization and, therefore, a presumptive identification. Media for culture of respiratory and genital mycoplasmas and identification procedures for *M. pneumoniae* and *U. urealyticum* are detailed in Charts 18-1, 18-2, 18-3, 18-4, 18-5, and 18-6.

Specimen Collection

M. pneumoniae may be recovered from both upper and lower respiratory tract specimens, including throat swabs, nasopharyngeal swabs, throat washings, sputum, tracheal and transtracheal aspirate, bronchoscopy, bronchoalveolar lavage, and lung tissue specimens. The organism may be recovered from these specimens throughout the course of the illness and for some time after symptomatic recovery. Because of the fastidious nature of these bacteria, culture media should be inoculated as soon after collection as possible. Culture media dispensed into small vials may be used for transport of swab specimens; other specimens (e.g., sputum, tissue, washings) may be transported to the laboratory in sterile screw-capped containers. Before inoculation of growth media, respiratory tract specimens should be homogenized by repeatedly drawing through a needle and syringe; sputolysin or other chemical treatments for sputum liquefaction are toxic to mycoplasmas.

Genital mycoplasmas may be isolated from a variety of specimens. These include urethral, vaginal, and cervical swab specimens; prostatic secretions, semen, urine, blood, miscellaneous body fluids (CSF, amniotic fluid, respiratory tract secretions, synovial fluid, pericardial fluid), and tissues (e.g., endometrial washings and biopsies, placental or amniotic tissues, fetal or abortus tissues, fallopian tube biopsies, uterine biopsies, wound biopsies, rectal tissues). Swab specimens should be obtained using Dacron, calcium alginate, or polyester swabs, with either plastic or aluminum shafts. Swabs with wooden shafts should not be used because the wood itself may be toxic to ureaplasmas. If other genital tract pathogens are being sought simultaneously, Rayon or Dacron swabs on plastic shafts are probably preferable because they are nontoxic to the other genital tract pathogens as well. Contact of the swab surfaces with antiseptic solutions, creams, jellies, or lubricants should be avoided. Swab specimens should not be allowed to dry and should be placed immediately into a transport or culture medium after collection. Other body fluids and tissue biopsy specimens should be submitted in sterile containers. Saline should not be used to moisten tissue specimens, for it may cause lysis of the organisms. In the laboratory, tissue specimens should be minced in sterile transport medium to produce a 10% (w/v)

suspension and serially diluted 10- and 100-fold. This is necessary to prevent inhibition of mycoplasmal growth by organic materials such as hemoglobin, toxic phospholipids, antibodies, or complement that may be present in the tissue specimen. These dilutions are then used to inoculate growth media.

Blood specimens can be cultured for mycoplasmas by inoculation of growth media at a ratio of one part blood to nine parts broth (1:10 dilution). Optimally, at least 10 ml of blood from adult patients should be cultured. Ideally, the growth medium should not contain sodium polyanethol sulfonate (SPS), which inhibits the growth of *Mycoplasma* species, but should be a medium specifically formulated for mycoplasmas (see below). As with *N. gonorrhoeae*, growth inhibition due to SPS can be overcome by adding sterile gelatin to the growth medium at a final concentration of 1% (wt/vol). Inoculated broth media should be subcultured blindly, since the automated, continuously monitored blood culture instruments are, for the most part, unable to detect growth of mycoplasmas.[472]

Transport Media

Mycoplasmas are very susceptible to adverse environmental conditions, so specimens should be placed into appropriate transport or growth media as soon after collection as possible. A variety of transport media may be used for genital mycoplasma cultures. These include trypticase-soy broth with 0.5% bovine serum albumin, 2SP broth (10% heat-inactivated fetal calf serum with 0.2 M sucrose in 0.02 M phosphate buffer, pH 7.2), or various types of mycoplasma growth media (e.g., SP-4, Shepard's 10B broth). Antibiotics and antifungal agents (penicillin, 100,000 U/ml; polymyxin B, 5,000 µg/ml; amphotericin B, 2 mg/ml, final concentrations) are generally added to decrease contamination by other bacterial and fungal organisms. Specimens should be transported to the laboratory immediately and may be held up to 24 hours at 4°C before inoculation of growth media. If culture is delayed beyond this time, the specimen should be frozen at −70°C. Prior to culture, these specimens should be thawed rapidly in a 37°C water bath. Urine specimens for culture should be centrifuged and the sediment diluted 1:1 with transport medium before freezing. The protein stabilizers in the transport medium prevent loss of organism viability that may occur if urine specimens are frozen without this protective measure.

Media for Culture of Mycoplasmas

Several types of media have been described in the literature for the cultivation of *M. pneumoniae* and the genital mycoplasmas.[471] As mentioned, most broth media are diphasic; that is, the tubes contain an agar phase that is overlaid with broth medium of similar composition. One medium recommended by the CDC for isolation of *M. pneumoniae* is methylene blue-glucose diphasic medium. This medium contains PPLO (pleuropneumonia-like organism) broth and agar, yeast extract, and serum supplements along with glucose, methylene blue, and phenol red. The methylene blue in the medium inhibits the growth of other human mycoplasmas that may be found in the respiratory tract, making the medium selective for *M. pneumoniae*. During growth of *M. pneumoniae*, the medium becomes more acidic and the phenol red turns color from salmon to yellow. At the same time, the organisms reduce the methylene blue and turn it from blue to colorless. Therefore, the color of the broth phase changes from purple to green or yellow-green, while the agar phase turns from a purple color to a yellow or yellow orange. This medium is used in conjunction with myco-plasma glucose agar medium. Colonies recovered either directly on this medium or from subcultures of positive broths are then subjected to inspection and identification procedures. The components and formulas for *M. pneumoniae* isolation medium are presented in Chart 18-4.

Another medium that is recommended for isolation of *M. pneumoniae* from clinical specimens is SP-4 broth and SP-4 agar containing glucose.[457] These media were originally formulated for the cultivation of spiraplasmas, but they also provide superior recovery of *M. pneumoniae* and other human mycoplasmas (e.g., *M. genitalium*). In a comparative study conducted by Tully and coworkers, diphasic SP-4 medium recovered *M. pneumoniae* from 69 of 200 specimens that were negative when cultured by other ''standard'' methods.[457] As with the methylene blue-glucose diphasic medium, growth is detected by the change of the phenol red indicator from red to yellow, indicating the production of acid from glucose. SP-4 agar and broth media can be used for isolation of *M. hominis* if the arginine is added instead of glucose.

Because *M. hominis* and *U. urealyticum* metabolize different substrates and differ in the pH for optimal growth, many laboratories use two types of agar medium for their cultivation. In addition, diphasic broth and agar formulations of each medium type should be inoculated for optimal recovery of mycoplasmas. H broth and H agar are used to isolate *M. hominis* and are buffered at a neutral pH (7.0). Some formulations may also contain arginine as the growth substrate, with both medium turbidity and a shift in the color of the phenol red indicator into the alkaline range being used to detect organism growth. U broth and U agar, used to isolate *U. urealyticum*, are buffered at a lower pH (5.5 to 6.0) and contain urea as the growth substrate. The latter media are also made more selective for *U. urealyticum* by the inclusion of lincomycin because ureaplasmas are resistant to this drug and *M. hominis* strains are susceptible. Medium formulations for isolation of genital mycoplasmas are found in Chart 18-5.

Several other media have been described in the literature for the isolation and identification of genital mycoplasmas. Broth media include the U-9 urease medium described by Shepard and Lunceford, bromthymol blue broth, S-2 Boston broth, and the SP-4 medium used for recovery of the respiratory tract mycoplasmas.[119,242,390,392,393,399,498] SP-4 medium should be supplemented with urea or arginine specifically to detect *U. urealyticum* and *M. hominis*, respectively. S-2 Boston broth is a single medium that contains enriched base medium, horse serum, yeast extract, phenol red indicator, L-cysteine, urea, and penicillin. Growth of *U. urealyticum* is detected by the appearance of a pink color in the medium, whereas growth of *M. hominis* is detected by a pale salmon-pink to orange color or by the appearance of slight turbidity.

Shepard's A7 differential agar medium and various modifications of it (e.g., A7B and A8) are particularly useful because both *M. hominis* and *U. urealyticum* grow well on them and can be easily differentiated from one another by colony morphology and by the direct detection of urease formation by the latter species (see discussion below).[390,392,393] As described below, presumptive identification of *M. hominis* and definitive identification of *U. urealyticum* can be attained with this medium, without the need for additional tests or reagents.

Isolation and Identification of *Mycoplasma pneumoniae*

In general, the growth of *M. pneumoniae* from clinical specimens is detected by the ability of these organisms to produce acid from glucose.[84] Methylene blue-glucose diphasic medium is inoculated with 0.2 mL of the specimen in transport fluid. Tubes of media are simultaneously inoculated with sterile transport medium and with a positive control culture and are incubated along with the specimens. Broth cultures are incubated at 35°C with the caps tightened. Tubes are inspected daily for color changes in the medium and for turbidity for 4 weeks. The development of gross turbidity and an acid or alkaline shift of the indicator within 1 to 5 days is generally due to bacterial contamination. A slight, gradual shift in the pH indicator over an 8- to 15-day period without gross turbidity suggests a true-positive culture. As soon as color changes in the medium are apparent, the broth must be subcultured to appropriate agar medium; as more acid accumulates in the medium, mycoplasmas rapidly become nonviable. At the earliest indication of growth, the broth is subcultured to agar medium (such as SP-4 agar) and incubated in air for 5 to 7 days. Inspection of the agar surface under the low power of the microscope will reveal small colonies of the organisms. In the absence of obvious color change in diphasic media, a blind subculture to agar media should be performed after 1 and 3 weeks of incubation. A general scheme for the isolation of *M. pneumoniae* is shown in Figure 18-1.

M. pneumoniae may be identified by a variety of procedures, some of which are more involved than others.[84] Tests that are easily adaptable to the clinical laboratory include the hemadsorption test (Chart 18-2) and the tetrazolium reduction test (Chart 18-6). In the hemadsorption procedure, colonies growing on the surface of the agar are flooded with a 0.2–0.4% suspension of washed guinea pig erythrocytes. After incubation, the surface of the plate is gently washed with sterile saline and examined under $50\times$ to $100\times$ magnification. Colonies of *M. pneumoniae* adsorb the erythrocytes to their surface and appear as round colonies studded with red blood cells (see Color Plate 18-1*A*). This procedure works best on colonies that are 5 to 7 days old; older colonies tend to lose their hemadsorbing properties. Other *Mycoplasma* species that inhabit the upper respiratory tract are negative in the hemadsorption test.

The tetrazolium reduction test exploits the unique ability of *M. pneumoniae* to reduce the colorless compound triphenyl tetrazolium to the red compound formazan. To perform the test, the agar surface bearing the suspected colonies is flooded with a solution of 2-(*p*-iodophenyl)-3-nitrophenyl-5-phenyl tetrazolium chloride (0.21%) and incubated at 35°C

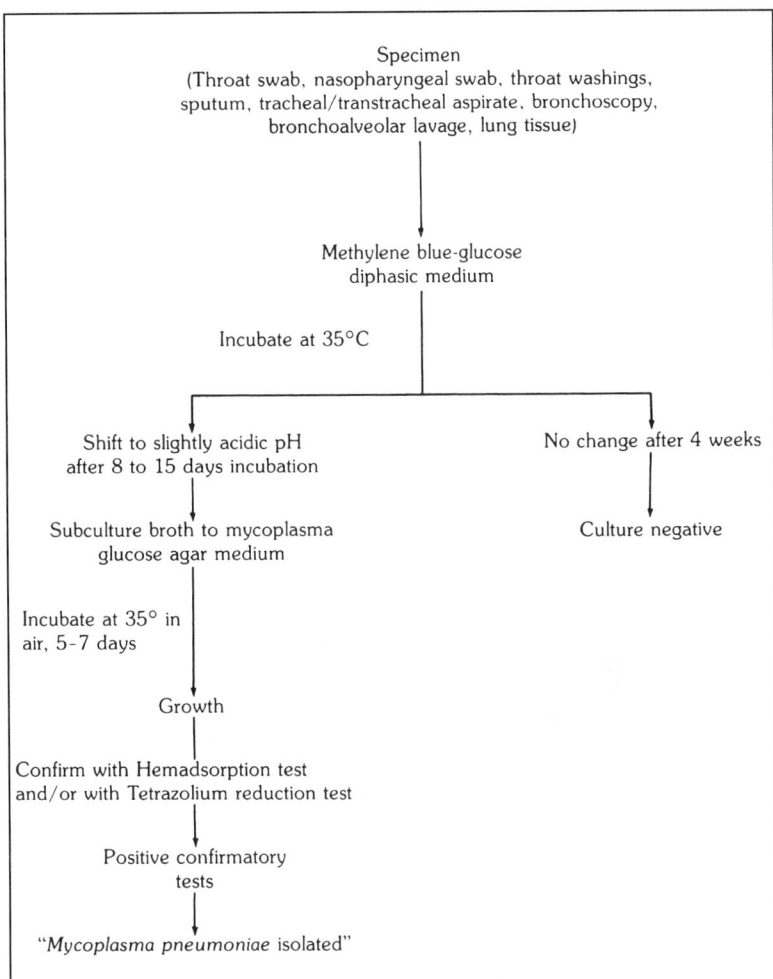

Specimen
(Throat swab, nasopharyngeal swab, throat washings, sputum, tracheal/transtracheal aspirate, bronchoscopy, bronchoalveolar lavage, lung tissue)

↓

Methylene blue-glucose diphasic medium

Incubate at 35°C

Shift to slightly acidic pH after 8 to 15 days incubation

No change after 4 weeks

Subculture broth to mycoplasma glucose agar medium

Culture negative

Incubate at 35° in air, 5-7 days

Growth

Confirm with Hemadsorption test and/or with Tetrazolium reduction test

Positive confirmatory tests

"*Mycoplasma pneumoniae* isolated"

Figure 18-1 Protocol for isolation of *mycoplasma pneumoniae* from respiratory tract specimens.

for 1 hour. Colonies of *M. pneumoniae* will appear reddish after 1 hour and may appear purple to black after 3 to 4 hours. Other mycoplasmas are negative with this test. The tetrazolium test can be performed even after the colonies are tested with the hemadsorption procedure.

Specific serologic methods may also be used for culture confirmation of *M. pneumoniae*. The more rapid of these is the epifluorescence procedure. Agar medium containing colonies is flooded with *M. pneumoniae*–specific antibodies conjugated to fluorescein isothiocyanate, washed to remove unbound conjugate, and subsequently examined with a microscope equipped for epifluorescence procedures. Colonies of *M. pneumoniae* will fluoresce. Although considered to be the reference procedure, the growth inhibition test for identification of *M. pneumoniae* is also the most time-consuming procedure. In this test, an agar plate is inoculated as a lawn from a broth suspension of the isolate to be identified. A piece of filter paper impregnated with anti–*M. pneumoniae* antibodies is then placed on the agar surface. After incubation, inhibition of colonial growth will be observed surrounding the filter paper that is saturated with the species-specific antibodies.

Other technologies have also been applied to the diagnosis of *M. pneumoniae* respiratory tract infections. Cimolai and associates described a novel culture-amplification technique similar to the shell vial methods currently used in virology.[66] Conventional agar and broth cultures were set up in duplicate. During each day of incubation, aliquots from one set of broth specimens were tested by an immunoblot technique using a monoclonal antigen-capture antibody directed against the 43-kDa membrane-associated adhesin of *M. pneumoniae*. The immunoblot method detected positive cultures in from 2 to 12 days (mean, 4.7), whereas conventional cultures were visibly positive in 7 to 14 days (mean, 8.3).

Noncultural Detection of *Mycoplasma pneumoniae*

Because of the slow growth of *M. pneumoniae*, non-growth-dependent, direct detection methods were developed and included antigen capture assays, direct immunofluorescence, immunoblot analysis, and nucleic acid probe methods.[224,272] In general, many of these tests lack sufficient sensitivity to be clinically useful. Marmion and colleagues described an antigen-capture enzyme immunoassay (EIA) using polyclonal antibodies directed against purified P1 antigen as the capture antibody.[283] In a study of respiratory tract specimens from 234 patients, the antigen test detected four of four patients who were positive by culture and serology and four of five patients who were positive by culture only.

Interestingly, 43% of 23 patients who were culture-negative but seropositive and 71% of patients who had a diagnostic rise in antibody titer and had no culture done were positive on the antigen EIA. These findings indicated that the antigen test and probably other direct tests need to be confirmed by an assessment of the serologic antibody response to verify that the infection diagnosed by the direct test is a current infection and not the result of prolonged or continuing carriage of the organism from a previous infection.[283] Assays for direct antigen detection have been largely replaced by molecular techniques.

Prior to the development of amplification-based methods, a direct, radiolabeled DNA probe was developed for the diagnosis of mycoplasmal respiratory tract infections. The *M. pneumoniae* DNA probe (Gen-Probe, San Diego CA) hybridized with the 16S rRNA of the organism and used a ^{125}I radioactive label to generate a detection signal. Tilton and coworkers compared the DNA probe with culture and found that the probe had a sensitivity of 100% and a specificity of 98% when compared with culture.[450] Dular and associates reported that the probe had both a sensitivity and a specificity of 89% compared with culture.[106] In both reports, the authors stressed the practical aspects of the probe as a rapid, sensitive, and timely approach to diagnosis because probe results are available in about 2 hours, whereas culture requires several weeks. In addition, the rapid diagnosis provided by the probe would eliminate the reliance on retrospective serologic testing (e.g., complement fixation) or nonspecific serologic markers (i.e., cold agglutinins) for diagnosis and would enable specific antimicrobial therapy to be initiated. The drawbacks of the probe included its relatively short 6-week shelf life, the need for additional equipment, the generation and disposal of radioactive wastes, and its expense. In addition, because the organisms may be harbored in the respiratory tract during convalescence, positive probe tests may be found in respiratory swab specimens collected from healthy individuals. The Gen-Probe test was withdrawn from the market in 1992.

Several molecular methods, including nested and seminested PCR, multiplex PCR assays, nucleic acid sequence–based amplification (NASBA), Qβ-replicase, and real-time PCR, have been developed since 1989 for the detection of *M. pneumoniae* in a variety of specimen types.[272,465] Specimen types include sputum, throat swabs, nasopharyngeal and tracheal aspirates, bronchoalveolar lavages, transthoracic needle aspirates, fixed lung tissues, and open lung biopsies. Major gene targets for these assays have included the P1 adhesin gene, species-specific 16S rRNA, the mycoplasmal ATPase operon genes, and the *tuf* gene, which codes for elongation factor 2, a factor that functions in protein synthesis at the ribosome-mRNA level.[46,48,71,86, 162,226,271–273,414,451,487,492] Buck and coauthors described a PCR test in which the amplified DNA segment was a 375-base pair (bp) segment of the *M. pneumoniae* P1 adhesin protein.[46] For simulated clinical specimens, this test was able to detect a lower limit of between 1 and 10 organisms, compared with a lower limit of 1,000 organisms for cultural detection. Similar sensitivity has been reported by others using the same target DNA sequence.[48,86] Several investigators have designed species-specific probes for *M. pneumoniae* based on *M. pneumoniae*–specific 16S rRNA sequences

and found that amplification and subsequent probe detection of these sequences in clinical specimens was more sensitive than culture.[451,469] By using PCR technology, Narita and coworkers detected *M. pneumoniae*-specific DNA in four of six CSF specimens and in three of four serum specimens from patients with clinically and serologically confirmed *M. pneumoniae* CNS infection.[316] PCR ''fingerprinting'' technology has also been used to subtype isolates of *M. pneumoniae* based on nucleotide sequence divergence of the P1 cytadhesin protein.[466]

Isolation and Identification of the Genital Mycoplasmas

Mycoplasmas that may be recovered from the genital tract include *M. hominis*, *M. genitalium*, *M. fermentans*, and *U. urealyticum*. Whereas *M. hominis* and *U. urealyticum* are easily cultivated and usually grow within 1 to 5 days, *M. genitalium* and *M. fermentans* grow much more slowly and are more difficult to detect in culture. Furthermore, culture systems that are in current use for the recovery of genital mycoplasmas may not support optimal growth of these species. For example, the SP-4 medium described above for the isolation of *M. pneumoniae* is the optimal medium for *M. genitalium* because this organism is a glucose metabolizer, yet most laboratories do not use glucose-containing culture media for culture of genital tract specimens. Furthermore, the slow growth of the organism on media precludes the clinical usefulness of such culture data. *M. fermentans* also uses glucose but is very slow growing. Because of these considerations, genital mycoplasmas other than *M. hominis* and *U. urealyticum* are generally not sought in genital tract specimens.

M. genitalium is exceeding difficult to recover using culture-based methods. Jensen and colleagues reported the successful isolation of *M. genitalium* from genital tract specimens.[193] From 11 specimens, 9 were successfully propagated in Vero cell cultures from PCR-positive urethral specimens from patients with urethritis. Growth in Vero cell culture was monitored by PCR. Of these nine isolates, six were adapted by serial passage to growth in Friis medium, a complex growth medium containing Hanks' balanced salts solution, brain-heart infusion broth, ''homemade'' yeast extract, and up to 20% (v/v) horse serum. These six isolates required from 1 to 19 serial passages in Vero cell cultures before they could be adapted to growth in broth, and from 2 to 6 passages in broth before visible colonies were produced on an agar medium similar in formulation to the broth. In this report, the authors point out that, although the development of a medium able to support the growth of *M. genitalium* represented a major breakthrough, PCR methods were essential for initial detection and for monitoring the cultures for growth. Molecular techniques that are highly sensitive and specific have been developed for detection of *M. genitalium* in genital tract specimens and first-pass urine specimens, but these assays are not widely available.[94,108–110,191,192,410, 483,506–508]

For culture of *M. hominis* and *U. urealyticum*, appropriate specimens received in transport media are inoculated onto both broth and agar media. In general, about 0.2 mL of the specimen should be streaked onto agar media and placed in broth media. Broths may be incubated aerobically at 35°C, but plates should be incubated in a CO_2 incubator or a candle jar. Both organisms may also be recovered under anaerobic conditions. Plated media should be inspected daily under $40\times$ magnification using oblique light to observe the "fried egg" colonies of *M. hominis* or the small, dense colonies of *U. urealyticum*. With broth cultures, any broths showing the slightest alkaline color change or turbidity should be subcultured to the appropriate plated media. In M broth, *M. hominis* produces a slight turbidity in addition to a change in color. In U broth, *U. urealyticum* will tend to produce a slight color change early in incubation with no distinct or obvious turbidity. In both cases, subcultures must be performed at these times to ensure recovery of viable bacteria because there is a rapid decrease in viability of the organisms once the pH has been elevated by substrate utilization and depletion. As with the primary culture plates, subcultures plates should be inspected daily. Most isolates of *M. hominis* and *U. urealyticum* will grow within 5 to 7 days. If growth is not detected on primary plates or broth subcultures after this time, the culture can be reported as negative for genital mycoplasmas. It is a good idea to freeze aliquots of positive broths at $-70°C$ in case problems are encountered with viability on direct agar cultures or subcultures. The general scheme for isolation of genital mycoplasmas is presented in Figure 18-2.

Identification of genital mycoplasmas is generally quite easy and straightforward. *M. hominis* colonies grow in 1 to 5 days, have the typical fried-egg colonial morphology, and are usually 50 to 300 fm in diameter. Colonies may be stained with the Diene's stain (Chart 18-1) to aid visualization (see Color Plate 18-1*B*). Further identification procedures are not necessary because rapidly growing, arginine-positive organisms exhibiting the typical colony morphology are invariably *M. hominis*. The small colonies of *U. urealyticum* may be difficult to distinguish from various artifacts, such as mammalian cells and cellular debris or materials present in serum. Because of these problems, suspect *U. urealyticum* colonies must be confirmed. This is done by exploiting the ability of *U. urealyticum* to hydrolyze urea. If the U agar medium contains urea and phenol red, the suspect ureaplasma colonies will be surrounded by a red halo.

Suspect *U. urealyticum* colonies may also be confirmed with the manganous chloride–urea test (Chart 18-3). In this test, an agar plate containing colonial growth is flooded with an aqueous solution of urea (1%) and 0.8% (w/v) manganous chloride. Hydrolysis of urea by urease liberates hydroxyl groups from water, and these hydroxyl moieties oxidize manganous chloride to insoluble manganese oxide, causing the deposition of a golden brown precipitate in the colonies themselves within a few minutes.

Shepard's A7 differential agar media and its modifications, A7B and A8 agars, have the urea and the urea-hydrolysis detection reagent incorporated in the medium already, so flooding the plate with manganous chloride is not required.[390,392,393] A7 agar contains manganous sulfate as the precipitating agent along with penicillin (1,000 U/ml) and amphotericin B (2.5 μg/ml). A7B differential agar is identical to A7 agar, except that the polyamine putrescine dihydrochloride (10 mM) is added to enhance the ureaplasma growth and development of the precipitate in the colonies. A8 differ-

ential agar incorporates calcium chloride (1 mM) as the divalent cation indicator for the detection of ammonia formation from urea, along with colistin (7.5 μg/mL), ampicillin (1 μg/mL, and amphotericin B (2.5 μg/mL). On all three medium formulations, *M. hominis* appears with the characteristic fried-egg morphology after 1 to 3 days on A7, A7B, and A8 differential agars. *U. urealyticum* colonies appear within 1 to 3 days, and they are 15 to 50 μm in diameter (depending on crowding). *U. urealyticum* colonies on A7 and A7B agars are dark brown owing to the accumulation of manganese oxide in the colony, whereas colonies on A8 differential agar are gold to light brown (see Color Plate 18-1*B*). Several comparative evaluations of A7, A7B, and A8 media indicate that they are probably the agar media of choice for culture of genital mycoplasmas and, when used with an appropriate broth medium (e.g., bromthymol blue broth, Boston broth), give the highest yield of positive cultures.[242,347,498] Because the growth characteristics of *U. urealyticum* on these media are unique, further testing is not necessary. Both A7 and A8 differential agars are commercially available from Remel Laboratories (Lenexa, KA).

Definitive identification of *M. hominis* may be made by growth inhibition using specific antisera. An indirect immunoperoxidase method has also been published for the identification of mycoplasmas.[179] This method uses filter paper strips that are impregnated with specific rabbit antisera to various mycoplasma species and are applied to mycoplasmal growth on an agar plate. After 1 hour, the papers are removed and the same spot is covered with another piece of filter paper impregnated with goat antirabbit antisera conjugated to horseradish peroxidase. After another hour of incubation, the filter papers are removed and the plate is flooded with the enzyme substrate (1% 4-chloro-1-naphthol). The identity of the isolate is indicated by the appearance of a deep blue color where the initial species-specific antisera was placed on the plate. This method produces results comparable with those of the antiserum growth inhibition procedure. Similar procedures, using both immunofluorescence and immunoperoxidase techniques, have been developed for use in mycoplasma studies in animals, where species having similar tissue tropisms may be present in mixed culture.[27]

Noncultural Detection of the Genital Mycoplasmas

Nonculture methods have also been examined for their ability to detect genital mycoplasmas. Hirai and colleagues developed an indirect fluorescence antibody (IFA) test for direct identification of *M. hominis* in vaginal specimens.[161] The staining of Vero cells that were infected with other *Mycoplasma* species, including *M. orale*, *M. salivarium*, and *M. fermentans*, demonstrated that the IFA procedure was specific for *M. hominis*. The IFA test was compared with culture on vaginal specimens collected from 193 healthy women. Among 22 culture-positive specimens, 17 were positive with the IFA test. Interestingly, 48 of 171 specimens that were negative by culture were positive with the IFA test, suggesting that the IFA method was more sensitive than culture. These workers also demonstrated that the location of granular aggregates that were observed on vaginal epithelial cells stained with the Papanicolaou stain frequently corre-

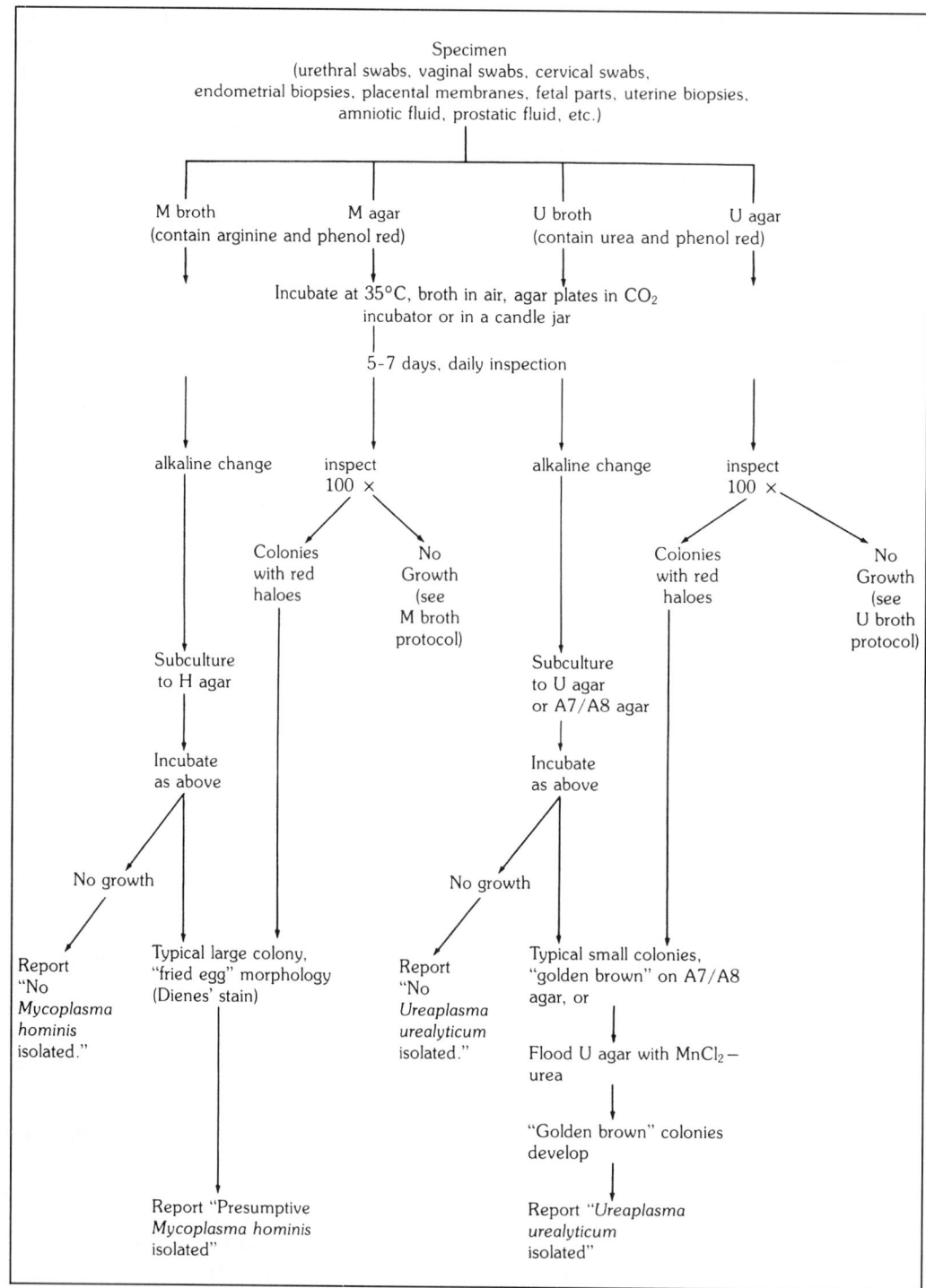

Figure 18-2 Protocol for isolation of *Mycoplasma hominis* and *Ureaplasma urealyticum* from genital specimens.

sponded to the areas of the smears that stained with the *M. hominis*-specific IFA reagents.[161]

Probe technology was initially exploited for detection of *M. genitalium* in urogenital specimens because this organism is very difficult to recover in culture. Because of the recognized antigenic cross-reactivity between *M. genitalium* and *M. pneumoniae* and similarities in certain nucleotide se-

quences between these organisms, nucleic acid probes for *M. genitalium* had to be constructed to exclude nucleotide sequences that are shared with *M. pneumoniae* in order to prevent false-positive results.[504] Such carefully constructed DNA probes were used along with gene amplification techniques and PCR to detect *M. pneumoniae*–and *M. genitalium*–specific nucleotide sequences directly in clinical specimens.[163,196] In one study, 10 of 150 genital specimens recovered from eight patients (three men and five women), were positive for M. genitalium.[196] These results were verified by Southern blot hybridization tests because cultures were not performed.

Molecular assays have also been developed for detection and specific identification of M. hominis and U. urealyticum in genital tract specimens, amniotic fluids, and respiratory tract specimens from newborns.[34,274,410,508] PCR assays for M. hominis have used M. hominis–specific 16S rRNA sequences as the target for amplification and detection, whereas similar assays for U. urealyticum have used organism-specific 16S rRNA sequences, the multiple banded (MB) antigen gene sequences, or urease gene sequences for detection and identification of this organism.[33,34,186,444] Some of these tests are able to detect as few as one colony-forming unit in specimens from the adult urogenital tract and amniotic fluids and endotracheal aspirates from newborn infants. Teng and coworkers examined 50 clinical specimens (8 urethral swab specimens, 8 urine specimens, 12 endocervical swab specimens, 8 prostatic fluid specimens, and 14 semen specimens) by both culture and PCR.[443] Cultures were positive for five specimens, and an additional four specimens produced appropriate pH changes in broth but did not grow on subculture to agar medium (''doubtful'' positives). PCR was positive for all five culture-positive specimens, all four doubtful-positive specimens, plus three specimens (one prostatic fluid and two endocervical specimens) that were culture-negative.

M. fermentans PCR methods detect a unique DNA sequence that appears repetitively in the genome of the organism, whereas those for detection of M. hominis, M. penetrans, and M. pirum detect unique nucleotide sequences within the 16S rRNA of these species.[133,134,484] Although serologic and genetic methods suggest that M. fermentans represents a homogeneous organism group, AIDS-associated strains, cell culture isolates, and other clinical isolates of M. fermentans can be differentiated from one another by pyrolysis mass spectrometry.[146]

Commercial Mycoplasma Culture Systems

The Mycotrim RS and Mycotrim Triphasic flask systems (Irvine Scientific, Irvine CA) are the only commercially available systems that have been used extensively for the cultivation of M. pneumoniae and the genital mycoplasmas, respectively. The Mycotrim GU system is available as an enrichment broth medium that can be used with conventional differential agars, such as A7 or A8 agars, or as a complete culture system, called the Mycotrim Triphasic flask system.

The Mycotrim RS system consists of a bottle containing a layer of enriched glucose agar medium containing phenol red indicator on one side and a broth of similar composition. Thirty minutes before inoculation with the specimen, disks that are saturated with cefoperazone, nystatin, and thallous acetate are added to the flasks to allow time for the antimicrobials to elute from the disk and diffuse into the agar. A pipette is used to add liquid specimens and to ''streak'' the agar surface. Swab specimens are rolled over the agar surface. The flask is incubated agar side up for 2 weeks at 35 to 37°C. Reinoculation after 3 days is performed by manipu-

lating the bottle so that the broth washes over part of the agar phase. Growth is first indicated by a change in the indicator from red to yellow-orange without noticeable turbidity. Definitive identification is made by placing the flask on the stage of a light microscope agar side up and inspecting the surface of the agar for mycoplasma colonies. This may be done with or without the addition of Diene's stain.

Mycotrim GU broth and the Mycotrim Triphasic flask system are the only widely used, commercially available systems for the isolation and identification of the genital mycoplasmas M. hominis and U. urealyticum. Mycotrim GU broth contains arginine, urea, and phenol red indicator. This broth is inoculated with 0.1 ml of the specimen and is incubated aerobically at 35°C. The medium is observed for changes in the color of the indicator to a more alkaline pH; subculture to solid media, such as A7 or A8 differential agar; and subsequent incubation allows the recovery and identification of both M. hominis and U. urealyticum.

The Mycotrim Triphasic flask (formerly called the Mycotrim GU system) system is a diphasic system that contains modified A8 differential agar with calcium chloride in a tissue culture flask and a broth medium containing arginine, urea, and phenol red indicator. Before inoculation, disks impregnated with cefoperazone (100 μg/mL) and nystatin (50 U/mL) are added and allowed to elute from the disk and diffuse into the agar phase. The flask is inoculated with 0.10 mL of the specimen, and the broth–specimen mixture is washed over the agar phase. The flask is incubated at 35°C aerobically. Subculture is achieved by allowing the broth to wash over part of the agar phase after 24 hours of incubation. With the appearance of a color change in the phenol red indicator from yellow to orange or orange-red, the agar phase is examined under the microscope for the typical fried-egg colonies of M. hominis or the small, brown calcium oxide–stained colonies of U. urealyticum. Cultures are inspected daily and incubated for 7 days.

In a study published in 1985, Wood and associates found that the Mycotrim GU system performed as well as the conventional method using arginine broth, urea broth, glucose agar, and A7B differential agar.[497] A subsequent study comparing the Mycotrim GU system with culture on A7 medium found that the Mycotrim system detected 73% of the M. hominis strains and 84% of the U. urealyticum strains, compared with 93% and 89%, respectively, of the organisms being isolated on A7 agar.[347] A 1992 study of the Mycotrim Triphasic flask system from the same laboratory that performed the 1985 study compared the flask with a culture system using Mycotrim GU broth with A7 and A8 differential agars with 129 clinical specimens.[42] Of the 64 specimens that grew U. urealyticum, 25%, 98%, and 100% were detected on Mycotrim Triphasic agar, A7 agar, and A8 agar, respectively. Of the 18 specimens from which M. hominis was isolated, all 18 grew in the broth–A7 agar and broth–A8 agar cultures, and 94% were detected on the Mycotrim Triphasic agar. In laboratories doing a modest amount of mycoplasma work, it appears that the Mycotrim GU broth combined with a differential agar medium and the Mycotrim Triphasic flask system are fairly comparable, although the components for the ''conventional'' procedure may be less expensive.

Isolation of Mycoplasmas on Routine Culture Media

In general, *M. pneumoniae* and *U. urealyticum* are more fastidious in their growth requirements than *M. hominis*, and the latter species is the one that is most frequently recovered from sites other than the genital tract, such as blood, wounds, and joint fluids. Therefore, *M. hominis* may occasionally be isolated on routine bacteriologic culture medium. The clinical microbiologist must be able to recognize these organisms under these less-than-optimal conditions. *M. hominis* is able to grow on enriched media such as Columbia CNA agar and chocolate agar; the organism grows less well on tryptic soybased blood agar.[335] The organisms will grow best under anaerobic conditions, with less rapid growth in an aerobic, CO_2-enriched environment. Mycoplasmal growth may not be apparent until after prolonged incubation (i.e., 72 to 96 hours), depending on the conditions of incubation and the numbers of organisms present. Colonies of *M. hominis* are extremely small and may be detected only as a "film" or "speckling" of the agar surface when examined by strong, incident, reflected light. Examination of this type of growth is facilitated by using a dissecting microscope. The colonies are difficult to pick up with a loop and will not stain with the Gram stain.

Suspected mycoplasma colonies from routine agar medium can be subcultured by cutting out a block of the blood agar and rubbing the side with the growth across the surface of a mycoplasma growth medium such as A7 differential agar. Another block should be aseptically removed and immersed in a broth medium such as H broth or Boston broth. Both broth and agar subcultures are then incubated and processed as described in the foregoing. Inspection of colony morphology, along with the growth rate and assessment of optimal incubation conditions for growth, will allow presumptive identification of the species.

M. hominis may also be occasionally recovered from blood cultures, particularly in women with postpartum fever. Sodium polyanethol sulfonate (SPS), the anticomplementary and antiphagocytic additive that is present in most routine blood culture media, is toxic to mycoplasmas. In general, the higher the SPS content (0.025 vs. 0.050%), the more inhibitory the medium becomes for the recovery of mycoplasmas.[80] Mycoplasmas have been recovered from radiometric blood culture media (i.e., the BACTEC system), but the SPS will inhibit or delay organism recovery, depending on the SPS content of the broth. Smaron and coworkers isolated *M. hominis* from blood cultures using the radiometric BACTEC system with SPS-free media.[403] Organisms were detected in both aerobic and anaerobic blood culture vials after 3 to 7 days of incubation. Blood bottles did not appear grossly positive, and growth indices on the instrument increased slowly over time. In addition, Gram stains from positive bottles failed to reveal any organisms, but they were visible when examined with the acridine orange stain. The addition of 10 mg/mL of gelatin to blood culture media has been demonstrated to partially overcome the inhibitory effects of SPS.[80] Also, the presence of sucrose in hypertonic blood culture media retards the growth of mycoplasmas.[80] In the BACTEC system, mycoplasmal growth may occur to some extent, but the growth index for the cultures may not exceed the threshold growth index value for positivity. Pratt explained this phenomenon by pointing out that CO_2 production by *M. hominis* results from arginine deaminase activity, which is produced by the organism late in the logarithmic growth phase. Limiting levels of arginine may prevent mycoplasmal growth from reaching levels that "trip" the positive threshold of the BACTEC instrument.[355]

If *M. hominis* bacteremia is suspected, blood should optimally be inoculated at the patient's bedside into an SPS-free medium. Incubation of the cultures should be prolonged, and blind subcultures to appropriate agar and broth mycoplasma isolation medium, in addition to CNA agar, should be made at frequent intervals. Blood for recovery of mycoplasmas should be inoculated directly into the mycoplasma culture medium. The blood should be diluted 1:10 with growth medium, so culture of a substantial blood volume may require multiple vials of culture media.

Serologic Tests for Diagnosis of Mycoplasma pneumoniae Infections

Because of the limited availability of culture, the technical difficulties inherent in the culture techniques, and the amount of time required for culture results to become available, the diagnosis of *M. pneumoniae* infection is often made by a combination of clinical and serologic findings. Diagnosis on clinical grounds alone is difficult because many other pneumonic processes, particularly those caused by viruses, can present similarly. In addition, persistence of *M. pneumoniae* in the respiratory tract for variable periods after resolution of the disease process clouds the interpretation of positive growth-based and molecular detection methods. The most widely used serologic test for diagnosis of *M. pneumoniae* infection is the complement fixation (CF) test. The antigen used in the test is a glycolipid from the organism that is extracted by chloroform-methanol (2:1 v/v).[220] The CF test measures predominantly early IgM antibodies to *M. pneumoniae* and detects IgG antibodies to a comparatively minor extent.[182] IgM antibodies appear during the first week of illness, reach peak titers during the third week of illness, and decline to low levels within a few months. IgG antibodies increase slowly over the course of the illness and reach peak titers about 5 weeks after the onset of symptoms.[183] In most cases, anti–*M. pneumoniae* IgG antibodies are not found during the first week of illness, but, once elevated, may remain so for 3 to 4 years. Therefore, low levels of IgG may indicate a past infection or an early IgG response to recent infection. Because these complement-fixing antibodies can persist for years after infection, the greatest diagnostic accuracy with the CF test is obtained when acute and convalescent sera demonstrate a fourfold rise in titer when tested together, indicating recent or current infection with *M. pneumoniae*. The acute specimen should be collected as soon after disease onset as possible, with the convalescent specimen being collected 2 to 3 weeks later. Single CF titers of 32 or higher collected in the convalescent period are highly suggestive of recent infection.[220] CF titers begin to rise 7 to 10 days after infection with the organism and reach peak titers after 4 to 6 weeks.[182] The crude extract from *M. pneumoniae* that is used in the CF test is similar in structure to other bacterial and plant glycolipids, so cross-reactions of this antigen with other nonmycoplasmal antibodies may occur. CF titers for diagnosis of mycoplasmal pneumonia may be false-positive in individuals with bacterial meningitis. In addition, some autoimmune conditions may also cause false-positive mycoplasmal CF serologic results.[182] Although the serologic diagnosis of infection using the CF test is usually reliable in pediatric populations, this is not the case with adults.[488] IgM antibodies may not be consistently produced in older individuals as a result of multiple past infections. In addition, older immunocompromised hosts may not mount an immune response that is sufficient to generate a detectable, reproducible result in the CF test.

The sensitivity and the specificity of the CF test in retrospective diagnosis of *M. pneumoniae* infection varies depending on the time during the illness when specimens are collected, the availability of paired specimens, and the cutoff used for interpretation of titers from single serum specimens. In a study by Kenny and coworkers, a fourfold rise in titer showed a sensitivity of only 53% in patients who had pneumonia and were culture-positive.[220] This sensitivity increased to 90% when single titers higher than 32 were included. Specificity of the CF test using either a fourfold titer increase or a titer of 32 or higher was 89%. A large 12-year study of the CF test and culture for diagnosis of *M. pneumoniae* found that the sensitivity and specificity of the CF test were 90% and 94%, respectively, whereas the sensitivity of culture was 64%.[182] In addition, other *Mycoplasma* species (i.e., *M. genitalium*) engender the production of antibodies that cross-react in the *M. pneumoniae* CF test, further contributing to the specificity problems of the CF test. Western immunoblot procedures have been described that circumvent the specificity issues of the test, but these methods are not readily available to most clinical laboratories.

Serologic test methods using immunofluorescence and enzyme immunoassay approaches are currently available commercially. The *M. pneumoniae* Antibody Test System (Zeus Scientific, Raritan, NJ) uses indirect immunofluorescence for the separate detection of *M. pneumoniae*–specific IgG and IgM. In one evaluation of this assay, IFA for *M. pneumoniae*–specific IgM was compared with PCR, culture, and CF for diagnosis of mycoplasmal infection.[101] Based on the positivity of culture and CF as the criteria for a positive diagnosis of infection, the sensitivity of the IgM IFA test was 78% and the specificity 92%. The predictive value of a positive IgM IFA in this study was only 57%. In another evaluation that used consensus results defining true positives as those yielding positive results in two or more EIA or CF assays (plus chart reviews), the IgM IFA had a sensitivity and specificity of 89% and 99%, respectively.[7]

Enzyme immunoassays (EIAs) for the detection of *M. pneumoniae*–specific antibodies have also been developed. Microtiter EIA kits that are available include the *Mycoplasma pneumoniae* IgG/IgM antibody test system (Remel), ImmunoWELL *Mycoplasma pneumoniae* IgM EIA (Gen-Bio, San Diego, CA), the Zeus *Mycoplasma* IgM EIA (Zeus Scientific), the Incstar *Mycoplasma* IgM ELISA (Incstar, Stillwater, MN), the Platelia IgM and IgG *Mycoplasma* EIA (Sanofi-Diagnostica Pasteur, Marnes la Coquette, France), the Biotest anti–*M. pneumoniae* IgG and IgM ELISA (Biotest, Buc, Germany), and the ETI–*M. pneumoniae* IgM/IgG assay (Diasoren, Antony, France). The ImmunoWELL,

Zeus, and Incstar assays are microtiter plate methods that detect IgM antibodies against *M. pneumoniae* in serum specimens. The ImmunoWELL and Zeus assays use an IgG sorbent step to prevent interference from IgG in the specimen, whereas the Incstar and Platelia IgM assays are IgM capture assays. The Remel, Platelia, Biotest, and ETI EIAs detect both IgM and IgG. These microtiter-format assays vary in the type of antigen used in the solid phase. Antigens used in these assays include solubilized and purified ultrasonicates from *M. pneumoniae* cultures (e.g., Platelia and Biotest assays), purified *M. pneumoniae* glycolipids (e.g., ImmunoWELL assay), or purified membrane protein antigens that include the immunodominant *M. pneumoniae* cytadhesin P1 (e.g., the ETI assays) as the predominant antigen in the solid phase. The specificity of IgM testing by EIA is improved when an IgM capture method is used. In a comparative evaluation of several IgM assays, a specificity of 100% was noted only for the Platelia IgM EIA, which uses IgM capture (i.e., the solid phase is coated with anti–μ-chain antibodies), whereas assays that used IgG absorption or other IgG removal methods for IgM detection had specificities ranging from 90% (i.e., the ImmunoWELL IgM) to as low as 25% (ETI–*M. pneumoniae* IgM).[342] In general, the IgM assays are more sensitive and specific when testing sera from children, since adults may not mount a significant IgM response.[398] In addition, since adult populations tend to have higher backgrounds of specific anti–*M. pneumoniae* IgG from past or subclinical infections, testing of paired sera collected 1 to 3 weeks apart and documenting a fourfold or greater rise in antibody titer is most useful for determining acute infections in adults.[462]

In recent years, several rapid membrane-based serologic tests for *M. pneumoniae*–specific IgM and IgG have become commercially available. The Remel *M. pneumoniae* IgG/IgM antibody test system is a 5-minute EIA for simultaneous, qualitative detection of antibodies against *M. pneumoniae*. Patient serum is diluted and reacted with *M. pneumoniae* antigen that is immobilized on a permeable membrane. After rinsing, enzyme-labeled antihuman IgG/IgM is added and allowed to rinse through the membrane. After two washes, substrate-chromogen is added to the filter and allowed to react for 5 minutes. Thacker and Talkington evaluated this test with 50 paired serum samples and found that the Remel test detected antibodies in three specimens with CF titers of 32 and was positive for all but one specimen with CF titers of 64 or higher.[445] Another evaluation of this system reported a sensitivity of 91% and a specificity of 91%, with corresponding positive and negative predictive values of 87% and 93%, respectively.[115] The Meridian ImmunoCard Mycoplasma IgM assay (Meridian Biosciences, Cincinnati, OH) is a 10-minute, qualitative, membrane-based EIA in which test serum is allowed to react with *M. pneumoniae* antigen extracts impregnated into filter paper. This assay does not require IgM separation or IgG removal from the serum prior to test performance. Evaluations of this assay suggest that the ImmunoCard test is more sensitive than other serologic tests for detecting low levels of IgM antibodies.[7,107,286,446] In an evaluation of the assay using specimens from 40 pediatric patients, all acute-phase serum specimens were positive with the ImmunoCard, whereas the CF and particle agglutination tests were positive for 30% and 77.5% of the specimens, respectively.[286] In another comparative evaluation with 64 acute-phase sera from adults, the ImmunoCard detected specific IgM in 46% of the specimens, whereas the CF test, the Remel EIA, and the ImmunoWELL IgM EIA detected antibodies in 38%, 41%, and 23%, respectively.[446] A third evaluation using 145 acute-phase sera from children reported resolved sensitivity, specificity, and positive and negative predictive values of 85%, 97%, 93%, and 93%, respectively, when compared with both Remel and Zeus IgM microtiter EIAs.[107] The evaluations of the ImmunoCard *Mycoplasma* IgM assay suggest that this rapid test is highly reliable for establishing a diagnosis of recent *M. pneumoniae* infection in both children and adults.

Microparticle agglutination assays have also been marketed for detection of *M. pneumoniae* antibodies. The Serodyne Color Vue IgG/IgM test (Serodyne, Indianapolis IN) uses latex particles coated with *M. pneumoniae* lipid antigen, whereas the Serodia-Myco II test (FujireBio, Tokyo, Japan) uses similarly sensitized gelatin particles. Both tests are performed by serially diluting heat-inactivated patient serum in a microtiter plate and adding a fixed aliquot of the latex or gelatin particles that are coated with *M. pneumoniae* lipid antigen to each of the dilution wells. After mixing on a microwell shaker and incubation, the end point is determined as the final dilution of serum causing agglutination of the antigen-sensitized particles. Thacker and Talkington evaluated the Serodyne 40-minute passive agglutination test and found it less sensitive than the Remel EIA; only 68% of cases of mycoplasmal pneumonia could be serologically diagnosed with this kit, compared with 94% and 96% of cases being diagnosed by the CF and Remel tests, respectively.[445] Lieberman and colleagues evaluated the Serodia-Myco II gelatin agglutination test and found the sensitivity, specificity, and predictive values of positive and negative tests to be 48.1%, 86.9%, 49.3%, and 86.3%, respectively.[251] Inadequate specificity of the Serodia Myco II particle agglutination assay compared with an IgM-specific capture EIA and an IgM IFA has been noted by other researchers as well.[17]

The purification and sequencing of the P1 adhesin of *M. pneumoniae* and the recognition of immunodominant epitopes of P1 and other cell surface molecules may allow the manufacture of synthetic peptides that can be used as specific, chemically defined antigens in future serologic tests for *M. pneumoniae*.[185] Suni and colleagues evaluated a new EIA method (*M. pneumoniae* IgG, IgA, and IgM, Thermolabsystems, Helsinki, Finland) in which the solid-phase antigen is enriched for the P1 cytadherence protein antigen of *M. pneumoniae*.[417] When compared with the ImmunoWELL and Platelia EIAs, the sensitivity and specificity of this test were 100% and 96.5–100%, respectively. Another group investigated the performance of two novel EIAs in comparison with the CF test. In one assay, the solid phase contained recombinant P1 antigen; in the other assay, the solid phase contained recombinant p116 antigen.[102] Both of these antigens have demonstrable antigenicity and engender the formation of specific antibodies in infected patients.[104,105,175] This study found that the recombinant antigen assays showed good agreement with the CF test, with the recombinant P1 EIA showing the best discrimination between positive and negative specimens.[102] The use of species-specific antigenic epitopes in serologic tests for *M. pneumoniae* infection may help to eliminate false-positive serologic tests resulting from *M. genitalium* respiratory or urogenital tract infection, since these organisms are known to possess cross-reacting antigens.[254]

Serodiagnosis by detection of serum anti-*M. pneumoniae* IgA levels has also been investigated as a possible method for diagnosis of *M. pneumoniae* infection. Watkins-Riedel and colleagues evaluated a 3-hour IgA EIA method (SeroMP-IgA kit; Savyon Diagnostics, Ashdod, Israel) and compared it with the microparticle agglutination assay (Serodia Myco II; FujireBio), the CF test, an IgM-specific EIA (SeroMP-IgM kit; Savyon Diagnostics), and the rapid ImmunoCard IgM EIA (Meridian Diagnostics) on acute-phase serum samples from 23 patients with *M. pneumoniae* pneumonia.[490] The IgA assay performed with a sensitivity of 96% to 100% and a specificity of 91% to 100%. Sensitivity of the other assays ranged from 87% to 91%. During the course of this study, the investigators noted that younger patients tended to have higher levels of IgM than adults, whereas the adult patients tended to have higher levels of IgA antibodies. This assay appeared to address two of the recognized shortcomings of mycoplasma serology: the comparatively lower sensitivity and specificity of the CF test and the inconsistent presence of *M. pneumoniae*–specific IgM in infected adult patients.

A nonspecific serologic test that is often used to support the diagnosis of *M. pneumoniae* infection is the production of **cold agglutinins.** These agglutinins react in the cold with human erythrocyte I antigens. The I antigen is inactivated by α-glycosidase, and the binding of cold agglutinins to these cells is inhibited by galactose.[72,499] Furthermore, when erythrocytes containing the I antigen are subjected to chloroform–methanol extraction, an antigen is extracted that will fix complement in the presence of anti–*M. pneumoniae* antibodies.[499] These data indicate that the I antigen of erythrocytes detected by cold agglutinins is similar in structure to certain antigenic determinants in the glycolipid membrane antigen of *M. pneumoniae*.[189] Similar to other IgM antibodies, cold hemagglutinins appear about 7 days after infection and peak after 4 to 5 weeks. Following this, titers decline rapidly, becoming undetectable after about 5 months. As with the CF and other serologic tests, a fourfold rise in cold agglutinin titers in the presence of a compatible clinical illness is suggestive of *M. pneumoniae* infection. The major drawback of using this test alone for presumptive diagnosis is that only about 50–60% of individuals with acute *M. pneumoniae* infection will have demonstrable cold agglutinin titers.[172,182] In addition, several other conditions can cause increases in cold agglutinins, including infectious mononucleosis, mumps, influenza, rubella, respiratory syncytial virus infections, adenovirus infections, peripheral vascular disease, and psittacosis.

Serologic Tests for Genital Mycoplasmas

Serologic methods have also been investigated for the diagnosis of *M. hominis* infections. Lipid-associated membrane proteins (LAMPs) constitute a major group of cell surface proteins that are highly antigenic and are major targets in the immune response against mycoplasmas.[267]

LAMPs have been identified in several *Mycoplasma* species, including *M. salivarium*, *M. penetrans*, *M. pirum*, and *M. genitalium*, and these antigens have been used in serologic assays for testing patients with various types of infections.[483,485,486] Antibodies to these LAMP antigens appear to be highly species-specific, with no apparent cross-reactions with those of other species. Antibodies against LAMP antigens have also been used to delineate serotypes of *M. hominis*. In a recent study, the antigenicity and antibody profiles of 14 different *M. hominis* strains were compared by sodium dodecyl sulfate—polyacrylamide gel electrophoresis (SDS-PAGE) and Western immunoblot.[267] The LAMPs from these 14 strains showed similar SDS-PAGE profiles, and immunoblot analysis showed that these proteins were highly immunogenic when tested with sera from infected patients. These workers also demonstrated that sera from 28 of 31 HIV-positive patients with *M. hominis* culture-positive urine specimens reacted with every one of the 14 different *M. hominis* isolates on Western immunoblot examination. These studies showed that LAMPs from any isolate of *M. hominis* could be used as a target antigen in an EIA test format for detection of antibodies against *M. hominis*. This LAMP-derived EIA was used to demonstrate that the prevalence of *M. hominis*–specific antibodies was significantly greater among patients attending STD clinics (67.8% prevalence) than among healthy blood donors (34.4% prevalence) and that *M. hominis* infection occurred at a much younger age in women than in men. These EIAs for detection of serum antibodies against *M. hominis* are research-based assays and are not widely available.

Serologic methods have also been evaluated as a way to establish the presence of *U. urealyticum* infection. Serologic methods have included EIA techniques, with purified organism sonicates as the solid-phase antigen, or Western immunoblot techniques, where antigens were prepared by growing representative *U. urealyticum* serovars in culture, lysing the organisms with SDS, separating the antigens by electrophoresis, and transblotting of the antigens onto nitrocellulose paper. A study conducted in 1995 examined the presence of the *U. urealyticum* in amniotic fluids along with the serologic response as documented by EIA in women in their third trimester who were undergoing amniocentesis for genetic indications, women admitted for preterm labor with intact fetal membranes, and women with preterm rupture of the fetal membranes.[170] Although the prevalence of *U. ureaplasma* infection was 2.9%, 4.3%, and 17.8%, respectively, in the three groups the corresponding antibody prevalences were 50%, 86%, and 57%. These workers found that the incidence of adverse pregnancy outcomes—preterm birth, low birth weight, or fetal death—was significantly greater in women who had mounted an immune response against *U. urealyticum*.[170] In another study by the same group, 30% of women with postpartum endometritis had positive EIA serologies for *U. urealyticum*, compared with 6% of the control group.[55] A serologic study of women and infants using immunoblots for *U. urealyticum*–specific IgM and IgA found that 4.5% of infants born at less than 30 weeks of gestation, less than 1.7% of infants born between 30 and 34 weeks of gestation, and none of the infants born at 35 weeks or greater had detectable IgM or IgA specific antibodies, suggesting a possible role for the immune response in preg-

nancy outcome.[75] Serologic studies such as these may help to clarify the role of the specific immune response to *U. urealyticum* in the pathogenesis of infection and to provide information for the development of sensitive and specific serologic tests to augment cultural and molecular diagnostic approaches in the clinical laboratory. As with *M. hominis*, serologic tests for *U. urealyticum* are not widely available and are mainly used in research settings.

Antimicrobial Susceptibility and Treatment of Mycoplasma *Infections*

Atypical pneumonia cause by *M. pneumoniae* is generally treated with tetracycline or erythromycin.[69] Although the organism may still be present in the upper respiratory tract during and after treatment, clinical manifestations of infection generally improve, and infiltrates on chest radiography usually disappear during therapy. Because of the difficulty in culturing the organism, its slow growth rate, and the lack of a readily available method, antimicrobial susceptibility testing of *M. pneumoniae* is neither necessary nor appropriate. Antimicrobial susceptibility testing of *M. pneumoniae* strains indicate that this organism is susceptible to a wide variety of antimicrobial agents, including the quinolones (i.e., ciprofloxacin, levofloxacin, ofloxacin, gemifloxacin, moxifloxacin, garenoxacin, trovafloxacin, grepafloxacin, rufloxacin), clindamycin, lincomycin, tetracycline, doxycycline, minocycline, erythromycin, and certain aminoglycosides (streptomycin).[103,122,145,213,429,473–475] Some of the newer macrolide antibiotics, such as clarithromycin, azithromycin, and flurithromycin, are also highly active against *M. pneumoniae* and show a very narrow range of minimal inhibitory concentrations (MICs).[23,122,145,474] *M. pneumoniae* strains may demonstrate decreased susceptibility to gentamicin, chloramphenicol, clindamycin, and lincomycin and are frankly resistant to penicillins, cephalosporins, nalidixic acid, and rifampin.[429]

Most isolates of both *M. hominis* and *U. urealyticum* are susceptible to tetracyclines. *M. hominis* strains are usually susceptible to clindamycin and lincomycin, but not to erythromycin and other macrolides (i.e., azithromycin, clarithromycin). *U. urealyticum* strains are usually susceptible to erythromycin and azithromycin, but not to clindamycin and lincomycin. The growth of *M. hominis* and *U. urealyticum* is also inhibited by chloramphenicol, streptomycin, and gentamicin, but not by cell wall–active agents (i.e., cephalothin, ampicillin, and vancomycin). During the mid- to late 1970s and early 1980s, strains of both species that were resistant to tetracycline were isolated and found to contain a genetic antimicrobial resistance determinant called *tetM*.[365,366] This determinant has also been found in other genital tract microorganisms, including group B streptococci, *Gardnerella vaginalis*, and *Neisseria gonorrhoeae*.[367] Strains of *U. urealyticum* that are resistant or intermediate in susceptibility to erythromycin and newer macrolides (e.g., flurithromycin) have also been described.[122,218] Most *M. hominis* strains are now resistant to erythromycin, and some are resistant to tetracycline and clindamycin. Resistance to macrolides like erythromycin in *M. hominis* is usually due to mutations in the 23S rRNA.[340] Tetracycline resistance has also been reported in strains of *U. urealyticum;* these strains also contain the *tetM* resistance determinant.[365,366,413] Erythromycin remains the drug of choice for the treatment of *U. urealyticum* non-CNS infections in neonates; CNS infections in this group of patients are best treated with tetracycline or chloramphenicol.[477] Strains of *U. urealyticum* are generally less susceptible to the quinolone antibiotics than either *M. pneumoniae* and or *M. hominis*.[122,214,216,217,219]

The antimicrobial susceptibility profile of *M. genitalium* appears to be similar to that of *M. pneumoniae* in that isolates of this species are susceptible to tetracyclines and a variety of macrolides.[428,429] Renaudin and colleagues determined the susceptibilities of seven *M. genitalium* isolates using an agar dilution method and compared them with three *M. pneumoniae* strains.[361] Both species were susceptible to macrolides (i.e., erythromycin, spiramycin, roxithromycin, azithromycin, and clarithromycin), clindamycin, tetracycline, doxycycline, minocycline, and the fluoroquinolones (i.e., ofloxacin, ciprofloxacin, lomefloxacin, sparfloxacin).[92] Despite *in vitro* susceptibility of *M. genitalium* to the tetracyclines, several studies have shown that tetracycline therapy is often associated with treatment failures. A study by Johannison and colleagues found that 62% of 13 men with *M. genitalium* urethritis who were treated with tetracycline for 10 days still had the organism in the urethra at follow-up.[197] In another study, all of seven men with *M. genitalium* urethritis who were treated with doxycycline still had urethritis on follow-up.[164] In a treatment study comparing tetracyclines and azithromycin, all six patients who had received azithromycin were negative for *M. genitalium* by PCR after treatment, while 63% of 16 patients treated with tetracycline were still PCR-positive for *M. genitalium* after treatment.[114] The presence of the organisms in the urogenital tract with or without attendant symptoms following treatment with these agents may be directly related to the dosage and duration of treatment. According to the treatment guidelines for STDs, azithromycin for treatment of urethritis is administered in a single 1-g dose.[54] Patients with *M. genitalium* urethritis who have been treated with azithromycin according to these recommendation have had partial clinical responses and remained positive for *M. genitalium* by PCR a week after completion of therapy.[124] Whatley and colleagues found that 500 mg of azithromycin in a single dose followed by 250 mg of azithromycin once daily for 2 days was more effective in eradicating *M. genitalium* than 200 mg of doxycycline for 7 days or 1 g of azithromycin in a single dose.[493]

With use of a modified broth dilution procedure with SP-4 medium, Hayes and colleagues determined the antimicrobial susceptibilities of the *M. fermentans* incognitus strain along with reference strains of both *M. fermentans* (strain PG18 [ATCC 19989]) and *M. pneumoniae* (ATCC 15531).[153,155] As expected, all three mycoplasmas were resistant to cell wall–active agents (penicillin, ampicillin). Both the PG18 and the incognitus *M. fermentans* incognitus strains were resistant to erythromycin (mean MICs of erythromycin, 31.2 µg/mL and 43.0 µg/mL, respectively), whereas *M. pneumoniae* was susceptible to erythromycin (mean MIC, 0.0073 µg/mL). The *M. fermentans* incognitus strain was susceptible to tetracycline, doxycycline, clindamycin, lincomycin, chloramphenicol, and ciprofloxacin. Both *M. fermentans* strains tested in this study were resistant to the aminoglyco-

sides (gentamicin, kanamycin, streptomycin, and neomycin), whereas *M. pneumoniae* was susceptible. Aminoglycoside MICs for the incognitus strain of *M. fermentans* were higher than 1,000 µg/mL for all four of these drugs, while the MICs for gentamicin, kanamycin, streptomycin, and neomycin for the PG18 strain were 15.6, 20.8, 18.2, and 52.1 µg/mL, respectively. Subsequent antimicrobial susceptibility testing of 24 additional *M. fermentans* isolates also indicated that this species is resistant to erythromycin and the aminoglycosides.[153] This subsequent study also documented that only ciprofloxacin and levofloxacin, both fluoroquinolone antimicrobial agents, had a significant bactericidal effect.[153]

Using a modified dilution technique with Hayflick's broth, Hannon examined several *M. fermentans* strains isolated from human infections and from tissue culture cells.[143] These strains were much more susceptible to azithromycin than to either erythromycin or clarithromycin. Clindamycin and several tetracycline congeners also showed good activity against the *M. fermentans* strains, although mycoplasmacidal concentrations were severalfold greater than inhibitory concentrations of antibiotic. This study also demonstrated that *M. fermentans* strains isolated during the 1960s in cell-free media were susceptible to the aminoglycosides, while recent human isolates and strains obtained from tissue culture cells were often resistant to single or multiple aminoglycoside drugs, with MICs to these agents exceeding 500 µg/mL. Strains of *M. fermentans* developed resistance to the streptomycin and gentamicin within 5 passages in broth media containing these agents, while resistance to tobramycin, kanamycin and gentamicin developed after 7, 8, and 14 passages in media containing these agents, respectively. This induced aminoglycoside resistance remained stable for over 17 passages in broth lacking aminoglycosides. Azithromycin was more active against *M. fermentans* strains than either erythromycin or clarithromycin.[143]

In a subsequent study, Hannon examined the aminoglycoside susceptibility of several *M. fermentans* strains, including three AIDS-associated isolates (including one incognitus strain), six recent respiratory tract isolates, one leukemia-associated isolate from 1962, and eight tissue culture cell isolates.[144] Two of the three AIDS-associated isolates and all of the non-AIDS associated respiratory tract isolates were susceptible to the six aminoglycoside drugs tested, while the *M. fermentans* incognitus strain and all the recent tissue culture isolates were highly resistant to all six agents, with MICs exceeding 250 µg/mL. The strain isolated from tissue culture of leukemic bone marrow in 1962 was highly resistant to streptomycin (MIC, >250 µg/mL) but susceptible to the other five aminoglycosides. These results were consistent with Hannon's earlier studies, which established that *M. fermentans* incognitus was the only human strain of the nine examined that demonstrated multiple aminoglycoside resistance.[143] This resistance profile was identical to that of the cell culture isolates. These results led Hannon to postulate that the original *M. fermentans* incognitus isolate, which was recovered by direct transfection of NIH/3T3 cells with DNA extracted from Kaposi's sarcoma tissue of an AIDS patient, may have been a contaminant in either the transfected DNA or in the 3T3 tissue culture cells used at the NIH.[144] This is supported by the fact that prokaryotic DNA is not generally infective for eukaryotic cells in the same way that viral nucleic acids are, and that the ability of *M. fermentans* to grow intracellularly may have enabled this strain to develop cross-resistance to aminoglycosides that are used in tissue cultures to control contamination. This is also supported by the knowledge that *M. fermentans* is a frequent contaminant of tissue culture cells.[15] Studies by others have also shown that the original *M. fermentans* incognitus strain is more closely related genetically to cell culture–associated isolates.[383] Even though the original *M. fermentans* incognitus strain may have been a spurious contaminant, subsequent work has shown that *M. fermentans* is an important pathogen in AIDS and non-AIDS patients.

Using a macrodilution, metabolic inhibition assay, Poulin and colleagues examined the antimicrobial susceptibilities of several "AIDS-associated" mycoplasmas, including *M. fermentans* (a stock strain, two clinical isolates from AIDS patients, and the "incognitus" strain), *M. penetrans* (one strain), and *M. pirum* (one strain).[352] All isolates were susceptible to azithromycin, clarithromycin, clindamycin, doxycycline, ofloxacin, and tetracycline. *M. fermentans* strains and *M. pirum* were resistant to erythromycin, whereas *M. penetrans* was susceptible. These workers also found that dried Sensititre Gram-Positive MIC panels (BD Microbiology Systems, Irvine, CA) inoculated with a standardized suspension of the organisms in SP-4 broth produced results comparable with the metabolic inhibition method for all of the drugs tested by both methods. On the Sensititre panel, all strains tested were resistant to penicillin, ampicillin, cephalothin, imipenem, vancomycin, rifampin, and trimethoprim-sulfamethoxazole. *M. fermentans* strains and *M. penetrans* were resistant to gentamicin, whereas *M. pirum* was moderately susceptible.

Hayes and colleagues also examined the antimicrobial susceptibilities of *M. penetrans* isolates by a broth dilution procedure.[154] In their study of nine strains, all *M. penetrans* were susceptible to azithromycin, chloramphenicol, ciprofloxacin, clindamycin, doxycycline, erythromycin, levofloxacin, lincomycin, and tetracycline. All isolates were resistant to gentamicin and streptomycin. The fluoroquinolones were the only class of antimicrobial agents that demonstrated bactericidal, rather than bacteriostatic, activity against *M. penetrans*.[154]

Because of variability in antimicrobial susceptibility, methods for susceptibility testing on mycoplasmas have been devised, but are not widely available because they require special media and may incur considerable expense for routine clinical microbiology laboratories. Spaepen and Kundsin devised a relatively simple broth-disk elution procedure for susceptibility testing of ureaplasmas that is similar to those described in the past for testing anaerobic bacteria.[407] This procedure provided fairly reproducible results when inoculated with organisms grown in culture or with urine specimens containing organisms. Robertson and associates subsequently reported a standardized broth dilution method for determining MICs of antimicrobial agents for *U. urealyticum* strains.[368] In 1986, Kenny and associates published an agar dilution procedure for ureaplasma testing that appeared to yield more reproducible results that broth methods.[218] Side-by-side comparisons of microbroth dilution and agar dilution methods have indicated that either one

can provide similar results when testing *U. urealyticum* for susceptibility to tetracycline and erythromycin.[480]

Both agar dilution and broth dilution methods for antimicrobial susceptibility testing of mycoplasmas have been described.[24] H agar at a pH of 7.2 to 7.4 may be used for *M. hominis* and *M. pneumoniae*, while U agar at a pH of 6.3 to 6.5 is used for testing of *U. urealyticum*. Doubling dilutions of antimicrobial agents are incorporated into the medium when the agar dilution plates are prepared. Inoculation is performed using a Steer's replicator to deliver an inoculum of 30 to 300 colony-forming units (CFUs) per inoculum spot. This inoculum is determined by plating aliquots of 10-fold dilutions of a growing broth culture in triplicate, performing colony counts, and diluting the organism suspension appropriately so that the replicator delivers 30 to 300 CFUs per spot. Plates are incubated in air for 4 days (*U. urealyticum*), 5 days (*M. hominis*), or 14 days (*M. pneumoniae*).

Broth microdilution procedures usually use 10B broth for ureaplasma testing and SP-4 broth for testing of other mycoplasmas. The antimicrobial agents are solubilized and diluted in microtiter trays with the proper broth medium containing a phenol-red indicator to achieve a range of drug concentrations. The inoculum should be prepared from cultures that are in the exponential growth phase, where the numbers of organisms is generally about 10^7 CFU/mL for ureaplasmas and 10^8 to 10^9 CFU/mL for large-colony mycoplasmas, which are also expressed as color-changing units (CCUs) per milliliter. An inoculum of 10^4 to 10^5 CFU (CCU) of organism is added to each of the microtiter wells containing the antimicrobial dilutions, and then the plates are sealed and incubated aerobically at 35 to 37°C. The microtiter trays are examined daily until a color change due to a change in pH is detected in the drug-free growth control. The MIC is defined as the lowest concentration of antimicrobial agent at which the metabolism of the organisms is inhibited enough to prevent a change in the color of the medium (due to the pH indicator) at the time that the drug-free control first shows a color change. For *U. urealyticum*, growth will usually be present within the control well after 24 hours, while growth of *M. hominis* usually requires 48 hours. *M. pneumoniae* strains generally require 4 to 8 days of incubation before a change is noted in the control well. Bactericidal activity of antimicrobial agents can be assessed with the broth dilution approach by removal of an aliquot from the MIC well and the wells containing higher antibiotic concentrations, diluting the aliquot with drug-free medium, and observing for a color change in the medium on further incubation. With both agar and broth dilution procedures, strains with known susceptibilities and reproducible MICs must be included with each susceptibility test for validation of the results.

In all of these procedures, problems that relate to the biologic characteristics of the organisms and to the method itself may be encountered. Biologic problems include the possibility of mixed cultures (e.g., both mycoplasmas and ureaplasmas) and the coexistence of susceptible and resistant populations in the same culture. The latter problem may be detected only in agar dilution-based systems, because colonies growing on antibiotic-containing media can be directly reidentified by urea hydrolysis or by serologic methods. Problems relating to methodology include the lack of a standard medium for test performance, discrepancies related to the pH required for optimal mycoplasmal growth versus optimal antibiotic activity, the difficulty in standardization of inoculum size, the lack of standardized incubation times and conditions, and the lack of a standardized susceptibility breakpoints.[215,218] Because of these problems, susceptibility testing on mycoplasmas is usually performed only in larger institutions with special research interests in the therapy of genital mycoplasma infections.

Diagnosis and Treatment of Hemotrophic Mycoplasma *Infections in Animals*

Former members of the genera *Eperythrozoon* and *Haemobartonella* cannot be grown in culture, so diagnosis is based on the examination of blood smears stained by Romanowsky-type blood film stains, including Giemsa, May-Grünwald-Giemsa, Wright, and Wright-Giemsa stains or by the acridine orange stain.[301,302,424] Because the organisms display a cyclical parasitemia where they may be rapidly cleared from the blood, examination of multiple blood films collected over a 24-hour period increases the likelihood of a positive diagnosis in a clinically compatible host species. Blood films should be prepared immediately after collection using nonanticoagulated blood or blood collected in heparinized tubes; EDTA anticoagulant may cause detachment of the organisms from the red cell membrane, making microscopic diagnosis difficult.[301,424] The organisms appear as coccal forms that are 0.5 to 0.8 μm in diameter and adherent to the surfaces of the erythrocytes. They are usually found around the periphery of the erythrocyte and may appear singly or in pairs, clusters, and chains. With the acridine orange fluorescence stain, the organisms appear as bright orange to yellow-green. Molecular and serologic assays for the hemotrophic mycoplasmas have also been developed but are not widely available.[424] All species appear to be susceptible to tetracyclines and resistant to β-lactam antimicrobial agents. Treatment with erythromycin effectively controls acute infection, but treatment does not consistently clear animals of the infection.[301]

REFERENCES

1. Abele-Horn M, Wolff C, Dressel P, et al. Association of *Ureaplasma urealyticum* biovars with clinical outcomes for neonates, obstetric patients, and gynecological patients with pelvic inflammatory disease. J Clin Microbiol 1997;35:1199–1202.
2. Abu-Amero KK, Halablab MA, Miles RJ. Nisin resistance distinguishes *Mycoplasma* spp. from *Acholeplasma* spp. and provides a basis for selective growth media. Appl Environ Microbiol 1996;62:3107–3111.
3. Ainsworth JG, Easterbrook PJ, Clarke J, et al. An association of disseminated *Mycoplasma fermentans* in HIV-1 positive patients with non-Hodgkin's lymphoma. Int J STD AIDS 2001;12:499–504.
4. Ainsworth JG, Hourshid S, Easterbrook PJ, et al. *Mycoplasma* species in rapid and slow HIV progressors. Int J STD AIDS 2000;11:76–79.
5. Ainsworth JG, Hourshid S, Webster AD, et al. Detection of *Mycoplasma fermentans* in healthy students and patients with congenital immunodeficiency. J Infect 2000;40:138–140.
6. Ainsworth JG, Katseni V, Hourshid S, et al. *Mycoplasma fermentans* and HIV-associated nephropathy. J Infect 1994;29:323–326.
7. Alexander TS, Gray LD, Kraft JA, et al. Performance of Meridian ImmunoCard *Mycoplasma* test in a multicenter clinical trial. J Clin Microbiol 1996;34:1180–1183.
8. Alfa MJ, Robertson JA. The co-existence of genital mycoplasmas and *Neisseria gonorrhoeae* isolated from the male urethra. Sex Transm Dis 1984;11:131–136.
9. Alonso-Vega C, Wauters N, Vermeylen D, et al. A fatal case of *Mycoplasma hominis* meningoencephalitis in a full-term newborn. J Clin Microbiol 1997;35:286–287.
10. Andrade-Rocha FT. *Ureaplasma urealyticum* and *Mycoplasma hominis* in men attending for routine semen analysis: prevalence, incidence by age and clinical settings, influence on sperm characteristics, relationship with leukocyte count and clinical value. Urol Int 2003;71:377–381.
11. Andrews WW, Hauth JC, Cliver SP, et al. Randomized clinical trial of extended spectrum antibiotic prophylaxis with coverage for *Ureaplasma urealyticum* to reduce post-cesarean delivery endometritis. Obstet Gynecol 2003;101:1183–1189.
12. Andrews WW, Shah SR, Goldenberg RL, et al. Association of post-cesarean delivery endometritis with colonization of the chorioamnion by *Ureaplasma urealyticum*. Obstet Gynecol 1995;85:509–514.
13. Angulo AF, Reijgers R, Brugman J, et al. *Acholeplasma vituli* sp. nov., from bovine serum and cell cultures. Int J Syst Evol Microbiol 2000;50:1125–1131.
14. Armstrong D, Yu BH, Yagoda A, et al. Colonization of humans by *Mycoplasma canis*. J Infect Dis 1971;124:607–609.
15. Barile MF. Mycoplasma-tissue cell interactions. In: Tully JG, Whitcomb RF, eds. The Mycoplasmas. Vol. 2. Human and Animal Mycoplasmas. New York: Academic Press, 1979:425–474.
16. Barile MF. DNA homologies and serologic relationships among ureaplasmas from various hosts. Pediatr Infect Dis 1986;5:S296–S299.
17. Barker CE, Sillis M, Wreghitt TG. Evaluation of Serodia Myco II particle agglutination test for detecting *Mycoplasma pneumoniae* antibody: comparison with mu-capture ELISA and indirect immunofluorescence. J Clin Pathol 1990;43:163–165.
18. Baseman JB, Cagle M, Korte JE, et al. Diagnostic assessment of *Mycoplasma genitalium* in culture-positive women. J Clin Microbiol 2004;42:203–211.
19. Baseman JB, Cole RM, Krause DC, Leith DK. Molecular basis for cytoadsorption of *M. pneumoniae*. J Bacteriol 1982;151:1514–1522.
20. Baseman JB, Dallo SF, Tully JG, et al. Isolation and characterization of *Mycoplasma genitalium* strains from the human respiratory tract. J Clin Microbiol 1988;26:2266–2269.
21. Bauer FA, Wear DJ, Angritt P, et al. *Mycoplasma fermentans* (incognitus strain) infection in the kidneys of patients with acquired immunodeficiency syndrome and associated nephropathy: a light microscopic, immunohistochemical, and ultrastructural study. Hum Pathol 1991;22:63–69.
22. Bebear C, deBarbeyrac B, Clerc M-T, et al. Mycoplasmas in HIV-1 seropositive patients. Lancet 1993;341:758–758.
23. Bebear C, Dupon M, Renaudin H, et al. Potential improvements in therapeutic options for mycoplasmal respiratory infections. Clin Infect Dis 1993;17(Suppl 1):S202–S207.
24. Bebear C, Robertson JA. Determination of minimal inhibitory concentration. In: Tully JG, Razin S, eds. Molecular and Diagnostic Procedures in Mycoplasmatology. Vol. 2. San Diego, CA: Academic Press, 1996:189–197.
25. Beecham HJ III, Lo SC, Lewis DE, et al. Recovery from fulminant infection with *Mycoplasma fermentans* (incognitus strain) in non-immunocompromised host. Lancet 1991;338:1014–1015.
26. Bejar R, Curbelo V, Dairs C, et al. Premature labor: bacterial sources of phospholipase. Obstet Gynecol 1981;57:479–482.
27. Bencina D, Bradbury JM. Combination of immunofluorescence and immunoperoxidase techniques for serotyping mixtures of *Mycoplasma* species. J Clin Microbiol 1992;30:407–410.
28. Bencina D, Dove P, Mueller-Premru M, et al. Intrathecal synthesis of specific antibodies in patients with invasion of the central nervous system by *Mycoplasma pneumoniae*. Eur J Clin Microbiol Infect Dis 2000;19:521–530.
29. Benstein BD, Crouse DT, Shanklin DR, Ourth DD. Ureaplasma in lung. 2. Association with bronchopulmonary dysplasia in premature newborns. Exp Mol Pathol 2003;75:171–177.
30. Biscardi S, Lorrot M, Marc E, et al. *Mycoplasma pneumoniae* and asthma in children. Clin Infect Dis 2004;38:1341–1346.
31. Bitnun A, Ford-Jones E, Blaser S, Richardson S. *Mycoplasma pneumoniae* encephalitis. Semin Pediatr Infect Dis 2003;14:96–107.
32. Blanchard A, Hamrick W, Duffy L, et al. Use of the polymerase chain reaction for detection of *Mycoplasma fermentans* and *Mycoplasma genitalium* in the urogenital tract and amniotic fluid. Clin Infect Dis 1993;17(Suppl 1):S272–S279.
33. Blanchard A, Hentschel J, Duffy L, et al. Detection of *Ureaplasma urealyticum* by polymerase chain reaction in the urogenital tracts of adults, in amniotic fluid,

and in the respiratory tract of newborns. Clin Infect Dis 1993;17(Suppl 1): S148–S153.

34. Blanchard A, Yanez A, Dybvig K, et al. Evaluation of intraspecies genetic variation within the 16S rRNA gene of *Mycoplasma hominis* and detection by polymerase chain reaction. J Clin Microbiol 1993;31:1358–1361.

35. Blasco M, Torres L, Marco ML, et al. Prosthetic valve endocarditis caused by *Mycoplasma hominis*. Eur J Clin Microbiol Infect Dis 2000;19:638–640.

36. Bobade PA, Nash AS. A comparative study of the efficiency of acridine orange and some Romanowsky staining procedures in the demonstration of *Haemobartonella felis* in feline blood. Vet Parasitol 1987;26:169–172.

37. Bochud P-Y, Moser F, Erard P, et al. Community-acquired pneumonia: a prospective outpatient study. Medicine (Baltimore) 2001;80:75–87.

38. Boesen T, Emmersen J, Jensen LT, et al. The *Mycoplasma hominis vaa* gene displays a mosaic gene structure. Mol Microbiol 1998;29:97–100.

39. Boesen T, Fedosova NU, Kjeldgaard M, et al. Molecular design of *Mycoplasma hominis* Vaa adhesin. Protein Sci 2001;10:2577–2596.

40. Bonilla HF, Chenoweth CE, Tully JG, et al. *Mycoplasma felis* septic arthritis in a patient with hypogammaglobulinemia. Clin Infect Dis 1997;24:222–225.

41. Brihmer C, Kallings I, Nord CE, Brundin J. Salpingitis: aspects of diagnosis and etiology: a four-year study from a Swedish capital hospital. Eur J Obstet Gynecol Reprod Biol 1987;24:211–220.

42. Broitman NL, Floyd CM, Johnson CA, et al. Comparison of commercially available media for detection and isolation of *Ureaplasma urealyticum* and *Mycoplasma hominis*. J Clin Microbiol 1992;30:1335–1337.

43. Brooker RJ, Eason JD, Solimano A. *Mycoplasma* surgical wound infection in a neonate. Pediatr Infect Dis J 1994;13:751–752.

44. Brunner S, Frey-Rindova P, Altwegg M, Zbinden R. Retroperitoneal abscess and bacteremia due to *Mycoplasma hominis* in a polytraumatized man. Infection 2000;28:46–48.

45. Brus F, Van Waarde WM, Schoots C, et al. Fatal ureaplasmal pneumonia and sepsis in a newborn infant. Eur J Pediatr 1991;150:782–783.

46. Buck GE, O'Hara LC, Summersgill JT. Rapid, sensitive detection of *Mycoplasma pneumoniae* in simulated specimens by DNA amplification. J Clin Microbiol 1992;30:3280–3283.

47. Burdge DR, Reid GD, Reeve CF, et al. Septic arthritis due to dual infection with *Mycoplasma hominis* and *Ureaplasma urealyticum*. J Rheumatol 1988;15: 366–368.

48. Cadieux N, Lebel P, Brousseau R. Use of a triplex polymerase chain reaction for the detection and differentiation of *Mycoplasma pneumoniae* and *Mycoplasma genitalium* in the presence of human DNA. J Gen Microbiol 1993;139: 2431–2437.

49. Campo L, Larocque P, La Malfa T, et al. Genotypic and phenotypic analysis of *Mycoplasma fermentans* strains isolated from different host tissues. J Clin Microbiol 36:1371–1377, 1998.

50. Casin I, Vexiau-Robert D, De La Salmoniere P, et al. High prevalence of *Mycoplasma genitalium* in the lower genitourinary tract of women attending a sexually transmitted disease clinic in Paris, France. Sex Transm Dis 2002;29:353–359.

51. Cassell GH, Waites KB, Crouse DT, et al. Association of *Ureaplasma urealyticum* of the lower respiratory tract with chronic lung disease and death in very-low-birth-weight infants. Lancet 1988;2:240–244.

52. Cassell GH, Waites KB, Gibbs RS, et al. Role of *Ureaplasma urealyticum* in amnionitis. Pediatr Infect Dis 1986;5:S247–S252.

53. Castro-Alcaraz S, Greenberg EM, Bateman DA, Regan JA. Patterns of colonization with *Ureaplasma urealyticum* during neonatal intensive care unit hospitalizations of very low birth weight infants with the development of chronic lung disease. Pediatric 2002;110:1–7.

54. Centers for Disease Control and Prevention. Sexually transmitted disease treatment guidelines 2002. Morbid Mortal Weekly Rep 2002;51(RR-6):1–78.

55. Chaim W, Horowitz S, David JB, et al. *Ureaplasma urealyticum* in the development of postpartum endometritis. Eur J Obstet Gynecol Reprod Biol 2003;109: 145–148.

56. Chaudhry R, Nisar N, Malhotra P, et al. Polymerase chain reaction confirmed *Mycoplasma pneumoniae* arthritis: a case report. Indian J Pathol Microbiol 200346:433–436.

57. Chen CJ, Juan CJ, Hsu ML, et al. *Mycoplasma pneumoniae* infection presenting as neutropenia, thrombocytopenia, and acute hepatitis in a child. J Microbiol Immunol Infect 2004;37:128–130.

58. Cheng X, Naessens A, Lauwers S. Identification of serotype 1-, 3-, and 6-specific antigens of *Ureaplasma urealyticum* by using monoclonal antibodies. J Clin Microbiol 1994;32:1060–1062.

59. Cherry JD. Anemia and mucocutaneous lesions due to *Mycoplasma pneumoniae* infections. Clin Infect Dis 1993;17(Suppl 1):S47–S51.

60. Cherry JD, Hurwitz ES, Welliver RC. *Mycoplasma pneumoniae* infections and exanthems. J Pediatr 1975;87:369–371.

61. Chingbingyong MI, Hughes CV. Detection of *Mycoplasma fermentans* in human saliva with a polymerase chain reaction-based assay. Arch Oral Biol 1996;41: 311–314.

62. Chirgwin KD, Cummings MC, DeMeo LR, et al. Identification of mycoplasmas

in urine from persons infected with human immunodeficiency virus. Clin Infect Dis 1993;17(Suppl 1):S264–S266.

63. Choppa PC, Vojdani A, Tagle C, et al. Multiplex PCR for the detection of *Mycoplasma fermentans*, *M. hominis*, and *M. penetrans* in cell cultures and blood samples of patients with chronic fatigue syndrome. Mol Cell Probes 1998; 12:301–308.

64. Christiansen G, Andersen H. Heterogeneity among *Mycoplasma hominis* strains as detected by probes containing parts of ribosomal ribonucleic acid genes. Int J Syst Bacteriol 1988;38:108–115.

65. Cimolai N, Bryan LE, To M, et al. Immunological cross-reactivity of a *Mycoplasma pneumoniae* membrane-associated protein antigen with *Mycoplasma genitalium* and *Acholeplasma laidlawii*. J Clin Microbiol 1987;25:2136–2139.

66. Cimolai N, Schryvers A, Bryan LE, et al. Culture-amplified immunological detection of *Mycoplasma pneumoniae* in clinical specimens. Diagn Microbiol Infect Dis 1988;9:207–212.

67. Clausen HF, Fedder J, Drasbek M, et al. Serological investigation of *Mycoplasma genitalium* in infertile women. Human Reproduction 2001;16:1866–1874.

68. Clough W, Cassell GH, Duffy LB, et al. Septic arthritis and bacteremia due to *Mycoplasma* resistant to antimicrobial therapy in a patient with systemic lupus erythematosus. Clin Infect Dis 1992;15:402–407.

69. Clyde WA. Clinical overview of typical *Mycoplasma pneumoniae* infections. Clin Infect Dis 1993;17(Suppl 1):S32–S36.

70. Cohen CR, Manhart LE, Bukusi EA, et al. Association between *Mycoplasma genitalium* and acute endometritis. Lancet 2002;359:765–766.

71. Corsaro D, Valassina M, Venditti D, et al. Multiplex PCR for rapid and differential diagnosis of *Mycoplasma pneumoniae* and *Chlamydia pneumoniae* in respiratory infections. Diagn Microbiol Infect Dis 1999;35:105–108.

72. Costea N, Yakulis VJ, Heller P. The mechanism of induction of cold agglutinins by *Mycoplasma pneumoniae*. J Immunol 1971;106:598–604.

73. Coufalik ED. Taylor-Robinson, Csonka GW. Treatment of nongonococcal urethritis with rifampicin as a means of defining the role of *Ureaplasma urealyticum*. Br J Vener Dis 1979;55:36.

74. Crouse DT, Odrezin GT, Cutter GR, et al. Radiographic changes associated with tracheal isolation of *Ureaplasma urealyticum* from neonates. Clin Infect Dis 1993;17(Suppl 1):S122–S130.

75. Cunningham CK, Bonville CA, Hagen JH, et al. Immunoblot analysis of anti-*Ureaplasma urealyticum* antibody in pregnant women and newborn infants. Clin Diagn Lab Immunol 1996;3:487–492.

76. Dallo SF, Baseman JB. Intracellular DNA replication and long-term survival of pathogenic mycoplasmas. Microb Pathog 2000;29:301–309.

77. Dallo SF, Chavoya A, Su CJ, et al. DNA and protein sequence homologies between the adhesins of *Mycoplasma genitalium* and *Mycoplasma pneumoniae*. Infect Immun 1989;57:1059–1065.

78. Dallo SF, Horten JR, Su CJ, et al. Homologous regions shared by adhesin genes of *Mycoplasma pneumoniae* and *Mycoplasma genitalium*. Microb Pathog 1989; 6:69–73.

79. Dan M, Tyrrell DLJ, Stemke GW, et al. *Mycoplasma hominis* septicemia in a burned infant. J Pediatr 1981;99:743–745.

80. Davies S, Eggington R. Recovery of *Mycoplasma hominis* from blood culture media. Med Lab Sci 1991;48:110–113.

81. Davis CP, Cochran S, Lisse J, et al. Isolation of *Mycoplasma pneumoniae* from synovial fluid samples in a patient with pneumonia and polyarthritis. Arch Intern Med 1988;148:969–970.

82. Dawson MS, Hayes MM, Wang RY-H, et al. Detection and isolation of *Mycoplasma fermentans* from urine of human immunodeficiency virus type 1-infected patients. Arch Pathol Lab Med 1993;117:511–514.

83. Daxboeck F, Iro E, Tamussino K, et al. Bacteremia with *Mycoplasma hominis* and *Ureaplasma urealyticum* in patients undergoing hysterectomy. Eur J Clin Microbiol Infect Dis 22:608–611, 2003.

84. Daxboeck F, Krause R, Wenisch C. Laboratory diagnosis of *Mycoplasma pneumoniae* infection. Clin Microbiol Infect 2003;9:263–273.

85. Daxboeck F, Zedtwitz-Liebenstein K, Burgmann H, Graninger W. Severe hemolytic anemia and excessive leukocytosis masking *Mycoplasma pneumoniae*. Ann Hematol 2001;80:180–182.

86. deBarbeyrac B, Bernet-Poggi C, Febrer F, et al. Detection of *Mycoplasma pneumoniae* and *Mycoplasma genitalium* in clinical samples by polymerase chain reaction. Clin Infect Dis 1993;17(Suppl 1):S83–S89.

87. DeCordova CMM, Takei K, Rosenthal C, et al. Evaluation of IgG, IgM, and IgA antibodies to *Mycoplasma penetrans* detected by ELISA and immunoblot in HIV-1-infected and STD patients in Sao Paolo, Brazil. Microb Infect 1999; 1:1095–1101.

88. DeGirolami PC, Madoff S. *Mycoplasma hominis* septicemia. J Clin Microbiol 1982;16:566–567.

89. Deguchi T, Gilroy CB, Taylor-Robinson D. Failure to detect *Mycoplasma fermentans*, *Mycoplasma penetrans*, or *Mycoplasma pirum* in the urethra of patients with acute nongonococcal urethritis. Eur J Clin Microbiol Infect Dis 1996;15: 169–171.

90. Deguchi T, Komeda H, Yasuda M, et al. *Mycoplasma genitalium* in nongonococcal urethritis. Int J STD AIDS 1995;6:144–145.

91. Deguchi T, Maeda S-I. *Mycoplasma genitalium*: another important pathogen of nongonococcal urethritis. J Urol 2002;167:1210–1217.

92. Deguchi T, Maeda S-I, Tamaki M, et al. Analysis of the *gyrA* and *parC* genes of *Mycoplasma genitalium* detected in first-pass urine of men with non-gonococcal urethritis before and after fluoroquinolone treatment. J Antimicrob Chemother 2001;48:735–748.

93. Deguchi T, Yoshida T, Miyazawa T, et al. Association of *Ureaplasma urealyticum* (biovar 2) with non-gonococcal urethritis. Sex Transm Dis 2004;31:192–195.

94. Deguchi T, Yoshida T, Yokoi S, et al. Longitudinal quantitative detection by real-time PCR of *Mycoplasma genitalium* in first-pass urine of men with recurrent nongonococcal urethritis. J Clin Microbiol 2002;40:3854–3856.

95. Del Giudice RA, Carski TR, Barile MF, et al. Proposal for classifying human strain Navel and related simian mycoplasmas as *Mycoplasma primatum* sp. n. J Bacteriol 1971;108:439–445.

96. Del Giudice RA, Tully JG, Rose DL,, et al. *Mycoplasma pirum* sp. nov., a terminal structured mollicute from cell cultures. Int J Syst Bacteriol 1985;35:285–291.

97. De Silva NS, Quinn PA. Endogenous activity of phospholipases A and C in *Ureaplasma urealyticum*. J Clin Microbiol 1986;23:354–359.

98. Dimitrov DS, Franzoso G, Salman M, et al. *Mycoplasma fermentans* (incognitus strain) cells are able to fuse with T lymphocytes. Clin Infect Dis 1993;17(Suppl 1):S305–S308.

99. Dinsmoor MJ, Ramamurthy RS, Gibbs RS. Transmission of genital mycoplasmas from mother to neonate in women with prolonged membrane rupture. Pediatr Infect Dis J 1989;8:843–847.

100. Donders GGG, Van Bulck B, Caudron J, et al. Relationship of bacterial vaginosis and mycoplasmas to the risk of spontaneous abortion. Am J Obstet Gynecol 2000;183:431–437.

101. Dorigo-Zetsma JW, Zaat SAJ, Wertheim-van Dillen, et al. Comparison of PCR, culture, and serological tests for diagnosis of *Mycoplasma pneumoniae* respiratory tract infection in children. J Clin Microbiol 1999;37:14–17.

102. Drasbek M, Nielsen PK, Persson K, et al. Immune response to *Mycoplasma pneumoniae* P1 and P116 in patients with atypical pneumonia analyzed by ELISA. BMC Microbiol 2004;4:1–10.

103. Duffy LB, Crabb D, Searcey K, Kempf MC. Comparative potency of gemifloxacin, new quinolones, macrolides, tetracycline, and clindamycin against Mycoplasma spp. J Antimicrob Chemother 2000;45(Suppl S1):29–33.

104. Duffy MF, Walker ID, Browning GF. The immunoreactive 116 kDa surface protein of *M. pneumoniae* is encoded in an operon. Microbiology 1997;143:3391–3402.

105. Duffy MF, Whithear KG, Noormohammadi AH, et al. Indirect enzyme-linked immunosorbent assay for detection of immunoglobulin G reactive with a recombinant protein expressed from the gene encoding the 116-kilodalton protein of *Mycoplasma pneumoniae*. J Clin Microbiol 199937:1024–1029,.

106. Dular R, Kajioka R, Kasatiya S. Comparison of Gen-Probe commercial kit and culture technique for the diagnosis of *Mycoplasma pneumoniae* infection. J Clin Microbiol 1988;26:1068–1069.

107. Dunn JJ, Malan AK, Evans J, Litwin CM. Rapid detection of *Mycoplasma pneumoniae* IgM antibodies in pediatric patients using ImmunoCard Mycoplasma compared to conventional immunoassays. Eur J Clin Microbiol Infect Dis 2004;23:412–414.

108. Dupin N, Bijaoui G, Schwarzinger M, et al. Detection and quantitation of *Mycoplasma genitalium* in male patients with urethritis. Clin Infect Dis 2003;37:602–605.

109. Dutro SM, Hebb JK, Garub CA, et al. Development and performance of a microwell-plate-based polymerase chain reaction assay for *Mycoplasma genitalium*. Sex Transm Dis 2003;30:756–763.

110. Eastick K, Leeming JP, Caul EO, et al. A novel polymerase chain reaction assay to detect *Mycoplasma genitalium*. J Clin Pathol Mol Pathol 2003;56:25–28.

111. Embree J. *Mycoplasma hominis* in maternal and fetal infections. Ann NY Acad Sci 1988;549:56–64.

112. Eschenbach DA. *Ureaplasma urealyticum* as a cause of postpartum fever. Pediatr Infect Dis 1986;5:S258–S261.

113. Eschenbach DA. *Ureaplasma urealyticum* and premature birth. Clin Infect Dis 1993;17(Suppl 1):S100–S106.

114. Falk L, Fredlund H, Jensen JS. Tetracycline treatment does not eradicate *Mycoplasma genitalium*. Sex Transm Dis 2003;79:318–319.

115. Fedorko DP, Emery DD, Franklin SM, Congdon DD. Evaluation of a rapid enzyme immunoassay system for serologic diagnosis of *Mycoplasma pneumoniae* infection. Diagn Microbiol Infect Dis 1996;23:85–88.

116. Feldner J, Gobel U, Bredt W. *Mycoplasma pneumoniae* adhesion localized to tip structure by monoclonal antibody. Nature 1982;298:765–767.

117. Feng S-H, Lo S-C. Induced mouse spleen B-cell proliferation and secretion of immunoglobulin by lipid-associated membrane proteins of *Mycoplasma fer-*

mentans incognitus and *Mycoplasma penetrans*. Infect Immun 1994;62:3916–3921.

118. Fenkci V, Yilmazer M, Aktepe OC. Have *Ureaplasma urealyticum* and *Mycoplasma hominis* infections any significant effect on women infertility? Infect Med 2002;10:220–223.

119. Fiacco V, Miller MJ, Carney E, et al. Comparison of media for isolation of *Ureaplasma urealyticum* and genital *Mycoplasma* species. J Clin Microbiol 1984;20:862–865.

120. Fischman Marschall KE, Kislak W, et al. Adult respiratory distress syndrome caused by *Mycoplasma pneumoniae*. Chest 1978;74:471–473.

121. Foy HM. Infections caused by *Mycoplasma pneumoniae* and possible carrier state in different populations of patients. Clin Infect Dis 1993;17(Suppl 1):S37–S46.

122. Furneri PM, Bisignano G, Cerniglia G, et al. *In vitro* antimycoplasmal activity of flurithromycin. J Antimicrob Chemother 1995;35:161–165.

123. Gallily R, Salman M, Tarshis M, et al. *Mycoplasma fermentans* (incognitus strain) induces TNFα, and IL-1 production by human monocytes and murine macrophages. Immunol Lett 1992;34:27–30.

124. Gambini D, Decleva I, Lupica L, et al. *Mycoplasma genitalium* in males with nongonococcal urethritis: prevalence and clinical efficacy of eradication. Sex Transm Dis 2000;27:226–229.

125. Gauthier DW, Meyer WJ, Bieniarz A. Expectant management of premature rupture of membranes with amniotic fluid cultures positive for *Ureaplasma urealyticum* alone. Am J Obstet Gynecol 1994;170:587–590.

126. Geissdorfer W, Schorner C, Lohoff M. Systemic *Mycoplasma hominis* infection in a patient immunocompromised due to combined transplantation of kidney and pancreas. Eur J Clin Microbiol Infect Dis 2001;20:511–512.

127. Gibbs RS, Cassell GH, Davis JK, et al. Further studies on genital mycoplasmas in intra-amniotic infection: blood cultures and serologic response. Am J Obstet Gynecol 1986;154:717–726.

128. Gilbert GL, Drew JH. Chronic *Mycoplasma hominis* infection complicating severe intraventricular hemorrhage in a premature neonate. Pediatr Infect Dis J 1988;7:817–818.

129. Gilbert GL, Garland SM, Fairley KF, et al. Bacteriuria due to ureaplasmas and other fastidious organisms during pregnancy: prevalence and significance. Pediatr Infect Dis 1986;5:S239–S243.

130. Gilroy CB, Keat A, Taylor-Robinson D. The prevalence of *Mycoplasma fermentans* in patients with inflammatory arthritides. Rheumatology (Oxford) 2001;40:1355–1358.

131. Glaser JB, Engelberg M, Hammerschlag M. Scalp abscess associated with *Mycoplasma hominis* infection complicating intrapartum monitoring. Pediatr Infect Dis 1983;2:468–470.

132. Goulet M, Dular R, Tully JG, et al. Isolation of *Mycoplasma pneumoniae* from the human urogenital tract. J Clin Microbiol 1995;33:2823–2825.

133. Grau O, Kovacic R, Griffais R, et al. Development of a selective and sensitive polymerase chain reaction assay for the detection of *Mycoplasma pirum*. FEMS Microbiol Lett 1993;106:327–334.

134. Grau O, Kovacic R, Griffais, et al. Development of PCR-based assays for the detection of two human mollicute species: *Mycoplasma penetrans* and *Mycoplasma hominis*. Mol Cell Probes 1994;8:139–148.

135. Grau O, Slizewicz B, Tuppin P, et al. Association of *Mycoplasma penetrans* with human immunodeficiency virus infection. J Infect Dis 1995;172:672–681.

136. Grau O, Tuppin P, Slizewicz B, et al. A longitudinal study of seroreactivity against *Mycoplasma penetrans* in HIV-infected homosexual men: association with disease progression. AIDS Res Hum Retroviruses 1998;14:661–667.

137. Gravat MG, Eschenbach DA. Possible role of *Ureaplasma urealyticum* in preterm premature rupture of the fetal membranes. Pediatr Infect Dis 1986;5:S253–S257.

138. Gray DJ, Robinson HB, Malone J, Thomson RB Jr. Adverse outcome in pregnancy following amniotic fluid isolation of *Ureaplasma urealyticum*. Prenat Diagn 1992;12:111–117.

139. Gray GC, Kaiser KS, Hawksworth AW, Watson HL. No serologic evidence of an association found between Gulf War service and *Mycoplasma fermentans* infection. Am J Trop Med Hyg 1999;60:752–757.

140. Grullich C, Baumert TF, Blum HE. Acute *Mycoplasma pneumoniae* infection presenting as cholestatic hepatitis. J Clin Microbiol 2003;41:514–515.

141. Haller M, Forst H, Ruckdeschel G, et al. Peritonitis due to *Mycoplasma hominis* and *Ureaplasma urealyticum* in a liver transplant recipient. Eur J Clin Microbiol Infect Dis 1993;10:172.

142. Hannaford K, Todd DA, Jeffery H, et al. Role of *Ureaplasma urealyticum* in lung disease of prematurity. Arch Dis Child Neonatal Ed 1999;81:F162–F167.

143. Hannan PCT. Antibiotic susceptibility of *Mycoplasma fermentans* strains from various sources and the development of resistance to aminoglycosides *in vitro*. J Med Microbiol 1995;42:421–428.

144. Hannan PCT. Observations on the possible origin of *Mycoplasma fermentans* incognitus strain based on antibiotic sensitivity tests. J Antimicrob Chemother 1997;39:25–30.

145. Hannan PCT. Comparative susceptibilities of various AIDS-associated and

human urogenital tract mycoplasmas and strains of *Mycoplasma pneumoniae* to 10 classes of antimicrobial agents *in vitro*. J Med Microbiol 1998;47:1115–1122.

146. Hannan PCT, Kearns AM, Sisson PR, Freeman R. Differentiation of strains of *Mycoplasma fermentans* from various sources by pyrolysis mass spectrometry. J Med Microbiol 1997;46:348–353.

147. Harasawa R, Dybvig K, Watson HL, et al. Two genomic clusters among 14 serovars of *Ureaplasma urealyticum*. Syst Appl Microbiol 1991;14:393–396.

148. Harasawa R, Imada Y, Ito M, et al. *Ureaplasma felinum* sp. nov. and *Ureaplasma cati* sp. nov. isolated from the oral cavities of cats. Int J Syst Bacteriol 1990; 40:45–51.

149. Harasawa R, Imada Y, Kotani H, et al. *Ureaplasma canigenitalium* sp. nov., isolated from dogs. Int J Syst Bacteriol 1993;43:640–644.

150. Harasawa R, Stephens EB, Koshimizu K, et al. DNA relatedness among established *Ureaplasma* species and unidentified feline and canine serogroups. Int J Syst Bacteriol 1990;40:52–55.

151. Harrison HR. Cervical colonization with *Ureaplasma urealyticum* and pregnancy outcome: prospective studies. Pediatr Infect Dis 1986;266–S269.

152. Hawkins RE, Rickman LS, Vermund SH, et al. Association of mycoplasma and human immunodeficiency virus infection: detection of amplified *Mycoplasma fermentans* DNA in blood. J Infect Dis 1992;165:581–585.

153. Hayes MM, Foo H-H, Kotani H, et al. *In vitro* antibiotic susceptibility testing of different strains of *Mycoplasma fermentans* isolated from a variety of sources. Antimicrob Agents Chemother 1993;37:2500–2503.

154. Hayes MM, Foo H-H, Timenetsky J, et al. *In vitro* antibiotic susceptibility testing of clinical isolates of *Mycoplasma penetrans* from patients with AIDS. Antimicrob Agents Chemother 1995;39:1386–1387.

155. Hayes MM, Wear DJ, Lo S-C. *In vitro* antimicrobial susceptibility testing for the newly identified AIDS-associated mycoplasma. Arch Pathol Lab Med 1991; 115:464–466.

156. Heggie AD, Jacobs MR, Butler VT, et al. Frequency and significance of isolation of *Ureaplasma urealyticum* and *Mycoplasma hominis* from cerebrospinal fluid and tracheal aspirate specimens from low birth weight infants. J Pediatr 1994; 124:956–961.

157. Henrich B, Feldmann R-C, Hadding U. Cytoadhesins of *Mycoplasma hominis*. Infect Immun 1993;61:2945–2951.

158. Henrich B, Hoppe M, Kitzerow A, Hadding U. The adherence-associated lipoprotein P100, encoded by an *opp* operon structure, functions as the oligopeptide-binding domain OppA of a putative oligopeptide transport system in *Mycoplasma hominis*. J Bacteriol 1999;181:4873–4878,.

159. Hill AC. *Mycoplasma spermatophilum*, a new species isolated from human spermatozoa and cervix. Int J Syst Bacteriol 1991;41:229–233.

160. Hill GB, Livengood CH. Bacterial vaginosis–associated microflora and effects of topical intravaginal clindamycin. Am J Obstet Gynecol 1994;171:1198–1204.

161. Hirai Y, Kanatani T, Ono M, et al. An indirect immunofluorescence method for detection of *Mycoplasma hominis* in vaginal smears. Microbiol Immunol 1991; 35:831–839.

162. Honda J, Yano T, Kusaba M, et al. Clinical use of capillary PCR to diagnose *Mycoplasma pneumoniae*. J Clin Microbiol 2000;38:1382–1384.

163. Hooton TM, Roberts MC, Roberts PL, et al. Prevalence of *Mycoplasma genitalium* determined by DNA probe in men with urethritis. Lancet 1988;1: 266–268.

164. Horner PJ, Gilroy CB, Thomas BJ, et al. Association of *Mycoplasma genitalium* with acute non-gonococcal urethritis. Lancet 1993;342:582–585.

165. Horner PJ, Thomas B, Gilroy CB, et al. Role of *Mycoplasma genitalium* and *Ureaplasma urealyticum* in acute and chronic nongonococcal urethritis. Clin Infect Dis 2001;32:995–1003.

166. Horner PJ, Thomas B, Gilroy C, et al. Antibodies to *Chlamydia trachomatis* heat-shock protein 60 kDa and detection of *Mycoplasma genitalium* and *Ureaplasma urealyticum* are associated independently with chronic nongonococcal urethritis. Sex Transm Dis 2003;30:129–133.

167. Horowitz S, Evinson B, Borer A, Horowitz J. *Mycoplasma fermentans* in rheumatoid arthritis and other inflammatory arthritides. J Rheumatol 2000;27: 2747–2752.

168. Horowitz S, Horowitz J, Hou L, et al. Antibodies to *Mycoplasma fermentans* in HIV-positive heterosexual patients: seroprevalence and association with AIDS. J Infect 1998;36:79–84.

169. Horowitz S, Horowitz J, Mazor M, et al. *Ureaplasma urealyticum* cervical colonization as a marker of pregnancy complications. Int J Gynecol Obstet 1995; 48:15–19.

170. Horowitz S, Mazor M, Horowitz J, et al. Antibodies to *Ureaplasma urealyticum* in women with intraamniotic infection and adverse pregnancy outcome. Acta Obstet Gynecol Scand 1995;74:132–136.

171. Horowitz S, Mazor M, Romero R, et al. Infection of the amniotic cavity with *Ureaplasma urealyticum* in the midtrimester of pregnancy. J Reprod Med 1995; 40:375–379.

172. Hosker HSR, Tam JS, Chan CHS, Lai CKW. *Mycoplasma pneumoniae* infection in Hong Kong: clinical features during an epidemic. Respiration 1993;60: 237–240.

173. Howard CJ, Gourley RN. Proposal for a second species within the genus *Ureaplasma*, *Ureaplasma diversum* sp. nov. Int J Syst Bacteriol 1982;32:446–452.

174. Hu PC, Cole RM, Huang YS, et al. *Mycoplasma pneumoniae* infection: role of surface protein in the attachment organelle. Science 1982;216:1126–1131.

175. Hu PC, Huang CH, Collier AM, Clyde WA Jr. Demonstration of antibodies to *Mycoplasma pneumoniae* attachment protein in human sera and respiratory secretions. Infect Immun 1983;41:437–439.

176. Hussain AI, Robson WLM, Kelley R, et al. *Mycoplasma penetrans* and other mycoplasmas in urine of human immunodeficiency virus-positive children. J Clin Microbiol 1999;37:1518–1523.

177. Hyman HC, Yogev D, Razin S. DNA probes for detection of *Mycoplasma pneumoniae* and *Mycoplasma genitalium*. J Clin Microbiol 1987;25:726–728.

178. Ieven M, Ursi D, Van Bever H, et al. Detection of *Mycoplasma pneumoniae* by two polymerase chain reactions and role of *M. pneumoniae* in acute respiratory tract infections in pediatric patients. J Infect Dis 1996;173:1445–1452.

179. Imada Y, Uchida I, Hashimoto K. Rapid identification of mycoplasmas by indirect immunoperoxidase test using small square filter paper. J Clin Microbiol 1987;25:17–21.

180. Iyama K, Ono S, Kuwano K, et al. Induction of tumour necrosis factor-α (TNFα) and enhancement of HIV-1 replication in the J22HL60 cell line by *Mycoplasma penetrans*. Microbiol Immunol 1996;40:907–914.

181. Izraeli S, Samra Z, Sirota L, et al. Genital mycoplasmas in preterm infants: prevalence and clinical significance. Eur J Pediatr 1991;150:804–807.

182. Jacobs E. Serological diagnosis of *Mycoplasma pneumoniae* infections: a critical review of current procedures. Clin Infect Dis 1993;17(Suppl 1):S79–S82.

183. Jacobs E, Bennewitz A, Bredt W. Reaction patterns of human anti-*Mycoplasma pneumoniae* antibodies in enzyme-linked immunosorbent assays and immunoblotting. J Clin Microbiol 1986;23:517–522.

184. Jacobs E, Buchholz A, Kleinman B, et al. Use of adherence protein of *Mycoplasma pneumoniae* as antigen for enzyme-linked immunosorbent assay (ELISA). Isr J Med Sci 1987;23:709–712.

185. Jacobs E, Pilatschek A, Gerstenecker B, et al. Immunodominant epitopes of the adhesin of *Mycoplasma pneumoniae*. J Clin Microbiol 1990;28:1194–1197.

186. Jacobs E, Vonski M, Stemke GW, et al. Identification of *Ureaplasma* biotypes. Med Microbiol Lett 1994;3:31–35.

187. Jacobs F, Van de Stadt J, Gelin M, et al. *Mycoplasma hominis* infection of perihepatic hematomas in a liver transplant recipient. Surgery 1992;111:98–100.

188. Jalil N, Doble A, Gilchrist C, et al. Infection of the epididymis by *Ureaplasma urealyticum*. Genitourin Med 1988;62:367–368.

189. Janney FA, Lee LT, Howe C. Cold hemagglutinin cross-reactivity with *Mycoplasma pneumoniae*. Infect Immun 1978;22:29–30.

190. Jensen JS. *Mycoplasma genitalium*: the aetiological agent of urethritis and other sexually transmitted diseases. Eur Acad Dermatol Venereol 2004;18:1–11.

191. Jensen JS, Bjornelius E, Dohn B, Lidbrink P. Use of TaqMan 5′ nuclease real-time PCR for quantitative detection of *Mycoplasma genitalium* DNA in males with and without urethritis who were attendees at a sexually-transmitted disease clinic. J Clin Microbiol 2004;42:683–692.

192. Jensen JS, Borre MB, Dohn B. Detection of *Mycoplasma genitalium* by PCR amplification of the 16S rRNA gene. J Clin Microbiol 2003;41:261–266.

193. Jensen JS, Hansen HT, Lind K. Isolation of *Mycoplasma genitalium* strains from the male urethra. J Clin Microbiol 1996;34:286–291.

194. Jensen JS, Heilmann C, Valerius NH. *Mycoplasma pneumoniae* infection in a child with AIDS. Clin Infect Dis 1994;19:207.

195. Jensen JS, Orsum R, Dohn B, et al. *Mycoplasma genitalium*: a cause of male urethritis? Genitourin Med 1993;69:265–269.

196. Jensen JS, Uldum SA, Sondergard-Andersen J, Vuust J, et al. Polymerase chain reaction for detection of *Mycoplasma genitalium* in clinical samples. J Clin Microbiol 1991;29:46–50.

197. Johannisson G, Enstrom Y, Lowhagen GB, et al. Occurrence and treatment of *Mycoplasma genitalium* in patients visiting STD clinics in Sweden. Int J STD AIDS 2000;11:324–326.

198. Johansson KE, Tully JG, Bolske G, Pettersson B. *Mycoplasma cavipharyngis* and *Mycoplasma fastidiosum*, the closest relatives to *Eperythrozoon* spp. and *Haemobartonella* spp. FEMS Microbiol Lett 1999;174:321–326.

199. Johnson S, Sidebottom D, Bruckner F, Collins D. Identification of *Mycoplasma fermentans* in synovial fluid samples from arthritis patients with inflammatory disease. J Clin Microbiol 2000;38:90–93.

200. Johnston CLW, Webster ADB, Taylor-Robinson D, et al. Primary late-onset hypogammaglobulinemia associated with inflammatory polyarthritis and septic arthritis due to *Mycoplasma pneumoniae*. Ann Rheum Dis 1983;42:108–110.

201. Jordan JL, Berry KM, Balish MF, Krause DC. Stability and subcellular localization of cytadherence-associated protein P65 in *Mycoplasma pneumoniae*. J Bacteriol 2001;183:7387–7391.

202. Jorup-Ronstrom C, Ahl T, Hammarstrom L, et al. Septic osteomyelitis and polyarthritis with *Ureaplasma* in hypogammaglobulinemia. Infection 1989;17: 301–303.

203. Joste NE, Kundsin RB, Genest DR. Histology and *Ureaplasma urealyticum*

culture in 63 cases of first trimester abortion. Am J Clin Pathol 1994;102: 729–732.

204. Kakulphimp J, Finch LR, Robertson JA. Genome sizes of mammalian and avian ureaplasmas. Int J Syst Bacteriol 1991;41:326–327.

205. Kane JR, Shenep JL, Krance RA, et al. Diffuse alveolar hemorrhage associated with *Mycoplasma hominis* respiratory tract infection in a bone marrow transplant recipient. Chest 1994;105:1891–1892.

206. Kapatais-Zoumbos K, Chandler DKF, Barile MF. Survey of immunoglobulin A protease activity among selected species of *Ureaplasma* and *Mycoplasma*: specificity for host immunoglobulin A. Infect Immun 1985;47:704–709.

207. Kass EH, Lin J-S, McCormack WM. Low birth weight and maternal colonization with genital mycoplasmas. Pediatr Infect Dis 1986;5:S279–S281.

208. Katseni VL, Gilroy CB, Ryait BK, et al. *Mycoplasma fermentans* in individuals seropositive and seronegative for HIV-1. Lancet 1993;341:271–273.

209. Kaufmann A, Muhlradt PF, Gemsa D, Sprenger H. Induction of cytokines and chemokines in human monocytes by *Mycoplasma fermentans*-derived lipoprotein MALP-2. Infect Immun 1999;67:6303–5308.

210. Kayser S, Bhend HJ. Lumbar pain caused by *Mycoplasma* infection. Infection 1992;20:97–98.

211. Keane FE, Thomas BJ, Gilroy CB, et al. The association of *Mycoplasma hominis*, *Ureaplasma urealyticum* and *Mycoplasma genitalium* with bacterial vaginosis: observations on heterosexual women and their male partners. Int J STD AIDS 2000;11:356–360.

212. Kenney RT, Li JS, Clyde WA Jr, et al. *Mycoplasma* pericarditis: evidence of invasive disease. Clin Infect Dis 1993;17(Suppl 1):S58–S62.

213. Kenny GE, Cartwright FD. Susceptibility of *Mycoplasma pneumoniae* to several new quinolones, tetracycline, and erythromycin. Antimicrob Agents Chemother 1991;35:587–589.

214. Kenny GE, Cartwright FD. Susceptibilities of *Mycoplasma hominis* and *Ureaplasma urealyticum* to two new quinolones, sparfloxacin and WIN 57273. Antimicrob Agents Chemother 1991;35:1515–1516.

215. Kenny GE, Cartwright FD. Effect of pH, inoculum size, and incubation time on the susceptibility of *Ureaplasma urealyticum* to erythromycin *in vitro*. Clin Infect Dis 1993;17(Suppl):215–218.

216. Kenny GE, Cartwright FD. Susceptibilities of *Mycoplasma hominis*, *Mycoplasma pneumoniae*, and *Ureaplasma urealyticum* to a new quinolone, OPC 17116. Antimicrob Agents Chemother 1993;37:1726–1727.

217. Kenny GE, Cartwright FD. Susceptibilities of *Mycoplasma hominis*, *M. pneumoniae*, and *Ureaplasma urealyticum* to GAR-936, dalfopristin, dirithromycin, evernimicin, gatifloxacin, linezolid, moxifloxacin, quinupristin-dalfopristin, and telithromycin compared to their susceptibilities to reference macrolides, tetracyclines, and quinolones. Antimicrob Agents Chemother 2001;45:2604–2608.

218. Kenny GE, Cartwright FD, Roberts MC. Agar dilution method for determination of antibiotic susceptibility of *Ureaplasma urealyticum*. Pediatr Infect Dis 1986; 5:S332–S334.

219. Kenny GE, Hooten TM, Roberts MC, et al. Susceptibilities of genital mycoplasmas to the newer quinolones as determined by the agar dilution method. Antimicrob Agents Chemother 1989;33:103–107.

220. Kenny GE, Kaiser GG, Cooney MK, et al. Diagnosis of *Mycoplasma pneumoniae* pneumonia: sensitivities and specificities of serology with lipid antigen and isolation of the organism on two peptone medium for identification of infections. J Clin Microbiol 1990;28:2087–2093.

221. Kersten RC, Haglund L, Kulwin DR, et al. *Mycoplasma hominis* orbital abscess. Arch Ophthalmol 1995;113:1096–1097.

222. Kho SH, Hajia M, Storey CC, et al. Influenza-like episodes in HIV-positive patients: the role of viral and "atypical" infections. AIDS 1998;12:751–757.

223. Kitzerow A, Hadding U, Henrich B. Cyto-adherence studies of the adhesion P50 of *Mycoplasma hominis*. J Med Microbiol 1999;48:485–493.

224. Kok T-W, Vrkanis G, Marmion BP, et al. Laboratory diagnosis of *Mycoplasma pneumoniae* infection. I. Direct detection of antigen in respiratory exudates by enzyme immunoassay. Epidemiol Infect 1988;101:669–684.

225. Koletsky RJ, Weinstein AJ. Fulminant *Mycoplasma pneumoniae* infection. Am Rev Respir Dis 1980;122:491–469.

226. Kong F, Gordon S, Gilbert GL. Rapid cycle PCR for detection and typing of *Mycoplasma pneumoniae* in clinical specimens. J Clin Microbiol 2000;38: 4253–4259.

227. Kong F, James G, Ma Z, et al. Phylogenetic studies of *Ureaplasma urealyticum*: support for the establishment of a new species, *Ureaplasma parvum*. Int J Syst Bacteriol 1999;4:1879–1889.

228. Koshimizu K, Harasawa R, Pan I-J, et al. *Ureaplasma gallorale* sp. nov. from the oropharynx of chickens. Int J Syst Bacteriol 1987;37:333–338.

229. Kostyal DA, Butler GH, Beezhold DH. A 48-kilodalton *Mycoplasma fermentans* membrane protein induces cytokine secretion by human monocytes. Infect Immun 1994;62:3793–3800.

230. Kotecha S, Wilson L, Wangoo A, et al. Increase in interleukin (IL)-1-β and IL-6 in bronchoalveolar lavage fluid obtained from infants with chronic lung disease of prematurity. Pediatr Res 1996;40:250–256.

231. Kotikoski MJ, Kleemola M, Palmu AA. No evidence of *Mycoplasma pneumoniae* in acute myringitis. Pediatr Infect Dis J 2004;23:465–466.

232. Kountouras D, Deutsch M, Emmanuel T, et al. Fulminant *Mycoplasma pneumoniae* infection with multi-organ involvement: a case report. Eur J Intern Med 2003;14:329–331.

233. Kovacic R, Launay V, Tuppin P, et al. Search for the presence of six *Mycoplasma* species in peripheral blood mononuclear cells of subjects seropositive and seronegative for human immunodeficiency virus. J Clin Microbiol 1996;34: 1808–1810.

234. Kraft M, Cassell GH, Henson JE, et al. Detection of *Mycoplasma pneumoniae* in the airways of adults with chronic asthma. Am J Respir Crit Care Med 1998; 158:998–1001.

235. Krause DC. *Mycoplasma pneumoniae* cytadherence: organization and assembly of the attachment organelle. Trends Microbiol 1998;6:15–18.

236. Krause DC, Balish MF. Structure, function, and assembly of the terminal organelle of *Mycoplasma pneumoniae*. FEMS Microbiol Lett 2001;198:1–7.

237. Kreier JP, Ristic M. Genus III. *Haemobartonella*; Genus IV. *Eperythrozoon*. In: Krieg NR, Holt JG, eds. Bergey's Manual of Systematic Bacteriology. Vol. 1. Baltimore: Williams & Wilkins, 1984:724–729..

238. Krohn MA, Hillier SL, Nugent RP, et al. The genital flora of women with intraamniotic infection. J Infect Dis 1995;171:1475–1480.

239. Lamey JR, Eschenbach DA, Mitchell SH, et al. Isolation of mycoplasmas and bacteria from the blood of postpartum women. Amer J Obstet Gynecol 1982; 143:104–112.

240. LaScola B, Michel G, Raoult D. Use of amplification and sequencing of the 16S rRNA gene to diagnose *Mycoplasma pneumoniae* osteomyelitis in a patient with hypogammaglobulinemia. Clin Infect Dis 1997;24:1161–1163.

241. LeGrand-Poels S, Vaira D, Pincemail J, et al. Activation of human immunodeficiency virus type 1 by oxidative stress. AIDS Res Human Retroviruses 1990; 6:1389–1397.

242. Leland DS, Lapworth MA, Jones RB, et al. Comparative evaluation of media for isolation of *Ureaplasma urealyticum* and genital *Mycoplasma* species. J Clin Microbiol 1982;16:709–714.

243. Lemaitre M, Guetard D, Henin Y, et al. Protective activity of tetracycline analogs against the cytopathic effect of the human immunodeficiency viruses in CEM cells. Res Virol 1990;141:5–16.

244. Lemaitre M, Henin Y, Destouesse F, et al. Role of mycoplasma infection in the cytopathic effect induced by human immunodeficiency virus type 1 in infected cell lines. Infect Immun 1992;60:742–748.

245. Levi N, Prag J, Jensen JS, et al. Surgical infections with *Mycoplasma*: a brief review. JR Coll Surg Edinb 1997;41:107–109.

246. Levy M, Shear NH. *Mycoplasma pneumoniae* infection and Stevens-Johnson syndrome: report of eight cases and review of the literature. Clin Pediatr (Phila) 1991;30:42–49.

247. Levy R, Layani-Milon MP, D'Estaing G, et al. Screening for *Chlamydia trachomatis* and *Ureaplasma urealyticum* infection in semen from asymptomatic male partners of infertile couples prior to *in vitro* fertilization. Int J Androl 1999; 22:113–118.

248. Li Y-H, Brauner A, Jonsson B, et al. *Ureaplasma urealyticum*-induced production of proinflammatory cytokines by macrophages. Pediatr Res 2000;48: 114–119.

249. Li Y-H, Chen M, Brauner A, et al. *Ureaplasma urealyticum* induces apoptosis in human lung epithelial cells and macrophages. Biol Neonate 2002;82:166–173.

250. Li Y-H, Yan Z-Q, Jensen JS, et al. Activation of nuclear factor κB and induction of inducible nitric oxide synthase by *Ureaplasma urealyticum* in macrophages. Infect Immun 2000;68:7087–7093.

251. Lieberman D, Lieberman D, Horowitz S, et al. Microparticle agglutination versus antibody-capture enzyme immunoassay for diagnosis of community-acquired *Mycoplasma pneumoniae* pneumonia. Eur J Clin Microbiol Infect Dis 1995;14: 577–584.

252. Lieberman D, Schlaeffer F, Lieberman D, et al. *Mycoplasma pneumoniae* community-acquired pneumonia: a review of 101 hospitalized adult patients. Respiration 1996;63:261–266.

253. Lind K, Kristensen GB, Bollerup AC, et al. Importance of *Mycoplasma hominis* in acute salpingitis assessed by culture and serological tests. Genitourin Med 1985;61:185–189.

254. Lind K, Lindhardt BO, Schutten HJ, et al. Serological cross-reactions between *Mycoplasma genitalium* and *Mycoplasma pneumoniae*. J Clin Microbiol 1984; 20:1036–1043.

255. Lo S-C. Isolation and identification of a novel virus from patients with AIDS. Am J Trop Med Hyg 1986;35:675–676.

256. Lo S-C, Buchholz CL, Wear DJ, et al. Histopathology and doxycycline treatment in a previously healthy non-AIDS patient systemically infected with *Mycoplasma fermentans* (incognitus strain). Mod Pathol 1991;6:750–754.

257. Lo S-C, Dawson MS, Newton PB, et al. Association of the virus-like infectious agent originally reported in patients with AIDS with acute fatal disease in previously healthy non-AIDS patients. Am J Trop Med Hyg 1989;41:364–376.

258. Lo S-C, Dawson MS, Wong DM, et al. Identification of *Mycoplasma incognitus*

infection in patients with AIDS: an immunohistochemical, *in situ* hybridization and ultrastructural study. Am J Trop Med Hyg 1989;41:601–616.

259. Lo S-C, Hayes MM, Kotani H, et al. Adhesion onto and invasion into mammalian cells by *Mycoplasma penetrans*: a newly isolated mycoplasma from patients with AIDS. Mod Pathol 1993;6:276–280.

260. Lo S-C, Hayes MM, Tully JG, et al. *Mycoplasma penetrans* sp. nov., from the urogenital tract of patients with AIDS. Int J Syst Bacteriol 1992;42:357–364.

261. Lo S-C, Hayes MM, Wang RY-H, et al. Newly discovered mycoplasma isolated from patients infected with HIV. Lancet 1991;338:1415–1418.

262. Lo S-C, Lange M, Wang R, et al. Development of Kaposi's sarcoma is associated with serologic evidence of *Mycoplasma penetrans* infection: retrospective analysis of a prospective cohort study of homosexual men. First National Conference on Human Retroviruses and Related Infections, Program and Abstracts. 1993:67. Abstract 504.

263. Lo S-C, Levin L, Ribas J, et al. Lack of serological evidence for *Mycoplasma fermentans* infection in Army Gulf War veterans: a large scale case-control study. Epidemiol Infect 2000;125:609–616.

264. Lo S-C, Shih JW-K, Newton PB, et al. Virus-like infectious agent (VLIA) is a novel pathogenic mycoplasma: *Mycoplasma incognitus*. Am J Trop Med Hyg 1989;51:586–600.

265. Lo S-C, Shih JW-K, Yang N-Y, et al. A novel virus-like infectious agent in patients with AIDS. Am J Trop Med Hyg 1989;40:213–226.

266. Lo S-C, Tsai S, Benish JR, et al. Enhancement of HIV-1 cytocidal effects on CD4+ lymphocytes by the AIDS-associated mycoplasma. Science 1991;251:1074–1076.

267. Lo, S-C, Wang RY-H, Grandinetti T, et al. *Mycoplasma hominis* lipid-associated membrane protein antigens for effective detection of *M. hominis*-specific antibodies in humans. Clin Infect Dis 2003;36:1246–1253.

268. Lo S-C, Wang RY-H, Newton PB, et al. Fatal infection of silver leaf monkeys with a virus-like infectious agent (VLIA) derived from a patient with AIDS. Am J Trop Med Hyg 1989;40:399–409.

269. Lo S-C, Wear DJ, Green SL, et al. Adult respiratory distress syndrome with or without systemic disease associated with infections due to *Mycoplasma fermentans*. Clin Infect Dis 1993;17(Suppl 1):S259–S263.

270. Lo S-C, Wear DJ, Shih JW-K el al: Fatal systemic infections of nonhuman primates by *Mycoplasma fermentans* (incognitus strain). Clin Infect Dis 1993;17(Suppl):S283–S288.

271. Loens K, Ieven M, Ursi D, et al. Application of NucliSens basic kit for the detection of *Mycoplasma pneumoniae* in respiratory specimens. J Microbiol Methods 2003;54:127–130.

272. Loens K, Ursi D, Goossens H, Ieven M. Molecular diagnosis of *Mycoplasma pneumoniae* respiratory tract infections. J Clin Microbiol 2003;41:4915–4923.

273. Loens K, Ursi D, Ieven M, et al. Detection of *Mycoplasma pneumoniae* in spiked clinical samples by nucleic acid sequence-based amplification. J Clin Microbiol 2002 ;40:1339–1345.

274. Luki N, Lebel P, Boucher M, et al. Comparison of polymerase chain reaction assay with culture for detection of genital mycoplasmas in perinatal infections. Eur J Clin Microbiol Infect Dis 1998 ;17:255–263.

275. Luo D, Xu W, Chiang G, et al. Isolation and identification of *Mycoplasma genitalium* from high risk populations of sexually transmitted diseases in China. Chin Med J (Engl) 1999;112:489–492.

276. Luttrell LM, Kanj SS, Corey R, et al. *Mycoplasma hominis* septic arthritis: two case reports and review. Clin Infect Dis 1994;19:1067–1070.

277. Macon WR, Lo S-C, Poiesz BJ, et al. Acquired immunodeficiency syndrome-like illness associated with systemic *Mycoplasma fermentans* infection in a human immunodeficiency virus-negative homosexual man. Hum Pathol 1993;24:554–558.

278. Madoff S, Hooper DC. Nongenitourinary tract infections caused by *Mycoplasma hominis* in adults. Rev Infect Dis 1988;10:602–613.

279. Maeda SI, Tamaki M, Kojima K, et al. Association of *Mycoplasma genitalium* persistence in the urethra with recurrence of nongonococcal urethritis. Sex Transm Dis 2001;28:472–476.

280. Maede Y. Sequestration and phagocytosis of *Haemobartonella felis* in the spleen. Am J Vet Res 1979;40:691–695.

281. Manhart LE, Critchlow CW, Holmes KK, et al. Mucopurulent cervicitis and *Mycoplasma genitalium*. J Infect Dis 2003;187:650–657.

282. Markham JG, Markham NP. *Mycoplasma laidlawii* in human burns. J Bacteriol 1964;98:827–828.

283. Marmion BP, Worswick JWDA, Kok T-W, et al. Experience with newer techniques for the laboratory detection of *Mycoplasma pneumoniae* infection: Adelaide, 1978–1992. Clin Infect Dis 1993;17(Suppl 1):S90–S99.

284. Marston BJ, Plouffe JF, File TM, et al. Incidence of community-acquired pneumonia requiring hospitalization. Arch Intern Med 1997;157:1709–1718.

285. Martinez OV, Chan J, Cleary T, et al. *Mycoplasma hominis* septic thrombophlebitis in a patient with multiple trauma: a case report and literature review. Diagn Microbiol Infect Dis 1989;12:193–196.

286. Matas L, Dominguez J, DeOry F, et al. Evaluation of Meridian ImmunoCard *Mycoplasma* test for the detection of *Mycoplasma pneumoniae*-specific IgM in paediatric patients. Scand J Infect Dis 1998;30:289–293.

287. Matovina M, Husnjak K, Milutin N, et al. Possible role of bacterial and viral infections in miscarriages. Fertil Steril 2004;81:662–669.

288. McAuliffe L, Ellis RJ, Ayling RD, Nicholas RAJ. Differentiation of *Mycoplasma* species by 16S ribosomal DNA PCR and denaturing gradient gel electrophoresis fingerprinting. J Clin Microbiol 2003;41:4844–4847.

289. McCormack WM. *Ureaplasma urealyticum*: ecologic niche and epidemiologic considerations. Pediatr Infect Dis 1986;5:S232–S233.

290. McCormack WM, Almeida PC, Bailey PE, et al. Sexual activity and vaginal colonization with genital mycoplasmas. JAMA 1972;221:1375–1377.

291. McCormack WM, Lee Y-H, Zinner SH. Sexual experience and urethral colonization with genital mycoplasmas: a study in normal men. Ann Intern Med 1973;78:696–698.

292. McCormack WM, Rosner B, Alpert S, et al. Vaginal colonization with *Mycoplasma hominis* and *Ureaplasma urealyticum*. Sex Transm Dis 1986;13:67–70.

293. McCormack WM, Rosner B, Lee Y-H, et al. Isolation of genital mycoplasmas from blood obtained shortly after vaginal delivery. Lancet 1975;1:596–599.

294. McDonald JC, Moore DL. *Mycoplasma hominis* meningitis in a premature infant. Pediatr Infect Dis J 1989;7:795–798.

295. McDonald MI, Moore JO, Harrelson JM, et al. Septic arthritis due to *Mycoplasma hominis*. Arthritis Rheum 1983;26:1044–1047.

296. Meis JF, van Kuppeveld FJ, Kreme JA, et al. Fatal intrauterine infection associated with *Mycoplasma hominis*. Clin Infect Dis 1992;15:753–754.

297. Meloni F, Paschetto E, Mangiarotti P, et al. Acute *Chlamydia pneumoniae* and *Mycoplasma pneumoniae* infections in community-acquired pneumonia and exacerbations of COPD or asthma: therapeutic considerations. J Chemother 2004;16:70–76.

298. Mena L, Wang X, Mroczkowski TF, Martin DH. *Mycoplasma genitalium* infections in asymptomatic men and men with urethritis attending a sexually transmitted diseases clinic in New Orleans. Clin Infect Dis 2002;35:1167–1173.

299. Mernaugh GR, Dallo SF, Holt SC, et al. Properties of adhering and nonadhering populations of *Mycoplasma genitalium*. Clin Infect Dis 1993;17(Suppl 1):S69–S78.

300. Meseguer MA, Perez-Molina JA, Fernandez-Bustamante J, et al. *Mycoplasma pneumoniae* pericarditis and cardiac tamponade in a ten-year-old girl. Pediatr Infect Dis J 1996;15:829–831.

301. Messick JB. New perspectives about hemotrophic mycoplasma (formerly *Haemobartonella* and *Eperythrozoon* species) infections in dogs and cats. Vet Clin North Am Small Anim Pract 2003;33:1453–1465.

302. Messick JB. Hemotrophic mycoplasmas (hemoplasmas): a review and new insights into pathogenic potential. Vet Clin Pathol 2004;33:2–13.

303. Messick JB, Walker PG, Raphael W, et al. 'Candidatus Mycoplasma haemodidelphis' sp. nov., 'candidatus Mycoplasma haemolanae' sp. nov., and *Mycoplasma haemocanis* comb. nov., haemotrophic parasites from a naturally infected opossum (*Didelphis virginiana*), alpaca (*Lama pacos*) and dog (*Canis familiaris*): phylogenetic and secondary structural relatedness of their 16S sRNA genes to other mycoplasmas. Int J Syst Evol Microbiol 2002;52:693–698.

304. Meyer RD, Clough W. Extragenital *Mycoplasma hominis* infections in adults: emphasis on immunosuppression. Clin Infect Dis 1993;17(Suppl 1):S243–S249.

305. Milla E, Zografos L, Piguet B. Bilateral optic papillitis following *Mycoplasma pneumoniae* pneumonia. Ophthalmologica 1998;212:344–346.

306. Miranda C, Alados JC, Molina JM, et al. Posthysterectomy wound infection: a review. Diagn Microbiol Infect Dis 1993;17:41–44.

307. Miranda C, Carazo C, Banon R, et al. *Mycoplasma hominis* infection in three renal transplant patients. Diagn Microbiol Infect Dis 1990;13:329–331.

308. Moller BR, Taylor-Robinson D, Furr PM. Serological evidence implicating *Mycoplasma genitalium* in pelvic inflammatory disease. Lancet 1984;1:1102–1103.

309. Montagnier L, Blanchard A. Mycoplasmas as cofactors in infection due to human immunodeficiency virus. Clin Infect Dis 1993;17(Suppl 1):S309–S315.

310. Morrison-Plummer J, Lazzell A, Baseman JB. Shared epitopes between *Mycoplasma pneumoniae* major adhesin protein P1 and a 140-kilodalton protein of *Mycoplasma genitalium*. Infect Immun 1987;55:49–56.

311. Mossad SB, Rehm SJ, Tomford KW, et al. Sternotomy infection with *Mycoplasma hominis*: a cause of "culture-negative" wound infection. J Cardiovasc Surg (Torino) 1996;37:505–509.

312. Muhlradt PF, Frisch M. Purification and partial biochemical characterization of a *Mycoplasma fermentans*-derived substance that activates macrophages to release nitric oxide, tumor necrosis factor, and interleukin-6. Infect Immun 1994;62:3801–3807.

313. Muhlradt PF, Quentmeier H, Schmitt E. Involvement of interleukin-1 (IL-1), IL-6, IL-2, and IL-4 in generation of cytolytic T cells from thymocytes stimulated by a *Mycoplasma fermentans*-derived product. Infect Immun 1991;59:3962–3968.

314. Muhlradt PF, Schade U. MDHM, a macrophage-stimulatory product of *Mycoplasma fermentans*, leads to in vitro interleukin-1 (IL-1), IL-6, tumor necrosis factor, and prostaglandin production and is pyrogenic in rabbits. Infect Immun 1991;59:3969–3974.

315. Naessens A, Foulen W, Breynaert J, et al. Postpartum bacteremia and placental colonization with genital mycoplasmas and pregnancy outcome. Am J Obstet Gynecol 1989;160:647–650.

316. Narita M, Matsuzono Y, Togashi T, et al. DNA diagnosis of central nervous system infection by *Mycoplasma pneumoniae*. Pediatrics 1992;90:250–253.

317. Nasralla M, Haier J, Nicolson GL. Multiple mycoplasmal infections detected in blood of patients with chronic fatigue syndrome and/or fibromyalgia syndrome. Eur J Clin Microbiol Infect Dis 1999;18:859–865.

318. Neimark H, Hoff B, Ganter M. *Mycoplasma ovis* comb. nov. (formerly *Eperythrozoon ovis*), an epierythrocytic agent of haemolytic anaemia in sheep and goats. Int J Syst Evol Microbiol 2004;54:365–371.

319. Neimark H, Johansson K-E, Rikihisa Y, Tully JG. Proposal to transfer some members of the genera *Haemobartonella* and *Eperythrozoon* to the genus *Mycoplasma* with descriptions of "candidatus Mycoplasma haemofelis," "candidatus Mycoplasma haemomuris," "candidatus Mycoplasma haemosuis," and "candidatus Mycoplasma weyonii." Int J Syst Evol Microbiol 2001;51:891–899.

320. Neimark H, Johansson K-E, Rikihisa Y, Tully JG. Revision of haemotrophic *Mycoplasma* species names. Int J Syst Evol Microbiol 2002;52:683.

321. Neimark H, Kocan KM. The cell wall-less rickettsia *Eperythrozoon wenyonii* is a mycoplasma. FEMS Microbiol Lett 1997;156:287–291.

322. Neumayr L, Lennette E, Kelly D, et al. *Mycoplasma* disease and acute chest syndrome in sickle cell disease. Pediatrics 2003;112:87–95.

323. Nijs J, Nicolson GL, De Becker P, et al. High prevalence of *Mycoplasma* infections among European chronic fatigue syndrome patients: examination of four *Mycoplasma* species in blood of chronic fatigue syndrome patients. FEMS Immunol Med Microbiol 2002 ;34:209–214.

324. Nozaki-Renard J, Iino T, Sato Y, et al. A fluoroquinolone (DR-3355) protects human lymphocyte cell lines from HIV-1-induced cytotoxicity. AIDS 1990;4:1283–1286.

325. Nunez-Calonge R, Caballero P, Redondo C, et al. *Ureaplasma urealyticum* reduces sperm motility and induces membrane alterations in human spermatozoa. Hum Reprod 1998;13:2756–2761.

326. Ohkawa M, Yamaguchi K, Tokunaga S, et al. *Ureaplasma urealyticum* in the urogenital tract of patients with chronic prostatitis or related symptomatology. Br J Urol 1993;72:918–921.

327. Ohkawa M, Yamaguchi K, Tokunaga S, et al. Antimicrobial treatment for chronic prostatitis as a means of defining the role of *Ureaplasma urealyticum*. Urol Int 1993;51:129–132.

328. Ohlsson A, Wang E, Vearncombe M. Leukocytes counts and colonization with *Ureaplasma urealyticum* in preterm neonates. Clin Infect Dis 1993;17(Suppl 1):S144–S147.

329. Olson LD, Gilbert AA. Characteristics of *Mycoplasma hominis* adhesion. J Bacteriol 1993;175:3224–3227.

330. Orange GV, Jones M, Henderson IS. Wound and perinephric haematoma infection with *Mycoplasma hominis* in a renal transplant recipient. Nephrol Dial Transplant 1993;8:1395–1396.

331. Ovetchkine P, Brugieres P, Seradj A, et al. An 8-year-old boy with acute stroke and radiological signs of cerebral vasculitis after recent *Mycoplasma pneumoniae* infection. Scand J Infect Dis 2002;34:307–309.

332. Ozcan SA, Miles R. Biochemical diversity of *Mycoplasma fermentans* strains. FEMS Microbiol Lett 1999;176:177–181.

333. Palmer HM, Gilroy CB, Claydon EJ, et al. Detection of *Mycoplasma genitalium* in the genitourinary tract of women by the polymerase chain reaction. Int J STD AIDS 1991;2:261–263.

334. Parides GC, Bloom JW, Ampel NM, et al. Mycoplasma and ureaplasma in bronchoalveolar lavage specimens from immunocompromised hosts. Diagn Microbiol Infect Dis 1988;9:55–57.

335. Pasculle AW. Recognition of *Mycoplasma hominis* in routine bacteriology specimens. Clin Microbiol Newslett 1988;10:145–148.

336. Pastural M, Audard V, Bralet M-P, et al. *Mycoplasma hominis* infection in renal transplantation. Nephrol Dial Transplant 2002;17:495–496.

337. Payan DG, Seigal N, Madoff S. Infection of a brain abscess by *Mycoplasma hominis*. J Clin Microbiol 1981;14:571–573.

338. Payne NR, Steinberg SS, Ackerman P, et al. New prospective studies of the association of *Ureaplasma urealyticum* colonization and chronic lung disease. Clin Infect Dis 1993;17(Suppl 1):S117–S121.

339. Peeters MF, Polak-Vogelzang AA, Debruyne FM, Van der Veen J. Role of mycoplasmas in chronic prostatitis. Yale J Med Biol 1983;6:551.

340. Pereyre S, Gonzalez P, de Barbeyrac B, et al. Mutations in 23S rRNA account for intrinsic resistance to macrolides in *Mycoplasma hominis* and *Mycoplasma fermentans* and for acquired resistance in *M. hominis*. Antimicrob Agents Chemother 2002;46:3142–3150.

341. Perez CR, Leigh MW. *Mycoplasma pneumoniae* as the causative agent for pneumonia in the immunocompromised host. Chest 1991;100:860–861.

342. Petitjean J, Vabret A, Gouarin S, Freymuth F. Evaluation of four commercial immunoglobulin G (IgG)- and IgM-specific enzyme immunoassays for diagnosis of *Mycoplasma pneumoniae* infections. J Clin Microbiol 2002;40:165–171.

343. Petzel JP, Hartmen PA, Allison MJ. Pyrophosphate-dependent enzymes in walled bacteria phylogenetically related to the wall-less bacteria of the class *Mollicutes*. Int J Syst Bacteriol 1989;39:413–419.

344. Pflausler B, Engelhardt K, Kampfl A, et al. Post-infectious central and peripheral nervous system diseases complicating *Mycoplasma pneumoniae* infection: report of three cases and review of the literature. Eur J Neurol 2002;9:93–96.

345. Phillips DM, Pearce-Pratt R, Tan X, et al. Association of human mycoplasmas with HIV-1 and HTLV-I in human lymphocytes. AIDS Res Hum Retroviruses 1992;8:1863–1868.

346. Phillips LE, Faro S, Pokorny SF, et al. Postcesarean wound infection by *Mycoplasma hominis* in a patient with persistent postpartum fever. Diagn Microbiol Infect Dis 1987;7:193–197.

347. Phillips LE, Goodrich KH, Turner RM, et al. Isolation of *Mycoplasma* species and *Ureaplasma urealyticum* from obstetrical and gynecological patients by using commercially available medium formulations. J Clin Microbiol 1986;24:377–379.

348. Pigrau C, Almirante B, Gasser I, et al. Sternotomy infection due to *Mycoplasma hominis* and *Ureaplasma urealyticum*. Eur J Clin Microbiol Infect Dis 1995;14:597–598.

349. Pitcher D, Hilbocus J. Variability in the distribution and composition of insertion-like sequences in strains of *Mycoplasma fermentans*. FEMS Microbiol Lett 1998;160:101–109.

350. Pollack JD, Jones MA, Williams MV. The metabolism of AIDS-associated mycoplasmas. Clin Infect Dis 1993;17(Suppl 1):S267–S271.

351. Potts JM, Ward AM, Rackley RR. Association of chronic urinary symptoms in women and *Ureaplasma urealyticum*. Urology 2000;55:486–489.

352. Poulin SA, Perkins RE, Kundsin RB. Antibiotic susceptibilities of AIDS-associated mycoplasmas. J Clin Microbiol 1994;32:1101–1103.

353. Povlsen K, Bjornelius E, Lidbrink P, Lind I. Relationship of *Ureaplasma urealyticum* biovar 2 to nongonococcal urethritis. Eur J Clin Microbiol Infect Dis 2002;21:97–101.

354. Powell DA, Miller K, Clyde WA. Submandibular adenitis in a newborn caused by *Mycoplasma hominis*. Pediatrics 1979;63:798–799.

355. Pratt BC. Recovery of *Mycoplasma hominis* from blood culture media. Med Lab Sci 1991;48:350.

356. Quinn PA, Gillan JE, Markestad T, et al. Intrauterine infection with *Ureaplasma urealyticum* as a cause of fatal neonatal pneumonia. Pediatr Infect Dis 1985;4:538–543.

357. Razin S, Harasawa R, Barile MF. Cleavage patterns of the mycoplasma chromosome, obtained by using restriction endonucleases, as indicators of genetic relatedness among strains. Int J Syst Bacteriol 1983;33:201–206.

358. Razin S, Michmann J, Shimshoni Z. The occurrence of mycoplasma (pleuropneumonia-like organisms, PPLO) in the oral cavity of dentulous and edentulous subjects. J Dent Res 1964;43:402–405.

359. Razin S, Yogev D. Genetic relatedness among *Ureaplasma urealyticum* serotypes (serovars). Pediatr Infect Dis 1986;5:S300–S304.

360. Razin S, Yogev D, Naot Y. Molecular biology and pathogenicity of mycoplasmas. Microbiol Mol Biol Rev 1998;62:1094–1156.

361. Renaudin H, Tully JG, Bebear C. In vitro susceptibilities of *Mycoplasma genitalium* to antibiotics. Antimicrob Agents Chemother 1992;36:870–872.

362. Ridgway EJ, Allen KD. *Mycoplasma hominis* abscess secondary to respiratory tract infection. J Infect 1994;29:207–210.

363. Riedel K, Kempf VA, Bechtold A, Klimmer M. Acute disseminated encephalomyelitis (ADEM) due to *Mycoplasma pneumoniae* in an adolescent. Infection 2001;29:240–242.

364. Rikihisa Y, Kawahara M, Wenyon B, et al. Western immunoblot analysis of *Haemobartonella muris* and comparison of 16S rRNA gene sequences of *H. muris*, *H. felis*, and *Eperythrozoon suis*. J Clin Microbiol 1997;35:823–829.

365. Roberts MC, Kenny GE. Dissemination of the *tetM* tetracycline resistance determinant to *Ureaplasma urealyticum*. Antimicrob Agents Chemother 1986;29:350–352.

366. Roberts MC, Kenny GE. *TetM* tetracycline-resistant determinants in *Ureaplasma urealyticum*. Pediatr Infect Dis 1986;5:S338–S240.

367. Roberts MC, Koutsky LA, Holmes KK, et al. Tetracycline-resistant *Mycoplasma hominis* strains contain streptococcal *tetM* sequences. Antimicrob Agents Chemother 1985;28:141–143.

368. Robertson JA, Coppola JE, Heisler OR. Standardized method for determining antimicrobial susceptibility of strains of *Ureaplasma urealyticum* and their response to tetracycline, erythromycin, and rosaramicin. Antimicrob Agents Chemother 1981;20:53–58.

369. Robertson JA, Stemke GW. Expanded serotyping scheme for *Ureaplasma urealyticum* strains isolated from humans. J Clin Microbiol 1982;9:673–678.

370. Robertson JA, Vekris A, Bebear C, et al. Polymerase chain reaction using 16S rRNA gene sequences distinguishes the two biovars of *Ureaplasma urealyticum*. J Clin Microbiol 1993;31:824–830.

371. Rogers MJ, Simmons J, Walker RT, et al. Construction of the mycoplasma evolutionary tree from 5S RNA sequence data. Proc Natl Acad Sci USA 1995;82:1160–1164.

372. Roifman CM, Rao CP, Lederman HM, et al. Increased susceptibility to mycoplasma infections in patients with hypogammaglobulinemia. Am J Med 1986; 80:590–594.

373. Rudd PT, Waites KB, Duffy LB, et al. *Ureaplasma urealyticum* and its possible role in pneumonia during the neonatal period and infancy. Pediatr Infect Dis 1986;5:S288–S291.

374. Ruiter N, Wentholt HMM. Isolation of a pleuropneumonia-like organism from a skin lesion associated with a fusospirochetal flora. J Invest Dermatol 1955; 24:31–34.

375. Sadler JP, Gibson J. *Mycoplasma pneumoniae* infection presenting as Stevens-Johnson syndrome: a case report. Dent Update 1997;24:367–368.

376. Saillard C, Carle P, Bove JM,, et al. Genetic and serologic relatedness between *Mycoplasma fermentans* strains and a mycoplasma recently identified in tissues of AIDS and non-AIDS patients. Res Virol 1990;141:385–395.

377. Salzman MB, Sood SK, Slavin ML. Ocular manifestations of *Mycoplasma pneumoniae* infection. Clin Infect Dis 1992;14:1137–1139.

378. Sanchez PJ. Perinatal transmission of *Ureaplasma urealyticum*: current concepts based on review of the literature. Clin Infect Dis V;16(Suppl 1):S107–S111.

379. Sanchez PJ, Regan JA. *Ureaplasma urealyticum* colonization and chronic lung disease in low birth weight infants. Pediatr Infect Dis J 1988;7:542–546.

380. Sands MJ Jr, Rosenthal R. Progressive heart failure and death associated with *Mycoplasma pneumoniae* pneumonia. Chest 1982;81:763–765.

381. Sanyal D, Thurston C. *Mycoplasma hominis* infection of a breast prosthesis. J Infect 1991;23:210–211.

382. Sasaki T, Blanchard A, Watson HL, et al. *In vitro* influence of *Mycoplasma penetrans* on activation of peripheral T lymphocytes from healthy donors or human immunodeficiency virus-infected individuals. Infect Immun 1995;63: 4277–4283.

383. Sasaki T, Sasaki Y, Kita M, et al. Evidence that Lo's mycoplasma (*Mycoplasma fermentans* incognitus) is not a unique strain among *Mycoplasma fermentans* strains. J Clin Microbiol 1992;30:2435–2440.

384. Sasaki Y, Honda M, Naitou M, Sasaki T. Detection of *Mycoplasma fermentans* DNA from lymph nodes of acquired immunodeficiency syndrome patients. Microb Pathog 1994;17:131–135.

385. Sasaki Y, Ishikawa J, Yamashita A, et al. The complete genomic sequence of *Mycoplasma penetrans*, an intracellular bacterial pathogen in humans. Nucleic Acids Res 2002;30:5293–5300.

386. Savige JA, Gilbert GL, Fairley KF, et al. Bacteriuria due to *Ureaplasma urealyticum* and *Gardnerella vaginalis* in women with preeclampsia. J Infect Dis 1983; 148:605–607.

387. Schaeverbeke T, Clerc M, Lequen L, et al. Genotypic characterization of seven strains of *Mycoplasma fermentans* isolated from synovial fluids of patients with arthritis. J Clin Microbiol 1998;36:1226–1231.

388. Schaeverbeke T, Gilroy CB, Bebear C, et al. *Mycoplasma fermentans*, but not *M. penetrans*, detected by PCR assays in synovium from patients with rheumatoid arthritis and other rheumatic disorders. J Clin Pathol 1996;49:824–828.

389. Seto S, Miyata M. Attachment organelle formation represented by localization of cytadherence proteins and formation of the electron-dense core in wild-type and mutant strains of *Mycoplasma pneumoniae*. J Bacteriol 2003;185: 1082–1091.

390. Shepard MC. Culture media for ureaplasmas. In: Razin S, Tully JG, eds. Methods in Mycoplasmatology. Vol. 1. New York, Academic Press, 1983:137–146.

391. Shepard MC. *Ureaplasma urealyticum*: overview with emphasis on fetal and maternal infections. Ann NY Acad Sci 1988;549:48–55.

392. Shepard MC, Combs RS. Enhancement of *Ureaplasma urealyticum* growth on a differential agar medium (A7B) by a polyamine, putrescine. J Clin Microbiol 1979;10:931–933.

393. Shepard MC, Lunceford CD. Differential agar medium (A7) for identification of *Ureaplasma urealyticum* (human T mycoplasmas) in primary cultures of clinical material. J Clin Microbiol 1976;3:613–625.

394. Shepard MC, Lunceford CD, Ford DK, et al. *Ureaplasma urealyticum* gen. nov., sp. nov.: proposed nomenclature for the human (T-strain) mycoplasmas. Int J Syst Bacteriol 1974;24:160–171.

395. Shibata K, Kaga M, Kudo M, et al. Detection of *Mycoplasma fermentans* in saliva sampled from infants, preschool and school children, adolescents, and adults by a polymerase chain reaction-based assay. Microbiol Immunol 1999; 43:521–525.

396. Shibata K-I, Sasaki T, Watanabe T. AIDS-associated mycoplasmas possess phospholipase C in the membrane. Infect Immun 1995;63:4174–4177.

397. Shibata K-I, Watanabe T. *Mycoplasma fermentans* enhances concanavalin A-induced apoptosis of mouse splenic T cells. FEMS Immunol Med Microbiol 1997;17:103–109.

398. Sillis M. The limitations of IgM assays in the serological diagnosis of *Mycoplasma pneumoniae* infections. J Med Microbiol 1990;33:253–258.

399. Sillis M. Genital mycoplasmas revisited: an evaluation of a new culture medium. Br J Biomed Sci 1993;50:89–91.

400. Simms I, Eastick K, Mallinson H, et al. Associations between *Mycoplasma genitalium, Chlamydia trachomatis* and pelvic inflammatory disease. J Clin Pathol 2003;56:616–618.

401. Siomou E, Kollios KD, Papadimitriou P, et al. Acute nephritis and respiratory tract infection caused by *Mycoplasma pneumoniae*: case report and review of the literature. Pediatr Infect Dis J 2003;22:1103–1106.

402. Skerk V, Schonwald S, Krhen I, et al. Aetiology of chronic prostatitis. Int J Antimicrob Agents 2002;19:471–474.

403. Smaron MF, Boonlayangoor S, Zierdt CH. Detection of *Mycoplasma hominis* septicemia by radiometric blood culture. J Clin Microbiol 1985;21:298–301.

404. Smyth EG, Weinbren MJ. *Mycoplasma hominis* sternal wound infection and bacteremia. J Infect 1993;26:315–319.

405. Socan M, Ravnik I, Bencina D, et al. Neurological symptoms in patients whose spinal fluid is culture- and/or polymerase chain reaction-positive for *Mycoplasma pneumoniae*. Clin Infect Dis 2001;32:E31–E35.

406. Sotgui S, Pugliatti M, Rosati G, et al. Neurological disorders associated with *Mycoplasma pneumoniae* infection. Eur J Neurol 2003;10:165–168.

407. Spaepen MS, Kundsin RB. Simple, direct broth-disk method for antibiotic susceptibility testing of *Ureaplasma urealyticum*. Antimicrob Agents Chemother 1977;11:267–270.

408. Stadtlander CTK-H, Watson HL, Simecka JW, et al. Cytopathogenicity of *Mycoplasma fermentans* (including strain incognitus). Clin Infect Dis 1993;17(Suppl 1):S289–S301.

409. Stancombe BB, Walsh WF, Derdak S, et al. Induction of human neonatal pulmonary fibroblast cytokines by hyperoxia and *Ureaplasma urealyticum*. Clin Infect Dis 1993;7(Suppl 1):S154–S157.

410. Stellrecht KA, Woron AM, Mishrik NG, Venezia RA. Comparison of multiplex PCR assay with culture for detection of genital mycoplasmas. J Clin Microbiol 2004;42:1528–1533.

411. Stevens MK, Krause DC. Localization of the *Mycoplasma pneumoniae* cytadherence-accessory proteins HMW1 and HMW4 in the cytoskeletonlike triton shell. J Bacteriol 1991;173:1041–1050.

412. Stevens MK, Krause DC. *Mycoplasma pneumoniae* cytadherence phase-variable protein HMW3 is a component of the attachment organelle. J Bacteriol 1992; 174:4265–4274.

413. Stimson JB, Hale J, Bowie WR, et al. Tetracycline-resistant *Ureaplasma urealyticum*: a cause of persistent nongonococcal urethritis. Ann Intern Med 1981;94: 192–194.

414. Stone BB, Cohen SP, Breton GL, et al. Detection of rRNA from four respiratory pathogens using an automated Qβ replicase assay. Mol Cell Probes 1996;10: 359–370.

415. Storgaard M, Tarp B, Ovesen T, et al. The occurrence of *Chlamydia pneumoniae, Mycoplasma pneumoniae*, and herpesviruses in otitis media with effusion. Diagn Microbiol Infect Dis 2004;48:97–99.

416. Stuart PM. Mycoplasmal induction of cytokine production and major histocompatibility complex expression. Clin Infect Dis 1993;17(Suppl 1):S187–S191.

417. Suni J, Vainionpaa R, Tuominen T. Multicenter evaluation of the novel enzyme immunoassay based on P1-enriched protein for the detection of *Mycoplasma pneumoniae* infection. J Microbiol Methods 2001;47:65–71.

418. Svenstrup HF, Nielsen PK, Drasbek M, et al. Adhesion and inhibition assay of *Mycoplasma pneumoniae* by immunofluorescence microscopy. J Med Microbiol 2002;51:361–373.

419. Sweet RL. Colonization of the endometrium and fallopian tubes with *Ureaplasma urealyticum*. Pediatr Infect Dis 1986;5:S244–S246.

420. Swenson CE, VanHamont J, Dunbar BS. Specific protein differences among strains of *Ureaplasma urealyticum* as determined by two-dimensional gel electrophoresis and a sensitive silver stain. Int J Syst Bacteriol 1983;33:417–421.

421. Sykes JE. Feline hemotropic mycoplasmosis (feline hemobartonellosis). Vet Clin North Am Small Anim Pract 2003;33:773–789.

422. Syrogiannopoulos GA, Kapatais-Zoumbos K, Decavalas GO, et al. *Ureaplasma urealyticum* colonization of full term infants: perinatal acquisition and persistence during early infancy. Pediatr Infect Dis J 1990;9:236–240.

423. Takiguchi Y, Shikama N, Aotsuka N, et al. Fulminant *Mycoplasma pneumoniae* pneumonia. Intern Med 2001;40:345–348.

424. Tasker S, Helps CR, Day MJ, et al. Use of real-time PCR to detect and quantify *Mycoplasma hemofelis* and ''candidatus Mycoplasma haemominutum.'' J Clin Microbiol 2003;41:439–441.

425. Tasker S, Lappin MR. *Haemobartonella felis*: recent developments in diagnosis and treatment. J Feline Med Surg 2002;4:3–11.

426. Taylor-Robinson D. Evaluation of the role of *Ureaplasma urealyticum* in infertility. Pediatr Infect Dis 1986;5:S262–S265.

427. Taylor-Robinson D. Infections due to species of *Mycoplasma* and *Ureaplasma*: an update. Clin Infect Dis 1996;23:671–684.

428. Taylor-Robinson D. *Mycoplasma genitalium*: an up-date. Int J STD AIDS 2002; 13:145–151.

429. Taylor-Robinson D, Bebear C. Antibiotic susceptibilities of mycoplasmas and treatment of mycoplasmal infections. J Antimicrob Chemother 1997;40: 622–630.

430. Taylor-Robinson D, Davies HA, Sarathchandra P, et al. Intracellular location

of mycoplasmas in cultured cells demonstrated by immunocytochemistry and electron microscopy. Int J Exp Pathol 1991;72:705–714.

431. Taylor-Robinson D, Evans RT, Coufalik ED, et al. Effect of short-term treatment of non-gonococcal urethritis with minocycline. Genitourin Med 1986;62:19–21.

432. Taylor-Robinson D, Furr PM. Models of infection due to mycoplasmas, including *Mycoplasma fermentans*, in the genital tract and other sites in mice. Clin Infect Dis 1993;17(Suppl 1):S280–S282.

433. Taylor-Robinson D, Furr PM, Hanna NF. Microbiological and serological study of non-gonococcal urethritis with special reference to *Mycoplasma genitalium*. Genitourin Med 1985;61:319–324.

434. Taylor-Robinson D, Furr PM, Tully JG, et al. Animal models of *Mycoplasma genitalium* urogenital infection. Isr J Med Sci 1987;23:561–564.

435. Taylor-Robinson D, Furr PM, Webster ADB. *Ureaplasma urealyticum* in the immunocompromised host. Pediatr Infect Dis 1986;5:S236–S238.

436. Taylor-Robinson D, Gilroy CB, Hay PE. Occurrence of *Mycoplasma genitalium* in different populations and its clinical significance. Clin Infect Dis 1993; 17(Suppl 1):S66–S68.

437. Taylor-Robinson D, Gilroy CB, Horowitz S, et al. *Mycoplasma genitalium* in the joints of two patients with arthritis. Eur J Clin Microbiol Infect Dis 1994; 13:1066–1068.

438. Taylor-Robinson D, Gilroy CB, Keane FE. Detection of several *Mycoplasma* species at various anatomical sites of homosexual men. Eur J Clin Microbiol Infect Dis 2003;22:291–293.

439. Taylor-Robinson D, Gilroy CB, Thomas BJ, Hay PE. *Mycoplasma genitalium* in chronic non-gonococcal urethritis. Int J STD AIDS 2004;15:21–25.

440. Taylor-Robinson D, Gumpel JM, Hill A, et al. Isolation of *Mycoplasma pneumoniae* from the synovial fluid of a hypogammaglobulinaemic patient in a survey of patients with inflammatory polyarthritis. Ann Rheum Dis 1978;37:180–182.

441. Taylor-Robinson D, Sarathchandra P, Furr PM. *Mycoplasma fermentans*-HeLa cell interactions. Clin Infect Dis 1993;17(Suppl 1):S302–S304.

442. Taylor-Robinson D, Webster ADB, Furr PM, et al. Prolonged persistence of *Mycoplasma pneumoniae* in a patient with hypogammaglobulinemia. J Infect 1980;2:171–175.

443. Teng K, Li M, Yu W, et al. Comparison of PCR with culture for detection of *Ureaplasma urealyticum* in clinical samples from patients with urogenital infections. J Clin Microbiol 1994;32:2232–2234.

444. Teng L-J, Zheng X, Glass JI, et al. *Ureaplasma urealyticum* biovar specificity and diversity are encoded in multiple-banded antigen gene. J Clin Microbiol 1994;32:1464–1469.

445. Thacker WL, Talkington DF. Comparison of two rapid commercial tests with complement fixation for serologic diagnosis of *Mycoplasma pneumoniae* infections. J Clin Microbiol 1995;33:1212–1214.

446. Thacker WL, Talkington DF. Analysis of complement fixation and commercial enzyme immunoassays for detection of antibodies to *Mycoplasma pneumoniae* in human serum. Clin Diagn Lab Immunol 2000;7:778–780.

447. Tham TN, Ferris S, Bahraoui E, et al. Molecular characterization of the P1-like adhesin gene from *Mycoplasma pirum*. J Bacteriol 1994;176:781–788.

448. Thomas M, Jones M, Ray S, et al. *Mycoplasma pneumoniae* in a tubo-ovarian abscess. Lancet 1975;2:774–775.

449. Ti TY, Dan M, Stemke GW, et al. Isolation of *Mycoplasma hominis* from the blood of men with multiple trauma and fever. JAMA 1982;247:60–61.

450. Tilton RC, Dias F, Kidd H, et al. DNA probe versus culture for detection of *Mycoplasma pneumoniae* in clinical specimens. Diagn Microbiol Infect Dis 1988;10:109–112.

451. Tjhie JH, van Kuppeveld FJM, Roosendaal R, et al. Direct PCR enables detection of *Mycoplasma pneumoniae* in patients with respiratory tract infections. J Clin Microbiol 1994;32:11–16.

452. Totten PA, Schwartz MA, Sjostrom KE, et al. Association of *Mycoplasma genitalium* with nongonococcal urethritis in heterosexual men. J Infect Dis 2003; 183:269–276.

453. Tullus K, Noack GW, Burman LG, et al. Elevated cytokine levels in transbronchial aspirate fluids from ventilator treated neonates with bronchopulmonary dysplasia. Eur J Pediatr 1996;155:112–116.

454. Tully JG. Mollicute–host interrelationships: current concepts and diagnostic implications. In: Tully JG, Razin S, eds. Molecular and Diagnostic Procedures in Mycoplasmology. Vol 2. San Diego: Academic Press, 1996:1–21.

455. Tully JG, Bove JM, Laigret F, et al. Revised taxonomy of the Class *Mollicutes*: proposed elevation of a monophyletic cluster of arthropod-associated mollicutes to ordinal rank (*Entomoplasmatales* ord. nov.), with provision for familial rank to separate species with non-helical morphology (*Entomoplasmataceae* fam. nov.) from helical species (*Spiroplasmataceae*), and emended descriptions of the order *Mycoplasmatales*, Family *Mycoplasmataceae*. Int J Syst Bacteriol 1993;43:378–385.

456. Tully JG, Rose DL, Baseman JB, et al. *Mycoplasma pneumoniae* and *Mycoplasma genitalium* mixture in synovial fluid isolate. J Clin Microbiol 1995;33: 1851–1855.

457. Tully JG, Rose DL, Whitcomb RF, et al. Enhanced isolation of *Mycoplasma*

pneumoniae from throat washings with a newly modified culture medium. J Infect Dis 1979;139:478–482.

458. Tully JG, Taylor-Robinson D, Cole RM, Rose DL. A newly discovered mycoplasma in the human genital tract. Lancet 1981;1:1288–1291.

459. Tully JG, Taylor-Robinson D, Rose DL, et al. *Mycoplasma genitalium*, a new species from the human genital tract. Int J Syst Bacteriol 1983;33:387–396.

460. Tully JG, Whitcomb RF, Rose DL, et al. *Acholeplasma brassicae* sp. nov. and *Acholeplasma palmae* sp. nov., two non-sterol-requiring mollicutes from plant surfaces. Int J Syst Bacteriol 1994;44:680–684.

461. Tuppin P, Delamare O, Launay V, et al. High prevalence of antibodies to *Mycoplasma penetrans* in human immunodeficiency virus-seronegative and seropositive populations in Brazzaville, Congo. Clin Diagn Lab Immunol 1997;4: 787–788.

462. Uldum SA, Sondergard-Andersen J, Jensen JS, Lind K. Evaluation of a commercial enzyme immunoassay for detection of *Mycoplasma pneumoniae* specific immunoglobulin G antibodies. Eur J Clin Microbiol Infect Dis 1990;9:221–223.

463. Uno M, Deguchi T, Komeda H, et al. *Mycoplasma genitalium* in the cervices of Japanese women. Sex Transm Dis 1997;24:284–286.

464. Uphoff CC, Drexler HG. Comparative PCR analysis for detection of mycoplasma infections in continuous cell lines. In Vitro Cell Dev Biol 2002;38: 79–85.

465. Ursi D, Ieven M, Noordhoek GT, et al. An interlaboratory comparison for the detection of *Mycoplasma pneumoniae* in respiratory samples by the polymerase chain reaction. J Microbiol Methods 2003;53:289–294.

466. Ursi D, Ieven M, VanBever H, et al. Typing of *Mycoplasma pneumoniae* by PCR-mediated DNA fingerprinting. J Clin Microbiol 1994;32:2873–2875.

467. Uuskula A, Kohl PK. Genital mycoplasmas, including *Mycoplasma genitalium*, as sexually transmitted agents. Int J STD AIDS 2002;13:79–85.

468. Valencia GB, Banzon F, Cummings M, et al. *Mycoplasma hominis* and *Ureaplasma urealyticum* in neonates with suspected infection. Pediatr Infect Dis J 1993;12:571–573.

469. Van Kuppeveld FJ, Johansson K-E, Galama JM, et al. 16S rRNA based polymerase chain reaction compared with culture and serological methods for diagnosis of *Mycoplasma pneumoniae* infection. Eur J Clin Microbiol Infect Dis 1994; 13:401–405.

470. Vojdani A, Choppa PC, Tagle C, et al. Detection of *Mycoplasma* genus and *Mycoplasma fermentans* by PCR in patients with chronic fatigue syndrome. FEMS Immunol Med Microbiol 1998;22:355–365.

471. Waites KB, Bebear CM, Robertson JA, et al. Cumitech 34: laboratory diagnosis of mycoplasma infections. Washington, D.C.: ASM Press, 2001.

472. Waites KB, Canupp KC. Evaluation of BacT/ALERT system for detection of *Mycoplasma hominis* in simulated blood cultures. J Clin Microbiol 2001;39: 4328–4331.

473. Waites KB, Crabb DM, Bing X, Duffy LB. *In vitro* susceptibilities to and bactericidal activities of garenoxacin (BMS-284756) and other antimicrobial agents against human mycoplasmas and ureaplasmas. Antimicrob Agents Chemother 2003;47:161–165.

474. Waites KB, Crabb DM, Duffy LB. *In vitro* activities of ABT-773 and other antimicrobials against human mycoplasmas. Antimicrob Agents Chemother 2003;47:39–42.

475. Waites KB, Crabb DM, Duffy LB. Comparative *in vitro* susceptibilities and bactericidal activities of investigational fluoroquinolone ABT-492 and other antimicrobial agents against human mycoplasmas and ureaplasmas. Antimicrob Agents Chemother 2003;47:3973–3975.

476. Waites KB, Crouse DT, Cassell GH. Systemic neonatal infection due to *Ureaplasma urealyticum*. Clin Infect Dis 1993;17(Suppl 1):S131–S135.

477. Waites KB, Crouse DT, Cassell GH. Therapeutic considerations for *Ureaplasma urealyticum* infections in neonates. Clin Infect Dis 1993;17(Suppl 1): S208–S214.

478. Waites KB, Crouse DT, Philips JB III, et al. Ureaplasmal pneumonia and sepsis associated with persistent pulmonary hypertension of the newborn. Pediatrics 1989;83:79–85.

479. Waites KB, Duffy LB, Crouse DT, et al. Mycoplasmal infections of cerebrospinal fluid in newborn infants from a community hospital population. Pediatr Infect Dis J 1990;9:241–245.

480. Waites KB, Figarola TA, Schmid T, et al. Comparison of agar versus broth dilution techniques for determining antibiotic susceptibilities of *Ureaplasma urealyticum*. Diagn Microbiol Infect Dis 1991;14:265–271.

481. Waites KB, Tully JG, Rose DL, et al. Isolation of *Acholeplasma oculi* from human amniotic fluid in early pregnancy. Curr Microbiol 1987;15:327–327.

482. Walsh WF, Butler J, Coalson J, et al. A primate model of *Ureaplasma urealyticum* infection in the premature infant with hyaline membrane disease. Clin Infect Dis 1993;17(Suppl 1):S158–S162.

483. Wang RY-H, Grandinetti T, Shih JW-K, et al. *Mycoplasma genitalium* infection and host antibody response in patients infected by HIV, patients attending STD clinics and in healthy blood donors. FEMS Immunol Med Microbiol 1997;19: 237–245.

484. Wang RY-H, Hu WS, Dawson MS, et al. Selective detection of *Mycoplasma*

fermentans by polymerase chain reaction and by using a nucleotide sequence within the insertion sequence-like element. J Clin Microbiol 1992;30:245–248.

485. Wang RY-H, Shih JW-K, Grandinetti T, et al. High frequency of antibodies to *Mycoplasma penetrans* in HIV-infected patients. Lancet 1992;340:1312–1316.

486. Wang RY-H, Shih JW-K, Weiss SH, et al. *Mycoplasma penetrans* infection in male homosexuals with AIDS: high seroprevalence and association with Kaposi's sarcoma. Clin Infect Dis 1993;17:724–729.

487. Waring AL, Halse TA, Csiza CK, et al. Development of a genomics-based PCR assay for detection of *Mycoplasma pneumoniae* in a large outbreak in New York State. J Clin Microbiol 2001;39:1385–1390.

488. Waris ME, Toikka P, Saarinen T, et al. Diagnosis of *Mycoplasma pneumoniae* pneumonia in children. J Clin Microbiol 1998;36:3155–3159.

489. Watanabe T, Shibata K-I, Yoshikawa T, et al. Detection of *Mycoplasma salivarium* and *Mycoplasma fermentans* in synovial fluids of temporomandibular joints of patients with disorders in the joints. FEMS Immunol Med Microbiol 1998;22:241–246.

490. Watkins-Riedel T, Stanek G, Daxboeck F. Comparison of SeroMP-IgA with four other commercial assays for serodiagnosis of *Mycoplasma pneumoniae* pneumonia. Diagn Microbiol Infect Dis 2001;40:21–25.

491. Webster D, Windsor H, Ling C, et al. Chronic bronchitis in immunocompromised patients: association with a novel *Mycoplasma* species. Eur J Clin Microbiol Infect Dis 2003;22:530–534.

492. Welti M, Jaton K, Altwegg M, et al. Development of a multiplex, real-time quantitative PCR assay to detect *Chlamydia pneumoniae*, *Legionella pneumophila* and *Mycoplasma pneumoniae* in respiratory tract secretions. Diagn Microbiol Infect Dis 2004 ;45:85–95.

493. Whatley JD, Thin RN, Mumtaz G, Ridgway GL. Azithromycin vs doxycycline in the treatment of nongonococcal urethritis. Int J Std AIDS 1991;2:248–251.

494. Willby MJ, Krause DC. Characterization of a *Mycoplasma pneumoniae hmw3* mutant: implications for attachment organelle assembly. J Bacteriol 2002;184:3061–3068.

495. Woese CR, Maniloff J, Zablen LB. Phylogenetic analysis of the mycoplasmas. Proc Natl Acad Sci USA 1980;77:494–498.

496. Wolthers KC, Kornelisse RF, Platenkamp GJJM, et al. A case of *Mycoplasma hominis* meningo-encephalitis in a full-term infant: rapid recovery after start of treatment with ciprofloxacin. Eur J Pediatr 2003;162:514–516.

497. Wood JC, Lu RM, Peterson EM, et al. Evaluation of Mycotrim-GU for isolation of *Mycoplasma* species and *Ureaplasma urealyticum*. J Clin Microbiol 1985;22:789–792.

498. Yajko DM, Balston E, Wood D, et al. Evaluation of PPLO, A7B, E, and NYC agar media for the isolation of *Ureaplasma urealyticum* and *Mycoplasma* species from the genital tract. J Clin Microbiol 1984;19:73–76.

499. Yakulis VJ, Costea N, Heller P. α-Galactoside determinants of the I-antigen. Proc Soc Exp Biol Med 1966;121:812–816.

500. Yanez A, Cedillo L, Neyrolles O, et al. *Mycoplasma penetrans* bacteremia and primary anti-phospholipid syndrome. Emerg Infect Dis 1999;5:164–167.

501. Yang J, Hooper WC, Phillips DJ, Talkington DF. Cytokines in *Mycoplasma pneumoniae* infections. Cytokine Growth Factor Rev 15:157–168, 2004.

502. Yechouron A, Lefebvre J, Robson HG, et al. Fatal septicemia due to *Mycoplasma arginini*: a new human zoonosis. Clin Infect Dis 1992;15:434–438.

503. Yogev D, Halachmi D, Kenny GE, et al. Distinction of species and strains of mycoplasmas (*Mollicutes*) by genomic DNA fingerprints with an rRNA probe. J Clin Microbiol 1988;26:1198–1201.

504. Yogev D, Razin S. Common deoxyribonucleic acid sequences in *Mycoplasma genitalium* and *Mycoplasma pneumoniae* genomes. Int J Syst Bacteriol 1986;36:426–430.

505. Yoon BH, Romero R, Kom M, et al. Clinical implications of detection of *Ureaplasma urealyticum* in the amniotic cavity with the polymerase chain reaction. Am J Obstet Gynecol 2000;183:1130–1137.

506. Yoshida T, Degeuchi T, Ito M, et al. Quantitative detection of *Mycoplasma genitalium* from first-pass urine of men with urethritis and asymptomatic men in real-time PCR. J Clin Microbiol 2002;40:1451–1455.

507. Yoshida T, Maeda S-I, Degeuchi T, Ishiko H. Phylogeny-based rapid identification of mycoplasmas an ureaplasmas from urethritis patients. J Clin Microbiol 2002;40:105–110.

508. Yoshida T, Maeda S-I, Deguchi T, et al. Rapid detection of *Mycoplasma genitalium*, *Mycoplasma hominis*, *Ureaplasma parvum*, and *Ureaplasma urealyticum* organisms in genitourinary samples by PCR-microtiter plate hybridization assay. J Clin Microbiol 2003;41:1850–1855.

509. Zhang Q, Wise KS. Localized reversible frameshift mutation in an adhesin genes confers a phase-variable adherence phenotype in mycoplasma. Mol Microbiol 1997;25:859–869.

Trends in Clinical Tuberculosis

Worldwide Increase in the Incidence of Tuberculosis
Impact of Coinfection With HIV and *Mycobacterium tuberculosis*
Persons at Risk for Tuberculosis
Rapidly Progressive Disease
Implementation of More Aggressive Infection Control and Epidemiologic Measures

Trends in the Laboratory Diagnosis of Tuberculosis

Use of Molecular Techniques
Use of Automated Instruments
Use of Broth Culture Media
Inoculation of Clinical Specimens to Agar-Based Culture Media
Use of *p*-nitro-acetylamino-hydroxypropiophenone (NAP)
Applications of Gas-Liquid and High-Performance Liquid Chromatography
Use of the Lysis-Centrifugation System Blood Culture Tube

The Clinical Laboratory

Optimizing the Detection and Identification of Mycobacteria
Laboratory Safety

Specimen Collection

Respiratory Specimens
Blood Cultures
Stool Specimens

Miscellaneous "Sterile" Specimens

Laboratory Approach to the Recovery and Identification of Mycobacteria

Specimen Preparation
Digestion and Decontamination
Centrifugation
Bone Marrow and Biopsy Specimens
Miscellaneous Liquid Specimens
Staining of Acid-Fast Bacilli

Culture of Specimens for Recovery of Mycobacteria

Culture Media
Nonselective Culture Media for Recovery of Mycobacteria
Media of Cohen and Middlebrook
Selective Media
Incubation

Rapid Methods for Establishing a Diagnosis

Sensitivity of Acid-Fast Smears
Gas-Liquid and High-Performance Liquid Chromatography
Use of Broth Culture Medium

Automated Detection Systems

BACTEC AFB System
Mycobacteria Growth Indicator Tube (MGIT) and MGIT 960

MB/BacT Mycobacteria Detection System

The ESP Culture System II

The BACTEC MYCO/F LYTIC

Manual Detection Systems

Septi-Chek AFB System

Identification of Mycobacteria Using Conventional Methods

Optimal Temperature for Isolation and Rates of Growth

Pigment Production

Niacin Accumulation

Reduction of Nitrates to Nitrites

Tween 80 Hydrolysis

Catalase Activity

Arylsulfatase Activity

Urease Activity

Pyrazinamidase

Iron Uptake

Growth Inhibition by Thiophene-2-Carboxylic Acid Hydrazide

Growth in 5% Sodium Chloride

Growth on MacConkey Agar

Classification of Mycobacteria

Laboratory Identification of Mycobacteria and Related Clinical Syndromes

Review of *Mycobacterium* Species: Laboratory Aspects and Clinical Correlations

Mycobacterium tuberculosis Complex

Photochromogens

Scotochromogens

Nonphotochromogens

Rapid Growers

Other Mycobacteria

The Detection and Identification of Mycobacteria by Molecular Methods

Signal-Amplification Methods

Nucleic-Acid Probes

In Situ Hybridization

Nucleic-Acid Amplification Methods

Commercially Available Applications

Home-Brew PCR Assays, Including Real-Time PCR

Postamplification Analysis

Reverse Hybridization

DNA Sequencing

Microarray Analysis

Strain Typing and DNA Fingerprinting

Susceptibility Testing
Short-Course Therapy

American Thoracic Society Recommendations

Summary

New techniques and revised algorithms for the recovery, identification, and susceptibility testing of mycobacteria are being implemented in many clinical laboratories in view of changes in the clinical manifestations and epidemiology of tuberculosis. In the short term, conventional methods will continue to be used; however, rapid molecular-based techniques for the identification and susceptibility testing of *Mycobacterium* species recovered from clinical specimens are being introduced. At least two thirds of the basic and applied research papers relative to mycobacteriology and tuberculosis published in the current medical literature focus on potential laboratory applications of molecular techniques. Although the quest for pure research in molecular biology is an integral part of this evolution, the driving force for clinical laboratory personnel is to provide ever more rapid species identifications and antimycobacterial drug susceptibility profiles. As molecular-based procedures evolve from research laboratories into commercial products, many of which will receive Food and Drug Administration (FDA) approval, the ability to diagnose tuberculosis within days—or incredibly even hours—rather than weeks, will be possible in most diagnostic laboratories.

Trends in Clinical Tuberculosis

The following are trends in the epidemiology of tuberculosis that must be addressed by clinicians and infection control and laboratory personnel.

Worldwide Increase in the Incidence of Tuberculosis

The incidence of tuberculosis in the United States progressively declined during the first eight decades of the 1900s, but this trend changed in the early 1980s.[24] Complacency replaced vigilance as the incidence curve of tuberculosis approached zero in many parts of the world by the late

1970s, and many had confidence that tuberculosis was about to be conquered.[41,144,285] In fact, the opposite has happened. From 1985 to 1992 there was an increase in reported cases of tuberculosis in the United States.[144] In addition to complacency, a number of factors contributed to this trend, including changes in the means of federal funding for tuberculosis control, the HIV/AIDS epidemic, increased immigration of people from areas of high endemicity, overcrowding of the impoverished, and the emergence of multidrug-resistant strains of *M. tuberculosis*.[24–26,42,59,144,249,335,341,343] From 1992 to 2002 there was again a decreasing trend in the number of cases of tuberculosis in the United States because of improved public health measures, including directly observed therapy. Throughout the world, however, the impact of tuberculosis is worse than ever, particularly in areas with a large number of HIV-infected persons.

In 1993 the World Health Organization in an unprecedented step declared tuberculosis a global emergency. The fact sheet of global tuberculosis is stunning (http://www.who.int/mediacentre/factsheets/who104/en/) and contains the following information:

1. One third of the world's population is currently infected with *M. tuberculosis*.
2. A new infection with tuberculosis occurs every second, resulting in new tuberculosis infections in 1% of the world population annually.
3. The tuberculosis epidemic is growing; it kills approximately 2 million persons per year.
4. HIV is significantly contributing to the spread of tuberculosis.
5. Newly acquired infections between 2002 and 2020 are projected at 1 billion persons. Of these, 150 million will get sick and 36 million will die of tuberculosis.

In industrialized countries, 80% of cases occur in persons older than 50 years of age; in developing countries, 80% of cases occur between the ages of 15 and 50. It has been estimated that at least 15 million persons in the United States are skin-test-positive or have clinical disease. The rates of increase are even greater in developing countries, because of high rates of endemicity, declining or chronically poor socioeconomic conditions in densely populated cities, and the increasing number of HIV-infected individuals.

Impact of Coinfection With HIV and *Mycobacterium tuberculosis*

The HIV pandemic, which is largely uncontrolled in many parts of the world, has contributed significantly to the spread of tuberculosis. HIV infection and tuberculosis are synergistic diseases on the every level, from the molecular to the epidemiologic.[25,59] For instance, the presence of HIV promotes the intracellular replication of the tubercle bacillus and thereby promotes the transmission of *M. tuberculosis* to others. In many parts of the world, tuberculosis is the leading cause of death in persons infected with HIV. It has been estimated by the World Health Organization (WHO) that a third of the 36.1 million persons who are infected with HIV

also have tuberculosis.[279] The most powerful risk factor known for the reactivation of latent tuberculosis is coinfection with HIV.[31,88,181,310] Considering that the majority of people infected with HIV, *M. tuberculosis*, or both live in impoverished conditions with inadequate healthcare, this situation will only deteriorate.

Persons at Risk for Tuberculosis

The following high-risk groups, designated by the Centers for Disease Control and Prevention (CDC) Advisory Council for the Elimination of Tuberculosis, should be screened for tuberculosis[56]:

1. Close contacts (those sharing the same household or other enclosed environment) of persons known or suspected to have tuberculosis.
2. Persons infected with HIV.
3. Persons who inject illicit drugs or other locally identified high-risk substance users (such as crack-cocaine users).
4. Persons who have medical risk factors known to increase the chance for disease if infection occurs.
5. Residents and employees of high-risk congregate settings (such as correctional institutions, nursing homes, mental institutions, other long-term residential facilities, and shelters for the homeless).
6. Healthcare workers who serve high-risk clients.
7. Foreign-born persons, including children, recently arrived (within 5 years) from countries that have a high incidence or prevalence of tuberculosis.
8. Some medically underserved low-income populations.
9. High-risk racial or ethnic minority populations, as defined locally.
10. Infants, children, and adolescents exposed to adults in high-risk categories.

It is recommended that local or state tuberculosis programs take the lead in determining the groups to be screened. In some locales, the local health departments should conduct the screening, or they should discuss the need for screening with other appropriate persons, such as the staff of correctional facilities, hospital infection-control officers, and operators of shelters. The CDC provides several recommendations for conducting programs and handling specific high-risk groups.[56]

Rapidly Progressive Disease

Recently acquired infections with *M. tuberculosis* do not invariably follow the classic, slowly progressive course of secondary disease. Primary progressive tuberculosis or the rapidly spreading miliary type of tuberculosis is the rule rather than the exception in patients with profound immunosuppression, such as patients with AIDS. Progression of disease in such patients is no longer measured in terms of months and years but, rather, in weeks. The more rapid replication of mycobacteria at sites of infection, both of *M. tuberculosis* and particularly of strains belonging to the *M. avium-*

intracellulare (MAI) complex, leads not only to high concentrations of organisms at these sites, but also to septicemia, miliary spread, and potentially treatment failures secondary to the overwhelming burden of mycobacteria and possibly the emergence of multidrug-resistant strains.

Implementation of More Aggressive Infection Control and Epidemiologic Measures

More aggressive measures are also being instituted to ensure that patients with a high index of suspicion for tuberculosis are promptly placed in isolation. Hospital personnel involved in the direct care of patients with tuberculosis are at high risk for infection and are required to follow isolation procedures and wear protective clothing and high-filtering masks. Laboratory personnel who handle clinical specimens from patients with tuberculosis are also at risk for infection, but may work in a safe manner with these specimens using universal precautions, including specimen processing in laminar-flow biologic safety hoods. Ventilation systems in hospitals and in crowded settings, such as in prisons, nursing homes, and urban homeless shelters, where outbreaks of tuberculosis have been reported, are under intense scrutiny. Nardell and associates found that poor air quality contributed to airborne infection in buildings fitted with air duct systems that delivered an inadequate mixture of outside air.[241] Problems will remain in unsuspected settings, however, such as the outbreak of tuberculosis among 41 patrons of a local bar reported by Kline and coauthors.[180] The index case in this report was a homeless person who was a regular patron of the bar, who had a long asymptomatic interval before diagnosis. The possibility of heavy alcohol use among this population of patrons may also have contributed to the high rate of infectivity; others have shown this risk factor to be associated with tuberculosis transmission.

Trends in the Laboratory Diagnosis of Tuberculosis

In response to these altered clinical and epidemiologic situations, several changes in laboratory practice have evolved over the past several years. Several new techniques have been introduced that are directed toward the detection of *M. tuberculosis* directly in clinical specimens by nucleic-acid amplification, the more effective recovery of mycobacteria from clinical specimens, the rapid identification of mycobacteria, and the determination of drug susceptibility profiles. The following is a brief summary of several of these new methods:

Use of Molecular Techniques

Molecular methods have significantly changed the time to identification for laboratories that use these technologies (see below for more details). This began with the use of commercially available nucleic-acid probes for the identification of members of the *M. tuberculosis* complex, the MAI complex, *M. kansasii*, and *M. gordonae*. The use of these probes significantly reduced the time to identification for

these organisms and, most importantly, rapidly confirmed or excluded the presence of *M. tuberculosis*.

The detection of *M. tuberculosis* directly on clinical specimens is possible using nucleic-acid amplification tests. Two such methods have received approval by the FDA for use on clinical specimens; both are highly sensitive and specific for *M. tuberculosis* in smear-positive specimens. A variety of "home-brew" assays have also been described, most recently in several of the real-time formats. Although theoretically, DNA from a single mycobacterial cell may be detected after PCR amplification, in reality, more than one cell is required, given the presence of PCR inhibitors in clinical specimens. For example, Yajko and associates determined that 42 colony-forming units (CFU) was the lower cutoff concentration in direct sputum specimens with their assay, which corresponded to eight CFU that were be recovered in culture from *N*-acetyl-L-cysteine (NALC)-NaOH–processed specimens.[401]

Other molecular biology techniques, such as nucleic-acid sequencing, reverse hybridization, and microarray analysis have also been used successfully to rapidly characterize mycobacteria that grow in culture. These techniques will have considerable impact on the way we practice mycobacteriology in the future and are considered further below.

Use of Automated Instruments

The time to recovery of mycobacteria from sputum and other specimens, including blood cultures, has been shortened by as much as 2 to 3 weeks with the use of automated systems.[236,287] The BACTEC 460 (BD Diagnostic Systems, Sparks, MD), BACTEC Mycobacteria Growth Indicator Tube (MGIT) 960 (BD Diagnostic), and the ESP II (Trek Diagnostic Systems, Westlake, OH) are also cleared by the FDA for rapid drug susceptibility testing of front-line antituberculous drugs.[128,396] A rise in the growth index, as determined by the instrument, in the antibiotic-containing vial within 3 to 5 days following inoculation with the test strain indicates drug resistance.

Use of Broth Culture Media

The rate of recovery and time to positivity of mycobacteria from clinical specimens have also been improved through the use of broth culture media. Broth-based culture systems for mycobacteria include the manual and automated MGIT systems (BD Diagnostic), which use 7H9 broth and an O_2-sensitive fluorescent sensor to indicate microbial growth, the MB/BacT bottle (BioMérieux, Durham, NC), the BACTEC MYCO/F lytic bottle (BD Diagnostic), the manual Septi-Chek system (BD Diagnostic), and the ESP Culture System II (Trek Diagnostic).

Inoculation of Clinical Specimens to Agar-Based Culture Media

The inoculation of a clear, agar-based culture medium, such as Middlebrook 7H10 or 7H11 permits the microscopic observation for microcolonies. Growth of colonies may be observed microscopically as early as 5 to 7 days after inoculation of smear-positive specimens. The morphology of the microcolonies has been used by some for making early presumptive identifications of *M. tuberculosis* and members of the MAI. This information often provides a helpful guide to further workup of the isolate, particularly in selecting the appropriate nucleic-acid probe assay.

Use of *p*-nitro-acetylamino-hydroxypropiophenone (NAP)

NAP is an antimycobacterial agent that selectively inhibits the growth of *M. tuberculosis* in broth culture media. After inoculation of a BACTEC culture vial containing NAP and the test organism, any rise in the growth index, which indicates resistance to NAP, after 3 days of incubation excludes the possibility of *M. tuberculosis*.

Applications of Gas-Liquid and High-Performance Liquid Chromatography

The composition of cell wall mycolic acids and fatty acid constituents, as determined by gas-liquid chromatography (GLC) and high-performance liquid chromatography (HPLC), provides profiles that are helpful in making a rapid species identification of mycobacteria recovered from clinical specimens.

Use of the Lysis-Centrifugation System Blood Culture Tube

The recovery of mycobacteria from peripheral blood and bone marrow samples may be improved by releasing intracellular mycobacterial cells into the blood culture broth, increasing the rate and reducing the time of recovery.

Thus, a combination of improved traditional microbiologic techniques and applications of molecular diagnostic techniques are being used as tools for the rapid detection and identification of mycobacteria in clinical specimens and positive cultures. The more rapid identification of the mycobacteria present affords aggressive, directed antimycobacterial therapy, which helps to prevent the emergence of drug-resistant strains and has implications regarding the human-to-human transmission of tuberculosis.[262] The several new approaches outlined in the foregoing will be discussed in more detail later in this chapter.

The Clinical Laboratory
Optimizing the Detection and Identification of Mycobacteria

Salfinger outlines what he refers to as a ''fast-track'' program, in reference to the overall organization of clinical laboratories and the necessity to provide more laboratory services.[298,300] Three primary goals of the fast-track program are:

1. To use the most rapid and reliable technologies to achieve the shortest turnaround times possible for organism identification and susceptibility testing.
2. To centralize such services to control costs.

3. To have patients with non–*M. tuberculosis* infections confined to respiratory isolation rooms for as short a time as possible.

The traditional practice of waiting for bacterial colonies to appear on solid agar, making species identifications without probe technology, and performing drug susceptibility tests only on solid media is too time-consuming. Decisions regarding the procedures and tests that will be performed in the on-site laboratory and which will be sent to a qualified reference laboratory must be determined within each practice care community. In many practice settings, activities of the on-site laboratory may be limited to rapid-turnaround procedures, such as screening acid-fast smears or the inoculation and provisional assessment of cultures. Other procedures, again to be determined by local healthcare personnel, may be best performed in the regional reference laboratory. Most of the techniques involved in direct identifications, such as HPLC, nucleic-acid probe analysis, polymerase chain reaction (PCR), restriction endonuclease assays, and DNA sequencing, will be within the province of the reference laboratory, but are becoming more widely available. A team of healthcare workers, including clinicians, laboratory specialists, and support personnel must be established to determine how diagnostic approaches are to be coordinated within the fast-track program to ensure that the goals are attained. Early diagnosis, prompt appropriate therapy, and respiratory isolation are the major ingredients to ensure the cure of the infected patient, prevent the emergence of resistant strains, and interrupt person-to-person transmission.

Laboratory Safety

The inappropriate handling of infectious biologic material such as clinical specimens places laboratory personnel at risk for infection. There has been a growing national concern over biosafety relative to the handling of potentially infectious clinical specimens and cultures in clinical microbiology laboratories. Stringent safety control standards conforming to the biosafety level 3 (BSL3) standard are now being recommended in many instances, particularly when working with cultured isolates. Specifically, BSL3 practices are required for laboratories in which American Thoracic Society levels II and III activities are performed, which for mycobacteria are the propagation and manipulation of cultures for *M. tuberculosis* or *M. bovis*. The following are the proposed biosafety requirements as specified by the Department of Health and Human Services (*Biosafety in Microbiological and Biomedical Laboratories*, 3rd ed., 1993).

The BSL3 space, which includes the biologic safety cabinet (BSC) and centrifuge, should have nonpermeable walls and work surfaces, directional airflow (with the lowest air pressure in the laboratory), and a double-door air lock to prevent the backflow of air. Air from the BSL space should be vented through high-efficiency particulate air (HEPA) filters directly to the outside. Laboratories and hoods should be equipped with gauges to monitor air pressure.

Because equipment and the worker's arms placed in a BSC may disrupt the laminar airflow and deflect contaminated air out of the cabinet, anyone working in the laminar flow biologic safety cabinet and in the BSL3 space should also wear personal protective equipment, including a respirator. Personnel must be tested each year to ensure that the respirator fits correctly. Disposable gowns should be worn over a scrub suit (street clothes should not be worn into the BSL3 space because they may become contaminated), along with gloves, caps, and shoe protection to complete the protective personal accessories, since accidental splashes may occur. Protective clothing should be removed and placed in a bag for autoclaving when work in the BSL3 is completed.

Each laboratory director must determine the extent to which renovations in the current laboratory space may be required. Renovations may cost many thousands of dollars and may not be cost-effective in certain settings. In such instances, a decision must be considered about whether cultures for mycobacteria would be more effectively performed at another facility, such as a reference laboratory that can comply with the recommended standards.

Specimen Collection

Mycobacteria can be recovered from a variety of clinical specimens, including upper respiratory specimens (sputum, bronchial washes, bronchoalveolar lavage, and bronchial biopsies); urine, feces, blood, cerebrospinal fluid (CSF); tissue biopsies, and deep needle aspirations of virtually any tissue or organ.[184] Specimens that may contain normal bacterial flora should be processed as soon after collection as possible to minimize the degree of overgrowth with specimen contaminants.

Respiratory Specimens

Sputum samples collected by expectoration or by ultrasonic nebulization are best obtained shortly after the patient awakens in the morning, when mycobacteria are at their highest concentration. In the past, 24-hour sputum samples were required to have a sufficient concentration of mycobacteria present to maximize recovery; however, the extraction procedures currently being used are more efficient and require a smaller specimen to achieve the same degree of recovery. Twenty-four-hour collections are now discouraged because the sample containing the highest concentration of mycobacteria will be proportionally diluted by subsequent low-yield samples, and the chances for bacterial and fungal overgrowth during the prolonged collection process are significantly increased.[166]

The irregular and intermittent release of mycobacteria into the bronchial lumen from mucosal ulcers or loculated cavities often results in a variable pattern of recovery from respiratory secretions. Cultures obtained from patients with pulmonary or renal tuberculosis, in particular, may be positive one day but negative the next; thus, a minimum of three early-morning sputum or five early-morning urine specimens should be collected on successive 24-hour periods to maximize the chance of recovery of mycobacteria. All specimens should be transported promptly to the laboratory and refrigerated if processing is delayed.

Blood Cultures

Several approaches may be used for the recovery of mycobacteria from blood cultures. Berlin and associates report on the use of a biphasic system using modified 7H11 oleic acid albumin as the agar phase and brain-heart infusion as the broth phase. Positive cultures for MAI were obtained as early as 6 to 8 days.[20] However, Agy and coworkers report that only 43.8% of blood cultures from known blood culture–positive patients were recovered using a similar biphasic system.[3] The use of the lysis-centrifugation blood culture system (Isolator; Wampole Laboratories, Cranbury, NJ) has increased the yield and shortened the time of recovery of mycobacteria from blood cultures.[104,212] The lysis-centrifuge tube contains an anticoagulant and a lysing agent to effect rupture of both erythrocytes and neutrophils. Thus, intracellular mycobacteria are released into the broth milieu, further enriched by the lysis of the red blood cells. Each tube holds 5 mL of blood, and cell lysis can be enhanced by gently inverting the tube several times immediately after adding the sample. Following centrifugation of the tube at 3,000 g for 20 to 30 minutes, the eluate is discarded and 1.6 mL of sediment is divided into 0.2-mL aliquots for transfer to appropriate culture media.

One of the first semiautomated blood culture systems for the mycobacteria was the BACTEC (Becton Dickinson, Sparks, MD) system; the detection of positive bottles was based on the detection of radioactive $^{14}CO_2$ released in the blood culture vial from the metabolism of 1-[^{14}C]-palmitic acid that was included in the broth medium (Middlebrook).

It has been theorized that the lysis-anticoagulant reagent (LAR) contained within the Isolator tube may be toxic to MAI when the lysate is transferred to a closed liquid system, in contrast to subculture to solid media, for which the component is able to diffuse into the agar or evaporate into the overlying airspace. Whittier and associates conducted an Isolator recovery study in which recovery of MAI from Septi-Check AFB biphasic media was superior to their recovery from the BACTEC 12B bottles inoculated in parallel.[383a]

However, Doern and Westerling found that the inhibitory effect of LAR in BACTEC 12B bottles is minimized if a small inoculum (0.2 mL) of Isolator lysate is used.[77,78] Wasilauskas and Morrell, however, provide the counterargument that using a smaller inoculum may compromise recovery in light infections.[372] Perhaps, if a closed-liquid system is to be used for transfer of lysis-centrifuged-processed blood specimens, inoculation of solid media in parallel may be in order, particularly in AIDS patients, from whom the recovery of MAI organisms is highly likely.

The issue is avoided in many laboratories by using the lytic blood culture bottles, thereby bypassing the potential problems associated with the Isolator system. In a study of 32 cases of mycobacterial sepsis, growth was detected in 30 of the 13A vials (93.7%), on 27 Middlebrook 7H11 agar plates inoculated with sediment obtained from the Isolator tube (84.4%), and in 26 BACTEC 12B bottles inoculated with the Isolator sediment (81.2%).[3] Growth was detected in the 13B vial and in the 12B vials at 14.2 and 13.7 days, respectively, compared with 20.8 days for the M7H11 plates. This study concluded that the BACTEC 13A vial is equal to or better than the Isolator system, both in the rate and the time of recovery of mycobacteria from blood cultures, a conclusion also reached by others.[390] Strand and associates also found the BACTEC 13A vial comparable with the lysis-centrifugation/7H11 agar procedure in the rate of recovery (96.9% and 98.5%, respectively) and the time of detection of 64 blood cultures positive for *M. avium* and one for *M. tuberculosis.*[337] Details of the lytic blood culture bottles and their applications in the mycobacteriology laboratory will be presented later in this chapter.

There are several newer commercially available options for the culture of blood for mycobacteria, some of which contain lytic agents to aid in the release of the mycobacteria from phagocytes. These include the ESP Culture System II (Trek Diagnostic), the BACTEC MYCO/F lytic (BD Diagnostic Systems), and the MB/BacT bottle (BioMérieux) and are discussed further below.

Whatever blood culture system is used, the policy of routinely obtaining at least two culture sets may not be cost-effective for patients in whom mycobacteremia is suspected.[334] From a total of 1,047 mycobacterial blood cultures obtained from 273 patients with disseminated MAI, Stone and colleagues found that only one of the two bottles was positive in only four of 98 positive cultures (4%).[334] In 85%, both bottles were negative, and in 11%, both bottles were positive. Thus, as a routine they recommend obtaining only a single blood culture for the diagnosis of mycobacterial septicemia and ordering a repeat culture only if there is strong clinical evidence of disseminated infection. The importance of obtaining blood cultures in patients with suspected tuberculosis has been stressed.[29] Fourteen percent of patients with disseminated tuberculosis had positive blood cultures (intravenous-drug use and chronic alcoholism were risk factors); in the past, up to 26–42% of patients with AIDS had mycobacterial infections at some time during the course of their illness, and in 33%, positive blood cultures provided the initial recovery of the organism. Blood cultures positive for acid-fast bacilli, therefore, provide a noninvasive procedure for diagnosing disseminated disease.

Stool Specimens

In certain patients with AIDS, the concentration of mycobacteria, particularly MAI may be sufficiently high in the lower intestinal tract to be recovered in culture. Kiehn and associates have outlined a procedure for processing stool specimens for mycobacterial culture[170]:

- Stool specimens are collected in a clean (not necessarily sterile) container with a tightly fitting lid, as for routine bacterial cultures.
- A direct smear is first prepared from a small quantity of the specimen and stained for acid-fast bacilli, using either the Ziehl-Neelsen or Kinyoun carbolfuchsin techniques or the rhodamine-auramine fluorescence method.
- If the smears are negative for acid-fast bacteria, the specimen is not processed further.
- If acid-fast bacilli are seen in the smear, 1 g of feces is suspended in 5 mL of Middlebrook 7H9 broth or equivalent and subjected to the same NaOH digestion-decon-

tamination as used for sputum specimens, to be described below.
- Culture contamination with intestinal bacteria is significantly diminished during the digestion procedure.

One might raise a question about the significance of detecting mycobacteria in fecal samples. Conlon and coworkers, in a study of 89 patients with AIDS-related enteropathy in Lusaka, Zambia, found that the symptom of chronic diarrhea did not correlate with the presence of mycobacteria in stool specimens.[54] They concluded that mycobacteria play an insignificant role in the pathogenesis of enteropathy in AIDS patients. Alternatively, Chin and colleagues found that the recovery of MAI organisms from stool specimens is predictive of disseminated disease.[44] The technique described in the foregoing is workable; whether the procedure should be made available in a given laboratory must be an individual decision.

Miscellaneous "Sterile" Specimens

Specimens submitted for acid-fast culture that are normally sterile, such as cerebrospinal fluid, synovial fluid, and other body fluids, need not be decontaminated before culture. Processing can commence with centrifugation, as described below, and a small aliquot of the sediment transferred to an appropriate culture medium. Low-volume fluid samples can be added directly to approximately 10 mL of 7H9 or 7H11 broth and incubated directly. Urine samples can usually be processed without decontamination, centrifuged, and a portion of the sediment used for culture, as described above. The first morning sample rather than a 24-hour collection is preferred. It is the practice in some laboratories to set up bacterial cultures before culturing for mycobacteria to determine whether the specimens require decontamination. Also, 10 or 15 mL of 10% calcium chloride can be added to the urine sample until a precipitate forms to remove inhibitory factors. Following centrifugation, a portion of the sediment is cultured, as described above. Tissues and needle biopsy material should be placed in a small quantity of 7H9 or 7H11 broth as a holding medium. Depending on the size and nature of the material obtained, the specimen should be ground in a small amount of broth with a mortar and pestle and aliquots of the suspension transferred to appropriate culture media.

There is virtually no indication for obtaining material for mycobacterial culture with a swab because the hydrophobic nature of the lipid-containing cell wall of the bacteria inhibits transfer of the organisms from the swab to the aqueous culture medium. If a swab is received in the laboratory, the tip should be placed directly on the surface of the culture medium or into a tube containing approximately 5 mL of 7H9 broth and incubated for 4 to 8 weeks. Mycobacteria, if present, may be found forming colonies in the fibers of the swab at the junction with the culture media. Alternatively, the laboratory director may properly decide that a swab is an inappropriate specimen for mycobacteria and reject the specimen for mycobacterial culture. Decisions not to process these low-to-no-yield specimens can save the hospital a considerable amount of money over time. The medical staff should be educated regarding the reasoning of such decisions and notified prior to the implementation of specimen-rejection protocols.

Laboratory Approach to the Recovery and Identification of Mycobacteria

The classic laboratory approach to the diagnosis of mycobacterial infections involves the phenotypic characterization of colonies growing on Löwenstein-Jensen medium. Using a battery of biochemical tests is too time-consuming for current applications. Figure 19-1 is an algorithm that reflects the practice of processing sputum specimens in many clinical laboratories. Other specimens may require alternative treatments. The current recommendation is that a combination

of phenotypic and molecular assays are used for the rapid identification of mycobacteria, particularly for the identification of *M. tuberculosis*.

Smears should be prepared from the material submitted for acid-fast staining. Most laboratories use the auramine O stain for screening and follow up with a carbolfuchsin-based stain (Ziehl-Neelsen or Kinyoun) for confirmation of positive results. Most laboratories treat sputum specimens with NALC-NaOH, a decontamination-digestion procedure for concentrating any mycobacterial cells that may be present. It is currently recommended that all sputum digests and other specimens be inoculated to broth culture media in addition to Löwenstein-Jensen media or Middlebrook agar. The choices of broth cultures include the BACTEC 12A bottles in laboratories where a 460 BACTEC instrument is available or inoculation of the Septi-Chek (BD Diagnostic Systems,

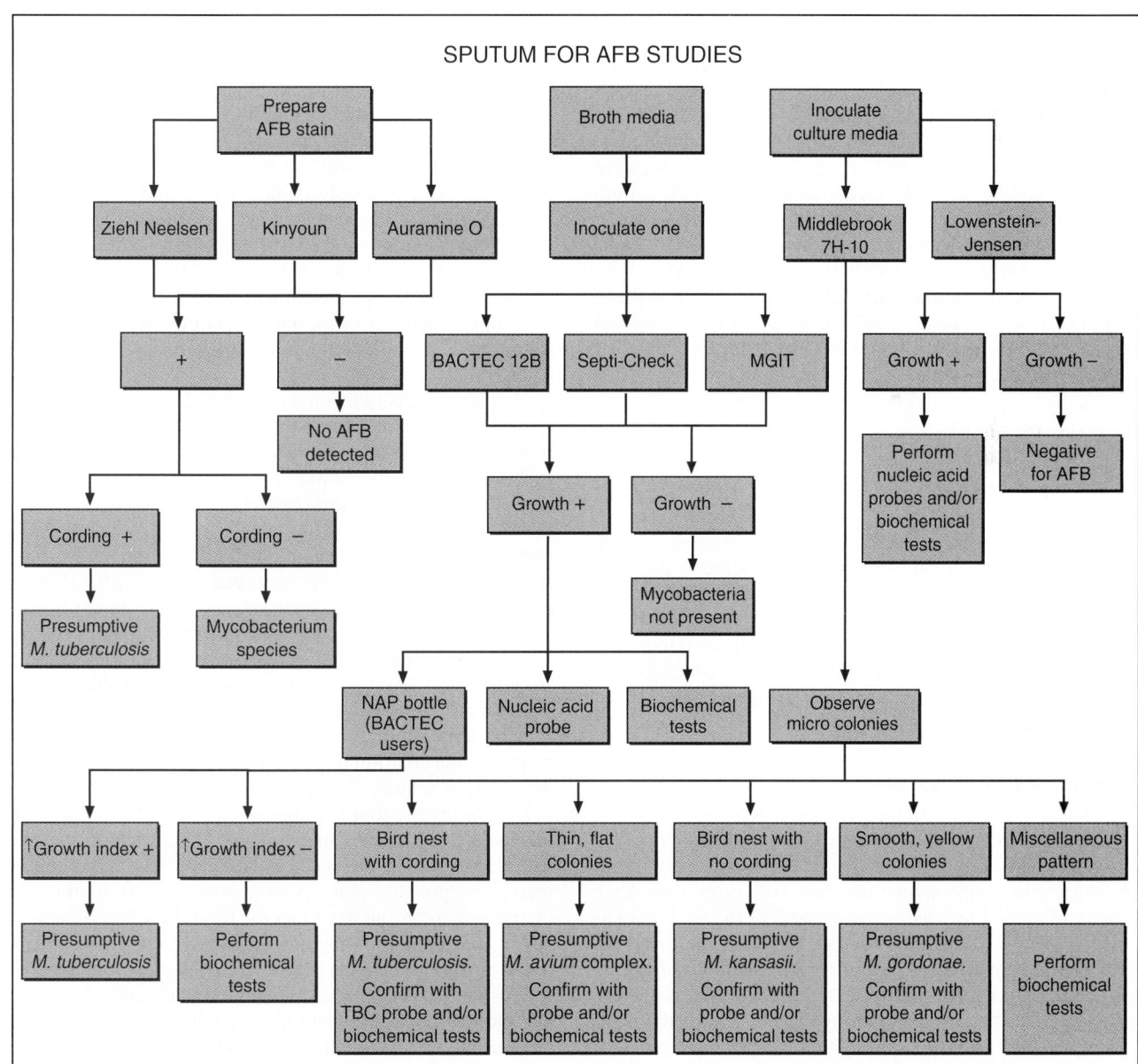

Figure 19-1 An algorithm reflecting the practice of processing sputum specimens.

Sparks, MD) or the MGIT (BD Diagnostic) culture system. If any of these cultures show evidence of growth, nucleic-acid probe studies should be done as soon as the concentration of organisms exceeds the threshold of sensitivity for the assay. In laboratories using the BACTEC system, a NAP bottle should be inoculated to rule out *M. tuberculosis*.

Observation of microcolonies on Middlebrook agar may serve as a guide as to which probe should be performed: if an interweaving pattern with cording is observed, a probe for *M. tuberculosis* should be performed; if the colonies are flat and transparent, the probe for MAI is in order. Metchock and Diem suggest that if smears are 3+ or 4+ and growth is detected within 5 days, a probe for *M. tuberculosis* should be done.[225] For 1+ or 2+ smears that grow in culture after 7 days, the MAI probe should be done. If all probes are negative and the isolate is considered clinically significant, conventional biochemical studies should be performed using the colonies grown on Löwenstein-Jensen medium if positive. *In vitro* drug susceptibility studies should also be performed if required.

By following the algorithm shown in Figure 19-1, the identification of *M. tuberculosis*, MAI, *M. kansasii*, and *M. gordonae* may be possible in smear-positive cases within 2 to 3 weeks. An additional 1 or 2 weeks may be required to recover and identify these four species in smear-negative cases. An additional week is required after the broth culture becomes positive for susceptibility test results against the four mainline drugs: isoniazid, *p*-aminosalicylic acid, ethambutol, and streptomycin. An additional 2 to 4 weeks will be required to identify mycobacterial species other than those just mentioned, depending on the results of biochemical tests, and to determine drug profiles using conventional agar growth methods.

Specimen Preparation

The high concentration of lipids in the cell wall of most mycobacteria makes them more resistant to killing by strong acid and alkaline solutions than other bacteria that may be present in the specimen. Consequently, specimens likely to contain a mixed bacterial flora are treated with a decontaminating agent to reduce undesirable bacterial overgrowth and to liquefy mucus. After treatment with the decontaminating agent for a carefully controlled period, the acid or alkali used is neutralized and the mixture is centrifuged at high speed to concentrate the mycobacteria.

Digestion and Decontamination

Some decontaminating solutions, such as 6% sodium hydroxide, are so strong that they may kill or seriously injure mycobacteria to the point that they will grow only very slowly, if at all. Decreasing the strength of the acid or alkaline decontamination solution has resulted in improved recovery of mycobacteria by culture, but frequently at the price of overgrowth of the culture with contaminants. Exposure of specimens to strong sodium hydroxide, 5% oxalic acid, or other agents must be carefully timed to prevent excessive chemical injury to the mycobacterial cells.

The use of mild decontaminating agents, such as trisodium phosphate (TSP) alone or combined with benzalkonium chloride (Zephiran; Winthrop Laboratories, New York, NY), is popular in some laboratories. Specimens containing a large quantity of *M. tuberculosis* can withstand the action of these agents for as long as overnight, and careful timing of exposure is not required.[75] Specimens treated with TSP-Zephiran should be inoculated onto an egg-based culture medium to neutralize the growth inhibition of the Zephiran. If agar-based media are used, neutralization of the Zephiran can be accomplished by adding lecithin. The standard digestion-decontamination procedure is shown in Box 19-1.

Usually, concentrated HCl or concentrated NaOH is used to neutralize the decontaminating agents. Because of the strength of these solutions, a neutral end point is sometimes difficult to achieve. One advantage of the NALC procedure is that the addition of a large volume of phosphate buffer makes strong shifts in pH less likely. The addition of buffer serves to "wash" the specimen, dilutes toxic substances, and decreases the specific gravity of the specimen so that centrifugation is more effective in sedimentation of organisms.

Table 19-1 lists additional agents for decontaminating and concentrating specimens, along with comments about their use. Each mycobacteriologist should select the agents to use in their laboratory on the basis of the number and types of specimens received and the time and technical staff available to process the specimens. As listed in Table 19-1, dithiothreitol is also an effective mucolytic agent when used with 2% NaOH. Cetylpyridium chloride has also been recommended for the decontamination of specimens, particularly those mailed from remote sites of collection.[321] The digestion-decontamination procedure is further described in Chart 19-1.

Ratnam and coauthors have described a simplified acetyl-cysteine-alkaline procedure that combines the decontamination and the concentration steps and the inoculation of the specimen to selective culture media (containing antibiotics, to be described later in this chapter).[278] Specimens are mixed with the NALC-NaOH solution on a vortex mixer and, without any waiting or addition of buffer or water to the digested specimens, the mixture is centrifuged at 3,000 g for 15 minutes. The supernatant is decanted, and the sediment is suspended in 1 to 2 mL of phosphate buffer (0.067 M, pH 5.3). The NaOH concentration in the solution may be reduced from the usual 2% to 1.5% if necessary or feasible.

The modified method eliminates two steps: the 15- to 20-minute decontamination time following digestion of specimens and the addition of phosphate buffer or water. According to these authors[278], the greatest killing of mycobacteria occurs during the first few minutes of exposure to the alkali digestion fluid, and as many as 10^4 mycobacteria may be lost, depending on the species. The modified method eliminates the potential for specimens to drip from the cap or run down the outer surface of the tube when diluent is added after vortex mixing and reduces the chance for cross-contamination. Thus, the authors found the modified method to be simpler, faster, and safer than the original procedure, and the reduced manipulation is also likely to minimize the chance for cross-contamination in sequential specimen processing. Eliminating the initial digestion step had no adverse effects on the recovery of mycobacteria. In fact, at times,

Box 19-1 The Standard Digestion-Decontamination Procedure Developed by Kubica et al. at the Centers for Disease Control and Prevention[190]

1. Prepare the acetylcysteine-alkali digestant as follows: Combine 50 mL of 2.94% trisodium citrate-3H$_2$O (0.1 M) with 50 mL of 4% NaOH. To this solution, add 0.5 g of powdered *N*-acetyl-L-cysteine (NALC) just before use. The NaOH (which becomes a 2% solution after mixing equal parts with the specimen) serves as a decontaminating agent. Occasionally, the concentration of NaOH must be increased to 3% (6% original solution) during warm weather or in treating specimens from patients with large pulmonary cavities associated with persistent bacterial contamination. The NALC is a mucolytic agent without bactericidal activity that liquefies mucus by splitting disulfide bonds. The mycobacteria are released when the mucus is liquefied, rendering them easy to concentrate by high-speed centrifugation.

2. Use 50-mL plastic centrifuge tubes with tightly fitting lids for the processing of all specimens. Add the NALC digestant mixture in a volume equal to that of the specimen. Typically, a volume of 10–15 mL of specimen is used. Tighten the screw cap.

3. Homogenize the mixture with a vortex mixer for 15–20 seconds or until well mixed and allow to stand at room temperature for 15–20 minutes, swirling the tubes periodically. Proper attention should be paid so that this digestion time does not exceed 20 minutes, because "overtreated" specimens result in fewer positive cultures.

4. After the digestion-decontamination step, add phosphate buffer, pH 6.8 (preferred over sterile water), up to the top ring in the tube. Mix well. The phosphate buffer makes strong shifts in pH less likely and also serves to "wash" the specimen, to dilute and neutralize toxic substances, and to reduce the specific gravity of the specimen so that centrifugation is more effective in the sedimentation of organisms.

5. Concentrate the specimen by centrifugation at 2,000–3,000 *g* for 15–20 minutes. A refrigerated centrifuge may be used at higher speeds to increase the yield of mycobacteria.

6. After centrifugation, decant all the supernatant carefully into a splashproof receptacle containing a phenolic disinfectant. Wipe the lip of the tube with a cotton ball soaked with 5% phenol. Add a small quantity of phosphate buffer, pH 6.8 (1–2 mL), and resuspend the sediment with a Pasteur pipette. Although addition of a small quantity of serum albumin has been advocated in the past, this is currently avoided because it increases the chances for contamination and a potential delay in the detection time.

7. Prepare smears on clean microscope slides for Ziehl-Neelsen (or Kinyoun) and/or fluorochrome staining. Use either a sterile applicator stick or a flamed, 3-mm diameter bacteriologic loop and smear a portion of the sediment over an area 1 × 2 cm. If the quantity of sediment is very small, delay making smears until after the next step (i.e., the addition of albumin). Add 1 mL of sterile 0.2% bovine albumin.

8. Transfer a small quantity (0.2–0.4 mL) of the concentrate to an appropriate culture medium. Inoculation of a 1 : 10 dilution of the concentrate in sterile water to a second culture medium set is also done in some laboratories. Löwenstein-Jensen slants and Middlebrook 7H10 or 7H11 agar plates are generally used.

Table 19-1 Agents Commonly Used for Decontamination and Concentration of Specimens

AGENT	COMMENTS
N-Acetyl-L-cysteine plus 2% NaOH	Mild decontamination solution with mucolytic agent NALC to free mycobacteria entrapped in mucus. Limit exposure to NaOH to 15 minutes.
Dithiothreitol plus 2% NaOH[a]	Very effective mucolytic agent used with 2% NaOH. Trade name of dithiothreitol is Sputolysin. Reagent is more expensive than NALC. Limit exposure to NaOH to 15 minutes.
Trisodium phosphate, 13% plus benzalkonium chloride (Zephiran)	Preferred by laboratories that cannot carefully control time of exposure to decontamination solution. Zephiran should be neutralized with lecithin and not inoculated onto egg-based culture medium.
NaOH, 4%	Traditional decontamination and concentration solution. Time of exposure must be carefully controlled to no more than 15 minutes. NaOH, 4%, effects mucolytic action to promote concentration by centrifugation.
Trisodium phosphate, 13%	Can be used for decontamination of specimens when exposure time can be completely controlled. Not as effective as TSP-Zephiran mixture.
Oxalic acid, 5%	Most useful in processing specimens that contain *Pseudomonas aeruginosa* as a contaminant.
Cetylpyridium chloride, 1%, plus 2% NaCl[b]	Effective as a decontamination solution for sputum specimens mailed from outpatient clinics. Tubercle bacilli have survived 8-day transit without significant loss.

[a] See Shah and Dye.[313]
[b] See Smithwick et al.[321]

the addition of phosphate buffer or water actually resulted in poorer recovery, owing to a greater dissolution of the particulate matter in the specimens. Alkali tolerance was not a consistent feature among the mycobacterial species and strains tested, with the rapid growers being the most susceptible to a high pH. By reducing or eliminating the standard treatment time of 15 to 20 minutes or by decreasing the concentration of NaOH in the digestant solution from the usual 2% to either 1.5% or 1%, the adverse effects can be easily overcome.

Because of the emergence of drug-resistant strains of *M. tuberculosis*, the performance of rapid laboratory tests to determine drug susceptibility profiles may be necessary to guide early therapy.[98] Many of the new tests for identifying drug-resistance profiles are based on nucleic-acid amplification procedures. Consequently, it may be necessary to store specimens or digested concentrates for future batch testing or for shipping to a distant reference laboratory. It may be advisable to render such samples noninfectious at early stages of processing to minimize the biohazard to laboratory workers. Williams and associates found that ethanol fixation of sputum sediments containing *M. tuberculosis* served to render the bacteria nonviable, while still preserving the integrity of genomic DNA in a state suitable for testing by PCR techniques.[387] In their studies, 0.25 mL of sputum sediments were diluted with 0.583 mL of 100% ethanol to bring the final ethanol concentration to 70%. They recommend storage of the ethanol-treated specimens at 4°C if PCR testing is to be delayed. Zwadyk and coworkers review several methods for rendering specimens safe for further testing.[411] They discuss the killing effects and preservation of genomic DNA of mycobacteria in specimens after treatment with several disinfectants. They also introduced the technique of heating the samples at 100°C for 30 minutes in a boiling water bath or a forced-air oven, which both killed and lysed the mycobacteria, releasing short DNA fragments suitable for amplification.

Centrifugation

Rickman and Moyer have called attention to the importance of carefully controlling centrifugal force in the recovery of mycobacteria from clinical specimens, particularly in the correlation of positive smears with positive cultures.[284] The focus of their study was to understand the unique physical characteristics conferred on mycobacteria by the high lipid content of the cell wall (up to 30% dry weight). The lipid has the effect of making the specific gravity of the organism very low. If the organism is to be maximally sedimented during the centrifugation of the specimen, the specific gravity of the suspending fluid should be kept as low as possible, and the centrifugal force applied to the specimen should be as high as practical. Improved recovery of mycobacteria by culture occurred as the relative centrifugal force (RCF) was increased from 1,260 to 3,000 *g* (Table 19-2).[284] When the RCF was increased to 3,800 *g*, a twofold increase in the correlation of positive smears to positive cultures from 40% to 82% was realized, or more than a threefold increase from the correlation when the RCF was only 1,260 *g*.

Subsequent evaluation for recovery of mycobacteria from sputum samples seeded with known concentrations of organ-

Table 19-2 Effect of Increasing Centrifugal Force on Positive Smears and Cultures for Mycobacteria

	RELATIVE CENTRIFUGAL FORCE (g)		
	1,260	**3,000**	**3,800**
Positive smears	1.8%	4.5%	9.6%
Positive cultures	7.1%	11.2%	11.6%
Correlation of positive smears/ cultures	25%	40%	82%

Adapted from reference[284].

isms following centrifugation has confirmed that the recovery rate increases with centrifugation time and speed.[277] However, the recovery rates in these experimental samples were not significantly lower when using an RCF of 2,074 *g* for 20 minutes (67–71%) compared with the recovery rates at RCFs of 3,005 *g* and 3,895 *g* for 15 minutes (76–80%). Acid-fast smear sensitivity for 25,000 specimens processed with an RCF of 3,800 *g* for 20 minutes was 71%. However, sensitivity was still 69%, as determined for an additional 30,000 specimens processed in a similar manner but with an RCF of 2,000 *g*. The authors conclude that the actual rates of recovery of viable mycobacteria from clinical specimens also depends on the method of treatment and individual species and strain differences of mycobacteria for alkali tolerance. Thus, although centrifugation at an RCF of 3,000 *g* for 15 minutes may be optimal for the recovery of mycobacteria from clinical specimens, the chances for recovery will not be substantially compromised in laboratories where lower-cost centrifuges attaining only a maximum of 2,074 *g* are available, if the time is increased to 20 minutes. As pointed out by Sommers and Good, with the centrifugation forces produced at RCFs of 3000 *g* or higher, glass or plastic centrifuge tubes may collapse and must be placed in sealed cups.[324] Also, considerable heat is generated at high speeds, and refrigerated centrifuges may be required when RCFs exceed 3,000 *g*.

Bone Marrow and Biopsy Specimens

Mycobacterium tuberculosis is a facultative intracellular parasite that may be present in macrophages of the bone marrow, liver, blood, and lymph nodes of patients with disseminated infections. Because tissue biopsies are usually not contaminated with other microorganisms, they can be homogenized and inoculated directly onto culture media without the use of a decontaminating solution. Draining sinuses or other cutaneous lesions suspected of harboring mycobacteria are best cultured by obtaining a small portion of infected tissue or drainage. Fine-needle biopsies are also being used with increased frequency to obtain material for tissue culture from a variety of subcutaneous and deep visceral lesions. In a study of 390 cases in which needle biopsy specimens were obtained to diagnose suspected tuberculous lymphadenitis, the overall rate of smear positivity was 23.6%, and culture positivity was 35%.[273] Caseating lesions were more likely to produce positive cultures (40%) than noncaseating ones (9%).

Miscellaneous Liquid Specimens

Liquid specimens (e.g., CSF, pleural fluid, or other) should be centrifuged, stained for acid-fast bacilli, and inoculated directly onto liquid or solid culture media. Pleural fluid specimens are diluted with buffer in some laboratories to lower the specific gravity, thereby improving sedimentation of mycobacteria. Liquid specimens with a low protein content, such as CSF, can be filtered through a 0.22-μm cellulose nitrate membrane. The membrane can be cut into pieces, which can then be placed on or in different types of solid and liquid culture media.

Centrifuges used for the processing of specimens potentially containing acid-fast bacilli should be equipped with 50- or 250-mL centrifuge cups with aerosol-free tops that can be adapted to hold 50-mL centrifuge tubes. Such centrifuges should not be vented to the outdoors because of the danger of reverse airflow through the vent during windstorms. Precautions should be taken to prevent the spontaneous rupture of fluid surface tension membranes when inoculating broth cultures or liquid specimens. If such a membrane in an inoculation loop breaks, for example, droplet aerosols may be created that can persist in the air for long periods. All such transfers must be performed in a biologic safety hood.

Staining of Acid-Fast Bacilli

The cell walls of mycobacteria, because of their high lipid content, have the unique capability of binding the fuchsin dye so that it is not removed (destained) by acid alcohol. This acid-fast staining reaction of mycobacteria, along with their characteristic size and shape, is a valuable aid in the early detection of infection and in the monitoring of therapy for mycobacterial disease. The presence of acid-fast bacilli in the sputum, combined with a history of cough, weight loss, and chest radiographic evidence of a pulmonary infiltrate, is still presumptive evidence of active tuberculosis.

It has been estimated that when using standard concentrating techniques, approximately 10,000 acid-fast bacilli per milliliter of sputum are required to be detected by routine microscopy.[134] Patients with extensive disease shed large numbers of mycobacteria, with a good correlation between a positive smear and a positive culture. Many patients have minimal or less-advanced disease, and the correlation of positive smears to positive cultures in this group may be only 25–40%.

Acid-fast smears are also useful in following response to treatment. After antimycobacterial drugs are started, cultures become negative before the smears do, suggesting that the organisms are not capable of replicating but are capable of binding the stain. With continued treatment, more organisms are killed and fewer shed, so assessing the number of organisms in the sputum during treatment can provide an early objective measure of response. Should the number of organisms fail to decrease after therapy is started, the possibility

of drug resistance must be considered, and additional cultures and susceptibility studies should be obtained.

Two types of acid-fast stains are commonly used (Table 19-3):

1. Carbolfuchsin stains: a mixture of fuchsin with phenol (carbolic acid)
   a. Ziehl-Neelsen (hot stain)
   b. Kinyoun (cold stain)
2. Fluorochrome stain: auramine O, with or without a second fluorochrome, rhodamine

The carbolfuchsin and auramine O dyes used in these techniques each function by binding to mycolic acids in the mycobacterial cell wall. Smears stained with the carbolfuchsin technique must be scanned with an oil-immersion objective. This limits the total area of a slide that can be viewed in a given unit of time. In contrast to the carbolfuchsin stains, smears stained by the auramine procedure can be scanned with a 25× objective, thereby increasing the field of view and reducing the time needed to scan a given area of the slide. Fluorochrome-stained smears require a strong light source—either a 1200-W mercury vapor burner or a strong blue light with a fluorescein isothiocyanate (FITC) filter.

Fluorochrome-stained bacteria are bright yellow (rhodamine) or orange-red (rhodamine) against a dark background, allowing the slide to be scanned under lower magnification without losing sensitivity. The sharp contrast between the brightly colored mycobacteria and the dark background offers a distinct advantage in scanning the slide (see Color Plate 19-1A). Modifications of the auramine fluorochrome stain include the addition of rhodamine, giving a golden appearance to the cells, or the use of acridine orange as a counterstain, resulting in a red to orange background. False-positive reactions may be due to fluorescence of nonspecific tissue or cellular debris that can be mistaken for bacilli with the 25× objective. The 40× objective should be used to confirm any suspicious forms. Dead mycobacterial cells will also stain with rhodamine and auramine, leading to a smear-positive, culture-negative situation about 10% of the time. This feature is also important to remember when using acid-fast smears to assess treatment efficacy—the presence of acid-fast bacilli in fluorochrome-stained smears does not necessarily indicate treatment failure—and carbolfuchsin stains should also be performed. Fluorochrome-stained smears can be stained subsequently with carbolfuchsin; the opposite situation does not apply.

With carbolfuchsin, the acid-fast bacteria (AFB) stain bright red against either a blue or a green background, depending on the counterstain used (see Color Plate 19-1B). Although the Ziehl-Neelsen and the Kinyoun techniques are theoretically the same, it has been the experience of some that the former is more sensitive in detecting lightly staining organisms, particularly some of the rapidly growing mycobacteria. The property of acid-fastness is due to the thick, waxy capsule that surrounds the mycobacterial cells. For aqueous carbolfuchsin to penetrate through the wax, the capsule must be "softened." This is done with heat in the Ziehl-Neelsen procedure, much like the melting of a paraffin film in the hot rays of the sun. Dye that penetrates the heat-softened capsule binds to the cell wall; then, when the bacte-

Table 19-3 Acid-Fast–Staining Procedure

ZIEHL-NEELSEN PROCEDURE	KINYOUN COLD PROCEDURE	AURAMINE FLUOROCHROME PROCEDURE
Carbolfuchsin: Dissolve 3 g of basic fuchsin in 10 mL of 90–95% ethanol. Add 90 mL of 5% aqueous solution of phenol.	**Carbolfuchisin:** Dissolve 4 g of basic fuchsin in 20 mL of 90–95% ethanol and then add 100 mL of a 9% aqueous solution of phenl (9 g of phenol dissolved in 100 mL of distilled water)	**Phenolic auramine:** Dissolve 0.1 g of auramine O in 10 mL of 90–95% ethanol and then add to a solution of 3 g of phenol in 87 mL of distilled water. Store the stain in a brown bottle.
Acid-alcohol: Add 3 mL of concentrated HCl *slowly* to 97 mL of 90–95% ethanol, in this order. Solution may get hot!	**Acid-alcohol:** Add 3 mL of concentrated HCl *slowly* to 97 mL of 90–95% ethanol, in this order. Solution may get hot!	**Acid-alcohol:** Add 0.5 mL of concentrated HCl to 100 mL of 79% alcohol.
Methylene blue counterstain: Dissolve 0.3 g of methylene blue chloride in 100 mL of distilled	**Methylene blue counterstain:** Dissolve 0.3 g of methylene blue chloride in 100 mL of distilled water.	**Potassium permanganate:** Dissolve 0.5 g potassium permanganate in 100 mL of distilled water.
Procedure	**Procedure**	**Procedure**
Cover a heat-fixed, dried smear with a small rectangle (2 × 3 cm) of filter paper.	Cover a heat-fixed, dried smear with a small rectangle (2 × 3 cm) of filter paper.	Cover a heat-fixed, dried smear with carbol auramine and allow to stain for 15 min. Do not heat or cover withh filter paper.
Apply 5–7 drops of carbolfuchisin stain to thoroughly moistened filter paper.	Apply 5–7 drops of carbolfuchsin stain to thoroughly moisten filter paper. Allow to stand for 5 min.	Rinse with water and drain.
Heat the stain-covered slide to steaming, but do not allow to dry.	Add more stain if paper dries. Do not steam!	Decolorize with acid-alcohol (2 min). Rinse with water and drain.
Heating may be done by gas burner or over an electric staining rack.	Remove paper with forceps, rinse slide with water, and drain.	Flood smear with potassium permanganate for at least 2 and not more than 4 min.
Remove paper with forceps, rinse slide with water, and drain.	Decolorize with acid-alcohol until no more stain appears in the washing (2 min).	Rinse with tap water. Drain.
Decolorize with acid-alcohol until no more stain appears in the washing (2 min).	Counterstain with methylene blue (1–2 min).	Examine with 253 objective using a mercury vapor burner and BG-12 filter or a strong blue light.
Counterstain with methylene blue (1–2 min).	Rinse, drain, and air dry (1–2 min).	Mycobacteria are stained yellow-orange against a dark background.
Rinse, drain, and air dry (1–2 min).	Examine with 100 3 oil-immersion objective. Mycobacteria are stained red and the background light blue.	
Examine with 100 × oil-immersion objective.		
Mycobacteria are stained red and the background light blue.		

ria cells cool after the heat is removed, the wax again hardens, protecting the bound dye from the action of the acid-alcohol decolorizer (''acid-fast''). In the Kinyoun, or ''cold'' technique, a surface-active agent is used to increase permeability of the dye through the waxy capsule; however, the re-formation of the waxy film may be incomplete, allowing most, if not all, of the bound dye to be extracted by the acid-alcohol decolorizer. Obviously, mycobacterial cells that are endowed with a thin waxy capsule will be more susceptible to decolorization, as may be the situation with many rapidly growing strains. In these circumstances, the use of a less stringent decolorizer, such as 1% HCl (''partial acid-fast'' procedure), may disclose the innate acid-fast property. The carbolfuchsin-based procedure is described in Chart 19-2.

Although workers in various laboratories may be partial to either the carbolfuchsin- or the fluorescent-staining method, the specificity for detecting mycobacteria of the two methods is approximately the same, with the possible exception of the staining of rapid growers. In one study of 15 strains of *M. fortuitum*, five of the strains did not stain with auramine, but all 15 stained with carbolfuchsin.[163] Uribe-Botero et al., who used Truant's auramine-rhodamine staining of routinely processed bone marrow aspirates and biopsies, describe considerable success in the detection of mycobacteria with this method.[357] In this study 51 bone marrow specimens from 47 HIV-positive patients were studied and mycobacteria were detected in 72%. If the fluorescent stain was positive, the positive predictive value for culturing mycobacteria was 87%. McCarter and Robinson studied 782 primary sputum smears evaluated blindly by the rhodamine-auramine method both at room temperature and at 37°C and found that the preparation stained at room temperature detected only 85.7% of the positive smears; 43.3% of the smears had more AFB in the 37°C stained smears, compared with only 13.3% more AFB in the room temperature–stained smears.[219] They concluded that staining at 37°C with this method enhances the detection of AFB. Regarding smears made from cytocentrifugation versus traditional NALC-NaOH concentration, Woods and coworkers found no increase in the detection of acid-fast bacilli in 844 auramine O–stained cytocentrifuged sputum smears when compared with the traditional NALC-NaOH concentration method.[398]

The fluorochrome stain offers the advantage of greater sensitivity compared with the carbolfuchsin method, since a significantly larger area of the smear can be scanned per unit of time with the auramine fluorochrome stain. Some workers use the fluorochrome method for scanning purposes and then confirm their findings by reexamining the preparation after destaining and restaining with the carbolfuchsin method. After laboratory workers have become familiar with the auramine fluorochrome method, most prefer it over the carbolfuchsin procedure. The introduction of relatively low-cost blue-light illuminators has made fluorescence microscopy available to clinical laboratories where the detection and recovery of mycobacteria is offered as a service.[267] In laboratories where expensive illuminators may not be affordable, use of the UV ParaLens adapter (Becton Dickinson, Sparks, MD), a lightweight, portable, inexpensive epi-illuminator offers an alternative possibility. Patterson and associates found a comparable sensitivity and specificity in the detection of fluorescing acid-fast bacilli using the UV ParaLens adapter when compared with Kinyoun-stained smears.[253] Implementation of such an adapter offers applications in the examination of specimen preparations for the detection of other microorganisms, such as *Giardia* and *Pneumocystis*, that have been stained with fluorescing reagents.

It should be emphasized that neither the auramine nor the auramine-rhodamine fluorochrome stain is a fluorescent antigen-antibody technique; rather, each is a direct physicochemical binding of the stain to the mycolic acid-rich cell wall. The use of fluorescence-tagged antibodies to aid in the identification of various species of mycobacteria has been described, but they are neither commonly used nor commercially available.

The recommendations of the American Lung Association for reporting mycobacteria seen on acid-fast-stained smears are given in Table 19-4. These recommendations are followed by many laboratories to provide consistency of observations between technologists in a given laboratory and uniformity of reporting from one laboratory to another. A summary of the carbolfuchsin-based and fluorescent techniques for the staining of mycobacteria can be found in Charts 19-2 and 19-3.

Culture of Specimens for Recovery of Mycobacteria
Culture Media

The recovery of mycobacteria from agar culture media was poor when the first attempts were made late in the 19th

Table 19-4 Method for Reporting Numbers of Acid-Fast Bacilli Observed in Stained Smears[a]

NUMBER OF BACILLI OBSERVED	CDC METHOD REPORT	
0	Negative	−
1–2/300 fields	Number seen[b]	±
1–9/100 fields	Average no./100 fields	1+
1–9/10 fields	Average no./10 fields	2+
1–9/field	Average no./field	3+
More than 9/field	More than 9/field	4+

[a] *Examination at 800× to 1,000× is assumed. Magnifications less than 800× should be clearly stated. If a microscopist uses a consistent procedure for smear examination, relative comparisons of multiple specimens should be easy for the clinician, regardless of the magnification used. To equate numbers of bacilli observed at less than 800× with those seen under an oil-immersion objective, adjust counts as follows: for magnifications about 650×, divide count by 2; near 450×, divide by 4; near 250×, divide by 10; e.g., if 8 bacilli per 10 fields were seen at 450×, the count at 1,000× would be equivalent to about 2/10 fields (8 ÷ 4).*
[b] *Counts less than 3/3000 fields at 800× to 1,000× are not considered positive; another specimen (or repeat smear of same specimen) should be processed if available.*
Adapted from the American Thoracic Society. Diagnostic standards and classification of tuberculosis and other mycobacterial diseases. Am Rev Respir Dis 1981;123:343–358.

century. Through experimentation it was found that a culture medium containing whole eggs, potato flour, glycerol, and salts solidified by heating to 85–90°C for 30–45 minutes was effective in isolating *M. tuberculosis*. The process of solidifying protein-containing medium by heat is known as inspissation. An inspissated culture medium is more subject to liquefaction from the effects of proteolytic enzymes produced by contaminating bacteria than a medium solidified by the addition of agar. However, it was soon discovered that the use of aniline dyes, such as malachite green or crystal violet, in the inspissated medium helped control contaminating bacteria. The concentration of dye must be carefully controlled; if the concentration is too high, the growth of mycobacteria may also be inhibited along with the contaminating bacteria. Malachite green is the dye most commonly incorporated into nonselective culture media, in concentrations ranging between 0.0025 g/100 mL and 0.052 g/100 mL (Table 19-5).

Nonselective Culture Media for Recovery of Mycobacteria

Several of the egg-based culture media for the recovery of mycobacteria are listed in Table 19-5. Löwenstein-Jensen (LJ) medium is most commonly used in most clinical diagnostic laboratories; it is less inhibitory to the growth of mycobacteria than is Petragnani medium, which is used primarily to recover mycobacteria from specimens heavily contaminated with bacteria. Conversely, the American Thoracic Society (ATS) medium, which contains only 0.02 g/100 mL of malachite green, is less inhibitory to the growth of

Table 19-5 Nonselective Mycobacterial Isolation Media

MEDIUM	COMPONENTS	INHIBITORY AGENT	MEDIUM	COMPONENTS	INHIBITORY AGENT
Löwenstein-Jensen	Coagulated whole eggs, defined salts, glycerol, potato flour	Malachite green, 0.025 g/100 mL	Middlebrook 7H10	Defined salts, vitamins, cofactors, oleic acid, albumin, catalase, glycerol, dextrose	Malachite green, 0.0025 g/100 mL
Petragnani	Coagulated whole eggs, egg yolks, whole milk, potato, potato flour, glycerol	Malachite green, 0.052 g/100 mL	Middlebrook 7H11	Defined salts, vitamins, cofactors, oleic acid, albumin, catalase, glycerol, 0.1% casein hydrolysate	Malachite green, 0.0025 g/100 mL
American Thoracic Society medium	Coagulated fresh egg yolks, potato flour, glycerol	Malachite green, 0.02 g/100 mL			

mycobacteria and is recommended for use in usually sterile specimens, such as CSF, pleural fluid, and tissue biopsies.

Because LJ medium is less sensitive in the recovery of mycobacteria from clinical specimens compared with broth culture media and Middlebrook 7H10 agar, and because detection of growth is delayed when positive, routine use of this medium is being discontinued in many laboratories. The use of broth culture media followed by molecular identification often establishes the identification of the organism before growth is visible on the LJ slant. Chromogenic studies and biochemical tests are most accurate when performed on subcultures from LJ medium. Thus, positive broth cultures are transferred to LJ medium when biochemical tests may be necessary.

Media of Cohen and Middlebrook

During the 1950s, Cohen and Middlebrook developed a series of defined culture media for use in both research and clinical laboratories. These media were prepared from defined salts and organic chemicals; some contained agar, but all were found to require the addition of albumin for optimal growth of mycobacteria. The Middlebrook media that contain agar are transparent and allow early detection of growth after 10 to 12 days, instead of the 18 to 24 days of incubation required with other media. This is partly due to the inclusion of biotin and catalase to stimulate revival of damaged bacilli in clinical specimens. Albumin is also incorporated to bind toxic amounts of oleate and other compounds that might be released from spontaneous hydrolysis of Tween 80. The albumin does not appear to be metabolized by the bacilli.[374]

Not many of the earlier Cohen and Middlebrook culture media are used today. However, 7H9 is a popular liquid medium, and both 7H10 and 7H11 agar media are widely used for isolation and susceptibility testing.[396] The antimycobacterial agents should be incorporated into the medium just before it solidifies to reduce the loss of activity known to occur with some drugs during the long heating period needed to prepare the inspissated egg-based media. This application will be discussed in more detail later in this chapter. 7H11 differs from 7H10 only in containing 0.1% casein hydrolysate, an additive that improves the rate and amount of growth of mycobacteria resistant to isoniazid (INH).[52] Both 7H10 and 7H11 contain malachite green but at one tenth the quantity of those usually used in egg-based media, explain-

ing in part the higher incidence of contamination than on egg-based media.

One other advantage of the use of Middlebrook agar is that experienced mycobacteriologists can often make a presumptive identification of *M. tuberculosis* and other groups of mycobacteria within 10 days by examining early microcolonies on Middlebrook agar and observing certain well-defined morphologic features.[296] Photomicrographs of representative microcolonies are illustrated in Color Plate 19-1C (*M. tuberculosis*) and Color Plate 19-2A and 2B (MAI complex).

Although essentially all culture media yield more growth and larger colonies of mycobacteria when incubated in 5–10% CO_2, the Middlebrook media absolutely require capneic incubation for proper performance. Exposure of 7H10 and 7H11 to strong light, or storage of the media at 4°C for more than 4 weeks may result in deterioration and release of formaldehyde, a chemical very inhibitory to mycobacteria.[231]

Selective Media

Culture media containing antimicrobial agents are used to suppress bacterial and fungal contamination. Although certain antimicrobial agents are known to reduce contamination, they may also inhibit the growth of mycobacteria. Therefore, the times of exposure must be carefully controlled. The use of selective media can result in greatly improved recovery of mycobacteria. Table 19-6 lists the names and components of several selective media.

Currently, the selective medium described by Gruft, which consists of Löwenstein-Jensen medium with penicillin, nalidixic acid, and RNA, is commonly used.[117] Petran subsequently described a selective medium containing cycloheximide, lincomycin, and nalidixic acid to control fungal and bacterial contaminants.[259] By varying the concentrations of these agents, the medium can be prepared with either Löwenstein-Jensen or 7H10 base.

Selective 7H11 is a modification of an oleic acid agar medium first described by Mitchison.[232] The medium was originally designed for use with sputum specimens without the use of a decontaminating agent. Mitchison's medium contains carbenicillin, polymyxin, trimethoprim lactate, and amphotericin B. McClatchy suggested reducing the concen-

Table 19-6 Selective Mycobacterial Isolation Media

MEDIUM	COMPONENTS	INHIBITORY AGENT	MEDIUM	COMPONENTS	INHIBITORY AGENT
Gruft modification of Löwenstein-Jensen	Coagulated whole eggs, defined salts, glycerol, potato flour, RNA, 5 mg/100 mL	Malachite green, 0.025 g/100 mL Penicillin, 50 U/mL Nalidixic acid, 35 mg/mL	Middlebrook 7H10	Defined salts, vitamins, cofactors, oleic acid, albumin, catalase, glycerol, glucose	Malachite green, 0.0025 g/100 mL Cycloheximide, 360 μg/mL Lincomycin, 2 μg/mL Nalidixic acid, 20 μg/mL
Löwenstein-Jensen	Coagulated whole eggs, defined salts, glycerol, potato flour	Malachite green, 0.025 g/100 mL Cycloheximide, 400 μg/mL Lincomycin, 2 μg/mL Nalidixic acid, 35 μg/mL	Selective 7H11 (Mitchison's medium)	Defined salts, vitamins, cofactors, oleic acid, albumin, catalase, glycerol, glucose, casein hydrolysate	Carbenicillin, 50 μg/mL Amphotericin B, 10 μg/mL Polymyxin B, 200 U/mL Trimethoprim lactate, 20 μg/mL

tration of carbenicillin from 100 μg/mL to 50 μg/mL and using 7H11 medium instead of oleic acid agar.[220] He called this modification selective 7H11, or S7H11. With use of S7H11 medium with Löwenstein-Jensen and 7H11, recovery of mycobacteria is definitely improved, particularly when the S7H11 medium is used with the NALC-1% NaOH decontamination procedure.[220]

Subsequent to this report, a 3-year study comparing the use of S7H10 medium with nondecontaminated specimens has shown significantly less contamination on S7H10 plates with homogenized specimens than on 7H10 medium with decontamination, using 2% NaOH with NALC. In addition, S7H10 medium recovered 18% more positive cultures, usually with more colonies per culture and with less contamination than did cultures inoculated onto 7H10 after 2% NALC-NaOH decontamination. In contrast to the recommendation in McClatchy's report, carbenicillin was held at 100 μg/mL instead of 50 μg /mL. Specimens inoculated directly to 7H10 plates were homogenized after the addition of equal quantities of NALC in 0.1 M sodium citrate at pH 8.1 and allowed to stand for 15 minutes before centrifugation. Inoculation of concentrated, but nondecontaminated specimens, should predispose to recovery of fastidious or partially injured mycobacterial cells, sparing the additional injury of exposure to NaOH. Although the nondecontaminated specimens on S7H10 recovered more mycobacterial species than the nonselective media, the antibiotics in the medium have a distinct inhibitory effect on the growth and colony appearance of some species. During the development of 7H12 1-[^{14}C]-palmitic acid broth medium, it was found that smaller amounts of the antibiotics were as effective as the higher concentrations used in S7H11. The antibiotics can be added to the broth culture before inoculation of the nondecontaminated specimen.

Incubation

Different species of mycobacteria show striking dependence on the temperature of incubation for optimal growth.

Species having a propensity for infecting skin (such as *M. marinum*, *M. ulcerans*, and *M. haemophilum*) grow best at the temperature of the skin (30–32°C) and very poorly or not at all at 37°C. *M. tuberculosis* grows best at 37°C and poorly or not at all at 30°C or 42–45°C (the body temperature of birds). *Mycobacterium xenopi*, a species not commonly found as a cause of infection in humans, grows best at 42°C and has been implicated as an environmental contaminant in the hot water system of a large hospital.[115]

Optimal recovery of different mycobacterial species depends on the incubation of at least part of the concentrated specimen at a temperature most likely to promote growth of that species. An incubator set at 30°C should be used for all specimens from suspected skin or subcutaneous mycobacterial infections. If a 30°C incubator is not available, the specimens can be held in a temperature-monitored, closed box placed in a sheltered area away from warm or cool drafts. The temperature in the box should be between 24 and 25°C and recorded daily. An incubator maintained at 42°C can be helpful in recovering *M. xenopi*.

Mycobacteria grow best in an atmosphere of 3–11% CO_2 (Fig. 19-2). Use of CO_2 is mandatory if Middlebrook 7H11 medium is used. However, if lack of incubator space to maintain cultures is a problem, cultures can be removed from the CO_2 atmosphere after 7–10 days, for organisms will be in a log phase of growth and are less dependent on CO_2. For reasons that are not well understood, mycobacteria do not grow well in candle extinction jars. The CO_2 concentration in incubators should be monitored daily and a record kept of both the incubator temperature and the CO_2 level.

Rapid Methods for Establishing a Diagnosis
Sensitivity of Acid-Fast Smears

One of the more practical and readily available methods to improve the rapid diagnosis of tuberculosis is to increase the RCF applied to clinical specimens to improve the sedimentation of the lipid-laden mycobacterial cells.[284] The improved correlation of positive smears to positive cultures has

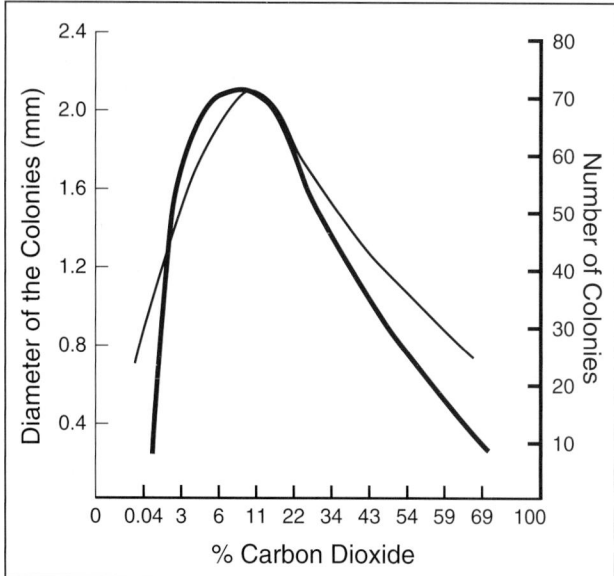

Figure 19-2 Effect of CO_2 on the growth (colony size and number of colonies) of *M. tuberculosis* after primary isolation from sputum. (Redrawn from David HL. Bacteriology of the Mycobacterioses. DHEW Publication No. [CDC] 76-8316, Atlanta: Centers for Disease Control and Prevention Mycobacteriology Branch, 1976.)

made the examination of an acid-fast-stained smear somewhat more reliable as an index of mycobacterial infection. Lipsky, in a review of factors affecting the clinical value of microscopy for acid-fast bacilli, concluded that when the results of all specimens from each patient are considered in total, the acid-fast smear has a predictive value higher than 96% and remains one of the most rapidly performed tests in the detection of mycobacterial infections.[207]

Gas-Liquid and High-Performance Liquid Chromatography

Analysis of cellular long-chain fatty acids by gas-liquid chromatography (GLC) has been used to aid in the characterization of mycobacteria. The pyrolysis gas-liquid method of Reiner, in which long-chain mycolic acids are split into characteristic cleavage products, is largely restricted to research laboratories.[280] Tisdall has developed a GLC procedure for saponifying organisms in methanolic NaOH that permits the correct identification of most mycobacterial species based on chromatogram tracings and colony characteristics.[346] Guerrant and associates have used acid methanolysis for isolating mycolic acid methyl esters from bacterial cells, a method that is not only less time-consuming than saponification techniques but is also more sensitive in detecting small numbers of cells.[118] As little as a 1-mm loopful of organisms can be used, and the total time for analysis is less than 2 hours.[288]

An FDA-cleared, commercial system, the MIDI Sherlock Microbial Identification System, (Microbial ID, Newark DE), consisting of an 1100 HPLC and a computer is a rapid and reliable method for the culture confirmation of mycobacteria. The computer system includes a library of 40 cell wall lipid profiles for the most medically important *Mycobacterium* species, derived from isolates acquired from the Ameri-

can Type Culture Collection and including numerous clinical isolates. The use of negative-ion mass spectrometry to detect tuberculostearic acid in clinical specimens also holds promise for the rapid detection of mycobacteria in such specimens for those equipped with the necessary instruments.[195]

High-performance liquid chromatography utilizing fluorescence detection (HPLC-FL) of mycolic acid 6,7-dimethoxycoumarin esters has been used for the rapid identification of *M. tuberculosis* and *M. avium* directly from fluorochrome-stained, smear-positive sputum specimens and BACTEC 12B cultures with early growth. In a study of 132 sputum specimens positive for *M. tuberculosis* and 48 positive for *M. avium-intracellulare*, HPLC-FL made direct identifications with sensitivities of 56.8% and 33.3%, respectively.[164] When performing HPLC-FL testing of cultures grown in BACTEC 12B bottles, sensitivities of 99.0% and 94.3% were achieved. The specificity was 100% in both evaluations. Cage also successfully identified to the species level 117 of 126 (93%) mycobacteria grown in BACTEC 7H12B medium supplemented with oleic acid.[36] Glickman and colleagues describe a computer-based file that contained the patterns of mycolic acids characteristic of 45 species of *Mycobacterium*.[107] By using their system in the evaluation of 1,333 strains representing 24 *Mycobacterium* species, 97% were correctly identified (identification of *M. tuberculosis* was 99.85% accurate; of MAI complex, 98% accurate). Thus, for those possessing the equipment and using computer-based pattern recognition files, mycobacteria can be identified accurately and rapidly using HPLC-generated chromatographic data. These systems are in direct competition with nucleic acid-based methods for the rapid identification of mycobacteria.

Use of Broth Culture Medium

For many years, those using the BACTEC 12B broth culture bottles have experienced a greater rate of recovery of *M. tuberculosis* and other *Mycobacterium* species 1 to 2 weeks earlier than groups who used only solid culture media. Therefore, the use of a broth culture medium for the early recovery of mycobacteria is now highly recommended; in fact, this has been added as a phase-deficiency item to the College of American Pathologists Inspection and Accreditation Checklist. The semiautomated, automated, and manual systems for the culture of mycobacteria are briefly described below.

Automated Detection Systems

Five semiautomated and automated mycobacteria detection systems are currently available: the time-honored and tested radiometric BACTEC 460 system (BD Diagnostic Systems, Sparks, MD), and newer nonradiometric systems, the MGIT 960 System (BD Diagnostic Systems), the MB/BacT System (BioMérieux, Durham, NC), the BACTEC MYCO/F Lytic blood culture bottle (BD Diagnostic Systems), and the ESP Culture System II (Trek Diagnostic). Two viable alternatives are the manual Septi-Chek System (BD Diagnostic) and the manual version of the MGIT system (BD Diagnostic) for use in laboratories without automated systems.

BACTEC AFB System

The components of the automated BACTEC 460 instrument (BD Diagnostic) include a scintillation counter, a needle aspiration assembly, and a movable track on which up to 60 culture bottles can be placed. The track is aligned so that each culture bottle passes, in turn, beneath the needle aspiration assembly at the rate of approximately one every 80 seconds. When the test bottle is immediately below the needle assembly, the needle is lowered through the rubber stopper into the headspace. A sample of the head gas is aspirated and delivered to the scintillation counter chamber. The head gas is replaced with a fresh bolus of 10% CO_2 immediately after the sample is aspirated. The instrument is fitted with a hood that provides HEPA-filtered air under negative pressure in the area of testing and a UV light source as an added safety feature. The needle is electrically heat-sterilized during the interval before the next bottle is to be sampled.

The BACTEC 12B broth culture bottle is the key to operation. The bottle consists of a 20-mL glass vial with a short neck, the mouth of which is sealed with a thin rubber stopper. It contains 4 mL of broth culture medium consisting of Middlebrook 7H9 broth base; bovine serum albumin (BSA); casein hydrolysate, catalase, and polyoxylene stearate as growth enhancers; small quantities of an antimicrobial mixture of polymyxin B, amphotericin B, nalidixic acid, trimethoprim, and azlocillin to suppress growth of contaminants; and ^{14}C-labeled palmitic acid as the growth detector. The vial is inoculated with 0.5 mL of the processed specimen and placed in a 35°C incubator. If mycobacteria are present in the inoculum, $^{14}CO_2$ is released into the headspace, the amount of which is proportional to the amount of growth in the vial. The very sensitive radioactive detector system is used because the slowly metabolizing mycobacteria produce only trace quantities of CO_2. When a designated period of incubation has passed, usually about 3 days, the vials are placed on the track of the BACTEC 460 instrument in preparation for reading. The amount of radioactivity is measured in the aspirated head gas, which is translated into a numerical value called the growth index (GI). A GI higher than 10 is considered positive; however, acid-fast stains must be performed on a small aliquot of broth, because other bacteria may break through the antibiotic inhibition.

Both an increase in the yield of positive cultures from clinical specimens and lessening of the time to detection is achieved with use of the BACTEC system, compared with conventional solid media.[246,308] The detection time for *M. tuberculosis* averages 9–14 days; it may be less than 7 days for some strains of mycobacteria other than *M. tuberculosis*. Disadvantages of the system include the cost of instrumentation, the inability to observe colony morphology and detect mixed cultures, overgrowth by contaminants, need for disposal of radioactive materials, and extensive use of needles. Cases of pseudomycobacterial infections have been reported when the needle is incompletely sterilized following aspiration of a vial with a high concentration of organisms.[57,239] Specimens processed using reagents other than NALC-NaOH (such as benzalkonium chloride or Zephiran-trisodium phosphate) cannot be used with the BACTEC system because residual quantities in the broth potentially inhibit the growth of mycobacteria.

Initial studies of the sensitivity of this system in monitoring mycobacterial growth showed that an inoculum of 200 viable *M. tuberculosis* bacilli could be detected in 12–13 days, whereas if one waited for 14–17 days, as few as 20 viable bacilli could be detected.[226]

The value of the BACTEC in the detection of mycobacteria from sputum, blood, and other clinical specimens has been demonstrated in several field trials and clinical correlation studies.[15,34,112,134] In a multicenter collaborative study, the recovery of *M. tuberculosis* from clinical specimens known to be smear-positive was accomplished by the BACTEC system in 14 days, compared with 21 days by the standard culture method.[287] In this same study, the total time for isolation and drug susceptibility testing of *M. tuberculosis* was completed in an average of 18 days by the radiometric method, compared with an average of 38 days using standard procedures. Similarly, smear-negative, culture-positive specimens were positive for growth of *M. tuberculosis* in an average of 14 days by the radiometric method, compared with 25 days by the standard culture procedure.[67,236]

The capability of performing rapid mycobacterial drug susceptibility studies is an additional advantage of the BACTEC system.[126] The BACTEC instrument can also be used to differentiate *M. tuberculosis* and *M. bovis* from nontuberculous mycobacteria using blood culture vials containing *p*-nitro-α-acetylamino-β-hydroxy-propiophenone (NAP). *M. tuberculosis* and *M. bovis* cannot grow in NAP-containing culture media and, therefore, will not produce a positive GI after several days of incubation. The NAP test is presented in Chart 19-4. Detection of *M. tuberculosis* in contaminated clinical specimens can also be accomplished by using a 7H12A culture vial containing the same antimicrobial agents used in S7H11 agar, only in smaller concentrations (polymyxin, 50 μg/mL; amphotericin, 5 μg/mL; carbenicillin, 25 μg/mL; and trimethoprim, 2.5 μg/mL (PACT).

Although the BACTEC 460 system represents possibly the best broth-based system developed to date for the rapid recovery of mycobacteria, it is being replaced by nonradiometric systems, largely because of the problems associated with maintaining radioactive materials and the disposal of radioactive waste.

Mycobacteria Growth Indicator Tube (MGIT) and MGIT 960

The MGIT system (BD Diagnostic) consists of a 16- × 100-mm round-bottomed glass tube that contains 4 mL of modified 7H11 broth base, to which has been added 0.5 mL of OADC enrichment (oleic acid, bovine albumin, dextrose, and catalase) and 0.1 mL of PANTA antibiotic mixture (polymyxin B, amphotericin B, nalidixic acid, trimethoprim, and azlocillin). The antibiotic mixture inhibits the growth of contaminating bacteria; the OADC supplement provides oleic acid, an important metabolic stimulant for mycobacteria; albumin, to bind toxic free fatty acids; dextrose, as an energy source; and catalase, to destroy toxic peroxides that may be present in the medium. A fluorescent compound is embedded in silicone on the bottom of the tube. The fluorescent compound is sensitive to dissolved oxygen in the broth; that is, the presence of oxygen in the uninoculated medium serves to quench the emission of fluorescent light. As the actively growing bacteria consume the dissolved oxygen, the fluorescence is unmasked and can be detected by observing the tube under long-wave ultraviolet light (Wood's lamp). Growth may also be detected by observing a nonhomogeneous turbidity or small grains or flakes in the culture medium.

In performing the test, the 0.1 mL of PANTA and 0.5 mL of OADC mixture are added aseptically to the tube, reconstituting the lyophilized medium. This is followed by 0.5 mL of specimen or specimen concentrate; adding more than 0.5 mL of specimen may adversely affect the performance of the tube. The cap is replaced, the ingredients mixed by inverting the tube several times, and the tube placed in a 37°C incubator. Tubes are read every other day starting on the second day after inoculation with the manual application. Tubes are read with a Wood's lamp, placing the tube with the test mixture between a positive (sodium sulfite solution) and a negative (uninoculated MGIT tube) control. UV-protective goggles are worn while looking for a bright orange color in the bottom of the positive tubes; an orange reflection is also seen at the meniscus. Positive tubes are stained for acid-fast bacilli, preferably using the Ziehl-Neelsen technique. Negative tubes are returned to the incubation rack and again observed at regular intervals for up to 6 weeks. An automated platform that examines each tube periodically for positivity is now available.

Hanna and coworkers used the MGIT system to test 193 specimens (44 patients) from various body sites for the presence of *Mycobacterium* species.[124] Sputum concentrations from 32 patients from whom at least one positive acid-fast smear was seen were studied. The MGIT cultures were positive in 31 (*M. tuberculosis* complex [MTB], 25; MAI, 4; and *M. haemophilum*, 2) cases. MGIT tubes were positive for an additional three smear-negative patients; the one false-negative MGIT test occurred in a patient with very few acid-fast bacilli seen on smear. The mean time to detection was 10.4 days (range, 4 to 26). The two *M. haemophilum* isolates were recovered by adding an X (hemin) disk to the MGIT tube and incubating at 30°C. All positive reactions with this system must be confirmed by an acid-fast stain, since other oxygen-consuming bacteria may occasionally break through the PANTA antibiotic mixture. One major disadvantage is the cost of each tube, but this may be offset to some degree because fluorescence is observed visually and does not require elaborate or costly equipment.

The MGIT 960 System is a nonradiometric, automated system that uses the BD BBL MGIT media and sensors to detect the fluorescence that is visually interpreted in the manual version described above. The system holds 960 plastic tubes, which are continuously monitored. In an early comparison of this technology with the BACTEC 460 and LJ medium using 2,567 clinical specimens, Tortoli and associates found that the MGIT 960 had the shortest mean time to positivity at 13.3 days, compared with 14.8 days for the BACTEC 460 system and 25.6 days for the LJ medium.[349] The best yield, however, was with the BACTEC 460 system (201 isolates), followed by 190 isolates with the BACTEC MGIT 960 system and 168 isolates with LJ medium. In this comparison, the MGIT 960 also had the highest contamination rate (10.0%), compared with the radiometric system (3.7%) and the LJ medium (17.0%). The contamination rate has been improved by others, with only a slight increase in the time to positivity.[384]

MB/BacT Mycobacteria Detection System

The MB/BacT is an automated system to detect mycobacteria, similar in design to the BacT/Alert blood culture system. The MB/BacT bottles contains 10 mL of enhanced Middlebrook 7H9 broth in an atmosphere of CO_2, nitrogen, and oxygen under vacuum. This bottle therefore provides suitable nutritional and environmental conditions to recover the more commonly encountered *Mycobacterium* species for clinical specimens other than blood. Reconstituted mycobacteria antibiotic supplement (MAS; 0.5 mL), containing amphotericin B, azlocillin, nalidixic acid, polymyxin B, trimethoprim, and proprietary growth factors, is added to each bottle just before use to enhance the growth of *Mycobacterium* species and curtail the growth of contaminating bacteria that may survive the decontamination and concentration procedure. The bottom of each broth bottle is fitted with a gas-permeable sensor that changes from dark green to bright yellow when CO_2 is produced in the broth by metabolizing mycobacteria. Bottles are placed bottom down within individual wells in the incubation chamber, and reflected light is used to continuously monitor the production of microbial-generated CO_2.

The multicenter field trials sponsored by the manufacturer indicate that the MB/BacT system recovered a higher percentage of mycobacteria with less time to detection when compared with conventional methods, and compared favorably in parallel cultures with the BACTEC 460 TB system. Gil-Setas and associates compared the MB/BacT system, Middlebrook 7H11 agar plates using the microcolony method for growth detection, and conventional LJ medium for the recovery of mycobacteria from 2101 consecutive, non-selected specimens.[105] Of the 111 specimens positive for *M. tuberculosis*, 100 were recovered with the MB/BacT system, 99 from the M7H1 agar plates, and 86 from the LJ medium. The time to detection was 11 days for the M7H11 agar plates, 16 days for the MB/BacT System, and 19.5 days for the LJ medium. This system may also be used as a reliable means of performing broth-based susceptibility testing.[18] The colorimetric, nonradiometric detection of mycobacterial growth, eliminating the need for handling and disposing of radioisotopes, is a distinct advantage. Several other studies have been performed examining the utility of this automated detection method.[9,19,142,202,265,291,388]

The ESP Culture System II

The ESP Culture System II (Trek Diagnostic) is an adaptation of the ESP Blood Culture System. Each culture bottle, when placed in a special drawer in the incubation module, is attached to a sensor, consisting of a plastic housing, a recessed needle, and a hydrophobic membrane. Thus, each bottle is continuously monitored for any change in gas pressure due to the metabolic activity of microorganisms in the culture bottle. Significant pressure change may be signaled early, from the consumption of oxygen, or later, with the production of gases by the metabolizing microorganisms.

The bottles contain modified Middlebrook 7H9 medium, Casitone, glycerol, and cellulose sponges. The sponges provide a growth platform for the mycobacteria, simulating the alveoli of the lungs. Immediately prior to specimen inoculation, each bottle is supplemented with an antibiotic mixture containing polymyxin B, vancomycin, nalidixic acid and amphotericin B (PVNA).

Field trials sponsored by the manufacturer indicate that the total percentage of positive cultures detected by the ESP MYCO System compared favorably with the BACTEC 460 system. Of note, specimens from patients receiving antituberculosis therapy were at times not positive in either broth system, indicating the need to inoculate solid culture media in parallel with the broth bottles. The results from this study further indicate that the ESP MYCO system detected positive cultures first about three times more frequently than the BACTEC 460 system and more than 7 days sooner in about half the cultures, presumably based on the early signal derived during the oxygen-consumption phase of the growth cycle. Williams-Bouyer et al. compared the ESP Culture System II with the BACTEC MGIT 960 and Middlebrook 7H11 and 7H11 selective agar, examining a total of 3,151 specimens.[388] The recovery rates for all mycobacteria were 71.2% for the ESP II, 63.9% for the MGIT 960, and 61.8% for the Middlebrook media. However, with the exclusion of *M. gordonae*, the recovery rates for the remaining mycobacteria were 70.2%, 72.6%, and 66.3%, respectively. These differences were not statistically significant.

For isolates recovered in both automated systems, the mean times to detection of all mycobacteria and members of the *M. tuberculosis* complex, respectively, were 15.8 and 17.4 days for ESP II and 12.5 and 11.9 days for BACTEC MGIT 960 (P < 0.05). False-positive signals occurred less frequently with the BACTEC MGIT 960 cultures (23 [0.7%]) compared with the ESP II cultures (84 [2.7%]) (P < 0.01). In a comparison with the BACTEC 460 system, the ESP II was found to be comparable for susceptibility testing.[295] The nonradiometric detection method used also precludes the need to handle and dispose of radioactive materials.

The BACTEC MYCO/F LYTIC

The BACTEC MYCO/F LYTIC culture bottle contains a lytic agent to release the mycobacteria that have been phagocytosed by white blood cells. It is incubated and monitored automatically in a manner similar to the other BACTEC blood culture bottles. In addition to growing mycobacteria, the BACTEC MYCO/F LYTIC is a good culture system for bacteria and fungi that may be present in the bloodstream.[100,361] In a direct comparison of many of the commercially available products, Crump et al. evaluated the performance of the BACTEC 13A (BD Diagnostic), BACTEC MYCO/F LYTIC (BD Diagnostic), BacT/ALERT MB (BioMérieux), and ISOLATOR 10 lysis-centrifugation (Wampole Laboratories) systems for detection of mycobacteremia in adults.[64] Of 600 patients tested, 85 (14%) yielded *M. avium/M. intracellulare* complex (MAI) and 9 (2%) yielded other species of mycobacteria. Of 26 complete (three bottles and one tube) and adequately filled (5 ± 1 mL) sets from which MAI was recovered, BACTEC 13A was positive for 19 (73%), BACTEC MYCO/F LYTIC was positive for 21 (81%), BacT/ALERT MB was positive for 22 (85%), and ISOLATOR 10 was positive for 21 (81%). Of the six possible two-way comparisons, the mean times to detection for the recovery of MAI from each bottle in adequately paired

sets were 15.3 days for BACTEC 13A versus 12.8 days for MYCO/F LYTIC for 33 of 340 pairs, 14.1 days for BACTEC 13A versus 11.6 days for BacT/ALERT MB for 38 of 380 pairs, 12.6 days for BACTEC 13A versus 20.0 days for ISOLATOR 10 for 26 of 261 pairs, 12.8 days for BACTEC MYCO/F LYTIC versus 11.0 days for BacT/ALERT MB for 33 of 340 pairs, 13.2 days for BACTEC MYCO/F LYTIC versus 20.4 days for ISOLATOR 10 for 24 of 230 pairs, and 9.9 days for BacT/ALERT MB versus 19.0 days for ISOLATOR 10 for 24 of 257 pairs. There were no significant differences found in yields between the systems. However, there were differences in the mean time to detection among the systems. The time to detection was shortest for BacT/ALERT MB, followed by BACTEC MYCO/F LYTIC and BACTEC 13A and then ISOLATOR 10. They found the continuously monitored systems (BACTEC MYCO/F LYTIC and BacT/ALERT MB) to be as sensitive and, on balance, faster for the detection of MAI bacteremia than the standard manual ISOLATOR 10 and radiometric BACTEC 13A systems. Others have also found this method to be superior to traditional methods.[216]

Manual Detection Systems

The manual MGIT and the Septi-Chek AFB systems are the two options for commercially available broth-based manual mycobacteria culture systems. The manual MGIT is described in conjunction with the automated version, the MGIT 960, above.

Septi-Chek AFB System

The Septi-Chek AFB System is a capped bottle that contains 20.0 mL of modified Middlebrook 7H9 broth under 20% CO_2. A second component is a plastic tube, fitted on one end with a removable screw cap, within which is enclosed a two-faced paddle, on both surfaces of which are embedded solid culture media. One surface of the paddle is covered with nonselective Middlebrook 7H11 agar; the reverse side is divided into two sections, one containing modified LJ medium and the other containing chocolate agar to detect the growth of contaminating bacteria. The system is processed by removing the cap from the bottle containing the culture medium, to which is added 1.0 mL of a reconstituted supplement also provided by the manufacturer, composed of glucose, glycerin, oleic acid, pyridoxine, HCl, catalase, albumin, azlocillin, nalidixic acid, trimethoprim, polymyxin B, and amphotericin B. The supplemented broth is next inoculated with 0.5 mL of a NALC-NaOH-processed specimen. The screw cap is removed from the bottom of the paddle, and the assembly is secured to the broth culture bottle. The solid culture media on the paddle are inoculated by inverting the assembly, permitting the broth culture mixture to bathe all surfaces of the agar. The system is then placed into a 35°C incubator in an upright position. The agar surfaces and the culture media are examined every third day for the appearance of growth, after which, if negative, the assembly is again inverted to reinoculate the agar media. If growth is observed, acid-fast smears can be performed from isolated colonies growing on the agar surface, and subcultures of the broth can be made to appropriate selective media or can be prepared for DNA probe analysis.

In a four-center study in which over 3,000 clinical specimens of various sources were studied, Isenberg and coworkers found that the Septi-Chek system was more sensitive than LJ, 7H11, and BACTEC broth in the percentage of mycobacterial isolates recovered.[150] The authors concluded that this better recovery rate could be attributed to the biphasic nature of the system and the advantage gained from repeated early exposure of the agar media to actively proliferating organisms in the broth phase. Compared with LJ and 7H11, the average number of days for recovery of mycobacteria was less for the Septi-Chek AFB system, averaging 3

days less for the detection of *M. tuberculosis* and 9 days less for MAC. Although the time of recovery for the BACTEC system was less by an average of 3 days for *M. tuberculosis* and 12 days for MAC compared with the Septi-Chek system, the former does not provide for isolated colonies; therefore, the time to final identification was about equal between the two systems. Similar results were found in a follow-up study by D'Amato and associates of the revised Septi-Chek AFB System, in which LJ agar was added to the paddle.[66] A later study also confirmed that both the rate and time of recovery of *M. tuberculosis*, MAC, and *M. gordonae* from smear-positive respiratory secretions were improved with the Septi-Chek AFB System compared with LJ me-

Table 19-7 Differential Characteristics of Mycobacteria

	OPTIMAL ISOLATION TEMPERATURE AND TIME FOR GROWTH	PIGMENTATION GROWTH IN		NIACIN TEST	NITRATE REDUCTION	TWEEN 80 HYDROLYSIS— 10 DAYS
		Light	Dark			
M. tuberculosis	37° C 12–25 d	Buff	Buff	+	+	V
M. africanum	37° C 31–42 d	Buff	Buff	V	V	−
M. bovis	37° C 24–40 d	Buff	Buff	V	−	−
M. ulcerans	32° C 28–60 d	Buff	Buff	−	−	−
M. kansasii	37° C 10–20 d	Yellow	Buff	−	+	+
M. marinum	30° C 5–14 d	Yellow	Buff	V	−	+
M. simiae	37° C 7–14 d	Yellow	Buff	+	−	+/−
M. asiaticum	37° C 10–21 d	Yellow	Buff	−	−	+
M. szulgai	37° C 12–25 d	Yellow to orange	Yellow—37° C Buff—25° C	−	+	V
M. scrofulaceum	37° C 10 d	Yellow	Yellow	−	−	−
M. gordonae	37° C 10 d	Yellow to orange	Yellow	−	−	+
M. thermoresistible	45° C 7 d	Yellow	Yellow	−	+	+
M. flavescens	37° C 7–10 d	Yellow	Yellow	−	+	+
M. xenopi	42° C 14–28 d	Yellow	Yellow	−	−	−
M. avium complex	37° C 10–21 d	Buff to pale yellow	Buff to pale yellow	−	−	−
M. haemophilum	30° C 14–21 d	Gray	Gray	−	−	−
M. malmoense	37° C 21–28 d	Buff	Buff	−	−	+
M. shimoidei	37° C 14–28 d	Buff	Buff	−	−	+
M. genavense	37° C 14–28 d	Buff	Buff	−	−	+
M. celatum	37° C 14–28 d	Buff	Buff	−	−	−
M. gasti	37° C 10–21 d	Buff	Buff	−	−	+
M. terrae complex	37° C 10–21 d	Buff	Buff	−	V	+
M. triviale	37° C 10–21 d	Buff	Buff	−	+	+
M. fortuitum	37° C 3–5 d	Buff	Buff	−	+	V
M. chelonei	28° C 3–5 d	Buff	Buff	V	−	V
M. abscessus	35° C 3–5 d	Buff	Buff	−	−	V
M. smegmatis	37° C 3–5 d	Buff to yellow	Buff to yellow	−	+	+

+, *positive;* −, *negative; V, variable; blank spaces, little or no data.*

dium.[311] In this study, BACTEC 12A bottles detected growth of these *Mycobacterium* species earlier than Septi-Chek; however, as found in the study by D'Amato et al., the latter provided isolated colonies earlier and did not require special equipment for detection of growth.

Identification of Mycobacteria Using Conventional Methods

Although the applications of molecular techniques are being used with increasing frequency for the direct detection of *M. tuberculosis* in clinical specimens, the identification of cultured mycobacteria, and in epidemiologic studies, the direct testing of clinical specimens by conventional methods remains the standard of practice in most clinical mycobacteriology laboratories.[134] Charts 19-1 through 19-16 provide a detailed presentation of the principles, reagents, procedures, and interpretation of various laboratory techniques, including digestion-decontamination methods, biochemical tests (included in Table 19-7), and drug susceptibility testing. The use of molecular assays, including nucleic-acid probe analysis, is covered separately.

Optimal Temperature for Isolation and Rates of Growth

Each *Mycobacterium* species has an optimal temperature for growth and a range of time for recovery in culture (Table

	CATALASE		ARYLSUL-FATASE 3 DAYS	UREASE	PYRAZIN-AMIDASE	IRON UPTAKE	GROWTH ON		
	Semi-quantitative	pH 7.0; 68° C					T₂H (1 µg/mL)	5% NaCl 28° C	MacConkey Agar
M. tuberulosis	<45	−	−	+	+	−	+	−	−
M. africanum	>45	−	−	V	−	−	+	−	−
M. bovis	<45	−	−	+	−	−	−	−	−
M. ulcerans	>45	+	−	V	−	−	+	−	−
M. kansasii	>45	+	−	+	+	−	+	−	−
M. marinum	>45	−	V	+	+	−	+	−	−
M. simiae	>45	+	−	+	−	−	+	−	
M. asiaticum	>45	+	−	−	−	−	+	−	
M. szulgai	>45	+	−	+	−	−	+	−	
M. scrofulaceum	>45	+	−	+	V	−	+	−	−
M. gordonae	>45	+	−	−	V	−	+	−	
M. thermoresistable	>45	+	−	+		−		+	
M. flavescens	>45	+	−	+	+	−	+	V	−
M. xenopi	<45	+	+	−	+	−	+	−	−
M. avium complex	<45	−	−	−	+	−	+	−	V
M. haemophilum	<45	−	−	−	+	−	+	−	
M. malmoense	<45	V	−	V	V	−	+	−	
M. shimoidei	<45	−	−	−	+	−	+	−	
M. genavense	>45	+	−	+	+	−	+	−	
M. celatum	<45	+	+	−	+	−	+	−	
M. gastri	<45	−	−	+	−	−	+	−	
M. terrae complex	>45	+	+	−	V	−	+	−	V
M. triviale	>45	+	V	−	V	−	+	+	
M. fortuitum	>45	+	+	+	+	+	+	+	+
M. chelonei	>45	+	+	+	+	−	+	−	−
M. abscessus	>45	+	+	+	+	−	+	+	+
M. smegmatis	>45	+	−			+	+	−	

19-7). The time to recovery varies depending on the type of media used—the average time of recovery of mycobacteria on egg-based media is about 21 days, but ranges from as short as 3–5 days to as long as 60 days, depending on the species. The time to recovery on solid media is generally shorter by several days when using 7H10 or 7H11 agar if the technique of microscopic observation for microcolonies is used (described below). The use of broth-based culture, for the inoculation of both blood cultures and other body fluids, can shorten the times of detection considerably.[66,177,287]

Any standard nonselective culture medium can be used when assessing the time of growth, either in tubed slants or in Petri plates. A well-isolated colony of the test organism is subcultured to a 7H9 broth containing Tween 80 and incubated for several days or until the medium is slightly turbid. The broth is diluted 1:100, and isolation streaks are made to the test medium, either in tubed slants or on Petri plates, to obtain isolated colonies. To determine the growth rate accurately, it is necessary to use an inoculum sufficiently diluted to produce individual colonies. An inoculum of large numbers of slow-growing mycobacteria may form a visible colony within a few days and give an erroneous impression of the growth rate. *M. tuberculosis* stock cultures of known growth rates should be used as a control for slow-growing organisms; similarly, stock cultures of *M. fortuitum* can be used as a control comparison for rapidly growing organisms.

Petri plates of 7H10 agar or equivalent are preferred to the use of tubed media because the appearance of developing microcolonies can be studied with a dissecting or low-power microscope. With experience, an assessment of the morphology of these microcolonies can be useful in the exclusion of certain mycobacteria, and potentially the preliminary classification of others. Runyon published guidelines by which the microcolonies of various species of mycobacteria can be distinguished by those who have gained experience with this approach.[296]

Koneman and associates in the clinical microbiology laboratory at the University of Illinois, Chicago, were able to detect the microcolonies of 29 smear-positive clinical sputum isolates of *Mycobacterium* species growing on 7H10 agar in an average of 6.1 days (range, 3 to 12) compared with average recovery times using standard visual observations of 32.4 days with Löwenstein-Jensen and 27.9 days with 7H11 agar (personal communication). The average detection time for these 29 isolates was 5.8 days by the BACTEC system, using radiometric 12B bottles. The results of this study indicate that mycobacteria can be detected by observing for microcolonies in the same shortened time period as that achieved with the BACTEC system. The microcolony method also allows an assessment of colony morphology, providing an additional piece of information not provided by the BACTEC system, which is helpful in making an early presumptive characterization of an unknown *Mycobacterium* species. In a study that examined the time to detection, the average time to detection of microcolonies of *M. tuberculosis* was 11 days on Middlebrook 7H11 agar, whereas it was 16 days with the MB/BacT bottles and 19.5 days with the LJ medium.[105]

Some *Mycobacterium* species, such as *M. marinum* and some of the rapid growers, grow better at temperatures that are slightly less than core body temperature. This may also be associated with the fact the disease produced by these organisms, particularly *M. marinum*, most commonly affects the extremities, which are slightly cooler than core body temperature. Therefore, laboratories should incubate mycobacterial cultures from specimens that may contain these organisms (e.g., skin biopsies from the extremities) at slightly reduced temperatures.

Pigment Production

The determination of whether an unknown *Mycobacterium* species isolate is capable of producing colony pigmentation in the dark (scotochromogen) or only after exposure to light (photochromogen) is not very helpful in making a final species identification, but may be useful in narrowing the possibilities (see Chart 19-6). *M. tuberculosis* fails to produce pigment, beyond a light buff color, even after exposure to light. The pigment-producing capabilities of other *Mycobacterium* species are listed in Table 19-7 (see Color Plate 19-2C–E).

Niacin Accumulation

All mycobacteria produce niacin; however, only *M. tuberculosis*, *M. simiae*, and occasional strains of *M. africanum*, *M. bovis*, *M. marinum*, and *M. chelonae* lack the enzyme necessary to further convert the niacin to niacin ribonucleotide. Thus, the determination of whether niacin has accumulated in the culture medium is a valuable differential test in identifying these species of mycobacteria, particularly *M. tuberculosis* (see Chart 19-11 for details). Reagent-impregnated filter paper strips have been developed that eliminate the need for using cyanogen bromide, a highly toxic substance, as required in the originally described method for performing this test. The development of a yellow color in the test medium incubated with a reagent strip is indicative of niacin accumulation and a positive test (see Color Plate 19-1D). It is essential to have sufficient growth on the primary egg-based medium, otherwise the risk of obtaining false-negative results is increased.

Reduction of Nitrates to Nitrites

Only a few species of mycobacteria, most notably *M. tuberculosis*, produce nitroreductase, which catalyzes the reduction of nitrate to nitrite. The development of a red color on addition of sulfanilic acid and *N*-naphthyl ethylenediamine to an extract of the unknown culture is indicative of the presence of nitrite and a positive test (see Chart 19-12). The test must be carefully performed using three control cultures—one known to give a strong positive reaction, one a weak reaction, and the last a negative reaction. In addition to supporting the identification of *M. tuberculosis*, the nitrate reduction test is also a key test in the identification of *M.*

kansasii and *M. szulgai* (see Table 19-7 and Color Plate 19-1*E*).

Tween 80 Hydrolysis

Tween 80 is the trade name of a detergent that can be useful in identifying mycobacteria that possess a lipase that splits the compound into oleic acid and polyoxyethylated sorbitol. This test is helpful in identifying *M. kansasii*, which can produce a positive result in as quickly as 3 to 6 hours. Two scotochromogens with similar-appearing colonies, *M. gordonae* (positive) and *M. scrofulaceum* (negative), can be differentiated using the Tween 80 hydrolysis test. The Tween 80 hydrolysis reactions for other mycobacteria are listed in Table 19-8; the test procedure is described in detail in Chart 19-15, and a positive reaction is illustrated in Color Plate 19-2*G*.

Catalase Activity

Most of the mycobacteria produce catalase; however, not all species are capable of producing a positive reaction after heating the culture at 68°C for 20 minutes (heat-stable catalase). Most strains of *M. tuberculosis* and other members of the *M. tuberculosis* complex do not produce heat-stable catalase, except for certain isoniazid (INH)-resistant strains, for which the results of this test are of particular value as a possible surrogate marker. Catalase activity is assessed semiquantitatively by measuring the height achieved by the column of bubbles produced when hydrogen peroxide is added to growing colonies in a tube culture (see Chart 19-7). To perform this test, tubes of Löwenstein-Jensen medium must be poured in an upright position to produce a flat rather than a slanted surface. This surface is heavily inoculated with the test organism and incubated for 14 days before adding the hydrogen peroxide reagent. A column higher than 45 mm is considered a positive test (see Color Plate 19-2*H*). A quick assessment of catalase activity can be determined by placing a few drops of hydrogen peroxide on colonies growing on the surface of Middlebrook 7H10 agar and observing for rapid effervescence of bubbles (Color Plate 19-2*I*).

Arylsulfatase Activity

Determination of the activity of the enzyme arylsulfatase in mycobacteria is helpful in identifying certain species, notably in differentiating the rapidly growing mycobacteria from group III nonphotochromogenic mycobacteria (see Color Plate 19-2*J*). Small quantities of this enzyme can also be produced by *M. marinum*, *M. kansasii*, *M. szulgai*, and *M. xenopi* (see Table 19-8). These slower-growing species, however, do not produce sufficient enzyme to give a consistently positive reaction. The development of a red color in the test medium, indicating a release of free phenolphthalein, is a positive result (see Chart 19-5).

Urease Activity

Assessment of urease activity is an important test to differentiate *M. scrofulaceum* (positive) from *M. gordonae* (negative). It is also useful in differentiating *M. gastri* (positive) from other members of the group III nonchromogenic mycobacteria (see Table 19-7). Determination of whether any given *Mycobacterium* species can produce urease can be performed either by inoculating the organism into distilled water containing a urea-base concentrate or by use of filter paper disks containing urea that are added to distilled water.[253,391] Details of the urease test as applied to the identification of *Mycobacterium* species are presented in Chart 19-16 (see also Color Plate 19-2*K*).

Pyrazinamidase

Another useful test in distinguishing *M. kansasii* and *M. marinum*, weakly niacin-positive *M. bovis* and *M. tuberculosis*, and members of the *M. avium* complex from other species is the test for pyrazinamidase (all positive). Pyrazinamidase is an enzyme that deaminates pyrazinamide to form pyrazinoic acid, which produces a red band in the culture medium.[373] Details of this test are presented in Chart 19-13, and the end reaction is illustrated in Color Plate 19-2*L*.

Iron Uptake

The rapidly growing mycobacteria have many similarities. The ability of *M. fortuitum* to take up soluble iron salts from the culture medium, and to produce a rusty brown appearance on addition of an aqueous solution of 20% ferric ammonium citrate, is a useful characteristic that differentiates this organism from both *M. chelonae* and *M. abscessus,* which lacks this property (see Chart 19-10).[374]

Growth Inhibition by Thiophene-2-Carboxylic Acid Hydrazide

Thiophene-2-carboxylic hydrazide (T2H) selectively inhibits the growth of *M. tuberculosis*, whereas most other mycobacteria can grow in a medium containing this compound; this is particularly helpful for differentiating certain strains of *M. bovis* (see Chart 19-9 and Color Plate 19-1*F*). For example, 30% of *M. bovis* BCG strains may be weakly niacin-positive, and others may be weak nitrate reducers, at times making differentiation of these strains from *M. tuberculosis* by these key tests somewhat difficult.

Growth in 5% Sodium Chloride

The ability to grow on an egg-based culture medium containing 5% NaCl when incubated at 28°C is a characteristic shared by *M. triviale,* some strains of *M. flavescens, M. fortuitum,* and *M. abscessus* (see Table 19-8). Other mycobacteria

Table 19-8 Nomenclature of Select Mycobacteria in Order of Presentation

LEGITIMATE SPECIES NAME	RELATIVE PATHOGENICITY FOR HUMANS	EQUIVALENT RUNYON GROUP	ACCEPTABLE COMMON NAME	NAMES WITHOUT LEGITIMATE STANDING AND COMMENTS
M. tuberculosis	+++		Human tubercle bacillus	Causes human tuberculosis—highly contagious
M. bovis	+++		Bovine tubercle bacillus	Causes bovine and human tuberculosis; avirulent strains are used for bacille Calmette-Guérin (BCG) vaccines.
M. ulcerans	+++			Associated with skin infections in tropics—M. buruli
M. africanum	+++			Intermediate form between M. bovis and M. tuberculosis. It is found in northern and central Africa.
M. kansasii	+++	I photochromogen		Rare, nonpigmented, scotochromogenic, and niacin-positive strains
M. marinum	+++	I photochromogen		M. balnei, M. platypeocilus associated with skin infections
M. simiae	++	I photochromogen		M. habana—facultatively pathogenic; photoreactivity may be unstable; niacin-positive
M. genavense	++			Grows only in broth culture. Propensity for causing pulmonary disseminated disease in patients with AIDS
M. asiaticum	++	I photochromogen		Similiar to M. simiae but differs antigenically
M. scrofulaceum	++	II scotochromogen		M. marinum and MAI—may cause cervical lymphadenitis
M. szulgai	+++	I photochromogen at 25° C II scotochromogen at 37° C		Associated with chronic pulmonary and extrapulmonary disease; distinctive lipid composition of cell walls
M. xenopi	++	III nonphotochromogen		M. littorale, M. xenopi grows slowly; best at 42° C; may contaminate hot-water systems

Species		Classification	Synonym	Comments
M. celatum	+			Propensity for causing respiratory infections in patients with AIDS. Closely resembles *M. xenopi*
M. gordonae	0/+	II scotochromogen	Tap-water scotochromogens	*M. aquae*—occasionally pathogenic for humans
M. thermoresistible	+	II scotochromogen		Growth at 52° C. Potentially pathogenic. Slow-growing
M. avium/*M. intracellulare*	+++	III nonphotochromogen[a]	Battey bacillus	*M. batteyi*, *M. battey*—frequently drug-resistant. Often complex cause of infection in patients with AIDS
M. terrae	Rare	III nonphotochromogen	Radish bacillus	May be closely related to *M. triviale*
M. shimoidei	+	III nonphotochromogen		Resembles *M. terrae* complex. Rare cases of pulmonary infections
M. triviale	0/+	III nonphotochromogen	V bacillus	Has been called atypical-atypical *Mycobacterium*
M. malmoense	+++	III nonphotochromogen		Slowly growing mycobacterium usually causing pulmonary disease
M. haemophilum	+++	III nonphotochromogen		Associated with skin lesions usually in immunosuppressed patients
M. fortuitum	++	IV rapid grower		*M. ranae*; *M. minetti*—skin and lung infections. It may cause disease in immunosuppressed host. May cause nosocomial infection
M. chelonae	++	IV rapid grower		May cause skin infections, particularly in persons with compromised cell-mediated immunity. An important cause of pulmonary disease in patients with chronic respiratory disease
M. abscessus	++	IV rapid grower		May cause skin infections, particularly in persons with compromised cell-mediated immunity. An important cause of pulmonary disease in patients with chronic respiratory disease

[a] Strains recovered from patients with AIDS are often scotochromogenic.
Adapted from Sommers HM. *The Clinically Significant Mycobacteria.* Chicago: American Society of Clinical Pathologists, 1974.

do not tolerate this increased salt concentration. Slants of Löwenstein-Jensen medium containing 5% NaCl are commercially available. The test cannot be performed in an agar-based medium (see Chart 19-14 for details).[189]

Growth on MacConkey Agar

MacConkey agar, from which the crystal violet has been removed, will support the growth of the rapidly growing mycobacteria. However, most other *Mycobacterium* species cannot grow on this medium. The test procedure is detailed in Chart 19-8.

Classification of Mycobacteria

The recognition that an unknown microorganism is "acid-fast" is usually the first clue that the organism may be a mycobacterium. *Acid-fast* is a term that is used to describe bacteria that resist decolorization with acidified alcohol once they have been stained with carbolfuchsin. Certain bacterial species, notably *Nocardia* species and *Rhodococcus* species, retain carbolfuchsin only if a less stringent decolorizing agent is used, such as a low-concentration inorganic acid like 1% H_2SO_4 or 1% HCl). These species are referred to as being "partially acid-fast."

Wayne and Kubica consider *Corynebacterium*, *Nocardia*, and *Rhodococcus* species to be clustered together in a supergenus based on many similarities.[375] They have designated this cluster of organisms the CNM group. Details for the identification of these nonmycobacterial species have been presented elsewhere. Slow growth, the presence of beaded gram-positive, slightly curved or straight rods that rarely branch, resistance to lysozyme, and the patterns of reactions in the biochemical tests presented in the foregoing are the characteristics by which the mycobacteria can generally be recognized and by which species identifications can be made. However, the taxonomy and classification of *Mycobacterium* species have become somewhat complex. The relationships and identity of these microorganisms are being redefined through DNA sequencing.

In the late 1950s, as species of mycobacteria other than *M. tuberculosis* were being encountered with increasing frequency in medical practices, Runyon proposed the grouping of these "atypical" organisms based on growth rate and pigment production (Box 19-2). Advances in our knowledge

of the genetics, cell structure, and aberrant phenotypic properties of previously known and newly discovered strains of the mycobacteria have advanced our knowledge beyond the neat packaging of species under the classic Runyon system of classification that has served clinical mycobacteriology laboratories for the past three decades. In addition, Sommers and Good point out that certain strains of *M. kansasii*, for example, are either pigmented in the dark or are nonpigmented (qualifying for Runyon group II or group III, respectively).[324] Pigmented species in the MAI complex have also been encountered. Therefore, a reliance on these phenotypic criteria may be misleading, and Sommers and Good advise that each isolate must be definitively identified and considered for its individual identity in light of the possible associated disease syndromes. Similarly, Woods and Washington have suggested a clinically oriented classification of mycobacteria (Box 19-3), refined from an earlier published proposal by Wolinski.[393,399]

Nevertheless, for the traditionally trained mycobacteriologist, the splitting off of *M. tuberculosis* (and *M. bovis*) from mycobacteria other than *M. tuberculosis* (MOTT) and the

---

Box 19-2 Runyon's Classification Scheme[a]

Group I: Photochromogens
Group II: Scotochromogens
Group III: Nonphotochromogens
Group IV: Rapid Growers

[a] *Does not include M. tuberculosis complex, including M. bovis.*

Box 19-3 Woods and Washington Classification Scheme, Updated

Species Potentially Pathogenic in Humans

M. avium/M. intracellulare complex
M. kansasii
Rapid growers: *M. fortuitum, M. chelonae, M. abscessus*
M. scrofulaceum
M. xenopi
M. szulgai
M. malmoense
M. simiae
M. genavense
M. marinum
M. ulcerans
M. haemophilum
M. celatum

Saprophytic Mycobacteria Rarely Causing Disease in Humans

M. gordonae
M. asiaticum
M. terrae
M. triviale
M. shimoidei
M. gastri
M. nonchromogenicum
M. paratuberculosis

Species With an Intermediate Growth Rate

M. flavescens

Other Rapidly Growing Species

M. thermoresistible
M. smegmatis
M. vaccae
M. parafortuitum complex
M. phlei

preliminary separation of MOTT into the four Runyon groups will continue to provide a meaningful initial orientation. The fact that certain strains of the usually photochromogenic *M. kansasii* may be nonpigmented or even scotochromogenic, that some strains of the MAI complex may be lightly pigmented, and even that *M. szulgai* is scotochromogenic at 37°C but photochromogenic at 25°C (certainly disruptive to the Runyon scheme) does not suggest that past orientations should be totally discarded, but rather that the phenotypic variability of these organisms should be recognized and incorporated into conventional identification schemes.

Laboratory Identification of Mycobacteria and Related Clinical Syndromes

The identification of mycobacteria by traditional methods is not difficult but requires patience, familiarity with the end points of different identification characteristics, and a collection of control strains. Not every laboratory needs the ability to identify all mycobacteria to the species level. The number of patients with tuberculosis in any given hospital in the United States is not large, and it may be prudent to use the services of a reference laboratory to provide definitive identifications and susceptibility testing of clinically important isolates recovered in the primary care laboratory. Each laboratory director or microbiology supervisor must determine the extent of services to be provided to meet the needs of the local clinical practice. Table 19-9 is a listing of the options for extent or level of services to be provided, in keeping with the inspection and accreditation guidelines provided by the College of American Pathologists.

Experience with the College of American Pathologists Special Mycobacterial Interlaboratory Survey over the many years has shown that increasing numbers of laboratories are restricting their services for mycobacterial infections to the preparation and interpretation of acid-fast stained smears, setting up primary cultures, and referring positive cultures to reference laboratories for identification and susceptibility testing.[323,397] Cost-containment measures imposed on most clinical laboratories and the commercial availability of nucleic-acid probes, which can provide more accurate and rapid results, are current forces that are prompting even more laboratories to provide services of no more than those required of level 1 or at the most level 2 laboratories.

Review of *Mycobacterium* Species: Laboratory Aspects and Clinical Correlations

Although a presumptive diagnosis of pulmonary tuberculosis can be made based on clinical history, presenting symptoms, physical examination, radiographic evidence of disease, and the presence of acid-fast bacilli in the sputum, the definitive diagnosis requires recovery of the causative organisms in culture or demonstration of these organisms by nucleic-acid amplification methods. Several *Mycobacterium* species other than *M. tuberculosis* are now recognized as important pulmonary pathogens, each with a different poten-

tial for producing disease and often with unique antimycobacterial drug susceptibility profiles that must be determined by laboratory tests. A wide variety of *Mycobacterium* species may be isolated from extrapulmonary sites, including blood, skin, soft tissues, and bones and joints. Laboratory culture characteristics and the clinical manifestations of select human mycobacterial diseases are listed in Box 19-4.

MYCOBACTERIUM TUBERCULOSIS COMPLEX

Mycobacterium tuberculosis. *Mycobacterium tuberculosis*, the most common cause of mycobacterial disease in humans, is often the major focus of definitive identification in many laboratories. Traditionally, it has been taught that classic strains of *M. tuberculosis* can be phenotypically differentiated from *M. bovis* and the intermediate species, *M. microti* and *M. africanum*.[375] However, several parameters, including analysis of antigenic extracts, target epitopes for monoclonal antibodies, and antigenic and DNA-relatedness studies, suggest that *M. tuberculosis*, *M. bovis*, *M. microti*, and *M. africanum* represent a single species and currently are considered under the general term "*M. tuberculosis* complex."

A few relatively simple tests are needed to identify most isolates of the *M. tuberculosis* complex. Some of these tests are to some extent made easier in laboratories where broth-based cultures are used. The following are phenotypic characteristics by which an identification of *M. tuberculosis* can be made:

1. Formation of nonpigmented, rough, buff colonies after 14 to 28 days of incubation at 37°C on Löwenstein-Jensen or Middlebrook media (see Color Plate 19-1*G* and *H*)
2. Appearance of microcolonies after 5 to 10 days incubation on Middlebrook 7H10 or 7H11 agars, with formation of serpentine cords owing to the production of "cording factor" (see Color Plate 19-1*C* and *I*).
3. Accumulation of niacin (*M. simiae*, certain strains of *M. bovis*, and occasional strains of *M. marinum* and *M. chelonae* may also be niacin-positive); therefore, this characteristic must be used in conjunction with the other findings (see Color Plate 19-1*D*).
4. Reduction of nitrates to nitrites (see Color Plate 19-1*E*).
5. Ability to grow in the presence of thiophene-2-carboxylic acid hydrazide (T2H; see Color Plate 19-1*F*).
6. Lack of catalase activity.
7. Selective inhibition of growth in broth culture media containing NAP (see Chart 19-4 for the details of this procedure).

The NAP inhibition of *M. tuberculosis* is used in many laboratories as a key test for making preliminary identifications, particularly for blood culture isolates. NAP selectively inhibits the growth of *M. tuberculosis*, and in the BACTEC system, the ability of the organism to release $^{14}CO_2$ from the radioactive 1-[^{14}C] palmitic acid contained in the me-

Table 19-9 Laboratory Self-Determined Extents or Levels of Service as Proposed by the College of American Pathologists and the American Thoracic Society

COLLEGE OF AMERICAN PATHOLOGISTS EXTENTS OF SERVICE FOR PARTICIPATION IN MYCOBACTERIAL INTERLABORATORY COMPARISON SURVEYS	AMERICAN THORACIC SOCIETY LEVELS OF SERVICE FOR MYCOBACTERIAL LABORATORIES
1. No mycobacterial procedures performed	**Level I** 1a. Collect adequate clinical specimens, including aerosol-induced sputa 1b. Transport specimens to a higher-level laboratory for isolation and identification. 1c. May prepare and examine smears for presumptive diagnosis or as a means of following the progress of diagnosed patients on chemotherapy
2. Acid-fast stain of exudates, effusions, and body fluids, with inoculation and referral of cultures to reference laboratories for further identification	**Level II** 2a. May perform all functions of level I laboratories, and process specimens as necessary for culture on standard agar- or egg-based media 2b. Identify *M. tuberculosis* 2c. May perform drug susceptibility studies against *M. tuberculosis* with primary antituberculosis drugs 2d. Retain mycobacterial cultures for a reasonable time
3. Isolation of mycobacteria; identification of *M. tuberculosis* and preliminary identification of the atypical forms such as photochromogens, scotochromogens, nonphotochromogens, and rapid growers. Drug susceptibility testing may or may not be performed 4. Definitive identification of mycobacteria isolated to the extent required to establish a correct clinical diagnosis and to aid in the selection of safe and effective therapy. Drug susceptibility testing performed	**Level III** 3a. May perform all functions of laboratories at lower levels, and identify all *Mycobacterium* species from clinical specimens 3b. Perform drug susceptibility studies against mycobacteria 3c. Retain mycobacterial cultures for a reasonable time 3d. May conduct research and provide training

dium. In broth culture systems NAP is also used for inoculation of other smear-positive specimens to enhance recovery and shorten the time for detection. Although the definitive identification of most NAP-negative mycobacteria strains still requires isolation and characterization by either the spectrum of tests discussed above or molecular methods, isolates that also produce microcolonies with serpentine cording on 7H10 agar can be presumptively identified as *M. tuberculosis* and subsequently confirmed by additional studies (see Color Plate 19-1*C*). The colonies appear "rough and buff" after 2–4 weeks of incubation on Löwenstein-Jensen (LJ) medium. These observations are sufficient criteria to warrant commencement of empiric therapy when clinically indicated.

The typical cell morphology of *M. tuberculosis* as seen in acid-fast stains is a thin, slightly curved, bacillus that measures 0.3–0.6 × 1–4 nm, deeply red staining (strongly acid-fast), with a distinct beaded appearance (see Color Plate 19-1*B*). In the preparation of smears from cultures, the individual cells are often difficult to disperse, appearing as irregular aggregates, or lying in parallel strands. Distinctive cord-

ing may be seen in preparations from broth cultures, wherein aggregates of the acid-fast bacilli form long serpentine cords. Mycobacteria may be seen in the Gram stain as gram-positive, beaded bacilli. The beading represents nonuniform staining of the bacillus. The presence of a *Mycobacterium* species can also be suspected in Gram stains if poorly or nonstaining bacilli are observed surrounded by a clear halo (see Color Plate 19-1*J*). The crystal violet dye in the Gram stain reagent does not penetrate the thick, waxy lipid cell wall of the organism, and they may appear as either beaded or almost as negative image against the counterstained background.

Mycobacterium bovis. *Mycobacterium bovis* is now included in the *M. tuberculosis* complex. Phenotypic characteristics by which *M. bovis* can be differentiated from classic strains of *M. tuberculosis* include the following:

1. Most strains are niacin-negative.
2. Nitrates are not reduced to nitrites.
3. Pyrazinamidase is not produced.

Box 19-4 *Mycobacterium* Species: Order of Presentation

Mycobacterium tuberculosis complex

M. tuberculosis
M. bovis
M. africanum
M. ulcerans (genetically related to *M. marinum*)

Photochromogens

M. kansasii
M. marinum
M. simiae
M. genavense (genetically related to *M. simiae* but not chromogenic)
M. asiaticum

Scotochromogens

M. scrofulaceum
M. szulgai (photochromogenic at 25°C)
M. xenopi
M. celatum
M. gordonae
M. flavescens

Nonphotochromogens

M. avium-intracellulare complex
M. paratuberculosis
M. terrae and *M. triviale*
M. shimoidae

Rapid Growers

M. fortuitum
M. chelonae
M. abscessus
M. thermoresistible

4. Selective inhibition of growth by T2H; *M. bovis* will not grow in medium containing T2H.

The classic human strains have a very slow growth rate, producing "dysgonic"-appearing colonies on LJ medium. Thus, a problem in recognizing *M. bovis* may arise in laboratories where LJ cultures are discarded after 4 weeks, because often 6 to 8 weeks are required for visible growth. Growth of most strains is better on LJ medium than on Middlebrook 7H11 or equivalents. The medium most favorable for *M. bovis* contains 0.4% pyruvate without glycerol. Typical colonies are buff, low, and small and may appear either smooth or rough on egg-containing medium. On Middlebrook 7H11 agar, colonies are very thin and often show little or no stranding (referred to as "water-droplet-like"). These colonies may also simulate dysgonic forms of organisms in the MAI complex. The latter, however, are 68°C catalase-positive, do not produce urease, and are pyrazinamidase-positive. If pyruvate has been added to the medium, colonies may show serpentine cords similar to those of eugonic *M. tuberculosis*.

Certain laboratory strains of *M. bovis*, known as BCG (bacille Calmette-Guérin), which have been used as a vaccine in highly endemic areas of the world, simulate *M. tuberculosis* by being "eugonic," or more rapidly growing (3 to 4 weeks on LJ medium), having a rough, buff appearance and, in some cases, accumulating niacin. However, these strains remain T2H-sensitive and can be differentiated on that basis.[116] The microscopic morphology of *M. bovis* cells in acid-fast-stained smears is not distinctive.

PHOTOCHROMOGENS

Mycobacterium kansasii. *M. kansasii* is an important cause of pulmonary disease that may clinically and histopathologically resemble tuberculosis. Pulmonary disease due to *M. kansasii*, however, does not have the same public health implications as tuberculosis and is not transmitted from person to person. Originally known as the "yellow bacillus" following the first description by Buhler and Pollak in 1953, *M. kansasii* is a photochromogen classified within the Runyon group I. Although infections occur throughout the United States, most cases have been reported from the southern states (Texas, Louisiana, and Florida), Midwest (Illinois), and California. Kim and associates report a decline in the overall incidence of disease in the United States over the past decade.[175] Males are infected more frequently than females, with a ratio of approximately 3:1. The disease is uncommon in children and individuals with higher incomes and better standards of living.[301]

Laboratory Aspects Typical strains of *M. kansasii* grow at approximately the same rate as or slightly more rapidly than *M. tuberculosis* at 37°C. The distinctive feature is the dependence on light exposure for the production of a visible yellow pigment (see Color Plate 19-2C and D) and the formation of reddish carotene crystals on prolonged incubation. The colonies are typically intermediate between fully rough and fully smooth, however certain strains are totally one or the other. The microcolonies typically show elevated centers and curving strands of bacilli in the outer, thinner margins that may be confused with the serpentine cording of *M. tuberculosis*. The group of phenotypic properties, in addition to photochromogenicity, by which the identification of *M. kansasii* can be confirmed include:

1. Rapid hydrolysis of Tween within 3 days
2. Strong reduction of nitrate to nitrite
3. Rapid catalase reaction, including 68°C test
4. Strong pyrazinamidase activity

Less commonly, scotochromogenic or nonchromogenic strains may be encountered, including some strains with low catalase activity. The bacterial cells in acid-fast smear preparations are characteristically long and broad and distinctly cross-banded or barred (see Color Plate 19-2M), presumably from utilization of the fatty material of the medium. Although experienced mycobacteriologists may make a presumptive identification based on acid-fast stain, determination of phenotypic properties is usually required and recommended before a definitive identification can be made.

Mycobacterium marinum. In 1926, while investigating infectious diseases in saltwater fish, Aronson discovered a new *Mycobacterium* species, later named *Mycobacterium mari-*

CLINICAL CORRELATION BOX 19-1 *Mycobacterium tuberculosis*

The recovery of *M. tuberculosis* from clinical specimens is almost always associated with infection, and tuberculosis is known to be a highly communicable disease. Most infections begin in the lungs, where diffuse, finely nodular, or patchy infiltrates may be seen, predominantly in the apical portions of the upper lobes, but also spreading to other foci in miliary form or as progressive exudative tuberculosis (see Color Plate 19-3*A*). Cavitary lesions, primarily in the apical portions of the upper lobes are common, and a solitary tuberculoma or "coin lesion" that may be part of an old Ghon complex may be seen (see Color Plate 19-3*B* and *C*). Outbreaks in closed populations, such as schools, ships, and crowded family groups are common. Disseminated or miliary spread of infection occurs in certain persons, usually those with malnutrition, immunosuppression, or other chronic debilitating diseases. Jereb and coworkers, using restriction-fragment-length polymorphism (RFLP) by PCR, were able to trace the source of an outbreak of *M. tuberculosis* among 10 kidney-transplant recipients in one hospital to a single patient who had posttransplantation exposure in another hospital before transfer.[158] The mean incubation time for the onset of tuberculosis in the newly infected kidney-transplant recipients was 7.5 weeks. This situation illustrates how new molecular techniques can be helpful in detecting point sources of tuberculosis so that early isolation can be implemented to prevent nosocomial transmission of disease.

   M. tuberculosis infections are most frequent among persons engaged in the following occupations[56]:

1. Persons with occupational tuberculosis exposure: funeral directors and health service personnel
2. Persons with occupational silica exposure: construction workers, brick and stone masons, carpenters, mining machine operators, and construction laborers
3. Low socioeconomic status occupations: food preparation and service workers
4. Unknown risk: farm operators, automobile racers and mechanics, butchers, entertainers

   Reactivation, or adult-type, tuberculosis is a slowly progressive inflammatory process in the lungs, characterized by intense chronic granulomatous inflammation, usually with the formation of many Langhans-type giant cells, necrosis, and caseation, with the propensity of the process to erode into bronchi (see Color Plate 19–3*D*). Large numbers of tubercle bacilli are spread to fresh foci within the lung when a cavity ruptures, and may be expectorated in profusion if the cavity breaks into a bronchus, potentially infecting others in close contact. Coughing, weight loss, low-grade fever, dyspnea, and chest pain are the usual clinical signs and symptoms of chronic progressive pulmonary tuberculosis. This is a description of the so-called secondary- or reactivation-type tuberculosis. In patients with AIDS, the disease is more reminiscent of a primary progressive tuberculosis, and is characterized by more rapid progression, septicemia, and miliary dissemination, less focal fibrosis and caseation, and miliary dissemination to involve virtually any organ in the body.

   Tuberculosis meningitis is a relatively rare disease in the United States, and it virtually always occurs as a complication of primary pulmonary tuberculosis. Patients may be asymptomatic, present with vague reports of headaches, change in mentation, or, uncommonly, progress to manifestations of severe meningitis. In most instances, one of three laboratory measurements of cerebrospinal fluid will be altered: an increase in cell count, usually a lymphocytosis; a decrease in glucose levels; or an increase in protein concentrations, although any one of these parameters may be normal. In rare instances, all three parameters may be normal, providing little objective evidence for establishing the diagnosis. Acid-fast organisms may be observed in centrifuged specimens in about 40% of cases, a yield that increases with the number of spinal examinations performed. Pathologically, the meningeal involvement is most pronounced at the base of the brain, where visible changes range from a diffuse opacity to the presence of a thick gelatinous exudate, seen primarily in the area overlying the pons and adjacent to the optic chiasm (see Color Plate 19–3*E*).

   Septicemia with *M. tuberculosis* is traditionally considered to be rare; however, Bouza and associates, in a study of 285 patients with culture-proved tuberculosis in whom blood cultures were obtained, found that 50 (14%) had bacteremia.[29] Of these, 81% were infected with HIV. In 14 patients, blood was the first specimen from which organisms were recovered. Archibald et al., when studying 517 patients with possible community-acquired bloodstream infections (BSI) in sub-Saharan Africa, found that of the 145 patients with a proven BSI, 81% of which were HIV-infected, the most frequently isolated pathogen was *M. tuberculosis*, at 39%.[8]

   More than 93% of *M. tuberculosis* strains isolated from untreated patients are susceptible to antituberculosis drugs and respond promptly to treatment with two, or preferably three, drugs. The susceptibility testing of mycobacteria is presented later in this chapter.

num ("of the sea").[10,376] The organism has also been called *M. platypoecilus* from infections observed in Mexican platyfish and also as *M. balnei* (a name referring to bath or spas). All are the same organism.

   Laboratory Aspects *M. marinum*, when recovered from clinical specimens, grows optimally at 30 to 32°C. Growth is poor, if it occurs at all, at 37°C. However, subcultures may grow at 37°C. Colonies appear in 8 to 14 days; those

grown in the dark may appear nonpigmented. When exposed to light, a deep yellow pigment develops. Colonies vary between wrinkled and rough to smooth and hemispheric, particularly if grown on 7H10 or 7H11 media (which contains oleic acid and albumin). Microscopically, the cells are relatively long rods with frequent cross-barring.

   Thus, photochromogenicity and preference for growth at 30°C are initial clues to the identification of *M. marinum*.

CLINICAL CORRELATION BOX 19-2
Mycobacterium bovis

M. bovis produces tuberculosis typically in cattle but may also infect other animals, including dogs, cats, swine, rabbits, and possibly, certain birds of prey. Fanning and Edwards traced 446 contacts of humans with domesticated elk in Alberta, Canada, 81 of whom were skin-test-positive for *M. bovis*.[90] Of these, 50 had been in contact with culture-positive animals, including one case of active *M. bovis* pulmonary infection diagnosed by a positive sputum specimen. With DNA fingerprinting assays with IS6110 as the genetic marker, van Soolingen et al. were able to determine that the strains of *M. bovis* causing human infection in Argentina were transmitted from cattle, whereas the strains causing human disease among persons living in The Netherlands were contracted from animals other than cattle (various wild and zoo animals).[360] In some areas in Scotland and in Eastern Europe, where cattle and dairy farming is still the chief livelihood, *M. bovis* still may constitute as many as 39% of all cases of tuberculosis.[386] Human bovine pulmonary tuberculosis closely resembles that caused by *M. tuberculosis*, in deference to Robert Koch, whose fame at the end dwindled among colleagues as he held firmly to the position that bovine tuberculosis caused only intestinal disease in humans. We now know that these two species are generally part of a complex, and *M. bovis* pulmonary tuberculosis is treated similarly to disease caused by *M. tuberculosis*.

During the time that humans physically milked cows much more frequently than today, cutaneous infections of the fingers were common, often with underlying osteomyelitis and osteoarthritis of the digits (see Color Plate 19-3F). A common site of recovery of *M. bovis* in clinical laboratories is from urine samples, as the bacille Calmette-Guérin (BCG) strain is used in bladder irrigations as an immunologic stimulant in the treatment of urothelial-cell carcinoma. This possibility should be considered when a slow-growing mycobacterium is recovered from urine samples, and any such isolate should not be passed off as a commensal. In some individuals, the BCG strain being used is not totally attenuated and may cause cystitis.

The following are additional characteristics by which a definitive identification can be made:

1. Some strains may accumulate niacin.
2. Nitrates are not reduced to nitrites.
3. Tween is hydrolyzed.
4. Urease is positive.
5. Pyrazinamidase is produced.
6. Heat-stable catalase is not produced.

Mycobacterium simiae. Weiszfeiler and Karczag named *M. simiae* in 1969,[379] in recognition of the first recovery of the organism four years earlier by Karassova and colleagues,[378a] from *Macaca* rhesus monkeys imported into Hungary from India. This organism was subsequently found to be identical to a niacin-positive strain of a group III mycobacterium re-

covered in Cuba by Valdivia and coworkers from patients with pulmonary tuberculosis. They named the organism *M. habana*, which subsequently has been shown to be the same organism as *M. simiae*.[375]

Laboratory Aspects Colonies of *M. simiae* develop within 2 to 3 weeks on egg-based media and are typically smooth. Most strains are photochromogenic. Prolonged exposure to light may be required for isolates that fail to produce pigment. The key identifying biochemical reactions are as follows:

1. Positive niacin accumulation
2. Hydrolysis of Tween (may be slow, requiring more than 10 days)
3. High thermostable catalase activity

Poor reproducibility of test reactions by some strains may make identification somewhat difficult. Some strains of *M. simiae* may be misidentified as members of the *M. avium/M. intracellulare/M. scrofulaceum* (MAIS) group.

Mycobacterium asiaticum. *Mycobacterium asiaticum* is in many ways phenotypically similar to *M. gordonae;* both have high catalase activity, hydrolyze Tween 80, and are negative for urease and nitrate reduction.[376] It, however, is photochromogenic. It is also biochemically similar to *M. simiae*, except it is niacin-negative. *M. asiaticum* has a distinct 16S rRNA profile, justifying a separate species status.[329]

Rare cases of human infection have appeared in the literature. The first indication that this organism could be pathogenic was in a report from Australia by Blacklock.[23] Two of the five patients had progressive cavitary pulmonary disease; three had no evidence of progressive pulmonary disease, and the sputum isolates were thought to represent secondary colonization. The first case of pulmonary infection caused by *M. asiaticum* in the United States was isolated from a 62-year-old man living in Los Angeles.[342] Four isolates have also been reported from Florida.[109] Dawson and coworkers have reported recovery of *M. asiaticum* from fluid aspirated from an olecranon bursa in a case of postsurgery infection.[69] The infection cleared with drainage, regular dressing changes, and immobilization, without the need for antimycobacterial therapy. *M. asiaticum* is photochromogenic and biochemically similar to *M. simiae* but is negative for niacin production.

SCOTOCHROMOGENS

Mycobacterium scrofulaceum. The species name *scrofulaceum*, derived from *scrofula* ("brood sow"), was named in 1956 by Prissick and Mason in reference to the most common form of disease by this organism, cervical lymphadenitis in children.[269] *M. scrofulaceum*, however, is not the only mycobacterium that causes cervical lymphadenitis. Gill et al. reviewed the cases of 16 children with this disease; 6 were caused by *M. scrofulaceum*, 4 by *M. tuberculosis*, and 4 by *M. avium* complex.[103] Therefore, culture and species identification of organisms isolated is required. *M. scrofulaceum* is uncommonly associated with AIDS. Mycobacteria recovered from cervical lymphadenitis in this patient population are much more likely to be *M. tuberculosis* or members of the MAI complex.

CLINICAL CORRELATION BOX 19-3 *Mycobacterium kansasii*

Chronic pulmonary disease simulating classic tuberculosis is the most common manifestation, classically involving the upper lobes. Cavitation with scarring is evident in most cases, and disease is slowly progressive.[301] Extrapulmonary or disseminated infections are less common, although cases of scrofula-like lymphadenitis, sporotrichosis-like cutaneous infections, osteomyelitis, soft-tissue infections, and tenosynovitis have been reported. Dillon et al. in particular cite the progressive damage to the deep structures of the wrist and hand that can occur in cases of tenosynovitis.[74] Disseminated disease may be seen in the presence of severe immunosuppression and has been reported in patients with AIDS. Jacobson and Isenberg report an AIDS-related case of diffuse granulomatous interstitial pneumonitis caused by *M. kansasii*, but report that only 0.2% of AIDS patients have superimposed *M. kansasii* infections.[153] However, Valainis and coworkers, reporting from Louisiana, a region endemic for *M. kansasii*, in a 60-month review of patients attending two major referral centers in New Orleans, found that 31.9% of HIV-1-infected patients were coinfected with *M. kansasii*.[359] In a retrospective study of 35 patients conducted in Kansas City, the incidence of *M. kansasii* infections in patients with AIDS was three times higher than *M. tuberculosis* infections.[14] Most patients responded to several different combinations of antituberculosis drugs that included isoniazid, rifampin, ethambutol, and ciprofloxacin. Some patients tolerated therapy poorly; isoniazid-induced hepatitis developed in one. The authors recommend that at least two active agents, such as ethambutol and rifampin, be used.

M. kansasii infections in patients with AIDS usually occur during the late stages, when CD4 lymphocyte counts are fewer than 50, with serious and life-threatening complications in many cases. Levine and Chaisson reviewed 19 patients with *M. kansasii* and HIV infection, 14 of whom had exclusive pulmonary infection, three pulmonary and extrapulmonary disease, and two extrapulmonary involvement exclusively.[203] All patients with pulmonary infection presented with fever and cough of at least 2 weeks' duration. Focal upper-lobe infiltrates, diffuse interstitial infiltrates, or thin-walled cavitary lesions, or a combination thereof, were seen on chest radiographs. Nine patients receiving antituberculosis therapy showed resolution of fever and respiratory symptoms, with clearing of the radiographic infiltrates. Other AIDS-related cases of *M. kansasii* infections have been reported.[137,306] In one case, caseating granulomas were seen in the bowel wall and in the mesenteric lymph nodes, with accumulation of foamy histiocytes resembling Whipple's disease. Giladi and coauthors report a case of catheter-associated *M. kansasii* peritonitis in a 62-year-old woman undergoing continuous ambulatory peritoneal dialysis, presumably the first such case report.[102] Good response was achieved with combination therapy with isoniazid and rifampin and removal of the catheter. Tortoli and coworkers found a cluster of *M. kansasii* strains that did not hybridize with the AccuProbe *M. kansasii* culture identification test (Gen Probe, San Diego, CA) and that were distinctly associated with AIDS status.[354] This suggests that *M. kansasii* may differ in virulence and that additional tests for identification may be required for AccuProbe-negative strains.

Strains of *M. kansasii* resistant to rifampin have been reported. Wallace and coauthors reported on 36 patients from whom rifampin-resistant *M. kansasii* had been isolated, 90% of whom had previously received therapy with this agent.[367] The majority of patients, however, responded to a four-drug regimen, based on *in vitro* susceptibility studies, and sputum cultures converted to negative in 90% of those treated in a mean of 11 weeks.

Kirschner and associates recovered large quantities of *M. scrofulaceum* from swamp water in several locations in Georgia, West Virginia, and Virginia, indicating that environmental water sources are likely connected with the increased incidence of scrofula infections seen in these regions.[179] High concentrations of organisms were found in warm water with low pH, low dissolved oxygen content, high soluble zinc levels, and high levels of humic and fulvic acids.

Laboratory Aspects Colonies of *M. scrofulaceum* grow slowly (4 to 6 weeks) at various temperatures (25, 31, and 37°C). They produce colonies that are typically smooth, buttery in consistency, and globoid, with pigmentation ranging from light yellow to deep orange (see Color Plate 19-2D). Pigment production is not dependent on light exposure; thus, the organism is included in the scotochromogen group II of Runyon.

Key biochemical test reactions include the following:

1. Failure to hydrolyze Tween.
2. Nitrates are not reduced to nitrites.
3. 68°C catalase test is positive.
4. Urease is produced.

Other slow-growing scotochromogens include certain strains of the MAI complex, *M. gordonae*, and *M. szulgai* Tween hydrolysis (the latter two are positive [*M. szulgai* may require 7 days or more], whereas *M. scrofulaceum* is negative) and urease activity (*M. scrofulaceum* hydrolyzes urea, whereas the other species, including pigmented strains of *M. avium* complex, are negative). Two groups of pigmented organisms within the MAI complex, intermediate in biochemical reactivity with *M. scrofulaceum*, have been designated with the term MAIS complex.[127] One group of MAIS organisms produces a column of foam higher than 45 mm in the semiquantitative catalase test and is urease-negative; the other is catalase-negative but urease-positive.

Mycobacterium szulgai. *M. szulgai*, officially reported as a species in 1972 by Marks and coworkers, is named after the Polish microbiologist T. Szulg.[215,375] The unique feature of this species is the temperature-dependent production of pigment. When grown at 37°C, the organism is scotochromogenic, whereas it is photochromogenic when grown at room temperature (25°C). Therefore, to assess the photochromogenicity of an unknown strain of *M. szulgai*, the light-exposed plates must be incubated at room temperature and not at 37°C. The scotogenic pigment produced at the higher

CLINICAL CORRELATION BOX 19-4
Mycobacterium marinum

Typical infections with *M. marinum* involve the skin, usually resulting when traumatized skin comes in contact with inadequately chlorinated freshwater or saltwater (swimming pools, tropical fish aquariums, water-cooling towers). Fisher has reported three cases of cutaneous skin infection in lifeguards, citing this infection as a hazard of the trade.[93] Included in Fisher's article are good color photographs of the skin lesions. Several cases were seen in Denver, Colorado, in the 1950s, secondary to massive contamination of a swimming pool spa in the mountain community of Glenwood Springs. Hoyt and associates report several deep-tissue infections and destructive tenosynovitis among fishermen in the Chesapeake Bay area.[141] Several other citations of deep cutaneous infections, usually of the hands, and commonly associated with aquatic activity, such as cleaning of fish, include a case of tenosynovitis, arthritis and bursitis, and osteomyelitis.[17,48,143] Chemotherapy with some combination of drugs, such as rifampin and ethambutol, may be effective, but frequently, surgery may be required. Chemotherapy is least likely to be effective in patients previously treated with steroid injection, and avoidance of steroid injections is key to successful management.[48,162]

Some patients present with sporotrichosis-like lesions, with central spread along the lymphatics emanating from an ulcerated area at the primary site of inoculation.[246] More typically, the lesions present as tender, red or blue-red subcutaneous nodules, usually involving the elbow, knee, toe, or finger ("swimming pool granuloma"). Such lesions may be mistaken for rheumatoid nodules.[11] These authors cite other cases of deep subcutaneous infections, in some instances involving subcutaneous bursae, tendon sheaths, joints, and bone.

Treatment is usually directed to resecting the primary lesions if possible (curettage, electrodesiccation, excision). Antituberculosis therapy may be required to cure chronic cases in which lymphatic spread is evident. Most strains are susceptible to rifampin and ethambutol but resistant to isoniazid and streptomycin.

CLINICAL CORRELATION BOX 19-5
Mycobacterium simiae

Reports of human infection with *M. simiae* are relatively few. Isolated case reports of pulmonary infections occurring in France, Israel, Thailand, and the United States have been cited.[204] These authors report a case of a 43-year-old man with AIDS in whom disseminated mycobacterial infection developed. Organisms were recovered from blood, jejunal fluid, and duodenal and rectal biopsies. Although a few other cases of *M. simiae* infections have been reported in patients with AIDS, the association is infrequent and does not serve as a marker.[257] The Israeli experience with *M. simiae* is interesting, in that 399 strains were isolated from 287 persons during the period 1975 to 1981, primarily among inhabitants of the coastal plain of Tel Aviv.[198] Most of the isolates were commensal organisms related to environmental water sources. A few pulmonary infections occurred among patients from whom multiple isolates were recovered, usually complicating preexisting chronic pulmonary conditions.

Two cases of disseminated disease, with renal involvement following pulmonary infection have been reported.[294] Although most strains of *M. simiae* are resistant to antituberculous drugs by *in vitro* testing, a case of intraabdominal disease that was successfully treated with combination chemotherapy has been reported.[132]

temperature will mask any chance to visualize any photogenetic pigment that may be produced (see Chart 19-6).

Laboratory Aspects Growth is relatively rapid, with either smooth or rough colonies developing within 2 weeks at 37°C. Orange pigment may be observed, intensifying with exposure to continuous light. In acid-fast smear preparations, the bacterial cells appear as moderately long bacilli, with some cross-barring, reminiscent of *M. kansasii*.

Key biochemical test reactions for *Mycobacterium szulgai* include the following:

1. Slow hydrolysis of Tween
2. Nitrates reduced to nitrites
3. Positive catalase activity
4. Intolerance to 5% NaCl

Mycobacterium xenopi. *M. xenopi* (*Xenopus*, a genus of frog), was first isolated from an African toad.[375] Hot and cold water taps, including water storage tanks and hot water generators of hospitals, are potential sources for nosocomial infections. Previously considered to be nonpathogenic, *M. xenopi* has been incriminated in several infections. Wolinski reported 50 cases of human *M. xenopi* infections, primarily in England, France, Denmark, Australia, and the United States.[393] Birds that frequent the costal regions in Great Britain constitute an important reservoir.

Laboratory Aspects *Mycobacterium xenopi* colonies are slow-growing, small, erect, and produce characteristic yellow pigment (occasional strains are nonpigmented). Growth is more rapid at 42°C than 37°C; growth is absent at 25°C. Although previously included with the nonphotochromogenic mycobacteria, the brightly pigmented yellow colonies usually found on primary isolation suggest that the organism would be better considered with the scotochromogens. Colonies tend to be rough, and an aerial mycelium may be evident. Examination of young microcolonies on 7H10 agar reveals a distinctive "bird's nest" appearance, with sticklike projections. Branching and filamentous extensions appear in older colonies, particularly those grown on cornmeal-glycerol agar. Microscopically, acid-fast-stained smears reveal long, filamentous rods that are tapered at both ends, tending to arrange in palisades.

Key biochemical test reactions for *Mycobacterium xenopi* include the following:

1. Optimal growth at 42°C
2. Yellow scotochromogenic pigment
3. No niacin accumulation
4. Nitrate reduction-negative

CLINICAL CORRELATION BOX 19-6
Mycobacterium scrofulaceum

Lymphadenitis is the classic presenting symptom of infection with *M. scrofulaceum*, occurring most commonly in children between 18 months and 7 years of age, during a time when a barrier break in the oral mucous membrane occurs during teething. The next higher incidence of disease occurs in young adults who are cutting molar teeth. The lymphadenitis is unilateral, involving nodes high in the neck adjacent to the mandible or posteriorly behind the ears (see Color Plate 19–3G and H). The nodes often drain from the surface of the skin without complications, except for varying degrees of residual scarring at the sites of surface penetration of sinus tracts. The disease often affects healthy children; pain is usually minimal, and constitutional symptoms are absent. Colonization of the organism in the mouth and throat is presumed to be the site of origin. The high incidence of disease among young children is thought to be related to disruption of the gums during tooth eruptions, during an age when the immune system is still relatively immature. Only a few cases of progressive pulmonary disease and dissemination to other organs, primarily in patients with serious debilitating illness, have been cited.[301] The local disease is best treated with surgical incision and drainage of the involved nodes; only rarely are antituberculous drugs necessary.

Susceptibility patterns vary to antituberculous drugs and other antibiotics, such as sulfonamides and erythromycin. Treatment of serious infections should involve use of at least three of the following drugs: INH, streptomycin, rifampin, and cycloserine.[301]

5. Catalase produced at 68°C only
6. Arylsulfatase-positive
7. Pyrazinamidase-positive

Mycobacterium celatum. *M. celatum* is the name proposed for this *Mycobacterium* species by Butler and coauthors.[35] It most closely resembles *M. xenopi* phenotypically (in fact, it was not discovered until recently because it was hidden

CLINICAL CORRELATION BOX 19-7
Mycobacterium szulgai

Maloney and associates present three cases of human infections with *M. szulgai* and reviewed 24 cases previously reported in the literature before 1987.[214] Lung infections were present in two thirds of the cases, and chest radiographs revealed unilateral or bilateral apical disease, with cavitation, simulating *M. tuberculosis*. A case of persistent lung infection caused by *M. szulgai* has also been reported.[53] Fever, cough, hemoptysis, and weight loss were common symptoms. Extrapulmonary infections with *M. szulgai* cited in the foregoing review include olecranon bursitis, tenosynovitis, and carpal tunnel syndrome, osteomyelitis, and localized cutaneous disease.

CLINICAL CORRELATION BOX 19-8
Mycobacterium xenopi

Most human cases of *M. xenopi* infections have been pulmonary, resembling those seen in patients with *M. tuberculosis*, *M. kansasii*, or MAI infections. Multinodular densities, often showing cavitation and fibrosis, are often seen radiologically. Infections usually occur in patients with preexistent lung disease or predisposing conditions (alcoholism, malignancy, diabetes mellitus). Contreras and coauthors, in reviewing 89 cases of adult patients with pulmonary infections, report that *M. xenopi* was the second most frequent isolate (38% of cases).[55] Similarly, in a review of cultures positive for nontuberculous mycobacteria, excluding MAI complex and *M. gordonae*, from 86 patients at the State University of New York Health Sciences Center at Brooklyn, *M. xenopi* was the species most commonly isolated (33 cases).[312] The majority of these isolates were recovered from respiratory specimens in patients with AIDS. The recovery of 28 isolates of *M. xenopi* from patients residing in the Ontario province of Canada has also been reported.[317] In 19 patients, the isolate was considered insignificant; nine isolates were from middle-aged men with other chronic pulmonary diseases. In the province of Ontario, *M. xenopi* has been the second most common nontuberculous mycobacterial pathogen, second only to the MAI complex.

Intrapulmonary spread usually occurs in patients with AIDS; in disseminated cases, organisms may also be recovered from bone marrow aspirates.[12] *M. xenopi* infections are uncommonly found in HIV-positive patients. In two cases of HIV-infected men with symptomatic pulmonary infection, night sweats, cough, and pleuritic pain were reported.[154] This organism grew in cultures of multiple respiratory specimens obtained from each patient. Both patients improved with multidrug therapy that included isoniazid and rifampin, which was unexpected, although in one case *in vitro* resistance to isoniazid and rifampin was demonstrated. A case of pulmonary infection in a 39-year-old kidney allograft recipient has been reported.[377] Isolated cases of extrapulmonary infection involving bone, lymph node, epididymis, sinus tract, and a prosthetic temporomandibular joint have also been cited.[393] Infections of the lumbar spine have been reported; one patient was a 77-year-old immunocompetent woman who presented with a paravertebral abscess.[270,274] An outbreak of 13 cases of pulmonary infection in residents of a housing project in Prague have been reported.[319] The point source was thought to be the local water supply, as organisms were recovered from water faucets in five of the flats. Tortoli and coauthors, reviewed the cases of 64 isolates of *M. xenopi* recovered from patients living in Florence, Italy, during a 15-year period.[353] The homogeneity of the biochemical, cultural, and antimicrobial sensitivity patterns of these isolates indicates there may be an endemic focus in the Florence area.

[*celatum*, ''to conceal''] among strains of MAI and *M. xenopi*), differing only in its poor growth at 45°C, growth of large colonies on 7H10 agar, and the production of only trace amounts of the fatty acid 2-docanosol.[246,353] This new species has been recovered from respiratory tract cultures, and less commonly from the blood, stool, and cerebrospinal fluid, in cultures obtained from patients residing in diverse geographic locations, including the United States, Finland, and Somalia. In the original report by Butler and coauthors, approximately one third of the isolates were recovered from patients with AIDS.[35] They also found cross-reactivity for 8 of 20 strains with *M. tuberculosis* using the acridinium ester–labeled DNA probe, AccuProbe (Gen-Probe, San Diego CA), a problem that, although addressed, remains unresolved. This cross-reactivity with *M. tuberculosis* and the need for genomic sequencing or high-performance liquid chromatography of cell wall mycolic acids to make a correct identification will pose problems for those working in clinical laboratories. Tortoli and associates reported two cases in patients with AIDS. In the first patient, *M. celatum* was recovered from multiple blood cultures, first a cluster of four positive cultures, followed by a cluster of three additional positive cultures 9 months later.[353] The second isolate was from a sputum culture, and the pulmonary condition of the patient improved following combined drug treatment with clarithromycin, ciprofloxacin, and amikacin. Haase and coworkers report a case of scrofula-like unilateral cervical lymphadenitis in an immunocompetent child.[121]

Mycobacterium gordonae. *Mycobacterium gordonae* is a *Mycobacterium* species that rarely causes human infections, but is possibly the mycobacterium that is recovered in clinical laboratories with greatest frequency. It is found particularly in aqueous environments, leading to the alternative designation of *M. aquae*, or the ''tap water bacillus.''[375]

Laboratory Aspects *Mycobacterium gordonae* is a scotochromogen, and it is readily recognized by the smooth, deeply yellow-orange pigmented colonies that develop after 7 days of incubation at 37°C (see Color Plate 19-2*E* and *M*). The organism hydrolyzes Tween 80 and produces heat-stable catalase; it is urease-negative and does not reduce nitrates to nitrites. *Mycobacterium gordonae* is resistant to isoniazid, streptomycin, and *p*-aminosalicylic acid but is susceptible to rifampin and ethambutol. An organism that may be phenotypically confused with *M. gordonae* is *M. flavescens*, which is a scotochromogen; however, *M. flavescens* possesses urease activity and reduces nitrates to nitrites, two characteristics not demonstrated by *M. gordonae*. *M. flavescens* is a commensal for humans and is not known to cause disease.[375]

NONPHOTOCHROMOGENS

Mycobacterium avium/M. intracellulare Complex. Strains of *M. avium* and *M. intracellulare* are also often referred to as the MAI complex (MAC). This is the same organism that caused an outbreak of pulmonary infections at the Battey State Hospital in Rome, Georgia, in the 1950s and for some time carried the designation ''Battey bacillus.'' MAI is widely distributed in water, soil, dust, animals, and poultry. For humans, the organism was considered of low pathogenicity and rarely caused disease. However, the AIDS epidemic has demonstrated the pathogenicity of these organ-

---

CLINICAL CORRELATION BOX 19-9
Mycobacterium gordonae

Several isolated reports of infections with *M. gordonae* have been cited by Woods and Washington: meningitis secondary to ventriculoatrial shunts, hepatoperitoneal disease, endocarditis in a prosthetic aortic valve, cutaneous lesions of the hand, and possible cases of pulmonary involvement.[399] The case of peritonitis in a patient undergoing peritoneal dialysis suggests that infections with *M. gordonae*, being so prevalent in the environment, may emerge as a significant problem.[209] It is believed that *M. gordonae* should not automatically be dismissed as a contaminant when isolated from clinical material.[378] The clinical characteristics of 23 reported human cases of *M. gordonae* infection that fit these criteria for inclusion had been tabulated from the literature as of June 1992.[378] The organ distribution of these previously reported cases was as follows: lungs in eight patients, soft tissue (seven), peritoneal cavity (three), the cornea (one), and disseminated disease (five). They reported an additional case of disseminated disease in an 11-year-old girl. Multiple round granular lesions were seen scattered in both lung fields during an open lung biopsy. Necrotizing granulomatous inflammation was seen on histologic examination of biopsy material, including numerous acid-fast bacilli in acid-fast smears. Smooth, yellow colonies, later identified as *M. gordonae*, grew on solid media after 14 days of incubation at 37°C in 8% CO_2. The patient recovered after 15 months of antituberculosis therapy, commencing with a combination of isoniazid, rifampin, amikacin, and ethambutol, followed by a 1-year course of rifampin and ethambutol.

Jarikre reported two cases of *M. gordonae* infection, each in 40-year-old housewives. One was a woman with a chronic urinary tract infection from whom *M. gordonae* was repeatedly recovered in urine specimens; the other was a Pakistani patient with systemic infection, from whom the organism was recovered from sputum and urine.[155,156] Liver biopsy revealed multiple granulomata from which *M. gordonae* was also recovered. The second patient responded dramatically on an antitubercular drug regimen of streptomycin, isoniazid, rifampin, and pyrazinamide. A case was reported of chronic nodular cutaneous infection that presented histologically as classic tuberculoid granulomas teeming with acid-fast bacilli from which *M. gordonae* was recovered.[409]

Wayne and Sramek, however, after reviewing many of the previously reported alleged cases of *M. gordonae* infection, caution that organism descriptions and convincing clinical correlations often are lacking in many of the papers, and that its true pathogenicity remains in question.[376] When recovered from specimens, each isolate must be accurately identified and a careful clinical correlation made to determine the clinical significance for what in most instances will be a contaminant.

CLINICAL CORRELATION BOX 19-10 *Mycobacterium avium/M. intracellulare*

Conditions predisposing individuals to pulmonary infections with members of the *M. avium/M. intracellulare* (MAI) complex include chronic obstructive pulmonary disease by whatever primary cause, bronchiectasis, chronic aspiration or recurrent pneumonia, inactive or active tuberculosis, pneumoconiosis, and bronchogenic carcinoma.[86] An association with cystic fibrosis has also been reported.[172] Pulmonary disease is also being seen in older women without predisposing conditions, the so-called Lady Windermere's syndrome, after Oscar Wilde's Victorian character who had the peculiar habit of suppressing a cough. In nonimmunosuppressed patients, pulmonary manifestations of MAI infections are similar to those of *M. tuberculosis:* cough, fatigue, weight loss, low-grade fever, and night sweats. Cavitary disease can usually be demonstrated radiologically, or solitary nodules or more diffuse infiltrates may be observed. Occasionally, patients may be asymptomatic.

The greatest upsurge in MAI infections during the past few decade has been in patients with AIDS, to the point that, in some settings, MAI is more frequently recovered than *M. tuberculosis*. In a review of MAI infections in HIV-positive patients before the widespread use of highly active antiretroviral therapy (HAART), it was found that the MAI infections were usually disseminated and occurred late in the course of HIV infection.[211] The risk of contracting MAI infections in AIDS patients with CD4 counts lower than 50 is high (45% within 1 year after diagnosis).[44] When organisms were found in the sputum or gastrointestinal tract, 60% of patients had disseminated disease. Thus, these authors advise that AIDS patients with sputum or stool positive for MAI should receive prophylactic therapy with rifabutin. Disseminated infections are characterized by intermittent fever, sweats, weakness, anorexia, and weight loss that is relatively rapidly progressive. Abdominal pain or diarrhea with malabsorption was seen in some. Significant pulmonary involvement was not seen, despite recovery of MAI organisms in sputum specimens. Bacteremia occurs in over 90% of patients with disseminated disease, with organisms found within the circulating monocytes; therefore, mycobacterial blood culture is the recommended specimen for culture in these patients. Colony counts as high as 10^6 colony-forming units (CFUs)/mL have been reported, although counts in the range of 10^1 to 10^2 are more common.[394]

In a study of mycobacterial infections in 94 patients with AIDS, significant pulmonary disease occurred in only about 25% of patients with MAI, in contrast to 83% of patients with *M. tuberculosis* infections who had pulmonary disease.[234] Also, classic tuberculosis caused by *M. tuberculosis* preceded the diagnosis of AIDS in two thirds of the cases, in contrast with MAI infections, which were secondary complications of AIDS in all cases studied. Members of the MAI complex have also been recovered from 15 of 16 cases of tuberculosis meningitis.[151] The recovery of organisms from the spinal fluid always indicated disseminated disease, and prognosis in this group of patients was poor. The recovery of MAI from sputum specimens in this patient population is also an indicator of disseminated disease.[152] Disseminated disease caused by MAI, however, has become much less common since the introduction of HAART for HIV infection.

From our experience, the following features of MAI infections in patients with AIDS seem evident. The organism load in biopsy or autopsy tissue sections is often extremely heavy, with intracellular bacterial aggregates often seen within large foamy macrophages, simulating the lepra cells seen in *M. leprae* infections (see Color Plates 19–2*P* and 19–3*I* and *J*). Involvement of the gastrointestinal tract also is often heavy. In some instances, large foamy macrophages, simulating the cells seen in Whipple's disease, seem to predominate in the areas of inflammation. Patients with histologic evidence of gastrointestinal (and pulmonary) involvement invariably have disseminated disease.[44] Ingestion of contaminated water or food could well be the major mode of transmission. Lesions in other organs, notably the lungs, liver, spleen, and lymph nodes may also show a massive invasion with acid-fast bacilli. In some cases, little inflammation may be seen at the time of death. Necrotizing inflammation, rather than granuloma formation and caseation necrosis, is more characteristic of the histologic appearance of these lesions. Other investigators also have found heavy organism loads and atypical inflammatory reactions in AIDS patients with mycobacterial infections, and particularly cite the high incidence of mycobacterial septicemia and positive blood cultures in these patients.[126,344,408]

The MAI organisms also cause a scrofula-like cervical lymphadenitis in children.[176,193] Woods and Washington cite several other MAI infections, including granulomatous synovitis, genitourinary tract disease, cutaneous lesions, osteomyelitis, meningitis and colonic ulcers.[399] Evidence is mounting[399] that for intestinal ulcer disease a causal relation exists between regional enteritis, or Crohn's disease, and mycobacteria, specifically a mycobacterium species closely related to *M. avium* and likely classified within the MAI complex, *M. paratuberculosis*.

isms in persons with depleted T-cell immunity, and currently only *M. tuberculosis* is recovered with more frequency than MAI.[110]

Members of the MAI complex of bacteria are ubiquitous, and they can be recovered from water estuaries, pools, soil, house dust, plants, and bedding materials. Natural sources of water, including potable water, pose considerable risk for acquiring human infections.[364] Waters that have moderate salinity (1–2% salt), have relatively high acidity (pH 4.5 to 6.5), and are located at lower altitudes are ideal for supporting the propagation of MAI organisms.[32] Human MAI infec-

tions may occur from ingestion of contaminated water and food (the intestinal tract is thought to be the primary route of infection in AIDS patients) or by inhalation of organisms contained within aqueous aerosols. Wendt and coworkers found MAI organisms in droplet sizes of 0.7 to 3.3 mm above freshwater surfaces, sufficiently small to reach the alveolar spaces, and organisms may become highly concentrated in jet streams emanating from air-seawater interfaces.[381] Although poultry, swine, and other species of birds and animals become infected and excrete organisms in the feces that can remain viable for long periods in soil, animal-to-human transmission is a rare event. Human-to-human transmission also is thought to be a minimal risk factor.[149]

The MAI complex has a worldwide distribution; however, endemic areas have been found in temperate geographic areas, including the United States, Canada, Great Britain, Europe, the Netherlands, and Japan.[149] From a 1979 survey in the United States, the overall prevalence of MAI was 3.2 cases per 100,000 population, with the highest incidences in Hawaii (10.8 cases), Connecticut (8.9 cases), Florida (8.4 cases), and Kansas (6.8 cases).[110] Although *M. gordonae* is the most frequent nontuberculous mycobacterium recovered from human sources, members of the MAI complex are the organisms most frequently associated with human disease. The rates of human infections in the population who do not have AIDS have remained stable or have decreased slightly; in San Francisco, the overall increase in the incidence of infections due to the MAI complex paralleled the incidence of AIDS cases early in the course of the epidemic.[199] For example, of the 161,073 cases of AIDS reported to the CDC by December 1990, more than 12,000 cases of nontuberculous mycobacterial infections were also reported; in 96% of these, the causative agent was a member of the MAI complex.[140] HIV infection is the primary risk factor for disseminated infections with this organism.[244] The incidence of disseminated MAI infections in HIV-infected patients has diminished dramatically since the introduction of highly active antiretroviral therapy.

Laboratory Aspects The members of the MAI complex may appear as one of three colony variants: 1) smooth, opaque, and dome-shaped; 2) smooth, transparent, and flat; and 3) rough (see Color Plate 19-2*N* and *O*). The isolates recovered from AIDS patients most commonly produce the smooth, transparent, flat colony variant, as seen in microcolony observations (see Color Plate 19-2*A* and *B*). These flat, translucent colony types are thought by some to be more virulent than strains that produce other colony types.[63,297,305] Although *M. avium* was originally classified in Runyon group III (nonchromogens), in the experience of many, most strains recovered from patients with AIDS have varying degrees of yellow pigmentation, intensifying as the colony ages. Doern and associates, however, found that most of their strains were nonpigmented.[77] Stormer and Falkingham have determined that the strains recovered from HIV-positive patients were nonpigmented and were more likely to be resistant to antimicrobial agents compared with pigmented strains.[336]

Microscopic examination of acid-fast smears reveals cells that are typically short and coccobacillary. Early in culture and under certain conditions, long, thin bacilli may be seen. Staining is usually uniform, without beading or banding. Although conventional carbolfuchsin-based stains, such as Ziehl-Neelsen and Kinyoun, are used in most laboratories, auramine-rhodamine staining with fluorescence microscopy may be helpful in some cases. Because mixed infections may occur, a predicted identification based on microscopic morphology alone is not recommended.

Phenotypically, MAI complex strains are best characterized by a battery of negative reactions (see Table 19-7). The organism does produce heat-stable catalase and has the ability to grow on T2H; otherwise, the biochemical reactions are inert. With the availability of a nucleic-acid probe for the culture confirmation of members of the MAI complex,

the delay in obtaining a species identification by conventional methods is no longer warranted. Although the applications of PCR for the direct identification of mycobacteria, including members of the MAI complex, in the sputum and other clinical specimens, is receiving much attention in research laboratories, a commercial product is not available for diagnostic laboratories. Although it is common to perform the combination probe for the MAI complex, it may be important to determine whether the causative agent is *M. avium* or *M. intracellulare*, since some suggest that disease with *M. avium* appears to be more severe than that caused by *M. intracellulare*.[404]

Most strains of the MAI complex are resistant to the commonly used antituberculosis drugs. The underlying mechanism of resistance is based on the impermeability of the cell wall.[276] The synthesis of aminoglycoside- and peptide-inactivating enzymes has not been demonstrated, although some strains do produce beta-lactamases.[233] The surfactant effect on the cell wall of Tween 80 may potentiate the effect of certain antimicrobial agents; ethambutol also has an effect on cell wall permeability, reflecting how this agent may work synergistically to potentiate the effect of certain other antituberculous drugs.[139] Thus, in the past, ethambutol was usually included in the battery of drugs, such as INH, rifabutin, clofazimine, and others, used to treat patients with infections caused by the MAI complex.[2] The addition of macrolides to treatment regimens has dramatically improved outcomes for non-HIV infected patients with MAI pulmonary disease.

Mycobacterium paratuberculosis *and Crohn's Disease.*
Hermon-Taylor and coauthors cite the work of a Glasgow surgeon, T.K. Dalziel, who in 1913 published a detailed description of chronic enteritis in humans.[136] He proposed that the disease was caused by the same microorganisms as those responsible for Johne's disease, an ulcerative intestinal condition associated with chronic diarrhea in cattle. Johne's disease had been known since 1895 and was thought to be associated with acid-fast bacilli, which could be seen in the tissues of infected animals but, in these early days, could not be cultured. Not long afterward, however, a slow-growing mycobacterium was finally recovered from the intestinal mucosa of infected animals, initially known simply as Johne's bacillus but later identified as *M. paratuberculosis*.

In 1984, Chiodini and associates, working with Hermon-Taylor and colleagues at St. George's Hospital in London, reported the recovery of an unclassified, extremely fastidious *Mycobacterium* species from three patients with Crohn's disease.[46] After considerable effort, these workers identified the organism as belonging to the Runyon group III, closely related to the MAI and *M. paratuberculosis* complexes. Several additional cases linking *M. paratuberculosis* and Crohn's disease have been cited from the United States, The Netherlands, Australia, and France.[45] Further evidence that the Crohn's disease mycobacterium and *M. paratuberculosis* are the same was provided in yet another publication from the St. George's hospital group, who demonstrated identical DNA restriction digests between these groups of organisms.[221]

Gitnick and coauthors report the recovery of fastidious mycobacteria, including *M. paratuberculosis*, from 5 of 82 surgically resected intestinal specimens from patients, 27 of whom had Crohn's disease.[106] These isolates required between 4 and 8 months for cultivation, which may be one reason why this organism has not been recovered in clinical laboratories. Prantera and coworkers provided indirect evidence of the association of Crohn's disease with *M. paratuberculosis* by demonstrating high serum levels of antimycobacterial antibody that was demonstrated in patients following successful dapsone therapy, a phenomenon similar to that observed after treatment of classic cases of tuberculosis.[268] With PCR and a portion of the *M. paratuberculosis* insertion sequence *IS900* as a probe, Sanderson and associates were able to identify *M. paratuberculosis* DNA in 65% of rectal biopsy specimens in patients with Crohn's disease, in comparison with only 4.3% and 12.5% of patients with ulcerative colitis and healthy persons, respectively.[302] Similarly, Fidler and colleagues found that the material obtained from granulomata of Crohn's disease tissues (31 biopsy samples in the study) were much more likely to amplify *M. paratuberculosis*–specific DNA on PCR than non–Crohn's disease tissues (10 biopsies of ulcerative colitis as negative controls).[92] If indeed mycobacteria are the cause of intestinal diseases, new methods for prevention and treatment of these conditions, notably Crohn's disease, may be in order. The association has not been proved by Koch's postulates (see Cocito and coauthors for a commentary on paratuberculosis[51]).

Mycobacterium terrae, M. gastri, and M. triviale. These mycobacteria are also slow-growing nonphotochromogenic bacteria that, in the past, have not generally been known as pathogens but are rarely encountered in the clinical laboratory. They can be differentiated by the characteristics listed in Table 19-7. *M. triviale* colonies may resemble those of MAI complex and in some instances may be so rough that they are confused with tubercle bacilli; however, these strains are niacin-negative and can grow in media containing 5% NaCl. *M. triviale* also hydrolyzes Tween 80 within 5 days, whereas the MAI complex organisms are Tween-negative. *M. gastri* and *M. terrae* are other nonphotochromogenic species that may require biochemical differentiation (see Table 19-7). *M. terrae* is also known as the "radish bacillus," since it was initially recovered from radish washings. Colonies of *M. terrae* tend to be smoother than the rough colonies of *M. triviale*.

Mycobacterium shimoidei. *M. shimoidei* has been proposed for an *M. terrae*–like organism recovered on multiple occasions over an 11-year period from a 56-year-old resident of Japan who had tuberculosis-like pulmonary disease.[375] In 1988, Imaeda and coworkers, based on DNA homology studies, officially established *M. shimoidei* as a distinct species.[148] It differs phenotypically from members of the *M. terrae* complex by negative catalase and positive beta-galactosidase reactions, and from *M. malmoense* by a positive acid phosphatase reaction. Because beta-galactosidase and acid phosphatase reactions are rarely performed in clinical laboratories, species identification based on phenotypic properties may be difficult to establish.

Additional clinical cases of infections caused by *M. shimoidei* have been reported since the report of the index case. This organism has been reported as the cause of pulmonary infections in patients living in Australia and in Germany, the latter case complicating long-standing silicosis.[129,376] Initial therapy with isoniazid, propionamide, and rifampin failed because the organism was both isoniazid- and rifampin-resistant; a cure was effected with a 14-day course of streptomycin and isoniazid. Therefore, when a *Mycobacterium* species phenotypically similar to *M. terrae* complex or *M. malmoense* is recovered from respiratory specimens obtained from patients with pulmonary infections, *M. shimoidei* should be considered, and a species identification should be attempted.

Mycobacterium malmoense. In 1977, Schroder and Juhlin recovered a new *Mycobacterium* species from four patients with pulmonary disease.[308] They called the organism *Mycobacterium malmoense*, after the Swedish city Malmo, in which these patients lived. The disease has also been noted to occur in Scotland.[96] The recovery of isolates has been reported from the United States: 12 strains by Good and associates in 1980,[110] and more recently, from four patients with chronic lung disease by Albers and coworkers,[6] in two of whom progressive disease developed.

Laboratory Aspects This organism typically grows slowly, some strains are seen as soon as 2 to 3 weeks of incubation at 37°C; however, some strains may require as long as 12 weeks before colonies become visible. This need for prolonged incubation, beyond a period used in most clinical laboratories, may lead to underdiagnosis. Typical colonies of *M. malmoense* are grayish white, smooth, glistening, opaque, and domed. They are colorless, and exposure to light does not produce pigment. On acid-fast smears, the organisms appear coccoid or as short rods without cross-bands.

CLINICAL CORRELATION BOX 19-11
Mycobacterium terrae and *Mycobacterium triviale*

M. terrae and *M. triviale*, although previously considered together in a complex, may also be considered separately. These mycobacteria have been incriminated in several cases of human infections, as cited by Woods and Washington: septic arthritis caused by *M. triviale* in an infant, synovitis and osteomyelitis caused by *M. terrae* in a young man with Fanconi's pancytopenia, and possible disseminated *M. terrae* infection in a young woman with previous miliary tuberculosis.[399] Several cases of pulmonary infection with *M. terrae* have been reported.[191,347] Krishner and coauthors report one case and cite six previous cases of respiratory infection.[187] Peters and Morice report a case of pulmonary *M. terrae* infection in a 64-year-old woman with ovarian carcinoma, presenting as caseating miliary infiltrates on chest radiographs and accompanied by a rash on the extremities.[256] The lung and skin lesions resolved after 6 weeks of therapy with isoniazid, rifampin, and pyrazinamide, despite "resistance" of these drugs, as determined by *in vitro* susceptibility testing. Petrini and coworkers report a case of *M. terrae* tenosynovitis of the hand.[120,261] Both the tendon and tendon sheaths were swollen and chronic inflammation, granuloma formation, and necrosis were seen histologically. A case of tenosynovitis of the finger was reported in a middle-aged fisherman who incurred puncture wounds while handling Crappie fins.[186]

CLINICAL CORRELATION BOX 19-12
Mycobacterium malmoense

In the past decade, *M. malmoense* has been reported with increasing frequency as a pulmonary pathogen. More than 180 cases have been reported, most affecting patients with previous lung diseases, often middle-aged men with pneumoconioses.[410] Roentgenograms typically show a picture indistinguishable from *M. tuberculosis*. Jenkins and Tsukamura[157] describe two cases of cervical adenitis, whereas Warren and associates[371] present a patient in the United States with chronic pulmonary disease. Albers and coworkers believe that *M. malmoense* infections may be more common in the United States than suspected and is underreported, as some strains require 8 to 12 weeks or more of incubation before visible growth occurs, a period longer than cultures are held in most laboratories.[6] Growth is significantly more rapid in specimens grown in BACTEC broth vials compared with delayed growth on Löwenstein-Jensen medium.[109] A broth culture medium should be used in parallel to improve the yield of particularly slow-growing strains.[138] Additional case reports include lymphadenitis in a 5-year-old girl, septic cutaneous infection in a patient with hairy-cell leukemia, and several cases of infection in HIV-positive patients.[37,49,60,264,389,407] In one case, the infection was successfully treated with ethambutol, cycloserine, and isoniazid, despite multiresistance in in vitro susceptibility tests.[37] The lack of a clear correlation between in vitro susceptibility tests and clinical response was reported over a decade ago.[15] In the experience of these authors, omission of ethambutol from the therapeutic regimen, even if it showed resistance in in vitro studies, led to an unsatisfactory response.

CLINICAL CORRELATION BOX 19-13
Mycobacterium haemophilum

Painful subcutaneous nodules, swellings, and ulcers that can progress into abscesses and draining fistulas are common clinical presentations of *M. haemophilum*. Rogers and coworkers report cases of disseminated disease in patients with AIDS, in whom the skin lesions were multiple, involving the upper arm, hands, and feet (refer to this paper for excellent color photographs of these lesions).[290] In a study of 13 patients with *M. haemophilum* infections culled from seven metropolitan hospitals in New York, clinical manifestations included disseminated cutaneous lesions, bacteremia, and diseases of the bones and joints, lymphatics, and lungs.[338] The authors of this study stress that improper culture techniques may delay or even miss making a laboratory diagnosis, and that infections may be more common than realized.

Additional cases in patients with AIDS have been reported. These include isolation from the wrist and ankle at sites of severe tenosynovitis, and recovery from a cutaneous lesion, lymph node, and eye of a male patient that represented the first reported case of *M. haemophilum* infection in Canada (a second case of lymphadenitis in a 3-year-old Canadian girl was also included in this report).[213,345] Patients with lymphopenia are at particularly high risk for infections; renal dialysis and corticosteroid therapy have been shown to be predisposing conditions of *M. haemophilum* infection.[113,237]

Key biochemical test reactions for *Mycobacterium malmoense* include the following:

1. No accumulation of niacin.
2. Nitrate is not reduced to nitrite.
3. Tween 80 is hydrolyzed.
4. Catalase is produced at 68°C.
5. Pyrazinamidase is positive.

Most strains are resistant to isoniazid, streptomycin, *p*-aminosalicylic acid, and rifampin but are susceptible to ethambutol (1 g/mL) and cycloserine (16 g/mL).

Mycobacterium haemophilum. Sompolinsky and associates first recovered *M. haemophilum* in 1978 from a subcutaneous lesion of an Israeli patient with Hodgkin's disease.[326] As the species name would indicate, *M. haemophilum* requires hemoglobin or hemin for growth. Chocolate agar, 5% sheep-blood Colombia agar, Mueller-Hinton agar with Fildes supplement, or LJ medium containing 2% ferric ammonium citrate are suitable for recovery of this organism.[399] McBride and associates report success in the recovery of *M. haemophilum* using a medium containing Casman base, 5% heated sheep blood, and crystal violet.[218] Because of the remote chance for recovery of this organism in most laboratories in the United States, use of an X factor strip in the area of

inoculation on 7H10 agar, as suggested by Vadney and Hawkins, offers a suitable alternative in suspected cases.[358]

Most infections involve the skin and underlying tissue, possibly reflecting the propensity of the organism to grow at lower temperature.[188] Gupta and coworkers report a case of osteomyelitis and skin infection in a patient with AIDS, which was successfully treated with minocycline.[120] Kiehn and associates reported four cases in immunocompromised patients, two had AIDS and two were allogeneic bone marrow transplant recipients.[171] Because of the unique requirements for iron and lower temperature for optimal growth, these authors suggest that *M. haemophilum* should be considered when specimens from immunocompromised patients with unexplained illness fail to grow mycobacteria under routine culture conditions or when acid-fast bacilli are seen on smears.

Laboratory Aspects Optimal growth occurs at 28–32°C; some strains grow at 20°C; little or no growth occurs at 37°C. Growth is stimulated by an incubation atmosphere of 10% CO_2. Typical colonies may be rough or smooth after 2 to 4 weeks of incubation at 32°C on egg medium or 7H10 agar (supplemented with hemin or on the surface of which an ''X-strip'' has been placed, as discussed earlier). Pigment does not develop, even after exposure to light. Under the microscope, the cells are short, curved, and strongly acid-fast, without banding or beading. This organism is also biochemically inert, with the production of pyrazinamidase the only positive reaction among the tests commonly used to identify mycobacteria.

RAPID GROWERS

Mycobacterium fortuitum, M. chelonae, *and* M. abscessus.

M. fortuitum was first described in 1938 by daCosta Cruz and was fully categorized in 1955 by Gordon and Smith.[375] This organism was noted to be unique among the known mycobacteria because of its comparatively rapid rate of growth (3 to 5 days). However, in the 1923 edition of *Bergey's Manual*, another rapidly growing organism called *M. chelonae* was described, which had several metabolic characteristics in common with daCosta Cruz's organism. These two organisms are two of the most important, and most commonly recovered, rapidly growing mycobacteria. The third rapidly growing mycobacterium that deserves mention is *M. abscessus*, which may be considered part of the *M. chelonae* complex. It is not difficult to differentiate this organism from *M. chelonae*, which is recommended here, since it may cause severe disease and is highly resistant to antimicrobial therapy.[33,65,303,402] These mycobacteria are ubiquitous land and aquatic organisms that contaminate water supplies, including reagents and wash solutions used in hospitals.

Laboratory Aspects An unknown isolate can be suspected of being a rapidly growing mycobacteria if growth of an acid-fast organism is observed after 2 to 4 days of incubation. However, growth may be delayed in some instances. Mycobacteria are categorized as rapid growers, by definition, if they grow within 7 days after subculture. The young colonies appear smooth and hemispherical, usually with a butyrous or waxy consistency. Colonies are typically nonchromogenic but may appear off-white or faintly cream-colored (see Color Plate 19-2*Q*). *M. fortuitum* may produce branching, filamentous extensions from 1- to 2-day-old colonies on cornmeal-glycerol or Middlebrook 7H11 agar. Some strains produce rougher colonies with short aerial hyphae, best observed under a stereomicroscope. *M. chelonae* lacks these filamentous extensions.

These mycobacteria often have the capability of growing on MacConkey agar without crystal violet. They also appear as smooth, dome-shaped colonies that may have a slight pink pigmentation (see Color Plate 19-2*R*). Growth may also be observed with some strains on routine 5% sheep blood agar, appearing as tiny pinpoint colonies (see Color Plate 19-2*S*). Microbiologists must be alert to this possibility and perform acid-fast stains in addition to Gram stains if the correct identification is to be made.

Microscopically, in acid-fast-stained preparations, the bacterial cells are generally pleomorphic, ranging from long filamentous forms to short, thick rods. Branching is absent or rudimentary; at times the cells may appear beaded or swollen, with nonstaining ovoid bodies present at one end. Some strains of *M. fortuitum* may grow within 48 hours on routine 5% sheep blood agar. The bacterial cells appear as short, slender, filamentous, faintly staining gram-positive bacilli (see Color Plate 19-2*T*).

Silcox and associates have identified the following characteristics for an isolate to belong to the rapidly growing mycobacteria[316]:

1. Acid-fast
2. Lack of pigment production
3. Growth in less than 7 days at its optimal temperature
4. Evidence of arylsulfatase activity at 3 days
5. Growth at 28°C on special MacConkey agar (devoid of crystal violet)

Additional tests for characteristics can be performed to differentiate *M. fortuitum*, *M. chelonae*, and *M. abscessus*:

1. *M. chelonae* and *M. abscessus* do not reduce nitrates (*M. fortuitum* is positive).
2. *M. chelonae* and *M. abscessus* are incapable of assimilating iron from ferric ammonium citrate, a property uniquely possessed by *M. fortuitum* (see Chart 19-10).
3. *M. fortuitum* is susceptible to ciprofloxacin and pipemidic acid but resistant to polymyxin B; *M. chelonae* has the opposite reactions.[332]
4. *M. chelonei* cannot grow on LJ medium containing 5% NaCl at 28°C, but can use citrate, whereas the opposite reactions define *M. abscessus*

Subspecies identification of *M. fortuitum* is possible, but has little clinical relevance; it may, however, be useful for certain epidemiologic applications. *M. fortuitum* exists in three biovariants: biovariant fortuitum, biovariant peregrinum, and an unnamed biovariant designated ''third group.''

M. smegmatis is another rapidly growing mycobacterium closely resembling *M. fortuitum*, differing only in its negative reaction in the 3-day arylsulfatase test, its ability to grow at 45°C, and delayed pigment production after 2 weeks of incubation.[243]

Mycobacterium thermoresistible.
As the species name would indicate, *M. thermoresistible* has the unique ability to grow at 52°C. This organism is potentially pathogenic; however, the infrequency of case reports indicates that exposure is either minimal or the organism is of very low virulence. Weitzman and coauthors reported a case of *M. thermoresistible* human infection in an immunocompromised white female with fever, cough, and weight loss.[380] Cavitary pulmonary disease was seen on radiographs. The organisms were recovered from sputum and a bronchoscopy specimen. Histologic examination of a lung biopsy revealed numerous microabscesses and granulomata with giant cells of the Langhans type, typical for tuberculosis. Wolfe and Moore reported a case of breast infection in a woman following augmentation mammoplasty.[392]

The organism may grow slowly as a scotochromogen on primary isolation medium and may be mistaken for *M. gordonae*. Most strains of *M. gordonae* are urease-negative and do not grow in medium containing 6.5% sodium chloride.

OTHER MYCOBACTERIA

Mycobacterium ulcerans.
Most cases of *M. ulcerans* infections have been reported from Central and West Africa, Malaysia, New Guinea, Guyana, Mexico, and Australia. The name ''Bairnsdale ulcer'' has been used for the cutaneous lesions of *M. ulcerans* infections, named after the Australian town where the organism was first recognized by Alsop and Searls in the 1930s.[272] Most human infections occur in the tropical regions following rain forest disturbance.[131] It is postulated that the mycobacteria are carried from the soil

CLINICAL CORRELATION BOX 19-14 Rapid Growers: *Mycobacterium fortuitum, Mycobacterium chelonae,* **and** *Mycobacterium abscessus*

M. fortuitum, M. chelonae, and *M. abscessus,* the latter of which is in the *M. chelonae* complex, are the most clinically important of the rapidly growing mycobacteria. A wide variety of infections have been associated with these mycobacteria, including infections of the lungs, skin, bone, central nervous system, prosthetic heart valves, and disseminated disease.[316,399] Skin infections are particularly common, often evolving into draining subcutaneous abscesses.[125] Wallace and Brown reviewed 100 isolates of *M. chelonae* from skin, soft tissue, and bone over a 10-year period.[366] Cutaneous infection (53%), localized cellulitis or osteomyelitis (35%), and catheter infections (12%) were most commonly found. Underlying risk factors for infections included organ transplantation, rheumatoid arthritis and other autoimmune disorders, trauma and invasive medical procedures. Previously, Wallace and coworkers had reviewed 125 human infections caused by rapidly growing mycobacteria.[368] Fifty-nine percent of these cases involved the skin (postsurgical wound infections, accidental trauma, and needle injections).

An outbreak on a hospital ward of skin infections caused by *M. fortuitum* from exposure to a contaminated ice machine and contamination of an automated bronchoscope disinfection machine have been reported as other sources of nosocomial infections.[97,197] A clinically distinctive cutaneous syndrome, associated with infections caused by the then *M. chelonae* complex (*M. abscessus* was not routinely distinguished from *M. chelonae* at that time) in kidney-transplant recipients, consisting of indolent, tender, nodular lesions, on the extremities has been reported.[58] Sporotrichoid spread of these infections may occur in immunosuppressed patients, and, rarely, cutaneous infections with rapidly growing mycobacteria may represent the extension of disseminated disease.[79,238]

Several other clinical entities caused by rapidly growing mycobacteria have been reported. Several cases of keratitis have been reported both in wearers of both soft and hard contact lens.[31,168] Most infections follow trauma, and topical antibiotic therapy is often not successful; therefore, keratoplasty is often required to effect a cure. It is recommended that acid-fast smears of corneal scrapings be performed on any patient with chronic corneal ulcers.[283] Patients receiving continuous ambulatory peritoneal dialysis are also at risk for acquiring peritonitis caused by rapidly growing mycobacteria.[47,84,182,224,327] The collective recommendations are that mycobacterial cultures be performed on patients with peritonitis associated with continuous ambulatory peritoneal dialysis when routine cultures fail to reveal organisms. Rapidly growing mycobacteria should be considered when examining culture plates and Gram stains prepared from isolates recovered from peritoneal or dialysis fluids that have the appearance of poorly characterized diphtheroids. Removal of the catheter, drainage of fluid collections, and appropriate use of antimicrobial agents usually results in rapid cure.

Any of these organism are important causes of pulmonary infections, but infections with *M. abscessus* may be particularly serious.[369] Rapidly growing mycobacteria are ubiquitous in many water sources and may colonize the respiratory tract of patients who have compromised local defense mechanisms or who are debilitated or immunocompromised or who have long-standing chronic obstructive pulmonary disease. Invasive respiratory tract procedures also put patients at risk for infection with *M. abscessus.* Burns and associates studied an outbreak of positive *M. fortuitum* sputum cultures among 16 patients being treated on an alcoholism rehabilitation ward.[34] Pulsed-field electrophoresis of large genomic DNA restriction enzyme fragments disclosed that the 16 isolates were identical. The point source was found to be a tap connected to the water line supplying the showers being used by these patients; no further cases occurred after the showers were disconnected and decontaminated.

Several cases of catheter infections caused by rapidly growing mycobacteria have been reported. Raad and coworkers reviewed 15 infected cancer patients at M.D. Anderson Cancer Center, 9 caused by *M. fortuitum* and 6 by *M. chelonae.*[271] Four patients with bacteremia and associated catheter infections recovered after removal of the catheter and prompt institution of antibiotic therapy. Bacteremia recurred in seven patients in whom the catheter was left in place and who were treated with antibiotics alone. Patients with infections of the catheter tunnel required surgery for cure. Three cases of *M. chelonae* infections were reported in febrile patients with neutropenia, which they consider a distinct risk factor for developing progressive and disseminated disease.[222]

Miscellaneous infections caused by the rapidly growing mycobacteria include an outbreak of *M. chelonae* otitis media in an office clinic setting, where transfer occurred between patients from contaminated instruments, aortitis following aortic-valve replacement, and sternal wound infection with *M. fortuitum; M. fortuitum* endocarditis in a 54-year-old woman with chronic renal failure receiving hemodialysis;, a series of cardiac bypass-related infections; rare cases of hepatitis and synovitis; a retroperitoneal abscess infected with *M. chelonae* complicating a gunshot wound to the flank; and a case of disseminated *M. fortuitum* infection in a patient with AIDS.[146,210,289,307,318,380,399] Two cases of *M. smegmatis* posttraumatic soft-tissue infections were reported in a 21-year-old man and a 29-year-old woman who were involved in separate motor vehicle accidents.[243] The former patient presented with a draining left leg lesion and inguinal adenopathy and the latter with a chronically draining subcutaneous area of cellulitis of the posterolateral thigh. The authors also cite 12 cases of *M. smegmatis* infections reported in the literature, dispelling some doubt that this organism is nonpathogenic. Newton and Weiss subsequently reported a case of aspiration pneumonia caused by *M. smegmatis.*[242]

The rapidly growing mycobacteria vary in their *in vitro* susceptibilities.[143] Amikacin is predictably active; other aminoglycosides, cefoxitin, doxycycline, and erythromycin have also been selectively active. Newer agents that have shown *in vitro* activity against some strains include imipenem-cilastatin, amoxicillin-clavulanate, and ciprofloxacin.[307]

Infection presents as a painless "boil" or lump under the skin, which typically develops at the site of previous trauma, and proceeds into a shallow, nonhealing ulcer, with a necrotic base within a few weeks. Some of the lesions studied by Igo and Murthy were quite severe, with avascular coagulation necrosis extending deep into the subcutaneous fat.[147] Satellite nodules that ulcerate may also develop. Successful therapy has been reported with application of local heat, excision, and grafting.[301] Igo and Murthy provide the clinical, histologic, and microbiologic features of 46 cases of *M. ulcerans* infections studied in several villages along the Sepik River in New Guinea.[147] Lesions are usually found on the lower extremities and consist of shallow ulcers that develop in areas of subcutaneous induration at sites of previous trauma. Satellite nodules and superficial ulcers may develop. These are usually nonpainful unless secondarily infected. Delaporte et al. report one of the first cases of *M. ulcerans* infections in a patient with AIDS.[72] The patient was a 30-year-old pregnant Zairian woman, with a chronic, painful, ulcerating lesion of the knee. A superficial punch biopsy grew no organisms; a deeper biopsy of the fascia, however, revealed numerous acid-fast bacilli. The lesion healed with a 2-month regimen of isoniazid, rifampin, and ethambutol. Despite the association of *M. ulcerans* infection and AIDS in this patient, the association is too infrequent to serve as a marker.

into draining lacustrine systems, where they multiply over a period of months or years. Humans become infected by contacting organisms from these contaminated estuaries.

Laboratory Aspects *M. ulcerans* grows optimally at 33°C and not at all at 37°C. Rough, lightly buff or nonpigmented, convex to flat colonies, with irregular outline, often simulating those of *M. tuberculosis*, develop after 6 to 12 weeks. Microscopically the acid-fast cells are moderately long and rod-shaped, without banding or beading. *Mycobacterium ulcerans* is biochemically inert, showing only heat-stable catalase activity among the several tests usually used to identify mycobacteria.

Mycobacterium genavense. *M. genavense* is an uncommonly recovered, slow-growing, nonpigmented, nontuberculous mycobacterium that causes infection in patients with AIDS. The organism was first recognized by Boettger and associates by finding a unique pattern using DNA extracted from mycobacteria growing in BACTEC 13A blood culture media.[28] Amplified gene fragments were sequenced directly, and electrophoretic profiles were determined in 0.8% agarose gel stained with ethidium bromide. The authors studied 16 cases whose organisms had this unique DNA sequence profile and officially designated the organism *M. genavense* after the 28-year-old AIDS patient living in Geneva from whom the first isolate was recovered. Subsequently, Coyle and associates, using assays for sequencing of the gene for 16S rRNA that had been extracted from unidentified mycobacterial isolates of 15 blood cultures obtained from seven patients with AIDS, also confirmed the identity of *M. gena-*

vense as a separate species.[61] The sequence pattern was most closely related to *M. simiae;* however, the clinical presentation, response to therapy, and autopsy manifestations more closely resemble infections with *M. avium* complex.[21] Histopathologically, *M. genavense* in HIV-positive patients produces lesions characterized by masses of foamy histiocytes and ill-defined granulomas, the development of which depends on the immunologic reactivity of the host.[217] In one autopsy series, the small intestine, spleen, liver, and lymph nodes were most commonly involved; the lungs, myocardium, and kidney were spared, a distribution similar to that seen in patients with disseminated disease caused by a member of the MAI complex.

The initial isolates were identified in samples obtained from AIDS patients in Switzerland (thus the species name *genavense*), but disseminated infections caused by *M. genavense* have been described from Europe, North America, and Australia.[28,255] This geographic distribution may reflect more the awareness by health workers of this new species rather than select areas of endemicity. *M. genavense* may be underrecognized because it grows only in broth culture media (such as BACTEC 13A broth, in which it was first discovered) and requires prolonged incubation.[246] Fever, weight loss, diarrhea, hepatosplenomegaly, and anemia are the most common symptoms.

The Detection and Identification of Mycobacteria by Molecular Methods

As indicated by the algorithm presented earlier in this chapter, there is a movement in clinical laboratories away from the time-consuming and tedious task of performing biochemical tests to make a species identification of mycobacteria recovered in culture. More and more often, nonculture methods based on molecular biology are being used in clinical laboratories for the culture confirmation of *Mycobacterium* species isolates recovered in culture. For example, the use of nucleic-acid probe assays has virtually replaced conventional biochemical testing in the identification of *M. tuberculosis* and the MAI complex. Nucleic-acid probes have also been produced for the identification of *M. kansasii* and *M. gordonae*. The usefulness of these probes in the clinical laboratory has been described by several groups.[62,227,282,304,352]

There are four major applications for molecular techniques that are available for use in clinical laboratories:

1. Culture confirmation of isolates recovered from clinical specimens using DNA probes.
2. The identification of mycobacteria through DNA sequencing.
3. The direct detection of *M. tuberculosis* in sputum and other clinical specimens using nucleic-acid amplification assays.
4. DNA fingerprinting and strain-typing of *Mycobacterium* species.

The medical literature relative to molecular diagnostics as applied to the identification of the mycobacteria is vast. It is difficult at this juncture to predict which of the several specific techniques will stand the test of time; therefore, it is equally difficult to determine what references and applications should be included in a general textbook. Although the precise molecular tools used in different mycobacteriology laboratories vary, virtually all modern mycobacteriology laboratories use molecular diagnostics to some extent. The standard for using molecular diagnostics are being determined. Regardless of the use of these technologies in the future, there remains a need for continued expertise with the conventional techniques that are still used in most clinical laboratories. Study of these techniques also provides a fundamental understanding of the basic biology of mycobacteria and helps to determine the best role for newer techniques when they are introduced into the clinical laboratory. The detection and characterization of mycobacteria by molecular methods may be separated into non-amplification- and amplification-based methods. After amplification, the product(s) of amplification may be analyzed by DNA sequencing to acquire identification information or by other techniques or typing. The salient features of these applications are described below.

Signal-Amplification Methods
NUCLEIC-ACID PROBES

Nucleic-acid probes were the first nucleic acid–based technology to be used routinely in the clinical microbiology laboratory for the identification of mycobacteria in positive cultures. These probes, which are initially radiolabeled, but are now nonisotopic, were pioneered and brought to market by Gen-Probe (San Diego, CA). The accuracy, sensitivity, and specificity of these probes is very high when used to identify mycobacteria in culture, according to the manufacturer's instructions, and has been authenticated in several studies.[80,112,169,199,227,240,304] Nucleic-acid probes are available for the identification of organisms in the *M. tuberculosis* complex, the *M. avium/M. intracellulare* complex, *M. kansasii*, and *M. gordonae*. Separate probes are also available for *M. avium* and *M. intracellulare* if the differentiation of these mycobacteria is desired.

In brief, this technology uses acridine ester-labeled single-stranded DNA probes that hybridize with the recombinant RNA (rRNA), which is released from the test bacterium through the action of a lysing agent, heat, and sonication. Ribosomal rRNA is a useful genetic target for the identification of microorganisms, since it often contains signature sequences and is present in the cells and culture in high quantities secondary to the growth of the organism (biologic amplification). The DNA probe and rRNA hybridize according to traditional Watson and Crick base pairing for a stable DNA:RNA complex.[288] After the inactivation of the unhybridized probe, a signal-generating step is performed and light is produced and recorded by an instrument. The light produced is proportional to the amount of probe present, and a predetermined threshold is used to determine positivity. The 2 hours required for the probe-based determination of the species for which genetic probes are available represents a significant advance compared with identification by traditional methods.[227,304] Probe-negative isolates still require identification using phenotypic methods for laboratories that do not use DNA sequencing, but this represents a distinct minority of isolates, usually <10%. The commercial kits

have an extended shelf-life, which also extends the usefulness to a large number of laboratories. See Chart 19-17 for a detailed description of this procedure.

One advantage recognized early was the use of these probes on positive broth cultures, which recover mycobacteria more rapidly than solid media in most instances. Because recovery of mycobacteria in culture requires 2 to 3 weeks, several studies indicated that probe assays could be performed on organisms recovered in broth culture, specifically in BACTEC bottles.[87,258] The technique involves aspirating 1.0 to 1.3 mL of fluid from a blood culture vial after a growth index of at least 100 is reached (GI = 999 achieves the highest level of sensitivity). The broth culture aliquot is placed into a 1.5-mL, screw-cap tube and placed into a microcentrifuge. Centrifugation at 9,000 g for 5 to 7 minutes is used to concentrate the bacteria. After discarding the supernatant, the pellet is suspended in a sonication-lysate reagent, and the procedure is completed as previously described in this chapter. Kiehn and Edwards combined the BACTEC TB system with the nucleic-acid probe targeted to the rRNA of *M. avium* to rapidly identify this species when recovered from blood cultures of patients with AIDS.[169] In a study conducted by Ellner and associates, the combination of BACTEC recovery and DNA probe assay identified 89% of 176 isolates of *M. tuberculosis* and 89% of 110 isolates of *M. avium*.[87] Most impressive was the reduction, by 5 to 7 weeks, of the time to final report compared with their conventional isolation and biochemical methods. Similarly, the rapid identification of *M. tuberculosis* was made with the BACTEC TB-DNA probe combination in 83% of 64 cases, and in 92% of *M. avium* and 86% of *M. intracellulare* isolates.[258]

In a study of 359 acid-fast-positive isolates in BACTEC 12 vials, the following percentages of organisms were identified on initial direct screening of centrifuged pellets with species-specific nonisotopic, chemiluminescent AccuProbes (Gen-Probe): *M. tuberculosis* complex, 87.2%; *M. avium* complex, 78.6%; *M. kansasii*, 91.7%; and *M. gordonae*, 85.9%.[281] The authors concluded that the lower percentage detection, when compared with previous studies, resulted in part from the centrifugal force used (3,000 g, rather than 9,000 to 10,000 g). When high-speed centrifuges are not available, extending the centrifugation time to 30 minutes may improve performance. In a similar effort to decrease the time of detection even further, Forbes and coworkers applied PCR amplification to detect *M. tuberculosis* recovered in BACTEC 12B broth cultures.[94] By using PCR, positive BACTEC 12B vials could be assayed when the GI reached 10, shortening the time of incubation required for the GI to reach 100 or more. The use of PCR in this study resulted in a mean time to detection of *M. tuberculosis* of 9 days, compared with 14 days using nucleic-acid probes from growth of BACTEC 12B subcultures on solid media. Kaminski and Hardy suggest that the observation of cord formation in acid-fast stains performed on positive BACTEC 12B bottles can be used as a guide to immediately select the *M. tuberculosis* probe assay.[165]

IN SITU HYBRIDIZATION

In situ hybridization is a molecular diagnostic tool that has been used for years in anatomic pathology, but has made little impact in clinical microbiology. This technology uses an oligonucleotide probe labeled with a detector molecule. If the detector molecule is fluorescein and interpretation is made by direct observation using a fluorescence microscopy, it is referred to as fluorescence *in situ* hybridization (FISH). If, however, detection of the hybridized probe is achieved through secondary reaction and color, rather than light produced, the reaction is termed chromogenic *in situ* hybridization (CISH). Both FISH and CISH reactions have been used by several investigators for the detection of infectious agents. More recently, FISH has been used to identify bacterial and yeast pathogens in positive blood cultures. This technology has been used to identify *M. tuberculosis* in cultures that become positive and in direct respiratory specimens that contain acid-fast bacilli. This technology has been used by pathologists to identify mycobacteria in formalin-fixed, paraffin-embedded tissues and to confirm the identity of *M. leprae*. Unfortunately, commercial kits are not available for mycobacteria, but may become available, as kits for *S. aureus* and *C. albicans* are commercially available.

Nucleic-Acid Amplification Methods
COMMERCIALLY AVAILABLE APPLICATIONS

The burden of organisms in rare instances is large enough in the clinical specimen to achieve detection with a chemiluminescent genetic probe. However, in most instances this method is too insensitive for direct use on clinical specimens.[43] A nucleic-acid-amplification–based assay is recommended if identification of mycobacteria is to be attempted directly from the clinical specimens. In the late 1990s two commercially available nucleic-acid amplification assays for the detection of *M. tuberculosis* received approval by the FDA for use on respiratory specimens. These tests, the Amplicor *M. tuberculosis* PCR assay (Roche Diagnostics, Indianapolis, IN) and the Amplified *Mycobacterium tuberculosis* Direct test (AMTD), which uses transcription-mediated amplification, have both been approved for use with smear-positive specimens, whereas only the latter has been approved for use on smear-negative respiratory specimens. This is the culmination of several developmental studies and field trials over several years, leading to products that are standardized and designed in such a way that problems of contamination with extraneous DNA and inhibition of amplification reactions by endogenous inhibitors are minimized. Nucleic-acid amplification assays perform well on smear-positive specimens, but suboptimally on smear-negative respiratory specimens, when compared with culture.[73,250,299]

It is beyond the scope of this textbook to review all the published works of other researchers in the evolution of AMTD and PCR applications to direct testing of specimens for mycobacteria, but there are many.[27,229,263] Several of the important studies for each of these FDA-approved technologies are described.

One of the early field trial studies of the Gen-Probe AMTD test (GenProbe, Inc., San Diego, CA) was published by Jonas and coauthors in 1993.[161] In a study of 758 processed sputum sediments, 119 (16%) of which were positive for *M. tuberculosis*, the Gen-Probe assay performed with a sensitivity, specificity, positive and negative predictive value of 82%, 99%, 97%, and 96%, respectively, which were comparable with the results derived from culture and better than from smear analysis.

Miller and coworkers performed a retrospective evaluation of three separate respiratory specimens from each of 250 patients using the AMTD, comparing the results with those of microscopy, culture, and patient chart review.[229] Of these patients, 198 (from whom 594 specimens were collected) were negative for *M. tuberculosis* by culture and clinical criteria and 52 were positive (156 specimens). The overall specificity of the AMTD was 98.5%. Of the 156 specimens obtained from the patients with tuberculosis, organisms were recovered from 142 (91%), acid-fast microscopy was positive for 105 (67.3%), and the AMTD was positive for 142 (91%). When all three specimens from each patient were tested, AMTD found all 52 patients positive for tuberculosis.

In a study of 938 respiratory specimens, Pfyffer and associates found that the AMTD test performed with a sensitivity of 93.9%, a specificity of 97.6%, a positive predictive value of 80.7%, and a negative predictive value of 99.3% after resolution of discrepant results by chart review.[263] These authors conclude that the AMTD is highly sensitive and specific for detecting *M. tuberculosis* complex organisms within a few hours. The results of another study, however, were less encouraging.[27] Of 617 respiratory tract specimens, 590 were culture- and AMTD-negative. Twenty-one cultures (3.4%) yielded *M. tuberculosis*; of these, 15 (71.4%) were detected by AMTD and 6 were missed. *M. tuberculosis* did not grow in culture from six AMTD-positive specimens (28.6%) obtained from three patients under treatment for tuberculosis. Thus, the sensitivity, specificity, and negative and positive predictive values for AMTD were 71.4%, 99%, 99%, and 71.4%, respectively. The test was judged to be easy to perform and highly specific by these authors, but lacking in sensitivity. They suggested that inclusion of an internal amplification control may be helpful.

Vuorinen and associates conducted studies that compared the performance of the Gen-Probe product with the Roche Amplicor *M. tuberculosis* Test (Roche Molecular Diagnostics, Indianapolis, IN), prior to FDA approval of the latter assay in the United States.[365] These authors tested 256 respiratory specimens obtained from 243 patients for the presence of *M. tuberculosis* complex with both the AMTD and PCR Roche Amplicor *Mycobacterium tuberculosis* Test (Amplicor PCR). When compared with the results of culture performed in parallel, the sensitivities of staining, AMTD and Amplicor PCR were 80.8%, 84.6%, and 84.6%, respectively. The specificities for these three tests were 99.1%, 98.7%, and 99.1%, respectively. The conclusions of these authors were that both nucleic-acid amplification methods were rapid, sensitive, and specific for the detection of *M. tuberculosis* in respiratory specimens.

The following are brief summaries of a few other studies of the PCR Roche Amplicor *Mycobacterium tuberculosis* Test. Ichiyama and associates, in a parallel study of 422 sputum samples obtained from 170 patients with mycobacterial infections, also found that the AMTD system and the Amplicor *Mycobacterium* system performed equally well, with 98.7% agreement.[145] D'Amato and colleagues tested the Roche Amplicor test on 985 specimens from 372 patients.[68] The sensitivity, specificity, and positive and negative predictive values compared with culture and clinical diagnosis were 66.7%, 99.6%, 91.7%, and 97.7%, respectively, comparable with culture results. The authors cite the great advantage of having test results available approximately 6.5 hours after the specimen arrives in the laboratory. Wobeser and coworkers found that the Amplicor PCR assay performed with sensitivity, specificity, positive and negative predictive values of 79%, 99%, 93%, and 98%, respectively, in a study of 1480 clinical specimens obtained from 1,155 patients.[391] In smear-positive specimens, the sensitivity was 98%, versus 59% for smear-negative specimens. The sensitivity and specificity of specimens demonstrating a positive growth index on the BACTEC 460 system were 98% and 100%, respectively. Delacourt and associates, in a study of 68 children with various stages of tuberculosis, found that PCR was positive in 83.3% of 199 specimens obtained from children with active disease, but also in 38.9% of children without symptoms.[71] The latter group may require renewal or continuation of therapy.

Two additional amplification assays for *M. tuberculosis* are available for use outside the United States; these have not been FDA-approved. They are the *M. tuberculosis* BD ProbeTec (BD Diagnostic) assay, which uses strand-displacement amplification, and the Abbott LCx *M. tuberculosis* assay (LCR; Abbott Laboratories, Chicago, IL), which uses the ligase chain reaction. The BD ProbeTec *M. tuberculosis* assay, which is not available in the United States has been used to study direct respiratory specimens, as well as positive cultures.[16,370] Barrett et al. studied the direct respiratory specimens of 205 patients who had a high probability of having tuberculosis. Of the 109 patients with culture-proven tuberculosis, 101 were positive by the BD ProbeTec assay, yielding a sensitivity of 92.7%.[16] There were three false-positive reactions reported in this study from patients with nontuberculous mycobacteria, giving a specificity of 96%. The studies using the Abbott LCx *M. tuberculosis* assay also demonstrated excellent sensitivities and specificities.[89,200,205,235] Lindbrathen and associates,[205] in a large study in Norway, examined 482 specimens from 457 patients with the Abbott LCx *M. tuberculosis* assay, and demonstrated a sensitivity of 90.2% and a specificity of 99.2%.

The use of commercial products does not preclude users from encountering problems in implementation and use of the test. Laboratory directors and supervisors who elect to implement one of these tests for the direct detection of mycobacteria in clinical specimens must ensure that the manufacturer's recommendations are closely followed and that quality-control standards are rigidly enforced. These tests are not yet a replacement for culture. There are still instances in which *M. tuberculosis* is recovered from culture but not detected by molecular methods. Furthermore, complete molecular profiling for all the determinants of resistance is not yet available, so routine susceptibility testing must be performed. Routine recovery methods must be run in parallel for each specimen received, and the clinical aspects of each case must be closely monitored, and communication between the laboratory and primary care physicians must be maintained throughout. With all of these provisions in place, the ability to diagnose new cases of tuberculosis early will have a major impact on therapy and infection control, with the prevention of human-to-human transfer of disease.

HOME-BREW PCR ASSAYS, INCLUDING REAL-TIME PCR

In addition to FDA-approved assays, numerous "home-brew" PCR, and more recently real-time PCR, assays have been developed and tested.[247] These applications, although not approved for use by the FDA, may be important diagnostic tools in the hands of the skilled user. The potential for shortening to hours, rather than days and weeks, the detection and identification of *Mycobacterium* species directly in a variety of clinical specimens makes these assays attractive. The cost of home-brew PCR is often considerably less than comparable commercially available products, but the appropriate validation of the assay resides with the user of the test. Those working in molecular diagnostics have an interesting and bright future and the day may well come when the tedious and often marginally accurate species identifications as described previously in some detail in this chapter will be relegated to the dust bins of antiquity.

Nolte et al. developed one of the earliest PCR assays for the rapid diagnosis of pulmonary tuberculosis; in this paper they described important background information that would be of interest to those who wish to learn more about developing and setting up a PCR assay.[247] Some of the potential problems that must be addressed with nucleic-acid-based amplification assays are inhibition of amplification and reproducibility of the assay. These were addressed in a multilaboratory study reported by Noordhoek and coauthors.[248] They circulated 200 sputum, saliva, and water samples containing known numbers of *M. bovis* BCG cells along with negative controls for PCR analysis, among seven laboratories that used the IS*6110* insertion sequence as the target for DNA amplification. Each laboratory used its own protocol for pretreatment, DNA extraction, and detection of the amplification product. High levels of false-positive PCR results were found among the participating laboratories, ranging from 3% to 20% (with an extreme of 77% in one laboratory). This relatively poor performance resulted from lack of monitoring of each step of the procedure and underscores the necessity for careful quality control during all stages of the assay. In addition, inhibition of amplification and the erroneous reporting of false-negative results may be a problem with PCR. For this reason, the use of an internal amplification control, or the documentation and monitoring of the false-negative rate of an assay, is required for laboratory accreditation by the College of American Pathologists for laboratories that use these tests.

Real-time nucleic-acid amplification is a more rapid method of performing PCR or other methods of amplification, wherein amplification and detection occur in the same reaction vessel. This vessel is closed, which significantly decreases the chance of amplicon contamination of the laboratory. Several assays have been designed for the rapid detection of *M. tuberculosis*, using most of the available formats.

Several assays have been described using the LightCycler system (Roche Diagnostics, Indianapolis, IN). Some of these are specific for *M. tuberculosis* using a single set of fluorescence resonance energy transfer (FRET) probes.[185,228] Miller et al. examined 135 AFB-positive specimens, of which 105 grew *M. tuberculosis*. Both the LightCycler assay and the Amplicor *M. tuberculosis* PCR test to which it was compared detected 103 of 105, yielding a sensitivity of

98.1%, each. They also studied 232 BacT/Alert MP culture bottles of respiratory specimens, 114 of which were positive for *M. tuberculosis*. All the positive cultures were detected by the LightCycler assay.[228]

Shrestha et al. took another approach and designed a broad-range PCR to detect all mycobacteria, but to differentiate *M. tuberculosis* from nontuberculous mycobacteria based on postamplification melt-curve analysis.[315] After amplification is complete, melt curves may be generated with some types of real-time amplification assays. Assays that use FRET probes produce very distinct melt curves that distinguish even a single nucleotide difference in the probe hybridization sites. Shrestha et al. used this feature to differentiate *M. tuberculosis* from nontuberculosis using both 186 cultured isolates and 50 clinical specimens that were culture positive for *M. tuberculosis*. Both the LightCycler assay and the Amplicor *M. tuberculosis* PCR test to which it was compared detected 48 of 50 specimens.

The results of real-time PCR assays are innately quantitative, and when used with standards the definitive amount of an organism present may be determined. Kramme and associates describe a real-time PCR assay, wherein not only the presence of the organism is detected, but an indication of the amount of organism present could be determined.[183] Similarly, Rondini et al. have developed a TaqMan-based assay for the detection of another important cutaneous mycobacterial pathogen, *M. ulcerans*.[293]

Postamplification Analysis
REVERSE HYBRIDIZATION

Reverse hybridization is similar in many ways to the traditional Southern blot, wherein the amplicon-probe hybridization reaction occurs on a nitrocellulose or similar substrate. In this technology, the multiple probes are immobilized on a nitrocellulose strip, and the amplicon is applied to the strip, which is the reverse of a Southern blot. Lines or dots form at the site of amplicon-probe hybridization. When this pattern is compared with a key, one can interpret the results of this reaction (Fig. 19-3). The advantage over traditional Southern blotting is that numerous probes are assayed simultaneously and radioisotopes are not used.

Reverse-hybridization technology is commercially available as line probe assays (LiPA) (Innogenetics, Gent, Belgium, and Bayer Diagnostics, Tarrytown) or reverse dot blot strips (Roche). In addition to assays for HCV genotyping, HIV genotyping for mutations associated with resistance to antiretroviral agents, subtyping human papillomavirus (HPV), and the detection of pathogenic fungi, an assay is available for the rapid identification of mycobacteria. The first-version reverse-hybridization assay examined was the LiPA Mycobacteria assay (Innogenetics). This assay used a broad-range PCR directed against the 16S to 23S spacer region and probes for *M. tuberculosis* complex, MAI complex, and the following mycobacterial species: *M. avium, M. intracellulare, M. kansasii, M. chelonae* group, *M. gordonae, M. xenopi,* and *M. scrofulaceum*.[230] Miller et al. studied 60 clinical isolates of mycobacteria from 59 patients using this product and found no discrepancies with routine laboratory identification with the majority of the isolates, although some were not identified to the species level.[230]

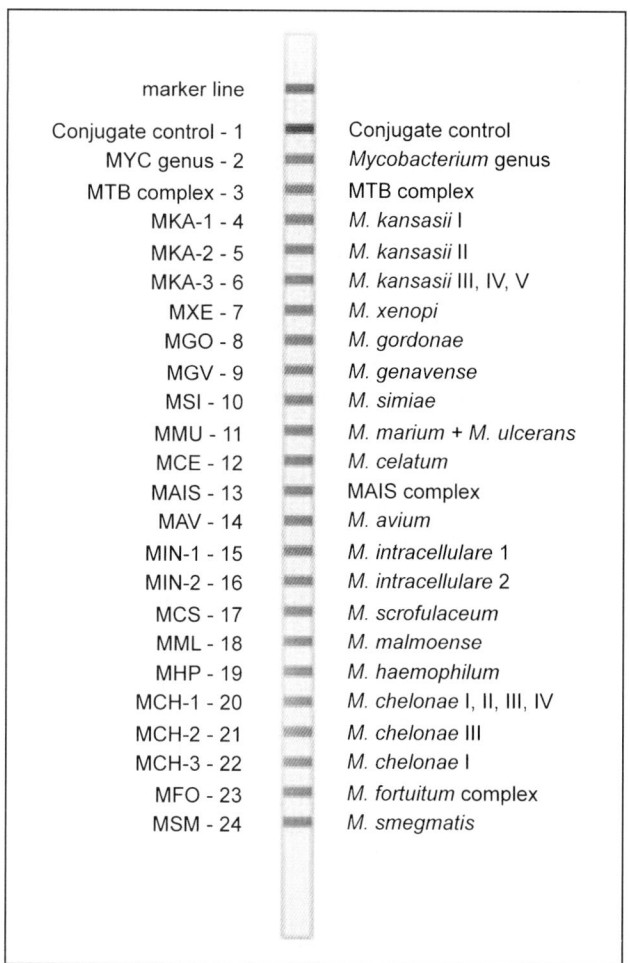

marker line	
Conjugate control - 1	Conjugate control
MYC genus - 2	*Mycobacterium* genus
MTB complex - 3	MTB complex
MKA-1 - 4	*M. kansasii* I
MKA-2 - 5	*M. kansasii* II
MKA-3 - 6	*M. kansasii* III, IV, V
MXE - 7	*M. xenopi*
MGO - 8	*M. gordonae*
MGV - 9	*M. genavense*
MSI - 10	*M. simiae*
MMU - 11	*M. marium + M. ulcerans*
MCE - 12	*M. celatum*
MAIS - 13	MAIS complex
MAV - 14	*M. avium*
MIN-1 - 15	*M. intracellulare* 1
MIN-2 - 16	*M. intracellulare* 2
MCS - 17	*M. scrofulaceum*
MML - 18	*M. malmoense*
MHP - 19	*M. haemophilum*
MCH-1 - 20	*M. chelonae* I, II, III, IV
MCH-2 - 21	*M. chelonae* III
MCH-3 - 22	*M. chelonae* I
MFO - 23	*M. fortuitum* complex
MSM - 24	*M. smegmatis*

Figure 19-3 The INNO-LiPA MYCOBACTERIA V2 (Innogenetics, Gent, Belgium) reverse-hybridization assay is demonstrated. This strip contains a conjugate control line, and hybridization probes to determine the presence of mycobacteria at the genus level and identification information for 16 different species. (The photograph is from the company package insert.)

Of the isolates tested, 26 were *M. tuberculosis* complex, 9 *M. avium*, 3 MAI complex, 3 *M. kansasii*, 4 *M. gordonae*, and 5 *M. chelonae* group isolates. Three patient samples had positive reactions for MAI complex, and were subsequently determined to have *M. intracellulare* by PCR-RFLP analysis. Seven additional mycobacterial species were identified only to the genus level (*Mycobacterium* spp.); six of these were *M. fortuitum*, and one was *M. szulgai*. Several other groups have examined this product with similar results, and during these studies they demonstrated minor problems that led to the development of a new, improved version.[304,339,351] PCR followed by reverse hybridization has also been used on direct clinical specimens, with excellent results from smear-positive specimens.[160] The newer version, the INNO-LiPA Mycobacteria v2, has expanded the number of identifiable mycobacterial species to 16. Tortoli et al. tested 197 mycobacteria belonging to 81 taxa with this product and found 100% specificity and sensitivity for 20 out of 23 probes.

The probes specific for *M. fortuitum* complex, for the MAI-scrofulaceum group, and for *M. intracellulare* type 2 demonstrated cross reactivity with several mycobacteria that are rarely isolated from clinical specimens. The overall sensitivity was 100%, and the overall specificity was 94.4%.[350]

Reverse-hybridization assays have also been shown to be useful for the detection of the genetic determinants of rifampin resistance.[4,40,70,159,314,325] As with species identification, detection of the genetic determinants of resistance has also been achieved directly from the clinical specimen.[159] In contrast to DNA sequencing described below, the LiPA is technically much easier to perform than DNA sequencing, with simpler postanalytic analysis.

DNA SEQUENCING

DNA sequencing for the analysis of an amplified product is now a common method of postamplification analysis. Although useful, this technology is more complicated than simple probe hybridization and often requires the user to have experience with sequence alignment and editing software, and genetic databases. Analysis of these variable regions interspersed between conserved regions that serve as broad-range primer hybridization sites becomes a powerful tool for microorganism identification.[30,101,108,114,194,208,275,309,363,382,400]

Traditional DNA sequencing, also known as Sanger sequencing, was once used solely in research laboratories, but it has also become commonplace in many molecular pathology and molecular microbiology laboratories (See the "DNA Sequencing" section in Chapter 4). These methods have been used successfully for the identification of bacteria, mycobacteria, nocardia, and fungi. The genes that encode for the ribosomal subunits of these organisms are the most commonly used genetic targets of sequence-based identification.

This technology is revolutionizing the laboratory identification of slow-growing microorganisms such as mycobacteria and nocardia.[50,122,167,223,254,260] One of the most useful regions of the 16S gene complex for the identification of mycobacteria involves the hypervariable A region. This has been used to achieve rapid and accurate sequenced-based identification of the most common clinically relevant mycobacteria.[76,123] It has also been used to help identify and differentiate more difficult to characterize isolates.[328] This region has also been used successfully for the identification of most clinically relevant mycobacteria using a newer technology, pyrosequencing or sequencing by synthesis (see Chapter 4).[356]

MicroSeq (Applied Biosystems, Inc. [ABI], Foster City, CA) is a commercially available system for the identification of microorganisms by DNA sequencing. After cultivation, a PCR is performed using the primers provided. The sequence is then determined through ABI capillary-based sequencing and the product is submitted as a query to a genetic database that is maintained and updated by the manufacturer. Hall et al.[122] examined this database using 59 American Type Culture Collection (ATCC) strains and 328 clinical isolates. Sequence-based identification correctly identified, based on what is called a distance score of <1%, 98.3% (58 of 59) of the ATCC strains to the correct group or complex and 90.1% (219 of 243) of the clinical isolates. Of the remaining isolates that had distance scores of >1%, 41.1% (35 of 85) were identified to the appropriate species, complex, or group level, whereas 15.3% (13 of 85) were identified to the species level. Most significantly, they report a turnaround time for mycobacteria identification of less than 24, which is phenomenal when one considers the time to identification of traditional phenotypic methods.

The *rpoB*, *hsp*, and *tuf* genes have also been used successfully as the genetic targets for sequence-based identification for a variety of bacteria.[81,82,95,167,192,251,252,286] The *rpoB* gene, which encodes for DNA-dependent RNA polymerase, has been used by several groups for the identification of mycobacteria.[173,174,201,355] Sequencing this genetic target is popular, since it not only provides identification information, but also provides information regarding the susceptibility of the isolate to rifampin.[325,362]

MICROARRAY ANALYSIS

Microarrays, devices commonly referred to as gene chips, have been used extensively for research. These have also been used for the identification of mycobacteria and the detection of the genetic determinants of resistance. Troesch et al. describe the use of a microarray that examined two genetic regions, the 16S rDNA and the *rpoB* gene.[355] They examined 70 mycobacteria representing 27 different species and 15 rifampin-resistant isolates of *M. tuberculosis* with this microarray and were able to identify 26 of 27 species and all of the resistant mutants. Microarrays hold great promise, but they are expensive, and currently remain a research tool. The precise role these will play in the routine mycobacteriology laboratory has yet to be determined.

Strain Typing and DNA Fingerprinting

The advent of molecular techniques permits strain-specific analysis of *M. tuberculosis* isolates for purposes of epidemiologic studies. The insertion sequence, IS*6110*, was specifically identified as the target of a DNA probe to be used in fingerprint analysis.[38,39] The IS*6110* was conserved in all of the *M. tuberculosis* strains studied and was present in high copy numbers. The specific fingerprint technique described involved digestion of the genomic DNA with the restriction endonuclease *Bam*HI, followed by separation of the fragments by agarose-gel electrophoresis, transferring the DNA fragments to a nylon membrane, and hybridizing the membrane with cloned DNA segments representing two different portions of IS*6110*.

Several workers have used the insertion sequence IS*6110* as the target for conducting epidemiologic studies. Yang and associates compared the fingerprinting patterns of 68 mycobacterial isolates obtained from HIV-seropositive patients with tuberculosis in the Dar es Salaam region of Tanzania, with 66 isolates recovered from HIV-negative patients living in the same region.[405] They observed 101 fingerprint patterns among this group of patients, with the level of diversity equal between the two. Of these isolates, 8.8% showed resistance to at least one drug, again, with no tendency to cluster within either of the groups. In a study of the IS*6110* fingerprint patterns of *M. tuberculosis* recovered from 64 patients living in French Polynesia, 11 separate clusters were identified.[348] Clustering of strains with identical patterns were identified among family groups, indicating that active transmission plays as significant a role as reactivation disease in French Polynesia. Similarly, in a subsequent study, a high degree of likeness was found in IS*6110* fingerprint patterns among closely related individuals.[406] One of the prevalent IS*6110*-defined clusters in Greenland accounted for 91% of 245 cases of tuberculosis in Denmark collected during the same period. These cases were traced to a group of immigrants from Greenland living in a small, defined geographic region in Denmark.

van Soolingen and associates detected 43 different IS*6110* fingerprint patterns of 153 *M. bovis* strains originating from cattle and humans in The Netherlands and Argentina, various animals in Dutch zoos, and in a wild park in Saudi Arabia, and from diseased seals and cats in Argentina.[360] Strains presenting only a single band were characteristic for the strains recovered from cattle. Of the 20 human isolates from Argentina, 18 showed a single band, similar to that seen in the cattle strains, strongly suggesting bovine-to-human transmission. The fingerprint patterns of human *M. bovis* isolates from The Netherlands were diffuse, except for similar patterns in five patients, all living in Amsterdam and three of whom were from the same family. Cave and coworkers found that the IS*6110* fragment-length polymorphism patterns among six *M. bovis* isolates from 1 patient and 42 *M. tuberculosis* repeat isolates from 18 patients remained stable over a period of 8 months to 4.5 years and were not altered by changes in drug-resistance profiles.[38] These studies illustrate the usefulness of restriction endonuclease analyses in epidemiologic studies of human and animal tuberculosis.

Several other DNA repetitive elements have been used as markers by a large number of researchers for the strain typing of *M. tuberculosis* and other *Mycobacterium* species. Space permits coverage of only a few such applications from the plethora of manuscripts that have been published over the past 10 years. Hermans and coworkers discovered a complex-specific mycobacterial DNA insert that hybridized specifically with DNA of *M. tuberculosis* complex strains.[135] A nonrepetitive 158-bp fragment of this sequence was amplified with PCR and used for the selective detection of mycobacteria from the *M. tuberculosis* complex directly in pleural fluid, bronchial washings, and biopsies, to a lower limit of sensitivity of 20 bacterial cells (about 10^3 cells in a sputum sample). Wiid and associates used oligonucleotide GTG5 as a marker for the identification of *M. tuberculosis* strains, which they found useful in cases in which certain *M. tuberculosis* strains have few or no insertion elements such as IS*6110*.[385] Friedman and colleagues used PCR amplification of DNA segments located between two copies of repetitive elements IS*6110* and the polymorphic GC-rich repetitive sequence (PGRS).[99] A PCR-amplified 439-bp segment of the 65-kDa heat-shock protein (HSP) gene was used to develop RFLP patterns of several rapidly growing *Mycobacterium* species, including *M. fortuitum*, *M. chelonae*, *M. smegmatis*, and *M. mucogenicum*.[333] The repetitive insertion sequence element IS*1245* was used in a study of human and animal isolates of *M. avium*.[119] In another study, the repetitive insertion sequences IS*1311* and IS*900* were used as DNA probes in assessing the RFLP of 75 clinical isolates of *M. avium*.[292]

Two markers, one of which encodes for a 40-kDa protein (p40) and the insertion sequence IS*901*-IS*902* have been used as molecular markers in the typing of 184 field strains of the *M. avium* complex.[5]

Pulsed-field electrophoretic separation of restriction fragments generated by digestion of chromosomal DNA was used in the typing of 16 strains of *M. haemophilum*, 12 of which showed similar patterns, including 6 from the same hospital.[403] This technique has also been used to identify several patients who were infected with more than one strain of MAI complex.[320] Random amplified polymorphic DNA (RAPD; also referred to as arbitrary primer PCR) was used in the study of several primers to determine which are most discriminatory in providing reproducible fingerprints in the strain typing of *M. tuberculosis*.[206] This technique has also been used to type 15 strains of *M. tuberculosis*, with a PCR-amplified region separating the genes coding for 16S and 23S rRNA serving as the marker.[1] These authors present molecular typing by RAPD as being more rapid and less technically demanding than most other molecular-typing methods. Also, smaller quantities of purified DNA are required than for other methods, allowing earlier analysis of young primary isolates of *M. tuberculosis*.

Kirschner and colleagues have developed libraries of restriction-fragment profiles of 16S rRNA subunits extracted from several *Mycobacterium* species that were previously characterized by biochemical tests or nucleic-acid probes.[178] The specific restriction endonuclease profile of an unknown *Mycobacterium* species can be easily compared with the library profile, providing a rapid nonculture means for making an accurate identification. Similarly, Avaniss-Aghajani and associates developed a method for identifying mycobacterial isolates directly from water and clinical specimens.[13] The PCR was first used to amplify a portion of the small-subunit rRNA (SSU) from 13 different species of mycobacteria, using a 5′ PCR primer that carried a fluorescent label to allow detection of the amplified product. The PCR product was digested with restriction endonucleases, and the sizes of the labeled restriction fragments were determined by an automated DNA sequencer. A library of 5′ restriction-fragment lengths produced by five restriction endonucleases has been developed that can categorize 20 *Mycobacterium* species. Each *Mycobacterium* species has a unique 5′ restriction-fragment length for each specific endonuclease, selections from which can be used to make identifications of unknown species. Advantages of this technique over rapid PCR methods include lower cost and the ability to characterize several *Mycobacterium* species and to detect more than one *Mycobacterium* species in the same sample.

Strain-typing methods have also been used in the detection of drug-resistant strains of *M. tuberculosis*. In separate studies, Whelen and coworkers[383] and Felmlee and associates[91] used unique methods to detect mutations in the beta subunit of *M. tuberculosis* RNA polymerase (*rpoB*) to detect mutations most frequently associated with rifampin resistance. Plikaytis and coworkers, in the study of an outbreak of multidrug-resistant tuberculosis in New York City, used a multiplex PCR assay targeting a direct repeat of IS*6110* with a 556-bp intervening sequence (NTF-1), to identify patients who were infected with what they designated the multidrug-resistant ''W'' strains of *M. tuberculosis*.[266] Their assay correctly identified all 48 strain W isolates of *M. tuberculosis*, among a total of 193 strains studied. These studies indicate the degree of sophistication achieved by molecular techniques and the practical applications for which they are being used.

Susceptibility Testing

The need for prompt and accurate antimycobacterial susceptibility testing for *M. tuberculosis* has become a necessity, since the emergence of multidrug-resistant strains. A nationwide survey performed by the CDC in the early 1990s showed that 14.9% of the isolates from patients with tuberculosis were resistant to at least one of the antituberculosis drugs and 3.3 % were resistant to both INH and rifampin.[56,83] At one point in New York City, isolates resistant to at least one drug, including emerging resistance to fluoroquinones were recovered from 33% of cases, and the incidence of resistance to INH and rifampin was 19%.[340] In addition to resistance associated with the misuse of antimicrobial therapy, the drug resistance of mycobacteria may occur as a process of random evolution, independent of exposure to the agents.

The frequency of drug-resistant mutants in a culture of tubercle bacilli has been estimated to be about $1:10^5$ bacteria for INH and $1:10^6$ for streptomycin. If two drugs (i.e., INH and streptomycin) are taken together, the incidence of resistance is $1:10^{11}$, which is the sum $(1:10^5 + 1:10^6)$ of the two taken separately. Knowledge of the incidence of mutants becomes important because it has been determined that patients with an open pulmonary cavity may have a total bacillary population of 10^7 to 10^9 bacteria. Therefore, if these patients are treated with a single antituberculosis agent, their cultures may soon show the emergence of the resistant phenotype to that agent, and thus treatment fails. Consequently, patients with tuberculosis must always be treated with two, or preferably three, drugs. Therefore, the failure of patients to take more than one of the drugs may lead to the rapid emergence of a specific drug-resistant tubercle bacillus (Fig. 19-4). After following a group of patients coinfected with *M. tuberculosis* and the AIDS virus, Nolan found that lack of compliance with antituberculosis drug therapy was the primary reason for treatment failure.[245] Lack of compliance may also contribute to therapeutic failure and the emergence of drug resistance.

A second principle of mycobacterial drug susceptibility testing, which is particularly germane to the testing of *M. tuberculosis*, is based on the *in vitro* correlation between the clinical response to an antimycobacterial agent and the result of *in vitro* susceptibility testing. If more than 1% of the tubercle bacilli present are resistant to a drug *in vitro*, therapy with that drug is not clinically useful. Therefore, most methods for drug susceptibility testing of mycobacteria must be capable of determining the proportion of bacilli susceptible and resistant to a given drug. When using agar dilution methods, the inoculum should be adjusted so that the number of spontaneously resistant mutants will not mislead the laboratory worker to interpret the culture as resistant. By the same token, there must be a sufficient number of colonies on the

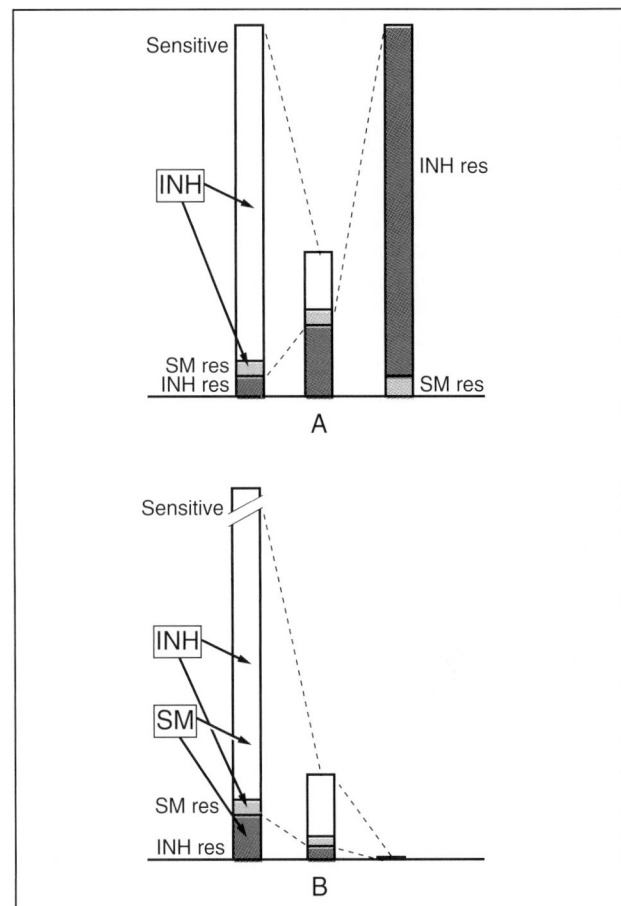

Figure 19-4 Emergence of mycobacterial antimicrobial resistance with one- and two-drug therapy. (**A**) The patient is treated with only isoniazid (INH). Although the small number of streptomycin-resistant mutants are inhibited by the INH, the INH-resistant mutants are refractory and, in time, make up the majority of the population. This represents drug failure. (**B**) The patient is treated with both streptomycin and INH. The streptomycin-resistant mutants are inhibited by the INH, and the INH-resistant mutants are inhibited by streptomycin. Thus, neither of these mutant strains can overgrow and drug therapy is successful. (Redrawn from Crofton J. Some principles in the chemotherapy of bacterial infections. BMJ 1969;2:209–212.)

plate that the incidence of drug resistance in the range of 1% can be determined. This is best accomplished when 100 to 300 CFUs are present on each quadrant of a four-quadrant Petri plate. To determine the incidence of resistance, it is usually necessary to inoculate two sets of susceptibility test plates, the second set with a 100-fold dilution of the inoculum used for the first set. This procedure is known as the proportional susceptibility testing method.

The test is performed in plastic Petri dishes divided into four quadrants. Five milliliters of agar medium are placed into each quadrant, the first with no antimycobacterial agent to act as a growth control, the other three with varying concentrations of the drug to be tested. Although in the past drugs have been incorporated in inspissated egg-based media, the use of 7H10 agar as the base is the current and recommended medium, if this type of testing is to be performed.[396] The drugs to be tested are added after the agar is cooled to 45°C, which diminishes any loss of activity that can occur during inspissation. An additional loss of drug activity may occur in egg-based media as the result of some agents binding to albumin and other proteins.

Because of the need for a more rapid turnaround time of results and to overcome certain problems inherent in *in vitro* agar dilution antituberculosis drug susceptibility testing, use of a test based on broth medium culture is currently recommended because results are more accurate, precise, and obtained sooner than with tests performed on solid media.[149] Heifets cites three disadvantages for the use of agar media[133]:

1. The activity of some antituberculosis drugs is compromised because of binding to the agar or to protein components in the medium.
2. The end results when using agar require prolonged incubation times, potentially reducing the potency of certain antimicrobials.
3. For unknown reasons, some *Mycobacterium* species lose their potency when tested in agar as opposed to growth in broth medium. For determining the end point of ''susceptible'' for *M. tuberculosis* tested in broth media, the 99% inhibition end point was equivalent to the failure of the growth index to increase in the test broth for at least 4 to 5 days following inoculation of a 1:100 dilution of the inoculum compared with an uninoculated broth control.

In the past, most broth-based antimicrobial susceptibility testing for mycobacteria used the BACTEC radiometric system, which includes the BACTEC 460 instrument fitted with a ''TB hood'' and BACTEC 12B bottles. The basis of this broth test is the radiometric detection of ^{14}C, released from 7H12 liquid medium containing 1-[^{14}C] palmitic acid by the metabolizing bacteria.[226] The BACTEC 460 instrument has been adapted in many laboratories to perform susceptibility tests. The principle of operation of the instrument involves aspiration of the headspace gas above the medium of an inoculated vial and quantitatively detecting the amount of radioactivity of the aspirate that, in turn, reflects the degree of growth in the vial. The headgas radioactivity counts are compared with a predetermined baseline level, and a growth index can be established. (See Chart 19-18 for details on the performance of this test.)

Several published studies confirm that the level of agreement between standard and radiometric susceptibility test methods exceeds 90%, at least for susceptible organisms.[196,287] Early problems in the accuracy of the radiometric detection of resistant strains was resolved by adjusting the concentration of antibiotic included in the culture vials.[126] For example, increasing the concentration of streptomycin from 4 to 6 g/mL improved the correlation with 10 g/mL in the 7H10 method; an adjustment of ethambutol to 2.5 g/mL correlates with 5 g/mL for resistant strains tested by the conventional method.[126,395] Regarding INH in the detection of resistance, Hawkins and coworkers determined that most discrepancies were caused by strains resistant to INH at 0.2

g/mL but not at 0.1 g/mL; therefore, reducing the concentration of drug in the INH vial to 0.1g/mL minimized the problem.[130]

The BACTEC MGIT 960 (BD Diagnostic) and the ESP II System (Trek Diagnostics) are nonisotopic, broth-based methods for performing mycobacterial susceptibility testing. These methods, as well as the BACTEC 460, are the only methods currently cleared by the FDA for this purpose, but other methods are in development.[396]

Currently, the drugs used in treating mycobacterial infections are those used primarily for classic tuberculosis, those for the nontuberculous mycobacteria (NTM), and those used for treating leprosy.[404] The first-line drugs for treating tuberculosis are isoniazid, rifampin, ethambutol, streptomycin, and pyrazinamide. The second-line drugs are *p*-aminosalicylic acid, cycloserine, ethionamide, kanamycin, amikacin, viomycin, and capreomycin.[322,331] The first-line drugs, except ethambutol, are considered bactericidal; the remaining included in the secondary list are to be used only when resistance to the primary drug develops. Table 19-10 lists the suggested concentrations of select drugs used for mycobacterial susceptibility testing from the approved Clinical Laboratory Standards Institute (formerly, the National Committee for Clinical Laboratory Standards, or NCCLS) document on susceptibility testing of mycobacteria.

Even if there is primary resistance to one drug, such as INH, treatment with the recommended triple-drug therapy provides adequate coverage. Susceptibility tests should be performed on all initial isolates of *M. tuberculosis* and on isolates from patients who remain culture-positive after 3 months or demonstrate clinical evidence of therapeutic failure.[396] The probability of induced resistance in the latter groups of patients is high. If these recommendations are not followed and susceptibility tests are not performed on isolates obtained from patients not previously seen by a laboratory, then at least one culture should be saved for 6 months to 1 year in the event the patient does not respond to therapy.

Control strains for susceptibility studies should be run with each set of isolates tested. The controls should include a susceptible strain, an intermediate susceptible strain (e.g., *M. kansasii* resistant to 0.2 g/mL INH, but susceptible to 1 g/mL of INH), and a resistant strain. There are no standard methods for testing agents in combination. Although interpretive criteria of susceptibility and resistance are not established for testing multiple drugs in combination, the rate of killing as determined by time/kill curves may have more clinical relevance than the degree of killing.[330]

The only drug for which *in vitro* susceptibility testing is recommended when testing members of the MAI is clarithromycin. The use of interpretive criteria applied to *M. tuberculosis* cannot be used as a guide for the treatment of patients with MAI disease.[149] Members of the MAI are predictably resistant to isoniazid and pyrazinamide and are susceptible to rifampin and ethambutol only to varying degrees. There is no correlation between *in vitro* susceptibility testing results and clinical outcome of patients with MAI for drugs other than clarithromycin. Furthermore, some believe that drug susceptibility profiles are more variable when testing MAI compared with *M. tuberculosis*. The translucent colony variants are thought to be more resistant to antimicrobial agents than the rough strains, and the nonpigmented strains

Table 19–10 Drug Concentration for Proportion Method of Susceptibility Testing Using Various Culture Media

	DRUG CONCENTRATIONS (µG/ML)	
DRUG	Middlebrook 7H10	Löwenstein-Jensen
Isoniazid	0.2, 1	0.2,1
Streptomycin	2	4
Rifampin	1	40
Ethambutol	2	2
Ethionamide	5	20
Kanamycin	5	20
Capreomycin	10	20
Cycloserine	20	30
Pyrazinamide	50	–

From McClatchy JK. In: Lorian V, ed. Antibiotics in Laboratory Medicine. Baltimore: Williams & Wilkins, 1980.

are thought to be more resistant than those producing pigment. However, the pigmented variants grow more rapidly, and it is possible that a slower-growing, nonpigmented strains, although present, may be masked by a more rapidly growing pigmented variant; thus, testing of the more obvious pigmented strains may lead to false-susceptible results.[336]

For the susceptibility testing of rapidly growing species, broth microdilution may be used, but the Etest (AB Biodisk North America, Piscataway NJ) may also be useful. Biehle and associates performed Etests for 100 clinical strains of rapidly growing mycobacteria against six drugs: amikacin, cefoxitin, ciprofloxacin, clarithromycin, doxycycline, and imipenem.[22] The Etest is an antibiotic-impregnated strip in which the test antibiotic is adsorbed to produce a concentration gradient from the top of the strip to the bottom, through at least 15 doubling dilutions. The diffusing antibiotic provides a continuous minimal inhibitory concentration (MIC) gradient in the agar, which can be interpreted by reading the meniscus of growth inhibition against a calibration scale printed on the strip. These authors found 85% agreement between the Etest results and agar dilution MICs within 1 log2 and a 97% agreement at 2 log2 dilutions. The rates of major and minor errors were 2.2% and 11.7%, respectively; there were no very major errors (disagreement of 3 log2 dilutions or more). Interlaboratory agreement between Etest MICs determined in two separate laboratories was 81% within 1 log2 dilution and 92% within 2 log2 dilutions. They concluded that Etest may be an accurate and reproducible method for determining susceptibility of rapidly growing mycobacteria.

The Clinical Laboratory Standards Institute has published a document that provides considerable guidance for the susceptibility testing of mycobacteria, nocardiae, and other aerobic actinomycetes.[49a] Recommendations for antimycobacterial susceptibility testing for mycobacteria not covered in this section are discussed in this document. We suggest that all laboratories that perform susceptibility tests familiarize themselves with this document.

In conclusion, the broth-based susceptibility testing for *M. tuberculosis*, when performed according to well-controlled test conditions with the appropriate concentrations of drugs, is reliable for the front-line drugs.[130] Several commercially available systems make this testing easier to perform. Results can be determined within 4 to 5 days, which is considerably shorter than the 3 to 7 weeks required using standard techniques.

Short-Course Therapy

Gosset has provided a graphic illustration of the three most important types of tuberculous lesions harboring viable mycobacteria and the activity of the most important tuberculocidal agents in these lesions. It is postulated that, in a patient with pulmonary tuberculosis, three populations of mycobacteria are present[111]:

1. Those located extracellularly in open cavities
2. Those located intracellularly in macrophages
3. Those in closed caseous lesions.

Organisms in each site have different metabolic activities and rates of replication.

The third characteristic listed is of considerable importance, because most mycobacteria are susceptible to the bactericidal effects of antibiotics only when they are preparing to divide. Because *M. tuberculosis* is an obligate aerobe, metabolic activity and the rate of replication will vary with the available oxygen supply. This rate may be high, as in a cavity in which bacilli are undergoing rapid division, or low, with only infrequent replication of bacilli, as in closed caseous lesions. A tuberculous cavity may contain 10^7 to 10^9 organisms actively multiplying in a neutral or slightly alkaline environment. Inasmuch as 1 of every 10^5 to 10^6 mycobacteria may be resistant to a single mycobacterial agent, the cavity may contain as many as 10^2 to 10^4 drug-resistant microorganisms. This potentially large population of drug-resistant bacilli underscores the need to use at least two bactericidal drugs for effective therapy of such lesions.

The second group of organisms found in a patient with

tuberculosis is located in the phagosomes of macrophages. The intracellular environment in macrophages is acidic (pH 5.5), resulting in slow growth of mycobacteria. It has been estimated that macrophage phagosomes contain no more than 10^4 to 10^5 organisms and, therefore, are not likely to contain many drug-resistant strains. Successful killing of mycobacteria in macrophages depends on the use of an antibiotic resistant to the acidic environment of macrophage phagolysosomes (e.g., pyrazinamide). This requirement excludes streptomycin and other aminoglycoside antibiotics that do not readily penetrate into macrophages and lose activity rapidly in a lower pH environment.

The third population of mycobacteria present in patients with chronic tuberculosis is in the closed caseous lesion. These organisms are present in areas of necrosis, where the blood supply is greatly diminished and the metabolic activity of any surviving organisms is presumably very low. There may be a total of 10^4 to 10^5 organisms in closed caseous

---

Box 19-5 Recommendations for the Prevention and Treatment of Tuberculosis

I. Preventive therapy for person with recent conversion of skin test.
  A. The criteria for interpretation of a positive skin test is:
    1. For adults and children with HIV infection, close contacts of infectious cases and those with fibrotic lesions on chest radiographs: a reaction of 5 mm or larger is considered positive.
    2. For other at-risk adults and children, a reaction of 10 mm or larger is considered positive.
    3. For persons without a defined risk factor for infection, a reaction of 15 mm or larger is considered positive. In general, persons not at risk for infection should not be skin tested.
  B. For persons with a positive skin test, and any of the following risk factors, administer isoniazid for 6–12 months to decrease risk of future tuberculosis:
    1. Those with HIV infection (12-month regimen recommended)
    2. Those at risk for HIV infection with unknown HIV status
    3. Close contacts of sputum-positive persons with newly diagnosed infectious tuberculosis
    4. Persons with any of the following conditions known to increase the risk for tuberculosis:
      a. Diabetes mellitus
      b. Adrenocorticosteroid and immunosuppressive therapy
      c. Intravenous-drug users
      d. Hematologic and reticuloendothelial malignancies
      e. End-stage renal disease
      f. Rapid weight loss or malnutrition
    5. In the absence of the foregoing risk factors, persons younger than 35 years with a positive skin test who belong to one or more of the following high-incidence groups should receive 6 months of prophylactic isoniazid therapy:
      a. Foreign born from a high-prevalence country
      b. Medically underserved, low-income persons from high-prevalence populations—persons of African descent, Hispanics, Native Americans
      c. Residents of facilities for long-term care
    6. Persons older than 35 should have liver-enzyme levels checked before commencement of therapy and monthly thereafter during the course of treatment
    7. Persons presumed to be infected with isoniazid-resistant organisms should be treated with rifampin

II. Therapy for persons with known tuberculosis by isoniazid-susceptible strains
  A. A 6-month regimen, beginning with isoniazid, rifampin, and pyrazinamide during the first 2 months, followed by isoniazid and rifampin for the next 4 months.
  B. Ethambutol should be included in the initial regimen until the results of drug susceptibility studies are available.
  C. The recommended regimen applies to both HIV-infected and noninfected persons. Therapy prolonged beyond the recommended period may be needed in HIV-infected persons, depending on the clinical and bacteriologic status.
  D. Alternatively, a 9-month regimen of isoniazid and rifampin is acceptable for persons who cannot, or should not, take pyrazinamide.
  E. Multidrug-resistant tuberculosis poses difficult treatment problems. Treatment must be individualized based on *in vitro* susceptibility studies.
  F. Extrapulmonary tuberculosis should be managed according to the principles and with drug regimens outlined for pulmonary tuberculosis.
  G. A 4-month regimen of isoniazid and rifampin is acceptable therapy for adults who have active tuberculosis, but who are smear- and culture-negative, if there is little possibility of drug resistance.
III. Compliance with drug therapy is mandatory: any regimen is irrelevant if drugs do not enter the patient's body. Consider the following techniques:
  A. Ask patients routinely about compliance.
  B. Periodic pill counts and urine tests may be used to monitor drug ingestion.
  C. Carefully track persons who fail to return for follow-up visits.
  D. Set hours of clinic visits to meet the needs of the patient.
  E. Give observed treatment in the clinic, home, work place, or other location.
  F. Offer incentives such as food, car fare, babysitting services, or small gifts.

lesions, where, although the pH is neutral, multiplication is slow or intermittent.

Streptomycin, the first of the mycobactericidal agents, is most effective in killing actively multiplying extracellular organisms found in cavities. In contrast with INH and rifampin, streptomycin has little effect against organisms in closed caseous lesions or those in the acid phagosomes of macrophages. Isoniazid is active against all groups of rapidly dividing mycobacteria as well as against the slowly dividing mycobacteria found in the acid environment of macrophages. Although not as active as rifampin against organisms in the closed caseous lesions, INH does have some bactericidal effect on this group of mycobacteria. Rifampin is effective against all groups of organisms, particularly those in closed caseous lesions, where the metabolic activity of the bacilli may be slow and episodic. Rifampin is the most universal antimycobacterial agent. Pyrazinamide is unique among the bactericidal agents effective against mycobacteria, in that it is active only at an acid pH and, hence, is effective only against those organisms in macrophage phagosomes.[85]

In contrast with the other agents just discussed, ethambutol is not considered to be a bactericidal drug and cannot be used with only one other drug in short-course therapy. It can, however, penetrate both the extracellular and intracellular environments of mycobacteria and can deter selection of resistant mutants. Recent studies have suggested that when ethambutol is used with three or four bactericidal drugs, it may play a role in shortening the duration of treatment.

In addition to the antituberculous drugs described, capreomycin, kanamycin, ethionamide, and cycloserine are also available in the United States. The first two agents are bactericidal to extracellular organisms in large cavities, whereas the second two are bacteriostatic to intracellular and extracellular organisms. However, when possible, therapy with streptomycin, isoniazid, and rifampin, pyrazinamide, or ethambutol, or a combination thereof, is preferred over the less commonly used agents.

The simplest regimen for the treatment of uncomplicated pulmonary tuberculosis is to administer INH and rifampin for a period of 9 months. Streptomycin or ethambutol may be added for the first 2 to 8 weeks. The 9-month period of therapy is in sharp contrast to the previously standard 18- to 24-month period necessary when using INH and ethambutol. The combination of INH and rifampin has introduced the concept of "short-course" therapy based on the ability of these two drugs to sterilize human tissue during a 9-month period.[96] One additional important aspect of short-course therapy is the finding that, following an initial month of therapy, both the INH and rifampin can be given twice weekly instead of daily. This schedule permits both a two-thirds savings on the use of the expensive drug, rifampin, and better compliance in patients taking the medication, particularly those considered to be unreliable. With this regimen, fewer than 3% of those who complete their course of therapy suffer a relapse. An important factor in the treatment of cavitary tuberculosis is the rapid elimination of organisms by the bactericidal action of INH and rifampin. This greatly reduces the emergence of drug-resistant organisms, which results all too often when only a single bacterial agent is used.

American Thoracic Society Recommendations

A committee of the scientific assembly of the American Thoracic Society (ATS) on microbiology, tuberculosis, and pulmonary infections has published recommendations for the treatment of tuberculosis in adults and children; these may be found at http://www.thoracic.org/statements/. A summary of recommendations for the treatment of tuberculosis are found in Box 19-5.

Summary

"The ultimate elimination of tuberculosis requires an organized and smoothly functioning network of primary and referral services based on cooperation between clinicians and public health officials, between health care facilities and community outreach programs, and between the private and public sectors of medical care."[7]

REFERENCES

1. Abed Y, Davin-Regli. A., Bollet C, De Micco P. Efficient discrimination of Mycobacterium tuberculosis strains by 16S–23S spacer region-based random amplified polymorphic DNA analysis. J Clin Microbiol 1995;33:1418–1420.
2. Agins BD, Berman DS, Spicehandler D, et al. Effect of combined therapy with ansamycin, clofazimine, ethambutol, and isoniazid for Mycobacterium avium infection in patients with AIDS. J Infect Dis 1989;159:784–787.
3. Agy MB, Wallis. CK, Plorde JJ, et al. Evaluation of four mycobacterial blood culture media: BACTEC 13A, Isolator/BACTEC 12B, Isolator/Middlebrook agar and biphasic medium. Diagn Microbiol Infect Dis 1989;12:303–308.
4. Ahmad S, Mokaddas E, et al. Characterization of rpoB mutations in rifampin-resistant clinical Mycobacterium tuberculosis isolates from Kuwait and Dubai. Diagn Microbiol Infect Dis 2002;44:245–252.
5. Ahrens P, Giese SB, Kauasen J, Inglis NF. Two markers, IS901-IS902 and p40, identified by PCR and by using monoclonal antibodies in Mycobacterium avium strains. J Clin Microbiol 1995;33:1049–1053.
6. Albers WM, Chandler KW, Solomon DA, Goldman AL. Pulmonary disease caused by Mycobacterium malmoense. Am Rev Respir Dis 1987;135:1375–1378.
7. Control of tuberculosis in the United States. Am Rev Respir Dis 1992;146:1623–1633.
8. Archibald LK, den Dulk MO, et al. Fatal Mycobacterium tuberculosis bloodstream infections in febrile hospitalized adults in Dar es Salaam, Tanzania. Clin Infect Dis 1998;26:290–296.
9. Ardito F, Posteraro B, et al. Evaluation of BACTEC Mycobacteria Growth Indicator Tube (MGIT 960) automated system for drug susceptibility testing of Mycobacterium tuberculosis. J Clin Microbiol 2001;39(12):4440–4444.
10. Aronson, JD. Spontaneous tuberculosis in salt water fish. J Infect Dis 1926;39:315–320.
11. Aubrey M, Fam AG. A case of clinically unsuspected Mycobacterium marinum infection. Arthritis Rheum 1987;30:1317–1318.
12. Ausina V, Barrio J., Luguin M, et al. Mycobacterium xenopi infections in AIDS. Ann Intern Med 1988;109:927–928.
13. Avaniss-Aghajani E, Jones K, Holtzman A, et al. Molecular technique for rapid identification of mycobacteria. J Clin Microbiol 1996;34:98–102.
14. Bamberger DM, Driks M., Gupta MR, et al. Mycobacterium kansasii among patients infected with human immunodeficiency virus in Kansas City. Clin Infect Dis 1994;18:395–400.
15. Banks J, Jenkins PA., Smith AP. Pulmonary infection with Mycobacterium malmoense—problems with treatment and diagnosis—a review of treatment and response. Tubercle 1985;66:197–203.
16. Barrett A, Magee JG, et al. An evaluation of the BD ProbeTec ET system for the direct detection of Mycobacterium tuberculosis in respiratory samples. J Med Microbiol 2002;51:895–898.

17. Beckman EN, Pankey GA, McFarland GB. The histopathology of Mycobacterium marinum synovitis. Am J Clin Pathol 1985;83:457–462.

18. Bemer P, Bodmer T, et al. Multicenter evaluation of the MB/BACT system for susceptibility testing of Mycobacterium tuberculosis. J Clin Microbiol 2004;42: 1030–1034.

19. Bemer P, Palicova F, et al. Multicenter evaluation of fully automated BACTEC Mycobacteria Growth Indicator Tube 960 system for susceptibility testing of Mycobacterium tuberculosis. J Clin Microbiol 2002;40:150–154.

20. Berlin OG, Zakowski. P., Bruckner DA, Johnson BL Jr. New biphasic culture system for isolation of mycobacteria from blood cultures of patients with the acquired immunodeficiency syndrome. J Clin Microbiol 1984;20:572–574.

21. Berman SM, Kim RC, Haghighat D, et al. Mycobacterium genavense infection presenting as a solitary brain mass in a patient with AIDS: case report and review. Clin Infect Dis 1994;19:1152–1154.

22. Biehle JR, Cavalieri SJ, Saubolle MA, Getsinger LJ. Evaluation of Etest for susceptibility testing of rapidly growing mycobacteria. J Clin Microbiol 1995; 33:1760–1764.

23. Blacklock, Z. Mycobacterium asiaticum as a potential pulmonary pathogen for humans: a clinical and bacteriological review of 5 cases. Am Rev Respir Dis 1983;127:241–244.

24. Bloch AB, Rieder HL, Kelly GD, Cauthen GM, Hayden CH, Snider DE Jr. The epidemiology of tuberculosis in the United States: implications for diagnosis and treatment. Clinics Chest Med 1989;10:297–313.

25. Bloom BR, Murray CJ. Tuberculosis: commentary on a reemergent killer. Science 1992;257:1055–1064.

26. Ho, M-J. Sociocultural aspects of tuberculosis: a literature review and a case study of immigrant tuberculosis. Soc Sci Med 2004;59:753–762.

27. Bodmer T, Gurtner A., Schopfer K, Matter L. Screening of respiratory tract specimens for the presence of Mycobacterium tuberculosis by using the Gen-Probe Amplified Mycobacterium tuberculosis Direct Test. J Clin Microbiol 1994;32:1483–1487.

28. Boettger EC, Teske A., Kirschner P, et al. Disseminated Mycobacterium genavense infection in patients with AIDS. Lancet 1992;340:76–80.

29. Bouza E, Diaz-Lopez. M, Moreno S, et al. Mycobacterium tuberculosis bacteremia in patients with and without human immunodeficiency virus infection. Arch Intern Med 1993;153:496–500.

30. Boye K, Hogdall E, et al. Identification of bacteria using two degenerate 16S rDNA sequencing primers. Microbiol Res 1999;154:23–26.

31. Broadway DC, Kerr-Muir M, Eykyn SJ, Pambakian H. Mycobacterium chelonei keratitis: a case report and review of previously reported cases. Eye 1994;8: 134–142.

32. Brooks RW, Parker BC, Gruft H, Falkingham JO III. Epidemiology of infection by nontuberculous mycobacteria. V. Numbers of eastern United States soils and correlation with soil characteristics. Am Rev Respir Dis 1983;130:630–633.

33. Brown-Elliott BA, Wallace RJ Jr. Clarithromycin resistance to Mycobacterium abscessus. J Clin Microbiol 2001;39:2745–2746.

34. Burns DN, Wallace R J, Schultz ME, et al. Nosocomial outbreak of respiratory tract colonization with Mycobacterium fortuitum: demonstration of the usefulness of pulsed-field gel electrophoresis in an epidemiologic investigation. Am Rev Respir Dis 1991;144:1153–1159.

35. Butler WR, O'Conner SP, Yakrus MA, Gross WM. Cross-reactivity of genetic probe for detection of Mycobacterium tuberculosis with newly described species Mycobacterium celatum. J Clin Microbiol 1994;32:536–538.

36. Cage G. Direct identification of Mycobacterium species in BACTEC 7H12B medium by high-performance liquid chromatography. J Clin Microbiol 1994; 32:521–524.

37. Castor B, Juhlin I, Henriques B. Septic cutaneous lesions caused by Mycobacterium malmoense in a patient with hairy cell leukemia. Eur J Clin Microbiol Infect Dis 1994;13:145–148.

38. Cave MD, Eisenach KD, McDermott PF, et al. IS6110: conservation of sequence in the Mycobacterium tuberculosis complex and its utilization in DNA fingerprinting. Mol Cell Probes 1991;5:73–80.

39. Cave MD, Eisenach KD, Templeton G. Stability of DNA fingerprint pattern produced with IS6110 in strains of Mycobacterium tuberculosis. J Clin Microbiol 1994;32:262–266.

40. Cavusoglu C, Hilmioglu S, et al. Characterization of rpoB mutations in rifampin-resistant clinical isolates of Mycobacterium tuberculosis from Turkey by DNA sequencing and line probe assay. J Clin Microbiol 2002;40:4435–4438.

41. Centers for Disease Control and Prevention. A strategic plan for the elimination of tuberculosis in the United States. MMWR Morb Mortal Wkly Rep 1989;38: 1–25.

41a. Centers for Disease Control/National Institutes of Health. Biosafety in microbiological and biomedical laboratories. 3 Ed. Atlanta: U.S. Department of Health and Human Services, Public Health Service, CDC/NIH, 1993; DHHS pub no. (CDC) 93-8395.

42. Centers for Disease Control and Prevention. Tuberculosis among foreign-born persons who had recently arrived in the United States—Hawaii, 1992–1993, and Los Angeles County. MMWR Morb Mortal Wkly Rep 1995;44:703–707.

43. Chemaly RF, Tomford JW, et al. Rapid diagnosis of Histoplasma capsulatum endocarditis using the AccuProbe on an excised valve. J Clin Microbiol 2001; 39:2640–2641.

44. Chin DP, Hopewell PC, Yajko DM, et al. Mycobacterium avium complex in the respiratory or gastrointestinal tract and the risk of M. avium complex bacteremia in patients with human immunodeficiency virus infection. J Infect Dis 1994;169:289–295.

45. Chiodini R. Crohn's disease and the mycobacterioses: a review and comparison of two disease entities. Clin Microbiol Rev 1989;2:90–117.

46. Chiodini RJ, van Kruiningen HJ, Merkal RS, et al. Characteristics of an unclassified Mycobacterium species isolated from patients with Crohn's disease. J Clin Microbiol 1984;30:966–971.

47. Choi CW, Cha DR, Kwon YJ, et al. Mycobacterium fortuitum peritonitis associated with continuous ambulatory peritoneal dialysis. Korean J Intern Med 1993; 8:25–27.

48. Chow SP, Ip FK, Lau JHK, et al. Mycobacterium marinum infection of the hand and wrists. J Bone Joint Surg Am 1987;679:1161–1168.

49. Claydon EJ, Coker RJ, Harris JR. Mycobacterium malmoense infection in HIV positive patients. J Infect Dis 1991;23:191–194.

49a. Clinical Laboratory Standards Institute. Susceptibility testing of mycobacteria, Nocardiae, and other aerobic aetinomycetes. Approved Standard M24-A. Vol. 23. Wayne, PA: CLSI, 2003.

50. Cloud JL, Conville PS, et al. Evaluation of partial 16S ribosomal DNA sequencing for identification of nocardia species by using the MicroSeq 500 system with an expanded database. J Clin Microbiol 2004;42:578–584.

51. Cocito C, Gilot P, Coene M, et al. Paratuberculosis. Clin Microbiol Rev 1994; 7:328–345.

52. Cohn ML, et al. The 7H11 medium for the culture of mycobacteria. Am Rev Respir Dis 1976;98:295–296.

53. Collazos J, Diaz F, Rodriquez J, Ayarza R. Persistent lung infection due to Mycobacterium szulgai. Tubercle Lung Dis 1993;74:412–413.

54. Conlon CP, Brandon HM, Luo NP, et al. Fecal mycobacteria and their relationship to HIV-related enteritis in Lusaka, Zambia. AIDS 1989;3:539–541.

55. Contreras MA, Cheung OT, Sanders DE, Goldstein RS. Pulmonary infections with nontuberculous mycobacteria. Am Rev Respir Dis 1988;137:149–152.

56. Centers for Disease Control and Prevention Advisory Council for the Elimination of Tuberculosis. Screening for tuberculosis and tuberculosis infection in high-risk populations. MMWR Morb Mortal Wkly Rep 1995;44(RR-11).

57. Conville PS, Keiser JF. Inter-bottle transfer of mycobacteria by the BACTEC 460. Diagn Microbiol Infect Dis 1989;460:401–405.

58. Cooper JF, Lichtenstein MJ, Graham BS, Schaffner W. Mycobacterium chelonae: a cause of nodular skin lesions with a proclivity for renal transplant recipients. Am J Med 1989;86:173–177.

59. Corbett E, Watt C, et al. The growing burden of tuberculosis: global trends and interactions with the HIV epidemic. Arch Intern Med 2003;163:1009–1021.

60. Cowling P, Glover S, Reeves DS. Mycobacterium malmoense type II bacteremia contributing to death in a patient with AIDS. Int J SID AIDS 1992;3:445–446.

61. Coyle MB, Carlson L, Wallis C, et al. Laboratory aspects of Mycobacterium genavense, a proposed species isolated from AIDS patients. J Clin Microbiol 1992;30:3206–3212.

62. Crawford, J. T. New technologies in the diagnosis of tuberculosis. Semin Respir Infect 1994;9:62–70.

63. Crowle AJ, Tsang AY, Vatter AE, May MH. Comparison of 15 laboratory and patient-derived strains of Mycobacterium avium for ability to infect and multiply in cultured human macrophages. J Clin Microbiol 1986;24:812–821.

64. Crump JA, Tanner DC, et al. Controlled comparison of BACTEC 13A, MYCO/F LYTIC, BacT/ALERT MB, and ISOLATOR 10 systems for detection of mycobacteremia. J Clin Microbiol 2003;41:1987–1990.

65. Daley CL, Griffith DE. Pulmonary disease caused by rapidly growing mycobacteria. Clin Chest Med 2002;23:623–632, vii.

66. D'Amato JJ, Collins MT, Rothlauf MV, et al. Detection of mycobacteria by radiometric and standard plate procedures. J Clin Microbiol 1983;17:1066–1073.

67. D'Amato RF, Isenberg HD, Hochstein L, et al. Evaluation of the Roche Septi-Check AFB system for recovery of mycobacteria. J Clin Microbiol 1991;29: 2906–2908.

68. D'Amato RF, Wallman AA, Hochstein LH, et al. Rapid diagnosis of pulmonary tuberculosis by using Roche AMPLICOR Mycobacterium tuberculosis PCR test. J Clin Microbiol 1995;33:1832–1834.

69. Dawson DJ, Blacklock ZM, Ashdown LR, Boettger EC. Mycobacterium asiaticum as the probable causative agent in a case of olecranon bursitis. J Clin Microbiol 1995;33:1042–1043.

70. de Oliveira MM, da Silva Rocha A, et al. Rapid detection of resistance against rifampicin in isolates of Mycobacterium tuberculosis from Brazilian patients using a reverse-phase hybridization assay. J Microbiol Methods 2003;53: 335–342.

71. Delacourt C, Poveda JD, Chureau C, et al. Use of polymerase chain reaction for improved diagnosis of tuberculosis in children. J Pediatr 1995;126(5 Part 1):703–709.

72. Delaporte E, Alfandari S, Piette F. Mycobacterium ulcerans associated with infection due to the human immunodeficiency virus. Clin Infect Dis 1994;18:839.

73. Della-Latta P, Whittier S. Comprehensive evaluation of performance, laboratory application, and clinical usefulness of two direct amplification technologies for the detection of Mycobacterium tuberculosis complex. Am J Clin Pathol 1998;110:301–310.

74. Dillon J, Misslon C, Morris I. Mycobacterium kansasii infection of the wrists and hand. Br J Rheumatol 1990;29:150–153.

75. Dixon JMS, Cithbert, EH. Isolation of tubercle bacilli from uncentrifuged sputum on pyruvic acid medium. Am Rev Respir Dis 1967;96:119–122.

76. Dobner P, Feldmann K, et al. Rapid identification of mycobacterial species by PCR amplification of hypervariable 16S rRNA gene promoter region. J Clin Microbiol 1996;34:866–869.

77. Doern GV, Westerling, JA. Optimum recovery of Mycobacterium avium complex from blood specimens of human immunodeficiency virus-positive patients by using small volumes of isolator concentrate inoculated into BACTEC 12B bottles. J Clin Microbiol 1994;32:2576–2577.

78. Doern GV, Westerling, JA. Optimum recovery of Mycobacterium avium complex from blood specimens of human immunodeficiency virus-positive patients by using small volumes of isolator concentrate inoculated into BACTEC 12B bottles. J Clin Microbiol 1995;33:784–785.

79. Drabick JJ, Duffy PE, Samlaska CP, Scherbenske JM. Disseminated Mycobacterium chelonei subspecies chelonei infection with cutaneous and osseous manifestations. Arch Dermatol 1990;126:1064–1067.

80. Drake TA, Hindler JA, Berlin OGW, Bruckner DA. Rapid identification of Mycobacterium avium complex in culture using DNA probes. J Clin Microbiol 1987;25:1442–1445.

81. Drancourt M, Raoult D. rpoB gene sequence-based identification of Staphylococcus species. J Clin Microbiol 2002;40:1333–8.

82. Drancourt M, Roux V, et al. rpoB gene sequence-based identification of aerobic Gram-positive cocci of the genera Streptococcus, Enterococcus, Gemella, Abiotrophia, and Granulicatella. J Clin Microbiol 2004;42:497–504.

83. Driver CR, Frieden TR, Bloch AB, et al. Drug resistance among tuberculosis patients, New York City, 1991 and 1992. Public Health Rep 1994;109:632–636.

84. Dunmire RB III, Breyer JA. Nontuberculous mycobacterial peritonitis during continuous ambulatory peritoneal dialysis: case report and review of diagnostic and therapeutic strategies. Am J Kidney Dis 1991;18:126–130.

85. Dutt AK, Snead WW. Present chemotherapy for tuberculosis. J Infect Dis 1982;146:698–705.

86. Edzkorn ET, Sigfredo A. McAllister CK, et al. Medical therapy of Mycobacterium avium-intracellulare pulmonary disease. Am Rev Respir Dis 1986134:442–445.

87. Ellner PD, Kiehn TE, Cammarata R, Hosmer M. Rapid detection and identification of pathogenic mycobacteria by combining radiometric and nucleic acid probe methods. J Clin Microbiol 1988;26:1349–1352.

88. Enarson DA, Fanning EA, Allen EA. Case-finding in the elimination phase of tuberculosis: high-risk groups in epidemiology and in clinical practice. Bull Int Union Tuberc Lung Dis 1990;65:73–75.

89. Fadda, G., F. Ardito, et al. Evaluation of the Abbott LCx Mycobacterium tuberculosis assay in comparison with culture methods in selected Italian patients. New Microbiol 1998;21:97–103.

90. Fanning A, Edwards S. Mycobacterium bovis infection in human beings in contact with elk (Cervus elaphus) in Alberta, Canada. Lancet 1991;338:1253–1255.

91. Felmlee TA, Liu Q, Whelen AC, et al. Genotypic detection of Mycobacterium tuberculosis rifampin resistance: comparison of single-strand conformation polymorphism and dideoxy fingerprinting. J Clin Microbiol 1995;33:1617–1623.

92. Fidler HM, Thurrell W, Johnson NM, et al. Specific detection of Mycobacterium paratuberculosis DNA associated with granulomatous tissue in Crohn's disease. Gut 1994;35:506–510.

93. Fisher A. Swimming pool granulomas due to Mycobacterium marinum: an occupational hazard of lifeguards. Cutis 1988;41:397–398.

94. Forbes BA, Hicks KE. Ability of PCR assay to identify Mycobacterium tuberculosis in BACTEC 12B vials. J Clin Microbiol 1994;32:1725–1728.

95. Fouad AF, Barry J, et al. PCR-based identification of bacteria associated with endodontic infections. J Clin Microbiol 2002;40:3223–3231.

96. France AJ, McLeod DT, Calder MA, Seaton A. Mycobacterium malmoense infections in Scotland: an increasing problem. Thorax 1987;42:593–595.

97. Fraser VJ, Jones M, Murray PR, et al. Contamination of flexible fiberoptic bronchoscopes with Mycobacterium chelonae linked to an automated bronchoscope disinfection machine. Am Rev Respir Dis 1992;145:853–85.

98. Frieden TR, Sterline R, Pablos-Mendez A, et al. The emergence of drug-resistant tuberculosis in New York City. N Engl J Med 1993;328:521–526.

99. Friedman CR, S. M., Johnson WD Jr, Riley LW. Double-repetitive-element PCR method for subtyping Mycobacterium tuberculosis clinical isolates. J Clin Microbiol 1995;33:1383–1384.

100. Fuller DD, Davis TE Jr, et al. Evaluation of BACTEC MYCO/F Lytic medium for recovery of mycobacteria, fungi, and bacteria from blood. J Clin Microbiol 2001;39:2933–6.

101. Gauduchon V, Chalabreysse L, et al. Molecular diagnosis of infective endocarditis by PCR amplification and direct sequencing of DNA from valve tissue. J Clin Microbiol 2003;41:763–766.

102. Giladi M, Lee BE, Berlin OG, Panosian CB. Peritonitis caused by Mycobacterium kansasii in a patient undergoing continuous ambulatory peritoneal dialysis. Am J Kidney Dis 1992;19:497–499.

103. Gill MJ, Fanning EA, Chomyc S. Childhood lymphadenitis in a harsh northern climate, due to atypical mycobacteria. Scand J Infect Dis 1987;19:77–83.

104. Gill VJ, Park CH, Stock F, et al. Use of lysis-centrifugation (Isolator) and radiometric (BACTEC) blood culture systems for the detection of mycobacteria. J Clin Microbiol 1985;22:543–546.

105. Gil-Setas A, Torroba L, et al. Evaluation of the MB/BacT system compared with Middlebrook 7H11 and Lowenstein-Jensen media for detection and recovery of mycobacteria from clinical specimens. Clin Microbiol Infect 2004;10:224–8.

106. Gitnick G, Collins J, Beaman B, et al. Preliminary report on isolation of mycobacteria from patients with Crohn's disease. Dig Dis Sci 1989;34:925–932.

107. Glickman SE, Kilburn JO, Butler WR, Ramos LS. Rapid identification of mycolic acid patterns of mycobacteria by high-performance liquid chromatography using pattern recognition software and a mycobacterium library. J Clin Microbiol 1994;32:740–745.

108. Goldenberger D, Kunzli A, et al. Molecular diagnosis of bacterial endocarditis by broad-range PCR amplification and direct sequencing. J Clin Microbiol 1997;35:2733–2739.

109. Good R. Opportunistic pathogens in the genus Mycobacterium. Annu Rev Microbiol 1985;39:347–369.

110. Good RC, Snider DE. Isolation of non-tuberculous mycobacteria in the United States. J Infect Dis 1980;146:829–833.

111. Gosset J. Bacteriologic basis of short course chemotherapy for tuberculosis. Clin Chest Med 1980;1:231.

112. Gotto M, Oka S, Okuzumi K, et al. Evaluation of acridinium-ester-labeled DNA probes for identification of Mycobacterium tuberculosis and Mycobacterium avium-intracellulare complex in culture. J Clin Microbiol 1991;219:2473–2476.

113. Gouby A, Branger B, Oules R, Ramuz M. Two cases of Mycobacterium haemophilum infections in a renal dialysis unit. J Med Microbiol 1988;25:299–300.

114. Greisen K, Loeffelholz M, et al. PCR primers and probes for the 16S rRNA gene of most species of pathogenic bacteria, including bacteria found in cerebrospinal fluid. J Clin Microbiol 1994;32:335–51.

115. Gross W, Hawkins JE, Murphy B. Mycobacterium xenopi in clinical specimens. I. Water as a source of contamination. Am Rev Respir Dis 1976;113:78 [abstract].

116. Gross WM, Hawkins J. Radiometric selective inhibition tests for differentiation of Mycobacterium tuberculosis, Mycobacterium bovis and other mycobacteria. J Clin Microbiol 1985;21:565–568.

117. Gruft H. Isolation of acid-fast bacilli from contaminated specimens. Health Lab Sci 1971;8:79–82.

118. Guerrant GO, Lambert MA, Moss CW 1981. Gas-chromatographic analysis of mycolic acid cleavage products in mycobacteria. J Clin Microbiol 1981;13:899–907.

119. Guerrero C, Bernasconi C, Burki D, et al. A novel insertion element from Mycobacterium avium, IS1245, is a specific target for analysis of strain relatedness. J Clin Microbiol 1995;133:304–307.

120. Gupta I, Kocher J, Miller AJ, et al. Mycobacterium haemophilum osteomyelitis in an AIDS patient. NJ Med 1992;89:201–202.

121. Haase G, Skopnik H, Batge S, Boettger EC. Cervical lymphadenitis caused by Mycobacterium celatum. Lancet 1994;344:1021.

122. Hall L, Doerr KA, et al. Evaluation of the MicroSeq system for identification of mycobacteria by 16S ribosomal DNA sequencing and its integration into a routine clinical mycobacteriology laboratory. J Clin Microbiol 2003;41:1447–1453.

123. Han XY, Pham AS, et al. Rapid and accurate identification of mycobacteria by sequencing hypervariable regions of the 16S ribosomal RNA gene. Am J Clin Pathol 2002;118:796–801.

124. Hanna BA, Walters SB, Kodsi SE, et al. Detection of Mycobacterium tuberculosis directly from patient specimens with the mycobacteria growth indicator tube; a new rapid method. Presented at the American Society for Microbiology Annual meeting, Las Vegas, 1994.

125. Hanson PJV, Thomas JM, Collins JV. Mycobacterium chelonei and abscess formation in soft tissue. Tubercle 1987;68:297–299.

126. Hawkins CC, Gold JWM, Whimbey E, et al. Mycobacterium avium complex infections in patients with the acquired immune deficiency syndrome. Ann Intern Med 1986;105:184–188.

127. Hawkins J. Scotochromogenic mycobacteria which appear intermediate between Mycobacterium avium-intracellulare and M. scrofulaceum. Am Rev Respir Dis 1977;116:963–964.

128. Hawkins J. Rapid mycobacterial susceptibility tests. Clin Microbiol Newslett 1986;8:101–104.

129. Hawkins JE, Gross JM. Program Abst 23rd Intersci Conf Microbial Newsletter. Chemother. 1983

130. Hawkins JE, Wallace RJ Jr, Brown BA. Antibacterial susceptibility tests: mycobacteria. In: Balows A, ed. Manual of Clinical Microbiology 5th ed. Chap 108, Washington DC: American Society for Microbiology, 1991

131. Hayman, J. Postulated epidemiology of Mycobacterium ulcerans infection. Int J Epidemiol 1991;20:1093–1098.

132. Heap B. Mycobacterium simiae as a cause of intra-abdominal disease: a case report. Tubercle 1989;70:217–221.

133. Heifets L. Qualitative and quantitative drug susceptibility tests in mycobacteriology. Am Rev Respir Dis 1988;137:1217–1222.

134. Heifets L. Gen-Probe test should not be considered final in Mycobacterium tuberculosis identification. J Clin Microbiol 1989;37:229.

135. Hermans PWM, Schuttema, ARJ, Van Soolsingen D, et al. Specific detection of Mycobacterium tuberculosis complex strains by polymerase chain reaction. J Clin Microbiol 1990;28:1204–1213.

136. Hermon-Taylor J, Moss M, Tizard M, et al. Molecular biology of Crohn's disease mycobacteria. Baillieres Clin Gastroenterol 1990;4:23–42.

137. Hirasuna J. Disseminated Mycobacterium kansasii infection in the acquired immunodeficiency syndrome (AIDS). Ann Intern Med 1987;107:784.

138. Hoffner SE, Henriques B, Petrini B, Kallenius G. Mycobacterium malmoense: an easily missed pathogen. J Clin Microbiol 1991;29:2673–2674.

139. Hoffner SE, Kratz M, Olsson-Liljequist B, et al. In-vitro synergistic activity between ethambutol and fluorinated quinolones against Mycobacterium avium complex. J Antimicrob Chemother 1989;24:317–324.

140. Horsburgh CR Jr, Chin DP, Yajko DM, et al. Environmental risk factors for acquisition of Mycobacterium avium complex in persons with human immunodeficiency virus infection. J Infect Dis 1994;170:362–367.

141. Hoyt RE, Bryant JE, Glessner SF, et al. Mycobacterium marinum infections in a Chesapeake Bay community. VA Med 1989;116:467–470.

142. Huang TS, Chen CS, et al. Comparison of the BACTEC MGIT 960 and BACTEC 460TB systems for detection of mycobacteria in clinical specimens. Ann Clin Lab Sci 2001;31:279–83.

143. Hurst LC, Amadio PC, Badalamente MA, et al. Mycobacterium marinum infections of the hand. J Hand Surg 1987;12:428–435.

144. Iademarco MF, Castro KG. Epidemiology of tuberculosis. Semin Resp Infect 2003;18:225–240.

145. Ichiyama S, Iinuma Y, Tawada Y, et al. Evaluation of the Gen-Probe amplified Mycobacterium tuberculosis direct test and Roche PCR-Microwell plate hybridization method (Amplicor Mycobacterium) for direct detection of mycobacteria. J Clin Microbiol 1996; 34:130–133.

146. Idemyor V, Cherubin CD. Retroperitoneal abscess caused by Mycobacterium chelonae and treatment. Ann Pharmacother 1993;27:178–179.

147. Igo JD, Murphy DP. Mycobacterium ulcerans infection in Papua New Guinea: correlation of clinical, histological and microbiologic features. Am J Trop Med Hyg 1988;38:391–392.

148. Imaeda T, Broslawski G, Imaeda S. Genomic relatedness among mycobacterial species by nonisotopic blot hybridization. Int J Syst Bacteriol 1988;38:151–156.

149. Interlied CB, Klemper CA, Bermudez LEM. The Mycobacterium avium complex. Clin Microbiol Rev 1993;6:266–310.

150. Isenberg HD, D'Amato RF, Heifets L, et al. Collaborative feasibility study of a biphasic system (Roche Septi-Check AFB) for rapid detection and isolation of mycobacteria. J Clin Microbiol 1991;129:1719–1722.

151. Jacob CN, Henein SS, Heurich AE, Kamholz S. Nontuberculous mycobacterial infection of the central nervous system in patients with AIDS. South Med J 86: 638–640.

152. Jacobson MA, Hopewell PC, Yajko DM, et al. Natural history of disseminated Mycobacterium avium complex infection in AIDS. J Infect Dis 1991;164: 994–998.

153. Jacobson MA, I. Isenberg, WM. kansasii diffuse pulmonary infection in a patient with acquired immune deficiency syndrome. Am J Clin Pathol 1989;91: 236–238.

154. Jacoby HM, Jivas TM, Kaminski DA, et al. Mycobacterium xenopi infection masquerading as pulmonary tuberculosis in two patients infected with the human immunodeficiency virus. Clin Infect Dis 1995;20:1299–1401.

155. Jarikre L. Case report: disseminated Mycobacterium gordonae infection in an immunocompromised host. Am J Med Sci 1991;302:382–384.

156. Jarikre L. Mycobacterium gordonae genitourinary disease. Genitourin Med 1992;68:445–446.

157. Jenkins PA, Tsukamura M. Infections with Mycobacterium malmoense in England and Wales. Tubercle 1979;60:71–76.

158. Jereb JA, Burwen DR, Dooley SW, et al. Nosocomial outbreak of tuberculosis in a renal transplant unit: application of a new technique for restriction fragment length polymorphism analysis of Mycobacterium tuberculosis isolates. J Infect Dis 1993;168:1219–1224.

159. Johansen IS, Lundgren B, et al. Direct detection of multidrug-resistant Mycobacterium tuberculosis in clinical specimens in low- and high-incidence countries by line probe assay. J Clin Microbiol 2003;41:4454–4456.

160. Johansen IS, Lundgren BH, et al. Rapid differentiation between clinically relevant mycobacteria in microscopy positive clinical specimens and mycobacterial isolates by line probe assay. Diagn Microbiol Infect Dis 2002;43:297–302.

161. Jonas V, Alden MJ, Curry JI, et al. Detection and identification of Mycobacterium tuberculosis directly from sputum sediments by amplification of rRNA. J Clin Microbiol 1993;31:2410–2416.

162. Jones MW, Wahid IA. Mycobacterium marinum infections of the hand and wrist: results of conservative treatment in twenty-four cases. J Bone Joint Surg 1988;70:631–632.

163. Joseph SW, Vaichulis EMK, Houk VN. Lack of auramine rhodamine fluorescence of Runyon group IV mycobacteria. Am Rev Respir Dis 1967;95:114–115.

164. Jost KC Jr, Dunbar DF, Barth SS, et al. Identification of Mycobacterium tuberculosis and M. avium complex directly from smear-positive sputum specimens and BACTEC 12B cultures by high-performance liquid chromatography with fluorescence detection and computer-driven pattern recognition models. J Clin Microbiol 1995;33:1270–1277.

165. Kaminski DA, Hardy DJ. Selective utilization of DNA probes for identification of Mycobacterium species on the basis of cord formation in primary BACTEC 12B cultures. J Clin Microbiol 1995;33:1548–1550.

166. Kestle DG, Kubica GP. Sputum collection for cultivation of mycobacteria: an early morning specimen or the 24 to 72 hour pool? Am J Clin Pathol 1967;48: 347–351.

167. Khamis A, Colson P, et al. Usefulness of rpoB gene sequencing for identification of Afipia and Bosea species, including a strategy for choosing discriminative partial sequences. Appl Environ Microbiol 2003;69:6740–6749.

168. Khooshabeh R, Grange JM, Yates MD, et al. A case report of Mycobacterium chelonae keratitis and a review of mycobacterial infections of the eye and orbit. Tubercle Lung Dis 1994;75:377–382.

169. Kiehn TE, Edwards FF. Rapid identification using a specific DNA probe of Mycobacterium avium complex from patients with acquired immunodeficiency syndrome. J Clin Microbiol 1987;25:1551–1552.

170. Kiehn TE, Edwards FF, Brannon P, et al. Infections caused by Mycobacterium avium complex in immunocompromised patients: diagnosis by blood culture and fecal examination, antimicrobial susceptibility tests and morphological and seroagglutination characteristics. J Clin Microbiol 1985;21:168–173.

171. Kiehn TE, White M, Pursell KG, et al. A cluster of four cases of Mycobacterium haemophilum infection. Eur J Clin Microbiol Infect Dis 1993;12:114–118.

172. Kilby JM, Gilligan PH, Yankaskas JR, et al. Nontuberculous mycobacteria in adult patients with cystic fibrosis. Chest 1992;102:70–75.

173. Kim BJ, Lee KH, et al. Differentiation of mycobacterial species by PCR-restriction analysis of DNA (342 base pairs) of the RNA polymerase gene (rpoB). J Clin Microbiol 2001;39:2102–2109.

174. Kim BJ, Lee SH, et al. Identification of mycobacterial species by comparative sequence analysis of the RNA polymerase gene (rpoB). J Clin Microbiol 1999; 37:1714–1720.

175. Kim TC, Arora NS, Aldrich TK, Rochester DF. Atypical mycobacterial infections: a clinical study of 92 patients. South Med J 1981;74:1304–1308.

176. Kinsella JP, Culver K, Jeffry RB, et al. Otomastoiditis caused by Mycobacterium avium-intracellulare. Pediatr Infect Dis J 1986;6:289–291.

177. Kirihara JM, Hillier SL, Coyle MB. Improved detection times for Mycobacterium avium complex and Mycobacterium tuberculosis with the BACTEC radiometric system. J Clin Microbiol 1985;22:841–845.

178. Kirschner P, Springer B, Vogel U, et al. Genotypic identification of mycobacteria by nucleic acid sequence determination: report of a 2-year experience in a clinical laboratory. J Clin Microbiol 1993;31:1189–2282.

179. Kischner RA Jr, Parker BC, Falkinham JO III. Epidemiology of infection by nontuberculous mycobacteria. Mycobacterium avium, Mycobacterium intracellulare and Mycobacterium scrofulaceum in acid, brown-water swamps of the southeastern United States and their association with environmental variables. Am Rev Respir Dis 1992;145:271–275.

180. Kline SE, Hedemark LL, Davies SF. Outbreak of tuberculosis among regular patrons of a neighborhood bar. N Engl J Med 1995;333:222–227.

181. Kochi A. The global tuberculosis situation and the new control strategy of the World Health Organisation. Tubercle Lung Dis 1991;72:1–6.

182. Kolmos HJ, Brahm M, Bruun B. Peritonitis with Mycobacterium fortuitum in a patient on continuous ambulatory peritoneal dialysis. Scand J Infect Dis 1992; 24:801–803.

183. Kramme S, Bretzel G, Panning M, et al. Detection and quantification of Mycobacterium leprae in tissue samples by real-time PCR. Med Microbiol Immunol (Berl) 2004;193:189–193.

184. Krasnow I, Wayne LG. Comparison of methods for tuberculosis laboratory. Appl Microbiol 1969;28:915–917.

185. Kraus G, Cleary T, et al. Rapid and specific detection of the Mycobacterium tuberculosis complex using fluorogenic probes and real-time PCR. Mol Cell Probes 2001;15:375–383.

186. Kremer LB, Rhame FS, House JH. Mycobacterium terrae tenosynovitis. Arthritis Rheum 1988;32:132–134.

187. Krishner KK, Kallay MC, Nolte FS. Primary pulmonary infection caused by Mycobacterium terrae complex. Diagn Microbiol Infect Dis 1988;11:171–175.

188. Kristjansson M, Bieluch VM, Byeff PD. Mycobacterium haemophilum infection in immunocompromised patients: case report and review of the literature. Rev Infect Dis 1991;13:906–910.

189. Kubica G. Differential identification of mycobacteria. VII. Key features for identification of clinically significant mycobacteria. Am Rev Respir Dis 1987; 107:9–21.

190. Kubica GP, et al. Laboratory services for mycobacterial diseases. Am Rev Respir Dis 1975;112:783–787.

191. Kuze F, Mitsouka W, Chiba W, et al. Chronic pulmonary infection caused by M. terrae complex: a resected case. Am Rev Respir Dis 1983;128:561–565.

192. Kwok AY, Su SC, et al. Species identification and phylogenetic relationships based on partial HSP60 gene sequences within the genus Staphylococcus. Int J Syst Bacteriol 1999;49(Part 3):1181–1192.

193. Lai KK, Stottmeier KD, Sherman IH, McCabe WR. Mycobacterial cervical lymphadenopathy: relation of etiologic agents to age. JAMA 1984;251: 1286–1288.

194. Lang S, Watkin RW, et al. Evaluation of PCR in the molecular diagnosis of endocarditis. J Infect 2004;48:269–275.

195. Larssons L, Odham G, Westerdahl G, Olsson B. Diagnosis of pulmonary tuberculosis by selected ion monitoring: improved analysis of tuberculostearate in sputum using negative-ion mass spectrometry. J Clin Microbiol 1987;25: 893–896.

196. Laszlo AP, Siddiqui SH. Evaluation of a rapid radiometric differentiation test for the Mycobacterium tuberculosis complex by selective inhibition with p-nitro-acetylamino- hydroxy-propiophenone. J Clin Microbiol 1984;19:694–698.

197. Laussuco S, Baltsch AL, Smith RW, et al. Nosocomial Mycobacterial fortuitum colonization from a contaminated ice machine. Am Rev Respir Dis 1988;138: 891–894.

198. Lavy A, Yoshpe-Purer Y. Isolation of Mycobacterium simiae from clinical specimens in Israel. Tubercle 1982;63:279–285.

199. Lebrun L, Espinasse F, Poveda JD, et al. Evaluation of nonradioactive DNA probes for identification of mycobacteria. J Clin Microbiol 1992;30:2476–2478.

200. Leckie GW, Erickson DD, He Q, Facey IE, Lin BC, Cao J, Halaka FG. Method for reduction of inhibition in a Mycobacterium tuberculosis-specific ligase chain reaction DNA amplification assay. J Clin Microbiol 1998;36:764–767.

201. Lee H, Bang HE, et al. Novel polymorphic region of the rpoB gene containing Mycobacterium species-specific sequences and its use in identification of mycobacteria. J Clin Microbiol 2003;41:2213–2218.

202. Leitritz L, Schubert S, et al. Evaluation of BACTEC MGIT 960 and BACTEC 460TB systems for recovery of mycobacteria from clinical specimens of a university hospital with low incidence of tuberculosis. J Clin Microbiol 2001;39: 3764–3767.

203. Levine B, Chaisson RE. Mycobacterium kansasii: a cause of treatable pulmonary disease associated with advanced human immunodeficiency virus (HIV) infection. Ann Intern Med 1991;114:861–868.

204. Levy-Frebault V, Pangon B, Bure A, et al. Mycobacterium simiae and Mycobacterium avium-intracellulare mixed infection in acquired immune deficiency syndrome. J Clin Microbiol 1987;25:154–157.

205. Lindbrathen A, Gaustad P, et al. Direct detection of Mycobacterium tuberculosis complex in clinical samples from patients in Norway by ligase chain reaction. J Clin Microbiol 1997;35:3248–3253.

206. Linton CJ, Jalal H, Leeming JP, Millar MR. Rapid discrimination of Mycobacterium tuberculosis strains by random amplified polymorphic DNA analysis. J Clin Microbiol 1994;32:2169–2174.

207. Lipsky BA, Gates JA, Tenover FC, et al. Factors affecting the clinical value of microscopy for acid-fast bacilli. Rev Infect Dis 1984;6:214–222.

208. Loeffler J, Hebart H, et al. Identification of rare Candida species and other yeasts by polymerase chain reaction and slot blot hybridization. Diagn Microbiol Infect Dis 2000;38:207–212.

209. London RD, Damsker B, Neibert EP, et al. Mycobacterium gordonae: an unusual peritoneal pathogen in a patient undergoing continuous ambulatory peritoneal dialysis. Am J Med 1988;85:703–704.

210. Lowry PW, Jarvis WR, Oberle AD, et al. Mycobacterium chelonei causing otitis media in an ear nose and throat practice. N Engl J Med 1988;31:978–982.

211. MacDonell KB, Glassroth J. Mycobacterium avium complex and other nontuberculous mycobacteria in patients with HIV infection. Semin Resp Infect 1989; 4:123–132.

212. Macher AM, Kovacs JA, Gill V, et al. Bacteremia due to Mycobacterium intracellulare in the acquired immunodeficiency syndrome. Ann Intern Med 1983; 99:782–785.

213. Males BM, West TE, Bartholomew WR. Mycobacterium haemophilum infection in a patient with acquired immune deficiency syndrome. J Clin Microbiol 1987; 25:186–190.

214. Maloney JM, Clark RG, Stephans DS, et al. Infections caused by Mycobacterium szulgai in humans. Rev Infect Dis 1987;9:1120–1126.

215. Marks J, Jenkins PA, Tsukamura M. Mycobacterium szulgai-a new pathogen. Tubercle 1972;53:210–214.

216. Martinez-Sanchez L, Ruiz-Serrano J, et al. Utility of the BACTEC Myco/F lytic medium for the detection of mycobacteria in blood. Diagn Microbiol Infect Dis 2000;38:223–226.

217. Maschek H, Gerogii A. Schmidt RE, et al. Mycobacterium genavense. Autopsy findings in three patients. Am J Clin Pathol 1994;101:95–99.

218. McBride JA, McBride MM, Wolf JE Jr, et al. Evaluation of commercial blood-containing media for cultivation of Mycobacterium haemophilum. Am J Clin Pathol 1992;98:282–286.

219. McCarter YS, Robinson A. Detection of acid-fast bacilli in concentrated primary specimen smears stained with rhodamine-auramine at room temperature and at 37 degrees C. J Clin Microbiol 1994;32:2487–2489.

220. McClatchy JK, et al. Isolation of mycobacteria from clinical specimens by use of selective 7H11 medium. Am J Clin Pathol 1976;65:412–415.

221. McFadden JJ, Butcher PD, Chiodini R, Hermon-Taylor J. Crohn's disease-isolated mycobacteria are identical to Mycobacterium paratuberculosis, as determined by DNA probes that distinguish between mycobacterial species. J Clin Microbiol 1987;25:796–801.

222. McWhinney PH, Yates M, Prentice HG, et al. Infection caused by Mycobacterium chelonae: a diagnostic and therapeutic problem in the neutropenic patient. Clin Infect Dis 1992;14:1208–1212.

223. Mellmann A, Cloud JL, et al. Evaluation of RIDOM, MicroSeq, and Genbank services in the molecular identification of Nocardia species. Int J Med Microbiol 2003;293:359–370.

224. Merlin TL, Tzamaloukas AH. Mycobacterium chelonae peritonitis associated with continuous ambulatory peritoneal dialysis. Am J Clin Pathol 1989;91: 717–720.

225. Metchock B, Diem I. Algorithm for use of nucleic acid probes for identifying Mycobacterium tuberculosis from BACTEC 12B bottles. J Clin Microbiol 1995; 33:1934–1937.

226. Middlebrook G, R3eggiardo Z, Tigertt WD. Automatable radiometric detection of growth of Mycobacterium tuberculosis in selective media. Am Rev Respir Dis 1977;115:1066–1069.

227. Middleton AM, Chadwick MV, et al. Detection of Mycobacterium tuberculosis in mixed broth cultures using DNA probes. Clin Microbiol Infect 1997;3: 668–671.

228. Miller N, Cleary T, et al. Rapid and specific detection of Mycobacterium tuberculosis from acid-fast bacillus smear-positive respiratory specimens and BacT/ALERT MP culture bottles by using fluorogenic probes and real-time PCR. J Clin Microbiol 2002;40:4143–4147.

229. Miller N, Hernandez SG, Cleary TJ. Evaluation of Gen-Probe Amplified Mycobacterium tuberculosis Direct Test and PCR for direct detection of Mycobacterium tuberculosis in clinical specimens. J Clin Microbiol 1994;32:393–397.

230. Miller N, Infante S, et al. Evaluation of the LiPA MYCOBACTERIA assay for identification of mycobacterial species from BACTEC 12B bottles. J Clin Microbiol 2000;38:1915–1919.

231. Millner R, Stottmeir KD, Kubica GP. Formaldehyde: a photothermal activated toxic substance produced in Middlebrook 7H10 medium. Am Rev Respir Dis 1969;99:603–607.

232. Mitchison DA, et al. A selective oleic acid albumin agar medium for tubercle bacilli. J Med Microbiol 1972;5:165–175.

233. Mizuguchi Y, Ogawa M, Odou T. Morphological changes induced by B-lactam antibiotics in Mycobacterium avium-intracellulare complex. Antimicrob Agents Chemother 1985;27:541–547.

234. Modilevsky T, Sattler FR, Barnes PF. Mycobacterial disease in patients with human immunodeficiency virus infection. Arch Intern Med 1989;149: 2201–2205.

235. Moore DF, Curry JI. Detection and identification of Mycobacterium tuberculosis directly from sputum sediments by ligase chain reaction. J Clin Microbiol 1998; 36:1028–1031.

236. Morgan MA, Horstmeier CD, DeYoung DR. Comparison of a radiometric method (BACTEC) and conventional culture media for recovery of mycobacteria from smear negative specimens. J Clin Microbiol 1983;18:384–388.

237. Moulsdale MT, Harper JM, Thatcher GN. Infection by Mycobacterium haemophilum, a metabolically fastidious acid-fast bacillus. Tubercle 1983;64:29–36.

238. Murdoch ME, Leigh IM. Sporotrichoid spread of cutaneous M. chelonei infection. Clin Exp Dermatol 1989;14:309–312.

239. Murray, P. Mycobacterial cross-contamination with the modified BACTEC 460 TB system. Diagn Microbiol Infect Dis 1991;14:33–35.

240. Musial CE, Tice LS, Stockman L, Roberts GD. Identification of mycobacteria from culture by using the Gen-Probe rapid diagnostic system for Mycobacterium avium complex and Mycobacterium tuberculosis complex. J Clin Microbiol 198826:2120–2123.

241. Nardell EA, Keegan J, Cheney SA, Etkind SC. Airborne infection: theoretical limits of protection achievable by building ventilation. Am Rev Respir Dis 1991; 144:302–306.

242. Newton JA, Weiss PH. Aspiration pneumonia caused by Mycobacterium smegmatis. Mayo Clin Proc 1994;69:296.

243. Newton JA, Weiss PH, Bowler WA, Oldfield EC III. Soft-tissue infection due to Mycobacterium smegmatis: report of two cases. Clin Infect Dis 1993;16:531–533.

244. Nightingale SD, Byrd LT, Southern PM, et al. Incidence of Mycobacterium avium-intracellulare complex bacteremia in human immunodeficiency virus-positive patients. J Infect Dis 1992;165:1082–1085.

245. Nolan, C. Failure of therapy for tuberculosis in human immunodeficiency virus infection. Am J Med Sci 1992;304:168–173.

246. Nolte FS, Metchock B. Mycobacterium. In: Murray PR, ed. Manual of Clinical Microbiology. 6th ed. Washington DC: ASM Press, 1995:Chapter 31.

247. Nolte FS, Metchock B, McGowan JE Jr, et al. Direct detection of Mycobacterium tuberculosis in sputum by polymerase chain reaction and DNA hybridization. J Clin Microbiol 1993;31:1777–1782.

248. Noordhoek GT, Kolk AH, Bjune G, et al. Sensitivity and specificity of PCR for detection of Mycobacterium tuberculosis: a blind comparison study among seven laboratories. J Clin Microbiol 1994;32:277–284.

249. World Health Organization Global Tuberculosis Control. WHO report Geneva: WHO, 2003.

250. O'Sullivan CE, Miller DR, et al. Evaluation of Gen-Probe amplified mycobacterium tuberculosis direct test by using respiratory and nonrespiratory specimens in a tertiary care center laboratory. J Clin Microbiol 2002;40:1723–1727.

251. Pai S, Esen N, et al. Routine rapid Mycobacterium species assignment based on species-specific allelic variation in the 65-kilodalton heat shock protein gene (hsp65). Arch Pathol Lab Med 1997;121:859–864.

252. Patel JB, Leonard DG, et al. Sequence-based identification of Mycobacterium species using the MicroSeq 500 16S rDNA bacterial identification system. J Clin Microbiol 2000;38:246–251.

253. Patterson KV, McDonald CL, Miller BF, Chapin KC. Use of UV ParaLens adapter for detection of acid-fast organisms. J Clin Microbiol 1995;33:239–241.

254. Pauls RJ, Turenne CY, et al. A high proportion of novel mycobacteria species identified by 16S rDNA analysis among slowly growing AccuProbe-negative strains in a clinical setting. Am J Clin Pathol 2003;120:560–566.

255. Perchere M, Opravil M., Wald A, et al. Clinical and epidemiologic features of infection with Mycobacterium genavense. Swiss HIV Cohort Study. Arch Intern Med 1995;155:400–404.

256. Peters EJ, Morice R. Miliary pulmonary infection caused by Mycobacterium terrae in an autologous bone marrow transplant patient. Chest 1991;100:1449–1450.

257. Peters M, Schurmann D, Mayr AC, et al. Immunosuppression and mycobacteria other than Mycobacterium tuberculosis: results from patients with and without HIV infection. Epidemiol Infect 1989;103:293–300.

258. Peterson EM, Lu R, Floyd C, et al. Direct identification of Mycobacterium tuberculosis, Mycobacterium avium, and Mycobacterium intracellulare from amplified primary cultures in BACTEC media using DNA probes. J Clin Microbiol 1989;27:1543–1547.

259. Petran EL, Vera HD. Media for selective isolation of mycobacteria. Health Lab Sci 1971;8:2245.

260. Petrini, B. 16S rDNA sequencing in the species identification of non-tuberculous mycobacteria. Scand J Infect Dis 2003;35:519–520.

261. Petrini B, Svartengren G, Hoffner SE, et al. Tenosynovitis of the hand caused by Mycobacterium terrae. Eur J Clin Microbiol Infect Dis 1989;8:722–724.

262. Pfaller M. Application of new technology to the detection, identification, and antimicrobial susceptibility testing of mycobacteria. Am J Clin Pathol 1994;101:329–337.

263. Pfyffer GE, Kissling P, Wirth R, Weber R. Direct detection of Mycobacterium tuberculosis complex in respiratory specimens by a target-amplified test system. J Clin Microbiol 1994;32:918–923.

264. Piersimoni C, Felici L, Penati V, Lacchini C. Mycobacterium malmoense in Italy. Tubercle Lung Dis 1995;76:171–172.

265. Pinheiro MD, Ribeiro MM. Comparison of the Bactec 460TB system and the Bactec MGIT 960 system in recovery of mycobacteria from clinical specimens. Clin Microbiol Infect 2000;6:171–173.

266. Plikaytis BB, Marden JL, Crawford JT, et al. Multiplex PCR assay specific for multidrug-resistant strain W of Mycobacterium tuberculosis. J Clin Microbiol 1994;32:1542–1546.

267. Pollock HM, Wieman EJ. Smear results in the diagnosis of mycobacteriosis using blue light fluorescence microscopy. J Clin Microbiol 1977;5:329–331.

268. Prantera C, Bothamley G, Levenstein S, et al. Crohn's disease and mycobacteria: two cases of Crohn's disease with high anti-mycobacterial antibody levels cured by dapsone therapy. Biomed Pharmacother 1989;43:295–299.

269. Prissick FH, Mason AM. Cervical lymphadenitis in children caused by chromogenic mycobacteria. Can Med Assoc J 1956;75:798–803.

270. Prosser A. Spinal infection with Mycobacterium xenopi. Tubercle 1986;67:229–232.

271. Raad II, Vartivarian S, Khan A, Bodey GP. Catheter-related infections caused by the Mycobacterium fortuitum complex: 15 cases and review. Rev Infect Dis 1991;13:1120–1125.

272. Radford A. Mycobacterium ulcerans in Australia. Aust NZ J Med 1975;5:162–169.

273. Radhika S, Gupta SK, Chakrabarti A, et al. Role of culture for mycobacteria in fine-needle aspiration diagnosis of tuberculous lymphadenitis. Diagn Cytopathol 1989;5:260–262.

274. Rahman MA, Phongsathorn V, Hughes T, Bielawska C. Spinal infection by Mycobacterium xenopi in a non-immunosuppressed patient. Tubercle Lung Dis 1992;73:392–395.

275. Rantakokko-Jalava K, Nikkari S, et al. Direct amplification of rRNA genes in diagnosis of bacterial infections. J Clin Microbiol 2000;38:32–39.

276. Rastogi N, Frehel C, Ryter A, et al. Multiple drug resistance in Mycobacterium avium: is the wall architecture responsible for the exclusion of antimicrobial agents? Antimicrob Agents Chemother 1980;20:666–677.

277. Ratnam SM, March SB. Effect of relative centrifugal force and centrifugation time on sedimentation of mycobacteria in clinical specimens. J Clin Microbiol 1986;23:582–585.

278. Ratnam SM, Stead FA, Howes M. Simplified acetylcysteine-alkali digestion-decontamination procedure for isolation of mycobacteria from clinical specimens. J Clin Microbiol 198725:1428–1432.

279. Narain JP, Raviglione MC, Kochi A. HIV-associated tuberculosis in developing countries: clinical features, diagnosis, and treatment. Bull WHO 1992;70:515–526.

280. Reiner E. Identification of bacterial strains by pyrolysis-gas-liquid chromatography. Nature 1965;206:1272–1274.

281. Reisner BS, Gatson AM, Woods GL. Use of Gen-Probe AccuProbes to identify Mycobacterium avium complex, Mycobacterium tuberculosis complex, Mycobacterium kansasii, and Mycobacterium gordonae directly from BACTEC TB broth cultures. J Clin Microbiol 1994;32:2995–2998.

282. Reisner BS, Gatson AM, et al. Use of Gen-Probe AccuProbes to identify Mycobacterium avium complex, Mycobacterium tuberculosis complex, Mycobacterium kansasii, and Mycobacterium gordonae directly from BACTEC TB broth cultures. J Clin Microbiol 1994;32:2995–2998.

283. Richardson P, Crawford GJ., Smith DW, Xanthis CP. Mycobacterium chelonae keratitis. Aust NZ J Ophthalmol 1989;17:195–196.

284. Rickman TW, Moyer NP. Increased sensitivity of acid fast smears. J Clin Microbiol 1980;11:618–620.

285. Rieder H, Cauthen GM, Kelly GD, et al. Tuberculosis in the United States. JAMA 1989;262:385–389.

286. Ringuet H, Akoua-Koffi C, et al. hsp65 sequencing for identification of rapidly growing mycobacteria. J Clin Microbiol 1999;37:852–857.

287. Roberts GD, Goodman NL, Heifets L, et al. Evaluation of the radiometric method for recovery of mycobacteria and drug susceptibility testing of Mycobacterium tuberculosis from acid-fast smear positive specimens. J Clin Microbiol 1983;18:689–696.

288. Roberts GD, Koneman EW, Kim YK. Mycobacterium. In: Balows A, ed. Manual of Clinical Microbiology. 5th ed. Washington DC: American Society for Microbiology, 1991:Chapter 34.

289. Rodriquez-Barradas MC, Clarridge J, Darouiche R. Disseminated Mycobacterium fortuitum disease in an AIDS patient. Am J Med 1992;93:473–474.

290. Rogers PL, Walker RE, Lane HC, et al. Disseminated Mycobacterium haemophilum infection in two patients with the acquired immunodeficiency syndrome. Am J Med 1988;84:640–642.

291. Rohner P, Ninet B, et al. Evaluation of the Bactec 960 automated nonradiometric system for isolation of mycobacteria from clinical specimens. Eur J Clin Microbiol Infect Dis 2000;19:715–717.

292. Rois MP, Palenque E, Guerrero C, Garcia MJ. Use of restriction fragment length polymorphism as a genetic marker for typing Mycobacterium avium strains. J Clin Microbiol 1995;33:1289–1391.

293. Rondini S, Mensah-Quainoo E, et al. Development and application of real-time PCR assay for quantification of Mycobacterium ulcerans DNA. J Clin Microbiol 2003;41:4231–4237.

294. Rose HD, Dorff GJ, Lauwasser M, et al. Pulmonary and disseminated Mycobacterium simiae infection in humans. Am Rev Respir Dis 1982;126:1110–1113.

295. Ruiz P, Zerolo FJ, et al. Comparison of susceptibility testing of Mycobacterium tuberculosis using the ESP culture system II with that using the BACTEC method. J Clin Microbiol 2000;38:4663–4664.

296. Runyon E. Identification of mycobacterial pathogens utilizing colony characteristics. Am J Clin Pathol 1970;54:578–586.

297. Saito H, T. H. Susceptibilities of transparent, opaque, and rough colonial variants of Mycobacterium avium complex to various fatty acids. Antimicrob Agents Chemother 1988;32:400–402.

298. Salfinger, M. Role of the laboratory in evaluating patients with mycobacterial disease. Clin Microbiol Newslett 1995;17:108–111.

299. Salfinger M, Hale YM, et al. Diagnostic tools in tuberculosis. Present and future. Respiration 1998;65:163–170.

300. Salfinger M, Morris AJ. The role of the microbiology laboratory in diagnosing mycobacterial diseases. Am J Clin Pathol 1994;101(Suppl 1):S6–S13.

301. Sanders WE Jr, Horowitz EA. Other mycobacteria species. In: Mandell GL, Bennett JE, eds. Principles and Practice of Infectious Diseases. New York: Churchill Livingstone, 1990: Chapter 231.

302. Sanderson JD, Moss MT, Tiozard ML, Hermon-Taylor. Mycobacterium paratuberculosis DNA in Crohn's disease tissue. Gut 1992;33:890–896.

303. Sanguinetti M, Ardito F, et al. Fatal pulmonary infection due to multidrug-resistant Mycobacterium abscessus in a patient with cystic fibrosis. J Clin Microbiol 2001;39:816–819.

304. Scarparo C, Piccoli P, et al. Direct identification of mycobacteria from MB/BacT alert 3D bottles: comparative evaluation of two commercial probe assays. J Clin Microbiol 2001;39:3222–3227.

305. Schaefer WB, Davis CL, Cohn ML. Pathogenicity of transparent, opaque and rough variants of Mycobacterium avium in chickens and mice. Am Rev Respir Dis 1970;102:499–506.

306. Scherer R, Sable R, Sonnenberg M, et al. Disseminated infection with Mycobacterium kansasii in the acquired immunodeficiency syndrome. Ann Intern Med 1986;105:710–712.

307. Schlossberg D, Aaron T. Aortitis caused by Mycobacterium fortuitum. Arch Intern Med 1991;151:1010–1011.

308. Schroder KH, Juhlin I. Mycobacterium malmoense sp. nov. Int J Syst Bacteriol 1977;27:241–246.

309. Schuurman T, de Boer RF, et al. Prospective study of use of PCR amplification and sequencing of 16S ribosomal DNA from cerebrospinal fluid for diagnosis of bacterial meningitis in a clinical setting. J Clin Microbiol 2004;42:734–740.

310. Selwyn PA, Hartel D, Lewis VA, et al. A prospective study of the risk of tuberculosis among intravenous drug users with human immunodeficiency virus infection. N Engl J Med 1989;320:545–550.

311. Sewell DL, Rashad AL., Rourke WJ, et al. Comparison of the Septi-Chek AFB and BACTEC systems and conventional culture for recovery of mycobacteria. J Clin Microbiol 1993;31:2689–2691.

312. Shafer RW, Sierra MF. Mycobacterium xenopi, Mycobacterium fortuitum, Mycobacterium kansasii, and other nontuberculous mycobacteria in an area of endemicity for AIDS. Clin Infect Dis 1992;15:161–162.

313. Shah RR, Dye WE. The use of dithiothreitol to replace N-acetyl-L-cysteine for routine sputum digestion-decontamination for the culture of mycobacteria. Am Rev Respir Dis 1966;94:454.

314. Sharma M, Sethi S, et al. Rapid detection of mutations in rpoB gene of rifampicin resistant Mycobacterium tuberculosis strains by line probe assay. Indian J Med Res 2003;117:76–80.

315. Shrestha NK, Tuohy MJ, et al. Detection and differentiation of Mycobacterium tuberculosis and nontuberculous mycobacterial isolates by real-time PCR. J Clin Microbiol 2003;41:5121–5126.

316. Silcox VA, Good RA, Floyd MM. Identification of clinically significant Mycobacterium fortuitum complex isolates. J Clin Microbiol 1981;14:686–691.

317. Simor WE, Salit IE, Vellend H. Role of Mycobacterium xenopi in human disease. Am Rev Respir Dis 1984;129:435–438.

318. Singh M, B. A., Cave G, Boyle P. Mycobacterium fortuitum endocarditis in a patient with chronic renal failure on hemodialysis. Pathology 1992;24:197–200.

319. Slosarek M, Kubin M, Jaresova M. Water-borne household infections due to Mycobacterium xenopi. Central Eur J Public Health 1993;1:78–80.

320. Slutsky AM, Arbeit RD, Barber TW, et al. Polyclonal infections due to Mycobacterium avium complex in patients with AIDS detected by pulsed-field gel electrophoresis of sequential clinical isolates. J Clin Microbiol 1994;32:1773–1778.

321. Smithwick RW, et al. Use of cetylpyridium chloride and sodium chloride for the decontamination of sputum specimens that are transported to the laboratory for the isolation of Mycobacterium tuberculosis. J Clin Microbiol 1975;1:411–413.

322. Snider DE Jr, Cohn DL, Davidson PT, et al. Standard therapy for tuberculosis. Chest 1985;87(Suppl):S117–S124.

323. Sommers H. Special Mycobacterial Survey. Skokie, IL: College of American Pathologists, 1976.

324. Sommers HM, Good RC. Mycobacterium. In: Lennette EH, ed. Manual of Clinical Microbiology. 4th ed. Washington, DC: American Society for Microbiology, 1985.Chapter 22.

325. Somoskovi A, Song Q, et al. Use of molecular methods to identify the Mycobacterium tuberculosis complex (MTBC) and other mycobacterial species and to detect rifampin resistance in MTBC isolates following growth detection with the BACTEC MGIT 960 system. J Clin Microbiol 2003;41:2822–2826.

326. Sompolinsky D, Lagziel A, Naveh D, Yankilevitz T. Mycobacterium haemophilum sp. nov., a new pathogen of humans. Int J Syst Bacteriol 1978;28:67–75.

327. Soriano F, Rodriquez-Tudela JL Gomez-Garces JL, Velo M. Two possibly related cases of Mycobacterium fortuitum peritonitis associated with continuous ambulatory peritoneal dialysis. Eur J Clin Microbiol Infect Dis 1989;8:895–897.

328. Springer B, Stockman L, et al. Two-laboratory collaborative study on identification of mycobacteria: molecular versus phenotypic methods. J Clin Microbiol 1996;34:296–303.

329. Stahl DA, Urbance JW: The division between fast- and slow-growing species corresponds to natural relationships among the mycobacteria. J Bacteriol 1990;172:116–124.

330. National Committee for Clinical Laboratory Standards. Methods for determining bactericidal activity of antimicrobial agents (M26P). Villanova PA: National Committee for Clinical Laboratory Standards, 1987.

331. Stead WW, Dutt D. Chemotherapy for tuberculosis today. Am Rev Respir Dis 1982;125(Suppl 3):94–101.

332. Steele LC, Wallace RJ. Ability of ciprofloxacin but not pipemidic acid to differentiate all three biovariants of Mycobacterium fortuitum from Mycobacterium chelonae. J Clin Microbiol 1987;25:456–457.

333. Steingrube VA, Gibson JL, Brown BA, et al. PCR amplification and restriction endonuclease analysis of a 65-kilodalton heat shock protein gene sequence for taxonomic separation of rapidly growing mycobacteria. J Clin Microbiol 1995;33:149–153.

334. Stone BL, Cohn DL, Kane MS, et al. Utility of paired blood cultures and smears in diagnosis of disseminated Mycobacterium avium complex infections in AIDS patients. J Clin Microbiol 1994;32:842.

335. Stone, R. Tuberculosis rebounds while funding lags. Science 1992;255:1064.

336. Stormer RS, Falkingham JO 3d. Differences in antimicrobial susceptibility of pigmented and unpigmented colonial variants of Mycobacterium avium. J Clin Microbiol 1989;27:2459–2465.

337. Strand CL, Epstein C, Verzosa S, et al. Evaluation of a new blood culture medium for mycobacteria. Am J Clin Pathol 1989;91:316–318.

338. Straus WL, Ostroff SM, Jernigan DB, et al. Clinical and epidemiologic characteristics of Mycobacterium haemophilum, an emerging pathogen in immunocompromised patients. Ann Intern Med 1994;120:118–125.

339. Suffys, P. N., A. da Silva Rocha, et al. Rapid identification of Mycobacteria to the species level using INNO-LiPA Mycobacteria, a reverse hybridization assay. J Clin Microbiol 2001;39:4477–4482.

340. Sullivan EA, Kreisworth BN, Palumbo L, Kapur V, et al. Emergence of fluoroquinolone-resistant tuberculosis in New York City. Lancet 1995;345:1148–1150.

341. Talbot E, Moore M, et al. Tuberculosis among foreign-born persons in the United States, 1993–1998. JAMA 2000;284:2894–2900.

342. Taylor S. Pulmonary disease caused by Mycobacterium asiaticum. Tubercle 1990;71:303–305.

343. Telzak E. Tuberculosis and human immunodeficiency virus infection. Med Clin North Am 1997;81:345–360.

344. Tenholder MF, Moser RJ, Tellis CJ. Mycobacteria other than M. tuberculosis. Pulmonary involvement in patients with AIDS. Arch Intern Med 1988;148:953–955.

345. Thibert L, Lebel F, Martineau B. Two cases of Mycobacterium haemophilum infection in Canada. J Clin Microbiol 1990;28:621–623.

346. Tisdall PA, Roberts GE, Anhalt JP. Identification of clinical isolates of mycobacteria with gas-liquid chromatography alone. J Clin Microbiol 1979;10:506–514.

347. Tonner JA, Hammond MD. Pulmonary disease caused by Mycobacterium terrae complex. South Med J 1989;82:1279–1282.

348. Torrea G, Levee G, Grimont P, et al. Chromosomal DNA fingerprinting analysis using the insertion sequence IS6110 and the repetitive element DR as strain-specific markers for epidemiological study of tuberculosis in French Polynesia. J Clin Microbiol 1995;33:1899–1904.

349. Tortoli E, Cichero P, et al. Use of BACTEC MGIT 960 for recovery of mycobacteria from clinical specimens: multicenter study. J Clin Microbiol 1999;37:3578–3582.

350. Tortoli E, Mariottini A, et al. Evaluation of INNO-LiPA MYCOBACTERIA v2: improved reverse hybridization multiple DNA probe assay for mycobacterial identification. J Clin Microbiol 2003;41:4418–4420.

351. Tortoli E, Nanetti A, et al. Performance assessment of new multiplex probe assay for identification of mycobacteria. J Clin Microbiol 2001;39:1079–1084.

352. Tortoli E, Simonetti MT, et al. Evaluation of a commercial DNA probe assay for the identification of Mycobacterium kansasii. Eur J Clin Microbiol Infect Dis 1994;13:264–267.

353. Tortoli E, Simonetti MT, Labardi C, et al. Mycobacterium xenopi isolation from clinical specimens in the Florence area: review of 46 cases. Eur J Epidemiol 1991;7:677–678.

354. Tortoli E, Simonetti MT, Lacchini C, et al. Tentative evidence of AIDS-associated biotype of Mycobacterium kansasii. J Clin Microbiol 1994;32:1779–1782.

355. Troesch A, Nguyen H, et al. Mycobacterium species identification and rifampin resistance testing with high-density DNA probe arrays. J Clin Microbiol 1999;37:49–55.

356. Tuohy MJ, Hall G, Procop GW. The Rapid Identification of Routine Clinical Mycobacteria by Pyrosequencing™. 42nd ICAAC Meeting, San Diego, CA, 2002.

357. Uribe-Botero G, Prichard JG, Kaplowitz HJ. Bone marrow in HIV infections: a comparison of fluorescent staining and cultures in the detection of mycobacteria. Am J Clin Pathol 1989;91:313–315.

358. Vadney FS, Hawkins JE. Evaluation of a simple method for growing Mycobacterium haemophilum. J Clin Microbiol 1985;22:884–885.

359. Valainis GT, Cardona LM, Greer DL. The spectrum of Mycobacterium kansasii disease associated with HIV-1 infected patients. J AIDS 1991;4:516–520.

360. van Soolingen D, de Haas PE, Haagsma J, et al. Use of various genetic markers in differentiation of Mycobacterium bovis strains from animals and humans and for studying epidemiology of bovine tuberculosis. J Clin Microbiol 1994;32:2425–2433.

361. Vetter E, Torgerson C, et al. Comparison of the BACTEC MYCO/F Lytic bottle to the isolator tube, BACTEC Plus Aerobic F/bottle, and BACTEC Anaerobic Lytic/10 bottle and comparison of the BACTEC Plus Aerobic F/bottle to the Isolator tube for recovery of bacteria, mycobacteria, and fungi from blood. J Clin Microbiol 2001;39:4380–4386.

362. Viader-Salvado JM, Luna-Aguirre CM, et al. Frequency of mutations in rpoB and codons 315 and 463 of katG in rifampin- and/or isoniazid-resistant Mycobacterium tuberculosis isolates from northeast Mexico. Microb Drug Resist 2003;9:33–38.

363. Voldstedlund M, Pedersen LN, et al. Different polymerase chain reaction-based analyses for culture-negative endocarditis caused by Streptococcus pneumoniae. Scand J Infect Dis 2003;35:757–9.

364. von Reyn CF, Maslow JN, Barber TW, et al. Persistent colonization of potable water as a source of Mycobacterium avium infection in AIDS. Lancet 1994;343:1137–1141.

365. Vuorinen P, Miettinen A, Vuento R, Hallstrom O. Direct detection of Mycobacterium tuberculosis complex in respiratory specimens by Gen-Probe Amplified Mycobacterium tuberculosis Direct Test and Roche Amplicor Mycobacterium tuberculosis Test. J Clin Microbiol 1995;33:1856–1859.

366. Wallace RJ, Brown B, et al. Skin, soft tissue, and bone infections due to Mycobacterium chelonae chelonae: importance of prior corticosteroid therapy, frequency of disseminated infections, and resistance to oral antimicrobials other than clarithromycin. J Infect Dis 1992;166:405–412.

367. Wallace RJ Jr, Dunbar D, Brown BA, et al. Rifampin-resistant Mycobacterium kansasii. Clin Infect Dis 1994;18:736–743.

368. Wallace RJ Jr, Swenson JM, Silcox VA, et al. Spectrum of disease due to rapidly growing mycobacteria. Rev Infect Dis 1983;5:657–679.

369. Wallace RJ Jr, Swenson JM, et al. Spectrum of disease due to rapidly growing mycobacteria. Rev Infect Dis 1983;5:657–679.

370. Wang SX, Sng LH, et al. Preliminary study on rapid identification of Mycobacterium tuberculosis complex isolates by the BD ProbeTec ET system. J Med Microbiol 2004;53(Part 1):57–59.

371. Warren NG, Body BA, Silcox VA, Matthews JH. Pulmonary disease due to Mycobacterium malmoense. J Clin Microbiol 1984;20:245–247.

372. Wasilauskas B, Morrell R Jr. Optimum recovery of Mycobacterium avium complex from blood specimens of human immunodeficiency virus-positive patients by using small volumes of isolator concentrate inoculated into BACTEC 12B bottles. J Clin Microbiol 1995;33:784–785.

373. Wayne, L. Simple pyrazinamidase and urease tests for routine identification of mycobacteria. Am Rev Respir Dis 1974;109:147–151.

374. Wayne, L. Microbiology of tubercle bacilli. Am J Respir Dis Suppl 1982;125:31–41.

375. Wayne LG, Kubica GP. Genus Mycobacterium. In: Sneath PHA, Sharpe ME, Holt JG, eds. Bergey's Manual of Systematic Bacteriology. Vol. 2. Baltimore: Williams & Wilkins, 1986:1436–1457.

376. Wayne LG, Sramek HA. Agents of newly recognized or infrequently encountered mycobacterial diseases. Clin Microbiol Rev 1992;5:1–25.

377. Weber J, Mettang T, Staerz E, et al. Pulmonary disease due to Mycobacterium xenopi in a renal allograft patient. Rev Infect Dis 1989;11:964–969.

378. Weinberger M, Berg SL, Feuerstein IM, et al. Disseminated infection with Mycobacterium gordonae: report of a case and critical review of the literature. Clin Infect Dis 1992;14:1229–1239.

378a. Weissfeiler J, Karassova V, Holland J. Atypical mycobacteria in monkeys. Acta Microbiologica Academiae Scientiarum Hungaricae 1964–65;11:403–407.

379. Weiszfeiler JG, Karczag E. Synonymy of Mycobacterium simiae Karasseva et al, 1965 and Mycobacterium habana Valdiva et al. Int J Syst Bacteriol 1971;26:474–477.

380. Weitzman I, Osadczyi K, Corrado ML, Karp D. Mycobacterium thermoresistible: a new pathogen for humans. J Clin Microbiol 1981;14:593–595.

381. Wendt SL, George KL, Parker BC, et al. Epidemiology of infection by nontuberculous mycobacteria. III. Isolation of potentially pathogenic mycobacteria from aerosols. Am Rev Respir Dis 1980;122:259–263.

382. Westergren V, Bassiri M, et al. Bacteria detected by culture and 16S rRNA sequencing in maxillary sinus samples from intensive care unit patients. Laryngoscope 2003;113:270–275.

383. Whelen AC, Feknkee TA, Hunt JM, et al. Direct genotypic detection of Mycobacterium tuberculosis rifampin resistance in clinical specimens by using single-tube heminested PCR. J Clin Microbiol 1995;33:556–561.

383a. Whittier PS, Westfall K, Setterquist S, Hopfer RL. Evaluation of the Septi-Chek AFB system in the recovery of mycobacteria. Eur J Clin Microbiol 1992;11:915–918.

384. Whyte T, Cormican M, et al. Comparison of BACTEC MGIT 960 and BACTEC 460 for culture of Mycobacteria. Diagn Microbiol Infect Dis 2000;38:123–126.

385. Wiid IJ, Werely C, Beyers N, et al. Oligonucleotide (GTS)5 as a marker for Mycobacterium tuberculosis strain identification. J Clin Microbiol 1994;32:1318–1321.

386. Wilkins EGI, Gruffutgs RH, Roberts C. Pulmonary tuberculosis due to Mycobacterium bovis. Thorax 1986;41:685–687.

387. Williams DL, Gillis TP, Dupree WG. Ethanol fixation of sputum sediments for DNA-based detection of Mycobacterium tuberculosis. J Clin Microbiol 1995;33:1558–1561.

388. Williams-Bouyer N, Yorke R, et al. Comparison of the BACTEC MGIT 960 and ESP culture system II for growth and detection of mycobacteria. J Clin Microbiol 2000;38:4167–4170.

389. Willocks L, Leen C, Brettle RP, et al. Isolation of Mycobacterium malmoense from HIV-positive patients. J Infect Dis 1993;26:345–346.

390. Witebsky FG, Keiser J, Conville P, et al. Comparison of BACTEC 13A medium and Du Pont Isolator for detection of mycobacteremia. J Clin Microbiol 1988;26:1501–1505.

391. Wobeser WL, Krajden M, Conly J, et al. Evaluation of Roche Amplicor PCR assay for Mycobacterium tuberculosis. J Clin Microbiol 1996;34:134–139.

392. Wolfe JM, Moore DF. Isolation of Mycobacterium thermoresistible following augmentation of mammaplasty. J Clin Microbiol 1992;30:1036–1038.

393. Wolinski, E. Nontuberculous mycobacteria and associated diseases. Am Rev Respir Dis 1979;119:107–159.

394. Wong B, Edwards FF, Kiehn TE, et al. Continuous high-grade Mycobacterium avium-intracellulare bacteremia in patients with the acquired immune deficiency syndrome. Am J Med 1985;78:35–40.

395. Woodley C. Evaluation of streptomycin and ethambutol concentrations for susceptibility testing of Mycobacterium tuberculosis by radiometric and conventional procedures. J Clin Microbiol 1986;23:385–386.

396. Woods GL, Brown-Elliott, BA, Desmond EP, et al. Susceptibility testing of mycobacteria, nocardiae, and other aerobic actinomycetes; approved standard. NCCLS 2003;23(18):1–68.

397. Woods GL, Pentony E, Boxley MJ, Gatson AM. Concentration of sputum by cytocentrifugation for preparation of smears for detection of acid-fast bacilli does not increase sensitivity of the fluorochrome stain. J Clin Microbiol 1995;33:1915–1916.

398. Woods GL, Witebsky FG. College of American Pathologists Mycobacteriology E Proficiency Testing Survey: summary of participant performance, 1979–1992. Arch Pathol Lab Med 1995;119:17–22.

399. Woods GL, Washington JA II. Mycobacteria other than Mycobacterium tuberculosis: review of microbiologic and clinical aspects. Rev Infect Dis 1987;9:275–294.

400. Xu J, Millar BC, et al. Employment of broad-range 16S rRNA PCR to detect aetiological agents of infection from clinical specimens in patients with acute meningitis—rapid separation of 16S rRNA PCR amplicons without the need for cloning. J Appl Microbiol 2003;94:197–206.

401. Yajko DM, Wagner C, Tevere VJ, et al. Quantitative culture of Mycobacterium tuberculosis from clinical sputum specimens and dilution endpoint of its detection by the Amplicor PCR assay. J Clin Microbiol 1995;33:1944–1947.

402. Yakrus MA, Hernandez SM, et al. Comparison of methods for Identification of Mycobacterium abscessus and M. chelonae isolates. J Clin Microbiol 2001;39:4103–4110.

403. Yakrus MA, Straus WL. DNA polymorphisms detected in Mycobacterium haemophilum by pulsed-field gel electrophoresis. J Clin Microbiol 1994;32:1083–1084.

404. Yamori S, Tsukamura M. Comparison of prognosis of pulmonary diseases caused by Mycobacterium avium and by Mycobacterium intracellulare. Chest 1992;102:89–90.

405. Yang ZH, de Haas PE, van Soolingen D, et al. Restriction fragment length polymorphism Mycobacterium tuberculosis strains isolated from Greenland during 1992: evidence of tuberculosis transmission between Greenland and Denmark. J Clin Microbiol 1994;32:3018–3025.

406. Yang ZH, Mtoni I, Chonde M, et al. DNA fingerprinting and phenotyping of Mycobacterium tuberculosis isolates from human immunodeficiency virus (HIV)-seropositive and HIV-seronegative patients in Tanzania. J Clin Microbiol 1995;33:1064–1069.

407. Yoganathan K, Elliot MW, Moxham J, et al. Pseudotumor of the lung caused by Mycobacterium malmoense infection in an HIV positive patient. Thorax 1994;49:179–180.

408. Young LS, Interlied CB, Berlin OG, Gottlieb MS. Mycobacterial infections in AIDS patients with emphasis on the Mycobacterium avium complex. Rev Infect Dis 1986;8:1024–1033.

409. Zala L, Nunzikere T, Braathen L. Chronic cutaneous infection caused by Mycobacterium gordonae. Dermatology 1993;187:301–302.

410. Zaugg M, Salfinger M, Opravil M, Luthy R. Extrapulmonary and disseminated infections due to Mycobacterium malmoense: case report and review. Clin Infect Dis 1993;16:540–549.

411. Zwadyk P Jr, Down JA, Myers N, Dey MS. Rendering of mycobacteria safe for molecular diagnostic studies and development of a lysis method for strand displacement amplification and PCR. J Clin Microbiol 1994;32:2140–2146.

CHAPTER 20

Spirochetal Infections

Taxonomy

Treponema

Treponema pallidum Subspecies pallidum

Incubation Period
Primary Syphilis
Secondary Syphilis
Latent Syphilis
Late Syphilis
Epidemiology
Immunity

Treponema pallidum Subspecies pertenue

Treponema pallidum Subspecies endemicum

Treponema carateum

Laboratory Diagnosis of Treponemal Diseases

Serologic Tests
Innovations: Provisional and Investigative Tests

Borrelia

Relapsing Fever

Epidemiology
Clinical Disease
Laboratory Diagnosis

Lyme Disease

Epidemiology
Clinical Disease
Laboratory Diagnosis

Leptospira

Leptospirosis

Epidemiology
Clinical Disease
Laboratory Diagnosis

Spirillum minor (Rat-Bite Fever)

The past several decades have been a good time to buy stock in spirochetes. At one extreme, *Treponema pallidum*, a scourge of humans for centuries, was almost eliminated by penicillin, but has staged a dramatic comeback that continues into the new century. At the other end of the spectrum *Borrelia burgdorferi*, recognized only 20 years ago, has become the most common spirochetal infection in the United States.[45,47]

This large and diverse group of bacteria includes pathogens and saprophytes. There are microaerophiles, strict anaerobes, species that have been cultured only in vivo, and some species that have never been cultured under any conditions. Some organisms have complex ecologic relations, and humans are only incidental victims. Other spirochetes infect only humans and must be transmitted directly from person to person.

Taxonomy

The order Spirochaetales contains the major human pathogens. They are all helically shaped, motile bacteria that measure 0.1 to 3.0 μm in diameter by 5 to 120 μm in length.[42] The flagella of most spirochetes are encased within the multilayered outer membrane, referred to as an outer sheath. The genus *Spirillum*, however, has external flagella. In contrast with other bacteria, the spirochetes propel themselves by rotation through a liquid environment and are able to maintain their motility, even in high-viscosity liquids.

The classification of the pathogenic spirochetes is detailed in Table 20-1. The pathogens are concentrated in three genera: *Treponema*, *Borrelia*, and *Leptospira*.

Treponema

The four major pathogens in the genus *Treponema* are genetically related, infect only humans, and have not been cultivated indefinitely in vitro. Despite these similarities they produce very different diseases.

Treponema pallidum Subspecies *pallidum*

T. pallidum subspecies *pallidum* (hereafter called *T. pallidum*) is the dominant pathogen among the spirochetes. *T.*

pallidum, the cause of venereal syphilis, has been infamous for 500 years. It shares "100%" genetic homology with *T. pallidum* subspecies *pertenue,* which causes a nonvenereal cutaneous disease that differs in most aspects from syphilis.[177] One group of investigators, who tested a reference strain of each organism, reported a difference of only one nucleotide in the gene coding for a 19-kDa protein,[192] but the immunoreactivity of this protein was identical in the two subspecies.[191] In 1998 the entire genome of *T. pallidum* was sequenced.[88]

The origin of *T. pallidum* is uncertain. The disease did not appear prominently in Europe until the 16th century. Fornaciari and colleagues studied a Renaissance mummy that contained structures identified by immunofluorescence and electron microscopy as *T. pallidum*.[86] Devotees of one school of thought believe that Columbus and his sailors brought the disease back from the New World.[22] These historians identify *T. pallidum* as the "Great Pox," whereas variola virus produced the "Small Pox." It is hypothesized that the Great Pox developed from a milder clinical disease in American Indians. There is abundant evidence of bone changes similar to those of syphilis in New World skeletons.[229] Similar lesions have also been noted in pre-Columbian skeletons from the Old World; the question has not been answered definitively because the osseous lesions of venereal and nonvenereal syphilis are difficult to differentiate. Rothschild and Rothschild have suggested discriminators among treponemal species if adequate material is avail-

Table 20-1 Classification of Spirochetes		
ORGANISM	GEOGRAPHIC LOCATION	DISEASE
Order Spirochaetales		
Family *Spirochaetaceae*		
Genus III. *Treponema*		
T. pallidum subspecies *pallidum*	Worldwide	Venereal syphilis
T. pallidum subspecies *pertenue*	Tropical Asia, Africa, South and Central America	Yaws
T. pallidum subspecies *endemicum*	Africa, SE Asia, Middle East, Yugoslavia	Endemic, nonvenereal syphilis
T. carateum	Central and South America	Pinta
"*T. pallidum*-like oral spirochetes"	Worldwide	Necrotizing gingivitis
Genus IV. *Borrelia*		
Borrelia spp.	Worldwide	Tick-borne relapsing fever
Borrelia recurrentis	South America, Europe, Africa, Asia	Louse-borne relapsing fever
Borrelia burgdorferi	North America, Europe	Lyme disease
Family *Leptospiraceae*		
Genus I. *Leptospira*		
Leptospira interrogans	Worldwide	Leptospirosis

Adapted from Krieg NR, Holt JR, eds.: Bergey's Manual of Systematic Bacteriology. Baltimore: Williams & Wilkins, 1984 : 38–64.

able.[230] Whatever the original source, each European country chose to associate the disease with its neighbor. To the English, syphilis was the "French disease." The French considered it the "Italian pox." It seems that no culture or country wants to claim this particular scourge.

The clinical presentation of venereal syphilis is varied and complex. Sir William Osler, one of the founders of modern medicine, referred to the disease as "the great imitator" and admonished students that if they knew syphilis, they would know medicine. The clinical disease has been somewhat arbitrarily divided into a series of stages, as outlined below.[115,259,291]

INCUBATION PERIOD

The treponemes are introduced into the body through a mucous membrane or a cut or abrasion on the skin. It has been estimated epidemiologically that as many as 50% of sexual contacts of infectious persons escape infection. Experimental studies in human volunteers have documented, however, that the ID_{50} (the number of organisms needed to infect 50% of those exposed) for *T. pallidum* is as few as 57 organisms.[166] Shortly after inoculation the spirochetes are disseminated throughout the body, where they may eventually cause disease. The incubation period varies from 3 to 90 days, with a mean of 3 weeks.

PRIMARY SYPHILIS

This phase encompasses the development of the primary lesion at the site of inoculation. The inflammatory reaction creates an ulcerated lesion, called a chancre. The chancre has a clean, smooth base, and the edge is raised and firm. The ulcer is usually painless, although slightly tender. There is scant exudate unless the chancre is secondarily infected. There is usually a single primary chancre, but multiple primary ulcers may occur in patients with the acquired immunodeficiency syndrome (AIDS). The base contains spirochetes that can be visualized by darkfield microscopy or immunofluorescence after scraping of the lesion.

The chancre occurs at the inoculation site, most commonly on the genitalia. Occasionally, syphilis may occur without a visible ulcer.[268] The regional lymph nodes are enlarged, but painless and firm. The chancre heals in 3 to 6 weeks (range, 1 to 12).

The laboratory diagnosis of primary syphilis depends on demonstration of spirochetes in the lesions by darkfield microscopy or direct immunofluorescence in addition to serology.[116] Nontreponemal tests for syphilis are negative in 10–30% of patients with primary syphilis.[146]

SECONDARY SYPHILIS

The secondary phase of dissemination is the most florid part of the disease and is the period when organisms are most numerous. The secondary phase begins 2 to 8 weeks after the appearance of the chancre and lasts for a few days to months. The most dramatic presentation is a widespread rash, which may be macular, maculopapular, or pustular, but not vesicular. The rash in syphilis characteristically involves the palms of the hands and soles of the feet. In moist intertriginous areas, broad, moist, gray-white plaques called condylomata lata are teeming with infectious spirochetes, which can be visualized by darkfield microscopy or immunofluorescence in scrapings of the lesions. Similarly, infectious lesions called mucous patches are found on mucous membranes. There may be loss of hair or thinning of the eyebrows.

Systemic symptoms include generalized lymphadenopathy, fever, and malaise. Virtually any organ may be involved in secondary syphilis. Keratitis, hepatitis, and osteitis can be found. Infection of the central nervous system occurs at any stage of syphilis, but is most common in the secondary phase.[239] Meningismus and headache are common. Aseptic meningitis may develop. Spirochetes can also be cultured from the cerebrospinal fluid (CSF), however, without any evidence of inflammation and without clinical disease.[160]

The borderline between the primary and secondary phases is not cleanly drawn. On occasion, the primary chancre may still be present when the secondary rash appears.

The laboratory diagnosis of secondary syphilis can usually be established easily by serologic techniques. The diagnosis of neurosyphilis is more difficult, as discussed below. Abnormalities of CSF in a patient with a serologic diagnosis of syphilis provide presumptive evidence that the nervous system has been involved.

LATENT SYPHILIS

Following the secondary phase, the disease becomes subclinical, although not necessarily dormant. The latent phase has been arbitrarily divided into an initial 4-year period, referred to as the early latent phase, and a subsequent late latent period.[44] During early latency, relapses may occur, and the patient is infectious. Ninety percent of the relapses occur within the first year. The late latent period is of indefinite duration, and complications may never appear. During the latent stage of syphilis the presence of the disease can be detected only serologically.

LATE SYPHILIS

Late complications of syphilis include central nervous system disease, cardiovascular abnormalities, and tumors, called gummas, in any organ. Late neurovascular syphilis may be symptomatic or asymptomatic.[117] Asymptomatic disease is characterized by CSF abnormalities in the absence of symptoms. Pleocytosis, elevated protein levels, or depressed glucose levels are usually found in the CSF. A positive serologic test, classically the VDRL assay, in the CSF defines the disease, although the spirochetes are rarely demonstrated by culture or, more recently, by molecular methods. Symptomatic infection is either meningovascular or parenchymatous, but there is considerable overlap in the categories. Meningovascular syphilis resembles the aseptic meningitis of the secondary stage. Any cranial nerve may be affected by the inflammation, and deafness or visual impairment may result. Parenchymatous disease may involve the neurons of either the cerebrum or the spinal cord. Cerebral involvement is manifested as a wide variety of neuropsychiatric disturbances, including physical changes, such as paralysis, and psychiatric problems, such as delusions of grandeur ("general paresis of the insane"). The posterior columns (sensory tracts) of the spinal cord are preferentially affected, causing severe pains and inability to perceive sensual impulses from the extremities. The disease, called tabes dorsalis, includes a peculiar "slapping" gait and deformed knees (Charcot's joints), which are caused by the lack of the feedback loop that tells the body to "go easy" on the joints.

The interval between primary disease and neurologic complication is 5 to 10 years for meningovascular syphilis, 15 to 20 years for general paresis, and 25 to 30 years for tabes dorsalis.

Cardiovascular Syphilis. The cardiovascular lesion in tertiary (late) syphilis, syphilitic aortitis, occurs in approximately 10% of untreated cases. It is caused by inflammation in the small vessels that feed the aorta (syphilitic endarteritis) and affects primarily the ascending aorta. Two complications may result: an aortic aneurysm and dilatation of the aortic ring causing insufficiency and regurgitation of blood through the aortic valve. Aortic aneurysms may grow to such a size that they erode through the sternum and are visualized under the skin of the chest.

Late "Benign" Syphilis. This phase is characterized by the formation of nonspecific granulomatous lesions called gummas. This lesion is the most common complication in late syphilis and occurs in approximately 15% of untreated patients. The formation of the granuloma indicates a fully active cellular immune response. The gumma, however, may destroy surrounding tissue as it enlarges.[222] Clinically, gummas are destructive mass lesions in virtually any organ and may be mistaken initially for carcinomas.

The laboratory diagnosis of late syphilis requires the demonstration of serologic reactivity with a treponemal or nontreponemal test. The only universally recognized test for the documentation of neurosyphilis is the nontreponemal VDRL test as adapted for spinal fluid. Unfortunately, this test is very insensitive, but other serologic tests are prone to nonspecificity. It has been suggested that the fluorescent treponemal antibody absorption (FTA-ABS) test be used as a more sensitive screening test to eliminate patients with nonreactive spinal fluids from further consideration, but there is no currently approved test in the United States for this purpose.

Congenital Syphilis. One of the greatest tragedies of syphilis is the intrauterine infection of the fetus.[302] Reflecting the increase in the general population, congenital syphilis has increased steadily since 1983.[63] Transplacental infection is most likely to occur during the primary or secondary stages of syphilis (see Color Plate 20-1*A*). The spirochetes may infect the fetus at any time during pregnancy, but the likelihood of clinical disease increases as the pregnancy progresses.

Many of the infected fetuses die. In some areas of the country congenital syphilis is the most common cause of nonimmune hydrops, a disease of the placenta that causes fetal death.[21] Of those who survive, half are asymptomatic and the remainder have the lesions of secondary syphilis without detectable primary lesions because they do not have a single primary portal of entry. Hepatosplenomegaly, meningitis, thrombocytopenia, anemia, and bone lesions characterize the infection.[154] Intrauterine infection of bone may result in visible abnormalities of bone and teeth, such as deformed tibias (saber shins) or teeth (mulberry molars). To prevent this tragedy, screening of women during pregnancy

has been recommended. In high-risk populations it is additionally necessary to test maternal and neonatal sera for antibody at delivery. Cord blood is inferior to neonatal sera.[50]

The interpretation of serologic tests in congenital infection is difficult. Symptomatic infants born to untreated seropositive mothers require antimicrobial therapy. If the mother has received adequate penicillin therapy, congenital infection is unlikely and it has been recommended that the infant be followed closely.[108] The VDRL test usually reverts to normal within 6 months and the FTA-ABS test within 1 year.[49] Traditional attempts to detect IgM antibody in the infant have floundered on the shoals of insensitivity and nonspecificity.

New approaches and variations of traditional approaches, however, provide additional means for evaluation of infants born to mothers who have positive syphilis serology. Modifications of methods for detection of IgM, use of immunoblots with defined antigens,[33] detection of spirochetes by direct immunofluorescence, and detection of nucleic acid with amplification techniques[237] have been used. Funisitis (inflammation of the umbilical cord) with or without necrosis may be documented in somewhat less than half of mothers with serologic evidence of syphilis.[101] The treponemal etiology can be documented by immunohistochemistry, but few laboratories will have such capability.

A combination of serology and detection of antigen or genome in the infant of an infected mother provides the best chance for documenting congenital syphilis, including neurosyphilis.[178] In the absence of clear evidence that the mother has been adequately treated, empiric treatment of the infant is indicated until tests with sufficient sensitivity to eliminate the possibility of intrauterine infection are widely available.

EPIDEMIOLOGY

Syphilis can be transmitted by only a few routes: sexual contact,[223] direct introduction into the vascular system by shared needles or transfusions,[48] direct cutaneous contact with infectious lesions, or transplacental transfer of spirochetes (Table 20-2).

Despite successful antitreponemal therapy and knowledge of the epidemiology for decades, the problem of syphilis remains and the incidence of infection is increasing. Between 1981 and 1989 the incidence of primary and secondary syphilis in the United States grew from 13.7 to 18.4 cases per 100,000 persons, an increase of 34%.[224] In 1987 the incidence of congenital syphilis increased by 21%.[43] During this decade prostitution and cocaine abuse were recognized as risk factors for syphilis. After an apparent reversal of these trends in the 1990s the rate increased again in 2001, caused primarily by a recurrence of unsafe sexual practices among homosexual/bisexual men.[6] Other recalcitrant pockets of disease persist. In 1997 women who were jailed multiple times in New York City had an incidence of syphilis that was more than 1,000-fold greater than that in women in the city at large.[28]

A national epidemiologic study of syphilis seroreactivity indicated that race, age, education, income, and place of residence correlated with positivity.[105] Men are usually diagnosed during the primary stage, whereas the primary lesion

Table 20-2 **Transmission of Spirochetes**

ORGANISM	TRANSMISSION
Treponema pallidum pallidum	Veneral
	Blood transfusion (human only)
T. pallidum pertenue	Direct skin contact (human only)
T. carateum	Direct skin contact (human only)
T. pallidum endemicum	Direct mucosal contact (human only)
	Contaminated eating or drinking vessels
Borrelia recurrentis	Human host, human louse vector (*Pediculus humanus humanus*)
Borrelia spp.	Rodents, primates, human host; tick vector (*Ornithodoros, Rhipicephalus*)
B. burgdorferi	Rodent, deer host; tick vector (*Ixodes*)
Leptospira interrogans	Rat hosts; contaminated water

is often not detected in women, who are diagnosed during the early latent phase.[148] It has been estimated that over a period of 6 years 1,200 cases of unsuspected syphilis were detected by screening donated blood, almost 60% of which was from volunteers.[92] Distressingly, 81% of volunteer donors and 64% of paid donors reported no risk factors for syphilis.

Reflecting major changes in American society in the past 50 years, a study of prenatal syphilis at Boston City Hospital documented a shift from married white women in 1951 to unmarried minority women in 1991. A positive serologic test was associated with substance abuse and the presence of other sexually transmitted diseases.[135] A very different manifestation of the impact of modern life on an old disease was the observation that at least one cluster of syphilis cases could be traced to contacts made through an internet chat room.[136]

Traditional epidemiologic techniques of partner notification are proving inadequate for changed socioeconomic circumstances of modern America.[14,94] Between 1983 and 1984 Alexander-Rodriguez and colleagues studied 285 girls and 2,236 boys, aged 9 to 18 years, who were entering a detention facility.[11] The prevalence rate for gonorrhea was 3% in boys and 18.3% in girls. For syphilis the rate was 0.63% in boys and 2.5% in girls.

Theoretically, modern molecular tools should make tracing of contacts and identification of focal hot spots more sophisticated. In several reported applications of molecular epidemiology, however, numerous genetic subtypes have been identified in a geographic area.[208,287]

T. pallidum and human immunodeficiency virus (HIV) interact in several ways. It has been suggested that genital ulcers of a variety of etiologies facilitate the acquisition of HIV.[271] The immunosuppression that accompanies HIV infection may affect the serologic response to syphilis. In immunocompetent individuals, serologic tests are uniformly reactive during the secondary phase of syphilis. Haas and

colleagues, however, observed 109 homosexual men who had been treated for syphilis.[103] All of the men who had not been infected with HIV virus maintained their reactivity to treponemal antigen. In contrast, 7% of the men who had subclinical HIV infection and 38% of those with HIV disease had lost reactivity to the treponemal antigens. To make matters worse, biologic false-positive reactions in nontreponemal tests appear to be more common in HIV-infected patients than in those without HIV infection.[16,227] The mechanism for the association is unclear, and there are many potential confounding factors in these complicated patients. For instance, an association of biologic false-positive reactions has also been described in patients who are infected with hepatitis C virus.[289] Most positive nontreponemal tests in HIV-infected patients, however, do indicate syphilis, and it has been suggested that the FTA-ABS confirmatory tests may, in fact, be false-negative.[73]

Patients who are infected with HIV are more likely to present with secondary syphilis and with persistent chancres than non-HIV-infected patients.[120] Some investigators have suggested that the HIV epidemic has been accompanied by an increase in neurosyphilis,[187] but other investigators have not identified HIV as a risk factor for infection of the nervous system. In any event, patients are usually detected in the early stages of neurosyphilis.[84] Unsuccessful treatment of syphilis in patients infected with HIV has been reported by several investigators.[27]

The standard of therapy for syphilis remains penicillin. Documentation of treatment failures, particularly in HIV-infected patients, has caused concern that the convenient regimen of long-lasting benzathine penicillin may be inadequate in some patients.[114,308] In certain situations it may be appropriate to administer more recently developed antibiotics.[15] One of the uncommon complications of therapy is the Jarisch-Herxheimer reaction, which is both local and systemic. This reaction, which is associated with circulating endotoxin released from damaged organisms,[93] was classically noted in treated louseborne relapsing fever.

IMMUNITY

Experimental studies have documented the importance of the cellular immune system in resistance to *T. pallidum*.[234] There is firm evidence in humans that immunity to *T. pallidum* is partial or delayed in development. Congenitally infected infants have been reinfected as adolescents.[81] Similarly, human volunteers who previously had natural syphilis have been successfully reinfected. The likelihood that reinfection will occur decreases with increasing time after primary infection.[82] A period of partial resistance develops, in which reinfection may occur without the presence of a chancre. By the late stage, the patient is completely immune to reinfection.

Treponema pallidum Subspecies *pertenue*

T. pallidum subspecies *pertenue* (hereafter called *T. pertenue*) is the cause of yaws, a chronic, nonvenereal treponemal disease (see Table 20-1).[139] Yaws is endemic in central Africa and parts of the Indian subcontinent, South America, and Southeast Asia. There are primary, secondary, and tertiary stages of the disease. The skin and bones are primarily affected. Disease begins in childhood and is transmitted by contact with infectious skin lesions (see Table 20-2). In the tertiary phase the lesions may be gummatous. Benzathine penicillin is curative, although it may take months for the lesions to regress. Antibodies to *T. pertenue* are indistinguishable from antibodies to *T. pallidum*.

Treponema pallidum Subspecies endemicum

T. pallidum subspecies *endemicum* (hereafter called *T. endemicum*) is the cause of endemic, nonvenereal syphilis, or bejel (see Table 20-1). It is endemic in parts of Africa, the Middle East, India, and Asia. Infection occurs in childhood in rural areas with poor standards of hygiene. It is transmitted by contact with mucosal lesions or through contaminated drinking and eating utensils (see Table 20-2). The primary lesion of endemic syphilis is rarely seen, but the disease is otherwise similar to venereal syphilis. Benzathine penicillin is the therapy of choice. Correction of poor sanitation and hygiene may be preventive. Antibodies from patients with endemic syphilis cross-react with *T. pallidum*.

Treponema carateum

T. carateum, the etiologic agent of pinta, is probably the oldest of the human treponemes. The disease is characterized by ulcerative or papulosquamous skin lesions that often depigment. Pinta is endemic in parts of South and Central America (see Table 20-1) and is spread by contact with infected skin lesions (see Table 20-2). There are no long-term systemic health effects, but the cosmetic disability is considerable. Antisera from patients with pinta cross-react with specific antigens of *T. pallidum*.[85]

Laboratory Diagnosis of Treponemal Diseases

The laboratory diagnosis of syphilis has been reviewed extensively by Larsen and colleagues,[146] and a cost-effective approach to diagnosis and therapy has been developed by Hart.[108]

The gold standard for diagnosis of syphilis is culture, which must be performed in vivo, usually by intratesticular inoculation of rabbits with clinical material (Table 20-3).

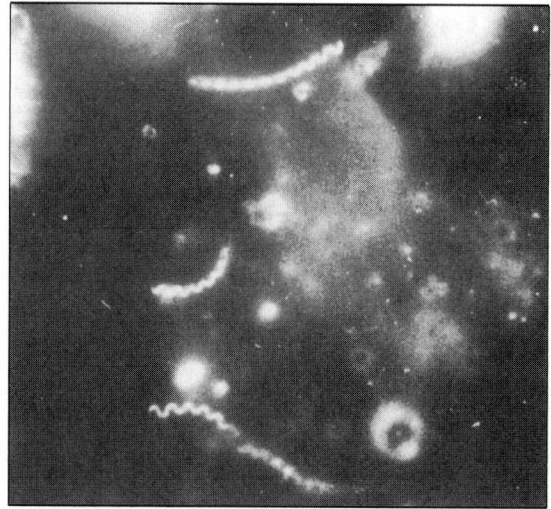

Figure 20-1 Positive darkfield examination for *Treponema pallidum.* The tightly coiled spiral nature of the organisms is evident. The background consists of debris and occasional red blood cells, indicating an adequate specimen. × 1000. (Photomicrograph courtesy of CDC, Atlanta GA.)

The procedure is expensive and time-consuming, requiring several months for subculture of testicular material if the original animal does not seroconvert. For obvious reasons, culture remains an investigative tool.

In primary syphilis, before the appearance of antibody, direct detection of spirochetes in chancres is the only means of diagnosis (Chart 20-1). The traditional method has been darkfield microscopy of material scraped from the surface of a lesion (Fig. 20-1). Observation of spirochetal motility is integral to differentiation of *T. pallidum* from saprophytic spirochetes, so that the microscopy must be accomplished immediately after collection of the specimen, a feat that is very difficult for most clinical laboratories to accomplish. Examination of oral lesions is not recommended because of the frequent presence of saprophytic treponemes in the mouth. Cutaneous and visceral lesions of secondary syphilis often contain large numbers of spirochetes, which can be

Table 20-3 Culture of Spirochetes

ORGANISM	IN VIVO	IN VITRO
Treponema pallidum pallidum	Rabbit testis; hamster; guinea pig	None
T. pallidum pertenue	Rabbit testis; hamster; guinea pig	None
T. pallidum endemicum	Rabbit testis; hamster; guinea pig	None
T. carateum	None (chimpanzee ±)	None
Borrelia recurrentis	Various	Modified Kelly medium
Borrelia spp.	Various	Modified Kelly medium
B. burgdorferi	Various	Modified Kelly medium
Leptospira interrogans	Various	Fletcher medium; Korthof's medium; Tween 80—albumin medium

demonstrated by darkfield microscopy of scrapings or imprints.

An alternative approach that is more satisfactory than darkfield microscopy is to demonstrate the presence of spirochetes in the lesions by immunofluorescence (see Color Plate 20-1*B*). Monoclonal reagents with greater specificity have now been developed.[122] Hook and colleagues[116] demonstrated fluorescent treponemes in 30 of 30 patients with primary syphilis, 29 of whom also had positive darkfield examinations. An oral spirochete that is antigenically related to *T. pallidum* has been described in cases of necrotizing gingivitis,[221] so the possibility of false-positive reactions exists when oral lesions are tested, even with a monoclonal antibody. Fluorescein-conjugated monoclonal antibody is currently available from the Centers for Disease Control and Prevention (Catalog Number: BE3051).

To perform the direct fluorescent antibody test for *T. pallidum* (DFA-TP), material from a lesion or tissue is collected as described for the darkfield examination, except that the material is allowed to dry on the slide (Chart 20-1). Alternatively, the dried smears may be sent to a reference laboratory or the exudate may be collected in capillary tubes, which are then sealed and stored at 4°C for mailing. The direct immunofluorescence method has been effective for *T. pertenue* as well as for *T. pallidum*.[205]

Spirochetes in formalin-fixed tissue can be demonstrated with one of several variations of a silver impregnation stain, such as the Steiner, Warthin-Starry, or Dieterle procedures (see Color Plate 20-1*A*).[295] Although finding spirochetes in the appropriate clinical situation is presumptive evidence of syphilis, the stain itself is nonspecific. Application of a fluoresceinated antibody provides specificity as well as sensitivity. Ito and colleagues have demonstrated *T. pallidum* in formalin-fixed tissues using either polyclonal antisera[123] or monoclonal antibodies after treatment with NH$_4$OH or trypsin to open antigenic sites.

SEROLOGIC TESTS

The serologic tests for syphilis can be divided into two groups: nontreponemal tests and treponemal tests. The two groups have distinctive characteristics that make them useful for different purposes. They are complementary, not mutually exclusive. The nontreponemal tests are most useful as screening tests. The treponemal tests should be reserved as confirmatory tests when a nontreponemal test is positive or

when clinical suspicion of syphilis is high despite a nonreactive nontreponemal test. Hart[108] has pointed out that the "greater" specificity of the treponemal tests is entirely an artifact of their current use as confirmatory tests after performance of a nontreponemal test. When the tests are compared head to head as the initial serologic procedure, the VDRL nontreponemal test is actually as specific as or more specific than the treponemal FTA-ABS test.[144] The general characteristics of these tests are summarized in Table 20-4.

The procedures for performance of these tests have been standardized and published in great detail by the U.S. Public Health Service.[145] Several of the procedures are summarized in the tables for pedagogic purposes. When these tests are performed in the laboratory, it is imperative that the manual or manufacturer's directions be consulted and followed exactly. The *Manual of Tests for Syphilis* even contains a classic typographic error: in Chapter 3 readers are instructed in the "Collection Procedure for Venus [sic] Blood."

Nontreponemal Tests. The nontreponemal tests take advantage of antibodies to a tissue lipid, called cardiolipin, that are produced as a byproduct of treponemal infection. The association was recognized early in this century when a variety of complement fixation tests was developed. The procedures in current use are predominantly flocculation tests. They use a form of cardiolipin that is complexed with cholesterol and lecithin. The most commonly used procedures are the Venereal Disease Research Laboratory (VDRL) and the rapid plasma reagin (RPR) tests. The RPR card tests achieved popularity because the VDRL test is technically very demanding and unforgiving. The cessation of manufacture of the bottles required for preparation of VDRL antigen prompted a scramble for an acceptable alternative.[211] Other tests that have been used are the reagin screen test (RST), the unheated serum reagin (USR) test, and the toluidine red unheated serum test (TRUST).

The nontreponemal tests have a sensitivity of 70–99%, depending on the stage of disease. The tests may not be positive in primary syphilis, so they should be repeated after 1 week, 1 month, and 3 months if a negative result is obtained in a patient in whom syphilis is suspected. The sensitivity of these tests approaches 100% during the secondary phase of the disease. Plasma and cord blood should not be used because borderline reactions may be obtained.[143]

The nontreponemal tests are affected by antitreponemal therapy. As a result they are useful for following the progres-

Table 20-4 Characteristics of Serologic Tests for Syphilis

| TEST | TYPE | % POSITIVE AT INFECTIOUS STAGES | | |
		Primary	Secondary	Late
VDRL	Nontreponemal	70	99	1
RPR	Nontreponemal	80	99	0
FTA-ABS	Treponemal	85	100	98
TPHA	Treponemal	65	100	95
TPI	Treponemal	50	97	95

Adapted from Tramont EC. Treponema pallidum (syphilis). In: Mandell GL, Douglas RG, Bennett JE (eds). Principles and Practice of Infectious Diseases. 3rd ed. New York: Churchill Livingstone, 1990.

sion of disease and response to therapy. The results of any positive test should be titered to an end-point dilution. In addition, serum from patients with large amounts of antibody may produce a prozone phenomenon. When a prozone occurs, the relative concentrations of antibody and antigen are not in balance, and precipitation or flocculation does not occur. The false-positive results caused by the prozone phenomenon continue to be a clinical concern. The prozone results are often marked by a "rough" appearance to the flocculated antigen. Any serum that produces this rough appearance should be titered. In addition, serum should be diluted and retested if it is strongly suspected on clinical grounds that a patient with negative test results has syphilis. In the general population the frequency of prozone reactions is sufficiently low that routine dilution of serum is not cost-effective.[70]

If the titer of the antibody does not fall progressively with treatment, the possibility of a treatment failure should be considered. There should be at least a fourfold decrease in antibody titer after 3 months of antitreponemal therapy. In patients who are treated in the late stages of syphilis or who are reinfected, titers that decline very slowly or remain stable may develop. Some of these "chronic persisters" may maintain positive nontreponemal tests for life.

The nontreponemal tests cannot be used to diagnose late syphilis, especially if treated, because the titer of antibody will eventually decline to undetectable levels.

The VDRL test has become the standard nontreponemal test. Preparation of the antigen must be done with great precision and attention to detail. It is the only serologic test that is universally accepted for the diagnosis of neurosyphilis. Examples of VDRL reactions are shown in Figure 20-2. The procedure is summarized in Chart 20-2.

The RPR test is an adaptation of the flocculation principle to a card format. The visibility of the flocculation is enhanced by incorporation of charcoal particles. The uses of the RPR test are similar to those of the VDRL test except that the RPR test cannot be used to test CSF. The simplicity of the RPR test has led most laboratories to adopt it as the primary screening test (Fig. 20-3). The procedure is described in Chart 20-3.

The specificity of the nontreponemal tests averages 98%, with a range from 93% to 99%. The lack of specificity is mostly a problem when the tests are used for screening populations with a low prevalence of syphilis, for whom positive reactions are likely to be false-positive. The false-positive reactions occur in patients who have other treponemal infections, but also in patients with diseases that elicit anticardiolipin antibodies. These "biologic false-positives" may be transient, usually from viral infections, or may be persistent, usually related to immunologically mediated diseases. Biologic false-positive reactions have been reported in drug addicts, a population at increased risk for contracting syphilis.[132] As discussed above, patients with HIV infection also have an increased frequency of biologic false-positive reactions. In one study, these positive reactions were associated with hepatitis C infection. It has also been suggested that an important determinant of biologic false-positive reactions is the use of illicit intravenous drugs.[112] A positive reaction in a nontreponemal test should be confirmed, therefore, with a more specific treponemal test. It should be noted, however,

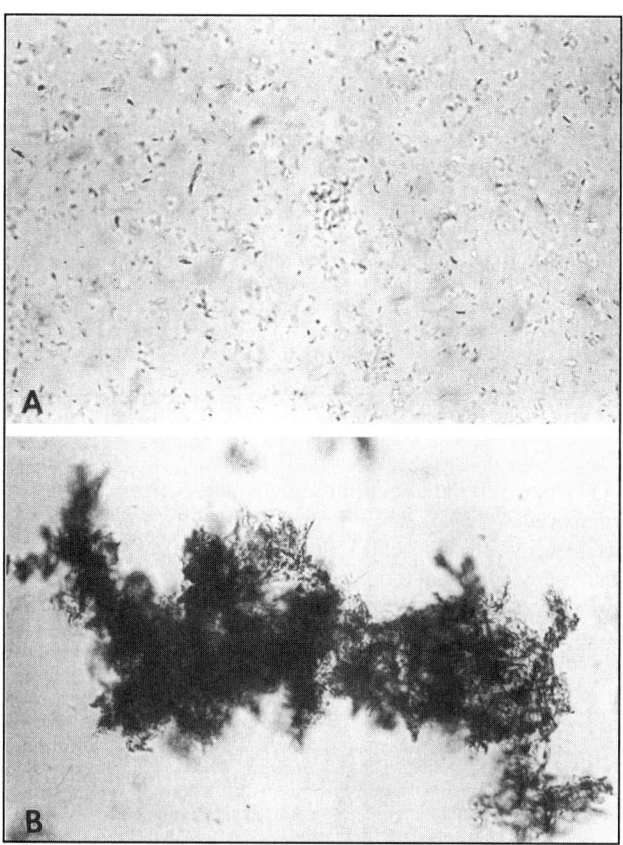

Figure 20-2 VDRL test: The reactions in this test are evaluated microscopically. **(A)** Nonreactive serum. The particles of VDRL antigen are uniform and freely dispersed without clumping. **(B)** Reactive serum: The VDRL antigen particles are strongly agglutinated by this syphilitic serum. The individual particles have aggregated into sheaves and large clumps. ×100. (Courtesy of Burton Wilcke, PhD and Mary Celotti.)

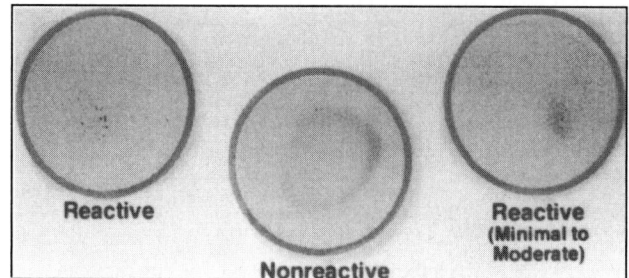

Figure 20-3 RPR card test: The reactions in this test are read with the naked eye, using incandescent light illumination. This control card contains *Reactive* (R), *Weakly reactive* (W), and *Nonreactive* (N) sera. The modified VDRL antigen is made visible by complexing with charcoal particles. The charcoal-antigen particles are evenly dispersed and finely distributed in the nonreactive serum and are grossly clumped. The serum with minimal to moderate activity produces small aggregates and clumps of charcoal-VDRL antigen particles.

that the possibility of false-negative results on treponemal tests must be considered.

Several new variations on the nontreponemal tests have been introduced, but they have not replaced the traditional tests.

Treponemal Tests. The treponemal tests incorporate specific treponemal antigens into the system. The traditional gold standard was the *T. pallidum* immobilization (TPI) test, in which the motility of live, virulent treponemes was inhibited by the presence of specific antibody. This expensive and cumbersome test has been replaced by the FTA-ABS test. Subsequently, another test specific for treponemal antigens, the microhemagglutination test for *T. pallidum* (MHA-TP) was developed.

The FTA-ABS test is summarized in Chart 20-4. The specificity of the assay is increased by absorption of the test sera with a nonpathogenic spirochete, the Reiter strain of *T. phagedenis*. The FTA-ABS test has a higher rate of positivity in early syphilis than do the nontreponemal tests (see Table 20-4). The positivity rate approaches 100% in the secondary stage and remains so for life. It is not affected by antitreponemal therapy. The FTA-ABS test is, therefore, a good test for screening late syphilis, but it cannot be used to follow treatment. The degree of positivity in the FTA-ABS test has no biologic meaning, so the intensity of fluorescence is not reported and positive sera are not titered. The specificity of the FTA-ABS test is high. With few exceptions, the biologic false-positive reactions of the nontreponemal tests do not occur. Sera from some patients, especially those with systemic lupus erythematosus or other connective-tissue diseases, may produce an unusual beaded staining reaction.[141] It has been estimated that 1% of the normal population will have a positive FTA-ABS test. Cross-reactions occur with other pathogenic treponemes. If the FTA-ABS test is used to screen populations with very low prevalences of syphilis, false-positive reactions may occur even with this very specific test.

A variation on the FTA-ABS test is the double-staining procedure. This test is very similar to the FTA-ABS, except that rhodamine-conjugated IgG antitreponemal antibody is used to locate the spirochetes. In the classic FTA-ABS test, darkfield illumination is used to locate the spirochetes. The results of the traditional and double-staining procedures are comparable.[220]

The FTA-ABS test can be adapted to detect either IgG or IgM antibody. One advantage of detecting IgM antibody is to document infection in utero. Immunoglobulins of the G class cross the placenta and enter the fetal circulation, but IgM antibodies do not cross the placenta. IgM antibodies are made by the fetus in utero; therefore, the detection of specific antitreponemal IgM antibodies in a neonate indicates intrauterine infection.[12] There are potential problems with the IgM assays, however, and great care must be taken to validate a given assay before use. If antiglobulins, such as rheumatoid factors or anti-idiotype antibodies, are present in fetal sera, they will produce false-positive reactions. If present in excessive amounts, IgG antibody may block the antigenic sites, producing false-negative reactions. Rosen and Richardson demonstrated good performance with a research assay, but encountered problems when commercial reagents were used.[228]

The microhemagglutination test uses antigens specific to *T. pallidum.* The test is considerably less complicated than the FTA-ABS test and does not require a fluorescence microscope. It is similar in performance to the fluorescence procedure, but it is less sensitive in early syphilis. The FTA-ABS test should be available to test sera that give equivocal reactions.[285]

INNOVATIONS: PROVISIONAL AND INVESTIGATIVE TESTS

Disappointment in the performance of the IgM FTA-ABS test has prompted the investigation of other approaches. The 19S IgM FTA-ABS test includes fractionation of serum to obtain IgM specificity, rather than depending on antiglobulin reagents.[283] This test appears to avoid the problems of nonspecificity, so it can be used as a confirmatory procedure, but insensitivity prevents its use as a screening test. Sequential evaluation with quantitative nontreponemal tests remains an important part of the laboratory evaluation of congenital syphilis.

Enzyme and particle agglutination immunoassays for detection of specific treponemal antigens have been developed.[67,75,104,212,235,245,306] These tests offer comparable sensitivity and specificity to reference tests, but are often presented in formats that are easier to use. With increasing use, the level of comfort in abandoning traditional approaches will undoubtedly increase.

Modern molecular techniques may facilitate dissection of the issues. Sanchez and colleagues used Western blot analysis (immunoblots; see Chapter 3) to identify a 47-kDa antigen that was not seen in control patients and was correlated with intrauterine infection.[236] The sensitivity of immunoblotting for detection of IgM antibodies in 14 symptomatic neonates was 92%, whereas 83% of 12 asymptomatic neonates who were later proved to be infected were detected by Western blotting. Twenty-seven of 30 (90%) uninfected infants were correctly characterized.[176] Dobson and colleagues[59] demonstrated reactivity to 47- and 37-kDa protein antigens in the serum of congenitally infected infants. Although rheumatoid factor could theoretically cause problems in the immunoblot assay, removing rheumatoid factor from the sera did not affect the results. Immunoblots have also been used successfully as a confirmatory test for syphilis.[39] An advantage of this technology is that purified antigen can be used as the substrate, and the pattern of reactivity of sera can be used to determine positivity. If the criteria for determining positive immunoblot tests are not standardized, however, the variation in interpretation among laboratories can cause diagnostic problems. As understanding of the nature of the protein antigens of *T. pallidum* increases,[270] the number and quality of tests available in future years will undoubtedly expand.

Molecular techniques have also been applied to the direct detection of spirochetes in tissues and fluids. Investigators have concentrated their attention on intrauterine and central nervous system infection, because serologic techniques are not adequate for these important clinical problems.[100,193] DNA probes have not been sufficiently sensitive, so efforts have been focused on amplification techniques, such as polymerase chain reaction.[155,168] Although the new technology is a valuable addition to the diagnostic armamentarium, the presence of inhibitors in clinical specimens may yield false-negative tests, especially in CSF. Treponemal DNA in spinal fluid appears stable, so negative results are probably not from deterioration of nucleic acids in the specimens.[296]

False-positive reactions from contamination have been minimal in the research protocols, but it was necessary to address problems of nonspecificity in one study. The close correlation of polymerase chain reaction and the impossibly impractical rabbit infectivity assays in other studies, however, suggests that this approach is the way of the future for difficult diagnostic problems.

Borrelia

Borrelia spp. are helical bacteria that measure 0.2 to 0.5 μm in diameter and 3 to 20 μm in length, with 3 to 10 loose coils and 15 to 29 periplasmic flagella (see Color Plates 20-1*C, D,* and *F*). Those species that have been cultivated in vitro are microaerophilic (see Table 20-3). The bacteria are gram-negative and stain well with Giemsa's stain.[134] The human pathogens are transmitted by insect vectors (see Table 20-2). Louseborne relapsing fever is caused by *B. recurrentis,* tickborne relapsing fever by a variety of species, and Lyme disease by *B. burgdorferi* and related species. Borrelial spirochetes also cause infection in animals, and some species have yet to be associated with a disease process. The relationships among the various species have been assessed by characterization of their flagellin genes.[90]

Relapsing Fever

Relapsing fever is a distinctive clinical disease that was probably recognized by Herodotus in ancient Greece. There are two forms: 1) epidemic louseborne disease and 2) endemic tickborne relapsing fever. The epidemiologic, ecologic, and clinical characteristics are compared and contrasted in Table 20-5. Several old but still pertinent reviews are available.[36,79,266]

EPIDEMIOLOGY

Louseborne relapsing fever is a disease fostered by poverty, crowding, and poor sanitation, as is louseborne typhus fever. It has occurred in Africa, the Middle East, and Asia, but not in the New World. The human body louse inhabits humans only, and *B. recurrentis* is not transmitted vertically to succeeding generations of lice. The organism must be maintained by passage from louse to a human host and then back to another louse. The louse remains infected for its entire life. Epidemic disease thus occurs only under conditions of extreme deprivation. For the first half of the last century epidemics occurred approximately every 20 years. In recent times, Ethiopia has been the only major geographic locus of infection.

Tickborne relapsing fever is distributed worldwide. Many soft-bodied ticks of the genus *Ornithodoros* carry distinctive borreliae. In the United States, taxonomists have attempted to use the same name for a tick and its associated spirochete. Thus *O. hermsii* is the vector for *B. hermsii.* The epidemiologic characteristics of tickborne relapsing fever depend on the habits of the local vector. *O. hermsii* is the most common vector and *B. hermsii* the most common *Borrelia* in California, the Pacific Northwest, and Canada.[66] *O. hermsii* lives in the remains of dead trees and parasitizes rodents, which often carry it into hunters' cabins. *O. parkeri* inhabits caves and burrows of ground squirrels and prairie dogs in the western United States. *B. parkeri* is a relatively infrequent pathogen of humans because of the inaccessibility of its vector. *O. turicata* inhabits caves and animal burrows in the western United States, Mexico, and South America, but it has also been found in closer association with humans under the foundations of houses in Texas. The tickborne borreliae have a solid ecologic niche with virtually no possibility of eradication. The spirochete can be passed from generation to generation of ticks without intervention of a vertebrate host. *O. turicata* has been reported to survive in a starving state for 5 years, and survival of borreliae in ticks without loss of infectivity has been reported for up to 12 years.

Table 20-5 **Characteristics of Relapsing Fever**

CHARACTERISTIC	LOUSE-BORNE	TICK-BORNE
Epidemiology	Epidemic	Usually endemic
Etiologic agent	*B. recurrentis*	Various; *B. hermsii, B. turicatae, B. parkeri* in U.S.
Vector	*Pediculus humanus* spp. *humanus*	Various; *Ornithodoros hermsii, O. turicatae, O. parkeri* in U.S.
Mean duration of primary attack	5.5 days	3.1 days
Mean duration (range) of asymptomatic interval	9.25 days (3–27)	6.8 days (1–63)
Mean number (range) of relapses	3 (0–13)	1 (0–3+)
Mean duration of relapse	1.9 days	2.5 days

Adapted from reference[266].

Most tickborne relapsing fever is endemic, afflicting the unfortunate person who becomes an incidental host. Under the right conditions, however, epidemic disease can occur. In 1968 there was an outbreak of tickborne relapsing fever among 42 Boy Scouts and scoutmasters who were camping near Spokane, Washington.[290] Clinical disease developed in 1 of the 42 persons at risk. In 9 cases an exact incubation period could be calculated because they were only at risk for one night (mean, 6.9 days; range, 3 to 9). The attack rate was higher in those who slept in abandoned cabins than in those who slept in tents, a fact that was also noted by Horton and Blaser in Colorado.[118] The authors noted poetic justice in the concentration of disease among scoutmasters and older scouts, who appropriated the cabins for themselves, leaving the younger scouts to "rough it."

In areas that have no indigenous relapsing fever spirochetes, importation of disease from endemic regions provides a diagnostic challenge.[51] Tickborne infection is a more likely infection than louseborne infection for tourists visiting Africa. Parasitologists should keep this diagnostic possibility in mind when examining smears collected for the detection of malaria parasites.

CLINICAL DISEASE

The clinical presentation of the two types of relapsing fever is similar. Differences in frequency and timing of relapses are noted in Table 20-5. *Ornithodoros* ticks feed on humans very inconspicuously and for short periods. Most patients, therefore, do not remember a tick bite. The onset of disease is typically abrupt, with a high fever, usually near 40°C (104°F), shaking chills, delirium, severe muscle aches, and pains in bones and joints. Hepatosplenomegaly and tenderness may be present, and the patient may be jaundiced. Neurologic complications, including lymphocytic meningitis and facial palsy, resemble those of *B. burgdorferi* infection.[41] Characteristically there is a crisis after which the fever remits and the patient feels well. Fatalities are very uncommon. When relapses occur, each cycle tends to be less severe than the preceding one. A rash may develop during the initial attack, but it does not usually appear in relapses. An outbreak of louseborne relapsing fever in Ethiopian troops after the cessation of civil war provided an unfortunate recent opportunity to review the clinical features.[29] The case fatality rate was 3.6%, and 1.8% of patients had recrudescent disease.

Although penicillin is effective against borreliae, tetracycline or erythromycin are more effective at eliminating the spirochetes. Jarisch-Herxheimer (JH) reactions may occur during treatment. In the recent Ethiopian epidemic of louseborne disease, 43% of patients experienced this complication. Use of low-dose penicillin leads to more frequent relapses but fewer JH reactions than with tetracycline or larger doses of penicillin.[250] Administration of acetaminophen and hydrocortisone modified the changes in vital signs during the JH reaction, but did not prevent the dramatic rigor that occurs.[38] Transient increases in tumor necrosis factor and interleukins-6 and -8 correlate temporally with the reaction,[190] although not all investigators have been able to detect elevations of these cytokines. Control of the vector is also essential for the control of epidemic louseborne infection.[286]

LABORATORY DIAGNOSIS

Relapsing fever borreliae can now be cultured in a modification[20] of Kelly's medium for borreliae,[133] but isolation is not a practical means of diagnosis in most situations. Similarly, although several serologic tests have been developed, they are not diagnostically useful. Approximately 5% of patients will have a positive VDRL test.

The mainstay of diagnosis is demonstration of the spirochetes in body fluids, usually in peripheral blood smears (see Color Plate 20-1*C*). The diagnosis is often made in the hematology laboratory, because the clinical presentation can be enigmatic for physicians unaccustomed to the disease. Horton and Blaser[118] report a case in which the spirochetes were missed by an automated differential scanner, but were noted by an astute technologist who reviewed the smear. In contrast to other spirochetes the relapsing fever borreliae are well stained by acid aniline dyes, such as Wright or Giemsa's stains. The borrelial spirochetes are thin, undulant, or overtly spiral organisms that are most visible when they are located between red blood cells (see Color Plate 20-1*C*). Felsenfeld[79] advocates staining with Wright's stain followed by application of a 1% solution of crystal violet for 10 to 30 seconds.

Borreliae are likely to be found in the blood during febrile episodes. The sensitivity of staining peripheral smears is estimated at 70%. Spirochetes are unlikely to be detected during the afebrile intervals between attacks, although they are still present in the body. Thick and thin films should be made as for malaria, because in some cases spirochetes will be detected only by examination of the thick film.

Goldschmid and Mahomed used a microhematocrit centrifugation technique to concentrate the borreliae in and above the buffy coat.[98] The buffy coat procedure has not been widely used, but has been confirmed in a study from West Africa that included isolation of *B. crocidurae*.[294] Sciotto and colleagues used the fluorescent acridine orange technique to demonstrate borreliae in peripheral smears (see Color Plate 20-1*D*).[249] The fluorescence procedure greatly enhances the visibility of the spirochetes.

A monoclonal antibody for the identification of *B. hermsii* in peripheral blood smears and amplification techniques for identification of borrelial nucleic acid have been described but are not generally available.[248]

Lyme Disease

In 1977, Steere and colleagues, at Yale University, reported that an epidemic of arthritis had been occurring in residents of several surrounding Connecticut communities since at least 1972.[278] The alarm had been sounded by two vigilant mothers. In 1975 a mother from Old Lyme, Connecticut, informed the State Health Department of 12 cases of childhood arthritis in her small community of 5,000 people. A second woman came to the Rheumatology Division at Yale University with a story of acute arthritis in herself, her husband, two children, and several neighbors. The disease in all the children had been diagnosed as juvenile rheumatoid arthritis, a clinical diagnosis that depends on exclusion of known causes of arthritis. The investigators at Yale believed that they were dealing with a new disease, which they named Lyme arthritis.

Steere and colleagues recognized that the arthritis was almost always preceded by a very distinctive skin rash, an erythematous papule that developed into a rapidly expanding annular lesion. Many of the physicians who examined the skin lesions believed that an insect bite had started the process, but an arthropod (in that case a tick) was recognized in only one patient. The nature of the primary lesion and the occurrence of cases in the summer and early fall suggested an arthropod vector. In that initial paper the authors noted the resemblance of the rash to a lesion called erythema chronicum migrans, which had been described in Europe, especially Scandinavia.

Little did the two mothers know what large waves would emanate from the rock they threw into their small Connecticut pool. Instead of discovering a new disease they had initiated an investigation that would unearth the cause of a century-old disease of worldwide proportions. The long history of European investigations is summarized in Box 20-1.[273] Lyme disease has been thoroughly reviewed in recent years.[256,274] Relevant web sites have been summarized by Sood.[264]

In 1982, only 5 years after the original description of Lyme arthritis, Burgdorfer and colleagues determined the etiology by isolating a spirochete from the implicated tick vector, demonstrating that the spirochetes produced cutaneous lesions in rabbits and that the serum of patients with Lyme arthritis contained antibodies to the spirochete.[37] The next year Steere and associates clinched the issue by isolating a spirochete from blood, skin lesions, or CSF of infected patients as well as from ticks.[276] Shortly thereafter spirochetes were isolated from the lesions of erythema chronicum migrans and Bannwarth's syndrome in Europe.[7,214]

The newly isolated spirochete is related to other *Borrelia* species,[243] but shares almost no homology with species of *Treponema* and *Leptospira*.[121] It has been named *Borrelia burgdorferi*, in honor of Willy Burgdorfer, who first isolated the organism.[127] *B. burgdorferi* is the longest and narrowest of the borreliae. Three genospecies are now recognized as definite human pathogens within the *B. burgdorferi* complex (*B. burgdorferi* sensu lato): *B. burgdorferi* sensu stricto, *B.*

Box 20-1 European Investigations of Lyme Disease

1921–1923	Afzelius in Sweden and Lipschütz in Austria described erythema chronicum migrans. Later the chronic atrophic skin lesion described by Herxheimer in 1902 was recognized as part of the same process.
1944	Bannwarth described a chronic radiculitis, sometimes preceded by erythema, accompanied by chronic lymphocytic meningitis, and cranial or peripheral neuritis. Later the disease was associated with ticks.
1948	Lennhoff described the presence of spirochetes in the lesion of erythema chronicum migrans.
1951	Hollström described the successful treatment of erythema chronicum migrans with penicillin.

---

garinii, and *B. afzelii*. An increasing number of other species, some as yet unnamed, have been documented within the *B. burgdorferi* sensu lato complex[213,298]; the extent of their association with human disease is not yet clear. Evidence of involvement in human disease is most compelling for *B. bissettii* sp. nov. and for *B. valaisiana*. In addition, a human disease that resembles Lyme disease has been associated with a noncultivable spirochete, named *B. lonestari*, because it is found in *Amblyomma americanum*, the "lone star tick."[125,184] This species may be responsible for many of the cases of Lyme disease found in the southeastern United States.

The complete genetic sequence of *B. burgdorferi* has now been determined.[87] It contains numerous antigens that may be important for pathogenesis and diagnosis, including numerous outer-surface proteins, the most important of which are OspA through OspF, that are located on plasmids, and a 41-kDa flagellar protein. *B. burgdorferi* sensu stricto is global in distribution. The other two pathogenic species are found in Europe[57] and Asia.[189] *B. garinii* appears to be particularly associated with neuroborreliosis, whereas *B. afzelii* is associated with arthritis and chronic skin lesions.[60] A significant minority of *I. ricinus* ticks in Europe are infected with more than one member of the *B. burgdorferi* complex.[218] Strains found in the United States are relatively homogeneous and conform to the definition of *B. burgdorferi* sensu stricto. The immunologic homogeneity of most American strains was demonstrated by analysis of borreliacidal antibodies in vitro.[158] Among strains of *B. burgdorferi* sensu stricto, however, some investigators have noted greater variation in strains from the United States than in those from Europe.[153] A potentially significant finding for studies of genetic homogeneity is the documentation of greater variation in *B. burgdorferi* when amplification products from skin lesions were compared to isolated spirochetes from the same lesions, suggesting that current culture techniques may select for certain genetic types.[156]

Outer-surface proteins A and C are particularly important in the biology of Lyme disease. OspA is expressed predominantly in the midgut of ticks, where it is responsible for adherence to epithelium.[202] After the tick takes a blood meal, the spirochetes migrate through the hemocele to the salivary glands. In the process the expression of OspA is downregulated and the amount of OspC produced increases dramatically.[217] Although cell-mediated and humoral immunity is mounted against multiple antigens, the predominant early antibody response is directed against OspC. It also appears that OspC is an important determinant of clinical disease, certain variants being associated with disseminated infection, others with limited or localized disease, and still others being found only in ticks.[252] Lin and associates[153] have suggested that the predominant isolates of *B. burgdorferi* sensu stricto found in the southeastern United States contain OspC variants that are not associated with invasive disease, possibly explaining, at least in part, the relative paucity of well-documented cases of classical Lyme disease in this region.

Retrospective examination of *Ixodes ricinus* ticks that had been preserved in Hungarian and Austrian museums in 1884 and 1888, respectively, has documented the presence of DNA from a member of the *B. burgdorferi* complex.[172] Similarly, OspA sequences from *B. burgdorferi* have been demonstrated by molecular techniques in white-footed mice that had been trapped in Massachusetts in 1894.[170] It appears, therefore, that the American and European foci have been independently present for at least a hundred years.

EPIDEMIOLOGY

Lyme disease is now the most common arthropodborne infection in the United States (Figure 20-4). From 1982 to 1989 there was an 18-fold increase in cases reported to the CDC. From 1986 to 1989 the number of cases doubled each year, after which the incidence appeared to have reached a plateau. In 1994, however, 13,083 cases were reported from 44 states, a 58% increase over 1993 (Figure 20-4). Cases have been reported in almost every state, but they are concentrated in the Northeast, the North Central region, and to a lesser extent the West Coast (Fig. 20-5). The infection is recognized around the entire northern hemisphere, including the Soviet republics.[56]

In the United States, the distribution of Lyme disease matches the distribution of ticks of the genus *Ixodes*. In the Northeast[277] and North Central[97] regions the vector is usually *I. scapularis* (see Color Plate 20-1*E*), whereas *I. pacificus* carries the spirochetes in the Northwest.[241] In Europe, *I. ricinus* is the most common vector, whereas *I. persulcatus* is the main arthropod host in Asia. These species share many characteristics and are also known as black-legged ticks or deer ticks. There has been controversy over the nomenclature of the black-legged ticks found in the eastern United States. *I. dammini* is now considered by most investigators to be synonymous with *I. scapularis*.[200,267]

A clinical illness that resembles Lyme arthritis has been reported in Australia.[89] Neither the vector nor the responsible infectious agent has yet been identified, despite extensive testing of ticks by culture and polymerase chain reaction.[232]

The frequency of tick infection in some areas is as high as 75%,[13] and the range of spirochetal load in adult ticks caught in several endemic areas was 950 to 4,350 spirochetes per tick in one study.[35]

Babesia microti and the newly recognized human granulocytic *Ehrlichia*, *Anaplasma* (*Ehrlichia*) *phagocytophila*, are also transmitted by the eastern deer tick and have a geographic distribution that matches that of *I. scapularis*. The cycle of both *B. burgdorferi*[151] and *Babesia microti*[269] in nature is maintained by a number of small rodents, notably the white-footed mouse (*Peromyscus leucopus*), which maintains an asymptomatic parasitemia or spirochetemia. Other small mammals, such as the Norway rat on Monhegan Island in Maine, may also serve as reservoirs.[260] White-tailed deer are important for the survival of the tick. Although deer are not directly involved in transmission of the infection, reduction of deer populations diminishes the number of vector ticks, after which the incidence of infection decreases.[55] It is not surprising that infection with various combinations of *Babesia microti*, *A. phagocytophila*, and *B. burgdorferi* has been documented in the same patient.[180] Although talk of ticks, mice, and deer conjures images of the countryside, or at least suburbia, all of the necessary components, including the infectious agents, have been found in New York City's Van Cortlandt Park.[54]

The importance of the environmental factors for development of human disease is illustrated by the geographic variation in the frequency of clinical Lyme disease. Most dramatically, an enzootic cycle of *B. burgdorferi* infection in *I. spinipalpus* ticks and wood rats exists in northern Colorado, an area in which Lyme disease has not been recorded.[174] It appears that lack of contact between humans and this species of ticks is the most likely explanation for the absence of human infection. Although clinical disease is present in the

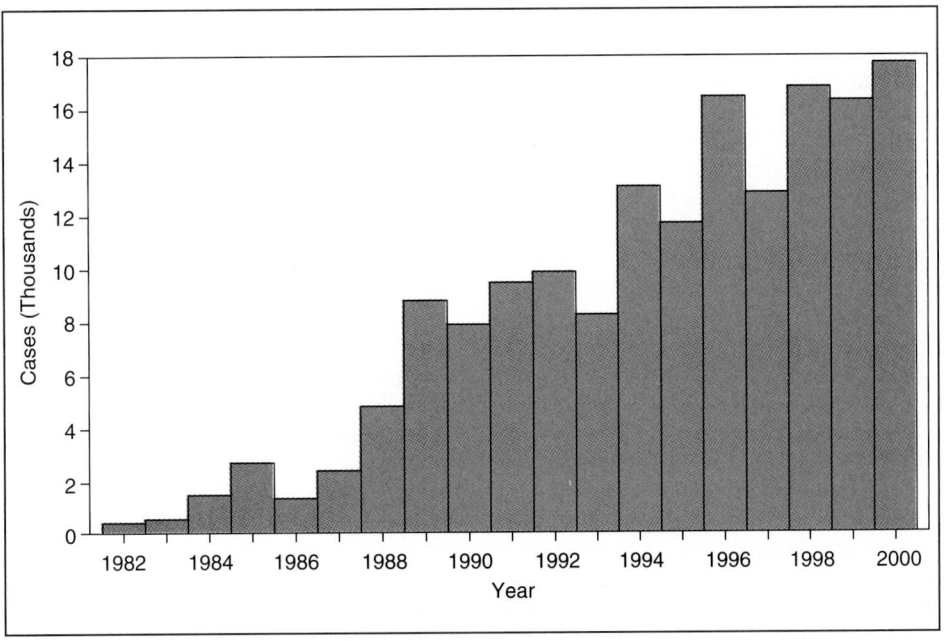

Figure 20-4 Number of reported Lyme disease cases by year in the United States, 1982–2000. (Adapted from reference [5].)

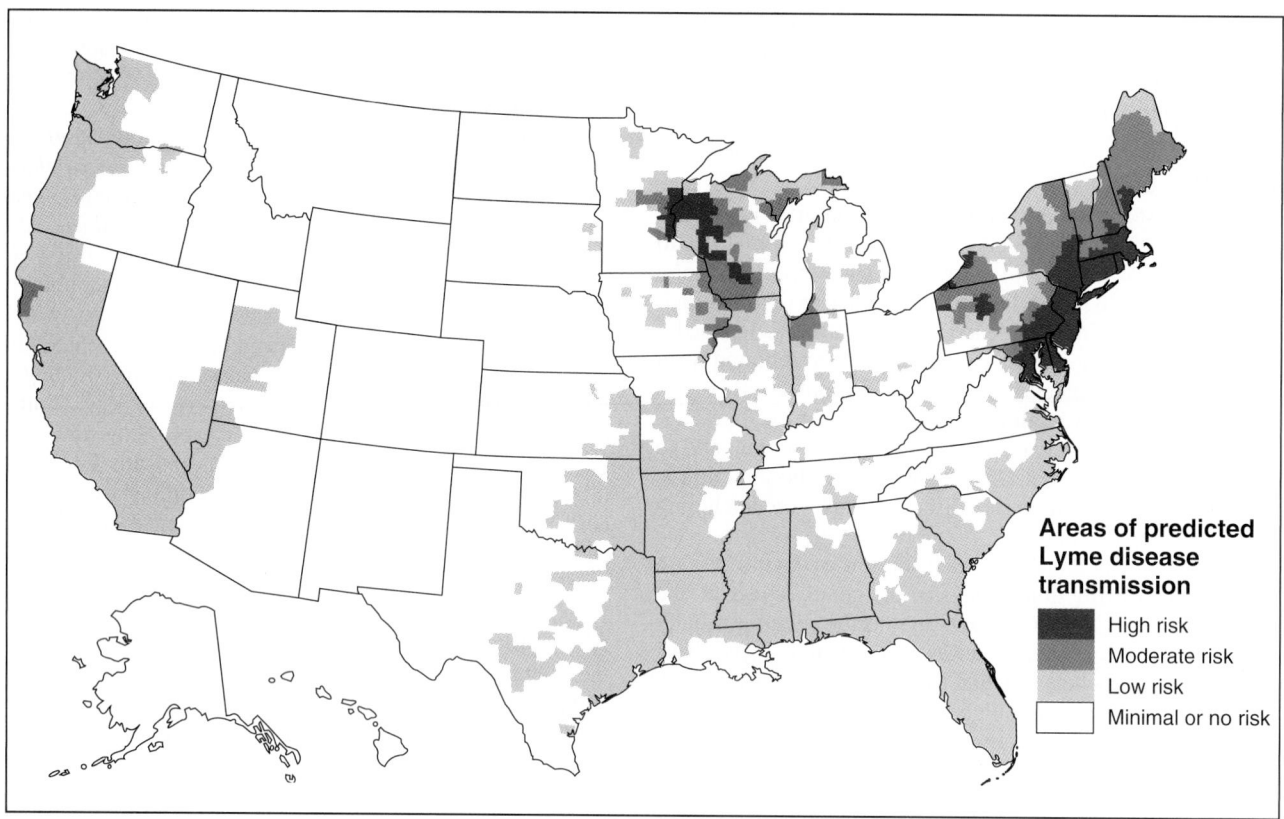

Figure 20-5 Geographic depiction of risk for contracting Lyme disease in the United States, compiled by CDC. http://www.cdc.gov/ncidod/dvbid/lyme/riskmap.htm

Pacific Northwest, where the vector is *I. pacificus*, it is much less frequent than in North Central and Northeastern states. One possible explanation is provided by the pertinent animal host. In the central and eastern states the white-footed mouse supports luxuriant growth of the spirochetes, providing ample material for a new stage of hungry ticks. In the Pacific states, on the other hand, the ticks feed on lizards, in which the borreliae multiply poorly, limiting the intensity of infection in the tick populations.[34,171] An unidentified borreliacidal chemical produced by the lizards may be the biologic explanation for this phenomenon. It has been noted that *I. scapularis* in southeastern states also feed preferentially on lizards, rather than mice, perhaps contributing to the infrequency of classical Lyme disease in this region also.

The life cycle of ixodid ticks involves three distinct stages and a life span of 2 years. Ticks feed in late summer as larvae and the next year as nymphs (early spring) and adults (late summer). A blood meal is required for the molts from larva to nymph and nymph to adult, as well as for oviposition (laying eggs) by the adult female. The larval and nymphal stages are so small that many patients do not recall having been bitten. In order to transmit the infection, however, a tick has to have fed on an infected rodent. *B. burgdorferi* is not transmitted vertically from parent to offspring, so the larval stages of ticks are never infected and cannot transmit the infection. The most effective tick stage for transmission is the nymph, which is prevalent during the late spring and early summer, when most cases of human disease occur.

Among other reasons for the efficacy of nymphal transmission is undoubtedly their small size, which allows them to escape detection for longer times than adult ticks. The adult male has the potential for transmission of infection, but they rarely feed on humans because they do not require a blood meal, as does the adult female before laying her eggs.

From experimental data the ticks must remain attached for at least 24 hours to transmit the spirochetes effectively.[207] During the first 12 hours after attachment the body of the tick remains flat. After feeding for 24 hours, when approximately 5% of infected ticks transmit spirochetes, the posterior body of the nymph begins to extend. After 48 hours of feeding the posterior body is fully distended and appears opalescent; at this point approximately 50% of infected ticks transmit *Borrelia*. After 4 days of feeding, almost all infected ticks will transmit spirochetes, at which point the ticks are opaque and so bloated that the body is as thick as it is wide.[173] Attempts to culture spirochetes from skin immediately after removal of an infected tick in a hyperendemic area were successful in only 2 of 48 patients, on both of whom the tick had been attached for approximately 24 hours.[25]

Assessment of the degree to which a tick is engorged is necessarily subjective. An attempt to make this determination more objective has been proposed as an "scutal index" (see Chapter 22).[74,197,265] This index is based on the fact that the body of a nymph or adult female will swell as the blood meal is taken, but the rigid scutum will remain unchanged. The ratio of the scutum to the body is, therefore, a rough indication of the degree of engorgement. The requirement for prolonged feeding before transmission comes from several factors: the spirochetes must pass from the midgut into the hemocele and thence into the salivary glands, and the spirochetes must downregulate the production of OspA and upregulate the production of OspC.

Careful epidemiologic study of several endemic areas has documented the magnitude of the problem. On Fire Island, New York, symptomatic disease developed in 0.7–1.2% of summer residents.[107] Antibodies developed in 4 (3.1%) of 129 persons studied serologically at the beginning and end of the summer, but only 2 of the persons were symptomatic. In Great Island, Massachusetts, Lyme disease developed in approximately 3% of the population each year, and the disease developed in 16% of the population over the 4-year period of study.[282] In retrospect, the earliest case occurred in 1962. The clinical:subclinical ratio was estimated to be 1:1.

Prevention is the best way to deal with any disease. Avoidance of exposure to the arthropod vectors is the logical way to prevent a tickborne infection.[209] Recommendations that wooded areas be avoided are logical, but probably ineffective because most people contract the infection in the yards of their homes. Common sense measures, such as wearing long-sleeved shirts and long pants and using insect repellents, are reasonable (http://www.cdc.gov/ncidod/dvbid/lyme/prevent.htm), but have not been documented to be effective in controlled studies. Prompt removal of embedded ticks with fine-tipped tweezers is recommended; the tick should be grasped firmly as close to the skin as possible, after which it should be carefully pulled away. The tick should be removed intact if possible, but leaving the mouthparts is not disastrous because the spirochetes are in the salivary gland of the tick. Use of a hot match, nail polish, petroleum jelly or other instruments of torture is not recommended. After removal of the tick, clean the area with an antiseptic (http://www.cdc.gov/ncidod/dvbid/lyme/prevent.htm).

The next logical step on the road to prevention was a vaccine. OspA was chosen as the immunizing antigen, because the borreliacidal antibodies that would be elicited could kill the spirochetes in the tick's salivary gland and/or at the bite site before disseminated infection had occurred. Two controlled studies documented an effectiveness of 49–68% in the first year after two doses of the vaccine. In the second year after a third injection the effectiveness was 76–92%.[258,280] Unfortunately, it appeared that a regular booster injection would be required to maintain efficacy. A national review panel recommended that use of the vaccine be limited to individuals between the ages of 15 and 70 years who were exposed to areas of high or moderate risk for considerable period of times.[3] Although side effects of the vaccine appeared minimal in the original reports, anecdotal reports of problems began to accumulate and concern grew. The manufacturer announced in February 2002 that it would discontinue manufacture of the vaccine. It is perhaps a commentary on our society that a search of the internet for references to the Lyme disease vaccine revealed predominantly the web sites of personal injury lawyers.

Antibiotic prophylaxis after tick bites remains controversial. Magid and colleagues, who attempted to quantify the analysis, recommended that patients not be treated if the risk of Lyme disease developing was less than 0.01.[162] Factors such as prolonged attachment of a feeding tick in an endemic region would increase the likelihood of transmission. If the tick is available for examination and is not an *Ixodes* species, or if Lyme disease is not endemic in the area, prophylaxis is clearly not indicated. Detection of *B. burgdorferi* by culture or molecular methods provides a possible means to make a rational decision about prophylaxis. Strong arguments can be marshaled, however, against such a course of action. Evaluation of the tick sufficiently quickly to allow a clinical decision about treatment will be difficult in most locales. If the tick does not contain borreliae, there is no assurance that another unobserved tick was infected. An infected tick may well not have transmitted the spirochetes, as discussed above. In a study of tick attachment, Sood and colleagues[265] found that duration of attachment and degree of engorgement as measured by the scutal index were predictors of the likelihood that *B. burgdorferi* was transmitted, but PCR evaluation of the tick did not predict transmission.

Des Vignes and colleagues investigated the transmission of *B. burgdorferi* from infected ticks removed from patients in an endemic area.[58] The removed ticks were fed on mice that were evaluated subsequently for infection. An overall transmission rate of 4.6% from these infected ticks was estimated.

The documentation that a single dose of doxycycline, given within 72 hours of the bite of *I. scapularis,* is as effective as longer courses of antibiotics in preventing the subsequent development of Lyme disease provides a new impetus for routine prophylaxis after tick bites in endemic areas.[188] The efficacy of treatment compared to placebo was 87%. On the other hand, side effects, however mild, were more common in patients who received even a single dose of doxycycline than in those who were given placebo, so the prophylactic choice remains a matter of judgment.[255]

CLINICAL DISEASE

The clinical manifestations of *B. burgdorferi* infection are protean. This spirochete has been referred to as the "latest great imitator,"[272] following in the tracks of its relative *T. pallidum.* As in syphilis, the manifestations of Lyme disease may be catalogued into three stages, as described below.

Stage one is the stage in which the tick bite elicits the classic lesion, erythema (chronicum) migrans. The expanding erythematous skin lesion presents in multiple anatomic locations and to varying extents.[24] In New Jersey, erythema migrans developed in 93% of the patients and approximately half had systemic symptoms, including lymphadenopathy.[31] Similarly, 90% of infected children in Connecticut displayed the skin rash.[95] Peripheral edema with central clearing of the lesion has been emphasized, but homogeneous or central redness was more characteristic in a large series of microbiologically confirmed cases.[261] Central clearing was more common in Slovenian patients who had been infected with *B. afzelii* than in New Yorkers who had been infected with *B. burgdorferi* sensu stricto.[284] At this stage of the infection the spirochete is most easily cultivated, and it may be visualized in as many as 40% of biopsy specimens by silver impregnation staining.

The second stage of Lyme disease results from dissemination of the spirochete throughout the body.[275] The polymerase chain reaction was approximately three times more sensitive for detecting spirochetemia than was culture of the organisms. Borrelial DNA was documented in the serum of 14 of 76 patients (18.4%) with erythema migrans. The number of clinical symptoms was the strongest independent predictor of spirochetemia.[99] It appears that the spirochetemia is both low level and intermittent.[297] Examination of CSF fluid of patients with erythema chronicum migrans documented borrelial DNA in 8 of 12 patients, 4 of whom had no neurologic abnormalities or symptoms. Spirochetal DNA was documented in the CSF taken from four of nine patients with neurologic symptoms.[159] The most common lesions are acute arthritis[279] and meningitis.[201] Bowen and colleagues[31] documented arthritis in 26% of their patients, meningitis in 10%, and cranial nerve palsies in 8%. The meningitis may appear purulent.[30] Secondary cutaneous lesions, infection of the eye, hepatitis, and myocardial damage may occur.

The third and chronic phase of the disease is characterized by chronic skin lesions, chronic neurologic symptoms, and chronic arthritis. The recurrent episodes of arthritis diminish in frequency and severity each year, but chronic synovitis and permanent disability develop in some patients.

As in syphilis, *B. burgdorferi* may be transmitted from mother to infant,[240,301] but the full effects of congenital infection are not yet known. Survival of the spirochete has been demonstrated experimentally for as long as 45 days in stored red blood cells, so transmission in blood transfusions is possible.[17] To date, however, the risk remains theoretical. No instances of transfusion-associated Lyme disease were encountered among 149 patients who received more than 600 units of blood in an area that is endemic for Lyme disease. One patient contracted babesiosis, for a risk of 0.17%.[96]

The manifestations of Lyme disease in Europe are similar to those in the United States, but arthritis may be relatively underrepresented and chronic meningitis relatively overrepresented, perhaps because of the presence of the neurotropic species, *B. garinii*, in Europe. Conversely, widespread disseminated infection appears to be more common in the United States than in Europe. As discussed above, clinical differences have been noted between patients infected in New York by *B. burgdorferi* sensu stricto and Slovenian patients infected by *B. afzelii*.

Prompt antimicrobial therapy in the initial stages of Lyme disease is usually effective in controlling symptoms and preventing progression of disease. Practice guidelines have been provided by the Infectious Diseases Society of America.[304] In the later stages of illness it is less clear that antimicrobial therapy is of use.[137]

Although apparently rare, there have been well-documented examples of reinfection with a new strain of *B. burgdorferi* (as determined by molecular analysis of sequential isolates) in patients who have been treated for erythema migrans.[195] It is not clear whether reinfections occur after untreated natural disease.

Symptomatic infection appears not to occur in wildlife, but disease may develop in domestic animals. Kornblatt and colleagues have described Lyme arthritis in dogs.[140] Duray has described the surgical pathology of Lyme disease.[65]

LABORATORY DIAGNOSIS

Lyme disease may be diagnosed by culture of the spirochete, by demonstration of the spirochetes in tissue using immunologic or molecular techniques, or by documentation of a serologic response. Recommendations for diagnostic methods that were provided by a consensus group in 1997[1,292] have not changed appreciably. It is recommended that testing be performed only when the pretest probability of Lyme disease, based on clinical symptoms and exposure history, ranges between 0.2 and 0.8. The fly in the pudding is, of course, the difficulty of calculating the pretest probability in an individual patient. Vague symptoms, such as fatigue or arthralgias, are not sufficient reason by themselves to initiate testing. The comparative efficacy of various laboratory techniques in the diagnosis of 47 patients with erythema migrans is summarized in Box 20-2. Laboratory diagnosis of Lyme disease has been reviewed by Reed.[219]

Although the erythema migrans lesion is not pathognomonic, it is present in a very high percentage of acute infections and is found in few other diseases. Lyme disease may be confidently diagnosed if this lesion is present, therefore, and further testing is probably not necessary. Even after more than two decades of experience, inappropriate use of diagnostic testing and inappropriate antimicrobial therapy remain problems.[83,186,215]

Culture. *B. burgdorferi* has been isolated in cell-free medium (see Table 20-3). The process is relatively easy when infected ticks are triturated and cultured (see Color Plate 20-1E). Subculture from broth to agar results in the formation of spirochetal colonies with varying morphology.[142] The medium of choice is a modification of Kelly's medium for spirochetes that was developed by Barbour (Box 20-3). Additional modifications to that medium have been suggested.[210]

Culture is most effective in early Lyme disease and is rarely positive in later stages. Even at the primary stage, however, spirochetes were isolated from skin lesions only in 51% and from blood in 45% of 47 adult patients with a clinical diagnosis of Lyme disease.[194] The yield appears to be higher when the lesions are large and multiple, as in the secondary disseminated phase of the disease.[181] Citrated blood should be cultured. Tubes are incubated at 34 to 37°C in the dark. They are examined by darkfield microscopy after incubation for 2 to 3 weeks. The identity of any spiral

Box 20-2 Laboratory Investigation of 47 Adult Patients with Erythema Migrans

Laboratory Procedure	Diagnostic Yield (%)
Quantitative PCR of skin biopsy	80.9
Two-stage serologic testing of convalescent specimens	66.0
Conventional nested PCR	63.8
Skin culture	51.1
Blood culture	44.7
Serologic testing of acute specimens	40.4

Adapted from reference[194].

organisms detected must be confirmed by specific immunofluorescence reagents.

Morphologic Detection. Visualization of spirochetes in tissues by morphologic means is also insensitive for most specimens and stages of the disease. Any of the silver impregnation methods for demonstration of spirochetes in tissue (Warthin-Starry, Steiner, Dieterle) may be used to stain the organisms, but specific identification must be confirmed with antisera, because the silver stains detect any type of bacterium.

Molecular Detection. Amplification techniques have demonstrated greater sensitivity than culture or morphologic detection in the skin of erythema migrans lesions,[157] in peripheral blood, and in joint fluid.[206] Results of molecular detection in CSF and urine have been disappointing.[62] The sensitivity of polymerase chain reaction (PCR) is less in CSF than in urine in patients with symptomatic neurologic disease.[147] Recommendations for increasing the yield of PCR testing in urine have been developed by Bergmann and colleagues.[26] Real-time PCR assays have been validated with a variety of clinical specimens.[106,247]

An extensive review of molecular amplification methods in the diagnosis of Lyme disease was provided by Schmidt.[244] A role exists for molecular techniques in documenting acute infection or sorting out difficult cases, but thoroughly validated amplification tests are not readily available to most laboratories. Amplification tests are susceptible to false-positive results from cross-contamination or from nucleic acid sequences shared with other organisms. A false-positive PCR for *B. burgdorferi* in a commercial laboratory has been documented.[183] Amplification tests do not add significant value for the diagnosis of early Lyme disease, but they may be of great help in the later stages of infection, particularly for the diagnosis of neuroborreliosis. Detection of borrelial DNA in CSF may be especially helpful because of the difficulty in interpretation of antibodies in the central nervous system. The specificity of the molecular tests can be increased, however, by first evaluating the patient for the presence of IgG antibody, which should be virtually uniformly present in serum at that stage of the infection.

A commercial kit for detection of spirochetal antigen in urine has been developed, but has received poor reviews.[138]

Serologic Detection. The diagnostic method of choice by default is serologic analysis. The CDC recommends a two-step approach to diagnosis. An enzyme immunoassay or immunofluorescence assay with high sensitivity should be used as the initial test. Negative sera need not be studied further, but convalescent sera should be collected if clinically indicated. Positive results should be confirmed with both IgM and IgG immunoblots.[46]

Immunofluorescence and enzyme immunoassays have been used most commonly. Indirect immunofluorescence,[165] quantitative fluorescence immunoassay,[204] and a fluoroimmunoassay[111] have been recommended, but many investigators have found the enzyme immunoassay to be more satisfactory.[52,231] Antibody may be absent early, but is usually present after several weeks. A response to OspA tends to occur late, but may be detected in low titer or complexed to spirochetes early in the course of infection if special techniques are used.[246] A response to the OspC protein or the less specific flagellin antigen occurs more commonly in early sera.[164] For maximum sensitivity in early Lyme disease, use of an IgM assay has been recommended, either by immunofluorescence[179] or immunoblot[9] techniques. Specific IgM titers may remain elevated throughout the course of illness and even years after treatment, so the presence of IgM cannot be used to establish acute infection.[130] Collection of a second specimen 8 to 14 days after the baseline sample has been recommended for documentation of seroconversion in early Lyme disease. If IgM alone is detected a month or more after infection, the IgM result is probably false-positive.

Examination of spinal fluid for intrathecally produced antibodies has been performed for the diagnosis of neuroborreliosis. The presence of higher titers of antibody in CSF than in peripheral blood theoretically documents infection of the nervous system.[307] Given the many difficulties with serologic analysis of peripheral blood, these approaches should be reserved for experienced reference laboratories that have documented the efficacy of their tests.

Most currently available assays use sonicated whole spirochetes, and the reagents are not standardized. As a result there have been serious problems with reproducibility and with accuracy, compounding the difficulties of clinical diagnosis. In a proficiency testing program as many as 21% of participants failed to recognize the presence of antibody at a titer of 512 or higher.[18] With lower concentrations of antibody, as many as 55% of participants failed to recognize the serum as positive. Conversely, the false-positive rate was up to 7% with a polyvalent conjugate and as high as 27% with an IgG conjugate. Reproducibility of results when the same serum was submitted as a challenge at different times was also suboptimal. The fact that these proficiency testing problems are present in the real world is emphasized by the report from a Lyme disease referral center, where 45% of patients who had been referred with an incorrect diagnosis of Lyme disease had had positive serologic tests for *B. burgdorferi* that could not be confirmed in the reference laboratory.[281] Furthermore, in a single laboratory only 16.3% of positive results using an enzyme immunoassay could be confirmed with an immunoblot.[53] The authors argue that insensitivity of the immunoblot does not explain the results, because more cases of erythema migrans were detected with the immunoblot than with the enzyme immunoassay.

Our clinical colleagues have not been successful in dealing with this enigmatic disease either. At one university Lyme disease clinic, 38% of children were overdiagnosed and 8% were underdiagnosed.[76] One quarter of the patients who had been diagnosed correctly were subsequently treated incorrectly. In a study of diagnostic tests at a prepaid health care plan in California, only 19% of laboratory tests were ordered because the physician suspected Lyme disease.[152] Fully 60% of the tests were ordered as a part of a battery of tests for patients with vague complaints. In an area where Lyme disease is uncommon, such indiscriminant test ordering stacks the deck against serologic tests that already have more than enough problems of their own.

Cross-reactions with a variety of infectious agents have been found in sera from patients in whom Lyme disease is suspected. Sera of patients with other borrelial infections,[163] treponemal infections,[23,119,216] HIV, Epstein-Barr virus, and rickettsial infections may react in assays for *B. burgdorferi*. Reports on cross-reaction with leptospira antisera are conflicting. Although cross-reactions develop with specific treponemal antigens, the VDRL test is not positive in patients with Lyme disease. The nonspecific reactions have been reported to be concentrated in the IgG2 class of antibodies in several instances.[254]

As often happens, interpretation of serologic results is most straightforward when it is least needed, that is, when the classic erythema chronicum migrans rash occurs. When the presentation is atypical, the diagnosis is usually serologic and the possibility of misleading results with serious consequences is magnified. Steere[273] has pointed out that serologic evidence of infection may be correct but that the Lyme disease may be subclinical and the patient's problems caused by another agent.

Kaell and colleagues described four patients from an area endemic for Lyme disease who had confusing multisystemic disease that was initially attributed to *B. burgdorferi*.[129] All four patients had antibodies to the spirochete, and three of the four had positive results on Western blot tests; however, continued study revealed that the cause of the illness in all four cases was subacute bacterial endocarditis. Subsequently, these investigators demonstrated increased antibodies to *B. burgdorferi* in 13 of 30 patients (43%) with nonspirochetal endocarditis.[128] The specificity of Lyme serology in this population was only 60%. When immunoblots were

performed, only one patient had a pattern of reactivity that suggested prior exposure to the spirochete. The authors hypothesize that cross-reactions with the infecting bacterium might be responsible for the high frequency of nonspecific results.

Two major types of approach to the serologic problems have been taken: development of immunoblots (Western blots) and a search for defined—and, therefore, reproducible—antigens that react with the sera of most infected patients.

The presence of positive Western blots in patients with bacterial endocarditis indicates that immunoblotting is not per se a guarantee of specificity. As in HIV infection the immunoblot can be used to improve the specificity of other immunoassays. Dressler and colleagues developed criteria for positive immunoblots in a retrospective study.[61] The best discrimination was obtained if detection of 2 of the 8 most common IgM bands (18, 21, 28, 37, 41, 45, 58, and 93 kDa) was required for positivity in early disease and detection of at least 5 of the 10 most common IgG bands (18, 21, 28, 30, 39, 41, 45, 58, 66, and 93 kDa) was required for diagnosis after the first weeks of infection. Application of these criteria to more than 300 patients in a prospective study yielded a sensitivity of 32% and a specificity of 100% for the IgM test. The sensitivity and specificity of the IgG test were 83% and 95%, respectively. Slightly different criteria have been suggested by Engstrom and colleagues.[72] Their criteria for positivity of IgM immunoblots include recognition of at least two of the following proteins: 24 (OspC), 39, and 41 (flagellin) kDa. The sensitivities of the IgG and IgM immunoblots in 55 patients with documented erythema migrans were 58.5% and 54.6%, respectively, at the time of diagnosis and 100% after an additional 8 to 12 days. Ma and associates have emphasized the importance of antibody to the 39-kDa antigen for specific diagnosis.[161]

The CDC and Association of State and Territorial Public Health Laboratory Directors currently recommend the IgM criteria of Engstrom and the IgG criteria of Dressler. By using these criteria Aguero-Rosenfeld and associates[10] observed positive IgM immunoblots at the time of initial study in 43% of a group of 46 patients with culture-positive erythema migrans and in 84% of the patients 8 to 14 days later. Although antibodies to *B. burgdorferi* developed in 89% of patients, IgG immunoblots were positive by the recommended criteria in only 22% of convalescent sera. After 1 year 38% of the IgM immunoblots were still positive. IgM antibodies reactive with 39-, 58-, 60-, 66-, and 93-kDa antigens were most often seen in the first month after diagnosis, and these investigators suggest that the presence of these bands may be helpful in suggesting recent infection in patients from endemic areas.

Hilton and colleagues suggest that two additional antigens be added to the criteria for IgG positivity: 31-kDa (OspA) and 34-kDa (OspB) antigens.[113] Of 136 patients evaluated for Lyme disease, 4 (8%) would have been considered positive only if these two antigens were included in the criteria. These 4 patients had erythema migrans or arthritis and lived in endemic zones. It is obvious that the criteria for interpretation of immunoblots are still evolving.

Fine-tuning of the criteria for positive serologic tests will undoubtedly continue, but confirmation of an indeterminate or questionable result with an enzyme immunoassay should be sought by performing an immunoblot in an experienced laboratory. Wormser and colleagues have noted, however, that the confirmatory aspects of the immunoblots are reduced because the two assays are not completely independent.[303]

Attempts to improve the specificity of serologic diagnosis also include development of recombinant antigens for enzyme immunoassays, predominantly OspA,[80] OspB, and OspC.[91] Recognition of antigenic diversity among strains may be important for greater sensitivity in certain regions.[288]

An additional problem has been presented by the Lyme disease vaccine, which contains OspA outer-surface protein. If the serologic assay detects OspA, it will be impossible to tell whether an immunized individual also has had an infection. The sera of vaccinees may produce positive reactions in enzyme immunoassays, but do not produce a sufficient number of bands in Western blots to yield positive results.[10] The development of enzyme immunoassays that do not contain OspA should also help to resolve this dilemma.[182]

Leptospira

Leptospira are motile, obligately aerobic helical rods that measure 0.1 μm in diameter and 6 to 12 μm in length. They are gram-negative and are only faintly stained by aniline dyes. Darkfield microscopy must be used to visualize unstained leptospira (Figure 20-6). Two species of *Leptospira* have been recognized classically: *L. interrogans,* which contains all of the human pathogens, and the saprophytic species, *L. biflexa. L. interrogans* contains many individual serotypes that cause human disease. Antigenically related serovars are collected into serogroups for classification pur-

poses. The type strain is *L. interrogans* serovar icterohaemorrhagiae,[126] and the clinical disease is leptospirosis. Several thorough reviews, although old, still reflect the state of knowledge in many areas.[68,77,109,110]

Yasuda and colleagues studied the DNA relatedness among serogroups and serovars of *Leptospira.*[305] On genetic grounds they proposed at least five new species among the human pathogens. The nucleic acid analysis did not correlate well with the serologic classification. A single serovar might be found in several species. Not surprisingly, the number of genomospecies continues to expand.[149] The currently recognized genomospecies and the corresponding serogroups are detailed in Table 20-6.

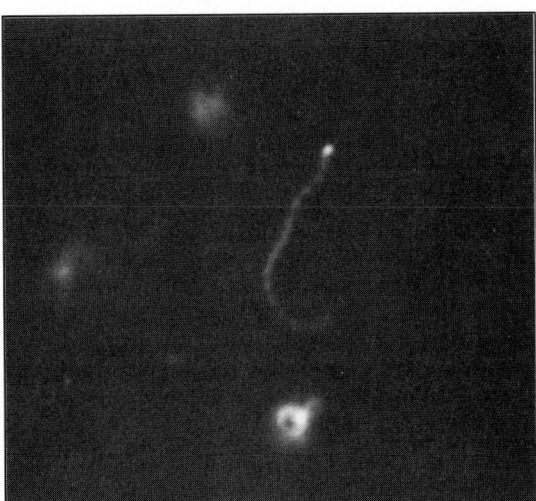

Figure 20-6 Darkfield examination of *Leptospira interrogans* culture. The spiral coils, which are not clearly demonstrated, appear as alternating bright and dark areas. The very bright upper end of the organism may represent the hooked end that many leptospira possess. It is easy for inexperienced observers to confuse cell debris and artifacts with leptospira in clinical specimens. × 1000. (Photomicrograph courtesy of David Miller, DVM, MS.)

Table 20-6 Genomospecies and Serogroups of *Leptospira*

GENOMOSPECIES	SEROGROUP
L. interrogans	Icterohaemorrhagiae, Canicola, Pomona, Australis, Autumnalis, Pyrogenes, Grippotyphosa, Djasiman, Hebdomadis, Sejroe, Bataviae, Ranarum, Louisiana, Mini, Sarmin
L. noguchii	Panama, Autumnalis, Pyrogenes, Louisiana, Bataviae, Tarassovi, Australis, Shermani, Djasiman, Pomona
L. santarosai	Shermani, Hebdomadis, Tarassovi, Pyrogenes, Autumnalis, Bataviae, Mini, Grippotyphosa, Sejroe, Pomona, Javanica, Sarmin, Cynopteri
L. meyeri	Ranarum, Semaranga, Sejroe, Mini, Javanica
L. wolbachii*	Codice
L. biflexa*	Semaranga, Andamana
L. fainei	Hurstbridge
L. borgpetersenii	Javanica, Ballum, Hebdomadis, Sejroe, Tarassovi, Mini, Celledoni, Pyrogenes, Bataviae, Australis, Autumnalis
L. kirschneri	Grippotyphosa, Autumnalis, Cynopteri, Hebdomadis, Australis, Pomona, Djasiman, Canicola, Icterohaemorrhagiae, Bataviae
L. weilii	Celledoni, Icterohaemorrhagiae, Sarmin, Javanica, Mini, Tarassovi, Hebdomadis, Pyrogenes, Manhao, Sejroe
L. inadia	Lyme, Shermani, Icterohaemorrhagiae, Tarassovi, Manhao, Canicola, Panama, Javanica
L. parva*	Turneria
L. alexanderi	Manhao, Hebdomadis, Javanica, Mini

* No pathogenic serogroups associated with this species to date
Adapted from reference[149].

Leptospirosis

An excellent review of all aspects of leptospirosis has been provided by Levett.[149]

EPIDEMIOLOGY

Leptospira are distributed worldwide and infect many types of domestic and wild animals. Humans become incidental, ''dead-end'' hosts because transmission from humans to animals or to other humans does not occur. Rats have been classically associated with this disease, but sheep, cattle, dogs, and other domestic animals may be infected. In the wild, foxes, raccoons, skunks, shrews, and hedgehogs carry the leptospires. Associations between serovars and animal species exist, such as *L. interrogans* sv. icterohaemorrhagiae and rats or *L. interrogans* sv. canicola and dogs. Several different serovars of *Leptospira* may be carried by a single animal genus, however, and a single serovar may be associated with more than one animal host. In general, the animal hosts are not symptomatic and antibody does not develop in them, despite overwhelming infection.

Leptospirosis has traditionally been considered an occupational disease, concentrated among workers in sewers, rice fields, sugar cane fields, and abattoirs. In the 1970s in the United States, however, only 30% of the persons for whom an occupation was reported to the CDC were exposed at work. There were children, homemakers, and retired or unemployed persons among the infected. It has been suggested that increasing leisure time and more frequent forays into the countryside have increased the likelihood of casual exposure. Leptospirosis has been reported in association with kayaking.[257] The recreational association continues to expand. Epidemic disease occurred during a triathlon in Illinois, where it was associated with even the briefest exposure to the water in a pond,[185] and among white water rafters in Costa Rica.[2] Most famously, participants in an Eco-Challenge race in Borneo got more of an ''Eco Challenge'' than they had bargained for when they contracted acute leptospirosis during the race.[4] Disease was associated with kayaking, spelunking, and swimming in or drinking water from the Segama River.

Epidemiologic factors that were associated with leptospirosis in Hawaii included catchment of rainwater for household use, contact with cattle and cattle urine, or handling of animal tissues.[238] Feigin and colleagues documented a small epidemic in University City, Missouri, an upper-middle-class suburb of St. Louis.[78] They were able to isolate *Leptospira interrogans* sv. icterohaemorrhagiae from rats and house pets and from soil in the yards of homes. Some of the dogs from whom they isolated leptospires had been immunized with commercially available anti-*Leptospira* vaccines. Epidemic disease may occur from a common source, as was recently found in a waterborne outbreak in Italy.[40] In that epidemic it was suggested that an outbreak associated with a town fountain was caused by a hedgehog trapped in a water reservoir. A recent outbreak in Illinois was traced to a contaminated pond; a drought was hypothesized to have increased the risk of exposure to infected animal excreta.[124] *Leptospira* are distributed worldwide, so that imported disease must be considered in travelers.[293]

CLINICAL DISEASE

Classic leptospirosis is a biphasic disease, which consists of an initial septicemic phase and a secondary immune phase. The severity ranges from subclinical infection to fatal systemic disease, known as Weil's disease, after the man who first described icterohemorrhagic fever in 1886. In severe cases the two phases merge together and an asymptomatic interval may not be recognized.

Surveys of workers at occupational risk have demonstrated antibodies without a recognized episode of leptospirosis in 5–16% of those tested. In patients who are recognized to have leptospiral infection, Weil's disease was described in 5–10% of cases in a classic review. More recently, however, jaundice was noted in 39% of cases from Hawaii between 1974 and 1998. Conjunctival suffusion was noted in 28% of cases.[131]

The initial septicemic phase of the disease is abrupt in onset, ushered in by high fever, severe headache, malaise, and muscle aches. Eye pain, photophobia, and conjunctival suffusion or even hemorrhage are characteristically present. It should be emphasized that inflammation or true conjunctivitis is conspicuously absent. Pulmonary infiltrates are relatively common. Disease is usually mild, but leptospirosis may present as adult respiratory distress syndrome[71,169,196] and pulmonary hemorrhage has been described.[251]

Patients may present with rashes that are macular, maculopapular, urticarial, or hemorrhagic. A distinctive pretibial rash accompanied an epidemic of *L. interrogans* sv. autumnalis infection and was named Fort Bragg fever. This pretibial rash has accompanied infections with other serovars.

After an asymptomatic interval of 1 to 3 days, the immune phase of the infection develops. The Jarisch-Herxheimer reaction has been reported after early treatment. Leptospires are rapidly cleared from the blood and CSF, and an inflammatory process develops. A CSF pleocytosis will develop in 90% of patients during the second week of illness, but only half of these patients have symptoms of aseptic meningitis. *L. interrogans* was responsible for 5–13% of cases of aseptic meningitis in one series.

The hallmarks of Weil's disease are jaundice and acute renal failure. The jaundice and other signs of liver dysfunction appear as early as the third week and as late as the ninth week after infection.

The diagnosis of classic infection is relatively straightforward, but the diagnosis is considerably more difficult in the average case without an occupational exposure. Schmid and associates reported a very unusual case of leptospirosis, in which the clinical symptoms mimicked Lyme disease. The etiologic agent was a previously unrecognized leptospira, which they named ''*L. inadai*'' sv. lyme.[242]

DuPont and colleagues evaluated prognostic factors in 68 patients from the French West Indies.[64] By multivariate analysis, five factors were associated with a fatal outcome: dyspnea, oliguria, white-blood-cell count >12,900/mm³, repolarization abnormalities on electrocardiograms, and alveolar infiltrates on chest radiographs.

LABORATORY DIAGNOSIS

Leptospirosis may be diagnosed by culture of the spirochete, by demonstration of the organisms in specimens, by detection of antigens or nucleic acid, or by serology.

Direct Detection. Direct demonstration of *Leptospira* may be attempted by darkfield examination of blood, CSF, or urine. Centrifugation at low speed of oxalated or heparinized blood to remove cellular elements and then at high speed to concentrate leptospira has been recommended. Unfortunately, the direct examination results in rapid but erroneous diagnoses, because fibrils or extrusions from red blood cells are misinterpreted as spirochetes. Although examination of CSF and urine are somewhat less treacherous, similar caveats apply.[262] Direct identification of leptospira with labeled antisera has been described, but reagents are not available commercially.

Culture. The most commonly used media for culture are Fletcher's semisolid medium, Korthof's liquid medium, and bovine serum albumin-Tween 80 medium, which may be either liquid or solid. The media may be stored at room temperature for long periods. Antibiotics are usually added when the specimen, such as urine, is likely to be contaminated with bacteria, but some of the antibiotics also inhibit leptospira at the required concentration. A combination of fosfomycin and 5-fluorouracil has been found effective when used with Korthof's medium, but the authors caution that the results cannot automatically be transferred to other *Leptospira* media.[198]

Leptospira can be isolated freely from blood and CSF during the first week of illness. During the immune stage the organisms disappear from the blood and CSF. The kidney, however, is a privileged site, and *Leptospira* are excreted in the urine for up to 1 month (see Color Plate 20-1*G*).

It is recommended that at least four 5-mL tubes of culture media from two different lots be inoculated with the clinical specimen. For recovery of fastidious serotypes, 0.4–1.0% sterile rabbit serum may be added to the bovine serum albumin-Tween 80 medium. Only small volumes of blood or urine should be inoculated, because larger volumes will introduce interfering substances. Media should be inoculated with one to two drops of specimen per tube. If the procedure cannot be done at the bedside, oxalated or heparinized blood may be sent to the laboratory. A triturated clot may also be inoculated, but citrated blood may be inhibitory. When urine is tested, an undiluted specimen and a 10-fold dilution should be inoculated. When CSF is used, 0.5 to 5.0 mL should be inoculated.

The cultures are incubated in the dark at 28 to 30°C for up to 6 weeks and examined weekly by darkfield microscopy for the presence of leptospira (see Fig. 20-6). Growth is often delayed for several weeks but occurs considerably earlier in Tween 80-albumin medium. Leptospira typically grow as a band 0.5 to 1.0 cm below the surface of semisolid media (see Color Plate 20-1*H*).

Manca and colleagues reported recovery of *L. interrogans* from simulated specimens and from human blood using a commercial radiometric blood culture system. They used Stuart's medium and Middlebrook TB (12A) medium that had been supplemented with bovine serum albumin, catalase, and casein hydrolysate and labeled with C-fatty acids. The time to recovery in human blood was 2 to 5 days.[167]

Serology. Diagnosis of leptospirosis by culture is definitive, but the techniques are specialized and difficult for most laboratories to maintain when the disease is of low prevalence. The mainstay of diagnosis in most hospitals is, therefore,

serologic analysis, and the gold standard is the microagglutination test, using live leptospira. The difficulty of maintaining large numbers of cultures of *Leptospira* is obvious. Formalin-killed leptospira are used as a practical compromise, but they result in somewhat lower sensitivity. The reference microagglutination test, often considered serovar-specific, is, in fact serogroup-specific. A large number of antigens must, nevertheless, be tested against the sera in order to detect local serovars with certainty. Commercially available serogroup-specific leptospiral antigens are used in a macroscopic agglutination test that may be used to screen sera. Positive reactions should be confirmed in a reference laboratory with the use of the microagglutination test.

Several versions of hemagglutination test have been less commonly used. Seki and colleagues described a rapid microcapsule agglutination test,[253] but this test has not been evaluated by other investigators. Several groups have reported enzyme immunoassays that appear promising.[8,203,300] IgM antibody is most specific for current infection. The assays appear to function well and may eventually replace the cumbersome microagglutination test, but cross-reactions do occur. More work is necessary before these procedures can be accepted as new gold standards, as demonstrated by two recent reports. Investigators in the West Indies noted a sensitivity of 100% for a commercially available indirect hemagglutination assay,[150] but investigators in Hawaii found only a 68% sensitivity in patients infected with serovar icterohaemorrhagiae and a 47% sensitivity in patients infected with serovar Australis.[69] The difference in sensitivity between the two studies may represent differing serovars in the two locations. This experience is a cautionary tale for all who attempt leptospiral serologic diagnosis.

Other serologic techniques, such as latex agglutination,[263] particle agglutination,[32] and a dipstick immunoblot,[102] have been reported. These assays are not commercially available and/or have not been evaluated extensively. Investigators at the CDC noted that a commercially available dipstick assay (Dip-S, PanBio INDX, Inc., Baltimore, MD) produced more positive results (apparently true-positives) than a commercial IgM enzyme-linked immunosorbent assay (P Brisbane, Australia).

The CDC has suggested a titer of >1:200 in a single serum by the microagglutination test as presumptive evidence of leptospirosis in a patient with a compatible clinical illness, but other experts have suggested a titer of 1:800 or 1:1600 as better cutoffs. Titers may reach extremely high levels and take months or years to decrease, so the height of the titer cannot be used for determination of recent infection.[226]

Detection of Antigen and Nucleic Acid. Monoclonal antibodies have been used to detect leptospiral antigen in urine in specimens from Thailand, with promising results.[233]

Molecular amplification techniques have been used successfully for the diagnosis of leptospirosis.[19,175] Leptospiral DNA was present in urine even in the early stages of infection, when spirochetemia predominates. A high percentage of patients with aseptic meningitis were found to have leptospiral DNA in CSF, but neither culture nor serologic analysis of blood specimens were done in this study, so it is difficult to interpret the results.[225] These assays are not widely available, but may find a place in reference laboratories.

Spirillium minor *(Rat-Bite Fever)*

Spirillum minor is a short, thick, tightly coiled spiral rod that measures 0.2 to 0.5 µm in diameter by 3 to 5 µm in length. It produces a large proportion of rat-bite fever in Asia, but rarely occurs in the United States. Transmission is, as the name implies, by rat bite. Human-to-human transmission has not been documented. One to four weeks after the bite, a systemic illness occurs, characterized by chills, headache, and fever. The site of the bite, which had healed, reactivates and is accompanied by regional lymphadenitis and a blotchy rash. Relapsing fever may occur for weeks, months, or years. The most serious complication is infectious endocarditis.[299] Although rare, this infection is still a threat when exposure to rats is a possibility.[199]

Spirillum minor cannot be cultured in vivo, and no specific serologic tests are available. As many as 50% of infected patients have false-positive serologic tests for syphilis. The spirochetes may be visualized in blood, exudates, or tissue using Giemsa's or Wright's stain or darkfield microscopy.

REFERENCES

1. Guidelines for laboratory evaluation in the diagnosis of Lyme disease. American College of Physicians. Ann Intern Med 1997;127:1106–1108
2. Outbreak of leptospirosis among white-water rafters-Costa Rica, 1996. MMWR Morb Mortal Wkly Rep 1997;46:577–579
3. Recommendations for the use of Lyme disease vaccine. Recommendations of the Advisory Committee on Immunization Practices (ACIP). MMWR Recomm Rep 1999;48:1–5
4. Centers for Disease Control and Prevention. Update: outbreak of acute febrile illness among athletes participating in Eco-Challenge-Sabah 2000-Borneo, Malaysia, 2000. JAMA 2001;285:728–730
5. Lyme disease-United States, 2000. MMWR Morb Mortal Wkly Rep 2002;51:29–31
6. Primary and secondary syphilis-United States, 2000–2001. MMWR Morb Mortal Wkly Rep 2002;51:971–973
7. Ackerman R, et al: Spirochäten-Ätiologie der Erythema-chronicum-migrans-Krankheit. Dtsch Med Wochenschr 1984;109:92–97
8. Adler B, et al: Detection of specific and antileptospiral immunoglobulins M and G in human serum by solid-phase enzyme-linked immunosorbent assay. J Clin Microbiol 1980;11:452–452
9. Aguero-Rosenfeld ME, et al: Evolution of the serologic response to *Borrelia burgdorferi* in treated patients with culture-confirmed erythema migrans. J Clin Microbiol 1996;34:1–9
10. Aguero-Rosenfeld ME, et al: Effects of OspA vaccination on Lyme disease serologic testing. J Clin Microbiol 1999;37:3718–3721
11. Alexander-Rodriguez T, Vermund Sh: Gonorrhea and syphilis in incarcerated urban adolescents: prevalence and physical signs. Pediatrics 1987;80:561–564
12. Alford CA, et al: Gamma-M-fluorescent treponemal antibody in the diagnosis of syphilis. N Engl J Med 1969;280:1086–1091
13. Anderson Jf: Epizootiology of *Borrelia* in *Ixodes* tick vectors and reservoir hosts. Rev Infect Dis 1989;11(Suppl 6):S1451–S1459
14. Andrus JK, et al: Partner notification: can it control epidemic syphilis? Ann Intern Med 1990;112:539–543
15. Augenbraun Mh: Treatment of syphilis 2001: nonpregnant adults. Clin Infect Dis 2002;35:S187–S190
16. Augenbraun MH, et al: Biological false-positive syphilis test results for women infected with human immunodeficiency virus. Clin Infect Dis 1994;19:1040–1044
17. Badon SJ, et al: Survival of *Borrelia burgdorferi* in blood products. Transfusion 1989;29:581–583
18. Bakken LL, et al: Performance of 45 laboratories participating in a proficiency testing program for Lyme disease serology. JAMA 1992;268:891–895
19. Bal AE, et al: Detection of leptospires in urine by PCR for early diagnosis of leptospirosis. J Clin Microbiol 1994;32:1894–1898
20. Barbour Ag: Isolation and cultivation of Lyme disease spirochetes. Yale J Biol Med 1984;57:521–525
21. Barton JR, et al: Nonimmune hydrops fetalis associated with maternal infection with syphilis. Am J Obstet Gynecol 1992;167:56–58
22. Benditt J: The syphilized world. Sci Am 1989;260:30–30
23. Berardi VP, et al: Serodiagnosis of early Lyme disease: analysis of IgM and IgG antibody responses by using an antibody-capture enzyme immunoassay. J Infect Dis 1988;158:754–760
24. Berger Bw: Erythema chronicum migrans of Lyme disease. Arch Dermatol 1984;120:1017–1021
25. Berger BW, et al: Cultivation of *Borrelia burgdorferi* from human tick bite sites: a guide to the risk of infection. J Am Acad Dermatol 1995;32:184–187
26. Bergmann AR, et al: Importance of sample preparation for molecular diagnosis of lyme borreliosis from urine. J Clin Microbiol 2002;40:4581–4584
27. Berry CD, et al: Neurologic relapse after benzathine penicillin therapy for secondary syphilis in a patient with HIV infection. N Engl J Med 1987;316:1587–1589
28. Blank S, et al: Incident syphilis among women with multiple admissions to jail in New York City. J Infect Dis 1999;180:1159–1163
29. Borgnolo G, et al: Louse-borne relapsing fever: a clinical and an epidemiological study of 389 patients in Asella Hospital, Ethiopia. Trop Geogr Med 1993;45:66–69
30. Bourke SJ, et al: Lyme disease with acute purulent meningitis. BMJ 1988;297:460
31. Bowen GS, et al: Clinical manifestations and descriptive epidemiology of Lyme disease in New Jersey, 1978 to 1982. JAMA 1984;251:2236–2240
32. Brandao AP, et al: Macroscopic agglutination test for rapid diagnosis of human leptospirosis. J Clin Microbiol 1998;36:3138–3142
33. Bromberg K, et al: Diagnosis of congenital syphilis by combining *Treponema pallidum*-specific IgM detection with immunofluorescent antigen detection for *T. pallidum*. J Infect Dis 1993;168:238–242
34. Brown RN, Lane RS: Lyme disease in California: a novel enzootic transmission cycle of *Borrelia burgdorferi*. Science 1992;256:1439–1442
35. Brunet LR, et al: Density of Lyme disease spirochetes within deer ticks collected from zoonotic sites. Am J Trop Med Hyg 1995;53:300–302
36. Bryceson ADM, et al: Louse-borne relapsing fever: a clinical and laboratory study of 62 cases in Ethiopia and reconsideration of the literature. Q J Med 1970;39:129–170
37. Burgdorfer W, et al: Lyme disease: a tick-borne spirochetosis. Science 1982;216:1317–1319
38. Butler T, et al: *Borrelia recurrentis* infection: single-dose antibiotic regimens and management of the Jarisch-Herxheimer reaction. J Infect Dis 1978;137:573–577
39. Byrne RE, et al: Evaluation of a *Treponema pallidum* western immunoblot assay as a confirmatory test for syphilis. J Clin Microbiol 1992;30:115–122
40. Cacciapuoti B, et al: A waterborne outbreak of leptospirosis. Am J Epidemiol 1987;126:535–545
41. Cadavid D, Barbour AG: Neuroborreliosis during relapsing fever: review of the clinical manifestations, pathology, and treatment of infections in humans and experimental animals. Clin Infect Dis 1998;26:151–164
42. Canale-Parola E: Spirochetales. In Krieg NR, Holt JR, eds.: Bergey's Manual of Systematic Microbiology. Baltimore: Williams & Wilkins, 1984
43. Centers For Disease Control: Syphilis and congenital syphilis-United States, 1985–1988. MMWR Morb Mortal Wkly Rep 1988;37:486–489
44. Centers For Disease Control: Comparison of early and late latent syphilis-Colorado, 1991. MMWR Morb Mortal Wkly Rep 1993;42:155–157
45. Centers For Disease Control And Prevention: Lyme disease—United States, 1994. MMWR Morb Mortal Wkly Rep 1995;44:459–462
46. Centers For Disease Control And Prevention: Recommendations for test performance and interpretation from the Second National Conference on Serologic Diagnosis of Lyme Disease. MMWR Morb Mortal Wkly Rep 1995;44:590–591
47. Centers For Disease Control And Prevention: Surveillance Summaries: Surveillance for Lyme Disease-United States, 1992–1998. MMWR Morb Mortal Wkly Rep 49:1–11, 2000
48. Chambers RW, et al: Transmission of syphilis by fresh blood components. Transfusion 1969;9:32–34
49. Chang SN, et al: Seroreversion of the serological tests for syphilis in the newborns born to treated syphilitic mothers. Genitourin Med 1995;71:68–70
50. Chhabra RS, et al: Comparison of maternal sera, cord blood, and neonatal sera for detecting presumptive congenital syphilis: relationship with maternal treatment. Pediatrics 1993;91:88–91
51. Colebunders R, et al: Imported relapsing fever in European tourists. Scand J Infect Dis 1993;25:533–536

52. Craft JE, et al: Antibody response in Lyme disease: evaluation of diagnostic tests. J Infect Dis 1984;149:789–795

53. Cutler SJ, Wright DJ: Predictive value of serology in diagnosing Lyme borreliosis. J Clin Pathol 47:344–349, 1994

54. Daniels TJ, et al: Deer ticks (*Ixodes scapularis*) and the agents of Lyme disease and human granulocytic ehrlichiosis in a New York City park. Emerg Infect Dis 1997;3:353–355

55. Deblinger RD, et al: Reduced abundance of immature *Ixodes dammini* (Acari: Ixodidae) following incremental removal of deer. J Med Entomol 1993;30:144–150

56. Dekonenko EJ, et al: Lyme borreliosis in the Soviet Union: a cooperative US-USSR report. J Infect Dis 1988;158:748–753

57. Demaerschalck I, et al: Simultaneous presence of different *Borrelia burgdorferi* genospecies in biological fluids of Lyme disease patients. J Clin Microbiol 1995;33:602–608

58. Des Vignes F, et al: Effect of tick removal on transmission of *Borrelia burgdorferi* and *Ehrlichia phagocytophila* by *Ixodes scapularis* nymphs. J Infect Dis 2001;183:773–778

59. Dobson SR, et al: Recognition of *Treponema pallidum* antigens by IgM and IgG antibodies in congenitally infected newborns and their mothers. J Infect Dis 1988;157:903–910

60. Dressler F, et al: Antibody responses to the three genomic groups of *Borrelia burgdorferi* in European Lyme borreliosis. J Infect Dis 1994;169:313–318

61. Dressler F, et al: Western blotting in the serodiagnosis of Lyme disease. J Infect Dis 167:392–400, 1993

62. Dumler JS: Molecular diagnosis of Lyme disease: review and meta-analysis. Mol Diagn 2001;6:1–11

63. Dunn RA, et al: Surveillance for geographic and secular trends in congenital syphilis-United States, 1983–1991. MMWR CDC Surveill Summ 1993;42:59–71

64. Dupont H, et al: Leptospirosis: prognostic factors associated with mortality. Clin Infect Dis 1997;25:720–724

65. Duray PH: The surgical pathology of human Lyme disease: an enlarging picture. Am J Surg Pathol 1987;11(Suppl 1):47–60

66. Dworkin MS, et al: Tick-borne relapsing fever in the northwestern United States and southwestern Canada. Clin Infect Dis 1998;26:122–131

67. Ebel A, et al: Evaluation of a new competitive immunoassay (BioElisa Syphilis) for screening for *Treponema pallidum* antibodies at various stages of syphilis. J Clin Microbiol 1998;36:358–361

68. Edwards GA, Domm BM: Human leptospirosis. Medicine (Baltimore) 1960;39:117–117

69. Effler PV, et al: Evaluation of the indirect hemagglutination assay for diagnosis of acute leptospirosis in Hawaii. J Clin Microbiol 2000;38:1081–1084

70. El-Zaatari MM, et al: Incidence of the prozone phenomenon in syphilis serology. Obstet Gynecol 1994;84:609–612

71. Emmanouilides CE, et al: Leptospirosis complicated by a Jarisch-Herxheimer reaction and adult respiratory distress syndrome: case report. Clin Infect Dis 1994;18:1004–1006

72. Engstrom SM, et,al: Immunoblot interpretation criteria for serodiagnosis of early Lyme disease. J Clin Microbiol 1995;33:419–427

73. Erbelding EJ, et al: Syphilis serology in human immunodeficiency virus infection: evidence for false-negative fluorescent treponemal testing. J Infect Dis 1997;176:1397–1400

74. Falco RC, et al: Duration of tick bites in a Lyme disease-endemic area. Am J Epidemiol 1996;143:187–192

75. Fears MB, Pope V: Syphilis fast latex agglutination test, a rapid confirmatory test. Clin Diagn Lab Immunol 2001;8:841–842

76. Feder HM, JR., Hunt MS: Pitfalls in the diagnosis and treatment of Lyme disease in children. JAMA 1995;274:66–68

77. Feigin RD, Anderson DC: Human leptospirosis. CRC Crit Rev Clin Lab Sci 1975;5:413–467

78. Feigin Rd, et al: Human leptospirosis from immunized dogs. Ann Intern Med 1973;79:777–777

79. Felsenfeld O: Borreliae, human relapsing fever, and parasite-vector-host relationships. Bacteriol Rev 1965;29:46–46

80. Fikrig E, et al: Serologic diagnosis of Lyme disease using recombinant outer surface proteins A and B and flagellin. J Infect Dis 1992;165:1127–1132

81. Fiumara NJ: Acquired syphilis in three patients with congenital syphilis. N Engl J Med 1974;290:1119–1120

82. Fiumara NJ: Reinfection primary, secondary, and latent syphilis: the serologic response after treatment. Sex Transm Dis 1980;7:111–115

83. Fix AD, et al: Tick bites and Lyme disease in an endemic setting: problematic use of serologic testing and prophylactic antibiotic therapy. JAMA 1998;279:206–210

84. Flood JM, et al: Neurosyphilis during the AIDS epidemic, San Francisco, 1985–1992. J Infect Dis 1998;177:931–940

85. Fohn MJ, et al: Specificity of antibodies from patients with pinta for antigens of *Treponema pallidum* subspecies *pallidum*. J Infect Dis 1988;157:32–37

86. Fornaciari G, et al: Syphilis in a Renaissance Italian mummy. Lancet 1989;2:614–614

87. Fraser CM, et al: Genetic sequence of a Lyme disease spirochete, *Borrelia burgdorferi*. Nature 1997;390:580–586

88. Fraser CM, et al: Complete genome sequence of *Treponema pallidum*, the syphilis spirochete. Science 1998;281:375–388

89. Fraser JR: Lyme disease challenges Australian clinicians: the implications of Australia's first reported case of Lyme arthritis. Med J Aust 1982;1:101–102

90. Fukunaga M, et al: Phylogenetic analysis of *Borrelia* species based on flagellin gene sequences and its application for molecular typing of Lyme disease borreliae. Int J Syst Bacteriol 1996;46:898–905

91. Fung BP, et al: Humoral immune response to outer surface protein C of *Borrelia burgdorferi* in Lyme disease: role of the immunoglobulin M response in the serodiagnosis of early infection. Infect Immun 1994;62:3213–3221

92. Gardella C, et al: Persons with early syphilis identified through blood or plasma donation screening in the United States. J Infect Dis 2002;185:545–549

93. Gelfand JA, et al: Endotoxemia associated with the Jarisch-Herxheimer reaction. N Engl J Med 1976;295:211–213

94. Gerber AR, et al: An outbreak of syphilis on an Indian reservation: descriptive epidemiology and disease-control measures. Am J Publ Health 1989;79:83–85

95. Gerber MA, et al: Lyme Disease in children in Southeastern Connecticut. N Engl J Med 1996;335:1270–1274

96. Gerber MA, et al: The risk of acquiring Lyme disease or babesiosis from a blood transfusion. J Infect Dis 1994;170:231–234

97. Godsey MS, Jr, et al: Lyme disease ecology in Wisconsin: distribution and host preferences of *Ixodes dammini*, and prevalence of antibody to *Borrelia burgdorferi* in small mammals. Am J Trop Med Hyg 1987;37:180–187

98. Goldschmid JM, Mahomed K: The use of the microhematocrit technic for the recovery of *Borrelia duttonii* from the blood. Am J Clin Pathol 1972;58:165–169

99. Goodman JL, et al: Bloodstream invasion in early Lyme disease: results from a prospective, controlled, blinded study using the polymerase chain reaction. Am J Med 1995;99:6–12

100. Grimprel E, et al: Use of polymerase chain reaction and rabbit infectivity testing to detect *Treponema pallidum* in amniotic fluid, fetal and neonatal sera, and cerebrospinal fluid. J Clin Microbiol 1991;29:1711–1718

101. Guarner J, et al: Testing umbilical cords for funisitis due to *Treponema pallidum* infection, Bolivia. Emerg Infect Dis 2000;6:487–492

102. Gussenhoven GC, et al: LEPTO dipstick, a dipstick assay for detection of *Leptospira*-specific immunoglobulin M antibodies in human sera. J Clin Microbiol 1997;35:92–97

103. Haas JS, et al: Sensitivity of treponemal tests for detecting prior treated syphilis during human immunodeficiency virus infection. J Infect Dis 1990;162:862–866

104. Hagedorn HJ, et al: Evaluation of INNO-LIA syphilis assay as a confirmatory test for syphilis. J Clin Microbiol 2002;40:973–978

105. Hahn RA, et al: Race and the prevalence of syphilis seroreactivity in the United States population: a national sero-epidemiologic study. Am J Publ Health 1989;79:467–470

106. Hammers-Berggren S, et al: Serological follow-up after treatment of patients with erythema migrans and neuroborreliosis. J Clin Microbiol 1994;32:1519–1525

107. Hanrahan JP, et al: Incidence and cumulative frequency of endemic Lyme disease in a community. J Infect Dis 1984;150:489–496

108. Hart G: Syphilis tests in diagnostic and therapeutic decision making. Ann Intern Med 1986;104:368–376

109. Heath CW, Jr, et al: Leptospirosis in the United States (concluded): analysis of 483 cases in man, 1949–1961. N Engl J Med 1965;273:915–922

110. Heath CW, Jr, et al: Leptospirosis in the United States: analysis of 483 cases in man. N Engl J Med 1965;273:857–864

111. Hechemy KE, et al: Fluoroimmunoassay studies with solubilized antigens from *Borrelia burgdorferi*. J Clin Microbiol 1989;27:1854–1858

112. Hernandez-Aguado I, et al: False-positive tests for syphilis associated with human immunodeficiency virus and hepatitis B virus infection among intravenous drug abusers. Valencian Study Group on HIV Epidemiology. Eur J Clin Microbiol Infect Dis 1998;17:784–787

113. Hilton E, et al: Recommendation to include OspA and OspB in the new immunoblotting criteria for serodiagnosis of Lyme disease. J Clin Microbiol 1996;34:1353–1354

114. Hook EW III: Treatment of syphilis: current recommendations, alternatives, and continuing problems. Rev Infect Dis 1989;11:S1511–S1517

115. Hook EW III, Marra CM: Acquired syphilis in adults. N Engl J Med 1992;326:1060–1069

116. Hook EW III, et al: Detection of *Treponema pallidum* in lesion exudate with a pathogen-specific monoclonal antibody. J Clin Microbiol 1985;22:241–244

117. Hooshmand H, et al: Neurosyphilis: a study of 241 patients. JAMA 1972;219:726–729

118. Horton JM, Blaser MJ: The spectrum of relapsing fever in the Rocky Mountains. Arch Intern Med 1985;145:871–875

119. Hunter EF, et al: Evaluation of sera from patients with Lyme disease in the

fluorescent treponemal antibody-absorption test for syphilis. Sex Transm Dis 1986;13:232–236

120. Hutchinson CM, et al: Altered clinical presentation of early syphilis in patients with human immunodeficiency virus infection. Ann Intern Med 1994;121:94–100

121. Hyde FW, Johnson RC: Genetic relationship of lyme disease spirochetes to *Borrelia, Treponema,* and *Leptospira* spp. J Clin Microbiol 1984;20:151–154

122. Ito F, et al: Specific immunofluorescent staining of pathogenic treponemes with a monoclonal antibody. J Clin Microbiol 1992;30:831–838

123. Ito F, et al: Specific immunofluorescence staining of *Treponema pallidum* in smears and tissues. J Clin Microbiol 1991;29:444–448

124. Jackson LA, et al: Outbreak of leptospirosis associated with swimming. Pediatr Infect Dis J 1993;12:48–54

125. James AM, et al: *Borrelia lonestari* infection after a bite by an *Amblyomma americanum* tick. J Infect Dis 2001;183:1810–1814

126. Johnson RC, Faine S: *Leptospira* Noguchi 1917. In: Bergey's Manual of Systematic Bacteriology Baltimore: Williams & Wilkins, 1984:62–67

127. Johnson RC, et al: *Borrelia burgdorferi* sp. nov.: etiologic agent of Lyme disease. Int J Syst Bacteriol 1984;34:496–497

128. Kaell AT, et al: Occurrence of antibodies to *Borrelia burgdorferi* in patients with nonspirochetal subacute bacterial endocarditis. Ann Intern Med 1993;119:1079–1083

129. Kaell AT, et al: Positive Lyme serology in subacute bacterial endocarditis: a study of four patients. JAMA 1990;264:2916–2918

130. Kalish RA, et al: Evaluation of study patients with Lyme disease, 10–20-year follow-up. J Infect Dis 2001;183:453–460

131. Katz AR, et al: Assessment of the clinical presentation and treatment of 353 cases of laboratory-confirmed leptospirosis in Hawaii, 1974–1998. Clin Infect Dis 2001;33:1834–1841

132. Kaufman RE, et al: Biological false positive serological tests for syphilis among drug addicts. Br J Vener Dis 1974;50:350–353

133. Kelly R: Cultivation of *Borrelia hermsii.* Science 1971;173:443–444

134. Kelly RT: *Borrelia* Swellengrebel 1907. In: Bergey's Manual of Systematic Bacteriology. Baltimore, Williams & Wilkins, 1984:57–62

135. Klass PE, et al: The incidence of prenatal syphilis at the Boston City Hospital: a comparison across four decades. Pediatrics 1994;94:24–28

136. Klausner JD, et al: Tracing a syphilis outbreak through cyberspace. JAMA 2000;284:447–449

137. Klempner MS, et al: Two controlled trials of antibiotic treatment in patients with persistent symptoms and a history of Lyme disease. N Engl J Med 2001;345:85–92

138. Klempner MS, et al: Intralaboratory reliability of serologic and urine testing for Lyme disease. Am J Med 2001;110:217–219

139. Koff AB, Rosen T: Nonvenereal treponematoses: yaws, endemic syphilis, and pinta. J Am Acad Dermatol 1993;29:519–535

140. Kornblatt AN, et al: Arthritis caused by *Borrelia burgdorferi* in dogs. J Am Vet Med Assoc 1985;186:960–964

141. Kraus SJ, et al: Fluorescent treponemal antibody-absorption test reactions in lupus erythematosus: atypical beading pattern and probable false- positive reactions. N Engl J Med 1970;282:1287–1290

142. Kurtti TJ, et al: Colony formation and morphology in *Borrelia burgdorferi.* J Clin Microbiol 1987;25:2054–2058

143. Larsen SA: Syphilis. Clin Lab Med 1989;9:545–557

144. Larsen SA, et al: Specificity, sensitivity, and reproducibility among the fluorescent treponemal antibody-absorption test, the microhemagglutination assay for *Treponema pallidum* antibodies, and the hemagglutination treponemal test for syphilis. J Clin Microbiol 1981;14:441–445

145. Larsen SA, et al: Manual of Tests for Syphilis. 8th Ed. Washington, D.C.: American Public Health Association, 1990

146. Larsen SA, et al: Laboratory diagnosis and interpretation of tests for syphilis. Clin Microbiol Rev 1995;8:1–21

147. Lebech AM, Hansen K: Detection of Borrelia burgdorferi DNA in urine samples and cerebrospinal fluid samples from patients with early and late Lyme neuroborreliosis by polymerase chain reaction. J Clin Microbiol 1992;30:1646–1653

148. Lee CB, et al: Epidemiology of an outbreak of infectious syphilis in Manitoba. Am J Epidemiol 1987;125:277–283

149. Levett PN: Leptospirosis. Clin Microbiol Rev 2001;14:296–326

150. Levett PN, Whittington CU: Evaluation of the indirect hemagglutination assay for diagnosis of acute leptospirosis. J Clin Microbiol 1998;36:11–14

151. Levine JF, et al: Mice as reservoirs of the Lyme disease spirochete. Am J Trop Med Hyg 1985;34:355–360

152. Ley C, et al: The use of serologic tests for Lyme disease in a prepaid health plan in California. JAMA 1994;271:460–463

153. Lin T, et al: Genetic diversity of the outer surface protein C gene of southern *Borrelia* isolates and its possible epidemiological, clinical, and pathogenetic implications. J Clin Microbiol 2002;40:2572–2583

154. Liu CC, et al: Congenital syphilis: clinical manifestations in premature infants. Scand J Infect Dis 1993;25:741–745

155. Liu H, et al: New tests for syphilis: rational design of a PCR method for detection of *Treponema pallidum* in clinical specimens using unique regions of the DNA polymerase I gene. J Clin Microbiol 2001;39:1941–1946

156. Liveris D, et al: Genetic diversity of *Borrelia burgdorferi* in Lyme disease patients as determined by culture versus direct PCR with clinical specimens. J Clin Microbiol 1999;37:565–569

157. Liveris D, et al: Quantitative detection of *Borrelia burgdorferi* in 2-millimeter skin samples of erythema migrans lesions: correlation of results with clinical and laboratory findings. J Clin Microbiol 2002;40:1249–1253

158. Lovrich SD, et al: Seroprotective groups of Lyme borreliosis spirochetes from North America and Europe. J Infect Dis 1994;170:115–121

159. Luft BJ, et al: Invasion of the central nervous system by *Borrelia burgdorferi* in acute disseminated infection. JAMA 1992;267:1364–1367

160. Lukehart SA, et al: Invasion of the central nervous system by *Treponema pallidum*: implications for diagnosis and treatment. Ann Intern Med 1988;109:855–862

161. Ma B, et al: Serodiagnosis of Lyme borreliosis by western immunoblot: reactivity of various significant antibodies against *Borrelia burgdorferi.* J Clin Microbiol 1992;30:370–376

162. Magid D, et al: Prevention of Lyme disease after tick bites: a cost- effectiveness analysis. N Engl J Med 1992;327:534–541

163. Magnarelli LA, et al: Cross-reactivity in serological tests for Lyme disease and other spirochetal infections. J Infect Dis 1987;156:183–188

164. Magnarelli LA, et al: Use of recombinant antigens of *Borrelia burgdorferi* in serologic tests for diagnosis of Lyme borreliosis. J Clin Microbiol 1996;34:237–240

165. Magnarelli LA, et al: Comparison of an indirect fluorescent-antibody test with an enzyme-linked immunosorbent assay for serologic studies of Lyme disease. J Clin Microbiol 1984;20:181–184

166. Magnuson HJ, et al: Inoculation syphilis in human volunteers. Medicine (Baltimore) 1956;35:33–82

167. Manca N, et al: Radiometric method for the rapid detection of *Leptospira* organisms. J Clin Microbiol 1986;23:401–493

168. Marfin AA, et al: Amplification of the DNA polymerase I gene of *Treponema pallidum* from whole blood of persons with syphilis. Diagn Microbiol Infect Dis 2001;40:163–166

169. Marotto PC, et al: Acute lung injury in leptospirosis: clinical and laboratory features, outcome, and factors associated with mortality. Clin Infect Dis 1999;29:1561–1563

170. Marshall Wf3, et al: Detection of *Borrelia burgdorferi* DNA in museum specimens of *Peromyscus leucopus.* J Infect Dis 1994;170:1027–1032

171. Matuschka FR, et al: Capacity of European animals as reservoir hosts for the Lyme disease spirochete. J Infect Dis 1992;165:479–483

172. Matuschka FR, et al: Antiquity of the Lyme-disease spirochaete in Europe. Lancet 1995;346:1367–1367

173. Matuschka FR, Spielman A: Risk of infection from and treatment of tick bite. Lancet 1993;342:529–530

174. Maupin GO, et al: Discovery of an enzootic cycle of *Borrelia burgdorferi* in *Neotoma mexicana* and *Ixodes spinipalpus* from northern Colorado, an area where Lyme disease is nonendemic. J Infect Dis 1994;170:636–643

175. Merien F, et al: Comparison of polymerase chain reaction with microagglutination test and culture for diagnosis of leptospirosis. J Infect Dis 1995;172:281–285

176. Meyer MP, et al: Analysis of western blotting (immunoblotting) technique in diagnosis of congenital syphilis. J Clin Microbiol 1994;32:629–633

177. Miao RM, Fieldsteel AH: Genetic relationship between *Treponema pallidum* and *Treponema pertenue* two noncultivable human pathogens. J Bacteriol 1980;141:427–429

178. Michelow IC, et al: Central nervous system infection in congenital syphilis. N Engl J Med 2002;346:1792–1798

179. Mitchell PD, et al: Comparison of four immunoserologic assays for detection of antibodies to *Borrelia burgdorferi* in patients with culture- positive erythema migrans. J Clin Microbiol 1994;32:1958–1962

180. Mitchell PD, et al: Immunoserologic evidence of coinfection with *Borrelia burgdorferi, Babesia microti,* and human granulocytic *Ehrlichia* species in residents of Wisconsin and Minnesota. J Clin Microbiol 1996;34:724–727, 1996

181. Mitchell PD, et al: Isolation of *Borrelia burgdorferi* from skin biopsy specimens of patients with erythema migrans. Am J Clin Pathol 1993;99:104–107

182. Molloy PJ, et al: Detection of multiple reactive protein species by immunoblotting after recombinant outer surface protein A Lyme disease vaccination. Clin Infect Dis 2000;31:42–47

183. Molloy PJ, et al: False-positive results of PCR testing for Lyme disease. Clin Infect Dis 2001;33:412–413

184. Moore VA IV, et al: Detection of *Borrelia lonestari,* putative agent of southern tick-associated rash illness, in white-tailed deer (*Odocoileus virginianus*) from the southeastern United States. J Clin Microbiol 2003;41:424–427

185. Morgan J, et al: Outbreak of leptospirosis among triathlon participants and com-

munity residents in Springfield, Illinois, 1998. Clin Infect Dis 2002;34: 1593–1599

186. Murray T, Feder HM Jr.: Management of tick bites and early Lyme disease: a survey of Connecticut physicians. Pediatrics 2001;108:1367–1370

187. Musher DM, et al: Effect of human immunodeficiency virus (HIV) infection on the course of syphilis and on the response to treatment. Ann Intern Med 1990; 113:872–881

188. Nadelman RB, et al: Prophylaxis with single-dose doxycycline for the prevention of Lyme disease after an *Ixodes scapularis* tick bite. N Engl J Med 2001;345: 79–84

189. Nakao M, Miyamoto K: Mixed infection of different *Borrelia* species among *Apodemus speciosus* mice in Hokkaido, Japan. J Clin Microbiol 1995;33: 490–492

190. Negussie Y, et al: Detection of plasma tumor necrosis factor, interleukins 6, and 8 during the Jarisch-Herxheimer reaction of relapsing fever. J Exp Med 1992;175:1207–1212

191. Noordhoek GT, et al: A new attempt to distinguish serologically the subspecies of *Treponema pallidum* causing syphilis and yaws. J Clin Microbiol 1990;28: 1600–1607

192. Noordhoek GT, et al: *Treponema pallidum* subspecies *pallidum* (Nichols) and *Treponema pallidum* subspecies *pertenue* (CDC 2575) differ in at least one nucleotide: comparison of two homologous antigens. Microb Pathog 1989;6: 29–42

193. Noordhoek GT, et al: Detection by polymerase chain reaction of *Treponema pallidum* DNA in cerebrospinal fluid from neurosyphilis patients before and after antibiotic treatment. J Clin Microbiol 1991;29:1976–1984

194. Nowakowski J, et al: Laboratory diagnostic techniques for patients with early Lyme disease associated with erythema migrans: a comparison of different techniques. Clin Infect Dis 2001;33:2023–2027

195. Nowakowski J, et al: Culture-confirmed infection and reinfection with *Borrelia burgdorferi*. Ann Intern Med 1997;127:130–132

196. O'neil KM, et al: Pulmonary manifestations of leptospirosis. Rev Infect Dis 1991;13:705–709

197. Obenchain FD, et al: Implications of tick size on the quantifications of engorgement in female *Dermacentor variabilis*. J Parasitol 1980;66:282–286

198. Oie S, et al: *In vitro* evaluation of combined usage of fosfomycin and 5- fluorouracil for selective isolation of *Leptospira* species. J Clin Microbiol 1986;23: 1084–1087

199. Ojukwu IC, Christy C: Rat-bite fever in children: case report and review. Scand J Infect Dis 2002;34:474–477

200. Oliver JH, Jr, et al: Conspecificity of the ticks *Ixodes scapularis* and *I. dammini* (*Acari: Ixodidae*). J Med Entomol 1993;30:54–63

201. Pachner AR, Steere AC: The triad of neurologic manifestations of Lyme disease: meningitis, cranial neuritis, and radiculoneuritis. Neurology 1985;35:47–53

202. Pal U, et al: Attachment of *Borrelia burgdorferi* within *Ixodes scapularis* mediated by outer surface protein A. J Clin Invest 2000;106:561–569

203. Pappas MG, et al: Rapid serodiagnosis of leptospirosis using the IGM-specific dot-ELISA: comparison with the microscopic agglutination test. Am J Trop Med Hyg 1985;34:346–354

204. Pennell DR, et al: Evaluation of a quantitative fluorescence immunoassay (FIAX) for detection of serum antibody to Borrelia burgdorferi. J Clin Microbiol 1987;25:2218–2220

205. Perine PL, et al: New technologies for use in the surveillance and control of yaws. Rev Infect Dis 1985;7:295–295

206. Persing DH, et al: Target imbalance: disparity of *Borrelia burgdorferi* genetic material in synovial fluid from Lyme arthritis patients. J Infect Dis 1994;169: 668–672

207. Piesman J, et al: Duration of tick attachment and *Borrelia burgdorferi* transmission. J Clin Microbiol 1987;25:557–558

208. Pillay A, et al: Molecular typing of *Treponema pallidum* in South Africa: cross-sectional studies. J Clin Microbiol 2002;40:256–258

209. Poland GA: Prevention of Lyme disease: a review of the evidence. Mayo Clin Proc 2001;76:713–724

210. Pollack RJ, et al: Standardization of medium for culturing Lyme disease spirochetes. J Clin Microbiol 1993;31:1251–1255

211. Pope V, Castro A: Replacement for 30-milliliter flat-bottomed, glass-stoppered, round bottles used in VDRL antigen preparation. J Clin Microbiol 1999;37: 3053–3054

212. Pope V, et al: Comparison of the Serodia *Treponema pallidum* particle agglutination, Captia Syphilis-G, and SpiroTek Reagin II tests with standard test techniques for diagnosis of syphilis. J Clin Microbiol 2000;38:2543–2545

213. Postic D, et al: Expanded diversity among Californian borrelia isolates and description of *Borrelia bissettii* sp. nov. (formerly *Borrelia* group DN127). J Clin Microbiol 1998;36:3497–3504

214. Preac-Mursic V, et al: Repeated isolation of spirochetes from the cerebrospinal fluid of a patient with meningoradiculitis Bannwarth. Eur J Clin Microbiol 1984; 3:564–565

215. Qureshi MZ, et al: Overdiagnosis and overtreatment of Lyme disease in children. Pediatr Infect Dis J 2002;21:12–14

216. Raoult D, et al: Cross-reaction with *Borrelia burgdorferi* antigen of sera from patients with human immunodeficiency virus infection, syphilis, and leptospirosis. J Clin Microbiol 1989;27:2152–2155

217. Rathinavelu S, De Silva AM: Purification and characterization of *Borrelia burgdorferi* from feeding nymphal ticks (*Ixodes scapularis*). Infect Immun 2001; 69:3536–3541

218. Rauter C, et al: Distribution of clinically relevant *Borrelia* genospecies in ticks assessed by a novel, single-run, real-time PCR. J Clin Microbiol 2002;40:36–43

219. Reed KD: Laboratory testing for lyme disease: possibilities and practicalities. J Clin Microbiol 2002;40:319–324

220. Riggsbee JH, Lamke CL: An evaluation of the double-staining procedure for the fluorescent treponemal antibody-absorption (FTA-ABS) test. Lab Med 1981; 12:232–234

221. Riviere GR, et al: Identification of spirochetes related to *Treponema pallidum* in necrotizing ulcerative gingivitis and chronic periodontitis. N Engl J Med 1991; 325:539–543

222. Rodriguez S, et al: Gummatous syphilis: a reminder. J Infect Dis 1988;157: 606–607

223. Rolfs RT, et al: Risk factors for syphilis: cocaine use and prostitution. Am J Publ Health 1990;80:853–857

224. Rolfs RT, Nakashima AK: Epidemiology of primary and secondary syphilis in the United States, 1981 through 1989. JAMA 1990;264:1432–1437

225. Romero EC, et al: Detection of *Leptospira* DNA in patients with aseptic meningitis by PCR. J Clin Microbiol 1998;36:1453–1455

226. Romero EC, et al: The persistence of leptospiral agglutinin titers in human sera diagnosed by the microscopic agglutination test. Rev Inst Med Trop Sao Paulo 1998;40:183–184

227. Rompalo AM, et al: Association of biologic false-positive reactions for syphilis with human immunodeficiency virus infection. J Infect Dis 1992;165: 1124–1126

228. Rosen EU, Richardson NJ: A reappraisal of the value of the IgM fluorescent treponemal antibody absorption test in the diagnosis of congenital syphilis. Pediatrics 1975;87:38–42

229. Rothschild BM, et al: First European exposure to syphilis: The Dominican Republic at the time of Columbian contact. Clin Infect Dis 2000;31:936–941

230. Rothschild BM, Rothschild C: Treponemal disease revisited: skeletal discriminators for yaws, bejel, and venereal syphilis. Clin Infect Dis 1995;20:1402–1408

231. Russell H, et al: Enzyme-linked immunosorbent assay and indirect immunofluorescence assay for Lyme disease. J Infect Dis 1984;149:465–470

232. Russell RC, et al: Lyme disease: a search for a causative agent in ticks in southeastern Australia. Epidemiol Infect 1994;112:375–384

233. Saengjaruk P, et al: Diagnosis of human leptospirosis by monoclonal antibody-based antigen detection in urine. J Clin Microbiol 2002;40:480–489

234. Salazar JC, et al: The immune response to infection with *Treponema pallidum*, the stealth pathogen. Microbes Infect 2002;4:1133–1140

235. Sambri V, et al: Evaluation of recomWell *Treponema*, a novel recombinant antigen-based enzyme-linked immunosorbent assay for the diagnosis of syphilis. Clin Microbiol Infect 2001;7:200–205

236. Sanchez PJ, et al: Molecular analysis of the fetal IgM response to *Treponema pallidum* antigens: implications for improved serodiagnosis of congenital syphilis. J Infect Dis 1989;159:508–517

237. Sanchez PJ, et al: Evaluation of molecular methodologies and rabbit infectivity testing for the diagnosis of congenital syphilis and neonatal central nervous system invasion by *Treponema pallidum*. J Infect Dis 1993;167:148–157

238. Sasaki DM, et al: Active surveillance and risk factors for leptospirosis in Hawaii. Am J Trop Med Hyg 1993;48:35–43

239. Scheck DN, Hook Ew3: Neurosyphilis. Infect Dis Clin North Am 1994;8: 769–795

240. Schlesinger PA, et al: Maternal-fetal transmission of the Lyme disease spirochete, *Borrelia burgdorferi*. Ann Intern Med 1985;103:67–68

241. Schmid GP, et al: Surveillance of Lyme disease in the United States, 1982. J Infect Dis 1985;151:1144–1149

242. Schmid GP, et al: Newly recognized *Leptospira* species ("*Leptospira inadai*" serovar *lyme*) isolated from human skin. J Clin Microbiol 1986;24:484–486

243. Schmid GP, et al: DNA characterization of the spirochete that causes Lyme disease. J Clin Microbiol 1984;20:155–158

244. Schmidt BL: PCR in laboratory diagnosis of human *Borrelia burgdorferi* infections. Clin Microbiol Rev 1997;10:185–201

245. Schmidt BL: Comparative evaluation of nine different enzyme-linked immunosorbent assays for determination of antibodies against *Treponema pallidum* in patients with primary syphilis. J Clin Microbiol 2000;38:1279–1282

246. Schutzer SE, et al: Early and specific antibody response to OspA in Lyme Disease. J Clin Invest 1994;94:454–457

247. Schwaiger M, et al: Routine diagnosis of *Borrelia burgdorferi* (sensu lato) infections using a real-time PCR assay. Clin Microbiol Infect 2001;7:461–469

248. Schwan TG, et al: Identification of the tick-borne relapsing fever spirochete

Borrelia hermsii by using a species-specific monoclonal antibody. J Clin Microbiol 1992;30:790–795

249. Sciotto CG, et al: Detection of *Borrelia* in acridine orange-stained blood smears by fluorescence microscopy. Arch Pathol Lab Med 1983;107:384–386

250. Seboxa T, Rahlenbeck SJ: Treatment of louse-borne relapsing fever with low dose penicillin or tetracycline: a clinical trial. Scand J Infect Dis 1995;27:29–31

251. Seijo A, et al: Lethal leptospiral pulmonary hemorrhage: an emerging disease in Buenos Aires, Argentina. Emerg Infect Dis 2002;8:1004–1005

252. Seinost G, et al: Four clones of *Borrelia burgdorferi* sensu stricto cause invasive infection in humans. Infect Immun 1999;67:3518–3524

253. Seki M, et al: One point method for serological diagnosis of leptospirosis: a microcapsule agglutination test. Epidemiol Infect 1987;99:399–405

254. Seppala IJ, et al: Diagnosis of Lyme borreliosis: non-specific serological reactions with *Borrelia burgdorferi* sonicate antigen caused by IgG2 antibodies. J Med Microbiol 1994;40:293–302

255. Shapiro ED: Doxycycline for tick bites-not for everyone. N Engl J Med 2001; 345:133–134

256. Shapiro ED, Gerber MA: Lyme disease. Clin Infect Dis 2000;31:533–542

257. Shaw RD: Kayaking as a risk factor for leptospirosis. Mo Med 1992;89:354–357

258. Sigal LH, et al: A vaccine consisting of recombinant *Borrelia burgdorferi* outer-surface protein A to prevent Lyme disease: Recombinant Outer-Surface Protein A Lyme Disease Vaccine Study Consortium. N Engl J Med 1998;339:216–222

259. Singh AE, Romanowski B: Syphilis: review with emphasis on clinical, epidemiologic, and some biologic features. Clin Microbiol Rev 1999;12:187–209

260. Smith RP, Jr., et al: Norway rats as reservoir hosts for Lyme disease spirochetes on Monhegan Island, Maine. J Infect Dis 1993;168:687–691

261. Smith RP, et al: Clinical characteristics and treatment outcome of early Lyme disease in patients with microbiologically confirmed erythema migrans. Ann Intern Med 2002;136:421–428

262. Smith TF, et al: Pseudospirochetes, a cause of erroneous diagnoses of leptospirosis. Am J Clin Pathol 72:459–463, 1979

263. Smits HL, et al: Simple latex agglutination assay for rapid serodiagnosis of human leptospirosis. J Clin Microbiol 2000;38:1272–1275

264. Sood SK: Effective retrieval of Lyme disease information on the Web. Clin Infect Dis 2002;35:451–464

265. Sood SK, et al: Duration of tick attachment as a predictor of the risk of Lyme disease in an area in which Lyme disease is endemic. J Infect Dis 1997;175: 996–999

266. Southern P, Sanford JP: Relapsing fever: a clinical and microbiological review. Medicine (Baltimore) 1969;48:129–149

267. Spach DH, et al: Tick-borne diseases in the United States. N Engl J Med 1993; 329:936–947

268. Sperling LC, et al: Occult primary syphilis: the nonerosive chancre. J Am Acad Dermatol 1990;23:514–515

269. Spielman A, et al: Human babesiosis on Nantucket Island, USA: description of the vector, *Ixodes (Ixodes) dammini, N. Sp. (Acarina: Ixodidae)*. J Med Entomol 1979;15:218–234

270. Stamm LV, et al: Identification, cloning, and purification of protein antigens of *Treponema pallidum*. Rev Infect Dis 1988;10(Suppl 2):S403–S407

271. Stamm WE, et al: The association between genital ulcer disease and acquisition of HIV infection in homosexual men. JAMA 1988;260:1429–1433

272. Stechenberg BW: Lyme disease: the latest great imitator. Pediatr Infect Dis J 1988;7:402–409

273. Steere AC: Lyme disease. N Engl J Med 1989;321:586–596

274. Steere AC: Lyme disease. N Engl J Med 2001;345:115–125

275. Steere AC, et al: The early clinical manifestations of Lyme disease. Ann Intern Med 1983;99:76–82

276. Steere AC, et al: The spirochetal etiology of Lyme disease. N Engl J Med 1983; 308:733–740

277. Steere AC, Malawista Se: Cases of Lyme disease in the United States: locations correlated with distribution of *Ixodes dammini*. Ann Intern Med 1979;91: 730–733

278. Steere AC, et al: Lyme arthritis: an epidemic of oligoarticular arthritis in children and adults in three Connecticut communities. Arthritis Rheum 1977;20:7–17

279. Steere AC, et al: The clinical evolution of Lyme arthritis. Ann Intern Med 1987; 107:725–731

280. Steere AC, et al: Vaccination against Lyme disease with recombinant *Borrelia*

281. Steere AC, et al: The overdiagnosis of Lyme disease. JAMA 1993;269: 1812–1816, 1993

282. Steere AC, et al: Longitudinal assessment of the clinical and epidemiological features of Lyme disease in a defined population. J Infect Dis 1986;154:295–300

283. Stoll BJ, et al: Clinical and serologic evaluation of neonates for congenital syphilis: a continuing diagnostic dilemma. J Infect Dis 1993;167:1093–1099

284. Strle F, et al: Comparison of culture-confirmed erythema migrans caused by *Borrelia burgdorferi* sensu stricto in New York State and by *Borrelia afzelii* in Slovenia. Ann Intern Med 1999;130:32–36

285. Su SJ, et al: Evaluation of the equivocal test results of *Treponema pallidum* haemagglutination assay. J Clin Pathol 1990;43:166–167

286. Sundnes KO, Haimanot AT: Epidemic of louse-borne relapsing fever in Ethiopia. Lancet 1993;342:1213–1215

287. Sutton MY, et al: Molecular subtyping of *Treponema pallidum* in an Arizona county with increasing syphilis morbidity: use of specimens from ulcers and blood. J Infect Dis 2001;183:1601–1606

288. Theisen M, et al: Polymorphism in OspC gene of *Borrelia burgdorferi* and immunoreactivity of OspC protein: implications for taxonomy and for use of OspC protein as a diagnostic antigen. J Clin Microbiol 1993;31:2570–2576

289. Thomas DL, et al: Association of hepatitis C virus infection with false-positive tests for syphilis. J Infect Dis 1994;170:1579–1581

290. Thompson RS, et al: Outbreak of tick-borne relapsing fever in Spokane County, Washington. JAMA 1969;210:1045–1050

291. Tramont EC: Syphilis in adults: from Christopher Columbus to Sir Alexander Fleming to AIDS. Clin Infect Dis 1995;21:1361–1371

292. Tugwell P, et al: Laboratory evaluation in the diagnosis of Lyme disease. Ann Intern Med 1997;127:1109–1123

293. Van Crevel R, et al: Leptospirosis in travelers. Clin Infect Dis 1994;19:132–134

294. Van Dam AP, et al: Tick-borne relapsing fever imported from West Africa: diagnosis by quantitative buffy coat analysis and in vitro culture of *Borrelia crocidurae*. J Clin Microbiol 1999;37:2027–2030

295. Van Orden AE, Greer PW: Modification of the Dieterle spirochete stain. Histotechnology 1977;1:51–53

296. Villanueva AV, et al: Effects of various handling and storage conditions on stability of *Treponema pallidum* DNA in cerebrospinal fluid. J Clin Microbiol 1998;36:2117–2119

297. Wallach FR, et al: Circulating *Borrelia burgdorferi* in patients with acute Lyme disease: results of blood cultures and serum DNA analysis. J Infect Dis 1993; 168:1541–1543

298. Wang G, et al: Molecular typing of *Borrelia burgdorferi* sensu lato: taxonomic, epidemiological, and clinical implications. Clin Microbiol Rev 1999;12: 633–653

299. Washburn RG: Spirillum minor (Rat-bite fever). In Mandell GL, Bennett JE, Dolin R, eds.: Principles and Practice of Infectious Diseases. 4th Ed. New York: Churchill Livingstone, 1995:2155–2156

300. Watt G, et al: The rapid diagnosis of leptospirosis: a prospective comparison of the dot enzyme-linked immunosorbent assay and the genus-specific microscopic agglutination test at different stages. J Infect Dis 1988;157:840–842

301. Weber K, et al: *Borrelia burgdorferi* in a newborn despite oral penicillin for Lyme borreliosis during pregnancy. Pediatr Infect Dis J 1988;7:286–289

302. Wendel GD: Gestational and congenital syphilis. Clin Perinatol 1988;15: 287–303

303. Wormser GP, et al: A limitation of 2-stage serological testing for Lyme disease: enzyme immunoassay and immunoblot assay are not independent tests. Clin Infect Dis 2000;30:545–548

304. Wormser GP, et al: Practice guidelines for the treatment of Lyme disease. The Infectious Diseases Society of America. Clin Infect Dis 2000;31(Suppl 1):1–14

305. Yasuda PH, et al: Deoxyribonucleic acid relatedness between serogroups and serovars in the family *Leptospiraceae* with proposals for seven new *Leptospira* species. Int J Syst Bacteriol 1987;37:407–415

306. Zarakolu P, et al: Preliminary evaluation of an immunochromatographic strip test for specific *Treponema pallidum* antibodies. J Clin Microbiol 2002;40: 3064–3065

307. Zbinden R, et al: Comparison of two methods for detecting intrathecal synthesis of *Borrelia burgdorferi*-specific antibodies and PCR for diagnosis of Lyme neuroborreliosis. J Clin Microbiol 1994;32:1795–1798

308. Zenker PN, Rolfs RT: Treatment of syphilis, 1989. Rev Infect Dis 1990;12(Suppl 6):S590–S609

Patients at Risk for Fungal Infections

General Signs and Symptoms Suggesting Fungal Infection

Clinical Categorization of Fungal Infections

Common Mycologic Terms

Laboratory Approach to the Diagnosis of Fungal Infections

Specimen Collection and Transport
Specimen Processing
Direct Examination

Preparation of Mounts for Study
Selection and Inoculation of Culture Media
Incubation of Fungal Cultures

Laboratory Approach to the Presumptive Identification of Fungal Isolates

Extent of Laboratory Genus/Species Identification
Genus and Species Identification of the Major Groups of Fungi

Zygomyces Species and Zygomycosis
Histopathology of Infections Caused by the Zygomycetes

Hyaline Molds and Hyalohyphomycosis

Aspergillus Species and Aspergillosis

Laboratory Presentation
Colony Morphology
Microscopic Features
Aspergillus fumigatus
Aspergillus flavus
Aspergillus niger
Aspergillus terreus
Aspergillus nidulans

Histopathology

Diagnosis Using Nonculture Techniques

Additional Rapidly Growing Hyaline Molds

Colony Characteristics

Genera of Hyaline Filamentous Molds Producing Conidia in Chains

Penicillium Species
Paecilomyces Species
Scopulariopsis Species

Identification of Hyaline Molds Producing Conidia in Clusters

Acremonium Species
Fusarium Species
Gliocladium Species
Trichoderma Species

Identification of the Genera of Hyalohyphomycetes Producing Conidia Singly

Scedosporium Species
Chrysosporium Species
Sepedonium Species
Beauveria Species

Identification of the Dermatophytes

Identification of *Microsporum* Species

Microsporum canis
Microsporum gypseum
Microsporum nanum

Identification of *Trichophyton* Species

Trichophyton mentagrophytes
Trichophyton rubrum
Trichophyton tonsurans
Trichophyton verrucosum
Epidermophyton floccosum

Diagnosis Using Nonculture Techniques

The Dimorphic Fungi

Blastomyces dermatitidis and Blastomycosis

Laboratory Presentation
Diagnosis Using Nonculture Techniques

Coccidioides immitis and Coccidioidomycosis

Laboratory Presentation

Histoplasma capsulatum and Histoplasmosis

Laboratory Presentation
Diagnosis Using Nonculture Techniques

Sporothrix schenckii and Sporotrichosis

Laboratory Presentation
Diagnosis Using Nonculture Techniques

Paracoccidioides immitis and Paracoccidioidomycosis

Laboratory Presentation
Diagnosis Using Nonculture Techniques

Dematiaceous Fungi

Agents of Phaeohyphomycosis

Laboratory Presentation

Macroconidia with Transverse and Longitudinal Septa (Muriform)

Alternaria Species
Ulocladium Species
Stemphylium Species
Epicoccum Species

Macroconidia With Transverse Septa

Bipolaris Species
Drechslera Species

Curvularia Species
Exserohilum Species

Macroconidia Borne Singly or Via Special Conidiation

Nigrospora Species
Phoma Species
Chaetomium Species

Agents of Chromomycosis and Mycetoma

Cladophialophora (Cladosporium) carrionii
Phialophora verrucosum
Phialophora richardsiae
Fonsecaea pedrosoi
Exophiala jeanselmei

The Laboratory Identification of Yeast

Germ Tube
Cornmeal Agar Preparations

Growth Patterns of Yeasts on Cornmeal Agar
CHROMagar
Candida albicans
Candida tropicalis
Candida parapsilosis
Candida kefyr (*pseudotropicalis*)
Other Emerging Pathogenic *Candida* Species
Candida Species and Candidiasis

Species That Produce True Hyphae
Species That Fail to Produce True Hyphae

Cryptococcosis and *Cryptococcus neoformans*
Diagnosis by Nonculture Methods

Miscellaneous Non-Hyphae-Forming Yeasts of Medical Importance

Candida (Torulopsis) glabrata
Rhodotorula Species
Saccharomyces Species
Hansenula anomala
Malassezia furfur

Laboratory Identification of "Black Yeasts"

Aureobasidium pullulans
Phaeoannellomyces werneckii

Packaged Yeast-Identification Systems
Antifungal Susceptibility Testing

Serologic Diagnosis of Fungal Diseases

The diagnosis of a fungal infection requires the co-operative efforts of the primary-care physician, the surgical pathologist, and the microbiologist. The primary-care physician is responsible for recognizing the signs and symptoms of fungal infections and for seeing that appropriate specimens are properly collected and transported to the laboratory in optimal condition without delay. The surgical pathologist must be alert to the tissue reactions that suggest a fungal infection and/or must be able to recognize fungal elements in stained tissue sections. The laboratory mycologist is responsible for implementing the laboratory techniques optimal for the recovery of fungi in culture and for making accurate genus/species identifications.

Patients at Risk for Fungal Infections

- Individuals who are immunosuppressed or who have reduced numbers or compromised function of the circulating polymorphonuclear leukocytes.
- Organ-transplant recipients, particularly during the post-transplantation period of immunosuppression.
- Patients with malignant neoplasms, particularly those with leukemia and lymphoma, particularly during periods of chemotherapy.
- Patients with a variety of debilitating immunologic and metabolic disorders, including systemic lupus erythematosus, and other collagen vascular diseases, diabetes mellitus, dysgammaglobulinemia, and alcohol or IV-drug abuse.
- Recipients of previous treatment with corticosteroids, cytotoxic agents, or prolonged antibiotic therapy.
- Travelers to or inhabitants of regions of the world known to be endemic for fungal infections.
- Participants in activities or occupations that bring them in direct skin contact with infected animals and/or contaminated materials or present the risk of ingestion or inhalation of aerosols or dust contaminated with fungal spores.

Within this background is a recent review by Nucci,[199] who emphasizes that the incidence of non-*Aspergillus* mold infections has particularly increased in transplant recipients over the past decade. Suggested by recent epidemiologic data, the greater depth of immunosuppression in changing transplant protocols seems to play a major role. These fungal infections tend to disseminate, and the prognosis is usually poor because the fungi are resistant to most of the available antifungal agents.

General Signs and Symptoms Suggesting Fungal Infection

- The early presenting symptoms leading to the suspicion of a fungal infection commonly are atypical, vague, and nonspecific, reducing the chance for making the correct clinical diagnosis.
- Low-grade fever, night sweats, weight loss, lassitude, easy fatigability, cough, and chest pain are common presenting symptoms.

- Deep-seated or disseminated fungal diseases may mimic other infections, such as tuberculosis, brucellosis, syphilis, sarcoidosis, and disseminated carcinomatosis.
- Careful examination of the skin and mucous membranes should always be performed, as systemic fungal infections often present with mucocutaneous lesions.
  - Ulcerating lesions in the intestine, larynx, pharynx, genitals, and tongue may complicate disseminated histoplasmosis in up to 50% of cases.
  - Patients with blastomycosis may initially present with verrucous or pustular lesions of the skin or ulcerating granulomas of mucous membranes including the larynx,[66] the esophagus, and the oral cavity, including the tongue.[207]
  - Coccidioidomycosis in AIDS may present as papular or macular skin lesions.[226]
- The signs, symptoms, and probable agents of pulmonary mycoses are listed in Table 21-1.
- The signs, symptoms, and probable agents of extrapulmonary mycoses are summarized in Table 21-2.
- Nonspecific laboratory findings, such as accelerated erythrocyte sedimentation rate, increase in C-reactive protein, elevations in γ-globulin, or low-grade and persistent elevations in the peripheral blood neutrophils and/or monocytes may provide initial clues to the presence of a fungal infection.

Clinical Categorization of Fungal Infections

From a broad perspective, fungal infections may be referred to as either ''superficial'' or ''deep-seated'' (or ''systemic''). However, this broad categorization no longer serves the needs of clinical practice, as several fungal species once thought to be ''superficial'' may cause disseminated disease. Therefore, several specific terms have evolved by which clinicians and mycologists can better communicate.

The terms **deep-seated** and **systemic** classically referred to a group of fungal infections caused by agents that inherently can be highly virulent, that can invade deeply into tissues, and organs, and that have the capability of spreading widely throughout the body. Until recently, most of these infections have been caused by the dimorphic fungi—that is, the species that exist in the form of mold in the environment (''room-temperature incubation'')—but as yeasts when incubated at 35–37°C (body temperature). Currently, because of the increase in the number of individuals who are immunosuppressed or who have severely compromised cellular immunity, other fungal agents, formerly considered only as ''saprobes'' or ''contaminants,'' are now agents of systemic disease. One prime example is the hyaline mold *Penicillium marneffii*, which causes a disseminated reticuloendothelial infection that resembles histoplasmosis clinically and pathologically.

The term **opportunistic** is now used to describe the ''nonpathogenic'' fungi that can cause subcutaneous and disseminated infections. These are fungi, usually of inherently low or limited virulence, that nevertheless can cause local or disseminated disease in intravenous-drug users, in the debili-

Table 21-1 Signs and Symptoms of Pulmonary Mycoses

TYPE OF INFECTION	SIGNS AND SYMPTOMS
General	A transient influenzalike syndrome or pneumonia that localizes in one lobe or spreads to other lobes seen in early infection.
	Cough, minimal sputum production, dyspnea, tachypnea, hemoptysis.
	Chest pain, frequently pleuritic in nature.
	Rales or rhonchi and a pleural friction rub may be detected on auscultation.
	Roentgenography of the chest may reveal small pulmonary infiltrates and hilar adenopathy or more diffuse and confluent opacities.
Allergic bronchopulmonary	Symptoms characteristic of asthma: nonproductive cough, wheezing, tightness in the chest.
	Episodic bronchospasm.
	Segmental atelectasis caused by plugging of bronchioles by mucus.
	Charcot-Leyden crystals and eosinophils in sputum; peripheral-blood eosinophilia.
	Cutaneous hypersensitivity reaction to antigens of *Aspergillus* spp.
	Elevated serum IgE concentration and IgG anti-*Aspergillus* antibodies.
Fungus ball	Growth of fungus colony within a pre-existing cavity.
	Hemoptysis, despite little or no invasion of cavity wall.
	Dissemination is rare, even in patients receiving corticosteroids.
Invasive	Symptoms of acute pneumonia.
	Low-grade, undulant fever.
	Cough may be productive or nonproductive; chest pain usually present.
	Progressive dyspnea and shortness of breath.
	Hemoptysis may indicate infarction and parenchymal necrosis.
	Chest radiography may reveal a diffuse infiltrate emanating from the hilum, finely nodular fibrosis, multifocal abscesses, or cavitation, depending on the fungus species. Clues to specific agents:
	"Millet seed" fibrosis: histoplasmosis
	Peripheral coin lesion: coccidioidomycosis
	Cavitary lesions: histoplasmosis or coccidioidomycosis
	Fungus ball: aspergillosis, pseudallescheriasis, zygomycosis
	Allergic bronchopulmonary disease: *Aspergillus fumigatus, A. flavus*

tated, in those who are immunosuppressed, or in those who wear intravascular or prosthetic devices. *Aspergillus* species, *Candida* species, and *Zygomyces* species (mucormycosis) are the three groups of fungi that classically were considered opportunistic. Recently, localized and deep-seated infections have been ascribed to several other species of light (hyaline) and dark (dematiaceous) rapidly growing molds that formerly were considered to be contaminants.

With the realization that a variety of fungal species can cause virtually all clinical forms of mycoses, Ajello[5,6]

Table 21-2 Signs, Symptoms, and Probable Agents of Extrapulmonary Mycoses

TYPE OF INFECTION	SIGNS AND SYMPTOMS
Cutaneous	Superficial scaling lesions—varying in size, shape, and color—of the thorax or back: tinea versicolor secondary to *Malassezia furfur* infection.
	Itching, scaling lesions known as tinea or ringworm: dermatophytosis
	Thickened, crusting, hyperkeratotic, exophytic fungoid affliction known as favus: *Trichophyton tonsurans, T. violaceum,* and *T. schoenleinii.*
	Scaling or crusting lesions confined to the moist intertriginous areas of skin suggest yeast infections: *Candida albicans.*
	Primary subcutaneous pustular infection at the site of inoculation, with proximal spread and evolution of secondary skin ulcers along the course of the lymphatics: *Sporothrix schenckii.*
	Nonhealing pustules, ulcers, or draining sinuses: disseminated dimorphic fungal diseases and mycetomas secondary to a variety of fungal agents.
	Purpuric lesions and subcutaneous cysts: phaeohyphomycosis.
	Fungating, discolored, hemorrhagic lesions: chromomycosis.
CNS	Insidious onset of headaches that increase in frequency and severity, accompanied by nausea, irritability, and clumsiness; cryptococcosis.
	Meningitis and meningoencephalitis: zygomycosis, particularly in diabetics. Brain abscesses: *Xylophyla bantiana,* other dematiaceous fungi; *Aspergillus* species.
Urinary tract	Pyelitis and pyelonephritis associated with long-term administration of antibiotics, corticosteroids, immunosuppressants, antineoplastic drugs, and prolonged insertion of indwelling catheters for urinary drainage, particularly in elderly women: candidiasis.
	Limited pyuria, lower abdominal pain, frequency of urination: nonbacterial cystitis in middle-aged women: *Torulopsis glabrata.*
Ocular infections	Conjunctivitis, corneal infections, and keratoconjunctivitis: *Fusarium* spp., *Aspergillus* spp., *Cladosporium* spp., *Acremonium* spp., and others. Intraocular infections, usually following trauma or eye surgery: *Candida albicans, Aspergillus* spp., or *Zygomyces* spp.
Endocarditis	Low-grade fever, cardiac murmurs, positive echogram: *Candida* spp., *Aspergillus* spp., *Paecilomyces* spp.
Sinusitis	Facial pain and cutaneous hyperemia, headache, low-grade fever, radiographic evidence of filling of a sinus or fluid levels: *Aspergillus fumigatus, Sporothrix schenckii, Alternaria* spp., and *Pseudallescheria boydii.*

has suggested the use of the generic terms **phaeohyphomycosis** and **hyalohyphomycosis** in reference to saprophytic fungi that appear dark or black in culture (dematiaceous) and that produce colorless, transparent (hyaline) hyphae, respectively. This terminology evolved to eliminate the need to use terms such as penicilliosis, fusariosis, and curvulariosis in reference to each of the myriad opportunistic fungal species that may occasionally serve as agents of mycotic infections. Thus, the all-encompassing terms phaeohyphomycosis and hyalohyphomycosis also relieve the clinician of having to recall the names of many specific fungal agents that are only rarely encountered in clinical practice.

Common Mycologic Terms

Before moving on, a few additional terms that will be used in this textbook should be defined. The term **mycology** itself is derived from the Greek word *mykes*, a direct counterpart of the Latin word *fungus*, which is in turn thought to be a modification of the Greek word *sponges*, from which our word ''sponge'' is derived. **Zygomycosis** has replaced the older term **phycomycosis** in reference to the fungal diseases caused by this important group of opportunistic fungi. The prefix ''zygo'' is derived from the Greek *zygon*, meaning a fusion or joining in the manner of a yoke. This derivation refers to the sexual phase of reproduction, in which there is a joining or fusion of the two independent sex cells to form a zygospore. The previous designation, *phycomycete* (from the Greek *phykos* = ''seaweed''), for this group of fungi has been more correctly replaced by the term *zygomycete*. **Mucormycosis** is also an older term for this group of fungal diseases, derived from the term for the Order ''*Mucorales*,'' from the Latin *mucere*, meaning ''moldy'' or ''musty.'' The term **anamorph** refers to nonsexual fungal reproduction, while **teleomorph** refers to the sexual form of reproduction, in which each new cell is derived from the joining of two separate cells. Most mycologists think that every fungus has a sexual phase that may manifest if the correct environmental conditions and nutritional requirements are provided.

In a broad context, fungi are members of the plant kingdom that are devoid of leaves, stems, or roots. Fungi are **eukaryotic;** that is, each cell possesses a nucleus, nuclear membrane, endoplasmic reticulum, Golgi apparatus, and mitochondria. They also possess a rigid cell wall composed of chitin (*N*-acetyl-D-glucosamine linked by β1-4 glycoside bonds), mannans (polymers of glucose in α- or β-glycoside bonds), and sometimes cellulose. These cell wall constituents adsorb several dyes, which provide for the application of special stains by which they can be identified in laboratory mounts and tissue sections.

Single cell fungus forms are known as **yeasts;** those with multiple cells forming a filamentous mycelium are known as **molds.** Fungi reproduce by **spores**, either sexually or asexually, that may be derived directly from the vegetative mycelium (**arthrospores, chlamydospores, blastospores**), or from the surface of special aerial fruiting bodies (**conidia**). The morphology, arrangement, and mode of derivation of spores serve as important criteria by which genus and species identifications can be made. Additional terms used in the laboratory workup of fungi are presented in Box 21-1.

Laboratory Approach to the Diagnosis of Fungal Infections

Once a fungus is recognized in culture, a presumptive identification is first made based on a visual examination of the colony morphology or from microscopic observations of a direct mount preparation. With a presumptive identification in mind, the primary physician may be consulted to determine if the clinical history warrants a full genus or species identification.

Although most fungal identifications are based primarily on the assessment of colony morphology and microscopic features, key biochemical tests may be required to differentiate between closely related genera or species within a given group. Nucleic-acid probe assays are being used with increasing frequency to provide an early culture confirmation in suspected cases of deep-seated mycoses. Serologic studies are required in some instances to establish a definitive clinical diagnosis, assess the status of a previously diagnosed mycosis, or determine the efficacy of therapy. Guidelines, therefore, will be set forth in this chapter to assist the mycologist in performing these various tasks, expanding from the laboratory observations to include assessments of the clinical parameters and the histopathologic criteria that must be interwoven to make a definitive diagnosis.

The final laboratory identification of a fungal isolate is dependent on visualization of the colony morphology and microscopic features, to be covered in detail later. Several previous practices and procedures must be in place to ensure that recovery in culture is optimal. Any break in a chain of events, beginning with improper collection of the specimen, failure of preservation during transit, a delay in processing on receipt in the laboratory, and finally, the inoculation to inappropriately selected primary fungal culture media will jeopardize the chances of making a final identification. Procedures must also be in place to provide guidelines for the microscopic study of an unknown isolate and the appropriate selection of differential tests when needed to make an important genus/species identification. The paragraphs that follow detail these steps.

When appropriate, sections will also be included to briefly describing nonculture methods for establishing the identity of a given fungal species, using antibody and antigen techniques, including conventional technologies and newer molecular-based approaches. Looking to the future, it must be mentioned that nucleic-acid sequencing offers promise of becoming the standard method for fungal identification in reference laboratories.[111] At this juncture, due to the technical expertise required and the cost of instrumentation and supplies, this technology will not be implemented in smaller laboratories in which only basic practices are performed.

The only current commercially available system is the Applied Biosystems (Foster City, CA) MicroSeq D2 large-subunit rDNA fungal sequencing kit. A study of the use of nucleic-acid sequencing for the identification of yeasts showed that it identified 98% of 19 different species of *Candida* seen in the clinical laboratory compared to identification by phenotypic methods.[110] DNA sequencing identified 32 isolates of yeasts belonging to nine genera, including *Trichosporon, Cryptococcus,* and others. Approximately 81% were correctly identified, and the primary reason for most incorrect identifications resulted from a lack of data entries in the library containing sequences for many yeasts.

In another study performed at the Mayo Clinic to determine the usefulness of sequencing in identifying filamentous molds, nucleic-acid sequencing, and phenotypic methods identified 234 isolates (67.5%) to the correct genus or species level.[111] Incorrect identifications were primarily due to an incomplete list of sequences in the database. Each laboratory can construct a custom database of sequences, greatly enhancing the accuracy of performance. This technology of-

Box 21-1 Terms Useful in the Examination of Fungi

The fundamental microscopic unit of a fungus is the threadlike structure called a **hypha.** Several hyphae combine to form the matt of growth known as the **mycelium.** Hyphae that are subdivided into individual cells by transverse walls or septate are called **septate;** those without walls are **aseptate.** Pseudohyphae form from elongation of budding yeast cells (**blastoconidia**), and show sausagelike constrictions between segments (Fig. 21-1).

The portion of the mycelium that extends into the substratum of the culture medium, and is responsible for absorbing water and nutrients, is the **vegetative mycelium;** the portion that projects above the substrate is the **aerial mycelium,** also called the **reproductive mycelium,** since special spore or conidia-bearing fruiting bodies derive from this portion.

The identification and classification of fungi are based primarily on the morphologic differences in reproductive structures and the manner in which spores or conidia are formed from specialized cells called **conidiogenous cells.**

Three general types of reproduction are commonly observed in the fungal species of medical importance, **vegetative** sporulation, **aerial** sporulation, and **sexual** sporulation.

Vegetative Reproduction

Three types of spores or conidia may form directly from the vegetative mycelium: **blastoconidia, chlamydoconidia**, and **arthroconidia** (the old term for vegetative spores was **thallospore**). The term **spore** should be reserved for reproductive elements that arise from meiosis (sexual reproduction), such as ascospores, oospores, or zygospores, or from mitosis (asexual reproduction) within a sporangium (as with the **Zygomycetes**). The term **endospore** is also used for spores produced within a confined space (the tissue form of *Coccidioides immitis*, for example). All other asexual "spores" are conidia.

Blastoconidia are the familiar budding forms characteristically produced by yeasts. A bud scar (dysjunctor) often remains at the point at which the conidium becomes detached.

Chlamydoconidia (chlamydospores) are formed from preexistent cells in the hyphae, which become thickened and often enlarged. Although *chlamydoconidia* is the correct terminology, the term *chlamydospores* is retained in most clinical laboratory circles. Chlamydospores may be found within (**intercalary**), along the side (**sessile**) or at the tip (**terminal**) of the hyphae. This type of conidiation is characteristic of *Candida albicans*.

Arthroconidia also are formed from preexisting cells in the hyphae, which become enlarged and thickened. On maturity, these conidia are released by lysis of adjacent hyphal cells. This type of sporulation is characteristic of the mold form of *Coccidioides immitis* and *Geotrichum* species, among others.

Aerial Reproduction

Emanating from the hyphae and extending from the mycelial surface are specialized fruiting bodies that give rise to a variety of spores or conidia. Fruiting bodies may form closed sacs called **sporangia,** within which spores called **sporangiospores** are produced. The specialized hyphal segment that holds up or supports the sporangium is called the **sporangiophore** (the suffix "phore" [Greek *phoros*] means "bearing") (Fig. 21-2). This type of sporulation is characteristic of the *Zygomycetes*. Many other fungi produce elaborate fruiting bodies that give rise to spores produced from the surface, to which the term *conidia* (dust) is applied. The specialized hyphal segment that supports a conidia-bearing fruiting head is called a **conidiophore** (Fig. 21-2).

The conidiophore may branch into secondary segments called **metulae,** which in turn produce conidia-producing segments, called **phialides.** This property of branching into metulae and phialides is characteristic of the fingerlike fruiting body of *Penicillium* species. Phialides by definition are conidiogenous cells that produce conidia from a locus inside its apex, which does not increase in width or length during conidiogenesis. This is in contrast to **annellide** formation, in which the tip of the phialide cyclically extends and retracts when conidia are formed, leaving a succession of scars or rings. The conidia of *Scopulariopsis* spp., for example, are **annelloconidia;** that is, form in basipetal sequence in which the conidiogenous part of each conidium elongates at the time a new one is formed, then contracting to form a **ringlike scar, annulus,** or **collarette** at the truncated base. Conidia may be borne singly, in long chains (**catenulate**), or in tightly bound clusters. **Acropetal** is a term used to describe the process of chain formation in which each new conidium is derived in sequence from the previous one, so that the youngest cell is at the tip (*Penicillium* spp., for example), in contrast to **basipetal sporulation,** in which each new conidium forms at the base of the chain, pushing all other conidia in the chain ahead, so that the oldest cell is at the tip (*Paecilomyces* species).

Tiny one-celled conidia, usually borne either directly from the sides of the hyphae or supported by a hairlike conidiophore, are called **microconidia,** in contrast to the much larger, multicelled **macroconidia,** which assume a variety of sizes and shapes. A multicelled macroconidia that is divided by both transverse and longitudinal septations, giving a mosaic appearance, is a **dictyospore,** more commonly referred to as **muriform** (resembling a stone wall). The term **aleuriospore** refers to a conidium, usually a macroconidium, that is attached to the hyphae by a supporting cell that fractures when the conidium is released (example, *Microsporum canis*).

(Continued)

Box 21-1 *Continued*

Sexual Sporulation

Sexual sporulation requires the merging and nuclear recombination of two specialized fertile cells (each having undergone meiosis) arising on the aerial hyphae. If the reproductive cells formed by fusion of morphologically identical cells, often from the same hyphae (homothallic), the spore is called a **zygospore,** characteristic of the *Zygomycetes.* If the fusing reproductive cells are derived from two different cells, often derived from separate hyphal segments, the resulting spore is called an **oospore** (Fig. 21-3).

The sexual spores of several members of the Class **Ascomycetes,** previously mentioned, which are of medical importance, are called **ascospores.** For example, certain strains of *Aspergillus* species, notably of the *A. nidulans* and *A. glaucus* groups, produce large closed, baglike structures called cleistothecia, which in turn contain smaller baglike structures called asci (Fig. 21-3). Within each ascus are four ascospores, the product of meiotic division. Medically important fungi, other than *Aspergillus* species, in which sexual sporulation may be observed include *Saccharomyces* spp. and *Pseudallescheria boydii* (Fig. 21-3).

The sexual form of a fungus is known as a **teleomorph,** in contrast to the term **anamorph,** which refers to the various asexual reproductive forms or structures produced by an imperfect fungus (such as phialides, annellides, branching chains, etc.). Thus, for example, *Pseudallescheria boydii* is the teleomorph of this species, and various "perfect" forms such as cleistothecia, asci, and ascospores may be observed. *Scedosporium monosporium* is the imperfect form of this species, producing primarily single-celled, anamorphic conidia.

fers great promise of simplifying the identification of yeasts and molds recovered from clinical specimens as well as those important to industry and agriculture. It may very well in the future become the standard for fungal identification.

Specimen Collection and Transport

General guidelines for the collection and transport of specimens for culture are given in Chapter 2 of this text. Guidelines for the collection of various types of specimens are presented in Table 21-3. Physicians, nurses, ward personnel, and laboratory technologists must work together in developing protocols that ensure the proper collection and prompt transport of specimens submitted for fungus culture. The selection of appropriate collection devices and transport containers, affixing labels that include pertinent patient information, and establishing a means of communication for special requests are possibly the most important considerations in ensuring the accurate diagnosis of fungal infections.

Specimens should be delivered to the laboratory promptly. Specimens that are not processed immediately should be held at room temperature. *Cryptococcus neoformans, Histoplasma capsulatum,* and *Blastomyces dermatitidis* do not survive well in frozen or iced specimens. Several fungal species, including the above-named species, and *Aspergillus* spp. can be recovered from samples that

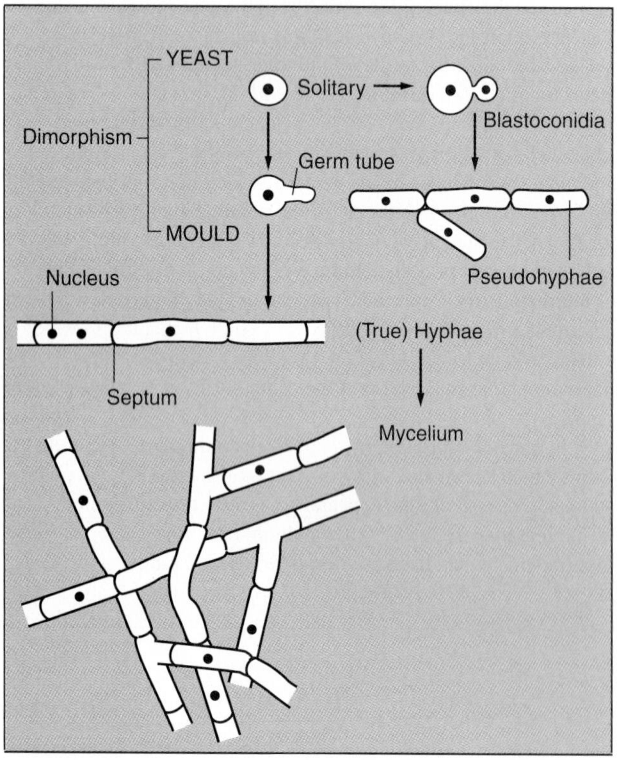

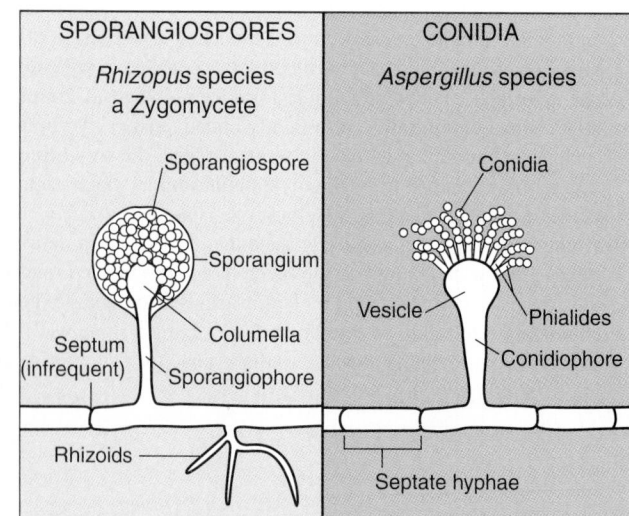

Figure 21-1 Sketches illustrating basic fungal structures.

Figure 21-2 Sketches illustrating structures of the aerial mycelium and asexual reproduction.

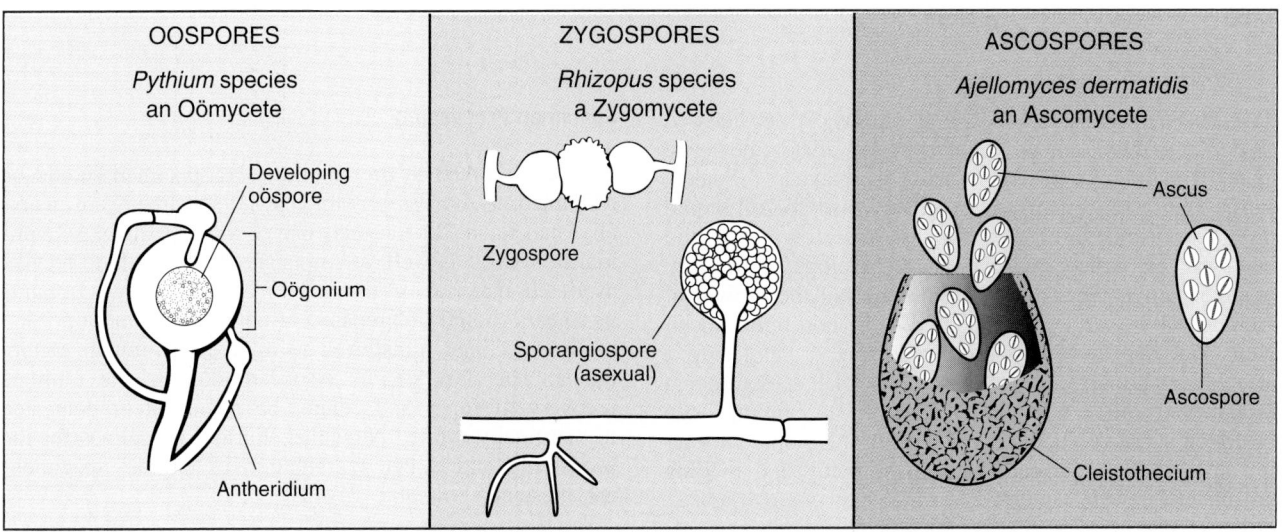

Figure 21-3 Sketches illustrating the structures of sexual reproduction.

Table 21-3 American Thoracic Society Recommendations for Collection of Specimen for Fungus Culture

SPECIMEN	RECOMMENDED PROCEDURE
Sputum	The first early-morning sample should be collected after rising, but before breakfast. Patients are instructed to vigorously rinse their mouths with water immediately before coughing 1/2 to 1 oz of sputum into a sterile, screw-capped container. Sputum induction with a heated aerosol saline suspension may be required if an adequate specimen cannot be obtained.
Bronchoscopy	Bronchial brushings, biopsy, or bronchoalveolar lavage fluid should be transported promptly to the laboratory in sterile, sealed containers.
	Middlebrook 7H11 broth is used in some laboratories as a transport medium because mycobacteria will also be preserved. A postbronchoscopy sputum sample should be collected when possible.
Cerebrospinal fluid	As much cerebrospinal fluid (CSF) as possible should be used for the culture of fungi. If processing is to be delayed, samples should be left at room temperature because CSF is an adequate fluid culture medium in which fungal elements can survive until subcultured.
Urine	The first early-morning urine sample is preferred; random samples are acceptable. Specimens should be collected aseptically in sterile, screw-cap containers and sent immediately for processing. If a delay in processing beyond 2 hours is anticipated, the urine sample should be refrigerated at 4°C to inhibit overgrowth by rapidly growing bacteria.
Prostatic secretions	Some deep-seated mycoses, notably blastomycosis and, less commonly, histoplasmosis or coccidioidomycosis, may be diagnosed by collecting prostatic secretions. The bladder is first emptied, followed by prostatic massage. Secretions should be inoculated directly into appropriate fungal culture media; also, 5–10 mL of urine should be collected in a separate container.
Exudates	The skin over pustular lesions should be disinfected and exudates aspirated using a sterile needle and syringe. The syringe may also serve as a transport container if the needle is capped. Biopsy of the lesion may be necessary if the aspirate fails to yield fungi.
Skin, nails, hair	First, swab the area of skin to be sampled with 70% alcohol to remove surface bacterial contaminants. Sample the peripheral, erythematous, growing margin of typical "ringworm" lesions, scraping with the side of a glass microscope slide or the edge of a scalpel blade. Infected nails should be sampled from beneath the nail plate to obtain softened material from the nail bed. If this is not possible, scrape away the surface of the nail before collecting shavings from the deeper portions. Hairs should be collected from areas of scaling or alopecia, or those that fluoresce when viewed under a Wood's (long-wavelength) ultraviolet lamp.
Tissue biopsies	Tissue biopsies of suspected sites of infection should be transported in a sterile gauze moistened with physiologic, nonbacteriostatic, sterile saline solution in a screw-cap container. The specimen should not be frozen or allowed to dehydrate prior to culture.
Blood	Biphasic agar-broth bottles designed specifically for fungal cultures are superior to routine bottles used for the recovery of bacterial pathogens. Lysis-centrifugation systems, such as the Isolator (Wampole Laboratories, Cranbury, NJ) are also highly recommended, particularly for the recovery of *H. capsulatum* and other yeasts.

have been in transit for as long as 16 days if not allowed to dry out; therefore, an attempt should always be made to recover fungi even if processing is delayed.[243] Sealed, sterile transport containers should be used for all liquid or moist specimens. Skin scrapings, nail fragments, and hairs can be transported dry in an envelope, Petri dish, or other convenient conveyance. To curtail the growth of commensal bacteria possibly present in nonsterile specimens that may be delayed in processing or mailed to a reference laboratory, penicillin (20 U/mL), streptomycin (100,000 μg/mL), or chloramphenicol (0.2 mg/mL) can be added to the specimen. Directions for the proper packaging and labeling of specimens for shipping and mailing are discussed in Chapter 2.

The criteria by which a specimen is judged unacceptable for culture and rejected should be written in the laboratory protocol. In Box 21-2 select rejection criteria and the actions to be taken for handling unacceptable specimens are presented. These criteria must also be understood by physicians, nurses, and other personnel who are assigned to collect the specimen, as not only will time and money be saved in the mycology laboratory, but an unacceptable delay in establishing the diagnosis can be avoided. Individual criteria must be established within each practice setting to accommodate to the local situation. With experience, the individual collecting the specimen can make a preliminary observation of the material obtained and immediately collect a second sample if necessary.

Specimen Processing

Once received in the laboratory, a specimen should be examined as soon as possible. Swab specimens are generally inadequate for the recovery of molds and are suboptimal for yeasts as well; attempts should be made to receive aspirated material or tissue biopsies. Direct wet mounts or smears should be prepared, if appropriate, and a portion of the specimen transferred to appropriate fungal culture media. This last step is also important in the ultimate recovery of fungi and cannot be neglected or delegated to marginally trained personnel. Further guidelines for the processing and direct examination of clinical specimens are presented in Table 21-4.

Direct Examination

It is highly recommended that a direct microscopic examination be made on most specimens submitted for fungal culture. Not only may this provide an immediate presumptive diagnosis for the physician, but it may also aid in the selection of appropriate culture media. Direct India ink and KOH/calcofluor mounts, lactophenol aniline blue–stained transparency tape preparations, and frozen sections of tissue biopsies are various methods by which rapid, direct microscopic examinations can be made.

A phase contrast microscope is a valuable adjunct in the direct examination of specimens. The advantages include:

Box 21-2 Criteria for Specimen Rejection

Situation: Absence of patient identification on the container, or a discrepancy between the information on the request form and the container label.
Action: Return to sender for resolution.

Situation: Sputum specimen with >25 squamous epithelial cells per low-power field (criteria for rejection of respiratory samples submitted for bacterial culture).
Action: The criteria for rejection of specimens submitted for bacterial culture may not necessarily pertain to fungal specimens. Pathogenic fungi may be recovered from such specimens in the face of oral contamination, particularly if an antibiotic-containing selective culture medium had been used. However, the final report should indicate that significant oral contamination was present, leaving the physician with the option of making an interpretation based on clinical information or obtaining a higher-quality specimen if a clearer differentiation between an upper and a lower respiratory infection is needed.

Situation: A dried-out swab is received or the material collected is insufficient in volume.
Action: Inform the person submitting the specimen to send a second sample if possible. As a general criterion, swab specimens are not suitable for the recovery of fungi and should be rejected, except in unusual circumstances. Rather, deep aspiration or biopsy of the affected site may be necessary, depending on the clinical presentation.

Situation: The sample is submitted in an improper container or in an unsuitable condition (evidence of drying, leakage, or lack of sterility).
Action: Notify the individual submitting the specimen that the chance for obtaining relevant results is compromised. If a second specimen cannot be conveniently obtained, process the specimen, but indicate on the final report that the quality of the specimen was compromised and that the result can be interpreted only in light of the clinical presentation.

Situation: A 24-hour sputum or urine specimen for fungal culture is received.
Action: It should be understood in the rejection protocol that 24-hour sputum and urine samples are suboptimal for the recovery and identification of fungi. Chances for contamination with bacteria and environmental molds are high, confusing any results that may follow. Establish in the protocol that first early-morning samples should be obtained on three successive days. As is the case with the culture recovery of mycobacteria, fungi also tend to be shed at intermittent intervals, thus making the chance of recovery much higher if successive samples over 3 days are collected.

Table 21-4 **Guidelines for Direct Examination and Processing of Specimens Submitted for Fungal Cultures**

Respiratory	The sputum quality-grading system described in Chapter 2 is not applicable to specimens submitted for fungal cultures. Select the most purulent or blood-flecked parts of the sample. If the sample is highly viscid, it should be homogenized by adding a small pinch of crystalline *N*-acetyl-L-cystine to the specimen. NaOH or other digesting agents, used for the processing of specimens for the recovery of mycobacteria, should not be used. Prepare a mount of the homogenized sample for direct microscopic examination and inoculate about 0.5 mL to each of the culture media to be used.
	Because respiratory secretions are often contaminated with bacteria, media containing antibiotics should be used. A combination of a nonselective agar, such as inhibitory mold agar or SABHI agar, and an inhibitory agar such as brain-heart infusion with chloramphenicol and cycloheximide are recommended.
Cerebrospinal fluid	CSF samples may be centrifuged at 1500–2000 *g* for 20 min and the sediment inoculated onto the surface of noninhibitory culture media, such as inhibitory mold agar or SABHI agar. Preferably, if more than 2 mL of fluid is available, pass fluid through a 0.45-μm membrane filter, using a Swinnex syringe attachment. Place the filtrate side of the filter paper face down on the surface of appropriate culture medium. The paper should be repositioned to other sites on the medium using sterile forceps on an every-other-day schedule. If only a scant amount of fluid is provided, spot-inoculate the surface of the agar medium directly in three- or four-drop aliquots.
	The India ink (nigrosin is an acceptable substitute) mounts may be prepared when *Cryptococcus neoformans* is suspected. To prepare the mount, either a drop of the centrifuged sediment or a small amount of material from the surface of the membrane is mixed with a drop of India ink on a microscope slide. A coverslip is applied and the mount microscopically examined for the presence of encapsulated, budding yeast forms.
Urine	Centrifuge about 10 mL of urine sample, then inoculate 0.5 mL of sediment to both a noninhibitory agar, such as inhibitory mold agar or SABHI agar, and to an inhibitory medium, such as brain-heart infusion agar, containing chloramphenicol and cycloheximide. Direct mounts can be prepared and examined microscopically for yeast or hyphal forms.
Skin, nails, hair	Skin scales, nail scrapings, and hairs should be examined after KOH treatment. The KOH preparation is made by emulsifying the specimen in a drop of 10% KOH on a microscope slide. The purpose of the KOH is to clear out any background scales or cell membranes that may be confused with hyphal elements. Clearing can be accelerated by gently heating the mixture over the flame of a Bunsen burner. A coverslip is applied, and the specimen is examined for the presence of narrow, regular hyphae that characteristically break up into arthroconidia. The visualization of hyphae is improved by adding calcofluor white to the potassium hydroxide reagent and examining with a fluorescence microscope fitted with filters of appropriate wavelengths. With hairs, mosaic arrangement of spores may be seen on the surface of the shaft (ectothrix infection) or hyphal fragments and arthroconidia may be seen internally (endothrix infection).
	Skin scales, nail scrapings, or hairs should be placed directly on the surface of the culture medium, such as brain-heart infusion agar with chloramphenicol and cycloheximide (commercially available as Mycosel or Mycobiotic agars). With a straight inoculating wire, submerge a few of the fragments beneath the agar surface. Examine in the areas of inoculation at frequent intervals for the appearance of surface colonies. Hold cultures for a minimum of 30 days before discarding as negative.
Tissue	When processing tissues for the recovery of fungi, the use of a mortar and pestle or a tissue grinder should be avoided. The hyphal forms can easily be destroyed by grinding, making it difficult to recover viable organisms in culture (particularly if the aseptate hyphae of one of the *Zygomycetes* are present). Rather, mince the tissue into 1-mm cubes with sterile scissors or a sharp scalpel blade and place the tiny fragments directly onto the agar, submerging them slightly beneath the surface with an inoculating needle.
	A 5- to 10-mL sample of tissue homogenate, bone marrow, or fluid specimen sediment should be placed onto the surface of appropriate culture media. Nonselective culture media, without antibiotics, such as inhibitory mold agar or SABHI, are probably adequate, as these specimens are usually sterile and antibiotic inhibition is not necessary.
Blood	Commercial blood culture bottles, designed for the recovery of bacteria from blood are not suitable for the recovery of many fungal species. The Isolator System (Wampole Laboratories, Cranbury, NJ) has shown much promise in the more direct recovery of fungi from blood samples obtained from patients with mycotic sepsis. If this system is used, carefully follow the instructions of the manufacturer. In particular, care must be taken during the subculture stage to avoid contamination with environmental organisms. Working in a laminar airflow hood during this procedure has been advocated.

Box 21-3 Procedure: The Tease Mount

- With a pair of dissecting needles or pointed applicator sticks, dig out a small portion of the colony to be examined, including portions of the subsurface agar.
- Place the colony fragment on a microscope slide in a drop of lactophenol aniline blue, tease the colony apart with the dissecting needles (Fig. 21–4), and overlay with a coverslip.
- Gentle pressure on the surface of the coverslip with the eraser end of a pencil may help to disperse the mount, particularly if small chunks of agar are present.
- Examine the preparation microscopically, first under the low-power (10×) objective and then under high-power (40×) or under oil immersion (100×) if suspicious fungal structures are seen.
- Teasing the colony often disrupts the delicate fruiting structures of the filamentous molds, making it difficult in some instances to observe the characteristic spore arrangements or hyphal attachments necessary for a definitive identification. In such cases, a transparency tape mount or microslide culture may be required.

Box 21-4 Procedure: Transparency Tape Preparation

- The transparency tape method of preparing cultures for microscopic examination is often helpful because the spore arrangements of the more delicate filamentous molds are better preserved.
- Press the sticky side of unfrosted, clear cellophane tape gently but firmly to the surface of the colony, picking up a portion of the aerial mycelium (Fig. 21–5A). This operation should always be performed under a biologic safety hood. Care must also be taken that exposed fingers do not come in contact with the mold surface. For maximum safety, gloves should be worn.
- The preparation is made by placing a drop of lactophenol aniline blue stain on a microscope slide.
- Stick one end of the tape to the surface of the slide adjacent to the drop of stain.
- Stretch the tape over the stain, gently lowering it so that the mycelium becomes permeated with stain (Fig. 21–5B).
- Pull the tape taught and stick the opposite end to the glass, avoiding as much as possible the trapping of air bubbles.
- Some practice may be needed in removing the sticky surface of the tape if gloves are worn.
- The preparation can now be examined microscopically in the same manner as described above for the tease mount preparation, with the exception that the use of oil immersion is generally less than satisfactory because of interference from the substance of the tape.
- The transparency tape method is inexpensive, rapid, simple to perform, and, with few exceptions, allows one to make an accurate identification.

1) mounts can be made and examined quickly; 2) there is no need for direct staining; and 3) the objects can be clearly visualized.

PREPARATION OF MOUNTS FOR STUDY

The tease mount, the transparency tape preparation, and the microslide technique are three commonly used methods for the microscopic examination of filamentous molds.[147] In each instance, a portion of the mold colony is mounted in a drop of lactophenol aniline (cotton) blue stain on a glass slide and examined microscopically. The technique for performing the tease mount is presented in Box 21-3, for the transparency tape mount in Box 21-4, and

for the microculture procedure in Box 21-5. Additional terms used in the laboratory workup of fungi are presented in Box 21-1.

SELECTION AND INOCULATION OF CULTURE MEDIA

The battery of culture media for the recovery of fungi from clinical specimens need not be elaborate. Although the recovery rate may be somewhat enhanced by using a variety of isolation media, considerations of cost, storage and incubator space, and demands on technologist time generally dictate a more conservative approach in most laboratories.

Two general types of culture media are essential to ensure the primary recovery of all clinically significant fungi from clinical specimens. One medium should be nonselective (such as brain-heart infusion agar); that is, one that will permit the growth of virtually all clinically relevant fungal species. The use of Sabouraud's dextrose agar as a primary recovery medium is discouraged because it is insufficiently rich to recover certain fastidious pathogenic species, particularly most of the dimorphic fungi. Rather, the use of potato flake agar (PFA), inhibitory mold agar (IMA), or combination Sabouraud's dextrose agar with heart infusion (SABHI) agar are recommended.[147] Sabouraud's dextrose agar is sufficient for the recovery of dermatophytes from cutaneous samples or yeasts from vaginal cultures. The use of either Mycosel or Mycobiotic

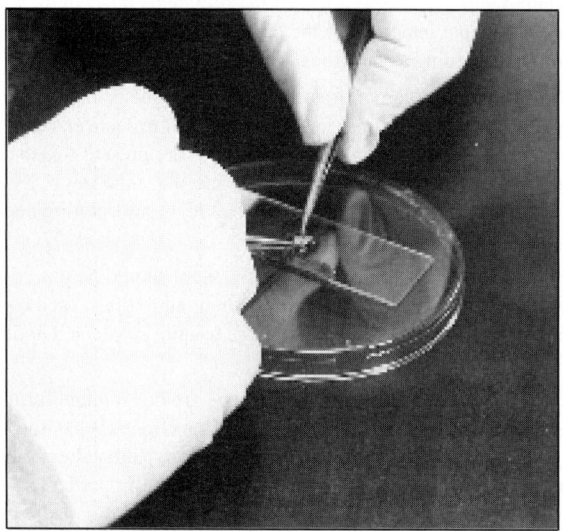

Figure 21-4 Tease mount preparation, illustrating dissection of the colony fragment with needles in a drop of lactophenol aniline blue prior to placement of the coverslip.

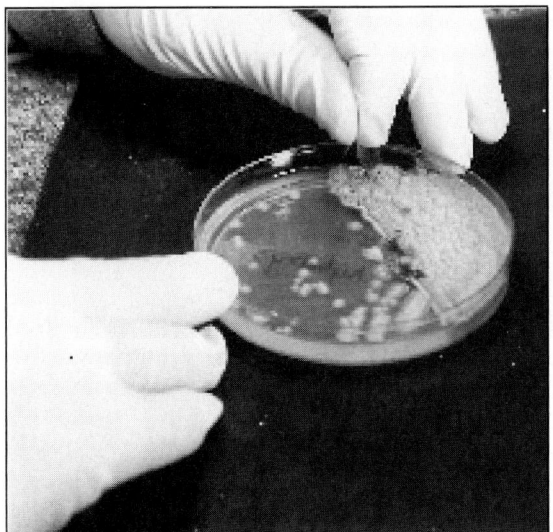
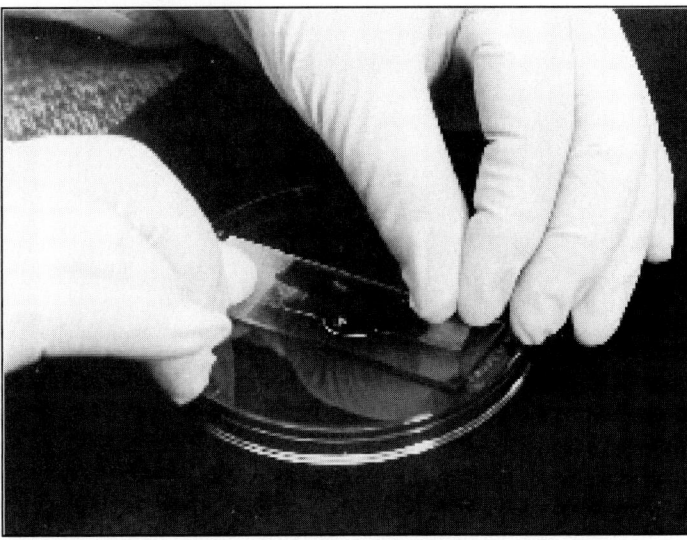

A   B

Figure 21-5 A. Transparency tape preparation: sticky side of tape being pressed to the surface of the fungus colony. **B.** Transparency tape preparation: stretching the inoculated tape over a drop of lactophenol aniline blue on the surface of a microscope slide.

Box 21-5 Procedure: The Microslide Culture Technique

In instances in which neither the tease mount nor the transparency tape preparation establishes an accurate identification, or when permanent slide mounts are desired for further study or for study use by students, the microslide culture technique is recommended. Although somewhat tedious to perform, high-quality preparations in which the spore structures and arrangements are beautifully preserved can be made. The technique is as follows:

1. Place a round piece of filter paper or gauze flat on the bottom of a sterile Petri dish. Place a pair of thin glass rods or applicator sticks cut to length to fit on top of the filter paper to serve as supports for a 3-in. × 1-in. glass microscope slide (Fig. 21-6A).
2. Place a block or plug of cornmeal or potato dextrose agar (Fig. 21-6B) on the surface of the microscope slide (Fig. 21-6C). Two blocks, separated by about 1 in., can be placed on the same microscope slide if more than one mount is desired.
3. Inoculate the margins of the agar plug in three or four places with a small portion of the colony to be studied, using a straight inoculating wire or the tip of a dissecting needle. (Fig. 21-6D and E).
4. Gently heat a coverslip by passing it quickly through the flame of a Bunsen burner and immediately place it directly on the surface of the inoculated agar block. Heating the coverslip produces a tight seal between the bottom of the coverslip and the surface of the agar, which is briefly melted by the warm glass.
5. Pipette a small amount of water into the bottom of the Petri dish to saturate the filter paper or the gauze. Place the lid on the Petri dish and incubate the assembly at room temperature (or 30°C) for 3 to 5 days.
6. When growth visually appears to be mature (Fig. 21-6F), the coverslip can be gently lifted from the surface of the agar with a pair of forceps, taking care not to disrupt the mycelium adhering to the bottom of the coverslip any more than necessary (Fig. 21-6G).
7. Place the coverslip on a small drop of lactophenol aniline blue applied to the surface of a second 3-in. × 1-in. glass slide (Fig. 21-6H). The mount can be preserved for future study by rimming the outside margins of the coverslip with mounting fluid or clear fingernail polish. This activity should be performed under a biologic safety hood.
8. After the coverslip has been removed from the agar block (or blocks), the agar block itself can be removed by prying it away from the glass slide with an applicator stick. This operation is performed over a beaker or pan containing 5% phenol decontamination fluid, into which the agar blocks are allowed to fall. The mycelium adhering to the surface of the original glass slide after the block is removed can also be stained with lactophenol aniline blue and a coverslip overlaid, serving as a second stained mount. Again, the mount can be preserved for future study by rimming the coverslip with mounting fluid or fingernail polish, as previously described.

One should not be concerned if the agar blocks completely dry out before harvesting the coverslip. Even if the coverslip is firmly adherent to the surface of the glass, a drop of lactophenol aniline blue can be placed adjacent to one margin of the slide. By capillary action the stain will diffuse between the undersurface of the coverslip and the glass slide. In fact, there is often less disruption of the mycelial elements, and superior preparations potentially are the result.

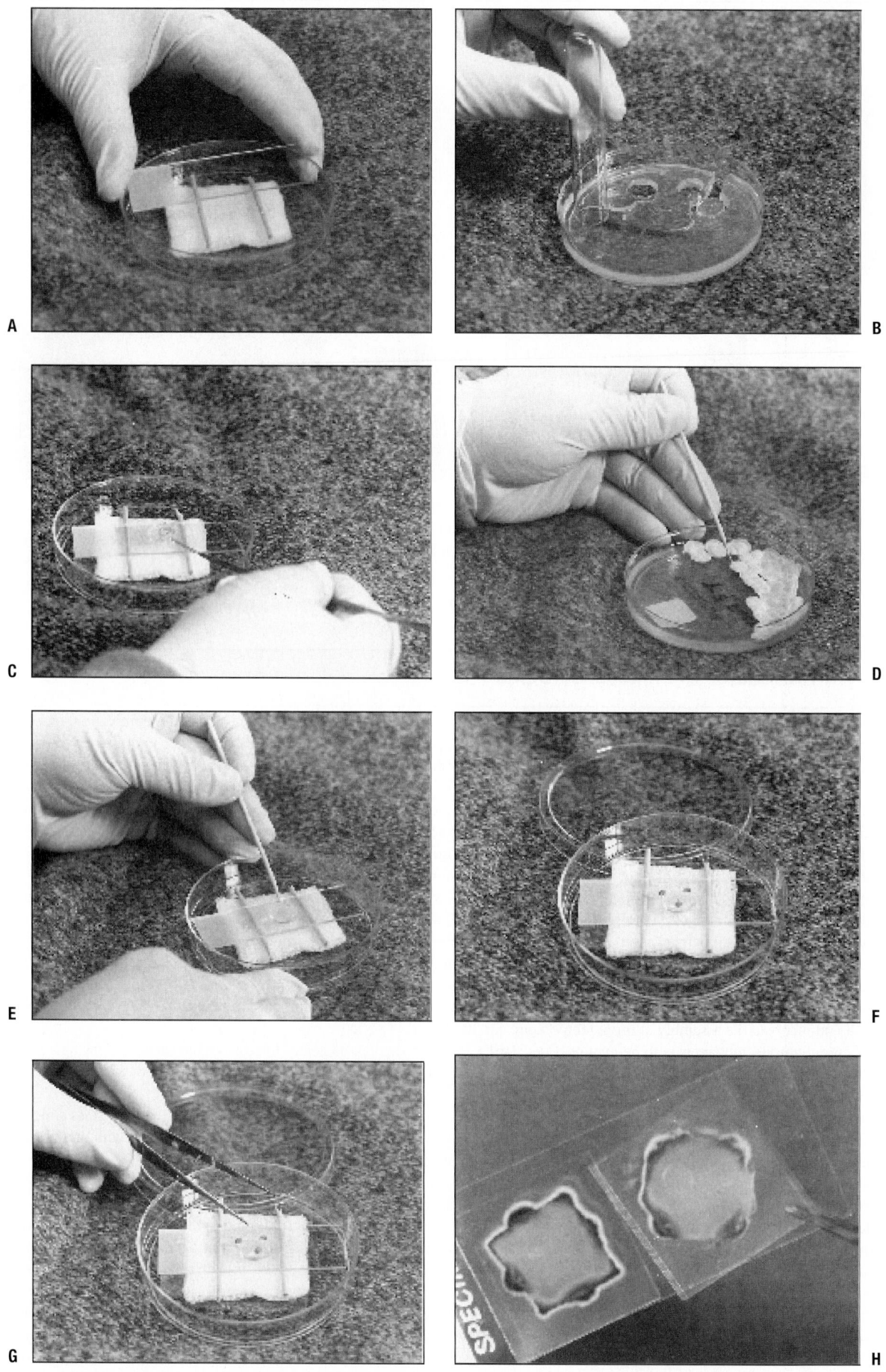

Figure 21-6 Series of photographs outlining the preparation of a microculture. See Box 21-4 for details.

agar, which essentially is Sabouraud's dextrose agar with cycloheximide and chloramphenicol added, may be considered for the recovery of dermatophytes.

Sabouraud's dextrose agar (2%) is most useful as a medium for the subculture of fungi recovered on enriched medium to enhance typical sporulation and provide the more characteristic colonial morphology. Czepak's agar should be used for the subculture of *Aspergillus* species if colony morphology is an important identifying criterion for any given unknown isolate.

For the recovery of the more fastidious dimorphic fungi, such as *Blastomyces dermatitidis* and *Histoplasma capsulatum*, an enriched agar base such as inhibitory mold agar, SABHI (Sabouraud's dextrose agar + heart infusion agar), or brain–heart infusion (with cycloheximide and chloramphenicol) must be used. Table 21-5 lists the more commonly used fungal isolation media, the key ingredients in each formula, and the specific applications for which each is designed. For optimal recovery of certain of these more fastidious strains, particularly for *Histoplasma capsulatum*, media with the addition of 5–10% sheep blood is recommended. If such blood-enriched media are used, it may be necessary to subculture to a less enriched medium such as Sabouraud's dextrose agar or potato dextrose agar so that the more characteristic colony morphology and modes of sporulation can be observed.

A second medium, more selective for the recovery of fungi, should also be used. The addition of one or more antibiotics, including penicillin (20 U/mL), streptomycin (40 U/mL), gentamicin (5 μg/mL), or chloramphenicol (16 μg/mL) may be used to inhibit the growth of bacteria. Cycloheximide (Acti-Dione) in a concentration of 0.5 μg/mL, may also be added to prevent the overgrowth of certain rapidly growing environmental molds. Opportunistic pathogenic fungi, including *Cryptococcus neoformans* and *Aspergillus fumigatus,* may be partially or totally inhibited by cycloheximide; therefore, a nonselective medium must always be used in parallel.

INCUBATION OF FUNGAL CULTURES

It is currently recommended that all fungal cultures be incubated at a controlled 30°C. Incubation of a second set of plates at 35°C for the recovery of the yeast forms of dimorphic fungi is not cost-effective. The previous practice of attempting to convert fungal isolates suspected of being dimorphic molds to their yeast form has largely been replaced by nucleic-acid probe assays. The probe assay can be performed as soon as colonies are visualized on the primary recovery media, prior to the observation of diagnostic sporulation.

All fungal cultures should be incubated for a minimum of

Table 21-5 Common Fungal Primary Recovery Culture Media and Indications for Use

CULTURE MEDIA	ESSENTIAL INGREDIENTS	INDICATIONS FOR USE
Brain–heart infusion agar	Calf brain and beef heart infusions; proteose peptone, NaCl, disodium phosphate, and agar (Cycloheximide and chloramphenicol may be added for selective recovery of dimorphic molds.)	Primary recovery of saprophytic and dimorphic fungi
Inhibitory mold agar (IMA)	Tryptone, beef extract, yeast extract, dextrose, starch, dextrin, chloramphenicol, gentamicin, and saline buffers	Primary recovery of dimorphic pathogenic fungi. Saprophytic fungi and dermatophytes will not be recovered.
Mycosel/Mycobiotic agars	Phytone peptone, dextrose, agar, cycloheximide, chloramphenicol	Primary recovery of dermatophytes
SABHI agar (Sabouraud's heart infusion agar)	Potato flakes, dextrose, agar	Primary recovery of saprophytic and dimorphic fungi, particularly fastidious strains
Sabouraud's dextrose agar	Dextrose, neopeptone, agar	Not recommended as a primary isolation medium. Best used for secondary workup of cultures.
Potato flake agar	Potato flakes, dextrose, agar	Primary recovery of saprophytic and dimorphic fungi, particularly fastidious and slow-growing strains

30 days before discarding as negative, even if plates appear contaminated with bacteria or other fungi. Colonies of *H. capsulatum*, for example, may be observed growing on the surface of colonies of *C. albicans* or on the top of contaminating molds.

The choice between the use of culture tubes or plates is optional. For low-volume laboratories, staffed with personnel who may not be as familiar with the handling of fungi, or where incubator and storage space may be at a premium, the use of tubes is recommended. Large culture tubes (150 mm × 25 mm) with tightly fitted, screw-cap lids are recommended. The media should be poured in thick slants to prevent dehydration during the prolonged incubation period. After the medium is inoculated, be sure not to screw down the cap too tightly because it is necessary for the fungi to ''breathe'' if they are to survive. The ease of transport of cultures recovered in tubes is an added advantage. The chief disadvantage is the difficulty in preparing stained mounts for microscopic examination.

Petri dishes have the advantage of providing a larger surface for growth, resulting in better colony separation and making the cultures easier to examine and subculture. Fungal colonies in mixed culture are easier to separate and work with as individual colonies. Tease mounts or transparency tape preparations are more effectively made from plate cultures, potentially leading to an improved chance for making a more rapid presumptive identification. Because plate cultures may become dehydrated during the prolonged incubation period, they may be placed into a sealed, moisturized polyester bag, or the edge of the Petri dish may be sealed with oxygen-permeable tape. If an incubator is used only for fungal cultures, placing a flat, open pan of water on the bottom shelf serves to provide the moisture needed for optimal recovery. Care must be taken, however, to control the growth of environmental mold in the water.

Laboratory Approach to the Presumptive Identification of Fungal Isolates

Once the observation of a culture plate reveals the growth of a probable fungus, several characteristics of the colony may be assessed to determine within which major group of fungi the isolate may belong. A guide to the genus and species identification of medically important fungi based on the colony morphology and microscopic features of clinical isolates is presented in Table 21-6, which is based on the observation of primary fungal isolates incubated at 30°C. If the fungal isolate presents a distinct wooly or cottony aerial mycelium, one of several species of molds must be considered. If the mold is rapidly growing, filling the Petri dish without an outer border within 48–72 hours, one of the Zygomycetes must be considered (see Display 21-1 at the end of this chapter).

Molds that grow within 3–5 days, have a distinct border, and are white or pastel on the surface, often with a white apron of new growth at the periphery, most likely belong to the hyaline group of molds. Keys to the identification of the hyaline molds are presented in Display 21-2, and for the identification of molds recovered from skin scrapings, nail shavings, or hairs, potentially belonging to the dermatophyte group in Display 21-3.

For molds that are generally slower-growing (7–14 days) or that have a delicate or cobweb aerial mycelium, usually gray or gray-brown, one of the dimorphic species should be considered. The dimorphic molds are in the filamentous form when incubated at ambient temperature (25–30°C), and in the yeast form when incubated at body temperature (35–37°C). At times, the colonies of certain dimorphic molds may appear focally yeastlike when incubated at 30°C. Dimorphic molds can be converted, sometimes with difficulty, from the mold to the yeast form by incubating a subculture on enriched agar at 35–37°C. The approach to the species identification of the dimorphic molds is presented in Display 21-4.

Colonies that develop a dark gray to black mycelium, particularly prominent when a black reverse of the colony is observed, one of the dematiaceous molds should be considered. The genus and species separation of the more rapidly growing saprophytic species of this group is shown in Display 21-5. The keys to the identification of the slower-growing, pathogenic dematiaceous species, associated with chromomycosis and mycetoma, are shown in Display 21-6.

If the colony has a smooth, creamy, viscous, or pasty appearance, a yeast must be considered. For the genus and species identification of common and less-commonly-encountered yeasts, including the yeastlike, arthroconidia-producing species that may produce a low aerial mycelium and the ''black yeasts,'' see Display 21-7.

Once the initial observations outlined in Table 21-6 are made, and a fungal isolate has been placed within one of the groups outlined therein, further studies will be required to make a final genus/species identification, using the following microscopic criteria:

* If hyphae are observed, determine the structure of the hyphae. Are they:
  * septate or aseptate?
  * branching (if so, at what angles), or not branching?
  * pigmented or not pigmented?
  * even or uneven in width?
  * composed of arthroconidia or pseudohyphae?
* Determine the structure and derivation of fruiting bodies.
* Visualize the type of conidiation:
  * The size and shape of the spores or conidia
  * The size, shape, and arrangement of the spores
* Look for the presence of special diagnostic structures: pycnidia, cleistothecia, Hülle cells.
* If only yeast cells are observed:
  * Note their size, shape, and arrangement.
  * Look for the presence or absence of capsules.
  * Determine the type of blastoconidiation—are daughter cells single or multiple?

Further guidelines for the presumptive identification of fungi based on direct microscopic examination of clinical specimens are presented in Table 21-7.

Extent of Laboratory Genus/Species Identification

Table 21-6 can also be used as a guide to the extent to which genera and species identifications are required in most

Table 21-6   Identification of Medically Important Fungi, Initial Growth at 30°C

HYALINE (MOLD COLONIES)				DEMATIACEOUS		YEAST COLONIES	YEAST-LIKE COLONIES
Growth <3 days Hyphae broad and aseptate **Suspect Zygomyces** *Rhizopus* *Absidia* *Syncephalastrum* *Circinella* *Cunninghamella* *Mucor* See Display 21-1 for species-identifying characteristics.	Growth 3–5 days Hyphae hyaline and septate **Suspect Agents of Hyalohyphomycosis** **Conidia in Chains:** *Aspergillus* *Penicillium* *Paecilomyces* *Scopulariopsis* **Conidia in Clusters:** *Acremonium* *Fusarium* *Trichoderma* *Gliocladium* **Conidia Borne Singly:** *Scedosporium apiospermum* *Scedosporium prolificans* (inflatum) *Chrysosporium* *Sepedonium* See Display 21-2 for species-identifying characteristics.	Growth >5 days Colonies often granular and pigmented; hyphae septate, hyaline **Suspect Dermatophyte** **Genus *Microsporum*** **Common:** *Microsporum canis* *Microsporum gypseum* **Uncommon:** *Microsporum audouinii* *Microsporum nanum* **Genus *Trichophyton*** **Common:** *Trichophyton rubrum* *Trichophyton mentagrophytes* *Trichophyton tonsurans* *Trichophyton verrucosum* **Uncommon:** *Trichophyton violaceum* *Trichophyton schoenleinii* **Genus *Epidermophyton*:** *Epidermophyton floccosum* See Display 21-3 for species-identifying characteristics.	Growth >5 days Hyphae hyaline and slender. Growth on cycloheximide agar. Yeast forms when incubated at 35°C **Suspect Dimorphic Fungi:** *Blastomyces dermatitidis* *Coccidioides immitis* *Histoplasma capsulatum* *Sporothrix schenckii* *Paracoccidioides brasiliensis* See Display 21-4 for species-identifying characteristics.	Growth 3–5 days Dark colony; black reverse; hyphae yellow-pigmented and septate **Suspect Agent of Phaeohyphomycosis** **Conidia Muriform:** *Alternaria* *Ulocladium* *Stemphylium* *Epicoccum* **Conidia Divided by Transverse Septa Only:** *Curvularia* *Bipolaris (Drechslera)* *Exserohilum* **Pycnidia Produced** *Phoma* *Chaetomium* See Display 21-5 for species-identifying characteristics.	Growth >5 days Dark colony; black reverse; hyphae yellow-pigmented and septate **Suspect Agent of Chromomycosis or Mycetoma** **Cladosporium-Type Sporulation:** *Cladophialophora carrionii* *Cladophialophora bantianum* **Phialophora-Type Sporulation:** *Phialophora verrucosa* *Phialophora richardsiae* *Exophiala jeanselmei* **Acrotheca-Type Sporulation:** *Fonsecaea pedrosoi* *Fonsecaea compacta* See Display 21-6 for species-identifying characteristics.	Growth 2–5 days Smooth, pasty, or mucoid colonies: **Suspect Yeast** **Common:** *Candida albicans* *Candida* *Cryptococcus neoformans* *Cryptococcus* *Rhodotorula* **Uncommon:** *Hansenula anomala* *Malassezia furfur* *Saccharomyces cerevisiae* **Rare:** *Basidiobolus* species *Conidiobolus* species **Black Yeasts:** *Pullularia pullulans* *Phaeoannellomyces werneckii* *Phaeococcomyces* species Yeast forms of dimorphic fungi (35°C incubation) See Display 21-7 for species-identifying characteristics.	Growth 2–5 days Yeastlike colonies with low aerial mycelium **Arthroconidia Produced** **Suspect:** *Geotrichum candidum* *Trichosporon beigelii* complex *Blastoschizomyces capitus* See Display 21-7 for species-identifying characteristics.

Table 21-7 Presumptive Identification of Fungi Based on Direct Microscopic Examination of Material From Clinical Specimens

DIRECT MICROSCOPIC OBSERVATIONS	PRESUMPTIVE IDENTIFICATION
Hyphae relatively small (3–6 µm) and regular in size, dichotomously branching at 45-degree angles with distinct cross-septa	*Aspergillus* spp.
Hyphae irregular in size (6–50 µm), ribbonlike, and devoid of septa	Zygomycetes (Phycomycetes) *Rhizopus–Mucor–Absidia*
Hyphae small (2–3 µm) and regular, some branching, with rectangular arthrospores sometimes seen; found only in skin, nail scrapings, and hair	Dermatophyte group *Microsporum* spp. *Trichophyton* spp. *Epidermophyton* spp.
Hyphae regular in diameter (3–6 µm), parallel walls, irregular branching, septate, dark yellow, brown, or hyaline	*Phaeohyphomyces* spp. *Hyalohyphomyces* spp.
Hyphae, distinct points of constriction simulating link sausages (pseudohyphae), with budding yeast forms (blastospores) often seen	*Candida* spp.
Yeast forms, cells spherical and irregular in size (5–20 µm), classically with a thick polysaccharide capsule (not all cells are encapsulated), with one or more buds attached by a narrow constriction	*Cryptococcus neoformans* *Cryptococcus* spp., nonencapsulated
Small budding yeast, relatively uniform in size (3–5 µm), with a single bud attached by a narrow base, extracellular or within macrophages	*Histoplasma capsulatum*
Yeast forms, large (8–20 µm), with cells appearing to have a thick, double-contoured wall, with a single bud attached by a broad base	*Blastomyces dermatitidis*
Large, irregularly sized (10–50 µm), thick-walled spherules, many of which contain small (2–4 µm), round endospores	*Coccidioides immitis*

clinical situations. As virtually any filamentous mold recovered in pure culture from normally sterile body sites may represent an opportunistic pathogen, clinical correlations are recommended before the isolate is discarded as insignificant. Species identifications need not go beyond those listed in the algorithm; other isolates not specifically identified should be reported with the appropriate genus name and species (for example, *Aspergillus* species).

Because yeasts are commonly recovered as commensals from skin and respiratory specimens, the definitive workup should be limited and performed only when clinically indicated. Clinically significant yeast isolates recovered from tissues (particularly if fungal elements are observed in stained tissue sections), normally sterile body fluids, and aspirates should be identified to both the genus and species level. The identification of certain species, *Candida krusei* for example, predict resistance to select antifungal agents, such as the imidazoles. If other organisms are also recovered, the possibility of contamination should be considered, and a clinical correlation is recommended before proceeding with further workup. Isolates recovered from swabs or superficial wounds must be evaluated as to their clinical significance. The criteria by which the fungi included in Table 21-6 can

be identified follow. The presentation of the several groups of fungi will follow the order in the columns of Table 21-6, with linkages to Displays 21-1 through 21-7 (located at the end of this chapter) for more detailed identification criteria.

Genus and Species Identification of the Major Groups of Fungi

ZYGOMYCES SPECIES AND ZYGOMYCOSIS

The fungi belonging to the subclass *Zygomycetes* are widely distributed environmental inhabitants of soil, dung, and vegetative matter. Humans usually become infected in the upper respiratory tract through the inhalation of airborne spores, although ingestion of contaminated foodstuffs may result in primary gastrointestinal disease. Direct inoculation of traumatic breaks in the skin and mucous membranes may lead to primary mucocutaneous infection. Most members of the Zygomycetes have a proclivity for hyphal invasion of the walls of blood vessels once a primary infection is established, often resulting in the dissemination of mycotic thrombi and the development of metastatic foci in many organs.

The medically important fungi within the subclass *Zygomycetes* include several genera, six of which are presented here, as outlined in Display 21-1. *Rhizopus* spp., *Absidia* spp., *Syncephalastrum* spp., *Circinella* spp., *Cunninghamella* spp., and *Mucor* spp. may be identified by the criteria outlined. *Rhizomucor pusillus, Saksenaea vasiformis, Apophysomyces elegans*, and the entomophthoromycotic agents, *Conidiobolomyces coronatus* and *Basidiobolobus* spp., are rarely encountered in clinical laboratories and will not be presented here.

As outlined in Display 21-1, the initial clue to the diagnosis of zygomycosis is the recovery of a rapidly growing colony on primary fungal recovery culture medium, usually within 48–72 hours, with the surface of the agar covered with a wooly mycelium that extends from border to border in the Petri dish (''lid-lifter'') (see Color Plate 21-1*A* and *B*). Microscopic examination of a mount made from the colony reveals broad, irregular width, ribbonlike, aseptate hyphae (sparsely septate in older cultures) (Fig. 21-7), and spores produced in saclike structures called sporangia (Fig. 21-8). The first step in making a genus identification is observing for the presence or absence of rootlike rhizoids (Fig. 21-9).

The genus identifications can then be made following the criteria outlined in Display 21-1; the descriptions and figure cross-references are presented below.

Rhizopus *Species.* Key to the identification of *Rhizopus* species is the production of distinct rootlike **rhizoids.** Rhizoids that are characteristically derived from the hyphae immediately adjacent to the sporangiophores are called ''**nodal**'' (Fig. 21-10). Sporangiophores measuring up to 1,000 μm terminate in a concave columella that extends into the saclike sporangium. The **umbrella-like collapse** of the **postmature sporangium,** is better illustrated in the close-up view in Figure 21-11. This collapse is often observed as a secondary feature in older cultures, particularly helpful in making a preliminary identification when rhizoids are poorly developed.

Absidia *Species.* *Absidia* spp. share with *Rhizopus* spp. the production of **rhizoids.** The rhizoids of *Absidia* spp., however, differ by generally being more delicate and taking origin from the hyphae between the conidiophores, a derivation

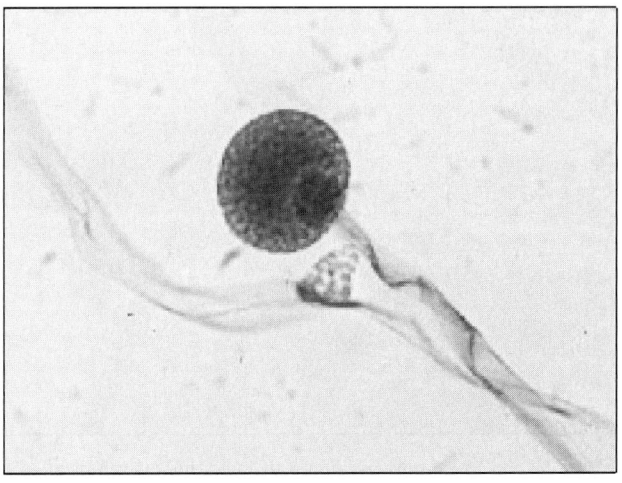

Figure 21-8 Photomicrograph of a sporangium of *Mucor* species, the asexual reproductive organ of the Zygomycetes. Note the extension of the columella into the sporangium and the aggregation of sporangiospores.

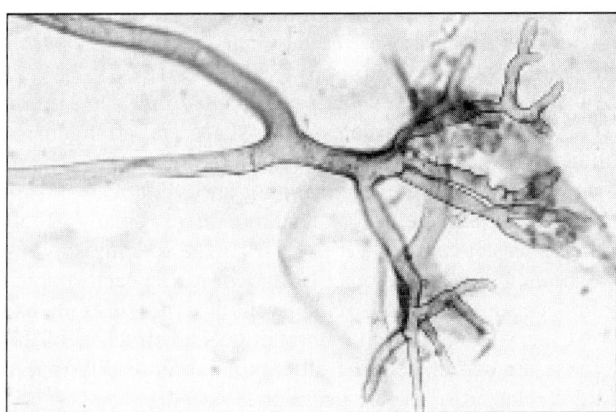

Figure 21-9 Photomicrograph of the rootlike rhizoids of *Rhizopus* species, characteristic of the Zygomycetes.

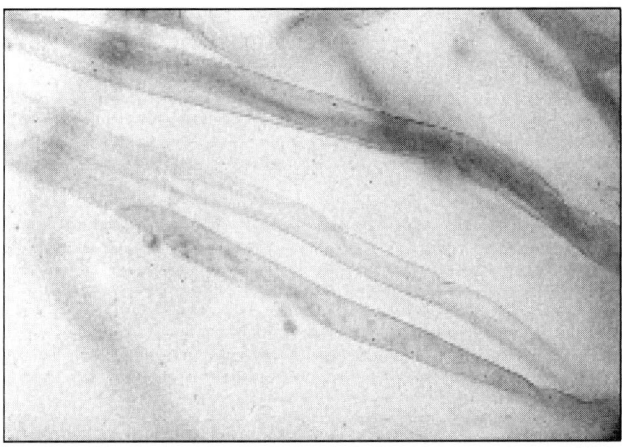

Figure 21-7 Photomicrograph of the broad, ribbon-like hyphae of *Zygomyces* species. Note the clear endoplasm and the absence of transverse septations.

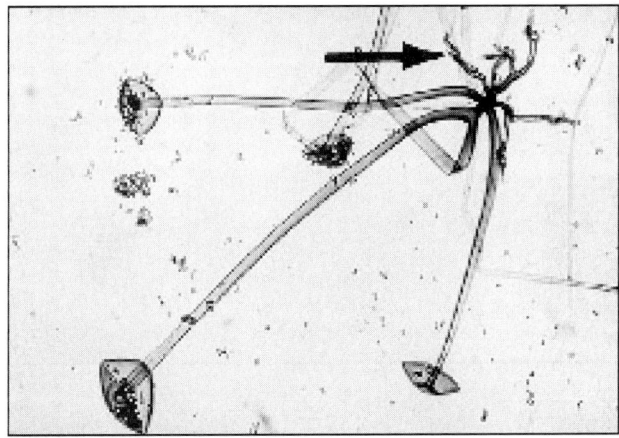

Figure 21-10 Photomicrograph of the fruiting structure of *Rhizopus* species. Note the derivation of the sporangiophores adjacent to the rootlike rhizoids (*arrow*), termed ''nodal.''

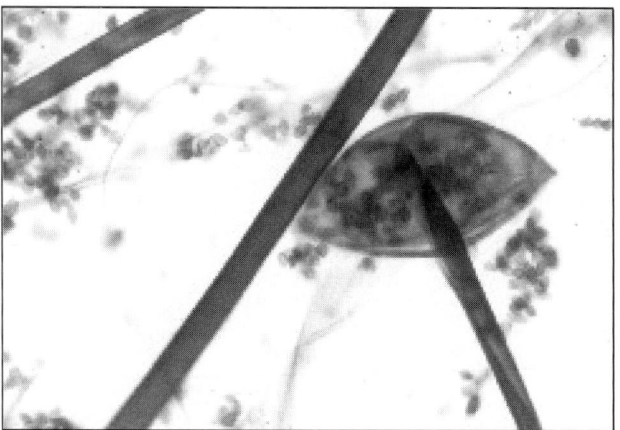

Figure 21-11 Close-up view of a post-mature sporangium of *Rhizopus* species illustrating the characteristic umbrella-like collapse.

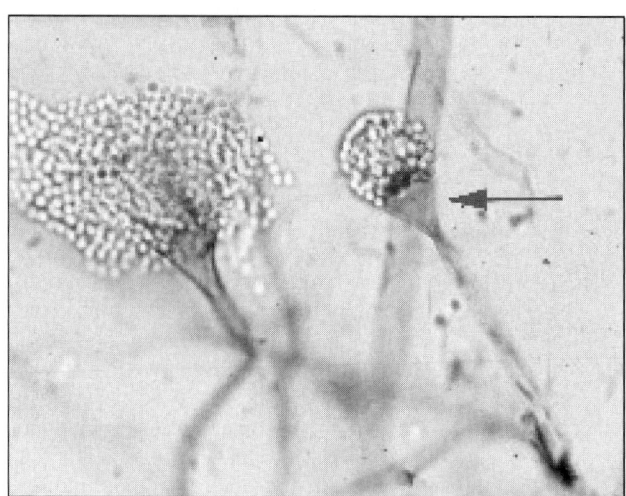

Figure 21-13 Close-up view of the apophysis of *Absidia* species, the funnel-like expansion of the terminal end of a sporangiophore.

known as "**internodal**" (Fig. 21-12). The sporangiophores may branch. A secondary feature of importance, particularly in strains in which the rhizoids are poorly developed, is the funnel-like expansion of the terminal conidiophore into a structure known as the **apophysis** (Fig. 21-13).

Syncephalastrum *Species.* *Syncephalastrum* spp. differ from the other Zygomycetes in the shape and arrangement of the sporangia. Rather than being in the shape of a sphere, *Syncephalastrum* "**merosporangia**" are cylindrical, and arranged as "**daisy petals**" around a relatively small (10–50 μm), spherical columella (Fig. 21-14). The sporangiospores are aligned one after another in tandem within each sporangium. This appearance is reminiscent of *Aspergillus flavus;* however, when the colony morphology and structure of the hyphae are scrutinized, the differentiation is readily made. Rudimentary rhizoids are occasionally seen.

Circinella *Species.* The key identifying feature of *Circinella* spp. is the distinctive **backward curve** of the **sporangiophores**. The sporangiophores are borne laterally from the hyphae, curve directly in reverse, and terminate in a **globose sporangium** that usually is filled with brown-staining sporangiospores (Fig. 21-15). *Circinella* spp. do not produce rhizoids.

Cunninghamella *Species.* The sporulation of *Cunninghamella* spp. differs from that of the other Zygomycetes by producing specialized spherical spores, called **sporangiola**, from the surface of a large, globose columella, without encasement within a sporangium (Fig. 21-16). With sharp focus of the microscope objective, a tiny hairlike **denticle** may be observed by which each sporangiole is attached to the columella.

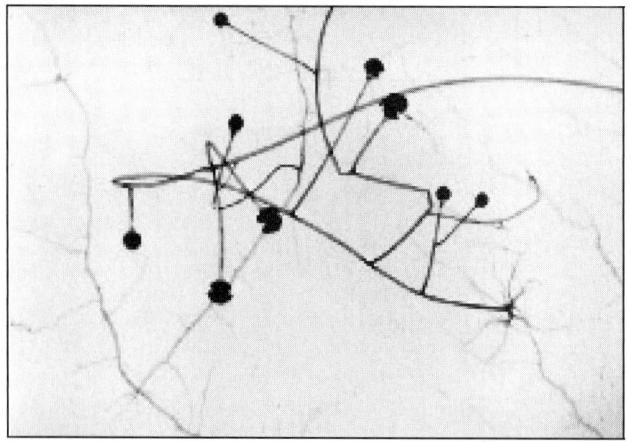

A

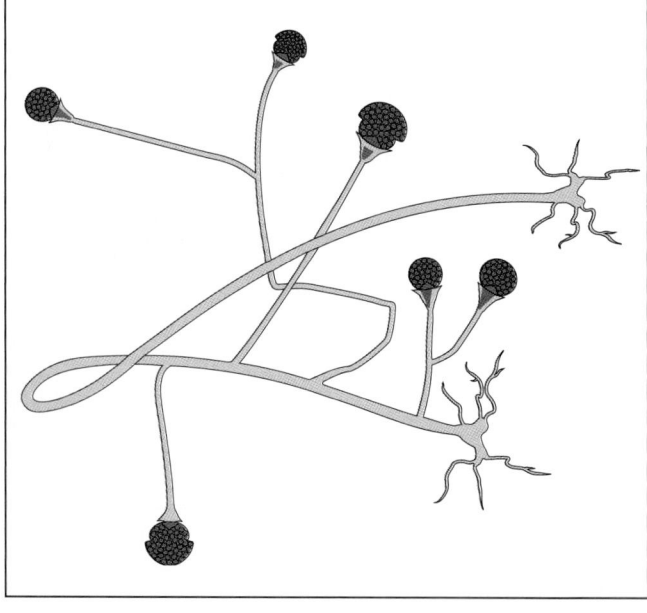

B

Figure 21-12 Photomicrograph and sketch of the fruiting structure of *Absidia* species, illustrating the characteristic internodal derivation of the conidiophores.

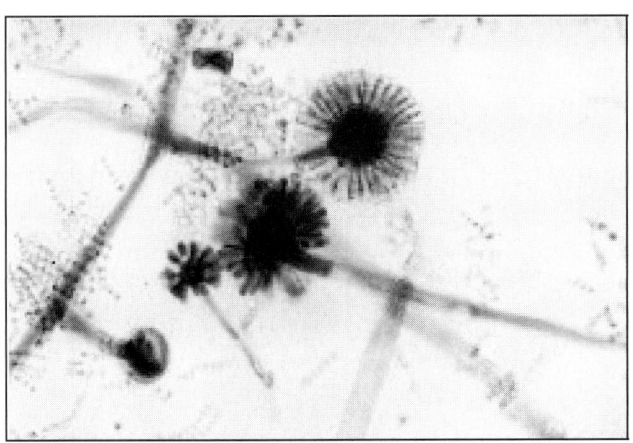

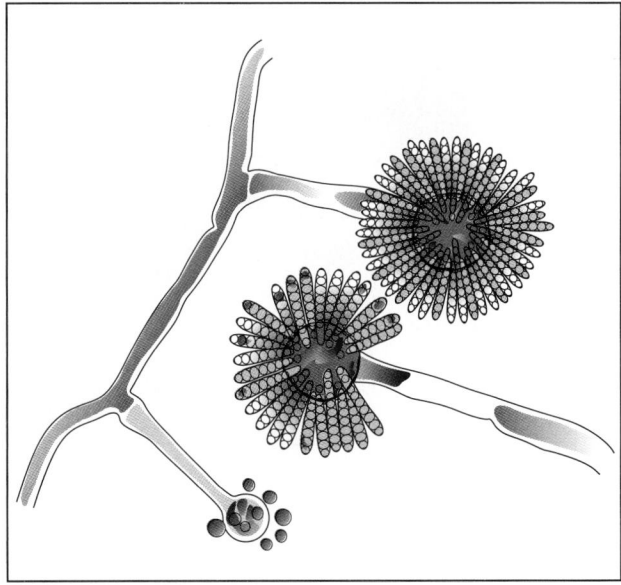

Figure 21-14 Photomicrograph and sketch of the fruiting structure of *Syncephalastrum* species, illustrating the radiating sporangia around a spherical columella.

Mucor *species*. The identification of *Mucor* spp. is often made after each of the above have been ruled out. *Mucor* spp. do not produce rhizoids. Sporangiophores are derived singly from the mycelium and are either branched or not branched. Each sporangiophore ends in a slightly bulbous columella, which extends within a spherical smooth-walled sporangium (Fig. 21-17). The sporangiospores are spherical or ellipsoid and may be hyaline or yellow-brown-pigmented.

Histopathology of Infections Caused by the Zygomycetes

The ribbonlike, broad, aseptate hyphae of the Zygomycetes are generally distinct from other hypha-producing fungi in tissue sections. The hyphae range from 3 to 25 μm in width, have nonparallel walls, and often tend to break up into small fragments (Fig. 21-18). The hyphae often do not stain well, even with periodic acid–Schiff (PAS) or Gomori methenamine silver (GMS) fungal stains. The background tissue reaction is typically purulent, and both intact and fragmented hyphae are usually seen amid a sea of segmented neutrophils. Occasional septa may be observed. Hyphae cut in cross section can also mimic spores or small immature spherules of *Coccidioides immitis*, potentially leading to an incorrect conclusion. The Zygomycetes also have a predilection for invading blood vessels, causing hemorrhagic infarction (one reason that the infected tissue often appears

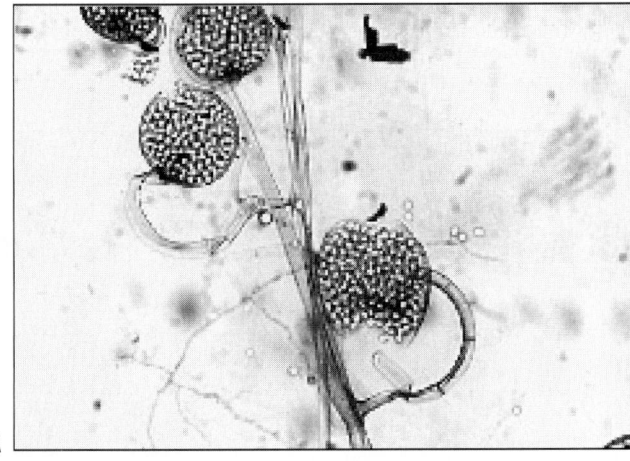

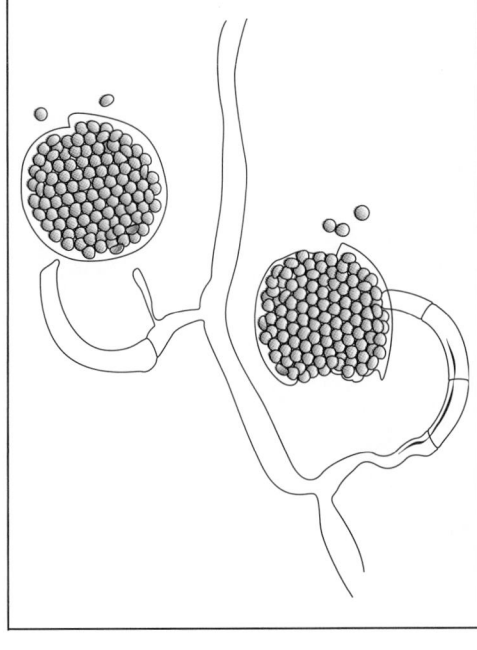

Figure 21-15 Photomicrograph and sketch of the fruiting structure of *Circinella* species, illustrating the characteristic backward curve of the sporangiophores.

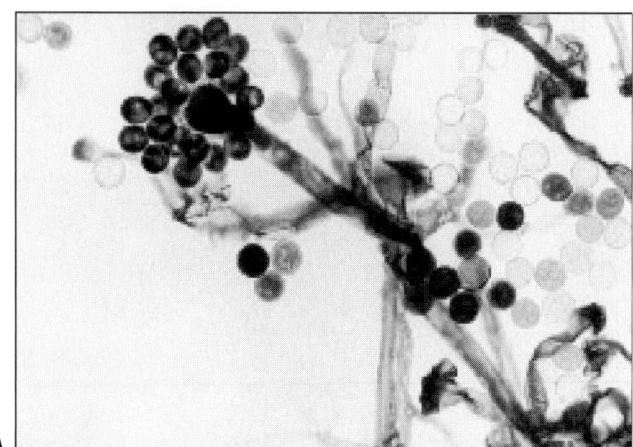

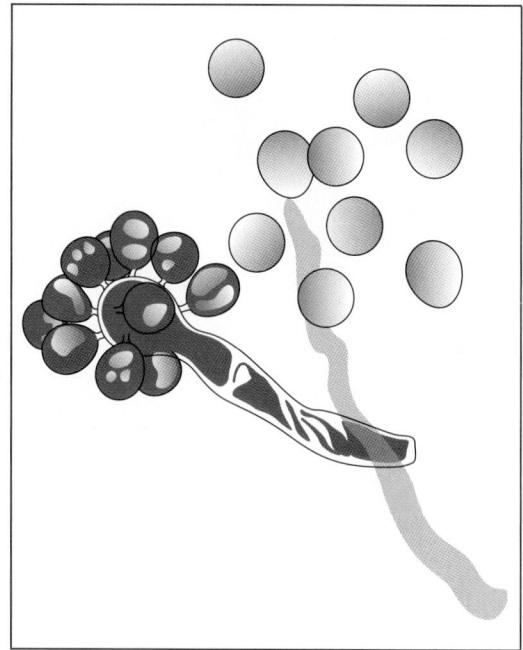

Figure 21-16 Photomicrograph and sketch of the fruiting structure of *Cunninghamella* species, illustrating spherical sporangiola from the surface of a globe-like columella.

charred). The Zygomycetes can also present as a fungus ball in body cavities and, occasionally, the typical fruiting heads, complete with sporangia and sporangiospores may be observed.

The clinical syndromes produced by the Zygomycetes is presented in Clinical Correlation Box 21-1.

Hyaline Molds and Hyalohyphomycosis

Ajello[6] originally coined the term "Hyalohyphomycosis" to represent a group of opportunistic fungal infections caused by a variety of rapidly growing, saprophytic molds. He thought this designation would be less confusing to physicians than using individual names, such as penicilliosis, paecilomycosis, scopulariopsis, and the like. Since that time, however, laboratory personnel have become more proficient in making genus identifications of the various fungi included in this group, and physicians have had additional experience in the clinical applications of laboratory reports that list the genus or species names of the more commonly recovered hyaline molds. Culture identification of *Scedosporium apiospermum* (and also its teleomorph, *Pseudallescheria boydii*) and *Fusarium* spp. in particular should be made. It is important to distinguish these fungi, many strains of which are resistant to amphotericin B, from *Aspergillus* spp. and other hyaline molds that may appear similar in tissue sections. Each mycologist must determine the extent to which genus/species identifi-

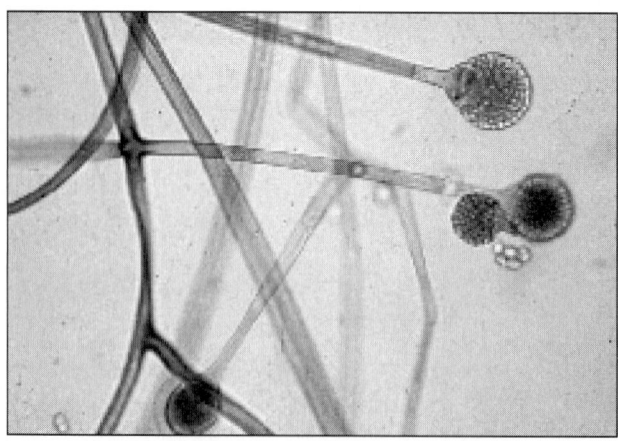

Figure 21-17 Photomicrograph of the fruiting structure of *Mucor* species. Note the lack of rhizoids and conidiophores terminating in a globe-like columella within sporangia containing sporangiospores.

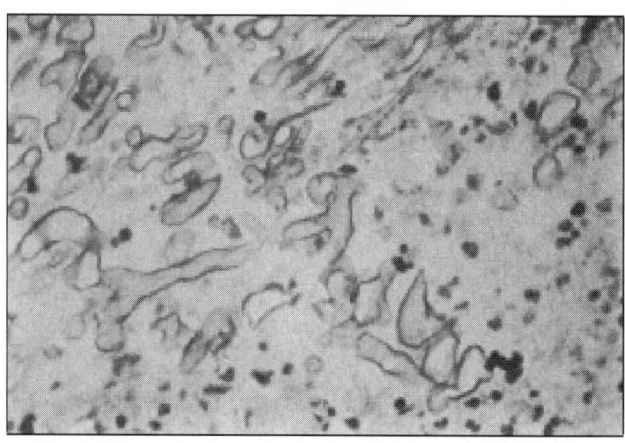

Figure 21-18 Photomicrograph of a tissue section illustrating irregular-sized, broad, fragmented aseptate hyphae characteristic of one of the *Zygomyces* species (H&E, ×400)

CLINICAL CORRELATION BOX 21-1 Zygomycosis

The fungi belonging to the Zygomycetes are widely distributed environmental inhabitants of soil, dung, and vegetative matter. Humans usually become infected in the upper respiratory tract through the inhalation of airborne spores, although ingestion of contaminated foodstuffs may result in primary gastrointestinal disease, or direct inoculation of traumatic breaks in the skin and mucous membranes may lead to primary mucocutaneous infection. A proclivity for the hyphae to invade the walls of blood vessels once a primary infection is established results in the dissemination of mycotic thrombi and the formation of metastatic foci in many organs.

Zygomycosis most commonly occurs as opportunistic infections in immunocompromised hosts. Host risk factors include diabetes mellitus, particularly during periods of acidosis, neutropenia, sustained immunosuppressive therapy (as may occur following bone marrow transplantation),[55] the prolonged use of antibiotics, and a breakdown in the integrity of the cutaneous barrier secondary to trauma, surgical wounds, needle sticks, or burns.[232] These authors also indicate that angioinvasive disease is a common complication, resulting in vascular thrombosis, infarction of the involved tissue, and tissue destruction from the action of proteases, lipases, and mycotoxins. Release of mycotic thrombi from primary sites may lead to disseminated disease. Rhinocerebral, pulmonary, cutaneous, and disseminated forms of disease are most commonly encountered.

A review by Prabhu and Patel[225] reiterates most of the background risk factors already mentioned. In particular, hematologic malignancy, bone marrow or peripheral blood stem cell transplantation, neutropenia, solid organ transplantation, diabetes mellitus with or without ketoacidosis, overuse of corticosteroids, and deferoxamine therapy for iron overload are cited as causing patients to be predisposed to infection. Emphasis is placed on reducing the high mortality rates, reaching as high as 100%, depending on underlying diseases. Successful outcomes depend on early diagnosis, treatment of the underlying medical condition, surgery when indicated, and amphotericin B therapy. High-dose lipid formulations of amphotericin B and the use of hyperbaric oxygen are the particular strategies that have shown potential value in the treatment of zygomycosis, as outlined by Gonzalez, Rinaldi, and Sugar.[97]

Rhizopus is the genus of *Zygomyces* recovered most frequently in culture from human infections, followed in incidence by *Mucor* species. Other *Zygomyces* species are less frequently encountered. *Cunninghamella* species are infrequently encountered in clinical laboratories. Nevertheless, several case reports indicate that this organism has been recovered as the causative agent of each of the more common forms of zygomycosis—rhinocerebral, pulmonary, cutaneous, and disseminated disease. Kontoyianis et al.[148] describe the common clinical predispositions of *Cunninghamella bertholetiae* infections; namely, previous corticosteroid therapy, prolonged severe granulocytopenia, and diabetes mellitus. Fever and pneumonia were the most common clinical presentations in this series of patients, usually an indication of disseminated disease. *Cunninghamella* infections are usually rapidly progressive, and the outcome in most cases reported in the literature has been almost uniformly fatal. Aggressive treatment with amphotericin B, resection of infected tissues, and control of the underlying disease may reverse this trend.

Rhinocerebral Disease

This form of infection often begins as sinusitis, progressing to local invasive disease, with edema of the eyelids, proptosis, malar anesthesia, and internal and external ophthalmoplegia. In many cases, infection is rapidly progressive, although slowly progressive, chronic forms have also been reported.[116] A thick, dark, blood-tinged nasal discharge may be observed; material débrided from the sinus may appear blackened and hemorrhagic because of vascular invasion and infarction. Meningitis and cerebritis may develop by direct extension, and are usually fatal. Localized cerebral disease is uncommon, occurring most frequently among intravenous-drug users.[182] Nenoff et al.[193] report a case of ascending cerebral infection in a patient after transplantation, in whom bilateral total amaurosis (blindness) developed. Cerebral disease has also been reported in patients with AIDS, presumably related to drug injection. Confusion and mood disturbances are more common presenting signs of cerebral involvement. Space-occupying lesions and brain abscesses are seen in drug addicts. Once cerebral symptoms set in, the process is often rapidly fatal, as occurred in the Nenoff case cited above. Noninvasive fungus ball infections of the nasal sinuses may also be seen.

Pulmonary Disease

Ill-defined, finely nodular or diffuse infiltrates may be seen radiologically.[189] **Fungus ball involvement** in preexisting natural or postinfection cavitary lesions may also be seen. Chest pain, hemoptysis, and cough productive of purulent or blood-tinged sputum are common clinical presentations. Subacute pulmonary disease is usually intrabronchial, with the formation of mucin plugs. The pleura may occasionally be involved.

Cutaneous Disease

Cutaneous disease usually occurs secondary to trauma and soil contamination,[276] in patients with burns,[51] and episodically, from direct implantation with Elastoplast bandages.[211] Occasionally, subcutaneous involvement via hematogenous spread may complicate disseminated disease. Lesions ranging from small violaceous plaques to cellulitis, ulceration, and gangrene may be seen. Zygomycetes belonging to the Order Entomophthorales have recently been cited in cases of subcutaneous disease, particularly in children and young adults. Gugnani[99] has reviewed infections caused by *Basidiobolus ranarum*, presenting as fluctuant granulomatous lesions primarily of the legs and trunk, secondary to skin trauma and/or bites of insects. Potassium iodide, amphotericin B, and azole drugs have been successfully used in treatment of these cases.

(continued)

CLINICAL CORRELATION BOX 21-1 *Continued*

Disseminated Disease

Virtually any organ may be involved, spreading from primary infections in the lung, sinuses, and gastrointestinal tract.[234] Most commonly affected are individuals who are immunosuppressed because of their age (the very young and the very old), drug therapy, or underlying diseases such as hematologic malignancies (particularly during periods of leukopenia), diabetes mellitus, and lupus erythematosus.[251] Although not an AIDS-defining illness, disseminated disease is more likely to occur in HIV-positive patients, as reviewed by Van den Saffele and Boelaert.[279] Metastatic spread occurs from the propensity of hyphae to invade the vasculature, resulting in thrombosis and the release of mycotic emboli into the circulation. Zygomycosis has also been reported in cases of **iron overload,** specifically in patients undergoing hemodialysis who are receiving **deferoxamine therapy.**[26] The growth of many microorganisms, including members of the Zygomycetes, are enhanced by an increased concentration of iron. The relationship between zygomycosis and deferoxamine therapy hinges on the primary chelating action of the drug, resulting in an increased local iron concentration that stimulates proliferation of the fungus.

---

cations are reported to best suit the needs of the physicians being served.

Aspergillus Species and Aspergillosis

Because of their ubiquity in nature and the frequency with which they are recovered in clinical laboratories as agents of mycotic diseases, *Aspergillus* species are commonly discussed as a separate subset of the hyaline molds.

Aspergillus spp. are widely distributed in nature; they are found in soil, on decaying vegetation, and on a wide variety of organic matter. The inhalation of spore-contaminated dust is the most common mode of infection in humans, resulting in sinusitis or bronchopulmonary disease. Schubert[248] describes three invasive (acute necrotizing, chronic invasive, and granulomatous invasive) and two noninvasive (fungal ball and allergic fungal) forms of fungal rhinosinusitis.

An increase in the rate of infection occurs during periods of building construction, particularly in zones surrounding hospitals. The report many years ago of an outbreak of aspergillosis among cancer patients, related to the fire-proofing operation in the resident hospital is apropos.[4] Surveillance studies should always include sampling of hospital air filters, which commonly reveal high fungal spore counts.[258] Ventilation ducts in particular may become contaminated with dirt and fragments of vegetative matter that become airborne from disruption of the soil and vegetative undergrowth.[205] The incidence of nosocomial aspergillosis is in direct proportion to the mean ambient airborne spore count, which is highest when mini-bursts of spores are released into the air via the shaking out of contaminated clothing or from disruption of accumulated contaminated dust on floors or other surfaces during cleanup operations.[231] Patients who are immunocompromised or who are receiving immunosuppressive drugs, notably bone marrow and organ transplant recipients, and those with hematologic malignancies, are particularly susceptible to infection.

LABORATORY PRESENTATION

The *Aspergillus* species most commonly encountered in clinical laboratories include *Aspergillus fumigatus, A. flavus, A. niger,* and *A. terreus.* The majority of serious infections are caused by *A. fumigatus.*[154] *A. nidulans* is also mentioned in this section because most strains readily produce the sex-

ual or telomorphic forms—cleistothecia enclosing species-specific ascospores.

COLONY MORPHOLOGY

Colonies of *Aspergillus* spp. can be suspected in culture if an isolate is rapidly growing (within 3–5 days) and has a distinct outer margin, often with a white apron at the advancing area of growth. The appearance as described below may vary depending on the culture medium being used. Early colonies may have a cottony consistency; however, with maturity, the surface becomes sugary or granular as conidia are produced. Descriptions of the colonies when grown on Sabouraud's dextrose agar, characteristic of each of the species mentioned above follow.

MICROSCOPIC FEATURES

Microscopically, *Aspergillus* species are characterized by the production of uniform, 4–6 μm in diameter, **hyaline, septate hyphae** with parallel walls. The **45-degree angle dichotomous branching** so characteristic of the invasive mycelium seen in tissue sections is less commonly seen in microscopic mounts made from culture plates. A specialized hyphal segment, known as a **foot cell,** serves as the base of origin of the **conidiophore** (Fig. 21-19).

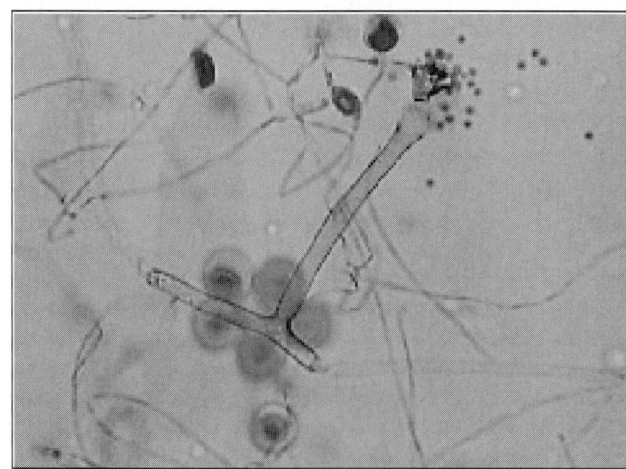

Figure 21-19 Photomicrograph of an *Aspergillus* species fruiting structure, illustrating the conidiophore being derived from a "foot cell."

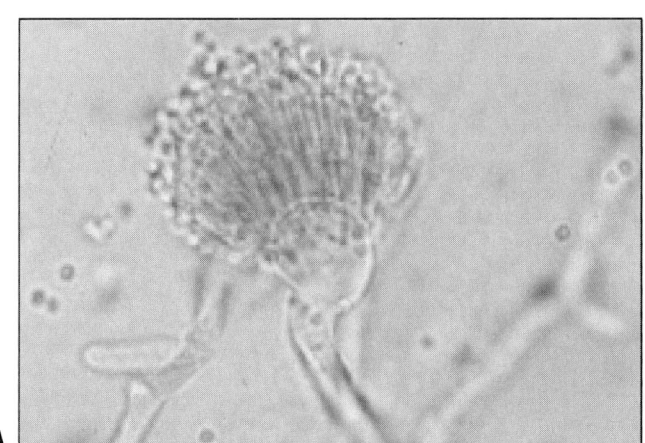
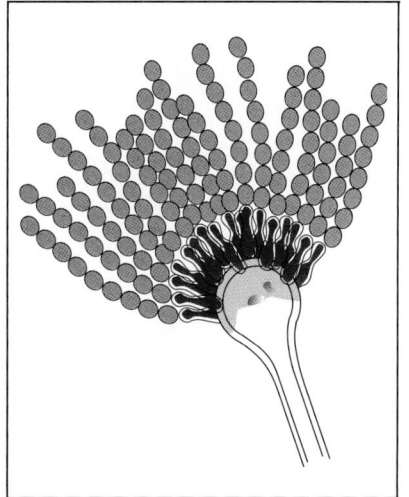

Figure 21-20 Photomicrograph and sketch of a generic fruiting head of *Aspergillus* species, illustrating the swollen vesicle giving rise to phialides from which chains of conidia are produced.

Conidiophores terminate in a swollen **vesicle,** from the surface of which are borne one (**uniseriate**) or two (**biseriate**) rows of **phialides** (technically, the inner row of cells are called metulae) giving rise to chains of pigmented conidia (Fig. 21-20). The length and width of the conidiophores, the size and contour of the vesicle, the arrangement of the phialides and the color, size, and chain-length of the conidia are features used in making species identifications. **Telomorphic cleistothecia** containing **ascospores** are produced by some species (Fig. 21-21).

ASPERGILLUS FUMIGATUS

Colonies of *A. fumigatus* are granular to cottony and usually have some shade of **blue-green, green-gray, or green-brown pigmentation** (see Color Plate 21-1*C*).

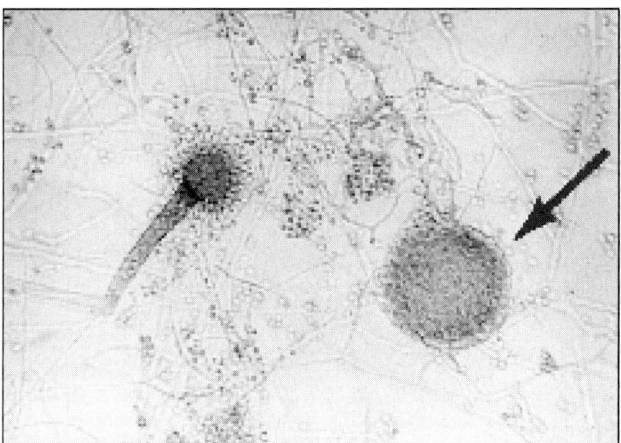

Figure 21-21 Photomicrograph of a cleistothecium (*arrow*) of *Aspergillus glaucus,* illustrating the sexual or telomorphic form of reproduction. A typical anamorphic fruiting head is seen to the left.

Microscopically, look specifically for the production of a **single row of phialides** over the **top half** of a **club-shaped vesicle** (Fig. 21-22). The **conidia are spherical**, usually smooth, and arranged in **long chains** that tend to **bend inward** toward a center axis. They may present a yellow-green or green pigmentation. The conidiophores are relatively long (300–500 μm), and each is derived from a special segment of a septate hypha known as a **foot cell** (Fig. 21-18).

ASPERGILLUS FLAVUS

Colonies of *A. flavus* are granular to wooly and present some shade of **yellow, yellow-green, or yellow-brown** (see Color Plate 21-1*D*).

On microscopic examination, what catches the eye immediately is the **daisy-petal-like** arrangement of the **chains of conidia,** which are derived from either a **single or a double row of phialides,** that cover the entire circumference of a spherical vesicle (Fig. 21-23). The conidiophore is relatively long (500–800 μm), with a **distinct roughening** of the wall just proximal to the junction of the vesicle. The conidia are spherical, smooth, or slightly roughened with maturity, and have a yellow-brown pigmentation.

ASPERGILLUS NIGER

The surface of a mature colony of *A. niger* is covered by a dense aggregate of **jet-black conidia,** giving a characteristic peppered effect (see Color Plate 21-1*E*). The reverse of the colony is buff or yellow-gray, in contrast to the deeper gray-black pigmentation of the dematiaceous fungi to be described below.

Microscopically, **sporulation** usually is **profuse,** with dense aggregates of single and short chains of jet-black conidia that usually **cover the surface of the vesicle** (Fig. 21-24, *upper frame*). On maturity, the conidia become distinctly roughened (**echinulate**). Bare vesicles, when observed, are

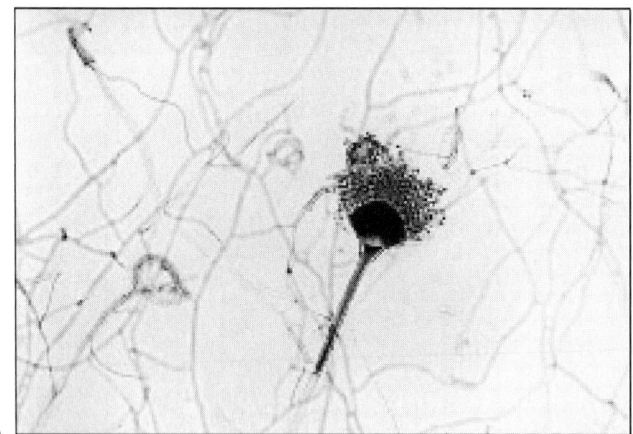

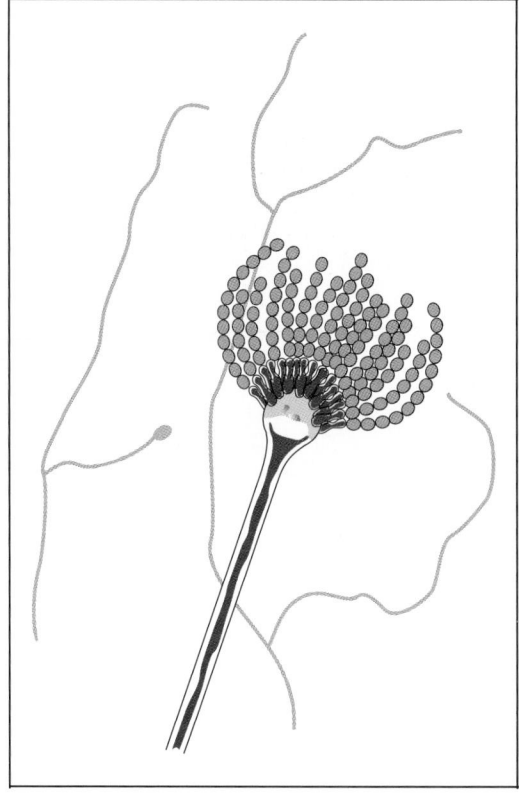

Figure 21-22 Photomicrograph and sketch of the fruiting structure of *Aspergillus fumigatus,* illustrating a single row of phialides derived from the top half of a vesicle from which chains of conidia are produced.

globose and cover the entire surface with a **double row of phialides** similar in appearance to *Aspergillus flavus*) (Fig. 21-24, *lower frame*).

ASPERGILLUS TERREUS

Colonies of *A. terreus* are granular, radially rugose, and **cinnamon buff, brown, or orange-brown** (see Color Plate 21-1*F*).

At first glance, the fruiting heads of *A. terreus* appear microscopically similar to those of *A. fumigatus* (sporulation from the **top half of a club-shaped vesicle**). Closer examination reveals that the vesicles of *A. terreus* are smaller, and the phialides are much longer, in fact representing a **double row,** and **interdigitated** so that the line of division between the two is often obscure (Fig. 21-25). The primary phialides (**metulae**) are shorter (5–8 μm) than the terminal ones (8–12 μm), which in turn give rise to the long chains of smooth, subspherical conidia. The identification of *A. terreus* can be confirmed by demonstrating in dig or tease mounts of the

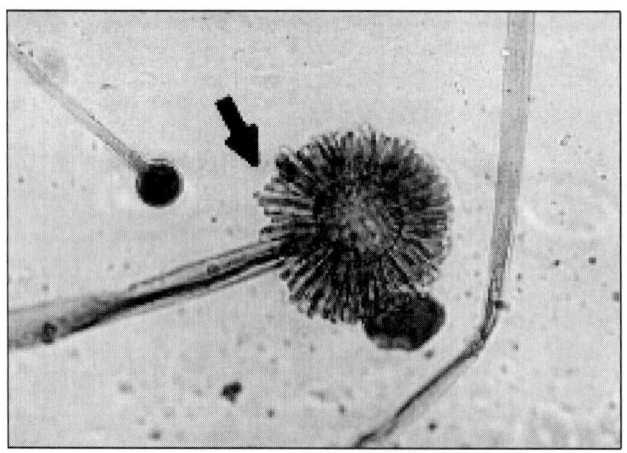

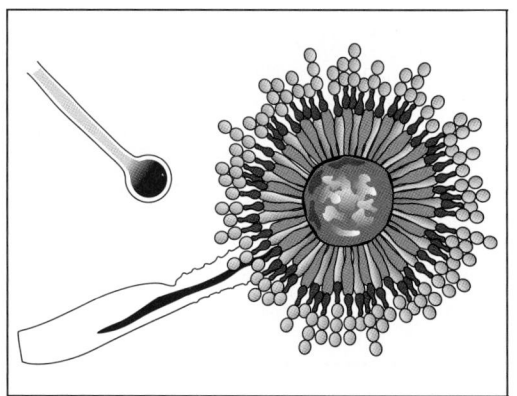

Figure 21-23 Photomicrograph and sketch of the fruiting structure of *Aspergillus flavus,* illustrating a central spherical vesicle supporting a double row of phialides derived from the entire surface.

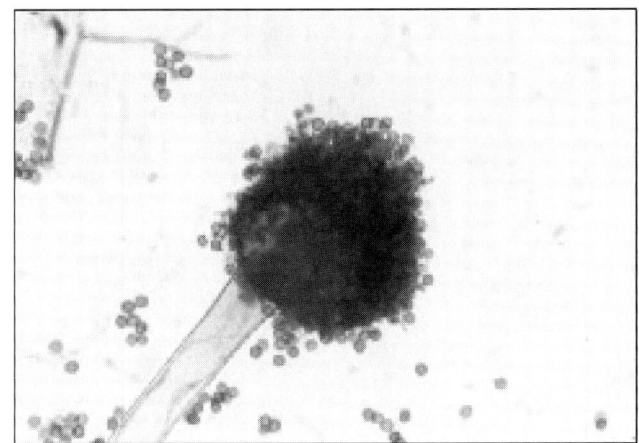

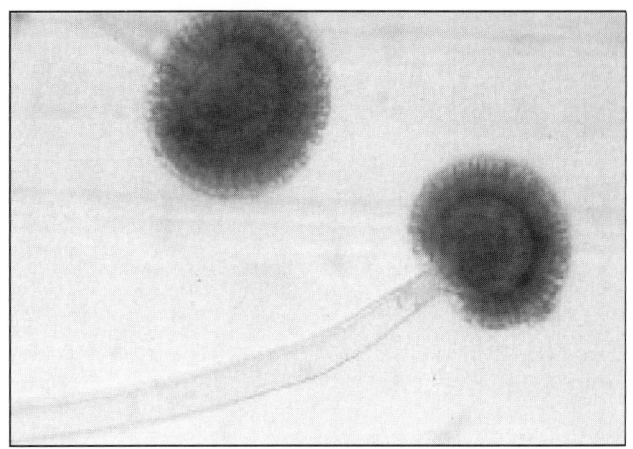

A

B

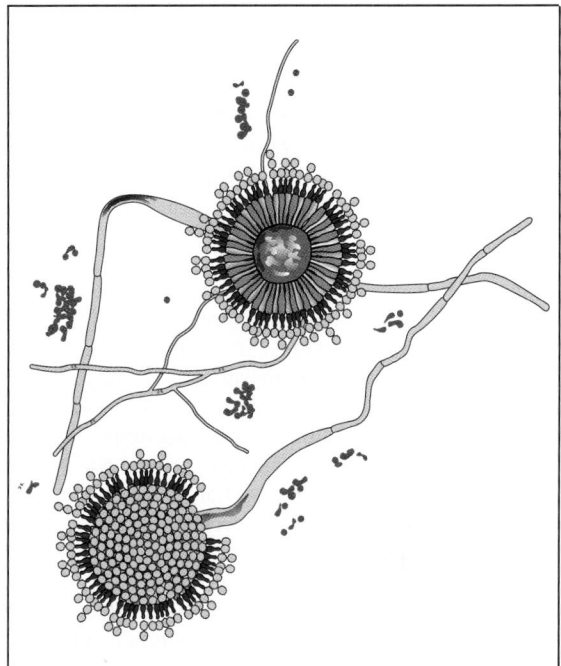

Figure 21-24 Photomicrographs and sketch of the fruiting structure of *Aspergillus niger.* Sporulation is often so dense as to cover the entire surface of the vesicle **(A)**. Bare fruiting heads consist of a spherical vesicle from which a double-row of phialides is derived off the entire surface **(B)**.

C

underlying mycelium, smooth, spherical **microconidia** attached laterally from the vegetative hyphae (Fig. 21-26).

ASPERGILLUS NIDULANS

A. nidulans is rarely encountered in clinical laboratories, but a brief discussion is included here because this species commonly produces sexual (telomorphic) reproductive structures (cleistothecia and ascospores), to be discussed below. The colonies are generally white or gray-white, cottony to granular in consistency, and may have radial rugae (see Color Plate 21-2*G*). A dark stippled effect may be noted with mature colonies as cleistothecia are produced. *Aspergillus glaucus* may also produce cleistothecia and ascospores. The colony generally is cottony to granular, and has a variegated green and yellow pigmentation (see Color Plate 21-1*H*).

The aspergilli, belonging to the **Class *Ascomycetes,*** are capable of reproducing "sexually" through the union of two cells, resulting in the production of a baglike structures

called the **cleistothecia** (see Fig. 21-21). Within each cleistothecium are myriad asci, each containing four or eight **ascospores** (myriad small baglike structures illustrated in Fig. 21-27). Some strains also produce spherical, hyaline bodies known as Hülle cells, illustrated in Fig. 21-28 (*large spherical bodies top and left*). These "**telomorphic**" **structures** are rarely seen in clinical specimens. *Aspergillus nidulans* and *Aspergillus glaucus* are two species, uncommonly recovered in clinical laboratories, that characteristically produce cleistothecia and ascospores. Ascospores are larger than conidia, are more deeply staining, and have a morphology unique to each species that can be recognized by experts in the field.

Histopathology

The hyphae of *Aspergillus* spp., as observed in stained tissue sections, are characteristically hyaline, septate, regular in outline, and have parallel walls. They average 3 to 6 μm

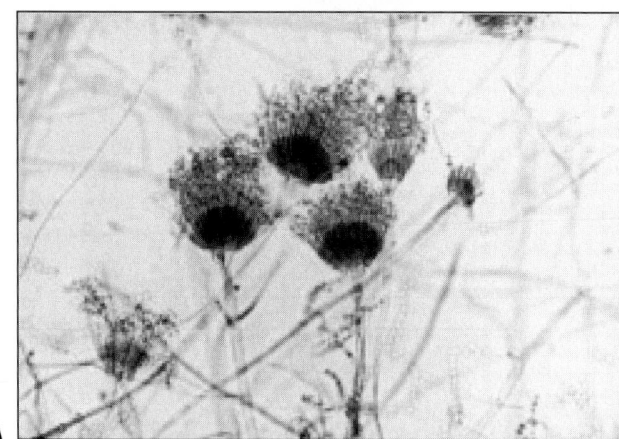

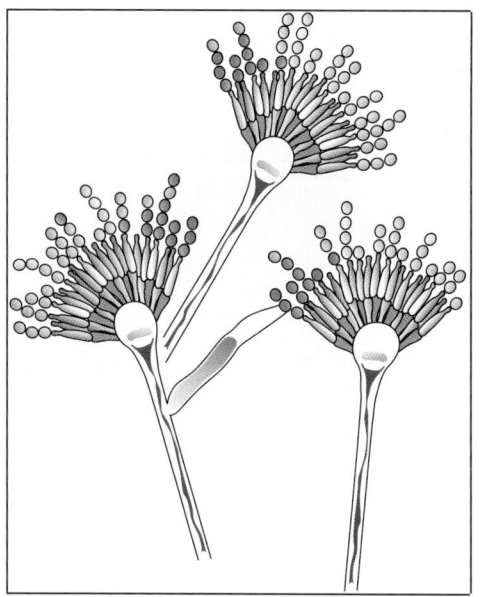

Figure 21-25 Photomicrograph and sketch of the fruiting structure of *Aspergillus terreus* revealing conidiophores terminating in a swollen vesicle from the top half of which are derived a double row of sterigmata giving rise to chains of conidia.

in diameter and are divided by transverse septa (Fig. 21-29). The regular dichotomous branching at 45-degree angles is helpful in differentiating these from other hyphae-producing fungi. The hyphae do not stain well in hematoxylin and eosin (H&E) sections, but are well outlined using PAS and GMS stains. The tissue reaction in immunocompetent hosts infected with these fungi may first be purulent and then granulomatous. More commonly, hyphal invasion of the tissues is not accompanied by a cellular response, and only varying degrees of necrosis are observed. *Aspergillus* species have a particular predilection to invade blood vessels, causing thrombosis and hemorrhagic infarction. Because certain strains produce oxalic acid, local deposits of calcium oxalate,

appearing as birefringent crystals, may be seen in the invaded tissue.

When a fungus colony grows within a preexisting cavity, such as in a nasal sinus or within a congenital or inflammatory lung cyst, the lesion is known as a "fungus ball." The hyphae often appear amorphous and stain poorly. Fruiting heads with well-formed vesicles and chains of conidia may be seen within cavities that are connected to open bronchi and exposed to air (Fig. 21-30). The lining of the cavity is often intact, with no evidence of extension into the surrounding tissue. In bronchopulmonary aspergillosis, bronchi and bronchioles often are dilated and filled with viscid, mucinous material in which are trapped cellular debris, many eosino-

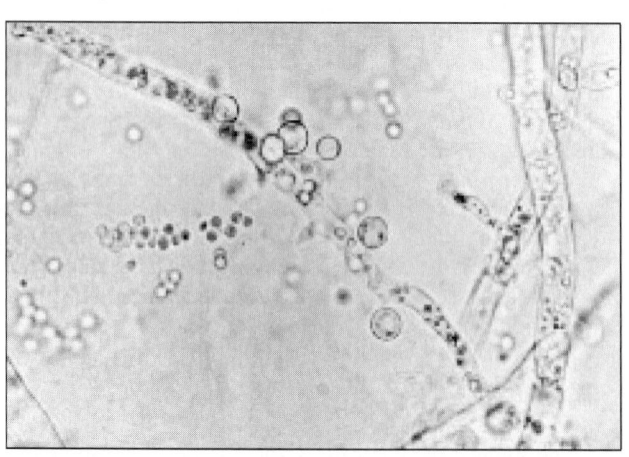

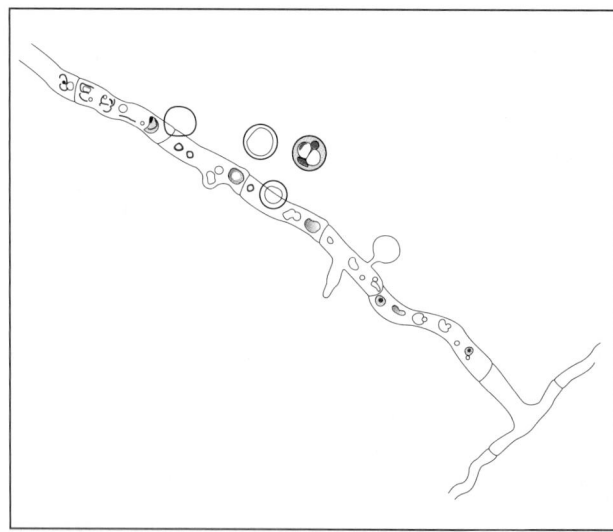

Figure 21-26 Photomicrograph and sketch of subsurface vegetative mycelia of *Aspergillus terreus*, illustrating spherical microconidia characteristic of the species.

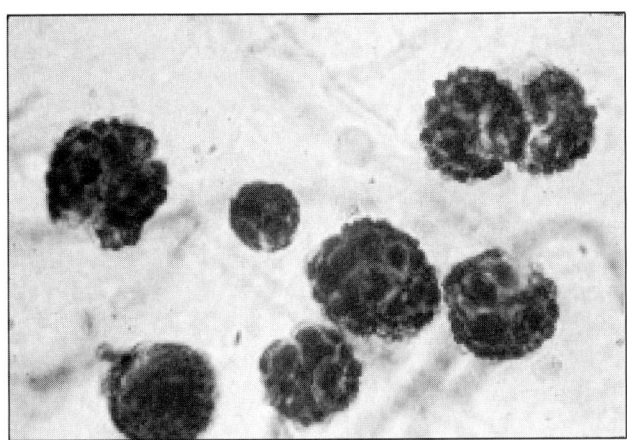

Figure 21-27 Photomicrograph of several cleistothecia of *Aspergillus nidulans* including smaller saclike asci that contain ascospores.

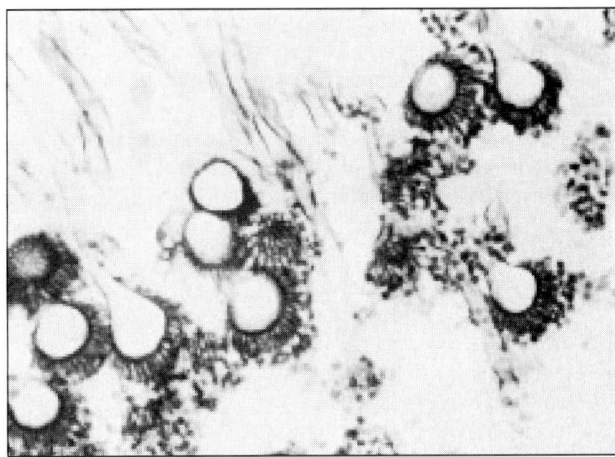

Figure 21-30 Photomicrograph of material from an *Aspergillus* fungus ball infection, illustrating club-shaped vesicles with sporulation only from the top half of the vesicles, characteristic of *Aspergillus fumigatus* (H&E, ×400).

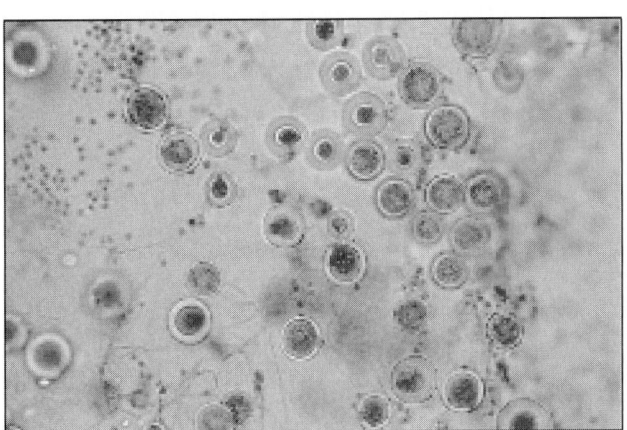

Figure 21-28 Photomicrograph of a cleistothecium of *Aspergillus nidulans* adjacent to which are clusters of thin-walled, spherical, hyaline Hülle cells.

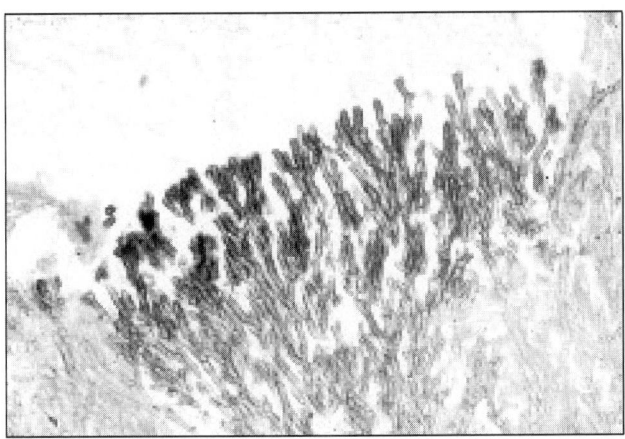

Figure 21-29 Photomicrograph of the dichotomously branching hyphae of *Aspergillus* species as observed in an H&E-stained tissue section.

phils, scattered neutrophils, lymphocytes, plasma cells, and hyphal fragments. Typical 45-degree branching hyphal fragments may be seen in direct mounts of sputum samples, which, when accompanied by eosinophils and Charcot-Leyden crystals, provide sufficient evidence to make a provisional diagnosis of aspergillosis.

DIAGNOSIS USING NONCULTURE TECHNIQUES

The Platelia Aspergillus test system is a sandwich enzyme-linked immunosorbent assay (ELISA) kit that is currently available in many reference laboratories, providing for a means for detection of aspergillus circulating galactomannan early in the course of progressive disease.[180] Although variation in sensitivity and specificity of this procedure has been found in different clinical trials and research studies, this procedure represents a major advance in the treatment of patients at risk for disseminated disease, particularly those with AIDS. Under study are the possible factors that affect the release of the *Aspergillus* antigen, the nature of the epitope that reacts with the monoclonal antibody used in the ELISA, its leakage from the site of infection, and the manner in which it binds to substances present in the blood. Once these issues are resolved, this ELISA system offers great hope for the future.

Musher et al.[191] evaluated the performance of the galactomannan assay (GM EIA, Bio-Rad, Benicia, CA) in the detection of *Aspergillus* antigen or DNA in bronchoalveolar lavage fluid obtained from patients with invasive pulmonary aspergillosis (IPA). In the study of 47 patients with IPA and 46 control patients, the GM EIA assay performed with a sensitivity of 76% and a specificity of 94%. These authors cite the relatively low cost, ease of processing, and rapid results yielded by this assay using bronchoscopy as a viable alternative to an invasive biopsy to establish a diagnosis of invasive aspergillosis, particularly in high-risk patients.

The several clinical presentations of aspergillosis are presented in Clinical Correlation Box 21-2.

CLINICAL CORRELATION BOX 21-2 Aspergillosis

Aspergillosis may present as well-defined clinical syndromes involving a variety of sites and organ systems: pulmonary, disseminated, central nervous system, cutaneous, endocardial, and nasoorbital. Pulmonary aspergillosis can be further divided into subgroups: saprophytic colonization, mycetoma, or "fungus ball" infection; allergic bronchopulmonary form; and invasive.[254] These clinical forms of pulmonary disease constitute a continuous spectrum, ranging from invasive disease in the severely immunosuppressed patient to hypersensitivity reactions in hyperactive patients to noninvasive colonization of the bronchial tree in otherwise normal persons with previously diseased areas of the lung. Disseminated aspergillosis most commonly occurs in severely immunosuppressed patients, and any organ in the body may be involved.

Allergic Bronchopulmonary Aspergillosis

This form chiefly involves the bronchi and bronchioles. Hallmarks include peribronchiolar inflammation, infiltrating eosinophils, and Charcot-Leyden crystals trapped within mucin plugs expectorated in sputum specimens. Lee et al.[156] suggest that the following criteria must pertain to make a diagnosis of allergic bronchopulmonary aspergillosis:

- episodic bronchial obstruction
- peripheral blood eosinophilia
- cutaneous reactivity to *A. fumigatus* antigen
- precipitating serum antibodies to *A. fumigatus*
- elevated total serum IgE
- history of pulmonary infiltrates
- elevated serum IgE and serum IgG to *A. fumigatus*
- proximal bronchiectasis

In cases of bronchopulmonary aspergillosis, serum IgE and IgG against *Aspergillus fumigatus* may be elevated in both serum and bronchoalveolar lavage specimens. The most common *Aspergillus* species causing allergic bronchopulmonary disease are *A. flavus* and *A. fumigatus*.

Fungus Ball Infections

Aspergilloma, or fungus ball, infections develop in preexisting cavities, either natural (sinuses) or acquired (inflammatory pseudocysts, commonly secondary to old tuberculosis). The fungus ball consists of a tangled mass of hyphae, often dead. In pulmonary aspergillomas, cavities in which air is supplied through an open bronchus may contain viable fruiting heads, the detection of which can lead to a definitive diagnosis. In most cases, the fungus ball remains confined to the cavity without invasion of the surrounding parenchyma. However, Nolan et al.[198] warn that aspergillomas should not be considered an indolent condition, as cases of intermittent or exsanguinating hemoptysis have been reported; and, on occasion, erosion into adjacent structures may result in morbidity or death.

Invasive Pulmonary Aspergillosis

This form occurs almost exclusively in patients who are immunosuppressed or have neutropenia, particularly in those with leukemias and lymphomas.[282] The disease often presents as pneumonia (cough, fever, signs of respiratory distress). Pleural invasion may result in chest pain and a pleural friction rub. Because of the propensity for advancing hyphae to invade blood vessels, disseminated disease with metastatic spread to the central nervous system and other organs is possible.

Although *Aspergillus fumigatus* and less commonly *Aspergillus flavus* are the two species most commonly involved,[154] *Aspergillus terreus* has also recently been incriminated. Woods and Goldsmith[301] reported four cases of disseminated disease caused by *A. terreus*, and reviewed five additional cases reported in the medical literature. In a more recent review of invasive *A. terreus* infections, Iwen et al.[127] culled 13 patients from the literature, 10 of whom died following distant dissemination of the disease. Most of the involved strains were resistant to amphotericin B.

Disseminated Aspergillosis

Because *Aspergillus* species has a propensity to invade into blood vessels, widespread dissemination into virtually any tissue or organ remains a threat in any cases of localized disease. Denning and Stephens,[61] in a review of over 2,000 cases of aspergillosis culled from the literature, found that aspergillosis in bone-marrow-transplant recipients is particularly devastating, with a mortality rate of 94% in reported cases, despite therapy. The overall rate of response to amphotericin B therapy of all cases reviewed in this series was 55%.

Ho and Yuen[121] postulate that the high mortality rate caused by invasive aspergillosis among bone-marrow-transplant recipients is the delay in diagnosis because an inflammatory response is blunted by immunosuppression.

Although the acquired immunodeficiency syndrome (AIDS) per se is not considered a risk factor for invasive pulmonary aspergillosis, the underlying risk factors, including neutropenia, use of corticosteroids, and intravenous-drug abuse puts these patients at particular risk. In a series of AIDS patients with aspergillosis reviewed by Singh et al.,[259] 79% were found to have one or more of these known predisposing risk factors. Invasive aspergillosis most commonly occurs in the later stages of AIDS, when the CD4+ count is low, and when diagnosed it has a dismal prognosis. Only early diagnosis can improve the prognosis.[138]

Miscellaneous conditions associated with *Aspergillus* infections include otitis externa ("swimmer's ear," a chronic local inflammation of the auditory canal characterized by itching, pain, and scaling), which is most commonly caused by *A. niger*. Most cases can be cured by topical antifungal therapy and avoiding water exposure. *Aspergillus* sinusitis, often indistinguishable clinically from viral, bacterial, or allergic sinusitis and occurring in immunocompetent hosts, has occurred in at least 29 reported cases since 1987.[46] Several isolated cases of aspergillosis involving virtually every organ system have been reported, with predisposing conditions in these studies most commonly related to prolonged neutropenia, hematologic malignancies, spinal trauma or surgery, and prolonged used of corticosteroids.

Additional Rapidly Growing Hyaline Molds
COLONY CHARACTERISTICS

As outlined in Display 21-2, a filamentous hyaline mold belonging to the general group called the hyalohyphomycetes, can be suspected if rapidly growing, cottony, wooly, or granular colonies are recovered in culture within 3–5 days, usually presenting with a variety of pale, pastel surface colors. The colonies are typically entire and have an outer margin, except for *Gliocladium* spp. and *Trichoderma* spp., the colonies of which grow border to border over the surface, forming a green or yellow "lawn." Colonies appear more or less granular on the surface, depending on the degree of sporulation. The reverse of the colonies remain light gray or buff in color.

Although generally considered to be nonharmful saprophytes, several of the hyaline molds have emerged during the past two decades as agents of opportunistic fungal infections with resulting morbidity and mortality in patients with severe underlying illnesses and compromised host defenses. Recent epidemiologic trends indicate a shift in the increase of infections caused by previously uncommon opportunistic fungi. such as *Fusarium* species, *Acremonium* species, *Paecilomyces* species, *Pseudallescheria boydii*, and *Scedosporium prolificans*. The striking increase in organ-transplant procedures and newer aggressive approaches to immunosuppression are in large part responsible for this shift.

The individual hyaline molds of medical significance, and most commonly recovered in clinical laboratories, are divided into three subgroups, depending on whether the conidia are:

- produced in chains from phialides,
- produced in clusters from conidiophores, or
- borne singly and directly from the hyphae (see Display 21-2).

Each of these subgroups is presented in the following paragraphs.

Genera of Hyaline Filamentous Molds Producing Conidia in Chains

The hyaline molds featured here are characterized by the production of conidia in chains.

Species of Laboratory Importance

Penicillium species
Paecilomyces species
Scopulariopsis species

The species featured here are characterized by the production of conidia in chains. Guidelines for the separation of these three species are outlined in Display 21-2.

PENICILLIUM SPECIES

The colonies of *Penicillium* spp. are granular, entire, generally with various shades of green, although yellow and yellow-brown variants are sometimes encountered (Color Plate 21-2*A*). One species, which has recently been involved in systemic infections, *Penicillium marneffei*, can be suspected if a wine-red pigment diffusing into the agar is detected (see Color Plate 21-2*B*).

As observed microscopically, the "**penicillus**" (brush) is produced by the branching of the conidiophore into primary metulae and secondary **phialides,** from the tips of which chains of conidia are produced (Fig. 21-31). It is important

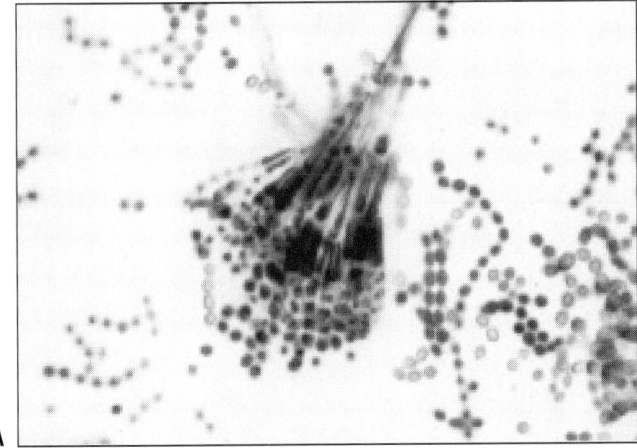

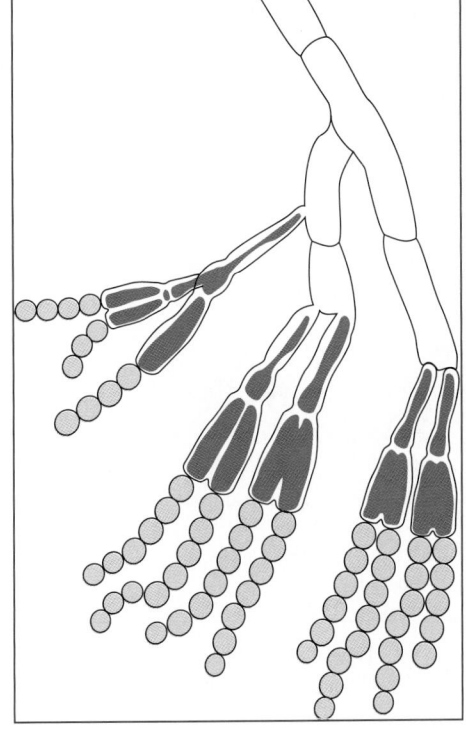

Figure 21-31 Photomicrograph and sketch of the fruiting structure of *Penicillium* species, illustrating the branching phialides from which are produced chains of spherical conidia.

to observe that the tips of the phialides are **blunt,** that is, as if cut off transversely with a cleaver, rather than being long and tapered. The conidia are **spherical, regular** in size, and **evenly staining,** representing an **acropetal** type of conidiation in which identical conidia are produced in sequence from the tips of the conidia previously formed (see Box 21-1).

PAECILOMYCES SPECIES

The colonies of *Paecilomyces* spp. may appear similar to those of *Penicillium* spp., although they generally are lighter pastel in color and yellow-brown or brown variants are more frequently encountered. The surface tends to be quite granular because of the production of myriad conidia (see Color Plate 21-2C).

Two important microscopic observations lead to the identification of *Paecilomyces* spp. The tips of the **phialides** are **long and tapered,** terminating in a "point," in contrast to the blunt ends of phialides seen with *Penicillium* spp. (Fig. 21-32). Secondly, the conidia are **oval to elliptical, irregular in size,** and **uneven in staining,** representing **basipedal** conidiation in which each new conidium is formed directly from the tip of the phialide, pushing the previous conidium ahead of it. The "older" conidia at the tips are larger and more deeply staining than those produced previously. Thus, even in the absence of characteristic phialides, the morphology of the conidia as described lead to an identification.

SCOPULARIOPSIS SPECIES

The colonies are characteristically yellow-brown to buff and granular and develop radial rugae emanating from the center to the periphery (see Color Plate 21-2D).

The identification of *Scopulariopsis* spp. can be made microscopically from observation of the size and morphology of the conidia. The conidia are **two to three times larger** than those of *Penicillium* spp. and *Paecilomyces* spp., are "**lemon-shaped,**" and have a distinct flat, **truncated base.** They are arranged in chains, with the truncated base of each

successive conidium attached to the round terminus of the previous one (Fig. 21-33). Initially, the conidia are smooth; however, as the colony matures, the outer wall becomes distinctly roughened (**echinulate**). Sharp focus of the microscope objective may reveal a short, **rodlike connection** between adjacent conidia. The production of conidia for *Scopulariopsis* spp. is **annellogenic;** that is, each new conidium is produced from an extension of the previous one, followed by a contraction, leaving the thickened truncated base or scar known as an **annellide.**

Identification of Hyaline Molds Producing Conidia in Clusters

Species of Laboratory Importance

Acremonium species
Fusarium species
Gliocladium species
Trichoderma species

This group of hyaline fungi is characterized by the formation of conidia in clusters. The conidia may be elongated or elliptical, as with *Acremonium* and *Fusarium* spp., or spherical, as with *Gliocladium* and *Trichoderma* spp. *Fusarium* spp. have the unique feature of producing both microconidia and macroconidia. Guidelines for the separation of these three species are outlined in Display 21-2.

ACREMONIUM SPECIES

The colonies of *Acremonium* spp. generally appear less wooly or granular than other hyaline molds, but rather are smooth or glabrous in appearance because of the production of a very delicate mycelium. Colonies may be white or various shades of light pastel green and yellow (see Color Plate 21-2E).

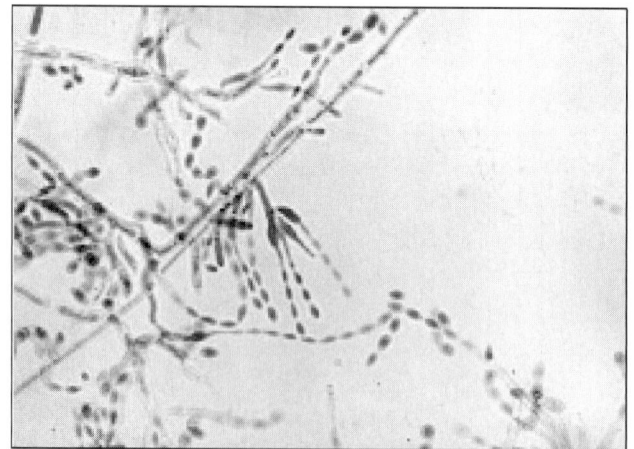
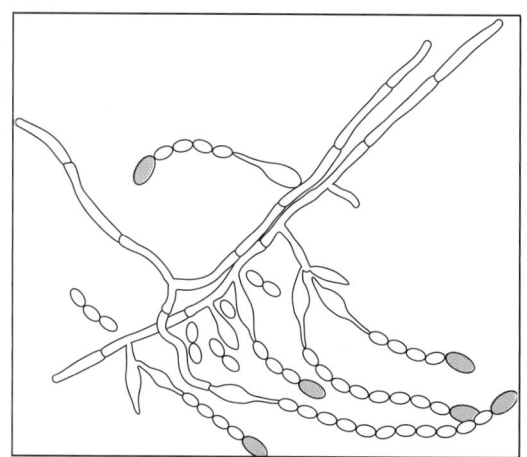

Figure 21-32 Photomicrograph and sketch of the fruiting structure of *Paecilomyces* species, illustrating the long tapered phialides from the tips of which are produced chains of elliptical conidia.

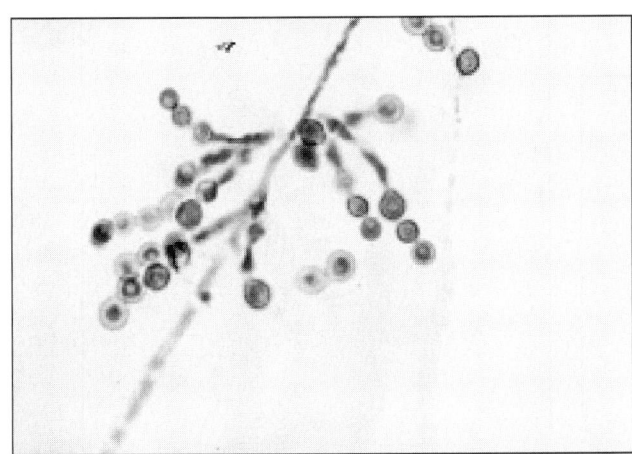
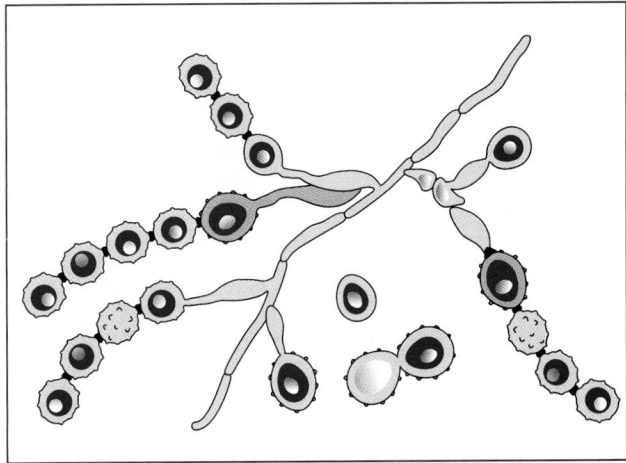

Figure 21-33 Photomicrograph and sketch of the fruiting structure of *Scopulariopsis* species, illustrating the chains of characteristic large, lemon-shaped annelloconidia.

As observed microscopically, the **conidia** of *Acremonium* spp. are **elongated,** and arranged in loose clusters in a **criss-cross formation,** simulating an **oriental letter** or **"diphtheroidal"** pattern (Fig. 21-34). Each cluster is borne at the tip of a long, slender, delicate conidiophore that ends in a blunt tip. **Macroconidia are not observed.**

FUSARIUM SPECIES

The colonies are generally cottony or wooly, and have a distinctive lavender, rose-red, or magenta surface and reverse-side pigmentation (see Color Plate 21-2*F*).

Of the hyaline filamentous molds, *Fusarium* spp. are unique in producing both **microconidia** and **macroconidia.** The microconidia are similar to those produced by *Acremonium* spp.; in fact, these two species are thought by some mycologists to be **genetically related** and probably species **variants within the same genus.** Key to the identification of *Fusarium* spp. is the observation of **long, sickle-form, multicelled macroconidia** separated by transverse septa

(Fig. 21-35). These macroconidia are sometimes described as "canoes" or "boats." Exact focusing on the hilar cell reveals a hairlike extension, called a **"foot cell."** The formation of this structure is helpful in separating *Fusarium* spp. (foot cell present) from *Cylindrocarpon* spp. (foot cell absent), the latter being a soil organism rarely encountered in clinical laboratories.

GLIOCLADIUM SPECIES

The colonies of *Gliocladium* spp. are green or green-yellow and extend from edge to edge of the agar plate as a "lawn" of growth, without a margin. The surface is generally powderlike (see Color Plate 21-2*H*).

The **regular-sized, spherical conidia** of *Gliocladium* spp. as observed microscopically are also **tightly clustered,** and appear similar to those produced by *Trichoderma* spp. However, in contrast to *Trichoderma* spp., in which each "ball" of conidia is derived at the tip of a single conidiophore, each cluster with *Gliocladium* spp. is supported at

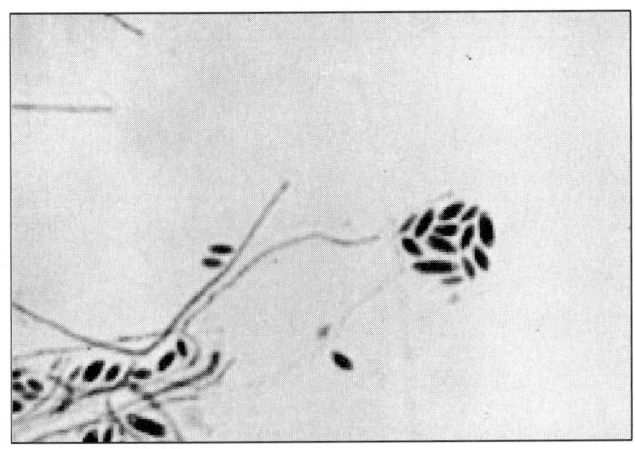
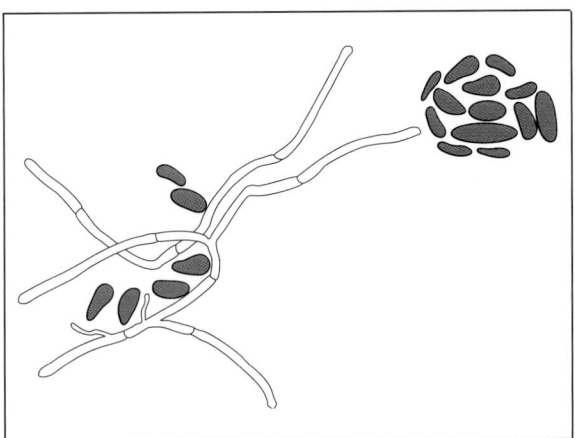

Figure 21-34 Photomicrograph and sketch of the fruiting structure of *Acremonium* species, illustrating the delicate conidiophore supporting a loose cluster of elliptical conidia arranged in a "diphtheroidal" pattern.

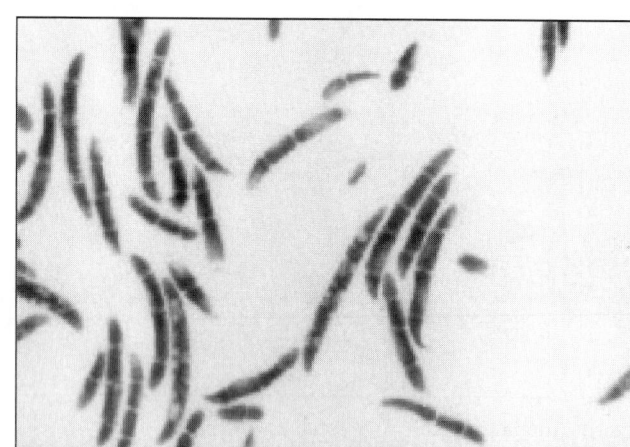
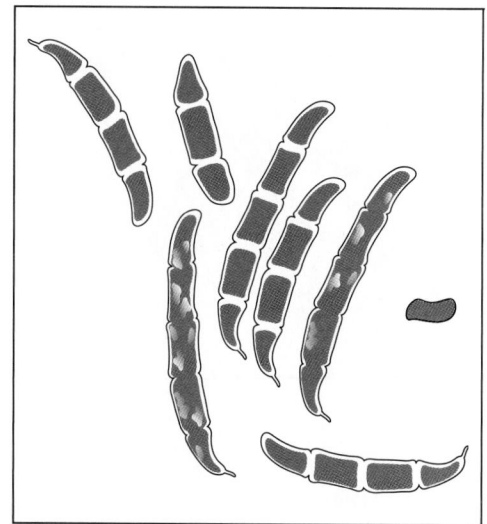

Figure 21-35 Photomicrograph and sketch of the long, multicelled, canoe-shaped macroconidia characteristic of *Fusarium* species.

the **tips of three or four tapered conidia,** much as a mulberry would be held at the tips of three fingers and a thumb of the human hand (Fig. 21-36).

TRICHODERMA SPECIES

The colonies are similar to those of *Gliocladium* spp., also producing a granular "lawn" of growth that extends from one edge of the agar plate to the other. Colors tend to be more yellow than green.

The conidia of *Trichoderma* spp. as observed microscopically are **regular in size, spherical,** and **tightly clustered** (Fig. 21-37). The adherence of these "balls" of conidia is thought to be secondary to the simultaneous production of a **mucinous substance** that makes them "stick together." Similar "balls" of conidia are also produced by *Gliocladium* spp.; however, with *Trichoderma* spp., these clusters are located at the **tips of tapered phialides** (appearing similar to

those of *Paecilomyces* spp.) that are derived laterally from the hyphae.

Identification of the Genera of Hyalohyphomycetes Producing Conidia Singly

Species of Laboratory Importance

Scedosporium species
Chrysosporium species
Sepedonium species
Beauveria species

The colony morphology of this group of hyaline molds is not distinctive, except for the house-mouse gray appearance of the mature colonies of *Scedosporium apiospermum*. The colonies of the other species are entire, white to gray,

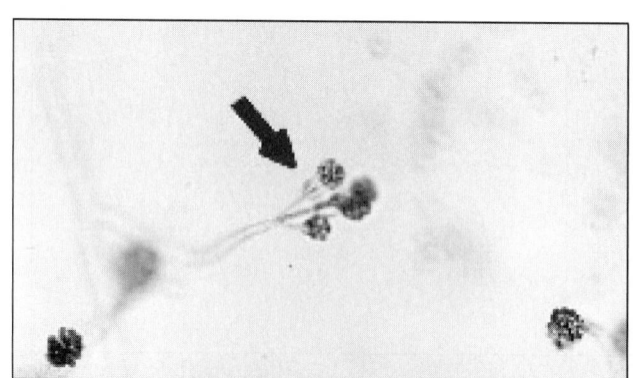
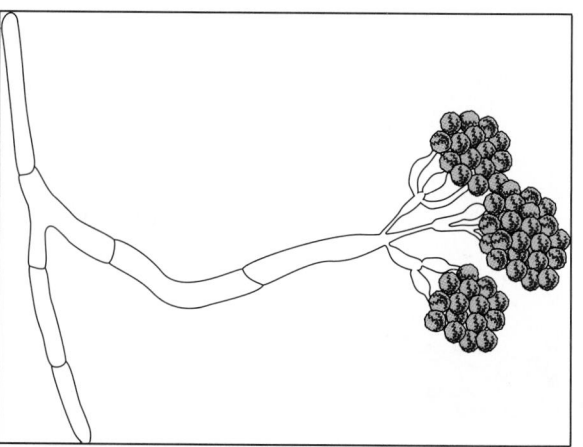

Figure 21-36 Photomicrograph and sketch of the fruiting structure of *Gliocladium* species, illustrating the fingerlike phialides supporting compact clusters of spherical conidia.

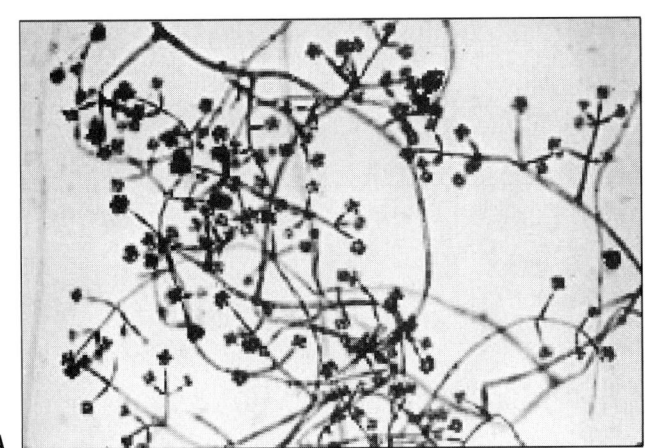
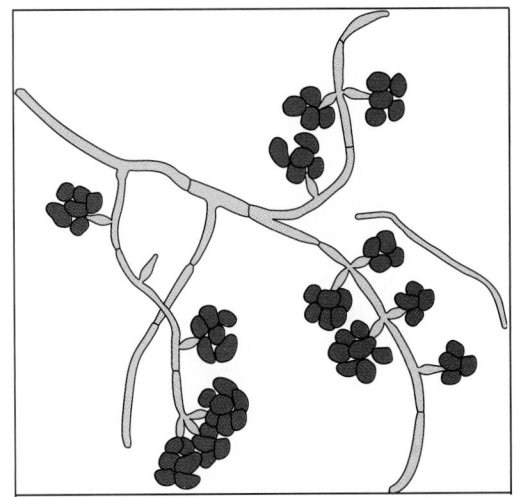

Figure 21-37 Photomicrograph and sketch of the fruiting structure of *Trichoderma* species, illustrating the laterally placed tapered phialides supporting compact clusters of spherical conidia.

smooth to slightly granular, and often rugose. Microscopic examination is required to make a genus separation.

Microscopically, this group of hyaline fungi is characterized by the formation of conidia singly from the tips of individual, straight or branched conidiophores. The unique microscopic features of each of these species are described below, as outlined in Display 21-2.

SCEDOSPORIUM SPECIES

Scedosporium apiospermum (**anamorphic form**), also known as *Pseudallescheria boydii* (sexual or "**telomorphic**" form) is the species of this group of hyaline molds most commonly encountered in clinical practices. *Scedosporium prolificans (inflatum)*, a newly designated species, also causes human infections. Both produce a char-

acteristic house-mouse gray, silky colony surface on which tiny water droplets tend to aggregate (see Color Plate 21-2*G*). Dark pigment may extend to the reverse surface, suggesting a dematiaceous fungus.

Microscopically, the hyphae of both species are hyaline and septate. Characteristic is the production of thin, smooth-walled, ovoid, conidia 3–5 μm in diameter from the tips of unbranched, irregularly spaced conidiophores (colloquially called "lollipops") (Fig. 21-38). The conidiophores of *S. apiospermum* are straight and narrow, in contrast to those of *S. prolificans,* in which the base is distinctly swollen, appearing as an urn (Fig. 21-39). Mature conidia take on a dark pigmentation with age, thus resulting in the house-mouse gray colony previously described. The tips of the conidiophores actually extend when a spore is produced,

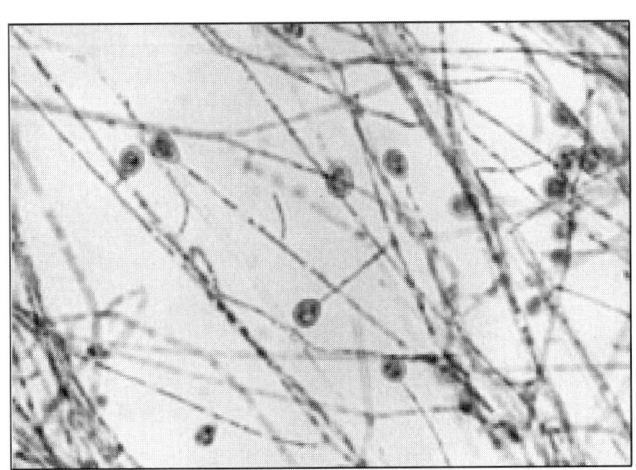
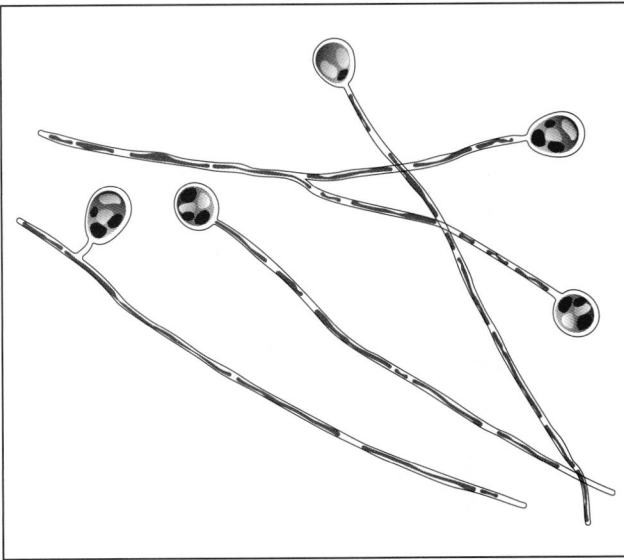

Figure 21-38 Photomicrograph and sketch of the long, straight, delicate conidiophores, each supporting a single oval, dark-staining conidium characteristic of *Scedosporium apiospermum*.

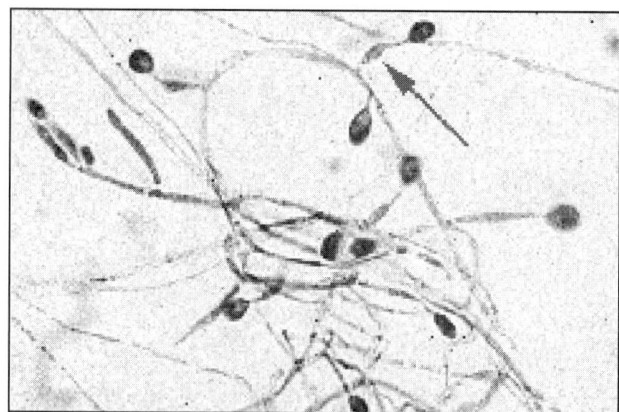

Figure 21-39 Photomicrograph of the conidia of *Scedosporium prolificans,* illustrating the characteristic urn-shaped swelling of the base of the conidiophore (see arrow).

with the formation of annelids, that are difficult to see with light microscopy, but are readily evident in scanning photomicrographs. The parallel bundling of conidiophores, the graphium morphotype may be seen with certain species (Fig. 21-40). Detached conidia may also aggregate in loose clusters.

CHRYSOSPORIUM SPECIES

The colonies of *Chrysosporium* spp. are not distinctive. A white to gray, cottony or wooly mycelium develops after 2–4 days of incubation. Microscopically subglobose to pyriform conidia are borne singly at the tips of long lateral conidiophores (''lollipops''), closely resembling the conidia of *Blastomyces dermatitidis* (Fig. 21-41). The bases of the conidia may appear flattened and scarred. The colonies of *Chrysosporium* spp. generally grow more rapidly than those of *B. dermatitidis,* do not grow on cycloheximide-containing selective culture media, and cannot be converted to a yeast

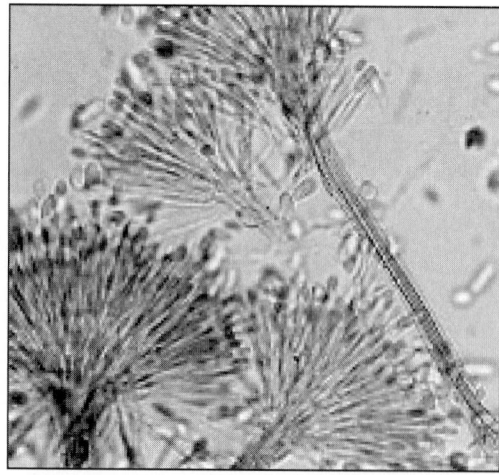

Figure 21-40 Photomicrograph of *Scedosporium* species, illustrating the graphium form in which the fruiting head is arranged in fan-like bundles simulating sheaves of wheat.

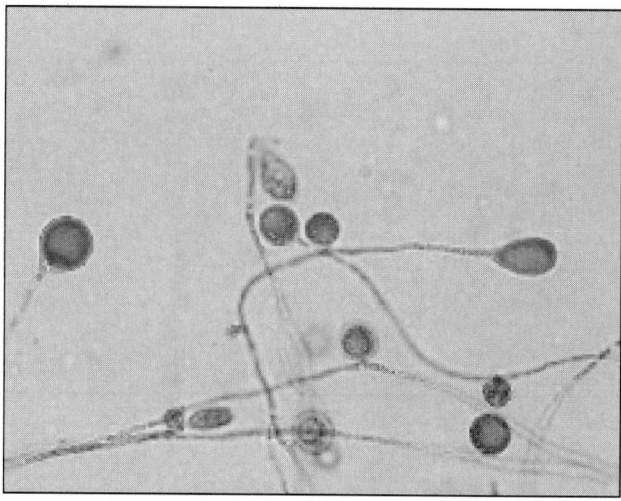

Figure 21-41 Photomicrograph of *Chrysosporium* spp., illustrating spherical to oval-shaped conidia each supported by a short, straight conidiophore (''lollipops'').

form on incubation at 35–37°C. In practice, either exoantigen extraction or nucleic-acid probe assays may be performed on colony extracts to establish a rapid identification to rule out blastomycosis.

SEPEDONIUM SPECIES

The colonies of *Sepedonium* spp. are similar to those of *Chrysosporium* spp. and cannot be distinguished visually. Microscopically, the observation of large, spherical, bluntly spiked macroconidia, simulating those of *Histoplasma capsulatum,* are characteristic (Fig. 21-42). The colonies of *Sepedonium* species grow more rapidly than those of *H. capsulatum,* are inhibited on selective media containing cycloheximide, and cannot be converted to a yeast form on incubation at 35–37°C. Smaller, ovate conidia, borne singly from short conidiophores, may also be observed in some strains. In cases of suspected histoplasmosis, nucleic-

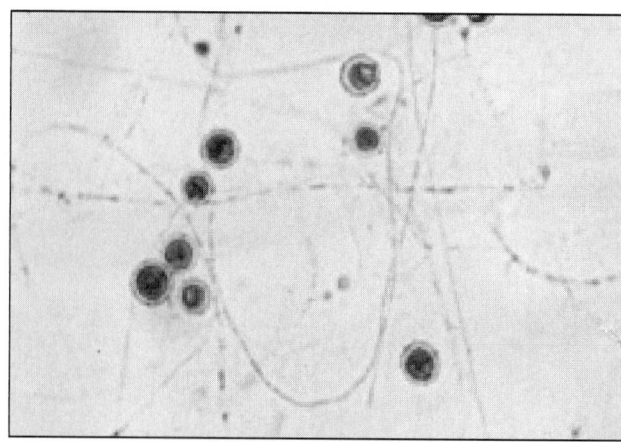

Figure 21-42 Photomicrograph illustrating large, spherical, finely echinulate conidia characteristic of *Sepedonium* species.

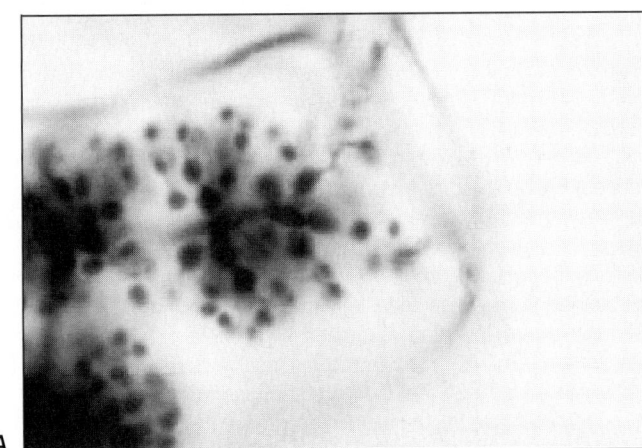
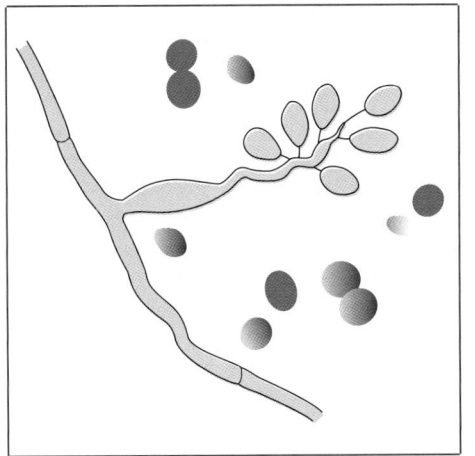

Figure 21-43 Photomicrograph and sketch illustrating the delicate, zigzag conidiophores of *Beauveria* spp., each supporting a single, oval-shaped conidium.

acid probe or exoantigen testing may be performed on mycelial extracts of young colonies to establish a rapid identification.

BEAUVERIA SPECIES

The colonies have a white, cottony, or wooly surface. The reverse of the colony is a light buff. Microscopically, tiny, globose microconidia are densely aggregated around delicate, short, branching conidiophores, that uniquely bend to form zigzag turns (a bent-knee, or **geniculate,** appearance) (Fig. 21-43). Each conidium is borne in one plane, after which the conidiophore turns before bearing another conidium in another plane, and so forth. This type of conidiation is called **sympodial.**

The various clinical manifestations of opportunistic infections with hyaline molds are presented in Clinical Correlation Box 21-3.

Identification of the Dermatophytes

The dermatophytes are a distinct group of fungi that infect the skin, hair, and nails of humans and animals, producing a variety of cutaneous infections, colloquially known as "ringworm." Any mold recovered in culture from specimens labeled skin, nail, or hair should be evaluated for the presence of a dermatophyte. One must be alert, however, that other pathogenic fungi, including the dimorphic molds, can also involve the skin and may have microscopic features similar to the dermatophytes. In addition, many saprophytic environmental molds may be recovered, especially from nails. Making a misidentification could have significant consequences. Observing typical hyphal segments in direct KOH mounts of skin scales (Fig. 21-44) or either ectothrix or endothrix invasion of infected hairs are helpful preliminary findings (Fig. 21-45). Because the colonies of the various strains of dermatophytes vary considerably in rates of growth, morphology, and pigment production, even within the same species,

the genus and species designations depend on observing microscopic features. However, a few colony characteristics, when present, may be helpful in identifying a given species. Representative dermatophyte colonies are illustrated in Color Plate 21-4. The species of medical importance more commonly encountered in clinical laboratories are:

Microsporum canis
Microsporum gypseum
Trichophyton mentagrophytes
Trichophyton rubrum
Trichophyton tonsurans
Trichophyton verrucosum
Epidermophyton floccosum

In a survey of dermatophyte infections in the United States between 1993 and 1995, conducted by Weitzman,[285] *Trichophyton tonsurans* was the dermatophyte species most frequently recovered (44.5% of cases) *Trichophyton rubrum* (41.3%) was next in frequency, followed less commonly by *Trichophyton mentagrophytes* (8.5%), *Microsporum canis* (3.5%), and *Epidermophyton floccosum* (1.1%).

The dermatophytes are separated into three genera, *Microsporum*, *Trichophyton*, and *Epidermophyton*, based primarily on differences in the microscopic morphology and modes of sporulation. An approach to the identification of the genera and species of the dermatophytes is presented in Display 21-3.

The genus *Microsporum* is characterized by the production of many macroconidia, and few or no microconidia. The macroconidia are multicelled, thick-walled, and have a thick, echinulate, or verrucose cell wall. The species identifications are based on differences in morphology of the macroconidia. The microconidia are small, hyaline, and tear-drop or elliptical in shape and attach directly to the sides of the hyphae.

The genus *Trichophyton* is characterized by the production of many microconidia, and few or no macroconidia.

Mycetoma, onychomycosis,[100] and mycotic keratitis[153] are the infections most commonly caused by this group of filamentous molds. Reports of other infections, including sinusitis (including fungus ball infections), meningitis, osteomyelitis, endocarditis, and otomycosis appear infrequently in the medical literature. Many of the earlier reports have been summarized by Rippon.[234]

Perhaps of most recent notoriety has been the emergence of *Penicillium marneffei* as an important human pathogen. Blum[24] reviewed 155 reported cases, concluding that *P. marneffei* is the third most common opportunistic infection in HIV-infected patients in certain parts of Southeast Asia, where the infection is endemic. *P. marneffei* can cause two types of disease—focal and a fatal progressive, disseminated form clinically simulating histoplasmosis.[197] The propensity for this fungus to invade and disseminate is based on its unique "dimorphic" property of converting into a yeastlike entity when found in diseased tissue or cultivated at 37°C.[50] In a report of five cases, Kurup et al.[152] found that fever, weight loss, anemia, and popular skin lesions were the more common clinical manifestations. The ability to recover the organism from blood cultures was an additional unique feature among the patients in this series.

Key to establishing the diagnosis of penicilliosis marneffei is the recognition of small intracellular bodies resembling the yeast forms of *Histoplasma capsulatum* in histologic sections obtained from typical focal lesions. Kaufman and associates at the Centers for Disease Control and Prevention[136] developed monoclonal antibodies against the yeastlike culture filtrate antigens of *P. marneffei* from which, after absorption with yeast forms of *H. capsulatum,* leading to a sensitive indirect fluorescent-antibody reagent. They were able to detect *P. marneffei* yeastlike forms in 43 isolates and in tissue sections from six humans with penicilliosis marneffei. No false-positive results were found in the study of tissue sections containing *H. capsulatum* yeast forms. Cooper and McGinnis,[50] in a comprehensive review, present the clinical presentation, differential diagnosis, mycology, histopathology, diagnostic serology, in vitro susceptibility testing, and therapy of *P. marneffei* infections in patients with AIDS.

Penicillium species other than *P. marneffei* only rarely cause opportunistic human infections. Chan et al.[39] report two cases of peritoneal dialysis–related peritonitis caused by *Paecilomyces variotii.* Each of these patients had received multiple antibiotics as a treatment for bacterial peritonitis, possibly contributing to the emergence of the opportunistic *Paecilomyces* infection.

Paecilomyces species–related infections have also been reported by Chan-Tack et al.[40] (fungemia in an adult bone marrow transplant recipient), Gucalp et al.[98] (amphotericin B–refractory sinusitis in an immunocompromised adult), Okhravi et al.[201] (endophthalmitis following penetrating keratoplasty), and Westenfeld et al.[286] (a case of subcutaneous infection with prepatellar bursitis). Castro et al.[37] reported a case of deep subcutaneous infection of the left forearm with *Paecilomyces lilacinus* in a kidney-transplant recipient, which responded to oral griseofulvin therapy. These authors reviewed 42 cases of human mycoses due to *Paecilomyces* species, usually in conjunction with prosthesis implants or immunosuppression. Most strains of *P. lilacinus* are resistant to amphotericin B; most strains of *P. variotii* are susceptible.

Scopulariopsis spp. have been reported to cause infections of nails, subcutaneous tissue, and the lungs.[274] Phillips et al.[222] report several human cases of *S. brevicaulis* mycosis involving the toenail in an allogeneic bone-marrow transplant recipient. Other infections cited were hypersensitivity pneumonitis, fungus ball formation in the lung, and deep subcutaneous infections in immunocompromised hosts. Miscellaneous *Scopulariopsis* infections include separate cases of invasive fungal sinusitis reported by Ellison et al.[73] and by Jabor et al.,[128] the latter involving invasive nasal destruction in a nonimmunocompromised host; a fatal case of *S. brevicaulis* prosthetic-valve endocarditis reported by Migrino et al.[181]; and a case of recurrent subcutaneous infection, occurring in a patient 6 years after liver transplantation, reported by Sellier et al.[250]

Schell and Perfect[246] report a case of disseminated infection with *Acremonium strictum* in a patient with neutropenia. In this case, the recovery of the organism from blood cultures after previous recovery from fecal specimens indicates the gastrointestinal tract as the primary source of infection. Vajpayee et al.[277] found *Fusarium* species to be the most common cause of mycotic keratitis among 156 patients with mycotic corneal ulcer disease, most commonly complicating allergic conjunctivitis and a combination of antibiotic and corticosterone therapy. A comprehensive review of the taxonomy, mycology, laboratory features, and clinical syndromes related to *Fusarium* species has been published by Nielsen et al.[194] These authors also cite *Fusarium* species as the most common cause of mycotic keratitis in the United States, usually following corneal trauma from ocular implantation of vegetable fragments or soil matter during outdoor activities. Fungal keratitis has been reported in 4–27% of contact lens wearers, with *Fusarium* species being recovered most frequently.[294] Low et al.[166] report a case of *Beauveria*-related keratitis that was cured with deep dissection. Predisposing conditions include improper lens care, the presence of an underlying corneal infection such as herpes simplex infection, and the prolonged use of local corticosteroid and antibiotic medication.

In a 10-year (1986–1995) retrospective study of patients with hematologic malignancy, Boutati and Anaissie[29] found cases of disseminated *Fusarium* species infection in 43 patients, 40 with disseminated disease and 3 with invasive pulmonary infection. Although drug therapy was efficacious in 13 of these patients, in the main, recovery from the infection occurred only on reversal of myelosuppression and neutropenia. The recovery of *Fusarium* species from the bloodstream in patients with a variety of malignancies has been reported by Krcmery et al.[150]

Cutaneous infections may occur from direct penetration of the skin by contaminated vegetative material. The author served as a consultant in an unreported case of posttraumatic *Fusarium* mycetoma in a 35-year-old woman. Initially, a species of *Alternaria* species, susceptible to amphotericin B by in vitro studies, was recovered from a superficial biopsy of the lesion. When the patient did not improve on amphotericin B therapy, a deeper biopsy was performed, from which an amphotericin B–resistant strain of *Fusarium* species was recovered. The condition regressed when itraconazole was administered.

CLINICAL CORRELATION BOX 21-3 *Continued*

Scedosporium apiospermum is one of the more common causes of subcutaneous mycetomas in the United States. Pulmonary infections with *S. apiospermum* often resemble infections with *Aspergillus* spp., and the hyphae have a similar appearance in stained tissue sections. The presence of soft to firm white to yellow, spherical grains points to *Scedosporium* species infection. Sinusitis, including fungus ball infections, meningitis, osteomyelitis, endocarditis, mycotic keratitis, endophthalmitis, and otomycosis are other *Scedosporium* infections extensively reviewed by Rippon.[234] Perez et al.[214] report a case of *Pseudallescheria boydii* brain abscess in association with an infected central venous catheter.

Tamm et al.[271] report infections with *Scedosporium apiospermum* (*Pseudallescheria boydii*) in seven lung-transplant recipients in whom pulmonary infection developed. *Scedosporium apiospermum* was documented in bronchoalveolar lavage (BAL) of all seven patients. All seven patients showed airway problems, including early ischemic airway stenosis in one and bronchiolitis obliterans syndrome in the other six. Combined treatment with itraconazole and fluconazole was not able to eradicate the scedosporium. Four of the seven patients died with advanced bronchiolitis obliterans 3–35 months after the diagnosis of pulmonary scedosporium infection.

Scedosporium prolificans (*inflatum*) is cited as an emerging pathogen by Salkin et al.,[240] who reported 15 cases of infection in humans. Wilson et al.[298] added another 11 cases of *Scedosporium prolificans* infection, almost always in patients who had penetrating trauma or surgery. *Scedosporium* species, in particular *S. prolificans* have been found to be resistant to amphotericin B, miconazole and ketoconazole and other antimycotic agents, one important reason for differentiating them from *Aspergillus* species. Pickles et al.,[223] however, report success in effecting cures through the use of fluconazole.

Alvarez et al.[10] report on a nosocomial outbreak of four fatal cases of *Scedosporium prolificans* (*inflatum*) in patients with severe neutropenia resulting from leukemia chemotherapy. The infections occurred sequentially within a 1-month period in two rooms during a phase of hospital reconstruction when the patients were housed in a provisional hematology unit. The authors conclude that, despite the inability to recover *S. proliferans* from the patients' rooms or adjacent corridors, circumstantial evidence indicated a nosocomial outbreak. Antifungal susceptibility tests performed on the isolates revealed resistance to amphotericin B, ketoconazole, and miconazole, confirming the resistance profile previously observed by others.

Two similar related cases have been reported by Simarro et al.[257] Both patients were admitted to the hematologic ward in nearby rooms during building work in the hospital. After a previous bacterial sepsis in the neutropenic phase, which improved with antibiotic treatment, the respiratory status in both patients deteriorated, presenting acute dyspnea, with a lung infiltrate in one of them. A few hours later both patients died. Blood cultures were positive for *S. prolificans*.

De Battle et al.[59] describe a case of disseminated *S. prolificans* infection in a patient with leukemia during a period of chemotherapy-induced neutropenia. *S. prolificans* was recovered from four blood cultures. At autopsy, generalized fungal infection was found, with multiple intravascular mycotic thromboses in the lungs, liver, spleen, and other organs. The authors make the plea that every effort be made to protect patients with leukemia from the invasion of saprophytic fungi during periods of therapy-induced neutropenia.

A recently recognized condition involving hyaline molds has been designated "sick building syndrome."[171] Physicians are being asked to evaluate patients with this environmentally related illness, commonly manifested in individual patients as stomatitis, rhinitis, conjunctivitis, pancytopenia, and neurologic disorders, both singly and in combinations. Death in horses and other animals has also been reported. *Stachybotrys chartarum* has been implicated as a common hyaline mold associated with this syndrome. This fungus is important because it produces trichothecene mycotoxins, which are biologically active and can produce the variety of pathologic conditions cited above both in humans and in animals. It can be recovered from contaminated grains, tobacco, insulation foams, and the walls of water-damaged buildings with high humidity.

Pieckova and Jesenska[224] have published a review of the quantitative and qualitative incidence of filamentous fungi in dwellings, the health problems of occupants of these "moldy homes," and approaches to the detection and recovery of these etiologic molds. Perfect and Schell[215] address several issues related to pathogenesis, epidemiology, diagnosis, and treatment of the frequent and prolonged exposure of immunocompromised patients to these molds in a variety of environmental conditions.

The macroconidia, when formed, in contrast to those of *Microsporum* spp. are thin-walled and smooth. The size and arrangement of the microconidia are important in making species identifications. The production of pigment, urease activity, hair baiting capabilities, and the differential growth patterns on culture media with and without thiamine and niacin (*Trichophyton* differential agars) are also helpful in making species identifications.

The genus **Epidermophyton** is characterized by the production of clavate, smooth-walled, two- to four-celled macroconidia that are borne either singly from the hyphae, or more characteristically, in clusters of two or three. Of prime importance in the identification of *Epidermophyton* is the absence of microconidia.

Identification of *Microsporum* Species
MICROSPORUM CANIS

Growth is rapid, within 3–5 days. The colonies are initially white and silky, later developing a lemon-yellow pigment at the colony peripheral apron (Color Plate 21-4A). The colony reverse becomes yellow-brown as the colony matures.

Microscopically, both macroconidia and microconidia may be observed, the former predominating. The production

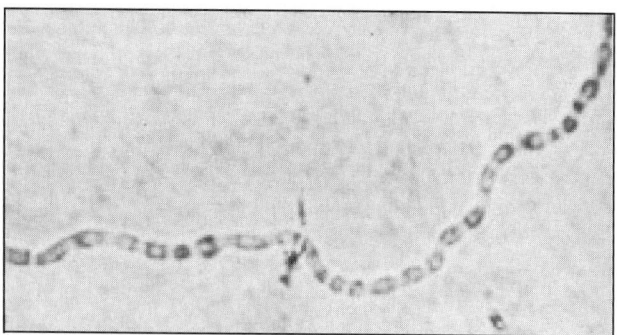

Figure 21-44 Photomicrograph of a KOH mount of skin scraping, illustrating a hyphal segment of one of the dermatophytic fungi. Note that the hyphal fragment is breaking up into tiny arthroconidia (oil immersion).

of spindle-shaped, multicelled macroconidia, pointed and slightly turned to one side at the tip, are characteristic of *Microsporum canis* (Fig. 21-46). Scattered microconidia may be seen borne laterally directly from the hyphae. In hair infections, mosaic clusters of microconidia develop on the outside of the shaft (**ectothrix**).

MICROSPORUM GYPSEUM

Growth is rapid, within 3–5 days. The colonies are flat, initially white but turning fawn-brown to reddish-brown on maturity (Color Plate 21-4*B*). The surface becomes sugary or granular as conidia are produced.

The macroconidia of *M. gypseum* generally are more numerous than found with *M. canis*, are less barrel-shaped, and have rounded tips (Fig. 21-47). These features are not always clear-cut and other criteria, such as the site and nature of the infection, a history of exposure to animals, and the colony morphology may be helpful in making the differential identification.

MICROSPORUM NANUM

Microsporum nanum macroconidia may resemble those of *Epidermophyton floccosum*. The colonies of *M. nanum*

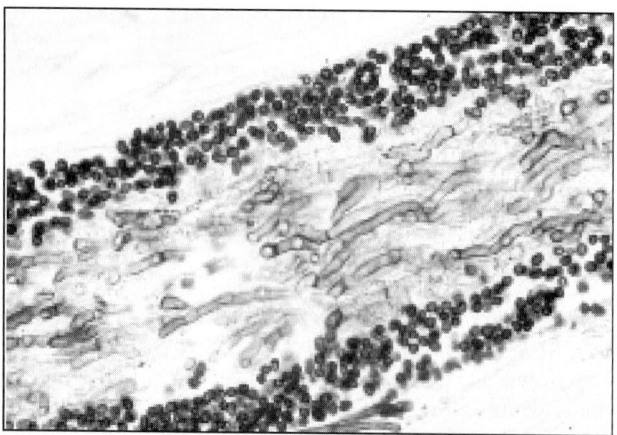

Figure 21-45 Photomicrograph taken through a longitudinal section of a hair shaft from a case of dermatophytosis. Note the endothrix invasion with septate hyphae centrally and conidia at the periphery. (Oil immersion, GMS stain × 400.)

grow rapidly, within 3–5 days. The surface is cottony, initially white, and later buff-colored, turning to brownish-red on the reverse side. Tufts may appear on the surface with maturity.

Microscopically, two- to three-celled, oval to clavate macroconidia are characteristically seen. The cell walls are finely verrucose (Fig. 21-48) in contrast to the conidia of *E. floccosum,* which have smooth walls. Small 3–5 μm clavate to cylindrical microconidia are derived from the sides of the hyphae, an additional important observation in differentiating *M. nanum* from *E. floccosum*. Only rare cases of *M. nanum* human infections have been reported, most commonly occurring in hog farmers.[235]

Identification of *Trichophyton* Species
TRICHOPHYTON MENTAGROPHYTES

Growth is relatively rapid, with maturation in 3–5 days. One of two colony types may be observed: cottony or granular. The cottony variants are initially white, but may become cream- to tan-colored with maturity. A central raised umbo of cobweblike sterile hyphae often develops. The periphery and reverse of the colony may be rose to tan (Color Plate 21-4*D*). The granular variants produce flat and spreading colonies with a fine to coarse granular surface. The colonies are initially white or off-yellow, but later become tan to brown. Red pigment similar to that seen with *T. rubrum* may be observed; however, the pigmentation is never as intense with *T. mentagrophytes*, particularly when colonies in parallel are grown on cornmeal or potato dextrose agars (Color Plate 21-4*F*)

The microconidia tend to form in loose grapelike clusters (*en grappe*) (Fig. 21-49). Macroconidia are typically absent or present in small numbers; they are more common in granular cultures and are long, multicelled, pencil-shaped, and have thin, smooth walls. Spiral hyphae and chlamydospores are often seen in the vegetative hyphae. Most strains have active urease activity, and in hair infections the hyphae invade the shafts (**endothrix**). Growth is equal on *Trichophyton* differential agars.

TRICHOPHYTON RUBRUM

Growth on Sabouraud's dextrose agar is relatively slow, requiring 4–7 days until maturity. The colony surface is initially white, and the consistency may be cottony, velvety, or granular, depending on the strain, the culture medium being used, and the magnitude of sporulation. As the species name indicates, a key observation is the production of a water-soluble, wine-red pigment on the reverse of the colony that diffuses into the agar (Color Plate 21-4*E* and *F*). Pigment production is more intense with colonies grown on cornmeal or potato dextrose agar than on Sabouraud's dextrose agar.

Microscopically, the microconidia of *T. rubrum* tend to be tear-shaped and are usually distributed on either side of the hyphal strands, producing a "birds-on-a-fence" appearance, rather than the loose clustering seen with *M. mentagrophytes* (Fig. 21-50). Multicelled macroconidia may rarely be observed—they are elongated and pencil-shaped, with smooth, thin walls, similar to those produced by *T. mentagrophytes*. Urease is not produced, the hair shaft is not in-

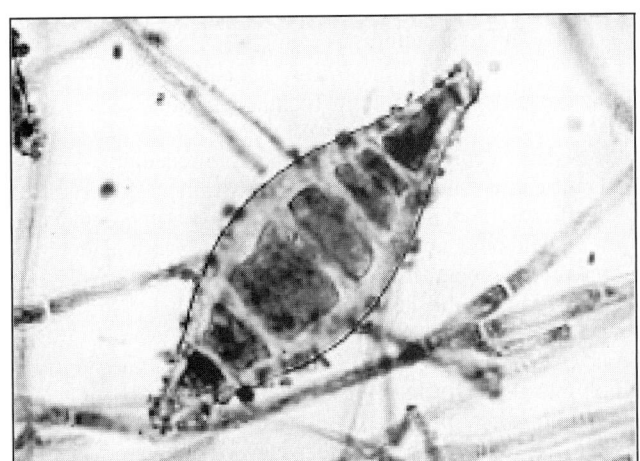
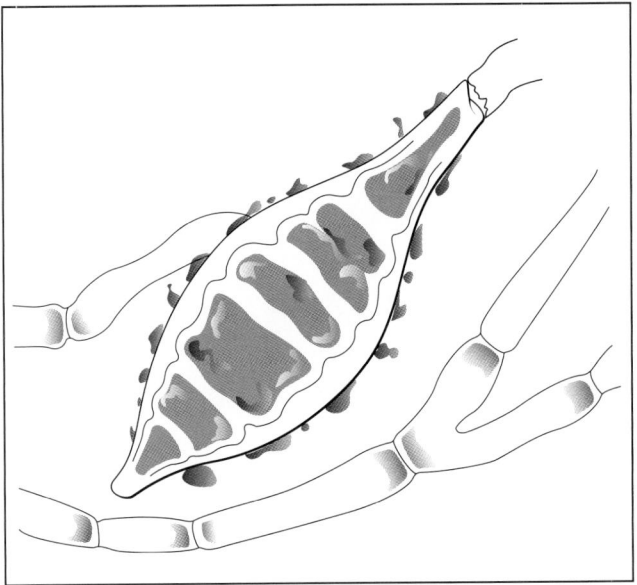

Figure 21-46 Photomicrograph and sketch of a multicelled macroconidium of *Microsporum canis,* illustrating the spindle shape, thick echinulate wall, cross septations, and tapered tip.

vaded in the hair-baiting test, and growth is equal on *Trichophyton* differential agars.

TRICHOPHYTON TONSURANS

Growth is slow, requiring 7–10 days to maturity. The colonies have a characteristic granular, buff surface, with the development of deep radial rugae on maturation (Color Plate 21-4*G*). Macroconidia are virtually never observed in laboratory isolates.

Microscopically, the microconidia are usually distinctive. They vary considerably in size, and are elongated, club-shaped, or large and balloon-shaped forms may be admixed with smaller oval or tear-shaped microconidia (Fig. 21-51). The identification can be confirmed by demonstrating poor growth on *Trichophyton* agar 1 (deficient in thiamine, which

is an absolute growth requirement for *T. tonsurans*), and good growth on *Trichophyton* agar 4 (rich in thiamine).

TRICHOPHYTON VERRUCOSUM

Growth is slow, requiring 7–14 days to maturity. Growth is poor in *Trichophyton* agar 1, which is deficient in thiamine and inositol. Growth will be observed on *Trichophyton* agars 2, 3, and 4, all of which contain either thiamine, inositol, or both. Colonies are small, circular, flat, glabrous initially or downy later, and white to off-yellow. The colony reverse remains nonpigmented.

Microscopically, sporulation is usually poor. Antler-type hyphae may be observed and also typical are the production of numerous chlamydospores typically arranged in chains

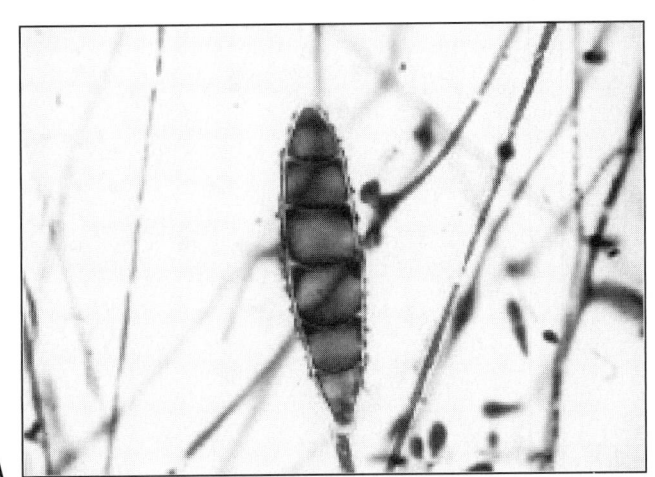
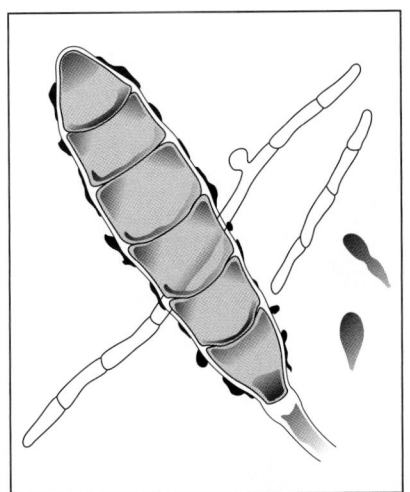

Figure 21-47 Photomicrograph and sketch of a multicelled macroconidium of *Microsporum gypseum,* revealing a thick, echinulate wall, cross septations, and a rounded terminal cell.

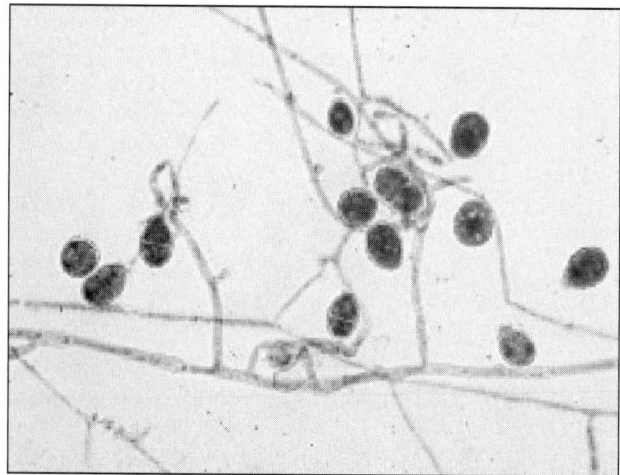

Figure 21-48 Photomicrograph of the macroconidia of *Microsporum nanum*. They differ from those of *E. floccosum* by being two-celled, having a thick, echinulate wall,

(Fig. 21-52). Macroconidia are rare, but are distinctive when present. They are multicelled, have thin, smooth walls, and are thin with a paddle, "string bean," or "rat tail" configuration. Microconidia, when present, are small, pyriform, and borne directly along the sides of the hyphae.

EPIDERMOPHYTON FLOCCOSUM

The colonies grow rapidly, within 3–5 days; initially they are gray-white and then develop a distinct, characteristic khaki-green pigment when mature. Yellow-white streamers of hyphae may be seen radiating from the center of the colony to the periphery (Color Plate 21-4*H*). The surface becomes granular on further maturity as conidia are produced.

Microconidia are never produced—a key observation. Thus, if microconidia are observed in an unknown culture

of a dermatophyte, *E. floccosum* can be eliminated from consideration. **Macroconidia** are usually produced in profusion, are typically club-shaped, have three to five cells and thin, smooth walls (Fig. 21-53). They often cluster in groups of three or four. Chlamydoconidia are typically present, particularly in older cultures.

Diagnosis Using Nonculture Techniques

Because conventional laboratory procedures for the identification of dermatophytes are either slow or lack specificity, brief mention is made here that the application of nucleic-acid amplification technology has made rapid and precise identification of dermatophytes possible. Recent studies published by Liu et al.[162] have shown that when one of the four random primers (OPAA11, OPD18, OPAA17, and OPU15) was used in arbitrarily primed polymerase chain reaction (AP-PCR), up to 20 of the 25 dermatophyte species or subspecies under investigation could be distinguished on the basis of characteristic band patterns detected in agarose gel electrophoresis. Although the use of such technology may be rarely required, reference is provided here for those instances when more exacting definition is needed.

The clinical manifestations of the various dermatophyte infections are in Clinical Correlation Box 21-4.

The Dimorphic Fungi

A subset of the hyaline molds, the dimorphic fungi, are usually considered separately because they have unique characteristics. First, they are dimorphic; that is, they exist in the mold form in the environment ("room-temperature incubation"), but as yeasts when incubated at 35–37°C (body temperature). The natural habitat for the dimorphic fungi is the soil, where, under ambient conditions, they exist as molds and undergo sporulation. The mold form is the

A
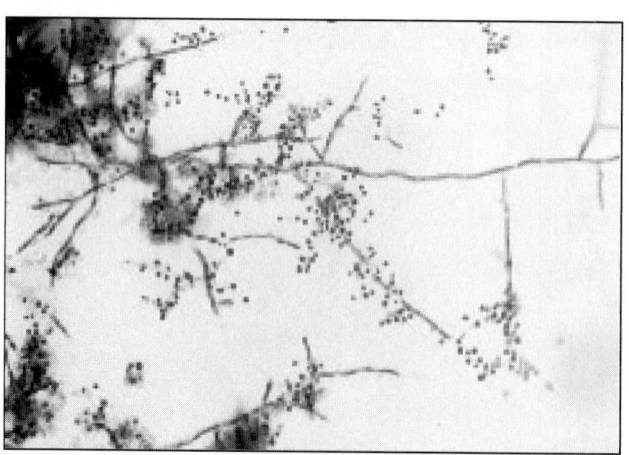

B
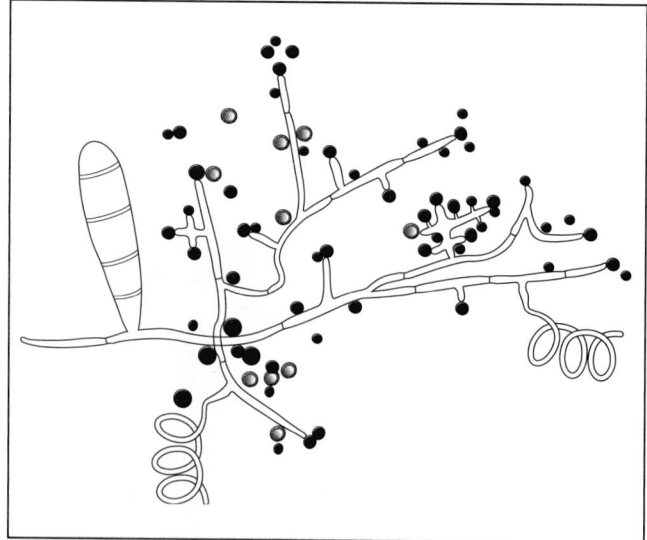

Figure 21-49 Photomicrograph and sketch of the microscopic forms of *Trichophyton mentagrophytes*, illustrating tiny, spherical conidia arranged in loose clusters.

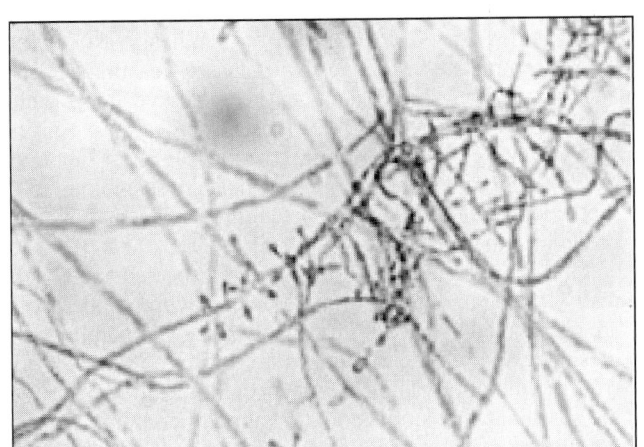
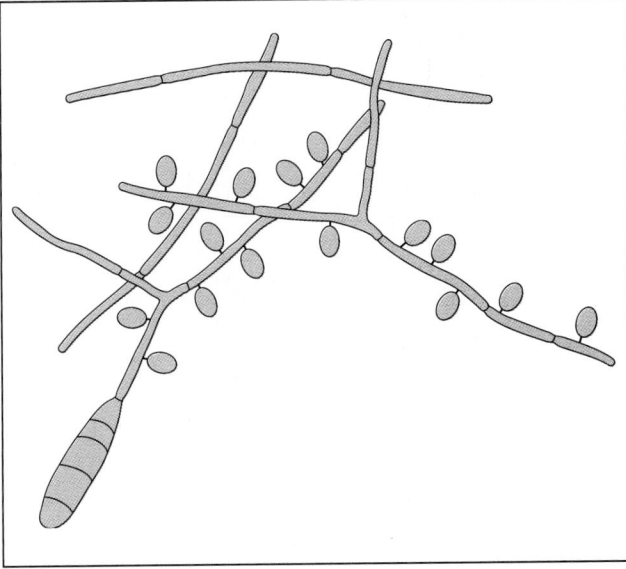

A   B

Figure 21-50 Photomicrograph and sketch of the microscopic forms of *Trichophyton rubrum*, illustrating the production of tiny conidia from the sides of the hyphae in a "birds on a fence" arrangement.

infective form. Humans and animals become infected either through inhalation or by direct traumatic implantation of material contaminated with conidia or hyphal elements. When incubated at 35–37°C or on access to the body temperature of human tissues, the conidia transform into a yeast form (or spherule form for *Coccidioides immitis*). Secondly, the dimorphic fungi are pathogens, causing "deep-seated" infections in humans. As a group, these fungi can be highly virulent in susceptible hosts and can invade deeply into tis-

sues and organs and have the capability of spreading widely throughout the body.

The species of medical importance include:

Blastomyces dermatitidis
Coccidioides immitis
Histoplasma capsulatum
Sporothrix schenckii
Paracoccidioides braziliensis

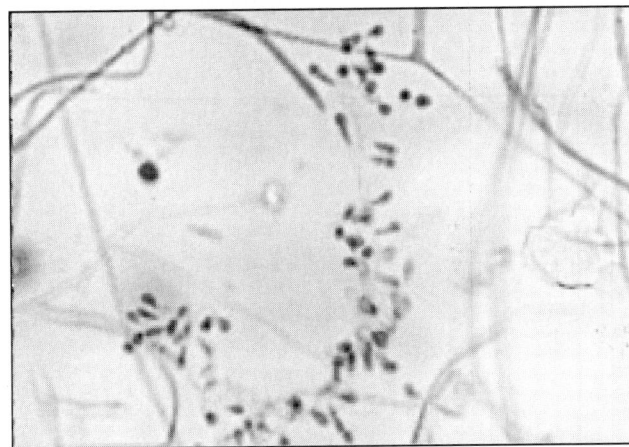
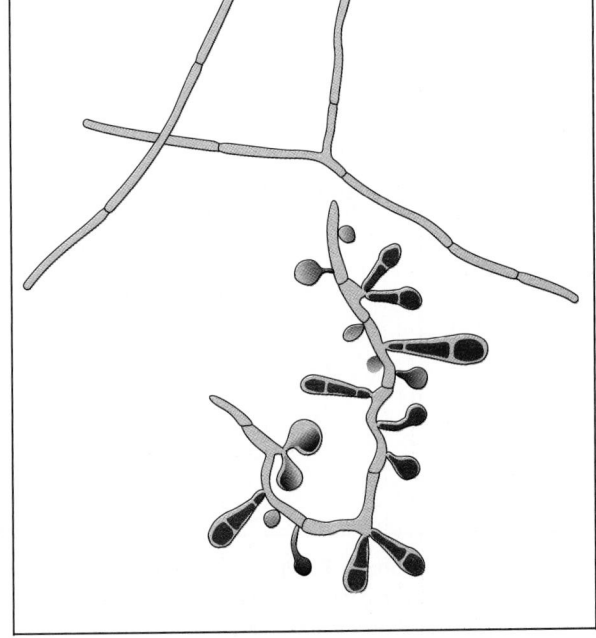

A   B

Figure 21-51 Photomicrograph and sketch of club-shaped and spherical conidia of *Trichophyton tonsurans* borne laterally from delicate, hyaline hyphae.

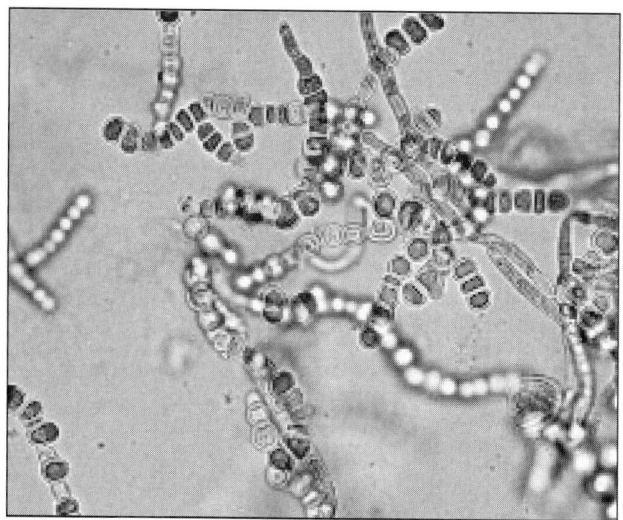

Figure 21-52 Photomicrograph of the microscopic appearance of chains of chlamydospores, characteristic of *Trichophyton verrucosum*.

The colonies typically grow slowly (10–30 days) when recovered in primary culture from clinical specimens. In cases in which the spore concentration in a clinical specimen is high, particularly in sputum, growth may be observed within 4–7 days. Rarely, a fine delicate growth may be observed in 24–72 hours on routine blood agar plates incubated at 35°C. At 30°C, the usual temperature of laboratory incubation, the colonies appear as a mold with a delicate, silky, hairlike, or cobweblike mycelium. In some cases, focal areas may appear yeastlike (Color Plate 21-5*A*). The colonies typically are gray-white or buff, although a few strains may show light pastel yellow shading into pink pigmentation. The dimorphic fungi as a group also have the capability of growing in culture media containing cycloheximide, a valuable property in separating out the saprophytic filamen-

tous molds, particularly their environmental look-alikes, which grow poorly or not at all.

If the temperature of incubation is increased, as in the process of conversion to the yeast form, a prickly stage of transformation may be observed before the typical yeastlike colonies develop (Color Plate 21-5*C*). When yeast conversion is complete, the colonies have a pasty, yeastlike appearance, are glabrous, are usually entire, and have an off-white to yellow pigmentation (Color Plate 21-5*E*). Yeast conversion of mold cultures is rarely attempted in most laboratories; rather, rapid identifications are made of suspicious colonies soon after they appear in culture, using nucleic-acid probe or exoantigen assays.

One of the dimorphic molds may be suspected microscopically if delicate hyaline, septate hyphae with parallel walls are observed. Commonly, the hyphae line up in parallel bundles. The species identifications are most commonly made from examination of colonies recovered in culture, based on the size, shape, position, and derivation of conidia. It is also possible to make an identification based on the morphology of the yeast forms as seen in stained tissue sections. The criteria for identification of the individual dimorphic molds will be presented in the paragraphs that follow.

Blastomyces dermatitidis and Blastomycosis

Blastomyces dermatitidis is a soil mold that is endemic in the states adjacent to the Mississippi and Ohio River valleys (Kentucky, Arkansas, Mississippi, North Carolina, Tennessee, Louisiana, Illinois, and Wisconsin). In contrast to histoplasmosis, in which the extent of the endemic zone has been clearly mapped based on positive skin tests, the regions of infection with blastomycosis are determined only on the basis of individual case findings because of the lack of a sensitive skin test.[57] Humans are presumed to become infected from inhalation of dust-contaminated spores; however, the mold form has only recently been recovered from

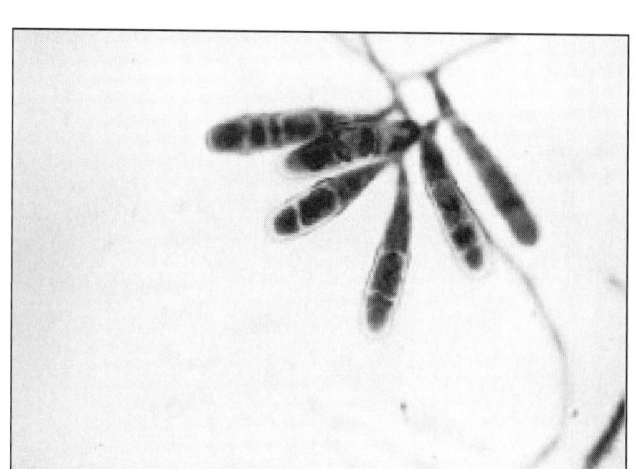

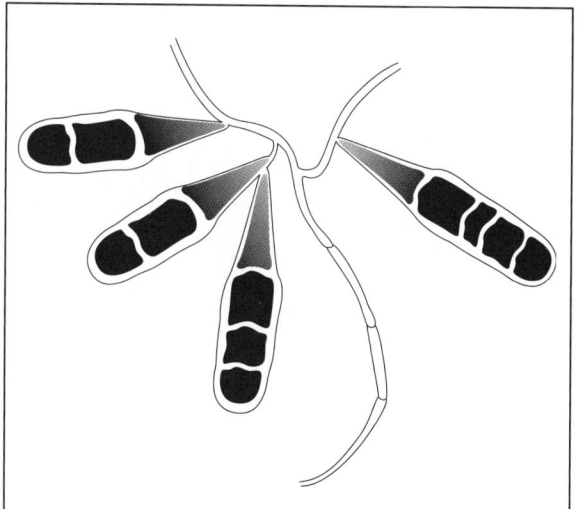

A   B

Figure 21-53 Photomicrograph and sketch of a cluster of elongated, cylindrical-shaped macroconidia of *Epidermophyton floccosum* with smooth walls and transverse septa. Microconidia are not observed.

CLINICAL CORRELATION BOX 21-4   The Dermatophytes

Tinea capitis, tinea corpora, tinea pedis, and tinea cruris are the names given to the various forms of dermatophyte infections. Onychomycosis refers to infections of the nails. With the advent of griseofulvin and topical antifungal compounds, the laboratory identification of the dermatophytes is now less frequently required. In most clinical practices, a KOH mount of skin scales, nail scrapings, or hairs are prepared in the physician's office and microscopically observed for the detection of typical hyphae that tend to break up into arthroconidia. Therapy is commonly instituted without obtaining a culture. This may change, however, as there have been reported cases of local invasive subcutaneous infections with *T. rubrum* and other dermatophyte species in rare cases of disseminated tinea infections.[249]

The term "tinea," dating back to the Middle Ages, refers to the circular holes in garments produced by the clothes moth, an appearance similar to the ringlike lesions of the skin produced by dermatophytic fungi. The term is now used to describe the various clinical syndromes caused by the dermatophytes. Tinea infections are also common in dogs, cats, horses, cattle, and other animals, providing a source for human zoophilic infections. The following is a brief summary of the several clinical types of tinea infections.

Tinea Capitis—Ringworm of the Scalp

Several types of infection may be observed:

(1) gray-patch ringworm, a communicable ectothrix infection of children caused by *Microsporum audouinii* or *M. canis*;

(2) inflammatory ectothrix infection with *T. mentagrophytes*, of animal origin;

(3) black-dot ringworm, an endothrix infection in which infected, degenerate hairs break off at the skin surface producing what appears to be a black dot, caused by *T. tonsurans*; and

(4) fungating exophytic masses (kerions) produced by *T. tonsurans*, or favus infections caused by *T. schoenleinii* (in Scandinavia and northern Europe) and by *T. violaceum* (in southern Mediterranean Europe).

During the past 50 years, *T. tonsurans* has replaced *T. audouinii as* the predominant etiologic agent of tinea capitis in the United States and Western Europe.[70,101,297] *T. tonsurans* infections are contagious, as evidenced by an outbreak of tinea corporis infections among four healthcare workers in an inpatient rehabilitation ward who contracted the disease from an infected patient.[160] Of recent interest, the contagious spread of *T. tonsurans* has become a nuisance among young competitive wrestlers. As the lesions appear somewhat different in a subset of youth wrestlers compared with the pediatric population as a whole, the term "tinea gladiatorum" has been applied to this form of infection.[146] Tinea capitis is most frequently obtained either from direct contact with an infected child or with a variety of fomites; an asymptomatic adult carrier state may contribute to persistence of infection in a given setting.[19] In a study of dermatophyte infection in 202 children residing in Kuwait, al-Fouzan et al.[7] found that tinea capitis was the most common infection and *M. canis* was the most prevalent species (96% of cases in this series). Although in the great majority of cases the infection remains confined to the superficial skin, reports have indicated that the fungus can invade deeper tissues in immunocompromised hosts. King et al.[142] report the case of subcutaneous papular infection in a kidney-transplant recipient, with invasive fungal elements seen in a deep biopsy of the skin. The second case was in a patient with AIDS and a CD4 count of 81, involving deep subcutaneous penetration of erythematous nodules of the scalp and face.

Tinea Corporis—Ringworm of the Body

Typical annular lesions on the skin of the smooth parts of the body that have a spreading, hemorrhagic border are caused most commonly by *T. rubrum*, *T. mentagrophytes,* and *T. tonsurans*. *T. tonsurans* is being recovered with increasing frequency as the cause of tinea corporis in the United States. *T. rubrum* in particular is well suited to survive on the surface of the skin, leading to chronic infection, often enduring for the patient's lifetime.[53] The mannans of *T. rubrum* appear to be better able to suppress cell-mediated immune reactions than are mannans from other fungi, thus evading host response and permitting survival. *T. rubrum* also can survive off the human body as spores in desquamated skin scales, promoting person-to-person transmission in various human habitats. Zoophilic *T. canis* and geophilic *T. gypseum* infections are also occasionally encountered in clinical practice.

Tinea Barbae—Ringworm of the Bearded Area

This zoophilic infection has most commonly been found in farm and dairy workers. *T. mentagrophytes* is the most common agent recovered from human infections, and the lesions tend to be inflammatory. *Trichophyton verrucosum* is also commonly associated with tinea barbae, acquired from the hide of dairy cattle. Sabota et al.[238] have reported *T. verrucosum* infection in five patients, three of whom had severe pustular tinea barbae and two of whom had eruptions of the forearms. All five patients were dairy farmers. A KOH preparation showed hyphae, and cultures yielded *T. verrucosum* in all three cases. *T. verrucosum* can cause pustular tinea barbae in farmers that may be mistaken for a *Staphylococcus aureus* infection by clinicians, including infectious-disease experts. The answer to the simple question "Are you a dairy farmer?" may suggest the diagnosis of *T. verrucosum* in the proper clinical setting.

Tinea Cruris—Ringworm of the Groin

The lesions tend to be circinate and serpiginous, with inflammatory, vesicular, enlarging margins, most commonly caused by *Epidermophyton floccosum*. This infection may reach epidemic proportions in athletes, soldiers, and ship's crews, among whom towels, linen, and clothing may be shared.

(continued)

Tinea Pedis—Ringworm of the Feet (Athlete's Foot)

This is the most common fungal infection in humans, typically manifesting as itching, scaling, or seeping skin lesions on the soles of the feet and/or between the toes. Infections are most common during the warm, humid months. *T. mentagrophytes, T. rubrum,* and *E. floccosum* are the dermatophyte species most commonly recovered. The increased amount of keratin on the soles of the feet and the palms of the hands makes these two sites selectively vulnerable to infection with *T. mentagrophytes* and other dermatophytes. The capability of *T. rubrum* to survive as spores in desquamated skin scales makes these hyperkeratotic areas particularly vulnerable to contracting infections from contaminated bath towels, locker room floors, and other human habitats.

Tinea Unguium—Ringworm of the Nails

Tinea unguium is the term used to describe involvement of the nails by dermatophyte fungi, to be differentiated from onychomycosis, which refers to nail infections caused by a wide variety of nondermatophytic fungi, including *Aspergillus* species, *Candida albicans, Geotrichum* species, and several species of hyaline and dematiaceous phaeohyphomycetes. Tinea unguium infections begin at the lateral or distal edge of the nail plate and result in paronychial inflammation. As the lesion progresses, the nail becomes thickened and brittle, with accumulation of subungual keratinized debris. The dermatophytes most commonly involved are *T. rubrum* and *T. mentagrophytes.*

Lugo-Somolinos and Sanchez,[168] in a study of 100 consecutive patients with diabetes, found no greater incidence of dermatophyte infections compared with a control population. Dermatophyte infections of one type or another were found in 31% of the diabetics and in 33% of the control group. Thus, contrary to popular notion, diabetes mellitus apparently does not predispose to dermatophytosis.

soil and decaying wood along riverways in Wisconsin.[21,144] A high incidence of infection exists in dogs.

LABORATORY PRESENTATION

The colonies typically grow slowly in primary culture (10–30 days), except in cases of heavy infections, when growth may be seen within 1 week. At 30°C, the colonies appear as a gray-white to light-buff-colored mold with a delicate, silky or hairlike mycelium (Color Plate 21-5*B*). In conversion to the yeast form, a prickly stage may be seen during transformation before the typical yeastlike colonies develop. The colonies become smooth and more yeastlike, except for the aerial protrusion of delicate spikes, appearing as hair standing on end (Color Plate 21-5*C*).

Microscopically, in the mold form, the hyphae are delicate (1–2 μm in diameter), hyaline, and septate. Oval or pyriform conidia measuring 1–4 μm in diameter are borne singly at the tips of long or short conidiophores (forming "lollipops") (Fig. 21-54). The conidia of the soil saprobe, *Chrysosporium* spp., have a similar appearance microscopically.

The yeast conversion colonies grown at 35°C on enriched agar are small, entire, slightly convex, smooth, and may have an off-yellow or buff pigmentation. Microscopically, the yeast forms are large (10–15 μm), and characteristically have a single bud attached by a broad base (Fig. 21-55). These broad-based budding yeast forms may also be observed in tissue sections against a purulent or granulomatous background cellular reaction (Fig. 21-56, *left*). These forms may be confused in tissue sections with the immature spherules of *Coccidioides immitis* that may be lying side by side.

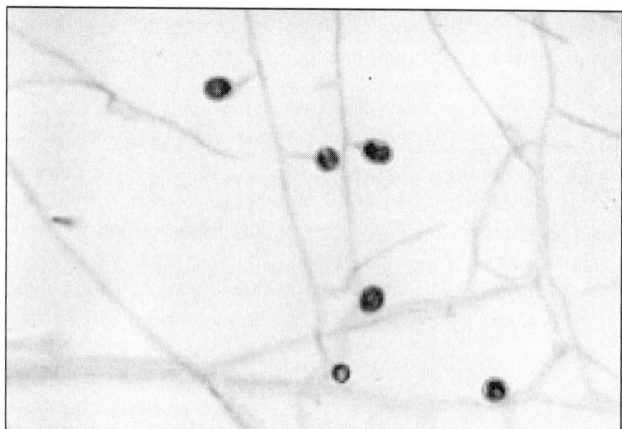

A

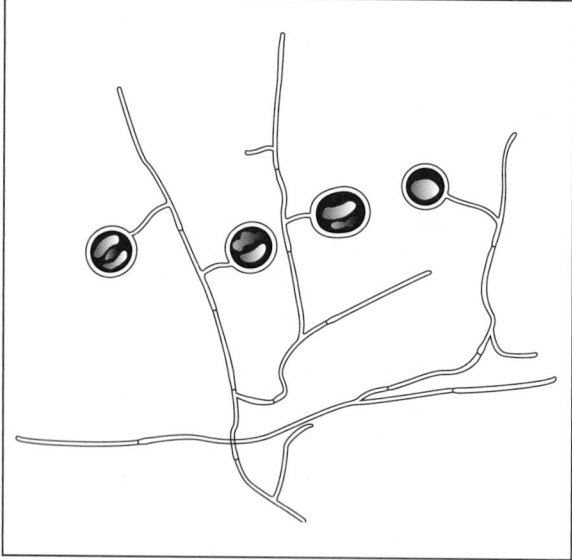

B

Figure 21-54 Photomicrograph and sketch of the small, single conidia of *Blastomyces dermatitidis* attached to the hyphae by delicate, short conidiophores.

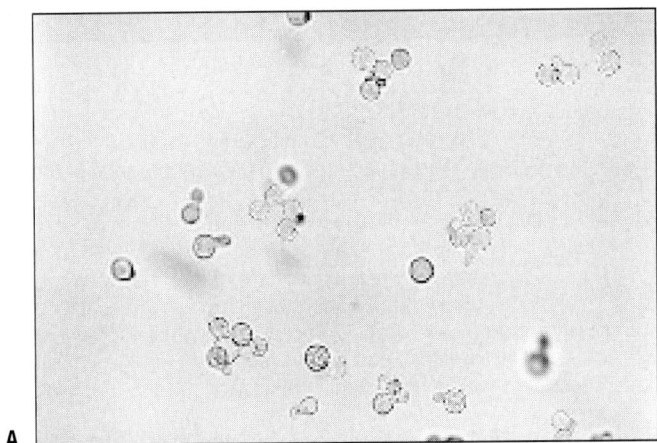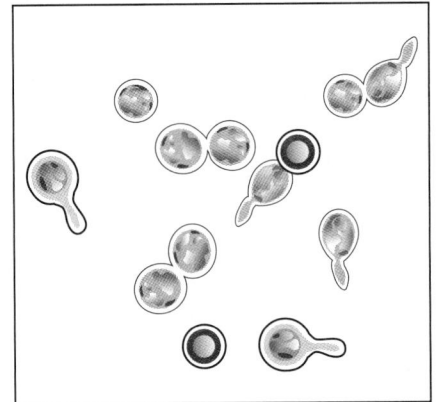

Figure 21-55 Photomicrograph and sketch of large yeast cells of *Blastomyces dermatitidis*, many producing a broad-based bud.

However, the development of endospores within the spherules provide for the true identification of *C. immitis* (Fig. 21-56, *right*).

The clinical manifestations of the various dermatophyte infections are in Clinical Correlation Box 21-4.

DIAGNOSIS USING NONCULTURE TECHNIQUES

Serologic tests for antibody detection are generally considered to be inadequate for use in diagnosis of blastomycosis. In only approximately 25% of known cases are immunodiffusion and complement fixation assays positive. Enzyme immunoassays (EIAs)are more sensitive than immunodiffusion (ID), but less specific. A large common-source outbreak is cited in which the sensitivity of EIA (77%) was higher than that of ID (28%) or complement fixation (CF) (9%), but its specificity was lower, 92%, compared to 100% for ID and CF.[67]

A recently developed test for *Blastomyces* antigen detected antigenuria in 92.9% of cases of blastomycosis, including 89.3% of disseminated and 100% of pulmonary forms of disease.[68] Other body fluids also may be suitable for antigen testing. Antigen has been detected in serum, cerebrospinal fluid (CSF), and bronchoalveolar lavage fluid (BALF). Detection of antigen in BALF may improve the sensitivity for diagnosis in patients with pulmonary disease, particularly in milder cases. Antigen detection in CSF may be helpful in establishing a diagnosis of *Blastomyces* meningitis, as yeast cells are not seen in direct examinations and cultures are negative in approximately 50% of cases. Failure of antigen to clear during a course of therapy may herald treatment failure; a recurrence of illness may be detected if antigen levels rise by two- or three-fold.[68]

The clinical manifestations of blastomycosis are presented in text in Clinical Correlation Box 21-5.

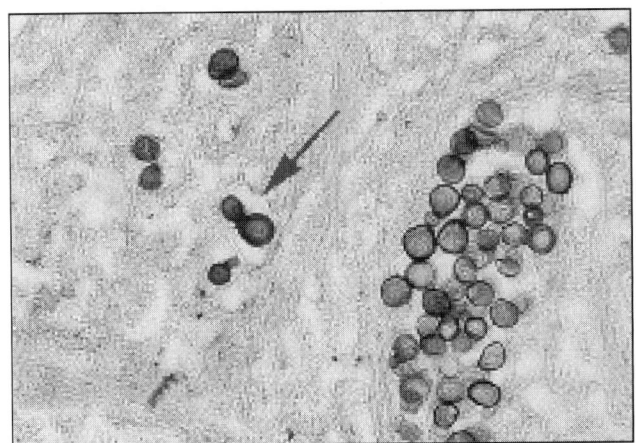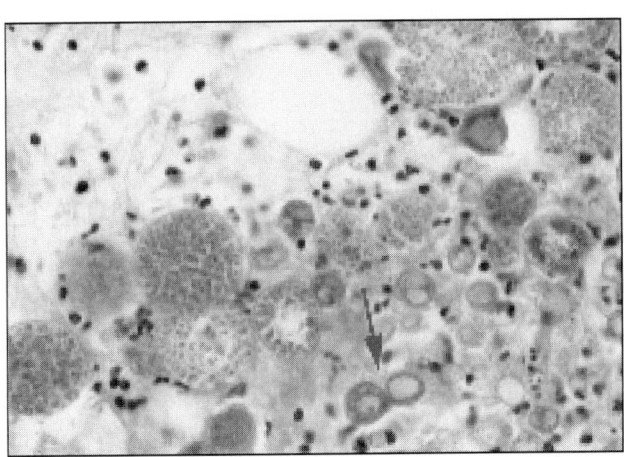

Figure 21-56 *Left,* Photomicrograph of a GMS-stained tissue section illustrating loose clusters of black-staining yeast cells of *Blastomyces dermatitidis*, some with a characteristic broad-based bud. *Right,* Photomicrograph of an H&E-stained tissue section, illustrating small empty immature spherules of *Coccidioides immitis*, along with large endospore-containing, mature forms. Empty spherules lying side by side may simulate the broad-based budding forms of *B. dermatitidis* (*arrow*).

CLINICAL CORRELATION BOX 21-5 Blastomycosis

The clinical presentations of blastomycosis have been categorized by Davies and Sarosi[57,58] as follows:

1. asymptomatic, currently discovered only in outbreak situations;
2. flulike illness of brief duration, resembling other upper respiratory infections;
3. illness resembling bacterial pneumonia, with acute onset of high fever, lobar infiltrates, and productive cough;
4. subacute or chronic respiratory illness with a symptom complex simulating tuberculosis or lung cancer, with radiographic presentation of fibronodular infiltrates or masslike lesions; and
5. fulminant infectious adult respiratory distress syndrome (ARDS) with high fever, diffuse infiltrates, and progressive respiratory failure.

In clinical settings, blastomycosis almost always begins in the lungs as the primary pulmonary form of the disease, with pneumonia being the most common initial clinical manifestation.[30] The pneumonia may be short term, mimicking bacterial pneumonia, or may become more indolent; occasionally, it may be progressive and severe. Most commonly, symptoms resolve spontaneously after a brief flulike syndrome. Dry cough, low-grade fever, weight loss, night sweats, pleuritic chest pain, and myalgias may be presenting symptoms early in acute infections. Persistent localized chest pain, weight loss, night sweats, and malaise may indicate progression to a chronic form of disease.

Mississippi has the highest prevalence of blastomycosis in North America.[158] Even in this endemic area of physician awareness, the diagnosis of blastomycosis was difficult to recognize. Blastomycosis was correctly suspected on initial examination in only 18% of 123 patients being evaluated at the University of Mississippi Medical Center in Jackson.[157] Nonspecific pneumonia (40%), malignant tumors (16%), and tuberculosis (14%) were the most frequent misdiagnoses. Only in the presence of cutaneous involvement was the initial suspicion raised to 64%. These misdiagnoses often led to unnecessary surgeries, delays in treatment, or the administration of ineffective antibiotic therapy for months. Immunosuppression (25% of cases) and diabetes mellitus (22%) were the more frequent predisposing conditions.

During the two decades prior to 2000, only three pregnancies were complicated by blastomycosis at the University of Mississippi Medical Center (a total of 120 patients with blastomycosis were treated during this period).[159] Fetal risk exceeded maternal risk. Of 20 babies born from mothers with blastomycosis, only two (10%) had transplacental infection and both died. Not only did none of the 18 affected mothers die from the disease, there was no progression with 14 complete cures and considerable postpartum regressions of lesions in the other four women.

Bone is a common site for extrapulmonary infection. From the older literature, a case of temporal bone osteomyelitis secondary to *B. dermatitidis* manifesting as serous otitis media was reported by Farr et al.[79] In a study of 17 patients by MacDonald et al.,[170] the metaphyses of long bones and small bones were most frequently involved. The metaphyseal lesions tend to be eccentric, well circumscribed, and lytic. More recently, Hadjupavlou et al.[103] reported a case of blastomycosis of the lumbar spine, causing severe and crippling deformity. The authors emphasize the importance of early, aggressive treatment to prevent deformity and disability.

The genitourinary tract, particularly the prostate gland, epididymis, and kidney; the brain, with local abscess formation; lymph nodes; and the adrenal gland are other extrapulmonary sites of involvement culled by Kwon-Chung and Bennett[153] from the earlier literature. The clinical manifestations commonly are those of nonspecific epididymitis and prostatitis, and the diagnosis must be made by demonstrating organisms in biopsy material, and may be missed in the absence of a high degree of suspicion.

A report by Hanson et al.[115] of two cases of laryngeal blastomycosis that were misdiagnosed as squamous-cell carcinoma is disturbing. In one of the cases, this misdiagnosis led to radiotherapy and laryngectomy. In the second case, although a clinical diagnosis of glottic squamous-cell carcinoma was rendered, the budding yeast forms of blastomycosis were identified in a biopsy specimen. Review of the English-language literature over the past 80 years revealed a number of cases that were misdiagnosed clinically and microscopically as squamous-cell carcinoma.

Reder et al.[228] reviewed a large series of blastomycosis diagnosed at the Mayo Clinic between 1960 and 1990. Involvement of the skin and mucous membranes (including the larynx) was quite common, often with clinical and histologic features resembling well-differentiated squamous-cell carcinoma. Skin or mucous membrane involvement usually indicates systemic disease, and in many instances these may be the initial lesions. The diagnosis of blastomycosis should be considered in the differential diagnosis of any patient with nonhealing skin lesions associated with risk factors such as living in an endemic area and having an occupation or vocation involving frequent contact with soil.[16] Single or multiple ulcerating papules or pustules of the skin, usually involving the face, hands, or lower legs, may slowly progress into an ulcerated verrucous granuloma with an advancing serpiginous border. Primary cutaneous lesions occurring at the site of penetrating injuries of the skin do not spread systemically. Cases of intraocular disease have also been reported.[165]

Blastomycosis is not considered as one of the AIDS-defining infections; nevertheless, in some practice settings, a distinct increase in incidence and in severity of disease occurring in immunocompromised hosts has been observed.[287] Disease is particularly progressive in AIDS patients when the CD4 count drops below 200/mL.[209] Fraser et al.[86] studied in parallel two friends, one with AIDS, who were infected with the same strain of *B. dermatitidis* (proven by restriction endonuclease analysis). In the patient with AIDS, severe, progressive fatal pulmonary blastomycosis developed despite aggressive treatment with fluconazole and amphotericin B; his HIV-negative friend responded completely to the same course of therapy. The authors concluded that cellular immunity plays a critical role in the progression of disease in patients with blastomycosis. Of interest is the review of 123 charts of patients with the diagnosis of blastomycosis at the University of Mississippi Medical Center from January 1980 through May 2000 to determine the role of wet preparation, cytology, histology, and culture in diagnosing this fungal disease.[157] The etiologic agent was detected by cytology in 56.1% of all cases, and in 71.8% of pulmonary cases. Wet preparation was second in line to uncover the fungus (37.4%); histology was the third (32.5%). Cultures were positive in 64.2% of all cases but provided the initial diagnosis in only 3.2% of all patients. There was pulmonary involvement in 87% of patients, cutaneous involvement in 20%, osseous involvement in 15%, and central nervous involvement in 3%.

Coccidioides immitis and Coccidioidomycosis

Coccidioides immitis is a dimorphic soil fungus native to the San Joaquin Valley of California, southern portions of Arizona, and northern regions of Mexico. Local regions of southern Utah, Nevada, southern New Mexico, and the western panhandle of Texas also serve as endemic areas of infection. The mycelial form grows beneath the hot desert sands, in which the elevated subsurface temperatures are ideal for propagation. The hyphae are branched, and fragment into individual arthroconidia when the soil is disturbed. These arthroconidia are tiny, light, and easily windborne in clouds of blowing sand and dust. On inhalation, these arthroconidia escape the mechanical defenses of the upper respiratory tract and reach deep into the bronchial tree. On arrival in the alveoli, the arthroconidia transform into thick-walled spherules within which, on maturity, thousands of endospores develop. Endospore-containing spherules are the diagnostic forms seen in stained tissue sections.

Hyphal forms may be found in tissue sections, particularly if the affected site has been exposed to air. Hagman et al.[104] reported five cases of coccidioidomycosis in which hyphae were found in brain tissue or spinal fluid. They theorized that in these cases the presence of central nervous system plastic devices appears to be associated with morphologic reversion to the saprophytic form.

The incidence of coccidioidomycosis in endemic areas has increased in the past several years, with peak rises in 1991 and 1992 during periods of interspersed heavy rainfall followed by drought.[185] A marked increase in incidence also occurred in the decade following the Simi Valley earthquake.[208] Kirkland and Fierer[143] have estimated that this outbreak cost more than $66 million in direct medical expenses and from time lost from work in Kern County, California, alone.

Recent reports indicate that coccidioidomycosis remains a growing problem in the southwestern United States.[12] Related is the parallel increase in individuals with depressed cellular immunity, particularly those with HIV infection, those who have undergone allogeneic transplantation, and others on immunosuppressive medications. Logan et al.[163] report that coccidioidomycosis remains the most common endemic mycosis in North America, largely related to the increase in solid-organ transplants. They cite underlying renal and liver disease, T-lymphocyte suppression from anti-rejection medication, and activation of immunomodulating viruses, such as cytomegalovirus, among these patients, as factors increasing the risk for coccidioidomycosis. Interestingly, reactivation of previously acquired coccidioidal infection was found to account for about half of all cases during the first year after transplantation.

Feldman and Snyder[80] also cite increased travel through the endemic regions in the southwestern Unites States as also contributing to persistence coccidioidomycosis. Patients with coccidioidomycosis are therefore likely to present with pulmonary manifestations, including pneumonia, cavities, and nodules, when they return home to nonendemic parts of the country. Thus, coccidioidomycosis is of nationwide importance. Physicians everywhere must maintain a heightened awareness of this disease and obtain a careful travel history of patients presenting with pulmonary signs and symptoms to avert delays in diagnosis and treatment.

In endemic areas, particular attention should be paid to ranchers, farmers, construction workers, and others engaged in outdoor activities requiring intimate exposure to dust and soil. Archeologists participating in excavations in endemic areas are at particularly high risk for infection. African and Filipino Americans and pregnant women remain at higher risk for disseminated disease.

LABORATORY PRESENTATION

The colonies of *C. immitis* vary in morphology but usually appear as delicate cobweblike, gray-white mycelium. Extreme care should be exercised when examining cultures suspicious for this fungus. When grown on blood agar, the colonies may appear dark green-black in areas where hemoglobin pigments have been adsorbed (Color Plate 21-5F).

Microscopically, in the mold form grown at 30°C, the hyphae are delicate and break up into barrel-shaped, arthroconidia that are separated by empty spaces (alternate staining) (Fig. 21-57). *Malbranchia* species and *Gymnoascus* species may appear similar.

A yeast form for *C. immitis* does not occur. As mentioned above, the diagnostic forms observed in tissue sections are spherules that range from 20 to 200 μm in diameter, filled with 2–4-μm diameter endospores when mature (Fig. 21-58).

The clinical manifestations of coccidioidomycosis are presented in Clinical Correlation Box 21-6.

Histoplasma capsulatum and Histoplasmosis

Histoplasmosis, caused by the dimorphic fungus, *Histoplasma capsulatum*, is a common systemic fungal disease in the United States. It also is the most common fungal infection in patients with AIDS.[183] The major endemic areas of histoplasmosis in North America are the drainage basins of the St. Lawrence, Ohio, Mississippi, and Missouri River valleys, where a high percentage of the native population is skin-test-positive, indicating past infection. Histoplasmosis is also found in Central America; only rare autochthonous cases have been reported from other parts of the world.

Isolated indigenous cases have been reported from Europe; in Germany, Belgium, Holland, and Denmark. Histoplasmosis is known as an "exo-European" disease, although a few cases have been reported from Italy. Confalonieri et al.[49] reported two new histologically documented disease in Italian patients who had never been abroad. A relatively high incidence of positive histoplasmin skin tests in a survey carried out in the Province of Cremona, Italy, confirmed the possibility of endogenous infections. A recent case of disseminated histoplasmosis with atypical, papular, and ulcerated skin lesions in an Italian patient with HIV, without a history of travel outside his native region, has been reported by Calza et al.[34] The authors cite this case as the fifth autochthonous case of AIDS-associated histoplasmosis described in Italy. O'Sullivan et al.[204] report a case of oral histoplasmosis in Brisbane, Queensland, indicating that this disease is increasingly being recognized in Australia, although the local source of infection remains obscure. The reality that

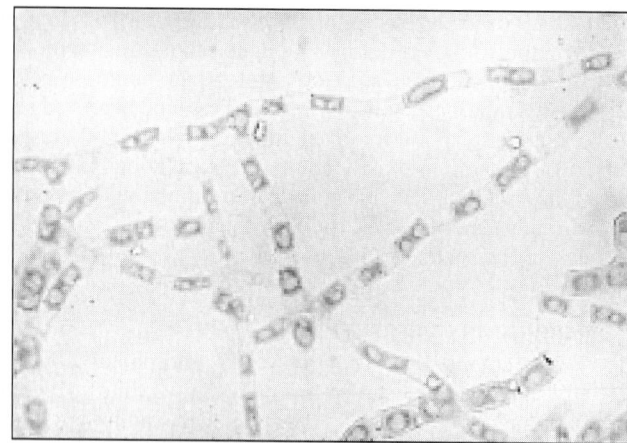

Figure 21-57 Photomicrograph and sketch of hyphal forms of *Coccidioides immitis,* illustrating the characteristic barrel-shaped arthroconidia, with individual cells separated by pale-staining empty spaces.

this infection may be underdiagnosed suggests a more widespread geographic distribution.

The mycelial form of *Histoplasma capsulatum* is present in warm, moist soil rich in organic content, such as that produced by heavy accumulation of bird or bat excreta. Bird roosts, chicken houses, caves, or old buildings frequented by bats are potentially highly infective areas. Patients with AIDS or who are otherwise severely immunocompromised are counseled to avoid working in these areas as much as possible. Disruption of these areas by bulldozing or cleanup efforts may expose humans to large numbers of airborne spores. Three large outbreaks of histoplasmosis in the Indi-

anapolis, Indiana, metropolitan area have been cited: in 1978 in conjunction with the demolition of an amusement park, in 1980 related to the building of a swimming pool, and in 1988–1993 during the time of the construction of a large tennis complex.[296]

During this outbreak, Williams et al.[296] detected antigen in 92%, 21%, and 39% of patients with the disseminated, chronic pulmonary, and self-limited forms, respectively. The authors conclude that tests for serum antigen are most useful in patients with clinical findings of disseminated infection or during the first month of illness in cases of severe pulmonary involvement when serologic tests for antibodies may be negative.

LABORATORY PRESENTATION

The mold form of *Histoplasma capsulatum* typically grows slowly (10–30 days), although from specimens with a heavy concentration of organisms, growth as early as 5 days may be observed. The observation of a delicate cobweblike or hairlike aerial mycelium, initially white but turning gray or gray-brown with age (Color Plate 21-5*D*) is typical.

Microscopically, the diagnostic structures seen in the mold form are large, roughened, or spiked macroconidia measuring 10 to 20 μm in diameter (Fig. 21-59). In earlier cultures, small oval microconidia may be seen borne laterally from the sides of delicate hyphae, in a sleevelike arrangement, simulating closely the microconidia seen in the mold cultures of *T. rubrum, B. dermatitidis,* and *S. schenckii.* The microscopic features of *Sepedonium* species appear similar.

The yeast colonies, whether grown from primary cultures incubated at 37°C or after conversion from the mold form,

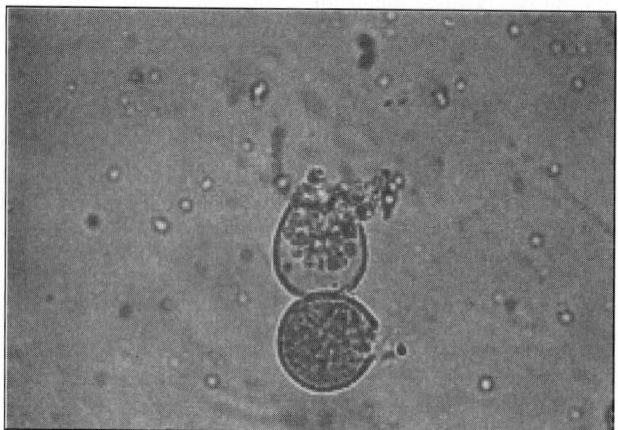

Figure 21-58 Photomicrograph of two spherules of *Coccidioides immitis* lying adjacent to one another, simulating the broad-based budding yeast cells of *Blastomyces dermatitidis.* Note the formation of endospores, particularly well illustrated in the upper spherule by their escape through a fracture in the wall.

CLINICAL CORRELATION BOX 21-6 Coccidioidomycosis

Following exposure to coccidioides arthroconidia, a "grippe" or influenzalike syndrome known as "valley fever" develops in the majority of individuals; in most cases, it is confined to the lung and self-limited, resolving over a period of weeks or months without therapy.[90] Sixty percent of infected individuals are asymptomatic; many skin-test-positive individuals do not recall having symptoms. Those who are symptomatic experience an acute, short-term, lower respiratory tract infection with varying degrees of cough, sputum production, chest pain, fever, and arthralgia. A bacterial-pneumonia-type syndrome is unusual, although two cases have been reported.[167] Chronic pulmonary disease with sequelae ultimately develops in only 2–5% of infected individuals. Solitary "coin lesions" or granulomas, solid or cavitary, usually located peripherally within the lung parenchyma, are common residual findings, primarily in individuals who do not reside permanently in the endemic area in which the infection was incurred.

In endemic areas, infection with human immunodeficiency virus (HIV) is also a risk factor for coccidioidomycosis.[12] Based on original work by Fish et al.[83] and later refined by Minamoto and Rosenberg,[183] six categories of disease based on primary clinical presentation are proposed:

Group 1, focal pulmonary disease—localized alveolar infiltrates; discrete lung nodules, solid and cavitary; hilar adenopathy.

Group 2, diffuse pulmonary disease—a clinical syndrome simulating *Pneumocystis carinii* infection

Group 3, cutaneous coccidioidomycosis—usually concomitant with pulmonary disease, with papules, pustules, nodules, subcutaneous abscesses, ulcers, and/or verrucous granulomas

Group 4, meningitis—CSF pleocytosis, chiefly lymphocytes, lowered glucose and elevated protein concentrations

Group 5, disseminated disease—extrathoracic lymph node (most commonly inguinal) or liver involvement; distant spread reported most commonly in kidneys, thyroid gland, heart, pituitary gland, esophagus, and pancreas

Group 6, positive coccidioidal serology without a clinical focus of infection.

In a study by Singh et al.[260] of 91 patients coinfected with AIDS and *C. immitis,* fever, chills, weight loss, and night sweats were the most common symptoms. The mortality rate in this group was 60%, with diffuse pulmonary disease and a CD4 lymphocyte count of $<5l0/\mu L$ were independent predictors of death. Coccidioidal serum serology titers were positive in two thirds (68%) of these patients, with negative results found in 23%. The highest percentage of false-negative serology reactions were in the group of patients with progressive, invasive pulmonary disease. Amphotericin B remains the treatment of choice, although azoles, particularly ketoconazole, is less toxic and equally effective.

Antoniskis et al.[15] found that two of eight patients in their study with coccidioidomycosis and HIV infection were repeatedly seronegative, concluding that histopathology and culture remain the most reliable methods for establishing the diagnosis in patients with AIDS. On the other side of the ledger, Arguinchona et al.[17] found that asymptomatic individuals with positive CF serum serology titers went on to have active coccidiomycosis. In reference to the accuracy of tissue biopsies, of 54 patients with coccidioidomycosis reported by diTomasso et al.,[62] transbronchial biopsy was 100% sensitive in yielding a rapid diagnosis, in contrast to cytologic examination of bronchial fluid or bronchoalveolar lavage, which provided a diagnosis in only 34% of cases.

The association of increased risk for disseminated coccidioidomycosis during pregnancy remains in doubt. Wack et al.,[281] refuting many previous studies in which coccidioidomycosis during pregnancy was considered a devastating disease with high mortality, found only 10 cases among 47,120 pregnancies among women living in Tucson, Arizona. The infection resolved in seven of the women in whom coccidioidomycosis was diagnosed during the first or second trimester; progressive disease developed in two of three women who were diagnosed in the third trimester. Improvement in medical care and the introduction of antifungal therapy relatively early in the course of coccidioidomycosis may account for the lower current mortality rate among pregnant women.

Although coccidioidomycosis is primarily a pulmonary disease, Arnold et al.[18] report that disseminated disease affecting skin, subcutaneous tissue, bone, joints, and meninges develops in approximately 0.5–1.0% of infected individuals. In a review of 47 cases from the medical literature, these authors found that virtually all head and neck manifestations in patients with disseminated coccidioidomycosis involved the skin, with a predilection for the central face. The lesions often tended to be multiple, including life-threatening airway lesions. A report of coccidioidal prostatitis by Truett and Crum[275] serve as a reminder that fungal agents must be included in the differential diagnosis of conditions in which they might be least expected. Persistent sterile pyuria, prostatitis, and granulomatous disease of the prostate were the presenting signs and symptoms in the cases reported.

are typically smooth, yellow-white, and somewhat glistening, with a pasty consistency (Color Plate 21-5*E*).

The yeast cells microscopically are small, 2–4 μm in diameter, and may show a single bud connected by a delicate filament. In tissue sections, the yeast cells are clustered within macrophages and are surrounded by a clear space, appearing pseudoencapsulated (Fig. 21-60). The background inflammatory reaction is granulomatous. Cavitation and caseation necrosis in older lesions may simulate tuberculosis.

The mold form of *H. capsulatum* is often difficult to convert to the yeast form in culture. For this reason, the exoantigen test or the nucleic-acid probe test is recommended to confirm the final identification, which may be made accurately within 1 day after the appearance of initial growth in

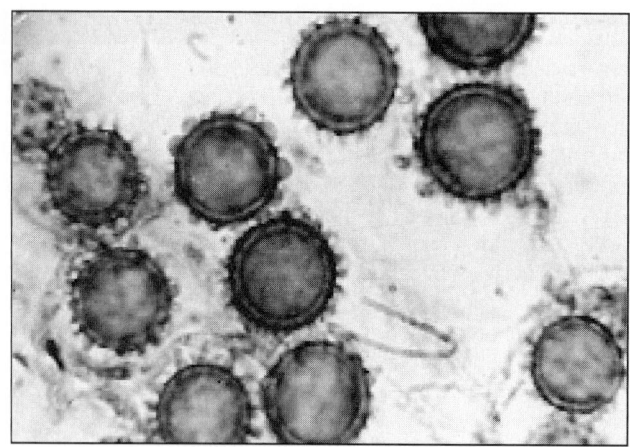

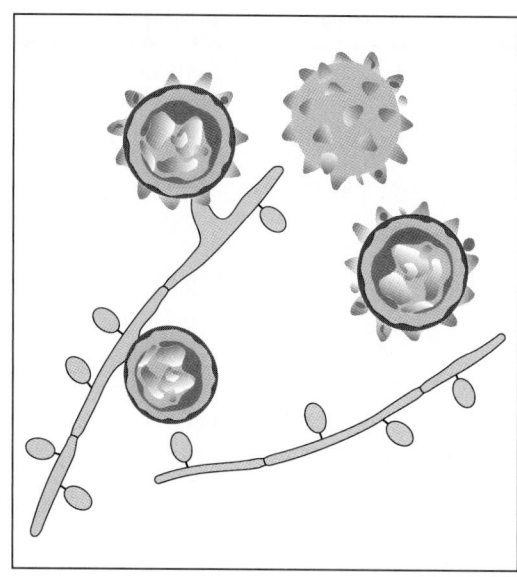

Figure 21-59 Illustrated in the photomicrograph and sketch is the mold form of *Histoplasma capsulatum* forming large, spherical, spiked macroconidia.

culture. The cultures need not be mature or have developed conidia for probe testing to be performed. Huffnagle and Gander[126] demonstrated 100% specificity and sensitivity in probing 95 mold-phase fungi, including 41 isolates of *H. capsulatum* and a variety of other molds. Using a chemiluminescent, acridinium ester-labeled, single-stranded DNA probe complementary to the rRNA of *H. capsulatum* mold forms (AccuProbe; Gene Probe, San Diego, CA), Padhye et al.[206] correctly identified 103 of 105 *H. capsulatum* cultures. Similarly, also using the AccuProbe assay, Hall et al.[109] correctly identified 53 of 54 isolates of *H. capsulatum,* and Stockman et al.[264] demonstrated 100% sensitivity and specificity in the study of 86 strains of *H. capsulatum* and 154 other nontarget fungi. The age of the culture, medium for isolation, and morphologic state did not affect the results, which indicates that an identification can be made before characteristic spores are produced.

The diagnosis of histoplasmosis may be made by identify-

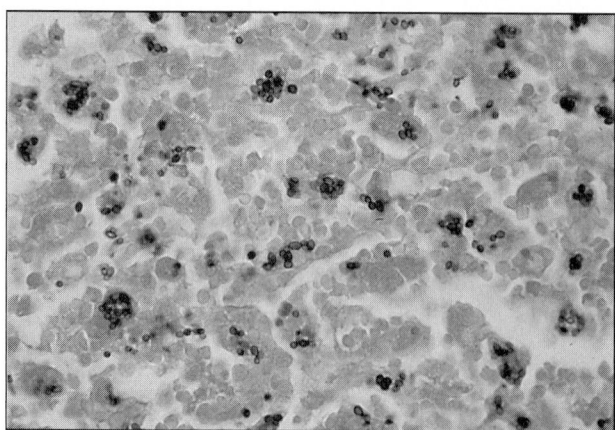

Figure 21-60 Photomicrograph of a tissue section revealing macrophages containing loose clusters of intracytoplasmic 2–3-μm diameter, black-staining pseudoencapsulated yeasts forms of *Histoplasma capsulatum* (H&E ×400, GMS stain).

ing the small, intracellular budding yeast cells in tissue sections or stained smears or by detecting antigen in body fluids. Blumenfeld et al.[25] were able to identify intracytoplasmic organisms in both Diff-Quik and Papanicolaou-stained smears of bronchoalveolar lavage fluid. Follow-up studies of tissue sections stained with methenamine silver revealed budding yeasts in an intracellular location, confirming that they were *H. capsulatum. H. capsulatum* antigen was detected in bronchoalveolar lavage fluid in 19 of 27 cases (70.3%) of pulmonary histoplasmosis studied by Wheat et al.[289]

DIAGNOSIS USING NONCULTURE TECHNIQUES

Molecular methods, particularly commercially available nucleic-acid probes, have been developed for the diagnosis of histoplasmosis. The time for the definitive identification of positive cultures has been reduced primarily because assays can be performed on mycelial elements, rather than waiting for the development of diagnostic spores. Research is in progress to detect *H. capsulatum* var. *capsulatum* DNA in body fluids and tissue sections, particularly to establish a definitive diagnosis of granulomatous disease when fungal stains fail to disclose diagnostic forms.[292]

Serologic tests for anti-*Histoplasma* antibodies are positive in over 90% of patients with cavitary or disseminated forms of histoplasmosis. These serologic tests, however, are less sensitive in immunosuppressed patients (50–80%), many of whom do not produce antibodies. Tests for antibody also have the disadvantage of a 4–6 week delay before a sufficiently high titer is achieved to be detected. *Histoplasma* antibodies may also be elevated in patients with blastomycosis, coccidioidomycosis, and paracoccidioidomycosis.[291]

The CF test using yeast and mycelial antigens is more sensitive than the ID test. In acute pulmonary histoplasmosis, the CF test is positive at titers of at least 1:8 in 90% of patients, M bands are present in about 76%, and H bands in 23%.[67] Titers in the range of 1:8–1:16 may be residual from past infection. A single titer of 1:32 or higher or a fourfold increase is diagnostic of active histoplasmosis. Immunodiffusion is sufficiently insensitive that other serologic tests are recommended.

Radioimmunoassay and enzyme immunoassay also cannot be recommended, although antibodies may be detected sooner and in a higher proportion of patients. These assays are poorly standardized and difficult to quantitate and interpret. Specificity is also low, with relatively high rates of false positivity in persons with other fungal or mycobacterial infections.[291]

Antigen detection provides a useful test in the diagnosis of pulmonary histoplasmosis in patients with AIDS and in the assessment of the efficacy of therapy in cases of progressive disease. In a study of 226 patients 18 years old or younger in whom *H. capsulatum* antigen was detected in urine specimens by radioimmunoassay, Fojtasek et al.[84] found that 85% had disseminated disease and 15% had self-limited pulmonary disease, when at least one other corroborating standard test was positive.

The several clinical manifestations of histoplasmosis are presented in Clinical Correlation Box 21-7.

Sporothrix schenckii and Sporotrichosis

Sporothrix schenckii is a fungus that is found worldwide in soil and in decaying vegetative matter, particularly plants, wood splinters, and rosebush thorns. It is the causative agent of sporotrichosis, a chronic infection of humans and animals. It also may be carried by certain wild and domestic animals and by rodents. Humans become infected when the organism penetrates the skin of individuals handling contaminated substances. The infection is characterized by the development of nodular lesions of the cutaneous and subcutaneous tissues, often with lymphatic involvement (lymphocutaneous disease). Systemic spread may occur with bone, muscle, central nervous system, and pulmonary involvement.

Certain occupations place workers at increased risk for infection. An outbreak of sporotrichosis occurred at a tree nursery in Florida, as reported by Hajjeh et al.[108] Lymphocutaneous sporotrichosis developed in 9 of 65 (14%) of workers involved in the production of sphagnum moss topiaries. The risk was directly related to the duration of working with sphagnum moss, in particular with the task of filling topiaries, and in individuals with less gardening experience. Those wearing gloves were protected.

An interesting outbreak was reported by Dooley et al.[65] Within a 5-week period, five patients living in Oklahoma presented with cutaneous sporotrichosis, four of whom had maintained hay bales in a Halloween haunted house. A fifth patient apparently contracted the disease while visiting the house. Thus, contact with hay, particularly when harvested from the Midwestern United States, may represent yet another risk factor.

A high area of endemicity for sporotrichosis has been recently reported by Pappas et al.[210] In a remote area of the south central highlands of Peru, 238 cases of culture-proven sporotrichosis were observed in a period of 3 years between 1995 and 1997. The incidence of sporotrichosis in this region was calculated at between 48 to 60 cases per 100,000 persons, with the highest incidence among children aged 7–14 years. The skin of the face was the most commonly affected site. The disease was clinically confined to the skin and subcutaneous tissue in all patients.

LABORATORY PRESENTATION

The growth of *Sporothrix schenckii* in culture is usually within 3–5 days at 30°C, although smooth, yeastlike colonies may develop as early as at 36–48 hours on 5% sheep blood agar incubated at 35°C. The colonies are usually smooth and may become tough and wrinkled or folded. A delicate, dark, fuzzy, aerial mycelium may develop when the colonies mature. The color is initially gray-white, but may turn buff, brown, or brown-black as the colony matures (Color Plate 21-5G). The colonies become distinctly yeastlike when incubated at 35–37°C, and may turn dark brown or black on maturity (Color Plate 21-5H).

The identification can be made microscopically by observing in the mold form delicate, hyaline, septate hyphae from which are borne oval, hyaline, smooth conidia measuring 2–4 μm in diameter. They are supported by a delicate, hairlike conidiophore, arranged either laterally along the side of the hyphae; or, more characteristically, in daisylike clusters from the tip of a straight, delicate conidiophore (Fig. 21-61). By exacting focus of the microscope and using an oil-immersion objective, it is possible to observe the characteristic hairlike attachments between the conidia and the conidiophore (from which the species name is derived). *Sporothrix cyanescens* has an appearance similar to *S. schenckii*, except that secondary conidia are formed, appearing as budding yeast cells borne from the tips of the primary conidia. The publication by Sigler et al.[255] includes excellent photomicrographs illustrating this microscopic feature.

The yeast forms are 2–4 μm in diameter and tend to be oval or elliptical, often with a single bud (Fig. 21-62). Most helpful in making the microscopic identification of *S. schenckii* yeast forms is the observation of cigar-shaped forms measuring 3 by 10 μm. These yeast forms may be difficult to see in stained human tissue sections, and animal inoculation may be required to demonstrate them. A methenamine silver–stained section of a subcutaneous granuloma that is packed with elliptical yeast cells is illustrated in Figure 21-63. Note the cigar-shaped daughter buds from a few of the mother cells.

DIAGNOSIS USING NONCULTURE TECHNIQUES

The application of serologic techniques have proven to be of minimal benefit in the diagnosis of sporotrichosis. Latex agglutination tests have been used in the past with limited success, particularly in the diagnosis of primary skin infections, in which results are usually negative. Agglutination titers of 1:80 or higher have been helpful in the diagnosis of active, extracutaneous infections.[56]

The clinical manifestations of sporotrichosis are presented in Clinical Correlation Box 21-8.

Paracoccidioides immitis and Paracoccidioidomycosis

Paracoccidioidomycosis is a progressive subacute to chronic systemic granulomatous fungal infection caused by the thermally dimorphic fungus, *Paracoccidioidomyces brasiliensis*. The mycelial form of this fungus resides in the soil, and pulmonary infection develops in humans by inhalation

CLINICAL CORRELATION BOX 21-7 Histoplasmosis

Most cases of histoplasmosis resolve after an acute pulmonary illness of varying degrees of severity, characterized by fever, headache, chills, cough, and chest pain. Underlying pneumonia and enlargement of the mediastinal lymph nodes are often seen. In less than 1% of cases, a chronic pulmonary form may develop, characterized by persistent cough, low-grade fever, and occasional episodes of hemoptysis. Cavitary lesions may develop in adults, or one or more thick, laminated, calcified "histoplasmomas" may be seen by x-ray examination. Mediastinal granuloma formation followed by fibrosing mediastinitis and esophagitis are rare complications, but cases have been reported.[175] Dyspnea, hemoptysis, postobstructive pneumonia, and superior vena cava obstruction are associated complications. The intense fibrosis found in these cases renders surgery difficult. A rare complication of pleural effusion and pericardial fibrosis has been reported by Kilburn and McKinsey.[141] Constrictive pericarditis later developed in this patient, confirmed at autopsy. Because *H. capsulatum* is an obligate intracellular organism residing in macrophages of the reticuloendothelial system, varying degrees of hepatomegaly, splenomegaly, and lymphadenopathy may be seen in cases of acute and chronic disseminated disease, which usually occurs in immunosuppressed hosts.

Progressive Disseminated Histoplasmosis

Progressive disseminated histoplasmosis is often an AIDS-defining illness, being the first manifestation in 50–75% of AIDS patients with histoplasmosis.[244,290] The clinical manifestations are fever, fatigue, and weight loss, the latter often presenting as a wasting disease.[107] Nightingale et al.[196] found a 4% prevalence of histoplasmosis among 980 AIDS patients seen in Dallas, Texas; examination of the peripheral smear and bone marrow established the diagnosis in 88% of these patients. In addition, Huang et al.[125] report five cases of disseminated histoplasmosis in patients with AIDS; all had fungemia, and three died within 4 weeks after the diagnosis was established.

The presence of AIDS typically renders histoplasmosis refractory to therapy. Kurtin et al.[151] reviewed bone marrow and peripheral blood specimens in 13 patients with AIDS and disseminated histoplasmosis. Anemia, leukopenia, and thrombocytopenia were found in 12, 10, and 7 patients, respectively. Circulating organisms in blood smears or buffy-coat preparations were seen in five patients, usually associated with the presence of circulating normoblasts and severe absolute monocytopenia. The marrow specimens revealed one of four morphologic patterns:

- no morphologic evidence of infection
- discrete granulomas
- lymphohistiocytic aggregates
- diffuse macrophage infiltrates.

Lysis centrifugation for recovery of organism from blood cultures and examination of the bone marrow, peripheral blood smear, and respiratory secretions may make the diagnosis.[190]

Other organ systems involved with histoplasmosis in patients with AIDS as recorded in the recent medical literature include the central nervous system, which may take the form of chronic meningitis, cerebral or spinal cord mass lesions simulating neoplasms, or encephalitis and an unusual case of sinusitis reported by Butt and Carreon.[13,33,288]

Wheat et al.[288] found CNS manifestations in 10–20% of patients with disseminated histoplasmosis, and the organism may be the cause of chronic meningitis with no other evidence of dissemination in select patients. Cerebral or spinal cord mass lesions resembling neoplasms or abscesses and encephalitis were the most common forms of presentation in this series.

Gastrointestinal Tract

Histoplasmosis of the gastrointestinal tract, usually of the small bowel, may present as ulcers or as a mass, often mimicking inflammatory bowel disease or carcinoma.[41] The gastrointestinal tract is secondarily involved in 70–90% of cases of disseminated histoplasmosis, although primary enteric disease per se is infrequently encountered.[266] Jain et al.[129] report a recent case of a 67-year-old man who presented with chronic diarrhea that did not respond to the conventional treatment, including detection of *Clostridium difficile*. He was found to have isolated colonic histoplasmosis infection, which was treated with itraconazole.

Cases of histoplasmosis of the oropharynx have also been reported, in which lesions may be mistaken for carcinoma on initial presentation,[120] particularly when the vocal cords are involved. Sataloff et al.,[245] in a review of the literature, found fewer than 100 cases of histoplasmosis presenting as laryngeal carcinoma, since the first case was reported in 1952. Perhaps of more significance, Economopoulou et al.[69] reviewed 20 case reports from the literature of oral histoplasmosis in HIV-infected patients, in many cases of which the oral lesions appear to be the primary or only manifestation of disease.

Cutaneous Histoplasmosis

Cutaneous lesions may be the initial presentation for histoplasmosis in about 10% of cases and may serve as a marker for AIDS. Erythematous or hyperpigmented papules, pustules, folliculitis, eczematous changes, erythema multiforme, and rosacea-like rashes are the more common skin manifestations.[287] Chalub et al.[38] reported four patients with disseminated histoplasmosis in AIDS patients. Multiple small (up to 3 mm in diameter) erythematous maculopapules on the extremities, face, and trunk, often centered around hair follicles were observed. Histologically, perivascular infiltrates with conspicuous leukocytoclasis, the lack of a macrophage response, and absence of granulomas and organisms lying free in the dermis, intraneurally and in skin appendages, were distinct differences from the presentations seen in patients who did not have AIDS.

CLINICAL CORRELATION BOX 21-7 *Continued*

Genitourinary Histoplasmosis

Although genitourinary tract fungal infections are more commonly seen in blastomycosis, cases of histoplasmosis have been reported, particularly in patients with AIDS. Kahn and Thommes[132] reported a case of massive granulomatous orchitis and epididymitis with caseous necrosis. Two additional current cases have been reported by Friskel et al.[87]

Ocular Histoplasmosis

The ocular histoplasmosis syndrome has been reviewed by Ciulla et al.[45] The classic clinical triad includes discrete atrophic choroidal scars in the macula or midperiphery known as histo spots, peripapillary atrophy, and choroidal neovascularization. Severe loss of central vision is a major complication.

Septicemia

Although septicemia with fungal agents is uncommon, the opportunity to establish an early diagnosis may be missed if the blood-culture techniques being used are inadequate. Paya et al.[212] found that the use of the lysis centrifuged blood-culture tubes was the optimal technique for recovering *H. capsulatum* yeast forms from the blood in suspected cases of disseminated disease, significantly increasing the yield of positive cultures and shortening the time of recovery. The superiority of this system is also supported by the observations of Murray,[190] who in a study of 182 fungal isolates of all types, found that *H. capsulatum* was recovered only in the lysis-centrifugation system. Early diagnosis is important, as dissemination can be rapidly progressive and fatal in patients with AIDS.

of the small (4-μm diameter) conidia or skin infections by direct inoculation of spore-contaminated dirt. In South America, 80% of cases have been reported from Brazil; followed in order of incidence by case reports from Colombia and Venezuela; endemic areas also exist in southern Mexico and in all countries in Central America except Belize and Nicaragua.[32]

The overall prevalence rate of paracoccidioidomycosis is difficult to derive. Although estimates of a million or more cases have been made, many cases either are not reported or remain undiagnosed. Botteon et al.[28] have published the analysis of a recent study of two groups of blood donors. One group consisted of donors living in a rural area where paracoccidioidomycosis is endemic, the other from a group of urban residents residing in Sao Paulo. The results showed that 21% of 700 samples drawn from those living in the

endemic rural areas, and 0.9% of 350 urban samples were serologically positive. Thus, with a population of approximately 150 million, even if the lower urban prevalence rate of paracoccidioidomycosis is used, well over 1 million residents of Brazil alone have been infected.

Countries in the Caribbean islands, the Guyanas, and Chile have been free of reported disease. In endemic areas, most cases occur in and around humid forested regions. The disease most frequently involves adults over 30 years of age, is rare in children, and occurs in males more often than females, with an overall ratio of 15:1. Although the majority of patients are agriculturists, cases have been reported in individuals with rare direct exposure to soil and vegetation as indicated by the report cited above. Whites are more prone to infections than Native Americans; more severe infections tend to develop in immigrants coming to endemic areas.[32]

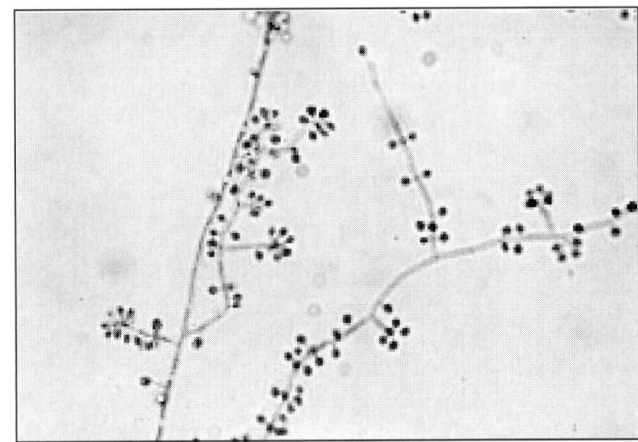

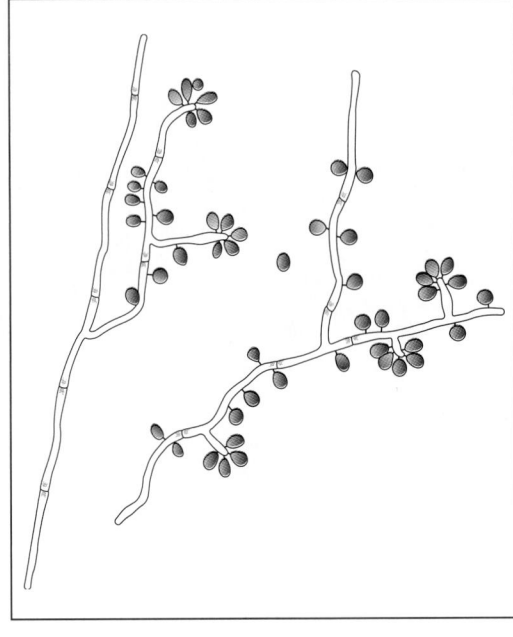

Figure 21-61 Photomicrograph and sketch of the mold form of *Sporothrix schenckii,* illustrating the delicate hyphae and daisylike clustering of small, oval conidia from the sides or the tips of straight conidiophores.

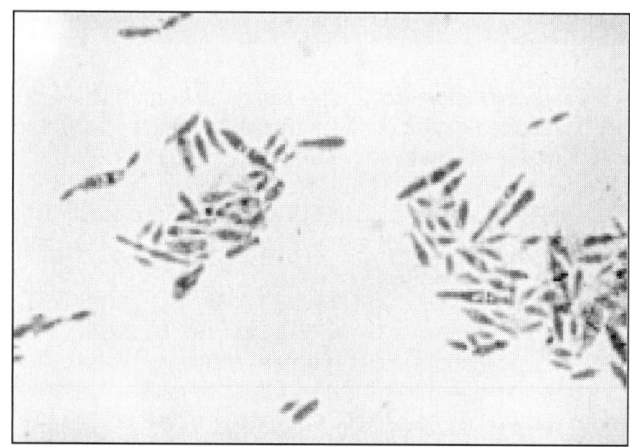

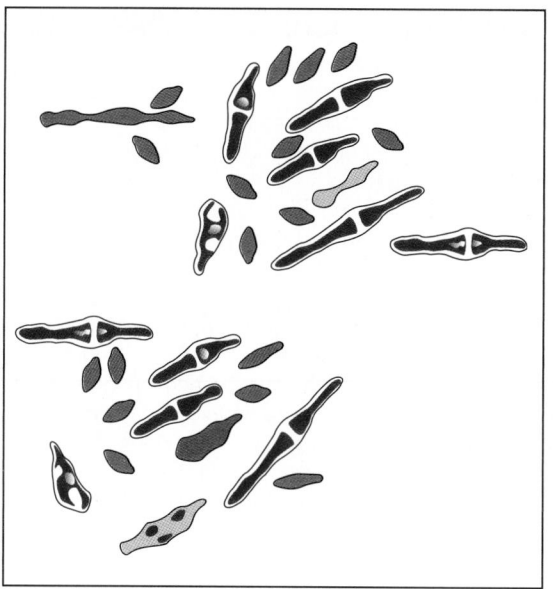

Figure 21-62 Photomicrograph and sketch of the yeast form of *Sporothrix schenckii,* revealing elongated, two-celled yeast cells, many with a "cigar body" form.

LABORATORY PRESENTATION

The colonies are similar in appearance to those of *Blastomyces dermatitidis.* They are slow-growing at 30°C, requiring 10–20 days to mature, are gray-white, and have a delicate silky or hairlike mycelium.

When incubated at 25–30°C, *P. brasiliensis* grows very slowly over 10–30 days as a silky, white to gray-tan mold. The identification and differentiation from other similar-appearing molds can be made by microscopically observing the delicate, hyaline, septate hyphae that make up the background mycelium. Characteristic oval, nonpigmented, 2–4 μm conidia are borne singly from short, slender conidiophores directly from the hyphae, in a "lollipop" fashion, similar in appearance to those produced by *Blastomyces dermatitidis* (Fig. 21-64).

The identification can be confirmed by converting the mold to the yeast form, which is accomplished by inoculating a small portion of the mold colony to enriched brain-heart infusion agar. Conversion to the yeast form is slow. The mother yeast cells of *P. brasiliensis* observed in culture are 6–15 μm in diameter and appear similar to those of *B. dermatitidis;* except that multiple narrow-necked buds of the former are easy to distinguish from the single, broad-based budding forms seen for the latter.

In the infective, or 37°C "body temperature" form, *Paracoccidioides brasiliensis* exists as a yeast. Therefore, the diagnosis of paracoccidioidomycosis can be most quickly established by demonstrating directly in clinical materials the characteristic 10–30 μm spherical, thick-walled yeast cells, with multiple daughter buds, each attached by a narrow-necked bud (likened to a "mariner's wheel") (Fig. 21-65). These yeast forms may be best observed in KOH mounts, either directly or using calcofluor white or immunofluorescence reagents. In some cases, the budding daughter cells may form short chains. In tissue sections, the background inflammation is usually granulomatous, admixed with varying concentrations of polymorphonuclear leukocytes. The diagnosis is established by finding the multibudding yeast forms described above, best seen in PAS- or GMS-stained sections.

DIAGNOSIS USING NONCULTURE TECHNIQUES

The exoantigen test, recently refined by Camargo et al.,[35] is a means for confirming the culture identification of unknown isolates. Indirect immunofluorescence techniques, immunoenzymatic assays, and, most recently, PCR amplification tests have been used by many investigators to establish the diagnosis of paracoccidioidomycosis. Current immunodiagnostic approaches to the diagnosis of paracoccidioidomycosis have been reviewed by Brummer et al.[32] Elevated serum levels of specific IgG antibodies can be detected for at least 1 year after infection. Elevated IgM antibody levels are usually not seen except in cases of extensive lymph node involvement.

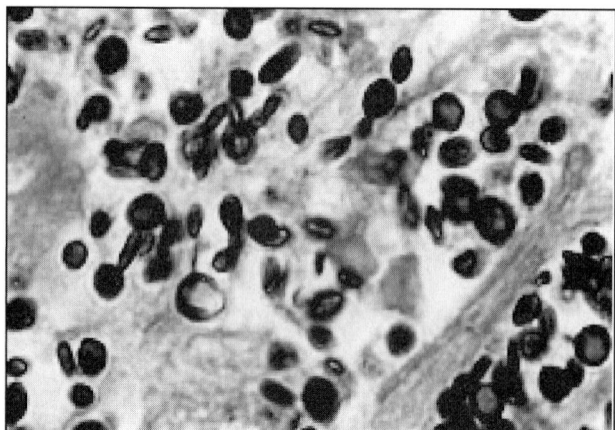

Figure 21-63 Photomicrograph of a cutaneous biopsy from a case of sporotrichosis revealing numerous spherical to oval yeast cells of *Sporothrix schenckii,* some of which show elongated, two-celled cigar-shaped buds (high-power, methenamine silver stain).

CLINICAL CORRELATION BOX 21-8 Sporotrichosis

In the United States, subcutaneous fungal infections are most commonly caused by *Sporothrix schenckii*.[11] The most common form of sporotrichosis is lymphocutaneous. The appearance of a small, red, painless pustule on an extremity, together with the appearance of multiple, linearly placed secondary pustular or ulcerating lesions along the proximal lymphatics is sufficient to suspect the diagnosis. The primary pustule may slowly enlarge, ulcerate, and discharge a small amount of serosanguineous exudate. Varying degrees of cellulitis with swelling and redness of the surrounding subcutaneous tissue may be observed. The secondary satellite lesions present initially as verrucous, erythematoid plaques or scaly patches, often developing into ulcers that also exude purulent material. Diagnosis is often delayed because associated secondary bacterial colonization may be mistaken for the primary infectious agent. Bacterial superinfections may confuse the gross appearance.

In cases of progressive disease, the infection may spread to joints, tendon sheaths, bursae, bone, and muscle.[300] Purvis et al.[227] report a case of bilateral polyarticular arthritis of the wrists and elbows. Although arthritis is an uncommon manifestation of sporotrichosis, this case points to the broadened spectrum of disease that may be caused by this fungus.[42]

Sporotrichal arthritis is an uncommon disease, with only 51 cases reported in the English literature. Howell and Toohey[123] report the findings of 13 patients with sporotrichal arthritis who had been treated in Wichita-area hospitals since 1979. The typical presentation was an afebrile patient with a mildly swollen warm joint without erythema. Seventeen joints were involved, including 10 knees, 3 interphalangeal joints, 1 elbow, 1 midtarsal, 1 intercarpal, and 1 metatarsophalangeal joint. Most of the patients were middle-aged men, and significant alcohol intake was noted in 77% of the patients. Wang et al.[283] report the case of a patient with a prepatellar bursa infected with *Sporothrix schenckii*. The infection persisted despite itraconazole therapy, and cure was achieved only after surgical excision of the bursa.

Primary pulmonary sporotrichosis is rare. However, England and Hochholzer[75] reported eight cases of primary pulmonary sporotrichosis in patients following inhalation of airborne conidia, an otherwise rare occurrence. Cough, sputum production, and low-grade fever are the usual presenting symptoms.

In patients infected with the human immunodeficiency virus, sporotrichosis may have atypical presentations, with the disease tending to become widespread and disseminated. Cutaneous disease beginning as localized lesions may disseminate to other skin sites, with dissemination to the meninges in one reported case.[64] Diagnosis may be difficult when sporotrichosis initially presents as fungemia and disseminated disease.[9] Although localized sporotrichosis is an innocuous disorder that responds well to therapy, these authors found in immunocompromised hosts that the disease is potentially life-threatening and often is difficult to treat, requiring prolonged therapy with potentially toxic medications such as amphotericin B. Progressive infection was most common in individuals with CD4 counts less than 100 cells/mm³.

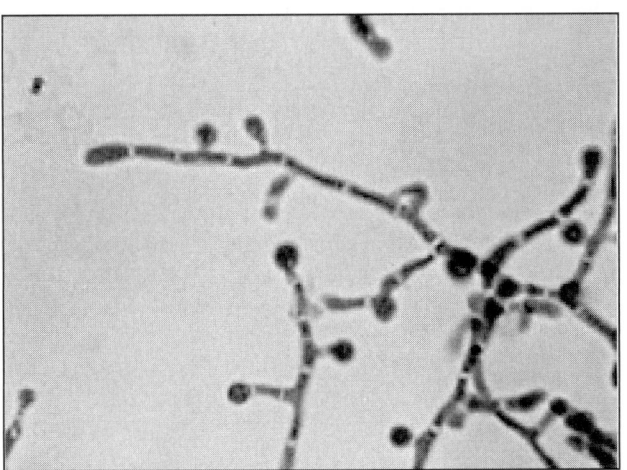

Figure 21-64 Photomicrograph of the mold form of *Paracoccidioides brasiliensis,* illustrating the small, smooth, spherical conidia borne laterally and terminally from short conidiophores derived from septate hyphae.

Mendes-Giannini et al.[179] demonstrated IgG-, IgA-, and IgM-specific antibodies to a 43-kDa antigen of *Paracoccidioides brasiliensis* in patients with paracoccidioidomycosis, and further demonstrated that a lowering of the titers during a course of treatment was correlated with an improvement in symptoms. Gomez et al.,[96] using a monoclonal antibody directed against the yeast form of *Paracoccidioides brasiliensis*, were able to develop an inhibition enzyme-linked immunosorbent assay (ELISA) test capable of detecting small quantities of circulating antigen in the serum of patients with active disease. Of 46 patients with paracoccidioidomycosis, 37 tested positive (80.4%). Sandu et al.[241] have developed a 14-base DNA probe specific for the 5′ terminus of fungal 28S ribosomal gene sequences of *P. brasiliensis*. Applying a uniform diagnostic protocol, consisting of common cell lysis and DNA purification procedures followed by PCR amplification, these authors demonstrated selective identification of *P. brasiliensis* from 47 other species of fungi representing 25 genera.

The results of these studies provide several alternative nonculture approaches in establishing the diagnosis of paracoccidioidomycosis.

The clinical manifestations of paracoccidioidomycosis are presented in Clinical Correlation Box 21-9.

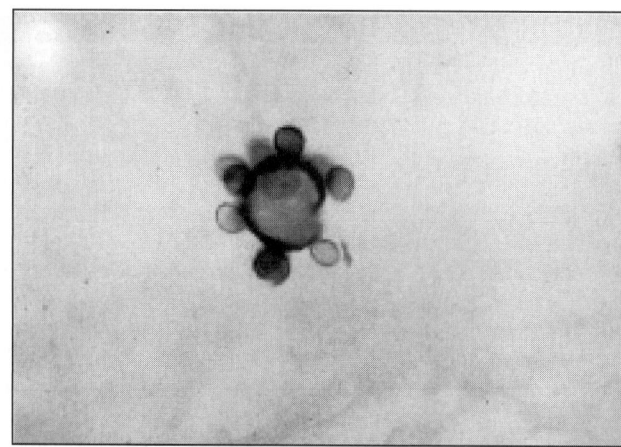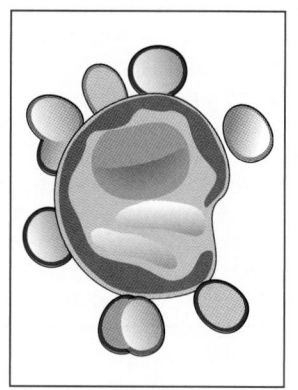

A   B

Figure 21-65 Photomicrograph and sketch of the yeast form of *Paracoccidioides brasiliensis,* illustrating the large central body giving rise to multiple buds, forming a ''mariner's wheel.''

Dematiaceous Fungi
Agents of Phaeohyphomycosis

In contrast to the hyaline group of fungi, a second large group of rapidly growing saprophytic molds produce a melaninlike pigment resulting in darkly pigmented hyphae, visually recognized as dark gray or black colonies, both on the surface and on the reverse side. The term phaeohyphomyces (Greek *phaeo* = dusky, gray) has been applied to this dematiaceous group of fungi.

The concept of ''phaeohyphomycosis'' was first proposed by Ajello et al.[6] in 1986 to ''cover all infections of a cutaneous, subcutaneous and systemic nature caused by hyphomycetous fungi that develop in the host tissues in the form of dark-walled, dematiaceous septate mycelial elements.'' Such dematiaceous mycelial elements are characteristically accompanied by granulomatous inflammatory reactions when observed in tissue sections. Thus, as originally described, ''phaeohyphomycosis'' was a term used to describe a histopathologic entity rather than representing any particular clinical disease or fungal species as identified in laboratory cultures. Nonetheless, the term *phaeohyphomycosis* currently applies to several clinical entities: sinusitis, keratitis, endocarditis, and pneumonia, among others. De Hoog[60] counsels that this term should be regarded strictly as an artificial descriptor, without biologic significance. Yet, many mycologists now recommend that the generic term be replaced with reports such as ''keratomycosis caused by *Bipolaris* species'' or ''mycetoma caused by *Phialophora richardsiae.*''[233] In this presentation, the agents of chromomycosis and mycetoma will be included under the general category of phaeohyphomycosis, referring in broader terms to the dark, dematiaceous fungi.

LABORATORY PRESENTATION

This dematiaceous group of fungi can be suspected in culture as agents of phaeohyphomycosis by observing the dark gray, brown, or black, wooly, hairy, or velvety surface with a smoky gray to jet black pigmentation on the reverse side (other fungi may produce black conidia that darkly pigment only the surface of the colony). Because the colony morphology is not distinctive among this group of fungi, microscopic examination is necessary to make a genus/species identification. The agents of chromomycosis and mycetoma are generally slower-growing and the colonies tend to be small. Representative colonies of the more rapidly growing, saprophytic dematiaceous molds are shown in Color Plate 21-3*A–D.*

Microscopically, the dematiaceous molds have a dark yellow-brown mycelium composed of uniform hyphae with parallel walls and distinct septations. The fungi included in this group of rapidly growing molds are characterized by the formation of darkly staining macroconidia. The genera of medical importance include:

Alternaria species
Ulocladium species
Stemphylium species
Epicoccum species
Bipolaris species
Drechslera species
Curvularia species
Exserohilum species
Nigrospora species
Phoma species
Chaetomium species

The identification of these fungi can be simplified by considering the following three subgroups based on the morphology of the macroconidia:

- Those in which the macroconidia are multicelled and divided by both longitudinal and transverse septa, called ''muriform'' (like a masonry wall);
- Those producing multicelled macroconidia divided by transverse septa only;
- Those belonging to a miscellaneous group in which the macroconidia are either single-celled or that manifest other specific modes of conidiation.

Macroconidia With Transverse and Longitudinal Septa (Muriform)

The genera of fungi of medical importance included in this group are:

CLINICAL CORRELATION BOX 21-9 Paracoccidioidomycosis

On inhalation of spore-contaminated dust, the small (4-μm diameter) conidia reach the distal portion of the pulmonary parenchyma, where they develop into yeast cells that may be confined locally, or where they may propagate and disseminate to distal organs in cases of progressive disseminated disease. In a competent host, local growth is retarded and the infection may end without development of a lesion. When symptomatic, Brummer et al.[32] have divided paracoccidioidomycosis into two general categories: 1) juvenile form, acute or subacute, and 2) chronic form, adult-type.

Juvenile Form, Acute or Subacute

The juvenile form of disease includes only 3–5% of all cases, primarily involving children or young adults, the majority of whom are immunosuppressed. The course of disease is relatively rapid (weeks to months), marked by diffuse involvement of the reticuloendothelial system. Hepatosplenomegaly, lymphadenopathy, and bone marrow hyperplasia are common clinical presentations. Dysfunction of the bone marrow may be so severe as to simulate a lymphoproliferative disorder.[164] Biopsies of the involved organs or tissues often reveal a large number of actively proliferating yeast cells, in the absence of granuloma formation. In this form of the disease, the lungs are seldom involved, although organisms may be detected in respiratory secretions. Mesenteric lymph nodes may on occasion become so enlarged as to cause bowel obstruction. Prognosis of the juvenile form of the disease is poor.

Chronic Form, Adult-type

Approximately 90% of patients have this form of disease, which occurs most commonly in adult men. The disease is slowly progressive, tends to remain confined primarily to the lungs, and may take months or years to become fully established. The lungs are involved in over 90% of infected patients, and in many cases the lungs are the sole site of infection. The pulmonary lesions as seen on x-ray films are nodular, infiltrative, fibrotic, or cavitary and are preferentially localized to the lower lobes of the lungs.[164] Cough, expectoration of sputum, and shortness of breath are the common symptoms, often accompanied by low-grade intermittent fever, weight loss, and anorexia. The pulmonary picture often mimics tuberculosis. The chronic disease may be mild, moderate, or severe, depending on the patient's general condition and immune status; severe fibrosis leading to chronic obstructive pulmonary disease and cor pulmonale are the fatal sequelae.

Brummer et al.[32] cite several case reports of extrapulmonary involvement, including the eyes, the central nervous system, bone, and the genital tract. Several reports also appear in the more recent literature, commonly from South America. Sant' Anna et al.[242] review the cases of seven patients with laryngeal disease. All these patients were middle-aged males, predominantly farm workers. Dysphonia, dysphagia, dyspnea, and cough were the main presenting symptoms. The first diagnostic impression was carcinoma in each of these patients.

Of most recent concern is the upsurge of oral involvement, and deep mycoses of the mouth.[8,94] Almeida et al.[8] report that oral fungal infections (mycoses) have come into particular prominence since the advent of HIV infections, as well as the phenomenal increase in world travel, with increased exposure to infections endemic in the tropics. Almeida et al. further report on 21 Argentinian patients living in the province of Corrientes who presented with oral manifestations of *Paracoccidioides brasiliensis*. All patients except one had detectable pulmonary involvement. The long-term administration of itraconazole provided for cure in these cases. The authors emphasize the need for early diagnosis and adequate therapy to prevent extensive tissue destruction. Long-term follow-up also is mandatory, as the recurrence rate is high.

The clinical manifestation encountered among the 27 AIDS patients reported by Goldani and Sugar[95] ran the spectrum from indolent infection to a rapidly progressive course. Disseminated disease was the most common form, with lung, skin, and lymph nodes being the most common sites of infection. Prolonged fever, lymphadenopathy, hepatosplenomegaly, and cutaneous lesions were most commonly encountered; in fact, they represent a cadre of symptoms that may serve as a marker for AIDS. The diagnosis is best made by direct examination and culture of sputum specimens, skin biopsies, and lymph-node aspirates. As mentioned before, PCR assays of these specimens promises to greatly enhance the chances for making a diagnosis. About half of the patients in this series died despite aggressive antifungal therapy.

Severo et al.[252] report a case of involvement of the male genital tract in a native of Brazil, including a review of 18 additional cases gathered from the Brazilian literature. Manns et al.[172] discuss a 59-year-old man who presented with paracoccidioidomycosis more than 15 years after leaving South America. Practitioners throughout the world must keep this infection in mind when evaluating a patient with appropriate travel history who has pulmonary, mucosal, or cutaneous manifestations suggestive of this disease, along with weight loss and other constitutional symptoms.

Alternaria species
Ulocladium species
Stemphylium species
Epicoccum species

ALTERNARIA SPECIES

The formation of short chains of large, smooth-walled, multicelled, macroconidia separated by both cross and longi-tudinal septa (**muriform**) are characteristic of *Alternaria* spp. The macroconidia are shaped like drumsticks, with the elongated beak of one conidium butting against the rounded, blunt end of the next (Fig. 21-66).

ULOCLADIUM SPECIES

Ulocladium spp. also produce muriform macroconidia; however, they are more spherical than those of *Alternaria*

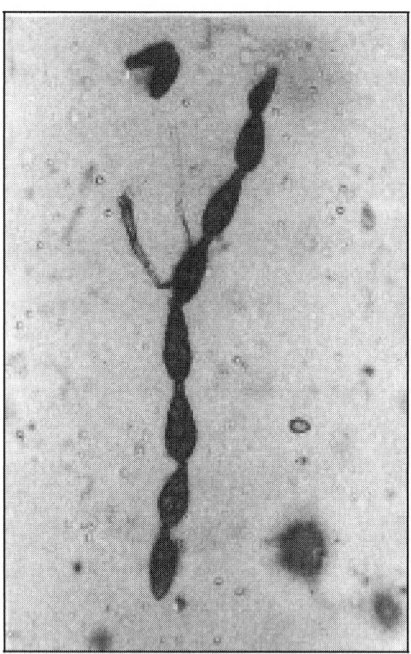

Figure 21-66 Photomicrograph of a short chain of dark-staining, muriform macroconidia characteristic of *Alternaria* species.

spp., do not arrange in chains, and are borne from short, twisted "bent-knee," or **geniculate,** conidiophores (Fig. 21-67). This **sympodial derivation** of the macroconidia is an important identifying characteristic.

STEMPHYLIUM SPECIES

Muriform macroconidia that appear similar to those of *Ulocladium* spp. are produced; however, they are borne singly at the apex of a short, straight **nongeniculate conidiophore.** The macroconidia are slightly swollen and rounded at the tip, which together with the supporting conidiophore,

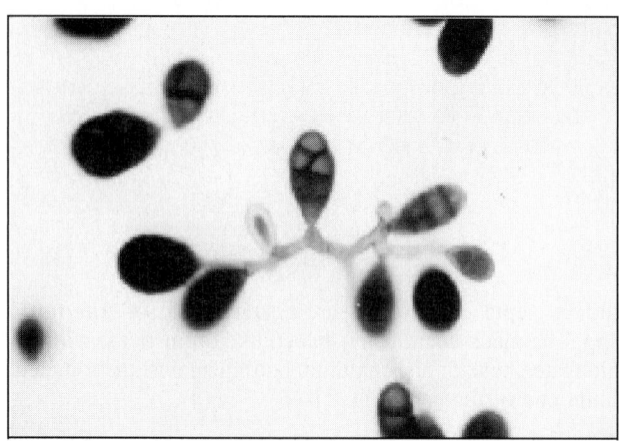

Figure 21-67 Photomicrograph of dark-staining, muriform macroconidia derived from geniculate conidiophores, characteristic of *Ulocladium* species.

has the appearance of a "**bale of cotton on a stick**" (Fig. 21-68).

EPICOCCUM SPECIES

The hyphae typically form focal repeated branching and rebranching of certain threads, forming masses known as **sporodochia.** Short conidiophores arise from these masses, bearing multicelled, muriform, spherical to slightly club-shaped macroconidia, that may be roughened on the surface, giving a blackish wartlike appearance (Fig. 21-69).

Macroconidia With Transverse Septa

BIPOLARIS SPECIES

The distinguishing feature of *Bipolaris* spp. is the production of multicelled, elliptical to oval, thick-walled macroconidia with smooth surfaces, borne from conidiophores that have knee-like bends (**geniculate**) in a **sympodial** arrangement (Fig. 21-70). The designation *Bipolaris* is derived from the property of producing germ tubes that **arise from both end cells of the macroconidia** in parallel with the long axis of the cell (when examined in direct water or saline mounts of the conidia are incubated at 25°C for 8–24 hours).

DRECHSLERA SPECIES

Drechslera spp. also produce cylindrical, multicelled macroconidia from geniculate conidiophores, indistinguishable from those of *Bipolaris* spp. The conidia have nonprotruding, rounded contours at the base cell. In saline mounts, a **single germ tube** derived midway between the base of the conidium and the septum and **extending at right angles to the long axis** is a key identifying feature. In practice, most clinical isolates having the conidia so described will belong to the genus *Bipolaris*.

CURVULARIA SPECIES

The macroconidia of *Curvularia* spp. are easy to recognize, having four to five cells separated by transverse septa, borne **sympodially** from twisted conidiophores. The **center cells grow more rapidly** and are larger than those at the ends, resulting in the characteristic curved or "**boomerang**" appearance (Fig. 21-71).

EXSEROHILUM SPECIES

The conidia of *Exserohilum* spp. are similar to those of *Bipolaris* spp., except that they are longer, pencil-shaped, have more cells, and characteristically have an **extended, prominent protruding hilum** from the hilar cell (Fig. 21-72).

Macroconidia Borne Singly or Via Special Conidiation

The genera of the dematiaceous molds included in this group are:

Nigrospora species
Phoma species
Chaetomium species

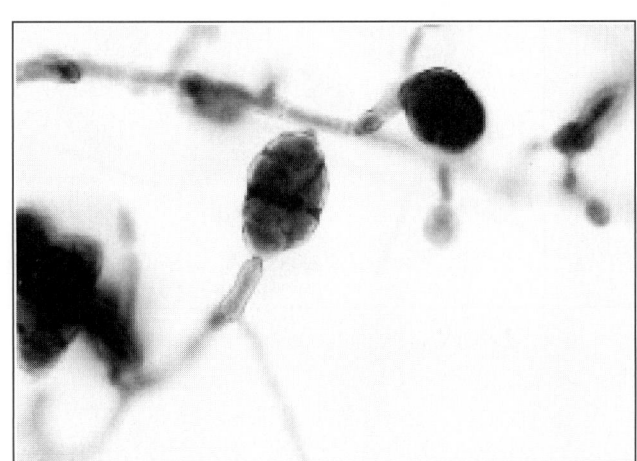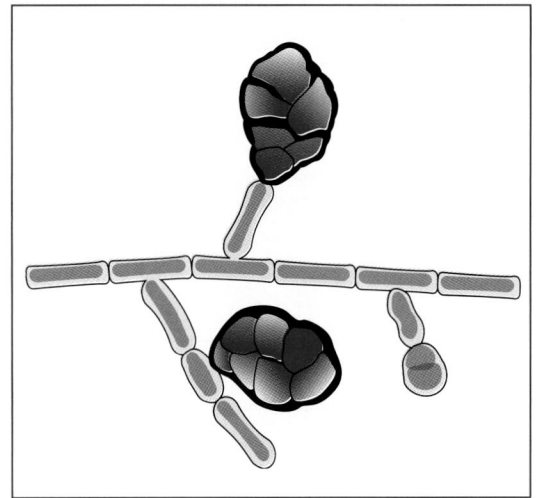

Figure 21-68 Photomicrograph and sketch of muriform macroconidia characteristically supported on the tip of a short, straight conidiophore, ''bale of cotton on a stick,'' characteristic of *Stemphylium* species.

NIGROSPORA SPECIES

The colonies of *Nigrospora* spp. are rapidly growing and cottony; initially they are dirty white, but turn gray with maturity as the vegetative hyphae become pigmented. The reverse of the colony also becomes darkly pigmented. Microscopically, the conidia are solitary, large, subglobose, smooth and jet black, and borne from the tips of inflated, urn-shaped, conidiophores (Fig. 21-73).

PHOMA SPECIES

The colonies of *Phoma* spp. are buff to dark brown, spreading over the surface with an indistinct outer margin. The con-

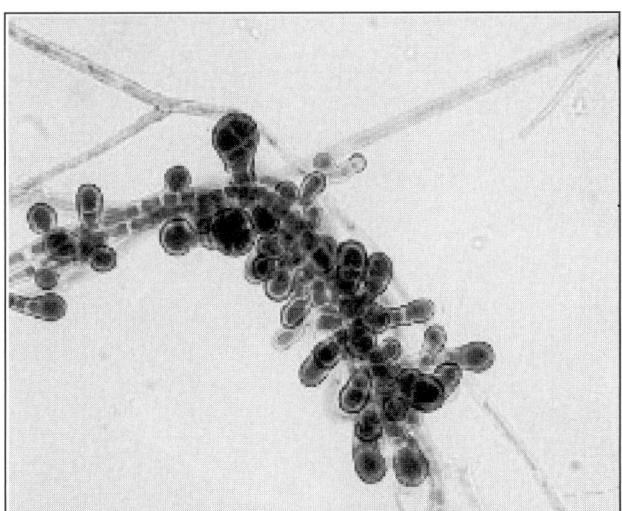

Figure 21-69 Photomicrograph of immature and mature muriform macroconidia of *Epicoccum* species, characteristically borne in loose clusters.

sistency is more glabrous than cottony because aerial hyphae develop poorly. Microscopically, large dark brown to black, smooth-walled, leathery, saclike structures called **pycnidia** are characteristically seen (Fig. 21-74). Within the pycnidia are borne myriad cylindrical, spindle-shaped or spherical, hyaline, one-celled conidia, which are released from a fracture in the cell wall. Because pycnidia may appear similar to the cleistothecia produced by *Aspergillus* spp. and other telomorphic fungi, one must determine if the spores contained are conidia (as is the case with *Phoma* spp.) or are the larger, darker-staining ascospores characteristic of the ascosporogenous fungi. This differentiation can be made in transparency tape mounts by gently pressing the surface of the tape with the tip of a pencil over the unknown baglike structure (visualized under the scanning objective of a microscope) until it breaks. The release of the one-celled hyaline conidia as described above confirms the identification of *Phoma* spp.

CHAETOMIUM SPECIES

The colonies of *Chaetomium* spp. are initially white, but may become yellow, yellow-green, or copper-colored on maturity. Microscopically, large, **spiked hyphae** may be observed extending through the wall of saclike cleistothecia, simulating the extending legs of a spider (Fig. 21-75).

Agents of Chromomycosis and Mycetoma

Chromomycosis is the term originally used to describe a cutaneous and subcutaneous infection characterized by the formation of elevated, roughened multicolored verrucous vegetations, most commonly spreading over the dorsal surfaces of the feet and lower leg, caused by a group of slow-growing, dematiaceous fungi belonging to the genera *Cladophialophora, Phialophora, Cladosporium,* and *Fonseceae.*[71]

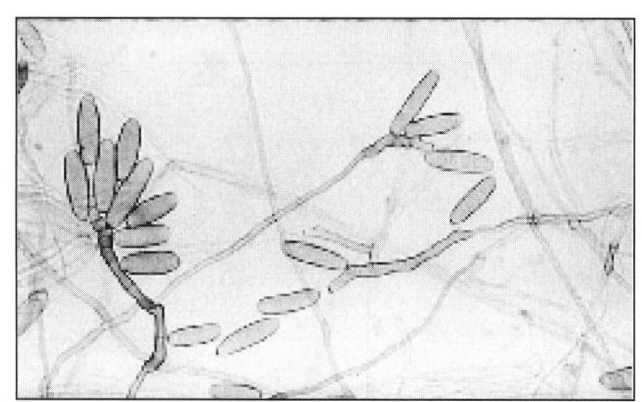
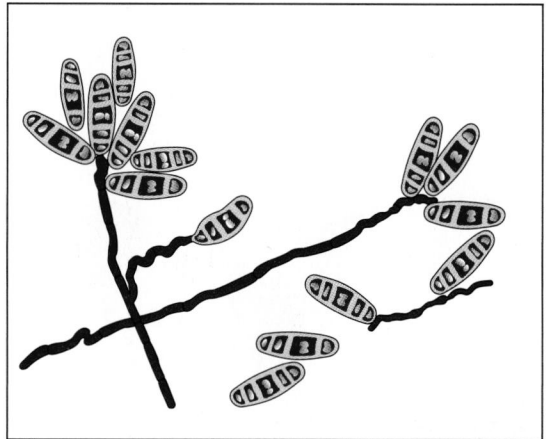

Figure 21-70 Photomicrograph and sketch of cylindrical, smooth-walled, multicelled macroconidia characteristic of *Bipolaris* species.

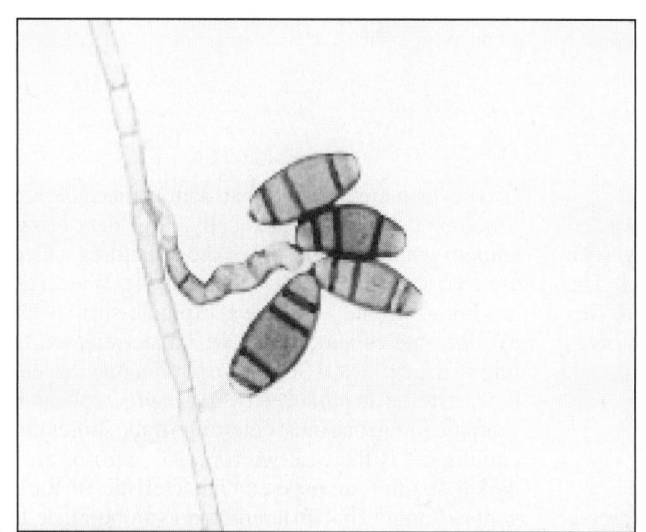
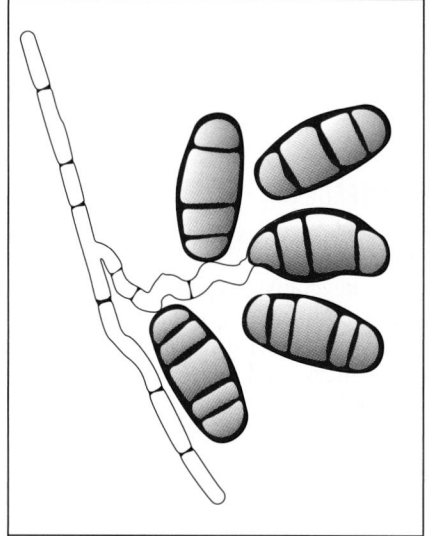

Figure 21-71 Photomicrograph and sketch of dark-staining, multicelled macroconidia divided by transverse septa and bent due to overgrowth of center cell, characteristic of *Curvularia* species.

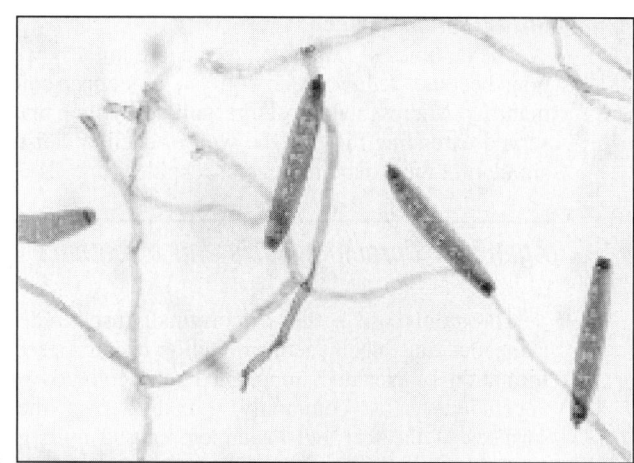
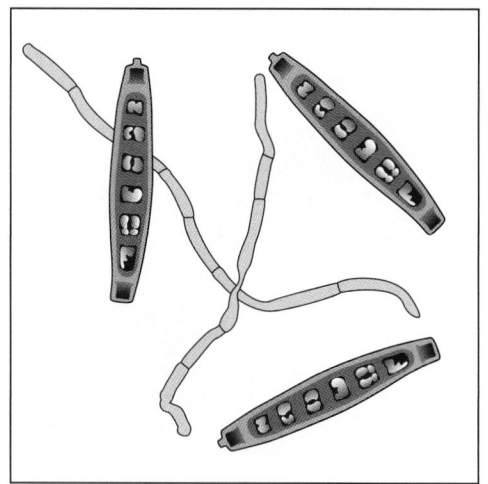

Figure 21-72 Photomicrograph and sketch of long, pencil-shaped macroconidia of *Exserohilum* species, characterized by a nipple-like protrusion from the hilar cell.

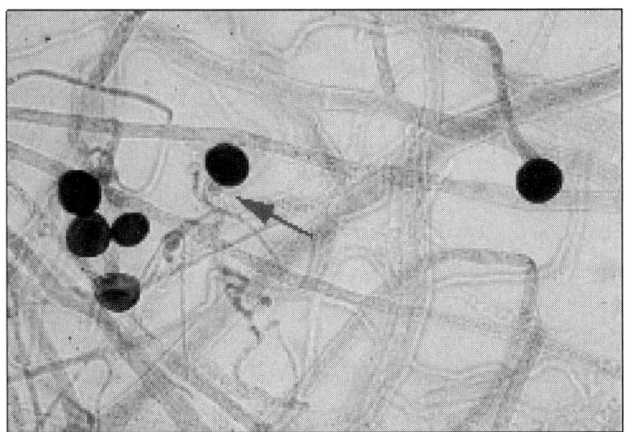

Figure 21-73 Photomicrograph of the mold form of *Nigrospora* spp., revealing background dematiaceous hyphae and spherical, jet-black conidia, each supported by a bulbous conidiophore (*arrow*).

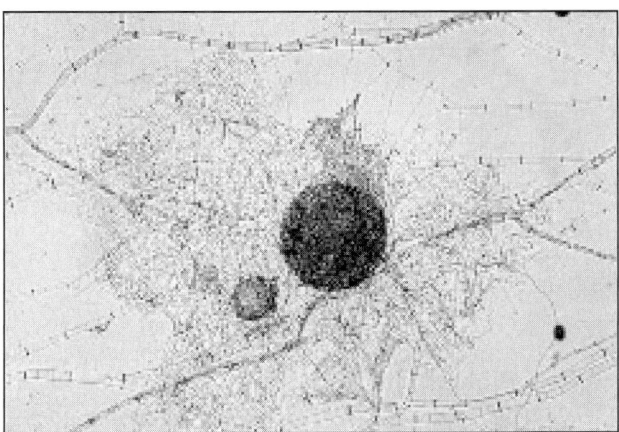

Figure 21-74 Photomicrograph of a large saclike pycnidium of *Phoma* species, with scattered tiny, hyaline conidia observed in the background.

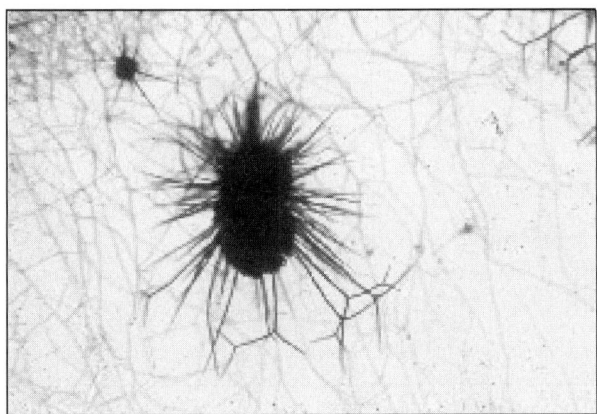

Figure 21-75 Photomicrograph of the spiderlike pycnidium of *Chaetomium* species, in which sprouting conidia extend through the wall.

The term *Mycetoma* refers to a condition in which the infection is located primarily in the subcutaneous tissue, forming an abscess or granulomatous mass with the formation of sinus tracts that reach the surface of the skin. Purulent material containing grains or granules of fungal elements are often discharged from these sinus tracts, and are also observed in histologic sections of the mass.

These agents gain entrance to the skin through traumatic wounds and penetrating injuries. Dematiaceous hyphal elements may be seen in the tissues. More diagnostic is the presence of muriform, light-yellow-staining yeast bodies grouped in clusters or in short chains, known as "Medlar bodies" or "copper pennies" (Fig. 21-76). Microabscesses, granulomatous nodules, extreme acanthosis, and pseudoepitheliomatous hyperplasia with varying degrees of fibrosis and scarring are the common histologic changes.

The following species of slow-growing dematiaceous fungi are the most common causes of chromomycosis, mycetoma, and other deep-seated mycotic infections:

Cladophialophora (Cladosporium) carrionii
Cladophialophora (Xylohypha) bantiana
Phialophora verrucosa
Phialophora richardsiae
Fonsecaea pedrosoi
Exophiala species
Wangiella species

The differentiation among each of the species listed above depends on the observation of key differences in the mode of conidiation, the structure of the conidiophores and phialides, and the morphology and arrangement of the conidia.

The fungi in this group causing chromomycosis and mycetoma produce four types of sporulation: cladosporium, phialophora, acrotheca, and rhinocladiella. The background

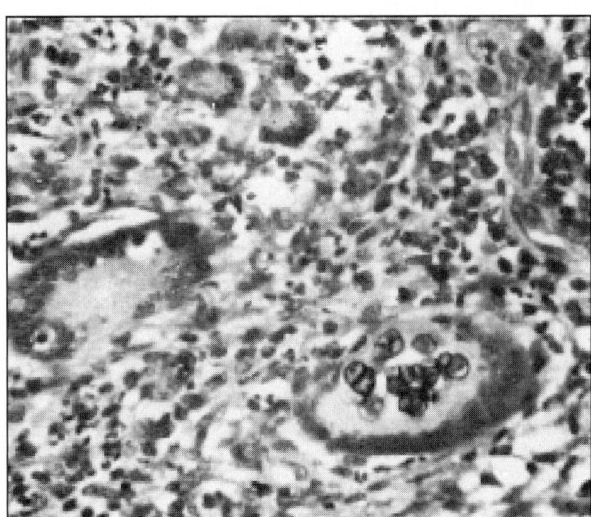

Figure 21-76 Photomicrograph of a tissue section from a case of subcutaneous chromomycosis. Note the inclusion of several spherical sclerotic bodies within the giant cell located in the lower right quadrant in the field of view (oil immersion, H&E).

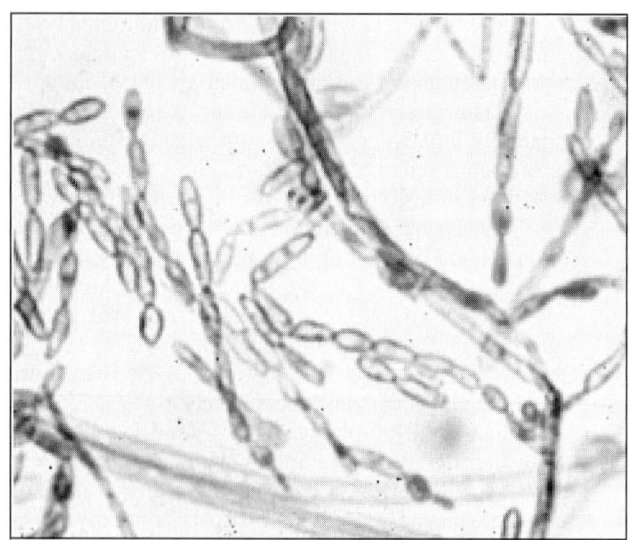

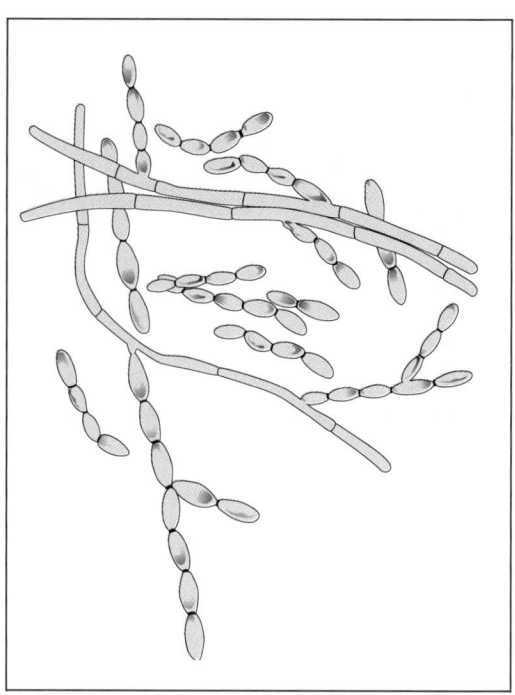

Figure 21-77 Photomicrograph and sketch illustrating cladosporium-type sporulation, in which chains of elliptical conidia are connected by dark-staining dysjunctors.

hyphae for each of these fungal species are distinctly dark and septate.

In the **cladosporium**-type sporulation, elliptical, dark-staining conidia are produced in long, branching chains, each separated by a delicate scar known as a dysjunctor (Fig. 21-77).

Phialophora-type sporulation is characterized by the production of single phialides that are either urn-shaped or long and tapered. Conidia are produced within the phialides and extruded in small clusters from the tips (Fig. 21-78).

In the **acrotheca**-type sporulation, sympodial branches of conidiophores are produced from the sides of the hyphae, simulating the prongs of a coat rack. Short chains of conidia

are borne from these clusters (Fig. 21-79). **Rhinocladiella**-type sporulation is a variant of acrotheca-type sporulation in which the conidia are produced singly, directly, and laterally from the sides of the hyphae (Fig. 21-80).

Cladophialophora (Cladosporium) carrionii

Freely branching hyphae give rise to long **chains of dark-staining, elliptical conidia**. The conidia often show scars or **dysjunctors** at the sites of attachment (see Fig. 21-77).

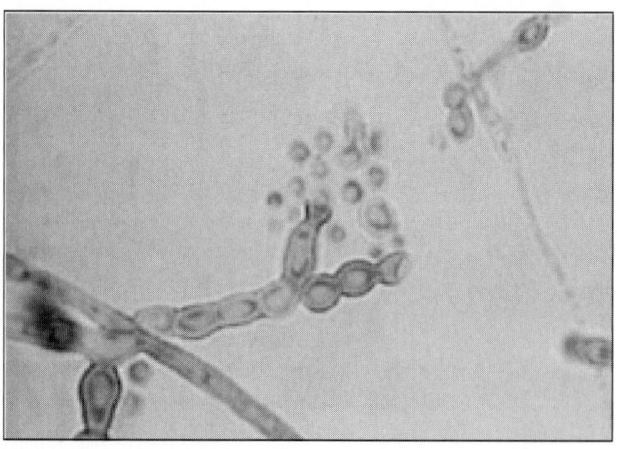

Figure 21-78 Photomicrograph of phialophora-type sporulation, illustrating short urn-shaped conidiophores, each with a narrow soda-bottle-like mouth from which spherical conidia are produced, arranging in loose clusters at the tip.

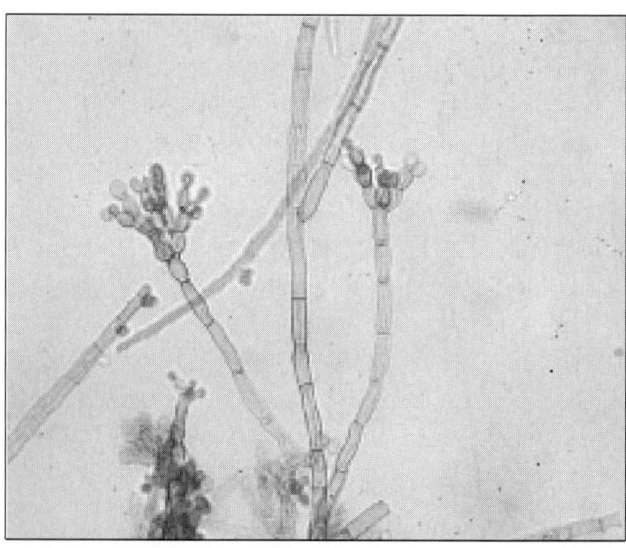

Figure 21-79 Photomicrograph of acrotheca-type sporulation, in which short chains of elliptical conidia are produced sympodially from the ends of conidiophores, a picture resembling a coat rack.

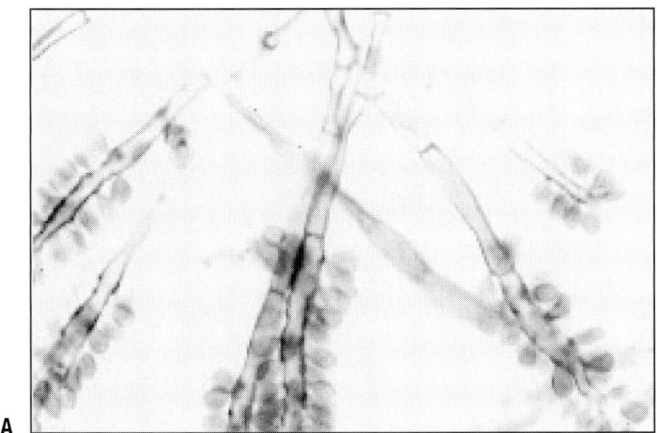

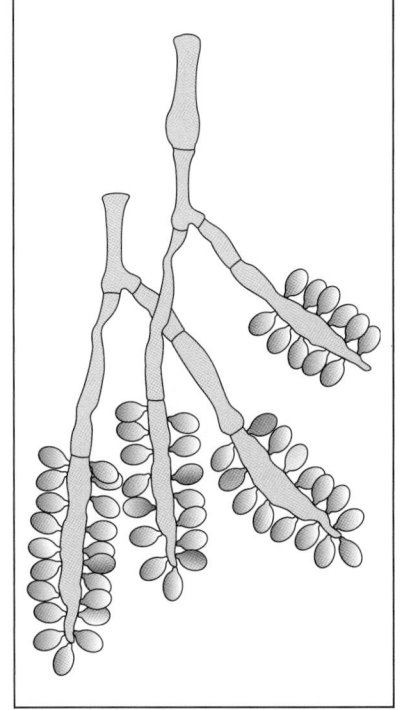

Figure 21-80 Photomicrograph and sketch of rhinocladiella-type sporulation in which elliptical conidia are borne directly and laterally in compact rows from the sides of the conidiophore.

Cladophialophora bantiana (formerly *Phialophora bantianum,* formerly *Cladosporium trichoides*) is a closely related species that also produces spores of the cladosporium type; however, the **chains of conidia are very long**, with as many as 30 cells each and producing nonpigmented conidia without dysjunctors. *Cladophialophora bantiana* **grows at 43°C** and **does not liquefy gelatin,** two additional characteristics by which it can be differentiated from *Cladophialophora carrionii,* which does not possess these properties.

Phialophora verrucosum

Flask-shaped or **urn-shaped phialides,** ranging from 4 to 7 μm in length, are borne directly from the sides of the hyphae (see Fig. 21-78). The terminal portion of the phialide is characteristically elongated, simulating the top of a **soda bottle.** Spherical to oval-shaped, yellow-pigmented conidia are produced from within each phialide, and aggregate in ball-like clusters at the terminal opening. These conidia may dislodge and aggregate along the sides of the phialides and along the adjacent supporting hyphae.

Phialophora richardsiae

In contrast to the narrow bottlelike phialides of *Phialophora verrucosum,* those of *Phialophora richardsiae* are flat and **saucer-shaped** (Fig. 21-81). *Phialophora richardsiae* is a common agent recovered from phaeohyphomycotic cysts. Spherical to elliptical, hyaline conidia are borne in **tight clusters at the tips of these phialides,** held together by a

mucinous material. These conidia may also dislodge and aggregate along the sides of the phialides.

Fonsecaea pedrosoi

Conidia arise from short denticles attached laterally to the sides of conidiogenous cells, which periodically swell, turn sympodially, and produce additional conidia that arrange in short chains at points of septation (see Fig. 21-79). This type of sporulation is known as "**acrotheca.**" Some strains produce conidia singly and laterally along the sides of the conidiophore, in a **rhinocladiella** arrangement (see

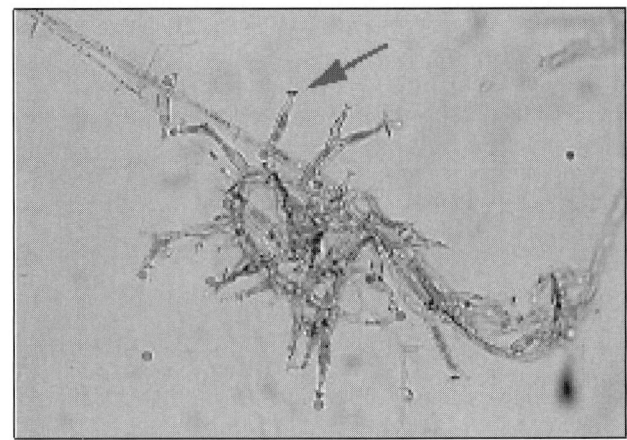

Figure 21-81 Photomicrograph of the long conidiophores of *Phialophora richardsiae,* illustrating the characteristic flat saucerlike terminal ending.

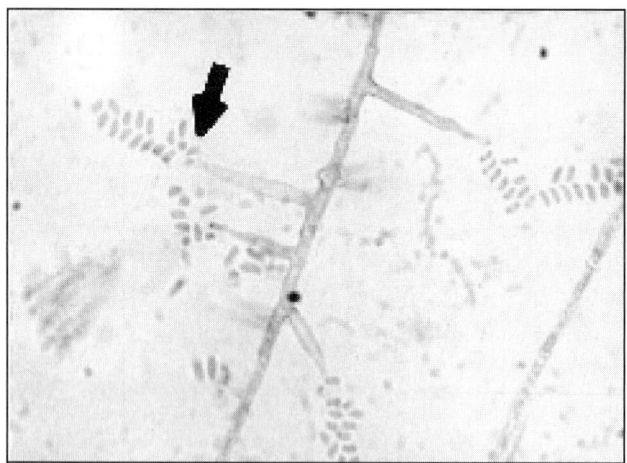
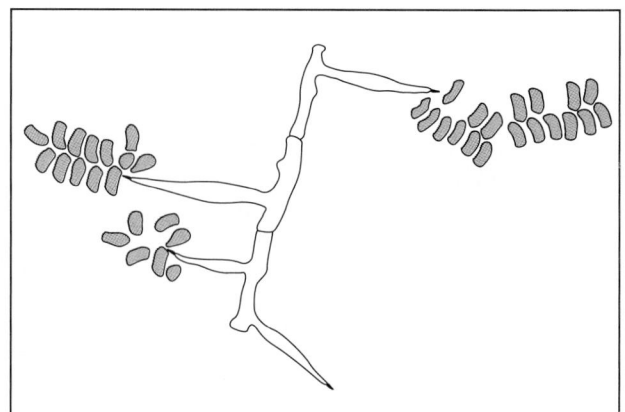

Figure 21-82 Photomicrograph and sketch of *Exophiala* species, illustrating the long, tapered conidiophores from the tips of which are released elongated annelloconidia that arrange in loose clusters.

Fig. 21-80). With certain strains of *F. pedrosoi*, cladosporium- and phialophora-type sporulations may be admixed. The conidia in a related, less-commonly-encountered species, *Fonsecaea compacta*, arrange in tight clusters.

Exophiala jeanselmei

This species, and the closely related "look-alike," *Wangiella dermatitidis,* produce **long, tapered conidiophores** that extend from the hyphae in right or obtuse angles. The tips of the conidiophores for *E. jeanselmei* may be **sharply pointed,** resulting from an extension involved in annellide formation (Fig. 21-82). **Rings or annellides** may be observed beneath the tapered tip of the phialide with exacting focusing of the microscope and diminution of the condenser light. Delicate scars or annellides will be observed with *E. jeanselmei;* they are absent in *W. dermatitidis.* Kwon-Chung and Bennett have found annellides to be produced by both these species, and believe *Wangiella* spp. is a variant of *Exophiala* spp.[153] Clusters of elliptical conidia may be seen at the tips of the phialides, falling off and aligning downward along the course of their long stems. The black yeasts of *Phaeoannellomyces* species, considered to be a synanamorph of *Exophiala* species, will be described below in the yeast section of this presentation.

The clinical manifestations of phaeohyphomycosis, including chromomycosis and mycetoma, are presented in Clinical Correlation Box 21-10.

The Laboratory Identification of Yeasts

The monomorphic yeast species of medical importance that are most commonly encountered in clinical microbiology laboratories include:

Candida albicans
Candida species
Cryptococcus neoformans
Cryptococcus species
Candida (Torulopsis) glabrata
Geotrichum species
Trichosporon species
Rhodotorula species
Saccharomyces species
Hansenula anomala
Malassezia furfur
Aureobasidium pullulans
Phaeoannellomyces werneckii

Display 21-7 provides a guide to the laboratory identification of these yeasts.

Most clinically significant yeast isolates grow within 36–72 hours in culture on sheep blood agar and most other nonselective primary isolation media. The colonies are typically white or yellow-white with a smooth or pasty consistency (Color Plate 21-6*A*). When an isolate presents with colonies suspicious for one of the monomorphic yeasts, the first step is to determine if pseudohyphae are being produced, and if so to set up a germ-tube preparation. If the isolate produces germ tubes under the conditions of the test, a presumptive identification of *Candida albicans* can be reported, and further workup is usually not necessary.

Germ Tube

A germ tube is defined as a filamentous extension from a yeast cell that is about half the width and three to four times the length of the mother cell (Fig. 21-83). The true germ tube produced by *Candida albicans* has no constriction at the neck. The germ tube is a true hyphal structure and therefore does not have the constriction characteristic of pseudohyphae. A description of the germ tube procedure is included in Box 21-6. As mentioned before, if germ tubes are present, a presumptive identification of *C. albicans* can be made. Because not all strains of *C. albicans* produce germ tubes, the culture should be inoculated to a cornmeal agar plate. At the end of the incubation period, observe the mount

As mentioned in the text, the clinical manifestations of chromomycosis and mycetoma will be included as subsets under the broader category of phaeohyphomycosis. Brandt and Warnock[31] from the Centers for Disease Control and Prevention have published a review covering the epidemiology, clinical manifestations, and therapy for infections caused by these dematiaceous fungi. They list *Alternaria* species, *Bipolaris* species, *Cladophialophora bantiana*, *Curvularia* species, *Exophiala* species, *Fonsecaea pedrosoi*, *Madurella* species, *Phialophora* species, *Scedosporium prolificans*, *Scytalidium dimidiatum,* and *Wangiella dermatitidis* as the more important human pathogens within this group. They go on to describe these fungi as being widespread in the environment, and found in soil, wood, and decomposing plant debris.

The cutaneous, subcutaneous, and corneal infections associated with these dematiaceous fungi occur worldwide, but are more common in tropical and subtropical climates. Infection most commonly results from traumatic implantation into the skin or other tissue. Most progressive cases occur in immunocompetent individuals. They also cite the dematiaceous molds as being important causes of invasive sinusitis and allergic fungal sinusitis, most commonly following inhalation of infective spores. Although cerebral infection is the most common form of systemic phaeohyphomycosis, other localized deep forms of the disease, such as arthritis, and endocarditis, have been reported. Disseminated infection is uncommon, but its incidence is increasing, particularly among immunocompromised individuals. *Scedosporium prolificans* is the most frequent agent involved in disseminated infection.

Literally hundreds of isolated cases of fungal infections caused by the rapidly growing, saprophytic species of dematiaceous molds have been reported in the recent medical literature. Space here allows for only a few examples. The three more common clinical manifestations of phaeohyphomycosis caused by the saprophytic fungi are keratitis, sinusitis, and onychomycosis.

As a recent example of keratitis, Wilhelmus and Jones[295] reported their laboratory experience with the isolation and identification of *Curvularia* species as a cause of keratitis over a 30-year period. The records for 32 individuals were available for analysis. It was determined that trauma, usually with plants or dirt, was the risk factor in half the cases. The majority of cases (69%) occurred during the hot, humid summer months along the U.S. Gulf Coast. Presenting signs varied from superficial, feathery infiltrates of the central cornea to suppurative ulceration of the peripheral cornea.

Sinusitis is also a common site of infection with dematiaceous fungi. From the older literature, Adam et al.[2] reported nine cases of sinusitis presenting as allergic rhinitis or nasal polyposis, caused by *Bipolaris* and *Exserohilum* species. More recently, Fernandez et al.[82] reported on the findings derived from a search of the literature for pediatric *Curvularia* infections between the years 1968 and 1998. Of 16 cases identified, 13 had allergic sinusitis, a unique form of sinusitis in which a history of asthma or nasal polyps are predisposing conditions. The patients in this review were usually immunocompetent teenagers who had a prolonged duration of symptoms, usually >3 weeks. Extensive surgical debridement combined with amphotericin B treatment has been recommended for the treatment of chronic invasive sinusitis.

Onychomycosis caused by *Alternaria* species is being reported with increasing frequency, particularly in patients with immunodeficiency. Romano et al.[236] reported nine cases of onychomycosis caused by *Alternaria alternata* observed in Tuscany, Italy, in the period 1985–1999. Diagnosis was made on the basis of repeated direct microscopic mycologic examination and culture. In most of the cases, dystrophy and distal subungual hyperkeratosis of one or two nails of the feet or hands were the primary clinical manifestations. Seven cases were treated with oral itraconazole; this treatment was successful in six cases.

A number of dematiaceous fungi are neurotropic, including *Cladophialophora bantiana*, *Ramichloridium mackenziei*, and *Wangiella dermatitidis*. Although cases have occurred in immunocompromised persons, cerebral phaeohyphomycosis is most common in immunocompetent individuals who may or may not have obvious risk factors.[63] Revankar et al.[229] reviewed 101 cases of culture-proven primary central nervous system phaeohyphomycosis reported in the English-language literature from 1966 to 2002. They found that the most frequently isolated species was *Cladophialophora bantiana*. The mortality rates were high among these reported cases, regardless of immune status. Therapy has not been standardized, although the combination of amphotericin B, flucytosine, and itraconazole along with an aggressive medical and surgical approach may improve survival rates.

Chromomycosis

Wortman[302] reported a case of chromomycosis caused concurrently by *Fonsecaea pedrosoi* and *Nocardia brasiliensis*, complicating a traumatic penetrating injury. Chromomycosis is widespread in tropical South America, occurring most commonly in male farm and plantation workers. Silva et al.[256] reviewed 325 cases reported in the Amazon river drainage region of Brazil. The data obtained revealed a mean age range of affected individuals between 41 and 70 years, 93.2% of whom were males. Agricultural workers comprised 86.1% of the total. Lesions on the lower limbs (feet and legs) were found in 80.7%. In 24% of patients (78 cases), the etiologic agent was isolated and identified through culture. *Fonsecaea pedrosoi* was present in 77 cases and *Phialophora verrucosa* in only one case.

Similar results were reported by Minotto et al.[184] in a study of 100 patients residing in Rio Grande do Sul, Brazil. Again, male patients predominated (4:1); the majority were white farmers ranging in age from 50 to 59 years. Most commonly, severe verrucous lesions appeared on their lower limbs, with the average time between the appearance of the disease and medical diagnosis being 14 years. Thorn wounds were associated with the disease in 16% of the cases. Statistical analysis showed recrudescence of the disease in 43% of cases despite the treatment used. *Fonsecaea pedrosoi* was recovered from 96% of the cases; *Phialophora verrucosa* in 4%.

(continued)

CLINICAL CORRELATION BOX 21-10 *Continued*

Mycetoma

Mycetoma refers to subcutaneous infections in which the tissue is markedly swollen with the formation of deeply penetrating sinus tracts that break through the superficial skin and discharge purulent material. The feet (Madura foot) and hands are most commonly involved, becoming markedly swollen and deformed in serious infections. Mycetomas have two primary causes—bacteria belonging to the family *Actinomycetales* (*Actinomyces, Nocardia,* and *Streptomyces* species), and the true fungi (eumycotic mycetomas), primarily the dematiaceous fungus *Exophiala jeanselmei* and the hyaline mold *Pseudallescheria boydii* in sporadic cases encountered in the United States.

Mycetoma is more commonly seen in other parts of the world, particularly western and eastern Africa. A history of prior injury is common. The lower extremities tend to be involved in the majority of cases, with the upper extremities and other sites such as the gluteal region, the lumbar area, submandibular area, and face less commonly.

The description many years ago of the presentation of a mycetoma by Thammayya et al.[273] of a patient who also lived in India remains classic for the condition: "The right lower leg and foot were irregularly swollen, firm, painless, and nontender and had many small nodules and sinuses all over the swelling. The lower end of the tibia and bones of the foot were affected. The discharge from the sinuses and nodules contained black-brown, soft, vermicular, crescent-shaped to irregular granules, measuring 0.5–2.00 mm and composed mostly of swollen spherical cells, 4–8 μm diameter, and a few hyphae, 2.5–3.0 μm diameter."

A relatively high incidence has also been encountered in Japan. Murayama et al.[187] report a case of mycetoma involving the lower leg of a 34-year-old woman with systemic lupus erythematosus (SLE). In an accompanying literature review of *Exophiala jeanselmei* infections in Japan , these authors found reference to 54 cases (24 in men and 30 in women). Fifty of these cases (21 men and 29 women, an interesting shift in the male: female ratio) were caused by dematiaceous fungi. About half of these patients had underlying diseases, and the sites of the lesions were mainly on the extremities.

Systemic disease occurs most commonly in immunocompromised hosts. Such infections commonly begin in the lungs after inhalation of conidia, which lead to invasive infections that may disseminate to distal organs. Several cases of invasive, systemic, and disseminated infections caused by many species of phaeohyphomycotic fungi listed by Rippon,[234] usually occurring in immunosuppressed patients, with the primary sites of infection being the lungs, sinuses, or sites of trauma to the skin. Included are cases of endocarditis resulting from implantation during surgery or intravenous injection of contaminated materials by drug users.

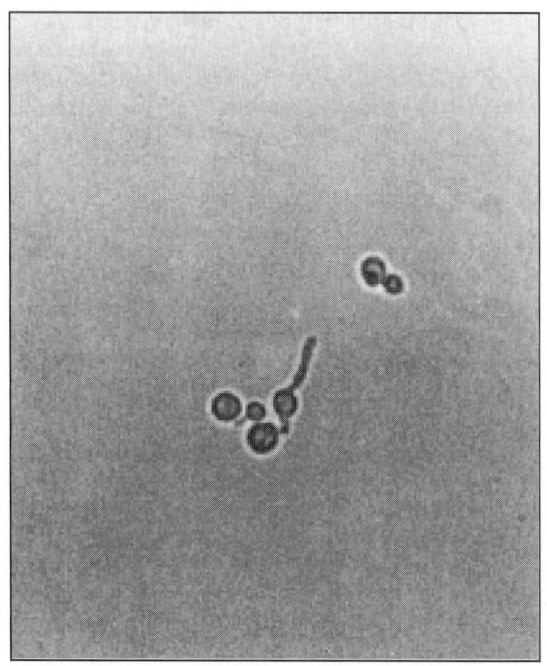

Figure 21-83 Photomicrograph of a germ tube, characteristic of *Candida albicans* (oil immersion).

microscopically for the presence of chlamydospores, which, if present, also allow for the presumptive identification of *Candida albicans.* (Fig. 21-84)

Cornmeal Agar Preparations

The preparation of the cornmeal agar mount is described in Box 21-7.

Again follow Display 21-7. If pseudohyphae and blastoconidia are present, a presumptive identification of *Candida* species can be made. The different patterns of growth in the cornmeal agar preparations often are sufficiently distinctive to establish a presumptive species identification.

Box 21-6 Procedure: Germ-Tube Test

1. A small portion of an isolate colony of the yeast to be tested is suspended in a test tube containing 0.5 mL of rabbit or human plasma or serum.
2. The test tube is inoculated at 35°C for no longer than 2 hours.
3. A drop of the yeast-serum suspension is placed on a microscope slide, overlaid with a coverslip, and examined microscopically for the presence of germ tubes (Fig. 15-83).
4. The test is not valid if examined after 2 hours.

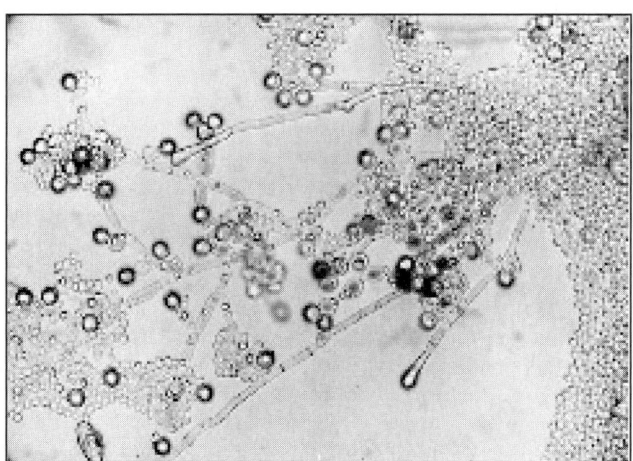
A

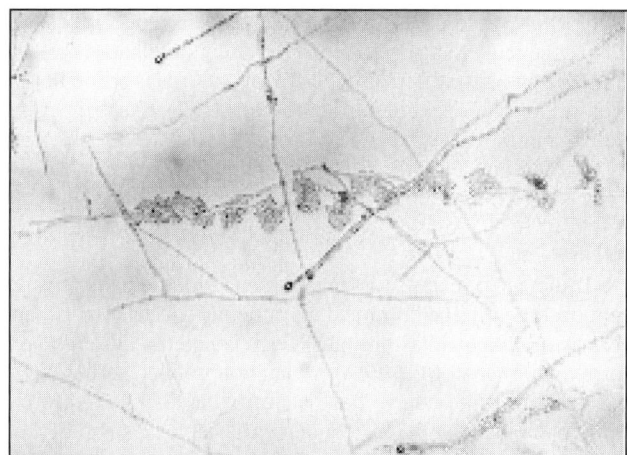
B

Figure 21-84 Photomicrographs of cornmeal agar preparations of *Candida albicans,* revealing the production of chlamydospores (*left*) and regular clustering of blastoconidia along the hyphae (*right*).

GROWTH PATTERNS OF YEASTS ON CORNMEAL AGAR

When observing the growth in a cornmeal agar preparation, determine at the onset if pseudohyphae are present. The observation of pseudohyphae and blastoconidia put an unknown isolate into the genus *Candida.* Most human infections are caused by *Candida albicans.* However, with the increase in immunosuppression related to organ transplantation and other related conditions, and the emergence of opportunistic fungal pathogens, the recovery of non-*albicans Candida* species in pure or predominant culture from blood or other sterile body sites cannot be ignored. A careful clinical correlation is necessary to determine if further workup is necessary. The patterns of growth on cornmeal agar are helpful in making a presumptive identification and in serving as a quality-control check on species identifications provided by the biocodes indicated by automated and kit systems. Because none of the cornmeal agar patterns are diagnostic (with the exception of the chlamydospore production by *C. albicans*), carbohydrate assimilation studies or the results derived from one of the commercial yeast identification systems are necessary before a definitive identification can be reported.

Box 21-7 Procedure for Inoculation of Cornmeal-Tween 80 Agar

1. Make three parallel cuts 1/4 in., or 1 cm, apart into the surface of cornmeal agar, holding the inoculating wire at about a 45-degree angle.
2. Lay a coverslip on the surface of the agar, covering a portion of the inoculated streaks.
3. Incubate the inoculated plates at 30°C for 24–48 hours in a closed, moisturized chamber. At the end of the incubation period, examine microscopically through the coverslip and observe the pattern of growth to make a presumptive identification.

If a presumptive identification cannot be made from the observation of the cornmeal agar preparation, tests for nitrate reduction, urease activity, inositol assimilation, nitrate reduction, and the production of caffeic acid (using a niger seed agar plate or performing a filter paper strip test), in addition to carbohydrate assimilation studies, are helpful in separating these various species. Although these studies can be accomplished by conventional techniques, packaged yeast identification kits or automated systems are currently used in most laboratories. In those rare instances in which referral to carbohydrate assimilation profiles are required, the reader is referred to Tables 19-8, 19-9, and 19-10 on pages 1045, 1050 and 1054 in the 5th edition of this textbook.

CHROMAGAR

CHROMagar, a chromogenic differential culture medium, is being used in many laboratories to facilitate the isolation and presumptive identification of certain clinically important yeast species, particularly *Candida albicans.* Observation of colony morphology and distinctive patterns of color are used to separate yeast species, particularly when observed in mixed cultures. *Candida albicans* forms distinctive yellow-green to blue-green colonies.

Ainscough and Kibbler[3] evaluated the cost-effectiveness and time advantage of CHROMagar in comparison with Sabouraud dextrose agar (SDA). An overall sensitivity of 95.2% was observed in the study of 21 yeast isolates recovered from 298 clinical samples from patients with neutropenia and those with AIDS. CHROMagar was found in this study to be 100% sensitive and 100% specific for *C. albicans.* It provided the most economical and least time-consuming approach to the initial culture and presumptive identification of yeast isolates. The authors also recommend the direct inoculation for blood cultures when yeast cells are seen on microscopy.

CANDIDA ALBICANS

Two patterns of growth on cornmeal agar are helpful in identifying *Candida albicans*: 1) the production of chlamydospores and/or 2) blastoconidia that arrange in dense clusters evenly distributed along the pseudohyphae (Fig. 21-84). A review for these cornmeal agar patterns is particularly helpful in making an identification for strains that are germ-tube-negative.

The colony growth of *Candida albicans* may also lead to a presumptive identification. The edges of the colonies often present radiating starburst spicules in older cultures (Color Plate 21-6*B*).

If the germ-tube test is negative and chlamydospores are not observed in the cornmeal agar mount, a yeast other than *Candida albicans* has probably been isolated. Although approximately 5% of *C. albicans* may not produce germ tubes, it would be quite rare to have a strain that also fails to produce chlamydospores. In keeping with Display 21-7, the next step is to observe the patterns of growth on cornmeal agar to presumptively identify other *Candida* spp. To reiterate, it is important to review the patterns of growth on cornmeal agar as a quality-control check on the species identifications provided by automated and kit systems, as they are not always correct. To this end, the classic patterns for these more commonly encountered non-*albicans Candida* species are discussed below.

CANDIDA TROPICALIS

Candida tropicalis produces pseudohyphae with blastoconidia either borne singly or in small irregular clusters along the pseudohyphae at points of constriction (Fig. 21-85). Because this pattern is not specific, carbohydrate-assimilation studies or identification through the use of one of the yeast identification systems is necessary.

CANDIDA PARAPSILOSIS

Key to the presumptive identification of *C. parapsilosis* in cornmeal agar preparations is the observation of multiple focal areas of satellite growth adjacent to the streak lines, forming what has been colloquially referred to as "sagebrush" or "cross matchstick" patterns (Fig. 21-86). Once

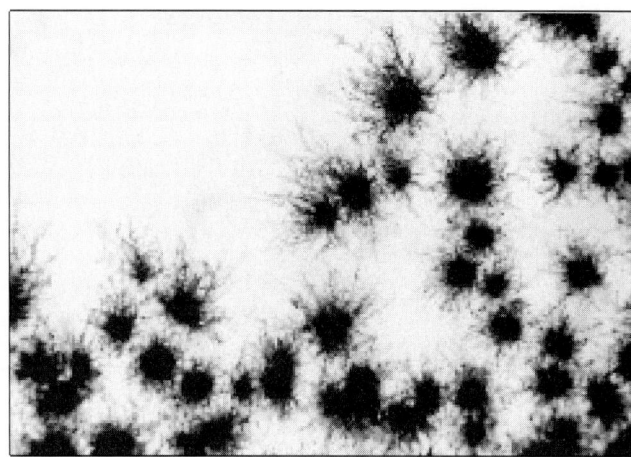

Figure 21-86 Photomicrograph of a cornmeal agar preparation of *Candida parapsilosis,* illustrating the characteristic formation of satelliting "spider colonies" along the streak line.

observed, this pattern will consistently match the identification codes obtained from commercial systems.

CANDIDA KEFYR (PSEUDOTROPICALIS)

Key here is the observation of the abundant production of elongated to rectangular blastoconidia that form distinct loose, criss-cross clusters, likened to the arrangement of "logs in a stream" (Fig. 21-87). *C. krusei* also produces a similar pattern, except that the points of derivation are sequentially clustered more as branches from a tree. Carbohydrate-assimilation studies may be required to differentiate these two species.

OTHER EMERGING PATHOGENIC CANDIDA SPECIES

The definitive identification of non-*albicans Candida* species is important to detect emerging pathogenic strains, particularly those that have acquired resistance to antifungal

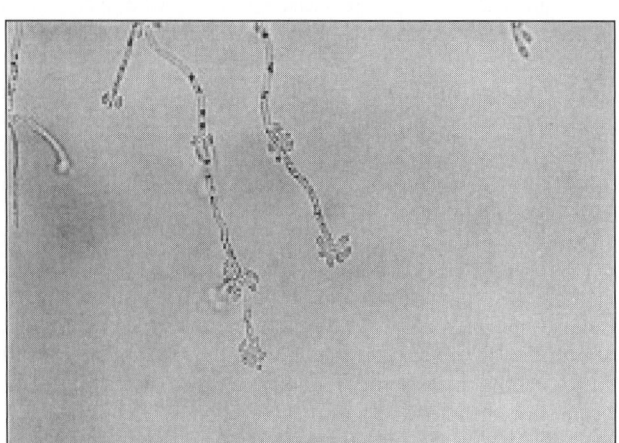

Figure 21-85 Photomicrograph of a cornmeal agar preparation of *Candida tropicalis,* illustrating light production of conidia irregularly along the hyphae.

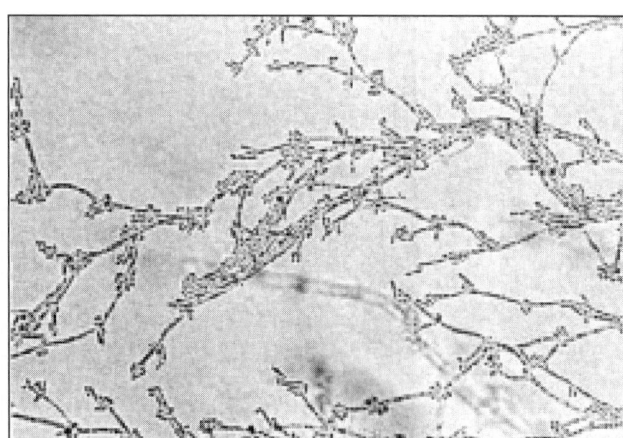

Figure 21-87 Photomicrograph of a cornmeal agar preparation illustrating the "log-in-stream" arrangement of elongated blastoconidia characteristic of *Candida kefyr.*

drugs.[200] *Candida krusei* has known resistance to ketoconazole.[299] *Candida dubliniensis*, phenotypically closely related to *Candida albicans*, particularly those strains recovered from patients with oropharyngeal thrush, has acquired induced resistance to fluconazole.[174] These strains can be identified in the laboratory by demonstrating the following characteristics[267]:

- Inability to grow at 45°C
- Appearance of rough colonies with ''feet'' on niger seed agar (*C. albicans* produce smooth-edged colonies)
- Production of pseudohyphae and chlamydospores on niger seed agar (*C. albicans* produce only round to oval blastoconidia)[262] (see Fig. 21-88)
- Production of dark blue colonies on CHROMagar *Candida*
- Carbohydrate-assimilation profiles using either the API 20C AUX or Vitek yeast identification systems. *C. dubliniensis*, in contrast to *C. albicans*, is not able to utilize D-xylose, trehalose, or methyl-D-glucosidase.[89]
- Species-specific DNA probes.[72]

Sporadic amphotericin B resistance has evolved in certain lineages of *Candida lusitaniae* through a mechanism of switching from previously susceptible colonies.[304] Again, it is important to identify these emerging pathogenic strains in the clinical laboratory to avoid empiric administration of resistant antifungal agents.

CANDIDA SPECIES AND CANDIDIASIS

From data obtained from 180 U.S. hospitals participating in the National Nosocomial Infections Surveillance (NNIS) system, 27,200 fungal isolates associated with nosocomial infections were reported in the United States between January 1980 and April 1990. Of these, *Candida* spp. accounted for 19,621 (72.1%).[130] Factors predisposing to this high frequency of yeast infections include:

- Increase in chemotherapy, and in bone-marrow and other organ transplantations, with accompanying profound immunosuppression

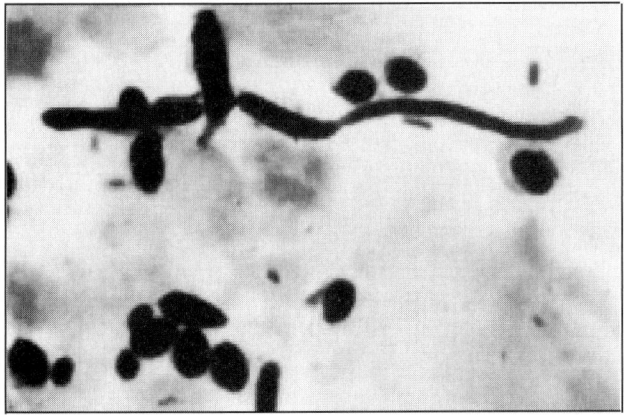

Figure 21-88 Photomicrograph of Gram-stained sputum, showing pseudohyphae and budding blastoconidia characteristic of *Candida* species (oil immersion).

- Prolonged stays in hospitals
- Vascular catheterizations
- Prolonged administration of broad-spectrum antimicrobial agents
- Extensive use of prophylactic antifungal drugs

Wright and Wenzel,[303] in a review of patients with nosocomial candidiasis, cite burns, artificial respiratory assistance, colonization with *Candida* species, and repeated transfusions as additional risk factors. These authors cite a 1996 nationwide study of participating hospitals, conducted under the Surveillance and Control of Pathogens of Epidemiologic Importance (SCOPE) program that *Candida* species has been established behind *Staphylococcus* species as the most frequent cause of septicemia in hospitalized patients.

Patients with cancer, particularly those with leukemia and lymphoproliferative disorders, in whom the peripheral white blood count is depressed, are also at increased risk. Kalin and Petrini[133] cite an increase in mortality in patients with leukemia caused by fungal infections from a low of 5% prior to the antibiotic era, to a current frequency of 40%. *Candida* species were recovered most frequently as the primary agents. Advanced age, although not directly related to yeast infections, nonetheless contributes to increased morbidity and mortality. For example, mucocutaneous candidiasis in the aged, including thrush and denture stomatitis, are commonly associated with local mechanical irritation of the oral mucosa.[118]

At the opposite end of the age spectrum, critically ill newborn babies also are at high risk for acquiring nosocomial yeast infections, with particular involvement of the central nervous system. Other conditions predisposing to yeast infections include altered host defenses due to compromised protein stores or antibody production, suppression of the normal bacterial flora, pregnancy, and diabetes mellitus or other chronic metabolic diseases.

In cases in which a clinical isolate is of high significance, or when an exacting species identification cannot be made using phenotypic characteristics, molecular techniques using species-specific DNA probes are available through Public Health Laboratories and the Centers for Disease Control and Prevention that provide rapid and unequivocal differentiation of these various *Candida* species.

The standardization of in vitro antifungal susceptibility testing, largely through the work of the Clinical Laboratory Standards Institute (formerly, the National Committee for Clinical Standards), has made it possible to determine the degree of resistance of yeast isolates.[220,230] Applications of the E test have also made available to clinical laboratories the ability to determine select antifungal susceptibility profiles.[218,221] Key clinical manifestations of candidiasis are presented in Clinical Correlation Box 21-11 (*Candida albicans*) and Clinical Correlation Box 21-12 (*Candida* spp., not *albicans*).

Species That Produce True Hyphae

Colonies of *Geotrichum* spp. and of *Trichosporon* spp. are white to gray, and are initially yeastlike but soon develop

CLINICAL CORRELATION BOX 21-11 Candidiasis (*Candida albicans*)

Human candidiasis is most commonly caused by *Candida albicans*. The rapid germination in tissues after seeding from the bloodstream; the production of proteases, adhesins to extracellular matrix proteins, and complement-binding receptors; and phenotypic switching are the most important virulence factors contributing to its increased infectivity.[52,200] The history, taxonomy, epidemiology, and virulence factors for *Candida albicans* have been reviewed by McCullough[176] and by Pfaller.[217] The clinical manifestations of *Candida albicans* are primarily of three types: mucocutaneous, cutaneous, and systemic.

Mucocutaneous Candidiasis

Candidiasis of the mucous membranes most commonly involves the oral cavity and the vaginal canal. Oral candidiasis, a condition known as thrush (a term derived from the Scandinavian word *trosk*), is the most common clinical manifestation of candidiasis in humans. The infection is manifested as white patches or plaques on the buccal mucosa and tongue,[20] which, in more serious infections, may coalesce into a membrane. These adhere firmly to the epithelium, revealing a reddened, edematous base when removed. The diagnosis can be made by observing microscopically the characteristic pseudohyphae and blastoconidia in Gram-stained preparations of smears prepared from some of the exudate (Fig. 21–88). Alteration of the normal flora after prolonged antibiotic therapy, low pH of the salivary secretions in newborns, hypertrophy of the papillae of the tongue ("black hairy tongue"), and chronic glossitis are predisposing causes.[25] Oral candidiasis is now recognized as an AIDS-defining condition, seen in virtually 100% of patients with AIDS.[270]

Although classically caused by *Candida albicans*, the closely related species, *Candida dubliniensis* has recently emerged as a more troublesome agent in many cases, expressing induced resistance to certain azole-derivative antifungal agents, particularly fluconazole.[174,267] Therefore, laboratory identification of *C. dubliniensis* may be indicated for isolates recovered from cases of oral thrush before empiric therapy with an azole antifungal agent is administered.

The mucous membranes of the trachea and bronchi, and virtually any part of the alimentary canal may harbor *Candida* infections, most commonly representing extensions of oropharyngeal disease. Cases of esophagitis, gastritis, enteritis, and perianal disease have been reported. The gastroesophageal junction in particular is a common site for *Candida* infections. A low-pH environment may explain this predisposition, particularly in patients with hematologic malignancy. Dysphagia, retrosternal pain, upper gastrointestinal bleeding, and nausea are associated symptoms. Esophageal candidiasis may also occur as an extension of oropharyngeal thrush, particularly in newborns.

Cutaneous Candidiasis

Infections of the skin commonly involve the moist, intertriginous areas, such as in the webs of the fingers and toes, beneath the female breasts, in the armpits, and in the folds of the groin. Infection of the nails proper is known as onychomycosis, or paronychia if the folds of skin encasing the nails are involved. Diaper rash infection of neonates is also a common manifestation. Chronic mucocutaneous candidiasis is an opportunistic infection of skin and mucous membranes associated with several genetic defects involving compromised function of leukocytes, or of the endocrine system. Thymic dysplasia with and without hypogammaglobulinemia, hypoparathyroidism, and chronic granulomatous disease, the latter involving a myeloperoxidase defect of phagocytes precluding postphagocytic killing of yeast forms, are among the predisposing conditions presented by Rippon.[234]

Disseminated Candidiasis

Systemic candidiasis is a relatively rare condition, occurring primarily as a terminal event in patients with debilitating, neoplastic (blast crisis of leukemias and lymphoma, for example), immunosuppressive diseases and following organ transplantation, particularly during an acute rejection syndrome. The conditions underlying hematogenous candidiasis is reviewed by Abi-Said.[1] Following are several organ systems that may be seeded after dissemination of *Candida* species from primary sites of mucocutaneous infections.

Candidiasis of the Urinary Tract

This presentation is relatively rare, manifesting as cystitis (more commonly caused by *Torulopsis (Candida) glabrata* and pyelonephritis, either ascending from a bladder infection or from hematogenous spread from a distant primary site of infection. Aggregates of pseudohyphae and blastoconidia may be seen histologically in glomeruli, presumably in a microenvironment conducive to growth because of the lowered pH from Na^+ and H^+ ion exchanges. Currently, *Candida (Torulopsis) glabrata* ranks second or third as the causative agent of superficial (oral, esophageal, vaginal, or urinary) or systemic candidal infections, as reported by Fidel et al.[81] The emergence of *C. glabrata* as a nosocomial pathogen may be related to its resistance to azole antimycotic agents, which has been effectively used in the treatment of other yeast infections. Zmierczak et al.[307] report a case of chronic, recurrent *C. glabrata* arthritis initially involving the right ankle. One year after successful treatment, the infection recurred in the left knee; this was thought to represent hematogenous dissemination.

CLINICAL CORRELATION BOX 21-11 *Continued*

Endocarditis

This infection is most often seen in people with preexisting valvular disease, particularly following episodes of septicemia associated with the use of indwelling catheters, prolonged intravenous infusions, and intravenous-drug abuse. Hogevik and Alestig[122] present seven cases of endocarditis occurring in western Sweden. In four cases the infections were associated with prosthetic-valve placements; in three cases the native valves were involved. Because of high mortality, the authors stress the need for early diagnosis, immediate antifungal therapy, and emergency surgery if sonography reveals a lack of response. *Candida* septicemia may also be seen in patients receiving long-term antibiotics and corticosteroids. Although most strains of *C. albicans* can be recovered from blood cultures in most commercially available blood culture bottles, Marcelis et al.[173] report that culture media containing resin (specifically, BACTEC PLUS high-blood-volume resin was used in their study) may enhance recovery, particularly in patients receiving antibiotics.

***Candida* Meningitis**

This rare condition is secondary to dissemination from sites of infection in the gastrointestinal or respiratory tracts, from septic emboli released from infected heart valves, from trauma, or as a complication of neurosurgery. In a retrospective review of 21 cases of *Candida* species isolated from cerebrospinal fluid following neurosurgery, Geers and Gordon[91] found that 86% of these patients had indwelling cerebrospinal devices (shunts). Gelfand et al.[92] reported cases of superinfection following acute bacterial meningitis in adults who incurred trauma to the central nervous system or surgical intervention. They counsel that any patient with bacterial meningitis who do not improve with antimicrobial chemotherapy should be examined for *Candida* superinfection, particularly patients with indwelling catheters.

CLINICAL CORRELATION BOX 21-12 Infections With *Candida* Species, Non-*albicans*

Species of *Candida* other than *C. albicans* are generally considered as normal flora of cutaneous and mucocutaneous surfaces and only rarely are incriminated as agents of infection. Yet, Wingard[299] found in a review of 1,591 cases of *Candida* infections published in 37 reports between 1952 and 1992 that non-*Candida albicans* species were the causative agents in 46% of systemic infections. *Candida tropicalis* accounted for 25% of the infections, *C. glabrata* for 8%, *C. parapsilosis* for 7%, and *C. krusei* for 4%. From these reports, patients with leukemia were more likely to be infected with *C. albicans* or *C. tropicalis;* bone-marrow-transplant recipients were more likely to be infected with *C. krusei* or *C. lusitaniae.*

In a similar, more recent study, Wright and Wenzel[303] found that *Candida albicans* was recovered from 58% of nosocomial infections, *C. tropicalis* in 25%, *C. parapsilosis* in 15%, *C. glabrata* in 6%, and *C. lusitaniae* in 2%. *C. tropicalis* and *C. krusei* were more frequently recovered from patients with neutropenia who had lymphoma or leukemia, *C. parapsilosis* from neonates receiving hyperalimentation fluids, and *C. glabrata* in postsurgical patients who had solid tumors removed. These non-*albicans* species are being encountered with increasing frequency as agents of other infections as well, making it important for the availability of accurate identifications in clinical laboratories.[47]

In an extensive review of new and emerging yeast pathogens, Hazen cross-linked 30 emerging yeast pathogens with 168 references.[117] Although among the non-*C. albicans* species, *C. parapsilosis*, *C. glabrata* (particularly isolates in blood cultures), *C. krusei*, *C. guilliermondii*, *C. lipolytica*, and *C. kefyr (C. pseudotropicalis)* were on the increase, Hazen also mentions the emergence and significant increase in incidence of *Malassezia*, *Rhodotorula*, *Hansenula*, and *Trichosporon* species as non-*Candida* species isolates from clinical materials, with several citations to specific case reports of infections caused by these agents.

Several causes have been proposed for the sudden emergence of species of yeasts as agents of invasive infections. Included are the use of broad-spectrum antibiotics and antineoplastic agents, the widespread administration of vancomycin, intravenous catheterization, and the increased number of patients with neutropenia and immunosuppression. The widespread use of fluconazole may account for the relative decrease in recovery of *C. albicans* from blood cultures relative to other *Candida* species. *Candida lusitaniae* in particular, many strains of which are resistant to antifungal drugs commonly used to treat *Candida albicans* infections, has emerged as an important opportunistic pathogen.[23]

Cross-contamination by hospital personnel may also account for increases in yeast infections in certain environments. For example, a recent survey of hospital personnel by Strausbaugh et al.[265] revealed that 70% of nurses and non-nursing hospital personnel carried yeasts on their hands, with *Rhodotorula* spp. and *C. parapsilosis* being the most frequently recovered. In this regard, newborn infants, who are intimately handled by nursing personnel, represent another population that is susceptible to candidiasis.[139] See Weems for a full review of the clinical pathology of *C. parapsilosis*.[284]

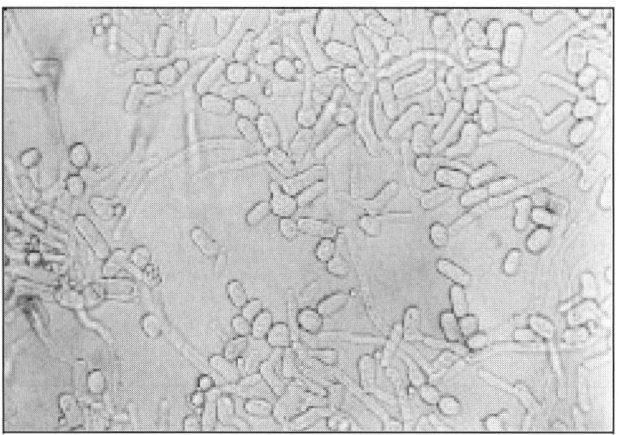

Figure 21-89 Photomicrograph of *Geotrichum candidum*, illustrating arthroconidia, a few of which present the characteristic germ-tube-like extension from one corner, simulating a "hockey stick."

a delicate, silklike surface as true hyphae and arthroconidia on maturity. In cornmeal agar mounts, **Geotrichum** and **Trichosporon spp.** produce true hyphae that become segmented and break up into arthroconidia. **Geotrichum spp.** can be differentiated because it produces a single germ tube from one corner of the arthroconidium, simulating a hockey stick (Fig. 21-89). In contrast, *Trichosporon* spp. typically form blastoconidia from both corners of an arthroconidium, simulating "rabbit ears" (Fig. 21-90). In cases in which these cornmeal agar identifying features are not evident, most strains of *Trichosporon* spp. produce a positive urease test, while *Geotrichum* spp. are universally negative.

The clinical manifestations of trichosporonosis and geotrichosis are presented in Clinical Correlation Box 21-13.

Species That Fail to Produce True Hyphae

Isolates that fail to form hyphae on cornmeal agar include *Cryptococcus* spp., *Candida (Torulopsis) glabrata*, *Rhodo-*

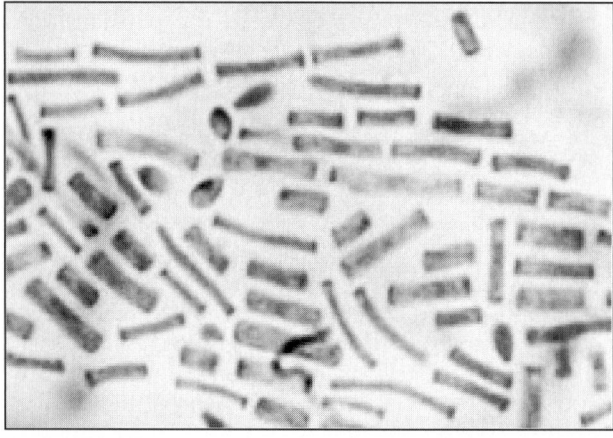

Figure 21-90 Photomicrograph of *Trichosporon beigelii*, illustrating arthroconidia, one of which presents the characteristic budding blastoconidia from two corners, simulating "rabbit ears."

torula spp., and *Saccharomyces* spp. The yeast cells of *Cryptococcus* spp. are spherical, vary in size, and are widely separated by capsular material. The yeast cells of *Candida glabrata* are smaller, regular in size, and tend to arrange in compact clusters. The genus characteristics will be discussed in more detail below, along with the differentiating features of other less commonly encountered genera, such as *Rhodotorula*, *Saccharomyces*, *Hansenula*, and *Malassezia*. Occasional strains of *Candida* spp. may produce only rudimentary pseudohyphae or none at all; therefore, cornmeal agar preparations should be set up for any colony that is suspicious for *Candida* spp.

CRYPTOCOCCOSIS AND *CRYPTOCOCCUS NEOFORMANS*

The recovery of *Cryptococcus neoformans* from clinical specimens must always be considered significant until proven otherwise. Until the onset of the AIDS epidemic early in the 1980s, the incidence of cryptococcosis in the United States was low (about 300 cases per year). Most of these early cases occurred in patients with cellular immunodeficiencies, particularly in individuals with Hodgkin's disease.[149] Currently, *C. neoformans* is one of a select group of microorganisms causing infection in patients with AIDS, occurring in 6–13% of cases, depending on the place of residence.[186] The incidence of cryptococcosis in patients with AIDS is as high as 15% or greater in some locales in Sub-Saharan Africa.[183]

Of the cryptococci, *Cryptococcus neoformans* is responsible for most human infections. This species is an encapsulated yeast with its natural habitat in the soil. Soil contaminated with pigeon, chicken, or turkey droppings, in which the pH is alkaline and the nitrogen concentration is increased, in particular promotes organism replication. Yeast cells may become airborne in clouds of dust created during sweeping, cleaning, and excavating projects. Therefore, poultry farm workers, groundskeepers of city parks frequented by starlings and other birds, and spelunkers, who may explore bat-infested caves, are particularly at risk for acquiring infection. Persons who are immunosuppressed, particularly those with AIDS, are advised not to participate in these activities. In cases in which an immediate exposure is not evident, the onset of acute cryptococcosis may represent unmasking of latent infections.

Capsule synthesis is a major virulence determinant, providing a mechanism for adherence to mucosal linings and protection from phagocytosis, both during transit through the bloodstream and at the sites of infection.[113] *Cryptococcus neoformans* has a particular tropism for the central nervous system, and many cases initially manifest clinically as meningitis. The production of melanin pigment also is a virulence determinant, protecting the yeast against oxidant-induced damage. The production of proteinases, mannoproteins, and release of polyol metabolites account for the invasion and cell destruction observed at the sites of infection.

Cryptococcus neoformans can be suspected if a yeast produces colonies that are distinctly mucoid. It should be mentioned, however, that not all strains may produce capsules. Nonencapsulated strains often elicit a more pronounced granulomatous reaction, as observed in tissue sections, in

CLINICAL CORRELATION BOX 21-13   Arthroconidia-Producing Yeasts

Trichosporonosis

Trichosporon beigelii, an arthroconidia-forming species most commonly encountered in clinical laboratories, classically causes white piedra. This fungus may be carried on the skin, particularly around the anus. White piedra is an infection involving the hair of the scalp, body, or pubic hairs, presenting as small, circumscribed nodules or concretions on the hair shafts. Each nodule contains twisted fungal hyphae, which can be readily observed in direct KOH preparations, and from which the organism can be readily recovered. The infection can often be eradicated simply by shaving; only rarely is the use of topical or systemic azoles necessary to eradicate the infection.

Disseminated disease, most likely endogenous in origin, representing extensions from colonized cutaneous or gastrointestinal sites, may develop in persons who are immunosuppressed, and become life-threatening in some cases.[76] Hoy et al.[124] reviewed 19 cases of disseminated *T. beigelii* infections in patients with a variety of neoplastic diseases being treated at M.D. Anderson Hospital in Houston over a 10-year period. A nonspecific febrile illness or pneumonia was the most common clinical manifestation among this group of patients. Three fourths of these patients died; in relation to the discussion elsewhere, the diagnosis was not suspected prior to death in 25% of the autopsied cases. Other *Trichosporon* species, may cause invasive infection, particularly in patients with hematologic malignancy.[135]

The report by Sweet and Reed[269] indicates that neonates are not immune to disseminated disease. Yoss et al.[305] found that low-birth-weight infants in particular were susceptible, a situation of great concern because most cases have been fatal. Unfortunately, in many cases the diagnosis is often delayed either because the condition may not be recognized or because the organism is not quickly identified in the laboratory. It is important that microbiologists recognize the characteristic arthroconidia in cornmeal mounts as the initial clue to the identification and perform appropriate confirmatory tests.

Trichosporon beigelii is rapidly urease-positive and quite saccharolytic, producing acid from most carbohydrates. As a precautionary note, *Trichosporon beigelii* shares antigenic determinants with *Cryptococcus neoformans*; therefore, serum and cerebrospinal fluid from patients with disseminated disease may give a false-positive reaction with the cryptococcal latex agglutination test.

Geotrichosis

Disseminated infections with *Geotrichum* species is less commonly encountered. Isolated cases of disseminated *Geotrichum candidum* infection have been reported, two in patients with acute leukemia.[247] In one of these patients renal failure developed 3 days before death. The glomeruli were blocked with hyphal segments of *Geotrichum candidum*. The most recent case, reported by Andre et al.,[14] was in a young girl being treated for hepatoblastoma. After complications with secondary bacterial infections, this patient survived following a 5-week course of intravenous amphotericin B followed by 6 months of oral itraconazole. Although treatment regimens in patients with disseminated *Geotrichum* infection have not been established, the use of high doses of itraconazole and liposomal amphotericin B are recommended.[247]

Although cases of pneumonitis secondary to *Geotrichum* species have been reported, its recovery from respiratory secretions usually represents either contamination or commensal habitation, and other causes should be ruled out. *G. candidum* assimilates only glucose, galactose, and xylose, which, except for the xylose utilization, is a pattern similar to that of *T. capitatus*. Most strains of *Geotrichum* are urease-negative.

---

contrast to the liquefaction necrosis that is more commonly associated with invasion by nonencapsulated strains. Growth is usually observed within 36–72 hours on 5% sheep blood agar and most other primary isolation media (Color Plate 21-6).

Microscopically, the identification of *Cryptococcus* species can be made by demonstrating irregularly sized (4–10 μm), spherical yeast cells surrounded by a thick polysaccharide capsule (cells may be as much as 20 μm or more in diameter if the capsule is included in the measurement). In cornmeal agar preparations, pseudohyphae are not produced; irregular-sized, spherical yeast cells are separated one from the other by spaces produced by the capsular material (Fig. 21-91). Encapsulated yeast cells, often with a single bud attached by a hairlike strand, may be also be seen in India ink preparations (Fig. 21-92). Because of its insensitivity, the India ink procedure is being performed less commonly on cerebrospinal fluid specimens submitted to clinical laboratories, giving way to the more sensitive cryptococcal antigen detection tests.

An isolate suspicious for *C. neoformans* can be confirmed

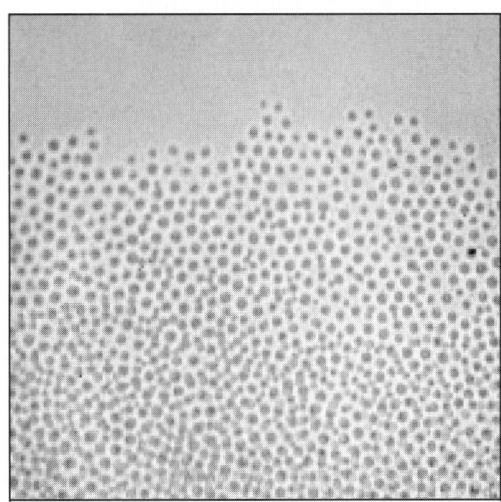

Figure 21-91 Photomicrograph of a cornmeal agar preparation of *Cryptococcus neoformans,* illustrating the irregular sized, spherical yeast cells separated by polysaccharide material.

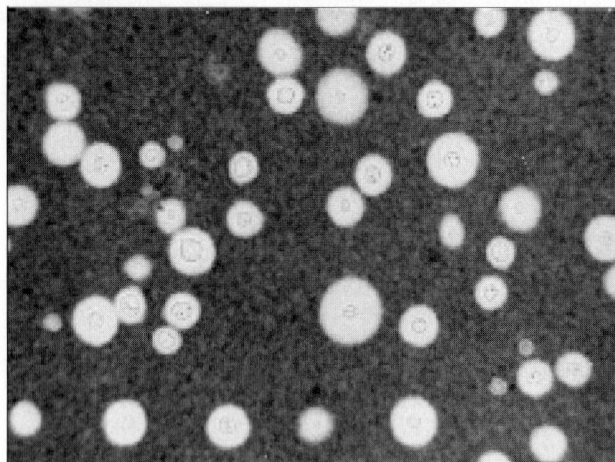

Figure 21-92 Photomicrograph of an India ink preparation, illustrating the irregular-sized, encapsulated, spherical yeast cells of *Cryptococcus neoformans.*

by demonstrating the production of caffeic acid, either through the production of a maroon-red pigment on "bird seed" agar (Color Plate 21-6*D*) or directly by inoculating a reagent-impregnated filter paper strip with a portion of the unknown colony and observing for the development of a black pigment.

Although other *Cryptococcus* spp. may be recovered from humans, their role as causative agents for infection is uncommon. The clinical presentations of such cases range from skin lesions to fungemia. Most cases of non-*neoformans* fungemia are nosocomially acquired, usually in patients with neutropenia, associated with indwelling intravascular catheters.[131] These authors also report two cases of fungemia caused by *Cryptococcus laurentii*, and warn that most non-*neoformans* cryptococci are more resistant to fluconazole and flucytosine than most *C. neoformans* isolates, thereby requiring a species identification in clinically relevant cases.

DIAGNOSIS BY NONCULTURE METHODS

Antigen detection assays on cerebrospinal fluid specimens are most commonly used to establish the diagnosis of cryptococcal meningitis, largely replacing the time-honored but less sensitive India-ink technique. The capsular material serves as the reactant, resulting in the agglutination reaction for the reagents used in these assays.[85] The latex agglutination assays currently available from several manufacturers are reliable, easy to perform, and sufficiently sensitive and specific to be implemented widely in most clinical mycology laboratories. Special equipment is not required, and the test procedure is easy to master. False-positive reactions can be minimized by boiling the fluid before testing or by pretreating with pronase to destroy extraneous proteins that may bind or block antigen-antibody coupling. Contaminating disinfectants and soaps may also cause false-positive reactions.[22] Syneresis fluid from agar plates may contaminate inoculating needles during colony sampling, leading to false-positive results. These false-positive reactions can often be detected by using control latex beads coated with normal globulins.

Additional clinical information on cryptococcosis is presented in Clinical Correlation Box 21-14.

Miscellaneous Non-Hyphae-Forming Yeasts of Medical Importance
CANDIDA (TORULOPSIS) GLABRATA

Candida glabrata is the currently accepted name for this organism. It is an agent of urinary tract infections, comprising about 20% of all yeast isolates from urine specimens.[88] Cases of endocarditis[36] and disseminated infection[119] caused by *C. glabrata* have been reported. *C. glabrata* assimilates both glucose and trehalose, an assimilation pattern that is helpful in making the laboratory identification.

Colonies of *C. glabrata* grow more slowly than other yeasts, often requiring 48–72 hours to evolve. Thus, if a slower-growing yeast is recovered on blood agar from a clinical specimen (particularly from the urine), that grows as small, entire, convex, glossy, smooth colonies (Color Plate 21-6*E*) and that microscopically appear as 2–3 μm in diameter, single-budding, regular-sized yeast cells, without the formation of pseudohyphae, *Candida (Torulopsis) glabrata* should be considered. On cornmeal agar preparations, the cells of *C. glabrata* arrange in relatively tight clusters, without the separation seen with *Cryptococcus* spp. (Fig. 21-93).

RHODOTORULA SPECIES

Rhodotorula spp. are airborne contaminants that may become commensal on the skin or may be recovered from the urine and feces. Recovery from respiratory secretions is usually of little significance. In the past, infections have been rare; however, currently, *Rhodotorula rubra* is listed among the "emerging" agents of infection. Fungemia is most often associated with colonized catheters or contaminated intravenous solutions.[43,140] *Rhodotorula* spp. have been recovered from shower curtains, bathtub grout, and toothbrushes. Septicemia related to indwelling catheters, meningitis, and peritonitis in patients receiving continuous peritoneal dialysis are among the uncommon infections caused by this organism.

The observation of yeastlike colony with a red or orange-red pigmentation (Color Plate 21-6*F*) is most likely *Rhodotorula* spp. The microscopic morphology is nondiagnostic. Pseudohyphae are not formed; rather, oval budding yeast cells in irregular, loose clusters are observed. Most strains are rapidly urease-positive.

SACCHAROMYCES SPECIES

The colonies, appearing within 36–48 hours, are gray-white and pasty in appearance, with irregular rugae. The appearance is nonspecific, and carbohydrate-assimilation studies may be required to confirm the identification. Failure to assimilate cellobiose and xylose are helpful in separating *Saccharomyces* spp. from other biochemically related species.

The microscopic morphology also is not specific. Loose clusters of large, oval, budding yeast forms are observed in cornmeal preparations, When colonies are grown on nutritionally poor ascospore agar (contains potassium acetate, yeast extract, glucose, water, and distilled water), the identification can be confirmed by observing ascospores. After incubation of an inoculated plate for 7–10 days, a smear can

CLINICAL CORRELATION BOX 21-14 Cryptococcosis

Following are the several clinical manifestations of cryptococcosis. Cryptococcosis currently is considered an AIDS-defining illness, and HIV testing should be performed whenever *C. neoformans* has been recovered from clinical specimens or when antigen-detection tests are positive. Nonetheless, recent cases of cryptococcosis in immunocompetent hosts have been reported as indicated below. Although rare, non-*neoformans Cryptococcus* species may also serve as agents of fungemia and disseminated disease.[131]

Central Nervous System

Central nervous system disease may occur without evidence of disease elsewhere. The onset of symptoms may be insidious, with mild headaches, memory lapses, or personality changes being the only clues. Low-grade fever may also be present. As the disease progresses, signs and symptoms suggestive of meningitis slowly develop—namely, nuchal rigidity, tenderness of the neck, and positive knee and leg flexion tests (Brudzinki's and Kernig's signs). In cases of localized cryptococcal granulomas, signs and symptoms such as paralysis, hemiparesis, and Jacksonian seizures may be evident. Blurring of vision, diplopia, ophthalmoplegia, slurred speech, double vision, and unsteadiness of gait are usually manifestations of an expanding lesion (cryptococcoma). Papilledema is generally a sign of increased intracranial pressure. Weight loss, malaise, persistence of fever, nausea, vomiting, and dizziness may be experienced as the disease progresses. In progressive fulminant or fatal cases, mental changes may be marked (agitation, irritability, confusion, hallucinations, psychosis), developing into delirium, coma, and finally death. Cerebrospinal fluid examination may reveal an increase in lymphocytes, low glucose levels, and elevated protein. Spontaneous onset of CNS cryptococcosis is an AIDS-defining illness.

Pulmonary Cryptococcosis

Localized or generalized pneumonia may be seen. A recently reported case by Sweeney et al.[268] indicates that pulmonary cryptococcosis may occur in immunocompetent hosts. They report the case of a 10-year-old boy with a malignant fibrous histiocytoma of bone and pulmonary nodule secondary to *C. neoformans* infection. This patient's diagnosis was suggested by the appearance of a pulmonary lesion on a computerized tomographic study. In a review of 13 cases, 6 were asymptomatic. Cryptococcal pulmonary disease is often recognized as a result of imaging done for other reasons. Zhu et al.[306] also report four cases of pulmonary cryptococcosis in non-HIV-infected patients, associated with cryptococcal meningitis. Again, all four patients had no apparent symptoms of pulmonary disease. Lee et al.[155] cite the Riu stain (commonly used to demonstrate bacterial flagellae) as an excellent way to demonstrate organisms in smears prepared from bronchoscopic brushings or needle aspirates in cases in which the diagnosis may not be made because of the lack of primary signs, symptoms, or x-ray findings.

The natural history, clinical presentation, diagnosis, and therapy of primary pulmonary cryptococcosis has been elucidated in a review of 41 patients by Kerking et al.[137] They were able to establish the diagnosis when an abnormal chest roentgenogram was associated with the isolation of *C. neoformans* from respiratory secretions and/or the observation of mucicarmine-positive, typical-appearing organisms in sections of lung tissue. The majority of the patients in their series had underlying conditions predisposing to cryptococcal infection: immunosuppressive therapy (28 of 41), diabetes mellitus (20 of 41), hematologic or lymphoreticular malignancies (12 of 41), recent renal transplantation (10 of 41), and connective-tissue diseases of chronic active hepatitis (5 of 41). Seven of the patients had no detectable underlying abnormalities. Constitutional symptoms predominated—fever and malaise occurred in over half the patients. Chest pain, dyspnea, weight loss, and night sweats in varying combinations were observed in from one fourth to one third of the patients. Only seven of the patients reported cough. Seven patients were asymptomatic and studied only because of abnormal roentgenograms. The abnormalities observed on chest x-ray examination included circumscribed mass lesions, alveolar or interstitial infiltrates, abscesses with air-fluid levels or cavitary lesions (7 of 41), solitary coin lesions, and multiple small rounded opacities.

Cutaneous Cryptococcosis

Primary cryptococcal infection of the skin is rare; usually cutaneous disease is a manifestation of systemic infection.[106] Murakawa et al.[186] found that in their institution 5.9% of patients treated with cryptococcal infection and AIDS also had skin lesions. The authors describe a variety of appearances of these lesions—umbilicated papules, nodules, and violaceous plaques, at times resembling molluscum contagiosum, or in other cases more reminiscent of Kaposi's sarcoma. Lesions were most commonly seen on the head and neck. A comparison of the clinical manifestations of cutaneous cryptococcosis in the pre-AIDS and AIDS era has been presented by Pema et al.[213] A case of primary cryptococcal cellulitis of the right arm in a 75-year-old man from Australia was described by Hamann et al.[112] The etiologic agent was *C. neoformans* var. *gattii*, a fungus that is endemic in Australia and may cause infections in immunocompetent humans.

Disseminated Cryptococcosis

Because strains of *C. neoformans* that produce capsular material can withstand the phagocytosis by segmented neutrophils, or can survive in the cytoplasm of mononuclear phagocytes, they may be distributed widely in the human host. In disseminated cases, virtually any viscera or organ system may be involved. As mentioned before, most cutaneous cryptococcal lesions represent disseminated disease. Even if an initial bout of meningitis is cured, symptoms may recur from reinfection from a remote site.

(continued)

CLINICAL CORRELATION BOX 21-14 *Continued*

Minamoto and Rosenberg[183] report that cryptococcal prostatitis persists after apparently successful therapy in 29% of males with disseminated disease and serves as a reservoir for ultimate meningitis relapse. Liu[161] culled from the literature 40 cases of cryptococcal osteomyelitis, which 75% of the time was limited to a single bone. The vertebrae were the most common site. Sarcoidosis, tuberculosis, and previous steroid therapy were the main predisposing causes of cryptococcosis in these cases. Cryptococcal myositis is only rarely reported, most commonly occurring in patients with HIV infection. O'Neill et al.[203] report an unusual non-AIDS case of cryptococcal myositis in a heart-transplant recipient undergoing immunosuppressive therapy. Primary liver disease may predispose to cryptococcal peritonitis, although it is a rare event.[263]

Cryptococcal infections of the urinary tract are also uncommon.[261] The kidneys, in particular the glomeruli, often harbor large numbers of organisms (may have to do with a slightly acid pH due to Na^+ and H^+ exchange. When *C. neoformans* is recovered from the urinary tract, a search for disseminated disease should be made. In cases of culture-negative meningitis, for example, the diagnosis of cryptococcosis may be made by recovering cryptococcal organisms being passed in the urine.

be prepared from one of the isolated colonies and stained with an acid-fast stain. Observe for ascospores, which appear as large, thick-walled, spherical cells with a distinct red pigment in an acid-fast preparation (Color Plate 21-6*H*).

Saccharomyces cerevisiae, the common "baker's" or "brewer's" yeast, usually colonizes the mucous membranes of humans but is not commonly considered pathogenic. Occasional cases of fungemia in immunosuppressed patients have been reported in the older literature.[44,77,194,272] Oliver et al.[202] describe three bone-marrow-transplant recipients on a hematology unit in whom invasive *S. cerevisiae* infection developed. Two of the patients died. Genotyping of the invasive and carriage strains demonstrated an indistinguishable strain from patients who had been on the unit at the same time, suggesting cross-infection.

HANSENULA ANOMALA

A rare isolate in clinical laboratories, *Hansenula anomala* is included here because, in addition to *Saccharomyces* spp., it also produces acid-fast ascospores when observed in an acid-fast smear. The ascospores of *Hansenula* differ from those of *Saccharomyces* by being flattened on one side rather than spherical, with a distinct outer rim or lip at the flat base, simulating the derby hat of an English bobby (Fig. 21-94). Isolated infections have been reported in immunosuppressed patients, commonly associated with indwelling catheters. Murphy and Buchanan[188] report 52 neonates who were colonized with *Hansenula anomala*, some of whom had evidence of systemic infection. Ma et al.[169] report a case of a premature infant with staphylococcal osteomyelitis who was found to have *Hansenula anomala* fungemia just before the initiation of the antimicrobial therapy with teicoplanin. The infant was cured after 10 days of antifungal therapy. Kalenic et al.[134] report a recent outbreak of *Hansenula* anomala infection in eight adult patients treated at a surgical intensive care unit. The source of the infections and route of transmission was not identified.

MALASSEZIA FURFUR

Recovery in culture may be difficult because the organism requires fatty acids for growth. When recovery of the organism is anticipated based on the clinical history, a few drops of virgin olive oil should be added to the surface of

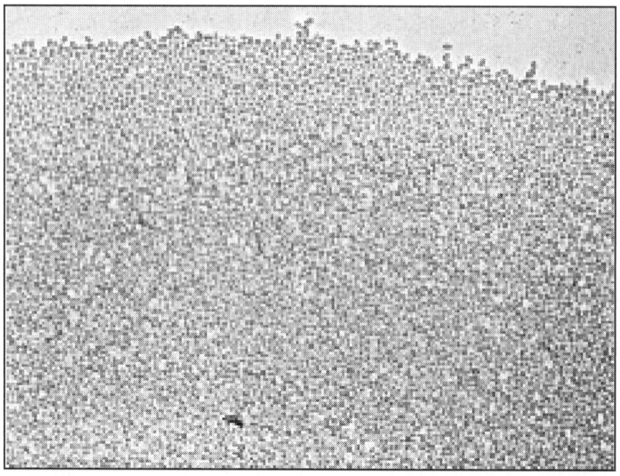

Figure 21-93 Photomicrograph of a cornmeal agar preparation of *Candida glabrata,* illustrating tight clusters of tiny, uniform yeast cells not separated by capsular material.

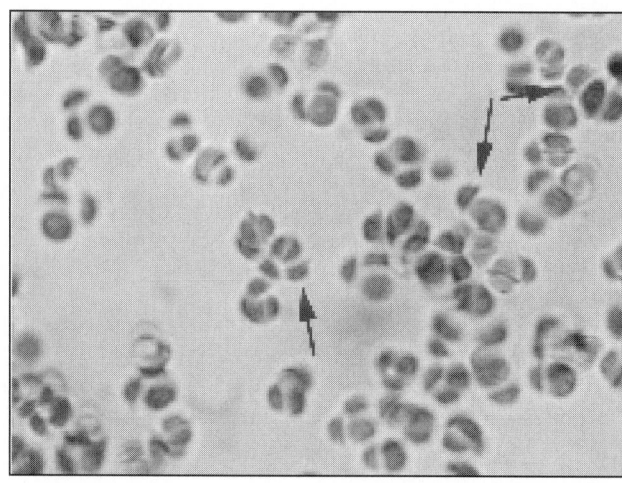

Figure 21-94 Photomicrograph of an acid-fast stained preparation, revealing acid-fast yeast cells on *Hansenula anomala*, characteristically shaped like an English bobby hat, complete with brim (*arrows*).

a sheep blood agar plate immediately after inoculation. In some mycology laboratories, it is common practice to overlay the agar plates prepared from all blood cultures received from the neonatal intensive-care ward because so many of these newborns are receiving total parenteral nutrition and are at high risk for malassezia septicemia.[54] The organisms grow well as small yeast colonies underneath the oil droplets (Color Plate 21-6G). Microscopically small budding yeast cells lying singly and in loose clusters are observed. The hyphal elements seen in direct KOH mounts of skin scrapings are not observed in microscopic mounts prepared from yeast cultures.

Malassezia furfur, a lipophilic yeast that is a common commensal of the skin, is the cause of a superficial cutaneous infection in persons with poor hygiene, known as tinea (pityriasis) versicolor. Tinea versicolor presents as scaling lesions of the skin, primarily of the thorax and back, at times extending to the neck, face, and arms. The lesions are flat, irregular in outline, and may have a tan or brown pigmentation, but often appear as white blotches of discoloration, particularly in skin exposed to sunlight. The fungal elements in these lesions produce a brick-red fluorescence when examined with long-wavelength ultraviolet light (Wood's lamp). Direct examination of skin scrapings reveal hyphal elements, and 3–5-μm diameter budding yeast cells (colloquially referred to as "spaghetti and meatballs"), with the formation of a distinct collarette at the margin between the mother and daughter cell.

Systemic infections and septicemia have also been reported, most commonly associated with deep-line vascular catheters, particularly in patients receiving long-term hyperalimentation therapy. The case report by Rosales et al.[237] of *Malassezia furfur* meningitis in a very-low-birth-weight infant receiving total parenteral nutrition and intralipid fluid infusion into the subarachnoid space via a peripheral scalp indicates that this source of fungemia has not been eliminated. Many of the hyperalimentation emulsions are rich in long-chain fatty acids. An ideal microenvironment is established at the catheter site, where a small amount of the oil-rich emulsion can pool, supporting growth of the endogenous lipophilic organisms present on the skin surface. The catheter provides a barrier break in the skin through which the proliferating organisms can enter the bloodstream.

Laboratory Identification of "Black Yeasts"
AUREOBASIDIUM PULLULANS

Aureobasidium spp. grow as smooth, moist colonies appearing as a "**black yeast.**" Microscopically, the dark, dematiaceous hyphae become thickened as the colony matures, appearing as arthroconidia. Myriad small, elliptical, single-celled, hyaline conidia are produced from buds from the centers of individual hyphal segments (Fig. 21-95). Occasional cases of cutaneous phaeohyphomycoses secondary to *Aureobasidium pullulans* have been reported in humans.[239] More recent case reports include rare case of disseminated nosocomial fungal infection due to *Aureobasidium pullulans* var. *melanigenum* in a severely traumatized patient by Bolignano and Criseo[27] and a 50-year-old patient with an infected corneal ulcer reported by Gupta and Elewski.[102] Scleritis developed 5 days after surgery, and the patient became asymptomatic after antifungal therapy, surgical debridement, and cryotherapy.

PHAEOANNELLOMYCES WERNECKII

The genus "*Phaeoannellomyces*" was created in 1985, by McGinnis et al.[177] "to accommodate those black yeasts that are characterized by the development of yeast cells that function as annellides" (*phaeo* = dark; *annello* = annellides; *myces* = fungus).

Phaeoannellomyces werneckii (*Exophiala werneckii*) microscopically produces two-celled yeast cells. The daughter cell is produced from an extension from the mother cell, which then contracts to form a scar (annellide), appearing as a deep-staining septum that separates the two cells (Fig. 21-96). It is this annellide formation that warrants inclusion in the new genus *Phaeoannellomyces*, according to the McGinnis scheme. Engleberg et al.[74] have reported a case of phaeohyphomycotic cyst caused by *Phaeoannellomyces elegans*. The

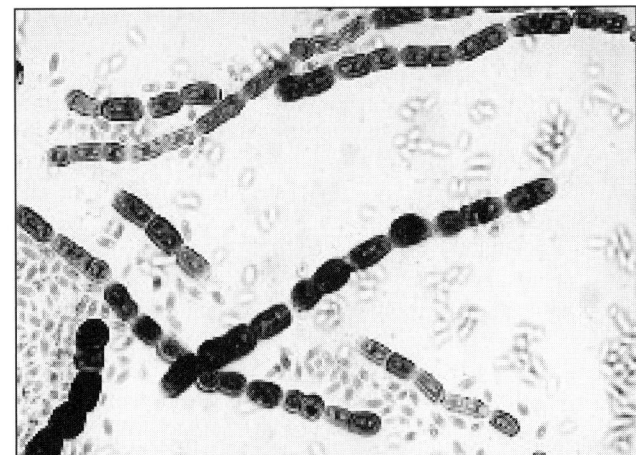
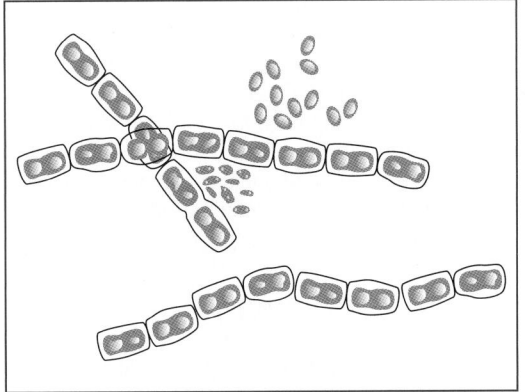

Figure 21-95 Photomicrograph and sketch of the microscopic appearance of *Aureobasidium pullulans,* illustrating chains of large, dark-staining arthroconidia-like cells with small, hyaline conidia in the background.

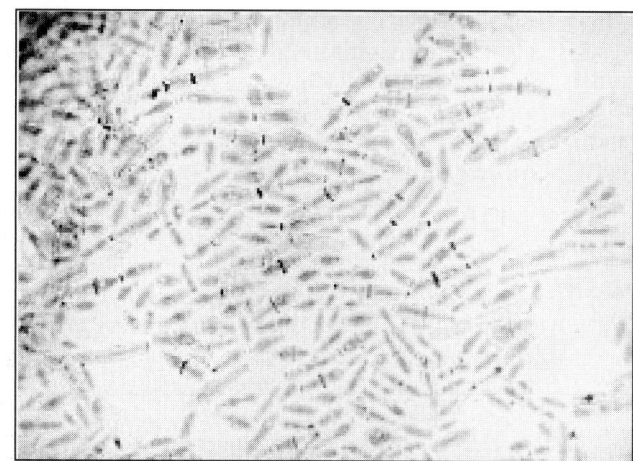
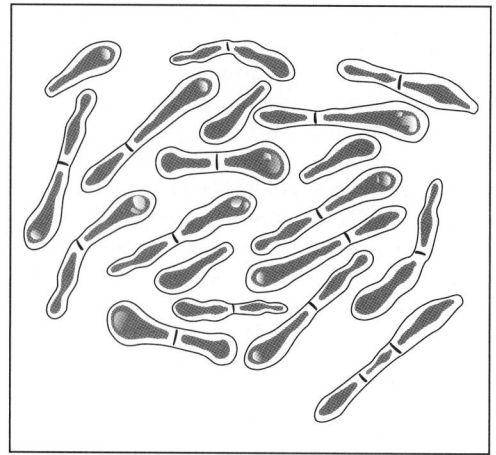

A   B

Figure 21-96 Photomicrograph and sketch of the yeast forms of *Phaeoannellomyces* species, revealing elongated double yeast cells separated by a distinct deeply staining transverse bar (annellide).

yeast cells with this species are unicellular and may develop thick dark walls and pseudohyphae on maturity.

Controversy still exists about whether the genus "*Phaeoannellomyces*" has taxonomic legitimacy. Kwon-Chung et al.[153] have found that "the yeastlike colonial characteristics are invariably unstable, and the colony becomes mycelial as the cultures are maintained in the laboratory." She goes on to describe a culture of *Phaeoannellomyces elegans* referred to her laboratory that, on arrival, had already taken on morphologic characteristics indistinguishable from those of *Exophiala jeanselmei*. Thus, based on these observations, Kwon-Chung argues against creating a separate genus designation for the yeast form as she feels they are synonymous. Perhaps in response to this finding, the McGinnis school cited above has suggested the term **synanamorph** to designate one of several anamorphic forms with which a fungus may present.

Packaged Yeast-Identification Systems

Several packaged kits for identifying yeasts have been introduced by commercial companies (Box 21-8).[280] The use of these systems requires technical skills and sufficient familiarity with each test performed to enable accurate interpretations. In each instance, the manufacturer's instructions must be closely followed. Each laboratory director or supervisor must weigh factors such as cost, availability and supply, shelf life and stability of reagents, adaptability to work flow, and the specific needs of the clinical services before a decision can be made to implement these systems in the home laboratory.

Antifungal Susceptibility Testing

Through a consensus process spanning the past decade, the Clinical Laboratory Standards Institute (formerly, the National Committee for Clinical Laboratory Standards) Subcommittee on Antifungal Susceptibility Testing has established standardized and reproducible methods for the antifungal susceptibility testing of yeasts.[192,219,220,230] Establishing these laboratory standards, particularly for the yeasts, has provided valuable guidelines for antifungal therapy with improved correlation with clinical outcomes.[93] The macrodilution method and its microdilution modification currently serve as the reference standards. It against this "gold standard" that other methods for performing antifungal susceptibility tests have evolved, now making it possible for many clinical microbiology laboratories to provide these services.

Sewell and coworkers,[253] in a comparative study of susceptibility tests for fluconazole, have shown that the Epsilometer "Etest®" (AB Biodisk, Solna, Sweden) compares favorably with the reference methods, with an overall 84% agreement, reaching as high as 90% for most *Candida* species, except for *C. tropicalis* (56%). *Candida* (*Torulopsis*) *glabrata* also had low comparison values in this study (34%).

The Etest® uses a plastic strip containing a defined continuous gradient of antimicrobial drug, which is placed on the surface of an agar plate after it has been evenly plated with an inoculum containing a standardized concentration of the yeast organisms to be tested (Fig. 21-97). Upon being hydrated, the plastic strip releases the antifungal agent into the surrounding agar, producing a logarithmic increase in the concentration of antibiotic from as low as 0.002 μg/mL to as high as 256 μg/mL, depending on the antifungal agent being tested. The details for performing the Etest®, including the recommended test medium, the preparation of the standard inoculum, the steps of the procedure, and the readout can be found in the publication by Colombo et al.[48] This report also included the results for the Etest® against 200 yeast isolates, compared with the standard methods for several individual drugs. The essential agreements between the two methods within a ± 1 dilution was 71% for ketoconazole, 80% for fluconazole, and 84% for itraconazole. Since the publication of this paper, the use of a standardized medium (RMPI 1640), a final reading at 48 hours, and other adjustments have raised the essential agreement percentage sufficient to establish the Etest® as an alternative method for the fungal susceptibility testing of most yeast species. As mentioned before, because the Etest® is less

Box 21-8 Study of Seven Yeast-Identification Systems

Vitek (BioMérieux Vitek, Hazelwood, MO)

The Vitek card used in this study comprises 30 wells that are inoculated with a suspension of the unknown yeast and incubated at 30°C for 24–48 hours in the instrument incubation chamber. Color changes are read spectrophotometrically and reported as a nine-digit numerical code. The database includes 36 yeast species. In this study, 59.6% of 52 isolates were identified without additional tests. However, with the use of the ID-YST card, which comprises 64 wells with 47 fluorescent biochemical tests, used in conjunction with the new VITEK 2 system, Graf et al. report that 92.1% of 222 strains were read unequivocally, with only 11 isolates identified with a low discrimination.

The API ID 32C and API 20C AUX Systems (BioMérieux, Lyon, France)

The API ID 32 C and 20C AUX contain 32 and 20 microtubes, respectively. The reactions are read visually after 24, 48, or 72 hours of incubation at 30°C by comparing the turbidity of the medium within each of the microtubes with that of controls. A profile number of 10 and 7 digits, respectively, can be calculated. The databases of API ID 32 includes 63 yeast species and that of API 20C AUX, 43. In the present study, the API ID 32C and API 20C Aux systems identified 63.5% and 59.6% of the 52 isolates without additional tests. These relatively low rates of performance, however, are much improved, to as high as 98%, if the final readings are made at 72 hours versus 24 hours. The major difficulty with this system is in the visual reading of the relative turbidities within each of the cupules, leading to considerable interobserver variability.

Yeast Star (CLARC Laboratories, Heerlen, The Netherlands)

The Yeast Star system relies on the inhibitory effects of specific dyes on yeast growth. A panel of six dyes is placed on top of an inoculated solid growth medium and incubated for 24–48 hours at 37°C. The results are recorded in the form of a six-digit code. The database contains 16 yeast species. In this study, the Yeast Star system identified 59.6% of the 52 isolates without the need for additional tests. The relatively low level of performance resulted primarily from nonidentification because of the small database. This system is not widely used.

Auxacolor (Sanofi Diagnostics Pasteur, Marnes-La-Coquette, France)

The Auxacolor identification system is based on carbohydrate utilization, and growth is visualized by color change of a pH indicator. The microtiter plate contains 16 wells, and the plates are read after 24–72 hours of incubation at 30°C. In addition, various other characteristics, such as the ability to grow at 37°C, the formation of mycelium or arthrospores, and the presence of a capsule are also included. The database contains 26 yeast species. In this study, the Auxacolor system correctly identified 80.8% of the 52 strains, the top performer among the systems studied. In a study by Campbell et al., the performance was 91.2%, with only 2 isolates of 146 being incorrectly identified.

RapID Yeast Plus system (Innovative Diagnostic Systems, Norcross, GA)

The RapID Yeast Plus system is based on the utilization of carbohydrate substrates, the hydrolysis of fatty acids and urea, and enzymatic hydrolysis of glycoside and aryl-amide substrates. A panel of 18 cavities is incubated for 4 hours at 30°C and read after adding specific reagents. A six-digit code is derived from the results and compared with those of a database that includes 43 yeast species. In the present study, 76.9% of 52 strains were identified without additional tests. Espinel-Ingroff et al. reported a performance of 79.1% in the identification of emerging species of *Candida*; however, the performance was 94.2% in the identification of the species more commonly encountered in clinical laboratories.

API Candida (BioMérieux, Lyon, France)

The API Candida system consists of 10 tubes containing dehydrated substrates and relies on sugar acidification or enzymatic reactions. The strips are read after 24–48 hours of incubation at 30°C. A four-digit numerical profile is obtained, which is compared with those in a database with 26 yeast species. In this study, 78.8% of 52 strains were correctly identified without additional tests. In a study by Frickler-Hidalgo et al., 75.2% of all yeast isolates studied were correctly identified without additional tests; however, 90% of the species commonly encountered in the clinical laboratories were correctly identified. The lower levels of performance resulted from difficulties in reading certain of the color reactions, particularly in the cupules containing *N*-acetyl-glucosamine and β-xylose.

Cited References

Campbell CK, Davey KG, Holmes AD. Comparison of the API Candida system with the Auxacolor system for identification of common yeast pathogens. J Clin Microbiol 1999;37:821–823.

Espenil-Ingroff A, Stockman L, Roberts G, et al. Comparison of the RapID Yeast Plus system with API 20C system for the identification of common, new, and emerging yeast pathogens. J Clin Microbiol 1998;36:883–886.

Fricker-Hidalgo H, Vandapel O, Duchesne MA. Comparison of new API Candida system to the ID 32C system for identification of clinically important yeasts. J Clin Microbiol 1996;36:1846–1848.

Graf B, Adam T, Zill E, Gopbel UB. Evaluation of the Vitek2 system for rapid identification of yeasts and yeastlike organisms J Clin Microbiol 2000;38:1782–1785.

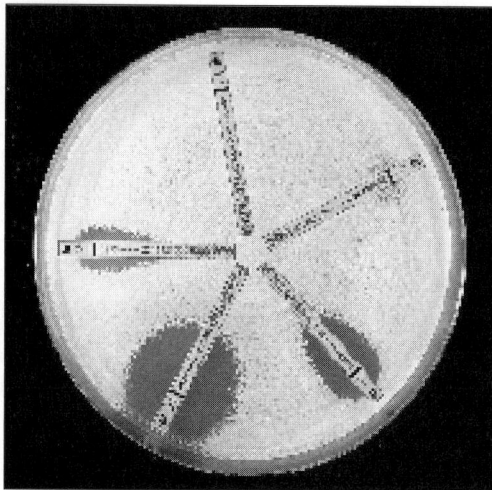

Figure 21-97 Photograph of the surface of an agar plate demonstrating an Etest®. Several gradient diffusion strips have been placed on a lawn of growth of *Candida kruzei*. The MIC interpretations of the strips reading clockwise beginning with fluconazole in the 11-o'clock position are: FL (fluconazole), >256 µg/ mL; FL (flucytosine) >32 µg/mL; IT (itraconazole), 0.38 µg/mL; VO (voriconazole) 0.38 µg/ mL, AP (amphotericin B), 2 µg/ mL.

labor intensive and easy to perform, in-house antifungal susceptibility testing is now within the reach of many clinical microbiology laboratories.

In a later multisite study, Pfaller et al.[218] demonstrated a high level of reproducibility of the Etest® minimal inhibitory concentration (MIC) method between four participating institutions. Each participating laboratory received subcultures of 2 American Type Culture Collection (ATCC) QC *Candida* strains (*C. parapsilosis*, ATCC 22019 and *C. krusei*, ATCC 6258), Etest® strips, and sufficient RPMI agar plates to perform 20 replicate tests with each of five drugs—amphotericin B, fluconazole, flucytosine, itraconazole, and ketoconazole. In almost all of the drug/bug combinations tested, a very tight distribution was observed, ranging between 98% and 100% of the MICs, falling within a three-dilution range. The selective discrepancies of results between the Etest® and the standard method for flucytosine and fluconazole against *C. krusei* was related to uneven growth between the glucose-enriched Etest® agar and the unsupplemented broth used in the reference macrobroth test.

The Etest® detected a resistant subpopulation of strains not picked up by the reference method. After analyzing all the data, the authors concluded that the study established excellent interlaboratory and intralaboratory levels of agreement between the two methods, providing further documentation of the utility of the Etest® in determining antifungal susceptibility profiles. This standardization of the test methods, the establishment of interpretive breakpoints for certain drug-yeast combinations, and reproducibility of results both within and between clinical laboratories will provide the basis on which clinical outcomes can be measured.[78]

The motivation to implement in vitro antifungal susceptibility tests in clinical laboratories goes beyond establishing

the resistance profiles of a given isolate. The emergence of antifungal resistance is becoming an issue of increasing concern. For example, with the more widespread use of fluconazole, reports of fluconazole resistance in *Candida* species and *Cryptococcus neoformans* have increased.[278] These workers also cite the increase in resistance of *Candida lusitaniae* and *Cryptococcus neoformans* to amphotericin B, presumably resulting from the use of single-drug therapy. Peyron et al.[216] have found that the Etest® provides the optimal means for discrimination between *C. lusitaniae* isolates that are amphotericin B–resistant and amphotericin B–susceptible. They found that putatively resistant isolates had an interpretive breakpoint MIC of ≥0.38 µg/mL using the Clinical Laboratory Standards Institute standard RPMI culture medium.

Decreased susceptibility to itraconazole has been observed against select *Aspergillus fumigatus* isolates. Azole resistance is also developing for *C. albicans* isolates from patients with AIDS, presumably resulting from the overuse of this drug in the treatment of oropharyngeal candidiasis (thrush). The intrinsic resistance of *Candida krusei* to the imidazoles and emerging resistance of *Candida glabrata* to this group of antifungal agents are also problematic. White et al.[293] have published a review of the clinical, cellular, and molecular factors that underlie the development of resistant strains, particularly of *Candida albicans*. In summary, it is becoming imperative that clinical microbiology laboratories provide in vitro antifungal susceptibility data in order to detect these emerging patterns of resistance.

Serologic Diagnosis of Fungal Diseases

Fungal serology is currently performed only in select reference laboratories. The time-honored procedures, including tube precipitin, immunodiffusion, latex agglutination, and complement fixation tests are giving way to newer, more sensitive technologies. Immunoassay (EIA) techniques that use species-specific monoclonal antibodies, nucleic-acid probe assays, and polymerase chain reaction (PCR) are being more widely used in clinical mycology laboratories.[114]

As a general rule, single species-specific serologic reactions in titers of 1:32 or greater indicate disease; however, demonstrating a rising titer fourfold or greater in samples drawn 3 weeks apart may be of greater significance.[56] Titers less than 1:32 or that do not show a fourfold increase between the paired samples usually indicate the presence of either early infection or nonspecific cross-reactivity with other antigens. The results from all serologic studies, nonetheless, must be considered presumptive.

Antibodies of the IgM class (using tube precipitin, latex agglutination, or immunodiffusion methods) are commonly detectable about 2 weeks after the disease is acquired, and indicate recent infection. Usually IgM antibodies are no longer detectable after 6 months. The presence of IgG antibodies (detected by complement fixation tests or by immunodiffusion) appear shortly after the rise in IgM titer, do not peak until about 6 to 12 weeks, and may remain elevated for many months after infection. Thus, a single elevated IgG antibody titer cannot be used to distinguish between recent and remote infections.

The nonculture serologic and new molecular techniques

have been reviewed in sections within the presentation of each fungus infection when helpful in establishing the diagnosis of invasive disease. Much attention is now shifting to sensitive assays being developed for the direct detection of fungal antigens in clinical specimens and in biologic fluids, often leading to same-day results. Breakthroughs in the practical applications of molecular techniques are being made monthly, making it mandatory for the directors and supervisors of clinical mycology laboratories to peruse the current medical literature to determine which of these techniques may be applicable to specific clinical settings.[145]

REFERENCES

1. Abi-Said D, Anaissie E, Uzur O, et al. The epidemiology of hematogenous candidiasis caused by different *Candida* species. Clin Infect Dis 1997;24: 1122–1128.
2. Adam RD, Piquin ML, Peterson EA, et al, Phaeohyphomycosis caused by the fungal genera *Bipolaris* and *Exserohilum*: a report of 9 cases and review of the literature. Medicine (Baltimore) 1986;65:203–217.
3. Ainscough S, Kibbler CC. An evaluation of the cost-effectiveness of using CHROMagar for yeast identification in a routine microbiology laboratory. J Med Microbiol 1998;47:623–628.
4. Aisner JA, Schimpff SC, et al. Aspergillus infection in cancer patients: association with fire-proofing materials in a new hospital. JAMA 1996;235:411–412.
5. Ajello L. Hyalohyphomycosis: a disease entity whose time has come. Newslett Med Mycol Soc NY 1982;10:305.
6. Ajello L. Hyalohyphomycosis and phaeohyphomycosis: two global disease entities of public health importance. Eur J Epidemiol 1986;2:243–251.
7. al-Fouzan AS, Nanda A, Kubec K. Dermatophytosis of children in Kuwait: a prospective survey. Int J Dermatol 1993;32:798–801.
8. Almeida OP, Jacks J Jr, Scully C. Paracoccidioidomycosis of the mouth: an emerging deep mycosis. Crit Rev Oral Biol Med 2003;14:377–383.
9. al-Tawfiq JA. Wools KK. Disseminated sporotrichosis and *Sporothrix schenckii* fungemia as the initial presentation. Clin Infect Dis 1998;26:1403–1406.
10. Alvarez M, Ponga BL, Rayon C, et al. Nosocomial outbreak caused by *Scedosporium prolificans* (*inflatum*): four fatal cases in leukemic patients. J Clin Microbiol 1995;33:3290–3295.
11. Amanio PC. Fungal infections of the hand. Hand Clin 1998;14:605–612.
12. Ampel NM, Dols CL, Galgiani JN. Coccidioidomycosis during human immunodeficiency virus infection: results of a prospective study in a coccidioidal endemic area. Am J Med 1993;94:235–240.
13. Anaissie E, Fainstein V, Samo T, et al. Central nervous system histoplasmosis. An unappreciated complication of the acquired immunodeficiency syndrome. Am J Med 1988;84:215–217.
14. Andre N, Coze C, Gentet JC, et al. *Geotrichum candidum* septicemia in a child with hepatoblastoma. Pediatr Infect Dis J 2004;23:86
15. Antoniskis D, Larsen RA, Akil B, et al. Sero-negative disseminated coccidioidomycosis in patients with HIV infection. AIDS 1990;4:691–693.
16. Areno JP IV, Campbell GD Jr, George RB. Diagnosis of blastomycosis. Semin Respir Infect 1997;12:252–262.
17. Arguinchona HL, Ampel NM, Dols CL, et al. Positive coccidioidal serologies in HIV-infected patients without evidence of active coccidioidomycosis. International Conference on AIDS, August 7–12, 1994. 10:160.
18. Arnold MG, Arnold JC, Bloom DC, et al. Head and neck manifestations of disseminated coccidioidomycosis. Laryngoscope 2004;114:747–752.
19. Babel DE, Rogers AL, Beneke ES. Dermatophytosis of the scalp: incidence, immune response, and epidemiology. Mycopathologia 1990;109:69–73.
20. Bassiouny A, El-Refai HA, et al. *Candida* infection of the tongue and pharynx. J Laryngol Otol 1984;98:609–611.
21. Baumgardner DJ, Buggy BP, Mattson RJ, et al. Epidemiology of blastomycosis in a region of high endemicity in north central Wisconsin. Clin Infect Dis 1992; 15:629–635.
22. Blevens LB, Fenn J, Segal H, et al. False positive cryptococcal antigen latex agglutination caused by disinfectants and soaps. J Clin Microbiol 1995;33: 1674–1675.
23. Blinkhorn RJ, Adelstein D, Spagnuolo PJ. Emergence of a new opportunistic pathogen, *Candida lusitaniae*. J Clin Microbiol 1989;27:236–240.
24. Blum HE. Infection due to *Penicillium marneffei*, an emerging pathogen: review of 155 reported cases. Clin Infect Dis 1996;23:125–130.
25. Blumenfeld W, Gan GL. Diagnosis of histoplasmosis in bronchoalveolar lavage fluid by intra-cytoplasmic localization of silver-positive yeast. Acta Cytol 1991; s35:710–712.
26. Boelaert JR, vanRoost GF, Vergauwe PL, et al. The role of desferrioxamine in dialysis-associated mucormycosis: report of three cases and review of the literature. Clin Nephrol 1988;29:261–266.
27. Bolignano G, Criseo G. Disseminated nosocomial fungal infection by *Aureobasidium pullulans* var. *melanigenum*: a case report. J Clin Microbiol 2003;41: 4483–4485.
28. Botteon FA, Camargo ZP, Benard G, et al. *Paracoccidioides brasiliensis*-reactive antibodies in Brazilian blood donors. Med Mycol 2002;40:387–391.
29. Boutati EI, Anaissie EJ. *Fusarium*, a significant emerging pathogen in patients with hematologic malignancy: ten years' experience at a cancer center and implications for management. Blood 1997;90:999–1008.
30. Bradsher RW. Clinical features of blastomycosis. Semin Respir Infect 1997;12: 229–34.
31. Brandt ME, Warnock DW. Epidemiology, clinical manifestations, and therapy of infections caused by dematiaceous fungi. J Chemother 2003;15:Suppl 2:36–47.
32. Brummer E, Castaneda E, Restrepo A. Paracoccidioidomycosis: an update. Clin Microbiol Rev 1993;6:89–117.
33. Butt AA, Carreon J. *Histoplasma capsulatum* sinusitis. J Clin Microbiol 1997; 35:2649–2650.
34. Calza L, Manfredi R, Donzelli C, et al. Disseminated histoplasmosis with atypical cutaneous lesions in an Italian HIV-infected patient: another autochthonous case. HIV Med 2003;4:145–148.
35. Camargo ZP, Taborda CP, Rodrequez EG, Travassos LR. The use of cell-free antigens of *Paracoccidioides brasiliensis* in serological tests. J Med Vet Mycol 1991;29:31–38.
36. Carmody TJ, Kane KK. *Torulopsis* (*Candida*) *glabrata* endocarditis involving a bovine pericardial xenograft heart valve. Heart Lung 1986;15:40–42.
37. Castro LG, Salebian A, Sotto MN. Hyalohyphomycosis by *Paecilomyces lilacinus* in a renal transplant patient and a review of human *Paecilomyces* species infections. J Med Vet Mycol 1990;28:15–26.
38. Chalub E, Sambuelli R, Armando R, Bistoni A. Histologic response of disseminated histoplasmosis in AIDS patients with skin lesions. International Conference on AIDS, August 7–12, 1994. 10:148.
39. Chan TH, Koehler A, Li PK. *Paecilomyces variotii* peritonitis in patients on continuous ambulatory peritoneal dialysis. Am J Kidney Dis 1996;27:138–142.
40. Chan-Tack RM, Thio CL, Miller NS, et al. *Paecilomyces lilacinus* fungemia in an adult bone marrow transplant recipient. Med Mycol 1999;37:57–60.
41. Chappell MS, Mandell W, Grimes MM, Neu HC. Gastrointestinal histoplasmosis. Dig Dis Sci 1988;33:353–360.
42. Chowdhary G, Weinstein A, Klein R, Mascarenhas BR. Sporotrichal arthritis. Ann Rheum Dis 1991;50:112–114.
43. Chung JW, Kim BN, Kim YS. Central venous catheter-related Rhodotorula rubra fungemia. J Infect Chemother 2002;8:109–110.
44. Cimolai N, Gill MJ, Church D. *Saccharomyces cerevisiae* fungemia: a case report and review of the literature. Diagn Microbiol Infect Dis 1987;8:113–117.
45. Ciulla TA, Piper HC, Xiao M, Wheat LJ. Presumed ocular histoplasmosis syndrome: update on epidemiology, pathogenesis, and photodynamic, antiangiogenic, and surgical therapies. Curr Opin Ophthalmol 2001;12:442–449.
46. Clancy CJ, Nguyen MH. Invasive sinus aspergillosis in apparently immunocompetent hosts. J Infect 1998;37:229–240.
47. Coleman DC, Rinaldi MG, Haynes KA, et al. Importance of *Candida* species other than *Candida albicans* as opportunistic pathogens. Med Mycol 1998;36: Suppl 1:156–165.
48. Colombo AL, Barchiesi F, McGough DA, Rinaldi MG. Comparison of Etest and National Committee for Clinical Laboratory Standards broth macrodilution method for azole antifungal susceptibility testing. J Clin Microbiol 1995;33: 535–540.
49. Confalonieri M, Nanetti A, Gandola L, et al. *Histoplasmosis capsulatum* in Italy: autochthonous or imported? Eur J Epidemiol 1994;110:435–439.
50. Cooper CR Jr, McGinnis MR. Pathology of *Penicillium marneffei*. An emerging acquired immunodeficiency syndrome-related pathogen. Arch Pathol Lab Med 1997;121:798–804.
51. Cooter RD, Lim IS, Ellis DH, Leitch IO. Burn wound zygomycosis caused by *Apophysomyces elegans*. J Clin Microbiol 1990;28:2151–2153.
52. Cutler JE. Putative virulence factors of *Candida albicans*. Annu Rev Microbiol 1991;45:185–218.
53. Dahl MV, Grando SA. Chronic dermatophytosis: what is special about *Trichophyton rubrum*? Adv Dermatol 1994;9:97–109.
54. Danker WM, Spector SA, Fierer J, Davis CD. *Malassezia* fungemia in neonates and adults: complication of hyperalimentation. Rev Infect Dis 1987;9:743–753.
55. Darrisaw L, Hanson G, Vesole DH, Kehl SC. *Cunninghamella* infection post bone marrow transplant: case report and review of the literature. Bone Marrow Transplant 2000;25:1213–1216.

56. Davies SF, Sarosi GA. Role of sero-diagnostic tests and skin tests in the diagnosis of fungal disease. Clin Chest Med 1987;8:135–146.

57. Davies SF, Sarosi GA. Blastomycosis. Eur J Clin Microbiol Infect Dis 1989;8: 474–479.

58. Davies SF, Sarosi GA. Epidemiological and clinical features of pulmonary blastomycosis. Seminars in Resp Infect 1997;12:206–218.

59. de Battle J, Motje M, Balanza R, et al. Disseminated infection caused by *Scedosporium prolificans* in a patient with acute multi-lineal leukemia. J Clin Microbiol 2000;38:1694–1695.

60. de Hoog GS. Significance of fungal evolution for the understanding of their pathogenicity, illustrated with agents of phaeohyphomycosis. Mycoses 1997;40: Suppl 2:5–8.

61. Denning DW, Stephens DA. Antifungal and surgical treatment of invasive aspergillosis: review of 2121 published cases. Rev Infect Dis 1990;12:1147–1201.

62. diTommasso JP, Ampel NM, Sobonya RE, Bloom JW. Bronchoscopic diagnosis of pulmonary coccidioidomycosis: comparison of cytology, culture, and transbronchial biopsy. Diagn Microbiol Infect Dis 1994;18:83–87.

63. Dixon DM, Walsh TJ, Merz WG, McGinnis MR. Infections due to *Xylohypha bantiana* (*Cladosporium trichoides*). Rev Infect Dis 1990;11:515–525.

64. Donabedian H, O'Donnell E, Olszewski C, et al. Disseminated cutaneous and meningeal sporotrichosis in an AIDS patient. Diagn Microbiol Infect Dis 1994; 18:2111–2118.

65. Dooley DP, Bostic PS, Beckius ML. Spook house sporotrichosis: a point-source outbreak of sporotrichosis associated with hay bale props in a Halloween haunted-house. Arch Intern Med 1997;157:1885–1887.

66. Dumich PS, Neel HB. Blastomycosis of the larynx. Laryngoscope 1983;93: 1266–1270.

67. Durkin MM, Connolly PA, Wheat LJ. Comparison of radioimmunoassay and enzyme-linked immunoassay methods for detection of *Histoplasma capsulatum* var. *capsulatum* antigen. J Clin Microbiol 1997;35:2252–2255.

68. Durkin M, Witt J, LeMonte A, et al. Antigen assay with the potential to aid in diagnosis of blastomycosis. J Clin Microbiol 2004;42:4873–4875.

69. Economopoulou P, Laskaris G, Kittas C. Oral histoplasmosis as an indicator of HIV infection. Oral Surg Oral Med Oral Pathol Oral Radiol Endodont 1998;86: 203–206.

70. Eleski BE. Tinea capitis: a current perspective. J Am Acad Dermatol 2000;42: 1–20.

71. Elgart GW. Chromomycosis. Derm Clin 1996;14:77–83

72. Ellepola AN, Hurst SF, Elie CM, Morrison CJ. Rapid and unequivocal differentiation of *Candida dubliniensis* from other *Candida* species using species-specific DNA probes: comparison with phenotypic identification methods. Oral Microbiol Immunol 2003;18:379–388.

73. Ellison MD, Hung RT, Harris K, Campbell BH. Report of the first case of invasive fungal sinusitis caused by *Scopulariopsis acremonium*: review of scopulariopsis infections. Arch Otolaryngol Head Neck Surg 1998;124.1014–1016.

74. Engleberg NC, Johnson J IV, Bleustein J, et al. Phaeohyphomycotic cyst caused by a recently described species, *Phaeoannellomyces elegans*. J Clin Microbiol 1987;25:605–608.

75. England DM, Hochholzer I. Primary pulmonary sporotrichosis: report of eight cases with clinicopathologic review. Am J Surg Pathol 1985;9:193–204.

76. Erer B, Galimberti M, Lucarelli G, et al. *Trichosporon beigelii*: a life-threatening pathogen in immuno-compromised hosts. Bone Marrow Transplant 2000;25: 745–49.

77. Eschete ML, West BC. *Saccharomyces cerevisiae* septicemia. Arch Intern Med 1980;140:1539.

78. Espenel-Ingroff A. Etest for antifungal susceptibility testing of yeasts. Diagn Microbiol Infect Dis 1994;19:217–220.

79. Farr RC, Gardner G, Acker JD, et al. Blastomycotic cranial osteomyelitis. Am J Otol 1992;13:580–586.

80. Feldman BS, Snyder LS. Primary pulmonary coccidioidomycosis. Semin Respir Infect 2001;16:231–237.

81. Fidel PL Jr, Vazquez JA, Sobel JD. *Candida glabrata*: review of epidemiology. pathogenesis, and clinical disease with comparison to *C. albicans*. Clin Microbiol Rev 1999;2:80–96.

82. Fernandez, M, Noyola, D, Rossmann, SN, Edwards, MS. Cutaneous phaeohyphomycosis caused by *Curvularia lunata* and a review of *Curvularia* infections in pediatrics. Pediatr Infect Dis J 1999;18:727–73.

83. Fish DG, Ampel NM, Galgiani JN, et al. Coccidioidomycosis during human immunodeficiency virus infection: a review of 77 patients. Medicine (Baltimore) 1990;69:384–391.

84. Fojtasek MF, Kleiman MB, Connolly-Stringfield P, et al. The *Histoplasma capsulatum* antigen assay in disseminated histoplasmosis in children. Pediatr Infect Dis J 1994;13:801–805.

85. Frank UJK, Nishimura SL, Li NC, et al. Evaluation of an enzyme immunoassay for detection of cryptococcal capsular polysaccharide antigen in serum and cerebrospinal fluid. J Clin Microbiol 1993;31:94–101.

86. Fraser VJ, Keath EJ, Powderly WG. Two cases of blastomycosis from a common

87. Friskel E, Klotz SA, Bartholomew W, Dixon A. Two unusual presentations of urogenital histoplasmosis and a review of the literature. Clin Infect Dis 2000; 31:189–191.

88. Frye RR, Donovan JM, Drach GW. *Torulopsis glabrata* urinary tract infections. J Urol 1988;139:1245–1249.

89. Gales AC, Pfaller MA, Houston, AK, et al. Identification of *Candida dubliniensis* based on temperature and utilization of xylose and α-methyl-D-glucoside as determined with the API 20C AUX and Vitek YBC systems. J Clin Microbiol 1999;37:3804–3808

90. Galgiani JN. Coccidioidomycosis: a regional disease of national importance: rethinking approaches for control. Ann Intern Med 1999;130:293–300.

91. Geers TA, Gordon SM. Clinical significance of *Candida* species isolated from cerebrospinal fluid following neurosurgery. Clin Infect Dis 1999;28:1139–1147.

92. Gelfand MS, McGee ZA, Kaiser AB, et al. Candidal meningitis following bacterial meningitis. South Med J 1990;83:567–570.

93. Ghannoum MA. Susceptibility testing of fungi and correlation with clinical outcome. J Chemother 1997;9 Suppl 1:19–24.

94. Godoy H, Reichart PA. Oral manifestations of paracoccidioidomycosis: report of 21 cases from Argentina. Mycoses 2003;46:412–417.

95. Goldani LZ, Sugar AM. Paracoccidioidomycosis and AIDS: an overview. Clin Infect Dis 1995;21:1275–1281.

96. Gomez BL, Figueroa JI, Hamilton AJ, et al. Use of monoclonal antibodies in diagnosis of paracoccidioidomycosis: new strategies for detection of circulating antigens. J Clin Microbiol 1997;35:3278–3283.

97. Gonzalez CE, Rinaldi MG, Sugar AM. Zygomycosis. Infect Dis Clin North Am 2002;16:895–914.

98. Gucalp R, Carlisle P, Gialanella P, et al. *Paecilomyces* sinusitis in an immuno-compromised adult patient: case report and review. Clin Infect Dis 1996;23: 391–393.

99. Gugnani HC. A review of zygomycosis due to *Basidiobolus ranarum*. Eur J Epidemiol 1999;15:923–929.

100. Gupta AK, Elewski BE. Non-dermatophyte causes of onychomycosis and superficial mycoses. Curr Top Med Mycol 1996;7:87–97.

101. Gupta AK, Summerbell RC. Increased incidence of *Trichophyton tonsurans* tinea capitis in Ontario, Canada between 1985 and 1996. Med Mycol 1998;36: 55–60.

102. Gupta V, Chawla R, Sen S. *Aureobasidium pullulans* scleritis following keratoplasty: a case report. Ophthal Surg Lasers 2001;32:481–482.

103. Hadjupavlou AG, Mader JT, Naua HJ. Blastomycosis of the lumbar spine: case report and review of the literature, with emphasis on diagnostic laboratory tools and management. Eur Spine J 1998;7:416–41, 1998.

104. Hagman HM, Madnick EG, D'Agostino AN, et al. Hyphal forms in the central nervous system of patients with coccidioidomycosis. Clin Infect Dis 2000;30: 349–353.

105. Hahn RC, Macedo AM, Fontes CJ. Randomly amplified polymorphic DNA as a valuable tool for epidemiological studies of *Paracoccidioides brasiliensis*. J Clin Microbiol 2003;41:2849–2854.

106. Haight DO, Esperanza LE, Greene JN. Case report: cutaneous manifestations of cryptococcosis. Am J Med Sci 1994;308:192–195.

107. Hajjeh RA. Disseminated histoplasmosis in persons infected with human immunodeficiency virus. Clin Infect Dis 1995;21 Suppl 1:S108–S110.

108. Hajjeh R, McDonnell S, Reef S, et al. Outbreak of sporotrichosis among tree nursery workers. J Infect Dis 1997;176:499–504.

109. Hall GS, Pratt-Rippin K, Washington JA. Evaluation of a chemiluminescent probe assay for identification of *Histoplasma capsulatum* isolates. J Infect 1991; 22:179–182.

110. Hall L, Wohlfiel SL, Roberts GD. Experience with MicroSeq D2 Large Subunit Ribosomal DNA Sequencing Kit for identification of commonly encountered clinically important yeast species. J Clin Microbiol 2003;41:5099–5102.

111. Hall L, Wohlfiel SL, Roberts GD. Experience with the MicroSeq D2 LSU rDNA Sequencing Kit for the identification of filamentous fungi encountered in the clinical laboratory. J Clin Microbiol 2004;42:622–626.

112. Hamann ID, Gillespie RJ, Ferguson JK. Primary cryptococcal cellulitis caused by *Cryptococcus neoformans* var. *gattii* in an immunocompetent host. Austral J Derm 1997;38:29–32.

113. Hamilton AJ, Goodley J. Virulence factors of *Cryptococcus neoformans*. Curr Topics Med Mycol 1996;7:19–42.

114. Hamilton AJ. Serodiagnosis of histoplasmosis, paracoccidioidomycosis and penicilliosis marneffei: current status and future trends. Med Mycol 1998;36: 351–364.

115. Hanson JM, Spector G, El-Mofty SK. Laryngeal blastomycosis: a commonly missed diagnosis: report of two cases and review of the literature. Ann Otol Rhinol Laryngol 2000;109:281–286.

116. Harril WC, Stewart MG, Lee AG, Cernoch P. Chronic rhinocerebral mucormycosis. Laryngoscope 1996;106:1292–1297.

source: use of DNA restriction analysis to identify strains. J Infect Dis 1991; 163:1278–1281.

117. Hazen KC. New and emerging yeast pathogens. Clin Microbiol Rev 1995;8: 462–478.
118. Hedderwick S, Kauffman CA. Opportunistic fungal infections: superficial and systemic candidiasis. Geriatrics 1997;52:50–54.
119. Hickey WF, Sommerville LH, Schoen FJ. Disseminated *Candida glabrata*: report of a uniquely severe infection and literature review. Am J Clin Pathol 1983; 80:724–727.
120. Hiltbrand JB, McGuirt WF. Oropharyngeal histoplasmosis. South Med J 1990; 83:227.
121. Ho PL, Yuen KY. Aspergillosis in bone marrow transplant recipients. Crit Rev Oncol Hematol 2000;34:55–69.
122. Hogevik H, Alestig K. Fungal endocarditis—a report on seven cases and a brief review. Infection 1996;24:17–21.
123. Howell SJ, Toohey JS. Sporotrichal arthritis in south central Kansas. Clin Orthop Relat Res 1998;346:207–214.
124. Hoy J, Hsu KC, Rolston K, et al. *Trichosporon beigelii* infection: a review. Rev Infect Dis 1986;8:959–967.
125. Huang CT, McGarry T, Cooper S, et al. Disseminated histoplasmosis in the acquired immunodeficiency syndrome: report of five cases from a non-endemic area. Arch Intern Med 1987;147:1181–1184.
126. Huffnagle KE, Gander RM. Evaluation of Gen-Probe's *Histoplasma capsulatum* and *Cryptococcus neoformans* AccuProbes. J Clin Microbiol 1993;312: 419–421.
127. Iwen PC, Rupp ME, Langnas AN, et al. Invasive pulmonary aspergillosis due to *Aspergillus terreus*: 12-year experience and review of the literature. Clin Infect Dis 1998;26:1092–1097.
128. Jabor MA, Greer DL, Amedee RG. Scopulariopsis: an invasive nasal infection. Am J Rhinol 1998;12:367–371.
129. Jain S, Koirala J, Castro-Pavia F. Isolated gastrointestinal histoplasmosis: case report and review of the literature. South Med J 2004;97:172–174.
130. Jarvis WR. Epidemiology of nosocomial fungal infections, with emphasis on *Candida* species. Clin Infect Dis 1995;20:1526–1530.
131. Johnson LB, Bradley SF, Kauffman CA. Fungemia due to *Cryptococcus laurentii* and a review of non-neoformans cryptococcemia. Mycoses 1998;41: 277–280.
132. Kahn DG, Thommes J. Granulomatous orchitis and epididymitis secondary to *Histoplasma capsulatum* and CMV in AIDS. International Conference on AIDS, July 19–24, 1992. 8:93.
133. Kalin M, Petrini B. Clinical and laboratory diagnosis of invasive candida infection in neutropenic patients. Med Oncol 1996;13:223–231.
134. Kalenic S, Jandrlic M, Vegar V, et al. *Hansenula anomala* outbreak at a surgical intensive care unit: a search for risk factors. Eur J Epidemiol 2001;17:491–496.
135. Kataoka-Nishimura S, Akiyama H, Saku K, et al. Invasive infection due to *Trichosporon cutaneum* in patients with hematologic malignancies. Cancer 1998;82:484–487.
136. Kaufman L, Standard PG, Anderson SA, et al. Development of specific fluorescent-antibody test for tissue form of *Penicillium marneffei*. J Clin Microbiol 1995;33:2136–2138.
137. Kerking TM, Duma RJ, Shadomy S. The evolution of pulmonary cryptococcosis: clinical implications from a study of 41 patients with and without compromising host factors. Ann Intern Med 1981;94:611–616.
138. Khoo SH, Denning DW. Invasive aspergillosis in patients with AIDS. Clin Infect Dis 1994;19:Suppl 1:S42–S48.
139. Khoory BJ, Vino L, Dall'Agnola A, Fanos V. *Candida* infections in newborns: a review. J Chemother 1999;11:367–378.
140. Kiehn TE, Gorey E, Browth AE, et al. Sepsis due to *Rhodotorula* related to use of indwelling central venous catheters. Clin Infect Dis 1992;14:841–846.
141. Kilburn CD, McKinsey DS. Recurrent massive pleural effusion due to pleural, pericardial, and epicardial fibrosis in histoplasmosis. Chest 1991;100: 1715–1717.
142. King D, Cheever LW, Hood A, et al. Primary invasive cutaneous *Microsporum canis* infection in immunocompromised patients. J Clin Microbiol 1996;34: 460–462.
143. Kirkland TN, Fierer J. Coccidioidomycosis: a re-emerging infectious disease. Emerg Infect Dis 1996;2:192–199.
144. Klein BSD, Vergeront JM, DiSlavo, et al. Two outbreaks of blastomycosis along rivers in Wisconsin. Isolation of *Blastomyces dermatitidis* from riverbank soil and evidence of transmission along waterways. Am Rev Respir Dis 1987;136: 1333–1338.
145. Kobayashi GS. Molecular genetics and the diagnostic mycology laboratory. Arch Med Res 1995;26:393–396.
146. Kohl TD, Lisney M. Tinea gladiatorum: wrestling's emerging foe. Sports Medicine 2000;29:439–47.
147. Koneman EW, Roberts GD. Practical Laboratory Mycology. 3rd ed. Baltimore: Williams & Wilkins, 1985.
148. Kontoyianis DP, Vartivarian S, Anaissie EJ, et al. Infections due to *Cunninghamella bertholletiae* in patients with cancer: report of three cases and review. Clin Infect Dis 1994;18:925–928.
149. Korfel A, Menssen HD, Schwartz S, Thiel E. Cryptococcosis in Hodgkin's disease: description of two cases and review of the literature. Ann Hematol 1998;76:283–286.
150. Krcmery V Jr, et al. Fungaemia due to *Fusarium* spp. in cancer patients. J Hosp Infect 1997;36:223–228.
151. Kurtin PJ, McKinsey DS, Gupta MR, Driks M. Histoplasmosis in patients with acquired immunodeficiency syndrome: hematologic and bone marrow manifestations. Am J Clin Pathol 1990;93:367–372.
152. Kurup A, Leo YS, Tan AL, Wong SY. Disseminated *Penicillium marneffei* infection: a report of five cases in Singapore. Ann Acad Med Singapore 1999; 28:605–609.
153. Kwon-Chung KJ, Bennett JE. Medical Mycology. Philadelphia: Lea & Febiger, 1992:136.
154. Latge JP. *Aspergillus fumigatus* and aspergillosis. Clin Microbiol Rev 1999;12: 310–350.
155. Lee CH, Lan RS, Tsai YH, et al. Riu's stain in the diagnosis of pulmonary cryptococcosis: introduction of a new diagnostic method. Chest 1988;93: 467–470.
156. Lee TM, Greenberger PA, Patterson R, et al. Stage V (fibrotic) allergic bronchopulmonary aspergillosis: a review of 17 cases followed from diagnosis. Arch Intern Med 1987;147:319–323.
157. Lemos LB, Guo M, Baliga M. Blastomycosis: organ involvement and etiologic diagnosis: a review of 123 patients from Mississippi. Ann Diagn Pathol 2000; 4:391–406.
158. Lemos LB, Baliga M, Guo M. Blastomycosis: the great pretender can also be an opportunist. Initial clinical diagnosis and underlying diseases in 123 patients. Ann Diagn Pathol 2002;6:194–203
159. Lemos LB, Soofi, M, Amir E. Blastomycosis and pregnancy. Ann Diagn Pathol 2002;6:211–215.
160. Lewis SM, Lewis BG. Nosocomial transmission of *Trichophyton tonsurans* tinea corporis in a rehabilitation hospital. Infect Contr Hosp Epidemiol. 1997;18: 322–325.
161. Liu PY. Cryptococcal osteomyelitis: case report and review. Diag Microbiol Infect Dis 1998;30:33–35.
162. Liu D, Coloe S, Baird R, Pedersen J. Application of PCR to the identification of dermatophyte fungi. J Med Microbiol 2000;49:493–497.
163. Logan JL, Blair JE, Galgiani JN. Coccidioidomycosis complicating solid organ transplantation. Semin Respir Infect 2001;16:251–256.
164. Londero AT, Melo IS. Paracoccidioidomycosis in childhood: a critical review. Mycopathologia 1983;82:49–55.
165. Lopez R, Mason JO, Parker JS, Pappas PG. Intraocular blastomycosis: case report and review. Clin Infect Dis 1994;18:805–807.
166. Low CD, Badenoch PR, Coster DJ. *Beauveria bassiana* keratitis cured by deep lamellar dissection. Cornea 1997;16:698–699.
167. Lopez AM, Williams PL, Ampel NM. Acute pulmonary coccidioidomycosis mimicking bacterial pneumonia and septic shock: a report of two cases. Am J Med 1993;95:236–239.
168. Lugo-Somolinos A, Sanchez JL. Prevalence of dermatophytosis in patients with diabetes. J Am Acad Dermatol 1992;26:908–910.
169. Ma JS, Chen PY, Chen CH, Chi CS. Neonatal fungemia caused by *Hansenula anomala*: a case report. J Microbiol Immunol Infect 2000;33:267–270.
170. MacDonald PB, Black GB, MacKenzie R. Orthopaedic manifestations of blastomycosis. J Bone Joint Surg 1990;72:860–864.
171. Mahmoudi M, Gershwin ME. Sick building syndrome. III. *Stachybotrys chartarum*. J Asthma 2000;37:191–198.
172. Manns BJ, Baylis BW, Urbanski SJ, et al. Paracoccidioidomycosis: case report and review. Clin Infect Dis 1996;23:1026–32.
173. Marcelis L, Verhaegen J, Vandeven J, et al. Evaluation of Bactec high blood volume resin media. Diagn Microbiol Infect Dis 1992;15:385–391.
174. Martinez M, et al. Replacement of *Candida albicans* with *C. dubliniensis* in HIV-infected patients with oropharyngeal candidiasis treated with fluconazole. J Clin Microbiol 2002;40:3135–3139.
175. Mathisen DJ, Grillo HC. Clinical manifestations of mediastinal fibrosis and histoplasmosis. Ann Thorac Surg 1992;54:1053–1057.
176. McCullough MJ, Ross BC, Reade PC. *Candida albicans*: a review of its history, taxonomy, epidemiology, virulence attributes, and methods of strain differentiation. Int J Oral Maxillofac Surg 1996;25:136–144.
177. McGinnis MR, Schell WA, Carson J. *Phaeoannellomyces* and the *Phaeococcomycetaceae*: new dematiaceous blastomycete taxa. J Med Vet Mycol 1985;232: 179–188.
178. McGinnis MR, Rinaldi MG. Selected medically important fungi and some common synonyms and obsolete names. Clin Infect Dis 1997;25:15–17.
179. Mendes-Giannini MJ, Bueno JP, Shikanai-Yasuda MA, et al. Antibody response to the 4ds kDa glycoprotein of *Paracoccidioides brasiliensis* as a marker for the evaluation of patients under treatment. Am J Trop Med Hyg 1990;43:200–206.
180. Mennink-Kersten MA, Donnelly JP, Verweij PE. Detection of circulating galactomannan for the diagnosis and management of invasive aspergillosis. Lancet Infect Dis 2004;4:349–357.

181. Migrino RQ, Hall GS, Longworth DL. Deep tissue infections caused by *Scopulariopsis brevicaulis*: report of a case of prosthetic valve endocarditis and review. Clin Infect Dis 1995;21:672–674.

182. Miller HS, Nance MA, Brummitt CF, et al. Fungal infections associated with intravenous drug abuse: a case of localized cerebral phycomycosis. J Clin Psychiatry 1988;49:320–322.

183. Minamoto GY, Rosenberg AS. Fungal infections in patients with acquired immunodeficiency syndrome. Med Clin North Am 1997;81:381–409.

184. Minotto R, Bernardi CD, Mallmann LF. Chromoblastomycosis: a review of 100 cases in the state of Rio Grande do Sul, Brazil. J Am Acad Dermatol 2001;44: 585–592.

185. MMWR. Coccidioidomycosis—United States, 1991–1992. MMWR Morb Mortal Wkly Rep 1993;22:21–24.

186. Murakawa GJ, Kerschmann R, Berger T. Cutaneous cryptococcus infection and AIDS: report of 12 cases and review of the literature. Arch Dermatol 1996;132: 545–548.

187. Murayama N, Takimoto R, Kawai M, et al. A case of subcutaneous phaeohyphomycotic cyst due to *Exophiala jeanselmei* complicated with systemic lupus erythematosus. Mycoses 2003;46:145–148.

188. Murphy N, Buchanan CR, et al. Infection and colonization of neonates by *Hansenula anomala*. Lancet 1986;1:290–293.

189. Murphy RA, Miller WT Jr. Pulmonary mucormycosis. Semin Roentgenol 1996; 31:83–87.

190. Murray PR. Comparison of the lysis-centrifugation and agitated biphasic blood culture system for detection of fungemia. J Clin Microbiol 1991;29:96–98.

191. Musher B, Fredricks D, Leisenring W, et al. Aspergillus galactomannan enzyme immunoassay and quantitative PCR for diagnosis of invasive aspergillosis with bronchoalveolar lavage fluid. J Clin Microbiol 2004;42:5517–5522.

192. National Committee for Clinical Laboratory Standards. Reference method for broth dilution antifungal susceptibility testing of yeasts: Approved standard M27-A. Wayne, PA: National Committee for Clinical Laboratory Standards, 1997.

193. Nenoff P, Kellermann S, Scholber R, et al. Rhinocerebral zygomycosis following bone marrow transplantation in chronic myelogenous leukemia: report of a case and review of the literature. Mycoses 1998;42:326–372.

194. Nielsen H, Stenderup J, Bruun B. Fungemia with *Sacharomycetaceae*: report of four cases. Scand J Infect Dis 1990;22:582–584.

195. Nielsen PG. Hereditary palmoplantar keratoderma and dermatophytosis in the northernmost country of Sweden (Norrbotten). Acta Derm Venereol Suppl (Stockh) 1994;1288:1–60.

196. Nightingale SD, Parks JM, Pou DK, et al. Disseminated histoplasmosis in patients with AIDS. South Med J 1990;83:624–630.

197. Nittayanama W. *Penicilliosis marneffei*: another AIDS defining illness in Southeast Asia. Oral Dis 1999;5:286–293.

198. Nolan MT, Long JP, Macrean DP, Fitzgerald MX. Aspergillosis and lung fibrosis. Irish J Med Sci 1985;154:336–342.

199. Nucci M. Emerging moulds: *Fusarium, Scedosporium* and Zygomycetes in transplant recipients. Curr Opin Infect Dis 2003;16:607–612.

200. Odds FC. Pathogenesis of *Candida* infections. 1994. J A Acad Dermatol 1994; 31(3 Pt 2):S2–S5.

200a. Odds FC. Prevalence of *Candida dubliniensis* isolates in a yeast stock collection J Clin Microbiol 1999;36:2869–2873.

201. Okhravi N, Dart JK, Towler HM, Lightman S. *Paecilomyces lilacinus* endophthalmitis with secondary keratitis: a case report and literature review. Arch Ophthal 1997;5:1320–1324.

202. Oliver WJ, James SA, Lennard A, et al. Nosocomial transmission of *Saccharomyces cerevisiae* in bone marrow transplant patients. J Hosp Infect 2002;52: 268–672.

203. O'Neill KM, Ormsby AH, Prayson RA. Cryptococcal myositis: a case report and review of the literature. Pathology 1998;30:317–318.

204. O'Sullivan MV, Whitby M, Chahoud C, Miller SM. Histoplasmosis in Australia: a report of a case with a review of the literature. Austral Dent J 2004;49:94–97.

205. Opal SM, Asp AA, et al. Efficacy of infection control measures during a nosocomial outbreak of disseminated aspergillosis associated with hospital construction. J Infect Dis 1986;153:634–637.

206. Padhye AA, Smith G, McLaughlin D, Standard PG. Comparative evaluation of a chemiluminescent DNA probe and an exoantigen test for rapid identification of *Histoplasma capsulatum*. J Clin Microbiol 1992;30:3108–3111.

207. Page LR, Drummond JF, et al. Blastomycosis with oral lesions: report of two cases. Oral Surg 1979;47:157–160.

208. Pappagianis D. Marked increase in cases of coccidioidomycosis in California, 1991, 1992, and 1993. Clin Infect Dis 1994;19:Suppl 1:S14–S18.

209. Pappas PG, Threlkeld MG, Bedsole GD, et al. Blastomycosis in patients with the acquired immunodeficiency syndrome. Medicine (Baltimore) 1993;72:322–325.

210. Pappas PG, Tellez I, Deep AE, et al. Sporotrichosis in Peru: description of an area of hyperendemicity. Clin Infect Dis 2000;30:65–70.

211. Patterson JE, Barden GE, Pia FJ. Hospital acquired gangrenous mucormycosis. Yale J Biol Med 1986;59:453–459.

212. Paya CV, Roberts GD, Cockerill FR III. Laboratory methods for the diagnosis of disseminated histoplasmosis: clinical importance of the lysis-centrifugation blood culture technique. Mayo Clin Proc 1987;62:480–485.

213. Pema K, Diaz J, Guerra LG, et al. Disseminated cutaneous cryptococcosis. Comparison of clinical manifestations in the pre-AIDS and AIDS eras. Arch Intern Med 1994;154:1032–1034.

214. Perez RE, Smith M, McClenndon J, et al. *Pseudallescheria boydii* brain abscess: complication of an intravenous catheter. Am J Med 1988;84:359–362.

215. Perfect JR. Schell WA. The new fungal opportunists are coming. Clin Infect Dis 1996;22:Suppl 2:S112–S118.

216. Peyron F, Favel A, Michel-Nguyen A, et al. Improved detection of amphotericin b-resistant isolates of *Candida lusitaniae* by E test. J Clin Microbiol 2001;39: 339–342.

217. Pfaller MA. Epidemiology of candidiasis. J Hosp Infect 1995;30:Suppl: 329–338.

218. Pfaller MA, Messer SA, Blomström A, et al. Multi-site reproducibility of the E-test MIC method for antifungal susceptibility testing of yeast isolates. J Clin Microbiol 1996;34:1691–1693.

219. Pfaller MA, Rex JH, Rinaldi MG. Antifungal susceptibility testing: technical advances and potential clinical applications. Clin Infect Dis 1997;24:776–784.

220. Pfaller MA, Bale M, Buchelman B, et al. Quality control guidelines for National Committee for Clinical Laboratory Standards recommended broth macrodilution testing of amphotericin B, fluconazole, and flucytosine. J Clin Microbiol 1995; 33:1104–1107.

221. Pfaller MA, Messer SA, Mills K, et al. Evaluation of Etest method for determining caspofungin (MK-0991) susceptibilities of 726 clinical isolates of *Candida* species J Clin Microbiol 2001;39:4387–4389.

222. Phillips P, Wood WS, Phillips G, Rinaldi MG. Invasive hyalohyphomycosis caused by *Scopulariopsis brevicaulis* in a patient undergoing allogeneic bone marrow transplant. Diagn Microbiol Infect Dis 1989;12:429–432.

223. Pickles RW, Pacey DE, Muir DB, Merrell WH. Experience with infection by *Scedosporium prolificans* including apparent cure with fluconazole therapy. J Infect Dis 1996;33:193–197.

224. Pieckova E, Jesenska Z. Microscopic fungi in dwellings and their health implications in humans. Ann Agricult Environ Med 1999;6:1–11.

225. Prabhu RM, Patel R. Mucormycosis and entomophthoramycosis: a review of the clinical manifestations, diagnosis and treatment. Clinical Microbiol Infect 2004;10:Suppl 1:31–47.

226. Prichard JB, Sorotzkin RA, Rames RE III. Cutaneous manifestations of disseminated coccidioidomycosis in the acquired immunodeficiency syndrome. Cutis 1987;39:203–205.

227. Purvis RS, Diven DG, Drechsel RD, et al. Sporotrichosis presenting as arthritis and subcutaneous nodules. J Am Acad Dermatol 1993;28:879–884.

228. Reder PA, Neel HB III, Neel HB. Blastomycosis in otolaryngology: review of a large series. Laryngoscope 1993;103:53–58.

229. Revankar SG, Sutton DA, Rinaldi MG. Primary central nervous system phaeohyphomycosis: a review of 101 cases. Clin Infect Dis 2004;38:206–216.

230. Rex JH, et al. Quality control guidelines for National Committee for Clinical Laboratory Standards: recommended broth macrodilution testing of ketoconazole and itraconazole. J Clin Microbiol 1996;34:816–817.

231. Rhame FS. Prevention of nosocomial aspergillosis. J Hosp Infect 1991;18: 466–467.

232. Ribes JA, Vanover-Sams CL, Baker DJ. Zygomycosis in human disease. Clin Microbiol Rev 2000;13:236–301.

233. Rinaldi MG. Phaeohyphomycosis. Derm Clin 1996;14:147–153.

234. Rippon RW. Medical Mycology: The Pathogenic Fungi and the Pathogenic Actinomyectes. 3rd ed. Philadelphia: WB Saunders, 1988.

235. Roller JA, Westblom TU. *Microsporum nanum* infection in hog farmers. J Am Acad Dermatol 1986;15:935–939.

236. Romano C, Paccagnini E, Difonzo EM. Onychomycosis caused by *Alternaria* spp. in Tuscany, Italy from 1985 to 1999. Mycoses 2001;44:73–76

237. Rosales CM, Jackson MA, Zwick D. *Malassezia furfur* meningitis associated with total parenteral nutrition subdural effusion. Pediatr Dev Pathol 2004;7: 86–90.

238. Sabota J, Brodell R, Rutecki GW, Hoppes WL. Severe tinea barbae due to *Trichophyton verrucosum* infection in dairy farmers. Clin Infect Dis 1996;23: 1308–1310.

239. Salkin IF, Martinez JA, Kemma ME. Opportunistic infection of the spleen caused by *Aureobasidium pullulans*. J Clin Microbiol 1986;23:828–831.

240. Salkin IF, McGinnis MR, Dykstra MJ, Renaldi MG. *Scedosporium inflatum*: an emerging pathogen. J Clin Microbiol 1988;26:498–503.

241. Sandhu GS, Aleff RA, Kline BC, da Silva Lacaz C. Molecular detection and identification of *Paracoccidioides brasiliensis*. J Clin Microbiol 1997;l35: 1894–1896.

242. Sant'Anna GD, Mauri M, Arrarte JL, Camargo H Jr. Laryngeal manifestations of paracoccidioidomycosis (South American blastomycosis). Arch Otolaryngol Head Neck Surg 1999;125:1375–1378.

243. Sarosi GA, et al. Laboratory diagnosis of mycotic and specific fungal infections. Am Rev Respir Dis 1985;132:1373–1379.

244. Sarosi GA, Johnson PC. Disseminated histoplasmosis in patients infected with human immunodeficiency virus. Clin Infect Dis 1992;14:Suppl 1:S60–S67.

245. Sataloff RT, Wilborn A, Prestipino A, et al. Histoplasmosis of the larynx. Am J Otolaryngol 1993;14:199–205.

246. Schell WA, Perfect JR. Fatal, disseminated *Acremonium strictum* infection in a neutropenic host. J Clin Microbiol 1996;34:1223–1336.

247. Schliemann R, Glasmacher A, Bailly E, et al. *Geotrichum capitatum* septicemia in neutropenic patients: case report and review of the literature. Mycoses 1998; 4:113–116.

248. Schubert MS. Allergic fungal sinusitis: pathogenesis and management strategies. Drugs 2004;64:363–374.

249. Seddon ME, Thomas MG. Invasive disease due to *Epidermophyton floccosum* in an immunocompromised patient with Behçet's syndrome. Clin Infect Dis 1997;25:153–154.

250. Sellier P, Monsuez JJ, Lacroix C, et al. Recurrent subcutaneous infection due to *Scopulariopsis brevicaulis* in a liver transplant recipient. Clin Infect Dis 2000; 30:820–823.

251. Sennesh J, Cooper JN, Perfect JR. Disseminated zygomycosis: report of four cases and review. Rev Infect Dis 1989;11:741–754.

252. Severo LC, Kauer CL, Oliveira FD, et al. Paracoccidioidomycosis of the male genital tract: report of eleven cases and review of Brazilian literature. Revista do Instituto de Medicina Tropical de Sao Paulo 2000;42:38–40.

253. Sewell DL, Pfaller MA, Barry AL. Comparison of broth macrodilution, broth microdilution, and E test antifungal susceptibility tests for fluconazole. J Clin Microbiol 1994;32:2099–2102.

254. Sharma OP, Chwogule R. Many faces of pulmonary aspergillosis. Eur Respir J 1998;12:705–715.

255. Sigler I, Harris JL, Dixon DM, et al. Microbiology and potential virulence of *Sporothrix cyanescens*, a fungus rarely isolated from blood and skin. J Clin Microbiol 1990;28:1009–1015.

256. Silva JP, de Souza W, Rozental S. Chromoblastomycosis: a retrospective study of 325 cases on Amazonic Region (Brazil). Mycopathologia 1998;143:171–175.

257. Simarro E, Marin F, Morales A, et al. Fungemia due to *Scedosporium prolificans*: a description of two cases with fatal outcome. Clin Microbiol Infect 2001;7: 645–647.

258. Simmons RB, Price DL, Noble JA, et al. Fungal colonization of air filters from hospital. Am Indust Hyg Assoc J 1997;58:900–904.

259. Singh G, Wijesurendra CS, Green JT. Disseminated aspergillosis in the acquired immunodeficiency syndrome. Int J STD AIDS 1994;5:63–66.

260. Singh VR, Smith DK, Lawrence J, et al. Coccidioidomycosis in patients infected with human immunodeficiency virus: review of 91 cases at a single institution. Clin Infect Dis 1996;23:563–568.

261. Sobel JD, Vazquez JA. Fungal infections of the urinary tract. World J Urol 1999;17:420–424.

262. Staib F, Arasteh K. Chlamydospore formation on Staib agar: observations made before *Candida dubliniensis* was described. Mycoses 2001;44:23–27.

263. Stiefel P, Pamies E, Miranda ML, et al. Cryptococcal peritonitis: report of a case and review of the literature. Hepato-Gastroenterol 1999;46:1618–1622.

264. Stockman L, Clark KA, Hung JM, Roberts GD. Evaluation of commercially available acridinium ester-labeled chemiluminescent DNA probes for culture identification of *Blastomyces dermatitidis, Coccidioides immitis, Cryptococcus neoformans,* and *Histoplasma capsulatum.* J Clin Microbiol 1993;31:845–850.

265. Strausbaugh LJ, Sewell DL, Ward T, et al. High frequency of yeast carriage on hands of hospital personnel. J Clin Microbiol 1994;32:2299–2300.

266. Suh KN, Anekthananon T, Mariuz PR. Gastrointestinal histoplasmosis in patients with AIDS: case report and review. Clin Infect Dis 2001;32:483–491.

267. Sullivan DJ, Westerneng TJ, Haynes KA, et al. *Candida dubliniensis* sp. nov.: phenotypic and molecular characterization of a novel species associated with oral candidosis in HIV-infected individuals. Microbiol 1995;141:1507–1521.

268. Sweeney, DA, Caserta, MT, Korones, DN. A ten year old boy with pulmonary nodule secondary to *Cryptococcus neoformans*: case report and review of the literature. Pediatr Infect Dis J 2003;22:1089–1093.

269. Sweet D, Reid M. Disseminated neonatal *Trichosporon beigelii* infection: successful treatment with liposomal amphotericin B. J Infect 1998;36:120–121.

270. Syrjanen S, Valle SL, Antonen J. Oral candidal infection as a sign of HIV infection in homosexual men. Oral Surg 1988;55:36–40.

271. Tamm M, Malouf M, Glanville A. Pulmonary scedosporium infection following lung transplantation. Transplant Infect Dis 2001;3:189–194.

272. Tawfick OW, Papasian CJ, Dixon AY, Potter LM. *Saccharomyces cerevisiae* pneumonia in a patient with acquired immune deficiency syndrome. J Clin Microbiol 1989;27:1689–1691.

273. Thammayya A. Sanyal M. *Exophiala jeanselmei* causing mycetoma pedis in India. *Sabouraudia* 1980;18:91–95.

274. Tosti A, Piraccini BM, Stinchi C, Lorenzi S. Onychomycosis due to *Scopulari-* *opsis brevicaulis*: clinical features and response to systemic antifungals. Br J Dermatol 1996;135:799–802.

275. Truett AA, Crum NF. Coccidioidomycosis of the prostate gland: two cases and a review of the literature. South Med J 2004;97:419–422.

276. Vainrub B, Macareno A, Mandel S, Musher DM. Wound zygomycosis (mucormycosis) in otherwise healthy adults. Am J Med 1988;84:546–548.

277. Vajpayee RB, Gupta SK, Bareja U, Kishore K. Ocular atopy and mycotic keratitis. Ann Ophthalmol 1990;22:369–372.

278. Vanden Bossche H, Dromer F, Improvisi I, et al. Antifungal drug resistance in pathogenic fungi. Med Mycol 1998;36:Suppl 1:119–128.

279. Van den Saffele JK, Boelaert JR. Zygomycosis in HIV-positive patients: a review of the literature. Mycoses 1996;39:44–84.

280. Verweiz PE, Breuker IM, Rijs ASMM, Maes JFGM. Comparative study of seven commercial yeast identification systems. J Clin Pathol 1999;52:271–273.

281. Wack EE, Ampel NM, Galgiani NJ, Bronnimann DA. Coccidioidomycosis during pregnancies. Chest 1988;94:376–379.

282. Walsh TJ. Invasive pulmonary aspergillosis in patients with neoplastic diseases. Semin Respir Infect 1990;5:111–122.

283. Wang JP, Granlund KF, Bozzette SA, et al. Bursal sporotrichosis: case report and review. Clinl Infect Dis 2000;31:615–616.

284. Weems JJ Jr. *Candida parapsilosis*: epidemiology, pathogenicity, clinical manifestations, and antimicrobial susceptibility. Clin Infect Dis 1992;14:756–766.

285. Weitzman I. A survey of dermatophytes isolated from human patients in the United States from 1993–1995. J Med Vet Mycol 1998;34:285–287.

286. Westenfeld F, Alston WK, Winn WC Jr. Complicated soft tissue infection with prepatellar bursitis caused by *Paecilomyces lilacinus* in an immunocompetent host: case report and review. J Clin Microbiol 1996;34:1559–1562.

287. Wheat J. Endemic mycoses in AIDS: a clinical review. Clin Microbiol Rev 1995;8:146–159.

288. Wheat LJ, Batteiger DE, Sathapatayavongs B. *Histoplasma capsulatum* in the central nervous system: a clinical review. Medicine (Baltimore) 1990;69: 244–260.

289. Wheat LJ, Connolly-Stringfield P, Williams B, et al. Diagnosis of histoplasmosis in patients with the acquired immunodeficiency syndrome by detection of *Histoplasma capsulatum* polysaccharide antigen in bronchoalveolar lavage fluid. Am Rev Respir Dis 1992;145:1421–1424.

290. Wheat LJ. Histoplasmosis in the acquired immunodeficiency syndrome. Curr Top Med Mycol 1996;7:7–18.

291. Wheat LJ. Laboratory diagnosis of histoplasmosis: a review. Semin Respir Infect 2001;16:131–140.

292. Wheat LJ, Kauffman CA. Histoplasmosis. Infect Dis Clin North Am 2003;17: 1–19.

293. White TC, Bowden RA, Marr KA. Clinical, cellular, and molecular factors that contribute to antifungal drug resistance. Clin Microbiol Rev 1998;11:382–402.

294. Wilhelmus DR, Robinson NM, Font RA, et al. Fungal keratitis in contact lens wearers. Am J Ophthalmol 1988;106:708–714.

295. Wilhelmus KR, Jones DB. *Curvularia* keratitis. Trans Am Ophthal Soc 2001; 99:111–130.

296. Williams B, Fojtasek M, Connolly-Stringfield P, Wheat J. Diagnosis of histoplasmosis by antigen detection during an outbreak in Indianapolis, Ind. Arch Pathol Lab Med 1994;118:1205–1208.

297. Wilmington M, Aly R, Frieden IJ. *Trichophyton tonsurans* tinea capitis in the San Francisco Bay area: increased infection demonstrated in a 20-year survey of fungal infections from 1974 to 1994. J Med Veterin Mycol 1996;34:285–287.

298. Wilson CM, O'Rourke EJ, McGinnis MR, Salkin IF. *Scedosporium inflatum*: clinical spectrum of a newly recognized pathogen. J Infect Dis 1990;161: 102–107. 1990.

299. Wingard JR. Importance of *Candida* species other than *C. albicans* as pathogens in oncology patients. Clin Infect Dis 1995;20:115–125.

300. Winn RE, Anderson J, Piper J, et al. Systemic sporotrichosis treated with itraconazole. Clin Infect Dis 1993;17:210–217.

301. Woods GL, Goldsmith JC. *Aspergillus* infection of the central nervous system in patients with acquired immunodeficiency syndrome. Arch Neurol 1990;47: 181–184.

302. Wortman PD. Concurrent chromoblastomycosis caused by *Fonsecaea pedrosoi* and actinomycetoma caused by *Nocardia brasiliensis*. J Am Acad Dermatol 1995;32:390–392.

303. Wright WL, Wenzel RP. Nosocomial candida: epidemiology, transmission, prevention. Infect Dis Clin North Am 1997;11:411–425.

304. Yoon SA, Vazquez JA, Steffan, PE, et al. High frequency, reversible switching of *Candida lusitaniae* clinical isolates from amphotericin B susceptibility to resistance. Antimicrob Agents Chemother 1999;43:836–845.

305. Yoss BS, Sautter RL, Brenker HJ. *Trichosporon beigelii*, a new neonatal pathogen. Am J Perinatol 1997;14:113–117.

306. Zhu LP, Shi YZ, Weng, XH, Mueller FM. Pulmonary cryptococcosis associated with cryptococcal meningitis in non-AIDS patients. Mycoses 2002;45:111–117.

307. Zmierczak H, Goemaere S, Mielants H, et al. *Candida glabrata* arthritis: case report and review of the literature of arthritis. Clin Rheumatol 1999;18:406–409.

Preliminary Observations Suggestive of the Zygomycetes

- Colonies rapidly growing with a poorly defined margin, filling the Petri dish in 48–72 hours
- Colony surface is wooly in consistency, and may become speckled as sporagnia are produced
- The hyphae are irregular in diameter, broad and ribbon-like, and aseptate
- Sporangiospores are borne within spherical or cylindrical, sack-like sporangia, supported at the tips of sporangiophores

Root-like rhizoids are formed

Yes			No		
Sporangiophores borne nodally	Sporangiophores borne internodally. Prominent flare-like apophysis	Spherical conidia borne from the surface of a globose sporangium.	Sporangia borne in cylindirical sporangia radiating in daisy-head fashion from the surface of a spherical columella.	Sporangiophores broadly curved back on themselves	Sporangiophores often branched, with no swelling where sporangiophore and sporangium merge.
***Rhizopus* sp.**	***Absidia* species**	***Cunninghamella* species**	***Syncephalastrum* species**	***Circinella* species**	***Mucor* species**

Display 21-1 Algorithm showing genus identification of the zygomycetes.

Preliminary Observations Suggestive of a Hyaline Mold

- Colonies rapidly growing, entire, cottony to granular, white or with varying pastel colors
- Hyphae are narrow, septate, hyaline, and have parallel walls

Conidia in Chains

Colonies green and granular; phialides branching and blunt; conidia 2-3 um, spherical.	Colonies green to green-yellow; phialides tapered; conidia 2-3 um elliptical, irregular in size and staining.	Colonies buff, granular, and radially rugose; 4-6 um, lemon-shaped, rough-walled alleureo-spores with truncated bases.
Penicillium species	*Paecilomyces* species	*Scopulariopsis* species

Conidia in Clusters

Colonies gray-white to salmon-colored, glabrous; elliptical conidia arranged in Oriental letter clusters.	Colonies fluffy, intense rose or purple pigment surface and reverse; large, multi-celled, sickle-form macroconidia.	Colonies spreading as green lawn without a border; balls of spherical conidia supported by tapered, finger-like phialides.	Colonies spreading as green or yellow lawn without a border; balls of spherical conidia borne laterally at tips of tapered phialides.
Acremonium species	*Fusarium* species	*Gliocladium* species	*Trichoderma* species

Conidia Borne Singly

Colonies house-mouse gray and cottony; elliptical conidia, turning dark with age, borne from tips of delicate conidiophores.	Colonies gray-white and cottony; elliptical non-pigmented conidia borne from tips of delicate conidiophores, resembling *Blastomyces dermatitidis*.	Colonies gray-white and cottony; large, spherical, rough-walled macroconidia resembling *Histoplasma capsulatum*.	Colonies gray-white and cottony; small elliptical conidia in loose clusters, each attached by a delicate, geniculate conidiophore.
Scedosporium species	*Chrysosporium* species	*Sepedonium* species	*Beauveria* species

GENUS ASPERGILLUS

Sporulation from Top Half of Vesicle

Phialides Uniseriate, Compact	Philides Biseriate, Compact	Phialides Biseriate Loose
Colonies green, granular and often rugose	Colonies buff, granular and radially rugose	Colonies gray-green to tan with yellow patches
Aspergillus fumigatus	*Aspergillus terreus*	*Aspergillus versicolor*

Phialides Circumferentially Placed

Conidia smooth and clear or buff	Conidia rough and black
Colonies buff, cottony or granular	Colony surface peppery black;
Aspergillus flavus	*Aspergillus niger*

Cleistothecia Seen

Colonies white and smooth:	Colonies variegated, green, yellow, white.
Aspergillus nidulans.	*Aspergillus glaucus*

Display 21-2 Algorithm showing laboratory identification of the rapidly growing hyaline molds.

Preliminary Observations Suggestive of the Dermatophytes

- Colonies grow in 3-5 days with distinct margins
- Colony surface is cottony to granular in consistency. Surface pigmentation ranging from gray white to yellow-buff
- Hyphae are narrow, septate, and hyaline
- Combinations of microconidia and macroconidia are produced, the size, shape, and arrangement of which provide for genus/species identifications

MICROSCOPIC EXAMINATION

Macroaleureospores large, club-shaped, walls thin and smooth, multi-celled, walls thin and smooth.	Macroaleureospores multi-celled, walls thick and rough. Microconida few or absent.		Microconidia abundant; macro-aleureospores few or absent, walls thin and smooth			Aleureospores usually not present; hyphae only observed.
	Macroaleureospores are spindle-shaped, pointed, curved tip.	Macroaleureospores are broad club-shape with rounded tip.	Microconidia spherical, uniform in loose clusters.	Microconidia tear-shaped, borne laterally from hyphae.	Microconidia irregular in size, balloon forms seen.	Antler hyphae and chlamydospores in chains observed.
Colony khaki-colored	Reverse of colony lemon-yellow	Colony cinnamon-colored		Wine-red pigment in agar	No growth on Trichophyton #1 agar	Slow-growing. Colony smooth on surface, heaped and partially submerged.
Epidermophyton flocossum	*Micrsporum canis*	*Microsporum gypseum*	*Trichophyton mentagrophytes*	*Trichophyton rubrum*	*Trichophyhton tonsurans*	*Trichophyton verrucosum*

Display 21-3 Algorithm showing genus identification of the commonly encountered dermatophytes.

Preliminary Observations Suggestive of a Dimorphic Fungus

- Colonies grow slowlyusually 7–14 days required for primary isolation
- Colony surface is gray-white and cob-web in consistency.
- Hyphae are delicate, septate, and hyaline. Arrangement in parallel bundles may be seen
- Species identification are made based on the size, shape, morphology, and arrangement of conidia

MICROSCOPIC EXAMINATION

Conidia, club-shaped, with thin-smooth walls, borne at the tips of long, straight conidiophores. (lollipops)	Hyphae segment into barrel-shaped arthroconidia, separated by non-staining cells. (alternate staining)	Tiny, microconidia produced early on. Later, large, spiked spherical macroconida are diagnostic.	Small, club-shaped conidia produced radially at the tip of a straight conidiophore, in a daisy head arrangement.	Small, thin-walled conidia borne at the tips of long, straight conidiophores.
Blastomyces dermatitidis	*Coccidioides immitis*	*Histoplasma capsulatum*	*Sporothrix schenckii*	*Paracoccidioides brasiliensis*

CONFIRM SPECIES IDENTIFICATION BY YEAST CONVERSION (OR NUCLEIC ACID PROBE)

Spherical yeast cells, 10–15 um in diameter, with a single broad-based bud.	Large spherules, 75–200um in diameter, containing 3-5um end-ospores observed in stained tissue sections.	Tiny, spherical, hyaline, smooth-walled conidia arranged in clusters. Seen intra-cellularly in stained tissue sections.	Elongated, 2–8 um in length, single-budding conidia, often referred to as cigar bodies.	Large, spherical, smooth, thick-walled mother cell with multiple buds, mariners wheel.

Display 21-4 Algorithm showing genus identification of the dimorphic fungi.

Preliminary Observations Suggestive of a Dematiaceous Mold

- Colonies grow in 3-5 days, are cottony or wooly, gray-brown or brown black; reverse jet black
- Hyphae are narrow, septate, brown-pigmented, and have parallel walls

Muriform Macroconidia				Transverse Macroconidia				Pycnidia or Conidia Single		
Multi-celled, muriform, macroconidia, beak or drumstick-shaped, borne in simple or branched chains, with the blunt end of one abutting the tapered end of the next.	Multi-celled muriform macroconidia borne singly from the tips of geniculate conidiophores, in a sympodial derivation.	Multi-celled muriform macroconidia, each borne singly from the tips of short conidiophores, simulating a bale of cotton on a stick.	Multi-celled muriform macroconidia, mature and immature, borne singly, aggregating in loose clusters.	3-4 -celled macroconidia divided by transverse septa only. The center cells grow more rapidly, become enlarged, resulting in a boomerang appearance.	Conidiophores dark, simple or branched, geniculate, bearing cylindrical conidia in a sympodial pattern. Conidia with multiple cells, encased in thickened septal walls. Germ tubes from each end of germinating conidia.	Conidiophores and conidia similar in appearance to those of *Bipolaris* species. A single germ-tube is observed emanating at right angles from the germinating conidia.	Conidiophores dark, erect, and geniculate. Multiseptate, elongated pencil-shaped conidia borne singly in a sympodial pattern. Each conidium has a dark, prominently protruding knob from the hilar cell.	Large, jet-black-spherical to oblong conidia borne singly from the tips of short, broad, conidiophores, each with a cup-like concavity within which the conidia rests.	Small, hyaline, spherical to elliptical conidia borne within sack-like, globose to subglobose pycnidia, scattered amid brown-staining septate hyphae with parallel walls.	Large perithecia, dark-brown to black, globose to flask-shaped, formed in the sub-stratum amid brown-staining, septate hyphae. Distinctive elongate, hairlike-hyphae protrude from the inside, simulating the legs of a spider
Alternaria species	*Ulocladium* species	*Stemphilium* species	*Epicoccum* species	*Curvularia* species	*Bipolaris* species	*Drechslera* species	*Exserohilum* species	*Nigrospora* species	*Phoma* species	*Chaetomium* species

Display 21-5 Algorithm showing laboratory identification of the rapidly growing dematiaceous molds.

Preliminary Observations Suggestive of the Agents of Chromomycosis/Mycetoma

- Colonies grow in 3–5 days with distinct margins
- Colony surface is cottony to granular in consistency. Surface pigmentation gray-white to brown black; reverse jet black
- Hyphae are relatively broad, have parallel walls, are distinctly septate, and are dark yellow to brown in color
- Conidia are borne in chains, clusters, or singly from the tips or sides of phialides distinctive for each genus

MICROSCOPIC EXAMINATION

Conidia borne in chains			Conidia borne in clusters			Conidia borne singly		
Short branching chains of elliptical conidia with dysjunctor scars	Long chains (35+ cells) of elliptical conidia without dysjunctor scars	Colonies rapidly growing; no growth at 42°C. Cladosporium type sporulation	Phialides short, urn-shaped		Phialide long and tapered	Sympodial phialides bearing elliptical conidia (acrotheca-type sporulation)		Conidia borne laterally from the hyphae (rhinocladiella-type sporulation)
			Tip of phialide bottle-shaped	Tip of phialide saucer-shaped		Conidia arranged loosely	Conidia arranged tightly	
Cladophialophora carrionii	*Cladophialophora bantiana*	*Cladosporium species*	*Phialophora verrucosa*	*Phialophora richardsiae*	*Exophiala jeanselmei*	*Fonsecaea* pedrosoi	*Fonsecaea compacta*	*Rhinocladiella species*

*Different *Fonsecaea* species may show several combinations of cladosporium,-phialphora, acrotheca, and cladosporium-types of sporulation.

Display 21-6 Algorithm showing genus identification of the agents of chromomycosis and mycetoma.

Preliminary Observations Suggestive of Yeasts

- Colonies grow in 24–72 hours
- Colony surface is smooth to mucoid; may develop feet or low aerial mycelium. Surface pigmentation ranging from white to yellow to rose red to black
- True hyphae are absent, except species that produce arthroconidia
- Pseudohyphae may or may not be present
- Blastoconidia are produced, the size, shape, and arrangement of which provide for genus/species identifications

MICROSCOPIC EXAMINATION

Pseudohyphae and blastoconidia produced		True hyphae and arthroconidia produced		Hyphae absent					Black Yeasts	
Germ Tube Test		Urease Test		Urease Test					Annelloconidia	
Pos	Neg	Pos	Neg	Pos				Neg	No	Yes
Chlamydospores on cornmeal Agar	No chlamydospores on cornmeal Agar	*Trichosporon sp.*	*Geotrichum sp.*	Caffeic Acid Test			Orange to red colonies		Dark-staining hyphae producing hyaline blastoconidia	Two-celled yeast cells with dividing cross septa (annellide)
				Pos		Neg				
					Pos	Neg	*Rhododorula species*			
				Cryptococcus neoformans		*Cryptococcus species*	Inositol Neg	*Saccharomyces sp.* *Hansenula sp.* *Malassezia sp.* *Blastoschizomyces sp.*		
Candida albicans	***Candida species***			Look for irregular-sized yeast cells surrounded by capsular material					***Aureobasidium pullulans***	***Phaeoannellomyces sp.***
	Make presumptive ID based on patterns of growth on cornmeal agar.	Look for blastoconidia on corners of arthroconidia—rabbit ears on cornmeal agar	Look for right angle germ tubes from corners of arthroconidia (hockey sticks) on cornmeal agar							May produce hyphae and phialides when mature

Display 21-7 Algorithm showing genus identification of the commonly encountered yeasts.

Risk and Prevention of Parasitic Infections

Clinical Manifestations of Parasitic Disease

Collection, Transport, and Processing of Specimens

Fecal Specimens

Preservation of Clinical Specimens
Visual Examination
Processing Fresh Stool Specimens for Ova and Parasite Examination

Examination of Intestinal Specimens Other Than Stool

Examination of Extraintestinal Specimens

Sputum
Urine and Body Fluids
Tissue Biopsies and Aspirates
Corneal Scrapings or Biopsy
Muscle Biopsy
Blood

Identification and Differentiation of Parasites

Life Cycles of Human Parasites

Intestinal Protozoa

The Intestinal Amoebae

Amebiasis and *Entamoeba histolytica*
Entamoeba histolytica Versus *Entamoeba coli*
Serologic Diagnosis of Amebiasis

Nonpathogenic *Entamoeba histolytica*: *Entamoeba dispar*
Other Intestinal Amoebae
Protozoa of Uncertain Classification

Intestinal Flagellates

Giardia lamblia
Other Intestinal Flagellates

Ciliates: *Balantidium coli*

Coccidia

Cryptosporidium parvum
Cyclospora cayetanensis
Isospora belli
Sarcocystis Species

Phylum *Microsporum*: *Microsporidium* Species

Nematodes

Ascariasis and *Ascaris lumbricoides*
Trichuriasis and *Trichuris trichiura* (Whipworm)
Enterobius vermicularis
Hookworms
Strongyloidiasis and *Strongyloides stercoralis*
Trichostrongylus Species
Capillaria philippinensis

Cestodes

Taenia solium and *Taenia saginata*
Diphyllobothrium latum: The Giant Fish Tapeworm
Hymenolepis Species
Dipylidium caninum

Trematodes

Schistosomes
Fasciola hepatica and *Fasciolopsis buski*
Clonorchis sinensis
Paragonimus westermani

Blood and Tissue Parasites

Malaria
Babesia
Hemoflagellates: *Leishmania* Species and
Trypanosoma Species

Leishmaniasis and *Leishmania* Species
Trypanosomiasis

Filarial Nematodes and Filariasis

Onchocerciasis and *Onchocerca volvulus*
Dracunculiasis
Dirofilariasis

Tissue Protozoan Infections

Toxoplasma gondii
Pneumocystis carinii

Miscellaneous Larval Tissue Parasite Infections

Trichinosis
Visceral Larval Migrans
Cutaneous Larva Migrans—Toxocara
Anisakiasis
Gnathostomiasis
Angiostrongyliasis
Echinococcosis (Hydatid Disease)
Multiceps Species—Coenurosis
Sparganosis: *Spirometra mansonoides*

Serologic Diagnosis of Parasitic Infections

Drugs Commonly Used in the Treatment of Parasitic Diseases

Knowledge of common parasites dates back to antiquity. Worms fitting the description of *Enterobius vermicularis*, *Ascaris lumbricoides*, and the tapeworms have been mentioned in the ancient writings from many countries—certain symptoms known to be caused by these worms have also been described.[135] Ectoparasites, such as, lice, fleas, and ticks could not have been overlooked. Ruffer[231] reported the observation of calcified *Schistosoma haematobium* eggs in the kidneys of two mummies of the 20th dynasty in Egypt, (1200–1090 B.C.), proving the existence of this infection in ancient Egypt. Chinese settlers in ancient times living in infected areas were familiar with the clinical picture of severe hookworm infection—it was called "lazy-yellow-disease."

Imaginary parasites have played an important role in medicine from ancient times. The pain of toothache was attributed to the work of a special boring "tooth-worm." Similarly, pus exuding from the ear and the eye resulted from the action of earworms and eyeworms, respectively. Heartworms were responsible for sudden death; echo worms, possibly related to ascaris balls in the intestine, were described, with the advice to those taking medication to remain silent during treatment for fear that the worm would be listening and not be removed.[135]

For centuries, spontaneous generation was thought to account for the origin of parasites, among other small creatures. It was commonly believed that out of a certain combination of the elements and proper contraries, parasites as well as other living organisms can be created. Tapeworms were known to be associated with the ingestion of raw meat—they were thought to take their origin in the stomach from macer-

ated food, before being passed out in the stool. Since Roman times, tapeworms were thought to be transformed strips of intestinal mucosa; according to many, ascaris worms originated in phlegm. According to ancient theorists, something imperceptible or invisible is endowed with all potentialities—then through the action of a metaphysical principle, or of a primordial force, visible living beings can be created.[25]

An understanding of the protozoan parasites developed closely with improvements in the compound microscope. van Leeuwenhoek is credited with making the first observation of protozoa, a "motile animalcule" in the gut of a horsefly, and shortly thereafter found to be present in his own feces. The current opinion is that he was looking at *Giardia lamblia*. After these observations, however, over a century passed before progress in the study of the protozoans was made. With the widespread use of the compound microscope, by the turn of the 20th century the morphology and life cycles of virtually all human parasites afflicting humans were well defined. The chronology of these advances is well presented in Foster's historical account.[84]

Despite the implementation of preventive measures to minimize the prevalence of parasitic diseases in most of the underdeveloped and many of the developing countries, human parasites still account for inestimable loss of life, widespread morbidity, and the retardation of economic development. To quote from a report of the distribution of human parasites in China, "prevalence rates (of parasitic diseases) are of such staggering magnitude that the mind has difficulty in conceiving the descriptive statistics."[295] As further stated in this report, "the total number of protozoan and helminthic infections currently existing worldwide far outnumbers the total world population since multiple infections is the rule rather than the exception.'' Box 22-1 lists the estimated worldwide prevalence of human parasitic diseases, based on statistics published by the World Health Organization and from other sources.

In the United States, certain parasite species are encountered more frequently than others, and expertise in their identification must remain foremost. From a Centers for Disease Control and Prevention (CDC) intestinal parasite surveillance program, parasitic forms were found in 64,901 (15.6%) of the over 400,000 stool samples examined.[29] *Giardia lamblia* was found in 3.8% of all stool specimens, *Trichuris trichiura* ova in 2.7%, *Ascaris lumbricoides* ova in 2.3%, *Enterobius vermicularis* ova in 1.6% (not a true reflection of the incidence of this disease, since stool specimen examination is not the most sensitive method for establishing a diagnosis), and *Entamoeba histolytica* in 0.6% of all stool specimens. Diphyllobothriasis, including sparganosis, and anisakiasis are also seen with increased frequency as ingestion of fresh fish becomes more in vogue. Private practitioners and public health officials must be on the alert for a possible increase in taenia infections, including neurocysticercosis and other parasitic diseases, with the advent of the North American Free Trade Agreement and a more free exchange of foodstuff between North American countries.[238]

Box 22-2 is a summary of the parasites found by Bruckner and associates in a 6-month survey of stool specimen examinations on outpatients treated at Olive View Medical Center and Harbor General Hospital in Los Angeles.[21]

In this study, other protozoa were identified in about 3% of all stool specimens; other nematodes were identified in 3% and cestodes in 0.5% of specimens. In a more recent study conducted through the Parasitology Center in Tempe, Arizona, Amin[7] reported that one third of 5,792 fecal specimens that were surveyed from 2,896 patients in 48 states and the District of Columbia during the year 2000 tested positive for intestinal parasites. Multiple infections with two to four parasitic species constituted 10% of 916 infected cases. *Blastocystis hominis* infected 662 patients (72% of the 916 cases), a prevalence that has appeared to be increasing in recent years. Eighteen other species of intestinal parasites were identified—*Cryptosporidium parvum* and *Entamoeba histolytica/E. dispar* ranked second and third in prevalence, respectively. Prevalence of infection was lowest (22–27%) in winter, gradually increased during the spring, reached peaks of 36–43% between July and October, and gradually decreased to 32% in December.

Malaria is uncommon in the United States, usually found in individuals who have traveled into endemic areas. The CDC received reports of 1,167 cases of malaria with onset of symptoms during 1995 among persons in the United States or one of its territories.[288] This number represents an increase of 15% from the 1,014 cases reported for 1994. *P. vivax*, *P. falciparum*, *P. malariae*, and *P. ovale* were identified in 48.2%, 38.6%, 3.9%, and 2.2% of cases, respectively. More than one species was present in three patients (0.3% of total). The infecting species was not determined in 80 (6.9%) cases. The number of reported malaria cases acquired in Africa ($n = 519$) remained approximately the same as in 1994 ($n = 517$); cases acquired in Asia increased by 32.4% ($n = 335$); and cases acquired in the Americas increased by 37.4 % ($n = 246$).

Because of expanded international travel, students and technologists working in diagnostic laboratories must maintain a broad acquaintance with all parasitic diseases. Trade

Box 22-1 Estimated Worldwide Prevalence of Parasitic Diseases*

Parasitic Disease	Global Prevalence (Millions of People)
Amebiases	500
Giardiasis	200
Ascariasis	800
Trichuriasis (whipworm)	800
Hookworm	900
Strongyloidiasis	50–100
Enterobius (pinworm)	42 (developed countries)
Taenia (cysticercosis)	1% of population in endemic countries
Diphyllobothriasis	5–10
Schistosomiasis	200
Fascioliasis	1–2
Clonorchiasis	20 (China)
Paragonimiasis	4–5
Malaria	100–270
Leishmaniasis	12
Trypanosomiasis (African)	20,00 new cases/year
Trypanosomiasis (Chagas' disease)	15
Onchocerciasis	20
Filariasis	90
Echinococcus disease	1/100,000–150/100,000

The incidence figures recorded here are rough estimates, intended only to illustrate the huge magnitude of infections. There are variations in numbers published in different sources, which probably reflect incomplete access to information or to differences in extrapolation of known data to the population at large.

Box 22-2 Incidence of Parasites in Stool Specimens[21]

Organism	Olive View (1350 Samples) %	Harbour General (493 Samples) %
Giardia lamblia	14.5	8.7
Endolimax nana	13.0	8.5
Entamoeba coli	10.5	7.7
Entamoeba histolytica	4.5	5.3
Ascaris lumbricoides	3.9	2.0
Hymenolepis nana	3.3	1.4
Dientamoeba fragilis	2.1	2.8

agreements between countries, some known to be endemic for parasitic diseases, also opens up borders to the influx of goods that potentially are contaminated with animal parasites. Travelers from the United States to foreign lands must also remember that a variety of parasitic diseases are endemic in most developing countries and that appropriate precautions must be taken. Unfortunately, accurate numbers of parasitic diseases and the prevalence of specific parasites is obscure in many countries because of the lack of a legal registration system requiring that certain diseases be reported. Parasitic diseases are often overlooked or left misdiagnosed since symptoms are frequently nonspecific and have similarities with other infectious diseases or cancer.

The frequent occurrence of certain parasitic infections in patients with AIDS has spurred a new interest in laboratory parasitology among laboratory workers in nonendemic areas. Vermud et al.[272] found that the AIDS epidemic has had a definite influence on the relative prevalence of parasitic diseases. For example, *Cryptosporidium* species, rarely recognized in humans before 1983, comprised 13.8% of all pathogenic protozoa in 1984. In a survey conducted at the New York Columbia–Presbyterian Medical Center of 41,958 stool specimens submitted for examination during the period 1971–1984, *Strongyloides stercoralis* was approaching the incidence of *Trichuris trichiura* as the most frequently identified nematode. In a recent report, Harms and Feldmeier[122] postulate that HIV and parasitic infections may interact and mutually affect one another. Although the natural history of parasitic diseases may be altered by coinfection with HIV, parasitoses may in turn facilitate the progression from asymptomatic infection to AIDS. According to these authors, the common immunopathogenetic basis for the deleterious effects that parasitic diseases may have on the natural history of HIV infection involves a preferential activation of the T helper (Th) 2 type process. They conclude that the control of parasitic diseases is also necessary to aid in combating the HIV pandemic

Risk and Prevention of Parasitic Infections

The risk factors in acquiring parasitic infections during travel to infested areas of the world and prophylactic measures have been reviewed by Warren and Mahmoud.[276] At lowest risk is the businessman who stays in first-class hotels in large cities for short periods. At the opposite end of the spectrum are volunteers and missionaries who live in tents or native dwellings in rural settings.

Most parasitic diseases are contracted either through ingestion of contaminated food or water or through the sting or bite of an arthropod vector. Drinking untreated water or brushing teeth with contaminated water can be particularly hazardous. Because most intestinal parasites withstand freezing, contaminated ice water is equally unsafe. Hot tap water is relatively safe because the infective forms of most intestinal parasites are heat-sensitive; however, tap water may not consistently exceed the critical temperature of 43°C (110°F); thus, its safety cannot be guaranteed. The ingestion of fresh, unpasteurized milk should also be avoided in endemic areas. Bottled milk and carbonated beverages are usually safe.

Ingestion of undercooked meats or raw freshwater fish can lead to infection with flukes, tapeworms, nematodes such as *Trichinella spiralis*, and the bradyzoites of *Toxoplasma gondii*. Raw vegetables are relatively safe if peeled before eating; however, lettuce and other leafy vegetables are particularly difficult to rid of infective parasitic eggs and cysts. Precautions should be taken to avoid insect bites in tropical regions. The use of screens, bug bombs, insect repellents, and long-sleeved protective clothing is highly recommended. Travelers to foreign countries, particularly to underdeveloped regions in the tropical or subtropical climates, should consult local health authorities concerning appropriate immunization programs. Travelers to areas where malaria is endemic should receive chemoprophylactic drugs. Individuals planning to visit certain countries should consult local state health authorities to learn of the magnitude and geographic distribution of the different malarial parasites, and which prophylactic regimen should be initiated.

Travelers to tropical regions should also be warned against swimming in natural freshwater estuaries. The infective cercariae of *Schistosoma* species abound in many freshwater rivers, lakes, and canals and can easily penetrate the unbroken skin of an unsuspecting wader. Chlorine in the concentration used in swimming pools may not make the water safe. Schistosomal cercariae that infest humans are not found in seawater; however, swimmer's itch may occur after wading in brackish water following penetration of the skin by cercariae of species that infect animals. Examining physicians should make an effort to obtain a history of recent travel into regions where parasitic diseases are endemic and question patients carefully about the conditions under which they lived. The laboratory should be informed if a physician suspects a parasitic disease so that relevant specimens can be collected and the proper procedures carried out for optimal recovery of the diagnostic forms. Depending on the presence of background immunosuppressive diseases and/or a history of recent travel to or from a region known to be endemic for parasitic diseases, stool examinations to screen for parasites, particularly the larval forms of *S. stercoralis*, should be considered for all patients before they receive immunosuppressive drugs.

Clinical Manifestations of Parasitic Disease

The most common symptom of intestinal parasitic infection is diarrhea that may be watery, bloody, and/or purulent. Cramping abdominal pain may be a prominent feature in diseases in which the bowel mucosa or wall is invaded by the parasite, such as in infections with hookworms, Manson's or oriental schistosomes, or intestinal flukes. Heavy infection with *Ascaris lumbricoides* can result in small-bowel obstruction. Patients with tapeworms may be symptomatic except for weight loss despite increased appetite and food intake. Bloating, belching, and steatorrhea may be seen in patients with giardiasis.

Peripheral blood eosinophilia (15–50% or higher) is one of the more important markers for parasitic infestation. Eosinophilia may also be seen in various body secretions, such as sputum, diarrheal stools, suppurative exudates, or fluids from pseudocysts or various body cavities. However, the lack of eosinophils in either the blood or body fluids does not preclude the diagnosis of parasitic diseases in which eosinophilia is not a common manifestation, or the load of parasites may be light. A generalized urticarial skin rash, thought to be a hypersensitivity reaction secondary to metabolic or lytic products of dead organisms that are absorbed into the circulation, may also suggest parasitic infection. Although nonspecific, elevation in serum immunoglobulin levels, particularly IgE may add support to the presence of a parasitic disease, particularly if coupled with eosinophilia.

Hepatosplenomegaly is a common manifestation of leishmaniasis (kala-azar) and liver fluke infection. Portal hypertension, in particular, can be caused by *Schistosoma japonicum*, and jaundice is a common presenting sign. Space-occupying cystic lesions of the liver, brain, and other organs can be found in amebiasis, echinococcosis, and cysticercus (larval stage of *Taenia solium*) infections.

Suprapubic pain, frequent urination, and hematuria are highly suggestive of *Schistosoma haematobium* infection. Transient pneumonitis may be experienced during the larval migratory phases of ascaris or hookworm infections. This condition can be suspected if large numbers of eosinophils are observed in the sputum. Cough, chest pain, and hemoptysis, together with the formation of parabronchial cysts, are common manifestations of the lung fluke, *Paragonimus westermani*. Low-grade fever, weight loss, facial edema, and skeletal muscle pain indicate possible infection with *Trichinella spiralis*. Focal itching of the skin may occur at the sites of penetration of hookworm larvae or the cercariae of *Schistosoma* species.

Generalized constitutional symptoms are more commonly experienced after infections with blood parasites. Fever, chills, night sweats, lassitude, myalgias, and weight loss are common manifestations of malaria, leishmaniasis, and trypanosomiasis. Varying degrees of hepatosplenomegaly and lymphadenopathy are also seen with these diseases. Neurologic signs and symptoms secondary to encephalitis, meningitis, or localizing neuropathies may be seen in a variety of parasitic diseases. Central nervous system (CNS) involvement is commonly diffuse in African trypanosomiasis (sleeping sickness), falciparum malaria, and toxoplasmosis, while space-occupying abscesses or cysts are more commonly seen with *Entamoeba histolytica*, *T. solium* (cysticercosis), and *Echinococcus granulosus* infections. Cardiac myopathy is one of the most serious complications of South American trypanosomiasis (*Trypanosoma cruzi*), of toxoplasmosis, and of several larval migratory infections. Huge swellings of the legs, arms, and scrotum (elephantiasis) are common symptoms of filariases because the adult worms block the lymphatic vessels, resulting in extensive chronic inflammation and fibrosis. Localized subcutaneous nodules or serpiginous inflammatory areas in the skin may be seen in diseases such as onchocerciasis, dracunculiasis, or cutaneous larva migrans, representing the larval migratory forms of hookworms of dogs and other animals.

A succinct overview of the clinical and laboratory aspects of several common and uncommon parasitic diseases has been published by Tan.[262]

Collection, Transport, and Processing of Specimens

Appropriate specimens must be collected from the patient and transported to the laboratory sufficiently preserved to allow for the detection and identification of any parasitic forms. The diagnosis of parasitic infections relies in large part on macroscopic or microscopic examination of feces, urine, blood, sputum, and tissues. The implementation of reliable laboratory processing techniques is an integral step. It is not possible to review more than a few of the commonly used laboratory procedures that can aid in the recovery and identification of parasitic forms in clinical specimens. For a succinct, current, and practical overview of these procedures, the reader is referred to the section, ''Diagnostic Procedures,'' found in the current edition of the classic text by Garcia.[96]

Fecal Specimens

Stool specimens should be collected in a clean, wide-mouthed container with a tightly fitted lid. Specimens that are mixed with water (i.e., contamination from the toilet bowel or bed pan) or urine are unsuitable because trophozoites may lose their motility or undergo lysis. Medications containing mineral oil, bismuth, antibiotics, antimalarials, or other chemical substances may compromise the detection of intestinal protozoa. Thus, examination of specimens must be delayed for 1 or more weeks after diagnostic procedures (barium enema) or therapy is stopped. Patients who have received a barium enema may not excrete organisms in their stools for at least 1 week following the enema. The container lid should be tightly affixed immediately after collection of the sample to maintain adequate moisture. Every specimen container must be properly labeled, as outlined in Chapter 1 of this text.

In obtaining fecal specimens for the examination of parasites, cathartics with an oil base should be avoided, since oils retard motility of trophozoites and distort the morphology of other forms. Specimens should also be collected before the administration of certain drugs and compounds that may compromise examination; or collection should be delayed until after the effects of such agents have passed. Such substances include antacids, kaolin, mineral oil and other oily materials, nonabsorbable antidiarrheal preparations, barium or bismuth (7–10 days needed for clearance of effects), antimicrobial agents (2–3 weeks), and gallbladder dyes (3 weeks).

The collection of three fecal specimens usually suffices to establish the diagnosis of intestinal parasitic diseases—two obtained on successive days during normal bowel movement and a third after a Fleet's phosphosoda or magnesium sulfate purge. No more than one fecal sample per day should be accepted. Some advocate that only a single specimen is required to diagnose most intestinal parasitic infections. This approach depends on the experience of the microscopist and the parasitic load in the specimen, or it may be implemented if the patient becomes asymptomatic between sample collections.[96] Hiatt et al.[132] found that, with additional examinations, the yield of *Entamoeba histolytica* increases by 22.7%, of *Giardia lamblia* by 11.3%, and of *Dientamoeba fragilis* by 31.1%. A total of six specimens, collected on successive days, may be required if intestinal amebiasis or giardiasis is suspected. Examination of more than six samples in a 10-day period rarely yields additional information. Posttherapy specimens should be examined 3–4 weeks after treatment of patients with protozoan infections and 5–6 weeks after therapy for *Taenia* infections.

If a PCR-based assay is requested on a stool specimen, implementation of the following protocol is recommended:

1. Collect the specimen in the absence of preservatives.
2. Store and ship the specimen either refrigerated (4°C) or frozen (shipped with dry ice).
3. Alternatively, stool specimens can be mixed in potassium dichromate (1:1 dilution with 5% w/v) or in absolute ethanol (1:1 dilution) and shipped refrigerated.

Trichrome and/or acid-fast stained smears should accompany the stool specimen when polymerase chain reaction (PCR) is requested for the detection of *G. lamblia* and *E. histolytica/dispar* or *Cryptosporidium parvum* or *Cyclospora cayetanensis*, respectively. All stained smears should first be thoroughly reviewed because the PCR assay is unnecessary if a parasite identification can be made. Details of the extraction procedure and steps to follow in the DNA amplification have been published by da Silva and associates.[54]

PRESERVATION OF CLINICAL SPECIMENS

Many stool specimens for examination of ova and parasites are collected either at home, in a physician's office, or in a clinic some distance from the laboratory that performs the examination. Because trophozoites disintegrate rapidly after defecation and do not encyst, liquid stool specimens should be examined within 30 minutes after collection (not 30 minutes after receipt in the laboratory), or semiformed stools within 60 minutes, in order to detect motile trophozoites, particularly in suspected infections with *E. histolytica*. Formed stools, in which trophozoites are not expected, may be examined up to 24 hours after passage. Stool specimens should never be frozen and thawed or placed in an incubator because parasitic forms may deteriorate rapidly.

Several preservatives are available for permanent fixation of stool specimens that are held for future teaching purposes, or that must be sent to reference laboratories for analysis. Box 22-3 presents the formulation and preparation of several currently used preservatives. Their advantages and disadvantages are summarized below.

Alternative Fixatives. Concerns over the toxicity of formalin and the difficulty of disposal of preservatives containing mercuric chloride, have led several commercial companies to market alternatives to the gold standard, low-viscosity polyvinyl alcohol reagent (LV-PVA). In a study of 68 fresh stool specimens, collectively containing 31 parasitic forms, Jensen and colleagues[146] concluded that Proto-Fix (Alpha-Tec Systems, Vancouver, WA) and EcoFix (Meridian Diagnostics, Cincinnati, OH) were environmentally safe substitutes for PVA, resulting in the least parasite distortion. In a study of 20 positive stool specimens containing one or more parasites with stages consisting of eggs, larvae, and cysts,

Pietrzak-Johnston et al.[215] also concluded that EcoFix is comparable to traditional LV-PVA for the visualization of protozoa in permanent-stained smears, confirming the earlier findings of Garcia and Shimizu.[94] In each of these studies, the parasitic forms had well-defined nuclear detail, with certain parasites even easier to identify in the EcoFix-preserved specimens than in the traditional PVA-fixed samples.

When properly stained by these techniques, the organisms have a blue-green to purple cytoplasm and red to purple-red chromatin against a green-staining background. Helminth eggs and larvae have a red or purple appearance. Remember that *Trichuris trichiura* eggs and *Giardia lamblia* cysts do not concentrate as well from PVA as from formalin-fixed material, that the morphology of larval forms of *Strongyloides stercoralis* is poor in PVA-fixed stools, and that *Isospora belli* may be missed completely.

Several commercially available fecal concentration devices, including the FPC JUMBO tube and the FPC HYBRID connecter systems (Evergreen Scientific, Los Angeles, CA), the PARA-SED concentration system (Medical Chemical, Torrance, CA), and the MACRO-CON concentration system (Meridian Diagnostics, Cincinnati, OH), in addition to an automated countertop workstation for the microscopic analysis of fecal concentrates (DiaSys., Waterbury, CT), have been presented by Garcia.[93] Each of these products, in current use in clinical laboratories, can be recommended.

VISUAL EXAMINATION

Freshly passed stool specimens submitted for the detection of parasites should be visually examined for the presence of barium, oils, or other materials that may render them unacceptable for further processing. Patches of blood or mucin should be specifically selected for microscopic study because they may be derived directly from ulcers or purulent abscesses, where the concentration of amoebae may be highest. Visual examination can also be used to determine the appropriate procedures to perform. Formed stools are unlikely to contain trophozoites; thus, wet mounts are usually unnecessary and only concentrates need to be prepared. Helminth eggs and larvae and protozoan cysts can be seen in the sediment of concentrates. The preparation of direct mounts should be limited to diarrheal stools, and stained smears should be prepared to better demonstrate the internal structures of any parasitic forms observed. These approaches are described in more detail in the sections to follow.

PROCESSING FRESH STOOL SPECIMENS FOR OVA AND PARASITE EXAMINATION

Liquid stool specimens should be examined within 30 minutes of passage (not within 30 minutes of arrival in the laboratory) in order to maximize the chance for observing motile trophozoites. Soft specimens, which may contain either trophozoites and/or cysts, should be examined within 1 hour of passage. In cases in which delays cannot be avoided, the specimen should be preserved as previously discussed to avoid possible disintegration of trophozoites. Formed stool specimens should either be rejected or, since they are less likely to contain trophozoites, can be kept for up to 1 day, with overnight refrigeration if needed.

Box 22-3 Common Fecal Specimen Fixatives: Formulations and Preparation

10% formalin-saline

In an appropriate storage container with a tightly fitting lid, add 100 mL of formaldehyde in 900 mL of 0.85% sodium chloride.

Advantages

- It is readily available, is easy to prepare, and serves as an all-purpose fixative.
- The prepared reagent has a long shelf life.
- The morphology of helminth eggs, larvae, protozoan cysts, and coccidial forms are well preserved.
- Formalin-preserved specimens are suitable for concentration procedures, epifluorescence microscopy, and performance of acid-fast, safranin, and chromotrope stains, and compatible with immunoassay kits.

Disadvantages

- Formalin-preserved specimens are not suitable for the preparation of trichrome-stained smears.
- Preservation is inadequate to maintain the morphology of protozoan trophozoites.
- The performance of PCR procedures may be hampered, particularly after extended fixation time.

Some parasitologists prefer a formula containing 5% formalin, which is purported to be less damaging to protozoa and emits less formalin vapor into the laboratory environment.

LV-PVA (low-viscosity polyvinyl alcohol)

Formulation
  Polyvinyl alcohol, 10.0 g
  95% ethyl alcohol, 62.5 mL
  Mercuric chloride, saturated aqueous, 125.0 mL
  Glycerin, 3.0 mL

Preparation
The liquid ingredients are mixed in a 500-mL beaker and the PVA powder added without mixing. Cover the beaker with paper or foil and allow the PVA to soak overnight. Slowly heat the mixture to 75°C and gently swirl for about 30 seconds until a light milky suspension is achieved.

Advantages

- The morphology of protozoan trophozoites and cysts are well preserved.
- Permanent smears stained with trichrome are easily prepared.
- Parasite forms are both preserved and adhere to the slide.
- Preserved samples remain stable for several months.

Disadvantages

- The morphology of helminth eggs and larvae, coccidian, and microsporidia are inadequately preserved.
- Mercuric chloride is the main ingredient, making it difficult and expensive to dispose of the fixative.
- The reagent is difficult to prepare in the laboratory.
- Cannot be used for concentration procedures or immunoassay kits.
- Unsuitable for acid-fast, safranin, and chromotrope stains.

MIF (Merthiolate-iodine-formaldehyde)

Formulation
The two solutions must be prepared and stored separately and mixed together only immediately before use.

Solution I
  Tincture of merthiolate, 1:1000, 40 mL
  Formaldehyde, 10% aqueous (USP), 5 mL
  Glycerol, 1 mL
  Distilled water, 50 mL

Solution II
  Potassium iodide crystals (KI), 10 g
  Iodine crystals (add after KI dissolves), 5 g of distilled water, 100 mL

Preparation
The shelf life of each solution is many months if stored at room temperature in a brown bottle. In a small vial, combine 9.4 mL of solution I with 0.6 mL of solution II just before use. Add the equivalent of about 1/4 teaspoon of fresh feces and thoroughly mix with an applicator stick. Allow the suspension to settle for 24 hours; then, with a pipette, remove a small portion of the pale orange middle layer and the deeper-staining lower layer for preparation of smears.

Box 22-3 *Continued*

Advantages

- The reagent components both fix and stain the parasitic forms.
- Preparation is easy and shelf life is long.
- Suitable for concentration procedures.

Disadvantages

- As with formalin preservative, it is not suitable for preparation of permanent trichrome smears.
- The morphology of protozoan trophozoites is poorly preserved.
- The iodine component may interfere with other stains and fluorescence and may cause distortion of protozoa.

Sodium acetate, acetic acid, formalin (SAF)

Formulation
   Formaldehyde (37–40% solution), 0.6 mL
   Glacial acetic acid, 0.3 mL
   Sodium acetate, 225.0 mg
   Distilled water, 13.88 mL
Preparation
Dissolve the sodium acetate in the distilled water, slowly add the glacial acetic acid and formalin solutions, mix, and store. The shelf life is several months.

Advantages

- Easy to prepare and reagent has long shelf life.
- Suitable for acid-fast, safranin, and chromotrope stains.
- No interference with immunoassay kit assays.
- Free of the toxic chemical mercuric chloride.

Disadvantages

- Albumin-glycerine or similar additive must be used for adhesion of specimen to slides.
- Permanent stains are inferior to those obtained with PVA or Schaudinn's fixative.

Schaudinn's Fixative

Formulation:
   Mercuric chloride, saturated aqueous solution (HgCl$_2$), 110 g
   Distilled water, 1,000 mL
Preparation
Into a beaker in a water bath placed in a hood, boil the mercuric chloride until dissolved, and let stand for several hours until crystals form.
Schaudinn's Fixative (Stock)
   Mercuric chloride, saturated aqueous solution, 600 mL
   Ethyl alcohol, 95%, 300 mL
Add 5 mL of glacial acetic acid per 100 mL of stock solution just before use.

Advantages

- Protozoan trophozoites and cysts are well preserved.
- Permanent stained smears are easily prepared.

Disadvantages

- Mercuric chloride is the main ingredient, making it difficult and expensive to dispose of the fixative.
- The morphology of helminth eggs and larvae, coccidian, and microsporidia are poorly preserved.
- Albumin-glycerine or a similar additive must be used for adhesion of the specimen to slides.
- Less suitable than other preservatives for concentration procedures.

Three types of preparation should be made for liquid and soft stool specimens that have been submitted for parasitic examinations: 1) direct wet mounts, 2) concentrates, and 3) permanent stained smears.

Direct saline mounts are valuable for the detection of motile trophozoites. Helminth eggs and larvae and protozoan cysts may also be observed in direct saline mounts; the addition of a drop of iodine may aid visualization of these forms.

For fecal specimens that are watery or liquid, centrifugation of the specimen alone may suffice because trophozoites do not concentrate well from liquid stools, and cysts that may be present will be seen in the sediment. The direct examination may be omitted for the processing of semiformed stools since any parasitic forms present will still be detected in the concentrated preparation.

Final identifications of parasites should not be made from

examination of direct mounts alone; rather, permanent stained smears should be prepared and examined to confirm the characteristic morphologic features. Permanent stains should be prepared on any specimens for which a delay in transport is anticipated. Mix one to two drops of the specimen with three to four drops of polyvinyl alcohol and spread over the surface of a glass slide and allow to air dry. Or, a small amount can be added to an equal volume of Schaudinn's fixatives in a capped tube.

Preparation of Direct Wet Mounts.
The wet mount procedure is useful for the identification of protozoan trophozoites, cysts, oocysts, and both helminth eggs and larvae. The saline mount is prepared by emulsifying a small portion of fecal material in a drop of physiologic saline on a microscope slide, then overlaying the mixture with a coverslip. Ideally, two mounts can be prepared on the same slide, the second one using iodine. Mounts should be just thick enough that newspaper print can be read through the slide. If the mounts are too thick, particularly iodine preparations, parasitic forms often stain poorly and may be difficult to differentiate from background debris. If the smear is too thin, parasitic forms in low numbers may be diluted out and missed during routine microscopic examination. Saline mounts are also prepared to observe the motility of trophozoites. Protozoan cysts also appear more refractile in saline than on iodine preparations. The internal structures of trophozoites or protozoan cysts are often poorly delineated in saline preparations making definitive identification difficult. Permanent stained smears should always be prepared, particularly if *Giardia lamblia* is suspected.

The oocysts of *Cyclospora* species may be observed microscopically in wet preparations using UV fluorescence microscopy, on which they appear intensely blue (UV excitation filter set at 330–365 nm). The use of both brightfield and fluorescence microscopy provides an efficient and reliable approach to diagnosis. Additional smears should also be prepared in the event that an identification is not made from the original preparations.

Iodine is used as a stain to highlight the internal structures of intestinal parasites. One percent solutions of iodine (for example, D'Antoni's iodine, prepared by adding 1.0 g of potassium iodide and 1.5 g of powdered iodine crystals to 100 mL of distilled water) should be used. Lugol's iodine, used for Gram stains, in full strength is too strong to stain protozoan forms but can be used if a freshly prepared solution is diluted 1:5 with distilled water (having the appearance of strong tea). Examination of iodine mounts alone, however, may not be satisfactory because trophozoites are no longer motile. Both saline and iodine mounts can be prepared on a single microscope slide, making it easy to compare any suspicious forms.

If desired the coverslip(s) may be sealed. A preparation of molten petroleum jelly and paraffin in a 1:1 ratio can be applied to the margins of the coverslip using the tip of a cotton-tipped swab. The paraffin and petroleum jelly must be heated to approximately 70°C to mix both just before use. The seal is made by first securing the four corners by placing a drop of hot sealant to anchor the coverslip. A thin layer of the mixture is then spread around the edges. Sealing the coverslip keeps organisms from moving when using oil-immersion objectives and prevents the preparation from drying out. Other suitable sealing preparations can be used if desired (clear nail polish, for example).

The entire coverslip area should be systematically scanned with an overlapping back and forth motion, using the $10\times$ objective. If a suspicious form is observed, a higher magnification may be necessary to study internal details.

Fecal Concentration Methods.
Eggs, cysts, and trophozoites are often in such low numbers in fecal material that they are difficult to detect in direct smears or mounts; therefore, concentration procedures should always be performed. The two most commonly used are: 1) flotation and 2) sedimentation. Both are designed to separate intestinal protozoa and helminth eggs from excess fecal debris. The details for these procedures are found in Chart 22-1.

Flotation Techniques Flotation techniques are less commonly used in clinical laboratories than the sedimentation procedure. The flotation method uses solutions that have higher specific gravity than the organisms to be floated so that certain parasitic forms rise to the top, while fecal debris sinks to the bottom. Most commonly, zinc sulfate with a specific gravity of 1.018 is used. In comparison, the specific gravity of protozoa and many of the helminth eggs is lower. For example, the specific gravity of a hookworm egg is 1.055, an *Ascaris* egg 1.110, a *Trichiura* egg 1.150, and *Giardia lamblia* cysts 1.060.

The chief advantage of the flotation technique is that it produces a cleaner material in which parasitic forms are easy to distinguish. The major disadvantages are that the walls of eggs and cysts will often collapse, thus hindering identification; also, some parasite eggs do not float. Also, operculated trematode and cestode eggs may not be detected because the high concentration of the zinc sulfate suspension causes the opercula to pop open and the egg to fill with fluid and sink to the bottom of the tube. For this reason, both the top filtrate and the bottom sediment should be examined microscopically.

Bartlett and associates[14] have described a modified zinc sulfate flotation technique that may be adapted for use with specimens that have been formalin-fixed. The formalin fixation not only prevents operculated eggs from popping so that they can be detected in flotation eluates, but it also prevents the distortion of parasitic forms caused by salt solutions of high specific gravity.

Sedimentation Techniques Solutions of a specific gravity lower than the parasitic organisms are used, thus concentrating the eggs, cysts, and other forms in the sediment. Sedimentation techniques are recommended for general diagnostic laboratories because they are easier to perform and less prone to technical errors.

Concentration of intestinal parasites by sedimentation techniques, using either gravity or centrifugation, leads to good recovery of protozoa, eggs, and larvae, although they may be more difficult to detect in microscopic mounts and in stained smears because of the comparatively large amount of background debris. Ethyl acetate has been substituted for diethyl ether in the formalin concentration procedure used in most laboratories. Young and associates[304] have demonstrated that ethyl acetate is less flammable and less hazardous to use than diethyl ether and that the capability to concentrate cysts and eggs is not compromised. Care must be taken during the washing steps in the procedure to decant the supernatant carefully; otherwise, a significant number of parasitic forms can be lost. Neimeister et al.[197] have demonstrated that Hemo-De (PMP Medical Industries, Irving, TX, and distributed by Fisher Scientific, Pittsburgh, PA) is an effective replacement for ethyl acetate. Hemo-De is a solvent with a specific gravity and solubility similar to that of ethyl acetate; it is nonflammable, nontoxic, and biodegradable (classified as GRAS [generally regarded as safe]) by the US Food and Drug Administration).

Permanent Stained Smears. Although temporary wet mounts of fecal material for direct microscopic examination facilitate the rapid detection of intestinal parasites in fecal specimens, smaller protozoan organisms may be missed. Therefore, Garcia[96] recommends that permanent stains be prepared as part of the examination of every stool specimen submitted for parasitologic examination. In particular, the detection and identification of *Entamoeba histolytica, Giardia lamblia,* and other protozoan infections can be greatly enhanced.[246] The morphology of cysts and trophozoites is better visualized in stained smears. Permanent mounts may also be prepared from stained smears, for future use in teaching collections, and for future consultation with experts when unusual forms are observed.

Two types of permanent stains are commonly used to visualize intestinal protozoa in fecal smears: 1) the iron hematoxylin stain and 2) the modified (Wheatley's) Gomori's trichrome stains. The iron hematoxylin stain is the time-honored technique used for the most exacting definition of the morphology of intestinal parasites. The staining procedure is somewhat difficult to control and is best performed by an experienced person to achieve optimum results. The trichrome stain is widely used in diagnostic laboratories because it is easy to perform and good results are obtained with both fresh and PVA-preserved fecal material. The trichrome staining procedure is reviewed in detail in Chart 22-2.

With the advent of diarrheal syndromes, particularly in patients who are immunosuppressed or infected with AIDS, involving new emerging pathogens—*Cryptosporidium* species, *Cyclospora* species, and *Microsporum* species—additional stains may be required in the examination of liquid and soft stools. The oocysts of *Cryptosporidium* species and *Cyclospora* species stain well with the modified acid-fast stain, in which 1% sulfuric acid is used as the decolorizer.

A fluorescent antibody method is also available for the detection of *Cryptosporidium* species, often in combination with a monoclonal antibody directed against *Giardia lamblia* cysts (discussed in detail later in his chapter). Remember that fresh or formalin-fixed material must be used to perform the acid fast and/or the monoclonal antibody techniques; PVA-preserved specimens cannot be used.[93]

The tiny organisms of *Microsporum* species do not stain well with most stains. The Weber stain[279] and the Ryan stain[232] have been used with success in clinical laboratories. More recently, the chromotrope R stain has been developed at the CDC. In this stain, the concentration of the chromotrope 2R component has been increased by 10 times to facilitate the penetration of dye into the minute parasitic forms. It is important to prepare a thin smear using approximately 10 µl of 10% formalin-fixed unconcentrated stool suspension on a glass slide (formalin concentrates may also be used, but the number of organisms, which do not concentrate well, per field of view is not substantially increased). The quick hot-gram-chromotrope procedure is an alternative stain that is fast, reliable, and simple to perform.[190] Using this technique, a routine Gram stain is first performed on the thin smear, but instead of safranin, the slide is placed in a warmed (50–55°C) chromotrope stain for at least 1 minute. The microsporidia spores appear as dark staining violet ovoid structures against a pale green background. A control slide of microsporidia spores from a 10% formalin-preserved specimen should be included for each staining run. This control provides a point of reference to distinguish true spores from other look-alike objects. These stains are described in more detail later in this chapter.

Examination of Intestinal Specimens Other Than Stool

Parasites such as *Giardia lamblia* and *Strongyloides stercoralis* commonly inhabit the duodenum and jejunum. Samples of duodenal contents may be required to demonstrate these organisms. A saline wet mount can be prepared from the aspirated material and examined microscopically. If motile organisms are seen, examination of a second iodine preparation may be helpful to highlight the internal structures so that a definitive identification can be made.

Duodenal contents can be examined by the string test.[148] The implement used is a weighted gelatin capsule containing a coiled length of nylon string (commercially available as Enterotest from Hedeco, Palo Alto, CA). One end of the string protrudes from the capsule, which is taped to the face of the patient. The capsule is swallowed and peristalsis carries the weighted string into the duodenum. After 4 to 6 hours, the string is removed and any bile-stained mucous adhering to the distal end is used to prepare direct mounts and stained smears for microscopic study. The examination of duodenal contents should be performed only on patients with signs and symptoms suggestive of giardiasis. McHenry et al.[184] obtained duodenal aspirates from 144 patients who were undergoing endoscopy for other reasons. *Giardia lamblia* was recovered in only one patient (0.7%).

Enterobius vermicularis infection of the rectal canal is best detected using cellulose tape. To perform the examination, the adhesive surface of a 3- or 4-inch strip of clear cellulose tape is applied to the perianal folds of a patient in whom pinworm infection is suspected. Specimens collected in the early morning, soon after the patient arises and before bathing, are optimal for detecting ova. A tongue blade can be used to provide a firm backing for the tape. The tape is then placed adhesive side down on a glass microscope slide and examined for the characteristic ova of *E. vermicularis*. A commercially available "paddle" with a flat, sticky surface ("Swube"-Falcon 2012 disposable applicator; Falcon, Oxnard, CA) can be used to obtain the specimen. The microscopic appearance of a positive preparation is illustrated in Figure 22-1.

Histologic examination of a sigmoid biopsy may be necessary in some cases of *Entamoeba histolytica* infection, when repeated stool examinations fail to reveal organisms. The processing of these specimens is described later in this chapter.

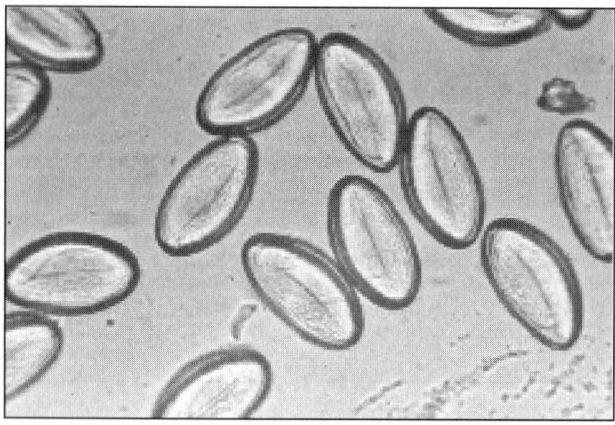

Figure 22-1 Photomicrograph of a positive cellulose tape preparation from a patient with suspected pinworm infection, illustrating several oval, thin-walled eggs of *Enterobius vermicularis*.

Examination of Extraintestinal Specimens
SPUTUM

On rare occasions, the larval stages of hookworm, *Ascaris lumbricoides* or *Strongyloides stercoralis*, or the eggs of *P. westermani* may be seen in sputum samples. The preparation of a direct saline mount is usually sufficient. If the sputum is unusually thick or mucoid, an equal quantity of 3% *N*-acetyl-L-cysteine or 3% sodium hydroxide (or undiluted chlorine bleach) can be added to liquefy the specimen, which is then mixed for 2 or 3 minutes and then centrifuged. After centrifugation, a wet mount of the sediment is prepared for microscopic examination. If examination of the sputum specimen is delayed for any reason, 10% formalin should be added to preserve helminth eggs or larvae.

URINE AND BODY FLUIDS

Samples of large volume should be allowed to settle for 1 or 2 hours. About 50 mL can then be taken from the bottom sediment for centrifugation. The highly concentrated sediment can then be examined by preparing a direct wet mount. If objects suggestive of parasites are seen, examination of an iodine mount or a stained preparation may be helpful in highlighting the diagnostic internal structures.

TISSUE BIOPSIES AND ASPIRATES

Cutaneous ulcers (as seen in leishmaniasis), skin nodules (seen in onchocerciasis and in *Mansonella streptocerca* infections), and lymph nodes may be either aspirated with a fine needle or biopsied. In suspected cases of cutaneous leishmaniasis, material should be aspirated with a needle and syringe from beneath the ulcer bed. A ''skin snip'' can be obtained to diagnose subcutaneous leishmanial disease by grasping a small portion of skin with a forceps or elevating it with the tip of a needle. The tip of the small ''cone'' of skin is then sliced with a sharp surgical instrument or razor blade. The snip should be sufficiently deep to include the dermal papillae; however, it should not be so deep as to

produce bleeding. Biopsies of rectal and bladder mucosa may be indicated to identify the characteristic ova in cases of suspected intestinal or urinary schistosomiasis.

All biopsy tissue must be submitted to the laboratory without the addition of formalin fixative. If a delay in processing cannot be prevented, the specimens should be placed in PVA fixative. If the specimen is soft, a small portion should be scraped free and placed in a drop of saline for wet mount examination. Impression smears should also be prepared, performed by pressing a freshly cut surface of the tissue against the surface of a glass slide and placing the slide immediately into a fixative, such as Schaudinn's solution. Trichrome and other stains can be applied. The remaining portion of the biopsy material should then be submitted for histologic examination.

CORNEAL SCRAPINGS OR BIOPSY

Corneal scrapings are helpful in making the diagnosis in suspected cases of *Acanthamoeba* keratitis. The corneal scrapings, obtained by a physician, are placed on a slide and fixed in methyl alcohol for 3–5 minutes. Garcia[96] suggests that staining should be done using calcofluor white, a commercially available textile whitener. A solution of 0.1% calcofluor white and 0.1% Evans blue are dissolved in distilled water. A few drops of this solution are placed on the methanol-fixed smear for 5 minutes. The slide is then tipped and the fluid drained into an absorbent paper towel; a coverslip is added and examined for apple-green amebic cysts (trophozoites do not stain), which will have an apple-green or blue-white fluorescence depending on the exciter light/filter combination used.

MUSCLE BIOPSY

The characteristic spiral larval forms of *Trichinella spiralis* are best demonstrated in a tease mount made from a skeletal muscle biopsy (see Color Plate 22-11G). Garcia[96] suggests that the biopsy material be treated with a digestion fluid before examination. The digestion fluid is prepared by adding 5 g of pepsin to a mixture of 1,000 mL of distilled water and 7 mL of concentrated HCl. The tissue is placed in a wide-mouth Erlenmeyer flask and digestion fluid is added in a ratio of 1 part tissue to 20 parts fluid. The digestion mixture is held at 37°C for 12 to 24 hours. After digestion, examine a few drops of the eluate under the microscope for the presence of larvae. If none are seen, centrifuge a 15-mL aliquot of the mixture and examine the sediment.

BLOOD

A drop of anticoagulated blood can be place on a microscope slide, a coverslip put in place and the specimen microscopically examined for large, often motile, extraerythrocytic forms, such as trypanosomes and microfilaria. The presence of microfilariae in the circulating blood exhibit a marked periodicity depending on the species involved; therefore, the time of specimen collection is critical. If a filarial infection is suspected, the optimal collection times for demonstrating microfilariae are: *Loa loa*—midday (10 A.M. to 2 P.M.); *Brugia* or *Wuchereria*—at night, after 8 P.M.; *Mansonella*—any time; *Onchocerca*—any time.

When first examining a stained blood film, screen the smear under low-power magnification ($\times 250$ or less) in search for these larger parasitic forms that may be missed if only oil immersion is used. The morphology of intraerythrocytic plasmodia (malaria, Babesia, Theileria) is best observed in Wright- or Giemsa-stained peripheral blood films.

Blood smears prepared for the detection of malaria should be collected specifically for that purpose and not allowed to remain on a blood collection tray during collection rounds. Smears should be prepared on anticoagulated blood specimens as soon after collection as possible since the long exposure to the anticoagulant may distort the morphology of mature schizonts and gametocytes. Also, sexual stages continue to develop during storage of the blood sample in a warm laboratory environment. Following exposure of the blood sample to air, gametocytes may exflagellate, releasing gametes into the plasma that can be confused microscopically with *Borrelia* species. Merozoites, particularly those of *Plasmodium vivax,* may be released from mature schizonts and reinvade erythrocytes, where they may appear similar to the small "accolade" ring forms of *Plasmodium falciparum.* Therefore, the collection of capillary blood samples is preferable.

Both thin and thick blood films should be prepared. The thin blood smear, used primarily for the definitive species identification of plasmodia and other intraerythrocytic parasites, is prepared exactly as for a differential blood count. At least two smears per patient should be prepared. Thin smears consist of blood spread in a layer such that the thickness decreases progressively toward the feathered edge, where the erythrocytes do not overlap. The thin-feathered edge should be 1.5–2.0 cm long. Care must be taken in preparing the thin film to see that the feathered edge is evenly spread and free of holes, streaks or other artifacts. The preparation of thin and thick blood smears is described in Chart 22-3.

Thick smears consist of a thick layer of dehemoglobinized (lysed) erythrocytes. A thick smear of proper density is one that allows one to barely read the words of newsprint through the film. Thick blood smears contain a $30 \times$ concentration of parasitic elements compared with an equal area of a thin smear. Thus, the preparation of thick smears is particularly useful in detecting malarial parasites in light infections; however, the morphology of trophozoites is often compromised, making it difficult to make a species identification. If elements suspicious for malarial parasites are observed, a thin smear should be prepared to make a species identification.

The thick smear is prepared by placing two or three drops of blood on the surface of a glass microscope slide to cover an area the size of a dime. Blood should be obtained from a fingerstick and allowed to flow freely; "milking" of the finger should be avoided. Continue stirring the drop for about 30 seconds to prevent formation of fibrin clots. Lay the slides flat on the tabletop and allow the smears to dry thoroughly, as any residual moisture may cause the film to detach. The time to drying will be at least 30 minutes, or much longer in a humid climate. The drying time can be shortened by ventilating the smear with a fan or hair dryer

(set on "cool"). The chance for detachment is increased with smears made from anticoagulated blood. Once the film is dry, the blood should be laked by placing the slide in water or a buffer solution immediately before staining.

If anticoagulated blood is used (which currently is almost the universal practice), stirring is not necessary because fibrin strands do not form. Potassium EDTA is the anticoagulant of choice. Garcia (personal communication) has described a technique by which both a thick and thin smear can be accomplished on the same slide. Place two or three drops of anticoagulated blood at one end of a glass slide, then with an applicator stick smear the drop over the surface of the remainder of the slide using a continuous rolling motion. Both thick and thin areas will develop where the concentric circles intersect. At least three specimens should be taken on successive days if initial samples are negative for parasites.

Both thin and thick smears should be stained as soon as possible after preparation (always within 48 hours) with Giemsa or Wright's stain. Remember that the pH of both the stain and the buffer must be carefully controlled between 7.0 and 7.2; the stains used in the routine hematology laboratory are closer to pH 6.8, eliminating any possibility of observing Schuffner's dots. The use of automated staining instruments is to be avoided. Thick smears may require a slightly longer exposure to the stain than the time used for the thin smear preparations.

It is recommended that at least 300 oil fields be microscopically examined at $1,000 \times$ magnification on the thin film and approximately 100 fields on the thick film. The number of organisms may be very few in patients in relapse, in those who have an early infection, or in those who have received inadequate treatment or partial prophylaxis. In these instances, the number of fields examined should be doubled. Proper interpretation of the thick smear requires considerable experience, and positive controls for comparison should be made available.

Identification and Differentiation of Parasites

Although certain clinical signs and symptoms may suggest the possibility of a parasitic disease, the final diagnosis is made by demonstrating the causative organism in properly collected specimens. Because many artifacts resemble parasitic forms, the final identification must always rest on well-established morphologic criteria. Microscopic interpretations, in particular, cannot be left to guesswork, and a laboratory diagnosis of a parasitic disease should not be rendered until adequate identifying features can be clearly and objectively demonstrated. Select artifacts that have features suggesting true parasites are illustrated in Color Plate 22-1.

One problem faced by both the new student and the teacher of clinical parasitology is the lack of a unified approach to the taxonomy of the parasites. The traditional approach of separating the parasites into various morphologic groups (protozoa, nematodes, cestode, trematodes, etc.) is followed in this textbook with the full realization that a certain degree of clinical and laboratory correlation may be lost. For example, even though hookworms and pinworms are taxonomically included with the nematodes, there are considerable differences in their life cycles, modes of infection, and the seriousness of the diseases they cause. In fact, each species of parasite is unique unto itself, and attempts to group them by whatever criteria will meet with some degree of failure.

The microscope to be used for the examination of parasites must have an eyepiece fitted with an accurately calibrated ocular micrometer. The procedure for calibrating an ocular micrometer is presented in Chart 22-4. The ability to measure exactly the size of parasitic forms encountered in clinical specimens is often vital to the correct identification of the parasites. In the discussions that follow, emphasis is placed on the size ranges of various diagnostic parasite forms that are reviewed.

Life Cycles of Human Parasites

Many of the life cycles of human parasites are included in the sections on the laboratory identification that follow. It is not intended that students memorize every phase of every life cycle; rather, these descriptions are helpful in pinpointing the infective, invasive, and diagnostic forms of each parasite, an awareness of which is necessary to make a diagnosis.

Figure 22-2 has been designed to provide an overall orientation to the life cycles of parasites of importance to humans. Parasites can be divided into three major groups on the basis of their life cycles: 1) those having no intermediate hosts, 2) those using one intermediate host and 3) those for which two intermediate hosts are necessary.

Parasites that have no intermediate host are transmitted directly between humans (or animal to animal) through fecally contaminated food or water. This is true for most of the protozoa and for nematodes such as *Enterobius vermicularis* and *Trichuris trichiura*. Human-to-human transmission occurs through the transfer of cysts or ova that can survive external environmental conditions and contaminate food and water supplies. The eggs of *Ascaris lumbricoides*, *Trichuris trichiura*, and the hookworms require a period of maturation after the stool is passed into the environment before they become infective. The life cycle of *Ascaris lumbricoides*, although following the fecal-to-oral route without the need for a secondary host, is more entailed because after hatching in the small intestine, the ingested larvae enter the circulation through the lymphatics and pass through the lungs before being swallowed with the oral secretions. The mode of infection for the hookworms and for *Strongyloides stercoralis* is not through the fecal–oral route; rather, is through the direct penetration of bare skin by filariform larvae lying in contaminated dung or soil.

Parasites requiring one intermediate host commonly involve either a large mammal, rodent, crustacean, or insect vector within which they complete their life cycle, a process that can be either simple or complex. For example, the human intestine serves as the primary host for the adult worms of *Taenia solium* and *Taenia saginata*. The pig and cow, respectively, are secondary hosts for these tapeworms, as the adults do not inhabit the intestine; rather, the larvae reside in skeletal muscle. Humans become infected by ingesting such flesh-infested, measly meat. The hatched larvae

ultimately find their way to the intestine to mature into adult worms. The larval form of select tapeworms may also cause a disease in humans called cysticercosis. If humans ingest the ova of *Taenia solium*, for example, these first stage larvae may encyst within the liver, brain, and other organs. Echinococcosis is a second example of cystic larval disease in humans, in which canines, as the primary host, harbor the adult echinococcal tapeworm in its intestine. In the normal life cycle of echinococcosis, sheep normally serve as the secondary host, in which, following ingestion of infective eggs, the cystic lesions develop primarily in the liver, and potentially in other organs as well. The life cycle of the parasite is completed when dogs and other carnivores ingest the larval-infected offal of dead sheep.

Parasites involving crustaceans and insects usually go through a complex series of developmental stages before the infective form is released. In malaria, for example, the plasmodia undergo sexual gametogenesis within the mosquito before infective sporozoites are injected back into a human host. A similar life cycle is characteristic of other blood parasitic infections such as trypanosomiasis, leishmaniasis, and filariasis. Parasites that require two intermediate hosts (*Diphyllobothrium latum* and most trematodes) follow similar life cycles.

Eggs that are passed from the adult parasite infecting the primary host hatch in a suitable aqueous environment and release ciliated, free-swimming forms called miracidia. The miracidia are highly motile and move very rapidly (2 mm/sec). Through the action of photoreceptors, touch receptors, and chemoreceptors, miracidia are attracted to their complementary snail host. Attachment must take place within a few hours because their life span is very short. They possess anteriorly placed glands that secrete proteolytic enzymes to penetrate into the snail's integument. Penetration into the snail takes about 30 minutes, during which time the miracidium loses its ciliated epithelium. Once in the snail, each miracidium rounds up and forms the sporocyst stage, in which multiplication division takes place in cystlike spaces known as rediae. Thus, a single miracidium is multiplied into numerous free-swimming, infective cercariae.

The cercariae, in a variety of shapes depending on the species, on release from the snail seek out and invade the flesh of crustaceans or fish, through the action of enzymes produced by several para-oral penetration glands. A second host, by ingesting the metacercaria contained in raw or inadequately cooked crab or fish meat, also becomes infected. In the life cycle of *Fasciola* and *Fasciolopsis* species, the cercariae become attached to water plants as inactive, encapsulated metacercaria. Humans are infected by ingesting raw or poorly cooked water plants on which these metacercaria are attached.

Intestinal Protozoa

Four broad groups of intestinal protozoa are currently recognized, as listed below: 1) the amoebae, 2) the flagellates, 3) the ciliates, and 4) the coccidia. The task of learning the differential features of these protozoa is somewhat lessened when one realizes that only a few species are of medical importance within each of these major groups. Following

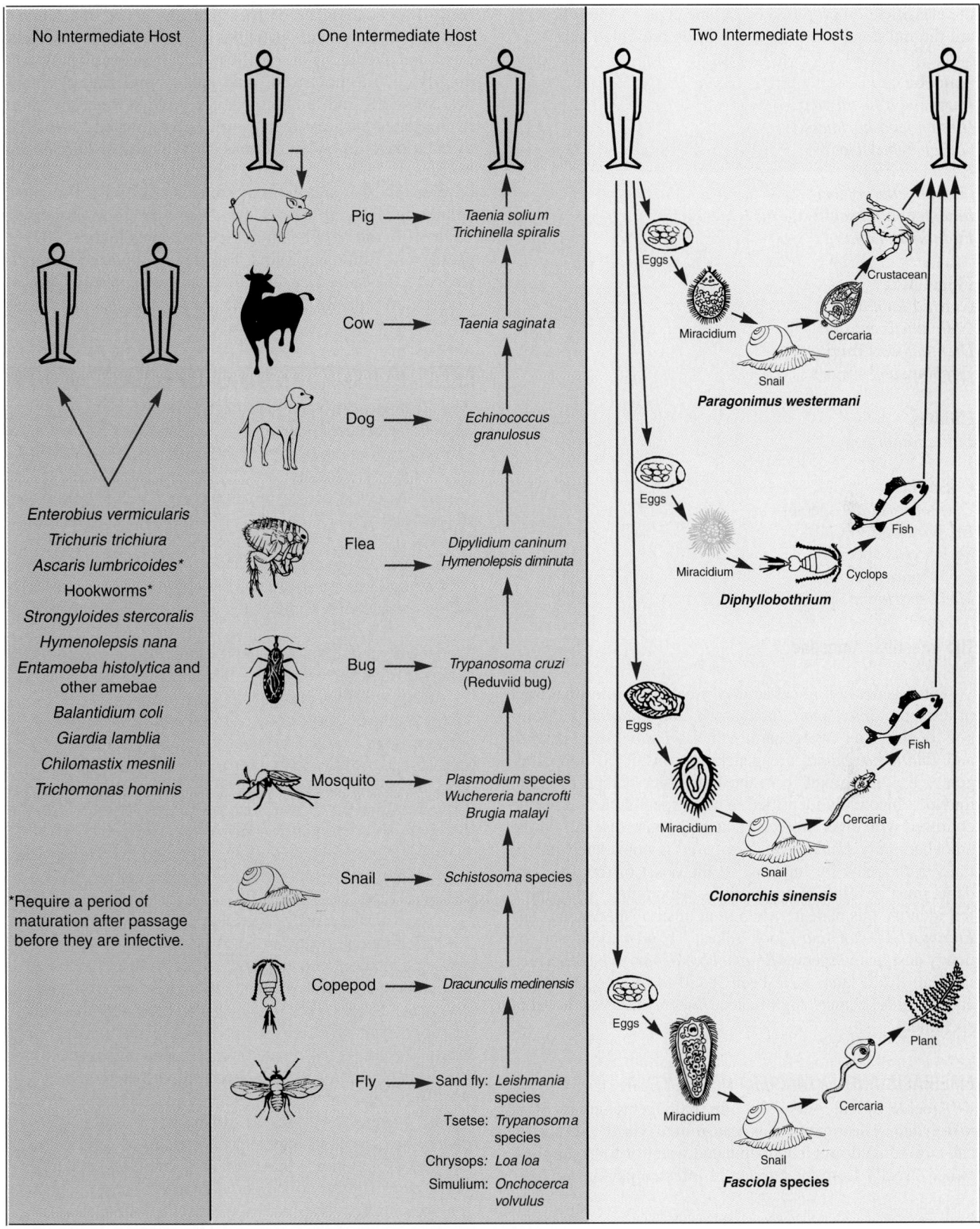

Figure 22-2 An overview of the life cycles of parasites of human importance. The parasite species are divided by their need for zero, one, or two intermediate hosts. Sketches of the common intermediate hosts are also included.

the classification proposed by Levine et al.,[163] the following are the intestinal protozoa that will be presented here:

Amoeba

Entamoeba histolytica
(*Entamoeba hartmanni*)
(*Entamoeba dispar*)
Entamoeba coli
(*Entamoeba polecki*)
Iodamoeba bütschlii
Endolimax nana

Flagellates

Giardia lamblia
Chilomastix mesnili
*Dientamoeba fragilis**
Trichomonas species

Ciliates

Balantidium coli

Coccidia

Cryptosporidium species
Isospora belli
Sarcocystis species
Cyclospora species
Microsporidium species

The Intestinal Amoebae

Three genera of amoebae may inhabit the intestinal tract of humans: *Entamoeba*, *Iodamoeba*, and *Endolimax*. Members of the latter two genera; namely, *Iodamoeba bütschlii* and *Endolimax nana*, are generally considered nonpathogenic. It is important from the laboratory perspective that they be objectively identified in stool specimens and not be confused with other protozoa that may cause disease. Of the amoebae, only *Entamoeba histolytica* is considered potentially pathogenic for humans. At the onset of training, students must develop an approach by which they can without fail identify this parasite when seen in stool specimens. The *Entamoeba histolytica* "look-alikes," *E. hartmanni*, and the newly designated species *Entamoeba dispar*, to be described in more detail later, have been found to be nonpathogenic and of little clinical significance when observed in stool specimens.

AMEBIASIS AND *ENTAMOEBA HISTOLYTICA*

Amebic dysentery is caused by pathogenic strains of *E. histolytica*. The organism is transmitted via the direct fecal–oral route through contaminated water or food supplies, either directly from the excreta of infected persons or indi-

rectly by cockroaches or flies that can act as mechanical vectors. Improvements in sanitation, socioeconomic conditions, and alterations in specific practices such as handwashing, fly control, improved water quality, and sanitary facilities are short- and long-term goals that fall woefully short in most endemic areas in the world. An estimated 5% to 50% of individuals in endemic areas carry intestinal *Entamoeba histolytica*. In these, invasive, dysenteric bowel disease will develop in 10% and extraintestinal disease in 0.5%, most commonly liver abscesses. Of those with liver abscesses, 2% to 10% die. The death rate can reach as high as 70% in people with fulminant colitis. The clinical syndromes associated with *E. histolytica* infections are presented in Clinical Correlation Box 22-1. The life cycle of *E. histolytica*, as

---

CLINICAL CORRELATION BOX 22-1 **Amebiasis**

The disease syndromes resulting from infection with *E. histolytica* have been outlined by Guerrant.[115] The majority of humans infected with *E. histolytica* (80–99%) are asymptomatic, as determined by observing for excreted cysts in fecal screening examinations or from the data of serologic surveys. A majority of those with symptoms have disease limited to the gastrointestinal tract, following an average incubation period of 1 to 4 weeks after infection. The typical large bowel lesions are called "button-hole" ulcers because the trophozoites that penetrate through the mucosa are incapable of digesting the musculature of the bowel wall, and therefore extend laterally along the submucosa. (Color Plate 22–2D illustrates several trophozoites in the submucosa.) Lower abdominal pain, low-grade fever, and bloody diarrhea with or without tenesmus are the usual presenting symptoms. Pregnancy, malnutrition, underlying metabolic diseases, and corticosteroid therapy predispose to more serious disease. Complications are relatively uncommon, developing in 1–4% of cases, and include bowel perforation and peritonitis. Cases of paracecal amebomas, at times forming an annular inflammatory mass simulating colonic carcinoma, have been reported.

Extraintestinal amebiasis occurs with varying frequency in different geographical areas. In Mexico, invasive disease develops in about one in every five infected individuals, compared with only 1 in 100–1,000 in the United States. The onset of symptoms may be within days after the acute bout of dysentery, or it may be delayed by months or even years. The liver is the most common organ of extraintestinal involvement. Adams and McLeod[3] report that in up to 50% of cases of amebic liver abscesses, a history of intestinal amebiasis is lacking and trophozoites or cysts cannot be detected in stool specimens. Symptoms include weight loss, low-grade fever, weakness, and vague right upper quadrant discomfort and elicitation of pain between the ribs on palpation. Anemia, leukocytosis, and an elevated alkaline phosphatase are other supporting findings. The diagnosis is usually made by observing the characteristic single, large defect in the right lobe with a liver scan. Direct extension into the pleura or pericardium or metastatic foci in the brain, lung, and kidney are uncommon events.

---

* *Dientamoeba fragilis*, formerly classified as an amoeba, is now thought to be a flagellate, specifically either in the genus *Histomonas* or in the genus *Trichomonas*, based on immunologic and ultrastructural studies performed over the past several years. Because the light microscope is most commonly used in clinical laboratories to examine specimens, the current shift in the classification of *Dientamoeba fragilis* is of more theoretical than practical value. The important task is to recover the organism from patients with intestinal symptoms and make an accurate identification.

a prototype for all intestinal amoeba, is shown in Figure 22-3.

Laboratory Identification. True parasitic forms must be differentiated from a variety of confusing background artifacts that may be present in microscopic mounts and smears of fecal material. Welsh[285] points out that the correct diagnosis of amebiasis rests with the accurate observations of skilled laboratory workers and laments the high frequency of both overidentification and underidentification of amoebae in stool specimens. Several studies were cited, indicating that in up to one third of laboratories in the United States and other countries, *E. histolytica* was not correctly identified; furthermore, several outbreaks of presumed amebiasis investigated by the CDC were false alarms because of laboratory misidentification errors. Pollen grains, incompletely digested vegetable elements, and host-derived somatic cells are among artifacts that can be confusing. Several commonly encountered artifacts are illustrated in Color Plate 22-1.

In particular, amebic cysts must be differentiated from active polymorphonuclear leukocytes that may have two or more lobes; however, the cytoplasm of leukocytes is coarse without evidence of a distinct karyosome, and the nuclear membrane is thick with no evidence of attached chromatin (Color Plate 2-2A). Microscopists can minimize the chances of error by making sure that parasitic structures are objectively identified before making a positive identification. If

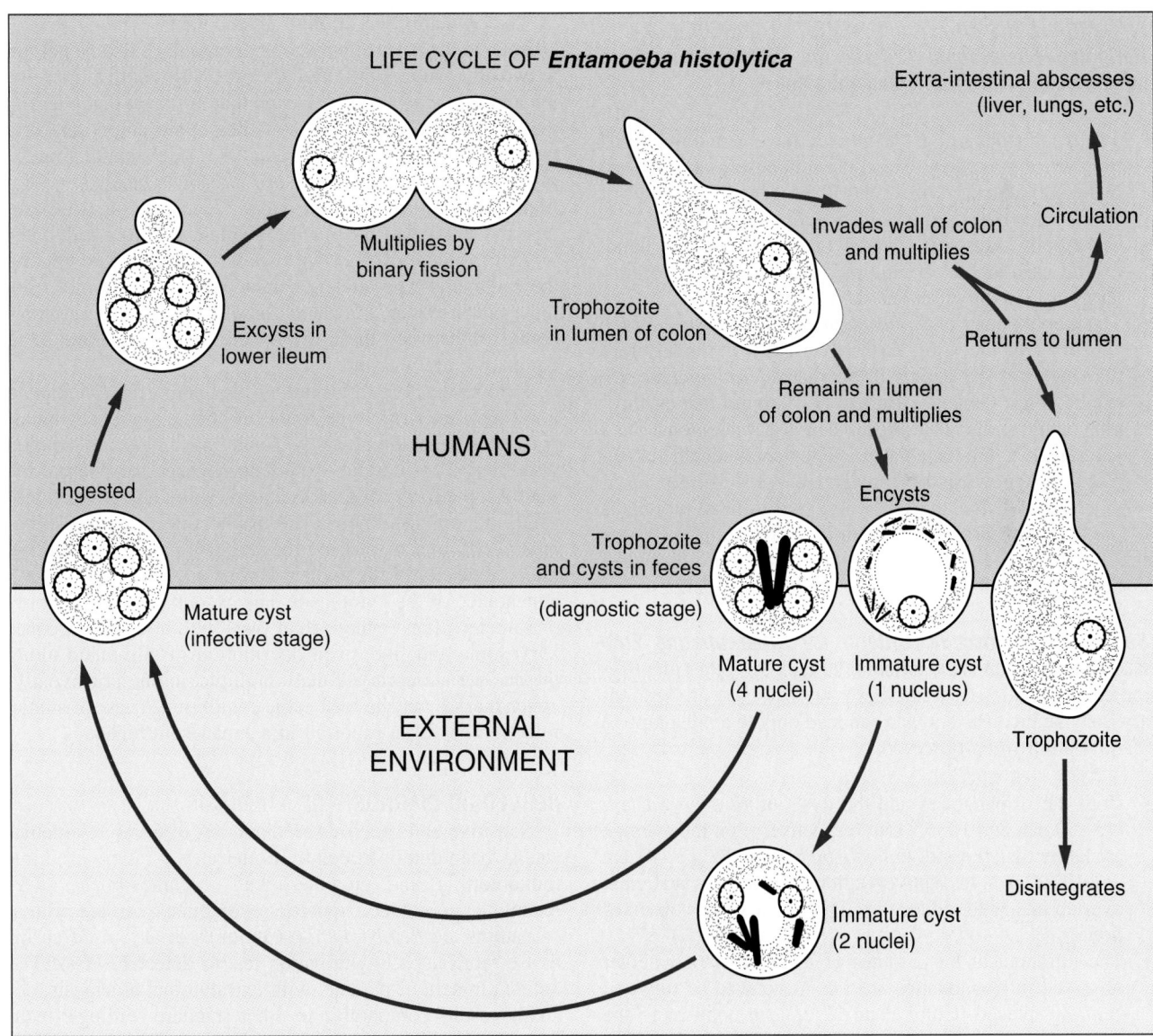

Figure 22-3 The life cycle of *Entamoeba histolytica* is simple, with no intermediate hosts required. Resistant cyst forms are found in the external environment, which, when ingested by a human in contaminated food or water, excyst in the intestine and develop into free-living, motile, feeding trophozoite forms. These trophozoites may invade the intestinal mucosa, and potentially can reach the circulation and cause extraintestinal abscesses in various organs, particularly the liver.

there is any doubt, one should back off and either look for more convincing forms in the same preparation, examine additional mounts from the same sample, or request that additional stool specimens be obtained.

Once it is determined that a form observed in a stool specimen is indeed an amoeba, either a trophozoite or a cyst, look to see if the nuclei have chromatin deposited on the outer membrane, giving the appearance of a densely stained ring (Color Plate 22-2B). This ring of chromatin is characteristic of an ''Entamoeba''-type nucleus. The nuclei of amoebae belonging to the other genera, *Iodamoeba* and *Endolimax*, are devoid of this peripheral placement of chromatin and appear more as a ''ball in socket'' (Color Plate 22-2I, J, and K).

ENTAMOEBA HISTOLYTICA VERSUS ENTAMOEBA COLI
Definitive Microscopic Criteria for Differentiating Entamoeba histolytica *From* Entamoeba coli

- The trophozoites of *E. histolytica* have a unidirectional motility; that is, they extend pseudopods along only one plane and actually will walk off the edge of the field of focus when observed in a microscopic mount.
- The trophozoites of *Entamoeba coli*, on the other hand, extend pseudopods in multiple planes and wander aimlessly in one direction and then another.
- The trophozoites of *E. histolytica* also have the unique capability of ingesting erythrocytes; it is extremely rare that ingested red cells will be seen in *Entamoeba coli* trophozoites. Gonzalez-Ruiz et al.[104] found that erythrophagocytic strains of *E. histolytica* always demonstrate a pathogenic zymodeme pattern. They conclude that erythrocyte phagocytosis is virtually 100% specific for *Entamoeba histolytica* and when observed in fecal mounts is predictive of infection with an invasive strain.
- An Entamoeba-type cyst that possesses more than four nuclei rules out *E. histolytica*. (Color Plate 22-2F)

Secondary Microscopic Criteria for Differentiating Entamoeba histolytica *From* Entamoeba coli. All other identifying characteristics between these two amoebae are secondary, may be inconsistent, and can lead only to a presumptive identification when observed.

- Both the trophozoites and the cysts of *Entamoeba coli* (15–50 μm and 10–35 μm, respectively) on the average are larger than those of *Entamoeba histolytica* (12–40 μm and 10–20 μm, respectively); however, there is sufficient overlap in size to reduce the significance of this observation.
- The intranuclear karyosomes of *E. histolytica*, whether observed in trophozoites or in cysts, tend to be tiny and centrally placed (Color Plate 22-2B), in contrast to the relatively larger and eccentrically positioned karyosomes of *Entamoeba coli* (Color Plate 22-2E).
- The ring of nuclear chromatin of *E. histolytica* is evenly dispersed and beadlike (Color Plate 22-2B), in contrast to the blotchy distribution seen in *Entamoeba coli* (Color Plate 22-2E).
- The cytoplasm of *E. histolytica* trophozoites tends to be smooth or finely granular (because powerful proteolytic enzymes completely digest phagocytized particles) (Color Plate 22-2B), in contrast to the ''junky'' cytoplasm seen in *Entamoeba coli* trophozoites (Color Plate 22-2E).
- Although chromatoid al bars are seen in only about 10–15% of cysts, when present, those of *E. histolytica* (and *E. hartmanni*) have smooth, rounded ends (Color Plate 22-2H) in contrast to the fragmented and frayed appearance of those seen in the cysts of *Entamoeba coli* (Color Plate 22-2F).

By combining two or more of these features when observing several amebic forms in a given microscopic mount, a highly presumptive if not definitive identification can usually be rendered.

The critical observation of an endameba-type nucleus of an amebic form in a microscopic mount may also be helpful in two other situations. Often the precysts of both *E. histolytica* and *Entamoeba coli* (intermediate forms at that phase in the life cycle when a trophozoite begins to encyst) can form prominent intracytoplasmic vacuoles, closely simulating the glycogen mass characteristic of *Iodamoeba bütschlii* (Color Plate 22-2I). *Entamoeba hartmanni* develops both trophozoites and cysts that are on the average smaller, within the 5–15 μm range of *Endolimax nana*. Again, differentiating the endameba-type nuclei characteristic of the former from the ''ball-in-socket'' presentation of the latter will minimize confusion between these two species. (In Color Plate 22-2, compare Frames B and K).

Entamoeba polecki is another member of the *Entamoeba* genus that may rarely be found in human stool specimens, particularly in individuals who may have close association with pigs. Considerable experience is necessary before the microscopic forms of this organism can be objectively identified in stool specimens. The trophozoite resembles *Entamoeba coli* in size, sharing the sluggish pattern of motility, the eccentricity of the nuclear karyosome, and the ''junky'' appearance of the cytoplasm. The cysts typically have only one nucleus (never more than two) with a small, eccentric karyosome and fine, even distribution of chromatin along the nuclear membrane. Small, multiple, iodine-positive glycogen masses may be seen in the cytoplasm. A case of human infection has been reported in a Japanese refugee.

SEROLOGIC DIAGNOSIS OF AMEBIASIS
Sensitive and specific serodiagnosis of invasive amebiasis has been demonstrated by Lotter et al.,[171] who used immunoblotting and enzyme-linked immunosorbent assay techniques to detect a specific recombinant surface protein of pathogenic *E. histolytica*. Cummins et al.[50] used an in-house rapid latex agglutination test to detect *E. histolytica* antigen in sera of patients with extraluminal amebiasis, deriving results comparable to other standard serologic techniques used in parallel. Haque and associates[119] recently reported that the TechLab *E. histolytica* II kit was able to detect serum antigen (Gal/GalNAc lectin) in almost all patients with amebic liver abscess who had not received treatment with metronidazole. Antigen-testing services are available through local state public health laboratories and through the CDC.

NONPATHOGENIC *ENTAMOEBA HISTOLYTICA*: *ENTAMOEBA DISPAR*

As early as 1925, Brumpt first recognized that severe dysentery or amebic liver abscess develops in only about 10% of individuals infected with *E. histolytica*, while 90% of intestinal carriers remain asymptomatic, prompting the hypothesis that amebic infections are caused by two species with the same morphology but with different pathogenicities.[22] Thus, the presence of *E. histolytica* cysts in stool specimens does not necessarily indicate active infection, indicating that only certain strains are capable of tissue invasion resulting in cytolysis.[249]

In 1978, Sargeaunt and Williams[234] used starch gel electrophoresis to demonstrate that extracts obtained from amoebae grown in axenic cultures had different isoenzyme patterns. Specifically, the reactivity of four enzymes: glucose phosphate isomerase, phosphoglucomutase, malate dehydrogenase, and hexokinase resulted in 18 so-called zymodeme patterns. This group of investigators later found that only *E. histolytica* strains demonstrating certain zymodeme patterns are associated with human infections. Furthermore, only nonpathogenic zymodeme patterns were found in the 20% of homosexual men attending sexually transmitted disease clinics who harbored intestinal *E. histolytica*.[6] The further demonstration by Weinke et al.[282] that only *E. histolytica* isolates with pathogenic zymodemes were recovered from five travelers returning from the tropics, in contrast with a group of 320 male homosexuals who had neither pathogenic zymodemes nor symptoms of amebiasis, led to the realization that methods must be developed by which these pathogenic and nonpathogenic strains could be differentiated.

During the late 1980s and early 1990s, many questions remained unanswered concerning the pathogenicity of certain strains of *E. histolytica*. The indigenous bacterial flora and the ability of *E. histolytica* to be able to modulate its virulence depending on culture conditions were thought to play a role.[185] Geurrant[115] and Ravdin[222] discuss other virulence mechanisms characteristic of *E. histolytica* to produce disease: 1) chemically defined adherence factors (galactose-specific adhesin) that determine whether the organism can attach to the bowel mucosa, 2) the secretion of cytotoxins, including hyaluronidase, trypsin, pepsin, gelatinase, and hydrolytic enzymes for casein, fibrin, and hemoglobin, and 3) the production of proteolytic enzymes. The host uses several defenses to protect against invasion by parasites.[212] Pancreatic proteases, bile salts, and bacterial glycosidases may destroy the galactose-specific adhesin on the amoeba surface and block adherence. Colonic mucins, produced in response to contact of the epithelial cells by amoebae, also can effectively block adherence by binding the carbohydrate-recognition domain of the galactose adhesin. Humans who have debilitating disease, are malnourished, or have defective immune responses are particularly prone to both intestinal and extraintestinal disease

The issue of the underlying mechanism for pathogenicity of *E. histolytica* was finally brought to conclusion by Clark and Diamond,[42] who used molecular methods based on analysis of stable DNA polymorphisms to identify the DNA patterns unique to different strains of *E. histolytica*. It was through these studies based on molecular biology, coupled with those of Orozco and colleagues,[203] who cloned, se-

quenced, and characterized various *E. histolytica* clones and strains, that the differences in pathogenic and nonpathogenic strains of *E. histolytica*, and the expression of their various differences in zymodeme patterns, were found to be based on encoded genetic differences. Clark and Diamond[42] have officially retained the name of the classic, pathogenic strain as *Entamoeba histolytica*, and given the nonpathogenic strain the designation *Entamoeba dispar*.[22]

Efficient techniques have been developed to differentiate between these two species. Antigen detection and PCR-based methods based on amplification of rRNA genes, are most commonly used. Antigen-detection tests are relatively simple to perform, provide for rapid results, and are best suited for use in most diagnostic parasitology laboratories, and for use in the field. Enzyme immunoassay (EIA) kits are commercially available for detection of fecal antigens for the diagnosis of intestinal amebiasis. These assays use monoclonal antibodies that detect the galactose-inhibitable adherence protein in the pathogenic *E. histolytica*. The primary drawback of these assays is the requirement for fresh, unpreserved stool specimens. Several EIA kits for antigen detection of the *E. histolytica/E. dispar* group are available in the U.S., but only the TechLab kit, to be discussed later, is specific for *E. histolytica*.

Yau et al.[302] developed monoclonal antibodies against a recombinant 170-kDa subunit of the Gal or GalNAc lectin of *Entamoeba histolytica* that specifically recognizes *E. histolytica* but not *Entamoeba dispar* in preserved stool samples. These antibodies were found not to cross-react with other bowel protozoa, including *Entamoeba coli*, *Giardia lamblia*, and *Dientamoeba fragilis*. Haque and colleagues[120] demonstrated that the performance of the antigen-detection kit, TechLab (Blacksburg, VA) *E. histolytica* test, designed to specifically identify *E. histolytica* and differentiate it from *E. dispar* in stool specimens, was comparable in sensitivity to a nested PCR procedure run in parallel. Although other antigen-detection kits are available at this time, only the TechLab product is specific for *E. histolytica*.

Other workers have found that PCR-based tests are more sensitive than antigen-detection procedures in the detection of *E. histolytica/dispar*. Katzwinkel-Wladarsch et al.,[149] using a simple DNA extraction method and PCR amplification, were able to detect *E. histolytica*–specific antigen directly in stool specimens containing as few as one trophozoite per milligram of feces. Acuna-Soto et al.[2] demonstrated that PCR techniques could also be used to detect *E. histolytica* antigen in formalin-fixed stool specimens. Most recently, Blessmann et al.,[19] using a real-time PCR technique, performed with the LightCycler system using fluorescence-labeled detection probes, was able to detect as little as 0.1 parasite per gram of feces. Of note, the sensitivity of this PCR procedure indicated that both microscopic examination of stool specimens, and culture, in particular, underestimate the presence of *E. histolytica* infections. Disadvantages of PCR procedures are the amount of time consumed in performing the test, its relative complexity, the cumbersomeness of performance, the requirement for special equipment, and the relatively high expense.

Thus, since a high percentage of persons in whom morphologic forms resembling *E. histolytica* are observed in stool specimens may not require treatment, follow-up antigen-detection or PCR-based procedures should be performed in the future to correctly identify the nonpathogenic *E. dispar* subgroup. The reagent kits currently available for transport of specimens to a reference laboratory require the processing of a fresh stool specimen. If therapy is not prescribed in cases in which *E. histolytica/dispar* organisms are identified in stool specimens, the patients should at least be informed that they are carrying potentially virulent organisms requiring that they practice preventive measures accordingly. Metronidazole (Flagyl) is the treatment of choice when indicated.

OTHER INTESTINAL AMOEBAE

As mentioned above, to other commonly encountered intestinal protozoa, *Iodamoeba bütschlii* and *Endolimax nana*, are not considered pathogenic. It is important from the laboratory perspective that they be objectively identified in stool specimens, and not be confused with other protozoa that may cause disease. Therefore, the identifying criteria for each are as follows.

Iodamoeba bütschlii. *Iodamoeba bütschlii* can be identified by demonstrating:

- The trophozoite, which ranges from 6–25 µm, possesses a "ball-in-socket"-type nucleus. The smaller forms are difficult to distinguish from *Endolimax nana,* and a search for the more distinctive cysts should be made. (See Color Plate 22-2*I*.)
- The cyst, which ranges from 6 to 15 µm, in addition to the "ball-in-socket" nucleus, possesses a unique, large, iodine-positive staining glycogen vacuole (the structure from which the genus name is derived). (See Color Plate 22-2*J*.)
- *Note:* Early precysts of *Entamoeba coli* and, less frequently, of *E. histolytica*, may also have a cytoplasmic inclusion that appears similar (Color Plate 22-2*G*). However, more than one nucleus may be observed, each with a ring of chromatin on the nuclear membrane, characteristic of the so-called Entamoeba-type nucleus.

Endolimax nana. *Endolimax nana* can be suspected on initial examination by:

- Its relatively small size, ranging from 5 to 8 µm.
- Observing trophozoites with sluggish motility, with a single nucleus devoid of peripheral chromatin, and a large "ball-in-socket" karyosome (Color Plate 22-2*K*.)
- Identifying the cysts, which are also small (5–14 µm), and have up to four nuclei, each with a relatively large, blotlike karyosome. (See Color Plate 22-2*L*.)
- *Entamoeba hartmanni*, although in the same size range as *E. nana*, can be distinguished primarily because both the trophozoite and the cysts possess an Entamoeba-type nucleus, in contrast to the "ball-in-socket" nucleus of *E. nana*.
- The cysts of *Entamoeba hartmanni* typically contain one or more chromatoid bars, with smooth, rounded end margins (Color Plate 22-2*H*.)

PROTOZOA OF UNCERTAIN CLASSIFICATION

Blastocystis hominis. *Blastocystis hominis*, once thought to be a yeast, has recently been classified as a protozoan, specifically an amoeba, based on the following characteristics outlined by Zierdt.[307] The organism:

- Has no cell wall.
- Grows only in the presence of bacteria and not on fungal media.
- Has a preference for alkaline pH and a mildly hypotonic environment.
- Reproduces by binary fission and not by budding.
- Extends and retracts pseudopods and ingests bacteria.
- Is optimally active at 37°C, does not grow at 25°C, and is killed at 4°C.

Yet, Stenzel and Boreham[258] point out that little is known of the basic biology of the organism, and controversy surrounds its taxonomy and pathogenicity. Three morphologic forms (vacuolar, granular, and ameboid) have been described, although additional forms (cyst, avacuolar, and multivacuolar) have also been observed. Little is known about the biochemistry of the organism, and organelles and structures of unknown function and composition are present in the cells. Several life cycles have been proposed, but none have been experimentally validated, and the form involved in transmission has not been defined.

Morphologically, the parasitic forms of *B. hominis*:

- Appear as irregularly sized spherical cells ranging from 5 to 15 µm in diameter, although smaller forms may occasionally be found (Color Plate 22-2*M*).
- Possess a homogeneous staining (green in trichrome stains) central body that occupies ≥70% of the cell.
- Have nuclear material either scattered in undefined fragments between the central body and the outer membrane. Or
- Appear as one or two elongated masses in a bipolar distribution.

MacPherson and MacQueen[173] point out the morphologic variability in size, shape, nuclear detail, and central body characteristics between cells, which may account to some extent for the differences in the incidence of detection of *B. hominis* in various reported case studies.

Based on early studies by Zierdt,[307] additional publications in the mid-1980s[90,161,269] were offered as evidence that *B. hominis* may be a cause of gastrointestinal disease. The potential pathogenic nature of *B. hominis* is supported by the cases of recurrent diarrhea reported by Vannatta[269] and Lebar.[161] In the latter study, numerous *B. hominis* (5 per high-power field) forms were seen in stool samples, and cultures for bacterial pathogens and tests for rotavirus particles were negative. The symptoms subsided when these patients received antiprotozoal therapy. Recurrent diarrhea without fever, episodes of vomiting and cramping abdominal pain have been the chief symptoms.

Blastocystis hominis may be a pathogen when no other agent is found, or when the parasite burden is high. Garcia and associates,[91] in a review of more than 6,000 stool specimens, found that 289 (4.8%) were positive for *B. hominis* (in two thirds of the cases, it was the only parasite found). Within this group, gastrointestinal symptoms were noted in 24 patients, the majority of whom had underlying debilitating disease or were immunosuppressed. The clinical picture of *B. hominis* consists of nonspecific abdominal pain, watery diarrhea, anorexia, vomiting, and weight loss. Rarely, a more invasive form of the disease with rectal bleeding can occur. Antonelli et al.[9] describe a case of a 10-year-old girl who was hospitalized for diarrhea, abdominal pain, and fever. Many *B. hominis* forms were demonstrated in her stools, and she responded favorably to treatment with metronidazole. The authors therefore cite this case as another in recognition of the fact that *B. hominis* should be considered a human pathogen.

In rebuttal, Markell and Udkow,[177] in a study of 32 persons with *B. hominis* infection, in whom at least 6 stool examinations were performed, found that 27 had other recognized pathogens—*E. histolytica, Giardia lamblia,* or *Dientamoeba fragilis*. In all of these cases, symptoms subsided with therapy. In the five remaining patients in whom only *B. hominis* was found, treatment with iodoquinol eradicated the organisms, but symptoms more consistent with irritable bowel syndrome persisted. Nagler et al.,[192] in a study of 12 patients with exacerbated inflammatory bowel disease in whom stool specimens were positive for *B. hominis*, also concluded that this organism is not a significant pathogen for this entity. All of their patients improved on medical therapy, three on treatment with corticosteroids alone and one on bowel rest without medication. Five patients failed to improve on metronidazole, but four responded to subsequent courses of corticosteroids. Keystone and Kozarsky,[152] applying antigen, isoenzyme, and DNA analyses, indicate that *Blastocystis hominis* may be more than one organism, with both virulent and avirulent strains identified. Such findings may account for the differences in apparent virulence as reported by various workers.

Until the issue of pathogenicity is settled, clinical laboratory parasitologists should still indicate the detection of *B. hominis* in stool specimens in the final report. Some form of quantitation should be made (rare, few, moderate, many); specifically, the presence of five or more *B. hominis* forms per high-power field is considered in the moderate-to-many category, and is reported by most laboratories. The clinician must evaluate whether such reports have clinical significance and decide whether to treat based on the clinical presentation.

Intestinal Flagellates

As the name implies, all flagellates possess an organelle of motility, the flagella, which serve as a means for locomotion. Other structures also serve as an integral part of the locomotor organelle, namely, the kinetoplast to which the flagella are attached and the axostyle and parabasal bodies. Therefore, when any of these structures are identified in a parasitic form, the parasite can be tentatively grouped with the flagellates. Unlike the amoebae, which assume variable shapes, the flagellates are more rigid and tend to retain distinctive shapes, a feature often helpful in their identification.

Giardia lamblia, Chilomastix mesnili, Trichomonas hominis, and *Dientamoeba fragilis* are the species of flagellates most commonly seen in human stool specimens submitted for examination.

GIARDIA LAMBLIA

By the late 1980s, *G. lamblia* had become the number one parasite-caused gastrointestinal disease in the United States,[214] and has become a major worldwide public health problem.[243] It was found in 3.8% of 414,820 stool specimens submitted to state health laboratories in the United States as part of a 1976 CDC intestinal parasitic surveillance study.[30] Over 50 waterborne outbreaks involving some 20,000 people were reported to the World Health Organization. Despite active surveillance programs in many states, the number of annually reported giardiasis cases doubled in the United States from 12,793 cases in 1992 to 27,778 cases in 1996.[89] The cases per 100,000 state population ranged from 0.9 to 42.3, with 10 states reporting >20.0 cases/100,000 population. New York State reported the highest number of total cases, 3,673 or 14.5% of all cases, and Vermont reported the highest incidence rate of 42.3/100,000 population.

The high prevalence of giardiasis is a worldwide problem, with endemic areas reported in England, Russia, several countries in Eastern Europe, and many coastal areas of the Mediterranean.[243] *Giardia lamblia* was found in 10% of children residing in the Ain-Shams and El-Mowassa orphanages in Cairo[237]; giardiasis was the most common parasitic disease (11.63%) found among Muslims coming for the annual ''Haj and Omra'' pilgrimages to Mecca.

The life cycle of *Giardia lamblia*, representative of the intestinal flagellates, is shown in Figure 22-4.

The clinical syndromes associated with *Giardia lamblia* infections are presented in Clinical Correlation Box 22-2.

Giardia lamblia is not difficult to identify in microscopic mounts of fecal specimens. The key identifying features are:

Trophozoite

- Ranges between 9 and 21 μm long by 5–15 μm wide, is bilaterally symmetrical, and has two nuclei, one on either side of a central axostyle (giving the appearance of a ''monkey face''). (Color Plate 22-2*O*.)
- Cytoplasm is finely granular. Two median parabasal bodies, simulating a ''mustache,'' are located on either side of the axostyle. Sucking disks occupy half of the ventral surface.
- Retains motility in the bowel lumen, and organisms attach to the surface of epithelial cells (Color Plate 22-2*N*).
- In wet preparations, has a graceful ''falling-leaf'' motility, a feature helpful in making an identification, distinguishing it from *C. mesnili*, which has a slower, stiff motion, and from *T. hominis*, the movement of which is quick, jerky and darting.

Cyst

- Measures from 8 to 12 μm, and is oval in outline, and may be lightly bile-stained.

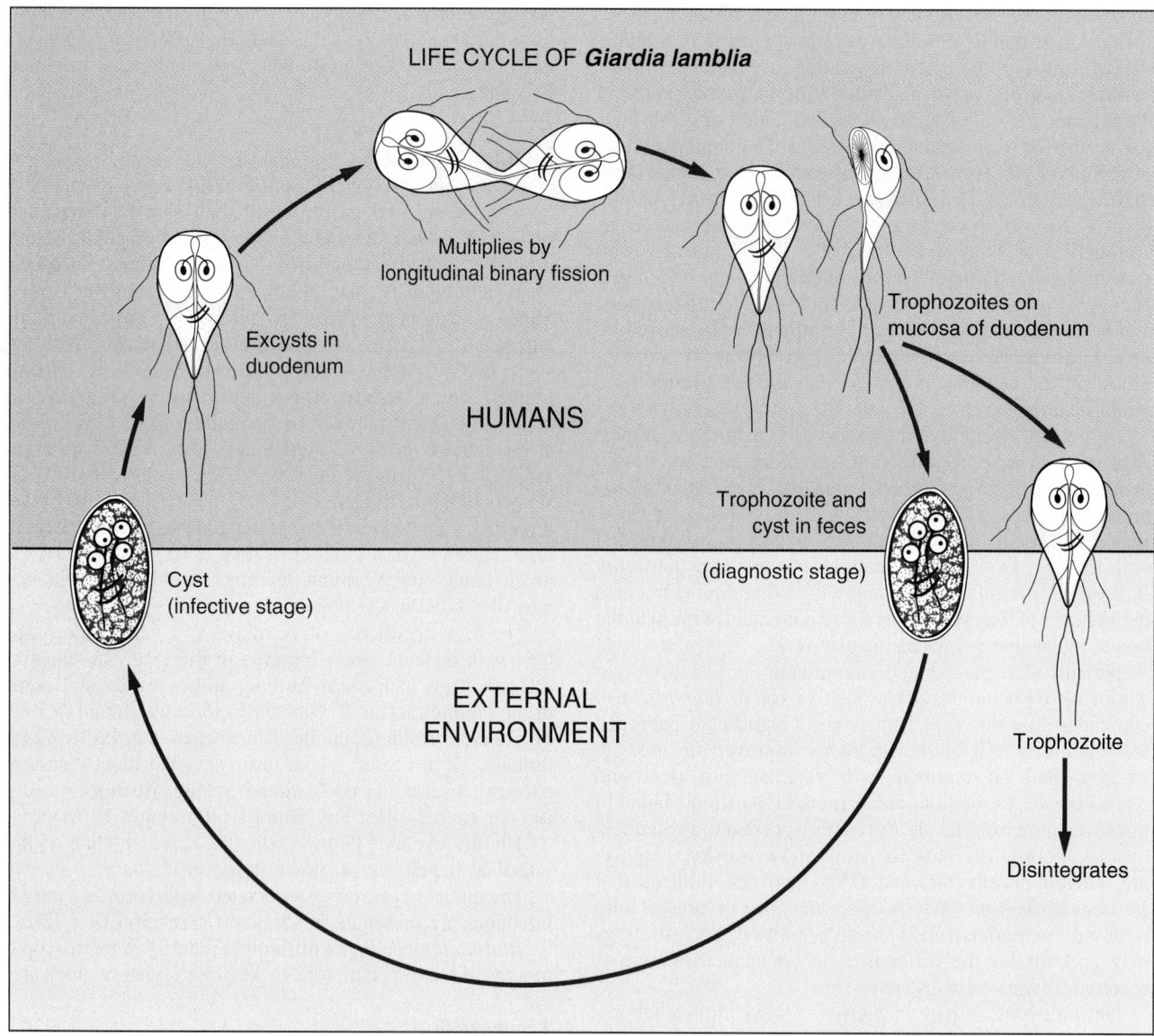

LIFE CYCLE OF *Giardia lamblia*

Multiplies by
longitudinal binary fission

Excysts in
duodenum

Trophozoites on
mucosa of duodenum

HUMANS

Cyst
(infective stage)

Trophozoite and
cyst in feces

(diagnostic stage)

EXTERNAL
ENVIRONMENT

Trophozoite

Disintegrates

Figure 22-4 The life cycle of *Giardia lamblia* is also simply completed by a fecal–oral route of transmission, with the cysts providing for a long-term survival in the external environment under adverse environmental conditions. Cysts commonly find their way into streams and wells from inadequately controlled sewer systems, and mountain streams downriver from residential areas are commonly contaminated. Humans become infected by ingesting fecally contaminated water or poorly washed fresh foods. In the human intestine, trophozoite multiplication occurs via binary fission. Trophozoites and cysts are passed in the feces to complete the life cycle.

- When mature, possesses four nuclei, with a small karyosome that is eccentrically placed.
- Has no peripheral chromatin on the nuclear membrane.
- Has a clear space beneath the thin cyst wall, producing an easy to recognize "halo" effect (Color Plate 22-2*P*).
- Has ill-defined longitudinal fibrils and four median bodies.

Because of irregular shedding of organisms in the feces, several samples obtained on nonsuccessive days may be required to establish a diagnosis in suspected cases, particularly in chronic disease. In a study reported by Heymans et

al.,[131] 53% of the patients had symptoms referable to giardiasis that existed for 6 months or more. The yield can be improved by preparing stained smears from concentrated fecal specimens, as organisms may often be missed if only saline mount procedures are performed.[95,246] Heymans and associates[131] also found that the "triple fecal test," (the examination of three stool specimens on nonconsecutive days) had a sensitivity of 95.7% in detecting organisms in known cases of giardiasis. Organisms were found in only 3 of 109 duodenal biopsies in patients whose stool examinations were negative (false-negative rate of 2.8%). Similarly, McHenry et al.[184] found only 1 positive aspirate in 144 duodenal aspirates in patients with nonspecific gastrointestinal symptoms. The conclusion can be drawn, therefore, that extraordinary procedures need not be performed to establish the diagnosis in the face of negative stool examinations.

In highly suspected cases in which a diagnosis has not been established, the string test is an alternative to duodenal aspiration or biopsy procedures.[148] The device consists of a weighted capsule containing gelatin and a tightly wound string (available as "Enterotest" from Hedeco, Mountain View, CA). The capsule is swallowed and the end of the string is taped to the side of the cheek. After approximately 5 hours the string is removed and the adherent material is stripped onto the surface of one or more glass slides. A small amount of material can be mixed with a drop or two of saline; a coverslip is applied and the specimen is examined directly for the presence of diagnostic forms. A permanent stained slide can be prepared if the wet mount results are equivocal.

Garcia et al.[93] reported 100% sensitivity and specificity in the detection of *Giardia lamblia* cysts and *Cryptosporidium* oocysts in fecal specimens, using the Merifluor (Meridian Diagnostics) direct immunofluorescence detection system. *Giardia* sp. cysts appeared as oval, apple-green fluorescing forms measuring 11–14 μm in diameter; the *Cryptosporidium* oocysts measured 4-6 μm in diameter and also displayed a bright apple green fluorescence. The authors cite the ability to screen smears under low-power magnification and the ability to detect forms in low concentration as major advantages of the direct fluorescence system. It is not uncommon to find organisms by the fluorescence procedure that are not observed by routine ova and parasite examination.

Antigen Detection. The detection of antigens on the surface of organisms in stool specimens is the current test of choice for diagnosis of giardiasis, and provides increased sensitivity over more common microscopy techniques. Fourteen commercial products (four direct fluorescence assays [DFAs], 11 EIAs, and three rapid tests) are available in the United States for the immunodiagnosis of giardiasis. Most of the EIA kits can be used on fresh or frozen stool samples, and those preserved in formalin, merthiolate-iodine-formaldehyde (MIF), and sodium acetate-acetic acid-formalin (SAF) fixatives, but not in PVA. The sensitivity and specificity of these kits approach 100% when compared with microscopy. They may be used for quantitation of cysts and oocysts, and thus may be useful for epidemiologic and control studies.

Three rapid immunochromatographic assays are available for the combined detection of either *Cryptosporidium* and *Giardia* or *Cryptosporidium parvum*, *Giardia lamblia*, and *Entamoeba. histolytica*. These offer the advantage of short test time and multiple results in one reaction device. Initial evaluations indicate sensitivity and specificity comparable to previously available tests.

By the early 1990s, the diagnosis of giardiasis had been established from the use of immunologic methods designed to directly detect *Giardia lamblia* antigen in fecal specimens.[157] Enzyme-linked immunosorbent assays (ELISAs) using antibodies prepared against a variety of *Giardia* antigens developed as the technology most often used. Knisley and colleagues,[157] using rabbit and goat antisera following immunization with *Giardia* trophozoites, reported sensitivities of 92% and 87% and specificities of 87% and 91%, respectively. Carlson and coworkers[29] reported a 97% correlation between enzyme immunoassay and direct microscopic examination on 353 specimens from human subjects in the U.S. Stibbs,[259] using a monoclonal antibody-based antigen-capture enzyme immunoassay for the detection of *Giardia lamblia* antigen in human stool specimens also found a 97% correlation with microscopic examinations, including formalin-fixed specimens (the absorbance was actually increased in 20 of 26 *G. lamblia*–positive specimens tested both for-malinized and unfixed).

Rostoff and associates[230] have evaluated a commercially available enzyme immunoassay (ProSpecT/Giardia; Alexon, Mountain View, CA) that detects Giardia-specific antigen 65 (GAS 65). All of 93 specimens obtained from symptom-atic and Giardia O- and P-positive stool specimens gave strongly positive visual and spectrophotometric results. Of 232 randomly collected specimens, 6 O- and P-negative specimens gave positive EIA results. Clinical evidence was strong that these six patients in fact had giardiasis. With these results taken into account, the EIA test performed with a sensitivity of 96% and a specificity of 100%. Scheffler and Van Etta[239] also demonstrated that antigen detection is also highly sensitive and specific when testing formalin-preserved stool samples. The ProSpecT/Giardia kit had a sensitivity of 95%, a specificity of 100%, positive predictive value of 99.5%, and a negative predictive value of 100% relative to conventional microscopy in the study of 223 for-malin-preserved stool specimens.

OTHER INTESTINAL FLAGELLATES

Chilomastix mesnili. *Chilomastix mesnili* is a flagellate of cosmopolitan distribution, more commonly found in persons living in warm climates. It is considered to be a nonpathogen, and treatment is not required when forms are found in fecal specimens. Infections are acquired through ingestion of feces-contaminated food and water; improved personal hy-giene and sanitation are paramount to reduce the incidence of infection.

Laboratory Identification Key to making an identifica-tion of forms seen in fecal specimens are the detection of:

Trophozoites

- Are pear-shaped in outline, measuring 6–24 μm in length and 4–8 μm in breadth (Color Plate 22-3*A*).
- Have a single large nucleus placed immediately beneath the outer membrane.
- Possess a prominent cytosome adjacent to the nucleus.
- Have three anterior flagella immediately adjacent to the nucleus, which are often difficult to visualize, but possi-bly seen by reducing the amount of condenser light and sharpening the focus.

Cysts

- Are pear to lemon-shaped and range from 6–10 μm long, by 4–6 μm wide (Color Plate 22-3*B*).
- Have a distinctive hyaline knob off to one side (Color Plate 22-3*C*).
- Possess a single nucleus with a small central karyosome.
- Characteristically have a curved cytostome, appearing as a "shepherd's crook," which is diagnostic when ob-served.

Dientamoeba fragilis. *Dientamoeba fragilis* is now classi-fied as a flagellate,[300] even though flagella are not observed with the light microscope. In practice, this organism may

appear as an amebic trophozoite, rather than as flagellate in microscopic mounts.

Dientamoeba fragilis produces a syndrome characterized by persistent diarrhea, abdominal pain, loss of appetite and weight loss, flatulence, and anal pruritus.[289] Microbiologists in clinical laboratories must be aware that *D. fragilis* is being recovered from stool specimens with increasing frequency. It has been reported in 1.4–19% of specimens submitted for routine examination and in up to 47% of defined populations, such as inmates in mental institutions.[300] A high prevalence has also been reported among certain groups of Indians resid-ing in Arizona. In some settings, identification of *D. fragilis* in stool specimens is as frequent as *Giardia lamblia;* in fact, in laboratories where *G. lamblia* is being identified to the exclusion of *D. fragilis*, a review of collection and diagnostic methods may be in order. Because the cytoplasm is so frag-ile, *Dientamoeba fragilis* may be difficult to identify in wet mounts, and study of a permanently stained preparation is virtually mandatory if morphologic details are to be studied.

Grendon et al.[110] warn that failure to use recommended stool fixation and permanent staining techniques virtually precludes identification of *D. fragilis*. To increase probabil-ity, they strongly recommend that all stools submitted for examination be fixed in polyvinyl alcohol, sodium ace-tate–acetic acid–formalin, or Schaudinn's fixatives, and that all specimens, regardless of consistency, should be perma-nently stained prior to microscopic examination. Chan et al.[34] successfully used an indirect fluorescence antibody assay to improve screening of preserved fecal specimens for *D. fragilis*, and further suggested that the development of ELISAs to detect *D. fragilis* antigens in fecal specimens would improve detection.

Laboratory Identification The identification of *D. frag-ilis* is made in fecal preparations by observing the trophozo-ite. A cyst stage has not been identified. The diagnostic mor-phologic features are:

- The appearance of an asymmetrical, "ameboid" form, measuring 5–12 μm in dimension.
- The presence of two nuclei (Color Plate 22-3*D*). Approxi-mately 20% of forms may possess only a single nucleus and may be difficult to differentiate from the trophozoites of *Endolimax nana*. Scanning of the smear will usually reveal the more diagnostic, double-nucleated forms.
- Prominent karyosomes that are fragmented into four to eight granules (difficult to see in most stained mounts).
- Relatively broad-lobed, clear pseudopods that provide purposeful motility when observed in wet mounts.

Because *D. fragilis* does not have an identified cyst state, direct foodborne or waterborne transfer from host to host is less likely. The nine times higher incidence of *D. fragilis* in patients with pinworm infection suggests that the *Enterobius vermicularis* eggs may be infected with the flagellate and serve as the chief vector for transfer to humans. This possi-bility may also explain why almost 50% of reported cases of dientamebiasis occur in patients under 20 years of age. The drugs of choice in the treatment of symptomatic cases include tetracycline and metronidazole.

Trichomonas hominis. *Trichomonas hominis* has been en-countered in all parts of the world. Although recovered from diarrheal stool specimens, it is not thought to be pathogenic. It may be somewhat more difficult to definitively identify in stained fecal preparations because the trophozoites are fragile and do not stain well. There is no cyst stage.

Laboratory Identification Identification is made by detecting trophozoites, which:

- Measure 7–15 μm long by 4–7 μm wide, are teardrop in shape and possess a single anterior-placed nucleus (which is slightly displaced from the outer membrane, helping to distinguish it from *Chilomastix mesnili*) (Color Plate 22-3*E*).
- Possess an undulating membrane that extends the full length of the organism (theoretically serving as a helpful feature in distinguishing *Trichomonas vaginalis*, the undulating membrane of which extends only half the distance of the body). In practice this is a moot point, as the undulating membranes are not seen in regular trichrome-stained smears; rather, they require mounts of anoxic cultures.
- In wet mounts, have a somewhat stiff, rotary motility, from the action of a single flagellum that is located along an undulating membrane that extends the full length of the body, in contrast to *Trichomonas vaginalis*, which extends along only half the body.
- Typical forms when observed in stool specimens are most likely T. *hominis;* although in females, *T. vaginalis* may be observed in some mounts as a contaminant.

Ciliates: *Balantidium coli*

Balantidium coli is the only member of the ciliates known to infect humans. The mode of transmission from humans to humans is via a simple fecal to oral route, and an intermediate host is not required for completion of the life cycle. The life cycle of *Balantidium coli* is shown in Figure 22-5.

Although *Balantidium coli* is found primarily in swine and less commonly in other animals, it has a worldwide distribution. Human balantidiosis is most prevalent where pigs are raised and slaughtered.[95] Reports of infection are uncommon, with most coming from Latin America, the Far East and New Guinea. Infestation in humans is generally noninvasive, asymptomatic, and self-limited. In debilitated patents carrying a heavy load of trophozoites, bloody dysentery, severe dehydration, or, in rare instances, death may result. In Color Plate 22-3*F* several *B. coli* trophozoites are observed invading the submucosa of the bowel. This photomicrograph was prepared from a rare fatal case of *Balantidium* infection. Intestinal ulcers, mesenteric lymphadenitis and rare extraintestinal extension to liver, lung and other organs have been reported in isolated autopsy cases.[156] Tetracycline or, alternatively, diiodohydroxyquin or metronidazole, is the drug of choice in cases of symptomatic infections.

Laboratory Identification. It is generally easy to recognize *Balantidium coli* in stool specimens because of its large size (100 μm or greater in diameter). Additional diagnostic features include:

Trophozoite

- An outer membrane covered throughout the circumference with short, delicate cilia.

- A large, kidney-shaped macronucleus (most visible in direct iodine-stained mounts) (Color Plate 22-3*G*).
- A small, spherical micronucleus adjacent to the macronucleus
- A rotary, boring motility when observed in wet mounts.

Cyst

- Spherical to ellipsoid in shape, measuring 50 μm to 65 μm.
- A single kidney-shaped macronucleus, within the hof of which is a small, spherical micronucleus (Color Plate 22-3*H*).
- Small vacuoles persist in the cytoplasm.
- Cilia are retracted within a thick, tough cyst wall.

Coccidia

The *Coccidia*, a subgroup of protozoa within the subphylum *Sporozoa*, are obligate tissue parasites with sexual and asexual stages in their life cycles. Included in this group are the malarial parasites in the blood, *Plasmodium* species, the tissue protozoan *Toxoplasma gondii* and the intestinal coccidia—*Isospora belli, Cryptosporidium* species, *Cyclospora* species, and *Sarcocystis* species.

The life cycle of most coccidia requires an external intermediate host, such as a cat, calf, or other animal, in which sporogenesis and oocyst formation take place. The life cycle of *Isospora belli* differs only in that both the sexual and asexual stages of gametogenesis can take place in the human host without the need for a second host. The life cycle of *Isospora belli*, as representative of the coccidia, is shown in Figure 22-6.

CRYPTOSPORIDIUM PARVUM

Cryptosporidia are minute coccidian protozoa that have been known to be associated with enterocolitis in a variety of domestic animals, including calves, pigs, and chickens.[8] With the spread of AIDS through the 1980s, cryptosporidiosis evolved as a new emerging infectious disease.[51,196] The detection of *Cryptosporidium* sp. or *Isospora belli* in patients in whom AIDS is not suspected should lead to testing for HIV infection. Humans become infected either from direct contact with infected animals or from ingestion of fecally contaminated food or water. Waterborne transmission is particularly troublesome for *Cryptosporidium* species because the oocysts are not eliminated by chlorination and may persist in posttreatment water supplies.[252] Two major outbreaks of gastroenteritis and diarrheal disease have been reported recently, one in Milwaukee,[172] involving over 300,000 people, the other in Carroll County, Georgia,[124] with an estimated 90,000 documented cases of acute gastroenteritis. The only collective risk factor determined in each of these outbreaks was exposure to the public water supply, which was filtered and chlorinated in compliance with Environmental Protection Agency guidelines.

The organism during all stages of development is confined to the microvilli of intestinal epithelial cells. Thus, the diagnosis can be made in hematoxylin and eosin (H &

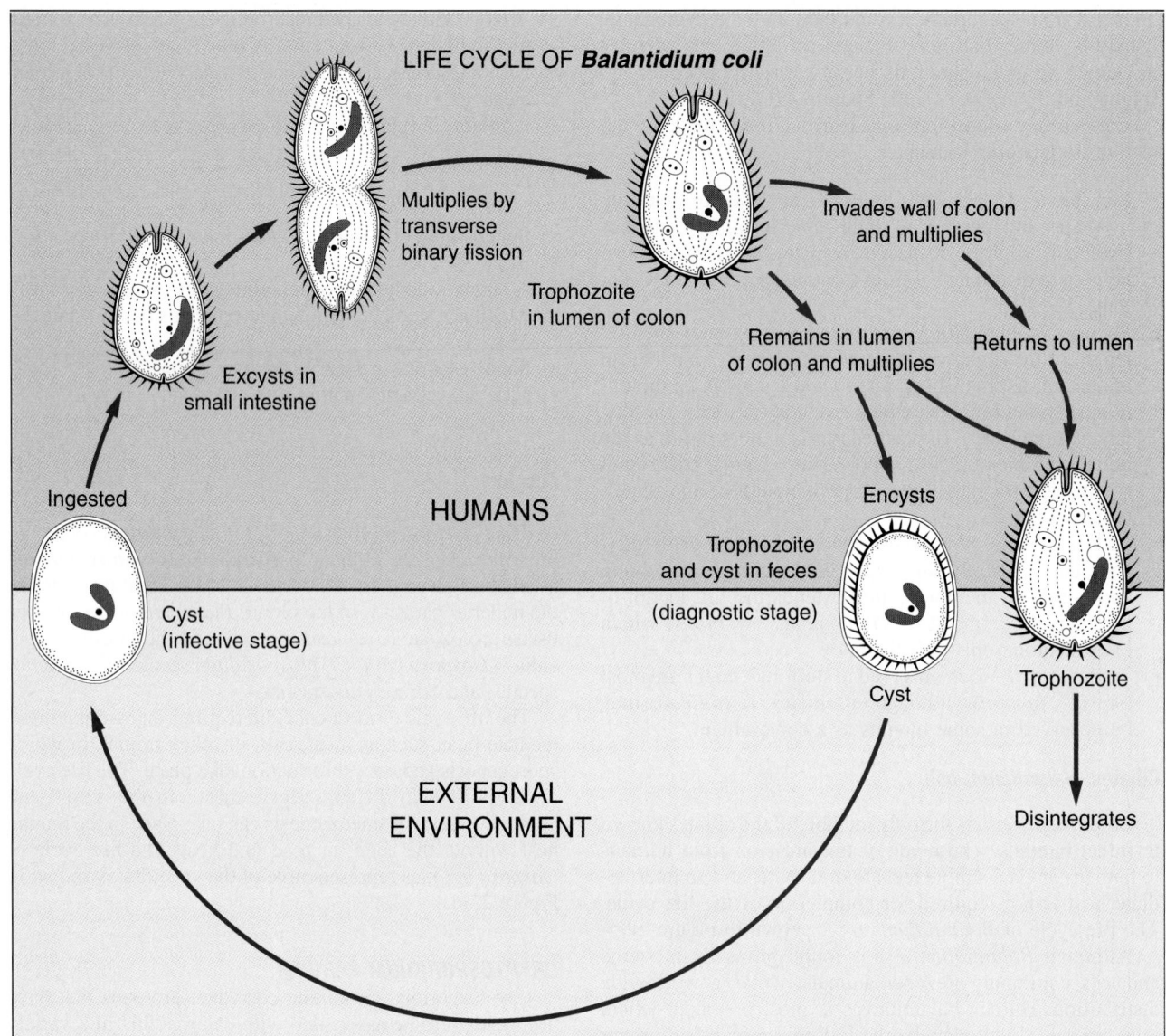

Figure 22-5 The life cycle of *Balantidium coli* is simple, requiring no intermediate host. Eggs pass in feces into the external environment, mature in soil under ideal conditions, and become infective. On ingestion of egg-contaminated food or water, excystation takes place in the small intestine, after which multiplication takes place by binary fission, and trophozoites take up residence in the lumen of the colon. On encystations, cysts are again passed in the feces to complete the life cycle.

E)–stained sections of small bowel by observing the tiny oocysts, often in huge numbers, attached to the surface of the epithelial cells lining the villi (see Color Plate 22-4*A*). Oocysts have a propensity to adhere to the brush border of the epithelial cells with loss or degeneration of the microvilli at the attachment zone.[196] The loss of microvilli may result in impaired digestion, malabsorption and diarrhea that make up the clinical syndrome. The clinical manifestations of cryptosporidiosis are presented in Clinical Correlation Box 22-3.

Laboratory Identification. The diagnosis is commonly made by identifying oocysts in fecal specimens. They have the following characteristics:

- They measure 5 to 6 μm in diameter, are ovoid to spherical, and appear highly refractile when observed in flotation preparations (Fig. 22-7).
- Small granules may be observed internally, or, with phase contrast microscopy, up to four slender, bow-shaped sporozoites may be seen in each oocyst.[51,196]
- They appear as homogeneous, red-staining spherical oocysts, 4–6 μm in diameter, when observed in acid-fast-stained stool preparations (Color Plate 22-4*B*).

Laboratory Notes. With heavy infections, the concentration techniques routinely used for the recovery of eggs and parasites in most laboratories are adequate for the recovery of

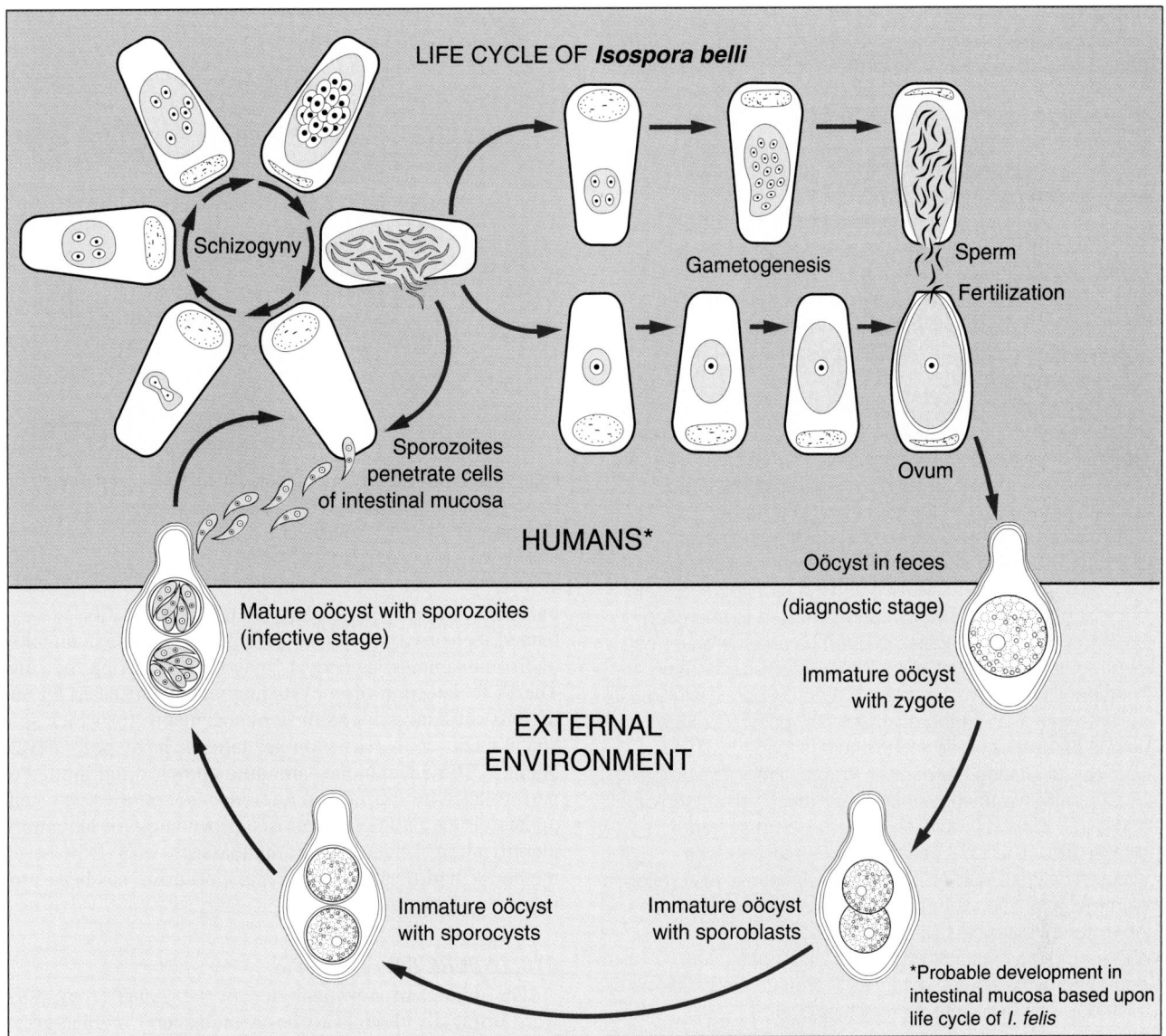

Figure 22-6 Life cycle of *Isospora belli*. Immature oocysts containing one sporocyst are released in the feces into the external environment. Under ideal environmental conditions, the oocyst matures and develops two sporozoites that serve as the infective form. On ingestion of infective oocysts in contaminated food or water by a human host, excystation takes place in the intestine. The released sporocysts invade the mucosal epithelial cells in which schizogony takes place. Mature sporozoites are released from the intestinal cells. In the process of gametogenesis male and female gametocytes are formed. After fertilization of the female gametocyte by sperm released from the sporozoite, an oocyst with a thick cell wall develops. Release of these immature oocysts into the external environment completes the life cycle.

Cryptosporidium oocysts. With light infections, Sheather's sugar flotation method is recommended and can be performed as described by Garza[98] (Box 22-4).

A modified formalin–ethyl acetate (FEA) stool concentration technique to detect cryptosporidium oocysts in stool specimens is in common use. Following the usual FEA procedure, the sediment was layered and floated over a hypertonic saline solution to separate parasites from stool debris. This technique showed the most significant improvement in the recovery of oocysts from stool specimens that were formed and not fatty.

A modified acid-fast stain can also be used to detect *Cryptosporidium* oocysts in air-dried, methanol-fixed smears prepared directly from a fecal sample.[98] The carbol fuchsin stain is applied to the smear in the same manner as the routine acid-fast stain; however, 1% H_2SO_4 is used as the decolorizer instead of acid alcohol. The oocysts appear pink-red against the light green background of the counterstain.

Several immunoassay kits are commercially available for the detection of *Cryptosporidium* oocysts in fecal specimens. In a recent comparative study, Garcia and Shimizu[94] found a sensitivity of 98–99% and a specificity of 100% in the

CLINICAL CORRELATION BOX 22-3
Cryptosporidiosis

The clinical syndrome of cryptosporidiosis includes a cholera-like, watery or mucous diarrhea, persistent gastroenteritis with varying degrees of vomiting and abdominal cramping, malabsorption, and low-grade fever. In immunocompetent patients, the syndrome is self-limited, with symptoms diminishing over 7–14 days. Cryptosporidiosis in AIDS patients, however, often is particularly troublesome because of the prolonged and progressively severe watery diarrhea that may last for months. In these patients, treatment must be aggressive, particularly if the CD4 count falls below 200 per cubic millimeter.

Oocyst-positive stools occur between 7 and 28 days of infection, with a mean incubation period of 7.2 days. In a study of 84 children with *Cryptosporidium*-related diarrhea, Stehr-Green and colleagues[256] found that shedding of oocysts ranged from 8 to more than 50 days, with no relationship between duration of shedding and severity of diarrhea. Shepherd and coworkers,[244] on the other hand, in a study of 49 patients, found that most stopped shedding oocysts by 20 days, with symptoms related to shedding in 25 of the 49. Thus, duration of diarrhea and the onset and length of time of oocyst shedding is patient-dependent.[147] Therapeutic regimens have largely been unsuccessful in patients with AIDS in the past, possibly because of the unique parasitophorous vacuole that is formed within the host cell, sheltering the parasite from antimicrobial drugs.[111]

Currently, treatment with azithromycin,[287] nitazoxanide,[72] and paromomycin[81] have shown promise in separate clinical trials. The ideal treatment in cryptosporidium-infected patients with AIDS also involves partial restoration of immune function with highly active antiretroviral therapy.[43] An excellent classical review of the clinical, epidemiologic, and parasitic aspects of cryptosporidiosis has been published by Navin and Juranek,[196] and more recently, as related to AIDS patients, by Whittner et al.[287]

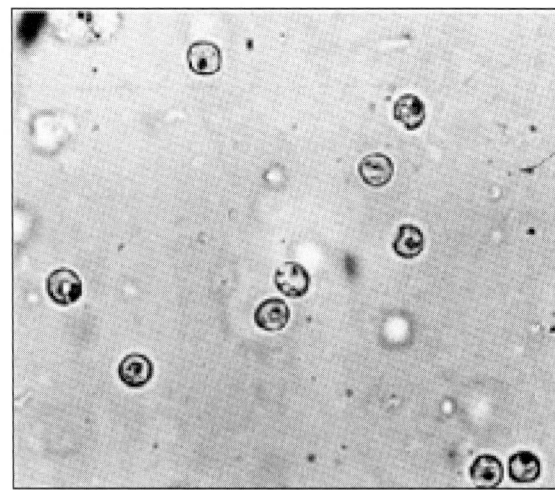

Figure 22-7 Oocysts of *Cryptosporidium parvum* as observed in a fecal flotation preparation (original magnification ×1280). (Courtesy of Bruce C. Anderson.)

buffered formalin, particularly if times of fixation are extended. Sensitivity may also be reduced in the examination of frozen samples, as oocysts may rupture during thawing. The PCR detection of oocysts may also be affected by numerous substances found in stool specimens, for which special nucleic acid extraction techniques have been developed.[306] These techniques are quite complex and limited to performance by specialized reference laboratories. A recent update on the biology, diagnosis, procedures for laboratory identification (including immunoassays and PCR-based methods), and treatment of cryptosporidiosis has been provided by Clark.[43]

CYCLOSPORA CAYETANENSIS

The organisms now included in the genus *Cyclospora* were originally thought to be cyanobacteria or blue-green algae-like organisms.[166,204] *Cyclospora* species have mor-

detection of *Cryptosporidium* oocysts using the ProSpecT (Alexon), and the Meridian Premier *Cryptosporidium* and the Meridian MERI*FLUOR Cryptosporidium/Giardia* EIA kits (Meridian Diagnostics). This affirms similar results previously reported by Kehl et al.,[150] who found that the Color Vue *Cryptosporidium* assay (Seardyn, Indianapolis, IN), and the ProSpecT *Cryptosporidium* microtiter assay and the Merifluor *Cryptosporidium* kit previously mentioned, were equally sensitive and specific for the detection of *Cryptosporidium* oospores, although in their experience, the immunofluorescence procedure was considered easiest to read and required the least hands-on technologist time.

The extreme sensitivity and specificity make several PCR-based methods for *Cryptosporidium* oocyst detection quite attractive, particularly in the analysis of drinking water. These PCR assays may detect as few as one oocyst in a sample, making them more sensitive than microscopic analysis of acid-fast smears.[88,189] However, the sensitivity of PCR-based methods is reduced in samples preserved in 10%

Box 22-4 Sheather's Flotation Technique for Recovery of *Cryptosporidium* Oocysts in Fecal Specimens

1. A heavy suspension of feces is made in physiologic saline solution and strained through gauze into a centrifuge tube to one-half full.
2. Add an equal volume of Sheather's sugar solution (500 g of sucrose, 320 mL of distilled water, and 615 g of melted phenol) to bring the surface of the liquid slightly above the top of the tube. Gently mix the suspension with an applicator stick.
3. Place an 18 mm² or 22 mm² coverslip on the surface of the suspension and let stand undisturbed for 45 minutes.
4. Gently remove the coverslip and mount it on a glass slide. Observe under phase contrast microscopy for the spherical, highly refractile 5 μm diameter oocysts (Fig. 22-7).[96]

phologic characteristics similar to *Isospora* species and *Cryptosporidium parvum*, except that they have two sporocysts per oocyst and two sporozoites per sporocyst (*Isospora belli* has two sporocysts per oocyst and four sporozoites per sporocyst; *Cryptosporidium* species have four "naked," or nonencysted, sporozoites per oocyst.) The species name, *Cyclospora cayetanensis*, honors the Universidad Peruana Cayetano Heredia in Lima, Peru, the institution where much of the original epidemiologic and taxonomic research was done.

In unstained, unconcentrated stool specimens, the oocysts of *Cyclospora* species appear as nonrefractile, spherical to oval, slightly wrinkled bodies, measuring 8–10 μm in diameter (almost twice the size of the oocysts of *Cryptosporidium* species), with an internal cluster of membrane-bound globules.[17] They are acid-fast and stain with a faint pink or pink-red color with darker staining internal structures (Color Plate 22-4C). Older cells may fail to stain. The oocysts stain orange red with safranin; they do not stain with iron hematoxylin, Grocott-Gomori methenamine silver, iodine, or periodic acid–Schiff (PAS).[166] The oocysts autofluoresce strong green (450–490 DM excitation filter), or intense blue (365 DM excitation filter) under epifluorescence. Directors and supervisors of microbiology laboratories must decide whether stool specimens are to be routinely examined for the presence of *Cryptosporidium* and *Cyclospora* organisms. In practice settings in which stool specimens are received from many AIDS patients, the preparation of routine acid-fast stains of fecal smears can be recommended.

The life cycle, although not completely worked out, is thought to be similar to that of *Cryptosporidium* species. Sporozoites excyst from oocysts in the digestive tract soon after ingestion in contaminated food or water. The sporozoites enter the epithelial cells in the small intestine. The mechanism by which diarrhea is produced is not known; endoscopy reveals moderate to marked erythema of the distal duodenum. Duodenal and jejunal biopsies reveal blunting of jejunal villi, villous atrophy, and crypt hyperplasia of varying degrees. The absence of fecal leukocytes and erythrocytes indicate that the process is not invasive; impaired D-xylose absorption implies a malabsorption type syndrome.

Illness usually follows ingestion of water and occurs primarily in the warm summer months. Powdered milk diluted with water before consumption has also been implicated.[297] In a Chicago outbreak at Cook County Hospital, diarrhea developed in house staff and employees in a dormitory following failure of the dormitory's water pump.[296] *Cyclospora*-linked disease often occurs as "traveler's diarrhea," with several literature citations of diarrhea occurring in travelers returning from Haiti, Mexico, Guatemala, Puerto Rico, Morocco, Cambodia, Pakistan, India, the Solomon Islands, and particularly Nepal.[136,218] Specifically, outbreaks in the United States and Canada during the spring months of 1996 and 1997 were related to the ingestion of raspberries imported from Guatemala.[128]

The incubation period is 2–7 days. Onset of diarrhea may be abrupt (68% of cases) or gradual (32%).[240] Watery diarrhea, which is self-limited in immunocompetent patients (rarely lasting more than 12 days), may be accompanied by mild nausea, abdominal cramping, fatigue, and malaise. In immunoincompetent patients, particularly in patients with AIDS, who are commonly infected, the diarrhea may be prolonged, lasting 4–6 weeks, may simulate tropical sprue, and may be associated with biliary disease. In 450 patients with AIDS, Pappe et al.[204] found *Cryptosporidium* species in the stool specimens of 135 (30%), *Isospora belli* in 12%, *Cyclospora* in 11%, *Giardia lamblia* in 3%, and *Entamoeba histolytica* in 1%.

Specific pharmacotherapy has proven to have limited effectiveness. Oral trimethoprim-sulfamethoxazole has been effective in the treatment of some cases; metronidazole, norfloxacin, quinacrine, nalidixic acid, and diloxanide furoate have been used with varying success in others.[204] In patients with AIDS, treatment is often limited to supportive care with hydration and nutritional supplements, although Pappe et al.[204] found trimethoprim-sulfamethoxazole effective in some cases, particularly when increased doses were prescribed. In a study conducted in Nepal, the shedding of oocysts and disappearance of symptoms occurred after 7 days of therapy.[136]

ISOSPORA BELLI

Isosporiasis, an illness characterized by diarrhea and malabsorption, was formerly only rarely encountered and was considered to be of limited clinical significance. Severe disease may be experienced in select cases, in which heavy concentrations of organisms may be seen in the intestine. Fever, headache, steatorrhea, and weight loss may occur in protracted cases; deaths due to water loss and electrolyte imbalance have been reported in overwhelming infections. The disease may persist for months, particularly in cases of AIDS, in which *Isospora belli* is being recovered with increasing frequency as one of the causes of the diarrheal syndrome. Garcia[96] reports several cases of debilitating intestinal and extraintestinal disease in patients coinfected with AIDS and *Isospora belli*, concluding with the recommendation that physicians consider this parasite in AIDS patients who have immigrated from or traveled to Latin America, or who are Hispanics born in the United States, particularly if they also are young adults. It is further recommended that AIDS patients traveling to Latin America and other developing countries be advised of the waterborne and foodborne transmission of *I. belli*, and consider the possibility of chemoprophylaxis. The drug of choice is trimethoprim-sulfamethoxazole; pyrimethamine is an alternative.

Human *I. belli* infections differ from those of other coccidians in that both the sexual and asexual forms inhabit the human intestine, and a second host is not required to complete the life cycle. Human-to-human transmission can occur after ingesting infective oocysts in fecally contaminated food and water; thus, the disease is not a zoonosis. The oocysts are the diagnostic forms observed in human fecal specimens. They measure 25–30 μm in diameter, have a thin, smooth wall, and are nonmotile. Immature oocysts contain a single sporocyst (Color Plate 22-4E); more typically the mature oocysts that contain two sporocysts are observed in fecal specimens (Color Plate 22-4F).

SARCOCYSTIS SPECIES

Sarcocystis species use two mammals for the sexual and asexual phases of their life cycles. Humans may serve as either the intermediate or the definitive host. As the definitive host, in which humans become infected by ingesting poorly cooked infected beef or pork, the sexual cycle of the organism develops in the subepithelial portion of the small bowel mucosa. Intestinal infections are associated with *S. hominis* or *S. suihominis* (formerly *Isospora hominis*) and are often asymptomatic, but may on occasion result in a diarrheal syndrome similar to that produced by *Isospora belli*. The diagnostic forms in stool specimens are broadly oval oocysts measuring between 10 and 20 μm. They contain two sporocysts, appearing similar to those of *I. belli*. Single sporocysts measuring 13–17 μm may also be seen.

Acting as intermediate host, which occurs when humans inadvertently ingest oocysts from other animal stool sources, sarcocysts develop in the skeletal musculature and may be observed in biopsies of skeletal muscle, or have been seen in skeletal muscle at autopsy.[15] The sarcocysts in skeletal muscle measure approximately 100×300 μm in dimension. (Color Plate 22-4*G*). This form is usually asymptomatic, although a history of polymyositis and eosinophilia has been reported in rare cases. Most recently, Arness et al.[10] reported on an outbreak of acute eosinophilic myositis among a 15-man U.S. military team working in rural Malaysia. Varying degrees of fever, myalgia, bronchospasm, fleeting pruritic rashes, transient lymphadenopathy, and subcutaneous nodules developed in seven soldiers; all of these are common for sarcocystosis. Laboratory abnormalities included eosinophilia, elevated erythrocyte sedimentation rates, and elevated levels of creatine kinase in muscle. *Sarcocystis* spp. were recovered from a skeletal muscle biopsy specimen obtained from the index case. Symptoms persisted in some soldiers for as long as 5 years. In such prolonged cases, chronic myositis, fasciulitis, and myonecrosis with calcification may be seen histologically.

Phylum *Microsporum: Microsporidium* Species

The microsporidia are obligate intracellular parasites that are sufficiently unique to be classified into a separate phylum, *Microspora*.[163] The unique feature of the *Microspora* is the production of spores that contain a complex tubular extrusion mechanism by which the infective material, "sporoplasm," is injected into host cells. This occurs after ingestion by the host, stimulated by changes in pH and in ionic concentration of the intestinal contents. The coiled tubule is everted and penetrates the host cell.

Approximately 80 genera and over 700 species are included in this collective catch-all group called *Microsporidium*, which primarily cause disease in a variety of nonhuman hosts of commercial import, including insects, fish, laboratory rodents, rabbits, fur-bearing animals, and primates.[23] They are true eukaryotes (perhaps arising as a very early branch of the eukaryotes), having a nucleus, a nuclear envelope, and an array of intracytoplasmic membranes. Within the phylum are several genera, only four of which cause disease in humans: *Encephalitozoon, Nosema, Pleistophora,* and *Enterocytozoon*. A fifth recently named genus, *Septata* has been found to be closely linked to *Enterocytozoon* and is no longer given separate genus status. Species differentiation is virtually impossible by light microscopy.

Laboratory Identification. The diagnosis of microsporidiosis can be made by identifying microsporidia spores in paraffin-embedded histologic sections. Although they may be seen in H & E–stained sections, they are better seen in PAS, silver (GMS), acid-fast, or Giemsa-stained sections. The spores appear within intestinal enterocytes, characteristically located between the cell nucleus and the lumen of the intestine. In PAS-stained preparations, a PAS-positive granule may be observed at the anterior end of each spore. These appear as dark-staining dots when stained with Giemsa. Several photomicrographs demonstrating these spores can be found in Garcia.[96]

Electron microscopy continues to serve as the gold standard. The identification of spores with a polar tube is characteristic of all genera. Members of the genus *Encephalitozoon* are enclosed in a host-produced, phagosome-like, limiting vesicle. Both *Enterocytozoon* species and *Nosema* species develop in direct contact with host-cell cytoplasm without a limiting vesicle; *Nosema* species are distinguished by having paired, abutted nuclei.[23]

The laboratory diagnosis is most commonly made in the clinical parasitology section by demonstrating spores in stained preparations of fecal specimens. They have the following characteristics:

- The spores are tiny, ranging from 1.5–2.5 × 2.5–4.0 μm.
- They are oval to cylindrical in shape and possess thick walls that render them environmentally resistant and difficult to stain.
- A transverse pink-staining band midway in the cells is a key identifying feature (Color Plate 22-4*H*).
- The spores stain poorly with H & E, but can be better visualized with Gram, acid-fast, PAS, Giemsa and a modified trichrome stain.
- They are gram-positive and acid-fast; in PAS stains an anterior PAS-positive granule is observed.
- The stain devised by Weber et al.[279] can be highly recommended for the detection of microsporidia spores in duodenal aspirates and in fecal material (Box 22-5).

DeGirolami et al.[60] found that both Weber's modified trichrome stain and the fluorochrome Uvitex 2B stains were equally and highly sensitive compared with duodenal biopsies in detecting microsporidia spores in smears of duodenal aspirates biopsy material from 43 patients. Ryan et al.[232] describe a modified stain in which the phosphotungstic acid is decreased in concentration to 0.25 g/dL and aniline blue instead of fast green was used as the counterstain. Each staining procedure requires 90 minutes, and selection between the Weber and the Ryan stain is one of personal preference. Kokoskin et al.[158] found that performing the stain at a temperature of 50°C and decreasing the time of staining to 10 minutes produced a deeper, easier-to-interpret stain. Because the microsporidia spores are very small and may resemble bacteria or very small yeast cells, staining of positive control material is always necessary when performing either of these stains.

Although all species of microsporidia may cause disseminated infections, and organisms may be found in several organs, including liver, kidney and brain, *Enterocytozoon*

Box 22-5 Weber Stain for the Detection of Microsporidia Spores in Stool and Duodenal Aspirates[280]

1. Prepare slides for light-microscopical examination of stool taking a 10-μL aliquot of unconcentrated liquid stool concentrate in 10% formalin (12:3 ratio), spread thinly over an area 45 × 25 mm
2. Fix smears in methanol for 5 minutes.
3. Stain for 90 minutes in the Weber chromotrope-based stain.
   To prepare the stain, mix:

Chromotrope 2R (Harleco, Gibbstown, NJ)	6.00 g
Fast green (Allied Chemical & Dye, New York)	0.15 g
Phosphotungstic acid	0.70 g

   Allow these ingredients to stand ("ripen") for 30 minutes in 3 mL of glacial acetic acid. Then mix with 100 mL of distilled water.
4. After staining, rinse slides in acid alcohol (4.5 mL of acetic acid and 995.5 mL of 90% ethyl alcohol) for 10 seconds and then rinse briefly in 95% alcohol.
5. Successively dehydrate smears in
   95% alcohol for 5 minutes
   100% alcohol for 10 minutes
   Hemo-De (xylene substitute, Fisher Scientific) for 10 minutes
6. Examine 100 oil-immersion fields per slide, a reading time of approximately 10 minutes. Look for the small 1–4 μm, cylindrical spores that stain bright pink-red.

---

bieneusi is the species that tends to preferentially infect enterocytes in the small bowel mucosa, particularly in patients with AIDS.[85] However, several case reports, as reviewed by Pol et al.,[216] indicate that *E. bieneusi* may colonize the bile-duct epithelium leading to cholangitis. The estimated prevalence of microsporidium intestinal infection in AIDS patients may be as high as 12%,[158] or even higher if special techniques including cytocentrifugation, fluorescent antibody detection, and serology are used. *Encephalitozoon cuniculi* is most commonly associated with disseminated infection, with a predilection for infecting the brain and kidneys. *Nosema corneum* has been found in several cases of keratoconjunctivitis[32]; however, *Encephalitozoon cuniculi* and *Encephalitozoon hellem* have also been recovered from the cornea and conjunctiva in AIDS patients with keratoconjunctivitis.[67] Conjunctivitis, scleritis, sensation of foreign body, and blurred vision are common presenting symptoms.

Those with experience may be able to identify the characteristic, tiny (2 μm in diameter) intracytoplasmic spores in stained tissue sections of intestinal biopsies. Spores are best demonstrated using Brown-Brenn or Brown-Hopps tissue Gram stains or Giemsa-stained touch preparations. Organisms may also be seen in semithin plastic sections stained with methylene blue-azure II with basic fuchsin or toluidine blue counterstains.[23] Positive control slides should always be prepared in parallel when using any of these stains. Spores have also been demonstrated in cerebrospinal fluid (CSF) and urine by the use of immunofluorescence light micros-

copy. As laboratory workers begin to use the various techniques described above and become more familiar with the morphology of *Microsporidium* species by light microscopy, the prevalence of infections will undoubtedly increase and the chances for underdiagnosis will be reduced.

Aldras et al.[5] demonstrated the superiority of detecting microsporidia spores in the stools of AIDS patients in indirect immunofluorescence antibody stains, using polyclonal antisera to *E. cuniculi* and *E. hellem* and monoclonal antibodies raised against *E. hellem*.

Several techniques for the nonmicroscopic detection of microsporidium spores are in the research laboratories, waiting for a time when the laboratory diagnosis may be simplified. Zierdt et al.[308] used a variety of polyclonal mouse and rabbit antisera raised against *E. cuniculi* and *Encephalitozoon hellem* spores in an indirect fluorescent-antibody assay to successfully identify microsporidial spores in 11 of 12 fecal samples, in addition to detection of antigen in colon and duodenal fluids and in duodenal biopsy touch preparations. Franzen et al.[85] successfully used microsporidian DNA amplification by PCR on six known positive duodenal biopsy specimens to detect a 353-bp DNA fragment specific for *Enterocytozoon bieneusi*. They suggest that PCR may be a useful approach to diagnosing microsporidiosis in HIV-infected patients. In fact, molecular diagnosis with species-specific PCR primers is commonly believed by the CDC to be the gold standard for identification of microsporidian species.[54] The PCR methods used in the CDC laboratory have been found to not cross-amplify some 20 other nonpathogenic *Microsporidian* species tested.

Effective therapy for microsporidiosis is limited. Treatment of intestinal infections due to *Enterocytozoon bieneusi* with pyrimethamine, metronidazole, or trimethoprim-sulfamethoxazole (SXT) may be effective. De Groote et al.[61] report successful treatment of an AIDS patient with albendazole, a case in which PCR was used to provide an early diagnosis. For a comprehensive review of human microsporidial infections, including over 250 references, see Weber et al.,[280] who introduce several new diagnostic techniques that will "facilitate future studies on the incidence, risk factors, origins of infection, modes of transmission, clinical manifestations, pathogenesis and treatment of this emerging pathogen."

Nematodes

The nematodes are helminth roundworms, the adults of which are characterized by a tapered, cylindrical body with longitudinally oriented muscles and a triradiate esophagus. The species of intestinal nematodes (roundworms) that most commonly infect humans include:

Ascaris lumbricoides
Trichuris trichiura
Hookworms:
   Necator americanus
   Ancylostoma duodenale
Strongyloides stercoralis
Enterobius vermicularis
Capillaria philippinensis
Trichostrongylus species

An estimated 3.2 billion people worldwide were infected with intestinal nematodes.[25,35] The magnitude of these figures reflects considerable human morbidity and mortality from the effects of this parasite, and also reflects the high probability that clinical laboratories will detect one or more of these parasitic forms in routine stool specimen examinations.

The life cycles of this group of helminths vary in complexity and modes of infection. These nematodes do not have an intermediate host in their life cycle, as shown in Figure 22-8; however, most require a stage outside the human host for the ova to develop into an infective form. The egg or ovum is a mature gamete produced by adult females residing in the intestine and passed with the feces. This form is the resting stage, serving as the diagnostic/and or infective form. The ova of most nematode species require intermediate stages of development in the external environment into a larval and often infective form, depending on the temperature, moisture, and nature of the soil into which they are passed. Life cycle drawings with legends are included for several of the nematode species to be presented in this chapter.

Ascariasis and *Ascaris lumbricoides*

It is estimated that *Ascaris lumbricoides* alone affects approximately 25%, or 1 billion, of the world's population.[25] The highest prevalence is in malnourished people residing in developing countries. Areas with modern water and waste treatment have a low incidence of disease. A life cycle drawing of *Ascaris lumbricoides*, representative of the nematodes as a group, is found in Figure 22-8.

The clinical manifestations of ascariasis are presented in Clinical Correlation Box 22-4.

Laboratory Identification. The laboratory diagnosis of ascariasis is made either by observing the adult worms as they protrude from body orifices, in situ in the intestine, or in contiguous duct systems such as the biliary or pancreatic ducts (as may be seen at surgery or at autopsy). Most commonly, the identification is made by detecting the characteristic ova in stool specimens. The key identifying characteristics of *Ascaris lumbricoides* are:

Adult Worms

- The adult worms measure between 15 and 35 cm in length.
- Male worms are smaller, and can be identified by their curved tail (Color Plate 22-5*A*).
- The cuticle is smooth and lacks the annular muscular striations characteristic of earth worms.

Ova

- Fertilized eggs measure between 45 and 60 μm; unfertilized eggs average 90 × 40 μm.
- They are yellow-brown (bile-stained), oval or spherical, and characteristically have a thick, transparent, hyaline shell, covered by an albuminous coat (Color Plate 22-5*B*).
- Eggs that have had prolonged exposure to pancreatic se-

cretions may be devoid of the albuminous coat (decorticoid).
- Fertilized eggs can be recognized by the cleavage of the internal yolk; internal organization is lacking in unfertilized ova. Embryonated eggs in later stages of development may contain a larval form (Color Plate 22-5*C*).
- Unfertilized, decorticate ova may resemble vegetable cells and can be extremely difficult to recognize in stool specimens (Color Plate 22-5*D*). In most instances, examination of additional fields will usually reveal the characteristic thick, outer mammillated albuminoid eggs.

Unfertilized *Ascaris lumbricoides* ova are too heavy to float in the zinc sulfate flotation procedure and may be missed if the sediment is not also examined. The presence of only unfertilized ova in stool specimens may indicate infection with a single female worm. One adult female *Ascaris lumbricoides* can produce about 200,000 ova per day; therefore, the enumeration of ova in fecal specimens using egg counts, a valuable procedure in evaluating the magnitude of hookworm infections, does not necessarily reflect the worm load.

Trichuriasis and *Trichuris trichiura* (Whipworm)

The overall incidence of *Trichuris trichiura* infections is not known, although a 90% prevalence has been cited in certain populations in Cameroon, Malaysia, and Caribbean countries. Vermud et al.,[272] found that *T. trichiura* was the most common nematode recovered from 41,958 stool specimens submitted to the Columbia-Presbyterian Medical Center in New York during 1971–1984.

The life cycle of *Trichuris trichiura* follows a simple fecal–oral route of transmission without an intermediate phase in an external host. The life cycle is illustrated in Figure 22-9.

The clinical manifestations of trichuriasis are presented in Clinical Correlation Box 22-5.

Laboratory Identification. The laboratory diagnosis of trichuriasis is most commonly made by observing characteristic barrel-shaped ova in fecal specimens. The adults measure 30–50 mm in length, with the males on the average being slightly smaller. The males can be recognized by their long, thin caudal extremity forming a 360-degree coil, from which the colloquial term "whipworm" is derived. In intestinal infections, the head is buried in the mucosa of the large bowel; therefore, adults are rarely seen in stool specimens. A magnified photograph of an adult worm is shown in Color Plate 22-5*E*.

Ova

- The eggs measure in the range of 54 × 22 μm.
- They are among the more easy parasitic forms to recognize in microscopic preparations by their distinct barrel shape and the refractile, convex, hyaline polar plugs at either end (Color Plate 22-5*F*).
- These eggs may be confused only with the eggs of *Capillaria philippinensis;* however, their polar plugs are less prominent, are flat, and the shell is thicker and striated (Color Plate 22-5*P*).

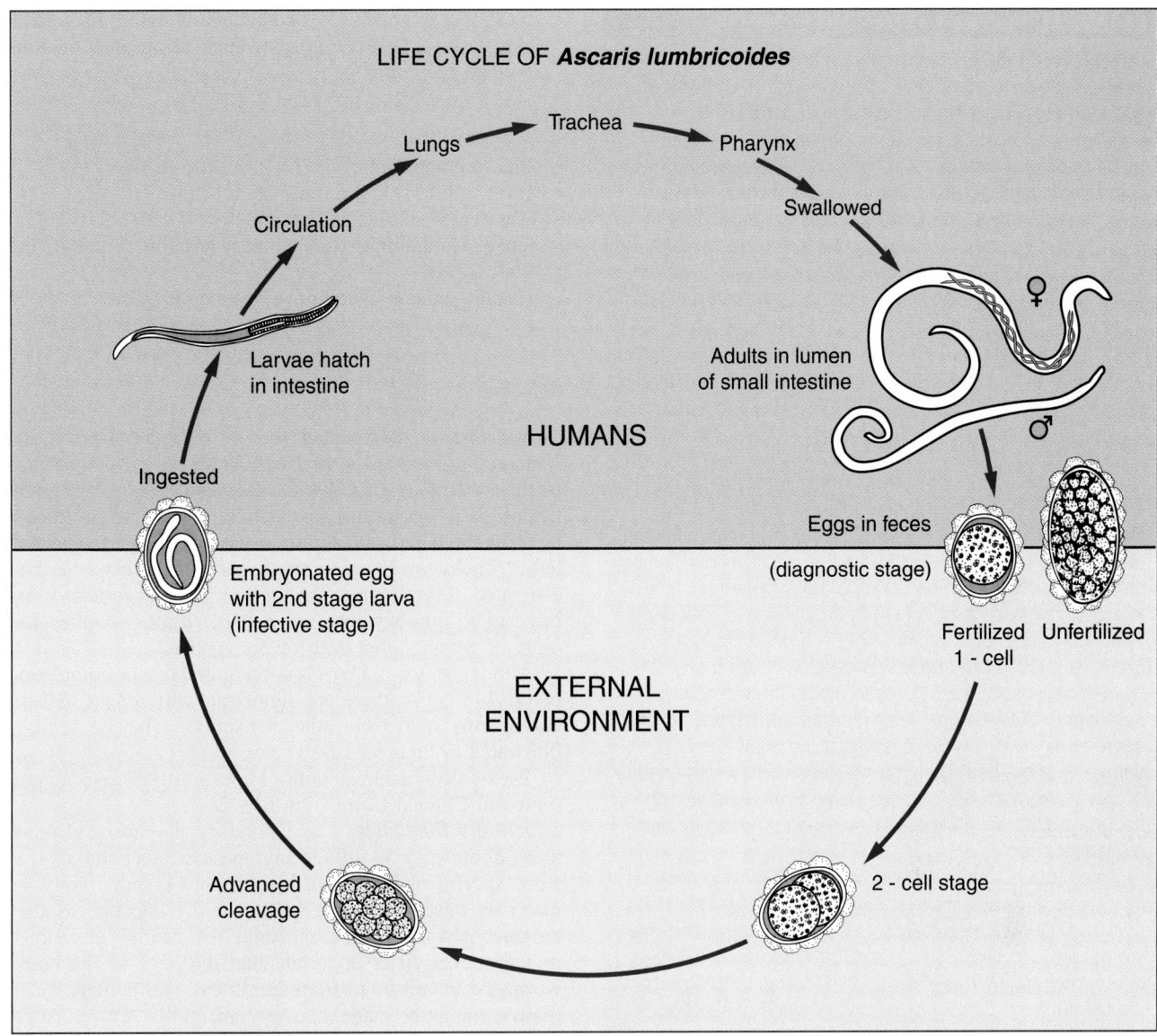

Figure 22-8 Life cycle of *Ascaris lumbricoides*. The life cycle does not involve an external intermediate host. It is somewhat complex, requiring a period for egg maturation in the external environment and a transpulmonary larval migratory phase in humans that may result in transient asthmalike symptoms in heavy infections. Fertilized eggs passed into the soil require 2 to 3 weeks under ideal conditions of moisture and temperature to develop from the initial two-cell stage to the advanced cleavage and the final infective embryonated stage. On ingestion of food or water contaminated with infective eggs by a human host, the larval forms hatch in the intestine and enter the circulation. After passage through the lung capillaries, the larvae break out into the pulmonary alveoli, then are coughed up and swallowed. In the intestine they mature into male or female adult worms, where they may remain confined to the lumen or migrate to various ducts or orifices. Gravid females lay a large number of eggs that are passed with the feces to complete the life cycle.

Enterobius vermicularis

"Pinworm" infections have been known since ancient times, and possibly represent the most common of all nematode infections. A well-known phrase is, "you may have had an infection as a child; or, if not, may likely get it when you have children." The life cycle of *Enterobius vermicu-* *laris* is quite simple, requiring no external host, with the fecal–oral route being the main means of direct finger-to-mouth human-to-human transmission, similar to that of the intestinal amebae. In most cases, eggs have matured at the time they are detected in stool specimens, or on mounts prepared from the perianal skin. Well-developed, highly infective larva are often observed in these specimens.

CLINICAL CORRELATION BOX 22-4 Ascariasis

Patients with light infections may be asymptomatic. In heavy intestinal infections, abdominal pain, discomfort, and diarrhea are common findings. In contrast to hookworms, for which a heavy worm load is prerequisite to the presence of disease, a human intestinal infestation with only one *A. lumbricoides* worm, because of its large size, may be important. Ascarid adults have the propensity to migrate and wander into the bile ducts, pancreatic duct, or lumen of the appendix, or may rarely penetrate the bowel. Maddern et al.[174] report a fatal case of pancreatitis in which a single *Ascaris lumbricoides* worm was found impacted within the ampulla of Vater. Appendicitis, pancreatitis, biliary obstruction, and hepatic abscess formation are all potential complications, even in light infections.[118]

This propensity for ascarids to wander from the lumen of the intestine, particularly during drug therapy, is one reason why inadequate or incomplete courses of treatment can be particularly dangerous. In heavy infections, adult worms may protrude from the rectum or be coughed up. Intestinal obstruction, intussusception, volvulus, or bowel perforation are other potential complications of heavy infection. Intestinal obstruction occurs in approximately 2 of every 1000 individuals infected; resulting in a fatality rate of 6 per 100,000 in children.[264] Baird et al.[13] report a fatal case of ascariasis in a 2-year-old black South African girl from whom 796 *Ascaris lumbricoides* worms, weighing an aggregate of 550 g were removed at autopsy. Torsion and gangrene of the heavily worm-infested ileum was the cause of death. Worms were also recovered from the stomach, esophagus, intrahepatic and extrahepatic bile ducts, and the gallbladder.

Treatment is with mebendazole (Vermox), which comes in 100-mg chewable tablets. Side effects include abdominal pain and diarrhea, particularly if infection is heavy and many worms are expelled. Use of the drug is contraindicated during pregnancy. There also is little indication that drugs are helpful during the larval migratory stage of infection.[96]

Laboratory Identification. The diagnosis of pinworm infection may be made by observing adult worms either visually on the anal opening, or microscopically in transparency (tape) mounts. These mounts are prepared by pressing the sticky side of a short segment of tape on the para-anal folds or perineal skin, then sticking the tape to the surface of a glass slide for microscopic study. The characteristic ova are uncommonly seen in stool specimens; however, they are usually observed in these same transparency tape preparations (Color Plate 22-4*F*). Yield of these diagnostic forms is best in children when the test is performed early in the morning when worm migration is maximal, immediately on waking and prior to a bowel movement. The clinical manifestations of enterobiasis are illustrated in Clinical Correlation Box 22-6. The identifying characteristics are:

Adult Worms

- The adult female worm measures approximately 8–13 mm long × 0.4 mm in diameter.

- It can be recognized by the cuticular, winglike alar expansion at the anterior end (Color Plate 22-5*G*) and the long pointed tail (''pin'').

Ova

- Measure approximately 30 × 50 μm in size.
- Have a thin, smooth, transparent shell.
- Are oval in outline and asymmetrical, with one side flattened, simulating a football that has lost its air (Color Plate 22-5*F*).
- Usually contain a well-developed larva. (Color Plate 22-5*F*, right)

Hookworms

Ancylostoma duodenale is the Old World hookworm, and *Necator americanus* is the New World species, as defined by the areas of endemic disease. Because the life cycle histories of these two species are essentially the same and cannot be differentiated by the appearance of their eggs, the general term ''hookworm'' is commonly used for both species. An estimated 700 million to 900 million people worldwide are infected with hookworm (mostly *Ancylostoma duodenale*), 0.2% of whom suffer from severe anemia.

Although a second host is not required for the completion of the life cycle, there are significant differences that set hookworms apart from other nematodes. The life cycle is illustrated in Figure 22-10.

The clinical manifestations of hookworm disease are presented in Clinical Correlation Box 22-7.

Laboratory Diagnosis. The laboratory diagnosis is made most commonly by observing the characteristic ova in stool specimens, although the diagnosis may rarely be made by observing adult worms in the intestine as they are anchored to the mucosal lining and are not discharged into the feces. It is important that the eggs of the hookworms be identified in stool specimens, and perhaps quantitative counts be made, because potentially severe disease may be associated with this nematode in heavy infections. The ova of both *A. duodenale* and *N. americanus* are identical, and also cannot be distinguished from those of *Strongyloides stercoralis*.

Adult Worms

- Measure up to 1.5 cm in length, and reside in the upper intestine, where they are firmly attached to the mucosa by the biting action of cutting mouth parts.
- Observation of the mouth parts can be used to distinguish between the two species.
  - *Ancylostoma duodenale* has two pairs of chitinous teeth (Color Plate 22-5*I*).
  - *Necator americanus* is fitted with a pair of cutting plates (Color Plate 22-5*J*).
- The male worms are distinguished by their frayed, posterior bursa.

Ova

- Measure approximately 60 × 40 μm, and are distinctly oval.

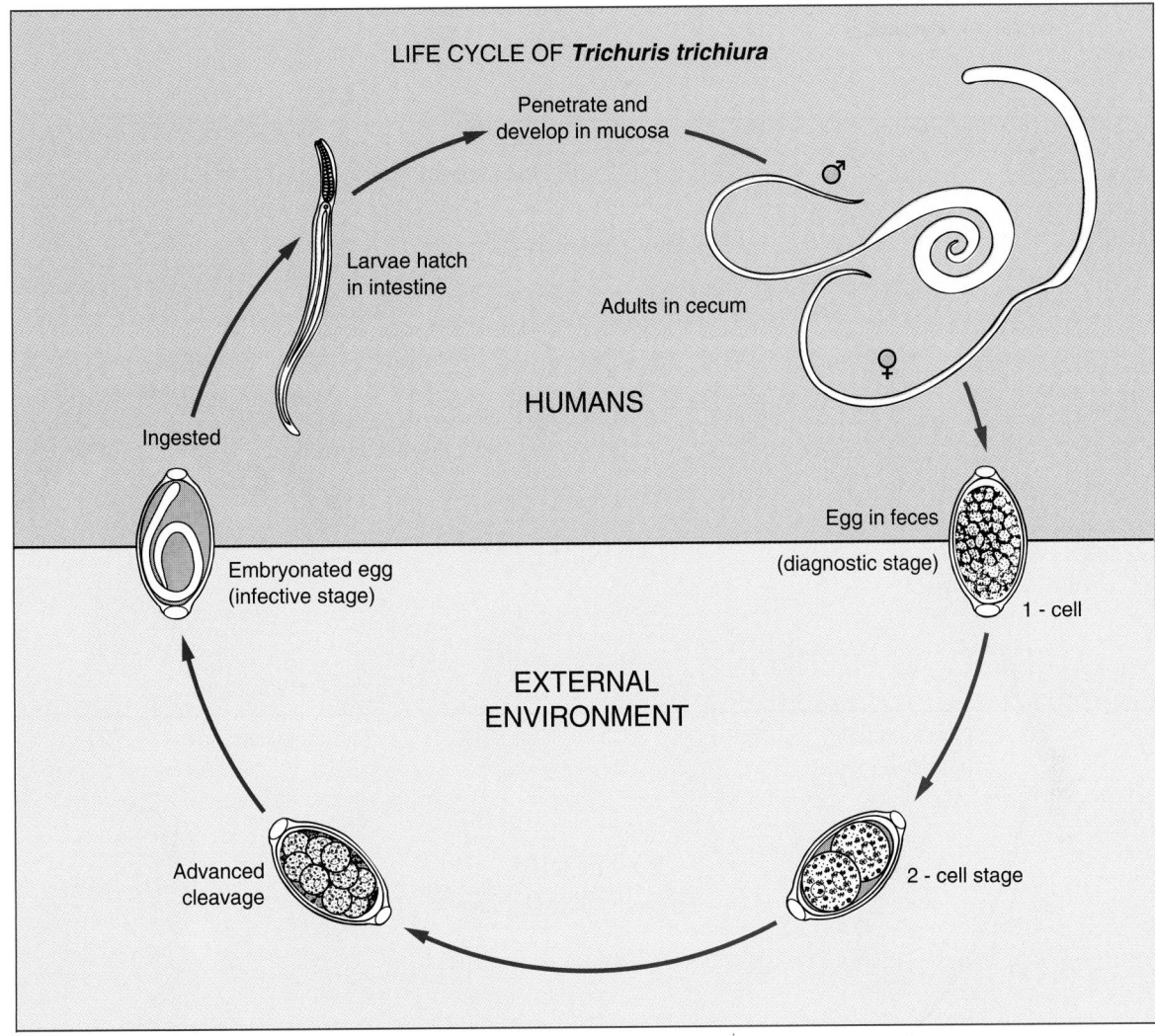

LIFE CYCLE OF *Trichuris trichiura*

Penetrate and
develop in mucosa

Larvae hatch
in intestine

Adults in cecum

♂

♀

HUMANS

Ingested

Embryonated egg
(infective stage)

Egg in feces
(diagnostic stage)

1 - cell

EXTERNAL
ENVIRONMENT

Advanced
cleavage

2 - cell stage

Figure 22-9 The life cycle of *Trichuris trichiura* is similar to that of *Ascaris lumbricoides*, except that a circulatory larval stage is absent. The eggs, after passage into the external environment, also require a period of about 21 days under favorable conditions before they become infective. On ingestion of embryonated eggs by a human host, larvae hatch in the intestine. However, in contrast to the ascarids, these larvae penetrate only into the mucosa of the intestine, primarily in the cecum, where they become anchored and develop into adult male and female worms. Gravid females pass eggs into the feces to complete the life cycle.

CLINICAL CORRELATION BOX 22-5 Trichuriasis

In light infections, patients are generally asymptomatic. The adult worms inhabit the large intestine. In heavy infections, diarrhea, dysentery, and abdominal discomfort, resulting largely from mechanical damage to the intestinal mucosa, may be experienced. Anemia, growth retardation, and intestinal leakiness have been identified as predictable consequences of heavy infection and may serve as an indication of the intensity of infestation.[44] Varying degrees of malabsorption may also be observed, and because the diarrhea tends to be watery, sodium and potassium electrolyte imbalances may be a problem. Rectal prolapse in children is one of the complications of heavy infection with *Trichuris*.[273] Because the tiny adult worms are visible with the naked eye, the term "coconut cake" prolapse has been used to describe this condition.

Mebendazole, 100-mg chewable tablet, is the treatment of choice.

CLINICAL CORRELATION BOX 22-6 Enterobiasis

The adult worms reside in the cecum and rectum. The diagnosis on occasion is made by observing worms in stained histologic preparations of the appendix or other portions of bowel. Symptoms occur when the gravid female deposits eggs in the folds of the perianal skin during the late evening hours. Nocturnal pruritus ani is the usual presenting symptom due to the irritation caused by the deposited eggs. Infections occur most commonly in children, and females are more prone to infection than males. In heavy infections, vaginitis with a mucoid discharge and/or urethritis may occur in young females.[96] Nervousness, insomnia, and nightmares are other presenting symptoms.

Pyrantel pamoate, or mebendazole, the latter in a single dose of 100 mg in the form of chewable capsules, are the treatments of choice. As infections may recur, repeat treatment after 1 or 2 weeks may be necessary if symptoms recur.

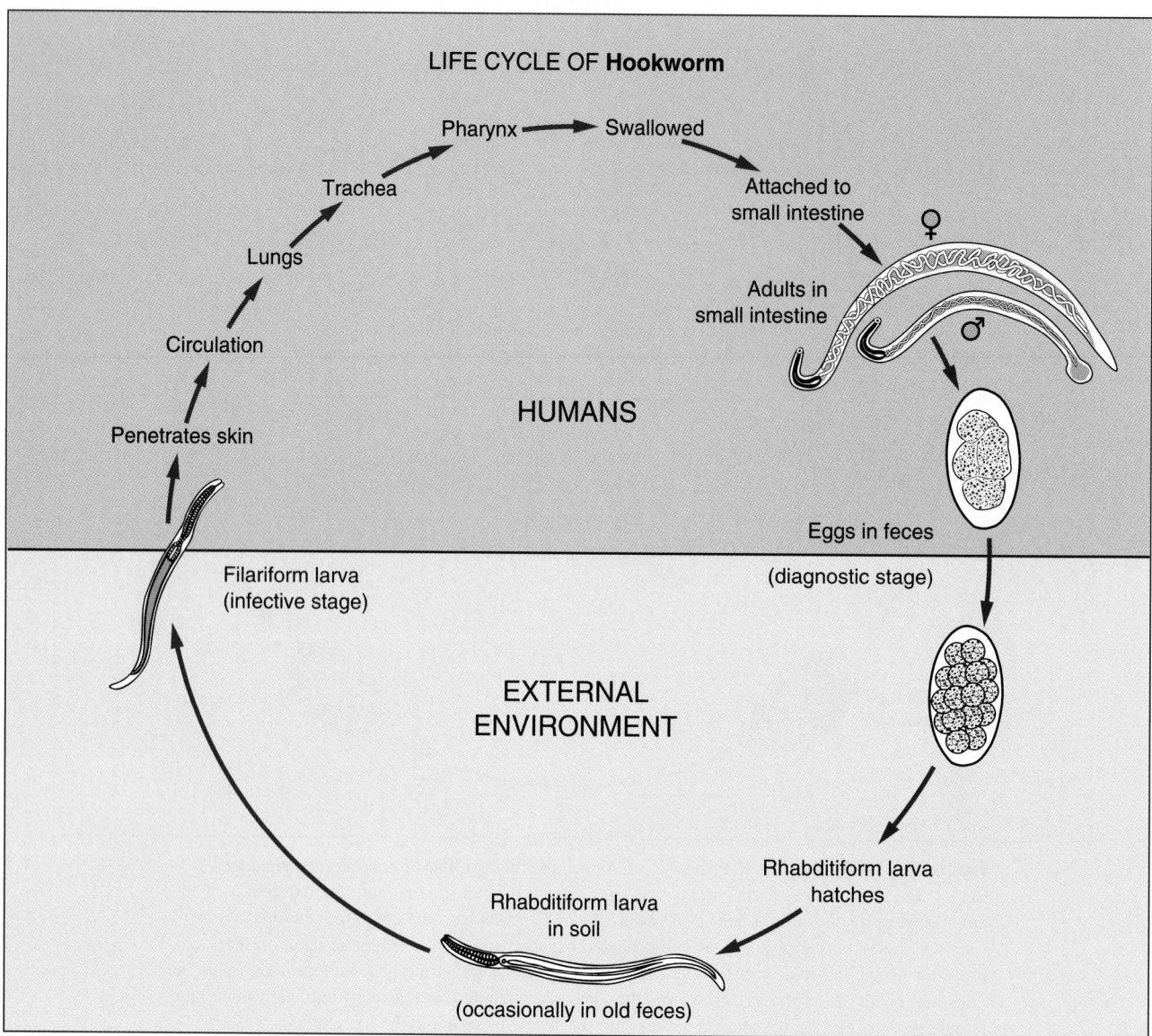

Figure 22-10 Life cycle of hookworm. Hookworm eggs are usually passed in early stages of cleavage into the feces from gravid female worms. In approximately 24 hours in soil of ideal temperature and moisture content, the eggs hatch into the first larval stage, the free-feeding rhabditiform larva. About 5–7 days later, the rhabditiform larva transforms into the third-stage filariform larva, the infective form for humans. Depending on the temperature and moisture content of the soil, filariform larva can remain infective for up to 6 weeks. Humans become infected by penetration of the filariform larva on skin contact, either of the hands when digging into larva-infested soil, or walking barefoot in soil contaminated with human feces. Similar to the ascarids, the hookworm larvae also penetrate the intestinal mucosa, enter the circulation, break out into the pulmonary alveoli, are coughed up, and swallowed. These "processed" larvae again burrow into the intestinal mucosa, where they develop into adult male and female worms. These adult worms remain firmly attached to the mucosa by either cutting plates or pairs of teeth depending on the species, in the meantime tapping into a constant supply of host blood. Female worms lay large numbers of eggs that pass in the feces to complete the life cycle.

CLINICAL CORRELATION BOX 22-7 Hookworm Infections

Symptoms may occur relative to various stages of the life cycle. Skin infections may be experienced at the penetration sites of filariform larvae, particularly when humans are infected with nonhuman hookworm species commonly involving other animals ("ground itch").[273] Loeffler's syndrome in lungs and eosinophilia may be seen during the pulmonary larval migratory stage. Adult female hookworms produce only about 2,500 to 5,000 eggs per day; thus, the fecal egg counts may reflect the number of adult hookworms and, in turn, indicate the severity of infection. The presence of more than 2,000 hookworm ova per milliliter of feces in women and children, and more than 5,000 per milliliter in males, is usually associated with anemia. Egg counting techniques are described by Garcia.[96]

In heavy infections of 500 or more worms, the host could lose the equivalent of 1/2 to 1 pint of blood per week, resulting in severe hypochromic, iron deficiency anemia, and marked erythroid hyperplasia of the bone marrow, which in turn may lead to osteoporosis and the formation of bone cysts. Weakness, fatigue, growth retardation, peripheral edema, and congestive heart failure may be complications in severe infections. Of major concern worldwide is the lack of mental development from anemia-associated hypoxia in millions of children infected with hookworms.[158] Diarrhea, abdominal pain, nausea are manifestations of the intestinal phase of infection. Kelley et al.[151] reported that hookworm infections developed in 35 of 684 soldiers who took part in the Grenada military operations; they were most commonly associated with ground exposure near homes where sanitation practices were minimal.

Mebendazole, 100 mg in chewable table form, every 12 hours for 3 days is the recommended treatment.

- The shells are thin, smooth, transparent, and nonpigmented.
- The yolk cells retract leaving a clear space beneath the shell (Color Plate 22-5*K*).

Rhabditiform Larvae

- In contrast to *Strongyloides* species in which the eggs hatch while still in the intestine and commonly are observed in microscopic mounts of fecal specimens, the rhabditiform larvae of hookworms are uncommonly present.
- The rhabditiform larvae of the hookworms possess a long buccal cavity (Color Plate 22-5*L*, left) a distinguishing feature from *Strongyloides stercoralis*. A hookworm ova rarely hatch within the intestine.
- The rhabditiform larvae of *Strongyloides stercoralis* that have a short buccal cavity (Color Plate 22-5*L*, right).

Strongyloidiasis and *Strongyloides stercoralis*

Peculiarities in the life cycle set infections with *Strongyloides stercoralis* apart from those of other nematodes. For example, the laboratory diagnosis of strongyloidiasis is usually made by observing motile rhabditiform larvae rather than ova in stool specimens (Color Plate 22-5*M*). The life cycle is illustrated in Figure 22-11.

Worldwide, the magnitude of strongyloidiasis is similar to that of the prevalence of hookworm infections, with upward of an estimated 800 million people being infected, involving up to 10% of the population in some locales. The incidence of infection in any given region is very spotty as the filariform larva require considerable moisture and grow best where the water table is high. In the United States, strongyloidiasis is endemic in the rural south and southeast, with 3–5% of people being infected in some locales.[273] Infections also have high prevalence in inmates in mental institutions and prisons and in immigrants who formerly resided in endemic tropical regions. The clinical manifestations of strongyloidiasis are presented in Clinical Correlation Box 22-8.

Laboratory Identification

Rhabditiform Larvae

- The rhabditiform larva of hookworms have a long buccal cavity (Color Plate 22-5*L*, left), in contrast to that of *S. stercoralis*, which is short (Color Plate 22-5*L*, right).
- *Strongyloides stercoralis* rhabditiform larvae also have a prominent genital primordium about one third the distance from the tail.

Often chronic infections are associated with light organism loads, making an objective diagnosis difficult. Examination of several stool specimens on successive days may be required; or the concentration procedure of Baermann may be indicated. In this procedure, active larvae are induced to migrate out of a fecal mass into a water reservoir through a wire screen covered with a pad of gauze, as described by Garcia.[96] DeKaminsky,[63] in a study of 427 stool samples, found that an additional 33 cases were diagnosed using a modified Baerman technique, and 28 additional cases were diagnosed using the agar plate culture method.

Trichostrongylus Species

Uncommonly detected in the United States, *Trichostrongylus* species are small adult nematodes similar to the hookworms that reside with heads buried in small intestinal epithelium. Adult worms typically inhabit the gastrointestinal tracts of sheep, cattle, goats, and other herbivores. Although third-stage larva lie on grass and vegetation, infection is by oral ingestion, as these larva lack the ability to invade skin. Also, in human infections, because they do not possess the special mouthparts characteristic of hookworms, leaching of blood does not occur. Heavy infections may produce abdominal pain, diarrhea, and mild eosinophilia, but for the most part symptoms are minimal. The ova resemble those of hookworm, but are longer (78–98 × 40–50 μm), with pointed ends. It is important to recognize these subtle differences in egg morphology so that an incorrect diagnosis of hookworm infection is not made. Thiabendazole, 25 mg/kg every 12 hours for 2 days, is the recommended treatment.

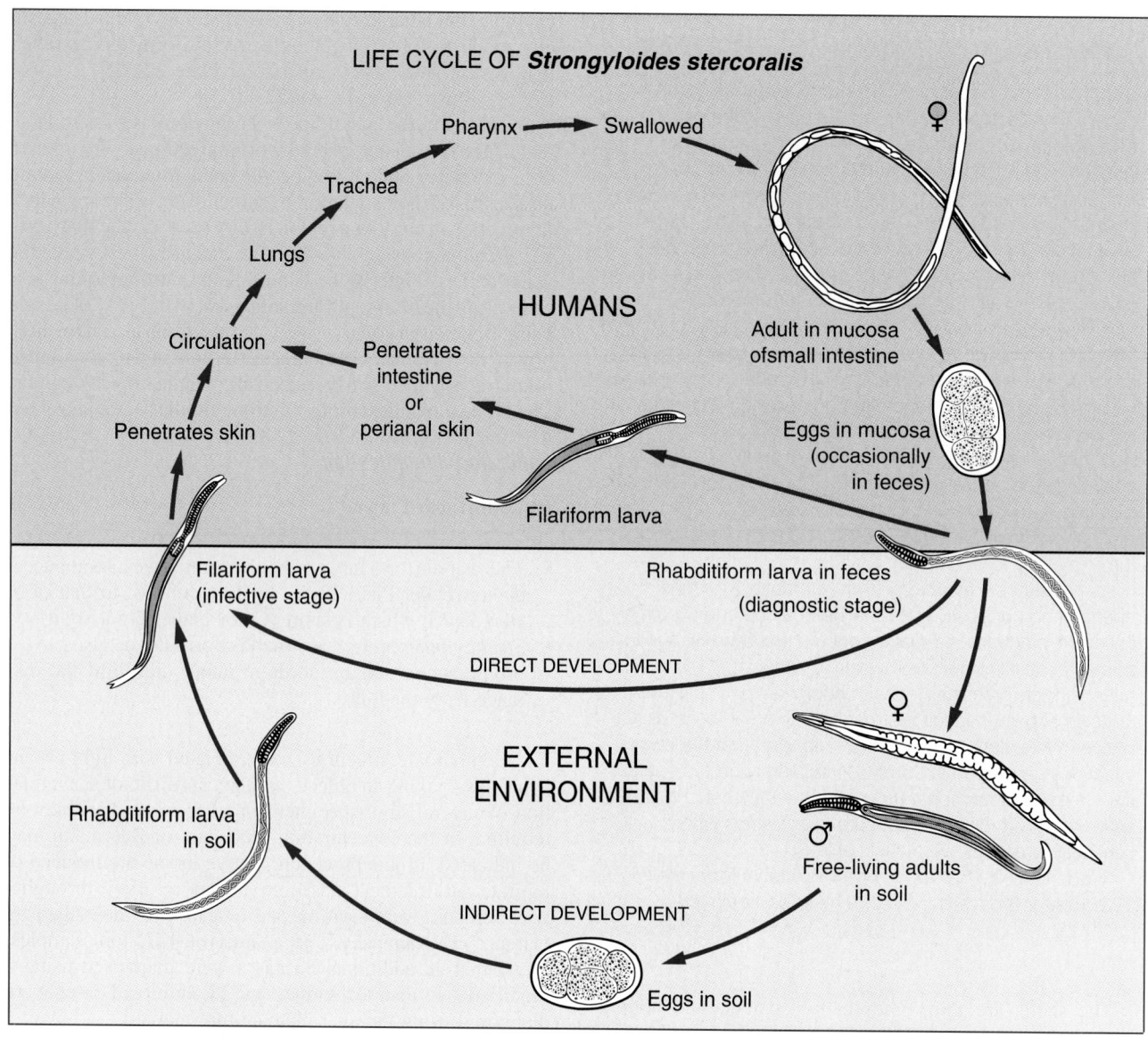

Figure 22-11 Life cycle of *Strongyloides stercoralis*. The life cycle of *Strongyloides stercoralis* is similar to that of the hookworms, except that the majority of eggs hatch into rhabditiform larvae while still in the intestinal lumen. In patients who have lost immunity, rhabditiform larvae may next hatch into filariform larvae within the intestinal lumen, from which they can directly invade the mucosa resulting in disseminated reinfection disease. In cases of diarrheal disease, eggs, indistinguishable from those of hookworm, may occasionally be observed in the feces. Under ideal conditions of moisture and temperature in the external environment, rhabditiform larvae hatch, and quickly transform into infective filariform larvae. Humans become infected by direct penetration of filariform larvae into the skin on direct contact. The migration of these invasive larvae into the circulation are similar to that of hookworms, ultimately resulting in the development of adult worms in the intestine.

Capillaria philippinensis

Capillaria philippinensis is an extremely small nematode; the adults measure 1.5–3.9 mm in length, and their width ranges from 5 μm at the filamentous head to 30 μm in midbody. After considerable research to find the reservoir hosts, it is now believed that fish-eating birds are natural hosts within a fish–bird life cycle.[47] Humans become in-

fected when they eat poorly cooked fish commonly consumed by birds.

The disease is endemic in the Philippines, Thailand, and regions adjacent to the South China Sea. Local eating habits include ingestion of raw animal organs and the use of intestinal juices from animals to season rice and other foodstuffs, and eating uncooked crabs and small freshwater fish is considered a delicacy in many indigenous populations. Infection

CLINICAL CORRELATION BOX 22-8   Strongyloidiasis

Skin irritation and pruritus in the form of low-grade chronic dermatitis may be seen at the portal of entry.[37] The full-blown ground itch characteristic for hookworm cutaneous infections usually does not occur. Leighton and MacSween,[162] however, report a case of a 74-year-old woman with a 65-year history of urticarial-like eruptions since childhood. These symptoms were finally correlated with long-term persistence of hyperinfection with strongyloidiasis. The case for making a diagnosis of disseminated strongyloidiasis through recognition of filariform larva in skin biopsies was also made by Gordon et al.[106]

The intestinal manifestations of strongyloides infections vary from few if any symptoms in light infections to severe necrotizing bowel disease in heavy infections. Symptoms may suggest peptic ulcer disease in some patients; in others, involvement of the small intestine may radiographically mimic Crohn's disease. A case of massive upper gastrointestinal hemorrhage involving a 29-year-old black immigrant from Africa, caused by a heavy infection of the duodenum with *S. stercoralis*, has been reported by Bhatt et al.[18]

With a heavy infective dose, pulmonary disease suggestive of Loeffler's pneumonia, manifested as wheezing and eosinophilia, may occur; or in cases of hyperinfection syndrome to be described later in this chapter, full-blown pneumonia, cough and shortness of breath may develop. Harris and associates[123] report two cases of disseminated strongyloidiasis in which the diagnosis was first made by observing larva in the sputum. They suggest that immunosuppressed patients in whom nonbacterial pneumonia develops, particularly in the presence of eosinophilia, should have both stool and sputum samples checked for infection with *S. stercoralis*.

Long-term corticosteroid therapy may also predispose to disseminated strongyloides infections. Chu et al.[39] describe a case of pneumonia developing in a 65-year-old man with steroid-dependent chronic obstructive pulmonary disease. *Strongyloides* rhabditiform larvae were detected in an expectorated sputum specimen. In general, the pneumonitis caused by nematode larvae is transient and characterized by cough and fever; in more severe cases, it is characterized by chest pain, dyspnea, and hemoptysis.

Immunosuppressed hosts are particularly vulnerable to disseminated strongyloides infections. The propensity for *S. stercoralis* eggs to hatch quickly and to product intraintestinal filariform larvae (Color Plate 22–5N) makes patients vulnerable to autoinfection, producing a condition known as hyperinfection syndrome.[143] Purtilo and associates,[220] after observing the absence of granulomatous tissue response to larvae in several autopsy cases of fatal strongyloidiasis, concluded that an intact cell-mediated immune system is necessary to keep the organism in check. Once immunity is compromised or abrogated, hyperinfection from direct invasion of the intestinal mucosa (Color Plate 22–5O) with dissemination of larvae to many organs and tissues is liable to occur in patients harboring the parasite. Genta[99] offers the alternative argument that corticosteroids, rather than working through suppression of immunity, may in fact act directly on the worm as "molting hormones" that directly promote organism proliferation, making disseminated disease a more likely possibility. Although strongyloides hyperinfection syndrome has not been specifically associated with HIV positivity and AIDS, a few cases have been reported.[121]

Because *S. stercoralis* can be carried by humans as a subclinical infestation for many years following initial contact, patients in whom disseminated strongyloidiasis develops need not have had a recent exposure. Klein and associates[155] reiterate the need to screen stool specimens for strongyloidiasis before treating patients living in endemic areas with a course of immunosuppressive therapy. Recipients of organ transplants represent another high-risk group who should have stool examinations to detect strongyloides larva before immunosuppressive therapy is begun.[56] Hyperinfection syndrome is further complicated because of the increased risk of gram-negative sepsis developing, presumably because intestinal bacteria can invade through mucosal breaks from the penetrating strongyloides larvae.

Thiabendazole, 25 mg/kg every 12 hours for 2 days, is the treatment regimen of choice.

with *C. philippinensis* always causes illness and may lead to death if untreated. From 1967 to 1990, 1,884 confirmed cases of intestinal capillariasis were documented, from which 110 people died.[47]

The gradual onset of abdominal pain, gurgling stomach, and intermittent diarrhea over a 4- to 8-week period is the common presenting clinical picture. Severe protein-losing enteropathy, malabsorption of fats and sugars, and low xylose excretion are commonly seen. Fluid loss and electrolyte imbalances characterized by low plasma levels of potassium, sodium, and calcium are seen. IgE is at high levels, and IgG, IgM, and IgA are at low levels. In fatal cases, heavy infection in the jejunum, fatty metamorphosis of the liver, and vacuolization of the cytoplasm of renal proximal convoluted tubular cells and of myocardial cells with heavy cytoplasmic deposition of lipochrome pigment were seen. Focal mucosal atrophy at sites of organism invasion were seen in histologic sections of the small intestine.[47]

Laboratory Identification

- Based on stool examination the condition may be confused with *Trichuris trichiura* because the ova have a similar appearance.
- The ova of *C. philippinensis* have less conspicuous polar plugs and a thick, striated shell (Color Plate 22-5P).
- A misidentification could lead to unnecessary morbidity or even death, as cases of *C. philippinensis* often go untreated.

Cestodes

The cestodes are a subclass of helminths comprising true tapeworms, which have a scolex and a series of hermaphroditic, egg-producing body segments called proglottids. The cestodes of human importance to be presented are:

Taenia saginata
Taenia solium
Diphyllobothrium latum
Hymenolepis nana
Hymenolepis diminuta
Dipylidium caninum

The body of an adult cestode or tapeworm, called the strobila, consists of two parts, a scolex and the proglottides (Color Plate 22-6*A*). The scolex is the anterior portion with hooklets and/or suckers by which the worm can attach and anchor to the intestinal mucosa. The crown of the scolex, called the rostellum may be fitted with hooklets (armed) (Color Plate 22-6*B*) or may be devoid of hooklets and smooth (unarmed). These morphologic differences are helpful in establishing a species identification.

The major portion of the body of a tapeworm is composed of a long series of segments called proglottides. Each proglottid possesses male and female reproductive structures, the uterine branches of which are packed with ova when mature (Color Plate 22-6*C*). The ova are passed in the feces, where they are observed in microscopic mounts in order to establish a laboratory diagnosis. Subtle differences in the size, shape, and internal structures of proglottides serve as aids in establishing a species identification.

With the exception of *Hymenolepis nana*, in which human-to-human transmission of infections may occur through ingestion of fecally contaminated food or water that contains infective eggs, the life cycles of the cestodes require one or more intermediate hosts to support stages of larval development. The life cycle of *Taenia solium*, representative of cestodes, is illustrated in Figure 22-12.

Taenia solium and *Taenia saginata*

Taenia infections have been known since biblical times, primitive knowledge of which may be related to the Judaic prohibition against the ingestion of pork. Differentiation of *Taenia saginata* from *Taenia solium* is more than an academic exercise. As mentioned above, humans acquire the intestinal infections with an adult *Taenia* tapeworm through ingestion of larval infected, poorly cooked pork (*T. solium*) or beef (*T. saginata*). (Color Plate 22-6*D*). Intestinal infections with the adult tapeworms of these two species produce similar symptoms in humans, as discussed below. However, humans may also serve as the intermediate host if the ova of *T. solium* are ingested. In this case, the larva travel widely in the circulation, with a propensity to lodge in the brain rather than in skeletal muscle, producing a disease called cysticercosis. (Color Plate 22-6*E*). Laboratory workers must be careful when handling the ova-packed proglottides of *T. solium* to avoid inadvertent hand-to-mouth transmission. Human cysticercosis does not occur with *T. saginata;* however, as the true identity may not be immediately known, care must be taken when handling any proglottides.

Cysticercosis has high prevalence in Mexico and Latin America, where an estimated 350,000 persons are infected. The disease has been found in 2–3% of autopsy cases in Mexico City, accounting for 25% of all intracranial masses found by computed tomography scans.[217] Until the past decade, neurocysticercosis has been uncommon in the

United States (only a few hundred cases recorded since surveillance began in 1957); however, a marked increase has been noted recently, in parallel with the increased immigration of peoples from Mexico, Central and South America, and Asia.[45] In 1989, cysticercosis became a reportable disease in California.[76] During the first year, 134 cases were reported, nearly all (117) from people of Hispanic background and most of whom had immigrated from countries where *T. solium* is endemic. In addition to the higher incidence of disease in California, several individual cases have also been reported from various diverse areas in the United States, including Texas, Colorado, Pennsylvania, and Missouri.[183] Perhaps because of this experience, Roman et al.[227] propose that neurocysticercosis be declared an international reportable disease. Several recent publications reflect high rates of incidence of symptomatic cysticercosis in many regions throughout the world, as exemplified by endemic areas in Andean communities and in Burundi, as reported by Cruz et al.[48] and by Newell et al.,[198] respectively. The clinical manifestations of taeniasis and cysticercus infections are presented in Clinical Correlation Box 22-9.

Laboratory Identification. The laboratory diagnosis of *Taenia* tapeworm infections is usually made by observing the characteristic eggs in microscopic mounts of fecal material; the adult worms or portions thereof are required to make a species identification. The eggs for the two species are morphologically identical.

The identifying characteristics of *Taenia* species are:

Ova

- Spherical in shape, measuring approximately 30 by 45 μm in diameter.
- Characteristic smooth, thick shell with radial striations (Color Plate 22-6*H*). A photograph of these eggs in situ within the uterus of a gravid female worm is illustrated in Color Plate 22-6*G*.
- Three pairs of hooklets may be observed internally, in a structure called an oncosphere.

Adult Worms

The features by which *T. saginata* and *T. solium* can be differentiated are:

	TAENIA SAGINATA	TAENIA SOLIUM
Strobila:	4–10 m long	2–4 m long
	Up to 2,000 proglottides	800–1,000 proglottides
Scolex:	Four suckers	Four suckers
	Unarmed rostellum	Armed rostellum (Color Plate 22-6*B*)
Proglottides:	More than 13 lateral uterine branches	Less than 13 lateral uterine branches (Color Plate 22-6*C*)

Chapman et al.[36] have developed a species-specific DNA probe that differentiates *T. solium* ova from those of *T. saginata*. The authors describe the isolation and characterization of recombinant clones that contain repetitive DNA sequences (a 158-bp sequence) for *T. solium* and an unrelated *T. saginata* sequence that encodes a

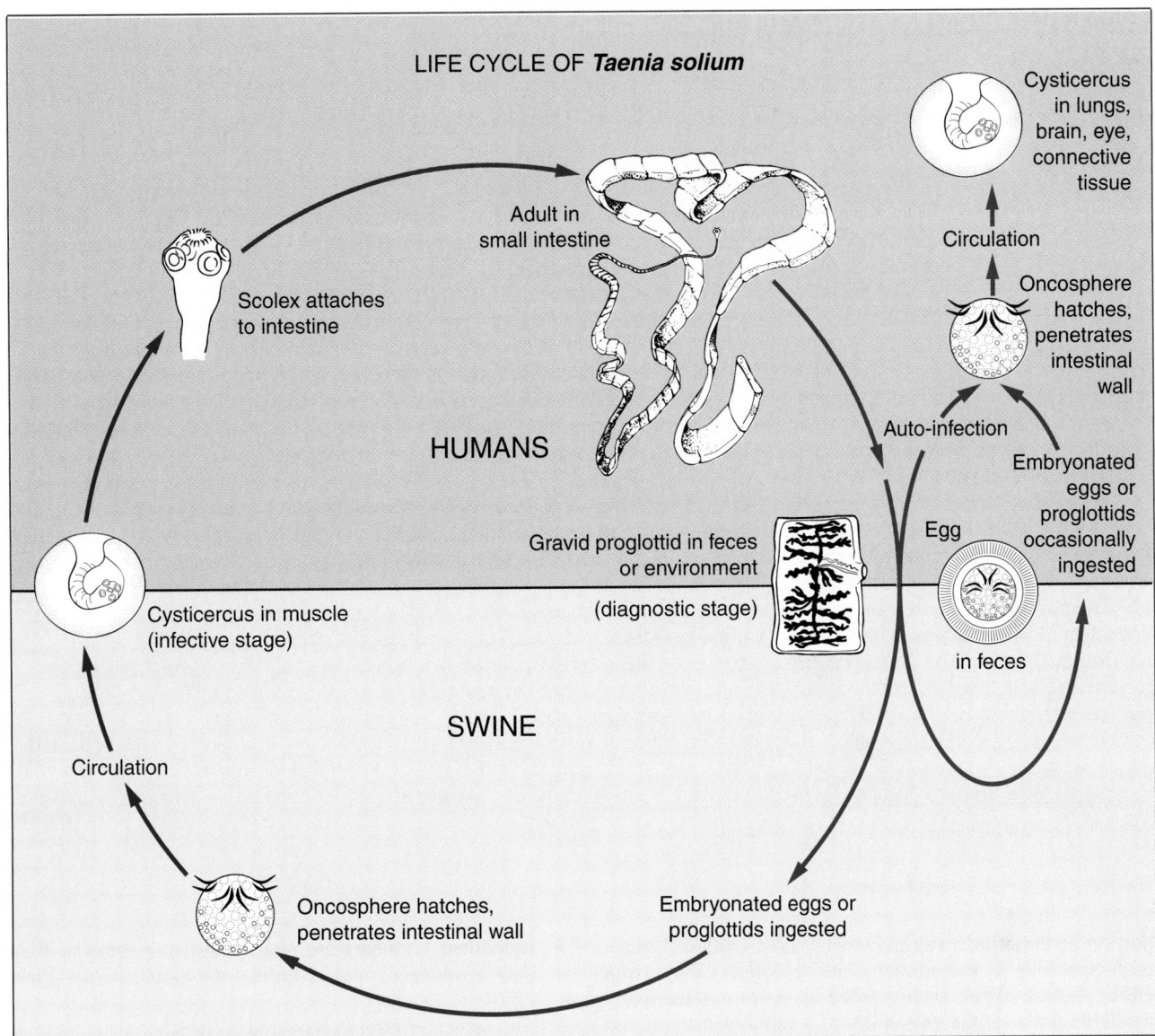

Figure 22-12 Life cycle of *Taenia solium*. A human infected with an intestinal tapeworm passes proglottids and/or mature ova into the external environment, where soil, water, and vegetative matter become contaminated with fecal matter. In the case of *Taenia solium*, the embryonated eggs are ingested by a pig, within the intestine of which an oncosphere hatches and penetrates the mucosa. The released larvae enter the circulation and migrate to the skeletal muscle to encyst in the form of a bladderlike cyst called a cysticercus. On ingestion of such cysticercus-infested measly pork by an unsuspecting human, the scolex evaginates in the intestine and the scolex attaches to the intestinal mucosa. In time the tapeworm grows through the proliferation of hundreds of proglottids, until a length of several meters is reached. Eggs and proglottids are again released into the intestinal lumen and passed with the feces to complete the life cycle.

CLINICAL CORRELATION BOX 22-9 Taeniasis and Cysticercosis

Taeniasis

Intestinal symptoms are usually insignificant. Passage of proglottides in stool may be the first indication of disease. Epigastric pain, vague abdominal discomfort, nervousness, and increase in appetite may be experienced. Weight loss is minimal. Eosinophilia is usually moderate.

Cysticercosis

Cysticercosis refers to the development of extraintestinal encysted larval forms of *T. solium* in various organs following the ingestion of gravid ova in fecally contaminated food or water. Although most human cases are caused by *T. solium*, other species of animal tapeworms can on rare occasions also produce morphologically similar cysticerci. The central nervous system is involved in 60–96% of patients, a condition known as neurocysticercosis (Color Plate 22–6E). The majority of patients with neurocysticercosis have more than one cyst, with as many as 200 found in one autopsy case.[183]

Symptoms vary considerably from patient to patient. Lesions in the cerebral cortex may result in seizures or localizing neurologic deficits. Cranial nerve palsies, in particular involving the fifth and seventh nerves, and abnormal reflexes are commonly found. Cysticercosis is the most frequently identified cause of epilepsy in young adults living in endemic areas, and it is the sole manifestation in up to one third of cases.[236] Focal seizures occur in up to three fourths of those infected. Intraventricular brain cysts may obstruct the flow of cerebrospinal fluid, leading to symptoms of acute intracranial hypertension (headache, vertigo, nausea, vomiting, papilledema, and visual disturbances); changes in personality and mental status are present in 40% of patients.[183]

The invasive larvae (onchospheres) are susceptible to circulating antibody and complement in the human host[286]; however, significant titers develop only after the larvae have transformed into the antibody-resistant metacestodes. In fact, antibody may bind via Fc receptors to the worm, which may use it as a source of protein. Taeniaestatin and other parasite molecules may interfere with lymphocyte proliferation and macrophage function, thus paralyzing the cellular immune response. Herrera et al.[127] report an increase in brain tumors and hematologic malignancies associated with cysticercosis, possible related to the induction of DNA damage in cells surrounding the cysticerci, and from a persistent host inflammatory response.

Praziquantel and albendazole have been extensively tested and successfully used for the treatment of neurocysticercosis, usually in combination with corticosteroids.[278] In a recent mass effort to treat cysticercosis in a rural community in Mexico (single dose of praziquantel of 5 mg/kg), human taeniasis was reduced by 56%, and late-onset seizures by 70% over a 42 month period.[236] In this same study, anticysticercus antibody levels were reduced in humans by 75%, and by 55% in treated pigs. Vaccines, using recombinant antigens, have been developed and found in experimental studies to induce over 90% protection for challenge infections for hydatid disease in sheep, providing encouragement for potential vaccine use in humans as well.[165]

---

portion of the mitochondrial cytochrome *c* oxidase I gene, each specifically hybridizing with genomic DNA from either species. When such a probe becomes commercially available, there is the possibility of a rapid, sensitive, and noninvasive diagnostic test for the detection of *T. solium* ova. Indirect hemagglutination serologic assays for confirming the diagnosis of cysticercosis in suspected cases are available through the CDC. Titers of 1:64 or greater is usually indicative of active infection.

Diphyllobothrium latum: The Giant Fish Tapeworm

D. latum, the human giant fish tapeworm, uses two intermediate hosts in the development of its larval forms. Endemic areas include the cold clear lake regions of Scandinavia, northern Europe, northern Japan, the upper Midwest of the United States, Canada, and Alaska. Figure 22-13 is an illustration of the life cycle.

The clinical manifestations of diphyllobothriasis are presented in Clinical Correlation Box 22-10.

Laboratory Identification

Adult Worm

Although the proglottides are rarely passed in the stool, they are distinctive.

- The strobila measures 3–10 m in length and has over 3,000 proglottides.

- Individual segments are characteristically broader than they are long (*latum* is Latin for *broad*). (Color Plate 22-6I)
- The scolex is rarely recovered from stool specimens. It is:
  - Almond-shaped and measures 2–3 × 1 mm.
  - Distinctive for its two deep dorsoventral suctorial grooves (*bothria* = pit), demarcated by lateral lip-like folds (*phyllon* = leaves) (Color Plate 22-6J).
- Each proglottid includes a nondescript coiled uterus in the form of a compact rosette (Color Plate 22-6K).

Ova

The laboratory diagnosis of human *D. latum* infection is commonly made by identifying the characteristic operculated eggs in stool specimens. These eggs:

- Measure approximately 55–75 × 40–55 μm and are elongated.
- Have a smooth shell with an inconspicuous nonshouldered operculum at one end and a knoblike thickening at the other (Color Plate 22-6L).
- Can be differentiated from those *Paragonimus westermani* (discussed later), which possess a distinct shouldered operculum (Color Plate 22-7P).

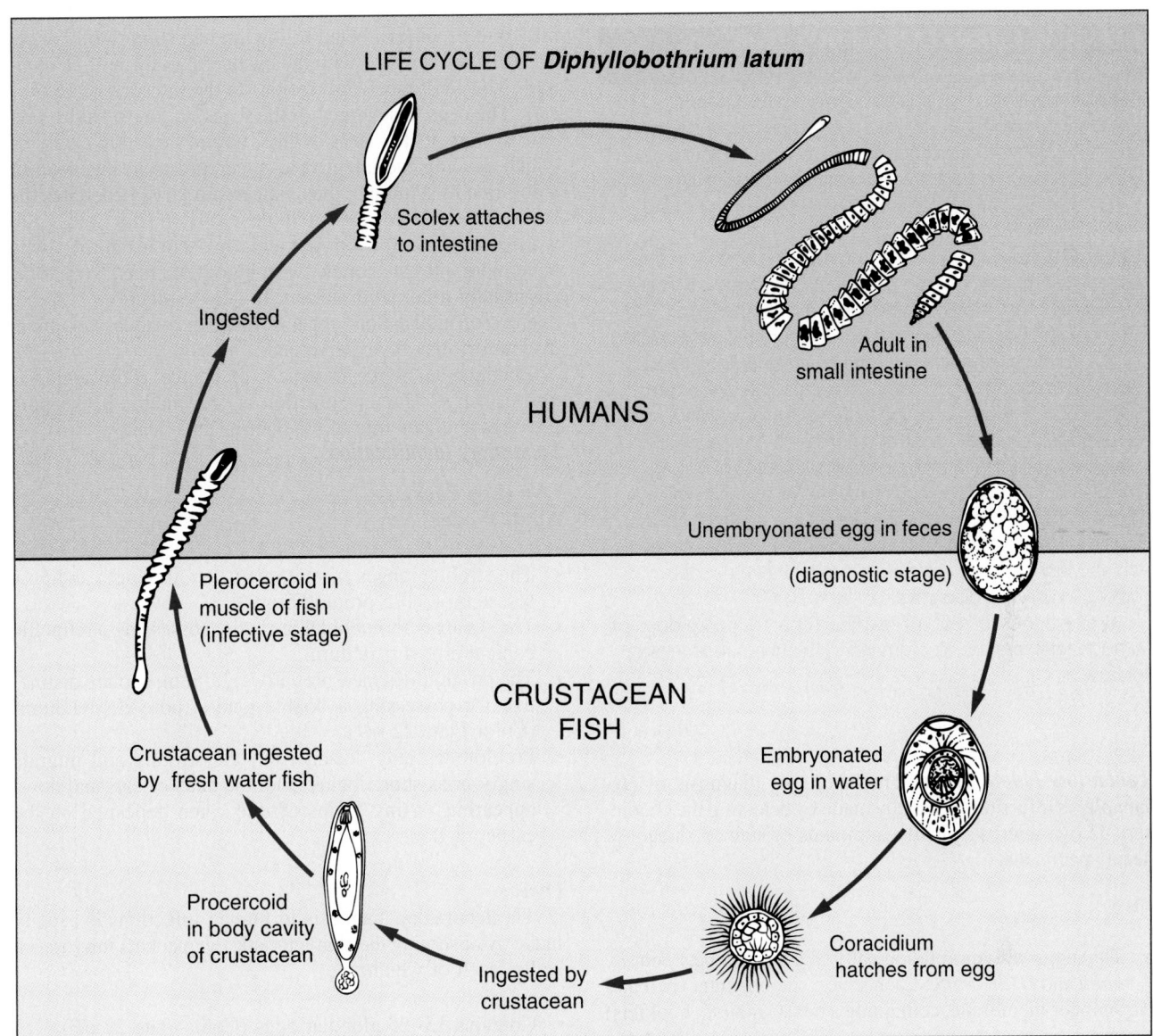

LIFE CYCLE OF *Diphyllobothrium latum*

Scolex attaches
to intestine

Ingested

HUMANS

Adult in
small intestine

Unembryonated egg in feces

(diagnostic stage)

Plerocercoid in
muscle of fish
(infective stage)

CRUSTACEAN
FISH

Embryonated
egg in water

Crustacean ingested
by fresh water fish

Procercoid
in body cavity
of crustacean

Ingested by
crustacean

Coracidium
hatches from egg

Figure 22-13 The life cycle of *Diphyllobothrium latum* involves two intermediate hosts. Unembryonated eggs, passed with the fecal material from an infected human into a freshwater estuary, undergo embryonation during a period of several days and hatch, releasing a free-swimming coracidium. These coracidia in turn are ingested by a crustacean (copepods or cyclops), within the body cavity of which develop procercoid larvae. Copepods serve as one of the major food sources for a variety of freshwater fish in North America. Following ingestion of the copepod by the fish, the plerocercoid larvae of the parasite (spargana) develop within the flesh of the fish. Humans ingest these plerocercoid larvae in raw or poorly cooked fish, where they develop into adult worms in the intestine. On maturation, the adult worm passes eggs into the feces, to complete the life cycle.

Hymenolepis Species

Hymenolepis nana, known as the dwarf tapeworm, has a worldwide distribution and is one of the more common causes of cestode infections in humans, particularly in children. In contrast, *Hymenolepis diminuta* is primarily a parasite of rats and mice, and is uncommonly found in humans. Various species of arthropod (''meal-beetles,'' for example), that harbor the infective larval forms, may serve as intermediate hosts. A photograph of an *Hymenolepis* cysticercus as

it may appear within the insect is illustrated in Color Plate 22-6*F*. Humans become infected through the ingestion of these larval-infected insects. Such an intermediate host is not obligatory for human-to-human transmission of *Hymenolepis nana*. Most commonly, humans become infected through the ingestion of food or water contaminated with *Hymenolepis* eggs. Figure 22-14 is an illustrated life cycle of *Hymenolepis diminuta*.

The clinical manifestations of hymenolepiasis are presented in Clinical Correlation Box 22-11.

CLINICAL CORRELATION BOX 22-10
Diphyllobothriasis

Patients may harbor an adult worm for up to 20 years. Intestinal symptoms are minimal. Large adult worms may cause mechanical bowel obstruction, accompanied by abdominal pain and diarrhea. In a minority of patients infected with *D. latum*, particularly in northern Europe and specifically in Finland, megaloblastic anemia secondary to vitamin B_{12} deficiency is not uncommon, secondary to the selective competition of the parasite for this essential vitamin.

Humans may also become infected with the larval plerocercoids of diphyllobothrioid tapeworms closely related to *D. latum*, causing an infection known as sparganosis. Adult worms are found in dogs and cats; the larval form develops in humans following ingestion of larval infected Copepoda or the raw flesh of amphibians and reptiles. The plerocercoid larvae (sparganum) develop into pruritic nodules in the subcutaneous tissues over a period of months. Peripheral blood eosinophilia is a nonspecific clue to the possibility of sparganosis; however, the characteristic larvae must be demonstrated in subcutaneous nodules before a definitive diagnosis can be made.

A single 2-g dose of niclosamide, or a 10 mg/kg dose of praziquantel, are the recommended treatment regimens of choice.

Laboratory Identification. The laboratory diagnosis of *Hymenolepis* infections is usually made by detecting the characteristic ova microscopically in mounts or stained smears of fecal specimens.

Ova

- The eggs are morphologically distinctive between *H. nana* and *H. diminuta*. Each have a smooth outer shell and an inner membrane, containing a hexacanth (six hooklets) embryo.
- The ova of *H. nana* are oval in outline and small (47×57 μm), and possess a characteristic pair of polar filaments that arise from thickenings on either side of the hexacanth membrane (Color Plate 22-6*M*)
- *H. diminuta* eggs are spherical, larger (58×86 μm) than those of *N. nana*, and are devoid of polar filaments (Color Plate 22-6*N*).

Adult Worms

- The adult worms of *H. nana* are small, measuring no longer than 1.5 in. when mature.
- They often simulate mucous threads; thus, they are not commonly seen in stool specimens.
- The tiny scolex has a protruding, armed scolex with a row of 20 to 30 hooklets.

Dipylidium caninum

The life cycle of *Dipylidium caninum* is similar to that of *Hymenolepis diminuta*. Humans serve as an accidental host, and become infected following ingestion of dog or cat fleas that are infected with the cysticercoid form of *D. caninum*. The adult tapeworm resides in the intestine of dogs or cats. The eggs, discharged in the feces, are ingested by several species of dog fleas or lice, within the body cavity of which develop the infective cysticercoids. On ingestion of a dog flea by a human, the cysticercoid larva penetrates the small intestinal mucosa and develops in situ into adult worms. Human infections particularly occur in children, who have more intimate contact with household pets. Symptoms are usually minimal or absent. In heavy infections, varying degrees of indigestion, appetite loss, and vague abdominal discomfort may be experienced.

Praziquantel is the treatment of choice; niclosamide is also effective. Human infection is preventable by keeping pet dogs and cats free of tapeworms and fleas.

Laboratory Identification

Ova (Egg Packets)
Adult Worm

- The strobila ranges from 15 to 70 cm in length and possesses 60 to 175 proglottides.
- The scolex is rhomboidal in shape, possessing a retractile conical armed rostellum.
- The proglottides measures 12×2.7 mm, and are distinctive for possessing a double genital pore (Dipylidium) (Color Plate 22-6*O*).
- Proglottides may detach from the strobila and migrate singly or as short chains from the anus of cats and dogs, appearing as tiny grains of rice when deposited on the carpet or floor.

Ova

The laboratory diagnosis in human infections is usually made by observing the characteristic egg packets microscopically, each of which:

- Contains 15–25 globular eggs (Color Plate 22-6*P*).
- Each egg measures 35–60 μm in diameter
- Each egg also contains an oncosphere with six hooklets.

Trematodes

The trematodes are a class of helminths including flukes that are parasites for humans. Flukes are leaflike and flat, hermaphroditic except for the Schistosomes, and possess two suckers—one oral, through which the digestive tract opens; the other ventral, for attachment. The trematodes of human importance to be presented in this chapter are:

The Schistosomes:	*S. mansoni, S. haematobium, S. japonicum*
Liver Flukes:	*Fasciola hepatica* and *Clonorchis sinensis*
Giant Intestinal Fluke:	*Fasciolopsis buski*
The Lung Fluke:	*Paragonimus westermani*

The life cycles of the flukes are similar, requiring two intermediate hosts before the stages infective for humans develop (*Schistosoma* species are an exception). The initial

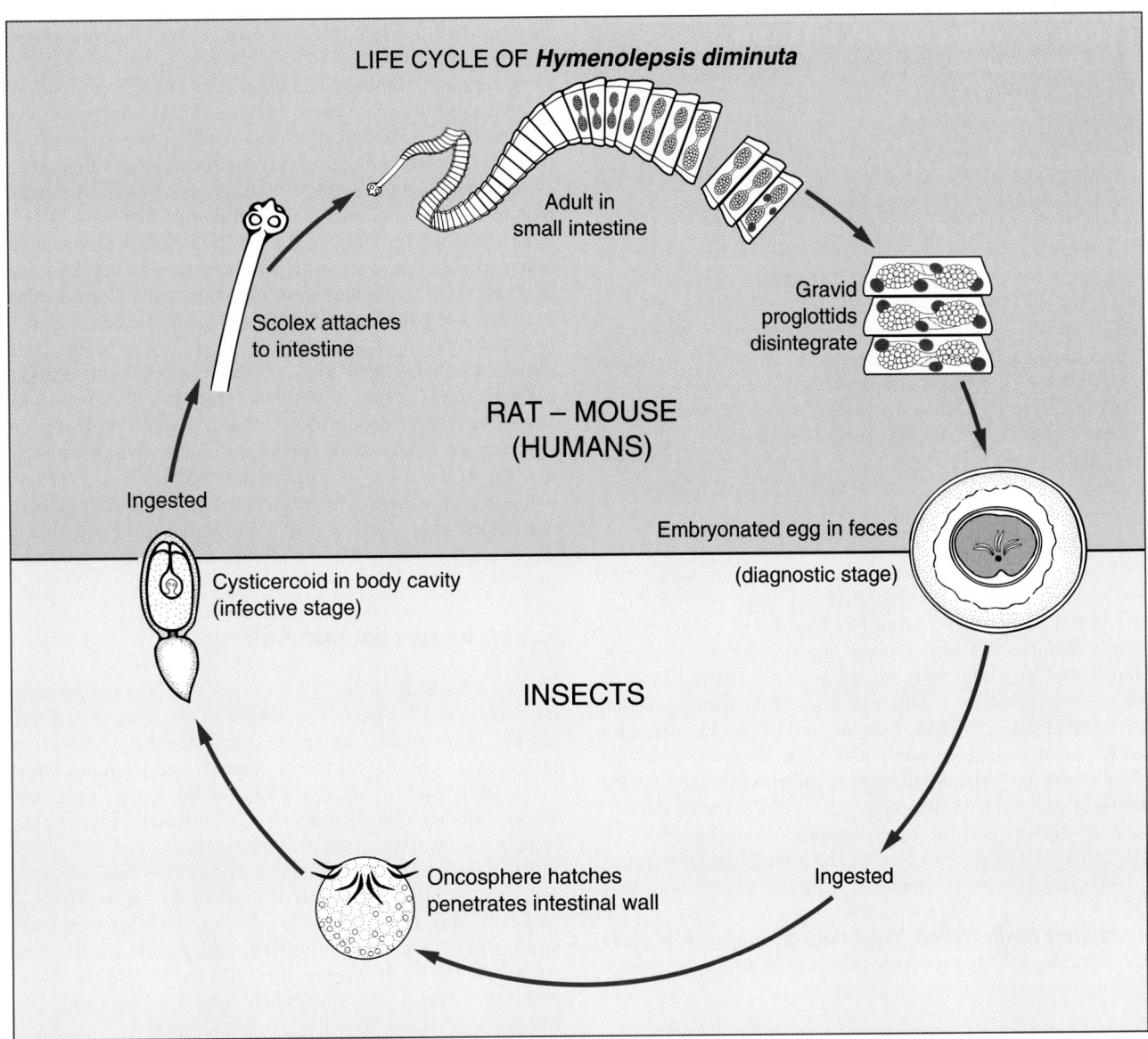

Figure 22-14 Life cycle of *Hymenolepis diminuta*. Embryonated eggs, passed into soil or water from an infected human via the feces, in turn are ingested by an insect. An oncosphere hatches in the intestine of the insect and penetrates the intestinal wall. An infective cysticercoid then develops in the body cavity. On the accidental ingestion of the infected insect by a human, larvae are released and penetrate the villi of the upper part of the small intestine. The scolex attaches to the intestinal mucosa, where they develop into adult worms. On maturity, embryonated eggs are released from gravid proglottids and passed in the feces, to complete the life cycle.

stages of the life cycles are virtually identical, with free-swimming miracidia released from gravid eggs discharged into appropriate water estuaries in the feces from an infected human. The developmental stages of the remaining stages in the life cycles of the trematode species included in this chapter are depicted in the life cycle drawings presented below.

Schistosomes

The name *schistosome* is derived from the appearance of the adult male, the body of which has a longitudinal genital groove, or canal, serving as a receptacle for the female during copulation (Color Plate 22-7A). Three *Schistosoma* species, *S. mansoni, S. haematobium,* and *S. japonicum,* cause the majority of human infections; *S. mekongi,* resembling *S. japonicum* and *S. intercalatum,* with ova resembling those of *S. haematobium* but a clinical illness mimicking *S. mansoni* infection, are two other species with limited geographic distributions in the Mekong basin and in Central and West Africa, respectively.[261] The life cycle is similar to that of other flukes except that a second intermediate host is not required to transmit disease. The *Schistosoma* life cycle is illustrated in Figure 22-15.

CLINICAL CORRELATION BOX 22-11
Hymenolepiasis

In contrast to infections with *Taenia* and *Diphyllobothrium* species, in which only one worm most commonly inhabits the intestine, up to 1,000 *H. nana* worms may be present. Symptoms in light infections may be absent or limited to mild, diffuse lower abdominal pain and loose stools. Anorexia, abdominal pain, diarrhea, headache, nervousness, and pruritus ani may be seen in heavy infections. Peripheral eosinophilia is mild to moderate (4–16%). Autoinfection, in which ova hatch in the intestine and reinfect via the normal life cycle described in the text, may result in a huge worm burden that can cause severe complications in immunosuppressed patients.

The treatment of choice is niclosamide, 2 g per day for 7 days, in adults, and 1 g initial dose, followed by 500 mg per day for 6 days in children.

Depending on the species, the schistosome adults may be in various locations in the portal vein system: 1) in the portal veins of the large intestine for *S. mansoni* and *S. intercalatum*, 2) in the small intestine for *S. japonicum* and *S. mekongi,* and 3) in the veins of the urinary bladder for *S. haematobium*. Although the adult worms, which measure about 2.5–3 cm in length and 0.5 mm in diameter when mature, may cause portal vein obstruction at the sites where they reside, disease is more commonly caused by the extensive tissue damage that results from the deposition of the myriad of eggs that are produced daily by the female.[261] A presentation of the clinical manifestations of schistosomiasis is found in Clinical Correlation Box 22-12.

Laboratory Identification. The laboratory diagnosis is made by detecting the characteristic ova in stool or, in cases of *S. haematobium* infections, in the urine.

Ova

- The eggs are very large. Following are the range of dimensions for each of three commonly encountered human species:
  - *Schistosoma mansoni*: 116–180 × 45–58 μm
  - *Schistosoma haematobium*: 112–180 × 40–70 μm
  - *Schistosoma japonicum*: 75–90 × 60–68 μm
- The eggs of *S. mansoni* and *S. haematobium* are distinctly oval.
  - The eggs of *S. mansoni* possess a prominent lateral spine (Color Plate 22-7*B*).
  - The eggs of *S. haematobium* possess a terminal spine (Color Plate 22-7*C*)
  - The eggs of the less commonly encountered species, *S. intercalatum,* also possess a terminal spine.
- The eggs of *S. japonicum* are broadly oval to semispherical; a small rudimentary, lateral, knoblike spine may be seen if the plane of focus is correct (Color Plate 22-7*D*).

A photomicrograph of a forked-tail cercaria, the infective form in the life cycle of Schistosoma species, is illustrated in Color Plate 22-7*E*.

Several immunologic techniques, including immunofluorescent antibody procedures, enzyme-linked immunosorbent assays, radioimmunoassays, and complement fixation are used in reference laboratories to help establish a diagnosis. Using a monoclonal antibody raised against a 15-kDa tegumental antigen of *S. mansoni* adult worms, Da Silva et al.[53] have developed a competitive enzyme-linked immunosorbent assay that they report as 94% sensitive in the detection of *S. mansoni* antibodies in infected patients. Considerable work has been done over the past decade by De Jonge et al.[62] in the serodiagnosis of schistosomiasis, using biotinylated monoclonal antibodies to detect both anodic and cathodic antigens in the serum of patients infected with *S. mansoni*. van Etten et al.[268] report 95.5% sensitivity and 96.7% specificity in the detection of schistosomal circulating cathodic antigen in the urine of patients infected with *S. mansoni,* using a monoclonal antibody-coated nitrocellulose/polyvinyl reagent strip. Such a strip is purported to be of value in the qualitative diagnosis of *C. mansoni* infections in control programs.

Fasciola hepatica and *Fasciolopsis buski*

Fascioliasis is primarily a cause of zoonotic parasitic liver disease in sheep. The adults of *Fasciolopsis buski,* on the other hand, remain in the intestine, where they attach to the mucosa of the duodenum and jejunum. Other herbivores, such as deer, rabbits, cattle, goats, pigs, and horses, among others, may also be infected. Flukes may remain in the bile ducts for many years, and can cause much damage from mechanical irritation at sites of local invasion, and the production of toxic by-products. *Fasciola hepatica* and *Fasciolopsis buski* are the two trematode species most commonly involved, and, except for the final habitat of the adult worms, their life cycles are the same. Both life cycles are somewhat complex, requiring two intermediate hosts. The life cycle of *Fasciola hepatica* is illustrated in Figure 22-16.

The clinical manifestations of fascioliasis and fasciolopsiasis are presented in Clinical Correlation Box 22-13.

Laboratory Identification

Adult Fluke

The adult flukes are seen only if removed at surgery. They can be recognized by:

- The *F. hepatica* adults, which measure 20–30 × 8–13 mm, are flattened and leaflike in appearance, having a cone-shaped anterior protrusion (Color Plate 22-7*F*); the adult flukes of *F. buski* have a rounded cephalic end (Color Plate 22-7*G*).
- Each adult fluke has an anterior and a ventral sucker and are hermaphroditic, with a convoluted uterus seen anteriorly.

Ova

The laboratory diagnosis is most commonly made by detecting eggs in fecal preparations. The eggs can be recognized by their:

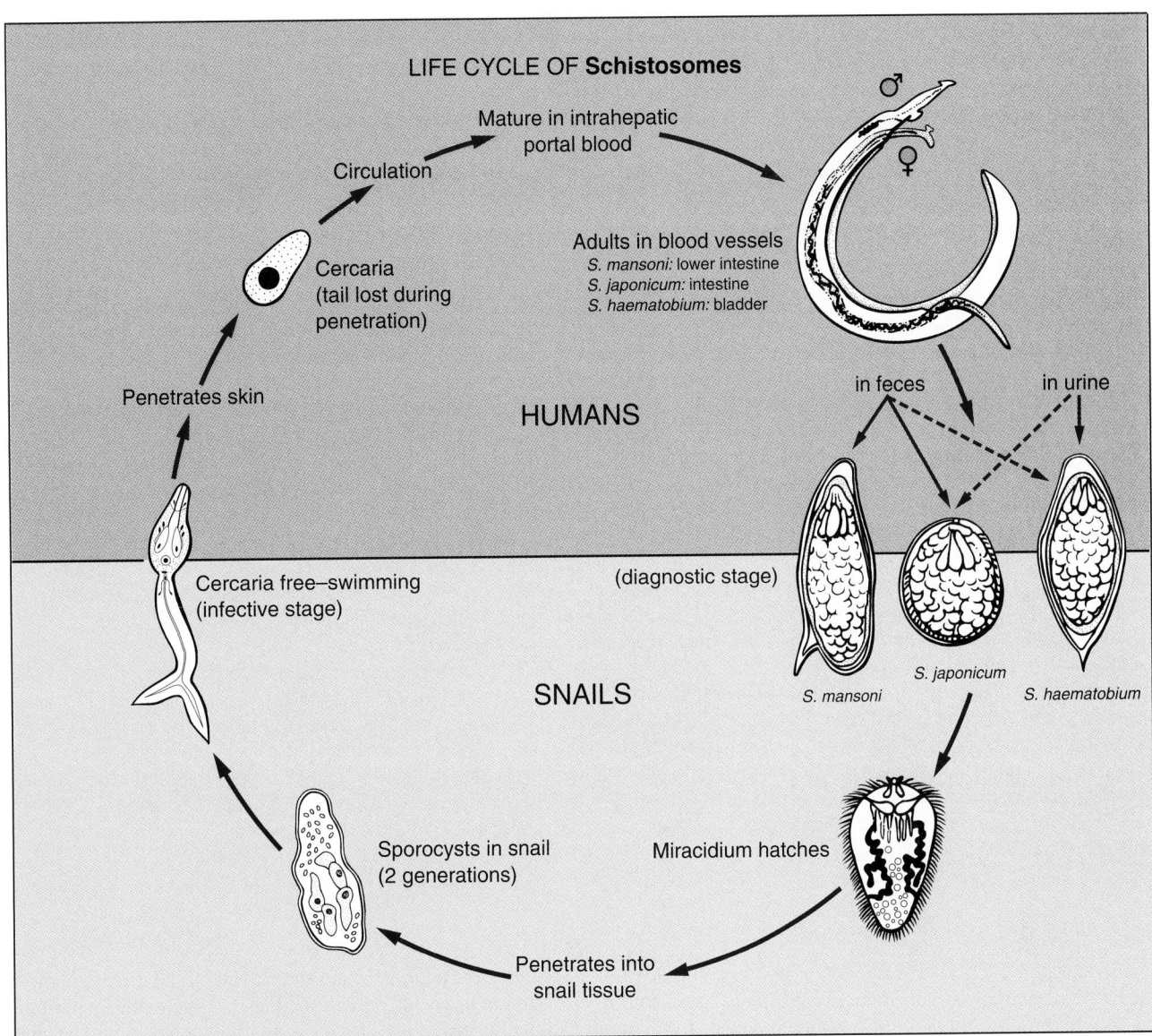

Figure 22-15 Life cycle of the schistosomes. Eggs that are passed in the feces into freshwater lakes, canals, and the like, hatch under suitable conditions, releasing a free-swimming miracidium. The miracidium penetrates the tissues of an appropriate species-specific snail, within which it undergoes maturation division to form hundreds of cercariae. The free-swimming cercaria, released from infected snails, have the capability to directly penetrate the water-softened skin of unsuspecting swimmers and waders in freshwater estuaries. Once in the subcutaneous tissues, the heads of the cercariae enter the circulation and migrate to the portal venous system, where they develop into adult male and female flukes. The females, occupying the gynecophoral canal of the male, produce a myriad of eggs that are released into an appropriate aquatic estuary to complete the life cycle.

- Very large size (150 × 80 μm), ovoid shape, and yellow-brown staining
- Thin, smooth shell, with an indistinct operculum at one of the narrow margins (Color Plate 22-7*H*).
- Internal cleavage material that is poorly organized and extends to the shell margin without leaving a clear space.

Because parasite eggs may be shed only after 8 weeks or more after infection or intermittently thereafter, sero-logic tests have been used in reference laboratories for the diagnosis of fascioliasis. Espino and Finlay[77] developed a mouse monoclonal antibody raised against *F. hepatica* excretory-secretory antigens, and a rabbit polyclonal antibody peroxidase conjugate detector to identify fasciola ES antigen in stool specimens. The authors indicated that their antigen-detection test had the advantage over several other antibody-detection methods because serum titers may re-

---

CLINICAL CORRELATION BOX 22-12 Schistosomiasis

Davis[57] has divided the clinical manifestations of schistosomiasis into four distinct stages, manifesting as symptoms that often overlap in individuals who are constantly reexposed to infection.

Stage 1: "Swimmer's Itch." Cercarial invasion early on produces a prickling sensation or itching of the involved skin. In nonimmune individuals, skin reactions, ranging from minute petechiae to urticaria or a pruritic papular eruption may be seen. The signs and symptoms of these eruptions are generally more severe in reaction to cercariae of nonhuman (bird) schistosomes. Davis-Reed and Theis[59] have reported a case of cutaneous *Schistosoma haematobium* infection that appeared as the sole clinical manifestation 3 years after exposure. These authors counsel that dermatologists should be reminded of schistosomiasis in patients who present with unusual skin lesions, particularly with a history of travel in endemic areas.

Stage 2: Katayama Syndrome. During the second, or maturation, stage, during which the schistosomes are migrating to their preferred anatomic sites and pairing preparatory to egg laying, symptoms may be minimal or develop into what has been referred to as the Katayama syndrome, characterized by varying degrees and combinations of fever, malaise, backache, arthralgia, anorexia, cough, headache, and toxemia. Mild hepatosplenomegaly may be detected, and peripheral blood eosinophilia may be significant. Because at this stage, eggs are often not yet excreted, the diagnosis may be dependent on eliciting a history of exposure, the presence of typical dermatitis, and one or more of the symptoms listed above.

Stage 3: Granulomatous Inflammation. The third stage involves the inflammatory reaction secondary to the deposition and migration of ova in the tissues. Egg deposition is approximately 300 per day for female *S. haematobium* and *S. mansoni* worms, and 3,000 per day for *S. japonicum*. After invading the wall of the veins in which the adult female resides, the ova have a propensity to penetrate into the adjacent viscera, eliciting a severe suppurative and granulomatous inflammation, ultimately resulting in fibrosis and scarring. Marked thickening of the walls of the intestine or urinary bladder, with loss of function, results. Bloody diarrhea, vague abdominal pain and in severe cases, bowel obstruction may be observed with *S. mansoni*, *S. japonicum*, and *S. mekongi* infections. *S. haematobium* produces inflammation of the urinary bladder, resulting in intermittent hematuria, lower abdominal pain, and ultimately, contraction.

Stage 4: Chronic Inflammation. In the fourth, or chronic, stage of disease, marked progressive fibrosis around the areas of granuloma occurs, with a marked decrease in the number of excreted ova. Patients with chronic *S. haematobium* infection have persistent urinary frequency and dysuria as the bladder continues to contract; and are also at high risk for carcinoma of the urinary bladder. In late-stage *S. mansoni* infections, hepatosplenomegaly, cirrhosis, and ascites are common complications, as the ova are swept upstream in the portal veins and lodge in the liver. Intestinal polyposis and inflammatory masses in the colon simulating carcinoma of the bowel may also be observed. *S. japonicum* may produce similar symptoms; however, because of its greater egg-laying capacity, morbidity may be much greater.

Praziquantel, 20 mg/kg taken orally for three doses spaced 8 hours apart, is the recommended treatment.

---

main elevated even after cure. They also cite the advantages of detecting antigen in stool specimens over serum as 1) avoiding the problem of immune complex formation that decreases the potential rate of detection, 2) circumventing venipuncture in many regions of the world where the procedure is objectionable, and 3) having a test readily available for cure.

Praziquantel, 25 mg/kg orally for three doses spaced 8 hours apart, is the recommended treatment.

Clonorchis sinensis

Clonorchis sinensis, the Chinese liver fluke, is a relatively small fluke that varies in size (12–20 × 3–5 mm) when mature and resides within the biliary ducts or in the gallbladder of humans. The life cycle is similar to that of *Fasciola hepatica*, except that a freshwater fish rather than water plants is used as the second intermediate host. Humans become infected with *C. sinensis* by ingesting the raw or poorly cooked flesh of several species of freshwater fishes. Figure 22-17 is an illustration of the life cycle.

The genus name (from the Greek *clon,* to divide, and *orchis,* testis) is derived from the freely branching testicular

organ in the adult hermaphroditic fluke. The disease is most common in a wide area of the Far East, particularly in Indochina, Japan, Korea, Formosa, and Southern China. The clinical manifestations of clonorchiasis are presented in Clinical Correlation Box 22-14.

Laboratory Identification

Adult Fluke

- The adult fluke is flat and flabby, ranging in size from 12–20 × 3–5 mm.
- A bottle-shaped, protruding head is seen at the cephalic end (Color Plate 22-7*I*).
- An anterior sucker leads to an esophagus that branches into blind ceca that extend laterally to the posterior end (Color Plate 22-7*J*).
- A ventral sucker is located just anterior to a loosely coiled uterus (Color Plate 22-7*K*).
- Immediately posterior to the uterus is the ovary connected to delicate vitelline ducts (Color Plate 22-7*L*).
- A highly branched testes, from which the genus name is derived, extends into the posterior part of the body (Color Plate 22-7*M*). The blind termination of the cecae and an ill-defined excretory bladder are also seen in this photograph.

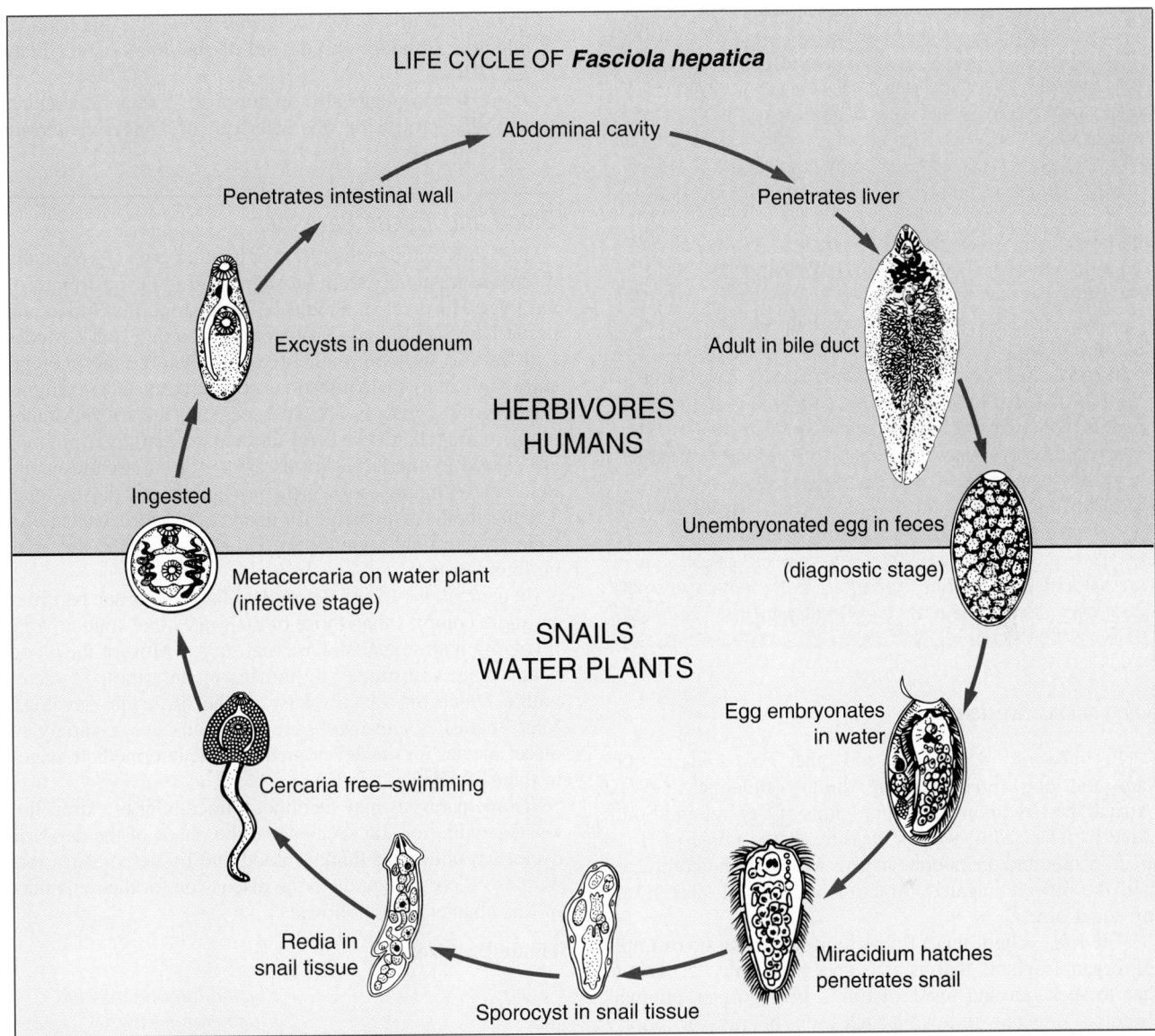

Figure 22-16 Life cycle of *Fasciola hepatica*. On discharge of mature ova into canals, lakes, streams, and the like, embryonated eggs hatch and release free-swimming miracidia. After burrowing into the flesh of an appropriate snail, sporocysts are formed in the tissue. Within the snail, maturation/multiplication takes place in the redia, ultimately leading to the release of hundreds of free-swimming, straight-tailed cercaria. The cercaria attach to water plants and encyst as infective metacercaria. Humans become infected by ingesting raw or undercooked, metacercaria-infested water plants. On ingestion, the metacercaria excyst in the human duodenum with the release of larval forms. These penetrate into the intestinal wall, transmigrate the abdominal cavity, and enter the liver, where mature flukes develop in the bile ducts. These flukes are hermaphroditic and release eggs into the lumen of the bile ducts. The eggs in turn are carried into the intestinal tract, where they are discharged in the feces, completing the life cycle.

The laboratory diagnosis is made by identifying the characteristic, small, urn-shaped eggs in stool specimens.

Ova

- The typical egg is relatively small, urn-shaped, and measures 27–35 × 14–16 μm.
- A light yellow-brown pigmentation is evident on bile staining.
- A prominent convex, shouldered operculum is a helpful identifying feature (Color Plate 22-7*O*).
- A small knob may be microscopically observed posteriorly when in the correct plane of focus.
- This egg is morphologically similar to those of *Heterophyes heterophyes* and *Metagonimus yokogawai*, two small intestinal flukes that are also prevalent in the Far East and infect humans who ingest raw or pickled fish.

CLINICAL CORRELATION BOX 22-13
Fascioliasis and Fasciolopsiasis

On ingestion of raw sheep or goat liver infected with adolescent worms, the flukes can attach to the pharyngeal mucosa and cause local laryngopharyngitis, called *halzoun*. Human fascioliasis is manifested by headache, chills, fever, and right upper quadrant pain. Hepatomegaly, jaundice, diarrhea, and anemia may occur in severe infections; hepatic biliary cirrhosis is a late complication. Praziquantel, 25 mg/kg three times a day for 6 days, is the recommended treatment regimen.

F. buski, a fluke similar to *F. hepatica* except that it is somewhat larger (20–75 mm × 8–20 mm) and has a rounded instead of a conical anterior portion (Color Plate 22–7G). These flukes reside in the small intestine and by means of a small oral sucker, attach to the intestinal mucosa. Local mucosal ulcers produce varying degrees of epigastric pain, nausea, and diarrhea, especially in the morning. Ascites and intestinal obstruction may be seen in heavy infections. Laboratory diagnosis is made by identifying the large eggs in the feces, which are identical in appearance to those of *F. hepatica*. Praziquantel in a single 25 mg/kg-dose is the recommended treatment.

Paragonimus westermani

Paragonimus westermani and other *Paragonimus* species are lung flukes causing disease endemic in West Africa, the Orient, and certain regions of Central and South America. The adult worms measure in the range of 8–16 × 4–8 mm and are spoon-shaped, with one end contracted and the other elongated. Anterior and ventral suckers are of equal size.

The life cycle of these flukes represent a classic example of organotropism; that is, the special affinity a parasite has to seek out and reside within a given organ. Humans become infected following ingestion of raw or poorly cooked crabmeat or crayfish, the flesh of which contain encysted metacercaria. Following ingestion, the metacercaria hatch in the duodenum, releasing larvae that attach to the duodenal mucosa. The larvae then penetrate the full thickness of the bowel wall and enter the abdominal cavity. They transmigrate the diaphragm and enter the pleural space. The larvae then bore into the peripheral lung tissue, where maturation takes place. Figure 22-18 is an illustration of the life cycle.

The clinical manifestations of paragonimiasis are presented in Clinical Correlation Box 22-15.

Laboratory Identification. The laboratory diagnosis is most commonly made by detecting the characteristics ova microscopically in stool preparations.

Ova

- The eggs range in size from 80 to 120 × 48 to 60 μm
- They are dark yellow-brown in color and have a thick, smooth shell with a prominent "shouldered" operculum.
- The shoulder serves to distinguish the *Paragonimus* ova

from those of *Diphyllobothrium latum*, the opercula of which are smooth and devoid of shoulders (Color Plate 22-7P).

- *P. westermani* eggs also do not possess an antiopercular, knoblike protrusion characteristic of *Diphyllobothrium* eggs.

Blood and Tissue Parasites

Parasites found in the blood or in other organs are usually discussed separately from those inhabiting the gastrointestinal tract. However, it should be understood that blood and tissue parasites include protozoa, nematodes, and cestodes with various forms of their life cycles that are morphologically similar to their intestinal counterparts. For example, *Toxoplasma gondii* is a tissue coccidia, the trypanosomes are hemoflagellates, visceral and cutaneous larval migrans are caused by the larval forms of dog or cat ascarid nematodes, and echinococcosis is the larval form of a dog cestode. The plasmodia responsible for malaria are sporozoa that also have an intestinal counterpart, *Isospora hominis*, that may be found in feces.

In general, the life cycles of the blood and tissue parasites are more complex than those of their intestinal counterparts, involving both sexual and asexual stages. Most of the blood parasites are transmitted to humans by an arthropod vector within which the sexual phase of the life cycle develops. Many parasites causing tissue infections use a variety of insect species for the development of the intermediate stages in their life cycles.

Tissue parasites may be either intracellular or extracellular, depending on the species and the phase of the parasitic cycle. An outline of human blood and tissue parasites that will also serve as a guide to the discussion for the remainder of this chapter, is as follows:

Tissue Protozoa

Malaria:	*Plasmodium falciparum*
	Plasmodium vivax
	Plasmodium malariae
	Plasmodium ovale
Babesia:	*Babesia microti*
Leishmaniasis:	*Leishmania donovani*
	Leishmania tropica
	Leishmania brasiliensis
	Leishmania mexicana
Trypanosomiasis:	*Trypanosoma brucei gambiense*
	Trypanosoma brucei rhodesiense
	Trypanosoma cruzi
	Trypanosoma rangeli
Filarial Nematodes:	*Wuchereria bancrofti*
	Brugia malayi
	Loa loa
	Mansonella ozzardi
	Mansonella perstans
	Onchocerca volvulus
	Dirofilaria immitis
Tissue Coccidia:	*Toxoplasma gondii*
	Pneumocystis carinii

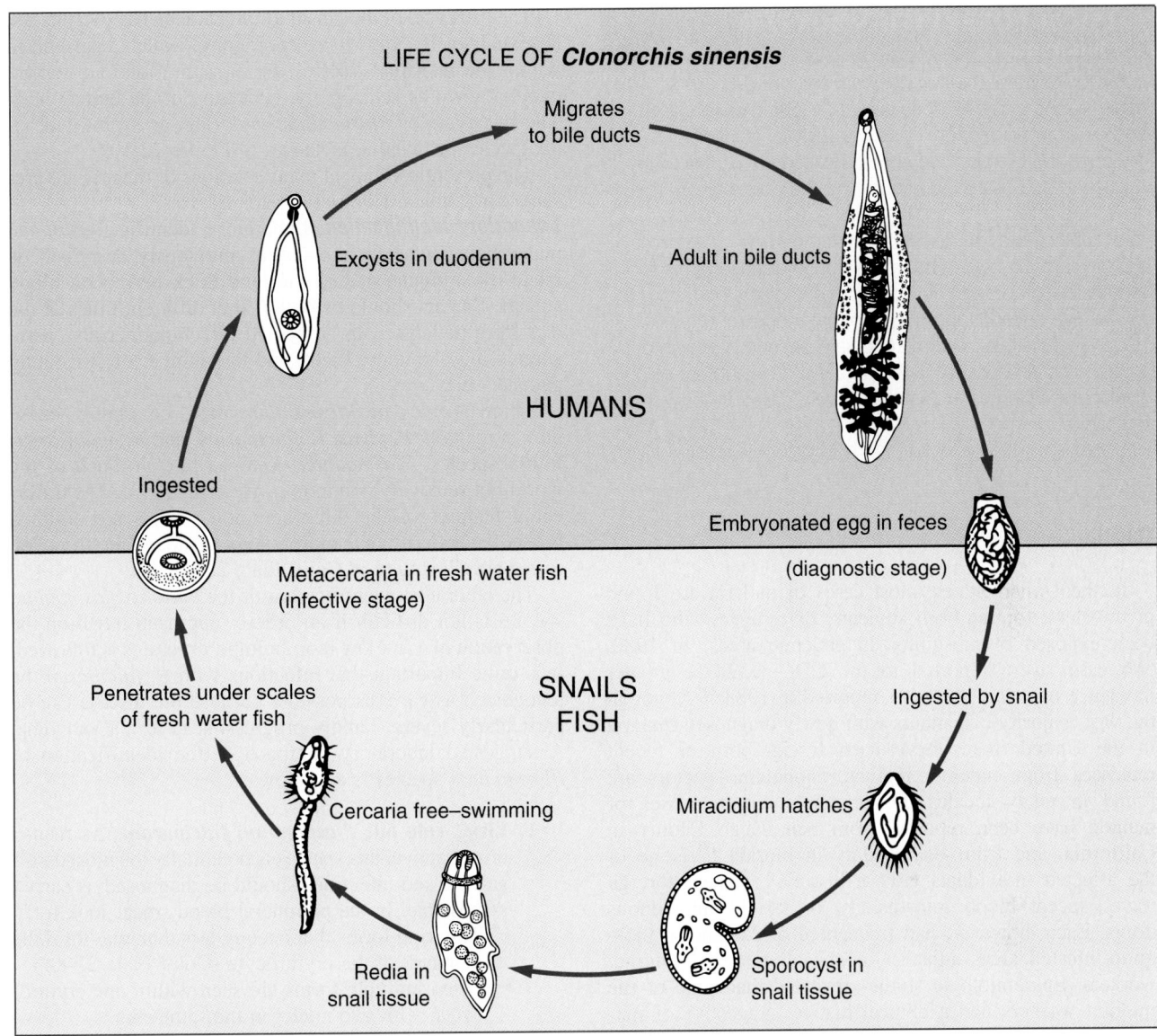

Figure 22-17 Life cycle of *Clonorchis sinensis*. On discharge of mature ova into canals, lakes, streams, and the like, embryonated eggs hatch and release free-swimming miracidia. The miracidia are ingested by an appropriate snail, within which it hatches and forms a sporocyst in the snail tissue. The sporocyst in turn matures into redia, within which maturation/multiplication takes place, leading to the release of hundreds of free-swimming, straight-tailed cercaria. The cercaria attach to and penetrate under the scales of several fresh-water fish species, forming metacercaria. Humans become infected by ingesting raw or undercooked, metacercaria-infested fish flesh. On ingestion, the metacercaria excyst in the human duodenum, with the release of larval forms that migrate into the bile ducts. These flukes are hermaphroditic and release eggs into the lumen of the bile ducts. The eggs in turn are carried into the intestinal tract, where they are discharged in the feces, completing the life cycle.

Tissue Nematodes:

Trichinella spiralis
Toxocara canis (visceral
    larva migrans)
Ancylostoma braziliensis or
    A. caninum
    (cutaneous larva migrans)
Dracunculus medinensis

Tissue Cestodes:

Anisakis species
Gnathostoma species
Echinococcus granulosus
Echinococcus multilocularis
Multiceps spp. (coenurosis)
Spirometra mansonoides
    (sparganosis)

CLINICAL CORRELATION BOX 22-14
Clonorchiasis

In light infections, the parenchymal liver cell damage is minimal, and cirrhosis does not occur. Slight leukocytosis and eosinophilia may be observed early in infection. Although the bile ducts in human infections may become thickened and dilated, particularly at the points where the flukes are attached to the inner lining, biliary obstruction and jaundice are rare except in extremely heavy infections (Color Plate 22–7N). In most cases, the disease tends to remain low-grade and chronic, with organisms persisting for four or five decades, producing only minor symptoms of abdominal distress, intermittent diarrhea, and liver pain or tenderness. Of concern is the potential development of cholangiocarcinoma in association with chronic Clonorchis infections[241,245]

Malaria

In the United States, most cases of malaria are found in travelers, foreign-born students, or refugees who have been exposed to mosquitos in endemic areas. In 1980, 566 cases were reported to the CDC, a 243% greater incidence over the 165 cases reported in 1988.[31] Although the vast majority of patients with newly diagnosed malaria in the United States have been foreign-born or recent returnees from endemic regions, anopheline vectors are found in many locales. For example, cryptic cases of malaria have been reported from San Diego County in California, and from Bay County in Florida.[100] None of the affected individuals gave a history of recent foreign travel, recent blood transfusions, or use of intravenous drugs. Each, however, had frequented or camped in mosquito-infested areas adjacent to encampments of migrant workers. Epidemiologic studies revealed that none of the migrant workers had a clinical history suggestive of malaria; however, the competent mosquito vector, *Anopheles hermsi*, was found along the San Luis Rey River in California. More recently, two cases of indigenous malaria were reported from Suffolk County, New York, in persons who had no history of travel outside the United States.[33] The conclusion from study of these isolated cases is that malaria must be included in the differential diagnosis of any patient with acute onset of cyclic fever, even if there is no history of recent foreign travel.

The worldwide prevalence of malaria is in the neighborhood of 100 million; 1 million deaths a year occur in Africa alone. Most cases occur in refugees, principally from Southeast Asia. Clinicians must, therefore, remain alert to the possibility of malaria in certain population groups. Although great progress in the elimination of malaria from certain locales has been made, malaria remains on the move, and reemergence of infection is of modern concern. Martens and Hall[179] attribute this resurgence in malaria to the relocation of poor people, often more likely to be infected with malaria, from endemic areas to malaria-free locales in search of a better life. The clinical manifestations of malaria are presented in Clinical Correlation Box 22-16.

The life cycle of the plasmodium parasite has two phases: a sexual cycle, known as sporogony, which takes place within the intestinal tract of the mosquito; and an asexual cycle, known as schizogony, occurring in the human host. The life cycle of *Plasmodium malariae*, as a prototype of all species of malaria, is shown in Figure 22-19.

The presenting clinical manifestations of malaria are presented in Clinical Correlation Box 22-16.

Laboratory Identification. Laboratory identification of the malarial parasites in humans, as previously described, is made by studying stained thin and thick peripheral blood smears. Smears should be obtained at different times of the day from patients with suspected infections because parasitemia may be intermittent, and the number of circulating parasites may vary.

Three species of *Plasmodium* most commonly cause human malaria; *P. vivax, P. falciparum,* and *P. malariae*. A fourth species, *Plasmodium ovale*, is rare in much of the world but relatively common in western Africa. The differential features of the three common species are outlined below. The microscopic morphology of the intraerythrocytic forms are illustrated in Color Plate 22-8.

The laboratory identification of the various *Plasmodium* species is not difficult if an orderly approach based on the observation of a few key morphologic structures is followed. It is quite important that infections with *P. falciparum* be recognized as early as possible because the disease can be particularly severe, rapidly progressing to a fatal outcome. A suggested laboratory approach to the identification of *Plasmodium* species is as follows:

1. **First, rule out *Plasmodium falciparum.*** As mentioned above, this species is potentially the most dangerous, and infections should be diagnosed as early as possible. In the peripheral blood smear look for:
   - Tiny ring forms that occupy less than one-third the diameter of the erythrocyte (Color Plate 22-8*A*).
   - Often multiple forms are seen within one erythrocytes; with two nuclei in the same ring.
   - Infections may be heavy, involving 20% or more of the erythrocytes, indicating a fulminant infection.
   - The tiny rings often are plastered on the erythrocyte cell membrane, known as an "appliqué" effect (Color Plate 22-8*B*).
   - Developing ring forms or schizonts are rarely observed in stained peripheral blood smears. The only forms usually seen, except in terminal, fulminant infections, are early ring forms and gametocytes.
   - The presence of banana- or crescent-shaped gametocytes is diagnostic (Color Plate 22-8*C*). These may be absent in early stages of infection and usually begin to appear only after 7–10 days after onset of fever.
2. If the above picture is not seen, next make an objective identification of *Plasmodium vivax.* Look for:
   - Infected erythrocytes that are somewhat irregular in shape, enlarged, pale, and contain prominent pink-red staining granules, called Schüffner's dots (Color Plate 22-8*D*).
   - Ring forms in all stages of development may be present.

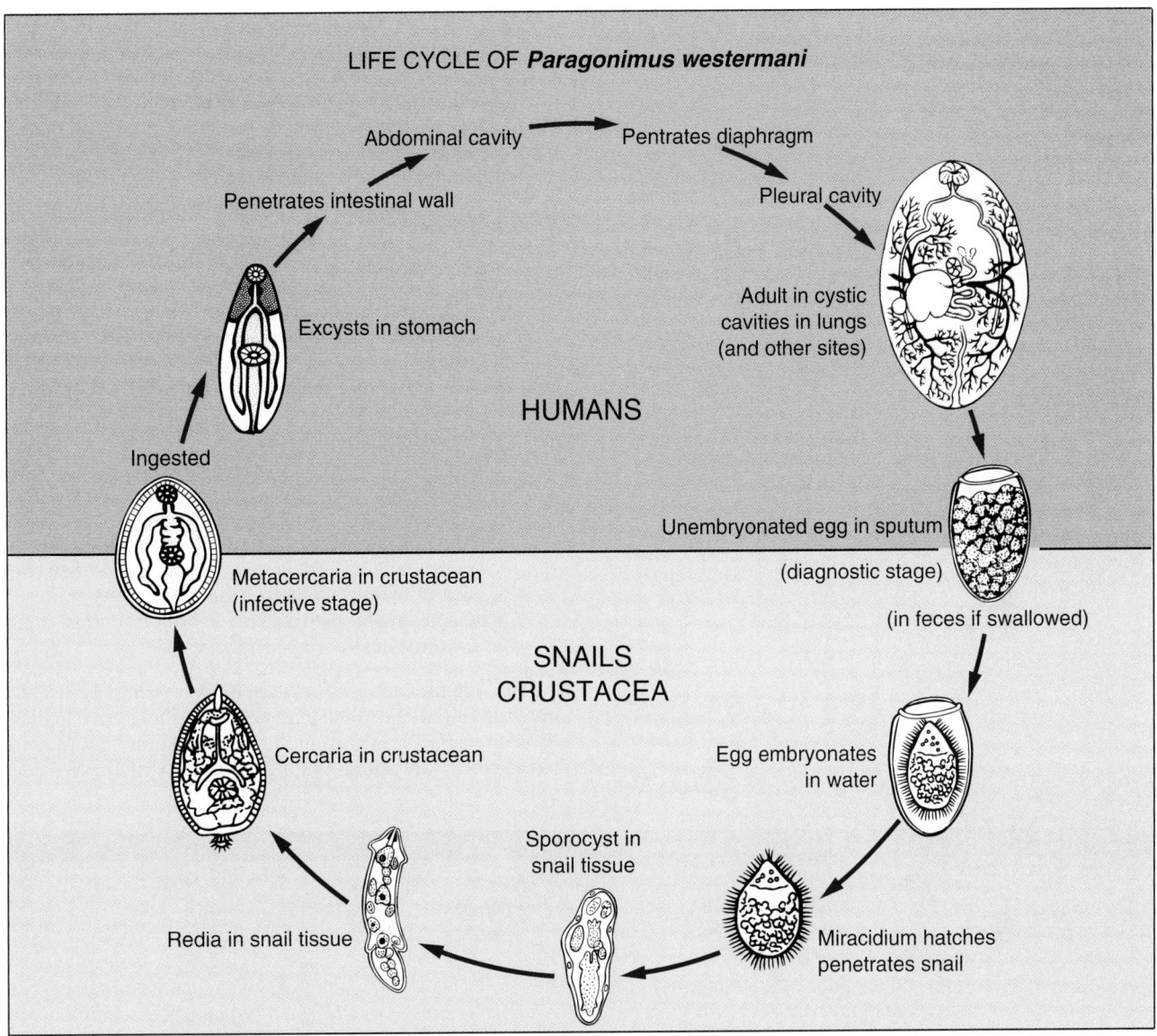

Figure 22-18 Life cycle of *Paragonimus westermani*. Nonembryonated eggs are discharged either in the sputum and/or in the feces into a water environment. These eggs then embryonate in the water, releasing a free-swimming miracidium that penetrates the tissues of a species-specific snail. Sporocysts and redia develop in the snail, within which cercaria replicate. When mature, free-swimming cercaria break out of the snail and penetrate the gills, muscles, or viscera of a freshwater crustacean, within which they encyst as dormant metacercaria. Humans become infected following ingestion of raw or poorly cooked metacercaria-infested crabmeat or crayfish. Following ingestion, the metacercaria hatch in the duodenum, releasing larvae that penetrate the full thickness of the bowel wall, enter the peritoneal cavity, transmigrate the diaphragm, and enter the pleural space. The larvae then bore into the peripheral lung tissue, where they mature into adult flukes that reside within parabronchial cysts. Eggs are released into the sputum, where they are either expectorated, or swallowed to ultimately pass in the feces, to complete the life cycle.

- Young rings measure greater than one-third the diameter of the infected erythrocyte.
- As the trophozoites mature, they begin to fill the erythrocyte with "flowing" or "ameboid" cytoplasm.
- The presence of more than one nucleus in a trophozoite indicates the formation of an early segmented

form, known as a schizont. The schizonts of *P. vivax* are comprised of 12–14 or more individual segments known as merozoites (Color Plate 22-8*E*).
- Gametocytes are large and circular (*Note:* Any single-celled nucleus occupying more than half the cell diameter is a gametocyte.)
- Trophozoites can always be distinguished from ga-

CLINICAL CORRELATION BOX 22-15
Paragonimiasis

Chills, fever, and marked eosinophilia may be seen during the migratory phase of the worm. In time, the adult fluke comes to reside within a small pseudocyst in the lung tissue. The cyst enlarges as the adult fluke grows and may break into an adjacent bronchiole. When a pseudocyst ruptures into a bronchus, coughing and hemoptysis are common symptoms. Eggs produced by mature flukes are discharged into the bronchi and are ultimately swallowed by the patient from secretions coughed into the oropharynx.

The disease tends to become chronic, leading to varying degrees of pulmonary fibrosis and scarring. Intermittent chest pain, fever, and chills may be late manifestations. Abdominal paragonimiasis may occur if the fluke remains localized to the abdomen. Dull abdominal tenderness and bloody diarrhea are the chief symptoms. Rare cases of cerebral disease have been reported, which must be differentiated from echinococcosis. Praziquantel, 25 mg/kg three times a day for 2 days, followed by 30–50 mg/kg every other day for 10–15 days, is recommended.

metocytes because, by the time it reaches the size of half the diameter of the cell, more than one nuclear segment would be observed (Color Plate 22-8*F*).
- Malarial pigment in the form of finely granular, brownish pigment may be abundant in both the gametocyte and the schizont.
3. Although the identification of *Plasmodium malariae* is often by exclusion after the characteristics of *P. falciparum* and *P. vivax*, as above described, have been ruled out, look for the following features by which an objective identification can be made:
    - The presence of developing trophozoites that extend to the borders of the erythrocyte membrane, producing bridging "bands" (Color Plate 22-8*G*).
    - The infected erythrocytes are neither enlarged nor pale.
    - Schüffner's dots are absent.
    - Schizonts comprised of no more than 6–12 segments, with the nuclear segments arranging to form a "rosette" (Color Plate 22-8*H*).
    - Malarial pigment is abundant and more coarse (or even "chunky") than seen with *P. vivax*, often condensed within the hof of the gametocytes.
    - Gametocytes are contained within normal-sized erythrocytes free of Schüffner's dots.

The identification of *Plasmodium* species is usually not difficult if the principles describe above are applied. Problems arise, however, in the interpretation of peripheral blood smears in patients who have been partially or inade-

CLINICAL CORRELATION BOX 22-16 Malaria

Fever is the constant presenting symptom of infections with all *Plasmodium* species. Temperature spikes commence 7 to 10 days following the bite of an infected anopheles mosquito during a period when the organisms are undergoing preerythrocyte multiplication in the cells of the liver. Prodromal symptoms of headache, myalgia, malaise, and fatigue suggestive of a flulike syndrome may be experienced during this period. However, once a brood of merozoites leaves the hepatic cells and invades the erythrocytes, the regularly spaced fever cycles begin. The periodicity of each episode of high fever is related to the rupture of erythrocytes as merozoites are released into the circulation. The designations of this fever cycle, "tertian" malaria, for *Plasmodium vivax* and *Plasmodium falciparum* malaria, and "quartan" malaria for *Plasmodium malariae* malaria is somewhat confusing. The fever spikes for tertian malaria occur on an every-other-day schedule; however, because any given fever episode is counted as day 1, the next spike will not occur until the third day (thus, tertian). Similarly, the fever spikes of quartan malaria occur on an every-three-day cycle; however, counting the first episode as day 1, the next spike will occur on the fourth day. Such classic fever patterns, however, may often be irregular and cannot be relied on exclusively to make a presumptive diagnosis.

Each fever episode is characterized by a short "cold" period lasting for approximately 1 hour, when the skin is cold and the lips and nailbeds appear cyanotic because of peripheral vasoconstriction. This short period is followed by the sudden onset of the "hot period," when the skin feels warm and dry and fever spikes up to 105 to 106°F are experienced, lasting 3–6 hours. Headaches, chest and back pain, tachycardia, cough, vomiting, and delirium of varying degrees of severity accompany the fever spikes. Fatigue and sleep follow each febrile episode. Patients are essentially asymptomatic between febrile episodes.

Hemolytic anemia, splenomegaly, and tender hepatomegaly are found to varying degrees. Patients are highly susceptible to rupture of the spleen, and deep palpation of the left upper abdomen and flank should be avoided during physical examination. Lymphadenopathy is absent and always points to some other condition if lymph nodes are enlarged. Of greatest concern are the central nervous system complications that may occur secondary to *P. falciparum* infections. The erythrocytes infected with *P. falciparum* trophozoites undergo membrane changes in which "knobs" appear on the surface, causing them to become "sticky" and adhere to specific receptors on the endothelial cell lining of capillaries.[40] The microcirculation of the brain is particularly vulnerable to blockage with *P. falciparum*–infected erythrocytes, resulting in small areas of cerebral infarction and hemorrhage.[4] Disturbances in consciousness ranging from somnolence to coma, behavioral changes, hallucinations, motor seizures, and occasionally tremors, focal muscle paralysis, and other localizing signs may be present. A rapidly progressive downhill course leading to death may occur in fulminant cases.

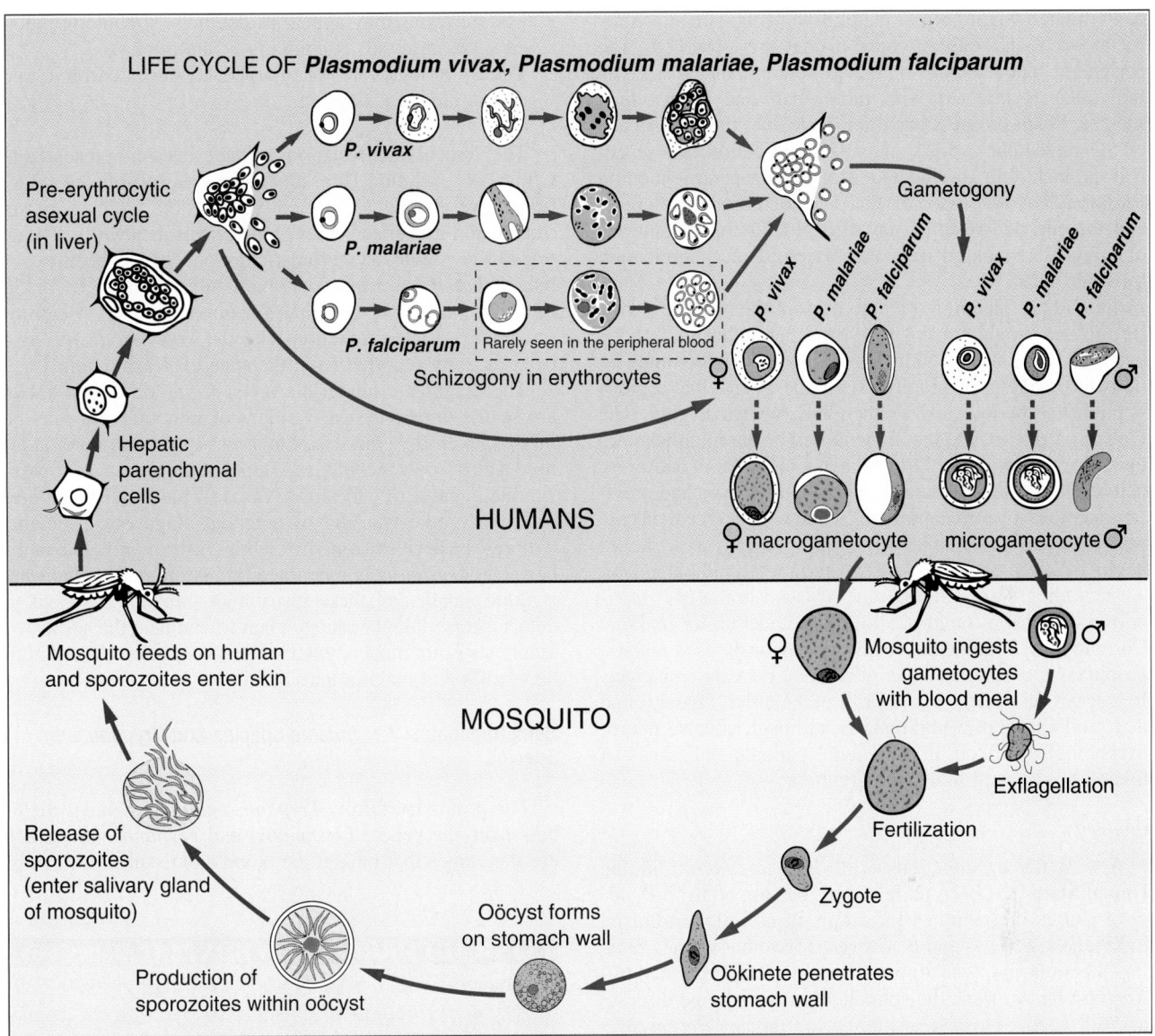

Figure 22-19 Life cycle of *Plasmodium malariae*. After several erythrocyte cycles have taken place, certain of the merozoites transform into sexual macrogametocytes (female) and microgametocytes (male). When a plasmodium-free mosquito bites a human infected with malaria), these gametocytes are ingested along with the trophozoite infected erythrocytes as part of the blood meal. In the stomach of the mosquito, the male microgametocytes develop six to eight flagella. The microgametocytes break free to penetrate the female macrogametocytes and produce fertilized zygotes. These zygotes then enter the wall of the mosquito stomach, where sporozoites eventually break out into the body cavity and migrate to the salivary glands. When the mosquito bites a new host, sporozoites are squeezed from the salivary glands and injected through the proboscis.

Sporozoites, the infective form for humans, are found in the salivary glands of female anopheline mosquitos. Saliva containing infective sporozoites is injected into the bloodstream of humans through the mosquito proboscis. After circulating in the peripheral blood for 20–30 minutes, the sporozoites enter the parenchymal cells of the liver, where they begin to multiply (the exoerythrocytic states). In about 10 days, multiple small forms, called merozoites, break out of the liver cells and are released into the circulation, where they seek out and penetrate erythrocytes. Within the erythrocytes (intraerythrocytic cycle), a series of developmental stages takes place (Color Plate 22-8). These organisms develop into a ''ring form'' known as the trophozoite, which, depending on the species, enlarges and divides into a segmented state known as the schizont. The individual segments of the schizonts are merozoites. When mature, the schizonts rupture the erythrocytes and merozoites are released into the circulation. These merozoites then seek out uninfected erythrocytes and the cycle continues.

quate treated when normal maturation of the parasites may be blocked and only atypical forms are observed. The peripheral blood picture may also be confusing if a given individual is infected with more than one *Plasmodium* species. Much progress has been made over the past decade in the molecular aspects of malarial infection. These advances, including an elucidation of the var genes encoding *Plasmodium falciparum* erythrocyte membrane protein 1, and the encoded rosettin and rifin proteins on the surface of infected red blood cells are reviewed in a publication by Chen et al.[38]

Individuals planning travel to parts of the world endemic for malaria should consult with local public health authorities for advice on protection and prophylaxis. Recommendations to travelers for prophylaxis while in endemic regions is published periodically by the CDC (www.cdc.gov). The type of prophylaxis to recommend will be based on whether the places of anticipated travel have a high risk of acquiring chloroquine-resistant malaria, whether the person had previous reactions to antimalarial drugs, and whether medical care will be readily available. Chloroquine prophylaxis should begin 1–2 weeks prior to anticipated travel and extend for 4 weeks after return. Chloroquine-resistant strains of *P. falciparum* have been found in all regions endemic for malaria. Currently, mefloquine has replaced previously used malaria prophylaxis drugs that have developed parasite resistance. In a series of clinical trials, Croft and Garner[46] have found that mefloquine prevents malaria, although adverse neuropsychological effects in occasional patients and issues of tolerability are still under investigation.

Babesia

The status of infections with *Babesia microti* in the United States has been reviewed by Persing et al.[209] *B. microti* causes most human infections in nonsplenectomized individuals; *B. bovis* and *B. divergens* are other species causing infections in splenectomized persons. *B. microti* shadows *Borrelia burgdorferi*, the spirochete causing Lyme disease, as both agents have the white-footed mouse, *Peromyscus leucopus*, as the main reservoir host. Most outbreaks have occurred in the northeastern regions of the United States, particularly in Connecticut, Nantucket Island, Long Island, and Cape Cod. The predominant vector for both agents is the *Ixodes dammini* tick, 40% of which are coinfected with both parasites. The much lower incidence of babesiosis relative to Lyme disease in humans living in endemic areas may reflect the tendency of *B. microti* to produce subclinical infections. Serologic studies indicate that 10% of *B. burgdorferi*–seropositive Connecticut natives also have antibodies against *B. microti*, indicating that infections are far more frequent than previously suspected.

Laboratory Identification.
The laboratory diagnosis is most commonly made by detecting the intraerythrocytic parasitic inclusions in stained peripheral blood smears. They have the following identifying characteristics:

- The ring forms are tiny, ranging between 1.0 and 3.0 μm, resembling the early trophozoites of *P. falciparum* (Color Plate 22-9*A*).
- The nuclei are very small, and one or two chromatin dots may be seen.

- Mature forms may appear as doublets, simulating rabbit ears; or, in tetrads resembling a Maltese cross.
- The erythrocytes are not enlarged, are normochromic, and do not develop stippling.

The clinical manifestations of babesiosis are presented in Clinical Correlation Box 22-17. Transfusion-related infections have also been reported; specifically, a cluster of six transfusion-associated cases of babesiosis in New York State traced to a single asymptomatic donor.[69] It has been established that *B. microti* can remain infective at 4°C for 30 days, the normal storage time for donor blood.[75] A case of transfusion-related infection with the WA1 strain has also been recently reported from the state of Washington.[130]

The diagnostic intraerythrocytic forms described above are scarce during the early stages of infection and may be missed, even by experienced microscopists. Mattia et al.[181] used a buffy-coat technique to improve the detection of parasitemia in cases of babesiosis. Garcia[96] has published a precautionary note warning of potential diagnostic problems with results derived from differential instruments. The number of fields routinely examined on instrument-read smears is quite small, and these instruments are not designed to detect intracellular parasites. Therefore, unless the suspected diagnosis is not made known to the laboratory, cases of both babesiosis and malaria may be missed.

Hemoflagellates: *Leishmania* Species and *Trypanosoma* Species

The protozoan family *Trypanosomatidae* includes members from the genera *Leishmania* and *Trypanosoma*, which are flagellates that inhabit the blood and tissues of humans.

CLINICAL CORRELATION BOX 22-17 Babesiosis

As pointed out by Persing et al.,[209] the symptoms in early babesiosis may be minimal: malaise, anorexia, and fatigue are nonspecific symptoms that are easily confused with other infectious diseases. Although the symptoms of infections incurred in the northeastern United States tend to be relatively mild, recent reports from case studies in California and other parts of the world indicate that fulminant, febrile, hemolytic disease presentations are more commonly encountered.[27,210] Genetic studies reveal that these more severe infections may be caused by a strain more closely related to a known canine pathogen, *B. gibsoni*, or to *Theileria* species, rather than *B. microti*.[209] This strain, designated WA1 (Washington 1), is currently under extensive investigation. Dorman et al.[71] report the case of a 58-year-old man, infected through a tick bite, in whom severe hemolytic anemia developed, followed by disseminated intravascular coagulation and acute renal and respiratory failure. Rapid clinical improvement was noted after treatment with clindamycin, 300 mg four times a day (started 2 days before admission), quinine (650 mg three times a day) on hospitalization, and an exchange transfusion, in which the proportion of parasitized red cells was reduced from 13.8% to 4.2%.

Four stages of development of the parasites may be observed. The adult, or trypanosomal, forms have an elongated body with a whiplike posterior flagellum attached by a delicate undulating membrane that runs the length of the body. Three species are associated with human disease, *Trypanosoma gambiense* and *Trypanosoma rhodesiense* cause African sleeping sickness, whereas *Trypanosoma cruzi* is responsible for South American trypanosomiasis. The least-developed form of these protozoa, called the amastigote or leishmanial forms, are devoid of flagella and are found as intracellular parasites in reticuloendothelial cells. *Leishmania donovani*, the cause of visceral kala-azar in humans, and *Leishmania tropica* complex, the agents of cutaneous tropical sores, are the leishmanial species most commonly associated with human diseases. *T. cruzi* also exists as a leishmanial form, infecting heart-muscle fibers or the cells of other visceral organs. The leptomonas and crithidial stages of development are harbored within the insect vector, the latter representing the infective form for humans.

LEISHMANIASIS AND *LEISHMANIA* SPECIES

Human leishmaniasis may take two forms, a disseminated disease, kala-azar, involving the liver, spleen and other parts of the reticuloendothelial system and a primary cutaneous form, clinically manifesting as ulcers or "sores" of the skin and mucous membranes (Color Plate 22-9*B*). Humans become infected through the regurgitation of the promastigotic infective forms of the parasite into the subcutaneous tissue at the time several species of *Phlebotomus* sandflies take a blood meal. Figure 22-20 depicts the life cycle of Leishmania species.

Visceral leishmaniasis is caused by several species belonging to the *Leishmania donovani* complex; namely, *L. donovani donovani*, *L. donovani infantum*, and *L. donovani chagasi*. When the flagellates gain access to humans, they first invade inflammatory monocytes in the subcutaneous tissue at the site of the bite. When these inflammatory cells rupture, they release free parasites that in turn invade other monocytes and macrophages, within which they are disseminated throughout the reticuloendothelial system. The incubation period is in the range of 3–8 months. Whether or not the disease progresses is dependent on the capability of the host's T-lymphocytes to activate macrophages to kill the parasites. The clinical manifestations of leishmaniasis are presented in Clinical Correlation Box 22-18.

Laboratory Identification. Disseminated leishmaniasis (kala-azar) is made by demonstrating amastigotes in stained smears, in imprints, or in biopsies of infected tissues. They have the following characteristics:

- The organisms are oval in shape, intracellular and very small, averaging 2–4 μm in size.
- They simulate the yeast cells of *Histoplasma capsulatum*.
- The leishmania amastigotes possess a barlike kinetoplast adjacent to the nucleus, a structure that is helpful in distinguishing these organisms from the yeast forms of *H. capsulatum* (Color Plate 22-9C, D, and *E*).

Cutaneous leishmaniasis The laboratory diagnosis is made by demonstrating intracellular leishmanial amastigotes in impression smears or tissue sections prepared from active lesions. Biopsies should be obtained from the elevated, inflamed margin of the lesion; aspirates should be obtained by extending the tip of the needle deep beneath the ulcer bed. Culture methods, used primarily in laboratories serving practices in endemic areas, are described in detail by Garcia.[96] Lopez-Velez et al.[170] also describe a culture method using buffy-coat samples from peripheral blood that was successful in diagnosing leishmaniasis in AIDS patients presenting with atypical clinical pictures. Animal inoculation techniques are also used in these laboratories for diagnosing infections when parasite concentrations are low.

ELISA techniques, using species-specific monoclonal antibodies and DNA probes have been successful in the direct detection of leishmania antigen in extracts of tissue samples in laboratories where reagents are available. Piarroux et al.[213] used a PCR assay amplifying a repeated sequence from the *Leishmania infantum* genome in a study of 73 patients with a working clinical diagnosis of visceral leishmaniasis; they demonstrated superior sensitivity of the method (82%) in making the diagnosis compared to examination of bone marrow aspirates (55%) and myeloculture (55%). They conclude that PCR may serve as an aid in diagnosing visceral leishmaniasis in immunocompromised patients. Rodriguez et al.,[226] using a PCR-hybridization technique, employing oligonucleotides directed against conserved regions of kinetoplast DNA, were able to detect the presence of Leishmania cells in 98% of patients clinically diagnosed as having cutaneous leishmaniasis by a positive Montenegro skin test. They further believe the technique is epidemiologically valuable in making the taxonomic discrimination between species.

TRYPANOSOMIASIS

Human trypanosomiasis is caused by a flagellate protozoan that inhabits the blood and tissues. The adult form, which measures 1.5–30 μm × 1.5–3.5 μm, has an elongated body with a whiplike posterior flagellum that is attached by a delicate undulating membrane that runs the length of the body. Wild game serve as the reservoir host. A central nucleus and a posterior kinetoplast are usually easily seen. These diagnostic forms can be readily seen in stained smears of peripheral blood (Color Plate 22-9*E*) and in the spinal fluid in cases of active infection. However, in chronic or light infections, Bailey and Smith,[12] in a study of blood samples obtained from 134 patients with *Trypanosoma gambiense* infection, found the quantitative buffy-coat test developed for malaria diagnosis to be the most sensitive diagnostic test for the detection of trypanosomal forms.

The life cycle involves animals and humans as the definitive hosts, in which the mature trypanosomes circulate and divide in the peripheral blood and ultimately invade the central nervous system; and an intermediate host, the tsetse fly, in which the immature forms develop in the salivary gland, ultimately forming infective metacyclic trypanomastigotes. The life cycle is illustrated in Figure 22-21.

The clinical manifestations of African trypanosomiasis are presented in Clinical Correlation Box 22-19.

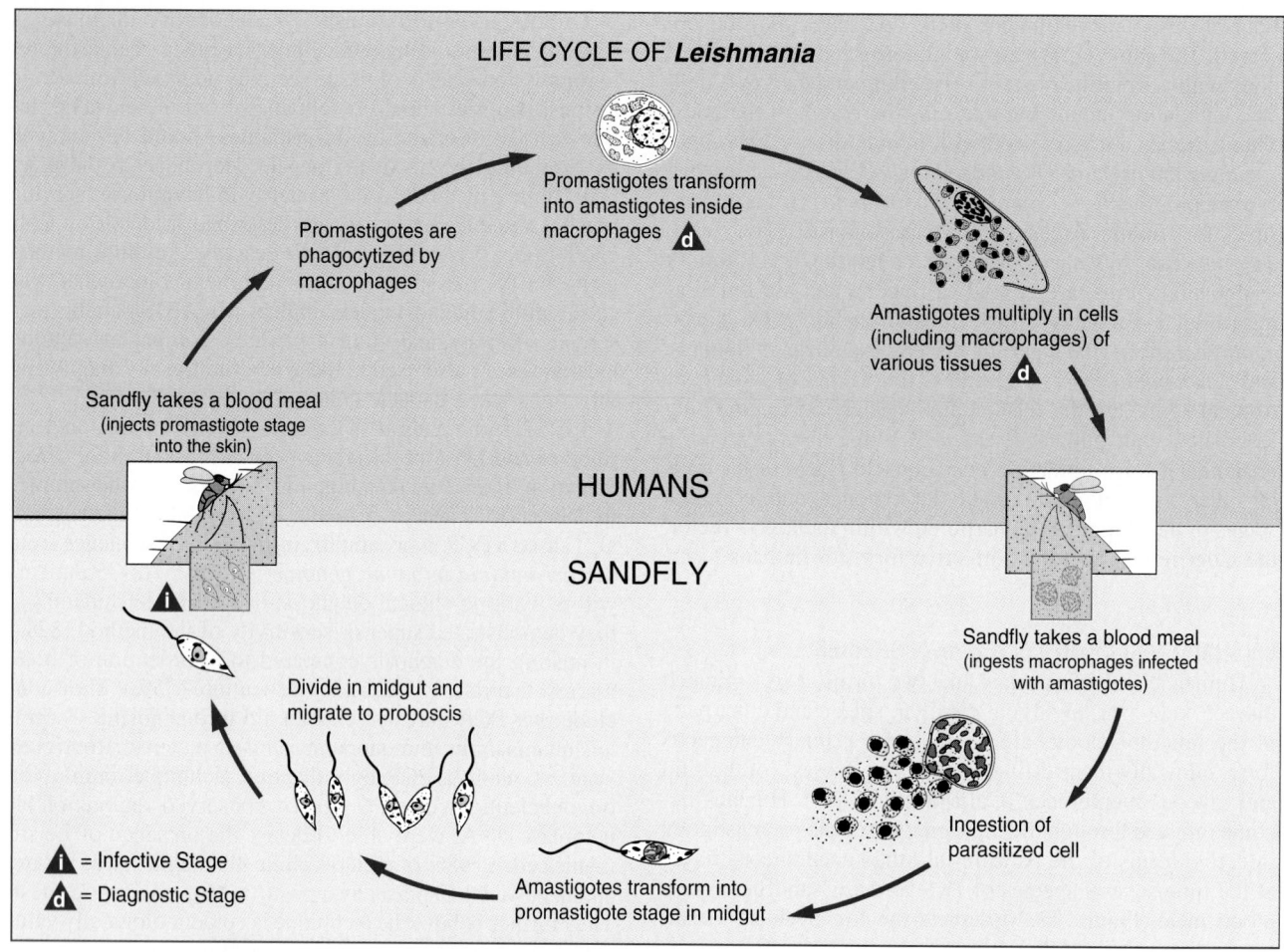

LIFE CYCLE OF *Leishmania*

Promastigotes transform
into amastigotes inside
macrophages **d**

Promastigotes are
phagocytized by
macrophages

Amastigotes multiply in cells
(including macrophages) of
various tissues **d**

Sandfly takes a blood meal
(injects promastigote stage
into the skin)

HUMANS

SANDFLY

Sandfly takes a blood meal
(ingests macrophages infected
with amastigotes)

Divide in midgut and
migrate to proboscis

Ingestion of
parasitized cell

i = Infective Stage

d = Diagnostic Stage

Amastigotes transform into
promastigote stage in midgut

Figure 22-20 Life cycle of *Leishmania* species. A small skin papule develops at the site of the sandfly bite, but rarely progresses to an ulcer. The promastigotes transform into amastigotes, which proliferate locally in the subcutaneous tissue into amastigotic forms that disseminate throughout the reticuloendothelial system to involve the spleen, liver, bone marrow and lymph nodes where the organisms are found as obligate intracellular parasites (Color Plate 22-9*C*). The simple life cycle is then completed when amastigotes are again taken up by a sandfly during a subsequent blood meal. The amastigotes transform into infective promastigotes in the midgut of the fly.

In a World Health Organization report issued in 1986, approximately 50 million people were considered to be at risk for African trypanosomiasis; 20,000 new cases were being diagnosed each year.[295] In the African form of the disease, humans become infected through the bites of infected *Glossina* tsetse flies that harbor the infective procyclic trypanomastigotes in their salivary glands. Tsetse flies are found only in Africa. This capacity of these organisms to remain viable in a population of chronically infected people is due to the unique property of periodically changing their antigenic structure of the glycoproteins within their surface membranes, thus bypassing the effects of host antibodies.[70]

Antigen-detection methods have been developed to diagnose African trypanosomiasis. In a field trial in Zaire, Nantulya et al.[195] effectively used an antigen ELISA in evaluating 77 parasitologically proven cases of Gambian trypanosomiasis. Of these patients, 69 (89.6%) had antigens in serum and 35 (45.5%) had antigens in the CSF. Of the latter, 34 (97.1%) had elevated CSF white-cell counts, 29 (82.9%) had elevated protein levels and 23 (65.7%) had trypanosomes microscopically identified in the CSF. The authors indicate that their ELISA test may be useful in staging disease and in follow-up to treatment. Kyambadde et al.[159] found that PCR demonstrated infection in 20 of 35 (57%) blood samples obtained from patients with suspected trypanosomiasis in Uganda, and in 21 of 34 CSF samples (61%). Of 21 blood samples negative for circulating diagnostic forms, 6 were positive by PCR (28.6%); and 8 of 21 CSF samples (38.0%) that were negative by double centrifugation were positive by PCR.

Either suramin or pentamidine is the drug of choice in the treatment of African trypanosomiasis. Melarsoprol may be used in later stages with CNS disease.

South American Trypanosomiasis: Chagas' Disease. South American trypanosomiasis, also known as Chagas' disease, caused by *Trypanosoma cruzi*, is found from the southern United States through Latin and South America to Argen-

CLINICAL CORRELATION BOX 22-18 Leishmaniasis

Disseminated Leishmaniasis: Kala-Azar

Symptoms may be mild and self-limited in light, contained infections. Or, there may be a sudden onset of symptoms, including spiking fevers (a pattern of two or three peaks per day), anorexia, malaise, and a feeling of ill health, simulating typhoid fever or malaria. If the disease progresses and becomes chronic, low-grade fever, vague abdominal pain, enlargement of the abdomen from hepatomegaly and splenomegaly (which can become enormous), generalized lymphadenopathy, anemia, and leukopenia may persist. Recently kala-azar has been recognized as an AIDS-related opportunistic infection.[191]

Primary Cutaneous Leishmaniasis

Disease is classified into Old World and New World forms. Old World disease, called Oriental sore, is caused most commonly by members of the *L. tropica* complex (including *L. major, L. tropica minor,* and *L. aethiopica).* This form of disease is endemic in the tropical and subtropical regions of Asia Minor, China, the Southern Mediterranean, India, and Africa. At the site of insect bites on exposed parts of the body, the promastigotes injected into the skin are taken up by the reticuloendothelial cells, where they develop into the amastigotes. The species causing cutaneous leishmaniasis do not circulate except in very rare instances. An intensely pruritic papule develops at the site of the bite, which in the course of several weeks or months progresses to a chronic well-circumscribed ulcer with a raised, erythematous margin and a shallow bed (Color Plate 22–6J). The ulcers caused by *L. major* tend to be moist and multiple; those of *L. tropica* minor are drier and tend to crust over. Most lesions are benign and self-healing, and permanent immunity develops. The cutaneous lesions of *L. aethiopica* may not ulcerate but often result in deep, spreading subcutaneous infections, and this species also has the predilection for causing disseminated disease indistinguishable from *L. donovani* infections.[207]

New World cutaneous leishmaniasis is caused by the *L. braziliensis* complex (also including *L. braziliensis guyanensis* and *L. braziliensis panamensis),* which is endemic in almost all states in South America and in several regions in Latin America, and by the *Leishmania mexicana* complex, including several separate species endemic in various regions in Mexico, Guatemala, Venezuela, and in the Amazon basin of Brazil. The *L. braziliensis* complex of organisms cause aggressive, chronic cutaneous ulcers, with mucous membrane (oral, nasal, pharyngeal) spread, a clinical picture called espundia. Organisms of the *L. mexicana* complex are more likely to produce self-limiting cutaneous ulcers (60% of lesions occur on the ear lobes[96] producing what are known as "Chiclero ulcers"). The mucous membranes are less commonly involved, although *L. peruviana* is likely to produce a more diffuse cutaneous disease known as "uta" in Peru.

Stibogluconate sodium is the treatment of choice.

---

tina. An estimated 10–12 million people are infected, approximately half of whom live in Brazil.[66] Although *T. cruzi* has been found in dogs, wild mammals, and insect vectors in the southern part of the United States, autochthonous human cases have been reported only very rarely.[117,263] The diagnosis may be made by observing circulating trypomastigotes in the peripheral blood, although the period of circulation is shorter than that observed in African trypanosomiasis. The trypomastigotes are similar in appearance to those of their African counterparts, except there is a distinct tendency to form the letter "C" (Color Plate 22-9G).

The latest reported case in the United States was in rural Tennessee, when a mother found a triatomine bug in the crib of her 18-month-old boy.[129] The gut content of the bug was found to be infected with *Trypanosoma cruzi* both by light microscopy and PCR. A buffy coat prepared from a blood sample from the child was negative for organisms; however, it was positive by PCR, indicating low-level parasitemia. Thus, this fifth reported case of autochthonous *T. cruzi* infection in the United States would have been missed without the mother's attentiveness and the highly sensitive PCR technique.

Both rodents and domestic animals, including dogs, cats, and pigs, serve as reservoir hosts for *T. cruzi.* In the United States, opossums and raccoons have been found to be infected. In the case reported above, three raccoons in the vicinity of the target case had positive hemocultures for *T. cruzi.* Houses built of adobe, mud, or vegetative material, in which there are numerous cracks in the walls, provide the optimal breeding places for the reduviid bugs (Color Plate 22-9H). The bugs are nocturnal and attack sleeping victims. Prevention of the disease is therefore aimed at improving housing conditions.

The life cycle of *T. cruzi* differs from the African species in that the triatomid (reduviid) bug serves as the arthropod vector and that visceral organs may be infected with the leishmanial form of the parasite. The life cycle is illustrated in Figure 22-22.

The clinical presentations of South American trypanosomiasis are found in Clinical Correlation Box 22-20.

Trypanosoma rangeli is another trypanosomal organism transmitted to humans by reduviid bugs. Human infections are usually asymptomatic. The trypanomastigotes can be identified in thick and thin smears of peripheral blood and morphologically resemble those seen in African trypanosomiasis. However, unless a careful clinical history is obtained, a misdiagnosis of *T. cruzi* infection may be made. Serologic testing may be of value in differentiating *T. rangeli* infections from Chagas' disease; however, double infections may occur producing confusing results.

Serodiagnostic methods are being developed to detect *T. cruzi* serum antibodies to aid in the diagnosis of Chagas' disease. Godsel et al.[101] identified in the serum of patients with Chagas' disease a new recombinant antigen called FCaBP, a 24-kDa flagellar calcium binding protein. This protein may be used as a component of a multiple-recombinant antigen preparation effective in screening for *T. cruzi* in donor blood supplies. Tantowitz et al.,[263] in a comprehensive

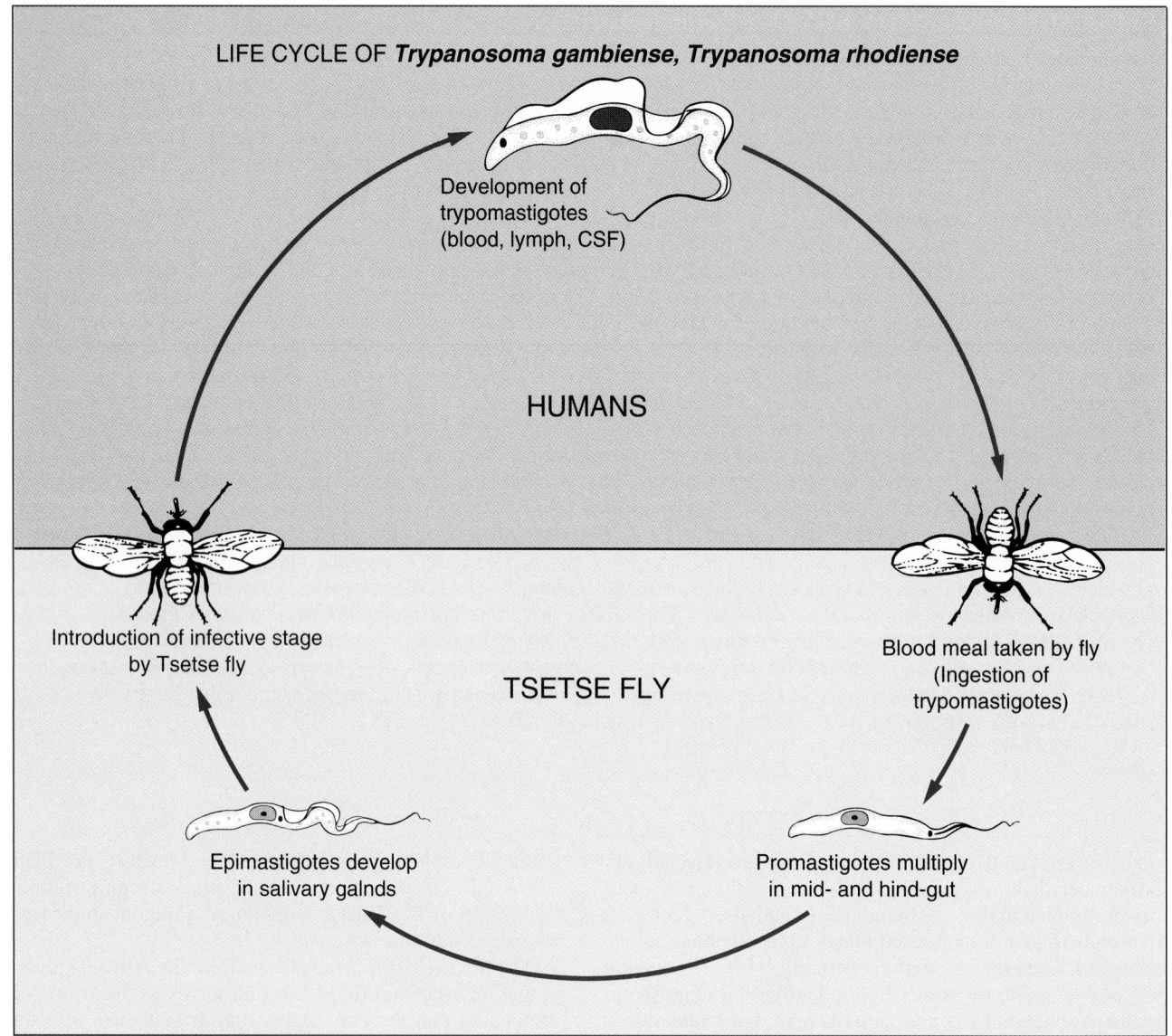

Figure 22-21 Life cycle of *Trypanosoma brucei gambiense*. The life cycle involves humans, and an insect, the tsetse fly. On ingestion of trypomastigotes from an infected human through a blood meal, promastigotes are released in the stomach of the fly, and multiply in the midgut and hindgut, finally migrating to the salivary glands as epimastigotes. Humans are infected in turn through the bite of an epimastigote-infected fly. A chancre develops at the site of the insect bite, within which over a period of several weeks, the trypanosomes undergo multiplication and maturation. Ultimately, they invade the lymphatics and bloodstream, widely disseminating to lymph nodes and ultimately to the central nervous system. Organism multiplication continues to take place in the bloodstream despite humoral immunity of the infected host, a fundamental difference from *T. cruzi*.

review, discuss the importance of screening donor blood for Chagas' disease. The issue affects not only individuals living in countries with endemic disease, but also is of concern in the United States, where upward of 50,000 immigrants from endemic countries may be infected. Avila et al.[11] also suggest a sensitive screening test for diagnosing chronic Chagas' disease in blood bank donors. They demonstrated 100% sensitivity compared with serologic tests in the detection of PCR-amplified products of *T. cruzi* kinetoplast minicircle

DNA in 114 blood samples obtained from chronic patients with and without Chagas' disease, using a specific digoxigenin-labeled oligonucleotide probe.

Because the number of circulating trypomastigotes is very low in chronic Chagas' disease, PCR-based detection of *T. cruzi* kinetoplast DNA provides a highly sensitive method for establishing a diagnosis. Many studies have shown a high degree of sensitivity, comparable to xenodiagnosis, capable of detecting as few as one circulating trypo-

African trypanosomiasis, also known as sleeping sickness,
is caused by one of two species, *Trypanosoma brucei
rhodesiense*, endemic in the savannah and woodland
regions of central and east Africa, and *Trypanosoma brucei
gambiense*, endemic in the tropical rain forests of Central
and Western Africa. The clinical disease caused by *T. brucei
rhodesiense* tends to be of more rapid onset with a greater
tendency to become rapidly progressive, even leading to
death. The more chronic picture of progressive neurologic
deterioration, culminating in "sleeping sickness,"
characteristic of Gambian trypanosomiasis often does not
have time to develop with the Rhodesian strains.

Patients infected with *T. brucei gambiense* first
experience intermittent recurring fever associated with
lymphadenopathy. Lymph nodes in the posterior cervical
region of the neck are frequently involved, producing a
lesion known as Winterbottom's sign. Ormerod[202] has
demonstrated experimental evidence of a physiologic
connection between cervical lymph glands and the
ventricles of the brain, suggesting that Winterbottom's sign
may be a marker for cerebral infection.

Hepatosplenomegaly may also be evident during this
early stage of infection. As the disease becomes chronic,
organism invasion of the central nervous system produces
the sleeping-sickness stage of the disease, characterized
initially by behavioral and personality changes, leading to
apathy, fatigue, confusion, and somnolence—signs of
progressive meningoencephalitis. Emaciation and profound
coma ultimately lead to death, often caused by
superinfections.

mastigote in 20 mL of blood.[20,103] This method also has
been found useful as a test for cure in the monitoring of
patients who are undergoing therapy.

Filarial Nematodes and Filariasis

The filarial parasites discussed here are threadlike worms.
The adults inhabit primarily the circulatory and lymphatic
channels, but may also be found in muscles, connective tissues, and serous cavities. Three species of filariae commonly
cause disease in humans: *Wuchereria bancrofti*, *Brugia malayi*, and *Loa loa*. As of 1989, an estimated 90 million to
150 million people were afflicted worldwide, over 90% of
whom have bancroftian and less than 10% of whom have
brugian filariasis.[193] As of 1999, an estimated 120 million
people were afflicted.[149a] Bancroftian filariasis is seen primarily in urban areas in Southeast Asia, due to poor sanitation and intense breeding of *Culex* mosquitos. Brugian filariasis is mainly a rural disease transmitted by *Anopheles* and
Aedes mosquitos. The number of infected persons is thought
to be on the rise worldwide because of the emergence of
shantytowns from rural to urban migrations, encouraging the
formation of favorable mosquito breeding sites.[275]

Humans acquire the disease following a bite from an infected mosquito (*W. bancrofti* and *B. malayi*) or tabanid flies

for *Loa loa*. Biting midges serve as the intermediate hosts
for the nonsheathed species, *M. perstans* and *M. ozzardi*.
The life cycle of *Wuchereria bancrofti* as a prototype for
the filarial worms is illustrated in Figure 22-23.

Laboratory Identification. The laboratory diagnosis is made
by observing circulating microfilaria in stained peripheral
blood smears.[112] Microfilaria circulate in the peripheral
blood with a regular periodicity. Those of *W. bancrofti* and
B. malayi are nocturnal; those of *Loa loa* are diurnal. Therefore, to diagnose bancroftian filariasis, optimally blood
should be obtained between midnight and 2:00 A.M. In cases
of light infections or when samples are collected at suboptimal times, membrane filtration, centrifugation, sedimentation (Knott's concentration), and preparation of thick smears
are techniques that may help to detect circulating microfilaria.[224] The use of polycarbonate filters (Nuclepore) to trap
microfilaria on a filter after the red blood cells have been
lysed is an alternative concentration technique.[64] Because
the 3–5 μm pore size filters are transparent when wet, they
can be directly examined for the presence of microfilaria on
a microscope slide.

Long et al.[168] describe an interesting approach to the laboratory diagnosis of filariasis using an acridine orange/micro-
hematocrit tube technique. A microhematocrit tube incorporating heparin, EDTA, and acridine orange serves as the
basis for this test. On centrifugation, parasites become concentrated in the buffy coat and can be visualized through
the clear glass wall of the tube. The acridine orange stains the
DNA of the parasites and the morphologic characteristics,
including the nuclear patterns in the tail sections, can be
examined by fluorescence microscopy in making a species
identification.

Mature female worms produce myriad prelarvae known
as microfilaria that circulate in the blood and serve as the
mode of transmission when the mosquito vector takes a
blood meal. An identification can be made by observing key
characteristics unique to each filarial species.
Microfilaria:

- Measure between 240–300 × 7–10 μm.
- Are ribbonlike and can be seen in microscopic mounts
  of anticoagulated blood by their undulating motion, dis-
  placing the red blood cells from side to side as they move.
- In stained peripheral blood smears of the pathogenic species a prominent sheath extends beyond the tail section.
  The sheath is a close-fitting membrane that envelops the
  microfilaria of pathogenic filarial worms, representing the
  remnants of the ovum membrane from which it was derived.
- Species can be differentiated by observing the size and
  the pattern of extension of nuclei into the tail sections:
  - *W. bancrofti:* the nuclei do not extend into the tail
    section (Color Plate 22-10*A*)
  - *B. malayi:* two nuclei extend into the tail, spaced about
    10 μm apart (Color Plate 22-10*B*)
  - *Loa loa:* an uninterrupted column of nuclei extend into
    the tail (Color Plate 22-10*C*).

The microfilaria of two other species, *Mansonella perstans* (formerly *Dipetalonema perstans* and *Mansonella ozzardi*, may also be seen in the peripheral blood; however,
patients with these infections are often asymptomatic. Occasionally eosinophilia, lymphadenitis, low-grade fever, macu-

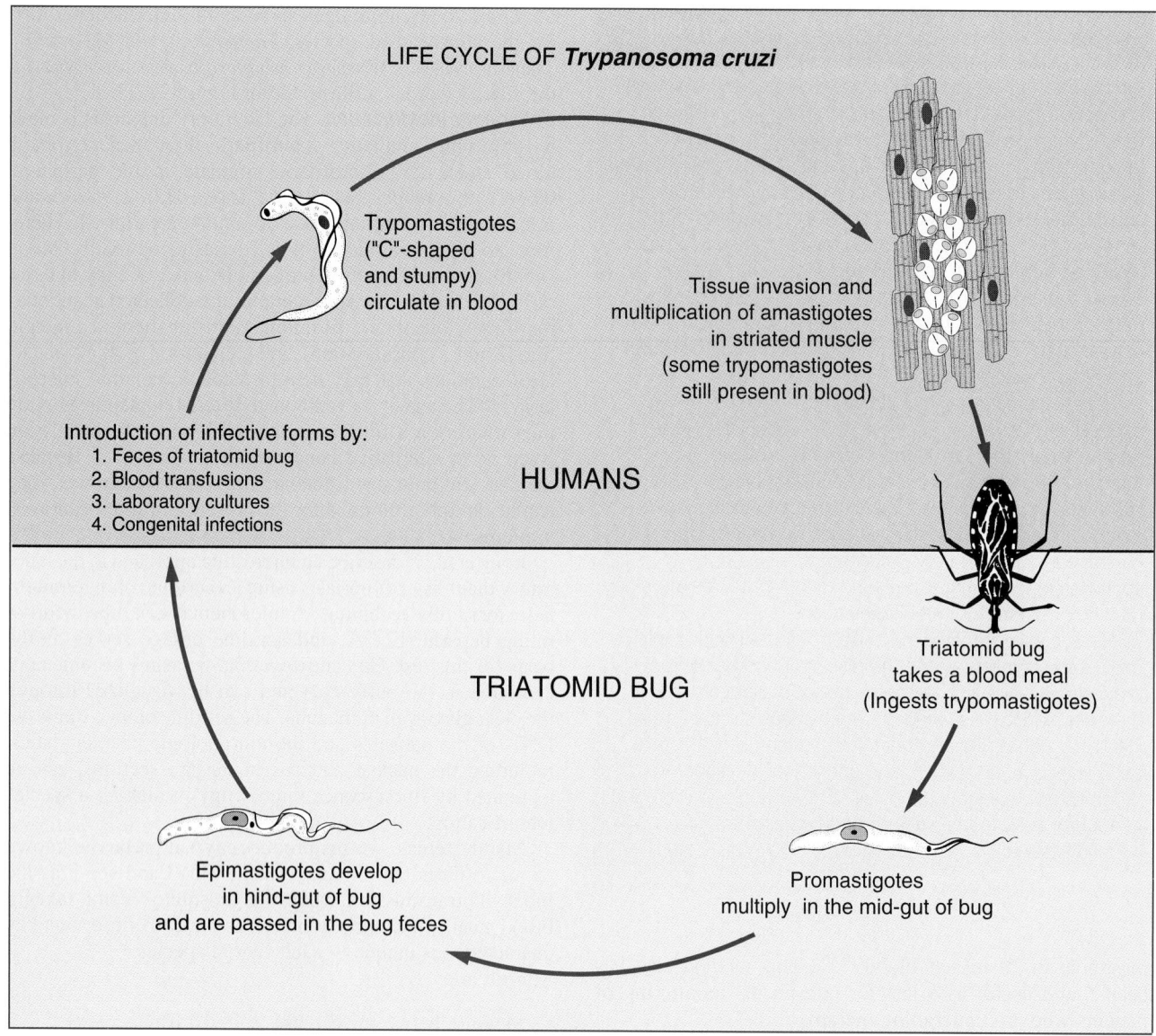

LIFE CYCLE OF *Trypanosoma cruzi*

Trypomastigotes
("C"-shaped
and stumpy)
circulate in blood

Tissue invasion and
multiplication of amastigotes
in striated muscle
(some trypomastigotes
still present in blood)

Introduction of infective forms by:
1. Feces of triatomid bug
2. Blood transfusions
3. Laboratory cultures
4. Congenital infections

HUMANS

Triatomid bug
takes a blood meal
(Ingests trypomastigotes)

TRIATOMID BUG

Epimastigotes develop
in hind-gut of bug
and are passed in the bug feces

Promastigotes
multiply in the mid-gut of bug

Figure 22-22 Life cycle of *Trypanosoma cruzi*. Humans become infected when the trypanosomal-infected fecal matter is discharged into the wound when the bug feeds. The bite is quite painful and the infected feces are rubbed into the wound. In the human host, the C-shaped trypanosomes circulate in the bloodstream during the early acute phase of the disease (Color Plate 22-9*G*), and intermittent febrile episodes are experienced. The cycle is completed when a reduviid bug (Color Plate 22-9*H*) again bites an infected host.

lopapular rash, and urticaria have been observed in infected individuals. The microfilariae of these species are devoid of a sheath.

Because the detection of circulating microfilaria by direct examination of blood is relatively insensitive in establishing a diagnosis of filariasis, and is dependent on the collection of specimens at specific times in the day, several antigen-detection procedures have been introduced. In a previous study, Weil et al.[281] demonstrated filarial antigen in the sera of 56 of 57 patients with bancroftian microfilaremia living in an endemic area in South India. Antigen shedding may be irregular, particularly during times when circulating microfilaria may not be detected; thus, even these approaches

lack sensitivity. The advent of PCR assays are proving to be useful not only in establishing a diagnosis in cases of light or amicrofilaremic infections, but also for use in monitoring therapy and in discriminating between past and present infection.[80] Of much current interest is the application of PCR technology in the diagnosis of bancroftian filariasis by examining diurnally collected sputum specimens.[1] Preliminary data from this initial study are quite encouraging and portend great potential in the future. Simonson and Dunyo[248] also have found that three recently introduced approaches for antigen detection also hold much promise—the ICT card test and the TropBio ELISA for serum specimens, and the TropBio ELISA for filter paper specimens.

CLINICAL CORRELATION BOX 22-20 American Trypanosomiasis

Children are most commonly infected, although adults are not excluded. In the acute form of disease, an inflamed and edematous chagoma may develop at the site of the bug bite. Because the bug often attacks during sleep, with the child in a reclining position, bites in the face area are common. When the conjunctiva is the portal of entry, painless edema of the periocular tissue develops, producing the classic Romana's sign. Local lymph nodes are commonly involved. Fever, malaise, anorexia, generalized lymphadenopathy, edema of the face and lower extremities, and hepatosplenomegaly of varying degrees of severity may be observed. The antiprotozoal Nifurtimox, a nitro-furfurylidene derivative, and benznidazole, an imidazole, are recommended drugs for the treatment of Chagas' disease. Both have potentially severe side effects, including polyneuropathy, skin allergies, gastric upset, and leukopenia.

In the chronic form, the leishmanial stage is more commonly found in tissues, usually either in the reticuloendothelial cells or in heart muscle (Color Plate 22–11A). Cardiomyopathy, secondary to swelling and destruction of myocardial fibers and an interstitial myocarditis, is the leading cause of death. Megaesophagus and megacolon are other complications of chronic Chagas' disease. Although central nervous system involvement is not typical; occasionally, meningoencephalitis progressing through confusion, apathy, stupor, coma, and death may occur.

Manzullo and Chuit,[176] in a study of 4,593 people with at least two positive serologic results for *T. cruzi* infection, found that 89 deaths occurred (1.5%). Of these fatal cases, three fourths died from cardiac insufficiency, and one fourth from severe ventricular arrhythmias. Those with low death risk had normal ECGs and clinical follow-up; high-risk patients were symptomatic and had abnormal ECGs, with right bundle-branch block and/or alterations of repolarization.

ONCHOCERCIASIS AND *ONCHOCERCA VOLVULUS*

Onchocerciasis is a filarial worm disease that involves primarily the subcutaneous skin in the form of dense, fibrous nodules ranging in diameter from 5–25 mm, at the sites of bites of the vector, the *Simulium* black or buffalo fly. It is estimated that 17.7 million people worldwide are infected with *Onchocerca volvulus*, of which 270,000 are blind and another 500,000 have visual impairment. Onchocerciasis is the leading cause of blindness in the world.

The *Simulium* fly has its main habitat in the underbrush lining the banks of fast-moving streams. African onchocerciasis occurs mainly in the Congo basin, Zaire, Angola. and the Sudan; in the Americas, it is found in the highlands of Guatemala, the states of Oaxaca and Chiapas in Mexico, in Colombia, and in northeastern Venezuela. The nodules are more likely to be distributed in the trunk, thighs, and arms in African subjects, but more likely are localized in the neck and shoulders in inhabitants of Central America. The life cycle of *Onchocerca volvulus* is illustrated in Figure 22-24.

The diagnosis is clinically suspected when a patient from an endemic area presents with pruritic subcutaneous nodules with associated dermatitis, loss of elasticity, and hyperpigmentation. Pruritus is a major symptom in some patients, resulting in fatigue, weakness, and inability to sleep to the point of being physically and socially debilitating. Affected areas of skin may become hot and edematous, discolored, and prematurely wrinkled, a condition known as mal morado in Central America. In Africa, involvement of the hip region, particularly around the inguinal lymph nodes, results in a condition known as "hanging groin," often leading to femoral and inguinal hernias. Several excellent photographs illustrating these clinical presentations have been published by Garcia.[96]

Color Plate 22-10*D* is an H & E–stained section through a nodule, including the cross section of a gravid worm within which many microfilaria are stored. Although the microfilaria may remain localized to the site of infection, they may wander through the adjacent skin and reach other tissues, including the eye. Ocular involvement is the most serious complication, often leading to varying degrees of loss of sight, known as "river blindness." The eye serves as a trap for wandering microfilaria, which may be found either dead or alive in the anterior chamber, cornea, choroid, and vitreous humor. The mechanical action and/or effects from secretory toxins released by the adult worm in a hypersensitive patient, and/or the production of antibodies to retinal antigens is thought to account for the development of bilateral blindness. The severity of blindness in various endemic regions is dependent on the *O. volvulus* strain involved, as determined by DNA sequence analyses.[200] The enzyme immunoassay described above may be helpful in establishing the diagnosis in patients presenting primarily with river blindness.

The laboratory diagnosis is established by demonstrating microfilaria in teased snips of skin. Examination of multiple strips may be necessary to establish a diagnosis. Zimmerman et al.[309] successfully used PCR to detect microfilariae in skin snips, providing significantly increased sensitivity in detecting active infection than that achieved by routine microscopic examination or serologic assays. Ogunrinade et al.[200] evaluated an enzyme immunoassay using recombinant *Onchocerca volvulus* antigens OC 3.6 and OC 9.3 as an aid in diagnosing patients with suspected onchocerciasis. Forty of 42 (95%) serum samples they tested from patients with known onchocerciasis were reactive with the OC 3.6 antigen, while 81% were positive for the OC 9.3 antigen. Additional studies revealed that the OC 3.6 antigen was most helpful in detecting prepatent infections in humans; the OC 9.3 antigen was more sensitive in patients with mature, patent infections.

Treatment consists of the surgical removal of detectable nodules when efficacious. Ivermectin is currently considered the drug of choice in the treatment of onchocerciasis when surgical removal of lesions is not possible. This drug reduces the numbers of microfilaria by blocking their release from the female worm. The drug is well tolerated, and side effects such as pruritus, arthralgia, and skin edema are usually minor. Diethylcarbamazine, beginning with small doses plus suramin are alternative drugs that have been used successfully, although side effects from death of the microfilaria

CLINICAL CORRELATION BOX 22-21 Filariasis[206]

Early in *W. bancrofti* and *B. malayi* infections, a bout of high fever and chills, lasting up to 5 days before subsiding, is usually associated with lymphadenitis. These febrile episodes may recur as the persistent lymphangitis extends distally from lymph nodes, as the adult worms migrate to take up final residence in the lymphatic channels. In contrast to the schistosomes, the adult filarial worms are sufficiently large to block the lymphatic channels. Lymphatic obstruction, inflammation, and swelling of the surrounding tissues evolve, producing extensive lymphedema, a condition known as elephantiasis. The characteristic clinical manifestation of *W. bancrofti* is genital disease with funiculitis, epididymo-orchitis and hydrocele, and less often elephantiasis.[201] In brugian filariasis, adenolymphadenitis of the inguinal region and elephantiasis, predominantly involving the leg below the knee, is more common, leaving the knee and elbow uninvolved, with normal contours. In lymphatic vessels that harbor the worms, a heavy infiltration of eosinophils, plasma cells, and macrophages are seen. The local damage to the vessels leads to increased vessel-wall permeability and the leaking of fluids of high concentrations of protein into the surrounding tissues into the surrounding tissue (lymphedema), ultimately leading to classic elephantiasis. Acute lymphangitis occurs when the adult worms die. Some patients may harbor adult worms without circulating microfilaria; others may have significant circulating microfilaremia without commensurate clinical symptoms.

Loa loa causes a disease in which the adult worms migrate through the subcutaneous tissue and may be observed as a small, serpiginous elevation of the thin parts of the skin or beneath the conjunctival lining of the eye. These migratory angioedematous skin lesions are known as Calabar swellings and serve as a diagnostic manifestation. Because of increased world travel, Rakita et al.[221] advise that *Loa loa* infection be considered in the differential diagnosis for patients presenting with migratory angioedema, urticarial vasculitis, and/or eosinophilia. The term "eye worm" was derived from this organism's propensity to infiltrate beneath the conjunctival epithelium. Fifty-six cases of human intraocular filariasis have been reviewed by Beaver.[16] In 10 cases, the filariae removed were identified as *Loa loa*. However, *W. bancrofti*, *Dipetalonema* sp. and *Dirofilaria* sp. were other filariae detected in the remaining cases.

may require coverage with antiinflammatory drugs. The administration of mebendazole or flubendazole (benzimidazole derivatives) has also been successful, with few side effects.

DRACUNCULIASIS

Dracunculus medinensis is a tissue roundworm often grouped with the filariae. *D. medinensis* is the guinea worm that probably represents the "fiery serpent" of biblical lore.[135] Hopkins et al.,[139] in a recent update, indicate that Asia is now free of dracunculiasis, with Pakistan, India, and Yemen having interrupted transmission in 1993, 1996, and 1997, respectively. The disease was also interrupted in Cameroon and Senegal during 1997, with only three cases reported in Chad during 1998. Dracunculiasis is now confined to only 13 countries in Africa, with the overall number of cases reduced from 3.2 million in 1986, to 78,557 cases in 1998 (97% decrease). This reduction resulted from an intensive program of case detection and containment, with rewards for reporting of cases.

Humans acquire the infection through ingestion of infected Copepoda. The larvae develop into adult worms in the serous cavities and the gravid females migrate to the subcutaneous tissue. These female worms can measure as long as 100 cm and cause a burning sensation and ulceration of the skin at the sites of infection. They can be removed surgically from the subcutaneous tissue by winding them slowly on a stick. The life cycle of the parasite is complete when the larvae produced by the female escape from the skin blister and are discharged into water in which the Copepoda live. Interruption of this part of the life cycle in infected populations as a whole promises to completely eradicate dracunculiasis within the next decade.

DIROFILARIASIS

Dirofilaria species, transmitted by mosquitos, are filarial parasites commonly infecting animals. In the definitive host, most commonly the dog, the infective larval forms injected into the subcutaneous tissue from the proboscis of the mosquito enter into the circulation and ultimately find their way to the heart, where they develop into adults (dog heart worms) (Color Plate 22-10*E*). The diagnosis is made in infected dogs by observing circulating microfilaria in the peripheral blood. When humans (acting as accidental hosts) are bitten by infected mosquitos, the larvae, because they are in the wrong host, are incapable of completing their life cycle. Rather, they lodge in and obstruct pulmonary arterioles, where they develop into local granulomatous nodules that may, on occasion, reach sufficient size to be diagnosed as "coin lesions" on x-ray examination. Microfilaria never circulate in human blood. The diagnosis is made by histologic observation of immature filarial larvae within the pulmonary granulomatous nodules. Flieder and Moran[82] recently reviewed 39 cases of histologically proven dirofilarial pulmonary infection. Approximately half of this group were asymptomatic, with only a pulmonary nodule detected on x-ray films obtained for routine physical examinations; the remaining half presented with respiratory symptoms. Only 10% presented with peripheral blood eosinophilia.

Tissue Protozoan Infections
TOXOPLASMA GONDII

Toxoplasma gondii is a protozoan parasite that has a particular predilection for infecting the CNS in humans. The life cycle of *Toxoplasma gondii* is illustrated in Figure 22-25.

Three modes of transmission lead to most human infections: 1) directly from ingestion of infective oocysts in food (e.g., unwashed leafy vegetables) or water contaminated with cat feces; 2) indirectly, from ingestion of the raw or undercooked meat of animals that had ingested oocysts (it is estimated that 25% of lamb and pork meat sold at supermarkets contain viable tissue cysts); and 3) transplacental

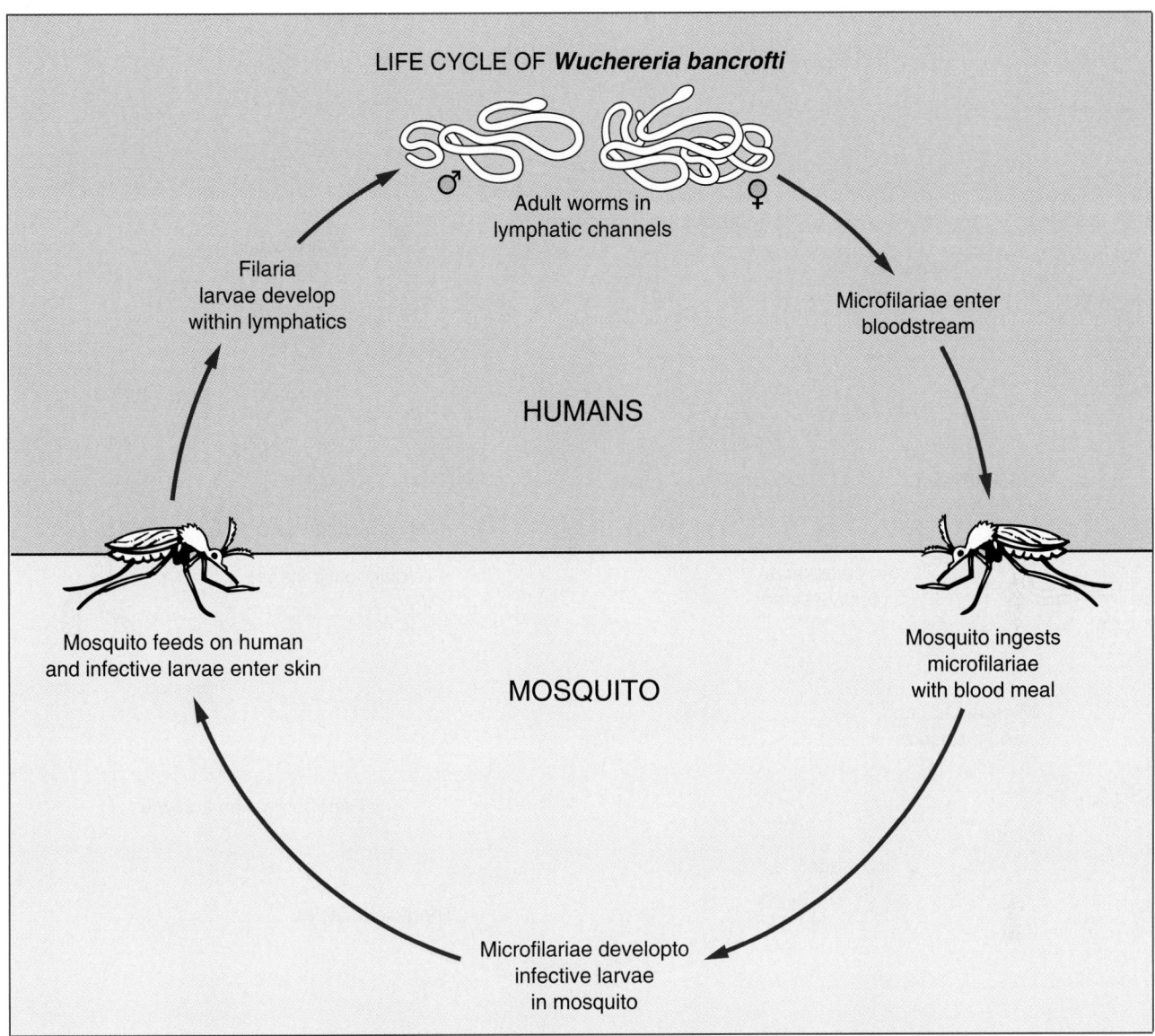

Figure 22-23 Life cycle of *Wuchereria bancrofti*. Humans acquire the disease following a bite from an infected mosquito (*W. bancrofti* and *B. malayi*) or tabanid flies (*Loa loa*). Biting midges serve as the intermediate hosts for the nonsheathed species, *M. perstans* and *M. ozzardi*. When the vector bites an infected human host, the infective microfilaria are ingested and penetrate the stomach wall of the insect. An infective third larval stage develops in the stomach, which in turn migrates to the thoracic muscles of the insect and then to the proboscis. When the insect bites a new human host, these infective larvae move down the proboscis and are injected into the cutaneous wound while the mosquito takes a blood meal. These infective larvae reproduce locally in the subcutaneous tissue and ultimately enter the peripheral lymphatics, where they find their way to lymph nodes and lymphatic channels in various parts of the body. Over a period of several weeks, the larvae develop into white, threadlike adult worms. The lymphatics of the lower extremities and the epitrochlear and femoral lymph nodes are the sites most commonly involved. Mature female worms release microfilaria that circulate in the blood, and are ingested by the appropriate insect during the next blood meal, to complete the life cycle.

transfer to the fetus from a mother infected during pregnancy. Maternal infection rates during the reproductive years is estimated to be between 3% and 5%.[87] Pregnant women should be strongly advised to avoid the handling of cats and the ingestion of undercooked meat. Clinical symptoms may

be minimal or absent in the acute stages of infection, and infants may not show the cardinal signs of infection—retinochoroiditis, cerebral calcification, hydrocephalus, or microcephaly—for several months or even years. Acquired infections in adults usually manifest as lymphadenitis and

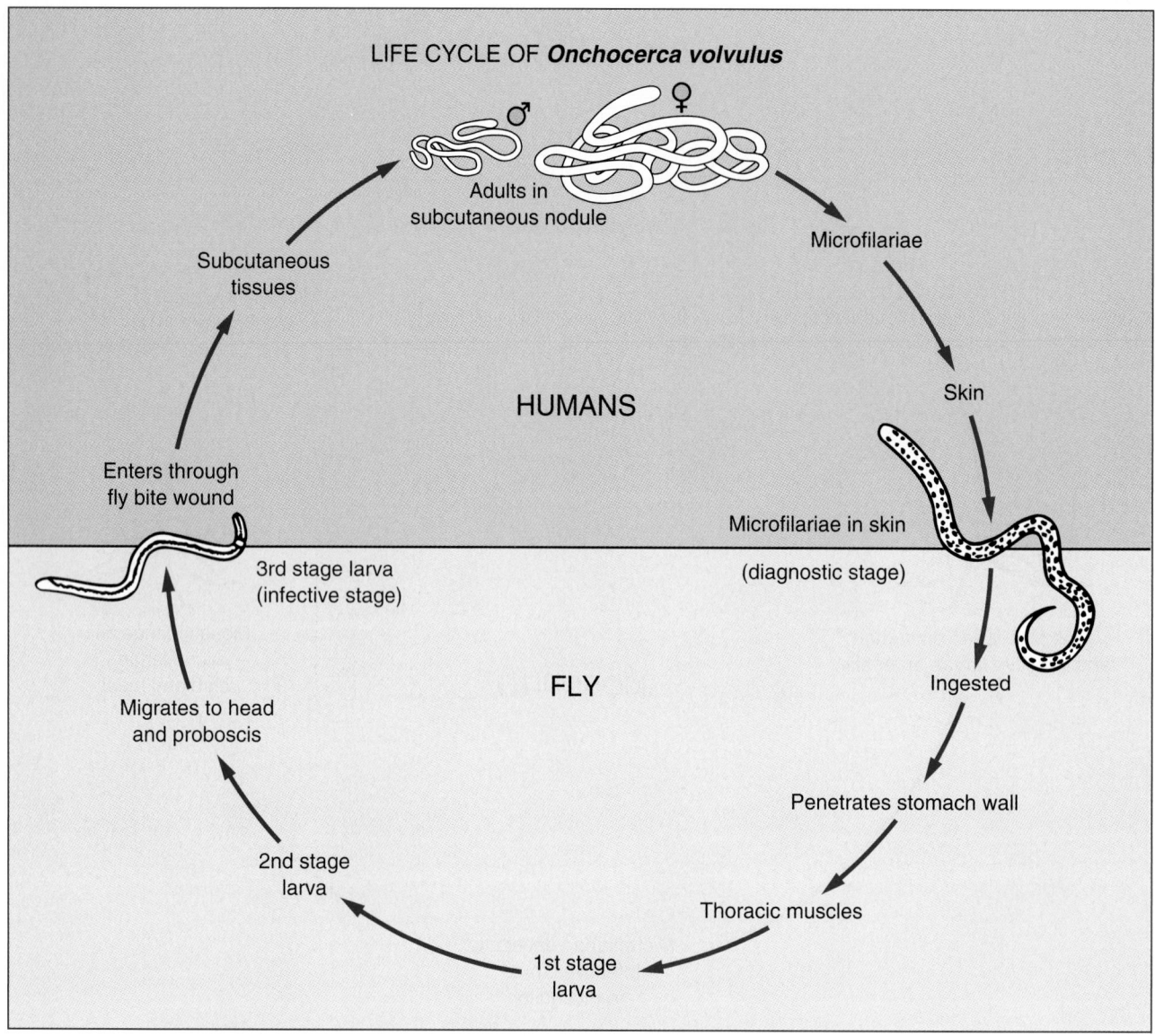

Figure 22-24 Life cycle of *Onchocerca volvulus*. In the life cycle, humans become infected by bites from a *Simulium* fly, the mouth parts of which possess the infective third-stage larval forms of the parasite. The adult worms develop in tangled masses within nodules beneath the skin and the females produce microfilaria (Color Plate 22-9D). The microfilaria remain localized to the infection sites and do not circulate in the peripheral blood except in rare instances. The life cycle is completed when a black fly again bites a diseased human at one of the infection sites, picking up the microfilaria in the mouth parts. The microfilaria then develop in the fly by penetrating the stomach wall, entering the thoracic muscles, and transforming through first- and second-stage larvae. They mature into the infective third-stage larval forms to complete the life cycle.

lymphadenopathy, varying degrees of myocarditis, meningoencephalitis, atypical pneumonia, and rhinochoroiditis.

Two parasitic stages may be involved in human infections. After ingestion of oocysts or the encysted infective forms in uncooked meat, tachyzoites (Color Plate 22-10F) are released in the small intestine and first invade the mucosal epithelial cells, from which they enter the circulation, and then are widely distributed throughout the body. Considerable tissue damage may occur as the tachyzoites destroy the cells they parasitize; however, as the immune response develops, the tachyzoites become less active and ultimately aggregate within a membrane-enclosed cyst (Color Plate 22-10G and H). Although inactive, the tachyzoites within these cysts may remain viable for weeks or for years. Most commonly, they ultimately disintegrate and become enmeshed in a hyaline scar and/or undergo calcification. The detection of intracerebral calcification in skull roentgenograms is one method for establishing previous infection.

CLINICAL CORRELATION BOX 22-22 Toxoplasmosis[154]

A broad spectrum of signs and symptoms may be encountered in cases of human toxoplasmosis. Based on the high prevalence of seropositivity in certain populations, as high as 90% in some regions of El Salvador, Tahiti, and France (an average of 20% in the United States),[182] millions of healthy people are or have been infected with *Toxoplasma gondii*. Yet, symptoms are absent or overlooked in all but about 10% of cases, and the incidence of progressive disease is very low.

Symptomatic acute toxoplasmosis in immunocompetent humans presents as generalized lymphadenopathy, particularly of the cervical area of the neck. If accompanied by sore throat, fever and myalgias, the disease complex may simulate infectious mononucleosis. The disease is self-limited in most cases; however, overt disseminated disease may rarely develop. Myocarditis, pneumonitis, and encephalitis may occur in varying degrees of severity and may mimic other disseminated diseases, such as tuberculosis, sarcoidosis, tularemia, lymphoma, or leukemia. The outcome may be fatal in severe cases.

A marked increase in the incidence of symptomatic disease has been found among homosexual men and individuals who intravenously inject illicit drugs. In fact, AIDS or drug abuse should be suspected in any patient diagnosed as having toxoplasmosis. The disease often localizes in the CNS with symptoms of encephalitis or meningoencephalitis, or manifestation as a space-occupying lesion.[114] The disease can progress rapidly and usually terminates in death if the compromised immune status remains unchanged. Pulmonary, cardiac, and lymphoreticular disease may also be present. The CSF typically shows high protein levels and an increase in mononuclear inflammatory cells.

Tachyzoites circulating in the blood of an infected pregnant woman transmigrate the placenta and are widely distributed in the fetal tissues. Term infants with a full component of maternal IgG antibody often withstand the infections; premature or antibody-deficient infants are more susceptible to progressive disease. General symptoms such as splenomegaly, jaundice, fever, and lymphadenopathy may be seen. The CNS is particularly susceptible, and symptoms may vary. Impaired vision, convulsions, mental retardation, spasticity, hydrocephalus, microcephalus, and deafness are among the more common symptoms. In newborns who are asymptomatic at birth late-onset disease may develop; spinal or subarachnoid punctures should be performed in suspected cases in order to make the diagnosis. Grover et al.[114] have applied PCR in the early diagnosis of congenital *Toxoplasma* infection. This technique is based on direct lysis of pelleted amniotic fluid cells followed by PCR amplification of a gene sequence specific for *T. gondii*. The PCR correctly identified the presence of *T. gondii* in five amniotic fluid samples obtained from four patients with proven congenital infection in the study cited.

Vitreous exudate and bilateral retinochoroiditis of the macula are common ocular signs of congenital toxoplasmosis. Symptoms may not manifest until the second or third decade of life. Chorioretinitis with blurred vision, photophobia, and ocular pain may be seen in acquired cases; however, it is usually unilateral.

The recommended treatment is pyrimethamine, 25–100 mg/day for 3–4 weeks plus spiramycin, 2–4 g/day for 3–4 weeks in adults. Children should receive doses of pyrimethamine, 2 mg/kg/day for 3 days (maximum, 25 mg/day), then 1 mg/kg/day for 4 weeks, plus, spiramycin 50–100 mg/kg/ day for 3–4 weeks.

Laboratory Diagnosis. The diagnosis of acute toxoplasmosis can be made by demonstrating clusters of tachyzoites in stained smears using the PAS and/or H & E stains. Fluorescent antibody staining and peroxidase–antiperoxidase techniques have been used to better demonstrate organisms in formalin-fixed and paraffin-embedded tissues. Tachyzoites are perhaps best seen in needle aspirates or impression smears stained with Wright-Giemsa.

- The tachyzoites are typically bow-shaped, measure 3–4 × 6–7 µm, and have a dark-staining central nucleus (Fig. 22-26 and Color Plate 22-10*F*).

One or more cysts, when observed in tissue sections of patients, usually indicates a chronic and usually inactive stage of infection, but serve as an important source of acute reactivation toxoplasmosis.

- Cysts measure up to 200 µm in diameter and contain several hundred bradyzoites 2–3 µm in diameter (Fig. 22-27 and Color Plate 22-10*G* and *H*).

The serologic diagnosis of toxoplasmosis is complex, and a full account is beyond the scope of this presentation. Pi-

oneering work has been done by McCabe and Remington,[182] a summary of which is included in Box 22-6. Because of the high prevalence of increased titers of *Toxoplasma* antibody in the general population, test results must be carefully interpreted before a definitive diagnosis can be established. The time-honored Sabin-Feldman dye test, based on the principle that live *Toxoplasma gondii* tachyzoites lose their affinity for methylene blue dye in the presence of immune serum, being both sensitive and specific, still serves as the reference method. Nonetheless, it has been replaced by newer techniques in most reference laboratories to bypass the necessity of having to work with live organisms. Also, this test measures IgG antibodies, which appear in the serum within 1–2 weeks following infection, peak in 6–8 weeks, and decline over the next few months, but never completely disappear after infection in most patients. Because serum titers as high as 1:512 can persist for may years in normal people, interpretations of single samples must be made with care.

Several new methods have been introduced in the past several years for the serologic diagnosis of toxoplasmosis. These include enzyme immunoassays, ELISAs, direct agglutination tests, indirect fluorescent assays (IFDA), and immunocapture and immunoblot techniques. Several of these have been reviewed by Cubitt et al.[49] Wong et al.[293] have evaluated the applications of determining toxoplasma immunoglobulin E

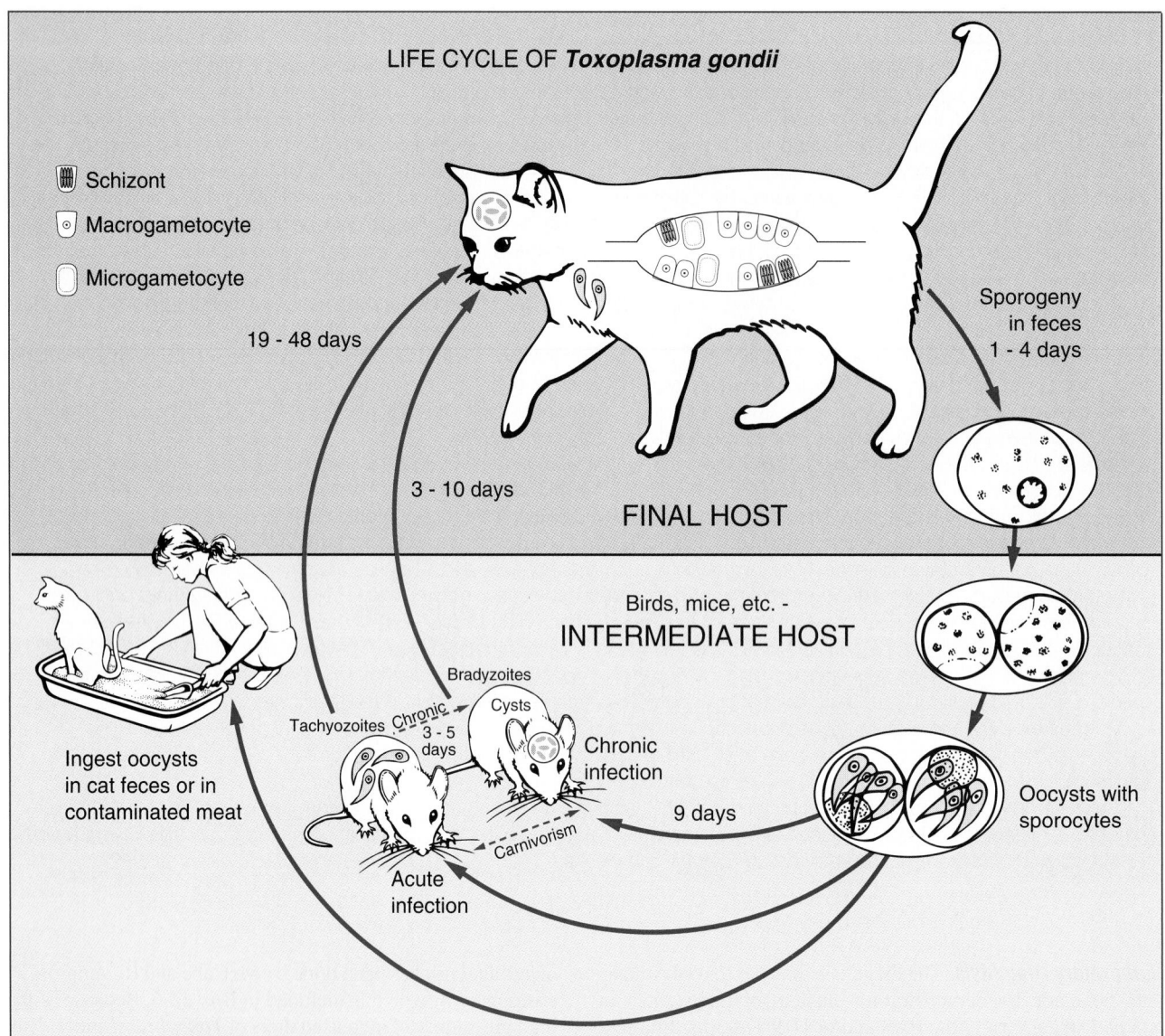

Figure 22-25 Life cycle of *Toxoplasma gondii*. The life cycle of *T. gondii* has both sexual and asexual stages. The sexual stage occurs in the intestine of cats, where infective oocysts, measuring 10–12 μm in diameter, replicate within the intestinal mucosal epithelial cells and are excreted in the feces. The asexual stage commonly occurs in a variety of herbivorous and carnivorous animals that ingest the infective oocysts when foraging through contaminated soil and vegetative matter. Humans also may become infected by ingesting food or water contaminated with oocysts. Cockroaches, earthworms, snails, and slugs may also serve as transport hosts for oocysts.

(IgE) antibodies as a diagnostic test. Using an immunosorbent agglutination assay (ISAGA) and an ELISA, serum IgE levels were determined on several groups of patients both with and without known toxoplasmosis. IgE antibodies were not detected in serum specimens from seronegative individuals, from those with chronic toxoplasma infection, or in infants without congenital toxoplasmosis. Pregnant women who seroconverted during gestation, patients with toxoplasmic lymphadenopathy, infants with signs of congenital toxoplasmosis, children and adults with toxoplasmic chorioretinitis, and adult patients with AIDS and toxoplasmic encephalitis all had

IgE titers above cutoff values. The authors conclude that recrudescence of serum IgE antibodies may be helpful in diagnosing patients with reactivated disease. Li et al.[164] have developed an ELISA test incorporating a recombinant protein (rP35 antigen of *Toxoplasma gondii*) that detects IgG antibodies produced only during the acute stage of infection, thereby serving as a serologic marker to differentiate between recently acquired and latent old infection.

Antigen-detection techniques have also improved significantly over the past several years, particularly with the introduction of PCR technology. Several reports describe

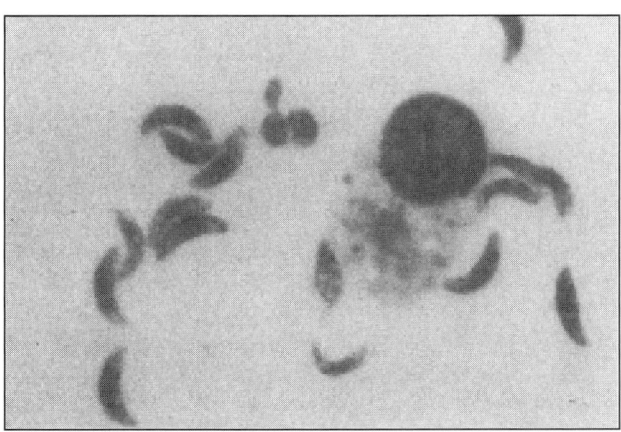

Figure 22-26 High-power view of Giemsa-stained impression smear demonstrating toxoplasma trophozoites. Note characteristic bow shape and central dark-staining nucleus (×1000).

the *T. gondii* B1 gene as the marker to be detected by gene amplification by PCR.[79,134,153,205] The B1 gene-amplification procedure is sufficiently sensitive to detect a single isolated parasite and as few as 10 parasites in a background of 100,000 leukocytes.[205] Gene-amplification techniques are more sensitive and may replace cell culture as the method of choice in detecting toxoplasma parasitemia.[134] The detection of toxoplasma parasitemia in AIDS patients with unexplained fever or central nervous system abnormalities by gene detection after PCR amplification has also been found promising.[79] Examination of blood by PCR may also be useful in diagnosing extracerebral toxoplasmosis from the local reactivation of latent brain cysts.[74] Dupon et al.[73] also found the PCR examination of CSF and/or blood to be a valuable adjunct in detecting reactiva-

tion of latent cerebral toxoplasmosis. In addition to detecting the *T. gondii* B1 nucleic acid sequences, they cite other studies successfully using p30, TGR1 genes, and the 18S rDNA as targets.

PNEUMOCYSTIS CARINII

Currently, based on DNA sequence analysis, *Pneumocystis carinii* is genetically more closely aligned with the fungi, and thus has been reclassified as an ascosporogenous yeast. The specific criteria for making this reclassification as cited by Hadley and Ng[116] is as follows:

- *P. carinii* and fungi have similar cell-wall ultrastructures.
- The cristae in the mitochondria of *P. carinii* is are lamellar (protozoans have tubular cristae).
- Cyst forms containing intracystic bodies resemble those of ascospores formed by the Ascomycetes.
- A high homology of the more conserved domains of the 16S rRNA subunit with that of Ascomycetes.
- The β-tubulin gene is 89–91% homologous with that of the filamentous fungi.
- *P. carinii* possesses separate proteins for thymidylate synthase and dihydrofolate reductase activities (protozoa produce a single bifunctional protein).
- NADH dehydrogenase subunits 1, 2, 3, and 6; cytochrome oxidase subunit II; and a small subunit of rRNA have an average similarity of 60% with fungi (only 20% with protozoa).

In keeping with these findings, *Pneumocystis carinii* is presented in Chapter 21 on mycology.

Miscellaneous Larval Tissue Parasite Infections

Humans may be inadvertent accidental hosts for several nematodes and cestodes that have life cycles in other animals. The adults of these species normally reside in the intestinal tract or select tissues of the definitive hosts; humans become infected by ingesting either the larvae in poorly cooked meat, or by the ingestion of fertile ova. Of particular concern in the United States is the potential increased exposure to a variety of helminthic parasites through the ingestion of uncooked seafood in the form of dishes such as sushi, sashimi, lomi lomi salmon, pickled herring, and the like. Because humans are not the natural definitive host for certain of these parasites, the larvae often aimlessly wander among tissues and organs, either forming cysticercoid lesions or areas of granulomatous inflammation. A brief discussion of the following larval parasitic diseases will follow.

Nematodes

Trichinella spiralis (pig, bear, walrus intestinal nematode)
Toxocara canis or *Toxocara cati* (dog and cat ascarids)
Ancylostoma braziliense or *A. caninum* (dog and cat hookworms)
Anisakis species (fish or sea mammal nematodes)
Gnathostoma spinigerum (dog and cat gastric nematode)
Angiostrongylus species (rats)

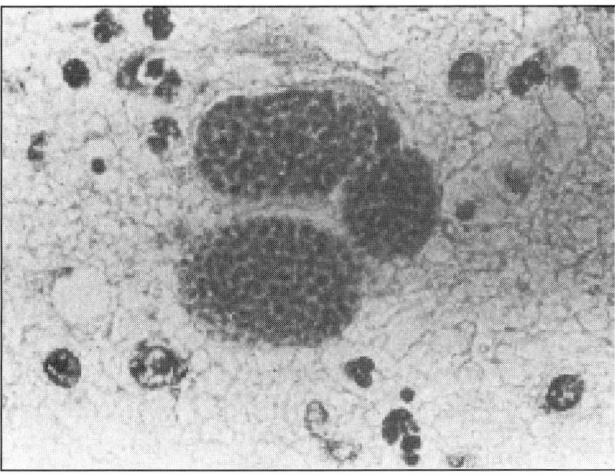

Figure 22-27 High-power view of the toxoplasmal pseudocysts illustrated in Fig. 22-25. Each pseudocyst contains several scores of trophozoites. These pseudocysts are most commonly seen in patients with latent disease. Note the absence of an inflammatory reaction adjacent to these pseudocysts (H & E ×1000).

Box 22-6 Interpretation of Serologic Results in Clinical Syndromes of Toxoplasmosis[182]

A. Acute acquired toxoplasmosis: immunocompetent patient

The diagnosis can be highly suspected if:

1. Seroconversion from negative to positive is demonstrated.

2. A twofold increase in titer between a baseline sample and a repeated test 3 weeks later.

3. A high IgM titer with a single high IgG titer ($>1:1000$).

4. A low IgM titer indicates that the infection was acquired 4 months or more before. The IGM titer usually reverts to normal within 9 months.

Note: A negative dye or immunofluorescence assay result in an immunocompetent person virtually precludes the diagnosis of acute toxoplasmosis.

B. Acute acquired toxoplasmosis: immunoincompetent patient

The criteria cited for immunocompetent patients apply to immunoincompetent individuals as well. However, IgM antibody or twofold rises in IgG antibody often is not detected; therefore, a negative test does not rule out acute toxoplasmosis. Organisms must be demonstrated in tissue biopsies or impression smears of aspirates before a secure diagnosis can be made in this group of patients.

C. Ocular toxoplasmosis

The diagnosis can be suspected if:

1. Low titers of IgG antibody in the presence of a typical retinal lesion

2. If "C" is equal to or greater than 8 using the following formula when testing aqueous humor fluid:

$$\frac{\text{Antibody titer in fluid} \times \text{concentration of gamma globulin in serum}}{\text{Antibody titer in serum} \times \text{concentration of } \gamma\text{-globulin in body fluid}}$$

D. Congenital toxoplasmosis

The diagnosis of toxoplasma infection in the neonate can be established if:

1. There is a persistent or rising titer in the dye or IFA test

2. A positive IgM test at any titer after birth in the absence of a placental leak (DS-IgM-ELISA test preferred) is demonstrated in tissue biopsies or impression smears of aspirates.

Cestodes

Echinococcus granulosus (dog tapeworm)
Echinococcus multilocularis (dog, fox, wolf, cat tapeworm)
Multiceps species (coenurosis)
Spirometra mansonoides (sparganum) (dog or cat *Diphyllobothrium* tapeworm)

TRICHINOSIS

Trichinosis is a disease of carnivores caused by infection with the nematode *Trichinella spiralis*, resulting from ingestion of raw or poorly cooked meat. Humans are accidental hosts and are most commonly infected through ingestion of pork or pork products that contain encysted larvae.[108] Infections have also been reported after ingestion of poorly cooked bear meat.[41] Smoking, salting, or drying the meat does not destroy the infective larval forms; however, prolonged freezing (20 days in the average home freezer) decontaminates the meat. The disease has a worldwide distribution; in the United States, 4% of human cadavers were found to be infected in 1968. By 1985, less than 50 new cases were being reported each year in the United States,[41] a tribute to the meat inspection program and the stringent laws against feeding uncooked garbage to pigs.

The life cycle in human infections is initiated by the ingestion of the infective larvae from poorly cooked meat. The life cycle is illustrated in Figure 22-28.

The clinical manifestations of trichinosis are presented in Clinical Correlation Box 22-23.

Laboratory Diagnosis. The laboratory diagnosis of trichinosis is most commonly made by detecting the spiral larvae in muscle tissue (Color Plate 22-11*G* and *H*). The deltoid muscle of the upper arm or the gastrocnemius muscle of the calf are usually selected for biopsy. The specimen may be examined microscopically by first digesting the muscle fibers with trypsin and then mounting some of the digested tissue on a microscope slide. Alternatively, a tease preparation may be prepared by squeezing a small fragment of muscle in a drop of saline solution between two glass slides, in each case looking microscopically for the coiled larval forms. Linear or spiral larval forms may also be observed in stained tissue sections, although their morphology often is not as well delineated.

Serologic tests are also helpful in establishing a diagnosis. Mahannop et al.,[175] using crude antigens obtained from the infective stage larvae of *Trichinella spiralis* in an ELISA system for detecting serum IgG antibodies to *T. spiralis*, reported a 100% sensitivity in a group of patients with confirmed trichinelliasis. They found cross-reactions in sera collected from patients with capillariasis, gnathostomiasis, opisthorchiasis, and strongyloidiasis.

VISCERAL LARVAL MIGRANS

Toxocara canis, the dog intestinal roundworm, with a life cycle similar to that of human *Ascaris lumbricoides*, is the most common cause of human larva migrans. Larva migrans

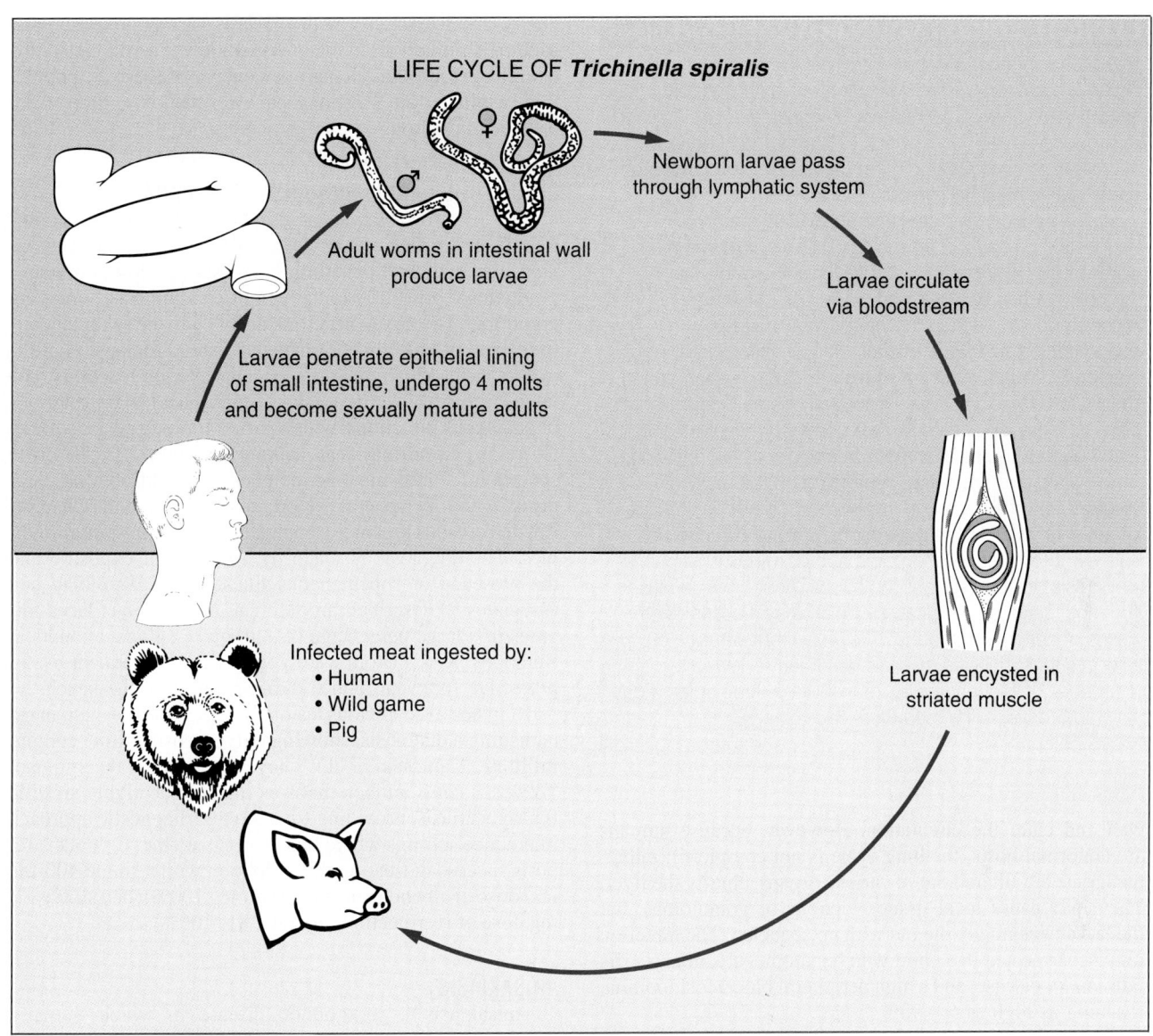

LIFE CYCLE OF *Trichinella spiralis*

Adult worms in intestinal wall produce larvae

Newborn larvae pass through lymphatic system

Larvae circulate via bloodstream

Larvae penetrate epithelial lining of small intestine, undergo 4 molts and become sexually mature adults

Larvae encysted in striated muscle

Infected meat ingested by:
• Human
• Wild game
• Pig

Figure 22-28 Life cycle of *Trichinella spiralis*. When humans ingest trichinosis-contaminated meat, the encysted larvae are released in the intestine and burrow into the villi. The larvae mature and mate, and develop into adult male and female worms, measuring from 2–4 mm in length. The average life span of the adults in the human intestine is about 1 month. During this time, each female releases as many as 3,000 larval offspring. These larvae pass through the lymphatic system and enter the circulation and are deposited throughout the tissues of the body. Most of these larvae are killed; however, many of those that reach the skeletal muscle become encysted and survive. The heaviest period of muscle invasion is around day 10 after infection. By days 17–20, these larval forms differentiate and become encapsulated, forming a coil two-and-a-half times on themselves, surrounded initially by an acute and later a chronic granulomatous inflammatory reaction. (Color Plate 20-11*G* and *H*). The adjacent muscle fibers undergo degeneration, leaving a cyst that measures about 0.25–0.50 mm. In approximately 3 months the worms die and the cystic lesions undergo a process of calcification, which is completed in 6–12 months.

is a condition in which the larvae of nematode parasites of lower animals migrate into the tissues of humans without further development. Larva migrans may be caused by many different species of parasites and may affect either cutaneous or visceral tissues, depending on the body areas affected and the parasites involved.

In *T. canis* infection, humans become an accidental host through ingestion of embryonated eggs in the soil. The disease is most common in children because of their inadvertent ingestion of soil and their close association with dogs. The embryonated eggs hatch in the intestine of the human host, liberating the larvae, which, in turn, penetrate the bowel

CLINICAL CORRELATION BOX 22-23 Trichinosis

Symptoms in most cases are mild, as the loading dose of larvae is commonly small. Many individuals have flulike symptoms. The minimal number of ingested larvae required to produce symptoms is about 100, and a fatal dose is estimated to be 300,000.[108] On ingestion of contaminated meat, gastrointestinal symptoms are the first to appear, including nausea, diarrhea, and abdominal cramps, suggesting acute food poisoning. These symptoms may persist with varying degrees of severity for as long as 10 weeks. Pain, swelling, and weakness of involved muscles develop during the larval invasion stage, accompanied by fever. Peripheral blood eosinophilia, with differential counts reaching as high as 50%, is seen during the muscle invasion stage. Periorbital edema is a diagnostic sign, as extraocular muscles are commonly involved. Damage to muscles may result in irregularities in chewing, swallowing, and breathing, depending on the muscles involved and the degree of involvement. In about 10–20% of patients, the CNS may be involved to varying degrees, with symptoms suggesting polyneuritis, myasthenia gravis, or paresis of localized muscle groups. Acute myocarditis is the most serious complication, which may result in death in cases of heavy worm loads. A review of antiparasitic drugs effective for trichinosis myositis has been reviewed by Watt et al.[277] Mebendazole, 200–400 mg three times a day for 3 to 5 days, is the recommended therapy.

wall and enter the circulation. However, because humans are abnormal hosts, the lung cycle is not completed; rather, the larvae are filtered out in various organs, chiefly the liver. They may cause local tissue reactions or granulomas, but the larvae eventually die out with no sequelae. The infection may be suspected in a child with hepatomegaly, nonspecific pulmonary disease, and a high peripheral blood eosinophilia, reaching as high as 50–90%.

Although a definitive diagnosis is confirmed only by the identification of larvae in autopsy or biopsy specimens, serologic testing is recommended to direct management and therapy. Serum titers of 1:32 or higher are indicative of visceral larval migrans; a titer of 1:8 is considered diagnostic of ocular larval migrans. Detecting elevated titers in ocular fluid specimens is confirmatory of the latter condition. Buijs et al.[24] report that the seroprevalence of *Toxocara* among young schoolchildren in the Netherlands as of 1994 was 11% in the Hague and 6% in Rotterdam. They found a significant correlation of recurrent asthma and bronchitis in *Toxocara*-seropositive children. They speculate that elevated allergen-specific IgE in these patients may account for the asthma. Jacquier et al.[145] evaluated a commercial ELISA kit marketed by Biokema-Affinity Products (Crissier-Lausanne, Switzerland), which is based on detection of excretory/secretory antigen derived from second-stage *T. canis* larvae. In a study of 1,000 serum samples randomly collected from healthy blood donors and children in Switzerland, the seroprevalence of toxocariasis was 2.7%. Of the positive samples, the Biokema kit had an overall diagnostic sensitivity of 91% and a specificity of 86%. The lower specificity was due to cross-reactivity with filariasis, strongyloidiasis, and trichinella infection. In the interpretation of serologic results one must recall that a small percentage of the U.S. population, estimated at 2%, may have residual low titers from previous infection.

CUTANEOUS LARVA MIGRANS—TOXOCARA

The filariform larvae of dog or cat hookworms, commonly of the species *Ancylostoma braziliense* and *A. caninum*, are capable of penetrating the exposed skin of humans, producing a pruritic, papular condition known as "creeping eruption." The larvae penetrate deeply into the subcutaneous tissue and produce linear tracts that extend for several millimeters each day. Impetigo, vesicular allergic reactions, and intense pruritus are the major local clinical manifestations of cutaneous infections, which persist for long periods. Deep tissue migration may lead to lung infections. *Ancylostoma* species infections must be included in the differential diagnosis when peripheral blood eosinophilia and Charcot-Leyden crystals are microscopically detected in sputum samples. The diagnosis is made by a history of exposure and the presence of subcutaneous linear tracts. Tremblay and associates[266] described an outbreak of cutaneous larva migrans in a large percentage of a group of 140 vacationers in Barbados. Risk factors were younger age, infrequent use of protective footwear, and walking barefoot to the beach.

Biopsies of suspicious lesions are often of little help in establishing a diagnosis, showing only an eosinophilic cellular infiltrate. Yamasaki et al.[299] have developed a recombinant *Toxocara canis* antigen that was found to be highly specific for toxocariasis, providing for a reliable diagnostic approach in practice settings where this test is available. Camous[28] reports success in treating this condition with a single 400-mg oral dose of albendazole (cure rate, 46–100%); or a single 12-mg dose of ivermectin (cure rate, 81–100%).

ANISAKIASIS

Anisakiasis is a zoonotic disease in which humans, through the ingestion of raw, pickled, smoked, or poorly cooked seafood such as sushi, sashimi, pickled herrings, and the like, become an accidental host for the larval nematodes belonging to the genera *Anisakis, Phocanema,* and *Contracaecum.* The number of infections in the United States has increased as raw fish such as lomi lomi salmon, sushi, and sashimi have become popular. Deardorff and Kent[68] report that only wild-caught salmon were infected; those pen-reared were free of infection. Thus, knowing the origin of fresh fish may help in avoiding infections.

On entering the stomach with the contaminated fish flesh, the larvae penetrate into the intestinal wall, forming small tunnels and burrows amid a dense granulomatous inflammatory reaction. In some cases, mucosal ulcers can be identified. Nausea and vomiting may be experienced within 24 hours after ingesting contaminated fish. Later manifestations include sharp, periodic, upper abdominal pain and diarrhea, at times simulating gastritis, duodenal ulcer, or on occasion, acute appendicitis. Daschner et al.[52] report hypersensitivity allergic manifestations in a series of 40 patients with anisakiasis. Urticaria, angioedema, erythema, bronchospasm, and varying degrees of anaphylaxis were the common presenting symptoms. Lopez-Serrano et al.[169] report an additional 22 patients with gastroallergic anisakiasis. Two or more worms were detected by gastroscopy in three of these patients. Moneo et al.[186] demonstrated that these allergic reactions are in response to a potent allergen (Ani S 1) produced in the excretory gland of the *Anisakis simplex* adult worm. Because these symptoms are often delayed, the diagnosis of anisakiasis may be difficult, but must be considered, particularly if there is a clinical history of ingestion of raw or undercooked fish. Anisakiasis larvae may on occasion migrate beyond the stomach, producing metastatic infections in the omentum, liver, pancreas, and lungs.[233] Ikeda et al.[142] report on the successful treatment of nine patients with gastric anisakiasis by removing the causative larval worms through an endoscope, which immediately alleviated the acute abdominal pain. Surgical removal of the worm granuloma and/or thiabendazole, 25 mg/kg three times a day for 3 days, is the recommended therapy.

Yaquihashi et al.[301] report on the successful diagnosis of anisakiasis using a microenzyme-linked immunosorbent assay, with a monoclonal antibody directed against a specific *A. simplex* larvae. However, this approach is limited to a few research or reference laboratories, as commercial reagents are not currently available.

GNATHOSTOMIASIS

Gnathostoma spinigerum is a nematode that normally infects the intestinal tract of cats and dogs; however, humans may become accidental hosts by ingesting poorly cooked or pickled seafoods containing immature larval forms. The disease is endemic in cats and dogs in the Far East. After ingestion of contaminated fish by a dog or cat, the released larvae develop in the stomach or intestinal wall into adults that become encased in granulomatous inflammatory nodules. In humans, however, the larvae do not mature; rather, they penetrate the gastric wall and migrate throughout the tissues. Deep cutaneous or subcutaneous tunnels may develop, simulating cutaneous larva migrans; or, hard, nonpitting painful swellings may occur. Hira et al.[133] reported a case in a Thai resident living in Kuwait, who presented with acute pain in the right iliac fossa. A mass of the terminal ileum and cecum was removed, revealing an immature male *G. spinigerum* worm. More recently, Grobusch and associates[113] reported the case of a cutaneous granuloma of the arm in a woman from Bangladesh living in Germany. Marked eosinophilia and a grossly elevated IgE were also observed. The diagnosis was made by demonstrating *Gnathostoma*-specific serum antibodies using an enzyme immunoassay.

ANGIOSTRONGYLIASIS

Human angiostrongyliasis is caused by the larvae of nematodes the adults of which live in rats as the definitive host. The disease presents in humans in two clinical forms, depending on the species: *A. cantonensis*, endemic in Thailand, Tahiti, and Taiwan among other South Pacific locales, causes a syndrome of meningitis, eosinophilic pleocytosis in the CSF and peripheral blood eosinophilia (known as eosinophilic meningitis). *A. costaricensis*, the rat lungworm, endemic primarily in Costa Rica, with cases also reported in Mexico and in Central and South America, causes abdominal disease primarily of the distal small intestine and ascending colon, the sites of penetration by the developing larvae.

The adult female produces eggs at the site of infection in the rat lung, which are then swallowed and passed in the feces. Slugs, land snails, and other mollusks (less commonly, also freshwater prawns, land crabs, and frogs) ingest these eggs and serve as an intermediate host within which the infective third-stage larvae develop. Humans acquire the infection by ingesting foods, usually leafy vegetables, contaminated with infected snails and slugs. After ingestion by humans, the larvae migrate to the brain causing eosinophilic meningitis. Symptoms vary from mild headache, stiff neck, and weakness to more full-blown symptoms, including nausea, vomiting, pruritic skin rash, and a variety of neurologic symptoms, including paresthesias, fourth and sixth cranial-nerve palsies, and in heavy infections, coma and death.

Witoonpanich et al.[291] report two fatal cases out of three infected in one family. Two days after ingestion of Pila snails, a generalized itchy maculopapular rash developed in all three patients, followed by myalgia, marked paresthesia, fever, and headache. Weakness of the extremities, urine retention, and cloudiness of consciousness progressing to coma was experienced by the two patients with a fatal outcome. Autopsy revealed multiple tracks and cavities with the presence of *A. cantonensis* in the brain and various levels of the spinal cord.

In the normal host, the rat, *A. costaricensis* adults occupy arteries and arterioles in the ileocecal part of the intestine. Eggs deposited in the rat tissue hatch and escape in the feces. Slugs also serve as intermediate hosts, and humans become infected by ingesting slug-contaminated foods. The larvae penetrate the tissues in the ileocecal portion of the human intestine, including the appendix, where a combination of the adult worms and the deposited eggs cause a severe granulomatous inflammatory reaction resulting in the formation of a tumorlike mass. Hulbert et al.[141] have reported two cases of *A. costaricensis* infections in children acquired within the United States. One patient presented with symptoms suggestive of acute appendicitis; the other with a possible Meckel's diverticulum.

The diagnosis is usually made in patients in endemic areas on the basis of the symptoms described together with increased eosinophils seen in the spinal fluid and in the peripheral blood. Larvae or young adult worms may be recovered in the CSF. A positive serologic ELISA titer, particularly when found in both serum and in the CSF, can also aid in the diagnosis.[301]

ECHINOCOCCOSIS (HYDATID DISEASE)

Echinococcosis, or hydatid disease, is possibly one of the more difficult parasitic diseases to understand because of the peculiar cystic lesions that form when the larval stages of the parasite invade the viscera. Two species with somewhat different morphology and patterns of behavior may be encountered, *Echinococcus granulosus* and *Echinococcus multilocularis*. Humans serve as accidental hosts for both species. The normal life cycle of *E. granulosa* involves dogs or foxes as the definitive hosts, within the intestines of which the adult tapeworms reside. They measure about 3–6 mm in length and possess three proglottides and a scolex armed with a double row of hooklets (Color Plate 22-11*F*). Sheep, cattle or swine serve as the intermediate hosts, and cystic larval disease develops, to be described below. *Echinococcus multilocularis* differs slightly in this regard as the definitive hosts are dogs, foxes, wolves, and cats, while the intermediate hosts are small rodents, including squirrels, field mice, and voles. If humans are infected, they are also intermediate hosts in whom the larval form of the parasite is harbored. The life cycle is illustrated in Figure 22-29.

The cysts of *E. granulosus* grow slowly and usually remain quiescent for many years. Only rarely do cysts rupture, at times into the biliary tract and at other times through the liver capsule into the peritoneal cavity. If the cyst should rupture, either spontaneously in the body or during surgery, the danger from death from anaphylactic shock is high. Metastatic cystic lesions can also develop in virtually any of the visceral organs if the primary cyst ruptures. If cyst material seeds the peritoneal lining, massive proliferation can occur with vascular invasion and spread to other organs. Brain cysts may also occasionally be found. The cysts of *E. multilocularis* grow more rapidly, with invasion of hepatic parenchyma simulating a carcinoma. Examples of hydatid cysts are illustrated in Color Plate 22-11*B* and *C*.

Laboratory Diagnosis. The laboratory diagnosis may be made by demonstrating the daughter cysts or brood capsules with protoscolices in surgically removed tissue. The inner lining of the cyst is a germinal membrane from which numerous daughter embryos develop. These form as tiny polypoid structures (brood capsules) that line the inner reproductive membrane from which large numbers of daughter cysts (hydatid sand) are produced (Color Plate 22-11*D*). When the embryos break free from the membrane and float in the fluid within the cyst, they are known as **hydatid sand** (Color Plate 22-11*E*). If examined under a microscope, each grain of sand is, in fact, a tiny embryonic beginning of a new tapeworm, complete with an inverted scolex and a rostellum armed with hooklets (Color Plate 22-11*H*).

Several immunodiagnostic techniques are available by which a clinical diagnosis may be confirmed. Gottstein[107] provides a comprehensive review of the molecular and immunologic approaches to the diagnosis of hydatid disease as of 1992. Most immunodiagnostic techniques involve the detection of echinococcus-specific antibody in the serum of suspected patients, using a variety of crude antigens. The problem with methods using crude antigens is the serologic cross-reactivity of echinococcal antibody tests with other parasite diseases, liver cirrhosis, and collagen diseases. Problems with cross-reactivity have been substantially improved with the development of a selected antigen called arc-5. In a study conducted by Schantz and McAuley,[238] a high percentage of the arc-5-positive persons subsequently were shown to harbor hydatid cysts. Cross-reactivity of the arc-5 antigen has been demonstrated in the sera of patients with cysticercosis; however, the differential diagnosis should be possible clinically in such cases.

Verastegui et al.[271] offer an enzyme-linked immunoelectrotransfer blot assay for the diagnosis of hydatid disease that circumvents the cysticercosis crossover problem. The antigen, prepared from lyophilized bovine hydatid fluid, was found to contain three 8-, 16-, and 21-kDa bands, that cross-reacted in only 12, 4, and 4%, respectively, of sera from patients with cysticercosis, a significant reduction from most ELISA assays. Newer enzyme immunoassays provide greater than 90% sensitivity and specificity in detecting echinococcus-specific antibodies. Using an ELISA procedure, Poretti et al.[219] demonstrated 91% sensitivity and 82% specificity for detecting *E. granulosus*–specific antigen in direct assay of cyst fluids, providing a 99% discrimination between seropositive cystic hydatid cases and noncestode parasitic infections or malignancies. Helbig et al.[126] were able to differentiate between cystic and alveolar disease with an assay using recombinant larval antigens, results of which proved to be more specific than radiologic imaging studies. The evolution of PCR coupled with the production of specific DNA probes has great promise in the diagnosis of echinococcal disease, particularly in the detection of target antigen in fine needle biopsy material obtained from suspicious lesions.[107]

MULTICEPS SPECIES—COENUROSIS

Coenurosis is another human disease related to a dog tapeworm, a Taenia-like cestode of the genus *Multiceps*, in which the normal intermediate host are sheep, cattle, horses, and other herbivorous animals. Humans become infected by ingesting food or water contaminated with dog feces containing *Multiceps* eggs. The disease in humans primarily involves the central nervous system, where the migrating larvae develop into echinococcal-type cysts individually known as a coenurus. These cysts differ from echinococcal cysts by having multiple scolices but no brood capsules or daughter cysts. Symptoms are often those of a space-occupying lesion, including headache, vomiting, and localizing neurologic symptoms such as hemiplegia, paraplegia, aphasia, and seizures. Basal arachnoiditis leading to the posterior fossa syndrome and internal hydrocephalus are also presenting symptoms. The diagnosis is usually made following surgical removal of the cyst and the histologic recognition of the coenurus.

SPARGANOSIS: *SPIROMETRA MANSONOIDES*

Dogs and cats serve as the definitive host for several species of diphyllobothroid tapeworms belonging to the genus *Spirometra*. *Spirometra* eggs passed in dog or cat feces into freshwater hatch and are ingested by minute *Cyclops* crustaceans, within which they develop into procercoid larvae. These larvae in turn develop into plerocercoid larvae, individually known as sparganum, in the flesh of a second intermediate host (fish, snakes, frogs) that feed on the *Cyclops*. Humans become infected either by ingesting an infected *Cyclops*, by eating the raw, infected flesh of the second intermediate host, or from the practice in certain cultures of applying raw fish to the skin, eyes, or vagina to heal other maladies. On ingestion, sparganum larvae penetrate the bowel wall and enter the circulation.

Most lesions in humans are subcutaneous, where slow-growing, painful, red, edematous nodules develop. The definitive diagnosis is made only after surgical removal of a sparganum and identifying the slender, delicate white worm that measures 60–80 × 1–2 mm wide. Aberrant spargana have been observed in the external eye, where edematous swelling of the eyelid simulating Romana's sign (Chagas' disease) has been reported, in lymph channels producing elephantiasis-

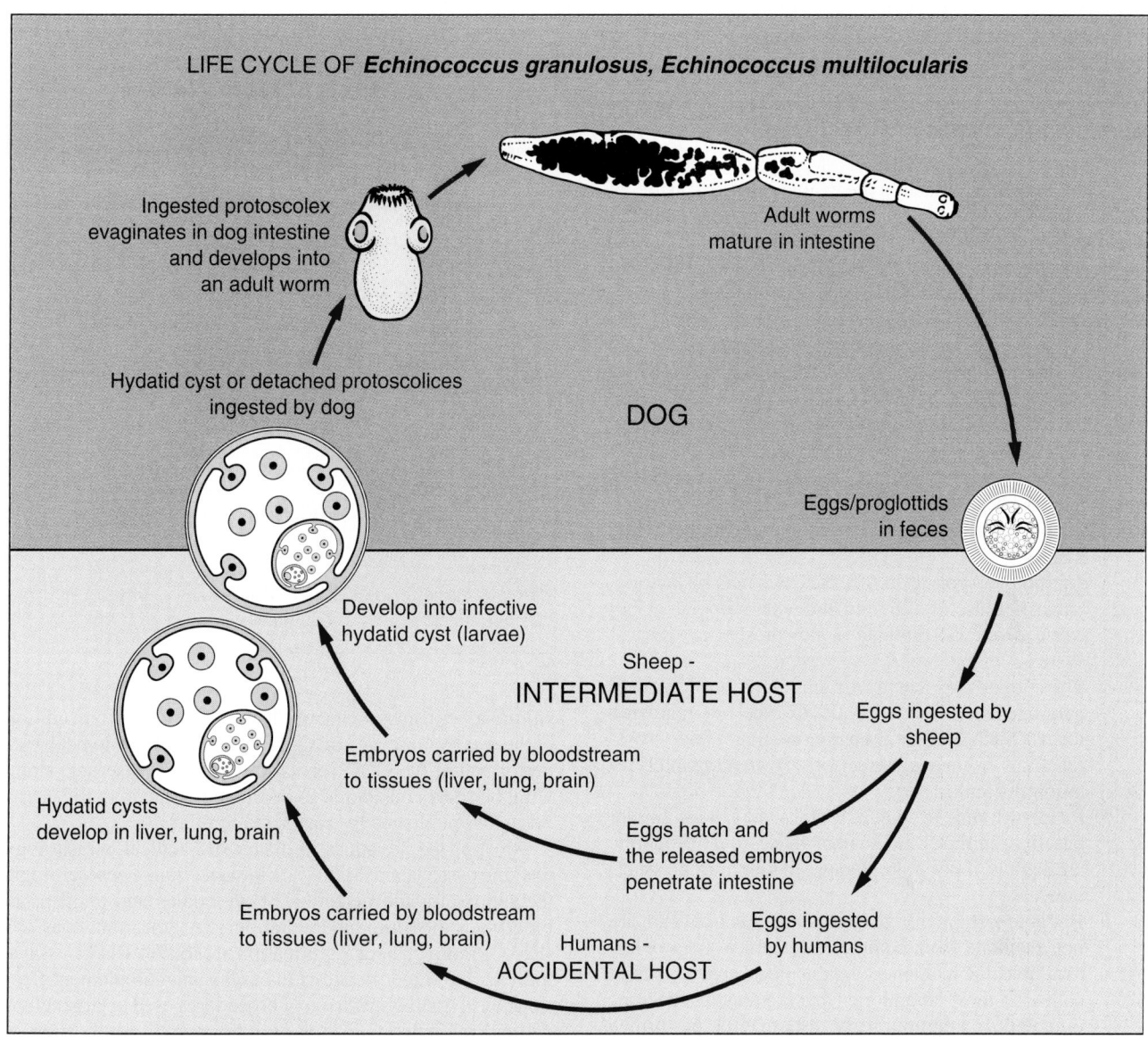

Figure 22-29 Life cycle of *Echinococcus granulosus*. Hexacanth eggs, either singly or within proglottids, closely resembling those of *Taenia* species, are passed in dog feces, and become embryonated in the soil. Under normal circumstances, these eggs are ingested by the natural intermediate hosts—sheep, cattle, or swine—or by the small rodents mentioned above in the case of *E. multilocularis*. The larvae are released from the eggs in the intestines of the intermediate hosts and, by means of their hooklets, bore through the bowel wall and enter the circulation.

The circulating embryos are filtered out in the capillaries of various organs, usually the liver because it is the first organ to drain the mesenteric blood. *Echinococcus granulosus* produces a single multilayered cyst from which small cysts called bladder worms may form (Color Plate 22-11*B*). The cysts of *E. multilocularis*, as the species name implies, have multiple locules. Multiple cysts up to 5 cm in diameter, resembling what Aristotle called hailstones, may be seen in some cases (Color Plate 22-11*C*). Humans may also become the intermediate host by ingesting the echinococcus eggs, the larvae of which also may migrate to various organs, particularly the liver, lung, and brain, and mature into cysticercoid lesions. The life cycle is complete when infected viscera of the definitive host are eaten by a dog, fox, or other related carnivore.

like swellings, and in the brain in the form of cerebral abscesses.

Serologic Diagnosis of Parasitic Infections

The serologic approach to the evaluation of parasitic diseases is most applicable when invasive techniques other than the routine examination of blood, feces, or other body fluids are required to establish a diagnosis. For example, the infective parasitic forms in toxoplasmosis, extraintestinal amebiasis, trichinosis, and cysticercosis are often lodged deep within tissues and organs, and either deep needle or open surgical biopsies are needed to confirm the diagnosis. In such cases, serologic diagnosis may be possible if several potential problems, as outlined by Garcia[96] are considered:

1. Certain parasites that pass through several developmental phases may not provide sufficiently constant or continuous antigenic stimuli to elicit antibody formation.
2. Antibody responses in specific cases may be lacking, either because of a limited antigenic stimulus or because a relevant antigen is not present in the test system.
3. The antigens used in assays are often poorly defined heterogeneous mixtures or extracts of parasitic forms. Such antigen preparations may show cross-reactivity or inadequate sensitivity, making interpretation difficult.
4. Patients living in endemic areas may have higher baseline antibody titers than those in nonendemic areas; thus, if possible, changes in titer must be ascertained.
5. Reliable test kits for general diagnostic use often are not available from commercial sources. Even when available, the incidence of parasitic disease is usually so low in most laboratories that the reagents become outdated. In addition, these tests may be performed too infrequently for laboratory personnel to feel comfortable in making interpretations.

Several of the applications of antibody and antigen detection provided in Garcia's review are reflected in short sections included within the discussion of each animal parasite in this textbook. We have elected to include such discussions within each section rather than having a stand-alone presentation here. Many of the details of the various methods currently being used in research laboratories are beyond the scope of this book. In a practical sense, the volume of parasitic diseases encountered in most practice settings in the United States is low to nonexistent, making serologic testing impractical in most diagnostic microbiology laboratories. In most instances, cases and specimens are referred to local and regional reference laboratories, including the various state public health laboratories. Each reference laboratory will have in operation a mixture of time-honored and newer technologies that is unique to that laboratory, and consultation is necessary to learn which application and the types of specimens required may be most applicable. Procedures for the detection of antigen and antibodies for the more commonly encountered parasitic diseases can be found in Chapter 22 of the current edition of the text by Garcia.[96] Box 22-7 is the list of serological tests performed at the CDC for various parasitic diseases, along with the titers considered to be diagnostically significant, as originally published by Walls and Smith.[274]

Most of the advances in diagnostic clinical parasitology over the past 5 years involve the introduction of new serologic techniques for the detection of antibodies and antigens in blood and other fluids and secretions. Enzyme immunoassays (EIAs), indirect hemagglutination inhibition (IHA) assays, indirect and direct fluorescent assays and complement fixation constitute the spectrum of procedures used in larger clinical and reference parasitology laboratories. Application of molecular biology into diagnostic parasitology, or to use Persing's sound bite,[208] "from trenches to the benches," is an exciting evolution coming from within research laboratories.

Enthusiasm, however, must be tempered by certain realities, as pointed out by Weiss.[283] A number of new molecular assays for the diagnosis of parasitic diseases have been included in this book as short segments in the sections on laboratory diagnosis of the various parasites discussed above. These citations focus on the work currently being performed in research laboratories; however, as pointed out by Weiss, very few of the new techniques have been subjected to field trials or large-scale clinical evaluations. The practical applications of PCR can be cited as an example. PCR provides a great increase in the sensitivity and specificity of DNA probe assays, resulting from the enhanced signals produced by the thousand times replication of targeted repetitive species-specific DNA sequences. This offers the possibility of quickly and directly identifying target antigens in very low concentrations or in trace amounts in clinical specimens. However, PCR is currently available in only a few diagnostic laboratories because of the great expense and technical demands of the method.

Box 22-7 Serologic Tests Performed at the Centers for Disease Control

Disease	Test	Diagnostic Titers
African trypanosomiasis	IFA	≥1:16
Amebiasis	IHA	≥1:256
Ascariasis	ELISA	≥1:32
Chagas' disease	CF, IHA	≥1:8; 1:64
Cysticercosis	IHA	≥1:64
Echinococcosis	IHA	≥1:256
Fascioliasis	IHA	≥1:128
Filariasis	IHA	≥1:128
Leishmaniasis	IIF	≥1:16
Malaria	IIF	≥1:64
Paragonimiasis	CF	≥1:8
Pneumocystosis	IIF	≥1:16
Schistosomiasis	IIF	≥1:16
Strongyloidiasis	IHA	≥1:64
Toxocariasis	ELISA	≥1:32
Toxoplasmosis	IIF, IgM-IIF	≥1:256; 1:16
Trichinosis	Bentonite Floc	≥1:16

Table 22-1 **Drugs Commonly Used in the Treatment of Parasitic Infections**

DRUG	TYPE OF AGENT	MODE OF ACTION	COMMENTS
Amphotericin B	Polyene macrolide	Increases cell membrane permeability leading to a loss by leakage, first of ions and then of other cellular contents. Binding is effected by sterols in membrane.	Mammalian cells may also be affected with severe side effects. Used in treatment of infections with *Acanthamoeba* species and in advanced cases of mucocutaneous leishmaniasis.
Chloroquine	4 amino quinoline (quinine)	The concentration of drug achieved in malarial parasitized erythrocytes is several hundred times greater than in normal erythrocytes. The drug binds to ferriprotoporphyrin IX (FP), a degradation product of the hemoglobin present in the parasite food vacuole. The complex of chloroquine is FP is lytic for the parasite.	Mainstay of malarial therapy for over two decades. *P. falciparum* drug resistance occurs in strains that can somehow sequester FP so that it does not bind to chloroquine. Chloroquine is not curative for *P. vivax*.
Emetine	Alkaloid (cycloheximide)	Directly lethal to trophozites of *E. histolytica* by causing degenerative changes in the trophozoites. The drug causes interruption of cell division by irreversibly inhibiting protein synthesis by preventing movement of mRNA along the 60s ribosomal subunit.	Used in the therapy for severe intestinal amebiasis or amebic liver abscess as an alternative to metronidazole. Mammalian cells are also affected, resulting in severe side effects and limiting its therapeutic use.
Diethylcarbamazine	Piperazine derivative (two nitrogens in benzene ring)	The drug is thought to alter surface properties and mobilization of microfilariae, causing them to leave the circulation through a specific neuromuscular effect. The microfilariae become trapped in the liver and are subject to phagocytosis.	Used primarily in the treatment of filarial infections. The drug is well absorbed, reaching peak serum concentrations within 3 hours, and is widely distributed throughout the body.
Ivermectin	A 22,23 dihydro derivative of avermectin B, a complex macrocyclic lactone produced by *Streptomyces avermitilis*	The drug acts on gamma-aminobutyric acid (GABA) receptors on the parasite musculature. Inhibitory neurons that cause release of GABA from presynaptic terminals are stimulated, in essence blocking signal transmission from interneurons to excitatory neurons. The effect is the loss of locomotor activity by the parasite, making normally motile parasites highly susceptible to various host defenses.	The drug has a broad spectrum of antinematodal activity but has no effects on flukes and tapeworms. It has been effectively used in onchocerciasis, cutaneous visceral larval migrans, *Angiostrongylus meningitis*, and various gastrointestinal nematode infections.
Mebendazole	Benzimidazole—benzine + five ring structure, including three carbon and two nitrogen molecules	Selective inhibition of glucose uptake in nematodes and cestodes, leading to increased utilization of parasite glycogen; parasites are thereby deprived of their main energy sources. Under action of the drug, the parasite is immobilized and in vitro larval development is interrupted.	Mebendazole is active against nematodes and used primarily in the treatment of trichuriasis, ascariasis, hookworm, and strongyloides infections. The drug is minimally absorbed from the gastrointestinal tract, thus being most effective in the treatment of intraintestinal worms.
Melarsoprol	Arsenical (a dimercaprol derivative of melarsen oxide)	Arsenoxides attach to trypanosomes by covalent bonding—sulfur groups in arsenoxide	Used in the treatment of trypsanosomiasis. The drug enters parasite cells more rapidly than

(Continued)

Table 22-1 *Continued*

DRUG	TYPE OF AGENT	MODE OF ACTION	COMMENTS
		exert lethal effect by blocking essential biologically active glycolytic enzymatic groups. Arsenicals react with sulfhydryl groups, leading to inactivation of various enzymes synthesized by the parasite for glycolysis.	human cells, and thus is more toxic to the parasite. The drug crosses the blood-brain barrier and enters the cerebrospinal fluid, making it highly effective in the treatment of CNS infection.
Metronidazole (Flagyl)	5-nitroimidazole	Metronidazole is metabolized into derivatives, including superoxide radicals, that interfere with DNA metabolism in parasites, causing extensive breaks in the DNA strands and interrupting the helical structure. Protein synthesis in the parasite is thus disrupted.	Used in the treatment of invasive amebiasis and also for infections with *Trichomonas vaginalis* and *Giardia lamblia*. Because only 10% of the drug is bound to serum proteins, it reaches high concentrations in the tissues, including lung, bile, bone, liver, and brain, exceeding levels required to inhibit the organisms against which it is active.
Niclosamide	Heterocyclic pyrazinoisoquinoline derivative	The oxidative phosphorylation of mitochondria of cestodes is interrupted. The effect on mature adult worms is lethal, inducing complete muscular paralysis in certain species. The drug induces the scoleces to detach and the worms to disintegrate before they are eliminated in the feces.	Niclosamide is an alternative drug for the treatment of tapeworms. Treatment for *Hymenolepsis* worms is increased to 5 days because onchospheres develop in the jejunal villi, and cysticercoids emerge into the intestinal lumen about 4 days later.
Praziquantel: (pyrazinoquinoline)	8-amino-quinoline derivative	The drug acts by increasing the membrane permeability to calcium, causing contractions and paralysis of the musculature of worms. Neuromuscular effects lead to increased motility and spastic paralysis, causing the worms to detach and disintegrate in the intestine.	Used for the treatment of schistosomiasis, cysticercosis, tapeworm infections, and liver, lung, and intestinal flukes. The drug achieves excellent therapeutic levels in the liver, bile, and muscle tissue, and crosses the blood-brain barrier to reach the brain and spinal fluid as well.
Primaquine	Tetrahydral pyrimidine	The drug is gametocidal and sporonticidal for all species of human malaria. Its mechanism of action is unknown, although inhibition of DNA synthesis is most likely.	Primaquine is a poor blood schizonticide but is effective against exoerythrocytic hypnozoites. Therefore, it is effective in preventing relapses due to *P. vivax* and *P. ovale*. Radical cure of malaria can be effected by a combination of chloroquine and primaquine therapy.
Pyrantel pamoate	Naphthylamine sulfonic acid, a polyanion dye	Pyrantel (and its analogues) acts as a cholinergic antagonist, causing the depolarization of muscle cells within the parasite, leading to irreversible contractures.	Used primarily in the treatment of infections with ascaria, hookworms, pinworms, and *Trichostrongylus*. The drug is insoluble in water and poorly absorbed from the gastrointestinal tract, leading to little toxicity.
Suramin		The drug inhibits glycerol 3-phosphate oxidase and glycerol	The drug is widely distributed in the body but, because of avid

Table 22-1 *Continued*

DRUG	TYPE OF AGENT	MODE OF ACTION	COMMENTS
		3-phosphate dehydrogenase, preventing reoxidation of nicotinamide-adenine dinucleotide and decreasing adenosine triphosphate synthesis. This interruption in metabolism is lethal to the parasite.	protein binding in the serum, does not pass the blood-brain barrier. The drug is used in the treatment of early trypanosomiasis; however, as it does not penetrate into the central nervous system, it is not effective in the treatment of progressive CNS disease.
Thiabendazole	Benzimidazole	Mechanism of action unknown.	The drug is well suited for the treatment of disseminated strongyloides infection and any larval forms causing visceral and cutaneous larval migrans. The bulk of absorbed drug is metabolized in the liver and excreted as metabolites in the urine.
Stibogluconate sodium	An antimony-containing compound	The drug is thought to act on sulfhydryl-containing enzymes within the parasite, decreasing the flow of glucose into the tricarboxylic acid cycle, resulting in the accumulation of glycolytic byproducts that are toxic to the developing amastigotes.	Used primarily in the treatment of leishmaniasis. After intramuscular or intravenous administration, a serum peak is achieved in 2 hours, and over 90% of the drug is excreted within 8 hours. However, the drug does gradually accumulate in the tissues, explaining why long courses of therapy are necessary.

A separate laboratory facility must be provided and great care must be taken in the handling of specimens to prevent contamination with extraneous DNA. High costs, the need for special training of personnel, and requirements for special equipment and reagents, will preclude widespread use of PCR in developing countries. However, the day when amplification methods become standard in many clinical laboratories is sooner rather than later. These direct diagnostic techniques will not only aid in the early diagnosis of parasitic diseases in humans, but will also provide the opportunity to study parasite-harboring vectors, leading to the prevention of parasitic diseases through more effective vector control. Automation, market forces, technical expertise, and the need for shortening the turnaround time to establish a diagnosis of parasitic disease are all working to bring molecular biology "to the benches."

parasitic diseases, particularly the larval forms. In some cases of extraintestinal amebiasis, a combination of a nonabsorbable drug to treat residual organisms in the intestine may be required. Many parasites exist in a cyst form, which may be poorly penetrated by many of the drugs, leading to potential reactivation of infection at a later date. A prime example is the inactive, encysted forms of *Toxoplasma gondii*, which are drug-resistant and prone to reactivate when immunity is lost, particularly in patients with AIDS, who are rarely cured.

Table 22-1 summarizes the mode of action and other attributes of select commonly used antiparasitic drugs. For a full review of all current drugs, including recommended drugs and dosages to be used for most human parasitic diseases, refer to Chapter 25 of the book by Garcia[96] and to the publication by Moore.[187]

Drugs Commonly Used in the Treatment of Parasitic Diseases

Drug therapy of parasitic diseases is directed to interrupting the invasive capabilities of parasites. Infections that occur primarily within the gastrointestinal tract are best treated with compounds that are poorly absorbed, resulting in high concentrations of active drug within the intestinal lumen. Agents that are well absorbed and achieve high serum and tissue levels are required for the treatment of invasive

REFERENCES

1. Abbasi I, Githure J, Ochola JJ, et al. Diagnosis of *Wuchereria bancrofti* infection by the polymerase chain reaction employing patients' sputum. Parasitology Res 1999;85:844–849.
2. Acuna-Soto R, Samuelson J, De Girolami P, et al. Application of the polymerase chain reaction to the epidemiology of pathogenic and nonpathogenic *Entamoeba histolytica*. Am J Trop Med Hyg 1993;48:48–70.

3. Adams EB, MacLeod IN. Invasive amebiasis: II. Amebic liver abscess and its complications. Medicine (Baltimore) 1977;56:325–334.

4. Aikawa M, Tseki M, Barnwell JW, et al. The pathology of human cerebral malaria. Am J Trop Med Hyg 1990;43:30–37.

5. Aldras AM, Orenstein JM, Kotler DP, et al. Detection of microsporidia by indirect immunofluorescence antibody test using polyclonal and monoclonal antibodies. J Clin Microbiol 1994;32:608–612.

6. Allason-Jones E, Mindel A. Sargeaunt P, Williams P. *Entamoeba histolytica* as a commensal intestinal parasite in homosexual men. N Engl J Med 1986;315:353–356.

7. Amin OM. Seasonal prevalence of intestinal parasites in the United States during 2000. Am J Trop Med Hyg 2002;66:799–803.

8. Anderson BX. Cryptosporidiosis. Lab Med 1983;14:55–56.

9. Antonelli F, Cantelli L, De Maddi F, Lamba M. *Blastocystis hominis* infection: a case report. Minerva Pediatrica 1996;48:571–573.

10. Arness M, Brown KJD, Dubey JP, et al. An outbreak of acute eosinophilic myositis attributed to human sarcocystis parasitism. Am J Trop Med Hyg 1999;61:548–553.

11. Avila HA, Pereira JB, Thiemann O, et al. Detection of *Trypanosoma cruzi* in blood specimens of chronic chagasic patients by polymerase chain reaction amplification of kinetoplast minicircle DNA: comparison with serology and xenodiagnosis. J Clin Microbiol 1993;33:2421–2426.

12. Bailey JW, Smith DH. The quantitative buffy-coat for the diagnosis of trypanosomes. Trop Doc 1994;24:54–56.

13. Baird JK, Mistrey M, Pimsler M, Connor DH. Fatal human ascariasis following secondary massive infection. Am J Trop Med Hyg 1986;35:314–318.

14. Bartlett MS, Harper K, Smith N, et al. Comparative evaluation of a modified zinc sulfate flotation technique. J Clin Microbiol 1977;7:524–528.

15. Beaver PC, Gadgel PK, Morera P. Sarcocystis in man: a review and report of five cases. Am J Trop Med Hyg 1979;28:819–844.

16. Beaver PC. Intraocular filariasis: a brief review. Am J Trop Med Hyg 1989;40:40–46.

17. Berlin OGW, Novak SM, Porchen RK. Recovery of *Cyclospora* organisms from patients with prolonged diarrhea. Clin Infect Dis 1994;18:606–609.

18. Bhatt RD, Chappell MS, Smilow PC, Das KM. Recurrent massive upper gastrointestinal hemorrhage due to *Strongyloides stercoralis* infection. Am J Gastroenterol 1990;85:1034–1036.

19. Blessmann J, Buss H, Non Nu, PA, et al. Real-time PCR for detection and differentiation of *Entamoeba histolytica* and *Entamoeba dispar* in fecal specimens. J Clin Microbiol 2002;40:4413–4417.

20. Britto C, Carsoso MA, Vanni CMM, et al. Polymerase chain reaction detection of *Trypanosoma cruzi* in human blood samples as a tool for diagnosis and treatment evaluation. Parasitology 1995;220:241–247.

21. Bruckner DA, Garcia LS, Voge M. Intestinal parasites in Los Angeles, California. Am J Med Technol 1979;45:1020–1024.

22. Brumpt E. Etude sommarie de l' ''*Entamoeba dispar*'' n. sp. Amibe á kystes quadrinuclées, parasite de l'homme. Bull Acad Med Paris 1925;94:943–952.

23. Bryan RT, Cali A, Owen RL, Spencer HC. *Microsporidia:* opportunistic pathogens in patients with AIDS. In: Sun T, ed. Progress in Clinical Parasitology, Vol 2. Philadelphia: Field and Wood, 1991;1–26.

24. Buijs J, Barsboom G, van Gemund J, et al. Toxocara seroprevalence in 5-year-old elementary schoolchildren: relation with allergic asthma. Am J Epidemiol 1994;140:839–847.

25. Bundy DA. Immunoepidemiology of intestinal helminthic infections: I. The global burden of intestinal nematode disease. Trans R Soc Trop Med Hyg 1994;88:259–261.

26. Bulloch W. The History of Bacteriology. London: Oxford University Press, 1938 (reprinted 1960).

27. California Department of Health Services. Babesiosis in California. Calif Morbid 1992;January.

28. Camous E. Treatment of cutaneous larva migrans. Clin Infect Dis 2000;30:811–814.

29. Carlson JR, Sullivan PS, Harryu DJ, et al. Enzyme immunoassay for the detection of *Giardia lamblia.* Eur J Clin Microbiol Infect Dis 1988;7:538–540

30. Centers for Disease Control and Prevention. Intestinal parasite surveillance: United States 1976. MMWR Morb Mortal Wkly Rep 1976;27:167.

31. Centers for Disease Control and Prevention. Summary of malarial diseases 1988. MMWR Morb Mortal Wkly Rep 1988;37:3.

32. Centers for Disease Control and Prevention. Microsporidian keratoconjunctivitis in patients with AIDS. MMWR Morb Mortal Wkly Rep 1991;39:188–189.

33. Centers for Disease Control and Prevention. Probable locally acquired mosquito-transmitted *Plasmodium vivax* infection—Suffolk County, New York, 1999. Morb Mortal Weekly Rep 2000;49:495–498.

34. Chan FT, Guan MX, Mackenzie AM. Application of indirect immunofluorescence to detection of *Dientamoeba fragilis* trophozoites in fecal specimens. J Clin Microbiol 1993;1:1710–1714.

35. Chan MS. The global burden of intestinal nematode infections—fifty years on. Parasitol Today 1997;13:438–443

36. Chapman A, Vallejo V, Mossie KG, et al. Isolation and characterization of species-specific DNA probes from *Taenia solium* and *Taenia saginata* and their use in an egg detection assay. J Clin Microbiol 1995;33:1283–1288.

37. Chaudhry AZ, Longworth DL. Cutaneous manifestations of intestinal helminth infection. Dermatol Clin 1989;7:275–290.

38. Chen Q, Schlichtherle M, Wahlgren M. Molecular aspects of severe malaria. Clin Microbiol Rev 2000;13:439–450.

39. Chu E, Whitlock WL, Dietrich RA. Pulmonary hyperinfection syndrome with *Strongyloides stercoralis.* Chest 1990;97:1475–1477.

40. Chuley JD, Ockenhouse CF. Host receptors for malaria-infected erythrocytes. Am J Trop Med Hyg 1990;43:6–14.

41. Clark PS, Brownsberger KM, Saslow AR, et al. Bear meat trichinosis: epidemiologic, serologic, and clinical observations from two Alaskan outbreaks. Ann Intern Med 1972;76:951–956.

42. Clark CG, Diamond LS. Differentiation of pathogenic *Entamoeba histolytica* from other intestinal protozoa by riboprinting. Arch Med Res 1992;23:15–16.

43. Clark DP. New insights into human cryptosporidiosis. Clin Microbiol Rev 1999;12:554–563.

44. Cooper ES, Thyte-Alleng CA, Finzi-Smith JS, MacDonald TT. Intestinal nematode infection in children: the pathophysiological price paid. Parasitology 1992;104(Suppl):S91–S103.

45. Couldwell WT, Apuzzo ML. Cysticercosis cerebri. Neurosurg Clin North Am 1992;3:471–481.

46. Croft AM, Garner P. Mefloquine for preventing malaria in non-immune adult travelers. Cochrane Database Syst Rev 2000;2:CD-000138.

47. Cross JH. Intestinal capillariasis. Clin Microbiol Rev 1992;5:120–129.

48. Cruz ME, Schantz PM, Cruz I, et al. Epilepsy and neurocysticercosis in an Andean community. Int J Epidemiol 1999;28:799–803.

49. Cubitt WD, Ades AE, Peckham CS. Evaluation of five commercial assays for screening antenatal sera for antibodies to *Toxoplasma gondii.* J Clin Pathol 1992;45:435–438.

50. Cummins AJ, Moody AH, Lalloo K, Chiodini PL. Rapid latex agglutination test for extra-luminal amoebiasis. J Clin Pathol 1994;47:647–648.

51. Current WL, Owens RL. Cryptosporidiosis and microsporidiosis. In: Farthing MJG, Keusch FT, eds. Enteric Infection: Mechanisms, Manifestations and Management. London: Chapman & Hall Medical, 1989:223–249.

52. Daschner A, Slonso-Gomez A, Cabanas R, et al. Gastroallergic anisakiasis: borderline between food allergy and parasitic disease: clinical and allergologic evaluation of 20 patients with confirmed acute parasitism by *Anisakis simplex.* J Allergy Clin Immunol 2000;105:176–181

53. Da Silva AJ, Piuverzam MR, De Moura H, et al. Rapid competitive enzyme-linked immunosorbent assay using a monoclonal antibody reacting with a 15-kilodalton tegumental antigen of *Schistosoma mansoni* for serodiagnosis of schistosomiasis. J Clin Microbiol 1993;31:2315–2319.

54. da Silva AJ, Bornay-Llinares FJ, del Aguila de la Puente C, et al. Diagnosis of *Enterocytozoon bieneusi* (Microsporidia) infections by polymerase chain reaction in stool samples using primers based on the region coding for small-subunit ribosomal RNA. Arch Pathol Lab Med 1997;121:874–879.

55. da Silva AJ, Bornay-Llinares FJ, Moura INS, et al. Fast and reliable extraction of protozoan parasite DNA from fecal specimens. Mol Diagn 1999;4:57–63.

56. Davidson RA, Fletcher RH, Chapman EE. Risk factors for strongyloidiasis—a controlled study. Arch Intern Med 1984;144:321–325.

57. Davis A. Recent advances in schistosomiasis. Q J Med 1986;226:95–110.

58. Davis CE. Laboratory diagnosis of parasitic diseases. In: Harrison's Principles of Internal Medicine. 15th Ed. New York, McGraw Hill, 2001:1186.

59. Davis-Reed L, Theis JH. Cutaneous schistosomiasis: report of a case and review of the literature. Am Acad Dermatol 2000;42:678–680.

60. DeGirolami PC, Ezratty CR, Desai G, et al. Diagnosis of intestinal microsporidiosis by examination of stool and duodenal aspirate with Weber's modified trichrome and Uvitex 2B stains. J Clin Microbiol 1995;33:805–810.

61. De Groote MA, Visvesvara GS, Wilson ML, et al. Polymerase chain reaction and culture confirmation of disseminated *Encephalitozoon cuniculi* in patient with AIDS: successful therapy with albendazole. J Infect Dis 1995;171:1375–1378.

62. De Jonge N, Rabello ALK, Kruger FW, et al. Levels of the schistosome circulating anodic and cathodic antigens in the serum diagnosis of schistosomiasis patients from Brazil. Trans Royal Soc Trop Med Hyg 1991;85:756–759.

63. DeKaminsky RG. Evaluation of three methods for laboratory diagnosis of *Strongyloides stercoralis* infection. J Parasitol 1993;79:277–280.

64. Dennis DT, Kean BH. Isolation of microfilariae: report of a new method. J Parasitol 1971;57:1146–1147.

65. Diamond LS, Clark CG. A re-description of *Entamoeba histolytica* Schaudinn, 1903 (Emended Walker, 1911) separating if from *Entamoeba dispar* Brumpt, 1925. J Eukaryotic Microbiol 1994;40:340–344.

66. Diaz JCP. Control of Chagas' disease in Brazil. Parasitol Today 1987;3:336–341.

67. Didier ES, Dider PJ, Friedberg DN, et al. Isolation and characterization of a

new human microsporidian, *Encephalitozoon hellem* (n. sp.), from three AIDS patients with keratoconjunctivitis. J Infect Dis 1991;163:617–621.

68. Deardorff TL, Kent ML. Prevalence of larval *Anisakis simplex* in pen-reared and wild-caught salmon (*Salmonidae*) from Puget Sound, Washington. J Wildlife Dis 1991;25:416–419.

69. Dobroszycki J, Herwaldt BL, Boctor F, et al. A cluster of transfusion-associated babesiosis cases traced to a single asymptomatic donor. JAMA 1999;281: 927–930.

70. Donelson JE. Antigenic variation in African trypanosomes. Contrib Microbiol Immunol 1987;8:138–175.

71. Dorman SE, Cannon ME, Telford SR III, et al. Fulminant babesiosis treated with clindamycin, quinine, and whole-blood exchange transfusion. Transfusion 2000;40:375–380.

72. Duombo O, Rossignol JF, Pichard E, et al. Nitazoxanide in the treatment of cryptosporidial diarrhea and other intestinal parasitic infections associated with acquired immunodeficiency syndrome in tropical Africa. Am J Trop Med Hyg 1997;56:637–639.

73. Dupon M, Cazenave J, Pellegrin JL, et al. Detection of *Toxoplasma gondii* by PCR and tissue culture in cerebrospinal fluid and blood of human immunodeficiency virus-seropositive patients. J Clin Microbiol 1995;33:2421–2426.

74. Dupouy-Camet J, De Souza SL, Maslo C, et al. Detection of *Toxoplasma gondii* in venous blood from AIDS patients by polymerase chain reaction. J Clin Microbiol 1993;31:1866–1869.

75. Eberhard ML, Walker EM, Steurer FJ. Survival and infectivity of Babesia in blood maintained at 25°C and 2-4°C. J Parasitol 1995;38:790–792.

76. Ehnert KL, Roberto RR, Barrett L, et al. Cysticercosis: first 12 months of reporting in California. Bull Pan Am Health Organ 1992;26:165–172.

77. Espino AM, Finlay CM. Sandwich enzyme-linked immunosorbent assay for detection of excretory secretory antigens in human fascioliasis. J Clin Microbiol 1994;32:190–193.

78. Esrey SA, Collett J, Mikoitis MD, et al. The risk of infection from Giardia lamblia due to drinking water supply, use of water and latrines among preschool children in rural Lesotho. Int J Epidemiol 1989;18:248–253.

79. Filice GA, Hitt JA, Mitchell CD, et al. Diagnosis of toxoplasma parasitemia in patients with AIDS by gene detection after amplification with polymerase chain reaction. J Clin Microbiol 1993;32:2327–2331.

80. Fischer P, Liu XL, Lizotte-Waniewski M, et al. Development of a quantitative, competitive polymerase chain reaction enzyme linked immunosorbent assay for the detection of Wuchereria bancrofti DNA. Parasitol Res 1999;85:176–183.

81. Flanigan TP, Ramratnam B, Graeber C, et al. Prospective trial of paromomycin for cryptosporidiosis in AIDS. Am J Med 1996;100:370–372.

82. Flieder DB, Moran CA. Pulmonary dirofilariasis: a clinicopathologic study of 41 lesions in 39 patients. Hum Pathol 1999;30:251–256.

83. Flynn PM. Emerging diarrheal pathogens: *Cryptosporidium parvum, Isospora belli, Cyclospora* species, and microsporidia. Pediatr Ann 1996;25:480–487.

84. Foster WE. A History of Parasitology. Edinburgh: E & S Livingstone, 1965.

85. Franzen C, Muller A, Hegener P, et al. Detection of microsporidia (*Enterocytozoon bieneuzi*) in intestinal biopsy specimens from human immunodeficiency virus-infected patients by PCR. J Clin Microbiol 1995;33:2294–2296.

86. Fraser GG, Cooke KR. Endemic giardiasis and municipal water supply. Am J Pub Health 1991;81:760–762.

87. Frenkel JK. Toxoplasmosis. Pediatr Clin N Am 1985;32:917–932.

88. Fricker CR, Crabb JH. Water-borne cryptosporidiosis: detection methods and treatment options. Adv Parasitol 1998;40:241–278.

89. Furness BW, Beach MJ, Roberts JM. Giardiasis surveillance—United States, 1992–1997. MMWR Morb Mortal Wkly Rep 2000;49:1.

90. Gallagher PG, Venglarcik JS III. *Blastocystis hominis* enteritis. Pediatr Infect Dis 1985;4:556–557.

91. Garcia LS, Bruckner DA, Clancy MN. Clinical relevance of *Blastocystis hominis*. Lancet 1984;1:1233–1234.

92. Garcia LS, Schum AC, Bruckner DA. Evaluation of a new monoclonal antibody combination reagent for direct fluorescence detection of Giardia cysts and Cryptosporidium oocysts in human fecal specimens. J Clin Microbiol 1992;30: 3255–3257.

93. Garcia LS, Shimizu RY. Evaluation of nine immunoassay kits (enzyme immunoassay and direct fluorescence) for detection of *Giardia lamblia* and *Cryptosporidium parvum* in human fecal specimens. J Clin Microbiol 1997;38:1526–1529.

94. Garcia LS, Shimizu RY. Evaluation of intestinal protozoan morphology in human fecal specimens preserved in EcoFix: comparison of Wheatley's trichrome stain and EcoStain. J Clin Microbiol 1998;36:1974–1976.

95. Garcia LS. Flagellates and ciliates 1999. Clin Lab Med 1999;19:621–638

96. Garcia LS. Diagnostic Medical Parasitology. 4th Ed. Washington, DC: ASM Press, 2001.

97. Garcia LS, Shimizu RY, Bernard CN. Detection of *Giardia lamblia, Entamoeba histolytica*/*E. dispar*, and *Cryptosporidium parvum* antigens in human fecal specimens using the EIA Triage parasite panel. J Clin Microbiol 2000;38:3337–3340.

98. Garza D. Diarrhea caused by a universal coccidian parasite. Lab Med 1983;14: 283–286.

99. Genta RM. Dysregulation of strongyloidiasis: a new hypothesis. Clin Microbiol Rev 1992;5:345–355.

100. Ginsberg M, Hung S, Bartzen M, et al. Mosquito-transmitted malaria—California and Florida. MMWR Morb Mortal Wkly Rep 1991;40:106–108.

101. Godsel LM, Tibbits RS, Olson CL, et al. Utility of recombinant flagellar calcium–binding protein for serodiagnosis of *Trypanosoma cruzi* infection. J Clin Microbiol 1995;33:2082–2085.

102. Gomes ML, Galvao LMC, Macedo AM, et al. Chagas' disease diagnosis: comparative analysis of parasitologic, molecular, and serologic methods. Am J Trop Med Hyg 1999;60:205–210.

103. Gomes ML, Macedo AM, Vago AR, et al. *Trypanosoma cruzi*: optimization of polymerase chain reaction for detection in human blood. Exp Parasitol 1998; 88:28–33.

104. Gonzalez-Ruiz A, Haque R, Rehman T, et al. Diagnosis of amebic dysentery by detection of *Entamoeba histolytica* fetal antigen by an invasive strain-specific monoclonal antibody-based enzyme-linked immunosorbent assay. J Clin Microbiol 1994;32:1964–1970.

105. Gonzalez-Ruiz A, Haque R, Aguirre A. et al. Value of microscopy in the diagnosis of dysentery associated with invasive *Entamoeba histolytica*. J Clin Pathol 1994;47:236–239.

106. Gordon SM, Gal AA, Solomon AR, Bryan JA. Disseminated strongyloidiasis with cutaneous manifestation in an immunocompromised host. J Am Acad Dermatol 1994;32:255–259.

107. Gottstein B. Molecular and immunological diagnosis of echinococcosis. Clin Microbiol Rev 1992;5:248–261.

108. Gould SE. The story of trichinosis. Am J Clin Pathol 1970;55:2–11.

109. Greensmith CT, Stanwick S, Elliot BE, Fast MV. Giardiasis associated with use of a water slide. Pediatr Infect Dis J 1988;7:91–94.

110. Grendon JH, Digiacomo RF, Frost FJ. *Dientamoeba fragilis* detection methods and prevalence: a survey of state public health laboratories. Pub Health Rep 1991;106:322–325.

111. Griffiths JK, Balakrishnan R, Widmer G, Tzipori S. Paromomycin and geneticin inhibit intracellular *Cryptosporidium parvum* without trafficking through the host cell cytoplasm: implications for drug delivery. Infect Immun 1998;66: 3874–3883.

112. Grimaldi G Jr, Tesh RB. Leishmaniasis of the New World: current concepts and implications for the future. Clin Microbiol Res 1993;6:230–250.

113. Grobusch MP, Bergmann F, Teishmann D, Klein E. Cutaneous gnathostomiasis in a woman from Bangladesh. Int J Infect Dis 2000;4:51–54.

114. Grover CM, Thulliez P, Remington JS, Boothroyd JC. Rapid prenatal diagnosis of congenital toxoplasma infection by using polymerase chain reaction and amniotic fluid. J Clin Microbiol 1990;28:2295–2301.

115. Guerrant RL. The global problem of amebiasis: current status, research needs, and opportunities for progress. Rev Infect Dis 1986;8:218–227.

116. Hadley WK, Ng V. Pneumocystis. In: Murray, PR, ed. Manual of Clinical Microbiology. Washington, DC: ASM Press, 1999:1200–1211.

117. Hagar JM, Rahimtoola SH. Chagas' disease in the United States. N Eng J Med 1991;325:763–768.

118. Hamalogue E. Biliary ascariasis in fifteen patients. Int Surg 1992;77:77–79.

119. Haque R, Ali IKM, Akther S, Petri WA Jr. Comparison of PCR, isoenzyme analysis, and antigen detection for diagnosis of *Entamoeba histolytica* infections. J Clin Microbiol 1998;136:449–452.

120. Haque R, Mollah NU, Ibne Karim M, et al. Diagnosis of amebic liver abscess and intestinal infection with the Tech Lab *Entamoeba histolytica* II antigen detection and antibody tests. J Clin Microbiol 2000;38:3235–3239.

121. Harcourt-Webster JN, Scaravilli F, Darwish AH. *Strongyloides stercoralis* hyperinfection in an HIV positive patient. J Clin Pathol 1991;44:346–348.

122. Harms G. Feldmeier H. HIV infection and tropical parasitic diseases: deleterious interactions in both directions. Trop Med Int Health 2002;7:479–488

123. Harris RA Jr, Musher DM, Fainstein V, et al. Disseminated strongyloidiasis: diagnosis made by sputum examination. JAMA 1980;244:65–68.

124. Hayes EB, Matte TD, O'Brien TR, et al. Large community outbreak of cryptosporidiosis due to contamination of a filtered public water supply. N Engl J Med 1989;320:1372–1376.

125. Hazll LR, Pearman F. Pathogenesis of onchocercal keratitis (river blindness). Clin Microbiol Rev 1999;12:445–453.

126. Helbig M, Frosch P, Kern P, Frosch M. Serological differentiation between cystic and alveolar echinococcus by use of recombinant larval antigens. J Clin Microbiol 1993;31:3211–3215.

127. Herrera LA, Ramirez T, Rodriquez U, et al. Possible association between *Taenia solium* cysticercosis and cancer: increased frequency of DNA damage in peripheral lymphocytes from neurocysticercosis patients. Trans R Soc Trop Med Hyg 2000;64:61–65.

128. Herwaldt BL, Akers ML, and the Cyclospora Working Group. An outbreak in 1996 of cyclosporiasis associated with imported raspberries. N Engl J Med 1997; 336:1548–1556.

129. Herwaldt BL, Grijalva MJ, Newsome AL, et al. Use of polymerase chain reaction

to diagnose the fifth reported US case of autochthonous transmission of *Trypanosoma cruzi* in Tennessee. J Infect Dis 1998;181:395–399.

130. Herwaldt BL, Kjemtrup AM, Conrad RC, et al. Transfusion-transmitted babesiosis in Washington state: first reported case caused by a WA1-type parasite. J Infect Dis 1997;175:1259–1262.

131. Heymans HS, Aronson DC, vanHooft MA. Giardiasis in childhood: an unnecessarily expensive diagnosis. Eur J Pediatr 1987;146:401–403.

132. Hiatt RA, Markell EK, Ng E. How many stool examinations are necessary to detect pathogenic intestinal protozoa? Am J Trop Med Hyg 1995;53:36–39.

133. Hira PR, Naefie R, Prakash B, et al. Human gnathostomiasis: infection with an immature male *Gnathostoma spinigerum*. Am J Trop Med Hyg 1989;41:91–94.

134. Hitt JA, Filice GA. Detection of *Toxoplasma gondii* parasitemia by gene amplification, cell culture, and mouse inoculation. J Clin Microbiol 1992;30:3181–3184.

135. Hoeppli R. Parasites and Parasitic Infections in Early Medicine and Science. Singapore: University of Malaya Press, 1959.

136. Hoge CW, Schlim DR, Rajah R, et al. Epidemiology of diarrhoeal illness associated with coccidian-like organisms among travelers and foreign residents in Nepal. Lancet 1993;349:1175–1179.

137. Hoge CW, Shlim DR, Ghimire M, et al. Placebo-controlled trial of cotrimoxazole for cyclospora infections among travelers and foreign residents in Nepal. Lancet 1995;345:691–693.

138. Holtan NR. Giardiasis. A crimp in the life-style of campers, travelers, and others. Postgrad Med 1988;83:54–57.

139. Hopkins DR, Ruiz-Tiben E, Reubush TK, et al. Dracunculiasis eradication: delayed, not denied. Am J Trop Med Hyg 2000;62:163–168.

140. Hotez PJ, Pritchard DI. Hookworm infection. Sci Am 1995;272:68–74.

141. Hulbert TV, Larsen RA, Chandrasoma PT. Abdominal angiostrongyliasis mimicking acute appendicitis and Meckel's diverticulum: report of a case in the United States and review. Clin Infect Dis 1992;14:836–840.

142. Ikeda K, Kumashiro R, Kifune T. Nine cases of acute gastric anisakiasis. Gastrointest Endosc 1989;35:304–308.

143. Ingra-Siegman Y, Kapila R, Sen P, et al. Syndrome of hyperinfection with *Strongyloides stercoralis*. Rev Infect Dis 1981;3:397–407.

144. Isaac-Renton JL. Immunological methods of diagnosis in giardiasis: an overview. Ann Clin Lab Sci 1991;21:116–122.

145. Jacquier P, Tottstein B, Stringelin Y, Eckert J. Immunodiagnosis of toxocariasis in humans: evaluation of a new enzyme-linked immunosorbent assay kit. J Clin Microbiol 1991;29:1831–1835.

146. Jensen B, Kepley W, Guarner J, et al. Comparison of polyvinyl alcohol fixative with three less hazardous fixatives for detection and identification of intestinal parasites. J Clin Microbiol 2000;138:1592–1598.

147. Jokiph I, Jokiph AM. Timing of symptoms and oocysts excretion in human cryptosporidiosis. N Engl J Med 1986;315:1643–1647.

148. Jones JE. String test for diagnosing giardiasis. Am Fam Physician 1986;34:123–126.

149. Katzwinkel-Wladarsch S, Loscher T, Rinder H. Direct amplification and differentiation of pathogenic and nonpathogenic *Entamoeba histolytica* DNA from stool specimens. Am J Trop Med Hyg 1994;52:115–118.

149a. Kazura, JW. *Filariasis*. In: Guerrant, RL, Walker DH, Weller PF. Tropical Infectious Diseases—Principles, Pathogens, and Practice. Philadelphia: Churchill Livingstone, 1999:852–860.

150. Kehl KSC, Cicirello H, Havens PL. Comparison of four different methods for detection of *Cryptosporidium* species. J Clin Microbiol 1995;33:416–418.

151. Kelley PW, Takafuji ET, Wiener H, et al. An outbreak of hookworm infection associated with military operations in Grenada. Mil Med 1989;154:55–59.

152. Keystone JS, Kozarsky P. *Blastocystis hominis*. In: Mandell GL, Bennett JE, Dolin R, eds. Principles and Practices of Infectious Diseases. 5th Ed. Philadelphia: Churchill Livingstone, 2000:2915.

153. Khalifa KES, Roth A, Roth B, et al. Value of PCR for evaluating occurrence of parasitemia in immunocompromised patients with cerebral and extracerebral toxoplasmosis. J Clin Microbiol 1994;32:2813–2819.

154. Kirchoff LV. Toxoplasmosis. In: Mandell GL, Bennett JE, Dolin R, eds. Principles and Practices of Infectious Disease. 5th Ed. Philadelphia: Churchill Livingstone, 2000:2858.

155. Klein RA, Cleri DJ, Doshi V, et al. Disseminated *Strongyloides stercoralis*: a fatal case eluding diagnosis. South Med J 1983;76:1438–1440.

156. Knight R. Giardiasis, isosporiasis, and balantidiasis. Clin Gastroenterol 1978;7:31–47.

157. Knisley CV, Englekirk PG, Pickering LK, et al. Rapid detection of Giardia antigen in stool with the use of enzyme immunoassays. Am J Clin Pathol 1989;91:704–708.

158. Kokoskin E, Gyorkos TW, Camus A, et al. Modified technique for efficient detection of microsporidia. J Clin Microbiol 1994;32:1947–1975.

159. Kyambadde JW, Enyaru JC, Motavu E, et al. Detection of trypanosomes in suspected sleeping sickness patients in Uganda using the polymerase chain reaction. Bull WHO 2000;78:119–124.

160. Lapham SC, Hopkins RS, White MC, et al. A prospective study of giardiasis and water supplies in Colorado. Am J Pub Health 1987;77:354–355.

161. Lebar WD, Larsen EC, Patei K. Afebrile diarrhea and *Blastocystis hominis*. Ann Intern Med 1985;103:806.

162. Leighton PM, MacSween HM. *Strongyloides stercoralis*. The cause of an urticarial-like eruption of 65 years' duration. Arch Intern Med 1990;150:1747–1748.

163. Levine ND, Corliss JO, Cox FEG, et al. A newly revised classification of the protozoa. J Protozool 1980;27:37–58.

164. Li S, Maine G, Yasuhiro S, et al. Serodiagnosis of recently acquired *Toxoplasma gondii* infection with recombinant antigen. J Clin Microbiol 2000;38:179–184.

165. Lightowlers MW, Flisser A, Gauci CG, et al. Vaccination against cysticercosis and hydatid disease. Parsitol Today 2000;16:191–196.

166. Long EG, Ebrahimzadeh A, White EH, et al. Alga associated with diarrhea in patients with acquired immunodeficiency syndrome and in travelers. J Clin Microbiol 1990;28:1101–1104.

167. Long EG, White EH, Charmichael WW, et al. Morphologic and staining characteristics of a cyanobacterium-like organism associated with diarrhea. J Infect Dis 1991;164:199–202.

168. Long GW, Rickman LS, Cross JH. Rapid diagnosis of *Brugia malayi* and *Wuchereria bancrofti* filariasis by an acridine orange/microhematocrit tube technique. J Parasitol 1990;76:278–281.

169. Lopez-Serrano MC, Gomez AA, Daschner A, et al. Gastroallergic anisakiasis: findings in 22 patients. J Gastroenterol Hepatol 2000;15:503–506.

170. Lopez-Valdez R, Laguna F, Alvar J, et al. Parasitic culture of buffy-coat for diagnosis of visceral leishmaniasis in human immunodeficiency virus-infected patients. J Clin Microbiol 1995;33:937–939.

171. Lotter H, Mannweiler E, Schreier M, Tahhich E. Sensitive and specific serodiagnosis of invasive amebiasis by using a recombinant surface protein of pathogenic *Entamoeba histolytica*. J Clin Microbiol 1992;30:3163–3167.

172. MacKenzie WR, Hoxie NJ, Proctor ME. Massive outbreak in Milwaukee of *Cryptosporidium* infection transmitted through the public water supply. N Engl J Med 1994;331:161–167.

173. MacPherson EW, MacQueen WM. Morphological diversity of *Blastocystis hominis* in sodium acetate-acetic acid-formalin-preserved stool samples stained with iron hematoxylin. J Clin Microbiol 1994;32:267–268.

174. Maddern GJ, Dennison AR, Blumgart LH. Fatal ascaris pancreatitis: an uncommon problem in the west. Gut 1992;33:402–403.

175. Mahannop P, Chaicumpa W, Setasuban P, et al. Immunodiagnosis of human trichinellosis using excretory-secretory (ES) antigen. J Helminthol 1992;66:297–304.

176. Manzullo EC, Chuit R. Risk of death due to chronic chagasic cardiopathy. Mem Inst Oswaldo Cruz 1999;94 (Suppl):S317–S320.

177. Markell EK, Udkow MP. *Blastocystis hominis*: pathogen or fellow traveler? Am J Trop Med Hyg 1986;35:1023–1026.

178. Marshall BG, Kropg P, Murray K, et al. Bronchopulmonary and mediastinal leishmaniasis: an unusual clinical presentation of *Leishmania donovani* infection. Clin Infect Dis 2000;30:764–769

179. Martens P, Hall L. Malaria on the move: human population movement and malaria transmission. Emerg Infect Dis 2000;6:103–109.

180. Marx JL. Spread of AIDS sparks new health concern. Science 1983;219: 42–43.

181. Mattia AR, Waldron MA, Sierra LS. Use of the quantitative buffy coat system for detection of parasitemia in patients with babesiosis. J Clin Microbiol 1993;32:2816–2818.

182. McCabe RE, Remington JS. *Toxoplasma gondii*. In: Mandell GI, Douglas RG Jr, Bennett JE., eds. Principles and Practice of Infectious Diseases. New York: Churchill Livingstone, 1990:2090–2101.

183. McCormick GF, Zee CS, Heiden J. Cysticercosis cerebri: review of 127 cases. Arch Neurol 1982;39:534–539.

184. McHenry R. Bartlett MS, Lehman GA, O'Conner KW. The yield of routine duodenal aspiration for *Giardia lamblia* during esophagogastroduodenoscopy. Gastrointest Endosc 1987;33:425–426.

185. Mirelman D, Bracha R, Chayen A. *Entamoeba histolytica*: effect of growth conditions and bacterial associates on isoenzyme patterns and virulence. Exp Parasitol 1986;621:142–148.

186. Moneo I, Caballero ML, Gomez F, et al. Isolation and characterization of a major allergen from the fish parasite *Anisakis simplex*. J Allergy Clin Immunol 2000;106:177–182.

187. Moore T. Therapy for parasitic infections. In: Harrison's Principles of Internal Medicine. 15th Ed. New York: McGraw Hill, 2001:1192.

188. Moorhead WP, Guasparini R, Donovan CA, et al. Giardiasis outbreak from a chlorinated community water supply. Can J Pub Health 1990;81:358–362.

189. Morgan UM, Thompson RCA. PCR detection of *Cryptosporidium*: the way forward? Parasitol Today 1998;14:241–246.

190. Moura H, Schwartz DA, Bornay-Llinares F, et al. A new and improved "quick-hot gram-chromotrope" technique that differentially stains microsporidian spores in clinical samples, including paraffin-embedded tissue sections. Arch Pathol Lab Med 1997;121:888–893.

191. Murray HS. Kala-azar as an AIDS-related opportunistic infection. AIDS Patient Care STS 1999;13:459–465.

192. Nagler J, Brown M, Soave R. *Blastocystis hominis* in inflammatory bowel disease. J Clin Gastroenterol 1993;16:109–112.

193. Nanduri J, Kazura JW. Clinical and laboratory aspects of filariasis. Clin Microbiol Rev 1989;2:39–50.

194. Nantulya VM, Doua F, Molisho S. Diagnosis of *Trypanosoma brucei gambiense* sleeping sickness using an antigen detection enzyme-linked immunosorbent assay. Trans R Soc Trop Med Hyg 1992;86:42–45.

195. Nantulya VM. TrypTect CIATT—a card indirect agglutination trypanosomiasis test for diagnosis of *Trypanosoma brucei gambiense* and *T. brucei rhodesiense* infections. Trans R Soc Trop Med Hyg 1997;91:551–553.

196. Navin TR, Juranek DD. Cryptosporidiosis: clinical, epidemiological and parasitic review. Rev Infect Dis 1984;6:313–317.

197. Neimeister R, Logan AL, Egleton JH. Modified trichrome staining technique with xylene substitution. J Clin Microbiol 1985;22:306–307.

198. Newell EF, Vyungimana S, Geerts IK, et al. Prevalence of cysticercosis in epileptics and members of their families in Burundi. Trans R Soc Trop Med Hyg 1997;92:389–391.

199. Orgeta YR, Sterling CR, Gilman RH, et al. *Cyclospora* species—a new protozoan pathogen of humans. N Eng J Med 1993;328:1308–1312.

200. Ogunrinade AF, Chandrashekar R, Ebberhard ML, Weil GK. Preliminary evaluation of recombinant *Onchocerca volvulus* antigens for serodiagnosis of onchocerciasis. J Clin Microbiol 1993;31:1741–1745.

201. Ogunrinade A, Boakye D, Merriweather A, Unnasch TR. Distribution of the blinding and nonblinding strains of *Onchocerca volvulus* in Nigeria. J Infect Dis 1999;179:1577–1579.

202. Ormerod WE. Hypothesis: the significance of Winterbottom's sign. J Trop Med Hyg 1991;94:338–340.

203. Orozco E, Baez-Camargo M, Gamboa L, et al. Molecular karyotype of related clones of *Entamoeba histolytica*. Mol Biochem Parasitol 1993;59:29–40.

204. Pappe JW, Verdier RI, Boney M, et al. *Cyclospora* infection in adults infected with HIV: clinical manifestations, treatment and prophylaxis. Ann Intern Med 1994;121:654–657.

205. Parmley SF, Goebel FD, Remington JS. Detection of *Toxoplasma gondii* in cerebrospinal fluid from AIDS patients by polymerase chain reaction. J Clin Microbiol 1992;30:3000–3002.

206. Partona F. The spectrum of disease in lymphatic filariasis. Ciba Found Symp 1987;127:15–31.

207. Pearson RDD, De Queiroz Sousa A. *Leishmania* species: visceral (kala-azar), cutaneous and mucosal leishmaniasis. In: Mandell GL, Bennett JE, Dolan R, eds. Principles and Practices of Infectious Diseases. 3rd Ed. New York: Churchill Livingstone, 1995:2067–2077.

208. Persing DH. Polymerase chain reaction: trenches to the benches. J Clin Microbiol 1991;29:1281–1285.

209. Persing DH, Mathiesen D, Marshall WF, et al. Detection of *Babesia microti* by polymerase chain reaction. J Clin Microbiol 1992;30:2097–2103.

210. Persing DH, Herwaldt BL, Glaser C, et al. Infection with a babesia-like organism in northern California. N Engl J Med 1995;332:298–303.

211. Peters CS, Kathpalia SB, Chitton-Swialto AL., et al. *Isospora belli* and *Cryptosporidium* spp. from a patient not suspected of having acquired immunodeficiency syndrome. Diag Microbiol Infect Dis 1987;8:197–199.

212. Petri WA Jr, Clark CG, Diamond LS. Host-parasite relationships in amebiasis: conference report. J Infect Dis 1994;169:483–484.

213. Piarroux R, Gambarelli F, Dumon H, et al. Comparison of PCR with direct examination of bone marrow aspiration, myeloculture, and serology for diagnosis of visceral leishmaniasis in immunocompromised patients. J Clin Microbiol 1994. 32:746–749.

214. Pickering LK, Engelkirk PG. *Giardia lamblia*. Pediatr Clin North Am 1988;35:536–577.

215. Pietrzak-Johnston SM, Bishop H, Wahlquist S, et al. Evaluation of commercially available preservatives for the laboratory detection of helminths and protozoa in human fecal specimens. J Clin Microbiol 2000;38:1959–1964.

216. Pol S, Romana CA, Richard S, et al. *Microsporidia* infection in patients with the human immunodeficiency virus and unexplained cholangitis. N Engl J Med 1993;328:95–99.

217. Polly SM. Neurocysticercosis. Infect Dis Newslett 1986;5:89–91.

218. Pollok RCG, Bendall RP, Moody A, et al. Traveler's diarrhoea associated with cyanobacterium-like bodies. Lancet 1992;340:556–557.

219. Poretti D, Felleisen E, Grimm F, et al. Differential immunodiagnosis between cystic hydatid disease and other cross-reactive pathologies. Am J Trop Med Hyg 1999;60:193–198.

220. Purtillo DT, Myers WM, Conner DH. Fatal strongyloidiasis in immunocompromised patients. Am J Med 1974;56:488–493.

221. Rakita RM, White AC Jr, Keilhofner MA. *Loa loa* infection as a cause of migratory angioedema: report of three cases from the Texas Medical Center. Clin Infect Dis 1993;17:691–694.

222. Ravdin JI. Pathogenesis of disease caused by *Entamoeba histolytica*: studies of adherence, secreted toxins, and contact-dependent cytolysis. Rev Infect Dis 1986;8:247–260.

223. Ravdin JI. *Entamoeba histolytica*—amebiasis. In: Mandell GL, Bennett JE, Dolin R, eds. Principles and Practices of Infectious Disease. 5th Ed. Philadelphia: Churchill Livingstone, 2000:2035–2049.

224. Rawlins SC, Chailett P, Ragoonanansingh RN, et al. Microscopical and serological diagnosis of *Wuchereria bancrofti*. West Indian Med J 1994;43:75–79.

225. Rinder H, Janitschke K, Aspöck H, et al. A blinded, externally controlled multicenter evaluation for the detection of microsporidia by light microscopy and PCR. J Clin Microbiol 1998;36:1814–1818.

226. Rodriguez N, Guzman B, Rodas A, et al. Diagnosis of cutaneous leishmaniasis and species discrimination of parasites by PCR and hybridization. J Clin Microbiol 1994;32:2246–2252.

227. Roman G, Sotelo J, Del Brutto O, et al. A proposal to declare neurocysticercosis an international reportable disease. Bull WHO 2000;78:399–406.

228. Rosenthal EP, Marty P, le Fichoux Y, Sassuto JP. Clinical manifestations of visceral leishmaniasis associated with HIV infection: a retrospective study of 91 French cases. Ann Trop Med Parasitol 2000;94:37–42.

229. Rossitch E Jr, Carrazana EJ, Samuels MA. Cerebral toxoplasmosis in patients with AIDS. Am Fam Physician 1990;42:867–873.

230. Rostoff JD, Sanders CA, Sonnad SS, et al. Stool diagnosis of giardiasis using a commercially available enzyme immunoassay to detect giardia-specific antigen 65 (GAS 65). J Clin Microbiol 1989;27:1997–2002.

231. Ruffer MA. Note on the Presence of *Bilharzia haematobia* in Egyptian mummies of the 20th dynasty (1250–1000 B.C.). BMJ 1910;16.

232. Ryan NJ, Sutherland G, Coughlan K, et al. A new trichrome-blue stain for detection of microsporidial species in urine, stool and nasopharyngeal specimens. J Clin Microbiol 1993;31:3264–3269.

233. Sakanari JA, McKerrow JH. Anisakiasis. Clin Microbiol Rev 1989;2:278–284.

234. Sargeaunt PG, Williams JE. Electrophoretic isoenzyme patterns of *Entamoeba histolytica* and *Entamoeba coli*. Trans R Soc Trop Med Hyg 1978;72:164–166.

235. Sargeaunt PG. The reliability of *Entamoeba histolytica* zymodemes in clinical diagnosis. Parasitol Today 1987;3:40–43

236. Sarti E, Schantz PM, Avila G, et al. Mass treatment against human taeniasis for the control of cysticercosis: a population-based intervention study. Trans R Soc Top Med Hyg 2000;94:85–89.

237. Sarwaut MA, alShaiby AL. Parasitic infections among patients of Al Nour specialized hospital. J Egypt Soc Parasitol 1993;23:821–827

238. Schantz PM, McAuley J. Current status of food-borne parasitic zoonoses in the United States. Southeast Asian J Trop Med Public Health 1991;22(Suppl):65–71.

239. Scheffler EH, Van Etta LL. Evaluation of rapid commercial enzyme immunoassay for detection of *Giardia lamblia* in formalin-preserved stool specimens. J Clin Microbiol 1994;32:1807–1808.

240. Schlim DR, Cohen MT, Eaton M, et al. An alga-like organism associated with an outbreak of prolonged diarrhea among foreigners in Nepal. Am J Trop Med Hyg 1991;45:383–389.

241. Schwartz DA. Cholangiocarcinoma with liver fluke infection: a preventable source for morbidity in Asian immigrants. Am J Gastroenterol 1986;81:76–79.

242. Shadduck JA, Greeley E. Microsporidia and human infections. Clin Microbiol Rev 1989;2:158–165.

243. Shandera WX. From Leningrad to the day-care center: the ubiquitous *Giardia lamblia*. West J Med 1990;153:154–159.

244. Shepherd RC, Reed CL, Sinha GP. Shedding of oocysts of Cryptosporidium in immunocompetent patients. J Clin Pathol 1988;42:1104–1106.

245. Sher L, Shunmzaburo I, Lebeau G, Zaiko AB. Hilar cholangiocarcinoma associated with *Clonorchis*. Dig Dis Sci 1989;34:1121–1123.

246. Shetty N, Brabhu T. Evaluation of fecal preservation and staining methods in the diagnosis of acute amoebiasis and giardiasis. J Clin Pathol 1988;412:694–699.

247. Sifuentesosornio J, Porrascortes G, Bendall RP, et al. *Cyclospora cayetanensis* infection in patients with and without AIDS: biliary disease as another clinical manifestation. Clin Infect Dis 1995;21:1092–1097.

248. Simonson PE, Dunyo SK. Comparative evaluation of three new tools for diagnosis of bancroftian filariasis based on detection of specific circulating antigens. Trans R Soc Trop Med Hyg 1999;93:278–282.

249. Singh BN. Pathogenic and Non-pathogenic Amoebae. New York: Wiley, 1975.

250. Sloan L, Schneider S, Rosenblatt J. Evaluation of enzyme-linked immunoassay for serological diagnosis of cysticercosis. J Clin Microbiol 1995;33:3124–3128.

251. Soave R. State of the art clinical article. *Cyclospora*: an overview. Clin Infect Dis 1996;23:429–437.

252. Smith JW, Patterson WJ, Hardie R, et al. 1989. An outbreak of waterborne cryptosporidiosis caused by post-treatment contamination. Epidemiol Infect 103:703–715.

253. Smith JW, Wolfe MS. Giardiasis. Annual Rev Med 1980;32:373.

254. Smith J. Institute of Parasitology at McGill. martin.parasitology.mcgill.ca/incidnec.htm 2003.

255. Starko KM, Lippy EC, Dominquez LB, et al. Campers' diarrhea outbreak traced to water-sewage link. Public Heath Rep 1986;101:527–531.

256. Stehr-Green JK, McCaig L, Remsen HM, et al. Shedding of oocysts in immunocompetent individuals infected with Cryptosporidium. Am J Trop Med Hyg 1987;36:338–342.

257. Steketee RW, Reid S, Cheng T, et al. Recurrent outbreaks of giardiasis in a child day center, Wisconsin. Am J Pub Health 1989;79:485–490.

258. Stenzel DJ, Boreham PF. *Blastocystis hominis* revisited. Clin Microbiol Rev 1996;9:563–584

259. Stibbs HH. Monoclonal antibody-based enzyme immunoassay for *Giardia lamblia* antigen in human stool. J Clin Microbiol 1989;27:2582–2588.

260. Steketee RW, Reid S, Cheng T, et al. Recurrent outbreaks of giardiasis in a child day care center, Wisconsin. Am J Pub Health 1989;79:485–490.

261. Strickland GT, Abdel-Wahab M. Schistosomiasis. In: Strickland GT, ed. Hunter's Tropical Medicine. 7th Ed. Philadelphia: Saunders, 1991:781–802.

262. Tan JS. Common and uncommon parasitic infections in the United States. Med Biomed Int 1978;62:1959–1081.

263. Tantowitz HB, Korchhoff LV, Simon D, et al. Chagas' disease. Clin Microbiol Rev 1992;5:400–419.

264. Tietze PE, Tietze PH. The roundworms. *Ascaris lumbricoides*. Primary Care 1991;18:23–41.

265. Todorov T, Bopeva V. Echinococcus in children and adolescents in Bulgaria: a comparative study. Ann Trop Med Parasitol 2000;94:135–144.

266. Tremblay A. MacLean JD, Gyorkos T, Macpherson DW. Outbreak of cutaneous larva migrans in a group of travelers. Trop Med Int Health 2000;5:330–334

267. Ungar BLP. Cryptosporidiosis. In: Mandell GL, Bennett JE, Dolin R, eds. Principles and Practices of Infectious Diseases. 5th Ed. Philadelphia: Churchill Livingstone, 2000:2903.

268. van Etten L, Folman CC, Eggelte TA. Rapid diagnosis of schistosomiasis by antigen detection in urine with a reagent strip. J Clin Microbiol 1994;2404–2406.

269. Vannatta JB, Adamson D, Mujllican K. *Blastocystis hominis* infection presenting as recurrent diarrhea. Ann Intern Med 1985;102:495–496.

270. Vargas MA, Orozco E. *Entamoeba histolytica*: changes in the zymodeme of cloned nonpathogenic trophozoites cultured under different conditions. Parasitol Res 1993;19:353–356

271. Verastegui M, Moro P, Guevera A, et al. Enzyme linked immunoelectrotransfer blot test for diagnosis of human hydatid disease. 1992;L30:1557–1561.

272. Vermud SH, Lalleur F, MacLoed S. Parasitic infections in a New York City hospital: trends from 1971 to 1984. Am J Pub Health 1986;76:1024–1026.

273. Walden J. Parasitic diseases: other roundworms: trichiuris, hookworm, and strongyloides. Primary Care 1991;18:53–74.

274. Walls KW, Smith JW. Serology of parasitic infections. Lab Med 1979;10:329–336.

275. Wamae CN. Advances in the diagnosis of human lymphatic filariasis: a review. E Afr Med J 1994;74:171–182.

276. Warren KS, Mahmoud AAF. Algorithms in the diagnosis and management of exotic diseases: XII. Prevention of exotic diseases: advice to travelers. J Infect Dis 1976;133:596–601.

277. Watt G, Saisorn S, Jongsakul K, et al. Blinded, placebo-controlled trial of antiparasitic drugs for trichinosis myositis. J Infect Dis 2000;182:371–374.

278. Webbe G. Human cysticercosis: parasitology, pathology, clinical manifestations and available treatment. Pharmacol Ther 1994;64:175–200.

279. Weber R, Bryan RT, Juranek DD. Improved stool concentration procedure for detection of *Cryptosporidium* oocysts in fecal specimens. J Clin Microbiol 1992;30:289–2873.

280. Weber R, Bryan RT, Schwartz DA, Owen RL. Human microsporidial infections. Clin Microbiol Rev 1994;7:426–461.

281. Weil GJ, Jain DC, Santhanasa S, et al. A monoclonal antibody-based enzyme immunoassay for detecting parasite antigenemia in bancroftian filariasis. J Infect Dis 1987;165:350–355.

282. Weinke T, Friedrich-Janichke B, Hopp P, Janitschke D. Prevalence and clinical importance of *Entamoeba histolytica* in two high-risk groups: travelers returning from the tropics and male homosexuals. J Infect Dis 1990;161:1029–1031.

283. Weiss JB. DNA probes and PCR for the diagnosis of parasitic infections. Clin Microbiol Rev 1995;8:113–130.

284. Welch TP. Risk of giardiasis from consumption of wilderness water in North America: a systematic review of epidemiologic data. Int J Infect Dis 2000;4:100–103

285. Welsh JA. Problems in recognition and diagnosis of amebiasis: estimation of the global magnitude of morbidity and mortality. Rev Infect Dis 1986;8:118–238.

286. White AC Jr, Tato P, Molinari JL. Host-parasite interactions in *Taenia solium* cysticercosis. Infect Agents Dis 1992;1:185–193.

287. Whittner M, Tanowitz HB, Weiss LM. Parasitic infection in AIDS patients: cryptosporidiosis, isosporiasis, microsporidiosis, cyclosporiasis. Infect Dis Clin 1993;7:569–586.

288. Williams HA, Roberts J, Kachur P. Malaria surveillance—United States, 1995. Atlanta: Centers for Disease Control and Prevention, Epidemiology Program Office, 1995.

289. Windsor JJ, Johnson EH. *Dientamoeba fragilis*: the unflagellated human flagellate. Br J Biomed Sci 1999;56:293–306.

290. Windsor JJ, Macfarlane L, Hughes-Thapa G, et al. Incidence of *Blastocystis hominis* in faecal samples submitted for routine microbiological analysis. Br J Biomed Sci 2002;59:154–157.

291. Witoonpanich R, Chuahirun S, Soranastaporn S, Rojanasunan P. Eosinophilic myelomeningoencephalitis caused by *Angiostrongylus cantonensis*: a report of three cases. Southeast Asian J Trop Med Public Health 1991;22:262–267.

292. Wolf MS. Giardiasis. Clin Microbiol Rev 1992;5:93–100.

293. Wong SY, Jaidu MP, Ramirez R, et al. Role of specific immunoglobulin E in diagnosis of acute toxoplasma infection and toxoplasmosis. J Clin Microbiol 1993;32:2952–2959.

294. Woo PT, Paterson WB. *Giardia lamblia* in children in day-care centers in southern Ontario, Canada, and susceptibility to animals to *G. lamblia*. Trans R Soc Trop Med Hyg 1986;80:56–59.

295. World Health Organization. Epidemiology and control of African trypanosomiasis: report of a WHO expert committee. WHO Tech Rep Ser 1986;739:36–58.

296. Wurtz R, Kocka FE, Peters CS, et al. Clinical characteristics of seven cases of diarrhea associated with a novel acid-fast organism in the stool. Clin Infect Dis 1991;16:136–138.

297. Wurtz R. *Cyclospora*: A newly identified intestinal pathogen of humans. Clin Infect Dis 1994;18:620–626.

298. Woo PT, Paterson WB. *Giardia lamblia* in children in daycare centers is southern Ontario, Canada, and susceptibility of animals to *G. lamblia*. Trans R Soc Trop Med Hyg 1986;80:56–59.

299. Yamasaki H, Araki K, Lim PK, et al. Development of a highly specific recombinant *Toxocara canis* second-stage larva excretory-secretory antigen for immunodiagnosis of human toxocariasis. J Clin Microbiol 2000;38:1409–1413.

300. Yang J, Scholton T. *Dientamoeba fragilis*: a review with notes on epidemiology, pathogenicity, modes of transmission, and diagnosis. Am J Trop Med Hyg 1979;26:16–22.

301. Yaquihashi A, Sato N, Takahashi S, et al. A serodiagnostic assay by microenzyme-linked immunosorbent assay for human anisakiasis using a monoclonal antibody specific for *Anisakiasis* larvae antigen. J Infect Dis 1990;161:995–998.

302. Yau YC. Crandall I. Kain KC. Development of monoclonal antibodies which specifically recognize *Entamoeba histolytica* in preserved stool samples. J Clin Microbiol 2001;39:716–719.

303. Yen C-M, Chen E-R. Detection of antibodies to *Angiostrongylus cantonensis* in serum and cerebrospinal fluid of patients with eosinophilic meningitis. Int J Parasitol 1991;21:17–21

304. Young DK, Bullock SL, Melvin DM, et al. Ethyl acetate as a substitute for diethyl ether in the formalin-ether sedimentation technique. J Clin Microbiol 1979;10:852–853.

305. Yu S, Xu L, Jiang Z, et al. Report on the first nationwide survey of the distribution of human parasites in China. Chin J Parasitol Dis 1994;12:241–247.

306. Zhu G, Marchweka MJ, Ennis JG, Keithly JS. Direct isolation of DNA from patient stools for polymerase chain reaction detection of *Cryptosporidium parvum*. J Infect Dis 1998;177:1443–1446.

307. Zierdt CH. *Blastocystis hominis*: an intestinal protozoan parasite of man. Pub Health Lab 1978;36:147–160.

308. Zierdt CH, Gill VJ, Zierdt WS. Detection of microsporidian spores in clinical samples by indirect fluorescent-antibody using whole-cell antisera to *Encephalitozoon cuniculi* and *Encephalitozoon hellem*. J Clin Microbiol 1993;31:3071–3074.

309. Zimmerman PA, Guderian RH, Araujo E, et al. Polymerase chain reaction-based diagnosis of *Onchocerca volvulus* infection: improved detection of patients with onchocerciasis. J Infect Dis 1994;169:686–689.

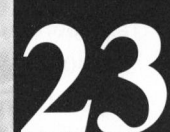
Diagnosis of Infections Caused by Viruses, *Chlamydia*, *Rickettsia*, and Related Organisms

Introduction

Historical Review
Evolution of Cell-Culture
  Techniques
Evolution of Diagnostic Virology
  Services
Levels of Service

**Taxonomy and
Nomenclature**

**Clinical Manifestations of
Viral Infections**

Orthomyxoviruses
Paramyxoviruses

  Parainfluenza Viruses
  Mumps Virus
  Measles Virus
  Respiratory Syncytial Virus
  Other Paramyxoviruses

Picornaviruses
Rhabdoviruses
Arenaviruses
Filoviruses
Togaviruses
Bunyaviruses

  California Encephalitis Viruses
  Hantaviruses

Human Gastroenteritis Viruses

  Rotaviruses
  Caliciviruses

Astroviruses
Enteric Adenoviruses

Coronaviruses
Coltiviruses
Retroviruses
Herpesviruses

  Herpes Simplex Virus
  Cytomegalovirus
  Epstein-Barr Virus
  Varicella-Zoster Virus
  Human Herpesviruses-6 and -7
  Human Herpesvirus-8
  B Virus

Adenoviruses
Poxviruses
Papovaviruses

  Papillomaviruses
  Polyomaviruses

Parvoviruses
Hepatitis Viruses

  Hepatitis A Virus
  Hepatitis B Virus
  Hepatitis C Virus
  Hepatitis D Virus
  Hepatitis E Virus

Prion Diseases (Transmissible
  Spongiform Encephalopathies)

**Clinical Classification of
Viral Infections**

Diagnosis of Viral Infections

Collection of Specimens for Diagnosis
Transportation and Storage of Specimens
Isolation of Viruses in Culture
Preparation and Maintenance of Cell Cultures
Contamination of Cell Cultures
Technical Aspects of Cell Culture
Selection of Cell Cultures for Isolation of Viruses
Inoculation and Incubation of Cell Cultures
Detection of Virus and Provisional Identification

Cytopathic Effect
Hemagglutination and Hemadsorption
Light Microscopy
Electron Microscopy
Biochemical Differentiation
Cell Association
Detection of Viral Antigens
Artifacts and Non–Virus-Induced Changes

Definitive Identification of Isolates
Storage of Viral Isolates
Summary of Detection and Identification of
Viruses in Culture

Direct Detection of Viruses in Clinical Specimens

Light Microscopic Detection of Inclusions
Electron Microscopic Detection of Viral Particles
Immunologic Detection of Viral Antigen

Respiratory Viruses
Herpes Group Viruses
Other Viruses

Molecular Techniques

Human Immunodeficiency Virus
Hepatitis C Virus
Hepatitis B Virus
Human Papillomaviruses
Parvovirus B19
West Nile Virus
Herpes Simplex Virus
Cytomegalovirus
Enteroviruses

SARS Coronavirus
Other Viral Infections

Selection of Tests for Rapid Diagnosis

Serologic Diagnosis of Viral Infections

Human Immunodeficiency Virus
Hepatitis B Virus and Epstein-Barr Virus
Hepatitis A Virus
Hepatitis C Virus
Parvovirus
Herpes Simplex Virus
Varicella-Zoster Virus
Cytomegalovirus
West Nile Virus
Rubella
SARS Coronavirus
Anti-IgM Antibodies
Miscellaneous Serologic Procedures
Diagnosis of Other Viral Infections
Antiviral Susceptibility Testing

Infections With *Chlamydia* Species

Chlamydia trachomatis

Clinical Features and Epidemiology
Collection of Specimens
Isolation of *Chlamydia trachomatis* in Cell Culture
Direct Detection of *Chlamydia trachomatis* in Clinical
Specimens
Serologic Diagnosis
Other Methods for Diagnosis
Diagnosis of Sexual Abuse

Chlamydia psittaci
Chlamydia pneumoniae

Infections With *Rickettsia*, *Coxiella*, *Ehrlichia*, and *Anaplasma*

Rickettsia and *Coxiella*

Clinical Features and Epidemiology
Collection of Specimens
Isolation of *Rickettsia* and *Coxiella* in Culture
Direct Detection of Antigen and Nucleic Acid in
Clinical Specimens
Serologic Diagnosis

Ehrlichia and *Anaplasma* Species

Introduction

Diagnostic virology is a recent addition to the services offered by clinical microbiology laboratories. Three distinct stages have evolved as laboratory workers have provided clinicians with objective data to evaluate patients with viral infections.

Historical Review

The first stage of historical interest spanned the years during which the existence of infection by submicroscopic particles was established. For many decades after Carlos Finlay hypothesized that yellow fever was transmitted by the bite of a mosquito, the only means available for isolation of viral agents was the inoculation of animals or embryonated eggs. Embryonated chicken eggs are still inoculated today for surveillance of infections caused by influenza A virus if cell culture is not available. New agents continue to be uncovered only by the use of subhuman primates (kuru and Creutzfeldt-Jakob viruses)[171] and even human volunteers (Norwalk agent of infectious gastroenteritis).[272]

Evolution of Cell-Culture Techniques

The next major breakthrough in diagnostic virology was provided by Enders and colleagues, who demonstrated that the virus that caused poliomyelitis could be isolated in nonneural cells in vitro.[143] In the 1950s and 1960s there was a rapid expansion of knowledge about clinical features, epidemiology, and diagnosis of common viral infections, largely provided by the expanding use of cell culture. Diagnostic efforts, which were an integral part of the clinical studies, were incorporated into university and government research laboratories. The high cost of definitive identification of isolates, the absence of effective antiviral chemotherapy, and the paucity of cell-culture facilities all combined to limit the importation of these tests into the diagnostic microbiology laboratory. A more detailed review of the historical development of virology is provided by Levine.[308]

Evolution of Diagnostic Virology Services

The first step was the incorporation of diagnostic services into clinical microbiology laboratories, many of which had previously limited their scope to bacteriology (including mycobacteriology), mycology, and parasitology. In Box 23-1 some of the factors that facilitated and encouraged this transfer from a research laboratory in a clinical department to a diagnostic laboratory, usually in a pathology or microbiology department, are summarized. A more detailed discussion of this transition can be found in previous editions of this book.

The complexity and sophistication of traditional viral diagnosis meant that most of the clinical laboratories able to take on the challenge were located in large medical centers, many of which were associated with academic centers. In the previous decade the pace of technologic development has accelerated so that some focused viral diagnostic testing can be introduced into community hospitals. In Box 23-1 there is a summary of some of the developments that encouraged even further concentration of diagnostic services in clinical laboratories, either based in hospitals or freestand-

---

Box 23-1 Some Factors That Facilitate the Transfer From a Research Laboratory to a Diagnostic Laboratory

Factors That Encouraged Transfer of Testing to the Clinical Laboratory	Recent Developments in Diagnostic Virology
Appearance of clinical scenarios in which viral diagnosis is essential; e.g., herpes simplex in pregnant women	Increasing frequency of clinical scenarios that depend on viral diagnosis; e.g., expanded capability in human immunodeficiency virology, monitoring of infection in transplant recipients
Development of antiviral chemotherapy	Increased number of diseases for which antiviral chemotherapy, including combination therapy, is possible
Availability of reliable commercial sources of mammalian cells for culture	Commercial sources of cells on coverslips for shell vial cultures; development of cell mixtures
Application of monoclonal antibody technology to diagnosis, with commercial availability of reliable reagents	Movement of nucleic-acid amplification technology from the research laboratory into the clinic; commercial availability of systems or validated reagents for amplification
Facilitation of more rapid diagnosis by application of monoclonal antibody and spin amplification (shell vial) technologies	Introduction of extremely rapid diagnosis by application of real-time PCR to detection of agents in clinical specimens
Application of enzyme immunoassays to direct diagnosis	Development of membrane immunoassays that can be performed quickly and simply
Regulation of hospital laboratories under CLIA '67	Extension of regulation to all laboratories, including physician offices, under CLIA '88
Support for public health epidemiology of transmissible disease	Support for investigation of bioterrorism threats

---

Box 23-2 Levels of Diagnostic Service

Level 1   No virology services performed. Specimens are collected for transfer to a reference laboratory.

Level 2   Limited virology procedures performed. Such laboratories may or may not also have the capability to detect viral or chlamydial antigens in body secretions and fluids. These laboratories also may or may not have the capability to inoculate specimens to tissue culture for transfer to reference laboratories.

Level 3   These laboratories are able to recover selected viral groups that grow in commonly used cell cultures. They may also perform limited identification of selected agents for which transportation, cell isolation, and simple immunologic confirmation systems are commercially available, with referral of other isolates to reference laboratories.

Level 4   These laboratories are expected to have personnel with a high degree of expertise in virology who are able to isolate all of the common viral groups and to perform clinically relevant identifications.

Level 5   Laboratories with the capability to perform sophisticated molecular amplification tests, including real-time amplification.

---

ing. In addition to the scientific issues an important determinant was the promulgation and enforcement of the CLIA '88 (Clinical Laboratory Improvement Amendments, 1988), the first major development in oversight of laboratories since the Clinical Laboratory Improvement Act of 1967 (CLIA '67). The numerous requirements for personnel and performance of tests were familiar to most clinical laboratories, but foreign (and extremely unwelcome) to most research laboratories, and essentially out of the reach of physician office laboratories.

Levels of Service

Each laboratory director or supervisor must decide the level of service that is appropriate for local clinical needs. It is far better to limit the scope of effort to tests that can be performed with high proficiency than to attempt broad coverage when resources are insufficient. Several likely levels of service can be imagined and are listed in Box 23-2.

Most small hospital laboratories will probably fit into level 1 or 2,[454] whereas larger community hospital and university laboratories may offer services at level 3, 4, or 5. These hospitals are most likely to serve the patients who need comprehensive virology services. It is feasible to use such laboratories as regional diagnostic resources.

Taxonomy and Nomenclature

Taxonomy is the science of systematic classification using general rules and principles; the term is most commonly used for the study of living things. Nomenclature is the activity of ascribing names to the taxonomic subjects.

Many viral infections, such as influenza, chickenpox, measles, and hepatitis, were well characterized clinically long before the etiologic agent was recognized. Once isolated, the virus was given the name of the corresponding clinical condition. In an attempt to bring order to the scheme of classification, taxonomists have used modern knowledge of viral structure and antigenic composition to construct a systematic classification.[107] Orders, families, and genera have Latin stems, but the concept of species has been more difficult for virologists.[56,491] Often the classic vernacular names are used as species designations.

The International Committee on Taxonomy of Viruses (ICTV) has proposed the ICTV Universal System of Virus Taxonomy. A summary of the conventions of viral nomenclature is provided in Box 23-3. The hierarchical names are italicized and may be preceded by the taxon, which is not italicized. In the case of the species names we are left with the peculiar situation that the same words may be italicized or not, depending on whether they are part of a taxonomic designation or are being used as the vernacular name. The taxonomic designation need be used only once in a scientific publication. For instance, a discussion might refer to measles virus (*Measles virus*, genus *Morbillivirus*, family *Paramyxoviridae*). At the moment this approach to taxonomy and nomenclature appears to have the upper hand, but the subject has not been settled definitively.

Much of viral taxonomy derives from detailed knowledge of viral structure. Viruses are among the smallest of infectious agents (Fig. 23-1). The poxviruses, which are the largest members of the virus family and similar in size to the smallest bacteria, are close to the resolution of the light microscope; an electron microscope is necessary to visualize all other viruses.

Almost without exception, viruses contain either DNA or RNA, but not both. The center of any viral particle, the ribonucleoprotein core, contains coiled nucleic acid and protein.[215] Around the core is a protective shell composed of repeating protein units called capsomeres, which, in the aggregate, make up the capsid shell. With the nucleoprotein core, the nucleocapsid unit is complete. The architecture of most viruses has a symmetry that is either helical, similar

---

Box 23-3 Conventions for Naming Viruses

Taxonomic Hierarchy	Ending	Example
Order	*-virales*	*Mononegavirales*
Family	*-viridae*	*Paramyxoviridae*
Subfamily	*-virinae*	*Pneumovirinae*
Genus	*-virus*	*Pneumovirus*
Species	None	Human respiratory syncytial virus

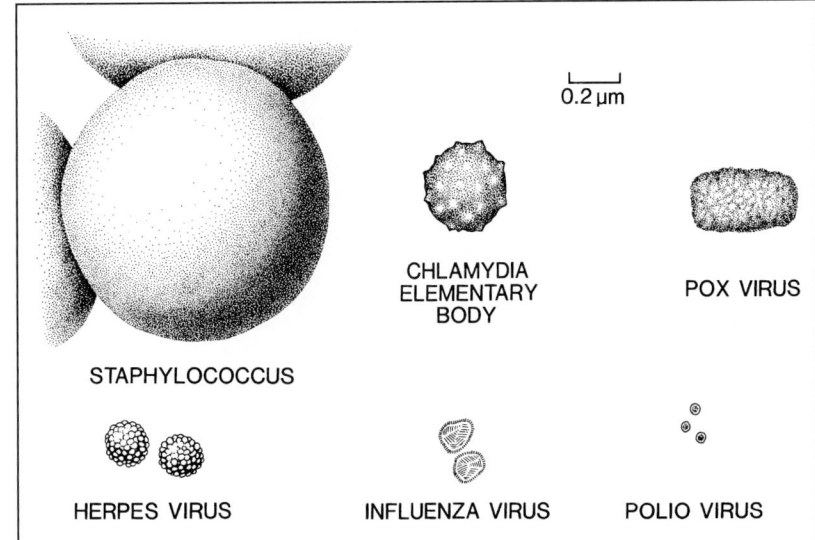

Figure 23-1 Viruses. Viruses are the smallest of infectious agents. The relative size of a bacterium, *Staphylococcus*, is compared with *Chlamydia*, with the largest virus group (poxvirus), and with one of the smallest viruses (poliovirus, a member of the enterovirus group).

to nucleic acid, or icosahedral, the architecture of a geodesic dome. These two symmetries, illustrated in Figure 23-2, provide the most efficient means for assembling the structural shells, an economy that is essential for these very small particles with limited genetic resources.

As a general rule, DNA viruses replicate and are assembled in the nucleus; RNA viruses are assembled in the cytoplasm. The complex events that occur after a virus infects a cell are reflected only incompletely in the morphologic cellular changes. In some instances, however, one can see

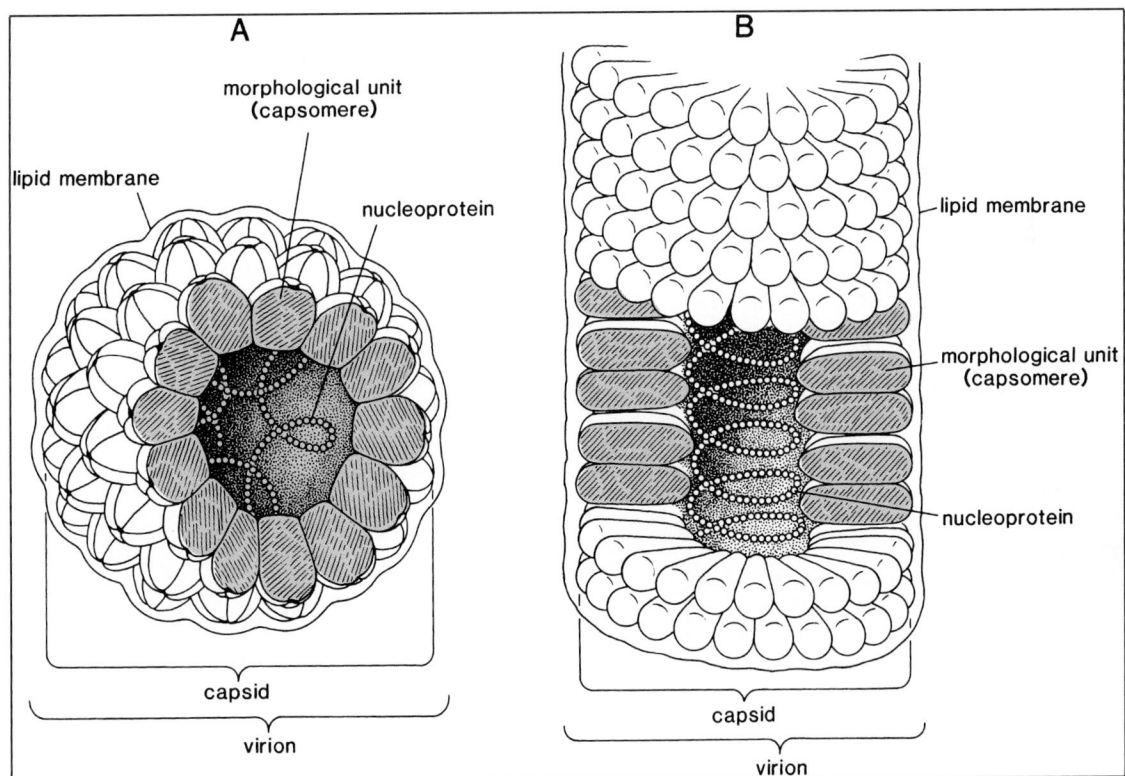

Figure 23-2 Virus construction. Viruses are constructed with great economy. A central nucleoprotein core is surrounded by a protein capsid, which is made up of individual capsomeres. Some viruses also have a lipoprotein membrane around the nucleocapsid. The two most common organizational patterns of symmetry are icosahedral (**A**) and helical (**B**). Ultrastructurally, the icosahedral viruses appear round, although the facets may occasionally be visualized (see the illustration of adenovirus in Table 23-2).

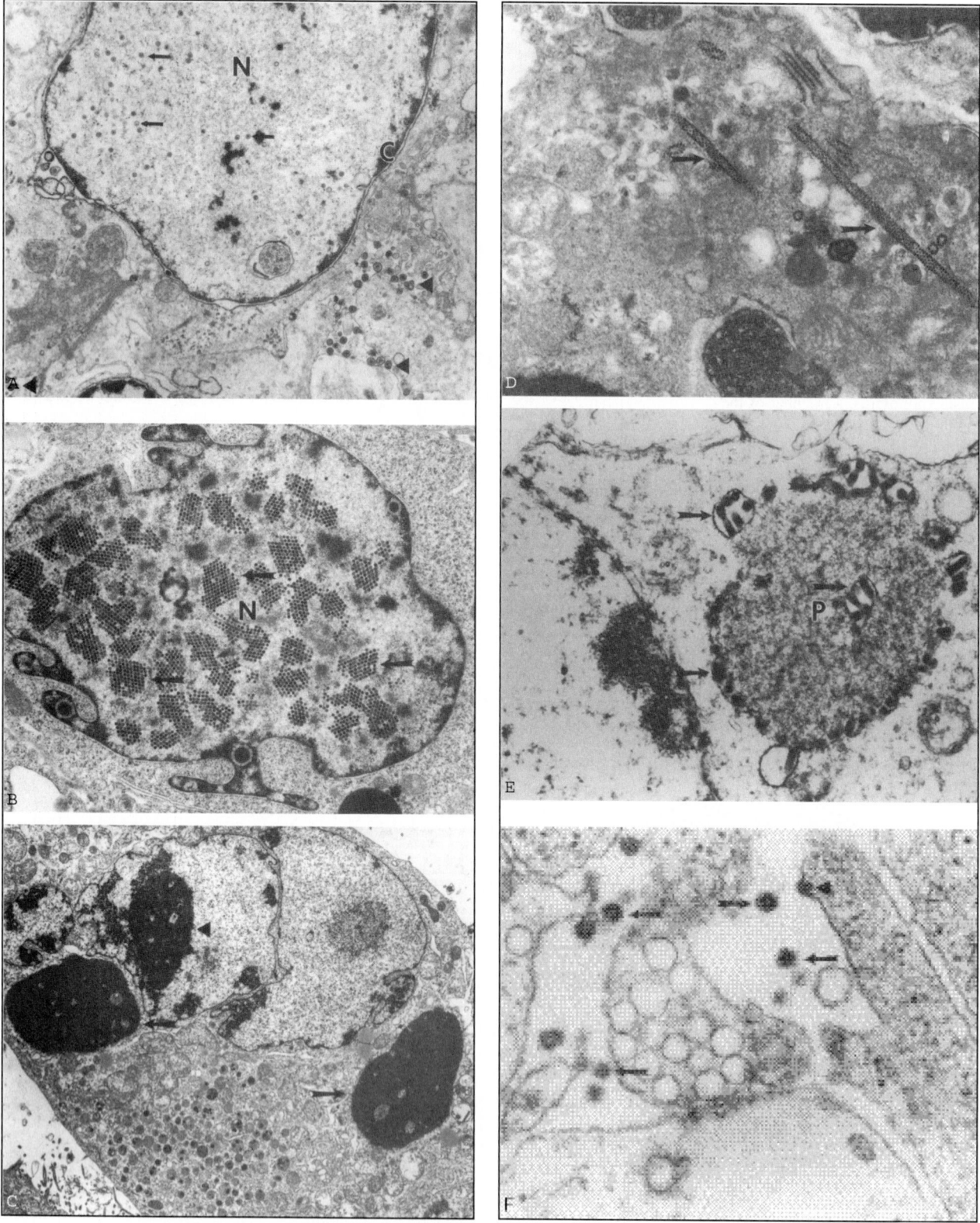

Figure 23-3 (**A**) Ultrastructure of viruses. Herpes simplex virus. The herpesviruses are assembled in the nucleus of the cell (*N*). The cellular chromatin (*C*) is pushed to the edge of the nucleus by the viral deoxyribonucleoprotein, which stains lightly in the micrograph. This material corresponds to the eosinophilic intranuclear inclusion seen with the light microscope (see Color Plate 23-1). Naked (nonenveloped) virions (*arrows*) are assembled in the nucleus. Outside the cell, some mature virions that have acquired a lipid envelope from the cell (*arrowheads*) are

clearly how the virus has appropriated the genetic resources of the cell (Fig. 23-3*A* and *B*). The final assembly of some viruses occurs at the nuclear or cytoplasmic membrane. As the virion moves from the nucleus to the cytoplasm or passes from the cytoplasm to the extracellular space, an external lipid-containing envelope is added to the nucleocapsid (see Figs. 23-2, 23-3*A* and *F*, and Table 23-2). Lipid solvents inactivate such enveloped viruses, whereas their nonenveloped counterparts are not affected. Replication of some viruses results in death of the cell, with release of the assembled nucleocapsids. The enveloped viruses that mature at the cytoplasmic membrane are released from the cell by ''budding'' through the membrane (see Figs. 23-3*F* and 23-16). In this process the envelope accumulates portions of the lipid membrane, as well as virus-specified glycoproteins that have been inserted into that membrane.

The major groups of viruses are summarized in Tables 23-1 and 23-2. Illustrative electron micrographs of negatively stained viral particles (provided by Frederick A. Murphy) are juxtaposed with a brief description of the families and genera. The list is not exhaustive, but it includes the most important human pathogens. The taxonomic characteristics are summarized in the tables, but the vernacular names are used subsequently in the text.

Structural and biochemical features that are used for classification include the characteristics of the nucleic acid, the configuration or symmetry of the nucleocapsid (helical, icosahedral, or complex), the presence or absence of a lipid envelope, the size of the virion, the number of capsomeres, the stability of the virion to chemical treatment, and the antigenic composition. Viruses contain either RNA or DNA. Most RNA viruses are single-stranded and repli-cate in the cytoplasm; DNA viruses are double-stranded and replicate in the nucleus. The major exceptions to the site of replication are influenza viruses (RNA), which begin replication in the nucleus, and poxviruses (DNA), which replicate in the cytoplasm. Reoviruses are double-stranded RNA viruses; parvoviruses are single-stranded DNA viruses.

The polarity of RNA viruses is considered positive if a virus can function as mRNA (i.e., proteins needed for construction of the virion can be synthesized directly from the viral nucleic acid once it is released into the cell by disruption of the virion capsid). An RNA virus with negative polarity must use an RNA-dependent RNA polymerase (an enzyme that must be packaged with the nucleic acid in the infecting virion) to make RNA with a positive polarity, after which the necessary proteins can be synthesized. The genome of most RNA viruses is contained in one linear segment, but there are multiple segments in a few cases. The segmented genome allows enhanced potential for genetic reassortments when two strains infect the same cell. One of the explanations for the amazing ability of influenza viruses to change and adapt is its segmented genome that facilitates recombination of segments when two different virions infect the same cell.

Clinical Manifestations of Viral Infections

The clinical manifestations of viral infection are legion. General symptoms include fever with or without chills, malaise, and myalgias. Specific symptoms derive primarily from the propensity of the virus to infect various cells and tissues

◄

visible (MRC-5 cells, infected with herpes simplex virus, type 1, X22,400). (**B**) Adenoviruses are assembled in the nucleus (*N*). They have icosahedral symmetry and are not enveloped. They are often closely packed in paracrystalline arrays (*arrows*). As the viruses accumulate, the whole nucleus may become filled with virions, producing the inclusions seen with the light microscope (see Color Plate 23-1*E*) (infected HEp-2 cells ×22,400). (**C**) Respiratory syncytial virus is assembled in the cytoplasm and matures at the cell membrane. Inclusions may be seen in the cytoplasm of infected cells, both in vivo and in vitro (see Color Plate 23-1*G*). The inclusions (*arrows*) are intracytoplasmic and are composed of fibrillar ribonucleoprotein. Contrast the density of the nucleolus (*arrowhead*) with that of the inclusions (infected HEp-2 cells, ×3,150). (**D**) Coxsackievirus B. The enteroviruses are small RNA-containing viruses that have icosahedral symmetry and are often packed in a paracrystalline array (*arrows*). They are assembled in the cytoplasm. Inclusions are not seen with the light microscope (infected rhesus monkey kidney cells, ×56,000). (**E**) Rabies virus. This bullet-shaped rhabdovirus is assembled in the cytoplasm. The fibrillar nucleoprotein (*P*) and the elongated viruses (*arrows*) are found together. The mass of viral material corresponds to the Negri body, which is seen with the light microscope (see Color Plate 23-1*H*). The internal structure that may be seen in classic Negri bodies comes from the incorporation of cytoplasmic material into the body of the inclusion (Infected human brain, ×25,000). (**F**) Eastern equine encephalitis virus. This togavirus illustrates the maturation of virus particles at the surface of the cell. Mature virions (*arrows*) are present in the extracellular space. A maturing (*budding*) virion is denoted by the dense nucleoprotein core and a condensation of the cellular membrane where the envelope is forming (*arrowhead*). Some viruses, such as the myxoviruses, insert their hemagglutinins into the membrane at this stage; they can be detected by the adherence of red blood cells to the viral hemagglutinin in the cell membrane (hemadsorption) (infected mouse brain, ×60,000). (**E**, courtesy of Daniel Perl; **F**, courtesy of Frederick Murphy).

Table 23-1 Classification of RNA Viruses (Selected Genera and Species that Infect Humans)

Family: *Orthomyxoviridae*
Genus *Influenza* virus A
Genus *Influenza* virus B
Genus *Influenza* virus C
Genus *Influenza* virus D
  (*Thogotovirus*)

Size: 100 nm, spherical or pleomorphic
Nucleic acid: Segmented, negative polarity, single stranded RNA
Symmetry: Helical
Lipid envelope: Present
Antigens: Hemagglutinin and neuraminidase
Natural habitat: humans and animals
Distribution: Worldwide

Mode of transmission: Aerosol droplet spread from person to person; rarely animal to person
Route of infection: Respiratory
Diseases: Respiratory infections including coryza (common cold), tracheobronchitis, and pneumonia. Extrapulmonary symptoms are prominent in the influenza syndrome; rarely, extrapulmonary disease such as myocarditis may be present

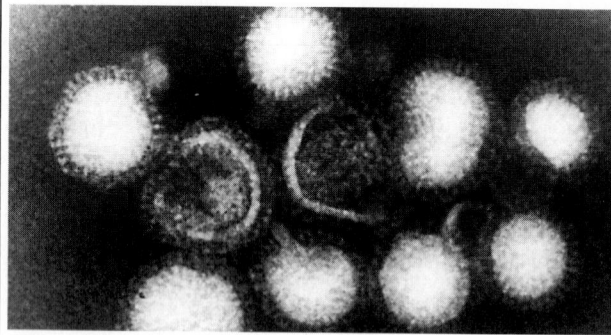

Influenzavirus A. The particles are roughly spherical but irregular. The internal helical structure is difficult to appreciate, but the fringe-like projections of hemagglutinin and neuraminidase are shown well. × 135,000

Family: *Paramyxoviridae*
Subfamily *Paramyxovirinae*
Genus *Respirovirus*
Species *Human parainfluenza virus 1*
Species *Human parainfluenza virus 3*
Genus *Rubulavirus*
Species *Human parainfluenza virus 2*
Species *Human parainfluenza virus 4*
Species *Mumps virus*
Genus *Morbillivirus*
Species *Measles virus*
Subfamily *Pneumovirinae*
Genus *Pneumovirus*
Species *Human respiratory syncytial virus*
Genus *Metapneumovirus*
Species *Human metapneumovirus*

Size: 150–300 nm, spherical or pleomorphic
Nucleic acid: Nonsegmented, negative polarity, single stranded RNA
Symmetry: Helical
Lipid envelope: Present
Antigens: Hemagglutinin, neuraminidase, fusion protein, nucleocapsid (depending on virus)
Natural habitat: Humans and animals
Distribution: Worldwide

Mode of transmission: Droplet aerosol or direct inoculation
Route of infection: Respiratory
Diseases: Common cold, tracheobronchitis, rarely pneumonia (parainfluenza); tracheobronchitis, bronchiolitis, and penumonia (respiratory syncytial virus); parotitis, pancreatitis, orchitis, meningitis (mumps); rash, pneumonia, encephalitis, subacute sclerosing panencephalitis (measles)

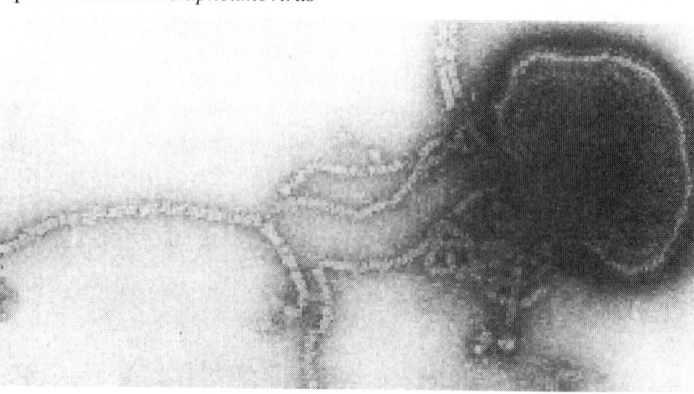

Parainfluenzavirus 1. The irregular virion has been disrupted, releasing a long strand of uncoiled RNA. The hemagglutinin fringes on the virion are evident. × 72,000.

Table 23-1 *Continued*

Family: *Rhabdoviridae*
Genus *Lyssavirus*
Species *Rabies virus*

Size: 50–95 nm by 130–389 nm, bullet-shaped
Nucleic acid: Nonsegmented, negative polarity, single stranded RNA
Symmetry: Helical
Lipid envelope: Present
Natural habitat: Wild and domestic animals
Distribution: Worldwide

Mode of transmission: Infected secretions, rabies usually transmitted by bites
Route of transmission: Cutaneous or respiratory
Disease: Encephalitis (rabies)

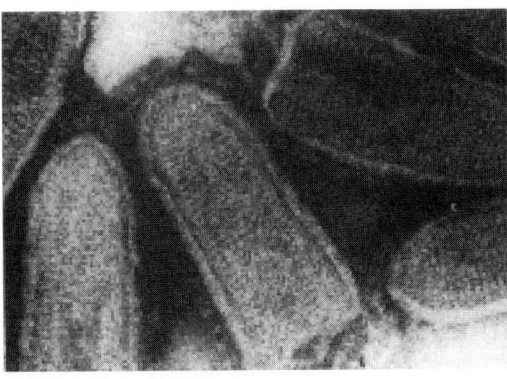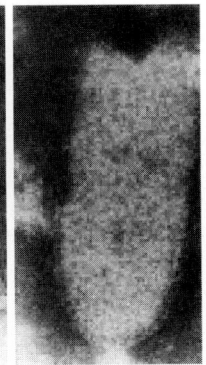

Vesicular stomatitis virus. The bullet shape of the virion is evident. The coiled helical nature of the internal ribonucleoprotein is reflected in the striations. × 216,000.

Family: *Filoviridae*
Genus "Marburg-like viruses," tentatively *Marburgvirus*
Species *Marburg virus*
Genus "Ebola-like viruses," tentatively *Ebolavirus*
Species *Zaire*
Species *Sudan*
Species *Reston*
Species *Cote d'Ivoire*

Size: 80 nm by 800–1000 nm, filamentous
Nucleic acid: Nonsegmented, negative polarity, single stranded RNA
Symmetry: Helical
Lipid envelope: Present
Natural habitat: Nonhuman primates
Distribution: Africa, Phillipines

Mode of transmission: Unknown, but close contact required
Diseases: Hemorrhagic fever with fatality rates as high as 90%

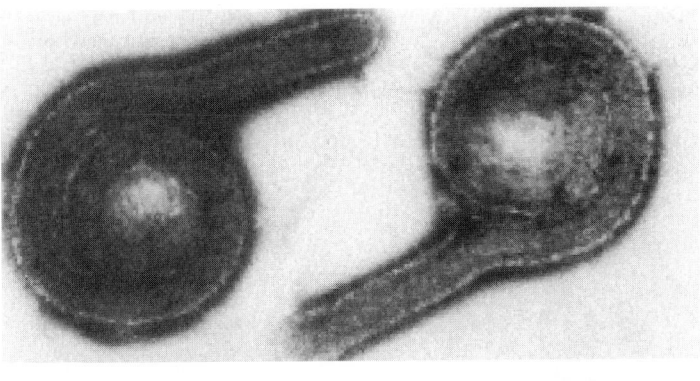

Ebola virus. Long, filamentous form has assumed a "crook" shape. × 59,000

(Continued)

(tropism), but may also depend on the route of infection, the virulence of the strain, the immunologic status of the patient, and other predisposing factors, such as underlying pulmonary or cardiac disease. The reader is referred to several excellent textbooks for additional details.[284,418]

Orthomyxoviruses

The orthomyxoviruses, which include influenza A, B, and C viruses, produce a wide variety of respiratory infections.[58,393] The influenza or "flu" syndrome begins with

Table 23-1 *Continued*

Family: *Bunyaviridae*
Genus *Bunyavirus*
Species *California encephalitis virus*
Species *La Crosse virus*
Genus *Hantavirus*
Species *Hantaan virus*
Species *Sin nombre virus*
Genus *Nairovirus*
Species *Crimean Congo Hemorrhagic Fever virus*
Genus *Phlebovirus*
Species *Rift Valley fever virus*
Species *Sandfly fever Sicilian virus*

Size: 90–120 nm
Nucleic acid: Segmented, single stranded RNA. May be negative polarity (Bunyavirus, Hantavirus, and Nairovirus) or contain examples of each polarity (Phlebovirus).
Symmetry: Helical
Lipid envelope: Present
Antigens: Surface hemagglutinin
Natural habitat: Small animals

Distribution: Worldwide
Mode of transmission: Bite of infected mosquitoes (Bunyavirus, Nairovirus, Phlebovirus); exposure to rodent excreta (Hantavirus)
Diseases: Febrile illness, aseptic meningitis (Bunyavirus); febrile illness, hemorrhagic fever, respiratory failure (Hantavirus); febrile illness, hemorrhagic fever (Nairovirus); febrile illness, encephalitis, hemorrhagic fever (Phlebovirus)

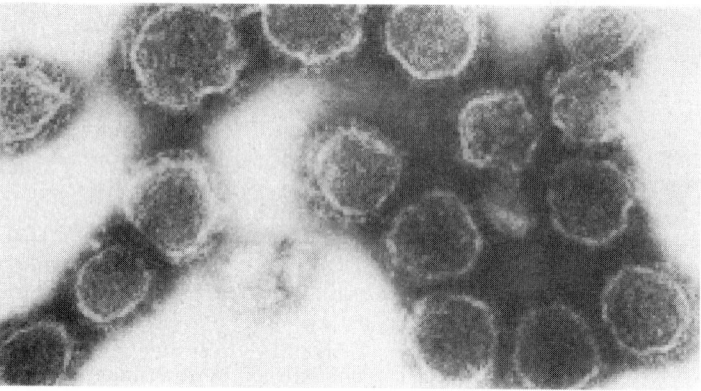

LaCrosse virus. Irregular virus particles; the lipid envelope and surface projections are evident. × 117,000

Family: *Coronaviridae*
Genus *Coronavirus*
Species *Human coronavirus 229E*
Species *Human coronavirus OC43*
Species *Human SARS virus* (tentative)

Size 80–130 nm
Nucleic acid: Nonsegmented, positive polarity, single stranded RNA
Symmetry: Helical
Lipid envelope: Present
Natural Habitat: Humans or animals (Coronaviruses)

Distribution: Worldwide
Transmission: Person-to-person, presumably by aerosol
Route of infection: Respiratory
Diseases: Common cold; rarely lower respiratory disease; severe acute respiratory syndrome

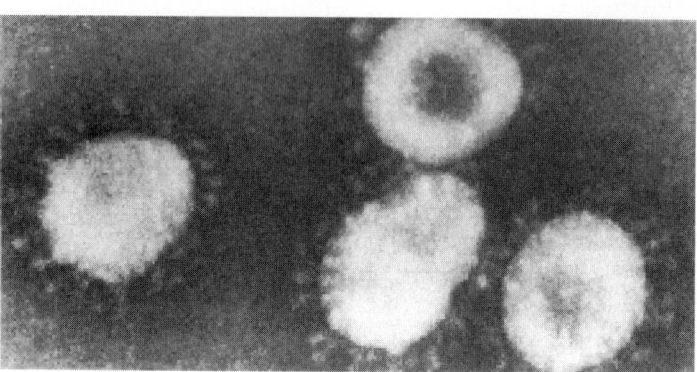

Human coronavirus OC43. The club-shaped projections are the most distinctive features of these pleomorphic particles. × 180,000.

Table 23-1 *Continued*

Family: *Picornaviridae*
Genus *Enterovirus*
Species *Poliovirus* (3 serotypes)
Species *Coxsackievirus* (23 serotypes)
Species *Echovirus* (28 serotypes)
Species *Enterovirus* (4 serotypes)
Genus *Hepatovirus*
Species *Human hepatitis A virus*
Genus *Parechovirus*
Species *Human parechovirus* (2 serotypes, formerly included in genus *Echovirus* as serotypes 22 and 23)
Genus *Rhinovirus*
Species *Human rhinovirus* (103 serotypes)

Size: 22–30 nm
Nucleic acid: Nonsegmented, positive polarity, single stranded RNA
Symmetry: Icosahedral
Lipid envelope: Absent
Natural habitat: Human gastrointestinal tract; survives in environment (Enterovirus, Hepatovirus, Parechovirus); human upper respiratory tract (Rhinovirus)

Distribution: Worldwide
Transmission: Fecal-oral from human-to-human or contaminated water (Enterovirus, Hepatovirus, Parechovirus); human respiratory tract by aerosol or on hands (Rhinovirus)
Route of infection: Gastrointestinal (Enterovirus, Hepatovirus, Parechovirus); respiratory (Rhinovirus)
Diseases: Febrile illness, meningitis, encephalitis, myocarditis (Enterovirus, Parechovirus); hepatitis (Hepatovirus); common cold (Rhinovirus)

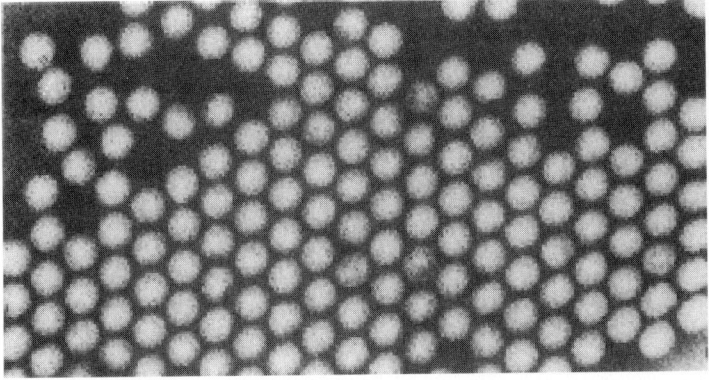

Poliovirus 1. The particles are small, regular, and nonenveloped. 3 180,000

Family: *Caliciviridae*
Genus *Norwalk-like viruses* (Tentative)
Genus *Sapporo-like viruses* (Tentative)

Size: 35–39 nm
Nucleic acid: Nonsegmented, positive polarity, single stranded RNA
Symmetry: Icosahedral
Lipid envelope: Absent
Natural habitat: Human gastrointestinal tract

Distribution: Worldwide
Transmission: Fecal-oral; contaminated water
Portal of entry: Gastrointestinal
Diseases: Gastroenteritis

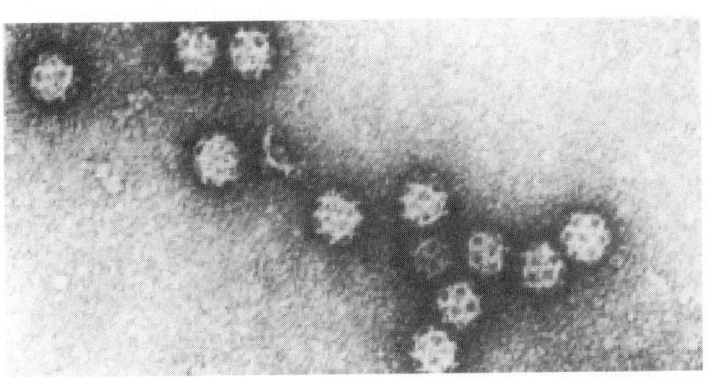

Swine exanthemata virus. Very small, regular particles with prominent cuplike depressions. The surface depressions of the human Norwalk-like viruses are not as pronounced.

(Continued)

Table 23-1 *Continued*

Family: *Reoviridae*
Genus *Orthoreovirus*
Serotypes 1–3
Genus *Rotavirus*
Serotypes A-G (D-G only in animals)
Genus *Coltivirus*
Type species *Colorado tick fever virus*

Size: 60–80 nm, variable morphology
Nucleic acid: Segmented, double stranded RNA
Symmetry: Icosahedral
Lipid envelope: Absent
Natural habitat: Gastrointestinal tract of humans (Reovirus and Rotavirus) and animals (Rotavirus)

Distribution: Worldwide
Transmission: Fecal-oral by direct contact; animal to human
Portal of entry: Gastrointestinal tract
Diseases: Gastroenteritis (Rotavirus); None (Reovirus)

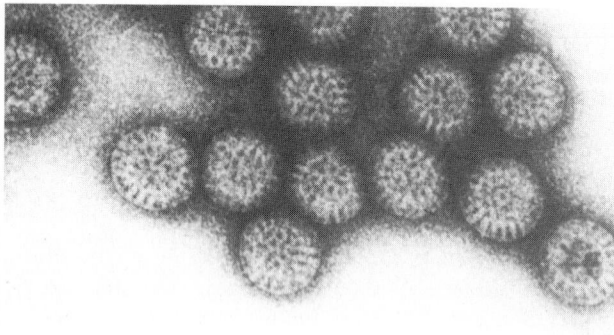

Human rotavirus. The distinctive feature of the Reoviridae is the presence of a double shell, each with icosahedral symmetry. × 135,000.

Family: *Astroviridae*
Genus *Astrovirus*
Species *Human Astrovirus*

Size: 28–30 nm
Nucleic acid: Nonsegmented, positive polarity, single stranded RNA
Symmtery: Icosahedral
Lipid envelope: Absent
Natural habitat: Gastrointestinal tract of human

Distribution: Worldwide
Transmission: Fecal-oral; contaminated water
Portal of entry: Gastrointestinal tract
Diseases: Gastroenteritis

Family: *Togaviridae*
Genus *Alphavirus*
Species *Eastern equine encephalitis virus*
Species *Venezuellan equine encephalitis virus*
(Other antropod-borne species)
Genus *Rubivirus*
Species *Rubella virus*

Size: 70 nm
Nucleic acid: Nonsegmented, positive polarity, single stranded RNA
Symmetry: Icosahedral
Lipid envelope: Present
Natural habitat: Small mammals and insects (Alphavirus); humans (Rubivirus)

Distribution: Worldwide
Transmission: By mosquito bites (Alphavirus); aerosols or transplacental (Rubivirus)
Portal of entry: Cutaneous (Alphavirus); respiratory or vascular (Rubivirus)
Diseases: Hepatitis, meningitis, encephalitis, arthritis, febrile illness (Alphavirus); rash illness, congenital infection (Rubivirus)

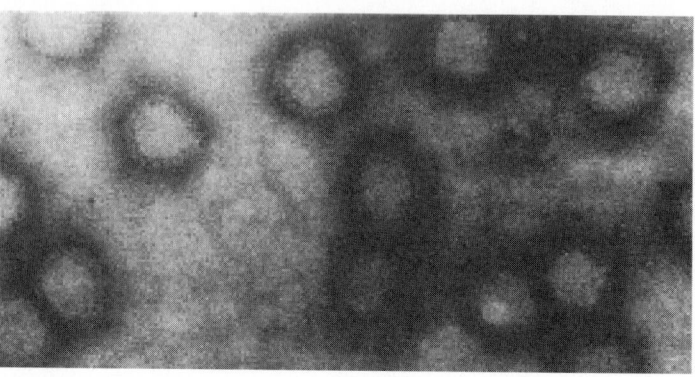

Rubella virus. The spherical virions have a lipid membrane and surface hemagglutinin projections. × 135,000.

Table 23-1 *Continued*

Family: *Flaviviridae* Genus *Flavivirus* Species *Yellow fever virus* Species *St. Louis encephalitis virus* Species *Japanese encephalitis virus* Species *West Nile virus* Species *Dengue virus* (Numerous other species, many arthropod-borne) Genus *Hepacivirus* Species *Hepatitis C virus* Unassigned viruses (GB agents)	Size: 40–60 nm Nucleic acid: Nonsegmented, positive polarity, single stranded RNA Symmetry: Icosahedral Lipid envelope: Present Natural habitat: Small mammals and insects (Flavivirus); humans (Hepacivirus)	Distribution: Worldwide Transmission: By bite of mosquito or tick (Flavivirus); by blood (Hepacivirus) Portal of entry: Cutaneous (Flavivirus); vascular; sexual (Hepacivirus) Diseases: Hepatitis, meningitis, encephalitis febrile illness, hemorrhagic fever (Flavivirus); hepatitis, cirrhosis, hepatocellular carcinoma (Hepacivirus)
Family: *Retroviridae* Genus *Deltaretrovirus* Species *Human T-cell lymphotrophic virus,* Types 1 and 2 (HTLV) Genus *Lentivirus* Species *Human immuno-deficiency virus,* Types 1 and 2 (HIV)	Size 100 nm Nucleic acid: Nonsegmented, positive polarity, single stranded RNA dimer (packaged with RNA-dependent DNA polymerase) Symmetry: Variable Lipid envelope: Present Natural habitat: Humans	Distribution: Worldwide Transmission: Sexual, contaminated needles, transfusions, maternal-fetal/neonate Portal of entry: Mucous membranes, vascular Diseases: T-cell leukemia and lymphoma (HTLV); acquired immunodefiency syndrome (HIV)

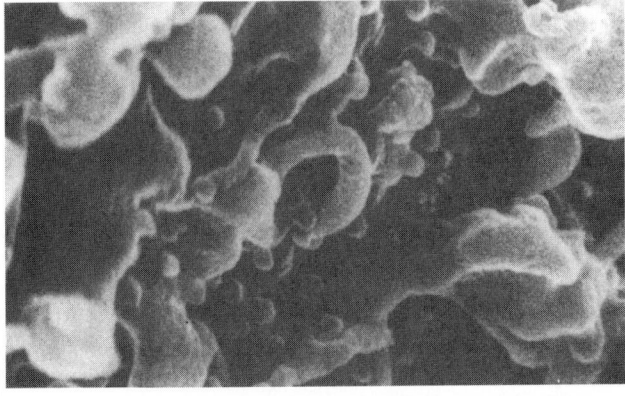

Human immunodeficiency virus. Scanning electron micrograph of human T lymphocyte with virus particles budding from surface.

(Continued)

the abrupt onset of headache, fever, chills, and dry cough; later, high fever, myalgias, malaise, and anorexia appear. In young children, gastrointestinal symptoms may be prominent. Almost all cases of influenza occur during the winter. Influenza A and B viruses account for most epidemic respiratory disease in which there is excess mortality. They are rarely isolated in the absence of infection. Influenza A virus infects a variety of mammalian and avian species. Transmission of swine influenza from pigs to humans has been described occasionally.[512] Concern about infection of humans with swine virus led to a nationwide immunization campaign in 1976, with unexpected and unwanted cases of Guillain-Barré syndrome resulting. Influenza C virus is an uncommon cause of human infection, but may produce bronchitis and pneumonia.[356] Influenza viruses may produce serious lower respiratory tract disease by themselves or, more commonly, may set up the patient for a secondary bacterial infection.[509] A twist on the secondary infection scenario has been the production of toxic-shock syndrome by the invading *Staphylococcus aureus*.[319] Other complications of influenza include myocarditis[144] and encephalopathy,[233,468] although the virus is not usually detected in these situations.

The structure and function of influenza virus are intimately related both to pathogenesis and to laboratory diagnosis.[294] The nucleoprotein antigen in the viral core defines the type of virus; for example, influenza A or B. This antigen is stable and is recognized by many of the diagnos-

Table 23-1 *Continued*

Family: *Arenaviridae*		
Genus *Arenavirus*	Size: 62–>200 nm	Distribution: Worldwide (LCM); South America
Old World Group	Nucleic acid: Bisegmented, ambi-	(Junin, Machupo, Sabia, Guanarito); Africa
Species *Lymphocytic*	polarity, single stranded	(Lassa)
choriomeningiti	Symmetry: Pleomorphic	Transmission: Contact with rodent or human
virus (LCM)	Lipid envelope: Present	secretions
Species *Lassa virus*	Naturally habitat: Rodents	Portal of entry: Respiratory, cutaneous (lacerations)
New World Group		Diseases: Febrile illness, meningitis (LCM);
Species *Junin virus*		Hemorrhagic fever (Lassa, Junin, Machupo,
Species *Machupo virus*		Sabia, Guanarito viruses)
Species *Sabia virus*		
Species *Guanarito virus*		

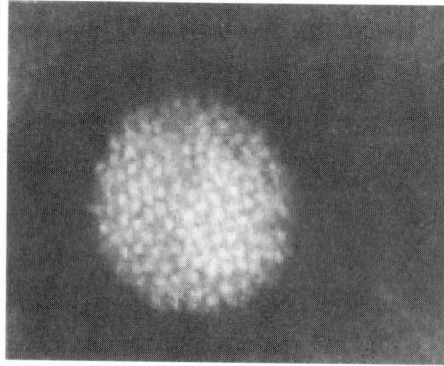 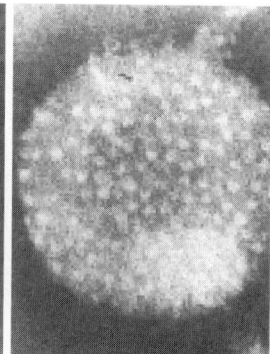

Lymphocytic choriomeningitis virus. The spherical virus has large surface projections. The name is derived from the Latin word arenosus (sandy), which was suggested by the internal ribosome-like particles that are seen by transmission electron microscopy, × 225,000.

tic antisera, which are able to detect all circulating strains of a particular type. Two glycoprotein antigens on the surface of the influenza virion are important for pathogenesis, epidemiology, and immunotherapy. The dominant antigen is the hemagglutinin, which is responsible for attachment to respiratory epithelial cells and therefore an important target for influenza vaccines. The surface neuraminidase enzyme participates in entry of the virus into the cell. These surface antigens are constantly changing, so that they are a moving target for therapeutic and diagnostic antibodies. It is the constant, incremental change (antigenic drift) and periodic, quantum change (antigenic shift) that allow recurring epidemics of influenza.

The viruses are named by their structure and geography. For instance, an isolate might be characterized influenza A/Leningrad/360/86 (H3N2). The name means that this strain was the 360th isolate of influenza A in Leningrad in 1986 and it contains the third antigenic type of hemagglutinin and the second type of neuraminidase. The hemagglutinin and neuraminidase are not useful antigens for diagnostic purposes, but they are essential for the epidemiologist to study so that the next year's vaccine can contain antibodies to currently circulating antigens. Although it has not yet been accomplished, attempts continue to predict the future drift of influenza A virus strains, so that the vaccine for the next flu season can be formulated more rationally.[50]

To date nine different hemagglutinins have been recog-

nized. The initial antigen (H1) was hypothesized to be a constituent of the strain that caused pandemic influenza in 1918, based on serologic analysis. Quite recently, independent evidence has been developed by using modern molecular techniques on tissue from influenza victims.[413] Two samples came from formalin-fixed lung tissue in England, but the sample that yielded the most complete sequence was taken from the body of an Inuit woman who had been buried in Alaskan permafrost. There was a remarkable homogeneity among the three samples from diverse geographic locations.

Subsequent major epidemics have been associated with major shifts in the hemagglutinin: H2 during the Asian influenza epidemic in 1957 and H3 during the Hong Kong influenza epidemic of 1968. Subsequently, strains with either the H1 or H3 hemagglutinin circulated until a new strain of avian influenza (H5 hemagglutinin) killed 6 of 18 individuals infected in Hong Kong. This virus, which was spread directly from chickens to humans without another intermediary, appears to have particularly virulent characteristics.[216] Fortunately, spread from human to human appeared limited. Subsequently, another strain (H9 hemagglutinin) appeared in Hong Kong with similar epidemiologic characteristics, but fortunately less mortality. More recently, the H5 virus has reappeared in Southeast Asia, once again with high mortality rates in patients who were exposed to poultry, but without significant person-to-person transmission.[224,282]

Table 23-2 Classification of DNA Viruses (Selected Genera and Species That Infect Humans)

Family: *Herpesviridae*
Subfamily: *Alphaherpesvirinae*
Genus: *Simplexvirus*
Species: *Herpes simplex virus 1*
    (HHV1)
Species: *Herpes simplex virus 2*
    (HHV2)
Genus: *Varicellovirus*
Species: *Varicella-zoster virus* (VZV)
Subfamily: *Betaherpesvirinae*
Genus: *Cytomegalovirus*
Species: *Human cytomegalovirus*
    (CMV)
Genus: *Roseolovirus*
Species: *Human herpesvirus 6A* (HHV6A)
Species: *Human herpesvirus 6B* (HHV6B)
Species: *Human herpesvirus 7* (HHV7)
Subfamily: *Gammaherpesvirinae*
Genus: *Lymphocryptovirus*
Species: *Epstein-Barr virus* (EBV)
Genus: *Rhadinovirus*
Species: *Human herpesvirus 8 (Kaposi's
    sarcoma–associated herpesvirus)* (HHV8)

Size: 120–300 nm
Symmetry: Icosahedral
Lipid envelope: Present
Natural habitat: Humans
Distribution: Worldwide
Transmission: By infected oral or
    genital secretions, by blood,
    or transplacentally
Portal of entry: Respiratory, cutaneous,
    intravascular, transplacental

Diseases: Pharyngitis, cervicitis, local skin
    lesions, pneumonia, esophagitis, encephalitis,
    disseminated infection (HSV1), skin lesions,
    meningitis, neonatal sepsis (HSV2); congenital
    infection, hepatitis, mononucleosis, pneumonia
    (CMV), chickenpox, disseminated
    infection, zoster/shingles (VZV), pharyngitis,
    mononucleosis, hepatitis (EBV); exanthem
    subitum (HHV6, HHV7), Kaposi's sarcoma,
    lymphoma (HHV8)

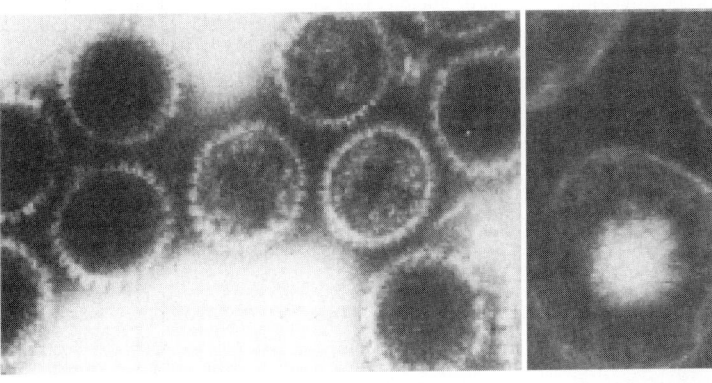

Herpes simplex virus. *(Left)* Naked nucleocapsids demonstrate the regular structure of the virion. Clearly defined structural units appear to have a central depression. *(Right)* Enveloped particle has, in addition, a lipid membrane derived from the infected cell. × 189,000

Family: *Adenoviridae*
Genus: *Mastadenovirus*
Species: *Adenovirus* (49 serotypes)

Size: 70-90 nm
Symmetry: Icosahedral
Lipid envelope: Absent
Natural habitat: Humans

Distribution: Worldwide
Transmission: Fecal-oral, ?aerosol droplet
Portal of entry: Respiratory, Gastrointestinal
Diseases: Conjunctivitis, keratitis, pharyngitis,
    tracheobronchitis, pneumonia, cystitis; gastro-
    enteritis (types 40 and 41)

Adenovirus, type 5. The regular arrangement of the structural units of the virion is clearly evident. × 234,000.

(Continued)

Table 23-2 *Continued*

Family: *Papovaviridae*
Genus: *Papillomavirus*
Species: *Human papillomavirus* (>100 genotypes)
Genus: *Polymavirus*
Species: *Simian virus 40* (SV40)
Species: *JC virus* (JCV)
Species: *BK virus* (BKV)

Size: 45-55 nm
Symmetry: Icosahedral
Lipid envelope: Absent
Natural habitat: Humans (papillomavirus, JCV, and BKV); monkeys (SV40)

Distribution: Worldwide
Transmission: Contact with infected secretions, sexual; viruses remain dormant in tissue and/or integrate into genome (pappilomavirus)
Portal of entry: Cutaneous, genital, respiratory (papillomavirus);? respiratory (polyomavirus)
Diseases: Cutaneous, genital, and respiratory papillomas (warts), epithelial neoplasia (papillomavirus); progressive multifocal leukoencephalopathy (PMLE) (polyomavirus)

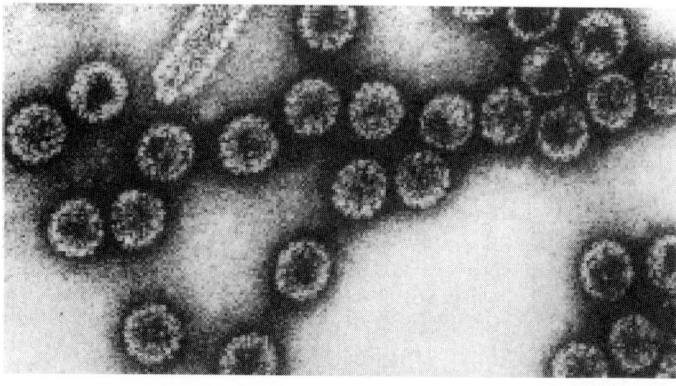

Human wart virus. These viruses have never been propagated successfully in cell cultures. The diseases have been associated by demonstration of virions, viral antigens, or nucleic acid in lesions. × 135,000.

Family: *Parvoviridae*
Subfamily *Parvovirinae*
Genus: *Erythrovirus*
Species: *B19 virus*

Size: 18–26 nm
Nucleic acid: Nonsegmented, single-stranded DNA
Symmetry: Icosahedral
Lipid envelope: Absent
Natural habitat: Humans

Distribution: Worldwide
Transmission: Person-to-person (route unknown); transfusion
Portal of entry: unknown; vascular
Diseases: Erythema infectiosum (fifth disease), hemolytic disease of newborn, anemia

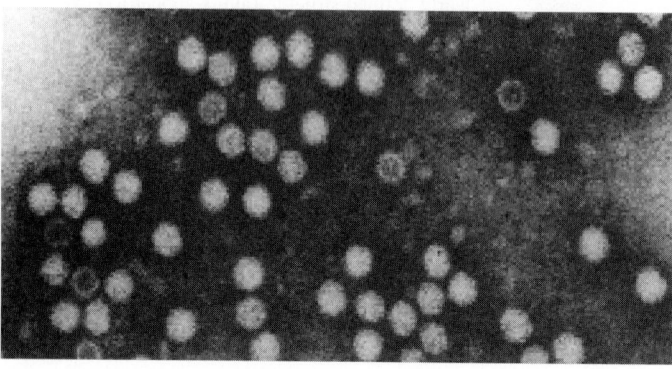

H-1 virus. The virions are very small and regular size and shape. Parvoviruses are unusual in that they contain single-stranded DNA.

The frequency with which avian influenza viruses have crossed the species barrier to infect humans is disconcerting. Clearly, devastating pandemic disease awaits only the combination of high virulence and efficient human-to-human transmission. The Centers for Disease Control and Prevention (CDC) has formulated interim recommendations for processing of specimens from patients with possible avian influenza. Use of Biosafety Level 3 facilities is recommended for some manipulations; submission of the specimens to an institution, such as the CDC, that has appropriate facilities is encouraged.[82]

Paramyxoviruses
PARAINFLUENZA VIRUSES

The paramyxoviruses are a varied group. The four serotypes of parainfluenza virus are important causes of respira-

Table 23-2 *Continued*

Family: *Hepadnaviridae*
Genus: *Hepadnavirus*
Species: *Hepatitis B virus*

Size: 42–47 nm
Nucleic acid: Nonsegmented
    circular DNA
Symmetry: Complex
Lipid envelope: Present
Natural habitat Humans
Antigens:
Surface antigen (HBsAg)
Core antige (HDcAg)
Early antigen (HBeAg)

Distribution: Worldwide
Transmission: Infected secretions and blood,
    sexual, transfusion
Portal of entry: Skin, vascular, genital
Diseases: Hepatitis, cirrhosis, hepatocellular
    carcinoma

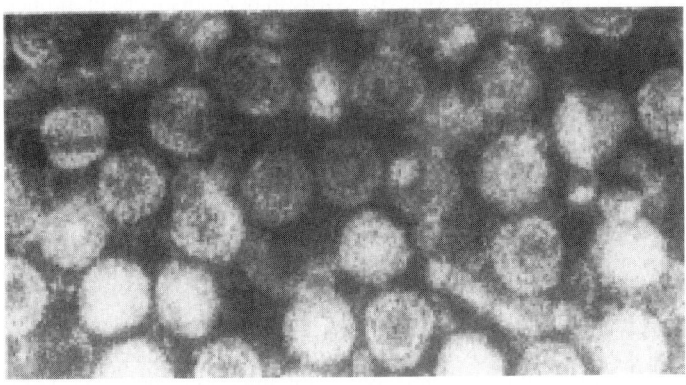

Hepatitis B virus. These 42-nm particles, which are the infectious agent, were originally known as Dane particles. × 225,000

Family: *Poxviridae*
Subfamily: *Chordopoxvirinae*
Genus: *Orthopoxvirus*
Species: *Variola virus (smallpox)*
Species: *Vaccinia virus*
Species: *Cowpox virus*
Species: *Monkeypox virus*
Genus: *Parapoxvirus*
Species: *Orf virus*
Genus: *Molluscipoxvirus*
Species: *Molluscum contagiosum virus*
Genus: *Yatapoxvirus*
Species: *Tanapoxvirus*

Size: 300–450 × 170–270 nm
Nucleic acid: Nonsegmented double-
    stranded DNA
Symmetry: Complex
Lipid envelope: Absent
Natural habitat: Humans and animals

Distribution: Worldwide; variola "extinct"
Transmission: Respiratory, cutaneous
Portal of entry: Respiratory, cutaneous
Diseases: Cutaneous ulcerative lesions, dissemi-
    nated disease (orthopoxvirus), cutaneous ulce-
    rative lesions (parapoxvirus, Yatapoxvirus);
    molluscum contagiosum (Molluscipoxvirus)

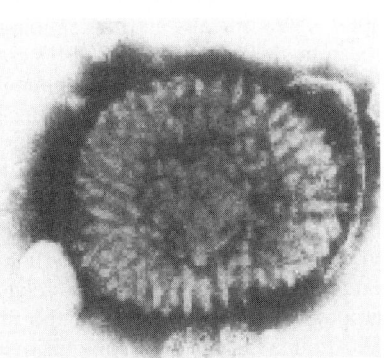

Vaccinia virus. The convoluted outer coat of these large, brick-shaped particles is evident. When smallpox existed, negative-stain electron microscopy was a useful tool for differentiation of the pocks from those of varicella. × 49,500

tory disease, which is usually mild in adults but may be severe in young children.[207] Parainfluenza viruses 1 and 2 cause croup (laryngotracheobronchitis) in children between ages 2 and 6 during the winter respiratory virus season. Parainfluenza virus 3 is an important cause of bronchiolitis in children younger than 2 years of age; infections occur all year long, with peaks in the fall and spring.

MUMPS VIRUS

Mumps virus produces infectious parotitis. It frequently causes aseptic meningitis, which is usually mild, and may also affect the pancreas, the gonads, and more rarely the joints. The introduction of effective vaccines has greatly reduced the incidence of mumps virus infection. At the Mayo Clinic, mumps virus was isolated 185 times in the 1960s but only 3 times in the 1970s.[453] Interestingly, after the introduction of mumps vaccine the circulating strains, which had been homogeneous, became more diverse.[259]

MEASLES VIRUS

Measles virus (rubeola virus) is unlikely to be encountered in the clinical laboratory,[453] but unfortunately the virus has made a clinical comeback. Laxity in monitoring and enforcing immunization practices has led to explosive outbreaks both in young adults, who may have waning immunity, and in children, especially in inner-city areas where levels of immunization are low.[64] The affliction of varsity sports teams and cancellation of highly visible sports contests are guaranteed to get the attention of the media and the public. Molecular analysis suggests the existence of multiple imported cases, rather than a single endemic strain.[423]

The public health implications of exposure in our mobile society was illustrated by an epidemic of 247 cases that began in a ski area in Breckenridge, Colorado.[69] After dispersal of infected individuals, cases of measles were detected in 10 states.

Two factors minimize the likelihood of isolating measles virus: the diagnosis is usually made on clinical grounds, and specimens are often not submitted to the laboratory. In addition, virus is isolated from respiratory secretions and urine only early in the course of the infection. The diagnostic rash is produced by complexes of viral antigen and antibody. Thus, at the time the diagnosis is made by a physician the virus is being neutralized and cultures are likely to be negative. Atypical clinical symptoms were seen formerly in patients who had received early inactivated measles vaccines,[12] but this phenomenon is no longer prevalent. Pneumonia and encephalitis are the most serious complications of measles.[142,265] In addition, measles virus (or a variant thereof) rarely produces a chronic encephalitis known as subacute sclerosing panencephalitis.[390]

RESPIRATORY SYNCYTIAL VIRUS

Respiratory syncytial virus (RSV) causes recurrent respiratory infections from infancy through adult life. Epidemics are common and may be hospital-associated. There are two distinct serologic groups of respiratory syncytial virus (A and B). A single group predominates in most epidemics,[364]

but the viral type does not correlate with severity of infection.[332] Disease is concentrated in the winter months, although summertime infection may occur in warm climates.[507]

Infection is spread by large particle droplets and by fomites (contaminated environmental particles, such as dust), rather than by small particle aerosols. This viral infection is a major cause of nosocomial infection; careful attention to the principles of infection control is essential.[192] Good laboratory diagnostic support is needed not only for treating the individual patient, but also for limiting nosocomial spread of the infection.

Respiratory syncytial virus may produce croup, bronchitis, bronchiolitis, or interstitial pneumonia.[207] It is the most common cause of respiratory disease in hospitalized infants younger than 1 year of age. Respiratory syncytial virus infections are often severe in young children. If congenital heart disease or immunologic deficiency is present, the disease may be especially lethal; in one study, 8 (73%) of 11 infants with congenital heart disease and pulmonary hypertension died.[320] Many previously normal children, especially infants, are sufficiently ill that ventilatory support is required. Apnea is a prominent part of the syndrome.

Immunity to respiratory syncytial virus is short-lived and incomplete. RSV was long thought to be a disease of infants and young children, but adult infection, including serious disease is now recognized to be an important clinical problem.[152,208] Epidemics in nursing homes have been reported.[153]

The serious nature of respiratory syncytial virus infection in immunocompromised adults has been recognized.[333] Serious respiratory syncytial virus infection occurs also in the elderly and in adults with chronic diseases, such as diabetes, cirrhosis, and chronic obstructive pulmonary disease.[205]

OTHER PARAMYXOVIRUSES

Several new paramyxoviruses have appeared in the past decade. Human metapneumovirus was initially recognized in Hong Kong, but has now been documented worldwide. It is a member of the subfamily *Pneumovirinae*, which includes RSV[345]; the human virus is closely related to two avian viruses. It resembles RSV clinically and epidemiologically.[34] Isolates have been made in LLC-MK2 cells (a continuous rhesus monkey kidney cell line that is not commonly used in diagnostic laboratories). The virus was recognized by cytopathic effect (CPE), but identification has been made by molecular techniques.

Two other newly recognized paramyxoviruses have been associated with severe neurologic disease, rather than respiratory infection. Nipah virus has caused encephalitis in pig farmers in Malaysia and Singapore.[191] It is closely related to Hendra virus, which produced equine disease and a few human infections in Australia. Laboratory-acquired infections have been noted.

Picornaviruses

The picornaviruses, which include the rhinoviruses and the enteroviruses, constitute the other large and important group of RNA viruses. The rhinoviruses are frequent causes of the common cold. They are acid-labile and do not infect the gastrointestinal tract. Transmission of rhinoviruses probably occurs by generation of respiratory aerosols,[110] as has been suggested for other respiratory viruses. These hardy viruses may also be transmitted through contact with contaminated inanimate surfaces.

There are so many rhinovirus serotypes (100 at present) that immunologic diagnosis is impractical. Culture is infrequently requested because rhinovirus infections are uncomfortable, but almost never life-threatening.

The classic enteroviruses are polioviruses 1 through 3, coxsackieviruses A and B, and echoviruses.[382] The Coxsackie group received its name from a small town in Upstate New York where the first isolates were recovered. "Echo" stands for *enteric cytopathic human orphan*, a name applied before the pathogenic potential of the viruses was appreciated. Subsequently, other members of the genus have been recognized and designated enteroviruses 68 through 71. Enteroviruses can be isolated from 40–80% of patients with aseptic meningitis.[96] Many more cases of sporadic and epidemic aseptic meningitis are probably caused by enteroviruses, based on the finding that the epidemic curve for all cases of aseptic meningitis parallels exactly the curve for cases from which enteroviruses have been isolated. The peak incidence is in the summer and early fall.

The enteroviruses, especially coxsackievirus B, also produce myocarditis, pericarditis, and epidemic pleurodynia. An association of these viruses with cardiomyopathy, a noninflammatory disorder of cardiac muscle, has also been suggested, but is controversial.[482] Coxsackievirus A causes herpangina and hand-foot-and-mouth disease. The enteroviruses also produce febrile disease with rash, which is usually maculopapular but rarely can be vesicular. Two recently recognized pathogenic enteroviruses are enterovirus 70, which causes epidemic hemorrhagic conjunctivitis, and enterovirus 71, which produces central nervous system (CNS) infection, including polio-like paralysis.

Enteroviral infection is most common in infants and young children. Paradoxically, paralytic poliovirus disease is most prevalent in young adults. Spread of enteroviruses is facilitated by poor hygiene and sanitation and by crowding. In populations among which virus spreads actively (low socioeconomic groups), infection occurs at an early age and paralytic disease is infrequent. Persons in high socioeconomic groups escape infection as infants and are more likely to experience paralysis after infection as a teenager. A similar phenomenon has been documented with varicella-zoster virus, Epstein-Barr virus, and rubella virus. Fortunately, paralytic disease was almost entirely caused by virulent poliovirus serotypes and has been virtually eliminated by immunization in most countries. Wild-type poliovirus has now been eradicated from three of the six World Health Organization (WHO) regions, with recalcitrant cases in Africa, the eastern Mediterranean, and Southeast Asia.[79] Paralytic disease may be caused by traditional coxsackieviruses and enteroviruses, but only very rarely. The production of paralytic disease by enterovirus 71 has been noted.

The pathogenesis of most enterovirus infections includes primary infection of the respiratory or gastrointestinal tracts followed by viremia and infection of a distant target organ, such as skin, heart, or meninges. The inactivated (Salk) poliovirus vaccine elicits neutralizing serum antibodies but not mucosal immunity. The vaccine works because the serum antibodies block the viremic spread to the meninges. The inability of the Salk vaccine to prevent mild gastrointestinal infection is not a serious problem for the individual patient, although it does allow continued circulation of the virulent strain.

In recent years most cases of paralytic poliomyelitis in developed countries have been caused by the attenuated (Sabin) vaccine strains. Consequently, inactivated (Salk) poliovirus vaccines are once again recommended for use in the United States.

The symptoms of most enterovirus infections are produced by direct viral cytopathic effect on the target organ. Meningoencephalitis is accompanied by productive infection of the CNS by actively replicating virus. The clinical syndrome of myocarditis, however, is caused by an immunologic reaction to enterovirus-infected cardiac tissue. By the time the patient becomes symptomatic the virus has usually been eliminated from the heart.

It is clear from the pathogenesis of enteroviral infection that culture of patients with aseptic meningitis (productive infection) makes sense, but culture of patients with myocarditis (immunopathologic disease) is unlikely to yield a viral isolate.

Rhabdoviruses

Many other important RNA viruses have been described, some of which cause highly lethal infections. These viruses are primarily tropical and are therefore less likely to be encountered by clinical laboratories than are the picornaviruses and the myxoviruses. Among these are the rhabdoviruses, including the agent of rabies, which is important worldwide.

The diagnosis of rabies is made by detection of viral antigen in clinical specimens from animals or humans. Culture of rabies virus is infrequently performed because of the simplicity, accuracy, and speed of direct immunofluorescence. This historical scourge is endemic in wild animals in the United States but is extremely uncommon in humans. Human exposure continues, however, from hunting dogs exposed to infected wild animals, from infected bats, and from domestic animals.[375] Bats may be insectivorous and the contact may be only casual. In some cases the only recognized contact was finding a bat in a bedroom in the absence of a recognized bite. It may be impossible to identify any source for human rabies. Not uncommonly the diagnosis is not suspected until autopsy.

Great anxiety is caused by possible exposures because of the lethality of the infection. The cost of preventing human disease can be enormous, as was shown in New Hampshire when a large number of individuals were potentially exposed to a rabid kitten in a pet store.[70] The estimated cost for epidemiologic investigation and prophylaxis was $1.5 million. Ongoing epizootic disease in raccoons in the eastern United States is of particular concern because of the frequency with which these aggressive animals invade human habitations. The molecular structure of rabies strains reflects their animal host. It is now possible to identify the likely source of a viral isolate from its nucleic-acid composition.

A case of inadvertent surgical transmission of rabies as a result of a corneal transplantation has been reported.[245]

Arenaviruses

The arenaviruses are a family of RNA viruses that share fascinating biologic characteristics.[48] Their natural host is a variety of rodents, which are persistently infected without an effective host response or symptomatic disease. Infectious virus is excreted in the urine, which is the source of human infection. Those at risk of infection are, therefore, individuals who come in contact with infected rodent excreta, either in their homes or at work in the fields. Person-to-person transmission occurs regularly only with Lassa virus, usually in healthcare workers who have been exposed to infected body fluids, especially at autopsy. Several of the hemorrhagic fever viruses appear to have been transmitted to sexual partners by convalescent men. The infected patient does not pose a significant risk to individuals with casual contact. Laboratory infections have been an uncommon, but regular risk of these agents. Most recently a laboratory worker was infected with Sabia virus.[67] The sources of infection have been aerosolization of culture fluids and probably rodent urine. Epidemics of lymphocytic choriomeningitis virus have occurred among laboratory workers who worked with hamsters and among individuals who owned hamsters as pets.[201]

The major human pathogens, the geographic distribution, rodent reservoir, clinical disease, and date of discovery are summarized in Table 23-3. Lymphocytic choriomeningitis (LCM) virus was discovered during investigation of the St. Louis encephalitis virus epidemic in 1933. It was soon recognized that the virus caused aseptic meningitis in humans. The frequency of infection is probably underestimated because clinicians do not suspect the infection and diagnostic tools are not readily available. Investigators found antibody to LCM virus in 5.1% of healthy women in Birmingham, Alabama.[469] Junin virus was the first recognized arenavirus

cause of hemorrhagic fever, Argentinian hemorrhagic fever in the pampas region. The mysteries of the epidemiology were unraveled a few years later by Karl Johnson et al. during investigation of an outbreak of Bolivian hemorrhagic fever in the Beni province, caused by Machupo virus.[261] Further notoriety for the viruses followed the recognition of severe hemorrhagic disease in several West African countries, caused by Lassa virus. The most recent additions come from South America: Guanarito virus in Venezuela and Sabia virus in Brazil. The old viruses are still with us: an outbreak of Bolivian hemorrhagic fever occurred in 1994 in the provinces of El Beni and Santa Cruz.[68]

The arenaviruses have a distinctive morphology (see Table 23-1) that led to the recognition of the group.[367] They are roughly spherical, enveloped particles with prominent ribosome-like structures in the center. The name of the group derives from the Latin *arenosus* (sandy), which was suggested by the internal particles. The original proposal, arenoviruses, was subsequently modified to arenaviruses to avoid confusion with adenoviruses.

Filoviruses

For many years the only known member of this group was Marburg virus, which caused a mysterious, fatal illness among monkey handlers in a laboratory in Marburg, Germany in 1967.[429] The source of the virus was African green monkeys, but attempts to identify the agent in freshly caught monkeys in Africa were unsuccessful. Over the next decade there were few isolations of the virus, which remained a curiosity, albeit a lethal one. In 1977 a new virus, designated Ebola virus, was isolated from simultaneous outbreaks of disease in Zaire and the Sudan. The outbreaks shared epidemiologic and clinical characteristics, and the viruses were closely related, although antigenically distinct. The disease was characterized by high fever, shock, involvement of multiple organ systems, and diffuse hemorrhage. The mortality rate for Marburg virus was 25%; for Ebola-Sudan, 50%, and

Table 23-3 Characteristics of Arenaviruses Pathogenic for Humans

VIRUS	GEOGRAPHIC DISTRIBUTION	RODENT HOST	HUMAN DISEASE	FATALITY RATE	YEAR OF DISCOVERY
Lymphocytic choromeningitis virus (LCM)	Europe, North and South America	*Mus domesticus; Mus musculus*	Aseptic meningitis	<1%	1939
Junin virus	Argentina	*Calomys musculinus*	Hemorrhagic fever	15–30%	1958
Machupo virus	Bolivia	*Calomys callosus*	Hemorrhagic fever	25%	1963
Lassa virus	West Africa	*Mastomys* spp.	Hemorrhagic fever	15%	1969
Guanarito virus	Venezuela	*Zygodontomys brevicauda; Sigmodon alsoni*	Hemorrhagic fever	25%	1990
Sabia virus	Brazil	Unknown	Hemorrhagic fever	Too few cases to determine	1990
White water arroyo virus	Southwestern United States	*Neotoma albicula*	Hemorrhagic Fever	Several cases presumptively identified	1999

for Ebola-Zaire, 90%. As with Marburg, the source of the infection was unknown, but transmission was clearly associated with exposure to body fluids of infected patients. The medical staff of some of the small mission hospitals were decimated by the mysterious disease.

The two epidemics in remote areas of Sudan and Zaire caused alarm in public health and infectious disease circles, but did not make an impact on the general public. That situation changed dramatically when a large outbreak occurred in 1995 in Kikwit, Nigeria. More than 300 cases occurred over a short period, approximately one third of the cases were in healthcare workers, and the fatality rate was approximately 80%. The epidemic was eventually controlled by introducing strict barrier precautions to prevent families and healthcare workers from having contact with secretions of infected patients. The source of this extensive epidemic was not clear.

A third strain of Ebola virus was identified in the Ivory Coast in 1994. Conjecture about the source in nature of Ebola virus had focused on monkeys because of the simian origins of Marburg virus, but no hard evidence had been found to support the hypothesis. A strain of Ebola virus most closely related to the Zaire type was isolated from the blood of a researcher, who probably acquired the infection while performing an autopsy on an infected chimpanzee. The highly lethal epidemic among chimpanzees was the first demonstration of natural infection in wild animals. Grooming and other close contact was not a risk factor for acquiring infection by a chimpanzee, but consumption of meat was a risk.[163] This observation bodes ill for the common practice of eating wild (bush) meat. The high mortality rate among the chimpanzees makes it unlikely that these primates are the natural reservoir of infection.

Additional evidence for a simian source of Ebola virus comes from an epidemic of lethal infection among cynomolgus monkeys in two animal holding facilities—the first in Reston, Virginia, the second in Texas. In both cases the animals had been imported from the Philippines, and the virus was antigenically distinct from the strains isolated in Zaire, Sudan, and the Ivory Coast. Only five cases of human infection with the Reston strain of Ebola virus have been documented, all of which were asymptomatic. There was evidence of transmission of infection from animal to animal by aerosols, a terrifying epidemiologic characteristic that has fortunately been missing from the human epidemics. Data indicating epidemic disease among captive cynomolgus monkeys in the Philippines before export have also been reported. The fatality rate among infected monkeys was 82%, and infection was more likely to develop in monkeys held in a group cage than those held in individual cages.

The filoviruses are RNA viruses with a characteristic ultrastructure (see Table 23-1) and a distinctive filamentous morphology that gives the family its name. The two viruses, Marburg and Ebola, can be distinguished by ultrastructural morphology, and the types of Ebola virus are antigenically distinct.

These Biosafety Level 4 agents are unlikely to be encountered by clinical diagnostic laboratories. Interested readers can consult several excellent reviews of the biology of these fascinating viruses and the diseases they produce.[394,429]

Togaviruses

The *Togaviridae* and *Bunyaviridae* now include most of the viruses that were previously known as arboviruses (arthropod-borne viruses).[55] Both groups are single-stranded RNA viruses with a lipid envelope.[437,439] The togaviruses were named for their lipid "toga" that surrounds the virus. These biologically diverse agents have a complex ecology; they usually infect small mammals or birds (reservoir) and are transmitted from animal to animal by ticks or mosquitoes (vector). Many of these viruses are also maintained by transovarial passage from insect to larva. Humans are accidental hosts when they are inadvertently infected instead of the usual animal reservoirs.

Two members of the family *Togaviridae* do not fit the traditional profile and will be discussed in their traditional context. They are rubella virus, an alphavirus, and hepatitis C virus, a flavivirus.

There are two divisions within the *Togaviridae*. The alphaviruses (formerly group A arboviruses) contain the agents of eastern equine encephalitis, western equine encephalitis, and Venezuelan encephalitis. The flaviviruses (formerly group B arboviruses) include the agents of St. Louis encephalitis, dengue (breakbone fever), yellow fever, and West Nile fever.

Small numbers of cases of eastern equine encephalitis and western equine encephalitis infections occur each year. Human disease may be presaged by an increased incidence of illness in horses. Epidemics of St. Louis encephalitis occur approximately every 10 years in the southern part of the United States, especially in Texas, in the Gulf Coast states, and in Florida. The reservoir for St. Louis encephalitis virus is birds, and the mosquito vectors vary with the geographic location. Disease is most severe in the elderly, and cases are concentrated in heavily wooded neighborhoods with poor screening of homes.

Dengue fever is prevalent in the Caribbean and in Southeast Asia. Imported cases are seen in the United States with increasing frequency, and indigenous transmission of the virus in the continental United States has been reported occasionally, most commonly in Texas. A most unusual route of entry into the United States was uncovered when infected mosquitoes were found in stagnant water that had accumulated in tires imported from Southeast Asia. Uncomplicated dengue infection is an undifferentiated febrile disease, sometimes accompanied by a rash and arthralgias or arthritis. The differential diagnosis includes other viral infections, such as rubella. There are four distinct serotypes of dengue virus. Halstead has hypothesized that serial infection with different serotypes triggers immunopathologic mechanisms that produce the dengue hemorrhagic fever syndrome.[210,327] Formerly limited to Southeast Asia, the lethal hemorrhagic form of the disease has occurred in the Caribbean with increasing frequency.

The most recent of these viruses to command attention is West Nile virus, which produces a spectrum of neurologic diseases, including encephalitis, meningitis, and a poliomyelitis-like syndrome.[443] Until 1999 it had produced localized infections in Africa, the Middle East, and Eastern Europe. In that year it made a surprise appearance in New York City and has subsequently spread throughout the United States.

The first cases of encephalitis were thought to be caused by St. Louis encephalitis virus, which is closely related immunologically to West Nile virus. These two viruses share other characteristics, including having birds as a frequent host (a characteristic that may be related to the rapid spread of the virus). Thus, in a few short years West Nile virus has gone from exotic trivia to everyday relevance.[396]

Bunyaviruses

The Bunyaviridae are a large and diverse group of viruses that are transmitted to humans by arthropod vectors, principally ticks and mosquitoes, and from the excreta of rodents. There are four medically important genera: 1) Bunyavirus, including the California encephalitis virus group; 2) Nairovirus, including Congo-Crimean hemorrhagic fever virus; 3) Phlebovirus, including Rift Valley fever virus and sandfly fever virus; and 4) Hantavirus, including the agents of Korean hemorrhagic fever, nephropathia epidemica, and hantavirus pulmonary syndrome.[55,374]

CALIFORNIA ENCEPHALITIS VIRUSES

The most important of the bunyaviruses in the United States is the California encephalitis group of viruses. Despite the name ''California,'' these viruses produce disease most commonly in Midwestern and north central states. The California encephalitis virus group commonly produce aseptic meningitis, a disease that occurs in the summer and is clinically indistinguishable from enteroviral disease.[55,374] California encephalitis virus itself is uncommon; LaCrosse virus is the most common human pathogen in the group. Most patients recover uneventfully from their infection.

HANTAVIRUSES

The hantaviruses are a steadily expanding group of viruses that have moved from exotic infectious agents to endemic threats in the United States.[439] The uniform characteristics of the group include asymptomatic, persistent infection of a rodent host, probable transmission to humans through infected rodent excreta, and infection of the vascular endothelium. The current status of the viruses, their rodent hosts, and associated clinical diseases are summarized in Table 23-4.

During the Korean War a severe hemorrhagic fever was recognized among American soldiers. Shock and renal failure, which were prominent symptoms, provided the descriptive name hemorrhagic fever with renal symptoms (HFRS). Fever, thrombocytopenia, and renal failure comprise the classic clinical picture. The return of platelets presages restoration of normal renal function. Shock and multiorgan failure, simulating bacterial sepsis, characterize the most severe cases. Less common manifestations include retroperitoneal hemorrhage and pulmonary edema. Some patients experience undifferentiated febrile illness with normal renal function. A clinical syndrome of severe hepatic disease has been described in Greece, where the prevalent strains resemble the virus associated with infections in Korea.

Subsequent to the documentation of disease in Korea, it was recognized that this severe clinical syndrome occurred in the eastern Soviet Union and Manchuria. The etiologic agent was not isolated until 1982, when Hantaan virus (named after a Korean river where epidemic disease had occurred) was isolated. This virus produces asymptomatic, persistent infection in its rodent host, *Apodemus agrarius*. Subsequently, a second, related agent, Seoul virus, which produces less severe infection, was isolated. The rodent hosts of Seoul virus are urban rats, *Rattus norvegicus* and *Rattus rattus*. Seoul virus has been found in laboratory rats and has produced infection in laboratory workers. There are no documented cases of Hantaan virus infection in the United States, but cases of Seoul virus-induced HFRS have been documented serologically in Baltimore. The rat-associated

Table 23-4 Selected Hantaviruses: Hosts and Clinical Diseases[a]

VIRUS	GEOGRAPHIC DISTRIBUTION	RODENT HOST	CLINICAL DISEASE
Hantaan	Far East	*Apodemus agrarius* (Eastern form)	Hemorrhagic fever with renal syndrome (HFRS)
Seoul	Worldwide	*Rattus rattus; Rattus norvegicus* (urban rats)	Mild HFRS
Dobrava	Balkans	*Apodemus flavicollis*	HFRS
Puumala	Scandinavia; Europe	*Clethrionomys glariolus* (vole)	Nephropathia endemica
Sin nombre	Southwestern United States	*Peromyscus maniculatus* (deer mouse)	Hantavirus pulmonary syndrome (HPS)
Bayou	Louisiana	*Oligoryzomys palustris* (rice rat)	HPS
Black Creek Canal	Florida	*Sigmodon hispidus* (cotton rat)	Unknown
New York	Northeastern United States	*Peromyscus leucopus* (white-footed mouse)	HPS
Monongahela	Eastern United States	*Peromyscus maniculatus nubiterrae* (forest form of deer mouse)	HPS
Andes	South and Central America	*Oligoryzomys longicaudatus*	HPS

[a] *For information on other viruses consult reference*[439].

hantaviruses in the United States have been associated with hypertensive renal disease but not with other chronic renal diseases.[186] Although hypertensive renal disease is not usually associated with infectious agents, the lesson of *Helicobacter pylori* and gastritis should caution us against dismissing the association out of hand.

A milder version of this infection, known as nephropathia epidemica, is produced by Puumala virus and occurs in Scandinavia (Table 23-4).[439] The virus produces asymptomatic infections in voles; in humans it is an acute febrile disease with lower back pain and polyuria but with mild or no hemorrhagic manifestations and without shock. Patients recover without sequelae. The symptoms are frequently nonspecific, and the clinical diagnosis was correct in only 28% of cases in one Finnish study.

The spotlight focused on hantaviruses in 1993, when an outbreak of severe respiratory disease occurred in the Four Corners area of the southwestern United States.[395,439] The patients had a prodromal syndrome of fever, myalgia, cough or dyspnea, gastrointestinal symptoms, and headache, which progressed rapidly to irreversible pulmonary edema. With amazing rapidity the causative agent was recognized as a new member of the hantavirus genus, named Sin Nombre virus (initially named Four Corners virus). The rodent host of Sin Nombre virus is the deer mouse, *Peromyscus maniculatus*. It is hypothesized that heavy rains increased food sources, causing a great increase in the number of rodents, increasing the frequency of contact between humans and mice, and altering the epidemiology from sporadic, endemic disease to epidemic infection. There is no evidence of human-to-human transmission of hantavirus pulmonary syndrome. Retrospective diagnosis of cases of infection with Sin Nombre or a related virus dating back as far as 1978 has been made by immunoperoxidase staining of stored paraffin-embedded tissue.[534] All of the 12 infections identified retrospectively had occurred west of the Mississippi River, most in the Far West.

Subsequent to the discovery of Sin Nombre virus, other related hantaviruses have been identified in the United States, including Louisiana, Florida, and the eastern United States (Table 23-4). The frequency of hantavirus infection outside of the endemic areas is unknown.

The lung is the target organ pathologically as well as clinically.[395] Edema and fibrin deposition with focal hyaline membranes in the airspaces are accompanied by an interstitial mononuclear exudate. Large immunoblastic cells infiltrate many organs. The hematologic findings include left-shifted neutrophilic leukocytosis, thrombocytopenia, circulating immunoblasts, and (in severe cases) hemoconcentration. Viral antigen is concentrated in endothelial cells, particularly in the pulmonary vasculature, and viruslike particles may be seen in those cells.[533] Hanta viral antigens are also found in follicular dendritic cells, macrophages, and lymphocytes.

Human Gastroenteritis Viruses

Viral gastroenteritis is second only to viral respiratory disease as a cause of morbidity in the United States. The incidence of viral gastroenteritis has been estimated at approximately 11% per year.[127] Mortality is rare. In the past decade much has been learned about the etiologic agents, but only approximately 50% of infectious gastroenteritis can be assigned an etiology. Most of these agents have been identified initially by immunoelectron microscopy. In this technique immune serum is mixed with a virus suspension or a stool specimen. Clumping of the submicroscopic viral particles can be observed when negatively stained preparations are examined with the electron microscope. Most of these agents cannot be cultivated easily. Therefore, details of their composition are not known; for convenience they will be discussed with the most common pathogen, the rotaviruses.

The agents of viral gastroenteritis can be divided into six groups. The classification is embryonic because of limited knowledge about some of the agents:

Rotaviruses
Caliciviruses (Small round-structured viruses)
Norwalk-like viruses (noroviruses)
Sapporo-like viruses
Astroviruses
Enteric adenoviruses

The frequency of these viruses in the United States is summarized in Table 23-5. The data come from a multicenter study, using electron microscopy.[309] The identification of agents in this study was entirely morphologic; adenovirus is likely overrepresented, because the ultrastructural approach did not distinguish between respiratory and gastrointestinal serotypes.

Many aspects of these viral gastrointestinal infections are similar. They produce acute vomiting or diarrhea, which is usually mild, self-limited, and noninflammatory. Bloody diarrhea does not occur. Microscopic analysis of biopsies from human volunteers who have been fed these infectious agents show blunting of intestinal villi and mild inflammatory changes in the submucosa, changes that are indicative of small-bowel malabsorption. Damaged cells at the tips of the villi are replaced by cells from the bases of the crypts over 5 to 10 days. Diarrhea that lasts more than 7 to 10 days is unlikely to be viral. Treatment is by replacement of lost

Table 23-5 Prevalence of Viral Agents of Gastroenteritis in the United States and Canada	
Number positive	8,262
Rotavirus	48%
Astrovirus	2.4%
Calicivirus	1.3%
SRV/SRSV[a]	10.0/0.4%
Adenovirus	17.2%[b]
Coronavirus	6.6%[b]
Other	14.6%

[a] *Small round virus/small round structured virus, including Norwalk-like agents.*
[b] *Includes both respiratory and intestinal strains.*
Adapted from reference[309].

fluid and electrolytes, usually caused by vomiting. Unfortunately immunity appears to be only partial.[127]

Of note is the absence of conventional intestinal viruses from the list of pathogens. There is little evidence that enteroviruses or respiratory adenoviruses cause gastrointestinal disease.

ROTAVIRUSES

Rotaviruses are the most important human pathogens in the Reoviridae. The reoviruses themselves are not associated with human disease, but they have been useful in the study of molecular mechanisms of viral pathogenesis. "Reo" stands for *respiratory-enteric orphan*, from the source of virus isolates and the lack of association with clinical disease. Rotavirus got its name from the wheel-like appearance of the virion in electron micrographs (see Table 23-1).

The rotaviruses contain both human and animal pathogens, but animal rotaviruses do not infect humans. Human rotaviruses have been classified serologically, with most pathogenic human strains in the United States and Europe falling into group A. Human rotavirus is a common cause of gastroenteritis in infants and young children.[271] The clinical presentation is varied, but vomiting and dehydration are prominent features in comparison to gastroenteritis produced by other viruses. The combination of vomiting and a seasonal occurrence in the winter months has led investigators to name the condition "winter vomiting disease." The frequency and specificity of respiratory symptoms in rotavirus infection is controversial. It is possible that the prevalence of vomiting in rotavirus infection reflects the age of the patient rather than a property of the virus, because Norwalk virus produces significantly more vomiting in infants than in adults. Uhnoo and Svensson studied the comparative features of group A, subgroups 1 and 2 in Swedish infants.[485] Patients with subgroup 1 strains developed fever up to 39°C significantly more often than those with subgroup 2, but infants who had subgroup 2 infections were sicker, hospitalized more frequently, and more likely to have respiratory symptoms. The frequency of diarrhea and vomiting in the two groups was similar.

Chronic rotavirus infection may occur in immunosuppressed children. In adults, rotavirus infection is usually asymptomatic. These viruses are notorious causes of nosocomial infection, including epidemics, in children.

CALICIVIRUSES

These viruses were originally identified by electron microscopy and characterized descriptively as small round-structured viruses.[200] There are two major groups of viruses within the calicivirus group, as described below.

Norwalk-Like Viruses (Norovirus). The Norwalk agent of gastroenteritis was recognized as a 27-nm particle in stool specimens from an outbreak of community gastroenteritis in Norwalk, Ohio. Subsequently, similar RNA viruses have been isolated from other epidemics. Molecular analysis has revealed that there are two main clusters.[11] These agents are also referred to as noroviruses.[274]

Norwalk-like viruses have frequently produced epidemics of disease and also cause sporadic infection.[200] These viruses produce infection and active disease in persons of all ages, in contrast to most of the other viral agents, which produce symptomatic disease predominantly in infants and young children. They are the predominant cause of infectious gastroenteritis in adults. The Norwalk-like agents have been associated with contaminated food and water and are one of the possibilities to consider when a patient has recently ingested shellfish. Epidemic disease has been described in venues that vary from football games to cruise ships or nursing homes.

Sapporo-Like Viruses (Classic Caliciviruses). These agents resemble the Norwalk-like viruses morphologically, but differ immunologically and genetically. Some authors view them as important agents of gastroenteritis in children, sometimes foodborne.[93] Other authorities reserve judgment.[200]

ASTROVIRUSES

The astroviruses also contain RNA and have been difficult to cultivate in vitro, although a few strains have been successfully grown.[339] They derive their name from their star-shaped ultrastructural appearance. Astroviruses are shed in large numbers in the stool but appear to be less pathogenic than the Norwalk-like agents. They have produced epidemic disease in young children, on pediatric wards, in day-care centers, and in nursing homes. Concurrent infection with astroviruses and caliciviruses has been described.

ENTERIC ADENOVIRUSES

A causative association of the classic adenovirus serotypes with diarrheal disease could not be established, but "noncultivable" serotypes were demonstrated by immuno-electron microscopy. Adenovirus types 40 and 41, which do not grow well in the usual tissue culture cells, are intestinal pathogens.[244] These enteric adenoviruses are the second most common cause of viral gastroenteritis in infants. They produce sporadic infection, although epidemics have been described. Most patients are younger than 2 years of age.

Coronaviruses

The classic coronaviruses are causes of the common cold.[236] Most require use of organ culture for reliable isolation and are unlikely to be encountered in the clinical laboratory.

A dramatic addition to the genus was recognized in 2003 when a novel coronavirus was identified as the cause of a mysterious new respiratory illness in China. This infection was called severe acute respiratory syndrome (SARS). In contrast to previously recognized coronavirus infections SARS is characterized by lower respiratory infection that often requires admission to an intensive care unit; it may be fatal.[36,94] Another troubling characteristic of this infection is the propensity for infection of hospital personnel, particularly those who have close patient contact.[230] With amazing rapidity and with the collaboration of scientists worldwide using molecular techniques the cause of the infection was identified as a novel coronavirus. The significance of a human metapneumovirus that was isolated from some patients is unclear.[86] It is of interest that a conventional coronavirus, OC243, recently produced an outbreak of respiratory infections that included pneumonia.

Coltiviruses

This group includes the virus of Colorado tick fever, an undifferentiated febrile illness that is usually mild and self-limited, but may on occasion be severe or even fatal.[424] It is transmitted by the bite of ticks. Previously this virus was included in the Orbivirus group, which is composed of animal pathogens. The orbiviruses are members of the family *Reoviridae*, along with rotaviruses.

Retroviruses

The retroviruses are RNA viruses; they were so named because they contain an enzyme that transcribes RNA into DNA, a reversal of the normal sequence in which DNA is transcribed into RNA. For many years, these viruses were known to cause tumors in animals. In the 1970s, two viruses that caused T-cell lymphocytic lymphomas in humans were recognized and named human T-cell lymphoma virus (HTLV-I and HTLV-II). This discovery was extremely important biologically, but the tumors are uncommon.[190]

The retrovirus group assumed sudden prominence and increased notoriety in 1983 when a third human retrovirus was identified as the cause of the acquired immunodeficiency syndrome (AIDS).[165] AIDS had been recognized clinically several years earlier when opportunistic infections were detected in young men who were homosexual, bisexual, or drug addicts, but did not have conventional risk factors for *Pneumocystis* pneumonia or candidiasis.

Similar viruses were isolated in several laboratories and named variously HTLV-III, lymphadenopathy-associated virus (LAV), and AIDS-related virus (ARV). An expert panel settled on the name, human immunodeficiency virus (HIV). Although HIV was first isolated in 1983, retrospective analysis of frozen serum and tissue suggested that a similar virus had infected a sexually active teenage boy in St. Louis in 1968.[176] Subsequently, a serologically related virus was isolated and named HIV-2. The distribution of HIV-1 is worldwide. HIV-2, found predominantly in West Africa, also produces an acquired immunodeficiency syndrome. Cases of HIV-2 infection have been reported in the United States, but most patients have had some connection with West Africa. There are immunologic cross-reactions between HIV-1 and HIV-2. Specific immunoassays must be performed both to distinguish between the two infections and also to detect the type-specific antigens with maximum sensitivity. To complicate matters further, at least one patient has been identified who was infected with both viruses. HIV is a member of the lentivirus (*lenti* = slow) subfamily of the *Retroviridae*. Other viruses in this group produce chronic infections with long periods of clinical latency. Some animal retroviruses also produce immunodeficiency, such as simian immunodeficiency virus and feline leukemia virus. Infection across species has not been demonstrated.

In contrast to the other lentiviruses HIV is genetically extremely heterogeneous, to the extent that virtually each isolate is unique (termed a quasispecies). There are, however, genetically related groups, which are in turn divided into clusters or clades. Group M (major) comprises 95% of global isolates and is divided into at least eight clades (A, B, C, D, F, G, H, and J). All clades are represented in Africa; in the United States and Europe Clade B is the dominant subtype. (It should be noted that genetic clades do not map to distinct viral serotypes.)

Group O (Other) strains, which are found predominantly in West Africa, share less than 50% homology with Group M strains. Group N (non-M or O) viruses are found in Cameroon.

To complicate matters even further, all retroviruses have a propensity for recombination when multiple strains are juxtaposed. It was assumed that patients infected with HIV virus would be resistant to infection with a second strain. Unfortunately, the absence of complete immunity and the frequency of multiple exposures to virus has resulted in infection with several strains, a situation in which recombination can occur.[30]

There is no question that HIV is the most devastating plague facing us as the 21st century begins. It has changed the face of our society and will continue to wreak havoc for many years to come, especially in the third world. Although the advent of effective antiretroviral chemotherapy has slowed the advance of infection and decreased mortalities in countries that can afford the drugs, the epidemic continues to spread. The current status of the global epidemic is summarized in Table 23-6.

The discussion below is a brief attempt to capture some of the most salient features of this multifaceted virus and the diseases it produces. It is a tribute to modern science that an infectious agent was reported only 3 years after the first reports of the clinical syndrome. Without the modern armamentarium of molecular biology and virology, we would still be defenseless against this scourge.

The HIV-1 virion is icosahedral and contains 72 external spikes.[165] It is considerably more complex than HTLV-1 and HTLV-2, consonant with its more complicated natural

Table 23-6 The Global HIV Epidemic in 2003

PARAMETER	GEOGRAPHIC REGION	PERSONS AFFECTED
Persons living with AIDS	Worldwide	34–46 million
	North America	790,000–1.2 million
	Sub-Saharan Africa	25.0–28.2 million
Adults and children newly infected with HIV	Worldwide	4.2–5.8 million
	North America	36,000–54,000
	Sub-Saharan Africa	3.0–3.4 million
Adult and child deaths due to AIDS	Worldwide	2.5–3.5 million
	North America	12,000–18,000
	Sub-Saharan Africa	2.2–2.4 million

Source: Annual UN AIDS Epidemic Update Report at http://www. unaids.org.

Table 23-7 Major Antigens of Human Immunodeficiency Virus, Type 1

GENE	GENE PRODUCTS
Group-specific antigen/core (*GAG*)	p(protein)18, p24, p55
Polymerase (*POL*)	p31, p51, p66
Envelope (*ENV*)	gp(glycoprotein)41, gp120, gp160

Adapted from reference[62].

history. The gene products can be divided into three groups. The viral proteins that represent the most important diagnostic antigens are summarized in Table 23-7.

The gp120 envelope protein holds the initial key for entry of HIV-1 virus into the patient.[165] This protein has a remarkable affinity for a complex of receptors on the surface of cells throughout the body. The primary component of the complex, the CD4 receptor, is found on T-helper lymphocytes, macrophages, and Langerhans cells in the skin. The second part of the receptor complex is a chemokine receptor. Viral strains that interact with the CXCR4 receptor (X4 virus) are most likely to infect T lymphocytes in vitro; strains that interact with the CCR5 receptor (R5 virus) are associated with macrophage cell lines in vitro. Some viruses, which interact with both chemokine coreceptors can infect both lymphocytes and macrophages.

It has been hypothesized that HIV infection is more likely to develop in uncircumcised men because the prepuce is a rich source of Langerhans cells as well as macrophages and lymphocytes.[3] The enhanced susceptibility to HIV infection in patients with genital ulcers may result from the accessibility of CD4 + macrophages and lymphocytes in the inflamed bases of the ulcers.[444]

The most important viral targets, however, are the CD4 + T lymphocytes.[103] These "helper" lymphocytes are the "Times Square" of the cellular immune system. Without them the body is at increased risk for many opportunistic infections. In addition to the T-cell abnormality, defective response of B cells to T-cell-independent antigens has also been documented. Macrophages are very important, because they provide a place for virus to be sequestered even after T cells have been destroyed and/or most virus has been killed by chemotherapy.

The initial encounter with HIV-1 virus produces a transient febrile disease, which may be accompanied by lymphadenopathy, pharyngitis, or a diffuse rash.[103] During the acute illness high levels of circulating virus are present in the absence of specific antibody. In the natural course of the infection antibody develops within several weeks to several months.

The ensuing subclinical phase of the disease is accompanied by antibody, circulating p24 antigen, immune complexes, and low levels of circulating virus. Testing blood products for virus, using molecular amplification technology, has been introduced in an attempt to reduce to a minimum the risk of transfusing infected units. During the chronic viremia, repetitive mutations in the viral genome thwart the attempts of the host immune system to eliminate the infection. The onset of clinical illness is associated with an increase in the quantity of virus, both within peripheral-blood mononuclear cells and in plasma.

A wide spectrum of clinical conditions may result after HIV-1 infection. The CDC classification of HIV disease is summarized in Tables 23-8, and 23-9.[61] Certain diseases (Group C in Table 23-9) are highly associated and are termed AIDS-defining conditions.

The infectious complications of HIV infection include viral, fungal, mycobacterial, bacterial, and parasitic infections. The practice of infectious disease and clinical microbiology has been irrevocably altered by HIV. Numerous previously uncommon or exotic infections have become commonplace in centers that have large numbers of HIV-infected patients. Old rules must be thrown out when the patient is as severely immunosuppressed as are patients with AIDS or patients with major organ transplants. Anything is possible, and the host inflammatory response that has been associated with a particular infectious agent may or may not

Table 23-8 1993 Revised Classification System among Adolescents and Adults Positive for HIV

CD4+ T-LYMPHOCYTE CATEGORIES	CLINICAL CATEGORIES		
	(A) Asymptomatic, Acute (Primary) HIV, or Persistent Generalized Lymphadenopathy	(B) Symptomatic, Not (A) or (C) Conditions (See Table 23-9)	(C) AIDS-Indicator Conditions (See Table 23-9)
(1) ≥500/μL	A1	B1	C1[a]
(2) 200–499/μL	A2	B2	C2[a]
(3) <200/μL	A3	B3	C3[a]

[a] These categories indicate AIDS.

The lowest accurate, but not necessarily the most recent CD4+ T-lymphocyte count should be used for classification.

From reference[61].

Table 23-9 Ancillary Conditions (Category B) and Conditions Included in the 1993 AIDS Surveillance Case Definition (Category C)

Category B

Bacillary angiomatosis

Candidiasis, oropharyngeal (thrush)

Candidiasis, vulvovaginal; persistent, frequent, or poorly responsive to therapy

Cervical dysplasia (moderate or severe)/carcinoma in situ

Constitutional symptoms, such as fever (38.5°C) or diarrhea lasting >1 month

Hairy leukoplakia, oral

Herpes zoster (shingles), involving at least two distinct episodes or more than one dermatome

Idiopathic thrombocytopenic purpura

Listeriosis

Pelvic inflammatory disease, particularly if complicated by tubo-ovarian abscess

Peripheral neuropathy

Other unspecified conditions

Category C[a]

Candidiasis of bronchi, trachea, or lungs

Candidiasis, esophageal

Cervical cancer, invasive

Coccidioidomycosis, disseminated or extrapulmonary

Cryptococcosis, extrapulmonary

Cryptosporidiosis, chronic intestinal (>1 month's duration)

Cytomegalovirus disease (except liver, spleen, lymph nodes)

Cytomegalovirus retinitis with loss of vision

Encephalopathy, HIV-related

Herpes simplex: chronic ulcers (>1 month's duration); or bronchitis, pneumonitis, or esophagitis

Histoplasmosis, disseminated or extrapulmonary

Isosporiasis, chronic intestinal (>1 month's duration)

Kaposi's sarcoma

Lymphoma, Burkitt's (or equivalent term)

Lymphoma, immunoblastic (or equivalent term)

Lymphoma, primary, of brain

Mycobacterium avium complex or *Mycobacterium kansasii*, disseminated or extrapulmonary

Mycobacterium tuberculosis, any site (pulmonary or extrapulmonary)

Mycobacterium, other species or unidentified species, disseminated or extrapulmonary

Pneumocystis carinii pneumonia

Pneumonia, recurrent

Progressive multifocal leukoencephalopathy

Salmonella septicemia, recurrent

Toxoplasmosis of brain

Wasting syndrome due to HIV

[a] *These categories indicate AIDS.*
From reference[61].

be present. What would be "shotgun" microbiology in a normal patient becomes good practice in this group of patients. Integration of clinical, epidemiologic, and laboratory data is needed to decide which laboratory resources must be tapped for an individual patient.

The most common opportunistic infections that afflict patients infected with HIV are among the AIDS-defining conditions that are listed in Table 23-9. Some of the infections are characteristic of a particular phase of the disease. For instance, oral candidiasis is often a presenting feature of the disease. *Pneumocystis jiroveci* (*carinii*) pneumonia first occurs when lymphocyte counts are relatively high early in the disease process. *Mycobacterium avium* complex infections tend to occur late in the disease, when the CD4 + lymphocyte count is low. Although infections with cell-associated pathogens (facultative intracellular organisms) are most closely associated with defects in cellular immunity, bacterial infections for which humoral immunity is an important host defense are also more common in HIV-infected patients. The search for the cause of an opportunistic infection should not stop when the first agent is identified because many of the infections in AIDS patients are polymicrobial.

Not all HIV-related diseases are caused by opportunistic infections. HIV itself is cytopathic and produces clinical disease such as encephalitis and AIDS-related dementia. Collapse of the cellular immune system and its surveillance mechanisms leads to neoplastic complications, some of which may be virus-induced. Lymphomas are frequently encountered.[350] A previously unusual neoplasm, Kaposi's sarcoma, has occurred frequently in patients with AIDS, often as an early manifestation of the disease. Other manifestations of disease may have an immunopathologic mechanism or the mechanisms are unknown. Some infections that might have been predicted to afflict AIDS patients, such as legionellosis and aspergillosis, are relatively uncommon. The cellular immune system undoubtedly contributes to the control of invasive aspergillosis and legionellosis, but other mechanisms, not destroyed by HIV-1, are presumably also important.

As therapy for HIV infection and for infectious complications of the immunodeficiency have improved, the pattern of infections encountered has changed. An analysis of autopsies from Los Angeles in 1982–1993 documented a decrease in the number of fatal infections caused by *Pneumocystis jiroveci*, bacterial sepsis, cytomegalovirus, *Mycobacterium avium* complex, and *Toxoplasma gondii* in 1989–1993 compared with 1982–1988.[281] Over time, institution of prophylaxis for AIDS-related infections and of more effective therapy have changed the causes of death in people with AIDS.[314] Although AIDS-defining conditions remain important, other chronic diseases and complications of chemotherapy have become more important.

These changes also affect the way surveillance for the infection is carried out.[72] The new case definition retains the clinical and immunologic criteria that were the backbone of the previous surveillance standards (Tables 23-8 and 23-9), but adds a virologic criterion (Table 23-10). Under the new approach patients who have been infected but in whom clinical disease has not yet developed are included. Guidelines for children are included in the new standard. Revised recommendations for screening of pregnant women have been published separately.[76]

HIV-1 is excreted in saliva, milk, semen, and other body fluids, but transmission of infection has been documented to occur only after exposure to blood or genital secretions. The importance of maternal milk in the transfer of virus from mother to child is unclear.

The most important groups at risk for HIV infection are those who have received blood products (recipients of blood transfusions, hemophiliacs), those who have shared contaminated needles (drug addicts), those who have had sexual intercourse with an infected individual, and children of an infected mother. At the outset of the epidemic, most of the sexually transmitted infections in the United States and Europe were between homosexual or bisexual men (presently described as men-who-have-sex-with-men [MSM]), but heterosexual transmission was soon documented. Heterosexual transmission of HIV-1 virus has been dominant in Africa from the beginning of the epidemic. The risk of transmission of HIV infection from mother to infant and the severity of disease in the infant are directly related to the severity of infection in the mother at the time of delivery.

Therapy for HIV infection has represented a constant battle between the virus and the pharmaceutical industry, resulting in alternating exhilaration and despair among patients and healthcare workers. By 1996, therapeutic efforts had concentrated on combination chemotherapy, using an inhibitor of RNA-dependent DNA polymerase (reverse transcriptase) along with an inhibitor of the viral protease.[139] The inhibitor of reverse transcriptase can be either nucleoside/nucleotide (NRTI) or nonnucleoside (NNRTI) in nature. Treating patients with these powerful drugs, known as highly active antiretroviral therapy (HAART), has become a subspecialty of infectious diseases. The virus, of course, has also been resilient, developing resistance to the major classes of antiviral drugs,[99] particularly if therapy is incomplete or inadequate.

Although no therapy has yet proved capable of eradicating HIV infection, the sentence of death that a diagnosis of HIV infection once connoted has been reversed by HAART in societies that can afford the expensive drugs. When combined with better education of high-risk groups, HAART resulted in a stable or decreasing incidence of new infections for the first time. The challenge seemed limited to finding resources to offer the new therapies to countries with meager financial reserves. Unfortunately, the epidemic curve has begun to creep back upward because of continuing appearance of drug resistance, difficulty in reaching users of intravenous drugs, and a resurgence in sexual activity once it was (incorrectly perceived) that the death sentence had been lifted.[80]

The risk of transmitting HIV in blood transfusions has been dramatically reduced by screening all units of blood for antibody and asking members of high-risk groups not to donate blood. The result has been a steadily decreasing incidence of transfusion-related HIV infection as the sensitivity of the tests used for screening blood products before transfusion has increased. The introduction of highly sensi-

Table 23-10 Revised Case Definitions for Surveillance of HIV Disease

PATIENT GROUP	LABORATORY CRITERIA	CLINICAL OR OTHER CRITERIA (IF LABORATORY CRITERIA NOT MET)
Adults, adolescents or children ≥18 months	Positive HIV serology[a] OR Positive viral assay[b]	Diagnosis of HIV infection, based on laboratory criteria, documented in medical record by a physician OR Conditions included in the case definition of AIDS (Tables 23–8 and 23–9)
Child <18 months	Positive viral assay on two separate occasions (cord blood excluded) OR (Presumptive) Positive viral assay on one occasion (cord blood excluded) and no subsequent viral assay or serology results	Diagnosis of HIV infection, based on laboratory criteria, documented in medical record by a physician OR Conditions that meet the 1987 pediatric surveillance case definition of AIDS[52]
Child <18 months born to an HIV-infected mother is considered not infected if the child does NOT meet the criteria for HIV infection but DOES meet the adjacent criteria	≥2 negative antibody tests from different specimens taken when the child is ≥6 months old OR At least two negative viral assays both performed at ≥1 month of age and one performed at ≥4 months of age AND No other laboratory or clinical evidence of HIV infection OR (Presumptive) One negative antibody test performed at ≥6 months of age and no positive viral assay OR One negative viral assay performed at ≥4 months of age and no positive viral assay OR One positive viral assay with ≥2 subsequent negative viral assays (at least one performed at ≥4 months of age) or negative antibody test (at least one performed at ≥6 months of age)	Determined by a physician to be "not infected" and the results of HIV diagnostic tests are noted in the medical record AND No other laboratory or clinical evidence of HIV infection
Child <18 months born to an HIV-infected mother is considered to have perinatal exposure if the child does not meet the criteria for HIV infection or the criteria for "not infected with HIV"		

[a] *Positive HIV serology = repeatedly reactive enzyme immunoassay followed by a positive confirmatory test; e.g., Western blot.*
[b] *Positive HIV viral assay = positive HIV nucleic-acid test, positive p24 antigen test, or positive viral culture.*
Adapted from reference[71].

tive amplification assays for screening all units of blood administered in the United States has probably reduced the risk of transfusion to an absolute minimum.

Occupational exposure to infectious agents is a fact of life for medical personnel. Blood-borne pathogens are a major part of the problem, because of the frequency of the pathogens and of exposure to blood. Sharp objects (e.g., needles and surgical instruments) are the most frequent vehicle for transmission. Viral agents represent the most serious occupational risks; among them, HIV tops the list. Recom-

Box 23-4 Management of Occupational Blood Exposures[a]

Provide immediate care to the exposure site
  Wash wounds and skin with soap and water
  Flush mucous membranes with water
Determine risk associated with exposure by
  Type of fluid (e.g., blood, visibly bloody fluid, other potentially infectious fluid or tissue, or concentrated virus) AND
  Type of exposure (i.e., percutaneous injury, mucous membrane or nonintact skin exposure, or bites resulting in blood exposure)
Evaluate exposure source
  Assess the risk of infection using available information
  Test known sources for HBsAg, anti-HCV, and HIV antibody (consider using rapid testing)
  For unknown sources, assess risk of exposure to HBV, HCV, or HIV infection
  Do not test discarded needles or syringes for virus contamination
Evaluate the exposed person
  Assess immune status for HBV infection (i.e., by history of hepatitis B vaccination and vaccine response)
Give postexposure prophylaxis for exposures posing risk of infection, according to current recommendations
Perform follow-up testing and provide counseling

[a] *Hepatitis B (HBV), hepatitis C (HCV), and human immunodeficiency virus (HIV)*

Adapted from references[73–75,77].

mendations for management, preferably by prevention, of occupational exposures have been formulated by the CDC.[73–75,77] A summary of the general recommendations is provided in Box 23-4.

Treatment of patients with HIV infection is complicated and requires support from many areas of the laboratory. In some ways the expansion of diagnostic possibilities has simplified the approach, as summarized in Table 23-11.

Herpesviruses

Viruses of the human herpesvirus group are the most frequent isolates in general laboratories. The group consists of the following:

Herpes simplex virus, type 1
Herpes simplex virus, type 2
Human cytomegalovirus
Epstein-Barr virus
Varicella-zoster virus
Human herpesvirus-6
Human herpesvirus-7
Human herpesvirus-8

Some members of the herpesvirus group can integrate their DNA with that of the host cell. Most produce a latent infection in lymphoid cells or ganglia of the CNS and subsequently reactivate to cause recurrent disease. In general, the primary infections are more severe than are recurrences. The primary infections produced by several viruses of this group are more severe when they occur during adolescence or adulthood, rather than childhood. The viruses circulate more freely and earlier in life among low socioeconomic groups and not until adolescence in more affluent society. The infections in high socioeconomic groups, therefore, tend to be more severe.

HERPES SIMPLEX VIRUS

Herpes simplex virus causes a wide variety of infections.[518] Two serotypes of the virus infect humans. Shared antigens between types 1 and 2 complicate serologic differentiation of antigens and antibodies, but reliable reagents are now commercially available. In healthy persons, infections of the oral cavity and genital tract predominate. Type

Table 23-11 Laboratory Support for Treating HIV-Infected Patients

PARAMETER	PRIMARY APPROACH	SECONDARY/ CONFIRMATORY APPROACH
Initial diagnosis	Enzyme immunoassay (repeatedly positive)	Western blot or immunofluorescence; nucleic-acid (viral load) testing for acutely symptomatic patients[269] and newborns of infected mothers
Prognosis and initiating therapy	Quantitative plasma viral concentration (viral load)	Ultrasensitive tests may be required
Initiating therapy and prophylaxis for opportunistic infections	Quantitation of CD4 lymphocytes	
Monitoring therapy	Quantitative plasma viral concentration (viral load)	Ultrasensitive tests may be required
Evaluating clinical or virologic relapse	Phenotypic or genotypic resistance testing	

1 infections are most common in the upper body, whereas type 2 infections produce genital lesions; but there are exceptions to the rule. As many as one third of isolates from the genital tract represent type 1 strains. In contrast, very few isolates from the oral cavity are type 2 strains.

Typing of herpes isolates from genital sites provides valuable prognostic information because genital infections caused by type 1 herpes simplex virus are less likely to recur than are those caused by type 2 virus.[292] In a group of 457 women who had a primary genital infection (defined by absence of antibody to type 2 virus and a positive culture of genital lesions), 89% had a recurrence after a median of 391 days.[26] There were at least six recurrences during the first year in 38% of patients, and 20% of individuals had more than 10 recurrences. A sequential study of patients with recurrent infection demonstrated that the patient was asymptomatic and lacked visible lesions during one third of the period during which the patient shed virus.[498] Genital infections with either viral type are more likely to recur than oral infections with the same type.[292] In addition, the mechanism of infection may be different for the two serotypes. Exposure to type 1 virus begins in childhood, with antibody having developed in 25–50% of college students. Acquisition of antibody to type 2 virus does not begin until the teens and continues throughout the period of sexual activity. Isolation of type 2 virus from a genital site implies sexual transmission, whereas the route of transmission for type 1 virus may be by autoinoculation with oral secretions.

Herpesvirus is passed from person to person by infected secretions or lesions. Infection is usually sporadic, but an epidemic of cutaneous infection at a wrestling camp (herpes gladiatorum) has been described.[24]

The most serious herpes simplex virus infections are encephalitis, which most commonly affects the temporal lobe and the orbital aspect of the frontal lobe in adults, and disseminated infection in newborn infants, which may be acquired either during or after birth. Herpes simplex virus causes sporadic encephalitis. In the neonatal period the infecting strains are type 2, reflecting their origin in the maternal genital tract. Type 1 strains are overwhelmingly predominant in older children and adults. The diagnosis can be made most definitively by brain biopsy and culture, but the availability of nontoxic antiviral chemotherapy has prompted clinicians to treat patients empirically, thus avoiding an invasive procedure. Unfortunately, other potentially treatable diseases may be missed as a result. Whitley and colleagues studied 432 patients who underwent brain biopsy for suspected herpes encephalitis as a part of a national collaborative chemotherapy trial.[519] Herpes simplex encephalitis was identified in 45% of the patients. Another 18% had other identifiable infectious diseases, half of which were treatable. Thus, 10% of the total population had a treatable infection that would have been missed without the brain biopsy. Until recently the only noninvasive diagnostic test was the electroencephalogram, in which abnormal temporal lobe discharges are characteristic if present. The advent of sophisticated imaging techniques has revolutionized the clinical approach. Magnetic resonance imaging (MRI) is more sensitive than computed tomography. Herpesvirus encephalitis occurs very rarely, if ever, in the presence of a normal MRI study. Lesions are not limited, however, to unilateral temporal lobe lesions. The abnormalities by MRI may be multifocal or diffuse.[438] At the beginning of the illness the only abnormalities may be in the electroencephalogram.[422]

Herpes simplex virus is infrequently isolated from cerebrospinal fluid (CSF). In the national collaborative study, an isolate was recovered from CSF in only 2 of 45 (4%) of biopsy-proven cases of herpes encephalitis.[370] Serologic diagnosis is too insensitive, nonspecific, and slow to be of use in therapeutic decisions. A major diagnostic advance has been the use of molecular amplification techniques for detection of the herpesvirus genome in the CSF of patients with encephalitis or meningoencephalitis.

Herpesvirus remains latent in spinal ganglia after the initial infection. Type 1 virus is recovered from thoracic ganglia and type 2 from sacral ganglia. Herpetic aseptic meningitis does occur uncommonly, usually caused by type 2 virus. Viral meningitis is characteristically associated with a normal level of glucose in the CSF, in contrast to the markedly diminished levels of glucose in bacterial meningitis. The cerebrospinal glucose level in herpes meningitis, however, may be very low, and the cell count may be in the thousands.[358] Early in the course of any viral meningitis, neutrophils may predominate and suggest the possibility of a bacterial process. Herpes simplex virus, usually type 2, also causes recurrent lymphocytic meningitis (Mollaret's meningitis); the culture is almost uniformly negative, but the viral genome can be demonstrated in the CSF by polymerase chain reaction (PCR).[477]

Neonatal herpes infection is estimated to occur in 1:2,000 to 1:5,000 deliveries. It is almost always symptomatic and is frequently fatal. In a collaborative study, the mortality rate was 50–60% in infants with disseminated infection who were treated with acyclovir or vidarabine.[517] In contrast, no fatalities occurred among infants with disease limited to the nose, eyes, or mouth. The diagnosis is suggested by the development of vesicular skin lesions, but these may be absent in 20% of patients. Poor prognostic factors include disseminated disease, comatose state at admission to the hospital, disseminated intravascular coagulation, or prematurity.

The high morbidity and mortality rates of infant disease has prompted great efforts to diagnose maternal infection. Most cases of neonatal herpes simplex virus infection are contracted during vaginal delivery and can be prevented by cesarean section. Complex protocols for screening pregnant women have been developed but unfortunately have not worked well. Asymptomatic maternal infection at the time of delivery occurs regularly, although the risk for infants appears to be low if the infection is recrudescent and maternal antibody to type 2 virus is present. Many women do not recognize their primary genital infection. In one study, specific antibody to type 2 herpes simplex virus was detected in 439 of 1,355 pregnant women who had no clinical history of genital herpes (32%).[167] Asymptomatic shedding of virus in late pregnancy and at delivery was detected in 5 of 1,160 cultures (0.43%). During the pregnancy, 43 of the women who had antibody to type 2 virus recognized their first symptomatic genital infection.

Efforts to prevent neonatal infection have shifted to assessment of antibody status in pregnant women and careful examination for active clinical disease at the time of delivery. The commercial availability of reliable assays for type-specific antibody facilitates identification of women who are at risk for primary infection.[359]

Persons with compromised defense mechanisms are predisposed to herpes simplex esophagitis, tracheobronchitis, or pneumonia and disseminated infection, including hepatitis. Herpes simplex infections may be necrotizing and may suggest a bacterial etiology if the characteristic inclusions are not recognized or viral cultures are not done.[372] Immunosuppression is not a prerequisite for lower respiratory tract infection or esophagitis. The risk factors for lower respiratory tract infection include intubation, suggesting that the pathogenesis may be similar to that of bacterial pneumonia—aspiration of contaminated oropharyngeal secretions.[408] Patients with extensive burns are at risk for infection both of the denuded skin and of the lower respiratory tract.[159]

Infection of the eye includes conjunctivitis, which may be accompanied by fever, photophobia, and regional lymphadenopathy. Herpetic keratitis, which has a branching or dendritic appearance, is the second most common cause of corneal blindness (after trauma) in the United States.

Herpes simplex virus is one of the viral causes of pharyngitis and tonsillitis, usually as a primary infection. The mucosa may be ulcerated, and lesions may be limited to the posterior pharynx.[189] Necrotizing tonsillitis may mimic bacterial peritonsillar abscess. Hemorrhagic cystitis has been reported as a part of disseminated infection,[121] and herpetic proctitis may occur in homosexual men.[193]

CYTOMEGALOVIRUS

Cytomegalovirus (CMV) is one of a family of related viruses that are specific for a particular species.[351] Mouse CMV does not infect humans, and vice versa. CMV was first isolated from mice by Margaret Smith, who subsequently isolated the human virus from the salivary gland tissues of an infected infant. She recognized the species specificity of the virus, although the reviewers of her initially rejected paper did not.[510] Isolation of the human virus was reported concurrently by Smith, Weller, and Rowe. With the generosity of a gentleman, who also happens to be a Nobel Prize winner, Dr. Weller gives Dr. Smith the credit for the primacy of her discovery. CMV is an opportunistic pathogen that may produce persistent, even lifelong, infections.[386] It was recognized many decades ago as a human pathogen by the peculiar cytopathology it produces (see Color Plate 23-1*D*). Initially, investigators considered CMV as a protozoan invader of human tissue.[258]

This virus is associated with leukocytes and may be transmitted with a blood transfusion or transplanted organ. When detected by monoclonal antibodies or genetic probes, CMV is concentrated in the neutrophil fraction of the buffy coat, rather than in the mononuclear fraction. Replicating virus is found in both fractions, so material for culture should include all leukocytes. Virus is also excreted in saliva and in semen. Venereal transmission has been strongly suggested by epidemiologically related clusters of cases. CMV may be passed from mother to offspring through the placenta, in cervical secretions during delivery, or in breast milk.

The variety of infectious diseases produced by this pathogen is great, and includes congenital infection, neonatal infection, heterophil-negative infectious mononucleosis, hepatitis, pneumonia in immunosuppressed patients, and disseminated infection in immunosuppressed patients.[386] At the same time it may be extremely difficult to decide whether an individual patient has CMV-induced disease or is only persistently infected, because replicating virus is found in normally sterile organs and body fluids in the absence of clinical disease. Multiple genetic variants of CMV have been found in a single infected patient.[97]

It is relatively easy to document infection by culturing the virus or demonstrating the presence of specific antibody. In contrast to documentation of CMV *infection*, proof that a particular *disease process* is caused by CMV often requires biopsy and histologic examination. Even then the assessment is not always easy. For instance, some patients excrete CMV in their urine for years without ill effect, especially those who were congenitally infected. Recovery of CMV from bronchoalveolar lavage correlates poorly with CMV pneumonia,[425] which ultimately must be diagnosed by putting all facts together, often including the results of lung biopsy. Detection of serum antibody is the most sensitive method for determining if the patient has ever been infected by CMV. The presence of serum antibody is of little use, however, in determining if the patient is currently infected or if CMV disease is present, although there is a presumption that virus may persist in some host cells or tissue. Quantitative assessment of viral antigen or DNA best differentiates infection from disease.

A latent virus or one that is clinically silent may reactivate to produce disease. An individual patient may experience CMV disease after reactivation of a latent infection or after a primary exposure to the virus. The distinction is prognostically important, because primary infections are clinically more severe and more likely to cause symptomatic disease in a neonate.

Some situations can be manipulated to increase the odds against primary infections. For example, transplant recipients can be screened so that seronegative patients do not receive blood or an organ from a seropositive donor.

Viral infection of previously healthy persons usually manifests as a self-limited mononucleosis syndrome. As in Epstein-Barr virus infection, there is evidence for CMV mononucleosis that the symptoms are produced by cytotoxic lymphocytes, which attempt to eliminate the CMV-infected cells.

The spectrum of disease is considerably broader in patients who are immunosuppressed, depending on the extent of immunocompromise. In patients who are moderately immunocompromised, such as kidney-transplant recipients, CMV pneumonia is a common manifestation. When immunosuppression is more extreme, extensive, overwhelming infection may result. Recipients of heart, liver, or bone marrow transplants or HIV-infected patients may experience hepatitis, or previously unheard of complications such as perforation through an infected intestinal wall.

An additional complication in organ recipients is the association of CMV infection with rejection of a kidney or heart transplant. The pathogenesis of the process is unclear. Although a glomerulopathy has been described in transplanted kidneys of CMV-infected patients, the pathology of the rejected kidneys usually suggests an immunologic rather than an infectious process. To complicate matters even further, evidence suggests that patients who receive a transplanted heart and are infected with CMV have more superinfections with bacteria and fungi than do transplant recipients who are free of CMV.

Most congenitally and neonatally acquired infection is asymptomatic, but subtle symptoms may develop in some infants who appear normal at birth. At the other extreme is disseminated infection with multiorgan disease and severe congenital abnormalities, such as microcephaly. The frequency of intrauterine transmission of CMV during a primary maternal infection has been estimated at 20–40%, and the risk of an adverse outcome is increased during the first half of the gestation.

EPSTEIN-BARR VIRUS

Epstein-Barr virus (EBV) is the primary cause of infectious mononucleosis.[419] This versatile virus produces disease that ranges from acute self-limited infection to malignant neoplasms. The mononucleosis syndrome consists of fever, malaise, exudative pharyngitis, lymphadenopathy, and atypical lymphocytes circulating in the peripheral blood. Splenomegaly is common, and rupture of the spleen is a serious complication. Acute hepatitis may also be a part of the syndrome.

The virus was originally recognized during studies of Burkitt's lymphoma in Africa and only later associated with mononucleosis.[419] The virus gains entry to the body by infecting the pharyngeal epithelium. Its primary target, however, is the circulating B lymphocyte, which it infects and then immortalizes. The activated B lymphoblast, along with its passenger EBV, matures into a long-lived memory lymphocyte in the germinal center of the lymph node.[481] The result of this interaction is a polyclonal stimulation of the humoral immune system, which produces an array of antibodies to many antigens. At the same time, the cellular immune system is triggered to fight the EBV infection. It is the activated T lymphocytes that are seen in the peripheral-blood smear as atypical lymphocytes. The circle is completed when virus is excreted through the oral mucosa into the saliva. Young children usually have an asymptomatic or minimally symptomatic infection, and the diagnostic heterophil antibody test is often negative.

If integration of the EBV genome into certain types of cells occurs, a neoplasm may result instead of an acute infection. The unregulated growth of EBV in patients with HIV infection, who have lost the regulatory control of cellular immunity, may lead to increased EBV-related tumors. Most of these tumors are of B-lymphocyte lineage, such as Burkitt's lymphoma and primary lymphoma of the brain, but nasopharyngeal carcinoma has also been associated strongly with EBV. A subset of gastric and colonic carcinomas has also been ascribed to infection with EBV. A variety of other processes include lymphocytic interstitial pneumonia and hemophagocytic syndrome. Establishing association of a latent or persistent virus such as EBV is not enough to prove a causal relationship, which can come only from repetitive association and careful molecular analysis. The relationship between EBV and lymphoma appears to be particularly complex.[481]

In the mid-1980s it was suggested that a poorly defined syndrome of chronic fatigue might represent chronic EBV infection. Chronic EBV infection does exist and may be troublesome, but the nonspecific syndrome of chronic fatigue does not appear to be EBV-related.[115]

The cells that best support viral replication with shedding of infectious particles are epithelial cells of the oropharynx. Saliva from acutely ill or chronically infected patients contains viable virus, which can be demonstrated by cocultivation with normal peripheral-blood lymphocytes. Alternatively, peripheral-blood lymphocytes of infected individuals can be cultured in the presence of an agent that depletes T lymphocytes, such as cyclosporine. The diagnosis of neoplastic manifestations must be by molecular demonstration that the virus has been integrated into the genome of the malignant cells. Cells from EBV-induced tumors can often be cultured as immortalized cell lines in vitro.

VARICELLA-ZOSTER VIRUS

Varicella-zoster virus (VZV) causes chickenpox as a primary infection.[13] The virus may remain latent in the sensory ganglia of the spinal cord for many years before reactivating and producing disease for a second time. The reactivated disease resembles chickenpox but is limited to the dermatome that is innervated by the infected nerve. The reactivation disease is known as shingles. The dermatome of most concern is the ophthalmic branch of the trigeminal nerve because destructive corneal infection may occur as part of the reactivation disease. Before the identity of the processes was recognized, the virus of chickenpox was called varicella virus and that of shingles was called herpes zoster.

Varicella-zoster virus produces considerable discomfort in healthy persons and may produce pneumonia, but in immunosuppressed individuals the disease can become a life-threatening disseminated infection. Pregnant women are at increased risk for severe varicella, and neonates who are born within 4 days of their mother's infection are at great risk because maternal antibodies have not yet developed. The risk of embryopathy in the fetus after maternal VZV infection in the first 20 weeks of pregnancy is approximately 2%.

Conventional wisdom states that immunity to varicella is lifelong and that all subsequent disease is recrudescent. Reinfection has been suggested, however, by careful serologic study of immune persons in a house with a fresh case of chickenpox.[14] Housemates who had preexisting antibody remained well but developed increased antibody titers, indicating subclinical infection.

There is great concern in hospitals for the safety of immunosuppressed patients who come in contact with an infected person. Exposure may occur unwittingly because patients with VZV are infectious shortly before the onset of the characteristic rash. Measures to reduce risk include use of immune healthcare personnel for immunosuppressed patients and limitation of visitors. Prompt administration of zoster immune globulin after inadvertent exposure has a protective effect.

HUMAN HERPESVIRUSES-6 AND -7

The next addition to the list of pathogens in the herpes group is human herpesvirus-6 (HHV-6). This virus was first isolated from patients with lymphoproliferative disorders and named human B-lymphotropic virus.[392] The virus has the morphologic structure of a herpesvirus but is genetically unrelated to the five previously identified herpesviruses. Thus, it was named human herpesvirus-6. There are two currently recognized subtypes, designated A and B; subtype B is predominant. This virus shares with EBV the ability to grow in human lymphocytes. In contrast to EBV, which infects lymphocytes in a latent stage and does not actively grow in the cells, HHV-6 appears to produce only productive infection in human lymphocytes (i.e., mature infectious viral particles are produced in the infected cells).

In 1990 a new herpesvirus was isolated from CD4+ T lymphocytes of a healthy individual, using techniques that cause activation of T cells. The virus, which was named human herpesvirus-7 (HHV-7), is distinct from but closely related to HHV-6. The two viruses do not produce cross-immunity.

HHV-6 and HHV-7 produce a common childhood disease called exanthem subitum (also known as roseola infantum, roseola subitum, Duke disease, or fourth disease). Exanthem subitum occurs in children between 6 months and 3 years of age. Almost all children over the age of 13 months have antibody to HHV-6. Antibody to HHV-7 appears at a slightly older age.

Exanthem subitum begins with an abrupt fever, which is followed by a rash as the fever subsides on the third or fourth day. Febrile convulsions occur in approximately 8% of acutely infected patients. This infection is very unlikely in an afebrile child. The illness usually resolves without sequelae, but serious disease may result on rare occasions. In immunosuppressed adults HHV-6 has produced serious disease after transplantation of bone marrow and solid organs and in patients who are infected with HIV. These viruses have been suggested as etiologic agents in chronic fatigue syndrome, multiple sclerosis, and neoplastic disease, but the issue has not been settled. The frequent reactivation of herpesviruses during the course of other diseases complicates definitive establishment of an etiologic role.

HUMAN HERPESVIRUS-8

The latest addition to the group of lymphotropic herpesviruses is the Kaposi's-sarcoma-associated herpesvirus, which has been named human herpesvirus-8 (HHV-8). As implied by the name, the virus was first detected in tissue from Kaposi's sarcoma in patients with HIV infection, using molecular techniques.[354] Subsequent investigation demonstrated that the viral gene sequences were present in several clinical types of Kaposi's sarcoma: that occurring in patients with AIDS, classic Kaposi's sarcoma unrelated to HIV infection, and Kaposi's sarcoma in homosexual men who are not infected with HIV. The sequences have been identified in AIDS-related body cavity–based lymphomas, which also contained genetic sequences from EBV. Finally (perhaps), HHV-8 sequences have been found in tissue from multicentric Castleman's disease, an atypical lymphoid hyperplasia, which may progress to lymphoma or Kaposi's sarcoma. The sequences are also found in nonneoplastic tissue of HIV-infected patients with Kaposi's sarcoma.

B VIRUS

In the 1930s a virus of the herpes group was isolated from a patient in whom a fatal neurologic disease developed after being bitten by a monkey. About the same time, Sabin isolated a virus from another patient in whom transverse myelitis developed after a monkey bite. He named the isolate B virus after the afflicted patient. It has also been called herpesvirus simiae, which is something of a misnomer because a variety of herpesviruses are found in monkeys. The recommended taxonomic name is cercopithecine herpesvirus 1. At least 25 cases of herpes B virus infection have been documented in humans, of which 16 were fatal.[520]

The B virus is unusual because it crosses species lines. It is indigenous to Old World monkeys, such as rhesus and cynomolgus, in which it establishes latency. Localized human infections have been reported, but most are severe and systemic. An animal bite is the usual means of transmission, but infection after a needle-stick injury has been reported. A vesicular eruption often develops around the bite and is followed by regional lymphadenopathy and fever. Encephalitis, transverse myelitis, or visceral necrosis accompanies systemic spread.

Two events have called renewed attention to B virus. The first documented episode of human-to-human transmission occurred as part of a cluster of cases at a research facility. The second event was the discovery that monkey kidney cells that had been commercially supplied for diagnostic laboratories were contaminated with B virus. No human infections resulted, but the cells were recalled.[513] The ability of B virus to replicate in monkey kidney monolayers has been known for years. In fact, the stress of processing the kidneys may stimulate activation of latent B virus. Cytopathic effect of the virus consists of cell enlargement and fusion, which may spread through the monolayer. Cowdry type A inclusions identical to those of herpes simplex virus or VZV will be seen in stained cell preparations. Subculture to other monkey kidney cells or to rabbit kidney cells (commonly used for isolation of herpes simplex virus) will transmit the virus.

Adenoviruses

Adenoviruses were originally recognized when spontaneous degeneration occurred in adenoidal tissue cultures. They were called adenoid degeneration (AD), adenoid-pharyngeal-conjunctival (APC), or acute respiratory disease (ARD) agents.[450] These viruses can be present in the pharynx and in the feces without causing disease. Designation of an infectious agent as the etiologic agent must be done carefully so that one is not misled by a fortuitous association. For instance, at one time adenoviruses were considered causes of the pertussis syndrome because they were isolated in the absence of the common bacterial cause, *Bordetella pertussis*. The role of adenovirus in a pertussis syndrome is controversial. It has been suggested that being fastidious, *B. pertussis* may not have been recovered in many cases of whooping cough while the adenoviruses represented incidental isolates or copathogens.[244]

Adenovirus disease may be sporadic or may occur in epidemics. These viruses produce approximately 5% of the acute respiratory disease in children younger than 5 years of age and may be responsible for 10% of childhood pneumonia. They produce an exudative pharyngitis that can mimic group A β-hemolytic streptococcal disease. Adenoviruses may cause otitis, pharyngitis, and gastroenteritis. Certain serotypes are associated with acute conjunctivitis, with or without pharyngitis. Adenovirus infections of the gastrointestinal tract were discussed earlier with the other viral causes of gastroenteritis. The major adenoviral infections and their associated serotypes are summarized in Table 23-12.

Poxviruses

The poxviruses are a diverse group.[168] Most are animal pathogens, but some can also infect humans. The king of the poxvirus group was the variola virus, the etiologic agent of smallpox and the sole member of the group that infects human only. It has now passed from endangered species status into extinction.[146] After the last natural case was recorded, stocks of viruses were restricted to the United States and Soviet Union; with the dissolution of Soviet Union, however, the possibility of dispersal of viral stocks beyond Moscow exists. The genome of variola and five other pox viruses has been sequenced.[362]

The recognition that variola poses a major threat as an agent of bioterrorism has stimulated renewed interest. The population of the world is now largely susceptible or only partially immune, and physicians are unfamiliar with its clinical presentation and diagnosis. The records of historical outbreaks, including an epidemic in Boston early in the 20th century, have been reexamined to refresh faded memories.[5,39] Immunization with vaccinia virus, one of the milestone achievements of modern medicine, was abandoned in the 1970s, because of well-characterized side effects of the vaccine.[41] The balance between cost and benefit of vaccination has clearly been affected by the altered circumstances,[169,170] but the proper course is disputed.[42,321] Resid-

ual antibody has been demonstrated in previously immunized individuals, but its efficacy is unclear.[173]

Orthopoxviruses of animals, such as cowpox and monkeypox viruses, can occasionally infect humans. These infections resemble smallpox clinically. A new dimension to the risk of monkeypox was added by the recognition of human infection that was acquired from pet prairie dogs.[412] The pets may have been infected by imported African rodents that are known to be susceptible to monkeypox virus. The differential diagnosis of all poxvirus infections includes varicella-zoster virus.[346] Laboratory support is, therefore, essential whenever the possibility of variola is raised.

The origin of vaccinia virus is unclear. It has many characteristics of a distinct species, but may have been derived from one of several candidate viruses (including cowpox virus) by mutation or recombination

Members of two other genera, *Parapoxvirus* and *Yatapoxvirus*, are animal pathogens, but can infect humans. Tanapox virus causes human infection in parts of Africa, but it has produced disease in travelers after they have returned from an endemic area.[124]

Molluscum contagiosum virus, the sole member of the Genus *Molluscipoxvirus*, causes a distinctive cutaneous lesion; like variola it infects only humans.[146]

The parapoxviruses include agents causing diseases in sheep (orf or contagious pustular dermatitis virus) and in cows (milker's node or pseudocowpox virus). They may also produce localized infections in humans who are occupationally exposed to the viruses. The poxviruses are unlikely to be isolated in the clinical laboratory.

Papovaviruses

The papovaviruses, a diverse group of DNA viruses, are made up of the papilloma (Pa), polyoma (PO), and vacuolating (VA) viruses. The subgroups differ greatly in their biol-

---

Table 23-12 Adenovirus Infections

SYNDROME	AGE GROUP	SEROTYPES
Acute febrile pharyngitis	Young children	1, 2, 3, 5, 6, 7
Pharyngoconjunctival fever	Young children and adolescents	3, 7, 14
Acute respiratory disease	Military recruits	3, 4, 7, 14, 21
Pneumonia	Young children	1, 2, 3, 7
	Military recruits	4, 7
Epidemic keratoconjunctivitis	All	8, 11, 19, 37
Acute hemorrhagic cystitis	Young children	11, 21
Gastroenteritis	Young children	39, 40
Meningoencephalitis	Children and immunocompromised patients	1, 2, 5
Hepatitis	Children and immunocompromised patients	1, 2, 5

Adapted from reference[244].

ogy. The vacuolating viruses are indigenous to animals and will be encountered by microbiologists only as contaminating agents in monkey kidney cell cultures.

PAPILLOMAVIRUSES

The human papillomaviruses (HPVs) cause common warts, sexually transmitted venereal warts, and tumors of the respiratory, intestinal, and genital tracts. The viral nature of warts was known early in the 20th century, when they were transferred with cell-free filtrates, and Shope defined the rabbit papillomavirus as the cause of papillomas in 1933.[315] Study of HPV was impeded until molecular techniques sufficient for the task were developed in the 1970s.

More than 60 genetic types of HPV have been described. There are strong associations between certain genotypes and clinical lesions (Table 23-13). The common wart is the most common lesion, but most attention has been focused on the genital infections, including the association with neoplasia. Sexual partners of patients who are infected with HPV are also frequently infected with the same genotype.

The association of HPV with cervical neoplasia has been constructed from many studies. Although HPV provides the major risk, other undefined factors appear to be necessary for the development of cancer. Rather than a dramatic shift from normal to neoplastic epithelium in the cervix, there is a continuous spectrum, recognized as increasingly severe

Table 23-13	Association of Selected Human Papillomaviruses (HPV) With Clinical Disease	
VIRAL TYPE	**CLINICAL DISEASE**	**NEOPLASTIC POTENTIAL**
HPV-1	Deep plantar wart	Not described
HPV-2	Common wart	Not described
	Mosaic wart	
	Lip lesions	
HPV-3	Flat wart	Not described
HPV-4	Common wart	Not described
HPV-5	Plaques in epidermodysplasia verruciformis	Squamous carcinoma may develop in sun-exposed areas
HPV-6	Genital: Exophytic condyloma; flat condyloma; giant condyloma	Weak association, especially in vulva
	Respiratory papillomas	
	Conjunctival papillomas	
HPV-7	Common butcher's warts	Not described
HPV-11	See HPV-6	See HPV-6
HPV-13	Focal epithelial hyperplasia of oral cavity	Not described
HPV-16	Anogenital: Bowenoid papulosis; flat condyloma	High association in cervix
		Moderate association in vagina, vulva, anus, and penis
		Also found in respiratory tract, including larynx, tonsils, and oral cavity
HPV-18	Genital: Flat condylomas	High association in cervix; infrequently found in precursor lesions
HPV-31	Genital: Flat condyloma	High association with cervical cancer
HPV-32	Focal epithelial hyperplasia in oral cavity	Not described
HPV-33, -35, -39, -51, -52, -56, -58, -59, -68	Genital	Moderate association with cervical cancer
HPV-45	Genital	High association with cervical cancer

Adapted from reference[315].

grades of cervical intraepithelial neoplasia. The final stage in the process is the development of overt malignancy, invasive carcinoma, which may be either glandular or squamous. Likewise, there is a continuum in the expression of HPV genes and antigens. In the normal epithelium the cells of the basal layer progressively differentiate to form nonkeratinized squamous epithelium at the surface. As the cervical epithelial changes progress from mildly dysplastic to severely dysplastic, the following changes occur: 1) the cells become less differentiated throughout the epithelium, 2) the chromosomal content of the nuclei becomes increasingly abnormal, 3) the expression of HPV gene products (antigens) becomes less intense, and 4) the expression of HPV genes is increasingly difficult to demonstrate. A characteristic of the HPV-infected cell is koilocytosis, a perinuclear clearing in the squamous epithelium accompanied by nuclear atypia, although this appearance is not present in all infected cells. The appearance of koilocytic atypia in exfoliated cervical cells is shown in Figure 23-4.

The cellular biology of HPV supports a primary role in the development of neoplasia.[315] The viral types most closely associated with cervical cancer, particularly HPV-16, are capable of transforming cells in culture so that they lose their normal growth control mechanisms. The DNA from these types integrates into host DNA, in one case near cellular oncogenes. The viral integration may cause chromosomal rearrangement and lead to abnormal cellular differentiation in vitro. Zur Hausen has put forth the hypothesis that cervical neoplasia is the result of failure of a primal cellular surveillance mechanism that was designed to control persisting viral genomes.[539]

Papillomavirus DNA has been demonstrated in normal cervical epithelium adjacent to genital warts and cancer. Failure to remove all the infected tissue may lead to recurrences. HPV DNA can also be demonstrated in 5–10% of women with normal cervical smears or biopsies. The infection may be transient; the association of even high-risk genotypes with cervical neoplasia is most dramatic when HPV DNA is persistently present.

National consensus recommendations for treatment of patients at risk for cervical neoplasia, which evolve continually, include morphologic parameters (cervical exfoliative cytology) and viral determinants (detection of HPV). The current approach to classifying endocervical cytology is the Bethesda System.[460] In Table 23-14 the current recommendations for treating patients with abnormalities are summarized[527]:

The role of the laboratory in the management of endocervical disease has many aspects.[1] Recommendations for man-

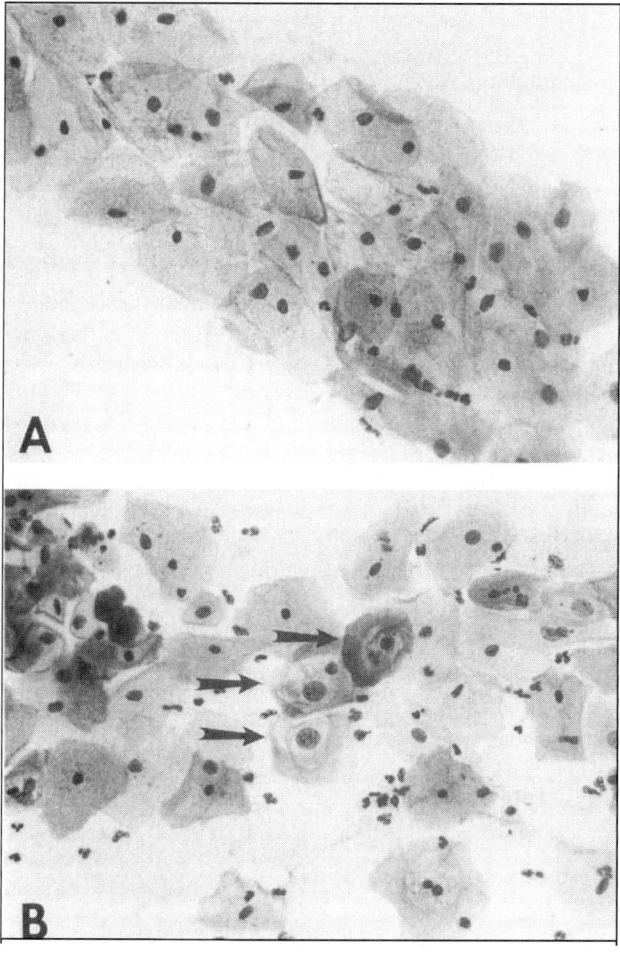

Figure 23-4 Papanicolaou stain. (**A**) Normal exfoliated cervical squamous epithelial cells. The nucleus is small and compact, and the cytoplasm is abundant in these mature, keratinized epithelial cells. (**B**) Koilocytic atypia. The nuclei in some of these superficial cells are enlarged with coarse, clumped chromatin, and there is a pallor or clearing in the cytoplasm (*arrow*) (×250).

Table 23-14	The Bethesda Classification of Cervical Cytology
CYTOLOGIC ABNORMALITY	**RECOMMENDED ACTION**
Negative for epithelial lesion or malignancy	Continue periodic cytologic testing
Atypical squamous cells of undetermined significance (ASC-US)[a]	Expedited cytologic testing OR HPV testing[b] OR Colposcopic examination
Atypical squamous cells, cannot rule out high-grade squamous intraepithelial lesion (ASC-H)	Colposcopic examination
Low-grade squamous intraepithelial lesion (LSIL)	Colposcopic examination
High-grade squamous intraepithelial lesion (HSIL)	Colposcopic examination
Squamous carcinoma	Biopsy confirmation

[a] *Consult references for recommendations on special circumstances: postmenopausal women, immunosuppressed women, and pregnancy.*
[b] *HPV testing recommended if material available from initial visit for testing (avoids repeat pelvic examination).*
Adapted from references[460,527].

agement of HPV disease continue to evolve. The American College of Obstetricians and Gynecologists suggests an option for combined cytology and HPV testing in women who are 30 years of age or older; if both tests are negative, repeat screening need be performed only every 3 years.

POLYOMAVIRUSES

The most important of the human polyomaviruses is the JC virus, which produces a destructive encephalitis (progressive multifocal leukoencephalopathy) in immunocompromised patients.[323] SV40 (simian virus 40) also produces the disease, another example of a monkey virus crossing species barriers. The histologic appearance, including intranuclear viral inclusions, of progressive multifocal leukoencephalopathy is diagnostic.

Polyomaviruses are frequently reactivated in recipients of transplants, often longer after transplantation than other latent human viruses. JC virus and BK virus are most frequently found. Both have been associated with a severe hemorrhagic cystitis in recipients of bone marrow transplants.

Parvoviruses

As the name implies, the parvoviruses are very small; they are unusual in that they contain single-stranded DNA. The only human parvovirus, known as B19, has been demonstrated to cause a common childhood febrile illness with rash. Erythema infectiosum is also known as fifth disease (the fifth childhood disease after rubeola, rubella, varicella, and roseola).[32,532] It is characterized by fever and a characteristic "slapped-cheek" rash in young children. Most persons are immune by the time they reach adulthood, but susceptible persons may experience arthritis or arthralgias. This pattern of mild rash illness in childhood and severe arthritis in adults resembles that of rubella virus. The rash in erythema infectiosum is maculopapular, but a vesiculopustular lesion has been reported in an adult.

Parvovirus B19 has an affinity for immature red-cell precursors. The receptor on human erythrocytes for parvovirus B19 is the P antigen; individuals who lack that antigen are naturally resistant to infection. Unfortunately, very few individuals lack the P erythrocyte antigen. Parvovirus B19 can produce transient anemia in normal persons and severe chronic anemia or aplastic crisis in patients with malignancies or hemoglobinopathies. If pregnant women undergo a primary parvovirus infection, fatal erythroblastosis fetalis with hydrops may result. In this case the virus produces severe chronic anemia, whereas in immunologic erythroblastosis (Rh disease) antibodies to the fetal red cells do the damage. A viral hemophagocytic syndrome in children and adults has been associated with human parvovirus. Transmission of parvovirus infection from heavily infected patients to susceptible healthcare workers has been documented.

The clinical manifestations of human parvovirus infection during an epidemic in Cadiz, Spain, included hematologic manifestations in 13.9% of 43 patients, dermatologic lesions in 53.4%, arthralgias or arthritis in 20.9%, and infection in pregnancy in 7.0% patients (two of these women suffered abortions). Fever and lymphadenopathy were presenting symptoms in 37% of the patients.[175]

Hepatitis Viruses

Many viruses can produce infectious damage to the liver. EBV and CMV occasionally cause symptomatic hepatitis as part of the mononucleosis syndrome. The primary hepatitis viruses are a diverse group. The "alphabet soup" of hepatitis is summarized in Table 23-15. Several other viruses have been described as possible agents of hepatitis, but the evidence is not conclusive that they are etiologic agents; they include hepatitis G virus (or GB variant of hepatitis C virus, a member of the family *Flavoviridae*[312]), as well as TT virus and SEN virus, both members of the family *Circoviridae*. Although hepatitis G virus has not been proven to cause hepatitis, patients with HIV infection who are coinfected with hepatitis G virus 5 to 6 years after seroconversion to HIV are less likely to die than HIV-infected patients who are not chronically infected with hepatitis G virus.[400,521]

Table 23-15	**Primary Viral Causes of Hepatitis**			
VIRUS	**TAXONOMY**	**TRANSMISSION**	**CHRONICITY**	**NEOPLASIA**
Hepatitis A	Hepatovirus RNA	Enteric: Water Food Shellfish	No	No
Hepatitis B	Hepadnavirus	Parental: Blood Sexual Needles Enteric	Yes	Yes
Hepatitis C	? Togavirus 27-nm virions RNA	Parental: Blood	Yes	Yes
Hepatitis D	42- to 47-nm virion RNA			
Hepatitis E	27- to 34-nm virion	Enteric	? No	? No

HEPATITIS A VIRUS

Hepatitis A virus produces sporadic and epidemic infectious hepatitis. The disease has been known since antiquity, but the virus was not identified until the 1970s. Hepatitis A virus was first classified as enterovirus 72 based on biochemical and physical features. Subsequently, it was recognized that there were considerable differences from classic enteroviruses. It has now been transferred into a new genus, *Hepatovirus*, within the family *Picornaviridae*.[234] There are seven genotypes of hepatitis A virus; most strains belong to genotype I.

Hepatitis A virus produces acute self-limited hepatitis. The incubation period between exposure and clinical disease is short (<1 month). For 7 to 10 days before clinical illness there is noncytopathic viral replication in hepatocytes, viremia, and fecal shedding of infectious virus. A period of viral replication with hepatocyte damage, including classic "ballooning" degeneration of liver cells, follows. At this point the communicable period is almost complete. Hepatitis A virus infection is rarely transmitted by blood transfusions because little virus is present in the blood and the duration of viremia is limited. Transmission of infection to patients with hemophilia in clotting factor concentrate, which contains samples from many donors, has been described in Europe and the United States. Massive hepatic necrosis and postinfectious cirrhosis are rare. Chronic hepatitis and neoplasia are not complications.

Hepatitis A is transmitted by contaminated food and water. Bivalve shellfish from contaminated waters have produced numerous outbreaks because they are often eaten raw or steamed to a temperature that does not kill the virus.[286] In one outbreak in Shanghai more than 300,000 individuals were infected after eating raw clams taken from contaminated water.[234] Sexual transmission also occurs.[268]

The transmission of hepatitis A virus, like EBV and poliovirus, is determined by sanitation and socioeconomic condition. Virus circulates freely under conditions of poor sanitation and infects humans at an early age, when the infection is usually asymptomatic. More affluent citizens escape infection until later in life, when symptomatic hepatitis results.[234] (See text on "Poliovirus" and "Epstein-Barr Virus".)

HEPATITIS B VIRUS

Hepatitis B virus is a DNA hepadnavirus. It produces acute and chronic hepatitis and is an etiologic agent of hepatocellular carcinoma.[174] Hepatitis B virus has a long incubation period (45–120 days) and is transmitted primarily by parenteral means.[235] Until routine screening of blood products for this virus was begun, hepatitis B was the most common cause of transfusion-associated hepatitis. Other parenteral routes have included acupuncture and tattooing. Hepatitis B antigen has been demonstrated in mosquitoes, but transmission of infection by arthropods has not been authenticated. This virus can be transmitted by sexual contact and has produced epidemic disease in male homosexuals, prostitutes, and abusers of intravenous drugs. Perinatal infection occurs, but breast milk does not appear to play a role in transmission. In contrast to hepatitis A virus, hepatitis B virus may produce fulminant fatal

acute hepatitis, called massive hepatic necrosis. It has been suggested that a mutation in the virus may cause this severe manifestation.

The array of mechanisms for transmission of hepatitis B virus infection recalls HIV. The concentration of hepatitis B virus in blood and body fluids is much greater than HIV, however, and nosocomial infection is consequently a greater problem. Hepatitis B has been an important cause of occupational infections in medical personnel, but the frequency has been greatly reduced by the widespread use of immunization in healthcare workers.

Hepatitis B virus is a 47-nm spherical virus that possesses several antigens of importance for diagnosis and pathogenesis. Several genotypes of hepatitis B virus have distinct clinical implications. Genotype A produces longer survival and less severe disease; genotype B is found more commonly in infections that result in hepatocellular carcinoma; genotype C produces severe disease; genotype D occurs in fulminant hepatitis.[235]

There are three envelope polypeptides that come under the designation HBsAg (hepatitis B surface antigen), HBcAg (hepatitis B core antigen), and HBeAg (hepatitis B e antigen). This virus has not been cultured in vitro, but the variety of antigens and corresponding antibodies provide ample tools for documenting clinical disease. Although not absolute, the presence of e antigen correlates well with the presence of DNA and DNA polymerase and with viral infectivity. The fascinating story of the discovery of Australia antigen (now known as HBsAg) and its relationship to hepatitis has been reviewed by Blumberg.[33] It serves as a reminder that no one can predict where basic research will have its impact. Who would have predicted that a research group interested in genetic polymorphisms of blood proteins would discover the key to an important cause of human hepatitis?

For reasons that are unclear, in some persons who are infected with hepatitis B virus antibody develops and clears the virus from their system, whereas other patients continue to have circulating viral antigens. Chronic liver disease develops in a subgroup of these chronic carriers. Another serious complication of this infection is the integration of viral DNA into the genome of the liver cells and the development of hepatocellular carcinoma.

HEPATITIS C VIRUS

After diagnostic reagents for hepatitis A and B viruses became available it became obvious that there were other causes of transfusion-associated hepatitis.[324] The unknown virus or viruses were dubbed non-A, non-B hepatitis. Thanks to the sophisticated technology of molecular biology we now recognize hepatitis C as the cause of most cases of transfusion-associated non-A, non-B hepatitis. The virus, which has not been cultivated, was eventually characterized by molecular techniques, one of the early triumphs of molecular biology. Surprisingly, the newly characterized agent was found to be most closely related to a group of viruses that are transmitted by arthropods; it is now a genus (*Hepacivirus*) in the family *Flaviviridae*. Concepts of genetic relationships among hepatitis C virus strains are evolving. At least 11 genotypes have been described, but other investigators assign the genotypes to six clades. Patients who are infected with strains of clades 1a and 1b (corresponding to genotypes 1a and 1b) respond less well to interferon treatment and progress more rapidly to chronic liver disease than do individuals who have been infected with other strains. Otherwise, there appear to be few phenotypic differences among genetically dissimilar strains.

The epidemiology of hepatitis C infections has many similarities to that of hepatitis B, but some significant differences are apparent. The most common route of spread is through blood products, including immune globulin, surgery, and intravenous-drug abuse. Screening of blood products for hepatitis C virus has substantially reduced the risk of transmission by this route. Sexual transmission occurs, but the frequency is much less than in hepatitis B infection. The prevalence of antibody to hepatitis C among healthcare workers in Baltimore was similar to that in the general population, suggesting that workers are exposed to low levels of virus or that the transmissibility is not great.[479]

Acute hepatitis C virus infection is often less severe than that of hepatitis B, but the frequency of chronic hepatitis C disease is high. The subject has been reviewed by Iwarson and colleagues.[255]

The long-term mortality of patients who are infected with hepatitis C virus is similar to that of controls, although infected patients have a slightly increased risk of dying from liver disease. Once a patient has documented chronic infection, however, the outlook is much worse. Cirrhosis is a significant complication of chronic infection. Hepatitis C infection is an independent risk factor for hepatocellular carcinoma after the development of cirrhosis. Extrahepatic immunologic manifestations, such as cryoglobulinemia and rheumatoid factors, are a prominent part of hepatitis C infection, as they are for hepatitis B.

HEPATITIS D VIRUS

Hepatitis D virus, also known as the delta agent, is a 35-nm double-shelled RNA virus that is incapable of multiplication without the surface antigen of hepatitis B.[182] The maturing delta virus covers itself in the HBsAg coat before infecting other cells. Thus, the biology of hepatitis D is inextricably tied to that of hepatitis B. Hepatitis D can produce infection and disease only in patients who are concurrently infected with hepatitis B or who are producing HBsAg from a previous infection. Not surprisingly, hepatitis D virus infection is concentrated in pockets of populations with hepatitis B virus infection, such as drug addicts and homosexual men.

When coinfection occurs, the clinical disease is similar to that of hepatitis B and is usually self-limited. When hepatitis D infects a patient who is a chronic carrier of hepatitis B, the clinical disease is much more severe, disease becomes chronic in as many as 80% of cases, and fatality rates may be dramatically increased to as high as 12%.

HEPATITIS E VIRUS

The newest addition to the alphabet soup of hepatitis viruses is a 27-nm labile RNA virus.[406] Hepatitis E virus produces an enterically transmitted acute hepatitis that most closely resembles that of hepatitis A. The viral genome has been cloned by techniques similar to those used to identify hepatitis C. The taxonomic status of this virus is not yet clear. It has similarities to the caliciviruses, but its closest genetic relative is rubella virus, currently classified as a togavirus. Large waterborne epidemics of disease are produced under conditions of poor sanitation, but the infection has not yet been recognized as a cause of indigenous disease in the United States. Travelers to endemic areas, however, have returned to the United States with the infection.

Prion Diseases (Transmissible Spongiform Encephalopathies)

The transmissible spongiform encephalopathies are a fascinating group of CNS infections. They are defined by a distinctive cellular pathology, characterized by a vacuolated appearance of the cerebral white matter. The infections and their natural hosts are summarized in Table 23-16. A molecular and clinical classification of prion diseases has been proposed.[495]

For decades it has been recognized that the scrapie agent

Table 23-16 Transmissible Spongiform Encephalopathies (Prion Diseases)		
AGENT	NATURAL HOST	HUMAN INFECTION
Scrapie	Sheep	No
Transmissible mink encephalopathy	Mink	No
Chronic wasting disease	Muler deer, elk	No
Kuru	Humans	Yes
Creutzfeldt-Jakob disease (CJD) (familial, sporadic, and iatrogenic forms)	Humans	Yes
Gerstmann-Straussler-Scheinker syndrome (GSS)	Humans	Yes
Fatal insominia (familial and sporadic forms)	Humans	Yes
Bovine spongiform encephalopathy (BSE)	Cattle	Yes

was novel—an apparently transmissible agent that contained no evidence of either type of nucleic acid. The responsible pathogen was originally considered a "slow virus," but the agent was more resistant to inactivation by x-rays, ultraviolet light, and harsh chemical treatment, including immersion in 10% formalin, than any other known infectious particle. In the 1960s, Pattison proposed that the agent was a basic protein and Griffith suggested several hypothetical mechanisms, one of which proved to be on target.[404] The nature of the infectious particles was painstakingly elucidated by Prusiner. He persisted in his battle to win over skeptical colleagues, but eventually won the Nobel Prize for his efforts. The unique infectious agent, which was named a prion, turned out to be a normal cellular protein (PrP^c) that was modified by a conformational change. The PrP^c protein is converted into the abnormal protein (PrP^{sc}) by refolding of a portion of its α-helical coil structure into a β-sheet.[403,404] Although the infectious-protein hypothesis has been generally accepted, agreement as to the nature of the infectious agent is not universal.[91]

The diseases produced by prions are referred to as transmissible spongiform encephalopathies (TSEs).[264,404,405] They were of veterinary interest until the first human TSE was recognized. Kuru occurred among a remote, isolated tribe of aborigines in the New Guinea highlands.[171] Gajdusek won a Nobel Prize for unraveling the mysterious disease that began with cerebellar ataxia and a shivering-like tremor, progressed to complete loss of motor and speech function, and resulted in death within a year. The agent was transmitted through the practice of ritual cannibalism as part of the mourning ritual for the dead. Transmission of the infection was stopped when the tribe was convinced to alter its practices. Subsequently, it was recognized that two rare human dementias—Creutzfeldt-Jakob disease (CJD) and a variant, Gerstmann-Sträussler-Scheinker syndrome (GSS)—were caused by a similar agent. These degenerative diseases, which occur in familial and sporadic forms, produce the rapid onset of dementia. Memory loss and behavioral problems ensue at some point in most patients. Death occurs within months to a year after onset.

Bovine spongiform encephalopathy (BSE) appeared in southern England in 1986, and approximately 100,000 cases had been documented by the end of 1993.[40] Scrapie has been passed from sheep to cattle experimentally,[184] and it has been conjectured that the disease was transmitted to cattle through sheep brains included in feed as a protein supplement.[40] Alternatively, BSE may have arisen by a chance mutation, as occurs in human CJD. Whatever the origin of the first case, the inclusion of animal products in animal feed allowed the widespread dissemination of the infection in cattle.[254]

What was an economic disaster turned into a political and scientific nightmare in 1996 when it was announced that some cases of "atypical Creutzfeldt-Jakob disease" in England may have been contracted by eating meat from cows with BSE. The British government underreacted, the European governments overreacted, and a crisis with more politics than science ensued. Soon it became clear that variant Creutzfeldt-Jakob disease (vCJD) was real. Several authors believe that it resulted from eating contaminated meat,[104,254,495] although Prusiner has been more circumspect in his analysis.[403–405] vCJD differs from the classic form in several ways, including onset at a young age. The epidemic of BSE and apparently of vCJD in Britain was eventually brought under control by widespread slaughter of cattle and prohibition of animal products in animal feeds. The long incubation periods of TSE make caution in declaring victory a wise policy.[254]

The BSE and vCJD saga shattered the previously held (and comforting) theory that prion diseases were species-specific. Although TSE had been recognized for many years, there had never before been transmission across species lines. It was devastating to realize that the species barrier may not be absolute and that humans may not be immune to risk. Additional concern was raised by the recognition that at least one victim of CJD had participated in wild game feasts.[78] It is not known whether the wild game were afflicted with chronic wasting disease, which afflicts herds of elk and deer in the Western and North Central United States. The potential for additional risks to humans is, however, all too obvious. Another comforting illusion was destroyed when BSE was identified in both Canada and the United States.[81,128]

To date all transmissions of prion disease have been through neural tissue, including transmission of CJD by hormones derived from human pituitary tissue, by transplantation of dura mater and corneas, and through contaminated electroencephalographic electrodes.[405] Cases have become clinically apparent more than 14 years after the putative exposure. Definitive evidence of transmission by extraneural tissue has not been forthcoming,[264] but prions have been documented outside the CNS in classic CJD[187] and in vCJD.[495]

When TSE is suspected clinically, elaborate precautions must be taken in the autopsy room and histology laboratory because the agents of these infections survive formalin fixation and are even demonstrable after tissue is embedded in paraffin blocks.

Clinical Classification of Viral Infections

Although virologic taxonomy is important scientifically, clinical schemes of classification have practical validity when considering an individual patient. The clinical syndromes and associated viruses that are most commonly encountered are summarized in Table 23-17. Note that viruses from varying taxonomic groups may produce the same symptoms.

Diagnosis of Viral Infections

The primary diagnostic technique for most viral infections is the isolation of the virus in cell culture. Serologic techniques may also be useful, especially if the virus was isolated from a nonsterile site. In some instances, serologic diagnosis is the only practical approach in a clinical laboratory. Direct detection of antigen in body fluids or tissues has also been effective for some viruses. The list of agents for which direct detection of antigen is useful will undoubtedly continue to expand. Molecular diagnosis is undoubtedly the

Table 23-17   Clinical Syndromes Associated With Viral Infections

CLINICAL SYSTEM	SYNDROME	MORE LIKELY AGENTS	LESS LIKELY AGENTS
Respiratory	Coryza (common cold)	Rhinovirus	Influenza A & B
		Coronavirus	Parainfluenza 1 &2
		Adenovirus	RSV
		Parainfluenza 3	Enterovirus
	Pharyngitis	Adenovirus	Influenza A &B
		Herpes simplex 1	RSV
		Enterovirus	Parainfluenza 1 &2
		EBV	Rhinovirus
			Coronavirus
	Croup	Parainfluenza 1	Influenza A
		Parainfluenza 2	RSV
		Parainfluenza 3	Measles
			Coronavirus
	Bronchiolitis	Parainfluenza 3	Adenovirus
		RSV	Parainfluenza 1 &2
			Influenza A & B
			Rhinovirus
	Pneumonia	Influenza A	Parainfluenza 1 &2
		RSV	Rhinovirus
		Parainfluenza 3	EBV
		Adenovirus	Influenza B
		CMV (in immuno-suppressed patients)	SARS coronavirus Metapneumovirus
	Pleurodynia	Coxsackievirus B	Coxsackievirus A
			Echovirus
Central nervous system	Aseptic meningitis	Echovirus	Mumps virus
		Coxsackievirus A	LCM
		Coxsackievirus B	Herpes simplex 2
			VZV
			Adenovirus
			Bunyaviruses
			Parainfluenza 3
			Polio virus (vaccine strains)
	Encephalitis	Herpes simplex 1	Togavirus
			Flavivirus
			Bunyavirus
			EBV
			Enterovirus
			Rabies
			CMV
Gastrointestinal	Diarrhea (infants)	Rotavirus	Calicivirus (Norwalk)
		Adenoviruses 40 & 41	
		Astrovirus	

Table 23-17 *Continued*

CLINICAL SYSTEM	SYNDROME	MORE LIKELY AGENTS	LESS LIKELY AGENTS
Gastrointestinal (continued)	Diarrhea (adults)	Calcivirus (Norwalk-like virus)	Rotavirus
			Adenoviruses 40 & 41
			Astrovirus
	Hepatitis	Hepatitis A	EBV
		Hepatitis B	CMV
		Hepatitis C	Hepatitis D
			Hepatitis E
	Parotitis	Mumps virus	Parainfluenza
Cutaneous	Vesicular rash	Herpes simplex 1 & 2	Echovirus
		VZV	Coxsackievirus A
			Vaccinia
	Maculopapular rash	Echovirus	Adenovirus
		Coxsackievirus	EBV
		Human herpesvirus 6 & 7	Dengue
			Measles
			Rubella
	Petechial rash	None frequent	Adenovirus
			Echovirus
			Coxsackievirus
			Hemorrhagic fever viruses
Urogenital	Hemorrhagic cystitis	None frequent	Adenovirus
			Herpes simplex 1
Cardiac	Myocarditis/pericarditis	Coxsackievirus A, B	Adenovirus
		Echovirus	Herpes simplex 1
			Influenza A
			Mumps
Ocular	Keratitis/conjunctivitis	Herpes simplex 1	Vaccinia
		VZV	Measles
		Adenovirus	

Adapted from McIntosh K. Diagnostic virology. In: Fields BN, Knipe DM, Melnick JL, et al., eds. Virology. 2nd Ed. New York: Raven Press, 1990:411–440.

approach of the future. In Table 23-18 the methods most commonly used in hospital laboratories to diagnose viral infections are summarized. The advantages and disadvantages of each of these approaches are compared and contrasted in Table 23-19. Interested readers should consult excellent general references for more detailed discussions.[248,462]

Collection of Specimens for Diagnosis

In general, an attempt should be made to obtain material from the organ or organs that are infected. For the most common viral infections of the skin, the cutaneous lesions are the best specimens for culture. For diagnosis of infections of the respiratory and gastrointestinal tracts, secretions from those regions should be cultured. Recommended specimens for viral culture are listed in Table 23-20.

Most viruses enter the body through the respiratory or gastrointestinal tracts. Although the most obvious clinical manifestations of disease may occur in a distant organ, it is often appropriate to collect a specimen from the point of entry. Sampling of multiple sites is particularly useful if it is difficult to obtain a specimen from an internal organ or if the virus is difficult to isolate from the target organ. For example, the skin is most dramatically involved in measles infection, but measles virus may be isolated from the respiratory tract or from the urine. Similarly, the cardiac and central nervous systems are commonly affected in serious enterovi-

Table 23-18   Methods for Diagnosis of Viral Infections

VIRUS	PRIMARY METHOD	EXPEDITED METHOD	ANCILLARY METHOD	COMMENTS
Adenovirus	Culture[a], MAT[b]	FA, EIA, RT-PCR[b]	Serology[c]	
Adenovirus, enteric	EIA, FA	RT-PCR[b]	IEM[b]	
Alphaviruses	Culture[b,c], MAT[b]	RT-PCR[b]	Serology	
Arenaviruses	Culture[b], MAT[b]	EIA[b], RT-PCR[b]	Serology	Test performed only in BSL-4 laboratories
Astroviruses	MAT[b]	RT-PCR[b]	EIA[b], IEM[b]	
Bunyaviruses	MAT[a,b]	RT-PCR[a,b]	Serology[a,b]	Both serology and molecular tests recommended for hantavirus
Calcivirus	MAT[b]	RT-PCR[b]	EIA[b], IEM[b]	
Coronavirus	Culture[b], MAT[b]	RT-PCR[b]	Serology[a,b]	Performed only in epidemics or possible SARS
Cytomegalovirus	Culture[a], MAT[a,b]	SV[a] FA blood antigen[a,b], QPCR[a,b]	Serology	Serology for immune status; antigenemia and QPCR for monitoring
Enteroviruses	Culture[a], MAT[b]	RT-PCR[b]	Serology[c]	Large number of serotypes make serology impractical
Epstein-Barr virus	Serology[a], MAT[b]	RT-PCR[b]	Culture[b,c]	
Filoviruses	Culture[b], MAT[b]	RT-PCR[b]	Serology[b]	Tests performed only in BSL-4 laboratory
Flaviviruses	Culture[a,b], MAT[b]	RT-PCR[b]	Serology[b], Histology	
Hepatitis A virus	IgM serology[a]		MAT[b]	
Hepatitis B virus	Serology[a]		MAT[b]	
Hepatitis C virus	Serology[a], MAT[a,b]			Serology for initial diagnosis; MAT for confirmation of active infection and monitoring
Hepatitis D virus	Serology[a,b]		MAT[b]	
Hepatitis E virus	Serology[a,b]	RT-PCR[b,c]	MAT[b,c]	All procedures investigational in United States
Herpes simplex virus	Culture,[a] MAT[a,b]	SV,[a] FA,[a] EIA,[a] RT-PCR[b]	Serology (type specific)[a]	Serology for immune status
Human herpesvirus 6 & 7	MAT[a,b]	RT-PCR[b]	Serology[b]	
Human herpersvirus8	MAT[a,b]	RT-PCR[b]		

Table 23-18 *Continued*

VIRUS	PRIMARY METHOD	EXPEDITED METHOD	ANCILLARY METHOD	COMMENTS
Human immuno-deficiency virus	Serology,[a,b] MAT[a,b]	Serology	Culture[b,c]	Serology for initial diagnosis; molecular monitoring
Influenza	Culture,[a] MAT[b]	SV,[a] FA,[a] EIA,[a] RT-PCR[b]	Serology[c]	Viral isolate required for typing
Measles	Serology[a]	FA,[c] RT-PCR[b]	Culture[c]	Rarely isolated
Metapneumovirus	Culture,[b] MAT[b]	RT-PCR[b]	Serology[b]	
Mumps	Culture[c] MAT[b]	RT-PCR[b]	Serology[c]	
Papillomaviruses	MAT[a]			
Parainfluenza	Culture,[a] MATb[2]	SV,[a] FA,[a] EIA,[c] RT-PCR[b]	Serology[3]	
Parvovirus B19	MAT[b]	RT-PCR[b]	Serology[b]	
Polyomaviruses	MAT[b]		Serology[b]	
Poxviruses	Culture,[a] MAT[a,b]	EM,[a,b] RT-PCR[a,b]	Serology[c]	Serology for immune status; tests performed only in BSL-4 laboratories
Rabies virus	Culture[a,b] MAT[b]	FA,[a,b] RT-PCR[a,b]		
Respiratory syncytial	Culture[a] MAT[b]	SV,[a] FA,[a] EIA,[a] RT-PCR[b]	Serology[c]	FA more sensitive than EIA
Rhinovirus	Culture,[c] MAT[b,c]	RT-PCR[b,c]		Rarely tested
Rotavirus	EIA[a]		Culture,[b,c] IEM,[b,c] Serology[b,c]	
Rubella virus	Serology[a]	RT-PCR[a]	Culture,[b,c] MAT[b]	
Varicella-zoster virus	Culture,[a] MAT[b,c]	SV,[a] FA,[a] RT-PCR[b]	Serology[a]	Serology for immune status

MAT, molecular-amplification test; FA, direct or indirect immunofluorescence; EIA, enzyme immunoassay; RT-PCR, real-time polymerase chain reaction; SARS, severe acute respiratory syndrome; SV, shell vial (spin amplification) culture; BSL-4, Biosafety Laboratory Level 4 (highest degree of containment); QPCR, quantitative polymerase chain reaction (including TaqMan); EM, electron microscopy; IEM, immune electron microscopy.
[a] Standard approach.
[b] Available in specialty or reference laboratories.
[c] Rarely performed.

ral infection, but the virus may be isolated from the upper airways or from the gastrointestinal tract.

If the virus is rarely isolated from these nonsterile sites (as is the case with measles), recovery of a virus establishes an etiologic diagnosis. If the virus is recovered from sites where it may be found in the absence of disease (e.g., the enteroviruses in throat or stool specimens), the recovery of a potentially pathogenic virus provides a presumptive diagnosis.

Viruses colonize mucosal surfaces less frequently than do bacteria, but may be present more commonly during the months when increased circulation of viruses occurs—the winter for respiratory viruses and the summer for enteroviruses. The frequency with which enteroviruses colonize the gastrointestinal tract is greatest in infants and least in adults.

In Cincinnati, the carrier rate for echoviruses was 5.2% among 1- to 4-year-old children, 2.6% in 5- to 9-year-old children, and only 0.2% in 10- to 14-year-old children.[428] Herpes simplex virus and CMV may produce chronic infections and be shed intermittently into secretions and fluids.[386,518]

The association of a clinical illness with a virus that has been recovered from a nonsterile site may be strengthened by demonstration of a serologic response to the isolated virus, although this inconvenient tack is rarely used.

The optimal specimens for viral culture are aspirates of fluids, exudates, or secretions; tissues; washings of the upper airways; or stool specimens. Swab specimens, which are convenient and more acceptable to patients than washings or aspirates, are acceptable in most situations. Swabs and

Table 23-19 Comparison of Diagnostic Methods

METHOD	TIME	ADVANTAGES	DISADVANTAGES
Culture	Days to weeks	Specificity maximum; sensitivity usually adequate; isolate available for characterization	Cell-culture facilities needed; time for diagnosis may be long (shortened by spin amplification)
Antigen detection	Hours to 1 day	Speed of diagnosis; used for viruses difficult to culture	False positives and false negatives; hard to batch tests
Molecular amplification	One to several days	Maximal sensitivity; specificity usually adequate	Molecular facilities needed; potential for cross-contamination; problems with inhibitors
Real-time amplification	Hours	Excellent sensitivity and specificity; speed of diagnosis; may be method of choice in future	Molecular facilities needed
Serology	Weeks	Assessment of immunity; used for viruses that are difficult to culture	Potential cross-reactions; need for acute and convalescent sera

Table 23-20 Recommended Specimens for Viral Culture

SYNDROME	OPTIMAL SPECIMENS	PERMISSIBLE ALTERNATIVES AND ADDITIONAL SPECIMENS
Coryza Croup	Nasopharyngeal aspirate	Nasopharyngeal swab
Pharyngitis	Throat washing or swab	
Bronchiolitis	Nasopharyngeal aspirate	Nasopharyngeal swab
Pneumonia	Tracheal aspirate Lung aspirate or biopsy	
Pleurodynia	Nasopharyngeal aspirate *plus* feces	Nasopharyngeal swab Rectal swab
Aseptic meningitis Encephalitis Transverse myelitis	Spinal fluid (use of feces, rectal swabs, and nasopharyngeal specimens controversial)	(Rectal swab) (Nasopharyngeal swab) Brain biopsy for herpes simplex; urine for measles or mumps
Gastroenteritis	Feces	Rectal swab
Parotitis	Nasopharyngeal aspirate *plus* urine	Nasopharyngeal swab
Vesicular rash	Aspirate or swab of vesicle	
Maculopapular rash	Nasopharyngeal aspirate *plus* feces	Nasopharyngeal swab Rectal swab
Hemorrhagic cystitis	Urine	
Myocarditis Pericarditis	Nasopharyngeal aspirate *plus* feces	Urine for mumps virus Nasopharyngeal swab Rectal swab
Keratitis Conjunctivitis	Conjunctival or corneal scraping plus nasopharyngeal aspirate	Conjunctival or corneal swab Nasopharyngeal swab

Adapted from McIntosh K. Diagnostic virology. In: Fields BN, Knipe DM, Melnick JL, et al., eds. Virology. Ed. 2. New York: Raven Press, 1990:411–440.

nasopharyngeal washings are generally equivalent for recovery of respiratory viruses. Some investigators have found that RSV is more reliably recovered from nasopharyngeal aspirates than from swabs,[222] but that experience has not been universal.[455] Virtually any material may be used for the swab tip, with the notable exception of calcium alginate (at least for herpes simplex virus).[455]

Viremia occurs frequently during viral infections but is not often detected. CMV viremia occurs regularly and can be detected by several methods. Blood may be a useful specimen for diagnosis of enteroviral infection in young children and infants.[401]

To culture vesicular skin lesions, the skin should be cleansed with an alcohol swab and allowed to dry for at least 1 minute. The vesicle should then be unroofed with a sterile scalpel and a sterile swab touched several times to the base. The swab should be placed in a viral transport medium, as described below. Alternatively, the contents of the vesicle may be aspirated with a tuberculin syringe and 26-gauge needle, if the vesicle is sufficiently large. Material for a Tzanck preparation can be collected by vigorously scraping the base of the lesion with the edge of a scalpel blade; the material on the blade is then touched to a glass slide and allowed to air dry.

As a general rule, the frequency with which viruses are recovered decreases as the duration of illness increases, so every effort should be made to obtain specimens as early in the infection as possible.

Transportation and Storage of Specimens

Aspirates, fluids, and tissues should be transported to the laboratory in a sterile, leakproof container. Every effort should be made to minimize the interval between collection of the specimen and its inoculation into cell culture. Inoculation of cell cultures at the bedside has been recommended for some fragile viruses, particularly RSV. Immediate inoculation is impractical in many practices; fortunately other investigators have not found a problem with transporting the specimen to the laboratory for inoculation, even in the case of RSV.[455]

Swabs should be placed into a transport medium that includes antibiotics; dry swabs are not acceptable. The type of transport medium is probably not critical, although it is difficult to conduct definitive comparative studies in which all variables are controlled. Data are most complete for herpes simplex virus. Commercial transport systems, such as the Culturette swab products (BD Diagnostics, Franklin Lakes, NJ), have been satisfactory. The sucrose-phosphate-glutamate medium (SPG) that was designed for *Chlamydia trachomatis* has been effective, as has been a variant without the glutamate (2SP medium).[260] Traditionally, a nutrient medium has been supplemented with a source of protein in an attempt to stabilize fragile viruses and with antibiotics to minimize bacterial contamination.

Specimens should be refrigerated until they are inoculated into cell cultures. To select the best temperature for storage, one must balance the decrease in viral titer that occurs progressively at 4°C against the sudden decrease that occurs when specimens are frozen and thawed. It is clear that 1) the specimens should be maintained at −70°C if they

are to be stored for a very long time (weeks or months) and 2) the best temperature is 4°C if the delay will be short (less than 24 hours). A reasonable recommendation is that specimens be refrigerated for up to 96 hours and frozen at −70°C if the delay will be longer. The worst temperature is −20°C, especially in a frost-free freezer, where repeated cycles of defrosting and freezing are extremely traumatic to all forms of life. Specimens should never be frozen in the freezing compartment of a standard refrigerator. Johnson has thoroughly reviewed the transport of specimens for viral diagnosis.[260]

Isolation of Viruses in Culture

Although a few of the largest hospital laboratories may have facilities for inoculation of animals, most diagnostic facilities are restricted to the use of in vitro analogs.

Preparation and Maintenance of Cell Cultures

Cell culture is the cultivation in vitro of dissociated single cells. Tissue and organ culture is the maintenance in vitro of a portion of an organ, usually for short, delimited periods of time. The use of organ culture has been restricted almost completely to the research laboratory. For example, cultures of trachea have been used to isolate human coronaviruses, most of which do not grow in cell culture. Occasionally, organ and cell cultures must be combined. For example, an explant of infected brain and an indicator monolayer of susceptible cells was used for the isolation of measles virus from patients with subacute sclerosing panencephalitis. Embryonated eggs are an inexpensive method for cultivating selected viruses, such as the orthomyxoviruses, but they are rarely used in diagnostic laboratories.[302]

Cell cultures are of three basic types (Table 23-21). Primary cell cultures consist of a mixture of cells, usually kidney, lung, or skin, obtained by dissociation of cells from the minced organ. These cells can be maintained in culture for a limited time only. Once subcultured repetitively in vitro, a primary cell culture becomes a cell line. The most commonly used cell lines are composed of fibroblasts, obtained from skin or embryonic lung. A cell line is diploid if at least 75% of the cells have a normal complement of chromosomes. A cell line is heteroploid if more than 25% of the cells have an abnormal complement of chromosomes. Some of the expanding choices of cell lines are detailed in Table 23-22.

Innovative thinking has produced even more variety in the choices for cell cultures. By combining cell lines the spectrum of viruses detected can be expanded while limiting the number of tubes required and even avoiding the need for primary cell cultures.[249] Some of the combinations of cell lines that have been developed as Fresh Cells or R-Mix (Diagnostic Hybrids, Athens, OH) are included in Table 23-21. The mixed cell lines may be combined with other approaches, such as spin amplification (shell vials) to enhance detection further.[21,137] A further innovation is the storage of the mixed cultures at −80°C for up to 4 months before inoculation.[251]

Still another innovation has been the engineering of cell cultures to facilitate isolation of particular viruses or to en-

Table 23-21   **Types of Cell Cultures**

TYPE OF CULTURE	CHARACTERISTICS	EXAMPLES	PRIMARY USE
Primary	Diploid; mixed cell types; 1 or 2 passages	Primary monkey kidney	Influenza; parainfluenza; some enteroviruses
		Primary rabbit kidney	Herpes simplex
Cell lines	Diploid; fibroblastic; limited passages (<50–70)	Human diploid fibroblast (WI-38, MRC-5, HEL, FS-9)	Herpes simplex; cytomegalovirus; varicella-zoster; rhinovirus
Established cell lines	Heteroploid; continuous passage in vitro	HeLa; HEp-2	Adenovirus; RSV; Coxsackie B virus
		A549	Herpes simplex; adenovirus; varicella-zoster; some enteroviruses
		MDCK	Influenza virus
		LLC-MK2	Parainfluenza virus
		Vero; ML cells	Herpes simplex
		RD cells	Some Coxsackie A viruses
		BGM cells	Coxsackie B viruses
		293 cells	Enteric adenovirus
Mixed cell lines	Combinations of established cell lines	MRC-5 + CV-1	Herpes simplex; varicella-zoster
		ML Cells + A549	Respiratory viruses
		RD +H292; BGMK + A549	Enteroviruses
Genetically modified cell lines	Introduction of a gene to produce a visible indicator after infection	Enzyme-linked-virus-inducible system (ELVIS)	Herpes simplex

hance their detection. One of the cell lines that has been used successfully for detection of enteroviruses is buffalo green monkey kidney (BGMK) cells. By engineering BGMK cells to express a receptor for enteroviruses (decay-accelerating factor, DAF) investigators were able to increase the diagnostic yield.[250]

A different approach to cellular engineering is the ELVIS (*e*nzyme-*l*inked *v*irus-*i*nducible *s*ystem) HSV test system (Diagnostic Hybrids). In this case, an HSV-specific gene promoter sequence in the baby hamster kidney (BHK) cell line is linked to a reporter gene, β-galactosidase. When the cells are infected with either serotype of HSV, the promoter gene is turned on and the reporter gene is then activated, producing a visible change in the color of the monolayer.[387] As with the mixed cell lines, the ELVIS cells can be stored at $-80°C$ until use.[251] HSV is the most common virus sought in diagnostic laboratories, and a targeted approach to detection of this agent is sensible.

The life expectancy of normal diploid cells is approximately 50 serial doublings in vitro[218]; those cell lines that have been transferred at least 70 times are considered to be established cell lines. These established or continuous lines

may be derived from normal tissue, as was the Vero cell line from African green monkey renal cells. Alternatively, they may originate from neoplastic epithelium, such as the HeLa cells that came from a cervical adenocarcinoma and the HEp-2 cells that were derived from a carcinoma of the larynx. The appearance of uninoculated cell cultures is illustrated in Figure 23-5. The fibroblastic cells are usually long, spindly, and oriented in parallel, whereas the established cell lines consist of polygonal epithelial cells. The primary cultures naturally contain a mixture of cell types.

Conditions for growth and maintenance of cell cultures vary considerably, and only a few generalizations are possible. The temperature of incubation is optimal at 36 to 37°C but may be lowered to 35°C after confluence of cells is achieved. This maneuver may facilitate isolation of viruses, such as myxoviruses and rhinoviruses, that grow optimally at 33°C. A physiologic pH must be maintained. Usually a CO_2-bicarbonate buffering system is used, with CO_2 being supplied by the metabolizing cells in a closed tube or flask. In an open system a CO_2-air mixture must be provided. Buffering compounds that do not depend on CO_2-bicarbonate, such as HEPES buffer (*N*-2-hydroxyethylpiperazine-*N*-2-

Table 23-22   Origins of Cell Lines

TYPE OF CELL LINE	NAME	ORIGIN OF CELLS
Established heteroploid	A549	Human alveolar cell carcinoma (type II epithelial cells)
Established heteroploid	BGM	Buffalo green monkey kidney cells
Established heteroploid	BHK	Baby hamster kidney cells
Established heteroploid	CV-1	African green monkey kidney cells
Diploid cell line	FS-9	Foreskin fibroblasts
Established heteroploid	Graham's 293 cells	Human embryonic kidney (HEK) cells transformed by sheared adenovirus type 5 DNA
Established heteroploid	HeLa	Adenocarcinoma of cervix; HPV-18 integrated into genome
Established heteroploid	HEp-2	Squamous cell carcinoma of larynx; transfected with HPV-16
Established heteroploid	LLC-MK2	Rhesus monkey kidney cells
Established heteroploid	McCoy	Mouse cell line of unknown origin
Established heteroploid	MDCK	Canine kidney cells with characteristics of tubular epithelium and papillary adenocarcinoma
Diploid cell line	MRC-5	Human embryonic lung fibroblasts
Established heteroploid	ML	Mink lung cells
Established heteroploid	RD	Human rhabdomyosarcoma cells
Established heteroploid	Vero	*Cercopithecus aethiops* (African green monkey) kidney cells
Diploid cell line	WI-38	Human embryonic lung fibroblasts

ethanesulfonic-acid), may be used in open systems if an incubator with CO_2 is not available. A pH indicator is often included in the media to monitor closely shifts in pH during incubation. Phenol red, which is red at physiologic pH, turning yellow at acidic pH and purple at alkaline pH, is frequently used.

Essential vitamins and amino acids must be supplied in viral culture media.[248] These compounds are stable when stored at 4°C, except for L-glutamine, which must be replenished periodically.[361] Eagle's Minimum Essential Medium

(MEM) is most commonly used, both for growth and for maintenance of cells. It is usually supplemented with small amounts of serum (up to 5%) for maintenance of a monolayer after cells have reached confluent growth. To enhance initial growth, larger amounts of serum (usually 10%) are used. It is important that the serum be free of infectious agents, including the mycoplasmas, and not contain antibodies to any viruses that might be present in clinical specimens. For this reason, either fetal, newborn, or agammaglobulinemic calf serum is most commonly used. Other formulations, such as Medium 199 or RPMI 1640, contain a richer mixture of nutrients and may be optimal for maintenance of some cell lines. Two forms of balanced salt solution are most frequently used, both for washing of cells and for incorporation into complete media. The formulations of Hanks' and Earle's solutions differ in several respects, notably the amount of buffering capacity. The two solutions are used virtually interchangeably, but Earle's balanced salt solution with its greater buffering power may be desirable for prolonged maintenance of monolayers.

Contamination of Cell Cultures

Contamination of media is reduced by inclusion of antibiotics. Penicillin (200 μg/mL) and streptomycin (200 μg/mL) or gentamicin (50 μg/mL) are commonly used for suppression of bacterial growth; amphotericin B (1.25 μg/mL) is used for inhibition of fungal growth.[248] The use of antibiotics does not substitute, however, for careful aseptic technique.

Contamination of culture media by *Mycoplasma* species is a common and troublesome problem.[344] *Mycoplasma* species usually are introduced in the serum additives or from contaminated stock viruses; once in the culture, they are very difficult to eradicate. The effects on the cells include suboptimal growth and disturbances in the interactions of cells and viruses. The presence of contaminating *Mycoplasma* species may be monitored by recovering them in culture, by staining for *Mycoplasma* DNA, by biochemical measurement of uracil incorporation, or by nucleoside phosphorylase activity techniques. Commercial suppliers of cells should be able to document their efforts at surveillance and quality control.

In addition, cell cultures may be contaminated with viruses (usually ones that were present in the original tissue)[248] or even with other cells.[373] The most frequent type of viral contamination is the presence of indigenous simian viruses in primary monkey cell cultures, such as the vacuolating agent (SV40), foamy viruses, or the monkey parainfluenza virus (SV5). Simian viruses that have hemagglutinins (e.g., SV5 virus) may produce misleading results if hemadsorption tests are performed. When myxoviruses are sought, it is important to perform control hemadsorption tests on uninoculated tubes from the same lot of cells that was used for the clinical specimens (see Chart 23-1; Figure 23-12*E*). The frequency with which tubes in a shipment of monkey kidney cells are contaminated may vary from 5–100%. Reserving a few uninoculated tubes for hemadsorption controls is not foolproof. If an unusual number of patients have hemadsorbing viruses on a given day, the possibility of simian virus contamination should be

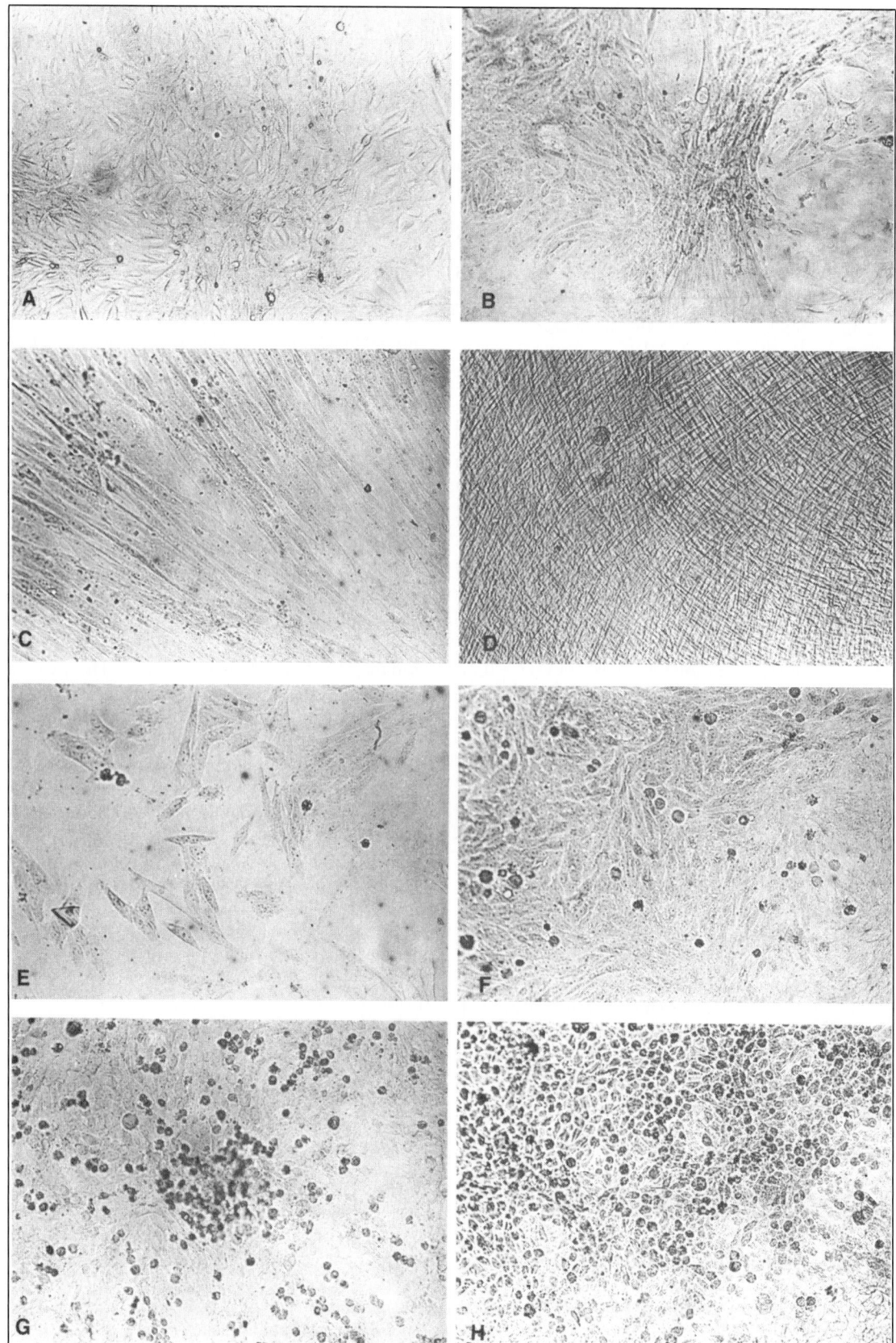

Figure 23-5 Normal cell cultures. (**A**) Normal rhesus monkey kidney monolayer. This primary culture is just at confluence—there are no spaces between the cells, but cells have not begun to pile on each other. The variability of the cells in the monolayer is a reflection of their origin

considered. Contamination of a commercial lot of A549 cells with infectious bovine rhinotracheitis virus has caused diagnostic problems in several laboratories.[161] Cytopathic effect in the contaminated monolayers resembled herpes simplex virus, but the agent could not be typed with available antisera. An additional problem was the inhibition by the contaminant virus of adenovirus that was in two of the specimens. The adenovirus isolates were subsequently recovered by inoculation of a new lot of A549 cells with residual specimen.

An extremely rare but potentially serious problem can be caused by the presence of pathogenic viruses in the tissues of monkeys. Although fortunately very rare, the simian herpes virus and Marburg virus, which produces a hemorrhagic fever, have caused lethal laboratory infections.[102,427,429] These agents provide justification for working with primary cell cultures of simian origin in a biologic safety cabinet.

Contamination of cell cultures with other cells has resulted in the erroneous supposition that a new cell line has been established in more than one research laboratory. In fact, a hardy HeLa cell may have found its way into the flask and taken over.[373] In the diagnostic laboratory, cross-contamination of an established cell line onto a diploid cell line or primary cell culture may give the appearance of cytopathic effects in the victimized cell culture (Fig. 23-6*D*).

Technical Aspects of Cell Culture

A variety of containers is used for the support of cell monolayers. The most common cell cultures in use are commercially available in tubes or vials that are ready for inoculation of specimens. Many laboratories may prefer, for reasons of economy, to maintain cell lines in their own laboratories. T-shaped plastic flasks have generally replaced glass bottles for the propagation of cell lines (Fig. 23-7).

Cell lines may be maintained in the laboratory by dissociation of cells, which are then distributed into new vessels (Box 23-5).

Established monolayers are dissociated by brief incubation in a solution of trypsin or a mixture of trypsin and ethylenediaminetetraacetic acid (EDTA), which is also known as Versene. Damage to cells may occur if the suspension of trypsin is too concentrated or if the contact is too prolonged. Neutralization of the trypsin is provided by serum in the growth medium that is added after cells have been dissociated. Detachment of the cells from the surface may be enhanced physically by agitation or by scraping with a rubber-tipped glass rod, a device known as a "rubber policeman" (see Fig. 23-7). The dissociated cells are then dispensed into tubes for inoculation of specimens or into additional flasks for continued propagation of stock cells. The density of the suspension can be adjusted to provide confluent monolayers after one or more days of incubation. After inoculation of clinical specimens, the same protocol may be used to prepare infected cells for subculture to additional monolayers.

Round-bottomed glass tubes (16 × 125 mm) are the containers most commonly used for viral isolation (Fig. 23-8). These tubes are incubated at a 5-degee fixed angle, so that the monolayer forms on one side of the tube. The heaviest aggregation occurs near the center and at the butt of the tubes; the thinnest layer is at the edges and toward the mouth. Round Petri dishes or glass slides, onto which are affixed plastic chambers, are less frequently used for diagnostic purposes. The slide-chamber system is expensive but useful if morphologic study of an undisrupted monolayer is planned.

Recently, shell vials, originally used for isolation of *Chlamydia trachomatis*, have been used to increase the frequency and speed with which viruses are isolated. A cell monolayer is prepared on a round glass coverslip that has been placed on the bottom of a flat-bottomed vial (Fig. 23-9). If the inoculum is centrifuged onto the monolayer, as is essential for the recovery of *C. trachomatis*, and the monolayer stained with fluorescein-conjugated antiserum or tested with a molecular probe, almost all isolates of herpes simplex virus

from diverse cell types (× 180). (**B**) Normal rhesus monkey kidney monolayer. After continued incubation, areas of more luxuriant growth have become evident. The variability of the cells in the monolayer can still be appreciated (× 180). (**C**) Normal MRC-5 fibroblast monolayer. These diploid fibroblastic cells have the elongated, spindly character of their type. They are just reaching confluence; a few spaces remain between some of the cells (× 180). (**D**) Normal MRC fibroblast monolayer. After continued incubation, the criss-cross pattern of fibroblasts piled one on top of the other is apparent. The detail of the individual cells is less apparent. Such senescent monolayers should not be inoculated (× 180). (**E**) Normal HEp-2 cells. An established cell line has been subcultured, and new cells have begun to grow. There are large spaces between individual cells, which have a spindle shape as they spread over the new glass surface (× 180). (**F**) Normal HEp-2 cells. The subcultured cells have now multiplied to the point of confluence but are still easily visible as distinct polygonal cells. The ideal point for inoculation of most viruses is at this stage or slightly earlier (× 180). (**G**) Normal HEp-2 cells. After continued incubation, the cell line has multiplied so that cells are piled one on top of the other. Cells that are dividing or detaching from the glass appear rounded. As the monolayers age, they become less susceptible to cytopathic effect of viruses, and it becomes increasingly difficult to detect cytopathic effect visually. (**H**) Normal McCoy cells. This established cell line, the origin of which is unknown, is pictured at a point at which confluent growth has been obtained. The cells are compact and polygonal. Specimens should be inoculated at this stage or when the cells are slightly less confluent (× 180).

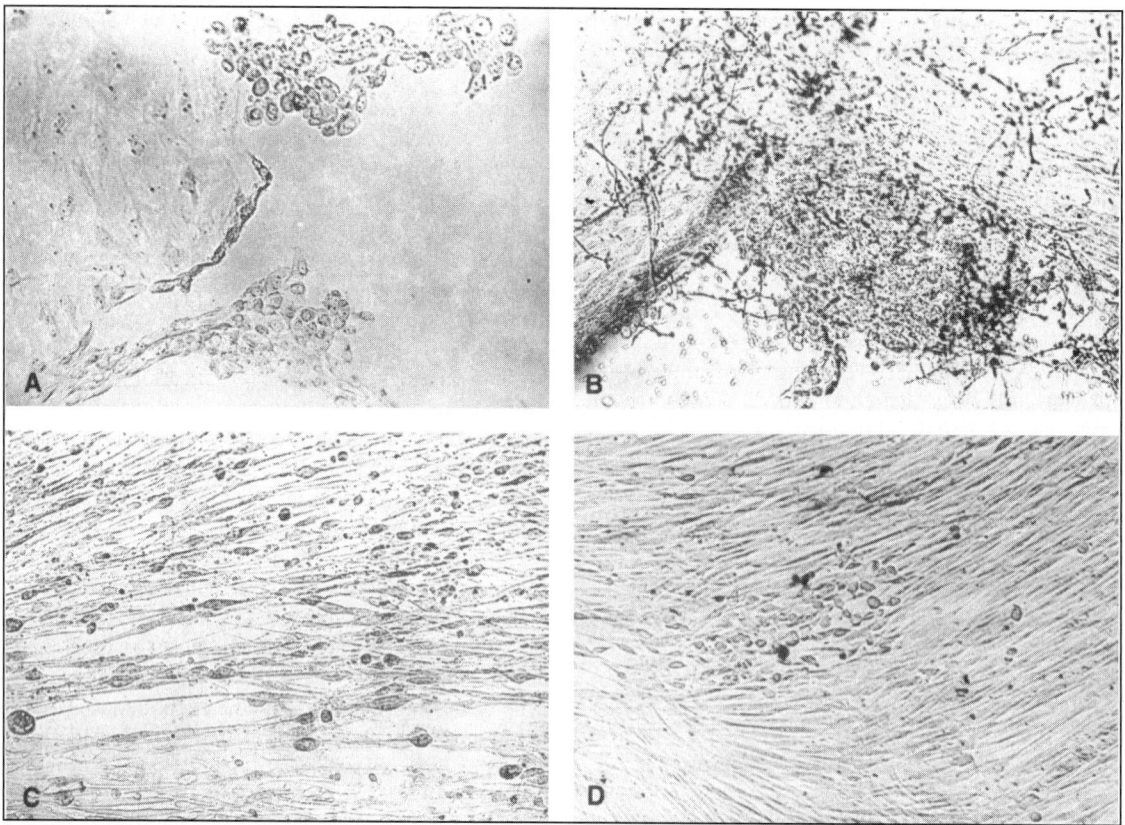

Figure 23-6 Artifacts in cell culture. (**A**) Rhesus monkey kidney cells. The tube has been inoculated with a specimen that contained nonspecific toxic material. Cells in the monolayer have rounded up focally, and many cells have detached from the glass. The nonviral effect can be distinguished from the viral cytopathic effect by the overall pattern, by the rapidity of occurrence, and by the inability to reproduce the nonspecific effect after subculture into fresh monolayers (×180). (**B**) Rhesus monkey kidney cell culture. A stool specimen was inadequately decontaminated before inoculation. Bacteria and fungal hyphae are evident on the monolayer, which is granular and will soon degenerate. The media may become acidic and cloudy. Retreatment of the specimen with additional antibiotics is necessary. The specimen may also be filtered, but cell-associated viruses may be lost (×180). (**C**) MRC-5 fibroblasts. A filtrate of stool that contained *Clostridium difficile* was inoculated onto the monolayer 24 hours earlier. The generalized disorganization of the monolayer with rounding and sloughing of cells is typical of this toxin. Specific identification of the cause of toxicity is provided by neutralization of the effect with specific antiserum. *C. difficile* toxin may give an initial impression of viral cytopathic effect, but the effect will not be reproduced when material from the suspect tube is subcultured onto additional monolayers (×180). (**D**) MRC-5 fibroblasts. Focal cell rounding and enlargement appeared on these fibroblasts that had been inoculated with CSF, suggesting viral cytopathic effect. The atypical progression of cytopathic effect and observation that some of the foci were superimposed on the fibroblasts suggested cellular contamination. HEp-2 cells were subsequently recovered from the tube and demonstrated to have a karyotype that was identical to that of the HEp-2 cells used in the laboratory. The mechanism by which the contamination occurred was never elucidated (×180).

can be detected within 24 hours.[148] The recovery of herpes simplex virus in conventional culture is sufficiently rapid that addition of an expensive procedure can be questioned.

A far more dramatic improvement in the speed of isolation has been reported for CMV.[162,388] The technique is more sensitive than conventional culture for most specimens other than blood, but use of both approaches maximizes results. The preferred method for detecting CMV in blood—and a

better way to differentiate infection from disease—is testing for viral antigen or nucleic acid. The gain from shell vial culture comes both from centrifugation and from the use of a fluoresceinated monoclonal antibody of high quality. Even supposedly uniform reagents, such as monoclonal antibodies, may vary from lot to lot. Nonspecific staining of cell nuclei may occur with some lots of antisera. The appearance of a shell vial culture containing CMV is shown in Color

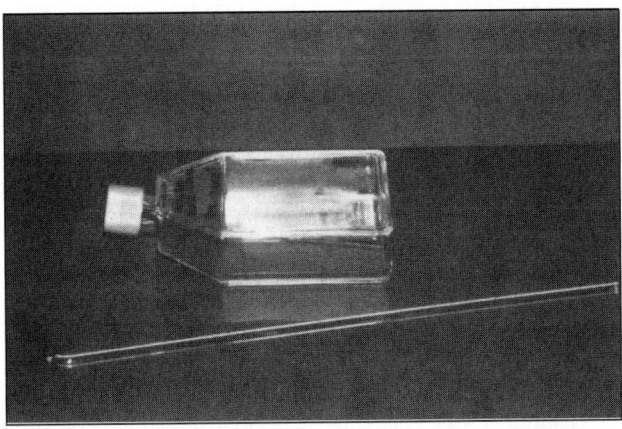

Figure 23-7 T-shaped plastic flask and rubber-tipped glass rod, known as a "rubber policeman." Monolayers of cell lines may be grown in large flasks. Many individual tubes for virus culture may be prepared from a single large flask. Mechanical disruption by pipetting or by the rubber policeman helps to dislodge the cells during trypsinization for subculture.

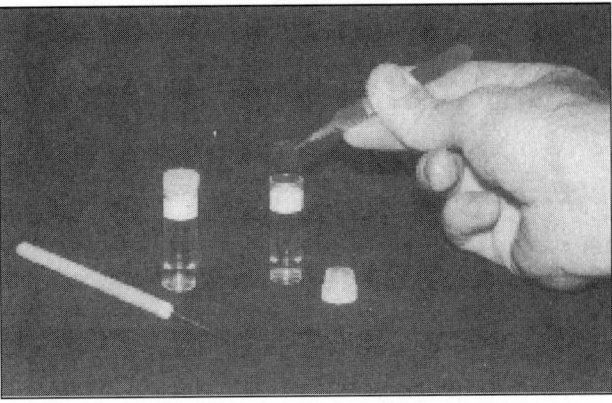

Figure 23-9 Shell vials for isolation of *Chlamydia trachomatis* and viruses. The vials are round with a flat bottom and contain a round coverslip on which the cells are grown. The top may be rubber or plastic as shown here. The coverslip is removed with forceps or with a needle.

Box 23-5 Procedure for Maintaining Cell Lines

1. The monolayer is washed with phosphate-buffered saline, pH 7.5.
2. A suspension of 0.25% trypsin or equal parts of 0.25% trypsin and 1 : 2,000 Versene is added for 15 to 30 seconds, then removed.
3. The monolayer is incubated at 35 °C until the cells have dissociated. Gentle shaking of the flask may enhance dissociation.
4. Growth medium is added and the cells resuspended at the concentration desired for subculture. Alternatively, the cells may be divided arbitrarily (1 : 2 or 1 : 3) as dictated by past experience.

Plate 23-2*F*. Paya and colleagues have studied the number of shell vials required for each specimen.[389] They found that three vials were required for maximal yield from blood specimens, whereas two vials were needed for urine, bronchoalveolar lavage, and tissue. Fedorko and colleagues found that the age of fibroblasts in the shell vials was important for recovery of cytomegalovirus. Old monolayers (8–15 days) were less sensitive for virus recovery but more sensitive to toxic components in the specimens than were young monolayers.[154] It is difficult for manufacturers to provide very young monolayers, and unfortunately most laboratories must depend on commercial suppliers for shell vials.

Gleaves and colleagues have reported success with still a third cell-associated herpesvirus, VZV.[188] They examined 68 specimens from 60 patients. VZV was identified by some method in 57% of patients. The sensitivity of diagnostic techniques in decreasing order was direct immunofluorescence of skin scrapings, shell vial culture, and conventional culture. Schirm and colleagues have confirmed the utility of

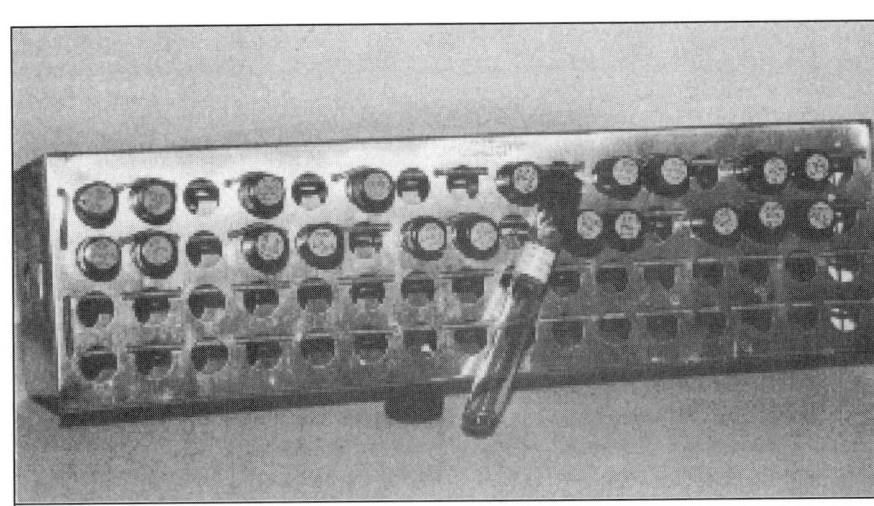

Figure 23-8 Viral culture tubes are slanted at a fixed angle of 5 degrees in a stationary rack. Metal springs hold the tubes in place. Round labels for the tops of the tubes facilitate identification of cultures without removing the tubes from the racks.

shell vial culture for VZV.[436] They were able to detect half of the positive patients within 3 days using shell vials and a monoclonal antibody, whereas the conventional tube method detected one third of the patients after a mean of 7.5 days. One factor in the yield of cell cultures is the choice of cell lines. Human diploid fibroblasts have been used most commonly, but the addition of rhesus monkey kidney cells[514] or A549 cells[44] substantially improves the recovery rate in conventional tube cultures. The enhanced recovery is less evident with shell vial cultures.[44] Presumably, the shell vial centrifugation technique increases contact of inoculum with monolayer, thus blunting the differences in sensitivity among cell lines, but the exact mechanisms are unknown. An additional manipulation that has been reported to be useful for VZV is freeze-thawing of the specimen before spin amplification.[45] The mechanism for the effect is not clear, as the speed of centrifugation is not sufficiently great to sediment free virus.

The shell vial technique has also been applied to viruses other than the herpes group, particularly influenza virus.[137] Other respiratory viruses are also detected using the shell vial technique, but experience is more limited and somewhat less satisfactory than with influenza. The shell vial technique has also been used for BK virus.[330]

Selection of Cell Cultures for Isolation of Viruses

The basic requirements for isolation of viruses in culture are a primary culture of simian kidney cells (for isolation of myxoviruses and enteroviruses) and a diploid cell line of human origin (essential for isolation of CMV, rhinovirus, and VZV; useful for isolation of herpes simplex virus). The addition of an established cell line of human origin (e.g., HEp-2 or A549) is also useful for isolation of adenovirus and respiratory syncytial virus.

Other cell lines may provide satisfactory substitutes for these three basic cell types if isolation of a specific virus is desired (Table 23-21). The additional cell lines may be used as substitutes for simian cells if simian cells are not available; alternatively, they may be used selectively to enhance the isolation rate of specific viruses during seasons when infections would be expected. There are no substitutes for human diploid fibroblasts.

The quality and provenance of the cells used for isolation are important. Careful studies of cloned fibroblasts from a single fetus demonstrated a large variation in the degree to which the clones supported the growth of respiratory viruses.[484] Variants of established cell lines, such as HeLa and HEp-2, differ also in the sensitivity with which they support some viruses. It is important to ensure that the selected cell variant is of adequate sensitivity.

Once a cell line has been found acceptable, multiple aliquots should be frozen in liquid nitrogen. Cells for daily use may be maintained in continuous culture. The original stock should be used periodically to replenish the working stock so that the cells do not mutate to a state that is less susceptible to viral growth.

Rhesus and cynomolgus monkey kidney cells are comparable for isolation of myxoviruses. MRC-5 fibroblasts, on the other hand, have been reported to be more sensitive than

WI-38 fibroblasts for the isolation of CMV.[202] The sensitivity of all diploid cell lines decreases as the number of passages increases. Some commercial suppliers are now using cells that have been subcultured as many as 30 times. The lowest passage level from a reliable supplier should be sought. If cell sheets, particularly those of established cell lines, are too thick, recovery of viruses may be reduced and evaluation of cytopathic effects is difficult. For some viruses, islands of cells or a barely confluent monolayer are preferable to a fully confluent cell sheet.[483]

In addition, the cells must be in sufficiently good condition to last the several weeks necessary for isolation of slowly growing viruses. Contamination with *Mycoplasma* species should be avoided if maximal isolation rates are to be ensured. Viruses, such as VZV, that spread directly from cell to cell rather than through the culture medium, require a healthy monolayer.

Use of growth medium with 10% serum may enhance development and progression of cytopathic effects caused by these viruses,[511] although we are not convinced that this manipulation is necessary. In contrast, serum contains inhibitors of myxoviruses and paramyxoviruses. The maintenance medium in the cells used for these viruses (usually primary monkey kidney) should be free of serum. Some manufacturers include (or offer) antisera to common endogenous simian viruses (e.g., SV5 or SV40). This approach is not uniformly accepted; in practice, the antisera will be eliminated when the shipping media are replaced with new media that lack the antisera.

Inoculation and Incubation of Cell Cultures

Transport vials that contain swabs should be vortexed and material from the swab expressed into the medium, which contains antibiotics. Tissues are minced and homogenized in a small volume of transport broth. It may be necessary to suspend fecal specimens in 10 volumes of transport medium. Feces, tissues, and respiratory aspirates that contain excessive debris or mucus may be clarified by low-speed centrifugation. Antibiotics are present in most transport and tissue culture media. If bacterial or fungal contamination of the specimen is expected, additional antibiotics should be added to the specimen before inoculation (penicillin and streptomycin or gentamicin plus amphotericin at twice the concentration used in cell culture media).[248] After processing, the specimen may be inoculated into the culture media. Alternatively, the inoculum may be placed directly onto the monolayer after most of the culture medium has been removed. The more direct contact of viral particles with cells enhances infectivity and may increase both the number of isolates and the speed with which they are recovered. After adsorption of the inoculum onto the monolayer for 30 to 60 minutes at 36 to 37°C, the medium is replaced and incubation of the culture is continued. Toxic substances in the specimen may also be more evident after adsorption of the inoculum. If two tubes of each cell type are used, one may be inoculated by introducing a specimen into the medium and the other by adsorption. Any remaining specimen should be retained at 4°C or frozen at −70°C in case toxicity or bacterial contamination occurs. If bacterial or fungal growth results, additional antibiotics may be added to the specimen. The specimen may be passed through a 0.45-μm micropore filter before additional cultures are inoculated, but viruses that are cell-associated, such as CMV and VZV, may be lost when infected cells are trapped in the filter.[307] Nonspecific toxicity to the monolayer is usually evident within 24 hours; the specimen may then be reinoculated after making a 1:10 dilution in balanced salt solution. The pH of the specimen should also be checked and adjusted to neutrality if the specimen is very acid or alkaline. If nonspecific degeneration of the monolayer occurs after incubation for several days, the cells and fluid may be subcultured onto fresh monolayer.

Monolayers should be incubated at 36 to 37°C for recovery of most viruses. The optimal temperature of incubation for respiratory viruses, especially rhinovirus, is 33°C, but recovery of other viruses may be reduced at this temperature. Use of a roller drum (Fig. 23-10) facilitates isolation of pathogens in primary monkey kidney and diploid fibroblast cells, especially from respiratory specimens.

Two weeks of incubation is adequate for the recovery of most other viruses. CMV may require longer incubation, but Gregory and Menegus found that 92% of CMV isolates were recovered within 14 days when MRC-5 fibroblasts were used.[202] If the recovery of only herpes simplex virus is sought, the period of incubation may be further abbreviated to 7 days. Centrifugation of the inoculum and detection of antigen will dramatically shorten the detection time for several viruses, including CMV and VZV. Hemadsorption tests should be performed after incubation of primary monkey kidney cells for 5 and 10 days.

Detection of Virus and Provisional Identification
CYTOPATHIC EFFECT

The most common method for detecting a virus is examination of cultures for virus-induced damage to the monolayers or cytopathic effect. Monolayers should be examined

daily if herpes simplex virus is sought and at least three times a week if more slowly growing viruses are suspected. Glass tubes can be examined with a conventional light microscope, using simple holders to prevent the round tubes from rolling on the microscope stage (Fig. 23-11). If the monolayer is to be examined in shell vials, an inverted microscope must be used.

Provisional identification of the specific virus (or at least the virus group) can often be provided on the basis of the type of cytopathic effect and the type of cell that is affected. Typical patterns of cytopathic effect and the rate of isolation for viruses most commonly isolated in hospital laboratories are summarized in Table 23-23.

When one examines a culture in the laboratory, the pattern of cytopathic effect is known but the name of the virus is not. A flow chart for analyzing cytopathic effect in a clinical specimen is presented in Table 23-24. This table represents the most common patterns of cytopathic effect. The inclusion of all possible combinations for all strains would make the table unwieldy and probably useless.

The effects of the virus on the cells may be subtle initially. Although quantitation of the viral inoculum based on the extent of cytopathic effect is not precise, it is useful to make a laboratory record of the semiquantitative estimate for comparative purposes (1+, <25% of the monolayer affected; 2+, 25–50%; 3+, 51–75%; 4+, >75%). These estimates make it easier to document progression of cytopathic effect and establish the presence of a cytopathic agent. It may be necessary to subculture the cells from a tube with a possible cytopathic effect onto fresh monolayers. If possible, such a subculture should be performed after cytopathic effect has reached 2+, using trypsinization, physical disruption of the

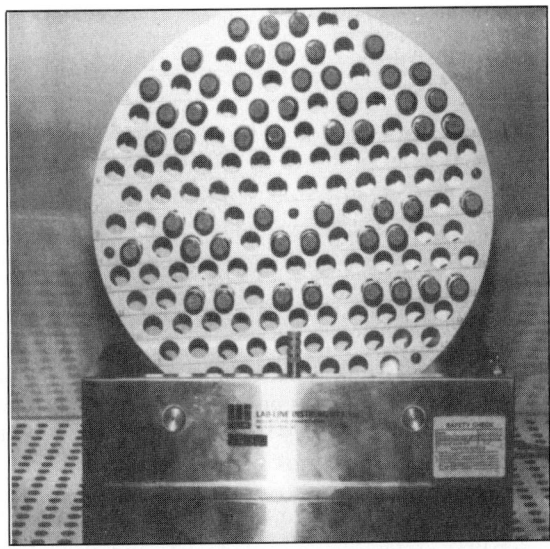

Figure 23-10 Roller drum for viral cultures. Cytopathic effect of many viruses, especially those that cause respiratory infection, is enhanced by slow rotation of the tubes, so that one revolution occurs every 3 minutes.

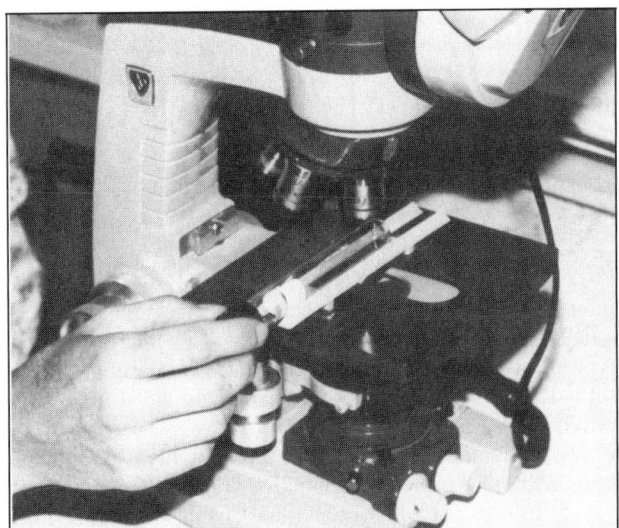

Figure 23-11 Examination of cultures for cytopathic effect. Examination of cultures for cytopathic effect can be performed with an inverted or a traditional microscope. A rack, which fits in the specimen holder of the microscope stage, prevents the round tubes from rolling. High magnification is not possible but is not needed for recognition and characterization of cytopathic effect.

Table 23-23   Differential Diagnosis of Viral Cytopathic Effect

| VIRUS | CELL CULTURE | | | DAYS TO ISOLATION | | DESCRIPTION |
	PMK	HDF	HEP-2	Mayo Mean[a]	Mt. Zion Mean[b]	
Influenza virus	+++	−	−	4	3.8	None or focal enlarged granular cells followed by sloughing; rapid progression
Parainfluenza virus	+++	+	+	11	6.4	None or focal rounding and multinucleated giant cells (types 2 and 3)
Respiratory syncytial virus	++	+	+++	8.3	6.1	Enlarged, glassy syncytial giant cells or granular, rounded cells
Mumps virus	+++	+	−	6.9		Enlarged, syncytial giant cells
Measles virus	+	−	+			Vacuolated, syncytial giants cells; rarely isolated
Poliovirus	+++	+++	+++	4.6		Random, swollen, glassy cells; rapid progression and detachment of cells from glass
Coxsackievirus B	+++	+	+++	3.5	4.2	Focal, swollen, glassy cells; detachment from glass
Echoviruses	+++	+++	+	3.9	4.2	Focal, swollen, glassy cells: detachment from glass
Rhinovirus	+	+++	−	6.6		Focal, swollen, or granular cells
Adenovirus	++	+	+++	6.2	6.4	Enlarged, clustered cells (bunches of grapes or lattice)
Herpes simplex virus	++	+++	++	3.5	2.7	Enlarged or shrunken granular cells starting at edge; rapid progression and sloughing; may have giant cells
Varicella-zoster virus	++	++	−	7.6	6.1	Discrete, elongated foci of enlarged or shrunken cells; slow contiguous progression enhanced by use of growth medium
Cytomegalovirus	−	+++	−	10	5.8	Compact foci of enlarged cells; slow, contiguous progression

+++, *Optimal cells for detection of cytopathic effect (CPE);* ++, *CPE frequent, may be best available system for detection of CPE;* +, *CPE occasionally be observed;* −, *CPE does not usually occur; PMK, primary monkey kidney cells; HDF, human diploid fibroblast cells; HEp-2, human continuous cell line*

[a] *From the Mayo Clinic, abstracted from Herrmann EC Jr. Experience in providing a viral diagnostic laboratory compatible with medical practice. Mayo Clin Proc 1967;42:112–123; and Herrmann EC Jr. Efforts toward a more useful viral diagnostic laboratory. Am J Clin Pathol 1971;56:681–686.*

[b] *From Mount Zion Hospital and Medical Center, San Francisco, abstracted from Drew WL. Controversies in viral diagnosis. Rev Infect Dis 1986;8:814–824.*

Adapted from McIntosh K. Diagnostic virology. In: Fields BN, Knipe DM, Melnick JL, et al., eds. Virology. Ed. 2. New York: Raven Press, 1990:411–440.

monolayer with a rubber policeman, or several cycles of quick freeze/thawing. Then, an aliquot is inoculated onto the type of cell in which cytopathic effect was originally observed and any other cell type that might aid in making a provisional diagnosis.

Viral cytopathic effects for three commonly used cell cultures are demonstrated sequentially in Figures 23-12 through 23-15. In most cases early and late changes have been depicted.

There are relatively few ways in which cells can express cytotoxicity. Rounding is a common expression of damage, but cells may appear either swollen or shrunken and granular or glassy. Some viruses produce factors that cause cell fusion, leading to the formation of multinucleated giant cells, which are also called syncytial cells; respiratory syncytial virus, parainfluenza viruses 2 and 3, measles virus, and

mumps virus can produce syncytial giant cells. In addition, herpes simplex virus and VZV produce smaller multinucleated giant cells.

Not all isolates of respiratory syncytial virus produce syncytial cells. Production of the F(usion) glycoprotein by the virus is required for cell fusion. Shahrabadi and Lee demonstrated that calcium must be present in the culture medium for respiratory syncytial virus-induced fusion of HEp-2 cells to occur.[449] The formation of syncytial giant cells also appears related, at least in part, to the concentration of glutamine in the culture medium.[328]

Cytopathic effect usually starts focally and often is most readily seen at the edges of the monolayer, where the density of cells is low. For viruses that spread from cell to cell through the culture media, cytopathic effect progresses from focality to totality, sometimes with great rapidity. If the num-

Table 23-24   Differential Diagnosis of Viral Cytopathic Effect

PRIMARY ISOLATION IN:			RBC HAD	CPE TYPE	VIRUS SUSPECTED	COMMENTS AND ANCILLARY TESTS	CONFIR- MATION
PMK	HDF	HEP-2					
+	+	+	−	Swelling/shrinking/ hyaline	Poliovirus		NT, FA
				Syncytium in HEp-2 and PMK	Respiratory syn- cytical virus		FA, NT, EIA
				Rounded, swollen, especially in fibroblasts	Herpes simplex	Growth in rabbit kidney	FA, EIA
				Swollen clusters/ lattice	Adenovirus		NT, FA, CF
+	+	−	−	Swelling/shrinking/ hyaline	Echovirus Cox- sackievirus A		NT, FA
				Focal, linear swelling/giant cells	Varicella-zoster	Cell association on passage	NT, FA
				Swelling/shrinking	Rhinovirus	pH 3 lability	NT
			+ (Guinea pig)	Large, granular syncytium	Mumps	Rarely isolated	HAI, NT
+	−	+	−	Swelling/shrinking/ hyaline/	Coxsackievirus B		NT, FA
				Swollen clusters/ lattice/	Adenovirus		NT, FA, CF
			+ (Monkey)	Vacuolated syncytium	Measles	Rarely isolated; clinical history; HAd	NT, FA
			+ (Guinea pig	Rounding, syncytium	Parainfluenza 2 and 3	HAd	FA, HAI
+	−	−	+ (Guinea pig	None/rounding	Influenza Parain- fluenza 1–3	HAd 4C = 20C HAd 4C = <20C	HAI, FA, CF HAI, FA, CF
				Syncytium	Parainfluenza 2 and	HAd	HAI, FA, CF
				Large, granular syn- cytium	Mumps	Rarely isolated	HAI, NT
			+ (Monkey)	Vacuolated syncyticum	Measles	Rarely isolated; clinical history; HAd	NT, FA
2	1	2	2	Focal/enlarged cells	Cytomegalovirus	Cell association	FA, H&E
				Focal, linear plaques	Varicella-zoster	Cell association; H&E	FA, CF
				Focal/swelling	Rhinovirus	pH 3 lability	NT

PMK, primary monkey kidney cells; HDF, human diploid fibroblast cells; HEp-2, human continuous cell line; CPE, cytopathic effect HAd, hemadsorption; FA, immunofluorescence; NT, neutralization test; CF, complement fixation; EIA, enzyme-linked immunosorbent assay; H&E, stain for inclusions.

ber of virions in the specimen is very large, most of the monolayer may be infected simultaneously; in this case, widespread degeneration must be differentiated from non-specific cytotoxicity by subculture of fluid to fresh cell cultures. For viruses that spread directly from cell to cell (CMV and VZV) cytopathic effect progresses more slowly and by local extension of the initial foci. We have, however, seen cultures in which a very large amount of CMV in the specimen produced cytopathic effect through the whole mono-layer, mimicking the effect produced by herpes simplex virus.

It is, of course, somewhat artificial to try to capture the considerable variability of a biologic process in a single pho-tographic frame. In a clinical laboratory, it will be possible to examine other parts of the monolayer, view other cell cultures, and even reexamine a suspicious culture after incu-bation for a few more hours. It will often be possible, there-fore, to detect cytologic changes that are even earlier than those that make convincing photographs.

HEMAGGLUTINATION AND HEMADSORPTION

Many viruses contain surface components that aggluti-nate red cells from various species of animals. Some viruses,

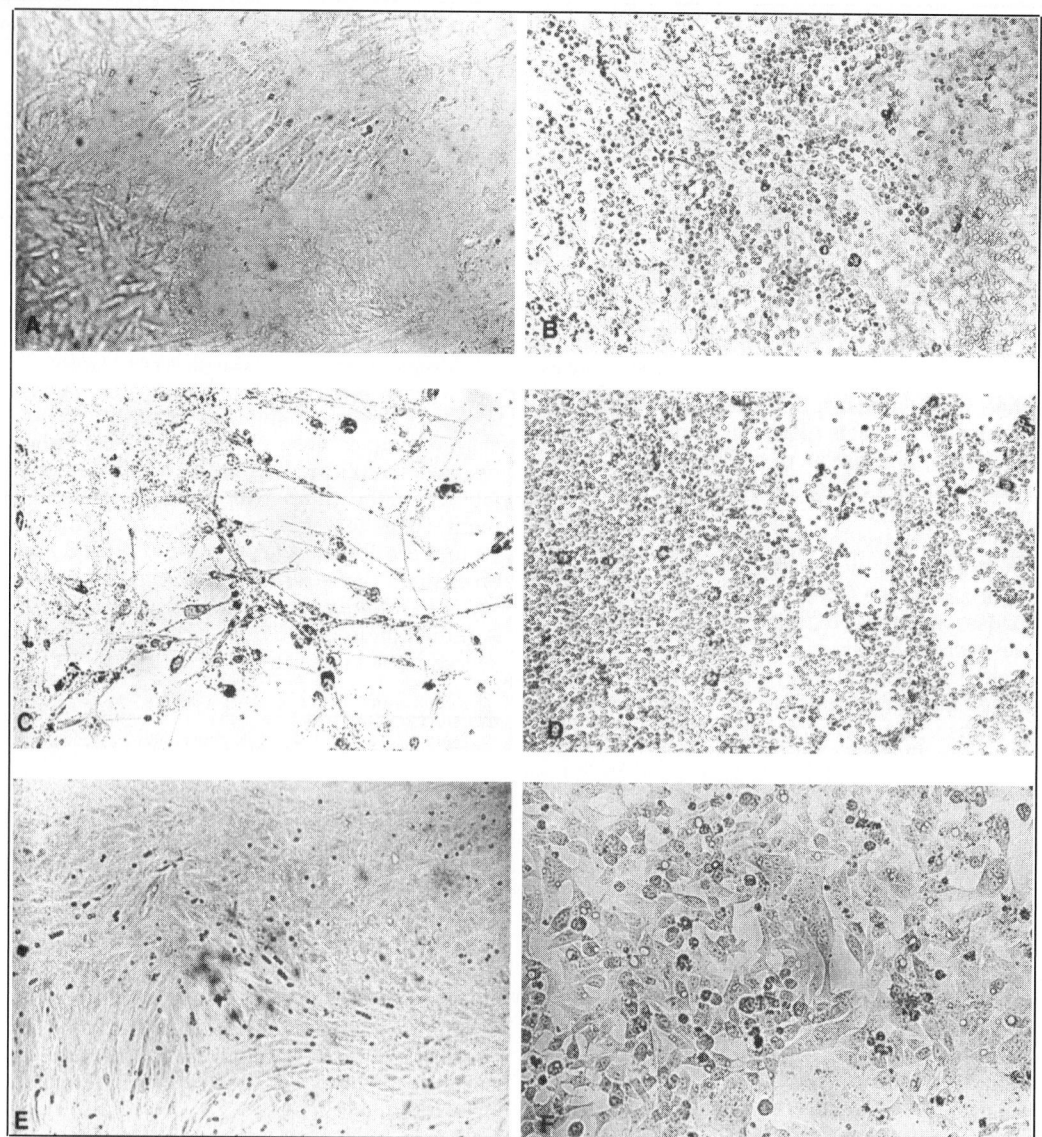

Figure 23-12 Cytopathic effect of myxoviruses. (**A**) Rhesus monkey kidney cells infected with influenza A virus. This isolate produces no cytopathic effect in the monolayer. A hemadsorption test identified the presence of a virus. Many of the current strains of influenza A virus and most strains of influenza B virus produce cytopathic effect, which often develops more rapidly than that produced by the parainfluenza viruses (×180). (**B**) Rhesus monkey kidney cells infected with influenza A virus. The monolayer is intact but is covered with numerous guinea pig red cells. The red cells have adhered to the viral hemagglutinins on the surface of the infected cells. Hemagglutination of red cells in the fluid phase by free virus can often be detected but is not shown in the photograph (×180). (**C**) Rhesus monkey kidney cells infected with parainfluenza virus 3. The monolayer has degenerated, and cells have fallen off the glass. Many of the remaining cells are enlarged or granular. Often, isolates of parainfluenza viruses do not produce obvious cytopathic effect and must be detected by hemadsorption (×180). (**D**) Rhesus monkey kidney cells infected with parainfluenza virus 3. A hemadsorption test has been performed. The remaining cells are covered with guinea pig red cells that have attached to the viral hemagglutinin on the cell membranes (×180). (**E**) Rhesus monkey kidney cells that are uninfected demonstrate a negative hemadsorption test. A few guinea pig red blood cells have stuck to the monolayer, but the massive adherence of red blood cells that characterizes a positive test is not present. The settled cells are also dislodged more easily from an uninfected monolayer than from a myxovirus-infected monolayer by shaking the tube. (**F**) HEp-2 cells infected with parainfluenza virus 3. Large multinucleated giant cells (known as syncytial cells) have formed in the monolayer by fusion of adjacent cells. This type of cytopathic effect is characteristic of parainfluenza viruses 2 and 3 in monkey kidney cells and parainfluenza virus 3 in HEp-2 cells. Syncytial cells are also formed by other viruses, notably respiratory syncytial virus. The parainfluenza viruses can be differentiated from respiratory syncytial virus easily by performance of a hemadsorption test (×180).

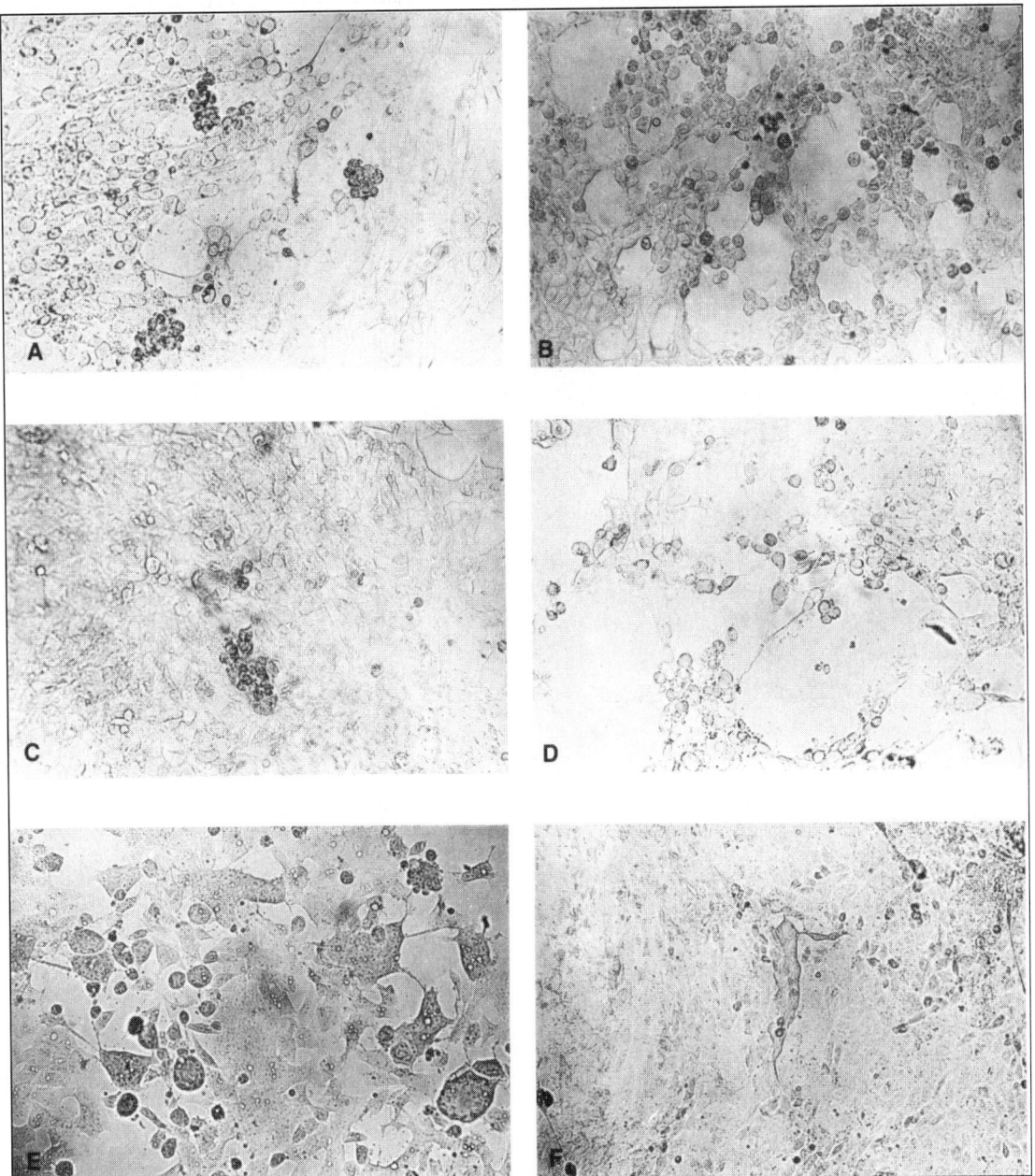

Figure 23-13 Cytopathic effect of other respiratory viruses. (**A**) HEp-2 cells infected with adenovirus. Several foci of enlarged, granular cells are evident. Adenovirus cells are often clustered like bunches of grapes, much as are staphylococci in a Gram stain ($\times$180). (**B**) HEp-2 cells infected with adenovirus. Most of the cells in the monolayer are now rounded; many cells have detached from the glass, leaving multiple holes. In several places, clustering of cells can be seen. Strands of cytoplasm connect some of the residual infected cells, producing the beginning of a lattice effect. ($\times$180). (**C**) Rhesus monkey kidney cells infected with adenovirus. One cluster of granular, enlarged cells is evident. A preliminary report could be issued if multiple foci were present in the culture. If only a few are present, it would be best to observe the monolayer for progression of cytopathic effect. ($\times$180). (**D**) Rhesus monkey kidney cells infected with adenovirus. The extent of cytopathic effect has increased considerably. Clustered, swollen cells with intercellular cytoplasmic bridges are evident. Many cells have detached from the glass. Eventually, there will be only scattered cells left on the glass tube as evidence that a monolayer was once present ($\times$180). (**E**) HEp-2 cells infected with respiratory syncytial virus. Many of the cells in the monolayer have been fused by the virus to form syncytial giant cells, much like those formed by parainfluenza viruses. Other cells are enlarged or have detached from the glass. A hemadsorption test on this monolayer would be negative. ($\times$180). (**F**) Rhesus monkey kidney cells infected with respiratory syncytial virus. One large syncytium has formed in the monolayer. One could differentiate this isolate from parainfluenza virus by hemadsorption or by identification of specific antigen.

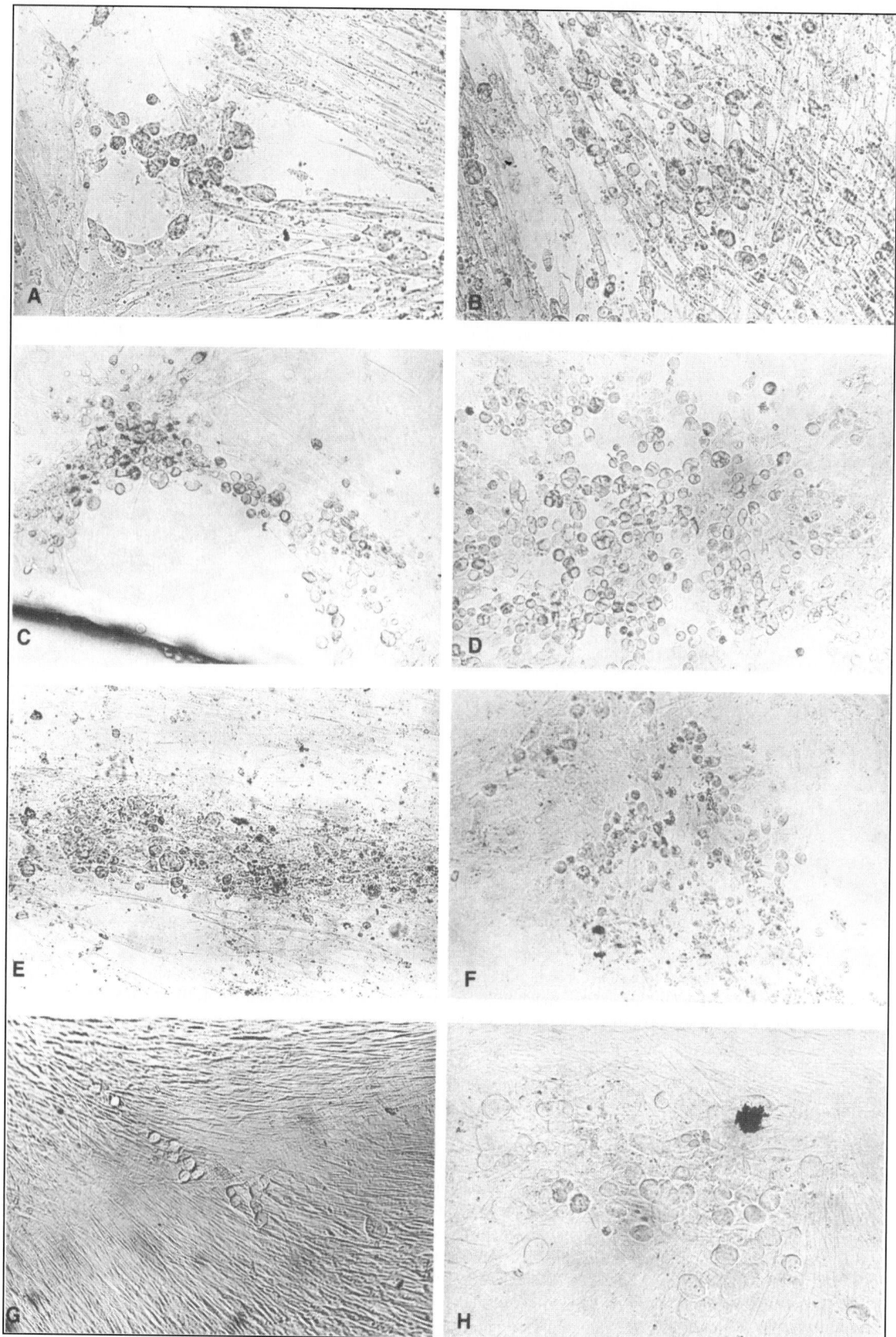

Figure 23-14 Cytopathic effect of herpesviruses. (**A**) MRC-5 fibroblasts infected with herpes simplex virus. There is a focus of enlarged, rounded cells in the monolayer. Many cells have detached from the glass. Such foci will enlarge rapidly, and the entire monolayer is usually

primarily those of the myxovirus and paramyxovirus groups, also insert the hemagglutinins into the membrane of the infected cell as the virus matures at the cytoplasmic membrane. Some isolates of influenza A virus and the parainfluenza viruses may be detected only by hemagglutination or hemadsorption (see Fig. 23-12A and B).

The hemagglutination test is performed less frequently than the hemadsorption test for detection of isolates in cell culture but is required if eggs have been inoculated. Hemagglutination of red cells is observed in tubes or microtiter plates after addition of fluid from infected cultures or eggs. If characterization of the strain is necessary, inhibition of viral hemagglutination by specific antiviral serum is the most economical procedure. New strains of influenza viruses are typed by this method in reference laboratories; cross-reacting inhibition by antisera against previous strains allows an assessment of how closely related the new strain is to previous isolates.

The hemadsorption test for myxoviruses (see Fig. 23-12A through E) is performed by adding fresh guinea pig red cells to an infected monolayer (see Chart 23-1).[493] The test can be performed without damage to the monolayer, after which incubation of the cell culture can be continued. Agglutination of the red cells in the fluid phase may be observed in addition to hemadsorption. The processes of hemadsorption and hemagglutination are shown in Figure 23-16.

Hemadsorption is more convenient than hemagglutination for testing the presence of virus in most clinical laboratories. Hemadsorption inhibition can also be used to identify

isolates, but it is much more wasteful of antisera than is hemagglutination inhibition.

LIGHT MICROSCOPY

As they replicate, some viruses produce masses of nucleoprotein and virions in various stages of assembly. The anatomic pathologist or cytologist uses these viral inclusions to detect the presence of a viral infection and identify the agent presumptively.[470,526] Although the characteristics of cytopathic effect in unstained monolayers are usually sufficient to render a provisional diagnosis, the virologist may gain additional information simply by staining the cells with hematoxylin and eosin, with the Papanicolaou stain, or with acridine orange (see Color Plate 23-1).

ELECTRON MICROSCOPY

For laboratories with access to an electron microscope, the ultrastructural morphology of an isolate may identify the group to which it belongs.[6,366] Negative-staining electron microscopy is simple and may be accomplished rapidly on supernatant fluid or lysed cells. This technique may be particularly useful for differentiation of nonspecific toxicity from a large viral inoculum.

BIOCHEMICAL DIFFERENTIATION

The cytolytic changes produced by rhinoviruses may resemble those of enteroviruses, although rhinoviruses repli-

---

involved within a few days (×180). (**B**) MRC-5 fibroblasts infected with herpes simplex virus. Cytopathic effect has progressed so that virtually every cell in the monolayer is affected. Again, the cells are enlarged, even ballooned, and granular. This type of generalized cytopathic effect can occasionally be seen with cytomegalovirus if very large quantities of virus are present, as in patients with AIDS. Cytomegalovirus can be distinguished from herpes simplex virus by identification of specific antigens and by demonstration that transfer of cells is necessary to transfer cytopathic effect to new cultures efficiently (×180). (**C**) Rhesus monkey kidney cells infected with herpes simplex. As often happens at the outset, this focus of cytopathic effect is at the edge of the monolayer. Enlarged, ballooned cells surround the center of the focus, where the cells have already detached from the glass (×180). (**D**) HEp-2 cells infected with herpes simplex virus. There is a large focus of swollen cells in the monolayer. Some of the cells have the appearance of multinucleated giant cells, although it is difficult to delineate the cellular structure in an unstained preparation at low magnification. (×180). (**E**) MRC-5 fibroblasts infected with varicella-zoster virus. A cytopathic focus consists of large swollen cells and granular degenerated cells. The focus is elongating in the direction of the underlying fibroblasts. The slow appearance and slow progression of the foci are characteristic. Transfer of cytopathic effect requires the inclusion of infected cells. Cytopathic effect has some similarities to that of cytomegalovirus; the foci of cytomegalovirus tend to be more compact and spread centrifugally without such a pronounced linear orientation (×180). (**F**) Rhesus monkey kidney cells infected with varicella-zoster virus. A focus of enlarged, swollen cells is less distinctive than cytopathic effect in MRC-5 cells. It can be differentiated from that produced by herpes simplex virus by the speed with which it appears and progresses. Cytomegalovirus does not produce cytopathic effect in monkey cells (×180). (**G**) WI-38 fibroblasts infected with cytomegalovirus. There is a small focus of enlarged, granular cells in the monolayer (×180). (**H**) MRC-5 fibroblasts infected with cytomegalovirus. A developing focus of cytopathic effect is evident. The cells are swollen, and the focus is quite compact. Cytopathic effect of cytomegalovirus appears late and progresses slowly. It tends to be more compact and less linear than that of varicella-zoster virus. Differentiation from varicella is by clinical history, by demonstration of multinucleated giant cells in varicella monolayers, and by demonstration of specific antigen (×180).

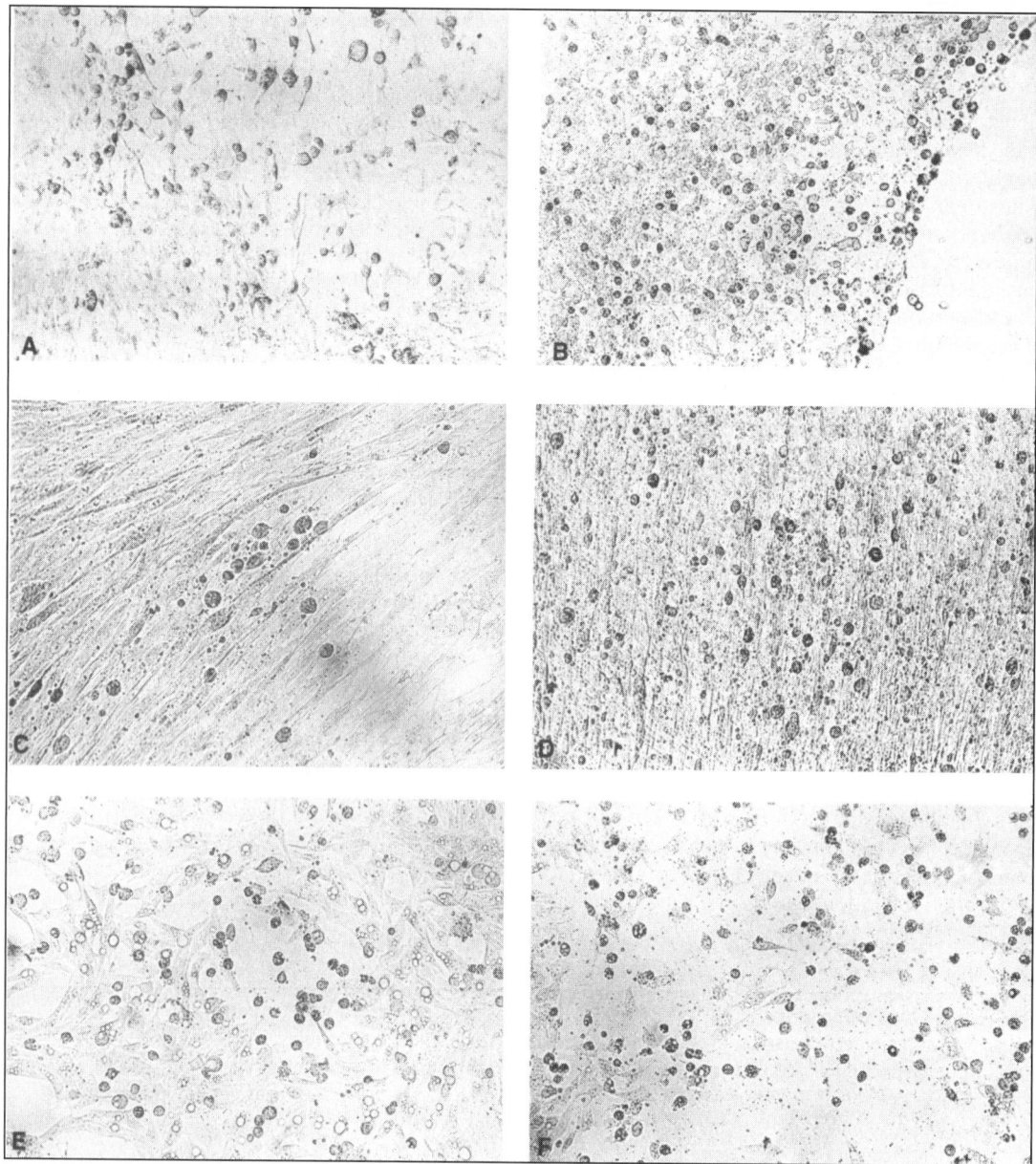

Figure 23-15 Cytopathic effect of enteroviruses. (**A**) Rhesus monkey kidney cells infected with coxsackievirus B. There is a focus of cytopathic effect in which cells are either small and shrunken or enlarged. Some of the cells have a refractile or glassy appearance that is typical of enteroviral cytopathic effect. Elongated "tadpole" cells are also typical of the cytopathology produced by this group of viruses ($\times$180). (**B**) Rhesus monkey kidney cells infected with coxsackievirus B. Cytopathic effect progresses relatively rapidly with the enteroviruses; poliovirus may cause complete destruction of the monolayer overnight. In this photomicrograph, virtually every cell in the monolayer has been damaged, and large segments of the cell sheet (*lower right*) have peeled off entirely ($\times$180). (**C**) MRC-5 fibroblasts infected with echovirus 11. An early focus of enteroviral cytopathic effect is evident. The cells appear enlarged and granular. It would be very difficult at this stage to guess the identity of the virus. Most isolates of echovirus grow well in human diploid fibroblasts, whereas isolates of coxsackievirus do not ($\times$180). (**D**) MRC-5 fibroblasts infected with echovirus 11. Cytopathic effect has extended to involve almost the entire monolayer. Virus is spread extracellularly through the medium so that cytopathic effect tends to change from focal to generalized in nature relatively rapidly ($\times$180). (**E**) HEp-2 cells infected with coxsackievirus B. A small focus of cytopathic effect in the HEp-2 cells is manifested by rounded, shrunken granular cells and detachment of cells from the glass. Early cytopathic effect is much more difficult to recognize if the cell sheet is too heavy and the cells are piled one on top of the other ($\times$180). (**F**) HEp-2 cells infected with coxsackievirus B. Almost all of the cells in the monolayer have detached from the glass. Those that remain are abnormal. Most coxsackievirus B isolates grow well in HEp-2 cells, whereas coxsackievirus A and echovirus do not ($\times$180).

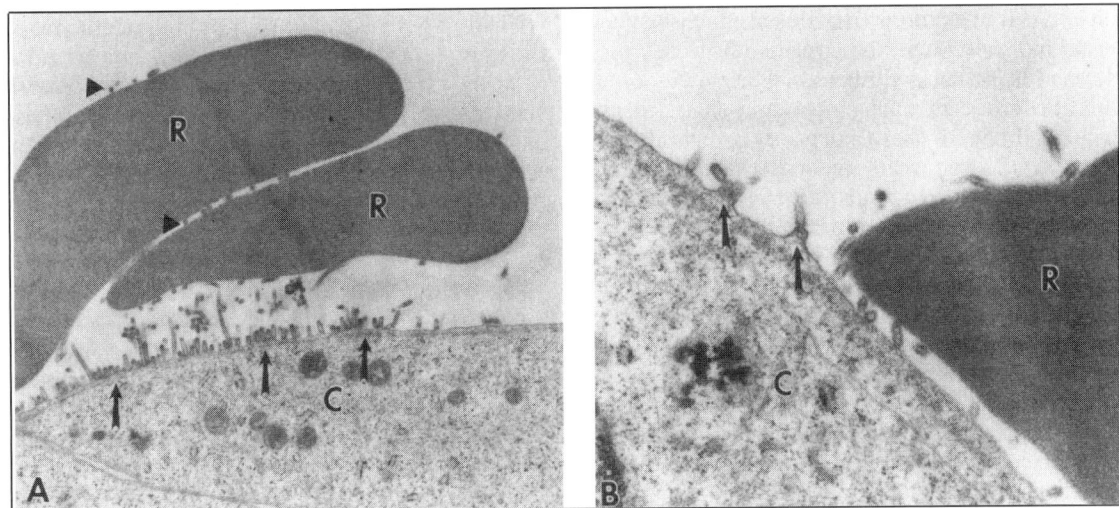

Figure 23-16 Electron microscopy of hemadsorption and hemagglutination of influenza A virus. (**A**) Two red cells (*R*) have adhered to a monolayer of rhesus monkey kidney cells (*C*). The glue that holds them together is the large number of influenza virions that are "budding" from the surface of the kidney cells (*arrows*) or adhering to the red blood cells (*arrowheads*) (×35,000). (**B**) At higher magnification, the bulges in the cell membrane at the point of budding can be seen clearly (*arrows*). The hemagglutinin and neuraminidase spikes on the virus particles appear as a "fringe" (×80,000).

cate less rapidly and demonstrate the lability of the rhinovirus group to an acid environment. To make this assessment, aliquots of infected cell culture are adjusted to pH 3.0 or 7.4 for 3 hours. Then an estimate of the infectivity is obtained by inoculating serial 10-fold dilutions of the aliquots into cell cultures. A reduction in infectivity of 2 to 4 $\log_{10}$ should be observed if the virus is a rhinovirus.[248] In practice, satisfactory demonstration of acid lability may be achieved without resorting to serial dilutions.

CELL ASSOCIATION

The demonstration of the association of virions with infected cells is useful to differentiate members of the herpesvirus group. Herpes simplex virus is released freely into the culture medium, whereas CMV and VZV remain cell-associated. Herpes simplex virus rapidly infects the whole monolayer (see Fig. 23-14*B*). Cytopathic effect of CMV and VZV is usually focal (see Fig. 23-14*E* through *H*), because virions do not spread through the medium. Occasionally, however, large numbers of viral particles in the inoculum may produce widespread cytopathic effect resembling that of herpes simplex. Subculture of the culture medium and disrupted cells separately documents the cell association of the isolate.

DETECTION OF VIRAL ANTIGENS

In addition to confirmation of the identity of a cytopathic agent, demonstration of specific antigens in culture has been used as a method for detecting the presence of a virus, even in the absence of cytopathic effect. Tests for antigen may be performed after a brief incubation if rapid diagnosis is

desired, an approach that has been used more commonly with spin amplification. The most dramatic improvements in the rapidity with which isolates are detected will occur with viruses that have the slowest growth in conventional systems, such as respiratory syncytial virus, cytomegalovirus, and varicella-zoster virus (Color Plate 23-2*D* and *F*).

The literature is replete with disparate reports on the sensitivity of such expedited approaches to viral diagnosis. For instance, the percentage of influenza virus isolates recovered after spin amplification, incubation overnight, and staining with monoclonal antibodies has ranged from 56%[149] to 98%.[137] Differences in operational variables, such as cell lines and source of monoclonal antibodies as well as varied patient populations, make universal recommendations treacherous. It is clear that expedited culture techniques can contribute useful information but that there is a tradeoff between sensitivity and rapidity when deciding on the length of incubation. Including conventional cultures and/or sampling shell vials at several times will increase sensitivity, but also increase costs. Although it is difficult to document, provision of results more rapidly may have clinical and financial impact.[20] In the future facilitated molecular detection, such as reverse transcriptase polymerase chain reaction (RT-PCR), may make the discussion moot.

Although most laboratories will not encounter rubella virus, Schmidt and colleagues have reported that immunoperoxidase staining of RK-13 or BSC-1 cells facilitated the detection of this fastidious virus.[440]

ARTIFACTS AND NON–VIRUS-INDUCED CHANGES

As cells age in culture, morphologic changes unrelated to viral infection may occur (see Fig. 23-5). The density of cells in diploid cell lines and, in particular, established cell lines may become very high; dying or dividing cells may appear rounded or granular. Scattered atypical cells occur in any culture and are especially noticeable in less-dense areas, such as the edge of the monolayer, where viral cytopathic effect may also become apparent first. It is important, therefore, to maintain uninoculated controls of cells from the same batch as those used for specimens.

Primary monkey kidney cells may be infected with simian viruses that produce a variety of degenerative changes,[248] including a foamy or vacuolated appearance in the monolayer.

The presence of extraneous cells that settle on the monolayer may also cause confusion (see Fig. 23-6*D*). Cytopathic effect may be mimicked because the contaminating cells differ in appearance from the original monolayer. Usually a virus that produces focal abnormalities in the monolayer, such as CMV, is simulated. The artifact may be suspected because the cells are on top of the monolayer, rather than becoming an integral part of it. Contaminating cells may be of human origin, such as epithelial or mesothelial cells present in the specimen, or may have originated in other cell cultures, particularly if a subculture from one cell line to another has been performed.

A variety of nonviral agents or substances in clinical specimens may be toxic to cell monolayers (see Fig. 23-6*A*). If bacterial or fungal growth occurs (see Fig. 23-6*B*), the nature of the problem is obvious; the specimen must then be treated again with antibiotics or filtered and inoculated into additional cell cultures.

Usually the nature of the cytotoxicity is unknown. The ordinary remedy is to dilute the specimen and inoculate additional monolayers. Howell and associates found that the toxicity of semen from patients with AIDS could be avoided by inoculating the monolayer with a cell pellet, obtained by high-speed centrifugation.[247] CMV, which is a frequent pathogen in patients with AIDS, is associated with leukocytes. On the other hand, toxic substances were concentrated in the supernatant fraction.

On occasion cytopathic effect may be "specific," although the cause is unexpected and perhaps unwanted. *Clostridium difficile* toxin in fecal specimens (see Fig. 23-6*C*) may produce cytopathic effect resembling enteroviral damage.[441]

Gentry and associates reported the isolation of *Trichomonas vaginalis* in BHK cell cultures.[181] The flagellates produced a cytopathic effect that mimicked that of herpes simplex virus; cytopathic effect was reproduced when viable *Trichomonas* or lysates from axenic cultures were added to cell cultures. Motile trichomonads could be seen when the cultures were inspected closely.

Isolation of *Pneumocystis jiroveci* (*carinii*) from patients with AIDS has been reported. It is difficult to propagate this protozoan parasite serially in the laboratory, but organisms have been grown in cell cultures, including MRC-5 human diploid fibroblasts.[303] The *P. jiroveci* isolates produced a cytopathic effect that resembled viral effects. *Toxoplasma gondii* may be recovered in cell culture lines, such as human diploid fibroblasts, although the sensitivity of culture has not been evaluated.[90]

Definitive Identification of Isolates

In a diagnostic laboratory the combination of clinical history and cytopathic effect provides sufficient information to identify some viruses, including herpes simplex virus, CMV, VZV, adenovirus, and respiratory syncytial virus. Enteroviruses can usually be identified to the genus level. Complete identification of isolates, including typing, requires immunologic characterization of the viral antigens or viral nucleic acid.

Immunologic tests can be adapted either for identification of antigens or antibodies against those antigens. Antisera, traditionally polyclonal, are increasingly monoclonal (see Chapter 3). The most specific immunologic test for the majority of viral infections is the neutralization assay. The identification of an unknown viral isolate is made by analyzing the degree to which antisera of known reactivity prevent the virus from infecting tissue culture cells, eggs, or animals. The disadvantages of the neutralization test are the time and expense required for its performance. It is most frequently used in a reference laboratory.

The hemagglutination inhibition test provides a convenient and economical alternative to the neutralization test for viruses that produce hemagglutinins. The principle is similar to that of the neutralization test, but the end point is inhibition of the virus-mediated agglutination reaction rather than inhibition of infectivity. Reference sera of known reactivity are used to characterize a viral isolate.

The complement-fixation test was the mainstay of viral diagnosis for many years. Other simpler and more reliable assays have now replaced it in most laboratories.

Many viral tests are important for epidemiologic analysis, but, with the exception of the myxoviruses, they are rarely necessary for routine diagnostic purposes. In instances in which complete characterization is necessary (e.g., paralytic disease), the isolate may be sent to a reference laboratory. A thorough discussion of antigenic characterization, which is beyond the scope of this chapter, may be found in textbooks of virology and viral diagnosis.[248,284,462]

For many hospital laboratories immunofluorescence and immunoenzyme assays provide a viable alternative by which definitive identification of many viruses to the genus and/or species level can be made. Fortunately, the expanding catalogue of commercially available reagents, which are of increasingly high quality, simplifies the task. The enteroviruses and rhinoviruses are notable exceptions because their complicated antigenic composition makes definitive identification difficult without neutralization tests.

Immunofluorescence and immunoenzyme assays are similar in principle, differing mainly in the detection system (see Chapter 3). The immunofluorescence test has been used for many years and in many variations. The direct fluorescent assay test is the simplest to perform, but specific conjugated antisera are required. Indirect immunofluorescent tests—using antiglobulin, staphylococcal protein A, or complement—are more sensitive but often suffer from lower specificity. In contrast to the direct test, multiple conjugated reagents are not needed to perform the indirect test, but the procedure is more time-consuming because of the serial steps required.

The solid phase of immunoenzymatic tests can be the

specimen itself, placed on a glass slide. In this case, the reaction is detected visually with a microscope. Solid-phase immunoassays can also be performed in tubes or microtiter trays.

Enzyme and fluorescence immunoassays can be considered equivalent for most applications, although the fluorescence tests have been more sensitive in some situations.[298] Nonspecificity has been a problem in some enzyme immunoassays, and controls for specificity should be available. On the other hand, visual assays, such as direct immunofluorescence, are subject to considerable viewer-to-viewer variation. Assays in which a positive reaction is determined microscopically have two advantages: 1) the cellularity (and the quality) of the specimen can be judged and 2) the relationship of the antigen to the cells can be assessed.[130]

The decision as to which assay to use will depend on local resources, experience, and the volume of tests. Immunofluorescence is simpler than classical enzyme immunoassays if a small number of specimens is to be tested. When the number of specimens increases and the tests can be performed in batches, immunoenzyme assays or newer molecular probes become more attractive because automated systems can be used. The advent of simple membrane immunoassays has made this technology quick and extremely convenient. These unit packages are designed for direct detection, but they may also be used for culture confirmation.

Positive and negative controls must be included in these tests, as indicated in the package insert. The specificity of the classical immunoenzyme assay can be enhanced by performing a blocking test.[46]

Identification of viral isolates by nucleic-acid hybridization with or without amplification has also been accomplished. Molecular approaches will undoubtedly continue to grow in popularity, but the extreme sensitivity provided by amplification is not essential when the culture has already provided amplified target.

Storage of Viral Isolates

If the necessity for additional characterization of an isolate seems probable, infected cell culture fluid should be frozen at −70°C. If the laboratory has the resources, it is good practice to retain all isolates for a period of time. A general rule is that mammalian cells should be frozen slowly, whereas infectious agents should be frozen quickly. The dramatic decrease in viability that accompanies the freezing process is minimized if the cultures are snap-frozen and if a stabilizing agent is included in the medium. A mixture of dry ice and alcohol is a convenient means for snap-freezing viral isolates. Many stabilizing agents have been used. Howell and Miller found that the sucrose phosphate broth that is used for transport of swabs for isolation of *Chlamydia* functioned as well as 70% sorbitol for maintenance of some of the most fastidious viruses, including cytomegalovirus and respiratory syncytial virus.[246]

Summary of Detection and Identification of Viruses in Culture

The orthomyxoviruses, paramyxoviruses, and respiratory syncytial virus (see Figs. 23-12 and 23-13) produce a variety

of cytopathic effects in cell culture. Many isolates of influenza and parainfluenza viruses produce no visible changes in the monolayer and must be detected by other means. Cytopathic strains can be differentiated from other viruses with similar effects by noting the restriction of cytopathic effect to monkey kidney cells and by demonstration of hemadsorption, as described above. Multinucleated giant cells occur in monolayers that have been infected with measles, respiratory syncytial (see Fig. 23-13E and F), parainfluenza (see Fig. 23-12F), and mumps viruses; they are produced by virus-directed fusion of adjacent cells (syncytium formation). Such cells may also be seen in infected patients (see Color Plate 23-1F and G).[470,526]

Isolates are definitively identified by immunologic means. Antisera of good quality are available for most of the common myxoviruses. The genus or type of virus (e.g., influenza A virus or respiratory syncytial virus) may be identified by immunofluorescence of infected cells. Characterization of strains of influenza viruses must be performed by hemagglutination inhibition.

Adenoviruses (see Fig. 23-13A through D) can be identified presumptively by observing the characteristic cytopathology in cell cultures. Clusters of swollen infected cells or a lattice appearance to the monolayer are typical. Group-specific antigens that are common to all adenovirus serotypes have been identified, and monoclonal antibodies to the common determinants have been prepared. For most clinical applications, confirmation of the genus of adenovirus by immunofluorescence is sufficient. If the type of adenovirus must be determined, neutralization tests are necessary.

The herpesvirus group produces a variety of cytopathic effects in cell culture. EBV does not grow in the cell cultures commonly used in clinical laboratories; human infections with this virus are usually diagnosed serologically. CMV and VZV are strongly cell-associated (see Fig. 23-14E through H). They are difficult to grow in cell culture, and they grow slowly. Successful subculture requires transfer of infected cells. Both CMV and VZV produce swollen cells in foci that slowly enlarge by direct spread; the plaques of VZV, in particular, tend to follow the orientation of the fibroblastic tissue culture cells. In contrast, herpes simplex virus is spread extracellularly (see Fig. 23-14A through D); cytopathic effect starts focally but spreads rapidly to affect other parts of the monolayer.

Centrifugation of the inoculum onto the monolayer has accelerated the recovery of herpes simplex, VZV, and CMV. Monoclonal antibodies have proved valuable for both detection and identification of CMV, VZV, and herpes simplex virus. Separation of isolates of herpes simplex into types 1 and 2 can be accomplished reliably with fluoresceinated monoclonal antibodies.[311]

Enteroviruses grow relatively rapidly in cell cultures, producing a widespread cytopathic effect (see Fig. 23-15). Affected cells may be shrunken and granular or may have a refractile, glassy appearance. Most serotypes of coxsackievirus A do not grow well in commonly used cell cultures. Isolates of coxsackievirus B usually do not grow well in human diploid fibroblast lines; echovirus strains do not grow well in HEp-2 cells. Definitive identification of an enterovirus requires immunologic identification. Fluoresceinated monoclonal antibodies directed against a genus-specific antigen and selected serotypes are available commercially. Immunofluorescence is not foolproof, especially for non-polio enteroviruses.[420] The reference method for identification is the neutralization test. Sequencing of the gene has been shown to correlate well with the serologic types.[326]

The SARS coronavirus was initially detected by isolation techniques, but molecular methods have superseded culture because of their rapidity and convenience. The virus is most readily detected in respiratory specimens during the first 2 weeks of illness and is infrequently recovered after 3 weeks, although viral RNA can still be detected.[85]

Direct Detection of Viruses in Clinical Specimens

The desire for greater rapidity in diagnosis of viral infections has been stimulated by the availability of rapid diagnostic methods in other areas of the laboratory and by the development of effective antiviral chemotherapy. A variety of methods is available, ranging from the traditional to the experimental.

Light Microscopic Detection of Inclusions

The detection of viral inclusions in smears or tissues by light microscopy has been the traditional means of directly demonstrating viral infections.[470,526] In general, viruses that are assembled in the nucleus (usually DNA viruses) produce intranuclear inclusions, whereas cytoplasmic assembly (predominantly RNA-containing viruses) yields cytoplasmic inclusions.

Intranuclear inclusions are produced in cells that have been infected by herpes simplex virus, VZV, CMV, adenovirus, and papovaviruses. The inclusions of herpes simplex (see Color Plate 23-1A, B, and C) and VZV are indistinguishable. Nuclei have a homogeneous, eosinophilic, or slightly basophilic appearance, and granular, basophilic nuclear chromatin is pushed against the edge of the nuclear membrane. Other infected cells may have a more eosinophilic inclusion that is accentuated by a halo between the inclusion and the nuclear membrane. This halo is an artifact of fixation but is useful diagnostically. Ultrastructurally, the inclusions are composed of a mixture of deoxyribonucleoprotein and assembled virions (see Fig. 23-3A); as the virions pass through the nuclear membrane, they pick up a lipid-containing membrane. The infected cells may be mononuclear or multinuclear.

Cytomegalovirus produces basophilic inclusions in an enlarged cell (see Color Plate 23-1D). These distinctive cells, which are pathognomonic of CMV infection, were originally believed to be protozoa that were invading tissue.[258] A halo is often present around the inclusion. Granular, basophilic inclusions may be found in the cytoplasm of some infected cells.

A variety of inclusions may be found in adenovirus infections. Early inclusions are eosinophilic and may closely resemble herpesvirus-infected cells. Inclusions become more basophilic as they mature and increasingly fill the nucleus (see Color Plate 23-1E). Eventually, they become extremely basophilic and may completely distort the cell; these diagnostic cells are referred to as "smudge cells" and must be

distinguished from uninfected cells with hyperchromatic nuclei. The adenovirus inclusions are composed of nucleoprotein and numerous virions, which often demonstrate a paracrystalline array because their icosahedral shape permits tight packing of the particles (see Fig. 23-3B).

The intranuclear inclusions of the papovavirus group will not be encountered frequently by clinical virologists because these viruses are difficult or impossible to grow in culture. The inclusions in human warts begin as granular eosinophilic matter, later condensing into rounded, basophilic masses; cytoplasmic inclusions in the epidermal cells of warts are condensed keratin and are not virus-specific. The inclusions in progressive multifocal leukoencephalopathy occur in astrocytes and oligodendroglia (nonnerve cells that perform a supportive function); the inclusions vary from small granular material to large basophilic masses that fill the nucleus.

Intracytoplasmic inclusions may be found in cells that have been infected by respiratory syncytial virus, rabies virus, and viruses of the pox group. The intracytoplasmic inclusions of respiratory syncytial virus are brightly eosinophilic (see Color Plate 23-1G); they are present regularly in cell culture but less frequently in clinical specimens. Ultrastructurally, the inclusions of respiratory syncytial virus consist of fibrillar ribonucleoprotein (see Fig. 23-3C). The intracytoplasmic inclusions of rabies virus are known as Negri bodies (see Color Plate 23-1H). They may be single or multiple and occur in neurons that look otherwise healthy. The edges of the inclusions are sharply defined, as if bounded by a membrane. Clear spaces or basophilic stippling, which may be seen within the inclusion, result from the incorporation of some cytoplasmic material into the mass of viral ribonucleoprotein (see Fig. 23-3E). Fortunately, the intracytoplasmic inclusions of the poxviruses, known as Guarneri bodies, are unlikely to be encountered today.

Intranuclear and intracytoplasmic inclusions are found in measles infection. During the prodromal stage of measles, giant cells appear in lymphoid tissue throughout the body. These so-called Warthin-Finkeldey giant cells contain as many as 100 nuclei and rarely may contain inclusion bodies. A second type of giant cell may arise later from epithelial tissue, such as that lining the lower respiratory tract. There are fewer nuclei in these giant cells, but inclusions are almost constant. The intranuclear inclusions resemble those produced by the herpesviruses, may be single or multiple, and vary in their degree of eosinophilia (see Color Plate 23-1F).

Detection of inclusions provides valuable information in selected clinical situations. The Tzanck test, performed by preparing a Giemsa-stained smear of vesicular scrapings, can be used to document the presence of a herpesvirus by demonstrating multinucleated giant cells (see Color Plate 23-1C). Hematoxylin-eosin or the Papanicolaou stain may also be used. The nuclei should have a ground-glass and molded or multifaceted appearance.[459] Intranuclear inclusions, which are accentuated in histologic sections by the artifactual halo produced by the fixation of tissues in formalin, may not always be visualized in the smears. A presumptive diagnosis of herpes infection can be made, although differentiation between herpes simplex virus and VZV is not possible by morphology alone.

Solomon and colleagues found positive Tzanck tests in 11 patients with clinical chickenpox (varicella virus) and in

12 of 15 patients (80%) with shingles (herpes zoster virus). However, varicella virus was recovered in only 7 of the 11 patients with chickenpox.[459] Multinucleated giant cells or inclusions or both have been demonstrated in skin lesions from 18 of 21 patients (86%) from whom herpes simplex virus was isolated.[363] An analysis of the proficiency with which dermatologists correctly interpreted a study set of 10 smears demonstrated a ''reverse learning curve'' (or loss of neuronal synapses with increasing age!).[203] Second- and third-year residents correctly interpreted a mean of 91% of the slides; dermatologists in practice for less than 10 years, 84%; and dermatologists in practice for more than 10 years, 67%.

Although the direct smears have worked well in the study of skin lesions, the sensitivity has unfortunately been low for other applications. Only a minority of culture-positive specimens from the genital tract[478] or the respiratory tract[371] contained inclusion-bearing cells. Similarly, Nahmias and colleagues found intranuclear inclusions in only 56% of 113 cases of herpes simplex encephalitis.[370] The specificity was considerably higher (86%) than the sensitivity in this collaborative study of antiviral chemotherapy, but false-positive results are potentially dangerous if therapy for another condition, such as bacterial brain abscess, is omitted. Intranuclear inclusions were reported in 10 patients from whom herpes simplex virus was not isolated; in 7 of these patients, an alternative diagnosis not associated with inclusions was established. These results emphasize the importance of careful and informed use of ''simple'' morphologic tests.

Histologic detection of CMV inclusions in tissue is less sensitive than culture, but may be equivalent to more ''sophisticated'' techniques, such as immunohistochemistry and in situ hybridization, for revealing cytomegalovirus in tissue.[471] Morphologic methods have the advantage of better correlation with disease produced by cytomegalovirus than does the more sensitive culture.

In parvovirus B19 infection, intranuclear inclusions are also found in giant pronormoblasts, which are found in the bone marrow.[288] These characteristic cells may also be seen in peripheral blood and other tissues in infected fetuses.

Electron Microscopic Detection of Viral Particles

Electron microscopy can be applied to the study of both clinical specimens and cell cultures, either in thin sections of tissue or by negative stain microscopy. The inaccessibility of electron microscopes to most clinical laboratories and the sampling errors inherent in the examination of small samples of tissue have deterred routine application of this technique in making diagnoses of viral disease. The use of electron microscopy was specific for the diagnosis of herpes simplex encephalitis in one study (98%), but herpes virions were detected in only 45% of the cases.[370] The technique has been used effectively in the detection of viral agents of gastroenteritis, especially those that are not recovered by conventional cell culture (rotavirus, Norwalk-like agents, and enteric adenoviruses). However, ultrastructural diagnosis remains a research technique in most laboratories.

Negative stain electron microscopy has drawn renewed interest as a result of increased concern about bioterrorism. When examining a specimen with the electron microscope, there is no requirement for predetermining the antigens or nucleic acids to be detected. The diagnosis of important viral infections, such as smallpox, can be made quickly and safely if the specimen can be inactivated before examination.[219]

Immunologic Detection of Viral Antigen

Immunologic and, more recently, molecular techniques have been used effectively to expedite diagnoses of certain viral infections. Immunofluorescence or immunoenzyme stains of clinical specimens or tissues are frequently used techniques. Increasingly, molecular assays are complementing or replacing immunologic approaches.

These techniques have many advantages and have functioned well when applied by trained persons. The risks of erroneous results are great in the absence of proper equipment and training.[130] For almost all procedures, culture of the infectious agent remains the standard. Whenever possible, cultures should be done in parallel with rapid immunologic tests, until proficiency at the technique is demonstrated.

RESPIRATORY VIRUSES

The most reliable antigenic method for detection of respiratory viruses is direct immunofluorescence (DFA). In one study DFA was as efficient as culture for all respiratory viruses except adenovirus. When the slides for immunofluorescence were prepared in a cytocentrifuge, less than 10% of the specimens had an inadequate number of respiratory cells.[297] In contrast, the sensitivity of enzyme immunoassays, particularly the rapid formats, has been considerably lower in most reports.[2,84,298,414] In addition, some immunoassays have yielded sufficient numbers of false-positive reactions that confirmation by a second method has been recommended.[2]

Although direct immunofluorescence is clearly the better of the two approaches, practical considerations often lead to the selection of enzyme immunoassays. These tests can be performed quickly and simply without the need for a fluorescent microscope or extensive training of personnel.

HERPES GROUP VIRUSES

Herpes Simplex Virus. Direct immunofluorescence has generally performed well in comparison with culture, particularly when performed on visible lesions and enhanced by cytocentrifugation.[299,415,430] Varying results may reflect different reagents, patient populations, types of lesions, and serotypes of virus. Herpes simplex virus grows quickly, however, so the gains from expedited diagnosis are not as great as with more slowly growing viruses.

Varicella-zoster Virus. VZV grows slowly in culture. Not surprisingly, direct immunofluorescence performs comparatively better with VZV than with herpes simplex virus. In fact, DFA of skin lesions may be the superior means for making this diagnosis.[111] In addition to direct examination of smeared material, staining of cytocentrifuged viral transport medium has proved useful.[342]

Cytomegalovirus. Monoclonal antibodies have facilitated the rapid immunologic diagnosis of CMV infections in patients' specimens as well as in cell culture. Hackman and colleagues were able to detect CMV by immunofluorescence in 25 of 27 lung biopsy specimens from which the virus was subsequently cultured[206]; light microscopic inclusions were demonstrated in only 20 of the specimens. Preliminary studies with bronchoalveolar lavage specimens from immunosuppressed patients[108,141,331] have yielded greatly differing estimates of sensitivity, varying from 31.6% to 100%. The numbers of patients in these studies were small, the antibodies were different, and the composition of the patient groups may have been different. The correlation of immunologic detection of viral antigen in tissue (without inclusions or histopathologic abnormalities) and clinical disease is not clear.

Detection of CMV antigenemia is more sensitive than viral culture,[31,508] is commercially available, and has replaced culture in many laboratories. The toxicity of blood for cell monolayers has limited the usefulness of culture. In the antigenemia assay the leukocyte-enriched fraction of peripheral blood is examined for the presence of pp65, an early-intermediate antigen in the course of cellular infection with CMV. One of the major drawbacks of the antigenemia assay—the amount of hands-on time required—has been considerably ameliorated by the development of commercially available expedited immunofluorescence procedures.[296,464] The test has proved useful for predicting clinical disease and monitoring the response to antiviral chemotherapy in patients at high risk, especially recipients of organ transplants.[54] The value of the test in patients who are infected with HIV is somewhat more controversial.[31,92] Protocols for timing and frequency of testing vary among major transplant centers. In some cases testing is performed routinely for a period after transplantation; in others, appearance of clinical symptoms initiates a request for the antigenemia test. When the density of the cell suspension is standardized, a quantitative assessment of the degree of antigenemia can be provided. Severe leukopenia sometimes makes examination of an adequate number of cells difficult. Quantitating the level of antigenemia is important; high-level antigenemia (>50 infected neutrophils per 2×10^5 cells) indicates the greatest risk of impending disease, ineffective antiviral chemotherapy, or potential relapse. The CMV antigenemia test remains a reference method and is particularly useful when small numbers of patients are tested.[341]

OTHER VIRUSES

Human rotavirus is difficult to recover in cell culture. Infections by these viruses can be diagnosed effectively either by an enzyme immunoassay or by latex agglutination. The sensitivity for both methods has ranged from 80% to 90%; the specificity has been 90% to 100%.[98,140,480] Krause and colleagues have questioned the reliability of the Rotazyme immunoassay in neonates.[289]

Molecular Techniques

The molecular era has been inextricably intertwined with infectious diseases from the outset, and the pace of innovation shows no sign of slowing. We have passed through several stages already, beginning with nucleic-acid hybridization and advancing to molecular amplification technology

(see Chapter 4). The polymerase chain reaction and other amplification approaches have made it into the mainstream of clinical laboratories for a few critical pathogens that have warranted the early introduction of commercial products.[492]

HUMAN IMMUNODEFICIENCY VIRUS

The only tests cleared by the Food and Drug Administration (FDA) for the initial diagnosis of HIV infections are tests for antibody. Molecular detection is not recommended for this purpose, because occasional false-positive reactions occur.[417] This policy is analogous to the approach to syphilis, in which the specificity of the fluorescent treponemal antibody absorption (FTA-ABS) test is safeguarded by using it only in a population of patients with a high prior probability of having syphilis because they have already had a positive VDRL or rapid plasma reagin (RPR) test (see Chapter 20).

Once the diagnosis has been made management of HIV-1 infection is based entirely on molecular methods. There are two situations, however, in which viral load testing is appropriate for initial diagnosis. In both cases there may not have been time for a serologic response to develop. The first situation is acute infection with HIV, which may manifest itself as a multifaceted febrile illness with symptoms referable to any organ system.[269] This initial illness is transient, usually lasting no longer than 14 days. Large quantities of virus may be present before the immune response has been generated. The second clinical scenario is neonatal infection when the mother is known to be infected. Molecular detection of virus is required, because antibody passively transferred across the placenta to the neonate complicates serologic analysis.

The backbone of monitoring the course of infection and response to antiviral chemotherapy is quantitative measurement of viral RNA, so-called viral load tests. Qualitative detection of RNA is the current method for screening blood products before transfusion, but is not used for managing patients' infections. Quantitative detection of viral RNA has been accomplished on a variety of specimens, including body fluids, serum, and peripheral-blood leukocytes. The standard specimen, however, is plasma. Three molecular approaches have been used in FDA-cleared viral load tests, and a fourth has been used as a qualitative assay to screen the blood supply.

The reverse transcriptase polymerase chain reaction (RT-PCR) has been the dominant platform. The Amplicor HIV-1 monitor and the COBAS Amplicor HIV-1 monitor test (Roche Diagnostics, Indianapolis, IN) comes in a standard format and as an ultrasensitive test, which was introduced to detect small (low) copy numbers after effective antiviral chemotherapy. The manual and automated versions perform similarly.[226,238] The dynamic range is 400 to 750,000 copies per milliliter (standard) and 50 to 75,000 copies per milliliter (ultrasensitive). The second approach uses branched-chain DNA (bDNA; Versant HIV-1 RNA Assay; Bayer Diagnostics, Tarrytown, NY), which provides reproducible results over a range of copy numbers from 75 to 500,000 per milliliter.[365]

Other approaches include nucleic-acid sequence–based amplification (NASBA; NucliSens HIV-1 QT; BioMérieux, Durham, NC)[185] for the quantitative determination of viral load and a qualitative transcription-mediated amplification assay (TMA; Gen-Probe, San Diego, CA).[183] These assays have not yet been cleared by the FDA for testing clinical specimens, although the TMA procedure has been licensed for screening of blood bank specimens. Real-time assays of several types have been described and will undoubtedly play a major role in the future.[118,383]

The two primary strategies (PCR and bDNA) perform equivalently for quantitation of group M strains (the predominant strains in the United States), but the PCR tests are less good at detecting group O strains[474] or non-clade B strains[256] than are the bDNA procedures. The coefficient of variation of the viral load tests is high, typically ranging from 30 to 40 (depending on the amount of virus present), and the copy numbers cannot be directly compared across molecular approaches. It is, therefore, essential that patients be followed sequentially with the same type of test; if the assay is switched to a different approach, a new baseline for the patient must be established.

Plastic and glass Vacutainer tubes for collecting blood to be tested in the viral load assays function equivalently.[300] Vacutainer plasma preparation (PPT) tubes are a convenient method for collecting blood if it is to be frozen and/or shipped to a reference laboratory for testing.[237] A wide variation in patient reports provided to physicians by clinical laboratories, including reports that were incomplete or unhelpful, has been noted.[164]

With the advent of effective antiviral chemotherapy, detection of resistance in clinical isolates became a priority. The clinical relevance of resistance testing soon became evident,[138] and evolving consensus recommendations have been promulgated.[229] Resistance testing is recommended in pregnant women and after failure of antiviral chemotherapy, either primary therapy or subsequent regimens. It is now clear that evaluation of resistance is useful for treating newly infected patients (infected within 12 months of testing), particularly if the individual who is the source of the infection is known to have been taking antiretroviral drugs. In addition, testing of patients who have been infected for up to 2 years (and perhaps longer) has been found to be useful for designing therapeutic regimens.[228]

Two approaches to the detection of resistance have been used. Evaluation of phenotypic resistance involves isolation of virus and traditional assessment of inhibition by antiviral dugs. The complexity of viral isolation has led to an alternative mechanism in which plasma RNA of the polymerase and protease genes is amplified and used to form a recombinant virus with laboratory constructs. By using a standard virus backbone into which the two most important genes of the patient strain have been inserted, standardization of the assay has been improved. Drug susceptibility testing can be performed within several weeks by using automated methods and reporter genes. Phenotypic assays include Pheno-Sense (ViroLogic, South San Francisco, CA) and The Antivirogram (VIRCO Lab USA, Raritan, NJ).

In contrast to phenotypic assays, which measure viral susceptibility, genotypic assays pinpoint the mutations that confer phenotypic resistance.[447] The initial step in PCR-based assays is similar to the recombinant phenotypic approach—amplification of HIV-1 sequences from plasma samples that contain 500 to 1,000 copies per milliliter. As a result, this genotypic approach will not work with samples that contain a small quantity of virus. The next step involves either genotyping all relevant codons or detecting selected codons by hybridization.[212,229] Several companies have attempted to predict the phenotype by analysis of the genotypic result, a so-called virtual phenotype. Genotypic assays include The VirtualPhenotype (VIRCO), GeneSeq HIV (ViroLogic), ViroSeq (Abbott Laboratories, Abbott Park, IL), and Trugene HIV-1 (Bayer Diagnostics, Tarrytown, NY).

Phenotypic assays have the attractiveness of more direct (and traditional) assessment of resistance, although the clinical interpretation of the results is neither completely defined nor straightforward. In patients in whom multiple treatment regimens have failed, genotypic assays may document many viral mutations, which are hard to interpret; in this situation phenotypic analysis may provide better guidance. The phenotypes have the considerable disadvantage of being time-consuming and expensive.

Genotypic assays are more straightforward, more rapid, and less expensive; the concern has been that important phenotypic resistance may not be pinpointed and that the significance of new mutations may not be clear. For both approaches, reproducibility and sophistication of analysis represent important factors. An additional concern is that a minority of resistant virions in the diverse population of virions that comprise the infecting strain in any individual patient may be missed (analogous to the problem with detecting resistant cells in a population of heteroresistant bacteria, as discussed in Chapter 17).[447]

Although the concern about genotypic assays has not been dissipated, comparative studies have demonstrated good correspondence of genotypic and phenotypic assays for the clinically important resistance mechanisms.[43] As experience has been gained and commercial products have been fine-tuned, the reproducibility and reliability of genotyping has been established.[172,197]

There is evidence that resistance testing can predict the response to antiviral therapy or time to suppression of virus.[196,538] The factors that determine success or failure in treatment of any infection are complex, however. As with all laboratory reports, the results of HIV resistance testing should be interpreted by an experienced clinician in light of all available data. Attempts to develop useful algorithms to facilitate clinical decisions continue.[447]

HEPATITIS C VIRUS

The diagnostic approach to hepatitis C virus and HIV infections is similar.[25,398] Identification of infected patients is best accomplished serologically. In order to differentiate patients who have cleared their infection from those who are chronically infected and at risk for chronic disease, however, it is necessary to determine if circulating virus is present.[398] Molecular detection is the only option, because hepatitis C virus has never been cultured in vitro.

Several qualitative assays are commercially available: Cobas Amplicor HCV test version 2.0 (Roche Diagnostics), which uses PCR technology, and Versant HCV RNA Qualitative Assay (Bayer Diagnostics), which uses TMA. The two assays perform similarly, although the TMA approach is somewhat more sensitive and less time-consuming.[287]

Quantitative (viral-load) assays are necessary for monitoring therapy. Commercial PCR assays (Cobas Amplicor HCV Monitor Test v2.0; Roche Diagnostics) and bDNA assays (Versant HCV RNA Test v3.0; Bayer Diagnostics) are available. The bDNA assay has a reputation for high reliability and reproducibility. It is less sensitive than the PCR test, but the PCR assay underestimates the viral load.[23,355] Real-time assays will likely become available in the future. As with HIV, individual patients should be followed with the same assay. Although useful for monitoring antiviral chemotherapy, neither test has been demonstrated to correlate with prognosis.

The third component of the molecular approach to hepatitis C virus is genotyping, which need be performed only once.[25] Several parts of the genome have been targeted; two commercial assays are directed at the 5′ noncoding region, by a standardized direct sequencing method (Trugene HCV 5′NC; Visible Genetics, Toronto, ON, Canada) or by a reverse-hybridization line probe assay (INNO-LiPA HCV II; Bayer Diagnostics). The two assays provided congruent genotypic results in 99.4% of 172 clinical samples, representing six genotypes of hepatitis C virus.[177,376] At the subtype level, however, there was only 68.2% agreement. No serotype or ambiguous subtype results were provided in approximately 15% of specimens with each assay. Thus, these two commercial methods are useful for genotyping, but should not be used for subtyping.

HEPATITIS B VIRUS

Molecular diagnostic tests for hepatitis B virus have not achieved the currency of those for hepatitis C, because the variety of serologic tests available for hepatitis B has served much of the need. Detection of viral DNA in blood, the definition of active infection, is more sensitive than the presence of HBeAg, however, and may be found with pre core mutants in the absence of seroconversion to HBeAg.[25] Molecular detection is not yet recommended for all infected patients, however; it should be reserved for patients who are candidates for antiviral chemotherapy. Commercially available methods, none of which has yet been cleared by the FDA for clinical use, include hybrid capture, bDNA, and PCR.[529] Assays that use TMA and real-time PCR are under development. Concern has been expressed that some of these assays are not sufficiently sensitive to monitor effective antiviral chemotherapy reliably.[487] In addition, several genotyping assays have been developed commercially. As experience with therapy of chronic hepatitis B infection expands and resistance becomes more prevalent, these tests will undoubtedly assume greater prominence.

HUMAN PAPILLOMAVIRUSES

Molecular diagnosis is the only practical approach to this group of viruses. Earlier use of labor-intensive techniques, such as nucleic-acid hybridization by the Southern blot method (see previous edition of this book), have been replaced by more convenient and sensitive methods. The only commercially available test that has been cleared by the FDA for diagnostic use at present is the hybrid capture assay (Hybrid Capture II HPV, Digene, Gaithersburg, MD). The second generation of this test has greatly improved sensitivity over the initial version; the results are reproducible,[59] although great care must be taken with the technical details of the procedure. It is cleared only for testing genital specimens and is available for two groups of HPV viruses—those with minimal risk for cervical neoplasia and genotypes with a moderate to high risk. The consensus recommendations for testing suggest using only the high-risk panel.[527]

A third generation of the hybrid capture assay, which is in development, may have slightly increased sensitivity and similar specificity.[60] Target amplification methods, such as PCR and real-time PCR, have been reported, but are not cleared for diagnostic use.[448]

PARVOVIRUS B19

Parvovirus infections are usually diagnosed clinically or serologically; assessment of risk is based on immunologic (i.e., immune) status. Occasionally, however, it is useful to document a serious infection virologically. Parvovirus does not grow in culture, so molecular detection is the only approach available. Several amplification assays have been developed[112,122,213]; although not cleared by FDA, molecular detection is provided by reference laboratories.

WEST NILE VIRUS

The newcomer to the roster of arthropod-borne viruses, West Nile virus, has become an important clinical problem in the United States. The preferred means of diagnosis is by serologic analysis of blood and CSF.[396] Molecular detection of viral nucleic acid in CSF is not sufficiently sensitive to substitute for serologic testing and remains in the research realm.[295,385]

HERPES SIMPLEX VIRUS

The primary diagnostic approach to herpes simplex virus infections is culture, which provides a relatively rapid result with this virus. Brain biopsy has been required to get an adequate specimen for culture diagnosis of encephalitis, the most serious herpetic infection in adults, because the virus is not reliably isolated from CSF. Amplified detection by PCR, however, is sufficiently sensitive to accomplish identification of viral DNA in CSF, both in encephalitis and in recurrent meningitis.[349,452] Although there are no commercial products that have been cleared by FDA, the test has been adapted to the real-time PCR protocol and is readily available as a validated test in several reference laboratories. Preparation of DNA for amplification can be accomplished equally well by manual or automated methods.[147] Fortunately, DNA is sufficiently stable that specimens can be stored without a decrease in sensitivity at 4°C, either as extracted DNA or as an unextracted specimen, for as long as 16 months before testing by real-time PCR.[257] The use of laboratory resources can be increased by screening specimens for pleocytosis in the CSF before testing, because neutrophils have been demonstrated in all positive specimens, at least in adults.[451] Children with encephalitis, however, may have very few neutrophils in CSF and initial PCR examinations may be negative if performed very early in the course of the infection.[119]

Although real-time PCR is most useful for diagnosing

herpetic encephalitis, molecular amplification has proved more sensitive than culture for detecting mucosal infections.[497] As these assays are simplified, it may be possible to provide screening of pregnant women near term with greater ease than is now possible.

CYTOMEGALOVIRUS

The antigenemia assay has become the reference method for monitoring CMV infections in immunosuppressed patients. Initial attempts to substitute molecular-amplification assays were hampered by poor correlation with clinical disease because of high sensitivity. Subsequently, quantitative assays of several varieties have correlated better with clinical disease and with the antigenemia assay. The methods that were used successfully include PCR, real-time PCR, and hybrid capture.[53,125,232,310,341] One of the factors that may be considered in selecting an assay is the volume of tests that is anticipated.[341]

One caveat must be kept in mind for users of molecular amplification. In contrast to herpes simplex virus, the quantity of CMV detected in plasma increased over time when the specimen was stored at 4°C, apparently by leakage of nucleic acid from infected leukocytes.[434] For specimens that were positive in the antigenemia assay there was little effect on the amplification result; if the patient was latently infected and the antigenemia test negative, however, the amount of plasma virus increased significantly over time.

ENTEROVIRUSES

Culture, which has been the mainstay of enteroviral diagnosis, has been suspected to be relatively insensitive. This impression has been validated by the appearance of amplified genetic tests, which are now available in many reference laboratories (although none has yet been cleared by the FDA for diagnostic use). Assays include PCR, real-time PCR, and NASBA.[37,293,301] As there are no generally used antiviral agents for enteroviral infection, prompt diagnosis is not quite as imperative as for herpes simplex virus, but prompt laboratory diagnosis would facilitate clinical management.

SARS CORONAVIRUS

Viral RNA is detectable in clinical specimens for more than 1 month in some patients. Recovery of nucleic acid increases progressively until a peak 11 days after the onset of clinical illness. Nucleic acid could be detected in 60% of patients with clinically diagnosed infection and in a very small number of patients without clinically evident disease. Nasopharyngeal aspirates, throat swabs, and sputum were the most useful specimens in the first 5 days. Later in the illness, virus was more readily detected in stool specimens.[85] Real-time PCR assays for this virus have also been developed.[537] At this juncture diagnostic tests are restricted to reference laboratories.

OTHER VIRAL INFECTIONS

Molecular-amplification assays have been developed for virtually every infectious agent, including real-time PCR assays for most. With the increasing availability of reliable commercial reagents (even in the absence of diagnostic instrument/reagent packages) we can expect the same kind of expansion that occurred after immunofluorescence and immunoenzyme reagents became widely available.

Assays for some of the agents will likely remain in the province of referral laboratories. Examples include exotic viruses, such as hemorrhagic fever viruses[131]; highly virulent agents that have potential for bioterrorism, such as smallpox[458]; and uncommonly considered viruses, such as JC and BK polyomaviruses,[515] measles,[122] rubella,[122] and mumps.[399]

Increasingly, many other agents that are now routinely detected by culture will be identified more rapidly by molecular methods. Examples include respiratory viruses and other herpes group viruses.[109,204,490,494,516]

Selection of Tests for Rapid Diagnosis

The choice of a technique for direct detection of virus must depend on the availability of equipment, the experience of personnel, and the number of specimens to be tested. Microscopic detection of inclusions is simple and inexpensive but relatively insensitive; it works well for documentation of herpetic skin lesions. Electron microscopy has restricted indications. Microscopic solid-phase immunoassays (immunofluorescence and enzyme assays) have advantages over assays for soluble antigens: 1) the location and type of staining can be assessed morphologically and 2) small numbers of specimens may be processed quickly. These attributes may be outweighed by the disadvantages of subjectivity in interpretation and the need to acquire an expensive microscope for fluorescence.

Enzyme immunoassay is most useful when a large number of specimens are to be tested or when the specimens can be collected and tested in a batch. The end point can be read with a spectrophotometer, eliminating subjective decisions. New membrane, single-use enzyme immunoassays have become the most convenient means of providing rapid results with minimal complexity, although usually there are compromises in sensitivity.

To study tissue sections for viral elements, immunoperoxidase has the advantage over other markers in that viral antigens are generally available for reaction without additional treatment. Endogenous peroxidases in the sections must be blocked completely. Before immunofluorescence for detection of some antigens can be performed, fixed, embedded tissue must be treated with a proteolytic agent, such as trypsin.[87,239]

There has been and will continue to be movement toward molecular detection as the procedure of choice, particularly real-time amplification technology. Within the next decade this approach will quite likely have replaced antigen detection in the most sophisticated laboratories—and perhaps in every venue.

Serologic Diagnosis of Viral Infections

Serologic tests are the mainstay of diagnosis for certain viral infections, such as those caused by hepatitis viruses, EBV, and rubella virus. Whenever recovery of the virus in culture is difficult or impossible, documentation of an immunologic response to the agent will continue to be important. In certain cases, such as the evaluation of rubella infections, serologic diagnosis may be as rapid as culturing the virus, even if one has to wait 2 or 3 weeks for collection of a convalescent serum specimen. In situations in which culture of the virus is reliable and readily available, serologic diagnosis has a supportive or adjunctive role.

General immunologic principles also apply when establishing a diagnosis of viral disease using serologic methods. Antibodies to many viral antigens remain for months or years after an acute infection. Demonstration of a significant increase (generally considered a fourfold rise) in titer of antibody is considered diagnostic of recent infection with the agent (unless the possibility of an immunologic cross-reaction exists).

If antibodies are not present in the initial specimen, this diagnostic increase in antibody titer is referred to as a seroconversion. In this case, the infection probably represents a primary encounter with the virus. The infection may be either a primary infection, a repeat infection, or reactivation of a latent infection if antibodies are present, even in low titer, at the time of initial testing.[370] The serologic diagnosis of herpes infections is frequently complicated by recrudescent disease. For example, in a patient with CNS disease, oral herpes lesions may be reactivated by the stress of the acute illness. A serologic response that may result from the reactivated oral lesions could be misinterpreted as evidence that the CNS disease was caused by herpesvirus.

Serologic cross-reactions within many virus groups and even across groups do exist, notably, among enteroviruses, paramyxoviruses, and togaviruses. Therefore, all serologic diagnoses must be considered presumptive to some degree.

A fourfold or greater decrease in antibody titer suggests an infection at some time in the past. Most antibodies disappear slowly, however, so that it is usually difficult to be sure how recent the infection was.

The clinical setting must be kept in mind when assigning a diagnosis. Even a seroconversion documents only a recent infection with the agent; association with the clinical illness is by inference.

Human Immunodeficiency Virus

Human immunodeficiency virus persists in patients in whom antibody to the virus has developed. Serologic tests for HIV have been used as a screening tool because isolation of the virus in cell culture is difficult and not readily available. The molecular tests for detection of viral nucleic acid are reserved for monitoring patients who already have serologically documented infection.

The reference serologic method is a Western blot procedure, in which sera are reacted with viral proteins that have been separated by polyacrylamide-gel electrophoresis and transferred onto nitrocellulose paper. This test requires considerable expertise and care in performance. Several other, more easily performed assay systems have been developed. An enzyme immunoassay has been evaluated most extensively. The test is both sensitive and specific for most HIV M strains found in the United States.[285] In patients with AIDS, the predictive value of a positive result is high. In

the general population of blood donors, among whom HIV infection is very infrequent, even a few false-positive test readings result in an unacceptably low predictive value. In most laboratories, a specimen that contains antibody to HIV by an enzyme immunoassay is first retested in the enzyme assay; if repeated positivity is demonstrated, the specificity of the reaction is documented by performing a Western blot.[106] Not all Western blots produce unequivocal results. The test is not interpreted as positive unless there are multiple protein bands that can be considered truly independent.[62] The criteria suggested by several expert groups for determination of positive Western blots are summarized in Table 23-25. The lack of uniformity among laboratories in applying criteria for interpretation of Western blots made comparison among test results difficult. In a 1990 survey, 22% of laboratories used multiple sets of criteria. Even among the 78% of laboratories that used a single criterion there were several standards.[65] For that reason considerable effort was made to promulgate national standards for interpretation.

An example of a positive Western blot is shown in Figure 23-17. Indeterminate Western blots occur in 10–20% of sera that are reactive by enzyme immunoassay.[83] The risk of AIDS for persons with a repeatedly reactive enzyme immunoassay and an indeterminate Western blot depends on the risk factors of the individual. If there are no risk factors for HIV infection and the validity of the Western blot is established, the patient or donor does not require further follow-up. There is a finite period shortly after infection with HIV when infectious virus may be present in the absence of detectable antibody.

There are several innovations in HIV serology. The Oral Fluid Vironostika HIV-1 Microelisa System (BioMérieux) uses oral secretions as the test medium, thus obviating a venipuncture and avoiding use of blood specimens. At present this assay is the only test that has been cleared by FDA for use on oral samples. It is not as sensitive as immunoas-

Table 23-25	Criteria for Positive Western Blot for Antibody to Human Immunodeficiency Virus
ORGANIZATION	**CRITERIA**
Association of State and Territorial Public Health Laboratory Directors/CDC	Any two of: p24 gp41 gp120/gp160
FDA Licensed DuPont Test	p24 and p31 and gp41 or gp120/ gp160
American Red Cross	≥3 bands: 1 from each gene product group: GAG and POL and ENV
Consortium for Retrovirus Serology Standardization	≥2 bands: p24 or p31 plus gp41 or gp120/ gp 160

Adapted from reference[62].

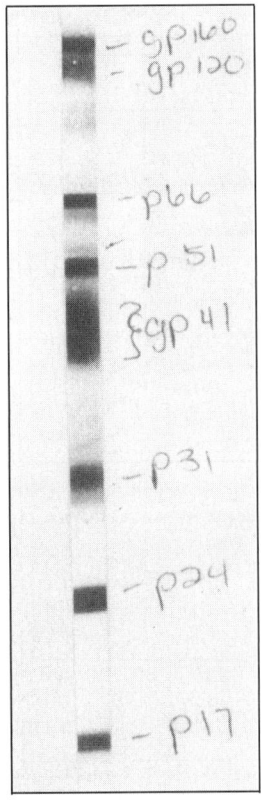

Figure 23-17 Western blot for HIV-1 antibody. Disrupted virus was electrophoresed through polyacrylamide gel, after which it was transferred (blotted) onto nitrocellulose paper. Patient's serum was then reacted with the nitrocellulose strips, after which enzyme-labeled anti–human immunoglobulin was added to the strips. Development of the enzyme reaction revealed multiple bands with this serum from an HIV-1-infected patient. The electrophoresis separated the various proteins and glycoproteins by molecular weight. The bands are labeled here according to the viral protein they have detected.

says performed on blood samples and cannot be used for screening blood donors.

Secondly, three rapid immunoassays: 1) the Orasure HIV-1 collection device for testing saliva and the Oraquick Rapid HIV-1 Antibody Test (OraSure Technologies, Bethlehem, PA) (a CLIA-waived test for use on whole blood), 2) the Reveal Rapid HIV Antibody Test (MedMira, Halifax, NS, Canada) (a CLIA moderate complexity test for use on serum or plasma), and 3) the Uni-Gold Recombigen®HIV Test (Trinity Biotech, Bray, Ireland) (a CLIA-waived test for use on whole blood, serum, or plasma) have been cleared by the FDA for clinical use (http://www.cdc.gov/hiv/pubs/rt-lab.htm).[377] The Oraquick test is approved for use with blood obtained by finger stick as well as by venipuncture; other manufacturers are seeking similar approval from the FDA.

The rapid tests should be treated in the same manner as conventional assays. Negative results should be followed with repeated tests, if indicated clinically. Positive results must be confirmed with either a fluorescence assay or a Western blot. A conventional immunoassay cannot be used for confirmation. Neither does a negative conventional assay prove that a positive rapid test was incorrect.

Not surprisingly, there have been multiple examples of unscrupulous individuals marketing tests that have not been approved by the FDA or even submitting false claims. In some instances criminal prosecutions have resulted (http://www.fda.gov/ora/about/enf_story/archive/2001/ch6/default.htm).

Hepatitis B Virus and Epstein-Barr Virus

There are a few exceptions to the general rule that a seroconversion must be documented to establish a diagnosis. In a few viral infections, antibodies to a variety of antigens appear at different times after infection and persist for varying lengths of time. It may be possible to establish a definitive diagnosis with a single serum when an antibody is detected that appears only acutely. The two prime examples are infectious mononucleosis caused by EBV (Fig. 23-18) and hepatitis B (Fig. 23-19) infections. In both cases, certain antibodies, such as IgG antibody to EBV persist for long periods; a seroconversion to these antigens must be detected. Other antibodies, such as those against the early antigen (EA) of EBV, appear transiently and may serve as markers of acute infection.[411]

If the infectious agent is not eliminated by the immune response, the presence of antibody means that the patient may still harbor the microbe. For instance, patients who have antibody to CMV, which often produces a latent infection, are more likely to transmit the virus if blood or an organ is transplanted than are seronegative individuals.[231]

Knowledge of the sequence of events is particularly important for the diagnosis of hepatitis B virus infection. Detection of viral antigen, especially the surface antigen (HBsAg), plays an important role in the diagnosis of acute infection. The e antigen of hepatitis B virus is detected at the same time as DNA polymerase activity, which is a marker for infectious virus; the presence of e antigen has correlated with acute, communicable disease in many studies,[368] as discussed above. Antibody to the viral core (HBc) is important diagnostically during the time when surface antigen has been cleared from the circulation and antibody to the surface antigen is not yet detectable. The presence of core antigen correlates with circulating viral DNA.[279] In some patients a chronic infection develops in which antigenemia persists in the absence of serum antibody; this group has an increased risk for the development of chronic liver disease. It is now apparent that many of these patients have circulating antibody, which is not detected by commercial systems because it is complexed with antigen.[335] In addition, it has been demonstrated that some patients who have circulating antibody and no detectable surface antigen have circulating viral DNA detectable by amplification techniques for as long as 5 years.[347]

Likewise the diagnosis of infectious mononucleosis can be made on a single serum if antibody to early antigen *and* IgM antibody to viral capsid antigen (VCA) are present. A high titer of IgG antibody to VCA in the absence of both antibody to EA and IgM antibody to VCA suggests a past infection. It is important to know the time course of the infection when interpreting the serologic results.[411]

The most common test for detecting infections by EBV is the heterophil antibody test. Heterophil antibodies are im-

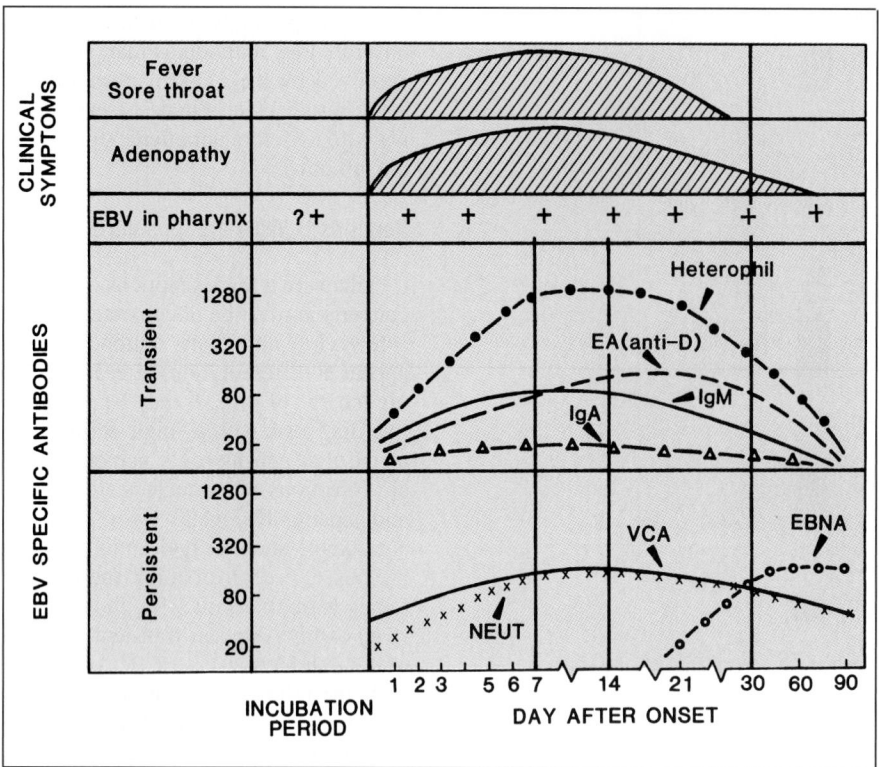

Figure 23-18 Time course of Epstein-Barr Virus (EBV) infections and serologic response. Although virus may be identified in oral secretions, the techniques for culture are difficult and are available only in research laboratories. The heterophil antibody response is the classic means of documenting infectious mononucleosis and is still the most useful test. The transient appearance of heterophil antibody, IgM antibody to viral capsid antigen, and antibody to EA allows one to associate the presence of antibody with the current illness. Neutralizing antibody and IgG antibody to viral capsid antigen (VCA) persist for months or years. These tests are useful to determine that the patient has been infected previously and is therefore immune; they may also be useful diagnostically if the first specimen is collected sufficiently early and a seroconversion is documented. If the patient is seen late in the course of the illness, diagnosis may be made by detection of a seroconversion to viral nuclear antigen (EBNA). (Modified with permission from James C. Niederman, Yale University School of Medicine, New Haven, CT.)

munoglobulins that react with substances from another species. In the course of an EBV infection, antibodies are produced to a variety of extraneous antigens. Agglutinins for sheep and horse red cells, hemolysins for beef red cells, and antibodies to the *Proteus* OX19 antigen of the Weil-Felix test are all produced. The heterophil antibodies that are very specific for infectious mononucleosis are absorbed by beef red cells but not by guinea pig kidney. The Paul-Bunnell-Davidsohn differential test for infectious mononucleosis is designed to characterize these heterophil antibodies; it is highly specific for EBV and confirmatory for making the laboratory diagnosis of infectious mononucleosis.[116] A variety of simplified tests for detecting the heterophil response in infectious mononucleosis are now available commercially; most test agglutination of horse red cells after appropriate absorption of the sera.[158,243] Results that do not conform to clinical or hematologic data should be evaluated by performing the differential tube test or testing for EBV-specific antibodies. The agglutination tests for heterophil antibody are "simple" tests, which can be performed by "anyone" with

no difficulty. In 1990 a pseudoepidemic of infectious mononucleosis was recognized in Puerto Rico.[66] Quality-control and proficiency-testing results gave no hint of problems, but careful investigation revealed that two technicians with limited experience had been reporting examinations as positive based on "weak reactivity," a category that did not exist for the method used.

Ninety percent of adults with infectious mononucleosis will have heterophil antibodies. The frequency with which these antibodies develop in young children is much lower. Heterophil antibodies developed in only 3 of 11 infants younger than 2 years of age after a primary EBV infection, whereas such antibodies developed in 16 of 21 children between the ages of 2 and 4 years.[241] Heterophil-negative infectious mononucleosis with circulating atypical lymphocytes is usually caused by EBV (demonstrable by specific antibodies to viral components) or by CMV.[242] Horwitz and colleagues found that sera from 38.1% of patients with heterophil antibody-positive mononucleosis cross reacted in an IgM-CMV test, but sera from patients with acute CMV in-

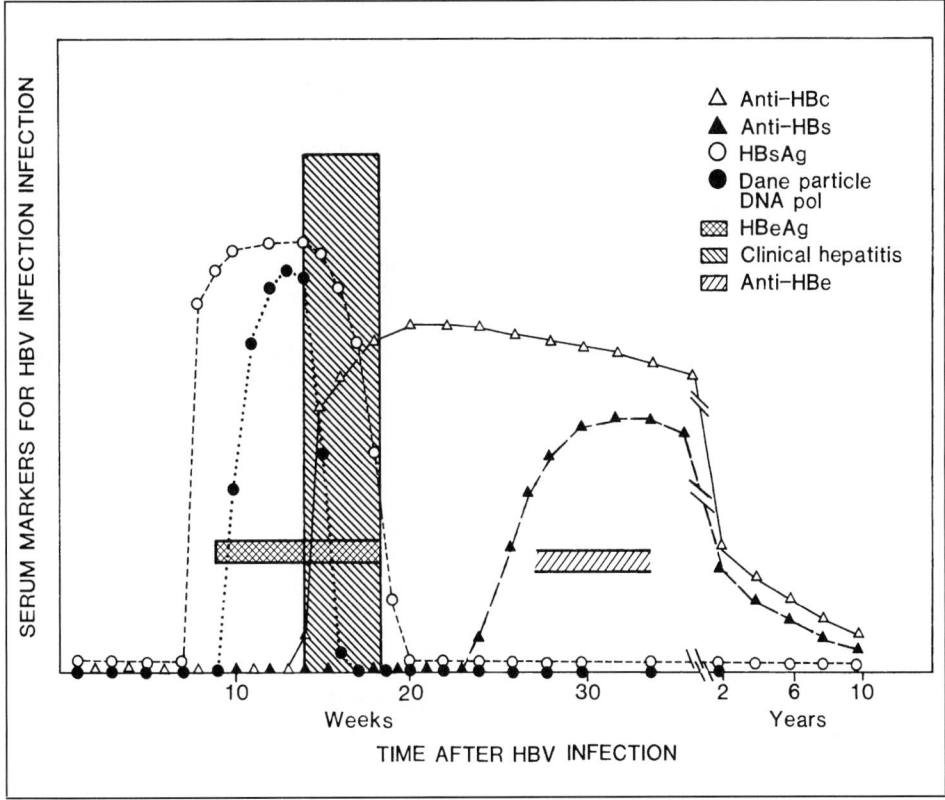

Figure 23-19 Antigens and antibodies after self-limited infection with hepatitis B virus. The appearance of antigens and antibodies after self-limited infection with hepatitis B virus is an example of how knowledge of the biology of infection led to very effective diagnostic strategies, although the virus itself was difficult or impossible to culture. One must look for both antigen and antibody to detect cases efficiently. Hepatitis B surface antigen (HBsAg) appears first; after it is cleared from the blood, antibody to that antigen can be detected (anti-HBsAg). There may be a time, however, when antigen has been cleared but antibody is not detectable; measurement of antibody to the core antigen (anti-HBc) will cover that possibility. The presence of HBs does not equal acute, self-limited infection because some persons become carriers. (Modified with permission from William S. Robinson, M.D., Stanford University Medical Center, Stanford, CA.)

fection did not react in the EBV VCA-IgM test.[242] Cross-reacting antibodies to either the D or R component of the early antigen were detected in sera from 9 of 36 patients (25%) with mononucleosis caused by agents other than EBV (six cases of CMV infection, one of toxoplasmosis, one of probable hepatitis, and one of unknown cause).

Hepatitis A Virus

Hepatitis A is the only primary hepatitis virus to have been cultured in vitro. The virus will grow in a variety of simian cells, most notably early passages of African green monkey kidney cells.[28] Culture is not a viable diagnostic option, however, because recovery from primary specimens is not reliable. Hepatitis A is diagnosed serologically by detection of specific IgM antibody.[407,457,472] Very early in the infection IgM antibody may not be detectable, so the test should be repeated 2 weeks later if clinical suspicion is high.[227]

Hepatitis C Virus

The laboratory diagnosis of hepatitis C infections requires a combination of serologic and molecular tests. The first generation of enzyme immunoassays lacked sensitivity and specificity, but the second and third generations have improved substantially on the early tests. An expert panel has recommended an approach to hepatitis C that is similar to that used for HIV. The initial evaluation is made with a sensitive enzyme immunoassay. If that screening test is positive, the result is confirmed, using a different method.[7]

Several immunoassays have been cleared by the FDA for diagnostic use: the Abbott HCV EIA 2.0 (Abbott Laboratories) and Ortho HCV version 3.0 Elisa (Ortho-Clinical Diagnostics, Raritan, NJ), and Vitros Anti-HCV Assay (an enhanced chemiluminescence assay; Ortho-Clinical Diagnostics). All three assays use HCV-encoded recombinant antigens.[7]

The only confirmatory assay that has been cleared by the FDA for diagnostic use in is an immunoblot assay, the Chiron RIBA HCV 3.0 SIA (Chiron, Emeryville, CA).

Once a serologic diagnosis of hepatitis C virus infection has been established, molecular tools are needed to characterize the infection fully.

Parvovirus

Parvovirus infections in children are usually transient and do not require laboratory support for diagnosis. Concern is focused on immunosuppressed patients, patients with sickle cell disease, and pregnant women. Enzyme immunoassays, immunoblot tests, and radioimmunoassay have been developed.[47] Determination of IgG is sufficient to determine immune status in a pregnant woman who has been exposed to the virus; measurement of IgM is necessary for documenting acute infection. If hydrops fetalis is feared or suspected, a combination of serologic and virologic approaches is complementary.[536]

Herpes Simplex Virus

The serologic diagnosis of herpes simplex virus infections was not useful because of the high prevalence of antibody to type 1 virus early in life and the inability of commercially available assays to distinguish between the two serotypes.

Glycoprotein G antigen of herpes simplex elicits type-specific antibodies, for which there are now commercially available enzyme and immunoblot assays for IgG. These assays provide a convenient way to document immune status in pregnant women and (with acute and convalescent specimens) recent infection in immunosuppressed patients and in pregnant women.[16,496] Although concern has been expressed about the time to seroconversion, using the gG protein, one of the commercial assays yielded similar results to an immunoblot reference procedure.[15]

When measured against culture-documented genital infections, the type-specific serologic assays have good sensitivity and specificity.[360] Assays are also available for type 1 virus, although the diagnostic imperative is less compelling than for type 2 virus.[496]

Potentially the greatest use for these serologic assays is defining the risk of a primary herpes infection developing in the near term in pregnant women, when it may be transmitted to the neonate. The highest risk is in a woman who lacks antibody (not previously infected) and a partner who is seropositive. Avoidance of a primary infection is imperative in that situation. It should be noted that recurrent shedding of virus is not uncommon in seropositive women,[499] although the risk for the neonate is less in recurrent infection than in primary disease.

Varicella-Zoster Virus

The place for serology in the diagnosis of VZV infections is for determination of immune status in patients or healthcare personnel. A latex agglutination assay compared favorably with the fluorescent test,[283,467] and was more sensitive than an enzyme immunoassay.[467] Enzyme immunoassays, however, have yielded satisfactory results.[126]

Cytomegalovirus

Serology is of secondary importance in the diagnosis of cytomegalovirus infection and disease.[329]

Serology does play an important role, however, in assessing risk for recipients of transplants. Infection with cytomegalovirus, which is often asymptomatic, may be accompanied by DNA in peripheral blood for many months after primary infection, even in the presence of a vigorous antibody response.[535] Recrudescence of this latent virus may be accompanied by an IgM response, so this usual marker of primary infection is flawed in this situation.[130] Problems in valid detection of IgM class antibodies complicate the picture. In one careful study of intrauterine CMV disease only 10% of women with IgM antibody as determined by an enzyme immunoassay delivered a congenitally infected fetus.[304] When the presence of IgM antibody was confirmed with a specific immunoblot assay,[305] however, the risk was similar to documented infection during the first trimester.

The highest risk for serious CMV infection developing is transplantation of an organ from a seropositive donor into a seronegative recipient.[473] When possible, attempts are made to avoid this combination.

West Nile Virus

As with other flaviviruses West Nile virus does not grow readily in the cell cultures used in most virology laboratories. The diagnosis of this infection is made by serology and, to a lesser extent at present, by molecular techniques. The clinical disease is primarily encephalitis, so the focus is on CSF. IgG and IgM antibody can be detected reliably in serum and CSF.[402] The presence of specific IgM antibody documents the infection. The initial outbreak was at first thought to be St. Louis encephalitis, because the two flaviviruses share common antigens. Positive antibody tests should, therefore, be confirmed with a different serologic approach. Until further experience is acquired it has been suggested that continuous validation of assays is a prudent course of action.[325]

Rubella

The traditional test for assessing immunity to rubella virus is hemagglutination-inhibition, but it has been replaced in most laboratories by more convenient assays, particularly enzyme immunoassays.[195] These tests work well for determining immune status. For diagnosis of congenital infection, measurement of IgM antibodies with a rigorously validated method is necessary.

SARS Coronavirus

Antibody to the SARS coronavirus can be detected in >90% of patients with clinically evident disease, using an indirect immunofluorescence technique.[85] A very small percentage of patients without clinically evident disease also had seroconversion. At present serologic diagnosis appears to be the most sensitive method for diagnosing the infection.

Anti-IgM Antibodies

In general, IgM antibody appears earlier than IgG after an acute infection and is more transient. In addition, IgM does not readily cross the placenta, so demonstration of this antibody in a neonate indicates a congenital or perinatal infection, rather than passive transfer of antibody from the mother.

Demonstration of IgM antibody to any antigen suggests, therefore, a recent infection. The test should be used only in laboratories in which the results have been carefully evaluated, because several theoretical and practical pitfalls may produce an erroneous interpretation. Most importantly, critical clinical decisions are often dependent on accurate results.

It is extremely important that the procedure for detection of the IgM class be demonstrably specific. The presence of IgM antibody is usually tested by demonstration of a decrease in titer after removal of IgM, by documenting residual activity after removal of IgG, by using specific antiglobulins directed against IgM, or by a combination of these approaches.

If an anti-IgM antibody is used to determine the acuteness of an infection, the specificity of the antiglobulin must be documented. False-negative results may be generated if there are very high levels of IgG, which may block the sites that would have reacted with IgM. False-positive results may be encountered if antiglobulins, such as rheumatoid factor, are present in the patient's serum. If a serum reacts with multiple antigens (i.e., rubella, CMV, herpes simplex virus, and *Toxoplasma gondii*), an antiglobulin should be suspected.

Finally, although IgM antibody in serum is usually transient, there are documented instances in which IgM antibody has persisted for months or even years. Furthermore, it is now recognized that IgM can be detected when some latent infections are reactivated.[130]

Miscellaneous Serologic Procedures

A wide variety of procedures can be used for serologic diagnosis of viral infections (Table 23-26). Enzyme immunoassay and immunofluorescence tests are gaining in popularity in clinical laboratories; many of these tests are available commercially in kit form.

Diagnosis of Other Viral Infections

Diagnosis of some viral infections is beyond the scope of most hospital laboratories because the infections are rare or exotic, the etiologic agents are hazardous, or special diagnostic facilities are necessary. Tests for rabies, arbovirus infections, and viral hemorrhagic fevers are usually performed in a reference laboratory, such as those in state departments of health or at the CDC.

Antiviral Susceptibility Testing

Resistance to antiviral agents is an unfortunate fact of life, although not yet in epidemic proportions. Evaluation of patients in whom antiviral therapy for HIV fails is a regular part of the treatment of patients, as discussed previously. Resistance in other viral agents, particularly the herpes group of viruses, is well recognized, but fortunately uncommon. Susceptibility testing of clinical isolates is available in selected reference laboratories.[475]

Infections With Chlamydia *Species*

Chlamydiae are obligately intracellular bacterial pathogens. Three species of *Chlamydia* produce human disease. *Chlamydia psittaci* causes acute respiratory infections, usually transmitted by infected birds.[435] Infections by *Chlamydia trachomatis*, which includes 15 serologic variants (serovars), are much more common.[432] Serovars L1, L2, and L3 produce a sexually transmitted disease, lymphogranuloma venereum. Trachoma, a chronic conjunctivitis often complicated by blindness, is associated with serovars A, B1, B2, and C. The newest member of the genus, *Chlamydia pneumoniae*, was originally referred to as the TWAR bacillus, using the initials of two patients from whom the bacterium was isolated. Genetic studies demonstrate that the three species are closely related.[178]

All of the chlamydia may be isolated in embryonated eggs and cell culture. Recovery of *C. psittaci* in cell culture should not be attempted unless stringent isolation facilities are available for protection of laboratory personnel. Care to prevent laboratory-acquired infections should also be exercised if the serovars that cause lymphogranuloma venereum are suspected.

Chlamydia trachomatis

CLINICAL FEATURES AND EPIDEMIOLOGY

Inclusion conjunctivitis (an infection distinguished from trachoma by the absence of corneal scarring), pneumonia in neonates, and sexually transmitted infections in adults, all of which are caused by serovars D through K, are the chlamydial diseases of most importance for diagnostic laboratories.[266] The sexually transmitted infections include urethritis, mucopurulent cervicitis, and salpingitis. The sexually transmitted and neonatal infections are, in fact, directly connected. Schachter and colleagues followed 131 infants born to mothers from whose cervix *C. trachomatis* was cultured.[433] Culture-confirmed inclusion conjunctivitis developed in 18% of the infants, and 16% had neonatal chlamydial pneumonia.

COLLECTION OF SPECIMENS

Cervical and ocular specimens are best collected by scraping the mucosa. Swabs are readily available and minimally traumatic. Wood-tipped swabs and swabs made of calcium alginate should be avoided; some cotton swabs have been toxic to *Chlamydia;* Dacron or rayon material is preferred.[101] Urethral and nasopharyngeal specimens may be collected with a fine swab on a flexible wire. The swab should be inserted 3 to 5 cm into the urethra. Semen and purulent urethral discharge are not considered adequate specimens for culture.[101] *C. trachomatis* can be detected in first morning urine specimens with amplification techniques, as discussed later.

Cervical specimens are collected from the endocervix after carefully removing mucus. The isolation rate is increased if a urethral and cervical swab are placed in the same transport vial.

Table 23-26 **Serologic Diagnosis of Viral Infections**

VIRUS	TESTS COMMONLY PERFORMED	COMMENTS
Respiratory Infections		
Influenza A & B	CF; HAI; EIA	HAI performed for strain-specific immunity
Parainfluenza	CF; HAI; EIA	
Respiratory syncytial	FA; EIA; IB	
Adenovirus	CF; HAI; EIA	Rhesus or rat RBC for HAI
Coronavirus	NT; EIA; FA; IB	Limited data for SARS virus
Central Nervous System Infections		
Enteroviruses	NT	Not commonly performed
Mumps	CF; HAI; FA; EIA	
Herpes simplex	EIA; IB	Type-specific reagents required
Rabies	NT; EIA	For immune status
Hepatitis		
Hepatitis A	EIA	
Hepatitis B	EIA; RIA	See text
Hepatitis C	EIA; IB	Screening test followed by confirmatory assay
Hepatitis D	EIA; RIA	Rarely performed
Hepatitis E	EIA	
Cutaneous Infections		
Measles	HAI; EIA	
Varicella-zoster	EIA; ACIF; FAMA; LA	For immune status
Genital Infections		
Herpes simplex	EIA; IB	Type-specific reagents necessary
HIV	EIA; IB	Screening test followed by confirmatory test
Other Infections		
Cytomegalovirus	EIA; IFA; Passive latex agglutination	Primarily for immune status
Rubella	HAI; EIA; LA; IB	HAI reference method
Epstein-Barr	CF; FA;EIA	See discussion
Parvovirus	RIA; EIA	
Human herpes 6 & 7	NT; FA; EIA; IB	

ACIF, anti-complement immunofluorescence; CF, complement fixation; EIA, enzyme immunoassay; FA, immunofluorescence; FAMA, fluorescent antibody staining of membrane antigens; HAI, hemagglutination-inhibition; IB, immunoblot or immunochromatograph; LA, latex agglutination; NT, neutralization test (the reference test for most viruses, although infrequently necessary); RIA, radioimmunoassay.

ISOLATION OF *CHLAMYDIA TRACHOMATIS* IN CELL CULTURE

Although chlamydiae are bacteria, they are obligate intracellular pathogens. Methods for isolation in culture are similar to those used in the virology laboratory. It is essential, however, that the infective elementary bodies of chlamydiae be centrifuged onto the monolayer in a shell vial (see Fig. 23-9). Isolation of the bacteria is optimized if a force of 3,000 *g* for 60 minutes can be achieved.[456] Cells that have been irradiated or treated with a metabolic inhibitor are used for culture. Cycloheximide-treated McCoy cells are the most commonly used cell line[531]; cycloheximide (1 μg/mL) is included in the tissue culture media that are used after infection of the monolayer. Polybrene, a poly cation that has been used to enhance the infectivity of retroviruses, also enhances the number of chlamydial inclusions and the rate of isolation from clinical specimens.[431] Sabet and colleagues successfully used HeLa 229 cells that had been treated with DEAE-dextran and cycloheximide for isolation of *C. trachomatis*.[426] Buffalo green monkey cells are reportedly superior to McCoy cells.[290]

Inclusion bodies of *C. trachomatis* contain glycogen, which may be stained with iodine. After incubation for 48 to 72 hours, the coverslips are removed and stained with iodine or, for somewhat greater sensitivity, with a fluoresceinated monoclonal antibody[465] (see Color Plate 23-2*C*). Species-specific monoclonal antibodies directed against outer-membrane proteins and genus-specific antibodies directed against lipopolysaccharide are available. Chlamydial inclusions are well-demarcated, cytoplasmic structures. Additional sensitivity may be achieved by subculturing growth in a vial if the culture is negative after a single passage, but the expense of the procedure is increased considerably.

Micromethods for culture have been described in which 96-well microplates are seeded with McCoy cells either before or at the time of inoculation with the clinical specimen.[476,531] The wells are examined microscopically after staining with iodine or fluorescein-conjugated antiserum. The microplates are considerably more economical than the individual shell vials and have been found to be of equivalent sensitivity by several investigators.[531] Other investigators, however, consider the micromethod less sensitive than conventional culture.[267] Much of the argument over whether blind subculture increases the recovery of *Chlamydia* probably derives from varying protocols for primary culture.[267] In general, there is little yield from blind subculture if vessels with a large surface are inoculated and a monoclonal antibody is used to detect inclusions. Micromethods benefit from routine subculture.

DIRECT DETECTION OF *CHLAMYDIA TRACHOMATIS* IN CLINICAL SPECIMENS

Morphologic Detection of Inclusions. If large numbers of chlamydial inclusion bodies are present, a diagnosis may be established easily by staining smears by the Giemsa or Gimenez methods. The Gimenez stain, which contains carbolfuchsin, is preferred because the inclusions are colored well, but the Giemsa stain is more generally available. The inclusions, which are located in the cytoplasm of epithelial cells, often have a perinuclear location and must be distinguished from artifacts, such as fragmented nuclei (see Color Plate 23-2*A*). The frequency with which inclusions are detected in smears is highest in neonatal conjunctivitis, lower in inclusion conjunctivitis of adults and in trachoma, and lowest in urethritis and cervicitis, where inclusions are rarely found. In practice, direct visualization is rarely attempted.

Detection of Antigen. The initial approaches to nonculture laboratory diagnosis were direct immunofluorescence (see Color Plate 23-2*B*) and subsequently enzyme immunoassay. Although commercial products for some of these tests are still available, they have been supplanted by molecular methods. Interested readers should consult the previous edition of this book.

Detection of Nucleic Acid. The first commercial molecular test applied to *C. trachomatis* was a DNA probe against rRNA (Pace 2 Systems Assays, Gen-Probe, San Diego, CA). The sensitivity of the test has ranged from approximately 80% to 95%, depending on the population of patients tested, the source of the specimen, the version of the test evaluated, and the "gold standard" applied.

The second generation of molecular tests are amplification tests of several kinds. Most comparative studies have evaluated either the hybridization assays (and/or antigen assays) and culture or amplification assays and culture. The cumulative evidence suggested that amplification assays were the most sensitive method, but the conclusions were indirectly derived. At least one study, however, compared all three approaches head to head, with amplification assays again being considerably more sensitive than the competition.[528]

The most commonly used molecular tests at present use polymerase chain reaction (Amplicor CT/NG Test and Cobas Amplicor Chlamydia trachomatis [CT]/Neisseria gonorrhoeae [NG] Test; Roche Diagnostics),[313] strand-displacement amplification (BD ProbeTec CT and CT/GC assays; BD Diagnostic),[488] transcription-mediated amplification (Gen-Probe Aptima Combo 2 assay; Gen-Probe)[179], and the hybrid capture method (Hybrid Capture 2 CT/NG DNA test; Digene).[113] One product, which used the ligase chain reaction, has been withdrawn from the market.

The various amplification methods appear to function in a similar fashion. All are more sensitive than other methods, but they are also more expensive. Price appears to be the most important factor that has deterred laboratories from adopting what is clearly the most sensitive approach to diagnosis.[22] In addition to sensitivity, the amplification methods also offer convenience. They can be applied to urine, which is a more acceptable alternative for male patients and for women who do not require a pelvic examination for other reasons. Research studies have documented the acceptability of self-collected vaginal swabs,[446] which may be an approved collection method in the future. In general, endocervical specimens are marginally more sensitive than urine in women, but urine is more sensitive than urethral swabs in asymptomatic men.[262]

There are also differences among the tests. Although not a problem for *C. trachomatis*, cross-reactions between *Neisseria gonorrhoeae* and commensal *Neisseria* spp. have been documented with tests that use polymerase chain reaction and strand-displacement methods,[263] leading one group of investigators to recommend that positive results be confirmed.[489] Cross-reactions have not been demonstrated with transcription-mediated amplification.

It should be noted that most authorities consider all positive screening tests to be presumptive,[263] requiring confirmation unless the specificity is absolute (a criterion that only culture fulfills). The issue is more pressing for *N. gonorrhoeae* than for *C. trachomatis*, because the prevalence of the former is less. Most assays for *C. trachomatis* are performed in the absence of clinical symptoms and are, therefore, screening tests. Each laboratory director must make a determination. If the economics of repeat testing make universal adoption of confirmatory testing unlikely, it is certainly true that repeat testing is indicated should there be any question about the validity of the result from a clinical perspective. The complexity of the issue has been carefully reviewed by an expert panel.[263] For instance, if the test is repeated, should a different method be used? A second specimen? If the two results differ, which is correct?

A significant problem for amplification tests is the presence of inhibitors of amplification in clinical specimens. Some commercial products offer, but do not necessarily require, an amplification control. If a substance normally present in the specimen (e.g., β-globin) is not amplified, a negative result must be considered suspect. Unfortunately, the cost of the test is increased by this manipulation. Transcription-mediated amplification appears not to be affected by inhibitors.[95] In at least one study, the results of testing by the strand-displacement method were not affected when an amplification control was used.[488] The issue is not academic, because the sensitivity of the test is, not surprisingly, increased by testing larger volumes of urine (thus increasing inhibitors if they affect the results of the assay).[352]

A common approach to endocervical cytology is the use of a liquid collection medium. This specimen can also be used for detection of human papillomavirus and appears to be useful for amplification of *C. trachomatis* DNA also.[27]

SEROLOGIC DIAGNOSIS

Antibodies to *C. psittaci* and the lymphogranuloma venereum serovars of *C. trachomatis* can be detected by the complement-fixation test. A microimmunofluorescence test for antibodies to *C. trachomatis* is more sensitive for diagnosis of lymphogranuloma venereum infections and can also be used to document infections by other serovars.[166] This test is less widely available, and multiple antigens must be tested. It is most useful for seroepidemiologic studies of populations at high risk for chlamydial infection.[263]

OTHER METHODS FOR DIAGNOSIS

Cytologic detection of *Chlamydia* has not generally been considered reliable. Kiviat and colleagues, however, have reported a cytologic inflammatory pattern that strongly suggested the presence of chlamydial infection.[280] If "transparent" lymphocytes and increased numbers of histiocytes were present, *C. trachomatis* was isolated in 53% of patients; in the absence of those findings *C. trachomatis* was isolated only from 4% of patients. If these cytologic features are noted in a cervical smear, specific tests for chlamydia should be considered.

Point-of-care tests with less restrictive testing require-

ments are available. They are less sensitive and more expensive than laboratory-based tests.[263]

DIAGNOSIS OF SEXUAL ABUSE

Among the less attractive aspects of *Chlamydia trachomatis* infections is the occurrence of the organism in sexually abused children.[114] The test of choice for investigation of suspected sexual abuse or when other legal considerations obtain is culture.[263]

Chlamydia psittaci

Chlamydia psittaci is the causative agent of psittacosis or ornithosis. The source of infection is a variety of birds, especially psittacine species such as parakeets.[214] An outbreak of psittacosis occurred at a turkey-processing plant in North Carolina.[63] Many organ systems may be affected in the natural host. In humans the primary infectious target is the lung.[435] The resulting pneumonia is usually subacute or chronic, but mild or inapparent infection[357] and acute, fulminating infection[51] can result. *C. psittaci* is also a cause of culture-negative endocarditis.[506]

The diagnosis of psittacosis is usually accomplished by serology. The traditional test was complement fixation, but the microimmunofluorescence test has become the reference serologic test.[166] Complement-fixing antibodies to *C. psittaci* were detected in 36 of 78 sera (46%) submitted for chlamydial serology.[524] An additional 12 sera (15%) were positive by microimmunofluorescence, and 9 more had antibodies to *C. pneumoniae* by microimmunofluorescence.

The organism can be isolated in cell culture using methods designed for *C. trachomatis*, but this agent has high potential for producing laboratory infections, so great care should be taken with the specimen. Species-specific antisera are necessary for definitive identification of the isolate. If the monolayer reacts with antibodies to the lipopolysaccharide, but not the outer-membrane protein of *C. trachomatis*, it suggests that another *Chlamydia* species is present. Presumptive identification of *C. psittaci* directly in respiratory secretions has been reported by using antisera to chlamydial lipopolysaccharide.[378] The PCR has been used to identify the organism directly in clinical specimens[120] and after isolation in culture.[150]

Chlamydia pneumoniae

Chlamydia pneumoniae was originally isolated from patients with respiratory infections and was first called TWAR after the source patients. It produces sporadic and epidemic lower respiratory disease characterized as atypical pneumonia.[199] It has been estimated that 10% of pneumonias worldwide are caused by *C. pneumoniae*,[277] but most infections do not require admission to the hospital. Asymptomatic infection occurs in 2–5% of individuals. *C. pneumoniae* was detected by culture or PCR in the nasopharynx of 2 of 104 (1.9%) asymptomatic adults.[253] The prevalence of antibody to *C. pneumoniae* in this population was 82%.

Primary infection occurs in children and young adults, but immunity is not solid and reinfections are common in adults.[277] The onset of pneumonia is often insidious, without purulent sputum or leukocytosis. The chest radiograph varies from normal to extensive involvement, and there are no diagnostic features. In primary infection the most common pattern is unilateral alveolar infiltrates.[343] Chronic pulmonary infections occur, and patients may be symptomatic for weeks or months.[211]

Chlamydia pneumoniae is a cause of pharyngitis alone and in combination with other agents[252] and is a cause of culture-negative endocarditis.[180] Multiple studies have documented an association between *C. pneumoniae* and atherosclerosis with or without coronary artery disease.[270] The organism has been demonstrated repeatedly in the pathologic lesions. The causality of the association, however, remains a matter for discussion and further investigation.[198]

Chlamydia pneumoniae can be cultured in the laboratory using HeLa 229 cells with dextran, HL cells,[100] HEp-2 cells,[318] or NCI-H 292 cells.[318,523] If HL cells or 292 cells are used, it may not be necessary to treat the monolayers or to perform blind passage.[523] Eagle's minimal essential medium or sucrose-phosphate-glutamate with an added protein source, such as fetal calf serum, as used for viruses and *C. trachomatis,* are useful transport media.[316] Laboratory-adapted strains of *C. pneumoniae* are relatively stable, but wild-type strains are more labile and do not survive well for more than a few hours even at 4°C. Samples should be frozen, preferably at −70°C if they cannot be processed on the day of collection. Fluorescein-conjugated monoclonal antisera are available for detection and identification of isolates in culture.[353] Cultures are incubated for 72 hours. Incubation in serum-free medium has been reported to increase the infectivity of laboratory-adapted strains for HL cells 10- to 50-fold and to increase the number of inclusions produced by a wild-type strain.[317]

The laboratory diagnosis of *C. pneumoniae* infections is complicated by the difficulty of culture and the absence of an alternative reliable gold standard. Most infections are diagnosed serologically. The serology may be more complicated than realized at present. Antigenic variation among isolates was sufficiently great in one study that some patients produced measurable antibody only against their own isolate.[29] The reference test is microimmunofluorescence. Enzyme immunoassays have been developed, but are variable in their performance.[223] Demonstration of seroconversion in acute and convalescent specimens is recommended[129] and represents the most reproducible serologic approach among laboratories.[391] Reproducibility of IgM determinations among collaborating laboratories was quite variable.[391]

Molecular-amplification methods for direct detection of *C. pneumoniae* in respiratory specimens have been developed because of the difficulties inherent in cultural and serologic approaches. Lack of standardization limits the utility of these potentially important assays at present.[35] Unfortunately less than 25% of PCR assays fulfilled the validation criteria suggested by expert panels.[129]

Infections With Rickettsia, Coxiella, Ehrlichia, and Anaplasma

The order *Rickettsiales* includes the families *Rickettsiaceae* and *Anaplasmataceae.*[135] The most numerous and important genus is *Rickettsia. Rickettsia tsutsugamushi* has been reclassified as *Orientia tsutsugamushi.* These organisms are found in the alpha-1 subgroup of *Proteobacteria. Coxiella,* once classified in the order *Rickettsiales,* is actually more closely related to *Legionella* and *Francisella,* members of the gamma subgroup of *Proteobacteria.*[340] Laboratory diagnosis of rickettsial infections and identification of rickettsia in ticks has been reviewed by La Scola and Raoult.[291] A century after the recognition of these infectious agents David Walker has described the origins of the field of rickettsiology and the life of Howard Ricketts, who ultimately died of typhus in Mexico City.[503]

Rickettsia and *Coxiella*

CLINICAL FEATURES AND EPIDEMIOLOGY

Rickettsia species infect vascular endothelial cells. The clinical manifestations of infection are consequently protean and may reflect damage to any organ system. The skin, lung, and brain are most frequently involved symptomatically. *Rickettsia* can be divided into the typhus, scrub typhus, and spotted fever groups (Table 23-27). The agent of Q fever, *Coxiella burnetii,* is also an obligate intracellular pathogen. The primary means of transmission of rickettsial infections is by the bite of an infected arthropod, with the exception of *C. burnetii,* which is most commonly transmitted through infected milk or by aerosol.

Epidemic typhus has been one of the great scourges of humankind, appearing during periods of crowding and starvation. *R. prowazekii* has been demonstrated in flying squirrels in the eastern United States,[525] and a small number of associated human infections have occurred. A case of epidemic typhus has also been recorded in the Southwest.[336]

Although epidemic (louse-borne) typhus is not a serious problem in North America, as recently as 1996–1997 this classic disease killed 6,000 people in Burundi. In the United States, endemic (flea-borne or murine) typhus has received renewed attention. A focus of murine typhus was identified in Southern California and in South Texas in the 1990s. It is transmitted by the cat flea and maintained in cats and opossums.[461] The etiologic agent is the classic *R. typhi*[461] and additionally a newly recognized rickettsia, initially named the ELB agent.[442,522] It is difficult to distinguish the two rickettsiae serologically, so molecular analysis is necessary.[442] The ELB rickettsia has now been classified as *R. felis.*[225] By molecular analysis it belongs in the spotted fever group, rather than the typhus group, of rickettsia.[38]

In the United States, the most important rickettsial infection is Rocky Mountain spotted fever, caused by *R. rickettsii.*[500] This multisystemic febrile disease is usually accompanied by a skin rash that begins on the extremities.[501] The infection is widely distributed throughout the country, wherever the tick vectors exist (see Chapter 22; Appendix I). Paradoxically, it is more common in the Midwestern and south central states than in the western and mountain states.[217] Similar infections, caused by other rickettsial species, are widely distributed around the world (Table 23-27).[409]

Scrub typhus is not endemic in the United States. The causative agent has been reclassified as *Orientia tsutsugamushi.* Scrub typhus is often accompanied by a primary es-

Table 23-27   Rickettsial Infections

DISEASE	SPECIES	INSECT VECTOR
Typhus Group		
Epidemic typhus[a]	*Rickettsia prowazekii*	Human body louse hause
Murine typhus[a]	*R. typhi*	Flea
Relapsing typhus (Brill-Zinsser disease)[a]	*R. prowazekii*	
Spotted fever group		
Rocky Mountain spotted fever[a]	*R. rickettsii*	*Dermacentor* spp.
Mediterranean spotted fever (Boutonneuse fever)	*R. conorii*	*Haemaphysalis* spp.
Siberian tick typhus	*R. sibirica*	*Haemaphysalis* spp., *Dermacentor* spp.
Queensland tick typhus	*R. australis*	*Ixodes holocyclus* *Ixodes tasmanii*
Israeli tick typhus	Israeli tick typhus rickettsia	*Rhipicephalus* spp.
Japanese (Oriental) spotted fever	*R. japonica*	*Haemaphysalis longicornis;* *Dermacentor taiwanensis*
Flinders Island spotted fever	*R. honei*	*Aponomma hydrosauri*
Astrakhan fever	Astrakhan fever rickettsia	*Rhipicephalus* spp.
African tick bite fever	*R. africae*	*Amblyomma* spp.
Rickettsialpox[a]	*R. akari*	*Allodermanyssus sanguineus* (mite)
"Cat flea typhus"	*R. felis*	*Ctenocephalides felis* (cat fleas)
Unnamed spotted fever	"*R. mongolotimonae*"	*Hyalomma* spp.
Scrub typhus group		
Scrub typhus	*Orientia tsutsugamushi*	*Leptotrombidium* chiggers (larval mites)
Q fever group		
Q fever[a]	*Coxiella burnetii*	Parturient animals, unpasteurized dairy foods

[a] Found in the United States.
Adapted from reference[409].

char, which is seen only rarely in Rocky Mountain spotted fever. Primary eschars are also seen in rickettsialpox, which is caused by *Rickettsia akari*. The infection was first documented in New York City and associated with the bites of blood-sucking mites. Rickettsialpox is a mild disease and is not commonly recognized, but occurs worldwide. It remains a presence in New York City.[275]

Q fever usually causes asymptomatic infection, undifferentiated febrile disease, granulomatous hepatitis, or atypical pneumonia.[340,410] It may be transmitted through milk, products of conception, or excreta of infected cattle, sheep, and goats. The organism is easily transmitted to susceptible humans, and epidemics have occurred in laboratories where sheep were used for research purposes.[209] A chronic form of the infection may result in subacute bacterial endocarditis. Rash is rare in Q fever.

COLLECTION OF SPECIMENS

Culture of *Rickettsia* is performed only in reference laboratories. Blood or biopsy tissue from a lesion should be frozen at $-70°C$. Direct immunofluorescence may be performed on a frozen or formalin-fixed biopsy or autopsy specimen. Rickettsial infections are usually diagnosed serologically, using acute and convalescent sera.

ISOLATION OF *RICKETTSIA* AND *COXIELLA* IN CULTURE

Rickettsia and *Coxiella* may be isolated in small laboratory animals or in embryonated eggs.[504] *Coxiella burnetii* has been isolated in shell vial cultures of human embryonic lung fibroblasts from blood of 17% of untreated patients with acute Q fever and 53% of untreated patients with chronic disease.[369] All of these bacteria are highly infectious when they are aerosolized. They have been responsible for many laboratory-acquired infections, some of which were fatal.[379] Isolation of the agents should be attempted only in laboratories where adequate containment of infection is possible. Whole blood or biopsied tissues may be cultured.

DIRECT DETECTION OF ANTIGEN AND NUCLEIC ACID IN CLINICAL SPECIMENS

Antigens of *Rickettsia rickettsii,* the cause of Rocky Mountain spotted fever, can be detected directly by staining sections of infected skin lesions using the direct or indirect immunofluorescence or immunoenzymatic techniques.[504] The sensitivity of the procedure is approximately 70%, and the specificity approaches 100%. Usually, petechial skin lesions are biopsied. The rickettsiae are most likely to be in the blood vessel at the center of the lesion, so it is important to ensure that such vessels are included in the tissue section. Antigens can also be demonstrated in paraffin-embedded, formalin-fixed specimens if the section is treated first with proteases to unmask antigens.[505] Although the immunofluorescence test is valuable for making an early diagnosis of Rocky Mountain spotted fever, it is available in very few laboratories.

Patients with fatal disease usually die before a serologic response develops. Identification of rickettsial antigens (and potentially nucleic acid) in tissue are the only methods available for making a specific etiologic diagnosis in that situation.[381]

Molecular-amplification assays for documentation of rickettsia in clinical specimens have been described, but are not widely available.[145,291]

SEROLOGIC DIAGNOSIS

Most diagnoses of rickettsial infections are made by serology.[132] In recent years, the microimmunofluorescence assay has become the reference test.[397] This procedure appears to be the most sensitive and specific method for the diagnosis of rickettsial infections.[273] The degree of cross-reaction among rickettsial species varies from patient to patient.[397] Cross-reactions are strongest within the rickettsial subgroups. It may be difficult to distinguish between epidemic and endemic typhus or between Rocky Mountain spotted fever and rickettsialpox.[504] Antibodies first appear 7 to 10 days after infection. A fourfold rise in serum antibody is desired for diagnosis, but a single titer of more than 1:64 is highly suggestive.

The microimmunofluorescence test requires highly trained personnel and a fluorescence microscope. Latex agglutination tests, which are now commercially available for Rocky Mountain spotted fever, are in more general use. The latex tests appear to produce positive reactions only during an acute infection, so a single positive test is diagnostic.[220] The sensitivity has ranged from 70% to 95%.[220,273] After infection by *Coxiella burnetii,* antibodies may be produced to two biologic phases of the organism. Antibodies to phase II are produced first. Antibodies to phase I, which appear weeks or months later, may reach high levels in patients with Q fever endocarditis. If antibodies to both phases of *Coxiella* are high in a patient with culture-negative endocarditis, a diagnosis of Q fever is likely.[278,463]

Historically, the most common diagnostic test for rickettsial disease has been the Weil-Felix test, in which antirickettsial antibodies that cross-react with strains of *Proteus* species are detected. The test originated from the chance observation that sera from patients with typhus agglutinated strains of *Proteus vulgaris.* As experience with immunologically specific serologic tests has been accumulated, it has become apparent that the Weil-Felix test is both insensitive and nonspecific.[221,273,504] In some populations, a positive Weil-Felix test result has been more common in those who did not have Rocky Mountain spotted fever than in those who were infected.[504] All of these facts argue strongly for the relegation of this test to the archives.

Ehrlichia and *Anaplasma* Species

The family Anaplasmataceae are rickettsia-like bacteria that can infect humans and a variety of animal species, producing diseases such as tropical canine pancytopenia and Potomac horse fever (Table 23-28).[421] They are obligate intracellular parasites and, like rickettsiae, grow in the cytosol of infected cells.

Human ehrlichial infection, which is a recently recognized phenomenon, is caused by several distinct species, of which two are most important: *Ehrlichia chaffeensis,* which infects human monocytic cells,[8,117] and a second species that infects granulocytic cells (*Anaplasma phagocytophilum,* originally designated the human granulocytic *Ehrlichia*).[88] Both species are transmitted to humans by ticks and produce febrile illness with leukopenia, thrombocytopenia, and elevated serum aminotransferase.[134]

Table 23-28 Some Ehrlichia and Related Organisms With Associated Diseases[a]

ORGANISM	DISEASE	HOST
Ehrlichia chaffeensis	Human monocytic ehrlichiosis	Human
	Canine monocytic ehrlichiosis	Dogs
Ehrlichia ewingii	"Ehrlichiosis ewingii"	Humans
	Canine granulocytic ehrlichiosis	Dogs
Ehrlichia canis	Canine monocytic ehrlichiosis	Dogs
Anaplasma phagocytophilum	Human granulocytic anaplasmosis	Humans
	Equine granulocytic anaplasmosis	Horses
	Canine granulocytic anaplasmosis	Dogs
Neorickettsia sennetsu	Sennetsus fever	Humans
Neorickettsia risticii	Potomac horse fever	Horses
Neorickettsia helminthoeca	Salmon poisoning disease	Salmon

[a] *Courtesy of J. Stephen Dumler, M.D.*

Human Monocytic Ehrlichiosis. The monocytic variety of ehrlichiosis, caused by *Ehrlichia chaffeensis,* was recognized first. It is distributed widely through the Southeast, Midwest, and Far West of the United States. Monocytic ehrlichiae have been documented worldwide. In areas where tick vectors are prevalent, seroconversions to *Rickettsia rickettsii* occurred in 2.5% and to *E. chaffeensis* in 1.3% of military personnel.[530] In southern Georgia, human monocytic ehrlichiosis was seven to eight times more prevalent than Rocky Mountain spotted fever.[157] Contact with ticks is a risk factor for both monocytic ehrlichiosis and Rocky Mountain spotted fever.[9] An outbreak of monocytic ehrlichiosis occurred in a golf-oriented retirement community (community A) that abutted a natural wildlife area.[466] Cases were not recognized at a nearby community and golf course (community B) that were not surrounded by a natural area. The prevalence of antibody to *E. chaffeensis* in community A was 12.5%, whereas in community B the prevalence was 3.3%. Thousands of *A. americanum* ticks were found in community A, but only three ticks were detected in community B. The risk factors for ehrlichiosis included tick bites, contact with wildlife, failure to use insect repellent, and golfing. Among golfers, those at greatest risk were the hookers and slicers, who were constantly retrieving their balls from the rough. The moral is that if you golf in a rural area, you should wear insect repellent and hit the ball straight.

The clinical symptoms of monocytic ehrlichiosis range from nonspecific febrile disease to severe systemic infection with multiorgan failure.[134,156] In one study of 237 infected patients, 60.8% were hospitalized.[156] Severe monocytic ehrlichiosis with failure of multiorgan systems has been mistaken for thrombotic thrombocytopenic purpura[334] and toxic-shock syndrome.[155] Life-threatening disease may occur in individuals who are infected with HIV.[380]

Masses of ehrlichiae (morula) may be seen within the cytoplasm of infected monocytes (Color Plate 23-2*G*), but these diagnostic structures are infrequently seen with *E. chaffeensis* infection.[134,136] The diagnosis is made serologically, by culture of the agent,[89] or by molecular methods.[10,151]

Human Granulocytic Anaplasmosis (Formerly, Human Granulocytic Ehrlichiosis). The second major pathogenic organism is the agent of human granulocytic anaplasmosis (HGA), which was first recognized in Minnesota and Wisconsin by an alert infectious disease physician, who recognized the similarity of the intracellular granulocytic inclusions to those described in *E. chaffeensis* infection.[18,88] The agent of human granulocytic anaplasmosis has been classified as *Anaplasma phagocytophilum;* it is considered conspecific with the human granulocytic agent, *E. phagocytophila,* and *E. equi.*[135] Although variants have been described,[337] *A. phagocytophilum* strains in the United States show a high degree of genetic uniformity.[133]

The most important vector in the United States is *Ixodes scapularis* (see Chapters 20 and 22 and Appendix I), the same tick that transmits the microbes that cause Lyme disease and babesiosis.[384] The duration of attachment required for transmission of *A. phagocytophilum* appears to be somewhat less than that required for infection with *Borrelia burgdorferi,*[123,276] but the exact dynamics are not yet clear. Patients in the North Central United States appear from serologic studies to have been infected with all three pathogens.[348] Not surprisingly, the distribution of human granulocytic anaplasmosis is expanding to cover the range of the host tick. Infections have now been reported from multiple areas in the North Central and Eastern United States. HGA has also been documented in California,[160] as well as in Europe and Asia. In some parts of the country, rickettsial and ehrlichial infections must all be included in the differential diagnosis of febrile disease.[57] Dual infections with ehrlichia and rickettsia have been described.[445] It may be important, therefore, to include antigens of all possible pathogens when attempting serologic diagnosis; demonstration of seroconversion assumes even greater importance.[105]

The clinical disease appears to be similar to that produced by *E. chaffeensis.* Thrombocytopenia is more common than leukopenia. Leukocytosis is accompanied by relative and absolute lymphopenia.[17] Cases of interstitial pneumonitis[416] and facial diplegia[306] also occur. Reinfection has been reported.[240]

Laboratory diagnosis is still in its infancy. Intracellular inclusions (morula) in granulocytes (Color Plate 23-2*H*) appear to be more common than are inclusions in monocytic ehrlichiosis,[18] but there may be an ascertainment bias without readily available laboratory diagnostic support. Culture of the organism in vitro has been reported,[194] but confirmation of most cases is by serologic techniques, which are available in reference laboratories.[502] The most common technique is indirect immunofluorescence. Antibodies reach their peak within a month after infection and are still detectable a year later in approximately half of patients.[4] The vast majority of patients seroconvert and a small percentage remain seropositive for years.[19] Although some bacterial antigens cross-react between the agents of monocytic and granulocytic ehrlichiosis/anaplasmosis, the major outer-membrane proteins do not share antigenic determinants.[486] Western blot analysis may help to resolve confusing serologic results.

Molecular-amplification assays for *A. phagocytophilum* have been described, and reagents are available commercially.[338] The assays, which are not widely available, should be considered to be in a developmental phase.

Other Ehrlichial Infections. A third ehrlichial agent infecting humans was identified as the cause of a disease that resembled ehrlichiosis in Missouri. The etiologic agent, *Ehrlichia ewingii,* had been recognized previously as a cause of canine ehrlichiosis.[49]

Two other bacteria can infect humans on occasion: *Ehrlichia canis,* which also infects dogs,[156,322] and *Neorickettsia* (formerly *Ehrlichia*) *sennetsu.*[421]

Chapter Update: Scientific and public concern about emerging and some re-emerging viral infections continues. Avian influenza viruses that have demonstrated the ability to infect humans are prime concerns (H5, H7, and H9 hemagglutin types) (http://www.cdc.gov/flu/avian/gen-info/). To date efficient transmission from humans has not occurred, but there is widespread fear that such a strain may be just around the corner. In addition, H2N2 viruses that have not circulated since the 1960s have attracted attention because they have not been included in vaccines and large segments of the population are susceptible. Use of an H2N2 strain (a laboratory-adapted strain that appears to have been nonpathogenic) brought the issue to the front burner. CDC now recommends that H2N2 strains and all avian strains be treated as biosafety level 3 agents, rather than the previously designated level 2 (http://www.cdc.gov/flu/han050305.htm). An epidemic of Marburg virus (a filovirus) in Angola (http://www/cdc.gov/mmwr/preview/mmwrhtml/mm5412a5.htm) and of lymphocytic choriomeningitis virus (an arenavirus) in immunosuppressed patients that was associated with pet hamsters (http://www.cdc.gov/mmwr/preview/mmwrhtml/mm54d526a1.htm) reinforce the continued relevance of "exotic" viruses. Although the SARS coronavirus has receded as a threat for the moment, it appears that the human metapneumovirus, which turned out *not* to be the cause of SARS, is a relatively common cause of respiratory infection in children and adults, but uncommon in asymptomatic individuals (Falsey, et al., J Clin Virol, in press, available online May 23, 2005). On a positive note several researchers have demonstrated the utility of screening patients for HIV infection (N Engl J Med, February 10, 2005).

REFERENCES

1. Strategic Science Symposium: human papillomavirus testing-are you ready for a new era in cervical cancer screening? Arch Pathol Lab Med 2003;127:927–996.
2. Abels S, et al. Reliable detection of respiratory syncytial virus infection in children for adequate hospital infection control management. J Clin Microbiol 2001; 39:3135–3139.
3. Ackerman SJ. HIV-1 link prompts circumspection on circumcision. J NIH Res 1991;3:44–46.
4. Aguero-Rosenfeld ME, et al. Serology of culture-confirmed cases of human granulocytic ehrlichiosis. J Clin Microbiol 2000;38:635–638.
5. Albert MR, et al. Smallpox manifestations and survival during the Boston epidemic of 1901 to 1903. Ann Intern Med 2002;137:993–1000.
6. Almeida JD. Uses and abuses of diagnostic electron microscopy. Curr Top Microbiol Immunol 1983;104:147–158.
7. Alter MJ, et al. Guidelines for laboratory testing and result reporting of antibody to hepatitis C virus. Centers for Disease Control and Prevention. MMWR Recomm Rep 2003;52(RR-03):1–15.
8. Anderson BE, et al. *Ehrlichia chaffeensis*, a new species associated with human ehrlichiosis. J Clin Microbiol 1991;29:2838–2842.
9. Anderson BE, et al. *Amblyomma americanum*: a potential vector of human ehrlichiosis. Am J Trop Med Hyg 1993;49:239–244.
10. Anderson BE, et al. Detection of the etiologic agent of human ehrlichiosis by polymerase chain reaction. J Clin Microbiol 1992;30:775–780.
11. Ando T, et al. Genetic classification of "Norwalk-like viruses." J Infect Dis 2000;181:Suppl:48.
12. Annunziato D, et al. Atypical measles syndrome: pathologic and serologic findings. Pediatrics 1982;70:203–209.
13. Arvin AM. Varicella-zoster virus. In: Fields BN, Knipe DM, Melnick JL, et al., eds. Virology. Ed. 2. New York: Raven Press, 1990:2731–2767.
14. Arvin AM, et al. Immunologic evidence of reinfection with varicella-zoster virus. J Infect Dis 1983;148:200–205.
15. Ashley RL, et al. Ability of a rapid serology test to detect seroconversion to herpes simplex virus type 2 glycoprotein G soon after infection. J Clin Microbiol 1999;37:1632–1633.
16. Ashley RL, Wald A. Genital herpes: review of the epidemic and potential use of type-specific serology. Clin Microbiol Rev 1999;12:1–8.
17. Bakken JS, et al. Serial measurements of hematologic counts during the active phase of human granulocytic ehrlichiosis. Clin Infect Dis 2001;32:862–870.
18. Bakken JS, et al. Human granulocytic ehrlichiosis in the upper Midwest United States: a new species emerging? JAMA 1994;272:212–218.
19. Bakken JS, et al. The serological response of patients infected with the agent of human granulocytic ehrlichiosis. Clin Infect Dis 2002;34:22–27.
20. Barenfanger J, et al. Clinical and financial benefits of rapid detection of respiratory viruses: an outcomes study. J Clin Microbiol 2000;38:2824–2828.
21. Barenfanger J, et al. R-Mix cells are faster, at least as sensitive and marginally more costly than conventional cell lines for the detection of respiratory viruses. J Clin Virol 2001;22:101–110.
22. Battle TJ, et al. Evaluation of laboratory testing methods for *Chlamydia trachomatis* infection in the era of nucleic acid amplification. J Clin Microbiol 2001; 39:2924–2927.
23. Beld M, et al. Performance of the new Bayer VERSANT HCV RNA 3.0 assay for quantitation of hepatitis C virus RNA in plasma and serum: conversion to international units and comparison with the Roche COBAS Amplicor HCV Monitor, Version 2.0, assay. J Clin Microbiol 2002;40:788–793.
24. Belongia EA, et al. An outbreak of herpes gladiatorum at a high-school wrestling camp. N Engl J Med 1991;325:906–910.
25. Bendinelli M, Pistello M, Maggi F, Vatteroni M. Blood-borne hepatitis viruses: hepatitis B, C, D, and G viruses and TT virus. In: Specter S, Hodinka RL, Young SA, eds. Clinical Virology Manual. Ed. 3. Washington, DC: ASM Press, 2000: 306–337.
26. Benedetti J, et al. Recurrence rates in genital herpes after symptomatic first-episode infection. Ann Intern Med 1994;121:847–854.
27. Bianchi A, et al. PreservCyt transport medium used for the ThinPrep Pap test is a suitable medium for detection of Chlamydia trachomatis by the COBAS Amplicor CT/NG test: results of a preliminary study and future implications. J Clin Microbiol 2002;40:1749–1754.
28. Binn LN, et al. Primary isolation and serial passage of hepatitis A virus strains in primate cell cultures. J Clin Microbiol 1984;20:28–33.
29. Black CM, et al. Antigenic variation among strains of *Chlamydia pneumoniae*. J Clin Microbiol 1991;29:1312–1316.
30. Blackard JT, et al. Human immunodeficiency virus superinfection and recombination: current state of knowledge and potential clinical consequences. Clin Infect Dis 2002;34:1108–1114.
31. Blank BS, et al. Value of different assays for detection of human cytomegalovirus (HCMV) in predicting the development of HCMV disease in human immunodeficiency virus-infected patients. J Clin Microbiol 2000;38:563–569.
32. Bloom ME, Young NS. Parvoviruses. In: Fields BN, Knipe DM, Melnick JL, et al., eds. Virology. Ed. 2. New York: Raven Press, 1990:2361–2379.
33. Blumberg BS. Australia antigen and the biology of hepatitis B. Science 1977; 197:17–25.
34. Boivin G, et al. Virological features and clinical manifestations associated with human metapneumovirus: a new paramyxovirus responsible for acute respiratory-tract infections in all age groups. J Infect Dis 2002;186:1330–1334.
35. Boman J, et al. Molecular diagnosis of *Chlamydia pneumoniae* infection. J Clin Microbiol 1999;37:3791–3799.
36. Booth CM, et al. Clinical features and short-term outcomes of 144 patients with SARS in the greater Toronto area. JAMA 2003;289:2801–2809.
37. Bourlet T, et al. New PCR test that recognizes all human prototypes of enterovirus: application for clinical diagnosis. J Clin Microbiol 2003;41:1750–1752.
38. Bouyer DH, et al. *Rickettsia felis*: molecular characterization of a new member of the spotted fever group. Int J Syst Evol Microbiol 2001;51:339–347.
39. Boylston AW. Clinical investigation of smallpox in 1767. N Engl J Med 2002; 346:1326–1328.
40. Bradley R, Wilesmith JW. Epidemiology and control of bovine spongiform encephalopathy (BSE). Br Med Bull 1993;49:932–959.
41. Bray M, Wright ME. Progressive vaccinia. Clin Infect Dis 2003;36:766–774.
42. Breman JG, et al. Preventing the return of smallpox. N Engl J Med 2003;348: 463–466.
43. Brindeiro PA, et al. Testing genotypic and phenotypic resistance in human immunodeficiency virus type 1 isolates of clade B and other clades from children failing antiretroviral therapy. J Clin Microbiol 2002;40:4512–4519.
44. Brinker JP, Doern GV. Comparison of MRC-5 and A-549 cells in conventional culture tubes and shell vial assays for the detection of varicella-zoster virus. Diagn Microbiol Infect Dis 1993;17:75–77.
45. Brinker JP, Doern GV. Enhancement of varicella-zoster virus detection in A-549 shell vials by use of freeze-thawed specimens, extended incubation, and "a centrifuged, not incubated" direct detection method. Diagn Microbiol Infect Dis 1998;31:555–558.
46. Bromberg K, et al. Comparison of Ortho respiratory syncytial virus enzyme-linked immunosorbent assay and HEp-2 cell culture. J Clin Microbiol 1985;22: 1071–1072.
47. Bruu AL, Nordbo SA. Evaluation of five commercial tests for detection of immunoglobulin M antibodies to human parvovirus B19. J Clin Microbiol 1995; 33:1363–1365.
48. Buchmeier MJ, Bowen MD, Peters CJ. *Arenaviridae:* the viruses and their replication. In: Fields BN, Knipe DM, Melnick JL, et al., eds. Virology. Ed. 2. New York: Raven Press, 1990:1635–1668.

49. Buller RS, et al. *Ehrlichia ewingii*, a newly recognized agent of human ehrlichiosis. N Engl J Med 1999;341:148–155.

50. Bush RM, et al. Predicting the evolution of human influenza A. Science 1999; 286:1921–1925.

51. Byrom NP, et al. Fulminant psittacosis. Lancet 1979;1:353–356.

52. Caldwell MB, et al. 1994 revised classification system for human immunodeficiency virus infection in children less than 13 years of age. MMWR Morb Mortal Wkly Rep 1994;43(RR 12):1–10.

53. Caliendo AM, et al. Distinguishing cytomegalovirus (CMV) infection and disease with CMV nucleic acid assays. J Clin Microbiol 2002;40:1581–1586.

54. Caliendo AM, et al. Comparison of quantitative cytomegalovirus (CMV) PCR in plasma and CMV antigenemia assay: clinical utility of the prototype AMPLICOR CMV MONITOR test in transplant recipients. J Clin Microbiol 2000;38: 2122–2127.

55. Calisher CH. Medically important arboviruses of the United States and Canada. Clin Microbiol Rev 1994;7:89–116.

56. Calisher CH, Mahy BW. Taxonomy: get it right or leave it alone. Am J Trop Med Hyg 2003;68:505–506.

57. Carpenter CF, et al. The incidence of ehrlichial and rickettsial infection in patients with unexplained fever and recent history of tick bite in central North Carolina. J Infect Dis 1999;180:900–903.

58. Carrat F, et al. Evaluation of clinical case definitions of influenza: detailed investigation of patients during the 1995–1996 epidemic in France. Clin Infect Dis 1999;28:283–290.

59. Castle PE, et al. Results of human papillomavirus DNA testing with the hybrid capture 2 assay are reproducible. J Clin Microbiol 2002;40:1088–1090.

60. Castle PE, et al. Comparison between prototype hybrid capture 3 and hybrid capture 2 human papillomavirus DNA assays for detection of high-grade cervical intraepithelial neoplasia and cancer. J Clin Microbiol 2003;41:4022–4030.

61. Castro KG, et al. 1993 revised classification system for HIV infection and expanded surveillance case definition for AIDS among adolescents and adults. MMWR Morb Mortal Wkly Rep 1992;41:(RR-17).

62. Centers for Disease Control and Prevention. Interpretation and use of the Western blot assay for serodiagnosis of human immunodeficiency virus type 1 infections. MMWR Morb Mortal Wkly Rep 1989;38(S7):1–7.

63. Centers for Disease Control and Prevention. Psittacosis at a turkey processing plant-North Carolina, 1989. MMWR Morb Mortal Wkly Rep 1990;39:460–469.

64. Centers for Disease Control and Prevention. Update: measles outbreak. MMWR Morb Mortal Wkly Rep 1990;39:317–326.

65. Centers for Disease Control and Prevention. Interpretive criteria used to report Western blot results for HIV-1-antibody testing—United States. MMWR Morb Mortal Wkly Rep 1991;40:692–695.

66. Centers for Disease Control and Prevention. Pseudo-outbreak of infectious mononucleosis—Puerto Rico, 1990. MMWR Morb Mortal Wkly Rep 1991;40: 552–555.

67. Centers for Disease Control and Prevention. Arenavirus infection—Connecticut, 1994. MMWR Morb Mortal Wkly Rep 1994;43:635–636.

68. Centers for Disease Control and Prevention. Bolivian hemorrhagic fever-El Beni Department, Bolivia, 1994. MMWR Morb Mortal Wkly Rep 1994;43:943–946.

69. Centers for Disease Control and Prevention. Interstate Measles Transmission from a Ski Resort—Colorado, 1994. MMWR Morb Mortal Wkly Rep 199443: 627–629.

70. Centers for Disease Control and Prevention. Mass treatment of humans exposed to rabies—New Hampshire, 1994. MMWR Morb Mortal Wkly Rep 1995;44: 484–486.

71. Centers for Disease Control and Prevention. Appendix: Revised surveillance case definition for HIV infection. MMWR Recomm Rep 1999;48(RR-13): 29–31.

72. Centers for Disease Control and Prevention. Surveillance for AIDS-defining opportunistic illnesses. MMWR CDC Surveill Summ 1999;48:1–22.

73. Centers for Disease Control and Prevention. Appendix A: practice recommendations for health-care facilities implementing the U.S. public health service guidelines for management of occupational exposures to bloodborne pathogens. MMWR Recomm Rep 2001;50(RR-11):43–44.

74. Centers for Disease Control and Prevention. Appendix B: management of occupational blood exposures. MMWR Recomm Rep 2001;50(RR-11):45–46.

75. Centers for Disease Control and Prevention. Appendix C: basic and expanded HIV postexposure prophylaxis regimens. MMWR Recomm Rep 2001;50(RR-11):47–52.

76. Centers for Disease Control and Prevention. Revised recommendations for HIV screening of pregnant women: perinatal counseling and guidelines consultation. MMWR Recomm Rep 2001;50(RR-19):59–66.

77. Centers for Disease Control and Prevention. Updated U.S. public health service guidelines for the management of occupational exposures to HBV, HCV, and HIV and recommendations for postexposure prophylaxis. MMWR Recomm Rep 2001;50(RR-11):1–42.

78. Centers for Disease Control and Prevention. Fatal degenerative neurologic illnesses in men who participated in wild game feasts—Wisconsin, 2002. MMWR Morb Mortal Wkly Rep 2003;52:125–127.

79. Centers for Disease Control and Prevention. Global progress toward certifying polio eradication and laboratory containment of wild polioviruses—August 2002–August 2003. MMWR Morb Mortal Wkly Rep 2003;52:1158–1160.

80. Centers for Disease Control and Prevention. Increases in HIV diagnoses-29 states, 1999–2002. MMWR Morb Mortal Wkly Rep 2003;52:1145–1148.

81. Centers for Disease Control and Prevention. Bovine spongiform encephalopathy in a dairy cow—Washington State, 2003. MMWR Morb Mortal Wkly Rep 2004; 52:1280–1285.

82. Centers for Disease Control and Prevention. Outbreaks of avian influenza A (H5N1) in Asia and interim recommendations for evaluation and reporting of suspected cases—United States, 2004. MMWR Morb Mortal Wkly Rep 2004; 53:97–100.

83. Celum CL, et al. Indeterminate human immunodeficiency virus type 1 western blots: seroconversion risk, specificity of supplemental tests, and an algorithm for evaluation. J Infect Dis 1991;164:656–664.

84. Chan KH, et al. Evaluation of the Directigen FluA + B test for rapid diagnosis of influenza virus type A and B infections. J Clin Microbiol 2002;40:1675–1680.

85. Chan KH, et al. Detection of SARS coronavirus in patients with suspected SARS. Emerg Infect Dis 2004;10:294–299.

86. Chan PK, et al. Human metapneumovirus detection in patients with severe acute respiratory syndrome. Emerg Infect Dis 2003;9:1058–1063.

87. Chandler FW, Gorelkin L. Immunofluorescence staining of adenovirus in fixed tissues pretreated with trypsin. J Clin Microbiol 1983;17:371–373.

88. Chen SM, et al. Identification of a granulocytotropic Ehrlichia species as the etiologic agent of human disease. J Clin Microbiol 1994;32:589–595.

89. Chen SM, et al. Cultivation of *Ehrlichia chaffeensis* in mouse embryo, Vero BGM, and L929 cells and study of Ehrlichia-induced cytopathic effect and plaque formation. Infect Immun 1995;63:647–655.

90. Chernin E, Weller TH. Serial propagation of *Toxoplasma gondii* in roller tube cultures of mouse and of human tissues. Proc Soc Exp Biol Med 1954;85:68–72.

91. Chesebro B. Introduction to the transmissible spongiform encephalopathies or prion diseases. Br Med Bull 2003;66:1–20.

92. Chevret S, et al. Usefulness of the cytomegalovirus (CMV) antigenemia assay for predicting the occurrence of CMV disease and death in patients with AIDS. Clin Infect Dis 1999;28:758–763.

93. Chiba S, et al. Sapporo virus: history and recent findings. J Infect Dis 2000; 181:Suppl 8.

94. Choi KW, et al. Outcomes and prognostic factors in 267 patients with severe acute respiratory syndrome in Hong Kong. Ann Intern Med 2003;139:715–723.

95. Chong S, et al. Specimen processing and concentration of *Chlamydia trachomatis* added can influence false-negative rates in the LCx assay but not in the APTIMA Combo 2 assay when testing for inhibitors. J Clin Microbiol 2003; 41:778–782.

96. Chonmaitree T, et al. Role of the virology laboratory in diagnosis and management of patients with central nervous system disease. Clin Microbiol Rev 1989; 2:1–14.

97. Chou S. Reactivation and recombination of multiple cytomegalovirus strains from individual organ donors. J Infect Dis 1989;160:11–15.

98. Christy C, et al. Comparison of three enzyme immunoassays to tissue culture for the diagnosis of rotavirus gastroenteritis in infants and young children. J Clin Microbiol 1990;28:1428–1430.

99. Clavel F, Hance AJ. HIV drug resistance. N Engl J Med 2004;350:1023–1035.

100. Cles LD, Stamm WE. Use of HL cells for improved isolation and passage of *Chlamydia pneumoniae*. J Clin Microbiol 1990;28:938–940.

101. Clyde WA, Kenny GE, Schachter J. Diagnosis of *Chlamydia* Infection. Washington DC: American Society for Microbiology, 1984.

102. Cohen JI, et al. Recommendations for prevention of and therapy for exposure to B virus (cercopithecine herpesvirus 1). Clin Infect Dis 2002;35:1191–1203.

103. Cohen OJ, Fauci AS. Pathogenesis and medical aspects of HIV-1 infection. In: Knipe DM, Howley PM, eds. Fields Virology. Ed. 4. Philadelphia: Lippincott Williams & Wilkins, 2001;2043–2094.

104. Collinge J. Variant Creutzfeldt-Jakob disease. Lancet 1999;354:317–323.

105. Comer JA, et al. Serologic testing for human granulocytic ehrlichiosis at a national referral center. J Clin Microbiol 1999;37:558–564.

106. Consensus Conference: The impact of routine HTLV-III antibody testing of blood and plasma donors on public health. JAMA 1986;256:1778–1783.

107. Condit RC. Principles of virology. In: Knipe DM, Howley PM, eds. Fields Virology. Ed. 4. Philadelphia: Lippincott Williams & Wilkins, 2001:19–51.

108. Cordonnier C, et al. Evaluation of three assays on alveolar lavage fluid in the diagnosis of cytomegalovirus pneumonitis after bone marrow transplantation. J Infect Dis 1987;155:495–500.

109. Cote S, et al. Comparative evaluation of real-time PCR assays for detection of the human metapneumovirus. J Clin Microbiol 2003;41:3631–3635.

110. Couch RB. Rhinoviruses. In: Knipe DM, Howley PM, eds. Fields Virology. Ed. 4. Philadelphia: Lippincott Williams & Wilkins, 2001:777–797.

111. Dahl H, et al. Antigen detection: the method of choice in comparison with

virus isolation and serology for laboratory diagnosis of herpes zoster in human immunodeficiency virus-infected patients. J Clin Microbiol 1997;35:347–349.

112. Daly P, et al. High-sensitivity PCR detection of parvovirus B19 in plasma. J Clin Microbiol 2002;40:1958–1962.

113. Darwin LH, et al. Comparison of Digene Hybrid Capture 2 and conventional culture for detection of *Chlamydia trachomatis* and *Neisseria gonorrhoeae* in cervical specimens. J Clin Microbiol 2002;40:641–644.

114. Dattel BJ, et al. Isolation of *Chlamydia trachomatis* from sexually abused female adolescents. Obstet Gynecol 1988;72:240–242.

115. David AS, et al. Postviral fatigue syndrome: time for a new approach. BMJ 1988;296:696–699.

116. Davidsohn I, Lee CL. The laboratory in the diagnosis of infectious mononucleosis with additional notes on epidemiology, etiology and pathogenesis. Med Clin North Am 1962;46:225–244.

117. Dawson JE, et al. Isolation and characterization of an *Ehrlichia* sp. from a patient diagnosed with human ehrlichiosis. J Clin Microbiol 1991;29:2741–2745.

118. de Baar MP, et al. Single rapid real-time monitored isothermal RNA amplification assay for quantification of human immunodeficiency virus type 1 isolates from groups M, N, and O. J Clin Microbiol 2001;39:1378–1384.

119. De Tiege X, et al. Limits of early diagnosis of herpes simplex encephalitis in children: a retrospective study of 38 cases. Clin Infect Dis 2003;36:1335–1339.

120. Dean D, et al. Molecular identification of an avian strain of *Chlamydia psittaci* causing severe keratoconjunctivitis in a bird fancier. Clin Infect Dis 1995;20:1179–1185.

121. DeHertogh DA, Brettman LR. Hemorrhagic cystitis due to herpes simplex virus as a marker of disseminated herpes infection. Am J Med 1988;84:632–635.

122. del Mar MM, et al. Simultaneous detection of measles virus, rubella virus, and parvovirus b19 by using multiplex PCR. J Clin Microbiol 2002;40:111–116.

123. des Vignes F, et al. Effect of tick removal on transmission of *Borrelia burgdorferi* and *Ehrlichia phagocytophila* by *Ixodes scapularis* nymphs. J Infect Dis 2001;183:773–778.

124. Dhar AD, et al. Tanapox infection in a college student. N Engl J Med 2004;350:361–366.

125. Diaz-Mitoma F, et al. Comparison of DNA amplification, mRNA amplification, and DNA hybridization techniques for detection of cytomegalovirus in bone marrow transplant recipients. J Clin Microbiol 2003;41:5159–5166.

126. Doern GV, et al. Comparison of the Vidas and Bio-Whittaker enzyme immunoassays for detecting IgG reactive with varicella-zoster virus and mumps virus. Diagn Microbiol Infect Dis 1997;28:31–34.

127. Dolin R, et al. Novel agents of viral enteritis in humans. J Infect Dis 1987;155:365–376.

128. Donnelly CA. Bovine spongiform encephalopathy in the United States-an epidemiologist's view. N Engl J Med 2004;350:539–542.

129. Dowell SF, et al. Standardizing assays: recommendations from the Centers for Disease Control and Prevention (USA) and the Laboratory Centre for Disease Control (Canada). Clin Infect Dis 2001;33:492–503.

130. Drew WL. Controversies in viral diagnosis. Rev Infect Dis 1986;8:814–824.

131. Drosten C, et al. Rapid detection and quantification of RNA of Ebola and Marburg viruses, Lassa virus, Crimean-Congo hemorrhagic fever virus, Rift Valley fever virus, dengue virus, and yellow fever virus by real-time reverse transcription-PCR. J Clin Microbiol 2002;40:2323–2330.

132. Dumler JS. Serodiagnosis of rickettsial infections. In: Isenberg HD, ed. Clinical Microbiology Procedures Handbook. Ed. 2. Washington, DC: ASM Press, 2004:11.7.1.1–11.7.4.3.

133. Dumler JS, et al. Analysis of genetic identity of North American *Anaplasma phagocytophilum* strains by pulsed-field gel electrophoresis. J Clin Microbiol 2003;41:3392–3394.

134. Dumler JS, Bakken JS. Ehrlichial diseases of humans: emerging tick-borne infections. Clin Infect Dis 1995;20:1102–1110.

135. Dumler JS, et al. Reorganization of genera in the families *Rickettsiaceae* and *Anaplasmataceae* in the order *Rickettsiales*: unification of some species of *Ehrlichia* with *Anaplasma*, *Cowdria* with *Ehrlichia* and *Ehrlichia* with *Neorickettsia*, descriptions of six new species combinations and designation of *Ehrlichia equi* and 'HGE agent' as subjective synonyms of *Ehrlichia phagocytophila*. Int J Syst Evol Microbiol 2001;51:2145–2165.

136. Dumler JS, et al. Persistent infection with *Ehrlichia chaffeensis*. Clin Infect Dis 1993;17:903–905.

137. Dunn JJ, et al. Sensitivity of respiratory virus culture when screening with R-mix fresh cells. J Clin Microbiol 2004;42:79–82.

138. Durant J, et al. Drug-resistance genotyping in HIV-1 therapy: the VIRADAPT randomised controlled trial. Lancet 1999;353:2195–2199.

139. Dybul M, et al. Guidelines for using antiretroviral agents among HIV-infected adults and adolescents: recommendations of the panel on clinical practices for treatment of HIV. MMWR Recomm Rep 2002;51(RR-07).

140. Eing BR, et al. Evaluation of two enzyme immunoassays for detection of human rotaviruses in fecal specimens. J Clin Microbiol 2001;39:4532–4534.

141. Emanuel D, et al. Rapid immunodiagnosis of cytomegalovirus pneumonia by

bronchoalveolar lavage using human and murine monoclonal antibodies. Ann Intern Med 1986;104:476–481.

142. Enders JF, et al. Isolation of measles virus at autopsy in cases of giant-cell pneumonia without rash. N Engl J Med 1959;261:875–881.

143. Enders JF, et al. Cultivation of the Lansing strain of poliomyelitis virus in cultures of various human embryonic tissues. Science 1949;109:85–87.

144. Engblom E, et al. Fatal influenza A myocarditis with isolation of virus from the myocardium. Acta Med Scand 1983;213:75–78.

145. Eremeeva ME, et al. Evaluation of a PCR assay for quantitation of *Rickettsia rickettsii* and closely related spotted fever group rickettsiae. J Clin Microbiol 2003;41:5466–5472.

146. Esposito JJ, Fenner F. Poxviruses. In: Knipe DM, Howley PM, eds. Fields Virology. Ed. 4. Philadelphia: Lippincott Williams & Wilkins, 2001:2885–2921.

147. Espy MJ, et al. Detection of herpes simplex virus DNA in genital and dermal specimens by LightCycler PCR after extraction using the IsoQuick, MagNA Pure, and BioRobot 9604 methods. J Clin Microbiol 2001;39:2233–2236.

148. Espy MJ, Smith TF. Detection of herpes simplex virus in conventional tube cell cultures and in shell vials with a DNA probe kit and monoclonal antibodies. J Clin Microbiol 1988;26:22–24.

149. Espy MJ, et al. Rapid detection of influenza virus by shell vial assay with monoclonal antibodies. J Clin Microbiol 1986;24:677–679.

150. Essig A, et al. Diagnosis of ornithosis by cell culture and polymerase chain reaction in a patient with chronic pneumonia. Clin Infect Dis 1995;21:1495–1497.

151. Everett ED, et al. Human ehrlichiosis in adults after tick exposure: diagnosis using polymerase chain reaction. Ann Intern Med 1994;120:730–735.

152. Falsey AR, Walsh EE. Respiratory syncytial virus infection in adults. Clin Microbiol Rev 2000;13:371–384.

153. Falsey AR, et al. Serologic evidence of respiratory syncytial virus infection in nursing home patients. J Infect Dis 1990;162:568–569.

154. Fedorko DP, et al. Effect of age of shell vial monolayers on detection of cytomegalovirus from urine specimens. J Clin Microbiol 1989;27:2107–2109.

155. Fichtenbaum CJ, et al. Ehrlichiosis presenting as a life-threatening illness with features of the toxic shock syndrome. Am J Med 1993;95:351–357.

156. Fishbein DB, et al. Human ehrlichiosis in the United States, 1985 to 1990. Ann Intern Med 1994;120:736–743.

157. Fishbein DB, et al. Human ehrlichiosis: prospective active surveillance in febrile hospitalized patients. J Infect Dis 1989;160:803–809.

158. Fleisher GR, et al. Limitations of available tests for diagnosis of infectious mononucleosis. J Clin Microbiol 1983;17:619–624.

159. Foley FD, et al. Herpesvirus infection in burned patients. N Engl J Med 1970;282:652–656.

160. Foley JE, et al. Human granulocytic ehrlichiosis in Northern California: two case descriptions with genetic analysis of the ehrlichiae. Clin Infect Dis 1999;29:388–392.

161. Fong CKY, Landry ML. An adventitious viral contaminant in commercially supplied A-549 cells: identification of infectious bovine rhinotracheitis virus and its impact on diagnosis of infection in clinical specimens. J Clin Microbiol 1992;30:1611–1613.

162. Forbes BA, Bartholoma NY. Detection of cytomegalovirus in clinical specimens using shell vial centrifugation and conventional cell culture. Diagn Microbiol Infect Dis 1988;10:121–124.

163. Formenty P, et al. Ebola virus outbreak among wild chimpanzees living in a rain forest of Cote d'Ivoire. J Infect Dis 1999;179:S120–S126.

164. Francis DP, et al. Viral load test reports: a description of content from a sample of US laboratories. Arch Pathol Lab Med 2001;125:1546–1554.

165. Freed ER, Martin MA. HIVs and their replication. In: Knipe DM, Howley PM, eds. Fields Virology. Ed. 4. Philadelphia: Lippincott Williams & Wilkins, 2001:1971–2041.

166. Freidank HM, et al. Evaluation of a new commercial microimmunofluorescence test for detection of antibodies to *Chlamydia pneumoniae*, *Chlamydia trachomatis*, and *Chlamydia psittaci*. Eur J Clin Microbiol Infect Dis 1997;16:685–688.

167. Frenkel LM, et al. Clinical reactivation of herpes simplex virus type 2 infection in seropositive pregnant women with no history of genital herpes. Ann Intern Med 1993;118:414–418.

168. Frey SE, Belshe RB. Poxvirus zoonoses-putting pocks into context. N Engl J Med 2004;350:324–327.

169. Fulginiti VA, et al. Smallpox vaccination: a review, part I. Background, vaccination technique, normal vaccination and revaccination, and expected normal reactions. Clin Infect Dis 2003;37:241–250.

170. Fulginiti VA, et al. Smallpox vaccination: a review, part II. Adverse events. Clin Infect Dis 2003;37:251–271.

171. Gajdusek DC. Unconventional viruses and the origin and disappearance of kuru. Science 1977;197:943–960.

172. Galli RA, et al. Sources and magnitude of intralaboratory variability in a sequence-based genotypic assay for human immunodeficiency virus type 1 drug resistance. J Clin Microbiol 2003;41:2900–2907.

173. Gallwitz S, et al. Smallpox: residual antibody after vaccination. J Clin Microbiol 2003;41:4068–4070.

174. Ganem D, Prince AM. Hepatitis B virus infection-natural history and clinical consequences. N Engl J Med 2004;350:1118–1129.

175. Garcia-Tapia AM, et al. Spectrum of parvovirus B19 infection: analysis of an outbreak of 43 cases in Cadiz Spain. Clin Infect Dis 1995;21:1424–1430.

176. Garry RF, et al. Documentation of an AIDS virus infection in the United States in 1968. JAMA 1988;260:2085–2087.

177. Gault E, et al. Evaluation of a new serotyping assay for detection of anti-hepatitis C virus type-specific antibodies in serum samples. J Clin Microbiol 2003;41:2084–2087.

178. Gaydos CA, et al. Phylogenetic relationship of *Chlamydia pneumoniae* to *Chlamydia psittaci* and *Chlamydia trachomatis* as determined by analysis of 16S ribosomal DNA sequences. Int J Syst Bacteriol 1993;43:610–612.

179. Gaydos CA, et al. Performance of the APTIMA Combo 2 Assay for detection of *Chlamydia trachomatis* and *Neisseria gonorrhoeae* in female urine and endocervical swab specimens. J Clin Microbiol 2003;41:304–309.

180. Gdoura R, et al. Culture-negative endocarditis due to *Chlamydia pneumoniae*. J Clin Microbiol 2002;40:718–720.

181. Gentry GA, et al. Isolation and differentiation of herpes simplex virus and Trichomonas vaginalis in cell culture. J Clin Microbiol 1985;22:199–204.

182. Gerin JL, Casey JL, Purcell RH. Hepatitis delta virus. In: Knipe DM, Howley PM, eds. Fields Virology. Ed. 4. Philadelphia: Lippincott Williams & Wilkins, 2001:3037–3050.

183. Giachetti C, et al. Highly sensitive multiplex assay for detection of human immunodeficiency virus type 1 and hepatitis C virus RNA. J Clin Microbiol 2002;40:2408–2419.

184. Gibbs CJ Jr, et al. Experimental transmission of scrapie to cattle. Lancet 1990;335:1275–1275.

185. Ginocchio CC, et al. Multicenter evaluation of the performance characteristics of the NucliSens HIV-1 QT assay used for quantitation of human immunodeficiency virus type 1 RNA. J Clin Microbiol 2003;41:164–173.

186. Glass GE, et al. Infection with a ratborne hantavirus in US residents is consistently associated with hypertensive renal disease. J Infect Dis 1993;167:614–620.

187. Glatzel M, et al. Extraneural pathologic prion protein in sporadic Creutzfeldt-Jakob disease. N Engl J Med 2003;349:1812–1820.

188. Gleaves CA, et al. Use of murine monoclonal antibodies for laboratory diagnosis of varicella-zoster virus infection. J Clin Microbiol 1988;26:1623–1625.

189. Glezen WP, et al. Acute respiratory disease of university students with special reference to the etiologic role of herpesvirus hominis. Am J Epidemiol 1975;101:111–121.

190. Goff SP. *Retroviridae:* the retroviruses and their replication. In: Knipe DM, Howley PM, eds. Fields Virology. Ed. 4. Philadelphia: Lippincott Williams & Wilkins, 2001:1871–1939.

191. Goh KJ, et al. Clinical features of Nipah virus encephalitis among pig farmers in Malaysia. N Engl J Med 2000;342:1229–1235.

192. Goldmann DA. Epidemiology and prevention of pediatric viral respiratory infections in health-care institutions. Emerg Infect Dis 2001;7:249–253.

193. Goodell SE, et al. Herpes simplex virus proctitis in homosexual men. Clinical, sigmoidoscopic, and histopathological features. N Engl J Med 1983;308:868–871.

194. Goodman JL, et al. Direct cultivation of the causative agent of human granulocytic ehrlichiosis. N Engl J Med 1996;334:209–215.

195. Grangeot-Keros L, Enders G. Evaluation of a new enzyme immunoassay based on recombinant rubella virus-like particles for detection of immunoglobulin M antibodies to rubella virus. J Clin Microbiol 1997;35:398–401.

196. Grant RM, et al. Time trends in primary HIV-1 drug resistance among recently infected persons. JAMA 2002;288:181–188.

197. Grant RM, et al. Accuracy of the TRUGENE HIV-1 genotyping kit. J Clin Microbiol 2003;41:1586–1593.

198. Grayston JT. Background and current knowledge of *Chlamydia pneumoniae* and atherosclerosis. J Infect Dis 2000;181:S402–S410.

199. Grayston JT, et al. Community- and hospital-acquired pneumonia associated with Chlamydia TWAR infection demonstrated serologically. Arch Intern Med 1989;149:169–173.

200. Green KY, Chanock RM, Kapikian AZ. Human caliciviruses. In: Knipe DM, Howley PM, eds. Fields Virology. Ed. 4. Philadelphia: Lippincott Williams & Wilkins, 2001:841–874.

201. Gregg MB. Recent outbreaks of lymphocytic choriomeningitis in the United States of America. Bull World Health Organ 1975;52:549–554.

202. Gregory WW, Menegus MA. Practical protocol for cytomegalovirus isolation: Use of MRC-5 cell monolayers incubated for 2 weeks. J Clin Microbiol 1983;17:605–609.

203. Grossman MC, Silvers DN. The Tzanck smear: can dermatologists accurately interpret it? J Am Acad Dermatol 1992;27:403–405.

204. Gu Z, et al. Multiplexed, real-time PCR for quantitative detection of human adenovirus. J Clin Microbiol 2003;41:4636–4641.

205. Guidry GG, et al. Respiratory syncytial virus infection among intubated adults in a university medical intensive care unit. Chest 1991;100:1377–1384.

206. Hackman RC, et al. Rapid diagnosis of cytomegaloviral pneumonia by tissue immunofluorescence with a murine monoclonal antibody. J Infect Dis 1985;151:325–329.

207. Hall CB. Respiratory syncytial virus and parainfluenza virus. N Engl J Med 2001;344:1917–1928.

208. Hall CB, et al. Respiratory syncytial virus infections in previously healthy working adults. Clin Infect Dis 2001;33:792–796.

209. Hall CJ, et al. Laboratory outbreak of Q fever acquired from sheep. Lancet 1982;1:1004–1006.

210. Halstead SB, Simasthien P. Observations related to the pathogenesis of dengue hemorrhagic fever. II. Antigenic and biologic properties of dengue viruses and their association with disease response in the host. Yale J Biol Med 1970;42:276–292.

211. Hammerschlag MR, et al. Persistent infection with *Chlamydia pneumoniae* following acute respiratory illness. Clin Infect Dis 1992;14:178–182.

212. Hanna GJ, et al. Comparison of sequencing by hybridization and cycle sequencing for genotyping of human immunodeficiency virus type 1 reverse transcriptase. J Clin Microbiol 2000;38:2715–2721.

213. Harder TC, et al. New LightCycler PCR for rapid and sensitive quantification of parvovirus B19 DNA guides therapeutic decision-making in relapsing infections. J Clin Microbiol 2001;39:4413–4419.

214. Harding HB. The epidemiology of sporadic urban ornithosis. Am J Clin Pathol 1962;38:230–243.

215. Harrison SC. Principles of virus structure. In: Knipe DM, Howley PM, eds. Fields Virology. Ed. 4. Philadelphia: Lippincott Williams & Wilkins, 2001:53–85.

216. Hatta M, et al. Molecular basis for high virulence of Hong Kong H5N1 influenza A viruses. Science 2001;293:1840–1842.

217. Hattwick MAW, et al. Rocky Mountain spotted fever: Epidemiology of an increasing problem. Ann Intern Med 1976;84:732–739.

218. Hayflick L. The limited in vitro lifetime of human diploid cell strains. Exp Cell Res 1965;37:614–636.

219. Hazelton PR, Gelderblom HR. Electron microscopy for rapid diagnosis of infectious agents in emergent situations. Emerg Infect Dis 2003;9:294–303.

220. Hechemy KE, et al. Detection of Rocky Mountain spotted fever antibodies by a latex agglutination test. J Clin Microbiol 1980;12:144–150.

221. Hechemy KE, et al. Discrepancies in Weil-Felix and microimmunofluorescence test results for Rocky Mountain spotted fever. J Clin Microbiol 1979;9:292–293.

222. Heikkinen T, et al. Nasal swab versus nasopharyngeal aspirate for isolation of respiratory viruses. J Clin Microbiol 2002;40:4337–4339.

223. Hermann C, et al. Comparison of eleven commercial tests for *Chlamydia pneumoniae*-specific immunoglobulin G in asymptomatic healthy individuals. J Clin Microbiol 2002;40:1603–1609.

224. Hien TT, de Jong M, Farrar J. Avian influenza-a challenge to global health care structures. N Engl J Med 2004;351:2363–2365.

225. Higgins JA, et al. *Rickettsia felis*: a new species of pathogenic *Rickettsia* isolated from cat fleas. J Clin Microbiol 1996;34:671–674.

226. Hill CE, et al. Assessment of Agreement between the AMPLICOR HIV-1 MONITOR Test Versions 1.0 and 1.5. J Clin Microbiol 2004;42:286–289.

227. Hirata R, et al. Patients with hepatitis A with negative IgM-HA antibody at early stages. Am J Gastroenterol 1995;90:1168–1169.

228. Hirsch MS, et al. Antiretroviral drug resistance testing in adults infected with human immunodeficiency virus type 1: 2003 recommendations of an International AIDS Society-USA Panel. Clin Infect Dis 2003;37:113–128.

229. Hirsch MS, et al. Antiretroviral drug resistance testing in adult HIV-1 infection: recommendations of an International AIDS Society-USA Panel. JAMA 2000;283:2417–2426.

230. Ho AS, et al. An outbreak of severe acute respiratory syndrome among hospital workers in a community hospital in Hong Kong. Ann Intern Med 2003;139:564–567.

231. Ho M, et al. The transplanted kidney as a source of cytomegalovirus infection. N Engl J Med 1975;293:1109–1112.

232. Ho SK, et al. Comparison of the CMV brite turbo assay and the digene hybrid capture CMV DNA (version 2.0) assay for quantitation of cytomegalovirus in renal transplant recipients. J Clin Microbiol 2000;38:3743–3745.

233. Hochberg FH, et al. Influenza type B-related encephalopathy. The 1971 outbreak of Reye syndrome in Chicago. JAMA 1975;231:817–821.

234. Hollinger FB, Emerson SU. Hepatitis A virus. In: Knipe DM, Howley PM, eds. Fields Virology. Ed. 4. Philadelphia: Lippincott Williams & Wilkins, 2001:799–840.

235. Hollinger FB, Liang TJ. Hepatitis B virus. In: Knipe DM, Howley PM, eds. Fields Virology. Ed. 4. Philadelphia: Lippincott Williams & Wilkins, 2001:2971–3036.

236. Holmes KV. Coronaviruses. In: Knipe DM, Howley PM, eds. Fields Virology. Ed. 4. Philadelphia: Lippincott Williams & Wilkins, 2001:1187–1203.

237. Holodniy M, et al. Stability of plasma human immunodeficiency virus load in

VACUTAINER PPT plasma preparation tubes during overnight shipment. J Clin Microbiol 2000;38:323–326.

238. Holzl G, et al. Entirely Automated Quantification of Human Immunodeficiency Virus Type 1 (HIV-1) RNA in Plasma by Using the Ultrasensitive COBAS AMPLICOR HIV-1 Monitor Test and RNA Purification on the MagNA Pure LC Instrument. J Clin Microbiol 2003;41:1248–1251.

239. Hondo R, et al. Enzymatic treatment of formalin-fixed and paraffin-embedded specimens for detection of antigens of herpes simplex, varicella-zoster and human cytomegaloviruses. Jpn J Exp Med 1982;52:17–25.

240. Horowitz HW, et al. Reinfection with the agent of human granulocytic ehrlichiosis. Ann Intern Med 1998;129:461–463.

241. Horwitz CA, et al. Clinical and laboratory evaluation of infants and children with Epstein-Barr virus-induced infectious mononucleosis: report of 32 patients (aged 10–48 months). Blood 1981;57:933–938.

242. Horwitz CA, et al. Heterophil-negative infectious mononucleosis and mononucleosis-like illnesses. laboratory confirmation of 43 cases. Am J Med 1977;63: 947–957.

243. Horwitz CA, et al. Spurious rapid infections mononucleosis test results in non-infectious mononucleosis sera: the role of high-titer horse agglutinins. Am J Clin Pathol 1982;78:48–53.

244. Horwitz MA. Adenoviruses. In: Knipe DM, Howley PM, eds. Fields Virology. Ed. 4. Philadelphia: Lippincott Williams & Wilkins, 2001:2301–2326.

245. Houff SA, et al. Human-to-human transmission of rabies virus by corneal transplant. N Engl J Med 1979;300:603–604.

246. Howell CL, Miller MJ. Effect of sucrose phosphate and sorbitol on infectivity of enveloped viruses during storage. J Clin Microbiol 1983;18:658–662.

247. Howell CL, et al. Elimination of toxicity and enhanced cytomegalovirus detection in cell cultures inoculated with semen from patients with acquired immunodeficiency syndrome. J Clin Microbiol 1986;24:657–660.

248. Hsiung GD. Diagnostic Virology Illustrated by Light and Electron Microscopy. Ed. 3. New Haven, CT: Yale University Press, 1982.

249. Huang YT, et al. Application of mixed cell lines for the detection of viruses from clinical specimens. Clin Microbiol Newslett 2000;22:89–92.

250. Huang YT, et al. Engineered BGMK cells for sensitive and rapid detection of enteroviruses. J Clin Microbiol 2002;40:366–371.

251. Huang YT, et al. Cryopreserved cell monolayers for rapid detection of herpes simplex virus and influenza virus. J Clin Microbiol 2002;40:4301–4303.

252. Huovinen P, et al. Pharyngitis in adults: the presence and coexistence of viruses and bacterial organisms. Ann Intern Med 1989;110:612–616.

253. Hyman CL, et al. Prevalence of asymptomatic nasopharyngeal carriage of *Chlamydia pneumoniae* in subjectively healthy adults: assessment by polymerase chain reaction-enzyme immunoassay and culture. Clin Infect Dis 1995;20: 1174–1178.

254. Irani DN, Johnson RT. Diagnosis and prevention of bovine spongiform encephalopathy and variant Creutzfeldt-Jakob disease. Annu Rev Med 2003;54: 305–319.

255. Iwarson S, et al. Hepatitis C. natural history of a unique infection. Clin Infect Dis 1995;20:1361–1370.

256. Jenny-Avital ER, Beatrice ST. Erroneously low or undetectable plasma human immunodeficiency virus type 1 (HIV-1) ribonucleic acid load, determined by polymerase chain reaction, in West African and American patients with non-B subtype HIV-1 infection. Clin Infect Dis 2001;32:1227–1230.

257. Jerome KR, et al. Quantitative stability of DNA after extended storage of clinical specimens as determined by real-time PCR. J Clin Microbiol 2002;40: 2609–2611.

258. Jesionek K. Über einen Befund von protozoenartigen Gebilden in den Organen eines Feten. Münch Med Wochenschr 1904;51:1905–1907.

259. Jin L, et al. Genetic heterogeneity of mumps virus in the United Kingdom: identification of two new genotypes. J Infect Dis 1999;180:829–833.

260. Johnson FB. Transport of viral specimens. Clin Microbiol Rev 1990;3:120–131.

261. Johnson KM, et al. Virus isolations from human cases of hemorrhagic fever in Bolivia. Proc Soc Exp Biol Med 1965;118:113–118.

262. Johnson RE, et al. Evaluation of nucleic acid amplification tests as reference tests for *Chlamydia trachomatis* infections in asymptomatic Men. J Clin Microbiol 2000;38:4382–4386.

263. Johnson RE, et al. Screening tests to detect *Chlamydia trachomatis* and *Neisseria gonorrhoeae* infections—2002. MMWR Recomm Rep 2002;51(RR-15):1–38.

264. Johnson RT, Gibbs CJ Jr. Creutzfeldt-Jakob disease and related transmissible spongiform encephalopathies. N Engl J Med 1998;339:1994–2004.

265. Johnson RT, et al. Measles encephalomyelitis—clinical and immunologic studies. N Engl J Med 1984;310:137–141.

266. Jones RB, Batteiger BE. Chlamydia trachomatis (trachoma, perinatal infections, lymphogranuloma venereum, and other genital infections). In: Mandell GL, Bennett JE, Dolin R, eds. Mandell, Douglas, and Bennett's Principles and Practice of Infectious Diseases. Ed. 5. Philadelphia: Churchill Livingstone, 2000: 1989–2004.

267. Jones RB, et al. Effect of differences in specimen processing and passage technique on recovery of *Chlamydia trachomatis*. J Clin Microbiol 1989;27: 894–898.

268. Kahn J. Preventing hepatitis A and hepatitis B virus infections among men who have sex with men. Clin Infect Dis 2002;35:1382–1387.

269. Kahn JO, Walker BD. Acute human immunodeficiency virus type 1 infection. N Engl J Med 1998;339:33–39.

270. Kalayoglu MV, et al. *Chlamydia pneumoniae* as an emerging risk factor in cardiovascular disease. JAMA 2002;288:2724–2731.

271. Kapikian AZ, Hoshino Y, Chanock RM. Rotaviruses. In: Knipe DM, Howley PM, eds. Fields Virology. Ed. 4. Philadelphia: Lippincott Williams & Wilkins, 2001:1787–1833.

272. Kapikian AZ, et al. Visualization by immune electron microscopy of a 27-nm particle associated with acute infectious nonbacterial gastroenteritis. J Virol 1972;10:1075–1081.

273. Kaplan JE, Schonberger LB. The sensitivity of various serologic tests in the diagnosis of Rocky Mountain spotted fever. Am J Trop Med Hyg 1986;35: 840–844.

274. Karim MR, et al. Detection of noroviruses in water-summary of an international workshop. J Infect Dis 2004;189:21–28.

275. Kass EM, et al. Rickettsialpox in a New York City hospital, 1980 to 1989. N Engl J Med 1994;331:1612–1617.

276. Katavolos P, et al. Duration of tick attachment required for transmission of granulocytic ehrlichiosis. J Infect Dis 1998;177:1422–1425.

277. Kauppinen M, Saikku P. Pneumonia due to *Chlamydia pneumoniae*: Prevalence, clinical features, diagnosis, and treatment. Clin Infect Dis 1995;21:S244–S252.

278. Kimbrough RC, et al. Q fever endocarditis in the United States. Ann Intern Med 1979;91:400–402.

279. Kimura T, et al. New enzyme immunoassay for detection of hepatitis B virus core antigen (HBcAg) and relation between levels of HBcAg and HBV rDNA. J Clin Microbiol 2003;41:1901–1906.

280. Kiviat NB, et al. Cytologic manifestations of cervical and vaginal infections. II. Confirmation of Chlamydia trachomatis infection by direct immunofluorescence using monoclonal antibodies. JAMA 1985;253:997–1000.

281. Klatt EC, et al. Evolving trends revealed by autopsies of patients with the acquired immunodeficiency syndrome. 565 autopsies in adults with the acquired immunodeficiency syndrome, Los Angeles, Calif, 1992–1993. Arch Pathol Lab Med 1994;118:884–890.

282. Klempner MS, Shapiro DS. Crossing the species barrier-one small step to man, one giant leap to mankind. N Engl J Med 2004;350:1171–1172.

283. Klevjer-Anderson P, Anderson LW. Comparison of a new latex agglutination assay with indirect immunofluorescence to detect varicella-zoster antibodies. Diagn Microbiol Infect Dis 1993;17:247–249.

284. Knipe DM, Howley PM, eds. Fields Virology. Ed. 4. Philadelphia: Lippincott Williams & Wilkins, 2001.

285. Koch WH, et al. Evaluation of United States-licensed human immunodeficiency virus immunoassays for detection of group M viral variants. J Clin Microbiol 2001;39:1017–1020.

286. Koff RS, et al. Viral hepatitis in a group of Boston hospitals. III. Importance of exposure to shellfish in a nonepidemic period. N Engl J Med 1967;276: 703–710.

287. Krajden M, et al. Qualitative detection of hepatitis C virus RNA: comparison of analytical sensitivity, clinical performance, and workflow of the Cobas Amplicor HCV test version 2.0 and the HCV RNA transcription-mediated amplification qualitative assay. J Clin Microbiol 2002;40:2903–2907.

288. Krause JR, et al. Morphological diagnosis of parvovirus B19 infection. A cytopathic effect easily recognized in air-dried, formalin-fixed bone marrow smears stained with hematoxylin-eosin or Wright-Giemsa. Arch Pathol Lab Med 1992; 116:178–180.

289. Krause PJ, et al. Unreliability of Rotazyme ELISA test in neonates. J Pediatr 1983;103:259–262.

290. Krech T, et al. Comparison of buffalo green monkey cells and McCoy cells for isolation of *Chlamydia trachomatis* in a microtiter system. J Clin Microbiol 1989;27:2364–2365.

291. La Scola B, Raoult D. Laboratory diagnosis of rickettsioses: current approaches to diagnosis of old and new rickettsial diseases. J Clin Microbiol 1997;35: 2715–2727.

292. Lafferty WE, et al. Recurrences after oral and genital herpes simplex virus infection. Influence of site of infection and viral type. N Engl J Med 1987;316: 1444–1449.

293. Lai KK, et al. Evaluation of real-time PCR versus PCR with liquid-phase hybridization for detection of enterovirus RNA in cerebrospinal fluid. J Clin Microbiol 2003;41:3133–3141.

294. Lamb RA, Krug RM. *Orthomyxoviridae:* the viruses and their replication. In: Knipe DM, Howley PM, eds. Fields Virology. Ed. 4. Philadelphia: Lippincott Williams & Wilkins, 2001:1487–1531.

295. Lanciotti RS, Kerst AJ. Nucleic acid sequence-based amplification assays for rapid detection of West Nile and St. Louis encephalitis viruses. J Clin Microbiol 2001;39:4506–4513.

296. Landry ML, Ferguson D. 2-Hour cytomegalovirus pp65 antigenemia assay for rapid quantitation of cytomegalovirus in blood samples. J Clin Microbiol 2000; 38:427–428.

297. Landry ML, Ferguson D. SimulFluor respiratory screen for rapid detection of multiple respiratory viruses in clinical specimens by immunofluorescence staining. J Clin Microbiol 2000;38:708–711.

298. Landry ML, Ferguson D. Suboptimal detection of influenza virus in adults by the Directigen Flu A + B enzyme immunoassay and correlation of results with the number of antigen-positive cells detected by cytospin immunofluorescence. J Clin Microbiol 2003;41:3407–3409.

299. Landry ML, et al. Detection of herpes simplex virus in clinical specimens by cytospin-enhanced direct immunofluorescence. J Clin Microbiol 1997;35: 302–304.

300. Landry ML, et al. Use of plastic Vacutainer tubes for quantification of human immunodeficiency virus type 1 in blood specimens. J Clin Microbiol 2001;39: 354–356.

301. Landry ML, et al. Comparison of the NucliSens Basic kit (Nucleic Acid Sequence-Based Amplification) and the Argene Biosoft Enterovirus Consensus Reverse Transcription-PCR assays for rapid detection of enterovirus RNA in clinical specimens. J Clin Microbiol 2003;41:5006–5010.

302. Landry ML, Hsiung GD. Primary isolation of viruses. In: Specter S, Hodinka RL, Young SA, eds. Clinical Virology Manual. Ed. 3. Washington, DC: ASM Press, 2000:27–42.

303. Latorre CR, et al. Serial propagation of *Pneumocystis carinii* in cell line cultures. Appl Environ Microbiol 1977;33:1204–1206.

304. Lazzarotto T, et al. Prenatal diagnosis of congenital cytomegalovirus infection. J Clin Microbiol 1998;36:3540–3544.

305. Lazzarotto T, et al. Development of a new cytomegalovirus (CMV) immunoglobulin M (IgM) immunoblot for detection of CMV-specific IgM. J Clin Microbiol 1998;36:3337–3341.

306. Lee FS, et al. Human granulocytic ehrlichiosis presenting as facial diplegia in a 42-year-old woman. Clin Infect Dis 2000;31:1288–1291.

307. Levin MJ, et al. Factors influencing quantitative isolation of varicella-zoster virus. J Clin Microbiol 1984;19:880–883.

308. Levine AJ. The origins of virology. In: Knipe DM, Howley PM, eds. Fields Virology. Ed. 4. Philadelphia: Lippincott Williams & Wilkins, 2001:1–18.

309. Lew JF, et al. Six-year retrospective surveillance of gastroenteritis viruses identified at ten electron microscopy centers in the United States and Canada. Pediatr Infect Dis J 1990;9:709–714.

310. Li H, et al. Measurement of human cytomegalovirus loads by quantitative real-time PCR for monitoring clinical intervention in transplant recipients. J Clin Microbiol 2003;41:187–191.

311. Liljeqvist JA, et al. Typing of clinical herpes simplex virus type 1 and type 2 isolates with monoclonal antibodies. J Clin Microbiol 1999;37:2717–2718.

312. Lindenbach BD, Rice CM. *Flaviviridae:* the viruses and their replication. In: Knipe DM, Howley PM, eds. Fields Virology. Ed. 4. Philadelphia: Lippincott Williams & Wilkins, 2001:991–1041.

313. Livengood CH III, Wrenn JW. Evaluation of COBAS AMPLICOR (Roche): accuracy in detection of *Chlamydia trachomatis* and *Neisseria gonorrhoeae* by coamplification of endocervical specimens. J Clin Microbiol 2001;39: 2928–2932.

314. Louie JK, et al. Trends in causes of death among persons with acquired immunodeficiency syndrome in the era of highly active antiretroviral therapy, San Francisco, 1994–1998. J Infect Dis 2002;186:1023–1027.

315. Lowy DR, Howley PM. Papillomaviruses. In: Knipe DM, Howley PM, eds. Fields Virology. Ed. 4. Philadelphia: Lippincott Williams & Wilkins, 2001: 2231–2264.

316. Maass M, Dalhoff K. Transport and storage conditions for cultural recovery of *Chlamydia pneumoniae*. J Clin Microbiol 1995;33:1793–1796.

317. Maass M, et al. Growth in serum-free medium improves isolation of *Chlamydia pneumoniae*. J Clin Microbiol 1993;31:3050–3052.

318. Maass M, Harig U. Evaluation of culture conditions used for isolation of *Chlamydia pneumoniae*. Am J Clin Pathol 1995;103:141–148.

319. MacDonald KL, et al. Toxic shock syndrome. A newly recognized complication of influenza and influenzalike illness. JAMA 1987;257:1053–1058.

320. MacDonald NE, et al. Respiratory syncytial viral infection in infants with congenital heart disease. N Engl J Med 1982;307:397–400.

321. Mack T. A different view of smallpox and vaccination. N Engl J Med 2003; 348:460–463.

322. Maeda K, et al. Human infection with *Ehrlichia canis*, a leukocytic rickettsia. N Engl J Med 1987;316:853–856.

323. Major EO. Human polyomavirus. In: Knipe DM, Howley PM, eds. Fields Virology. Ed. 4. Philadelphia: Lippincott Williams & Wilkins, 2001:2175–2196.

324. Major ME, Rehermann B, Feinstone SM. Hepatitis C viruses. In: Knipe DM, Howley PM, eds. Fields Virology. Ed. 4. Philadelphia: Lippincott Williams & Wilkins, 2001:1127–1161.

325. Malan AK, et al. Evaluations of commercial West Nile virus immunoglobulin G

326. (IgG) and IgM enzyme immunoassays show the value of continuous validation. J Clin Microbiol 2004;42:727–733.

326. Manayani DJ, et al. Comparison of molecular and conventional methods for typing of enteroviral isolates. J Clin Microbiol 2002;40:1069–1070.

327. Marchette NJ, et al. Studies on the pathogenesis of dengue infection in monkeys. III. Sequential distribution of virus in primary and heterologous infections. J Infect Dis 1973;128:23–30.

328. Marquez A, Hsiung GD. Influence of glutamine on multiplication and cytopathic effect of respiratory syncytial virus. Proc Soc Exp Biol Med 1967;124:95–99.

329. Marsano L, et al. Comparison of culture and serology for the diagnosis of cytomegalovirus infection in kidney and liver transplant recipients. J Infect Dis 1990; 161:454–461.

330. Marshall WF, et al. Rapid detection of polyomavirus BK by a shell vial cell culture assay. J Clin Microbiol 1990;28:1613–1615.

331. Martin WJ, Smith TF. Rapid detection of cytomegalovirus in bronchoalveolar lavage specimens by a monoclonal antibody method. J Clin Microbiol 1986;23: 1006–1008.

332. Martinello RA, et al. Correlation between respiratory syncytial virus genotype and severity of illness. J Infect Dis 2002;186:839–842.

333. Martino R, et al. Respiratory virus infections in adults with hematologic malignancies: a prospective study. Clin Infect Dis 2003;36:1–8.

334. Marty AM, et al. Ehrlichiosis mimicking thrombotic thrombocytopenic purpura. Case report and pathological correlation. Hum Pathol 1995;26:920–925.

335. Maruyama T, et al. The serology of chronic hepatitis B infection revisited. J Clin Invest 1993;91:2586–2595.

336. Massung RF, et al. Epidemic typhus meningitis in the southwestern United States. Clin Infect Dis 2001;32:979–982.

337. Massung RF, et al. Genetic variants of *Ehrlichia phagocytophila*, Rhode Island and Connecticut. Emerg Infect Dis 2002;8:467–472.

338. Massung RF, Slater KG. Comparison of PCR assays for detection of the agent of human granulocytic ehrlichiosis, *Anaplasma phagocytophilum*. J Clin Microbiol 2003;41:717–722.

339. Matsui SM, Greenberg HB. Astroviruses. In: Knipe DM, Howley PM, eds. Fields Virology. Ed. 4. Philadelphia: Lippincott Williams & Wilkins, 2001:875–893.

340. Maurin M, Raoult D. Q fever. Clin Microbiol Rev 1999;12:518–553.

341. Mazzulli T, et al. Multicenter comparison of the digene hybrid capture CMV DNA assay (version 2.0), the pp65 antigenemia assay, and cell culture for detection of cytomegalovirus viremia. J Clin Microbiol 1999;37:958–963.

342. McCarter YS, Ratkiewicz IN. Comparison of virus culture and direct immunofluorescent staining of cytocentrifuged virus transport medium for detection of varicella-zoster virus in skin lesions. Am J Clin Pathol 1998;109:631–633.

343. McConnell CT Jr, et al. Radiographic appearance of *Chlamydia pneumoniae* (TWAR strain) respiratory infections. CBPIS Study Group. Community-based Pneumonia Incidence Study. Radiology 1994;192:819–824.

344. McGarrity GJ, et al. Cell culture techniques. ASM 1985;51:170–183.

345. McIntosh K, McAdam AJ. Human metapneumovirus-an important new respiratory virus. N Engl J Med 2004;350:431–433.

346. Meyer H, et al. Outbreaks of disease suspected of being due to human monkeypox virus infection in the Democratic Republic of Congo in 2001. J Clin Microbiol 2002;40:2919–2921.

347. Michalak TI, et al. Hepatitis B virus persistence after recovery from acute viral hepatitis. J Clin Invest 1994;93:230–239.

348. Mitchell PD, et al. Immunoserologic evidence of coinfection with *Borrelia burgdorferi*, *Babesia microti*, and human granulocytic *Ehrlichia* species in residents of Wisconsin and Minnesota. J Clin Microbiol 1996;34:724–727.

349. Mitchell PS, et al. Laboratory diagnosis of central nervous system infections with herpes simplex virus by PCR performed with cerebrospinal fluid specimens. J Clin Microbiol 1997;35:2873–2877.

350. Mitsuyasu R. Oncological complications of human immunodeficiency virus disease and hematologic consequences of their treatment. Clin Infect Dis 1999;29: 35–43.

351. Mocarski ES Jr, Courcol R. Cytomegaloviruses and their replication. In: Knipe DM, Howley PM, eds. Fields Virology. Ed. 4. Philadelphia: Lippincott Williams & Wilkins, 2001:2629–2673.

352. Moncada J, et al. Volume effect on sensitivity of nucleic acid amplification tests for detection of *Chlamydia trachomatis* in urine specimens from females. J Clin Microbiol 2003;41:4842–4843.

353. Montalban GS, et al. Performance of three commercially available monoclonal reagents for confirmation of *Chlamydia pneumoniae* in cell culture. J Clin Microbiol 1994;32:1406–1407.

354. Moore PS, Chang Y. Kaposi's sarcoma-associated herpesvirus. In: Knipe DM, Howley PM, eds. Fields Virology. Ed. 4. Philadelphia: Lippincott Williams & Wilkins, 2001:2803–2833.

355. Morishima C, et al. Strengths and limitations of commercial tests for hepatitis C virus RNA quantification. J Clin Microbiol 2004;42:421–425.

356. Moriuchi H, et al. Community-acquired influenza C virus infection in children. J Pediatr 1991;118:235–238.

357. Moroney JF, et al. Detection of chlamydiosis in a shipment of pet birds, leading

to recognition of an outbreak of clinically mild psittacosis in humans. Clin Infect Dis 1998;26:1425–1429.

358. Morrison RE, et al. Adult meningoencephalitis caused by herpesvirus hominis type 2. Am J Med 1974;56:540–544.

359. Morrow RA, Friedrich D. Inaccuracy of certain commercial enzyme immunoassays in diagnosing genital infections with herpes simplex virus types 1 or 2. Am J Clin Pathol 2003;120:839–844.

360. Morrow RA, et al. Performance of the Focus and Kalon enzyme-linked immunosorbent assays for antibodies to herpes simplex virus type 2 glycoprotein G in culture-documented cases of genital herpes. J Clin Microbiol 2003;41: 5212–5214.

361. Morton HJ. A survey of commercially available tissue culture media. In Vitro 1970;6:89–108.

362. Moss B. *Poxviridae:* the viruses and their replication. In: Knipe DM, Howley PM, eds. Fields Virology. Ed. 4. Philadelphia: Lippincott Williams & Wilkins, 2001:2849–2883.

363. Motyl MR, et al. Diagnosis of herpesvirus infections: correlation of Tzanck preparation with viral isolation. Diagn Microbiol Infect Dis 1984;2:157–160.

364. Mufson MA, et al. Respiratory syncytial virus epidemics: variable dominance of subgroups A and B strains among children, 1981–1986. J Infect Dis 1988; 157:143–148.

365. Murphy DG, et al. Reproducibility and performance of the second-generation branched-DNA assay in routine quantification of human immunodeficiency virus type 1 RNA in plasma. J Clin Microbiol 1999;37:812–814.

366. Murphy FA. Virus taxonomy. In: Fields BN, Knipe DM, Howley PM, et al., eds. Fields Virology. Ed. 3. Philadelphia: Lippincott-Raven,1996:15–57.

367. Murphy FA, et al. Morphologic comparison of Machupo with lymphocytic choriomeningitis virus: Basis for a new taxonomic group. J Virol 1969;4: 535–541.

368. Mushahwar IK, et al. Radioimmunoassay for detection of hepatitis B e antigen and its antibody: results of clinical evaluation. Am J Clin Pathol 1981;76: 692–697.

369. Musso D, Raoult D. *Coxiella burnetii* blood cultures from acute and chronic Q-fever patients. J Clin Microbiol 1995;33:3129–3132.

370. Nahmias AJ, et al. Herpes simplex virus encephalitis: laboratory evaluations and their diagnostic significance. J Infect Dis 1982;145:829–836.

371. Naib ZM, et al. Cytological features of viral respiratory tract infections. Acta Cytol 1968;12:162–171.

372. Nash G. Necrotizing tracheobronchitis and bronchopneumonia consistent with herpetic infection. Hum Pathol 1972;3:283–291.

373. Nelson-Rees WA, et al. Banded marker chromosomes as indicators of intraspecies cellular contamination. Science 1974;184:1093–1096.

374. Nichol ST. Bunyaviruses. In: Knipe DM, Howley PM, eds. Fields Virology. Ed. 4. Philadelphia: Lippincott Williams & Wilkins, 2001:1603–1633.

375. Noah DL, et al. Epidemiology of human rabies in the United States, 1980 to 1996. Ann Intern Med 1998;128:922–930.

376. Nolte FS, et al. Clinical evaluation of two methods for genotyping hepatitis C virus based on analysis of the 5′ noncoding region. J Clin Microbiol 2003;41: 1558–1564.

377. O'Connell RJ, et al. Performance of the OraQuick rapid antibody test for diagnosis of human immunodeficiency virus type 1 infection in patients with various levels of exposure to highly active antiretroviral therapy. J Clin Microbiol 2003; 41:2153–2155.

378. Oldach DW, et al. Rapid diagnosis of *Chlamydia psittaci* pneumonia. Clin Infect Dis 1993;17:338–343.

379. Oster CN, et al. Laboratory-acquired Rocky Mountain spotted fever. The hazard of aerosol transmission. N Engl J Med 1977;297:859–863.

380. Paddock CD, et al. Infections with *Ehrlichia chaffeensis* and *Ehrlichia ewingii* in persons coinfected with human immunodeficiency virus. Clin Infect Dis 2001; 33:1586–1594.

381. Paddock CD, et al. Hidden mortality attributable to Rocky Mountain spotted fever: immunohistochemical detection of fatal, serologically unconfirmed disease. J Infect Dis 1999;179:1469–1476.

382. Pallansch MA, Roos RP. Enteroviruses: Polioviruses, coxsackieviruses, echoviruses, and newer enteroviruses. In: Knipe DM, Howley PM, eds. Fields Virology. Ed. 4. Philadelphia: Lippincott Williams & Wilkins, 2001:723–775.

383. Palmer S, et al. New real-time reverse transcriptase-initiated PCR assay with single-copy sensitivity for human immunodeficiency virus type 1 RNA in plasma. J Clin Microbiol 2003;41:4531–4536.

384. Pancholi P, et al. *Ixodes dammini* as a potential vector of human granulocytic ehrlichiosis. J Infect Dis 1995;172:1007–1012.

385. Parida M, et al. Real-time reverse transcription loop-mediated isothermal amplification for rapid detection of West Nile virus. J Clin Microbiol 2004;42: 257–263.

386. Pass RF. Cytomegalovirus. In: Knipe DM, Howley PM, eds. Fields Virology. Ed. 4. Philadelphia: Lippincott Williams & Wilkins, 2001:2675–2705.

387. Patel N, et al. Confirmation of low-titer, herpes simplex virus-positive specimen

388. Paya CV, et al. Rapid shell vial culture and tissue histology compared with serology for the rapid diagnosis of cytomegalovirus infection in liver transplantation. Mayo Clin Proc 1989;64:670–675.

389. Paya CV, et al. Evaluation of number of shell vial cell cultures per clinical specimen for rapid diagnosis of cytomegalovirus infection. J Clin Microbiol 1988;26:198–200.

390. Payne FE, et al. Isolation of measles virus from cell cultures of brain from a patient with subacute sclerosing panencephalitis. N Engl J Med 1969;281: 585–589.

391. Peeling RW, et al. *Chlamydia pneumoniae* serology: interlaboratory variation in microimmunofluorescence assay results. J Infect Dis 2000;181:Suppl 9.

392. Pellett PE, Dominguez G. Human herpesviruses 6A, 6B, and 7. In: Knipe DM, Howley PM, eds. Fields Virology. Ed. 4. Philadelphia: Lippincott Williams & Wilkins, 2001:2769–2801.

393. Peltola V, et al. Influenza A and B virus infections in children. Clin Infect Dis 2003;36:299–305.

394. Peters CJ. Ebola virus. J Infect Dis 1999;179:S1–S288.

395. Peters CJ, Khan AS. Hantavirus pulmonary syndrome: the new American hemorrhagic fever. Clin Infect Dis 2002;34:1224–1231.

396. Petersen LR, Marfin AA. West Nile virus: a primer for the clinician. Ann Intern Med 2002;137:173–179.

397. Philip RN, et al. Microimmunofluorescence test for the serological study of Rocky Mountain spotted fever and typhus. J Clin Microbiol 1976;3:51–61.

398. Podzorski RP. Molecular testing in the diagnosis and management of hepatitis C virus infection. Arch Pathol Lab Med 2002;126:285–290.

399. Poggio GP, et al. Nested PCR for rapid detection of mumps virus in cerebrospinal fluid from patients with neurological diseases. J Clin Microbiol 2000;38: 274–278.

400. Pomerantz RJ, Nunnari G. HIV and GB virus C-can two viruses be better than one? N Engl J Med 2004;350:963–965.

401. Prather SL, et al. The isolation of enteroviruses from blood: a comparison of four processing methods. J Med Virol 1984;14:221–227.

402. Prince HE, et al. Utility of the focus technologies West Nile virus immunoglobulin m capture enzyme-linked immunosorbent assay for testing cerebrospinal fluid. J Clin Microbiol 2004;42:12–15.

403. Prusiner SB. Prions. Proc Natl Acad Sci USA 1998;95:13363–13383.

404. Prusiner SB. Prions. In: Knipe DM, Howley PM, eds. Fields Virology. Ed. 4. Philadelphia: Lippincott Williams & Wilkins, 2001:3063–3087.

405. Prusiner SB. Neurodegenerative diseases and prions. N Engl J Med 2001;344: 1516–1526.

406. Purcell RH, Emerson SU. Hepatitis E virus. In: Knipe DM, Howley PM, eds. Fields Virology. Ed. 4. Philadelphia: Lippincott Williams & Wilkins, 2001: 3051–3061.

407. Rabinowitz M, et al. A modified, solid phase radioimmunoassay for the differential diagnosis of acute and convalescent phases of hepatitis A infection. Am J Clin Pathol 1987;88:738–742.

408. Ramsey PG, et al. Herpes simplex virus pneumonia: clinical, virologic, and pathologic features in 20 patients. Ann Intern Med 1982;97:813–820.

409. Raoult D, Roux V. Rickettsioses as paradigms of new or emerging infectious diseases. Clin Microbiol Rev 1997;10:694–719.

410. Raoult D, et al. Q fever 1985–1998. Clinical and epidemiologic features of 1,383 infections. Medicine (Baltimore) 2000;79:109–123.

411. Rea TD, et al. A systematic study of Epstein-Barr virus serologic assays following acute infection. Am J Clin Pathol 2002;117:156–161.

412. Reed KD, et al. The detection of monkeypox in humans in the Western Hemisphere. N Engl J Med 2004;350:342–350.

413. Reid AH, et al. 1918 influenza pandemic caused by highly conserved viruses with two receptor-binding variants. Emerg Infect Dis 2003;9:1249–1253.

414. Reina J, et al. Evaluation of a new dot blot enzyme immunoassay (directigen flu A + B) for simultaneous and differential detection of influenza A and B virus antigens from respiratory samples. J Clin Microbiol 2002;40:3515–3517.

415. Reina J, et al. Evaluation of a direct immunofluorescence cytospin assay for the detection of herpes simplex virus in clinical samples. Eur J Clin Microbiol Infect Dis 1997;16:851–854.

416. Remy V, et al. Human anaplasmosis presenting as atypical pneumonitis in France. Clin Infect Dis 2003;37:846–848.

417. Rich JD, et al. Misdiagnosis of HIV infection by HIV-1 plasma viral load testing: a case series. Ann Intern Med 1999;130:37–39.

418. Richman DD, Whitley RJ, Hayden FG. Clinical Virology. Ed. 2. Washington, DC: ASM Press, 2002.

419. Rickinson AB, Kieff E. Epstein-Barr virus. In: Knipe DM, Howley PM, eds. Fields Virology. Ed. 4. Philadelphia: Lippincott Williams & Wilkins, 2001: 2575–2627.

420. Rigonan AS, et al. Use of monoclonal antibodies to identify serotypes of enterovirus isolates. J Clin Microbiol 1998;36:1877–1881.

421. Rikihisa Y. The tribe *Ehrlichieae* and ehrlichial diseases. Clin Microbiol Rev 1991;4:286–308.

422. Rose JW, et al. Atypical herpes simplex encephalitis: clinical, virologic, and neuropathologic evaluation. Neurology 1992;42:1809–1812.

423. Rota PA, et al. Molecular epidemiology of measles viruses in the United States, 1997–2001. Emerg Infect Dis 2002;8:902–908.

424. Roy P. Orbiviruses. In: Knipe DM, Howley PM, eds. Fields Virology. Ed. 4. Philadelphia: Lippincott Williams & Wilkins, 2001:1835–1869.

425. Ruutu P, et al. Cytomegalovirus is frequently isolated in bronchoalveolar lavage fluid of bone marrow transplant recipients without pneumonia. Ann Intern Med 1990;112:913–916.

426. Sabet SF, et al. Enhancement of *Chlamydia trachomatis* infectious progeny by cultivation in HeLa 229 cells treated with DEAE-Dextran and cycloheximide. J Clin Microbiol 1984;20:217–222.

427. Sabin AB. Studies of B virus. I. the immunological identity of a virus isolated from a human case of ascending myelitis associated with visceral necrosis. Br J Exp Pathol 1934;15:248–268.

428. Sabin AB. The significance of viruses recovered from the intestinal tracts of healthy infants and children. Ann NY Acad Sci 1956;66:226–230.

429. Sanchez A, Khan AS, Zaki SR, et al. *Filoviridae:* Marburg and Ebola viruses. In: Knipe DM, Howley PM, eds. Fields Virology. Ed. 4. Philadelphia: Lippincott Williams & Wilkins, 2001:1279–1304.

430. Sanders C, et al. Cytospin-enhanced direct immunofluorescence assay versus cell culture for detection of herpes simplex virus in clinical specimens. Diagn Microbiol Infect Dis 1998;32:111–113.

431. Sankar-Mistry P, et al. Effect of polybrene on isolation of *Chlamydia trachomatis* from clinical specimens. J Clin Microbiol 1985;22:671–673.

432. Schachter J. Chlamydial infections. N Engl J Med 1978;298:428–434.

433. Schachter J, et al. Prospective study of perinatal transmission of *Chlamydia trachomatis.* JAMA 1986;255:3374–3377.

434. Schafer P, et al. False-positive results of plasma PCR for cytomegalovirus DNA due to delayed sample preparation. J Clin Microbiol 2000;38:3249–3253.

435. Schaffner W, et al. The clinical spectrum of endemic psittacosis. Arch Intern Med 1967;119:433–443.

436. Schirm J, et al. Rapid detection of varicella-zoster virus in clinical specimens using monoclonal antibodies on shell vials and smears. J Med Virol 1989;28:1–6.

437. Schlesinger S, Schlesinger MJ. *Togaviridae:* the viruses and their replication. In: Knipe DM, Howley PM, eds. Fields Virology. Ed. 4. Philadelphia: Lippincott Williams & Wilkins, 2001:895–916.

438. Schlesinger Y, et al. Expanded spectrum of herpes simplex encephalitis in childhood. J Pediatr 1995;126:234–241.

439. Schmaljohn CS, Hooper JW. *Bunyaviridae:* the viruses and their replication. In: Knipe DM, Howley PM, eds. Fields Virology. Ed. 4. Philadelphia: Lippincott Williams & Wilkins, 2001:1581–1602.

440. Schmidt NJ, et al. Application of immunoperoxidase staining to more rapid detection and identification of rubella virus isolates. J Clin Microbiol 1981;13:627–630.

441. Schmidt NJ, et al. *Clostridium difficile* toxin as a confounding factor in enterovirus isolation. J Clin Microbiol 1980;12:796–798.

442. Schriefer ME, et al. Identification of a novel rickettsial infection in a patient diagnosed with murine typhus. J Clin Microbiol 1994;32:949–954.

443. Sejvar JJ, et al. Neurologic manifestations and outcome of West Nile virus infection. JAMA 2003;290:511–515.

444. Serwadda D, et al. Human immunodeficiency virus acquisition associated with genital ulcer disease and herpes simplex virus type 2 infection: a nested case-control study in Rakai, Uganda. J Infect Dis 2003;188:1492–1497.

445. Sexton DJ, et al. Dual infection with *Ehrlichia chaffeensis* and a spotted fever group rickettsia: a case report. Emerg Infect Dis 1998;4:311–316.

446. Shafer MA, et al. Comparing first-void urine specimens, self-collected vaginal swabs, and endocervical specimens to detect *Chlamydia trachomatis* and *Neisseria gonorrhoeae* by a nucleic acid amplification test. J Clin Microbiol 2003;41:4395–4399.

447. Shafer RW. Genotypic testing for human immunodeficiency virus type 1 drug resistance. Clin Microbiol Rev 2002;15:247–277.

448. Shah KV. Papovaviruses. In: Specter S, Hodinka RL, Young SA, eds. Clinical Virology Manual. Ed. 3. Washington, DC: ASM Press, 2000:374–383.

449. Shahrabadi MS, Lee PW. Calcium requirement for syncytium formation in HEp-2 cells by respiratory syncytial virus. J Clin Microbiol 1988;26:139–141.

450. Shenk TE. *Adenoviridae:* the viruses and their replication. In: Knipe DM, Howley PM, eds. Fields Virology. Ed. 4. Philadelphia: Lippincott Williams & Wilkins, 2001:2265–2300.

451. Simko JP, et al. Differences in laboratory findings for cerebrospinal fluid specimens obtained from patients with meningitis or encephalitis due to herpes simplex virus (HSV) documented by detection of HSV DNA. Clin Infect Dis 2002;35:414–419.

452. Smalling TW, et al. Molecular approaches to detecting herpes simplex virus and enteroviruses in the central nervous system. J Clin Microbiol 2002;40:2317–2322.

453. Smith TF. Clinical uses of the diagnostic virology laboratory. Med Clin North Am 1983;67:935–951.

454. Smith TF. Diagnostic virology in the community hospital. Extent and options. Postgrad Med 1984;75:215–223.

455. Smith TF. Specimen requirements: selection, collection, transport, and processing. In: Specter S, Hodinka RL, Young SA, eds. Clinical Virology Manual. Ed. 3. Washington, DC: ASM Press, 2000:11–26.

456. Smith TF, et al. Diagnosis of *Chlamydia trachomatis* infections by cell cultures and serology. Lab Med 1982;13:92–100.

457. Snydman DR, et al. Use of IgM-hepatitis A antibody testing. Investigating a common-source, food borne outbreak. JAMA 1981;245:827–830.

458. Sofi IM, et al. Real-time PCR assay to detect smallpox virus. J Clin Microbiol 2003;41:3835–3839.

459. Solomon AR, et al. A comparison of the Tzanck smear and viral isolation in varicella and herpes zoster. Arch Dermatol 1986;122:282–285.

460. Solomon D, et al. The 2001 Bethesda System: terminology for reporting results of cervical cytology. JAMA 2002;287:2114–2119.

461. Sorvillo FJ, et al. A suburban focus of endemic typhus in Los Angeles County: association with seropositive domestic cats and opossums. Am J Trop Med Hyg 1993;48:269–273.

462. Specter S, Lancz GJ. Clinical Virology Manual. Ed. 3. Washington, DC: ASM Press, 2000.

463. Spelman DW. Q fever: a study of 111 consecutive cases. Med J Aust 1982;1:547–553.

464. St George K, et al. A multisite trial comparing two cytomegalovirus (CMV) pp65 antigenemia test kits, biotest CMV brite and Bartels/Argene CMV antigenemia. J Clin Microbiol 2000;38:1430–1433.

465. Stamm WE, et al. Detection of *Chlamydia trachomatis* inclusions in McCoy cell cultures with fluorescein-conjugated monoclonal antibodies. J Clin Microbiol 1983;17:666–668.

466. Standaert SM, et al. Ehrlichiosis in a golf-oriented retirement community. N Engl J Med 1995;333:420–425.

467. Steinberg SP, Gershon AA. Measurement of antibodies to varicella-zoster virus by using a latex agglutination test. J Clin Microbiol 1991;29:1527–1529.

468. Steininger C, et al. Acute encephalopathy associated with influenza A virus infection. Clin Infect Dis 2003;36:567–574.

469. Stephensen CB, et al. Prevalence of serum antibodies against lymphocytic choriomeningitis virus in selected populations from two U.S. cities. J Med Virol 1992;38:27–31.

470. Strano AJ. Light microscopy of selected viral diseases (morphology of viral inclusion bodies). Pathol Annu 1976;11:53–75.

471. Strickler JG, et al. Comparison of in situ hybridization and immunohistochemistry for detection of cytomegalovirus and herpes simplex virus. Hum Pathol 1990;21:443–448.

472. Supran EM, et al. Report of a joint DMRQC/Organon field trial to detect hepatitis A IgM by ELISA. J Clin Pathol 1983;36:1111–1115.

473. Sutherland S, et al. Donated organ as a source of cytomegalovirus in orthotopic liver transplantation. J Med Virol 1992;37:170–173.

474. Swanson P, et al. Comparative performance of three viral load assays on human immunodeficiency virus type 1 (HIV-1) isolates representing group M (subtypes A to G) and group O. LCx HIV RNA quantitative, AMPLICOR HIV-1 MONITOR Version 1.5, and Quantiplex HIV-1 RNA Version 3.0. J Clin Microbiol 2001;39:862–870.

475. Swierkosz EM. Antiviral drug susceptibility testing. In: Specter S, Hodinka RL, Young SA, eds. Clinical Virology Manual. Ed. 3. Washington, DC: ASM Press, 2000:154–168.

476. Tam MR, et al. Culture-independent diagnosis of *Chlamydia trachomatis* using monoclonal antibodies. N Engl J Med 1984;310:1146–1150.

477. Tedder DG, et al. Herpes simplex virus infection as a cause of benign recurrent lymphocytic meningitis. Ann Intern Med 1994;121:334–338.

478. Thin RNT, et al. Value of Papanicolaou-stained smears in the diagnosis of trichomoniasis, candidiasis, and cervical herpes simplex virus infection in women. Br J Vener Dis 1975;51:116–118.

479. Thomas DL, et al. Viral hepatitis in health care personnel at The Johns Hopkins Hospital. The seroprevalence of and risk factors for hepatitis B virus and hepatitis C virus infection. Arch Intern Med 1993;153:1705–1712.

480. Thomas EE, et al. The utility of latex agglutination assays in the diagnosis of pediatric viral gastroenteritis. Am J Clin Pathol 1994;101:742–746.

481. Thorley-Lawson DA, Gross A. Persistence of the Epstein-Barr virus and the origins of associated lymphomas. N Engl J Med 2004;350:1328–1337.

482. Tracy S, et al. Molecular approaches to enteroviral diagnosis in idiopathic cardiomyopathy and myocarditis. J Am Coll Cardiol 1990;15:1688–1694.

483. Treuhaft MW, et al. Practical recommendations for the detection of pediatric respiratory syncytial virus infections. J Clin Microbiol 1985;22:270–273.

484. Tyrrell DAJ, et al. Clones of cells from a human embryonic lung: their growth and susceptibility to respiratory viruses. Arch Virol 1979;61:69–85.

485. Uhnoo I, Svensson L. Clinical and epidemiological features of acute infantile gastroenteritis associated with human rotavirus subgroups 1 and 2. J Clin Microbiol 1986;23:551–555.

486. Unver A, et al. Western blot analysis of sera reactive to human monocytic ehrlichiosis and human granulocytic ehrlichiosis agents. J Clin Microbiol 2001; 39:3982–3986.

487. Valentine-Thon E, et al. European proficiency testing program for molecular detection and quantitation of hepatitis B virus DNA. J Clin Microbiol 2001;39: 4407–4412.

488. Van Der PB, et al. Multicenter evaluation of the BDProbeTec ET system for detection of *Chlamydia trachomatis* and *Neisseria gonorrhoeae* in urine specimens, female endocervical swabs, and male urethral swabs. J Clin Microbiol 2001;39:1008–1016.

489. Van Der PB, et al. Enhancing the specificity of the COBAS AMPLICOR CT/NG Test for *Neisseria gonorrhoeae* by retesting specimens with equivocal results. J Clin Microbiol 2001;39:3092–3098.

490. van Elden LJ, et al. Simultaneous detection of influenza viruses A and B using real-time quantitative PCR. J Clin Microbiol 2001;39:196–200.

491. van Regenmortel MHV, Mahy BMJ. Emerging issues in virus taxonomy. Emerg Infect Dis 2004;10:8–13.

492. Versalovic J. Diagnostic molecular microbiology: nucleic acid probes and microbes. Pathol Case Rev 2003;8:137–144.

493. Vogel J, Shelokov A. Adsorption-hemagglutination test for influenza virus in monkey kidney tissue culture. Science 1957;126:358–359.

494. Wadowsky RM, et al. Measurement of Epstein-Barr virus DNA loads in whole blood and plasma by TaqMan PCR and in peripheral blood lymphocytes by competitive PCR. J Clin Microbiol 2003;41:5245–5249.

495. Wadsworth JD, et al. Molecular and clinical classification of human prion disease. Br Med Bull 2003;66:241–254.

496. Wald A, Ashley-Morrow R. Serological testing for herpes simplex virus (HSV)-1 and HSV-2 infection. Clin Infect Dis 2002;35:2–82.

497. Wald A, et al. Polymerase chain reaction for detection of herpes simplex virus (HSV) DNA on mucosal surfaces: comparison with HSV isolation in cell culture. J Infect Dis 2003;188:1345–1351.

498. Wald A, et al. Virologic characteristics of subclinical and symptomatic genital herpes infections. N Engl J Med 1995;333:770–775.

499. Wald A, et al. Reactivation of genital herpes simplex virus type 2 infection in asymptomatic seropositive persons. N Engl J Med 2000;342:844–850.

500. Walker DH. Rocky Mountain spotted fever: a disease in need of microbiological concern. Clin Microbiol Rev 1989;2:227–240.

501. Walker DH. Rocky Mountain Spotted Fever: A Seasonal Alert. Clin Infect Dis 1995;20:1111–1117.

502. Walker DH. Diagnosing human ehrlichioses: current status and recommendations. Despite shortcomings, immunofluorescence testing remains the best choice, with PCR and culture methods being valuable adjuncts. Task Force on Consensus Approach for Ehrlichiosis. ASM 2001;66:287–291.

503. Walker DH. Ricketts creates rickettsiology, the study of vector-borne obligately intracellular bacteria. J Infect Dis 2004;189:938–955.

504. Walker DH, et al. Laboratory diagnosis of Rocky Mountain spotted fever. South Med J 1980;73:1443–1447.

505. Walker DH, Cain BG. A method for specific diagnosis of Rocky Mountain spotted fever on fixed, paraffin-embedded tissue by immunofluorescence. J Infect Dis 1978;137:206–209.

506. Ward C. Acquired valvular heart-disease in patients who keep pet birds. Lancet 1974;2:734–736.

507. Washburne JF, et al. Summertime respiratory syncytial virus infection: epidemiology and clinical manifestations. South Med J 1992;85:579–583.

508. Weinberg A, et al. Comparison of PCR, antigenemia assay, and rapid blood culture for detection and prevention of cytomegalovirus disease after lung transplantation. J Clin Microbiol 2000;38:768–772.

509. Weingarten S, et al. Influenza surveillance in an acute-care hospital. Arch Intern Med 1988;148:113–116.

510. Weller TH. Cytomegaloviruses: the difficult years. J Infect Dis 1970;122: 532–539.

511. Weller TH. Varicella and herpes zoster. In: Lennette EH, Schmidt NJ, eds. Diagnostic Procedures for Viral, Rickettsial and Chlamydial Infections. Ed. 5. Washington, DC: American Public Health Association, 1979:375–398.

512. Wells DL, et al. Swine influenza virus infections: transmission from ill pigs to humans at a Wisconsin agricultural fair and subsequent probable person-to-person transmission. JAMA 1991;265:478–481.

513. Wells DL, et al. Herpesvirus simiae contamination of primary rhesus monkey kidney cell cultures. CDC recommendations to minimize risks to laboratory personnel. Diagn Microbiol Infect Dis 1989;12:333–336.

514. Westenfeld FW, Winn WC Jr. Recovery of varicella-zoster virus in diploid fibroblast and monkey kidney cell cultures. Am J Clin Pathol 1994;102:733–735.

515. Whiley DM, et al. Detection and differentiation of human polyomaviruses JC and BK by LightCycler PCR. J Clin Microbiol 2001;39:4357–4361.

516. Whiley DM, et al. Detection of human respiratory syncytial virus in respiratory samples by LightCycler reverse transcriptase PCR. J Clin Microbiol 2002;40: 4418–4422.

517. Whitley R, et al. Predictors of morbidity and mortality in neonates with herpes simplex virus infections. N Engl J Med 1991;324:450–454.

518. Whitley RJ. Herpes simplex viruses. In: Knipe DM, Howley PM, eds. Fields Virology. Ed. 4. Philadelphia: Lippincott Williams & Wilkins, 2001:2461–2509.

519. Whitley RJ, et al. Diseases that mimic herpes simplex encephalitis: diagnosis, presentation, and outcome. NIAD Collaborative Antiviral Study Group. JAMA 1989;262:234–239.

520. Whitley RJ, Hilliard JK. Cercopithecine herpesvirus (B virus). In: Knipe DM, Howley PM, eds. Fields Virology. Ed. 4. Philadelphia: Lippincott Williams & Wilkins, 2001:2835–2848.

521. Williams CF, et al. Persistent GB virus C infection and survival in HIV-infected men. N Engl J Med 2004;350:981–990.

522. Williams SG, et al. Typhus and typhuslike rickettsiae associated with opossums and their fleas in Los Angeles County, California. J Clin Microbiol 1992;30: 1758–1762.

523. Wong KH, et al. Efficient culture of *Chlamydia pneumoniae* with cell lines derived from the human respiratory tract. J Clin Microbiol 1992;30:1625–1630.

524. Wong KH, et al. Utility of complement fixation and microimmunofluorescence assays for detecting serologic responses in patients with clinically diagnosed psittacosis. J Clin Microbiol 1994;32:2417–2421.

525. Woodman DR, et al. Biological properties of Rickettsia prowazekii strains isolated from flying squirrels. Infect Immun 1977;16:853–860.

526. Woods GL, Walker DH. Detection of infection or infectious agents by use of cytologic and histologic stains. Clin Microbiol Rev 1996;9:382–404.

527. Wright TC Jr, et al. 2001 Consensus guidelines for the management of women with cervical cytological abnormalities. JAMA 2002;287:2120–2129.

528. Wylie JL, et al. Comparative evaluation of Chlamydiazyme, PACE 2, and AMP-CT assays for detection of *Chlamydia trachomatis* in endocervical specimens. J Clin Microbiol 1998;36:3488–3491.

529. Yao JD, et al. Multicenter Evaluation of the VERSANT Hepatitis B Virus DNA 3.0 Assay. J Clin Microbiol 2004;42:800–806.

530. Yevich SJ, et al. Seroepidemiology of infections due to spotted fever group rickettsiae and Ehrlichia species in military personnel exposed in areas of the United States where such infections are endemic. J Infect Dis 1995;171: 1266–1273.

531. Yoder BL, et al. Microtest procedure for isolation of *Chlamydia trachomatis*. J Clin Microbiol 1981;13:1036–1039.

532. Young NS, Brown KE. Parvovirus B19. N Engl J Med 2004;350:586–597.

533. Zaki SR, et al. Hantavirus pulmonary syndrome. Pathogenesis of an emerging infectious disease. Am J Pathol 1995;146:552–579.

534. Zaki SR, et al. Retrospective diagnosis of hantavirus pulmonary syndrome, 1978–1993: implications for emerging infectious diseases. Arch Pathol Lab Med 1996;120:134–139.

535. Zanghellini F, et al. Asymptomatic primary cytomegalovirus infection: virologic and immunologic features. J Infect Dis 1999;180:702–707.

536. Zerbini M, et al. Comparative evaluation of virological and serological methods in prenatal diagnosis of parvovirus B19 fetal hydrops. J Clin Microbiol 1996; 34:603–608.

537. Zhai J, et al. Real-time polymerase chain reaction for detecting SARS coronavirus, Beijing, 2003. Emerg Infect Dis 2004;10:300–303.

538. Zolopa AR, et al. HIV-1 genotypic resistance patterns predict response to saquinavir-ritonavir therapy in patients in whom previous protease inhibitor therapy had failed. Ann Intern Med 1999;131:813–821.

539. zur Hausen H. Intracellular surveillance of persisting viral infections. Human genital cancer results from deficient cellular control of papillomavirus gene expression. Lancet 1986;2:489–491.

Ectoparasites and Other Invertebrates in the Clinical Laboratory: A Brief Guide

With Contributions by Fred Westenfeld and Fred Patterson

Submission of Specimens to the Laboratory

Arachnida: Ticks, Mites, and Spiders

Ixodidae

Biology of Hard Ticks
Relation to Disease
Geographic Distribution
Identification
Summary of Identification

***Ornithodoros* Species**

Relation to Disease
Identification
Geographic Distribution

Mites

Sarcoptes scabiei (Scabies)

Relation to Disease
Identification
Geographic Distribution

Demodex folliculorum (Hair Follicles) and *Demodex brevis* (Sebaceous Glands)

Relation to Disease
Identification
Geographic Distribution

Spiders

Loxosceles reclusa

Relation to Disease
Identification
Geographic Distribution

Latrodectus mactans

Relation to Disease
Identification
Geographic Distribution

Tegenaria agrestis

Relation to Disease
Identification
Geographic Distribution

Insecta: Flies, Bugs, Fleas, and Lice

Myiasis-Producing Fly Larvae

Dermatobia hominis (Human Bot Fly)

Relation to Disease
Identification
Geographic Distribution

Cordylobia anthropophaga (Tumbu Fly)

Relation to Disease
Identification
Geographic Distribution

Other Flies
Mosquitoes

Relation to Disease
Identification
Geographic Distribution

"Bugs"

Cimex lectularius
Kissing Bugs: *Panstrongylus, Rhodnius,* and
     Triatoma Species

Fleas

Relation to Disease
Identification
Geographic Distribution

Lice

Pediculus humanus
Pediculus capitis
Phthirus pubis

Ectoparasites are organisms that live in or on the skin of a host, from which they receive nourishment. The relation is, therefore, parasitic or possibly symbiotic. Intimacy of contact varies from the time required for a blood meal to days, weeks, or even months of association. Organisms that contact a host casually (e.g., houseflies) or without deriving benefit (e.g., scorpions, bees, and spiders) are not, strictly speaking, ectoparasites.[64]

Arthropods are invertebrates with jointed appendages (hence the name) and a chitinous exoskeleton. They have long been recognized as direct or indirect causes of human disease and may produce damage to the human host in their own right. Alternatively, they may serve as the vectors for transmission of infectious agents and entry of the agent into the human host. In some instances, the arthropod serves as a mere carrier, depositing the infectious agent in the proximate environment, where it can contact the potential victim. An example of such a scenario is the transmission of bacterial pathogens from one site to another on the bodies of flies or cockroaches.[2,45] A much more intimate relationship occurs when the arthropod is the direct mediator of cellular damage or when a biting insect transmits an infectious agent into the tissue of the victim. Most biting insects ingest the infectious agent when they take a blood meal from an infected human or from an infected nonhuman mammal, which is referred to as a **reservoir of infection.** When an insect bites an animal or human, it often injects salivary secretions that contain enzymes and anticoagulants designed to permit the ingestion of a blood meal. If the infectious agent has moved from the gut of the insect into the hemolymph and subsequently made its way to the salivary glands, the infection is transmitted in the salivary secretions at the time of the bite.[43] If the infectious agent is present in the gut—with or without infectious material in the saliva—the microbial agent may be excreted in the feces when the arthropod defecates after ingestion of the blood meal. Entry of the agent from the feces into the injection site is facilitated when the host scratches the site of irritation.

The list of medically significant arthropods continues to expand, as does the list of diseases they can produce. At the same time, clinical laboratories are receiving increasing numbers of specimens for identification. Many arthropods that are very important in human infectious disease are rarely, if ever, seen in clinical microbiology laboratories because the insects were not seen, were exterminated, or were not collected for examination. Other important insects, such as scorpions, are seen in localized geographic distributions. On the other hand, clinical microbiologists may be called on to identify insects that caused alarm at their presence even though they have done no harm.

This section is designed to assist the reader in understanding the medical significance and laboratory identification of some arthropods that may be encountered in the clinical laboratory. An abbreviated classification schema is detailed in Table A-1 and select definitions and related taxonomy of the ectoparasites of importance to humans are listed in Box A-1. The reader is referred to several excellent reference textbooks for more detailed information.[17–20,40,49,54,56]

Submission of Specimens to the Laboratory

Because of the diversity of specimens dealt with in medical entomology, it is difficult to recommend a single method for submission of specimens. In general, 70% ethanol will work well as a preservative for most specimens, also preventing escape or autoinfection. It should be added to the specimen in a clean container so that the arthropod is completely submersed. Specimens can darken after extended periods of preservation, negating the utility of color differences for identification after long periods of fixation. We have observed no degradation of color in specimens preserved in 70% ethanol over a period of days, which is the usual time from collection to processing.

Formalin and sterile saline may be satisfactory but generally have more disadvantages when compared with ethanol. Flying insects should be killed using gases, such as chloroform, and then preserved as a dry mount.[18] Garcia lists a recipe for Berelese's medium, which she suggests is a good solution to use for most specimens.[18] Killing in hot water has been suggested for examination of fly larvae.[17] If in doubt, check with the facility that will be handling the specimen for specific recommendations.

The preferred method for removal of ticks is to grasp the tick with fine tweezers as close to the site of penetration as possible without pinching the skin. Steady outward pressure, while lifting the tick upward and forward, usually removes the specimen intact.[36] The capitulum of hard ticks is an important identifying feature. Specimens that are degraded because of improper removal are more difficult to identify.

Table A-1 Classification of Arthropods of Medical Importance

CLASS	ORDER OR SUBCLASS	EXAMPLES	DIRECT INJURY OR INFECTIONS TRANSMITTED
Diplopoda		Millipedes	Direct
Chilopoda		Centipedes	Direct
Hexapoda (Insecta)	Hemiptera	Bedbugs	Direct
		Kissing bugs	
Hexapoda (Insecta)	Siphonaptera	Fleas	Direct
Hexapoda (Insecta)	Anoplura	Sucking lice	Direct; typhus; trench fever; relapsing fever
Hexapoda (Insecta)	Dictyoptera	Cockroaches	Sanitation problems; allergic reactions
Hexapoda (Insecta)	Hymenoptera	Ants, wasps, bees	Direct
Hexapoda (Insecta)	Coleoptera	Beetles	Direct
Hexapoda (Insecta)	Diptera	Flies, mosquitoes, midges	Direct; arboviruses; parasitic infection; *Bartonella; Francisella*
Hexapoda (Insecta)	Lepidoptera	Moths, butterflies, caterpillars	Direct
Pentastomida		Tongue worms	Direct
Arachnida	Subclass: Scorpiones	Scorpions	Direct
Arachnida	Subclass: Araneae	Spiders	Direct
Arachnida	Subclass: Acari	Ticks, mites, chiggers	Direct; *Borrelia;* arboviruses; *Ehrlichia; Anaplasma, Rickettsia; Francisella*

The materials and techniques required for examination of arthropods are simple. Low magnification can be obtained with a hand lens or optimally with a stereomicroscope. Low- to moderate-power magnification can also be obtained with a low-power objective (e.g., 2× or 4×) and a compound microscope. A good light source is essential for observation. Fiberoptic lights provide excellent illumination without heating and excessive drying of the specimen. Lights with flexible arms allow maximal control of the illumination angle. The specimen can be manipulated best with a pair of dissecting needles.

In the exceptional circumstance that culture of the potential pathogen from the vector is under consideration, the insect must be unfixed. If the specimen was fixed before submission to the laboratory, modern molecular methods allow specific identification of infectious agents by amplification of nucleic acids.

Arachnida: Ticks, Mites, and Spiders

Ticks are arthropods in the Suborder *Ixodida*, which is divided into three families, two of which, *Ixodidae* (Hard Ticks) and *Argasidae* (Soft Ticks), have been established as

vectors for human disease.[36,51] In *Ixodidae* the anterior portion of the body is sclerotized and includes a scutum ("dorsal shield") and an anterior facing capitulum ("head"), thus the term, "hard tick."[51] The genera most commonly submitted to microbiology laboratories are *Ixodes, Dermacentor,* and *Amblyomma. Argasidae* have a leatherlike outer surface with no scutum and have ventrally located mouthparts.[51] Increasingly in past decades hard ticks have been recognized as important vectors for a wide variety of human diseases, the diversity of which is greater than for any other group of arthropods.[51] In the United States hard ticks are more prevalent than soft ticks and are more important vectors of human pathogens. Identification of a submitted tick should include description of the species, life-cycle stage, gender for adults, level of engorgement, and status of mouthparts.

Ixodidae
BIOLOGY OF HARD TICKS

Hard ticks have a life cycle that consists of four stages (instars): egg, larva, nymph, and sexually dimorphic adult. Larval ticks have six legs, a key identifying feature (Color Plate A-1*A*), whereas nymphs and adults have eight. Immature stages lack a genital aperture but otherwise resemble adult females. Both have a scutum that covers one-third to

Box A-1 Ectoparasites: Definitions and Taxonomy

Arthropoda: Phylum organisms having a hard, jointed exoskeleton and symmetrical paired, jointed legs. Of the five classes of arthropods, only the *Arachnida* and the *Insecta* serve as vectors of human disease.

Class *Arachnida* (ticks, mites, and spiders): a class of arthropods characterized by the absence of wings, presence of four pairs of legs, and fusion of the head and thorax into a cephalothorax.

Ticks are larger than mites, have a leathery body that is either hairless or covered with short hairs, an exposed hypostome and a pair of spiracles near the coxae of the fourth pair of legs. They are divided into the argasid, or soft ticks (*Ornithodoros* species being of human importance), and the ixodid, or hard ticks, including the genera *Dermacentor, Amblyomma* and *Ixodes,* which are responsible for transmitting the agents of several rickettsial, viral, bacterial, and spirochetal diseases.

Mites are smaller than ticks, do not have a leathery covering, and have a hypostome that may be unarmed. Of importance to humans are the trombiculid mites, causing chiggers, and the mange mites of the family *Sarcoptidae,* which include *S. scabiei,* the agent of scabies, and *Demodex folliculorum,* which infest the hair follicles and sebaceous glands.

Spiders are unsegmented, have a hairy abdomen to which are attached four pairs of legs through a slender constriction. They also possess a pair of poisonous jaws through which venom flows from a pair of glands in the cephalothorax. The brown recluse, black widow, and hobo spiders most commonly cause painful and toxic bites in humans.

Class *Insecta* (flies, mosquitoes, bugs, fleas, and lice): a class of arthropods, including organisms with a body divided into three parts, head, thorax, and abdomen, and possessing three pairs of legs. The order *Hemiptera* includes winged or wingless bugs and lice that have mouth parts adapted for piercing and sucking; the order *Diptera* (two winged) include flies, gnats, and mosquitos, and the order *Siphonaptera* includes the fleas, which are wingless and have mouth parts adapted for sucking blood.

Flies are two-winged insects that serve as vectors for the transmission of several agents of human disease. Included are the *Phlebotomus* sandflies (leishmaniasis), *Simulium* black fly (onchocerciasis), Chrysops deer fly (*Loa loa*), and the *Glossina* or tsetse fly (trypanosomiasis). Mosquitos transmit a variety of viral, protozoan, and helminth diseases, most notably malaria and filariasis. Humans may also be infested with the larval forms of flies, a condition known as myiasis.

The biting and blood-sucking "bugs" of importance in human disease include *Cimex lectularius,* the common bedbug, and the "kissing bugs" of the family *Reduviidae,* which transmit the causative agent of South American trypanosomiasis (Chagas' disease).

Fleas are small, brown, wingless, laterally compressed, blood-sucking insects most notably cited as vectors for transmission of the agents of bubonic plague and murine typhus. Fleas are also involved in the transmission of parasitic diseases, including the dog tapeworm, *Dipylidium caninum,* and the rat tapeworm, *Hymenolepis diminuta.*

Lice are dorsoventrally flattened, wingless insects that include three species of importance to humans: *Pediculus humanus* var. *capitis* (head louse), *Pediculus humanus* var. *corporis* (body louse) and *Phthirus pubis* (crab louse). The order includes both biting and sucking lice; however, only the latter, in the suborder *Anoplura,* are ectoparasitic for humans. Lice are important vectors for epidemic typhus and relapsing fever.

---

one-half of the dorsum and allows the prolific intake of blood and tissue fluids (Color Plate A-1*B*). Feeding is necessary for females to achieve fertility, and their body weight can increase as much as 100 times while feeding.[36,51] Males have a scutum that covers almost the entire dorsum (Color Plate A-1*B*) as well as sclerotized ventral plates that limit engorgement in most species, if the male tick feeds at all.

The important vectors of human disease in the United States are three-host ticks, meaning each instar feeds once on a host, after which the tick leaves the host to molt into the next instar in a suitable microenvironment, such as leaf litter or a nest.[51] The process proceeds until adult mating takes place. Mating can occur on the host or off, depending on the species. After mating, the female finds a suitable environment, lays hundreds to thousands of eggs depending on the species,[36,51] then dies. The duration of a life cycle, averaging 1 to 2 years, varies with the presence or absence of suitable environmental conditions and availability of a suitable host.[51] In adverse conditions ticks are capable of long periods of diapause, a torpid phase in which the tick secretes a hygroscopic saliva that allows them to absorb

moisture, enhancing survival until host-seeking conditions improve.

Most hard ticks are burrow or nest dwellers, living out their lives in a closed environment, feeding on a readily available host. In these species human contact is rare or nonexistent.[51] *Ixodes spinipalpus* and wood rats perpetuate an enzootic cycle of *B. burgdorferi* infection in Colorado.[31] The absence of human infection can be attributed to the lack of contact between *I. spinipalpus* and humans.

In only few instances does host specificity place infected ticks in an environment that promotes human contact, which makes them more competent as vectors for disease. The preferred host of *I. scapularis* in early life stages is *Peromyscus leucopus,* the white-footed mouse, known to be the reservoir for *Babesia microti* as well as *Borrelia burgdorferi* in these locations. Although the reservoir for *Anaplasma* (*Ehrlichia*) *phagocytophila* remains unclear, *I. scapularis* is the documented vector. The preferred host of adult ticks is the white-tailed deer (*Odocoileus virginianus*), a far-ranging animal with a distribution that is expanding to include areas of dense human population. With the ability to harbor and transmit multiple pathogens and the willingness to feed on humans, *I. scapularis*'s grades for vector competence are high. In contrast, *I. scapularis* in the Southeast and *I. pacificus* in the Northwest are less competent as vectors of Lyme borreliosis. Host selectivity appears to be the reason. The preferred hosts in both cases are lizards, in which the spirochetes multiply poorly. This biologic phenomenon could account for fewer cases reported in the West and the virtual absence of reported cases in the Southeast.[31,55]

Ticks seek their host by questing, a passive ambush style of host-seeking, in which they climb low grasses and herbaceous vegetation, waiting to attach themselves to a passing host.[51] A few species, on the other hand, actively seek their prey. *Amblyomma americanum* is the only species in the group of ticks discussed here that actively seeks a host.[36] The species that commonly seek human hosts appear to have anatomic preferences for their attachment.[14] *Dermacentor variabilis* prefers the head and neck, whereas *Amblyomma americanum* is more likely to attach to the buttocks, groin, or legs. *Ixodes scapularis* is ubiquitous, attaching to all parts of the body without any obvious preference for a particular site.

The geographic ranges of ticks seem to be expanding. The explosion in the white-tailed deer population into areas of dense human population may be one reason. Another explanation could be that current lifestyles in the United States promote outdoor activities that place people in the way of ticks that have been there all along. This phenomenon brings to mind young urban professionals moving to farm country and then complaining about the smell!

Within the life cycle of a tick a pathogen may be acquired in one of two ways: 1) transstadial (horizontal; i.e., larva to nymph, nymph to adult) or 2) transovarial (vertical; i.e., mother to egg).[51] Larval *Ixodes scapularis* are unable to transmit Lyme disease because *B. burgdorferi* is not transmitted vertically, but is acquired from a reservoir host.[36,51,54] The preferred host for *I. scapularis* larvae and nymphs is the white-footed mouse (*Peromyscus leucosis*), a principle reservoir for *B. burgdorferi*, *B. microti*, and *A. phagocytophilum* in endemic areas. A parallel cycle for *A. phagocytophilum* has been documented between cottontail rabbits and *Ixodes dentatus*,[21] although this species feeds on humans much less frequently than does *I. scapularis*. Ticks acquire *B. burgdorferi* or *A. phagocytophilum* while feeding. In contrast, *Rickettsia rickettsii*, the agent of Rocky Mountain spotted fever, is transmitted vertically from infected *Dermacentor variabilis* females to their progeny,[36,51] making larvae potential vectors.

The level of engorgement gives a rough estimate of feeding time. *B. burgdorferi* dwells in the midgut of infected *I. scapularis*. When the tick feeds, the spirochete multiplies and begins to migrate via the hemolymph. It requires 2 to 3 days for the spirochete to reach the tick's salivary glands,[13,41,52] where in the process of shedding excess water to make room for the blood meal the tick "spits" into the feeding site, thus inoculating the spirochete.[50] In experimental studies, *I. scapularis* nymphs and females were allowed to feed on rodent hosts for defined periods. Given the fact that body length increases while the size of the rigid scutum remains constant, regression equations based on a ratio of body length to scutum width, termed the "scutal index," were developed. The scutal index is considered a more accu-

rate predictor of feeding time than subjective visual estimates.[13,52] In the case of Lyme borreliosis, the identification of an unengorged specimen of *I. scapularis* with intact mouthparts would suggest brief host contact and would make transmission doubtful even if the patient had traveled to an endemic area. *Anaplasma* (*Ehrlichia*) *phagocytophilum* appears to be transmitted somewhat more quickly than is *B. burgdorferi*, so the degree of engorgement and scutal index may be less useful for assessing the likelihood that the pathogen has been inoculated into the patient.[10,26] More studies are required to elucidate this issue.

Nymphs are considered the most likely instar to transmit disease because their small size often allows them to complete feeding undetected (Color Plate A-1*B*). A high percentage of tick-related diseases present in late spring and the summer months because of increased nymph activity.

RELATION TO DISEASE

The history of *Ixodidae* is long in veterinary medicine and more recently intense in human disease. *Ixodidae* (hard ticks) are vectors for a wide variety of pathogens associated with human disease,[51] including spirochetes, rickettsia, gram-negative bacilli, viruses, protozoa, and neurotoxins. The species described here are associated with one or a combination of these agents (Table A-2).

Infections transmitted by ticks may present with similar vague early symptoms of fever, fatigue, and other flulike symptoms that make quick accurate diagnosis problematic,[11,32,36,54] considering that antibiotic therapy differs depending on the agent involved. In most cases, tick-transmitted diseases are mild and resolve with an early accurate diagnosis, followed by proper treatment. Misdiagnosis can lead to increased morbidity, chronic infection and in rare cases, death.

Coinfection after tick bites seems likely.[32,39] Although not proof of coinfection as opposed to sequential infection, serologic studies have shown that, in overlapping endemic areas, patients with clinical Lyme disease have antibodies to *Babesia* or *Ehrlichia* as well.[32] At one point *Babesia* was considered the agent of Lyme disease because patients diagnosed as having babesiosis presented with erythema migrans, which is characteristic of *B. burgdorferi* infection.

Certain species are the vectors for specific pathogens. For instance, Lyme borreliosis is well documented worldwide. *Ixodes scapularis* is defined as the vector for *Borrelia burgdorferi*, the Lyme disease spirochete, in the northeastern and upper Midwestern sections of the United States. Elsewhere *I. ricinus* (Europe), *I. persulcatus* (Asia), and *I. pacificus* (northwestern U.S.) are vectors. Currently other *Ixodes* species are not considered competent vectors. In the eastern United States, identification of an *Ixodes* sp. other than *I. scapularis* would all but rule out Lyme disease, although if the clinical presentation were classic (erythema migrans present)[35,50,54] the presence of a second unnoticed tick would need to be considered. Recently, in the southern United States, a Lyme-like borreliosis caused by *Borrelia lonestari*, similar to *B. theileri* (the agent of bovine borreliosis), has been attributed to exposure to *Amblyomma americanum* (the Lonestar tick).[24]

Tick paralysis is a fascinating disease of unknown pathogenesis.[12,15,46] The acute flaccid paralysis can mimic botulism and Guillain-Barré syndrome; removal of the tick pro-

Table A-2 Hard Ticks and Associated Disease With Geographic Distribution

TICK SPECIES	DISEASE	GEOGRAPHIC RANGE
Ixodes scapularis	Lyme disease	Eastern and upper midwestern U.S.
	Human granulocytic anaplasmosis	
	Babesiosis	
Ixodes pacificus	Lyme disease	Northwest U.S.
Dermacentor variabilis	Rocky Mountain spotted fever	Eastern two thirds of the U.S., West coast of the U.S.
	Tularemia	
	Tick paralysis	
Dermacentor andersoni	Rocky Mountain spotted fever, Colorado tick fever	Rocky Mountain states
	Tick paralysis	
Amblyomma americanum	Human monocytic ehrlichiosis	South Central U.S., southeastern U.S., Mid-Atlantic states as far north as southern New York State
Ixodes cookei	Tularemia Powassan virus	Northeastern U.S. and southeastern Canada
Ixodes marxi	Powassan virus	Northeastern U.S. and southeastern Canada

duces a rapid and dramatic reversal of the paralysis. There are no sequelae. Although over 60 species of tick can produce tick paralysis in animals, only *Dermacentor andersoni*, *Dermacentor variabilis*, and *Ixodes holocyclus* (the Australian marsupial tick) bite humans. In North America the disease occurs most commonly in the southeastern and northwestern states of the United States and in British Columbia.

GEOGRAPHIC DISTRIBUTION

The geographic distribution of the hard ticks in summarized in Table A-2.

Ixodes scapularis. Once referred to as *Ixodes dammini* in the Northeast and *Ixodes scapularis* elsewhere, the two are now considered by most authorities to be a northern and southern variety of the same species because of their ability to mate successfully.[34,54] The name *Ixodes scapularis* has precedence. *I. scapularis* occupies a wide range east of the Rocky Mountains, although infectious populations appear to be focal in the upper Midwest and in the Northeast from Maryland to southern New England.

Ixodes cookei. The range of *Ixodes cookei* (the woodchuck tick) overlaps that of *I. scapularis;* it is found primarily in the northeastern United States and southeastern Canada.

Ixodes marxi. *Ixodes marxi*, (the squirrel tick) also has a range that overlaps *I. scapularis* in the northeastern United States and southeastern Canada.

Dermacentor spp. *Dermacentor variabilis* (the dog tick) is widely distributed throughout the United States east of the Rocky Mountains. The wide range and host-seeking habits of *D. variabilis* increase the incidence of contact with humans when compared with other *Dermacentor* spp.

Dermacentor andersoni is distributed in the Rocky Mountain states and is the tick that was described by Ricketts as the vector of Rocky Mountain spotted fever in the Bitter Root Valley of Idaho.[60]

Amblyomma americanum. *Amblyomma americanum* (the Lonestar tick) is widely distributed in the South (east of the Rocky Mountains) and in the East to southern New York State. There are indications that the range may be extending into New England. *A. americanum* is unique among the tick species described here in that it actively seeks a host.[36,51]

IDENTIFICATION

Acari (ticks and mites) are distinguished from other arachnids by the absence of obvious segmentation. An anterior prosoma (appendages) is fused with the opisthosoma (abdomen). A gnathosoma (capitulum) bearing the mouthparts is unique to Acari.[51] Figures A-1 and A-2 represent the dorsal and ventral view, respectively, of a generic hard tick. The drawings were made to place as many key features in view as possible. A glossary of identifying features depicted in these figures follows. All features are useful for identification of ticks; size, placement, color, and presence or absence of each characteristic may be important.

A. Capitulum: The anterior portion of the body, including the basis capituli, hypostome, chelicerae, and palpi
B. Basis capituli: The base of the capitulum to which the mouthparts are attached. (The length of the capitulum in proportion to the basis capituli is useful in identification.)

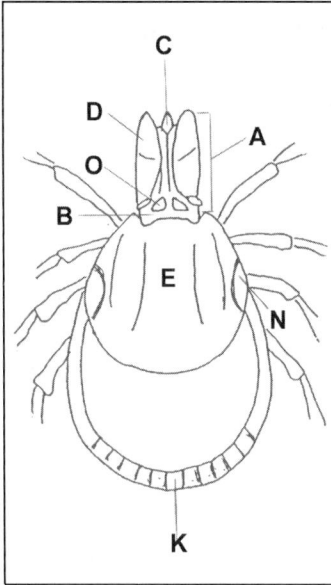

Figure A-1 Generic diagram of the dorsum of a hard tick.

C. Hypostome: The median structure of the mouthparts parallel to and between the palpi. The hypostome holds teethlike structures called denticles. Denticles appear on the hypostome in a specific arrangement called the "dentition formula" (ratio of left denticles to right denticles). *Ixodes scapularis*, for instance, has a dentition formula of 3/3, becoming 2/2 as it progresses posteriorly.

D. Palpi: Paired movable appendages lying parallel to the hypostome.

E. Scutum: The sclerotized dorsal plate posterior to the capitulum.

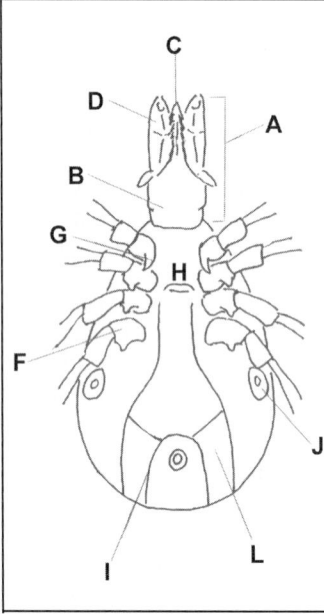

Figure A-2 Generic diagram of the ventral aspect of a hard tick.

F. Coxa: The basal segment of the legs. Coxa are numbered I through IV, with coxa I located closest to the capitulum.

G. Coxal spurs: Projection on the posterior margin of the coxa. Spurs on the median side are called internal spurs while those on the lateral side are external spurs. There is little or no variation in spur size or configuration from specimen to specimen of the same species.

H. Genital aperture: External opening of the genital organs, located ventrally on the median axis between the coxae.

I. Anal groove: Semicircular groove curving around the anus of some species. In *Ixodes* spp. the curve is anterior to the anus. In other genera the curve is posterior or absent.

J. Spiracular plates: External opening of the respiratory system, located ventrally, posterior to coxa IV on the lateral margins (useful in differentiating male *I. scapularis* from male *I. cookei* and male *I. marxi*)

K. Festoons: Rectangular areas separated by distinct grooves located on the posterior margin of some hard ticks. Festoons are absent in *Ixodes* spp.

L. Ventral plates: A group of plates of definite shape and size on the ventral surface of adult males. We will specifically refer to the anal plate when describing *Ixodes* spp.

M. Ornamentation: Some ticks are referred to as ornate ticks based on the presence of colorful markings distinct to certain species. *D. variabilis* and *A. americanum* are ornate ticks.

N. Eyes: Ornate ovoid markings on the lateral margins of the scutum of some ticks.

O. Porose areas: Areas resembling "eyes" found on the dorsal basis capituli of adult ticks.

Ixodes scapularis. An important feature of all *Ixodes* spp. is an anterior facing U-shaped groove that surrounds the anus and terminates at the posterior margin of the ventral surface (Figure A-3 and Color Plate A-1*C*). Other genera of hard ticks lack this feature.[51] *I. scapularis* nymphs and adult

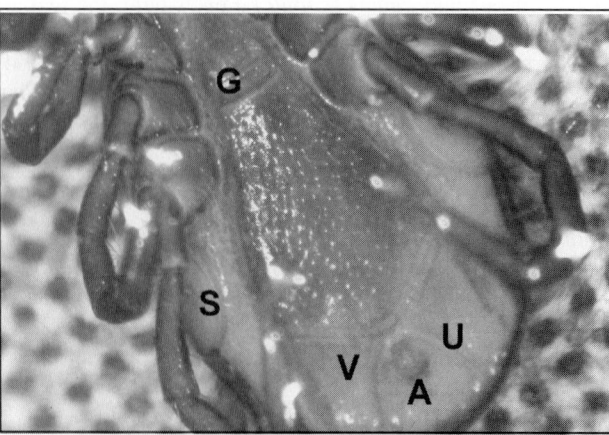

Figure A-3 Ventral aspect of adult male *Ixodes scapularis*, demonstrating the anus (*A*), U-shaped anal groove (*U*), genital pore (*G*), ventral plates (*V*), and spiracular plates (*S*).

females have an oval-shaped scutum (Color Plate A-1*B*) that is approximately half the size of the dorsum in unengorged specimens. The scutum of adult males covers essentially the entire dorsum (Color Plate A-1*B*), a characteristic of all hard ticks that will not be mentioned in further descriptions. The presence of coarse hairs over the entire scutum is one of the characteristics that distinguish *I. scapularis* males from *I. cookei* and *I. marxi* specimens, in which they are fine or absent. When viewed ventrally (Color Plate A-1*C*), mouthparts appear twice as long as the basis capituli. The hypostome of nymphs and adult females has a dentition formula of 3/3, progressing to 2/2 anterior to posterior. Adult males have a more ''businesslike'' hypostome than most other *Ixodes* spp., with severe lateral denticles that get blunt to crenulated as they approach the median.

Color can help in distinguishing *I. scapularis* from other *Ixodes* spp. The sclerotic anterior portion of nymphs and adult females (includes the capitulum, legs, and scutum) is dark brown, in sharp contrast to the abdomen, which appears reddish-brown in unengorged specimens (Color Plate A-1*B*) to gray-tan in engorged specimens, thus the name *black-legged tick*. Adult males appear entirely dark brown (Color Plate A-1*B*). Coxal spurs (Color Plate A-1*D* and Figure A-4) are present, with coxa I having a severe internal spur that overlaps coxa II. Coxa I through IV have blunt external spurs. The internal spur on coxa I appears less severe in nymphs. The spiracular plates of nymphs and females are round (Color Plate A-1*C*); in males they are elongated anterior to posterior (Fig. A-3). The spiracular plates in males of *I. cookei* and *I. marxi* appear round. The anal plate in males is short anterior to posterior in comparison to *I. cookei* and *I. marxi* (Fig. A-3).

Ixodes cookei. The scutum of nymphs and female adults is angular from the posterior apex to the midlateral margins (Color Plate A-1*E*). In adult females, the scutum appears about as wide to the lateral margins as it is anterior to posterior, whereas in nymphs the scutum appears wider laterally than anteriorly to posteriorly. The mouthparts of all life stages appear proportional in length to the basis capituli (Color Plate A-1*E*). When compared to *I. scapularis*, the hypostome of females and nymphs is similar, with a dentition formula of 3/3, progressing to 2/2, although in *I. cookei* females the apex is more rounded. The hypostome of nymphs is more rounded still. The hypostome in males is short, round, and crenulated. An interesting feature, most pronounced in the nymph of this species, is the projection of the first segment of the palpi laterally from the posterior margin. These projections have a spurlike appearance and are often referred to as palpal spurs. In all stages, color is a lightly-creamed-coffee brown. Color is consistent over the entire tick. The arrangement of coxal spurs is similar to that of *I. scapularis,* with a pronounced internal spur on coxa I and blunt external spurs on coxae I through IV. Spiracular plates in nymphs and females are similar to *I. scapularis*. In males they appear more round, not elongated, as is the case in *I. scapularis* males. The anal plate in males of this species appears twice as long anterior to posterior in proportion to lateral width, which helps distinguish this species from *I. scapularis*.

Ixodes marxi. The scutum of nymphs and females of this species is similar to *I. cookei* in that it is angular from the midlateral margin to the posterior apex (Color Plate A-1*F*). That fact can confuse the identification of these species. In females there are differences in length and width. The scutum of *I. marxi* females is noticeably longer anterior to posterior in relation to lateral width. In *I. cookei,* length and width are equally proportional. In *I. marxi* nymphs length and width are basically equal, whereas in *I. cookei*, the scutum appears laterally wider than it is long anterior to posterior. Given the similarity in scutal proportion of an *I. marxi* nymph and an *I. cookei* adult female, identification should be made by observing the presence or absence of a genital aperture. The male scutum appears to be absent of hair.

When viewed ventrally, the mouthparts of all three stages appear proportional in length to the basis capituli. The hypostome of nymphs and females is similar to *I. scapularis*, with a dentition formula of 3/3 at the apex then 2/2 as it approaches the posterior end. The apex in females is severely pointed. The male hypostome appears short, rounded at the apex, and crenulated. Color in this species is similar to *I. cookei*, in which the entire body of all three stages appears a lightly-creamed-coffee brown. The arrangement of coxal spurs is a key characteristic in the identification of *I. marxi*. Nymphs and females have a blunt internal spur and the hint of an external spur on coxa I. The notable absence of spurs on coxae II through IV distinguishes the females and nymphs of this species from the other *Ixodes* described here. The coxal spur arrangement of males is similar to that of *I. cookei,* with the exceptions of a less severe internal spur on coxa I and the notable absence of spurs on coxa IV. Round spiracular plates in all stages help distinguish males of this species from *I. scapularis*, in which they appear elongated. The anal plate in male *I. marxi* is longer anteriorly to posteriorly in proportion to lateral width than in *I. scapularis*, in which proportions appear equal.

Dermacentor variabilis. *D. variabilis* is an ornate tick, meaning the tick is quite colorful, with contrasting markings. Coloration in ornate ticks is described as the base color (the predominant overall color of the tick) and the pattern color (contrasting markings) (Color Plate A-1*G* and Color Plate A-1*H*).[8] Pattern color is present on the scutum as well as the legs of *D. variabilis*. Eleven festoons are arranged in a

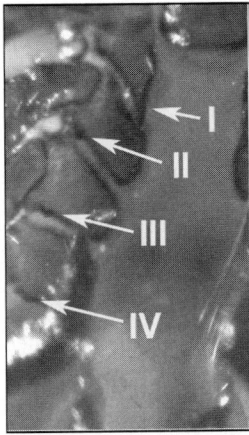

Figure A-4 Detail of Color Plate A-1*D*. Coxal spurs of adult *Ixodes scapularis*. The spur on coxa I is long, pointed, and oriented internally. The spurs on coxae II through IV are short, blunt, and oriented externally.

semicircle around the posterior margin (Color Plate A-1*G*). They can be observed in both the dorsal and ventral view of all stages. The scutum of females is angular and appears roughly equal in length anteriorly to posteriorly as side to side. Pattern color is predominantly pearl-white to gray and appears in stark contrast to the rest of the tick, in which the base color is chestnut brown. Brown lines and spots in random patterns, not consistent from specimen to specimen, are present. The presence of ''eyes'' can be observed at the midlateral margins (Color Plate A-1*H*). Color and contrast are similar in males and females. Ornamental markings cover the entire dorsum because of the nature of the male scutum. Base color areas appear larger as they approach the midlateral and posterior margins. Markings on each side of the median axis are roughly mirror-imaged. The scutum of nymphs is long and does not appear as angular as it is in the female; from the midlateral margins it is rounded to the posterior median. Pattern color appears to be more prominent. ''Eyes'' are present at the angles of the lateral margins, as they proceed to the posterior apex. (note: nymphs have not been seen in our laboratory and are known to have infrequent human contact).[8]

The basis capituli of all stages appears wider than it is deep (Color Plate A-1*H*). The basis capituli of nymphs in the dorsal view have pronounced posterior lateral spurlike projections that make the basis look triangular. The hypostome in all stages is short and rounded. Palpi appear short and thick in adults, but narrow in nymphs. Coxal spurs are similar in adults. Coxa I has large internal and external spurs that converge in the median, conveying a notched appearance. Coxae II though IV have smaller external spurs. Nymphs have a predominant external spur and less dominant internal spur on coxa I, with unremarkable external spurs on coxae II and III and no spurs on coxa IV. In the Northeast, *D. variabilis* must not be confused with *Dermacentor albipictus* (the moose tick, also called the winter tick). Just as a moose is bigger than a dog or a deer, *D. albipictus* is appreciably larger than *D. variabilis* or *I. scapularis* (Fig. A-5). A mean of 2 mm divides unengorged specimens of

these species.[8] A fed *D. variabilis* can achieve impressive dimensions (Color Plate A-1*G*), but a fully engorged *D. albipictus* female can achieve the size of an adult's fourth fingernail. In optimal environmental conditions *D. albipictus* has been known to exsanguinate a moose because of the number of ticks feeding simultaneously. Fortunately, human contact with *D. albipictus* is minimal to absent.

Amblyomma americanum. *A. americanum* is another ornate tick (Color Plate A-2*A*). Eleven festoons are present. Base color is more predominant than in *D. variabilis,* and pattern colors are more consistent. The scutum in females is angular and about as long as wide. Approaching the lateral margins it becomes darker than the base color, which is red-tan. ''Eyes'' are present at the lateral apices (Color Plate A-2*B*). The remarkable scutal pattern in females is an iridescent patch at the posterior apex (Color Plate A-2*A*). Depending on the angle of the light source this marking appears bluegreen to pearl-pink and brings to mind gasoline on water. This appearance characterizes all pattern color markings on *A. americanum* in all stages. The scutum of nymphs appears wider than long, with ''eyes'' at the lateral apices. The iridescent patch found at the posterior apex of females is missing. The male scutum is most remarkable for the presence of two, inverted, pattern-colored ''horse shoes'' at the posterior margin (Color Plate A-2*C*). ''Eyes'' are present at the lateral margins. Pattern color markings proceed below the ''eyes'' toward the median and give the appearance of a pseudoscutum resembling that of the female. Male and female specimens may be confused by an inexperienced observer. Random pattern color markings follow the posterior lateral margins as well.

The mouthparts on all stages are long in proportion to the basis capituli. The hypostome appears bulbous in that it is narrow posteriorly and is wide and rounded anteriorly. Coxal spur arrangement is similar in all stages. There is a severe internal spur and a short, rounded external spur on coxa I. A short, pointed spur on coxae II though IV appears closer to the median, though is most likely an internal spur. Males have a long severe internal spur on coxa IV (Color Plate A-2*D*). All stages have an anal groove. The groove appears as a semicircle posterior to the anus. From the median of the semicircle a single groove descends toward the posterior margin. The overall appearance is that of a wineglass or chalice (Color Plate A-2*D*)

SUMMARY OF IDENTIFICATION

The descriptions above follow a sequence of observation used in our laboratory. When a specimen is presented with an anterior facing U-shaped groove, *Ixodes scapularis* must be identified or ruled out. When distinguishing *I. cookei* from *I. marxi,* coxal spur arrangement and scutal configuration are key. When the tick is ornate, distinctions are made based on scutal configuration, pattern color markings versus base color, configuration of pattern color markings, the length of the mouthparts in relation to the basis capituli, and coxal spur arrangement. The diagnostic features are summarized in Table A-3.

Good reference books make these descriptions more comprehensive.[8,9,27,37] The envelope continues to be pushed in regard to diseases transmitted by ticks. Emergent disease as well as established disease, now being associated with tick

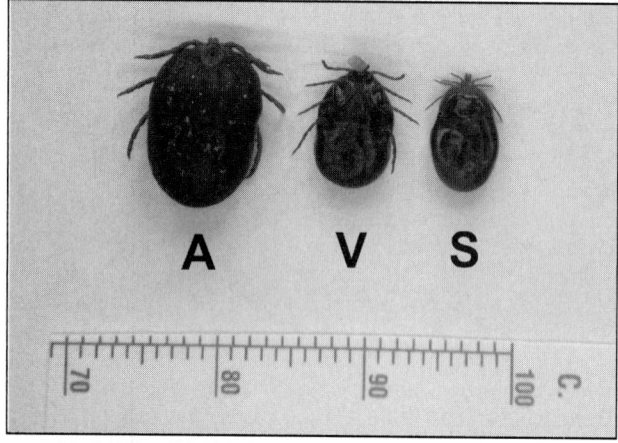

Figure A-5 Size comparison of engorged ticks. An engorged moose tick, *Dermacentor albopictus* (*A*), dwarfs an engorged American dog tick, *Dermacentor variabilis* (*V*), which in turn is larger than the enlarged deer tick, *Ixodes scapularis* (*S*). All are adult females.

Table A-3 Diagnostic Features of Hard Ticks

SPECIES	STAGE	SCUTUM	ANAL GROOVE	COXAL SPURS	MOUTHPARTS/ BASIS CAPITULI	EYES	FESTOONS	COLOR
Ixodes scapularis	Nymph	Oval; covers one third of the dorsum and is dark in contrast to the abdomen	Anterior facing U-shaped; surrounding the anus	Prominent internal spur on coxa I; blunt external spurs on I through IV	Mouthparts twice as long as basis capituli when viewed ventrally	No	Absent	Capituli, legs, and scutum are black coffee brown with contrasting red-tan abdomen
	Adult female	Covers half the dorsum, otherwise resembles nymph	Same as nymph	Same as nymph	Same as nymph	No	Absent	Same as nymph
	Adult male	Covers entire dorsum; hairy	Same as nymph	Same as nymph	Same as nymph; more "businesslike" hypostome than other *Ixodes* spp.	No	Absent	Overall black-coffee brown
Dermacentor variabilis	Nymph	Covers half the dorsum; predominant pattern color	Absent	Prominent external spur on coxa I; less blunted external spurs on II and III	Dorsal basis capituli looks triangular; palpi are narrow	Yes	Present	Pattern colors more predominant
	Adult female	Angular; as long as wide; pattern-colored with random base color markings	Absent	Prominent internal and external spurs on coxa I, giving a notched appearance	Thick palpi; basis capituli wider than mouthparts are long	Yes	Present	Base color is chestnut brown; pattern color is gray-white
	Adult male	Base color and pattern color roughly equal	Chalice-shaped	Same as female	Same as female	Yes	Present	Same as female
Amblyomma americanum	Nymph	Angular; wider than long; predominant base color; "eyes" at lateral apices	Chalice-shaped	Spurs appear at the posterior median of all four coxa; spur on coxa I is more pronounced	Mouthparts appear much longer than the basis capituli; hypostome is bulbous	Yes	Present	Predominant caramel base color; pattern color is iridescent blue-green to yellow
	Adult female	Angular; about as wide as long; predominant base color with "eyes"; pattern colored patch at posterior apex	Chalice-shaped	Coxa I has a prominent median spur; spurs appear absent on II through IV	Same as nymph	Yes	Present	Same as nymph

(Continued)

Table A-3 *Continued*

SPECIES	STAGE	SCUTUM	ANAL GROOVE	COXAL SPURS	MOUTHPARTS/ BASIS CAPITULI	EYES	FESTOONS	COLOR
	Adult male	Predominant base color; inverted pattern color "horseshoes" at posterior margin	Chalice-shaped	Similar to the female with a severe internal spur on coxa IV	Same as nymph	Yes	Present	Same as nymph
Ixodes cookei	Nymph	Angular; wider than long	Anterior facing U-shaped; surrounding the anus	Similar to *I. scapularis*	Mouthparts equal in length to the basis capituli; hypostome similar to *I. scapularis*, though more rounded at the apex; palpal spurs present	No	Absent	Lightly-creamed-coffee brown
	Adult female	Angular; as wide as long	Same as nymph	Same as nymph	Same as nymph	No	Absent	Same as nymph
	Adult male	Less hairy in comparison with *I. scapularis*	Same as nymph	Same as nymph	Proportional to nymph; hypostome rounded and crenulated	No	Absent	Same as nymph
Ixodes marxi	Nymph	Angular; as wide as long	Anterior facing U-shaped; surrounding the anus	Blunt internal spur and presence of external spur on coxa I; absence of spurs on II through IV	Mouthparts equal in length to the basis capituli	No	Absent	Lightly-creamed-coffee brown
	Adult female	Angular; longer than wide	Same as nymph	Same as nymph	Same as nymph; hypostome is severely pointed	No	Absent	Same as nymph
	Adult male	Appears hairless	Same as nymph	Coxa I has prominent internal spur and blunt external spur; II through IV have blunt external spurs; spurs absent on coxa IV	Proportional to nymph; hypostome rounded and crenulated	No	Absent	Same as nymph

transmission, is the subject of wide study. An accurate identification of a recovered tick from a patient who presents with vague flulike symptoms can and should influence early therapy.

Ornithodoros Species

Relation to Disease

Ornithodoros spp. transmit the *Borrelia* spp. that cause endemic relapsing fever.

Identification

Ornithodoros spp. are soft ticks. By definition, their mouthparts are not visible from above, and they do not have a scutum. They have a prominent hypostome covered with teeth (see Color Plate A-2*E*).

Geographic Distribution

It is difficult to differentiate among the several species that may transmit relapsing fever. In the northwestern United States and western Canada *O. hermsi* is the primary vector. This species feeds on small rodents as well as humans and typically inhabits cracks and crevices in shacks and cabins. A famous outbreak in a Boy Scout troop was concentrated in senior scouts and scoutmasters, who commandeered an abandoned cabin, leaving the younger scouts to spend their night unbitten under the stars.[58]

In the Southwest and southern Midwest the common vector is *O. turicata*, which is found on a variety of small and large mammals, rodents, birds, and reptiles. This species is often found in animal burrows.

Mites

Numerous species of mites exist in nature. Species of the family *Trombiculidae* (chigger mites) produce intense itching or dermatitis as they feed transiently. Members of the genus *Leptotrombidium* transmit scrub typhus in Southeast Asia and Australia.[65] House-dust mites in the genus *Dermatophagoides* serve as allergens for certain individuals. The mouse mite, *Liponyssoides* (*Allodermanyssus*) *sanguineus*, transmits *Rickettsia akari*, the agent of rickettsialpox. Rickettsialpox was first described in New York City and continues to be a problem there.[25]

The itch mite, *Sarcoptes scabiei*, and the follicle mite, *Demodex folliculorum*, are the two mites that have an intimate and prolonged parasitic association with humans.

Sarcoptes scabiei (Scabies)

RELATION TO DISEASE

Sarcoptes scabiei is known as the "itch mite." The mite causes mange by burrowing into the skin and laying eggs in the burrows. Resulting larval and nymphal stages of the mite live in the burrows and adjacent hair follicles. Fecal deposits left by the mites provoke intense itching, leading

to significant irritation and hair loss. Recurrence of disease is usually by reinfestation from mites on inadequately treated contacts, but relapse may also occur even after a standard course of treatment.[61]

IDENTIFICATION

Microscopic examination of skin scrapings reveals the characteristic mite (which measures 0.2 to 0.4 mm in length), eggs, or fecal pellets (scybala) (see Color Plate A-2*F*). Specimens are collected after placing a drop of mineral oil on a sterile scalpel blade and allowing some of the oil to cover the papule. Scrape the papule vigorously six or seven times to remove the top; then transfer the scraped material, which should contain some flecks of blood in the oil, to a glass slide, using an applicator stick if necessary. After adding a couple of drops of mineral oil to the preparation and mixing, place a glass coverslip on top.[18]

GEOGRAPHIC DISTRIBUTION

Itch mites are distributed worldwide.

Demodex folliculorum (Hair Follicles) and *Demodex brevis* (Sebaceous Glands)

RELATION TO DISEASE

Infections are usually found on the face. Organisms can cause pruritus and local tissue reaction as they burrow in the skin. They are also found, however, in asymptomatic individuals.

IDENTIFICATION

Microscopic examination of specimens from skin reveals the characteristic mite, which measures 0.1 to 0.4 mm in length.

GEOGRAPHIC DISTRIBUTION

Follicle mites are distributed worldwide.

Spiders

Thousands of species of spiders exist in nature. Most possess potent toxins, but only a small number are capable of penetrating human skin when biting.[17]

Loxosceles reclusa

RELATION TO DISEASE

Loxosceles reclusa, known commonly as the brown recluse spider, prefers to exist in stored clothes and sleeping bags, basements, closets, and other sites with reduced human activity.[17,18] Their venom is injected through biting, and can cause serious desquamation and necrosis of skin. Large doses of venom are associated with dissemination and significant mortality. The bite of the brown recluse spider does not produce a diagnostic lesion; several reports suggest that dermonecrotic lesions are incorrectly attributed to spiders on a regular basis.[59]

IDENTIFICATION

The brown recluse spider is characterized by its yellow to brown coloration, 1- to 2-cm size, and a violin- or fiddle-shaped marking on its head (see Color Plate A-2G).[17,18] There are several related species, which may require expert help for correct identification.

GEOGRAPHIC DISTRIBUTION

The brown recluse spider is found in most of the continental United States except for the extreme western sections.

Latrodectus mactans

RELATION TO DISEASE

Several species of widow spiders exist. *Latrodectus mactans*, the most common black widow spider, may cause a serious systemic reaction, even death, after injection of its venom. Fortunately, most patients do not become gravely ill and recover quickly.[17,18] Most bites occur on the hands.[56] Male spiders produce mild or no symptoms after their bite.[20]

IDENTIFICATION

The black widow female is 3 cm long (including legs), glossy black, and displays a characteristic red hourglass marking on her abdomen (see Color Plate A-2H).[17,18,56] Differentiation among related species is difficult and best left to experts.

GEOGRAPHIC DISTRIBUTION

Different species of widow spiders exist throughout the entire continental United States. *Latrodectus mactans* occurs from southern New England south to Florida and west to California and Oregon; it is more common in the southern part of the range. The northern black widow spider, *L. variolus* is present in New England and southern Canada south to Florida and west to eastern Texas, Oklahoma, and Kansas; it is more common in the northern part of its range.

Tegenaria agrestis

RELATION TO DISEASE

In recent years, there have been increasing reports of toxic reactions to the bite of the hobo spider, *T. agrestis*. Many bites are not followed by serious reactions, but some bites may produce a dermonecrotic lesion similar to that of the brown recluse spider. Erythema is followed by blistering and then ulceration. An eschar forms and subsequently sloughs, with or without formation of a scar. Systemic effects are usually mild but may be severe. The male spider is more venomous than the female.[7]

IDENTIFICATION

Hobo spiders are brown with gray markings. They are moderately large, measuring 7 to 14 mm in body length and 27 to 45 mm in leg span.

GEOGRAPHIC DISTRIBUTION

Tegenaria agrestis is distributed throughout the Pacific Northwest, southwestern Canada, and the Alaskan panhan-

dle. The distribution of this spider does not overlap that of *Loxosceles reclusa*. The hobo spider builds funnel-shaped webs in damp, moist places, such as wood piles and crawl spaces. It is rarely found above foundation or ground level.

Insecta: Flies, Bugs, Fleas, and Lice

Myiasis-Producing Fly Larvae

Myiasis occurs when fly larvae infect humans either accidentally or by penetrating skin directly to form subcutaneous skin lesions, for the purpose of feeding on tissue. Imported cases of myiasis are increasing because of more frequent travel to endemic areas.[4,62] The two most common genera that parasitize humans are *Dermatobia* and *Cordylobia*. Flies in the genera *Wohlfahrtia*, *Cochliomyia*, *Hypoderma*, and *Oestrus* affect humans much less commonly and will not be discussed here.[17,20,49]

Dermatobia hominis (Human Bot Fly)

RELATION TO DISEASE

The fascinating life cycle of this organism requires some discussion to understand infection. The female attaches her eggs to another insect vector, often a mosquito. While the insect is biting a host, the eggs release larvae, which immediately penetrate the skin. Larvae mature in the skin for approximately 6 to 12 weeks, after which they leave the subcutaneous tissue for the soil, where they require another 3 weeks of maturation before an adult fly emerges.[4,49,62]

While in the skin, the larvae produce a lesion that resembles a "boil," which is often quite pruritic and occasionally painful. Complete excision of the larvae eliminates the disease and allows confirmation of the diagnosis. Secondary bacterial infections of the lesions occur occasionally.

IDENTIFICATION

Larvae range in size from several millimeters to 18 to 25 mm, depending on maturity at the time of excision. Rows of spines that are easily visible with a dissecting microscope encircle them (see Color Plate A-3A). Larval stages may have a distinct "flask" shape, with a long tapered neck. Microscopic examination of the spiracles (stigmal plates) are useful when making an identification.[17,18]

GEOGRAPHIC DISTRIBUTION

Dermatobia hominis is common in Central and South America.[4,17,47]

Cordylobia anthropophaga (Tumbu Fly)

RELATION TO DISEASE

Larvae emerge from eggs that have contaminated bed linen, clothing, or other materials and penetrate the host's skin shortly after contact.[4,28] Development in the subdermal layer occurs much faster than with *Dermatobia hominis*, usually within 2 weeks,[4] reducing the relative number of imported cases.[28] Patients are generally exposed to a larger number of eggs, so numerous lesions are more likely with *Cordylobia* infection than with *Dermatobia*.[4]

IDENTIFICATION

Larvae reach 7 to 12 mm at maturation. Their more conical shape readily distinguishes them from *Dermatobia*.[28] Spiracles appear at the widest end.

GEOGRAPHIC DISTRIBUTION

Cordylobia is found primarily in sub-Saharan Africa.

Other Flies

Several other medically important flies warrant brief discussion, although specimens are rarely submitted to clinical laboratories.

Sandflies belonging to the genera *Lutzomyia* and *Phlebotomus* are responsible for transmission of leishmaniasis. These flies are hairy, small, and tend to have wings held in an erect V shape. *Chrysops* spp., commonly known as deer flies, are involved in transmission of *Loa loa*, the African eye worm. Black flies (*Simulium* spp.) are the vectors for the microfilariae causing onchocerciasis. Different *Simulium* species exist in distinct geographic regions, but all reproduce in fast-flowing waterways near which the largest number of bites occur. Tsetse flies (*Glossina* spp.) exist only in tropical Africa and transmit African trypanosomiasis (sleeping sickness). These elongated flies possess a powerful proboscis capable of inflicting painful bites.[56]

Mosquitoes

Mosquitoes are responsible for transmitting diseases causing greater morbidity and mortality than any other arthropod.[17,18,20,56]

RELATION TO DISEASE

Mosquitoes produce pruritic skin lesions that appear shortly after they take a blood meal. They are also capable of transmitting serious infections. *Anopheles* spp. are the arthropod vectors responsible for transmitting malaria. Filariasis is spread by some *Aedes* spp., *Mansonia* spp., and *Anopheles* spp. A variety of arthropodborne viruses (arboviruses) use *Aedes* spp., *Culex* spp., *Culiseta* spp., *Haemagogus* spp., and *Sabethes* spp. as vectors of serious infections, such as equine encephalitis, West Nile fever, yellow fever, and dengue.[5,42,56] Both male and female mosquitoes feed on nectar and pollinate flowers. The female mosquito must take a blood meal to complete development of eggs.[20]

Mosquitoes use olfactory clues to find their human targets. A specific component of human sweat has been identified as an important compound for *Anopheles gambiae*, an important vector for *Plasmodium falciparum*.[22] For those of us who are unable to stop sweating, a variety of insect repellents is available to discourage mosquitoes from biting. Products based on botanicals are attractive options for those who wish to avoid chemical deterrents; unfortunately the options that are available currently are not as effective as products that contain *N,N*-diethyl-3-methylbenzamide

(DEET).[16] Perhaps in the future compounds that block relevant components in sweat will make effective deterrents.

IDENTIFICATION

Mosquitoes are dainty-appearing, flying insects easily recognized by most. Identification to genus and species level requires significant experience and should be left to the experts. Mosquito bites are sufficiently common that patients rarely bring specimens to the clinical laboratory for identification.

GEOGRAPHIC DISTRIBUTION

Mosquitoes are found worldwide, but individual species have well-defined environmental niches. For instance, classic yellow fever was an urban disease because the primary vector, *Aedes aegypti*, was limited to standing water in the vicinity of human dwellings. It was hoped that the disease could be completely eliminated by controlling the mosquito vector. Unfortunately, control of urban yellow fever revealed a sylvatic cycle among monkeys and several forest mosquito species, and it soon became clear that the virus could be controlled but never eliminated (unless we are successful at destroying all of the rain forests).[56]

Mosquitoes are one of the beneficiaries of global commerce. *Aedes albopictus*, also known as the ''tiger mosquito,'' is a resident of Southeast Asia, but it hitched a ride to the United States by laying eggs in accumulated water in automobile tires.[33] This aggressive mosquito species is a competent vector for important human pathogens, although only eastern equine encephalitis and Cache Valley viruses have been isolated from naturally infected mosquitoes.

"Bugs"

Bedbugs (*Cimex* spp.) and reduviid (Family *Reduviidae*) bugs suck the blood of vertebrates, including humans, and may act as important vectors in transmission of disease.[17,56] They are nocturnal, feeding at night and hiding and resting during the day. The common bedbug (*C. lectularius*) is occasionally submitted to microbiology laboratories for identification.

CIMEX LECTULARIUS

Relation to Disease. The common bedbug can cause numerous small lesions on the skin wherever a blood meal is taken. The severity of the lesions is related to the sensitivity of the individual. Bedbugs feed primarily at night, otherwise hiding in the bed linen, loose wallpaper, and mattresses.[17] They do not act as vectors of infectious agents.

Identification. Bedbugs are light to orange-brown, 5 mm long by 3 mm wide.[17,18,20] Adults have small, nonworking wing appendages (Color Plate A-3*B*).

Geographic Distribution. *Cimex lectularius* is distributed worldwide, although more common in temperate zones, whereas *C. hemipterus* is more common in tropical climates.[56]

KISSING BUGS: *PANSTRONGYLUS, RHODNIUS,* AND *TRIATOMA* SPECIES

Relation to Disease. The family *Reduviidae* has several popular names. These bugs are sometimes known as ''cone-nose bugs'' because of the elongated shape of the head. The majority of the group are known as assassin bugs from their lethal aggression against other insects. Assassin bugs may also bite humans and cause painful lesions.[20]

Medically, the most important group are the ''kissing bugs,'' so-named because they may take their blood meals from the skin around the lips. Kissing bugs transmit the causative agent of Chagas; disease, *Trypanosoma cruzi*. They are unable to bite through clothing, so lesions are most common on exposed parts of the body.[20] Feces containing *T. cruzi* are deposited on the host while the bugs feed. Subsequent scratching of pruritic skin at the bite site introduces organisms into the wound. Transmission also occurs when fecally contaminated fingers are rubbed in the eyes, nose, or mouth.[56]

Identification. Unlike bedbugs, reduviid (triatomid) bugs possess functioning wings. They range in size from 1 to 4 cm, are more elongated than bedbugs, and have relatively long, thin heads (see Color Plate A-3*C*).[17,18,20,56]

Geographic Distribution. Kissing bugs occur in southern portions of the United States and in Central and South America.

Fleas

RELATION TO DISEASE

Fleas may cause irritating, itchy bites after sucking blood from a host. The species that transmit the most serious human infections most commonly are considered here. The Oriental rat flea, *Xenopsylla cheopis*, is the classic vector of plague[30] and murine typhus.[20] *Tunga penetrans*, the ''jigger'' flea found in Africa and in Central and South America, penetrates the skin and lays eggs inside the host (Color Plate A-3*D*).

The cat flea, *Ctenocephalides felis*, and the dog flea, *Ctenocephalides canis*, can infect either species of domestic animal (Color Plate A-3*E*). In North America, the dog flea is uncommon, and most human disease is caused by the cat flea.[20] Either species can bite humans. The dog tapeworm, *Dipylidium caninum*, may occasionally infect humans when a flea containing the cysticercoid stage of the tapeworm is accidentally ingested.[17,18] Several species of fleas, in addition to other insects, may transmit the larvae of the rat tapeworm, *Hymenolepis diminuta,* to humans. Recently it has been recognized that endemic plague may be associated with exposure to cats, and endemic typhus, caused by *Rickettsia typhi*, may be transmitted by the cat flea.[53] A newly described rickettsia, known as the ELB agent,[48,63] also infects the cat flea and causes an illness that resembles murine typhus. This new rickettsial organism can be maintained by transovarial transmission in cat fleas.[1] The ELB agent has now been classified as *Rickettsia felis*.[23] In developed countries cats may be more important than rats in transmission of these infections.

IDENTIFICATION

Recognition of fleas is relatively easy. They are wingless, and have long, muscular legs[17,18,56] hanging down from a body that looks ''hunched over'' (Color Plates A-3*D* and *E*). Speciation of fleas is very difficult, usually requiring considerable expertise.

GEOGRAPHIC DISTRIBUTION

Fleas are found worldwide, following the distribution of the mammalian host. *Xenopsylla cheopis* is associated primarily with brown rats (*Rattus norvegicus*, also known as Norwegian sewer rats) and black rats (*Rattus rattus*, also known as house or roof rats). *Ctenocephalides* spp. are found on cats and dogs.

Lice

Lice are a considerable public health concern, producing diseases that range from relatively benign to life-threatening. As agents of direct injury they cause minor, yet irritating, skin and hair infestations. As arthropod vectors they are capable of transmitting important bacterial pathogens. Although individual species are associated with different parts of the body, some overlap does occur.

PEDICULUS HUMANUS

Relation to Disease. *Pediculus humanus* (the human body louse) parasitizes most parts of the human body other than the head. Body lice are primarily found in the hairier regions, where they migrate back and forth from clothing to skin to take blood meals.[17] Feeding causes irritating, pruritic bite wounds, a general characteristic of infestations with lice. Most eggs, called nits, are laid on clothing.

Body lice transmit *Borrelia recurrentis*, the causative agent of relapsing fever,[3,57] and *Rickettsia prowazekii* and *Bartonella* (*Rochalimaea*) *quintana*,[29] which cause epidemic typhus and trench fever, respectively.[17,56] In relapsing fever, crushed lice release organisms onto the skin that then enter through abrasions. Typhus and trench fever agents, which are present in louse feces, enter when scratched into the skin by the host.[56] The mortality rate in untreated epidemic typhus may be as high as 60%,[56] perhaps because of the presence of other complicating factors, but antimicrobial therapy effectively controls the infection.[38]

Body lice are spread by fairly close contact with infected individuals. Shared clothing, bedding, and close communal habitation are associated with transmission.[17] Not surprisingly, louseborne infections occur under conditions of extreme privation, such as war and famine.

Identification. Body lice reach 2 to 4 mm in length, with a relatively long, slender abdomen. They have three pairs of legs, with clawlike hooks on the ends that aid in securing the louse to its host (Color Plate A-3*F*).

Geographic Distribution. Body lice occur worldwide.

PEDICULUS CAPITIS

Relation to Disease. Head lice produce irritating infections of the head, hair, and neck regions.[44] They infect only humans; pets and other animals are not susceptible. Unlike the body louse, head lice do not serve as vectors for transmission of bacteria, although secondary bacterial infection of the bite wound may occur.[6] The 1-mm-sized nits (eggs) are most often glued to a hair shaft near the scalp (Color Plate A-3*G*).

Infestations are most common in children.[6] They occur through close contact and sharing of fomites such as combs, hats, and scarves.[17]

Identification. Head lice closely resemble body lice. Although size overlap does occur, they may be slightly shorter than body lice, averaging 1 to 3 mm.[17,18,20] The elongated abdomen and the three pairs of legs with hooks are virtually identical to those found on the body louse. Nits are easily confused with dandruff, seborrheic scales, hair spray, or fungal infection (Color Plate A-3*G*).[6] Specimens should be submitted to experts for confirmation.

Geographic Distribution. The head louse is found throughout the world.

PHTHIRUS PUBIS

Relation to Disease. *Phthirus pubis*, also known as the crab or pubic louse, causes an irritating infection of the pubic area. It may be found less frequently in the armpits, chest, thighs, and short facial hairs of mustaches, eyebrows, and eyelashes.[17,18,20] The lice leave a pruritic bite wound on the skin after taking a blood meal. Secondary infection of the bite wound may occur, but is uncommon. Nits are laid on the lower portion of hair shafts as with head lice. Pubic lice do not transmit infectious agents. Transmission occurs primarily through intimate contact.

Identification. Pubic lice are 1 to 2 mm long and have a short, round abdomen. Their shape has been described as ''turtlelike.'' Pubic lice possess three pairs of legs, with claws that appear larger and thicker than those of the body or head louse (Color Plate A-3*H*).

Geographic Distribution. Pubic lice can be found worldwide.

REFERENCES

1. Azad AF, et al. Genetic characterization and transovarial transmission of a typhus-like rickettsia found in cat fleas. Proc Natl Acad Sci USA 1992;89:43–46.
2. Bennett G. Cockroaches as carriers of bacteria. Lancet 1993;341:732–732.
3. Borgnolo G, et al. Louse-borne relapsing fever: a clinical and an epidemiological study of 389 patients in Asella Hospital, Ethiopia. Trop Geogr Med 1993;45:66–69.
4. Brewer TF, et al. Bacon therapy and furuncular myiasis. JAMA 1993;270:2087–2088.
5. Calisher CH. Medically important arboviruses of the United States and Canada. Clin Microbiol Rev 1994;7:89–116.
6. Carson DS. Detection and treatment of pediculosis capitis. IM 1990;11:74–86.
7. Centers for Disease Control and Prevention. Necrotic arachnidism—Pacific northwest, 1988–1996. MMWR Morb Mortal Wkly Rep 1996;45:433–436.
8. Cooley RA. The genus *Dermacentor* and *Otocenter* (*Ixodidae*) in the United States, with studies in variation. National Institutes of Health Bulletin No. 171, United States Government Printing Office, Washington, DC, 1938.
9. Cooley RA, Kohls GM. The genus *Ixodes* in North America. National Institutes of Health Bulletin No. 184, United States Government Printing Office, Washington, DC, 1945.
10. des Vignes F, et al. Effect of tick removal on transmission of *Borrelia burgdorferi* and *Ehrlichia phagocytophila* by *Ixodes scapularis* nymphs. J Infect Dis 2001;183:773–778.
11. Dumler JS, Bakken JS. Ehrlichial diseases of humans: emerging tick-borne infections. Clin Infect Dis 1995;20:1102–1110.
12. Dworkin MS, et al. Tick paralysis: 33 human cases in Washington State, 1946–1996. Clin Infect Dis 1999;29:1435–1439.
13. Falco RC, et al. Duration of tick bites in a Lyme disease-endemic area. Am J Epidemiol 1996;143:187–192.
14. Felz MW, Durden LA. Attachment sites of four tick species (*Acari: Ixodidae*) parasitizing humans in Georgia and South Carolina. J Med Entomol 1999;36:361–364.
15. Felz MW, et al. A six-year-old girl with tick paralysis. N Engl J Med 2000;342:90–94.
16. Fradin MS, Day JF. Comparative efficacy of insect repellents against mosquito bites. N Engl J Med 2002;347:13–18.
17. Fritsche TR. Arthropods of medical importance. In: Murray PR, Baron EJ, Jorgensen JH, et al., eds. Manual of Clinical Microbiology. 8th Ed. Washington, DC: ASM Press, 2003:2061–2078.
18. Garcia LS. Diagnostic Medical Parasitology. 4th Ed. Washington, DC: ASM Press, 2001.
19. Goddard J. Arthropods, tongue worms, leeches, and arthropod-borne diseases. In: Guerrant RL, Walker DH, Weller PF, eds. Tropical Infectious Diseases. Principles, Pathogens, & Practice. Philadelphia: Churchill Livingstone, 1999:1325–1342.
20. Goddard J. Physician's Guide to Arthropods of Medical Importance. 4th Ed. Boca Raton, FL: CRC Press, 2003.
21. Goethert HK, Telford SR III. Enzootic transmission of the agent of human granulocytic ehrlichiosis among cottontail rabbits. Am J Trop Med Hyg 2003;68:633–637.
22. Hallem EA, et al. Olfaction: mosquito receptor for human-sweat odorant. Nature 2004;427:212–213.
23. Higgins JA, et al. *Rickettsia felis*: a new species of pathogenic *Rickettsia* isolated from cat fleas. J Clin Microbiol 1996;34:671–674.
24. James AM, et al. *Borrelia lonestari* infection after a bite by an *Amblyomma americanum* tick. J Infect Dis 2001;183:1810–1814.
25. Kass EM, et al. Rickettsialpox in a New York City hospital, 1980 to 1989. N Engl J Med 1994;331:1612–1617.
26. Katavolos P, et al. Duration of tick attachment required for transmission of granulocytic ehrlichiosis. J Infect Dis 1998;177:1422–1425.
27. Keirans JE, Litwak TR. Pictorial key to the adults of hard ticks, Family *Ixodidae* (*Ixodida:Ixodoidea*), east of the Mississippi river. J Med Entomol 1989;26:435–448.
28. Lane RP, et al. Human cutaneous myiasis: a review and report of three cases due to *Dermatobia hominis*. Clin Exp Dermatol 1987;12:40–45.
29. Logan JS. Trench fever in Belfast, and the nature of the ''relapsing fevers'' in the United Kingdom in the nineteenth century. Ulster Med J 1989;58:83–88.
30. Mann JM, et al. Endemic human plague in New Mexico: risk factors associated with infection. J Infect Dis 1979;140:397–401.
31. Maupin GO, et al. Discovery of an enzootic cycle of *Borrelia burgdorferi* in *Neotoma mexicana* and *Ixodes spinipalpus* from northern Colorado, an area where Lyme disease is nonendemic. J Infect Dis 1994;170:636–643.
32. Mitchell PD, et al. Immunoserologic evidence of coinfection with *Borrelia burgdorferi*, *Babesia microti*, and human granulocytic *Ehrlichia* species in residents of Wisconsin and Minnesota. J Clin Microbiol 1996;34:724–727.
33. Moore CG, Mitchell CJ. Aedes albopictus in the United States: ten-year presence and public health implications. Emerg Infect Dis 1997;3:329–334.
34. Oliver JH Jr, et al. Conspecificity of the ticks *Ixodes scapularis* and *I. dammini* (*Acari: Ixodidae*). J Med Entomol 1993;30:54–63.
35. Orloski KA, et al. Surveillance for Lyme disease—United States, 1992–1998. MMWR CDC Surveill Summ 2000;49:1–11.
36. Parola P, Raoult D. Ticks and tickborne bacterial diseases in humans: an emerging infectious threat. Clin Infect Dis 2001;32:897–928.
37. Patterson FC, Winn WC Jr. Practical identification of hard ticks in the parasitology laboratory. Pathol Case Rev 2003;8:187–198.
38. Perine PL, et al. A clinico-epidemiological study of epidemic typhus in Africa. Clin Infect Dis 1992;14:1149–1158.
39. Persing DH. The cold zone: a curious convergence of tick-transmitted diseases. Clin Infect Dis 1997;25:Suppl 42.
40. Peters W. A Colour Atlas of Arthropods in Clinical Medicine. London: Wolfe,1992.
41. Piesman J, et al. Duration of tick attachment and *Borrelia burgdorferi* transmission. J Clin Microbiol 1987;25:557–558.
42. Ramirez-Ronda CH, Garcia CD. Dengue in the Western Hemisphere. Infect Dis Clin North Am 1994;8:107–128.
43. Ribeiro JM, et al. Dissemination and salivary delivery of Lyme disease spirochetes in vector ticks (*Acari: Ixodidae*). J Med Entomol 1987;24:201–205.
44. Roberts RJ. Head lice. N Engl J Med 2002;346:1645–1650.
45. Rosef O, Kapperud G. House flies (*Musca domestica*) as possible vectors of *Campylobacter fetus* subsp. *jejuni*. Appl Environ Microbiol 1983;45:381–383.
46. Schaumburg HH, Herskovitz S. The weak child: a cautionary tale. N Engl J Med 2000;342:127–129.
47. Schembre DB, et al. *Dermatobia hominis* myiasis masquerading as an infected sebaceous cyst. CJS 1990;33:145–146.
48. Schriefer ME, et al. Identification of a novel rickettsial infection in a patient diagnosed with murine typhus. J Clin Microbiol 1994;32:949–954.
49. Service MW. A Guide to Medical Entomology. London: Macmillan, 1980.
50. Shapiro ED, Gerber MA. Lyme disease. Clin Infect Dis 2000;31:533–542.
51. Sonenshine DE, Azad AF. Ticks and mites in disease transmission. In: Strickland GT, ed. Hunter's Tropical Medicine. 8th Ed. Philadelphia: Saunders, 2000:992–999.
52. Sood SK, et al. Duration of tick attachment as a predictor of the risk of Lyme disease in an area in which Lyme disease is endemic. J Infect Dis 1997;175:996–999.

53. Sorvillo FJ, et al. A suburban focus of endemic typhus in Los Angeles County: association with seropositive domestic cats and opossums. Am J Trop Med Hyg 1993;48:269–273.

54. Spach DH, et al. Tick-borne diseases in the United States. N Engl J Med 1993; 329:936–947.

55. Steere AC. Lyme disease. N Engl J Med 2001;345:115–125.

56. Strickland GT. Hunter's Tropical Medicine and Emerging Diseases. 8th Ed. Philadelphia: Saunders, 2000.

57. Sundnes KO, Haimanot AT. Epidemic of louse-borne relapsing fever in Ethiopia. Lancet 1993;342:1213–1215.

58. Thompson RS, et al. Outbreak of tick-borne relapsing fever in Spokane County, Washington. JAMA 1969;210:1045–1050.

59. Vetter RS, Bush SP. Reports of presumptive brown recluse spider bites reinforce improbable diagnosis in regions of North America where the spider is not endemic. Clin Infect Dis 2002;35:442–445.

60. Walker DH. Ricketts creates rickettsiology, the study of vector-borne obligately intracellular bacteria. J Infect Dis 2004;189:938–955.

61. Walton SF, et al. Crusted scabies: a molecular analysis of *Sarcoptes scabiei* variety *hominis* populations from patients with repeated infestations. Clin Infect Dis 1999;29:1226–1230.

62. Westenfeld F. Cutaneous myiasis caused by *Dermatobia hominis*. Clin Microbiol Newslett 1993;15:3.

63. Williams SG, et al. Typhus and typhuslike rickettsiae associated with opossums and their fleas in Los Angeles County, California. J Clin Microbiol 1992;30: 1758–1762.

64. Wilson BB. Ectoparasites: introduction. In: Mandell GL, Bennett JE, Dolin R, eds. Principles and Practice of Infectious Diseases. 4th Ed. New York: Churchill Livingstone,1995:2258–2258.

65. Yamashita T, et al. Transmission of *Rickettsia tsutsugamushi* strains among humans, wild rodents, and trombiculid mites in an area of Japan in which tsutsugamushi disease is newly endemic. J Clin Microbiol 1994;32:2780–2785.

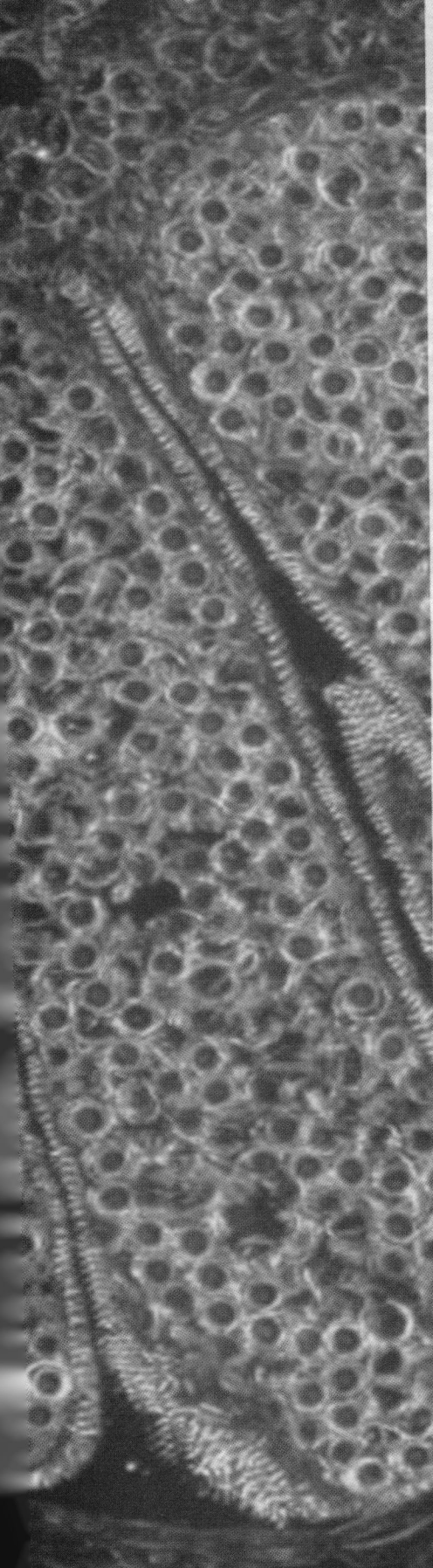

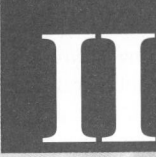

Free-Living Amebae

Ecology, Epidemiology, Pathogenesis, and Disease

Primary Amebic
   Meningoencephalitis
Acanthamoeba Keratitis

Laboratory Investigation

Collection and Transport of
   Specimens

Direct Microscopic Examination
Culture of Free-Living Amebae
Tissue Culture
Morphologic Features

Interpretation of the Significance of Free-Living Amebae Isolated in Culture

Treatment

S mall, free-living water and soil amebae of the genera *Naegleria* and *Acanthamoeba* are capable of producing opportunistic infections in humans. The major diseases produced by this group are forms of devastating, usually fatal meningoencephalitis and *Acanthamoeba* keratitis, an ulcerative, vision-threatening infection involving the cornea of the eye, caused by certain species of *Acanthamoeba* but not *Naegleria*.[28] The free-living amebae are not related to the intestinal amebae discussed previously and do not inhabit the intestines of humans or other mammals.

Ecology, Epidemiology, Pathogenesis, and Disease

Naegleria and *Acanthamoeba*, along with many other genera of free-living amebae, have a worldwide distribution in various freshwater habitats, including rivers, lakes, ponds, hot springs and spas, domestic water systems, air-conditioning systems, humidifiers, and cooling towers.[18,19] They are believed to play a role in a hypersensitivity pneumonitis known as humidifier fever.[39] They are ubiquitous in soils, dust, air, and composts; have been found on the surfaces of vegetables; and have been isolated from sewage sludge and fresh water polluted by domestic or industrial waste. *Acanthamoeba* species have been isolated from sea water, especially associated with discharges of inadequately treated sewage from hotels and municipal sewage effluents (D. A. Munson: personal communication, 1991).[19] *Naegleria* and *Acanthamoeba* have also been found associated with thermally polluted discharges in ponds and lakes connected with electric power plants, nuclear power plants, or thermal polluting factories.[18,19]

In nature, free-living amebae feed on bacteria, including *Legionella* species,[3,35,39,42] and the amebae form cysts that tend to be more resistant to adverse environmental conditions (such as drying in soil) than the vegetative ameboid forms. De Jonckheere and Van de Voorde reported that the cysts of some strains of *Acanthamoeba* are highly resistant to chlorine and not killed by the usual concentrations of chlorine maintained in municipal or domestic water supplies or in chlorinated swimming pools.[20] On the other hand the cysts of *Naegleria fowleri* were more sensitive to chlorine; these authors concluded that viable *N. fowleri* are not likely to be found in clean water where low concentrations of chlorine (e.g., 0.5 μg free available chlorine per milliliter) are maintained.[20] Rowbotham was the first to point out that *L. pneumophila* can grow within *Acanthamoeba* species, thus providing an explanation of how nutritionally fastidious legionellae can maintain viability in pristine, low-nutrient waters.[39] *Legionella* species also proliferate within various other free-living amebae.[42] It has been speculated that legionellae could be aerosolized through the air to humans in droplets of water while residing within amebae.[39] This makes sense, especially if amebic cysts could protect legionellae from chlorine in domestic water supplies (see Chapter 10).

In addition, free-living amebae, including *Naegleria fowleri*, *Hartmanella* species, and various *Acanthamoeba* species, have been isolated from the throats and nasal passages of humans[1,6,26,38,42,43]—probably as cysts that were inhaled with dust in the air, in aerosols, or were present in ingested food or water.[16] Trophozoites of *Naegleria* or *Acanthamoeba* have not been demonstrated in the human nasopharynx in absence of CNS disease.[16]

Primary Amebic Meningoencephalitis

Prior to 1958, none of the free-living water and soil amebae were recognized as pathogenic. Then Culbertson and associates observed an ameba contaminant in tissue culture cells.[17] This strain, now called *Acanthamoeba culbertsoni* strain A-1, when instilled intranasally into young mice or various other animals, produced infection within the nasal mucosa and submucosa that spread from there along the olfactory nerve through the cribriform plate of the skull to produce invasion of the brain and a rapidly fatal meningoencephalitis.[12,13,17] Based on his experimental work with animals, Culbertson predicted that similar disease could occur in humans.[12,15,17] In 1965, the first human case was reported in a child from Australia by Fowler and Carter.[22] The following year, three additional cases were reported by Butt from Florida, who called the disease "primary amebic meningoencephalitis."[9] Thus, conceptually, primary amebic meningoencephalitis differed from amebic disease of the CNS involving *Entamoeba histolytica* because primary amebic meningoencephalitis was *not* "secondary" to amebic disease of the colon.

It is now known that the portal of entry for *Naegleria* is the nose and the true "primary" site of the infection is the upper respiratory tract.[10,13,16] Most patients with *Naegleria* CNS infections have been children or young adults who were swimming in lakes or rivers or otherwise had an opportunity for water (containing *Naegleria*) to enter the nose.[3,4,29,31] After infecting the nasal mucosa, *N. fowleri* then spread along the olfactory nerve, through the cribriform plate into the brain via the route originally observed in animals by Culbertson and colleagues.[12,17] Pathologic findings in humans with acute meningoencephalitis caused by *N. fowleri* have been remarkably similar to those seen originally in the experimental animal models by Culberston and associates

with *Acanthamoeba culbertsoni* strain A-1 (the most virulent of the *Acanthamoeba* species).[9,10,13–16,23,28,30] Other *Acanthamoeba* species are not so virulent and tend to produce subacute or chronic brain abscesses, with or without granulomas.

In humans, CNS disease associated with *Acanthamoeba* species have not been as common as that produced by *N. fowleri*. More than 140 cases of primary amebic meningoencephalitis have been estimated to have occurred worldwide, whereas only 40 or more cases of *Acanthamoeba* CNS infections have been reported.[28] Most patients with *Acanthamoeba* CNS disease have been immunocompromised and have not had a history of exposure to water.[16,28,30,31] However, since *Acanthamoeba* cysts may be present in soil or dust, it is possible that the organisms could have been inhaled into the nasal cavity or even the lower respiratory tract.[16] It is conceivable that in humans *Acanthamoeba* species might spread either from the nasal cavity to the brain by way of the olfactory nerve or intravascularly from the lungs or possibly from skin lesions (reported rarely) to the brain.[16,31]

N. fowleri produces a diffuse and fulminant meningoencephalitis characterized by large areas of hemorrhagic necrosis, especially involving the olfactory bulbs, frontal lobes, base of the brain, proximal spinal cord, and/or temporal lobes of the brain. The parietal lobes and occipital cortex may also be involved. Acute purulent exudate is found in the leptomeninges and within the cortex. Amebic trophozoites are scattered or may be seen focally in clusters within necrotic cortex. They especially show a predilection for blood vessels; small arteries, arterioles, veins, venules, and capillaries may be surrounded by 10- to 15-μm *Naegleria* trophozoites containing large prominent nucleoli.[13,15,31]

Within the brain, *Acanthamoeba* species produce acute inflammation in early stages of the disease in animals. However, species less virulent than *A. culbertsoni* strain A-1 tend to produce focal or multifocal chronic abscesses, with or without granulomas (including presence of foreign body giant cells). Trophozoites and cysts may be focal or scattered in small numbers throughout involved areas but may be located in perivascular spaces and can be seen within the walls of small vessels in association with perivascular hemorrhage and intravascular thrombosis. Amebic cysts are seen within tissue in *Acanthamoeba* infections but have not been observed in tissues infected with *Naegleria*.[13,15,31]

Acanthamoeba Keratitis

Acanthamoeba keratitis is a serious, often devastating infection of the cornea involving certain species of *Acanthamoeba* (e.g., *A. polyphaga*, *A. castellanii*, *A. rhysodes*, *A. culbertsoni*, and *A. hatchetti*).[5,28,33] Since the first case was described in 1975,[24] more than 200 cases have been reported worldwide.[28] Until about 1984, the majority of infections were associated with trauma to the cornea and exposure to contaminated water; more recently, many cases have been associated with the use of contact lenses, especially daily-wear or extended-wear soft contact lenses.[5,11,33,41] Other factors involved in *Acanthamoeba* keratitis include trauma to the cornea and the use of contaminated homemade saline or tap water rinses to clean lenses, the failure to disinfect lenses properly or as often as recommended by manufacturers, and wearing lenses while swimming.[8,28,41] Acanthamoebae may be present in contact lens cases and contact lens wash solutions, and they are capable of adhering to contact lens surfaces.[8,27,33,41,44] *Acanthamoeba* keratitis presents as an ophthalmologic emergency. It occurs commonly in children, mostly in persons 12 years of age and older, but also is common in young adults and less common in older persons.[41] The infection progresses relentlessly with corneal ulceration and may result in blindness. It is difficult to diagnose and treat. The disease has often been misdiagnosed as herpes simplex keratitis, fungal keratitis, or bacterial (or mycobacterial) infection, sometimes resulting in delays of weeks or months before a diagnosis has been made and proper treatment is begun. Detailed clinical findings have been published elsewhere in several excellent reviews.[27,33,37,41,44]

Laboratory Investigation

Collection and Transport of Specimens

When amebic disease is suspected, fresh cerebrospinal fluid or tissue (e.g., corneal biopsy, corneal scrapings, CNS tissue) should be collected aseptically and examined immediately. Specimens intended for culture must never be frozen or refrigerated and should be maintained at 20°C to 30°C during transport to the laboratory or prior to processing within the laboratory.[3,14] If immediate examination is not possible or not practical, amebae have survived in sterile fluid or otherwise sterile tissue for several days at room temperature prior to processing in the laboratory. If a transport medium is needed for transport of tissue biopsy samples or corneal scrapings, the minimal essential medium used in virology laboratories is preferred (see Chapter 23) over Page's ameba saline (D. Place, F. Curtis, E. Powell, and A. Newsome: personal communication, 1991).

Direct Microscopic Examination

Small drops of cerebrospinal fluid, other body fluids, or tissue suspensions should be examined in wet mounts (on slides under coverslips) by light microscopy under reduced light, or by phase microscopy for motile trophozoites (using a 40× objective). Keeping the microscope stage warmed to 30°C to 37°C may enhance motility, especially of *Acanthamoeba* species.[14] *Naegleria* may be actively motile at 22°C to 25°C, but the motility of *Acanthamoeba* species at room temperature is very sluggish. These amebae tend to be more actively motile than leukocytes, and the nuclei and nucleoli of *Naegleria* and *Acanthamoeba* species differ from those of granulocytes or macrophages.

Material to be stained on slides should first be fixed in 10% neutral buffered formalin. After the slide is air-dried it can then be stained with trichrome, the Papanicolaou stain, or hematoxylin and eosin.[3,14] Tissue sections should be stained with hematoxylin and eosin. Other stains preferred for direct examination preparations by some include lactophenol cotton blue, Giemsa's, acridine orange, and calcofluor white.[28] Certain reference and research laboratories, such as those of the CDC and of the Department of Pathology

at the Indiana University Medical Center have developed specific indirect fluorescent antibody procedures or indirect immune coagglutination procedures that provide rapid direct immunologic identification of amebae in specimens.[3,28]

Culture of Free-Living Amebae

Culbertson's method for culturing amebae with *Escherichia coli* on salt-free, water agar,[14] a slight modification of Singh's original procedure, has proven to be useful for culturing body fluids, suspensions of eye tissue, and other specimens. Agar plates are prepared with 20 to 25 mL of 1.5% agar in distilled water (without nutrients and no salt added). A loopful or one drop of a heavy suspension of *E. coli*, from a 24- to 48-hour blood agar plate culture, is spread in the center of the plate in an area 1 cm in diameter.

Alternatively, the *E. coli* can be spread as an X-streak (with 2 streaks of *E. coli* suspension that intersect in the middle of the plate) (C. G. Culbertson: personal communication, 1989). The inoculum (a drop of cell suspension, sediment, or tissue fragments) is placed on top of the center of the bacterial spot and the plate is sealed with tape. Duplicate plates are incubated at 30°C and 37°C, or a single plate is incubated at 34°C to 35°C. After 18 to 24 hours of incubation, the plate is kept sealed and examined agar side up with a 10× objective. Alternatively, an inverted microscope can be used. If no amebae are seen, the plate is reincubated and examined daily for 10 days. The amebae may be in clusters of cells or will appear as small refractile bodies that migrate from the inoculum, often leaving irregular trails or tortuous tracks behind them where they have moved through the bacteria.[14] Individual amebae can be transferred from the agar to a slide to view as a wet mount or stained preparation. Subculture can be made by cutting out a plug of agar at the "front" containing amebae (using a sterile scalpel) from outside the zone of bacteria, where the amebae are more likely to be free of bacteria, and then transferring the amebae to another water agar plate containing *E. coli* (the addition of amphotericin B in final concentration of 2.5 mg/mL in the agar aids in minimizing fungal contaminants) (E. Powell: personal communication, 1991). From there, the amebae are transferred to a broth medium (e.g., trypticase-soy broth) containing antibiotics (e.g., penicillin 1,000 μ/mL and streptomycin 0.1 mg/ml final concentration).

After the amebae are free of bacteria (axenic), they can be transferred to trypticase-soy broth without antibiotics to be used as a growth medium.[3,14] *Naegleria* will not grow in trypticase-soy broth unless it contains 10% sterile fetal calf serum. The growth of amebae in trypticase-soy broth is optimized by using plastic tissue culture tubes so that the amebae will attach to the tubes.[3,14] The cultures are incubated at 35°C almost horizontally at a 15° to 20° angle, analogous to what is often done with cell cultures in virology laboratories. Not all amebae grow in trypticase-soy broth. Alternative media include Plate Count Broth (Difco Laboratories, Detroit, MI) and broth media recommended in the American Type Culture Collection Catalogue (www.atcc.org) including *Acanthamoeba* medium, PYNFH medium, and Fresh Water Amoeba medium (E. Powell: personal communication, 1991). Neroad and co-workers[34] have also described a chemically defined medium for cultivating pathogenic and high temperature tolerant species of *Naegleria*.

Tissue Culture

The more virulent free-living amebae (e.g., *A. culbertsoni* strain A-1) grow in mammalian cell cultures including monkey kidney, McCoy cells, and others, and may produce cytopathogenic effects (CPE) resembling those seen with viruses.[17,43] Less virulent amebae may grow poorly in tissue (cell) culture without producing CPE. Amebae can be extremely difficult to see when growing with tissue culture cells; fluid should be removed from a tissue culture tube or flask, centrifuged at 500–800 g (×5 min), or can be prepared using a Cytospin™, then the sediment is used to prepare a wet mount that is examined by phase or light microscopy using low illumination. Alternatively the slide preparation can be dried, fixed in formalin, and stained with H&E to aid in observing amebic features.[3] Once isolated in tissue culture, isolates can be transferred to a broth medium and/or to water agar with *E. coli* (as described in the preceding section).

Morphologic Features

When rounded up, the trophozoites of *Naegleria* are 8 to 15 μm and usually smaller than those of *Acanthamoeba* species, which are usually 10 to 25 μm in diameter.[2,4] The nuclei of both genera are similar and contain large, prominent nucleoli. *Naegleria* have one or more smooth, lobate pseudopodia and are actively motile at room temperature or 35°C to 37°C. *Acanthamoeba* species are very sluggish at 22°C to 25°C but may become more actively motile at 35°C and 37°C. Acanthamoebae have numerous, spiny pseudopodia on their surface called acanthopodia. *Naegleria* species are characterized by a temporary ameboflagellate stage; when *Naegleria* trophozoites are put in distilled water, they may develop pear-shaped, actively motile forms containing two or more flagella (within 1 to 3 hours). The cysts of acanthamoebae are more thick-walled than those of *Naegleria* and have distinctive appearances that aid in identification of the species level.[36] In addition, *Naegleria* species produce a distinctive form of mitosis (promitosis) in which the nuclear membrane remains intact.[36] In contrast, acanthamoebae produce a more classic type of mitosis (metamitosis) in which the nucleolus and nuclear membrane disappear and the mitotic spindle appears with the chromosomes in metaphase.[14,36,59,194] For more detailed descriptive information, readers are referred to references[3,14,16,25,28,36].

Identification of *Naegleria* and *Acanthamoeba* beyond the genus level requires not only a detailed morphologic study but also the use of other procedures, including tests with species-specific immunologic reagents (e.g., immunofluorescent antibody tests, coagglutination tests) and tests for pathogenicity (in mice). Identification of *Naegleria* or *Acanthamoeba* to species level may be useful in an epidemiologic investigation or research projects, but its practical value for the clinical laboratory to assist clinicians in the management of patients has not been demonstrated. Looking to the future, Flores and associates have described the use of specific monoclonal antibodies and applications of flow cytometry as an aid in the separation of *Naegleria fowleri* and *Acanthamoeba* species; experimental nucleic acid probes are also available to make this separation (see Chapter 1).[21]

Interpretation of the Significance of Free-Living Amebae Isolated in Culture

Because free-living amebae are ubiquitous in water, soil, dust, and the air, it is possible that cysts, carried about in the air, could contaminate the surface of a corneal scraping, tissue biopsy, or fluid specimen during the time of specimen collection, processing, inspection of primary plates for growth, or following prolonged incubation. Amebae could also be on the skin, lid margin, or in the conjunctival sac of an eye without causing keratitis, although this has not been demonstrated. Thus, as emphasized by Allen and Culbertson, personnel should not accept positive cultures of amebae, by themselves, as being clinically significant with respect to causing disease, unless trophozoites can be demonstrated on direct microscopic examination of the specimen or can be seen microscopically within the tissue by histopathologic examination.[3]

Treatment

At least two patients with *Naegleria* meningoencephalitis have survived. Each received amphotericin B. One of the patients, in addition to receiving amphotericin B, also received miconazole, rifampin, and sulfasoxazole.[3,7,37,40] The treatment of choice for *Acanthamoeba* CNS disease has not been established, since most cases have been diagnosed at autopsy. However, Culbertson and associates found that sulfadiazine was highly active against some strains of *Acanthamoeba* in animal models *in vivo*.[3,16] The treatment of *Acanthamoeba* keratitis has been successful in several patients using an intensive treatment protocol involving topical propamidine isethionate (Brolene drops) and neomycin sulfate–polymyxin B sulfate–gramicidin drops (Neosporin Ophthalmic Solution).[32,33,37,45]

REFERENCES

1. Abraham SN, Lawande RV. Incidence of free-living amoebae in the nasal passages of local population of Zaria, Nigeria. J Trop Med Hyg 1982:85:217–222.
2. Adams EB, MacLaud IN. Invasive amebiasis: II. Amebic liver abscess and its complications. Medicine 1977:56:325–334.
3. Allen SD, Culbertson CG. *Naegleria* and *Acanthamoeba*. In: Feigin R, Cherry J (eds.). *Textbook of Pediatric Infectious Diseases*, 3rd Ed. Philadelphia: WB Saunders, 1992.
4. Arrowood MJ, Sterling CR. Comparison of conventional staining methods and monoclonal antibody-based methods for *Cryptosporidium* oocyst detection. J Clin Microbiol 1989:27:1490–1495.
5. Auran JD, Starr MB, Jakobiec FA. *Acanthamoeba* keratitis: A review of the literature. Cornea 1987:6:2–26.

6. Badenoch PR, Grimmond TR, Cadwgan J, et al. Nasal carriage of free-living amoebae. Microb Ecol Health Dis 1988:1:209–211.
7. Blackett K. Amoebic pericarditis. Int J Cardiol 1988:21:183–187.
8. Brandt FH, Ware DA, Visvesvara GS. Viability of *Acanthamoeba* cysts in ophthalmic solutions. Appl Environ Microbiol 1989:55:1144–1146.
9. Butt CG. Primary amebic meningoencephalitis. N Engl J Med 1966:274:1473–1476.
10. Carter RF. Description of a *Naegleria* sp. isolated from two cases of primary amoebic meningoencephalitis, and of the experimental pathological changes induced by it. J Pathol 1970:100:217–244.
11. Centers for Disease Control: *Acanthamoeba* keratitis associated with contact lenses—United States. MMWR 1986:35:405–408.
12. Culbertson CG. Pathogenic *Acanthamoeba* (*Hartmanella*). Am J Clin Pathol 1961:35:195–202.
13. Culbertson CG. The pathogenicity of soil amebas. Ann Rev Microbiol 1971:25:231–254.
14. Culbertson CG. Soil amoeba infection. In: Lennette EH, Spaulding EH, Truant JP (eds.). *Manual of Clinical Microbiology.* 2nd Ed. Washington, DC: American Society for Microbiology, 1974.
15. Culbertson CG. Amebic meningoencephalitides. In: Binford CH, Connoe DH (eds.). *Pathology of Tropical and Extraordinary Diseases, An Atlas,* Vol. 1. Washington, DC: Armed Forces Institute of Pathology, 1976.
16. Culbertson CG. Amebic meningoencephalitis. Antibiot Chemother 1981:30:28–53.
17. Culbertson CG, Smith JW, Minner JR. *Acanthamoeba*: Observations on animal pathogenicity. Science 1958:127:1506.
18. Dejonckheere JF. Epidemiology. In: Rondanelli EG (ed.). *Amphizoic Amoebae Human Pathology.* Padua, Italy: Piccin Nuova Libraria, 1987.
19. De Jonckheere JF. Ecology of *Acanthamoeba.* Rev Infect Dis 1991:13(suppl 5):S385–S387.
20. De Jonckheere JF, Van De Vorde H. Differences in destruction of cysts of pathogenic and nonpathogenic *Naegleria* and *Acanthamoeba* by chlorine. Appl Environ Microbiol 1976:31:294–297.
21. Flores BM, Garcia CA, Stamm WE, Torian BE. Differentiation of *Naegleria fowleri* from *Acanthamoeba* species by using monoclonal antibodies and flow cytometry. J Clin Microbiol 1990:28:1999–2005.
22. Fowler M, Carter RF. Acute pyogenic meningitis probably due to *Acanthamoeba* sp.: A preliminary report. Br Med J 1965:2:740–742.
23. John DT: Primary amoebic meningoencephalitis and the biology of *Naegleria fowleri.* Ann Rev Microbiol 1982:36:101–123.
24. Jones DB, Visvesvara GS, Robinson NM. *Acanthamoeba polyphaga* keratitis and *Acanthamoeba* uveitis associated with fatal meningoencephalitis. Trans Ophthalmol Soc UK 1975:95:221–232.
25. Kilvington S, Larkin DFP, White DG, Beeching JR. Laboratory investigation of *Acanthamoeba* keratitis. J Clin Microbiol 1990:28:2722–2725.
26. Lawande RV, Abraham SN, John I, Egler LJ. Recovery of soil amebas from the nasal passages of children during the dusty harmattan period in Zaria. Am J Clin Pathol 1979:71:201–203.
27. Lindquist TD, Sher NA, Doughman DJ. Clinical signs and medical therapy of early *Acanthamoeba* keratitis. Arch Ophthalmol 1988:106:73–77.
28. Ma P, Visvesvara GS, Martinez AJ, et al. *Naegleria* and *Acanthamoeba* infection: Review. Rev Infect Dis 1990:12:490–513.
29. Marciano-Cabral F. Biology of *Naegleria* spp. Microbiol Rev 1988:52:114–133.
30. Martinez AJ. Is *Acanthamoeba* encephalitis an opportunistic infection? Neurology 1980:30:567–574.
31. Martinez AJ. *Free-Living Amebas: Natural History, Prevention, Diagnosis, Pathology, and Treatment of Disease.* Boca Raton, FL: CRC Press, 1985.
32. Moore MB. Parasitic infections. In: Kaufman HE, Barron BA, McDonald MB, et al. (eds.). *The Cornea.* New York: Churchill Livingstone, 1988.
33. Moore MB, McCulley JP. *Acanthamoeba* keratitis associated with contact lenses: Six consecutive cases of successful management. Br J Ophthalmol 1989:73:271–275.
34. Neroad TA, Visvesvara GS, Daggett PM. Chemically defined media for the cultivation of *Naegleria*: Pathogenic and high temperature tolerant species. J Protozool 1983:30:383–387.
35. Newsome AL, Baker RL, Miller RD, et al. Interactions between *Naegleria fowleri* and *Legionella pneumophila.* Infect Immun 1985:50:449–452.
36. Page FC. A *New Key to Freshwater and Soil Gymnamoebae.* Ambleside, Cumbria: Freshwater Biological Association, The Ferry House, 1988.
37. Petri WA Jr, Rardin JI. Free-living amebae. In: Mandell GL, Douglas RG Jr, Bennett JE (eds.). *Principles and Practices of Infectious Diseases.* New York: Churchill Livingstone, 1990.
38. Rivera F, Rosas I, Castillo M, et al. Pathogenic and free-living protozoa cultured from the nasopharyngeal and oral regions of dental patients: II. Environmental Research 1986:39:364–371.
39. Rowbotham TJ. Preliminary report on the pathogenicity of *Legionella pneumophila* for freshwater and soil amoebae. J Clin Pathol 1980:33:1179–1183.
40. Seidel JS, Harmatz P, Visvesvara GS, et al. Successful treatment of primary amebic meningoencephalitis. N Engl J Med 1982:306:346–348.
41. Stehr-Green JK, Bailey TM, Visvesvara GS. The epidemiology of *Acanthamoeba* keratitis in the United States. Am J Ophthalmol 1989:107:221–336.
42. Wadowsky RM, Butler LJ, Cook MK, et al. Growth-supporting activity for *Legionella pneumophila* in tap water cultures and implication of Hartmannellid amoebae as growth factors. Appl Environ Microbiol 1988:54:2677–2682.
43. Wang SS, Feldman HA. Isolation of *Hartmannella* species from human throats. N Engl J Med 1967:277:1174–1179.
44. Wilhelmus KR, Jones DB (eds.). International symposium on *Acanthamoeba* and the eye. Rev Infect Dis 1991:13(suppl 5):S450.
45. Wright P, Warhurst D, Jones BR: *Acanthamoeba* keratitis successfully treated medically. Br J Ophthalmol 1985:69:778–782.

Charts

CHART 1-1

CATALASE

I. Principle
Catalase is an enzyme that decomposes hydrogen peroxide (H_2O_2) into water and oxygen. Chemically, catalase is a hemoprotein, similar in structure to hemoglobin, except that the four iron atoms in the molecule are in the oxidized (Fe^{3+}), rather than the reduced (Fe^{2+}), state. Excluding the streptococci, most aerobic and facultative bacteria possess catalase activity.

Hydrogen peroxide forms as one of the oxidative end products of aerobic carbohydrate metabolism. If allowed to accumulate, it is lethal to bacterial cells. Catalase converts hydrogen peroxide into oxygen and water as shown by the following reaction:

$$2H_2O_2 \rightarrow 2H_2O + O_2 \text{ (gas bubbles)}$$

The catalase test is most commonly used to differentiate members of the *Micrococcaceae* from members of the *Streptococcaceae*.

II. Reagents
   A. Hydrogen peroxide 3% stored in a brown bottle under refrigeration
   B. An 18- to 24-hour culture of the organism to be tested

III. Quality Control
The hydrogen peroxide reagent must be tested with positive and negative control organisms each day or immediately before unknown bacteria are tested.
   A. Positive control: *Staphylococcus aureus*
   B. Negative control: *Streptococcus* species

IV. Procedure
   1. With an inoculating needle or a wooden applicator stick, transfer growth from the center of a colony to the surface of a glass slide.
   2. Add one drop of 3% hydrogen peroxide and observe for bubble formation.

V. Results
   A. Interpretation
   The rapid and sustained appearance of bubbles or effervescence constitutes a positive test. Because some bacteria possess enzymes other than catalase that can decompose hydrogen peroxide, a few tiny bubbles forming after 20 to 30 seconds is not considered a positive test. In addition, catalase is present in red cells, so care must be taken to avoid carryover of red cells with the colony material.

CHART 1-2

BILE-SOLUBILITY TEST

I. Principle
Bile salts, specifically sodium deoxycholate and sodium taurocholate, have the capability to lyse *Streptococcus pneumoniae* selectively when added to actively growing bacteria in agar or broth media. *S. pneumoniae* produces autolytic enzymes (autolysins) that account for the central depression or umbilication characteristic of older pneumococcal colonies on agar media. The addition of bile salts activates the autolysins and accelerates the natural lytic reaction observed with cultures or pneumococci.

The bile-solubility test can be performed either with a broth culture of the organism or with colonies growing on agar media. The turbidity of a broth suspension visibly clears on addition of bile salts if the organism is soluble. On agar medium, bile-soluble colonies "disappear" when drops of the reagent are placed on them. Because sodium deoxycholate may precipitate at a pH of 6.5 or less, the broth culture medium used must be adjusted to pH 7.0 to prevent false-negative reactions.

II. Media and Reagents
   1. A pure culture of the test organism grown at 35°C for 18 to 24 hours in Todd-Hewitt broth (or equivalent)
   2. Sheep blood agar plate
   3. Sodium deoxycholate (10% for tube test, 2% for plate test)
   4. Phenol red solution (1% aqueous)
   5. Sodium hydroxide (NaOH) solution, 0.10 N

III. Quality Control
   A. Positive (bile-soluble) control: *Streptococcus pneumoniae*
   B. Negative (bile-insoluble) control: Viridans streptococcus

CHART 1-2

BILE-SOLUBILITY TEST *continued*

IV. Procedure
    A. *Broth Test*
      1. Transfer approximately 0.5 mL of an 18- to 24-hour broth culture to two clean test tubes. Alternatively, a suspension of the organism may be prepared from growth on agar media in phosphate-buffered saline, pH 7.0. If the latter is done, the pH need not be readjusted.
      2. Add one drop of the phenol red indicator to each tube.
      3. Add 0.10 N NaOH to adjust the pH to 7.0 (indicator a light pink color).
      4. Add 0.5 mL of 10% sodium deoxycholate to one of the tubes (labeled ''test'').
      5. Add 0.5 mL sterile normal saline to the other tube (labeled ''control'').
      6. Gently agitate both test tubes and place them in an incubator or a water bath at 35°C for 3 hours, checking hourly.
    B. *Plate Test*
      1. To a few well-isolated colonies on the test organism growing on sheep blood agar, place a drop of 2% sodium deoxycholate.
      2. Without inverting the plate, place it in a 35°C incubator for 30 minutes.
V. Results
    A. Interpretation
      1. Broth Test
        Bile-soluble (positive reaction): there is visible clearing of the suspension in the tube containing the sodium deoxycholate, with no change in the saline control suspension.
        Bile-insoluble (negative reaction): there is no change in the turbidity of the sodium deoxycholate–containing tube relative to the control saline suspension.
      2. Plate Test
        Bile-soluble (positive reaction): colonies on which the reagent was placed disappear, leaving a partially hemolyzed area where the colony had been.
        Bile-insoluble (negative reaction): colonies where the reagent was placed remain intact and visible.
VI. Limitations of Test
    Only 86% of pneumococcal strains will lyse completely, and additional testing (e.g., Quellung tests) may be required for the remaining, incompletely lysed strains.

CHART 1-3

THE SLIDE COAGULASE TEST

  I. Principle
    Staphylococcal coagulase is a protein of unknown chemical composition that has a prothrombin-like activity, which can convert fibrinogen into fibrin. A visible clot will result. Coagulase is believed to function in vivo by producing a fibrin barrier at the site of staphylococcal infection. This enzyme probably plays a role in localizing the abscesses (e.g., carbuncles and furuncles). In the laboratory, the coagulase test is used to identify *Staphylococcus aureus* and differentiate it from most other species of staphylococci.
    Coagulase is present in two forms, bound and free, each having different properties that require the use of separate testing procedures.
    Bound coagulase (slide test): Bound coagulase, also known as clumping factor, is attached to the bacterial cell wall and is not present in culture filtrates. Fibrin strands are formed between the bacterial cells when suspended in plasma (fibrinogen), causing them to clump into visible aggregates.
    Free coagulase (tube test): Free coagulase is a thrombin-like substance present in culture filtrates. When a suspension of coagulase-producing organisms is prepared in plasma in a test tube, a visible clot forms as the result of coagulase reacting with a serum substance (coagulase-reacting factor) to form a complex that, in turn, reacts with fibrinogen to produce the fibrin clot.
 II. Media and Reagents
    Rabbit plasma with EDTA (commercially available in lyophilized form). Reconstituted plasma should be refrigerated.
III. Quality Control
    Coagulability of plasma may be tested by adding one drop of 5% calcium chloride to 0.5 mL of the reconstituted plasma. A clot should form within 10 to 15 seconds. A known *Staphylococcus aureus* strain and a *Staphylococcus*

CHART 1-3

THE SLIDE COAGULASE TEST *continued*

epidermidis strain serve as positive and negative controls, respectively. Each reconstituted vial of rabbit plasma with EDTA should be tested with 18- to 24-hour cultures of the control strains.

IV. Procedure
1. *Slide test* (bound coagulase): Place two drops of sterile water or saline in two circles drawn on a glass slide with a wax pencil. Gently emulsify colony material from the organism to be identified in liquid in each of the circles. Place a drop of coagulase plasma in the suspension in one of the circles and mix with a wooden applicator stick. Place another drop of water or saline in the other circle as a control. Rock the slide back and forth, observing for agglutination of the test suspension.
2. *Tube test* (free coagulase): Emulsify a small amount of the colony growth of the organism in a tube containing 0.5 mL of coagulase plasma. Incubate the tube at 35°C for 4 hours and observe for clot formation by gently tilting the tube. If no clot is observed at that time, reincubate the tube at room temperature and read again after 18 hours.
V. Results
A. Interpretation
1. *Slide test:* A positive reaction will be detected within 10 to 15 seconds of mixing the plasma with the suspension by the formation of a white precipitate and agglutination of the organisms in the suspension. The test is considered negative if no agglutination is observed after 2 minutes. The saline control should remain smooth and milky. If the control suspension agglutinates as well, the test is uninterpretable. All strains that are coagulase-positive can be reported as coagulase-positive *Staphylococcus* or, less precisely, *Staphylococcus aureus*. All strains producing negative slide tests must be tested with the tube coagulase test.
2. *Tube test:* The tube coagulase test is considered positive if any degree of clotting is noted. The tube should be gently tilted and not agitated, because this may disrupt partially formed clotted material. Fibrinolysins produced by the organism may also dissolve the clot soon after formation. Tube tests that are negative after 4 hours should be incubated at room temperature overnight and read after 18 hours.

CHART 1-4

INDOLE TEST

I. Principle
Indole, a benzyl pyrrole, is one of the metabolic degradation products of the amino acid tryptophan. Bacteria that possess the enzyme tryptophanase are capable of hydrolyzing and deaminating tryptophan with the production of indole, pyruvic acid, and ammonia. Indole production is an important characteristic in the identification of many species of microorganisms, being particularly useful in separating *Escherichia coli* (positive) from members of the *Klebsiella-Enterobacter-Hafnia-Serratia* group (mostly negative).

The indole test is based on the formation of a red complex when indole reacts with the aldehyde group of *p*-dimethylaminobenzaldehyde. This is the active chemical in Kovac and Ehrlich reagents. A medium rich in tryptophan must be used. In practice, combination media such as sulfide indole motility (SIM), motility indole ornithine (MIO), or indole nitrate are used. Rapid spot tests, using filter paper strips impregnated with *p*-dimethylaminocinnamaldehyde reagent, are useful in screening for bacteria that are prompt indole producers.

II. Media and Reagents
A. Tryptophan broth (1% tryptophan)

Peptone or pancreatic digest of casein (trypticase)	2 g
Sodium chloride	0.5 g
Distilled water	100 mL

B. Kovac reagent

Pure amyl or isoamyl alcohol	150 mL
p-Dimethylaminobenzaldehyde	10 g
Concentrated HCl	50 mL

CHART 1-4

INDOLE TEST *continued*

C. Ehrlich's reagent
    p-Dimethylaminobenzaldehyde   2 g
    Absolute ethyl alcohol   190 mL
    Concentrated HCl   40 mL

III. Quality Control
Each new batch of medium or reagent should be tested for positive and negative indole reactions. The following organisms serve well as controls:
   A. Positive control: *Escherichia coli*
   B. Negative control: *Klebsiella pneumoniae*

IV. Procedure
Inoculate tryptophan broth (or other suitable indole media) with the test organism and incubate at 35°C for 18 to 24 hours. At the end of this time, add 15 drops of reagent down the inner wall of the tube. If Ehrlich reagent is used, this step should be preceded by the addition of 1 mL xylene. This is not necessary with Kovac reagent.

V. Results
   A. Interpretation
      The development of a bright fuchsia red color at the interface of the reagent and the broth (or the xylene layer) within seconds after adding the reagent is indicative of the presence of indole and is a positive test (see Color Plates 6-4*C* and 7-2*C*).

VI. Bibliography
Blazevic DJ, Ederer GM. Principles of Biochemical Tests in Diagnostic Microbiology. New York: Wiley, 1975: 63–67.

Isenberg HD, Sundheim LH. Indole reactions in bacteria. J Bacteriol 1958;75:682–690.

MacFaddin JF. Biochemical Tests for Identification of Medical Bacteria. Ed. 2. Baltimore: Williams & Wilkins, 1980:173–183.

Miller JM, Wright JW. Spot indole test: evaluation of four reagents. J Clin Microbiol 1982;15:589–592.

Vracko R, Sherris JC. Indole-spot test in bacteriology. Am J Clin Pathol 1963;39:429–432.

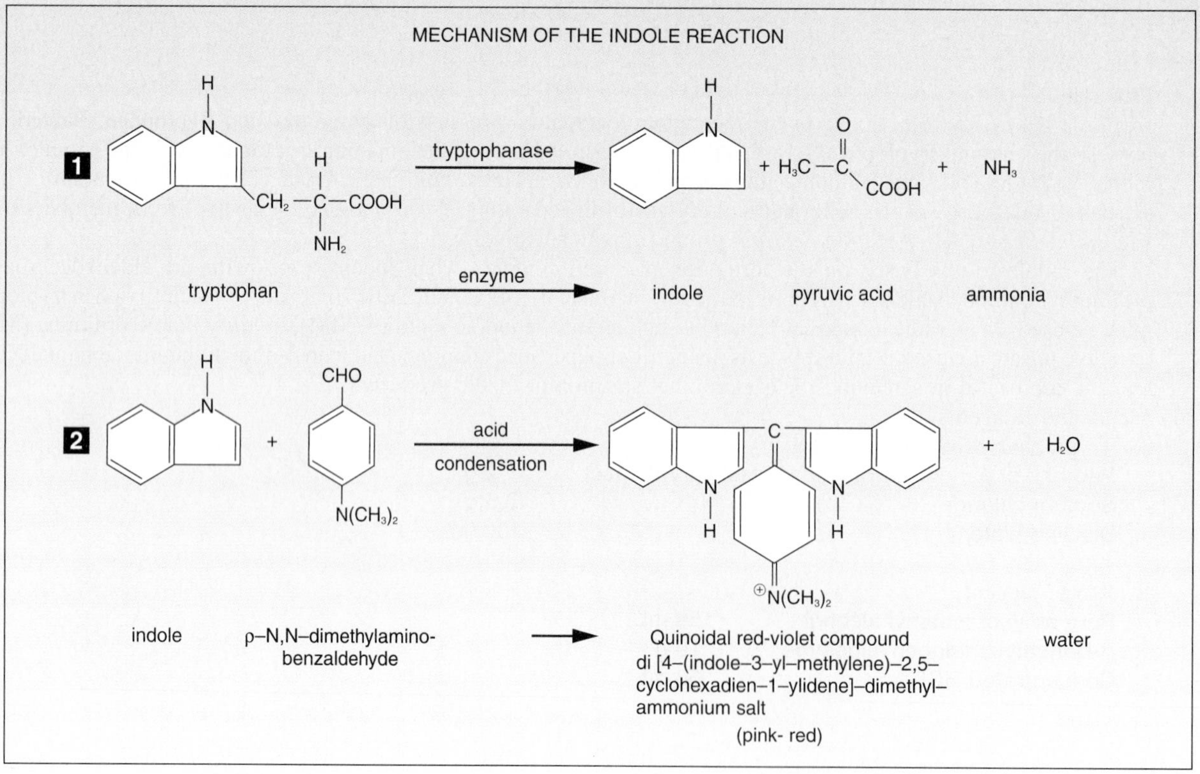

MECHANISM OF THE INDOLE REACTION

1 tryptophan →(tryptophanase / enzyme)→ indole + pyruvic acid + ammonia

2 indole + p–N,N–dimethylamino-benzaldehyde →(acid condensation)→ Quinoidal red-violet compound di [4–(indole–3–yl–methylene)–2,5–cyclohexadien–1–ylidene]–dimethyl–ammonium salt (pink- red) + water

CHART 1-5

CYTOCHROME OXIDASE TEST

I. Principle

The cytochromes are iron-containing hemoproteins that act as the last link in the chain of aerobic respiration by transferring electrons (hydrogen) to oxygen, with the formation of water. The cytochrome system is found in aerobic, or microaerophilic, and facultatively anaerobic organisms, so the oxidase test is important in identifying organisms that either lack the enzyme or are obligate anaerobes. The test is most helpful in screening colonies suspected of being one of the *Enterobacteriaceae* (all negative) and in identifying colonies suspected of belonging to other genera such as *Aeromonas, Pseudomonas, Neisseria, Campylobacter,* and *Pasteurella* (positive).

The cytochrome oxidase test uses certain reagent dyes, such as *p*-phenylenediamine dihydrochloride, that substitute for oxygen as artificial electron acceptors. In the reduced state, the dye is colorless; however, in the presence of cytochrome oxidase and atmospheric oxygen, *p*-phenylenediamine is oxidized, forming indophenol blue.

II. Media and Reagents

A. Tetramethyl-*p*-phenylenediamine dihydrochloride, 1% (Kovac's reagent)

B. Dimethyl-*p*-phenylenediamine dihydrochloride, 1% (Gordon and McLeod's reagent)

III. Quality Control

Bacterial species showing positive and negative reactions should be run as controls at frequent intervals. The following are suggested:

A. Positive control: *Pseudomonas aeruginosa*

B. Negative control: *Escherichia coli*

IV. Procedure

The test is commonly performed by one of two methods: 1) the direct plate technique, in which two to three drops of reagent are added directly to isolated bacterial colonies growing on plate medium; and 2) the indirect paper strip procedure, in which either a few drops of the reagent are added to a filter paper strip or commercial disks or strips impregnated with dried reagent are used. The tetramethyl derivative of *p*-phenylenediamine is recommended because the reagent is more stable in storage and is more sensitive to the detection of cytochrome oxidase and is less toxic than the dimethyl derivative. In either method, a loopful of suspected colony is smeared into the reagent zone of the filter paper.

V. Results

A. Interpretation

Bacterial colonies having cytochrome oxidase activity develop a deep blue color at the inoculation site within 10 seconds (Color Plate 6-1G). Any organism producing a blue color in the 10- to 60-second period must be further tested because it probably does not belong to the *Enterobacteriaceae*. Stainless steel or Nichrome inoculating loops or wires should not be used for this test because surface oxidation products formed when flame-sterilizing may result in false-positive reactions.

VI. Bibliography

Gordon J, McLeod JW. The practical application of the direct oxidase reaction in bacteriology. J Pathol Bacteriol 1928;31:185–190.

MacFaddin JF. Biochemical Tests for Identification of Medical Bacteria. Ed. 2. Baltimore: Williams & Wilkins, 1980:249–260.

Steel KJ. The oxidase reaction as a taxonomic tool. J Gen Microbiol 1961;25:297–306.

Weaver DK, Lee EKH, Leahy MS. Comparison of reagent impregnated paper strips and conventional methods for identification of *Enterobacteriaceae*. Am J Clin Pathol 1968;49:494–499.

MECHANISM OF THE CYTOCHROME OXIDASE REACTION

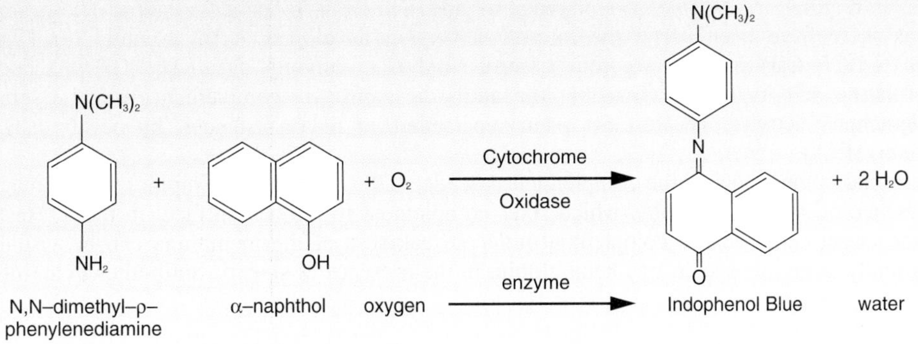

CHART 1-6

PYR TEST

I. Principle

The PYR test was first described by Facklam and coauthors in 1982; since that time, it has gained acceptance as a rapid test for the presumptive identification of both group A β-hemolytic streptococci and enterococci. Whereas the original test was described as a 16- to 20-hour agar test, subsequent PYR test formats included a 4-hour broth assay and several rapid (10- to 15-minute) tests in which the PYR reagent is impregnated in filter paper disks or strips that are inoculated with the organism to be tested. The PYR test also appears on several of the kit systems for identification of streptococci and streptococcus-like bacteria. This chart describes the 4-hour broth PYR test. Disks impregnated with the PYR substrate can also be used for an even more rapid test.

The substrate used for the PYR test is L-naphthylamide-β-naphthylamide. This compound is hydrolyzed by a specific bacterial aminopeptidase enzyme. Hydrolysis of the substrate by this enzyme releases free β-naphthylamide, which is detected by the addition of N,N-dimethylaminocinnamaldehyde. This detection reagent couples with the naphthylamide to form a red Schiff base.

II. Media and Reagents
1. PYR broth (Todd-Hewitt broth with 0.01% L-pyrrolidonyl-β-naphthylamide) dispensed into sterile tubes in 0.20-mL volumes
2. PYR reagent (0.01% p-dimethylaminocinnamaldehyde)

III. Quality Control
A. Positive control: *Enterococcus faecalis* or *Streptococcus pyogenes*
B. Negative control: *Streptococcus agalactiae*

IV. Procedure
1. With a sterile bacteriologic loop, pick up the growth of two to three morphologically similar colonies and emulsify them in the small volume of PYR broth.
2. Incubate the tube at 35°C for 4 hours.
3. Add one drop of the PYR reagent and observe for color change. The reaction should be read and recorded 1 minute after the addition of reagent.

V. Results
A. Interpretation
1. Positive: the development of a deep cherry red color within a minute of addition of the reagent
2. Negative: a yellow or orange color

VI. Procedure Notes

It is essential that testing be performed before the PYR test to determine that the organism is a streptococcus (i.e., gram-positive cocci, catalase-negative). Other organisms (e.g., some aerococci, staphylococci, nutritionally variant streptococci, *Arcanobacterium haemolyticum*) may also be PYR-positive.

CHART 3-1

COMPLEMENT FIXATION (CF) TEST

I. Principle

The complement fixation test is one of the major traditional tests for demonstration of infectious antigens and antibodies. It requires a veritable zoo of reagents and numerous preparatory steps. There are almost as many versions as there have been users; the microtiter version developed at the Centers for Disease Control and Prevention (LBCF test) includes rigorous controls and is commonly used. The CF test does not depend on hemagglutinating activity of the virus, but the antibodies must fix complement, and the sera must be free of anticomplementary activity. The test has been superseded, in many instances, by newer tests, such as enzyme immunoassay (EIA).

The terminal components of the complement cascade, C789 (the attack complex), can damage cell membranes in the presence of specific antibody, which fixes complement to the cell surface. In the CF test, erythrocytes are used as the target cell, because complement-induced leakiness of the membrane can be visualized or measured colorimetrically as an increase in free hemoglobin. In the presence of specific antibodies to an infectious agent, any

CHART 3-1

COMPLEMENT FIXATION (CF) TEST *continued*

complement in the system is bound, leaving no residual complement for reaction with antibodies to the indicator erythrocytes. Thus, the presence of specific antibody is indicated by the absence of hemolysis.

II. Materials and Reagents

Sheep erythrocyte suspension

Hemolysin (rabbit anti-sheep red-cell antibody)

Guinea pig complement, free of antibodies to the agent of interest

Barbital-buffered diluent

Plastic microtiter plate

Centrifuge adapter for microtiter plates

Water bath for incubation of plates

Color standards for judging hemolysis (prepared by lysing various concentrations of red cells)

III. Quality Control

Known positive antibody or antigen

Known negative antibody or antigen

Serum control without antigen (to detect anticomplementary activity)

Antigen controls without serum (to detect anticomplementary activity)

Tissue control (the cells or tissue in which the antigen was prepared)

Buffer control without antigen or antibody

Back titration of complement to document the use of 5 CH_{50} units

Cell control to demonstrate absence of hemolysis

Reference hemolysis standards

IV. Procedure

1. *Sensitization of Erythrocytes*

Serial dilutions of hemolysin are incubated with a 2.8% solution of sheep red cells in barbital buffer. As the concentration of hemolysin increases, the percentage hemolysis will increase to a plateau level. The concentration of hemolysin that represents the second point on the plateau is used for the test.

2. *Quantitation of Complement*

Varying amounts of a 1:400 dilution of cold, reconstituted guinea pig complement are incubated with sensitized cells. The volume of complement that produces 50% lysis of the red cells (CH_{50} unit) is calculated from the graphed results of the hemolysis. The complement stock may be aliquoted and frozen at $-70°C$, but adequate reactivity must be demonstrated before use in the test.

3. *The Complement Fixation Test*

A block titration of serial dilutions of both antigen and antibody is performed in the presence of 5 CH_{50} units of complement at 4°C for 18 hours. Serum is heated at 56°C for 30 minutes to inactivate any endogenous complement. The characteristics of either the antigen or antibody will be known; the serial dilutions of the known reagent may be abbreviated to include the dilution on each side of the expected optimum. Subsequently, sheep red cells that have been sensitized with the optimal dilution of hemolysin are incubated at 37°C for 30 minutes. Plates are centrifuged at low speed to sediment the unlysed erythrocytes.

V. Results

A. Interpretation

The highest dilution of antigen or antibody that provides 3+ to 4+ fixation of complement (<30% hemolysis) is the end point. All reagents must be free of anticomplementary activity, the correct quantity of complement must have been added, and the control specimens must react as expected.

VI. Bibliography

Hsiung GD. Diagnostic Virology. Ed. 3. New Haven, CT: Yale University Press, 1982.

Standardized diagnostic complement fixation method and adaptation to microtest. Atlanta: Public Health Service, 1965. Publication no. 1228 (Public Health Monograph 74).

CHART 3-2

HEMAGGLUTINATION INHIBITION (HAI) TEST

I. Principle
The nucleic acids of many viruses encode surface proteins that agglutinate the red cells of a variety of species. The phenomenon is most commonly used for diagnosis of infections produced by orthomyxoviruses, paramyxoviruses, and the arboviruses-togaviruses (including rubella), flaviviruses, and bunyaviruses. The presence of virus in infected cell cultures can be detected by hemagglutination; the identity of the virus or of antibodies in a patient's serum can be determined by specific inhibition of that hemagglutination. Although influenza viruses can be detected by hemadsorption (see Chart 23-1) typing of the isolate is done most efficiently by hemagglutination inhibition. Reagents and conditions for the test vary by virus.

Reaction of viral hemagglutinins with red cells results in a lattice of agglutinated cells which settle irregularly in a tube or microtiter well. Unagglutinated cells settle in a compact button.

II. Materials and Reagents
    1. Red cells from an appropriate species (chicken, goose, guinea pig, trypsinized human O) collected in Alsever's solution or heparin
    2. Diluent at appropriate pH
    3. Solutions to remove nonspecific hemagglutinins from serum
    4. Infected culture fluid or standard antigen for serology

III. Quality Control
    A. Known positive serum
    B. Known negative serum
    C. Serum and cells without antigen (to detect nonspecific agglutination)
    D. Back titration of hemagglutination activity of the antigen (to ensure that 4 hemagglutinating units [HAU] were tested)

IV. Procedure
    A. Determination of Hemagglutinating Titer
        1. A diluted suspension of red cells is incubated at 4°C or room temperature with serial dilutions of antigen until red cells in tubes without virus settle in a compact button (1 to 4 hours). The highest dilution that produces partial or complete agglutination represents 1 HAU.
    B. Treatment of Sera
        1. Removal of nonspecific inhibitors in sera is necessary for most viruses. Removal may be accomplished by physical means, such as kaolin; by enzymes, such as neuraminidase or the receptor-destroying enzyme (RDE) of *Vibrio cholerae*; or by a combination. The choice varies with the virus to be tested.
    C. Inhibition Test
        1. A dilution of antigen that contains 4 HAU is mixed with appropriate red cells and serial twofold dilutions of treated serum. The suspension is incubated as for the hemagglutination test.

V. Results
    A. Interpretation
    The end point is the last well at which partial or complete agglutination of the red cells occurs. A smooth or jagged shield of cells or an irregular button indicates agglutination. Observation of the movement of the button of red cells when the plate is tilted may help to clarify the end point.

VI. Bibliography
Hsiung GD. Diagnostic Virology. Ed. 3. New Haven, CT: Yale University Press, 1982.
Lennette EH, Schmidt NJ, eds. Diagnostic Procedures for Viral, Rickettsial, and Chlamydial Infections. Ed. 5. Washington DC: American Public Health Association, 1979.
Smith TF. Viruses. In: Washington JA, ed. Laboratory Procedures in Clinical Microbiology. Ed. 2. New York: Springer-Verlag, 1985.

CHART 6-1

o-NITROPHENYL-β-D-GALACTOPYRANOSIDE

I. Principle

o-Nitrophenyl-β-D-galactopyranoside (ONPG) is structurally similar to lactose, except that orthonitrophenyl has been substituted for glucose, as shown in the following chemical reaction:

ORTHONITROPHENYL-β-D-GALACTOPYRANOSIDE

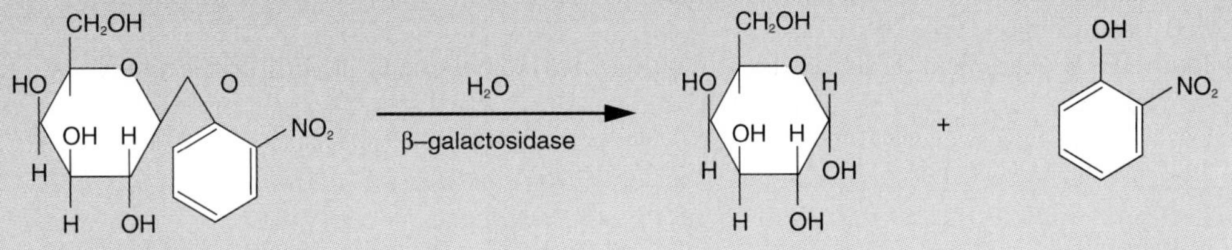

Orthonitrophenyl-β-D-Galactopyranoside (ONPG) (colorless) + H₂O / β-galactosidase → Galactose + Orthonitrophenol (yellow)

On hydrolysis, through the action of the enzyme β-galactosidase, ONPG cleaves into two residues, galactose and *o*-nitrophenol. ONPG is a colorless compound; *o*-nitrophenol is yellow, providing visual evidence of hydrolysis.

Lactose-fermenting bacteria possess both lactose permease and β-galactosidase, two enzymes required for the production of acid in the lactose fermentation test. The permease is required for the lactose molecule to penetrate the bacterial cell where the β-galactosidase can cleave the galactoside bond, producing glucose and galactose. Non–lactose-fermenting bacteria are devoid of both enzymes and are incapable of producing acid from lactose. Some bacterial species appear to be non-lactose-fermenters because they lack permease, but do possess β-galactosidase and give a positive ONPG test. So-called late lactose fermenters may be delayed in their production of acid from lactose because of sluggish permease activity. In these instances, a positive ONPG test may provide a rapid identification of delayed lactose fermentation.

II. Media and Reagents
  1. Sodium phosphate buffer, 1 M, pH 7.0
  2. *o*-Nitrophenyl-β-D-galactopyranoside (ONPG), 0.75 M (Buffered ONPG tablets are commercially available.)
  3. Physiologic saline
  4. Toluene

III. Quality Control
  A. Positive control: *Escherichia coli*
  B. Negative control: *Proteus* species

IV. Procedure

Bacteria grown in medium containing lactose, such as Kligler iron agar (KIA) or triple-sugar iron (TSI) agar, produce optimal results in the ONPG test. A loopful of bacterial growth is emulsified in 0.5 mL of physiologic saline to produce a heavy suspension. One drop of toluene is added to the suspension and vigorously mixed for a few seconds to release the enzyme for the bacterial cells. An equal quantity of buffered ONPG solution is added to the suspension, and the mixture is placed in a 37°C water bath.

When using ONPG tablets, a loopful of bacterial suspension is added directly to the ONPG substrate resulting from adding 1 mL of distilled water to a tablet in a test tube. This suspension is also placed in a 37°C water bath.

V. Results

A. Interpretation

The rate of hydrolysis of ONPG to *o*-nitrophenol may be rapid for some organisms, producing a visible yellow color reaction within 5 to 10 minutes (see Color Plate 6-4*A*). Most tests are positive within 1 hour; however, reactions should not be interpreted as negative before 24 hours of incubation. The yellow color is usually distinct and indicates that the organism has produced *o*-nitrophenol from the ONPG substrate through the action of β-galactosidase.

CHART 6-1

o-NITROPHENYL-β-D-GALACTOPYRANOSIDE *continued*

VI. Bibliography

Belliveau RR, Grayson JW Jr, Butler TJ. A rapid, simple method of identifying *Enterobacteriaceae*. Am J Clin Pathol 1968;50:126–128.

Blazevic DJ, Ederer GM. Principles of Biochemical Tests in Diagnostic Microbiology. New York: Wiley, 1975: 83–85.

Lederberg J. The beta-*d*-galactosidase of *Escherichia coli*, strain K-12. J Bacteriol 1950; 60:381–392.

Lowe GH. The rapid detection of lactose fermentation in paracolon organisms by the demonstration of β-galactosidase. J Med Lab Technol 1962;19:21–25.

MacFaddin JF. Biochemical Tests for Identification of Medical Bacteria. Ed. 2. Baltimore: Williams & Wilkins, 1980:120–128.

CHART 6-2

NITRATE REDUCTION: GENERAL APPLICATIONS

I. Principle

The capability of an organism to reduce nitrates to nitrites is an important characteristic used in the identification and species differentiation of many groups of microorganisms. All *Enterobacteriaceae* except certain biotypes of *Pantoa agglomerans* and certain species of *Serratia* and *Yersinia* demonstrate nitrate reduction. The test is also helpful in identifying members of the *Haemophilus*, *Neisseria*, and *Moraxella* genera.

Organisms demonstrating nitrate reduction have the capability of extracting oxygen from nitrates to form nitrites and other reduction products. The chemical equation is

$$NO_3^- + 2e^- + 2H \rightarrow NO_2 + H_2O$$
$$\text{Nitrate} \qquad\qquad\qquad \text{Nitrite}$$

The presence of nitrites in the test medium is detected by the addition of α-naphthylamine and sulfanilic acid, with the formation of a red diazonium dye, *p*-sulfobenzeneazo-α-naphthylamine. See Figure in Chart 19-12.

II. Media and Reagents

A. Nitrate Broth or Nitrate Agar (Slant)

Beef extract	3 g
Peptone	5 g
Potassium nitrate (KNO$_3$)	1 g
Agar (nitrite-free)	12 g
Distilled water to	1 L

B. Reagent A

α-Naphthylamine	5 g
Acetic acid (5 N), 30%	1 L

C. Reagent B

Sulfanilic acid	8 g
Acetic acid (5 N), 30%	1 L

III. Quality Control

It is important to test each new batch of medium and each new formulation of test reagents for positive and negative reactions. The following organisms are suggested:

A. Positive control: *Escherichia coli*

B. Negative control: *Acinetobacter baumannii*

IV. Procedure

1. Inoculate the nitrate medium with a loopful of the test organism isolated in pure culture on agar medium and incubate at 35°C for 18 to 24 hours.

2. At the end of incubation, add 1 mL each of reagents A and B to the test medium, in that order.

CHART 6-2

NITRATE REDUCTION: GENERAL APPLICATIONS *continued*

V. Results
  A. Interpretation
  The development of a red color within 30 seconds after adding the test reagents indicates the presence of nitrites and represents a positive reaction for nitrate reduction (see Color Plate 6-1*H*). If no color develops after adding the test reagents, this may indicate either that nitrates have not been reduced (a true negative reaction) or that they have been reduced to products other than nitrites, such as ammonia, molecular nitrogen (denitrification), nitric oxide (NO) or nitrous oxide (N_2O), and hydroxylamine. Because the test reagents detect only nitrites, the latter process would lead to a false-negative reading. Thus, it is necessary to add a small quantity of zinc dust to all negative reactions. Zinc ions reduce nitrates to nitrites, and the development of a red color after adding zinc dust indicates the presence of residual nitrates and confirms a true negative reaction.

VI. Bibliography
Finegold SM, Martin WJ, Scott EG. Bailey and Scott's Diagnostic Microbiology. Ed. 5. St Louis: Mosby, 1978: 490.

MacFaddin JF. Biochemical Tests for Identification of Medical Bacteria. Ed. 2. Baltimore: Williams & Wilkins, 1980:236–245.

Wallace GI, Neave SL. The nitrite test as applied to bacterial cultures. J Bacteriol 1927;14:377–384.

CHART 6-3

METHYL RED

I. Principle
Methyl red is a pH indicator with a range between 6.0 (yellow) and 4.4 (red). The pH at which methyl red detects acid is considerably lower than the pH for other indicators used in bacteriologic culture media. Thus, to produce a color change, the test organism must produce large quantities of acid from the carbohydrate substrate being used.

The methyl red test is a quantitative test for acid production, requiring positive organisms to produce strong acids (lactic, acetic, formic) from glucose through the mixed acid fermentation pathway (see Fig. 6-2). Because many species of the *Enterobacteriaceae* may produce sufficient quantities of strong acids that can be detected by methyl red indicator during the initial phases of incubation, only organisms that can maintain this low pH after prolonged incubation (48 to 72 hours), overcoming the pH-buffering system of the medium, can be called methyl red–positive.

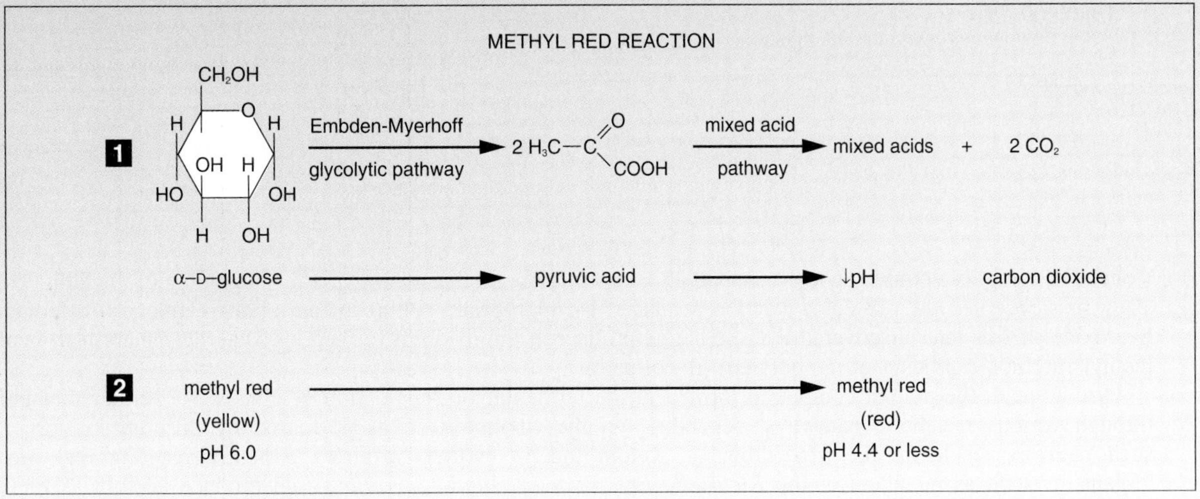

METHYL RED REACTION

II. Media and Reagents
The medium most commonly used is methyl red–Voges-Proskauer (MR/VP) broth, as formulated by Clark and Lubs. This medium also serves for the performance of the Voges-Proskauer test.

CHART 6-3

MᴇᴛHʏʟ Rᴇᴅ *continued*

    A. MR/VP broth

Polypeptone	7 g
Glucose	5 g
Dipotassium phosphate	5 g
Distilled water to	1 L
Final pH = 6.9	

    B. Methyl red pH indicator
    Methyl red, 0.1 g, in 300 mL of 95% ethyl alcohol
    Distilled water, 200 mL

III. Quality Control
Positive and negative controls should be run after preparation of each lot of medium and after making each batch of reagent. Suggested controls include the following:
    A. Positive control: *Escherichia coli*
    B. Negative control: *Enterobacter aerogenes*

IV. Procedure
    1. Inoculate the MR/VP broth with a pure culture of the test organism. Incubate the broth at 35°C for 48 to 72 hours (no fewer than 48 hours).
    2. At the end of this time, add 5 drops of the methyl red reagent directly to the broth.

V. Results
    A. Interpretation
    The development of a stable red color in the surface of the medium indicates sufficient acid production to lower the pH to 4.4 and constitutes a positive test (see Color Plate 6-4C). Because other organisms may produce smaller quantities of acid from the test substrate, an intermediate orange color between yellow and red may develop. This does not indicate a positive test.

VI. Bibliography
Barry AL, et al. Improved 18-hour methyl red test. Appl Microbiol 1970; 20:866–870.
Blazevic DJ, Ederer GM. Principles of Biochemical Tests in Diagnostic Microbiology. New York: Wiley, 1975: 75–77.
Clark WM, Lubs HA. The differentiation of bacteria of the colon-aerogenes family by the use of indicators. J Infect Dis 1915;17:160.
MacFaddin JF. Biochemical Tests for Identification of Medical Bacteria. Ed. 2. Baltimore: Williams & Wilkins, 1980;209–214.

CHART 6-4

Vᴏɢᴇs-Pʀᴏsᴋᴀᴜᴇʀ Tᴇsᴛ

I. Principle
Voges-Proskauer is a double eponym, named after two microbiologists working at the beginning of the 20th century. They first observed the red color reaction produced by appropriate culture media after treatment with potassium hydroxide. It was later discovered that the active product in the medium formed by bacterial metabolism is acetyl methyl carbinol, a product of the butylene glycol pathway.

    Pyruvic acid, the pivotal compound formed in the fermentative degradation of glucose, is further metabolized through various metabolic pathways, depending on the enzyme systems possessed by different bacteria. One such pathway results in the production of acetoin (acetyl methyl carbinol), a neutral-reacting end product. Organisms such as members of the *Klebsiella-Enterobacter-Hafnia-Serratia* group produce acetoin as the chief end product of glucose metabolism and form smaller quantities of mixed acids. In the presence of atmospheric oxygen and 40% potassium hydroxide, acetoin is converted to diacetyl, and α-naphthol serves as a catalyst to bring out a red complex.

CHART 6-4

VOGES-PROSKAUER TEST *continued*

II. Media and Reagents
   A. Media
      1. The medium is the MR/VP broth described in Chart 6-3.
   B. Reagents
      1. α-Naphthol, 5% color intensifier

α-Naphthol	5 g
Absolute ethyl alcohol	100 mL

      2. Potassium hydroxide, 40%, oxidizing agent

Potassium hydroxide	40 g
Distilled water to	100 mL

III. Quality Control
   Positive and negative controls should be run after preparation of each lot of medium and after making each batch of reagent. Suggested controls include the following:
   A. Positive Control: *Enterobacter aerogenes*
   B. Negative Control: *Escherichia coli*
IV. Procedure
   Inoculate a tube of MR/VP broth with a pure culture of the test organism. Incubate for 24 hours at 35°C. At the end of this time, aliquot 1 mL of broth to a clean test tube. Add 0.6 mL of 5% α-naphthol, followed by 0.2 mL of 40% KOH. It is essential that the reagents be added in this order. Shake the tube gently to expose the medium to atmospheric oxygen and allow the tube to remain undisturbed for 10 to 15 minutes.

CHART 6-4

VOGES-PROSKAUER TEST *continued*

V. Results
   A. Interpretation
      A positive test is represented by the development of a red color 15 minutes or more after addition of the reagents, indicating the presence of diacetyl, the oxidation product of acetoin (see Color Plate 6-4*D*). The test should not be read after standing for over 1 hour because negative Voges-Proskauer cultures may produce a copper-like color, potentially resulting in a false-positive interpretation.
VI. Bibliography

Barritt MM. The intensification of the Voges-Proskauer reaction by the addition of α-naphthol. J Pathol Bacteriol 1936;42:441–454.

Barry AL, Feeney KL. Two quick methods for Voges-Proskauer test. Appl Microbiol 1967;15:1138–1141.

Blazevic DJ, Ederer GM. Principles of Biochemical Tests in Diagnostic Microbiology. New York: Wiley, 1975:105–107.

MacFaddin JF. Biochemical Tests for Identification of Medical Bacteria Ed. 2. Baltimore: Williams & Wilkins, 1980:308–320.

Voges O, Proskauer B. Beitrag zue Ernährungsphysiologie und zur Differential-diagnose der Bakterien der hämorrhagischen Septicamia. Z Hyg 1898;28:20–32.

CHART 6-5

CITRATE UTILIZATION

I. Principle
   Sodium citrate is a salt of citric acid, a simple organic compound found as one of the metabolites in the tricarboxylic acid cycle (Krebs cycle). Some bacteria can obtain energy in a manner other than by the fermentation of carbohydrates by using citrate as the sole source of carbon. The measurement of this characteristic is important in the identification of many members of the *Enterobacteriaceae*. Any medium used to detect citrate utilization by test bacteria must be devoid of protein and carbohydrates as sources of carbon.

   The utilization of citrate by a test bacterium is detected in citrate medium by the production of alkaline by-products. The medium includes sodium citrate, an anion, as the sole source of carbon, and ammonium phosphate as the sole source of nitrogen. Bacteria that can use citrate can also extract nitrogen from the ammonium salt, with the production of ammonia (NH^+), leading to alkalinization of the medium from conversion of the NH_3^{2+} to ammonium hydroxide (NH_4OH). Bromthymol blue—yellow below pH 6.0 and blue above pH 7.6—is the indicator.

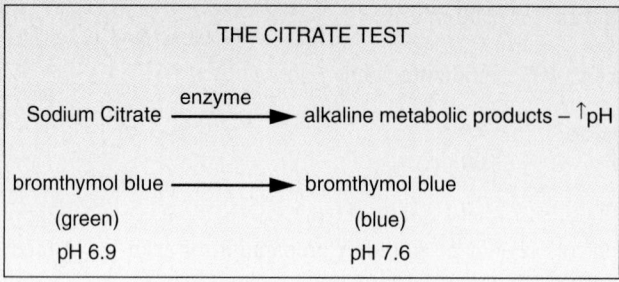

II. Media and Reagents
   The citrate medium most commonly used is the formula of Simmons. The medium is poured into a tube on a slant. The formula of Simmons citrate medium is shown below:

CHART 6-5

CITRATE UTILIZATION *continued*

Ammonium dihydrogen phosphate	1 g
Dipotassium phosphate	1 g
Sodium chloride	5 g
Sodium citrate	2 g
Magnesium sulfate	0.20 g
Agar	15 g
Bromthymol blue	0.08 g
Distilled water to	1 L

Final pH = 6.9

III. Quality Control
Each new batch of medium should be tested with a positive- and a negative-reacting organism. The following species are suggested controls:
A. Positive control—*Enterobacter aerogenes*
B. Negative control—*Escherichia coli*

IV. Procedure
    1. A well-isolated colony is picked from the surface of a primarily isolation medium and inoculated as a single streak on the slant surface of the citrate agar tube. The tube is incubated at 35°C for 24 to 48 hours.

V. Results
    A. Interpretation
    A positive test is represented by the development of a deep blue color within 24 to 48 hours, indicating that the test organism has been able to utilize the citrate contained in the medium, with the production of alkaline products (see Color Plate 6-4*D*). A positive test may also be read without a blue color if there is visible colony growth along the inoculation streak line. This is possible because, for growth to be visible, the organism must enter the log phase of growth, possible only if carbon and nitrogen have been assimilated. A positive interpretation from reading the streak line can be confirmed by incubating the tube for an additional 24 hours, when a blue color usually develops.

VI. Bibliography
BBL Manual of Products and Laboratory Procedures. Ed. 5. Cockeysville MD: BioQuest, 1968:115, 138.

Blazevic DJ, Ederer GM. Principles of Biochemical Tests in Diagnostic Microbiology. New York: Wiley, 1975: 15–18.

Koser SA. Utilization of the salts of organic acids by the colon-aerogenes groups. J Bacteriol 1923;8:493–520.

MacFaddin JF. Biochemical Tests for Identification of Medical Bacteria. Ed. 2. Baltimore: Williams & Wilkins, 1980:59–63.

Simmons JS. A culture medium for differentiating organisms of typhoid-colon aerogenes groups and for isolation of certain fungi. J Infect Dis 1926;39:209–214.

CHART 6-6

UREASE: CONVENTIONAL

I. Principle
Urea is a diamide of carbonic acid with the formula

$$NH_2 - \overset{\overset{\displaystyle O}{\|}}{C} - NH_2$$

All amides are easily hydrolyzed with the release of ammonia and carbon dioxide.

Urease is an enzyme possessed by many species of microorganisms that can hydrolyze urea following the chemical reaction

$$NH_2 - \overset{\overset{\displaystyle O}{\|}}{C} - NH_2 + 2HOH \xrightarrow{\text{Urease}} CO_2 + H_2O + 2NH_3 \rightleftharpoons (NH_4)_2CO_3$$

CHART 6-6

UREASE: CONVENTIONAL *continued*

The ammonia reacts in solution to form ammonium carbonate, resulting in alkalinization and an increase in the pH of the medium.

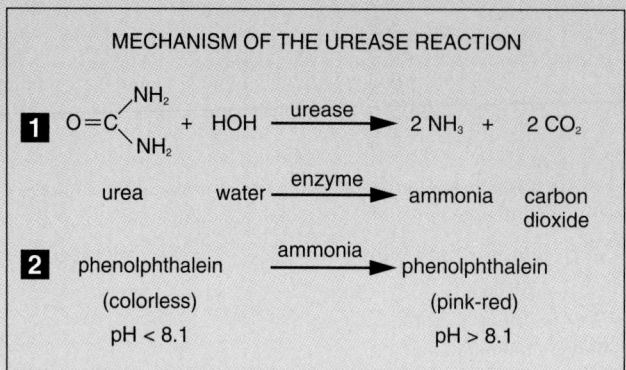

II. Media and Reagents
Stuart's urea broth and Christensen's urea agar are the two media most commonly used in clinical laboratories for the detection of urease activity.

STUART'S UREA BROTH

Yeast extract	0.1 g
Monopotassium phosphate	9.1 g
Disodium phosphate	9.5 g
Urea	20 g
Phenol red	0.01 g
Distilled water to	1 L

Final pH = 6.8

CHRISTENSEN'S UREA AGAR

Peptone	1 g
Glucose	1 g
Sodium chloride	5 g
Monopotassium phosphate	2 g
Urea	20 g
Phenol red	0.012 g
Agar	15 g
Distilled water to	1 L

Final pH = 6.8

III. Quality Control
Positively and negatively reacting control organisms should be run with each new batch of medium. The following organisms are suggested:
A. Positive control: *Proteus* species
B. Positive control (weak): *Klebsiella* species
C. Negative control: *Escherichia coli*
IV. Procedure
The broth medium is inoculated with a loopful of a pure culture of the test organism; the surface of the agar slant is streaked with the test organism. Both media are incubated at 35°C for 18 to 24 hours.
V. Results
A. Interpretation
Organisms that hydrolyze urea rapidly may produce positive reactions within 1 or 2 hours; less active species may require 3 or more days. The reactions are as follows:
1. Stuart's broth
Red color throughout the medium indicates alkalinization and urea hydrolysis
2. Christensen's agar
Rapid urea splitters (*Proteus* species): red color throughout medium
Slow urea splitters (*Klebsiella* species): red color initially in slant only, gradually converting the entire tube
3. No urea hydrolysis: medium remains original yellow color (see Color Plate 6-4E).

CHART 6-6

UREASE: CONVENTIONAL *continued*

VI. Bibliography
    BBL Manual of Products and Laboratory Procedures. Ed. 5. Cockeysville MD: BioQuest, 1968:154.
    Christensen WB. Urea decomposition as a means of differentiating *Proteus* and paracolon cultures from each other and from *Salmonella* and *Shigella* types. J Bacteriol 1946;52:461–466.
    MacFaddin JF. Biochemical Tests for Identification of Medical Bacteria. Ed. 2. Baltimore: Williams & Wilkins, 1980:298–308.
    Stuart CA, Van Stratum E, Rustigian R. Further studies on urease production by *Proteus* and related organisms. J Bacteriol 1945;49:437–444.

CHART 6-7

DECARBOXYLASES

I. Principle
   Decarboxylases are a group of substrate-specific enzymes that are capable of reacting with the carboxyl (COOH) portion of amino acids, forming alkaline-reacting amines. This reaction, known as decarboxylation, forms carbon dioxide as a second product. Each decarboxylase enzyme is specific for an amino acid. Lysine, ornithine, and arginine are the three amino acids routinely tested in the identification of the *Enterobacteriaceae*. The specific amine products are as follows:

   Lysine   →   Cadaverine
   Ornithine   →   Putrescine
   Arginine   →   Citrulline

   The conversion of arginine to citrulline is a dihydrolase, rather than a decarboxylase reaction, in which an NH_2 group is removed from arginine as a first step. Citrulline is next converted to ornithine, which then undergoes decarboxylation to form putrescine.

   Moeller decarboxylase medium is the base most commonly used for determining the decarboxylase capabilities of the *Enterobacteriaceae*. The amino acid to be tested is added to the decarboxylase base before inoculation with the test organism. A control tube, consisting of only the base without the amino acid, must also be set up in parallel. Both tubes are anaerobically incubated by overlaying with mineral oil. During the initial stages of incubation, both tubes turn yellow, owing to the fermentation of the small amount of glucose in the medium. If the amino acid is decarboxylated, alkaline amines are formed and the medium reverts to its original purple color.

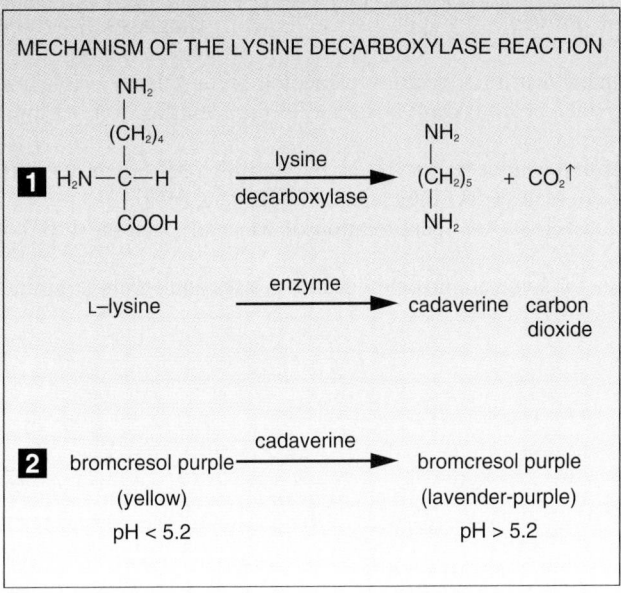

CHART 6-7

DECARBOXYLASES *continued*

II. Media and Reagents
A. *Møller Decarboxylase Broth Base*

Peptone	5 g
Beef extract	5 g
Bromcresol purple	0.01 g
Cresol red	0.005 g
Glucose	0.5 g
Pyridoxal	0.005 g
Distilled water to	1 L
Final pH = 6.0	

B. Amino Acid
Add 10 g (final concentration = 1%) of the L (*levo*)-form of the amino acid (lysine, ornithine, or arginine). Double this amount if the D (*dextro*)-L-form is to be used, because only the L-form is active.

III. Quality Control
The following organisms are suggested for positive and negative controls:

AMINO ACID	POSITIVE CONTROL	NEGATIVE CONTROL
Lysine	*Enterobacter aerogenes*	*Enterobacter cloacae*
Ornithine	*Enterobacter cloacae*	*Klebsiella pneumoniae*
Arginine	*Enterobacter cloacae*	*Enterobacter aerogenes*

IV. Procedure
From a well-isolated colony of the test organism previously recovered on primary isolation agar, inoculate two tubes of Moeller decarboxylase medium, one containing the amino acid to be tested, the other to be used as a control tube devoid of amino acid. Overlay both tubes with sterile mineral oil to cover about 1 cm of the surface and incubate at 35°C for 18 to 24 hours.

V. Results
A. Interpretation
Conversion of the control tube to a yellow color indicates that the organism is viable and that the pH of the medium has been lowered sufficiently to activate the decarboxylase enzymes. Reversion of the tube containing the amino acid to a blue-purple color indicates a positive test owing to the formation of amines from the decarboxylation reaction (see Color Plate 6-4*F*).

VI. Bibliography
Blazevic DJ, Ederer GM. Principles of Biochemical Tests in Diagnostic Microbiology. New York: Wiley, 1975; 29–36.

Carlquist PR. A biochemical test for separating paracolon groups. J Bacteriol 1956;71:339–341.

Falkow S. Activity of lysine decarboxylase as an aid in the identification of salmonellae and shigellae. Am J Clin Pathol 1958;29:598–600.

Gale EF. The bacterial amino acid decarboxylases. In: Nord FF, ed. Advances in Enzymology and Related Subjects of Biochemistry. Vol. 6. New York: Interscience Publishers, 1946.

MacFaddin JF. Biochemical Tests for Identification of Medical Bacteria. Ed. 2. Baltimore: Williams & Wilkins, 1980;78–93

Møller V. Simplified tests for some amino acid decarboxylases and for the arginine dihydrolase system. Acta Pathol Microbiol Scand 1955;36:158–172.

CHART 6-8

PHENYLALANINE DEAMINASE

I. Principle
Phenylalanine is an amino acid that on deamination forms a keto acid, phenylpyruvic acid. Of the *Enterobacteriaceae*, only members of the *Proteus, Morganella,* and *Providencia* genera possess the deaminase enzyme necessary for this conversion.

   The phenylalanine test depends on the detection of phenylpyruvic acid in the test medium after growth of the test organism. The test is positive if a visible green color develops on addition of a solution of 10% ferric chloride.

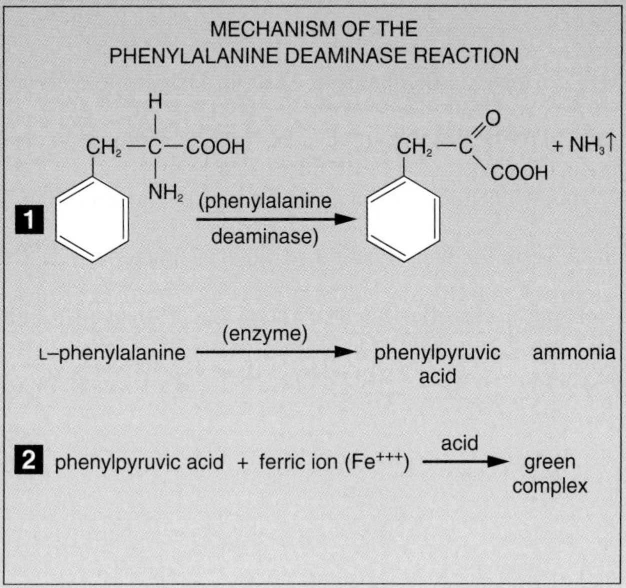

MECHANISM OF THE
PHENYLALANINE DEAMINASE REACTION

1 L–phenylalanine $\xrightarrow{\text{(enzyme)}}$ phenylpyruvic acid + ammonia

2 phenylpyruvic acid + ferric ion (Fe^{+++}) $\xrightarrow{\text{acid}}$ green complex

II. Media and Reagents
Phenylalanine agar is poured as a slant into a tube. Meat extracts or protein hydrolysates cannot be used because of their varying natural content of phenylalanine. Yeast extract serves as the carbon and nitrogen source. The formula is shown below:
Medium:

DL-Phenylalanine	2 g
Yeast extract	3 g
Sodium chloride	5 g
Disodium phosphate	1 g
Agar	12 g
Distilled water to	1 L
pH = 7.3	

Reagent:

Ferric chloride	12 g
Concentrated HCl	2.5 mL
Distilled water to	100 mL

III. Quality Control
Each new batch of medium or reagent must be tested with positive- and negative-reacting organisms. The following are suggested:
A. Positive control: *Proteus* species
B. Negative control: *Escherichia coli*

CHART 6-8

PHENYLALANINE DEAMINASE *continued*

IV. Procedure
The agar slant of the medium is inoculated with a single colony of the test organism isolated in pure culture of primary plating agar. After incubation at 35°C for 18 to 24 hours, 4 or 5 drops of the ferric chloride reagent are added directly to the surface of the agar. As the reagent is added, the tube is rotated to dislodge the surface colonies.

V. Results
   A. Interpretation
      The immediate appearance of an intense green color indicates the presence of phenylpyruvic acid and a positive test (see Color Plate 6-4*E*).

VI. Bibliography

Blazevic DJ, Ederer GM. Principles of Biochemical Tests in Diagnostic Microbiology. New York: Wiley, 1975: 23–28.

Hendriksen SD. A comparison of the phenylpyruvic acid reaction and unrease test in the differentiation of *Proteus* from other enteric organisms. J Bacteriol 1950; 60:225–231.

Hendriksen SD, Closs K. The production of phenylpyruvic acid by bacteria. Acta Pathol Microbiol Scand 1938;15: 101–113.

MacFaddin JF. Biochemical Tests for Identification of Medical Bacteria. Ed. 2. Baltimore: Williams & Wilkins, 1980;269–274.

Shaw C, Clarke PH. Biochemical classification of *Proteus* and *Providencia* cultures. J Gen Microbiol 1955;13: 155–161.

CHART 7-1

OXIDATIVE-FERMENTATIVE TEST (HUGH AND LEIFSON)

I. Principle
Saccharolytic microorganisms degrade glucose either fermentatively or oxidatively, as shown in Figure 7-1. The end products of fermentation are relatively strong mixed acids that can be detected in a conventional fermentation test medium. However, the acids formed in oxidative degradation of glucose are extremely weak, and the more sensitive oxidation-fermentation medium of Hugh and Leifson (OF medium) is required for their detection.
    The OF medium of Hugh and Leifson differs from carbohydrate fermentation media as follows:
The concentration of peptone is decreased from 1% to 0.2%.
The concentration of carbohydrate is increased from 0.5% to 1.0%.
The concentration of agar is decreased from 1.5% to 0.3%, making it semisolid.
The lower protein/carbohydrate ratio reduces the formation of alkaline amines that can neutralize the small quantities of weak acids that may form from oxidative metabolism. The relatively larger amount of carbohydrate serves to increase the amount of acid that can potentially be formed. The semisolid consistency of the agar permits acids that form on the surface of the agar to permeate throughout the medium, making interpretation of the pH shift of the indicator easier to visualize. Motility can also be observed in this medium.

II. Media and Reagents
For comparison, the formulas for a conventional carbohydrate fermentation medium and OF medium are as follows:

CARBOHYDRATE FERMENTATION MEDIUM		OF MEDIUM OF HUGH AND LEIFSON	
Peptone	10 g	Peptone	2 g
Sodium chloride	5 g	Sodium chloride	5 g
D-glucose	5 g	D-glucose	10 g
Bromcresol purple	0.02 g	Bromthymol blue	0.03 g
Agar*	15 g	Agar	3.0 g
Distilled water to	1 L	Dipotassium phosphate	0.30 g
pH = 7.0		Distilled water to	1 L
		pH = 7.1	

CHART 7-1

OXIDATIVE-FERMENTATIVE TEST (HUGH AND LEIFSON) *continued*

The OF sugar reactions listed in the Weaver CDC tables, described in Chapter 7, are based on tests using a ''special'' base with phenol red as the indicator:

Bacto casitone, 2 g
Bacto agar, 3 g
Phenol red, 1.5% aqueous, 2 mL
Distilled water to equal 1 L

The basal medium is adjusted to a pH of 7.3 and autoclaved. Carbohydrate solutions are passed through a Seitz filter and added to the basal medium to a final concentration of 1.0%. Studies at the CDC revealed that the correlation of test results between the Difco and the special CDC OF basal media are excellent and that either can be used when making interpretations from the Weaver tables.

OF medium should be poured without a slant into tubes with an inner diameter of 15 to 20 mm to increase surface area.

III. Quality Control
   A. Glucose fermenter: *Escherichia coli*
   B. Glucose oxidizer: *Pseudomonas aeruginosa*
   C. Nonsaccharolytic: *Moraxella* species

IV. Procedure
Two tubes are required for the OF test, each inoculated with the unknown organism, using a straight needle, stabbing the medium three to four times halfway to the bottom of the tube. One tube of each pair is covered with a 1-cm layer of sterile mineral oil or melted paraffin, leaving the other tube open to the air. Incubate both tubes at 35°C and examine daily for several days.

V. Results
   A. Interpretation
      Acid production is detected in the medium by the appearance of a yellow color. In the case of oxidative organisms, color production may be first noted near the surface of the medium. Following are the reaction patterns:

OPEN TUBE	COVERED TUBES	METABOLISM
Acid (yellow)	Alkaline (green)	Oxidative
Acid (yellow)	Acid (yellow)	Fermentative
Alkaline (green or blue)	Alkaline (green or blue)	Nonsaccharolytic

These color reactions are shown in Color Plate 7-1*D*. For slower-growing species, incubation for 3 days or longer may be required to detect positive reactions.

VI. Bibliography
BBL Manual of Products and Laboratory Procedures. Ed. 5. Cockeysville MD: BioQuest, 1973:129–130.
Hugh R, Leifson E. The taxonomic significance of fermentative versus oxidative metabolism of carbohydrates by various gram-negative bacilli. J Bacteriol 1953;66:24–26.
MacFaddin JF. Biochemical Tests for Identification of Medical Bacteria. Ed. 2. Baltimore: Williams & Wilkins, 1980:260–268.

CHART 7-2

FLAGELLAR STAIN

I. Principle
Most motile bacteria possess flagella, the shape, number, and position of which are important characteristics in the differentiation of genera and species identification, particularly when biochemical reactions are weak or equivocal. The Leifson staining technique (or modification) is most commonly used in clinical laboratories and is not difficult to perform, providing exact details are followed in each step of the procedure.

Bacterial flagella can be stained by alcoholic solutions of rosaniline dyes that form a precipitate as the alcohol evaporates in the staining procedure. Basic fuchsin (pararosaniline acetate) serves as the primary stain with tannic acid added to the solution as a mordant. A counterstain, such as methylene blue, may be used to better visualize the bacteria in instances in which the primary stain is weak or does not react at all with the bacterial cell wall.

CHART 7-2

FLAGELLAR STAIN *continued*

II. Media and Reagents
  A. Leifson method
    1. Basic fuchsin, 1.2% in 95% alcohol
      a. Commercial product must be certified for flagellar stain.
      b. Pararosaniline acetate is preferred. If the dye solution is a mixture of pararosaniline acetate and pararosaniline hydrochloride, the hydrochloride compound must not compose more than two thirds of the solution.
      c. The stain must have the odor of acetic acid to be satisfactory.
      d. When new stain is prepared, at least 1 day must be allowed for the dye to enter completely into solution.
    2. Tannic acid, 3% in water
      a. The suspension must have a light yellow color to be satisfactory.
      b. Add phenol in a 1:200 concentration to discourage emergence of molds during storage.
    3. Sodium chloride, 1.5% in water
    4. Final stain
      a. Combine the three stock solutions in equal volumes. The stain is ready for use immediately after preparation and should be stored in a tightly stoppered bottle.
      b. A precipitate will form during storage. This should not be disturbed; rather, remove the staining solution from the top with a pipette.
      c. Shelf life of the staining solution is 1 week at room temperature, 1 month in the refrigerator, and indefinite if frozen.
  B. Ryu method
    1. Solution I
      a. 5% phenol, 10.0 mL
      b. Powdered tannic acid, 2.0 g
      c. Saturated aluminum potassium sulfate 12-hydrate (crystals) (prepare 14 g potassium alum in 100 mL distilled H_2O), 10.0 mL
    2. Solution II
      a. Saturated solution of crystal violet in alcohol (prepare 12 g in 100 mL of 95% ethanol)
    3. Final stain
      a. Ten parts of solution I (mordant) are mixed with one part of solution II and stored in a plastic bottle at room temperature.
III. Quality Control
  The following bacterial species may serve as controls:
  A. Positive: peritrichous, *Escherichia coli*; polar, monotrichous, *Pseudomonas aeruginosa*; multitrichous, *Burkholderia cepacia*
  B. Negative: *Acinetobacter baumannii*
IV. Procedure
  A. Leifson method
    1. Using a young culture on an appropriate agar medium, prepare a light suspension of the bacteria in water.
    2. Place 2 drops of the bacterial suspension toward one end of an acid-cleaned microscope slide. Allow to air-dry. With a wax pencil, draw a perpendicular line on the glass surface toward the opposite end from the dried suspension.
    3. Place the slide on a tilted rack and overlay the dried bacterial suspension with a thin film of stain. The wax pencil mark prevents the stain from running off the end of the slide.
    4. Stain for 5 to 15 minutes, allowing a precipitate to form as the alcohol evaporates. The staining time is decreased if the stain is fresh, if the room temperature is high, if there are air currents in the laboratory, or if the layer of stain is thin. The opposite effects increase the staining time.
    5. When a precipitate forms, rinse the slide gently with distilled water, drain off excess water, and allow to air dry.
  B. Ryu method
    1. Prepare the smear by picking up some young growth from carbohydrate-free culture medium on an inoculating needle and lightly touching the center of each of 2 drops of distilled water on a new, precleaned slide. Let the drops air dry at room temperature.
    2. Flood the air-dried smears with the staining solution for 1 to 5 minutes (some trial and error may be needed to determine the time that best produces satisfactory staining of the flagella, but avoids excessive debris in the background). Wash the staining solution off in tap water.

CHART 7-2

FLAGELLAR STAIN *continued*

3. After the smears have dried, examine them under the oil-immersion objective of the microscope. Cell bodies and flagella stain violet.

V. Results
A. Interpretation
Observe the stained slide under the oil-immersion (100×) objective of the microscope. Dark-staining red to blue-black flagella should be observed. Compare morphology with the photomicrographs provided in Leifson's *Atlas of Bacterial Flagellation*, cited in the bibliography, and see also, Fig. 7-3.

VI. Bibliography

Clark WA. A simplified Leifson flagella stain. J Clin Microbiol 1976;3:632–634.
Leifson E. Atlas of Bacterial Flagellation. New York: Academic Press, 1960.
Ryu E. A simple method of staining bacterial flagella. Kitasato Arch Exp Med 1937;14:218–219.

CHART 7-3

FLUORESCENCE-DENITRIFICATION

I. Principle
The ability to produce fluorescein pigment and to reduce nitrate or nitrite completely to nitrogen gas are two important characteristics in the identification of the pseudomonads and other nonfermentative bacilli. Fluorescence denitrification (FN) medium is formulated to detect these two characteristics. Fluorescence-lactose nitrate (FLN) medium is a modification in which lactose and phenol red indicator are added to permit detection of acid formed from utilization of lactose, which is helpful in identifying the strongly lactose-positive group of nonfermenters.

A. Fluorescence test
Fluorescein is an organic luminescent pigment that on excitation with ultraviolet light emits a green-yellow fluorescence. A few of the nonfermentative bacilli, notably *Pseudomonas aeruginosa*, are capable of producing fluorescein, detection of which is helpful in their identification. Fluorescence of colonies may not be detected on an ordinary isolation medium, such as blood agar or MacConkey agar; rather, media containing cationic salts, such as magnesium sulfate (included in FN medium), which act as activators or coactivators to intensify luminescence, often must be used.

B. Denitrification test
The reduction of nitrate to nitrogen gas (N_2) or nitrous oxide (N_2O) is called denitrification and is shown by the following chemical equation:

$$2\ NO_3^- + 10\ e^- + 12\ H^- \longrightarrow N_2 \uparrow + 6\ H_2O$$

In this reduction process, five electrons are accepted by the nitrate radical, resulting in formation of nitrogen gas and six molecules of water. The denitrification test is helpful in the separation of *Pseudomonas stutzeri* group (most strains are positive) from other nonfermentative bacilli (see Table 7-5).

II. Media and Reagents
A. The formula for FN medium is as follows:

Proteose peptone 3 (Difco Laboratories, Detroit MI)	1 g
Magnesium sulfate · 7H$_2$O	0.15 g
Dipotassium hydrogen phosphate	0.15 g
Potassium nitrate	0.2 g
Sodium nitrite	0.05 g
Agar	1.5 g
Distilled water to	100 mL

pH = 7.2

1. Suspend all the ingredients except the magnesium sulfate in distilled water. The magnesium sulfate is dissolved separately in a small amount of water before adding to the agar medium to avoid the formation of an insoluble precipitate.

2. If FLN medium is to be prepared, add 2 g of lactose and 0.002 g of phenol red indicator. Dispense 4 mL of medium into 13-mm screw-cap tubes and let solidify to give a deep and a slant of approximately equal length.

CHART 7-3

FLUORESCENCE-DENITRIFICATION *continued*

3. Sellers medium, available commercially, is also suitable for determination of fluorescence and denitrification by nonfermentative bacteria.

B. The formula for nitrate/nitrite reduction medium is as follows:

Heart infusion broth (Difco Laboratories, Detroit MI)*	25 g
Potassium nitrate C.P.	2 g
Distilled water to	1 L
pH = 7.0	

III. Quality Control

The following organisms are appropriate controls:

Positive fluorescence/positive denitrification: *Pseudomonas aeruginosa*

Negative fluorescence/positive denitrification: *Pseudomonas stutzeri*

Negative fluorescence/negative denitrification: *Escherichia coli*

IV. Procedure

Inoculate the medium by stabbing the deep with a heavy suspension of the culture and then streaking the slant. Incubate at 35°C for 24 to 48 hours.

V. Results

A. Interpretation

Examine the tube for fluorescence with an ultraviolet light source (Wood's lamp). A bright yellow-green glow constitutes a positive test. The presence of gas bubbles in the deep of the medium indicates that nitrogen gas has been produced from denitrification, and a yellow slant with FLN medium indicates acid has been produced from the utilization of lactose by the microorganism. In broth medium, nitrogen gas formation is detected by noting the presence of a gas bubble in the upper portion of the inverted Durham tube, Color Plate 7-2B.

VI. Bibliography

Pickett MJ, Pedersen MM. Screening procedure for partial identification of nonfermentative bacilli associated with man. Appl Microbiol 1968;16:1631–1632.

---

* Agar is omitted from broth medium and inverted Durham tubes added to detect gas.

CHART 7-4

ESCULIN HYDROLYSIS TEST

I. Principle

Esculin medium without bile is useful in differentiating several species on nonfermenting bacilli. Esculin is a substituted glucoside that can be hydrolyzed by certain bacteria to yield glucose and esculetin. Esculin is a fluorescent compound that fluoresces under long-wave UV light at 360 nm. When esculin is hydrolyzed, fluorescence is lost, and the medium turns black due to the reaction of esculetin with the ferric ions in the medium. Several species of *Chryseobacterium, Sphingobacterium,* as well as *C. luteola, B. vesicularis, S. paucimobilis, S. maltophilia, R. radiobacter,* and some species of *B. cepacia, B. pseudomallei,* and *O. anthropi* are esculin-positive.

II. Media and Reagents

The formula for esculin medium is as follows:

Esculin Agar Modified:

Esculin	1 g
Ferric citrate	0.5 g
Heart infusion agar	40 g
Distilled water to	1 L

CHART 7-4

ESCULIN HYDROLYSIS TEST *continued*

Esculin Broth:

Heart muscle, infusion	10 g
Peptic digest of animal tissue	10 g
Sodium chloride	5 g
Esculin	1 g
Distilled water to	1 L

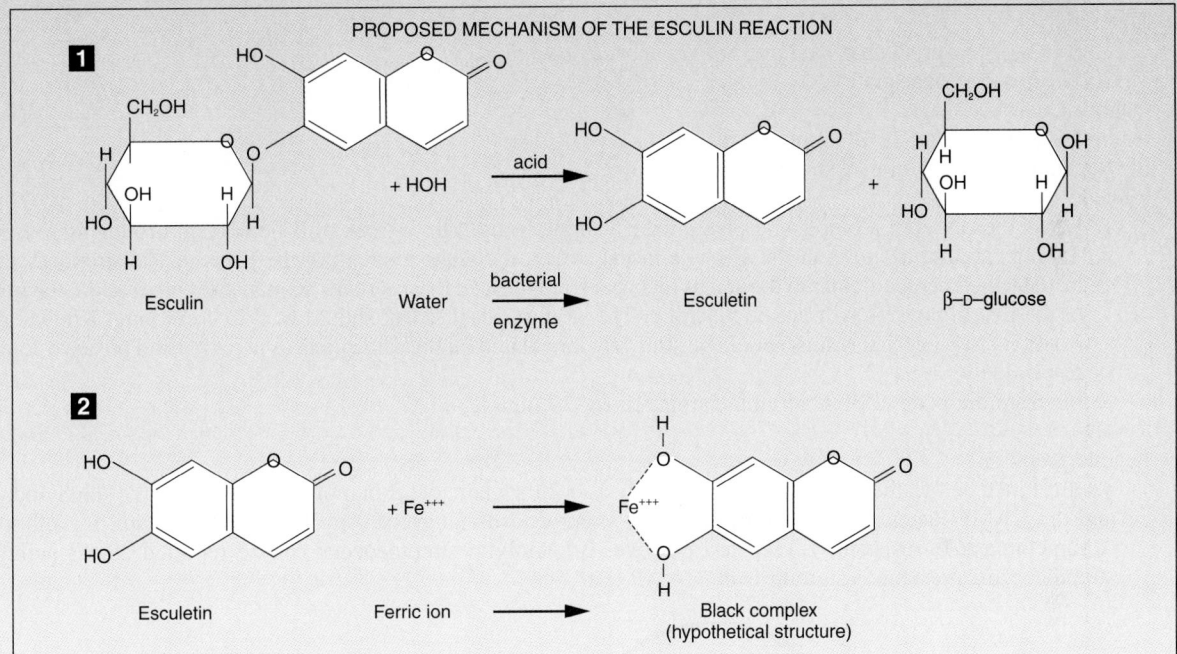

PROPOSED MECHANISM OF THE ESCULIN REACTION

1 Esculin + Water → (acid / bacterial enzyme) → Esculetin + β–D–glucose

2 Esculetin + Ferric ion → Black complex (hypothetical structure)

III. Quality Control
   A. Positive control: *Aeromonas hydrophila* ATCC 7965
   B. Negative control: *P. aeruginosa* ATCC 27853
IV. Procedure
   After touching the center of one well-isolated colony with a sterile inoculation loop or wooden stick, inoculate the organism onto the surface of the agar slant or into the broth. Incubate for 18 to 24 hours at 35°C.
 V. Results
   A. Interpretation
      The development of a black color or the loss of fluorescence under UV light (360 nm) is interpreted as a positive test. Fluorescence or lack of a black color is interpreted as a negative test (Color Plate 7-2 E).
VI. Bibliography
   MacFaddin JF. Biochemical Tests for Identification of Medical Bacteria. Ed. 2. Baltimore: Williams & Wilkins, 1980:4–12.
   Shigei J. Test methods used in the identification of commonly isolated aerobic gram-negative bacteria. In: Isenberg HH, ed. Clinical Microbiology Procedures Handbook. Vol. 1. Washington DC: American Society for Microbiology, 1992;1.19.38–1.19.40.

CHART 8-1

THE CAMP TEST

I. Principle

The presumptive identification of group B β-hemolytic streptococci can be done with the CAMP test, which is reliable and easy to perform. The hemolytic phenomenon was first described in 1944 by Christie, Atkins, and Munch-Petersen, and it is their names that provide the acronym (CAMP) for the test.

   The hemolytic activity of the β-hemolysin produced by most strains of *Staphylococcus aureus* is enhanced by an extracellular protein produced by group B streptococci. Interaction of the β-hemolysin with this factor causes "synergistic hemolysis," which is easily observed on a blood agar plate. This phenomenon is seen with both hemolytic and nonhemolytic isolates of group B streptococci.

II. Materials
   1. β-hemolysin-producing strain of *Staphylococcus aureus*
   2. Sheep blood agar plate

III. Quality Control
   A. Positive control: group B streptococcus
   B. Negative control: group A streptococcus

IV. Procedure
   1. Down the center of a blood agar plate, make a single straight line streak of β-hemolysin-producing *S. aureus*.
   2. Taking care not to intersect the staphylococcal streak, inoculate a streak of the β-hemolytic streptococcus to be identified perpendicular to the staphylococcal streak. Make these streaks so that, after incubation, the growth of the two organisms will not be touching. The streptococcal streak should be 3 to 4 cm long. Known group A and B streptococcal strains should be similarly inoculated on the same plate as negative and positive controls, respectively.
   3. Incubate the plate at 35°C in ambient air for 18–24 hours.

V. Results
   A. Interpretation
   As illustrated below, the area of increased hemolysis occurs where the β-hemolysin secreted by the staphylococcus and the CAMP factor secreted by the group B streptococcus intersect. Any bacitracin-resistant, trimethoprim-sulfamethoxazole–resistant, CAMP test-positive, β-hemolytic streptococcus can be reported as "β-hemolytic streptococcus, presumptive group B by CAMP test."

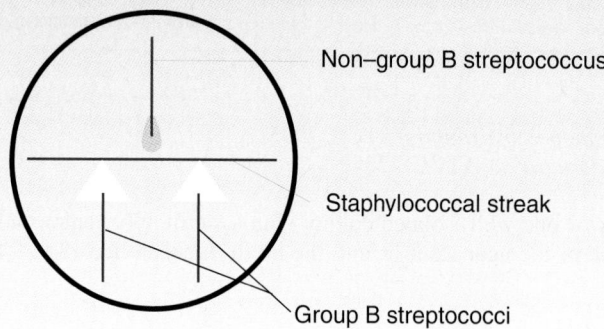

Non–group B streptococcus

Staphylococcal streak

Group B streptococci

VI. Limitations

Some group A streptococci will be CAMP test–positive if the test plate is incubated in a candle jar, in a CO_2 atmosphere, or under anaerobic conditions. Therefore, ambient-air incubation should be used.

CHART 9-1

TEST FOR X AND V FACTOR REQUIREMENTS

I. Principle

X factor (hemin, hematin) and V factor (NAD) are required either singly or in combination to support the growth of various species of *Haemophilus* on agar media. Filter paper strips or disks impregnated with X and V factors are commercially available.

X and V factors, each being water-soluble, readily diffuse in agar culture media. Filter paper disks or strips impregnated with these factors are placed on the surface of a medium deficient in these factors, such as trypticase-soy or brain-heart infusion agar, which has been inoculated as a lawn with the test organism. Factor requirements of the organism are then determined, after overnight incubation, by observing the patterns of growth around the paper strips or disks (see following illustration).

II. Media and Reagents

    1. Paper strips or disks impregnated with X and V factors

    2. An agar medium deficient in X and V factors. Trypticase-soy or brain-heart infusion agars are suitable

    3. Brain-heart infusion broth

III. Quality Control

    A. *Haemophilus parainfluenzae:* requires V factor only

    B. *Haemophilus influenzae:* requires both X and V factors

IV. Procedure

    1. From a pure culture of the organism to be identified, prepare a light suspension of the growth in the brain-heart infusion broth. Be careful when transferring the growth not to pick up any of the hemin-containing medium from the culture plate. From this suspension, inoculate the surface of the factor-deficient agar medium.

    2. Place an X and a V factor strip on the surface of the agar in the area of inoculation.

    3. Position the strips about 1 cm apart.

    4. Incubate the plate in 3–5% CO_2 at 35°C for 18 to 24 hours.

V. Results

    A. Interpretation

Visually inspect the agar surface, observing closely for visible growth between or around one or more of the strips or disks. The following patterns indicate the need for X factor only (*left*), V factor only (*center*), or both X and V factors (*right*):

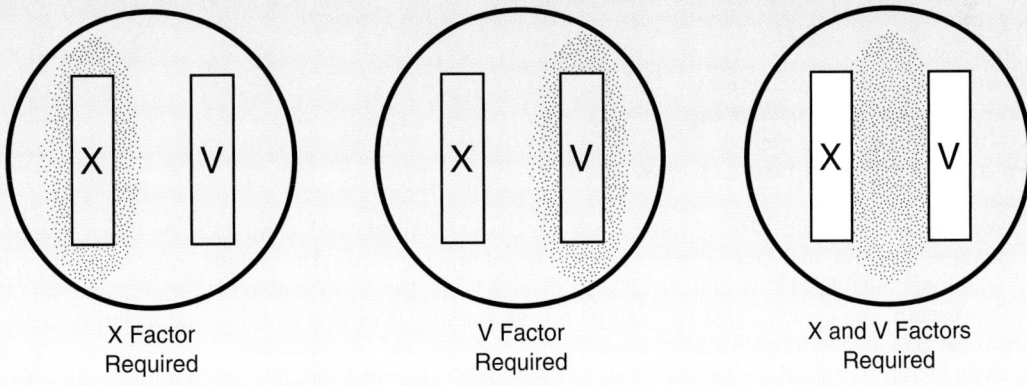

| X Factor Required | V Factor Required | X and V Factors Required |

VI. Bibliography

Parker RH, Hoeprich PD. Disk method for rapid identification of *Haemophilus* sp. Am J Clin Pathol 1963;37: 319–327.

CHART 11-1

RAPID CARBOHYDRATE UTILIZATION TEST FOR IDENTIFICATION OF *NEISSERIA* SPECIES

I. Principle

The rapid carbohydrate utilization test procedures have largely supplanted the use of cystine-tryptic digest semisolid agar with carbohydrates for the identification of *Neisseria* species. The procedure described is a modification of the procedure described in *Cumitech 4* from the American Society for Microbiology.

The rapid carbohydrate utilization test uses a balanced phosphate-buffered saline solution containing phenol red indicator. Small (0.10-mL) aliquots of the buffer are distributed in a series of tubes, one for each carbohydrate tested. Single drops of the individual carbohydrates (20% w/v) are added to individual tubes. A heavy suspension of the organism to be tested is prepared in the buffer without carbohydrates, and one drop of this suspension is added to each of the carbohydrate tubes. After 4 hours of incubation, the reactions are interpreted. Production of acid from carbohydrates is indicated by a change in the color of the phenol red indicator from red to yellow.

II. Media and Reagents

A. Phosphate balanced salts solution (BBS): a 10× stock solution having the following formula:

K_2HPO_4	0.40 g
KH_2PO_4	0.10 g
KCl	8.0 g
Distilled water	100 mL

Filter sterilize and store at 4 to 8°C

B. Working Solution

Add 10 mL of the 10× BSS to 90 mL of distilled water. After this, 0.5 to 0.8 mL of a 1% aqueous solution of phenol red is added to the solution, so that the final product is "cherry red." This working solution is then filter-sterilized. To ensure that the distilled water is the proper pH, the use of pharmacy-grade sterile distilled water is recommended.

C. Stock Carbohydrate Solutions

Weigh out 10 g each of glucose, maltose, sucrose, and lactose (and, if desired, fructose) individually. Each is dissolved in 50 mL of distilled water. The solutions are filter-sterilized, dispensed into sterile vials, and frozen at 20°C. It is important that "reagent-grade" carbohydrates be used, because the maltose from some bacteriologic media vendors may be contaminated with glucose. Carbohydrates may be obtained from Sigma Chemical Company (St. Louis, MO), Fisher Scientific Company (Fairlawn, NJ), or Mallinckrodt Chemical Works (St Louis, MO).

III. Quality Control

A. Positive glucose: *N. gonorrhoeae*

B. Positive maltose: *N. meningitidis*

C. Positive lactose: *N. lactamica*

D. Positive sucrose and fructose: *N. mucosa*

IV. Procedure

1. A series of nonsterile 12 × 75-mm tubes are labeled with the carbohydrate to be tested. Generally, glucose, maltose, sucrose, and lactose are tested. Some laboratories will also include fructose in the test battery. An additional tube, labeled with the isolate or specimen number, is also included for preparation of the inoculum.

2. For each of the carbohydrate tubes, 0.10 mL of working BSS is added. For the inoculum tube, 0.30 to 0.40 mL of BSS is placed in the tube.

3. A single drop of each of the carbohydrates is added to the appropriately labeled tube with a Pasteur pipette.

4. A heavy suspension of the organism to be tested is prepared in the inoculum tube using a sterile bacteriologic loop. The inoculum is prepared from an 18- to 24-hour, pure chocolate agar subculture of the organism. The inoculum suspension is carefully vortexed to obtain a uniform, heavy suspension.

5. Single drops of the inoculum suspension are added to each of the carbohydrate-containing tubes. The tubes are briefly agitated to ensure thorough mixing and are placed in an incubator or water bath at 35°C for 4 hours.

V. Results

A. Interpretation

The development of a yellow color in any of the carbohydrate-containing tubes indicates utilization of that carbohydrate by the organism. Negative carbohydrate-utilization tests remain red or red-orange.

VI. Bibliography

Janda WM. Identification of *Neisseria* species and *Branhamella catarrhalis.* In: Identification of Aerobic Gram-Positive and Gram-Negative Cocci. Washington DC: American Society for Microbiology, 1986:115–131.

Kellogg DS, Holmes KK, Hill GA. Cumitech 4. In: Marcus S, Sherris JC, eds. Laboratory Diagnosis of Gonorrhea. Washington DC: American Society for Microbiology, 1976.

CHART 12-1

FURAZOLIDONE DISK TEST

I. Principle
There are several methods available for differentiation of staphylococci from micrococci (Table 12-1). One of these is susceptibility to the compound furoxone (also called furazolidone). This test is performed as a disk susceptibility procedure: staphylococci are susceptible to this compound, whereas micrococci are resistant.

II. Reagents
1. Furazolidone disks, 100 μg (FX 100, BD Microbiology Systems, Franklin Lakes, NJ)
2. Sheep blood agar plate

III. Quality Control
Known strains of *Staphylococcus* (either *S. aureus* or a coagulase-negative strain) and *Micrococcus* species should be tested with each new lot of disks, or on a weekly basis.

IV. Procedure
1. Prepare a suspension of the organism to be tested in sterile distilled water or broth. The suspension should be equivalent to a 0.5 MacFarland turbidity standard.
2. With a swab, spread the organism suspension onto one-half of a blood agar plate.
3. Aseptically place an FX disk in the center of the inoculated area, and gently tamp the disk so it adheres to the agar surface.
4. Incubate the plate at 35°C in an ambient-air incubator for 18 to 24 hours.

V. Results
A. Interpretation
1. *Micrococcus* species are FX-resistant and will have zones of 6 mm (no zone) to 9 mm.
2. *Staphylococcus* species are FX-susceptible and will have zones of inhibition of 15 mm or larger.

CHART 12-2

NOVOBIOCIN DISK TEST

I. Principle
Coagulase-negative staphylococci can be divided into novobiocin-susceptible and novobiocin-resistant species. Among the novobiocin-resistant species, *S. saprophyticus* is the one commonly recovered from humans as a cause of urinary tract infections. Therefore, screening coagulase-negative staphylococci isolated from quantitative urine cultures for susceptibility to novobiocin provides a reliable presumptive identification of this species.

II. Reagents
1. Novobiocin disks, 5 μg (NB 5, BD Microbiology Systems, Franklin Lakes, NJ)
2. Sheep blood agar plate

III. Quality Control
A known *S. saprophyticus* strain and a *S. epidermidis* strain should be tested with each new lot of novobiocin disks or on a weekly basis.

IV. Procedure
1. Prepare a suspension of the organism to be identified in sterile distilled water or broth.
2. The suspension should be equivalent in turbidity to a 0.5 McFarland standard.
3. With a sterile swab, spread some of the suspension over half of a blood agar plate.
4. Aseptically place a novobiocin disk on the inoculated area. Susceptibility to furazolidone (see Chart 12-1) may be assessed on the same plate by placing the disks about 4 cm apart on the inoculated area. Gently tamp the disk(s) with sterile forceps to assure contact with the agar surface.
5. Incubate the plate aerobically for 18 to 24 hours at 35°C.

V. Results
A. Interpretation
1. *S. saprophyticus* are novobiocin-resistant and will show zones of inhibition of 6 mm (no zone) to 12 mm.
2. Other coagulase-negative staphylococci and *S. aureus* are novobiocin-susceptible and will show zones of 16 mm or larger.

CHART 13-1

BACITRACIN AND SXT SUSCEPTIBILITY TESTS

I. Principle

Susceptibility to low concentrations of the polypeptide antibiotic bacitracin and to the combination sulfonamide trimethoprim-sulfamethoxazole (SXT) provides an easy and inexpensive method for the presumptive identification of both group A and group B β-hemolytic streptococci. Although still used in many laboratories, this test has largely been supplanted by reliable and relatively inexpensive serologic procedures.

Group A streptococci are susceptible to relatively low concentrations of bacitracin and are resistant to SXT. Group B streptococci are resistant to both antibiotics. Other β-hemolytic streptococci show varying susceptibility to bacitracin, but these organisms are usually susceptible to SXT. Therefore, the performance of the SXT test along with the bacitracin test increases the sensitivity and predictive value of the bacitracin test.

II. Reagents
   A. Sheep blood agar plate
   B. Taxo ''A'' bacitracin differential disks (0.04 units/disk)
   C. SXT disks (trimethoprim-sulfamethoxazole, 1.25 μg/23.75 μg)

III. Quality Control
   A. Bacitracin S, SXT R: Group A streptococcus
   B. Bacitracin R, SXT R: Group B streptococcus
   C. Bacitracin S or R, SXT S: β-Hemolytic streptococcus, groups C, F, or G

IV. Procedure
   1. Pick three to four isolated colonies of the β-hemolytic streptococcus and streak the inoculum down the center of half of a blood agar plate.
   2. Using a sterile swab or a bacteriologic loop spread the inoculum as a lawn over the entire half of the plate.
   3. Aseptically place a Taxo ''A'' bacitracin disk and an SXT disk on the inoculated area. Make sure that the disks are spaced evenly. Using flamed forceps, gently tamp down the disks so that they adhere to the agar surface.
   4. Incubate the plate in ambient air at 35°C.

V. Results
   A. Interpretation
      1. Susceptible (S): Any zone around either of the disks
      2. Resistant (R): Growth up to the edge of the disk

Bacitracin	SXT	Identification
S	R	Presumptive Group A
R	R	Presumptive Group B
S/R	S	Not groups A or B

   3. Results should be reported as ''β-hemolytic streptococci, presumptive group A, by bacitracin/SXT,'' or ''β-hemolytic streptococci, presumptively not group A by bacitracin/SXT.''
   4. Because these tests are generally performed on throat isolates, for which group A streptococci are being sought, the presumptive group B is generally not reported.

VI. Limitations of Test

Only β-hemolytic streptococci should be tested, because many α-hemolytic streptococci (including pneumococci) are susceptible to low concentrations of bacitracin.

No data are available to indicate that zones of inhibition should be measured. Interpretation of SXT susceptibility may be difficult, because the organisms may grow slightly before total inhibition of growth occurs.

The lawn of bacterial inoculum should be confluent. Too light an inoculum will cause non-group A streptococci to appear susceptible to bacitracin.

CHART 13-2

BILE-ESCULIN TEST

I. Principle

The bile-esculin test is based on the ability of certain bacteria, notably the group D streptococci and *Enterococcus* species, to hydrolyze esculin in the presence of bile (4% bile salts or 40% bile). Esculin is a glycosidic coumarin derivative (6-β-glucoside-7-hydroxy-coumarin). The two moieties of the molecule (glucose and 7-hydroxycoumarin) are linked together by an ester bond through oxygen. For this test, esculin is incorporated into a medium containing 4% bile salts.

Bacteria that are bile-esculin-positive are, first of all, able to grow in the presence of bile salts. Hydrolysis of the esculin in the medium results in the formation of glucose and a compound called esculetin. Esculetin, in turn, reacts with ferric ions (supplied by the inorganic medium component ferric citrate) to form a black diffusible complex.

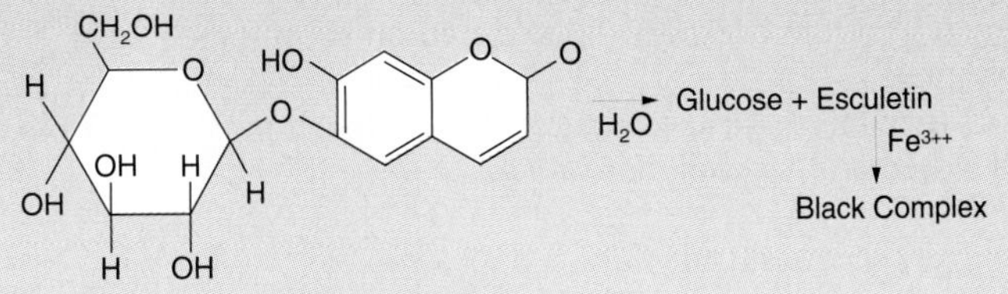

Esculin

II. Materials

A. Medium

Bile-esculin agar medium is prepared as agar slants or plates. The medium has the following formula:

Peptone	5 g
Beef extract	3 g
Oxgall (bile)	40 g
Esculin	1 g
Ferric citrate	0.5 g
Agar	15 g
Distilled water	1 L
pH = 7.0	

III. Quality Controls

A. Positive control: *Enterococcus* species (e.g., *E. faecalis*)

B. Negative control: Viridans streptococcus, not group D

IV. Procedure

1. With an inoculating wire or loop, touch two or three morphologically similar streptococcal colonies and inoculate the slant of the bile esculin medium with an S-shaped motion, or streak the surface of a bile esculin plate for isolation.

2. Incubate the tube or plate at 35°C for 24–48 hours in an ambient air incubator.

V. Results

A. Interpretation

Diffuse blackening of more than half of the slant within 24–48 hours indicates esculin hydrolysis. On plates, black haloes will be observed around isolated colonies and any blackening is considered positive. All group D streptococci will be bile-esculin-positive within 48 hours.

VI. Limitations of Test

Some viridans streptococci (approx. 3%) may also hydrolyze esculin in the presence of bile.

CHART 13-3

OPTOCHIN SUSCEPTIBILITY TEST

I. Principle

Ethylhydrocupreine hydrochloride (optochin), a quinine derivative, selectively inhibits the growth of *Streptococcus pneumoniae* at very low concentrations (5 µg/mL or less). Optochin may also inhibit other viridans streptococci, but only at much higher concentrations. The test has a sensitivity of more than 95%, is simple to perform, and is inexpensive.

Optochin is water-soluble and diffuses readily into agar medium. Therefore, filter paper disks impregnated with optochin can be used in a disk diffusion test format to determine susceptibility of suspected pneumococci and, thereby, confirm their identity as such. *S. pneumoniae* cells surrounding the disk are lysed owing to changes in the surface tension, and a zone of inhibition is produced.

II. Media and Reagents

    1. Well-isolated colonies of the organism to be tested on sheep blood agar

    2. Sheep blood agar plate

    3. Optochin disks (5 µg): Bacto Differentiation Disks, Optochin (Difco) Taxo ''P'' disks (BD Microbiology)

    4. Disks should be stored at 4°C when not in use.

III. Quality Control

    A. Positive control: *Streptococcus pneumoniae*

    B. Negative control: Viridans streptococcus or *Enterococcus faecalis*

IV. Procedure

    1. Using an inoculating loop or wire, select three to four well-isolated colonies of the organism to be tested and streak onto one-half to a one-third of a blood agar plate. The inoculated area should be about 3 cm².

    2. Place an optochin disk in the upper third of the streaked area. Tamp down the disk with flamed forceps so that the disk adheres firmly to the agar surface.

    3. Incubate the plate at 35°C for 18 to 24 hours in a candle jar or in 5–7% CO_2.

V. Results

    A. Interpretation

    A viridans streptococcus can be presumptively identified as *S. pneumoniae* if it shows a zone of inhibition of 14 mm or more around a 6-mm (Taxo A) disk, or a zone of 16 mm or more around a 10-mm disk (Bacto). Organisms showing zones smaller than these should be tested for bile solubility.

VI. Limitations of Procedure

Occasionally, viridans streptococci will show small zones of inhibition around the optochin disk. These organisms, however, will not be bile-soluble.

CHART 13-4

SALT-TOLERANCE TEST

I. Principle

Ability to grow in the presence of variable amounts of sodium chloride (NaCl) is a test that has been used to characterize several bacteria, including the viridans streptococci. It is particularly useful, however, for presumptive identification of the enterococcal group D organisms, which have the specific ability to grow in the presence of 6.5% NaCl incorporated into either a broth or an agar medium. This test, along with the bile-esculin test, is used in many laboratories to distinguish *Enterococcus* species from the group D streptococci, *S. bovis* and *S. equinus*.

Heart infusion broth is a general-purpose nutritional broth that is used for the cultivation of many bacteria. It normally contains 0.5% NaCl. By increasing the salt concentration to 6.5%, the medium becomes semiselective for the growth of enterococci.

II. Medium

    1. 6.5% NaCl broth has the following formula:

Heart infusion broth	25 g
Sodium chloride	60 g
Indicator (1.6 g of bromcresol purple in 100 mL of 95% ethanol)	1 mL
Glucose	1 g
Distilled water	1 L

CHART 13-4

SALT-TOLERANCE TEST *continued*

    2. The indicator may be omitted.

    3. Dispense into tubes in 3- to 5-mL volumes and autoclave at 121°C for 15 minutes.

III. Quality Control

    A. Positive growth: *Enterococcus faecalis*

    B. Negative growth: *Streptococcus bovis*

IV. Procedure

    1. Inoculate two or three colonies into broth.

    2. Incubate overnight at 35°C in ambient-air incubator.

V. Results

    A. Interpretation

    A positive test is the presence of obvious bacterial growth in the medium, with or without a color change in the indicator. If the organism is bile-esculin-positive and grows in the 6.5% NaCl broth, the organism is an *Enterococcus* species. If the organism is bile-esculin-positive and fails to grow in the 6.5% NaCl broth, the organism is a group D streptococcus.

VI. Limitations of Procedure

    1. If the medium is inoculated too heavily, inoculum may be interpreted as growth, resulting in a false-positive reaction.

    2. To prevent interpretation of the test falsely as negative, agitate the tube gently before reading, as the growth may settle out during incubation.

    3. Up to 80% of group B streptococci may be salt-tolerant, as will occasional isolates of group A streptococci. Aerococci may also be bile-esculin–positive and may grow in 6.5% NaCl.

CHART 14-1

LOEFFLER'S METHYLENE BLUE STAIN

I. Principle

Methylene blue is a simple stain that is particularly useful in the identification of *Corynebacterium* species.

    The metachromatic granules of *C. diphtheriae* readily take up methylene blue dye and appear deep blue. Although some authors have stated that the cytoplasmic granule formation characteristic of *C. diphtheriae* is rarely seen with saprophytic species of *Corynebacterium,* this criterion is unreliable and cannot be used for definitive identification of *C. diphtheriae* without further studies.

II. Media and Reagents

Methylene blue (80% dye content)	0.3 g
Ethyl alcohol (95%)	30 mL
Distilled water	100 mL

III. Procedure

    1. Heat-fix the smear. Flood the surface of the smear with the methylene blue-staining solution for 1 minute. Wash the slide with water and blot dry.

    2. In the past it was necessary to add alkali to the above solution before use. However, methylene blue dyes prepared in recent years do not require this additional step because acid impurities found in older stains have been removed.

IV. Results

    A. Interpretation

    The corynebacteria are pleomorphic bacilli that range in size from 0.5 to 1.0 μm in width and from 2 to 6 μm in length and appear as straight, curved, or club-shaped rods. Characteristic for the microorganisms are the metachromatic granules that take up the methylene blue stain and appear dark blue. Although this finding is characteristic of the corynebacteria, species of *Propionibacterium,* some of the actinomycetes, pleomorphic strains of streptococci, and other bacteria may also morphologically resemble the corynebacteria and must be differentiated by other cultural and biochemical characteristics.

CHART 14-2

LOEFFLER'S SERUM MEDIUM

I. Principle

Loeffler's serum medium is used primarily for the recovery of *C. diphtheriae* from clinical specimens. Because of this serum content, the medium may also be used more generally to determine the proteolytic activity of various microorganisms.

C. diphtheriae produces cells with characteristic morphologic features on Loeffler medium. The medium is also helpful in the determination of pigment production by some bacteria.

II. Media and Reagents

A. Formula

Beef serum	70 g/L
Infusion dextrose broth (dry powder)	2.5 g/L
Egg (whole, dried)	7.5 g/L
Final pH = 7.6	

B. Preparation

1. To rehydrate the medium, dissolve 80 g of Loeffler medium (BBL) in 1 L of distilled water and warm to 42 to 45°C. The powder should be gradually added while the flask is gently rotated to minimize mixing air into the suspension.

2. The medium should be dispensed in tubes and coagulated-sterilized in the autoclave as follows:

   a. When the suspension is uniform, dispense in tubes.

   b. Arrange the tubes in a slant position not more than four deep with several layers of newspaper or paper towels below and above the tubes to prevent rapid coagulation.

   c. Tightly close the autoclave, turn on the steam, and allow pressure to remain at 10 psi for 20 minutes.

   d. During this time allow no air or steam to escape.

   e. Adjust the steam-inlet valve and open the air-escape valve such as to maintain a pressure of 10 psi. Abrupt changes in pressure may cause the medium to bubble.

   f. Close the outlet valve when all air has been replaced by steam and allow the pressure to reach 15 psi and hold there for 15 minutes.

   g. Allow the autoclave to cool slowly. When properly prepared the slants are smooth and grayish white. Before inoculation, the slants should be incubated for 24 hours at 35°C as a sterility check.

III. Procedure

1. When *C. diphtheriae* is suspected, inoculate the Loeffler medium as soon as possible after collection of the specimen.

2. Examine the slants for growth after 8 to 24 hours of incubation.

3. Prepare smears and stain with methylene blue.

IV. Results

A. Interpretation

See Chart 14-1 for interpretation of these stained smears.

V. Comment

Because Loeffler's medium is difficult to prepare, purchase of commercially prepared medium in sealed tubes is recommended.

VI. Bibliography

BBL Manual of Products and Laboratory Procedures. Ed. 5. Cockeysville, MD: BBL, Division of Becton, Dickinson, and Co, 1973:118–119.

Buck T. A modified Loeffler's medium for cultivating *Corynebacterium diphtheriae*. J Lab Clin Med 1949;34: 582–583.

CHART 14-3

TINSDALES' AGAR (AS MODIFIED BY MOORE AND PARSONS)

I. Principle

Tinsdale medium supports the growth of all species of *Corynebacterium* while inhibiting the growth of normal inhabitants of the upper respiratory tract. Moore and Parsons modified the original Tinsdale formula, simplifying the composition, but retaining the specificity for the recovery of *C. diphtheriae* and *C. ulcerans*.

The potassium tellurite is deposited within the colonies of *Corynebacterium*, turning them black. Tinsdale medium is cystine-sodium thiosulfate tellurite, which is specifically helpful in the identification of *C. diphtheriae*, colonies of which are surrounded by a brown halo (see Color Plate 14-2*F*).

II. Media and Reagents
   A. Formula (modified Tinsdale base)

Thiotone peptone	20 g
Sodium chloride	5 g
Agar	14 g
L-Cystine	0.24 g
Sodium thiosulfate	0.24 g
Distilled water	1 L

   B. Preparation
      1. Suspend 39 g of powder in 1 L of distilled water and heat with agitation. Boil for 1 minute. Autoclave for 15 minutes at 121°C.
      2. Cool the modified base to 50°C and add:

Sterile bovine serum	100 mL
Tellurite solution, 1%	30 mL

      3. Pour 15 to 20 mL of this medium into petri dishes and allow to harden.
      4. The Tinsdale agar base medium without serum and tellurite is stable indefinitely if stored in closed screw-capped tubes or bottles. However, the medium is ordinarily stable for only 2 or 3 days when stored in the refrigerator following the addition of serum and tellurite.

III. Procedure

Streak the plate so as to obtain well-isolated colonies. It is recommended that the agar be stabbed at intervals, because browning of the medium can be detected early in the stab areas.

IV. Results
   A. Interpretation

   A brown halo around the colony is considered presumptive evidence of *C. diphtheriae*. This can sometimes be seen after 10 to 12 hours of incubation, although 48 hours may be required for the appearance of typical dark-brown halos. The only related species other than *C. diphtheriae* that produces this halo is *C. ulcerans*. Other bacteria, such as coagulase-positive staphylococci, grow well on this medium, but do not have a brown halo. Bacteria, such as species of *Proteus* that produce a heavy, diffuse blackening of the medium, can be distinguished by their Gram stain reaction and biochemical characteristics.

V. Bibliography

Moore MS, Parsons EI. A study of modified Tinsdale's medium for the primary isolation of *Corynebacterium diphtheriae*. J Infect Dis 1958;102:88–93.

Tinsdale GFW. A new medium for the isolation and identification of *C. diphtheriae* based on production of hydrogen sulfide. J Pathol Bacteriol 1947;59:61–66.

CHART 14-4

CYSTINE-TELLURITE BLOOD AGAR

I. Principle
Cystine-tellurite blood agar is a medium used for the primary isolation of *Corynebacterium diphtheriae*. It has advantages over Tinsdale medium in being easier to prepare and having a longer shelf life.

The potassium tellurite in this medium serves to inhibit growth of most normal bacterial inhabitants of the upper respiratory tract, including most species of *Streptococcus* and *Staphylococcus*. *C. diphtheriae* grows well, producing grayish or black colonies after 24 to 48 hours of incubation.

II. Media and Reagents
   A. *Formula*

Heart infusion agar, 2% solution	100 mL
Potassium tellurite, 0.3% solution	15 mL
L-Cystine	5 mg
Sheep blood	5 mL

   B. *Preparation*
   Melt the sterile heart infusion agar solution and cool to 45°C or 50°C. Carefully maintain this temperature while performing subsequent steps. Aseptically add the sterile potassium tellurite solution (previously sterilized by autoclaving) and the sheep blood. Mix thoroughly. Add the cystine powder, mix well, and pour the medium into sterile petri dishes. Rotate the flask frequently while pouring into plates because the cystine does not go entirely into solution.

III. Procedure
Streak the plate with the clinical material to be cultured to obtain well-isolated colonies.

IV. Results
   A. Interpretation
   C. diphtheriae develops gray or black colonies after 24 to 48 hours of incubation. On occasion, colonies of staphylococci not inhibited by the medium also appear black; however, these can be distinguished by their characteristic Gram stain reaction.

   Three biotypes of *C. diphtheriae* can be distinguished on cystine-tellurite blood agar: 1) biotype *gravis* colonies are flat, dark gray with radial striations, and dry and have an irregular edge; 2) biotype *mitis* colonies are small, black, shiny, and convex with an entire edge and have a moist appearance; 3) biotype *intermedius* colonies are small and flat and have a raised, black center.

V. Bibliography
Frobisher M Jr. Cystine-tellurite agar for *C. diphtheriae*. J Infect Dis 1937;60:99–105.

CHART 15-1

HYDROLYSIS OF XANTHINE, HYPOXANTHINE, TYROSINE, AND CASEIN

I. Principle
Aerobic actinomycetes may be characterized by their ability to hydrolyze xanthine, hypoxanthine, tyrosine, and casein. These compounds are incorporated into nutrient agar, and the organisms are seeded heavily on the agar surface. Results are interpreted by observing for clearing of the medium under and around the bacterial growth, indicating hydrolysis.

II. Media and Reagents
   A. Xanthine, hypoxanthine, and tyrosine suspensions
      1. Basal Medium

Beef extract	3.0 g
Peptone	5.0 g
Agar	15.0 g
Distilled water	1 L

CHART 15-1

HYDROLYSIS OF XANTHINE, HYPOXANTHINE, TYROSINE, AND CASEIN *continued*

2. Suspensions

Tyrosine	0.5 g
Xanthine	0.4 g
Hypoxanthine	0.4 g
Distilled water	100 mL

Heat the basal medium to bring the ingredients into solution and place 100-mL aliquots into 250-mL flasks. Sterilize by autoclaving at 15 psi for 15 minutes. Allow medium to cool almost to solidification. To each aliquot, add 10 mL of xanthine, hypoxanthine, or tyrosine suspensions. The suspensions are autoclaved before adding to the basal media. It is essential that the granules of xanthine, tyrosine, and hypoxanthine be kept in suspension until the medium solidifies; hence, the addition of the biochemical granules and the pouring of the medium into Petri dishes should be done when the basal medium has cooled just short of solidification. The media are poured into sterile 15 × 100-mm Petri dishes.

3. Casein Medium
   a. Solution A

(1) Skim milk (powdered)	10.0 g
(2) Distilled water	100 mL

   b. Solution B

(1) Agar	2.0 g
(2) Distilled water	100 mL

Autoclave solutions A and B separately, allow each to cool to about 50°C, and combine A with B and pour into 15 × 100-mm Petri dishes.

III. Quality Control
    A. Negative control: *Nocardia asteroides*
    B. Positive control: *Streptomyces* species
IV. Procedure
    Each xanthine, hypoxanthine, tyrosine, and casein plate is commonly divided into wedge-shaped thirds, providing an area to inoculate positive and negative controls along with the organism to be identified. The plates are incubated at 30°C and read at the following times:
    A. Casein hydrolysis: Read after 2 weeks
    B. Xanthine hydrolysis: Read after 3 weeks
    C. Hypoxanthine hydrolysis: Read after 3 weeks
    D. Tyrosine hydrolysis: Read after 3 weeks
 V. Interpretation
    Casein hydrolysis is read by observing for a complete clearing to transparency of the white, milky medium. The other three hydrolysis tests are read by observing the dissolution of the crystalline compounds around the colonies growing on the media.
VI. Bibliography
    Gordon RE, Mihm JM. Identification of *Nocardia caviae* (Erickson) nov. comb. Ann NY Acad Sci 1962;98:628–636.

CHART 17-1

DISK DIFFUSION (BAUER-KIRBY) SUSCEPTIBILITY TEST FOR NONFASTIDIOUS BACTERIA

I. Principle

Continued evaluation and revision of the disk diffusion procedure has been performed by a committee of the Clinical Laboratory Standards Institute (formerly, the National Committee for Clinical Laboratory Standards). Designating a national standard test for disk diffusion has not only permitted more exacting quality control, but has also allowed valid comparison of results among different laboratories using the procedure. The committee publishes periodic updates that incorporate new information and changes that have been suggested by users. It is important to maintain currency of the procedure. This chart summarizes the basic procedure; consult the referenced Clinical Laboratory Standards Institute document for variation used to test fastidious bacteria.

The principle of the disk diffusion procedure has been discussed in the text. The zone diameters that are generated by the test are meaningless without reference to the minimum inhibitory concentration (MIC) correlates and interpretive guidelines published by the Clinical Laboratory Standards Institute.

II. Media and Reagents
   A. Bacterial isolate from an infectious process
   B. Nutrient broth (tryptic soy broth is recommended) for growth of the inoculum
   C. McFarland 0.5 standard for adjusting the turbidity of the inoculum
   D. Vortex mixer for suspension of the inoculum
   E. Viewbox for comparison of broth with standard. A photometer may be used if satisfactory results are documented.
   F. Mueller-Hinton agar plates (100-mm diameter for a maximum of five disks; 150-mm diameter for a maximum of 12 disks) from a lot that produces satisfactory quality control results. The pH must be 7.2 to 7.4, and the depth must be approximately 4 mm.
   G. Calipers, ruler, or template for measuring the diameters of inhibitory zones

III. Quality Control

Reference strains of *Staphylococcus aureus*, *Escherichia coli*, and *Pseudomonas aeruginosa* should be tested each time a new batch of disks or agar is used. Additional controls should be performed each day the test is done, unless the laboratory can justify weekly quality control by conformance to published criteria (see Table 17-14).

IV. Procedure
   A. Preparation of Inoculum (Growth Method)
      1. With a wire loop touch the tops of four or five similar-appearing, well-isolated colonies on an agar plate culture. Transfer the growth to a tube that contains 4 to 5 mL of a suitable broth medium.
      2. Allow the culture to incubate at 35°C until it matches the turbidity of the standard prepared in the foregoing (usually 2 to 6 hours). Vigorously agitate the standard on a mechanical vortex mixer immediately before use. Use adequate light to read the tube against a white background with a contrasting black line. Add sterile saline or broth if necessary to obtain a turbidity that is visually comparable with that of the standard. For the *E. coli* quality control strain approximately 1 to 2×10^8 colony-forming units (CFU)/mL should result. Alternatively, a direct broth or saline suspension of colonies from an 18- to 24-hour agar plate may be adjusted to the standard. In this case, the bacteria must have been grown on a nutrient, nonselective medium, such as blood agar. Commercially available devices to standardize the inocula without adjustment of turbidity and without preincubation in broth media have also performed acceptably.
      3. Within 15 minutes after adjusting the turbidity of the inoculum suspension to that of the standard, dip a sterile nontoxic cotton swab into the inoculum suspension and rotate the swab several times with firm pressure on the inside wall of the tube to remove excess fluid.
      4. Inoculate the dried surface of a Mueller-Hinton agar plate that has been brought to room temperature by streaking the swab three times over the entire agar surface, rotating the plate approximately 60 degrees each time to ensure an even distribution of the inoculum. Finally swab the rim of the agar. Replace the lid of the dish. Allow at least 3 to 5 minutes but no longer than 15 minutes for the surface of the agar to dry before adding the antibiotic disks.
   B. Alternative Inoculum Preparation (Direct Colony Suspension; DCS)
      1. Make a direct saline or broth suspension of colonies from a nutrient nonselective agar plate (e.g., blood agar) that has been incubated for 18 to 24 hours.
      2. Immediately adjust the inoculum to the standard density, as for the growth method.
      3. This method is recommended for *Haemophilus* species, *Neisseria gonorrhoeae*, *Streptococcus pneumoniae*, and *Staphylococcus* species when testing susceptibility to oxacillin.
   C. Testing of Antibiotics
      1. Place the appropriate antimicrobial-impregnated disks on the surface of the agar, using either forceps or a multidisk dispenser.

CHART 17-1

DISK DIFFUSION (BAUER-KIRBY) SUSCEPTIBILITY TEST FOR NONFASTIDIOUS BACTERIA *continued*

2. Gently tamp each disk down onto the agar to provide uniform contact. Do not move a disk once it has contacted the agar, because some of the drug diffuses almost immediately. Disks must be evenly distributed on the agar so that they are no closer than 24 mm from center to center.
3. Invert the plates and place them in a 35°C air incubator for 16 to 18 hours (24 hours when testing staphylococci against methicillin or oxacillin or enterococci against vancomycin).

V. Results
  A. Interpretation
    Measurement of zone diameters: Examine the plates after overnight incubation. With the use of sliding calipers, a ruler, or a template, the zones of complete growth inhibition around each of the disks are carefully measured to within the nearest millimeter; the diameter of the disk is included in this measurement.

    All measurements are made with the unaided eye while viewing the back of the Petri dish with reflected light against a black, nonreflecting background. The plates should be viewed from a directly vertical line of sight to avoid any parallax that may result in misreadings. Susceptibility plates prepared with blood must be viewed from the agar surface and measurements made with the cover of the Petri dish removed, again using reflected light to illuminate the plate. Common problems in delineation of zone sizes are discussed in the text.

    An interpretive correlate (susceptible, moderately susceptible, intermediate, or resistant) is provided by reference to published guidelines (see Table 17-17). Zones that fall into the intermediate range should be considered equivocal; if therapy with the drug is desired, a dilution susceptibility test should be performed to clarify the issue.

VI. Bibliography
  1. National Committee for Clinical Laboratory Standards. Performance standards for antimicrobial disk susceptibility tests: Approved standard (M2-A8). Wayne, PA: National Committee for Clinical Laboratory Standards, 2003.
  2. National Committee for Clinical Laboratory Standards: Disk Diffusion. Supplemental Tables, M100-S13 (M2). Wayne, PA: National Committee for Clinical Laboratory Standards, 2003.

CHART 17-2

PERFORMANCE OF MICROBROTH DILUTION SUSCEPTIBILITY TESTS WITH NONFASTIDIOUS BACTERIA

I. Principle
The microdilution test is an adaptation of the reference macroscopic test. Large numbers of isolates can be tested against multiple drugs easily, so the procedure is well adapted to routine use. This test generates more quantitative information, which may be useful or even essential in certain circumstances, than does the disk diffusion test. This chart summarizes the basic procedure; consult the referenced Clinical Laboratory Standards Institute (formerly, the National Committee for Clinical Laboratory Standards) document for the variation used to test fastidious bacteria.

    The principle of the microdilution test is the same as that of the macroscopic test. Bacterial isolates are exposed to serial dilutions of each antimicrobial agent, after which the concentration of drug that inhibits growth is determined by visual inspection.

II. Media and Reagents
  A. Nutrient broth (tryptic soy broth is recommended)
  B. 0.5 McFarland standard for adjusting inoculum
  C. White background with black lines for comparison of turbidity of inoculum with 0.5 McFarland standard
  D. Frozen or lyophilized microtiter plates containing antibiotics in cation-supplemented Mueller-Hinton broth
  E. Multiprong inoculators—either wire loops or disposable plastic pins
  F. Viewing mirror and template for visualization of endpoints. A photometric or fluorometric analysis of endpoints may be done if demonstrated to be equivalent to visual inspection.

III. Quality Control
Quality control should be performed with each new lot of plates. During use, controls may be performed daily or at weekly intervals if strict criteria have been fulfilled.

    The organisms used for the dilution test are *Staphylococcus aureus* (American Type Culture Collection [ATCC] 29213), *Enterococcus faecalis* (ATCC 29212), *Escherichia coli* (ATCC 25922), *Pseudomonas aeruginosa* (ATCC 27583), *Neisseria gonorrhoeae* (ATCC 49226), and *Haemophilus influenzae* (ATCC 49247). Note that the *S. aureus*

CHART 17-2

PERFORMANCE OF MICROBROTH DILUTION SUSCEPTIBILITY TESTS WITH NONFASTIDIOUS BACTERIA *continued*

strain differs from that used in the disk diffusion test. *E. coli* (ATCC 35218) may be used to control combinations that include clavulanic acid, a β-lactamase inhibitor (see Table 17-22).
IV. Procedure
  A. Preparation of Inoculum: Proceed as for the disk diffusion test (see Chart 17-1).
  B. Inoculation of Plates
  Inoculate the bacterial suspension into each well of the microplate within 15 minutes of adjusting the density of the inoculum. One well should contain bacteria without antibiotic (growth control) and one should contain broth only (sterility control). If the volume of the inoculum exceeds 10% of the volume of the well, the dilution effect on the antimicrobial agent must be calculated. To prevent drying, seal the plates in a plastic bag, with plastic tape, or with a tight-fitting plastic cover. A portion of a nutrient agar plate, such as blood agar, should be inoculated to detect contamination.
  C. Incubation
  Incubate the plates at 35°C for 16 to 20 hours (24 hours when testing staphylococci against oxacillin, methicillin, or vancomycin or when testing enterococci against vancomycin) in a forced-air incubator. Do not place more than four plates in a stack, so that a uniform temperature of incubation is maintained.
V. Results
  A. Interpretation
  The minimum inhibitory concentration (MIC) is the lowest concentration of antibiotic that inhibits growth of the isolate. It may be determined by viewing the wells with the unaided eye, comparing the growth in the wells that contain antibiotics with that in the growth control well. A viewing mirror, with which the bottom of the microtubes may be visualized, facilitates observation. A template on which the contents of each well are detailed is useful. For a test to be valid, adequate growth must be present (diffuse turbidity or at least a 2-mm button). For trimethoprim-sulfamethoxazole, the endpoint is at least 80% inhibition of growth. A single skipped well may be ignored; if there are more skipped wells, the test should be repeated.
  Refer to the guidelines for interpretation of MIC results as susceptible, moderately susceptible, intermediate, or resistant (see Table 17-16).
  Examine the purity plate and repeat the test if contamination is present.
VI. Bibliography
  1. National Committee for Clinical Laboratory Standards. M7-A6 methods for dilution antimicrobial susceptibility tests for bacteria that grow aerobically: Approved standard. Ed. 6. Wayne, PA: National Committee for Clinical Laboratory Standards, 2003.
  2. National Committee for Clinical Laboratory Standards. M100-S13 (M7) MIC Testing. Supplemental Tables. Wayne, PA: National Committee for Clinical Laboratory Standards, 2003.

CHART 17-3

GRADIENT DIFFUSION TEST (ETEST) FOR BACTERIAL SUSCEPTIBILITY

I. Principle
  The gradient diffusion test uses a nonporous plastic strip that has been calibrated with minimum inhibitory concentration (MIC) values that cover 15 twofold dilutions. A predefined antibiotic gradient is immobilized on the surface of the strip that is opposite the MIC scale. When transferred to agar, antibiotic diffuses from the strip (similar to the disk diffusion test). This chart summarizes the general procedure, which should be used only for combinations of antibiotic and organism that have been validated by comparison to reference methods.
II. Materials and Reagents
  A. Nutrient broth or 0.85% saline
  B. Sterile swabs (not too tightly spun)
  C. 0.5 and/or 1.0 McFarland standard
  D. Etest strips
  E. Etest applicator kit or forceps
  F. Mueller-Hinton agar plates (100 mm or 150 mm) with supplements if appropriate
III. Quality Control is performed using strains appropriate for dilution tests (see Chart 17-2).

CHART 17-3

GRADIENT DIFFUSION TEST (ETEST) FOR BACTERIAL SUSCEPTIBILITY *continued*

IV. Procedure
   A. Allow the Etest strips to reach room temperature (approximately 30 minutes after removal from a $-20°C$ freezer).
   B. Preparation of inoculum is performed as for the disk diffusion or microbroth dilution tests (see Charts 17-1 and 17-2).
   C. Inoculate the agar plate as for the disk diffusion test (see Chart 17-1).
   D. Allow the agar surface to dry 10 to 15 minutes at room temperature or in the incubator before proceeding.
   E. Open the Etest package and place the strip(s) in a dry Petri dish or applicator tray.
   F. Apply the strip(s) to the surface of the agar with forceps or an applicator, with the MIC scale facing up. If the strip is positioned upside down, the positioning can be corrected if the error is recognized immediately. If the strip is incubated in the inverted position, the test is invalid.
   G. Incubate as appropriate for the organism being tested.
V. Results
   A. After the appropriate incubation period interpret the test only if there is adequate growth and the ellipse of inhibition is clearly visible.
   B. Read the MIC where a clearly defined zone of inhibition intersects the strip. Factors to be considered when determining the MIC are discussed in the text and in Box 17-7.
   C. As the antibiotic gradient is continuous (linear) and the interpretive criteria are discontinuous (twofold dilutions), round up the MIC value to the next twofold dilution when reporting the result.
VI. Reference
   Etest Technical Guide 3B. Solna, Sweden: AB Biodisk.

CHART 18-1

DIENE'S STAIN PROCEDURE FOR IDENTIFICATION OF MYCOPLASMAS

I. Principle
   Mycoplasma colonies from genital cultures are easily identified by observing typical colonies on agar medium. Visualization of colony morphology is facilitated by application of Diene's stain directly to the agar surface.
   Diene's stain is a nonspecific stain that imparts a contrasting appearance to *Mycoplasma* colonies on agar, allowing easier visualization of colony morphology and characteristics.
II. Reagents
   A. Modified Diene's Stain (stock solution)

Methylene blue	2.5 g
Azure II	1.25 g
Maltose	10.0 g
Na_2CO_3	0.25 g
Distilled water	100 mL

   Diene's stain working solution is prepared by diluting an aliquot of the stock solution 1:3 with distilled water.
III. Procedure
   1. Flood an agar plate containing mycoplasmal growth with 1 mL of Diene's stain working solution.
   2. *Immediately rinse the agar surface with distilled water to remove the stain.*
   3. Decolorize the medium by adding 1 mL of 95% ethanol. Leave in contact with the agar for 1 minute, then remove. Repeat the wash step a second time.
   4. Rinse the plate with distilled water and allow to dry.
   5. Observe for colonies under the low power of a microscope (50 to 100×).
IV. Results
   A. Interpretation
      Mycoplasmas with the "fried-egg" colony morphology will stain with a dark blue center and a light blue periphery and will appear highly granular. The agar background will be clear or slightly violet.

CHART 18-1

DIENE'S STAIN PROCEDURE FOR IDENTIFICATION OF MYCOPLASMAS *continued*

Mycoplasmas other than *M. pneumoniae* will remain stained; *M. pneumoniae* reduces the methylene blue after a time and will become colorless. If the isolate is from the genital tract and produces typical colonies and staining, the isolate can be reported as *M. hominis.*

V. Bibliography

Velleca WM, Bird BR, Forrester FT. Laboratory Diagnosis of Mycoplasma Infections. Atlanta: Department of Health and Human Services, 1980.

CHART 18-2

HEMADSORPTION TEST FOR IDENTIFICATION OF *MYCOPLASMA PNEUMONIAE*

I. Principle

Among the respiratory mycoplasmas, *M. pneumoniae* is the only species that will specifically absorb red blood cells. This property, therefore, provides a method for the presumptive identification of *M. pneumoniae.*

When colony growth is noted on mycoplasma isolation media inoculated with respiratory tract specimens a suspension of guinea pig erythrocytes is placed on the agar surface for a given time and then washed off. *M. pneumoniae* colonies will adsorb some of the red cells to the colony surface.

II. Reagents

A. Mycoplasma glucose agar with suspicious colonies present.

B. Washed guinea pig erythrocytes (0.2–0.4%) suspended in mycoplasma broth medium.

III. Quality Control

A. Positive control: *M. pneumoniae*

B. Negative control: *Mycoplasma* species

IV. Procedure

1. Flood the surface of the agar plate with 2 mL of the red-cell suspension.

2. Incubate the plate at 35°C for 30 minutes and rotate the plate occasionally to prevent the red cells from settling out.

3. Wash the surface of the plate three times with 3 mL of mycoplasma broth by gently rotating the plate. Remove wash fluid by aspiration with a pipet.

4. Examine the colonies at 50 to 100× magnification under a dissecting microscope.

V. Results

A. Interpretation

1. Positive test: Colonies with red cells adsorbed onto the surface = *M. pneumoniae.*

2. Negative: Colonies with no red cells adsorbed = *Mycoplasma* species, not *M. pneumoniae.*

VI. Bibliography

Manchee RJ, Taylor-Robinson D. Hemadsorption and hemagglutination by mycoplasmas. J Gen Microbiol 1968; 50:465.

CHART 18-3

MANGANOUS CHLORIDE-UREA TEST FOR IDENTIFICATION OF *UREAPLASMA UREALYTICUM*

I. Principle

Of the human mycoplasmas, *U. urealyticum* is the only species that is able to hydrolyze urea to ammonia. This property not only facilitates isolation of the organism, but also provides a rapid and convenient way to identify the species in culture. The manganous chloride ($MnCl_2$)–urea test provides a visual method for detecting ammonia formation by *U. urealyticum.*

Urease activity of *U. urealyticum* is detected by exposing the colonies to a solution of $MnCl_2$ in the presence of urea. The urease of the organism hydrolyzes urea to ammonia, and then the following reaction occurs:

$$2NH_3 + 2 H_2O \longrightarrow 2NH_4OH \longrightarrow 2NH_4^+ + 2OH^-$$
$$MnCl_2 + 2OH^- \longrightarrow MnO_2 + 2 HCl$$

CHART 18-3

MANGANOUS CHLORIDE-UREA TEST FOR IDENTIFICATION OF *UREAPLASMA UREALYTICUM continued*

The manganese oxide formed in the reaction is insoluble and forms a dark brown precipitate around the colonies. This reaction is then detected under a dissecting microscope.

II. Reagents
   A. $MnCl_2$-urea Reagent

Urea (Sigma, St Louis, MO)	1.0 g
$MnCl_2$ (Fisher Scientific, Hampton, NH)	0.8 g
Distilled water	100 mL

   B. Sterilize by filtration, dispense in 3-mL aliquots, and freeze at $-20°C$
   C. Growth of suspect colonies on agar medium
III. Quality Control
   A. Positive control: *U. urealyticum*
   B. Negative control: *M. hominis*
IV. Procedure
   1. Flood the plate with 2 to 3 mL of the $MnCl_2$-urea reagent.
   2. After 5 minutes at room temperature, examine the colonies under 50 to $100\times$ magnification with a dissecting microscope.
V. Results
   A. Interpretation
      Colonies of *U. urealyticum* will stain a dark brown. Other mycoplasmas (e.g., *M. hominis*) will remain unstained.
VI. Comments
   This test works optimally on colonies that are not too crowded together on agar medium. Colonies should not be older than 48 hours when the test is performed.
VII. Bibliography
   Shepard MC, Howard DR. Identification of ''T'' mycoplasmas in primary agar cultures by means of a direct test for urease. Ann NY Acad Sci 1970;174:809.

CHART 18-4

MEDIUM FOR ISOLATION OF *MYCOPLASMA PNEUMONIAE*

I. Base reagents for preparation of complete media
   A. Mycoplasma base agar: This medium may be prepared using commercial PPLO agar as directed according to the package insert, or may be prepared from raw materials using the following formula:

Beef heart infusion	50 g
Peptone	10 g
NaCl	5 g
Purified agar	14 g
Distilled water	1 L

   Mix together and melt the agar in a boiling water bath. Dispense in 70-mL aliquots and autoclave at 15 psi for 15 minutes. Store at 4°C.
   B. Yeast Extract
   1. Purchase commercial 25% yeast extract or prepare as follows: Weigh out 250 g of active bakers' yeast and place in 1 L of distilled water. Heat to boiling, cool, and filter to remove particulate matter. Adjust the pH to 8.0, and filter-sterilize.
   2. Yeast extract (20 mL) is then mixed with uninactivated horse serum (10 mL) in a 2:1 ratio and frozen in 30-mL aliquots at $-20°C$.
   C. Phenol red solution (0.4%): Phenol red (1 g) is dissolved in 3 mL of 1 N NaOH and then 247 mL of distilled water is added. Solution is filter-sterilized and stored at 4 to 8°C.
   D. Methylene blue solution (1%): Methylene blue (1 g) is dissolved in 100 mL distilled water and autoclaved for 15 minutes.

CHART 18-4

MEDIUM FOR ISOLATION OF *MYCOPLASMA PNEUMONIAE continued*

E. Thallium acetate solution (10%): Thallium acetate (10 g) is dissolved in 100 mL of distilled water and filter-sterilized.

F. Glucose solution: Glucose (50 g) is dissolved in 100 mL distilled water and filter-sterilized.

G. Penicillin solution: Penicillin powder is dissolved in distilled water to achieve a concentration of 100,000 units/mL.

II. Methylene Blue-Glucose Diphasic Medium

    1. Melt 70 mL of mycoplasma agar in a boiling water bath. Cool to 50°C and add 30 mL prewarmed yeast extract-serum.

    2. Add the following:

Methylene blue solution (1%)	0.1 mL
Phenol red solution (0.4%)	0.5 mL
Glucose solution	2.0 mL
Thallium acetate solution (10%)	0.25 mL
Penicillin solution	3.0 mL

    3. Adjust the pH to 7.8 with sterile 1 N NaOH.

    4. Dispense agar in 1-mL aliquots into sterile 13 × 100-mm screw-capped tubes.

    5. Mix 140 mL of mycoplasma broth (A, above, without agar) with 60 mL of the yeast extract-serum. Add the following to this mixture:

Methylene blue solution (1%)	0.2 mL
Phenol red solution	1.0 mL
Glucose solution	4.0 mL
Thallium acetate solution (10%)	6.0 mL
Penicillin solution	0.5 mL

    Adjust the pH to 7.8 with sterile 1 N NaOH. Dispense 2.0 mL into each of the tubes containing the solidified agar medium.

III. Mycoplasma Glucose Agar Medium

    1. Melt 70 mL of mycoplasma agar in a boiling water bath. Cool to 50°C.

    2. Prewarm 30 mL of yeast extract-serum and mix with the agar medium.

    3. Aseptically add the following reagents:

Glucose solution	2.0 mL
Thallium acetate solution (10%)	0.25 mL
Penicillin solution	3.0 mL

    4. Adjust the pH to 7.8 with sterile 1N NaOH.

    5. Dispense 6 mL of medium into 60 × 15-mm petri dishes. Allow to cool. Store media at 4°C.

IV. SP-4 Medium (also used for culture of *M. pneumoniae,* but mostly for culture of highly fastidious species)

    A. Basal medium

Mycoplasma Broth Base (BBL)	3.5 g/L
Bacto Tryptone (Difco)	10.0 g/L
Bacto Peptone (Difco)	5 g/L
Glucose	5.0 g/L
Deionized water	615 mL
Adjust to pH 7.5 to 7.6	
Autoclave at 121°C, 15 minutes	

CHART 18-4

MEDIUM FOR ISOLATION OF *MYCOPLASMA PNEUMONIAE continued*

   B. Sterile supplements

CMRL 1066 Tissue Culture Supplement with glutamine (Gibco)	50.0 mL
Fresh yeast extract (25% solution)	35.0 mL
Yeastolate (2% solution)	100.0 mL
Fetal bovine serum (heated to 56°C for 1 hour)	170.0 mL
Penicillin (100,000 U/mL stock)	10 mL
Phenol red solution (0.1%, aqueous)	20 mL

   C. Final formulation
      Combine basal medium (615 mL) with supplements (385 mL) and dispense aseptically in 3-mL volumes into 4-mL, screw-capped vials.
   V. Bibliography
      Velleca WB, Bird BR, Forrester FT. Laboratory Diagnosis of *Mycoplasma* Infections. Atlanta: Department of Health and Human Services, 1980.

CHART 18-5

MEDIUM FOR ISOLATION OF THE GENITAL MYCOPLASMAS

   I. U Broth and U agar for isolation of *Ureaplasma urealyticum*
      A. U broth
         1. Add the following to 70 mL of Mycoplasma broth base (BBL) (see Chart 18-4):

Yeast extract-horse serum	30 mL
Urea solution (50%)	0.1 mL
Phenol red solution (0.4%)	0.5 mL
Penicillin solution	0.5 mL
Polymyxin B solution (5000 μg/mL)	0.5 mL
Lincomycin solution (1500 μg/mL)	1.0 mL
Amphotericin B solution (5000 μg/mL)	0.1 mL

         2. Adjust the pH to 6.0 with 1N HCl.
         3. Dispense in 2-mL aliquots into sterile 12 × 75-mm screw-capped tubes or sterile 1-dram vials. Store at 4 to 8°C.
      B. U agar
         1. Add 30 g of trypticase-soy broth to 1 L distilled water. Add 11.3 g of purified agar (e.g., Noble agar, Ion agar 2) and heat to boiling to dissolve. Dispense into 80-mL aliquots and store refrigerated.
         2. Melt 80 mL of the agar base in a boiling water bath and cool to 50°C. Adjust the pH to 6.0 with 1N HCl.
         3. In a separate sterile flask, combine the following:

Horse serum	2.0 mL
Phenol red solution (0.4%)	0.5 mL
Urea solution (50%)	0.1 mL
Penicillin solution	0.5 mL
Lincomycin solution (1500 μg/mL)	1.0 mL

         4. Add the agar to the contents of the flask, mix, and dispense 3-mL aliquots into 60 × 15-mm petri plates. Place in plastic bags and store at 4 to 8°C.

CHART 18-5

MEDIUM FOR ISOLATION OF THE GENITAL MYCOPLASMAS *continued*

II. H broth and H agar for isolation of *Mycoplasma hominis*
   A. H broth
      1. Add the following to 70 mL of Mycoplasma broth base (BBL) (see Chart 18-4).

Yeast extract/horse serum	30 mL
L-Arginine hydrochloride (30%)	0.66 mL
Phenol red solution (0.4%)	0.5 mL
Penicillin solution	0.5 mL
Polymyxin B (5000 μg/mL)	1.0 mL
Amphotericin B (5000 μg/mL)	0.1 mL

      2. Adjust the pH to 7.0 with 1N HCl.
      3. Dispense in 2-mL aliquots into sterile 12 $\times$ 75-mm screw-capped tubes or 1-dram vials. Store at 4 to 8°C.
   B. H agar
      1. Melt 70 mL of mycoplasma agar base in a boiling water bath and let cool to 50°C.
      2. Adjust the pH of the agar to 7.0 with 1N HCl.
      3. Prewarm 30 mL of yeast extract-serum and add the following:

L-Arginine hydrochloride (30%)	0.66 mL
Phenol red solution (0.4%)	0.5 mL
Penicillin solution	0.5 mL

      4. Mix the agar base with the yeast extract-serum and additives and dispense 3-mL aliquots into 60 $\times$ 15-mm agar plates. Store in plastic bags at 4 to 8°C.
III. Bibliography
   Velleca WM, Bird BR, Forrester FT. Laboratory Diagnosis of Mycoplasma Infections. Atlanta: Department of Health and Human Services, 1980.

CHART 18-6

TETRAZOLIUM REDUCTION TEST FOR THE PRESUMPTIVE IDENTIFICATION OF *MYCOPLASMA PNEUMONIAE*

I. Principle
   M. pneumoniae is able to reduce the colorless compound tetrazolium to the red-colored compound formozan. Among the large-colony mycoplasmas, this is a unique feature of *M. pneumoniae* and provides the laboratory with a rapid and easy method for identification of *M. pneumoniae* colonies directly on isolation medium.
      By using enzymes that are associated with the cell membrane of the organism, *M. pneumoniae* can reduce the compound 2-(*p*-iodophenyl)-3-nitrophenyl-5-phenyl tetrazolium chloride to formozan, a red-insoluble compound that precipitates in the cells and renders the colony red to purple-black on prolonged exposure to the substrate.
II. Reagents
      1. Isolated colonies on mycoplasma glucose agar
      2. 2-(*p*-iodophenyl)-3-nitrophenyl-5-phenyl tetrazolium chloride (Aldrich Chemical)–0.21 g/100 mL distilled water. Sterilize by filtration and store in brown-glass bottle at room temperature.
III. Quality Control
   A. Positive control: *M. pneumoniae*
   B. Negative control: *Mycoplasma* species
IV. Procedure
      1. Flood the surface of the agar plate containing the colonies of the organism with 2 mL of the tetrazolium reagent.
      2. Incubate the plate at 35°C for 30 to 60 minutes (incubation for 60 minutes intensifies reactions that are already apparent at 30 minutes).
      3. Examine the colonies under 50 to 100$\times$ magnification with a dissecting microscope.

CHART 18-6

TETRAZOLIUM REDUCTION TEST FOR THE PRESUMPTIVE IDENTIFICATION OF *MYCOPLASMA PNEUMONIAE* *continued*

V. Results
   A. Interpretation
      1. Positive test: Colonies of *M. pneumoniae* will visibly darken, becoming red to purple after 60 minutes. On prolonged incubation (3 to 4 hours), the colonies will become black.
      2. Negative test: No color change will be noted after 60 minutes.
VI. Comments
   Although equivalent to the hemadsorption test, tetrazolium reduction can be performed on the same plate after doing the hemadsorption procedure.
VII. Bibliography
   Johnson JE, Smith TF. A simplified tetrazolium reduction test for *Mycoplasma pneumoniae*. Med Lab Sci 1976; 33:235.

CHART 19-1

DIGESTION AND DECONTAMINATION: *N*-ACETYL-L-CYSTEINE–SODIUM HYDROXIDE (NALC)

I. Principle
   Mycobacteria are optimally recovered from clinical specimens when they are released from mucin, body fluids, and cells (digestion.) *N*-acetyl-L-cysteine (NALC) is a mucolytic agent that in concentrations of 0.5–2% can rapidly digest tenacious sputum and other mucoid specimens within 2 minutes. Growth of mycobacteria in culture media is also enhanced when the concentration of competing organisms is minimal (decontamination). The addition of 4% sodium hydroxide to the digestion mixture to reach a final concentration of 2% is the most commonly used decontaminating agent.
II. Specimen
   A. Type of Specimen
      Any specimen that is mucoid in consistency or is known to be contaminated with bacteria should undergo digestion and decontamination. Included are all respiratory specimens, gastric lavage fluid, stools, urine (when Gram stain shows the presence of bacteria), postmortem tissue, and biopsy samples.
   B. Patient Preparation
      When collecting specimens through a contaminated area, such as collection of expectorated sputum, every effort should be made to cleanse or decontaminate the area. For example, before patients are asked to produce expectorated sputum, they should rinse out their mouth two or three times with water or a proprietary mouth wash. The skin adjacent to a biopsy site should be carefully cleaned with iodine followed by an alcohol swab.
   C. Special Collection Procedures
      In patients in whom pulmonary tuberculosis is suspected and who cannot produce adequate sputum, induced sputum should be collected. In instances in which diagnosis has been difficult to establish, invasive procedures, such as bronchial brush biopsies, bronchial washings, or bronchoalveolar lavage may be required.
   D. Special Handling Conditions
      All specimens submitted for the culture of mycobacteria must be handled in a properly functioning biohazard hood. Care must also be taken in the preparation, examination, and storage of stained smears, as all acid-fast bacilli may not be killed in the fixation and staining procedure. Care must be taken not to produce aerosols when subcultures are made, when specimens are centrifuged, and when various biochemical tests are performed.
III. Materials
   A. Equipment
      1. Centrifuge with aerosol-free centrifuge cups
      2. Vortex mixer
   B. Supplies
      1. Discard container containing disinfectant solution
      2. Sterile 50-mL conical polypropylene screw-capped tubes (aerosol-free and graduated)
      3. 10 mL sterile transfer pipette
      4. Clean, unscratched, 1″ × 3″ microscope slides
   C. Reagents
      1. *N*-acetyl-L-cysteine (NALC) digestant-decontaminant: TB base digestant, 50 mL (available commercially)

CHART 19-1

DIGESTION AND DECONTAMINATION: *N*-ACETYL-L-CYSTEINE–SODIUM HYDROXIDE (NALC) *continued*

    2. TB phosphate buffer: 0.067 M, pH 6.8, 250 mL (commercially available)
    3. *N*-acetyl-L-cysteine (NALC): Mucomyst, 20% solution (commercially available from Bristol Laboratories, Evansville, IN)

IV. Quality Control

The percentage of clinical specimens that grow bacterial contaminants in TB cultures following the digestion and decontamination procedure should average about 3%. A contamination rate significantly less than 3% may indicate overly harsh decontamination, and the concentration of NaOH should be reduced. A contamination rate significantly greater than 5% suggests either too weak a decontamination or incomplete digestion. Increasing the concentration of NaOH or the time of exposure, or both, may correct this problem.

V. Procedure

    1. Add 1.5 mL NALC to 50 mL TB base digestant to make a working solution.
    2. Add a volume of working NALC-NaOH solution (no more than 24 hours old) equal to the volume of specimen in a sterile 50-mL conical polypropylene screw-capped centrifuge tube. If more than 20 mL of specimen is submitted, use a sterile transfer pipette to select 10 mL of the most purulent blood, or mucoid portion. Secure the cap tightly.
    3. Agitate the tube on a vortex mixer for not more than 30 seconds. Be sure to move the tube so that the NALC-NaOH comes in contact with the entire inner surface of the tube.
    4. Let the tube stand for 15 minutes at room temperature to decontaminate the specimen.
    5. Dilute the mixture to the 50-mL mark with either sterile distilled water or sterile 0.067 phosphate buffer (pH 6.8). This will reduce the continued action of the NaOH and lower the viscosity of the mixture.
    6. Recap the tube tightly and invert several times to mix the contents.
    7. Centrifuge the tube at 3000 *g* for 15 to 20 minutes. Use aerosol-free sealed centrifuge cups.
    8. Pour the supernatant into a splash-proof discard container filled with disinfectant.
    9. Use a sterile 3-mm–diameter bacteriologic loop or the end of two sterile wooden applicator sticks to remove a portion of the sediment, and prepare a smear over an area 1 × 2 cm on a new, clean, unscratched glass slide.
    10. Suspend the remaining sediment in 1 to 2 mL of TB buffer or sterile distilled water if media are to be inoculated immediately. Otherwise, suspend the sediment in 1 to 2 mL of sterile 0.2% bovine albumin fraction V. If the amount of the sediment is very small, reconstitute the sediment in 1 mL only.
    11. Add three drops to each side of a 7H11 agar slant.
    12. Inoculate 0.5 mL into BACTEC vial

VI. Results

Not applicable

VII. Procedure Notes

    1. Excessive agitation of the NALC-NaOH solution should be avoided because NALC is unstable in the presence of oxygen.
    2. Bovine serum albumin serves to buffer the inoculum and enhance adhesion of the sample to solid media.
    3. Sterile water only should be used: Tap water may contain environmental mycobacteria that can confuse observations of stained smears and contaminate culture media.

VIII. Limitation of Procedure

The concentration of NaOH and the time of exposure of specimen to reagent during the decontamination procedure must be carefully controlled to avoid undue loss of mycobacterial cells during this procedure.

IX. Bibliography

Good RC, Silcox V, Kilburn JO. Tuberculosis and other mycobacterioses. In: Balows A, Hausler WJ, eds. Diagnostic Procedures for Bacterial, Mycotic and Parasitic Infections. Ed. 6. Washington DC: American Public Health Association, 1985:675–703.

Kubica GP, Dye WE, Cohn ML, Middlebrook G. Sputum digestion and decontamination with *N*-acetyl-L-cysteine-sodium hydroxide for culture of mycobacteria. Am Rev Respir Dis 1963;87:775–779.

Strong BE, Kubica GP. Isolation and Identification of *Mycobacterium tuberculosis:* A Guide for the Level II Laboratory. Atlanta: Centers for Disease Control, 1976. Public Health Service publication no. 81-8390.

CHART 19-2

CARBOL FUCHSIN STAINS

I. Principle

The carbolic acids within the lipid-rich, waxy cell wall of mycobacteria have the unique capability of binding fuchsin dye so that it is not destained by acid alcohol. The Ziehl-Neelsen stain is known as a "hot stain," as heat is used for the dye to penetrate through the cell wall. The Kinyoun stain is known as a "cold stain" because the high concentration of phenol in the reagent serves to "dissolve" the lipid material in the cell wall, allowing penetration of the carbol fuchsin dye without the use of heat. Once stained, the cell wall holds the dye "fast," giving the characteristic red color.

II. Specimen

A smear is prepared either directly from the specimen or from a suspension of organisms obtained from colonies grown on primarily culture media.

III. Materials

A. Equipment: 3″ × 1″ glass slides and reagents

B. Media: Not applicable

C. Reagents

1. Carbolfuchsin (commercially available)

2. Acid-alcohol (commercially available)

3. Methylene blue counterstain (commercially available)

IV. Quality Control

A. Unstained positive control smears (*M. tuberculosis*) and negative control smears (*Nocardia asteroides*) have been prepared.

B. Control smears are reviewed before the patient smears are read to confirm that the mycobacteria stain acid-fast:

1. Positive: *Mycobacterium* spp.; magenta red against blue background

2. *N. asteroides:* no acid-fast cells; background blue

C. If control slide is unacceptable, review procedures and reagent preparation. Unacceptable control slides include the following:

1. Bacilli in positive control do not stain red.

2. Negative control remains red after destaining.

3. Background is not properly decolorized.

V. Procedure

A. Ziehl-Neelsen

1. Place a 2 × 3-cm filter paper strip on the slide to help hold the stain on the slide and filter undissolved crystals.

2. Flood the paper strip with Ziehl-Neelsen carbol fuchsin.

3. Using a Bunsen burner or electric staining rack, heat the slide slowly until steaming, but short of boiling.

4. Stain for 5 minutes. If the stain dries, add more stain without heating.

5. Carefully remove the paper slip from the slide using forceps.

6. Rinse the slide thoroughly with water.

7. Flood the smear with 3% acid-alcohol decolorizer for 2 minutes.

8. Rinse with water and drain excess water.

9. Flood the slide with methylene blue-counterstain for 1 minute. Do not blot.

10. Examine the smear with a 100× oil-immersion objective.

B. Kinyoun

1. Heat-fix smears on slide warmer at 72–75°C.

2. Cover the smear with the Kinyoun's carbol fuchsin reagent. A small 2″ × 3″ rectangular piece of filter paper can be placed over the smear and the stain applied to the filter paper to avoid spilling over the sides of the smear. Do not steam.

3. Stain for 5 minutes.

4. Remove the filter paper with forceps, rinse the stain off the slide with distilled water.

5. Decolorize for 3 minutes with acid-alcohol or until no red stain appears.

6. Flood smear for 3–4 minutes with methylene blue counterstain.

7. Rinse dry and examine under a 100× oil-immersion objective.

CHART 19-2

CARBOL FUCHSIN STAINS *continued*

VI. Results
Examine smears with a $100\times$ oil-immersion objective and report as follows:

Smear Observation	Report
1 or 2 per 300 fields (3 sweeps)	(Doubtful, repeat and report the result of the repeat)
1–9 per 100 fields	Rare, 1+
1–9 per 10 fields	Few, 2+
1–9 per immersion field	Numerous, 3+
9 per field	4+

VII. Procedure Notes
1. Avoid underdecolorization with acid-alcohol. Organisms that are truly acid-fast are difficult to overdecolorize.
2. Avoid making thick smears, which may interfere with proper decolorization.
3. If an inordinate number of smear-positive, culture-negative results are encountered, check water reservoirs for contaminating acid-fast organisms. Transfer of material from slide to slide and from immersion oil are other possible sources of false-positive smear results.
4. Strong counterstains may mask the presence of acid-fast bacilli. Brilliant green may have a slight advantage over methylene blue as a counterstain.

VIII. Limitation of Procedure
1. Acid-fast smears do not stand alone, and final interpretation must always be correlated with culture results.
2. Organisms other than mycobacteria may demonstrate various degrees of acid-fastness: *Rhodococcus* spp., *Nocardia* spp. *Legionella micdadei,* and the cysts of *Cryptosporidium* spp. Use differences in smear morphology and correlation with culture appearance and other biochemical tests.
3. Rapidly growing mycobacteria may stain poorly or not at all. The Ziehl-Neelsen stain may provide better staining than the Kinyoun method for weak acid-fast organisms.

IX. Bibliography
Berlin OGW. Mycobacteria. In: Baron EJ, Finegold SM, eds. Bailey and Scott's Diagnostic Microbiology. St. Louis: Mosby, 1990: 597–640.

Ebersole LL. Acid-fast stain procedures. In: Isenberg HD. Mycobacteriology Section, Clinical Microbiology Procedure Handbook, Washington, DC: American Society for Microbiology, 1992.

Kent PT, Kubica GP. Public Health Mycobacteriology: A Guide for the Level III Laboratory. Atlanta: Centers for Disease Control, 1985. Department of Health and Human Services Publication no. 86-21654.

CHART 19-3

FLUORESCENT STAIN: AURAMINE O; AURAMINE-RHODAMINE

I. Principle
Acid-fast organisms emit a bright yellow fluorescence when activated with a short-wave ultraviolet light. The potassium permanganate counterstain causes the nonspecific background debris to fluoresce a pale yellow, in contrast with the bright yellow appearance of acid-fast bacilli.

II. Specimen
Smear prepared either directly from the specimen or from a suspension of organisms obtained from colonies grown on primary culture media.

III. Materials
A. Equipment
1. $3'' \times 1''$ glass slides
B. Reagents
1. Auramine O
a. Solution 1: Dissolve 1.5 g of Auramine O in 10 mL of 95% ethanol.
b. Solution 2: Dissolve 3.0 g of phenol crystals in 87 mL of distilled water
c. Working solution: Combine solutions 1 and 2. Label with name of reagent and dates of preparation and expiration. Shelf life is 3 months if stored in a brown bottle.

CHART 19-3

FLUORESCENT STAIN: AURAMINE O; AURAMINE-RHODAMINE *continued*

    2. Auramine-rhodamine
       a. Solution 1: Dissolve 1.5 g of Auramine O and 0.75 g of rhodamine B in 75 mL of glycerol
       b. Solution 2: Mix 10 mL of phenol with 50 mL distilled water
       c. Working solution: Combine solutions 1 and 2 and mix for 24 hours with a magnetic stirrer. Filter stain through glass wool and store in a glass bottle. Affix a label with the name of the reagent and dates of preparation and expiration. Shelf life is 3 months if stored in a brown bottle.
    3. Permanganate counterstain: 0.5%
       a. Dissolve 0.5 g of potassium permanganate in 100 mL distilled water.
       b. Affix a label with the name of the reagent and dates of preparation and expiration.
    4. 0.5% acid alcohol decolorizer
       a. Add 0.5 mL of concentrated hydrochloric acid to 100 mL of 70% ethanol.
       b. Affix label with name of reagent and dates of preparation and expiration.
       c. Shelf life is 3 months when stored at room temperature.
  C. Special Supplies
    1. Fluorescence microscope fitted with a BG-12 or 52112 primary filter and an OG-1 barrier filter.
  D. Biosafety Instructions
    1. Handle all slides carefully. Heat-fixing may not kill all of the mycobacteria. Dispose of all slides in a biohazard container.
    2. Heat-sterilize bacteriologic loops in the electric incinerator contained in the biologic safety hood.
    3. Perform all operations in a biosafety hood. Place a paper towel soaked with disinfectant under the field of operation. Thoroughly clean all work surfaces with a disinfectant solution before and after use.
    4. Carcinogenic
    5. Work under the hood in the special chemistry laboratory.
IV. Quality Control
  A. Control Materials To Be Used
  A positive and negative control smear for mycobacteria is included with each run of stains. Control slides are reviewed before the patient smears are read to confirm that the positive control contains mycobacteria that fluoresce and that the negative smear has no fluorescing cells.
    1. Positive control: *Mycobacterium* spp.; bacilli with yellow to orange fluorescence
    2. Negative control: *Nocardia asteroides*; no fluorescing cells
  If either of the control smears is unacceptable, reagent preparations and procedure are checked
V. Procedure
    1. Heat-fix smears on slide warmer at 72 to 75°C.
    2. Flood surface of the smear with Auramine O stain. Let stand at room temperature for 15 minutes.
    3. Rinse with tap water. Drain.
    4. Decolorize with 0.5% acid alcohol for 2 minutes.
    5. Rinse with tap water. Drain.
    6. Flood smear for 2 minutes with 0.5% potassium permanganate counterstain.
    7. Rinse with tap water. Drain.
    8. Air dry. *Do not blot.*
    9. Observe the smear as soon as possible using the fluorescence microscope. If there is a delay, refrigerate the smears at 4°C in the dark.
VI. Results
  A. Interpretation (Readout or Calculations)
  Acid-fast bacilli (AFB) are 1 to 10 μm long, and appear as slender, rod-shaped bacilli emitting a bright yellow fluorescence against the pale yellow background. First scan the smears briefly with the 25× objective; move to the 63× objective to confirm the bacterial morphology of any suspicious fluorescing forms. Thoroughly examine each slide for the presence of acid-fast bacilli. Mycobacteriologists recommend that a minimum of 100 fields be examined before a smear is reported as negative. Three passes along the long axis of the slide or nine passes along the short axis usually provide ample area for reading this technique minimizes the possibility of reading the same area more than once.

CHART 19-3

FLUORESCENT STAIN: AURAMINE O; AURAMINE-RHODAMINE *continued*

B. Reporting Format
The American Lung Association recommends the following method for fuchsin stains, also applicable to fluorescent stains:

Number of Bacilli	Report
0	No AFB seen
1–2 on entire smear	Report number seen and ask for repeat
1–9 per 10 fields	Rare or 1+
1–9 per field	Few or 2+
10–90 per field	Numerous or 3+
>90 per field	4+

VII. Procedure Notes
Fluorochrome-stained smears may be directly restained with any of the carbol fuchsin staining procedures. This is done to confirm positive slides and to study the morphology of the organisms present.

VIII. Limitation of Procedure
Organisms other than mycobacteria, including *Rhodococcus* spp., *Nocardia* spp., *Legionella micdadei,* and the cysts of *Cryptosporidium* and *Isospora* spp. may demonstrate varying degrees of acid-fastness. These can often be suggested by differences in morphology; recovery of contaminating bacteria in subcultures may be necessary in equivocal cases.

Rapidly growing mycobacteria may vary in their abilities to retain acid-fast dyes. Most species will not fluoresce in fluorochrome-stained smears and a carbol fuchsin procedure is recommended.

Dead acid-fast bacilli may still stain positive in fluorescent stains, a feature that must be considered when using smears to assess efficacy of treatment.

IX. Bibliography

Joseph SW, Vaichulis EMK, Houk VN. Lack of Auramine Rhodamine fluorescence of Runyon Group IV mycobacteria. Am Rev Respir Dis 1967;95:114–115.

Koneman EW, Allen SD, Janda WM, Schreckenberger PC, Winn WC Jr. Color Atlas and Textbook of Diagnostic Microbiology. Ed. 4. Philadelphia: Lippincott, 1992:713–715.

Pollock HM, Wieman EJ. Smear results in the diagnosis of mycobacteriosis using blue light fluorescence microscopy. J Clin Microbiol 1977;5:329–331.

Uribe-Botero G, Prichard JG, Kaplowitz HJ. Bone marrow in HIV infections: a comparison of fluorescent staining and culture in the detection of mycobacteria. Am J Clin Pathol 1989;91:313–315.

CHART 19-4

NAP TEST (*p*-NITRO-α-ACETYLAMINO-β-HYDROXYPROPIOPHENONE); (BACTEC)

I. Principle
Members of the *Mycobacterium tuberculosis* complex do not grow in the presence of *p*-nitro-α-acetylamino-β-hydroxypropiophenone (NAP). Each BACTEC vial contains 5 μg of NAP. When 1 mL of an actively growing culture in 12B medium is added to this vial, the growth of mycobacteria belonging to the *M. tuberculosis* complex is inhibited. Mycobacteria other than tuberculosis (MOTT) do not demonstrate significant inhibition. The presence of growth is detected by monitoring $^{14}CO_2$ production by the radioactive detector of the instrument, the absence of which (no increase in the growth index) is consistent with the *M. tuberculosis* complex.

II. Specimen
BACTEC 12B medium with a growth index > 50

III. Materials
A. Equipment
1. BACTEC 560 instrument (Becton Dickinson, Sparks, MD)
2. Carbon dioxide tank containing 5–10% CO_2 and 90–95% air attached to the instrument
3. BACTEC TB hood (Becton Dickinson)

CHART 19-4

NAP TEST (*p*-NITRO-α-ACETYLAMINO-β-HYDROXYPROPIOPHENONE); (BACTEC) *continued*

    4. Biologic safety cabinet
    5. Incubator, well calibrated at 37 ± 1°C
    6. Vortex mixer
  B. Supplies
    1. Disposable tuberculin syringes with permanently attached needles
    2. Amphyl disinfectant
    3. Gloves, masks, gowns
    4. Cotton or gauze pads
    5. Alcohol swabs
  C. Media and Reagents
    1. Middlebrook 7H12 (BACTEC 12B) medium (contains 7H9 broth base, bovine serum albumin, casein hydrolysate, catalase, and ^{14}C-labeled substrate)
    2. BACTEC NAP vials

IV. Quality Control
  A. Medium: Quality control of the 12B medium is done by the manufacturer.
  B. Include *M. tuberculosis* American Type Culture Collection (ATCC) 27294 and *M. kansasii* ATCC 35775 as controls.
  C. Test the control organisms along with test cultures at least once a month and each time a new lot of NAP is used. The growth index of *M. tuberculosis* should be flat; that of *M. kansasii* should show an ascending curve with time of incubation.

V. Procedure
  1. Read vials positive for AFB daily until the growth index (GI) reaches approximately 50 to 100.
  2. Mix medium well and aseptically transfer 1 mL of the culture medium from this vial into a NAP vial.
  3. Clean the vial tops with Amphyl then with 70% ethyl alcohol.
  4. Shake vial to mix.
  5. Read both the original and inoculated NAP vials daily for 2 to 5 days and record the GI reading.
  6. For cultures in which the GI has passed 100, dilution is necessary before performing the NAP test. The following table should be used to determine the dilution:

GI Reading	Dilution
50–100	No dilution
101–200	0.8 mL into 4 mL 7H12/12B
201–400	0.6 mL into 4 mL 7H12/12B
401–600	0.4 mL into 4 mL 7H12/12B
601–800	0.3 mL into 4 mL 7H12/12B
801–999	0.2 mL into 4 mL 7H12/12B

Mix the dilution thoroughly and transfer 1.0 mL of the contents to a NAP test vial. Incubate the remaining dilution and test as a control for the assay.

VI. Results
  A. Reporting
    1. Reporting is done within 2 to 7 days, with an average of 4 days.
      Report as: NAP test indicates *M. tuberculosis* complex, if growth index is flat; NAP test indicates MOTT, if growth index increases.
    2. The *M. tuberculosis* complex should not be reported in less than 4 days.
    3. Among mycobacteria other than the *M. tuberculosis* complex, certain strains of *M. kansasii, M. gastri, M. szulgai, M. terrae,* and *M. triviale* are partially inhibited by NAP. In such instances, there is a longer lag phase in the presence of NAP, and results interpreted in the first 2 to 4 days may be misleading. Incubate further, and test for an additional 2 to 3 days before reporting.
    4. Optimal incubation temperature is critical for the NAP test. Some mycobacteria (*M. marinum, M. chelonae*) grow at 30°C. There will be inhibition by NAP at 37°C in such cases. The test results will be clear and can be reported within 4 days if the cultures are incubated at 30°C. The NAP test for specimens originating from wounds or skin should be incubated at 37 and 30°C.

CHART 19-4

NAP TEST (*p*-NITRO-α-ACETYLAMINO-β-HYDROXYPROPIOPHENONE); (BACTEC) *continued*

    B. Interpretation
        1. Interpretation of NAP results: The daily GI of the control vial (original culture vial) will continue to increase or decrease. In the NAP vial, increase or decrease depends on the species of mycobacteria:
           a. TB complex: Two consecutive significant decreases in GI after the inoculation = TB complex; slight but not significant increase in the first 2 days and then no increase, or as a decrease in GI = TB complex
           b. MOTT: Daily GI reading increase to over 400 within 4 days = MOTT; no increase or slight decrease in the first 1 or 2 days after inoculation and then two consecutive daily significant increases following day 2 = MOTT
  VII. Limitations of the Procedure
    The NAP test is successful in differentiating the *M. tuberculosis* complex from MOTT only if pure isolated cultures are used. A mixed culture of TB and MOTT will result in an increase of GI indicating MOTT only. Contamination with bacteria can also result in false increases in GI; therefore, acid-fast and in some cases a Gram stain should be performed to confirm a mixed culture or bacterial contamination.
  VIII. Bibliography
    Siddiqi SH. BACTEC NAP test. In: Isenberg HD, ed. Clinical Microbiology Procedure Handbook, Mycobacteriology Section. Washington DC: American Society for Microbiology, 1992.

CHART 19-5

ARYLSULFATASE

    I. Principle
    Arylsulfatase is an enzyme that splits free phenolphthalein from the tripotassium salt of phenolphthalein disulfite. The test for the identification of *Mycobacterium* species is performed in a tube containing a substrate of phenolphthalein in oleic acid agar. After 3 (or 14) days of incubation of a subculture of the unknown species, the appearance of a pink color after addition of sodium carbonate indicates a positive reaction.
  II. Specimen
    Mature colony of the unknown *Mycobacterium* species recovered from clinical material, grown on an Löwenstein-Jensen slant or on Middlebrook 7H-10 agar. Prepare a suspension of the organism in sterile water and incubate for 3 days (14 days).
  III. Materials
    A. Equipment
        1. Biologic safety cabinet
    B. Media
        1. Arylsulfatase stock substrate
           a. Dissolve 2.6 g of phenolphthalein disulfate tripotassium salt in 50 mL of sterile deionized water.
           b. Sterilize by membrane filtration (0.22-μm–pore size filter)
           c. Store in the refrigerator at 2–8°C
           d. Shelf life is indefinite if stored properly. Discard if solution becomes cloudy.
        2. Arylsulfatase broth: 3-day test
           a. Aseptically add 2.5 mL of stock substrate to 200 mL of sterile Dubos Tween broth.
           b. Aseptically dispense 2.0 mL amounts into screw-capped test tubes (16 × 125 mm)
           c. Store at 2–8°C. Discard if the solution becomes cloudy.
        3. Arylsulfatase broth: 2-week test
           a. Aseptically add 7.5 mL of stock substrate to 200 mL of sterile Dubos Tween broth.
           b. Aseptically dispense 2.0 mL amounts into screw-capped test tubes (16 × 125 mm).
           c. Store at 2–8°C.
    Wayne's arylsulfatase agar is commercially available from several sources.
    C. Reagents
        1. 2 N sodium carbonate (Na_2CO_3): Dissolve 10.6 g of anhydrous sodium carbonate in 100 mL of distilled water.

CHART 19-5

ARYLSULFATASE *continued*

IV. Quality Control
   A. Three-Day Test
      1. Positive Control: *Mycobacterium fortuitum* American Type Culture Collection (ATCC) 6841 (if positive control is negative, repeat tests with a fresh subculture of the positive organism. If the negative controls are positive, repeat the tests with a new lot of media).
      2. Negative Control: *Mycobacterium intracellulare* ATCC 13950
      3. Uninoculated medium and reagent only: No color
   B. Fourteen-Day Test
      1. Positive control: *Mycobacterium fortuitum* ATCC 23292
      2. Negative control: *Mycobacterium intracellulare* ATCC 13950
      3. Uninoculated medium and reagent only: No color
V. Procedure
      1. Inoculate each tube of substrate with a slightly turbid suspension of the test organism in sterile water. Thoroughly emulsify the culture in the broth.
      2. Incubate tube for 3 days or 14 days (2-week test) at 35°C in the non-CO_2 incubator
      3. Following incubation, add 1 mL of the 2 N sodium carbonate reagent, mix, and observe for color change.
VI. Results
   A. Interpretation (Readout or Calculations)
   Visually observe for a color change from pale pink to deep red. The lack of color change indicates a negative reaction.
VII. Procedure Notes
   Include an actively growing control organism with each batch of test. For slow growers, use a 3- to 5-week subculture; for rapid growers, a 1- to 3-week subculture. If the positive control is negative, repeat the tests with a fresh subculture of the positive organism. If the negative controls are positive, repeat the tests with a new lot of media.
VIII. Limitation of Procedure
   A. False-negative results can be due to control cultures that are too old.
   B. False-positive results may occur if medium contains free phenolphthalein.
IX. Bibliography
   Kubica GP, Ridgon AL. The arylsulfatase activity of mycobacteria. III. Preliminary investigation of rapidly growing mycobacteria. Am Rev Respir Dis 1961;83:737–740.
   Kubica GP, Vestal AL. The aryl sulfatase activity of acid-fast bacilli: I. Investigation of stock cultures of mycobacteria. Am Rev Respir Dis 1961;83:728–732.
   Lutz B. Arylsulfatase test. In: Isenberg HD. Mycobacteriology Section, Clinical Microbiology Procedure Handbook. Washington, DC: American Society for Microbiology, 1992.
   Wayne LG. Recognition of *Mycobacterium fortuitum* by means of a three-day phenolphthalein sulfatase test. Am J Clin Pathol 1961;36:185–187.

CHART 19-6

ASSESSMENT OF PHOTOREACTIVITY OF MYCOBACTERIA

I. Principle
   The appearance of yellow pigment in the colonies of photochromogenic mycobacteria is the result of yellowish-orange carotene crystals that are produced by actively metabolizing microorganisms after exposure to bright light. Scotochromogenic species have the capability of producing yellow pigment without exposure to light; however, the type of pigment is unknown. The pigmentation of young colonies of mycobacteria after growth in the dark or following exposure to light can be an important aid in the identification of certain *Mycobacterium* species.
II. Specimen
   A primary broth culture of the test organism, diluted sufficiently to produce isolated colonies when inoculated to agar culture

CHART 19-6

ASSESSMENT OF PHOTOREACTIVITY OF MYCOBACTERIA *continued*

III. Materials
    A. Equipment
        1. Biologic safety cabinet
        2. 37°C incubator
    B. Supplies
        1. Sterile screw-capped test tubes, 20 × 110 or 20 × 125 mm
        2. Sterile Pasteur pipettes
        3. Inoculating wires and loops
    C. Medium
        1. Three slants of Löwenstein-Jensen medium
        2. Three Middlebrook 7H10 agar plates
IV. Standards and Controls (include controls with each batch of tests)
    A. Positive photochromogen: *M. kansasii* ATCC 12478
    B. Positive scotochromogen: Stock strains of *M. scrofulaceum* or *M. gordonae*
    C. Negative chromogen: *M. tuberculosis* ATCC 25177
V. Procedure
    1. Inoculate the surfaces of three Löwenstein-Jensen slant media or three Middlebrook 7H11 agar plates with fluid from a dilute broth culture of the organism to be tested. Wrap two of the tubes or plates with aluminum foil; leave the third exposed to the ambient light in the incubator.
    2. Incubate one of the wrapped tubes or plates at 25–30°C; the other wrapped tubes or plates at 37°C.
    3. Several days after growth is noted in the light-exposed control tube or plate, examine the wrapped tubes or plates for growth.
    4. If early growth is detected in the wrapped tubes or plates, expose one of each pair to a strong light for approximately 5 hours. A 100-W tungsten bulb or fluorescent equivalent is adequate. Loosen the cap of the culture tube during this period of light exposure.
    5. Following exposure to light, the tube or plate is returned to the incubator and inspected after 24 to 48 hours for the appearance of yellow pigment.
VI. Results
    A. Interpretation
    Mycobacteria that are scotochromogenic produce an equal amount of pigment whether light-exposed or left in the dark. *M. scrofulaceum, M. gordonae, M. flavescens, M. xenopi,* and *M. szulgai* (the latter is scotochromogenic only when incubated at 37°C) compose the scotochromogenic group.
        Mycobacteria that are photochromogenic produce yellow pigment only after exposure to light. The more commonly encountered photochromogens include *M. kansasii, M. marinum, M. simiae,* and *M. asiaticum.*
        Nonchromogenic mycobacteria are incapable of producing pigment either in the dark or after exposure to light. *M. tuberculosis, M. bovis, M. ulcerans, M. fortuitum, M. chelonae,* and classic strains of *M. avium* are the more commonly encountered nonchromogens.
VII. Procedure Notes
    When *M. szulgai* is suspected, the light-exposed tubes or plates should be incubated at 25°C for 3–5 days. If incubated at 37°C, the photochromogenic potential will be masked by the development of the scotochromogenic pigment at that temperature.
VIII. Limitation of Procedure
    Currently, a high proportion of strains of *M. avium/M. intracellulare* recovered from patients with AIDS show pigment production. Thus, certain strains previously classified as nonchromogens may indeed be chromogenic. This departure, along with the temperature-dependent chromogenicity of *M. szulgai,* are reasons currently brought forth against the validity of the classic Runyon classification of the mycobacteria.
IX. Bibliography
    Wayne LG, Doubek SR. The role of air in the photochromogenic behavior of *M. kansasii. Am J Clin Pathol* 1964; 42:431–435.

CHART 19-7

CATALASE 68°C

I. Principle
Catalase splits hydrogen peroxide into water and oxygen. The evolution of oxygen appears as bubbles. Some forms of catalase are inactivated by heating at 68°C for 20 minutes, a valuable identifying feature for certain *Mycobacterium* species. The hydrogen peroxide used for the identification of *Mycobacterium* species differs from that used to detect catalase in other types of bacteria, by using a 30% concentration (Superoxol) in a strong detergent solution (10% Tween 80). The detergent helps disperse the hydrophobic tightly clumped mycobacteria from large aggregates to individual bacilli, maximizing the detection of catalase.

II. Specimen
Mature colony of the unknown *Mycobacterium* species recovered from clinical material, grown on an Löwenstein-Jensen slant or on Middlebrook 7H-10 agar.

III. Materials
   A. Equipment
      1. 68°C water bath or heat block
   B. Media
      1. Middlebrook 7H9 broth
      2. Löwenstein-Jensen deeps in 25- × 150-mm screw-capped test tubes
   C. Reagents
      1. 30% hydrogen peroxide (commercially available as Superoxol)
      2. 10% Tween 80
      3. M/15 phosphate buffer (0.067 M)

IV. Quality Control
   A. Negative control: *M. tuberculosis* American Type Culture Collection (ATCC) 15177, bubbles at 22–25°C, but not at 68°C.
   B. Positive control: *M. fortuitum* ATCC 6841, bubbles at 22–25°C and at 68°C.
   C. Controls are included with each batch of tests.

V. Procedure
   A. Heat-stable catalase test
      1. Set up one screw-capped tube per organism specimen to be tested in sterile water.
      2. Label each tube with the number of the specimen.
      3. Add 0.5 mL of sterile 0.067 M phosphate buffer to each tube.
      4. Inoculate the buffer with a spadeful of growth from an actively growing subculture of the organism to be tested (2–4 weeks old).
      5. Thoroughly emulsify the culture in the buffer.
      6. Incubate the tubes in a 68°C water bath for exactly 20 minutes.
      7. Remove the tubes from the water bath. Cool to room temperature.
      8. Add 0.5 mL of freshly prepared Tween 80-hydrogen peroxide reagent.
      9. Allow the tubes to sit at room temperature for 20 minutes. Do not shake the tubes.
      10. Visually observe for the evolution of bubbles.
   B. Semiquantitative catalase test
      1. Inoculate a liquid medium, such as Dubos Tween broth or Middlebrook 7H9 broth with a spadeful or loopful of the culture to be tested. Include controls.
      2. Incubate for 7 days at 37°C.
      3. Mix for 5–10 seconds on a vortex mixer.
      4. Transfer six drops to a Löwenstein-Jensen deep (prepared in 25- × 150-mm tubes).
      5. Incubate the deeps for 14 days at 37°C. Be sure caps are loose.
      6. Add 1 mL of freshly prepared Tween 80-hydrogen peroxide reagent. Avoid contact of reagent with skin.
      7. Allow tests to sit at room temperature for 5 minutes.
      8. Measure the column of bubbles.

VI. Results
   A. Interpretation (Readout or Calculations)
      1. Heat-stable catalase test: The appearance of bubbles indicates a positive test; lack of bubbles is a negative reaction. *M. tuberculosis* and other mycobacteria lose their catalase activity when heated to 68°C.
      2. Semiquantitative catalase test:
         High catalase reaction: >45 mm of foam
         Low catalase reaction: <45 mm of foam

CHART 19-7

CATALASE 68°C *continued*

VII. Procedure Notes
Failure of control cultures to give expected results is usually due to the use of cultures that are too old—use only actively growing cultures.
VIII. Limitation of Procedure
False-negative results can be due to use of cultures with inadequate growth, the use of cultures that are too old, or reagents that are outdated. Inadequate growth may result from an inadequate inoculum or from screwing lids too tightly.
False-positive results may occur if the culture contains catalase-positive, contaminating bacterial species.
IX. Bibliography
Kubica GP, et al. Differential identification of mycobacteria: I. Tests on catalase activity. Am Rev Respir Dis 1966;95:400–405.
Lutz B. Catalase tests. In: Isenberg HD, ed. Clinical Microbiology Procedure Handbook, Mycobacteriology Section. Washington, DC: American Society for Microbiology, 1992.

CHART 19-8

GROWTH ON MACCONKEY AGAR

I. Principle
The ability to grow on special MacConkey agar, formulated without crystal violet, differentiates *M. fortuitum*, *M. chelonae* and *M. abscessus*, which can grow within 5 days, from other rapidly growing mycobacteria that show only slight growth after 11 days.
II. Specimen
A mature colony of the unknown *Mycobacterium* species recovered from clinical material, grown on a Löwenstein-Jensen slant or on Middlebrook 7H-10 agar is tested.
III. Materials
A. Equipment: None
B. Media: MacConkey agar without crystal violet. Purchased from Remel Laboratories (Lenexa, KS). Stored in the walk-in refrigerator at 4°C.
C. Reagents: None
D. Supplies: None
IV. Quality Control
A. Positive control: *M. fortuitum* American Type Culture Collection (ATCC) 6841
B. Negative control: *M. phlei* ATCC 11758; uninoculated medium and reagent only
V. Procedure
1. Inoculate a fresh MacConkey plate with three drops of the organism grown for 7 to 10 days in 7H9 broth and streak for isolation.
2. Incubate at 28 to 30°C for 11 days without CO_2.
3. At 5 and 11 days, visually observe the surface of the agar plate for the presence of colony growth.
VI. Results
A. Interpretation (Readout or Calculations)
A positive test for *M. fortuitum* will show growth along the entire streak area and possibly a color change in the medium in 5 days. The absence of growth indicates a negative test.
VII. Procedure Notes
Include controls with each batch of tests. If results are not as expected, repeat tests with fresh control organisms and a new lot of media.
VIII. Limitation of Procedure
About 25% of *M. smegmatus* strains grow on MacConkey agar without crystal violet. To obviate any diagnostic difficulties, the 3-day arylsulfatase test may be used to separate *M. smegmatus* (negative) from *M. fortuitum*, *M. chelonae,* and *M. abscessus* (positive).
IX. Bibliography
Jones WD, Kubica GP. The use of MacConkey agar for differential typing of *M. fortuitum*. Am J Med Technol 1946;30:182–195.
Lutz B. Nitrate reduction. In: Isenberg HD, ed. Clinical Microbiology Procedure Handbook, Mycobacteriology Section. Washington, DC: American Society for Microbiology, 1992.

CHART 19-9

INHIBITION BY THIOPHENE-2-CARBOXYLIC ACID HYDRAZIDE (T$_2$H, 1 μg/mL)

I. Principle
Thiophene-2-carboxylic acid hydrazide has the property of inhibiting *Mycobacterium bovis*, but not other species of mycobacteria, a helpful feature differentiating *M. bovis* from *M. tuberculosis*.
II. Specimen
A 3- to 4-week-old culture of the test organism growing on Löwenstein-Jensen medium or Middlebrook 7H10 agar.
III. Materials
   A. Equipment
      1. Biologic safety cabinet
      2. 10% CO$_2$ incubator at 37°C
   B. Supplies
      1. Sterile applicator sticks
      2. Sterile 9.0 mL water blanks
      3. Sterile deionized water
      4. Quadrant petri dishes
   C. Media
      1. Thiopene-2-carboxylic acid hydrazide (T$_2$H) (also known as TCH) susceptibility medium (10 μg/mL)
         a. Make two 200-mL batches of Middlebrook 7H10 medium in separate flasks.
         b. Sterilize by autoclaving. Cool to 50°C in a water bath.
         c. Pipette 5.0 mL of cooled medium from one of the flasks into quadrants I and III of a quadrant petri dish.
         d. Add 2.0 mL of a 1000 μg/mL TCH stock solution into the remaining flask (final concentration of 10 μg/mL). Swirl well to mix.
         e. Dispense 5.0 mL of this medium into quadrants II and IV of each plate.
         f. Protect the plates from light by covering with brown paper. Store plates at 2 to 8°C; shelf life is approximately 1 month.
IV. Quality Control
   A. Positive control: *M. bovis* American Type Culture Collection (ATCC) 35734 (susceptible to TCH at 10 μg/mL)
   B. Negative control: *M. tuberculosis* ATCC 25177 (resistant)
V. Procedure
      1. Prepare a suspension of the unknown mycobacterium in sterile water equivalent to a McFarland 1 standard.
      2. Dilute to make a suspension of 10^{-3} to 10^{-4} in sterile deionized water.
      3. Inoculate three drops of each dilution onto a control quadrant and a TCH quadrant on the quadrant plates.
      4. Cover the plates with brown paper to prevent exposure to light, letting the plates sit at room temperature to allow adsorption of the inoculum.
      5. Place each plate into a CO$_2$-permeable zipper bag, invert the plates, and incubate at 37°C in 8–10% CO$_2$ for 3 weeks.
      6. After incubation, count the colonies on the control quadrant and on the quadrant that contains the TCH at 10 μg/mL.
VI. Results
   A. Calculate the percentage of resistance as follows:
$$\textit{Number of colonies on quadrant containing TCH} \times 100 =$$
percentage of colonies resistant on control quadrant
   B. Record the test culture as resistant to TCH if the derived number is higher than 1%.
VII. Bibliography

Harrington R, Karlson AG. Differentiation between *M. tuberculosis* and *M. bovis* by in vitro procedures. Am J Vet Res 1967;7:1193–1196.
Lutz B. Identification tests for mycobacteria: inhibition by thiophene-2-carboxylic acid hydrazide. In: Isenberg HD, ed. Clinical Microbiology Procedure Handbook. Washington, DC: American Society for Microbiology, 1992.
Wayne LG, et al. Highly reproducible techniques for use in systematic bacteriology in the genus *Mycobacterium*: tests for niacin and catalase and for resistance to isoniazid, thiophene 2-carboxylic acid hydrazide, hydroxylamine and *p*-nitrobenzoate. Int J Syst Bacteriol 1976;26:311–318.

CHART 19-10

IRON UPTAKE

I. Principle
   The ability to take up iron from an inorganic iron-containing reagent helps to differentiate *Mycobacterium fortuitum* and *M. phlei* (positive) from *M. chelonae* and *M. abscessus* which do not take up iron.
II. Specimen
   Mature colony of the unknown *Mycobacterium* species recovered from clinical material, grown on an Löwenstein-Jensen slant.
III. Materials
   A. Equipment
      1. Biologic safety hood
      2. 28 to 30°C incubator
      3. Sterile Pasteur pipettes
   B. Media
      1. Löwenstein-Jensen slants (purchased from Remel Laboratories, Lenexa, KS)
   C. Reagents
      20% ferric ammonium citrate
      1. Add 20 g of ferric ammonium citrate to 100 mL of deionized water
      2. Swirl to dissolve
      3. Autoclave for 15 minutes at 121°C
      4. Store in the refrigerator at 2 to 8°C
IV. Quality Control
   A. Positive control: *M. fortuitum,* American Type Culture Collection (ATCC) 6841
   B. Negative control: *M. chelonae,* ATCC 35751; uninoculated medium and reagent only
V. Procedure
      1. Use an actively growing (1- to 2-week-old) subculture of a rapidly growing mycobacterium on a Löwenstein-Jensen slant.
      2. Add as many drops of sterile 20% ferric ammonium citrate as there are milliliters of medium in the slant. For example, for 8 mL of medium, add eight drops of ferric ammonium citrate.
      3. Reincubate the slant at 28 to 30°C for up to 3 weeks.
      4. Visually examine the surface of the slants for the presence of a dark, rust brown color.
VI. Results
   The color of a truly positive iron uptake test will be very dark rust. A positive reaction seen in a rapidly growing strain of mycobacteria is indicative of *M. fortuitum.*
VII. Procedure Notes
   If the results are not as expected, check the ages and purity of the control and test cultures. Repeat the tests with new ferric ammonium citrate reagent and new control cultures.
VIII. Limitation of Procedure
   Some isolates of *M. chelonae* will turn tannish brown, a color sometimes referred to as ''turtlelike,'' giving a false-positive reaction. Look for a very dark rust color.
IX. Bibliography
   Lutz B. Iron uptake. In: Isenberg HD, ed. Clinical Microbiology Procedure Handbook, Mycobacteriology Section. Washington, DC: American Society for Microbiology, 1992.
   Silcox VA, Good RA, Floyd MM. Identification of clinically significant *Mycobacterium fortuitum* complex. J Clin Microbiol 1981;14:686–691.

CHART 19-11

NIACIN ACCUMULATION

I. Principle
   All *Mycobacterium* species produce niacin ribonucleotide; however, virtually all strains of *M. tuberculosis* and *M. simiae* and some strains of *M. chelonae* lack the enzymes to further convert niacin to nicotinamide adenine dinucleotide (NAD). Niacin accumulates in the culture medium, from which it can be extracted with sterile water or physiologic saline. The extract is placed in a small test tube to which is added a reagent-impregnated niacin filter strip.

CHART 19-11

NIACIN ACCUMULATION *continued*

II. Specimen

A longer than 3-week-old heavy growth on Löwenstein-Jensen of the organism to be tested. Growth on other culture media do not produce sufficient niacin to produce a positive test reaction by this method.

III. Materials
   A. Equipment
      1. Biologic safety cabinet
      2. 37°C incubator
   B. Supplies
      1. Sterile screw-capped test tubes, 20 × 110 or 20 × 125 mm
      2. Sterile Pasteur pipettes
      3. Sterile 5 mL pipettes
   C. Reagents
      1. Niacin filter paper strips (Difco)
      2. Sterile H_2O

IV. Standards and Controls (include controls with each batch of tests):
   A. Positive control: *M. tuberculosis* American Type Culture Collection (ATCC) 25177
   B. Negative control: *M. intracellulare* ATCC 13950

V. Procedure
   1. Flood the surface of the Löwenstein-Jensen slant over the heavy growth of the test organism with 1 mL sterile H_2O. Stab the medium with the tip of the pipette to allow access of the water to the underlying medium.
   2. Tilt the tube so the water covers the surface of the slant. Let stand for 20 to 30 minutes.
   3. Rotate the tube so that the slant faces downward. Carefully remove 0.6 mL of extract without touching the slant and transfer to the screw-capped test tube.
   4. Using a pair of forceps, drop a niacin test strip with the arrow pointing downward into the tube. Stopper the tube immediately.
   5. Gently shake the tube and repeat shaking after 5 and 10 minutes.
   6. After 12 to 15 minutes, and not longer than 30 minutes, read the test for the presence of a yellow color.

VI. Results
   A. Interpretation
      The development of a yellow color indicates a positive test. If a culture resembles *M. tuberculosis,* but the niacin test is negative, reincubate the slant for an additional 2 to 4 weeks and repeat the test.

VII. Limitation of Procedure
   False-negative reactions may occur. Reasons include 1) an insufficient amount of growth on the slant, 2) failure to stab the agar if the growth is confluent, and 3) the presence of contaminating bacteria that may have metabolized any niacin that may have accumulated.
   M. simiae and occasional strains of *M. bovis, M. marinum,* and *M. chelonae* may accumulate niacin in the test medium. These species can be readily differentiated from *M. tuberculosis* by several key characteristics described in the interpretation section of this manual.

VIII. Bibliography

Gangadharam PR, Droubi DSA. A comparison of four different methods for testing the production of niacin by mycobacteria. Am Rev Respir Dis 1971;104:434–437.

Kilburn JO, Kubica GP. Reagent impregnated paper for detection of niacin. Am J Clin Pathol 1968;50:530–531.

Konno K, et al. Niacin metabolism in mycobacteria. Am Rev Respir Dis 1966;93:41–46.

Lutz B. Nitrate reduction. In: Isenberg HD, ed. Clinical Microbiology Procedure Handbook, Mycobacteriology Section. Washington, DC: American Society for Microbiology, 1992.

Runyon EH, Selin MJ, Hawes HW. Distinguishing mycobacteria by the niacin test. Am Rev Tubercu 1959;79:663–665.

Young WE Jr, et al. Development of paper strip test for the detection of niacin produced by mycobacteria. Appl Microbiol 1970;20:949–945.

CHART 19-12

NITRATE REDUCTION: MYCOBACTERIA

I. Principle

Mycobacteria producing nitroreductase are capable of catalyzing the reduction of nitrate to nitrite. In the reaction, oxygen is extracted from nitrate according to the following formula:

$$NO_3 + 2e^- + 2H \longrightarrow NO_2 + H_2O$$

The nitrate produced is detected by the addition of α-naphthalamine and sulfanilic acid, forming the red diazonium dye, p-sulfobenzene-azo-α-naphthalamine.

II. Specimen

A 3- to 4-week-old culture of the test organism growing on Löwenstein-Jensen medium or other coagulated egg medium.

III. Materials

A. Equipment
   1. Biologic safety hood
   2. 37°C water bath or heating block

B. Supplies
   1. Sterile Pasteur pipettes
   2. Sterile forceps

C. Reagents
   1. Nitrate test substrate (0.01 M) in M/45 phosphate buffer (0.02 M, pH 7.0)

$NaNO_3$	0.8 g
$KH2PO_4$	1.17 g
Na_2HPO_4	1.93 g
H_2O	999 mL (final volume)

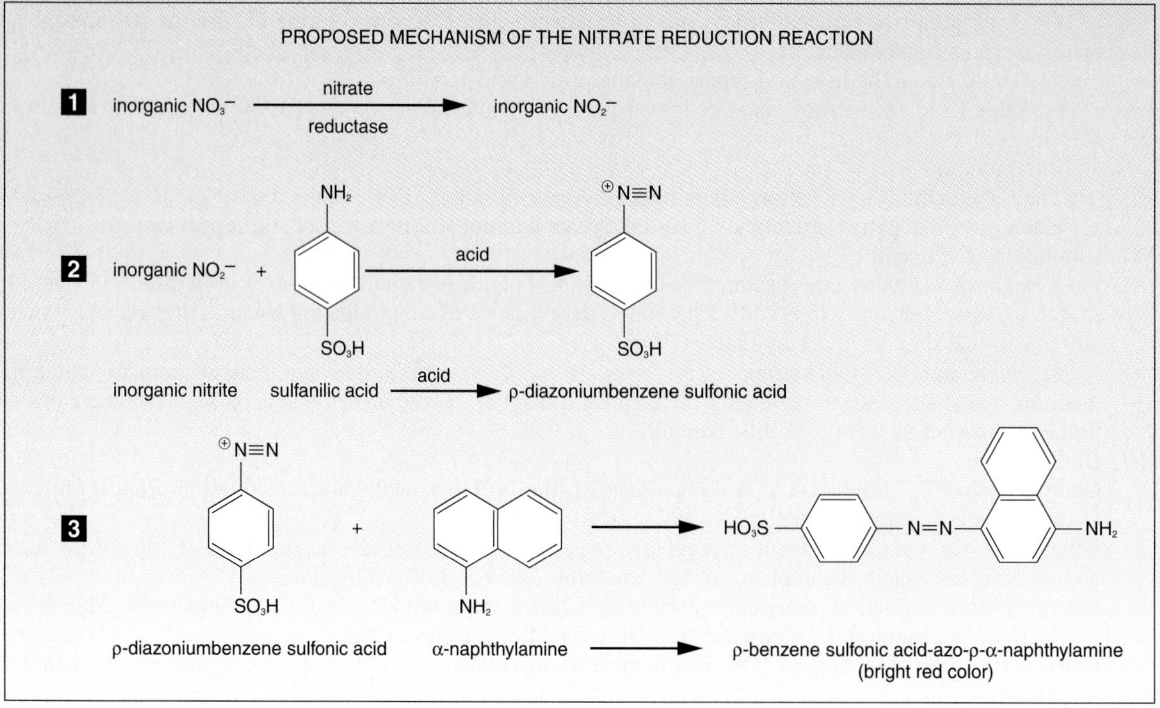

PROPOSED MECHANISM OF THE NITRATE REDUCTION REACTION

CHART 19-12

NITRATE REDUCTION: MYCOBACTERIA *continued*

> Dissolve and mix the chemicals. Adjust pH to 7.0. Autoclave and store and dispense in 2.0-mL aliquots in sterile tubes. When stored at 2 to 8°C, the shelf life is 1 to 2 months.
> 2. 0.2% sulfanilimide: Completely dissolve 0.1 g of sulfanilamide in 50 mL of deionized water. It may be necessary to warm the water to 47 to 50°C for complete solubility. If stored in brown-glass bottles at 2 to 8°C, the shelf life is about 1 month.
> 3. 0.1% *N*-(1-naphthyl)ethylenediamine dihydrochloride: Dissolve 0.05 g of *N*-(1-naphthyl)ethylenediamine dihydrochloride in 50 mL of deionized water. The shelf life is 1 month if stored in a brown-glass bottle at 2 to 8°C.

IV. Quality Control
   A. Positive control: *M. tuberculosis* American Type Culture Collection (ATCC)
   B. Negative control: *M. avium* complex ATCC
   C. Negative reagent control: Uninoculated tube containing appropriate substrate

V. Procedure
   1. Emulsify one loopful or spadeful of colonies from solid medium into 2 mL of nitrate substrate.
   2. Shake by hand to mix and incubate at 35 to 37°C for 2 hours.
   3. Add reagents to mixture in the following order:
      1 drop concentrated HCl
      2 drops of 0.2% sulfanilamide
      2 drops of 0.1% *N*-(1-naphthyl)ethylenediamine dihydrochloride
   4. Allow mixture to sit at room temperature for 5 minutes.
   5. Read for the development of a pink to red color.

VI. Results
   The appearance of a red or pink color is indicative of a positive test. A quantitative reading can be made by comparing with nitrate reduction standards. Quantitation is not performed in most laboratories.

VII. Procedure Notes
   If no color change occurs, confirm negative results by adding a small amount of zinc dust. A deep red to pink color after the addition of zinc dust indicates that nitrate was reduced. Reagents are stored at 2 to 8°C in the refrigerator, away from direct light.

VIII. Limitation of Procedure
   The color may fade rapidly in some instances and can lead to a false-negative test if a reading is not made soon after the reagents are added.

IX. Bibliography
   Master RN. Nitrate reduction. In: Isenberg HD, ed. Clinical Microbiology Procedure Handbook, Mycobacteriology Section. Washington, DC: American Society for Microbiology, 1992.
   Virtanen S. A study of nitrate reduction of mycobacteria. Acta Tuberc Scand Suppl 1960;418:119.
   Wayne LC, Doubek SR. Classification and identification of mycobacteria: II. Tests employing nitrite as substrates. Am Rev Respir Dis 1965;91:478–745.

CHART 19-13

PYRAZINAMIDASE

I. Principle
   The deamidation of pyrazinamide to pyrazinoic acid in 4 days is a useful phenotypic characteristic by which *M. marinum* (positive) can be differentiated from *M. kansasii* (negative) and by which weakly niacin-positive strains of *M. bovis* (negative) can be distinguished from *M. tuberculosis* complex (positive).

II. Specimen
   Mature colonies of the unknown *Mycobacterium* species recovered from clinical material, grown on a Löwenstein-Jensen slant or on Middlebrook 7H-10 agar.

III. Materials
   A. Equipment: None
   B. Medium
      1. Pyrazinamidase substrate medium
         a. Dissolve 6.5 g of Dubos broth base in 1 L distilled water.

CHART 19-13

PYRAZINAMIDASE *continued*

b. Add

Pyrazinamide	0.1 g
Sodium pyruvate	2.0 g
Agar	15 g

c. Heat to dissolve. Dispense in 50.0-mL amounts into screw-cap tubes.
d. Autoclave for 15 minutes at 121°C.
e. Allow agar to harden with tubes in upright position.
f. Shelf life is 6 months when stored at 2 to 8°C. Discard if agar appears dehydrated or contaminated.

C. Reagents
1% ferrous ammonium sulfate (prepare immediately before use): Place 0.1 g of ferrous ammonium sulfate in sterile screw-capped test tubes. Add 10 mL of sterile deionized water immediately before use, and allow the crystals to dissolve.

D. Supplies
1. Sterile applicator sticks
2. Sterile 1.0- or 5.0-mL pipettes

IV. Quality Control
A. Positive control: *M. intracellulare* American Type Culture Collection (ATCC) 13950
B. Negative control: *M. kansasii* ATCC 12478

V. Procedure
1. Inoculate a large loopful of growth from an actively growing subculture to the surface of two pyrazinamidase agar deeps.
2. Incubate the tubes with caps loose at 37°C.
3. Remove one of the tubes from the incubator after 4 days. Remove one of the control tubes also.
4. Add 1.0 mL of freshly prepared 1% ferrous ammonium sulfate to each tube.
5. Examine the tubes for a pink band in the agar after 30 minutes at room temperature.
6. Refrigerate any negative tubes for 4 hours more and reexamine for the presence of a pink band.

VI. Results
A. Interpretation
After 4 hours, examine the tubes for a pink band in the reagent layer on the surface of the agar (positive reaction), using incident room light against a white background. Repeat the procedure with the remaining tube after 7 days of incubation.

VII. Procedure Notes
Perform all tests under a biologic safety hood.

VIII. Bibliography
Wayne LG. Simple pyrazinamidase and urease tests for routine identification of mycobacteria. Am Rev Respir Dis 1974;109:147–151.

Lutz B. Identification tests for mycobacteria: Pyrazinamidase. In: Isenberg HD, ed. Clinical Microbiology Procedure Handbook. Washington, DC: American Society for Microbiology, 1992.

CHART 19-14

SODIUM CHLORIDE TOLERANCE: MYCOBACTERIA

I. Principle
Of the slowly growing mycobacteria, only *M. triviale* grows in media containing 5% NaCl; of the medically significant rapidly growing mycobacteria, only *M. chelonae* subsp. *chelonae* fail to grow in such media.

II. Specimen
A 3- to 4-week-old culture of the test organism growing on Löwenstein-Jensen medium or other coagulated egg medium.

CHART 19-14

SODIUM CHLORIDE TOLERANCE: MYCOBACTERIA *continued*

III. Materials
  A. Equipment
    1. Biologic safety hood
    2. Slant racks
  B. Supplies
    1. Sterile applicator sticks
    2. Sterile 1.0-mL pipettes
    3. McFarland 1 standard
  C. Media
    1. Löwenstein-Jensen without 5% NaCl in slants
    2. Löwenstein-Jensen with 5% NaCl in slants
    3. Dubos Tween or Middlebrook 7H9 broth
IV. Quality Control
  A. Positive control: *M. fortuitum* American Type Culture Collection (ATCC) 6841
  B. Negative control: *M. gordonae* ATCC 14470
  Set up controls for each new lot number of medium received. Reject medium if results on control organisms are not as expected. Purchase Löwenstein-Jensen with and without NaCl in the same size tubes for consistency in interpretation.
V. Procedure
  1. Use an actively growing culture (2 to 4 weeks for slow growers; 1 to 2 weeks for rapid growers). Make a suspension of organisms in Middlebrook 7H9 broth equal to a McFarland 1 standard.
  2. Take one Lowenstein-Jensen slant with 5% NaCl and one slant without 5% NaCl and inoculate into each tube, 0.1 mL of the described suspension.
  3. Incubate the slants with the caps loose in a 5 to 10% CO_2 incubator. Lie slants flat in a rack during incubation. Incubate for 1 week at 29 to 30°C for rapid growers and 37°C for slow growers. Stand negative tubes up straight; incubate 3 more weeks. Visually examine slants weekly for growth.
VI. Results
  1. When numerous colonies are seen on the control slant and more than 50 colonies on the medium containing 5% NaCl, record the test as positive.
  2. When there are colonies on the control slant and no visible growth on the slant containing NaCl, continue incubation for up to 4 weeks.
VII. Procedure Notes
  Use the slant without 5% NaCl to check for viability of the organism. It is not necessary to have equal growth in both tubes. If the organism does not grow on the slant without 5% NaCl, repeat the test.
VIII. Limitation of Procedure
  Some strains of *M. fortuitum* and *M. chelonae* grow on an NaCl-containing media only at temperatures lower than 35°C. For this reason all test specimens should be incubated at 29 to 30°C.
IX. Bibliography
  Lutz B. Sodium chloride tolerance. In: Isenberg HD, ed. Clinical Microbiology Procedure Handbook, Mycobacteriology Section. Washington, DC: American Society for Microbiology, 1992.
  Silcox VA, Good RA, Floyd MM. Identification of clinically significant *Mycobacterium fortuitum* complex. J Clin Microbiol 1981;4:686–691.

CHART 19-15

TWEEN-80 HYDROLYSIS

I. Principle
  Tween 80 is the trade name of the polyethylene derivative of sorbitan mono-oleate. Some *Mycobacterium* species possess an enzyme that releases oleic acid from the Tween 80. The color change from orange to pink is due to hydrolysis of Tween 80, which modifies the optical rotation of light passing through the substrate.
II. Specimen
  Mature colony of the unknown *Mycobacterium* species recovered from clinical material, growth on a Löwenstein-Jensen slant.

CHART 19-15

TWEEN-80 HYDROLYSIS *continued*

  III. Materials
     A. Supplies
       1. Sterile applicator sticks
       2. Screw-capped tubes (12 × 100 mm) containing 2.0 mL of deionized water per tube
     B. Media
       1. Löwenstein-Jensen slants
     C. Reagents
       1. Tween-80 hydrolysis reagent
       2. 2 drops of Difco (Detroit, MI) reagent added to distilled water in screw-capped tubes.
     D. Equipment
       1. Biohazard hood
  IV. Quality Control
     A. Positive control: *M. kansasii,* American Type Culture Collection (ATCC) 12478 incubated for 12 days
     B. Negative control: Stock culture of *M. intracellulare* ATCC 13950
     C. Negative reagent: Uninoculated tube of substrate, incubated for 12 days
  V. Procedure
     1. Add two drops of Tween reagent to 1 mL of sterile distilled water in screw-capped tubes.
     2. Inoculate a loopful of the organism to be tested.
     3. Incubate at 35°C in the dark with caps tight.
     4. Visually read tubes at 24 hours. If negative, read again at 5 and 10 days. Compare the color of the liquid with that in the control tubes.
  VI. Results
     A positive result is recorded when the liquid, not the cells, turns from light orange to pink or red. *M. kansasii* usually turns positive within 24 hours. Read again at 3, 5, and 10 to 12 days. Record results and discard positives. Discard all tubes at 12 days.
  VII. Procedure Notes
     Keep Tween hydrolysis reagent in the dark. Do not store or incubate tubes in the light. The red color of a positive reaction is not due to a pH change, rather to release of neutral red.
  VIII. Bibliography
     Lutz B. Tween-80 hydrolysis. In: Isenberg HD, ed. Clinical Microbiology Procedure Handbook, Mycobacteriology Section. Washington, DC: American Society for Microbiology, 1992.
     Kilburn JO, et al. Preparation of a stable mycobacterial Tween hydrolysis test substrate. Appl Microbiol 1973;26: 826.
     Wayne LG, Doubek JR, Russell RL. Classification and identification of mycobacteria: I Tests employing Tween-80 as substrate. Am Rev Respir Dis 1964;90:588–597.

CHART 19-16

UREASE: MYCOBACTERIA

  I. Principle
     Urease is an enzyme possessed by many *Mycobacterium* species that can hydrolyze urea to form ammonia and carbon dioxide. The ammonia reacts in solution to form ammonium carbonate, resulting in alkalinization and an increase in the pH of the medium.
  II. Specimen
     A. Type of Specimen
       Mature colony of the unknown *Mycobacterium* species recovered from clinical material, grown on a Lowenstein-Jensen slant.
  III. Materials
     A. Equipment
       1. Biologic safety hood
       2. 37°C incubator

CHART 19-16

UREASE: MYCOBACTERIA *continued*

    B. Medium
        1. Urea broth
           a. Add 10 g of Difco (Detroit, MI) Bacto urea agar base concentrate to 90 mL of sterile deionized water. Mix well to dissolve.
           b. Aseptically aliquot 3.0 mL portions into sterile screw-capped test tubes.
           c. Store at 2 to 8°C; shelf life is 1 month.
 IV. Quality Control
    A. Positive control: *M. kansasii* American Type Culture Collection (ATCC) 12478
    B. Negative control: *M. avium/M. intracellulare* ATCC 13950
  V. Procedure
        1. Inoculate each substrate tube with a spadeful of growth from an actively growing culture. Thoroughly emulsify the culture in the broth.
        2. Incubate at 35°C for 5 days.
        3. Visually read the tubes at 1, 3, and 7 days.
 VI. Results
    Color change from yellow to dark pink or red indicates a positive reaction. No color change is a negative reaction.
 VII. Procedure Notes
    Repeat tests that appear slightly pink; if the repeat test result is still ±, report as negative.
VIII. Limitation of Procedure
        1. False-positive tests are usually due to incorrect interpretation of results, incubation beyond 5 days, or contaminated test or control cultures.
        2. False-negative results are due to the use of an incorrect medium (i.e., one used for testing bacteria other than acid-fast bacilli), insufficient inoculum, or cultures that are too old.
 IX. Bibliography

Kent PT, Kubica GP. Public Health Mycobacteriology: A Guide for the Level III Laboratory. Atlanta: Centers for Disease Control, 1985. Department of Health and Human Services publication no. 86-21654-6.

Lutz B. Identification tests for mycobacteria: urease. In: Isenberg HD, ed. Clinical Microbiology Procedure Handbook. Washington, DC: American Society for Microbiology, 1992.

Murphy DB, Hawkins JE. Use of urease disks in the identification of mycobacteria. J Clin Microbiol 1975;1: 465–468.

CHART 19-17

DNA PROBES FOR THE IDENTIFICATION OF MYCOBACTERIA

  I. Principle
    A commercially manufactured system, AccuProbe Culture Confirmation Tests (GenProbe, Inc., San Diego, CA), is available for identification of isolates of several species of mycobacteria (*M. tuberculosis* complex, *M. avium*, *M. intracellulare*, *M. gordonae*, *M. avium* complex, and *M. kansasii*). The system is based on the use of DNA probes that are complementary to species-specific rRNA. The mycobacterial cells are lysed by sonication, heat-killed, and exposed to DNA that has been labeled with a chemiluminiscent tag. The labeled DNA probe combines with the organism's rRNA to form a stable DNA-RNA hybrid. A selection reagent "kills" the signal on all unbound DNA. Chemiluminescence produced by DNA-RNA hybrids is measured in a luminometer.
  II. Specimen
    Any actively growing culture less than 1 month old recovered on solid or broth medium (Middlebrook 7H9, 7H10, 7H11, 7H11 Selective or Löwenstein-Jensen) may be used.

CHART 19-17

DNA PROBES FOR THE IDENTIFICATION OF MYCOBACTERIA *continued*

III. Materials
   A. Reagents

Reagent	Description	Storage Temperature (°C)
Lysing tubes	Lyophilized glass beads and buffer	23–25
Probe reagent	Tubed lyophilized species-specific DNA	4
Reagent 1	Specimen diluent	23–25
Reagent 2	Probe diluent	23–25
Reagent 3	Selection reagent	23–25
Detection I	H_2O_2 in nitric acid solution containing 1 N NaOH	23–25
Detection II	H_2O_2 in nitric acid solution containing 1 N NaOH	23–25
Ultrasonic enhancer	Detergent-like solution to increase sonication	23–25

   B. Supplies
      1. Micropipettes (100 μL)
      2. Micropipettor (300 μL)
      3. Repipettor (300 μL)
      4. Repipettor syringes
      5. Plastic sterile inoculating loops (1 μg)
   C. Equipment
      1. Luminometer (Leader 1, Leader 250, or PAL)
      2. Vortex mixer
      3. Water or dry bath, 90 ± 5°C
      4. Water or dry bath, 60 ± 5°C
IV. Quality Control
   A. Frequency and tolerance of controls
      1. Run a positive and negative control with each batch of organisms to be tested.
      2. If controls are not set within limits, check age of culture (should be less than 2 months old), level of water in sonicator, quality of sonicator (by observing waving water patterns while sonicator is on; water should "dance"), and temperature of hybridization; if necessary, run a tritium standard.
   B. Control Organisms

Probe to be Tested	Control	
	Positive	Negative
M. avium	*M. avium* American Type Culture Collection (ATCC) 25291	*M. intracellular* ATCC 13950
M. intracellulare	*M. intracellulare* ATCC 13950	*M. avium* ATCC 25291
M. tuberculosis complex	*M. tuberculosis* ATCC 14470	*M. avium* ATCC 25291
M. gordonae	*M. gordonae* ATCC 14470	*M. scrofulaceum* ATCC 19073
M. avium complex	*M. intracellulare* ATCC 13950	*M. gordonae* ATCC 14470
M. kansasii	*M. kansasii* ATCC 12478	*M. tuberculosis* ATCC 25177

V. Procedure
   1. Add 1 cup of ultrasonic enhancer to the water in the sonicator. Degas the water for 15 minutes. Turn on 95°C water bath (or heat block) and 60°C water bath (or heat block).
   2. Add 100 mL of reagent 1 (specimen diluent) and 100 mL of reagent 2 (probe diluent) to each lysing tube.
   3. Working in a biologic safety cabinet, transfer a loopful (1 mL) of test organism into the lysing tube. Twirl the loop against the side of the tube to remove the entire inoculum.
   4. Place the lysing tubes in the sonicator. Ensure that the water level is high enough to cover the contents of the tube. Do not allow the tubes to touch the sides of the sonicator. Sonicate at room temperature for 15 minutes.

CHART 19-17

DNA PROBES FOR THE IDENTIFICATION OF MYCOBACTERIA *continued*

      5. Place the lysing tubes in the 95°C water bath (or heat block) for 15 minutes.
      6. Allow the tubes to cool at room temperature for 5 minutes.
      7. Pipette 100 mL of the killed lysate into the probe reaction tube.
      8. Incubate the tubes for 15 minutes at 60°C in the water bath (or heat block).
      9. Pipette 300 mL of reagent 3 (selection reagent) into each tube. Recap and vortex the tubes, and immediately place them back into the 60°C water bath (or heat block). Incubate for 5 minutes.
     10. Prepare the luminometer for operation by completing a wash cycle. To prevent static buildup and to ensure that no residue is present on the outside of the tube, wipe each tube with a damp tissue before inserting it into the luminometer. Read each tube and controls. The luminometer records relative light units (RLU).

  VI. Results
     A. A positive result is >30,000 RLU.
     B. Signals lower than 30,000 RLU are considered negative.
     C. Repeat any test with a result between 20,000 and 29,999 RLU.
 VII. Procedure Notes
     A. It is important to maintain the 60 ± 1°C dry bath, because annealing of the DNA-RNA hybrid is temperature-sensitive.
     B. The water level of the sonicator should be sufficiently high to cover the hybridization buffer, beads, and organism.
     C. Other sources of error include failure to vortex after addition of the organism-buffer mixture to the probe tube and after addition of reagent 3, which inactivates the acridinium ester not bound to rRNA.
     D. This method is currently being evaluated for use with BACTEC bottles.
VIII. Limitations of the Procedure
     A. This method cannot be used directly on fresh clinical specimens; it is for culture confirmation only.
     B. A small number of biochemically determined *M. avium* complex isolated will not produce a positive result with the *M. avium* complex probe. The taxonomic status of these strains is currently uncertain.
     C. The *M. tuberculosis* complex culture confirmation test does not differentiate between *M. tuberculosis, M. bovis, M. bovis* BCG, *M. africanum,* and *M. microti.*
     D. The *M. avium* complex culture confirmation does not differentiate between *M. avium* and *M. intracellulare.*
  IX. Bibliography
     Gen-Probe. Product Information: AcuProbe Mycobacterium Culture Confirmation Tests. San Diego, CA: Gen-Probe, 1990.
     Stockman L. Identification of Mycobacteria in DNA probes. In: Isenberg HD, ed. Clinical Microbiology Procedure Handbook. Washington, DC: American Society for Microbiology, 1992.

CHART 19-18

DETECTION, IDENTIFICATION, AND DRUG SUSCEPTIBILITY TESTING OF *M. TUBERCULOSIS* BY RADIOMETRIC INSTRUMENTATION

   I. Principle
     The metabolism of [^{14}C]palmitic acid to $^{14}CO_2$ by members of the genus *Mycobacterium* is a sensitive and specific method to recover, identify, and test mycobacteria for drug susceptibility. $^{14}CO_2$ is detected in the ion chamber of the BACTEC 460 (Becton Dickinson Instruments Systems, Sparks, MD). Because of the sensitivity of the instrument to detect $^{14}CO_2$, the ability to assess growth in the presence of one of several antituberculosis drugs incorporated into the media provides a rapid method to determine drug resistance. Clinical specimens can be scanned for activity every day. Growth is determined by finding increasing readings for $^{14}CO_2$ in the ion chamber.
  II. Specimen
     A positive culture for suspected *M. tuberculosis* (as determined by growth inhibition in a NAP bottle run in parallel, or by observing cord formation in acid-fast stain or on examination of microcolonies on a clear Middlebrook 7H10 plate) from a BACTEC 12A blood culture vial that has reached a growth index of 500 or more is used.

CHART 19-18

DETECTION, IDENTIFICATION, AND DRUG SUSCEPTIBILITY TESTING OF *M. TUBERCULOSIS* BY RADIOMETRIC INSTRUMENTATION *continued*

III. Materials
A. Equipment: BACTEC 460 instrument
B. Media
1. BACTEC 12A broth culture vials (two per unknown)
2. BACTEC NAP vial
3. BACTEC 12A broth culture vials, one each including the following antituberculous drugs:
a. Isoniazid
b. Streptomycin
c. Rifampin
d. Ethambutol
IV. Quality Control
Quality control of the antibiotic-containing vials is performed by the manufacturer before shipment. Local practice must dictate whether it is necessary to perform a quality control check on each new lot of antibiotic-containing vials with a strain of *M. tuberculosis* that has a known resistance profile.
V. Procedure
1. The procedure starts by detecting a BACTEC-positive 12A vial that has reached a growth index of 100 and determining that acid-fast bacilli are present.
2. Inoculate 1 mL of the culture into a vial containing 12A medium plus *p*-nitroacetyl-aminohydroxypropiophenone (NAP; see Chart 19-4). Also inoculate 1 mL of the positive culture into a third vial containing 12A medium only.
3. If growth is inhibited after 3 to 5 days of incubation, the isolate is either *M. tuberculosis* or *M. bovis*; no inhibition of growth indicates that the organism is a *Mycobacterium* species other than *M. tuberculosis,* in which case a BACTEC susceptibility test cannot be performed.
4. If growth is inhibited in the NAP bottle, observe the growth index in the 12A vial without NAP that had been inoculated in parallel. When the growth index reaches 500, the concentration is sufficient to perform antimycobacterial susceptibility studies against the unknown strain of *M. tuberculosis.*
5. Inoculate 0.1 mL of the positive culture into each of the drug-containing vials provided by the manufacturer (currently isoniazid, streptomycin, rifampin, and ethambutol) and with representative control strains.
6. At the same time, inoculate another vial of 12A medium without drugs with 0.1 mL of a 1:100 dilution of the positive culture used to inoculate the drug-containing vials. This will be equivalent to 1% growth in the proportion method for drug susceptibility testing.
7. Incubate the vials and read daily until the growth index of the control vial reaches 30. Then record the growth index of the drug-containing vials.
VI. Results
A. Interpretation
If the increase in growth index in drug-containing medium is more than the change in growth index in the control (30 or greater), the *M. tuberculosis* strain is growing in the presence of that drug and is considered resistant.
VII. Procedure Notes
The final drug concentrations in each of the drug-containing vials is 90% of the stated concentration because of the dilution factor (2.0 mL of medium plus 0.1 mL of drug solution plus 0.1 mL of inoculum = 2.2 mL).
VIII. Bibliography

Damato JJ, Collins MT, Rothlauf MV, et al. Detection of mycobacteria by radiometric and standard plate procedures. J Clin Microbiol 1983;17:1066–1073.

Gross WM, Hawkins JE. Radiometric selective inhibition tests for differentiation of *Mycobacterium tuberculosis, Mycobacterium bovis* and other mycobacteria. J Clin Microbiol 1985;21:565–568.

Morgan MA, Horstmeier CD, DeYoung DR. Comparison of a radiometric method (BACTEC) and conventional culture media for recovery of mycobacteria from smear-negative specimens. J Clin Microbiol 1983;18:384–388.

Roberts GD, Goodman NL, Heifets L, et al. Evaluation of the radiometric method for recovery of mycobacteria and drug susceptibility testing of *Mycobacterium tuberculosis* from acid-fast smear positive specimens. J Clin Pathol 1983;18:689–696.

CHART 20-1

DARKFIELD MICROSCOPY OF GENITAL LESIONS

I. **Principle**

Darkfield detection of spirochetes allows presumptive diagnosis of syphilis during the primary phase before antibody has developed. There are few contaminating spirochetes in genital sites, so detection of spirochetes with a morphology compatible with *Treponema pallidum* subsp. *pallidum* provides a solid diagnosis. The prevalence of spirochetes in the oral cavity necessitates caution. The test is best not performed in the oral cavity; if spirochetes are seen there, their identity must be established by specific immunologic means.

II. **Equipment and Reagents**

Microscope with transmitted light and a darkfield conser. Use a $10\times$ objective to focus the specimen and center the darkfield condenser. Use a $40\times$ to $63\times$ objective to search the specimen. Final identification is made with a $100\times$ objective.

Microscope slides, $1'' \times 3''$. Thickness should match that recommended in microscope manual.

Coverglass #1, 22 mm $\times$ 22 mm

Immersion oil, nondrying, Cargille type A or equivalent

Lens paper and lens cleaner

Applicator sticks

Sterile saline

Disinfectant, such as iodine or 70% alcohol

III. **Quality Control**

A scraping of gingival mucosa may be used as a control with which to set up the darkfield condenser.

IV. **Procedure**

A. *Collection of Specimen*

1. General
   a. Remove any scab or crust covering the lesion.
   b. Remove any exudate with a gauze sponge.
   c. If necessary, compress the base of the lesion or apply a suction cup to promote accumulation of tissue fluid on the ulcer surface.
   d. Apply a glass slide with a sterile bacteriologic loop.
   e. Place a glass coverslip on the specimen and press it down to remove bubbles.
   f. Examine immediately.

2. Dry papulosquamous lesions of the skin
   a. Gently remove the superficial layer of skin, trying not to cause bleeding.
   b. Compress the lesion if very little fluid appears.
   c. Touch a microscope slide to the lesion or transfer a small amount of fluid to a slide with a bacteriologic loop.
   d. Alternatively, a small amount of sterile saline can be injected into the lesion, aspirated back, and placed on a slide.
   e. Place a coverslip on the slide and examine immediately.

3. Cervical/vaginal lesions
   a. Under visualization with a bivalve speculum, remove any cervical or vaginal discharge.
   b. Obtain serous exudate with a bacteriologic loop.
   c. If necessary, serous exudate can be produced by compressing the lesion with a Kelly clamp.
   d. Prepare slides as above.

4. Mucous patches
   a. Using a sterile bacteriologic loop, collect some of the mucus and place it on a glass slide.
   b. Place a coverslip on the slide and examine immediately.

V. **Examination of the Specimen**

Prepare the darkfield microscope before collection of the specimen.

Using a $40\times$ to $63\times$ objective, search the slide systematically.

When a suspicious structure is found, examine under $100\times$ magnification.

When observation is completed, discard the slide in disinfectant.

Characteristics of *T. pallidum* and saprophytic genital species, *T. refringens.*

CHART 20-1

DARKFIELD MICROSCOPY OF GENITAL LESIONS *continued*

Characteristic	*T. pallidum*	*T. refringens*
Morphology		
Shape	Delicate corkscrew shape	Loose coiled, coarse
Length	6–14 μm	8–20 μm
Width	0.25–0.3 μm	0.4–0.75 μm
Spiral wavelength	Approx. 1.0–1.5 μm	
Motility		
Translation	Slow, deliberate back and forth movement	Rapid, writhing motion
Rotation	Slow to rapid rotation (corkscrew); may rotate in place	Active serpentine rotation
Flexion	Rotation accompanied by soft bending and twisting. Bending occurs stiffly in middle of organism	Marked flexion
Distortion	May occur as a ring or attached to cells	None noted

VI. Results
    A. Interpretation
        False-positive results may occur if oral spirochetes are not confirmed or if characteristic motility of genital spirochetes is misinterpreted.
        A few red cells in the preparation are a sign that exudate was obtained, but the specimen should not be bloody. Bubbles should be carefully removed.
        False-negative results may be obtained if insufficient exudate was obtained, if there was too long an interval between collection and examination, if the lesion is late, or if the patient has been treated with antitreponemal drugs.

VII. Bibliography
    Larson SA, Hunter EF, Kraus SJ, eds. Manual of Tests for Syphilis. Ed. 8. Washington, DC: American Public Health Association, 1990.

CHART 20-2

VENEREAL DISEASE RESEARCH LABORATORY (VDRL) SLIDE TEST ON SERUM

  I. Principle
    The VDRL slide test is the reference nontreponemal antibody test for syphilis. It is the only generally recognized test for diagnosing neurosyphilis.
    The VDRL is a nontreponemal microflocculation test. It uses an antigen that contains cardiolipin, lecithin, and cholesterol. The antigen forms microscopic clumps when mixed with antibodies to cardiolipin complex.
 II. Equipment and Reagents
    A. Equipment
        1. Nondisposable needles without a bevel
           a. Serum test: 18 gauge
        2. Bottles: 30-mL, round, narrow-mouthed, 35 mm in diameter, with glass or equivalent stoppers and *flat inner-bottom surface* (Corning Glass Works, Corning, NY, cat. no. LG-1 MW-90530).
        3. Safety pipetting device with disposable tip to deliver 50 μL.
        4. Pipettes, serologic, graduated to tip:
           a. 1.0 mL, graduated in 1/100 mL
           b. 5.0 mL, graduated in 1/10 mL
           c. 10.0 mL, graduated in 1/10 mL

CHART 20-2

VENEREAL DISEASE RESEARCH LABORATORY (VDRL) SLIDE TEST ON SERUM *continued*

    5. Slides
       a. Serum test: 2×3 in., with 12 paraffin or ceramic rings approximately 14 mm in diameter (rings must be high enough to prevent spillage during rotation).
       b. 12 concavities measuring 16 mm in diameter and 1.75 mm in depth.
    6. Slide holder for 2×3-in. slides.
    7. Ringmaker to make paraffin rings if ceramic rings not used.
    8. Mechanical rotator adjustable to 180 ± 2 rpm, circumscribing a circle 19 mm in diameter on a horizontal plane.
    9. Discard containers or disinfectants, disposable latex gloves.
   10. Humidifying covers (in dry climates).
  B. Reagents
    1. VDRL antigen: Store in the dark at room temperature or in refrigerator. Discard vials that contain a precipitate.
    2. VDRL-buffered saline, pH 6.0 ± 0.1 (1.0% NaCl) (purchased or prepared)
    3. Control serum samples: reactive (R), weakly reactive (W), nonreactive (N)
    4. 0.9% saline
    5. 10.0% saline
III. Procedures for Serum Tests
  A. Preparing the Antigen Suspension
    1. Prepare a fresh VDRL antigen suspension each day. The temperature of all reagents should be at 23 to 29°C.
    2. Pipette 0.4 mL of VDRL-buffered saline to the bottom of a round, 30-mL, glass-stoppered bottle with a flat inner surface.
    3. Add 0.5 mL VDRL antigen directly into the saline while continuously but gently rotating the bottle on a flat surface. Add antigen drop by drop at a rate allowing approximately 6 seconds for each 0.5 mL of antigen. Keep the pipette tip in the upper third of the bottle and do not splash saline onto the pipette tip. The proper speed of rotation is obtained when the center of the bottle circumscribes a 2-in.-diameter circle approximately three times per second.
    4. Expel the last drop of antigen from the pipette without touching the pipette to the saline. Continue rotation of the bottle for 10 seconds.
    5. Add 4.1 mL buffered saline from a 5-mL pipette.
    6. Cap the bottle and shake it from bottom to top and back approximately 30 times in 10 seconds. The antigen suspension must be used within 8 hours.
    7. Mix the suspension by gently swirling it each time it is used. Do not mix it by forcing it back and forth through the syringe and needle.
  B. Testing Accuracy of Antigen Suspension Needle
    1. The accuracy of the test depends on the amount of antigen dispensed. Check the calibrated needle periodically for accuracy.
    2. For the qualitative and quantitative tests on serum, dispense the antigen suspension from a syringe fitted with an 18-gauge needle without a bevel, which will deliver 60 ± 2 drops of antigen suspension per milliliter (17 µL/drop) when held vertically.
    3. Place the needle on a 2-mL syringe or on a 1-mL pipette and fill the syringe or pipette with VDRL antigen suspension. Holding the syringe or pipette vertically, count the number of drops delivered in 0.5 mL. The needle is correctly calibrated if 30 ± 1 drop are delivered in 0.5 mL. Adjust or replace the needle if it does not meet the specifications.
  C. Testing and Storing the VDRL Antigen Suspension
    1. Prepare a fresh antigen suspension each day. Store the suspension at room temperature, 23 to 29°C.
    2. Test the antigen suspension with control sera that are reactive, weakly reactive, and nonreactive.
    3. Use only suspensions that reproduce the established reactivity pattern of the controls.
    4. After completing the day's tests, discard the antigen suspension and clean the dispensing needle and syringe by rinsing with water, alcohol, and acetone, in that order. Remove the needle from the syringe after cleaning.
  D. Preparing and Storing Specimens
    1. Observe recommended safety precautions for handling human sera.
    2. Centrifuge clotted blood at room temperature at 1500 to 2000 rpm for 5 minutes to sediment the cellular elements.
    3. Transfer the serum to a clean, dry test tube and heat it in a 56°C water bath for 30 minutes.

CHART 20-2

VENEREAL DISEASE RESEARCH LABORATORY (VDRL) SLIDE TEST ON SERUM *continued*

4. Recentrifuge any specimen that contains debris after heat-inactivation.
5. Reheat the serum at 56°C for 10 minutes if testing is delayed more than 4 hours.
6. Specimens must be at room temperature (23 to 29°C) at the time of testing.

E. Performing the Qualitative Test on Serum
   1. With all reagents at room temperature, place 50 μL of serum into one ring of a paraffin- or ceramic-ringed slide, using a safety pipetting device. Do not use glass slides with concavities, wells, or glass rings.
   2. Gently resuspend the VDRL antigen suspension.
   3. Holding the VDRL antigen suspension dispensing needle and syringe in a vertical position, dispense several drops to clear the needle of air. Then add exactly 1 free-falling drop (17 μL) of antigen suspension to each circle that contains serum.
   4. Place the slide on a mechanical rotator. Rotate for 4 minutes at 180 ± 2 rpm. In a dry climate, cover the slide with a moist humidifying cover during rotation.
   5. Immediately after the completion of rotation, remove the slide from the rotator and read the test results microscopically, using a 10× ocular and a 10× objective.
   6. Report the results as follows:

Reading	Report
Medium or large clumps	Reactive (R)
Small clumps	Weakly reactive (W)
No clumping or slight roughness	Nonreactive (N)

   7. Test quantitatively to an endpoint all serum specimens that produce reactive, weakly reactive, or "rough" nonreactive results in the qualitative test.

F. Performing the Quantitative Test in Serum
   1. Quantitate the serum samples to an endpoint titer. Quantitative tests through the 1:8 dilution for three serum specimens may be performed on one slide.
   2. Place 50 μL of 0.9% saline in circles numbered 2 through 4, but do not spread the saline.
   3. Using a safety pipetting device, place 50 μL of serum in both circle 1 and circle 2.
   4. Mix the saline and the serum in circle 2 by drawing the mixture up and down in the safety pipette eight times. Avoid formation of bubbles.
   5. Transfer 50 μL from circle 2 (1:2) to circle 3 and mix.
   6. Transfer 50 μL from circle 3 to circle 4 and mix. Discard the last 50 μL.
   7. Gently resuspend the VDRL antigen suspension.
   8. Holding the VDRL antigen suspension–dispensing needle and syringe in a vertical position, dispense several drops to clear the needle of air. Then add exactly 1 free-falling drop (17 μL) of antigen suspension to each circle.
   9. Place the slide on the mechanical rotator. Rotate the slide for 4 minutes at 180 ± 2 rpm. Add a humidifying cover in dry environments.
   10. Immediately after rotation, read the test microscopically using a 10× ocular and a 10× objective.
   11. If the highest dilution tested (1:8) is reactive, proceed as follows:
       a. Prepare a 1:8 dilution of the test specimen. Add 0.1 mL serum to 0.7 mL of 0.9% saline and mix thoroughly.
       b. Place 50 μL of 0.9% saline into the second, third, and fourth paraffin rings in a row on the slide. Prepare additional serial dilutions for strongly reactive specimens.
       c. Add 50 μL of the 1:8 dilution of the test specimen to paraffin rings 1 and 2.
   12. Report titers in terms of the highest dilution that produces a reactive (not a weakly reactive) result:

Serum Dilutions						Report
Undiluted	1:2	1:4	1:8	1:16	1:32	
R	W	N	N	N	N	Reactive, undiluted, 1 dil.
R	R	W	N	N	N	Reactive, 1:2 dilution, 2 dils
R	R	R	W	N	N	Reactive, 1:4 dilution, 4 dils
W	W	R	R	W	N	Reactive, 1:8 dilution, 8 dils
N (Rough)	W	R	R	R	N	Reactive, 1:16 dilution, 16 dils
W	N	N	N	N	N	Weakly reactive, undiluted, 0 dil

CHART 20-2

VENEREAL DISEASE RESEARCH LABORATORY (VDRL) SLIDE TEST ON SERUM *continued*

IV. Results
  A. Interpretation
    1. The VDRL test is an aid in the diagnosis of syphilis. A positive test may indicate a past or present infection. False-positive results occur because of laboratory error, infection with other treponemes, or the presence of antibodies unrelated to treponemal infection. The predictive value of a positive VDRL result is increased when combined with a reactive treponemal test, such as the fluorescent treponemal antibody absorption test (see Chart 20-4) or the microhemagglutination test.
    2. A nonreactive result may indicate no infection, adequately treated infection, or infection in the remote past. A nonreactive result may be obtained in incubating or early primary syphilis. Prozone phenomena occur, especially with high titers in secondary syphilis. Sera should be diluted if a rough result is obtained or if clinical information indicates the likelihood of syphilis.
    3. A fourfold increase in titer may indicate a reinfection or treatment failure. A four-fold decrease in titer in early syphilis usually indicates adequate therapy.
    4. All sera should be titered to the endpoint. Unusually high titers may be seen in some patients who are concurrently infected with human immunodeficiency virus, type 1. Unusually high false-positive titers may be seen in some patients with lymphomas.
  V. Sources of Error
    1. Reactivity is decreased if the specimen, testing area, or reagents are at temperatures lower than 23°C. Reactivity is increased if any of these are at temperatures higher than 29°C.
    2. Test results are unpredictable if hemolyzed, contaminated, or extremely turbid sera are tested.
    3. Reactivity will be unpredictable if reagents are outdated, inadequately tested, or if procedures are not followed strictly. Forcing the VDRL antigen through the needle and syringe repetitively will cause the suspension to lose reactivity.
  VI. Test Limitations
    1. The prozone phenomenon described in the foregoing may produce false-negative results on high-titered sera.
    2. The VDRL antigen suspension must be prepared daily.
    3. The VDRL cerebrospinal fluid (CSF) test should be performed only if the serum test is reactive.
    4. Plasma cannot be used for the VDRL test.
    5. Biologic false-positive results occur with cardiolipin antigens, especially in specimens from persons who abuse drugs; who have diseases such as lupus erythematosus, mononucleosis, malaria, leprosy, or viral pneumonia; or who have recently been immunized.
    6. Note: The VDRL slide test on CSF is similar to the serum test, but there are important methodologic differences (see bibliography). Only reactive and nonreactive results are reported on CSF.
  VII. Bibliography
    Larson SA, Hunter EF, Karus SJ, eds. Manual of Tests for Syphilis. Ed. 8. Washington, DC: American Public Health Association, 1990.

CHART 20-3

RAPID PLASMA REAGIN (RPR) CARD TEST

  I. Principle
  The RPR (circle) Card Test was instituted as the routine screening test in the Maryland State Department of Health Laboratories on January 13, 1964. The main advantages of the RPR over the VDRL test are that the serum does not have to be heat-treated, interpretations are made macroscopically instead of microscopically, the antigen is stable, and components are disposable. Tests can be performed rapidly and inexpensively, thereby making the technique suitable for large-volume operations. The sensitivity and specificity of the RPR test are equal to those of the VDRL and other nontreponemal serologic tests.
  The RPR antigen suspension is a carbon-containing cardiolipin antigen that detects "reagin," an antibody-like substance present in the plasma and sera of persons with syphilis or previous exposure to the treponema spirochete. When a specimen contains specific antibody, flocculation occurs with coagglutination of the carbon particles of the RPR card antigen, appearing as black clumps against a white background of the plastic-coated card. This coagulation can be read macroscopically; nonreactive specimens have a smooth, milky light-gray color.

CHART 20-3

RAPID PLASMA REAGIN (RPR) CARD TEST *continued*

II. Equipment, Supplies, and Reagents
    1. Disposable, calibrated 20-gauge needle without bevel, silicone-treated
    2. Plastic antigen dispensing bottle, 1 dram
    3. Plastic-coated RPR cards with 10 circles, each approximately 18 mm in diameter
    4. Dispenstirs, a disposable (plastic) dispensing-stirring device that delivers 50 μL
    5. Mechanical rotator, fixed speed or adjustable to 100 ± 2 rpm, circumscribing a circle 3/4 in. in diameter on a horizontal plane
    6. Humidifying cover for rotator
    7. High-intensity incandescent lamp
    8. Safety pipetting device with disposable tip that delivers 50 μL
    9. Discard containers and disinfectants
    10. Disposable latex gloves, safety glasses, and protective clothing
    11. RPR antigen suspension (a variation of the VDRL antigen): a stabilized combination of 0.003% cardiolipin, 0.020–0.022% lecithin, 0.09% cholesterol, 10% choline chloride, 0.0125 M EDTA, 0.1875% charcoal, 0.1 M Na_2HPO4, 0.01 M KH_2PO_4, 0.1% thimerosal, and distilled water
    12. Control serum samples: lyophilized reactive (R), minimally reactive (MR), and nonreactive (N) control serum specimens on a card
    13. 0.9% saline as a diluent
III. Procedures
    A. Testing Accuracy of Antigen Needle
        1. Check the calibrated needle periodically to be sure that it delivers 60 ± 2 drops/mL (17 μL). The accuracy of the test depends on the amount of antigen used.
        2. Consult the procedure for calibrating needles in the VDRL test (see Chart 20-2).
    B. Testing and Storing the Antigen Suspension
        1. Store ampules of antigen at 2 to 8°C. Do not store in the bright sunlight. Do not store above 29°C and do not freeze. Antigen in an opened ampule is stable for up to 12 months.
        2. Attach the needle hub to the fitting on the plastic dispensing bottle. Open the ampule after shaking it to resuspend the particles. Squeeze the dispensing bottle to collapse it, insert the needle into the ampule, and withdraw all the antigen suspension into the dispensing bottle. Shake the dispensing bottle gently before each series of antigen drops is delivered.
        3. Test each lot of antigen suspension in parallel with an antigen of known standard reactivity before putting it into use.
        4. At each routine test run, test the reactivity of the antigen with control cards or sera of known reactivity. Use only suspensions that produce appropriate activity.
        5. After completion of the day's work, remove the needle from the antigen-dispensing bottle, rinse in distilled water, and air-dry. Do not wipe the needle (an action that will remove the silicone coating).
    C. Preparing and Storing Specimens
        1. Either serum or plasma may be tested. Plasma is obtained by collecting blood into a tube that contains EDTA as an anticoagulant.
        2. Do not test specimens that are grossly contaminated, excessively hemolyzed, or chylous.
    D. Performing the Qualitative Test
        1. All reagents should be at room temperature (23 to 29°C) before tests are performed.
        2. Place 50 μL of serum or plasma into an 18-mm circle of the RPR test card, using a disposable Dispenstir or a safety pipetting device.
        3. With the inverted Dispenstir (closed end) or flat toothpicks, spread the serum or plasma to fill the entire circle, but not to extend beyond the bounds of the circle.
        4. Gently shake the antigen-dispensing bottle to resuspend the particles.
        5. While holding the dispensing bottle and needle in a vertical position, dispense several drops to clear the needle of air. Then add exactly 1 free-falling drop (17 μL) of antigen suspension to each circle containing serum or plasma. Do not mix the antigen and serum or plasma.
        6. Place the card on the mechanical rotator under a humidifying cover. Rotate the card for 8 minutes at 100 ± 2 rpm.
        7. Immediately remove the card from the rotator. Briefly rotate and tilt the card by hand to aid in differentiating nonreactive from minimally reactive results. Read the test reactions in the "wet" state, using a high-intensity incandescent light, without magnification.

CHART 20-3

RAPID PLASMA REAGIN (RPR) CARD TEST *continued*

8. Report the results as follows:

Reading	Report
Characteristic clumping ranging from marked and intense (reactive) to slight but definite (minimally reactive)	Reactive (R)
Slight roughness or no clumping	Nonreactive (N)

9. Perform the quantitative test on serum specimens showing any degree of reactivity or "roughness."

IV. Performing the Quantitative Test

1. Quantitate to an endpoint all serum specimens with reactive or rough nonreactive results in the qualitative test. Test each specimen undiluted (1:1) and in 1:2, 1:4, 1:8, and 1:16 dilutions.
2. Place 50 μL of 0.9% saline in circles numbered 2 through 5. Do not spread the saline.
3. Using a safety pipette device, place 50 μL of serum in circle 1 and 50 μL of serum in circle 2. Mix the saline and the serum in the circle by drawing the mixture up and down in the safety pipette eight times. Avoid forming bubbles.
4. Transfer 50 μL from circle 2 (1:2) to circle 3 and mix.
5. Transfer 50 μL from circle 3 (1:4) to circle 4 and mix.
6. Transfer 50 μL from circle 4 (1:8) to circle 5 (1:16) and mix. Discard the last 50 μL.
7. With the broad end of a clean Dispenstir, spread the serum dilution to fill the entire surface of circle 5, the highest dilution (1:16). With the same Dispenstir, do the same for circles 4 (1:8), 3 (1:4), 2 (1:2), and 1 (undiluted).
8. Gently shake the dispensing bottle to resuspend the antigen particles.
9. Holding the antigen-dispensing bottle in a vertical position, dispense 1 or 2 drops to clear the needle of air. Then add exactly 1 free-falling drop (17 μL) of antigen suspension in each circle. Do not mix.
10. Place the card on the rotator under the humidifying cover and rotate the card for 8 minutes at 100 ± 2 rpm.
11. Immediately remove the card from the rotator; briefly rotate and tilt the card by hand (three or four to-and-fro motions) to aid in differentiating nonreactive from minimally reactive results. Read the results in the wet state with the unaided eye, using a bright incandescent light.
12. Report the results in terms of the highest dilution that has given a reactive result, including a minimally reactive result, as follows:

Serum Dilutions					Report
Undiluted	1:2	1:4	1:8	1:16	
RM	N	N	N	N	Reactive, undiluted
R	R	R	N	N	Reactive, 1:4 dilution
R	R	R	RM	N	Reactive, 1:8 dilution

R, Reactive; RM, Reactive, minimally; N, nonreactive
Note: Report the result as either reactive or nonreactive; there is no minimally reactive report in the RPR card test

V. Results

A. Interpretation

1. Clinicians must combine the results of this test with the clinical and epidemiologic information. The predictive value of a positive RPR test is increased if the specimen is also reactive in a specific treponemal test, such as the fluorescent treponemal antibody absorption test (FTA-ABS).
2. A reactive test indicates present or past inadequately treated infection or a false-positive reaction. Technical false-positive reactions may be detected by a negative RPR test when repeated. Biologic false-positive reactions are detected by a negative specific treponemal test, such as the FTA-ABS test.
3. A negative test in the absence of clinical symptoms may indicate no infection or adequately treated infection in the past. A negative test may also occur during the incubation period before the first symptoms have manifested. A negative test in the presence of clinical symptoms may occur during early primary syphilis, as a prozone during secondary syphilis, or occasionally in tertiary syphilis.

CHART 20-3

RAPID PLASMA REAGIN (RPR) CARD TEST *continued*

4. When the quantitative RPR test is performed on patients with syphilis, a fourfold rise in titer may indicate an active infection, a reinfection, or failure of therapy. A fourfold fall in titer usually means adequate syphilis therapy.

5. All reactive qualitative RPR tests should be titered to an endpoint and the endpoint titer reported. Very high RPR card titers may occur in patients with HIV infection. Very high false-positive titers may occur in patients with lymphomas.

B. Acceptable Variations

1. Prepare a 1:16 dilution for further quantitation, using 50 μL of specimen to 750 μL of 0.9% saline.

2. If, after screening, the serum to be quantitated seems likely to exceed 1:16, prepare all dilutions directly on the card, using a 1:50 nonreactive serum as the diluent beginning with circle 6 (1:32) and continuing for the remainder of the card.

VI. Sources of Error

1. If the temperatures of the sera, reagents, or testing area are lower than 23°C, test reactivity decreases; if temperatures are higher than 29°C, test reactivity increases.

2. If the speed of the mechanical rotator is too fast or too slow, improper mixing of antigen and antibody will yield unpredictable results.

3. If the card is excessively rotated and tilted by hand after removal from the rotator, a false-positive reaction may occur.

4. If lighting produces a glare on the card, results may be obscured.

5. If the antigen is outdated or not tested for standard reactivity, results may be unpredictable.

6. If the serum is unevenly spread in the circle, the antigen and antibody may not mix properly.

7. If hemolyzed, contaminated, or improperly collected serum or plasma samples are tested, the reaction may be masked.

8. If plasma specimens are stored at −20°C for longer than 1 week, the specimens become unsuitable for testing.

9. If the moistened humidifying cover is not used to cover tests as they are being rotated, proper humidity will not be maintained, and test components may dry on the card, causing false-positive reactions to occur.

VII. Test Limitations

1. The RPR card tests cannot be used to test spinal fluids.

2. A prozone reaction may be encountered occasionally. In a prozone reaction, complete or partial inhibition of reactivity occurs with undiluted serum. The prozone phenomenon may be so pronounced that only a rough reaction is produced in the qualitative test by a serum that will be strongly positive in the quantitative test. Any specimen that produces any degree of roughness or reactivity in the qualitative test should be retested in the quantitative test.

3. The RPR test may be reactive in persons from areas where yaws, pinta, or nonvenereal syphilis is endemic. As a general rule, residual titers from these infections will be less than 1:8.

4. Biologic false-positive reactions occur occasionally, particularly in persons who abuse drugs; who have diseases such as lupus erythematosus, mononucleosis, malaria, leprosy, or viral pneumonia; or who have been vaccinated recently.

5. Nontreponemal test titers of persons who have been treated in latent or late stages of syphilis or who have been reinfected do not decrease as rapidly as those who are treated in early primary infection. Some of these individuals may become "serofast," retaining their reactivity for life.

VIII. Bibliography

Fiumara NJ. Serologic responses to treatment of 128 patients with late latent syphilis. Sex Transm Dis 1979;6: 243–246.

Larson SA, Hunter EF, Karus SJ, eds. Manual of Tests for Syphilis. Ed. 8. Washington, DC: American Public Health Association, 1990.

CHART 20-4

FLUORESCENT TREPONEMAL ANTIBODY ABSORPTION TEST (FTA-ABS)

I. Principle

The fluorescent treponemal antibody-absorption test (FTA-ABS) is an indirect fluorescent antibody technique (see Chap. 3). The patient's serum, which has been diluted 1:5 in sorbent (an extract from cultures of *Treponema phagadenis,* the Reiter treponeme), is layered on a microscope slide to which *T. pallidum* subsp. *pallidum* has been fixed. If the patient's serum contains antibody to *T. pallidum*, it will coat the treponeme. When fluorescein isothiocyanate (FITC)-labeled antihuman globulin is added, it will fix to any antibodies that have become affixed to the spirochete. The fluorescent reaction is visible when viewed by fluorescence microscopy.

II. Materials

A. Equipment

Incubator, 35 to 37°C

Water bath, adjustable to 56°C

Safety pipetting devices

Micropipettors delivering 10 to 200 μL

Loop, bacteriologic standard, 2 mm, 26-gauge, platinum

Bibulous paper

Slide board with moist chamber and paper towels

Staining dishes, glass or plastic, with removable slide carriers

Microscope slides, 1 × 3 in., with frosted end, 1-mm thick, with two etched circles, 1-cm inside diameter

Coverslips, No. 1, 2-mm square

Test tubes (12 × 75 mm) and holders

Discard containers and disinfectants

Disposable latex gloves, safety glasses, and protective clothing

Fluorescence microscope set up for fluorescein microscopy

Mixer; Vortex Jr. or equivalent

B. Reagents

1. Purchased

a. *T. pallidum* antigen: A suspension of *T. pallidum* (Nichols strain) extracted from rabbit testicular tissue and washed in phosphate-buffered saline to remove rabbit globulin.

b. FITC-labeled antihuman IgG.

c. Sorbent: Prepared from cultures of nonpathogenic Reiter treponemes, usually with no preservative added. Frequently dispensed in 5-mL amounts and freeze-dried, but also sold in liquid state.

d. Reactive control serum: A pool of human serum samples obtained from syphilitic donors that are 4+ reactive. Used to prepare 4+ serum controls and minimally reactive 1+ control. The 1+ control demonstrates the minimal degree of fluorescence reported as reactive and is used as a reading standard.

e. Nonspecific control serum: A serum pool obtained from nonsyphilitic individuals. No preservative is added. This control demonstrates a ≥2+ nonspecific reactivity at a 1:5 dilution in phosphate-buffered saline (PBS) and essentially no staining when diluted 1:5 in sorbent.

f. Oil: Low fluorescence, nondrying, immersion oil, type A, Cargille No. 1248

g. Acetone: ACS reagent grade

2. Prepared

a. PBS, pH 7.2

b. 2% Tween 80 (polysorbate 80) in PBS. Heat the reagents in a 56°C water bath. To 49 mL of sterile PBS, add 1 mL of Tween 80, by measuring from the bottom of a pipette and rinsing the pipette in the mixture. Check pH and adjust to pH 7.2 with 1 N NaOH. Discard if a precipitate develops or the pH changes.

c. Mounting medium: Add 1 part PBS to 9 parts glycerin (reagent grade).

d. Distilled water

III. Preparing Test Reagents

A. *T. pallidum* Antigen

1. Rehydrate antigen according to manufacturer's instructions. Opened vials, stored at 2 to 8°C, are stable for 1 week.

2. To prepare slides, mix antigen suspension thoroughly on a mixer for 10 seconds. Determine by darkfield examination that treponemes are adequately dispersed before making slides for the FTA-ABS test.

3. Wipe slides with clean gauze to remove dust particles. Clean slides by sonic vibration or alcohol wiping if treponemes are not clearly observed after staining.

CHART 20-4

FLUORESCENT TREPONEMAL ANTIBODY ABSORPTION TEST (FTA-ABS) *continued*

    4. Prepare very thin *T. pallidum* antigen smears within each circle by using a 2-mm wire loop. Place one loop of antigen within the two 1-mm circles. Allow to air-dry at least 15 minutes.

    5. Fix slides in acetone for 10 minutes and air-dry. Fix no more than 60 slides with 200 mL of acetone. Store acetone-fixed smears at −20°C. Do not thaw and refreeze smears.

    6. Store unopened vials of antigen at 2 to 8°C. The unopened antigen is stable until the expiration date.

  B. *Titration of Antihuman IgG Globulin*

    1. Rehydrate conjugate according to directions. If the conjugate is cloudy, centrifuge it at 500 *g* for 10 minutes. Aliquot in small volumes and store at −20°C. Do not refreeze thawed conjugate, but store at 2 to 8°C.

    2. Prepare 4+ and 1+ dilutions of the reactive control serum to determine conjugate working dilution.

    3. Run the control pattern with a reference or a known conjugate. An example is shown:

Conjugate Dilutions	Nonspecific Staining Control (PBS)	Reactive (4+) Control Serum (1:5 in PBS)	Reaction (1+) Control Serum
Reference Conjugate			
Dilution 1:400	−	4+	1+
New Conjugate			
1:12.5	<1+	4+	3+
1:25	−	4+	3+
1:50	−	4+	3+
1:100	−	4+	2+
1:200*	−	4+	1+
1:400	−	4+	<1+
1:800	−	3+	±

    * The dilution selected for the working titer is 1:200, one doubling dilution below the 4+ endpoint (1:400), 1+ staining with the 1+ control dilution (1:200), and no nonspecific staining for three doubling dilutions below the working dilution (1:25).

  C. *Sorbent*

    1. Rehydrate freeze-dried material with sterile distilled water or according to manufacturer's instructions. The rehydrated sorbent may be stored at 2 to 8°C or at −20°C. It can be used as long as acceptable reactivity is obtained and the product is not contaminated.

  D. *Test Serum*

    1. Observe recommended safety precautions for handling human serum.

    2. Heat the test and control sera at 56°C for 30 minutes before testing.

    3. Reheat previously heated test sera for 10 minutes at 56°C on the day of testing.

  E. *Control Test*

    1. Rehydrate serum according to manufacturer's instructions.

    2. Aliquot in 0.25 mL amounts and store at −20° for as long as acceptable reactivity is obtained.

    3. Prepare the following controls for each test run:

      a. Reactive (R) 4+ control serum: a syphilitic serum showing 4+ fluorescence in the unabsorbed test and only slightly reduced fluorescence in the absorbed test. To produce unabsorbed serum, add 50 μL of reactive control serum to a tube containing 200 μL PBS and mix well. To produce absorbed serum, transfer 50 μL of reactive control serum to a tube containing 200 μL PBS and mix well. To produce absorbed serum, transfer 50 μL of reactive control serum to a tube containing 200 μL of sorbent and mix well.

      b. Minimally reactive (MR) control serum: This is a dilution in PBS of the reactive control serum, which will give the minimal degree of fluorescence (1+) considered reactive.

      c. Nonspecific (NS) control serum: a nonsyphilitic serum showing ≥2+ fluorescence in the unabsorbed test. To produce the unabsorbed serum, transfer 50 μL of nonspecific control serum to a tube containing 200 μL of PBS and mix well. To produce the absorbed serum, transfer 50 μL of nonspecific control serum to a tube containing 200 μL of nonspecific control serum into a tube containing 200 μL of sorbent and mix well.

      d. Controls for nonspecific staining by conjugate consist of an antigen smear overlaid with 30 μL of PBS in place of serum and an antigen smear overlaid with 30 μL of sorbent in place of serum.

CHART 20-4

FLUORESCENT TREPONEMAL ANTIBODY ABSORPTION TEST (FTA-ABS) *continued*

F. *The FTA-ABS Test*
1. Identify previously prepared antigen slides by numbering the frosted end.
2. Number each tube and slide to correspond to the test serum and the control serum to be used.
3. Prepare reactive (4+), minimally reactive (1+), and nonspecific control serum dilutions in sorbent or PBS according to the directions.
4. Pipette 200 μL of sorbent into a test tube for each test serum.
5. Add 50 μL of the heated test serum to the appropriate tube and mix eight times.
6. Cover the appropriate antigen smears with 30 μL of the reactive (4+), minimally reactive (1+), and nonspecific control serum dilutions.
7. Cover the appropriate antigen smears with 30 μL of the PBS and 30 μL of the sorbent for nonspecific-staining controls a and b. The controls should give the following pattern:

CONTROL PATTERN FOR THE FTA-ABS TEST

Reactive control	a. 1:5 PBS dilution	R4+
	b. 1:5 Sorbent dilution	R(4+ −3+)
Minimally reactive control	1+ Control dilution	R1+
Nonspecific serum	a: 1:5 PBS dilution	R(2+ −4+)
controls	b. 1:5 Sorbent dilution	N−±
Nonspecific-staining	a. Antigen, PBS, conjugate	N
controls	b. Antigen, sorbent, conjugate	N

8. Cover the appropriate antigen smears with 30 μL of the test serum dilutions.
9. Prevent evaporation by placing slides in a moist chamber and incubate at 35 to 37°C for 30 minutes.
10. At the completion of the incubation perform the following rinses:
    a. Place slides in slide carriers and rinse 5 seconds with running PBS.
    b. Place slides in staining dish containing PBS for 5 minutes.
    c. Agitate slides by dipping them into the PBS at least 30 times.
    d. Using fresh PBS, repeat the above two steps.
    e. Rinse slides for 5 seconds in running distilled water and gently blot with bibulous paper.
11. Dilute FITC-labeled antihuman IgG to its working titer in PBS containing 2% Tween 80 and place approximately 30 μL of the diluted conjugate on each smear.
12. Repeat incubation and rinsing of slides.
13. Mount slides immediately by placing a small drop of mounting medium on each smear and applying a cover glass.
14. Place slides in a darkened room and read within 4 hours.
15. Check smear by darkfield microscopy using the tungsten lamp first, to verify the presence of treponemes on the smear, then read FITC (test) fluorescence.
16. Using the minimally reactive (1+) control slide as the reading standard, record the intensity of fluorescence of the treponemes:

RECORDING INTENSITY OF FLUORESCENCE

Reading	Intensity of Fluorescence
2+ to 4+	Moderate to strong
1+*	Equivalent to minimally reactive (1+) control
± to <1+	Visible staining but less than 1+
−	None or vaguely visible but without distinct fluorescence
Atypical**	Varied: treponemes appear to be ''moth-eaten'' or to have ''beads'' of fluorescence throughout their length

* Retest all specimens that initially give a 1+ intensity of fluorescence.
** Atypical or beaded pattern of fluorescence has been described in patients with lupus and other autoimmune diseases.

CHART 20-4

FLUORESCENT TREPONEMAL ANTIBODY ABSORPTION TEST (FTA-ABS) *continued*

17. Report the result as follows:

REPORTING SYSTEM FOR FTB-ABS TEST

Initial Test Reading	Repeat Test Reading	Report
4+		Reactive
3+		Reactive
2+		Reactive
1+	>1+	Reactive
1+	1+	Reactive minimal*
1+	<1+	Nonreactive
<1+		Nonreactive
N		Nonreactive
Beaded fluorescence		Atypical Fluorescence Observed**

* In the absence of evidence of treponemal infection, this test result should be considered equivocal. A second specimen should be obtained 1–2 weeks after the initial specimen and submitted to the laboratory for serologic testing.

** Beaded fluorescence has been observed in serum from patients with active systemic lupus erythematosus and from patients with other autoimmune diseases. The DNA absorption procedure can be requested from the Treponemal Pathogenesis and Immunobiology Branch, Division of Sexually Transmitted Diseases, CDC, Atlanta, GA 30333. The request must be routed through the appropriate State Health Department.

IV. Acceptable Variations
  1. Reading of slides may be delayed beyond 4 hours if slides are protected from light and stored at 2 to 8°C. For the test to be valid with a delayed reading, *the complete control pattern must be clearly satisfactory when the slides are read.*
  2. Conjugate that has been filter-sterilized and contains a preservative, such as sodium azide, to prevent bacterial contamination may be stored at 2 to 8°C. Any precipitate or cloudiness must be removed by centrifugation.
  3. Slides may be held from 30 minutes to 1 hour in PBS if the test is interrupted. For the results to be valid, control slides must react appropriately when the test is read.
  4. Multicircle slides may be used rather than the two-circle slide. Add only 10 μL volumes to the antigen smears. Exercise care in handling and washing slides to prevent serum runover.
  5. With accurate micropipettors, the 1:5 test dilution may be prepared by pipetting 25 μL of serum into 100 μL of diluent.
V. Sources of Error
  1. If reagent evaluation procedures are not strictly followed, results will be unreliable.
  2. If multicircle slides are used and serum from one well is allowed to run onto another well, serum from a person without syphilis may appear reactive.
  3. If microscope slides are not clean, the test may be difficult to read and the results unreliable.
  4. If the FTA-ABS test is used as a screening procedure, rather than to confirm the reactive results of a nontreponemal test, or as a specific diagnostic test in patients with signs or symptoms of late syphilis, the positive predictive value of the FTA-ABS test is decreased.
  5. If the microscope is not properly aligned and the control pattern is not obtained, the test results are invalid.
  6. If reagents become contaminated with bacteria, the antibody may be reduced and the results may be invalid.
  7. If reagent storage instructions are not followed, the reagents will not produce satisfactory control results.
  8. If frozen antigen slides are thawed and refrozen, the treponemes will be difficult to see and the test results will be unsatisfactory.
  9. If a serum is contaminated with bacteria or is excessively hemolyzed, the test results may be invalid.
  10. If antigen slides are not dried and stored according to the procedure or if too much volume is placed on the slide, the antigen may wash off. One loop of antigen is sufficient for two 1-cm circles.
  11. If too many smears are fixed in a given volume of acetone, the background staining may be increased.
  12. If rehydrated antigen does not adhere to the slide, too few treponemes may be observed.

Chart 20-4

Fluorescent Treponemal Antibody Absorption Test (FTA-ABS) *continued*

13. If a precipitate is observed in conjugate preparation, nonspecific staining may be observed.
14. If the atypical staining pattern of beaded fluorescence is not recognized, these specimens may be incorrectly reported as reactive.
15. If FTA-ABS slides are read on a microscope equipped with incident illumination, the nonreactive slides must be examined by darkfield examination for the presence of treponemes.

VI. Test Limitations
1. The FTA-ABS test is not intended for routine use or as a screening procedure. Its greatest value is in distinguishing true-positive nontreponemal results from false-positive results and to establish the diagnosis of late latent or late syphilis.
2. Problems arise when the FTA-ABS test is used as a screening procedure, because approximately 1% of the general population will be falsely positive.
3. Although false-positive results in the FTA-ABS test are often transient and the cause is unknown, a definite association has been made between false-positive FTS-ABS results and the diagnosis of discoid, systemic, and drug-induced varieties of lupus erythematosus.
4. Unexplained FTA-ABS reactive results may occur in elderly patients.

VII. Bibliography
Larson SA, Hunter EF, Kraus SJ, eds. Manual of Tests for Syphilis. Ed. 8. Washington, DC: American Public Health Association, 1990.

Chart 22-1

Fecal Concentration Techniques for the Recovery of Intestinal Parasites

I. Principle
The number of parasitic forms in fecal specimens is often too low to be observed microscopically in direct wet mounts or in stained smear preparations. Concentration procedures must therefore be used for their detection. The two most commonly used techniques are sedimentation and flotation.

A. Sedimentation Techniques
Sedimentation techniques are performed most commonly in general diagnostic microbiology laboratories because they are easier to perform and less prone to technical errors. Sedimentation takes advantage of the high specific gravity of protozoan cysts and helminth eggs compared to water. Their natural tendency to settle out in aqueous solutions can be accelerated by light centrifugation. A formalin-ethyl acetate mixture, or other preservative that avoids the problems of the potential flammability of ether, may be added to the final suspension to clear out fecal debris and fix any parasitic forms that may be present.

B. Flotation Techniques
The main advantage of the flotation technique is that preparations for microscopic study have a cleaner background. Flotation takes advantage of the property of many protozoan cysts and helminth eggs to float to the surface of a solution of high specific gravity. A zinc sulfate solution with a specific gravity of 1.180 is most commonly used. The parasites that float to the top can be harvested by skimming the surface layer of solution with a wire loop. Flotation techniques have the disadvantages that some parasite eggs do not float, and of those that do, the walls of eggs and cysts will often collapse, compromising their identification.

II. Reagents
1. Sedimentation procedure:
Ethyl acetate
10% buffered formalin
0.85% NaCl
D'Antoni's or Lugol's iodine
2. Flotation procedure:
10% buffered formalin
0.85% NaCl
Zinc sulfate (33% aqueous solution)
Zinc sulfate 330 g
Distilled water 670 mL

CHART 22-1

FECAL CONCENTRATION TECHNIQUES FOR THE RECOVERY OF INTESTINAL PARASITES *continued*

Dissolve zinc sulfate in distilled water in an appropriate flask with a magnetic stirrer. Adjust the specific gravity to 1.20 by adding more zinc sulfate or distilled water as needed. Store in a bottle with a glass-stopper. Shelf life is 2 years.

III. Procedure

A. Sedimentation Technique

1. Wear gloves when handling stool specimens.
2. In a suitable container, thoroughly mix a portion of stool specimen about the size of a walnut into 10 mL of saline solution. Mix thoroughly.
3. Filter the emulsion through fine mesh gauze into a conical centrifuge tube.
4. Centrifuge the suspension at relative centrifugal force (RCF) of 600 g (about 2000 rpm) for no less than 10 minutes. The suspension should yield about 0.75 mL of sediment for fresh specimens and 0.5 mL for formalinized feces.
5. Decant the supernatant and wash the sediment with 10 mL of saline solution. Centrifuge again and repeat washing until the supernatant is clear.
6. After the last wash, decant the supernatant and add 10 mL of 10% formalin to the sediment. Mix and let stand for 5 minutes to effect fixation.
7. Add 1 to 2 mL of ethyl acetate, Stopper the tube and shake vigorously.
8. Centrifuge at 450 g RCF (about 1500 rpm) for 10 minutes. Four layers should result as follows: 1) a top layer of ethyl acetate; 2) plug of debris); 3) layer of formalin; and 4) sediment.
9. Free the plug of debris from the side of the tube by ringing with an applicator stick. Carefully decant the top three layers.
10. With a pipette, mix the remaining sediment with the small amount of remaining fluid and transfer one drop each to a drop of saline and iodine on a glass slide. Cover with a coverslip and examine microscopically for the presence of parasitic forms. Systematically examine the entire surface of each coverslip with the 10× objective; if nothing is seen, scan about half of each coverslip with the 40× objective.

B. Flotation Technique

1. Add 1 part feces (a quantity sufficient to yield about 0.75 mL of sediment) to 3–5 parts of 10% formalin. Mix thoroughly and allow to stand for 30 minutes to effect fixation.
2. Strain the well-mixed fecal-formalin suspension through one layer of gauze into a round-bottom tube (100 × 26 mm) to within 3/4 inch (19.05 mm) of the top of the rim.
3. Centrifuge the suspension at 600 g RCF (about 2000 rpm) for 3 to 5 minutes. Let centrifuge come to rest without mechanical braking.
4. Decant the supernatant and drain the last drop onto a clean section of paper towel.
5. Add $ZnSO_4$ solution to within 1 inch (25 mm) of the rim of the tube.
6. With two applicator sticks, resuspend the packed sediment until no coarse particles remain.
7. Immediately centrifuge the suspension for 1.5 minutes at 450 g RCF (about 1500 rpm). Again, allow the centrifuge to stop without mechanical braking.
8. Carefully transfer the tube to a rack that will hold it in a straight, upright position. Allow the tube to stand for 5–10 minutes.
9. With a 7-mm-diameter wire loop bent at a right angle at the stem, transfer two loops of surface film to a drop of 0.85% saline and to a drop of D'Antoni's or Lugol's iodine reagent on a glass slide, separated sufficiently so that the fluids do not mix when a coverslip is added. Mix each suspension with an applicator stick.
10. Place a clean #1 coverslip on each fluid mount. Examine each preparation within 1 hour. Systematically examine the entire surface of each cover slip with the 10× objective; if nothing is seen, scan about half of each coverslip with the 40× objective.

IV. Quality Control

1. Check solutions with each use to be sure they are clear and free of any bacterial contamination.
2. Run known positive specimens through the procedure to verify organism recovery. This should be done at least two times per year.

V. Results

Report protozoan cysts, trophozoites, and helminth eggs and/or larvae as may be appropriate. Semiquantitation of results may be helpful in some cases. A permanently stained smear may be required to confirm the species identification of parasitic forms seen in the sediment or flotation preparations.

CHART 22-1

FECAL CONCENTRATION TECHNIQUES FOR THE RECOVERY OF INTESTINAL PARASITES *continued*

VI. Procedure Notes
   A. Sedimentation
      1. The sedimentation procedure can also be used to process polyvinyl alcohol (PVA)-fixed specimens. Alter the procedure by filling one half of a tube with the stool-PVA mixture and add 0.85% NaCl almost to the top of the tube. Then filter the mixture through wet gauze into a 15-mL centrifuge tube and follow the remaining standard procedure.
      2. If ethyl acetate is used, swab the insides of the tube with a cotton-tipped applicator stick after the plug of debris is rimmed and the excess fluid is decanted. Excess ethyl acetate in the sediment at the time smears are prepared will lead to bubbles that may obscure parasitic forms one is attempting to observe.
      3. Errors in interpretation may occur if too much or too little feces is used in the sedimentation procedure. Adhere to the recommended formula of 0.75 mL of sediment for fresh specimens and 0.5 mL for formalinized feces as outlined in step 4 of the procedure.
      4. Allow the centrifuge to reach maximum speed before the time is monitored. If the centrifugation time is too little, certain smaller parasitic forms, such as the oocysts of *Cryptosporidium* species, may not reach the sediment.
   B. Flotation
      1. Zinc sulfate flotation techniques have the general advantage that the background fecal debris is eliminated, exposing any cysts or eggs that may be present.
      2. The flotation mount should be prepared within 12 hours after preparation because cysts and ova begin to resettle after that time.
      3. In preparing the mount, do not use the wire loop as a ''dipper.'' Only the very surface of the flotation mixture should be touched; make sure the loop is not below the surface film.
      4. An alternative procedure for preparing the mount is to add a small amount of zinc sulfate to the tube after the final centrifugation step to form a slightly convex meniscus. A coverslip can be gently placed on top of the meniscus and left undisturbed for 5 minutes. Carefully remove the coverslip and place it on a glass slide for examination.
      5. When calibrating the specific gravity of the zinc sulfate, spin the hydrometer lightly to free it from the sides of the tube. Read the bottom of the meniscus and correct for temperature (add or subtract 0.001 for each degree above or below the calibration temperature of hygrometer, which is usually 20°C).

VII. Limitation of Procedure
   Certain parasites, such as *Giardia lamblia*, hookworm eggs, and *Trichuris* eggs may not concentrate well from PVA-preserved specimens. The oocysts of *Isospora belli* do not routinely appear in concentrates. Therefore, examination of permanently stained smears is highly recommended.

   Protozoan cysts and helminth eggs with thin shells may collapse on prolonged exposure to the high-specific-gravity environment of the zinc sulfate solution. Therefore, preparations should be made as soon as possible after the centrifuge stops. Operculated eggs may pop, causing them to sink to the bottom. Thus, both the surface film and the sediment should be examined to ensure that no forms are being missed.

   With both the sedimentation and the flotation techniques, species identification may not be possible in all cases, depending on the clarity of the forms observed. Permanently stained smears are usually required to make the final identification, particularly when attempting to confirm the identity of *Entamoeba histolytica* cysts.

VIII. Bibliography
   Bartlett MS, Harper K, Smith N, et al. Comparative evaluation of a modified zinc sulfate flotation technique. J Clin Microbiol 1977;7:524–528.
   Garcia L. Examination of Fecal Specimens. In: Diagnostic Medical Parasitology. Washington, DC: American Society for Microbiology, 2001.
   Smith JW, Gutierrez Y. Medical parasitology. In: Henry JB, Clinical and Diagnosis Management by Laboratory Methods. Ed. 18. Philadelphia: Saunders, 1992.
   Young KH, Bullock SL, Melvin DM, et al. Ethyl acetate as a substitute for diethyl ether in the formalin-ether sedimentation technique. J Clin Microbiol 1979;10:852–853.

CHART 22-2

TRICHROME-STAINING TECHNIQUE FOR FECAL SMEARS

I. Principle

Because the refractive index of protozoan cysts and some helminth eggs is near that of water, staining procedures are required for detailed study of their internal structures. Permanent stains enhance the identification of *Entamoeba histolytica* and the detection of *Giardia lamblia*, two of the more commonly encountered and important protozoa. The Wheatley trichrome technique, a modification of the original Gomori technique, which contains chromotrope 2R and light green SF as the primary staining agents, is the stain used in most clinical parasitology laboratories. It is easy to perform and rapid and it produces uniformly excellent staining of most parasitic forms. Smears made from fresh fecal material must be fixed; polyvinyl alcohol (PVA) samples are already fixed and need no additional treatment.

II. Reagents

Chromotrope 2R	0.6 g
Light green SF	0.3 g
Phosphotungstic acid	0.7 g
Acetic acid (glacial)	1.0 mL
Distilled water	100 mL

Add 1.0 mL of acetic acid to the dry components. Allow the mixture to ripen for 15–30 minutes at room temperature before adding 100 mL of distilled water. The stain should appear purple. When properly stored in glass or plastic bottles at room temperature, the shelf life is 2 years.

Iodine-Alcohol Solution.

70% ethanol plus iodine

Add sufficient iodine crystals to 70% alcohol to make a dark, concentrated stock. At the time of use, dilute the desired amount of stock solution with 70% alcohol until a port-wine working solution is obtained. The exact concentration is not critical.

III. Quality Control

1. It is recommended that several smears of material containing parasitic organisms of known staining properties be stained in parallel with each unknown smear. If staining is of poor quality, the smears may have been too thick or poorly fixed, or residual $HgCl_2$ may not have been removed owing to the use of an alcohol-iodine mixture that was too weak. Properly fixed smears produce a blue-green cytoplasm of protozoan trophozoites with a slight tinge of purple. Nuclei and inclusions are red, tinged with purple. Cloudy preparations may result if dehydration is incomplete owing to failure to change alcohol solutions that may have become contaminated with water. Staining quality can be improved by draining slides between transfers from one reagent to another.

IV. Procedure

1. Wear gloves when handling stool specimens.
2. With a small portion of the fresh stool specimen, prepare two smears on a microscope slide by using an applicator stick or brush.
3. Immerse smears immediately in Schaudinn's fixative and allow to fix for a minimum of 30 minutes. Overnight fixation is preferred.
4. If the specimen is liquid, mix several drops of fecal material with three or four drops of PVA on a glass slide and let it dry for several hours in a 37°C incubator.
5. If the specimen is in PVA, pour some of the mixture onto a paper towel to absorb out the PVA. Prepare slides of the material from the paper towels as described.

V. Staining Procedure

1. After smears are properly fixed and dried, place slides in the 70% ethyl alcohol for 3 minutes.
2. Place slides in alcohol-iodine working solution for 2–5 minutes.
3. Wash with two changes of 70% alcohol, one for 5 minutes and one for 2–5 minutes.
4. Place in trichrome staining solution for 10 minutes.
5. Place in acidified 90% ethyl alcohol for 5 seconds.
6. Dip slides several times in 100% ethanol.
7. Place in two changes of 100% ethyl alcohol.
8. Remove alcohol with two changes of xylene or toluene for 2–5 minutes each.
9. Add mounting medium and overlay with a #1 coverslip. Allow to dry overnight.
10. Examine under oil immersion for parasitic forms.

CHART 22-2

TRICHROME-STAINING TECHNIQUE FOR FECAL SMEARS *continued*

VI. Results

The cytoplasm of thoroughly fixed and well-stained cysts and trophozoites is blue-green, tinged with purple. The nuclear chromatin, chromatoid bodies, and ingested red cells appear red or red-purple. Background material is green.

VII. Procedure Notes

1. If specimens are improperly fixed, protozoan forms may take on a dirty red color.
2. Incomplete removal of mercuric chloride (Schaudinn's fixative) may result in the deposit of highly refractive granules that may interfere with detection of parasitic forms. Be sure to change the 70% ethanol-iodine solution regularly so this does not happen.
3. Smears that are too green may indicate inadequate removal of iodine by 70% ethanol. Lengthening the time of wash in 70% alcohol and frequent changes of solution will minimize this problem.

VIII. Bibliography

1. Garcia L. Examination of fecal specimens. In: Diagnostic Medical Parasitology. Washington, DC: American Society for Microbiology, 2001:759–764.
2. Gomori G. A rapid one-step trichrome stain. Am J Clin Pathol 1950;20:661–663.
3. Wheatley W. A rapid staining procedure for intestinal amoebae and flagellates. Am J Clin Pathol 1951;21: 990–991.

CHART 22-3

PREPARATION OF THIN AND THICK BLOOD SMEARS

Preparation of Thin Blood Film

I. Principle

The thin blood film, prepared similarly to that for the differential white-cell count, allows optimal assessment of the morphology of any parasitic forms that may be present.

II. Specimen

The blood smear may either be prepared from fresh blood obtained by a finger prick or from an EDTA-anticoagulated specimen collected by venipuncture.

III. Materials

A. Equipment: None

B. Supplies

1. 3 × 1-in. microscope slides, alcohol-washed
2. Glass marker
3. Blood-collection supplies

C. Reagents

1. Absolute methanol for Giemsa stain

IV. Quality Control

A. Visually, the smear should appear even, without ridges, smudges, or streaks, and gradually thin out to a rounded, feather edge.

V. Procedure: Thin Film

1. Blood from finger stick:

Puncture the skin of the side of the finger with a sharp lancet and carefully wipe away the first drop of blood. Then touch the next small drop of blood to the surface of a clean glass microscope slide about 1 cm from one end. Turn the slide blood side up and place on a horizontal surface.

2. Venipuncture specimen:

Place a clean glass slide on a horizontal surface. With the tip of the needle, place a small drop of blood on the surface of the glass slide about 1 cm from one end.

3. With a second glass slide held at an angle of 40 degrees to the glass with the blood drop, back into the drop of blood, hesitate momentarily while the blood extends to both margins of the spreader slide, then quickly and steadily advance the angled slide to the opposite end. The result is a thin, feathered film that becomes progressively thinner.

CHART 22-3

PREPARATION OF THIN AND THICK BLOOD SMEARS *continued*

4. Label the smear and allow it to air-dry for about 10 minutes.
5. Stain the smear either with Giemsa or Wright's. If the Giemsa stain is used, the smear must first be fixed in absolute alcohol.
6. Procedure notes
   a. Use a diamond marking pen to label the smear.
   b. Make sure films are protected during drying from the deposition of dust from the air.
7. Limitations of the procedure
   a. Parasitic forms may be missed in light infections. In such instances, a thick film must be examined.
   b. Smears must be prepared from anticoagulated blood within 1 hour after venipuncture. The morphology of parasitic forms and the erythrocytes become atypical after that time from direct action of the anticoagulant.

Preparation of Thin Blood Film
I. Principle
The thick blood film samples a relatively large volume of blood providing a better opportunity to recover parasitic forms in light infections. Red cells are lysed, providing a better opportunity to detect parasitic forms against a more transparent background.
II. Specimen
The blood smear may either be prepared from fresh blood obtained by a finger prick or from an EDTA-anticoagulated specimen collected by venipuncture. Heparin or sodium citrate anticoagulated blood samples may be used if the presence of trypomastigotes or microfilaria are suspected.
III. Materials
   A. Equipment: None
   B. Supplies
      1. 3 × 1-in. microscope slides, alcohol-washed
      2. Glass marker
      3. Blood-collection supplies
      4. Newspaper
      5. Applicator sticks
   C. Reagents
      1. Absolute methanol for Giemsa stain
IV. Quality Control
   A. Visually, the smear should appear as a round to oval smear of blood about 2 cm in diameter. It should be of such thickness that newsprint can barely be seen through the wet or dry smear.
   B. The spread of blood should be even, without ridges, smudges, or streaks.
V. Procedure
   1. Blood from finger stick:
   Puncture the skin of the side of the finger with a sharp lancet and carefully wipe away the first drop of blood. Then touch a large drop of blood to the surface of the middle of a clean glass microscope slide. Without breaking contact with the blood, rotate the slide on the finger to make a circle about the size of a nickel. Remove the slide and place it on a horizontal surface. The thickness should be such that newsprint can barely be seen through the slide. If it is too thick, spread it with a circular motion using an applicator stick until the correct thickness is achieved. If too thin, a second slide must be prepared.
   2. Venipuncture specimen:
   Place a clean glass slide on a horizontal surface. With the tip of the needle, place a large drop of blood on the surface of the glass slide.
   3. With the tip of an applicator stick, spread the blood into a circle about the size of a dime or nickel, to achieve a thickness through which newsprint can barely be seen.
   4. Label the smear and allow it to air-dry for several hours or overnight.
   5. Stain the smear either with Giemsa or Wright's. If the Giemsa stain is not to be performed until 3 days or more after preparation; or, if the Wright's stain is used, lyse the red cells by placing the thick film in buffered water (pH 7.2) for 10 minutes. Then place the slide in a vertical position to let it drip dry. Do not fix the thick smear.
   6. Procedure notes:
      a. Use a diamond marking pen to label the smear.
      b. Make sure films are protected during drying from the deposition of dust from the air.

CHART 22-3

PREPARATION OF THIN AND THICK BLOOD SMEARS *continued*

7. Limitations of Procedure
   a. Making a species identification of malarial parasites may be difficult to impossible, even for experienced workers.
   b. A thin film should always be examined if a definitive identification based on morphology is required.
   c. Smears must be prepared from anticoagulated blood within 1 hour after venipuncture. The morphology of parasitic forms and the erythrocytes become atypical after that time from direct action of the anticoagulant.

VI. Bibliography
   Garcia L. Examination of Fecal Specimens. In: Diagnostic Medical Parasitology. Washington, DC: American Society for Microbiology, 2001:759–764.
   Garcia L. Parasitology. In: Isenberg HD, ed. Clinical Microbiology Procedure Handbook. Washington, DC: American Society for Microbiology, 1992.

CHART 22-4

CALIBRATION OF THE OCULAR MICROMETER

I. Principle
Ocular micrometers are etched with a fixed scale, usually consisting of 50 parallel lines. Depending on the magnifying power of the set of objectives used in a compound microscope, each division in the ocular micrometer scale represents different measurements. Therefore, for each set of oculars and objectives used, the ocular scale must be calibrated using a stage micrometer etched with a scale (0.1-mm divisions are commonly used). It is important to remember that a calibration for a given set of oculars and objectives cannot be interchanged with corresponding components from another microscope.

II. Specimen: Not applicable

III. Materials
   A. Equipment
      1. Binocular microscope with $10\times$, $40\times$, and $100\times$ objectives. Other objective magnifications may be used as required.
      2. Oculars should be $10\times$. A single ocular may be used to calibrate all laboratory microscopes.
   B. Supplies
      1. An ocular micrometer disk, with scale-line divisions of 50 U. These are available from several laboratory supply companies.
      2. A stage micrometer with scale divisions of 0.1 and 0.01 mm
      3. Immersion oil
      4. Lens paper
   C. Reagents: Not applicable

IV. Quality Control
   1. All microscopes used for parasitology examinations should be recalibrated at a minimum of once per year.
   2. The width of red cells can be used to check the calibrations at various magnifications.
   3. Latex or polystyrene beads of standardized diameter can be used to check calculations and measurements. Beads with diameters of 10 and 90 μm are recommended. These are available from several laboratory supply companies.

V. Procedure
   1. Remove the ocular from the microscope to be used. If a binocular microscope is used, it is customary to remove the right $10\times$ ocular.
   2. Unscrew the eye lens (top lens) of the ocular and insert the micrometer wafer so that it rests on the diaphragm ring inside the ocular. Place the micrometer with the engraved side down. The micrometer should be handled with lens paper and every effort made to prevent lint from adhering to the surface.
   3. Replace the ocular in the housing. When viewed through the ocular, the micrometer scale appears as a series of lined division, illustrated in **A**.

CHART 22-4

CALIBRATION OF THE OCULAR MICROMETER *continued*

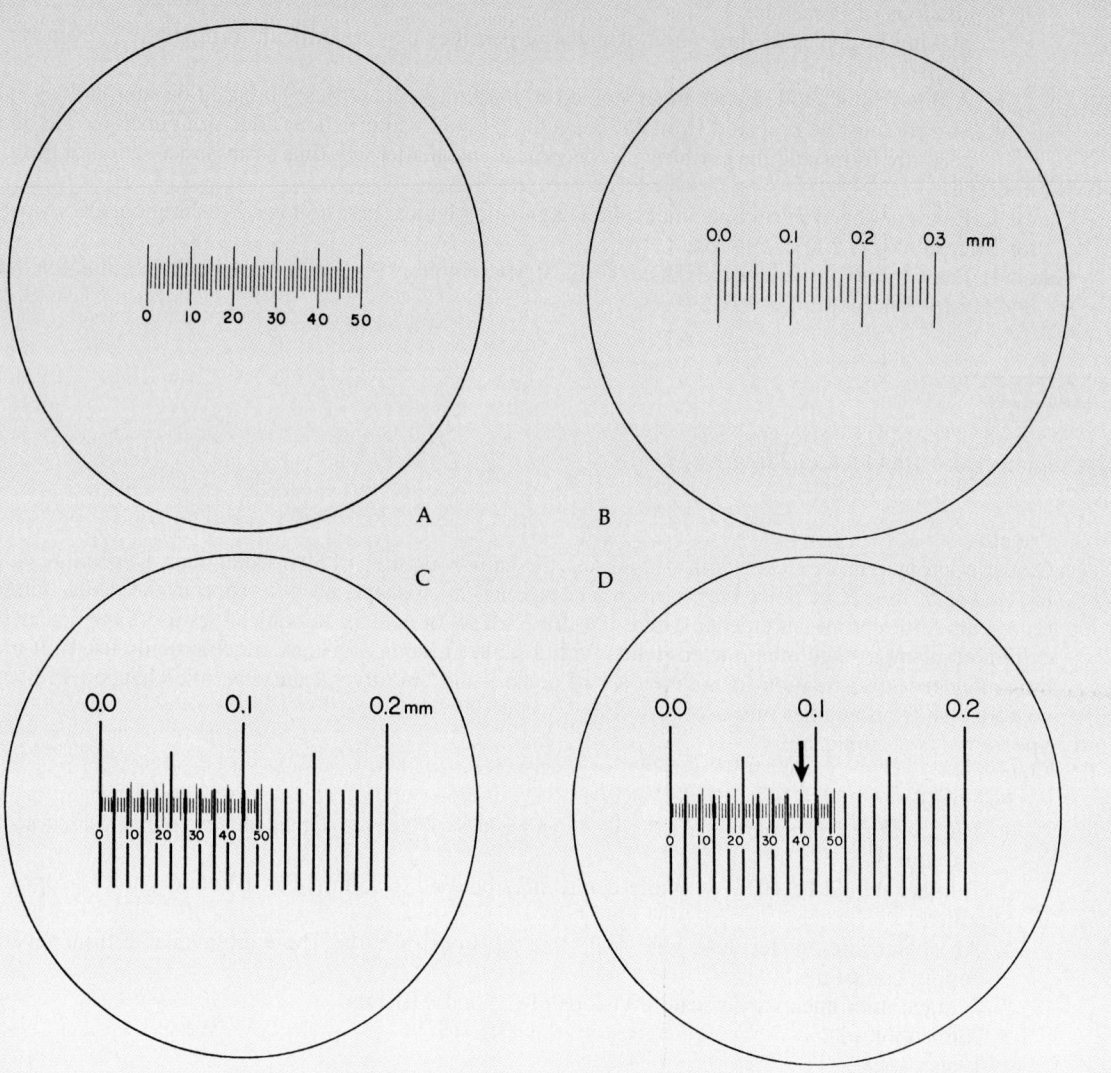

4. Place the stage micrometer under the objective of the microscope that is to be calibrated. Bring into view the stage micrometer scale, which appears as a series of lines divided into 0.1-mm and 0.01-mm divisions, as shown in the simulated view through the microscope in **B.**
5. Adjust the stage micrometer so that the 0 line on the ocular micrometer is exactly superimposed with the 0.0 line on the stage micrometer scale. When viewed under high magnification (450×), the superimposition of the two scales appears as in the simulated view through the microscope shown in **C.**
6. Without further manipulation, look across the two scales and find the next pair of lines that exactly coincide. In **D** (a simulated high-power 450× view), the coinciding lines are the 40 mark on the ocular scale and the 0.09-mm mark on the stage micrometer (*arrow*).
7. The object of the calibration is to determine the width in micrometers of each ocular scale division, when calibrated against the stage micrometer scale. Determine the calibration as follows:
   a. As illustrated in **D,** 40 units on the ocular scale are equal to 0.09 mm on the stage micrometer scale.
   b. Therefore, each ocular division is equal to 0.09 mm/40, or 0.00225 mm. Since there are 1,000 μm in each millimeter, each ocular micrometer division in the calibration illustrated in **D** is equal to 0.00225 × 1000, or 2.25 μm.

CHART 22-4

CALIBRATION OF THE OCULAR MICROMETER *continued*

VI. Results
Thus, based on the procedure just described, if an object viewed under the microscope occupies 10 ocular scale divisions, it would measure 2.25×20, or 22.5 μm. These same interpolations can be made for other magnifications. Once the number of ocular lines per width and length of the organism is measured, then, depending on the objective lens being used, the ocular/microns multiplication factor can be applied to the number of ocular scale lines spanning the length and width of the organism being viewed. Comparison of these measurements for any given parasitic form can be compared with published results in standard textbooks in making a final identification.

VII. Procedure Notes
   1. As a rule of thumb, the high dry objective ($40\times$) factor should be approximately 2.5 times the factor obtained from the oil immersion objective ($100\times$). Likewise, the $10\times$ low-power objective should be about 10 times that of the oil immersion objective.
   2. The multiplication factors for each objective should be posted on the base of each microscope to be used for parasitology examinations.

VIII. Bibliography
   Garcia L. Examination of Fecal Specimens. In: Diagnostic Medical Parasitology. Washington, DC: American Society for Microbiology, 2001:759–764.
   Garcia L. Parasitology. In: Isenberg HD, ed. Clinical Microbiology Procedure Handbook. Washington, DC: American Society for Microbiology, 1992.

CHART 22-5

CELLULOSE TAPE PREPARATION FOR PINWORM EXAMINATION

   I. Principle
   The eggs discharged by adult female *Enterobius vermicularis* worms are characteristically deposited on the perianal skin during periods of extraintestinal migration. These eggs stick to the glued surface of cellulose tape. By applying the sticky surface of the tape to a glass slide, the mount can be examined under a microscope.

   II. Specimen
   The specimen is collected from the perianal skin. An early-morning sample, before the patient has bathed or used the toilet, is optimal. Up to 6 successive daily morning samples should be collected before a negative result is issued.

   III. Materials
   A. Equipment
      1. Binocular microscope with $10\times$, $40\times$, and $100\times$ objectives. Other objective magnifications may be used as required.
      2. Oculars should be $10\times$. A single ocular may be used to calibrate all laboratory microscopes.
   B. Supplies
      1. Clear cellulose tape
      2. Tongue depressors
      3. 3×1-in. glass microscope slides
   C. Reagents
      1. Xylene or xylene substitute

   IV. Quality Control
      1. All microscopes used for parasitology examinations should be recalibrated at a minimum of once per year.
      2. The availability of a textbook or atlas with photomicrographs and/or illustrations of *E. vermicularis* eggs may be helpful to confirm suspected results.

   V. Procedure
      1. Prepare the microscope slide by attaching a piece of transparent cellulose tape sticky side down about 1.5 cm from one end of the slide. Run the tape over the edge and along the entire length of the opposite side and cut it even with the distal end. Place a paper label under the edge just cut to serve as a tab for removing the tape.

CHART 22-5

CELLULOSE TAPE PREPARATION FOR PINWORM EXAMINATION *continued*

  2. To obtain the specimen from the perianal skin, grip the paper label and tear the tape from the glass slide. Rest the glass slide on a tongue blade in such a way that the tape can be looped sticky side out over and extending beyond the end of the tongue blade by about 2.5 cm. The tongue blade then serves as a support as the sticky side of the tape is pressed in several areas against the perianal skin.
  3. Once the sample is obtained, remove the slide from the tongue depressor and affix the tape sticky side down on the glass slide. Label the slide with the patient name and date of collection.
  4. Examine the slide under a microscope using the low power (10×) objective. The eggs can be made more visible by detaching the tape from the slide, adding a drop of xylene or toluene, and again affixing the tape.
 VI. Results
    The eggs of *E. vermicularis* measure about 50–60 μm × 20–30 μm and have a relatively thick, smooth shell and an ovoid shape flattened on one side, much like a flattened, partially inflated football. Adult worms may occasionally be seen in transparency tape preparations. They measure about 1 cm long, have a pointed tail posteriorly and transparent wings flanking the anterior end.
VII. Procedure Notes
  1. The person obtaining the specimen must take care, as the eggs are infectious if swallowed. Gloves can be worn or the hands thoroughly washed following the procedure. A paddle with a sticky adhesive coat is commercially available (BD Falcon™, Swube™, Pinworm Paddle, BD Diagnostic Systems, Sparks, MD), serving as a less cumbersome collection device that is also safer to use.
  2. If an opaque tape has been used by mistake, adding immersion oil to the surface will facilitate microscopic examination.
VIII. Limitations of the Procedure
  1. Female *E. vermicularis* worms deposit eggs on an irregular schedule. Thus, several daily samples must be obtained before ruling out infection.
 IX. Bibliography
    Garcia L. Examination of Fecal Specimens. In: Diagnostic Medical Parasitology. Washington, DC: American Society for Microbiology, 2001:759–764.
    Garcia L. Parasitology. In: Isenberg HD, ed. Clinical Microbiology Procedure Handbook. Washington, DC: American Society for Microbiology, 1992.

CHART 23-1

HEMADSORPTION (HAD) TEST

  I. Principle
    The hemadsorption test is the simplest method of identifying the presence of an orthomyxovirus or paramyxovirus. Identification of the isolate may also be accomplished by testing inhibition of hemadsorption, but the hemagglutination inhibition (HAI) test is less cumbersome and is cheaper to perform.
      Among the viruses that produce agglutination of red cells, the orthomyxoviruses and paramyxoviruses mature at the plasma membrane of infected cells. As they "bud" at the plasma membrane, they insert virally specified hemagglutinins into the membrane. The presence of infected cells in a monolayer can be detected by adherence of the red cells to the monolayer. Because some simian viruses that may be present in monkey tissue also produce hemagglutinins, it is important to include uninfected monolayers as controls.
 II. Materials and Reagents
    A. Infected and control primary monkey kidney cells
    B. 0.4% solution of fresh, washed guinea pig erythrocytes in serum-free medium
III. Quality Control
    A. Positive control (hemagglutinating virus)
    B. Negative control (uninfected monolayer)
 IV. Procedure
  1. Add 0.2 mL of guinea pig erythrocytes for each 1 mL of medium.
  2. Incubate in a slanted rack for 1 hour at 4°C.
  3. Observe microscopically for agglutination in the fluid phase and adherence of erythrocytes to the monolayer.
  4. Incubate the cultures for an additional 1 hour at 20°C.
  5. Observe again for agglutination and adherence.

CHART 23-1

HEMADSORPTION (HAD) TEST *continued*

V. Results
    A. Interpretation
        Agglutination of erythrocytes in the fluid phase or adherence of red cells to the monolayer. If HAD occurs in the negative control, the test is invalid. Elution of erythrocytes at 20°C suggests the presence of parainfluenza virus 1–3.
VI. Bibliography
        Smith TF. Viruses. In: Washington JA, ed. Laboratory Procedures in Clinical Microbiology. Ed. 2. New York: Springer-Verlag, 1985.

CHART A-1

FORMULATIONS OF COMMONLY USED STOOL PRESERVATIVES

   I. Merthiolate-Iodine-Formalin (MIF)
      A. Solution I
         Tincture of merthiolate, 1:1000, 40 mL
         Formaldehyde, 10% aqueous (USP), 5 mL
         Glycerol, 1 mL
         Distilled water, 50 mL
      B. Solution II
         Potassium iodide crystals (KI), 10 g
         Iodine crystals (add after KI dissolves), 5 g
         Distilled water, 100 mL
         The shelf life of each solution is many months if stored at room temperature in a brown bottle. In a small vial, combine 9.4 mL of solution I with 0.6 mL of solution II just before use. Add the equivalent of about 1/4 teaspoon of fresh feces and thoroughly mix with an applicator stick. Allow the suspension to settle for 24 hours; then, with a pipette, remove a small portion of the pale orange middle layer and the deeper staining lower layer for preparation of smears.
  II. LV-PVA
      A. Formulation
         Polyvinyl alcohol, 10.0 g
         95% ethyl alcohol, 62.5 mL
         Mercuric chloride, saturated aqueous, 125.0 mL
         Glycerin, 3.0 mL
         The liquid ingredients are mixed in a 500 mL beaker and the polyvinyl alcohol (PVA) powder added without mixing. Cover the beaker with paper or foil and allow the PVA to soak overnight. Slowly heat the mixture to 75°C and gently swirl for about 30 seconds until a light milky suspension is achieved.
  III. Sodium Acetate-Acetic-Acid-Formalin (SAF)
      A. Formulation:
         Formaldehyde (37–40% solution), 0.6 mL
         Glacial acetic acid, 0.3 mL
         Sodium acetate, 225.0 mg
         Distilled water, 13.88 mL
         Dissolve the sodium acetate in the distilled water, slowly add the glacial acetic acid and formalin solutions, mix, and store. The shelf life is several months.
  IV. Schaudinn's Fixative (mercuric chloride in ethyl alcohol and glacic acetic acid)
      A. Formulation:
         Mercuric chloride, saturated aqueous solution ($HgCl_2$), 110 g
         Distilled water, 1,000 mL
         Into a beaker in a water bath placed in a hood, boil the mercuric chloride until dissolved, and let stand for several hours until crystals form.
  V. Schaudinn's Fixative (stock)
     Mercuric chloride, saturated aqueous solution, 600 mL
     Ethyl alcohol, 95%, 300 mL
     Add 5 mL of glacial acetic acid per 100 mL of stock solution just before use.

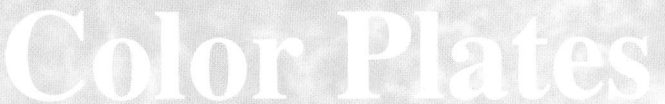

Color Plates

GRAM STAIN EVALUATION OF SPUTUM SMEARS

The quality of sputum samples can be evaluated by counting the relative numbers of squamous epithelial cells and segmented neutrophils per low-power field in a Gram-stained smear. The presence of squamous epithelial cells indicates contamination with oropharyngeal secretions. In contrast, bacterial pneumonia will produce large numbers of segmented neutrophils that can be detected in sputum samples. The following are photomicrographs of Gram-stained smears of sputum samples illustrating the relative presence of the various cellular components.

A. Low-power view of Gram-stained sputum smear revealing full field of squamous epithelial cells and absence of segmented neutrophils. This specimen represents saliva, would give a low quality score, and is not acceptable for culture.

B. The squamous epithelial cell shown here is heavily colonized with Gram-positive bacteria. The overgrowth of bacterial cells in sputum specimens generally indicates that the specimen has been delayed in transit to the laboratory and that any semiquantitative results will be of little value.

C. This Gram-stained sputum smear shows a mixture of squamous cells and segmented neutrophils. The presence of segmented neutrophils indicates that a nidus of infection exists somewhere in the respiratory tract; however, the squamous epithelial cells indicate contamination with upper respiratory tract secretions. This type of sputum smear is difficult to interpret because upper respiratory tract infections cannot be distinguished from lower respiratory tract infections.

D. Full field of neutrophils and virtual absence of squamous epithelial cells. This is a high-quality sputum sample that provides a good chance for producing relevant results.

E. Higher-power view of sample in **D,** revealing scattered segmented neutrophils against a background of pink-staining mucus threads.

F. Smear of an induced sputum sample stained with Diff-Quik, illustrating several ciliated, columnar epithelial cells. These cells have their origin in the lower respiratory tract and, when present in a sputum smear such as seen here, indicate a high-quality specimen from which relevant results can potentially be obtained.

G. High-power view of a Gram-stained sputum specimen illustrates the morphology of a ciliated columnar epithelial cell. Note the distinct cilia atop the flared terminal end of this eosinophilic-staining columnar epithelial cell.

H. Toluidine blue stain of an induced sputum specimen revealing mononuclear inflammatory cells consistent with alveolar macrophages. As in columnar epithelial cells, alveolar macrophages have their origin deep within the lower respiratory tract, and their presence in sputum samples increases the significance of any bacterial species recovered.

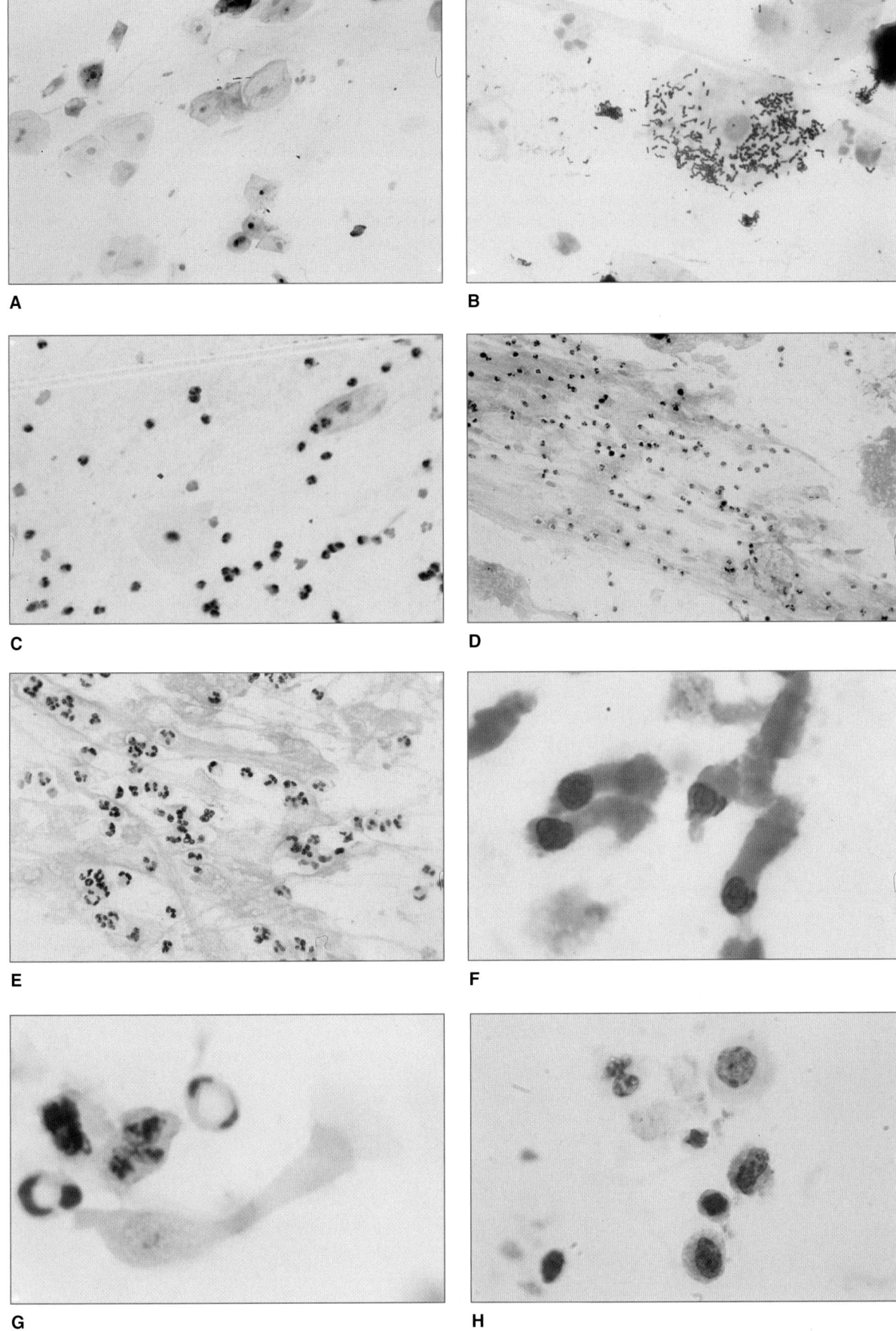

A

B

C

D

E

F

G

H

MISCELLANEOUS STAINS USED IN MICROBIOLOGY

Because many of the microbes of medical importance have refractive indices near that of water, stains are needed to make possible their detection and study. A variety of stains have been developed over the years, each designed to highlight internal organelles or specific components of the cell wall. The following are illustrations of selected stains and some of their applications.

A. *Gram's stain.* The most common stain used in the microbiology laboratory is designed to differentiate between bacteria that can retain crystal violet dye and appear deep blue-black after decolorization (gram-positive) and those that cannot and stain red (gram-negative). Illustrated here is a Gram-stained preparation revealing red-staining, gram-negative bacilli.

B. *Acid-fast.* This stain is commonly used to demonstrate a variety of acid-fast organisms, including *Nocardia* species in sputum specimens and *Cryptosporidium* oocysts in fecal samples. Shown here are clusters of red-staining, acid-fast bacilli in a liver biopsy specimen from a patient with AIDS. The organisms stain red with the acid-fast stain, and those shown here were identified as belonging to the *Mycobacterium avium-intracellulare* complex.

C. *Direct fluorescence.* Fluorescent dyes (rhodamine and auramine) react directly with the cell wall of mycobacteria. Fluorescein-conjugated antibodies are also available to demonstrate a variety of microbial agents using the direct fluorescent antibody test. Shown here are yellow-green, fluorescing mycobacteria in a sputum concentrate from a patient with pulmonary tuberculosis.

D. *Acridine orange.* This rapid fluorescent stain is used to demonstrate bacterial forms in direct smears and mounts of biologic fluids. It is particularly useful in detecting gram-negative bacteria in positive blood culture broths, which may be missed in Gram stains because of the deep red-staining debris in the background. Shown here is a long, rod-shaped bacterium, with a characteristic orange glow, when microscopically observed with a fluorescence microscope.

E. *Methylene blue.* This nonspecific, rapid stain is used to demonstrate bacteria and other microbes in direct smears. Illustrated here are bacilli that have taken the blue stain. One important application is in the detection of bacteria in direct smears of cerebrospinal fluid in cases of suspected acute meningitis, particularly gram-negative species, that may be obscured by the red background staining of the proteinaceous material.

F. *Calcofluor white.* This autofluorescent whitening agent has the property of coupling with carbohydrate moieties in the cell walls of fungi. Shown here are brilliant yellow-green staining hyphae in a direct calcofluor white–stained mount as observed with a fluorescence microscope.

G. *Wright-Giemsa.* This stain is commonly used to demonstrate the cellular elements in peripheral blood and bone marrow smears. In microbiology, the stain is most commonly used to detect intraerythrocytic (plasmodia, babesiae) and exoerythrocytic (trypanosomes, microfilaria) parasites, chlamydial inclusions, and, as shown here, the intracellular yeast forms of *Histoplasma capsulatum*.

H. *Periodic acid–Schiff (PAS).* This general stain is used to demonstrate polysaccharide-rich cell walls. It has specific applications in detecting fungi in tissue sections and smears. Recognized here is the fruiting body of *Aspergillus* species in an aspirate of a fungus ball lesion of the lung surrounded by red-staining *Aspergillus* spores.

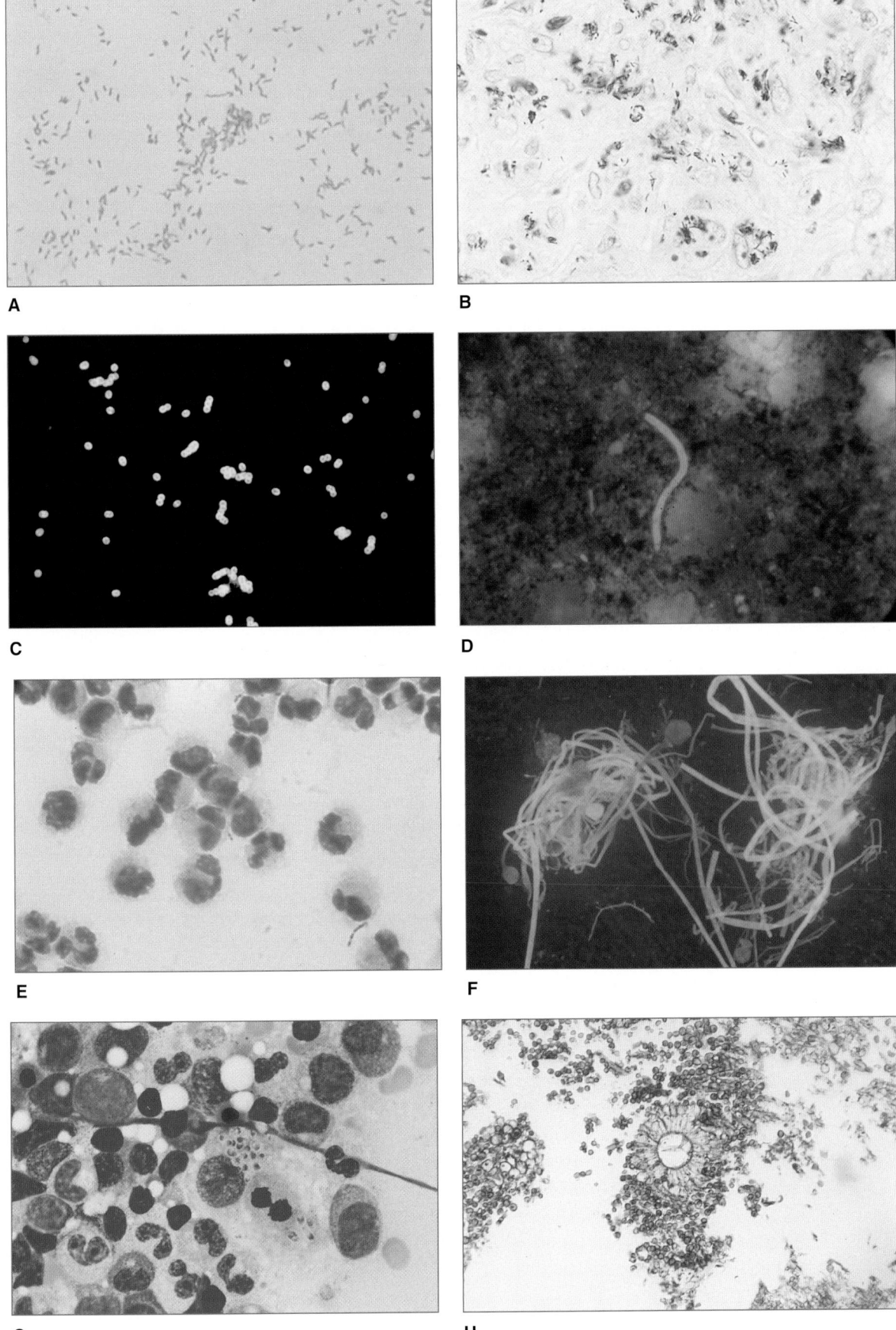

A

B

C

D

E

F

G

H

PRESUMPTIVE BACTERIAL IDENTIFICATION BASED ON OBSERVING MICROSCOPIC CELLULAR MORPHOLOGY IN STAINED SMEAR PREPARATIONS

The Gram stain of bacteria, in addition to other staining techniques, is one of the more important determinations in the presumptive identification of microorganisms. The morphology of the bacterial cells, their arrangement, and their staining characteristics are often distinctive enough to allow a presumptive identification in a Gram-stained smear. The microscopic characteristics suggestive of several groups of bacteria are included in this plate.

A. Relatively slender, gram-positive bacilli arranged in a Chinese letter pattern, suggesting one of the coryneform (diphtheroid) bacteria.

B. Gram-positive, spore-forming bacilli. The aerobic spore formers belong to the genus *Bacillus;* the anaerobic spore formers belong to the genus *Clostridium.* Illustrated here are spore-forming cells of *Bacillus sphaericus.*

C. Direct Gram's stain of purulent exudates illustrating gram-positive cocci arranged in small clusters, characteristic of *Staphylococcus* species.

D. Direct smear of necrotic exudates from a case of myonecrosis. The tiny, gram-positive cocci seen in this photomicrograph are streptococci.

E. Direct Gram's stain of a smear of purulent sputum demonstrating gram-positive diplococci, characteristic of *Streptococcus pneumoniae.*

F. Purulent exudates from the chest wall of a patient with acute, suppurative empyema. Against the background of segmented neutrophils are numerous gram-positive, branching bacilli. *Actinomyces* species and *Nocardia* species can produce a picture similar to this; however, in this case, a pure culture of *Bifidobacterium* species was recovered in anaerobic culture.

G. Gram-stained preparation of a direct smear of urine sediment from a case of acute cystitis. Note the several gram-negative bacilli amid the background segmented neutrophils. *Escherichia coli* was recovered in pure culture.

H. Gram-stained preparation of a direct smear prepared from purulent urethral exudates of a sexually active male, illustrating the intracellular, gram-negative, diplococci characteristic of *Neisseria gonorrhoeae.* The bacterial cells in this photograph are paler staining than normally seen by direct microscopic examination.

I. Photomicrograph of a sputum smear illustrating a few segmented neutrophils in the background and a diffuse infiltration with many short, gram-negative bacilli some of which appear to be surrounded by a halo. *Klebsiella pneumoniae* grew out in culture.

J. Photomicrograph of delicate, branching gram-positive filaments suggestive of *Actinomyces* species. *Propionibacterium acnes* grew out in culture.

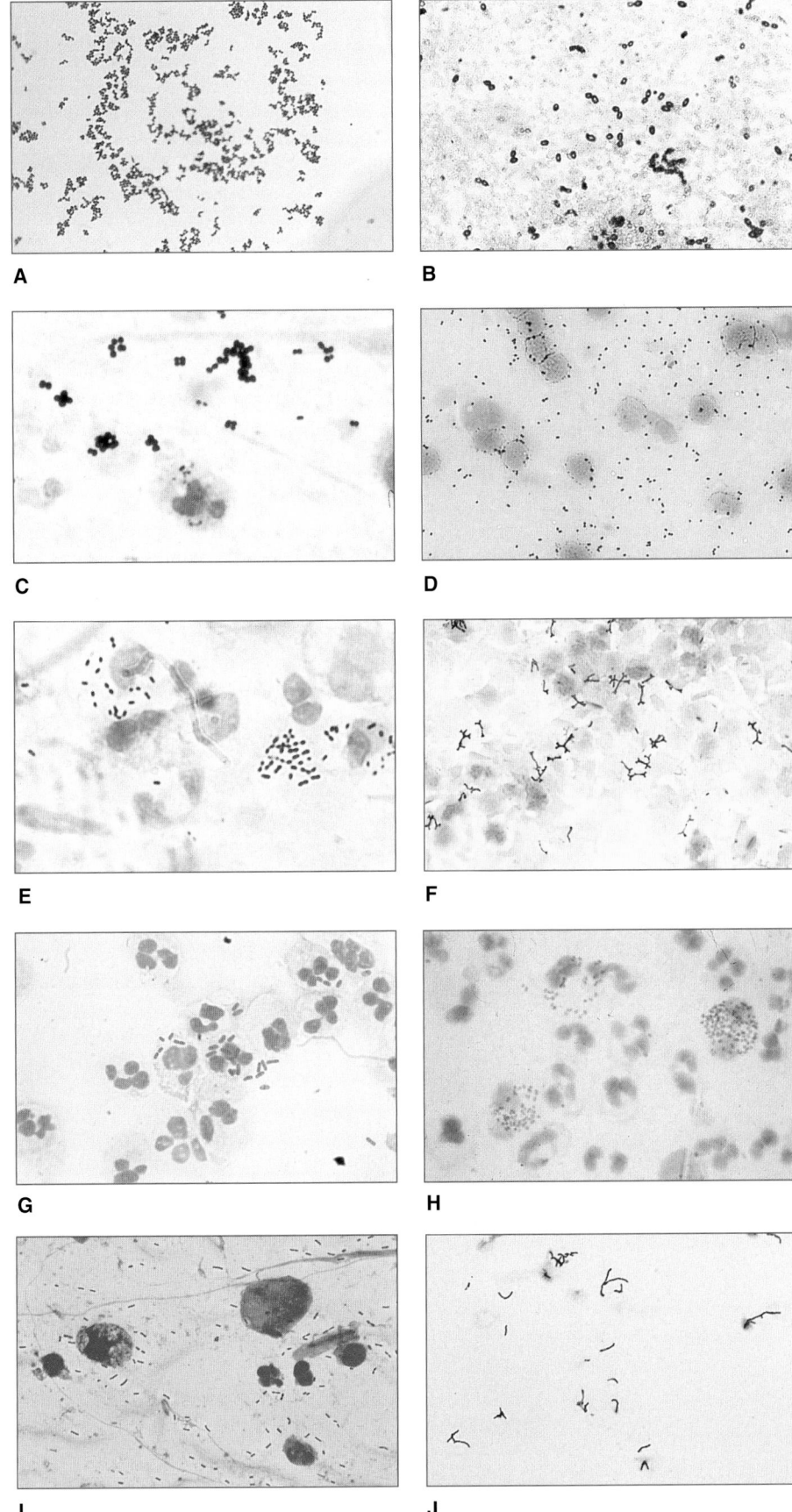

A

B

C

D

E

F

G

H

I

J

PITFALLS AND ARTIFACTS IN GRAM'S STAIN

A. *Acinetobacter* sp. in a blood culture. This genus is coccobacillary and tends to retain the crystal violet. Thus, a Gram stained smear may be misinterpreted as gram-negative cocci, gram-positive cocci (arrows), or gram-positive bacilli. The microscopist must evaluate the pattern of all the bacterial cells in the smear. The presence of cells that stain magenta is one clue that the true reaction may be gram-negative. Original magnification, ×1000.

B. Overdecolorized staphylococci in a genital specimen misinterpreted as gram-negative cocci. Although both gonococci and staphylococci may appear as diplococci, with a rare exception (*arrow*) the "kidney bean" shape of gonococci is not present here, and the bacterial cells are not intracellular. It is important not to imply the presence of *Neisseria gonorrhoeae* unless the morphology is characteristic. Original magnification, ×1000.

C. Elongated cells of *Streptococcus pneumoniae* (arrows) in a sputum smear may be misinterpreted as gram-positive bacilli, and their importance as a major respiratory pathogen may be missed. Other cells in the smear had the characteristic "lancet-shaped" appearance of pneumococci. The microscopist must assess the overall pattern and not be misled by occasional outliers. Original magnification, ×1000.

D. *Clostridium perfringens* decolorizes easily and may appear gram-negative. Clues to the true nature of the bacterial cells is provided by the occasional gram-positive cells (*arrow*) and the large "boxcar" appearance that does not resemble a typical enteric bacillus. *Bacillus* spp. may also decolorize and appear gram-negative. Original magnification, ×1000.

E. Gram stain debris masquerading as gram-positive cocci. The true nature of the material is suggested by the small size and the marked variation in size. Artifactual material often appears refractile when the focus is varied. Original magnification, ×1000.

F. Retinal rods and cones masquerading as gram-positive cocci and bacilli in a vitreous specimen. The true nature of the structures is suggested by the anatomical site and their refractile appearance. Original magnification, ×1000.

G. Conidia of *Aspergillus fumigatus* mimicking gram-positive cocci in a sputum specimen. The true nature of the structures is suggested by the enlarged size and by roughened edges of the conidia if present. Search of the smear may reveal hyphae. Original magnification, ×1000.

H. Exfoliated cilia from a respiratory cell (*arrow*) resembling gram-negative bacilli. A pale-staining bacillus such as *Fusobacterium nucleatum* may be suggested. On closer inspection, however, the structures do not have the morphologic detail of a bacterium. Further search will usually reveal intact cells with their attached cilia. Original magnification, ×1000. (Image enhanced.)

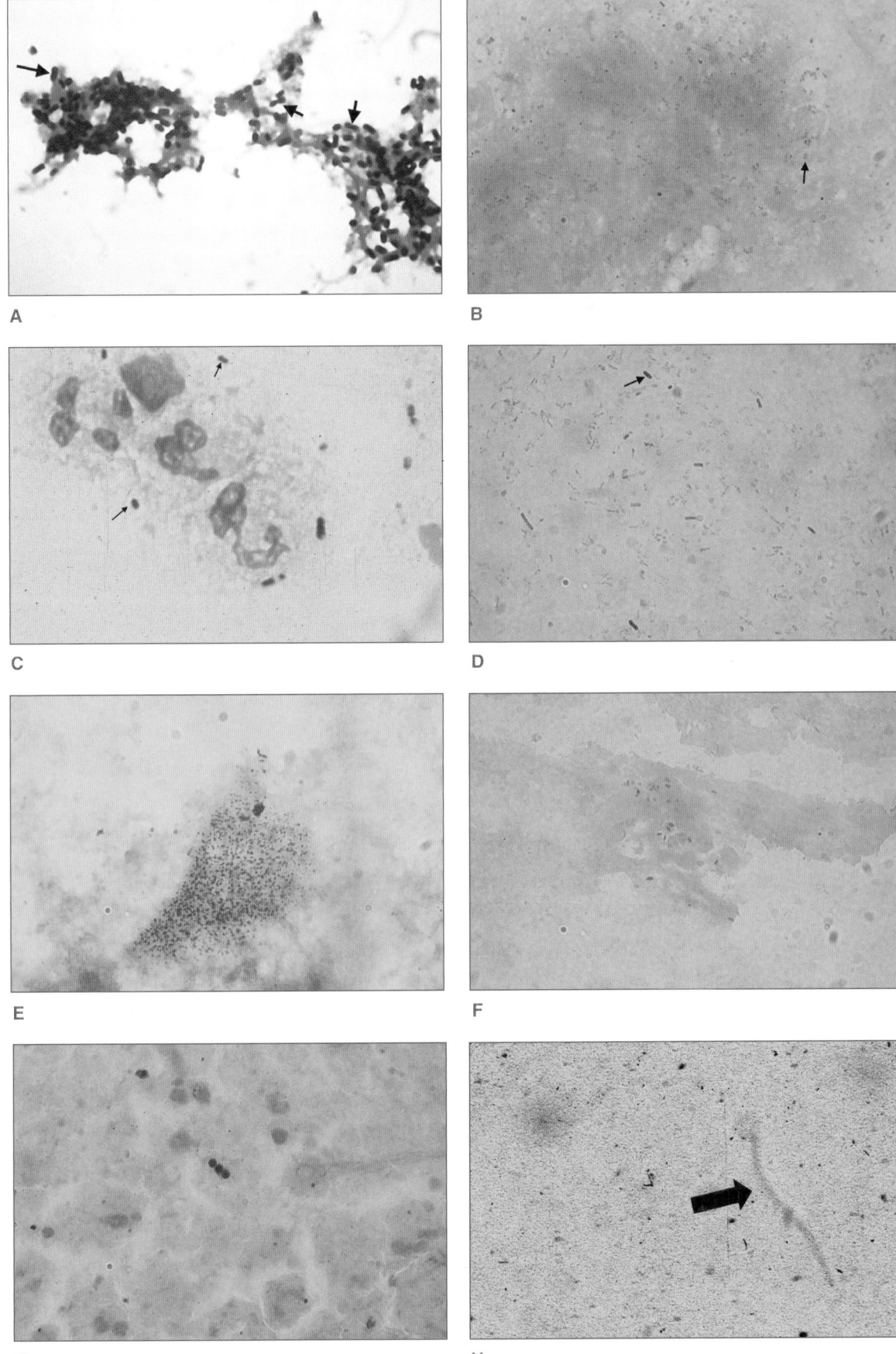

A

B

C

D

E

F

G

H

PRESUMPTIVE BACTERIAL IDENTIFICATION BASED ON OBSERVING COLONIAL MORPHOLOGY

Microbiologists use various characteristics of bacterial colonies that grow on the surface of agar culture media to make a presumptive identification of the group or genus and as a guide in selecting differential tests to make the final species identification. Size, shape, consistency, color, and pigment production by the colonies, as well as the presence of hemolytic reactions on blood agar, are the criteria commonly used.

A. Blood agar plate on which are growing round, yellow-white, entire, convex, nonhemolytic colonies of *Staphylococcus* species.

B. Colonies growing on blood agar illustrating distinct zones of β-hemolysis around the colonies. The relation between the size of the colonies and the zones of hemolysis is used to differentiate between certain species. Shown here are *Streptococcus* species, which commonly have a lower ratio of colony size to hemolytic zones, in contrast with *Staphylococcus* species, in which the relative size of the colonies is generally larger.

C. Blood agar plate demonstrates the greenish discoloration of the agar, characteristic of α-hemolysis. Growing on this plate are tiny, clear colonies of viridans streptococci, with larger zones of α-hemolysis.

D. Opaque, dull gray, somewhat moist colonies growing on blood agar (*right*) and MacConkey agar (*left*), suggestive of one of the members of the family *Enterobacteriaceae*. The growth on MacConkey agar shows no red pigmentation, indicating that the organism is a non–lactose fermenter. The bacteria shown here are *Salmonella* species.

E. Dry, wrinkled colonies of a *Bacillus* species. Similar-appearing, wrinkled colonies are also seen with *Pseudomonas stutzeri*.

F. Yellow-pigmented colonies on blood agar. Pigment production is an important feature in the differential identification of many bacterial species, particularly those belonging to several groups of nonfermentative bacilli. The colonies shown here are those of *Flavobacterium* species after 48 hours of incubation, with the last 24 hours of incubation being at room temperature. The intensity of pigment is often accentuated after additional incubation at room temperature.

G. Distinctly mucoid colonies growing on blood agar. The mucoid consistency of colonies is generally secondary to the production of capsules, a protective mechanism used by several bacterial species in defense against phagocytosis. *Pseudomonas* species, *Klebsiella pneumoniae*, *Streptococcus pneumoniae*, and *Cryptococcus neoformans* are among the more commonly recovered microbial species producing mucoid colonies. The colony shown here is *Streptococcus pneumoniae*.

H. Gray semitranslucent colonies of *Eikenella corrodens* growing on blood agar. Note the halo appearance around the colonies, illustrating the "pitting" characteristic of the species.

I. Gray, smooth, semitransparent colonies of *Capnocytophaga ochracea*. Note the mistlike extension of the colonies, illustrating the gliding motility characteristic of *Capnocytophaga* species.

J. White, dry, chalky colony of *Nocardia* species. *Streptomyces* species produce similar-appearing colonies. These presumptive identifications can be confirmed if the musty basement odor characteristic of these species can be detected.

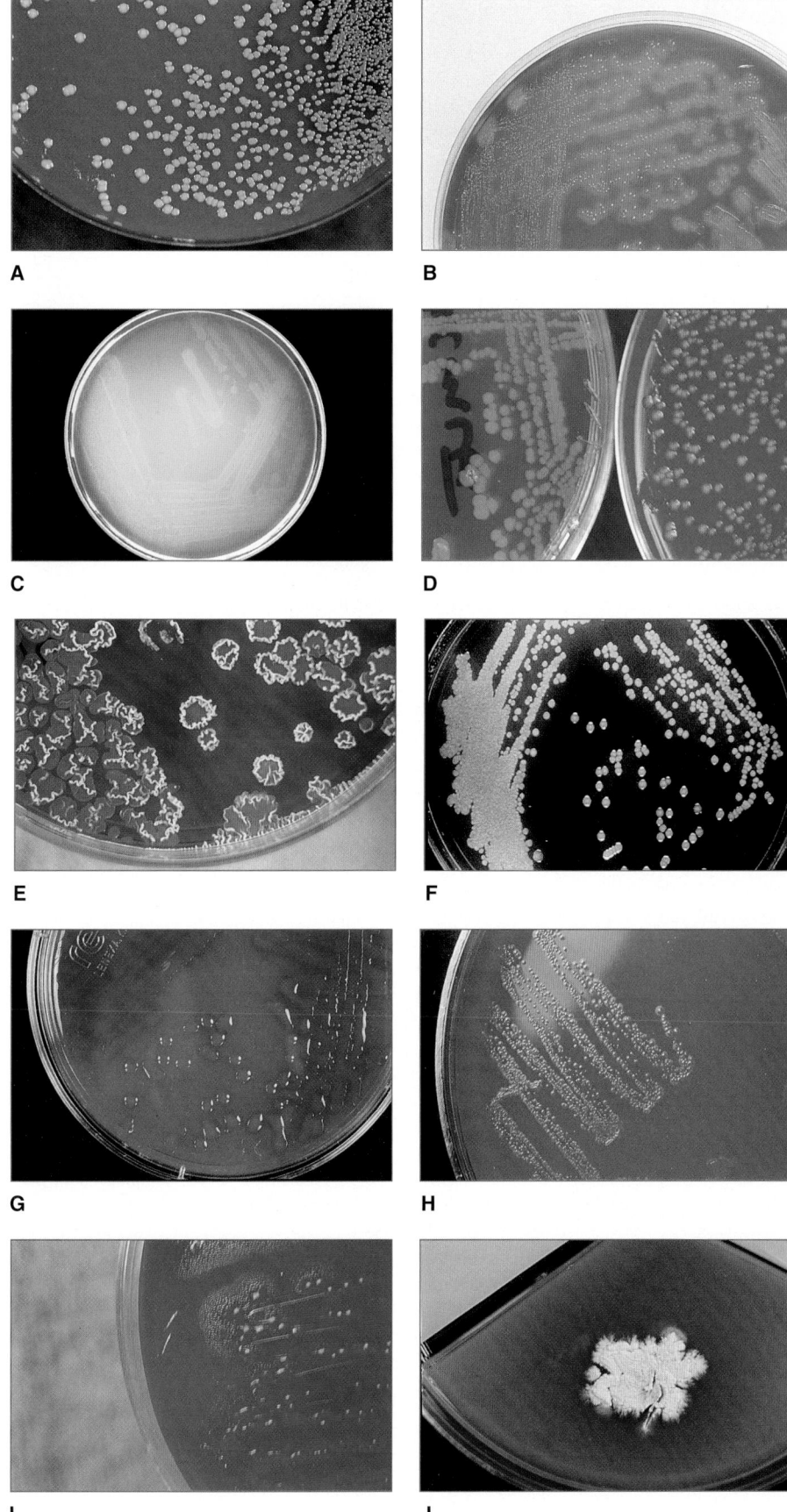

A

B

C

D

E

F

G

H

I

J

PRESUMPTIVE IDENTIFICATION OF THE *ENTEROBACTERIACEAE*

Presumptive identification of the *Enterobacteriaceae* is based on the appearance of colonies growing on primary isolation media and on an assessment of certain biochemical reactions. By definition, for an organism to be classified within the *Enterobacteriaceae*, it must ferment glucose, producing acid or acid and gas; reduce nitrates to nitrites; and exhibit no cytochrome oxidase activity.

A. A Gram stain of a sputum smear showing characteristic short, plump, gram-negative rods that are typical for members of the *Enterobacteriaceae*. Also depicted are two polymorphonuclear leukocytes, suggesting an ongoing infectious process in this patient. In this case the culture confirmed the organism to be *K. pneumoniae*.

B. Mixed culture showing 24-hour growth on blood agar of two morphotypes of large gram-negative rods and a third morphotype of a smaller organism that can be suspected to be a gram-positive species. One morphotype can be seen as large, shiny, white colonies while the other appears as large, gray colonies with irregular edges. Both of these colony types can be suspected to be gram-negative rods typical for members of the *Enterobacteriaceae*. Also present are many small, white, entire colonies typical of one of the gram-positive cocci.

C. Large, mucoid, glistening, pink colonies on MacConkey agar typical of many *Klebsiella* and *Enterobacter* species. By their appearance alone, these colonies can be suspected to be one of the species of *Enterobacteriaceae*.

D. Swarming pattern of a motile strain of *Proteus* species on chocolate agar plate.

E. Series of Kligler iron agar (KIA) slants illustrating several reaction patterns. The tube on the far left illustrates an acid (yellow) slant and acid (yellow) butt, indicating both glucose and lactose fermentation. Also note the space at the bottom of the tube and the split in the agar in the middle of the tube which indicates gas (CO_2) production by the organism. Copious amounts of CO_2, such as seen here, are usually produced only by organisms belonging to Tribe V (*Klebsielleae*). The second tube from the left shows an acid/acid reaction, but without the presence of gas, typical of the type of reaction seen with *E. coli*. The third tube from the left illustrates an alkaline (red) slant/acid butt characteristic of a non–lactose fermenter. The fourth tube illustrates a red slant/black butt, indicating hydrogen sulfide (H_2S) production. When this type of reaction is seen with an oxidase-negative organism, the assumption is made that the butt portion of the tube is acid (yellow), indicating glucose fermentation even though the yellow color is masked due to the H_2S production. The reaction in the fifth tube (*far right*) red/red is typical of nonfermenting gram-negative bacilli that ferment neither lactose nor glucose.

F. Three tubes of purple broth media containing Durham tubes to demonstrate gas formation. The two tubes on the right illustrate acid from glucose (yellow color), compared with the negative control on the left. The tube on the far right shows the collection of gas within the Durham tube, characteristic of an organism that produces both acid and gas from glucose.

G. Cytochrome oxidase test revealing a positive purple color reaction (*left*) compared with a negative reaction (*right;* no blue color within 10 seconds—see Chart 1-5). Any organism giving a positive reaction can be excluded from the family *Enterobacteriaceae*.

H. Nitrate test media containing Durham tubes to demonstrate nitrogen gas formation. The tube on the left shows a positive (red) reaction after addition of α-naphthylamine and sulfanilic acid. The test organism had reduced the nitrates in the medium to nitrites, which reacted with the reagents to form the red pigment *p*-sulfobenzene-azo-α-naphthylamine (see Chart 6-2). The tube in the middle also depicts a positive nitrate reaction, but in this case all the nitrate was first reduced to nitrite and then further reduced to nitrogen gas, indicated by the collection of gas within the Durham tube. Since there is no nitrite in the tube, there is no red color when the reagents are added. The tube on the far right shows no red color and no gas and depicts a negative test for nitrate reduction.

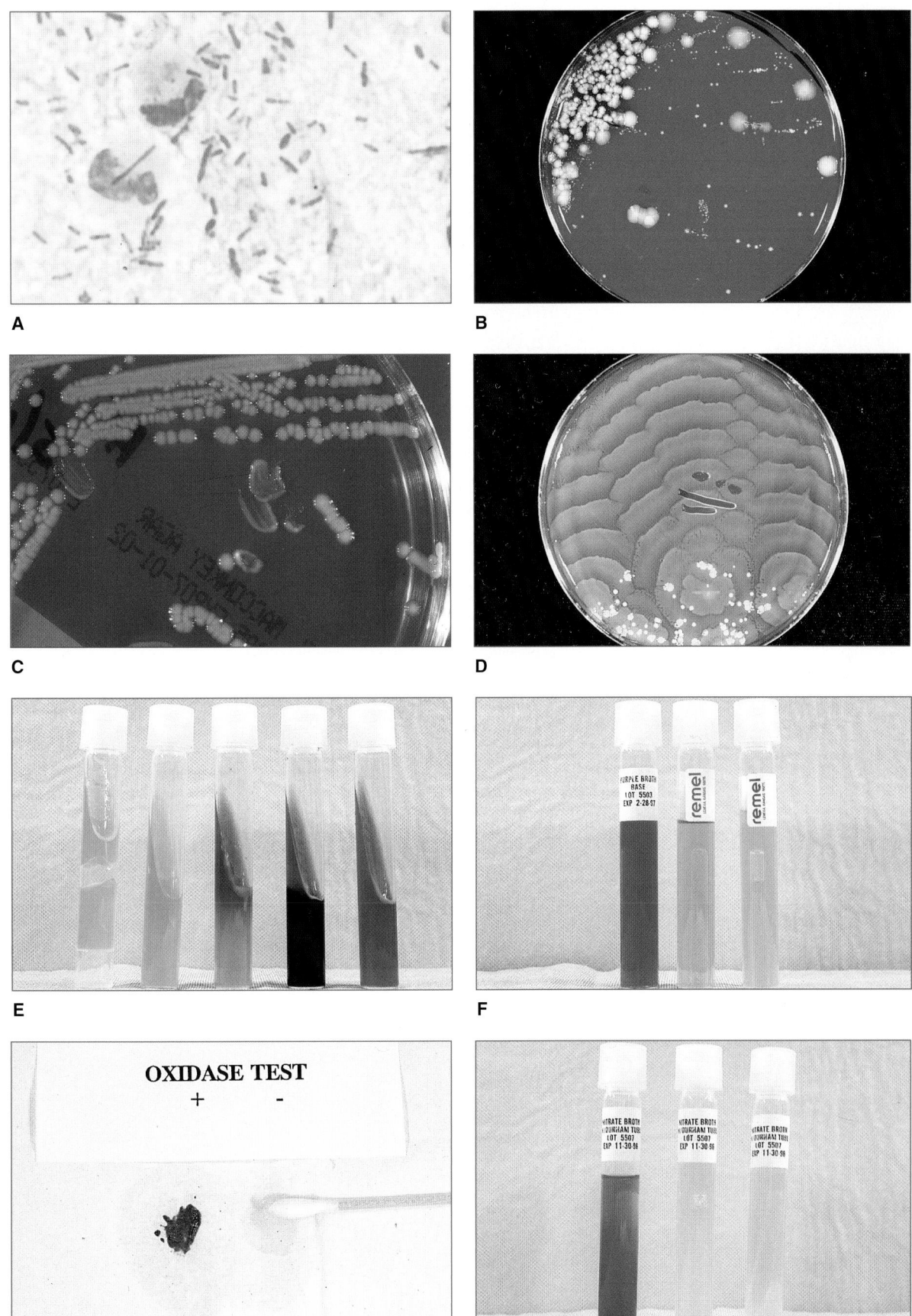

A

B

C

D

E

F

OXIDASE TEST

+   –

G

H

APPEARANCE OF THE *ENTEROBACTERIACEAE* COLONIES ON MACCONKEY AND EMB AGARS

MacConkey and eosin methylene blue (EMB) agars are two commonly used selective primary isolation media for the presumptive differentiation of lactose-fermenting from non–lactose-fermenting members of the *Enterobacteriaceae*. On MacConkey agar, lactose-fermenting colonies appear red because of the acid conversion of the indicator, neutral red. On EMB, a green metallic sheen is produced by avid lactose fermenters when the production of acid is sufficient to lower the pH to approximately 4.5 or below.

A. Surface of MacConkey agar with 24-hour growth of red, lactose-fermenting colonies. The diffuse red color in the agar surrounding the colonies is produced by organisms that avidly ferment lactose, producing large quantities of mixed acids, and cause precipitation of the bile salts in the medium surrounding the colonies (e.g., *Escherichia coli*).

B. Surface of MacConkey agar illustrating both red, lactose-fermenting colonies and smaller, clear non–lactose-fermenting colonies.

C and **D.** Surface of EMB agar plates illustrating the green sheen produced by avid lactose- (or sucrose-) fermenting members of the *Enterobacteriaceae*. Most strains of *E. coli* produce colonies with this appearance of EMB agar, and since *E. coli* is among the most frequent isolates from clinical specimens, the appearance of such colonies can often serve as presumptive identification of *E. coli*. However, characteristics other than the production of a green sheen on EMB must be assessed before an organism can be definitely identified as *E. coli*, since other lactose-fermenting *Enterobacteriaceae* can have a similar appearance.

E and **F.** Surface of EMB agar plates illustrating a mixed culture of *E. coli* (green sheen colonies) and *Shigella* species. Most *Shigella* species do not ferment lactose, and thus produce nonpigmented, semitranslucent colonies on EMB agar. Other species incapable of fermenting lactose produce colonies that appear similar to those illustrated in these photographs.

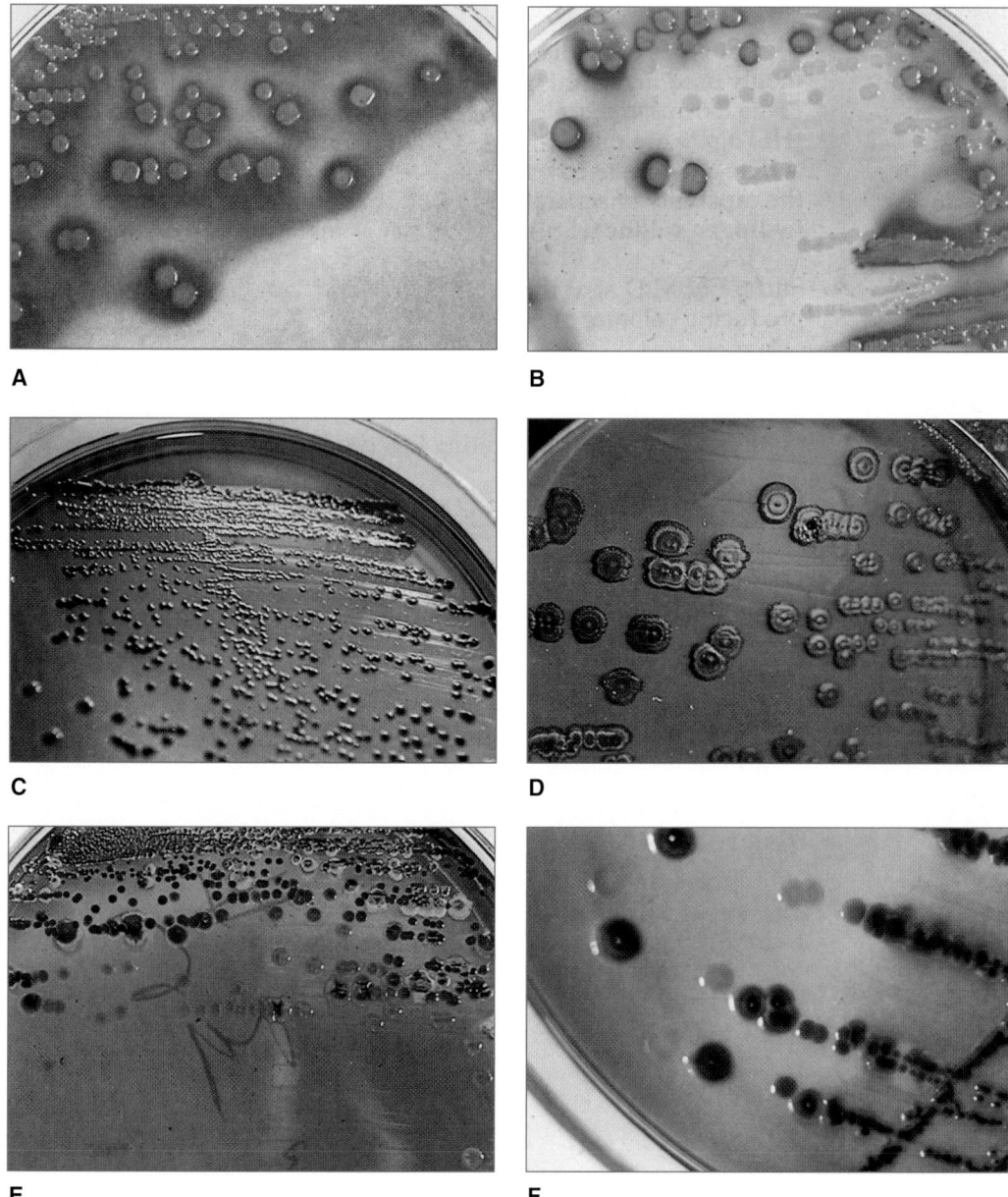

A

B

C

D

E

F

APPEARANCE OF THE *ENTEROBACTERIACEAE* ON XLD AND HE AGAR PLATES

Several types of media more selective than MacConkey or EMB agars are commonly used in clinical microbiology laboratories for recovering select members of the *Enterobacteriaceae*. Xylose-lysine-deoxycholate (XLD) and Hektoen enteric (HE) agars are most commonly used; highly selective media such as bismuth sulfate agar are used only for special applications. These media not only have the capability of separating lactose fermenters from non–lactose fermenters but can detect hydrogen sulfide (H_2S)-producing microorganisms as well.

A. Surface of XLD agar illustrating yellow conversion of the medium from acid-producing colonies of *E. coli*.

B. Non–lactose-fermenting colonies (no acid conversion of the medium) of *Salmonella* species growing on the surface of XLD agar. Note the black pigmentation of some of the colonies, indicating H_2S production.

C. Photograph illustrating an XLD agar plate inoculated with a 50/50 mixture of *E. coli* and *Salmonella* species. Note the preponderant growth of the *Salmonella* species (red colonies) compared with the few yellow, lactose-fermenting colonies of *E. coli* that have been effectively inhibited. The distinct pink halo around the *Salmonella* colonies indicates the decarboxylation of lysine, a helpful feature in differentiating *Salmonella* species (positive) from H_2S-producing colonies of *Proteus* species.

D. XLD agar plate inoculated with an H_2S-producing strain of a *Proteus* species. Note the lack of a light pink halo around the colonies, indicating the lack of lysine decarboxylation (compare with the colonies shown in panel **C**).

E. Surface of HE agar illustrating yellow acid production by colonies of *E. coli*.

F. Surface of HE agar illustrating the faint green (colorless) colonies of non–lactose-fermenting members of the *Enterobacteriaceae*.

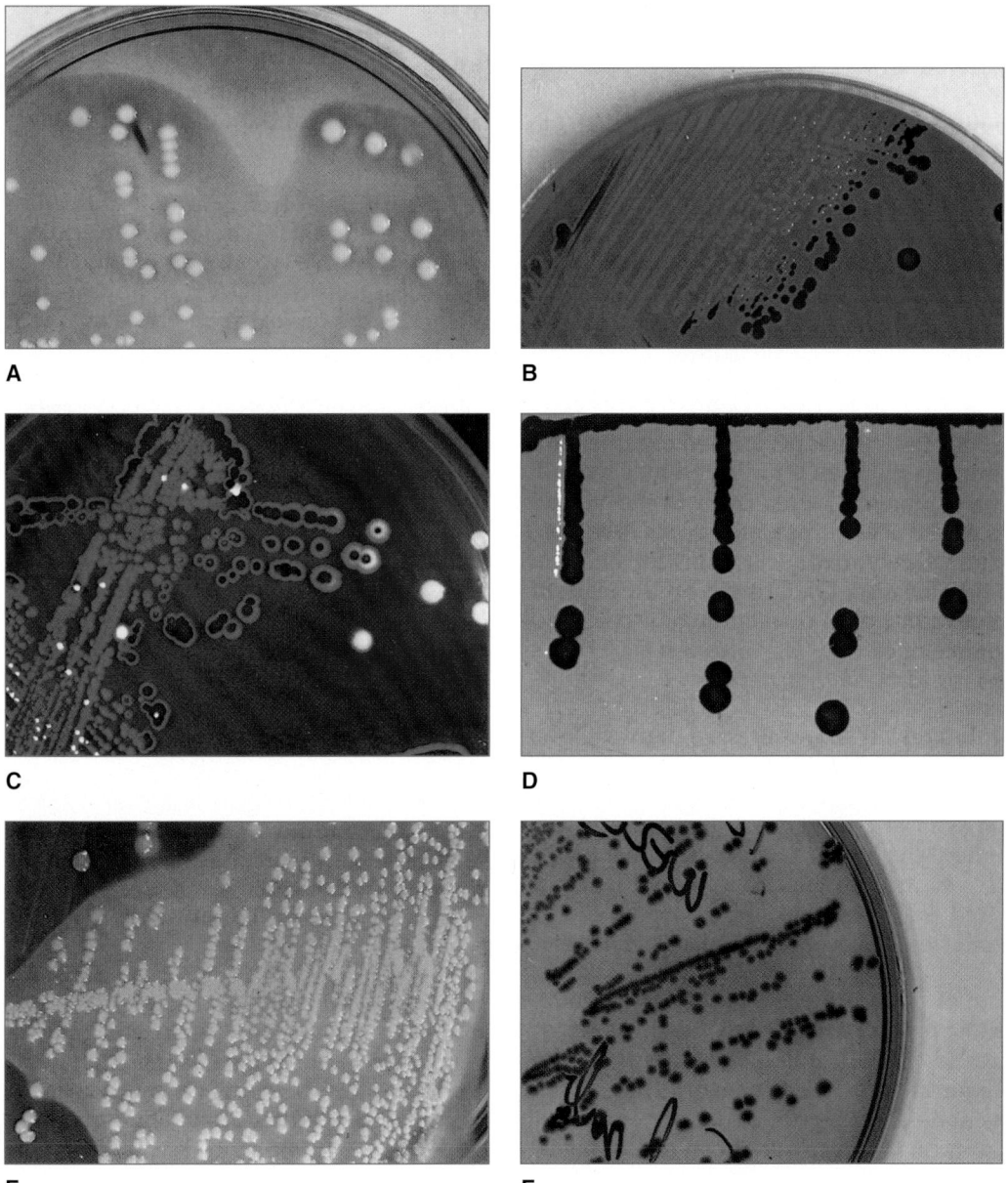

A

B

C

D

E

F

DIFFERENTIAL CHARACTERISTICS OF THE *ENTEROBACTERIACEAE*

A. *Ortho*-nitrophenyl-β-D-galactopyranoside (ONPG) test showing a positive (yellow) reaction (*left*) compared with the negative control (*right*). A positive reaction indicates that the organism is capable of producing β-galactosidase, an enzyme required for the initial degradation of lactose, releasing the yellow-colored *ortho*-nitrophenol.

B. Sulfide indole motility (SIM) semisolid agar tube (*right*) and Kligler iron agar (KIA) slant (*left*), illustrating the differences in sensitivity in detecting hydrogen sulfide (H_2S) by different media. The diffuse delicate blackening in the SIM tube is produced by a motile, weak H_2S-producing organism (in this case *S. typhi*). Note that the H_2S produced in the less sensitive KIA tube appears only in the middle of the tube at the interface of the slant and butt and is the typical appearance of *S. typhi* in this medium.

C and **D.** Four tubes demonstrating the indole (I), methyl red (MR), Voges-Proskauer (VP), and citrate (C) tests. These four tests when performed together constitute the classic IMViC reactions. The formation of indole from tryptophan is indicated by a red color on the addition of Kovac's reagent (*far left tube,* panel **C**). The development of a red color in the MR tube indicates a drop in pH to 4.4 or below, indicative of strong mixed acid fermenters (*second tube from left,* panel **C**). A red color in the VP tube indicates the presence of acetoin (acetylmethylcarbinol) formed from pyruvate in the butylenes glycol metabolic pathway (*third tube from left,* panel **D**). Growth on the slant of Simmon's citrate agar and conversion of the bromthymol blue indicator to an alkaline blue color indicates that the organism can utilize sodium citrate as the sole source of carbon (*rightmost tube,* panel **D**). C shows the reactions for *E. coli* (+ + − −). Panel **D** shows the reactions for *Klebsiella/Enterobacter* (− − + +).

E. The two tubes on the left show negative (light yellow) and positive (dark green) phenylalinine deaminase reactions. The green color is produced by the reaction between the $FeCl_3$ reagent and phenylpyruvic acid in the medium, resulting from the deamination of phenylalinine (see Chart 6-8). The three tubes on the right are Christensen's urea agar slants. The third from the right shows a strong positive reaction (red color throughout the medium, indicating an alkaline reaction from the degradation of urea), compared with the negative control on the far right (yellow color throughout). The reaction in the second tube from the right (red color in slant only) is produced by organisms such as *Klebsiella* species and certain *Enterobacter* species that are weak urease producers.

F. Four tubes containing Møller decarboxylase medium covered with a layer of mineral oil to effect an anaerobic environment (see Chart 6-7). *From left to right:* A growth control tube devoid of the amino acids (growth is indicated by conversion to a yellow color due to the fermentation of glucose in the medium), arginine, lysine, and ornithine. The bromcresol purple indicator is yellow at an acid pH and purple at an alkaline pH. Thus, any tube that appears purple indicates an alkaline pH, the reaction produced by organisms that can decarboxylate the amino acid contained in the medium. The organism pictured here is arginine-negative and lysine- and ornithine-positive and is the typical reaction seen with *E. aerogenes.*

G. Lysine iron agar (LIA) is used to differentiate enteric organisms based on their ability to decarboxylate or deaminate lysine and to form H_2S. Organisms that decarboxylate lysine produce an alkaline (purple) reaction in the butt of the tube (*middle tube*). Organisms that deaminate lysine produce a red slant over an acid (yellow) butt (*leftmost tube*). Bacteria that produce H_2S cause blackening of the medium mainly in the middle and the butt of the tube (*also seen in tube on far left*). The tube on the far left is lysine deaminase positive and lysine decarboxylase negative. The middle tube is lysine deaminase–negative and lysine decarboxylase–positive. The tube on the far right is negative for both lysine deaminase and lysine decarboxylase. (Butt reddish but not yellow.)

H. Tubes of motility medium. Motile organisms will show diffuse growth away from the line of inoculation (*left tube*); nonmotile organisms show growth only along the stab line (*right tube*). Also available is motility medium to which 2,3,5-triphenyltetrazolium chloride (TTC) is added. Growth of organisms capable of reducing TTC will appear red along the stab line as well as in the area into which the cells have migrated, making it easier to differentiate between motile and nonmotile bacteria (see Color Plate 7.1*E*). (Photo courtesy of Health and Education Resources, Bethesda, MD.)

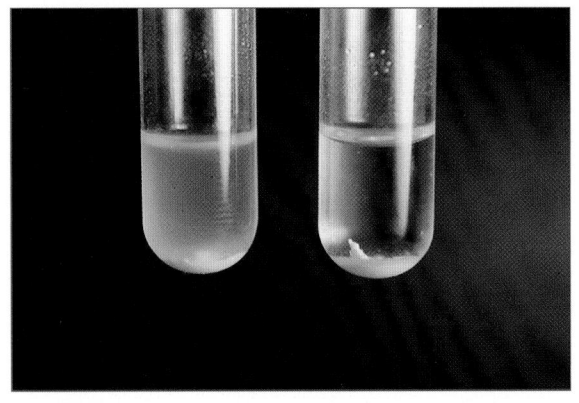

A

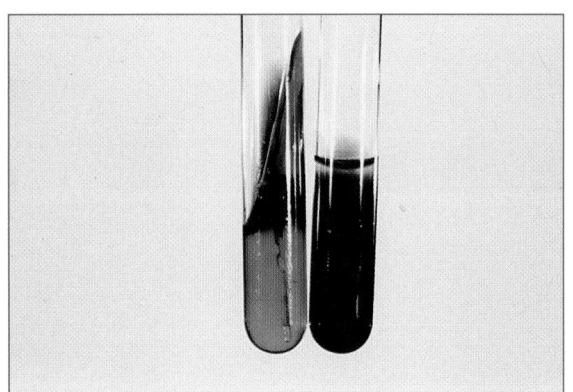

B

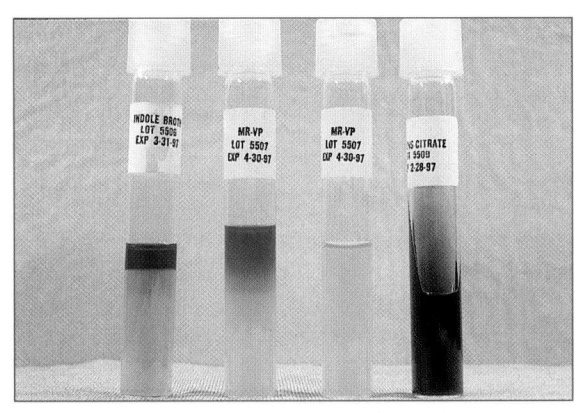

C

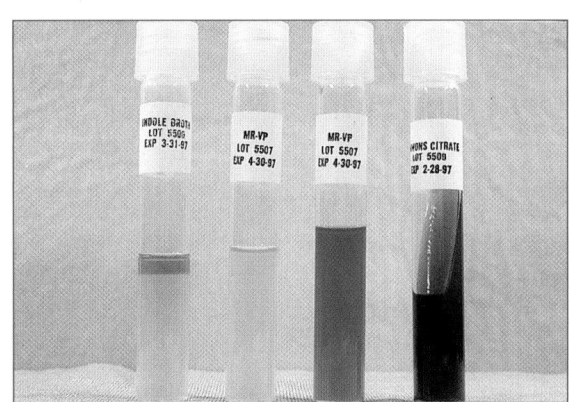

D

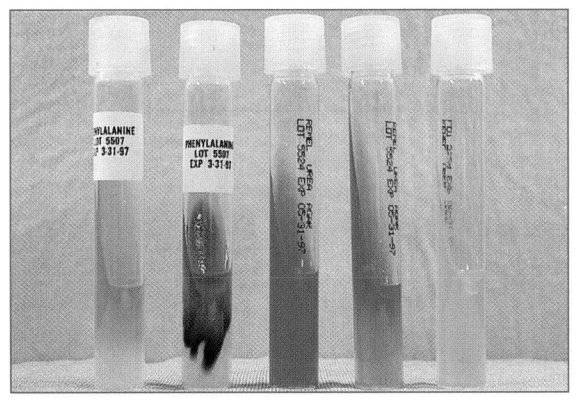

E

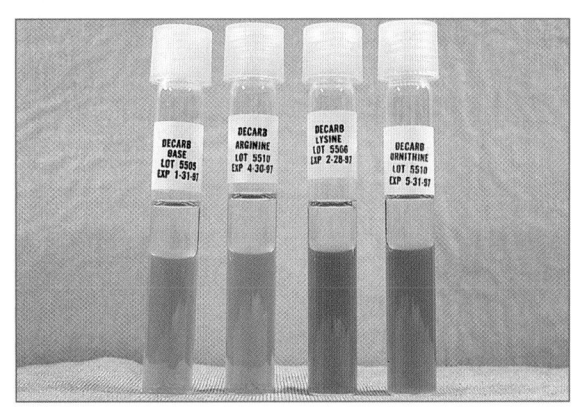

F

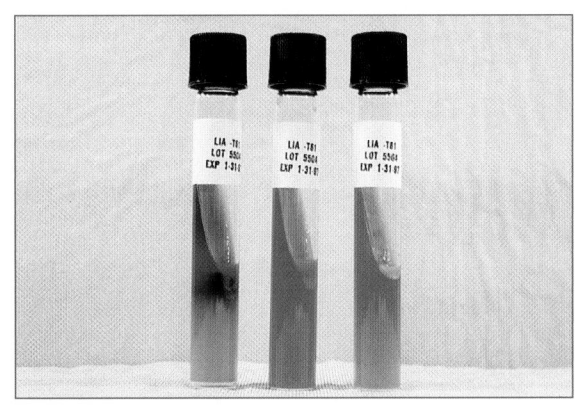

G

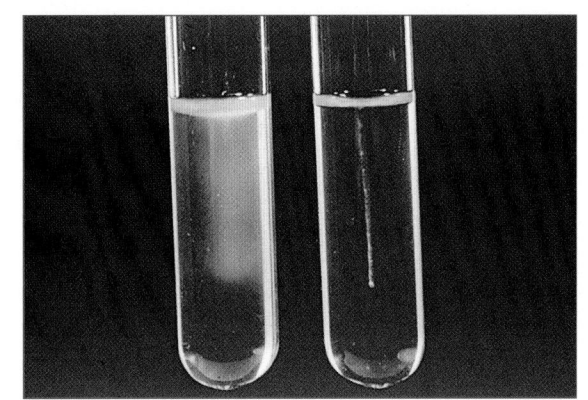

H

HUMAN PLAGUE

A. Hematogenous dissemination of *Y. pestis* from the portal of entry to other organs and tissues may cause intravascular coagulation and endotoxic shock, producing small hemorrhages on the skin. (CDC, Public Health Image Library)

B. Gram stain of *Y. pestis* showing short, plump, gram-negative rods with biopolar staining. Organisms appear pink at the polar ends with a white area or non-staining in the center.

C. Peripheral blood smear stained with Wright's stain showing "safety pin" appearance of *Y. pestis*. Bacteria stain dark blue, leukocytes stain light blue with purple-staining nuclei, erythrocytes stain light tan. (CDC, Public Health Image Library)

D. Colonies of *Y. pestis* growing on a blood agar plate at 72 hrs. *Yersinia pestis* grows well on most standard laboratory media, after 48–72 hours, showing grey-white to slightly yellow opaque raised, irregular "fried egg" morphology; alternatively colonies may have a "hammered copper" shiny surface. (CDC, Public Health Image Library)

CHROMOGENIC AGAR

E. BBL™ CHROMagar™ O157 is designed for use as a primary plate for stool cultures when screening for *E. coli* O157. Distinguishes *E. coli* O157 (mauve colonies) from *E. coli* non-O157 (blue colonies). Also inhibits most *Proteus*, *Pseudomonas* and *Aeromonas* strains using selective agents. (Courtesy of BD Diagnostic Systems.)

F and **G.** BBL™ CHROMagar™ Orientation medium is a non-selective, differential medium for presumptively identifying bacterial isolates from primary clinical specimens. Allows isolation and presumptive identification of both gram-positive and gram-negative pathogens with a single plate. Useful for identification and enumeration of urinary tract pathogens. Identifies *E. coli* (pink colonies) and *Enterococcus* (blue or turquoise colonies, small) from primary plate. Frame F shows Orientation agar with a pure culture of *E. coli*. Frame G shows a mixed culture of *E. coli* and *Enterococcus* together with some colonies of *Proteus* spp. (beige with brown halo) (Courtesy of BD Diagnostic Systems.)

H. BBL™ CHROMagar™ Salmonella is designed for use in *Salmonella* screening of either clinical or industrial samples. Detects *Salmonella* with a highly specific chromogenic reaction (purple colonies with purple halo), while minimizing interference from other hydrogen sulfide-producing colonies such as *Proteus* and *Citrobacter* spp. (Courtesy of BD Diagnostic Systems.)

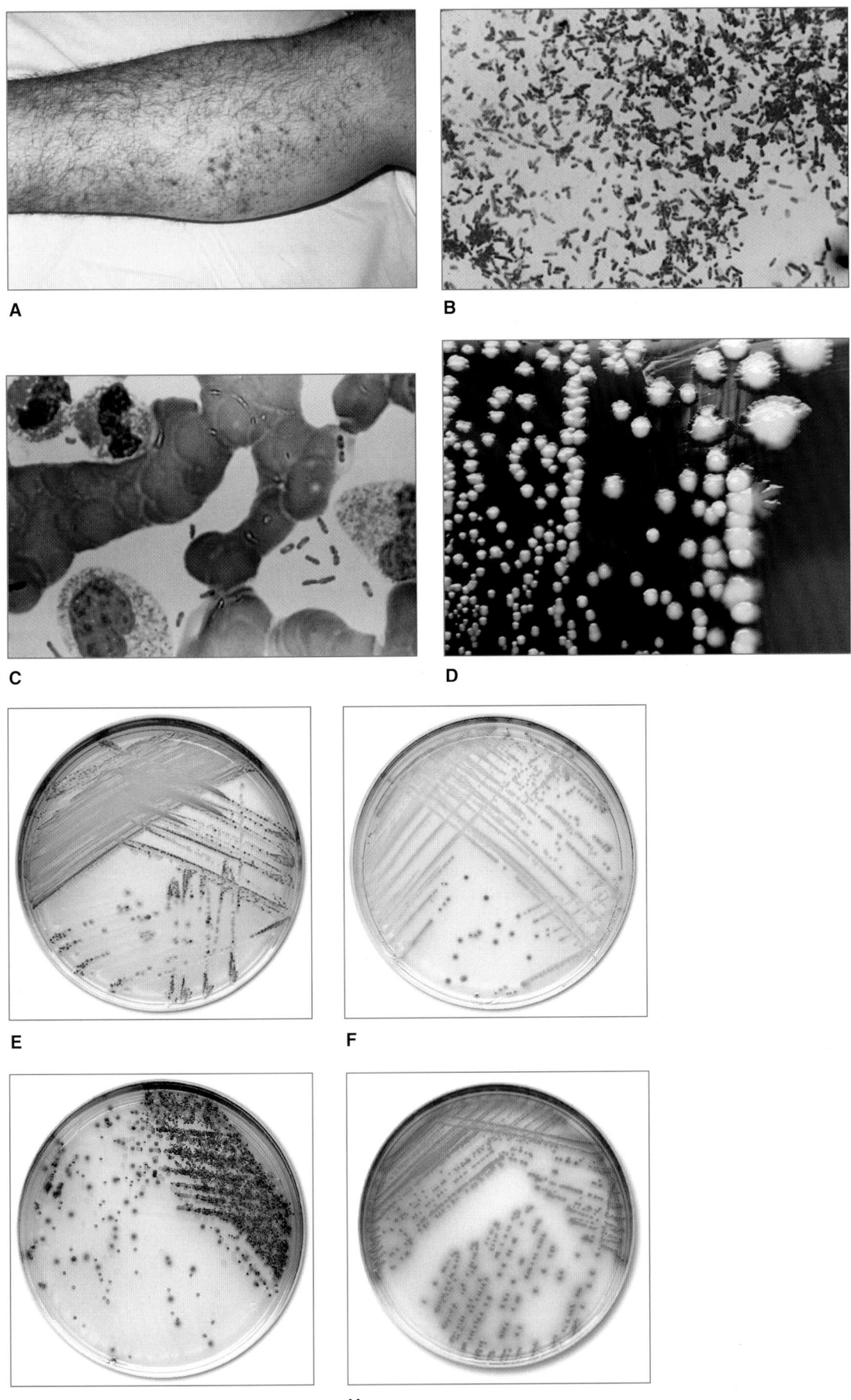

A

B

C

D

E

F

G

H

COMMERCIAL IDENTIFICATION SYSTEMS

A number of commercially manufactured identification systems are currently available that contain stable reagents and media designed for determining biochemical characteristics. These products range from those that are inoculated and reading manually to those that are fully automated.

A. API 20E strips illustrating method of inoculation and the appearance of a strip following inoculation and incubation. A suspension of the organism to be tested is transferred with a pipette into each of the 20 media compartments. Color reactions are read after 18 to 24 hours of incubation at 35°C. The manufacturer supplies worksheets for recording the visual interpretation of the color reactions, which are then converted into a seven-digit biotype number.

B. The BBL Crystal Enteric/Nonfermenter identification system contains a lid with 30 dehydrated substrates on the tips of the plastic prongs. A test suspension is prepared and added to all 30 wells in the base unit. The lid is then aligned with the base and snapped in place, whereby the test inoculum rehydrates the dried substrates and initiates test reactions. After incubation, panels are read upside-down using the BBL Crystal light box. The wells are examined for color changes and a 10-digit profile number is generated and entered on a personal computer in which the BBL Crystal Electronic codebook has been installed, to obtain the identification.

C. The REMEL RapID ONE (Oxidase Negative Enterobacteriaceae) panel has 19 substrates for identification of over 70 organisms belonging to the family Enterobacteriaceae. The system consists of a plastic tray with 18 reaction cavities. Reaction cavities contain dehydrated reactants, and the tray allows the simultaneous inoculation of each cavity with a predetermined amount of inoculum. Test 18 is bifunctional, containing two separate tests in the same cavity. Each test is interpreted visually for color changes after 4 hours of incubation at 35°C. The 19 test results plus oxidase are scored in the appropriate boxes of the report form and a seven-digit profile code is generated similar to that shown in A. The biocode number is entered on a PC in which the ERIC (Electronic RapID Compendium) has been installed, to obtain the identification.

D. Biolog GN Microplate system consisting of a 96-well microtiter plate containing 95 carbon substrates and a redox indicator-tetrazolium dye. If a carbon substrate is utilized by the inoculated bacteria, the colorless dye is irreversibly reduced and forms a purple color. With the use of a computer screen, purple wells are coded as positive and colorless wells are coded as negative. The computer then matches the "metabolic fingerprint" of the inoculated organism with those in the database and generates the most likely identification.

E and **F.** In the MicroScan gram-negative ID panel, the microtiter wells are inoculated with a heavy suspension of the organism to be identified and incubated at 35°C for 15 to 18 hours. The panels can be interpreted visually (Frame E), after which the biochemical results are converted into a seven- or eight-digit biotype number that is looked up in a codebook that is supplied by the manufacturer. An automated tray reader, autoSCAN®-4 System, can also be used along with the LabPro information manager. Some trays also include antibiotics for performing both microdilution susceptibility testing and bacterial identification in the same panel. The same panels can also be used with the fully automated WalkAway® System. (Frame F) The instrument processes both rapid and conventional overnight panels on one system and is available in both 40 and 96 panel capacity models. (Courtesy of Dade Behring.)

G. The VITEK®2 is a new system from bioMérieux that performs bacterial identification and susceptibility testing analyses using a standardized inoculum. The VITEK 2 features the AES (Advanced Expert System) that integrates artificial intelligence technologies in the VITEK 2 instrument. AES interprets the results of the antibiotic susceptibility test using a highly developed knowledge database. This base contains most of the known resistance mechanisms (approximately 2,000 phenotypes, 20,000 MIC distributions). (Courtesy of bioMérieux.)

H. The BD PHOENIX™ Automated Microbiology System for Identification and Susceptibility Testing offers fully automated ID and susceptibility testing with no off-line tests, handwritten labels or reagent additions required. The sealed test panel never moves once placed inside, so it can't dislodge, jam, crack or leak while in the instrument. The PHOENIX comes with integrated software combined with the BD EpiCenter™ (Courtesy of BD Diagnostic Systems.)

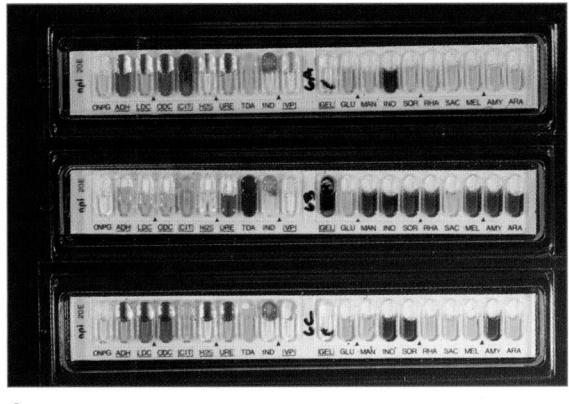

A

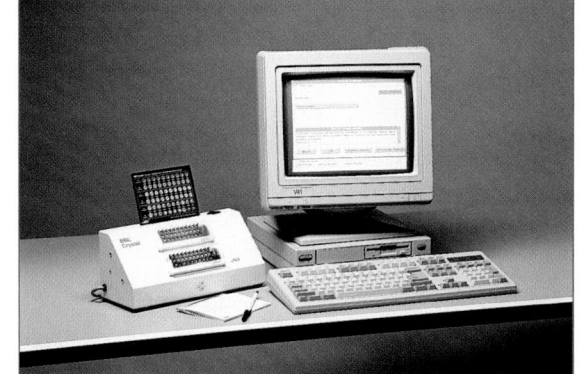

B

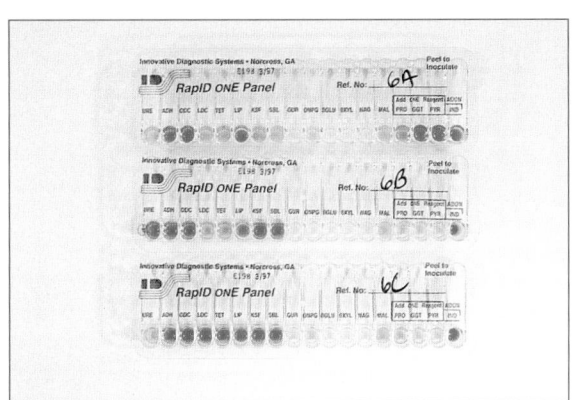

C

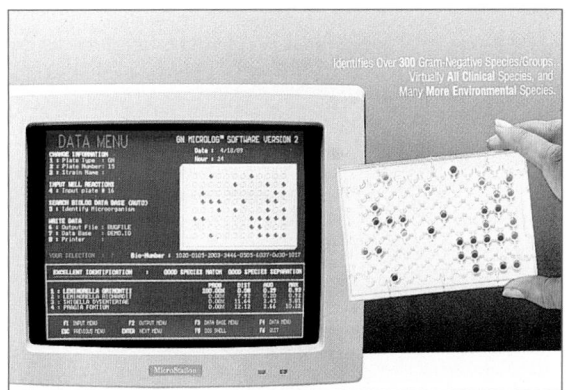

D

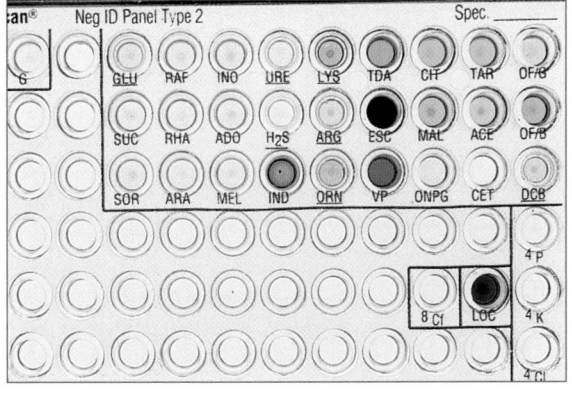

E

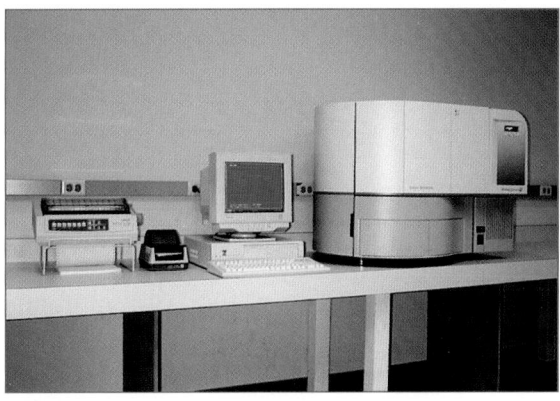

F

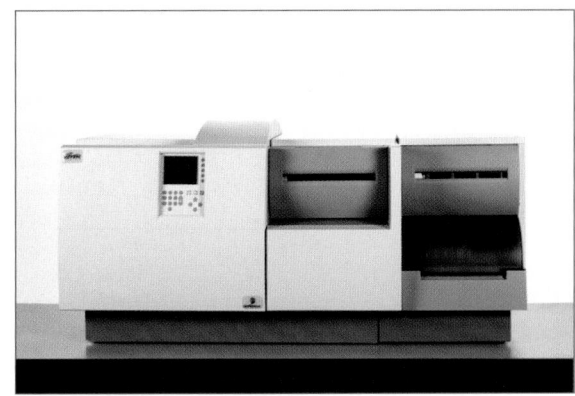

G

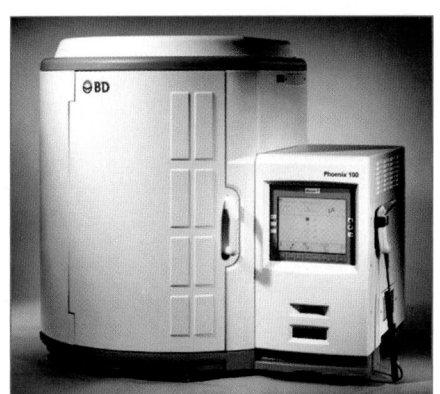

H

IMPORTANT CHARACTERISTICS FOR DISTINGUISHING NONFERMENTATIVE GRAM-NEGATIVE BACILLI

A. Detection of fermentation. The Kligler's Iron agar (KIA) tube on the right shows an alkaline slant/alkaline butt reaction characteristic of a nonfermenting organism; the tube on the left shows an alkaline slant/acid deep reaction indicating fermentation of dextrose but non-fermentation of lactose (characteristics of lactose-negative species of the *Enterobacteriaceae*). No acid production in KIA or in triple sugar iron (TSI) agar indicates the inability of nonfermenting bacteria to utilize the lactose or dextrose in KIA (or the lactose, dextrose or sucrose in TSI).

B. Cytochrome oxidase test. The formation of a blue color within 10 seconds after smearing a test colony on filter paper saturated with the oxidase reagent (tetramethyl-*p*-phenylenediamine dihydrochloride) indicates cytochrome oxidase activity, a characteristic helpful in identifying many species of nonfermenters. All members of the *Enterobacteriaceae* are cytochrome oxidase--negative.

C. Failure to grow on MacConkey agar or inhibited growth on MacConkey agar is a clue that a gram-negative rod may be a nonfermenter. Although many species of nonfermenters are capable of growing on MacConkey agar, the lack of growth on this medium, as illustrated on the right side of this split frame, excludes the *Enterobacteriaceae*, all members of which grow well on MacConkey (*left side*).

D. Oxidative utilization of glucose. Illustrated here are two tubes of Hugh-Leifson oxidative-fermentative (OF) medium. The tube on the right is open to the atmosphere, whereas the tube on the left is covered with mineral oil to exclude exposure to atmospheric oxygen. Acid (yellow color) is seen only in the top portion of the open tube, indicating that the organism is capable of oxidizing glucose but incapable of fermenting glucose.

E. Tubes of Motility B medium containing 2,3,5-triphenyltetrazolium chloride (TTC). Motility is often difficult to observe with nonfermentative bacteria since the organisms tend to grow only in the upper (most aerobic) portion of the tube. The addition of tetrazolium aids in detecting motility because organisms capable of reducing TTC will appear red along the stab line as well as in the area into which the cells have migrated, making it easier to differentiate between motile (*left*) and non-motile (*right*) bacteria.

F. Blood agar plate inoculated with a yellow pigment-producing bacterium. Pigment production is an important differential characteristic in identifying nonfermenative gram-negative bacilli. The organism depicted here is *Sphingomonas paucimobilis*.

G. Tubes of Flo and Tech agar inoculated with *Pseudomonas aeruginosa* viewed under visible light. These media are used to enhance the production of two pigments: pyoverdin (fluorescein), which appears as a yellow diffusible pigment on Flo agar (*left*) in visible light, and pyocyanin, which appears as a turquoise-blue pigment on Tech agar (*right*) in visible light. Although three species of nonfermenting bacilli produce pyoverdin (*P. aeruginosa*, *P. fluorescens*, and *P. putida*), only one species (*P. aeruginosa*) produces pyocyanin.

H. Tubes of Flo and Tech agar inoculated with *Pseudomonas aeruginosa* viewed under ultraviolet (UV) light using a Wood's lamp. Note that the Flo agar tube (*on the left*) fluoresces, while the Tech agar tube (*on the right*) does not fluoresce under UV light. Only pyoverdin pigment, which is enhanced by growing the organism on Flo agar, fluoresces under UV light.

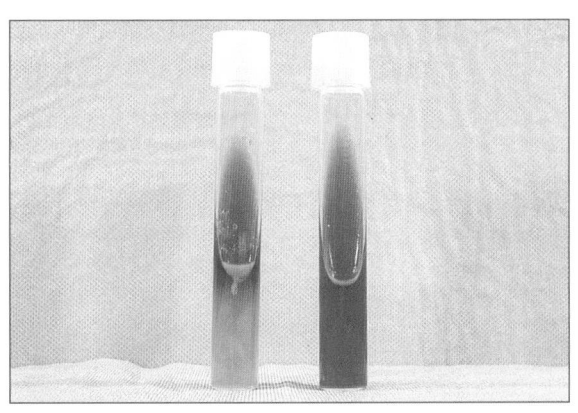

A

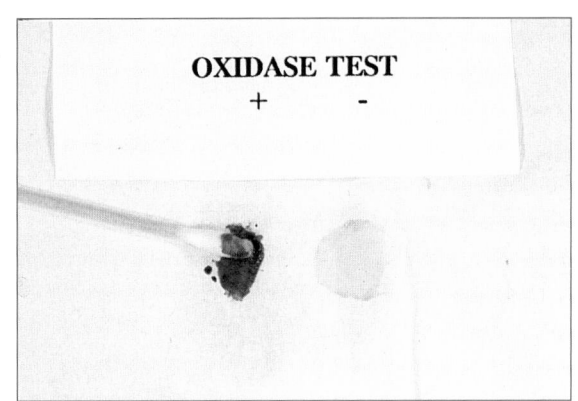

OXIDASE TEST

\+ –

B

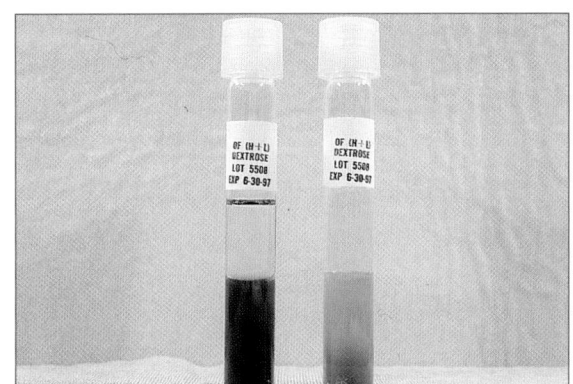

1 2

C

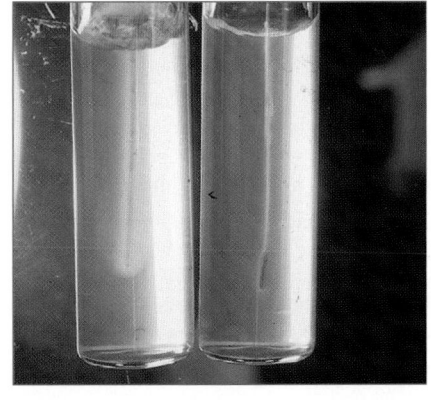

OF (H+L) DEXTROSE LOT 5508 EXP 6-30-97 OF (H+L) DEXTROSE LOT 5508 EXP 6-30-97

D

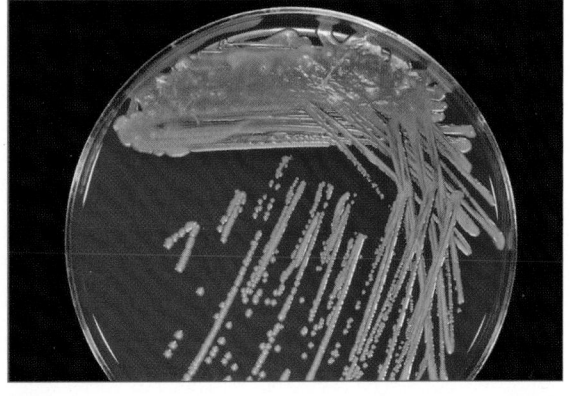

E

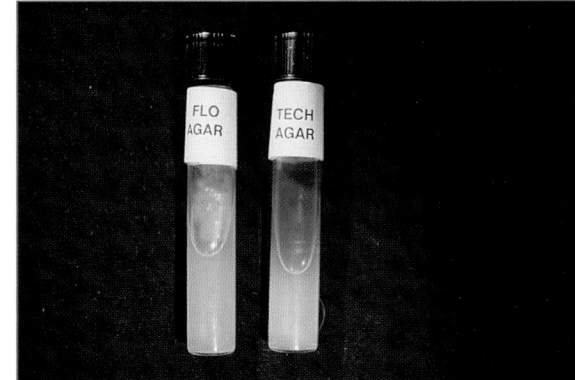

F

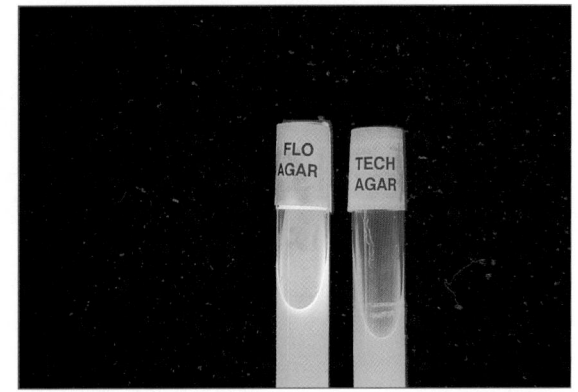

FLO AGAR TECH AGAR

G

FLO AGAR TECH AGAR

H

TESTS USED IN THE IDENTIFICATION OF NONFERMENTATIVE GRAM-NEGATIVE BACILLI

A. Two tubes of Christensen's urea illustrating the fuchsia red color of a positive test (*right*) compared with a negative control (*left*). A rapid positive urease reaction (<4 hr) is seen with the following species of nonfermentative bacilli: *Bergeyella zoohelcum*, *Bordetella bronchiseptica*, *Cupriavidus pauculus*, and *Oligella ureolytica*.

B. Two tubes demonstrating nitrate reduction (*left*) and nitrite reduction (*right*). Both tubes contain a Durham tube to demonstrate nitrogen gas formation. The tube on the left depicts the reduction of nitrate to nitrogen gas and the tube on the right demonstrates the reduction of nitrite to nitrogen gas. Note that there is more gas formed in the tube on the right indicating that quantitatively more nitrogen gas is formed from nitrite than nitrate during the same incubation period. Production of gas from both nitrate and nitrate is typical of the *Pseudomonas stutzeri* group and *Alcaligenes denitrificans*.

C. Three tubes of Heart Infusion broth showing a positive indole reaction (*left*), an orange indole reaction (*center*), and a negative indole reaction (*right*). The reactions shown here were obtained using the xylene extraction method followed by the addition of Ehrlich's reagent (see Chart 1-4). A positive indole reaction is noted by the appearance of a red band at the interface of the tryptophane broth and the xylene layer. The indole positive nonfermentative bacilli include: *Balneatrix*, *Bergeyella*, *Chryseobacterium*, *Empedobacter*, *Weeksella* and some unnamed CDC groups. A peculiar orange indole reaction (*center tube*) is observed with *Delftia acidovorans* and is due to the formation of anthranilic acid from tryptophane by this bacterium. An orange pigment is produce upon the addition of either Ehrlich's of Kovac's reagent. The reaction may take over 1 hour to develop following the addition of reagents.

D. Four tubes of Møller decarboxylase medium covered with a layer of mineral oil. Reading from left to right: lysine, arginine, ornithine, and control tube devoid of amino acid. With the nonfermentative bacilli, negative tests remain the same color as the original uninoculated tubes, while positive decarboxylation reactions appear darker purple owing to the formation of alkaline amines causing a more alkaline ph in the tube. The positive lysine decarboxylase reaction illustrated here occurs with only two species of nonfermenting bacilli: *Stenotrophomonas maltophilia* and *Burkholderia cepacia* complex.

E. Split frame showing two tubes of esculin agar viewed under visible light (*on the left*), and the same two tubes viewed under ultraviolet light from a Wood's lamp (*on the right*). When esculin is hydrolyzed by a microorganism, the glycoside esculin is converted to esculetin and glucose. The esculetin reacts with an iron salt (ferric citrate) in the medium to form a dark brown of black complex (*second tube from left*). The production of a dark brown of black pigment may be difficult to discern if the organism itself produces a brown or deep-colored pigment. Since esculin is a fluorescent compound, true esculin hydrolysis can be determined by observing for the absence of fluorescence. The brightly fluorescing tube in the right frame (*second tube from the far right*) depicts the reaction observed with a negative esculin reaction. The tube on the far right shows marked squelching of fluorescence, particularly in the slant, indicating that the test organism is capable of hydrolyzing esculin.

F. Blood agar plate demonstrating the typical appearance of *Pseudomonas aeruginosa* after 24 hr incubation at 35°C. Colonies are large with a spreading periphery and are frequently beta hemolytic. Colonies in the heaviest area of growth appear to have a metallic sheen and a scaling appearance sometimes describe as alligator skin morphology. Colonies appearing like this typically produce a sweet grape-like odor.

G. MacConkey agar plate demonstrating growth of two colony types. The dark purple colonies are lactose-positive and have the typical appearance of *E. coli*. The lactose-negative colonies are producing a turquoise-blue diffusible pigment noted best in the area of heaviest growth. This is the typical appearance of colonies of *Pseudomonas aeruginosa* that are producing pyocyanin.

H. MacConkey agar plate demonstrating growth of a mucoid variety of *Pseudomonas aeruginosa* typical of the strains isolated from the sputum of patients with cystic fibrosis. Colonies can be extremely mucoid and runny. Note that several colony variants can be seen which is the typical presentation for these mucoid variants of *P. aeruginosa*. Note that in the heaviest growth area there appears to be some pyocyanin pigment developing.

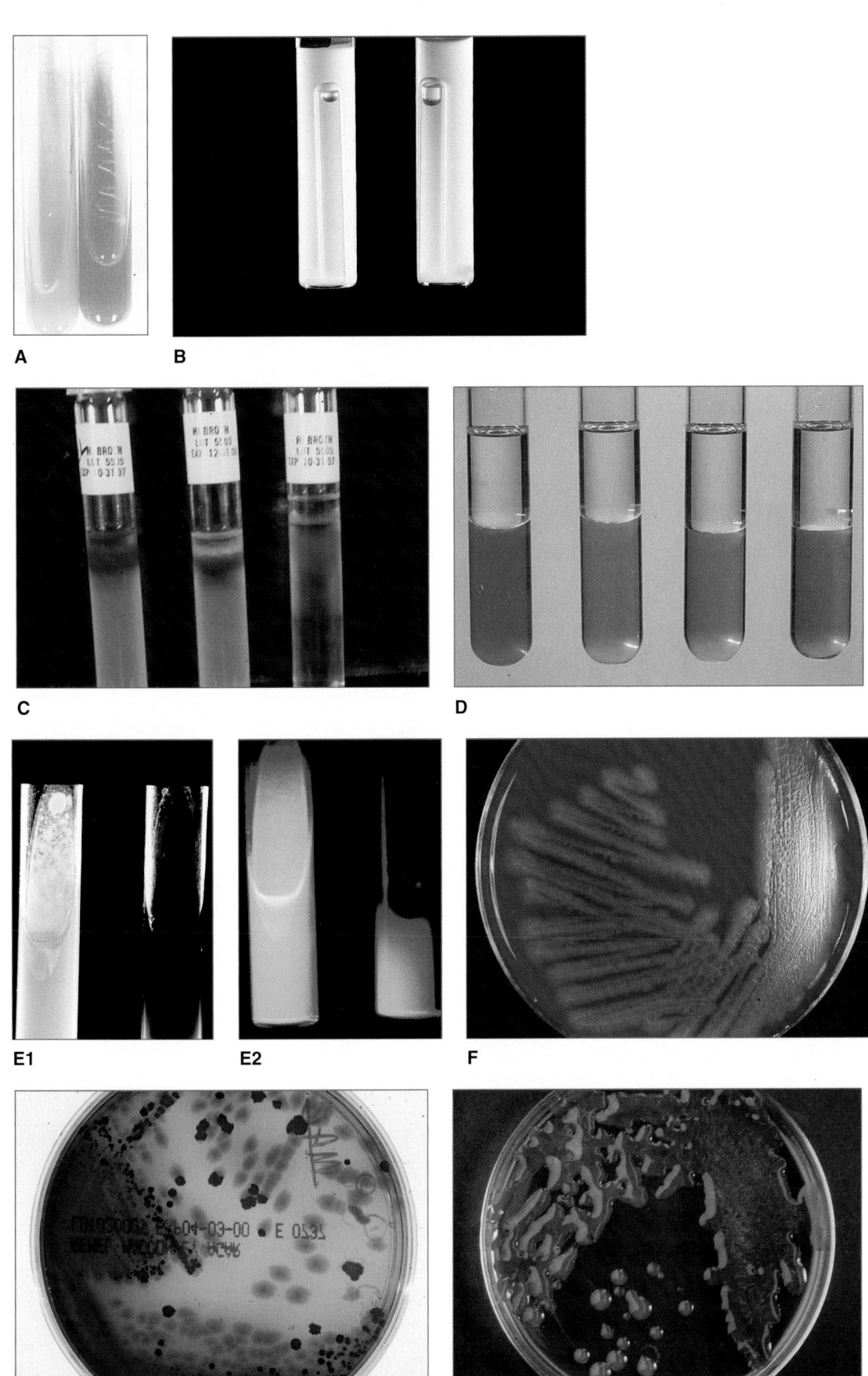

A

B

C

D

E1

E2

F

G

H

COLONIAL AND MICROSCOPIC MORPHOLOGY OF CERTAIN NONFERMENTATIVE BACILLI

Some species of nonfermentative gram-negative bacilli have characteristic features that can be observed on growth media or in Gram-stained preparations. An awareness of these functions can be an aid in making a correct species identification.

A. *Pseudomonas stutzeri* on blood agar medium. Note the characteristic dry, wrinkled colonies that are typical of this species. One should immediately think of *P. stutzeri* when an oxidase-positive, nonfermenting bacillus produces this type of colony on blood agar.

B. Blood agar plate showing the yellow, dry and wrinkled appearance of *Pseudomonas luteola*. Colonies are often adherent to the agar and difficult to remove. Colonial morphology resembles that of *Pseudomonas oryzihabitans* and *Pseudomonas stutzeri*. Both *P. luteola* and *P. oryzihabitans* are oxidase negative, while, *P. stutzeri* is oxidase-positive.

C. MacConkey agar (*left*) and BAP (*right*) inoculated with a pure culture of *Brevundimonas vesicularis*. Note that this organism fails to grow on MacConkey agar and appears as deeply yellow-colored, slightly wrinkled colonies on BAP. This organism is also sensitive to vancomycin and resistant to polymyxin B, additional features that can help in identification.

D. Blood agar plate illustrating growth of *Stenotrophomonas maltophilia*. The dull yellow pigment is distinctive for this species but at times may be difficult to visualize. Colonies may also appear dark tan to lavender upon continued incubation, particularly if left at room temperature.

E. *Methylobacterium* species growing on Sabouraud dextrose agar. Colonies appear dry and exhibit a deep pink or coral pigmentation. These colonies absorb ultraviolet light and appear dark when held under a Wood's lamp.

F. Gram stain of Methylobacterium species showing characteristic gram-negative bacilli containing vacuoles.

G. Gram stain of *Roseomonas* species showing characteristic faint-staining, gram-negative coccoid forms, some containing vacuoles.

H. *Roseomonas* species growing on Sabouraud dextrose agar. They appear as light pink, mucoid, almost runny colonies. Like *Methylobacterium* species, *Roseomonas* species grow best on Sabouraud's agar, however, they do not absorb UV light and do not appear dark when held under a Wood's lamp.

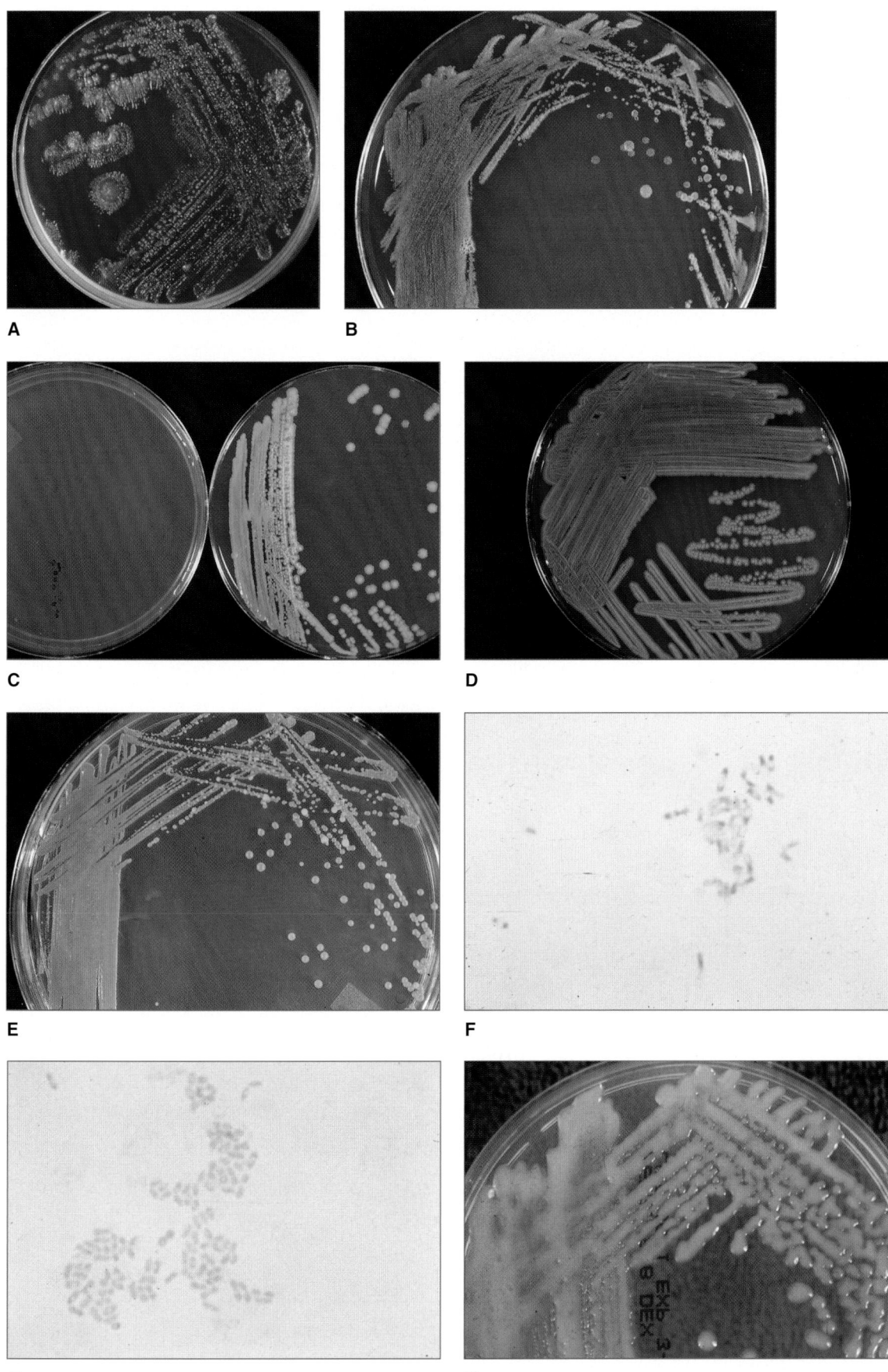

A

B

C

D

E

F

G

H

COLONIAL AND MICROSCOPIC MORPHOLOGY OF CERTAIN NONFERMENTATIVE BACILLI (*CONTINUED*)

A. Blood agar plate demonstrating growth of *Alcaligenes faecalis* after 48 hours incubation at 35°C. Colonies are white and glistening; in older cultures colonies tend to spread at the outer border of the colonies and turn the agar green. This species typically gives off a fruity odor sometimes described as smelling like green apples.

B. MacConkey agar plate showing growth of *Rhizobium radiobacter*. Even though these bacteria are nonfermenters, they rapidly oxidize lactose and consequently appear as pink-colored, extremely mucoid colonies on MacConkey agar. These organisms can be easily confused with a lactose-positive fermenter, however, they are oxidase-positive, which automatically excludes any members of the *Enterobacteriaceae*.

C. Blood agar plate showing growth of *Chryseomonas indologenes*. Colonies have a deep yellow to orange appearance after 48 hours of incubation particularly if incubated at 30°C. Phenotypically these organisms are difficult to distinguished from *Chryseomonas gleum* and some laboratories choose to report such isolates as *C. indologenes/gleum*.

D. Blood agar plate showing characteristic growth of *Myroides odoratus*. Colonies are yellow and spready. Most strains exhibit a characteristic fruity odor like that of *Alcaligenes faecalis*.

E and **F.** A useful test for distinguishing between *Neisseria* species and *Moraxella* species is to grow the organisms on blood agar around a penicillin disk. Both organisms are susceptible to penicillin and will demonstrate a zone of inhibition around the penicillin disk (E). After overnight incubation, a Gram stain can be performed on colonies taken from the edge of the zones of inhibition. *Neisseria* species are true cocci and in the presence of subinhibitory concentrations of penicillin will continue to stain as gram-negative diplococci (*left side*, F). *Moraxella* species are coccobacilli and in the presence of subinhibitory concentrations of penicillin will form bizarre rod-shaped cells (*right side*, F).

G. Blood (left) and MacConkey agar plates showing growth of *Paracoccus yeei* (CDC group EO-2) after 72 hours incubation at 30°C. Colonies appear white and mucoid in appearance. On MacConkey agar they appear slightly pink in color.

H. Gram stain of *Paracoccus yeei* (CDC group EO-2) prepared from broth culture. These organisms stain peripherally giving the appearance of "O-shaped" cells.

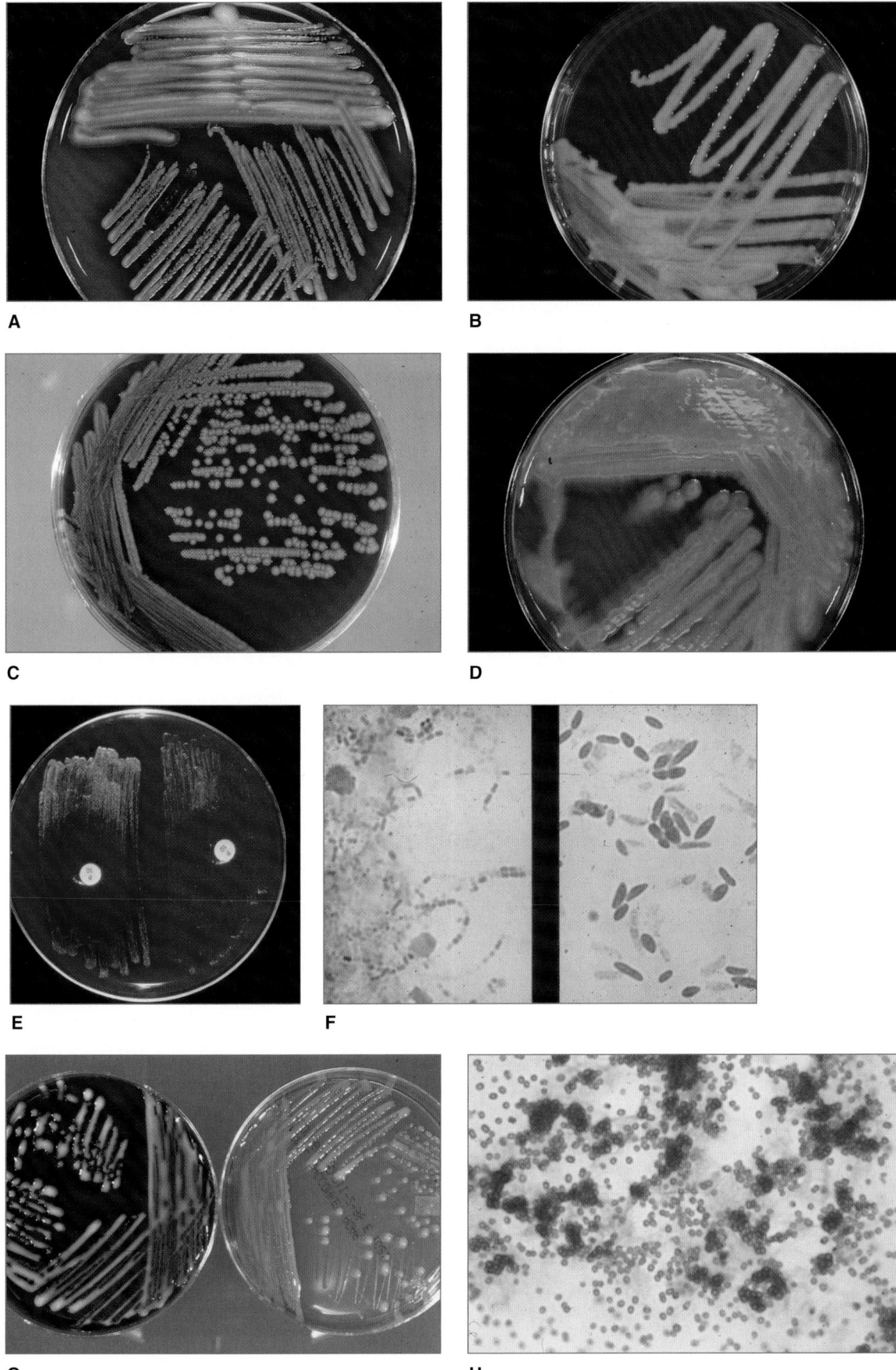

A

B

C

D

E

F

G

H

COLONIAL AND MICROSCOPIC MORPHOLOGY OF CERTAIN NONFERMENTATIVE BACILLI
(*CONTINUED*)

A. Gram stain illustrating gram-negative coccobacilli. *Acinetobacter* and *Moraxella* species are the nonfermentative bacilli that characteristically have this staining morphology. The smear depicted here was made from a broth culture of *A. baumannii*. *Acinetobacter* species have a tendency to retain crystal violet and may appear gram-positive in some gram stain preparations particularly those made directly from positive blood culture bottles.

B. Acinetobacter baumannii on MacConkey agar showing a pink to light lavender appearance that is typical for this species. Often a bluish pigmentation may be observed, particularly striking in colonies grown on EMB agar, where it is described as a "cornflower blue" in appearance.

C. Certain glucose-oxidizing acinetobacters may produce a unique brown discoloration of heart infusion agar with tyrosine or blood agar into which glucose is incorporated. This phenomenon may also be observed on MacConkey and Mueller-Hinton agars. Shown here is a clinical isolate of *A. baumannii* producing a brown diffusible pigment on MacConkey agar.

D. API 20 NE strips illustrating the 24-hour (*top*) and 48-hour (*bottom*) reactions. Note that the first eight tests (reading left to right) are conventional colorimetric reactions, while the remaining 12 tests are carbon assimilation reactions that are read as positive if turbid and negative in the absence of turbidity. Users of this system should note that the strip is incubated at 30°C rather than the usual 35°C used for most other commercial identification kits. (Photographed by Leon J. LeBeau, University of Illinois at Chicago)

E. Remel Uni-N/F system illustrating the circular plate containing 11 independently sealed peripheral wells and a center well containing medium for detecting indole and hydrogen sulfide production. The constricted GNF tube (*second tube from the left*) is used for detection of glucose fermentation and nitrogen gas (below the constriction) and fluorescein production on the slant (above the constriction). The nonconstricted 42P tube (*first tube from the left*) is used to test for growth at 42°C and pyocyanin pigment production.

F. The Remel RapID NF Plus system consists of a plastic tray containing 10 reactions cavities. Seven of the reaction cavities (4 through 10) are bifunctional, containing two separate tests in the same cavity. The system is inoculated with a heavy suspension of the test organism and incubated for 4 hours at 35°C. Following incubation, bifunctional tests are first scored before the addition of reagent, providing the first test result (*top row*). The same cavities are scored again after the addition of reagent to provide the second test result (*bottom row*). The reactions obtained with these 17 tests plus oxidase provide 18 test scores.

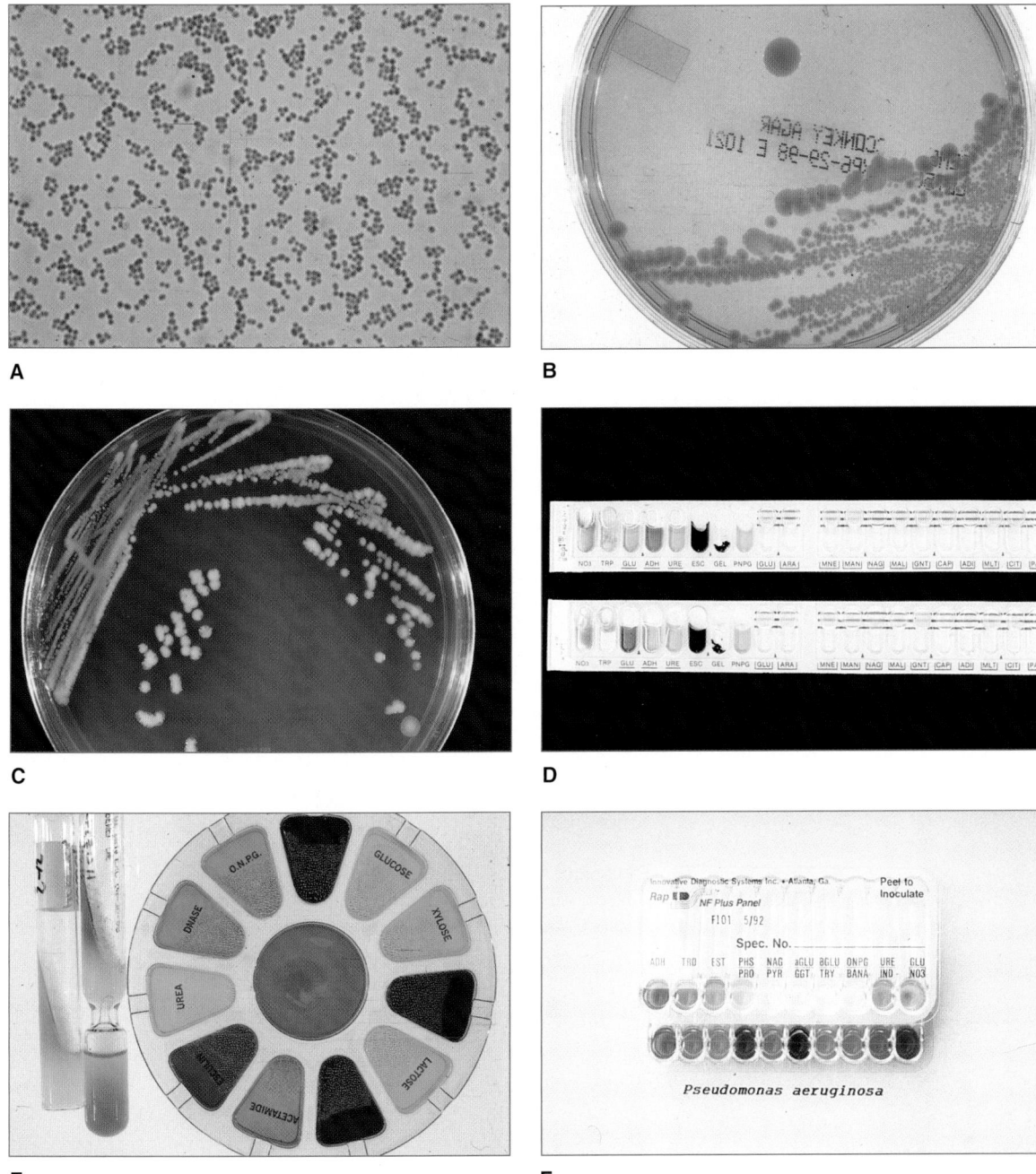

A

B

C

D

E

F

LABORATORY IDENTIFICATION OF *CAMPYLOBACTER* SPECIES

A. Gram stain of *Campylobacter jejuni* illustrating pleomorphic gram-negative bacilli, with short, curved, and spiral forms. Note that some cells connect to form gull-winged and "S" shapes.

B. *C. jejuni* growing on nonselective *Brucella* agar plate following isolation from stool using the membrane filter technique (described in text). Note that growth has occurred only in the area of the plate underneath where the filter had been placed.

C. Close-up view of *C. jejuni* on blood agar, illustrating raised, gray-white, and somewhat mucoid colonies.

D. Growth of *C. jejuni* on Campy BAP agar illustrating the tendency of the organism to grow along the streak lines.

E. Tubes showing the rapid hippurate reaction. Purple color develops with the addition of Ninhydrin when hippurate has been hydrolyzed to form glycine and benzoic acid (*positive tube on left compared with negative control on right*). Of the *Campylobacter* species, only *C. jejuni* gives a positive hippurate reaction.

F. *Brucella* blood agar plate showing growth of *C. jejuni* around cephalothin and nalidixic acid disks. Note that with *C. jejuni* a zone of inhibition forms around the nalidixic acid disk (*right*), indicating that this species is susceptible to nalidixic acid but resistant to cephalothin. This test is easy to perform and allows presumptive identification of *C. jejuni.*

G. Triple sugar iron (TSI) agar slant reactions illustrating the hydrogen sulfide (H_2S) reactions of several species. The tube to the extreme left illustrates the lack of H_2S, characteristic of *C. jejuni, C. fetus* subsp. *fetus*, and *C. fetus* subsp. *venerealis*. Tubes 2, 4, and 5 (*reading from left*) illustrate a strong butt reaction, characteristic of *C. sputorum* biovar *bubulus*, *C. sputorum* biovar *fecalis*, or *C. sputorum* biovar *sputorum*. Tube 3 illustrates a strong slant reaction characteristic of *C. mucosalis.*

H. Silver-stained tissue section of superficial gastric mucosa demonstrating clusters of blue-black staining bacilli along the epithelial lining, consistent with the bacillary forms of *Helicobacter pylori*. When observed in a Gram-stained preparation, the individual cells are long, thick, and curved.

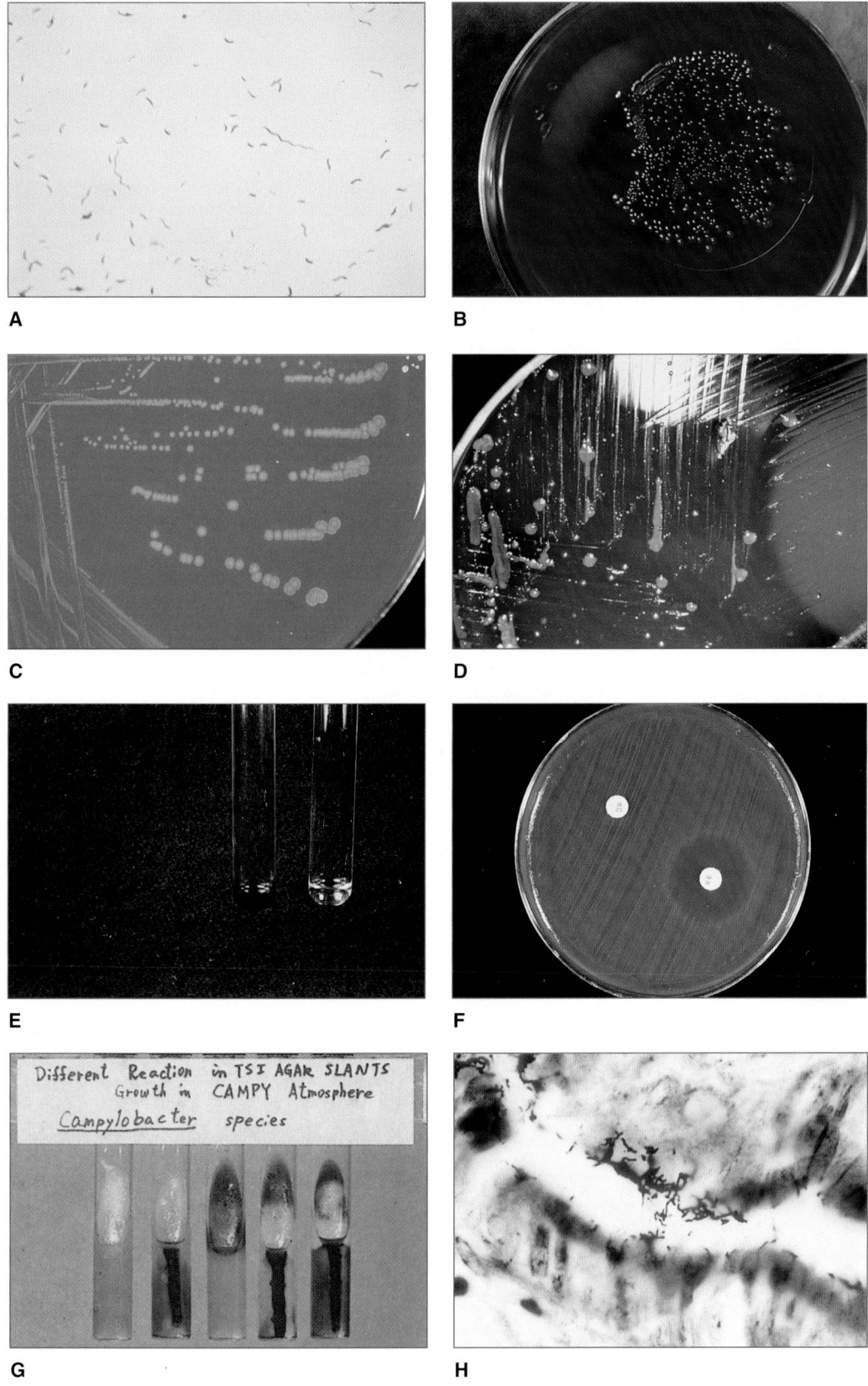

A

B

C

D

E

F

G Different Reaction in TSI AGAR SLANTS
Growth in CAMPY Atmosphere
Campylobacter species

H

LABORATORY IDENTIFICATION OF *VIBRIO CHOLERAE* AND OTHER *VIBRIO* SPECIES

A. Appearance of *Vibrio cholerae* on thiosulfate citrate bile sucrose (TCBS) agar. The yellow colonies result from citrate utilization and the formation of acid from utilization of the sucrose in the medium. The appearance of yellow colonies on this medium is virtually diagnostic of *V. cholerae.*

B. Colonies of *V. parahaemolyticus* growing on TCBS agar illustrating the characteristic semi-translucent, green-gray appearance.

C. Gelatin agar with white, opaque colonies of *V. cholerae.* Note the opalescence of the agar adjacent to the colonies, indicating hydrolysis and denaturation of the gelatin.

D. Gram stain of *V. vulnificus* illustrating gram-negative bacterial cells with the curved, rod-shaped morphology typical of *Vibrio* species.

E. Positive string test with *V. cholerae.* When colonies of *V. cholerae* are mixed in a drop of 0.5% sodium deoxycholate, they produce a viscous suspension that can be drawn into a string when the inoculating loop is slowly raised from the side.

F. Positive slide agglutination test for *V. cholerae* using polyvalent O antiserum.

G. Blood agar plate illustrating the relatively large, intensely β-hemolytic colonies of the El Tor biotype of *V. cholerae.*

H. Chicken erythrocyte agglutination test. Classic strains of *V. cholerae* do not agglutinate chicken erythrocytes (*top*), in contrast to the El Tor biotype (*bottom*), which is capable of agglutinating the erythrocytes.

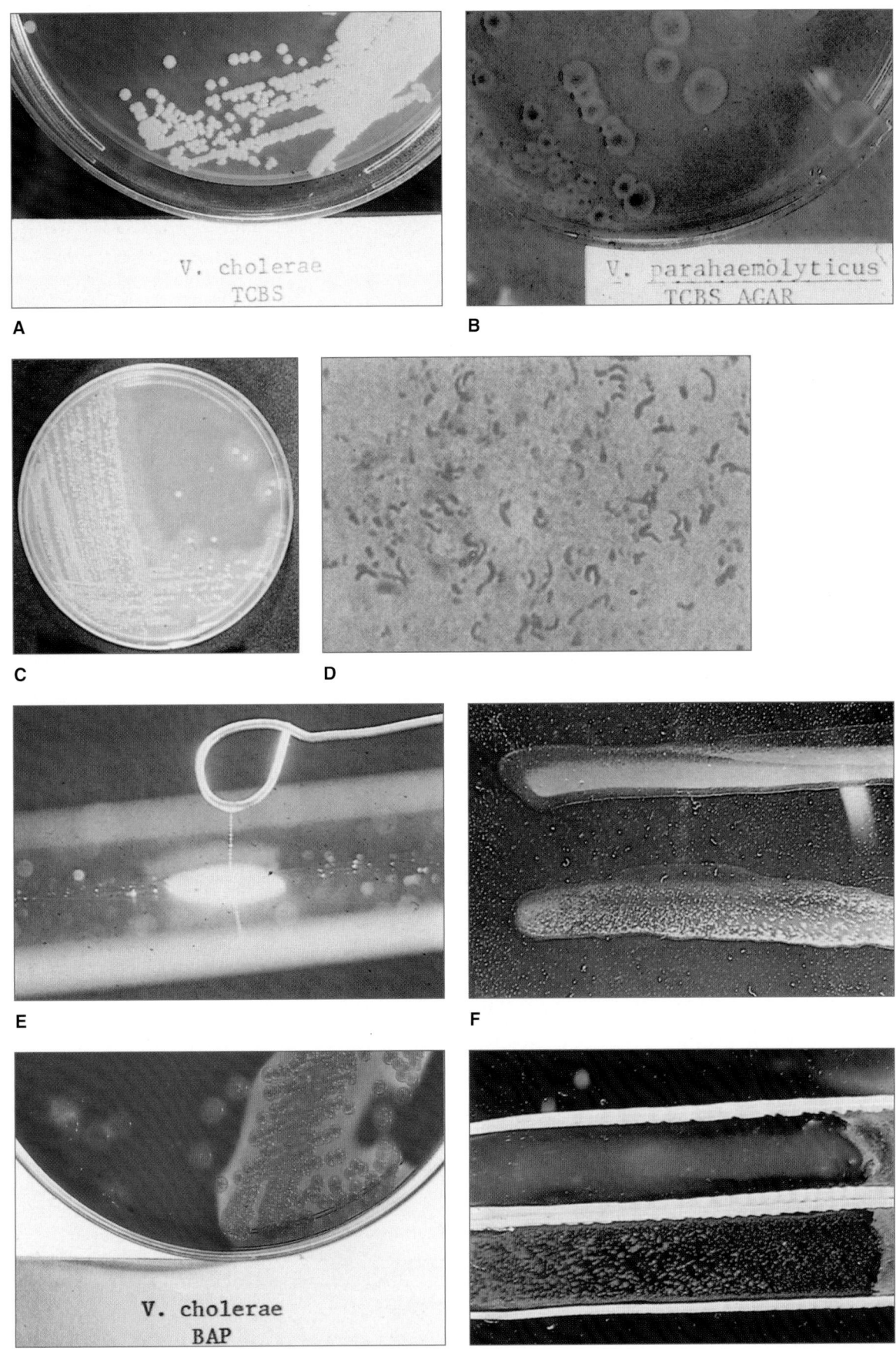

A   V. cholerae TCBS

B   V. parahaemolyticus TCBS AGAR

C

D

E

F

G   V. cholerae BAP

H

IDENTIFICATION OF *HAEMOPHILUS* SPECIES

A. A Gram-stained smear of centrifuged cerebrospinal fluid showing polymorphonuclear cells and scattered gram-negative bacilli of *Haemophilus influenzae*. These organisms characteristically appear as small, poorly staining coccobacilli on Gram stains of clinical specimens. Occasionally, longer, filamentous bacilli may be seen.

B. Growth of moist, smooth, gray colonies of *H. influenzae* type b on chocolate agar after 24 hours of incubation at 35–37°C in 5–7% CO_2. This medium contains hematin (X factor) and is enriched with other cofactors, such as NAD (V factor) that allow the growth of *Haemophilus* and other fastidious microorganisms.

C. Satellite growth of *Haemophilus* around streaks of *Staphylococcus aureus* on sheep blood agar. X factor, or hemin, is provided by the lysed sheep erythrocytes surrounding the *Staphylococcus* streak, while the staphylococci themselves provide the V factor, or NAD. These factors enable the tiny, dew-drop colonies of *Haemophilus* to grow adjacent to the staphylococcus streak.

D. Growth factor test for identification of *H. influenzae*. The organism is inoculated onto a plate of trypticase-soy or brain-heart infusion agar, and disks containing X factor and V factor are placed in proximity to one another on the inoculated plate surface. After incubation in a CO_2-enriched environment at 35–37°C, factor requirements are determined by observing the pattern of organism growth relative to the two disks. In this picture, growth is observed between the X factor and V factor disks, indicating that the organism requires both exogenous X and exogenous V factors for growth.

E. Growth factor test for *Haemophilus parainfluenzae*. The organism is inoculated as described for **D** above, but in this photograph, filter paper strips that are impregnated with X factor, V factor, and both X and V factors are placed on the lawn of inoculum. After incubation in a CO_2-enriched environment at 35–37°C, growth is observed around the V factor strip and around the XV factor strip, but not around the X factor strip. This growth pattern indicates that the organism requires only V factor for growth.

F. The ALA-porphyrin agar test. This is an alternative method for determining the X factor requirements of *Haemophilus* isolates. The agar medium contains δ-aminolevulinic acid (ALA). Organisms are inoculated onto the medium and, after overnight incubation at 35–37°C in a CO_2-enriched environment, the growth is observed under a Wood's (ultraviolet) light. If the colony growth fluoresces "brick-red," the organism is able to synthesize X factor (hemin) from ALA and does not require exogenous X factor. This picture shows growth of both *H. influenzae* (*left*), with its negative ALA-porphyrin test (i.e., requires exogenous hemin for growth), and *H. parainfluenzae* (*right*), with its positive ALA-porphyrin test (i.e., synthesizes hemin from ALA).

G. ALA-porphyrin disk method. This picture also shows the ALA-porphyrin test, but in this approach, a δ-aminolevulinic acid-impregnated disk is used. The disk is moistened with water, and some of the colony growth is rubbed onto the surface of the disk. After incubation for 4 hours at 35–37°C, the disks are observed in the dark under a Wood's light. If the disk fluoresces "brick-red," the organism is able to synthesize its own X factor. If no fluorescence is observed, the organism requires exogenous X factor. In this picture, *H. influenzae* (*left*) shows no fluorescence (i.e., requires exogenous X factor) while *H. parainfluenzae* (*right*) shows fluorescence (i.e., synthesizes X factor from ALA).

H. Nitrate reduction and biotyping reactions for *H. influenzae* biotype I. Isolates of *H. influenzae* and *H. parainfluenzae* reduce nitrate to nitrite and can be grouped into distinct biotypes by their reactions in three biochemical tests: production of indole, ornithine decarboxylase, and urease. This picture shows the nitrate and biotyping reactions of *H. influenzae* biotype I. Tests shown (*left to right*) are a positive nitrate reduction test, indole production in tryptone broth following Xylene extraction (positive), Moeller's decarboxylase broth base (negative), Moeller's ornithine decarboxylase broth (positive), and a urea slant (positive).

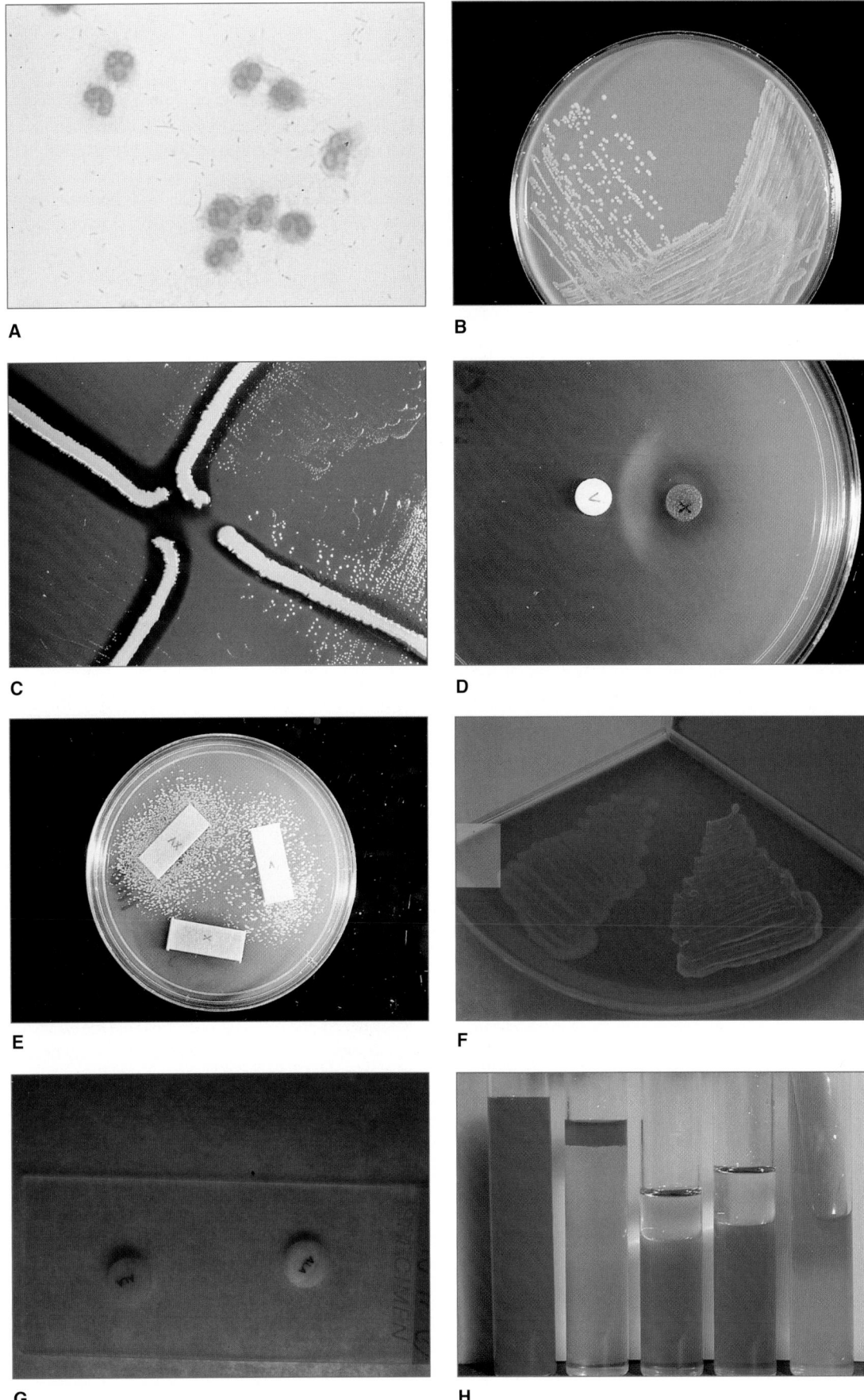

A

B

C

D

E

F

G

H

IDENTIFICATION OF *HAEMOPHILUS* SPECIES (*CONTINUED*)

A. The MicroScan *Haemophilus-Neisseria* Identification (HNID) panel (Dade-MicroScan, West Sacramento, CA). The manual microtiter format system identifies both *Haemophilus* and *Neisseria* species and provides biotype designations for *H. influenzae* and *H. parainfluenzae*. This picture shows a panel inoculated with *H. influenzae* biotype I (urease [URE]-positive, ornithine decarboxylase [ODC]-positive, and indole [IND]-positive. (Courtesy of Dade-MicroScan)

B. A lesion of chancroid on the external female genitalia. Lesions of chancroid may resemble chancres of syphilis, however, chancroid lesions are usually painful and soft, while lesions of primary syphilis are usually painless and indurated. The etiologic agent of chancroid, *Haemophilus ducreyi*, may be cultured from these lesions.

C. RapID NH panel (Remel) inoculated with *H. ducreyi*. The top panel is before addition of reagents to the three bifunctional wells of the cuvette (PO4/NO2, ORN/NO3, and URE/IND), while the bottom panel is after reagent addition for development of the NO_2, NO_3, and IND reactions. The only positive reactions observed with *H. ducreyi* on the RapID NH panel are the phosphatase reaction (*top, eighth reaction from the left [yellow]*) and the nitrate reductase reaction (*bottom, ninth reaction from the left [red]*).

D. Gram-stained smear of *Haemophilus aphrophilus*, showing small, pale-staining coccobacilli.

E. Growth of *H. aphrophilus* on sheep blood agar (*left*) and chocolate agar (*right*) after 48 hours of incubation at 35–37°C in 5–7% CO_2. *H. aphrophilus* is the only *Haemophilus* species that does not require either exogenous X or V factors and, consequently, is able to grow on sheep blood agar. Colonies are characteristically small and have a slight yellowish pigmentation.

F. *Haemophilus paraphrophilus* on sheep blood agar (*left*) and chocolate agar (*right*) after 48 hours of incubation at 35–37°C in 5–7% CO_2. *H. paraphrophilus* is biochemically identical to *H. aphrophilus,* but it requires V factor for growth. Consequently, *H. paraphrophilus* grows on chocolate agar (*right*) but not on sheep blood agar (*left*).

G. Biochemical tests for identification of *H. aphrophilus*. The tubes shown in this photograph (*left to right*) include nitrate broth, indole-tryptone broth, Moeller's decarboxylase base broth, Moeller's lysine decarboxylase broth, Moeller's ornithine decarboxylase broth, and a urea agar slant. As shown here, *H. aphrophilus* is nitrate-positive, but negative for indole, lysine decarboxylase, ornithine decarboxylase, and urease.

H. Rapid carbohydrate utilization tests for *H. aphrophilus*. In this procedure, a balanced salts-phenol red solution (BSS) is dispensed in a series of tubes in 0.10-ml aliquots. A single drop of a filter-sterilized carbohydrate solution (20% w/v) is added to each tube. A heavy suspension of the organism is prepared in the BSS without added carbohydrate, and a single drop of this suspension is added to each of the BSS-carbohydrate tubes. After 4 hours of incubation at 35–37°C, the reactions are interpreted. With the production of acid, the phenol red indicator turns from red to yellow. In this frame, the tubes (*left to right*) are the BSS organism suspension (without added carbohydrate), BSS with glucose (G), maltose (M), sucrose (S), lactose (L), mannitol (MN), xylose (X), and mannose (MA). As can be seen from these reactions, *H. aphrophilus* produces acid from glucose, maltose, sucrose, lactose and mannose, but not from mannitol or xylose. Details of this procedure, which can also be used for identifying *Neisseria* species, are presented in Chart 11-1.

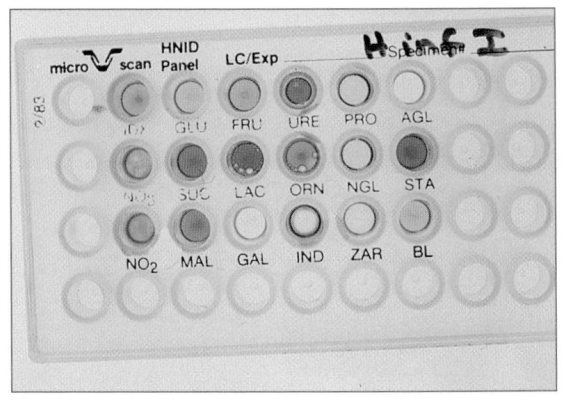

A

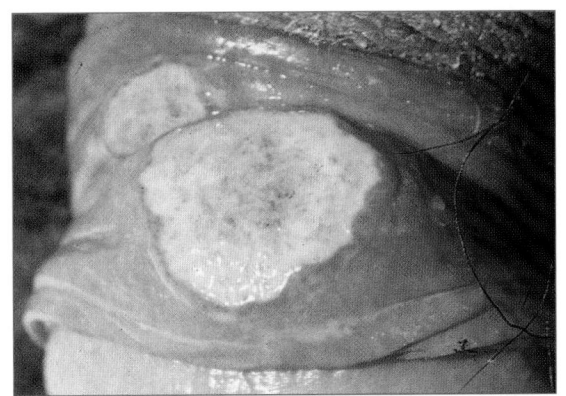

B

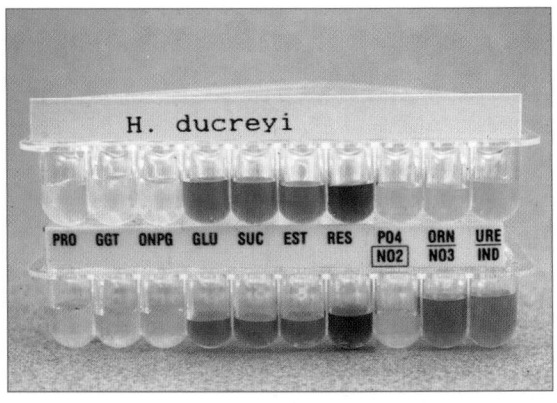

C

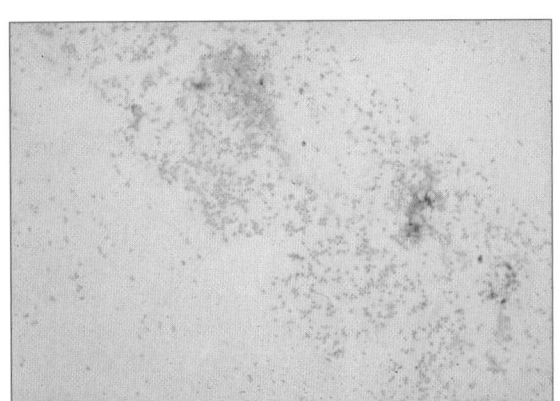

D

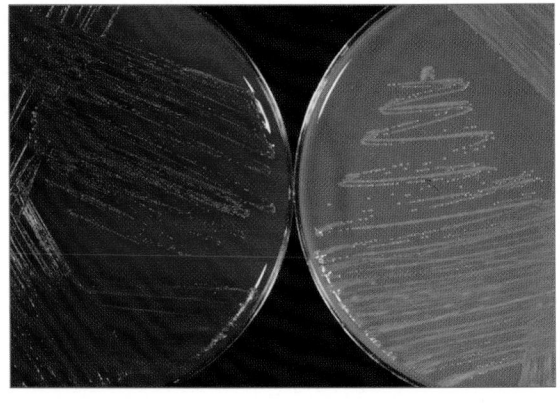

E

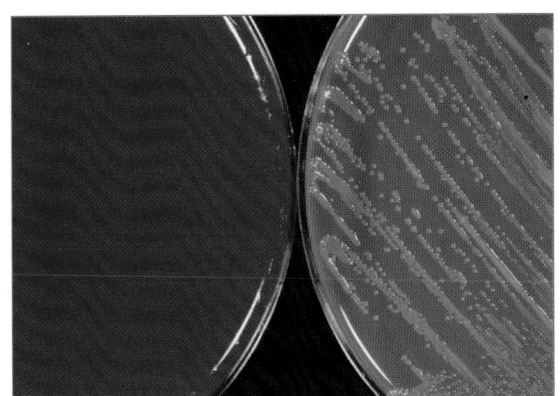

F

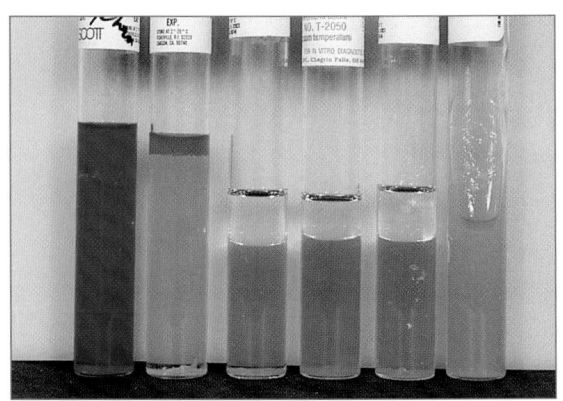

G

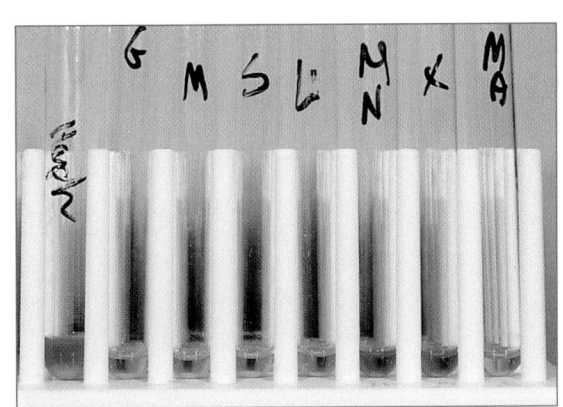

H

ACTINOBACILLUS, CARDIOBACTERIUM, AND EIKENELLA SPECIES

A. Gram-stained smear of *Actinobacillus actinomycetemcomitans*, showing the pale staining, gram-negative bacilli and coccobacilli of this species.

B. *A. actinomycetemcomitans* growing on chocolate agar after 72 hours of incubation at 35–37°C in 5–7% CO_2.

C. Rapid carbohydrate utilization tests for *A. actinomycetemcomitans*. As shown here, *A. actinomycetemcomitans* produces acid from glucose (G), mannitol (MN) and mannose (MA), but not from maltose (M), sucrose (S), lactose (L), or xylose (X). Failure to produce acid from lactose, along with a positive catalase test, helps to differentiate *A. actinomycetemcomitans* from *H. aphrophilus* (see Color Plate 9-2*H* above) Nitrate reduction, lysine and ornithine decarboxylases, and urease reactions are the same for both *A. actinomycetemcomitans* and *H. aphrophilus* (see Color Plate 9-2*G* above).

D. Gram-stained smear of *Cardiobacterium hominis*. These organisms are often gram-variable, but are staining uniformly gram-negative in this photograph. The cells of *C. hominis* are generally longer than the other HACEK bacteria and show considerable pleomorphism (e.g., cells with pointed or swollen ends, teardrop-shaped and dumbbell-shaped cells, etc.). The characteristic palisading of the cells in "picket fence" arrangements and the clustering of cells to form compact rosettes are also evident in this picture.

E. Growth of *C. hominis* on sheep blood agar after 72 hours of incubation at 35–37°C in 5–7% CO_2. Colonies of this organism are small, opaque and glistening. Some strains may also pit the agar like *E. corrodens*.

F. Gram-stained smear of *Eikenella corrodens*. The cells of *E. corrodens* appear as "regular" gram-negative bacilli, and are not coccobacillary or pleomorphic like other members of the HACEK bacteria.

G. Growth of *E. corrodens* on sheep blood agar after 72 hours of incubation at 35–37°C in 5–7% CO_2. The incident light on the plate in this photograph demonstrates the pitting of the agar surface that is characteristic of most strains. Nonpitting strains may also be identified, and both pitting and nonpitting variants may be observed in the same culture.

H. Biochemical tests for identification of *E. corrodens*. The tubes shown here are (*left to right*) nitrate broth, indole-tryptone broth, Moeller's decarboxylase base, Moeller's lysine decarboxylase broth, Moeller's ornithine decarboxylase broth, and a urea slant. *E. corrodens* is nitrate-positive, urease-negative, and is the only HACEK member that is both lysine and ornithine decarboxylase-positive. *E. corrodens* also differs from the other HACEK bacteria in not producing acid from carbohydrates either fermentatively or oxidatively.

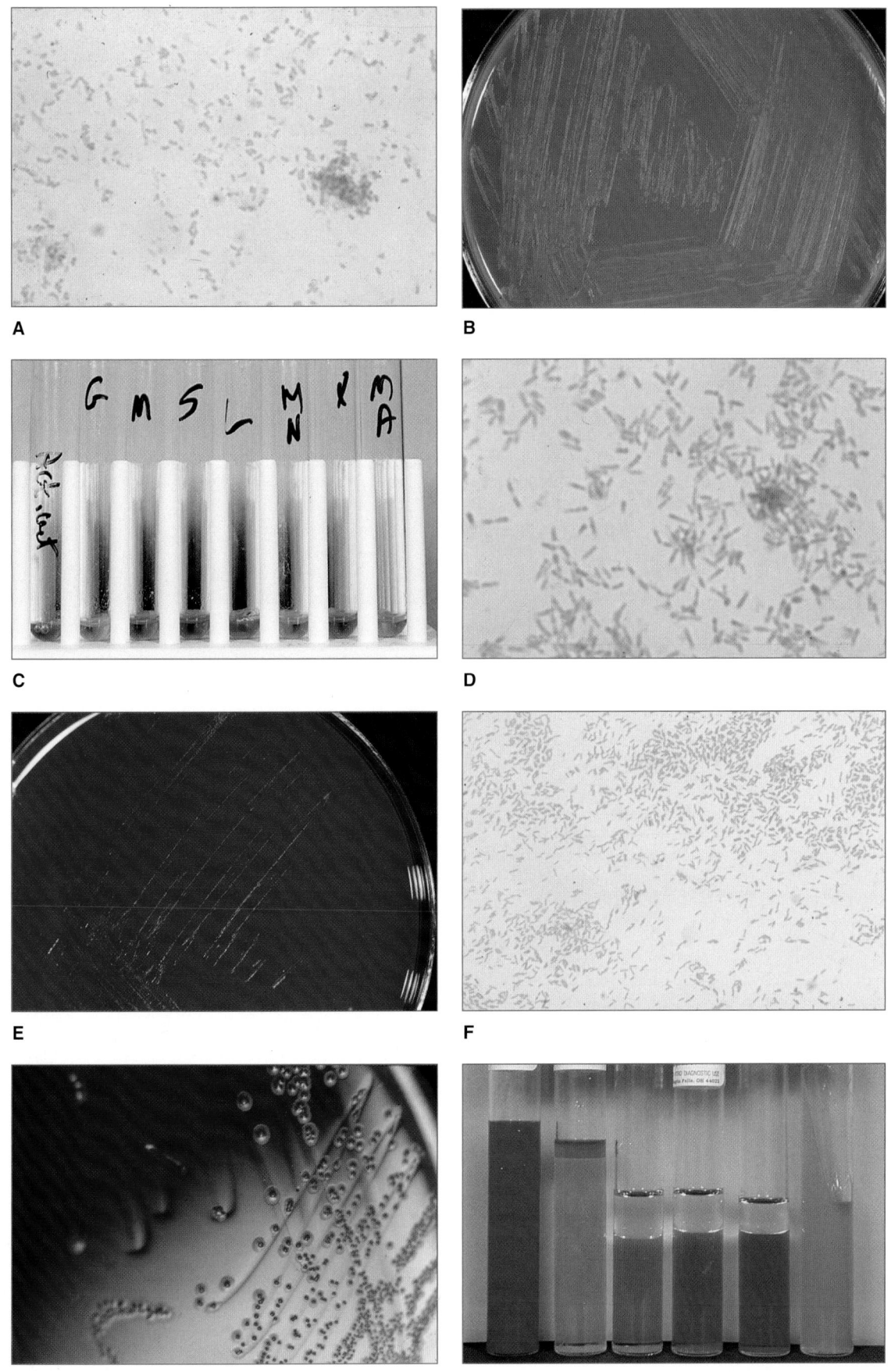

A

B

C

D

E

F

G

H

KINGELLA, CAPNOCYTOPHAGA, AND *DYSGONOMONAS* SPECIES

A. *Kingella kingae* on sheep blood agar. The plate on the left is after 24 hours of incubation at 35–37°C in 5–7% CO_2, while the plate on the right is the same isolate after 48 hours of incubation. The β-hemolysis produced by this organism may be apparent only underneath and immediately adjacent to the colony after 24 hours of incubation, but after 48 hours of incubation, the β-hemolysis is more apparent.

B. Colonies of *Kingella denitrificans* on chocolate agar after 24 hours of incubation at 35–37°C in 5–7% CO_2. Colonies of this organism resemble the small colony types of *Neisseria gonorrhoeae.*

C. RapID NH panel (Remel) inoculated with *K. denitrificans.* Two identical panels are depicted in this photograph. The upper panel is before the addition of nitrate and indole reagents to the appropriate bifunctional cuvette wells. Positive reactions on the panel for this oxidase-positive, catalase-negative organism include prolyl aminopeptidase (PRO), glucose fermentation (GLU), and positive nitrite reduction (NO_2), and nitrate reduction (NO_3) tests. All other test results are negative.

D. Human isolate of *Capnocytophaga* species on sheep blood agar after 48 hours of incubation at 35–37°C in 5–7% CO_2. This photograph shows the characteristic colony morphology of these organisms and illustrates the fringe of "gliding motility" at the periphery of the colonies. Toward the centers of the areas of growth, the colonies have a mottled appearance.

E. Gram-stained smear of human *Capnocytophaga* species. These organisms characteristically appear as gram-negative, slightly curved, fusiform bacilli with pointed ends. In this respect, these bacteria resemble the obligately anaerobic species *Fusobacterium nucleatum.*

F. Colonies of *Capnocytophaga canimorsus* on sheep blood agar after 5 days of incubation at 35°C in 5–7% CO_2. Colonies of this species are entire, circular, convex, and shiny, as shown here.

G. Gram-stained smear of *C. canimorsus.* This photograph shows the fusiform cells typical of the genus. Like the *Capnocytophaga* species that are found in the human oropharynx, some of the cells of this species are also slightly curved.

H. Colonies of *Dysgonomonas capnocytophagoides* (formerly CDC group DF-3). This organism grows as pinpoint colonies after 24 hours of incubation that subsequently form larger, gray to white colonies. This photograph shows a 48-hour culture of *D. capnocytophagoides* growing on sheep blood agar after incubation at 35–37°C in 5–7% CO_2. Colonial growth of this organism has been reported to have a characteristically "sweet" odor.

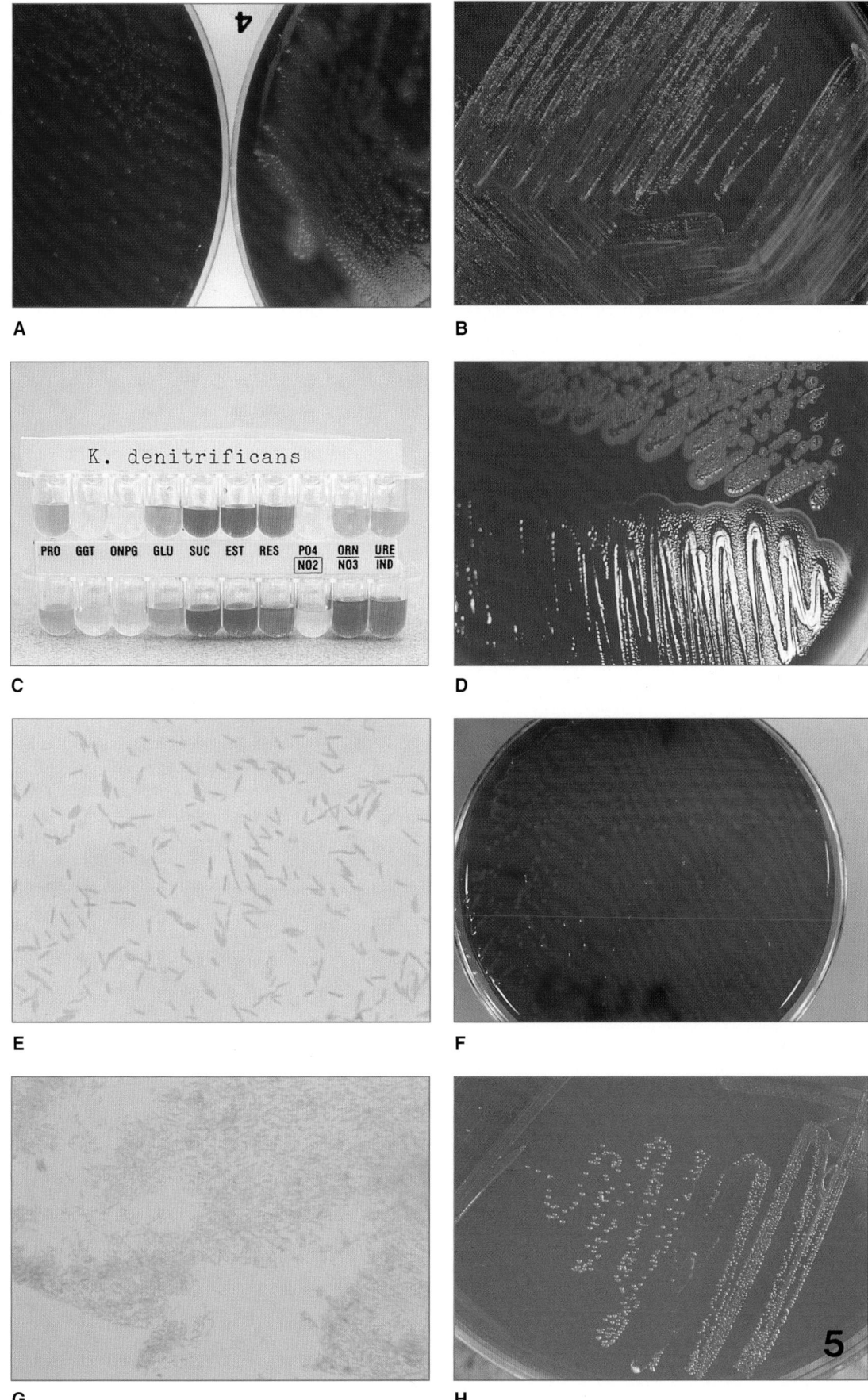

C

K. denitrificans

| PRO | GGT | ONPG | GLU | SUC | EST | RES | PO4 NO2 | ORN NO3 | URE IND |

A

B

D

E

F

G

H

5

PASTEURELLA, BRUCELLA, AND BORDETELLA SPECIES

A. Colonies of *Pasteurella multocida* growing on sheep blood agar after 48 hours of incubation at 35–37°C in 5–7% CO_2. The organism is nonhemolytic and does not grow on MacConkey, EMB, or other selective/differential enteric media. *P. multocida* is most frequently isolated from bite wounds from domesticated animals, especially cats and dogs.

B. Gram-stained smear of *P. multocida*, showing the small, gram-negative coccobacilli that are characteristic of this species and other species in the genus *Pasteurella*.

C. Positive spot-indole reaction of *P. multocida*. A piece of filter paper is saturated with a few drops of *p*-dimethylaminocinnamaldehyde reagent, and colony growth of the organism is removed from the agar surface and rubbed onto the reagent along with a negative control organism. The appearance of a teal-blue color on the filter paper is a positive test, whereas the negative control organism results in a pale pink color, as shown here. *P. multocida* is also oxidase-positive.

D. *Brucella melitensis* growing on sheep blood agar after 48 hours of growth in 5–7% CO_2-enriched atmosphere at 35–37°C. The colonies are small, nonpigmented, nonhemolytic, entire, and convex.

E. Direct fluorescence antibody (DFA) test for *Bordetella pertussis*. The DFA test is an important adjunct to culture for the detection of *B. pertussis* in nasopharyngeal specimens. This photograph shows a positive DFA preparation, with the organisms appearing as apple-green fluorescent coccobacilli. As demonstrated here, the bacteria may appear singly or in clusters resulting from the trapping of bacteria in mucous strands. (Photo courtesy of Marty Roe, Children's Hospital, Denver, CO).

F. Gram-stained smear of *B. pertussis*, showing the characteristic, small, coccobacillary morphology.

G. Growth of *B. pertussis* on Regan-Lowe agar without (*left*) and with (*right*) cephalexin incorporated into the medium. The small white colonies present on both plates are colonies of *B. pertussis*, while the large colonies on the medium lacking cephalexin represent contaminant organisms present in the specimen. Culture for pertussis should include media with and without antibiotics, since some strains of both *B. pertussis* and *B. parapertussis* may be inhibited by cephalexin.

H. Colonies of *B. pertussis* on Regan-Lowe agar after 72 hours of incubation at 35–37°C in 5–7% CO_2. This medium contains horse blood (10% w/v) in a charcoal agar base. The high concentration of blood and the incorporation of activated charcoal in the medium help to neutralize any toxic materials that may be presence in the specimen and to facilitate recovery of the bacteria.

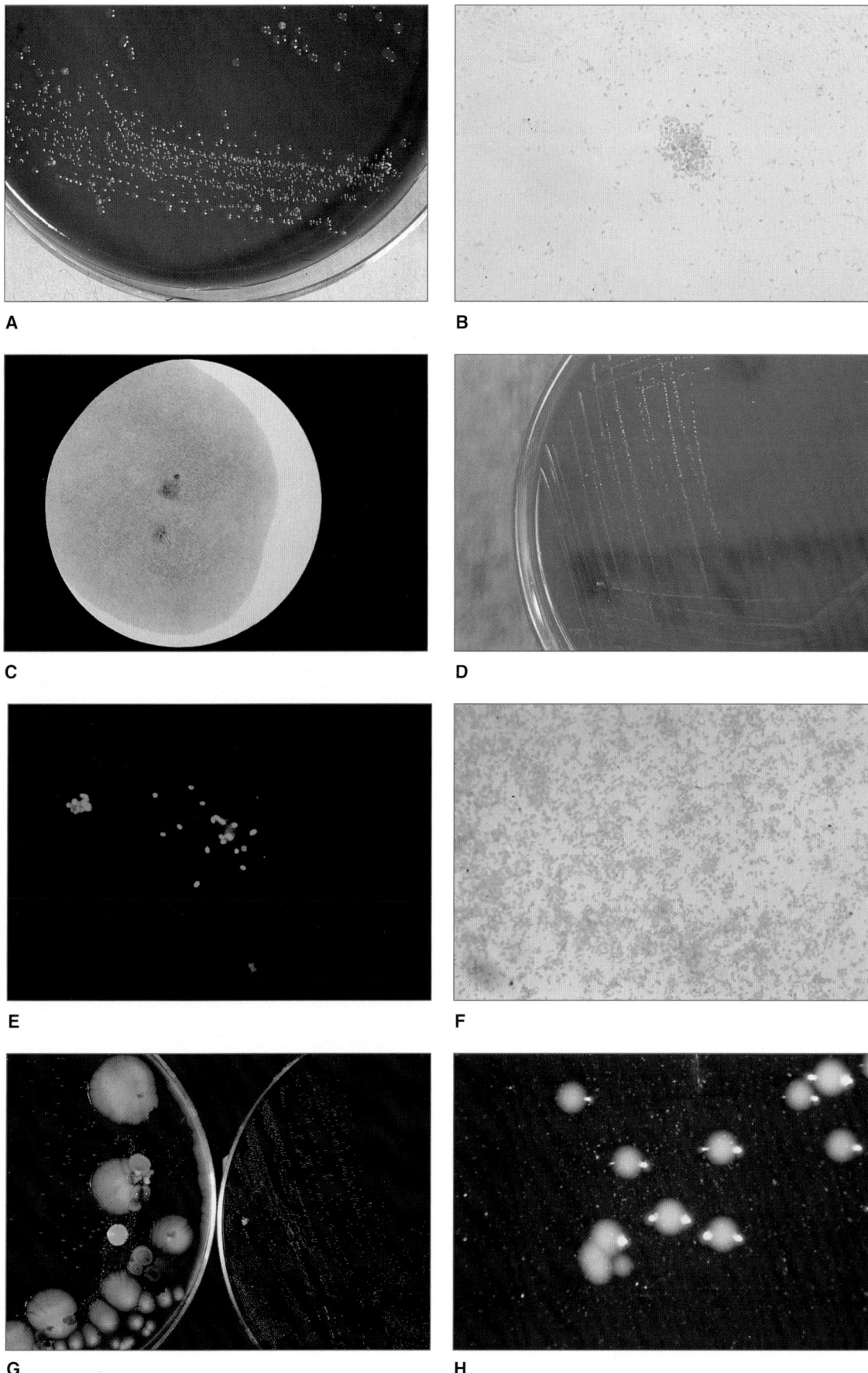

A

B

C

D

E

F

G

H

LABORATORY DIAGNOSIS OF LEGIONELLOSIS

A. Gram stain of *Legionella pneumophila* culture using basic fuchsin instead of safranin for the counterstain. The organisms are thin rods of various lengths.

B. Gram-Weigert–stained touch preparation of open-lung biopsy specimen revealing small, thin intracellular and extracellular bacilli (original magnification, ×100; objective lens). Note the short, blunt rods in the macrophage nearest the center of the slide. *L. pneumophila* serogroup 1 was the only organism isolated in culture; a tissue imprint of the lung was DFA-positive when stained with the conjugate specific for this organism.

C. Heavy growth on buffered charcoal yeast extract agar (BCYEa) after 3 or more days of incubation and no growth on blood agar are characteristic of *Legionella* species.

D. Dissecting microscopic view of *L. pneumophila* colonies on BCYEa. Note the crystalline-like internal structures within 3–5 mm colonies that have entire margins (original magnification, approximately ×40).

E. Blue-white autofluorescence of *L. bozemanii* on BCYEa; photographed under long-wave ultraviolet light. Other species that autofluoresce blue-white include *L. dumoffii, L. gormanii, L. anisa, L. tucsonensis, L. cherrii, L. parisiensis,* and *L. steigerwaltii.* This characteristic is absent in *L. pneumophila, L. micdadei, L. feeleii, L. longbeachae, L. oakridgensis,* and many other *Legionella* species.

F. Modified-Kinyoun acid-fast stain of *L. micdadei* grown on BCYEa. Some of the rod-shaped bacteria in the preparation are acid-fast (red), whereas some are not acid-fast (blue); thus, they are "partially acid-fast." Using the traditional Ziehl-Neelsen stain, or an auramine-rhodamine stain, they are not likely to be acid-fast (see text for details).

G. Paraffin section of lung tissue from a patient with acute Legionnaires' disease. The section shows an area of consolidation. Inflammatory exudates consisting of fibrin, many neutrophils, few macrophages, and some erythrocytes fills alveolar spaces and alveolar ducts (hematoxylin and eosin stain; original magnification, approximately ×200).

H. Paraffin section of lung from a different patient with a more chronic form of Legionnaires' disease. Alveoli are filled with prominent, foamy macrophages, and the interstitium is edematous. A silver impregnation stain (e.g., Dieterle or Warthin-Starry [not shown]) aids in demonstrating the organisms.

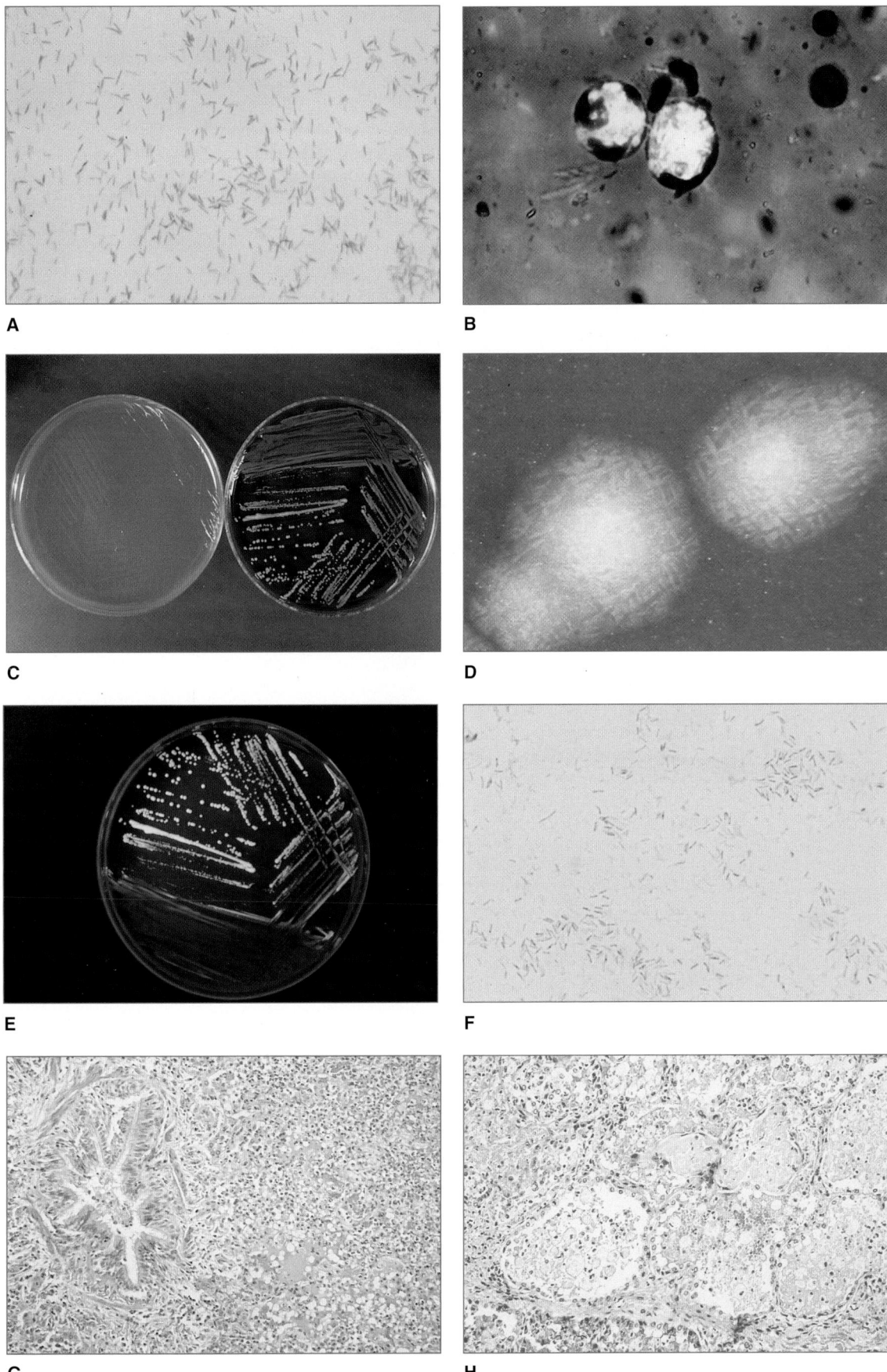

A

B

C

D

E

F

G

H

IDENTIFICATION OF *NEISSERIA* SPECIES

A. Gram-stained smear of a urethral discharge from a male with gonococcal urethritis. Note the presence of intracellular gram-negative diplococci within pale-staining segmented neutrophils.

B. Skin lesion of disseminated gonococcal infection (DGI) on the index finger of the left hand. Skin lesions associated with DGI are usually located on the extremities.

C. Typical colonies of *Neisseria gonorrhoeae* on modified Thayer-Martin (MTM) medium after 24 hours of incubation at 35–37°C in 5–7% CO_2. MTM is a chocolate agar-based formulation that contains vancomycin, colistin, and nystatin to inhibit gram-positive, gram-negative, and fungal organisms, respectively. Pathogenic *Neisseria* species, notably *N. gonorrhoeae* and *N. meningitidis*, grow well on MTM medium.

D. Close-up view of colonies of *N. gonorrhoeae* growing on MTM agar after 24 hours of incubation at 35–37°C in 5–7% CO_2.

E. Conventional cystine-tryptic digest semisolid agar (CTA) for identification of *Neisseria* species. This photograph shows the typical battery of carbohydrates used for identification. The battery includes (*left to right*) CTA-glucose, CTA-maltose, CTA-sucrose, and CTA-lactose (the control CTA tube without carbohydrate is not shown). The CTA basal medium contains a phenol-red indicator, and a change in the color of the medium from red to yellow indicates acid production from the respective carbohydrate. In this photograph, acid has been produced from glucose only, identifying the organism as *N. gonorrhoeae*.

F. Close-up view of colonies of *Neisseria meningitidis* growing on sheep blood agar after incubation for 24 hours at 35–37°C in 5–7% CO_2.

G. Rapid carbohydrate utilization test for identification of *Neisseria* species (see Chart 11-1). The rapid carbohydrate utilization test is performed using a balanced salts-phenol red solution (BSS, 0.10 mL per tube), with a single drop of carbohydrate (20% w/v aqueous solution, filter-sterilized) added for each carbohydrate tested. A dense suspension of the organism is prepared in BSS without carbohydrate, and a single drop of this heavy suspension is added to each of the BSS-carbohydrate tubes. The inoculated tubes are incubated at 35°C for 4 hours. This photograph shows a set of BSS-carbohydrates composed of (*left to right*) BSS only (for the organism suspension), BSS-glucose, BSS-maltose, BSS-fructose, BSS-sucrose, and BSS-lactose. Because acid has been produced in the BSS-glucose and BSS-maltose tubes (color change from red to yellow), the organism is identified as *N. meningitidis*.

H. GONOCHEK II (EY Laboratories, San Mateo, CA). Three chromogenic substrates are included in a single plastic tube to detect glycosidase and aminopeptidase enzymes specifically found in *N. meningitidis*, *N. lactamica*, and *N. gonorrhoeae*. Hydrolysis of substrates in the tube results in the small inoculum volume turning various colors. Identification patterns observed are: blue (*upper left*)—*N. lactamica* (β-galactoside hydrolysis); yellow (*upper right*)—*N. meningitidis* (γ-glutamyl-*p*-nitroanilide hydrolysis); and red (*lower left*)—*N. gonorrhoeae* (prolyl-β-naphthylamide hydrolysis). Lack of a color reaction (*lower right*) following the 30-minute incubation presumptively identifies the organism as *Moraxella catarrhalis*.

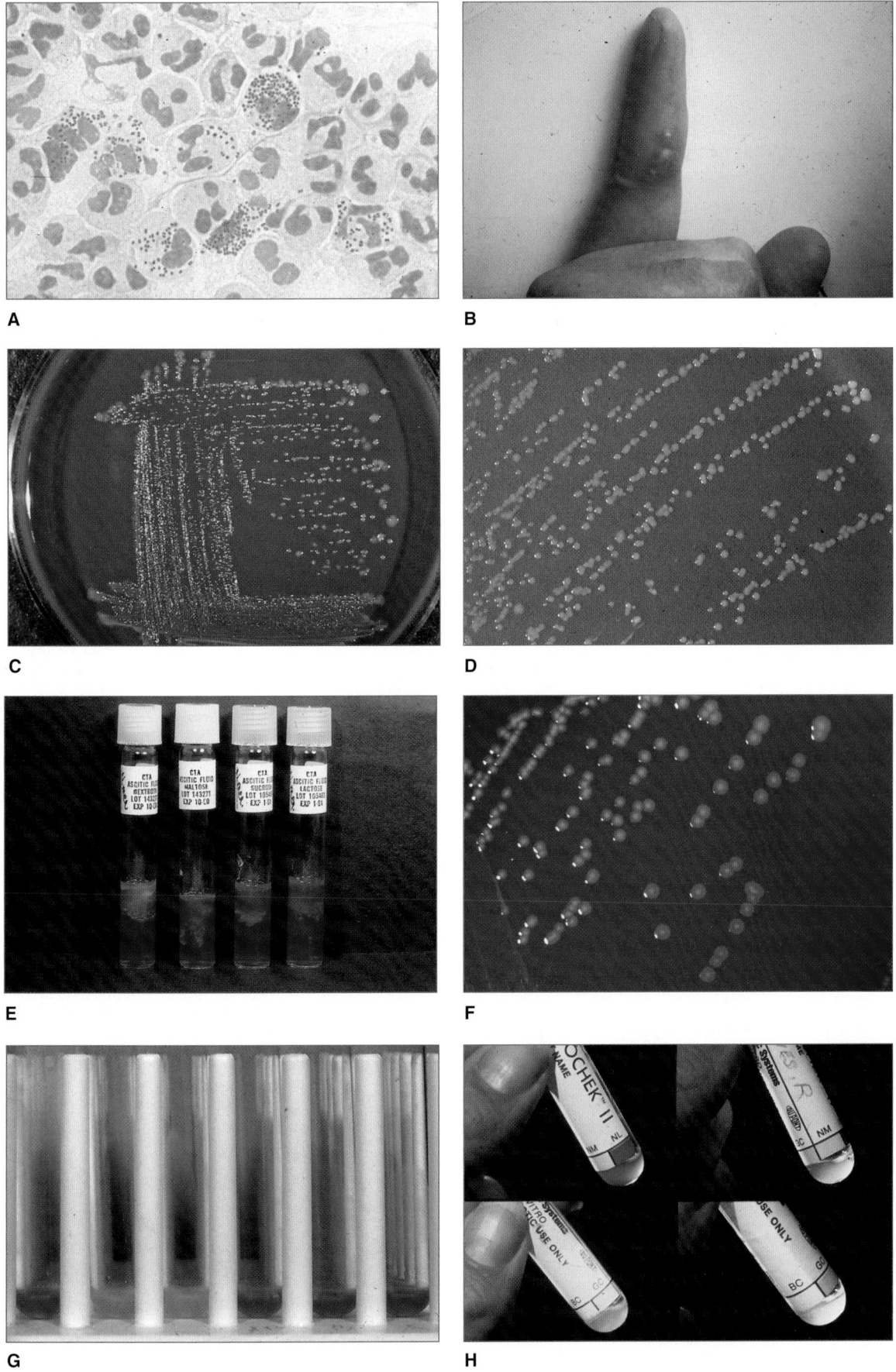

A

B

C

D

E

F

G

H

IDENTIFICATION OF *NEISSERIA* SPECIES AND *MORAXELLA CATARRHALIS*

A. BactiCard *Neisseria* (Remel Laboratories, Lenexa KS). This identification strip contains four chromogenic enzyme substrate tests for identification of the pathogenic *Neisseria* species and *Moraxella catarrhalis*. After hydration of each of the four test circles with a drop of buffer, growth from selective media or a suitable subculture is applied onto each of the four test areas. If a blue-green color develops in the IB (butyrate esterase) test area within 2 minutes (*strip at left*), the organism is identified as *M. catarrhalis*. If no color develops in this area, the strip is incubated for an additional 13 minutes. If a blue-green color develops in the BGAL (β-galactosidase) test area (*strip at far right*) during this time, the organism is identified as *N. lactamica*. If no color reaction develops in this area during the incubation period, a single drop of color-developing reagent is added to the PRO and GLUT test areas. The appearance of a red color in the PRO (prolyl aminopeptidase) test area identifies the isolate as *N. gonorrhoeae* (*second strip from the left*), whereas the development of a red color in the GLUT (γ-glutamyl aminopeptidase) test area identifies the isolate as *N. meningitidis* (*third strip from the left*)

B. Fluorescent antibody (FA) test for culture confirmation of *N. gonorrhoeae* (Microtrak *N. gonorrhoeae* Culture Confirmation Kit, Wicklow, Ireland). In a positive test, apple-green fluorescent diplococci are observed, as shown in this photograph.

C. RapID NH system (Remel). The RapID NH system is a 4-hour commercial system for identification of *Neisseria* species, *Haemophilus* species, and several other species of fastidious gram-negative bacteria. The photograph actually shows two duplicate panels inoculated with *N. meningitidis*. The top panel in the photo is the system prior to the addition of reagents, while the bottom panel is the system after the addition of reagents to the last three bifunctional test wells. The reactions that identify the isolate as *N. meningitidis* are the positive prolyl aminopeptidase (PRO) and γ-glutamyl aminopeptidase (GLUT) reactions, the positive glucose (GLU) reaction, and the positive NO$_2$ (reduction of nitrite) test.

D. MicroScan HNID panel (Dade-MicroScan, West Sacramento, CA). The MicroScan HNID panel is a 4-hour test panel for the identification of *Haemophilus* and *Neisseria* species, Positive tests on the panel shown in the photograph include the nitrate reduction (NO$_3$) and nitrite reduction (NO$_2$) tests, production of acid from glucose (GLU), sucrose (SUC), maltose (MAL), fructose (FRU), and prolyl aminopeptidase (PRO). These characteristics identify this isolate as *N. mucosa*.

E. API NH panel (BioMérieux, Durham, NC). The API NH is a strip format identification system for the 2-hour identification of *Neisseria* and *Haemophilus* species. The strip include seven single-substrate cupules and three bifunctional cupules. The single substrate tests include (*left to right*), a β-lactamase-test (PEN), acid production from glucose (GLU), fructose (FRU), maltose (MAL), sucrose (SAC), ornithine decarboxylase (ODC), and urease (URE). The bifunctional cupules include butyrate esterase plus prolyl aminopeptidase (LIP/PRO A), alkaline phosphatase (PAL) plus γ-glutamyl aminopeptidase (PAL/GGT), and β-galactosidase plus indole (βGAL/IND). The entire strip is read first, including the LIP, PAL, and βGAL tests, and then a color development reagent is added to the PRO A and GGT wells, and indole reagent is added to the IND well. These last three cupules are then reread to provide the fourth number of a 4-digit biocode. The carbohydrate cupules, LIP, PRO A, GGT, and βGAL address the identification of *Neisseria* species and *Moraxella catarrhalis*, while the carbohydrate cupules, ODC, URE, PAL, βGAL, and IND are used for identifying and biotyping *Haemophilus* species. In this photograph, the GLU and PRO A tests are positive, providing a biocode of 1001. Consultation with the API NH database provides an identification of *N. gonorrhoeae*. The PEN well is an acidometric β-lactamase detection cupule that is not used for identification purposes. The PEN test is positive here, indicating that the isolate is β-lactamase positive.

F. API NH inoculated with *N. meningitidis*. Positive tests on the strip include glucose (GLU), maltose (MAL), prolyl aminopeptidase (PRO A), and GGT (γ-glutamyl aminopeptidase). These reactions result in an API biocode of 5003, which provides an identification of *N. meningitidis*. This isolate is β-lactamase-negative, as indicated by the blue color in the PEN cupule.

G. The *M.cat* butyrate disk test (Carr-Scarborough Microbiologicals, Decatur, GA). *M. catarrhalis* strains produce a butyrate esterase enzyme that is able to hydrolyze indoxyl butyrate. An indoxyl butyrate–impregnated filter paper disk is moistened with water, and growth from a colony is rubbed onto the disk. The butyrate esterase enzyme hydrolyzes the compound and a blue-green color appears on the disk within 2 minutes. This figure shows three positive *M.cat* butyrate disks on a glass slide.

H. API NH inoculated with *M. catarrhalis*. In this photograph, the only positive test is the LIP cupule (blue is a positive reaction). The API biocode for these reactions is 0010, which identifies it as *M. catarrhalis*. The PEN cupule is not used to determine the API biocode, but only to detect β-lactamase production. The blue color in the PEN cupule indicates that this strain is β-lactamase-negative.

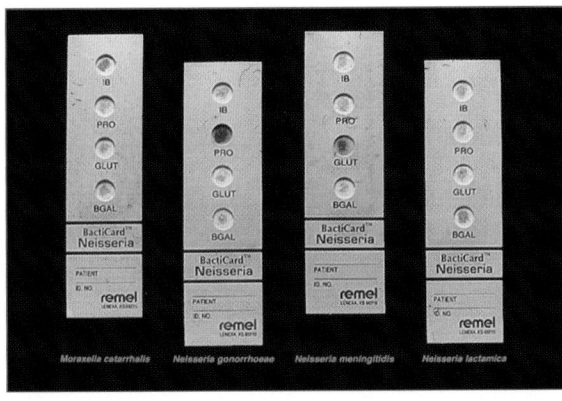

A

B

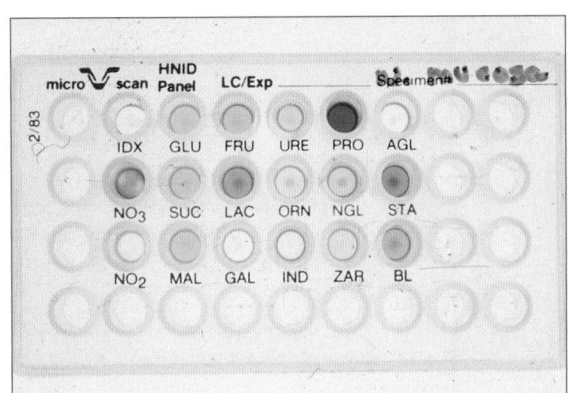

C

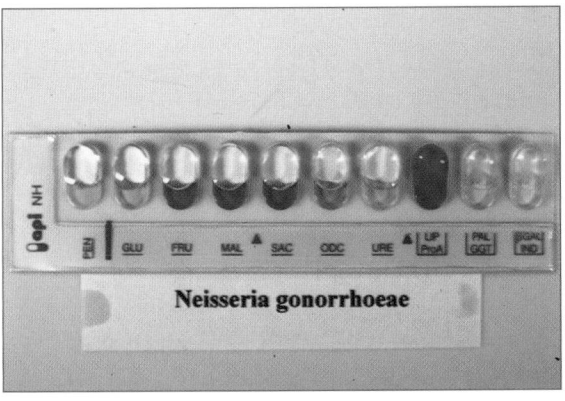

D

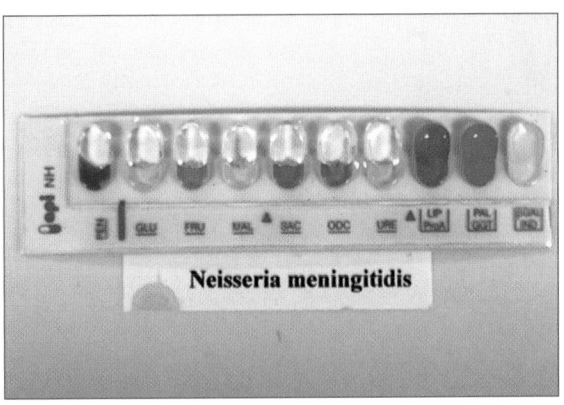

E

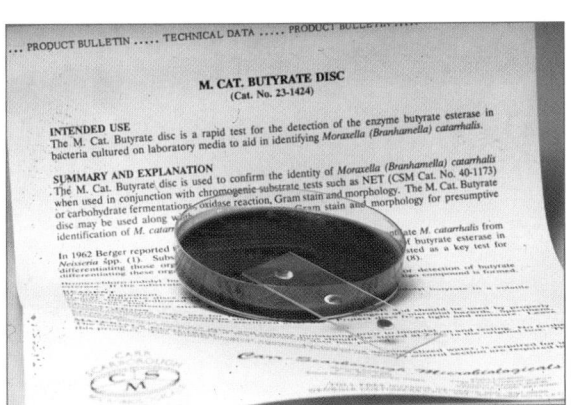

F

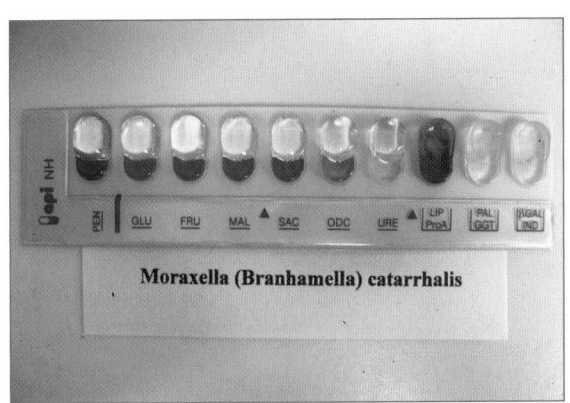

G

H

IDENTIFICATION OF STAPHYLOCOCCI AND RELATED SPECIES

A. Adult patient with staphylococcal cellulitis of the upper lip

B. Adult patient with the bullous, vesicular lesions of facial staphylococcal impetigo. Culture of the serosanguinous fluid within these vesicles reveals large numbers of *Staphylococcus aureus*.

C. Neonate with staphylococcal scalded skin syndrome. This syndrome is seen in newborns infected with *S. aureus* strains that produce exfoliatins (i.e., epidermolytic toxins). These toxins dissolve the mucopolysaccharide matrix of the epidermis, resulting in intraepithelial splitting of the cellular linkages in the stratum granulosum. Bullous formation occurs over large areas of the body, with subsequent sloughing of the superficial skin layers, as shown here.

D. Gram-stained smear from a lesion of staphylococcal cellulitis. The organisms appear as small extracellular gram-positive cocci arranged in clusters along with the pink-staining polymorphonuclear leukocytes.

E. Colonies of *S. aureus* on sheep blood agar. This photograph shows typical colonies of *S. aureus* after 24 hours of incubation at 35–37°C. A zone of β-hemolysis owing to the hemolytic activity of the staphylococcal α-hemolysin is seen immediately surrounding the colonies. The darker red area outside the hemolyzed area around each colony represents the action of the β-hemolysin (or "hot/cold" hemolysin). It is the β-hemolysin that interacts with the CAMP factor produced by group B streptococci to produce the synergistic hemolysis seen in the CAMP test for presumptive identification of group B streptococci (see Chapter 13).

F. Gram-stained smear from a broth culture of *S. aureus*, showing the typical gram-positive cocci in grape-like clusters.

G. Positive catalase test. The catalase test differentiates staphylococci and micrococci from the streptococci, enterococci, and the streptococcus-like bacteria (Chapter 13). The test is performed by placing growth from a colony onto a glass slide and adding a drop of 3% hydrogen peroxide to the inoculum. Immediate and vigorous bubbling owing to the production of oxygen gas, as shown here, indicates a positive test. Micrococci and staphylococci are catalase-positive, whereas streptococci and enterococci are catalase-negative. *Rothia mucilaginosa*, another organism that grows as gram-positive cocci in clusters, is weakly catalase-positive or may be catalase-negative.

H. Colonies of *Micrococcus luteus* on sheep blood agar. This species produces yellow-pigmented colonies. Other micrococci and organisms in related genera may be nonpigmented or may produce orange- or red-pigmented colonies on agar media. Micrococci and related organisms may be differentiated from staphylococci by resistance to furazolidone, susceptibility to bacitracin, or other methods as shown in Table 12-1.

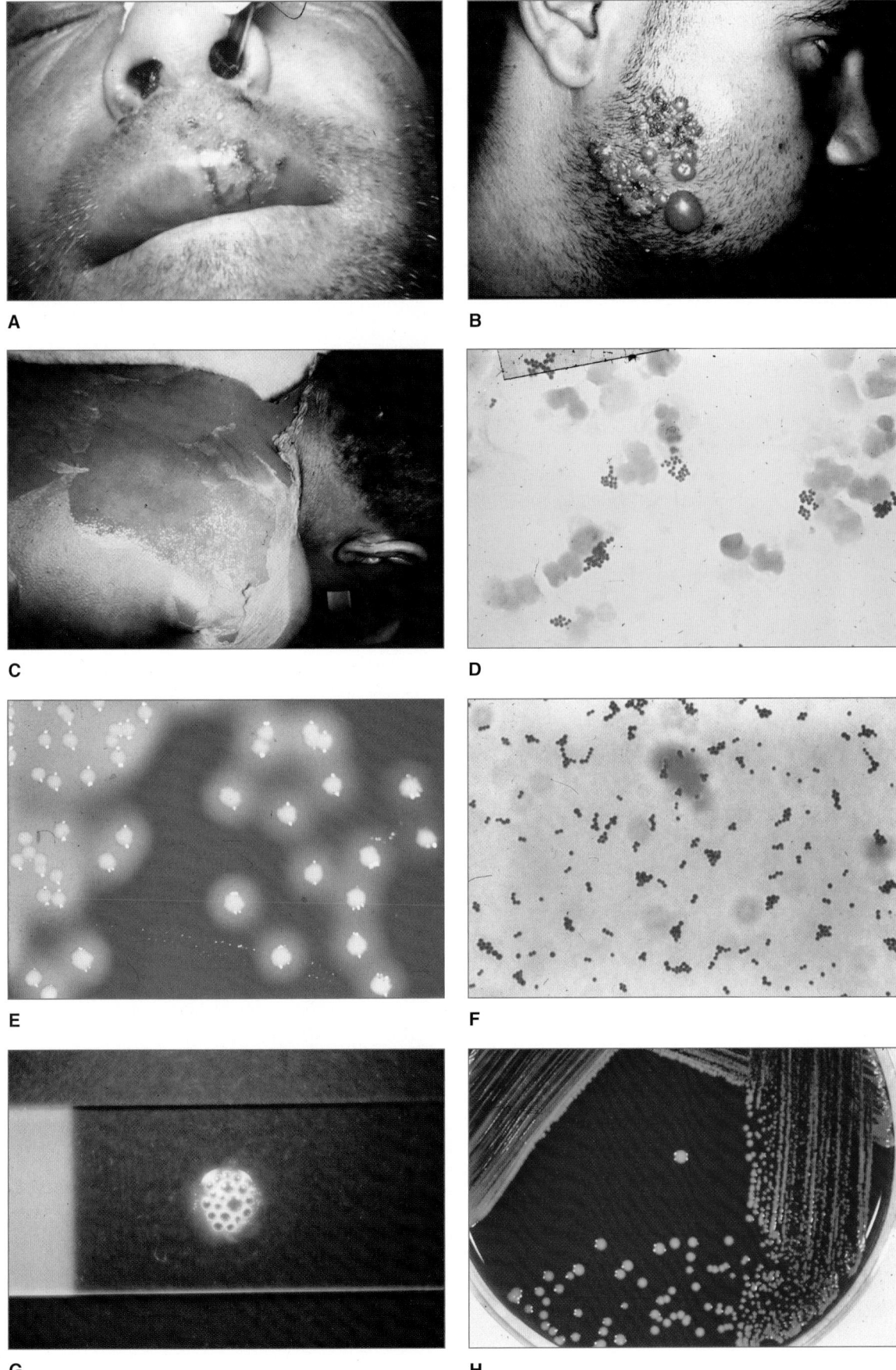

A

B

C

D

E

F

G

H

IDENTIFICATION OF STAPHYLOCOCCI

A. Furazolidone disk test with a *Micrococcus* species. Several tests are available for differentiating micrococci and related genera from staphylococci. The furazolidone susceptibility test is a reliable overnight method for making this differentiation. Micrococci are resistant to furazolidone and will usually grow right up to the edge of the 6 mm furazolidone disk (FX, 100 μg, BD Biosciences, Franklin Lakes, NJ).

B. Furazolidone disk test with a *Staphylococcus* species. The growth of staphylococci is inhibited by furazolidone and will show an area of growth inhibition around the disk, as depicted in this figure.

C. Modified oxidase test. (Remel, Lenexa, KS) This test is a rapid, 30-second method for differentiating staphylococci from micrococci and related species. The oxidase reagent (tetramethyl-*p*-phenylenediamine dihydrochloride) is made up of dimethyl sulfoxide (DMSO), which allows the reagent to penetrate the staphylococcal cell wall. The test is performed by rubbing a portion of colony growth from a plate onto a filter paper disk that is impregnated with the reagent. Most micrococci and related species are modified oxidase-positive, producing a blue-purple color on the disk within 30 seconds, whereas most *Staphylococcus* species are modified oxidase-negative.

D. Slide coagulase test. This test is a rapid method for identifying *S. aureus*. Most strains of this species produce a cell-bound coagulase or "clumping factor" that is detected by mixing a saline suspension of the organism with EDTA-rabbit plasma. A saline control (*left*) must be included with each test to assess autoagglutination. Not all *S. aureus* strains possess clumping factor, so negative slide coagulase tests must be confirmed with the tube coagulase test (see Color Plate 12-2*E*).

E. Tube coagulase test. In this test, extracellular coagulase produced by *S. aureus* forms a complex with a component in plasma, called coagulase-reacting factor. This complex, in turn, reacts with fibrinogen in the plasma to form fibrin and, consequently, the development of a visible clot in the tube. A positive test is shown at the *bottom* of the figure, and a negative test is shown at the *top* of the figure.

F. Latex agglutination test for identification of *S. aureus*. This alternative coagulase test procedure uses latex beads that are coated with plasma. Fibrinogen bound to the latex detects clumping factor, and the immunoglobulins, also present on the latex, detect protein A on the surface of the *S. aureus* cell. Newer formulations of these tests also contain latex beads coated with antibodies against *S. aureus* capsular types 5 and 8, which enable more reliable detection of oxacillin-resistant *S. aureus* strains. Mixing of colonial growth of *S. aureus* with the latex reagent results in rapid agglutination (*left*). A coagulase-negative staphylococcus, which produces a negative latex agglutination reaction, is also shown (*right*).

G. DNase medium with toluidine-blue. This medium detects the production of deoxyribonuclease by *S. aureus*. The organisms are spot-inoculated heavily onto the agar surface and the plate is incubated at 35–37°C for 24 hours. A positive test is indicated by the appearance of a pink color under and around the inoculum. As shown here, *S. aureus* ("SA" on plate) is DNase-positive, while the control (*S. saprophyticus*, "SS" on plate) is DNase-negative. The DNase test serves as a helpful adjunct test for *S. aureus* strains that have weak or equivocal coagulase test results.

H. API ID32 Staph system (BioMérieux) for identification of staphylococci and micrococci. This strip-format identification system contains 26 biochemical substrates. Positive and negative reactions are recorded to generate a biotype number that is used along with a computerized database (the APIWEB) to identify the organism. This system has the most complete database of all the commercially-available identification products for staphylococci.

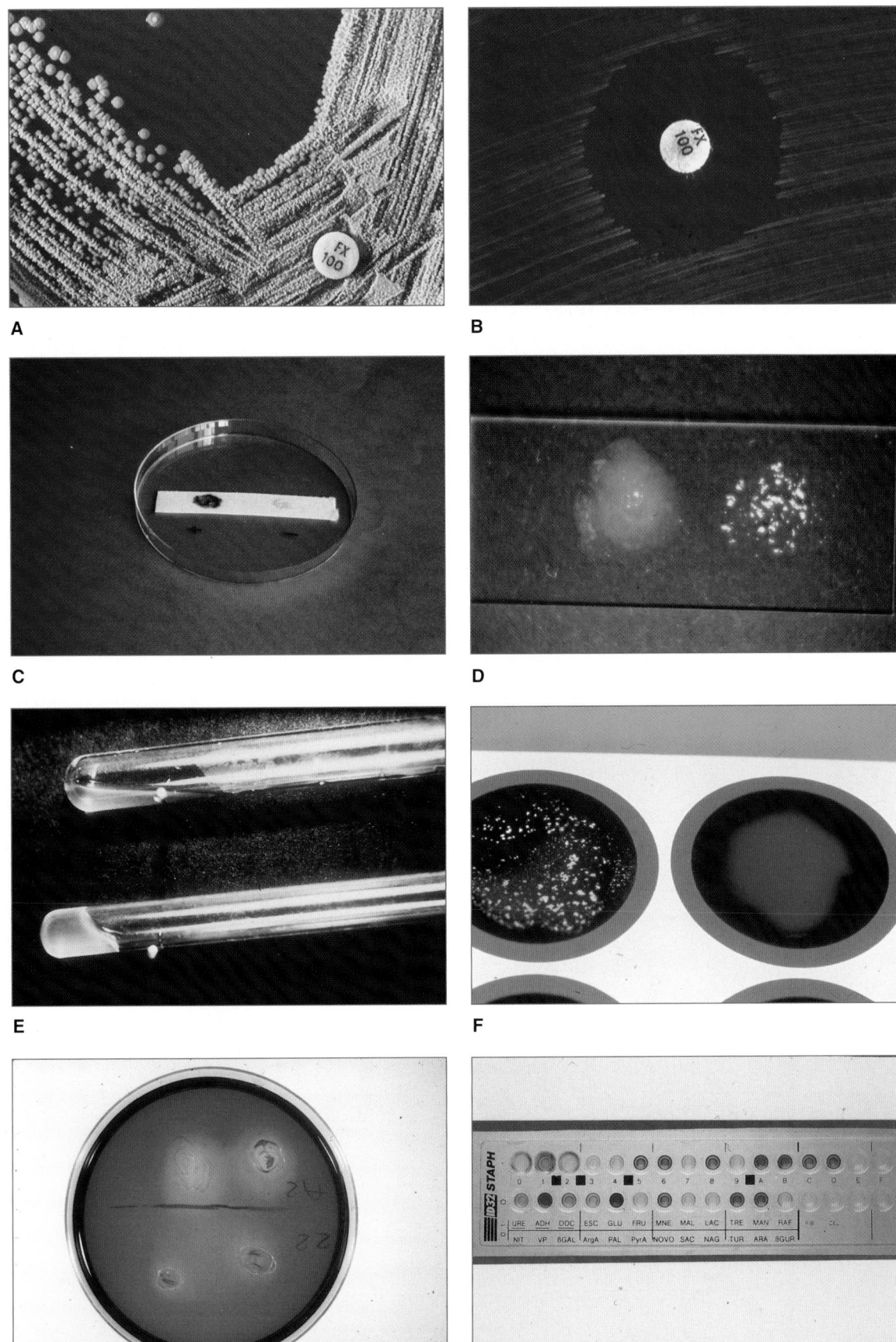

A

B

C

D

E

F

G

H

IDENTIFICATION OF STAPHYLOCOCCI (*CONTINUED*)

A. Colonies of *Staphylococcus epidermidis* on sheep blood agar (SBA) after 24 hours of incubation at 35–37°C.

B. *S. saprophyticus* on SBA with furazolidone and novobiocin disks. *S. saprophyticus* is a cause of urinary tract infections in young women. Like other staphylococci, this species is susceptible to furazolidone (FX), as shown by the zone of inhibition around the FX disk. The other disk (designate c-) on this slide is a novobiocin disk. *S. saprophyticus* is one of several staphylococcus species that is resistant to novobiocin.

C. API Staph identification panel inoculated with *S. saprophyticus*. This picture shows the reactions on the first half of the panel. The interpretations of the test reactions shown are as follows:

CHO Control	Negative	GLU	Positive	FRU	Positive
MNE	Negative	MAL	Positive	LAC	Positive
TRE	Positive	MAN	Positive	XLT	Negative
MEL	Negative				

D. API Staph identification panel inoculated with *S. saprophyticus*. This picture shows the second half of the panel. The interpretations of the test reactions shown are as follows:

		NIT	Negative	PAL	Positive
VP	Positive	RAF	Negative	XYL	Negative
SAC	Positive	MDG	Negative	NAG	Negative
ADH	Negative	URE	Positive		

The API biocode numbers for these reactions, shown in Color Plate 12-3*C* and *D*, is 6634112. Consultation with the computer-assisted API Staph database provides a list of possible identifications, including *S. saprophyticus* (71.9% likelihood), *S. warneri* (19.3% likelihood), or *S. hominis* (6.6% likelihood). Since *S. saprophyticus* is the only species that is novobiocin-resistant, the organism can be identified as *S. saprophyticus*.

E. This slide shows an isolate growing on sheep blood agar after incubation at 35–37°C for 24 hours. This isolate was recovered from several blood cultures of a 38-year-old patient with presumed staphylococcal endocarditis. This isolate is nonpigmented and nonhemolytic, and was also furazolidone- and novobiocin-susceptible (not shown).

F. This photograph shows the latex agglutination reaction of the isolate from Color Plate 12-3*E*. The isolate is coagulase-positive by the latex test. Since the isolate did not "look" like *S. aureus*, the technologist inoculated an API Staph identification strip. These reactions are shown in Color Plate 12-3*G* and *H*.

G. API Staph identification strip inoculated with the blood culture isolate shown in Color Plate 12-3*E*. This photograph shows the reactions on the first half of the strip. The interpretations of these test reactions are as follows:

CHO Control	Negative	GLU	Positive	FRU	Negative
MNE	Positive	MAL	Negative	LAC	Negative
TRE	Positive	MAN	Negative	XLT	Negative
MEL	Negative				

H. API Staph identification strip inoculated with the blood culture isolate from Color Plate 12-3*E*. This photograph shows the reactions on the second half of the strip. The interpretations of these test reactions are as follows:

		NIT	Positive	PAL-Positive
VP	Positive	RAF	Negative	XYL-Negative
SAC	Negative	MDG	Negative	NAG-Positive
ADH	Positive	URE	Negative	

The API biocode for the reactions shown in Color Plate 12-3*G* and *H* is 2116141. Consultation with the API Staph computer-assisted database provides an identification of this isolate as *S. schleiferi*. This is consistent with the positive latex reaction shown in Color Plate 12-3*F*, as this species can be slide-, latex-, and/or tube coagulase-positive.

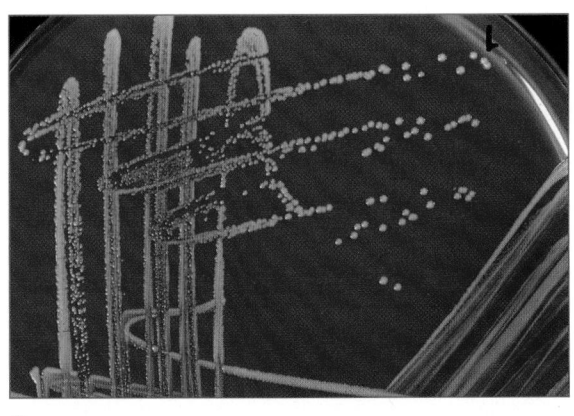

A

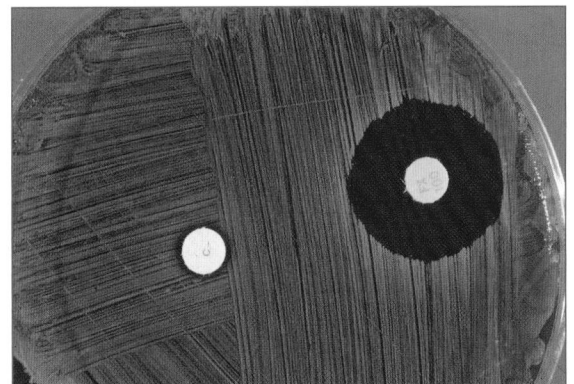

B

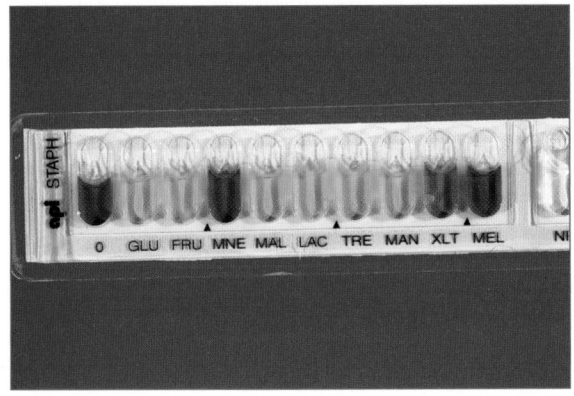

C

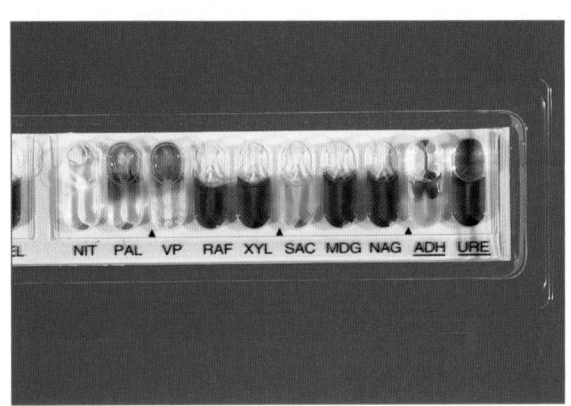

D

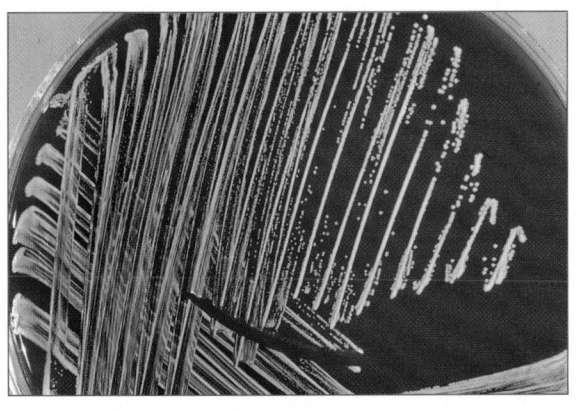

E

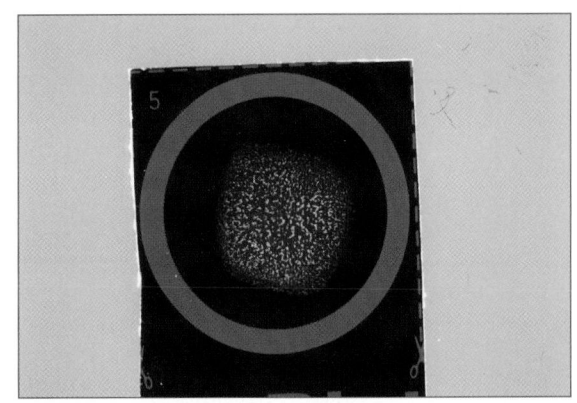

F

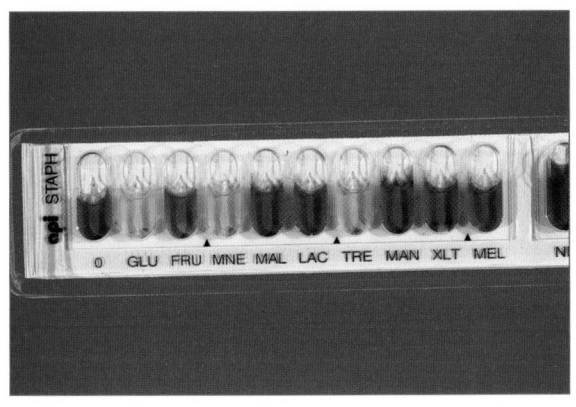

G

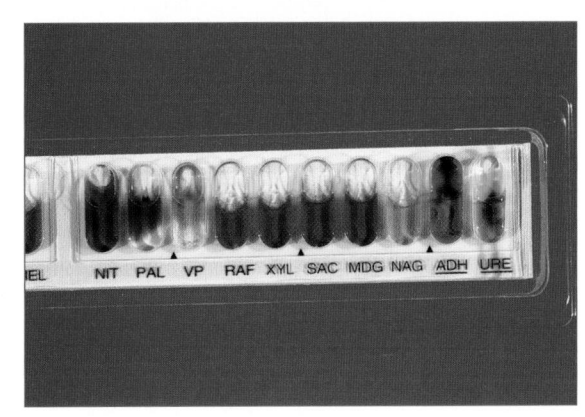

H

IDENTIFICATION OF STREPTOCOCCI

A. Patient with erysipelas due to group A β-hemolytic streptococci. This infection involves the soft tissues and cutaneous lymphatics and results in systemic manifestations of infection, including fever. Note the bullous lesions adjacent to the chin.

B. Gram-stained smear of streptococci growing in a broth culture. As their name suggests, streptococci characteristically grow in chains. These chains are most frequently seen when the organisms are grown in broth. On Gram-stained smears prepared from growth on agar media, the organisms usually appear in pairs or in shorter chains.

C. Gram-stained smear of *Streptococcus pneumoniae*. This photograph shows the typical appearance of pneumococci in blood culture broth. These bacteria characteristically grow in pairs in which the cells have a slightly elongated "lanceolate" morphology. With some cells in this photograph, a clear area or "halo" may be observed surrounding the organism pairs, indicating the presence of the polysaccharide capsule of *S. pneumoniae*.

D. β-Hemolytic streptococci on sheep blood agar. β-Hemolytic streptococci produce hemolysins that lyse the sheep erythrocytes, resulting in a clearing of the medium surrounding the colonies. The group A streptococcus shown here demonstrates this type of hemolysis, as do groups B, C, and G streptococci. The zones of β-hemolysis surrounding colonies of group B streptococci, however, are not as large relative to the size of the colony as those seen with groups A, C, and G β-hemolytic streptococci.

E. α-Hemolytic streptococci on sheep blood agar. Streptococci initially may be classified on the basis of their hemolytic properties on sheep blood agar. Partial hemolysis of the erythrocytes results in a "greening" of the agar medium surrounding the colonies (α-hemolysis). Streptococci that are α-hemolytic include *S. pneumoniae*, the viridans group of streptococci, and most *Enterococcus* (formerly *Streptococcus*) species.

F. β-Hemolytic streptococci on sheep blood agar. More intense β-hemolysis is noted in areas where the medium has been "stabbed," pushing some of the bacteria under the medium surface. The β-hemolysis in these areas is due to the combined activities of streptolysin O and streptolysin S, the principal hemolysins of group A streptococci. Streptolysin O is oxygen-labile and does not show maximal activity on the surface of the agar; the surface β-hemolysis is largely due to streptolysin S, which is oxygen-stable.

G. Direct latex agglutination test for group A streptococci. Both latex agglutination and rapid enzyme immunoassays are currently available for the direct detection of group A streptococci in throat swab specimens. With the latex agglutination method shown here, the throat swab is enzymatically treated to extract the group A antigen and the extract is reacted with a latex bead suspension coated with anti–group A streptococcal antibodies and with a control, uncoated latex suspension. Agglutination of the latex with the test latex reagent (*left*) but not the control latex (*right*) is a positive test. Although most of these tests are highly specific for the group A cell wall antigen, the sensitivities of these assays vary widely.

H. Strep OIA (Biostar, Boulder, CO). The Strep OIA is an immunoassay for direct detection of group A streptococci in throat swab specimens. The swab is extracted with acetic acid, neutralized, and then mixed with anti–group A antibodies bound to horseradish peroxidase (HRP). A drop of this mixture is placed on the surface of an OIA slide, which is coated with anti–group A streptococcal antibodies. After a 2-minute incubation, the slide is rinsed and HRP substrate is added and allowed to react on the slide for 4 minutes. After rinsing, the slide is read by examining the hue of light reflected from the reaction area on the OIA slide. If group A streptococcal antigen is present, the slide shows a purple spot (*left*). If no antigen is present, the slide surface retains its gold color, with or without a tiny blue dot, as shown here (*right*).

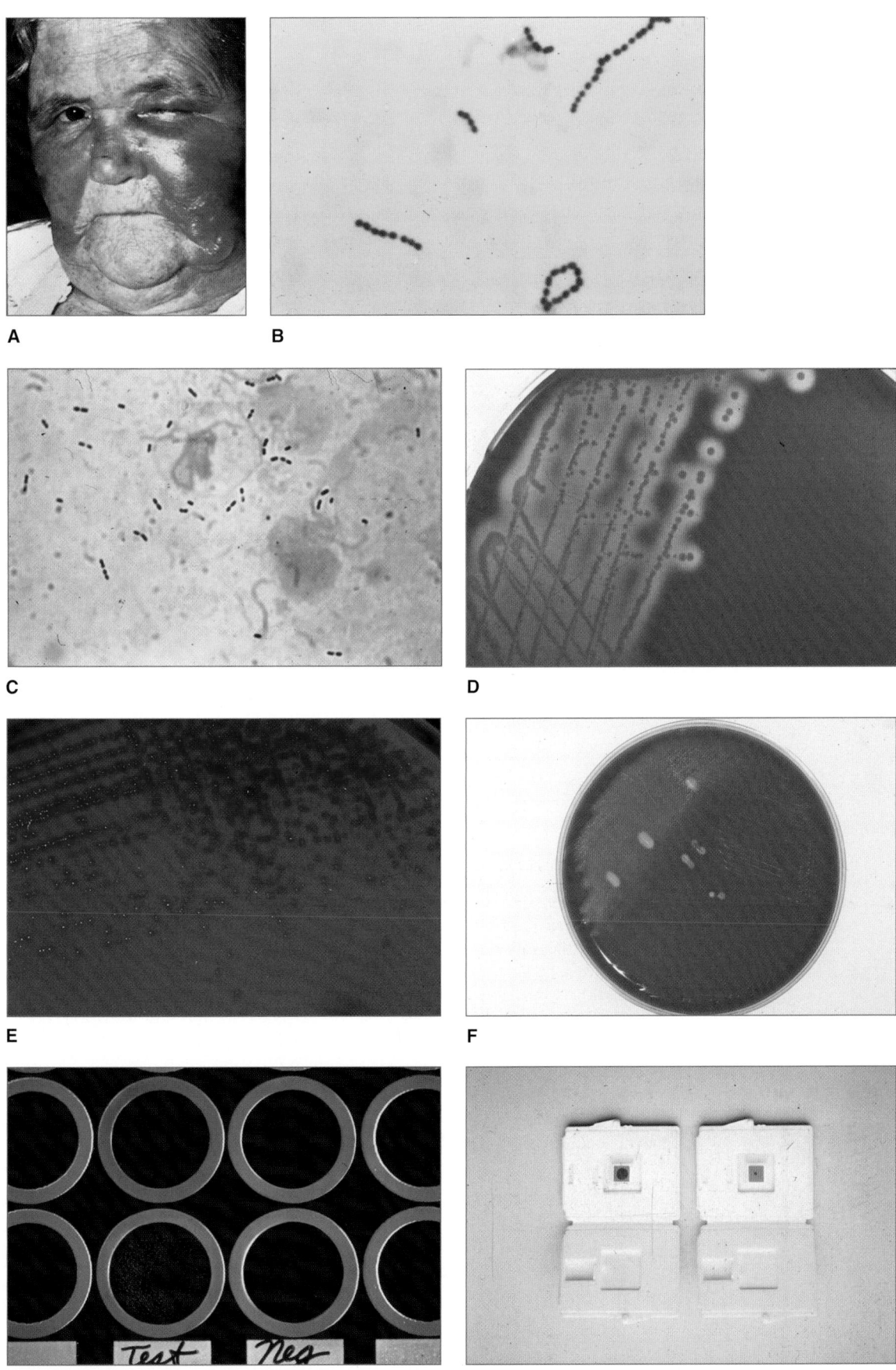

A

B

C

D

E

F

G

H

IDENTIFICATION OF STREPTOCOCCI AND ENTEROCOCCI

A. *S. pneumoniae* colonies on sheep blood agar. Two characteristics of *S. pneumoniae* can be used for presumptive identification. On the *left* is shown a typical α-hemolytic, mucoid strain of *S. pneumoniae* growing on sheep blood agar. Its appearance is due to the production of large amounts of capsular polysaccharide. On the *right* is a close-up photograph illustrating the collapse of the central portion of the colonies owing to organism autolysis, resulting in the so-called checker-piece and nail-head colony morphologies shown here.

B. Bacitracin susceptibility test. Group A streptococci are susceptible to low concentrations of bacitracin. The Taxo A bacitracin disk (BD Microbiology Systems) shown here contains 0.04 unit of bacitracin. This photograph shows the bacitracin test reactions for a group A β-hemolytic streptococcus (*left*) and a group B β-hemolytic streptococcus (*right*). Any zone of inhibition around the bacitracin disk is considered a positive test.

C. Susceptibility to bacitracin and sulfamethoxazole-trimethoprim. The β-hemolytic streptococcus shown here is susceptible to bacitracin (*right*), but also shows a large zone of growth inhibition around the sulfamethoxazole-trimethoprim (SXT) disk (*left*). Group A β-hemolytic streptococci are susceptible to bacitracin, but are resistant to SXT, while group B β-hemolytic streptococci are resistant to both bacitracin and SXT. Some non–group A β-hemolytic streptococci (e.g., groups C, F and G) are susceptible to bacitracin, but will also be susceptible to SXT, as shown here. Therefore, the performance of these two tests together increases the specificity of the presumptive identification that would be obtained by using the bacitracin test alone. This isolate would be called "presumptive β-hemolytic streptococcus, not groups A or B, by bacitracin/SXT."

D. CAMP test for presumptive identification of group B β-hemolytic streptococci. The CAMP test reaction depends on the interaction between CAMP factor, a product of the group B streptococcus, with the β-hemolysin of *Staphylococcus aureus*. Possible group B streptococci are streaked at right angles to a streak of *S. aureus* (without the streaks touching) on a sheep blood agar plate. Following overnight incubation at 35–37°C, an arrowhead-shaped area of synergistic hemolysis is found in the intersecting area where the CAMP factor and the β-hemolysin have diffused into the medium. Nonhemolytic variants of group B streptococci will also be CAMP test–positive. This photograph shows three positive CAMP tests.

E. Susceptibility to optochin for identification of *S. pneumoniae*. Susceptibility to ethyl hydrocuprene hydrochloride (optochin) is used to differentiate *S. pneumoniae* from other viridans streptococci. α-Hemolytic colonies are subcultured onto a sheep blood agar plate and an optochin disk (P disk; BD Microbiology Systems) is placed on the inoculum. The presence of a zone of growth inhibition of 14 mm around a 6-mm optochin disk after overnight incubation at 35–37°C identifies the organism as *S. pneumoniae*.

F. Bile-esculin hydrolysis and salt-tolerance tests. These tests are used for the presumptive identification of *Enterococcus* species and group D streptococci. The bile-esculin test (*right*) is performed by inoculating a slant of bile-esculin medium and incubating it overnight at 35–37°C. Enterococci and group D streptococci are able to grow in the presence of 40% bile and to hydrolyze esculin to esculetin (which forms the black precipitate). The salt-tolerance test (*left*) is performed with a broth medium containing 6.5% NaCl. *Enterococcus* species will grow, whereas nonenterococcal group D streptococci will not grow in this medium. The photograph shows a positive reaction for both tests, identifying this organism as a group D *Enterococcus* species.

G. PYR test. Hydrolysis of L-pyrrolidonyl-α-naphthylamide (PYR) is a presumptive test for identification of group A β-hemolytic streptococci and *Enterococcus* species that can replace the bacitracin-SXT disk tests and the salt-tolerance tests, respectively. In the disk test shown, colony growth is applied to a moistened disk impregnated with the PYR substrate. After 2 minutes, a drop of dimethylaminocinnamaldehyde reagent is placed on the disk to detect the free naphthylamide that is released on hydrolysis of PYR (*red*).

H. Tri-Plate for presumptive identification of streptococci. This single plate is designed to provide the results of several tests for the presumptive identification of streptococci and enterococci. The three sectors of the plate contain sheep blood agar, bile-esculin agar, and PYR agar, respectively. Determination of hemolysis and a CAMP test are performed in the blood agar sector, and the bile-esculin and PYR reactions are read in the other two sectors. This photograph shows the triplate inoculated with an *Enterococcus* species: α-hemolytic, CAMP test-negative, bile-esculin–-positive, and PYR-positive.

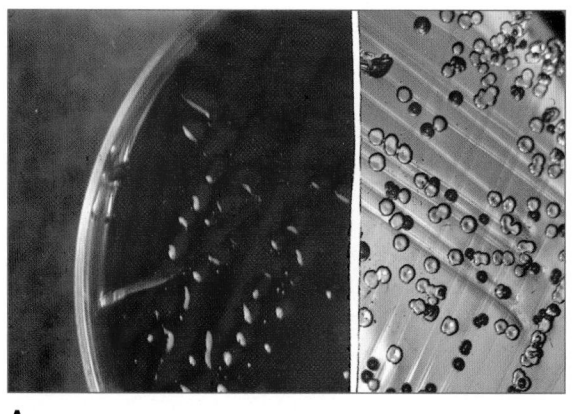

A

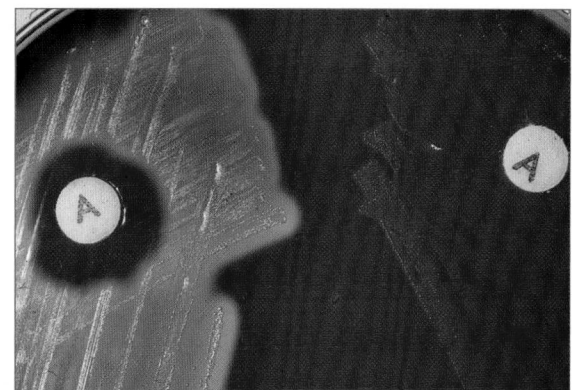

B

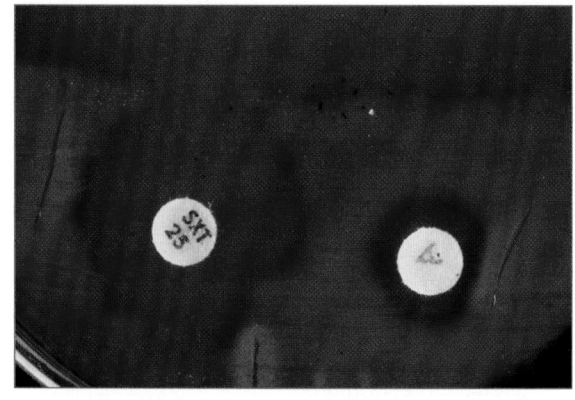

C

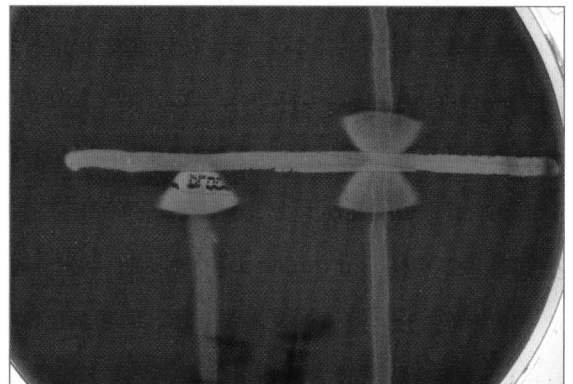

D

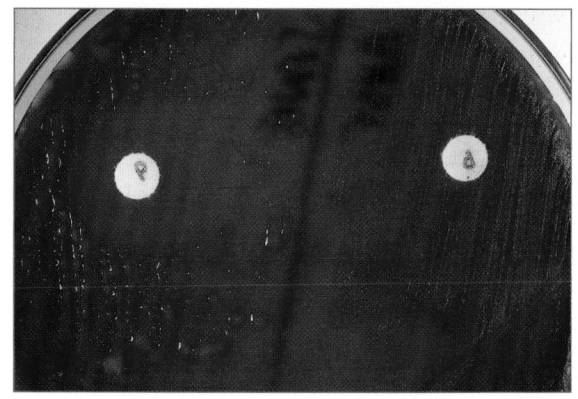

E

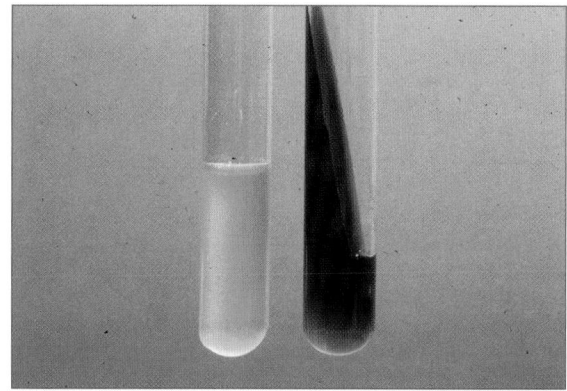

F

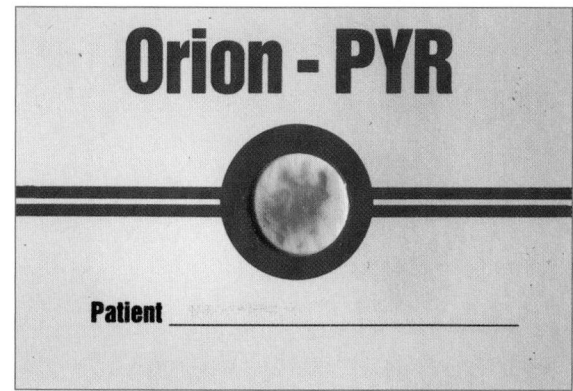

G

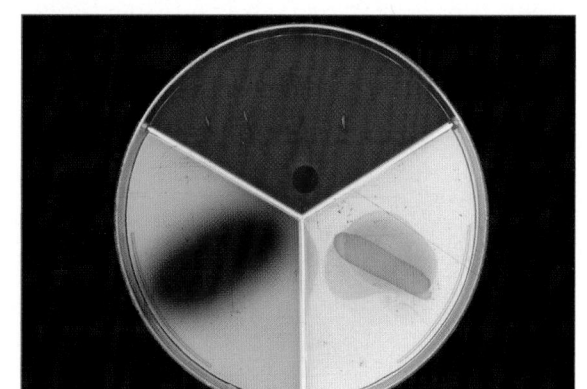

H

IDENTIFICATION OF STREPTOCOCCI AND ENTEROCOCCI AND STREPTOCOCCUS-LIKE BACTERIA

A. Latex agglutination test for serologic grouping of β-hemolytic streptococci. Although the Lance-field extraction method and the capillary precipitin tests are the time-honored techniques for definitive identification of the groupable streptococci, other methods, such as the one shown here, have been adopted in most laboratories and are considered standard procedures. In this test, the cell-wall grouping antigen is extracted from the bacterial cell wall enzymatically, and the extract is subsequently reacted with latex beads to which group-specific antibodies are bound. A positive test is indicated by agglutination of the latex beads in the homologous latex reagent. As shown here, agglutination has occurred with the group A reagent, but not with the group B, C, D, F, or G reagents, thereby identify the isolate as a group A β-hemolytic streptococcus.

B. Quellung test for identification of *S. pneumoniae*. This microscopic "precipitin test" can be used to identify pneumococci or to determine the capsular serotype of individual pneumococcal iso-lates. Reaction of the anticapsular antibodies with the carbohydrate material of the capsule causes a microprecipitin reaction on the surface of the organism and a change in the refractive index of the capsule itself. Microscopically, the capsule appears to "swell." A small amount of methylene blue is added to the preparation to allow visualization of the cells and to provide contrast so that subtle refractile changes in the capsule can be more easily discerned.

C. Pneumoslide latex agglutination test (BD Microbiology Systems). The Pneumoslide test uses la-tex beads that are sensitized with antipneumococcal antibodies. Mixture of the sensitized latex with colony material from a culture plate results in visible agglutination of the suspension, thereby identifying the isolate as *S. pneumoniae*.

D. *Abiotrophia/Granulicatella* species. These organisms were formerly called satelliting or nutri-tionally variant streptococci because they require thiol compounds, cysteine, or the active form of vitamin B_6 (pyridoxal or pyridoxamine) for growth on media. This requirement may be met by cross-streaking a staphylococcus across an inoculum of the probable nutritionally variant isolate, as shown in this photograph. The small colonies of the organism are observed growing adjacent to the staphylococcus streak following incubation in a manner similar to the satellite test for pre-sumptive identification of *Haemophilus* species. Members of the satelliting streptococci have now been placed in either the genus *Abiotrophia* or the genus *Granulicatella*.

E. *Enterococcus faecium*. This photograph shows a sheep blood agar plate inoculated with *E. fae-cium*. Colonies of this organism are smooth, gray, and nonhemolytic or α-hemolytic. The swab, which was used to pick up some of the colony growth from the plate, shows that the organism is nonpigmented. This becomes important for the identification of certain other enterococcal species.

F. API Strep identification panel (BioMérieux) inoculated with *E. faecium*. This photograph shows the first half of the identification panel. Interpretations of the reactions shown are as follows:

VP	Positive	HIP	Negative	ESC	Positive
PYRA	Positive	α-GAL	Positive	β-GUR	Negative
β-GAL	Positive	PAL	Negative	LAP	Positive

G. API Strep identification panel inoculated with *E. faecium*. This photograph shows the second half of the identification panel. Interpretations of the reactions shown are as follows:

ADH	Positive	RIB	Positive	ARA	Positive
MAN	Positive	SOR	Positive	LAC	Positive
TRE	Positive	INU	Negative	RAF	Positive
AMD	Negative	GLYG	Negative	HEM	Negative

The API biocode for the reactions shown in Color Plate 13-3*F* and *G* is 5357750. Consultation with the API computer-assisted database provides an identification of *E. faecium*, with 99% likelihood.

H. Vancomycin screening agar. Vancomycin screening agar consists of brain-heart infusion agar con-taining vancomycin (6 μg/mL). This medium can be used to detect vancomycin-resistant entero-cocci, the majority of which are *E. faecium*. As shown in this photograph, isolates A, B, C, and D are vancomycin-resistant and are able to grow on this medium. Isolate E is a strain of *E. faecalis*, most of which are vancomycin-susceptible, as indicated by growth inhibition on this medium.

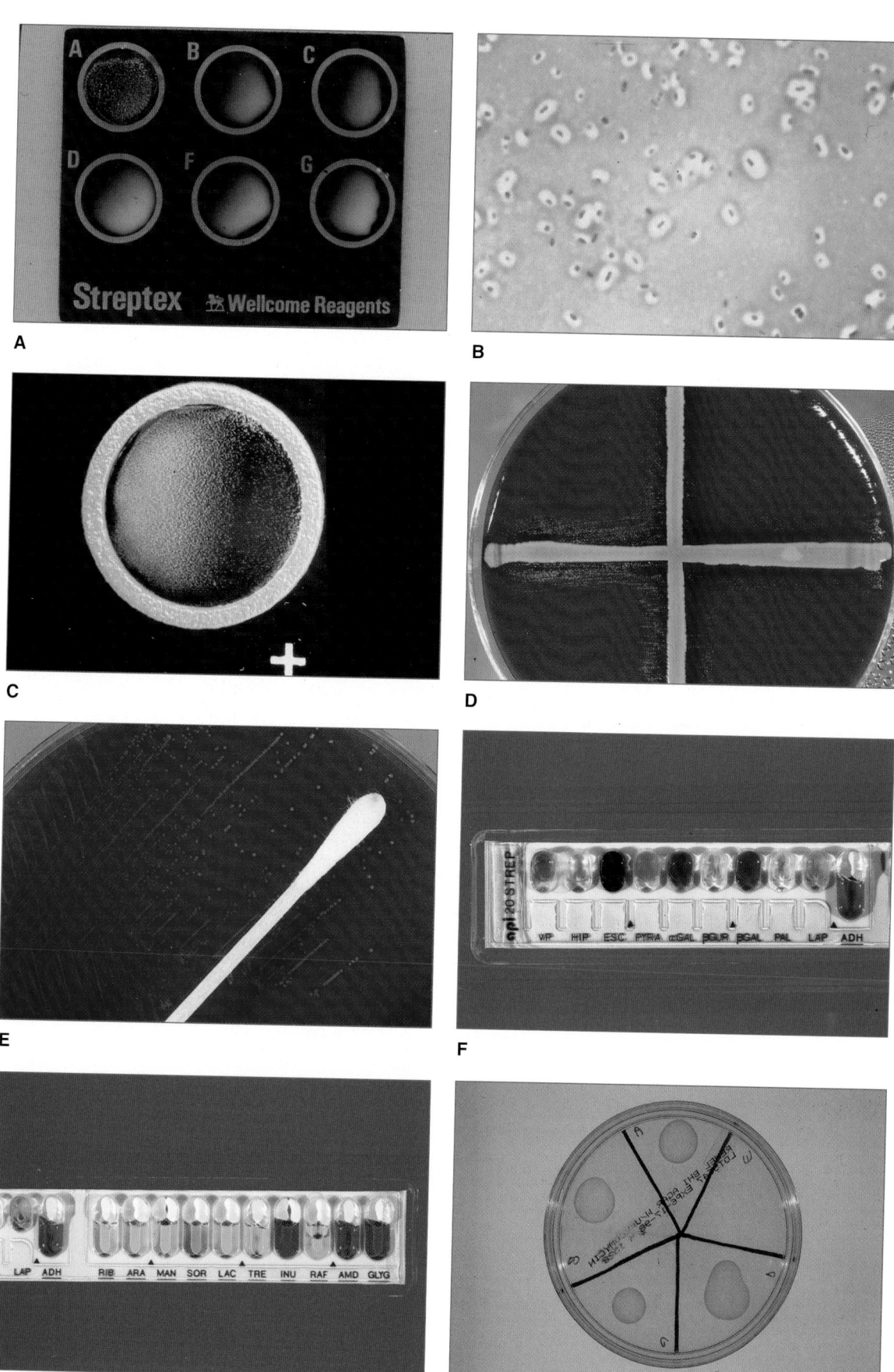

A

B

C

D

E

F

G

H

IDENTIFICATION OF ENTEROCOCCI AND VIRIDANS GROUP STREPTOCOCCI

A. *Enterococcus casseliflavus* on sheep blood agar. *E. casseliflavus* is one of two motile *Enterococcus* species. In addition, *E. casseliflavus* produces a yellow pigment. This pigment is evident on inspection of the swab in the photograph, which has been used to pick up some of the colony growth.

B. *Enterococcus gallinarum* in semisolid motility agar. As mentioned above, *E. gallinarum* and *E. casseliflavus* are the two motile *Enterococcus* species. In this photograph, *E. gallinarum* has been stab-inoculated into a tube of semisolid motility medium containing tetrazolium. On incubation of the inoculated tube, the motile organisms move out from the streak line to create turbidity in the medium. The purple color results from the motile organisms reducing the tetrazolium to formazan, which appears as a purple precipitate anywhere that viable organisms are found.

C. *Streptococcus bovis* on sheep blood agar. *S. bovis* is a nonenterococcal group D streptococcus. This organism is bile-esculin–positive, but does not grow in 6.5% NaCl broth and is PYR-negative. Isolation of *S. bovis* from blood cultures is associated with colonic neoplasia.

D. API Strep identification panel inoculated with *S. bovis*. This photograph shows the first half of the identification panel. The interpretations of the reactions shown are:

VP	Positive	HIP	Negative	ESC	Positive
PYRA	Negative	α-GAL	Positive	β-GUR	Negative
β-GAL	Positive	PAL	Negative	LAP	Positive

E. API Strep identification panel inoculated with *S. bovis*. This photograph shows the second half of the identification panel. The interpretations of the reactions shown are:

ADH	Negative	RIB	Negative	ARA	Negative
MAN	Positive	SOR	Negative	LAC	Positive
TRE	Positive	INU	Positive	RAF	Positive
AMD	Positive	GLYG	Positive	βHEM	Negative

The API biocode for the reactions shown in Color Plate 13-4D and E is 5250573. Consultation with the API computer-assisted database provides an identification of this isolate as *S. bovis* I (99.9% probability). According to the new nomenclature for this organism complex, *S. bovis* I is now called *Streptococcus gallolyticus* subsp. *gallolyticus* (Table 13-7).

F. *Streptococcus mitis* growing on sheep blood agar after 24 hours of incubation. This particular isolate appears to be γ-hemolytic or nonhemolytic. Other strains of this species may be α-hemolytic.

G. API Strep identification panel inoculated with *S. mitis*. This photograph shows the first half of the identification panel. Interpretations of the reactions are as follows:

VP	Negative	HIP	Negative	ESC	Negative
PYRA	Negative	α-GAL	Negative	β-GUR	Negative
β-GAL	Negative	PAL	Positive	LAP	Positive

H. API Strep identification panel inoculated with *S. mitis*. This photograph shows the second half of the identification panel. The interpretations of the reactions are as follows:

ADH	Negative	RIB	Negative	ARA	Negative
MAN	Negative	SOR	Negative	LAC	Positive
TRE	Positive	INU	Negative	RAF	Negative
AMD	Positive	GLYG	Negative	βHEM	Negative

The biocode for the reactions shown in Color Plate 13-4G and H is 0060411. Consultation with the API computer-assisted database provides an identification of *S. mitis* (80%)/*oralis* (20%). *S. mitis* and *S. oralis* belong to the "mitis group" of viridans streptococci. Some isolates of *S. mitis* have been shown to be resistant to penicillin and may be resistant to other antimicrobial agents as well.

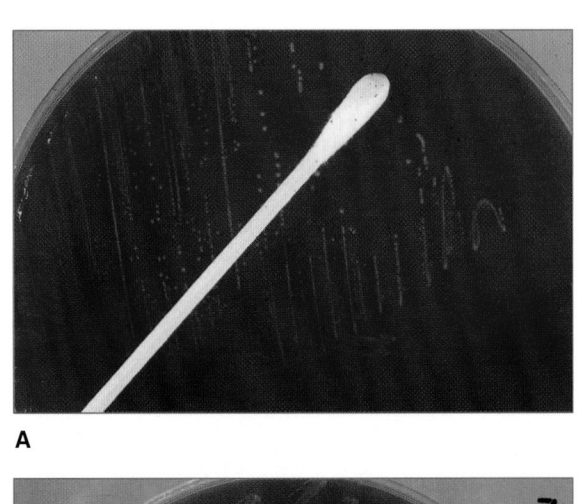

A

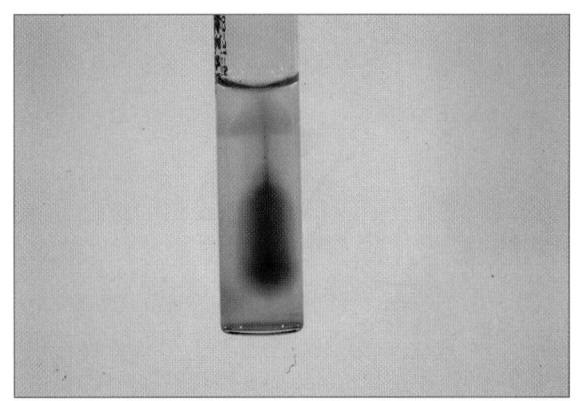

B

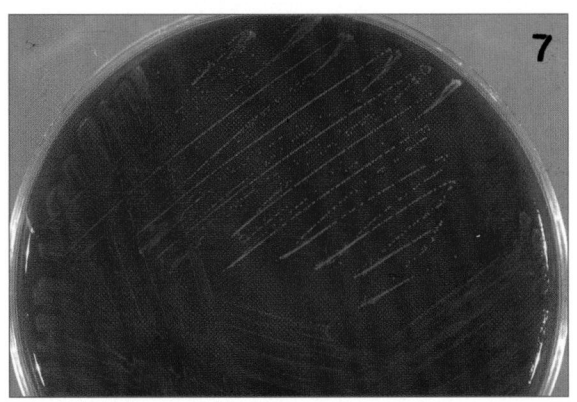

C

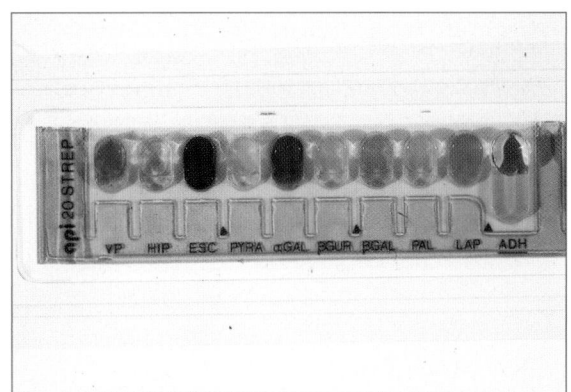

D

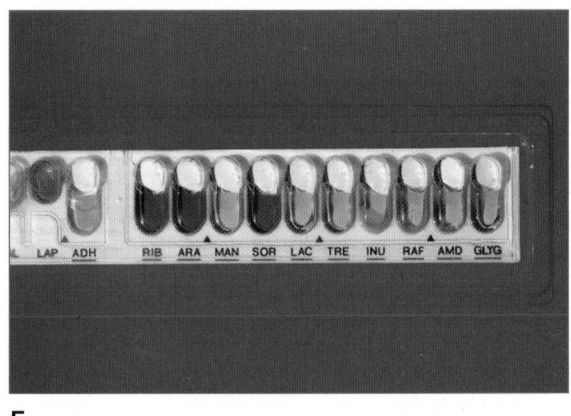

E

F

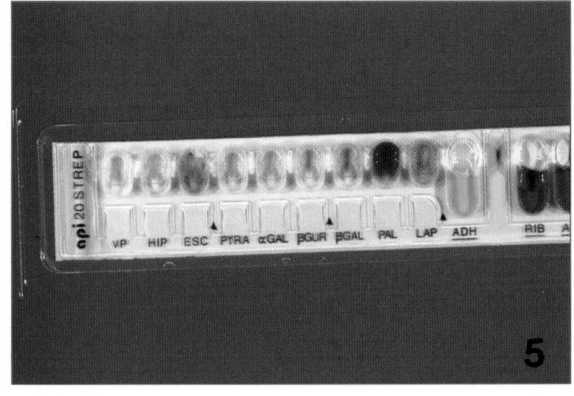

G

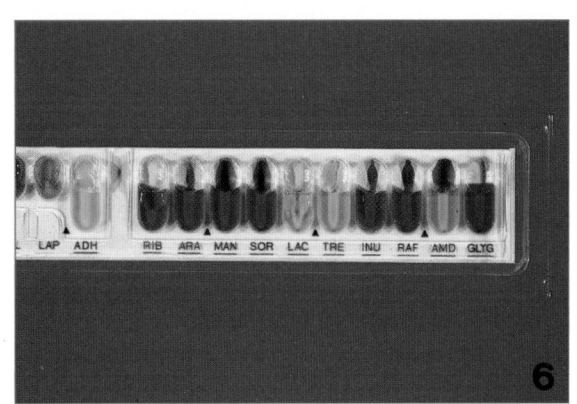

H

LISTERIA AND ERYSIPELOTHRIX SPECIES

A. Gram-stained smear of *Listeria monocytogenes*, showing short, gram-positive bacilli.

B. Small, β-hemolytic colonies of *L. monocytogenes* on sheep blood agar (SBA) after 72 hours of incubation at 35–37°C.

C. *L. monocytogenes* growing on SBA after 24 hours (*left*) and 48 hours (*right*) of incubation. After 24 hours, the β-hemolytic nature of the organism may not be obvious. After 48 hours, the zone of hemolysis extends beyond the margin of the colony, but is still rather subtle.

D. *L. monocytogenes* on bile-esculin agar (right). The tube on the left is an uninoculated bile-esculin agar slant. Like the enterococci, *L. monocytogenes* is able to hydrolyze esculin in the presence of 40% bile. Esculin hydrolysis is indicated by blackening of the medium.

E. Umbrella-shaped zone of motile growth produced *by Listeria monocytogenes* after 24 hours of growth in semisolid motility medium at 25°C.

F. API Coryne inoculated with *Listeria monocytogenes*. The API biocode of the isolate shown is 0170164. Consultation with the API Profile Index provides an identification as "*Listeria monocytogenes/innocua*, 97.1% likelihood." Differentiation of *L. monocytogenes* and *L. innocua* is determined by assessment of hemolysis on sheep blood agar and by reactivity of *L. monocytogenes* in the CAMP test with *S. aureus*.

G. Gram-stained smear of *Erysipelothrix rhusiopathiae*, showing the long, thin, gram-positive rods of this species.

H. Colonies of *Erysipelothrix rhusiopathiae* on SBA after 24 hours of incubation at 35°C.

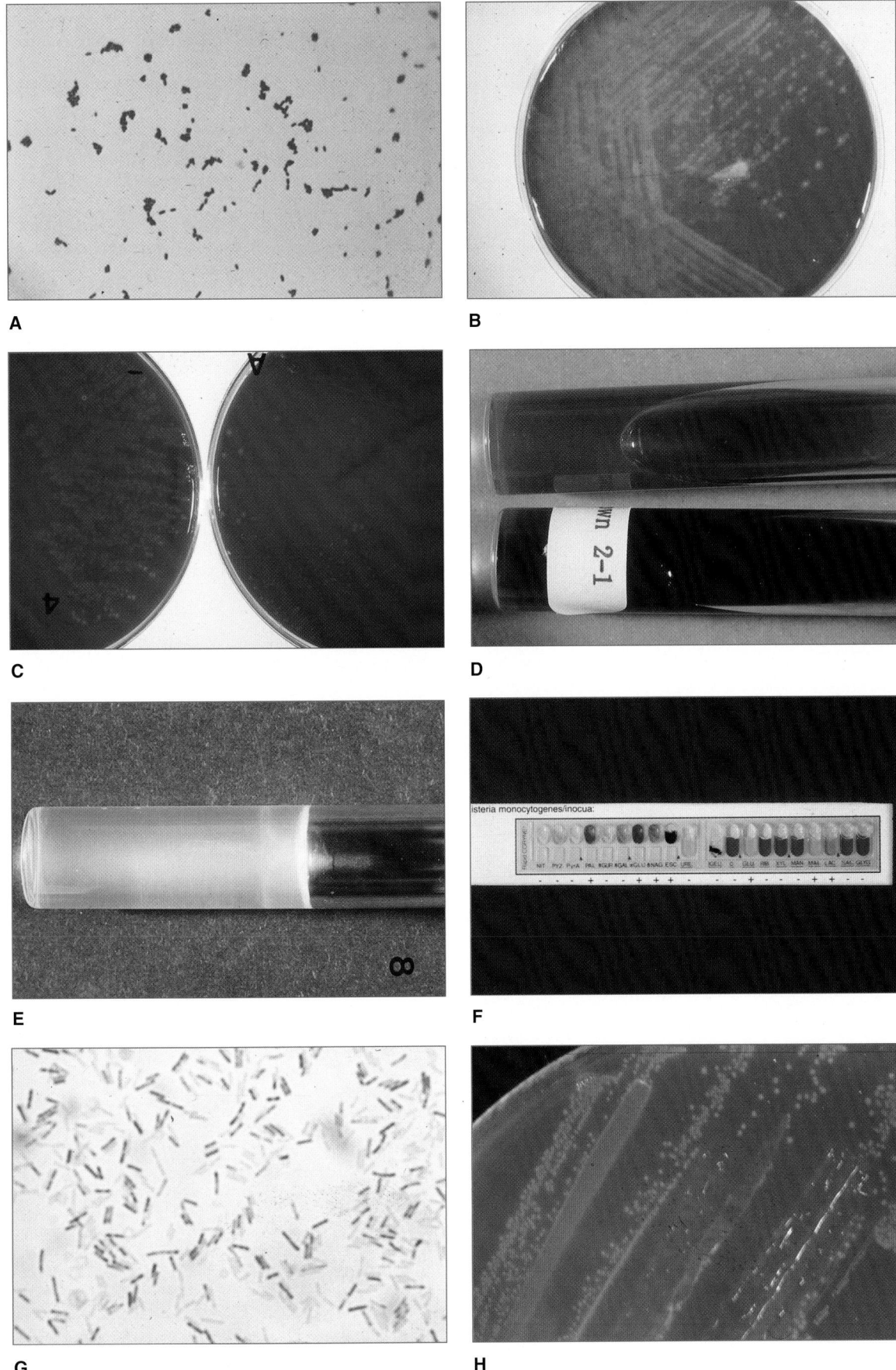

A

B

C

D

E

F

G

H

ERYSIPELOTHRIX AND *BACILLUS* SPECIES

A. *Erysipelothrix rhusiopathiae* after overnight growth in a streak-and-stab inoculated tube of Kligler's iron agar. Note the production of H_2S along the line of the stab in the butt of the tube.

B. Gram-stained smear of a *Bacillus* species. Note the presence of central/subterminal, nonstaining endospores that do not swell the cell.

C. Gross specimen of intestinal tract from a patient who died of gastrointestinal anthrax. The appendix is noted in the lower left portion of the photograph. Lesions of gastrointestinal anthrax are usually noted in the cecum and adjacent areas of the bowel. Symptoms include abdominal pain, hematemesis, and bloody diarrhea.

D. Gram stain (*left*) and malachite-green spore stain (*right*) of *B. anthracis*. *B. anthracis* grows as rather large gram-positive bacilli, with the individual cells having squared-off or slightly concave ends. Often the organisms are arranged in chains that have the appearance of bamboo as depicted here. The spore stain shows the ovoid spores that do not swell the cell. (Courtesy of Elmer W. Koneman.)

E. Off-white, dull, nonhemolytic colonies of *Bacillus anthracis* on SBA.

F. Close-up of *B. anthracis* colonies on SBA. Colonies of *B. anthracis* have a ground-glass morphology with comma-shaped outgrowths along the colony margins as shown here. These outgrowths are even more apparent microscopically. Such colonies have been described as "Medusa-head" colonies, after the Greek sorceress who had hair composed of serpents. (Courtesy of Elmer W. Koneman.)

G. Close-up of the rough, nonhemolytic colonies of *B. anthracis*. A few of the colonies have been touched with an inoculating loop, resulting in the colonies "standing up" like beaten egg whites.

H. Large, β-hemolytic colonies of *Bacillus cereus* on SBA. *B. cereus* is one of the more frequently isolated *Bacillus* species in the clinical laboratory. Unlike *B. anthracis*, this species is β-hemolytic, motile, and β-lactamase-positive

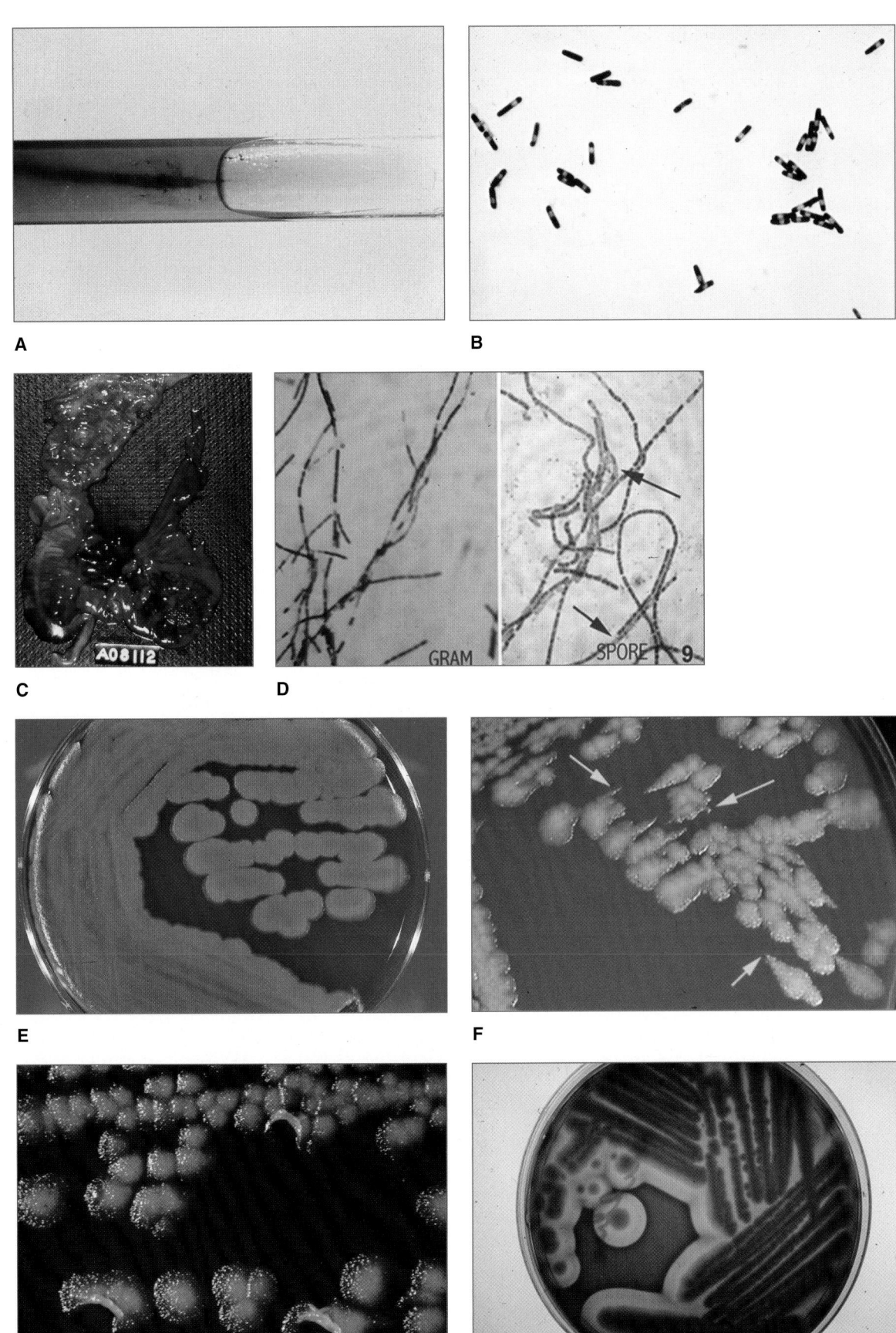

A

B

C

D

E

F

G

H

CORYNEBACTERIUM SPECIES

A. Gram-stained smear showing the typical morphology of members of the genus *Corynebacterium*. Regularly shaped rods, club-shaped bacilli, "Chinese-letter" and "picket-fence" cellular arrangements can be observed in this photograph.

B. BHI agar inoculated with a lipophilic and a nonlipophilic *Corynebacterium* species. On the right side of the plate, a lipophilic species has been inoculated as a lawn on the plate, and a drop of 0.1% Tween 80 has been placed in the center of the inoculum. A nonlipophilic *Corynebacterium* species is inoculated as a lawn on the left half of the plate. After incubation for 24 hours at 35–37°C, growth of the lipophilic species is only observed where the drop of Tween 80 was placed, while the nonlipophilic species grows all over the surface of the medium on the right side of the plate.

C. *Corynebacterium amycolatum* growing on SBA after 3 days of incubation at 35°C. Note the dry, matte appearance of the colonies and the "wrinkling" of the growth in confluent areas. *C. amycolatum* is the most frequently isolated *Corynebacterium* species and is found on the skin.

D. API Coryne panel inoculated with *Corynebacterium amycolatum*. The photograph shows first half of the identification panel. The interpretations of the reactions shown are:

NIT	Positive	PYZ	Positive	PYRA	Negative
PAL	Positive	β-GUR	Negative	β-GAL	Negative
α-GLU	Negative	β-NAG	Negative	ESC	Negative
URE	Negative				

E. API Coryne panel inoculated with *Corynebacterium amycolatum*. This photograph shows the second half of the identification panel The interpretations of the reactions shown are:

GEL	Negative	CHO Control	Negative		
GLU	Positive	RIB	Positive	XYL	Negative
MAN	Negative	MAL	Negative	LAC	Negative
SAC	Positive	GLYG	Negative	CAT	Positive

The API Coryne biocode for the reactions shown in Color Plate 14-3D and E is 3100305, which gives a cross-call identification of *Corynebacterium* group G, *C. striatum*, or *C. amycolatum*. *C. amycolatum* is nonlipophilic, while group G coryneform strains are lipophilic, so this isolate is not a group G coryneform. Additional tests (e.g., gas-liquid chromatography of glucose broth cultures), are needed to differentiate *Corynebacterium amycolatum* and *Corynebacterium striatum* from one another. This isolate produced propionic acid from glucose as determined by gas-liquid chromatographic analysis of culture broth, so this organism can be identified as *C. amycolatum*.

F. Local inflammation and pseudomembrane formation in the oropharynx produced by toxigenic strains of *Corynebacterium diphtheriae*.

G. Growth of *Corynebacterium diphtheriae* on modified Tinsdale agar. On this medium, *C. diphtheriae* grows as black colonies with brown halos. Isolates with this colonial morphology are first identified biochemically as *C. diphtheriae*, and subsequent testing involves demonstrating the production of diphtheria toxin.

H. Growth of *C. diphtheriae* from Loeffler's coagulated serum medium. This medium is inoculated with material from the posterior pharynx (i.e., the diphtheritic pseudomembrane), and a smear is prepared after about 8 hours of incubation and stained with methylene blue. As shown here, *C. diphtheriae* appears as pleomorphic beaded bacilli. The beaded appearance is due to the production of metachromatic granules by the organism on this medium.

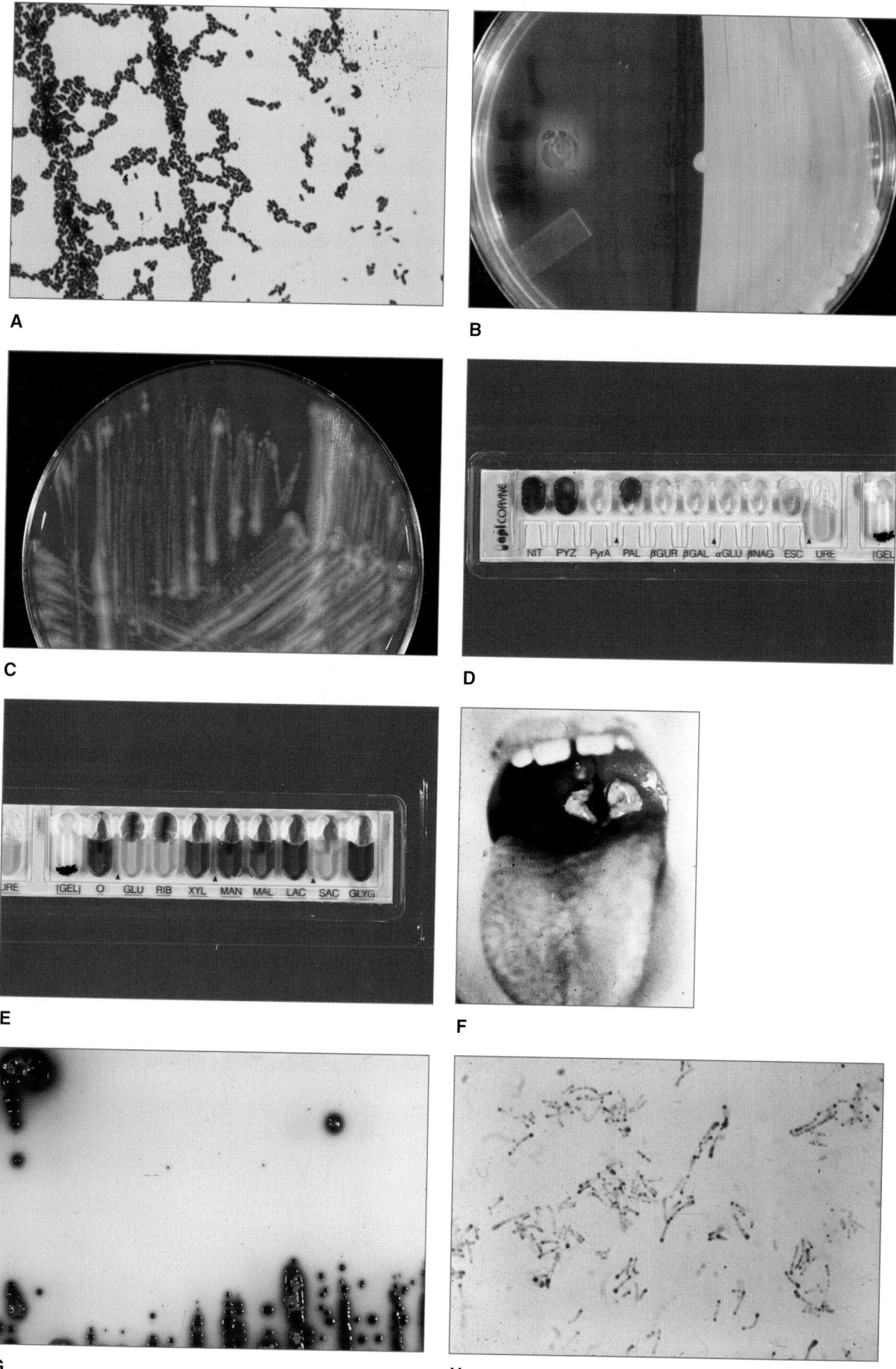

A

B

C

D

E

F

G

H

CORYNEBACTERIUM SPECIES (*CONTINUED*)

A. Growth of *C. diphtheriae* on SBA after 24 hours of incubation at 35°C. Colonies of this organism are nonlipophilic, white, and creamy. This isolate was inoculated onto the API Coryne identification kit, and the biochemical reactions for identification are shown in **B** and **C** below.

B. API Coryne inoculated with *C. diphtheriae*. This photograph shows the first half of the identification panel. The interpretations of the reactions shown are:

NIT	Positive	PYZ	Negative	PYRA	Negative
PAL	Negative	β-GUR	Negative	β-GAL	Negative
α-GLU	Positive	β-NAG	Negative	ESC	Negative
URE	Negative				

C. API Coryne inoculated with *C. diphtheriae*. This photograph shows the other half of the identification panel. The interpretations of the reactions shown are:

GEL	Negative	CHO Control	Negative		
GLU	Positive	RIB	Negative	XYL	Negative
MAN	Negative	MAL	Positive	LAC	Negative
SAC	Negative	GLYG	Negative	CAT	Positive

The API Coryne biocode for these reactions is 1010124, which corresponds to an identification of *Corynebacterium diphtheriae* (97.8% probability). Additional testing must be performed to determine whether the isolate produces diphtheria toxin.

D. *Corynebacterium jeikeium* on SBA after 48 hours of incubation at 35–37°C. This lipophilic species produces small, nonhemolytic colonies on SBA.

E. API Coryne inoculated with *Corynebacterium jeikeium*. This photograph shows the first half of the identification panel. The interpretations of the reactions shown are:

NIT	Negative	PYZ	Positive	PYRA	Negative
PAL	Positive	β-GUR	Negative	β-GAL	Negative
α-GLU	Negative	β-NAG	Negative	ESC	Negative
URE	Negative				

F. API Coryne inoculated with *C. jeikeium*. This photograph shows the second half of the identification panel. The interpretations of the reactions shown are:

GEL	Negative	CHO Control	Negative		
GLU	Positive	RIB	Positive	XYL	Negative
MAN	Negative	MAL	Negative	LAC	Negative
SAC	Negative	GLYG	Negative	CAT	Negative

The API Coryne biocode for these reactions is 2100304, which corresponds to an identification of *C. jeikeium* (93.6% probability).

G. Gram-stained smear showing the rather plump, gram-positive bacilli of *Corynebacterium glucuronolyticum* ("*C. seminale*").

H. *C. glucuronolyticum* on SBA after 24 hours of incubation at 35–37°C.

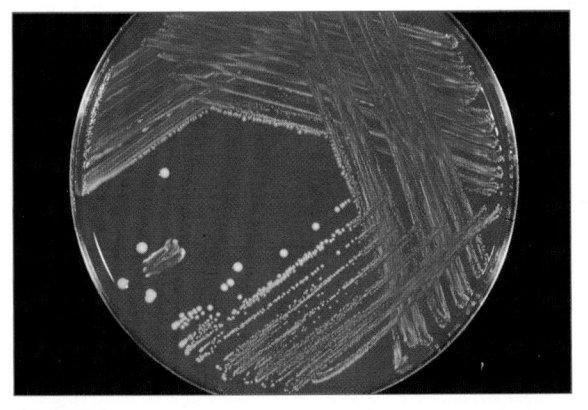

A

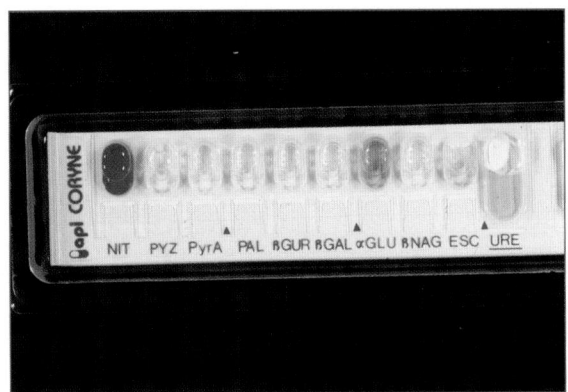

B

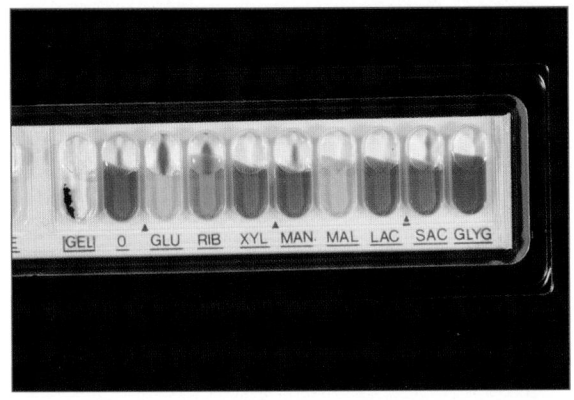

C

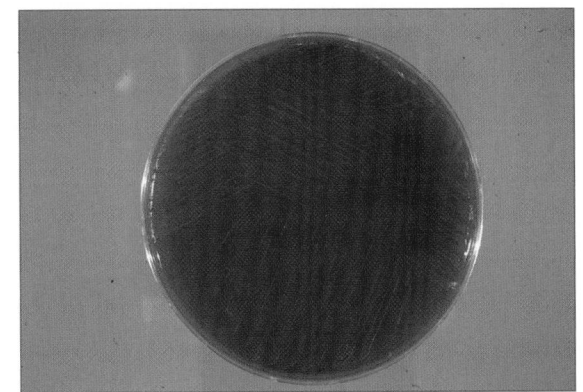

D

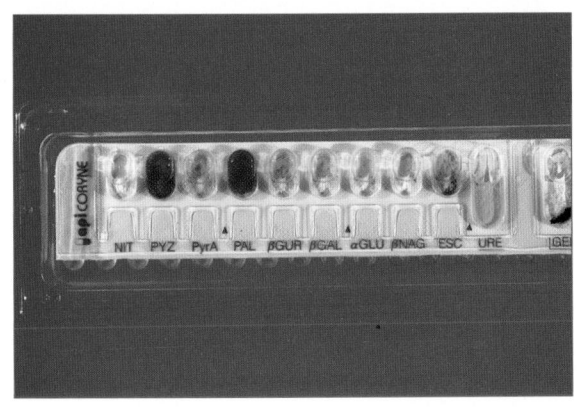

E

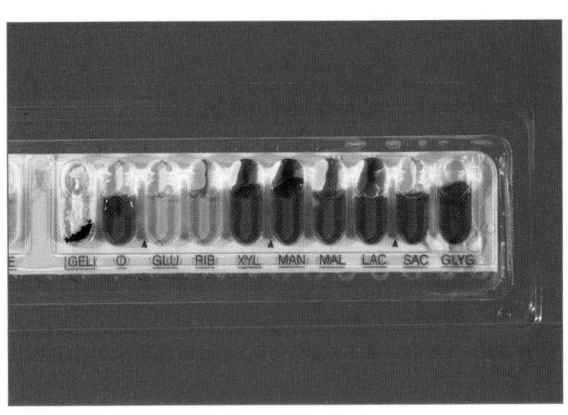

F

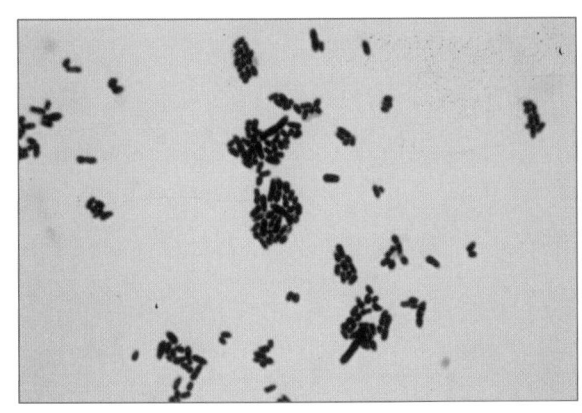

G

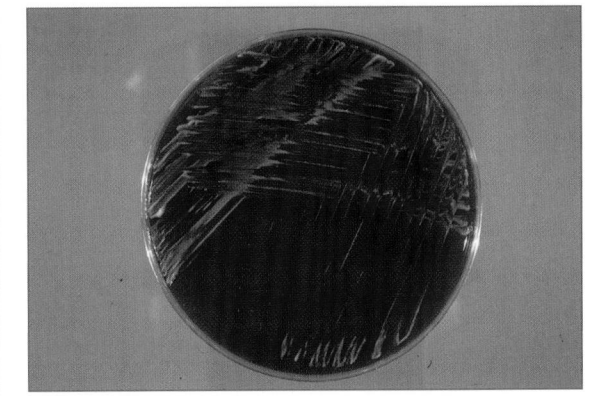

H

CORYNEBACTERIUM SPECIES (*CONTINUED*)

A. API Coryne inoculated with *C. glucuronolyticum*. This photograph shows the first half of the identification panel. The interpretations of the reactions shown are:

NIT	Negative	PYZ	Positive	PYRA	Negative
PAL	Negative	β-GUR	Positive	β-GAL	Negative
α-GLU	Negative	β-NAG	Negative	ESC	Positive
URE	Positive				

B. API Coryne inoculated with *C. glucuronolyticum*. This photograph shows the second half of the identification panel. The interpretations of the reactions shown are:

GEL	Negative	CHO Control	Negative		
GLU	Positive	RIB	Negative	XYL	Negative
MAN	Negative	MAL	Positive	LAC	Negative
SAC	Positive	GLYG	Negative	CAT	Positive

The API biocode for these reactions is 2241125, which corresponds to an identification of *C. glucuronolyticum* (99.9% probability). This species has been recovered from semen specimens and is the only *Corynebacterium* species that is β-glucuronidase (β-GUR)-positive. This species was also described by another research group and was given the name "*C. seminale*." However, the name "*C. glucuronolyticum*" has taxonomic precedence.

C. Creamy, smooth, nonlipophilic, nonhemolytic colonies of *Corynebacterium pseudodiphtheriticum* growing on SBA after 24 hours at 35–37°C.

D. API Coryne inoculated with *Corynebacterium pseudodiphtheriticum*. The interpretations of the reactions shown are:

NIT	Positive	PYZ	Positive	PYRA	Negative
PAL	Negative	β-GUR	Negative	β-GAL	Negative
α-GLU	Negative	β-NAG	Negative	ESC	Negative
URE	Positive	GEL	Negative	CHO Control	Negative
GLU	Negative	RIB	Negative	XYL	Negative
MAN	Negative	MAL	Negative	LAC	Negative
SAC	Negative	GLYG	Negative	CAT	Positive

The API Coryne biocode for these reactions is 3001004, which corresponds to an identification of *C. pseudodiphtheriticum* (96.7% probability).

E. Creamy, nonlipophilic, nonhemolytic colonies of *C. riegelii* on SBA after 24 hours of incubation at 35–37°C.

F. Rapid urease reaction of *C. riegelii*. *C. riegelii*, like *C. urealyticum*, is rapidly urease-positive. This photograph shows an uninoculated urea agar slant (*top*) and a urea agar slant inoculated with *C. riegelii* (*bottom*). This reaction was photographed after the slant on the right was incubated for 30 minutes at 35–37°C.

G. API Coryne inoculated with *C. riegelii*. This photograph shows the first half of the identification panel. The interpretations of the reactions shown are:

NIT	Negative	PYZ	Positive	PYRA	Negative
PAL	Negative	β-GUR	Negative	β-GAL	Negative
α-GLU	Negative	β-NAG	Negative	ESC	Negative
URE	Positive				

H. API Coryne inoculated with *C. riegelii*. This photograph shows the second half of the identification panel. The interpretations of the reactions shown are:

GEL	Negative	CHO Control	Negative		
GLU	Negative	RIB	Positive	XYL	Negative
MAN	Negative	MAL	Positive	LAC	Negative
SAC	Negative	GLYG	Negative	CAT	Positive

The API biocode for these reactions is 2001204. This biocode is not included in the API Coryne database at present, but it is the same biocode that was published with the original description of this new species. *C. riegelii* is associated with urinary tract infections. Besides being rapidly urease-positive, this species is also atypical in that it produces acid from maltose and ribose, but not from glucose, as shown here.

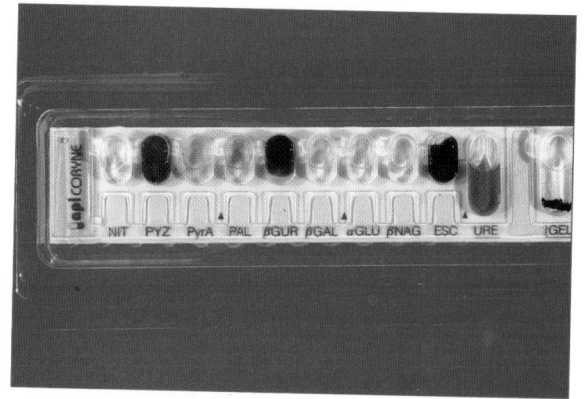

A

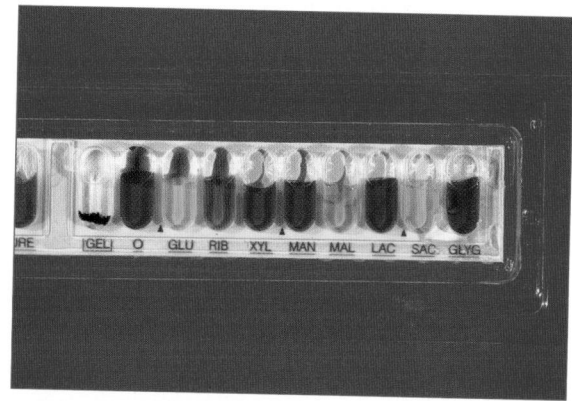

B

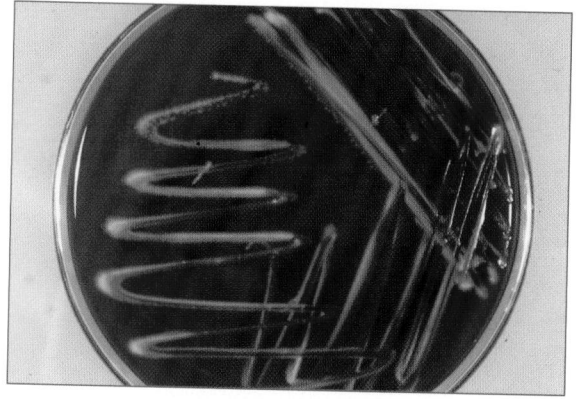

C

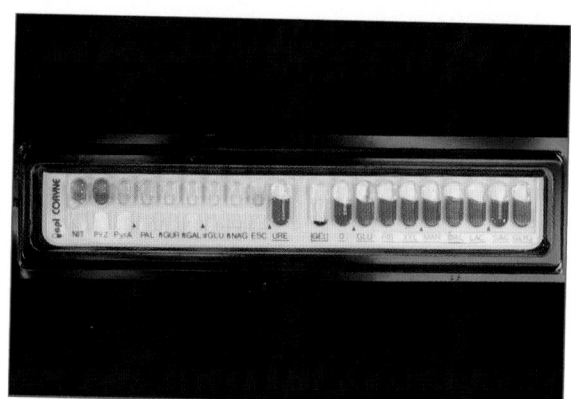

D

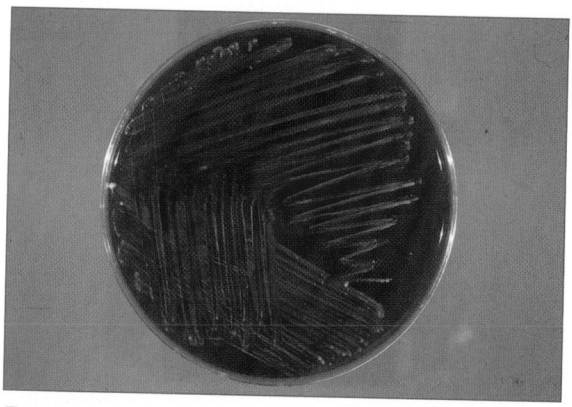

E

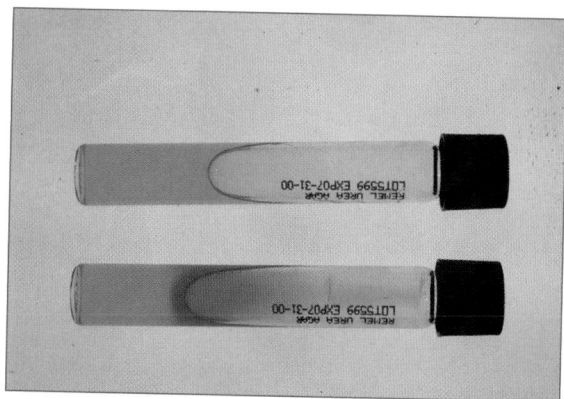

F

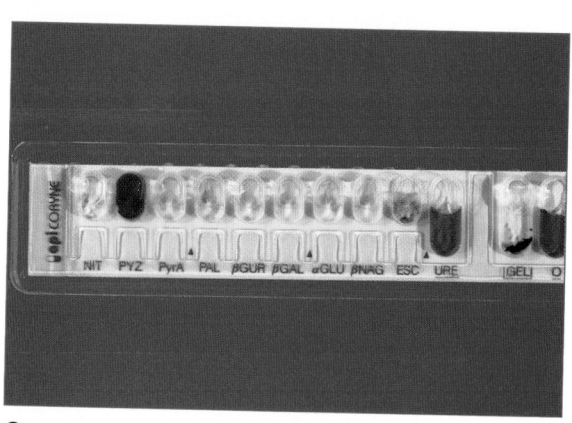

G

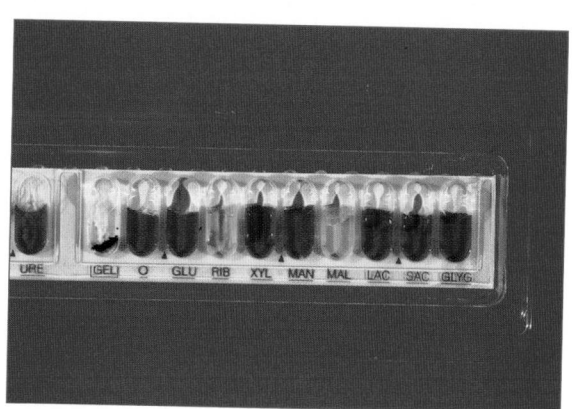

H

CORYNEBACTERIUM, ARCANOBACTERIUM, AND *BREVIBACTERIUM* SPECIES

A. Creamy, nonlipophilic, nonhemolytic colonies of *Corynebacterium striatum* on SBA after 48 hours of incubation at 35–37°C. Note the "target" morphology of the individual colonies.

B. API Coryne inoculated with *C. striatum.* The interpretations of the reactions shown are:

NIT	Positive	PYZ	Positive	PYRA	Negative
PAL	Positive	β-GUR	Negative	β-GAL	Negative
α-GLU	Negative	β-NAG	Negative	ESC	Negative
URE	Negative	GEL	Negative	CHO Control	Negative
GLU	Positive	RIB	Negative	XYL	Negative
MAN	Negative	MAL	Negative	LAC	Negative
SAC	Positive	GLYG	Negative	CAT	Positive

The API Coryne biocode for these reactions is 3100105, which corresponds to an identification of *Corynebacterium* group G, 55.5%/*C. striatum-amycolatum,* 43.6%. Since group G strains are lipophilic, this organism is either *C. striatum* or *C. amycolatum.* This isolate did not produce propionic acid from glucose on gas-liquid chromatographic analysis, so this isolate is identified as *C. striatum.*

C. *Corynebacterium* group G after 24 hours of incubation at 35–37°C. After 24 hours, individual colonies are extremely small, with good growth occurring only in the heavily inoculated areas. This lipophilic species has been isolated from vitreous, blood, cerebrospinal fluid, and urogenital tract specimens.

D. API Coryne inoculated with *Corynebacterium* group G. The interpretations of the reactions shown are as follows:

NIT	Negative	PYZ	Positive	PYRA	Negative
PAL	Positive	β-GUR	Negative	β-GAL	Negative
α-GLU	Negative	β-NAG	Negative	ESC	Negative
URE	Negative	GEL	Negative	CHO Control	Negative
GLU	Positive	RIB	Positive	XYL	Negative
MAN	Negative	MAL	Positive	LAC	Negative
SAC	Positive	GLYG	Negative	CAT	Positive

The API biocode for these reactions is 2100325. Consultation with the computer-assisted database provides an identification of *Corynebacterium* group G (76.6% likelihood)/*C. striatum/amycolatum* (22.7% likelihood). Since this organism is lipophilic and both *C. striatum* and *C. amycolatum* are nonlipophilic, this isolate can be identified as *Corynebacterium* group G.

E. Growth of *Arcanobacterium haemolyticum* on SBA after 48 hours of incubation at 35–37°C. Note the zone of β-hemolysis surrounding the colonies.

F. API Coryne inoculated with *A. haemolyticum.* The interpretations of the reactions shown are:

NIT	Negative	PYZ	Positive	PYRA	Positive
PAL	Positive	β-GUR	Negative	β-GAL	Positive
α-GLU	Positive	β-NAG	Positive	ESC	Negative
URE	Negative	GEL	Negative	CHO Control	Negative
GLU	Positive	RIB	Positive	XYL	Negative
MAN	Negative	MAL	Positive	LAC	Positive
SAC	Negative	GLYG	Negative	CAT	Negative

The API Coryne biocode for these reactions is 6530360, which corresponds to an identification of *A. haemolyticum* 99.9% (excellent identification)

G. Growth of *Brevibacterium casei* on SBA after 24 hours of incubation at 35–37°C. Colonies of this organism are pigmented a pale yellow, which intensifies during incubation beyond 24 hours. These isolates also have a strong odor reminiscent of "stinky feet." This particular isolate was recovered from multiple blood culture of a patient with AIDS who had a central-line–associated infection.

H. API Coryne inoculated with *B. casei.* The interpretations of the reactions shown are:

NIT	Negative	PYZ	Positive	PYRA	Positive
PAL	Positive	β-GUR	Negative	β-GAL	Negative
α-GLU	Positive	β-NAG	Negative	ESC	Negative
URE	Negative	GEL	Positive	CHO Control	Negative
GLU	Negative	RIB	Negative	XYL	Negative
MAN	Negative	MAL	Negative	LAC	Negative
SAC	Negative	GLYG	Negative	CAT	Positive

The API Coryne biocode for these reactions is 6112004, which corresponds to an identification of *Brevibacterium* species. Additional testing confirmed that this blood culture isolate was indeed *B. casei.*

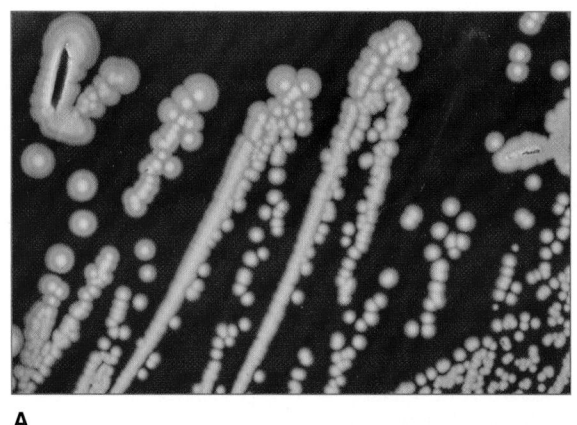

A

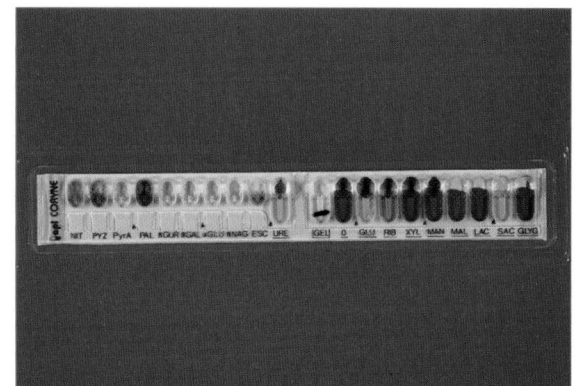

B

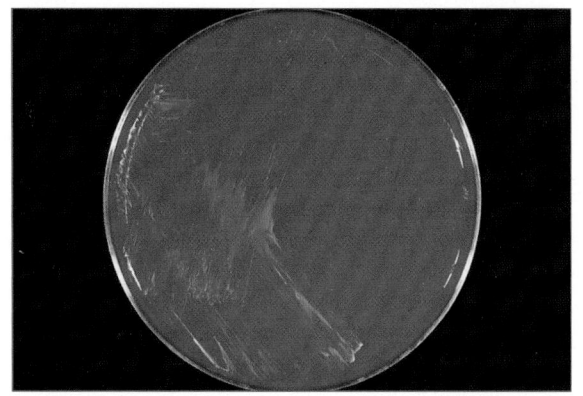

C

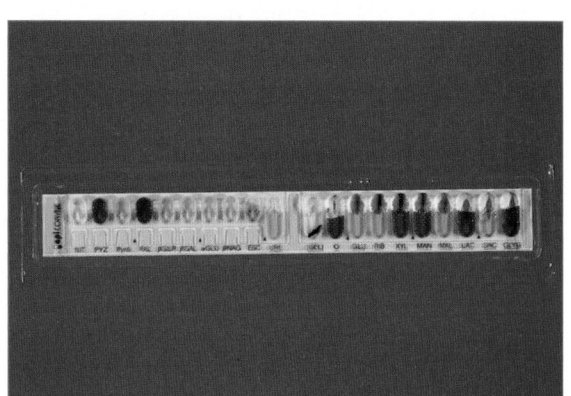

D

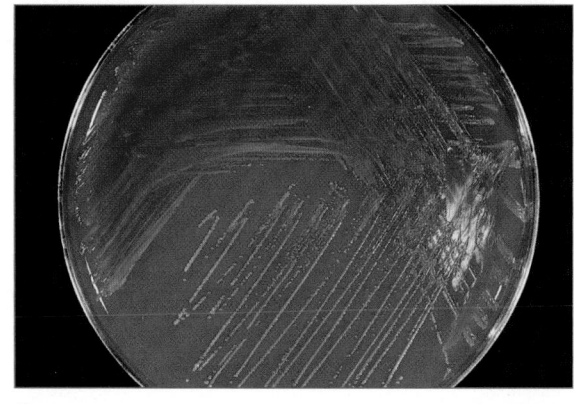

E

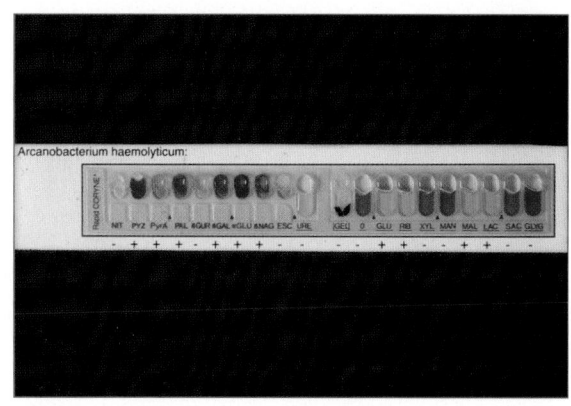

F

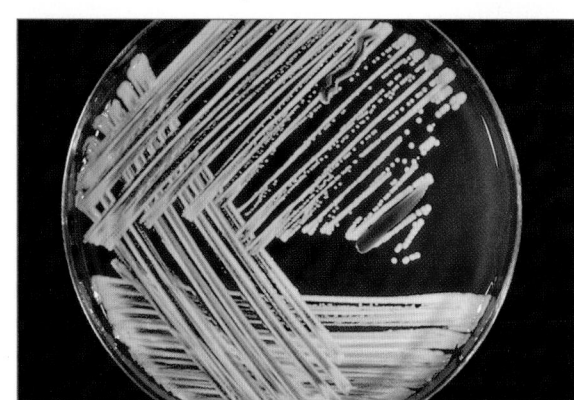

G

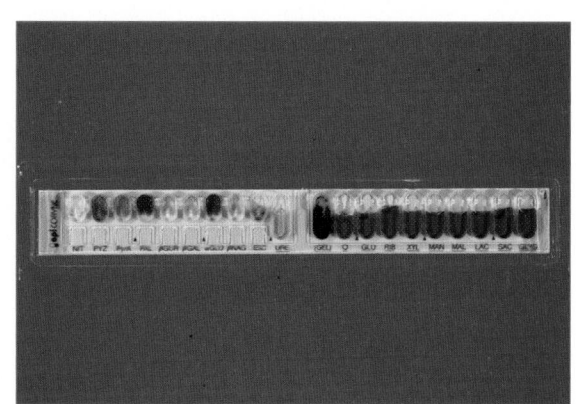

H

Rothia, *Cellulosimicrobium*, *Cellulomonas*/*Microbacterium*, and *Lactobacillus* Species

A. Growth of *Rothia dentocariosa* on SBA after 48 hours of incubation at 35–37°C. This gram-positive bacillary organism is related to the nocardioform organisms and forms dry, white, cerebriform colonies on agar media, as shown here.

B. API Coryne inoculated with *R. dentocariosa*. The interpretations of the reactions shown are:

NIT	Positive	PYZ	Positive	PYRA	Positive
PAL	Negative	β-GUR	Negative	β-GAL	Negative
α-GLU	Positive	β-NAG	Negative	ESC	Positive
URE	Negative	GEL	Negative	CHO Control	Negative
GLU	Positive	RIB	Negative	XYL	Negative
MAN	Negative	MAL	Positive	LAC	Negative
SAC	Positive	GLYG	Negative	CAT	Positive

The API biocode for these reactions is 7050125, which corresponds to an identification of *R. dentocariosa*, 99.5% likelihood.

C. Growth of *Cellulosimicrobium cellulans* on SBA after 24 hours at 35–37°C. This bright yellow-pigmented organism was formerly called *Oerskovia xanthineolytica*.

D. API Coryne inoculated with *C. cellulans*. The interpretations of the reactions shown are:

NIT	Positive	PYZ	Positive	PYRA	Positive
PAL	Positive	β-GUR	Negative	β-GAL	Positive
α-GLU	Positive	β-NAG	Positive	ESC	Positive
URE	Negative	GEL	Positive	CHO Control	Negative
GLU	Positive	RIB	Positive	XYL	Positive
MAN	Negative	MAL	Positive	LAC	Negative
SAC	Positive	GLYG	Positive	CAT	Positive

The API biocode for these reactions is 7572727, which corresponds to an identification of *Oerskovia xanthineolytica* (*C. cellulans*), 99.9% probability.

E. Growth of a yellow-pigmented *Microbacterium* species on SBA after 24 hours at 35–37°C.

F. API Coryne inoculated with *Microbacterium* species. The interpretations of the reactions shown are:

NIT	Negative	PYZ	Positive	PYRA	Negative
PAL	Positive	β-GUR	Negative	β-GAL	Positive
α-GLU	Positive	β-NAG	Positive	ESC	Positive
URE	Negative	GEL	Negative	CHO Control	Negative
GLU	Positive	RIB	Positive	XYL	Positive
MAN	Positive	MAL	Positive	LAC	Negative
SAC	Positive	GLYG	Positive	CAT	Positive

The API biocode for this organism is 2570737, which corresponds to an identification of *Cellulomonas* spp./*Microbacterium* spp. (99.9% likelihood). Additional tests are needed to separate these two genera.

G. Gram-stained smear of a blood culture that grew *Lactobacillus* species. These organisms are regular, gram-positive bacilli that occur singly, in pairs, or in short chains.

H. Small colonies of a nonhemolytic *Lactobacillus* species growing on SBA after 24 hours of incubation at 35–37°C.

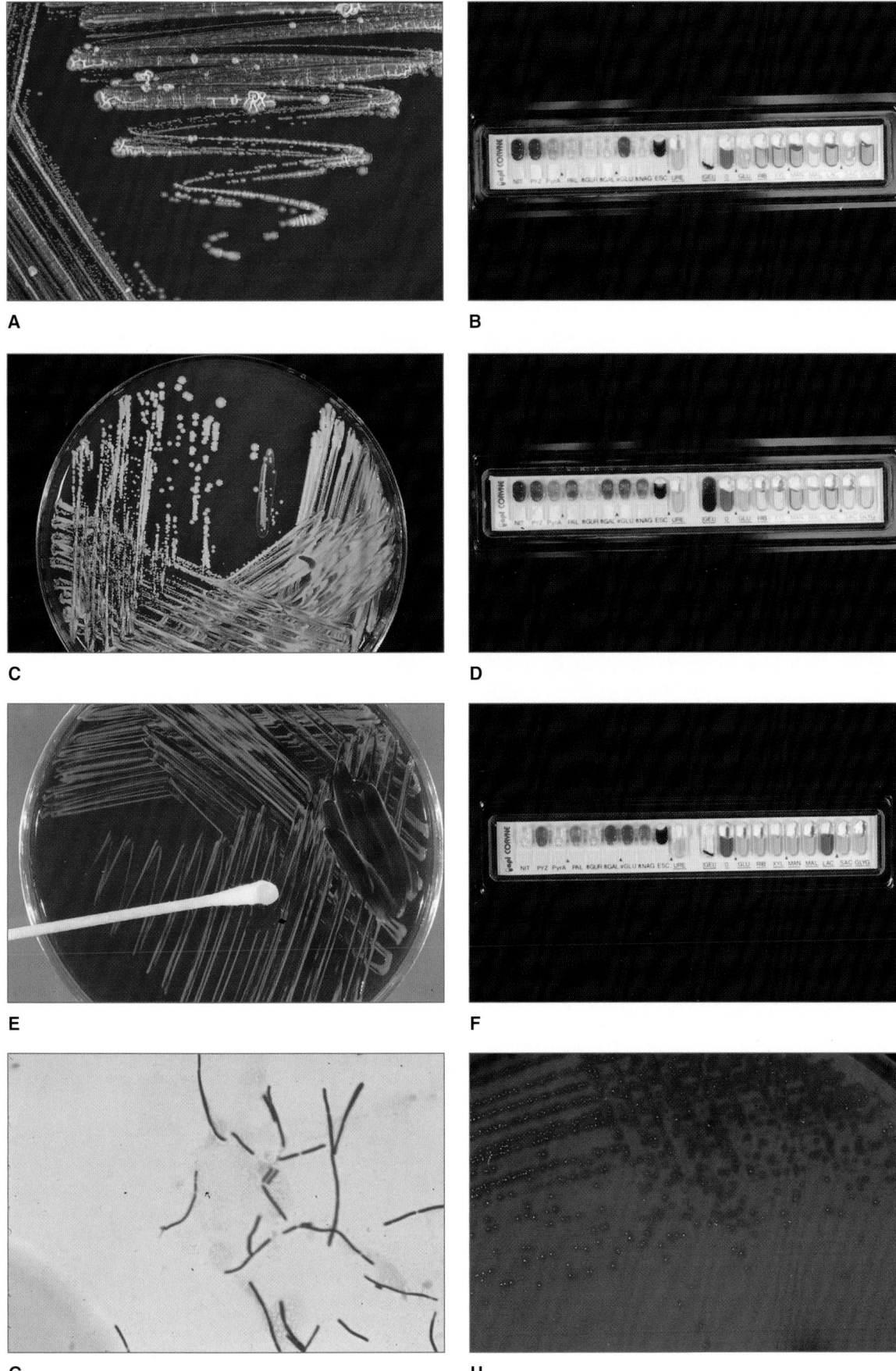

A

B

C

D

E

F

G

H

LACTOBACILLUS AND GARDNERELLA SPECIES

A. *Lactobacillus* species inoculated as a lawn on a SBA plate with a vancomycin disk. Some lactobacilli are resistant to the glycopeptide antibiotics vancomycin and teicoplanin, as indicated by growth of the organisms to the edge of the vancomycin disk, as shown here.

B. Gram-stained smear of a normal vaginal specimen. Note the presence of the large epithelial cells and the gram-positive bacilli that correspond to the "lactobacillus morphotype."

C. Gram-stained smear of material collected from the vagina of a patient with bacterial vaginosis. The epithelial cell shown in the slide is covered with a preponderance of gram-negative bacilli and coccobacilli, which represent anaerobic gram-negative bacilli and "*Gardnerella* morphotypes."

D. Growth of *G. vaginalis* on CNA blood agar 48 hours of incubation at 35–37°C in 5–7% CO_2. After this time, colonies are very small and are best observed in areas of confluent growth.

E. Small, β-hemolytic colonies of *Gardnerella vaginalis* growing on HBT (human blood bilayer-Tween) medium after 72 hours of incubation at 35–37°C in 5–7% CO_2. This organism is β-hemolytic on medium containing human blood (like HBT agar).

F. Rapid carbohydrate utilization technique for identification of *G. vaginalis*. This 4-hour identification procedure is similar to that used for identification of *Neisseria* species (Chapter 11). A balanced salt solution with phenol red and no carbohydrates (BSS) is dispensed in small tubes in 0.10-mL volumes, and single drops of 20% filter-sterilized carbohydrates are added to the BSS. A dense suspension of the organism is prepared in BSS with no carbohydrate (0.5 mL), and single drops of this suspension are added to the carbohydrate-containing tubes. In the photograph, the individual tubes are (*left to right*) the BSS organism suspension, BSS-glucose, BSS-maltose, and BSS-mannitol. The last tube (*far right*) is a hippurate hydrolysis test. As shown, *G. vaginalis* produces acid from glucose and maltose, but not mannitol, and is strongly hippurate-hydrolysis–positive.

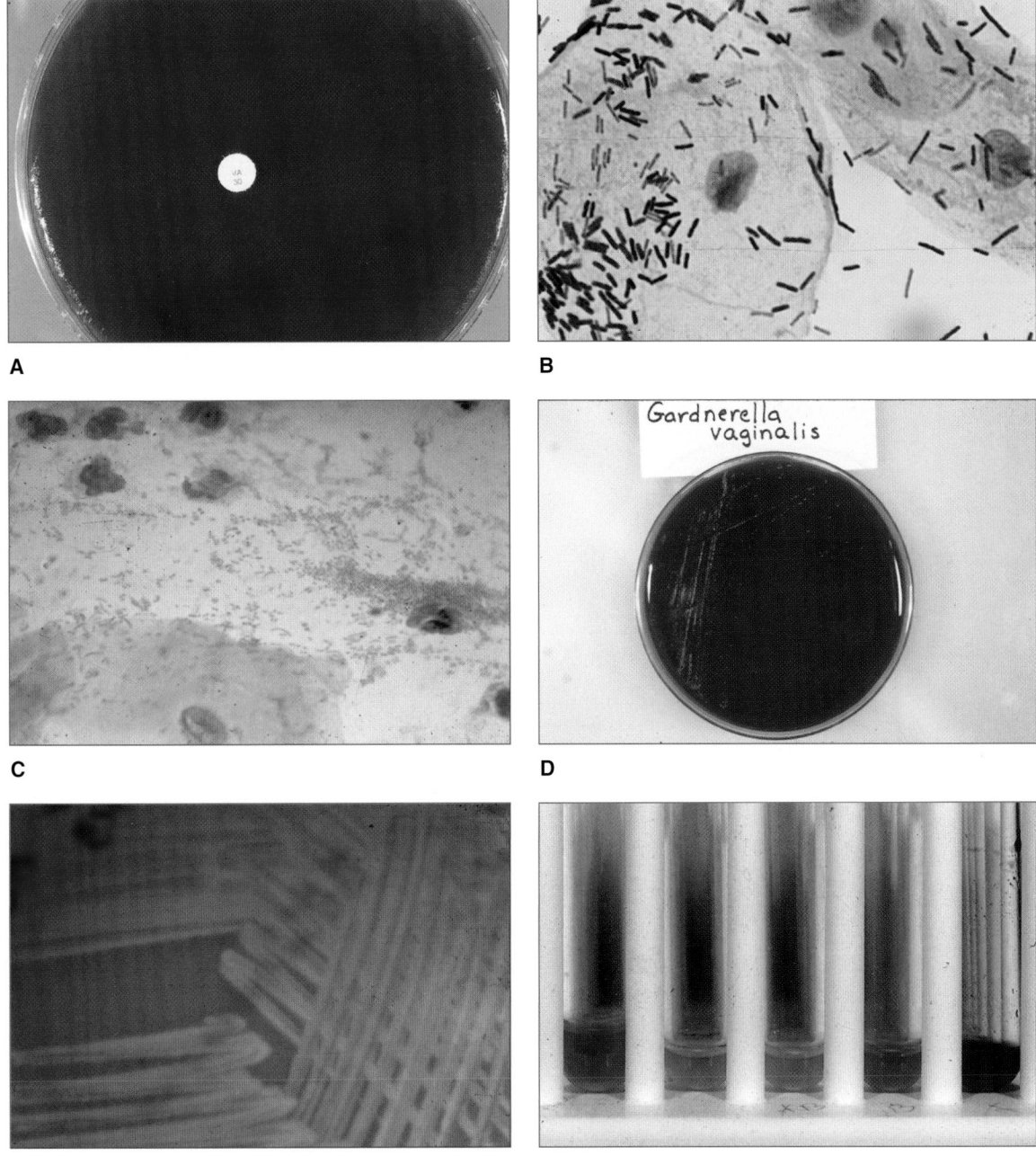

A

B

C

D Gardnerella vaginalis

E

F

Identification of Aerobic and Facultatively Anaerobic Gram-Positive Bacilli

A. Close-up view of *Nocardia asteroids* after 7 days of incubation at 30°C on Middlebrook 7H11 agar. Seen here is the typical orange, glabrous, wavy colonies that tend to be adherent to the agar surface. Other species produce white, dry, chalky colonies (see Color Plate 1-5*J*). it is noteworthy that *Nocardia* species will grow on the selective isolation media used for the recovery of *Mycobacterium* species; in fact, the laboratory diagnosis of nocardiosis is often first suspected in the mycobacteriology section of the laboratory. The detection of a distinct musty basement odor is an initial clue to the identification.

B. Middlebrook 7H11 agar plate on which a 48-hour culture of *Rhodococcus* species is growing. The colonies are relatively large, ranging from 2 to 4 mm in diameter, and are entire and smooth. Note the salmon-pink pigmentation, an initial clue to the identification of this species.

C. Partial acid-fast stain of an exudate containing acid-fast, delicate, branching filaments characteristic of *Nocardia* species. *Nocardia asteroides* was recovered from the culture obtained from this specimen.

D. Gram-stain of *Rhodococcus* species illustrating short gram-positive coccobacilli arranged singly and in Chinese letter clusters.

E. Acid-fast stain of *Rhodococcus* species showing short coccobacilli, many of which are acid-fast positive.

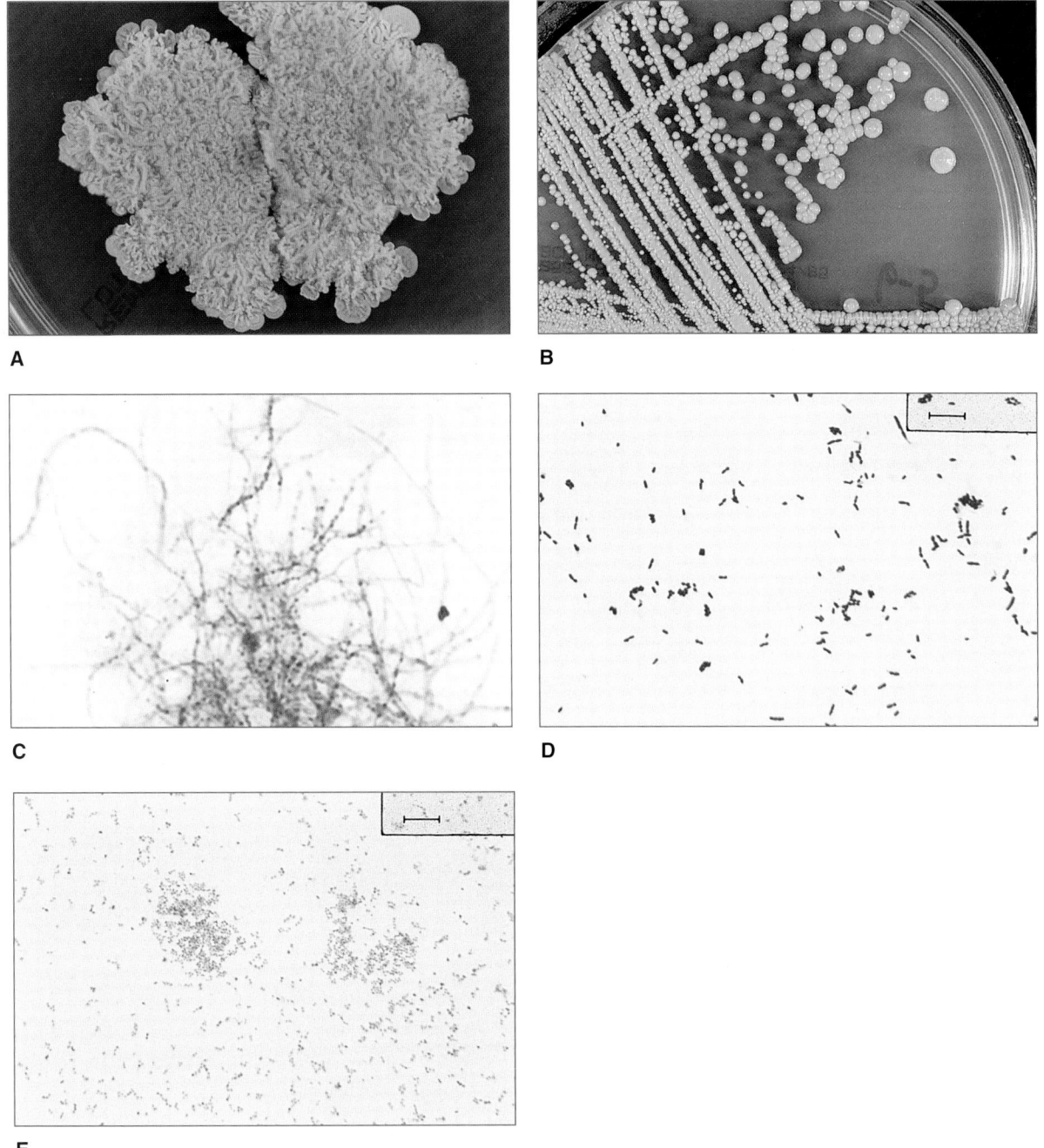

A

B

C

D

E

IDENTIFICATION OF ANAEROBIC BACTERIA: GRAM-NEGATIVE BACILLI

A. *Bacteroides fragilis.* Gram stain of cells in 48-hour thioglycolate broth culture.

B. *B. fragilis.* Colonies on anaerobic blood agar after 48 hours of incubation at 35°C.

C. *Prevotella melaninogenica.* Gram stains of cells from a 48-hour colony on blood agar.

D. *P. melaninogenica.* Black colonies on blood agar after 5 days of incubation at 35°C.

E. *Fusobacterium nucleatum.* Gram stain of cells from a 48-hour colony on anaerobic blood agar. Note long, gram-negative bacilli with pointed ends.

F. *F. nucleatum.* Characteristic colonies on anaerobic blood agar after 48 hours of incubation at 35°C, illustrating the opalescent effect.

G. *F. necrophorum.* Gram stain of cells from a 48-hour colony on anaerobic blood agar. Note pleomorphism.

H. *F. necrophorum.* Colonies on anaerobic blood agar after 48 hours of incubation at 35°C.

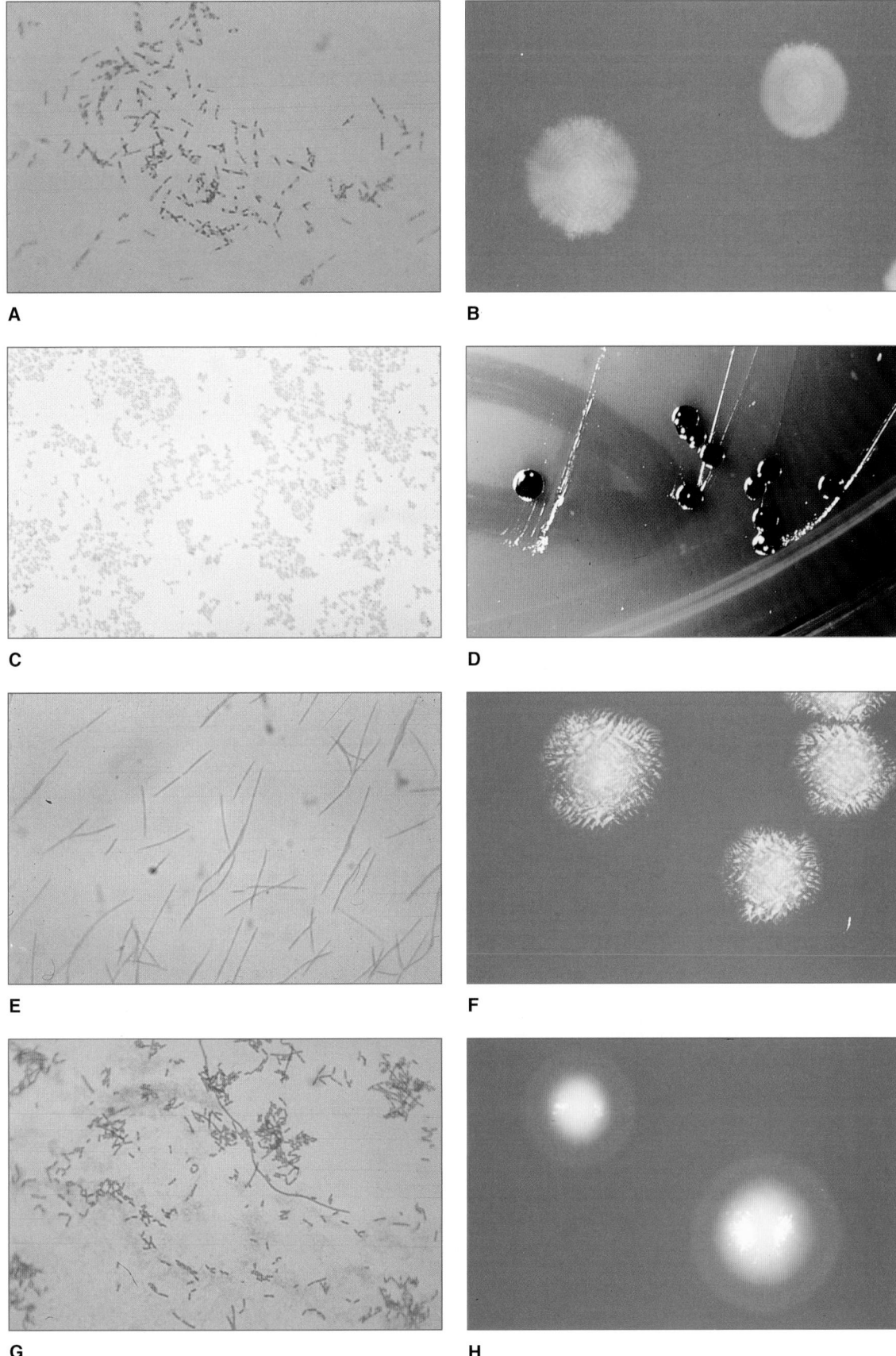

A

B

C

D

E

F

G

H

IDENTIFICATION OF ANAEROBIC BACTERIA: GRAM-POSITIVE, NON–SPORE-FORMING ORGANISMS

A. Gram-stained direct smear of a purulent exudate showing degenerated neutrophils and a mixture of gram-negative rods of different sizes. The smallest coccobacilli suggest one of the pigmented *Prevotella-Porphyromonas* species; the larger, pleomorphic rods suggest a member of the *Bacteroides fragilis* group.

B. Gram-stained direct smear of a purulent exudate from an intraabdominal abscess, showing segmented neutrophils, gram-positive cocci in pairs and short chains, and tiny gram-negative rods. Anaerobic infections usually contain a mixed bacterial flora.

C. Dissecting microscope view of actinomycotic "sulfur granules" (×10). (Exudate from an abdominal wound infection was photographed within a Petri dish.)

D. Appearance of a Gram-stained smear from the same specimen as in **C,** showing "sulfur granule" with thin, branching filaments of an *Actinomyces* species (×800).

E. *Actinomyces israelii.* Gram-stained preparation of growth from a colony on blood agar. Note branching of cells.

F. *A. israelii.* Characteristic "molar tooth" colonies produced on brain-heart infusion agar after 7 days of anaerobic incubation at 35°C.

G. *Eubacterium alactolyticum.* Gram stain of cells from growth in enriched thioglycolate broth after 48 hours of incubation at 35°C.

H. *E. alactolyticum.* Forty-eight-hour colonies on anaerobic blood agar.

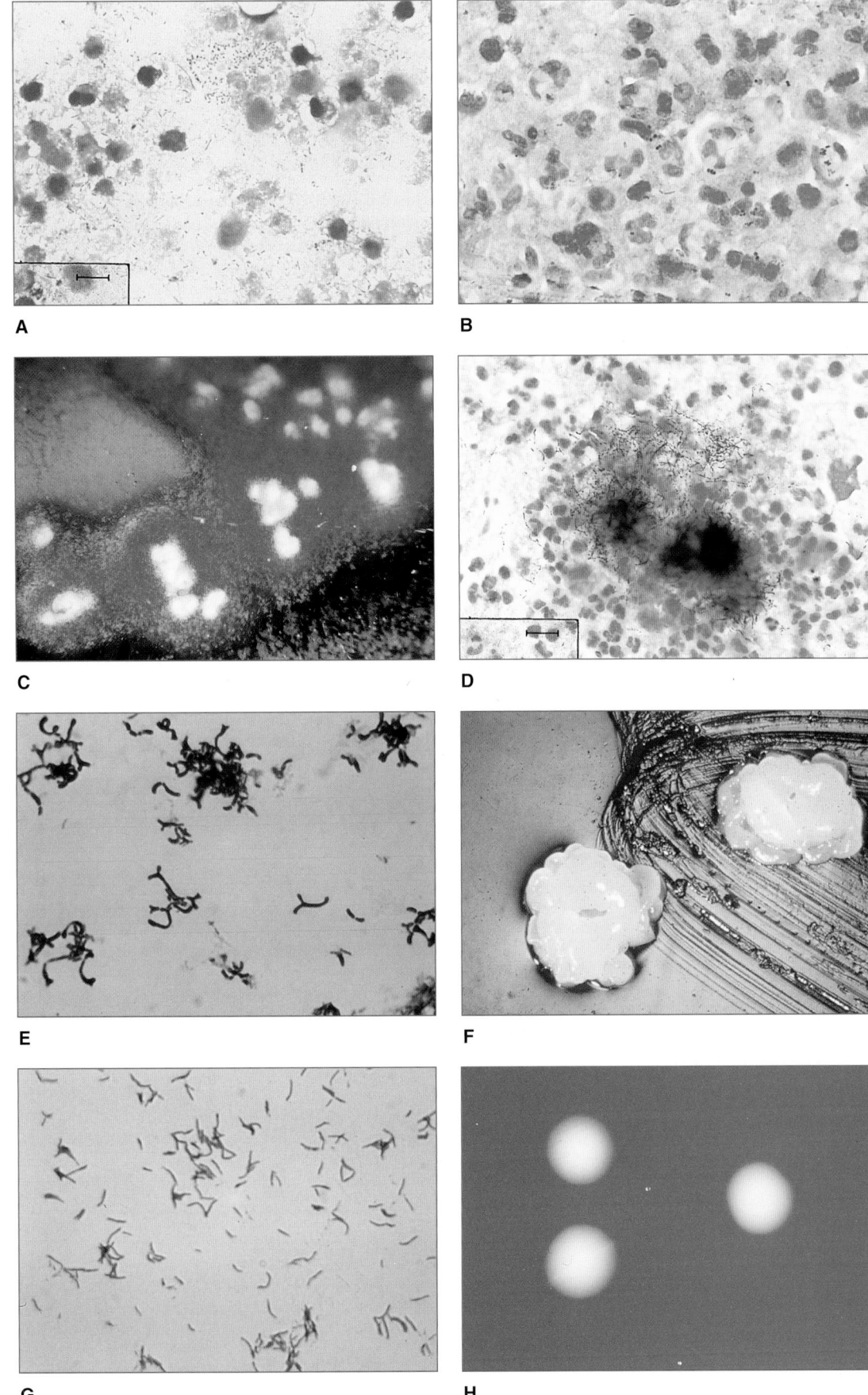

A

B

C

D

E

F

G

H

IDENTIFICATION OF ANAEROBIC BACTERIA: CLOSTRIDIA

A. *Clostridium perfringens.* Gram stain of cells from a 24-hour colony on blood agar. Note lack of spores and of some cells that tend to stain red (gram-negative).

B. *C. perfringens.* Gram stain of cells from a 24-hour thioglycolate broth culture. Note lack of spores and presence of a few filamentous forms.

C. Typical appearance of *C. perfringens* on blood agar after 24 hours of incubation at 35°C. Note the double zone of hemolysis. The inner zone of complete hemolysis is due to theta-toxin and the outer zone of incomplete hemolysis to alpha-toxin (lecithinase activity).

D. *C. perfringens.* Direct Gram stain of a muscle tissue aspirate from a patient with gas gangrene my-onecrosis. There is a necrotic background, without intact inflammatory cells or muscle cells, and relatively large "box car"-shaped gram-positive rods and a gram-negative rod that is either a gram-variable *C. perfringens* cell or another organism.

E. Colonies of *C. perfringens* on modified McClung egg yolk agar. The precipitate surrounding the colonies indicates lecithinase activity of alpha-toxin produced by the organism.

F. Lipase production on egg yolk agar. A few clostridia, such as *C. botulinum, C. sporogenes,* and *C. novyi* type A, exhibit lipase activity on egg yolk agar, as shown here. Note the iridescent pearly layer on the surface of the colonies extending onto the surface of the medium immediately surrounding them.

G. *C. septicum.* Rough, irregular, flat, rhizoid, spreading colony on a 48-hour anaerobic blood agar plate.

H. Direct Gram-stained smear of a positive blood culture that contained *C. septicum.* Numerous ovoid or citron-shaped, subterminal spores are present.

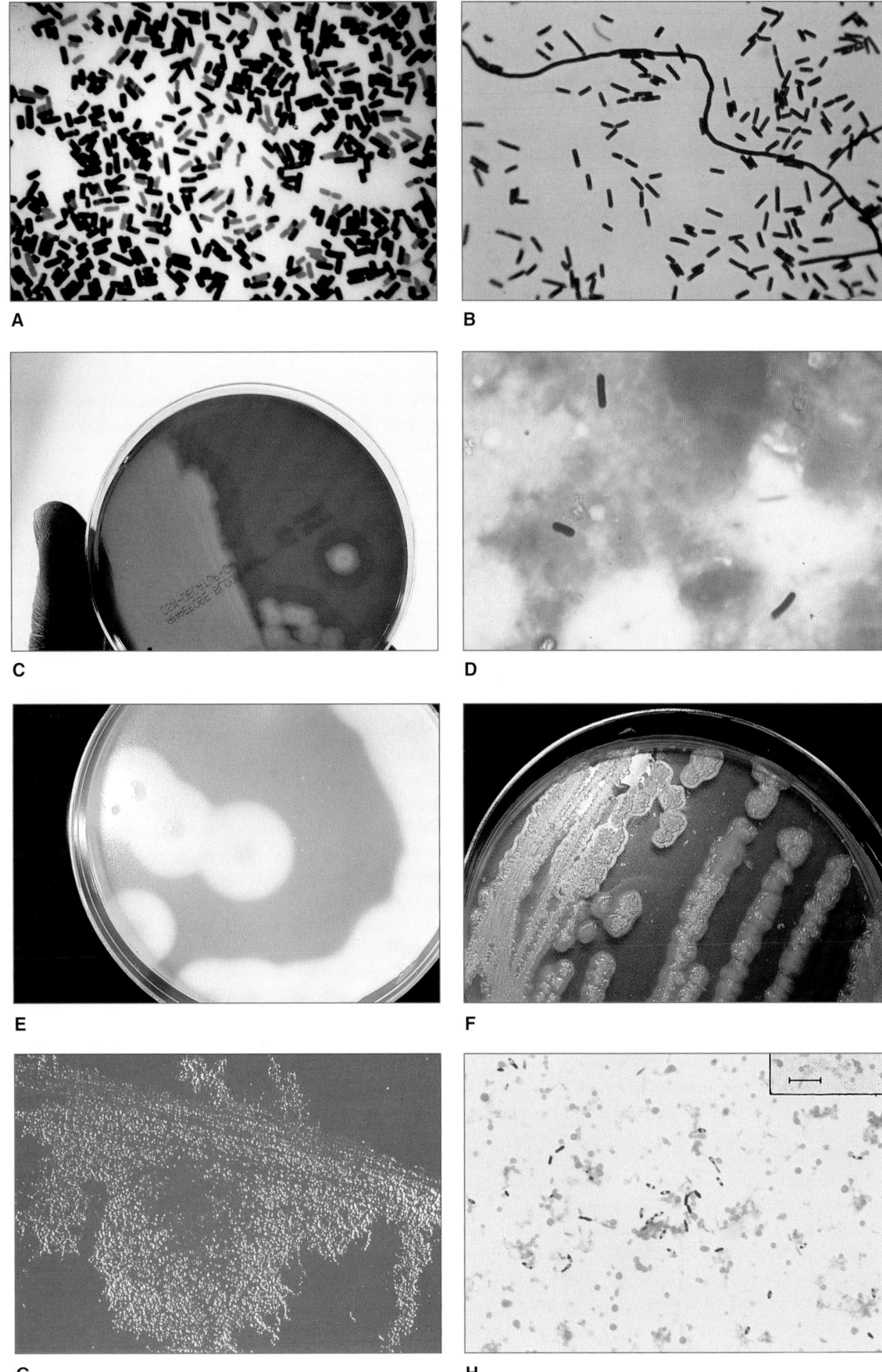

A

B

C

D

E

F

G

H

IDENTIFICATION OF ANAEROBIC BACTERIA: CLOSTRIDIA (CONTINUED)

A. Colonies of *C. tetani* on stiff blood agar (4% agar), which is used to inhibit the swarming of the microorganism so that it can be isolated from other bacteria present in mixed cultures.

B. *C. tetani.* Gram stain of cells from a chopped meat glucose broth culture. Some of the cells have round, terminal spores, which are characteristic of *C. tetani.*

C. *C. sporogenes.* "Medusa-head" colonies on 48-hour anaerobic blood agar.

D. *C. ramosum.* Gram stain from a thioglycolate broth culture after 48 hours of incubation.

E. *C. difficile* on anaerobe blood agar after 48 hours of incubation (original magnification ×2.8).

F. *C. difficile* on cycloserine-cefoxitin fructose agar after 48 hours of incubation.

G. *C. sordellii* on anaerobe blood agar following prolonged anaerobic incubation. Colony is 5 × 10 mm.

H. *C. sordellii.* Gram stain from 2-day-old blood agar plate reveals clumps of free spores and bacteria distended with ovoid subterminal spores.

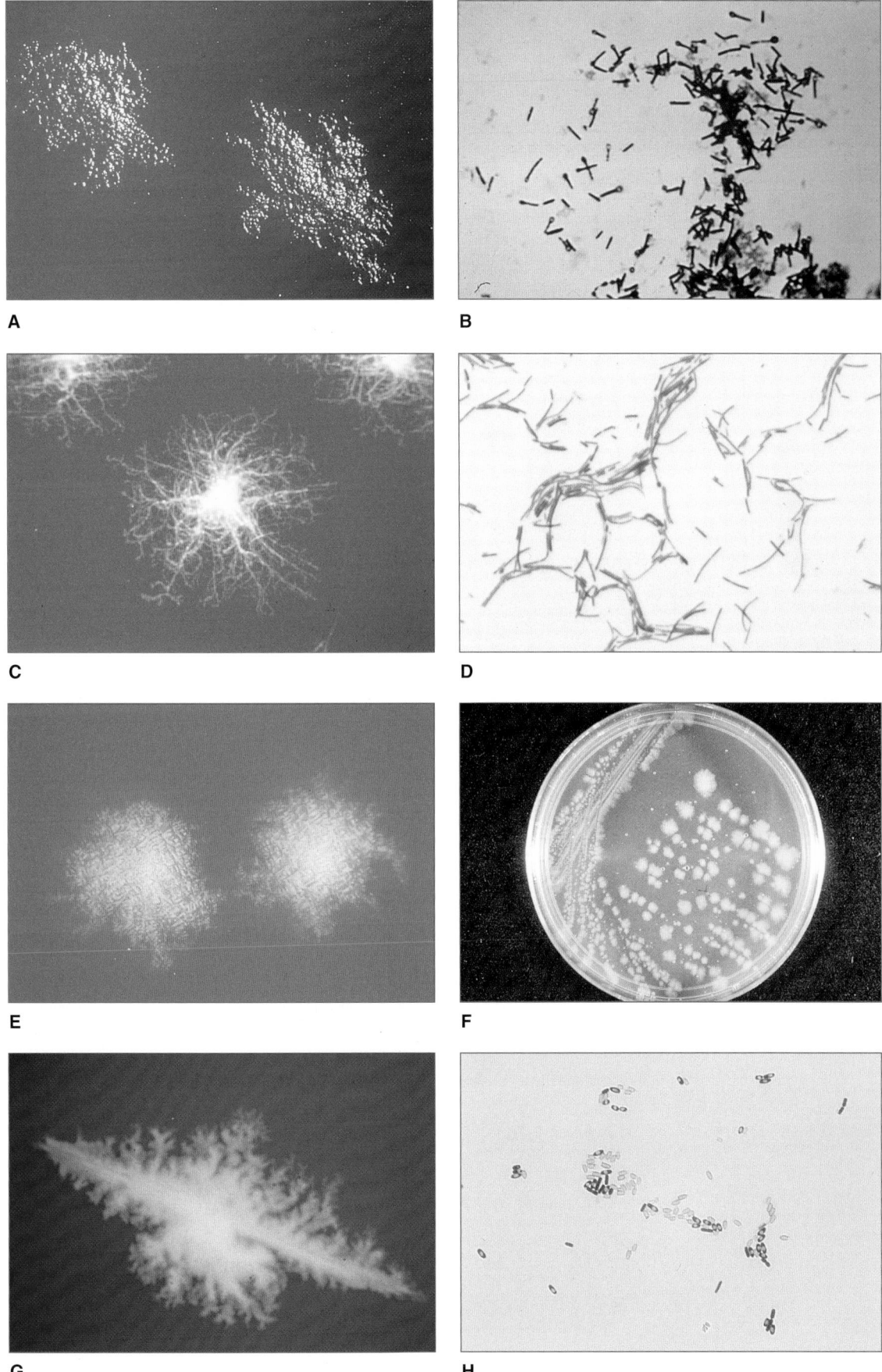

A

B

C

D

E

F

G

H

IDENTIFICATION OF ANAEROBIC BACTERIA: USE OF PRESUMPTO QUADRANT PLATES AND DISKS ON ANAEROBE BLOOD AGAR

A. Overview appearance of three quadrant plates (described in detail in the text).

B. A Presumpto 1 quadrant plate and a plate of CDC anaerobe blood agar. After inoculation with an active broth culture or cell suspension of the isolate to be identified, antibiotic disks (penicillin, 2 units; rifampin, 15 g; kanamycin, 1,000 g) are placed on the blood agar medium, and a blank filter-paper disk is placed on the LD agar portion of the quadrant plate for use in detection of indole production. The Presumpto 1 plate contains the following media: LD agar, LD esculin, LD egg yolk agar, and LD bile agar.

C. Growth of *Bacteroides fragilis* on Presumpto 1 plate after 48 hours of incubation at 35°C. On the first quadrant (*top, far right*), LD agar shows moderate growth. Indole production can be detected by adding a drop of para-dimethylaminocinnamaldehyde to the paper disk (see **F**). The LD esculin agar to the left of the LD agar is diffusely dark because of the hydrolysis of the esculin.* The LD egg yolk agar underneath the esculin agar shows good growth but no lecithinase, lipase, or proteolytic activity. There is abundant growth in the LD bile agar (*bottom, far right*), and a characteristic precipitate was produced in the medium by this strain.

D. Antibiotic disk tests. A zone of growth inhibition is seen around the 15-g rifampin disk, but no growth inhibition is seen around the 2-unit penicillin disk or the 1,000-g kanamycin disk. This pattern is characteristic of the *B. fragilis* group.

E. Reactions of *B. thetaiotaomicron* of the Presumpto 1 quadrant plate. The first quadrant (*top, far right*) shows a weak, positive indole reaction, as indicated by the pale blue color of the disk on LD agar after addition of para-dimethylaminocinnamaldehyde reagent. Black (amber) appearance of esculin agar (*left of first quadrant*) indicates esculin hydrolysis. There is adequate growth but no lecithinase, lipase, or proteolysis on LD egg yolk agar (*bottom, far left*). There is good growth on LD bile agar but no precipitate as exhibited by *B. fragilis* (*bottom, far right*).

F. Reactions of *Fusobacterium necrophorum* on the Presumpto 1 quadrant plate after 48 hours of incubation at 35°C. The first quadrant (*bottom, far right*) shows strong indole reaction as evidenced by the dark blue color of the paper disk on LD agar after the addition of para-dimethylaminocinnamaldehyde reagent. Growth is inhibited on LD bile agar (*top, right*). Although not visible in this photograph because of the lighting arrangement, there is good growth in LD egg yolk agar (*top, far left*) and characteristic lipase activity as evidenced by an iridescent sheen—a pearly layer—on the surface of the colonies and in the medium immediately surrounding the bacterial growth. This is best demonstrated with reflected light. On LD esculin agar (*bottom, left*), the *F. necrophorum* shows good growth and hydrogen sulfide production, as evidenced by the black appearance of the colonies, but no darkening of the medium to suggest esculin hydrolysis.

G. Presumpto 2 quadrant plate (uninoculated). The plate contains the following quadrants(clockwise, starting at 12 o'clock): LD starch agar, LD glucose agar, LD-DNA agar, and LD milk agar.

H. Presumpto 2 quadrant plate following inoculation, incubation, and addition of reagents. Note positive reactions for hydrolysis, deoxyribonuclease activity, and glucose fermentation.

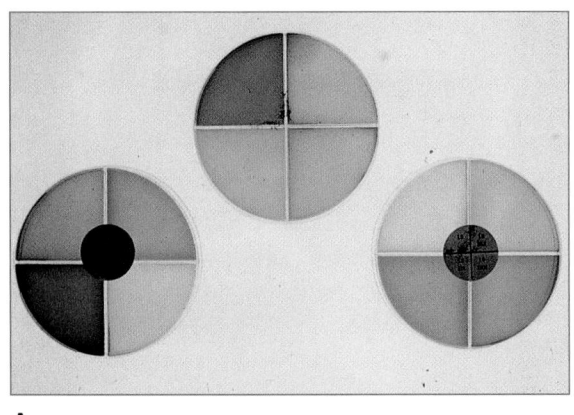

A

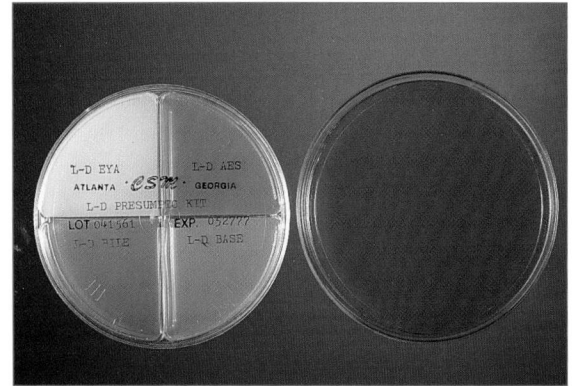

B

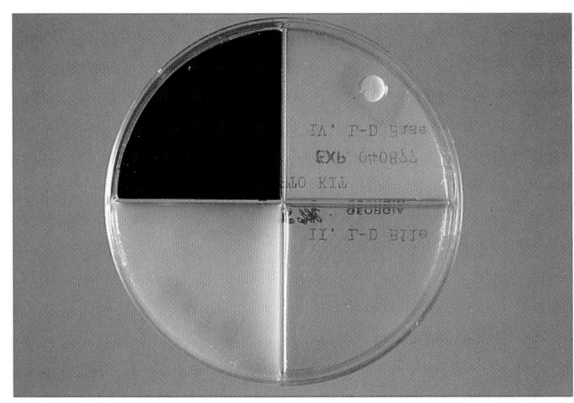

C

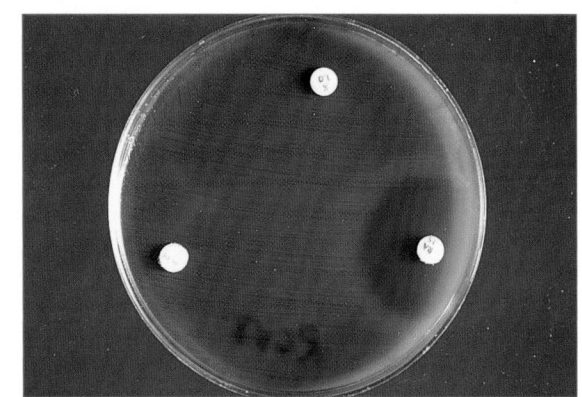

D

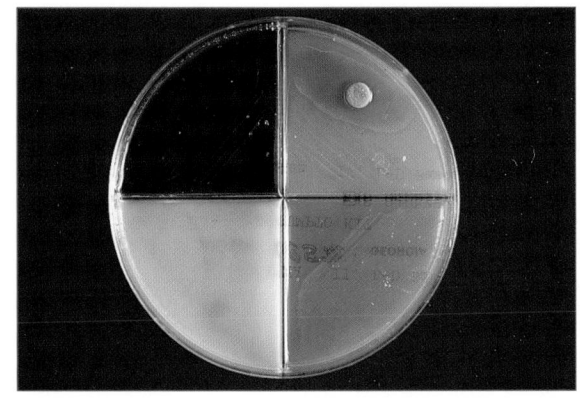

E

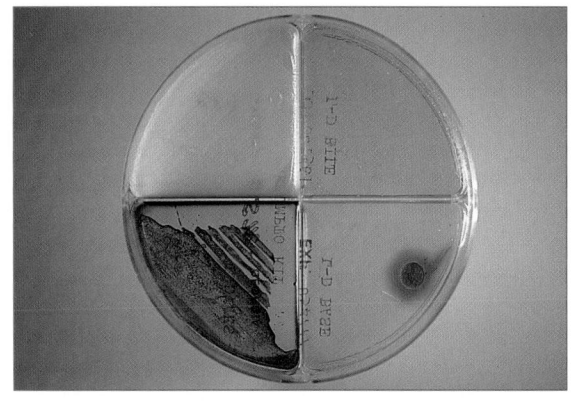

F

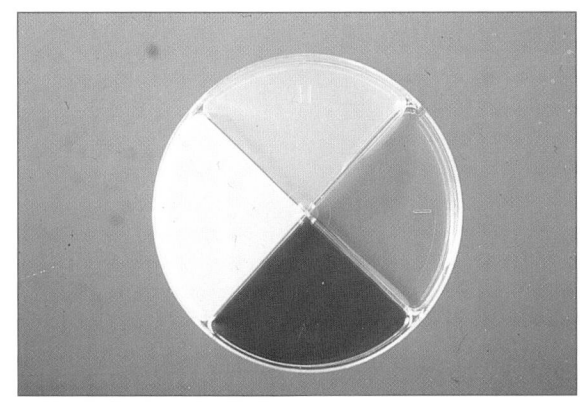

G

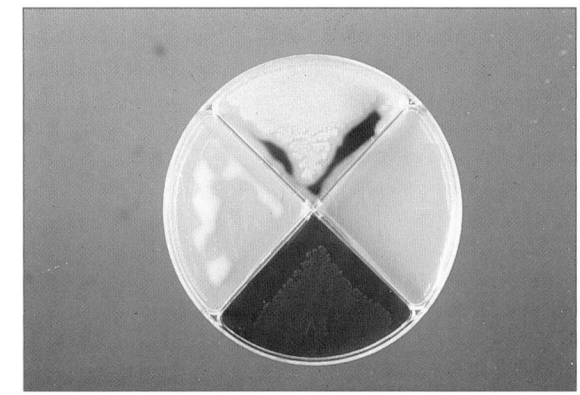

H

MYCOPLASMAS AND UREAPLASMAS

A. Colony of *M. pneumoniae* on mycoplasma glucose agar. This photograph shows a single colony of the organism to which guinea pig erythrocytes have become adsorbed. *M. pneumoniae* is the only species that demonstrates this hemadsorbing property. (Photograph courtesy of Health and Education Resources, Bethesda, MD.)

B. Colonies of *M. hominis* and *U. urealyticum* growing on Shepard's A7B differential agar. *M. hominis* colonies have the typical fried egg morphology; the blue color is due to the Diene's stain. *U. urealyticum* colonies are smaller, denser, and have a brownish pigmentation because of precipitation of manganese oxide in the colony due to the action of urease enzymes. (Photograph courtesy of Health and Education Resources, Bethesda, MD.)

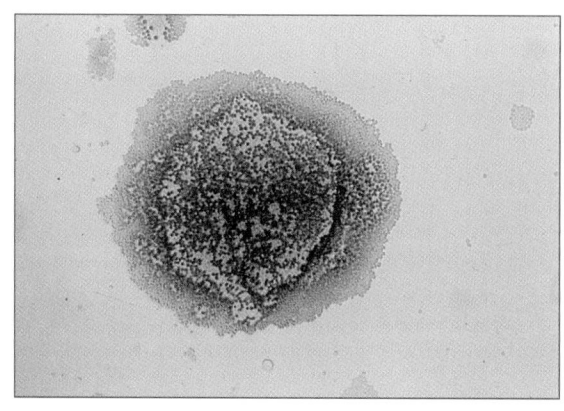

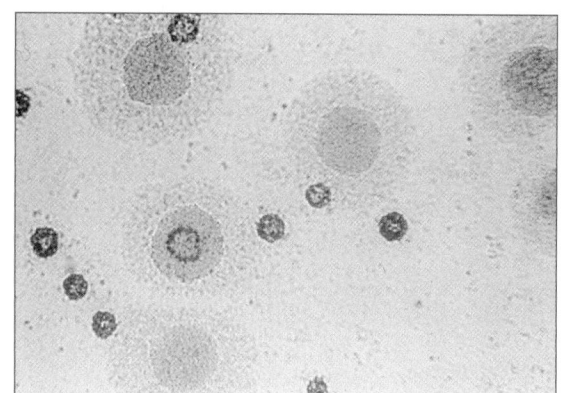

A   B

THE LABORATORY IDENTIFICATION OF *MYCOBACTERIUM TUBERCULOSIS*

A. Photomicrograph of a smear prepared from a colony similar to that illustrated in Color Plate 19-1**C,** stained with auramine-rhodamine. Note the bright yellow fluorescence of the very short, slightly curved bacilli. Although the cellular morphology is suggestive of *M. tuberculosis*, examination under higher-power optics and culture confirmation must be made before a definitive species identification can be made.

B. Photomicrograph of a Kinyoun acid-fast stain of a smear prepared from material obtained from a necrotic tuberculoma of the lung. Note the relatively short, thin, beaded, slightly curved, red-staining acid-fast bacilli. Although species identifications cannot be made from acid-fast smears alone, the appearance here is highly consistent with *M. tuberculosis*.

C. A microcolony growing on the surface of Middlebrook 7H10 agar, observed microscopically under low-power optics. Note that the bacterial cells are arranged in an undulating, serpiginous pattern. This indicates the production of cording factor, as illustrated in the acid-fast stain shown in Color Plate 19-1*I.*

D. A niacin-accumulation test. The tubes contain a filter paper strip impregnated with cyanogen bromide. The fluid in the tube on the *right* had been extracted from the surface of Löwenstein-Jensen culture medium after colonial growth of an unknown *Mycobacterium* species, compared with a negative water control on the left. The development of a yellow color on the strip and in the underlying fluid indicates the presence of niacin. *M. tuberculosis* has the unique property of accumulating niacin when colonies are grown on Löwenstein-Jensen medium, a property shared by the less commonly encountered *M. simiae* and occasional strains of *M. marinum*.

E. Tubes illustrating the nitrate-reduction test. The tube on the *right* had been inoculated with an unknown *Mycobacterium* species, compared with an uninoculated control on the *left*. The development of a red color after addition of sulfonamide and α-naphthylethylenediamine reagents indicates the presence of nitrites and a positive test. *M. tuberculosis* is an active nitrate reducer.

F. A quadrant plate containing Middlebrook 7H10 agar in which thiophene-2-carboxylic acid hydrazide (T_2H) had been incorporated. The three quadrants in which growth is observed are different strains of *M. tuberculosis* (resistant to T_2H); the quadrant without growth was inoculated with a strain of *M. bovis*. The ability to grow or not grow on medium containing T_2H is helpful in separating *M. tuberculosis* from *M. bovis*, respectively.

G. A flask of Löwenstein-Jensen medium on which are growing colonies of *M. tuberculosis* after a 22-day incubation at 35°C in a 10% CO_2 incubator. The colonies seen here are distinctly rough in consistency; however, they have more of a yellow pigmentation than the buff-colored colonies usually observed.

H. Colonies of a subculture of *M. tuberculosis* growing on Middlebrook 7H10 agar after a 25-day incubation at 35°C in 10% CO_2 incubator. The colonies have a rough, buff appearance, characteristic for the species.

I. Photomicrograph of a Kinyoun acid-fast stain prepared from the broth of a BACTEC 12A blood culture vial after a 10-day incubation at 35°C. Numerous acid-fast bacilli are seen, arranged in parallel sheaths. When the aggregate of bacterial cells, as illustrated here, is observed in smears prepared from a broth preparation, one can make a presumptive identification of *M. tuberculosis*, because the phenomenon is due to the production of cording factor, thought to be a virulence factor.

J. Photomicrograph of a Gram stain prepared from a smear of pleural fluid from a case of empyema in a patient with AIDS. Note the relatively long, slender, delicately beaded, poorly staining bacilli. Because of their thick waxy outer coating, the bacterial cells of mycobacteria do not stain well with gentian violet, the primary stain used in the Gram stain. Note the distinct halo around the bacilli, a clue that the organism is encapsulated and suggestive of a *Mycobacterium* species. *M. tuberculosis* grew out in culture in this case.

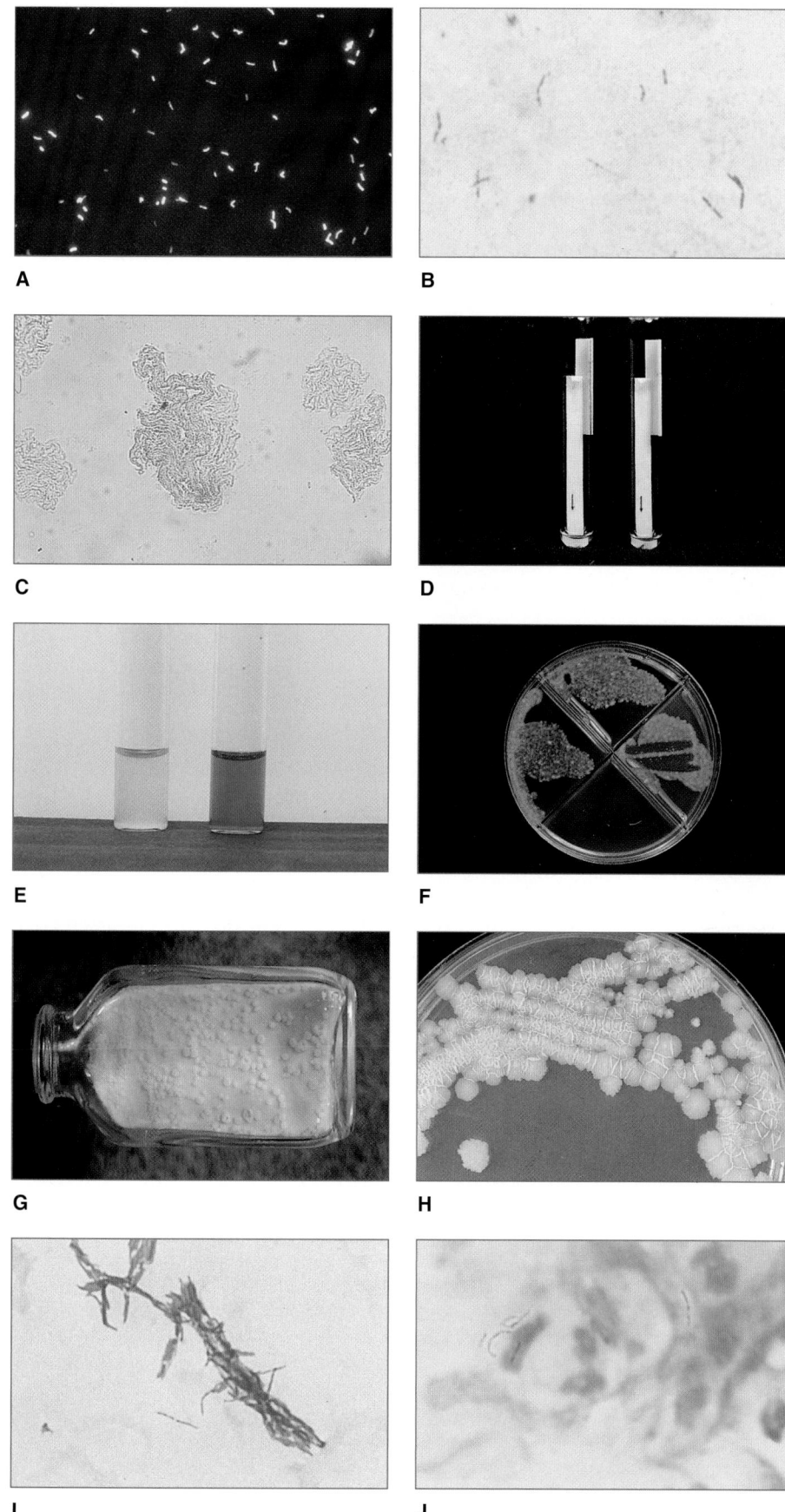

A

B

C

D

E

F

G

H

I

J

LABORATORY IDENTIFICATION OF *MYCOBACTERIUM* SPECIES OTHER THAN *M. TUBERCULOSIS*

A. Photomicrograph of microcolonies of *M. avium* growing on Middlebrook 7H10 agar after a 6-day incubation at 35°C in 10% CO_2. The flat, thin, translucent microcolonies, with a central darker umbonate elevation, suggestive of a fried egg, are characteristic of the smooth strains of *M. avium* commonly recovered from patients with AIDS. The observation of this type of microcolony may be helpful in directing one to perform an *M. avium/M. intracellulare* complex nucleic acid probe in the rapid culture confirmation of an unknown isolate.

B. Close-up photomicrograph of a single microcolony of *M. avium/M. intracellulare* complex, again illustrating the thin, translucent colony described in Color Plate 19-2*A*. The rhizoid-like peripheral extensions, as illustrated here, are often seen and provide an added clue to the presumptive identification of *M. avium/M. intracellulare* complex organisms.

C. Two Middlebrook 7H10 agar plates, each inoculated with the same subculture of *M. kansasii*. The plate on the *left* was exposed to light; the one on the *right* remained in the dark until just before the photomicrograph was taken. The yellow pigment of the colonies in the light-exposed plate is characteristic of a photochromogen.

D. Two Middlebrook 7H10 agar plates each inoculated with the same subculture of *M. scrofulaceum*. The plate on the *left* was exposed to light; the one on the *right* remained in the dark until just before the photograph was taken. The yellow pigment of the colonies in both the light-exposed and non–light-exposed plates is characteristic of a scotochromogen.

E. A Middlebrook 7H10 agar plate previously inoculated with a strain of *M. gordonae*: *M. gordonae* is a scotochromogen and characteristically produces a deep yellow pigment, as illustrated here.

F. Several tubes containing varying concentrations of buffered sodium nitrate inoculate with various strains of *Mycobacterium* species to illustrate 1+ (*second tube from left*) through 4+ (*rightmost tube*) reactions. Red color develops after the addition of sulfanilamide and *N*-naphthylethylene-diamine reagents; the intensity of color reflects the concentration of nitrites produced. The quantitative nitrate-reduction test may be helpful in differentiating strains of *M. tuberculosis* (4+ positive) from *M. bovis* (1+ positive) and *M. kansasii* (4+ positive) from other photochromogens (negative to 1+ positive).

G. Two tubes containing Tween 80 reagent. The *left* tube had been inoculated with a negative control strain, the tube on the *right* with a subculture of *M. kansasii*. The development of a red color (*right tube*) after incubation for 3 to 10 days is a positive test, indicating the ability of the test strain to hydrolyze Tween 80. The color change from yellow to red in this assay is not due to a shift in pH, rather it results from a change in optical density as oleic acid and polyoxyethylated sorbitol are produced as breakdown products of Tween hydrolysis.

H. Two tubes of Löwenstein-Jensen deeps previously inoculated with a catalase-negative control (*left tube*) and a subculture of *M. kansasii* (*right tube*). Note the tall area of bubble formation in the right tube after the addition of hydrogen peroxide to the surface of the agar, exceeding 45 mm, indicative of a positive test and strong catalase activity.

I. A positive catalase test. Immediately before the photomicrograph was taken, a few drops of hydrogen peroxide were placed on isolated colonies of the photochromogenic colonies of *M. kansasii*. The evolution of rapid bubbles, as illustrated here, indicates a positive test, indicating active catalase activity.

J. Two tubes of Dubos broth base, the *right* containing tripotassium phenolphthalein disulfate reagent (arylsulfatase reagent) compared with a negative control tube on the *left* devoid of reagent. Both tubes had been previously inoculated with a subculture of a strain of *M. fortuitum*. The development of a pink color after the addition of sodium carbonate reagent in the *left* tube indicates a positive test and arylsulfatase activity of the test strain.

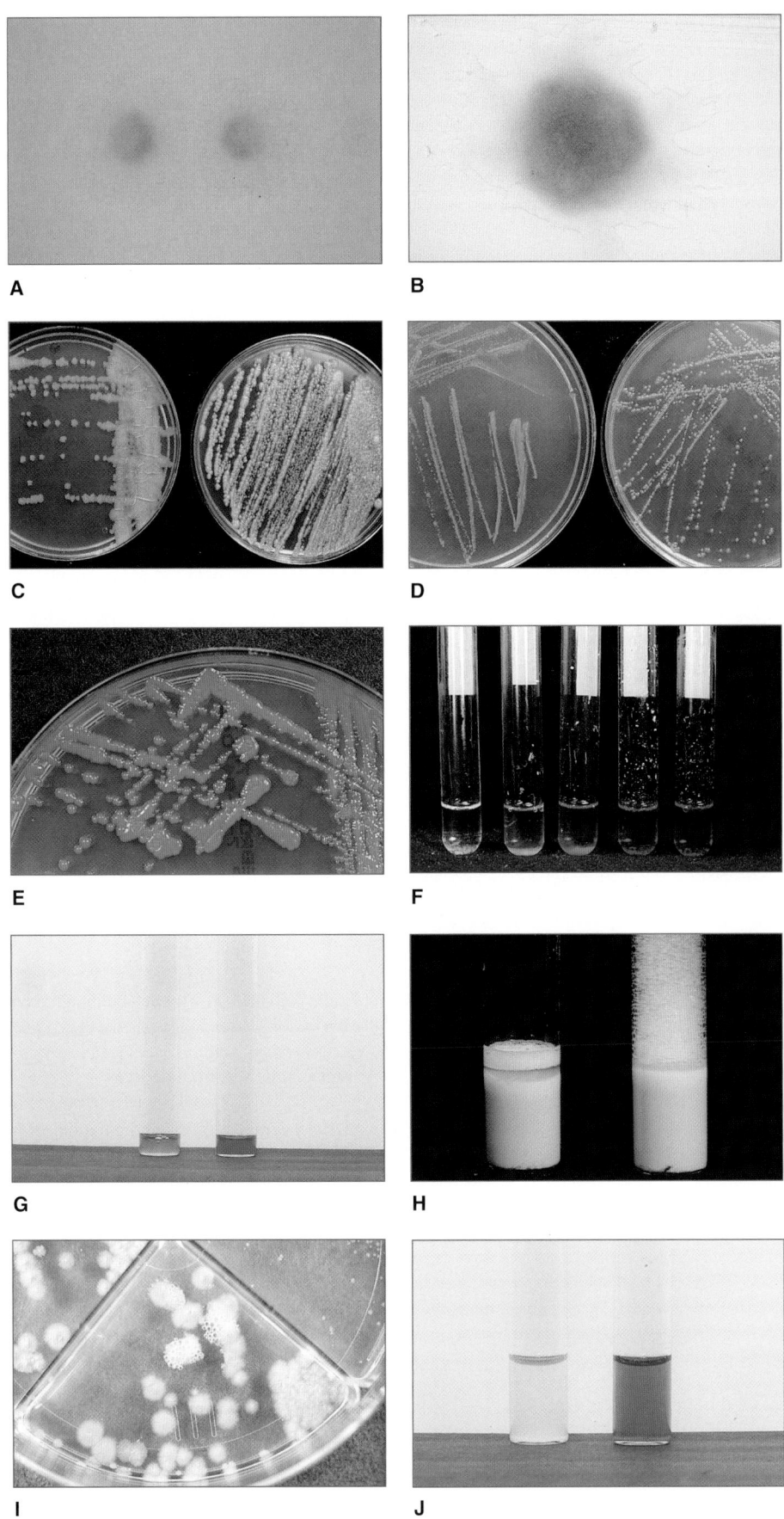

A

B

C

D

E

F

G

H

I

J

K. Two tubes of urea broth previously inoculated with a negative control (*left tube*) and a subculture of *M. gordonae* (*right*). Mycobacterial strains having urease activity will turn the broth pink within several hours (strong positive) to a few days, owing to the release of ammonia and alkalinization of the medium. Assessment of urease activity may be helpful in separating *M. gordonae* (strong positive) from other scotochromogens, and *M. fortuitum-chelonae* complex from other rapid growers.

L. Two tubes of Dubos broth base, the *left* containing pyrazinamide and the *right* a negative control devoid of reagent. Both tubes had previously been inoculated with a subculture of a strain of *M. avium*. The development of a pink-red band at the reagent layer toward the surface of the agar in the *left* tube, after addition of ferrous ammonium sulfate reagent, indicates a positive test and the ability of this strain to deaminate pyrazinamide.

M. Photomicrograph of an acid-fast smear prepared from a subculture of *M. kansasii*. The bacterial cells of *M. kansasii* are described as rectangular, straight, and banded, which is reasonably represented here. Because of variation between strains and between other species, a presumptive identification of *Mycobacterium* species based on acid-fast stain morphology is risky at best.

N. A Middlebrook 7H10 agar plate previously inoculated with a subculture of a classic strain of *M. avium*. The classic strains of *M. avium* were originally included in the group III nonphotochromogens in the Runyon classification. Note that the colonies here are relatively small, smooth, and gray-white, without evidence of pigmentation.

O. A Middlebrook 7H10 agar plate previously inoculated with a strain of *M. avium-intracellulare* (MAI) complex recovered from a patient with AIDS. Many of the MAI strains recovered from patients with AIDS have this distinct yellow pigmentation. The peculiar doughnut-shaped colonies have been produced by most of the strains recovered at the Denver Veterans Hospital during the early 1990s, but is probably not a distinctive characteristic for all strains.

P. Low-power photomicrograph of a liver biopsy from a patient with AIDS also infected with *M. avium-intracellulare*. Note the tight intracellular clusters of short, acid-fast bacilli in the central part of the photograph.

Q. A Middlebrook 7H10 agar plate inoculated 3 days before with a strain of *M. fortuitum* and incubated at 35°C in 10% CO_2. The colonies average 1 to 2 mm in diameter and are entire, smooth, moist, and devoid of pigmentation. The *M. fortuitum-chelonae* complex of organisms were originally assigned to Runyon group IV, the rapid growers.

R. A modified MacConkey agar plate (devoid of crystal violet) on which are growing colonies taken from a subculture of *M. fortuitum*. Strains belonging to the *M. fortuitum-chelonae* have the unique ability to grow on modified MacConkey agar. The colonies average 2 mm in diameter and are entire, moist, and have a slight pink-yellow tinge due to pigment derived from the agar.

S. A 5% sheep blood agar plate with a 48-hour growth on *M. fortuitum*. Strains belonging to the *M. fortuitum-chelonae* complex will grow on routine 5% sheep blood agar within 48 to 72 hours and may cause confusion with other gram-positive bacillary organisms if a partial acid-fast stain is not performed.

T. Photomicrograph of a Gram stain of a smear prepared from an isolated colony illustrated in Color Plate 19-2*S*. The bacterial cells appear as short, slender almost filamentous, faintly staining gram-positive coccobacilli. Microscopists must be alerted to this microscopic picture and not make a presumptive misidentification of an *Actinomyces* species or atypical corynebacterium. A partial acid-fast stain of a second smear will be helpful in making the correct identification.

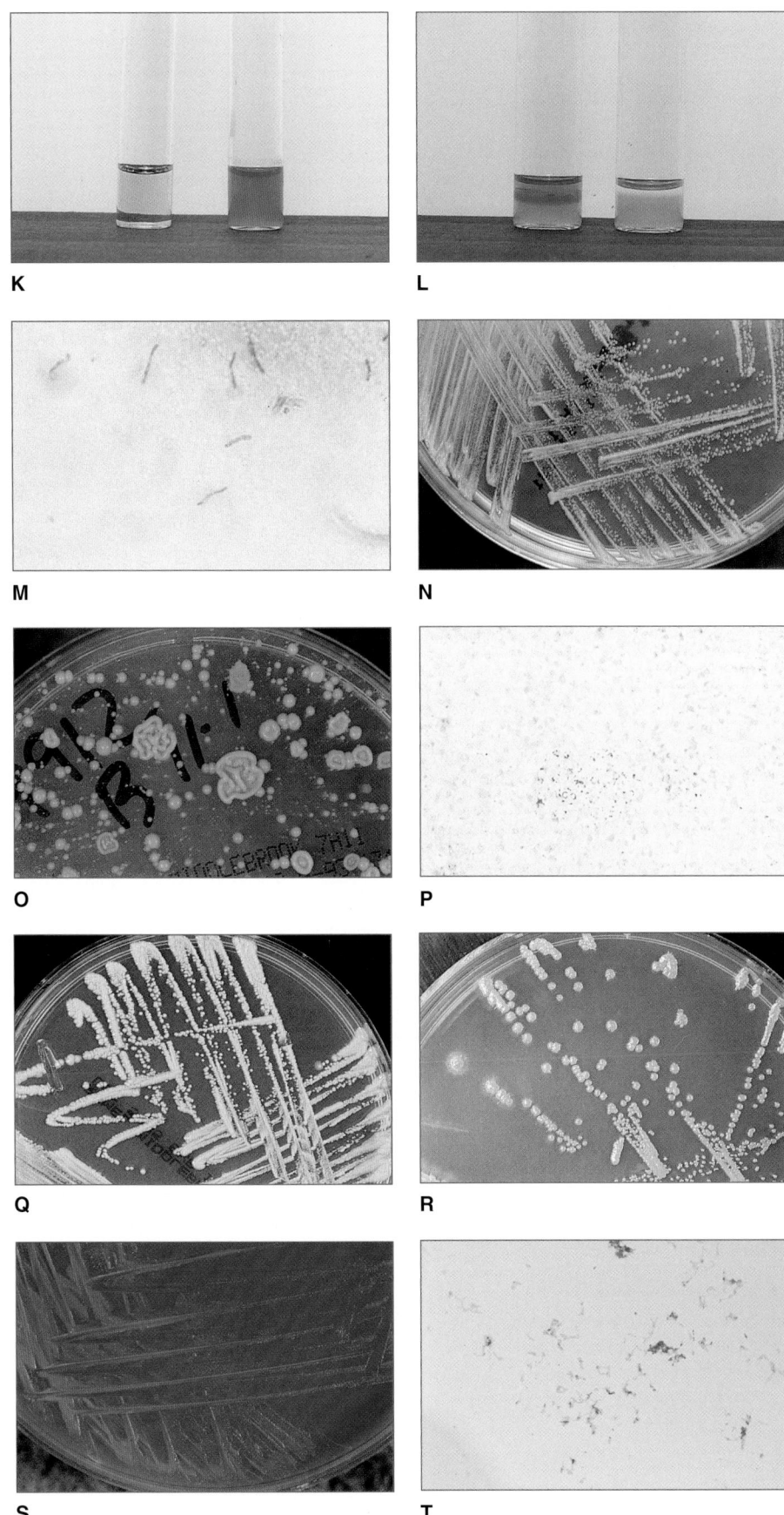

K

L

M

N

O

P

Q

R

S

T

CLINICAL MANIFESTATIONS OF SELECT MYCOBACTERIAL DISEASES

A. X-ray film of the chest from a patient with pulmonary tuberculosis. Note the extensive area of dense infiltration of the right upper lobe.

B. A solitary nodular lesion with well-defined margins is seen in the upper segment of the left lower lung field. A coin lesion of pulmonary coccidioidomycosis must be included in the differential diagnosis of such a lesion. This turned out to be a tuberculoma.

C. A resected lobe of lung illustrating centrally a well-circumscribed, 2.5-cm-diameter, white, firm-appearing nodule. This histologically was a tuberculoma, similar to what may have been removed from the patient whose chest radiograph is shown in Color Plate 19-3*B*.

D. Photomicrograph of a hematoxylin and eosin–stained section taken through a tuberculoma, illustrating varying degrees of background fibrosis and a cellular infiltration composed of lymphocytes and macrophages, many of the latter forming characteristic Langhans giant cells.

E. The base of the brain in a patient dying from tuberculous meningitis. The pia arachnoid covering the base of the brain, particularly in the area of the optic chiasm, appears cloudy, as a manifestation of the chronic inflammatory reaction.

F. A case of cutaneous tuberculosis of the fifth digit. The lesion shown here appears active and inflammatory. In fact, a radiograph revealed bone and joint involvement of the middle and distal phalanx. Lesions of the fingers similar to that shown here were, at one time, common among individuals who milked cows.

G. This posterior neck demonstrates an enlarged, postauricular lymph node with healed draining sinuses along the route of the lymphatic drainage. This is a classic picture of "scrofula" or tuberculous lymphadenitis, typically caused by *M. scrofulaceum* and mycobacteria other than *M. tuberculosis*. The route of infection is oral, and commonly occurs in two age groups during periods of teething—in children 3 to 7 years of age, when secondary teeth are coming in, and in persons in their late teen years, when molars are being cut.

H. The anterior portion of the neck, illustrating multiple healed sinus tracts in a case of chronic tuberculous lymphadenitis. Again, the route of infection is oral, with drainage of infecting mycobacteria along the lymphatic channels.

I. Low-power photomicrograph of a section of small bowel stained with a carbol-fuchsin-based acid-fast stain. The pink mottling seen in the submucosa is dense aggregates of acid-fast bacilli from a case of intestinal infection caused by *M. avium/M. intracellulare* complex in a patient with AIDS.

J. High-power photomicrograph of an area shown in Color Plate 19-3*I*, better illustrating the dense intracellular aggregates of acid-fast bacilli. This histopathologic picture is similar to the "lepra cells" seen in patients with Hanson's disease (leprosy).

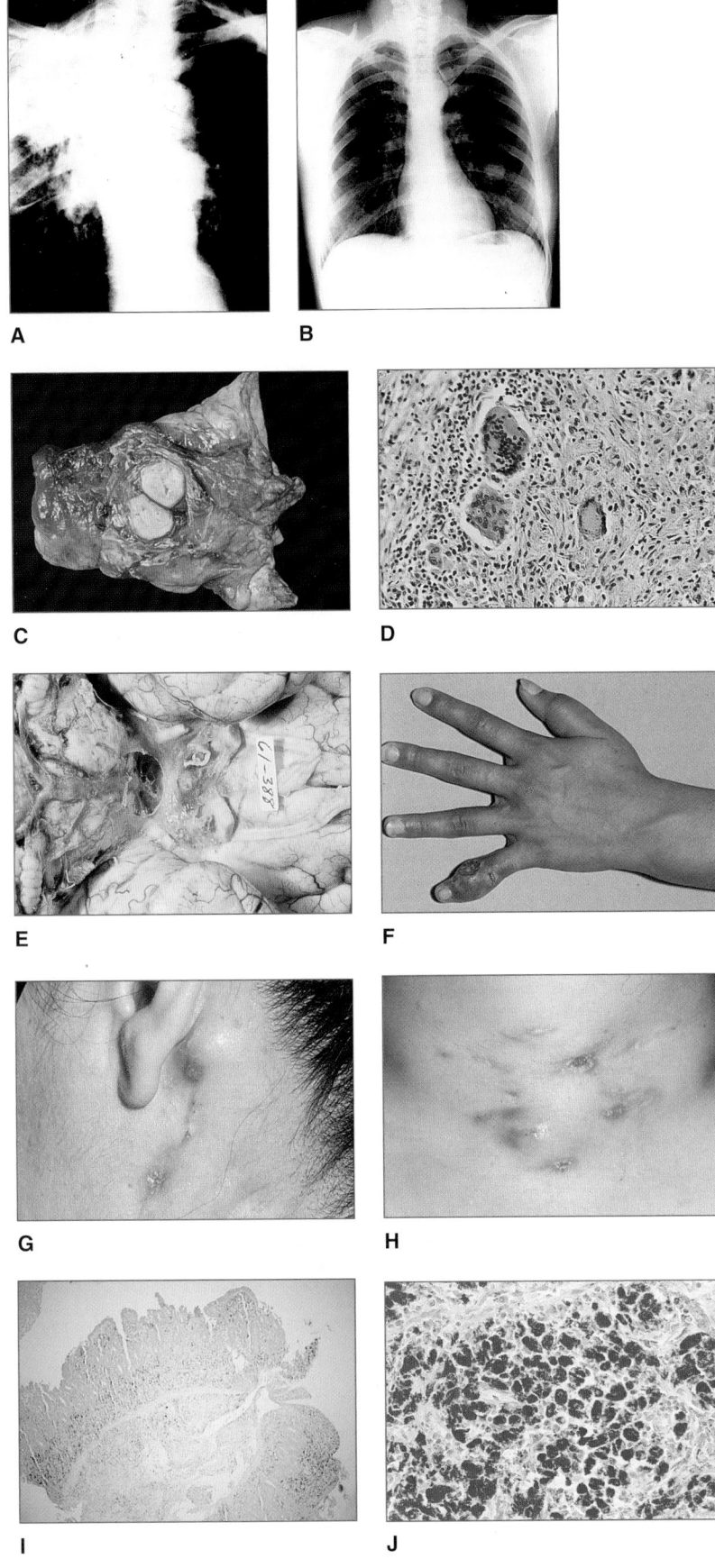

LABORATORY DIAGNOSIS OF SPIROCHETAL DISEASES

A. *Treponema pallidum.* This photomicrograph shows a Warthin-Starry stain of a histologic section of placenta from a patient with congenital syphilis. The tight spiral coils of the spirochete are clearly evident (original magnification, ×1,000).

B. *Treponema pallidum.* This control for the FTA-ABS test demonstrates 4+ staining of the spirochetes. The helical shape is evident, and the tightly coiled spirals can be visualized in some of the bacterial cells. This photomicrograph is an indirect immunofluorescence preparation of *T. pallidum* using fluorescein-conjugated antihuman globulin (original magnification, ×600). (Courtesy of Burton Wilcke, Ph.D., and Mary Celotti, Vermont Department of Public Health, Burlington, VT.)

C. Wright-stained peripheral blood smear from a case of *Borrelia* infection. The loose coils of the *Borrelia* organisms are evident, but the thin structure is easy to overlook. These spirochetes may be detected when examining smears for malaria or for cellular morphology, even if the physician does not suspect the diagnosis (original magnification, ×1,000). (Courtesy of Thomas Fritsche, M.D., Ph.D.)

D. An acridine orange stain of peripheral blood demonstrates *Borrelia* spp. dramatically. If the diagnosis is suspected, this technique, which may be more sensitive than Giemsa or Wright's stains, may be used (original magnification, ×1000). (Courtesy of Brian Lauer, M.D.)

E. *Ixodes scapularis* (*dammini*) ticks. These dark-colored hard ticks, also known as black-legged ticks or deer ticks, contain a dorsal scutum that covers the whole back on the male (M) but only a portion of the back on the female (F), nymph (N), and larva (L). It is the principle vector of *Borrelia burgdorferi*, the agent of Lyme disease, in the eastern United States. *Ixodes pacificus*, the vector in the Pacific region, looks very similar. The primary vectors are nymphs and adult females. Adult males bite only rarely, and the larval stage has not usually been infected when it bites humans. Nymphal ticks are a particular problem, because their small size makes it difficult to detect their presence.

F. *Borrelia burgdorferi* in a culture pellet stained with a monoclonal antibody to OspA protein conjugated to streptavidin–alkaline phosphatase. The typical polymorphism of *B. burgdorferi* is demonstrated. (Courtesy of Paul Duray, M.D.)

G. A histologic section of dog kidney stained with a silver impregnation stain (Warthin-Starry) demonstrates several renal tubules in longitudinal orientation. Even at low power, the masses of *Leptospira* organisms are evident as blackening of the surface of the tubular epithelium. It is clear that this privileged site, where the leptospires are protected from host defenses, can serve as a productive source for spread of infection as the leptospira-contaminated urine is passed onto the ground (original magnification, ×1000). (Courtesy of David Miller, D.V.M., M.S.)

H. Tubes of polysorbate 80–bovine albumin (PSO-BA) semisolid medium. An uninoculated tube is shown on the *left*. The tube on the *right* was inoculated with *Leptospira interrogans*. The subsurface growth in semisolid culture media is typical of leptospires, such as *L. interrogans* sv. *pomona*. Growth appears as a gray-white horizontal band about 1 cm below the medium surface after incubation for 2 to 6 weeks at room temperature. The band grows denser with continued incubation, but may be very scant with fastidious isolates, such as with *L. interrogans* sv. *hardjo*. (Courtesy of David Miller, D.V.M., M.S.)

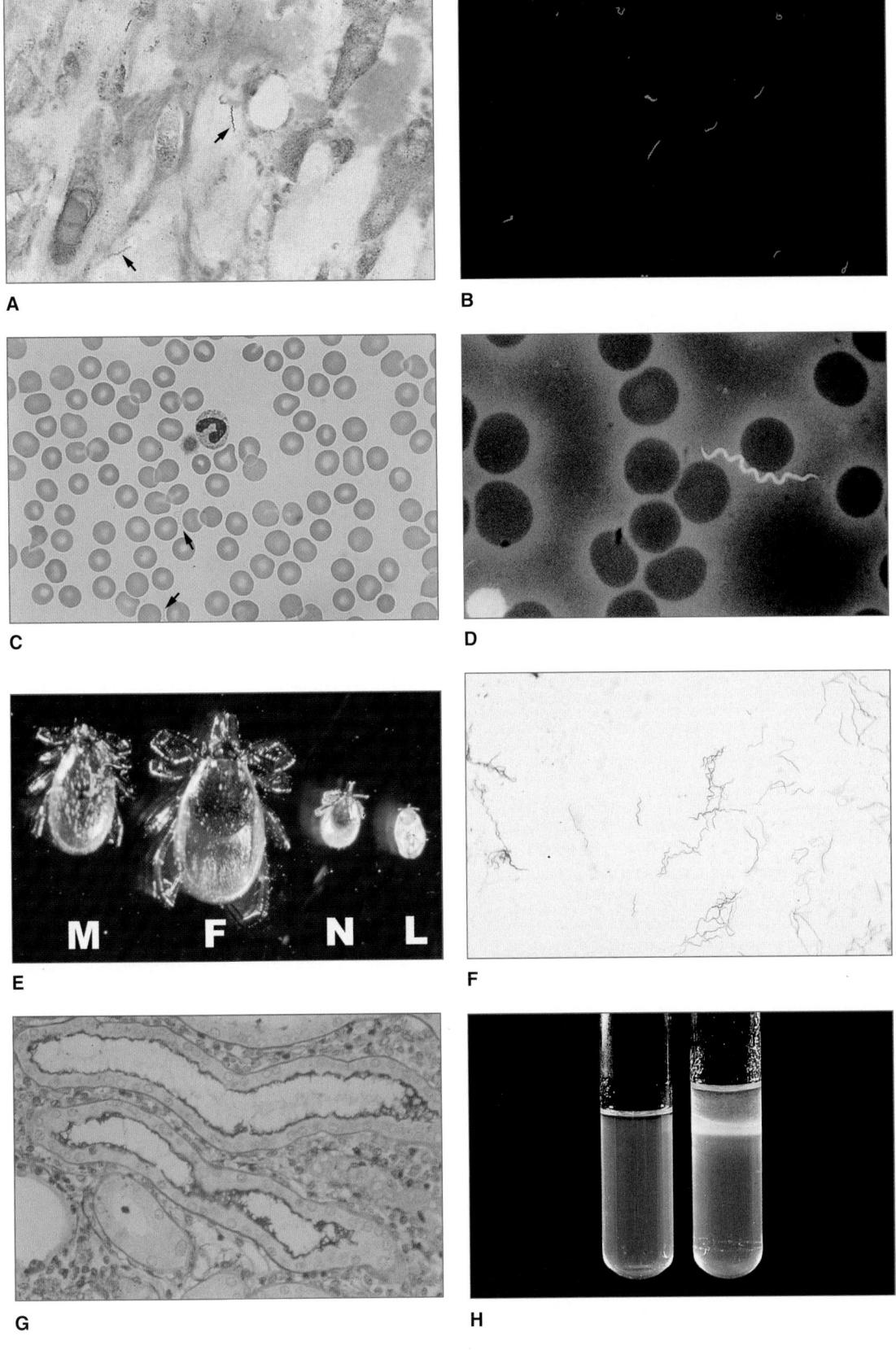

A

B

C

D

E

M F N L

F

G

H

COLONY MORPHOLOGY OF *ZYGOMYCETES* SPECIES AND SELECT *ASPERGILLUS* SPECIES

Members of the *Zygomycetes* and certain *Aspergillus* species are commonly encountered in clinical laboratories as agents of opportunistic infections. These fungi grow rapidly in culture, particularly the *Zygomycetes* species, which can fill a culture plate within 48 hours. Of the aspergilli, *A. fumigatus, A. flavus, A. niger,* and *A. terreus* are most commonly recovered from specimens obtained from patients with aspergillosis. Other species, when recovered, are usually not identified to the species level. *A nidulans* and *A. glaucus* are two uncommonly encountered species that often produce cleistothecia, the telemorphic form that contains ascospores.

A. Sabouraud's dextrose agar plate inoculated with a *Zygomyces* species. Notice that the entire plate is filled with a wooly, gray-white surface mycelium.

B. Close-up view of a colony of a *Zygomyces* species after 96 hours of incubation. As a *Zygomyces* species colony matures, it takes on a gray-brown color, often with black, pepperlike stipples, indicating the production sporangia.

C. The surface of a colony of *Aspergillus fumigatus* after a 5-day incubation on Sabouraud's dextrose agar. Mature colonies of *A. fumigatus* are generally powdery or granular, and have some shade of green from the production of pigmented conidia. The growing margin often appears as a white apron, as illustrated here.

D. The surface of a colony of *Aspergillus flavus* growing on Sabouraud's dextrose agar. The texture of mature colonies is usually granular from the production of conidia, and as the species name suggests, some shade of yellow pigmentation is characteristic.

E. The surface of a colony of *Aspergillus niger* after a 4-day incubation on Sabouraud's dextrose agar. The deep brown to black, densely stippled surface is characteristic. The black surface pigmentation of *A. niger* can be distinguished from one of the dematiaceous fungi by observing the reverse side. The reverse of *A. niger* is a light gray or buff color, as the pigmentation is caused by surface conidia; the reverse of dematiaceous fungi is jet black, as the vegetative hyphae carry the pigment.

F. The surface of a colony of *Aspergillus terreus* after a 6-day incubation on Sabouraud's dextrose agar. *A. terreus* characteristically has a granular surface and some shade of yellow or brown pigmentation. Rugae radiating from the center are often seen, and the concentric zones of light and dark pigmentation as seen here are not unusual.

G. The surface of an albino strain of *Aspergillus nidulans*. Although most strains have some light pigmentation, albino strains of most *Aspergillus* species may occasionally be encountered and must be kept in the differential identification. The granular surface, with radiating rugae, is also common.

H. The surface of a colony of *Aspergillus glaucus*. The green and yellow variegated appearance seen here is not specific, because other *Aspergillus* species may have a similar appearance. Microscopic examination is necessary to make a species identification.

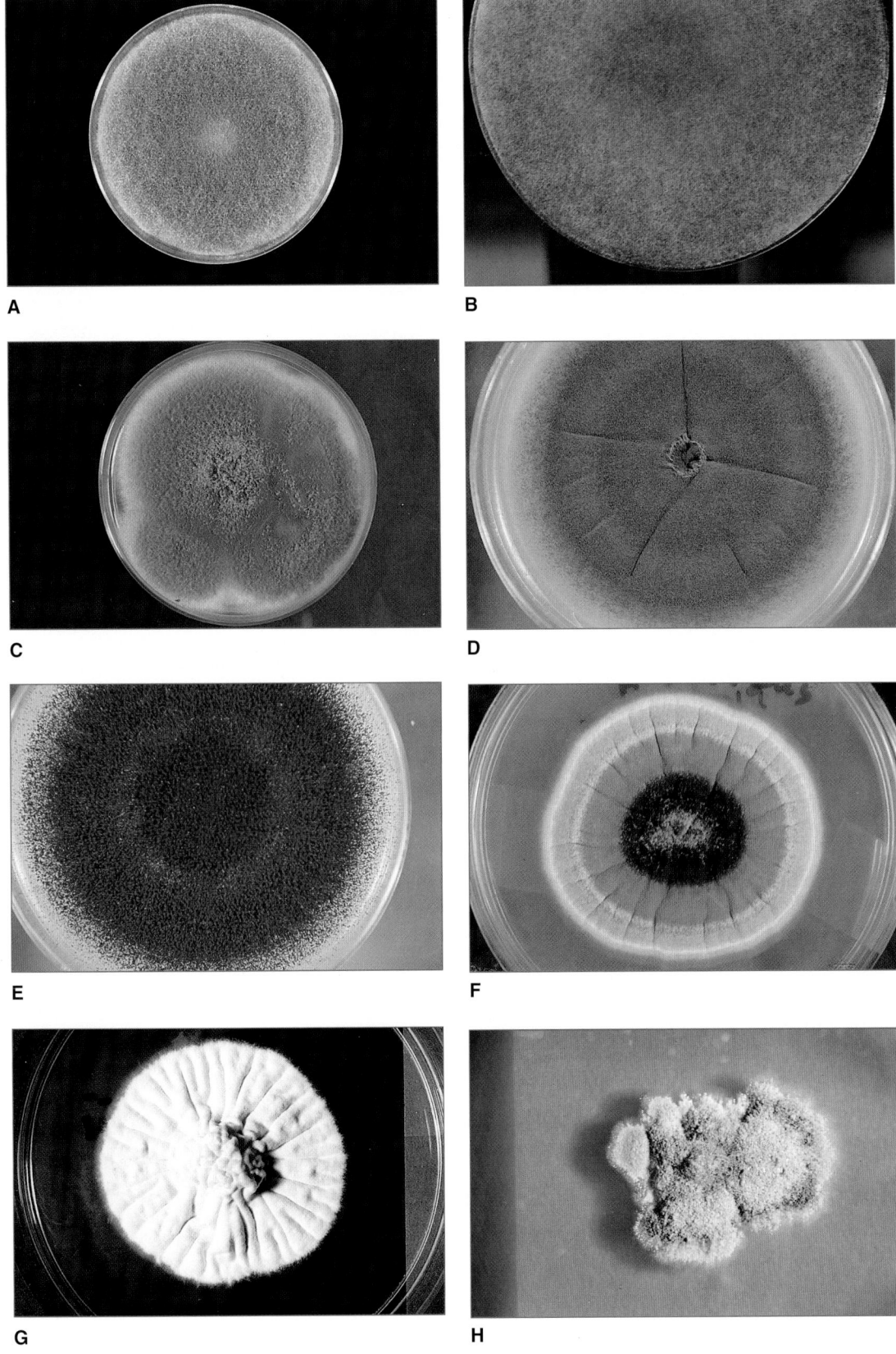

A

B

C

D

E

F

G

H

COLONY MORPHOLOGY OF COMMONLY ENCOUNTERED HYALINE MOLDS

The colonies of the hyaline fungi have a varied appearance. Most display light pastel or deeper pigmentation, with combinations of green, yellow, orange, and brown hues commonly observed. The texture of the colonies may be smooth (glabrous), granular, cottony, or wooly, depending on their maturity and degree of sporulation. Microscopic studies must be performed to confirm the genus and species identification.

A. The surface of a colony of *Penicillium* species after a 5-day incubation on Sabouraud's dextrose agar, illustrating the distinctive green color, granular surface, radial rugae and white apron at the periphery. Although most strains of *Penicillium* species display some shade of green, yellow variants are sometimes seen.

B. The surface of a colony of *Penicillium marneffei* after a 4-day incubation on Sabouraud's dextrose agar, illustrating the distinctive red pigmentation of a portion of the colony. Note that the pigment has leached out into the agar, which has a light wine-red coloration. The surface tends to be granular to fluffy, depending on the degree of sporulation; note the distinct white apron at the margin of peripheral new growth.

C. The surface of a colony of *Paecilomyces* species. The colonies of *Paecilomyces* species are usually granular and often have a yellow-brown pigmentation, as illustrated here. Other strains, however, may have a light pastel green, green-yellow, or bluish appearance.

D. The surface of a colony of *Scopulariopsis* species after 5 days of growth on Sabouraud's dextrose agar. The yellow pigmentation, granular texture, and radiating rugae, as illustrated here, are hallmarks of *Scopulariopsis* species.

E. The surface of a colony of *Acremonium* species after 5 days of incubation on Sabouraud's dextrose agar. The colonies of *Acremonium* species usually have a smooth, almost yeastlike appearance, as illustrated here, owing to the extremely delicate nature of the hyphae and fruiting bodies. Light pastel yellow, light green, and peach-red hues may be observed.

F. The surface of a typical colony of *Fusarium* species after 6 days of growth on Sabouraud's dextrose agar. *Fusarium* species can be suspected when a rapidly growing granular or fluffy colony, with a distinct rose-red, lavender, or purple pigmentation, is observed.

G. The surface of a typical fluffy, "house mouse gray" colony of *Scedosporium apiosperum* (anamorphic form of *Pseudallescheria boydii*) after 5 days of incubation on Sabouraud's dextrose agar. A rapidly growing colony with the mouse gray appearance, as illustrated here, always suggests *Scedosporium* species. The unique pigmentation is caused by darkly pigmented conidia.

H. A colony of *Gliocladium* species after 5 days of growth on Sabouraud's dextrose agar. The green pigment, extension of the colony from border to border without a well-defined growing margin and granular texture (so-called green lawn) is unique for *Gliocladium* and *Trichoderma* species. The latter more frequently may show a yellow, rather than a green, pigmentation.

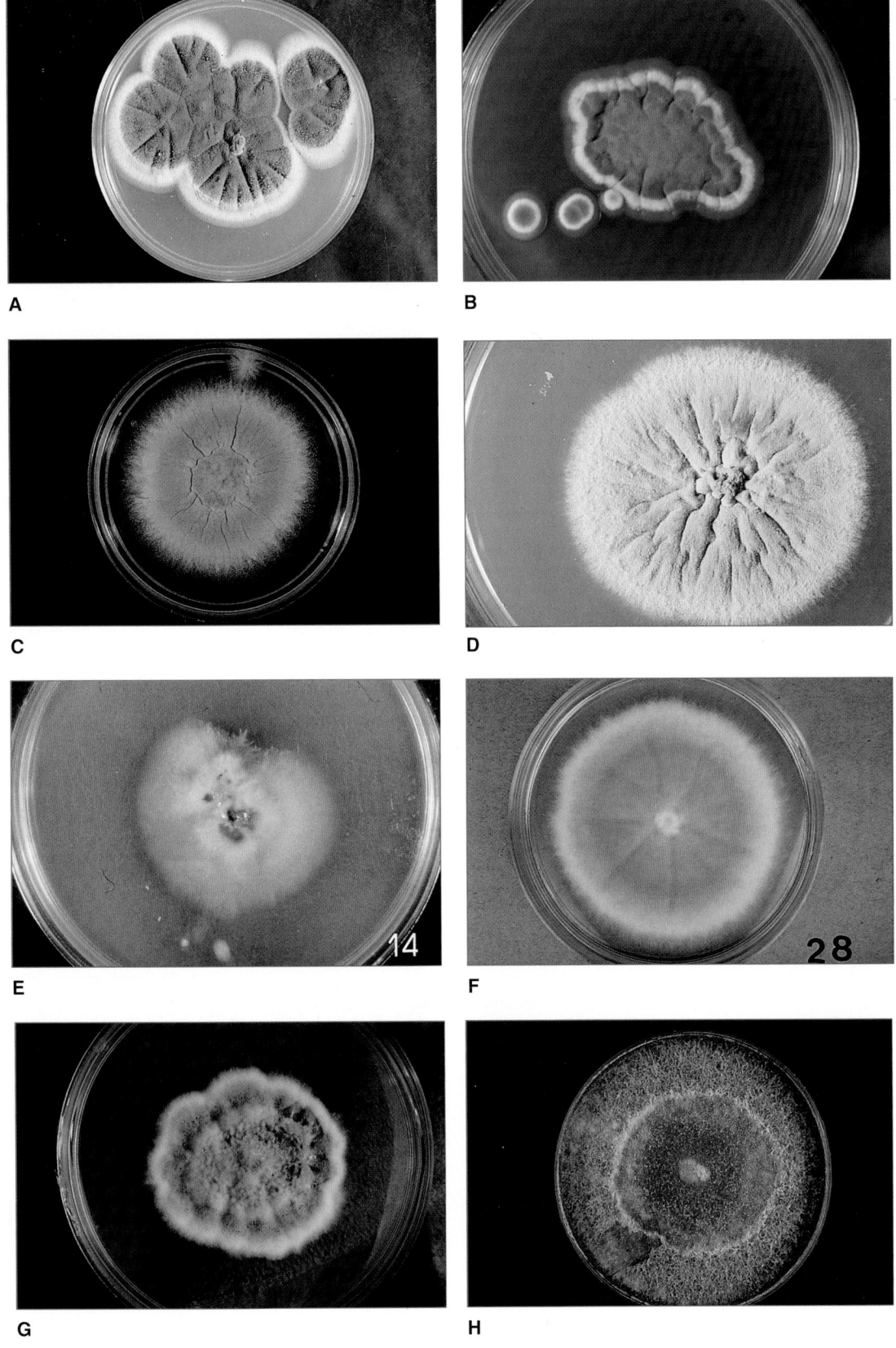

A

B

C

D

E

14

F

28

G

H

COLONY MORPHOLOGY OF COMMONLY ENCOUNTERED DEMATIACEOUS MOLDS

The dematiaceous (dark) molds are characterized by the growth of deep green, brown, or black colonies, with black pigmentation on the reverse surface. Most environmental species grow rapidly, producing mature colonies within 5 days. Slower-growing species, at times requiring 2 weeks or more before mature colonies are observed, are often recovered from clinical specimens taken from patients with mycetomas or chromomycosis. Photographs of representative colonies of select dematiaceous molds growing on Sabouraud's dextrose agar are illustrated here.

A. Fluffy, gray-black surface of a colony of *Alternaria* species after 6 days of growth. The appearance shown here is not distinctive for *Alternaria* species, but may also be observed with other species of environmental dematiaceous molds.

B. Reverse surface of a dematiaceous mold, illustrating the dark appearance caused by the dark brown pigmentation of the vegetative hyphae.

C. Surface view of a subculture of *Ulocladium* species, illustrating a wooly, dark brown to black pigmentation. Although frequently seen with certain strains of dematiaceous fungi, the light and darker concentric rings observed here are not distinctive for any given species.

D. Surface view of a colony of *Phialophora verrucosum* after 14 days of incubation. This particular strain has a dark gray-black hue, with a hairlike texture. Microscopic study is necessary, because other slow-growing species may produce similar-appearing colonies.

E. Surface view of a colony of *Fonsecaea pedrosoi* after 16 days of incubation. The colony is quite small, typical for the species, and the typical dark brown-black pigmentation is evident. This strain has a flatter, almost suedelike consistency.

F. Surface view of a colony of a more rapidly growing (5 days), environmental strain of *Cladosporium* species, illustrating a dark green, suedelike surface interrupted by irregular rugae. Environmental strains of *Cladosporium* species may appear dark green, as shown here, or may be gray, gray-brown, or brown-black, simulating other dematiaceous fungi.

G. Surface view of another variant of an environmental *Cladosporium* species showing a dark gray, leatherlike consistency. Colony texture among the dematiaceous molds range from wooly, to downy or hairlike, to suedelike, to leathery.

H. Appearance of the flat, smooth, yeastlike surface of *Aureobasidium pullulans* after 6 days of incubation. *Aureobasidium* spp. should be first on the list when a "black yeast," similar to that illustrated here, is observed; however, certain strains of *Exophiala wernickii* (so-called *Phaeoannelomyces* synanamorphs) must also be considered, which will develop a low, hairlike mycelium with true hyphae after several additional days of incubation.

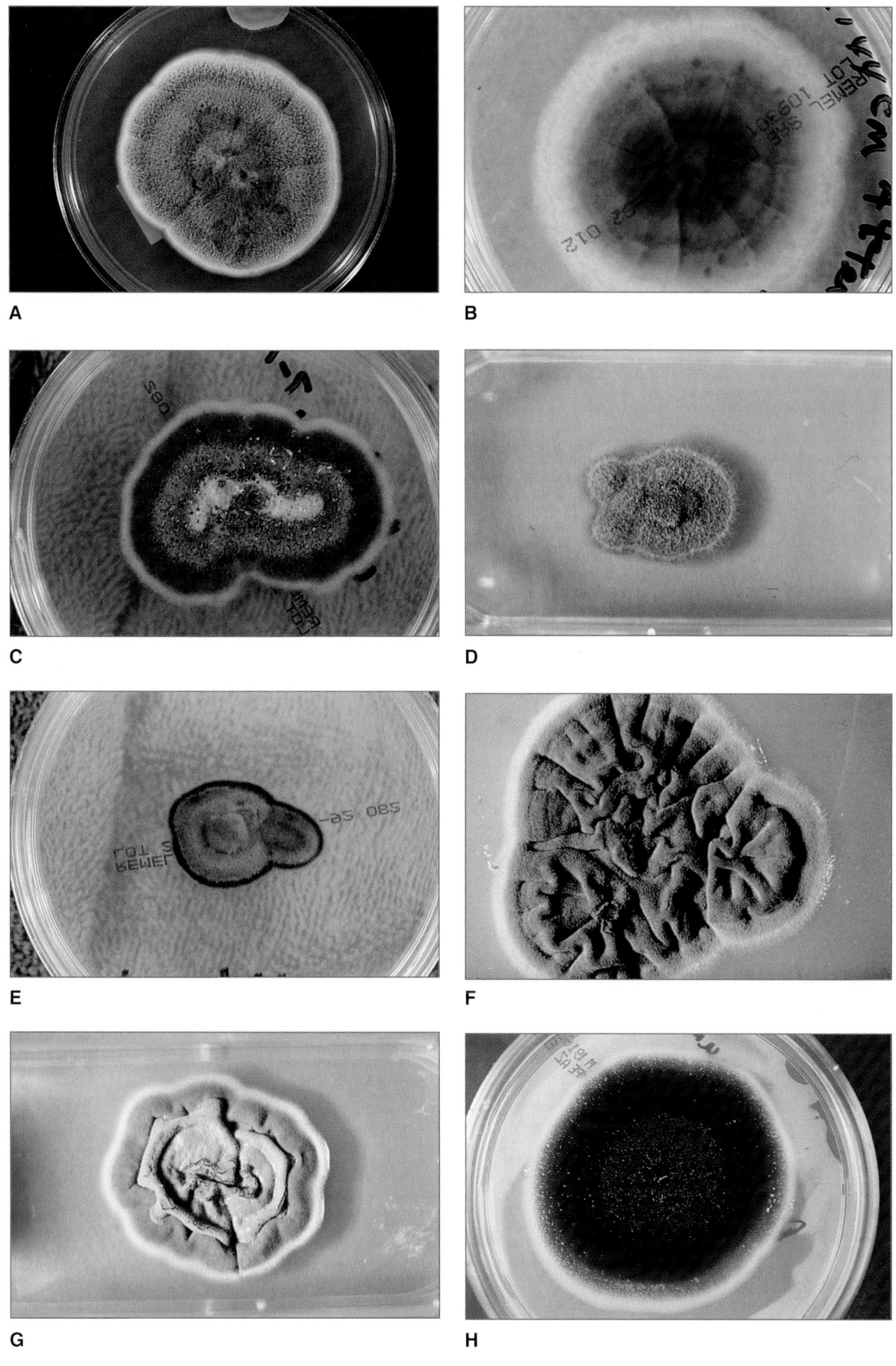

A

B

C

D

E

F

G

H

COLONY MORPHOLOGY OF DERMATOPHYTES

The colonies representative of the dermatophytic molds on artificial culture media are not distinctive. There is sufficient strain variation and differences in appearance of the same strain, depending on the type of culture medium used and the environmental conditions during incubation, that colonial morphology is not a reliable criterion for making presumptive identifications. Microscopic studies are almost always necessary to derive a definitive identification. Illustrated here are photographs of the colonies of select dermatophytes growing on Sabouraud's dextrose agar at 30°C, chosen to show certain characteristics that may offer clues to making a presumptive identification.

A. Colony of *Microsporum canis* after 5 days of incubation. The colonies tend to be fluffy or, at times, granular if conidiation is heavy. The lemon-yellow apron seen here, with pigment also extending to the reverse surface, is one clue suggesting *M. canis.*

B. Surface of a powdery, off-yellow colony of *Microsporum gypseum* after 6 days of incubation. *M. gypseum* tends to sporulate heavily; therefore, it is more prone to produce granular colonies than *M. canis.*

C. Surface of a smooth, white variant of *Trichophyton mentagrophytes,* with no evidence of background pigmentation of the agar. The colony illustrated here is not distinctive, and microscopic study is required to make an identification.

D. Surface of a fluffy variant of *Trichophyton mentagrophytes* demonstrating a reddish pigmentation of the background agar. Wine-red pigmentation is one feature that suggests *T. rubrum;* however, certain strains of *T. mentagrophytes* may also produce reddish pigment when growing on Sabouraud's dextrose agar. Pigmentation, however, is never as intense as with *T. rubrum* when colonies are grown on cornmeal or potato dextrose agar.

E. Reverse of a colony of *Trichophyton rubrum* growing on potato dextrose agar. The deep wine-red pigmentation is characteristic of the species, and is particularly intense when the colony is grown on potato dextrose or cornmeal agar.

F. Comparative growth of *T. mentagrophytes* (*bottom*) and *T. rubrum* (*top*) on cornmeal agar, illustrating the distinct difference in pigmentation between the two species.

G. Surface of a small colony of *Trichophyton tonsurans* after 14 days of incubation *T. tonsurans* grows slower on Sabouraud's dextrose agar. Most strains produce some shade of yellow-brown pigment. The surface tends to be granular, and radial rugae are frequently seen. Except for the slower growth, the colonies of *T. tonsurans* appear similar to *Scopulariopsis* species and *Aspergillus terreus.*

H. Surface of *Epidermophyton floccosum* after 6 days of incubation. This colony appears more fluffy than granular and has an off-yellow pigmentation. Classic colonies of *E. floccosum* are described as khaki green. The colony texture tends to be more fluffy than granular, as microconidia are not produced by this genus.

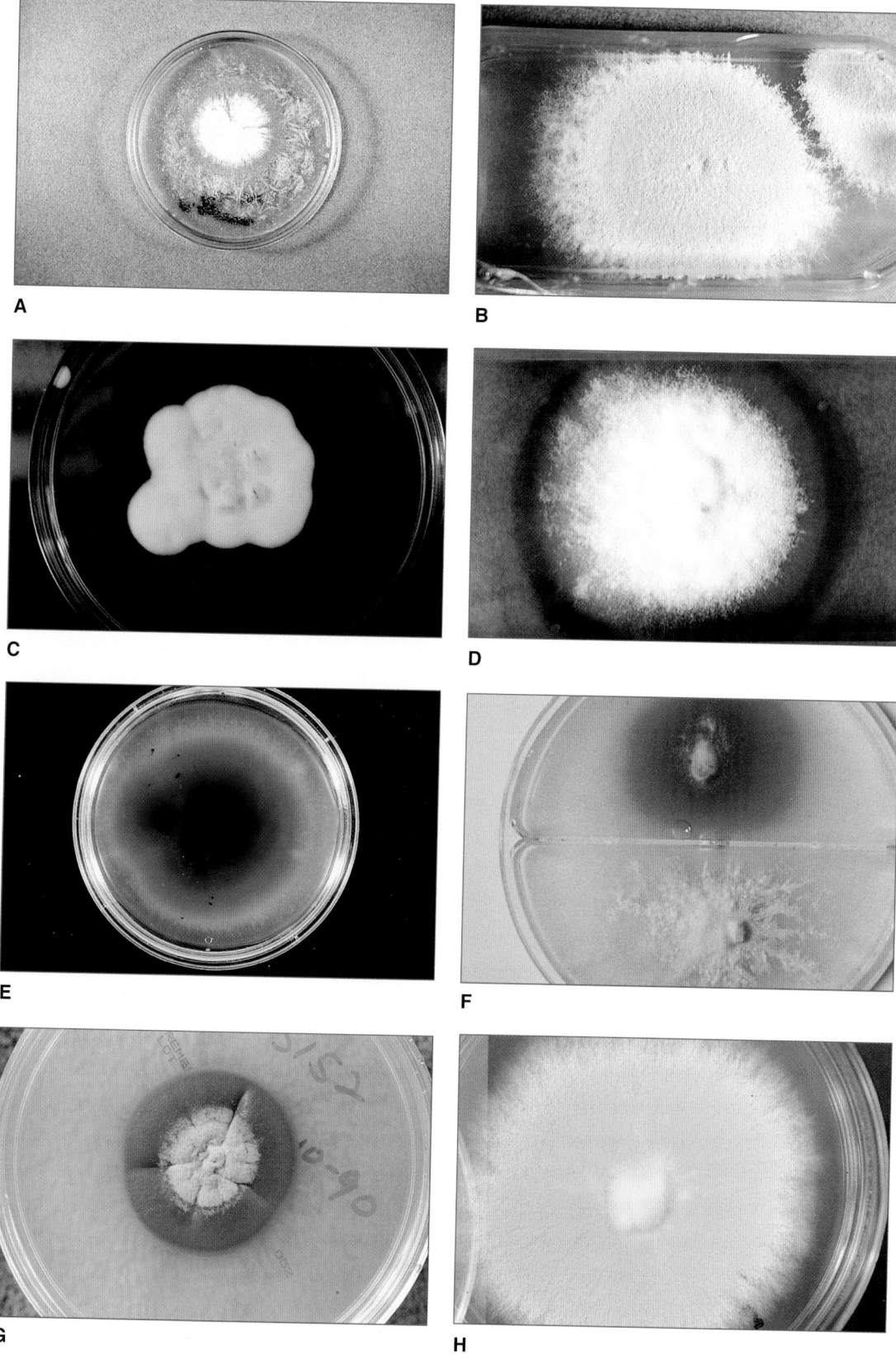

COLONY MORPHOLOGY OF DIMORPHIC FUNGI

The dimorphic fungi, so called because they grow in a mold form at 25 to 30°C (room temperature) and a yeast form at 37°C, are pathogenic in humans and are the agents of the deep-seated mycoses. Although definitive species identification depends on microscopic study, conformation that a given species belongs to the dimorphic group depends on demonstrating both the mold and yeast forms in laboratory isolates. The mold form may be converted to the yeast form by incubating subcultures on enriched media at 37°C and observing microscopically for the appearance of yeast forms typical of the species. With the advent of exoantigen extraction techniques and nucleic-acid probe assays, conversion tests are performed only infrequently in most clinical laboratories.

A. Surface colony of a dimorphic mold, illustrating both the yeast form (*centrally*) and the mold form (*peripherally*). This colony was incubated for 14 days at 30°C. When this mixture of yeast and mold texture is observed, one of the dimorphic fungi can be suspected, particularly if the colony is relatively slow-growing and the mold appears more hairlike or cobweblike in consistency.

B. Colonies of *Blastomyces dermatitidis* growing on 5% sheep blood agar after 5 days of incubation. Note the cobweblike appearance of these colonies, one clue that the isolate may be a dimorphic fungus, and alerting one to take special precautions when preparing subcultures or microscopic mounts to avoid a laboratory-acquired infection.

C. Appearance of colonies of *Blastomyces dermatitidis* incubated at 37°C, during a mold-to-yeast conversion. There is an intermediate form of the colonies between mold and yeast, known as the "prickly stage." Note the rather coarse spicules formed by these white colonies.

D. Colonies of *Histoplasma capsulatum* on brain-heart infusion agar after 25 days of incubation at 30°C. The colonies appear white and cobweblike in consistency. These colonies are nondescript, and microscopic examination is necessary to make an identification.

E. Surface of a 5% sheep blood agar plate incubated at 37°C on which are growing small, yellowish yeast colonies of *Histoplasma capsulatum* after successful conversion from the mold form. The yeast forms are similar to other true yeasts, except that growth is very slow and the colonies remain quite small.

F. Surface of colonies of *Coccidioides immitis* growing on 5% sheep blood agar after 7 days of incubation. The colonies are gray-white and have a delicate hairlike texture. Colonies of *C. immitis* growing on blood agar often show a red discoloration from leaching of hemoglobin from the culture medium (not shown here).

G. Surface of a smooth, gray-brown yeast colony of *Sporothrix schenckii*. Because of the extremely delicate sporulation of *S. schenckii*, colonies often appear more yeastlike than moldlike, even when incubated at 25 to 30°C. After prolonged incubation, colonies of *S. schenckii* tend to darken considerably, becoming almost jet black with some strains (see Color Plate 21-5*H*).

H. Tubes of brain-heart infusion agar, one containing cyclohexiide, on which are growing the yeast (*top*) and mold (*bottom*) forms of *S. schenckii*. Because of the delicate nature of the hyphae and fruiting structures, the mold colony appears quite yeastlike. The colonies tend to darken with maturity, becoming distinctly black in some cases, as illustrated here.

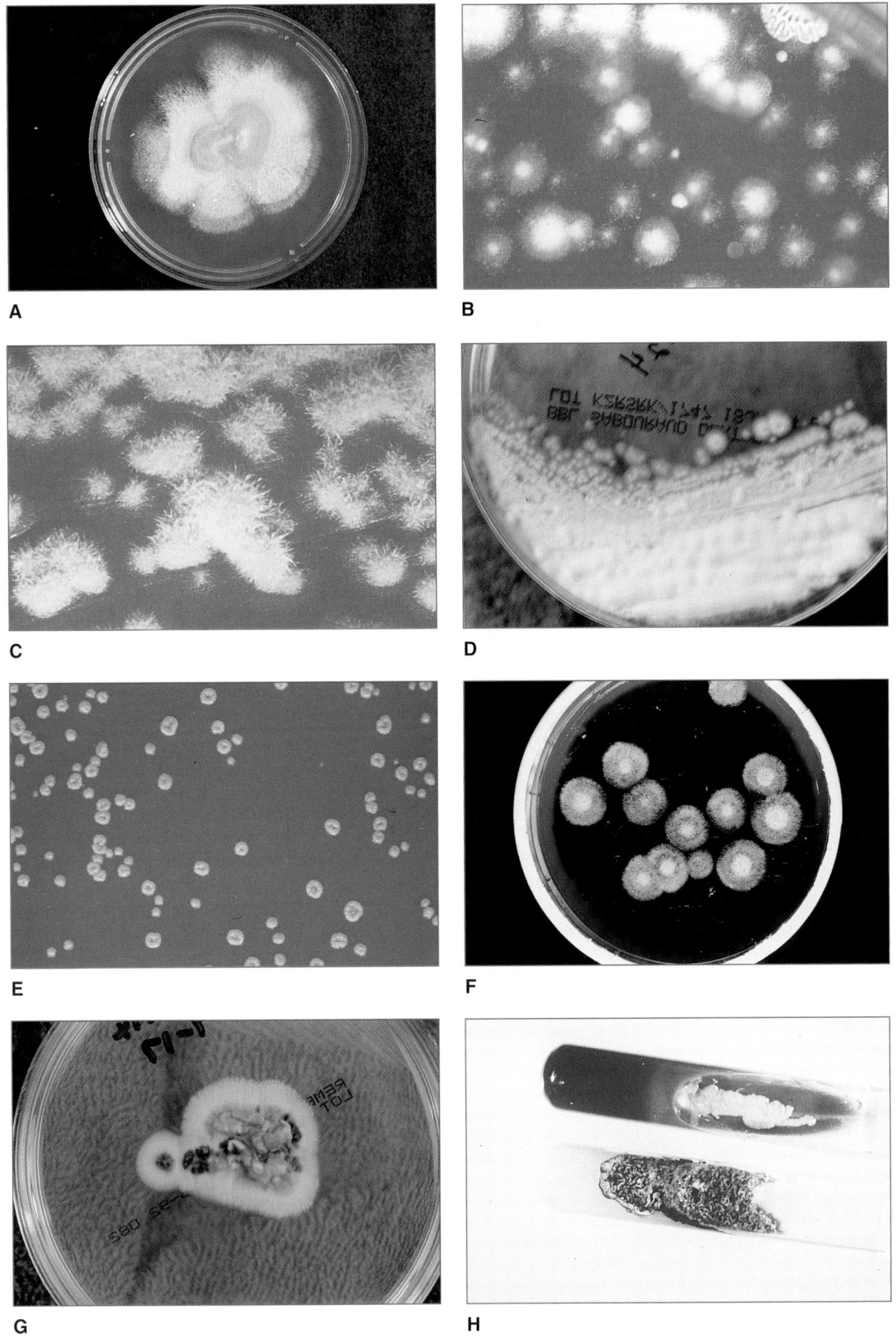

A

B

C

D

E

F

G

H

Morphology of Commonly Recovered Yeasts

The laboratory identification of medically important yeasts involves visual assessment of colony characteristics and the interpretation of results of carbohydrate fermentation and assimilation tests.

A. Surface of a smooth, off-white yeast colony obtained from a subculture of *Candida albicans* after 3 days of incubation. The colony shown here is not distinctive for *C. albicans*, but may be seen with other *Candida* species and yeasts of other species. Additional studies are required when a yeastlike colony, as illustrated here, is recovered in the microbiology laboratory.

B. Surface of 5% sheep blood agar plate on which are growing white colonies of a yeast. The foot-like extensions from the margins of the colonies are typically produced by *C. albicans*.

C. Colonies of *Cryptococcus neoformans* on Sabouraud's dextrose agar after 4 days of incubation. The distinct mucoid consistency of the colonies is indicative of a capsule-forming yeast, suggesting *Cryptococcus* species. Additional tests are required to identify *C. neoformans*.

D. Colonies of *Cryptococcus neoformans* growing on niger seed (birdseed) agar. The maroon-red pigmentation of the colonies when growing on this medium is characteristic of *C. neoformans*, distinguishing this species from other *Cryptococcus* species that are incapable of producing darkly pigmented colonies.

E. Colonies of *Torulopsis* (*Candida*) *glabrata* growing on Sabouraud's dextrose agar after 3 days of incubation at 30°C. *T. glabrata* is suggested when small, more translucent yeast colonies are observed, although additional studies are necessary to confirm the identification.

F. Colonies of *Rhodotorula* species, illustrating the distinctive orange-red pigmentation characteristic of this genus. Some strains of *Cryptococcus* species may also produce a reddish pigmentation; therefore, additional studies may be necessary to make a definitive identification.

G. Surface of a blood agar plate on which are growing the yeastlike colonies of *Malassezia furfur* only in the area where virgin olive oil had been spread. *M. furfur* is a lipophilic yeast commonly found on human skin. A medium rich in oil (such as spreading virgin olive oil on the surface, as shown here) is necessary for the recovery of this yeast. Laboratory personnel must be notified if cases of tinea versicolor are suspected so that an oil overlay preparation can be made.

H. Photomicrograph of an acid-fast–stained smear prepared from an isolated colony of *Saccharomyces cerevisiae* growing on the surface of ascospore agar. The spherical, red-staining (acid-fast) bodies seen here are ascospores. *Hansenula anomala* also produces acid-fast–staining ascospores when grown on ascospore agar; however, they are cap-shaped, rather than spherical, in outline.

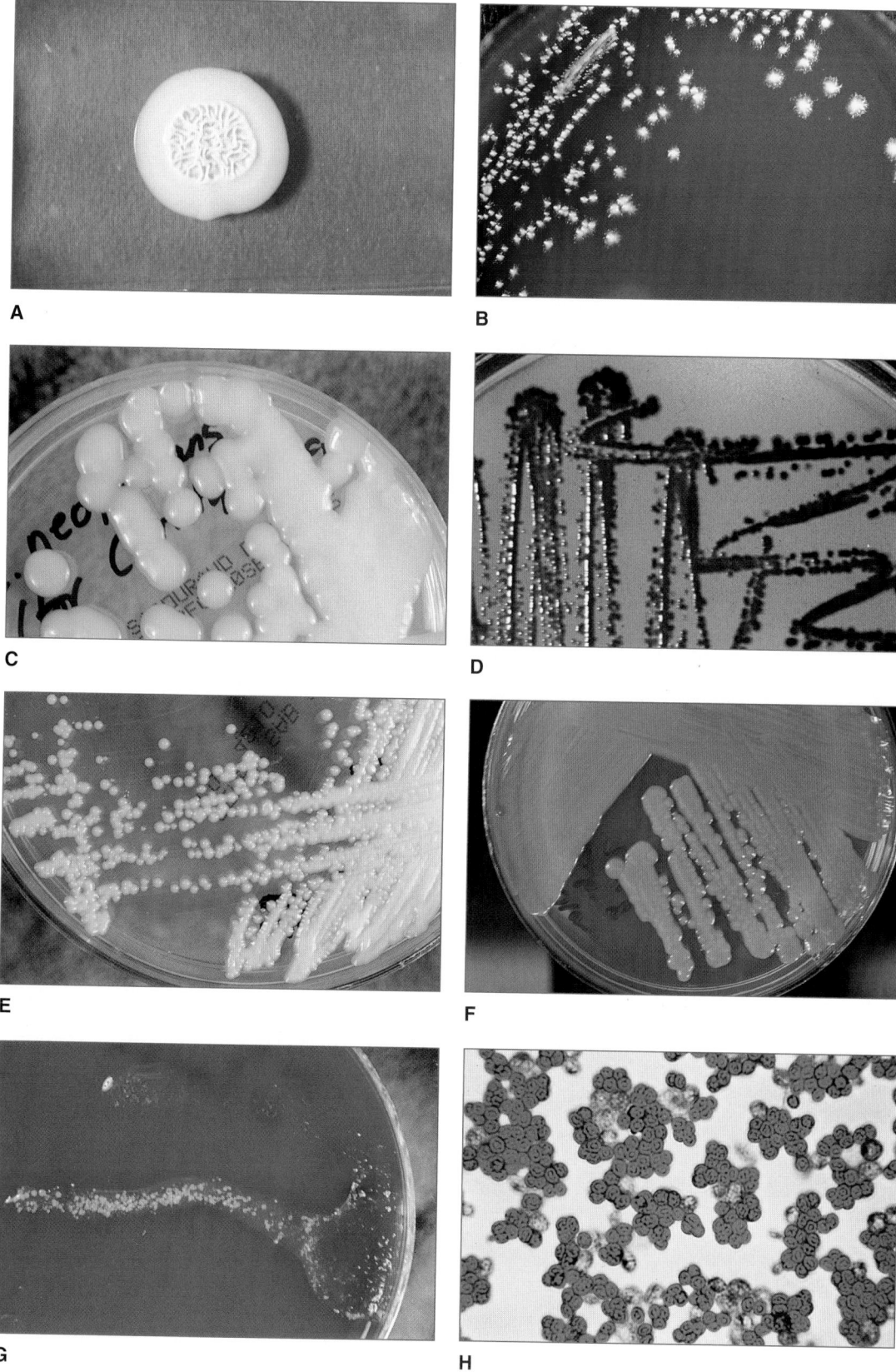

A

B

C

D

E

F

G

H

ARTIFACTS: "NOBODY KNOWS THE RUBBLE I'VE SEEN"

A. Vegetable matter simulating decorticate *Ascaris lumbricoides* egg.

B. Skeletal muscle fiber from ingested red meat simulating a parasitic larval form.

C. Talc powder fragments, often contaminating specimens collected while wearing rubber gloves, simulating amebic cysts.

D. Crystals simulating parasite eggs.

E. Vegetable strand simulating rhabditiform larva.

F. Echinulate pollen grain simulating egg of *Taenia* species.

G. Pollen grain simulating hookworm, *Strongyloides*, or decorticate *Ascaris* egg.

H. Peach hair simulating filariform larva.

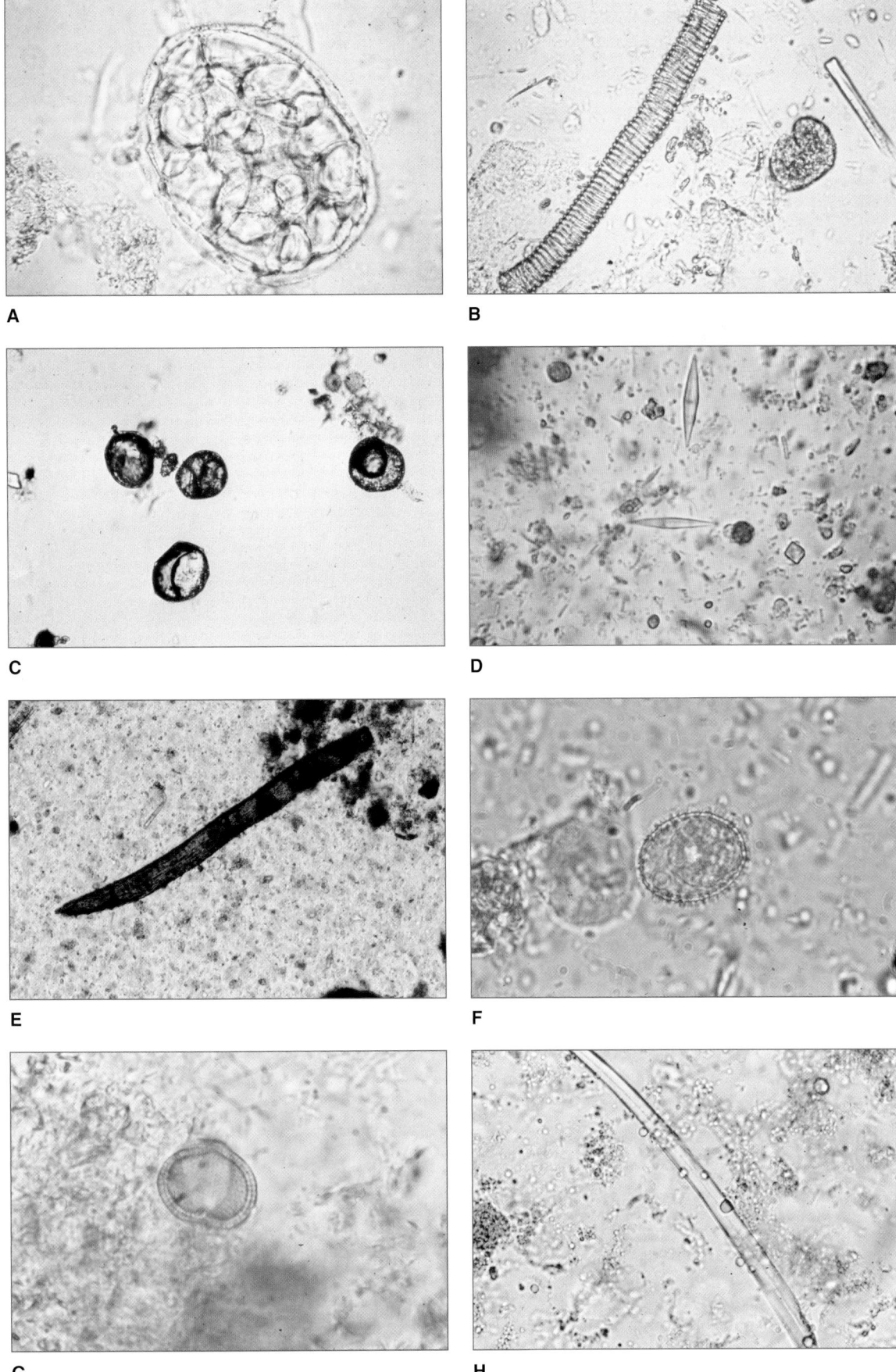

A

B

C

D

E

F

G

H

INTESTINAL AMOEBA/FLAGELLATES

A. Photomicrograph of fecal smear stained with trichrome. In the center of the field is a two-lobed segmented neutrophil simulating an *Entamoeba*-type cyst. Care must always be taken to be sure that polymorphonuclear leukocytes in fecal specimens are not mistaken for amebic cysts.

B. Photomicrograph of a fecal smear stained with iron hematoxylin, illustrating a single trophozoite of *Entamoeba histolytica*, measuring 10 μm in greatest dimension. Note the spherical nucleus containing a tiny, compact, centrally placed karyosome, and even, beadlike distribution of chromatin along the nuclear membrane (the *Entamoeba*-type nucleus). The extension of a single pseudopod reflects a purposeful, directional motility.

C. Photomicrograph of a direct iodine mount of a cyst of *Entamoeba histolytica*, measuring 12 μm in diameter. Four nuclei are observed, each of which contains a small centrally placed karyosome and a fine, even band of nuclear chromatin around the nuclear membrane.

D. Hematoxylin and eosin–stained section of colon mucosa, illustrating many infiltrating *Entamoeba histolytica* trophozoites. The trophozoites are the light-staining, irregularly spherical bodies, some of which show an *Entamoeba*-type nucleus. (×400.)

E. Iron-hematoxylin–stained fecal smear illustrating a single trophozoite of *Entamoeba coli*. Note the large karyosome, the uneven distribution of the chromatin along the nuclear membrane, and the coarse "junky" cytoplasm containing undigested debris and several irregular-sized vacuoles. The trophozoites of *E. coli* tend to be larger than those of *E. histolytica*, ranging, on average, between 14 and 25 μm in diameter.

F. Trichrome-stained cyst of *Entamoeba coli* illustrating five nuclei, each containing a relatively large centrally or slightly eccentrically placed karyosome. The presence of more than four nuclei rules out *Entamoeba histolytica*. A single red-staining intracytoplasmic chromatoidal bar with pointed ends is seen in the 2 o'clock position.

G. Iron-hematoxylin stain of a precyst of *Entamoeba histolytica*, measuring 8 μm in diameter. Precysts often have a single vacuole, simulating a cyst of *Iodamoeba bütschlii*. Note in the photograph the distinct "*Entamoeba*-type" distribution of chromatin around the nuclear membrane, ruling out *I. bütschlii*.

H. Iron-hematoxylin stain of a small (6 μm in diameter) cyst of *Entamoeba hartmanni*. The size is in the range of *Endolimax nana;* however, the *Entamoeba*-type nucleus and the chromatoidal bars with rounded ends rules out that possibility.

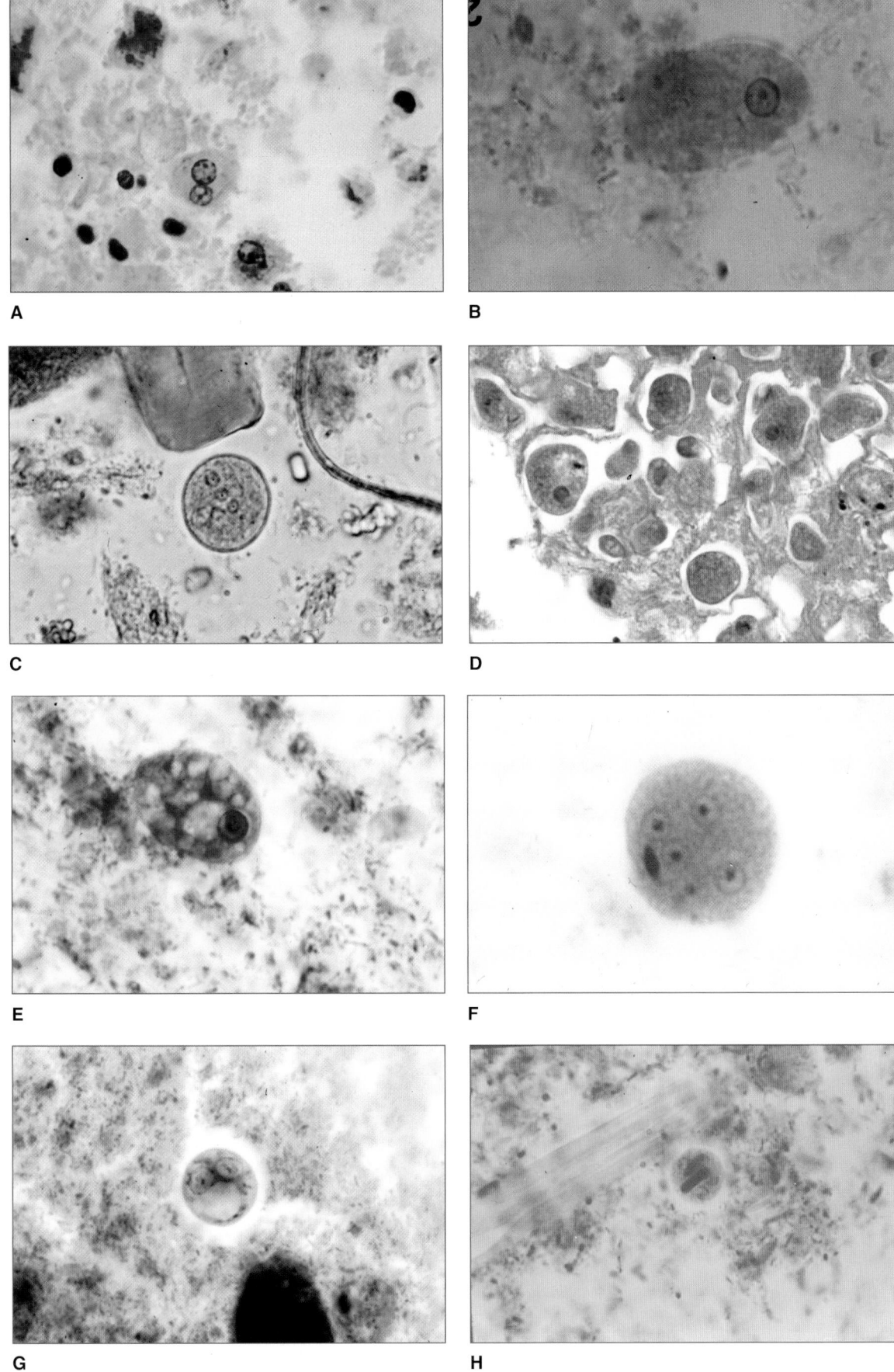

A

B

C

D

E

F

G

H

I. Trichrome-stained fecal smear illustrating a trophozoite of *Iodamoeba bütschlii*. This form measures approximately 14 μm um in diameter; the size range is 6–25 μm. Note the nucleus with a large karyosome surrounded by an empty space, with no visible nuclear membrane (so-called ball-in-socket nucleus). The smaller trophozoites are difficult to distinguish from those of *Endolimax nana;* other fields must be examined to detect the more characteristic cysts in making a final diagnosis.

J. Trichrome-stained fecal smear illustrating a cyst of *Iodamoeba bütschlii*, measuring 10 μm in diameter. The nucleus has a large central karyosome surrounded by a clear area with absence of peripheral chromatin (ball-in-socket nucleus). Note the single large vacuole in the cytoplasm, that stains positive with an iodine stain, indicating glycogen content.

K. Trichome-stained fecal smear illustrating a small trophozoite of *Endolimax nana* (*arrow*), measuring 8 μm in diameter. Note the small central nucleus with a prominent karyosome, and a narrow surrounding clear space and absence of nuclear chromatin.

L. Methylene-blue stained preparation illustrating a cyst of *Endolimax nana*, measuring 6 × 8 μm in diameter. Note the four tiny nuclei, each of which contains a minute karyosome, surrounded by a clear space.

M. Trichrome-stained fecal smear illustrating a single, spherical form of *Blastocystis hominis*, with a prominent central body surrounded by nuclear material that is plastered in clumps against the inner membrane of the cyst wall. The form here measures 10 μm; however, they vary considerably in size between 5 and 20 μm, with a mixture within any given preparation.

N. Photomicrograph of a hematoxylin-and-eosin–stained section of small bowel epithelium. Note the small, pear-shaped trophozoite of *Giardia lamblia*, with its familiar "monkey face," appearing almost as an aircraft looking for a place to land. In fact, the *Giardia* trophozoites attach to the mucosa, where they cause local damage, leading to the characteristic symptoms of diarrhea and flatulence.

O. Trichrome-stained smear illustrating a *G. lamblia* trophozoite recognized by its distinctly oval to elliptical shape, the two nuclei, with prominent contral karyosomes, lying anteriorly on either side of the rodlike axostyle, which runs the length of the organism. Note also the eosinophilic staining parabasal body (the "mustache") lying posteriorly on the axostyle. These features provide for the so-called monkey face appearance. *G. lamblia* trophozoites have six flagella, two each at anterior, posterior, and caudal positions; only three of these are visible in the photograph.

P. Trichrome-stained smear of intestinal debris including a *Giardia lamblia* cyst. The cyst is typically oval and has a thin, smooth outer wall. The cyst ranges from 9 to 12 μm in diameter, and typically includes double the number of organelles seen in the trophozoite. Each cyst typically has four nuclei, only two or three of which are usually seen in a single plane of focus, two axostyles, multiple parabasal bodies, and flagella that are wrapped beneath the smooth-walled cyst, all of which may not be observed in a single plane of focus.

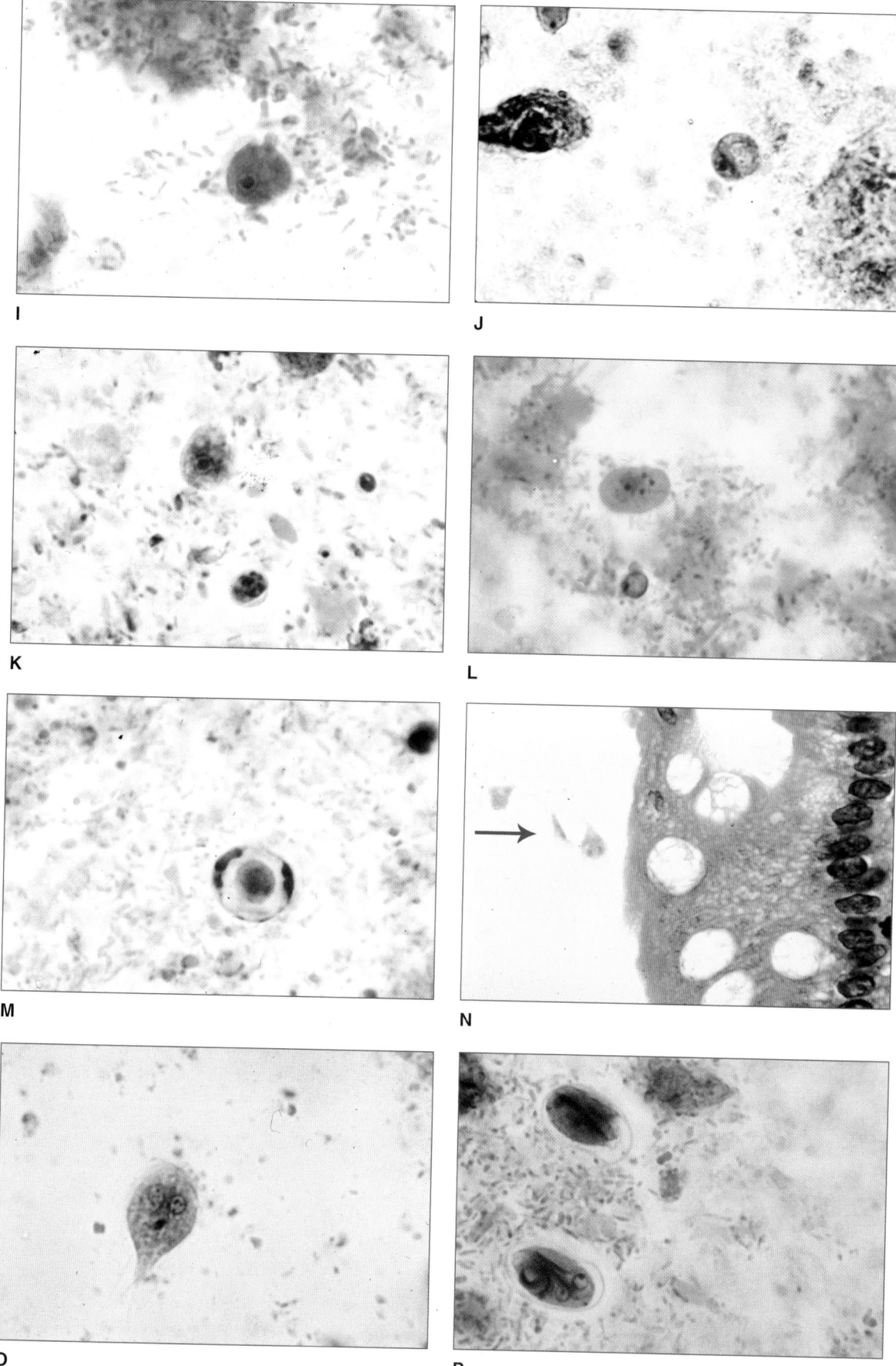

I

J

K

L

M

N

O

P

FLAGELLATES

A. Photomicrograph of two trophozoites of *Chilomastix mesnili*, one seen on end, the other from a lateral view. The trophozoite is typically pear-shaped and can be readily identified by observing the extreme anterior placement of a single nucleus, the posterior protrusion of the axostyle, and a spiral groove, which is difficult to observe in most preparations. A tuft of three anterior flagella, adjacent to the nucleus, is an additional identifying feature that is difficult to observe in most microscopic mounts.

B. Photomicrograph of a cyst of *C. mesnili*. A single nucleus, with central karyosome and a distinct cytostome, appearing as a well-outlined clear area in the cyst shown here, are easily observed. The outline of the cytostome, described as appearing as a shepherd's crook, is seen in this photomicrograph. Cysts typically are lemon-shaped, have a smooth cell wall, range from 6 to 70 μm in diameter and, in addition to the cytostome, often have an anterior knob that, when seen, is helpful in making an identification (see Color Plate 22-3C).

C. View of another cyst of *Chilomastix mesnili*, in which the anterior hyaline knob is better seen (*arrow*). The nucleus and cytostome are also visible.

D. Trichrome-stained fecal smear highlighting a single trophozoite of *Dientamoeba fragilis*. This cyst measures 8 × 12 μm, and one can readily observe the characteristic double nucleus, each with a large karyosome and indistinct nuclear membrane. The cytoplasm of this trophozoite is finely granular and shows early evidence of disintegration, as reflected by the species name.

E. Iron-hematoxylin preparation illustrating a single trophozoite of *Trichomonas hominis*. Note the typical tear-drop shape and single nucleus placed anteriorly, but not against the cell wall, as is characteristic of the trophozoite of *Chilomastix mesnili* (Color Plate 22-3A). The longitudinally running axostyle is visible in this photomicrograph, as is a single posterior flagellum. Typically *T. hominis* has three to five anterior flagella and one posterior flagellum and an undulating membrane that runs along the full length of the body, a structure that is readily seen only in preparations made from cell cultures.

F. Photomicrograph of a hematoxylin-and-eosin–stained section of an intestinal biopsy, illustrating many invading trophozoites of *Balantidium coli*. Note the distinct rod- or horseshoe-shaped macronucleus, a feature that along with its large size (80 μm in diameter), is helpful in making an identification.

G. View of a trophozoite of *Balantidium coli*, illustrating an oval outline with a smooth wall that is covered throughout the circumference with short, delicate cilia. These trophozoites range between 40 and 70 μm wide by 50 and 100 μm long. The presence of an anterior cytostome and the circumference of cilia and large rod- or horseshoe-shaped macronucleus are the key characteristics leading to an identification.

H. A cyst of *Balantidium coli* is illustrated in this trichrome-stained mount. These cysts range from 50 to 75 μm in diameter, are spherical to ellipsoid, and have a characteristic dumbbell-shaped macronucleus, clearly observed in this photograph. A single indistinct nucleus is observed adjacent to the macronucleus, and the cytoplasm includes a metabolic vacuole.

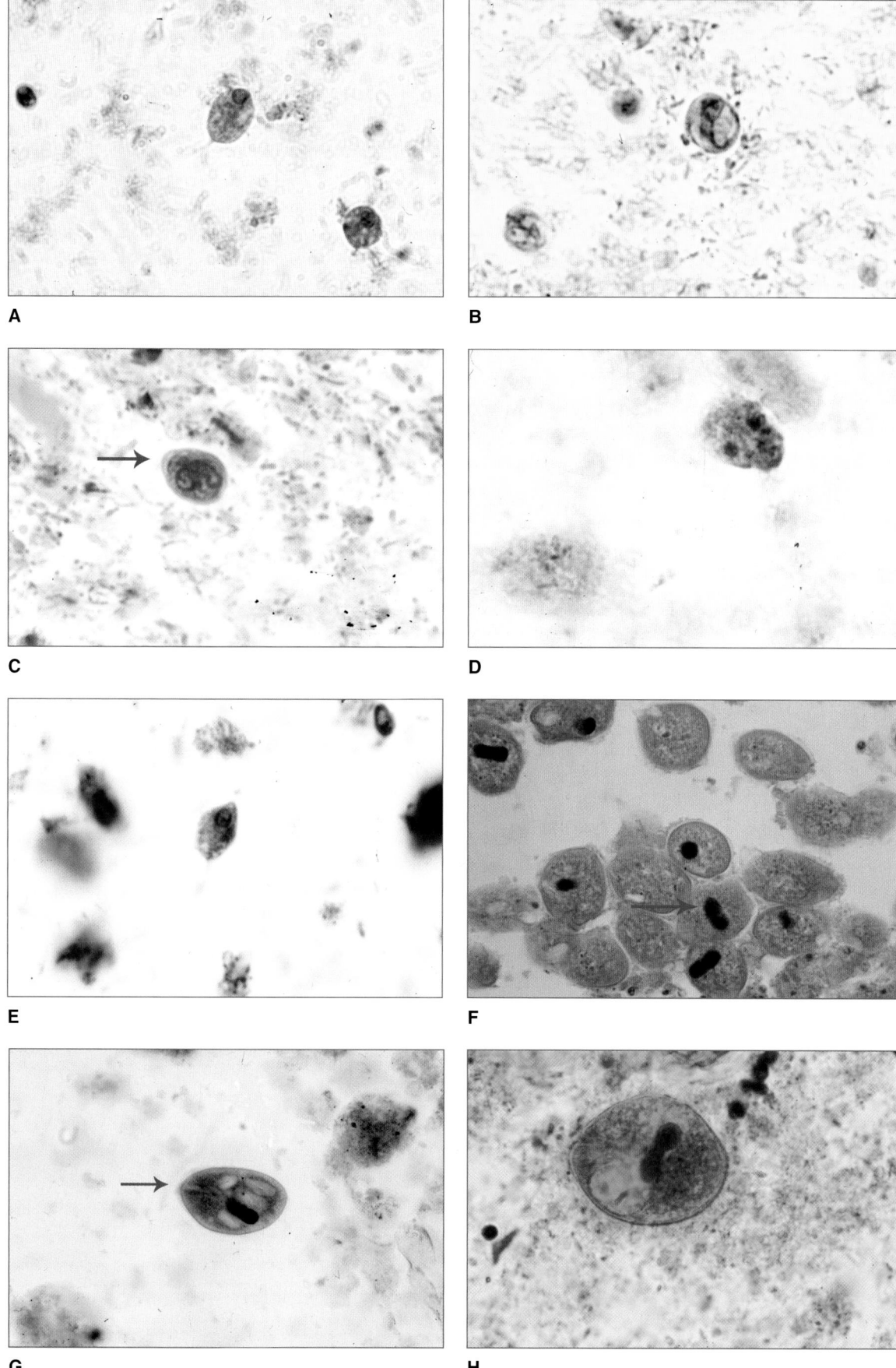

A

B

C

D

E

F

G

H

COCCIDIA

A. Photomicrograph of a hematoxylin-and-eosin–stained section of bowel mucosa along the brush border of which are attached many tiny, 2-to-3-μm-diameter oocysts of *Cryptosporidium* species. A histologic diagnosis is possible when these aggregates of oocysts are observed.

B. Acid-fast stain of fecal smear illustrating two red-staining, acid-fast, spherical, homogeneous staining, 4-to-5-μm-diameter oocysts of *Cryptosporidium* species. These forms are diagnostic when seen in acid-fast smear preparations.

C. Photomicrograph of an acid-fast-stained fecal smear illustrating a single spherical, acid-fast oocyst of *Cyclospora* species. These oocysts are about two times the size of the oocysts of *Cryptosporidium* species, ranging from 8 to 10 μm in diameter. Also in contrast, the *Cyclospora* oocysts have an ill-defined internal structure, instead of the homogeneous staining of *Cryptosporidium* oocysts.

D. Low-power (×250) view of an acid-fast-stained spindle-shaped oocyst of *Isospora belli* located in the center field of view. These oocysts measure 25 to 30 μm in length, a relatively large size that cannot be appreciated by this low-power view, except when compared with the very tiny, almost dotlike, 5 μm-diameter oocysts of *Cryptosporidium* species that are scattered in this field of view. The coexistence of these two species in the same stool specimen is highly suggestive of a person with HIV infection, and AIDS should always be ruled out when this picture is observed.

E. Photomicrograph of a direct mount preparation illustrating an elliptical-shaped, immature oocyst of *Isospora belli*. These oocysts measure 25–30 μm in the long axis, and when immature, enclose only a single spherical sporocyst, as illustrated in the photograph. Compare with the mature oocyst illustrated in Color Plate 22-4*F*.

F. View of a direct mount of fecal material illustrating a mature oocyst of *Isospora belli*, enclosing two spherical sporocysts. The sporocysts, now mature, are infective for a second host, and ready to release sporozoites into the intestine on ingestion.

G. Hematoxylin-and-eosin–stained section of skeletal muscle within which are two cysts of *Sarcocystis* spp. These cysts measure as large as 300 μm in diameter, and are filled with inactive, encysted bradyzoites. Humans are infected with this form if, as accidental intermediate hosts, infective oocysts are ingested in contaminated food or water.

H. Weber stain of a stool preparation illustrating many small, 2-to-3-μm, rod-shaped spores of *Microsporidium* species. With this stain, the spores stain a salmon-yellow. Note the characteristic thin, transverse septum that divides some of the spores (*arrow*) seen in this field of view, a helpful feature in making a genus identification.

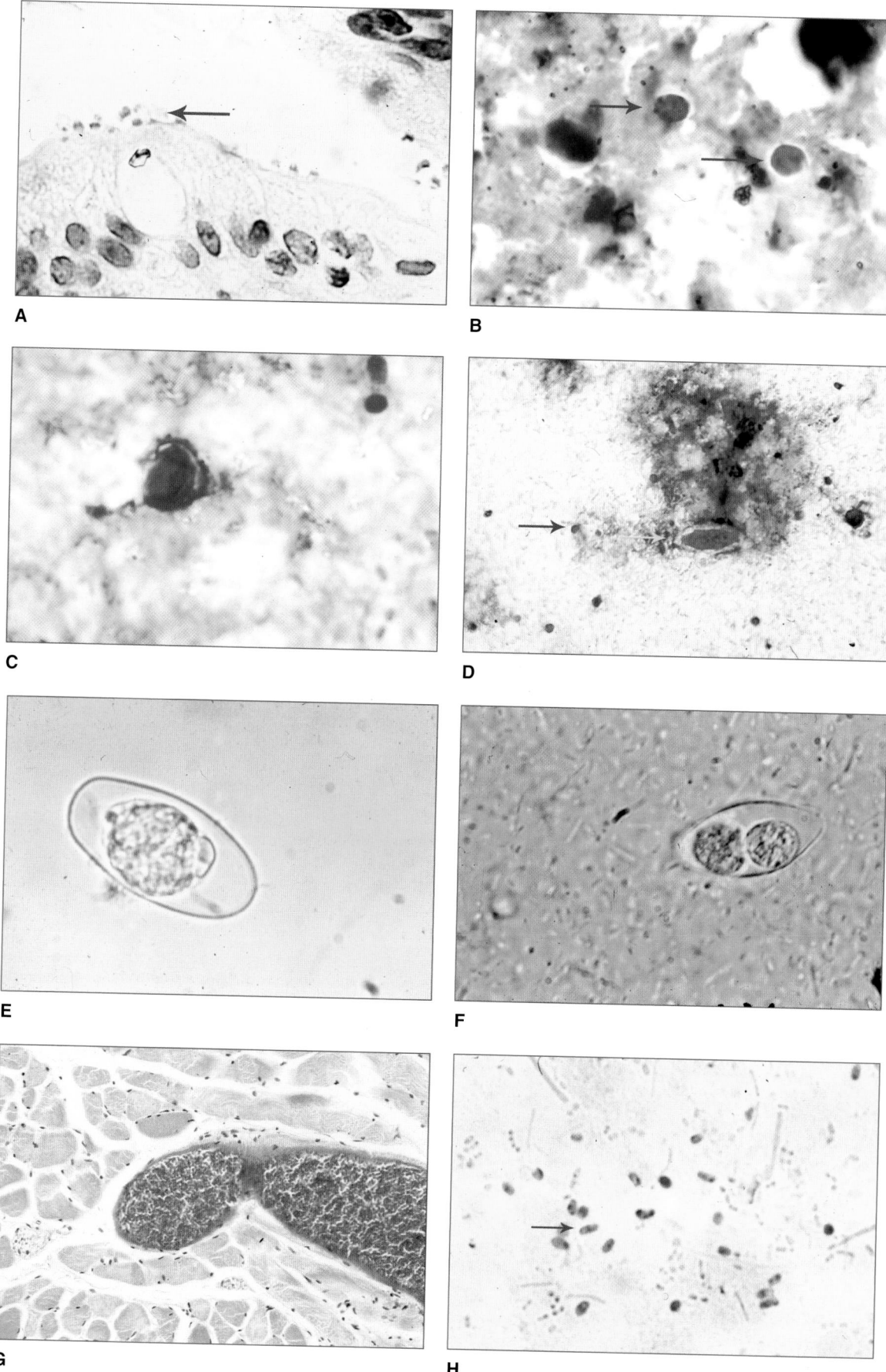

A

B

C

D

E

F

G

H

NEMATODES

A. Adult male and female worms of *Ascaris lumbricoides*. The adult males are generally shorter (20–25 cm) than the females (25–30 cm) and have a curved tail (lower worm in the photograph). The smooth, nonsegmented cuticle is a helpful feature in distinguishing adult ascarids from common earthworms, which on occasion may find their way into toilets and sewage systems, where they may be mistaken for worms passed in the feces.

B. Bile-stained, yellow-brown, slightly ovoid egg of *Ascaris lumbricoides*, which range in size from 45 to 60 μm in diameter. They possess a thick shell covered by a characteristic undulating albuminous coat. The retraction and development of the internal cleavage indicates fertilization and potential infectivity.

C. Illustrated is a spherical, decorticate egg of *Ascaris lumbricoides* featuring a well-developed larva that is at the stage of near hatching. This egg obviously is highly infective.

D. Fertilized egg of *Ascaris lumbricoides* showing a smooth outer shell. When exposed to bile within the intestinal lumen, the albuminous outer coat is dissolved, leaving a decorticate surface as seen here.

E. Composite photograph illustrating an adult worm of *Enterobius vermicularis* in the upper frame. These worms, measuring 0.3 to 0.5 mm in diameter and between 8 and 1.3 mm long, have a well-developed intestinal tract and internal reproductive organs. The pointed tail and paraoral alae (*arrow* in the left photograph) are diagnostic. The close-up view in the right frame better demonstrates the paraoral alae.

F. Split-frame photograph illustrating gravid *Enterobius vermicularis* eggs, the one to the right possessing a well-developed larva. These eggs have a thin, smooth wall, and measure approximately 55 × 25 μm. Each egg is elongated, asymmetrical, and flattened on one side, resembling an underinflated football.

G. Photograph of adult *Trichuris trichiura* worms demonstrating the characteristic long, attenuated whiplike anterior segment and the shorter, thicker more handlelike posterior body. These worms are relatively small, measuring 35–45 mm in length. The slolex with four suckers and a protruding armed postellum is illustrated in the left frame.

H. Photomicrograph of a typical bile-stained, yellow-brown egg of *Trichuris trichiura* with a relatively thick, smooth wall. Note the characteristic barrel-shape and the distinctive, dome-shaped, hyaline plug at each polar extremity. From "A Pictorial Presentation of Parasites" by H. Zaiman.

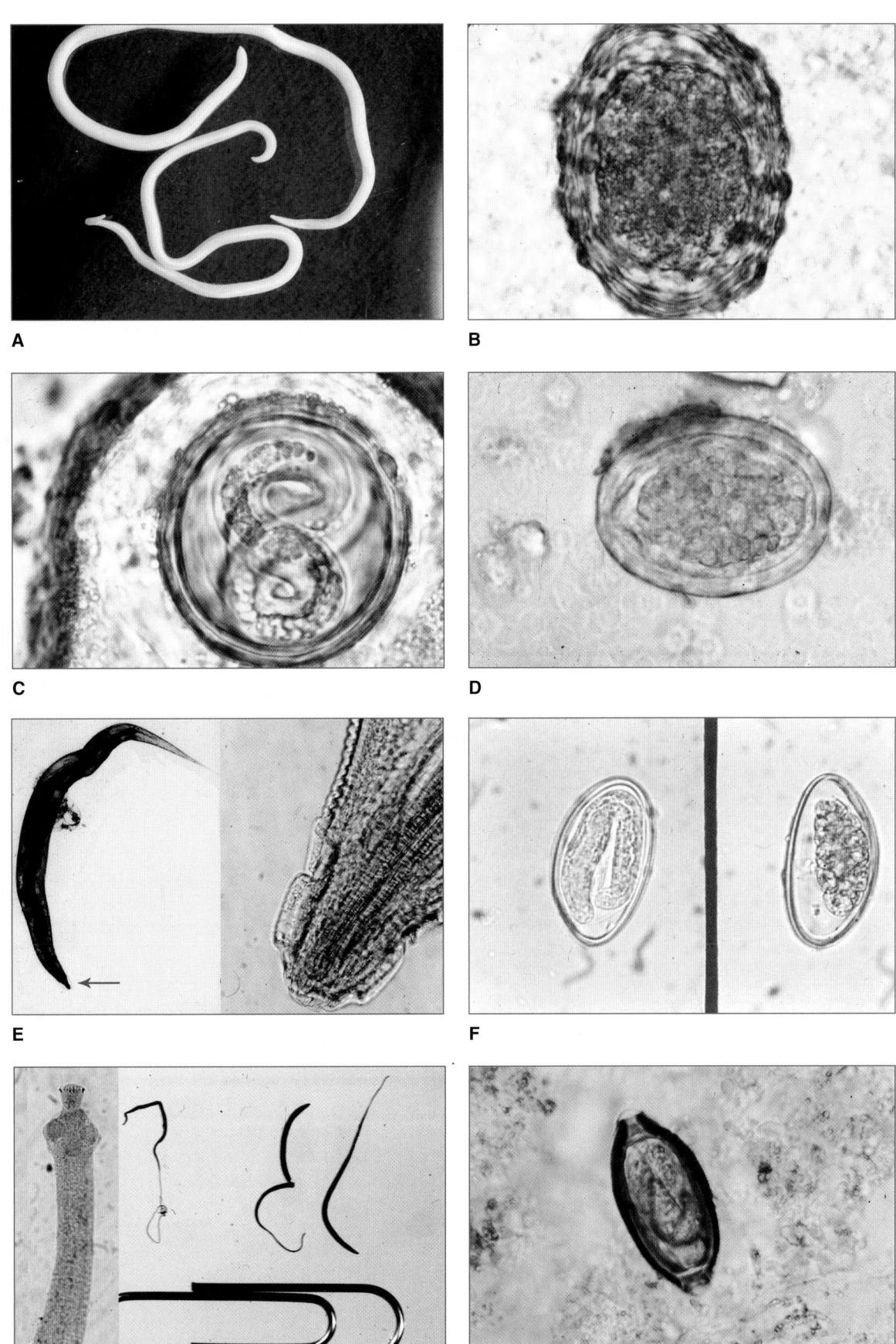

A

B

C

D

E

F

G

H

I. Photograph of the mouthpart of an adult hookworm. The chitinous teeth observed here are characteristic of the old-world hookworm, *Ancylostoma duodenale*. This mouthpart is well suited for the deep attachment of the worm to the intestinal mucosa and the fracture of capillaries enabling the milking of blood from the circulation.

J. Similar view of the mouthpart of the new-world hookworm, *Necator americanus*, illustrating the characteristic cutting plates. As with *Ancylostoma duodenale*, this mouthpart is also well suited for the deep attachment of the worm to the intestinal mucosa.

K. Photomicrograph of a direct iodine mount of fecal material within which is contained a typical oval-shaped hookworm egg measuring approximately 40×60 μm, with its characteristic thin, smooth wall, and the pulling away of the internal cleavage, leaving a clear space beneath the shell. These eggs cannot be distinguished from those of *Strongyloides stercoralis*. This differential identification is generally not necessary as *S. stercoralis* rarely passes eggs in the feces.

L. Split-frame photomicrograph in which the buccal cavities of the rhabditiform larvae of hookworm (*left*) and strongyloides (*right*) are compared. The buccal cavity of the hookworm rhabditiform larva is characteristically long compared with the shorter distance observed with strongyloides. Hookworm rhabditiform larvae are rarely seen in fecal specimens.

M. Microscopic field of view of a direct mount of fecal material, within which a small, coiled rhabditiform larva of *Strongyloides stercoralis* is present, as it would be observed under low magnification ($\times 100$). These larvae are highly motile when observed in direct mounts. Observation of the buccal cavity as described before is necessary to confirm the identification. These larvae average 15 μm in diameter and over 200 μm long.

N. Rhabditiform larvae, after a short feeding period of 2 to 3 days, develop into long, slender, nonfeeding, infective filariform larvae, that can reach 700 μm in length. These filariform larvae can penetrate directly into the skin of a human host on direct contact.

O. Hematoxylin-and-eosin–stained section of small intestine in which round, smooth filariform larvae of *Strongyloides stercoralis*, characteristic of the histologic findings of individuals with reinfection strongyloidiasis, can be observed burrowing into the lamina propria. In patients with strongyloides in whom a compromised immune system develops, the life cycle from oviposition to rhabditiform larva to filariform larva formation may be sufficiently short that autoinfection may occur within the intestine before stools are formed, as observed in this photograph.

P. Photomicrograph of a yellow-brown, bile-stained egg of *Capillaria philippinensis*. These eggs are lemon-shaped or elongated, measure approximately 60×35 μm, and resemble those of *Trichuris trichiura*, except that the shell is striate and the polar protuberances are broad and flat.

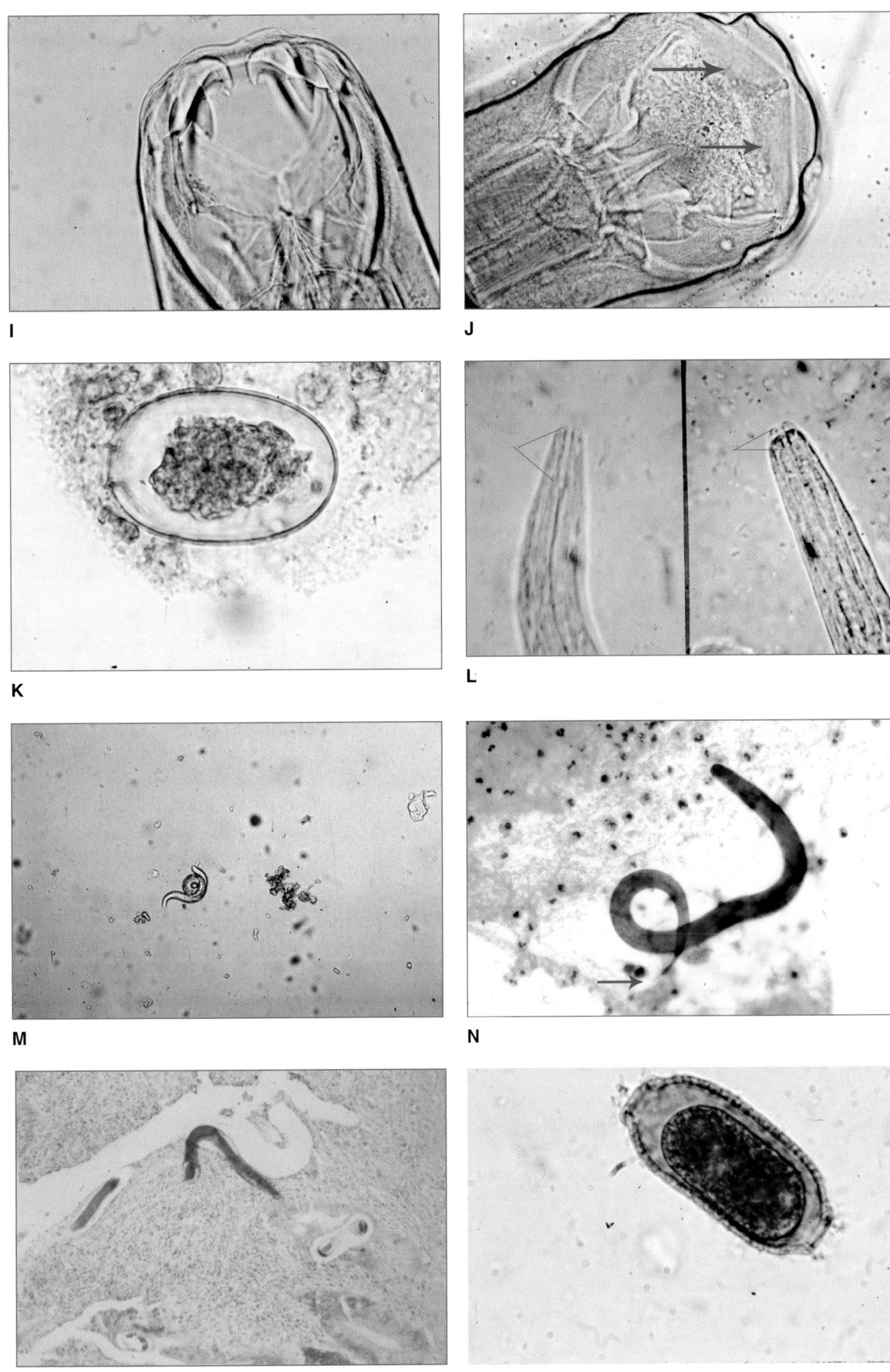

I

J

K

L

M

N

O

P

CESTODES

A. An adult *Taenia saginata* tapeworm illustrating the small scolex (*white arrow*) and a strobila extending several feet long, and composed of a long chain of proglottids.

B. Close-up view of the scolex of a *Taenia solium* tapeworm demonstrating the four suckers characteristic of the genus. The protruding, rostellum armed with a circular row of hooklets, permits the identification of *Taenia solium*. The scolex of *Taenia saginata* is not armed.

C. Close-up view of a single *Taenia saginata* proglottid that has been injected with India ink through the genital pore to outline the branching uterine segments. The proglottids of *T. saginata* possess more than 13 lateral uterine branches, as shown in the photograph, to distinguish them from the proglottids of *Taenia solium*, that typically have fewer than 13 branches. This observation permits a species identification based on an examination of proglottids that may have been passed intact in the feces.

D. Split-frame photographs of a piece of measly pork (*left*) including several small cystic spaces, each inhabited by a cysticercus larva of taenia solium. A cysticercus is illustrated in more detail in the right frame. Within the fluid-filled sac is contained an invaginated scolex. The suckers and hooklets are obscured by the stain.

E. Hematoxylin-and-eosin–stained section of brain illustrating a cystic space occupied by a *Taenia solium* cysticercus. The cyst has two walls, the outer composed of reactive fibrous tissue produced by the host tissue, and the second an inner thin membrane produced by the worm (bladder worm). The invaginated scolex is cut in cross section in this photograph and the internal structures are not identifiable.

F. Photograph of a cysticercus of the rat tapeworm, *Hymenolepis diminuta*. The invaginated scolex is better visualized in this field of view. These cysticerci form in an intermediate insect host, including fleas, cockroaches, and beetles. Humans are infected through ingestion of insect-contaminated foods, and the adult worms develop in the intestine after evagination and attachment of the scolex to the mucosa.

G. Photograph of the uterus of a gravid female of the *Taenia* species, illustrating the dense aggregation of thick-walled, spherical eggs, some of which show the characteristic striations.

H. Close-up view of *Taenia* species eggs as they would be observed microscopically in direct mounts of infected material. These eggs average 30–45 μm in diameter and have a thick, smooth wall, interrupted by distinctive radial striations. Many eggs also enclose three pairs of hooklets (hexacanth embryo) not observed in this photograph, but similar in appearance to those seen within the inner membrane of the *Hymenolepis diminuta* egg included in Color Plate 22-6*N*. These eggs are not species-specific, and also are similar in appearance to those of *Echinococcus* species.

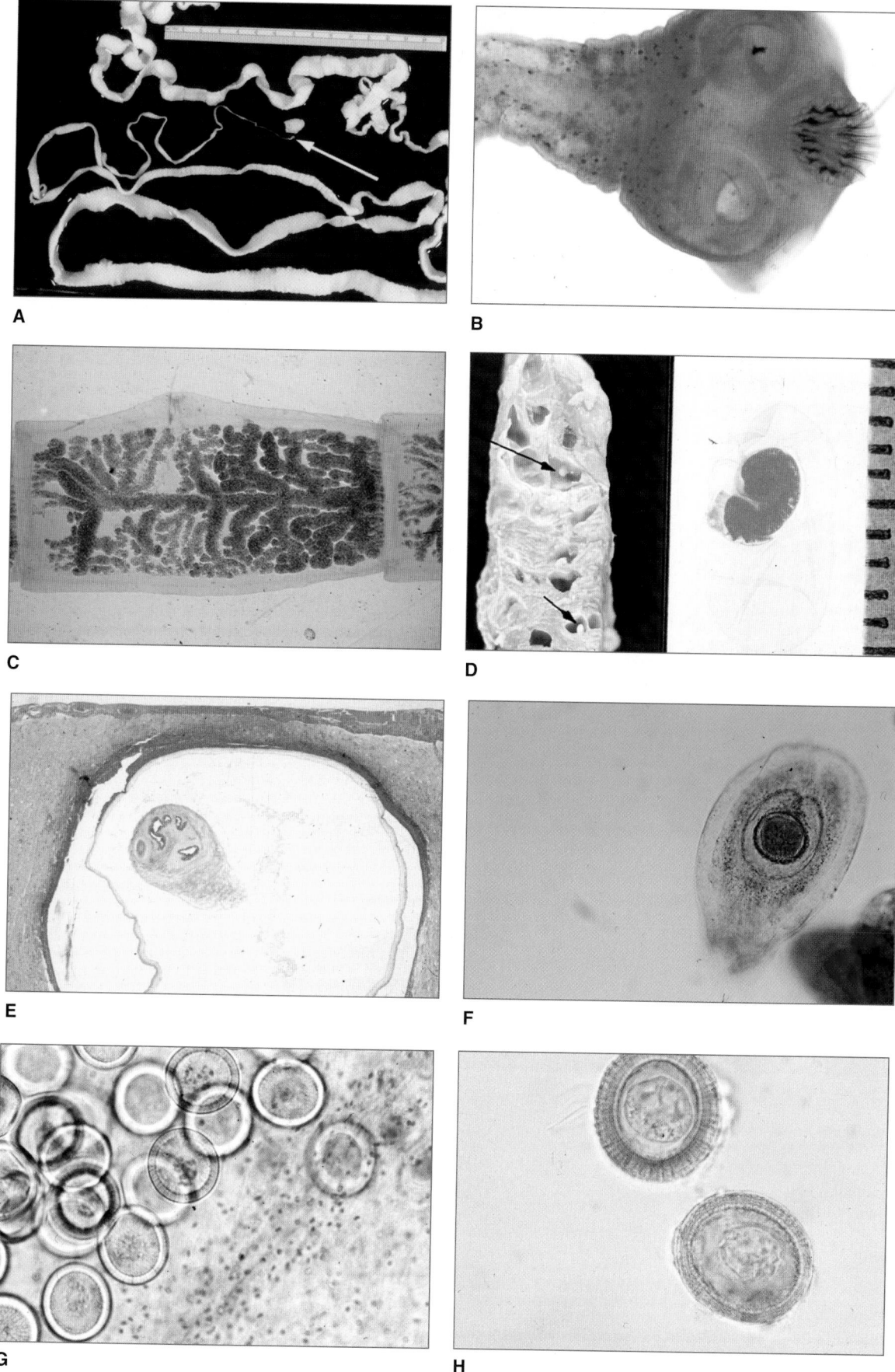

A

B

C

D

E

F

G

H

I. Photograph of the tiny scolex and the broad and narrow proglottids of *Diphyllobothrium latum*, the giant adult tapeworm. This tapeworm is the longest that infests humans, reaching between 3 and 10 m in length, often including more than 3,000 proglottids.

J. Close-up view of the spatula-shaped scolex of *D. latum*, demonstrating the characteristic central, longitudinal groove (bothrium), flanked on either side by a distinctive fold (*phyllo* = "leaf"), the structures from which the genus name, *Diphyllobothrium*, is derived.

K. Close-up view of a proglottid of *Diphyllobothrium*, demonstrating its characteristic width-over-length dimensions, from which the genus name "latum" is derived. Note the nondescript centrally and linearly placed branching uterus, appearing as a compact rosette.

L. Photomicrograph of an egg of *Diphyllobothrium latum*. These eggs are relatively large, measuring from 60 to 75 μm long by 40 to 50 μm wide. They are oval in shape and have a thin, smooth shell, and the cleavage extends to the inner shell membrane. Characteristic is the presence of an inconspicuous, non-shouldered operculum, separating it from the "look-alike" egg of *Paragonimus westermani*, the operculum of which is distinctly shouldered (Color Plate 22-7*P*).

M. Photomicrograph of a *Hymenolepis nana* egg, comprised of a double membrane—an outer thin, smooth shell, and an inner membrane enclosing an oncosphere. Three pairs of hooklets are commonly contained (hexacanth), as illustrated in this photograph. These eggs range between 40 and 60 μm in diameter and are usually oval to subspherical in outline. The eggs of *H. nana* are also distinctive for the presence of polar thickenings on either side of the inner hexacanth membrane, from which four to eight slender filaments are derived, extending into the intermembrane space (see photograph).

N. Photograph of an egg of *Hymenolepis diminuta*. These eggs are larger than those of *Hymenolepis nana*, with an average diameter of 60–80 μm, and usually are distinctively spherical in outline. The absence of polar thickenings and intermembrane filaments also distinguish this egg from those of *H. nana*. The six hooklets are clearly illustrated (arrow).

O. Photograph of a *Dipylidium caninum* proglottid, demonstrating a genital pore on either side, into which flow the delicate vitelline ducts. This double-pore arrangement is unique to *D. caninum* (from which the genus name is derived, *pyle* = "gate or orifice"), in that the proglottids of other tapeworms possess only one lateral genital pore that alternates from one side to the other on adjacent segments. The proglottids are vase-form in shape, being longer than wide.

P. Photomicrograph of an egg packet of *D. caninum*, demonstrating an aggregate of spherical eggs held in a matrix. The eggs shown in the photograph are immature, as the presence of internal hooklets indicate maturity and infectivity.

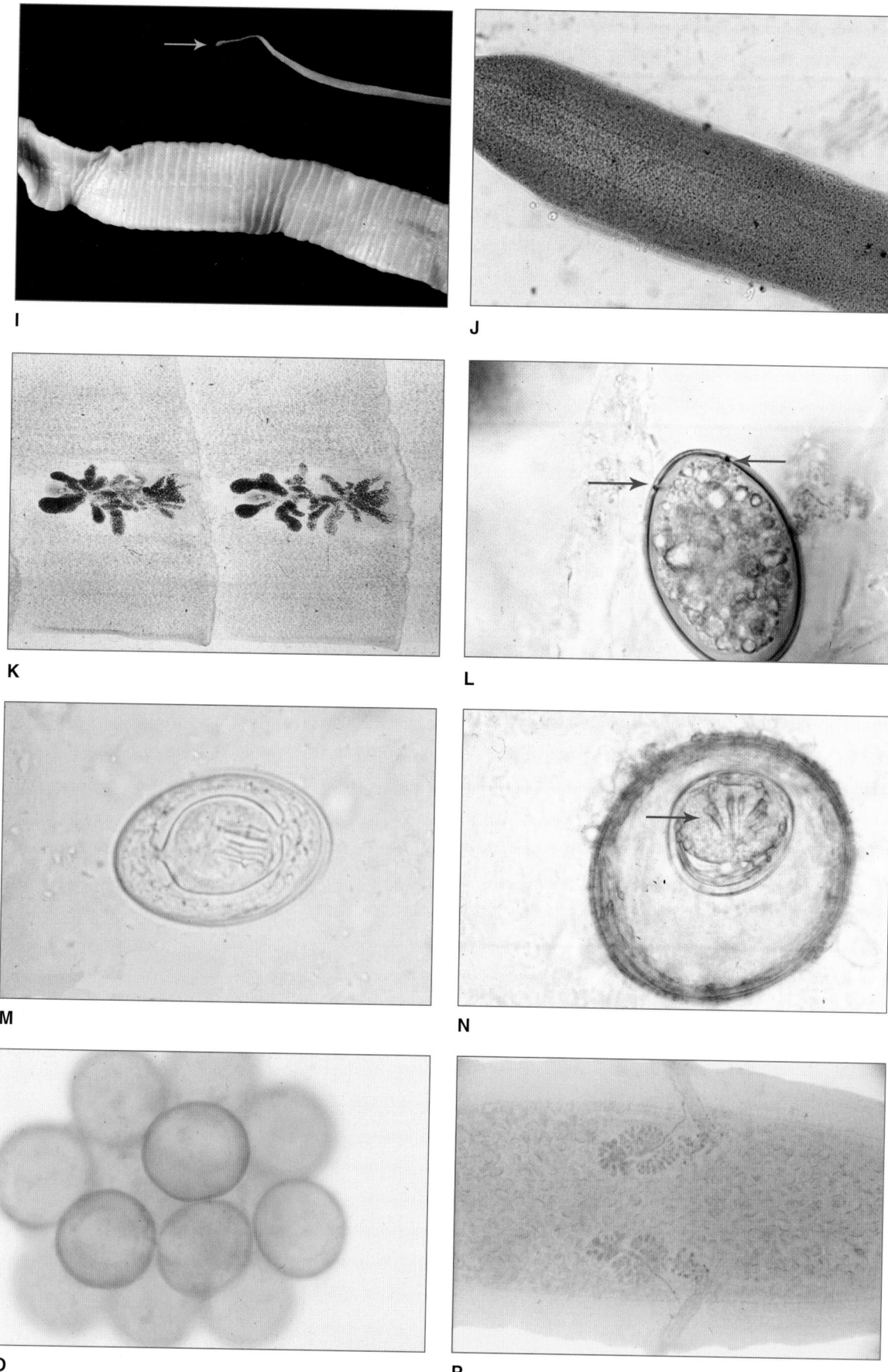

I

J

K

L

M

N

O

P

TREMATODES

A. Photograph of adult male and female *Schistosoma* adults. The male in this photograph is lighter-staining and possesses a gynecophoric canal from which the copulating female, darker in staining, has become detached. Adult males average 20–30 mm in length, females 17–14 mm. These flukes are threadlike in diameter, allowing them to occupy the lumina of venules without causing blockage of the blood flow, thus resulting in minimal edema.

B. Photomicrograph of an egg of *Schistosoma mansoni*, with its characteristic smooth, thin wall and oval outline with a prominent lateral spine. These eggs are relatively quite large, ranging from about 115 to 180 μm long by 45 to 70 μm wide. On maturity, the larval miracidium hatches intact, precluding a period of development in the external environment.

C. Photomicrograph of an egg of *Schistosoma haematobium*, also having a thin, smooth shell and an oval outline, but differing from the egg of *S. mansoni* by possessing a terminal, rather than a lateral spine. These eggs also are relatively large, ranging from 110 to 170 μm long, and 40 to 70 μm wide.

D. Illustrated here is an egg of *Schistosoma japonicum*, which is smaller (80–100 μm in diameter), more oval to spherical in outline, and has an internal cleavage that extends to the inner shell. Although a spine is not observed, a small lateral knob (not seen in this photograph), is distinctive.

E. Photomicrograph of a forked-tail cercaria, the infective stage in the life *Schistosoma* life cycle. These free-swimming cercaria are released from the rediae of infected snails and have the capacity, through enzymatic activity, to directly penetrate the skin of an unsuspecting human, who may be wading or swimming in infested freshwater estuaries.

F. An adult fluke of *Fasciola hepatica*. These flukes are hermaphroditic and possess both female and male reproductive organs. The anterior portion of *F. hepatica* projects into a cone-shaped nose, just posterior to which is the anterior sucker. Immediately posterior to the sucker, and darkly staining in this photograph, is the branching convoluted uterus. Immediately posterior to the uterus is the ventral sucker. The bulk of the posterior portion of the fluke includes the testes, appearing as a pink-staining meshwork in this photograph. These flukes measure about 3×1 cm (about the size of a glass microscope slide). From "A Pictorial Presentation of Parasites" by H. Zaiman.

G. An adult fluke of *Fasciolopsis buski*, the giant intestinal fluke, which is also hermaphroditic and has structures similar to those described for *F. hepatica*. In contrast, the cephalic end is rounded and devoid of the conical protrusion. These flukes range from about 2 to 7.5 cm long, by 0.8 to 2 cm wide.

H. Photomicrograph of an egg of *F. hepatica* (which cannot be distinguished from those of *F. buski*), demonstrating a thin, smooth wall and an internal cleavage that extends to the inner shell membrane. Notice the nick on either side of the shell toward the narrow end, representing the operculum, a lidlike structure that opens at the time the larva hatches. These eggs are large, averaging approximately 150×80 μm in greatest dimensions.

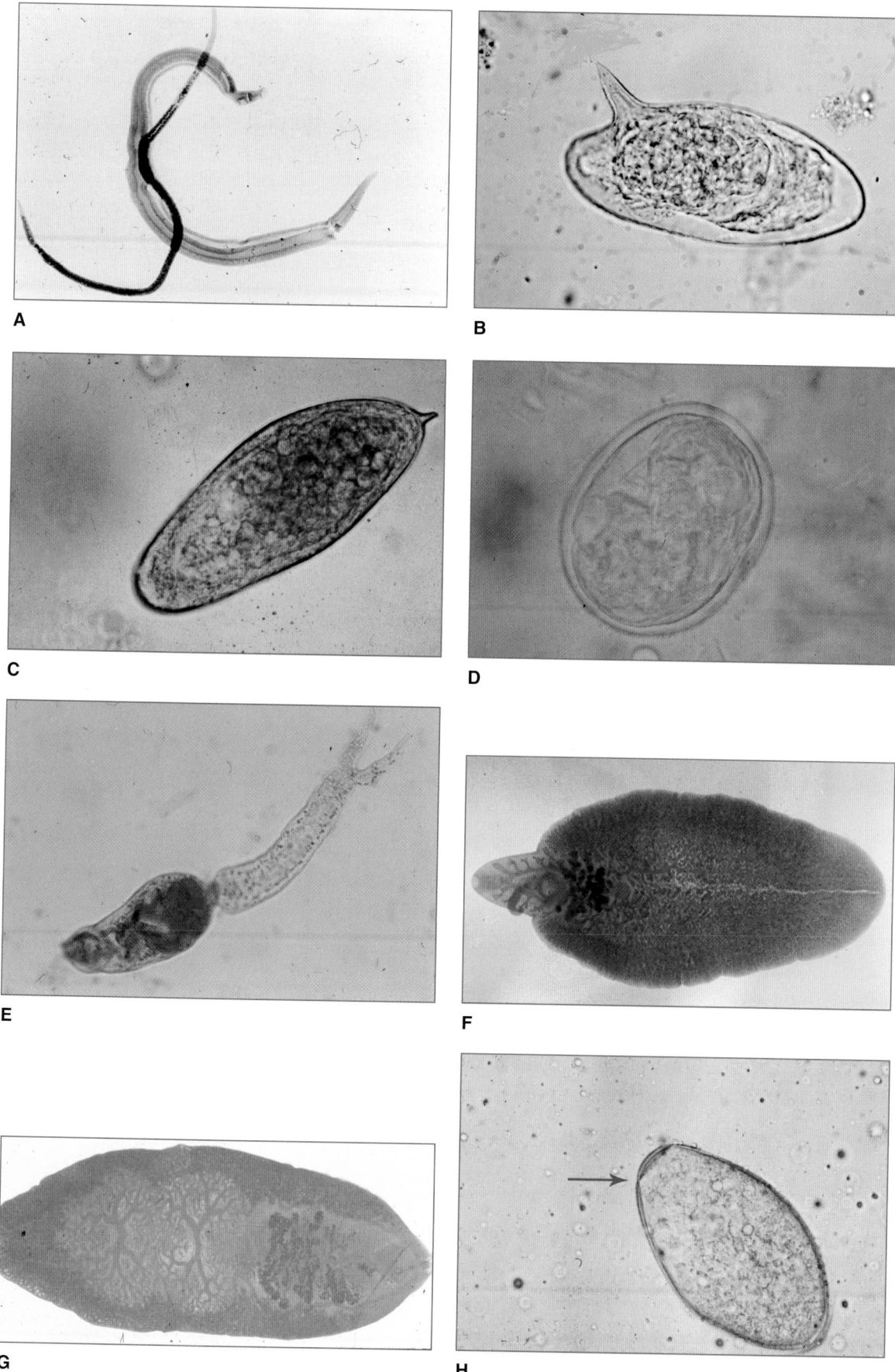

A

B

C

D

E

F

G

H

I. Photograph of an adult fluke of *Clonorchis sinensis*, demonstrating the long, bottle-shaped cephalic end with a prominent terminal sucker, dark brown-staining uterus, and the extensively branched, lighter pink-staining testes posteriorly. These internal structures, moving from mouth to tail, are illustrated in greater detail in Color Plates 22-7*J–M*.

J. Illustrated in this photograph is the anterior mouth or oral sucker, which leads to a blind digestive tract, called the ceca, a branch of which runs along the lateral margins of the worm.

K. Posterior to the oral sucker is the ventral sucker, which is placed immediately in front of the dark-staining uterus, flanked on either side by the branches of the ceca. The delicate-staining vitelline glands are seen at the upper margin of the worm between the ceca and the outer integument. These glands produce the yolk for the eggs produced in the ovaries.

L. This field of view is just posterior to the uterus illustrating the ovary. Note the delicate vitelline duct entering the ovary on the right side.

M. This field of view is the posterior part of the worm, highlighting the extensively branching tests, from which the genus name (*clon* = divided; *orchis* = testes) is derived. Note that the ceca end in blind alleys. The excretory bladder is the ill-defined white space at the immediate posterior margin.

N. Hematoxylin-and-eosin–stained section through a dilated bile duct within which resides three *Clonorchis sinensis* adult flukes cut in cross section. Although a mild chronic inflammatory infiltrate is noted in the surrounding submucosa, extensive fibrosis and lumen occlusion is not evident.

O. Photomicrograph of an egg of *Clonorchis sinensis*, illustrating a thin, smooth wall. Characteristic is the prominent, shouldered operculum at the broader end. A tiny knob, not visible in this photograph, may be seen at the narrower, antiopercular end of the egg. These eggs are relatively small, ranging from 25 to 35 μm long by 14 to 17 μm wide.

P. Photomicrograph of an egg of *Paragonimus westermani*. The shell is smooth, relatively thin, and interrupted at one end by a prominent shouldered operculum. This egg appears morphologically similar to that of *Clonorchis sinensis;* however, these comparative photographs are deceiving, as *P. westermani* eggs are two to three times the size, ranging from 65 to 120 μm long by 40 to 70 μm wide. With this larger size, *P. westermani* eggs appear similar to those of *Diphyllobothrium latum,* which, however, can be distinguished by its flat rather than raised, shouldered operculum.

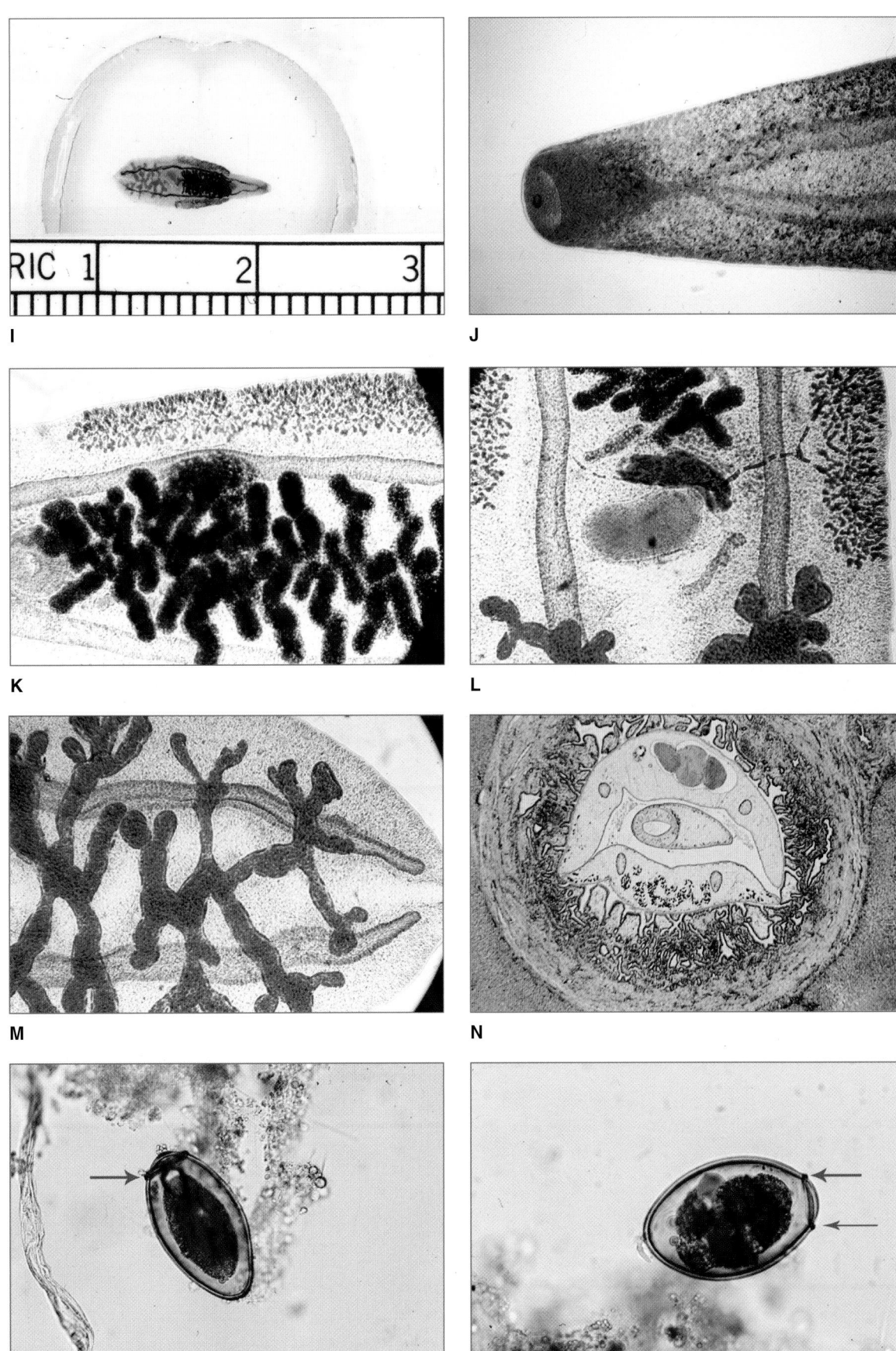

I

J

K

L

M

N

O

P

PLASMODIUM

A. Photomicrograph of a Wright-Giemsa–stained peripheral blood smear illustrating several erythrocytes that are infected with ring forms of *Plasmodium* species. The infected erythrocytes are no larger in size than the surrounding cells, and Schüffner's dots are not present. The small size of the rings without development into trophozoite forms and the heavy infection point to an infection with *Plasmodium falciparum*.

B. The infected erythrocytes in this photomicrograph of a stained peripheral smear also point to *Plasmodium falciparum*, both for the heavy involvement, and also the peripheral placement of tiny rings along the inner cell membranes, a so-called accolade effect. Indeed, this smear was obtained from a patient with fulminant falciparum malaria.

C. Falciparum malaria can be definitively identified in the peripheral blood smear if the large, sickle-form gametocyte as illustrated in the lower part of this photograph (*blue arrow*) is observed. Also note the small plasmodium ring in the cell near the top of the field of view (*red arrow*), again consistent with *Plasmodium falciparum*.

D. The infected erythrocyte illustrated in this stained peripheral smear is distinctly larger and paler than the surrounding cells and also has a distinctly stippled cytoplasm from the presence of Schüffner's dots. Note also that the ringed trophozoite is relatively large. These features are diagnostic for *Plasmodium vivax* infection.

E. *Plasmodium vivax* can be further suspected if a multicelled schizont, as illustrated by the enlarged erythrocyte in the center of this photomicrograph, is observed in a stained peripheral blood smear. These schizonts typically have more than 13 segments.

F. Illustrated in this stained peripheral smear is an enlarged, pale erythrocyte containing a uninucleated gametocyte of *Plasmodium vivax*.

G. Illustrated in this photomicrograph of a Wright-Giemsa–stained peripheral blood smear is an erythrocyte infected with a trophozoite *Plasmodium malariae*. Note that the cytoplasm is condensed, does not develop into an ameboid form, and bridges in a band form from one side of the cell membrane to the other. The red cell is not enlarged and Schüffner's dots are absent.

H. *Plasmodium malariae* can also be suspected if one observes a multinucleated schizont with less than 13 segments. Characteristically, the segments are arranged in a circular rosette pattern as seen in this photograph, often surrounding a coarse mass of malarial pigment that is absent in this particular infected cell.

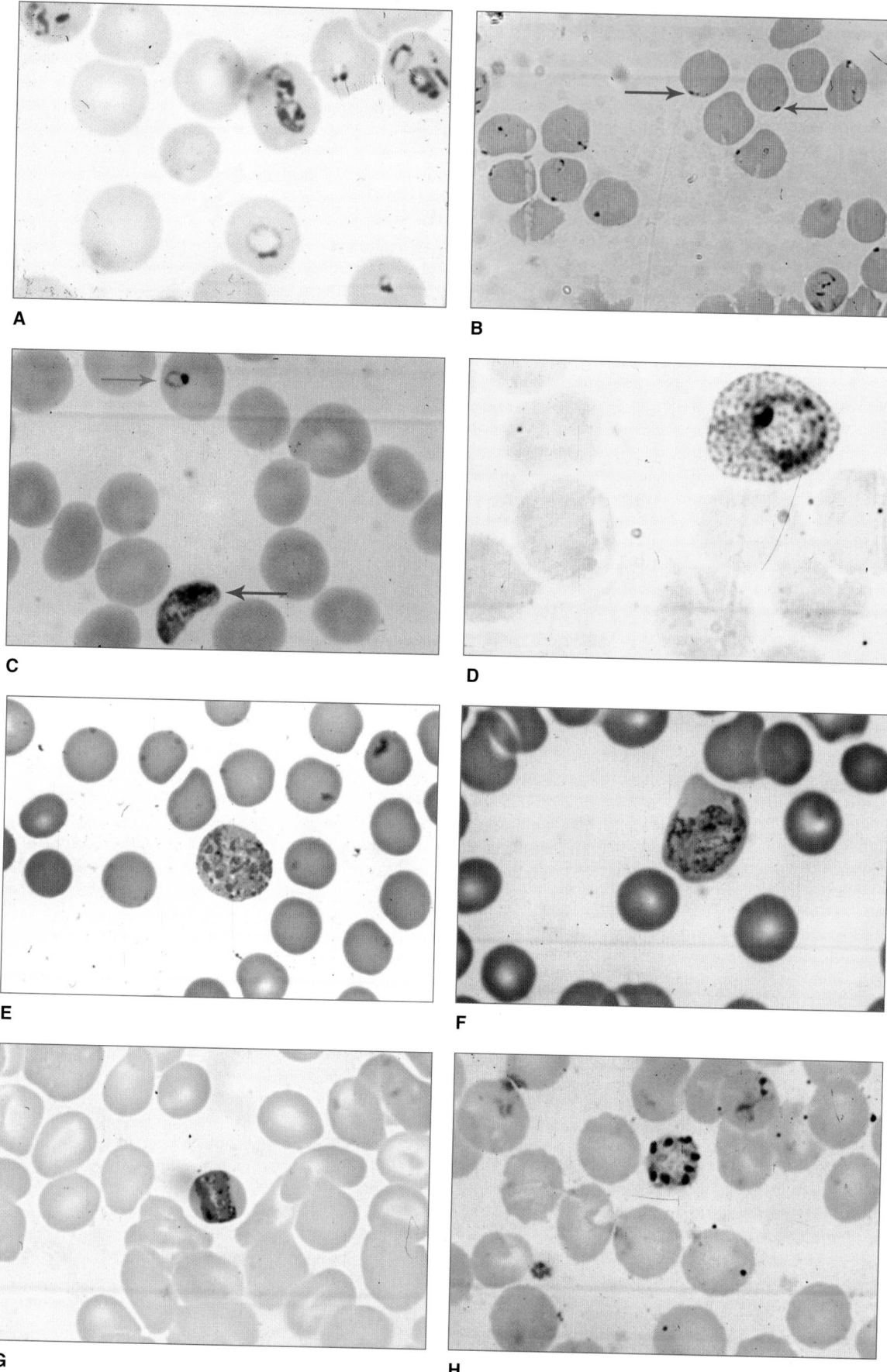

A

B

C

D

E

F

G

H

BABESIOSIS/LEISHMANIASIS/TRYPANOSOMIASIS

A. Illustrated in this photomicrograph of a Wright-Giemsa–stained peripheral blood smear are several erythrocytes that are infected with the tiny pleomorphic ringlike forms of *Babesia* species. Tiny rings may be observed, suggestive of *Plasmodium falciparum*, as seen in one of the erythrocytes in the lower center field of view. The infected erythrocytes are not enlarged, are not pale, and never accumulate malarial pigment. Noteworthy is the arrangement of these forms into doublets resembling rabbit ears; or, more characteristically, into tetrads resembling a Maltese cross.

B. Photograph of the lower legs of a patient infected with *Leishmania tropica*, a species that typically causes cutaneous leishmaniasis, also called Chiclero ulcers. The ulcerating lesions as seen in this photograph result from the granulomatous inflammation caused by the infiltrating amastigotes.

C. Hematoxylin-and-eosin–stained section from subcutaneous tissue taken from the margin of an ulcer similar to that shown in Color Plate 22-9*B.* Note the tiny yeastlike forms seen in the cytoplasm of many of the infiltrating histiocytes and macrophages. These represent the amastigotes, the infective forms seen both in visceral and cutaneous leishmaniasis. These forms are difficult to differentiate from the intracytoplasmic yeast cells of *Histoplasma capsulatum,* but they often can be differentiated in stained smears of aspirates by demonstrating the rodlike kinetoplasts, as illustrated in Color Plate 22-9*D* and *E.*

D. Wright-Giemsa–stained impression smear illustrating a few background macrophages and numerous tiny 2-to-3 μm amastigotes of *Leishmania* species. As mentioned before, these forms are often difficult to differentiate from the yeast cells of *Histoplasma capsulatum.* Careful observation, however, will reveal that many of these forms have a small, rod-shaped kinetoplast (*blue arrow*), characteristic of *Leishmania* amastigotes.

E. Close-up view of a stained aspirate illustrating amastigotes of *Leishmania* species, identified by the distinctive kinetoplasts included within many of these forms.

F. Photomicrograph of a Wright-stained peripheral blood smear in which several extracellular trypanosomes are observed. This smear was obtained from a patient with African trypanosomiasis. Each individual organism is long, slender, spindle-shaped, and ranges from 15 to 30 μm long by 1.5 to 4 μm wide. The darker-staining, dotlike structure seen posteriorly in each trypanosome is the kinetoplast, from which a single flagellum originates. Each flagellum follows the outer contour of an undulating membrane that runs the length of the body, and then extends for some distance from the anterior end.

G. Photomicrograph of a Wright-stained peripheral smear obtained from a patient with American trypanosomiasis, also known as Chagas' disease. Note the characteristic "C"-form trypanosomes. Each trypanosome has a deep-staining, dotlike structure posteriorly, the kinetoplast, from which a single flagellum originates.

H. Photograph of a triatomid (reduviid) bug, the vector for transmission of Chagas' disease. Metacyclic trypanosomes develop in the hindgut of this bug, following ingestion of trypanosomes through the bite of an infected patient. The trypanosomes reenter the subcutaneous tissue after the bite of the second human host, not from the bite itself, but when contaminated fecal material discharged from the bug is scratched by the fingernails into the painful bite wound.

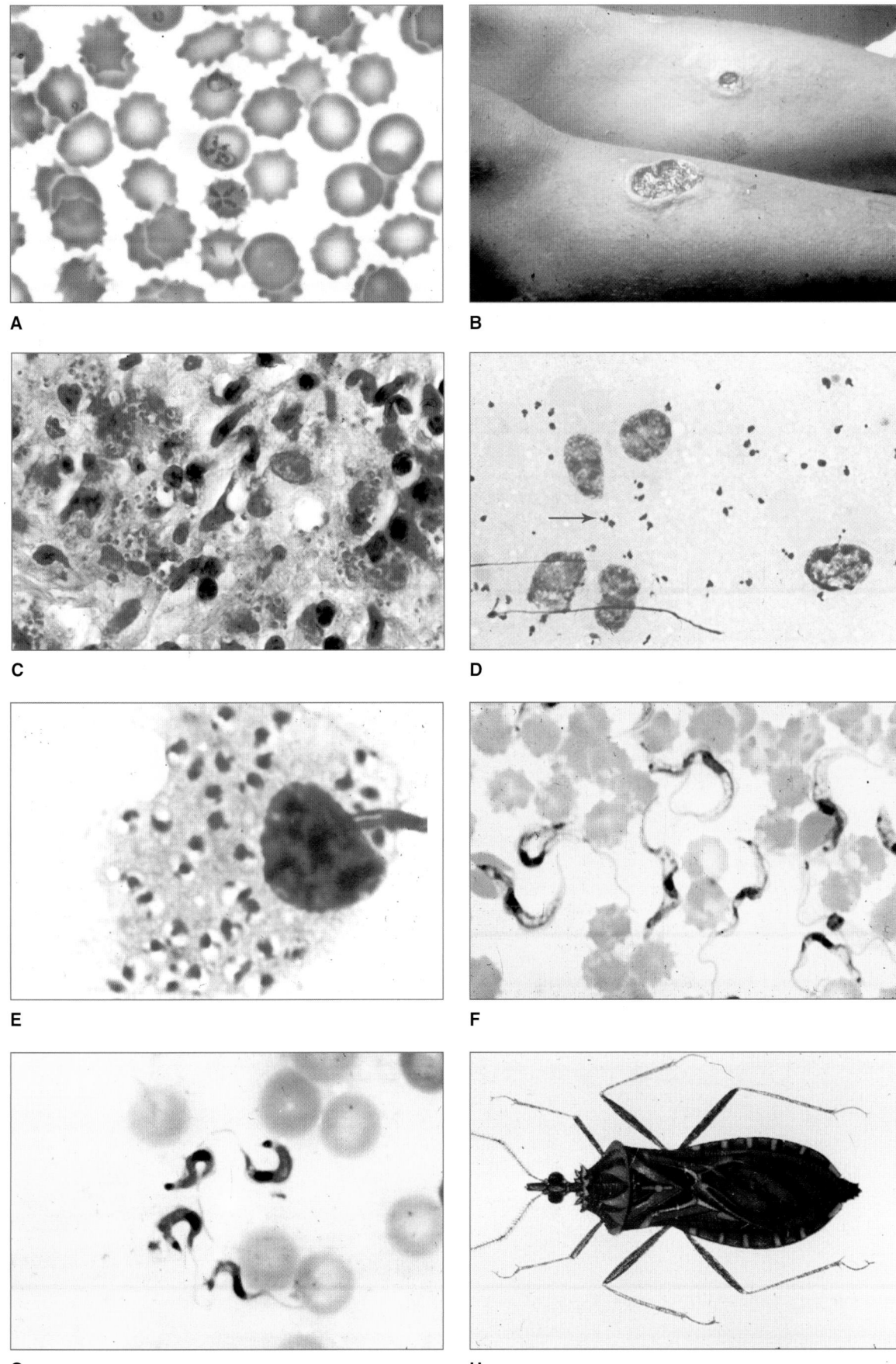

A

B

C

D

E

F

G

H

Filaria

A. Photomicrograph of a peripheral blood smear demonstrating a sheathed microfilaria. Microfilaria are extracellular parasites that measure about 245–295 μm in length and between 7 and 10 μm wide. They are released into the circulation from gravid female worms that reside within lymphatic channels in infected parts of the body. The microfilaria released by species pathogenic for humans have a sheath, as illustrated in this photograph (arrow). As the column of nuclei seen in the parasite illustrated in this photograph does not appear to extend to the tip of the tail, the most likely species is *Wuchereria bancrofti*.

B. Photomicrograph of a peripheral blood smear illustrating the tail section of a microfilaria, highlighting the nuclear arrangement. Note that two detached nuclei extend into the tail, a feature characteristic of *Brugia malayi*.

C. A column of nuclei that extends into the tail section of a microfilaria, as illustrated in this photomicrograph, is characteristic of *Loa loa*.

D. Photomicrograph of an hematoxylin-and-eosin–stained section of a subcutaneous nodule, to include the cross section through the body of a female filarial worm, *Onchocerca volvulus*. Within the cavity of this organism are numerous microfilariae, which ultimately are released into the surrounding tissue, where they cause an inflammatory reaction ending in fibrosis. The microfilaria of *O. volvulus* rarely circulate in the peripheral blood, or they circulate in such small quantities that they virtually are never detected in stained smears.

E. Photograph of a dog heart heavily infested with the adult worms of *Dirofilaria immitis*. Canines serve as the definitive host for this tissue nematode. In humans, who may serve as inadvertent hosts, the larval forms never reach the heart, being filtered out in the lungs, where they produce multifocal inflammatory granulomata.

F. Photomicrograph of a Giemsa-stained impression smear demonstrating numerous blue-staining, bow-shaped tachyzoites of *Toxoplasma gondii*. Each tachyzoite measures approximately 3×6 μm, is pyriform or bow-shaped, and has a nucleus and various internal organelles, including mitochondria, endoplasmic reticulum, and a Golgi apparatus, observed only in electron micrographs. The tachyzoites are the infective form of the parasite, which enter the circulation and are carried to various organs, particularly the central nervous system, where they cause microfocal inflammatory lesions. Tachyzoites can also transmigrate the placenta of pregnant women, enter the circulation of the developing fetus, and cause congenital infections in newborns.

G. Photomicrograph of a Giemsa-stained histologic section of a brain biopsy obtained from a patient with cerebral toxoplasmosis. Demonstrated are three cysts, ranging between 15 and 30 μm in diameter, within which are packed myriad tiny blue-staining bradyzoites. In humans with a competent immune system, the tachyzoites encyst and become inactive in the cyst forms shown in the photograph.

H. A close-up view of a toxoplasma cyst filled with bradyzoites. While the disease is arrested in this cyst form, on suppression of immunity in a previously infected person, these cysts can break down, again releasing active tachyzoites, again free to produce reinfection toxoplasmosis.

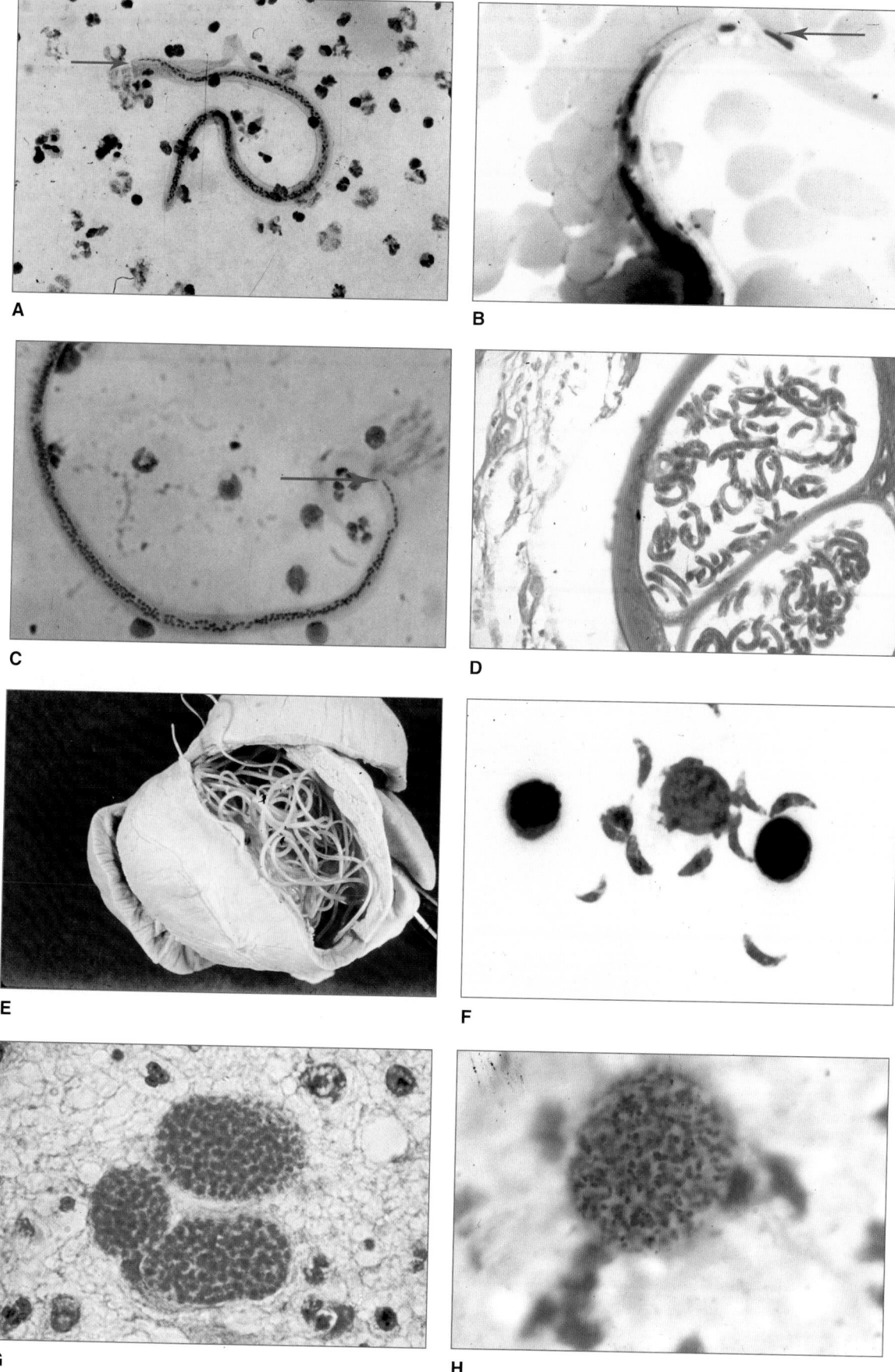

A

B

C

D

E

F

G

H

TISSUE PARASITES

A. Hematoxylin-and-eosin–stained section of heart muscle, including a swollen fiber from top to bottom along the center of the field of view that is inhabited by dense collections of the amastigotic forms of *Trypanosoma cruzi*. Cardiac involvement in patients with Chagas' disease commonly results in heart failure and death.

B. Photograph of a liver cyst from which multiple small, variable in size, hydatid cysts were contained.

C. Close-up view of two hydatid cysts removed from the mesentery of a person with echinococcal disease, illustrating a thin, smooth outer membrane to the outer surface of which aggregates of fat are attached.

D. Hematoxylin-and-eosin–stained section taken through an echinococcal cyst. The cyst wall is composed of a layer of dense fibrous tissue derived from the host reaction. The inner parasite membrane is germinal, from which three daughter embryos (brood capsules), each with an inverted scolex, have been produced. On breaking free from the germinal membrane, these daughter cysts, along with released protoscolices, form free-floating hydatid sand.

E. Illustrated are single protoscolices (fragments of "hydatid sand"), each containing an inverted rostellum with a prominent row of hooklets, representing the anlage of the protruding armed rostellum of the adult worm.

F. Photomicrograph of an adult *Echinococcus granulosus* tape worm. These adult worms, which reside in the intestinal tract of dogs and other canines, are very small, measuring no more than 6 mm long, and are composed of only three segments—an armed scolex, a neck, and a single proglottid, from which a relatively small number of eggs are released. However, as several hundred such worms may occupy the dog intestine, and the times of survival for each worm can reach 20 months, the total number of eggs released over a long period of time can be enormous, thereby guaranteeing completion of the life cycle.

G. Hematoxylin-and-eosin–stained section of skeletal muscle, including an encysted, coiled larval form of *Trichinella spiralis*. The dense infiltration of inflammatory cells into the tissue surrounding the cyst indicates relatively recent infection, most likely associated with local and possibly constitutional symptoms.

H. A second view of a muscle biopsy specimen including a coiled *Trichinella spiralis* larva. The absence of an inflammatory reaction and the laying down of dense fibrous tissue around the cyst indicates a chronic infection. In time this inactive cyst may become calcified, representing the last stage of infection.

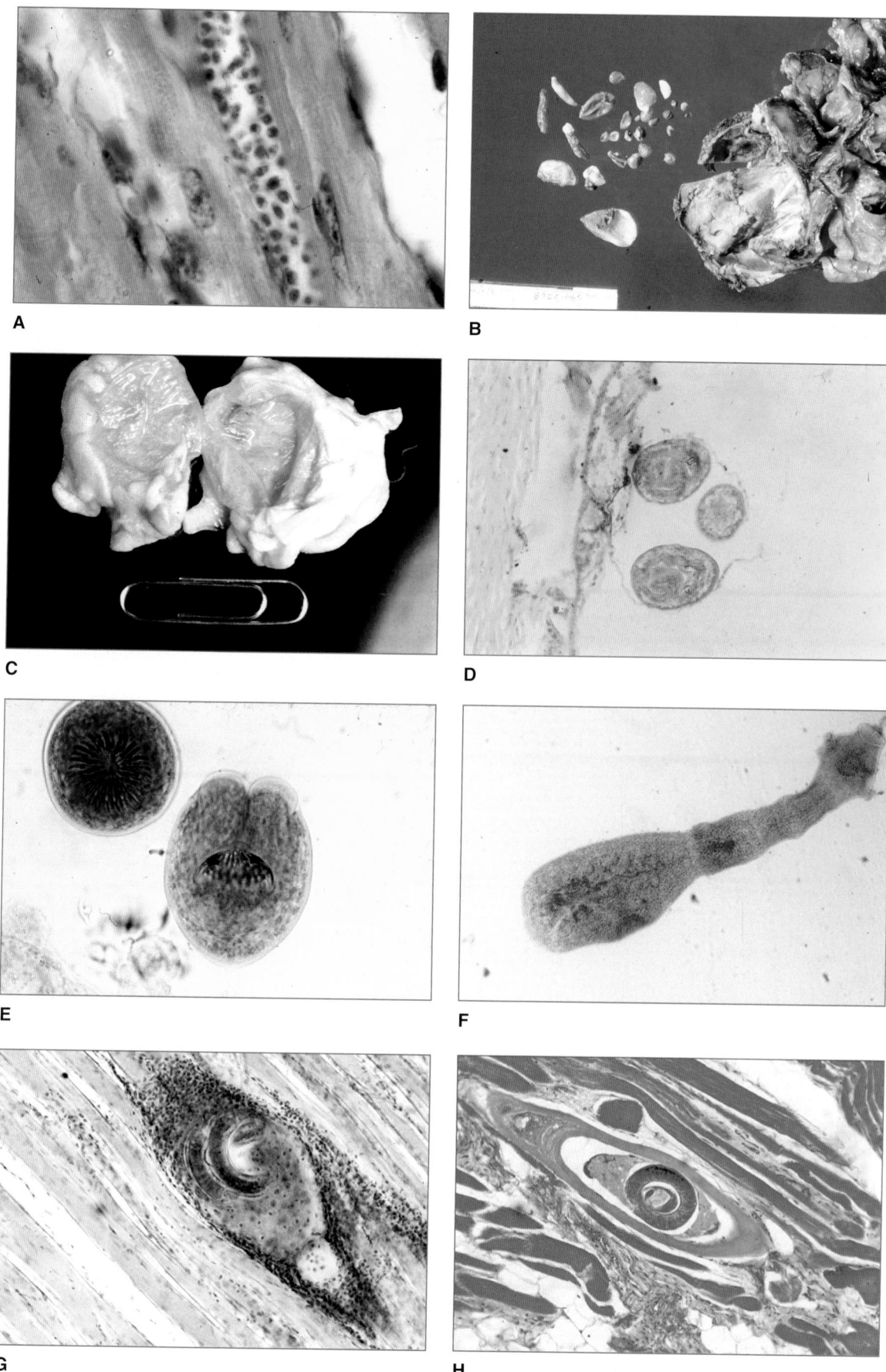

A

B

C

D

E

F

G

H

VIRAL INCLUSION

A. Varicella-zoster virus hepatitis. The nuclei of several hepatocytes contain typical herpes virus inclusions. The mass of the inclusion is eosinophilic and colored red, and the residual nuclear chromatin, which is basophilic and colored blue, is crowded around the rim of the nuclear membrane. The inclusion stands out because of an artifactual clear halo between the inclusion and the peripheralized nuclear chromatin. This artifact is caused by formalin fixation. The inclusions of herpes simplex virus and varicella-zoster virus cannot be distinguished. (Hematoxylin and eosin stain.)

B. Herpes simplex cervicitis. The Papanicolaou stain demonstrates numerous multinucleated giant cells in a cervical scraping. The nuclei are molded against each other, and inclusions are present. The inclusions appear homogeneous, and nuclear chromatin is peripheralized to the rim of the nuclear membrane. The cytologic preparation was fixed promptly in ethanol, and the formalin halo artifact is not present. A mature squamous epithelial cell stains pink.

C. Herpes simplex vesicular lesion—Tzanck test. These cells were scraped from the base of a herpetic vesicle. The multinucleated cell is characteristic of herpes infection, but one cannot differentiate the effects of herpes simplex virus from those of varicella-zoster virus. The multiple nuclei are molded and homogeneous, but inclusions are difficult to see in air-dried smears that have been stained with a Giemsa or similar stain. The direct scrapings can also be stained by the Papanicolaou method or with hematoxylin and eosin.

D. Cytomegalovirus sialadenitis. The epithelial cells of a salivary gland contain the inclusions of cytomegalovirus. The large basophilic (blue or purple) inclusions fill much of the nucleus. In some cells there are artifactual clear halos between the inclusion and the nuclear membrane that are produced by formalin fixation. Granular cytoplasmic inclusions are also visible in some cells. The architecture of the salivary gland is distorted by an intense lymphocytic infiltrate. Enlargement of the infected cells and nuclei inspired the name of the virus. Salivary gland virus was the original name for the virus, and salivary gland inclusion disease was the original name for the infection, because of the prominence of infection of this organ in neonatal disease. (Hematoxylin and eosin stain.)

E. Adenovirus pneumonia. In this case of adenovirus infection there is a large amount of proteinaceous exudate (which is eosinophilic) in the air spaces, but there are few inflammatory cells. The nuclei of the infected respiratory epithelial cells are completely replaced by viral DNA, which produces a dense basophilic inclusion. Early inclusions may resemble those of herpes simplex virus. The mature inclusions, as seen here, fill the nucleus and obliterate the outline of the nuclear membrane. They are referred to as *smudge cells.* (Hematoxylin and eosin stain.)

F. Measles virus pneumonia. Several large multinucleated giant cells are in the airways of this patient with measles pneumonia. The multiple nuclei contain eosinophilic nuclear inclusions that resemble those of herpes simplex virus. The nuclear chromatin is pushed to the rim of the nuclear membrane, but the formalin clear halo artifact is not present in this section. In addition, in this case there are also eosinophilic cytoplasmic inclusions, some of which are coalescent and/or surrounded by a clear space. (Hematoxylin and eosin stain.)

G. Respiratory syncytial virus infection. Monolayer of HEp-2 cells infected with respiratory syncytial virus. Two large syncytial giant cells have formed in the monolayer. There are no inclusions in the nuclei of the cells, but several brightly eosinophilic intracytoplasmic inclusions can be seen. (Hematoxylin and eosin stain.)

H. Rabies encephalitis. Two neurons each have an eosinophilic intracytoplasmic inclusion, which is known as a *Negri body.* Some vacuoles are evident in the inclusion. The irregular appearance comes from an admixture of normal cytoplasmic structures with masses of viral ribonucleic acid (Hematoxylin and eosin stain.). (Courtesy of Daniel Perl, M.D.).

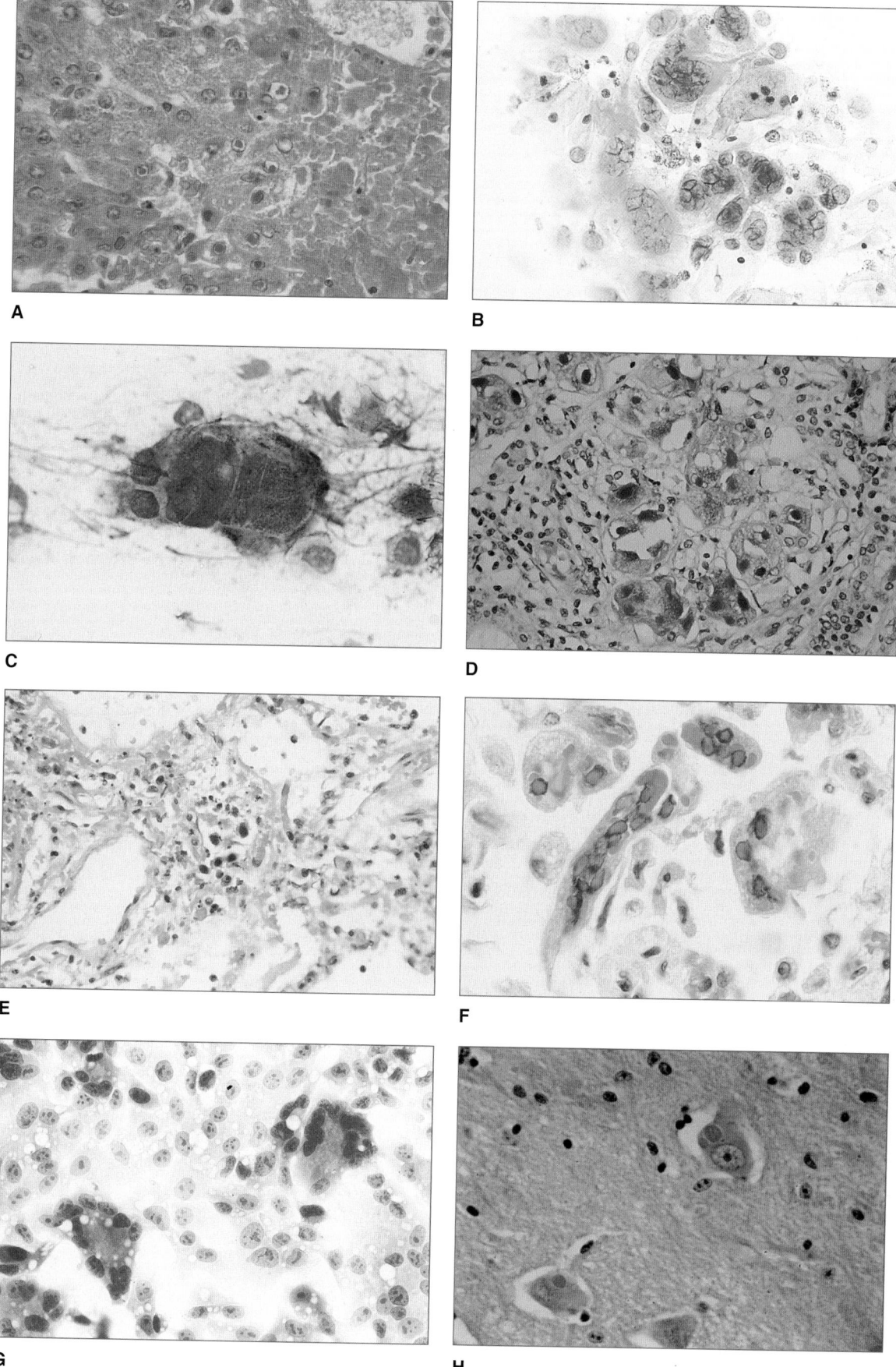

A

B

C

D

E

F

G

H

DIAGNOSIS OF INFECTIONS CAUSED BY VIRUSES, *CHLAMYDIA*, AND *EHRLICHIA*

A. *Chlamydia trachomatis* inclusion conjunctivitis. An epithelial cell that contains a chlamydial inclusion body is depicted. The cell has degenerated, leaving only the nucleus and the large inclusion. The large inclusion is molded around or capped over the underlying nucleus. Smear stained by the Giemsa method. (Photograph reproduced with permission of Julius Schachter and PSG Publishing Company, Inc., Littleton, MA.)

B. *C. trachomatis* cervicitis. Innumerable elementary bodies are present in this very heavy infection. The Evans blue counterstain causes the cells to fluoresce red, and the inclusions appear yellow in the photomicrograph. In areas with less background material or without a counterstain, the fluoresceinated antibody causes the elementary bodies to fluoresce apple green. A very heavily infected cell is present in the center of the photograph. Such cases are little challenge, but detecting positive specimens in which only a few elementary bodies are present is considerably more difficult.

C. McCoy cell monolayer infected with *C. trachomatis*. The specimen was centrifuged onto this monolayer of cycloheximide-treated McCoy cells, which were incubated for 48 hours. The cells have been stained with a fluorescein-conjugated monoclonal antibody to a major outer-membrane protein (MOMP) of *C. trachomatis*. Multiple intracytoplasmic inclusions, which correspond to the inclusion demonstrated in Color Plate 23-2A, stain bright green.

D. HEp-2 cells infected with herpes simplex virus, type 1. When a cytopathic effect became evident, the cells were scraped from the monolayer and placed on a slide. The cells have been stained with a fluorescein-conjugated monoclonal antibody to herpes simplex virus, type 1. There is bright, specific fluorescence, which is both nuclear and cytoplasmic.

E. Nasal aspirate infected with respiratory syncytial virus. Two cells in the smear show bright green cytoplasmic fluorescence. In addition to diffuse fluorescence, the discrete, punctate fluorescence represents viral inclusions, which are characteristic of this virus and help to confirm the specificity of the fluorescence. (Fluorescein isothiocyanate–conjugated monoclonal antibody to respiratory syncytial virus.)

F. Cytomegalovirus-infected human diploid fibroblasts in a shell vial. The elongated fibroblast cells are colored by the counterstain. The infected cells are distinguished by the bright green fluorescence of the oval nuclei. (Fluorescein isothiocyanate–conjugated antibody to cytomegalovirus early-intermediate antigen.)

G. Human monocytic ehrlichiosis caused by *Ehrlichia chaffeensis*. A circulating mononuclear cell contains a distinct cytoplasmic inclusion (morula) that is made up of individual bacterial cells. Inclusions are rarely seen in cases of monocytic ehrlichiosis (Wright stain. Slide contributed by J. Stephen Dumler, M.D.)

H. Human granulocytic ehrlichiosis caused by an unnamed *Ehrlichia* sp. A distinct bluish inclusion is present in the cytoplasm of a circulating neutrophil. The frequency with which inclusions are found in human granulocytic ehrlichiosis is unclear. (Wright stain. Slide contributed by J. Stephen Dumler, M.D.)

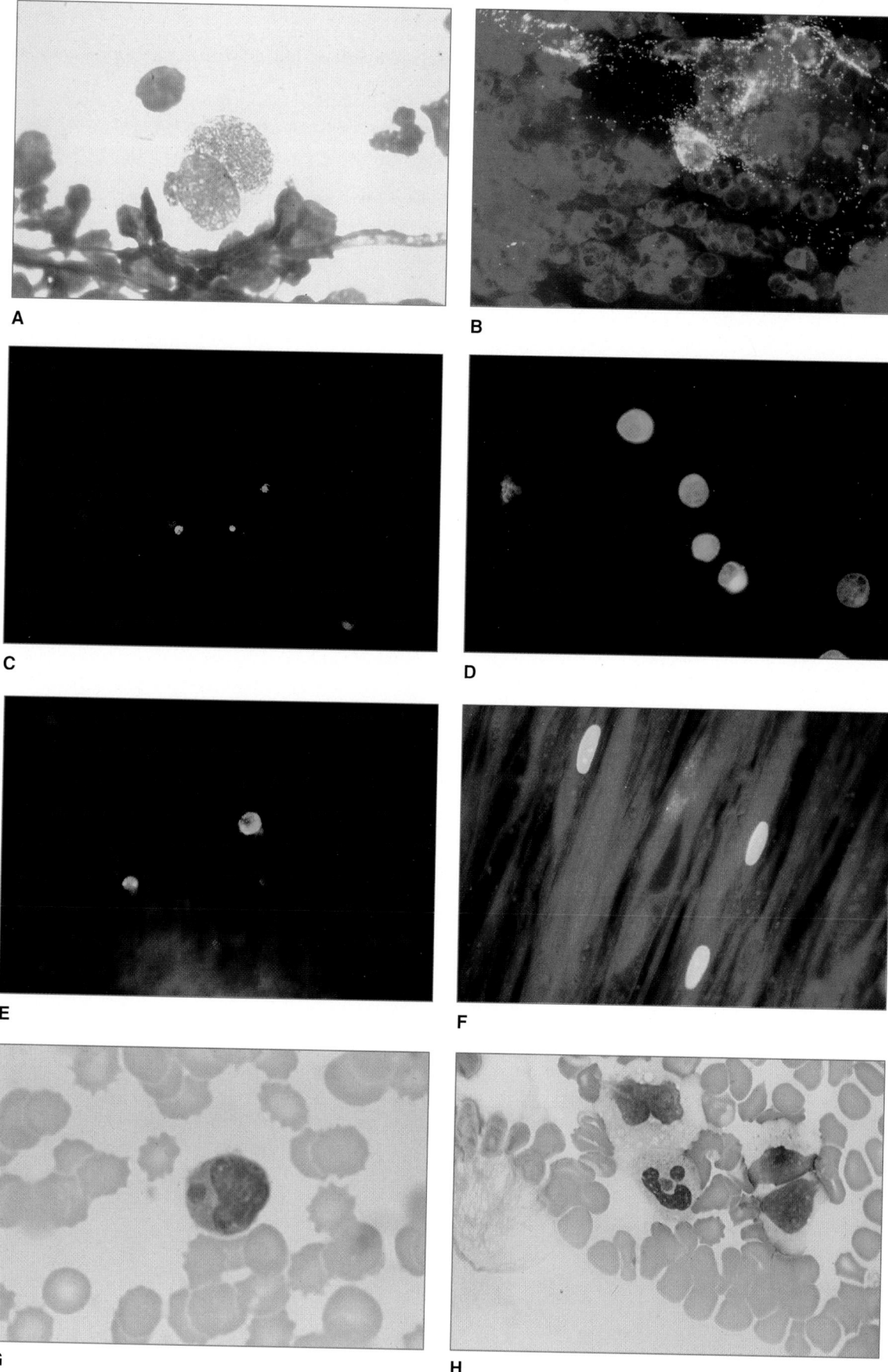

A

B

C

D

E

F

G

H

IDENTIFICATION OF TICKS

A. Larval ticks, in this case *Ixodes scapularis*, are distinguished by the presence of six legs, three on each side. Nymphs and adults have a total of eight legs.

B. Instars (life stages) of *Ixodes scapularis* on a dime for comparison of size. From left to right: adult female (*F*), adult male (*M*), nymph (*N*), larva (*L*).

C. Ventral aspect adult female *Ixodes scapularis*, demonstrating relationship of mouthparts to basis capituli. (*B*) Palp (*P*), hypostome (*H*), genital pore (*G*), anus (*A*), anal groove (*U*), spiracular plate (*S*). Inset shows detail of mouthparts, Note the teethlike denticles protruding from the lateral edges of the hypostome.

D. Coxal spurs of adult *Ixodes scapularis*. The spur on coxa I is long, pointed, and oriented internally. The spurs on coxae II through IV are short, blunt, and oriented externally.

E. *Ixodes cookei* female dorsum. The scutum (*S*) is angular. The length of the palps (*P*) is approximately the same as the basis capituli (*B*). In this specimen the hypostome (*H*) is broken.

F. *I. marxi* female dorsum. The scutum (*S*) is angular and resembles that of *I. cookei* (compare Color Plate A-1*F*), but the scutum of *I. marxi* is longer than it is wide in comparison to *I. cookei*.

G. *Dermacentor variabilis* adult females. The scutum demonstrates ornamentation (*O*). Festoons (*F*) are present at the posterior margin. One of the specimens is considerably engorged (*E*), changing the color of the dorsum from brown to cream.

H. *Dermacentor variabilis* adult female. The scutum is intensely ornamented (*O*). The basis capituli (*B*) is wider than it is tall. Note the "eyes" at the lateral margin bilaterally (*arrows*).

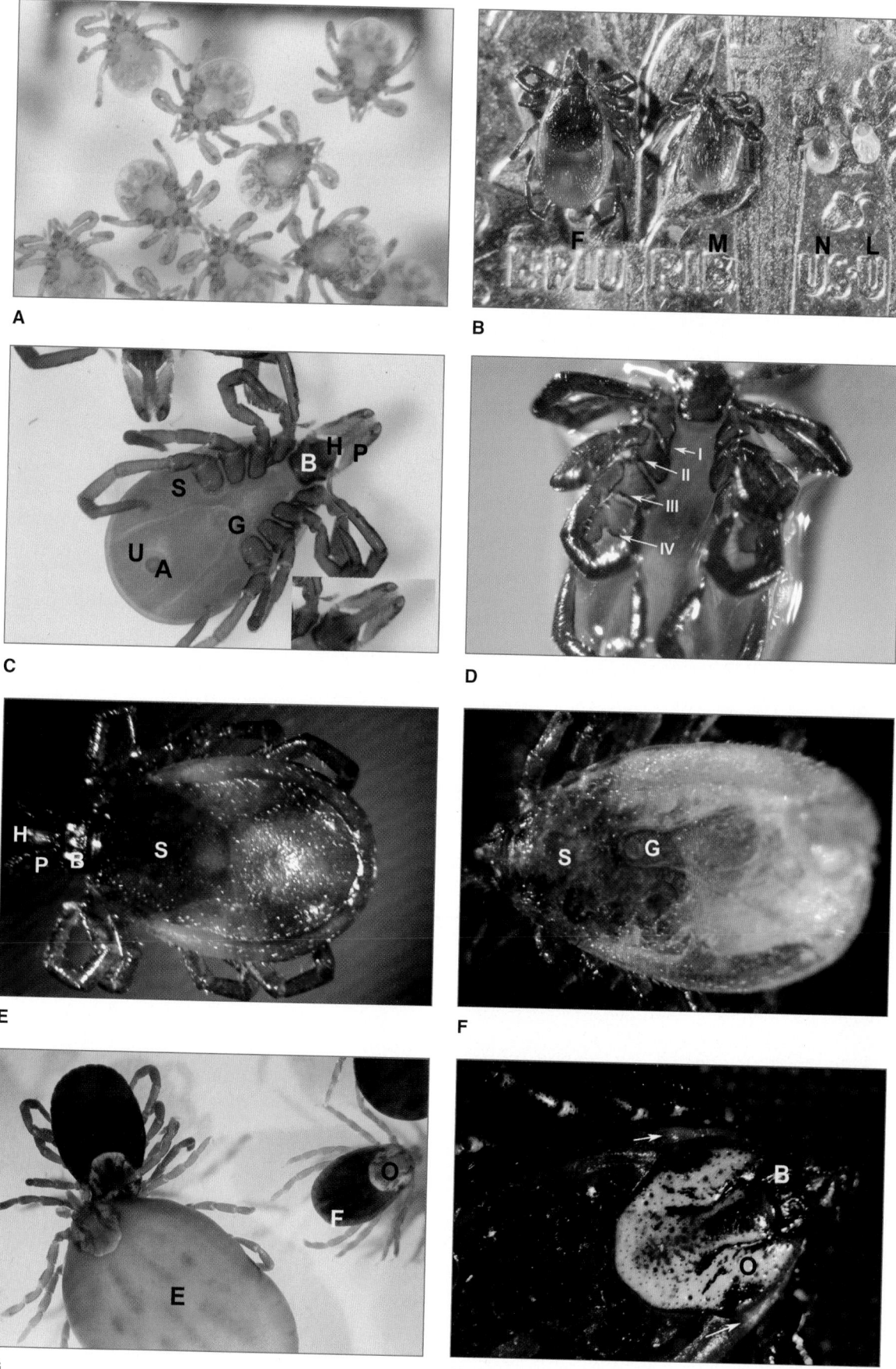

A

B

F   M   N   L

C

H
P
B
S
G
U
A

D

I
II
III
IV

E

H
P
B
S

F

S
G

G

O
F
E

H

B
O

IDENTIFICATION OF TICKS AND OTHER ARTHROPODS

A. *Amblyomma americanum* female dorsum. The ornamentation on the scutum (*S*) takes the form of a patch at the posterior edge—the lone star (arrow). Festoons (*F*) are present around the posterior edge of the tick. "Eyes" are present, but are difficult to see in this partially engorged specimen.

B. *Amblyomma americanum* male dorsum. A very prominent "eye" (*arrow*) is present at the lateral edge of the scutum, which covers the entire dorsum. The mouthparts are missing.

C. *Amblyomma americanum* male dorsum. The prominent festoons (*F*) are evident at the posterior margin. The arrows delineate two horseshoe-shaped markings just lateral to the midline bilaterally.

D. *Amblyomma americanum* male ventral surface. A prominent internal spur is evident on coxa IV (*arrows*). A detail of the spur is shown in the inset (*I*). The anus (*A*) is surrounded by a posterior facing groove (*GR*), in contrast to the anterior facing groove of *Ixodes* spp. The genital pore (*G*) is prominent. All of the mouthparts and the basis capituli are missing from this specimen.

E. Dorsal view of *Ornithodoros* spp. This soft tick lacks a scutum, and the mouthparts are not visible from above.

F. *Sarcoptes scabiei* in its burrow. The mite has deposited eggs and defecated in its newfound home, adding to the discomfort of the victim.

G. *Loxosceles reclusa*, the brown recluse spider. The brown color and characteristic head marking distinguish this venomous spider. (Photograph courtesy of Robert Suter, Ph.D.)

H. Black widow spider. The deep black color and characteristic red, hourglass-shaped marking on the ventral side are clearly visible. (Photograph courtesy of Robert Suter, Ph.D.)

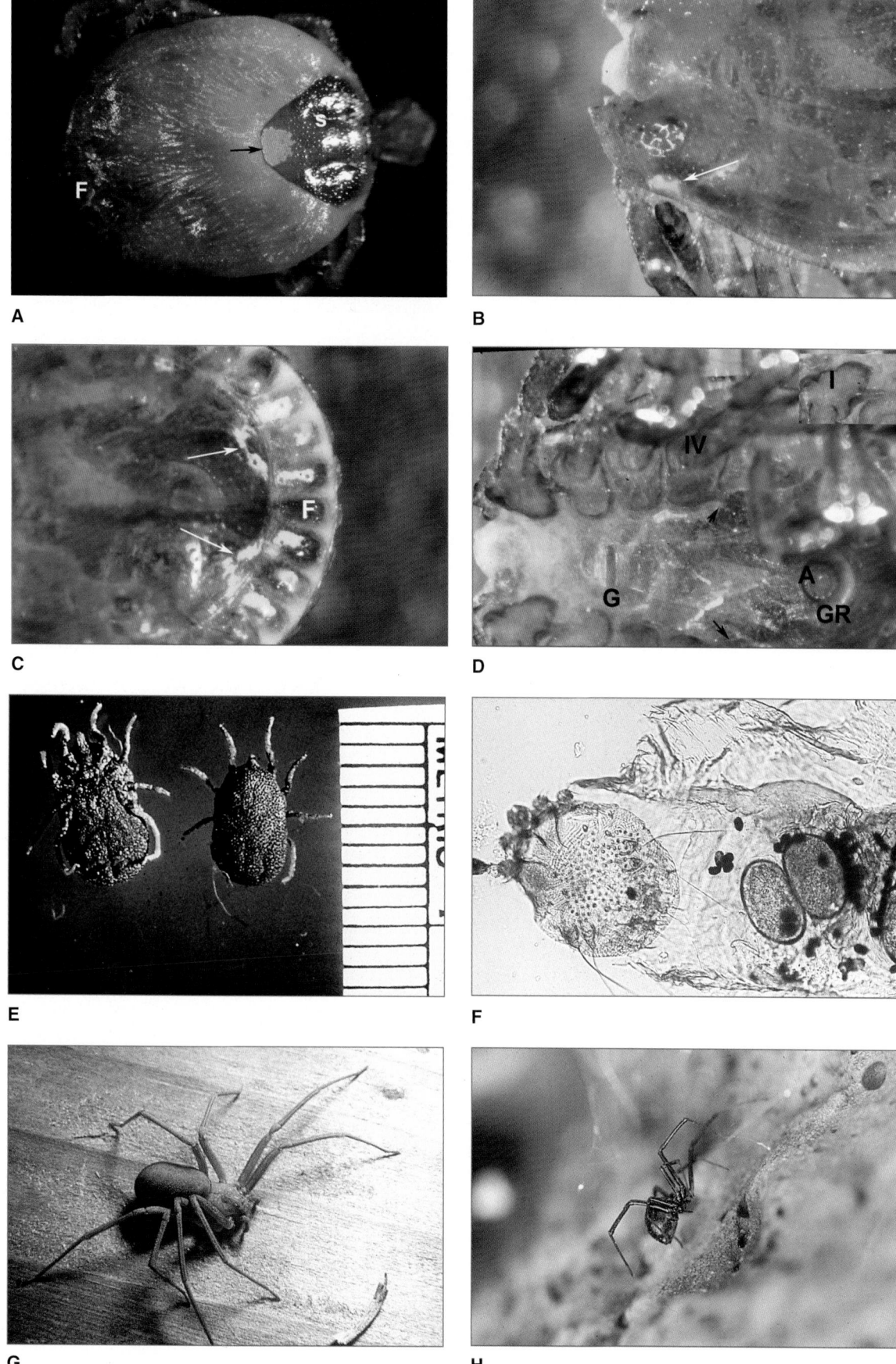

A

B

C

D

E

F

G

H

Identification of Miscellaneous Arthropods

A. *Dermatobia hominis*. The human botfly has been extracted from a pustular lesion. The flask shape, tapered neck, and encircling spines of the larva are evident. The neck was damaged at the time of surgical extraction.

B. Ventral view of *Cimex* spp., the bedbug. The orange-brown color and characteristic shape provide identifying features.

C. Dorsal view of *Triatoma* spp., a reduviid or kissing bug. The elongated body and long, thin head are characteristic. A pair of wings is evident.

D. *Tunga penetrans*, the jigger flea. Most fleas bite their host quickly and depart for completion of their life cycle, but the jigger flea remains embedded in the skin, where its eggs develop.

E. Female *Ctenocephalides* spp., the dog or cat flea. The long, muscular legs hang from the body and make the flea a prodigious jumper. The "hunched" appearance of the body is evident.

F. Female *Pediculosis humanus*, the human body louse. The long slender body supports three pairs of legs, each of which has clawlike hooks at the terminus.

G. Nit of a head louse. The egg is firmly attached to a hair shaft.

H. Female *Phthirus pubis*, the crab louse. The squat body and awesome pincers on three pairs of legs make the derivation of the popular name clear. The louse hangs onto a hair shaft, which also supports a nit.

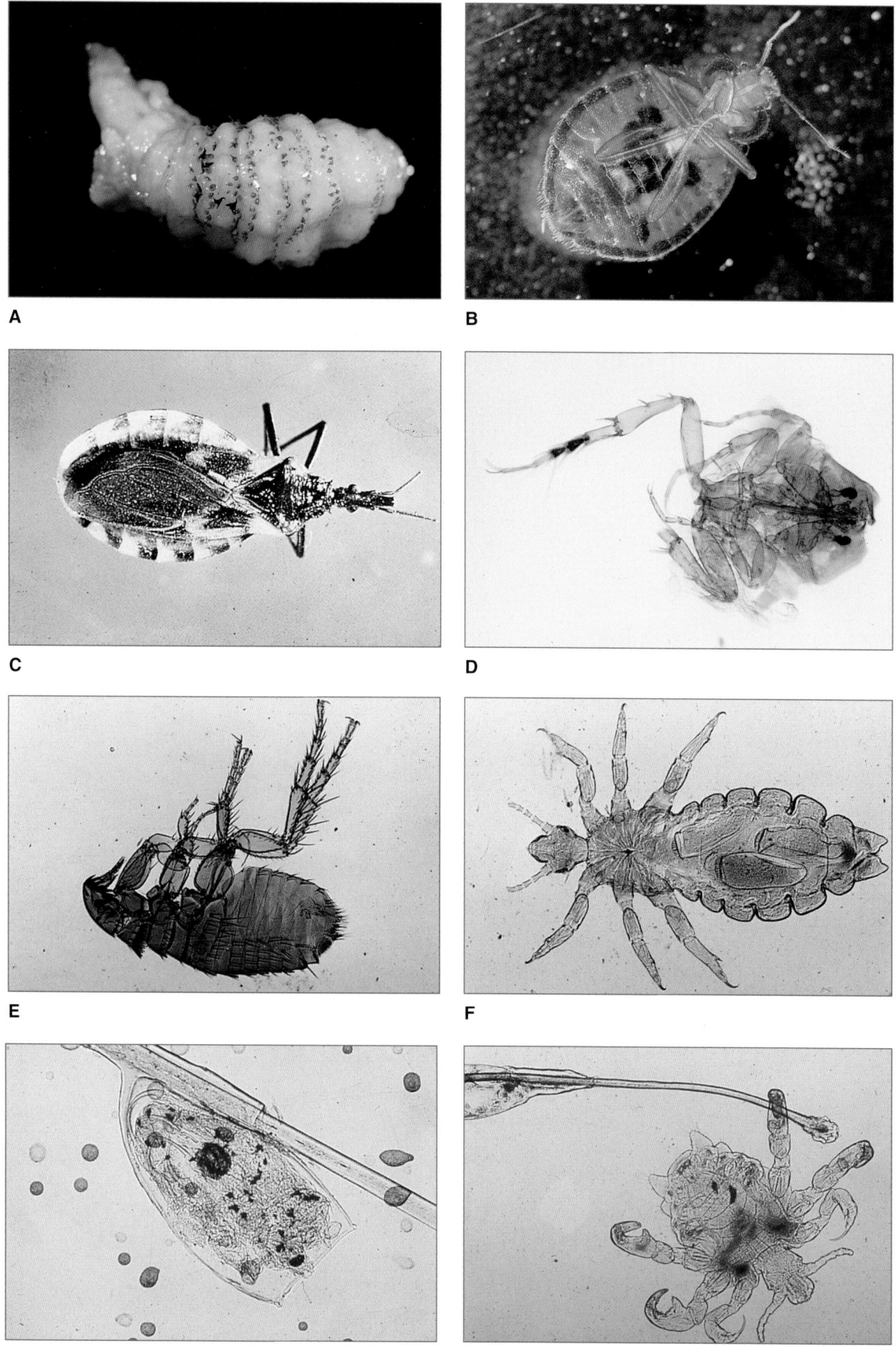

A

B

C

D

E

F

G

H

Index

Note: Page numbers followed by a ''b'' indicate material in boxes; page numbers followed by an ''f'' indicate figures; page numbers followed by a ''t'' indicate tables; ''CP'' refers to color plates; Charts follow the appendix.

Abbott LCx *M. tuberculosis* assay, in mycobacterial identification, 1109
Abdominal actinomycosis, 817
Abiotrophia sp., 704–705
  identification of, CP 13-3D, 731, 734t
Abscess(es), 7, 95–96
  brain, 93
  clinical presentation of, 95
  diagnosis of, 95–96
  lung, 76
Absidia sp., identification of, 1169–1170, 1170f
Abuse, sexual, in children, *C. trachomatis* infections and, 1406
Acari, identification of, C, CP A-1B, E–H, 1425–1428, 1426f–1428f
AccuProbe *Neisseria gonorrhoeae* culture confirmation test, in *N. gonorrhoeae* identification, 597
Acetoin production, in coagulase-negative staphylococci identification, 655
Achromobacter sp., 340–343, 341t, 342t
  asaccharolytic, 340, 341t
  groups B, E, and F, 306t
  saccharolytic, 340, 342t, 343
Acid(s)
  dipicolinic, 190
  fatty
    cellular, of *Legionella* sp., 559, 560t
    volatile, identification of, in determination of metabolic products of anaerobes, 906, 908, 909b, 909f–911, 915t
    from glycerol in presence of erythromycin, in differentiation of micrococci and staphylococci, 645
  lipoteichoic, 684
    of *S. pneumoniae*, 690
    as virulence factor in *Enterococcus* sp., 701
  meso-diaminopimelic, 785
  mycolic, 188
  nonvolatile, in determination of metabolic products of anaerobes, 908–909, 911b
  nucleic. *See* Nucleic acid(s)
  teichoic
    of *S. aureus*, 630b
    of *S. pneumoniae*, 690
Acid-fast bacilli, staining of, in mycobacteria recovery and identification, Charts 19-1–19-3, CP 19-1A–B, 1075–1077, 1076t, 1077t
''Acid-fast'' bacterial cell walls, 188–189, 189f
Acid-fast smears, in mycobacteria recovery, 1079–1080
Acid-fast stains
  in microscopic examination of specimens, CP 1-2, 25
  Ziehl-Neelsen, in microscopic examination of specimens, 20t
Acidovorans group of comamonadaceae, CP 7-2C, 331–332
ACIF test. *See* Anticomplement immunofluorescence (ACIF) test
Acinetobacter sp., CP 7-5A–B, 353–355, 354t
  A. baumannii, CP 7-5A–B, 353–355, 354t
  identification of, CP 7-5A, 357
Acremonium sp., clusters of conidia produced by, CP 21-2E, F, H, 1182–1184, 1183f–1185f
Acridine orange, in microscopic examination of specimens, CP 1-2D, 25–26, 26b
Acropetal, 1157b

Acrotheca, 1215, 1215f
Actinobacillus sp., 452–457
  A. actinomycetemcomitans, 452–455, 454b
    antimicrobial susceptibility of, 455
    clinical significance of, 452–453, 454b
    cultural characteristics of, CP 9-1E, 453, 455, 456t
    virulence factors of, 454b
  A. hominis, 458
  A. ureae, 455, 457
  animal species in, 457t, 458
  described, 452
  identification of, biochemical characteristics for, 457t
Actinobacteria, 175b–176b
Actinobaculum sp., 810–811, 812t
  identification of, flow chart for, 822f
Actinomadura sp., 864, 864t
  clinical disease due to, 864, 864t
  epidemiology of, 864
  pathology of, 864, 864t
Actinomyces sp.
  A. bovis, 813b
  A. cardiffensis, 813b
  A. europaeus, 813b
  A. funkei, 813b
  A. georgiae, 813b
  A. gerencseriae, 813b
  A. graevenitzii, 814b
  A. hongkongensis, 814b
  A. houstonensis, 814b
  A. israelii, 814b
  A. meyeri, 814b
  A. naeslundii, 814b
  A. nasicola, 814b
  A. neuii, subsp. *neuii*, 814b
  A. odontolyticus, 815b
  A. oricola, 815b
  A. radicidentis, 815b–816b
  A. radingae, 816b
  A. turicensis, 816b
  A. urogenitalis, 816b
  A. viscosus, 816b
  identification of, CP 16-2, 930
    flow chart for, 822f
  isolated from animals, 817, 818t–821t
  isolated from humans, 811–817, 813b–816b, 818t–821t, 822f
  members of, 813b–814b
  taxonomy of, CP 14-2A–D, 783, 785, 786t–787t
Actinomycete(s), 865–866, 866b
  aerobic, 858–876
    cell wall composition of, 860, 861t
    classification of, 858–860, 859f, 859t
    infections due to, laboratory diagnosis of, Chart 15-1, CP 15-1A–E, 866–875, 868t–870t, 871b, 871f, 872t–874t
      biochemical and physiologic tests in, 867, 868t–869t
      primary isolation in, 866–867
    introduction to, 858–860
    Nocardia sp., laboratory diagnosis of, in vitro antimicrobial susceptibility profiles in, 873t
    phenotypic grouping of, 859, 859t
    taxonomy of, 858–860, 860b
    terminology related to, 860, 860t
  epidemiology of, 861–862
  pathogenesis of, 861–862

  pathology of, 861–862
  thermophilic, 865
    identification of, 871
Actinomycosis
  abdominal, 817
  cervicofacial, 817
  CNS, 817
  pelvic, 817
  thoracic, 817
Acute glomerulonephritis, streptococci and, 680–681
Acute pharyngitis, *Haemophilus* sp. and, 434t
Acute rheumatic fever (ARF), streptococci and, 680
Acute suppurative inflammation, 7
Adaptive immunologic cellular defenses, 7–8
Adaptive immunologic noncellular (humoral) defenses, 8
Adenosine triphosphate (ATP), 196
Adenoviridae sp., described, 1341t
Adenovirus(es)
  clinical manifestations of, 1360–1361, 1361t
  enteric, clinical manifestations of, 1349t, 1350
  type 5, 1341f, 1341t
Adhesin(s), 192
  as virulence factors, 204
Adolescent(s), HIV in, revised classification system for, 1352, 1352t, 1353t
Adult(s), HIV in, revised classification system for, 1352, 1352t, 1353t
Aerial mycelium, 1157b
Aerobe(s)
  described, 878
  obligate, 195
Aerobic pathway, 311–312, 311f
Aerococcus sp., 705–706
  identification of, 731, 734, 735t
Aeromonas sp., 416t, 417, 419–422, 419t, 420b, 421t
  characteristics of, 416t
  clinical significance of, 419–420
  culturing of, agars in, 420, 420b
  laboratory identification of, 420–422, 421t
  laboratory recovery from clinical specimens, 420, 420b
  medicinal leeches, 420
  taxonomy of, 419, 419t
Aerotolerance tests, 900–901, 900f
Aerotolerant anaerobes, 195, 878–879
AFIP. *See* Armed Forces Institute of Pathology (AFIP)
Afipia sp., 510, 511t
  antimicrobial susceptibility of, 510
  clinical significance of, 510, 511t
  identification of, 510, 511t
    biochemical characteristics for, 511t
  isolation of, 510, 511t
  taxonomy of, 510
African trypanosomiasis, 1303b
Agar(s)
  in *Aeromonas* sp. culturing, 420, 420b
  blood, cystine-tellurite, 1478
  brain–heart infusion, uses of, 1159t
  chocolate, in *Haemophilus* sp. infection diagnosis, 445
  Christensen's urea, 225
  chromogenic, in *Enterobacteriaceae* identification, CP 6-5E–H, 283–284
  cornmeal, in yeast identification, CP 21-6B, 1218–1221, 1219b, 1220f, 1221f
  differential, 28t–29t, 30–31, 30f–32f

Agar(s) (*Continued*)

EMB, in *Enterobacteriaceae* recovery, CP 6-2C–F, 219t

Haemophilus isolation, in *Haemophilus* sp. infection diagnosis, 446

Hektoen enteric, in *Enterobacteriaceae* recovery, CP 6-3E–F, 220t

inhibitory, 28t–29t, 30–31, 30f–32f

inhibitory mold, uses of, 1159t

Kliger iron, in carbohydrate fermentation detection, CP 6-1E, CP 6-4B, 216–217, 217b, 217f

MacConkey

in *Enterobacteriaceae* recovery, CP 6-2A–B, 219t

growth on, 1500

failure of, CP 7-1C, 313

in mycobacteria identification, Chart 19-8, 1090

mannitol salts, 648

mycosel/mycobiotic, uses of, 1159t

NBG, in *Salmonella* sp. recovery and characterization, 256t

NBGL, in *Salmonella* sp. recovery and characterization, 256t

potato flake, uses of, 1159t

Rambach, in *Salmonella* sp. recovery and characterization, 256t

reactions in, in bacteria identification, 35b

SABHI, uses of, 1159t

Sabouraud's dextrose, uses of, 1159t

Sabouraud's heart infusion, uses of, 1159t

Salmonella-Shigella, in *Enterobacteriaceae* recovery, 220t

Skirrow's blood, in *C. jejuni* isolation, 397t

SM-ID, in *Salmonella* sp. recovery and characterization, 256t

Tinsdales', 1477

TSI, in carbohydrate fermentation detection, CP 6-1E, CP 6-4B, 216–217

XLD, in *Enterobacteriaceae* recovery, CP 6-3A–D, 220t

Agar dilution susceptibility test, in testing inhibitory activity of antimicrobial agents, 982–983, 988f

Agar plate, 30f, 33, 33f, 34f

Agar-based culture media, in tuberculosis diagnosis, 1067–1068

Agglutination, latex, in streptococci identification, CP 13-3A, 718

Agglutinin(s), cold, 1050

Aggregation substances, 194

as virulence factor in *Enterococcus* sp., 701

Aggressin(s), as virulence factors, 204–205

Agrobacterium sp., CP 7-4B, 342t, 344–345

Agrobacterium yellow group, 339

Alcaligenaceae, 340–343, 341t, 342t

Alcaligenes faecalis, 306t

Alcaligenes group of pseudomonads, 321–323, 322t

Alcaligenes sp., CP 7-4A, 340, 341t

Aleuriospore(s), 1157b

Alishewanella fetalis, 337, 337t

Alkaline encrusted cystitis, 809

Alkaline pseudomonads, characteristics of, 322t

Allergic bronchopulmonary aspergillosis, 1180b

Allergic bronchopulmonary disease, 76

Alloiococcus sp., 708

identification of, 738, 741t

Alternaria sp., 1209, 1210f

Alteromonadaceae, 336–337, 340t

Amblyomma americanum

geographic distribution of, 1425, 1425t

identification of, CP A-2A–D, 1428, 1429t–1430t

Amebiasis, B, CP 22-1, CP 22-2A, I–K, 1258–1260, 1258b, 1259f

serologic diagnosis of, 1260

American Society of Clinical Pathologists (ASCP), 47

American Thoracic Society (ATS), tuberculosis treatment recommendations of, 1116b, 1117

American trypanosomiasis, 1305f

American Type Culture Collection (ATCC), 167

Aminoglycoside(s), *Enterococcus* sp. resistant to, 1012

Amoeba(ae), intestinal, B, CP 22-2A, E–M, 1258–1263, 1258b, 1259f

Amphotericin B, for parasitic infections, 1319t

AMPLICOR *N. gonorrhoeae* PCR assay, in *N. gonorrhoeae* identification, 598

Amplification

nucleic acid, 141–147, 142f, 143f. *See also* Nucleic-acid amplification

transcription-mediated, 143, 144

Amplification test, in *N. gonorrhoeae* identification, 597–599

Anaerobe(s)

aerotolerant, 195, 878–879

described, 878–879

facultative, 195, 879

obligate, 195

oxygen tolerance of, 879

Anaerobic bacteria, 877–944. *See also* Bacteria, anaerobic

Anaerobic Bag Culture Set, 898, 899f

Anaerobic cocci, identification of, 924–947, 925t, 926t

Anaerobic disposable plastic bags, 898

Anaerobic fermentation, pyruvate formed during, fate of, 198, 202f

Anaerobic glove box, 897, 897f, 898f

Anaerobic specimens, transport containers for, 12, 12t, 13, 13f

Anamorph, 1158b

defined, 1156

Anaplasma sp., 1409–1410, 1409t

Anaplasmosis, granulocytic, 1410

Angiomatosis, bacillary, *Bartonella* sp. and, 501

Angiostrongyliasis, 1315

Anisakiasis, 1314–1315

Annellide(s), 1157b, 1182

Annelloconidia, 1157b

Annulus(i), 1157b

Anthrax. *See also Bacillus* sp., *B. anthracis*

clinical presentations of, 777–778

cutaneous, 777

epidemiology of, 776–777

gastrointestinal, 778

industrial, 776

inhalational, 778

nonindustrial, 776–777

oropharyngeal, 778

prevention of, 778

pulmonary, 778

treatment of, 778

Antibiotic(s). *See* Antimicrobial agents

Antibiotic-modifying enzymes, 958–959, 960t, 961t

Antibody(ies)

anti-Igm, serologic diagnosis of, 1402–1403

defined, 112

detection of

EIAs for, 119–122, 120f, 121f

immunofluorescence techniques in, 125–128, 126f, 127f

monoclonal, 113–114, 115b

production of, 114, 115b

Anticomplement immunofluorescence (ACIF) test, 127–128, 127f

Antifungal susceptibility testing, 1230, 1232, 1232f

Antigen(s)

C, 684

in clinical specimens of *C. trachomatis*, detection of, 1405

in clinical specimens of *Coxiella* sp., direct detection of, 1409

in clinical specimens of *Rickettsia* sp., direct detection of, 1409

in CNS infections, detection of, 94–95

defined, 112

detection of

EIAs for, CP 13-1, 122, 124–125, 124f

immunofluorescence techniques in, 125, 125f, 126f

in *Legionella* sp. examination, 557

O, 186–187

polysaccharide capsular, 683

protein, 683

somatic, 186–187

structures of, 113

violence-associated, of *N. meningitis*, 574b–575b

viral, in detection and provisional identification of viral infections, CP 23-2D, F, 1389

virulence-associated

of *Moraxella catarrhalis*, 586b–587b

of *N. gonorrhoeae*, 573b–574b

Antigen variation, 192

Antigen-antibody reaction, in diagnostic serology

complement fixation, Chart 3-1, 116, 117f

HAI test, Chart 3-2, 116, 118f

precipitin reactions, 114, 116

types of, 114, 116–119, 117f, 118f

Anti-Igm antibodies, serologic diagnosis of, 1402–1403

Antimicrobial agents. *See also* Antimicrobial susceptibility tests (testing); Antimicrobial therapy

active transport out of bacterial cell, 952–953

bacterial resistance to, 947, 949–963

mechanisms of resistance in, 949–963, 949t, 950f, 951t, 952f–957t, 960t, 961t, 962b, 964f, 965f

mechanistic variables in, 947, 949t

classification of, 948t

for *Enterococcus* sp., resistance to, 1011–1013

for *Haemophilus* sp., resistance to, 1008–1009

cephalosporins, 1009

chloramphenicol, 1009

S. pneumoniae, 1009

for *Haemophilus* sp. resistant to, resistance to, penicillin, 1009

inhibitory activity of, tests in determination of, 968–996

agar dilution susceptibility test, 982–983, 988f

agent selection, 970, 971t–976t

atmosphere, 975

cation concentration, 975

commercial systems, 993, 996

disk diffusion susceptibility test, 983, 986–992, 989b, 989f, 990f, 991t–992t

Etest, 996, 1001f, 1002b

grouping of agents, 975t

growth medium, 970

indications for, 968, 969t

inoculum, 975

interpretation of results, 977, 979–982, 980t–982t, 983b, 984t–986t

macrodilution broth susceptibility test, 982, 987f, 988f

microbroth dilution susceptibility test, 989–990, 993, 993f, 994t–995t, 996f, 997t–1000t

pH, 970

quality assurance, 977

quality control, 976–977, 977t, 978t

serum, 970, 975

situations for testing, 968, 969t

standardization of, 970, 975–976

temperature, 975

test selection, Charts 17-1–17-3, 966

interactions among resistance mechanisms, 963, 963f, 964f

in interference with formation of bacterial cell walls, 955, 957–961, 957f, 960t, 961t, 962b

laboratory guidance of, 963, 966–968, 966b, 966t, 967b
for *N. gonorrhoeae,* resistance to, 1011
for *N. meningitidis,* resistance to, 1011
not exerting effect on cell walls, 961–963
pathogen susceptibility to, testing of, 39, 39b
for *S. pneumoniae,* resistance to
   β-lactams, 1009–1010, 1010f
   lincosamides, 1010–1011
   macrolides, 1010–1011
   penicillin, 1009–1010, 1010f
for *Staphylococcus* sp., resistance to
   fluoroquinolones, 1008
   β-lactams, 1004–1007, 1006b, 1006f, 1007f
   lincosamides, 1008
   macrolides, 1008
   streptogramins, 1008
   vancomycin, 1007–1008, 1008b
test procedures, 967, 967b
transport across cell wall and cell membranes, 949–955, 952f–956f
Antimicrobial susceptibility plates, in anaerobic bacteria differentiation, 904
Antimicrobial susceptibility tests (testing), 92–102. *See also* Antimicrobial agents
   of anaerobic bacteria, 939–940
   direct, 1014–1015
   formatting summaries of, recommendations for, 983t
   historical introduction to, 946–947, 946f, 948t
   β-lactamases in, 996, 1001–1007
   of mycoplasma infections, 1051–1054
   special issues in, 996, 1001–1015
Antimicrobial therapy
   cations in, 967
   clinical pharmacology, 967
   guidance of, 966, 966t
   inoculum in, 964f, 965
   laboratory guidance of, 963, 966–968, 966b, 966t, 967b
   pH in, 967
Antiviral susceptibility testing, in serologic diagnosis of viral infections, 1403
API 20E identification system, CP 6-6A, 289, 290t
   in nonfermenter identification, 362, 372b
API 20E strip, 285–287, 286t
API 20NE system, in nonfermenter identification, CP 7-5D, 362, 372b
API Coryne, 785
API Rapid Strep, in identification of streptococci, enterococci, and selected ''*Streptococcus*-like'' bacteria, CP 13-3C, 743
API Staph, in coagulase-negative staphylococci identification, CP 12-2G, 656
API Staph-IDENT, in coagulase-negative staphylococci identification, 656
APTIMA assays, 144
APTIMA Combo 2 assay, in *N. gonorrhoeae* identification, 599
Arabinogalactan(s), 189
Arachnida sp., 1422–1435. *See also* Spider(s); Tick(s); specific types, e.g. Mite(s)
Arcanobacterium sp., CP 14-2G, 817, 820, 822–823, 824t
   A. haemolyticum pharyngitis, 72
   identification of, flow chart for, 822f
Arcobacter sp., 400t, 403
   A. butzleri, 400t, 403
   A. cryaerophilus, 400t, 403
   A. nitrofigilis, 400t, 403
   A. skirrowii, 400t, 403
Arenaviridae sp., described, 1338t
Arenavirus(es), clinical manifestations of, 1346, 1346t
ARF. *See* Acute rheumatic fever (ARF)
Arginine, decarboxylation of, in *Enterobacteriaceae* identification, Chart 6-7, CP 6-4F–G, 225–226

Armed Forces Institute of Pathology (AFIP), 1037
Arsenophonus nasoniae, 275t
Arthritis, septic
   S. aureus and, 635b
   symptoms of, 91
Arthrobacter sp., 823, 825t
Arthroconidia, 1157b
Arthropod(s). *See also* Mite(s); specific types, e.g., Arachnida
   Arachnida sp., 1422–1435. *See also* Spider(s); Tick(s); specific types, e.g., Mite(s)
   classification of, 1421, 1422t, 1423b
   described, 1421, 1422t, 1423b
   specimens of, laboratory submission of, 1421–1422
Arthrospore(s), defined, 1156
Artifact(s)
   in cell cultures, 1378f
   in detection and provisional identification of viral infections, 1389–1390
Arylsulfatase, 1496–1497
Arylsulfatase activity, in mycobacteria identification, Chart 19-5, CP 19-2J, 1087, 1088t–1089t
Asaccharolytic nitrate-positive species, 922
Ascariasis, CP 22-5A–D, 1274, 1275f, 1276b
Ascaris lumbricoides, CP 22-5A–D, 1274, 1275f, 1276b
   life cycle of, 1275f
Ascomycete(s), 1158b, 1159f
Ascospore(s), 1158b, 1159f
ASCP. *See* American Society of Clinical Pathologists (ASCP)
Aseptate, 1157b
Aseptic meningitis, viral infections and, 1368t
Aspergilloma, 1180b
Aspergillosis, 1174–1180, 1180b. *See also* *Aspergillus* sp.
   allergic bronchopulmonary, 1180b
   disseminated, 1180b
   fungus ball infections with, 1180b
   invasive pulmonary, 1180b
Aspergillus sp., 1174–1180
   A. flavus, CP 21-1D, 1175, 1176f
   A. fumigatus, CP 21-1C, 1175, 1175f, 1176f
   A. nidulans, CP 21-1G, 1177, 1189f
   A. niger, CP 21-1E, 1175–1176, 1187f
   A. terreus, CP 21-1F, 1176–1177, 1178f
   colony morphology of, 1174
   described, 1174
   histopathology of, 1177–1179, 1179f, 1180b
   laboratory presentation of, 1174
   microscopic features of, 1174–1175, 1174f, 1175f
Aspirate(s)
   duodenal, microsporidia spores in, Weber stain in detection of, 1272, 1273b
   endotracheal, in lower respiratory tract infection diagnosis, collection of, 77
   for parasite detection, 1254
   stool, microsporidia spores in, Weber stain in detection of, 1272, 1273b
   transtracheal, direct examination of, in infectious disease diagnosis, 22t
Aspiration
   suprapubic, 85–86, 85f
   translaryngeal, in lower respiratory tract infection diagnosis, 77
Aspiration pneumonia, 76
Assimilatory nitrate reduction, 196
Astroviridae sp., described, 1338t
Astrovirus(es), clinical manifestations of, 1349t, 1350
ATCC. *See* American Type Culture Collection (ATCC)
Atmosphere, in testing inhibitory activity of antimicrobial agents, 975
Atopic inflammation, 7
ATP. *See* Adenosine triphosphate (ATP)
ATP synthase, 200
ATS. *See* American Thoracic Society (ATS)
Auramine O, 1492–1494

Auramine-rhodamine, 1492–1494
Aureobacterium sp., 830–832, 831t
Aureobasidium pullulans, 1229, 1229f
Autolysin, of *S. pneumoniae,* 690
Autoscan-4 System, in nonfermenter identification, 375
Auxotrophic organisms, 196
Auxotype(s), 600
Aztreonam, screening tests for, 1003t

B. parapertussis, clinical significance of, 516, 520t
B virus, clinical manifestations of, 1360
Babesia sp., CP 22-9A, 1288, 1288b
Babesiosis, 1298b
Bacillary angiomatosis, *Bartonella* sp. and, 501
Bacillary dysentery, 249b
Bacillus(i), 174b–175b
   acid-fast, staining of, in mycobacteria recovery and identification, Charts 19-1–19-3, CP 19-1A–B, 1075–1077, 1076t, 1077t
   defined, 178, 179f
   gram-negative. *See* Gram-negative bacilli
   gram-positive. *See also* Gram-positive bacilli
   rod-shaped, nonmotile, oxidase-positive, in nonfermenter identification, 364t
Bacillus sp., CP 14-1H–J, 775–783
   antimicrobial susceptibility of, 783
   B. anthracis, 776–778. *See also* Anthrax
      identification of, 781–783, 782t, 783t
      virulence factors of, 777
   B. cereus, 778–779
      gastroenteritis due to, 779
      identification of, CP 14-1J, 781–783, 782t, 784
      virulence factors of, 778–779
   B. mycoides, identification of, 781–783, 782t
   B. thuringiensis, identification of, 781–783, 782t
   bacteremia due to, 779–780
   endocarditis due to, 779–780
   identification of, CP 14-1J, 781, 782t–784t, 782–783
      laboratory safety in, 781, 783t
      specimen collection in, 781, 783t
      specimen processing in, 781, 783t
   infections in compromised hosts due to, 780
   isolation of, CP 14-1J, 781–783, 782t–784t
   musculoskeletal infections due to, 780
   nosocomial infections due to, 780–781
   ocular infections due to, 780
   opportunistic infections due to, 779–781
   taxonomic dissection of, 775–776
   taxonomy of, 775–776
Bacitracin, susceptibility to
   in differentiation of micrococci and staphylococci, 645
   in streptococci identification, Chart 13-1, CP 13-2A, 715
Bacitracin susceptibility tests, 1472
BacT/Alert Blood Culture System, in blood culture processing, 103–104
BACTEC, 1494–1496
BACTEC 9240/9120 Blood Culture System, in blood culture processing, 104
BACTEC AFB System, in mycobacteria detection, Chart 9-4, 1085
BACTEC MYCO/F LYTIC, in mycobacteria detection, 1083
BACTEC system, 1048
BACTEC TB system, in mycobacterial identification, 1107
BACTEC TB-DNA probe combination, in mycobacterial identification, 1107
Bacteremia
   B. henselae, 502
   Bacillus sp. and, 779–780
   catheter-associated, 100
      special considerations related to, 105
   described, 97
   Haemophilus sp. and, 441

Bacteremia (*Continued*)
mortality rates due to, 98, 99t, 177, 178b
postpartum, *Haemophilus* sp. and, 434t, 441–442
prognosis of, 98, 99t
risk factors for, 98, 99t, 177, 178b
S. aureus and, 634b
S. epidermidis and, 640b
types of, 97–98, 99t
Bacteria
anaerobic, 877–944
antimicrobial susceptibility testing of, 939–940
characteristics of, 901, 902b
characterization of, 901, 901b
conventional biochemical tests in large tubes in, 904–905
classification of, 881t
cultivation of
anaerobic bag system in, 898
anaerobic glove box in, 897, 897f, 898f
anaerobic holding jar in, 898, 899b, 899f
anaerobic jar techniques in, 895–897, 895f, 896f
anaerobic systems for, 895–899, 895b, 895f–899f, 898b
optimal recovery in, 895b
results of, preliminary reporting of, 901
roll-streak system in, 897–898
defined, 878
described, 878
determination of metabolic products of, GLC in, 906–909, 907t, 908t, 909b, 909f–911f, 911b, 915t
differentiation of
antimicrobial susceptibility plates in, 904
CAMP test in, 905
determination of cultural and biochemical characteristics in, 901–906, 901b, 902b, 903t, 904b
differential agar media in, 901–904, 903t, 904b
Nagler test in, 905
packaged microsystems in, 905
presumptive identification in, 901, 902b
presumpto plates in, CP 16-5, 901–904, 902t, 903b
habitats of, 880, 880b
human infections due to, 887–890, 889f, 890b, 890t
described, 887–890, 889f, 890b, 890t
of endogenous origin, 890b
of exogenous origin, 890b
incidence of, 890b
sites of, 889f
identification of, 909–939
anaerobic non—spore-forming gram-positive bacilli, CP 16-2, 924, 927t, 928t, 929–931
Bacteroides sp., CP 16-1, 913–914, 915t–920t, 920b
cocci, 924–927, 925t, 926t
commercial packaged kits in, 905–906
gram-negative non—spore-forming bacilli, 912–924
isolation of, 890–895, 891t, 894t, 895b
aerotolerance tests in, 900–901, 900f
blood culture in, 891–892
CDC anaerobic blood agar in, 895b
direct examination of clinical materials in, CP 16-1–16-3, 892–893
incubation of cultures in, 898–899
inspection and subculture of colonies in, CP 16-1–16-3, 899–900
media in, CP 16-1–16-4, 893–895, 894t, 895b
specimen collection and transport in, 891
specimen selection for culture in, 890–891, 891t
specimens that should not be cultured, 891t

nomenclature associated with, 880–881, 881t–888t
present and former names of, 882t–887t
taxonomic classification of, 880–881, 881t–888t
anatomy of, 177–201
antimicrobial resistance to, mechanisms of, 951t
capsules of, 190
chemolithotrophic, 195
classification of, phylogenetic criteria, 168, 170–177, 171b–177b
coryneform, 785, 788b–796b, 796–797, 798t, 810–834
antimicrobial susceptibility testing of, 797, 798t
cytoplasm of, 181–182
described, 3
energy generation of, 196, 198–201, 199f–203f
fermentation of, 196, 198, 199f–201f
fimbriae of, 191–192
flagella of, 190–191, 191f
genetic exchange in, 192–195, 193f
gram-negative, cell membrane of, components of, 954t
gram-positive
antimicrobial therapy for, resistance to, 1014
cell wall of, components of, 953f
growth of, kinetics of, 196, 198f
hierarchical classification of, in *Bergey's Manual of Systematic Bacteriology,* 171b–177b
identification of
abbreviated, 40t–41t
colonial types in, 36t
colonies used in, characteristics of, 33, 35b
reactions in agar in, 35b
metabolism of, 196, 198–201, 199f–203f
requirements for, 195–196, 195t, 197f
morphologies of, 179f
naming of, 167, 168b
nocardioform, 860–864
nonfastidious
disk diffusion susceptibility test for, 1480–1481
microbroth dilution susceptibility test for, performance of, 1481–1482
phenotypic identification of, 168, 169b
photolithotrophic, 195
physiology of, 177–201
pili of, 191–192
pyruvate utilization effects on, 198–201, 202f, 203f
recombination in, 192–195, 193f
relationships to oxygen, 878–880
requirements for, 195–196, 195t, 197f
"*Streptococcus*-like," 672–764. *See also* "*Streptococcus*-like" bacteria
surface structures of, 190–192, 191f
taxonomy of, 167–177, 167b–169b, 171b–177b
ultrastructure of, 952f
Bacterial cell(s)
cytoplasmic membrane of, 182
DNA replication in, 178–179
growth of, kinetics of, 196, 198f
nuclear structure of, 178–181, 181f–183f
shape of, 177–178, 179f, 180f
size of, 177–178, 179f, 180f
transcription in, 180–181
translation in, 180–181
Bacterial cell walls
"acid-fast," 188–189, 189f
formation of, antibiotics interfering with, 955, 957–961, 957f, 960t, 961t, 962f
gram-negative, 185–188, 186f, 187f
gram-positive, 184–185, 186f
structure of, 182–189, 184f–187f, 189f
Bacterial endospores, 189–190
Bacterial exotoxins, 205
Bacterial infections, site-related, diagnosis of, 69t–71t
Bacterial isolates, preliminary identification of, procedures for, 38–39
Bacterial morphotypes, in mixed cultures, separation of, 36, 37t

Bacterial motility, in *Enterobacteriaceae* identification, CP 6-4H, 227–228, 227b
Bacterial products, tests for, 86
Bacterial resistance
to antimicrobial agents, 947, 949–963. *See also* Antimicrobial agents, bacterial resistance to
expression and transfer of, variables in, 949t
Bacterial species
CDC alphanumeric designations for, 310t
defined, 170
Bacterial superantigens, 207
Bacterial susceptibility, gradient diffusion test for, 1482–1483
Bacterial vaginosis, 88–89, 835–836
identification of, 931
Bacterial virulence
factors affecting, 201–207
pathogenicity of, requirements for, 203–204
Bacteriophage(s), lysogenic, 194
Bacteriuria
detection of, culture in, 86
microscopic examination of, 86
screening tests for, 86
Bacteroides, 176b–177b
Bacteroides sp.
B. fragilis
differential characteristics of, 917t
identification of, 913–914, 915t–917t
B. ureolyticus, 403, 922
identification of, CP 16-1, 913–914, 915t–920t, 920b
characteristics in, 920t
metabolic products of, 919t
BactiCard, in *Neisseria* sp. identification, CP 11-2A, 595–596
Balantidium coli, CP 22-3F–H, 1267, 1268f
life cycle of, 1268f
Balneatrix sp., 334, 335t
Barbour-Stoenner-Kelly medium, for *B. burgdorferi* culture, 1140, 1141b
Bartlett, Raymond, 15
Bartlett's grading system, in sputum assessment, 17, 17b
Bartonella sp., 497–510
B. bacilliformis
Oroya fever due to, 500
verruga peruana due to, 500
B. henselae
bacillary angiomatosis due to, 501
bacteremia due to, 502
peliosis due to, 501
B. quintana
bacillary angiomatosis due to, 501
endocarditis due to, 502–503
trench fever due to, 500
cat-scratch disease due to, 503–504
clinical significance of, 499–500
described, 497–499
detection of, 505
endocarditis due to, 502–503
epidemiology of, 497–499
geographic distribution of, 498
history of, 497–499
identification of, 505–507, 506t
biochemical characteristics for, 506t
isolation of, 505
colony morphology in, 505
culture in, 505
Gram stain in, 505
miscellaneous infections due to, 504–505
neuroretinitis due to, 504
recovery of, specimen types in, 505
serologic diagnosis of, 507–509
taxonomy of, 497–499
in vitro antimicrobial susceptibility of, 509–510
Basipetal sporulation, 1157b
Bauer-Kirby test, 966

BBL CHROMagar Salmonella, in *Salmonella* sp. recovery and characterization, 257t

BBL crystal enteric nonfermenter ID system, CP 6-6B, 289

BBL Crystal Gram-Positive Identification System, in coagulase-negative staphylococci identification, 657–658

BBL Septi-Chek Blood Culture System, in blood culture processing, 103

BD ProbeTec ET system, in *N. gonorrhoeae* identification, 598–599

BD ProbeTec *M. tuberculosis* assay, in mycobacterial identification, 1109

BD ProbeTec-SDA assay, 144

B-D Urine Collection Kit, 84

Beauveria sp., conidia produced singly by, 1187, 1187f, 1188b–1189b

Bedbugs, CP A-3B–C, 1423–1434

Bergeyella sp., 347t, 348
   B. zoohelcum, 306t

Bergey's Manual of Systematic Bacteriology, hierarchical classification of clinically significant bacteria in, 171b–177b

Bethesda classification of cervical cytology, 1363t

Bifidobacterium sp., identification of, 927, 930

Bile Solubility Test, Chart 1-2, 38

Bile-esculin test, 1473
   in streptococci identification, Chart 13-2, CP 13-2D, 717

Bile-solubility test, 1443–1444
   in streptococci identification, Chart 1-2, 718

Bilophila sp., 922, 922b

BioBASE, 285

Biochemical differentiation, in detection and provisional identification of viral infections, 1387, 1389

Biohazard(s), physical containment of, 20, 52t, 53f–56f

Biolog GN2 microplate, CP 6-6D, 291

Biolog Microplate Identification System, in coagulase-negative staphylococci identification, 658

Biolog System, in nonfermenter identification, 373

Biologic agents
   classification of, 50, 51t
   safety precautions for, 50–51, 51t, 52t, 53f–56f
   terrorism potential of, 58, 59t

Biologic safety cabinets, comparison of, 52t, 53f–55f

Biologic stains, 19, 20t–21t

Biopsy(ies)
   handling of, 105
   muscle, in parasite detection, CP 22-11G, 1254
   tissue, in parasite detection, 1254

Biopsy specimens, in mycobacteria recovery and identification, 1074–1075

Biopsy urease test (CLO test), in *H. pylori* identification, 408

Bioterrorism, in microbiology laboratory, 58, 59t, 60t

Biotype numbers, 286

Bipartite toxins, 206

Bipolaris sp., 1210, 1212f

Blaser's medium, in *C. jejuni* isolation, 397t

Blastoconidia, 1157b, 1158f

Blastocystis hominis, CP 22-2M, 1262–1263

Blastomyces sp., *B. dermatitidis*, 1194, 1196–1197, 1196f, 1197f, 1198b

Blastomycosis, 1194, 1196–1197, 1196f, 1197f, 1198b
   diagnosis using nonculture techniques, 1197, 1198b
   laboratory presentation of, CP 21-5B–C, 1196–1197, 1196f, 1197f, 1198b

Blastospore(s), defined, 1156

Blood
   direct examination of, in infectious disease diagnosis, 23t

needle stick exposure to, risks of contracting blood-borne viral infections after, 52, 55t
   occupational exposures to, management of, 1354–1356, 1356b

Blood agar, cystine-tellurite, 1478

Blood agar–MacConkey agar biplate, 31f

Blood cultures
   collection of, in blood-related infections, 100–102, 101f, 102b
      guidelines for, 102b
      media in, 101–102, 102b
      number of cultures in, 101
      timing of, 101
   systems for processing, in blood-related infections, 102–104
      automated and computerized blood culture systems, 103–104
      BacT/Alert Blood Culture System, 103–104
      BACTEC 9240/9120 Blood Culture System, 104
      BBL Septi-Chek Blood Culture System, 103
      comparative studies, 104–105
      Lysis-Centrifugation Blood Culture System, 103
      manual blood culture systems, 102–103
      Oxoid Signal System, 102–103
      TREK ESP Culture System II, 104
      Wampole Isostat/Isolator Microbial System, 103
   in tuberculosis diagnosis, 1069–1070

Blood infections, 70t–71t, 97–105
   bacteremia, 97–100, 99t
   clinical presentation of, 97–100
   collection of blood cultures in, 100–102, 101f, 102b. See also Blood cultures, collection of, in blood-related infections
   intravascular, 98–100
   pathogenesis of, 97–100, 99t
   special considerations related to, 105

Blood parasites, 1248, 1292–1318

Blood smears
   thick, preparation of, 1530–1531
   thin, preparation of, 1529–1530

Blood specimens, in parasite detection, Chart 22-3, 1254–1255

Body fluids, in parasite detection, 1254

Bond(s), galactoside, 214–215, 216f

Bone(s), infections of, 91

Bone marrow cultures, 105

Bone marrow specimens, in mycobacteria recovery and identification, 1074–1075

Bordetella sp., CP 7-2A, 306t–307t, 341t, 343–344, 354t, 510, 512–523. See also Pertussis
   antimicrobial susceptibility testing of, 522–523
   B. bronchiseptica, clinical significance of, 516–517, 520t
   B. hinzii, clinical significance of, 517, 520t
   B. holmesii, 354t, 355
      clinical significance of, 517, 520t
   B. pertussis
      clinical significance of, 512–513, 514b–515b
      detection of, new technologies in, 519, 521
      identification of, 519, 521
      isolation of, culture media in, 517–518, 518b
      virulence factors of, 514b–515b
   B. trematum, clinical significance of, 517, 520t
   background of, 510, 512
   cultural characteristics of, CP 9-4G, CP 9-5F, 515, 516t, 518, 519t
   detection of, DFA test in, 518–519
   identification of, CP 9-4G, CP 9-5F, 515, 516t, 518, 519t
      biochemical characteristics in, 520t
   isolation of, 517–519, 518b, 520t
      culture media in, 517–518, 518b
      specimens in, 517–518
   taxonomy of, 510, 512

Borrelia sp., 1126t, 1129t, 1130t, 1134–1143
   B. burgdorferi, Barbour-Stoenner-Kelly medium for culture of, 1140, 1141b
   described, CP 20-1C, D, F, 1134

epidemiology of, 1134–1135
   Lyme disease due to, 1135–1143. See also Lyme disease
   relapsing fever due to, 1134–1135

Botulism, 937–938
   causes of, 206

Brain abscess, 93

Brain–heart infusion agar, uses of, 1159t

Branched DNA, 139

Brazilian purpuric fever, *Haemophilus* sp. and, 434t, 442–443

Brevibacterium sp., 823–826, 827t

Brevundimonas sp., CP 7-3C, 307t, 332
   B. diminuta, CP 7-3C, 332
   B. vesicularis, CP 7-3C, 332

Broad-range PCR, 145–146

Brochothrix sp., characteristics of, 767t

Bronchial washings, direct examination of, in infectious disease diagnosis, 22t

Bronchiolitis, 75
   viral infections and, 1368t

Bronchitis, *Haemophilus* sp. and, 434t, 440

Bronchoalveolar lavage, in lower respiratory tract infection diagnosis, 77

Bronchopulmonary disease, allergic, 76

Bronchoscopy
   flexible, in lower respiratory tract infection diagnosis, 77
   rigid, in lower respiratory tract infection diagnosis, 77

Broth(s)
   enrichment, in *Enterobacteriaceae* recovery, 222, 223t
   selenite, in *Enterobacteriaceae* recovery, 222, 223t

Broth culture medium
   in mycobacteria recovery, 1080
   in tuberculosis diagnosis, 1067

Brucella sp., 482–491. See also Brucellosis
   cultural characteristics of, CP 9-5D, 485
   identification of, 488–490, 489t
   isolation of, CP 9-5D, 484
   taxonomy of, 484
   virulence of, 484–486

Brucellaceae, 342t, 345

Brucellosis. See also *Brucella* sp.
   clinical spectrum of, 486, 487b
   epidemiology of, 482–484
   geographic distribution of, 483–484
   incidence of, 483
   in laboratory workers, 484
   serologic diagnosis of, 486, 488
   transmission of, 482–483
   treatment of, 490–491

Bubonic plague, 271b, 275b

Budvicia aquatica, 275t
   biochemical reactions of, 236t–237t

Bug(s), CP A-3B–C, 1423–1434
   kissing, CP A-3B–C, 1423–1434
   reduvid, CP A-3B–C, 1423–1434

Bunyaviridae sp., described, 1336t

Bunyavirus(es), clinical manifestations of, 1348–1349, 1348t

Burkholderia sp., 307t
   B. cepacia, 326–328, 327t
   B. cepacia complex, 326–328, 327t
   B. gladioli, 327t, 328
   B. pseudomallei, 323–326, 324t, 325b

Burkholderiaceae, 323–331, 324t, 325b, 327t, 328b, 330t

Bush-Jacoby-Medeiros Functional Classification Scheme, for β-lactamases, 959, 960t

Butanediol fermentation, 199–200

Butanol fermentation, 200

Buttiauxella sp.
   biochemical reactions of, 236t–237t
   newer, 275t
   differentiating characteristics of, 278t, 281

Butzler selective medium, in *C. jejuni* isolation, 397t

Butzler virion medium, in *C. jejuni* isolation, 397t

C antigen, 684
C5a peptidase, 683–684
 as streptococcal virulence factor, 679
Calcofluor white stain, in microscopic examination of
 specimens, CP 1-2, 26
Calculation of frequency of occurrence and
 percentage likelihood, 288t
Caliciviridae sp., described, 1337t
Calicivirus(es), clinical manifestations of, 1349t, 1350
California encephalitis viruses, clinical manifestations
 of, 1348
CAMP test, 1468, 1469f
 in anaerobic bacteria differentiation, 905
 in streptococci identification, CP 13-2C, 717
Campylobacter sp.
 C. coli, 398, 399t
 C. concisus, 398, 399t, 401
 C. curvus, 399t, 402t, 403
 C. fetus
  subsp. *fetus*, 399t, 401
  subsp. *venereal*, 399t, 401
 C. gracilis, 399t, 402–403, 402t
 C. helveticus, 399t, 401
 C. hyoilei, 399t, 401
 C. hyointestinalis, 399t, 401
 C. jejuni
  historical background of, 393
  subsp. *doylei*, 399t, 401
  subsp. *jejuni*, 395–398, 396t, 397t, 398b,
   399t–400t
   clinical significance of, 395
   identification from culture, CP 8-1C–F, 398,
    399t–400t
   laboratory isolation of, CP 8-1B–F, 395–398,
    396t, 397t, 398b
   presumptive identification from stool, CP 8-
    1A, 395
 C. lari, 399t, 401
 C. mucosalis, 399t, 401
 C. rectus, 399t, 402t, 403
 C. showae, 399t, 401–402
 C. sputorum, 399t, 402
 C. upsaliensis, 399t, 402
 characteristics of, 394t, 398, 399t–400t
 classification of, 393–406, 394t, 396t, 397t, 398b,
  399t–400t, 402t, 405t
 described, 395
 enterohepatic, identification of, 408
 identification of, 406–408, 406b, 407t
  colonies and stool specimens in, 406–407, 406b
  direct detection methods in, 407
Campylobacteraceae, former *Wolinella* and
 Bacteroides sp., 402–403, 402t
Candida sp., 1221, 1222b–1223b
 C. albicans, identification of, cornmeal agar in, CP
  21-6B, 1219–1220
 C. glabrata, CP 21-6E, 1226, 1228f
 C. kefyr, 1220, 1220f
 C. parapsilosis, 1220, 1220f
 C. tropicalis, 1220, 1220f
 emerging pathogenic, 1220–1221, 1221f
 infections with, 1223b
Candidiasis, 1221, 1222b–1223b
 cutaneous, 1222b
 disseminated, 1222b
 mucocutaneous, 1222b
 of urinary tract, 1222b
CAP. *See* College of American Pathologists (CAP)
Capillaria philippinensis, CP 22-5P, 1280–1281
Capillary precipitin test, in streptococci identification,
 718
Capnocytophaga sp.
 canine, CP 9-3H, CP 9-4A, 476–478, 477t
  antimicrobial susceptibility of, 475
  biochemical characteristics of, 478t
  cultural characteristics of, CP 9-3H, CP 9-4A,
   476–478, 477t

 identification of, CP 9-3H, CP 9-4A, 476–478,
  477t
 taxonomy of, 474
 human, 474–476
  antimicrobial susceptibility of, 475
  biochemical characteristics of, 469t
  clinical significance of, 474–475
  cultural characteristics of, CP 9-3F–G, 474, 475
  taxonomy of, 474
Capsular polysaccharides
 of *N. meningitis*, 573b
 of *S. aureus*, 630b
Capsule(s)
 bacterial, 190
 polysaccharide, 689
Carbohydrate(s)
 CTA, conventional, in *Neisseria* sp. identification,
  CP 11-1C, 594
 oxidative metabolism of, 312
Carbohydrate fermentation, detection of
 biochemical principles in, CP 6-1E, CP 6-4A–C,
  CP 7-1A, 217–218, 217f, 218b
 culture media in, 216–218, 217b, 217f, 218b
Carbohydrate utilization
 in *Enterobacteriaceae* identification, 213–215,
  214f–216f
 fermentation in, 213
Carbohydrate utilization tests, in *Neisseria* sp.
 identification, CP 11-1C–E, 594
Carbol fuchsin stains, 1491–1492
Carbon, in bacterial growth and metabolism, 195,
 195t
Carbon dioxide, in bacterial growth and metabolism,
 195
Carbuncle(s), *S. aureus* and, 634b
Cardiobacterium hominis, 467–470, 469t
 antimicrobial susceptibility of, 468, 470
 clinical significance of, 468
 cultural characteristics of, CP 9-3A–B, 467–469,
  468t
 identification of, CP 9-3A–B, 467–469, 468t
  biochemical characteristics for, 469t
 taxonomy of, 467–468
Cardiovascular syphilis, 1128
Casein, hydrolysis of, 1478–1479
Catalase, 205, 1443
Catalase 68-degree C, 1499–1500
Catalase activity, in mycobacteria identification, Chart
 19-17, CP 19-2H–I, 1087
Catalase test, Chart 1-1, 38
 in *Staphylococcus* sp. isolation and preliminary
  differentiation, CP 12-1F, 644
 in streptococci identification, CP 13-1H, 713
Catheter(s)
 bacteremia due to, 100
  special considerations related to, 105
 infections due to, intravenous, *S. epidermidis* and,
  639b
 sepsis due to, 100
  special considerations related to, 105
Catheter collections, 85
Cation(s)
 in antimicrobial therapy, 967
 concentration of, in testing inhibitory activity of
  antimicrobial agents, 975
Cat-scratch disease (CSD), *Bartonella* sp. and,
 503–504
Caulobacteraceae, CP 7-3C, 332
 Brevundimonas diminuta group of, CP 7-3C, 332
 rRNA group of, 332
CCIS. *See* Computer-coding and identification system
 (CCIS)
CD protein, of *Moraxella catarrhalis*, 586b
CDC. *See* Centers for Disease Control and Prevention
 (CDC)
CDC bacterial groups
 EF-4A, 479–481, 480t
 EF-4B, 479–481, 480t

 identification of, biochemical characteristics for,
  489t
CDC eugonic oxidizers (EO) groups, 350, 352–353,
  352t
CDC group 1c, 339
CDC group 4, 832–834, 833t
CDC group EF-4b, 352–353
CDC group EO-5, 354t, 355
CDC group NO-1, 354t, 355
CDC group NO-2, 354t, 355
CDC group(s) O-1, O-2 and O-3, 339
CDC group WO-1, 339
CDC scheme, in nonfermenter identification, 358
Cedecea sp.
 biochemical reactions of, 236t–237t
 newer, 275t
 differentiating characteristics of, 278t, 281
Cefipime, screening tests for, 1003t
Cefotaxime, screening tests for, 1003t
Cefoxitin, screening tests for, 1003t
Cefpodoxime, screening tests for, 1003t
Ceftazidime, screening tests for, 1003t
Ceftriaxone, screening tests for, 1003t
Cell(s)
 bacterial. *See* Bacterial cell(s)
 conidiogenous, 1157b
 eukaryotic, 177, 178b
 foot, 1183
 Hfr, 194
 prokaryotic, 177, 178b
Cell association, in detection and provisional
  identification of viral infections, 1389
Cell cultures
 artifacts in, 1378f
 C. trachomatis isolation in, 1405
 in diagnostic virology, evolution of, 1329
 normal, 1374, 1376f
 roller drum for, 1381, 1381f
 types of, 1374, 1374t
 in viral infection diagnosis
  containment of, 1375, 1377, 1378f
  inoculation and incubation of, 1380–1381, 1381f
  preparation and maintenance of, 1373–1375,
   1374t, 1375t, 1376f
  selection of, 1380
  technical aspects of, CP 23-2F, 1377–1380,
   1379b, 1379f
Cell lines
 maintenance of, procedure for, 1379b
 origins of, 1373, 1375t
Cell membrane(s)
 antibiotics active at, 955, 957–961, 957f, 960t,
  961t, 962b
 of gram-negative bacteria, components of, 954t
 penicillin-recognizing enzymes active at, 955,
  957–961, 957f, 960t, 961t, 962b
 transport of antimicrobial agents across, 949–955,
  952f–956f
Cell wall
 of aerobic actinomycetes, 860, 861t
 antimicrobial agents not exerting effect on,
  961–963
 bacterial, formation of, antibiotics interfering with,
  955, 957–961, 957f, 960t, 961t, 962b
 of gram-positive bacteria, components of, 953f
 transport of antimicrobial agents across, 949–955,
  952f–956f
Cell-surface penicillin-binding protein (PBPIa), 684
Cellular defenses
 immunologic, adaptive, 7–8
 innate, 7
Cellulitis, 7, 95–96
 clinical presentation of, 95
 diagnosis of, 95–96
 Haemophilus sp. and, 443
 streptococci and, 680
Cellulomonas sp., 826, 828, 829t

Cellulose tape preparation, for pinworm examination, 1533–1534

Cellulosimicrobium sp., 828, 829t

Centers for Disease Control and Prevention (CDC), alphanumeric designations for bacterial species, 310t

Centers for Disease Control and Prevention (CDC) Advisory Council for the Elimination of Tuberculosis, 1066

Central nervous system (CNS) infections, 70t, 92–95. *See also specific type, e.g.,* Meningitis
  brain abscess, 93
  diagnosis of, 93–95, 94f
    antigen and nucleic acid detection in, 94–95
    by culture, 94
    microscopic techniques in, 93–94
    serologic, 95
  encephalitis, 93
  inflammatory response in, assessment of, 93–94
  meningitis, 92–93, 92t, 434t, 435, 439, 634b, 1223b, 1368t
  specimen collection in, 93, 94f

Centrifugation
  in mycobacteria recovery and identification, 1074, 1074t
  safety precautions for, 48

Cephalosporin(s), *Haemophilus* sp. resistant to, 1009

Cerebrospinal fluid (CSF)
  direct examination of, in infectious disease diagnosis, 22t
  in meningitis, 92, 92t

Cerebrospinal fluid (CSF) shunt infections, *S. epidermidis* and, 640b

Cereolysin, 779

Cereulide, 779

Cervical cytology, Bethesda classification of, 1363t

Cervical discharge, purulent, direct examination of, in infectious disease diagnosis, 22t

Cervicitis, 87–88
  diagnosis of, 89

Cervicofacial actinomycosis, 817

Cestode(s), 1281–1286
  described, CP 22-6A–C, 1281–1282, 1283f
  Diphyllobothrium latum, CP 22-6I–L, P, 1284, 1285f, 1286b
  Dipylidium caninum, CP 22-6O–P, 1286
  giant fish tapeworm, CP 22-6I–L, P, 1284, 1285f, 1286b
  H. nana, CP 22-6M–N, 1285, 1286
  Hymenolepis sp., CP 22-6F, M, N, 1285–1286, 1287f, 1288b
  Taenia sp., CP 22-6D, E, G, H, 1282–1284, 1283f, 1284b

Chaetomium sp., 1211, 1213f

Chancroid, *Haemophilus* sp. and, 434t

Charcoal-based blood-free selective, in *C. jejuni* isolation, 397t

Charts, 1442–1535

Checkerboard matrix, in *Enterobacteriaceae* identification, 284

Chemical(s)
  safety precautions for, 56–58
  terrorism potential of, 58, 59t

Chemolithotroph(s), 309

Chemolithotrophic bacteria, 195

Chemoorganotroph(s), 305

Children
  infections in, *S. epidermidis* and, 640b
  sexual abuse in, *C. trachomatis* infections due to, 1406

Chilomastix mesnili, CP 22-3A–C, 1266

Chlamydia sp.
  C. pneumoniae, infections with, 1406–1407
  C. psittaci, infections with, 1406
  C. trachomatis, 1403, 1405–1406
    antigen detection in, 1405
    cytologic detection of, 1406

direct detection in clinical specimens, 1405–1406
  infections with
    clinical features of, 1403
    epidemiology of, 1403
    in sexually abused children, 1406
    specimen collection in, 1403
  isolation in, in cell culture, 1405
  morphologic detection of inclusions in, 1405
  nucleic acid detection in, 1405–1406
  serologic diagnosis of, 1406
  infections with, 1403, 1405–1407

Chlamydiae, 176b

Chlamydoconidia, 1157b

Chlamydospore(s), defined, 1156

Chloramphenicol, *Haemophilus* sp. resistant to, 1009

Chloroquine, for parasitic infections, 1319t

Chocolate agar, in *Haemophilus* sp. infection diagnosis, 445

Cholera
  in Bengal, 410
  causes of, 409–411, 409t, 411b
  toxin for, action of, 411b, 412f
  in western hemisphere, 410
  world history of, 410

Choriomeningitis virus, lymphocytic, 1340f, 1340t

Christensen's urea agar, 225

CHROMagar, 1219

Chromobacterium sp., 422

Chromogenic agar, in *Enterobacteriaceae* identification, CP 6-5E–H, 283–284

Chromogenic enzyme substrate tests, in *Neisseria* sp. identification, 594–596, 595t

Chromogenic in situ hybridization (CISH), 139

Chromogenic media, in *Salmonella* sp. recovery and characterization, 255, 256t–257t, 258f

Chromogenic reaction, 255, 258f

Chromomycosis, 1217b
  agents of, 1211, 1213–1216
  defined, 1211

Chromomycosis/mycetoma, preliminary observations suggestive of agents of, 1242

Chronic obstructive pulmonary disease (COPD), *Haemophilus* sp. and, 440

Chryseobacterium sp., 307t, 346, 347t, 348

Chrysosporium sp., conidia produced singly by, 1186, 1186f

CIE. *See* Countercurrent immunoelectrophoresis (CIE)

Ciliate(s), intestinal, CP 22-3F–H, 1267, 1268f

Cimex lectularius, CP A-3B, 1433

Circinella sp., identification of, 1170, 1171f

CISH. *See* Chromogenic in situ hybridization (CISH)

Citrate utilization, 1456–1457, 1456f

Citrate utilization test, in *Enterobacteriaceae* identification, Chart 6-5, CP 6-4C–D, 225

Citrobacter sp., 259t
  biochemical reactions of, 236t–237t
  identification characteristics for, 234t
  species within, differentiation of, 260t

Citrobactereae (tribe), 229t–230t, 258–259, 259t, 260t
  identification characteristics for, 234t

Cladophialophora (Cladosporium) carrionii, 1214–1215, 1214f

Classification, defined, 167

Clean-catch urine collection, midstream, 83, 84b, 84f

Cleistothecia, 1177, 1179f

CLO test, in *H. pylori* identification, 408

CLO-3, 400t, 404–405, 405t

Clonorchiasis, 1294b

Clonorchis sinensis, CP 22-7I–N, O, 1290–1291, 1293f, 1294b

Clostridia, 173b–174b
  histotoxic, in clostridial myonecrosis or gas gangrene, 932, 935

Clostridium sp.
  C. botulinum, 937–938

C. difficile
  collection and transport of specimens containing, 936–937
  intestinal disease associated with, 936–937, 937b
  laboratory diagnosis of, 937, 937b

C. perfringens
  CAMP test for, 905
  intestinal diseases involving, 932, 935

C. ramosum, 935–936

C. tetani, 938–939

identification of, CP 16-3, 931–939, 933t–935t, 937b

CMV. *See* Cytomegalovirus (CMV)

CNS actinomycosis, 817

Coagglutination, in streptococci identification, 718–719

Coagglutination tests, in *Neisseria* sp. identification, 596

COBAS AMPLICOR, in *N. gonorrhoeae* identification, 598

Coccidia, intestinal, CP 22-4A–C, E–G, 1267–1272, 1269f, 1270b, 1270f

Coccidioides sp., *C. immitis,* CP 21-5F, 1199, 1200f, 1201b

Coccidioidomycosis, CP 21-5F, 1199, 1200f, 1201b

Coccobacillary, defined, 178, 179f

Coccobacillus(i), nonmotile, oxidase-positive, in nonfermenter identification, 363t

Coccolysin, as virulence factor in *Enterococcus* sp., 701

Coccus(i)
  anaerobic, identification of, 924–927, 925t, 926t
  defined, 178, 179f
  gram-positive
    staphylococci, 623–671
    streptococci, 672–764

Coenurosis, 1316

Cold agglutinins, 1050

Colistin susceptibility test, in *N. cinerea* identification, 603

Colitis, hemorrhagic, 247b

College of American Pathologists (CAP), Commission on Laboratory Inspection and Accreditation of, 60

College of American Pathologists (CAP) Special Mycobacterial Interlaboratory Survey, 1091

Colonizing flora, 4

Colony(ies), macroscopic, characteristics of, CP 1-5, 33–36, 34f, 35b, 35t, 36t

Coltivirus(es), clinical manifestations of, 1351

Comamonadaceae, CP 7-2C, 331–332
  acidovorans group of, CP 7-2C, 331–332
  facilis–delafieldii group of, 332

Comamonas sp., 307t

Comidia, defined, 1156

Commensal, 4

Commensalism, 4

Commercial kit systems, in nonfermenter identification, 359, 362, 367, 372b–374b, 373

Commercial systems, in testing inhibitory activity of antimicrobial agents, 993, 996

Commission on Laboratory Inspection and Accreditation, of College of American Pathologists (CAP), 60

Committee on Child Abuse and Neglect, of American Academy of Pediatrics, 602

Communicable disease, defined, 6b

Competent, defined, 192

Complement fixation (CF) test, Chart 3-1, 116, 117f, 1448–1449

Compound(s), in selective media in *Enterobacteriaceae* recovery, 219, 221b

Computer-aided schemes, in nonfermenter identification, 359

Computer-coding and identification system (CCIS), 291

Confidentiality, patient-related, in microbiology laboratory, 47
Congenital syphilis, 1128
Conidia
    hyaline molds producing chains of, CP 21-2B–D, 1181–1182, 1181f, 1182f
    hyaline molds producing clusters of, CP 21-2E, F, H, 1182–1184, 1183f–1185f
    hyaline molds producing single, CP 21-2G, 1184–1187, 1185f–1187f, 1188b–1189b
Conidiogenous cells, 1157b
Conidiophore(s), 1157b, 1158f, 1174, 1174f
Conjugation, 194
Conjugative plasmids, 182
Conjunctivitis
    clinical presentation of, 96
    Haemophilus sp. and, 434t, 442
Contagious disease, defined, 6b
CopB protein, of *Moraxella catarrhalis*, 587b
COPD. *See* Chronic obstructive pulmonary disease (COPD)
Cord factor, 188, 189f
Cordylobia anthropophaga, 1432–1433
Corneal scrapings, for parasite detection, 1254
Cornmeal agar, in yeast identification, CP 21-6B, 1218–1221, 1219b, 1220f, 1221f
Coronaviridae sp., described, 1336t
Coronavirus(es)
    clinical manifestations of, 1349t, 1350–1351
    OC43, human, 1336f, 1336t
    SARS
        molecular detection of, 1397
        serologic diagnosis of, 1404
Corridor(s), safety precautions for, 49
''*Corynebacterium seminale*,'' 791b
Corynebacterium sp., 783, 785–810
    animal-related, 809–810, 810t–811t
    antimicrobial susceptibility testing of, 797, 798t
    C. accolens, 788b
    C. afermentans, 788b
    C. amycolatum, 788b, 798, 800t, 801
    C. appendicis, 788b
    C. argentoratense, 788b
    C. atypicum, 789b
    C. aurimucosum, 789b
    C. auris, 789b
    C. bovis, 789b
    C. confusum, 789b–790b
    C. coyleae, 790b
    C. diphtheriae, Charts 14-1–14-4, CP 14-2B, 790b, 799t, 801–805, 804f, 805f
        flowchart for, identification of, 806f
        isolation of, 807f
    C. durum, 790b
    C. freneyi, 790b–791b
    C. glucuronolyticum, 791b
    C. imitans, 791b
    C. jeikeium, CP 14-2E–F, 791b, 800t, 807–808
    C. kroppenstedtii, 791b
    C. lipophiloflavum, 791b–792b
    C. macginleyi, 792b
    C. matruchotii, 792b
    C. minutissimum, 792b
    C. mucifaciens, 792b–793b
    C. nigricans, 793b
    C. propinquum, 793b
    C. pseudodiphtheriticum, 793b–794b, 801t, 808
    C. riegelii, 794b
    C. sanguinis, 794b
    C. simulans, 794b
    C. singulare, 794b
    C. striatum, 794b–795b, 801t, 808
    C. sundsvallense, 794b–795b
    C. thomssenii, 795b
    C. ulcerans, 795b–796b
    C. urealyticum, 796b, 801t, 809
    C. xerosis, 796b

characteristics of, 786t–787t
    group F1, 796b
    group F2, 796b
    group G, 796b
    group I, 796b
    identification of, 785, 788b–796b, 796–797, 798t
    isolated from foods and environment, 810
    members isolated from humans, Charts 14-1–14-4, CP 14-2B, E, F, 797–807, 799t–801t, 804f, 805f
Coryneform, defined, 178, 179f
Coryneform bacteria, 785, 788b–796b, 796–797, 798t, 810–834
    antimicrobial susceptibility testing of, 797, 798t
Coryza, viral infections and, 1368t
Countercurrent immunoelectrophoresis (CIE), 114
Coxiella sp.
    clinical features of, 1407–1409
    direct detection of antigen and nucleic acid in clinical specimens of, 1409
    epidemiology of, 1407–1409
    infections with, 1407–1409
        serologic diagnosis of, 1409
    isolation in culture, 1408–1409
CPT. *See* Current Procedural Terminology (CPT) codes
Crohn's disease, *M. paratuberculosis* and, 1101–1102
Croup, viral infections and, 1368t
Cryptococcosis, 1224–1226, 1225f, 1226f, 1227b–1228b
    cutaneous, 1227b
    disseminated, 1227b
    pulmonary, 1227b
Cryptococcus sp.
    C. neoforman, meningitis due to, 92
    C. neoformans, 1224–1226, 1225f, 1226f, 1227b–1228b
Cryptosporidiosis, 1270b
Cryptosporidium oocysts, in fecal specimens, Sheather's flotation technique in recovery of, 1270b
Cryptosporidium sp., *C. parvum*, CP 22-4A–B, 1267–1270, 1269f, 1270b, 1270f
    described, CP 22-4A, 1267–1268, 1270b
    laboratory identification of, CP 22-4B, 1268, 1270f
    laboratory notes, 1268–1270, 1270b
Crystal Enteric/Nonfermenter system, in nonfermenter identification, 367
Crystal Gram-Positive identification system, in identification of streptococci, enterococci, and selected ''*Streptococcus*-like'' bacteria, 743–744
CSD. *See* Cat-scratch disease (CSD)
CSF. *See* Cerebrospinal fluid (CSF)
Culture(s)
    bacteriuria detection by, 86
    blood, collection of, in blood-related infections, 100–102, 101f, 102b. *See also* Blood cultures, collection of, in blood-related infections
    bone marrow, 105
    cell. *See* Cell cultures
    in CNS infection diagnosis, 95
    in eye infections, 97
    Gram's stain in, CP 1-3, 36–38, 37f
    in *Haemophilus* sp. infection diagnosis, 445–446
    interpretation of, CP 1-5, 33–38, 33f, 35b, 35t–37t, 34f, 37f
    mixed, separation of bacterial morphotypes in, 36, 37t
    nasopharyngeal, 74
    quantitative microbial, 96
    sputum, interpretation of, 78, 78b
    throat
        collection of, 73–74, 73f
        direct examination of, in infectious disease diagnosis, 22t
    tissue samples for, handling of, 105

of urine specimens, 85–86
    viral, roller drum for, 1381, 1381f
    virus isolation in, in viral infection diagnosis, 1373
Culture media
    monitoring of, in quality control, 61–64, 62t–63t
    in specimen evaluation, 27, 28t–29t
Culture media transport systems, in *N. gonorrhoeae* isolation, 590
Culture medium
    Eh of, 879–880
    in *Enterobacteriaceae* recovery, CP 6-1C, CP 6-2A–D, CP 6-3A–F, 218–223, 219t, 220t, 221b, 223b, 223t
        chemicals and compounds in, 219, 221b
        enrichment media, 222, 223t
        selective isolation media, CP 6-1C, CP 6-2A–D, CP 6-3A–F, 221–223, 223b
    in *Salmonella* sp. recovery and characterization, 255–258, 256t–257t, 258f
Cunninghamella sp., identification of, 1170, 1172f
Cupriavidus sp., 328b, 328–329, 330t
    C. pauculus, 307t
Current Procedural Terminology (CPT) codes, 47
Curved rods, 393–408
Curvularia sp., 1210, 1212f
Cutaneous anthrax, 777
Cutaneous infections, *S. epidermidis* and, 640b
Cutaneous leishmaniasis, 1299
    primary, 1301b
Cyclospora cayetanensis, CP 22-4C, 1270–1271
Cystic fibrosis, pneumonia in, 76
Cysticercosis, 1284b
Cystine-tellurite blood agar, 1478
Cystitis
    alkaline encrusted, 809
    hemorrhagic, viral infections and, 1369t
Cytochrome oxidase activity, in *Enterobacteriaceae* identification, Chart 1-5, CP 6-1G, 215–216
Cytochrome oxidase reaction, positive, in nonfermenter identification, Chart 1-5, CP 7-1B, 312–313
Cytochrome oxidase test, Chart 1-5, 38, 1447, 1447f
Cytokine(s), 7, 8
Cytology
    in *C. trachomatis* detection, 1406
    cervical, Bethesda classification of, 1363t
Cytolysin/hemolysin, as virulence factor in *Enterococcus* sp., 701
Cytolytic toxins, 205–206
Cytomegalovirus (CMV)
    clinical manifestations of, 1358–1359
    immunologic detection of, 1393–1394
    molecular detection of, 1397
    serologic diagnosis of, 1402
Cytopathic effect
    in detection and provisional identification of viral infections, 1381–1383, 1381f, 1382t, 1383t, 1384f–1388f
        enteroviruses, 1388f
        examination of cultures, 1381, 1381f
        herpesviruses, 1397f
        myxoviruses, 1384f
        respiratory viruses, 1385f
    viral, differential diagnosis of, 1382t–1383t
Cytoplasm, bacterial, 181–182
Cytoplasmic membrane, of bacterial cells, 182

Darkfield examination, in microscopic examination of specimens, 18t–19t
Darkfield microscopy, of genital lesions, 1513–1514
Decarboxylase(s), 1459–1460, 1459f
Decarboxylation, in nonfermenter identification, Chart 6-7, CP 7-2D, 315
Decontamination
    digestion and, 1489–1490
    types of, 49t

Defense(s)
cellular, immunologic, adaptive, 7–8
humoral, innate, 6–7
Deferoxamine, susceptibility to, in coagulase-negative staphylococci identification, 655
Delftia acidovorans, 307t
''Delhi belly,'' 81
Dematiaceous fungi, 1208–1211
Dematiaceous mold, preliminary observations suggestive of, 1241
Demodex brevis, 1431
Demodex folliculoroum, 1431
Dengue fever, clinical manifestations of, 1347
Dental caries, 73
Dental infections, 74–75
3-Deoxy-D-mannooctulosonate, 187
Deoxyribonuclease(s), as streptococcal virulence factor, 679
Deoxyribonuclease (DNase) test, in *S. aureus* identification, 647–648
Deoxyribonucleic acid (DNA). *See also under* DNA
branched, 139
described, 133
function of, 135, 135f
nucleotide bases of, 133, 134f
nucleotide monophosphates in, 133, 134f
replication of, 135, 135f
bacteria and, 178–179
structure of, 133–134, 134f
Department of Transportation (DOT), 55
Dermabacter sp., 828, 829t
Dermacentor sp.
D. variabilis, identification of, CP A-1G–H, 1427–1428, 1428f, 1429t
geographic distribution of, 1425, 1425t
Dermatobia hominis, CP A-3A, 1432
Dermatophilus sp., 865
Dermatophyte(s), 1195b–1196b
described, 1187
identification of, 1187, 1189–1192, 1190f–1194f, 1195b–1196b
nonculture techniques in, 1192, 1195b–1196b
preliminary observations suggestive of, 1240
DFA techniques. *See* Direct fluorescent antibody (DFA) techniques
DFA test. *See* Direct fluorescent antibody (DFA) test
Diagnostic cycle
analysis of results in, 44, 44b
cost-effective approaches in, 15, 16t
criteria for rejection of specimens in, 14–15, 15b
interactions with epidemiologists in, 44
maintenance of samples and records in, 44
microscopic examination in, 15, 17–26, 17b, 18t–24t, 24b, 26b
phases of, 9f–13f, 9–44, 12t, 14b, 15b, 16t, 17b, 18t–24t, 24b, 26b, 28t–29t, 30f–34f, 35b, 35t–37t, 37f, 39b, 40t–43t, 44b
analytic phase, 15, 17–43, 17b, 18t–24t, 24b, 26b, 28t–29t, 30f–34f, 35b, 35t–37t, 37f, 39b, 40t–42t
postanalytic phase, 43–44, 43t, 44b
preanalytic phase, 9f–13f, 10–15, 12t, 14b, 15b, 16t
preliminary observations of specimen in, 14
reporting results in, 43–44, 43t
specimen collection in, 9f–13f, 10–14, 12t
specimen receipt in, 14
specimen transport in, 10, 12, 12t, 14, 14b
Diagnostic virology, 1327–1419. *See also specific virus types*
cell-culture technique in. *See also* Cell cultures
evolution of, 1329
historical review of, 1329
services for
evolution of, 1329–1330, 1329b
levels of, 1330, 1330b
Diarrhea
inflammatory, causes of, 80t

noninflammatory, causes of, 80t
with systemic disease, causes of, 80t
traveler's, 81
viral infections and, 1368t–1369t
Dictyospore(s), 1165b
Diene's stain, for mycoplasma detection, 1483–1484
Dientamoeba fragilis, CP 22-3D, 1266
Diethylcarbamazine, for parasitic infections, 1319t
Dietzia sp., 864
Differential media, changes in, 35b
Diffusion, double, 114
Digene Hybrid Capture test, in *N. gonorrhoeae* identification, 598
Digestion, decontamination and, 1489–1490
Digestion–decontamination procedure, Chart 19-1, 1072–1074, 1073b, 1073t
agents used in, 1072, 1073t
Dimorphic fungus, 1192–1194, 1196–1207
described, C, CP 21-5A, E, 1199–1200
preliminary observations suggestive of, 1240
Diphtheria, 72
causes of, 206
Diphtheritic pseudomembrane, 804
Diphyllobothriasis, 1286b
Diphyllobothrium latum, CP 22-6I–L, P, 1284, 1285f, 1286b
Dipicolinic acid, 190
Dipylidium caninum, CP 22-6O–P, 1286
Direct fluorescent antibody (DFA) procedure, 125, 125f, 126f
in *Legionella* sp. examination, 556–557
Direct fluorescent antibody (DFA) test
in *Bordetella* sp. detection, 518–519
in *N. gonorrhoeae* identification, CP 11-2B, 596
Direct Spot Indole Test, Chart 1-4, 38
Direct susceptibility testing, 1014–1015
Dirofilaria sp., CP 22-10E, 1306
Dirofilariasis, CP 22-10E, 1306
Disease(s)
communicable, defined, 6b
contagious, defined, 6b
infectious, defined, 6b
Disinfection, types of, 49t
Disk diffusion susceptibility test
for nonfastidious bacteria, 1480–1481
in testing inhibitory activity of antimicrobial agents, 983, 986–992, 989b, 989f, 990f, 991t–992t
development of standardized disk diffusion procedure, 984–985, 989b
interpretation of results, 987, 989, 990f
limitations of, 989
quality control in, 989, 991t–992t
Disseminated aspergillosis, 1180b
Disseminated leishmaniasis, 1301b
Dissimilatory nitrate reduction, 196
DNA. *See* Deoxyribonucleic acid (DNA)
DNA fingerprinting, in mycobacterial identification, 1111–1113
DNA gyrase enzyme, 181
DNA probe(s), in mycobacteria identification, 1509–1511
DNA Probe, in mycobacterial identification, 1107
DNA probe test, in *N. gonorrhoeae* identification, 597
DNA sequencing
described, 148
from HIV, 149, 149f
microarray analysis, 150–151
in mycobacterial identification, 1111
in postamplification analysis, 148–151, 149f, 150f
pyrosequencing, 149–150, 150f
by synthesis, 149–150, 150f
traditional, 149, 149f
DNA viruses, classification of, 1341t–1343t
DNA-DNA hybridization, 170
DNase test. *See* Deoxyribonuclease (DNase) test

Dolosicoccus sp., 709
identification of, 741t, 742
Dolosigranulum sp., 709
identification of, 741t, 742
Domain(s), defined, 170
DOT. *See* Department of Transportation (DOT)
Double diffusion, 114
Dracunculiasis, 1306
Dracunculus medinensis, 1306
Drechslera sp., 1210
Drug(s), for parasitic diseases, 1319t–1321t, 1321
Drug susceptibility testing, of *M. tuberculosis,* radiometric instrumentation in, 1511–1512
Duodenal aspirates, microsporidia spores in, Weber stain in detection of, 1272, 1273b
Dysentery, 249b
defined, 79, 80t
Dysgonomonas sp., 479, 480t

E protein, of *Moraxella catarrhalis,* 587b
Ebola virus, 1335f, 1335t
clinical manifestations of, 1346–1347
EBV. *See* Epstein-Barr virus (EBV)
E-cadherin, as virulence factor for *L. monocytogenes,* 768
Echinococcosis, CP 22-11B–F, H, 1315–1316, 1317f
Echinococcus granulosus, life cycle of, CP 20-11B–C, 1311f
Ecthyma diphtheriticum, 804
Ectoparasite(s), 1245, 1420–1436
definitions associated with, 1423b
described, 1421
insects, CP A-3A–H, 1432–1435
mites, CP A-2F, 1431
Ornithodoros sp., 1431
spiders, CP A-2G–H, 1431–1432
taxonomy related to, 1423b
ED pathway. *See* Entner–Doudoroff (ED) pathway
Edema toxin (ET), 777
edi*Campylobacter* sp., identification of, nonculture tests in, 406–407
EDTA. *See* Ethylenediaminetetraacetic acid (EDTA)
Edwardsiella sp.
biochemical reactions of, 236t–237t
E. tarda, 250–251, 251t
identification characteristics for, 234t
Edwardsielleae (tribe), 229t, 250–251, 251t
identification characteristics for, 234t
species within, differentiation of, 251t
Eh. *See* Oxidation-reduction potential (Eh)
Ehrlichia sp., infections with, 1409–1410, 1409t
Ehrlichiosis, monocytic, 1410
Eikenella corrodens, 470–472
antimicrobial susceptibility of, 474
clinical significance of, 470–471
cultural characteristics of, CP 9-3C–D, 468t, 470–471
identification of, CP 9-3C–D, 468t, 470–471
biochemical characteristics for, 469t
taxonomy of, 470
virulence factors of, 470
Elderly, pneumonia in, 76
Electrical safety, 48
Electron microscopy
in detection and provisional identification of viral infections, 1387
in direct detection of viruses in clinical specimens, 1393
immune, 119
Electron transport chain, 200
Electrophoresis, gel
in postamplification analysis, 147
pulsed-field, 156–157, 157f
Electroporation, 193
EMB agar. *See* Eosin methylene blue (EMB) agar
Embden–Meyerhof pathway, 213, 214f

Embden–Meyerhof–Parnas (EMP) pathway, 196, 198, 199f, 309–311, 310f

Emetine, for parasitic infections, 1319t

EMP pathway. *See* Embden–Meyerhof–Parnas (EMP) pathway

Empedobacter brevis, 307t, 347t, 348

Empyema, 76

Encephalitis, 93
viral infections and, 1368t

Encephalitis viruses, California, clinical manifestations of, 1348

Encephalopathy(ies), transmissible spongiform, 1366–1367, 1366t

Endocarditis, 1223b
Bacillus sp. and, 779–780
Bartonella sp. and, 502–503
fastidious organisms and, special considerations related to, 105
Haemophilus sp. and, 434t, 441
native-valve, *S. epidermidis* and, 639b
prosthetic-valve, *S. epidermidis* and, 639b
S. aureus and, 634b
viridans streptococcal, 693–695

Endolimax nana, CP 22-2H, K, L, 1262

Endometrial culture technique, 91, 91f

Endophthalmitis, clinical presentation of, 97

Endospore(s), 1157b
bacterial, 189–190

Endotoxic shock
diagnosis of, limulus lysate assay in, 212
gram-negative bacteria and, 212

Endotoxin(s)
described, 207
as virulence factors, 205–207

Endotracheal aspirate, in lower respiratory tract infection diagnosis, collection of, 77

Enrichment broths, in *Enterobacteriaceae* recovery, 222, 223t

Entamoeba sp.
E. coli, vs. *E. histolytica,* CP 22-2B, E, F, H, I, K, 1260
E. dispar, 1261–1262
E. histolytica, B, CP 22-1, CP 22-2A, I–K, 1258–1260, 1258b, 1259f
laboratory identification of, B, CP 22-1, CP 22-2A, I–K, 1259–1260
life cycle of, 1259f
nonpathogenic, 1261–1262
vs. E. coli, CP 22-2B, E, F, H, I, K, 1260

Enteric adenoviruses, clinical manifestations of, 1349t, 1350

Enteric fever, causes of, 80t

Enterobacter sp.
biochemical reactions of, 236t–239t
E. aerogenes, 264, 264t
E. amnigenus, 264t, 265
E. asburiae, 264t, 265
E. cancerogenus, 264t, 265
E. cloacae, 264, 264t
E. cowanii, 264t, 265
E. gergoviae, 264t, 265
E. hormaechei, 264t, 265
E. intermedius, 264t, 265
E. sakazakii, 264–265, 264t
identification characteristics for, 234t
species within, differentiation of, 264, 264t

Enterobacteriaceae, 211–302
antibiotics resistant to, 212
biochemical reactions of, 236t–249t
classification of, by tribes, 228, 229t–233t
genera of, established, important recent changes in, 229t–233t
gram-negative bacilli of, 212
identification of, 234t
arginine decarboxylation in, Chart 6-7, CP 6-4F–G, 225–226
automated systems in, 292–294
branching flow diagrams in, 284, 285f

carbohydrate fermentation in, culture media in, 216–218, 217b, 217f, 218b
carbohydrate utilization in, 213–215, 214f–216f
checkerboard matrix in, 284
chromogenic agar in, CP 6-5E–H, 283–284
citrate utilization test in, Chart 6-5, CP 6-4C–D, 225
classic systems in, 284–285, 285f
commercial screening kits in, 282–283
computer-aided schemes in, 285
cytochrome oxidase activity in, Chart 1-5, CP 6-1G, 215–216
differential characteristics for, 223–228, 224b, 224f, 227b, 227t
hydrogen sulfide production in, CP 6-4B, 226–227, 227b, 227t
indole production in, Chart 1-4, 224, 224f
key facts to remember in, 235, 235b
KIA in, CP 6-1E, CP 6-4B, 216–217, 217b, 217f
lysine decarboxylation in, Chart 6-7, CP 6-4F–G, 225–226
methyl red test in, Chart 6-3, CP 6-4C, 224
motility in, CP 6-4H, 227–228, 227b
nitrate reduction in, Chart 6-2, CP 6-1H, 216
numeric coding systems in, 285–287, 286t, 288t
OmniLog ID System in, 293–294
ornithine decarboxylation in, Chart 6-7, CP 6-4F–G, 225–226
packaged systems in, 287, 289–292, 290t. *See also* Packaged systems
phenylalanine deaminase production in, Chart 6-8, CP 6-4E, 226
Phoenix System in, CP 6-6H, 293
presumptive, characteristics for, Chart 6-1, CP 6-1A-H, 213–216, 214f–216f
quick screening methods for, 282–284, 283f
screening characteristics in, CP 6-1H, 213–216, 214f–216f
semiautomated systems in, 292–294
Sensititre gram-negative autoidentification system in, 293
TSI agar in, CP 6-1E, CP 6-4B, 216–217
urease production in, Chart 6-6, CP 6-4E, 225
Vitek System in, CP 6-6G, 292–293
Voges–Proskauer test in, Chart 6-4, CP 6-4C–D, 225
Walkaway, CP 6-6F, 292
key identification characteristics for most common species, 228, 234t, 235, 235b, 236t–245t
MIC interpretive standards for, 979t, 980t
newer, 274–277, 275t–277t
clinical significance of, 277, 281t–282t
differentiating characteristics of, 278t–280t
identification characteristics of, 277, 277t–278t
recovery of
enrichment broths for, 222, 223t
from gastrointestinal specimens, selective media for, CP 6-3A–F, 220t, 222
isolation media for, CP 6-1C, CP 6-2A–D, CP 6-3A–F, 218–223, 219t, 220t, 221b, 223b, 223t
taxonomy of, 228–282
zone diameter interpretive standards and equivalent MIC breakpoints for, 981t

Enterobiasis, 1277b

Enterobius vermicularis, CP 22-5F–G, 1275–1276

Enterococcus(i), 672–764
classification of, 674b
described, 674
identification of, commercially available systems for, 742–745

Enterococcus sp., 700–704, 702b–703b
antimicrobial resistance in, mechanisms of, 951t
antimicrobial therapy for, resistance to, 1011–1013
clinical significance of, 701, 703–704
identification of, 726, 731, 732t, 733f
β-lactamases of, induction of, 1002–1003
members of, 701, 702b–703b

taxonomy of, 700–701
testing methods for, 998t–999t
virulence factors of, 701

EnteroScreen4, 283

Enterotube II, 290–291

Enterovirus(es)
cytopathic effect of, 1388f
molecular detection of, 1397

Entner–Doudoroff (ED) pathway, 198, 200f, 311–312, 311f

Environment
in infectious diseases, 2
Legionella sp. in, 553–554
virulence and, 5, 6b, 6t

Environmental microbiology studies, of *Legionella* sp., 561–562, 562t

Enzyme(s)
antibiotic-modifying, 958–959, 960t, 961t
DNA gyrase, 181
neuraminidase, of *S. pneumoniae,* 690
penicillin-recognizing, active at cell membrane, 955, 957–961, 957f, 960t, 961t, 962b
of *S. aureus,* 631b
target, modification of, 958

Enzyme immunoassay(s) (EIAs)
antibody capture method, in IgM detection, 122, 123f
in antibody detection, 119–122, 120f, 121f
in antigen detection, CP 13-1, 122, 124–125, 124f

Enzyme immunoassay technology, in postamplification analysis, 147–148, 147f

Enzyme-linked immunosorbent assay (ELISA), in hyaline mold diagnosis, 1179

Eosin methylene blue (EMB) agar, in *Enterobacteriaceae* recovery, CP 6-2C–F, 219t

Epicoccum sp., 1218, 1219f

Epidemiologists, interactions with, in diagnostic cycle, 44

Epidermophyton sp., *E. floccosum,* identification of, CP 21-4H, 1192, 1194f

Epiglottis, *Haemophilus* sp. and, 434t

Epiglottitis, 74
Haemophilus sp. and, 439

Epsilometer test (Etest), in testing inhibitory activity of antimicrobial agents, Chart 17-3, 994, 1001f, 1002b

Epstein-Barr virus (EBV), 5
clinical manifestations of, 1359
serologic diagnosis of, 1399–1401, 1401f

Eremococcus sp., 709

Erwinieae (tribe), 274

Erysipelas, 774
streptococci and, 680

Erysipelothrix sp., 773–774, 774t
characteristics of, 767t
E. rhusiopathiae
clinical significance of, 774–775
virulence factors of, 774
taxonomy of, 773–774, 774t

Erythromycin, *S. pyogenes* resistant to, 1013

Escherichia sp.
biochemical reactions of, 236t–239t
E. adecarboxylata, described, 249
E. albertii
biochemical reactions of, 238t–239t
described, 248
E. blattae
biochemical reactions of, 238t–239t
described, 249
E. coli, 235, 250–252, 250t, 251b, 253t
biochemical reactions of, 238t–239t
diarrheagenic, features of, 246t
diffusely adherent, features of, 246t
enteroaggregative, features of, 246t
enterohemorrhagic
detection of, 248
epidemiology of, 247–248

features of, 246t
pathophysiology of, 235, 250–251
enteroinvasive, features of, 246t
enteropathogenic, features of, 246t
enterotoxigenic, features of, 246t
gastroenteritis due to, 235, 250t
meningitis due to, 92
structure of peptidoglycan, 185f
structure of repeating peptidoglycan unit of, 183, 184f
E. fergusonii
biochemical reactions of, 238t–239t
described, 248
E. hermanii
biochemical reactions of, 238t–239t
described, 248
E. vulneris
biochemical reactions of, 238t–239t
described, 248
identification characteristics for, 234t
species within, differentiation of, 249b
Escherichieae tribe, 229t, 235, 250–254, 250t, 251b, 253b, 253t, 254b, 254t
identification characteristics for, 234t
Esculin hydrolysis, in nonfermenter identification, Chart 7-4, CP 7-2E, 315
Esculin hydrolysis test, 1466–1467, 1467f
ESP Culture System II, in mycobacteria detection, 1082–1083
ET. *See* Edema toxin (ET)
Etest, in testing inhibitory activity of antimicrobial agents, Chart 17-3, 994, 1001f, 1002b
Ethylenediaminetetraacetic acid (EDTA), trypsin and, in viral infection diagnosis, 1377
Eubacterium sp., 928t, 929t, 930–931
Eukaryotic, defined, 1156
Eukaryotic cells, 177, 178b
Ewingella sp.
E. americana, 275t
biochemical reactions of, 238t–239t
newer, differentiating characteristics of, 278t, 281
Exiguobacterium sp., 828, 830, 831t
Exophiala jeanselmei, 1216, 1216f
Exotoxin(s)
bacterial, 205
as virulence factors, 205–207
Exserohilum sp., 1210, 1212f
Extracellular surface protein (Esp), as virulence factor in *Enterococcus* sp., 701
Eye(s), direct examination of, in infectious disease diagnosis, 23t
Eye infections, 70t, 96–97
Bacillus sp. and, 780
clinical presentation of, 96–97
conjunctivitis, 96
cultures of, 97
diagnosis of, 97
endophthalmitis, 97
Haemophilus sp. and, 433t, 442
keratitis, 97
microscopic examination of, 97
S. epidermidis and, 640b
specimen collection in, 97
uveitis, 97

F plasmid, 194
Facilis–delafieldii group of comamonadaceae, 332
Facklamia sp., 708–709
identification of, 741t, 742
Facultative anaerobes, 195, 879
FAMA test. *See* Fluorescent antibody to membrane antigen (FAMA) test
Family(ies), defined, 168
Fasciola hepatica, CP 22-7F–H, 1288–1290, 1291f, 1292b
Fascioliasis, CP 22-7F–H, 1288–1290, 1291f, 1292b
Fasciolopsiasis, 1292b
Fasciolopsis buski, CP 22-7F–H, 1288–1290, 1292b

Fastidious gram-negative bacilli, 429–548
Fatty acids
cellular, of *Legionella* sp., 559, 560t
volatile, identification of, in determination of metabolic products of anaerobes, 906, 908, 909b, 909f–911f
Fecal concentration techniques, for intestinal parasite recovery, 1525–1527
Fecal smears, trichrome-staining technique for, 1528–1529
Fecal specimen
collection of, 81
Cryptosporidium oocysts in, Sheather's flotation technique in recovery of, 1270b
medium for, 223, 223b
Feces, direct examination of, in infectious disease diagnosis, 23t
Federal agencies, in laboratory and medical practice, 45, 45b
Fermentation
anaerobic, pyruvate formed during, fate of, 198, 202f
bacterial, 196, 198, 199f–201f
basic principles of, CP 6-1F, 213–216, 214f–216f
butanediol, 199–200
butanol, 200
carbohydrate, detection of
biochemical principles in, CP 6-1E, CP 6-4A–C, CP 7-1A, 217–218, 217f, 218b
culture media in, 216–218, 217b, 217f, 218b
in carbohydrate utilization, 213
defined, 213
glucose
in differentiation of micrococci and staphylococci, 644–645
lack of evidence for, in nonfermenter identification, CP 7-1A, 312
heterolactic, 198
homolactic, 198
mannitol, in *S. aureus* identification, 648
mixed acid, 198–199
propionic acid, 200–201
Fermentative pathway, 309–311, 310f
Fermenter(s), oxidase-positive, 408–421
Fever
Brazilian purpuric, *Haemophilus* sp. and, 434t, 442–443
dengue, clinical manifestations of, 1347
enteric, causes of, 80t
Oroya, *B. bacilliformis* and, 500
Pontiac, 551, 551t
rat-bite, 1146
relapsing, *Borrelia* sp. and, 1136–1137
trench, *B. quintana* and, 500
typhoid, diagnosis of, culture and serology in, 10, 10f
Fibrosis, cystic, pneumonia in, 76
Filarial nematodes, CP 22-10A–C, 1303–1304, 1306b, 1307f
Filariasis, CP 22-10A–C, 1303–1304, 1306b, 1307f
Filoviridae sp., described, 1335t
Filovirus(es), clinical manifestations of, 1346–1347
Fimbriae (pili)
bacterial, 191–192
of *Moraxella catarrhalis,* 586b
of *N. gonorrhoeae,* 573b
of *N. meningitis,* 574b
Fimbrillin, 192
Fingerprinting, DNA, in mycobacterial identification, 1111–1113
Firmicutes, taxonomy of, 1024b
FISH. *See* Fluorescence in situ hybridization (FISH)
Fitz-Hugh-Curtis syndrome, 89
5% sodium chloride, growth in, in mycobacteria identification, Chart 19-14, 1087, 1090
Flagella
arrangements of, 316
bacterial, 190–191, 191f

morphology of, in nonfermenter identification, 316
peritrichous, organisms motile with, 340–345
polar, organisms motile with, 316–339
Flagella stains, in nonfermenter identification, Chart 7-2, 315–316, 320b
Flagellar stain, 1463–1465
Flagellate(s), intestinal, CP 22-2N–P, CP 22-3A–H, 1263–1267, 1264f, 1265b, 1268f
Flagellin, 191
Flaviviridae sp., described, 1339t
Flavobacteria, 177b
Flavobacteriaceae, CP 7-2C, CP 7-4C, 345–348, 346b, 348t
Flavobacterium sp., 307t
Flea(s), CP A-3D–E, 1434
Fleming, A., in penicillin discovery, 946–947, 946f
Flexible bronchoscopy, in lower respiratory tract infection diagnosis, 77
''Flexispira,'' characteristics of, 394t
''*Flexispira rappini,*'' 400t, 405, 405t
Flora
colonizing, 4
indigenous, of upper respiratory tract, 71–72
skin, contamination with, in blood culture collection, 100–101, 101f
Flow diagrams, in *Enterobacteriaceae* identification, 284, 285f
Fluid(s), body, for parasite detection, 1254
Fluorescence in situ hybridization (FISH), 137, 139–141, 141f
Fluorescence resonance energy transfer (FRET) probes, in real-time nucleic-acid amplification, 151, 152–154, 153f, 154f
Fluorescence-denitrification, 1465–1466
Fluorescent antibody to membrane antigen (FAMA) test, 128
Fluorescent nonfermenters, in nonfermenter identification, 365t
Fluorescent pseudomonads, CP 7-1G, CP 7-2F–H, 319–321, 320b, 320t
Fluorescent stains, 1492–1494
in microscopic examination of specimens, 25
Fluorescent treponemal antibody absorption test (FTA-ABS), Chart 20-4, 1133, 1521–1525
Fluorochrome stains
in microscopic examination of specimens, 20t
for mycobacteria, CP 1-2J, 25
Fluoroquinolone(s)
S. pyogenes resistant to, 1013–1014
Staphylococcus sp. resistant to, 1008
Fly(ies)
human bot, CP A-3A, 1432
tumbu, 1432–1433
Fly larvae, myiasis-producing, CP A-3A, 1432–1433
Follicle(s), hair, 1431
Follicle mites, 1431
Folliculitis, *S. aureus* and, 634b
Fonsecaea pedrosoi, 1215–1216
Food poisoning, staphylococcal, *S. aureus* and, 635b
Foot cell, 1183
Forma Model 1024 anaerobic glove box, 897, 898f
Francisella tularensis, 491–497. *See also* Tularemia
cultural characteristics of, CP 9-4E, 493–496, 495t
described, 491–497
history of, 491–492
identification of, biochemical characteristics for, 496t
isolation of, CP 9-4E, 493–496, 495t
taxonomy of, 491–492
virulence of, 492–493
FRET probes. *See* Fluorescence resonance energy transfer (FRET) probes
Fructosyltransferase(s), 190
FTA-ABS. *See* Fluorescent treponemal antibody absorption test (FTA-ABS)
Fungal diseases, serologic diagnosis of, 1232–1233

Fungal infections
  clinical categorization of, 1153–1156
  deep-seated, 1153
  diagnosis of, laboratory approach to, 1156–1166
    culture media in, selection and inoculation of, 1162, 1165, 1165f
    direct examination in, 1160, 1162–1166, 1162b, 1162f–1164f, 1163b, 1165t
    incubation of fungal cultures in, 1165–1166
    mounts for study in, preparation of, 1160b, 1162, 1162b, 1162f–1164f, 1163b
    specimen collection and transport in, 1158–1160, 1159t, 1160b
    specimen processing in, 1160, 1161t
    specimen rejection in, criteria for, 1160t
  patients at risk for, 1153
  signs and symptoms of, 1153, 1154t, 1155t
  superficial, 1153
Fungal isolates, laboratory approach to presumptive identification of, 1166–1172, 1167t, 1169f–1172f, 1173b–1174b
  Absidia sp., 1169–1170, 1170f
  Circinella sp., 1170, 1171?f
  Cunninghamella sp., 1170, 1172f
  extent of, 1166–1168, 1167t, 1238–1243
  genus and species identification, 1168–1171, 1169f–1172f
  Mucor sp., 1171, 1172f
  Rhizopus sp., 1169, 1169f, 1170f
  Syncephalastrum sp., 1170, 1171f
  Zygomycete sp., 1168–1171, 1169f–1172f
Fungus(i)
  culture of, American Thoracic Society recommendations for collection of specimen for, 1158–1160, 1159t, 1160b
  dematiaceous, 1208–1211
  described, 3
  dimorphic, 1192–1194, 1196–1207
    described, C, CP 21-5A, E, 1199–1200
    preliminary observations suggestive of, 1240
  medically important, identification of, 1167t
  opportunistic, 1153–1154
  preliminary identification of, 39
  preliminary observations suggestive of, based on direct microscopic examination of material from clinical specimens, 1168t
  terminology related to, 1157b–1158b
Fungus ball infections, 1180b
Furazolidone, susceptibility to, in differentiation of micrococci and staphylococci, Chart 12-1, CP 12-1G–H, 645
Furazolidone disk test, 1471
Furuncle(s), S. aureus and, 634b
Fusarium sp., clusters of conidia produced by, CP 21-2F, 1183, 1184f
Fusobacteria, 177b
Fusobacterium sp., 922–924
  differential characteristics of, 915t
  identification of, characteristics in, 920t
  metabolic products of, 919t

Galactomannan assay (GM EIA), in hyaline mold diagnosis, 1179
Galactoside bond, 214–215, 216f
β-Galactoside test, in Enterobacteriaceae identification, Chart 6-1, CP 6-4A, 215
Gangrene, gas, clostridia in, 932, 935
Gardnerella sp., G. vaginalis, 834–838, 836t
  antimicrobial susceptibility of, 838
  cellular morphology of, 834–835
  clinical significance of, 835–836
  described, 834–835
  identification of, 836–838, 837t
  isolation of, 836–838, 837t
  taxonomy of, 834–835
  virulence factors of, 835
Gas gangrene, clostridia in, 932, 935
Gas vesicles, 181

Gas-liquid chromatography (GLC)
  controls for, 909, 909f–911f, 915t
  in determination of metabolic products of anaerobes, 906–909, 907t, 908t, 909b, 909f–911f, 911b, 915t
    in analysis of nonvolatile acids, 908–909, 911b
    in identification of volatile fatty acids, 909, 909f–911f, 915t
  in mycobacteria recovery, 1080
GasPak anaerobic system, 895–897, 895f
Gastroenteritis
  B. cereus and, 779
  E. coli and, 235, 246t
  evaluation of, epidemiologic considerations in, 81, 81t
  V. cholerae and, pathophysiology of, 410, 411b, 412f
  viral, clinical manifestations of, 1349–1350, 1349t
Gastroenteritis syndromes, causes of, 80, 80t
Gastroenteritis viruses, human, clinical manifestations of, 1349–1350, 1349t
Gastrointestinal anthrax, 778
Gastrointestinal system, Enterobacteriaceae in, recovery of, selective media for, CP 6-3A–F, 220t, 222
Gastrointestinal tract infections, 79–82, 80t, 81t
  diagnosis of, 69t–70t
  lower, 69t–70t, 79–81, 80t, 81t
    causes of, 81, 81t
    clinical symptoms of, 79–81, 80t
    fecal specimen collection in, 81
  upper, 81–82
    clinical symptoms of, 81–82
    specimen collection in, 82
"Gastrospirillum hominis," 405, 405f
Gel electrophoresis
  in postamplification analysis, 147
  pulsed-field, 156–157, 157f
Gemella sp., 707
  identification of, 736, 739t
Genera, defined, 168
Generalized transduction, 194
Genetic exchange, in bacteria, 192–195, 193f
Genetic recombination, in bacteria, 192–195, 193f
Genital lesions, darkfield microscopy of, 1513–1514
Genital mycoplasmas
  isolation and identification of, Charts 18-1, CP 18-1B, 18-3, 1044–1045, 1046f
  noncultural detection of, 1045–1047
  serologic tests for, 1050–1051
Genital specimens, 90–91, 91f
Genital tract, commensal flora and pathologic agents in, 87t
Genital tract infections, 70t, 87–91, 87t, 91f. See also specific type, e.g., Vaginitis
  causes of, 87, 87t
  diagnosis of, 89–91, 91f
  Haemophilus sp. and, 434t, 441–442
  STDs, 87–88
  systemic complications of, 89
  transmission of, nonsexual, 88–89
  upper, infections of, 89
Genital ulcer(s), 88
  HIV infection and, interactions between, 88
  specimens from, collection of, 91
Genital ulcer disease, 88
  diagnosis of, 90
Genome(s), 178
Gen-Probe AMTD, in mycobacterial identification, 1108
Gen-Probe test, 1044
Germ tube
  defined, 1216, 1218f
  in yeast identification, 1216, 1218, 1218b, 1218f, 1219f
Germ tube test, 1218b
Giant fish tapeworm, CP 22-6I–L, P, 1284, 1285f, 1286b

Giardia sp., G. lamblia, CP 22-2N–P, 1263–1266, 1264f, 1265b
  antigen detection in, 1265–1266
  life cycle of, 1263, 1264f
Giardiasis, 1265b
Gilardi identification scheme, in nonfermenter identification, 358
Gilardi rod group 1, 351t, 353
Gingivitis, 73
Gingivostomatitis, ulcerative, necrotizing, 73
Glandular tularemia, 493
Glassware, safety precautions for, 48
GLC. See Gas-liquid chromatography (GLC)
Gliocladium sp., clusters of conidia produced by, CP 21-2H, 1183–1184, 1184f
Globicatella sp., 708
  identification of, 738, 741t, 742
Glomerulonephritis, acute, streptococci and, 680–681
Glucose, fermentation of
  in differentiation of micrococci and staphylococci, 644–645
  lack of evidence for, in nonfermenter identification, CP 7-1A, 312
Glucose utilization test, in nonfermenter identification, Chart 7-1, CP 7-1D, 313, 313f
Glucosyltransferase(s), 190
Glycocalyx, 190
Glycolytic pathway, 198, 199f
GM EIA. See Galactomannan assay (GM EIA)
Gnathostoma spinigerum, 1315
Gnathostomiasis, 1315
Gonochek II test, in Neisseria sp. identification, 595
Gonococcal pharyngitis, 72
GonoGen II test, in Neisseria sp. identification, 596–597
Gonorrhea, historical background of, 567–568
Gordonia sp., 863
Government regulations, in microbiology laboratory, 45–47, 45b, 46t
Gradient diffusion test, for bacterial susceptibility, 1482–1483
Gram-negative bacilli
  anaerobic
    non–spore-forming
      classification of, 912–913
      identification of, 912–924
      nomenclature associated with, 912–913
      pigmenting, identification of, CP 16-1, 913–914, 915t–920t, 920b
  curved, 392–408
  endotoxic shock due to, 212
  of Enterobacteriaceae, 212
  fastidious, 429–548
  nonfermentative, 303–391. See also Nonfermentative gram-negative bacilli
Gram-negative bacteria, cell membrane of, components of, 954t
Gram-negative bacterial cell walls, 185–188, 186f, 187f
Gram-negative broth, in Enterobacteriaceae recovery, 222, 223t
Gram-positive bacilli
  aerobic and facultative, 765–855
    in domain bacteria, classification of, 767b
  anaerobic, non–spore-forming, identification of, CP 16-2, 924, 927t, 928t, 929–931
Gram-positive bacteria
  antimicrobial therapy for, resistance to, 1014
  cell wall of, components of, 953f
Gram-positive bacterial cell walls, 184–185, 186f
Gram-positive cocci
  staphylococci, 623–671
  streptococci, 672–764
Gram's stain
  in Bartonella sp. isolation, 505
  in culture examination, CP 1-3, 36–38, 37f
  in Haemophilus sp. infection diagnosis, 444–445

in microscopic examination of specimens, CP 1-1, CP 1-3, CP 1-4, 16, 17, 20t, 21, 23–25, 24b, 24t
  interpretation of, pitfalls in, 24, 24t
  technique for, 21, 24b
Gram's stain reaction, 188
Granule(s), metachromatic, 181
Granulicatella sp., 705
  identification of, CP 13-3D, 731, 734t
Granuloma(s), 7
Granuloma inguinale, 89
Granulomatous inflammation, 7
Growth factors, in bacterial growth and metabolism, 196
Growth medium, in testing inhibitory activity of antimicrobial agents, 970

H-1 virus, 1342f, 1342t
H.8 protein, of *N. gonorrhoeae,* 572b
Habitat(s), of anaerobic bacteria, 880, 880b
HACCP. *See* Hazard Analysis at Critical Control Points (HACCP)
HAD test. *See* Hemadsorption (HAD) test
Haemophilus isolation agar, in *Haemophilus* sp. infection diagnosis, 446
Haemophilus sp., 431–452
  antimicrobial susceptibility of, 451–452
  antimicrobial therapy for, resistance to, 1008–1009
    cephalosporins, 1009
    chloramphenicol, 1009
    penicillin, 1009
    trimethoprim-sulfamethoxazole, 1009
  H. aphrophilus, infections caused by, 443–444
  H. ducreyi
    antimicrobial susceptibility of, 452
    infections caused by, 444
    laboratory diagnosis of, 449–451, 450f
  H. influenzae, 433–435, 433b, 434b, 435f, 436b–438b
    antimicrobial susceptibility of, 451–452
    bacteremia due to, 434t, 441
    biotyping of, 448–452, 449b
    Brazilian purpuric fever due to, 434t, 442–443
    bronchitis due to, 434t, 440
    cellulitis due to, 443
    conjunctivitis due to, 434t, 442
    COPD due to, 440
    endocarditis due to, 434t, 441
    epiglottitis due to, 434t, 439
    genital tract infections due to, 434t, 441–442
    infections caused by, 434t, 435, 439–443
    meningitis due to, 434t, 435, 439
    neonatal sepsis due to, 434t, 441–442
    ocular infections due to, 434t, 442
    otitis media due to, 434t, 439–440
    pneumonia due to, 434t, 440–441
    postpartum bacteremia due to, 434t, 441–442
    serotyping of, 448
    sinusitis due to, 434t, 440
    urethritis due to, 434t, 441–442
    virulence factors of, 436b–438b
  H. influenzae type B, vaccines for, 433, 435, 438b
  H. parainfluenzae
    biotyping of, 448–449, 449b
    infections caused by, 443
  H. paraphrophilus, infections caused by, 443–444
  infections caused by
    Gram's stain in identification of, Chart 9-1, CP 9-1A–D, 446–449, 447t, 449b
    laboratory diagnosis of, 444–451, 447t, 449b, 450f
      biochemical and kit methods in, 449, 456t
      biochemical characteristics in, 446, 447t
      chocolate agar in, 445
      culture in, 445–446
      detection of type b capsular antigen in, 445
      Haemophilus isolation agar in, 446

identifying characteristics in, 442, 443t
    Staphylococcus streak technique in, 446
  infectious diseases caused by, 434t, 435, 439–444.
    See also specific infection, e.g., Meningitis, *Haemophilus* sp. and
  β-lactamases of, induction of, 1002
  members of, 431, 433, 433b
  taxonomy of, 431–433, 432t, 433b
  testing methods for, 999t
Hafnia sp., 266
  biochemical reactions of, 238t–239t
  H. alvei, 266
  identification characteristics for, 234t
HAI test. *See* Hemagglutination inhibition (HAI) test
Hair(s), plucked, direct examination of, in infectious disease diagnosis, 23t
Hair follicles, 1431
Halomonadaceae, 337, 337t
Halomonas venusta, 337, 337t
Hanging-drop procedure, in microscopic examination of specimens, 18t
Hansenula anomala, 1228, 1228f
Hantavirus(es), clinical manifestations of, 1348–1349, 1348t
Hazard Analysis at Critical Control Points (HACCP), 770
Hazardous material, handling of, safety precautions for, 50
HBV. *See* Hepatitis, B
HE agar. *See* Hektoen enteric (HE) agar
Health Insurance Portability and Accountability Act of 1996 (HIPAA), 47
Hektoen enteric (HE) agar, in *Enterobacteriaceae* recovery, CP 6-3E–F, 220t
Helcococcus sp., 706
  identification of, 731, 734, 735t
Helicobacter sp., 400t, 403–405, 405t
  characteristics of, 394t
  H. cinaedi, 400t, 404, 405t
  H. fennelliae, 400t, 404, 405t
  H. heilmannii, 405, 405t
  H. pylori, 400t, 405, 405t
    culture and isolation of, 407–409, 407t
    historical background of, 393
    identification of, 407–408
      accuracy of invasive and noninvasive tests in, 408
      antigen detection in, 408
      biopsy urease test in, 408
      noninvasive tests in, 408
      serologic methods in, 408
      urease method in, 408
    recovery of, specimens for, 407
  nonhuman, 405
  strain flexispira, 400t, 405, 405t
Hemadsorption (HAD) test, 1534–1535
  in detection and provisional identification of viral infections, Chart 23-1, 1383, 1387, 1389f
  in *M. pneumoniae* identification, 1484
Hemagglutination
  in detection and provisional identification of viral infections, Chart 23-1, 1383, 1387, 1389f
  passive
    in *S. aureus* identification, CP 12-2E, 646
    test for, 117
Hemagglutination inhibition (HAI) test, Chart 3-2, 116, 118f, 1450
Hemagglutinin(s), of *Moraxella catarrhalis,* 586b
Hemoflagellate(s), CP 22-9B–E, G, H, 1288–1303, 1300f, 1301b, 1302f, 1303b
Hemolysin(s), of *S. aureus,* 631b–632b
Hemolysin II, 779
Hemolysin III, 779
Hemolysis, identification of, 710, 711b
β-Hemolysis/cytolysin, 684
Hemolytic-uremic syndrome, 247
Hemorrhagic colitis, 247b
Hemorrhagic cystitis, viral infections and, 1369f

Hendra virus, 1344
Hepadnaviridae sp., described, 1343t
Hepatitis
  A
    clinical manifestations of, 1364t, 1365
    serologic diagnosis of, 1401
  B, 1343f, 1343t
    clinical manifestations of, 1364t, 1365
    molecular detection of, 1396
    serologic diagnosis of, 1399–1401, 1401f
  C
    clinical manifestations of, 1364t, 1365–1366
    molecular detection of, 1395–1396
    serologic diagnosis of, 1401–1402
  causes of, 1364, 1364t
  clinical manifestations of, 1364–1366, 1364t
  D, clinical manifestations of, 1364t, 1366
  E, clinical manifestations of, 1364t, 1366
  viral infections and, 1369t
Hepatosplenomegaly, 1248
Herbaspirillum sp., 334, 336, 336t
Herpes simplex virus (HSV) infection, 73, 88, 1341f, 1341t
  clinical manifestations of, 1356–1358
  immunologic detection of, 1393
  molecular detection of, 1396–1397
  serologic diagnosis of, 1399
Herpesviridae sp., described, 1341t
Herpesvirus(es). *See also specific types and* Human herpesvirus
  clinical manifestations of, 1356–1361
  cytopathic effects of, 1397f
Heterolactic fermentation, 198
Heteroresistance, 637
Hexose diphosphate, defined, 196
Hfr cells, 194
HHV-6. *See* Human herpesvirus-6 (HHV-6)
HHV-7. *See* Human herpesvirus-7 (HHV-7)
HHV-8. *See* Human herpesvirus-8 (HHV-8)
High-performance liquid chromatography (HPLC)
  in mycobacteria recovery, 1080
  in tuberculosis diagnosis, 1068
High-performance liquid chromatography utilizing fluorescence (HPLC-FL), in mycobacteria recovery, 1080
HIPAA. *See* Health Insurance Portability and Accountability Act of 1996 (HIPAA)
Hirudo medicinalis, Aeromonas sp. in, 420
Histoplasma sp., *H. capsulatum,* CP 21-5D–E, 1199–1203, 1202f, 1204b–1205b
  described, 1199–1200
  diagnosis using nonculture techniques, 1202–1203, 1204b–1205b
  laboratory presentation of, CP 21-5D–E, 1200–1202, 1202f
Histoplasmosis, CP 21-5D–E, 1199–1203, 1202f, 1204b–1205b
HIV infection. *See* Human immunodeficiency virus (HIV) infection
Homolactic fermentation, 198
Hookworm(s), CP 22-5K–L, 1276, 1278f, 1279
  life cycle of, 1278f
Hookworm infections, 1279b
Host(s)
  infected, virulence and, 5–6
  infectious agents and, interactions between, 4, 4t
HPLC. *See* High-performance liquid chromatography (HPLC)
HPLC-FL. *See* High-performance liquid chromatography utilizing fluorescence (HPLC-FL)
HPVs. *See* Human papillomaviruses (HPVs)
HSV. *See* Herpes simplex virus (HSV)
HSV infection. *See* Herpes simplex virus (HSV) infection
Human bot fly, CP A-3A, 1432
Human coronavirus OC43, 1336f, 1336t

Human gastroenteritis viruses, clinical manifestations of, 1349–1350, 1349t
Human herpesvirus-6 (HHV-6), clinical manifestations of, 1359–1360
Human herpesvirus-7, clinical manifestations of, 1360
Human herpesvirus-8 (HHV-8), clinical manifestations of, 1360
Human immunodeficiency virus (HIV) infection, 1339f, 1339t
 DNA sequence from, 149, 149f
 genital ulcers and, interactions between, 88
 global epidemic of, 1351–1354, 1351t–1353t, 1355t, 1356b, 1356t
 M. tuberculosis with, impact of, 1066
 molecular detection of, 1394–1395
 revised classification system among adolescents and adults positive for, 1352, 1352t, 1353t
 serologic diagnosis of, 1398–1399, 1398t, 1399f
 surveillance of, revised case definitions for, 1355t
 treatment of, laboratory support for, 1356t
Human immunodeficiency virus type 1 (HIV-1) infection
 clinical manifestations of, 1352, 1352t, 1354
 Western blot procedures for, 120–121, 121f
Human infections, anaerobic bacteria and, 887–890, 889f, 890b, 890t
Human metapneumovirus, 1344
Human papillomaviruses (HPVs), 88
 clinical manifestations of, 1362t, 1362–1364, 1363f, 1363t
 molecular detection of, 1396
Human polyomaviruses, clinical manifestations of, 1364
Human rotavirus, 1338f, 1338t
 immunologic detection of, 1394
Human wart virus, 1342f, 1342t
Humoral defenses, innate, 6–7
Hyaline molds, 1172, 1174–1187
 Aspergillus sp., 1174–1180. *See also Aspergillus* sp.
 colony characteristics of, 1181
 conidia in chains produced by, CP 21-2B–D, 1181–1182, 1181f, 1182f
 conidia in clusters produced by, CP 21-2E, F, H, 1182–1184, 1183f–1185f
 described, 1172, 1174
 diagnosis of, nonculture techniques in, 1179, 1180b
 histopathology of, 1177–1179, 1179f, 1180b
 preliminary observations suggestive of, 1239
 rapidly growing, 1181
Hyalohyphomycete(s), conidia produced singly by, CP 21-2G, 1184–1187, 1185f–1187f, 1188b–1189b
Hyalohyphomycosis, 1155, 1172, 1174–1187, 1188b–1189b
Hyaluronic acid lyase, 205, 684
Hyaluronidase
 of *S. pneumoniae*, 690
 as streptococcal virulence factor, 677, 679
Hybrid Capture, 137–139, 138f
Hybridization
 DNA-DNA, 170
 reverse
  in mycobacterial identification, 1110–1111, 1110f
  in postamplification analysis, 148, 148f
 in situ, in mycobacterial identification, 1107–1108
Hybridization probes
 FRET probes, 151, 152–154, 153f, 154f
 hydrolysis probes, 151–152, 152f
 molecular beacons, 154, 155f
 in real-time nucleic acid amplification, 151–154, 152f–154f
 TaqMan probes, 151–152
Hydatid disease, CP 22-11B–F, H, 1315–1316, 1317f
Hydradenitis suppurativa, *S. aureus* and, 634b

Hydrogen sulfide, production of, in *Enterobacteriaceae* identification, CP 6-4B, 226–227, 227b, 227t
Hydrolysis
 esculin, in nonfermenter identification, Chart 7-4, CP 7-2E, 315
 Tween 80, in mycobacteria identification, Chart 19-15, CP 19-2G, 1087
 Tween-80, 1507–1508
 of urea, in nonfermenter identification, Chart 6-6, CP 7-2A, 314–315
Hydrolysis probes, in real-time nucleic acid amplification, 151–152, 152f
Hymenolepiasis, 1288b
Hymenolepis sp., CP 22-6F, M, N, 1285–1286, 1287f, 1288b
 H. diminuta, CP 22-6M, N, 1285–1286, 1287f
Hyphae, 1157b–1158b
 species failing to produce, 1224–1226, 1225f, 1226f, 1227b–1228b
 species producing, 1221, 1224, 1224f, 1225b
Hypoxanthine, hydrolysis of, 1478–1479

IATA. *See* International Air Transport Association (IATA)
Iatrogenic infection, defined, 6b
ID32 Staph, in coagulase-negative staphylococci identification, CP 12-2H, 656–657
IEM. *See* Immune electron microscopy (IEM)
IFA procedure. *See* Indirect fluorescent antibody (IFA) procedure
IgA1 protease
 of *N. gonorrhoeae*, 573b
 of *N. meningitis*, 575b
IgA₁ protease, of *S. pneumoniae*, 690
IgM. *See under* Immunoglobulin(s)
Ignavigranum sp., 709
 identification of, 741t, 742
Immune electron microscopy (IEM), 119
Immunoassay(s)
 enzyme, for antibody detection, 119–122, 120f, 121f
 solid-phase, methods of, 119–125, 120f, 121f, 123f, 124f. *See also* Solid-phase immunoassay
Immunocompromised patients, *Bacillus* infections in, 780
Immunodiffusion, radial, 114
Immunoelectrophoresis, countercurrent, 114
Immunofluorescence
 described, 125
 techniques for, 125–128, 125f–127f
  in antibody detection, 125–128, 126f, 127f
  in antigen detection, 125, 125f, 126f
Immunofluorescent antibody (IFA) test, serum indirect, in *Legionella* sp. examination, 560
Immunoglobulin(s)
 classes of, 112, 113f
 defined, 112
 IgM, detection of, EIA antibody capture method for, 122, 123f
Immunologic cellular defenses, adaptive, 7–8
Immunologic detection, of viruses in clinical specimens, 1393–1394
Immunologic methods, 111–131. *See also specific method, e.g.,* Enzyme immunoassays (EIAs)
Immunosuppressed patients, pneumonia in, 76
Impetigo, *S. aureus* and, 634b, 680
In situ hybridization, 139–141, 141f
 in mycobacterial identification, 1107–1108
Inclusion(s), in *C. trachomatis*, morphologic detection of, 1405
Incubation, in mycobacteria recovery, 1079, 1080f
India ink preparation, in microscopic examination of specimens, 18t
Indigenous flora, of upper respiratory tract, 71–72

Indirect fluorescent antibody (IFA) procedure, 125, 126f
Indole, production of, in *Enterobacteriaceae* identification, Chart 1-4, 224, 224f
Indole production test, 1445–1446, 1446f
 in nonfermenter identification, Chart 1-4, CP 7-2C, 315
Indole-positive nonfermenters, characteristics of, 347t
Industrial anthrax, 776
Infection(s). *See also Infectious diseases; specific sites and types and* Infectious agents
 of blood, 97–105
 of bones and joints, 91
 CNS, 92–95
 dental, 74–75
 eye, 96–97
 gastrointestinal tract, 79–82, 80t, 81t
 genital tract, 87–91, 87t, 91f
 hookworm, 1279b
 human, anaerobic bacteria and, 887–890, 889f, 890b, 890t
 iatrogenic, defined, 6b
 nosocomial, defined, 6b
 opportunistic, defined, 6b
 "pinworm," 1275
 reservoir of, defined, 1421
 respiratory tract, 68, 69t, 71–79
 subclinical, defined, 6b
 urinary tract, 70t, 82–87, 83t, 84b, 84f, 85f
 wound, 71t, 95–96
Infectious agents
 adaptive immunologic cellular defenses, 7–8
 adaptive immunologic noncellular defenses, 8
 cellular, innate, 7
 classes of, 3–4
 environment and, 5, 6b, 6t
 hosts and, interactions between, 4, 4t
 indirect effects on humans, 9
 infectious diseases due to, 2, 3t
 inflammation and, 7
 innate cellular defenses, 7
 innate humoral defenses, 6–7
 newly identified, 3t
 portals of entry for, 5, 6t
 purpose in nature, 4
 routes of transmission for, 5, 6t
 virulence and, 4–6, 5t, 6b, 6t
Infectious diseases. *See also* Infection(s); Infectious agents
 affected host in, 2
 categories of, defined, 6b
 clinical signs and symptoms of, 8–9
 defined, 6b
 diagnosis of
  direct examination of culture specimens in, 21, 22t–23t
  microbiology laboratory in, role of, 1–66
 diagnostic cycle of, phases of, laboratory tests in, 9f–13f, 9–44, 12t, 14b, 15b, 16t, 17b, 18t–24t, 24b, 26b, 28t–29t, 30f–34f, 35b, 35t–37t, 37f, 39b, 40t–43t, 44b. *See also* Diagnostic cycle, phases of
 environment and, 2
 infectious agents in. *See* Infectious agents
 triad of, 2–9, 3t–6t
 world of, 2
Infectious materials, cleaning spills of, 53, 55
Infectious parotitis, 1344
Infectivity, defined, 201
Inflammation, 6
 acute suppurative, 7
 atopic, 7
 granulomatous, 7
 lymphohistiocytic, 7
 types of, 7
Inflammatory diarrhea, causes of, 80t
Inflammatory response, in CNS infections, assessment of, 93–94

Influenza (flu) syndrome, 1335, 1339–1340, 1342
Influenza viruses
  A, 1334f, 1334t
  clinical manifestations of, 1335, 1339–1340, 1342
Inhalational anthrax, 778
Inhibitory mold agar, uses of, 1159t
Innate cellular defenses, 7
Innate humoral (noncellular) defenses, 6–7
Inoculum
  in antimicrobial therapy, 964f, 965
  in testing inhibitory activity of antimicrobial
    agents, 975
Inquilinus limosus, 327t, 331
Insect(s), CP A-3A–H, 1432–1435
  bugs, CP A-3B–C, 1423–1434
  fleas, CP A-3D–E, 1434
  flies, CP A-3A, 1432–1433
  lice, CP A-3F–H, 1434–1435
  mosquitoes, 1433
Insertion sequences, defined, 182, 194
Insoluble glucan matrix, 190
Intermedilysin, 696
Internalin, 204
  as virulence factor for L. monocytogenes, 768
International Air Transport Association (IATA), 55
Intestinal parasites, recovery of, fecal concentration
    techniques for, 1525–1527
Intestinal protozoa, 1256, 1258–1273
  amoebae, B, CP 22-2A, E–M, 1258–1263, 1258b,
    1259f
  Balantidium coli, CP 22-3F–H, 1267, 1268f
  Blastocystis hominis, CP 22-2M, 1262–1263
  C. parvum, CP 22-4A–B, 1267–1270, 1269f,
    1270b, 1270f
  Chilomastix mesnili, CP 22-3A–C, 1266
  ciliates, CP 22-3F–H, 1267, 1268f
  coccidia, CP 22-4A–C, E–G, 1267–1272, 1269f,
    1270b, 1270f
  Cyclospora cayetanensis, CP 22-4C, 1270–1271
  Dientamoeba fragilis, CP 22-3D, 1266
  E. histolytica, B, CP 22-1, CP 22-2A, I–K,
    1258–1260, 1258b, 1259f
  Endolimas nana, CP 22-2H, K, L, 1262
  flagellates, CP 22-2N–P, CP 22-3A–H,
    1263–1267, 1264f, 1265b, 1268f
  G. lamblia, CP 22-2N–P, 1263–1266, 1264f, 1265b
  Iodamoeba bütschlii, CP 22-2G, I, J, 1262
  Isospora belli, CP 22-4E–F, 1271
  Microsporidium sp., 1272–1273, 1273b
  Sarcocystis sp., CP 22-4G, 1271–1272
  Trichomonas hominis, CP 22-3E, 1266–1267
Intravascular infection, 98–100
Intravenous catheter infections, S. epidermidis and,
    639b
Invasive pulmonary aspergillosis, 1180b
Iodamoeba bütschlii, CP 22-2G, I, J, 1262
Iodine mount, in microscopic examination of
    specimens, 18t
Iron uptake, 1502
  in mycobacteria identification, Chart 19-10, 1087
Iron-binding/acquisition proteins, of N. meningitis,
    575b
Isolate(s)
  definitive identification of, 1390–1391
  viral, storage of, CP 23-1F–G, 1391
Isolator system, 91
Isospora belli, CP 22-4E–F, 1271
  life cycle of, 1269f
Isosporiasis, 1271
Itch, "swimmer's," 1290b
"Itch" mite, CP A-2F, 1431
Ivermectin, for parasitic infections, 1319t
Ixodes ricinus ticks, 1136–1143
Ixodida sp., 1422–1435. See also Tick(s)
  diagnostic features of, 1429t–1430t
  I. cookei
    geographic distribution of, 1425, 1425t
    identification of, CP A-1E, 1427, 1430t

I. marxi
  geographic distribution of, 1425, 1425t
  identification of, CP A-1E, 1427, 1430t
I. scapularis
  geographic distribution of, 1425, 1425t
  identification of, CP A-1B–C, 1426–1427,
    1426f, 1427f, 1429t
  relation to disease, 1424–1425, 1425t

Joint(s), infections of, 91

Kala-azar, 1301b
Katayama syndrome, 1290b
KDO. See 2-Keto-3-deoxyoctonoic acid (KDO)
Keratitis, clinical presentation of, 97
Keratitis/conjunctivitis, viral infections and, 1369t
Kersteria sp., 341t, 344
2-Keto-3-deoxyoctonoic acid (KDO), 187
KIA. See Kligler iron agar (KIA)
Kingella sp., 472–474
  antimicrobial susceptibility of, 474
  clinical significance of, 472–473
  cultural characteristics of, CP 9-3E, 468t, 472–473
  identification of, CP 9-3E, 468t, 472–473
    biochemical characteristics for, 469t
  taxonomy of, 472
Kissing bugs, CP A-3C, 1433–1434
Klebsiella sp.
  described, 259, 262, 264
  identification characteristics for, 234t
  K. granulomatis, 262
  K. oxytoca, biochemical reactions of, 238t–239t
  K. ozaenae, 262
  K. pneumoniae, 262
    biochemical reactions of, 238t–239t
  K. rhinoscleromatis, 262
  species within, differentiation of, 263t
  taxonomic changes in, 259, 262, 263t
Klebsiella-Enterobacter-Hafnia-Serratia group, 214,
    215f, 225
Klebsielleae (tribe), 230t–232t, 259, 261t, 262–267,
    263t, 264t, 266t
  identification characteristics for, 234t
  species within, differentiation of, 261t
Kligler iron agar (KIA), in carbohydrate fermentation
    detection, CP 6-1E, CP 6-4B, 216–217,
    217b, 217f
Kluyvera sp.
  biochemical reactions of, 238t–239t
  newer, 275t
    differentiating characteristics of, 278t, 281
Koneman, E.W., 2
Koserella trabulsii, differentiating characteristics of,
    280t, 282
Krebs tricarboxylic acid cycle, 198, 203f

Labeling, of specimens, 13–14
Laboratory, microbiology. See Microbiology
    laboratory
Laboratory equipment, monitoring of, in quality
    control, 60–61, 61t
Laboratory identifications, optimization of,
    approaches to, 42t
Laboratory workers, brucellosis in, 484
LaCrosse virus, 1336f, 1336t
β-Lactam(s)
  Enterococcus sp. resistant to, 1012
  S. pneumoniae resistant to, 1009–1010, 1010f
  Staphylococcus sp. resistant to, 1004–1007, 1006b,
    1006f, 1007f
β-Lactamase(s), 958–959, 960t, 961t
  Bush-Jacoby-Medeiros Functional Classification
    Scheme, 959, 960t
  characteristics of, 962b
  extended-spectrum
    confirmatory tests for, 1004t

screening tests for, 1003t
  in susceptibility testing, 1003–1004, 1003t,
    1004f, 1004t
in susceptibility testing, 996, 1001–1007
  described, 996, 1001
  Enterococcus sp.-related, 1002–1003
  Haemophilus sp.-related, 1002
  Moraxella catarrhalis-related, 1002
  N. gonorrhoeae-related, 1002
  Staphylococcus sp.-related, 1001–1002
  wide-spectrum, plasmid-mediated, characteristics
    of, 959, 961t
β-Lactamase inhibitors, 959
Lactobacillus sp., 838–840
  characteristics of, 767t
  clinical significance of, 839–840
  epidemiology of, CP 14-2H–I, 838–839
  identification of, 840, 930
  isolation of, 840
  taxonomy of, CP 14-2H–I, 838–839
Lactococcus sp., 709
  identification of, 742, 743t
Lactophenol, 21t
LAMPs. See Lipid-associated membrane proteins
    (LAMPs)
LAP test. See Leucine aminopeptidase (LAP) test
Laribacter hongkongensis, 336t, 339–340
Larva(ae), fly, myiiasia-producing, CP A-3A,
    1432–1433
Larval migrans
  cutaneous, 1314
  visceral, 1312–1314
Laryngitis, 74
Laryngotracheobronchitis, Haemophilus sp. and,
    434t
Latex agglutination, in streptococci identification, CP
    13-3A, 719
Latex agglutination test, in S. aureus identification,
    CP 12-2D, 646
Latrodectus mactans, CP A-2H, 1432
Lautropia mirabilis, 331
LE. See Leukocyte esterase (LE)
LeClercia sp., L. adecarboxylata, 276t
  biochemical reactions of, 240t–241t
Leclercia sp., newer, differentiating characteristics of,
    279t, 281
Leech(es), medicinal, Aeromonas sp. and, 420
Legionella sp., 549–565. See also Legionellosis
  antimicrobial susceptibility of, 558, 560
  cellular fatty acids of, 559, 560t
  characteristics of, 550–551, 550t, 558, 559t
  clinical manifestations of, 551, 551t
  in environment, 553–554
  environmental microbiology studies of, 561–562,
    562t
  identification of, CP 10-1C–D, 558, 559t, 560t
  isolates of, typing of, 561–562, 562t
  isolation of
    from blood cultures, 557–558
    from clinical specimens, 557–558, 558t
    from environmental samples, 561
    from pleural fluid and transtracheal aspirates,
      557
    from sputum and other contaminated specimens,
      557
    from tissues, 557
  in man-made (artificial) aquatic habitats, 554
  molecular diagnosis of, 560
  natural habitats for, 553–554
  serum indirect IFA test for, 560
  taxonomy of, 550–551, 550t
Legionellaceae, in environment, 553–554
Legionellosis. See also Legionella sp.
  clinical spectrum of, 551–553, 551t
  ecologic aspects of, 553–555
  epidemiology of, 553
  incidence of, 553
  laboratory diagnosis of, 555–557

Legionellosis (Continued)
  clinical specimens in
    antigen detection in urine and body fluids in, 557
    DFA procedure in, 556–557
    direction examination of, 556–557
    Legionella sp. isolation from, 557–558, 558t
    microscopic examination of, 556
    molecular detection of nucleic acids in, CP 10-1A–D, 557–560, 558b, 559t, 560t
    selection, collection, and transport of, 555–556
  nosocomial outbreaks of, 555
  pathogenesis of, 552–553
  pathology of, 552–553
  predisposing factors for, 552
  in travelers, 554–555
  treatment of, 558, 560
Legionnaires' disease, clinical manifestations of, 551, 551t
Leifson staining method, in nonfermenter identification, Chart 7-2, 315, 316b
Leifsonia sp., 830, 831t
Leishmania sp., CP 22-9B–E, 1299, 1300b, 1301b
  laboratory identification of, CP 22-9C–E, 1299
  life cycle of, 1300f
Leishmaniasis, CP 22-9B–E, 1248, 1299, 1300b, 1301b
  cutaneous, 1299
    primary, 1301b
  disseminated, 1301b
Leminorella sp.
  biochemical reactions of, 240t–241t
  newer, 276t
    differentiating characteristics of, 279t, 281
Leptospira sp., 1143–1145
  described, 1143, 1143f, 1143t
  genomospecies of, 1143t
  leptospirosis due to, 1144–1145
  serogroups of, 1143t
Leptospirosis, 1144–1145
  causes of, 1144–1145
  clinical manifestations of, 1144
  epidemiology of, 1144
  laboratory diagnosis of, CP 20-1G–H, 1144–1145
Lesion(s), genital, darkfield microscopy of, 1513–1514
Lethal toxin, 777
Leucine aminopeptidase (LAP) test, in streptococci identification, CP 13-2F, 718
Leuconostoc sp., 706
  identification of, 734, 736, 737t
Leukocyte esterase (LE), 86
Lice, CP A-3F–H, 1434–1435
Lifting, safety precautions for, 49
Ligase chain reaction, 143–144
Light microscopy
  in detection and provisional identification of viral infections, Chart 23-1, 1387
  in direct detection of viruses in clinical specimens, CP 23-1A–F, 1392–1393
LightCycler system, 1109–1110
Limulus lysate assay, in endotoxic shock diagnosis, 212
Lincosamide(s)
  S. pneumoniae resistant to, 1010–1011
  Staphylococcus sp. resistant to, 1008
Lipid(s), defined, 187
Lipid-associated membrane proteins (LAMPs), 1050–1051
Lipoarabinomannan, 189
Lipo-oligosaccharide(s), 188
  of *Moraxella catarrhalis*, 586b
  of *N. gonorrhoeae*, 573b
  of *N. meningitis*, 574b
Lipopolysaccharide(s) (LPS), 186, 187f
Lipoprotein(s), murein, 186
Lipoteichoic acid, 684

of *S. pneumoniae*, 690
as virulence factor in *Enterococcus* sp., 701
Liquid specimens, in mycobacteria recovery and identification, 1075
Listeria sp., 766–773
  antimicrobial susceptibility of, 773
  characteristics of, 767t
  E. rhusiopathiae
    antimicrobial susceptibility of, 775
    identification of, CP 14-1E–G, 775
    isolation of, CP 14-1E–G, 775
  identification of, CP 14-1B–D, 770–773, 772t
  L. monocytogenes, 766–773
    antimicrobial therapy for, resistance to, 1013
    clinical significance of, 768–770
    epidemiology of, 768
    isolation of, from clinical specimens, 770
    meningitis due to, 92
    virulence factors of, 768
  pathogenicity of, 773
  taxonomy of, CP 14-1A, 766–768, 767b, 767t
  testing methods for, 1000t
  treatment of, 773
Listeriolysin O, 204
  as virulence factor for *L. monocytogenes,* 768
Listonella sp., 417
Liver fluke infection, 1248
LJP. *See* Localized juvenile periodontitis (LJP)
Localized juvenile periodontitis (LJP), 453
Loeffler's methylene blue stain, 1475
  in microscopic examination of specimens, 20t
Loeffler's serum medium, 1476
Loxosceles reclusa, CP A-2G, 1431–1432
LpbA protein, of *Moraxella catarrhalis,* 587b
LpbB protein, of *Moraxella catarrhalis,* 587b
LPS. *See* Lipopolysaccharide (LPS)
Lung abscess, 76
Lung puncture and biopsy, in lower respiratory tract infection diagnosis, 77–78
LV-PVA, formulations of, 1535
Lyme disease
  Borrelia sp. and, 1135–1143
  clinical manifestations of, 1139–1140
  described, 1136–1138, 1136b
  epidemiology of, CP 20-1E, 1137–1139, 1137f, 1138f
  European investigations of, 1136, 1136b
  laboratory diagnosis of, 1140–1143, 1140b, 1141b
    culture in, 1140–1141, 1141b
    molecular detection in, 1141
    morphologic detection in, 1141
    serologic detection in, 1141–1143
  ticks and, 1424
Lymphadenopathy, of upper respiratory tract, 73
Lymphocytic choriomeningitis virus, 1340f, 1340t
Lymphohistiocytic inflammation, 7
Lysine, decarboxylation of, in *Enterobacteriaceae* identification, Chart 6-7, CP 6-4F–G, 225–226
Lysis-Centrifugation Blood Culture System, in blood culture processing, 103
Lysis-centrifugation system blood culture tube, in tuberculosis diagnosis, 1068
Lysogenic bacteriophages, 194
Lysostaphin, susceptibility to, in differentiation of micrococci and staphylococci, 645

M protein, as streptococcal virulence factor, 679
MacConkey agar
  in *Enterobacteriaceae* recovery, CP 6-2A–B, 219t
  failure to grow on, in nonfermenter identification, CP 7-1C, 313
  growth on, 1500
    in mycobacteria identification, Chart 19-8, 1090
MacConkey agar plate–blood agar, 31f
Macroconidia, 1157b, 1183, 1184f, 1192, 1194f
  borne singly or via special conidiation, 1210–1211, 1213f

with transverse and longitudinal septa, 1208–1210, 1210f, 1211f
  with transverse septa, 1210, 1212f
Macrodilution broth susceptibility test, in testing inhibitory activity of antimicrobial agents, 982, 987f, 988f
Macrolide(s)
  S. pneumoniae resistant to, 1010–1011
  Staphylococcus sp. resistant to, 1008
Macroscopic colonies, characteristics of, CP 1-5, 33–36, 34f, 35b, 35t, 36t
Maduromycete(s), 864–865, 864t
Magnetosome(s), composition of, 181
Malaria, CP 22-8A–H, 1294–1298, 1296b, 1297f
  described, 1294
  laboratory identification of, CP 22-8A–H, 1294–1296, 1298
  prevalence of, 1294
Malassezia furfur, CP 21-6G, 1228–1229
Manganous chloride-urea test, in *U. urealyticum* identification, 1484–1485
Mannheimia sp., 459b, 467
  currently recognized, 459b
  identification of, biochemical characteristics for, 462t
  M. haemolytica, 459b, 467
Mannitol fermentation, in *S. aureus* identification, 648
Mannitol salts agar, 648
Mannoside(s), phosphatidylinositol, 189
Mass spectrometry, in tuberculosis diagnosis, 1068
Massilia sp., 334, 335t
Mastitis, *S. aureus* and, 634b
MB/BacT Mycobacteria Detection System, in mycobacteria detection, 1082
Measles virus, clinical manifestations of, 1344
Mebendazole, for parasitic infections, 1319t
Medicinal leeches, *Aeromonas* sp. in, 420
Medium(a). *See specific type, e.g.,* Chromogenic media
Melarsoprol, for parasitic infections, 1319t–1320t
Melioidosis, 323–326, 324t, 325b
Melissococcus sp., 704
Meningitis, 92–93, 92t
  aseptic, viral infections and, 1368t
  Candida, 1223b
  causes of, pathogens as, 92–93
  CSF in patients with, 92, 92t
  Haemophilus sp. and, 434t, 435, 439
  neonatal sepsis with, *Haemophilus* sp. and, 434t
  S. aureus and, 634b
  signs and symptoms of, 92
Meningococcal disease
  prevention of, 582–584
  vaccines against, 582–584
Meso-diaminopimelic acid, 785
Mesosome(s), defined, 182
Messenger RNA (mRNA), 179–180
Metabolism, of nonfermenters, 305–316. *See also* Nonfermenter(s), metabolism of
Metachromatic granules, 181
Metapneumovirus, human, 1344
Methicillin resistance, in *S. aureus,* detection of, 648
Methyl red test, 1453–1454, 1453f
  in *Enterobacteriaceae* identification, Chart 6-3, CP 6-4C, 224
Methylene blue, Loeffler's, in microscopic examination of specimens, 20t, 1475
Methylene blue stain, in microscopic examination of specimens, CP 1-2, 26
Methylobacteriaceae, CP 7-3F, 337–339, 338t
Methylobacterium sp., CP 7-3E–F, 337–338, 338t
  M. mesophilicum, 307t
4-Methylumbelliferyl caprylate (MUCAP) test, in *Salmonella* sp. recovery and characterization, 255, 258
Metronidazole, for parasitic infections, 1320t

Metulae(ae), 1157b
MGIT 960 System, in mycobacteria detection, 1082
MGIT System. *See* Mycobacteria Growth Indicator Tube (MGIT) System
Microaerophile(s), 879
Microaerophilic organisms, 195
Microarray analysis, 150–151
    in mycobacterial identification, 1111
Microbact Staphylococcal 12S, in coagulase-negative staphylococci identification, 658
Microbacterium sp., 830–832, 831t
Microbe(s), odors of, 35, 35t
Microbial Identification System, in coagulase-negative staphylococci identification, 658
Microbial typing, clinical applications of, 158
Microbiology, introduction to, 1–66
Microbiology laboratory
    accreditation and inspection of, 46
    administrative aspects of, 45–64
    bioterrorism in, 58, 59t, 60t
    government regulations in, 45–47, 45b, 46t
    patient confidentiality in, 47
    personnel qualifications in, 46
    procedure manuals for, 46–47
    proficiency testing in, 46
    quality assurance in, 58–59
    quality control in, 59–64. *See also* Quality control, in microbiology laboratory
    reference or referral laboratories, 47
    risk management in, 47
    role of, 1–66
    safety in, 47–58. *See also* Safety, in microbiology laboratory
    space requirements for, 47
Microbroth dilution susceptibility tests
    for nonfastidious bacteria, performance of, 1481–1482
    in testing inhibitory activity of antimicrobial agents, 989–990, 993, 993f, 994t–995t, 996f, 997t–1000t
Micrococcus sp., 642
    described, 625
    identification of, phenotypic characteristics for, 659t–660t, 661
    Staphylococcus sp. *vs.*, Chart 12-1, CP 12-1G–H, 644–645, 644t
Microconidia, 1157b, 1183, 1192
Micro-ID, 291
Micrometer(s), ocular, calibration of, 1531–1533, 1532f
Microorganism(s), 204–207
    characterization of, methods for, 169b
MicroScan identification panels, in identification of streptococci, enterococci, and selected "*Streptococcus*-like" bacteria, 745
MicroScan POS ID Panel, in coagulase-negative staphylococci identification, 657
MicroScan products, in testing inhibitory activity of antimicrobial agents, 993, 996
MicroScan Rapid POS Combo Panel, in coagulase-negative staphylococci identification, 657
MicroScan System, CP 6-6E, 291
MicroScan systems, in nonfermenter identification, 375
MicroScan Walkaway, CP 6-6F, 292
Microscopic examination of specimens, 15, 17–26, 17b, 18t–24t, 24b, 26b
    acid-fast stains, CP 1-2B, 25
    acridine orange, CP 1-2D, 25–26, 26b
    calcofluor white stain, CP 1-2F, 26
    cost-effective approaches to, 39–43, 40t–42t
    culture interpretation in, CP 1-5, 33–38, 33f, 35b, 35t–37t, 34f, 37f
    direct stains, 19–21, 20t–21t
    fluorescent stains, 25
    fluorochrome stains, CP 1-2, 25
    Gram's stain, CP 1-3, CP 1-4, 21, 23–25, 24b, 24t

identification of organisms other than bacteria in, 39
    methylene blue stain, CP 1-2, 26
    periodic acid-Schiff stain, CP 1-2H, 26
    procedures for preliminary identification of bacterial isolates in, 38–39
    silver impregnation stains, 26
    stains in microbiology, use of, 21, 22t–23t
    techniques for, 17–19, 18t–19t
    testing of susceptibility to antimicrobial agents in, 39, 39b
    toluidine blue stain, CP 1-2E, 26
    Wright's-Giemsa's stain, CP 1-2, 26
Microscopy
    darkfield, of genital lesions, 1513–1514
    electron. *See* Electron microscopy
    light. *See* Light microscopy
MicroSeq, 1111
Microslide culture technique, 1162, 1163b, 1164f
Microsporidia spores, in stool and duodenal aspirates, Weber stain in detection of, 1272, 1273b
Microsporidium sp., 1272–1273, 1273b
Microsporum sp.
    identification of, CP 21-4A–B, 1189–1190, 1190f
    M. canis, identification of, CP 21-4A–B, 1189–1190, 1190f
    M. gypseum, identification of, CP 21-4B, 1190, 1191f
    M. nanum, identification of, 1190, 1192f
MIF, formulations of, 1535
Mims, Cedric, 2
Mite(s), CP A-2F, 1431
    follicle, 1431
    "itch," CP A-2F, 1431
    species of, 1431
Mixed acid fermentation, 198–199
Mobiluncus sp., identification of, 931
Modified ABC medium, in *Salmonella* sp. recovery and characterization, 257t
Modified oxidase test, in differentiation of micrococci and staphylococci, CP 12-2A, 645
Modified Preston, in *C. jejuni* isolation, 397t
Modified semisolid Rappaport-Vassiliadis (MSRV) medium, in *Salmonella* sp. recovery and characterization, 256t–257t
Moellerella sp.
    M. wisconsensis, 276t
        biochemical reactions of, 240t–241t
    newer, differentiating characteristics of, 279t, 281
Mold(s)
    defined, 1156
    dematiaceous, preliminary observations suggestive of, 1241
    described, 3
    hyaline. *See* Hyaline molds
        preliminary observations suggestive of, 1239
Molecular beacons, 154, 155f
Molecular methods, in mycobacterial identification, 112f, 1108–1115
Molecular microbiology, 132–165
Molecular techniques, in direct detection of viruses in clinical specimens, 1394–1397
Molecule(s), 16S rRNA, 170
Molluscum contagiosum virus, clinical manifestations of, 1361
Monoclonal antibodies, 113–114, 115b
    production of, 114, 115b
Monophosphate(s), nucleotide, in DNA, 133, 134f
Montezuma's revenge, 81
Moraxella sp., 307t–308t, 349–350, 351t
    M. catarrhalis, 566–622
        antimicrobial susceptibility of, 608–609
        clinical significance of, 585–588, 586b–587b
        cultural characteristics of, CP 11-2A, F, H, 600–604, 600t–601t
        identification of, 600t–601t
            characteristics for, 600t–601t
        β-lactamases of, induction of, 1002

virulence factors of, 586b–587b
        virulence-associated antigens of, 586b–587b
Moraxellaceae, 349–350, 351t
    classification of species within, 568, 569b
    taxonomy of, 568–569, 569b
Morganella sp., 268, 268t
    identification characteristics for, 234t
    M. morganii, biochemical reactions of, 240t–241t
Morphotype(s), bacterial, in mixed cultures, separation of, 36, 37t
Mosquitoes, 1433
Motility, bacterial, in *Enterobacteriaceae* identification, CP 6-4H, 227–228, 227b
Motility test
    medium for, 227, 227b
    in nonfermenter identification, CP 7-1E, 313–314, 314f
Mouth, trench, 73
mRNA. *See* Messenger RNA (mRNA)
MSRV medium. *See* Modified semisolid Rappaport-Vassiliadis (MSRV) medium
MUCAP test, in *Salmonella* sp. recovery and characterization, 255, 258
Mucor sp., identification of, 1171, 1172f
Mucormycosis, defined, 1156
MUG Disk, 282–283
MUG Test, 38
Multiceps sp., 1316
Multiplex PCR, 146
Mumps virus, clinical manifestations of, 1344
Murein lipoproteins, 186
Muriform, 1157b
Murray and Washington's grading system, in sputum assessment, 17, 17b
Muscle biopsy, in parasite detection, CP 22-11G, 1254
Musculoskeletal infections, *Bacillus* sp. and, 780
Mutualism, 4
Mycelium, 1157b, 1158f
    aerial, 1157b
    reproductive, 1157b
    vegetative, 1157b
Mycetoma(s), 864, 1218b
    agents of, 1211, 1213–1216
    causes of, 864, 864t
    defined, 1213
Mycobacteria, 1064–1124. *See also* *Mycobacterium* sp.
    classification of, 1090–1106
        history of, 1090, 1090b
    detection of
        automated detection systems for, 1080–1083
        BACTEC AFB System in, Chart 9-4, 1085
        BACTEC MYCO/F Lytic in, 1083
        ESP Culture System II in, 1082–1083
        manual detection systems in, 1083–1085
        MB/BacT Mycobacteria Detection System in, 1082
        MGIT 960 System in, 1082
        MGIT System in, 1081–1082
        Septi-Chek AFB System in, 1083–1085
    differential characteristics of, 1084t–1085t
    fluorochrome stains for, CP 1-2, 25
    identification of, 1091, 1092t
        arylsulfatase activity in, Chart 19-5, CP 19-2J, 1087, 1088t–1089t
        catalase activity in, Chart 19-17, CP 19-2H–I, 1087
        conventional methods in, Charts 19-1–19-16, 1084–1090, 1088t–1089t
        DNA fingerprinting, 1111–1113
        DNA probes for, 1509–1511
        growth in % sodium chloride, Chart 19-14, 1087, 1090
        growth inhibition by T2H in, Chart 19-9, CP 19-1F, 1087
        growth on MacConkey agar in, Chart 19-8, 1090
        iron uptake in, Chart 19-10, 1087

Mycobacteria (*Continued*)
molecular methods in, 1106–1113, 1110f
Abbott LCx *M. tuberculosis* assay, 1109
BD ProbeTec *M. tuberculosis* assay, 1109
DNA sequencing, 1111
Gen-Probe AMTD, 1108
nucleic-acid amplification methods, 1108–1110
nucleic-acid probes in, 1107
PCR assays, 1109–1110
postamplification analysis, 1110–1111, 1110f
reverse hybridization, 1110–1111, 1110f
Roche Amplicor *Mycobacterium tuberculosis* Test, 1108–1109
signal-amplification methods, 1107–1108
in situ hybridization in, 1107–1108
niacin accumulation in, Chart 19-11, CP 19-1D, 1086
pigment production in, Chart 19-6, CP 19-2C–F, 1086
pyrazinamidase in, Chart 19-13, CP 19-2L, 1087
reduction of nitrates to nitrites in, Chart 19-12, CP 19-1E–F, 1084t–1085t, 1086–1087
strain typing in, 1111–1113
Tween 80 hydrolysis in, Chart 19-15, CP 19-2G, 1087
urease activity in, Chart 19-16, CP 19-2K, 1084t–1085t, 1087
M. shimoidei, 1102
nitrate reduction in, 1504–1505, 1504f
nomenclature of, 1088t–1089t
photoreactivity of, assessment of, 1497–1498
preliminary identification of, 39
recovery of
acid-fast smears in, sensitivity of, 1079–1080
broth culture medium in, 1080
culture media in, 1077–1078, 1078t
culture of specimens for, 1077–1796, 1078t, 1079t, 1080f
GLC in, 1080
HPLC in, 1080
HPLC-FL in, 1080
incubation in, 1079, 1080f
media of Cohen and Middlebrook in, 1078
nonselective culture media in, 1077–1078
rapid methods for, 1079–1080
selective media in, 1078–1079, 1079t
sodium chloride tolerance in, 1506–1507
in tuberculosis diagnosis, recovery and identification of, 1071–1077, 1071f, 1073t, 1074t, 1076t, 1077t, 1708b. *See also* Tuberculosis, laboratory diagnosis of, in mycobacteria recovery and identification
urease in, 1508–1509
Mycobacteria Growth Indicator Tube (MGIT) System, in mycobacteria detection, 1081–1082
Mycobacterium sp.. *See also* Mycobacteria
M. abscessus, CP 19-2Q–T, 1104, 1105b
M. asiaticum, 1095
M. avium-intracellulare, CP 19-2A–B, CP 19-2N–O, 1099–1101
M. bovis, 1092–1093
M. celatum, 1098–1099
M. chelonae, CP 19-2Q–T, 1104, 1105b
M. fortuitum, CP 19-2Q–T, 1104, 1105b
M. gastri, 1102
M. genavense, 1106
M. gordonae, 1099, 1099b
M. haemophilum, 1103, 1103b
M. kansasii, 1093, 1096b
M. malmoense, 1102–1103, 1103b
M. marinum, 1093–1095, 1097b
M. paratuberculosis, 1101–1102
M. scrofulaceum, 1095–1099
M. simiae, 1095, 1097b
M. szulgai, Chart 19-6, 1096–1097, 1098b
M. terrae, 1102, 1102b

M. thermoresistible, 1104
M. triviale, 1102, 1102b
M. tuberculosis, Chart 19-4, CP 19-1B–J, 1094, 1095–1096
detection of, radiometric instrumentation in, 1511–1512
drug susceptibility testing of, radiometric instrumentation in, 1511–1512
HIV with, 1066
identification of, radiometric instrumentation in, 1511–1512
meningitis due to, 92
short-course therapy for, 1115–1117, 1116b
susceptibility testing for, 1113–1115, 1113f, 1115t
M. tuberculosis complex, Chart 19-4, CP 19-1B–J, 1095–1096
M. ulcerans, 1104, 1106, 1106b
M. xenopi, 1097–1098, 1098b
nomenclature of, 1088t–1089t
nonphotochromogens, CP 19-2A–B, CP 19-2N–O, 1099–1103
order of presentation of, 1093b
photochromogens, CP 19-2C–D, CP 19-2M, 1093–1095
rapid growers, CP 19-2Q–T, 1104, 1105b
review of, 1091–1106
scotochromogens, CP 19-2D, 1095–1099
Mycolic acids, 188
Mycology, 1151–1243
terminology related to, 1155–1154
Mycoplasma(s), 1022–1063
of animal origin, human infections due to, 1039
central, isolation of, medium for, 1487–1488
culture of
from clinical specimens, Charts 18-1–18-6, 1040–1048, 1043f, 1044f
media for, Charts 18-4–18-5, 1041–1042
specimen collection in, 1041
transport media in, 1041
described, 1023
detection of, Diene's stain for, 1483–1484
genital
isolation and identification of, Charts 18-1, CP 18-1B, 18-3, 1044–1045, 1046f
noncultural detection of, 1045–1047
serologic tests for, 1050–1051
isolation of
from humans, 1025b
on routine culture media, 1048
taxonomy of, 1023–1026, 1024b, 1025b, 1025t
Mycoplasma culture systems, commercial, 1047
Mycoplasma infections
antimicrobial susceptibility of, 1051–1054
hemotrophic, in animals, diagnosis and treatment of, 1054
treatment of, 1051–1054
Mycoplasma sp.
clinical significance of, 1027–1039
hemotrophic, 1039–1040
identification of, characteristics for, 1025b
M. fermentans, clinical significance of, 1034–1035
M. genitalium, clinical significance of, 1033–1034
M. hominis, clinical significance of, 1028–1033
M. penetrans, clinical significance of, 1037–1038
M. pirum, clinical significance of, 1038–1039
M. pneumoniae
clinical significance of, 1027–1028
identification of, Charts 18-2, CP 18-1A, 18-6, 1042–1043, 1043f
hemadsorption test in, 1484
presumptive, tetrazolium reduction test in, 1488–1489
infections due to, diagnosis of, serologic tests for, 1048–1050
isolation of, Charts 18-2, CP 18-1A, 18-6, 1042–1043, 1043f
medium for, 1485–1487
noncultural detection of, 1043–1044

M. primatum, clinical significance of, 1039
M. spermatophilum, clinical significance of, 1039
virulence factors of, 1026–1027
Mycosel/mycobiotic agars, uses of, 1159t
Mycoses
extrapulmonary, signs, symptoms, and probable agents of, 1155t
pulmonary, signs and symptoms of, 1154t
Mycotrim GU system, 1047
Mycotrim RS system, 1047
Mycotrim Triphasic flask, 1047
Myocarditis/pericarditis, viral infections and, 1369t
Myonecrosis, clostridial, 932, 935
Myroides sp., CP 7-4D, 308t, 348, 349t
Myxovirus(es), cytopathic effect of, 1384f

N-Acetylglucosamine, 183, 184f
N-Acetyl-L-cysteine–sodium hydroxide (NALC), 1489–1490
N-Acetylmuramic acid, 183, 184f
Naegleria sp., *N. fowleri,* meningitis due to, 93
Nagler test, in anaerobic bacteria differentiation, 905
Nail fragments, direct examination of, in infectious disease diagnosis, 23t
NALC. *See N*-acetyl-L-cysteine–sodium hydroxide (NALC)
Nanaerobe(s), 881, 888t
NAP. *See p*-Nitro-acetylamino-hydroxypropiophenone (NAP)
NAP test, 1494–1496
NASBA. *See* Nucleic acid sequence-based amplification (NASBA)
Nasopharynx
cultures of, 74
infections of, 74
National Type Culture Collection (NTCC), 167
Native-valve endocarditis, *S. epidermidis* and, 639b
NBG agar. *See* Novobiocin-brilliant green-glucose (NBG) agar
NBGL agar. *See* Novobiocin-brilliant green-glycerol-lactose (NBGL) agar
Necrosis, 7
Necrotizing bowel disease, *C. perfringens* and, 932, 935
Needle(s), safety precautions for, 48
Needle stick exposure to blood, risks of contracting blood-borne viral infections after, 52, 55t
Neisseria sp., 308t, 351t, 353, 566–622
antimicrobial susceptibility of, 605–608
atypical, cultural characteristics of, 600t–601t
characteristics of, 569–570, 571b–574b, 575f
clinical significance of, 570, 575–584, 575f, 576f
cultural characteristics of, 600–604, 600t–601t
identification of, CP 11-1B–E, CP 11-2A–E, 592–600, 595t

BactiCard in, CP 11-2A, 595–596
carbohydrate-utilization tests in, CP 11-1C–E, 594
characteristics for, 600t–601t
chromogenic enzyme substrate tests in, 594–596, 595t
coagglutination tests in, 596
colony morphology in, CP 11-1B, 592–593
confirmatory tests in, 593–594
differentiation of other organisms on selective media in, 593
''false'', characteristics for, 600t–601t
Gram's stain in, 593
multitest identification systems in, CP 11-2D–E, 597
oxidase test in, 593
rapid carbohydrate utilization test for, 1470
superoxol test in, 593
isolation of, CP 11-1A, 588–592, 589b, 589t, 590t, 592b
N. cinerea, 584
cultural characteristics of, 600t–601t, 603

N. elongata
    subsp. *elongata,* cultural characteristics of, 600t–601t, 604
    subsp. *glycolytica,* cultural characteristics of, 600t–601t, 604
N. flavescens, cultural characteristics of, 600t–601t, 603
N. gonorrhoeae
    antigens of, virulence-associated, 573b–574b
    antimicrobial susceptibility of, 605–607
    antimicrobial therapy for, resistance to, 1011
    clinical significance of, 570, 575–584, 575f, 576f
    cultural characteristics of, 600–604, 600t–601t
    culture confirmation of
        DNA probe test for, 597
        immunologic methods for, 596–597
    epidemiology of, 570, 575
    historical background of, 567–568
    identification of
        DFA test in, 596
        nucleic acid hybridization and amplification tests in, 597–599
        presumptive criteria for, 593
    infections caused by, 573, 576–578, 576f, 577f, t
    isolation of, CP 11-1A, 588–591, 589b, 589t, 590t
        direct Gram's-stained smears in, CP 11-1A, 588
        selective culture media in, inoculation and incubation of, 590t, 590–591
        specimen collection in, 588–591, 589b, 589t
        specimen transport in, 589–590
    β-lactamases of, induction of, 1002
    subsp. *kochii,* cultural characteristics of, 600t–601t, 604
    testing methods for, 999t
    virulence factors of, 573b–574b
N. lactamica, 584
    cultural characteristics of, 600t–601t, 603
N. meningitidis
    antigens of, virulence-associated, 574b–575b
    antimicrobial susceptibility of, 607–608
    antimicrobial therapy for, resistance to, 1011
    cultural characteristics of, 600t–601t, 602–603
    epidemiology of, 578–580
    historical background of, 567–568
    identification of, molecular methods for, 600
    infections caused by, 580–582
    isolation of
        direct capsular antigen tests in, 591
        direct Gram's-stained smears in, 591
        isolation and incubation in, 591–592
        laboratory safety in, 591
        specimen collection and transport in, 591
    meningitis due to, 92
    testing methods for, 999t
    virulence factors of, 574b–575b
N. polysaccharea, cultural characteristics of, 600t–601t, 604
N. sicca, 584
N. subflava, 584
non-human, cultural characteristics of, 600t–601t, 604
nonpathogenic, identification of, 600t–601t, 603–604
Neisseriaceae, 351t, 353
    classification of species within, 568, 569b
    taxonomy of, 568–569, 569b
Neisseria-Kwik test kit, in *Neisseria* sp. identification, 594
Nematode(s), 1273–1281
    Ascaris lumbricoides, CP 22-5A–D, 1274, 1275f, 1276b
    Capillaria philippinensis, CP 22-5P, 1280–1281
    described, 1273–1274, 1275b
    Enterobius vermicularis, CP 22-5F–G, 1275–1276

filarial, CP 22-10A–C, 1303–1304, 1306b, 1307f
hookworms, CP 22-5K–L, 1276, 1278f, 1279
Strongyloides stercoralis, CP 22-5L–M, 1278f, 1279, 1281b
Trichostrongylus sp., 1279
Trichuris trichuria, CP 22-5E, F, P, 1274, 1277b, 1277f
Neonatal sepsis, *Haemophilus* sp. and, 434t, 441–442
Nested PCR, 146–147
Neufeld's quellung reaction, in microscopic examination of specimens, 19t
Neuraminidase enzymes, of *S. pneumoniae,* 690
Neuroretinitis, *Bartonella* sp. and, 504
Niacin, accumulation of, 1502–1503
    in mycobacteria identification, Chart 19-11, CP 19-1D, 1086
Niclosamide, for parasitic infections, 1320t
Nigrospora sp., 1211, 1213f
Nipah virus, 1344
Nitrate(s)
    denitrification of, in nonfermenter identification, Chart 7-3, CP 7-2B, 315
    to nitrites, in mycobacteria identification, Chart 19-12, CP 19-1E–F, 1084t–1085t, 1086–1087
    in nonfermenter identification, Chart 7-3, CP 7-2B, 315
Nitrate reduction, 1452–1453
    in *Enterobacteriaceae* identification, Chart 6-2, CP 6-1H, 216
    mycobacterial, 1504–1505, 1504f
Nitrate reduction test, in nonfermenter identification, Chart 6-2, 315
Nitrite(s), nitrates to, in mycobacteria identification, Chart 19-12, CP 19-1E–F, 1084t–1085t, 1086–1087
p-Nitro-α-acetylamino-β-hydroxypropiophenone, 1494–1496
p-Nitro-acetylamino-hydroxypropiophenone (NAP), in tuberculosis diagnosis, 1068
Nitrogen
    assimilation and metabolism of, 196, 197f
    in bacterial growth and metabolism, 195–196, 197f
o-Nitrophenyl-β-D-galactopyranoside (ONPG), 1451–1453, 1451f
    in *Enterobacteriaceae* identification, Chart 6-1, CP 6-4A, 215
Nocardia(ae), described, 861
Nocardia sp., 860–863
    bacterial cells of, 862
    carbohydrate utilization by, patterns in, supplemental tests in resolution of, 873t
    clinical disease due to, 862–863
    described, 862
    differentiation of, Chart 15-1, CP 15-1A–E, 867–871, 868t–870t, 871b, 871f, 872t, 873t
        key tests for, 872t
    identification of
        API 20C AUX strips in, 872t
        lysozyme test in, 867, 871b
        modified acid-fast stain for, 867, 871b
    N. asteroides, 860–861
        isolates of, antimicrobial susceptibility profiles of, 861, 862t
    N. brasiliensis, 861
    N. otitidiscaviarum, 861
    taxonomy of, 860
    in vitro susceptibility of, 871–872, 874t, 875
Nocardioform bacteria, 860–864
Nocardioform group, 860–864
Nocardiopsis sp., 864–865
Nocardiosis, 861–862
Nomenclature
    defined, 1330
    viral infections-related, 1330–1333, 1330b, 1331f, 1332f, 1334t–1335t
Nonbiologic hazards, safety precautions for, 56–58

Nonfastidious bacteria
    disk diffusion susceptibility test for, 1480–1481
    microbroth dilution susceptibility test for, performance of, 1481–1482
Nonfermentative gram-negative bacilli, 303–391. *See also* Nonfermenter(s)
    defined, 305
    identification of
        decarboxylation in, Chart 6-7, CP 7-2D, 315
        denitrification of nitrates and nitrites in, Chart 7-3, CP 7-2B, 315
        esculin hydrolysis in, Chart 7-4, CP 7-2E, 315
        failure to grow on MacConkey agar in, CP 7-1C, 313
        flagella morphology in, 316
        glucose utilization test in, Chart 7-1, CP 7-1D, 313, 313f
        indole production in, Chart 1-4, CP 7-2C, 315
        lack of evidence for glucose fermentation in, CP 7-1A, 312
        Leifson staining method in, Chart 7-2, CP 7-2B, 315
        motility in, Chart 7-2, CP 7-1E, 313–314, 314f
        nitrate reduction in, Chart 6-2, 315
        pigment production in, CP 7-1F–H, 314
        positive cytochrome oxidase reaction in, Chart 1-5, CP 7-1B, 312–313
        Ryu staining method in, Chart 7-2, 316
        tests in, Charts 1-4, CP 7-1D–H, CP 7-2A–E, 6-2, 6-6, 6-7, 7-1–7-4, 314f, 313–316, 313f, 316b
        urea hydrolysis in, Chart 6-6, CP 7-2A, 314–315
        wet-mount technique in, Chart 7-2, 316
    nomenclature for, 306t–309t
Nonfermenter(s), 218
    acetamide-positive, in nonfermenter identification, 366t
    denitrifying, in nonfermenter identification, 369t
    described, 316
    dextrose-negative, in nonfermenter identification, 371t
    dextrose-positive, in nonfermenter identification, 370t
    fluorescent, in nonfermenter identification, 365t
    identification of
        API 20E system in, in nonfermenter identification, 362, 372b
        API 20NE system in, CP 7-5D, 362, 372b
        approach to, 355–376
        automated identification system in, 373–375
        Autoscan-4 System in, 375
        Biolog System in, 373
        commercial kit systems in, 359, 362, 367, 372b–374b, 373
        computer-aided schemes in, 359
        conventional tests in, 357–359, 358b, 360t–371t
        Crystal Enteric/Nonfermenter system in, 367
        initial clues in, Chart 1-5, CP 7-1A–C, 312–313
        levels of service in, 355–356, 355b
        oxidase-negative nonmotility in, 361t
        oxidase-positive motility in, 365t
        Oxi/Ferm tube in, 359, 362
        P. aeruginosa, 356–357
        Phoenix Automated Microbiology System in, 375
        pigmentation in, 368t
        practical approach to, 358–359, 360t
        problems associated with, 355, 355b
        RapID NF Plus System in, CP 7-5F, 367, 373, 374b
        Remel N/F system in, 362, 367, 373b
        Sensititre AP80 System in, 375
        systems in, selection of, 375–376
        Vitek 2 System in, 374–375
        Vitek Legacy System in, 373–374
        Walkaway-40 in, 375
        Walkaway-96 in, 375

Nonfermenter(s) (*Continued*)
  indole-positive, characteristics of, 347t
  lactose-positive, in nonfermenter identification, 365t
  lysine-positive, in nonfermenter identification, 367t
  medically important genera of, taxonomy, biochemical characteristics, and clinical significance of, 316–355, 317b
  metabolism of, 305–316
    ED pathway in, 311–312, 311f
    EMP pathway in, 309–311, 310f
    fermentative, 309–312, 311f
    oxidative, 309–312, 311f
    Warburg-Dickens Hexose Monophosphate pathway in, 311f, 312
  motile, oxidase-positive, in nonfermenter identification, 365t
  nomenclature for, 306t–309t
  nonmotile, oxidase-negative, in nonfermenter identification, 361t
  pigmented, in nonfermenter identification, 368t
  recovery of, guidelines for, 356
Nonindustrial anthrax, 776–777
Noninflammatory diarrhea, causes of, 80t
Nonmotile organisms
  oxidase-negative, CP 7-5A–B, 353–355, 354t
  oxidase-positive, 345–353
Non-nutritive swab transport systems, in *N. gonorrhoeae* isolation, 589–590
Nonphotochromogen(s), CP 19-2A–B, N–O, 1099–1103
Nonvolatile acids, analysis of, in determination of metabolic products of anaerobes, 908–909, 911b
Norwalk-like viruses, clinical manifestations of, 1350
Nosocomial infections
  Bacillus sp. and, 780–781
  defined, 6b
Novobiocin, susceptibility to, in *S. saprophyticus* identification, 655
Novobiocin disk test, 1471
Novobiocin-brilliant green-glucose (NBG) agar, in *Salmonella* sp. recovery and characterization, 256t
Novobiocin-brilliant green-glycerol-lactose (NBGL) agar, in *Salmonella* sp. recovery and characterization, 256t
NTCC. *See* National Type Culture Collection (NTCC)
Nuclear membrane, 179
Nucleic acid(s), 133–137, 134f–136f. *See also specific types, e.g.,* Deoxyribonucleic acid (DNA)
  in *C. trachomatis,* detection of, 1405–1406
  categories of, 133
  in CNS infections, detection of, 94–95
  in *Coxiella* sp., direction detection of, 1409
  in *Legionella* sp. examination, CP 10-1A–D, 557–560, 558b, 559t, 560t
  in *Rickettsia* sp., direction detection of, 1409
Nucleic acid amplification, 141–147, 142f, 143f
  ligase chain reaction, 143–144
  methods of, in mycobacterial identification, 1108–1110
  NASBA, 143, 144
  PCR in, 141–143, 142f, 143f
  postamplification analysis, 147–151, 147f–150f. *See also* Postamplification analysis
  real-time, 151–156, 152f–156f. *See also* Real-time nucleic acid amplification
  TMA, 143, 144
Nucleic acid bases, molecular structure of, 181f
Nucleic acid hybridization test, in *N. gonorrhoeae* identification, 597–599
Nucleic acid probes, 137
  molecular methods in, 1107
Nucleic acid sequence-based amplification (NASBA), 143, 144, 1044
Nucleoid(s), 179

Nucleotide monophosphates, in DNA, 133, 134f
Nuclisens HIV-1 QT, 144
Number(s), biotype, 286
Numeric code registers, octal codes in, reading of, 286–287
Numeric coding systems, 285–287, 286t, 288t
  calculation of likelihood in, 287, 288t
  estimated frequency of occurrence in, 287
  octal codes in, reading of, 286–287
  resolving discrepancies in, 287
Nymph(s), CP A-1B, 1424

O Antigens, 186–187
Obesumbacterium sp.
  newer, differentiating characteristics of, 279t
  O. proteus, 276t
    biochemical reactions of, 240t–241t
Obligate aerobes, 195
Obligate anaerobes, 195
Occupational blood exposures, management of, 1354–1356, 1356b
Oceanospirillaceae, 334, 335t
Ochrobactrum sp., 342t, 345
Ochrobactrum anthropi, 308t
Ocular infections. *See* Eye infections
Ocular micrometer, calibration of, 1531–1533, 1532f
Oculoglandular tularemia, 493
ODC test. *See* Ornithine decarboxylase (ODC) test
Odor(s), of microbes, 35, 35t
Oerskovia sp., 828, 829t, 865
OFBA-1, 339
Oligella sp., 308t, 344
OmniLog ID System, 293–294
OMP and NGP Wee-Tabs, 283
OMPs. *See* Outer membrane proteins (OMPs)
Onchocerca volvulus, CP 22-10D, 1305–1306, 1308f
  life cycle of, 1308f
Onchocerciasis, CP 22-10D, 1305–1306, 1308f
ONPG. *See* *o*-Nitrophenyl-β-D-galactopyranoside (ONPG)
Oocyst(s), *Cryptosporidium,* in fecal specimens, Sheather's flotation technique in recovery of, 1270b
Oospore(s), 1158b, 1159f
Opa protein
  of *N. gonorrhoeae,* 572b
  of *N. meningitis,* 575b
Opacity factor (OF), as streptococcal virulence factor, 678
Opc protein, of *N. meningitis,* 575b
Opportunistic infection, defined, 6b
Optochin, susceptibility to, in streptococci identification, Chart 13-3, CP 13-2G, 718
Optochin susceptibility test, 1474
Oral cavity, infections of, 73–74, 73f
Organelle(s), locomotor, 191
Ornithine, decarboxylation of, in Enterobacteriaceae identification, Chart 6-7, CP 6-4F–G, 225–226
Ornithine decarboxylase (ODC) test, in coagulase-negative staphylococci identification, 652, 655
Ornithodoros sp.
  geographic distribution of, 1431
  identification of, CP A-2E, 1431
Oropharyngeal anthrax, 778
Oropharyngeal tularemia, 493
Oropharyngeal ulcers, direct examination of, in infectious disease diagnosis, 22t
Oroya fever, *B. bacilliformis* and, 500
Orthomyxoviridae sp., described, 1334t
Orthomyxovirus(es), clinical manifestations of, 1335, 1339–1340, 1342
Orthopoxvirus(es), clinical manifestations of, 1361
Osteomyelitis
  diagnosis of, 91
  S. aureus and, 635b

  S. epidermidis and, 639b
  symptoms of, 91
Other End of the Microscope: The Bacteria Tell Their Story, The, 2
Otitis media, 74
  Haemophilus sp. and, 434t, 439–440
Outer membrane, 186
Outer membrane proteins (OMPs), 188
Oxalobacteraceae, 334, 335t
Oxidase-negative nonmotile organisms, CP 7-5A–B, 353–355, 354t
Oxidase-positive fermenters, 408–421
Oxidase-positive nonmotile organisms, 345–353
Oxidation-reduction potential (Eh), of culture medium, 879–880
Oxidative-fermentative test, 1462–1463
Oxi/Ferm tube, in nonfermenter identification, 359, 362
Oxoid anaerobic jar, 895–896, 896f
Oxoid Signal System, in blood culture processing, 102–103
Oxygen
  bacteria relationships to, 878–880
  in bacterial growth and metabolism, 195
Oxygen tolerance, to anaerobes, 879

PACE 2 system, 597, 598
  in *N. gonorrhoeae* identification, 598
Packaged systems, 287, 289–292, 290t
  API 20E, CP 6-6A, 289, 290t
  BBL crystal E/NF identification system, CP 6-6B, 289
  Biolog GN2 microplate, CP 6-6D, 291
  Enterotube II, 290–291
  Micro-ID, 291
  MicroScan System, CP 6-6E, 291
  overview of, 287, 289
  RapID onE system, CP 6-6C, 289–290
  Sensititre system, 291–292
Paecilomyces sp., chains of conidia produced by, CP 21-2C, 1182, 1182f
Pandoraea sp., 308t, 327t, 329–331
Pantoea sp., 265–266
  biochemical reactions of, 240t–241t
  identification characteristics of, 234t
Papanicolaou stain, 1363, 1363f
Papillomavirus(es), human
  clinical manifestations of, 1362t, 1362–1364, 1363f, 1363t
  molecular detection of, 1396
Papovaviridae sp., described, 1342t
Papovavirus(es), clinical manifestations of, 1361–1364, 1362t, 1363f, 1363t
Paracoccidioides sp., *P. immitis,* 1203, 1205–1207, 1207f, 1208f, 1209b
Paracoccidioidomycosis, 1203, 1205–1207, 1207f, 1208f, 1209b
Paracoccus yeei, CP 7-4G–H, 352, 352t
Paragonimus westermani, CP 22-7P, 1292, 1295f, 1296b
Parainfluenza virus(es)
  clinical manifestations of, 1342, 1344
  parainfluenza virus 1, 1334t
Paralysis, tick, 1424–1425
Paramyxoviridae sp., described, 1334t
Paramyxovirus(es), clinical manifestations of, 1342, 1344
Parasite(s), 4. *See also specific types, e.g.,* Intestinal protozoa
  blood, 1248, 1292–1318
  cestodes, 1281–1286
  described, 3
  differentiation of, Chart 22-4, CP 22-1, 1255–1256, 1257f
  history of, 1245
  human, life cycles of, 1256, 1257f
  identification of, Chart 22-4, CP 22-1, 1255–1256, 1257f

imaginary, 1245
intestinal, recovery of, fecal concentration
    techniques for, 1525–1527
nematodes, 1273–1281
    filarial, CP 22-10A–C, 1303–1304, 1306b,
        1307f
    preliminary identification of, 39
    prevalence of, 1245–1246, 1246b
    protozoan, 1245, 1256, 1258–1273
        intestinal, 1256, 1258–1273
    in stool specimens, incidence of, 1246, 1246b
    tissue, 1292–1318
    trematodes, 1286–1292
    types of, 1245
Parasitic diseases. See also Parasitic infections
    clinical manifestations of, 1247–1248
    specimens in, 1248–1255
        aspirates, 1254
        blood, Chart 22-3, 1254–1255
        body fluids, 1254
        collection of, 1248–1255
        corneal scrapings, 1254
        extraintestinal, examination of, 1254–1255
        fecal, 1248–1253, 1250b–1251b
            preservation of clinical specimens, 1249,
                1250b–1251b
            processing for ova and parasite examination,
                Charts 22-1–22-2, 1249, 1251–1253
            visual examination of, 1249
        muscle biopsy, CP 22-11G, 1254
        other than stool, examination of, Chart 22-5,
            1253–1254, 1254f
        processing of, 1248–1255
        sputum, 1254
        tissue biopsies, 1254
        transport of, 1248–1255
        urine, 1254
    treatment of, drugs in, 1319t–1321t, 1321
Parasitic infections. See also Parasitic disease
    prevention of, 1247
    risk factors for, 1247
    serologic diagnosis of, 1318, 1318b, 1321
Parasitism, 4
Parasitology, 1244–1326
Parotitis
    infectious, 1344
    viral infections and, 1369t
Parvoviridae sp., described, 1342t
Parvovirus(es)
    B19, molecular detection of, 1396
    clinical manifestations of, 1364
    molecular detection of, 1396
    serologic diagnosis of, 1402
Passive hemagglutination (PHA), in S. aureus
        identification, CP 12-2E, 646
Passive hemagglutination (PHA) test, 117
Pasteurella sp., 458–461
    antimicrobial susceptibility of, 464–465
    characteristics of, 432t, 457
    cultural characteristics of, CP 9-1H, 463–464
    currently recognized, 459b
    described, 458–459, 459b, 460t–462t
    identification of, CP 9-1H, 463–464
        biochemical characteristics for, 460t–461t
    P. aerogenes, 459b, 460t–461t, 465
    P. bettyae, 459b, 460t–461t, 466
    P. caballi, 459b, 460t–461t, 466
    P. canis, 459b, 460t–461t, 466
    P. dagmatis, 459b, 460t–461t, 465–466
    P. gallinarum, 459b, 460t–461t, 466–467
    P. multicoda
        antimicrobial susceptibility of, 464–465
        clinical significance of, 459, 463b–464b, 464
        cultural characteristics of, CP 9-1H, 463–464
        identification of, CP 9-1H, 463–464
            biochemical characteristics for, 460t–461t
        infections due to, clinical spectrum of, 458,
            463b–464b, 464
    virulence of, 459, 464

P. multocida, pathogenic isolate of, 157, 157f
P. pneumotropica, 459b, 460t–461t, 465
P. stomatis, 459b, 460t–461t, 466
taxonomy of, 458
Pasteurellaceae, differentiation of members of,
    characteristics for, 432t
Pathogen(s), 4
    defined, 201
    potential, 4
Pathogenicity
    bacterial virulence and, 203–204
    defined, 201
Patient confidentiality, in microbiology laboratory, 47
PCR. See Polymerase chain reaction (PCR)
PCR assays
    in mycobacterial identification, 1109–1110
    in N. gonorrhoeae identification, 599
PCR-RFLP, 157–158
Pediatric infections, S. epidermidis and, 640b
Pediculus sp.
    P. capitis, CP A-3G, 1434–1435
    P. humanus, CP A-3F, 1434
Pediococcus sp., 706–707
    identification of, 736, 738t
Pedobacter sp., 348–349, 349t
Peliosis, B. henselae and, 501
Pelvic actinomycosis, 817
Penicillin
    discovery of, 946–947, 946f
    S. pneumoniae resistant to, 1009–1010, 1010f
    S. pyogenes resistant to, 1013
Penicillin antibiotics, Haemophilus sp. resistant to,
    1009
Penicillin binding proteins, 184
Penicillin disk test, in Neisseria sp. identification, 593
Penicillin-recognizing enzymes, active at cell
        membrane, 955, 957–961, 957f, 960t,
        961t, 962b
Penicillium sp., chains of conidia produced by, CP
        21-2B–D, 1181–1182, 1181f, 1182f
Penicillus, 1181
Penile ulcer, direct examination of, in infectious
        disease diagnosis, 23t
Pentose phosphate pathway, 198, 201f
Peptidoglycan, 183, 955, 957–958, 957t
    of S. aureus, 630b
Pericarditis, S. aureus and, 634b
Periodic acid–Schiff stain, in microscopic
        examination of specimens, CP 1-2H, 26
Periodontitis, localized juvenile, 453
Peripheral proteins, 188
Periplasmic space, 186
Peritoneal dialysis catheter-associated infections, S.
        epidermidis and, 640b
Permease(s), 182
Pertussis. See also Bordetella sp.
    diagnosis of, serologic tests for, 521–522
    epidemiology of, 512
    stages of, 512–513
    treatment of, 522
    vaccines for, 513, 515–516
Petechial rash, viral infections and, 1369t
pH
    in antimicrobial therapy, 967
    in testing inhibitory activity of antimicrobial
        agents, 970
PHA test. See Passive hemagglutination (PHA) test
Phaeoannellomyces werneckii, 1229–1230, 1230f
Phaeohyphomycosis, 1155, 1217b–1218b
    agents of, CP 12-3A–D, 1208
Pharyngitis, 72–73
    acute, Haemophilus sp. and, 434t
    Arcanobacterium haemolyticum, 72
    causes of, infectious, 73
    culture for, 73–74, 73f
    gonococcal, 72
    streptococcal, 72, 679
    viral, 72–73
    viral infections and, 1368t

Phase variation, 191, 192
Phenylalanine deaminase, 1461–1462, 1461f
Phenylalanine deaminase determination, in
        Enterobacteriaceae identification, Chart
        6-8, CP 6-4E, 226
Phialide(s), 1157b, 1175, 1175f
Phialophora sp.
    P. richardsiae, 1215, 1215f
    P. verrucosa, 1215
Phoenix Automated Microbiology System, CP 6-6H,
        293
    in nonfermenter identification, 375
Phoma sp., 1211, 1213f
Phosphatase, production of, in S. epidermidis
        identification, 650
Phosphatidylinositol mannosides, 189
Phosphorylation, substrate level, 198
Photobacterium sp., 417
Photochromogen(s), CP 19-2C–D, M, 1093–1095
Photolithotrophic bacteria, 195
Photoreactivity, of mycobacteria, assessment of,
        1497–1498
Photorhabdus sp., 281–282
    biochemical reactions of, 240t–241t
    newer, 276t
Phthirus pubis, CP A-3H, 1435
Phycomycosis, defined, 1156
Pibwin (Probabilistic Identification of Bacteria for
        Windows), in nonfermenter identification,
        359
Pickett identification scheme, in nonfermenter
        identification, 358
Picornaviridae sp., described, 1337t
Picornavirus(es), clinical manifestations of,
        1344–1345
Pigment production, in streptococci identification, CP
        13-2C, 717
Pigment production test, in nonfermenter
        identification, CP 7-1F–H, 314
Pigmentation, in mycobacteria identification, Chart
        19-6, CP 19-2C–F, 1086
Pili
    bacterial, 191–192
    of Moraxella catarrhalis, 586b
    of N. gonorrhoeae, 573b
    of N. meningitis, 574b
Pilin, 192
Pinworm examination, cellulose tape preparation for,
        1533–1534
''Pinworm'' infections, 1275
Plague, CP 6-5A–D, 269–272, 271b, 272b, 272f
    bubonic, 271b, 275b
    classification of, phenotypic, 319b
    clinical findings of, 276b
    defined, 269
    diagnosis of, 271b, 272f
    epidemiology of, 269, 271–272, 272b, 272f
    history of, 271b
    laboratory diagnosis of, CP 6-5B–D, 272
    laboratory testing of, 272b
    number of cases of, 272f
    pandemics of, 271b
    pneumonic, 271b
    prevention of, 272b
    reporting of, 272b
    septicemic, 271b
    treatment of, 271b, 272b
    types of, 271b
    Y. enterocolitica, infections caused by, 273
    Y. frederiksenii, 274
    Y. pseudotuberculosis, infections caused by, 273
    Yersinia sp. and, CP 6-5A–D, 269–272, 271b,
        272b, 272f
Plasmid(s), 182
    conjugative, 182
    F, 194
    of N. gonorrhoeae, 573b
    of N. meningitis, 575b

Plasmodium sp.
  P. falciparum, CP 22-8A–C, 1294, 1298
  P. malariae
    identification of, 1296
    life cycle of, 1297f
  P. vivax, CP 22-8D–F, 1294–1296
Plesiomonas sp., 416t, 421t, 422
  laboratory isolation and identification of, 421t, 422
  P. shigelloides, 416t, 421t, 422
Pleurodynia, viral infections and, 1368t
Pneumococcal polysaccharide vaccines, for *S. pneumoniae*, 690–691
Pneumocystis sp., *P. carinii*, 1311–1312
Pneumolysin, of *S. pneumoniae*, 690
Pneumonia(s), 75–76
  acute, 76
  aspiration, 76
  atypical, 75–76
  chronic, 76
  clinical manifestations of, 1368t
  in cystic fibrosis patients, 76
  in the elderly, 76
  Haemophilus sp. and, 434t, 440–441
  in immunosuppressed patients, 76
  laboratory diagnosis of, 78–79, 78b, 79t
  in special populations, 76
Pneumonic plague, 271b
Pneumonic tularemia, 493
Pneumovirinae sp., 1344
Poisoning, food, *S. aureus* and, 635b
Poliovirus 1, 1337f, 1337t
Poly-beta hydroxybutyrate, 181
Polyclonal antisera, 114
Polymerase chain reaction (PCR)
  basics of, 141–143, 142f, 143f
  broad-range, 145–146
  clinical applications of, 143
  defined, 141
  methods for, 141–143
  modifications of, 144–147
  multiplex, 146
  nested, 146–147
  reverse transcriptase, 144–145
Polymyxin B, susceptibility to, in coagulase-negative staphylococci identification, 652
Polynucleotide(s), 179, 181f
  molecular structure of, 181f
Polyomavirus(es), clinical manifestations of, 1364
Polyribosome(s), defined, 180
Polysaccharide(s), capsular
  of *N. meningitis*, 573b
  of *S. aureus*, 630b
Polysaccharide capsular antigens, 683
Polysaccharide capsule, 689
Polysaccharide synthesis, in *Neisseria* sp. identification, 603
Polysome(s), defined, 180
Pontiac fever, clinical manifestations of, 551, 551t
PorA protein, of *N. meningitis*, 575b
PorB protein, of *N. meningitis*, 575b
Porin proteins, 188
  in transport of antimicrobial agents across cell membrane, 950–952, 954f, 955f
Porphyromonas sp.
  identification of, characteristics in, 920b, 920t
  metabolic products of, 919t
Postamplification analysis, 147–151, 147f–150f
  DNA sequencing in, 148–151, 149f, 150f
  enzymatic detection of amplified products in, 147–148, 147f
  gel electrophoresis in, 147
  reverse hybridization in, 148, 148f
  Southern blot analysis in, 148
Postpartum bacteremia, *Haemophilus* sp. and, 434t, 441–442
Potassium hydroxide (KOH) mount, in microscopic examination of specimens, 18t

Potato flake agar, uses of, 1159t
Potential pathogen, 4
Poxvirus(es), clinical manifestations of, 1361
Poxviridae sp., described, 1343t
Pragia fontium, 276t
  biochemical reactions of, 240t–241t
Praziquantel, for parasitic infections, 1320t
Precipitin reactions, 114, 116
Preston *Campylobacter* blood-free medium, in *C. jejuni* isolation, 397t
Presumpto plates, in anaerobic bacteria differentiation, CP 16-5, 901–904, 902t, 903b
Prevotella sp.
  characteristics of, 918t
  identification of, characteristics in, 920t
  metabolic products of, 919t
  P. oralis, 921–922
  types of, 921
Primaquine, for parasitic infections, 1320t
Prion(s), described, 4
Prion diseases, clinical manifestations of, 1366–1367, 1366t
Probe(s)
  DNA, for mycobacteria identification, 1509–1511
  FRET, in real-time nucleic acid amplification, 151, 152–154, 153f, 154f
  hybridization. *See* Hybridization probes
  hydrolysis, in real-time nucleic acid amplification, 151–152, 152f
  TaqMan, 151–152
Prokaryotic cells, 177, 178b
Prokaryotic organisms, replication, transcription, and translation of genetic code in, 183f
Propionibacterium sp.
  identification of, 927
  P. propionicum, identification of, 927
Propionic acid fermentation, 200–201
Prosthetic-valve endocarditis, *S. epidermidis* and, 639b
Protease(s)
  IgA1
    of *N. gonorrhoeae*, 573b
    of *N. meningitis*, 575b
  IgA$_1$, of *S. pneumoniae*, 690
Proteeae (tribe), 232t–233t, 267t, 267–269
  identification characteristics for, 234t
Protein(s)
  A, of *S. aureus*, 630b
  CD, of *Moraxella catarrhalis*, 586b
  cell-surface penicillin-binding, 684
  CopB, of *Moraxella catarrhalis*, 587b
  E, of *Moraxella catarrhalis*, 587b
  extracellular surface, as virulence factor in *Enterococcus* sp., 701, 703–704
  H.8, of *N. gonorrhoeae*, 572b
  iron-binding/acquisition, of *N. meningitis*, 575b
  LpbA, of *Moraxella catarrhalis*, 587b
  LpbB, of *Moraxella catarrhalis*, 587b
  M, as streptococcal virulence factor, 679
  Opa
    of *N. gonorrhoeae*, 572b
    of *N. meningitis*, 575b
  Opc, of *N. meningitis*, 575b
  outer membrane, 188
    of *N. gonorrhoeae*, 572b
  outer-membrane
    of *Moraxella catarrhalis*, 586b–587b
    of *N. meningitis*, 575b
  penicillin binding, 184
  peripheral, 188
  PorA, of *N. meningitis*, 575b
  PorB, of *N. meningitis*, 575b
  porin, 188
    in transport of antimicrobial agents across cell membrane, 950–952, 954f, 955f
  Rmp, of *N. gonorrhoeae*, 572b
  TbpA, of *Moraxella catarrhalis*, 587b

TbpB, of *Moraxella catarrhalis*, 587b
  transmembrane, 188
  UspA, of *Moraxella catarrhalis*, 586b
  vancomycin-binding, 955, 957–958, 957t
Protein antigen, 683
Proteobacteria, 171b–173b
Proteus sp., CP 6-1D, 267–268, 268t
  biochemical reactions of, 240t–241t
  identification characteristics for, 234t
  P. mirabilis, 267, 268t
  P. penneri, 267–268, 268t
  P. vulgaris, 267–268, 268t
Prototrophic organisms, 196
Protozoa, intestinal, 1256, 1258–1273. *See also* Intestinal protozoa
Protozoan infections, tissue, CP 22-10F–H, 1306–1312, 1310f, 1311f, 1312b
Providencia sp., 268–269, 269t
  biochemical reactions of, 240t–241t
  identification characteristics for, 234t
Pseudomembrane, diphtheritic, 804
Pseudomonad(s), 316–339. *See also Pseudomonas* sp.
  alkaline, characteristics of, 322t
  characteristics of, 318t
  curved, 336t
  halophilic–positive, 337t
  hydrogen sulfide–positive, 337t
  Stutzeri group of, CP 7-3A, 321, 321t
  yellow-pigmented, characteristics of, 323, 335t
Pseudomonadaceae, 317–323, 317b, 318t, 319b, 320b, 320t–323t. *See also Pseudomonas* sp.
  characteristics of, 318t
Pseudomonas sp., 308t
  alcaligenes group of, 321–323, 322t
  characteristics of, 318t
  fluorescent group of, CP 7-1G, CP 7-2F–H, 319–321, 320b, 320t
  P. aeruginosa, CP 7-1G, CP 7-2F–H, 319–321, 320b, 320t
    characteristics of, 320t
    identification of, CP 7-1G–H, 356–357
    minimum requirements for, 319, 320b
    virulence factors of, 319, 320b
  P. fluorescens, 320t, 321
  P. luteola, CP 7-3B, 323
  P. oryzihabitans, 323, 335t
  P. putida, 320t, 321
  rRNA group 1, 317–323, 317b, 318t, 319b, 320b, 320t–323t
  stutzeri group of, CP 7-3A, 321, 321t
  yellow-pigmented group of, CP 7-3B, 323, 335t
Pseudomonas-like group 2, 339
PspA, gA$_1$, 94, 690
Pseudomonad(s), fluorescent, CP 7-1G, CP 7-2F–H, 319–321, 320b, 320t
Psychrobacter sp., 350, 352–353, 352t
  P. immobilis, 352, 352t
  P. phenylpyruvicus, 308t, 350–352, 351t
Puerperal sepsis, streptococci and, 680
Pulmonary anthrax, 778
Pulmonary infections, *S. aureus* and, 635b
Pulsed-field gel electrophoresis, 156–157, 157f
Purpura fulminans, *N. meningitidis* and, 581
Purulent urethral discharge, direct examination of, in infectious disease diagnosis, 22t
Purulent vaginal discharge, direct examination of, in infectious disease diagnosis, 23t
Pus, aspirated, swab specimens *vs.*, 11, 11f
Pycnidia, 1211
Pyomyositis, *S. aureus* and, 635b
Pyrantel pamoate, for parasitic infections, 1320t
Pyrazinamidase, 1505–1506
  in mycobacteria identification, Chart 19-13, CP 19-2L, 1087
Pyrosequencing, 149–150, 150f

Pyrrolidonyl arylamidase (PYR) test, Chart 1-6, 38–39, 1448
  in coagulase-negative staphylococci identification, 650, 652
  in streptococci identification, Chart 1-6, CP 13-2E, 718
Pyruvate, utilization of, bacterial effects of, 198–201, 202f, 203f
Pyuria, screening tests for, 86

Q-probes, 58–59
Q-tracks program, 59
Quality assurance
  in microbiology laboratory, 58–59
  in testing inhibitory activity of antimicrobial agents, 977
Quality control
  in development of standardized disk perfusion procedure, 989, 991t–992t
  in identification of antimicrobial susceptibility results, 39
  in microbiology laboratory, 59–64
    monitoring culture media, reagents, and supplies in, 61–64, 62t–63t
    monitoring laboratory equipment in, 60–61, 61t
    program for, components of, 60
  in testing inhibitory activity of antimicrobial agents, 976–977, 977t, 978t
Quality control program, components of, 60
Quellung test, 190
Quorum sensing, 202–203

R factors, 205
Radial immunodiffusion, 114
Radioimmunoassay (RIA), 119
Rahnella sp.
  newer, 276t
    differentiating characteristics of, 280t, 282
  R. aquatilis, biochemical reactions of, 240t–241t
Ralstonia sp., 308t, 328b, 328–329,, 330t
Rambach agar, in Salmonella sp. recovery and characterization, 256t
Random amplified polymorphic DNA (RAPD), 1112
Raoultella sp., biochemical reactions of, 238t–239t
RAPD. See Random amplified polymorphic DNA (RAPD)
Rapid carbohydrate utilization test, in Neisseria sp. identification, 1470
Rapid carbohydrate-utilization test, in Neisseria sp. identification, CP 11-1D–E, 594
RapID CB Plus, 785
Rapid ID 32 Strep, in identification of streptococci, enterococci, and selected "Streptococcus-like" bacteria, CP 13-3G, 744
RapID NF Plus System, in nonfermenter identification, CP 7-5F, 367, 373, 374b
RapID onE system, CP 6-6C, 289–290
Rapid plasma reagin (RPR) test, 1517–1520
  for syphilis, Chart 20-2, 1131, 1132, 1132f
RapID SS/u System, 283
RapID STR system, in identification of streptococci, enterococci, and selected "Streptococcus-like" bacteria, CP 13-3H, 744
RapiDEC Staph, in coagulase-negative staphylococci identification, 656
Rash(es)
  maculopapular, viral infections and, 1369t
  petechial, viral infections and, 1369t
  vesicular, viral infections and, 1369t
Rat-bite fever, 1146
Reagent(s), monitoring of, in quality control, 61–64, 62t–63t
Real-time nucleic acid amplification, 151–156, 152f–156f
  clinical applications of, 154–156, 156f
  FRET probes in, 151, 152–154, 153f, 154f
  hybridization probes in, 151–154, 152f–154f

hydrolysis probes in, 151–152, 152f
molecular beacons, 154, 155f
products of, methods of detecting, 151–156, 152f–156f
SYBR green in, 151, 152f
TaqMan probes in, 151–152
Rectal swab, medium for, 223, 223b
Reduvid bugs, CP A-3B–C, 1423–1434
Relapsing fever
  Borrelia sp. and, 1134–1135
  characteristics of, 1134, 1134t
  clinical presentation of, 1135
  laboratory diagnosis of, CP 20-1C–D, 1135
Remel N/F system, in nonfermenter identification, 362, 367, 373b
Reoviridae sp., described, 1338t
Replication, defined, 180, 183f
Report(s), microbiology culture results, 43–44, 43t
Rep-PCR, 158, 158f
Reproductive mycelium, 1157b
Reservoir of infection, defined, 1421
Respiratory specimens, in tuberculosis diagnosis, 1069
Respiratory syncytial virus (RSV), clinical manifestations of, 1344
Respiratory tract, commensal flora and potential pathogens in, 78, 79t
Respiratory tract infections, 68, 71–79
  diagnosis of, 69t
  lower, 69t, 75–79, 78b, 79t
    bronchiolitis, 75
    diagnosis of, specimen collection for, 76–78
    pneumonia, 75–76
    tracheobronchitis, 75
  upper, 69t, 71–75, 73f
    dental infections, 74–75
    epiglottitis, 74
    laryngitis, 74
    nasopharyngeal, 74
    otitis media, 74
    pharyngitis, 72–73
    sinusitis, 74
Respiratory virus(es)
  cytopathic effect of, 1385f
  immunologic detection of, CP 23-2E, 1393
Retroviridae sp., described, 1339t
Retrovirus(es), clinical manifestations of, 1351–1354, 1351t–1353t, 1355t, 1356b, 1356t
Reverse hybridization
  in mycobacterial identification, 1110–1111, 1110f
  in postamplification analysis, 148, 148f
Reverse transcriptase (RT)–PCR, 144–145
Rhabdoviridae sp., described, 1335t
Rhabdovirus(es), clinical manifestations of, 1345–1346
Rhizobiaceae, 342, 344–345
Rhizobium sp., CP 7-4B, 342t, 344–345
  R. radiobacter, 308t
Rhizoid(s), 1169
Rhizopus sp., identification of, 1169, 1169f, 1170f
Rhodococcus sp., 863
  clinical disease due to, 863
  epidemiology of, 863
  pathogenesis of, 863
  pathology of, 863
Rhodotorula sp., CP 21-6F, 1226
RIA. See Radioimmunoassay (RIA)
Ribonucleic acid (RNA). See also under RNA
  function of, 135–137, 136f
  nucleotide bases of, 133, 134f
  structure of, 134
Ribosomal RNA (rRNA), 180
Ribosome(s), defined, 180
Rickettsia sp.
  clinical features of, 1407–1409
  direct detection of antigen and nucleic acid in clinical specimens of, 1409

epidemiology of, 1407–1409
infections with, 1407–1409
  serologic diagnosis of, 1409
isolation in culture, 1408–1409
specimen collection for, 1408
types of, 1407, 1408t
Rigid bronchoscopy, in lower respiratory tract infection diagnosis, 77
RIM-Neisseria test, in Neisseria sp. identification, 594
Risk management, in microbiology laboratory, 47
Rmp protein, of N. gonorrhoeae, 572b
RNA. See Ribonucleic acid (RNA)
RNA viruses, classification of, 1334t–1340t
Roche Amplicor Mycobacterium tuberculosis Test, in mycobacterial identification, 1108–1109
Roller drum, for viral cultures, 1381, 1381f
Roll-streak system, 897–898
Roseomonas sp., CP 7-3G–H, 308t, 338–339
Rotavirus(es)
  clinical manifestations of, 1349t, 1350
  human, 1338f, 1338t
  immunologic detection of, 1394
Rothia sp., 625, 832–834, 833t
  R. mucilaginosa, 642–643
    identification of, phenotypic characteristics for, 661, 661t
"Rothia-like" sp., 832–834, 833t
RPR test. See Rapid plasma reagin (RPR) test
rRNA. See Ribosomal RNA (rRNA)
rRNA group 1, 317–323, 317b, 318t, 319b, 320b, 320t–323t. See also Pseudomonas sp.
rRNA group II, 323–331, 324t, 325b, 327t, 328b, 330t
rRNA group of caulobacteraceae, 332
rRNA group of xanthomonadaceae, 332–334, 333t
RSV. See Respiratory syncytial virus (RSV)
Rubella virus, 1338f, 1338t
  serologic diagnosis of, 1402
Rubeola virus, 1344
Runyon's classification scheme, 1090, 1090b
Ryu staining method, in nonfermenter identification, Chart 7-2, 316

SABHI agar (Sabouraud's heart infusion agar), uses of, 1159t
Sabouraud's dextrose agar, uses of, 1159t
Saccharomyces sp., CP 21-6H, 1226, 1228
SAF, formulations of, 1535
Safety
  in microbiology laboratory, 47–58
    biologic agents, 50–51, 51t, 52t, 53f–55f
    centrifugation, 48
    chemicals, 56–58
    cleaning spills of infectious materials, 53, 55
    corridor cautions, 49
    electrical, 48
    fire, 58
    general rules and regulations, 47–48, 49t
    glassware, 48
    handling of wastes and hazardous material, 50
    handling specimens and spills, 49–50
    lifting, 49
    needles, 48
    nonbiologic hazards, 56–58
    routine precautions, 48–50
    shipping of specimens and etiologic agents, 55–56, 56f, 57f
    universal precautions, 51–53, 55, 55t
  in tuberculosis diagnosis, 1068–1069
Saline mount, in microscopic examination of specimens, 18t
Salmonella sp.
  biochemical reactions of, 242t–243t
  differential characteristics of, 253t
  identification characteristics for, 234t
  multidrug-resistant, emergence of, 254

Salmonella sp. (*Continued*)
  recovery and characterization of, new methods for, 255–258, 256t–257t, 258f
  S. arizonae
    biochemical reactions of, 242t–243t
    infections due to, 254, 254b
  S. enterica
    biochemical reactions of, 242t–243t
    infections due to, 254, 254b
  S. typhi
    biochemical reactions of, 242t–243t
    identification of, CP 6-4B, 255–256
  taxonomy of, 251, 251b
Salmonella sp. infection, 252, 253b
Salmonella-Shigella (SS) agar, in *Enterobacteriaceae* recovery, 220t
Salmonelleae (tribe), CP 6-4B, 229t, 251–258, 252b–254b, 253t, 256t–257t, 258f
  classification of, 251, 252b, 253t
  identification characteristics for, 234t
  nomenclature associated with, 251, 253b
Salmonellosis(es)
  incidence of, 252, 253b, 254
  sources of, 252, 253b, 254
Salt-tolerance test, 1474–1475
  in streptococci identification, Chart 3-4, CP 13-2D, 717
Sapporo-like viruses, clinical manifestations of, 1350
Saprobe, 4
Sarcocystis sp., CP 22-4G, 1271–1272
Sarcoptes scabiei, CP A-2F, 1431
  geographic distribution of, 1431
  identification of, CP A-2F, 1431
SARS. *See* Severe acute respiratory syndrome (SARS)
SARS coronavirus
  molecular detection of, 1397
  serologic diagnosis of, 1402
Scabies, CP A-2F, 1431
Scalded skin syndrome, staphylococcal, *S. aureus* and, 635b
Scedosporium sp., conidia produced singly by, CP 21-2G, 1185–1186, 1185f, 1186f
Schaudinn's Fixative, formulations of, 1535
Schistosome(s), CP 22-7A–E, 1287–1288, 1289f, 1290b
Schistosomiasis, 1290b
Scopulariopsis sp., chains of conidia produced by, CP 21-2D, 1182, 1183f
Scotochromogen(s), CP 19-2D, 1095–1099
SDA. *See* Strand-displacement amplification (SDA)
Selenite broth, in *Enterobacteriaceae* recovery, 222, 223t
Sensititre AP80 System, in nonfermenter identification, 375
Sensititre Automated Reading and Incubation System (ARIS), 293
Sensititre AutoReader, 293
Sensititre system, 291–292
Sepedonium sp., conidia produced singly by, 1186–1187, 1186f
Sepsis
  catheter-associated, 100
    special considerations related to, 105
  neonatal, *Haemophilus* sp. and, 434t, 441–442
  puerperal, streptococci and, 680
Septate, 1157b
Septic arthritis
  S. aureus and, 635b
  symptoms of, 91
Septicemic plague, 271b
Septi-Chek AFB System, in mycobacteria detection, 1083–1085
Serologic tests, in viral infections diagnosis, 1388t, 1397–1403, 1399f–1401f, 1404t. *See also* Viral infections, serologic diagnosis of
Serratia sp., 266–267, 266t
  biochemical reactions of, 242t–243t

identification characteristics for, 234t
  S. marcescens, 266–267, 266t
  S. rubidaea, 266t, 267
  species within, differentiation of, 266t
Serum
  in testing inhibitory activity of antimicrobial agents, 970, 975
  VDRL slide test on, 1514–1517
Severe acute respiratory syndrome (SARS), clinical manifestations of, 1350
Sexual abuse, in children, *C. trachomatis* infections and, 1406
Sexually transmitted infections (STDs), 87–88
  cervicitis, 87–88, 89
  genital ulcer disease, 88
  HIV infection, 88
  HPVs, 88
  HSV, 88
  urethritis, 87–88, 89
  vaginitis, 88–90
  vaginosis, 88–89
  venereal warts, 88
Sheather's flotation technique, for recovery of *Cryptosporidium* oocysts in fecal specimens, 1270b
Shewanella sp., 309t, 336–337, 340t, 417
Shigella sp.
  biochemical reactions of, 242t–243t
  identification characteristics for, 234t
  infections due to
    described, 249b
    incidence of, 249–250
    sources of, 249–250
  species within, differentiation of, 250t
  subgroups of, 249, 250t
Shock, endotoxic
  diagnosis of, limulus lysate assay in, 212
  gram-negative bacteria and, 212
Siderophore(s), 205
Signal transduction, two-component, 202
Signal-amplification methods, 137–141, 138f
  branched DNA, 139
  FISH, 137, 139–141, 141f
  Hybrid Capture, 137–139, 138f
  in mycobacterial identification, 1107–1108
  nucleic acid probes, 137
  in situ hybridization, 139–141, 141f
Silver impregnation stains, in microscopic examination of specimens, 26
Simonsiella sp., 481
Single-diffusion system, 114
Sinusitis, 74
  acute, *Haemophilus* sp. and, 434t, 440
16S rRNA molecule, 170
Skin flora, contamination with, in blood culture collection, 100–101, 101f
Skin infections, *S. epidermidis* and, 640b
Skin scrapings, direct examination of, in infectious disease diagnosis, 23t
Skirrow's blood agar, subsp. *jejuni*, 397t
Slide Coagulase Test, Chart 1-3, 38, 1444–1445
  in *S. aureus* identification, Chart 1-3, CP 2-2B, 645–646
Slime layer, 190
Small colony variants, 643
Smear(s)
  acid-fast, in mycobacteria recovery, 1079–1080
  blood
    thick, preparation of, 1530–1531
    thin, preparation of, 1529–1530
  fecal, trichrome-staining technique for, 1528–1529
  with specimen collection, 13
SM-ID agar, in *Salmonella* sp. recovery and characterization, 256t
Sodium chloride tolerance, in mycobacteria, 1506–1507
Sodium hippurate, hydrolysis of, in streptococci identification, 717

Solid-phase immunoassay
  defined, 119
  methods of, 119–125, 120f, 121f, 123f, 124f
    EIA antibody capture methods, 122, 123f
    EIA antibody detection methods, 119–122, 120f, 121f
Somatic antigens, 186–187
South American trypanosomiasis, CP 22-9G–H, 1300–1303
Southern blot analysis, in postamplification analysis, 148
Sparganosis, 1316–1318
Specialized transduction, 194
Species
  bacterial, defined, 170
  defined, 168
Specimen(s). *See also Specimen transport; specific type and* Specimen collection
  culturing of
    in mycobacteria recovery, 1077–1796, 1078t, 1079t, 1080f
    techniques for, 27, 29–33, 30f–32f
  ectoparasite, laboratory submission of, 1421–1422
  fecal. *See* Fecal specimens
  genital, 90–91, 91f
  handling of, safety precautions for, 49–50
  liquid, in mycobacterial recovery and identification, 1075
  microscopic examination of, 15, 17–26, 17b, 18f–24f, 24b, 26b, 96. *See also* Microscopic examination of specimens
  in parasitic diseases, 1248–1255. *See also* Parasitic disease, specimens in
  primary culture media selection of, 27, 28t–29t
  processing of, 26–33, 28t–29t, 30–32
    parasitic disease-related, 1248–1255
  receipt and preliminary observations of, 14
  rejection of, criteria for, 14–15, 15b
  stool. *See* Stool specimens
  transfer technique for, 27
  transport of, 10, 12, 12t, 14, 14b
    containers for, 12, 12t, 13, 13f
    parasitic disease-related, 1248–1255
    safety precautions for, 55–56, 56f, 57f
  urine, voided, 84–85
  in viral infection diagnosis
    storage of, 1373
    transport of, 1373
    types of, 1372t
Specimen collection, 9f–13f, 10–14, 12t
  for abscesses, 95–96
  in *C. trachomatis*-related infections, 1403
  in cellulitis, 95–96
  in CNS infections, 93, 94f
  collection of, 10
  cost-effective approaches in, 15, 16t
  in *Coxiella* sp., 1408
  devices for, 11–13, 12t, 11f–13f
  in eye infections, 97
  fecal, collection of, 81
  genital, 90–91, 91f
  labeling of, 13–14
  in lower respiratory tract infection diagnosis, 76–78
  quantities needed in, 11
  in *Rickettsia* sp., 1408
  sites for, 10
  smears with, 13
  timing of, 10–11, 10f, 13
  in tuberculosis diagnosis, 1069–1071
  from upper gastrointestinal tract, 82
  in viral infection diagnosis, 1369, 1371, 1372t, 1373
  in wound infections, 95–96
Spectrometry, mass, in tuberculosis diagnosis, 1068
Sphingobacteria, 177b
Sphingobacteriaceae, 348–349, 349t
Sphingobacterium sp., 309t, 348–349, 349t

Sphingomonadaceae, 334
Sphingomonas sp., 309t, 334
Spider(s), CP A-2G–H, 1431–1432
    geographic distribution of, 1432
    identification of, CP A-2G, 1432
Spill(s), handling of, safety precautions for, 49–50
Spinal tap, technique of, 93, 94f
Spirilla, defined, 178, 179f
Spirillum minor, 1146
Spirochetal infections, 1125–1150. *See also special*
        infection or pathogen, e.g., Lyme disease;
        Treponema sp.
    Borrelia sp., 1134–1143
    Leptospira sp., 1143–1145
    Spirillum minor, 1146
    taxonomy of, 1126, 1126t
    Treponema sp., 1126–1134
Spirochete(s), 176b
    culture of, 1130, 1130t
    transmission of, 1129t
Spirometra mansonoides, 1316–1318
Sporangia, 1157b
Sporangiola, 1170, 1172f
Sporangiospore(s), 1157b, 1158f
Spore(s)
    defined, 1156
    microsporidia, in stool and duodenal aspirates,
        Weber stain in detection of, 1272, 1273b
Sporodochia, 1210
Sporothrix sp., *S. schenckii,* CP 21-5G–H, 1203,
        1205f, 1206f, 1207b
Sporotrichosis, CP 21-5G–H, 1203, 1205f, 1206f,
        1207b
Sputum
    direct examination of, in infectious disease
        diagnosis, 22t
    expectorated, in lower respiratory tract infection
        diagnosis, collection of, 76–77
Sputum cultures, interpretation of, 78, 78b
Sputum samples, quality of, assessment of
    Bartlett's grading system for, 17, 17b
    Murray and Washington's grading system for, 17,
        17b
Sputum specimens, in parasite detection, 1254
Staf-System 18-R, in coagulase-negative
        staphylococci identification, 658
Stain(s)
    acid-fast, CP 1-2B, 25
        Ziehl-Neelsen, 20t
    acridine orange, CP 1-2, 25–26, 26b
    biologic, 19, 20t–21t
    calcofluor white, CP 1-2F, 26
    carbol fuchsin, 1491–1492
    Diene's, for mycoplasma detection, 1483–1484
    direct, 19–21, 20t–21t
    flagella, in nonfermenter identification, Chart 7-2,
        315–316, 316b
    fluorescent, 25, 1492–1494
    fluorochrome, 20t
        for mycobacteria, CP 1-2J, 25
    Gram's. *See* Gram's stain
    methylene blue, CP 1-2, 26
        Loeffler's, 1475
    in microscopic examination of specimens, CP 1-2,
        19–26, 20t–23t
    Papanicolaou, 1363, 1363f
    periodic acid-Schiff, CP 1-2H, 26
    silver impregnation, 26
    toluidine blue, CP 1-2E, 26
    Weber, in detection of microsporidia spores in
        stool and duodenal aspirates, 1272, 1273b
    Wright's-Giemsa, CP 1-2G, 21t, 26
    Ziehl-Neelson acid-fast, 20t
Stain typing, 156–158, 157f, 158f
    amplification-based, 157–158, 158f
    clinical applications of, 158
    non-amplification-based, 156–157, 157f

PCR-RFLP, 157–158
Rep-PCR, 158, 158f
Staphylococcal food poisoning, *S. aureus* and, 635b
Staphylococcal scalded skin syndrome, *S. aureus* and,
        635b
Staphylococcal toxic shock syndrome
    case definition of, 636b
    S. aureus and, 635b–636b
Staphylococci, 623–671
    clinical significance of, CP 12-1A, 625–643,
        626b–636b, 639b–640b
    coagulase-negative, 638–641, 639b–640b
        identification of, 649–661
            acetoin production in, 655
            API Staph in, CP 12-2G, 656
            API Staph-IDENT in, 656
            Biolog Microplate Identification System in,
                658
            commercial systems in, 655–658
            conventional methods in, 649–655, 650b, 651,
                652f, 653t–654t
            Crystal GP Identification System in, 657–658
            dichotomous key for, 652f
            ID32 Staph in, CP 12-2H, 656–657
            Microbact Staphylococcal 12S in, 658
            Microbial Identification System in, 658
            MicroScan Pos ID Panel in, 657
            MicroScan Rapid Pos Combo Panel in, 657
            molecular, 658, 661
            ODC test in, 652, 655
            phenotypic and genotypic tests in, 649, 650b,
                651t, 653t–654t
            phosphatase production in, 650
            pyrrolidonyl arylamidase activity in, 650, 652
            RapiDEC Staph in, 656
            Staf-System 18-R in, 658
            Staph-Zym in, 658
            susceptibility to, deferoxamine in, 655
            susceptibility to polymyxin B in, 652
            typing methods for, 658, 661
            urease production in, 655
            Vitek GPI card in, 657
    coagulase-positive, differentiation of, 648–649
    defined, 178, 179f
    identification of, laboratory approach to, 661–662
    isolation of, Chart 12-1, CP 12-1C–H, 643–645,
        644t
        catalase test in, CP 12-1F, 644
        from clinical specimens, 643
        colony morphology in, CP 12-1D–E, 643–644
    maximizing detection of methicillin resistant,
        1006b
    micrococci *vs.,* Chart 12-1, CP 12-1G–H, 644–645,
        644t
    preliminary differentiation of, 643–645, 644t
    taxonomy of, 624–625
Staphylococcus sp., 623–671. *See also* Staphylococci
    in animals, 628b–629b
    antimicrobial resistance in, mechanisms of, 951t
    antimicrobial therapy for, resistance to
        β-lactams, 1004–1007, 1006b, 1006f, 1007f
        lincosamides, 1008
        macrolides, 1008
        streptogramins, 1008
        vancomycin, 1007–1008, 1008b
    clinical significance of, CP 12-1A, 625–643,
        626b–636b, 639b–640b
    in differentiation of micrococci and staphylococci,
        passive hemagglutination in, CP 12-2E,
        646
    environmental, 629b
    in human and nonhuman primates, 626b–628b
    identification of, phenotypic characteristics for,
        650b, 651t, 653t–654t
    isolation of, Chart 12-1, CP 12-1C–H, 643–645,
        644t
        catalase test in, CP 12-1F, 644
        from clinical specimens, 643
        colony morphology in, CP 12-1D–E, 643–644

β-lactamases of, induction of, 1001–1002
preliminary differentiation of, 643–645, 644t
S. arlettae, in environment, 629b
S. aureus
    clinical significance of, 625–637, 626b–636b
    identification of, 645–649
        DNase test in, 647–648
        latex agglutination test in, CP 12-2D, 646
        mannitol fermentation in, 648
        slide coagulase test in, Chart 1-3, CP 2-2B,
            645–646
        thermostable endonuclease test in, 648
        tube coagulase test in, Chart 1-3, CP 12-2C,
            646
    impetigo due to, 680
    infections associated with, CP 12-1A, 629,
        634b–636b
    methicillin resistance in, detection of, 648
    structure of peptidoglycan in, 185f
    virulence factors of, 625, 630b–633b
        capsular polysaccharides, 630b
        enzymes, 631b
        hemolysins, 631b–632b
        peptidoglycans, 630b
        protein A, 630b
        superantigens, 632b–633b
        teichoic acids, 630b
        toxins, 632b
S. auricularis, in human and nonhuman primates,
    627b
S. capitis, in human and nonhuman primates, 627b
S. caprae, in human and nonhuman primates, 627b
S. carnosus, in environment, 629b
S. chromogenes, in animals, 628b
S. cohnii, in human and nonhuman primates, 628b
S. condimenti, in environment, 629b
S. delphini, in animals, 629b
S. epidermidis, 638–641, 639b–640b
    identification of, phosphatase production in, 650
    infections associated with, 638–641, 639b–640b
S. equorum, in animals, 629b
S. felis, in animals, 629b
S. fleurettii, in environment, 629b
S. gallinarum, in animals, 628b
S. haemolyticus, in human and nonhuman primates,
    626b
S. hominis, in human and nonhuman primates,
    626b
S. hyicus, in animals, 628b
S. intermedius, in animals, 628b
S. kloosii, in environment, 629b
S. lentus, in animals, 628b
S. lugdunensis, in human and nonhuman primates,
    627b
S. lutrae, in animals, 629b
S. muscae, in animals, 629b
S. pasteuri, in human and nonhuman primates,
    627b
S. piscifermentans, in environment, 629b
S. saccharolyticus, in human and nonhuman
        primates, 628b
S. saprophyticus
    identification of, susceptibility to novobiocin for,
        655
    subsp. *saprophyticus,* 641–642
S. schleiferi, in human and nonhuman primates,
    627b
S. sciuri, in animals, 628b
S. simulans, in human and nonhuman primates,
    626b
S. succinis, in environment, 629b
S. vitulinus, in animals, 629b
S. warneri, in human and nonhuman primates,
    626b
S. xylosus, in human and nonhuman primates, 628b
taxonomy of, 624–625
testing methods for, 998t

Staphylococcus streak technique, in *Haemophilus* sp. infection diagnosis, 446

Staph-Zym, in coagulase-negative staphylococci identification, 658

STDs. *See* Sexually transmitted infections (STDs)

Steele and McDermott membrane filter technique, 396, 398b

Stemphylium sp., 1210, 1211f

Stenotrophomonas sp., CP 7-3D, 332–334, 333t
  S. maltophilia, 332–334, 333t
    identification of, 357

Sterilization, types of, 49t

Stibogluconate sodium, for parasitic infections, 1321t

Stomatitis virus, vesicular, 1335f, 1335t

Stomatococcus mucilaginosus, 625

Stool aspirates, microsporidia spores in, Weber stain in detection of, 1272, 1273b

Stool preservatives, commonly used, formulations of, 1535

Stool specimens
  parasites in, incidence of, 1246, 1246b
  of parasitic diseases, 1248–1253
  in tuberculosis diagnosis, 1070

Strain, defined, 168

Strain typing, in mycobacterial identification, 1111–1113

Strand-displacement amplification (SDA), 143, 144

Streptobacillus moniliformis, 481–482, 482t
  antimicrobial susceptibility of, 482
  clinical significance of, 481
  cultural characteristics of, 481–482, 482t
  identification of, 481–482, 482t
  taxonomy of, 481

Streptococcal pharyngitis, 72, 679

Streptococcal pyrogenic exotoxins (SPEs), as streptococcal virulence factor, 678–679

Streptococci, 672–764. *See also Streptococcus* sp.
  anginosus group of, 695–697
  classification of, 674b
  defined, 178, 179f
  described, 674
  general characteristics of, 674, 676
  β-hemolytic
    group C, 688–689
    group D, 697–698
    group F, 689
    group G, 688–689
    groupable, identification of, biochemical characteristics for, 719, 720t
  β-hemolytic
    group A, 676–683, 677f
      clinical significance of, 679–683
      M protein of, 679
      pharyngeal specimens in identification of, nonculture direct detection techniques for, CP 13-1F–G, 711–712
      virulence factors for, 676–677
    group B, 683–688, 686b
      clinical significance of, 684–688, 686b
      evaluation of, collecting and processing clinical specimens for, 686b
      identification of, nonculture direct detection techniques for, 712–713
      late-onset disease due to, 685
      virulence factors for, 683–684
    identification of
      phenotypic characteristics for, 720t
      serologic, CP 13-3A–B, 718–719
    identification of, Charts 13-1–13-4, CP 13-1A–H, CP 13-1H, 709–745, 713
    bile-esculin test in, Chart 13-2, CP 13-2D, 717
    bile-solubility test in, Chart 1-2, 718
    CAMP test in, CP 13-2C, 717
    capillary precipitin test in, 718
    catalase testing in, CP 13-1H, 713
    coagglutination in, 718–719
    commercially available systems for, 742–745
    culture media in, 710

direct Gram's-stained smears in, CP 13-1A, 709–710
hemolysis on blood agar in, CP 13-1E, 710–711, 711b, 711f
hydrolysis of sodium hippurate in, 717
LAP test in, CP 13-2F, 718
pigment production in, CP 13-2C, 717
presumptive, Charts 1-2, 1-6, 8-1, 13-1–13-4, 715–718, 716t
  commercial, Chart 13-2H, 718
  phenotypic criteria for, 715, 716t
PYR test in, Chart 1-6, CP 13-2E, 718
salt-tolerance test in, Chart 3-4, CP 13-2D, 717
susceptibility to bacitracin in, Chart 13-1, CP 13-2A, 715
susceptibility to Optochin in, Chart 13-3, CP 13-2G, 718
susceptibility to SXT in, Chart 13-1, CP 13-2B, 715, 721
isolation of, Charts 13-1–13-4, CP 13-1A–H, 709–745
miscellaneous, 700
preliminary characterization of, 713–715, 714t
recognition of, 713–715, 714t
S. agalactiae, 683–688, 686b
viridans, 693–695
  antimicrobial therapy for, resistance to, 1014
  identification of, 719, 721t, 722–726, 723t–724t, 725f, 727t, 728t
    flow chart for, 725f
    S. anginosus group, 725–726, 727t
    S. bovis group, 726, 728t
    S. mitis group, 722, 723t–724t
    S. mutans group, 722, 723t–724t
    S. salivarius group, 722–725, 723t–724t
    S. sanguis group, 722, 723t–724t
  isolated from animals, 700
  phenotypic differentiation of, 721t

Streptococcus bovis/streptococcus equinus complex, 697–698

Streptococcus sp., 672–764. *See also* Streptococci
  classification of, 674b
  described, 674
  group(s) of, based on small-subunit rRNA sequence analysis, 675b–676b
  β-hemolytic, group B, early-onset disease due to, 684–685
  S. agalactiae
    antimicrobial therapy for, resistance to, 1014
    clinical significance of, 684–688, 686b
    early-onset disease due to, 684–685
    evaluation of, collecting and processing clinical specimens for, 686b
    late-onset disease due to, 685
    meningitis due to, 92
    virulence factors for, 683–684
  S. anginosus, 695–697
  S. anginosus group, identification of, 725–726, 727t
  S. bovis group, identification of, 726, 728t
  S. constellatus, 695–697
  S. intermedius, 695–697
  S. mitis group, identification of, 722, 723t–724t
  S. mutans group, identification of, 722, 723t–724t
  S. pneumoniae, 689–693
    antimicrobial resistance in, mechanisms of, 951t
    antimicrobial therapy for, resistance to, 1009–1011, 1010f
    clinical significance of, 691–693
    identification of, serologic, CP 13-3B, 719
    meningitis due to, 92
    pneumococcal vaccines for, 690–691
    testing methods for, 999t–1000t
    virulence factors for, 689–690
  S. pyogenes, 676–683, 677f
    antimicrobial therapy for, resistance to, 1013–1014
    clinical significance of, 679–683

M protein of, 679
virulence factors for, 676–679, 677f
S. salivarius group, identification of, 722–725, 723t–724t
S. sanguis group, identification of, 722, 723t–724t
S. suis, 698–700
  identification of, 726, 729t–730t
  testing methods for, 1000t
"*Streptococcus*-like" bacteria, 677f
Tetragenococcus sp., 706–707
"*Streptococcus*-like" bacteria, 672–764, 704–709
  Abiotrophia sp., 704–705
  Aerococcus sp., 705–706
  Alloiococcus sp., 708
  classification of, 674b
  described, 674
  Dolosicoccus sp., 709
  Dolosigranulum sp., 709
  Eremococcus sp., 709
  Facklamia sp., 708–709
  Gemella sp., 707
  Globicatella sp., 708
  Granulicatella sp., 705
  Helcococcus, sp., 706
  identification of, Charts 13-1–13-4, CP 13-1A–H, 709–745
    commercially available systems for, 742–745
  Ignavigranum sp., 709
  isolation of, Charts 13-1–13-4, CP 13-1A–H, 709–745
  Lactococcus sp., 709
  Leuconostoc sp., 706
  Pediococcus sp., 706–707
  preliminary characterization of, 713–715, 714t
  Vagococcus sp., 707–708

Streptogramin(s), *Staphylococcus* sp. resistant to, 1008

Streptokinase(s), as streptococcal virulence factor, 679

Streptolysin O (SLO), as streptococcal virulence factor, 678

Streptolysin S (SLS), as streptococcal virulence factor, 678

Streptomyces sp., 865

Streptomycete(s), 865

Strongyloides stercoralis, CP 22-5L–M, 1278f, 1279, 1281b
  life cycle of, 1280f

Strongyloidiasis, CP 22-5L–M, 1278f, 1279, 1281b

Stuart's transport medium, 14, 14b

Stutzeri group of pseudomonads, CP 7-3A, 321, 321t

Subclinical infection, defined, 6b

Substrate level phosphorylation, 198

Sulfamethoxazole-trimethoprim (SXT), susceptibility to, Chart 13-1, CP 13-2B, 715, 717

Superantigen(s)
  bacterial, 207
  of *S. aureus*, 632b–633b
  as streptococcal virulence factor, 679

Supercoiled, 179

Superoxide dismutase, 205

Superoxol test, in *Neisseria* sp. identification, 593

Supply monitoring, in quality control, 61–64, 62t–63t

Suprapubic aspiration, 85–86, 85f

Suramin, for parasitic infections, 1320t–1321t

Suttonella sp., 472–474
  antimicrobial susceptibility of, 474
  clinical significance of, 472–473
  identification of, 469t, 473–474
    biochemical characteristics for, 469t
  S. wadsworthensis, 406
  taxonomy of, 472

Svedberg unit, 180

Swab(s)
  aspirated pus *vs.*, 11, 11f
  rectal, medium for, 222, 223b

Swab transport systems, 12, 12f

Swarming, defined, 213

"Swimmer's itch," 1290b
Swine exanthemata virus, 1337f, 1337t
SXT. See Sulfamethoxazole-trimethoprim (SXT)
SXT susceptibility tests, 1472
SYBR green, in real-time nucleic acid amplification, 151, 152f
Symbiosis, 4
Synanamorph, 1230
Syncephalastrum sp., identification of, 1170, 1171f
Syphilis
  cardiovascular, 1128
  congenital, 1128
  epidemiology of, 1128–1129, 1129t
  FTA-ABS test for, Chart 20-4, 1133
  laboratory diagnosis of, Chart 20-1, CP 20-1A–B, 1130–1134, 1130t, 1131t, 1132f
  late "benign," 1128
  nontreponemal tests for, 1131–1133, 1132f
  provisional and investigative tests for, 1133–1134
  RPR test for, Chart 20-3, 1131, 1132, 1132f
  serologic tests for, 1131–1133, 1131t, 1132f
  T. pallidum subsp. pallidum and, 1127–1129, 1129t
  TPI test for, 1133
  treponemal tests for, 1133
  VDRL test for, Chart 20-2, 1131, 1132, 1132f

T2H. See Thiopene-2-carboxylic acid hydrazide (T2H)
Taenia sp.
  T. saginata, CP 22-6D, E, G, H, 1282, 1284
  T. solium, CP 22-6D, E, G, H, 1282–1284, 1283f, 1284b
    life cycle of, 1283f
Taeniasis, 1284b
Tanapox virus, clinical manifestations of, 1361
Tapeworm(s), giant fish, CP 22-6I–L, P, 1284, 1285f, 1286b
TaqMan probes, 151–152
Target enzymes, modification of, 958
Tatumella sp.
  newer, differentiating characteristics of, 280t, 282
  T. pytseos, 276t
    biochemical reactions of, 244t–245t
Taxonomy
  of bacteria, 167–177, 167b–169b, 171b–177b
  defined, 1330
  viral infections-related, 1330–1333, 1330b, 1331f, 1332f, 1334t–1335t
TbpA protein, of Moraxella catarrhalis, 587b
TbpB protein, of Moraxella catarrhalis, 587b
Tease mount preparation, 1162, 1162b, 1162f
Tegenaria agrestis, 1432
Teichoic acids
  of S. aureus, 630b
  of S. pneumoniae, 690
Teleomorph, 1158b
  defined, 1156
Temperature, in testing inhibitory activity of antimicrobial agents, 975
Terrorism, biologic and chemical agents with potential for, 58, 59t
Tetanus, 938–939
  causes of, 206
Tetragenococcus sp., identification of, 736, 738t
Tetrazolium reduction test, in presumptive identification of M. pneumoniae, 1488–1489
Thallospore(s), 1157b
Thermomonospora(s), 864–865, 864t
Thermostable endonuclease test, in S. aureus identification, 648
Thiabendazole, for parasitic infections, 1321t
Thiophene-2-carboxylic acid hydrazide (T2H)
  growth inhibition by, in mycobacteria identification, Chart 19-9, CP 19-1F, 1087
  inhibition by, 1501
Thoracic actinomycosis, 817

Throat culture
  collection of, 73–74, 73f
  direct examination of, in infectious disease diagnosis, 22t
Tick(s), C, CP A1-B, CP A-2A–D, E–H, 1422–1431, 1422t, 1423b, 1425t, 1426f–1428f, 1429t–1430t. See also Ixodida sp.
  described, 1422
  geographic distribution of, 1425, 1425t
  geographic ranges of, 1424
  hard
    diagnostic features of, 1429t–1430t
    identification of, C, CP A-1B, E–H, 1425–1428, 1426f–1428f
  identification of, C, CP A-1B, E–H, 1425–1428, 1426f–1428f
  Ixodes ricinus, 1136–1143
Tick paralysis, 1424–1425
Tinea barbae, 1195b
Tinea capitis, 1195b
Tinea corporis, 1195b
Tinea cruris, 1195b
Tinea pedis, 1196b
Tinea unguium, 1196b
Tinsdales' agar, 1477
Tissue(s), for culture, handling of, 105
Tissue biopsy, in parasite detection, CP 22-11G, 1254
Tissue parasites, 1292–1318
Tissue protozoan infections, CP 22-10F–H, 1306–1312, 1310f, 1311f, 1312b
TMA. See Transcription-mediated amplification (TMA)
Togaviridae sp., described, 1338t
Togavirus(es), clinical manifestations of, 1347–1348
Toluidine blue stain, in microscopic examination of specimens, CP 1-2, 26
"Tooth-worm," 1245
Toxic shock syndrome, staphylococcal
  case definition of, 636b
  S. aureus and, 635b–636b
Toxic shock syndrome toxin-1, 632b
Toxic shock-like syndrome (TSLS), group A streptococcal, 681–682
Toxin(s)
  bipartite, 206
  cytolytic, 205–206
  edema, 777
  lethal, 777
  of S. aureus, 632b
Toxocara canis, 1314
Toxoid development, 205
Toxoplasma sp., T. gondii, CP 22-10F–H, 1306–1311, 1310f
  life cycle of, 1310f
Toxoplasmosis, 1309b
  clinical syndromes of, serologic results in, 1312b
  laboratory diagnosis of, CP 22-10F–H, 1309–1311, 1311f, 1312b
TPI test. See Treponema sp., T. pallidum immobilization (TPI) test
Trabulsiella sp.
  newer, differentiating characteristics of, 280t, 282
  T. guamensis, 276t
    biochemical reactions of, 244t–245t
Tracheobronchitis, 75
Transcription, 180–181, 183f
  by DNA-dependent RNA polymerase, 180
  of genetic message, 136, 136f
Transcription-mediated amplification (TMA), 143, 144
Transduction
  defined, 193–194, 193f
  generalized, 194
  specialized, 194
Transfer RNA (tRNA), 180
Transformation, defined, 192
Translaryngeal aspiration, in lower respiratory tract infection diagnosis, 77

Translation, 180–181, 183f
  of genetic message, 136, 136f
Transmembrane proteins, 188
Transmissible spongiform encephalopathies (TSEs), clinical manifestations of, 1366–1367, 1366t
Transparency tape preparation, 1162, 1162b, 1163f
Transport of specimens, 10, 12, 12t, 14, 14b
  containers for, 12, 12t, 13, 13f
  safety precautions for, 55–56, 56f, 57f
Transposable genetic elements, defined, 194
Transposon(s), defined, 182, 194–195
Transtracheal aspirates, direct examination of, in infectious disease diagnosis, 22t
Traveler(s), legionellosis in, 554–555
Traveler's diarrhea, 81
TREK ESP Culture System II, in blood culture processing, 104
Trematode(s), 1286–1292
  Clonorchis sinensis, CP 22-7I–N, O, 1290–1291, 1293f, 1294b
  described, 1286–1287
  Fasciola hepatica, CP 22-7F–H, 1288–1290, 1291f, 1292b
  Fasciolopsis buski, CP 22-7F–H, 1288–1290, 1292b
  Paragonimus westermani, CP 22-7P, 1292, 1295f, 1296b
  schistosomes, CP 22-7A–E, 1287–1288, 1289f, 1290b
Trench fever, "classical" and "urban," B. quintana and, 500
Trench mouth, 73
Treponema sp., 1126–1134
  T. carateum, 1126t, 1129t, 1130
  T. pallidum
    subsp. endemicum, 1126t, 1129t, 1130
    subsp. pallidum, 1126–1129, 1126t, 1129t
      described, 1126–1127
      immunity against, 1129
      incubation period for, 1127
      syphilis due to
        late, 1127–1128
        latent, 1127
        primary, 1127
        secondary, 1127
    subsp. pertenue, 1126t, 1129–1130, 1129t
  T. pallidum immobilization (TPI) test, for syphilis, 1133
Tribe(s), in Enterobacteriaceae classification, 228, 229t–233t
Trichinella spiralis, life cycle of, CP 22-11G–H, 1311f
Trichinosis, CP 22-11G–H, 1312, 1313f, 1314b
Trichoderma sp., clusters of conidia produced by, 1184, 1185f
Trichomonas hominis, CP 22-3E, 1266–1267
Trichophyton sp.
  identification of, CP 21-4D–H, 1190–1192, 1192f–1999f
  T. mentagrophytes, identification of, CP 21-4D, F, 1190, 1997f
  T. rubrum, identification of, CP 21-4E–F, 1190–1191, 1193
  T. tonsurans, identification of, CP 21-4G, 1191, 1193
  T. verrucosum, identification of, 1191–1192, 1194f
Trichostrongylus sp., 1279
Trichrome-staining technique, for fecal smears, 1528–1529
Trichuriasis, CP 22-5E, F, P, 1274, 1277b, 1277f
Trichuris trichiura, CP 22-5E, F, P, 1274, 1277b, 1277f
Trimethoprim-sulfamethoxazole, Haemophilus sp. resistant to, 1009

Triple sugar iron (TSI) agar, in carbohydrate fermentation detection, CP 6-1E, CP 6-4B, 216–217

tRNA. *See* Transfer RNA (tRNA)

Tropheryma whipplei, 865–866
  identification of, 871

Trypanosoma sp.
  T. brucei gambiense, life cycle of, 1302f
  T. cruzi, life cycle of, 1304f

Trypanosomiasis, CP 22-9E, G, H, 1299–1303, 1302f, 1303b
  African, 1303b
  American, 1305f
  South American, CP 22-9G–H, 1300–1303

Trypsin, EDTA and, in viral infection diagnosis, 1377

TSEs. *See* Transmissible spongiform encephalopathies (TSEs)

TSI agar. *See* Triple sugar iron (TSI) agar

Tsukamurella sp., 863

Tube coagulase test, in *S. aureus* identification, Chart 1-3, CP 12-2C, 646

Tuberculosis
  clinical, trends in, 1065–1067
  control of, 1067
  incidence of, worldwide increase in, 1065–1066
  laboratory diagnosis of, 1067–1068
    automated instruments in, 1067
    broth culture media in, 1067
    gas-liquid chromatography in, 1068
    high-performance liquid chromatography in, 1068
    inoculation of clinical specimens to agar-based culture media in, 1067–1068
    laboratory safety in, 1068–1069
    lysis-centrifugation system blood culture tube in, 1068
    mass spectrometry in, 1068
    molecular techniques in, 1067
    in mycobacteria recovery and identification, 1071–1077, 1071f, 1073t, 1074t, 1076t, 1077t, 1708b
      acid-fast bacilli staining, Charts 19-1–19-3, CP 19-1A–B, 1075–1077, 1076t, 1077t
      bone marrow specimens, 1074–1075
      centrifugation, 1074, 1074f
      decontamination procedure, Chart 19-1, 1072–1074, 1073b, 1073t
      digestion procedure, Chart 19-1, 1072–1074, 1073b, 1073t
      liquid specimens, 1075
      specimen preparation, 1072
    NAP in, 1068
    optimizing detection and identification of mycobacteria in, 1068
    specimen collection in, 1069–1071
      blood cultures, 1069–1070
      respiratory specimens, 1069
      ''sterile'' specimens, 1070–1071
      stool specimens, 1070
  person at risk for, 1066
  prevention of, 1115–1117, 1116b
  rapidly progressive, 1066–1067
  treatment of, 1115–1117, 1116b
    American Thoracic Society recommendations for, 1116b, 1117

Tularemia. *See also Francisella tularensis*
  clinical spectrum of, 493–494
  cultural characteristics of, CP 9-4E, 490–491, 492t
  described, 491
  epidemiology of, 491
  glandular, 493
  history of, 491–492
  isolation of, CP 9-4E, 490–491, 492t
  oculoglandular, 493
  oropharyngeal, 493
  pneumonic, 493
  serologic diagnosis of, 495
  taxonomy of, 491–492

treatment of, 495, 497
  typhoidal, 493
  ulceroglandular, 493

Tumbu fly, 1432–1433

Turicella sp., 834, 834t

Tween-80 hydrolysis, 1507–1508
  in mycobacteria identification, Chart 19-15, CP 19-2G, 1087

Two-component signal transduction, 202

Type strain, defined, 168

Typhoid fever, diagnosis of, culture and serology in, 10, 10f

Typhoidal tularemia, 493

Tyronsine, hydrolysis of, 1478–1479

Ulcer(s)
  genital, 88
    HIV infection and, interactions between, 88
    specimens from, collection of, 91
  oropharyngeal, direct examination of, in infectious disease diagnosis, 22t
  penile, direct examination of, in infectious disease diagnosis, 23t
  vulvar, direct examination of, in infectious disease diagnosis, 23t

Ulcerative gingivostomatitis, necrotizing, 73

Ulceroglandular tularemia, 493

Ulocladium sp., 1209–1210, 1210f

UNI-N/F Tek plate, in nonfermenter identification, 367

Urea, hydrolysis of, in nonfermenter identification, Chart 6-6, CP 7-2A, 314–315

Ureaplasma(s), 1022–1063
  described, 1023
  isolated from humans, 1025b
  taxonomy of, 1023–1026, 1024b, 1025b, 1025t

Ureaplasma sp.
  identification of, characteristics for, 1025b
  U. urealyticum
    clinical significance of, 1028–1033
    identification of, manganous chloride-urea test in, 1484–1485
    virulence factors of, 1026–1027

Urease
  activity of, in mycobacteria identification, Chart 19-16, CP 19-2K, 1084t–1085t, 1087
  conventional, 1457–1459, 1458f
  in mycobacteria, 1508–1509
  production of
    in coagulase-negative staphylococci identification, 655
    in *Enterobacteriaceae* identification, Chart 6-6, CP 6-4E, 225

Urethral discharge, purulent, direct examination of, in infectious disease diagnosis, 22t

Urethritis, 87–88
  diagnosis of, 89
  Haemophilus sp. and, 434t, 441–442

Urinary tract, candidiasis of, 1222b

Urinary tract infections (UTIs), 70t, 82–87, 83t, 84b, 84f, 85f
  diagnosis of, 70t
  host factors in, 83
  S. epidermidis and, 639b
  screening tests for, 86–87
  signs and symptoms of, 70t, 82–83
  urine sample collection in, 83, 83t

Urine specimens
  clean-catch, instructions for obtaining, 83, 84b, 84f
  culture of, 85–86
  direct examination of, in infectious disease diagnosis, 22t
  midstream, 83–84, 84b, 84f
  in parasite detection, 1254
  in UTI diagnosis, 83–84, 84b, 84f
  voided, 84–85

UspA proteins, of *Moraxella catarrhalis,* 586b

UTIs. *See* Urinary tract infections (UTIs)

Uveitis, clinical presentation of, 97

Vaccine(s)
  H. influenzae type B, 433, 435, 438b
  for meningococcal disease, 582–584
  pertussis, 513, 515–516
  pneumococcal polysaccharide, for *S. pneumoniae,* 690–691

Vacinnia virus, 1343f, 1343t

Vaginal discharge, purulent, direct examination of, in infectious disease diagnosis, 23t

Vaginitis, 88–90
  diagnosis of, 88–90

Vaginosis, 88–89
  bacterial, 88–89, 835–836
    identification of, 931

Vagococcus sp., 707–708
  identification of, 736, 738, 740t

Vancomycin
  Enterococcus sp. resistant to, 1012
  Staphylococcus sp. resistant to, 1007–1008, 1008b

Vancomycin-binding proteins, 955, 957–958, 957t

Varicella-zoster virus (VZV)
  clinical manifestations of, 1359
  immunologic detection of, 1393
  serologic diagnosis of, 1402

Vascular graft infections, *S. epidermidis* and, 640b

VDRL test. *See* Venereal Disease Research Laboratory (VDRL) test

Vegetative mycelium, 1157b

Venereal Disease Research Laboratory (VDRL) slide test on serum, 1514–1517

Venereal Disease Research Laboratory (VDRL) test, for syphilis, Chart 20-3, 1131, 1132, 1132f

Venereal warts, 88
  diagnosis of, 90

Verruga peruana, *B. bacilliformis* and, 500

Vesicular rash, viral infections and, 1369t

Vesicular stomatitis virus, 1335f, 1335t

Vibrio sp., 408–417, 409t, 411b, 412f, 413t–414t, 416t–418t
  biochemical characterization of, CP 8-2E–H, 416–417, 416t–418t
  described, 409–414, 409t, 411b, 412f, 413t–414t
  differential tests for, 418t
  historical background of, 408–409
  laboratory identification of, CP 8-2E–H, 416–417, 416t–418t
  laboratory isolation of, methods for, CP 8-2A–D, 414–415
  non-cholera, 412–414, 413t–414t
  presumptive identification of, CP 8-2A–D, 415
  taxonomy of, 409
  V. alginolyticus, 411, 413t
  V. carchariae, 411
  V. cholerae, 409–411, 409t, 411b, 412f
    biotypes of, differentiation between, 416, 417t
    characteristics of, 409, 409t
    cholera due to, 409–411, 409t, 411b
    gastroenteritis due to, 410, 411b, 412f
    infections due to, treatment and prevention of, 410–411
    strains of, 409–410
    testing methods for, 1000t
    toxigenic, 409t, 410
  V. cincinnatiensis, 411
  V. damsela, 411–412, 413t
  V. fluvialis, 412, 413t
  V. furnissii, 412, 413t
  V. hollisae, 412, 413t
  V. metschnikovii, 412, 413t
  V. mimicus, 413t–414t, 414
  V. parahaemolyticus, 414, 414t
  V. vulnificus, 414, 414t

Vibrionaceae, phylogeny of, 408–417, 409t, 411b, 412f, 413t–414t, 416t–418t

Vibrios, defined, 178, 179f
Vincent's infection, 73
Viral antigens, in detection and provisional
        identification of viral infections, CP 23-
        2D, F, 1389
Viral cultures, roller drum for, 1381, 1381f
Viral gastroenteritis, clinical manifestations of,
        1349–1350, 1349t
Viral infections. See also Virus(es)
    Anaplasma sp., 1409–1410, 1409t
    Chlamydia sp. and, 1403, 1405–1407. See also
            Chlamydia sp.
    clinical classification of, 1367, 1368t–1369t
    clinical manifestations of, 1333, 1335, 1339–1340,
            1342–1367. See also specific infection
    clinical syndromes associated with, 1368t–1369t
    Coxiella sp., 1407–1409
    detection of, 1381–1390
    diagnosis of, 1367, 1369–1392
        artifacts in, 1389–1390
        biochemical differentiation in, 1387, 1389
        cell association in, 1389
        cell cultures in
            contamination of, 1375, 1377, 1378f
            inoculation and incubation of, 1380–1381,
                    1381f
            preparation and maintenance of, 1373–1375,
                    1374t, 1375t, 1376f
            selection of, 1380
            technical aspects of, CP 23-2F, 1377–1380,
                    1379b, 1379f
        cytopathic effect in, 1381–1383, 1381f, 1382t,
                1383t, 1384f–1388f. See also Cytopathic
                effect, in detection and provisional
                identification of viral infections
        electron microscopy in, 1387
        hemadsorption in, Chart 23-1, 1383, 1387, 1389f
        hemagglutination in, Chart 23-1, 1383, 1387,
                1389f
        isolates in, definitive identification of,
                1390–1391
        isolation of viruses in culture in, 1373
        light microscopy in, Chart 23-1, 1387
        methods for, 1370t–1372t
        non–virus-induced changes in, 1389–1390
        specimens in
            collection of, 1369, 1371, 1372t, 1373
            storage of, 1373
            transport of, 1373
            types of, 1372t
        viral antigen detection in, CP 23-2D, F, 1389
    Ehrlichia sp., 1409–1410, 1409t
    isolation of, in culture, 1373
    nomenclature related to, 1330–1333, 1330b, 1331f,
            1332f, 1334t–1335t
    provisional identification of, 1381–1390
    Rickettsia sp., 1407–1409
    serologic diagnosis of, 1395–1401, 1396t,
            1397f–1399f, 1402t
        anti-Igm antibodies, 1402–1403
        antiviral susceptibility testing in, 1403
        CMV, 1402
        EBV, 1399–1401, 1401f
        HAV, 1401
        HBV, 1399–1401, 1401f
        HCV, 1401–1402
        HIV, 1398–1399, 1398t, 1399f
        HSV, 1399
        parvovirus infections, 1402
        rubella, 1402
        SARS coronavirus, 1404
        VZV. See Varicella-zoster virus (VZV)
        West Nile virus, 1402
    taxonomy related to, 1330–1333, 1330b, 1331f,
            1332f, 1334t–1335t
Viral pharyngitis, 72–73
Viridans streptococcal endocarditis, 693–695

Viridans streptococci
    identification of, 719, 721t, 722–726, 723t–724t,
            725f, 727t, 728t. See also Streptococci,
            viridans, identification of
    isolated from animals, 700
Virulence, defined, 4, 201
Virulence factors, 5, 5t
    of microorganisms, 204–207
Virus(es). See also specific types and Viral infections
    adenoviruses, 1360–1361, 1361t
    arenaviruses, 1346, 1346t
    astroviruses, 1349t, 1350
    B, 1360
    bunyaviruses, 1348–1349, 1348t
    caliciviruses, 1349t, 1350
    California encephalitis, 1348
    in clinical specimens, direct detection of,
            1392–1397
        CMV, 1393–1394, 1397
        electron microscopy in, 1393
        enteroviruses, 1397
        HBV, 1396
        HCV, 1395–1396
        HIV, 1394–1395
        HPVs, 1396
        HSV, 1393, 1396–1397
        human rotavirus, 1394
        immunologic, 1393–1394
        light microscopy in, CP 23-1A–F, 1392–1393
        molecular techniques in, 1394–1397
        parvovirus B19, 1396
        rapid diagnostic tests in, 1397
        SARS coronavirus, 1397
        VZV, 1393
        West Nile virus, 1396
    CMV, 1358–1359, 1393–1394, 1397
    coltiviruses, 1351
    construction of, 1331, 1331f
    coronaviruses, 1349t, 1350–1351
    described, 3, 1330, 1331f
    diagnosis of, 1327–1419
    DNA, 1341t–1343t
    Ebola, 1335f, 1335t, 1346–1347
    EBV, 1359
        serologic diagnosis of, 1399–1401, 1401f
    enteric adenoviruses, 1349t, 1350
    filoviruses, 1346–1347
    gastroenteritis, human, 1349–1350, 1349f
    H-1, 1342f, 1342t
    hendra, 1344
    hepatitis, 1364–1366, 1364t. See also Hepatitis
    herpesviruses, 1356–1361
    HHV-6, 1359–1360
    HHV-7, 1360
    HHV-8, 1360
    HIV. See Human immunodeficiency virus (HIV)
            infection
    HPVs, 1362–1364, 1362t, 1363f, 1363t
    HSV. See Herpes simplex virus (HSV) infection
    human wart, 1342f, 1342t
    influenza, 1335, 1339–1340, 1342
    LaCrosse, 1336fm1336t
    measles, 1344
    molluscum contagiosum virus, 1361
    mumps, 1344
    naming of, 1330, 1330b
    Nipah, 1344
    Norwalk-like, 1350
    orthomyxoviruses, 1335, 1339–1340, 1342
    orthopoxviruses, 1361
    papillomaviruses, 1362–1364, 1362t, 1363f, 1363t
    papovaviruses, 1361–1364, 1362t, 1363f, 1363t
    parainfluenza, 1342, 1344
    paramyxoviruses, 1342, 1344
    parvoviruses, 1364, 1396, 1402
    picornaviruses, 1344–1345
    polyomaviruses, 1364
    poxviruses, 1361

preliminary identification of, 39
respiratory
    cytopathic effects of, 1385f
    immunologic detection of, CP 23-2E, 1393
retroviruses, 1351–1354, 1351t–1353t, 1355t,
        1356b, 1356t
rhabdoviruses, 1345–1346
RNA, classification of, 1334t–1340t
rotaviruses, 1349t, 1350
rubella, 1338f, 1338t
    serologic diagnosis of, 1402
rubeola, 1344
sappora-like, 1350
stomatitis, vesicular, 1335f, 1335t
swine exanthemata, 1337f, 1337t
tanapox, 1361
togaviruses, 1347–1348
ultrastructure of, 1332f, 1333
vaccinia, 1343f, 1343t
vesicular stomatitis, 1335f, 1335t
VZV. See Varicella-zoster virus (VZV)
wart, human, 1342f, 1342t
West Nile. See West Nile virus
Vitek, in testing inhibitory activity of antimicrobial
        agents, 993, 996
Vitek 2 System, in nonfermenter identification,
        374–375
Vitek Gram-Positive Identification (GPI) card
    in coagulase-negative staphylococci identification,
            657
    in identification of streptococci, enterococci, and
            selected ''Streptococcus-like'' bacteria,
            744–745
Vitek Legacy System, 284
    in nonfermenter identification, 373–374
Vitek System, CP 6-6G, 292–293
Voges–Proskauer test, 199, 1454–1456, 1455f
    in Enterobacteriaceae identification, Chart 6-4, CP
            6-4C–D, 225
Volatile fatty acids, identification of, in determination
        of metabolic products of anaerobes, 906,
        908, 909b, 909f–911f, 915t
Volutin, 181
Vulvar ulcer, direct examination of, in infectious
        disease diagnosis, 23t
VZV. See Varicella-zoster virus (VZV)

Walkaway, CP 6-6F, 292
Walkaway-40, in nonfermenter identification, 375
Walkaway-96, in nonfermenter identification, 375
Wampole Isostat/Isolator Microbial System, in blood
        culture processing, 103
Warburg-Dickens Hexose Monophosphate pathway,
        311f, 312
Wart(s), venereal, 88
    diagnosis of, 90
Wart virus, human, 1342f, 1342t
Waste(s), handling of, safety precautions for, 50
Weber stain, in detection of microsporidia spores in
        stool and duodenal aspirates, 1272, 1273b
Weeksella sp., 347t, 348
    W. virosa, 309t
West Nile virus
    clinical manifestations of, 1347–1348
    molecular detection of, 1396
    serologic diagnosis of, 1402
Western blot procedures, for anti-HIV-1 antibodies,
        120–121, 121f
Wet-mount technique, in nonfermenter identification,
        Chart 7-2, 316
Weyant identification scheme, in nonfermenter
        identification, 358
Whipple's disease
    described, 866
    extraintestinal sites of, 866t
    pathology of, 866
Whipworm, CP 22-5E, F, P, 1274, 1277b, 1277f

Wolinella sp., 405–406
    characteristics of, 394t
    W. succinogenes, 405–406
Woods and Washington classification scheme, 1090,
        1090b
Wound infections, 71t, 95–96
    clinical presentation of, 95
    diagnosis of, 95–96
    S. aureus and, 634b
Wright's–Giemsa stain, in microscopic examination
        of specimens, CP 1-26, 21t, 26
Wuchereria sp., *W. bancrofti,* CP 22-10A–C,
        1303–1304, 1306b, 1307f
    life cycle of, 1307f

X factor requirements, 1469, 1469f
Xanthine, hydrolysis of, 1478–1479
Xanthomonadaceae, CP 7-3D, 332–334, 333t
    rRNA group of, CP 7-3D, 332–334, 333t
Xenorhabdus sp.
    newer, 277t
    X. nematophilus, biochemical reactions of,
        244t–245t
XLD agar. *See* Xylose lysine deoxycholate (XLD)
        agar

XLT4. *See* Xylose-lysine-tergitol 4 (XLT4)
Xylose lysine deoxycholate (XLD) agar, in
        Enterobacteriaceae recovery, CP 6-
        3A–D, 220t
Xylose-lysine-tergitol 4 (XLT4), in *Salmonella* sp.
        recovery and characterization, 256t–257t

Y factor requirements, 1469, 1469f
Yeast(s)
    arthroconidia producing, 1225b
    black, laboratory identification of, 1229–1230,
        1229f, 1230f
    defined, 1156
    described, 3
    identification of, abbreviated, 40t–41t
    laboratory identification of, 1216, 1218–1232
        cornmeal agar preparations in, CP 21-6B,
            1218–1221, 1219b, 1220f, 1221f
        germ tube in, 1216, 1218, 1218b, 1218f, 1219f
        non-hyphae-forming, CP 21-6E–H, 1226,
            1228–1229, 1228f
    preliminary observations suggestive of, 1243
Yeast-identification systems, packaged, 1230, 1231f
Yellow-pigmented pseudomonads, characteristics of,
        323, 335t

Yersinia sp., CP 6-5A–D, 269–274, 270t, 271b, 272b
    biochemical reactions of, 244t–245t
    identification characteristics of, 234t
    species within, differentiation of, 270t
Yersinieae (tribe), CP 6-5A–D, 233t, 269–274, 270t,
        271b, 272b, 272f
    identification characteristics for, 234t
Yokenella sp.
    newer, differentiating characteristics of, 280t, 282
    Y. regensburgei, 277t
        biochemical reactions of, 244t–245t

Ziehl-Neelsen acid-fast stain, in microscopic
        examination of specimens, 20t
Zygomycete(s), 1157b, 1158f
    histopathology of, infections caused by,
        1171–1172, 1172f, 1173b–1174f
    preliminary observations suggestive of, 1238
Zygomycete sp., identification of, 1168–1171,
        1169f–1172f
Zygomycosis, 1173b–1174b
    defined, 1156
    identification of, 1168–1171, 1169f–1172f
Zygospore(s), 1158b, 1159f